Y0-BXI-581

ONCOLOGY NURSING

ASSESSMENT AND CLINICAL CARE

ONCOLOGY NURSING

ASSESSMENT AND CLINICAL CARE

Christine Miaskowski, RN, PhD, FAAN

Professor and Chair
Department of Physiological Nursing
University of California at San Francisco
San Francisco, California

Patricia Buchsel, RN, MSN

Clinical Instructor
School of Nursing
University of Washington
Seattle, Washington

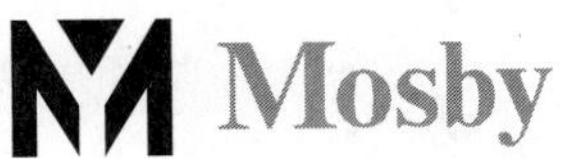

St. Louis Baltimore Boston Carlsbad Chicago Minneapolis New York Philadelphia Portland
London Milan Sydney Tokyo Toronto

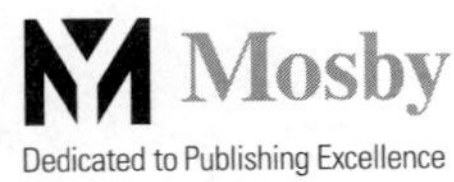

Editor-in-Chief: Sally Schrefer
Executive Editor: Barbara Nelson Cullen
Associate Developmental Editor: Eric Ham
Project Manager: Deborah L. Vogel
Production Editors: Mamata Reddy, Sarah Fike
Designer: Bill Drone
Cover Photograph: SPL/Photo Researchers

FIRST EDITION

A NOTE TO THE READER

The authors and publisher have made every attempt to check dosages and nursing content for accuracy. Because the science of pharmacology is continually advancing, our knowledge base continues to expand. Therefore we recommend that the reader always check product information for changes in dosage or administration before administering any medication. This is particularly important with new or rarely used drugs.

Composition by Clarinda Company
Printing/binding by Maple-Vail Book Mfg. Group

Mosby, Inc.
11830 Westline Industrial Drive
St. Louis, Missouri 63146

International Standard Book Number 0-8151-6990-6

99 00 01 02 03 / 9 8 7 6 5 4 3 2 1

To my mother, my dearest friend, who provided me with the ongoing love and support that I needed to see this text to completion.

Christine Miaskowski

To my family, especially my husband, whose patience and understanding guided and nurtured me through the process of this text.

Patricia Buchsel

Contributors

Sharon Aronovitch, PhD, RN, CETN
Regents College
Albany, New York

Theresa Atilio, MSW
Memorial Sloan Kettering Cancer Center
New York, New York

Susan Weiss Behrend, RN, MSN
Radiation Oncology
Fox Chase Cancer Center
Philadelphia, Pennsylvania

Karen Belford, RN, MS
Memorial Sloan Kettering Cancer Center
New York, New York

Laura Benson, RN, MS, AOCN
Schering Oncology Biotech
Yonkers, New York

Theresa Bredereck Boggs, PAC, MHS
St. Jude's Children's Research Hospital
Memphis, Tennessee

Jeannine Brant, RN, MS, AOCN
St. Vincent Hospital and Health Center
Billings, Montana

Tamie R. Bressler, RN, MN, OCN
Tulane University
New Orleans, Louisiana

Catherine C. Burke, RN, MS, CS, ANP
M. D. Anderson Cancer Center
Houston, Texas

Kathryn Ann Caudell, PhD, RN, AOCN
School of Nursing
University of New Mexico
Albuquerque, New Mexico

Margaret Cawley, RN, MS
Booth Memorial Hospital
Queens, New York

Deborah Chielens, RN, OCN
Department of Medicine
University of Washington
Seattle, Washington

Patricia Collins, RN, MS
South Miami Hospital
Miami, Florida

Tricia Corbett, MSPH
Corbett Consulting, Inc.
Issaquah, Washington

Nessa Coyle, RN, MS, FAAN
Memorial Sloan Kettering Cancer Center
New York, New York

Frances Crighton, RN, PhD(c), OCN
The Cancer Institute
Health Midwest
Kansas City, Missouri

Deborah B. Crom, RN, PhD
St. Jude's Children's Research Hospital
Memphis, Tennessee

Georgia Decker, RN, MS, ANP, AOCN
The Center for Progressive Medicine
Albany, New York

Elaine S. DeMeyer, RN, MSN, OCN
Trinity Valley Community College
Kaufman, Texas

Kathleen Dietz, RN, MA, MS, AOCN
Oncology Nurse Educator
Marston Mills, Maine

Peggy J. Eldredge, RN, MS, AOCN
The Cancer Institute
Health Midwest
Kansas City, Missouri

Noreen Facione, RN, PhD
University of California-San Francisco
San Francisco, California

Nellee M. H. Fine, RN, MA, AOCN
Oncology Nurse Consultant
St. Louis, Missouri

Eva Gallagher, RN, MS, AOCN
Methodist Hospital
Minneapolis, Minnesota

Ruth Gargon-Klinger, RN, MSN, ANP
Memorial Sloan Kettering Cancer Center
New York, New York

Edithe C. Garvey, RN, MN, OCN
Carolinas Homecare
Charlotte, North Carolina

Vivian Gates, RN, CS, MSN, AOCN
Oncology Consultant
Teanek, New Jersey

Myra Glajchen, DSW, ACSW, MSW, BSW
Beth Israel Medical Center
New York, New York

Cecilia Gatson Grindel, RN, PhD
Northeastern University
Boston, Massachusetts

Deborah Hamolsky, RN, MS
University of California-San Francisco Cancer Center
San Francisco, California

Barbara Hawkins, RN, MS, OCN
Cancer Center of Southwest Washington
Vancouver, Washington

Denise K. Hogan, RN, MS, OCN
Oncology Clinical Nurse Specialist
Carolinas Medical Center
Charlotte, North Carolina

Linda A. House RN, BSN
Medical Information Administrator
Eli Lilly and Company
Indianapolis, Indiana

Catherine Hydzik, RN, MS
Memorial Sloan Kettering Cancer Center
New York, New York

Jane Ingham, MD
Georgetown University Hospital
Washington, District of Columbia

Catherine Jansen, RN, MS
Kaiser Permanente Medical Center
San Francisco, California

Pamela Kapustay, RN, MS
Amerimmune Pharmaceuticals
Woodland Hills, California

Catherine H. Kelley, MSN, RN, OCN
Chimeric Therapies, Inc.
Laguna Niguel, California

Ellen W. Leum, ARNP, MSN, OCN
Coram Healthcare
Boynton Beach, Florida

Frances Marcus Lewis, RN, MN, PhD, FAAN
University of Washington
School of Nursing
Seattle, Washington

Kathy Lilleby, RN
Fred Hutchinson Cancer Research Center
Seattle, Washington

Lorie Precht Lindsey, RNC, FNP, OCN
Oncology Nurse Educator
Richardson, Texas

Mary P. Lovely, RN, PhD
University of California-San Francisco
San Francisco, California

Sandra Malamed, RN, MS, OCN
Oncology Nurse Educator
Birchville, Pennsylvania

Belinda N. Mandrell, RN, CPNP, MSN
St. Jude's Children's Research Hospital
Memphis, Tennessee

Marnie McHale, RN, MS, AOCN
Oncology Nurse Education
Chicago, Illinois

Kathleen McNamara, RN, BS, OCN
Oncology Nurse Education
New York, New York

Mary Monaghan, RN, APN, AOCN
Adult Nurse Practitioner
Gainesville, Florida

Theresa A. Moran, RN, MS, FNP
San Francisco General Hospital
San Francisco, California

Jamie S. Myers, RN, MN, AOCN
Research Medical Center
Kansas City, Missouri

Brenda Marion Nevidjon, RN, MSN
Duke University Hospital
Durham, North Carolina

Robbie Norville, RN, MSN, CPON, OCN
St. Jude's Children's Research Hospital
Memphis, Tennessee

Mikaela Olsen, RN, MS
Stanford University Hospital
Palo Alto, California

Nancy Oksenholt, RN, MSN, CCRN
Oregon Health Sciences University
Portland, Oregon

Judith A. Paice, RN, PhD, FAAN
Rush Neuroscience Institute
Chicago, Illinois

Julie Painter, RN, MSN, OCN
Community Hospital
Indianapolis, Indiana

Carolyn K. Pittinger, RN, MS, AOCN
Hematologic Product Specialist
OrthoBiotech
Portland, Oregon

Susan Rudder Randolph, RN, MSN, CS
Corem Healthcare, Inc.
Denver, Colorado

Denise K. Reinke, RN, BSN, OCN
Oncology Nurse Educator
Canton, Michigan

Mary Garlick Roll, RN, MSN
Magnet Therapy
Buffalo, New York

Gail Egan Sansivero, MS, ANP, AOCN
Albany Medical College
Albany, New York

Lynn E. Scallion, RN, MSN, AOCN
University of North Carolina-Chapel Hill
Chapel Hill, North Carolina

Sue M. Schlesselman, RN, MSN, OCN
Augusta State University
St. Joseph's Hospital
Augusta, Georgia

Lisa Karlin Schulmeister, RN, MS, CS, OCN
Louisiana State University Medical Center
School of Nursing
New Orleans, Louisiana

Florence Seelig, RN, OCN
Oregon Health Sciences University
Portland, Oregon

Gayle H. Shiba, RN, PhD, OCN
University of Tennessee-Memphis
Memphis, Tennessee

Betsy A. Stein, BA, CCRN
Bone Marrow Transplant Program
Baylor University Medical Center
Dallas, Texas

Roberta Strohl, RN, MSN, AOCN
University of Maryland-Baltimore
Baltimore, Maryland

Diva Thielvoldt, RN, MN, CNS, NP
Adult Nurse Practitioner
M. D. Anderson
Houston, Texas

Robbie Thomas, RN, MS, OCN
St. Joseph Mercy-Oakland
Pontiac, Michigan

Susan T. Tinley, RN, MS, CGC
Creighton University
Omaha, Nebraska

Amy Strauss Tranin, RN, MS, OCN
The Cancer Institute
Health Midwest
Kansas City, Missouri

Carol Viele, RN, MS
University of California/Stanford Health Care
San Francisco, California

Constance G. Visovsky, RN, MS, ACNP
Case Western Reserve University
Cleveland, Ohio

Dianna Wellen, RN, MS, OCN
IMPAC Medical Systems, Inc.
Mountain View, California

M. Linda Workman, PhD, RN, FAAN
Frances Payne Bolton School of Nursing
Case Western Reserve University
Cleveland, Ohio

Linda Worrall, RN, MSN, OCN
Oncology Nursing Society
Pittsburgh, Pennsylvania

Stacey Young-McCaughan, RN, PhD, OCN, Lt. Col.
Congressionally Directed Medical Research Programs
Fort Detrick, Maryland

Reviewers

Patricia Carter, RN, MSN, AOCN
El Paso Cancer Treatment Center
El Paso, Texas

Sharon Forester, RN, BSN, OCN
Saint Anthony's Health Center
Alton, Illinois

Carolyn Harvey, RN, PhD
University of Texas-Tyler
Tyler, Texas

Ann O'Mara, PhD, RN
School of Nursing
University of Maryland
Baltimore, Maryland

Virginia Sicola, BS, MS, PhD, CS, OCN, RN
Veteran Affairs Medical Center
Amarillo, Texas
West Texas A&M University
Amarillo, Texas

Susan Sturgeon, RN, BS, OCN
Community Cancer Care, Inc.
Indianapolis, Indiana

Julia Anne Walsh, RN, MSN, OCN
Hematology Medical Oncology Services
Cancer Management Center
Holy Family Hospital and Medical Center
Methuen, Massachusetts

About the Authors

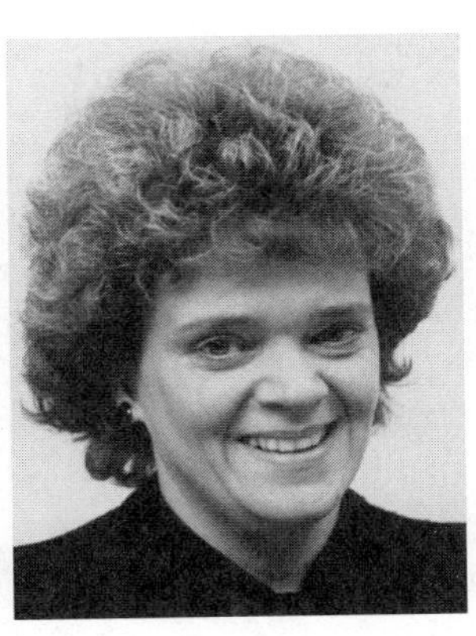

Christine Miaskowski, RN, PhD, FAAN, is professor and chair of the Department of Physiological Nursing at the University of California in San Francisco. She received her undergraduate nursing education at Molloy College in New York. She holds a Master's degree in biology and a PhD in physiology from St. John's University in New York. Christine Miaskowski has extensive clinical experience in oncology nursing, having worked as a staff nurse, a nurse manager, and an Oncology Clinical Nurse Specialist. Currently, she teaches in the oncology program at the University of California. She is an internationally recognized expert in pain management and oncology nursing. She served as chair of the Clinical Practice Committee and on the Board of Directors of the Oncology Nursing Society. Her program of research focuses on improving the management of acute and chronic pain by demonstrating to health care professionals the negative outcomes that occur in patients with unrelieved pain. In addition, she works on developing new and innovative behavioral and pharmacologic approaches to improving pain management.

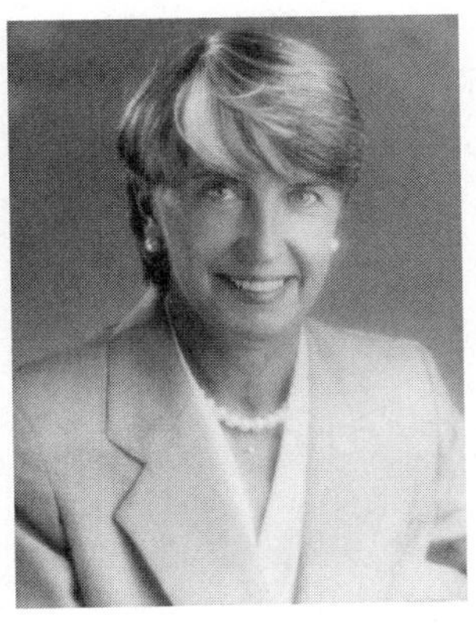

Patricia Buchsel, RN, MSN, is a clinical instructor at the University of Washington School of Nursing Education in Seattle, Washington, and a consultant in oncology care. She received her undergraduate in nursing at Seattle University, in Seattle, Washington. She holds a Master's degree in nursing from Seattle Pacific University in Seattle, Washington. Patricia Buchsel has extensive clinical experience in oncology nursing and has practiced as a staff nurse, a nursing director, and as an educator to health care professionals, patients, and their family caregivers. Her work also extends to symptom management in the oncology population, with an emphasis on fatigue issues. She is widely recognized as an expert in the nursing care of bone marrow and stem cell transplantation recipients, and has edited and written extensively in this area. She serves on numerous medical and nursing boards, and currently serves as the president of the Oncology Nursing Society Press.

Preface

The scope and nature of oncology nursing practice has expanded exponentially in the past five years. The majority of cancer care is being delivered in the outpatient and home care settings. Oncology nurses need to be able to understand a patient's disease trajectory (i.e., from the time of diagnosis to the time of death), determine the appropriate interventions throughout the course of the disease, predict and manage the most common complications of the disease and treatment, develop specific plans of care for patients with specific cancers, and teach patients and family members how to manage their disease and the side effects of cancer treatment in inpatient, outpatient, and home care settings.

In Part I of this comprehensive text, we provide an overview of the major principles governing cancer and cancer treatment. These chapters provide fundamental knowledge about such concepts as cancer pathophysiology, cancer treatments, genetic counseling, and palliative care. The information contained in these chapters applies to all patients who are living with the chronic illness of cancer.

Oncology nurses need a comprehensive reference book that provides precise management strategies for patients with specific cancer diagnoses. Therefore we organized this textbook around those specific diagnoses. Each chapter in Part II is organized in exactly the same way. Each disease-specific chapter includes a detailed discussion of the pathophysiology of the disease, the diagnostic workup, staging of the disease, the course of treatment, the patient problems associated with the disease and treatment, and oncologic emergencies. Each chapter has a number of special features, including standards of patient care for a certain cancer diagnosis, patient teaching guides, a section on home care needs of the patient, and quality improvement tools for monitoring the quality of care that patients are receiving in inpatient and outpatient settings. It is our goal that this user-friendly format will improve the care of oncology patients.

Our hope is that oncology nurses will find this comprehensive text extremely useful in their clinical practice. Patients with cancer require a great deal of care and information. We hope that nurses using this text will take the assessment tools and standards of care directly to the patient and review this information with both the patient and family caregivers to improve the care of these individuals.

We would like to acknowledge the superb support of Barbara Cullen, our executive editor. She supported us through all of the "ups and downs" of this huge undertaking. Her guidance, wisdom, and experience are unparalleled in the publishing industry. This text would never have been completed without Eric Ham, our developmental editor. Eric provided words of encouragement on an ongoing basis. He is extremely skilled and gifted in this type of work. Lastly, we would like to thank Mamata Reddy, our production editor, who made this project a reality. Her patience and support are greatly appreciated.

Christine Miaskowski

Patricia Buchsel

Contents

Principles of Cancer and Cancer Treatment

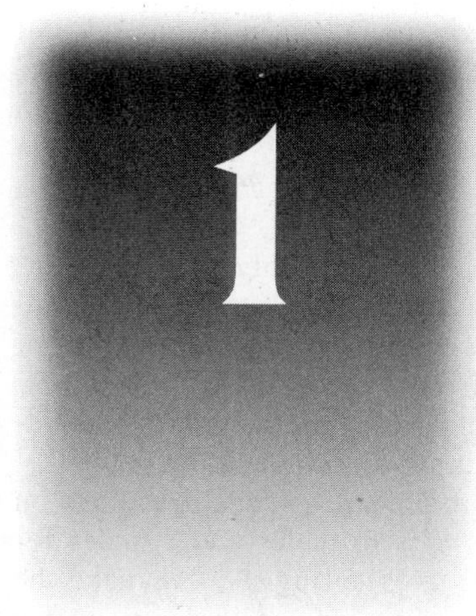

Cancer Epidemiology

Christine Miaskowski, RN, PhD, FAAN

In an editorial published with the American Cancer Society's (ACS's) 1998 Cancer Statistics (Landis, Murray, Bolden, & Wingo, 1998), Dr. David Rosenthal, President of the ACS, states that "the data in 'Cancer Statistics 1998' are both unique and encouraging. For the first time, the ACS's Department of Epidemiology and Surveillance reports a favorable change in direction, with a reduction in the total number of new cancer cases and declining cancer death rates in the United States. In addition, 5-year survival rates continue to improve for most cancers (except those of the lung and bronchus; Rosenthal, 1998, p. 3)." These data represent the results of a multitude of efforts in prevention and early detection, advances in medical and surgical approaches to cancer treatment, advances in symptom management and supportive care, and increased understanding of the basic mechanisms underlying the disease process itself. However, much more work needs to be done before cancer incidence and mortality rates can be reduced by a significant percentage.

This chapter provides an overview of cancer statistics and trends. Since each disease-specific chapter in this text provides detailed information on statistical trends and risk factors for a specific cancer, this chapter focuses on overall cancer incidence and mortality rates. In addition, differences in the magnitude and patterns of cancer by age and by race and ethnicity are reviewed.

EPIDEMIOLOGY

Epidemiologic studies are done to provide descriptions of patients who develop cancer. Often these studies assess the demographic characteristics, health histories, occupations, habits, and lifestyles that may predispose an individual to cancer. Epidemiologic studies report on the association between specific variables and the risk for or rate of occurrence of a particular cancer (e.g., differences in the incidence rates of cancer by gender or ethnicity). Several terms related to epidemiology are defined in Box 1-1.

According to the Surveillance, Epidemiology, and End Results (SEER) program, the impact of cancer in a population is measured and described by looking at a combination of three elements: incidence rates, mortality rates, and survival rates. Cancer incidence is monitored by population-based tumor registries throughout the world. Not all countries maintain population-based tumor registries; and in many countries, including the United States, these registries monitor considerably less than the entire population. Incidence data from existing population-based registries from around the world are compiled by the International Agency for Research on Cancer, a part of the World Health Organization. To make meaningful comparisons among the data from different countries, the rates are age adjusted to the world standard population. The effect of age adjustment is to eliminate differences in rates when a population of one country has an age distribution that differs from that of another country.

Data on cancer incidence, mortality, and survival rates are published on an annual basis by the American Cancer Society. These rates are calculated from a variety of data sources, including the SEER program (Landis et al., 1998). In 1973 the National Cancer Institute began the SEER program to estimate cancer incidence and patient survival in the United States. SEER collects incidence data in nine geographic areas (Fig. 1-1). The geographic areas comprising the SEER program's database represent an estimated 13.9% of the U. S. population. The database contains information on 2.2 million in situ and invasive cancers diagnosed between 1973 and 1995. Approximately 125,000 new cases are accessioned from the nine geographic areas. Areas were selected primarily for their ability to operate and maintain a population-based cancer-reporting system and for their epidemiologically significant population subgroups. With respect to selected demographic and epidemiologic factors, these areas provide a reasonably representative subset of the U. S. population.

INCIDENCE

The number of new cases of invasive cancer that are estimated to be diagnosed in the United States in 1998 is

1,228,600. This estimate does not include basal and squamous cell cancers of the skin (Table 1-1; Landis et al., 1998) or carcinoma in situ of any site except urinary bladder. The current estimate of new cancer cases for 1998 is more than 11% lower than the estimate for 1997 (i.e., 1,382,400; Parker, Tong, Bolden, & Wingo, 1997). The estimates suggest that approximately 51% of the new cases of cancer will be diagnosed in men (i.e., 627,900), and the remainder in women (i.e., 600,700).

Box 1-1
Epidemiology Terms

Incidence rate: The number of new cases per year per 100,000 persons
Mortality rate: The number of deaths per 100,000 cases per year
Survival rate: A determination of the proportion of patients alive at some point after their diagnosis of cancer
Prevalence: Measures the proportion of the population who have cancer at a specified point or during an interval of time; cancer prevalence reflects both the incidence of cancer and survival and provides a measure of cancer burden within a population

From Li, F. P., & Kantor, A. F. (1997). Cancer epidemiology. In J. F. Holland et al (Eds.), *Cancer Medicine* (4th ed.). Baltimore: Williams & Wilkins.

Among men the most common cancers diagnosed will continue to be cancers of the prostate, lung and bronchus, and colon and rectum. These three cancers make up approximately 54% of all new cancer cases in men. Prostate cancer remains the leading cancer site, accounting for 29% of the new cancer cases (Landis et al., 1998).

Among women the three most commonly diagnosed cancers are expected to be cancers of the breast, lung and bronchus, and colon and rectum. These cancers will account for approximately 54% of all new cancer cases in women. Breast cancer diagnoses will account for the largest percentage (i.e., 30%) of new cancer cases in women.

Data from the SEER program provide information on trends in cancer incidence rates in males and females for the period of time from 1973 to 1995 (Fig. 1-2). In males the three cancers with the largest percentage increases in the years 1973 to 1995 were melanomas of the skin, prostate cancer, and non-Hodgkin's lymphoma. In females, during the same time period, the largest increases were noted in lung cancer, melanomas of the skin, and non-Hodgkin's lymphoma (Ries, Kosary, Hankey, & Edwards, 1998).

MORTALITY

In 1998 564,800 Americans are expected to die of cancer—more than 1500 people per day (Table 1-2; Landis et al., 1998). The number of deaths is approximately the same as that predicted for 1997 (i.e., 560,000; Parker et al., 1997).

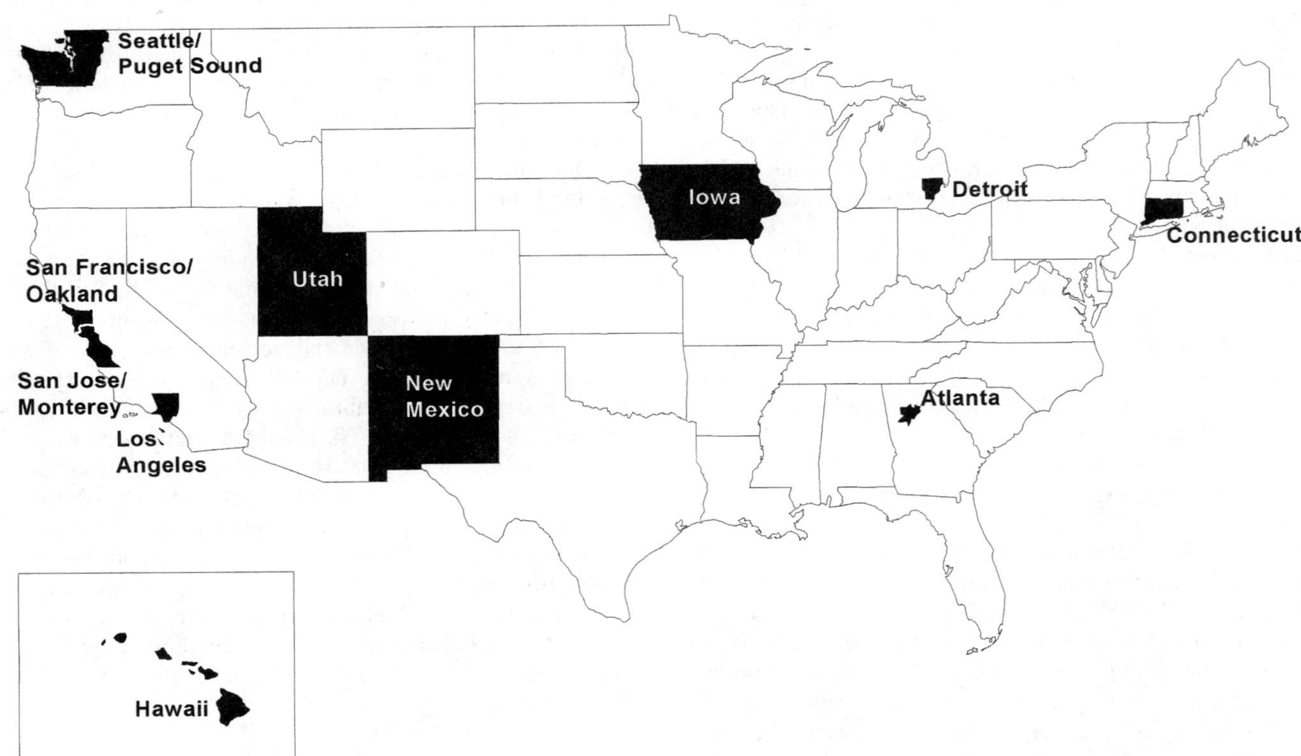

Fig.1-1 Surveillance, Epidemiology, and End Results program. (From Ries, L. A. G., Kosary,, C. L., Hankey, B. F., &Edwards, B. K. [Eds.]. [1998]. *SEER cancer statistics review, 1973-1995.* Bethesda: National Cancer Institute.)

Table 1-1 Estimated New Cancer Cases by Sex, United States, 1998*

	Total	Male	Female
All Sites	1,228,600	627,900	600,700
Oral cavity and pharynx	30,300	20,600	9,700
Tongue	6,700	4,300	2,400
Mouth	10,800	6,500	4,300
Pharynx	8,600	6,500	2,100
Other oral cavity	4,200	3,300	900
Digestive system	227,700	119,200	108,500
Esophagus	12,300	9,300	3,000
Stomach	22,600	14,300	8,300
Small intestine	4,500	2,400	2,100
Colon	95,600	44,400	51,200
Rectum	36,000	20,200	15,800
Anus, anal canal, and anorectum	3,300	1,400	1,900
Liver and intrahepatic bile duct	13,900	9,300	4,600
Gallbladder and other biliary	6,700	2,600	4,100
Pancreas	29,000	14,100	14,900
Other digestive organs	3,800	1,200	2,600
Respiratory system	187,900	104,500	83,400
Larynx	11,100	9,000	2,100
Lung and bronchus	171,500	91,400	80,100
Other respiratory organs	5,300	4,100	1,200
Bones and joints	2,400	1,300	1,100
Soft tissue (including heart)	7,000	3,700	3,300
Skin (excluding basal and squamous)	53,100	33,800	19,300
Melanomas—skin	41,600	24,300	17,300
Other nonepithelial skin	11,500	9,500	2,000
Breast	180,300	1,600	178,700
Genital system	274,000	193,600	80,400
Cervix (uterus)	13,700		13,700
Endometrium (uterus)	36,100		36,100
Ovary	25,400		25,400
Vulva	3,200		3,200
Vagina and other genital organs, female	2,000		2,000
Prostate	184,500	184,500	
Testis	7,600	7,600	
Penis and other genital organs, male	1,500	1,500	
Urinary system	86,300	58,400	27,900
Urinary bladder	54,400	39,500	14,900
Kidney and renal pelvis	29,900	17,600	12,300
Ureter and other urinary organs	2,000	1,300	700
Eye and orbit	2,100	1,100	1,000
Brain and other nervous system	17,400	9,800	7,600
Endocrine system	18,800	5,500	13,300
Thyroid	17,200	4,700	12,500
Other endocrine	1,600	800	800
Lymphoma	62,500	34,800	27,700
Hodgkin's disease	7,100	3,700	3,400
Non-Hodgkin's lymphoma	55,400	31,100	24,300
Multiple myeloma	13,800	7,200	6,600
Leukemia	28,700	16,100	12,600
Acute lymphocytic leukemia	3,100	1,700	1,400
Chronic lymphocytic leukemia	7,300	4,100	3,200
Acute myeloid leukemia	9,400	4,700	4,700
Chronic myeloid leukemia	4,300	2,500	1,800
Other leukemia	4,600	3,100	1,500
Other and unspecified primary sites	36,300	16,700	19,600

From Landis, S. H., Murray, T., Bolden, S., & Wingo, P. A. (1998). Cancer statistics, 1998. *CA: A Cancer Journal for Clinicians, 48,* 6-29.
*Excludes basal and squamous cell skin cancers and in situ carcinomas except urinary bladder.

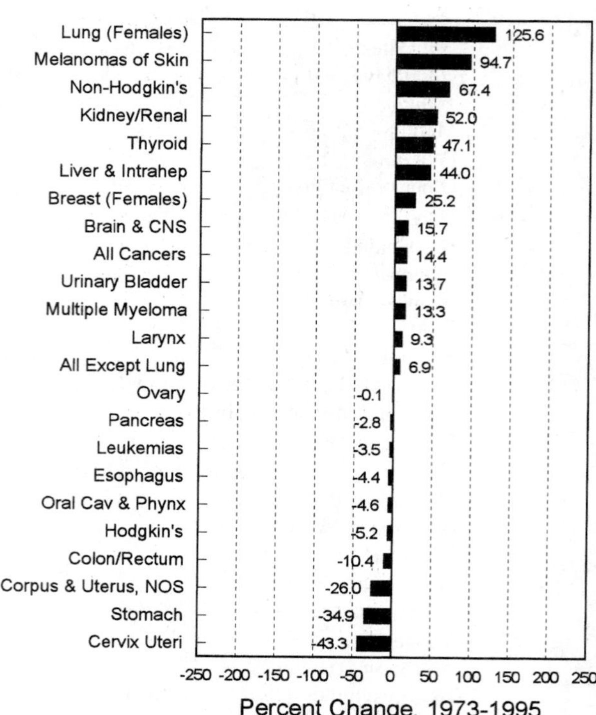

Fig. 1-2 Trends in SEER incidence rates by primary cancer site 1973-1995. (From Ries, L. A. G., Kosary, C. L., Hankey, B. F., & Edwards, B. K. [Eds.]. [1998]. *SEER cancer statistics review, 1973-1975.* Bethesda: National Cancer Institute.)

Most 1998 cancer deaths in men (54%) are expected to be from cancers of the lung and bronchus, prostate, and colon and rectum. However, the number of deaths from these sites appears to be leveling off and may be beginning to decline. This change is consistent with the overall decline in cancer mortality rates (Kramer & Klausner, 1997; Ries, Kosary, Hankey, Miller, & Edwards, 1997). Between 1990 and 1994, mortality rates for men decreased about 1.4% per year for lung cancer, 0.5% per year for prostate cancer, and 1.9% per year for colorectal cancers (Ries et al., 1997).

In women cancers of the lung and bronchus, breast, and colon and rectum are expected to account for more than 50% of the cancer deaths in 1998. In 1987 lung cancer surpassed breast cancer as the leading cause of cancer deaths in women, and that trend is expected to continue into 1998. It should be noted that between 1990 and 1994 the lung cancer mortality rate in women increased by about 1.7% per year (Landis et al., 1998; Ries et al., 1997). In contrast, the number of deaths of women from breast and colorectal cancer appear to be leveling off and may be beginning to decline. Between 1990 and 1994, mortality rates in women decreased about 1.8% per year for breast cancer and about 1.5% per year for colorectal cancers (Landis et al., 1998; Ries et al., 1997).

AGE-RELATED PATTERNS

SEER data on cancer incidence from 1973 to 1991 demonstrates an increase in cancer incidence for the five age groups depicted in Fig. 1-3. However, the largest increases in incidence were seen for the older groups (65 to 74 and 75 and over), where rates increased 35% and 28%, respectively, during this time period. Older people have the highest cancer incidence rates. The incidence rates range from less than 15 per 100,000 for those under 15 years of age to more than 2000 per 100,000 for those 75 and over (Ries et al., 1998).

Fig. 1-4 displays trends between 1973 and 1991 in cancer mortality rates in the United States in five different age groups. Unlike the incidence graph (see Fig. 1-3) that shows increasing trends for all age groups, the data on mortality rates indicate some downward trends among younger Americans. The decrease in mortality rates in children ages 0 to 14 is dramatic, with a greater than 40% decrease since 1973. The 15- to 44-year age group also shows a decrease, but it is not as large. The 45- to 64-year age group showed no change in cancer mortality rates. However, data on this age group are masking an 11% decrease for individuals between 45 and 54 years of age and a 4% increase in individuals between 55 and 64 years of age. In addition, increases of 13.7% and 18.5% are noted for the age groups of 65 to 74

TABLE 1-2 Estimated Cancer Deaths by Sex, United States, 1998*

	Total	Male	Female
All Sites	564,800	294,200	270,600
Oral cavity and pharynx	8,000	5,300	2,700
Tongue	1,700	1,100	600
Mouth	2,300	1,300	1,000
Pharynx	2,100	1,500	600
Other oral cavity	1,900	1,400	500
Digestive system	130,300	69,400	60,900
Esophagus	11,900	9,100	2,800
Stomach	13,700	8,100	5,600
Small intestine	1,200	600	600
Colon	47,700	23,100	24,600
Rectum	8,800	4,800	4,000
Anus, anal canal, and anorectum	500	200	300
Liver and intrahepatic bile duct	13,000	7,900	5,100
Gallbladder and other biliary	3,500	1,200	2,300
Pancreas	28,900	14,000	14,900
Other digestive organs	1,100	400	700
Respiratory system	165,600	97,200	68,400
Larynx	4,300	3,400	900
Lung and bronchus	160,100	93,100	67,000
Other respiratory organs	1,200	700	500
Bones and joints	1,400	800	600
Soft tissue (including heart)	4,300	2,000	2,300
Skin (excluding basal and squamous)	9,200	5,800	3,400
Melanomas—skin	7,300	4,600	2,700
Other nonepithelial skin	1,900	1,200	700
Breast	43,900	400	43,500
Genital system	66,900	39,800	27,100
Cervix (uterus)	4,900		4,900
Endometrium (uterus)	6,300		6,300
Ovary	14,500		14,500
Vulva	800		800
Vagina and other genital organs, female	600		600
Prostate	39,200	39,200	
Testis	400	400	
Penis and other genital organs, male	200	200	
Urinary system	24,700	15,800	8,900
Urinary bladder	12,500	8,400	4,100
Kidney and renal pelvis	11,600	7,100	4,500
Ureter and other urinary organs	600	300	300
Eye and orbit	300	200	100
Brain and other nervous system	13,300	7,300	6,000
Endocrine system	2,000	800	1,200
Thyroid	1,200	400	800
Other endocrine	800	400	400
Lymphoma	26,300	13,700	12,600
Hodgkin's disease	1,400	700	700
Non-Hodgkin's lymphoma	24,900	13,000	11,900
Multiple myeloma	11,300	5,800	5,500
Leukemia	21,600	12,000	9,600
Acute lymphocytic leukemia	1,300	700	600
Chronic lymphocytic leukemia	4,800	2,800	2,000
Acute myeloid leukemia	6,600	3,600	3,000
Chronic myeloid leukemia	2,400	1,400	1,000
Other leukemia	6,500	3,500	3,000
Other and unspecified primary sites	35,700	17,900	17,800

From Landis, S. H., Murray, T., Bolden, S., & Wingo, P. A. (1998). Cancer Statistics, 1998. *CA: A Cancer Journal for Clinicians, 48,* 6-29.
*Excludes basal and squamous cell skin cancers and in situ carcinomas except urinary bladder.

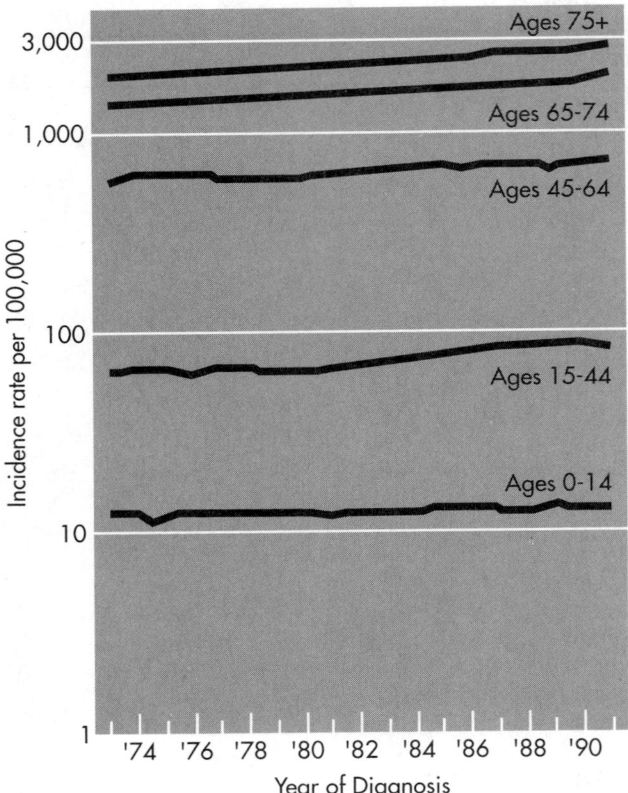

Fig.1-3 Cancer incidence rates by age group from 1973 to 1991. Ries, L. A. G., Kosary, C. L., Hankey, B. F., & Edwards, B. K. (Eds.), (1998). *SEER cancer statistics review, 1973-1995.* Bethesda: National Cancer Institute.

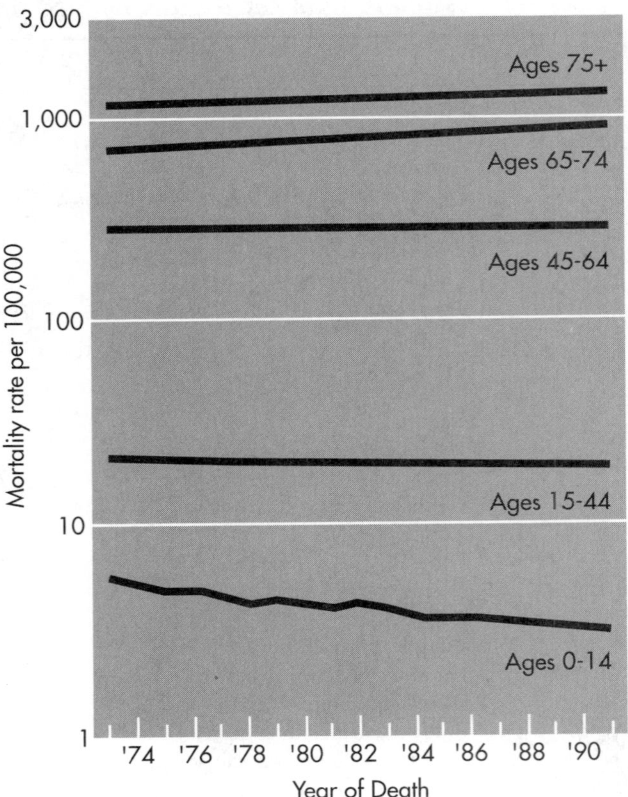

Fig.1-4 Cancer mortality rates by age group from 1973 to 1991. (From Ries, L. A. G., Kosary,, C. L., Hankey, B. F., & Edwards, B. K. [Eds.]. [1998]. *SEER cancer statistics review, 1973-1995.* Bethesda: National Cancer Institute.)

years and 75 years and over, respectively, for the same time period. These figures demonstrate the dramatic impact that cancer has on the elderly population in the United States (Ries et al., 1998).

ETHNIC/RACIAL PATTERNS

Incidence Rates

As shown in Fig. 1-5, overall cancer incidence rates in SEER regions are higher in men than in women. Black men have the highest incidence rate of cancer. Non-Hispanic white men have the next highest rate, which is 14% lower than the rate for black men. Rates for Alaska native men and Hawaiian men follow those for whites and are over one third lower than the rate for black men. The rate for white Hispanic men is similar to that for Hawaiian men. American Indians in New Mexico have the lowest overall cancer incidence rate among men, nearly two thirds lower than the rate for black men. Among the Asian subgroups, Vietnamese men have the highest cancer incidence rate, followed by Japanese, Chinese, Filipino, and Korean men (Ries et al., 1998).

Among women the racial/ethnic differences in cancer incidence rates for all cancers is not as extreme as the rates for men (see Fig. 1-5). The rate is highest in non-Hispanic white women, followed by Alaska Native (less than 2% lower), white (2% lower), black (8% lower), and Hawaiian (9% lower) women. The lowest cancer incidence rates occur in American Indian women in New Mexico and Korean women. Similar to the pattern in men, cancer incidence rates among women are low for Koreans, Chinese, and Filipinos. The incidence rate for all cancers in Vietnamese women is the highest among the Asian women and is higher than the rate for white Hispanic women. Alaska Natives have the highest rate among women 30 to 54 years and 70 years and older. Non-Hispanic white rates are highest among women 55 to 69 years of age (Ries et al., 1998).

Mortality Rates

Similar to the SEER area incidence rates, U.S. mortality rates are highest for blacks, non-Hispanic whites, Alaska Natives, and Hawaiians, although the relative rankings among these four groups differ somewhat from the incidence rate rankings (see Fig. 1-5). Among men blacks have the greatest risk of dying from cancer, whereas for women the highest mortality rate occurs in Alaska Natives. Mortality rates are not currently available for Koreans and Vietnamese. Among groups with relatively low mortality rates, Filipino men and women rank substantially below American Indians, Japanese, Chinese, and white Hispanics (Ries et al., 1998).

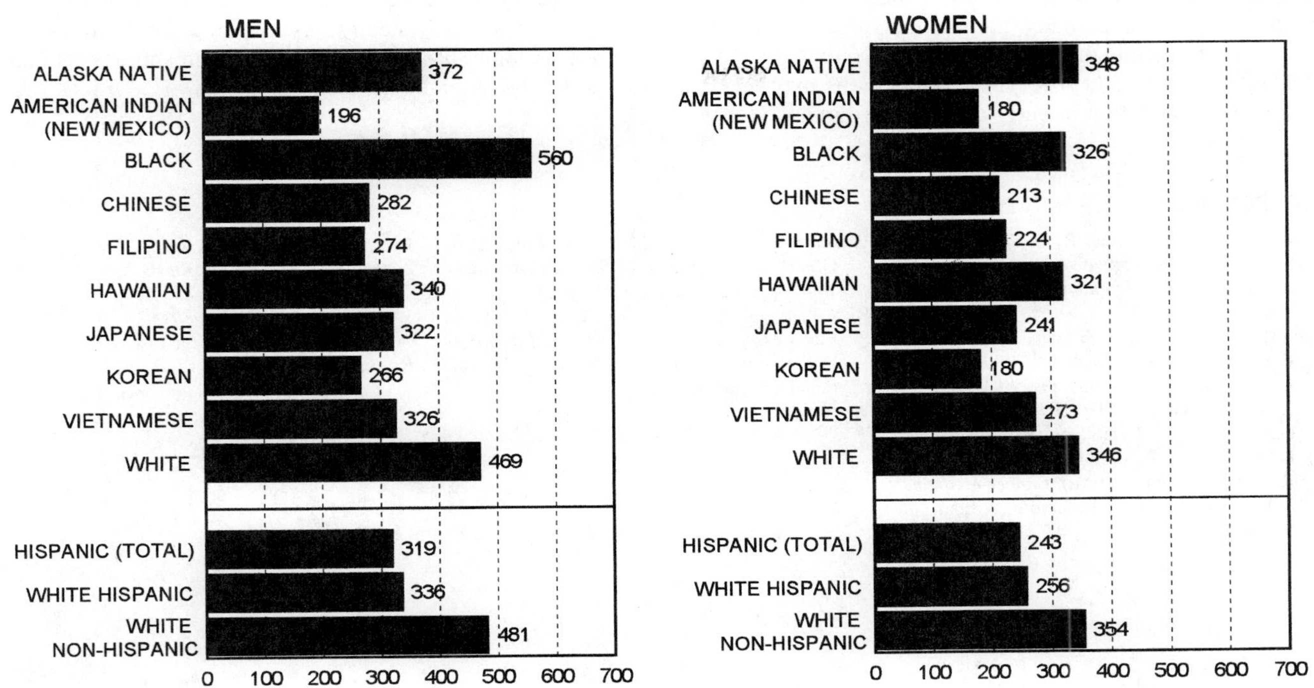

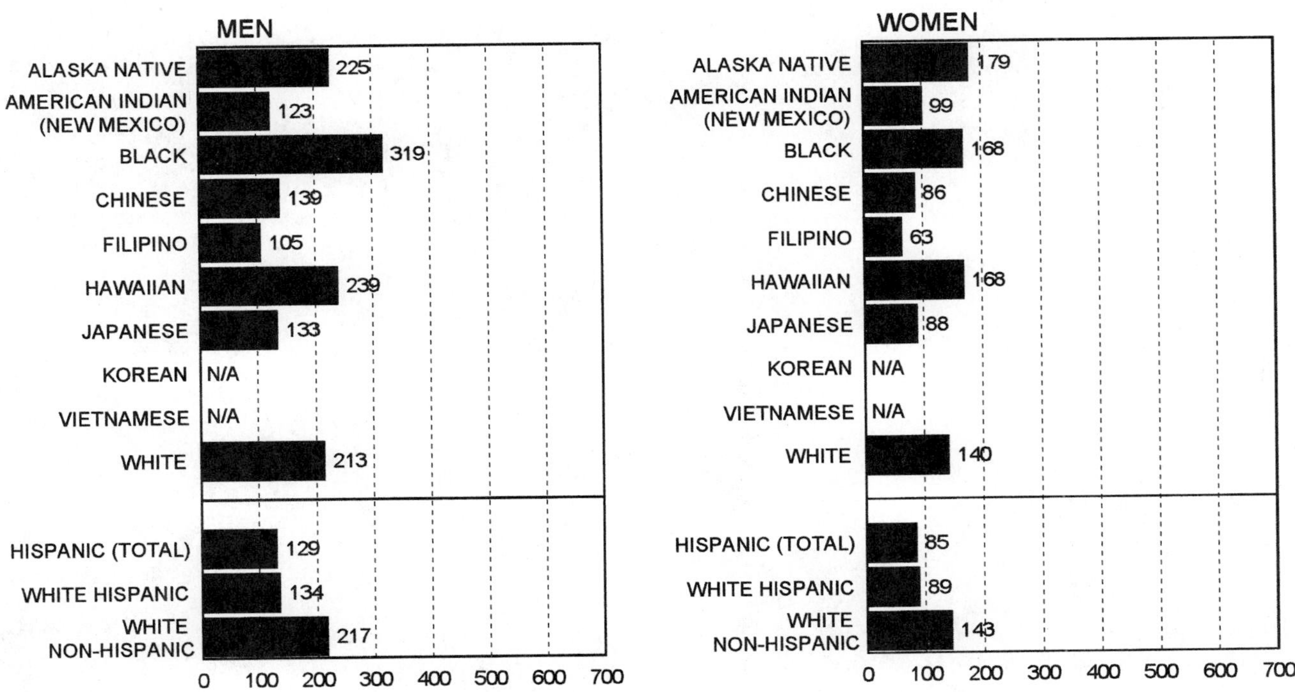

Fig. 1-5 SEER incidence rates 1988-1992 for all cancers combined compared with U.S. mortality rates from 1988 to 1992. (From Ries, L. A. G., Kosary, C. L., Hankey, B. F., & Edwards, B. K. [Eds.]. [1998]. *SEER cancer statistics review, 1973-1995.* Bethesda: National Cancer Institute.) (NOTE: Rates are "average annual" per 100,000 population, age-adjusted to 1970 U.S. standard; N/A = information not available.)

CONCLUSION

A knowledge of the overall trends in cancer incidence and mortality rates, particularly among individuals in certain age groups or racial/ethnic groups, can help oncology nurses identify populations at risk. These populations may require specialized prevention or early detection programs. If these individuals live within certain communities, efforts can be made to provide more targeted prevention and early detection intervention strategies. As noted earlier, more specific epidemiologic information is provided in subsequent chapters that focus on specific cancers.

REFERENCES

Kramer, B. S., & Klausner, R. D. (1997). Grappling with cancer: defeatism versus the reality of progress. *New England Journal of Medicine, 337,* 931-934.

Landis, S. H., Murray, T., Bolden, S., & Wingo, P. A. (1998). Cancer statistics, 1998. *CA: A Cancer Journal for Clinicians, 48*(1), 6-29.

Li, F. P., & Kantor, A. F. (1997). Cancer epidemiology. In J. F. Holland, R. C. Bast, Jr., D. L. Morton, E. Frei III, D. W. Keefe, & R. R. Weichselbaum (Eds.), *Cancer Medicine* (4th ed., pp. 411-420). Baltimore: Williams & Wilkins.

Parker, S. L., Tong, T., Bolden, S., & Wingo, P. A. (1997). Cancer statistics, 1997. *CA: A Cancer Journal for Clinicians, 47*(1), 5-27.

Ries, L. A. G., Kosary, C. L., Hankey, B. F., & Edwards, B. K. (Eds.). (1998). *SEER cancer statistics review, 1973-1995.* Bethesda: National Cancer Institute.

Ries, L. A. G., Kosary, C. L., Hankey, B. F., Miller, B. A., & Edwards, B. K. (1997). *SEER cancer statistics review, 1973-1994: Tables and graphs. (NIH Publication 97-2789).* Bethesda: National Cancer Institute.

Rosenthal, D. S. (1998). Changing trends. *CA: A Cancer Journal for Clinicians, 48*(1), 3-4.

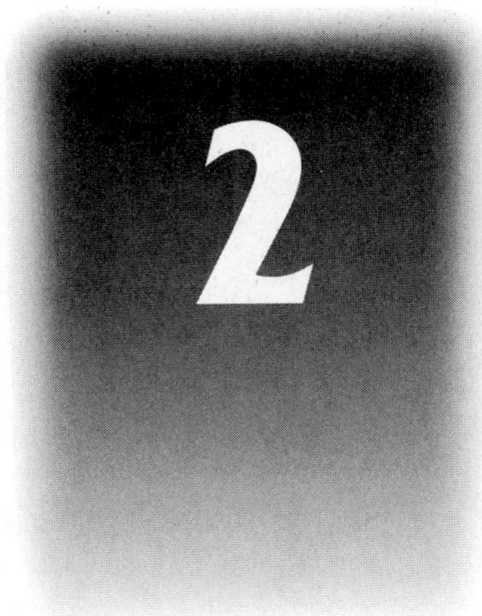

Cancer Pathophysiology

M. Linda Workman, PhD, RN, FAAN
Constance G. Visovsky, RN, MS, ACNP

INTRODUCTION

Cancer is a disorder in which differentiated body cells undergo changes at the molecular level resulting in loss of normal cell regulation, characteristics, and functions. Therefore, although cancer is classified according to organ systems, such as breast cancer, lung cancer, and colorectal cancer, *cancer is really a disease of cells*. Cancer cells actually have reverted to a less differentiated state reminiscent of embryonic development (Cooper, 1995). Biologic regulation of these cells is altered dramatically, allowing cancer cells a significant selection advantage over normal differentiated body cells and, without treatment, progression to the extent that vital physiologic functions are disrupted, leading to death. The molecular changes that transform normal cells to cancer cells are exerted at the level of the genes. Thus, all cancer is genetic in origin; however, few human cancers are heritable.

Every malignancy arises from one cell or one group of cells that were originally normal in appearance, function, regulation, genetic content, and gene expression. The concept that groups of cancer cells can arise from a single transformed normal cell is the *monoclonal origin of cancer.* The development of a recognizable tumor from one transformed cell requires a series of conditions occurring over time to a susceptible host. Such conditions include exposure to events or substances that mutate genetic content (quantitatively or qualitatively), enhanced expression of genetic changes, insufficient immunosurveillance, and other host factors.

Normal Cellular Biology

The pathophysiology of cancer is based on genetic and external factors inducing changes in normal cell biology. The regulatory, anatomic, and functional characteristics of normal cells, embryonic cells, nonmalignant neoplastic cells (benign cells), and malignant cells are compared.

Normal Cells.

Growth Characteristics. Regulation of cell division is strictly controlled for normal cells. Normal cells capable of mitosis divide only for one of two reasons: to develop normal tissue (such as breast development in a prepubescent girl), and to replace lost or damaged normal tissues (such as new skin growth after a partial-thickness burn injury). Among tissues capable of mitosis, even when cell loss has occurred and tissue replacement is needed, normal cells will divide only if conditions for optimum growth are present. These conditions include adequate nutrition, available blood supply, presence of specific cell growth factors, presence of inducing tissues, and appropriate space. If even one of these requirements is missing or less-than-optimum, cell division is minimal or absent. Once the reason for cell division no longer exists (e.g., the skin lost in a partial-thickness burn injury has been replaced with new skin growth), cell division stops so that redundant tissues do not form. This characteristic is demonstrated in vitro as density-dependent contact inhibition of cell growth in tissue culture. Once a cell is in direct contact on all sides with like cells, mitosis ceases, rendering normal cell division contact inhibited.

Cell Cycle. Normal cells undergoing mitosis do so in a predictable sequence with considerable regulation involved in leaving the usual reproductive resting state, G_0, and entering the reproductive cycle (cell cycle) (Fig. 2-1). Cells incapable of mitosis, such as neurons and myocardial cells, never leave the reproductive resting state. Cells capable of cell division enter the cell cycle periodically, spending the majority of their life spans in G_0. In the reproductive resting state, the cell functions normally and to its fullest physiologic capacity. In the cell cycle, the cell does not perform its standard differentiated functions; it only prepares itself for actual cell division, mitosis.

The point at which cells leave the reproductive resting state and enter the cell cycle is an area for regulation and control. For any cell to be able to enter the cell cycle, a variety of metabolic conditions must be met. Thus, in regulatory terms, entrance of the cell into the cell cycle is regulated by restriction point control factors. If conditions are not met, the cell cannot overcome the restrictions and reproduce at this time.

Entering the cell cycle is an irreversible act and commits the cell to mitosis. Cells can become trapped or arrested in

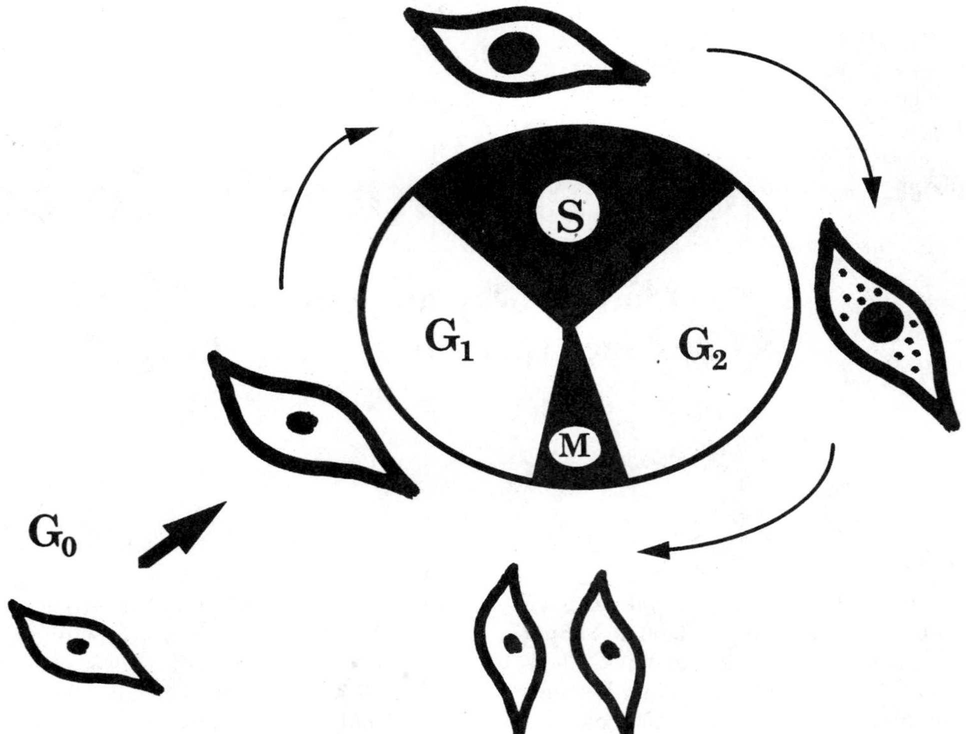

Fig. 2-1 The cell cycle.

any stage of the cell cycle, but they do not reverse the process back to G_0. The purpose of mitosis is to perform a duplication cell division in which the resulting two cells (daughter cells) are identical to each other and identical to the parent cell. Thus the activities of the cell in most phases of the cell cycle include the synthesis of twice as much cellular components to allow a complete duplication division. The cell cycle is divided into four distinct, sequential phases, each characterized by specific biologic tasks leading to cell division. The phase of G_1 usually lasts 4 to 6 hours and is characterized by membrane synthesis, production of increased amounts of cytoplasm, increased uptake of nutrients, and increased energy metabolism. The S phase usually lasts 4 to 6 hours and is characterized by deoxyribonucleic acid (DNA) synthesis, in which the cell exactly duplicates its DNA content. The phase of G_2 is the most variable in length, lasting from 2 to 8 hours. This phase is characterized by intense protein synthesis and synthesis of cellular organelles. The actual phase of cellular division is the M phase. This phase is the shortest, usually 1 hour, and has subphases describing the movement and final separation of all intracellular components, including the DNA, into the two daughter cells.

Phenotypic Characteristics. Mature normal cells are functionally and morphologically differentiated. Each cell type has a specific morphology and at least one specific function. Erythrocytes synthesize hemoglobin; myocytes contract in response to nerve stimulation; pancreatic endocrine cells secrete insulin.

Except for erythrocytes, leukocytes, and thrombocytes, which are supposed to be mobile, normal cells within a tissue are tightly adherent to one another, preventing migration. Normal cells secrete the glycoprotein, fibronectin, and retain it as a cell surface component. Fibronectin forms part of the extracellular matrix that binds normal cells of one type tightly together. Thus each cell type remains within its organ of origin and does not migrate from one organ to another.

Genotypic Characteristics. The nucleus is the site of gene storage and activity. All normal cells contain the total amount of genetic material (DNA), genes, that is appropriate for the species. During the M phase of the cell cycle, the genes can be viewed as condensed matter termed *chromosomes.* Normal human cells contain 46 chromosomes, 22 pairs of autosomes, and 1 pair of sex chromosomes, The number 46 is known as the *diploid* number because it represents all the normal chromosome pairs. Cells containing the right amount of chromosome material for the species are known as *euploid.* In the normal healthy human, all cells, with the exception of the sex cells (oocytes and spermatocytes) and mature erythrocytes, should be euploid. Sex cells are considered *haploid* because they contain only half of each pair of chromosomes. Mature erythrocytes have extruded their nuclei during the maturation process and contain no chromosomes.

Even though all normal cells each contain a full complement of human genes, not all genes in every cell are active. For example, only the beta cells of the pancreas synthesize insulin, although all cells have the gene for insulin. The insulin gene is suppressed or maintained in an inactive state in all cells except the pancreatic beta cells, where the insulin gene is permitted to be expressed.

The nucleus size of normal cells is relatively small, because each cell contains one copy of each pair of genes. In contrast, the cytoplasmic areas of normal differentiated cells are large, as this is the location of much intracellular activity. Thus normal differentiated cells have a small nuclear/cytoplasmic ratio.

Embryonic Cells. The concept of each normal, mature cell having a specific morphology and function (or set of functions) is interesting when one considers that all human beings started life as a single cell. Although human embryonic cells, those present from conception until postconception day 8, are clearly normal, for a narrow time frame their behavior and characteristics are very different from mature differentiated cells.

Growth Characteristics. The main focus of action for an early embryonic cell is to undergo mitosis, expanding the size and cell numbers of the embryo. Cell division for early embryonic cells is controlled but very rapid.

Cell Cycle. Early embryonic cells complete each phase of the cell cycle in the proper sequence. Conditions surrounding the embryo are so favorable that as quickly as an early cell completes mitosis, it is ready to re-enter the cell cycle. Thus these cells, while under restriction point control, do not spend significant time in the reproductive resting state of G_0. It appears that early embryonic cells do continue to enter the cell cycle even when contacted on all surfaces by other cells. Thus these cells do not exhibit density-dependent contact inhibition of cell growth.

Phenotypic Characteristics. Early embryonic cells are functionally and morphologically undifferentiated. No anatomic features are present that distinguish the future neuron from the future toenail. They all have a small, round appearance, or anaplastic morphology. These early embryonic cells cannot perform any differentiated functions. In addition, they do not synthesize any of the intracellular or cell-surface proteins found on normal differentiated cells. Early embryonic cells have no fibronectin. As a result, these cells are loosely adherent to each other and continually reposition themselves within the growing embryonic ball. At this developmental stage, embryonic cells have full potential to mature into any differentiated cells. This flexible state is referred to as *pluripotent, multipotent,* or *totipotent.*

The characteristic of pluripotency coupled with rapid mitosis allows early embryonic cells to survive and progress even when conditions are unfavorable. If exposed to lethal conditions at this stage, resulting in the destruction of 90% of the embryo, the remaining 10% continue mitosis and simply replace the lost cells. Such a situation would result in delay of development but would not result in disruption of development.

Genotypic Characteristics. All normal human early embryonic cells are euploid, containing only the normal diploid chromosome number. However, because these cells are in an almost constant state of mitosis in which the DNA content must be duplicated, the nuclei of embryonic cells appear larger than those of normal differentiated cells. In addition, because the embryonic cells have no differentiated function, the cytoplasmic space of the cells is smaller than that of differentiated cells. Thus the early embryonic cells have a large nuclear/cytoplasmic ratio.

In the early embryonic cell, all genes are duplicated during cell division. Although these early embryonic cells contain the same genes that mature, differentiated human cells contain, only a relatively few genes in the early embryo are expressed. The expressed genes are believed to regulate the growth and characteristics of the embryo at this stage. All other genes are suppressed at this time.

Commitment. At a defined point in early embryonic development, the cells initiate the steps to become differentiated. Commitment of human cells is thought to occur on postconception day 8. In response to an unknown signal(s), each cell commits itself to a specific maturational outcome. At the time of commitment, the cell has not taken on any differentiated features or functions, but it now positions itself within a group that will eventually take on a specific morphology and functional behavior. Differentiation does not involve the loss of any genes; all committed cells retain the same number of genes present in the fertilized egg. Differentiation is a function of the selective suppression and selective expression of individual genes. The process of commitment involves turning off (suppressing) specific genes that regulated and directed the early rapid growth and turning on (expressing) other individual specific genes that control the expression of specific differentiated functions. Which genes are selectively expressed determines what specific type of tissue each embryonic cell will complete maturation and differentiation to become.

Neoplastic Cell Biology

Neoplasia is the growth of new cells not required for normal development or for replacement of damaged or lost cells. All types of neoplasia are considered examples of abnormal cell growth. However, whether neoplasia leads to pathology or physiologic disruption depends on the location, growth rate, and characteristics of the neoplastic tissue.

Benign Neoplasia.

Growth Characteristics. Benign neoplastic cells arise from normal differentiated cells. These cells tend to retain most of the morphologic and functional characteristics of the totally normal cells from which they arose. However, benign cells represent populations of abnormal cells. Some examples of benign neoplastic tissues include hypertrophic scars, nevi, endometriosis, and a wide variety of benign (nonmalignant) tumors, such as myomas, lipomas, and hemangiomas.

Cell Cycle. Benign cells are capable of mitosis. They enter the cell cycle and progress through all phases in the same way and at the same general rate as normal cells. The major difference in growth characteristics between benign cells and normal cells is that the benign cells undergo mitosis either when there is no need or where there is no need. Thus benign cells have lost some degree of density-

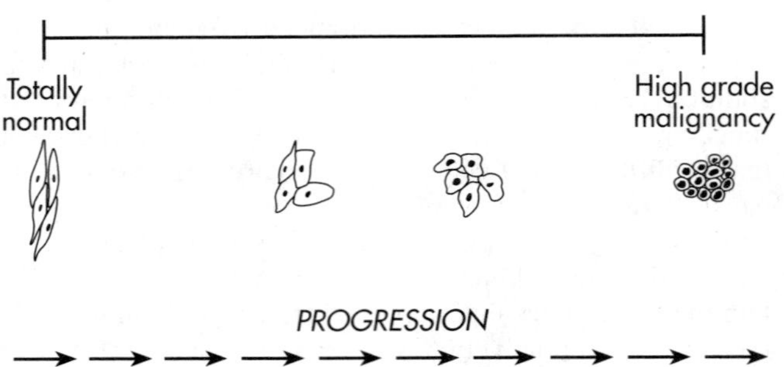

Fig. 2-2 Continuum of cancer development from totally normal to highly malignant.

dependent contact inhibition of cell growth and continue to grow by expansion.

Phenotypic Characteristics. Benign neoplastic tissues are morphologically and functionally similar, and often identical, to the normal tissues from which they arose. Identifying the tissue of origin for benign cells and tumors is not difficult because these cells and tumors continue to perform the parent tissue's differentiated function. They have a small nuclear/cytoplasmic ratio and continue to synthesize fibronectin. Thus benign cells adhere tightly together and do not migrate within the body or within any organ. Benign tumors are not capable of metastasis.

Even though benign cells and tumors do not invade surrounding tissue and do not metastasize to distant sites, at times their continued presence and growth can cause physiologic dysfunction and death. For example, a benign tumor in the trachea or mainstem bronchus might grow to such a size that complete airway obstruction could occur.

Genotypic Characteristics. At the microscopic level, benign cells are euploid, containing the normal chromosome complement. However, because their behavior is not totally normal, it is likely that at the molecular level, some alteration in gene regulation is present.

Malignant Neoplasia. Malignant neoplastic cells are cancer cells and have no beneficial purpose. These cells also arise from normal differentiated cells. However, over time and through many steps, they lose most normal cell characteristics and acquire new characteristics. The new characteristics that persist usually confer some type of advantage to the malignant cell that allows it and its progeny to survive and thrive even when environmental conditions are less than favorable. Some of the new characteristics appear to be reactivation of embryonic characteristics, especially the synthesis of proteins and enzymes, such as telomerase, important for embryonic development but that have no role in the maintenance of differentiated functions (Coursen, Bennett, Gollahon, Shay, & Hassis, 1997).

Cancer development and progression actually represent a continuum, with the totally normal cell at one end and the most malignant cancer cell at the other (Fig. 2-2). Most cancers are diagnosed somewhere along the continuum, not at the final or most malignant end. As a result, the biologic features of any cancer tend to change over time.

Growth Characteristics. To successfully divide and result in the formation of two functional daughter cells, a cancer cell must complete all phases of the cell cycle. Early in cancer development, malignant cells do not divide more rapidly than the parent tissue from which they arose. The major change in growth characteristics among cancer cells is the gradual loss of restriction point control. Eventually, nothing prevents cancer cells in the reproductive resting state of G_0 from entering the cell cycle. Thus cancer cells speed up the rate of tissue growth by largely spending very little time in G_0 and exhibit no density-dependent contact inhibition of cell division (Pitot, 1986).

In cell culture, malignant cells are considered to be immortal. For example, normal cells cultured in a flask grow to cover the surface of the flask over time and can be divided among a number of flasks. Each division is considered a passage. Normal cells can be passaged only a limited number of times before they enter a quiescent state and no longer engage in mitosis. Malignant cells can be grown in the same type of flask and possess the capability to be passaged an infinite number of times, maintaining their malignant functional characteristics.

Malignant cells are capable of growing without a supporting substratum. Such cells grow easily in semisolid agar or in a suspension culture. Thus malignant cells are considered to have a loss of anchorage dependence. This ability to grow in such diverse media correlates with the ability of the cells to produce tumors in experimental animals.

Phenotypic Characteristics. The further along the continuum of malignancy a cancer cell is, the less it has in common with the parent tissue from which it arose (Fidler & Hart, 1982). As cancer progresses, the cells become more anaplastic in appearance until they no longer resemble the parent tissue. Most differentiated functions are lost. Because the cancer cells continually undergo mitosis and perform fewer and fewer differentiated functions, the cytoplasmic volume decreases. Thus cancer cells have a large nuclear/cytoplasmic ratio.

Functional Membrane Changes. Some of the acquired characteristics of cancer cells involve cell surface and membrane changes. Cancer cells synthesize little if any fibronectin. Therefore cancer cells adhere loosely together. They can easily separate from the original site, enter the vascular system, and migrate throughout the body. Additional membrane surface enzymes enhance metastasis by digesting the extracellular matrix of normal cells, allowing tumor extension and/or invasion into surrounding normal tissues. These same enzymes loosen vascular cells in blood vessel walls, enhancing cancer cell penetration into the vascular system and contributing to metastasis.

Another membrane surface change that occurs in cancer cells is the increased permeability or enhanced uptake mechanisms of the cancer cell membrane for glucose, proteins, and other nutrients. For example, most cancer cells do not require the presence of insulin for glucose to enter the cell. If insulin is present, cancer cell uptake of glucose is even more rapid. This change ensures that cancer cells receive available nutrients before normal cells. Cancer cells in vitro demonstrate this characteristic by continuing to divide and grow even when the culture medium contains few nutrients.

Some malignant cells express (actually overexpress) specific receptor sites. This situation is thought to play an important role in cancer development by increasing the production or reception of signals that increase the proliferation rates of malignant cells (Baron & Borgen, 1997).

Anatomic Membrane Changes. Cancer cells express different membrane surface components, particularly receptors and proteins (antigens), than do the normal cells from which they arose. Most cancer cells have increased numbers of lectin binding sites and, as a result, are more easily stimulated to engage in mitosis. Some cancer cells express different cell surface antigens compared to surface antigens of normal differentiated cells. Some antigens are normal protein products synthesized by normal cells at an earlier developmental period but either are not expressed by mature cells or are expressed only in small quantities. Such antigens are alpha-fetoprotein (α-FP), carcinoembryonal antigen (CEA), human chorionic gonadotropin (HCG), lactate dehydrogenase (LDH), and alkaline phosphatase (AP).

In addition, different cancer cells may express surface antigens that are completely new and are found only on the cancer cells. Such proteins are termed *tumor-specific antigens* (TSAs). These antigens can be used as a marker to identify and quantify the amount of tumor present. More recently, antibodies directed against TSAs are being used for cancer therapy and cancer prevention.

Not all cancer cells express TSAs. They are found most frequently on tumors arising from chemical or viral carcinogenesis. Some TSAs are common to all tumors of the same type. Others are unique to the tumor of an individual.

Genotypic Characteristics. The genetic content of cancer cells differs quantitatively and qualitatively from normal cells (Mitelman, 1994). Such differences, initially arising as gene mutations, are largely responsible for cancer development. In the progression from beginning cancer development to the state of greatest or highest degree of malignancy, the genes of cancer cells continue to undergo changes. Thus the more malignant a cancer cell, the more abnormal the genetic material (Piao, Kim, Jeon, Lee & Park, 1997).

Quantitative Changes. Chromosomes of most cancer cells are seldom normal or euploid. Instead, cancer cell chromosomes may have additions or deletions of whole chromosomes, as well as structural rearrangements of other chromosomes. This abnormal gene/chromosome content is called *aneuploidy* and is used as a prognostic indicator. Overall, less aneuploidy is indicative of a lower level of malignancy. Additionally, because some chromosomal aberrations are specific for a type of cancer, aneuploidy can be used as a diagnostic indicator. For example, most chronic myelogenous leukemia cells demonstrate a specific chromosomal rearrangement in which chromosome 22 has lost part of its DNA. This specific chromosomal aberration is called the *Philadelphia chromosome.* Table 2-1 lists specific cancers frequently associated with a specific chromosomal aberration.

TABLE 2-1 Examples of Malignancies Associated With Specific Chromosomal Aberrations

Malignancy	Chromosomal Aberration
Acute myelogenous leukemia	t(8;21)
Acute promyelocytic leukemia	t(15;17)
Burkitt lymphoma	t(8;14)
Chronic myelogenous leukemia	t(9;22)
Ewing's sarcoma	t(11;22)
Neuroblastoma	1q+
Retinoblastoma	13q−
Small cell lung cancer	3p−
T-cell leukemia	t(10;14)
Wilms' tumor	11p−

The genetic mutations of cancer cells reflect losses of normal genes important for homeostatic regulation and function, or reflect amplification of those genes that direct the cancer cell to express a malignant phenotype. It is likely that both conditions are necessary to some degree for malignancy to occur and progress (Cohen & Geradts, 1997).

Qualitative Changes. The mechanism of converting normal cells into cancer cells is the changing of gene activity so that embryonic characteristics are expressed after cells have differentiated. The early embryonic genes that regulated embryonic growth for the first 8 days postconception have no known purpose beyond commitment. Therefore these early embryonic genes, known as *proto-oncogenes,* are part of the normal genetic complement (genome) of all human cells and should remain in a suppressed state forever after commitment occurs. The regulator genes that provide the continuing suppressive influence over proto-oncogenes are the suppressor genes. Cancer development involves the activation (lack of suppression) of proto-oncogenes into actively expressed genes termed *oncogenes.* When a normal cell is exposed to any carcinogen, the normal cell's DNA can be mutated, causing the proto-oncogenes, which should be repressed forever, to be expressed at an inappropriate time. Continued oncogene expression causes normal differentiated cells to revert to a less differentiated state and express malignant characteristics (Cooper, 1995; Macgrogan, Pegram, Slamon, & Bookstein, 1997).

More than 50 different proto-oncogenes have been identified, and more are suspected to exist (Cooper, 1995; Weinberg, 1994). Carcinogenic or mutational events can directly activate the proto-oncogene or can damage the associated suppressor gene, removing suppressor influence from the proto-oncogene and allowing oncogene activation and cancer development (Bosnar et al., 1997; Powell, Harper, Hamilton, Robinson, & Cummings, 1997). Table 2-2 lists known oncogenes, known suppressor genes, and their associated malignancies.

TABLE 2-2 Malignancies Associated with Altered Gene Activity

Gene	Malignancies
Oncogenes	
abl	Chronic myelogenous leukemia, other leukemias
c-myc	Burkitt's lymphoma; T-cell and B-cell neoplasms; breast, stomach, and lung carcinomas
erb B	Glioblastomas, squamous cell carinoma
erb B-2	Breast, salivary gland, ovarian carcinomas
ets	Lymphoma
hst	Breast carcinoma, squamous cell cancers
int-2	Breast carcinoma, squamous cell cancers
L-*myc*	Lung carcinomas
met	Osteosarcoma
myb	Colorectal carcinomas, leukemia
PRAD-1	Breast carcinoma, squamous cell cancers
ras K	Prostate; multiple carcinomas, sarcomas, neuroblastoma, leukemias, lymphomas
ret	Thyroid carcinomas
trk	Colorectal and thyroid carcinomas
Suppressor Genes	
APC	Colorectal, stomach, and pancreatic carcinomas
c-fos	Lung carcinoma
DCC	Colorectal carcinomas
EXT1	Hepatocellular carcinomas, hereditary multiple exostoses
MTS-1	Melanoma; brain tumors; leukemias; sarcomas; breast, bladder, ovarian, lung, and kidney carcinomas
NF1	Neurofibroma, colon, astrocytoma
NF2	Neurofibroma, meningioma, schwannoma
nm23-H1	Testicular carcinomas
p53	Breast, bladder, colorectal, esophageal, liver, lung, and ovarian carcinomas; brain tumors; sarcomas; leukemias and lymphomas
Rb	Retinoblastomas; sarcomas; breast, bladder, esophageal, and lung carcinomas
Smad4	Gastric adenocarcinomas, colorectal carcinomas
VHL	Renal cell carcinoma, pheochromocytoma, hemangioblastoma
WT1	Wilms' tumor

MOLECULAR GENETICS

The controlling factors for cellular development and function are the genes. A gene is a specific segment of DNA that codes for or has the pattern for a specific gene product (a protein). All cells make substances that are used for the normal "housekeeping" duties of the cell. In addition, some cells make at least one specific substance that leaves the cell and is either used by other cells or controls the activity of other cells. All of these substances are proteins, and the processes involved in making these proteins are termed *protein synthesis.* Protein synthesis involves the DNA and specific genes.

DNA Synthesis

The nucleus of a cell contains the DNA, which contains the codes or patterns for construction of every protein made by every cell within the body. DNA is composed of two very long chains (strands) of interlocking nucleotides. Each nucleotide is composed of a molecule of any one of the following four bases: adenine (A), guanine (G), thymine (T), or cytosine (C). Adenine and guanine are purines; thymine and cytosine are pyrimidines. These bases are attached to a five-carbon sugar (a pentose arrangement called a *ribose*). These ribose-base complexes are linked together by phosphate groups. This linkage between the individual bases allows polymerization of the complexes, forming long strands of DNA.

In humans, DNA is double-stranded in antiparallel arrangements. The two strands are held in close, but not direct, proximity by a number of relatively weak ionic forces. These ionic forces are easily disrupted when the cell needs to undergo either DNA synthesis or protein synthesis. The bases in the two adjoining strands have a special and specific affinity for each other. Adenine pairs with thymine, and guanine pairs with cytosine. Thus the two strands of DNA are lined up together, composed of interacting bases that form base pairs. Because the bases are specific in their attractions, the two strands of DNA are complementary to each other in terms of their nucleotide sequence (Fig. 2-3). Therefore if the sequence of one DNA strand is known, the sequence of the complementary DNA strand can be predicted with accuracy.

When cells are not dividing, the double-stranded DNA has a loosely coiled helical arrangement, which cannot be delineated with standard light microscopy. Late in the cell cycle, the DNA becomes more tightly condensed, coiling the DNA at well-regulated intervals around protein substances called *histones,* eventually forming chromosomes. Chromosomes are visible under standard light microscopy.

During mitosis, the DNA content of the dividing cell must first replicate (duplicate) through the process of DNA synthesis. This process occurs entirely within the nucleus. The new DNA is made by using the original strands of DNA as templates. The original strands of DNA temporarily loosen and separate from the tight helical arrangement, under the influence of a series of enzymes. The DNA relaxes, unwinds from the histones, slightly straightens, and separates the two strands over a limited area. A polymerizing enzyme attaches itself to one strand, travels down the strand (from the 5′ to 3′ direction), "reads" the base sequence of this strand, and forms a new strand of DNA complementary to the template strand (Fig. 2-4). The DNA synthesis process is called the *semiconservative method* because it results in the formation of two identical double helices, each containing one original strand of DNA, and one newly created strand of DNA. After the strands of DNA have been replicated, they condense into supercoiled chromosomes sets that split to become part of two new daughter cells.

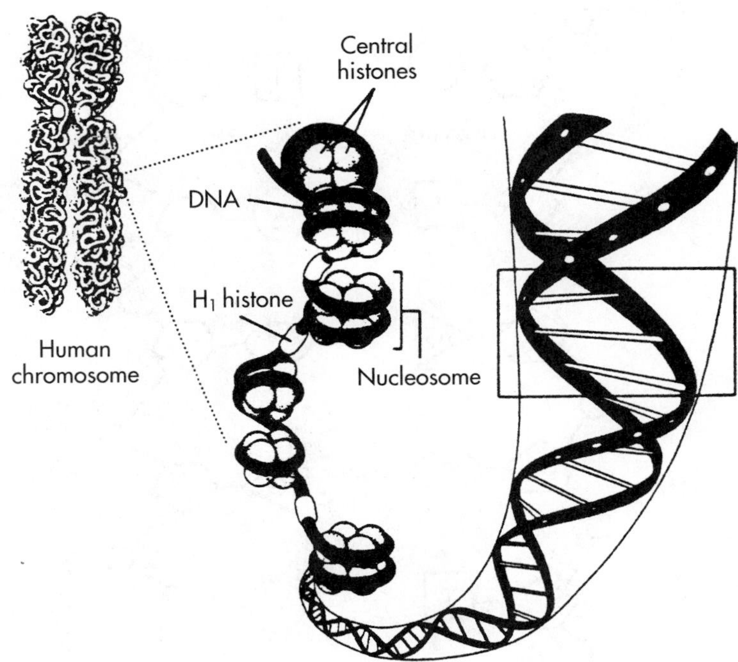

Fig. 2-3 Double-stranded DNA. (From McCance, K., & Huether, S. [1994]. *Pathophysiology: The biologic basis for disease in adults and children.* [2nd ed.]. St. Louis, Mosby.)

Protein Synthesis

Cells have DNA genes that serve as codes for individual proteins. The unique DNA gene sequence for a specific protein is first transcribed into a piece of ribonucleic acid (RNA). RNA is similar to DNA, but instead of containing thymine (T), RNA contains uracil (U).

Proteins are formed by linking individual amino acids together in a linear strand. There are 22 different amino acids. Each amino acid has a unique three-base code sequence, called a *codon,* which identifies the DNA and RNA segments specific for that amino acid. Some amino acids have only one codon, whereas others have as many as four distinct but closely related codons. Table 2-3 lists specific RNA codons for each amino acid.

The total number of amino acids in a specific protein and the exact code in which they are linked together determine the nature and activity of the protein. Protein synthesis is similar to some of the steps in DNA synthesis, but instead of completely separating and replicating the entire double helix containing all the genes (genome), only the DNA area containing the actual gene for the specific protein to be synthesized is separated and transcribed into a complementary RNA strand. The newly transcribed RNA, messenger RNA (mRNA), leaves the nucleus and enters the endoplasmic reticulum where the mRNA is processed and translated into protein.

In an active cell, messenger RNA interacts with two other types of RNA, ribosomal RNA (rRNA) and transfer RNA (tRNA). These substances literally build a protein by linking the specified individual amino acids in the correct sequence (Fig. 2-5).

TABLE 2-3 Amino Acid RNA Codons

Amino Acid	RNA Codons
Alanine	GCU, GCC, GCA, GCG
Arginine	CGU, CGC, CGA, CGG
Asparagine	AAU, AAC
Aspartic acid	GAU, GAC
Cysteine	UGU, UGC
Glutamic acid	GAA, GAG
Glutamine	CAA, CAG
Glycine	GGU, GGC, GGA, GGG
Histidine	CAU, CAC
Isoleucine	AUU, AUC, AUA
Leucine	CUU, CUC, CUA, CUG, UUA, UUG
Lysine	AAA, AAG
Methionine	AUG
Phenylalanine	UUU, UUC
Proline	CCU, CCC, CCA, CCG
Serine	UCU, UCC, UCA, UCG
Threonine	ACU, ACC, ACA, ACG
Tryptophan	UGG
Tyrosine	UAU, UAC
Valine	GUU, GUC, GUA, GUG

MALIGNANT TRANSFORMATION: CARCINOGENESIS

The transformation of normal cells to cells with malignant characteristics is called *malignant transformation* or *carcinogenesis.* Carcinogenesis is a multistep process that occurs

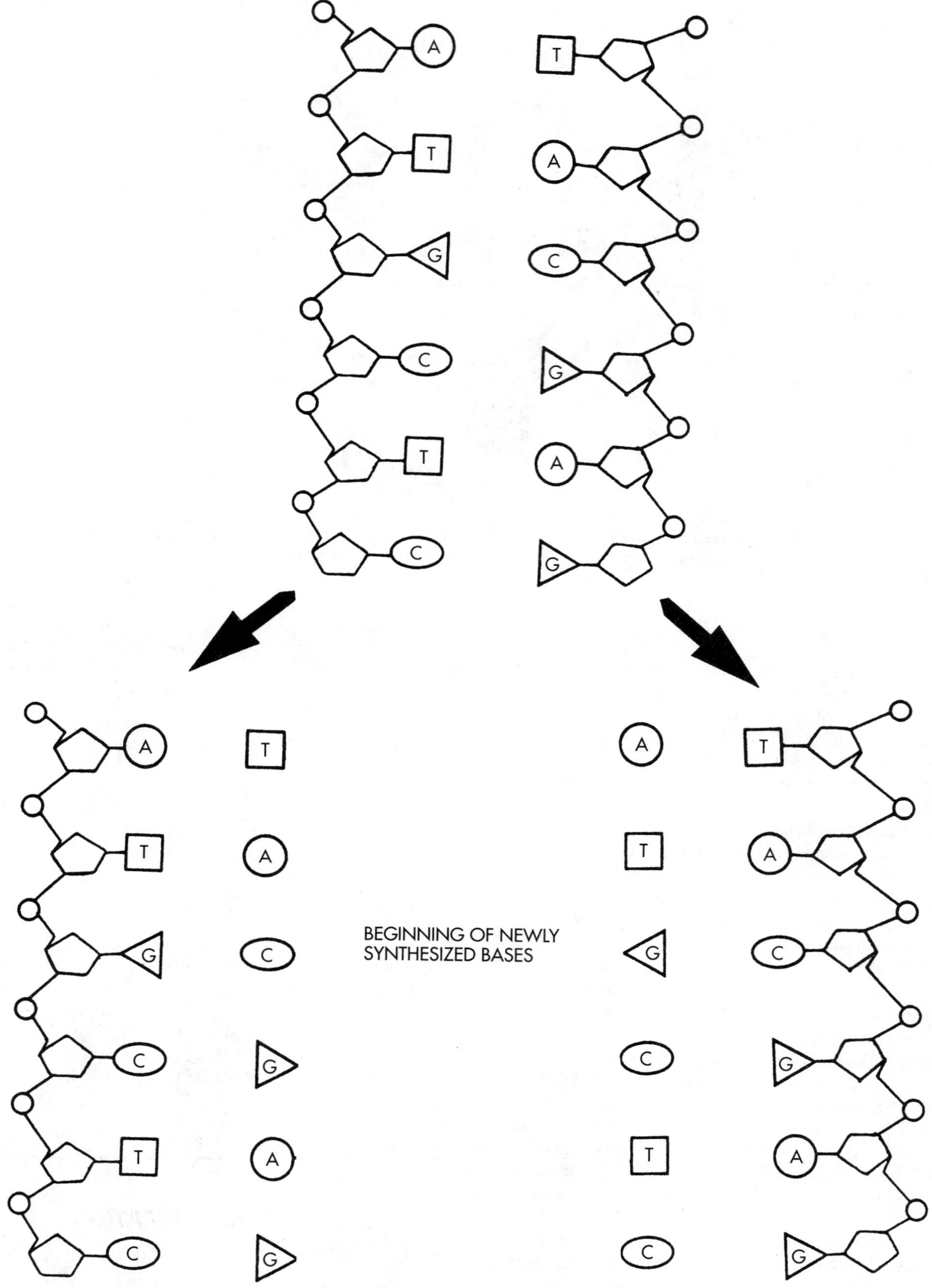

Fig. 2-4 Semiconservative model of DNA replication.

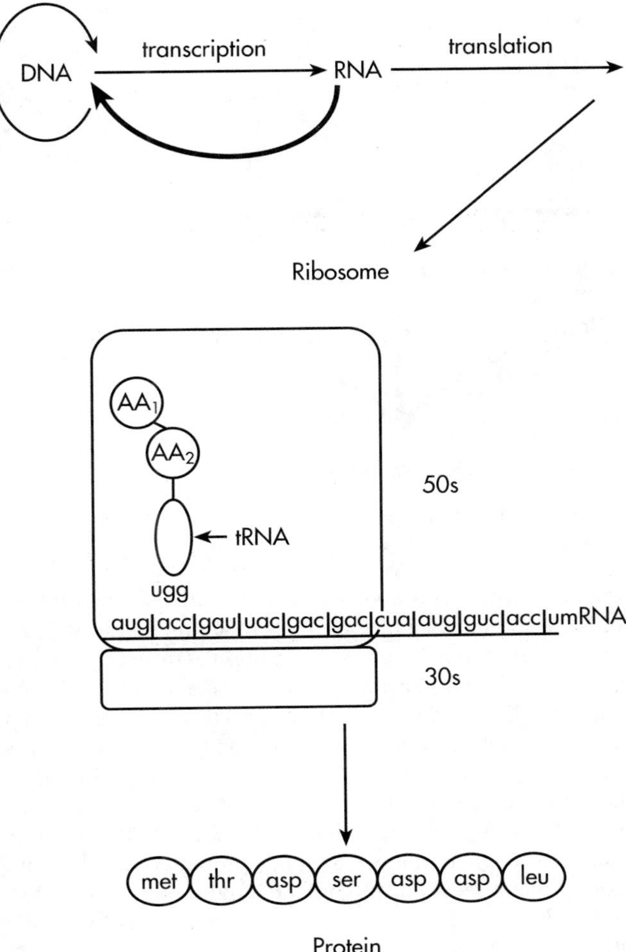

Fig. 2-5 Steps involved in protein synthesis.

over months to years. The underlying cause of carcinogenesis is damage or mutation of genetic material by physical, environmental, or chemical agents, or by viruses, or inherited factors in the germ line (Bishop, 1982, 1995). The normal regulatory genes, proto-oncogenes, and anti-oncogenes (suppressor genes) are most affected by genetic damage. Proto-oncogenes are structural genes that direct the synthesis of enzymes and protein growth factors; suppressor genes (anti-oncogenes) are regulatory genes that suppress the expression of structural gene products needed for growth and proliferation. Four critical events are associated with carcinogenesis: initiation, promotion, progression, and metastasis (Fig. 2-6).

Initiation

To become initiated, normal cells must be exposed to a carcinogen. A carcinogen is any agent or substance (living and nonliving) that causes malignant transformation. The mechanism of initiation is either a direct mutation of one or more proto- oncogenes (resulting in the replication of multiple copies of the genes and enhancing their oncogenic expression), or mutation of one or more suppressor genes, eliminating suppressor activity and allowing oncogene expression (Weinberg, 1996). The effects of initiation can lead to cancer development only if the mutation does not interfere with the cell's ability to divide and if the mutation is successfully transmitted to succeeding generations of cells. Thus for a malignancy to result from initiation, the effects of initiation must be irreversible.

There are two types of carcinogens: incomplete and complete. An incomplete carcinogen requires that the same cells be subsequently exposed to a promoter after initiation in order for a malignancy to develop. Initiators can be physical agents, such as asbestos, chemical agents, such as benzene, or viruses, such as hepatitis B. Some substances act together as co-carcinogens. For instance, alone, either smoking or daily alcohol intake increases the risk of developing head and neck cancers. The risk of cancer development by smoking 1 pack/day or consuming 2 ounces of alcohol/day is approximately 3/1000. Combining these substances by smoking and consuming alcohol daily gives rise to a 15/1000 risk of head and neck cancer developing. This is known as a *synergistic effect.*

Initiation from a carcinogen, for example, ultraviolet radiation, causes permanent damage to cellular DNA. Although the cell is forever altered, this damage alone may not be expressed and does not necessarily lead to the formation of a cancer. To become cancerous, cellular initiation must be followed by a continued promotion.

It is likely that many normal body cells become initiated daily. However, few of these initiations develop into recognizable malignancies. Several factors work together to prevent cancer development. These factors are ineffective initiation, DNA repair, removal/destruction of initiated cells, and insufficient promotion.

Ineffective Initiation. Not all mutational events result in sufficient gene damage to permit initiation. Sometimes a mutational event replaces one base with another (point mutation) and does not alter the coding region. Mutational events can occur in areas of the genome that are "silent" or do not contain important genes. Even when a mutational event alters a proto-oncogene or a suppressor gene, the alteration may not be significant enough to activate the proto-oncogene or deactivate the suppressor gene.

DNA Repair. Normal cell mitosis and activity are dependent on faithful, accurate transcription of DNA. Because this accuracy is so critical, redundant molecular genetic "backup" mechanisms exist to examine newly transcribed DNA and ensure that accurate transcription has occurred. These backup mechanisms literally repair DNA that has been transcribed inaccurately. These same repair mechanisms can examine cellular DNA that has undergone mutation as a result of exposure to a carcinogen and repair the mutated area(s). Thus cancer development is somewhat dependent on a lack of a balance between initiating events and DNA repair.

The effectiveness of DNA repair mechanisms varies among different people. This personal characteristic appears to be heritable. However, environmental insults can decrease the effectiveness of DNA repair mechanisms. Among people with active, well-functioning DNA repair mecha-

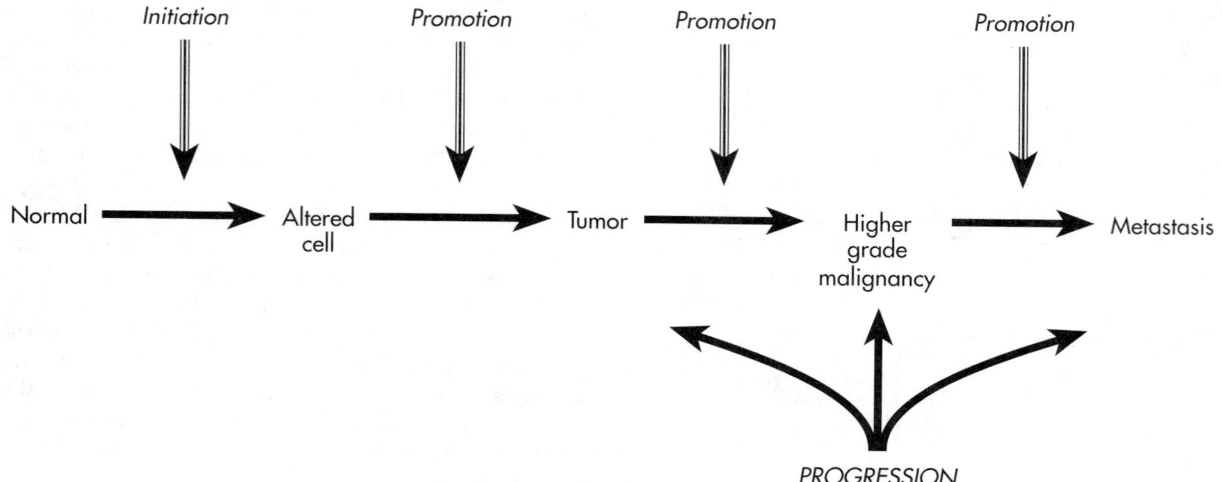

Fig. 2-6 Steps involved in cancer development. (From M. Linda Workman, 1994.)

nisms, the normal aging process is slow and cancer rates are low. Among people with less active or faulty DNA repair mechanisms, effects of the aging process appear earlier and cancer rates are higher. When exposure to initiating events occurs so frequently than even well-functioning DNA repair mechanisms cannot keep pace with the mutations, cancer is more likely to develop.

Removal/Destruction of Initiated Cells. Initiated cells as well as phenotypic cancer cells usually express some changes in the cell membrane properties or on the cell surface compared to normal cell membranes and surfaces. Such changes can be recognized by certain immunoreactive and inflammatory cells, which take actions to eliminate or destroy the initiated cells. Thus immunocompetence plays an important role in protection against cancer development (Applebaum, 1992).

Insufficient Promotion. Initiation alone, even when proto-oncogenes are activated to oncogene status, is not always sufficient to sustain cancer development. Most frequently, the initiated cell must be regularly and continually exposed to promoters (promoting substances or conditions) to have its growth rate enhanced to a point where proliferation of the initiated cell population occurs faster than the body's normal defenses are able to destroy or eliminate it.

Latency. Between initiation and promotion is a latency period. Latency is the period of time from the carcinogenic exposure and initiation to the expression of a full-blown recognizable malignant state. Latency is a general feature of malignancy, although the time lag is multifactorial and varies with genetic make-up, type of carcinogen, environmental factors, and dose of the carcinogen. Years can pass between exposure to a promoter and the subsequent development of cancer.

Promotion

A promoter is an agent or condition capable of altering the expression of genetic information in the cell. Examples of promoters include hormones (especially estrogen), plant products, drugs (psoralin, oral contraceptives, anabolic steroids), chemicals, and viruses. As much as initiation is the first step in carcinogenesis, promotion is a necessary secondary effect. This secondary effect results in the enhancement of cellular growth and division. Promotion in itself appears to be a reversible event, requiring two stages. The first stage involves fixation. In this stage of cellular proliferation, the promoter acts to increase the number of cells that have been previously initiated, thus fixing the genetic alteration caused through initiation. Second, promoters act to cause more direct effects on subsequent cellular populations. Promoters in this stage act to depress certain genes by turning off suppressor genes that have been functioning since the completion of embryonic development.

The promoting agents do not react directly with the genes (genetic material), but rather they affect the expression of the genetic material in a variety of ways. Promoters interact with cell surface receptor sites, activating enzyme systems and increasing the concentration of second messengers such as cyclic adenosine monophosphate, which in turn activates the nucleus of the cell. Changing the activity of the nucleus and cytoplasmic proteins increases protein synthesis and cell division. Some promoters alter the structure and function of other cellular components.

Exposure to promoters alone does not result in cancer development. For cancer to develop, promotion must follow initiation. Timing of promotion is a key element in malignant transformation. Early animal model experimentation and the well-documented sequence of events related to cervical cancer development provide evidence to support the role of promotion in cancer development.

Early studies of carcinogenesis in animals indicated that direct skin exposure to some chemicals eventually resulted in cancer development and that exposure to other chemicals did not result in a malignancy. Chemicals that caused cancer were designated as carcinogens (now known as *complete carcinogens*) and those that did not were considered safe. Further experimentation revealed that sometimes two safe chemicals applied together would cause cancer and that when the application of some safe chemicals followed the application of established carcinogens, tumors developed more quickly. Thus, these chemicals were termed *promoters*. However, it was noted that application of promoters before the application of the carcinogen (initiator) had no influence on subsequent tumor development. Additionally, it was noted that even if the application of the promoting agent occurred years after the initiator, malignant transformation still occurred.

Mass screening of women for cervical cancer has served as a human in vivo model of the steps involved in malignant transformation. Cervical cells are considered to be a part of the woman's external environment and are exposed to initiating conditions. One type of initiating condition is infection with viruses such as the human papilloma virus or herpes simplex virus type 2. These viruses infect cervical cells and induce DNA mutations when they intercolate the viral genomes into the DNA of the cervical cells. Thus these viruses can initiate cervical cells. For months to years after the cervical cells have been initiated, there is no phenotypic change in the appearance or function of the cervical cells. However, if the woman begins taking oral contraceptives or becomes pregnant (both conditions expose the woman to increased concentrations of estrogen), promotion occurs. The cervical cells undergo phenotypic changes that first are manifested as dysplasia; the cells have an abnormal appearance but continue to function normally. Often, when either the pregnancy is over or if the woman stops taking the oral contraceptives within only a few months, the cervical cells revert back to a normal appearance (morphology), but remain initiated. Subsequent pregnancies or other hormonal exposures promote the initiated cervical cells beyond dysplasia into frankly malignant cells, capable of progressing to a higher state of malignancy and undergoing metastasis.

Progression

Through initiation and promotión, cellular genetic material is altered, and there is enhancement of growth and cell division. As progression takes place, different cellular populations arise within one neoplasm. The cell lines with the most malignant characteristics tend to be the ones that survive. In this stage, neoplastic growth is characterized by an increased growth rate, increased invasiveness, metastases, and morphologic changes in the clonal cells (Liotta, 1992).

One normal cell that is altered (initiated) under the right conditions (promotion) will produce a colony or population of cells just exactly like itself, cloned cells. Because the cells are all exactly alike, they are homogeneous. The original altered cell is called the *main stem–line progenitor.* The expression of the original gene changes continues to vary with time so that subpopulations of cells within a tumor begin to appear, and these subpopulations differ in some ways from the stem-line progenitor (Fidler & Hart, 1982). Most of the differences in the subpopulations that survive long enough to be observed provide these subclones with certain advantages that enable them to survive no matter what or how the environmental conditions change. These advantages are thus called *selection advantages.*

The exact mechanism(s) of malignant cell progression has yet to be elucidated. However, theories for this process include hybridization, gene transfection, and gene amplification. Hybridization, or fusion of the malignant cell's nucleus with one of a normal cell, may occur as malignant cells interact with normal support cells of a tumor (stroma, blood vessels, connective tissues). Fusion with a normal cell has been postulated to help the malignant cell survive by allowing it to escape immunosurveillance, or to increase its response to normal growth factors. The process of transfection, or the insertion of other DNA sequences into the cancer cell's genome, may occur more easily than the same process in normal cells. This process may be one through which virally induced tumors continue their malignant progression. The theory with the greatest support is the gene amplification theory, in which loss of regulatory gene influence (suppressor gene activity) allows the systematic replication of oncogene DNA sequences (Renshaw, McWhirter, & Wang, 1995; Schmidt, Ackermann, Hartmann, & Strohmeyer, 1997). This action would result not only in enhanced transcription of an oncogene, but also in an actual increase in the number of oncogene copies. Conditions both internal and external to the malignant cell may result in enhanced gene activation and replication.

Metastasis

Metastasis is the spreading of a malignancy beyond the tissue from which it arose. It is the ability to metastasisze that makes cancer lethal and difficult to treat successfully (Nicolson, 1979). With progression, the ultimate stage of malignancy is metastasis, indicating the success of the malignant cell in overcoming host defenses. However, further progression can occur during the metastatic state.

Malignant cells can move from the original group of transformed cells (primary site) by direct extension (remaining in direct contact with the original group), invasion, and by severing connections with the original group and establishing colonies at remote or distant sites (Ruoslahti, 1996). Metastasis is neither a random event nor an early step in cancer development. It is an ability of malignant cells acquired through progression and involves significant sequential interactions and cooperativity with normal cells. The processes requisite for metastasis are neovascularization, extension into surrounding tissues and blood vessels, circulation, arrest, extravasation, and proliferation (Fig. 2-7).

Neovascularization. Although a requisite for metastasis, neovascularization must occur relatively early in progression after a tumor has formed. Initially, tumors derive their nutrients by diffusion from the extracellular fluid. As the tumor increases in size, diffusion to the innermost areas of the tumor is minimal, and the cells become hypoxic as well as deprived of other nutrients. The hypoxic tumor cells secrete tumor angiogenesis factor (TAF), which is similar to other tissue angiogenesis factors and which diffuses to nearby vasculature. TAF stimulates cell division in the vasculature and the extension of new blood vessels that grow from the normal vasculature into the tumor. This process

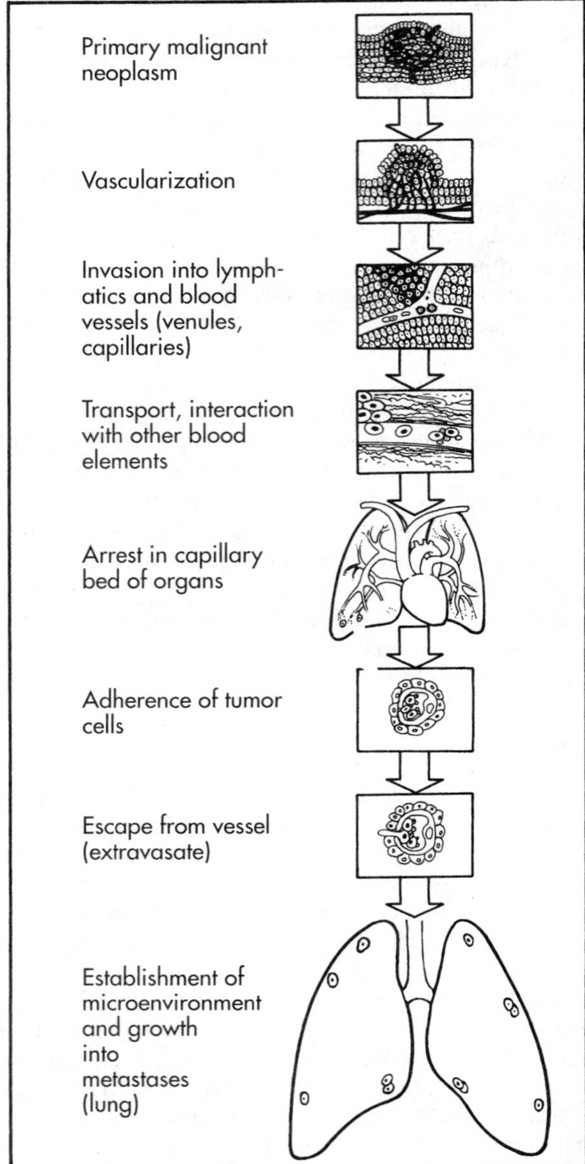

Fig. 2-7 Pathogenesis of metastasis. (From McCance, K., & Huether, S. [1998]. *Pathophysiology: The biologic basis for disease in adults and children.* [3rd ed.]. St. Louis, Mosby.)

provides the tumor with a blood supply, contributing to its successful progression.

Extension. Malignant cells within the tumor secrete enzymes to loosen areas of surrounding tissue. Mechanical pressure, created as the tumor increases in size, allows tumor cells to penetrate between the cells of neighboring tissue. Pieces of the tumor separate from the primary tumor. Some of these clumps of cells remain in or seed neighboring tissues with new colonies of cancer cells. Other clumps penetrate blood vessels and lymph channels, enter the systemic circulation, and metastasize to distant sites by the hematogenous and lymphatic routes.

Circulation. Once malignant cells are in the circulatory system, they have the potential to spread nearly everywhere. However, the blood, although the most common medium of transport for the tumor cells and the major mechanism for metastasis, is also a relatively hostile environment. Immune and inflammatory cells can attack and destroy the cancer cells. Some tumor cells are thought to protect themselves by surrounding their membranes with plasma proteins, such as fibrin, to prevent exposure and potential recognition of the tumor cell–specific surface antigens. With access to the circulatory system, tumor cells can circulate through all or most tissues. Thus by the hematogenous route, cancer cells have the potential to metastasize anywhere. However, cancer spread is not a random event. Table 2-4 lists usual sites of distant metastasis for common malignancies.

Table 2-4 Usual Sites of Metastasis for Common Malignancies

Malignancy	Usual Sites of Metastasis
Breast carcinoma	Adjacent lymph nodes, bone marrow, lung, liver, brain
Cervical carcinoma	Clavicular lymph node, adjacent pelvic structures
Colorectal carcinoma	Adjacent lymph nodes, liver, bone marrow
Leukemia	Central nervous system, visceral organs
Lung carcinoma	Liver, brain, bone marrow, adjacent structures
Prostate carcinoma	Bone, pelvic structures

Arrest and Extravasation. An early hypothesis for metastasis was that circulating tumor cells were trapped in fine capillary meshes of highly vascular organs. If metastasis were only just such a physical/mechanical event, all highly vascular organs would be at equal risk for becoming metastatic sites. Such is not the case. For example, the kidney is one of the most vascular organs in the body, normally receiving at least 20% of cardiac output. However, metastasis to the kidney is a relatively rare event.

More recent evidence indicates that although tumor cells probably enter all tissues/organs, there is some selection about which tissues provide the best secondary site for that malignant cell population. Studies by Fidler and Hart (1982) in animal models demonstrated metastatic selection. Metastatic melanoma cells that had colonized the brain were injected into the tail veins of mice (where they had the opportunity to circulate to almost all areas before reaching the brain). These "brain-specific" melanoma cells continued to establish metastatic sites almost exclusively in the brain. As a result of these heavily reproduced studies and results, Fidler put forth the "good soil" theory, which proposes that each subpopulation of tumor cells has specific growth requirements and will only colonize a body area that can provide the specific requirement. Essentially, this theory suggests that as tumor cells progress and the various subpopulations become heterogeneous within the primary tumor, each subpopulation of the tumor has different growth requirements and each subpopulation metastasizes separately.

Proliferation. Once malignant cells have left the circulation at remote sites, they are under the same constraints for growth that the primary tumor was at an earlier stage of development. These secondary tumor cells must manipulate the new environment to promote tumor cell survival, vascularization, and tumor growth. However, because these cells have already undergone progression to some degree and have developed selection advantages, their chance for successful colonization at the remote site is high ("practice makes perfect").

CAUSES OF CARCINOGENESIS

The complete carcinogenic/oncogenic process leading to oncogene activation and expression requires time and an interaction among three primary environmental and personal factors. These factors are environmental exposure to carcinogens, genetic predisposition, and immune function (Ames, Gold, & Willett, 1995). These interactions account for variation in cancer development among groups of people exposed to the same or similar known carcinogenic events.

Environmental (External) Factors

Most cancer development in North America is the result of exposure to environmental or extrinsic factors (Trichopoulos, Li, & Hunter, 1996). Environmental carcinogens include chemical, physical (such as radiation and chronic exposure), or viral agents. Exposures to these agents can occur anywhere—in the home, in the workplace, in almost any geographic setting (Stellman & Stellman, 1996).

Chemical Carcinogenesis. Most incidences of chemical carcinogenesis were identified through clinical observations. Current knowledge concerning the induction of cancer by certain exogenous substances can be traced to the observation associating the use of tobacco snuff with the occurrence of nasal polyps (Hill, 1961). In 1775, Percival Pott, an English physician, noted an unusually high incidence of scrotal cancer in men employed as chimney sweeps in childhood. He correctly surmised that the cancer was directly attributable to soot exposure and suggested chimney sweeps bathe daily as a means of prevention. More than a century later, Japanese pathologists induced skin tumors in rabbits by the repeated application of coal tar to the ears. Such early experiments gave rise to the notion that environmental factors can be responsible for the development of cancer, especially with repeated exposures over time.

Additional evidence in support of chemically induced carcinogenesis has been demonstrated through comparisons of cancer incidences in different parts of the world. Some cancers are more prevalent in certain geographic locations. Gastric cancer is a relatively rare cancer in the United States, but is common in Japan. However, studies over two generations of Japanese individuals who have immigrated to the United States found that patterns of cancer development became similar to those prevalent in Western society. This change implicates environmental factors in the pattern of cancer development.

Today, there is epidemiologic evidence of chemically induced carcinogenesis. Chemical carcinogens can react with the cell's DNA to induce certain genetic mutations through initiating events, altering the function of regulatory genes. Some chemicals act to cause cancer through promotion. These agents stimulate cell proliferation through increased cell division. Many chemical carcinogens act both as initiators and promoters; inducing genetic mutation and cell proliferation. Chemicals capable of inducing carcinogenesis can be direct acting or indirect acting. Direct-acting chemicals do not require a chemical transformation to induce carcinogenesis. Indirect-acting chemicals, or procarcinogens, require metabolic conversion in the host to be capable of malignant transformation. Both direct-acting and metabolically converted chemicals have electron-deficient atoms that react with electron-rich sites within the cell, including the DNA and RNA. Examples of chemicals capable of inducing carcinogenesis include tobacco and ethanol.

Smoking. Long after evidence was produced linking smoking of cigarettes to the development of lung cancer, smoking remains the number one cause of cancer in humans. Smoking can be linked to nearly one third of all cancer deaths. In addition, smoking has been linked to a variety of cancers, including lung, oral cavity, larynx, esophagus, kidney, pancreas, and bladder. Tobacco is a potent carcinogen, containing benzo(a)pyrene, dimethylnitrosamine, and nickel compounds, all of which act as both initiators and promoters of malignant transformation.

Despite warnings from the U.S. Surgeon General, the prevalence of tobacco use, in the form of cigarettes, pipes, cigars and chewing tobacco, has increased steadily over the years. In 1998, cancer of the lung and bronchus accounted for approximately 32% of cancer-related deaths (American Cancer Society, 1998). Although the occurrence of breast cancer in women has received much attention, cancer of the lung and bronchus has exceeded breast cancer as a cause of mortality in women. In fact, from 1990 to 1994, the risk of lung cancer–related deaths in women increased approximately 1.7% per year (Landis, Murray, Bolden, & Wingo, 1998).

The risk of developing lung cancer depends largely on the quantity and duration of tobacco use. There is a relatively long latency period between the onset of smoking and the development of lung cancer that can span 20 years. There is also evidence to suggest that passive smoking is also associated with an increased risk of lung cancer development.

Alcohol. The exact mechanism by which excessive alcohol intake is implicated in the subsequent development of cancer is uncertain. Experimental evidence suggests that ethanol is weakly carcinogenic in animals. However, it may act to potentiate the action of other carcinogens. Ingestion of excessive ethanol has been linked to the development of cancers of the liver, esophagus, oral cavity, and larynx. There has also been evidence to suggest cancers of the colon, rectum, breast, and thyroid may be associated with excessive alcohol intake. As a co-carcinogen, alcohol acts in conjunction with tobacco to greatly increase the risk of cancer development. The combination of tobacco and alcohol use can be attributed as a cause of 75% of all cancers of the oral cavity.

Radiation Carcinogenesis. Radiant energy is able to induce malignant transformation in experimental animals and humans. The two most common forms of radiant energy are ionizing radiation and ultraviolet radiation.

Ionizing Radiation. This type of radiation creates energy by removing electrons from atoms. Examples of ionizing radiation include x-rays, gamma rays, and particulate radiation. Sources of exposure to ionizing radiation include nuclear accidents, occupational exposure, and medical treatments. The effects of nuclear explosions have been seen in the survivors of the atomic bomb blasts in Hiroshima and Nagasaki, who developed acute and chronic myelocytic leukemias as long as 7 years later. In the early part of the twentieth century, radiologists who had frequent exposure to x-rays incurred a threefold to fourfold risk of developing leukemia. High-dose radiation therapy is a common treatment for cancer. However, it can induce the development of secondary cancers.

Ionizing radiation appears to exert its effects directly on the double helix, causing demethylation of DNA proteins and breaks (with subsequent rearrangements) of both the nucleotide and phosphate backbone. Radiation exposure is measured in *rads* (radiation absorbed doses). In living systems, the radiation is absorbed randomly by atoms and molecules in cells. With few exceptions, extended exposure to ionizing radiation can induce practically all types of human cancers. The risk of cancer development as a result of exposure to ionizing radiation depends on: the type of radiation, the total amount of energy deposited per unit volume of tissue (dose), and the rate of energy deposition (related to duration and intensity of exposure). Ionizing radiation has a temporal relationship of exposure, meaning the effects of this type of radiation are cumulative.

Ultraviolet Radiation. The primary source of ultraviolet radiation is from the sun. Solar radiation is the major cause of skin cancer worldwide. Ultraviolet (UV) rays exert several effects on the cells of the skin. The UV rays can inhibit cell division, inactivate cellular enzymes, and induce mutations through the formation of pyrimidine dimers in DNA. Unrepaired dimers in turn can lead to transcriptional errors and cancer development. Epidemiologic evidence suggests that the risk of developing cancer of the skin depends on the intensity and type of exposure and the quantity of melanin in the skin. The effects of UV exposure tends to be cumulative. Individuals with fair skin who experience repeated sunburn and live close to the equator have the highest incidence of melanoma. It is estimated that 1 million cases of basal and squamous cell cancers of the skin and 21,100 cases of melanoma can be expected to be diagnosed in 1998 (Landis et al., 1998). Although basal and squamous cell carcinomas occur fairly frequently, they are highly curable, as they metastasize very slowly. On the other hand, melanomas are far more deadly, as they tend to invade visceral organs and metastasize rapidly.

Chronic Irritation. Chronic irritation and tissue trauma have been suspected as predisposing physical agents to cancer development, but this theory has not been supported directly. The incidence of skin cancer is higher in people with burn scars and other tissues that have sustained severe injury. Chronically irritated tissues may undergo frequent mitosis and, thus, are at an increased risk for spontaneous DNA mutation (Pitot, 1986).

Viral Agents. Relatively few viruses have been proven to be carcinogenic to humans, although they are suspected to play major roles in the development of cancer. When viruses infect body cells, they break the DNA chain and insert their own genetic material into the human DNA chain. Breaking the DNA along with viral gene insertion mutates the normal cell's DNA and can either activate an oncogene or repress a suppressor gene. Viruses capable of causing cancer are known as *oncoviruses.* Although any type of virus has the potential to enter a cell and mutate the DNA, leading to oncogene activation, infection with retroviruses is more likely to be oncogenic.

Dietary Influences. Many dietary practices or combinations of dietary practices and environmental exposures are thought to be related to carcinogenesis, particularly diets consistently high in fat (especially animal fat) and low in fiber. In addition, preservatives, contaminants, preparation methods, and additives (dyes, flavorings, and sweeteners) have the potential for carcinogenic effects. However, the relationship of diet to carcinogenesis is poorly understood. Usually, dietary considerations are not independent of other possible carcinogenic agents and personal influences. Therefore, the contributions of diet to the process of carcinogenesis are not completely clear.

Personal (Internal) Factors

Immune Function. The immune system provides continual protection against the development of cancer. Malignant cells are considered nonself because they are no longer completely normal. Often malignant cells express some cell surface antigens different from normal cells, allowing recognition by macrophages, helper/induce T lymphocytes, and natural killer cells. These cells, once the malignant cell has been recognized as nonself, initiate defensive and offensive actions to eliminate or destroy the malignant cell. This continuing protection, or immunosurveillance, is crucial in suppressing cancer development.

The essential role of the immune system in preventing cancer development is supported by cancer incidence statistics in immunosuppressed people. Children younger than 2 years and adults older than 60 have immune systems that function at less than optimal levels, and both groups have a higher incidence of cancer compared with that of the general population. People on chronic immunosuppressive therapy, such as would be needed among organ transplant recipients to reduce the risk of organ rejection or among people with significant autoimmune disease in which chronic immunosuppression is the only means of controlling disease progression, also have higher incidences of cancer. Among people with human immunodeficiency virus (HIV)/acquired immunodeficiency syndrome (AIDS), who are immnocompromised, the actual incidence of cancer development may be as high as 70%.

Therefore anyone whose immune system functions at less than optimum levels has an increased risk for the development of cancer. In addition to people who may have inherited a faulty immune system, immune function can be decreased as a result of aging, cytotoxic therapy, injury to marrow forming bone areas, surgical removal of primary or secondary lymphoid tissues (thymectomy, splenectomy), or exposure to chronic low-dose radiation.

Advancing age is probably the most common risk factor related to the development of cancer. More than 50% of all malignancies in the United States occur in people over 65 years of age (American Cancer Society, 1998). The higher incidence of cancer in this age group reflects both the lifelong accumulation of DNA mutations resulting in transformation and the diminishing immune response. Additionally, DNA repair mechanisms also become reduced in efficiency. The body may no longer be able to repair even basal level mutations.

Surveillance Failure. The immune system constantly keeps the body under surveillance and detects the presence of foreign invaders and altered self-cells, which include malignant cells. The most active cell types involved in this function are the macrophages, T lymphocytes, and the natural killer cells. However, even when this system appears to be functioning at an optimal level, the functioning is not always perfect. The immune surveillance system is most effective at identifying and attacking those cancer cells that have been induced by viral and chemical carcinogenic events. The system appears to have little protective value against those tumors that are a result of inheritance of spontaneous DNA replication error. A likely explanation for this selectivity in the immune surveillance system is the difference in cell surface properties of malignant cells caused by different types of carcinogenic or mutational events. Malignancies arising from viral or chemical carcinogenesis have new cell surface proteins unique to the cancer cells and are more easily recognized by immunoreactive cells as nonself. Many mechanisms have been proposed for cancer surveillance failure among immunocompetent individuals (Pitot, 1986). These proposed mechanisms include those discussed in the next sections.

Malignant Cell "Mimic." Some types of cancer cells initially have a less malignant phenotype and more normal cell surface characteristics. Such properties may not be sufficient to trigger an immune response. Thus these cancer cells might go undetected by the immune system until significant proliferation has occurred.

Decoy Jamming. Some cancer cells that synthesize novel surface proteins capable of stimulating an immune response shed these tumor-specific antigens. Thus any immune response is directed toward the loose antigens rather than toward the malignant cell.

Bone Marrow Invasion. Invasion of the bone marrow by cancer cells makes the bone marrow far less able to carry on normal immune and inflammatory functions. Therefore, the number of cells that can be involved in an immune response is decreased, generally resulting in both lymphopenia and neutropenia.

Enhanced Lymphocyte Suppression Activity. Some tumors release factors that selectively enhance the activity and number of T-suppressor cells so that the T suppressors constitute a larger percentage of circulating leukocytes. These T suppressors function in at least two ways that cause an overall immunosuppression and favor tumor growth: (1) they suppress the proliferative response of other T lymphocytes, macrophages, and natural killer cells; and (2) they suppress immunoglobulin production.

Immune Blockade. Some cancer cells are capable of releasing factors that specifically suppress natural killer cells.

Subclinical Dose. The initial malignant colony contains so few cells that they are not capable of signalling or triggering the immune system initially. This delay in the signal allows the original cells to become well established and grow unnoticed until they reach a size that is noticed by the immune system and may be so large that the immune system cannot effectively destroy or inactivate these cells.

Promoter Enhancement. Exposure to promoters (as the second stage of carcinogenesis) may enhance the proliferative powers of cancer cells to such an extent that their ability to divide far outpaces the ability of the immune system to recognize and eliminate them.

Increased Protein Synthesis. Certain cancers are able to increase production and release of various prostaglandins (either directly in the cancer cells or by stimulating some normal tissue to increase the production and release of prostaglandins). Prostaglandins from any source inhibit the ability of most lymphocytes to respond to lectins and other mitogenic agents so that there is a decrease in the production of lymphocytes and an overall immunosuppressive effect.

Some cancer cells secrete a thromboplastin-like substance that splits fibrinogen (inactive) into fibrin and fibrin degradation products. These substances can surround the cancer cells, preventing lymphocyte recognition.

Down-Regulation of Tumor-Specific Antigens. As cancer cells progress toward an increased malignant state, some cells undergo antigenic modulation as part of malignant evolution. This modulation may involve loss of tumor-specific antigens, thereby decreasing the likelihood of an immune response. Another type of modulation is to continually change the nature of the tumor-specific antigens, requiring a corresponding change in immune surveillance before recognition and elimination can occur.

Immunoprivileged Sites. The original site of the malignant transformation occurs in special areas of the body that have less active immune functions compared to the rest of the body. These immunoprivilegded sites may differ with the developmental stage of the host. Initiation or metastasis in such a place would allow good establishment of cancer cells and a relatively large tumor burden before recognition by the immune system.

Genetic Predisposition. Although activation of proto-oncogenes to oncogene status and/or the decreased expression of suppressor genes can be the result of exposure to carcinogens, genetic predisposition has an influence on the efficiency of the carcinogenic process. First, the efficiency of DNA repair mechanisms is an inherited trait. Although this efficiency can be decreased over time as a result of exposure to disease, toxins, aging, and other genotoxic events, a person who inherits a faulty or inefficient DNA repair mechanism cannot do anything to increase its efficiency.

Second, proto-oncogenes, precursors of oncogenes, are passed from generation to generation. The development of cancer, however, depends on more than these genes. The proto-oncogene needs to be damaged or altered to allow for expression of the oncogene. In some people, the location of specific proto-oncogenes within the genome is different and may provide an increased susceptibility to mutation or activation (Cooper, 1995). In other people, the position of the oncogene may be normal, but the gene controlling the oncogene's activity, the suppressor gene, may be abnormal or out of place (Baron & Borgen, 1997; Calzone, 1997).

All genes exist in pairs, and their activity is dependent on how well one or both genes of a pair functions. For example, the BRCA1 gene is a suppressor gene. Faulty functioning of this gene is associated with the development of an inherited form of breast cancer. If both BRCA1 genes of this pair are normal in structure and location, the woman is not at greater than normal risk for the development of breast cancer. If a woman inherits one faulty gene and one normal gene (is heterozygous for a BRCA1 mutation), then her risk for developing breast cancer increases to between 25% and 50%. If a woman inherits two faulty BRCA1 genes (is homozygous for the mutation), her risk of developing breast cancer ranges from 60% to nearly 100%. Essentially, when a person has inherited one or more genes that are abnormal (mutated), the person has already undergone initiation. Thus, promotion is all that is needed to cause cancer.

For other types of cancer, a familial tendency may be noted, but no specific pattern of inheritance has been identified. These familial cancers may all be of one type, such as colorectal cancer or breast cancer, or there may be an excessively high incidence of all types of cancers within one family, called *cancer family syndromes.* The ontogeny of this type of genetic predisposition is more difficult to elucidate and may be multifactorial. It is possible that multiple small gene mutations may be responsible, or that even normal exposure to carcinogenic events enhances a basal level of genetic predisposition.

Race is a genetically determined characteristic, and racial differences for the incidence of different types of cancer do exist. For example, in the United States, the incidence of prostate cancer is higher among African Americans than among white Americans. Breast cancer rates are higher among European Americans than among Asian Americans. Esophageal and gastric cancer rates are higher among Asian Americans than among any other American population (Wingo et al., 1996). The overall cancer incidence among African Americans has increased 27% since 1960; it has increased 12% in that same period for whites. Cancer sites and cancer-related mortality vary along racial lines as well.

Table 2-5 Grading System for Malignancy

Grade	Characteristics
GX	Grade cannot be determined.
G1	Cells are well-differentiated, closely resembling the tissue from which it arose. Considered a "low grade" tumor.
G2	Cells are moderately differentiated, still resemble normal cells somewhat, but exhibit more malignant characteristics.
G3	Cells are poorly differentiated, few normal cellular characteristics are retained, but the tissue of origin may still be established.
G4	Cells are undifferentiated, no normal cellular characteristics can be found, and determining the tissue of origin is very difficult.

When risks for cancer development are assessed, however, race and genetic predisposition cannot be considered alone. Behavior related to culture or ethnic group, geographic location, diet, and socioeconomic factors must also be assessed. The American Cancer Society (1998) has reported that cancer incidence and survival are often related to socioeconomic factors, such as the availability of health care services or the belief that seeking early health care has a positive effect on the outcome of a cancer diagnosis.

QUANTIFICATION OF MALIGNANCY

Grading of Malignancy

To accurately qualify the malignant characteristics that a particular tumor possesses, a system of grading tumor cells was established. This system compares cancer cells with their normal counterparts on appearance and cellular activity. Some cancer cells retain more of their normal appearance and functions and are thus considered low-grade, whereas others appear to be more aggressive and treatment resistant, and are considered high-grade tumors. Table 2-5 shows an example of such a grading system.

Staging of Malignancy

The purpose of staging a cancer is to determine the bodily location of the cancer and the degree to which spread has occurred. For most cancers, the smaller the tumor at the time of diagnosis and the less it has spread, the greater the potential for cure or control. Therefore, to decide the amount and duration of treatment given for a specific malignancy, the stage of that malignancy must be determined. Three methods are used to stage a malignancy: clinical staging, surgical staging, and pathologic staging.

Clinical Staging. In clinical staging, the size of the tumor (in centimeters) and degree of metastasis (by number of sites) are determined by clinical tests and measurements such as a biopsy, but do not include major surgery.

Surgical Staging. Surgical staging reports the size of a tumor, the number of sites, and the degree of metastasis by appearance at surgery.

Pathologic Staging. Tumor size, number of sites, and degree of metastasis are determined by pathologic examination of tissue obtained at surgery. Pathologic examination provides the clinician with information about the cellular characteristics of the tumor.

The TNM System for Staging of Malignancy. In an attempt to qualify the characteristics of a malignancy, a unified system of staging cancer was established. It had been shown that survival rates tended to be higher for tumors that were localized. This finding gave rise to the notion that there is tumor progression over time, perhaps influenced by the type of cancer and other host factors.

Although several systems for grading tumor cells exist, the following is a fairly common example of such a system. The TNM (tumor, node, metastases) is an example of a system that attempts to capture this pattern of growth and spread as a means of tumor classification. The T indicates the extent of the tumor, the N indicates the presence or absence of lymph node involvement, and the M denotes the presence or absence of metastases. Additionally, subscript numbers assigned to any of these components is indicative of an increase in tumor size, nodal involvement, or metastases. This classification system serves several purposes: to examine the extent of the particular cancer as related to the natural course of the disease, to provide standardization on which to base treatment options, and to indicate prognosis (Beahrs, Henson, Hutter, & Myers, 1988). Table 2-6 is an example of the TNM staging system.

TABLE 2-6 TNM Staging System

Stage	Characteristics
Primary Tumor (T)	
TX	No primary tumor can be assessed
T0	No evidence of primary tumor
TIS	Carcinoma in situ
T1, T2, T3, T4	Increasing size and extent of the primary tumor
Regional Lymph Nodes (N)	
NX	Cannot be assessed
N0	No regional lymph node involvement
N1, N2, N3	Increasing involvement of regional lymph nodes
Distant Metastasis (M)	
MX	Presence of metastasis cannot be assessed
M0	No distant metastasis
M1	Distant metastasis

CONCLUSION

The process of carcinogenesis is multifactorial, with significant interactions between personal and environmental factors. Not all people are at equal risk for the development of cancer. The roles played by immune function, genetic predisposition, and environmental exposure to mutagenic events vary widely among individuals. Immune and genetic factors cannot, as of yet, be altered to prevent cancer development. However, manipulation of environmental exposure to carcinogenic events could reduce the incidence of cancer by as much as 50% (American Cancer Society, 1998).

REFERENCES

American Cancer Society. (1998). *Cancer facts & figures—1998.* Atlanta: American Cancer Society, Inc. (98-300M-No. 5008.98).

Ames, B., Gold, L., & Willett, W. C. (1995). The causes and prevention of cancer. *Proceedings of the National Academy of Sciences, 92*(12), 5258-5265.

Applebaum, J. (1992). The role of the immune system in the pathogenesis of cancer. *Seminars Oncology Nursing, 8*(1), 51-62.

Baron, R., & Borgen, P. (1997). Genetic susceptibility for breast cancer: Testing and primary prevention options. *Oncology Nursing Forum, 24*(3), 461-468.

Beahrs, O., Henson, D., Hutter, R., & Myers, M. (Eds.). (1988). *Manual for staging of cancer* (3rd ed.). Philadelphia: J. B. Lippincott.

Bishop, J. (1982). Oncogenes. *Scientific American, 246*(3), 80-92.

Bishop, J. (1995). Cancer: The rise of the genetic paradigm. *Genes and Development, 9*(11), 1309-1315.

Bosner, M., Pavelic, K., Hrascan, R., Zeljko, Z., Krhen, I., Krizanac, Z., & Pavelic, J. (1997). Loss of heterozygosity of the nm23-H1 gene in human renal cell carcinomas. *Journal of Cancer Research and Clinical Oncology, 123*(9), 485-488.

Calzone, K. (1997). Genetic predisposition testing: Clinical implications for oncology nurses. *Oncology Nursing Forum, 24*(4), 712-718.

Cohens, J., & Geradts, J. (1997). Loss of RB and MTS1/CDKN2 (p16) expression in human sarcomas. *Human Pathology, 28*(8), 893-898.

Cooper, G. (1995). *Oncogenes* (2nd ed.). Boston: Jones & Bartlett Publishers.

Coursen, J., Bennett, W., Gollahon, L., Shay, J., & Hassis, C. (1997). Genomic instability and telemerase activity in human bronchial epithelial cells during immortalization by human papillomavirus-16 E6 and E7 genes. *Experimental Cell Research, 235*(1), 245-253.

Fidler, I., & Hart, I. (1982). Biological diversity in metastatic neoplasia: Origins and implications. *Science, 217*(4564), 998.

Hill, J. (1961). *Cautions against the immoderate use of snuff* (2nd ed.) London: R. Baldwin.

Landis, S., Murray, T., Bolden, S., & Wingo, P. (1998). Cancer statistics, 1998. *CA: A Cancer Journal for Clinicians, 48*(1), 6-29.

Liotta, L. (1992). Cancer cell invasion and metastasis. *Scientific American, 266*(2), 54-62.

Macgrogan, D., Pegram, M., Slamon, D., & Bookstein, R. (1997). Comparative mutational analysis of DPC4 (Smad4) in prostatic and colorectal carcinomas. *Oncogene, 15*(9), 1111-1114.

Mitelman, F. (1994). Chromosomes, genes, and cancer. *CA: A Cancer Journal for Clinicians, 44*(3), 133-135.

Nicolson, G. (1979). Cancer metastasis. *Scientific American, 240,* 66-79.

Piao, Z., Kim, H., Jeon, B., Lee, W., & Park, C. (1997). Relationship between loss of heterozygosity of tumor suppressor genes and histologic differentiation in hepatocellular carcinoma. *Cancer, 80*(5), 865-872.

Pitot, H. (1986). *Fundamentals of Oncology* (2nd ed.). New York: Marcel Dekker.

Powell, S., Harper, J., Hamilton, S., Robinson, C., & Cummings, O. (1997). Inactivation of Smad4 in gastric carcinomas. *Cancer Research, 57*(19), 4221-4224.

Renshaw, M., McWhirter, J., & Wang, J. (1995). The human leukemia oncogene *bcr-abl* abrogates the anchorage requirement but not the growth factor requirement for proliferation. *Molecular and Cellular Biology, 15*(3), 1286-1293.

Ruoslahti, E. (1996). How cancer spreads. *Scientific American, 275*(3), 72-77.

Schmidt, B., Ackermann, R., Hartmann, M., & Stohmeyer, T. (1997). Alterations of the metastasis suppressor gene nm23 and the proto-oncogene c-myc in human testicular germ cell tumors. *Journal of Urology, 158*(5), 2000-2005.

Stellman, J., & Stellman, S. (1996). Cancer and the workplace. *CA: A Cancer Journal for Clinicians, 46*(2), 70-92.

Trichopoulos, D., Li, F., & Hunter, D. (1996). What causes cancer? *Scientific American, 275*(3), 80-87.

Weinberg, R. (1996). How cancer arises. *Scientific American, 275*(3), 62-70.

Weinberg, R. (1994). Oncogenes and tumor suppressor genes. *CA: A Cancer Journal for Clinicians, 44*(3), 160-170.

Wingo, P., Bolden, S., Tong, T., Parker, S., Martin, L., & Heath, C. (1996). Cancer statistics for African Americans, 1996. *CA: A Cancer Journal for Clinicians, 46*(2), 113-125.

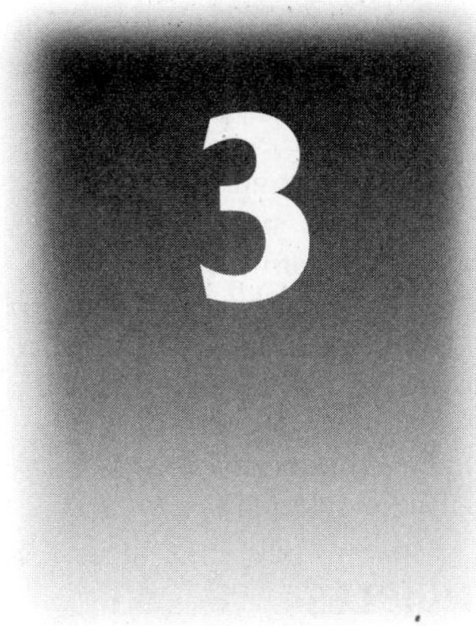

Surgical Treatment

Catherine C. Burke, RN, MS, CS, ANP

INTRODUCTION

Surgery, the oldest method of cancer treatment, did not become a distinct oncologic specialty until after the development of chemotherapy and radiation therapy. In this sense, modern surgical oncology represents one of the newest approaches for the treatment of cancer. A more scientific understanding of tumor behavior, coupled with the development of multimodal therapy, expanded the role of surgery. Originally used solely for the radical removal of obvious cancers, surgical therapy now has applications ranging from diagnosis to treatment to palliation.

The surgical care of the cancer patient is a complex process that requires the expertise of a multidisciplinary team. Successful surgical therapy requires preoperative preparation, a well-executed operation, vigilant postoperative care, and a complete program for recovery.

The majority of cancer patients receive some form of surgical therapy during the course of their disease. An understanding of the rationale, benefits, and potential complications of a given procedure enables the oncology nurse to provide both physical and psychologic support to patients and their families. As advances in research and technology continue to broaden the scope and practice of surgery, surgical oncology will continue its process of evolution. Oncology nurses will be challenged to assimilate this knowledge and incorporate it into their daily practice.

HISTORICAL PERSPECTIVE

The curative role of surgery in the treatment of cancer developed rapidly over the last 150 years. Although anecdotal reports of surgical therapy for cancer date back to ancient Egypt, as documented in the Edwin Smith Papyrus (circa 1600 BC), the development of surgical oncology as a major component of cancer therapy depended on the introduction of general anesthesia and an understanding of aseptic technique. Before these developments, major elective surgery was virtually impossible because of operative pain and sepsis. The development of general ether anesthesia is credited to American dentists William Morton and Crawford Long. The technique was first reported in 1846, when Dr. John Collins Warner excised a submaxillary gland at the Massachusetts General Hospital. The second major development occurred in 1867 when John Lister, applying the concepts of Louis Pasteur, introduced bactericidal therapy with carbolic acid and published an article describing the principles of antisepsis. William Stewart Halsted (1852-1922), the first Professor of Surgery at the Johns Hopkins University, introduced these principles in the United States (Hill, 1979).

Building on these milestones, surgeons of the late 1800s and early 1900s developed a number of radical surgical approaches for the treatment of primary malignancies. This era is best known for its emphasis on en bloc tumor resections because no other effective form of therapy existed. Examples include Kocher's thyroidectomy, Halstead's radical mastectomy, Young's radical prostatectomy, Wertheim's radical hysterectomy, Miles' abdominoperineal resection, and A. O. Whipple's pancreaticoduodenectomy (Hill, 1979; Rosenberg, 1997). Albert Theodor Billroth was another major figure in the evolution of surgery, performing the first successful gastrectomy, laryngectomy, and esophagectomy. In addition to his pioneering work in gastroenterology, he was one of the first surgeons to carefully document patient outcomes, both positive and negative, making comparative analyses between surgeons and centers possible (Rutledge, 1995).

Although it is impossible to list all of the contributions and technologic innovations (e.g., the development of surgical clamps, retractors, or electrocautery) that allowed for advances in surgery, scientific research that advanced our understanding of human anatomy and physiology was important for the development of modern surgical oncology. The loop colostomy by Bricker and the introduction of intratracheal insufflation by Metzler and Auer are two examples of where knowledge of anatomy and physiology led to advances in surgical oncology. Bricker's ileal conduit made the first total pelvic exenteration by Brunschwig possible. Intratracheal insufflation was the forerunner of mechanical ventilation, that permitted the development of modern thoracic surgery (Dobell, 1994; Hill, 1979).

The development of blood transfusions and the discovery of antibiotics in the 1940s and 1950s greatly expanded the role of surgical oncology by reducing operative mortality. In turn, the rapid growth of basic physiologic research and technology in the 1960s and 1970s led to the emergence of sophisticated critical care units capable of even greater perioperative support. These developments made radical surgery safer and available to a wider spectrum of cancer patients. Another significant achievement was the introduction of total parenteral nutrition. With the advent of central venous catheters, Dudrick and colleagues were able to administer intravenous (IV) hyperalimentation with minimal phlebitis and thrombosis. These catheters allowed for the delivery of high-tech nutritional support to patients unable to tolerate enteral feedings (Wretlind, 1992). Current innovations such as automatic stapling devices, endoscopic surgical equipment, and microsurgical instrumentation permit an even greater range of oncologic procedures. Table 3-1 outlines selected major achievements in surgical oncology.

Today, an understanding of tumor biology and tumor spread, coupled with effective chemotherapeutic, radiotherapeutic, and biologic treatments, form the basis of modern oncologic practice. Conservative surgical approaches for cancer therapy are currently under investigation. Research findings have demonstrated that for many tumors, tissue-sparing surgeries are equally effective to radical resections, while reducing operative morbidity and promoting overall quality of life. The ability of alternative therapies to control residual disease has also prompted surgeons to reevaluate the magnitude of surgical resections. Approximately 70% of patients with solid tumors have micrometastases beyond the primary site at the time of diagnosis (Rosenberg, 1997). Therefore many treatment programs involve the sequential use of multiple treatment modalities in addition to surgery. Multimodal therapy improves long-term survival and cure rates for patients with disease outside the operative field who would fail with resection alone. This approach requires interdisciplinary collaboration and treatment planning tailored to the individual patient.

CONCEPTS AND PRINCIPLES OF SURGICAL ONCOLOGY

Although many nurses view surgical oncology as the straightforward removal of tumor to achieve a cure, surgical procedures are also used in a variety of other ways. In addition to primary treatment, classic applications include diagnosis, staging, and cytoreduction (i.e., debulking). Surgical techniques are also used to prevent cancer, to relieve its symptoms, and to enhance functional and cosmetic outcomes. New technologies such as laser therapy, cryotherapy, ultrasonic aspiration, and the concomitant use of surgery with chemotherapy and/or radiation therapy have also expanded the role of surgery in cancer treatment. This section reviews these major clinical applications.

TABLE 3-1 Selected Achievements in the Development of Modern Surgical Oncology

Developer	Year	Event	Significance
Anton Lembert	1826	Described serosal-to-serosal suture technique	Allowed gastrointestinal resection and reanastamosis
John C. Warner	1846	Administration of ether anesthesia	Elimination of operative pain
Joseph Lister	1867	Outlined the principles of antisepsis	Reduced perioperative infections
A.T. Billroth	1872-81	First successful esopohagectomy, laryngectomy, and gastrectomy	
Richard von Volkman	1878	Rectal excision for cancer	
Theodore Kocher	1880	Development of thyroid surgery	
W.S. Halsted	1890	Radical mastectomy	
Hugh Young	1904	Radical prostatectomy	
Ernest Wertheim	1906	Radical hysterectomy	
W. Ernest Miles	1908	Abdominoperineal resection	
S.J. Metzler & J. Auer	1909	Intertracheal insufflation (forerunner of mechanical ventilation)	Permitted the development of modern thoracic surgery
Harvey Cushing	1910-1930	Development of surgery for brain tumors	
Alexis Carroll	1912	Described vascular anastomosis	Foundation for modern vascular surgery
E. Martin	1912	Cordotomy	Palliation of pain
H. Cushing and W.T. Bovie	1928	Introduction of the electrocautery	Control of operative bleeding
Evarts Graham	1933	Pneumonectomy for lung cancer	
A.O. Whipple	1935	Pancreaticoduodenectomy	
Alexander Brunschwig	1947	Total pelvic exenteration	
S. Dudrick, D. Wilmore, H. Vars, and J. Rhoads	1968	Intravenous hyperalimentation	

Diagnosis

A pathologic examination of a tissue sample is necessary to confirm the suspicion of cancer. Often, information obtained from the tissue sample is used to select therapy and predict prognosis. Diagnostic biopsy typically involves excision of a portion of tumor that provides a histologic diagnosis. More recently, cytologic techniques have been used to identify tumors using material obtained from needle aspirations, effusions, or washes from various body cavities. With experience, such cytologic techniques are often as accurate and reliable as surgical biopsy (Hindle, Payne, & Pan, 1993; Staerkel, 1993; Westcott, 1980).

The technique used to obtain a diagnostic biopsy depends on the size and location of the tumor. Incisional, excisional, and needle approaches can be used to obtain biopsy materials from superficial tumors that are visualized or readily palpated. For an incisional biopsy, a small portion of tumor is removed from a larger mass. This approach is commonly used to provide an initial diagnosis of large lesions that are likely to require complex treatment planning. Incisional biopsies, obtained by scalpel, skin punch, or specialized biopsy forceps, are taken from the most suspicious areas of the tumor.

Complete removal of a grossly identified tumor is termed an *excisional biopsy* (Fig. 3-1). This technique is commonly applied in the diagnosis of small superficial lesions. Although excisional biopsy may occasionally be therapeutic, wide excision margins are not usually obtained, and a more radical repeat excision may be required. When feasible, excisional biopsy is preferred over incisional biopsy because it allows pathologic examination of the entire tumor (Fig. 3-2).

Two techniques are available for needle biopsy. Fine needle aspiration (FNA) is used when a cytologic sample will provide adequate diagnostic material. A small-gauge needle is placed into the tumor mass, and cellular material is collected either directly into the needle's hub, or into a syringe by applying suction. Multiple passes are usually made to ensure that the sample is representative of the tumor (Fig. 3-3). The aspiration biopsy specimen contains individual cells and small tissue fragments (Fig. 3-4). A cytologic diagnosis depends on the identification of malignant characteristics within these cells. The advantages of this procedure are its ease of application, low cost, minimal morbidity, and rapid diagnosis (Staerkel, 1993). Although a positive aspiration biopsy provides valuable information, a negative biopsy cannot be used to rule out the presence of cancer. In this setting, alternative diagnostic approaches must be considered if clinical suspicion of a cancer diagnosis is high.

Core needle biopsy can be used to obtain a tissue specimen with intact cellular architecture. A specialized large-gauge needle is placed into the tumor mass to obtain a histologic sample. When a cytologic specimen is inconclusive or when tumor architecture is necessary for a definitive diagnosis, a core needle biopsy should be performed. A common application for core needle biopsy is to obtain bone marrow specimens for the diagnosis of hematologic malignancies. Tumors arising in the intraluminal portions of the respiratory, genitourinary, and gastrointestinal tracts can be easily visualized and biopsied using flexible endoscopy. A

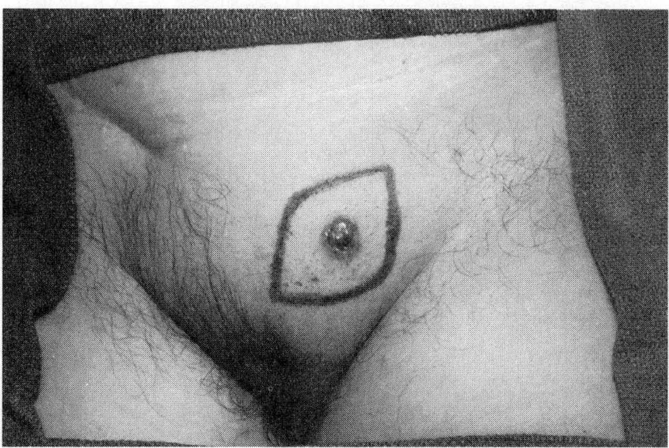

Fig. 3-1 Planned resection margins for an excisional biopsy of a basal cell carcinoma. A wide local excision with an elliptical incision is used. An excisional biopsy involves complete tumor removal and allows complete histologic evaluation.

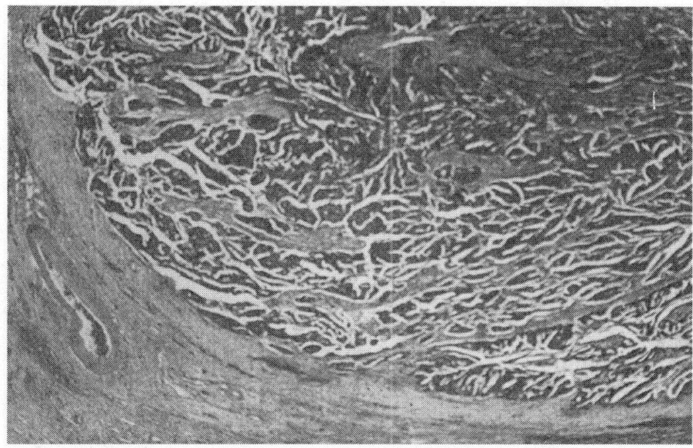

Fig. 3-2 A microscopic view of a metastatic omental nodule. The patient had a prior history of breast cancer and, at exploration, was found to have carcinomatosis. With a tissue sample, histologic examination is possible.

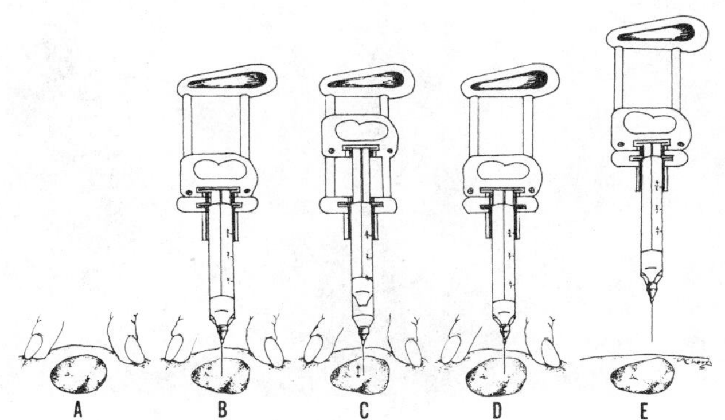

Fig. 3-3 Technique for fine needle aspiration. (From Staerkel, G. A. [1993]. Fine needle aspiration. Technique and application in the evaluation of malignancies. *Cancer Bulletin, 45,* 8-12.)

fiberoptic scope introduced into a lumen is used to view tumors, and specialized instruments are passed through an operating channel to obtain the tissue biopsy. Fiberoptic biopsies (e.g., endoscopy, bronchoscopy) are typically well tolerated with the use of IV sedation and are the diagnostic methods of choice for cancers of the bladder, stomach, colon, and lung (Kurtz & Ginsberg, 1997).

Tumors located in internal organs are often identified by imaging studies (e.g., computed tomography scanning, magnetic resonance imaging, and ultrasound). Because these tumors are not palpable, deep biopsy techniques must be used to establish a diagnosis. Options for deep tissue biopsy include directed FNA, open biopsy, or minimally invasive operative biopsy. For directed FNA, the target site for the biopsy is imaged first, enabling the physician to place a long, small-gauge needle directly into the tumor mass. A cytologic specimen is collected in the same manner as described for superficial FNA. This technique can be used to reach virtually any body site. A recent refinement of directed FNA is stereotactic biopsy, which allows placement of the biopsy needle with the help of a three-dimensional imaging technique (Ranjan, Rajshekhar, Joseph, Chandy, & Chandi, 1993; Schmidt, 1994).

When tissue samples from a tumor in a body cavity are required, a major surgical procedure under general anesthesia, called *open biopsy,* is performed. Examples of open biopsies are diagnostic thoracotomy and laparotomy. In many cases, open biopsy has been replaced by minimally invasive procedures (e.g., laparoscopy, thoracoscopy) that provide equivalent information (Kurtz & Ginsberg, 1997). A small incision is used to introduce a rigid fiberoptic scope connected to a television monitor. Under direct vision, additional instruments are inserted through separate punctures to permit examination of organs and to obtain biopsy materials. Although performed with the patient under general anesthesia, these operations can be accomplished in an outpatient setting with rapid recovery and minimal morbidity.

Although the physician selects the biopsy technique most appropriate for the clinical situation, the simplest procedure that provides an adequate diagnostic tissue sample should be chosen. Factors to be considered in selecting a specific biopsy technique include the site to be biopsied, the size of the tumor, the suspected diagnosis, and the patient's physical status. The advantages and disadvantages of various biopsy techniques are outlined in Table 3-2.

Staging

An important aspect of the pretreatment evaluation of the patient with cancer is to determine the extent of disease. Staging usually begins with a physical examination, laboratory studies, and imaging procedures that are tailored to the tumor site and patient symptoms. When the extent of disease is completely evaluated by noninvasive techniques, the tumor is said to be clinically staged. Many cancers cannot be accurately assessed clinically. Staging accomplished by an operative procedure provides more accurate information in these cases. Precise knowledge of the extent of disease permits (1) selection of an appropriate treatment plan; (2) a reliable estimate of prognosis; and (3) comparison of treatment results between health care centers and over time. Patients with high-risk or advanced cancers may be candidates for multimodal therapy. The information gained from the staging evaluation has important implications because inadequate or inaccurate staging results in compromised treatment planning and may jeopardize the opportunity for cure (Rosenberg, 1997). Fig. 3-5 illustrates a solitary lung metas-

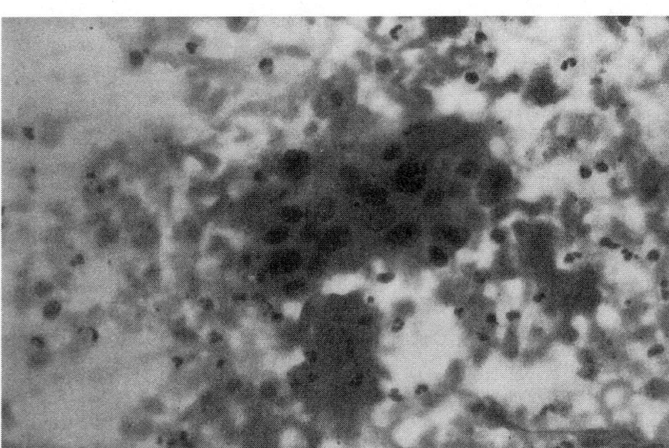

Fig. 3-4 The fine needle aspiration specimen contains individual cells and tissue fragments for a cytologic evaluation. This sample was taken from an enlarged scalene lymph node in a woman with a history of cervical cancer. A cluster of malignant squamous cells is evident.

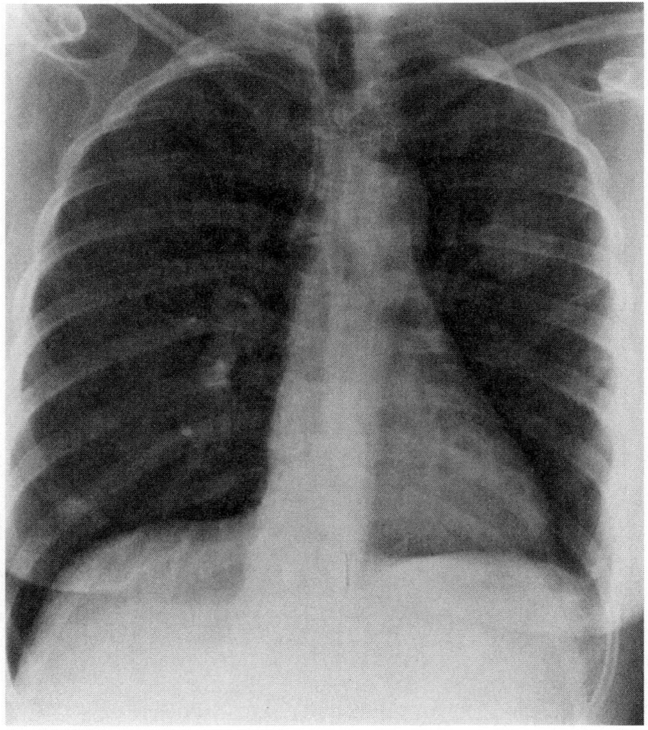

Fig. 3-5 The chest radiograph is a common component of cancer staging. A solitary lung metastasis is seen in an otherwise asymptomatic patient.

tasis found on a staging chest radiograph in an otherwise asymptomatic patient.

The components of a staging operation are specified by the type of cancer and the tumor site. The surgical procedure is designed to evaluate typical areas of disease spread, usually through observation, palpation, and biopsy of common sites for regional and distant metastases. Surgical staging procedures tend to focus on the abdominal (peritoneal) cavity because tumors and metastases located here are difficult to detect and evaluate by nonsurgical techniques (Fig. 3-6).

A general staging laparotomy is used to evaluate abdominal disease and involves several sequential steps. First, the peritoneal cavity is opened and its organs are exposed using a large midline incision. Before exploration, the peritoneal surfaces are irrigated with saline to provide samples for cytologic analysis. This technique collects cells from a large surface area to detect microscopic, serosal, and peritoneal metastases. The second step involves visual inspection and palpation of the organs and peritoneal surfaces to identify and target suspicious sites for biopsies. Finally, retroperito-

TABLE 3-2 Advantages/Disadvantages of Biopsy Techniques

Technique	Tissue Sample Obtained	Advantages	Disadvantages
Fine Needle Aspiration			
1. Superficial	Cytologic	Simple Low cost Rapid results Local anesthesia Outpatient procedure Minimal morbidity Avoids operative procedure	Negative findings are non-diagnostic Cellular samples difficult to interpret
2. Directed	Cytologic	Rapid results	Requires special expertise and equipment
3. Stereotactic		Local/intravenous (IV) sedation Outpatient procedure Avoids surgical procedure Low-cost compared with operative procedure Minimal morbidity	May require overnight hospitalization
Core needle biopsy	Histologic (small)	Simple Low cost Local anesthesia Outpatient procedure Low morbidity	Pain at biopsy site pain Rare organ injury/hematoma
Incisional Excisional	Histologic (small) Histologic (large)	Simple Low cost Local anesthesia Outpatient procedure Low morbidity	Pain at biopsy site pain Rare hematoma/infection
Fiberoptic	Histologic (small)	Low cost IV sedation Outpatient procedure Low morbidity	Requires special expertise and equipment Rare organ injury/bleeding
Minimally invasive	Histologic Cytologic	Outpatient procedure Multiple sites sampled Provides staging information Avoids open biopsy Some morbidity; rapid recovery	High cost General anesthesia May require overnight or short-stay hospitalization Requires special expertise and equipment Moderate pain (3-5 days recovery) Rare organ injury, bleeding
Open (surgical) biopsy	Histologic Cytologic	Accurate staging Multiple sites sampled	High cost General anesthesia Hospitalization required Significant pain (2-3 weeks recovery) Occasional organ injury/bleeding Increased morbidity and mortality

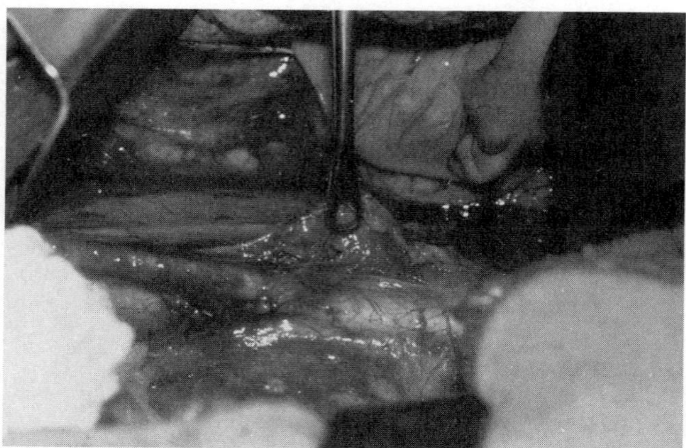

Fig. 3-6 Most staging operations include an assessment of tumor spread to retroperitoneal lymph nodes. This external iliac lymph node is being excised to look for microscopic metastases.

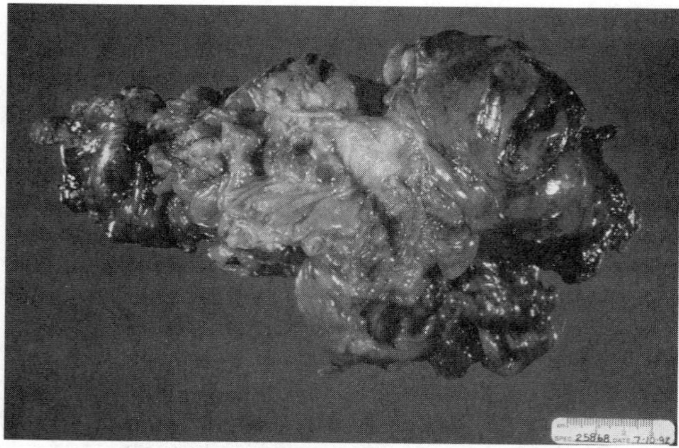

Fig. 3-7 Surgical specimen following total pelvic exenteration includes the bladder, genital tract, and rectum. Radical en bloc resection involves complete excision of tumor with an adequate margin of normal tissue.

neal lymph nodes in the drainage routes of the primary tumor are exposed and biopsied (Burke, 1994). When biopsy of regional lymph nodes is combined with a resection of the primary tumor (e.g., melanoma, breast cancer, vulvar cancer), the lymph node dissection is considered to be a staging procedure because nodal status affects subsequent therapeutic decisions. Examples of surgically staged cancers include cancers of the lymph nodes, testicles, endometrium, and ovary (Burke & Morris, 1993; Watson, Kantoff, & Richie, 1996). Some surgeons currently use laparoscopy as an alternative to laparotomy for staging. The peritoneal cavity and its contents can be visualized well with the laparoscope, but accurate lymph node evaluation is technically difficult. However, laparoscopy is often used in patients with pancreatic and gastric cancers to evaluate resectability, avoiding the morbidity of laparotomy in patients with unresectable disease (Cuschieri, 1995; Fernandez-del Castillo, Rattner, & Warshaw, 1995; Greene & Dorsay, 1993).

Second-look operations are sometimes used after primary therapy to measure tumor response (Griffiths, Parker, & Fuller, 1979). The second-look surgical technique is identical to that used for laparotomy. It is most often associated with the management of ovarian cancer, but its value in treatment planning has not been established. It may be offered in conjunction with protocol therapy and should be considered experimental (Gershenson, 1993).

Primary Treatment

Local resection may be the treatment of choice for small tumors confined to the site of origin. These resections are performed with curative intent by completely removing the tumor with an adequate margin of normal tissue. Cancers of the skin, breast, colon, prostate, and uterus are frequently treated by primary resection; however, the radicality of the surgery varies greatly (Fig. 3-7). For example, a small cutaneous squamous cell cancer of the skin can be easily and curatively excised by removing the lesion with a surrounding margin of normal skin. In contrast, a radical prostatectomy involves removing the prostate gland, including the prostatic capsule, the seminal vesicles, a portion of the bladder neck, and possible pelvic lymph node dissection. This operation is extensive and may be associated with significant postoperative morbidity (Held, Osborne, Volpe, & Waldman, 1994).

A major focus of modern oncologic surgery is to achieve equivalent cure rates with less radical primary resection. Most of these efforts attempt to maintain cosmetic appearance and functional integrity by combining tissue-sparing surgery with radiation therapy and/or chemotherapy. Strategies to accomplish this goal include preoperative therapy to shrink large tumors, thus making surgical excision possible or simpler. For example, preoperative chemoirradiation has been used successfully in the treatment of both breast and colorectal cancer (Lowy, Rich, Skibber, Dubrow, & Curley, 1996). Intraoperative therapy aimed at reducing the incidence of local recurrence is currently being explored in patients with pancreatic cancer (Kinsella & Sindelar, 1996; Staley et al., 1996). Postoperative adjuvant therapy is given to limit the extent of resections and to reduce the risk of recurrence in high-risk patients. It is often offered to patients with colorectal and breast cancer (Clahsen et al., 1996; Recht, 1996; Schmoll, 1994). For some tumors (e.g. melanoma, vulvar cancer), a better understanding of prognostic factors (e.g., depth of invasion, lesion size) and spread patterns has resulted in the use of conservative surgical approaches without additional therapy in selected patients (Burke et al., 1995; Homesley, 1995; Urist, 1996).

Cytoreductive Surgery

When complete removal of the primary tumor is not technically possible, cytoreductive or debulking operations may be attempted. This approach is useful for tumors in which other nonsurgical therapies are effective in eradicating remaining tumor. Because such postoperative therapies are most effective in eliminating small tumor masses, the goal of cytoreduction is to leave as small a volume of residual disease as possible (Fig. 3-8). Cytoreductive surgeries are technically difficult operations, requiring a skilled surgical team. Because cytoreductive operations are attempted in already compromised patients with bulky primary tumors and substantial regional metastases, intensive postoperative support is essential.

Cytoreduction is most widely applied for women with advanced cancer of the ovary (Gershenson, 1993). Survival advantages have been clearly documented for women who are left with small tumor volumes following primary cytoreduction. The success of cytoreduction is directly related to the high sensitivity of these tumors to postoperative chemotherapy. A survival benefit has also been documented in some patients with lymphoma, testicular germ-cell tumor, neuroblastoma, and rhabdomyosarcoma who undergo primary cytoreductive procedures (Silberman, 1982; Wong & DeCosse, 1990). Local control rates in patients with advanced breast and rectal cancers have been improved by cytoreduction, but survival benefits have not been achieved because control of distant metastases is poor.

Major cytoreductive procedures can cause significant postoperative morbidity; consequently candidates should be carefully selected. In general, such operations should be limited to patients who can tolerate an extensive procedure, to clinical situations in which tumor removal offers a survival advantage, and to tumors in which optimal cytoreduction is technically possible.

Palliation

Palliative surgical procedures can sometimes be used to relieve suffering, minimize symptoms, or improve quality of life (Table 3-3). Although these operations are not curative, they may achieve a specific short-term goal. Palliative operations should be considered only if the patient's symptoms cannot be relieved by more conservative means. Patient and family education that realistically addresses the goals and anticipated outcomes of the palliative operation is critical. It is also important to evaluate the patient's overall life expectancy before deciding to undertake a palliative procedure. A relatively minor procedure aimed at relieving intractable pain is quite reasonable, but offering a major operation to a patient with little survival time may prolong life without providing a tangible benefit.

A variety of palliative operations can be offered to cancer patients. Operative stabilization of pathologic fractures may be used to relieve pain, restore function of an extremity, or prevent loss of organ function from denervation (Dyck, 1991; Held & Peahota, 1993). When nerve compression by tumor causes pain and dysfunction, limited removal of the tumor mass can provide significant relief of symptoms and maintain function of the entrapped nerve. Other neurologic procedures designed to interrupt pain pathways can be valuable in controlling severe pain. Palliative interventions can be used to relieve obstructions and resect or bypass fistulas. In these situations, surgical intervention is often unavoidable because symptoms are severe and more conservative measures are ineffective. Bowel obstructions may be decompressed by resection, diversion to an ostomy, or placement of a drainage tube. Fistulas require operative resection or bypass proximal to the fistula tract. In selected patients, a surgically placed feeding tube or central venous catheter may be used to provide nutritional support. Although nutritional support of the terminal patient is controversial, if a realistic quality of life can be achieved (e.g., allowing a hospitalized patient to move to home care), such support is a reasonable palliative option.

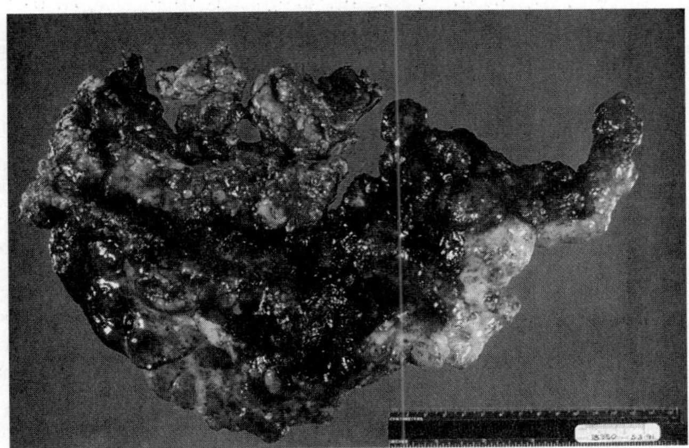

Fig. 3-8 This tumor-filled omentum was removed during a cytoreductive operation for advanced ovarian cancer. The goal is to remove as much tumor as possible, leaving a small volume of residual disease, which is treated with postoperative therapy.

Adjuvant Therapy

Although primary surgical resection is commonly intended as a cure, it is being combined increasingly with other treatment modalities to improve cure rates and increase disease-free intervals (Schabel, 1977). These additional therapies, termed *adjuvant,* are given to patients at risk for disease recurrence following presumed curative surgery. The term *adjuvant* is often used inappropriately. Although some clinicians use the term to refer to any postoperative therapy, treatment given to patients with known residual disease is better termed *adjunctive.* Additionally, treatments (e.g., chemotherapy, radiation therapy) given before surgical resection are best categorized as *neoadjuvant* (Frei, 1988).

Nonsurgical therapies can be classified by the timing of treatment relative to surgery and by the type of treatment. Preoperative neoadjuvant therapy may improve tumor resectability by shrinking the primary tumor before an attempted resection. This approach has important applications in settings where tumor resection is likely to be technically difficult, where organ function might be preserved, or where a less extensive procedure might have significant cosmetic benefits. Neoadjuvant therapy is currently used for cancers such as those of the pancreas, colon, rectum, ovary, and breast (Coia et al., 1994; Lowy et al., 1996; Staley et al., 1996). Intraoperative adjuvant therapy is largely limited to irradiation of the tumor bed to enhance local control. This technique requires a specialized operating suite equipped with a linear accelerator.

TABLE 3-3 Examples of Palliative Surgical Procedures

Procedure	Indication	Desired Outcome
Diverting colostomy	Large bowel obstruction	Maintain bowel function Prevent perforation and sepsis
Gastrostomy tube placement	Small bowel obstruction	Relieve nausea/vomiting by decompression Allows enteral nutrition
Internal fixation	Pathologic fracture Spinal cord compression	Relieve pain Maintain function
Chordotomy	Intractable pain	Relieve pain
Electrocautery fulgeration	Tumor bleeding	Control of bleeding
Tracheostomy	Upper airway obstruction	Maintain patent airway
Debulking of recurrent tumor mass	Pain Pressure Ulceration	Symptom control Maintain skin integrity
Ileostomy	Small bowel fistula	Eliminate chronic drainage Prevent local tissue breakdown

Radiosensitive organs are moved out of the treatment field and a single, large dose of radiation is given. At present, intraoperative therapy is best considered investigational (Kinsella & Sindelar, 1996; Zerbi et al., 1994). Postoperative adjuvant therapy is the most common method for additional treatment. This approach allows a complete pathologic assessment of risk factors before selection of a specific treatment plan. An important corollary is that low-risk patients can be identified so as to avoid the morbidity and expense of unnecessary treatment. Adjuvant therapy has revolutionized the surgical approach to cancer by augmenting the survival rates of primary resection and by fostering the development of less radical surgical procedures to preserve function and limit deformity.

Ablative Techniques

New ablative techniques designed to destroy tumor masses without excision can be used with or without exploratory surgery when classic resection is not practical. Laser therapy, cryotherapy, and ultrasonic aspiration are current examples of ablative technology.

Lasers destroy tissue by focusing a high-energy light beam in the area selected for destruction. Cellular absorption of the light energy results in tissue vaporization. Lasers are categorized on the basis of the beam-generating element. The CO_2, argon, and neodymium YAG lasers are in common clinical practice. (Dixon, 1988; Lehr, 1989). The CO_2 laser is adept at vaporization of surface lesions and is therefore frequently used for lesions occurring on the head, neck, and genital tract. In these areas, tissue destruction occurs with minimal blood loss and rapid healing. Because the argon laser has shallow penetration, it has been used in the treatment of vascular lesions and the palliative control of bleeding. In contrast, the neodymium YAG laser has deeper tissue penetration for coagulation of bleeding tumors and relief of intraluminal obstructions.

For cryotherapy, a probe is placed into the central portion of a tumor mass. A refrigerant circulated through the probe causes freezing and ultimate necrosis of adjacent tissue. The zone of tissue destruction is determined by the freezing time. A freeze-thaw-refreeze sequence provides the most effective tissue destruction. Current applications of cryotherapy include tumors of the skin, genital tract, prostate, and liver (Gage, 1992; Hacker, Browder, & Ramos-Caro, 1993; Onik, Atkinson, Zemel, & Weaver, 1993; Wieder et al., 1995; Zippe, 1995). Cryotherapy has also been used for palliation of airway obstruction in patients with endobronchial carcinomas (Maiwand & Homasson, 1995).

Occasionally, ultrasonic aspiration can be used to enhance the effects of cytoreductive operations. The ultrasonic probe produces high-frequency vibrations that fragment tumor but leave vascular structures unaffected. Its most common clinical application is the destruction of implant metastases on peritoneal or organ surfaces and is used in conjunction with cytoreductive surgery (Deppe, Malviya, Boike, & Malone, 1989).

Prophylactic Surgery

Prophylactic surgery for cancer is usually done in only two instances: in individuals from cancer-prone families and in individuals with certain rare hereditary conditions. Detailed analysis of family trees in certain cancer-prone individuals has led to the identification of several cancer family syndromes (Lynch, Krush, Thomas, & Lynch, 1976). Members of these families may have a lifetime cancer risk that exceeds 50%. Therefore prophylactic surgery to remove the organ at risk may be offered. Tumors with such inheritance patterns include colon, breast, ovary, thyroid, and endometrium. However, prophylactic surgery should be considered only in well-documented cases. Genetic testing may assist in the diagnosis of inherited cancer syndromes.

In addition, certain rare heredity or developmental conditions carry such a high predisposition for the development of cancer that prophylactic surgery is usually offered to individuals with these diseases. Examples are cryptorchidism (testicular cancer), hereditary colonic polyposis (colon carcinoma), ulcerative colitis (colon carcinoma), and multiple endocrine neoplasia (thyroid cancer).

Patients undergoing prophylactic surgery require expert counseling and emotional support. Any prophylactic operation is a major procedure and is performed in a patient who is asymptomatic and does not have cancer. Furthermore, removal of a major organ may necessitate lifestyle changes or chronic medication. An important part of therapy is to provide genetic testing and counseling for other family members.

Reconstruction

Emphasis on plastic and reconstructive procedures is a recent development in surgical oncology. During the development of en bloc resection, the primary concern was curative resection rather than long-term cosmetic and functional results. Even when available, reconstruction was commonly delayed to allow healing from the primary operation and a disease-free interval. Modern reconstructive surgery has flourished for a variety of reasons:

- Improved treatment plans that have increased survivals so that there are more long-term cancer survivors
- The development and refinement of plastic surgery techniques that have enhanced the number and quality of reconstructive options
- A greater focus on quality of life issues for cancer patients
- Patient interest in reconstructive procedures

Today, reconstruction is an integral part of primary therapy for many cancers because operations that produce major anatomic or structural deformities must have a reconstructive phase to produce an acceptable cosmetic and/or functional outcome. To ensure that the most appropriate reconstructive procedure is selected and that primary resection facilitates reconstruction, the reconstructive surgeon must participate in preoperative planning. Although most reconstructive procedures are performed or initiated during the primary surgery, reconstruction is not an option in situations when a prolonged recovery would interfere with curative postoperative therapy.

In many situations, primary resections cannot be accomplished without simultaneous reconstruction to maintain anatomic integrity and function (Fig. 3-9). In other situations when reconstruction is not anatomically required (e.g., mastectomy, pelvic exenteration), the restoration of function and preservation of normal appearance lessen the negative impact of treatment and enhance the patient's return to normal psychosocial and sexual functioning (Bostwick, 1995; Ratliff et al., 1996). A photograph of a breast reconstruction performed in conjunction with primary surgery is shown in Fig. 3-10.

FACTORS THAT INFLUENCE THE USE OF SURGERY AS A TREATMENT OPTION

The decision to use surgical therapy in the treatment of cancer must take into account several important factors. These factors include the growth rate, invasiveness, and metastatic potential of the tumor; the accessibility of the tumor for resection; the patient's ability to tolerate surgery; and the capabilities of the surgical team. An evaluation of these basic concepts lays the groundwork for every operation.

Tumor Characteristics

The tumor's growth rate, invasiveness, and metastatic potential must be assessed to determine whether surgery is a viable treatment and to plan the surgical resection procedure. *Growth rate* refers to the proliferation of tumor cells. Slow-growing tumors with prolonged cell cycles, such as sarcomas, nonmelanoma skin cancers, and colorectal cancers, are more amenable to surgical resection because they tend to be confined locally or regionally at the time of presentation.

The invasive growth pattern of the tumor must be evaluated carefully. Because curative surgical resection attempts to remove the entire tumor, tumors that have a compact and predictable pattern of invasion can be readily treated by standard primary resection. However, resection of tumors with extensive local spread and adjacent tissue invasion may not be technically possible. In this setting, the use of surgical adjuvants such as chemotherapy and radiation therapy may make less radical or incomplete resections a legitimate option. When effective, adjuvant treatment given preoperatively or postoperatively can reduce tumor mass and eliminate micrometastases. A major tenant of cancer therapy is that the first treatment offers the best chance for cure. Careful pretreatment planning that addresses eradication of all areas of known tumor is essential.

The treatment plan must consider the metastatic potential of the tumor, particularly at what point in the course of disease metastases typically occur, and the most common sites of metastases. Curative surgical resection is usually not possible for cancers that disseminate early in the course of disease or those that have a tendency for lymphatic or vascular spread beyond the primary site. Curative resection is best used when tumors have a long local growth phase characterized by infrequent or late metastases. A thorough search for metastases should be performed before primary surgical treatment is recommended. This workup includes a detailed history, physical examination, laboratory studies, and additional diagnostic procedures tailored to the individual patient and the specific tumor type. When metastatic disease is detected, surgical therapy may be offered to provide local disease control, prevent disease complications, or lessen morbidity. For example, removal of a primary breast tumor prevents skin ulcerations and breakdown while systemic therapy can be given to treat distant disease. When surgical resection of an advanced gastric cancer is not possible, operative placement of a gastrostomy tube can provide decompression of obstruction and can be used for elemental feedings.

Tumor Location

Another major issue in assessing resectability is the site of the tumor. Features that influence resectability include surgical access to the tumor, absence of involvement of adjacent vital structures, and the patient's ability to compensate for the organ or tissue removed. To be resectable, the tumor

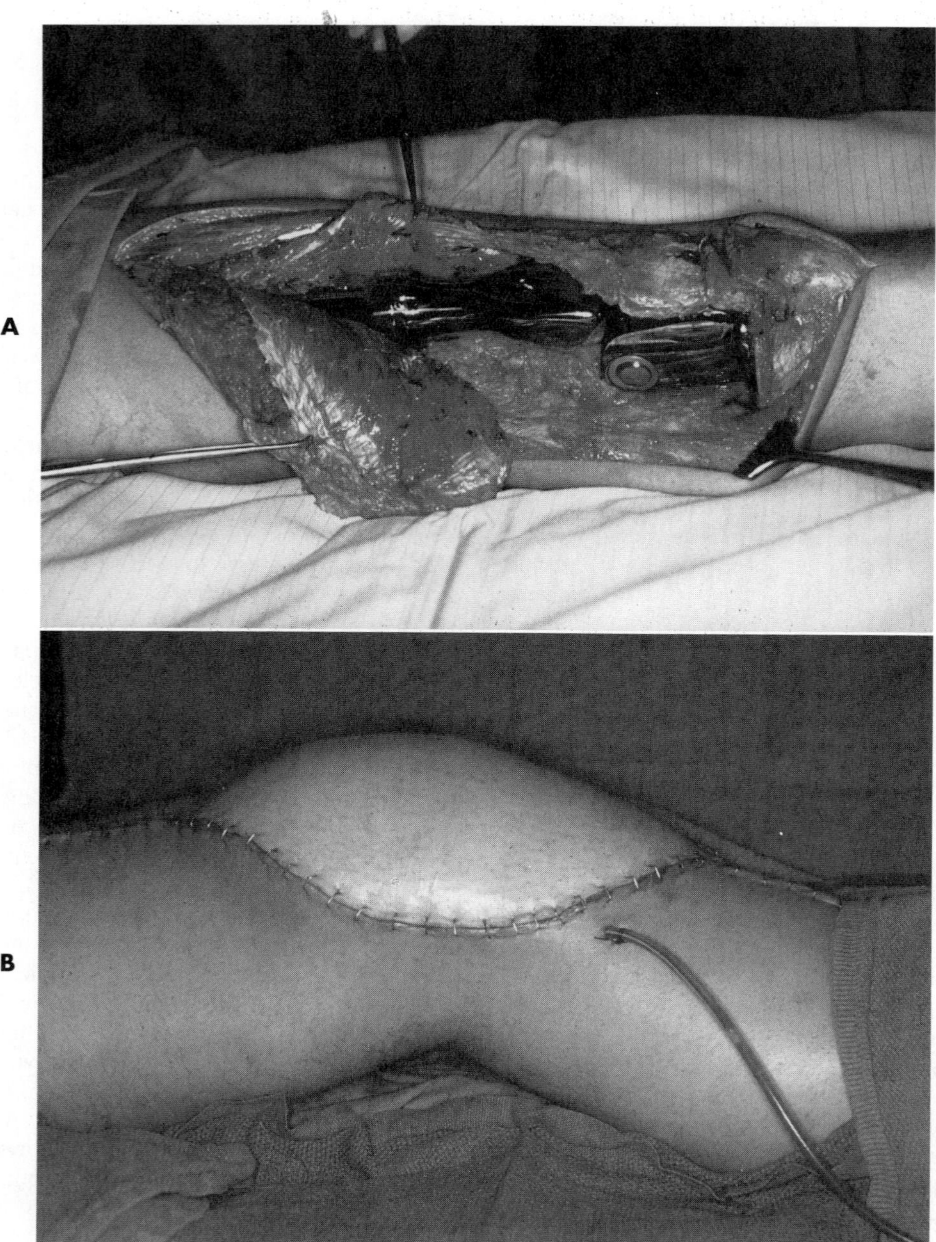

Fig. 3-9 Anatomic integrity and function were preserved in this patient diagnosed with a sarcoma in his leg, avoiding amputation of the extremity. Resection of the sarcoma required removal of the patient's knee. **A,** Surgical defect (with a rod in place) before reconstruction. **B,** Free transverse rectus abdominis myocutaneous (TRAM) flap was used to fill the defect. (Photographs courtesy Michael J. Miller, MD, and Alan W. Yasko, MD.)

Continued

must be anatomically accessible for a surgical resection. When local tumor growth encompasses adjacent vital structures or occurs in a difficult anatomic site, resection may be impossible. An example that illustrates all of these aspects of operability is pancreatic cancer (Fig. 3-11). The pancreas is an organ with important physiologic functions situated in the retroperitoneal space. It is surrounded by the duodenum, stomach, biliary ducts, gallbladder, spleen, lymph nodes, and major vascular structures including the hepatic and superior mesenteric arteries, and the portal and superior mesenteric veins. Because of these close anatomic relationships around the pancreas, local tumor growth frequently encases the vascular structures, rendering the tumor inoperable (McGrath, Sloan, & Kenady, 1996).

Host Characteristics

In addition to assessing tumor resectability, the patient's ability to withstand the proposed operation must also be determined. Major surgery is a physiologic stress that carries

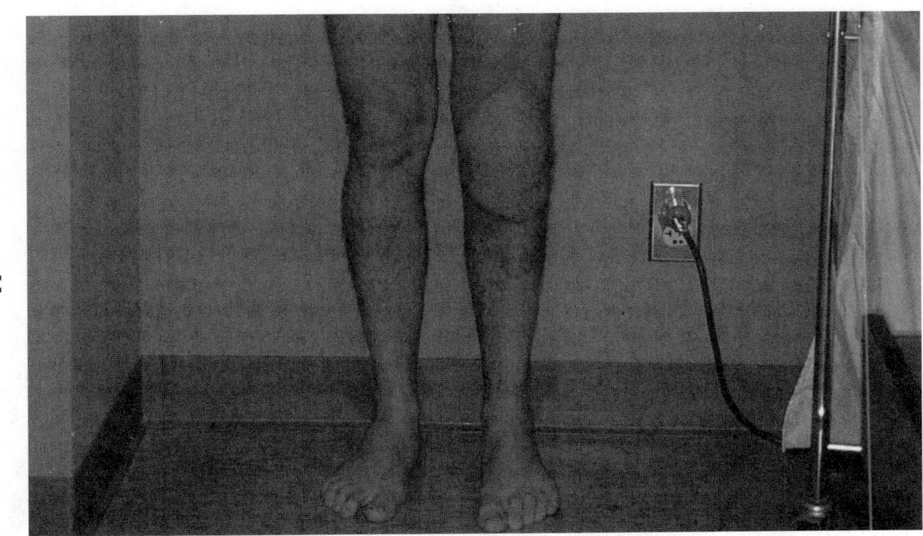

Fig. 3-9, cont'd C, Results were excellent.

an associated risk for morbidity and mortality. Determinants of operative risk include age, current health status, presence and severity of concomitant illnesses, and extent of the proposed surgery. Cancer is commonly diagnosed in individuals over the age of 65. Although age alone does not preclude an operation, patients in this upper age bracket are more likely to have medical illnesses and less physiologic tolerance that affect their ability to withstand surgical therapy (Derby, 1991; Patterson, 1989). However, improvements in perioperative care have reduced the morbidity and mortality associated with cancer surgery, making radical procedures more accessible to elderly patients.

A thorough preoperative evaluation should assess the function of the patient's major organ systems, including cardiovascular, pulmonary, renal, endocrine, nutritional, and immunologic (Polomano, Weintraub, & Wurster, 1994). Information obtained from the medical history and physical examination can be used to tailor laboratory and diagnostic testing required for risk evaluation (Ewer & Ali, 1990). Healthy patients with a negative medical history and normal physical examination require minimal preoperative testing compared with those who have an existing chronic illness. Detailed studies such as arterial blood gases, spirometry, and echocardiogram help evaluate organ function and estimate surgical risk (Box 3-1).

When organ dysfunction can be corrected or improved by medical therapy, preoperative management may reduce surgical risks. Examples include correction of fluid and electrolyte imbalances, control of hyperglycemia and hypertension, and reversal of malnutrition. For all operations, the estimated surgical risks must be balanced against the potential for cure or control of disease. When the potential for cure is high and patient risk is mild or moderate, surgical resection is clearly indicated. If, however, the cure rate is modest and significant organ impairment is present, alternate treatment options should be considered.

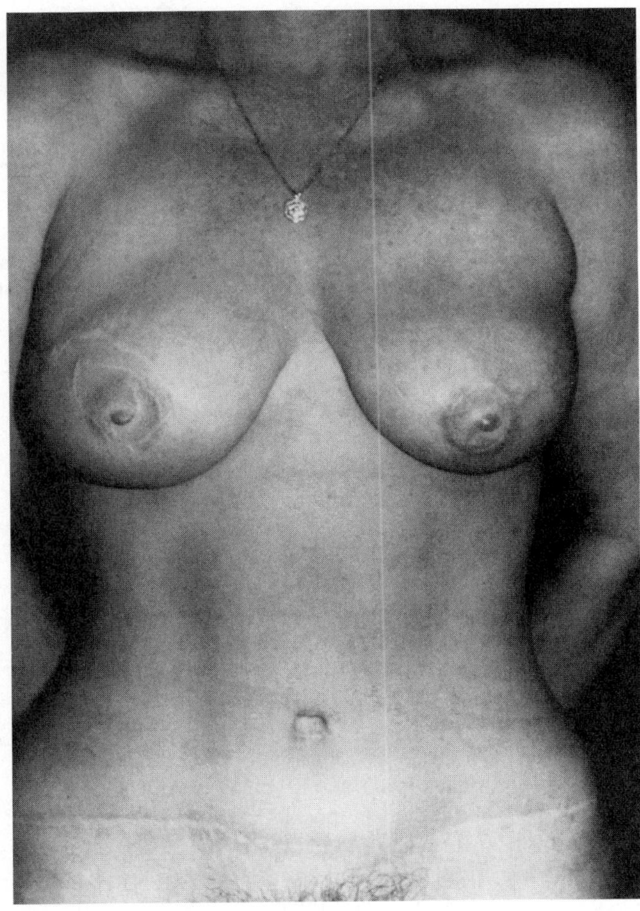

Fig. 3-10 Favorable cosmetic outcome of a breast reconstruction, performed in conjunction with primary surgery. (Photograph courtesy of Stephen S. Kroll, MD, FACS.)

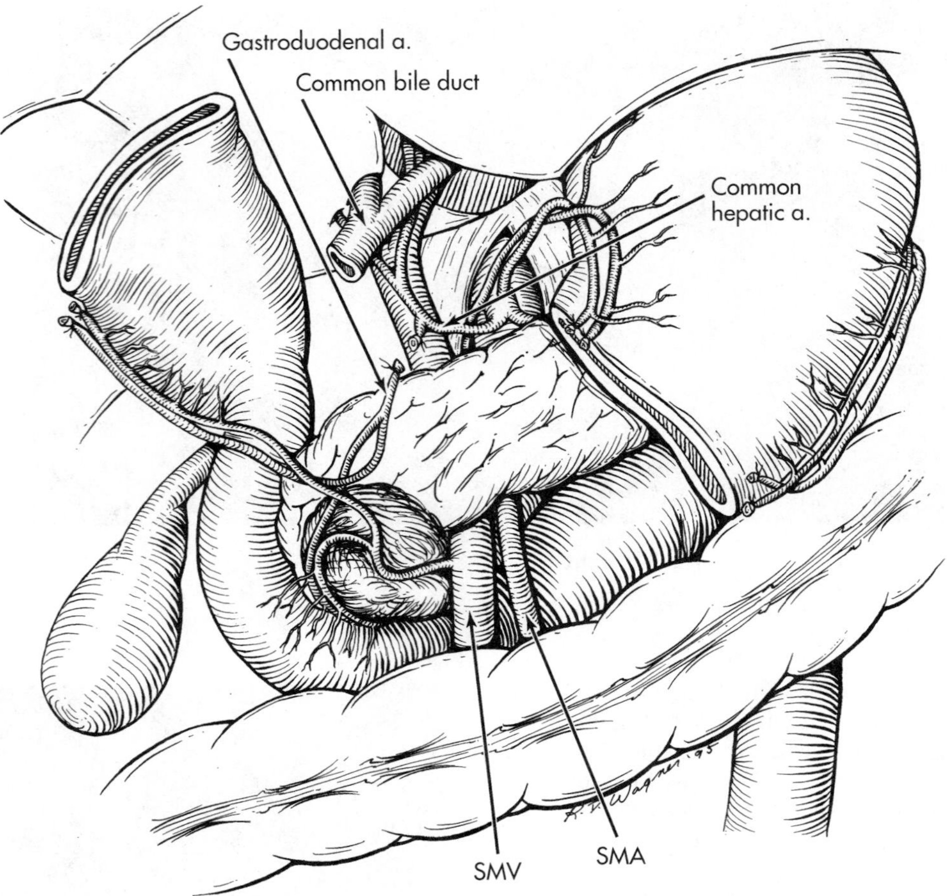

Fig. 3-11 The close anatomic relationships between the pancreas and other organs and vascular structures in the retroperitoneal space make surgical resection of pancreatic cancer a technically difficult procedure. (Courtesy of Douglas B. Evans, MD.)

The Operative Team

The skill of the personnel providing preoperative, intraoperative, and postoperative care is an essential component of any major surgical procedure. The team includes those performing the preoperative evaluation and teaching, those providing the surgical and anesthetic care, and those responsible for postoperative care both before and after discharge from the hospital. A smooth operation and recovery limit morbidity and return the patient to a functional status as rapidly as possible. Major cancer surgery should be performed only by surgeons with the expertise and experience to perform the given tumor resection. They must be adequately supported by an anesthesia team well versed in the care of high-risk patients and an intensive care service geared to provide high level physiologic support. Expert surgical technique and vigilant postoperative care reduce the incidence of postoperative complications. Miller and colleagues (1995), for example, observed that the incidence of postoperative fistula development was dramatically reduced from 16% to 4.5% with the advent of routine pelvic floor reconstruction following pelvic exenteration. Early and aggressive treatment of postoperative infections is also important to reduce the incidence of early fistula formation.

Failure at any point of the surgical experience increases the patient's potential for morbidity and delays ultimate recovery. This point is particularly critical when a multimodal treatment plan is being used. In addition to the heightened risk for postoperative complications as a result of prior therapy (e.g., immunosuppression), postoperative therapy cannot be instituted until recovery has progressed to a point at which additional therapy is possible.

DISEASES TREATED BY SURGERY

Curative surgical resection is primarily used for solid tumors that have not progressed beyond the site of origin. This clinical setting permits complete tumor removal with a normal tissue margin. When assessment of prognostic factors permits stratification of risk, patients in high-risk subsets may also be offered adjuvant therapy. Although surgical therapy may be part of the treatment of tumors with regional or distant spread, its use in these situations usually requires additional therapeutic modalities. Representative outcomes

Box 3-1
Preoperative Assessment of Surgical Risk

General

1. Medical history
2. Physical examination

Cardiovascular

1. Electrocardiogram
2. Echocardiogram
3. Stress test
4. Coronary angiogram
5. Complete blood count

Pulmonary

1. Arterial blood gases
2. Spirometry
3. Chest radiograph

Renal

1. Serum electrolytes, blood urea nitrogen, creatinine
2. Creatinine clearance
3. Urinary protein measurement
4. Urinalysis

Endocrine

1. Serum glucose
2. Thyroid function studies
3. Serum calcium, phosphorus

Hepatic

1. Serum liver enzymes
2. Bilirubin
3. Coagulation profile

Nutritional

1. Anthropometric measurements
2. Serum albumin
3. Total lymphocyte count
4. Skin test reactivity

*Extent of testing is determined by the findings of the history and physical examination.

for surgical resection of common solid tumors are summarized in Table 3-4.

THE SURGICAL EXPERIENCE

In addition to the routine perioperative care required by all patients undergoing surgery, the surgical oncology patient presents some unique challenges. In general, oncologic procedures are more likely to be complex, producing major physiologic alterations that may be temporary or permanent. Patients and caregivers are often faced with learning how to perform new tasks and to manage postoperative problems. These postoperative requirements are further complicated by the growing trend to reduce each patient's length of hospital stay. Not only are major postoperative stays shorter, but many procedures that previously required hospitalizations (e.g., mastectomy, lymph node biopsy, simple hysterectomy) are now performed in an outpatient or short-stay setting (Burke, Zabka, McCarver, & Singletary, 1997; Hunt, Feig, & Ames, 1995; Morris et al., 1997).

To accomplish patient education and care goals, the multidisciplinary team must develop and implement a detailed plan. Successful implementation of this plan must incorporate the combined efforts of the clinic nurse, inpatient staff nurse, and home health care nurse to promote continuity of care. An additional challenge is presented by the patient who receives other forms of therapy either preoperatively or postoperatively. For many patients, the operation is just one part of the total treatment plan. Therefore, an understanding of the complete treatment plan by the nurse, including the potential and anticipated impact of nonsurgical therapy, is critical. This knowledge can be used to minimize postoperative complications and avoid treatment delay. It also makes the nurse more sensitive to the patient's and family's psychosocial needs.

Table 3-4 Common Cancers Treated by Primary Surgical Resection

Site of Cancer	Percentage of Patients Diagnosed with Localized Disease	5 Year Survival of Patients with Localized Disease
Lung		
Small cell	30%-40%	7%
Non–small cell	20%-25%	60%-80%
Breast	58%	90%-95%
Gastrointestinal		
Colon/rectum	37%	85%-90%
Pancreas	8%	12%
Gastric	18%	57%
Esophagus	40%	20%
Liver	20%	12%
Genitourinary		
Prostate	57%	>90%
Bladder	74%	80%-90%
Renal cell	45%	65%
Testis	66%	>90%
Gynecologic		
Ovarian	23%	85%-90%
Cervix	51%	90%
Uterine corpus	73%	85%-90%
Head and Neck Cancers		
Oral cavity/pharynx	36%	70%-80%
Larynx	25%	85%
Thyroid	60%	90%
Skin		
Melanoma	82%	>90%
Non-melanoma	Near 100%	Near 100%
Sarcoma	80%	90%

From DeVita V. T., Jr., (1997). *Cancer: Principles and practice of oncology* (5th ed.). Philadelphia: Lippincott-Raven.

Preoperative Preparation

A thorough examination that includes the patient's physical and psychosocial health is performed after the surgical procedure is planned. The patient's general health status is assessed first, with information about concomitant disease and existing organ impairment elicited.

Patients with more advanced tumors tend to require more extensive operations. For this reason, the severity of the patient's existing medical problems should be correlated with the extent of the proposed surgery.

Box 3-2
Factors that Increase Surgical Risk

Age > 65
Concimitant medical illness
History of smoking
Obesity
Immunosuppression
Malnutrition
Large tumor burden
Extensive planned procedure
Prior cancer therapy

Special attention should then be directed toward factors most likely to negatively influence the surgical course and recovery (Box 3-2). Wound healing is impaired by factors such as diabetes, obesity, malnutrition, prior radiation therapy to the surgical field, cardiovascular disease, and recent treatment with cytotoxic drugs or steroids (Barber & Brown, 1993; Ehrlichman, Seckel, Bryan, & Moschella, 1991; Falcone & Nappi, 1984). Patients with chronic lung disease and those with radiation or bleomycin therapy-induced pulmonary fibrosis are at greater risk for the pulmonary complications associated with anesthesia. Patients with preexisting cardiovascular problems such as coronary artery disease, congestive heart failure, valvular prolapse, or prior anthracycline-based chemotherapy may have a diminished cardiac reserve. The risk of perioperative infection is higher in patients who are immunosuppressed by prior cancer therapy, advanced age, or by the tumor itself. Preoperative malnutrition may contribute to postoperative complications such as poor wound healing, sepsis, and ileus.

The patient's ability to deal with surgically induced changes in physical function must be determined before surgery. Arthritis, visual impairments, learning disabilities, neurologic deficits, or lack of an available caretaker has a direct bearing on many postoperative care requirements. Specific examples include ostomy care, self-injections, central venous catheter care, specialized feedings (enteral or IV), management of percutaneous tubes and drains, and complicated wound care.

A psychosocial evaluation is as important as the physical assessment. The patient and family must have the emotional stability and motivation to overcome the stress of a cancer diagnosis, the surgical procedure, and potentially lifelong alterations in physical status. The nursing assessment should evaluate the patient's normal coping mechanisms, existing support systems, and the availability of community resources.

Every operation has a standard set of requirements for patient education and preoperative preparation. The preoperative assessment provides the information needed to individualize these requirements for a particular patient. A plan to deal with identified deficits must be developed. For example, all patients undergoing large bowel resection require preoperative directions for mechanical and antibiotic bowel preparation. Fragile patients may require preoperative admission to monitor fluid and electrolyte status. Consequently, a meticulous preoperative assessment is used to develop a teaching plan that covers both standard requirements and individual needs. Basic patient education guidelines for surgery are outlined in Table 3-5.

Preoperative teaching must begin by determining the patient's understanding of the surgery and rehabilitation. Barriers to learning, such as anxiety, language differences, low intelligence, or illiteracy, must also be identified and addressed. The patient's family members or significant others should participate in the teaching program. The teaching plan should include a detailed explanation of the surgical procedure, the expected hospital course, and the requirements during the home recovery period. These explanations must include a step-by-step description that takes them from entry into the hospital through postoperative rehabilitation. For example, if an intensive care stay is anticipated, this should be discussed with the patient.

The benefits of preoperative education, in promoting a patient's physical and psychological recovery, are well documented in the literature (Devine & Cook, 1986). Patients who know what to expect tend to be less anxious, develop fewer postoperative complications, use fewer pain medications, and are better able to participate in their postoperative care. Basic preoperative teaching for the patient should include preparation for surgery and expectations for postoperative care: early ambulation; turning, coughing, and deep breathing procedures; and a description of the equipment that will be used (e.g., IV pumps, compression boots, nebulizers, Foley catheter, drains, incentive spirometers). The patient should also be given a realistic description of the expected degree of postoperative pain and how it will be controlled. Pain education should include the way in which the patient's pain will be assessed and managed with medication (e.g., oral, epidural, patient-controlled device, intermittent IV). The patient should be told that the goal of postoperative pain control is to facilitate the patient's ability to perform necessary recovery activities in reasonable comfort.

Teaching is most effective when several educational approaches are used. Oral explanations may be supplemented with written instructions, task demonstrations, diagrams, videotapes, and computer-assisted instruction to provide repetition and enhance patient comprehension (Doak, Doak, & Meade, 1996; Meade, 1996). The nurse must verify that the patient understands what has been taught and provide an opportunity for the patient and family to verbalize their feelings and ask questions (Padberg & Padberg, 1990).

Many institutions are developing and using clinical care pathways for surgical care. These pathways provide a comprehensive "roadmap" of the patient's perioperative care. Typically, care pathways are designed by a multidisciplinary group and incorporate patient education, physical care, laboratory studies, medications, and discharge planning. The advantages of such pathways are standardization of care, better overall planning, shorter hospitalizations, fewer

Table 3-5 Basic Patient Education Guidelines for Surgery

Guideline	Rationale
A. These general preoperative instructions are common for all surgical procedures:	A. These activities reduce the incidence of postoperative complications.
1. Do not eat or drink after midnight on the night before surgery.	
2. On the evening before surgery, take a shower, cleansing the surgical site with antiseptic soap.	
3. Your nurse will teach you how to perform coughing and deep breathing exercises. These must be done every hour postoperatively while you are awake.	
4. Your nurse will give you specific preoperative instructions for the type of surgery you will have.	4. Surgical patients who know what to expect postoperatively tend to be less anxious and are more able to participate in postoperative care.
5. Your doctor or nurse will discuss the plan for your postoperative pain management. This discussion includes how much pain is expected and how your pain will be controlled.	
6. Your nurse will describe the equipment that will be used for your postoperative care (e.g., Foley catheter, nasogastric tube, surgical drains).	
7. Your doctor will describe the surgical procedure that is planned for you and will outline the expected hospital course.	
8. Your doctor or nurse will discuss home care requirements to enhance your recovery after your discharge from the hospital.	8. Allows the patient and family an opportunity to coordinate resources so that home care is facilitated after discharge.
9. You and your family members should feel free to ask questions or express concerns to your doctor or nurse. Other support persons (e.g., chaplain, social worker) are available to you as needed.	9. Psychological support to the patient and family is imperative both pre- and postoperatively.
	During times of stress, patient and family comprehension of teaching instructions may be diminished. Repetition using multiple educational approaches enhances understanding.
B. These general postoperative instructions are common for all surgical procedures:	
1. Coughing and deep breathing exercises should be performed every hour while you are awake.	1. These actions reverse atelectasis and help prevent pneumonia.
2. Turn in bed at frequent intervals.	
3. Your nurse will teach you how to exercise your arms and legs (range-of-motion exercises) while you are in bed.	3. Frequent turning and exercise improve circulation and ventilation and help prevent pressure injuries.
4. Your nurse will help you get out of bed and walk as soon as possible. If you are unable to get out of bed, your doctor may order compression stockings and boots, or a special medicine that prevents blood clots to help promote circulation in your legs.	4. Patients with cancer are at higher risk for developing deep thrombosis and pulmonary embolus.
5. Your nurse will give you specific postoperative instructions according to the type of surgery you will have.	
C. Pain Management	
1. Your nurse will ask you to describe, locate, and rate the severity of your pain (using a pain scale) at regular intervals.	1. Adjustments to the pain management plan are based on subjective patient reports of comfort. Acceptable control of pain allows the patient to perform required tasks during the postoperative period.
2. Use a small pillow to splint your incision during coughing and deep breathing exercises.	2. This technique improves pain control.
3. You may be given a discharge prescription for pain medications. Take your pain medication as needed. Do not wait until your pain becomes severe or unbearable. Call your doctor or nurse if your pain medication is not providing you with satisfactory pain relief.	

Continued

TABLE 3-5 Basic Patient Education Guidelines for Surgery—cont'd

Guideline	Rationale
D. Discharge Instructions	
1. It is important for you to recognize the following signs and symptoms of infection. The following should be reported to your doctor or nurse immediately: Temperature >101.3° F (38.5° C) Redness, swelling, purulent (puslike) drainage, foul odor and/or increased tenderness at your surgical incision or drain site.	1. Ensures prompt intervention for postoperative infection.
2. Your nurse will teach you how to care for your surgical incision/drain site.	
3. Your nurse will give you specific discharge instructions according to the type of surgery you have had.	
4. You will be given an appointment for your first follow-up evaluation. If you have questions or concerns, call your nurse or doctor at the number given to you.	

documentation requirements, and lower cost. An example of a clinical pathway for abdominal hysterectomy is provided in Fig. 3-12.

Basic Postoperative Care

Meticulous postoperative nursing care seeks to return the patient to optimal function by providing physical and psychosocial support during the immediate recovery phase. Care focuses on monitoring vital functions, maintaining tubes and drains, providing pain control, reestablishing nutritional balance, and preventing surgical complications. Attention to detail may be more critical for the cancer patient who may be at greater risk for postoperative complications owing to immunosuppression, prior treatment, organ dysfunction, or an extensive surgical procedure.

Vital Signs. Monitoring vital functions includes serial measurement of temperature, pulse rate, respiratory rate, and blood pressure. A change in vital signs may provide the first clue that a postoperative problem is developing. For example, fever in this setting may indicate atelectasis or infection. Tachycardia may be due to pneumonia, pulmonary edema, or hypoxia. Any alteration in baseline vital signs requires further investigation to determine the underlying cause and to direct corrective intervention.

Body Fluid Shifts. Patients who undergo a major operative procedure often experience dramatic shifts in body fluids. Typical sources of fluid loss are blood loss, nasogastric suction drainage, increased sensible loss, and the movement of body fluid to the extracellular compartment. Fluid gains are caused by replacement therapy with blood products and IV fluids. The restoration of normal fluid balance is a dynamic process occurring over the first 3 to 5 postoperative days. Accurate measurement of input and output is used to guide adjustments in fluid replacement. When the intake and output indicate excess fluid load, early intervention by fluid restriction and diuretic therapy may prevent pulmonary edema. Conversely, excessive output should be treated with additional fluid to expand intravascular volume and maintain renal perfusion (Clark-Pearson, Olt, Rodriguez, & Boente, 1993). Optimal postoperative hydration ensures tissue perfusion and cellular function.

Serum Electrolytes. Serum electrolytes, particularly sodium and potassium, may be depleted by intraoperative losses, continuous output from nasogastric suction, or inadequate replacement. Hypokalemia is the most common postoperative electrolyte disturbance. Failure to detect and correct this abnormality may cause serious cardiac arrhythmias (Mahon & Casperson, 1993). Occasionally, hyponatremia may also be caused by inappropriate secretion of the antidiuretic hormone. Operative procedures that interfere with normal regulatory mechanisms can also cause electrolyte imbalances. For example, after thyroidectomy, calcium and magnesium levels must be monitored carefully to ensure normal function of the parathyroid glands. After most operations, a serum electrolyte panel should be obtained in the immediate postoperative period. The frequency of subsequent testing depends on the clinical situation.

Blood Component Therapy. The need for blood component therapy is directly related to operative blood loss and any ongoing losses after surgery. If surgical blood loss is significant, blood is replaced in the operating room under the direction of the anesthesia team. Blood losses of less than 20% of total volume generally do not require transfusion. For intermediate losses, replacement with packed red cells is appropriate. When blood loss is substantial, transfusion of additional components such as platelets, plasma, and cryoprecipitate may be necessary.

After major operations, a complete blood count is obtained periodically to assess circulating hemoglobin levels. Stable values indicate that intraoperative blood replacement and hemostasis are adequate. Falling levels suggest ongoing blood loss from the operative site. Postoperative bleeding may be exacerbated by thrombocytopenia or coagulopathy. Postoperative transfusion therapy must be individualized and is usually guided by the patient's symptoms and labora-

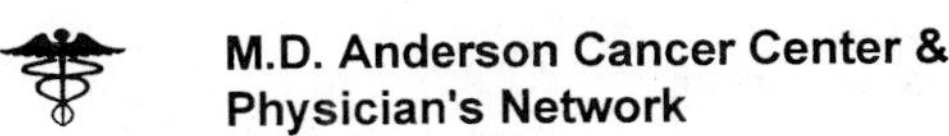

M.D. Anderson Cancer Center &
Physician's Network

MRN:
Name:
DOB:
Admit Date:
Path Entry:

Pathway:GynS2 Total Abdominal Hysterectomy

THIS PATH IS A GENERAL GUIDELINE: CARE IS REVISED TO MEET THE INDIVIDUAL PATIENT'S NEEDS BASED ON MEDICAL NECESSITY.

Date			
Category of Care	Pre-Operative Visit	Same Day Admit Surgery	Post-Op Day #1
Consult	Special Consults as needed Obtain insurance authorization Surgery Scheduling		
Diagnostic Test	T Protein, Alb, Ca, Phos, Gluc, BUN, Uric Acid, Creat, T Bili, Alk Phos, LDH, SGPT (within 30 days) CBC (within 14 days) CXR (if over 60 years old) ECG (if over 40 years old)	CBC if blood loss > 1,000cc or Hgb preop < 11 gm	CBC this AM
Treatment	Fleets enema	Compression boots TCDB q2h Observe for excessive bleeding Foley BSD Incentive Spirometer	Incentive Spirometer continued D/C Foley at 6 AM Remove O.R. Dressing Inspect Incision line Observe for excessive bleeding
Medication	Meds as per anesthesia Magnesium Citrate 1 bottle po 48 hrs. before surgery	IV Fluids at 100 cc/hr PCA pump basal Prophylactic antibiotic immediately preop: Ancef or Cefoxitin	PCA pump basal discontinue IV Fluids at 75 cc/hr PCA PRN dose
Performance Status / Activity	Activities of daily living		Ambulate in halls QID
Nutrition	NPO after midnight prior to surgery		Clear liquids
Teaching / Psychosoc	Provide educational materials Instructions on use of incentive spirometer Pre-op educational materials per standard Clarify any concerns Review care path		Review care path
Discharge Planning	Needs assessment	TCDB q2h	Needs assessment reviewed Discharge plan agreed upon
Outcome Criteria	Vital signs stable(within pt's normal range) Afebrile; physical exam at pre-op baseline and without any pulmonary complications. Incision line clean, intact and without signs of infection; no s/s of excessive bleeding; tolerating regular diet, activity appropriate for discharge.		
Followup Criteria			

Version:0 Approved:11/15/96 12:10:18 PM

Fig. 3-12 Surgical care pathways provide a comprehensive overview of the perioperative requirements for a given operation. A pathway for total abdominal hysterectomy with or without bilateral salpingo-oophorectomy (BSO)/unilateral salpingo-oophorectomy (USO) is illustrated. (Courtesy University of Texas M. D. Anderson Cancer Center.)

Continued

tory values. If coagulopathy is suspected, coagulation profiles must be monitored in addition to blood counts. The decision to transfuse must balance the risks of complications (e.g., congestive heart failure, hepatitis, human immunodeficiency virus infection, transfusion reaction) against the anticipated benefits of transfusion (Clark-Pearson et al., 1993).

Basic Nursing Interventions. Some of the simplest nursing interventions are key factors in the prevention of major postoperative complications. Frequent coughing and deep breathing exercises or oropharyngeal suctioning helps to expand pulmonary alveoli and clear respiratory secretions (O'Donohue, 1992; Orr, Holloway, & Orr, 1994). These actions reverse atelectasis and help prevent pneumonia. Early

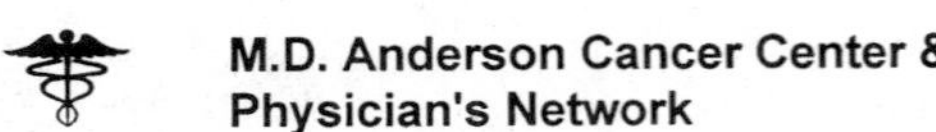

M.D. Anderson Cancer Center &
Physician's Network

MRN:
Name:
DOB:
Admit Date:
Path Entry:

Pathway:GynS2 Total Abdominal Hysterectomy

THIS PATH IS A GENERAL GUIDELINE: CARE IS REVISED TO MEET THE INDIVIDUAL PATIENT'S NEEDS BASED ON MEDICAL NECESSITY.

Date			
Category of Care	Post-Op Day #2	Post-Op Day #3	Post-Op Day #4/Discharge Day
Consult			
Diagnostic Test			
Treatment	Incentive Spirometer continued Inspect Incision line Observe for excessive bleeding	Incentive Spirometer continued Inspect incision line Observe for excessive bleeding	Staples removed in AM; steristrips applied
Medication	D/C PCA pump, heparin lock IV Oral pain meds (Lortab 7.5/500mg)	Oral pain meds (Lortab 7.5/500mg)	FeSo4 375 mg po q day until followup visit if Hgb < 10
Performance Status / Activity	Increase ambulation in halls	Increase ambulation in halls	Increase ambulation in halls
Nutrition	Soft/bland diet No bacon or milk products	Regular diet	Regular diet
Teaching / Psychosoc	Start discharge teaching with patient and significant other	Reinforce discharge teaching with patient and significant other	Checked off on discharge teaching
Discharge Planning	Discharge plan agreed upon	Discharge orders and meds written for Lortab & Senokot if needed	Discharge to home before 11 AM. Verify correct telephone number for followup
Outcome Criteria	Vital signs stable(within pt's normal range) Afebrile; physical exam at pre-op baseline and without any pulmonary complications. Incision line clean, intact and without signs of infection; no s/s of excessive bleeding; tolerating regular diet, activity appropriate for discharge.		
Followup Criteria			

Version:0 Approved:11/15/96 12:10:18 PM

Fig. 3-12, cont'd For legend see p. 45.

ambulation is encouraged in the patient to correct venous stasis in the lower extremities. Postoperative patients with cancer are at higher risk for developing deep vein thrombosis and pulmonary embolus. When ambulation is contraindicated, other prophylactic aids such as compression stockings and boots or low-dose anticoagulants can be used. Regular position changes and range-of-motion exercises should also be encouraged to prevent pressure injuries, venous pooling, and hypoventilation (Kemp, Keithley, Smith, & Morreale, 1990; Allman et al., 1986).

Perioperative Infections. Reducing the rate of postoperative infections is an important goal in postoperative care. The oncology patient is especially prone to developing infections. The combination of surgical manipulation and contamination of normally sterile tissues, disruption of the skin barrier, and the general debilitation of the cancer patient (e.g., malnutrition, immunosuppression, large tumor burden) contribute to this increased risk. Many routine surgical practices have been specifically designed to reduce postoperative infection.

Prevention should begin preoperatively. Showering with an antibacterial soap the evening before surgery reduces the concentration of bacterial flora on the skin surface. Traditionally, body hair at the operative site was removed by shaving to provide a smooth surface for the incision. The microtrauma associated with the use of prep razors actually increased the risk of local infection. When possible, shaving of body hair should be avoided. When necessary, the use of a hair clipper is preferable to use of a razor. Removal of body hair should be performed immediately before the operation to avoid local inflammation at the time of incision.

Surgical procedures may have specific preoperative requirements to reduce infections. For example, preoperative bowel preparation that includes mechanical cleansing and broad-spectrum antibiotics with aerobic and anaerobic activity has been shown to greatly reduce postoperative infections after colorectal surgery (Nichols & Holmes, 1995).

The prophylactic administration of parenteral antibiotics is commonly used to prevent wound and operative site infections. The benefits of prophylaxis have been well established by large randomized clinical trials that demonstrated a 50% reduction in postoperative infections when antibiotics were used (Ulualp & Condon, 1992). First- and second-

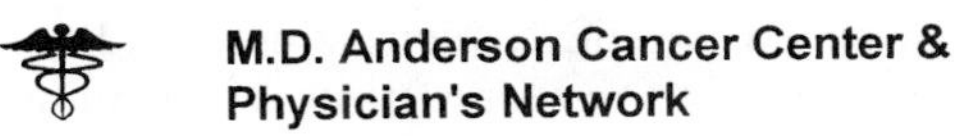
M.D. Anderson Cancer Center &
Physician's Network

MRN:
Name:
DOB:
Admit Date:
Path Entry:

Pathway:GynS2 Total Abdominal Hysterectomy
THIS PATH IS A GENERAL GUIDELINE: CARE IS REVISED TO MEET THE INDIVIDUAL PATIENT'S NEEDS BASED ON MEDICAL NECESSITY.

Date			
Category of Care	Post Discharge		
Consult	Follow-up phone call on POD #5 or #6 by Advanced Practice Nurse; Station 82 (4 weeks)		
Diagnostic Test			
Treatment			
Medication			
Performance Status / Activity			
Nutrition			
Teaching / Psychosoc			
Discharge Planning			
Outcome Criteria	Vital signs stable(within pt's normal range) Afebrile; physical exam at pre-op baseline and without any pulmonary complications. Incision line clean, intact and without signs of infection; no s/s of excessive bleeding; tolerating regular diet, activity appropriate for discharge.		
Followup Criteria			

Version:0 Approved:11/15/96 12:10:18 PM

Fig. 3-12, cont'd For legend see p. 45.

generation cephalosporins are commonly selected as prophylactic agents because of their broad spectrum of coverage, low toxicity, and low cost. The greatest impact is seen in clean-contaminated operations (no existing infection but exposure to host flora) or clean operations (no existing infection and no exposure to host flora) that involve implantation of a prosthetic device.

The general principles of antibiotic prophylaxis include (1) use of an agent with activity against the anticipated contaminating organisms; (2) administration of the agent just before surgery to ensure a high tissue concentration at the time of incision; and (3) maintenance of therapeutic tissue concentrations throughout the period of potential bacterial contamination but not beyond 24 hours after surgery (Ludwig, Carlson, & Condon, 1993; Sheridan, Tompkins, & Burke, 1994). The indiscriminate use of prophylactic antibiotics is unwarranted because it does not provide additional benefit, increases the incidence of resistant organisms, and is more expensive (Leaper, 1994).

External drainage is commonly used to remove fluid accumulation from the surgical site. Drains are left in place until the amount of collected fluid is minimal. Because a collection of undrained serous fluid is an excellent growth medium for bacteria, maintenance of drain patency is important.

Surgical infection rates have dramatically decreased over the last 25 years (Leaper, 1994). Although surgical skill is difficult to measure and is often overlooked, operative technique plays an important role in the prevention of infection. The lowest rates of infection are associated with shorter operation times and meticulous surgical technique that minimizes tissue damage, hematomas, and surgical dead space. Other obvious aspects of surgical technique include the maintenance of asepsis and the use of nonreactive suture materials that prevent localized inflammation (Leaper, 1995).

Because surgical infections develop after the operation, postoperative nursing care should focus on prevention and early recognition of infection. Preventive measures include regular cleansing of the surgical incision, topical care of drain sites, and provision of standard patient care activities (e.g., Foley catheter care, care of the IV site, handwashing). Prompt identification of operative site infections allows for early interventions and a reduction in morbidity. A comprehensive assessment that evaluates all possible sites for infection should be performed regularly.

Pain Management. A patient's ability to participate in his or her postoperative care requires adequate pain control. Postoperative pain is most intense during the first 48 to 72 hours, after which it gradually resolves over days to weeks. The intensity of the patient's pain should be regularly assessed and documented. Pain assessment should include the patient's description of the pain, the location of the pain, and the intensity of the pain using a standardized pain rating scale. The goals of pain control are to ensure patient comfort as well as the patient's ability to perform required tasks while avoiding sedation (Boysen, 1993). Nonsteroidal anti-inflammatory drugs (NSAIDs), splinting techniques, and relaxation therapies (e.g., hypnosis, music therapy) may be used to further enhance patient comfort.

The basic pain management plan is determined preoperatively and is based on the anticipated severity of the pain, prior experience of the operative team, and patient preferences. Computerized and programmable pumps for epidural or IV infusions are now routinely used to manage postoperative pain. Because continuous around-the-clock dosing provides superior pain control, these techniques have replaced the old standard of "as needed" (i.e., prn) injections (Polomano et al., 1994). In studies that compared patient controlled analgesia (PCA) usage to conventional opioid therapy, patients treated with PCA had shorter hospital stays, experienced less sedation and anxiety, and reported equal or improved pain relief and greater overall satisfaction (Lindley, 1994; Smythe, 1992). Epidural anesthesia is an alternative continuous infusion technique for controlling postoperative pain. It can be administered safely on any surgical unit with few reported complications (de Leon-Casasola, Parker, Lema, Harrison, & Massey, 1994).

A typical plan for pain control following an abdominal operation includes the use of a PCA pump. The pump can be programmed to deliver a continuous (basal) opioid infusion and, at the same time, allows the patient to administer additional bolus doses on an as-needed basis. The strength and frequency of bolus doses are controlled to prevent overdosing. If the patient is sedated or requiring too many bolus doses, the basal rate is adjusted. As pain begins to subside, the basal infusion is withdrawn, and the patient uses the as-needed dose for pain control. When oral intake is established and pain levels have decreased further, the PCA pump is replaced by oral pain medications. These medications are then gradually decreased and withdrawn as recovery progresses (Kane, Lehman, Dugger, Hansen, & Jackson, 1988; Lubenow & Ivankovich, 1991).

Nutrition. Most people, even those with cancer, can tolerate brief periods of inadequate nutrition. When the surgical recovery allows resumption of oral intake within 5 to 7 days, nutritional supplementation is probably not necessary. However, if the patient was malnourished before surgery or has difficulty reestablishing an oral diet, nutritional support should be considered. Complete nutritional requirements can be provided by either total parenteral nutrition or by liquid elemental diets through a feeding tube. If the upper gastrointestinal tract is capable of absorption, an enteral approach should be used. The advantages of enteral feedings are ease of administration, lower cost, fewer complications, and maintenance of intestinal villous structures. Parenteral nutrition is the only option for patients who require complete bowel rest (e.g., patients with fistulas or bowel obstructions) or for those who are unable to absorb nutrients (e.g., patients with short bowel syndromes) (Chen, Souba, & Copeland, 1991; Daly, Redmond, & Gallagher, 1992).

Psychosocial Care. Postoperative nursing care must also be directed toward the patient's psychosocial recovery. Listening is an underrated skill. Nurses must give patients and their family members opportunities to voice concerns, ask questions, and communicate feelings about the cancer diagnosis and various aspects of their treatment. Special attention should be given to helping patients and family members reduce anxiety, develop effective coping strategies, adjust to changes in body image, and maintain sexuality. Although frequently ignored, these psychosocial issues contribute to the patient's overall sense of well-being. Psychosocial rehabilitation can be facilitated by using specially trained resource persons, patient support groups, and other available hospital and community resources.

Postdischarge Care

Because the current trend is to shorten the length of the postoperative stay, some postoperative care must be delivered out of the hospital. Consequently, discharge planning must be integrated into the overall care plan of the surgical patient. The goal of discharge planning is to assess and coordinate resources so that care is not compromised when the patient moves from the hospital to home. The discharge plan should be initiated during the preoperative surgical assessment. Points to be addressed include the following:

1. Who will function as the primary caregiver?
2. What are the specific needs of the patient?
3. Can the caregiver meet the identified needs?
4. Will the caregiver require special training or education to function as the primary caregiver?
5. Will the caregiver require home care resources (e.g., homecare nursing services), and if so, how will these resources be delivered?

Nursing care should be coordinated to ensure implementation of the discharge plan. Because most patients and their caregivers require limited teaching and have adequate resources after discharge, the primary nurse can often perform the discharge planning independently. When patients have more complicated discharge needs, a discharge planning nurse should be consulted. Patients who have excessive care requirements or inadequate home resources may require an intermediate care facility before going home.

All patients return to the clinic shortly after hospital discharge (2 to 4 weeks) to evaluate their recovery process and detect potential complications. If adjuvant or adjunctive therapy will be part of the treatment plan, it is usually arranged and initiated during this interval. If the surgical procedure is the only therapy, then the patient enters a surveillance phase of care. The goals of surveillance are to detect recurrence and monitor for late complications of treatment. Most surveillance schedules are tailored to the tumor type, with the frequency of examinations and testing based on the natural history of the tumor and its known patterns of recurrence. For example, malignant melanomas typically recur early, with common sites of metastasis being the regional lymph nodes, lung, and liver. A typical postoperative surveillance schedule might include full body examinations every 3 months for 2 years, every 6 months for up to 5 years, and annually thereafter. In addition to the examinations, chest radiographs and hepatic enzymes are also monitored regularly. The time intervals for surveillance should be adjusted according to the patient's individual risk for recurrence (Ketcham & Loescher, 1993; Urist, 1996) (see standard of care, Table 3-6).

ACUTE SURGICAL COMPLICATIONS

Major surgery represents an acute physiologic stress. Consequently most surgical complications occur in the perioperative period. Many of the practices described in the postoperative care section of this chapter are performed to prevent common surgical complications. Prevention is always easier than treatment of a major postoperative complication. Despite attentive postoperative care, some patients develop perioperative problems. A review of the diagnosis and management of surgical complications is provided in Table 3-7.

CHRONIC SURGICAL COMPLICATIONS

Many cancer operations produce a loss of organ function or anatomic deformity. Compensation for these losses is an anticipated component of surgical therapy. Although adjustment to surgical deficits may be problematic and/or require lifelong therapy, these do not represent true surgical complications. Such problems are generally procedure specific and predictable. Some examples of resections that produce long-term sequelae include colectomy with ostomy placement; pancreatectomy requiring insulin therapy; amputation of an extremity; and short-gut syndrome following removal of the small intestine, leading to malabsorption and dehydration. Late complications directly attributable to surgical therapy are rare and are more frequently seen in patients who receive chemotherapy or radiotherapy in addition to surgery.

Bowel Obstructions

Bowel obstruction is the most common late complication associated with abdominal surgery. Typically, a loop of small bowel becomes kinked or entrapped by scarring or adhesion months or years after the initial operation. The clinical presentation includes abdominal pain, nausea and vomiting, abdominal distension, and absence of bowel sounds. Nasogastric decompression and bowel rest can be used to treat a partial obstruction, but a complete obstruction is an emergency that must be corrected surgically. The entire intestinal tract should be evaluated at the time of surgery because concurrent large and small bowel obstructions may be present (Tang, Davis, & Silberman, 1995).

Late bowel obstruction is four to five times more common in patients treated with postoperative pelvic or abdominal radiation. In a Gynecologic Oncology Group study, Weiser and colleagues (1989) compared the incidence of postoperative complications of advanced cervical cancer patients who received either transperitoneal or extraperitoneal lymphadenectomy before radiation. Patients who received lymphadenectomy through transection of the peritoneal cavity experienced significantly more bowel obstructions than those who did not.

Chronic Pain Syndromes

Postoperative scarring that compresses visceral or peripheral nerves may produce a chronic pain syndrome. The onset of pain tends to be gradual and is usually limited to the distribution of the involved nerve. Chronic pain is most often associated with extensive retroperitoneal dissections and is more common in patients who receive radiation therapy or develop a postoperative infection. A multimodal treatment plan that includes pharmacologic agents, neural blockades, physical therapy, and cognitive and behavioral interventions produces the most effective pain control for patients experiencing chronic pain (Barkin et al., 1996).

Lymphedema

Lymphedema is the gradual accumulation of protein-rich fluid in the interstitial spaces of an extremity, causing chronic inflammation and fibrosis of the surrounding tissue. When the lymphatic system is intact, serous fluid and proteins in the interstitial space are reabsorbed by the lymphatic capillaries and are ultimately returned to the intravascular space. Normal pressure gradients and one-way valves in the lymphatic vessels allow fluid to travel in this manner without backflow. Surgical lymph node dissection can disrupt the pressure gradients and patency of the valves, causing fluid and proteins to leak out into the interstitial space. The resulting fluid accumulation and fibrosis cause pain, numbness, decreased range of motion, and worsening lymphedema.

Although lymphedema has been reported in as many as 70% of patients after axillary node dissection, the incidence is greatest in patients who have received extensive lymph node dissections followed by radiation therapy. Other risk factors for lymphedema include metastatic disease, prolonged immobility or dependency of an extremity, obesity, and recurrent infections with lymphangitis. Although sometimes improved by elevation, massage, and compression garments, lymphedema tends to be gradually progressive. Therefore all patients who receive lymph node dissection should be educated about the risk factors for lymphedema, preventive measures (e.g., protect extremity from trauma, routine skin care), and signs and symptoms of lymphedema (Humble, 1995).

Fistulas

Although most fistulas occur in the perioperative period, they are occasionally seen as a delayed surgical complication. The fistula represents an abnormal connection between

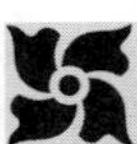

TABLE 3-6 Standard of Care for the Surgical Patient

Patient Problems and Outcomes	Nursing Interventions and Rationales	Patient Education Instructions
Knowledge Deficit Patient will: • Verbalize knowledge of pre/postoperative expectations before surgery.	1. Assess patient/family for barriers to learning. 2. Determine knowledge base and major concerns about surgery. 3. Orient to hospital environment and postoperative routine. 4. Encourage patient/family to verbalize questions, fears, anxieties.	1. Review surgical care pathway with patient and family to include the following: • Preoperative preparation specific to the procedure. • Equipment that will be used postoperatively. • Pain management plan. 2. Provide educational materials about the diagnoses, surgery, and follow-up care. 3. Provide copy of surgical pathway and patient information packet.
Ineffective Breathing Pattern Patient will: • Identify measures to prevent respiratory impairment. • Maintain effective breathing pattern within functional limitations.	1. Obtain history of past or coexisting pulmonary disease, smoking, chemotherapy, or radiation therapy to the head and neck or chest area. 2. Assess pulmonary status at necessary intervals to include rate, depth, character of breathing, presence of dyspnea or cough, and auscultation or breath sounds. 3. Monitor vital signs at necessary intervals. 4. Encourage coughing and deep breathing exercises to reverse atelectasis. 5. Encourage position changes, out-of-bed activities, and progressive ambulation to reduce risk of clots and mobilize secretions. 6. Administer prescribed medications and treatments (e.g., oxygen, suctioning) as indicated to promote gas exchange and evaluate results. 7. Evaluate test results (e.g., ABG, pulse oximetry, chest x-ray) when ordered. 8. Evaluate home care needs and initiate referrals if indicated.	1. Instruct patient on measures to promote respiratory function (e.g., smoking cessation, positioning, coughing, and deep breathing exercises). 2. Instruct patient in the use of prescribed medications and treatments.
Altered Fluid and Electrolyte Balance • Normal fluid balance will be maintained within physiologic limitations. • Early signs and symptoms of fluid and electrolyte imbalance will be recognized and treated.	1. Administer intravenous (IV) fluids as ordered. 2. Maintain intake and output as a guide to fluid status. 3. Assess weights daily. 4. Monitor vital signs at necessary intervals. 5. Evaluate serum electrolytes (K, Na, Cl, CO_2, BUN, CR, Ca) and supplement/restrict as indicated. Mild electrolyte imbalances are common following major surgery. 6. Provide skin care and oral hygiene as appropriate. 7. Assess for signs and symptoms of fluid overload (rales, dependent edema, decreased urine output) or dehydration (tachycardia, dry mucous membranes, loss of skin turgur, decreased urine output). 8. Administer prescribed therapy and evaluate results.	1. Explain rationale for nursing interventions and causes of fluid/electrolyte imbalances.

TABLE 3-6 Standard of Care for the Surgical Patient—cont'd

Patient Problems and Outcomes	Nursing Interventions and Rationales	Patient Education Instructions
Altered Nutrition: Less than Body Requirements		
Patient will:		
• Return to optimal nutritional status. • Demonstrate ability to administer nutritional supplements if needed.	1. Obtain baseline nutritional assessment. 2. Assess weights daily. 3. Assess for bowel sounds and abdominal distention at regular intervals. 4. Advance diet gradually as tolerated. 5. Promote out-of-bed activities and progressive ambulation to encourage return of bowel function. 6. Assess need for nutritional supplementation as indicated. Patients unable to achieve adequate oral intake may be candidates for parenteral or enteral supplementation. 7. Initiate nutritional consult if indicated. 8. Evaluate home care needs and initiate referrals if indicated.	1. Teach patient/caregiver caloric and nutrient requirements. 2. Teach patient/caregiver specific dietary restrictions/ modifications if required.
Pain		
Patient will:		
• Report acceptable pain control.	1. Assess pain at regular intervals to include disruption, location, and intensity (using a pain scale). 2. Administer pain medications. 3. Assess patient response to pain-relief measures and for side effects of medications. 4. Notify physician of inadequate pain control and adjust medications accordingly. 5. Assess for possible oversedation. Overmedication produces respiratory and cardiovascular depression.	1. Explain function of patient-controlled analgesia (PCA) epidural. 2. Teach patient effective strategies for pain control. 3. Before discharge, instruct patient on prescribed pain medications, side effects, and schedule of administration. Clarify misconceptions.
Impaired Tissue Integrity		
• Wound healing is promoted. • Postoperative morbidity is avoided.	1. Identify factors that may predispose the patient to impaired wound healing. 2. Assess incisional sites, wounds, and drains for signs and symptoms of infection at regular intervals. 3. Monitor vital signs at necessary intervals.	1. Teach patient/caregiver: • Signs and symptoms of infection to report. • How to measure temperature and report fever >101.3° F (38.5° C). • Incision and drain care.
Patient/caregiver will: • Demonstrate local wound care techniques as indicated by surgical procedure. • Verbalize signs and symptoms of infection to be reported.	4. Evaluate laboratory and diagnostic studies as ordered. 5. Obtain specimens for culture and sensitivity before the initiation of antibiotics and as needed. 6. Perform regular incision and drain care. 7. Maintain drain patency. 8. Evaluate home care needs and initiate referral if indicated.	

K, potassium; *Na,* sodium; *Cl,* chloride; *CO_2,* carbon dioxide; *BUN,* blood urea nitrogen; *Cr,* creatinine; *Ca,* calcium.

a hollow viscous and a body cavity or the skin. Most surgically related fistulae originate in the urinary or gastrointestinal tracts and ultimately drain onto a skin surface. The vast majority of late fistulae are associated with recurrent cancer. Consequently, a search for new disease should be part of the workup of every patient who develops a fistula. Late fistulae usually begin in an area of necrosis, infection, or inadequate blood supply. Miller and colleagues (1995), in a review of 533 patients who underwent pelvic exenteration for advanced cervical cancer, found that early fistulae were mainly related to infectious complications, and late fistulae were caused by delayed wound healing. Expert surgical

Table 3-7 Potential Postoperative Complications

System	Clinical and Diagnostic Manifestations	Treatments	Prognosis
Pulmonary			
1. Atelectasis	Shortness of breath Cough Fever Tachycardia Rales Abnormal chest x-ray	Coughing and deep breathing Progressive ambulation	Usually responds to treatment
2. Pneumonia (bacterial)	Fever, chills Pleuritic chest pain Productive cough Tachycardia Evidence of consolidation: • Percussion dullness • Bronchial breath sounds, egophany • Rales • Increased vocal fremitus • Shortness of breath Abnormal chest x-ray (infiltrate) Elevated white blood cell (WBC) count, positive blood culture Abnormal sputum gram stain, culture	Antimicrobial therapy Bronchodilators Frappage Intravenous (IV) hydration	Usually responds to treatment Mortality rates high in immunologically compromised host (Polmono et al., 1994)
3. Pulmonary embolism	Anxiety, restlessness Pleuritic chest pain Dyspnea (sudden onset) Respiratory distress Tachycardia, tachypnea Respiratory crackles/wheezing (initial) Diminished breath sounds (±) Abnormal electrocardiogram (ECG) (±) Abnormal chest x-ray Abnormal ventilation-perfusion scan	Anticoagulant therapy Oxygen	Usually responds to treatment High mortality rate associated with large or multiple emboli
4. Pleural effusion	Dyspnea, tachypnea Pleuritic chest pain Dry cough Fever Hypoxia Decreased breath sounds Percussion dullness Decreased vocal fremitus Abnormal chest x-ray	Identify and treat the underlying cause Thoracentesis (severe symptoms) Consider pleurodesis if refractory	Resolves with effective treatment of the underlying cause
5. Pneumothorax	Shortness of breath (sudden onset) Hypoxia Chest pain Diminished breath sounds Resonant percussion Decreased vocal fremitus Decreased respiratory motion on affected side Abnormal chest x-ray	*Small:* No treatment *Symptomatic:* • Chest tube placement • Oxygen	Usually resolves with treatment

TABLE 3-7 Potential Postoperative Complications—cont'd

System	Clinical and Diagnostic Manifestations	Treatments	Prognosis
Pulmonary—cont'd			
6. Adult respiratory distress syndrome (ARDS)	Dyspnea, tachypnea Dry cough Retrosternal discomfort Agitation Cyanosis Bronchial breath sounds Coarse crackles Abnormal chest x-ray Abnormal blood gases (severe hypoxemia)	Determine and treat the underlying disorder *Supportive Therapy* • Mechanical ventilation with positive end expiratory pressure (PEEP) • Vigilance against concomitant infections • Hemodynamic monitoring • Strict fluid control • Frequent monitoring of electrolytes, BUN, creatinine • Enteral nutrition	Mortality 50% to 70% Primary cause of death is multiple organ failure rather than pulmonary dysfunction (Petty, 1994; Varon, 1995)
Cardiovascular			
1. Pulmonary edema/congestive heart failure	Dyspnea, orthopnea, tachypnea Cough Tachycardia S_3 gallop Confusion Unilateral or bilateral crackles Abnormal chest x-ray Abnormal ECG	Diuretics Strict fluid maintenance Monitoring of electrolytes Pharmacologic agents to improve myocardial function, decrease cardiac workload and eliminate fluid congestion (e.g., digoxin, calcium channel blockers)	Usually resolves with treatment
2. Myocardial infarction	Severe, constricting retrosternal pain (onset usually at rest) with radiation to shoulder, arms, neck Anxiety restlessness Diaphoresis Dyspnea Abnormal ECG Elevated cardiac enzymes	*Pharamcologic agents:* • Morphine • Antiarrythmics • Vasodilators Oxygen Rest	Recovery depends on the magnitude of the infarct and preexisting cardiac disease
3. Thromboembolism	Swollen, reddened extremity Localized pain Abnormal Doppler study Abnormal venogram	Anticoagulants Rest Elevation of extremity	Usually resolves with treatment
4. Arrhythmias	Weakness, dizziness Shortness of breath Irregular pulse Hypotension Abnormal ECG	Correct electrolyte imbalance if present Antiarrhythmic agents	Usually resolves with treatment
5. Coagulopathy	Bleeding from wounds and puncture sites, purpura, petecchia *Abnormal coagulation studies:* • Prolonged prothrombin time (PT); partial thromboplastin time (PTT) • Decreased fibrinogen • Decreased platelets • Increased fibrin split products	Determine and treat the underlying cause Replace deficient factors	Resolves if underlying cause is effectively treated

Continued

TABLE 3-7 Potential Postoperative Complications—cont'd

System	Clinical and Diagnostic Manifestations	Treatments	Prognosis Pulmonary
Surgical			
1. Wound infection	Fever Tachycardia Localized redness, swelling, pain, foul smelling or purulent drainage Elevated WBC	Wound culture Antimicrobial therapy Open wound	Resolves with treatment
2. Abscess	Fever Tachycardia Pain Elevated WBC Abnormal CT scan (imaging method of choice)	Culture Antimicrobial therapy Operative or computed tomography (CT) guided percutaneous drainage (Fry, 1994)	Resolves with treatment
3. Ileus	Nausea, vomiting Decreased or absent bowel sounds Abdominal distention, pain Abnormal x-ray	NPO, IV fluids Nasogastric decompression	Resolves with treatment
4. Bowel obstruction	Nausea, vomiting Decreased or absent bowel sounds Abdominal distention Colicky abdominal pain Abnormal x-ray	NPO Parenteral nutrition Nasogastric decompression Operative correction	Resolves with treatment
5. Bleeding from operative site	Anemia Tachycardia Hypotension Clinically evident blood loss	Transfusion Surgical correction	Resolves with treatment
6. Hematoma	Anemia Detectable mass	Transfusion Observation if stable Percutaneous or operative drainage if enlarging or infected	Resolves with treatment
7. Wound separation/dehiscence	Localized (wound) pain Serosanguinous drainage Obvious wound separation	Open wound, localized wound care Surgical repair if fascial separation is present	Usually resolves with treatment
8. Pressure injuries	Absence of skin blanching Obvious skin breakdown on dependent skin surface	Eliminate pressure source (e.g., turning, ambulation) Topical wound care Debridement if necrosis present	Resolves with treatment
9. Malnutrition	Weight loss Muscle wasting Weakness, fatigue Decreased serum albumin and protein	Enteral/parenteral supplementation	Resolves with treatment
10. Fistula (intestinal tract)	Obvious drainage of bowel contents Defect in skin or mucous membrane Localized pain Fever Abnormal radiographic study	*Conservative treatment:* • Parenteral nutrition • Local skin care • Infection control • Ocreotide Surgical correction	Usually effective (65%-75%), but prolonged therapy may be required (Spiliotis et al., 1993)

technique, with recognition and intraoperative repair of tissue injuries, is also imperative to reduce the incidence of fistula.

Localized injuries result in breakdown of the organ wall and release of urine or stool into the adjacent peritoneal cavity. Further inflammatory reactions allow tracking to and breakdown of the connecting skin surface. Typically, this process produces a continuously draining tract or sinus. Because the fistula drainage is an intense irritant, it produces further maceration of adjacent skin.

Most fistulae have a clinically obvious presentation that can be readily confirmed by radiographic dye studies (e.g., barium enema, upper gastrointestinal study, IV pyleogram) and usually occur when there has been an operative repair of the bowel or bladder, followed by radiation therapy to the same area. Fistulae are a serious complication that require aggressive management. Small enteral fistulae in nonradiated tissues may heal with conservative therapy consisting of bowel rest, antibiotic therapy, parenteral nutrition, and local wound care. Somatostatin or octreotide (a somatostatin analog) may be added to the treatment plan because they are effective in reducing fistula output and accelerate spontaneous fistula closure (Kocak, Bumin, Karayalcin, Alacayir, & Aribal, 1994; Spiliotis et al., 1993; Torres-Garcia, Arguello, & Balibrea, 1994). Large fistulae and those associated with radiation require surgical correction. Previous treatment with chemotherapy and poor nutritional status also impede closure. Conservative therapy should precede operative repair to reduce local inflammation and enhance healing.

ETHICAL ISSUES

Many of the ethical issues that apply to an individual patient undergoing surgical treatment are well established. The patient must be given an understandable explanation of the proposed procedure, including the anticipated outcome, potential risks and complications, and alternative treatment options. The patient must then give consent for the procedure. There are special requirements for obtaining consent for patients who are incompetent, minors, or non-English speaking, or those who refuse blood transfusions.

Perhaps the greatest ethical challenge facing our society is providing quality oncologic care to all individuals with cancer. Surgical treatment is a limited and expensive resource. Financial, geographic, and insurance coverage constraints may prevent cancer patients from getting the care that they need. A substantial proportion of Americans are either indigent or uninsured. Although many have the option to obtain medical care at government-financed institutions, the facility may not employ a surgical oncologist. Consequently, the patient may not receive optimal care. Most surgical oncology services are concentrated in large, metropolitan areas. Patients residing in rural areas must overcome considerable obstacles to obtain care at a site distant from their home. While the patient's medical care may be covered by insurance, the patient must bear the financial costs associated with travel and living expenses.

Recent changes in the way medical insurance is approved and provided may prevent some insured patients from receiving the care they wish at a specific facility. Authorization issues have arisen for patients seeking reconstructive, experimental, and palliative operations. In some cases, patients may be limited to a fixed list of physicians or facilities for their care. If they choose to seek care outside their network, they incur a greater financial responsibility.

These issues related to access to care are complex and difficult to resolve on an individual basis. Ideally, every patient with cancer should receive the best possible oncologic care. Patients should be apprised of current standards of care as well as experimental options from which they are able to select the physician and medical facility of their choice. Resolution of these conflicts will require large-scale policy decisions.

FUTURE TRENDS

Much of the current focus of surgical research is aimed at refinement of current standards and techniques. Further improvements in diagnostic and imaging modalities are likely to provide a more accurate assessment of tumor extent and spread before determining a management plan. As a result, the selection of candidates and the design of the operation used for surgical therapy will continue to become more precise. This approach ensures that each patient gets the most appropriate surgery at the time of initial diagnosis. Patients who are not surgical candidates are spared the morbidity of a nontherapeutic resection and can be offered alternative therapy without delay.

New technology and instrumentation will also have a major role in defining future surgical applications. Just as lasers, minimally invasive surgery, and stereotactic radiosurgery moved from experimental programs to standard practice, current investigational technology such as photodynamics and three-dimensional and virtual reality imaging are likely to become a part of routine practice.

Photodynamic therapy (PDT) involves the concentration of a photosensitizer within the tumor followed by exposure of an appropriate wavelength of light. This process causes activation of the sensitizer and selective tissue destruction (Popovic, Kaye, & Hill, 1995). PDT has been used for the palliation of advanced esophageal cancers to relieve dysphagia and prolong survival. Additional current investigational uses for PDT include pleural mesotheliomas and cancers of the gastrointestinal tract, skin, and head and neck (Biel, 1995; Marcon, 1994). Computer imaging techniques such as three-dimensional reconstruction and virtual reality imaging have applications in both surgical training and treatment planning (Satava, 1994). Using virtual reality, surgical trainees have the opportunity to gain expertise before operating on patients (Ota, Loftin, Saito, Lea, & Keller, 1995). Three-dimensional reconstruction has been used to visualize tumor extent and location within organs such as the liver and brain, facilitating preoperative treatment planning (Sawaya, Rambo, Hammoud, & Ligon, 1995; van Leeuwen, Obertop, Hennipman, & Fernandez, 1995). As yet unidentified surgical applications of other new technologies are also likely to be developed.

Because surgical oncology has rapidly expanded as an academic and research-directed specialty, the clinical practice of surgery will continue to be enhanced. These improvements in clinical practice will come from a variety of areas (e.g., anesthesia, surgery, critical care, pharmacology, and nursing) and will ultimately result in more sophisticated tumor resections, wider applications for surgical therapy, greater reconstructive options, and supportive resources that will enhance a patient's quality of life. The impetus for any improvements in standard practice is further reduction in patient mortality and morbidity. A good example of this process can be seen in the surgical treatment of pancreatic cancer, where better patient selection, improved surgical technique, and perioperative support has reduced the mortality rates associated with pancreatoduodenectomy from 20% in 1935 to less than 5% today. The 5-year survival rate after resection has increased from 3.5% to more than 20% in some studies (McGrath et al., 1996).The goal of treatment is to always strive for better patient outcomes. Surgeons will continue to use their knowledge of tumor behavior to design and implement modifications of existing therapies. A surgical technique that illustrates a refined approach to the management of regional lymph nodes is intraoperative lymphatic mapping. Dye injected into the tumor provides a visual map of the unique lymphatic drainage pattern of the tumor. This dye collects in the "sentinel node," providing a precise target for biopsy. Complete lymphatic resection can thus be eliminated in patients whose sentinel node is negative. Originally developed for the treatment of cutaneous melanomas (Morton, Wen, & Cochran, 1992), lymphatic mapping is now being considered for patients with vulvar and breast cancer (Burke et al., 1995; Giuliano et al., 1995).

The care of the oncologic patient will continue to be a collaborative effort involving surgical, medical, and radiotherapeutic modalities. Clinical research involving all specialties will be needed to produce the next generation of adjunctive therapies. This knowledge will further refine the application of surgery in the treatment of cancer.

NURSING RESEARCH

The current trend to develop care pathways for surgical patients and to provide a critical analysis of treatment outcomes offers an unprecedented opportunity for nurses to become involved in clinical research. Many of the key areas of evaluation such as patient satisfaction, symptom management, and quality of life have been strong interests of surgical oncology nurses. Additionally, the multidisciplinary development of comprehensive surgical pathways must directly involve the nurses providing care if successful implementation is to occur.

When viewed from an overall perspective, the surgical experience provides many specific opportunities for nursing research projects. Every surgical procedure has unique patient and family educational requirements. The development, use, and evaluation of educational materials are fertile areas for investigation. Projects might focus on patient comprehension, evaluation of ethnically oriented and multilingual teaching tools, and application of video and computer technology.

Because many of the traditional nursing care practices are being challenged, research studies that evaluate simpler or less expensive alternatives must be performed. This area lends itself to straightforward prospective randomized investigations of nursing care. Specific areas to consider include wound and drain care, the need for and frequency of laboratory studies, postoperative feeding regimens, and the effectiveness of symptom management. Nurses should continuously challenge "routine" practices to ensure that they are research based and contribute to optimum patient care.

Shorter hospitalizations have increased the need for nurses to become involved in the postdischarge monitoring of patients. Telephone contact that reinforces education, answers questions, and verifies an uncomplicated recovery process is a new area of nursing practice. Research designed to evaluate all aspects of the postdischarge process is needed. Posttreatment surveillance protocols have been developed for a number of cancer types. Most involve a streamlined examination and testing schedule that are supplemented by nursing contacts by telephone for symptom evaluation and triage. Evaluation of the success of such programs is yet another excellent research opportunity.

CONCLUSION

Surgery is the oldest treatment for cancer. After the development of the principles of antisepsis and general anesthesia, a host of radical operations were designed to provide the curative resection of malignant disease. Modern surgical oncology has expanded into numerous other applications including diagnosis, staging, cytoreduction, palliation, prophylaxis, and reconstruction. Other factors that influence the choice of surgical treatment include tumor characteristics and location, the condition of the host, and the experience of the operative team. In general, surgical therapy is used in the treatment of localized solid tumors. It is also included as one component of a more complex multimodal treatment plan. Optimal care of the surgical patient requires adequate preoperative preparation, meticulous perioperative care, and careful coordination of postdischarge rehabilitation. Most complications of surgical therapy occur during the perioperative period. Emphasis on prevention and early symptom recognition has dramatically reduced postoperative morbidity. Future trends in surgical oncology are likely to focus on further applications of conservative resection, more intense emphasis on reconstruction and quality of life issues, and the application of new technology.

REFERENCES

Allman, R. M., Laprade, C. A., Noel, L. B., Walker, J. M., Moorer, C. A., Dear, M. R., & Smith, C. R. (1986). Pressure sores among hospitalized patients. *Annals of Internal Medicine, 105,* 337-342.

Barber, G. R., & Brown, A. E. (1993). Surveillance of surgical wound infections in cancer patients. *Cancer Practice, 1,* 72-76.

Barkin, R. L., Lubenow, T. R., Bruehl, S., Husfeldt, B., Ivankovich, O., & Barkin, S. J. (1996). Management of chronic pain. Part I. *Disease-A-Month, 42* (7), 389-454.

Biel, M. A. (1995). Photodynamic therapy of head and neck cancers. *Seminars in Surgical Oncology, 11,* 355-359.

Bostwick, J., III. (1995). Breast reconstruction following mastectomy. *CA-A Cancer Journal for Clinicians, 45*(5), 289-304.

Boysen, P. G. (1993). Perioperative management of the thoracotomy patient. *Clinics in Chest Medicine, 14*(2), 321-333.

Burke, C. C., Zabka, C. L., McCarver, K. J., & Singletary, S. E. (1997). Patient satisfaction with 23-hour "short stay" observation following breast cancer surgery. *Oncology Nursing Forum, 2*(4), 645-651.

Burke, T. W. (1994). Ovarian staging laparotomy. In M. S. Roh, & F. C. Ames (Eds.), *Advanced oncologic surgery.* St Louis: Mosby.

Burke, T. W., Levenback, C., Coleman, R. L., Morris, M., Silva, E. G., & Gershenson, D. M. (1995). Surgical therapy of T1 and T2 vulvar carcinoma: Further experience with radical wide excision and selective inguinal lymphadenectomy. *Gynecologic Oncology, 57,* 215-220.

Burke, T. W., & Morris, M. (1993). Adenocarcinoma of the endometrium. In L. J. Copeland (Ed.), *Textbook of gynecology.* Philadelphia: W. B. Saunders Company.

Chen, M. K., Souba, W. W., & Copeland, E. M. (1991). Nutritional support of the surgical oncology patient. *Hematology/Oncology Clinics of North America, 5,* 125-140.

Clahsen, P. C., van de Velde, C. J., Julien, J. P., Floiras, J. L., Delozier, T., Mignolet, F. Y., & Sahmoud, T. M. (1996). Improved local control and disease-free survival after perioperative chemotherapy for early-stage breast cancer: A European organization for research and treatment of cancer (Breast Cancer Cooperative Group Study. *Journal of Clinical Oncology, 14,* 745-753.

Clarke-Pearson, D. L., Olt, G. J., Rodriguez, G., & Boente, M. (1993). Preoperative and postoperative care. In D. M. Gershenson, A. H. DeCherney, & S. L. Curry (Eds.), *Operative gynecology.* Philadelphia: W. B. Saunders Company.

Coia, L., Hoffman, J., Scher, R., Weese, J., Solin, L., Weiner, L., Eisenberg, B., Paul, A., & Hanks, G. (1994). Preoperative chemoradiation for adenocarcinoma of the pancreas and duodenum. *International Journal of Radiation Oncology, Biology, Physics, 30*(1), 161-167.

Cuschieri, A. (1995). Laparoscopic management of cancer patients. *Journal of the Royal College of Surgeons of Edinburgh, 40*(1), 1-9.

Daly, J. M., Redmond, H. P., & Gallagher, H. (1992). Perioperative nutrition in cancer patients. *Journal of Parenteral and Enteral Nutrition, 16*(Suppl. 6), 100S-105S.

de Leon-Casasola, O. A., Parker, B., Lema, M. J., Harrison, P., & Massey, J. (1994). Postoperative epidural bupivacaine-morphine therapy. Experience with 4,227 surgical cancer patients. *Anesthesiology, 81,* 368-375.

Deppe, G., Malviya, V. K., Boike, G., & Malone, J. M., Jr. (1989). Use of cavitron surgical aspirator for debulking of diaphragmatic metastasis in patients with advanced carcinoma of the ovaries. *Surgery, Gynecology, & Obstetrics, 168,* 455-456.

Derby, S. E. (1991). Ageism in cancer care of the elderly. *Oncology Nursing Forum, 18,* 921-926.

Devine, E. C., & Cook, T. D. (1986). Clinical and cost-saving effects of psychoeducational interventions with surgical patients: A meta-analysis. *Research in Nursing & Health, 9,* 89-105.

De Vita, V. T., Jr., Hellman, S., & Rosenberg, S. A. (Eds.). (1997). *Cancer Statistics, 1996 and Cancer: Principles and practice of oncology* (5th ed.). Philadelphia: Lippincott-Raven Company.

Dixon, J. A. (1988). Current laser applications in general surgery. *Annals of Surgery, 207,* 355-370.

Doak, L. G., Doak, C. C., & Meade, C. D. (1996). Strategies to improve cancer education materials. *Oncology Nursing Forum, 23,* 1305-1312.

Dobell, A. R. C. (1994). The origins of endotracheal ventilation. *Annals of Thoracic Surgery, 58,* 578-584.

Dyck, S. (1991). Surgical instrumentation as a palliative treatment for spinal cord compression. *Oncology Nursing Forum, 18,* 515-521.

Ehrlichman, R. J., Seckel, B. R., Bryan, D. J., & Moschella, C. J. (1991). Common complications of wound healing: Prevention and management. *Surgical Clinics of North America, 71*(6), 1323-1348.

Ewer, M. S., & Ali, M. K. (1990). Surgical treatment of the cancer patient: Preoperative assessment and perioperative medical management. *Journal of Surgical Oncology, 44,* 185-190.

Falcone, R. E., & Nappi, J. F. (1984). Chemotherapy and wound healing. *Surgical Clinics of North America, 64,* 779-790.

Fernandez-del Castillo, C., Rattner, D. W., & Warshaw, A. L. (1995). Further experience with laparoscopy and peritoneal cytology in the staging of pancreatic cancer. *British Journal of Surgery, 82,* 1127-29.

Frei, E., III. (1988). What's in a name: Neoadjuvant. *Journal of the National Cancer Institute, 80,* 1088-1089.

Fry, D. E. (1994). Noninvasive imaging tests in the diagnosis and treatment of intra-abdominal abscesses in the postoperative patient. *Surgical Clinics of North America, 74,* 693-709.

Gage, A. A. (1992). Cryosurgery in the treatment of cancer. *Surgery, Gynecology, & Obstetrics, 174,* 73-92.

Gershenson, D. M. (1993). Epithelial ovarian cancer. In L. J. Copeland (Ed.), *Textbook of gynecology.* Philadelphia: W. B. Saunders Company.

Giuliano, A. E., Dale, P. S., Turner, R. R., Morton, D. L., Evans, S. W., & Krasne, D. L. (1995). Improved axillary staging of breast cancer with sentinel lymphadenectomy. *Annals of Surgery, 222,* 394-399.

Greene, F. L., & Dorsay, D. (1993). Laparoscopic evaluation of abdominal malignancy. *Cancer Practice, 1,* 29-34.

Griffiths, C. T., Parker, L. M., & Fuller, A. F., Jr. (1979). Role of cytoreductive surgical treatment in the management of advanced ovarian cancer. *Cancer Treatment Reports, 63,* 235-240.

Hacker, S. M., Browder, J. F., & Ramos-Caro, F. A. (1993). Basal cell carcinoma: Choosing the best method of treatment for a particular lesion. *Postgraduate Medicine, 93*(8), 101-104, 106-108, 111.

Held, J. L., Osborne, D. M., Volpe, H., & Waldman, A. R. (1994). Cancer of the prostate: Treatment and nursing implications. *Oncology Nursing Forum, 21,* 1517-1529.

Held, J. L., & Peahota, A. (1993). Nursing care of the patient with spinal cord compression. *Oncology Nursing Forum, 20,* 1507-1514.

Hill, G. J., II. (1979). Historic milestones in cancer surgery. *Seminars in Oncology, 6,* 409-426.

Hindle, W. H., Payne, P. A., & Pan, E. Y. (1993). The use of fine-needle aspiration in the evaluation of persistent palpable dominant breast masses. *American Journal of Obstetrics and Gynecology, 168,* 1814-1819.

Homesley. H. D. (1995). Management of vulvar cancer. *Cancer, 76*(Suppl. 10), 2159-2170.

Humble, C. A. (1995). Lymphedema: Incidence, pathophysiology, management, and nursing care. *Oncology Nursing Forum, 22,* 1503-1511.

Hunt, K. K., Feig, B. W., & Ames, F. C. (1995). Ambulatory surgery for breast cancer. *The Cancer Bulletin, 47,* 292-297.

Kane, N. E., Lehman, M. E., Dugger, R., Hansen, L., & Jackson, D. (1988). Use of patient-controlled analgesia in surgical oncology patients. *Oncology Nursing Forum, 15,* 29-32.

Kemp, M. G., Keithley, J. K., Smith, D. W., & Morreale, B. (1990). Factors that contribute to pressure sores in surgical patients. *Research in Nursing and Health, 13,* 293-301.

Ketcham, M., & Loescher, L. (1993). Skin cancers. In S. L. Groenwald, M. H. Frogge, M. Goodman, & C. H. Yarbro (Eds.), *Cancer nursing: Principles and practice* (3rd ed.). Boston: Jones & Bartlett.

Kinsella, T. J., & Sindelar, W. F. (1996). Intraoperative radiotherapy for pancreatic carcinoma: Experimental and clinical studies. *Cancer, 78*(Suppl. 3), 598-604.

Kocak, S., Bumin, C., Karayalcin, K., Alacayir, I., & Aribal, D. (1994). Treatment of external biliary, pancreatic and intestinal fistulas with a somatostatin analog. *Digestive Diseases, 12*(1), 62-68.

Kurtz, R. G., & Ginsberg, R. J. (1997). Endoscopy. In V. T. DeVita, Jr., S. Hellman, & S. A. Rosenberg (Eds.), *Cancer: Principles and practice of oncology* (5th ed.). Philadelphia: Lippincott-Raven Company.

Leaper, D. J. (1995). Risk factors for surgical infection. *Journal of Hospital Infection, 30*(Suppl.), 127-139.

Leaper, D. J. (1994). Prophylactic and therapeutic role of antibiotics in wound care. *American Journal of Surgery, 167*(Suppl.), 15S-19S.

Lehr, P. S. (1989). Surgical lasers: How they work, current applications. *AORN Journal, 50,* 972-977.

Lindley, C. (1994). Overview of current development in patient-controlled analgesia. *Supportive Care in Cancer, 2,* 319-326.

Lowy, A. M., Rich, T. A., Skibber, J. M., Dubrow, R. A., & Curley, S. A. (1996). Preoperative infusional chemoradiation, selective intraoperative radiation, and resection for locally advanced pelvic recurrence of colorectal adenocarcinoma. *Annals of Surgery, 223,* 177-185.

Lubenow, T. R., & Ivankovich, A. D. (1991). Patient-controlled analgesia for postoperative pain. *Critical Care Nursing Clinics of North America, 3,* 35-41.

Ludwig, K. A., Carlson, M. A., & Condon, R. E. (1993). Prophylactic antibiotics in surgery. *Annual Review of Medicine, 44,* 385-393.

Lynch, H. T., Krush, A. J., Thomas, R. J., & Lynch, J. (1976). Cancer family syndromes. In H. T. Lynch (Ed.), *Cancer genetics.* Springfield, IL: Charles C. Thomas.

Mahon, S. M., & Casperson, D. S. (1993). Pathophysiology of hypokalemia in patients with cancer: Implications for nurses. *Oncology Nursing Forum, 20,* 937-946.

Maiwand, M. O., & Homasson, J. P. (1995). Cryotherapy for tracheobronchial disorders. *Clinics in Chest Medicine, 16,* 427-443.

Marcon, N. E. (1994). Photodynamic therapy and cancer of the esophagus. *Seminars in Oncology, 21*(Suppl. 6), 20-23.

McGrath, P. C., Sloan, D. A., & Kenady, D. E. (1996). Surgical management of pancreatic carcinoma. *Seminars in Oncology, 23,* 200-212.

Meade, C. D. (1996). Producing videotapes for cancer education: Methods and examples. *Oncology Nursing Forum, 23,* 837-846.

Miller, B., Morris, M., Gershenson, D. M., Levenback, C. L., & Burke, T. W. (1995). Intestinal fistulae formation following pelvic exenteration: A review of the University of Texas M. D. Anderson Cancer Center experience, 1957-1990. *Gynecologic Oncology, 56,* 207-210.

Morris, M., Levenback, C., Burke, T. W., DeJesus, Y. A., Lucas, K. R., & Gershenson, D. M. (1997). An outcomes management program in gynecologic oncology. *Obstetrics and Gynecology.*

Morton, D. L., Wen, D., & Cochran, A. J. (1992). Management of early-stage melanoma by intraoperative lymphatic mapping and selective lymphadenectomy. *Surgical Clinics of North America, 1*(2), 247-259.

Nichols, R. L., & Holmes, J. W. (1995). Prophylaxis in bowel surgery. *Current Clinical Topics in Infectious Diseases, 15,* 76-96.

O'Donohue, W. J., Jr. (1992). Postoperative pulmonary complications. *Postgraduate Medicine, 91*(3), 167-175.

Onik, G. M., Atkinson, D., Zemel, R., & Weaver, M. L. (1993). Cryosurgery of liver cancer. *Seminars in Surgical Oncology, 9,* 309-317.

Orr, J. W., Jr., Holloway, R. W., & Orr, P. J. (1994). Pulmonary complications. In J. W. Orr, Jr., & H. M. Shingleton (Eds.), *Complications in gynecologic surgery: Prevention, recognition, & management.* Philadelphia: J. B. Lippincott Company.

Ota, D., Loftin, B., Saito, T., Lea, R., & Keller, J. (1995). Virtual reality in surgical education. *Computers in Biology and Medicine, 25*(2), 127-137.

Padberg, R. M., & Padberg, L. F. (1990). Strengthening the effectiveness of patient education: Applying principles of adult education. *Oncology Nursing Forum, 17,* 65-69.

Patterson, W. B. (1989). Surgical issues in geriatric oncology. *Seminars in Oncology, 16,* 57-65.

Petty, T. L. (1994). The acute respiratory distress syndrome: Historic perspective. *Chest, 105*(Suppl.), 44S-47S.

Polomano, R., Weintraub, F. N., & Wurster, A. (1994). Surgical critical care for cancer patients. *Seminars in Oncology Nursing, 10,* 165-176.

Popovic, E. A., Kaye, A. H., & Hill, J. S. (1995). Photodynamic therapy of brain tumors. *Seminars in Surgical Oncology, 11,* 335-345.

Ranjan, A., Rajshekhar, V., Joseph, T., Chandy, M. J., & Chandi, S. M. (1993). Nondiagnostic CT-guided stereotactic biopsies in a series of 407 cases: Influence of CT morphology and operator experience. *Journal of Neurosurgery, 79,* 839-844.

Ratliff, C. R., Gershenson, D. M., Morris, M., Burke, T. W., Levenback, C., Schover, L. R., Mitchell, M. F., Atkinson, E. N., & Wharton, J. T. (1996). Sexual adjustment of patients undergoing gracilis myocutaneous flap vaginal reconstruction in conjunction with pelvic exenteration. *Cancer, 78,* 2229-2235.

Recht, A. (1996). Selection of patients with early stage invasive breast cancer for treatment with conservative surgery and radiation therapy. *Seminars in Oncology, 23*(Suppl. 2), 19-30.

Rosenberg, S. A. (1997). Principles of surgical oncology. In V. T. DeVita, Jr., S. Hellman, & S. A. Rosenberg (Eds.), *Cancer: Principles and practice of oncology* (5th ed.). Philadelphia: Lippincott-Raven Company.

Rutledge, R. H. (1995). Theodor Billroth: A century later. *Surgery, 118,* 36-43.

Satava, R. M. (1994). Emerging medical applications of virtual reality: A surgeon's perspective. *Artificial Intelligence in Medicine, 6,* 281-288.

Sawaya, R., Rambo, W. M., Jr., Hammoud, M. A., & Ligon, B. L. (1995). Advances in surgery for brain tumors. *Neurologic Clinics, 13,* 757-771.

Schabel, F. M., Jr. (1977). Rationale for adjuvant chemotherapy. *Cancer, 39,* 2875-2882.

Schmidt, R. A. (1994). Stereotactic breast tissue biopsy. *CA-A Cancer Journal for Clinicians, 44,* 172-191.

Schmoll, H. J. (1994). Colorectal carcinoma: Current problems and future perspectives. *Annals of Oncology, 5*(Suppl. 3), 115-121.

Sheridan, R. L., Tompkins, R. G., & Burke, J. F. (1994). Prophylactic antibiotics and their role in the prevention of surgical wound infection. *Advances in Surgery, 27,* 43-65.

Silberman, A. W. (1982). Surgical debulking of tumors. *Surgery, Gynecology and Obstetrics, 155,* 577-584.

Smythe, M. (1992). Patient-controlled analgesia: A review. *Pharmacotherapy, 12,* 132-143.

Spiliotis, J., Briand, D., Gouttebel, M. C., Astre, C., Louer, B., Saint-Aubert, B., Kalfarentzos, F., Androulakis, J., & Joyeux, H. (1993). Treatment of fistulas of the gastrointestinal tract with total parenteral nutrition and octreotide in patients with carcinoma. *Surgery, Gynecology, & Obstetrics, 176,* 575-580.

Staerkel, G. A. (1993). Fine needle aspiration: Technique and application in the evaluation of malignancies. *Cancer Bulletin, 45,* 8-12.

Staley, C. A., Lee, J. E., Cleary, K. R., Abbruzzese, J. L., Fenoglio, C. J., Rich, T. A., & Evans, D. B. (1996). Preoperative chemoradiation, pancreaticoduodenectomy, and intraoperative radiation therapy for adenocarcinoma of the pancreatic head. *American Journal of Surgery, 171,* 118-124.

Tang, E., Davis, J., & Silberman, H. (1995). Bowel obstruction in cancer patients. *Archives of Surgery, 130,* 832-836.

Torres-Garcia, A. J., Arguello, J. M., & Balibrea, J. L. (1994). Gastrointestinal fistulas: Pathology and prognosis. *Scandinavian Journal of Gastroenterology, 207* (Suppl.), 39-41.

Ulualp, K., & Condon, R. E. (1992). Antibiotic prophylaxis for scheduled operative procedures. *Infectious Disease Clinics of North America, 6,* 613-625.

Urist, M. M. (1996). Surgical management of primary cutaneous melanoma. *CA-A Cancer Journal for Clinicians, 46,* 217-224.

van Leeuwen, M. S., Obertop, H., Hennipman, A. H., & Fernandez, M. A. (1995). 3-D reconstruction of hepatic neoplasms: A preoperative planning procedure. *Baillieres Clinical Gastroenterology, 9*(1), 121-133.

Varon, J. (1995). Acute respiratory distress syndrome in the postoperative cancer patient. *The Cancer Bulletin, 47,* 38-42.

Watson, D. L., Kantoff, P. W., & Richie, J. P. (1996). Staging and imaging of testis cancer. In N. J Vogelzang, W. U. Shipley, P. T. Scardino, & D. S. Coffey (Eds.), *Comprehensive textbook of genitourinary oncology.* Baltimore: Williams & Wilkins.

Weiser, E. B., Bundy, B. N., Hoskins, W. J., Heller, P. B., Whittington, R. R., DiSaia, P. J., Curry, S. L., Schlaerth, J., & Thigpen, J. T. (1989). Extraperitoneal versus tranperitoneal selective para-aortic lymphadenectomy in the pretreatment surgical staging of advanced cervical carcinoma (A Gynecologic Oncology Group Study). *Gynecologic Oncology, 33,* 283-289.

Westcott, J. L. (1980). Direct percutaneous needle aspiration of localized pulmonary lesions: Results in 422 patients. *Radiology, 137,* 31-35.

Wieder, J., Schmidt, J. D., Casola, G., van Sonnenberg, E., Stainken, B. F., & Parsons, C. L. (1995). Transrectal ultrasound-guided transperineal cryoablation in the treatment of prostate carcinoma: Preliminary results. *Journal of Urology, 154,* 435-441.

Wong, R. J., & DeCosse, J. J. (1990). Cytoreductive surgery. *Surgery, Gynecology, and Obstetrics, 170,* 276-281.

Wretlind, A. (1992). Recollections of pioneers in nutrition: Landmarks in the development of parenteral nutrition. *Journal of the American College of Nutrition, 11(4),* 366-373.

Zerbi, A., Fossati, V., Parolini, D., Carlucci, M., Balzano, G., Bordogna, G., Staudacher, C. & Di Carlo, V. (1994). Intraoperative radiation therapy adjuvant to resection in the treatment of pancreatic cancer. *Cancer, 73,* 2930-2935.

Zippe, C. D. (1995). Cryosurgical ablation for prostate cancer: A current review. *Seminars in Urology, 13,* 148-156.

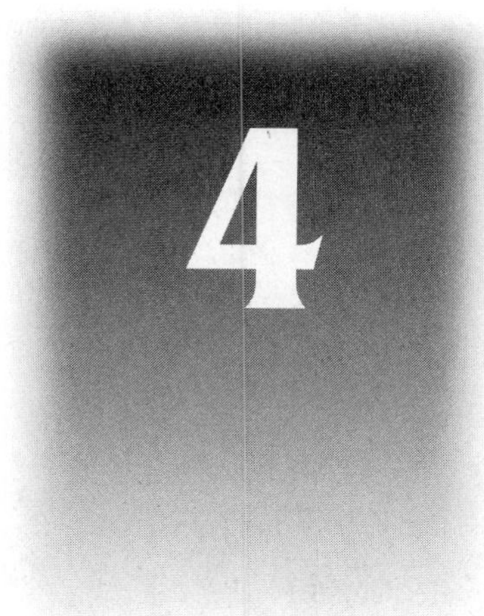

Radiation Therapy

Roberta Anne Strohl, RN, MN, AOCN

INTRODUCTION

Radiation therapy is a local treatment for cancer. It is used throughout the disease trajectory. Recent estimates suggest that 60% of persons with cancer will receive radiation at some point during the course of treatment for their disease. Prophylactic radiation therapy is indicated to prevent development of disease in known high-risk areas such as the delivery of cranial radiation in small cell lung cancer and in adults with leukemia. Palliative radiation therapy provides symptomatic relief of bony pain, bleeding, obstruction, and seizures. Primary therapy is used with curative intent in early stage cervical and prostate cancer, Hodgkin's disease, and head and neck cancer (Perez & Brady, 1992).

Combined modality therapy is the treatment of choice for many individuals. Radiation therapy is given concomitantly or sequentially with chemotherapy to address the local and systemic components of cancer.

Radiation therapy is a frightening modality for persons with cancer to face. The images of radiation as a dangerous commodity associated with war and nuclear accidents confound the therapeutic explanations. The fact that radiation cannot be felt or seen contributes to its mystery. Being alone in a room with thick lead or concrete walls isolates the individual and further vilifies the modality as something extremely powerful. Radiation therapy is often viewed as a modality used only if curative surgery cannot be done. The nurse has the formidable responsibility of clarifying misconceptions by explaining the treatment in terms that patients can understand. Fears of being radioactive are still prevalent and need to be addressed with every patient. Symptom management and patient/family education during therapy are the major components of the nursing role.

HISTORICAL PERSPECTIVE

Radiation therapy is one of the oldest treatments for cancer. Roentgen discovered x-rays in 1895, and the Curies reported the discovery of radium in 1898. The first reported cure using radiation therapy was of a basal cell cancer in 1899. Technologic strategies evolved more rapidly than biologic knowledge. The early history of radiation was a challenging period because the primitive equipment was able to treat superficial cancers but was not adequate to treat deeper lesions. The doses needed to penetrate deeper tissues resulted in unacceptable morbidity (Perez & Brady, 1992).

In 1913, Coolidge developed an x-ray tube with a peak energy of 140 kV, and by 1922, 200 kV x-rays were available for deep therapy. Coutard and Hautant presented a case of advanced laryngeal cancer that was treated successfully without significant sequelae at the International Congress of Paris in 1922. Coutard is also credited with having developed the concept of delivering incremental daily doses or fractions, a strategy that is still the standard of care (Perez & Brady, 1992).

Ionizing radiation became more precise as high-energy protons and electrons became available along with advances in treatment planning and knowledge of radiation biology and physics. The use of computers has produced an exponential growth in the capabilities of treatment and planning systems to deliver more precise and reproducible therapy (Perez & Brady, 1992).

CONCEPTS AND PRINCIPLES OF RADIATION THERAPY

An understanding of the basic principles of radiation physics and biology is necessary to describe the effects of radiation on normal and tumor cells. The atom has a central core, the nucleus, surrounded by orbiting particles known as *electrons.* The dense nucleus is made up of protons and neutrons. In 1913, Niels Bohr proposed a model of a nucleus surrounded by electrons in concentric shells or energy levels. Energy is released when an electron is moved closer to the nucleus, and energy is required to move an electron into a higher orbit (Bomford, Kunkler, & Sherriff, 1993; Purdy, Glasgow, & Lightfoot, 1992).

An electron in an inner shell of an atom is attracted to the nucleus by a force greater than that which the nucleus exerts on an electron in an outer shell. This process means that moving an electron from an inner to an outer shell requires energy and is known as *excitation*. To remove an electron completely from an atom requires energy and is known as *ionization*. The amount of energy that is needed to remove an electron from an atom is known as the *binding energy* of that electron (Bomford et al., 1993).

X-Rays

When energetic electrons impinge on a target and interact with orbital electrons or their nuclei, x-rays are produced. Thermal energy or electromagnetic energy formed from the kinetic energy of electrons results in x-rays by the interaction of incoming electrons with outer shell electrons within the atom. This energy, although not sufficient to result in ionization, creates excited electrons that in time return to normal energy levels, emitting low-energy infrared electromagnetic radiation (Bomford et al., 1993; Purdy et al., 1992).

Radioactivity

Investigations of x-rays resulted in the discovery of radioactivity. Roentgen found that passing electricity through a tube of gas at low pressure caused a paper screen coated with a fluorescent material to glow. In 1896, Henri Becquerel wrapped a photographic plate in black paper to keep out the light and placed various elements on the paper. If elements emitted x-rays, the rays would pass through the paper and blacken the plate. He discovered that the mineral pitch blend did emit x-rays. Elements, such as radium and polonium discovered by the Curies, were also able to emit x-rays (Hall & Cox, 1994; Withers, 1992).

The radioactive elements emitted three types of radiation; α-particles having a positive electrical charge, β-particles having a negative electrical charge, and γ-rays having no electrical charge. It is now known that α-particles are a helium nucleus, β-particles are electrons, and γ-rays are a form of electromagnetic radiation originating from within the nucleus of an atom (Bomford et al., 1993).

X-rays and γ-rays are considered bundles of energy known as *photons*. Before 1951, most radiation treatment units were x-ray machines capable of producing photon beams having only limited penetrability. The first $Cobalt^{60}$ unit was developed in Canada in 1951. $Cobalt^{60}$ is a manufactured radioisotope that emits high-energy γ-rays in sufficient amounts for use in treatment units. In 1953, the first microwave electron linear accelerator for clinical use was commissioned in London (Withers, 1992) (Fig. 4-1).

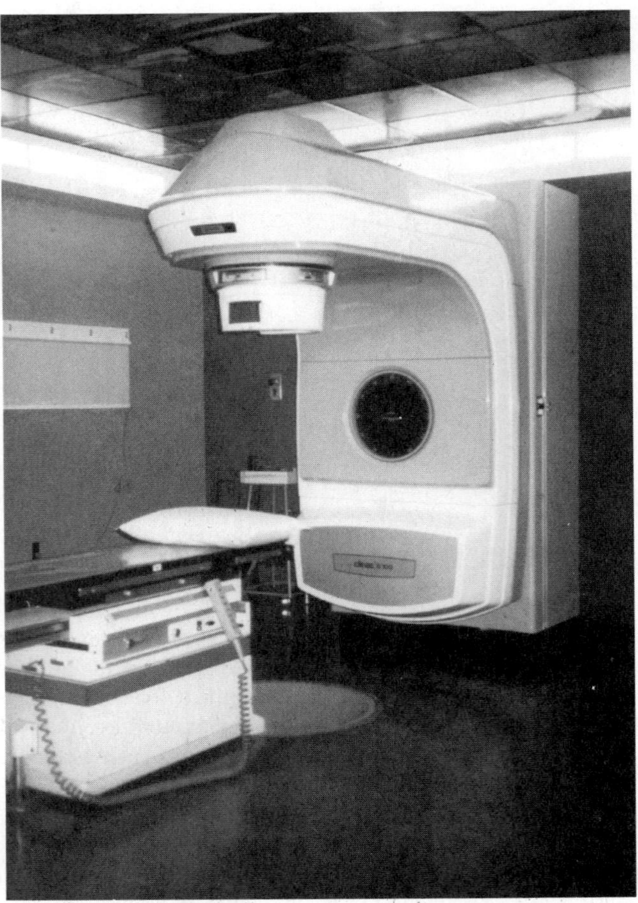

Fig. 4-1 Linear accelerator.

Unlike the Cobalt units, the linear accelerator uses a high-frequency electromagnetic wave to accelerate electrons to high energy through a microwave accelerator structure. The high-energy electron beam can be used to treat superficial lesions, or it can be made to strike a target to produce an x-ray beam for the treatment of deeper tumors. The interaction of x-rays or γ-rays with tissue results in a biologic effect (Withers, 1992).

When x-rays are absorbed in biologic material, a chain of events is initiated. The photon energy creates a fast-moving electron, which with sufficient energy, can completely remove an orbital electron, resulting in ionization. The average energy needed to remove an electron in air is 34 eV, with about 15% to 20% of this energy actually needed for ionization with the rest dissipated as excitation energy. If the ejected electron leaves the atom with 100 eV of kinetic energy, it may cause further ionization and excitation. The biologic effects of radiation are produced by direct and indirect effects, the latter mediated through the production of free radicals. The target of damage within the cell is deoxyribonucleic acid (DNA). Radiation damage results in the breaking of chemical bonds within DNA disrupting the reproductive integrity of the cell. Cellular death is therefore mitotically linked in that the cell dies after it attempts to divide. Cells in G_2/M are the most sensitive to radiation, and those in late S-phase are the most resistant (Hall & Cox, 1994).

Radiochemical lesions in DNA are the result of the direct action of charged particles or the indirect effects of free radicals produced by ionization of cellular water. These radicals are able to diffuse far enough to damage critical targets. A free radical is an atom or molecule that carries an unpaired electron in its outer shell, the most important being the hydroxyl radical (OH). A free radical has a lifetime of about 10 to 15 seconds, and it is estimated that about two thirds of the damage caused by γ-rays or x-rays is the result of the action of free radicals. The component of damage caused by free radicals is amenable to modification by the presence or absence of oxygen or chemical compounds. This mechanism is the impetus for research with radiosensitizers. Direct damage cannot be modified. Oxygen is a potent sensitizer, and hypoxic cells are significantly less sensitive to x-rays (Hall & Cox, 1994).

The structure and function of DNA require that it is loosely bound so that it can separate at an appropriate time for cell division to occur. When cells are irradiated, many single-strand breaks in DNA occur. These breaks may be readily repaired using the opposite strand as a template. A double-strand break in a chromosome is believed to be the most important lesion produced by radiation. A double-strand break is important when, after the break occurs, the chromosome rejoins in an incorrect way. Then, when the cell attempts to divide, the damage produced by radiation is manifested.

The rate at which injury develops is related to the proliferative activity of the tissue. This concept is known as *radiosensitivity*. Actively proliferating tissues manifest evidence of radiation effects in a matter of hours or days. These acutely responding tissues are listed in Box 4-1. Tissues that exhibit damage within weeks to months after irradiation include lung, liver, kidney, heart, spinal cord, and brain. Given sufficient doses of radiation, all tissues will manifest late effects. Tissues that show few acute effects but may evidence late effects include lymphatic vessels, thyroid, pituitary, breast, bone, cartilage, pancreas, uterus, and bile ducts (Hall & Cox, 1994; Withers, 1992).

Malignant cells differ little from normal tissues in their response to ionizing radiation. Tumors are able to undergo repair of sublethal damage if sufficient time is permitted between doses. Tumor cells that are hypoxic are not sensitive to radiation. However, inherent sensitivity of tumor cells to radiation seems to exist. The rapidly proliferating cells within a tumor show an early response. Other factors that contribute to sensitivity include the tumor's hypoxic fraction and vascularity (Withers, 1992).

Not all cells within a tumor are proliferating. The fraction of cells within a tumor that are detected to be in cycle is called the *growth fraction*. The growth fraction of solid tumors is estimated to be about 20%. Solid tumors grow at a slower rate as they enlarge. These slower-growing cells are, unlike normal cells, able to reoxygenate after exposure to radiation. The fractionated approach in radiation therapy addresses the concepts of repair, repopulation, and reoxygenation. Daily fractions are more likely to kill a larger number of tumor cells than is a single dose (Fajardo, 1994; Withers, 1992).

Dividing the total radiation dose into a number of fractions spares normal tissues because of the repair of sublethal damage between doses and the repopulation of normal cells. Tumor cells reoxygenate between fractions, and this process increases their sensitivity to radiation. Allowing too much time between treatments can alter a patient's outcome. Therefore, nurses need to spend a great deal of time and effort to explain to patients and families why radiation treatments cannot be missed on a routine basis. Future trends in radiation therapy, discussed later in this chapter, include the use of alterations in fraction schedules as a means of increasing cell kill in resistant tumors (Peters, Ang, & Thames, 1992).

Box 4-1
Tissues that Respond Acutely* to the Effects of Radiation Therapy

- Bone marrow
- Ovary
- Testis
- Lymph nodes
- Salivary glands
- Small bowel
- Stomach
- Colon
- Oral mucosa
- Esophagus
- Arterioles
- Skin
- Bladder
- Capillaries
- Vagina

*Respond within a matter of hours or days

As the number of surviving clonogenic cells decreases with increasing doses of radiation, the probability of tumor control increases. The probability of tumor control must be balanced against the risk of damage to normal tissues in the treatment field. For each normal cell type, there is information about the total radiation dose that can be given without causing irreversible damage. Information also exists about the standard dose needed to treat tumors. These issues are discussed in the complex treatment planning process. The result is a plan of care that allows for an effective dose within the tolerable range for the surrounding normal structures (Hall & Cox, 1994; Peters, Ang, & Thames, 1992).

DISEASES TREATED WITH RADIATION THERAPY

Radiation therapy plays an important role in the treatment of many cancers. As it is a local treatment, it remains a primary therapy for most solid tumors with the exception of colorectal cancer that remains a surgical disease. It is beyond the scope of this chapter to describe all of the cancers treated with radiation therapy. However, the role of radiation in the treatment of the most common cancers is discussed in the next section of this chapter.

Skin Cancer (Nonmelanoma)

Skin cancer is the most common cancer, with 500,000 new cases estimated to occur each year. Basal cell and squamous cell cancers make up about 95% of all skin cancers. For most skin lesions, surgical excision or radiation therapy is curative. Factors to be considered in the selection of therapy include the size and anatomic location of the lesion,

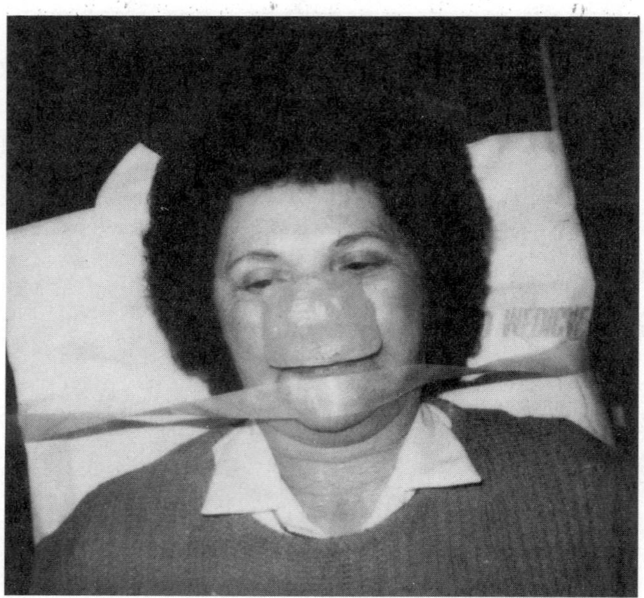

Fig. 4-2 Treatment setup for skin cancer.

involvement of cartilage or bone, depth of invasion, grade of the lesion, and previous treatment modalities. As mentioned previously, the first reported cure using radiation therapy was of a skin cancer in 1899. Tumor control is related to the size of the lesion. With lesions less than 1 cm, control is 97% (Fig. 4-2). Skin cancers are treated with superficial x-rays or electron beam therapy (Shimm & Cassady, 1994; Solan, Brady, Binnick, & Fitzpatrick, 1992).

Lung Cancer

Patients with stages I and II non-small–cell lung cancer are treated primarily with surgery. The remainder of patients are considered inoperable and usually are treated with radiation therapy despite poor 5-year survival rates (i.e., 5% at 5 years RTOG*). Recent clinical trials have added chemotherapy (i.e., vinblastine and cisplatin) to the radiation therapy regimen in an attempt to reduce the incidence of metastatic disease. Failure to control the disease is usually related to the large size of the tumor at the time of diagnosis. Advances in treatment planning, such as three-dimensional planning that allows for sophisticated spatial views of the tumor, are being used with the belief that more accurate coverage of the tumor volume may contribute to better local control.

Due to high incidence of metastatic disease at diagnosis, small cell lung cancer is primarily treated with chemotherapy. Radiation therapy may be given to consolidate response in the chest. Radiation therapy may also be given prophylactically to prevent cranial disease (Sause & Turrisi, 1996).

Prostate Cancer

An estimated 184,500 new cases of prostate cancer were diagnosed in 1998. Radiation therapy plays a major role in the management of prostate cancer. Stage A1 disease may be treated with radiation. In stage A2 or B prostate cancer, tumors may be treated with radical prostatectomy, with interstitial radiation, or with external beam radiation. Stage C tumors may be treated primarily with external beam radiation with or without hormonal manipulation. Stage D disease is managed primarily with hormones with radiation therapy used to palliate bony metastases or local growth. Five-year disease-free survival for patients with disease localized to the prostate is 60% to 75% at 10 years. With extracapsular extension, 5-year survival ranges from 30% to 50% at 10 years (Hanks, 1994; Perez, 1992).

Breast Cancer

Radiation therapy plays a major role throughout the treatment of breast cancer. In early stage disease, primary radiation following lumpectomy has proven to be an effective treatment for lesions less than 5 cm (Fig. 4-3). Veronesi reported on 701 patients with tumors less than 2 cm, who were randomized to receive either quadrantectomy and axillary dissection plus irradiation (5000 cGy in 5 weeks plus 1000 cGy boost) or a radical mastectomy. All of the women with positive lymph nodes received chemotherapy. The actuarial and disease-free survival rates were comparable in both groups. Fisher and the National Surgical Adjuvant Breast Project (NSABP) published similar results (Perez, Garcia, Kuske, & Levitt, 1992).

Radiation therapy may also be useful in the management of chest wall recurrence following mastectomy and with inoperable disease. Palliative radiation is beneficial for the relief of bone pain and in the management of brain metastases (Monyak & Levitt, 1992).

Benign Diseases

In its early history, radiation therapy was used for a number of benign conditions. As knowledge grew about the sequelae of treatment in normal tissue, this practice decreased. However, a number of benign diseases are treated with radiation therapy. The risks versus benefits are always considerations when planning radiation treatments. When treating nonmalignant disease with radiation therapy, the benefit must far outweigh the risk, and other treatment options must be explored (Hoppe & Strober, 1992).

The immunosuppressive effect of radiation has been used in the treatment of a number of diseases. Post-transplant organs have been treated with radiation in an attempt to prevent rejection. Patients have been treated prior to transplantation to a dose of 2000 cGy. Autoimmune diseases that cause significant morbidity have also undergone trials of radiation therapy. Rheumatoid arthritis has been treated to doses of 2000 cGy with relief of morning stiffness, joint tenderness, and joint swelling within 3 months after treatment. Multiple sclerosis has also undergone clinical trials with total lymphoid irradiation showing a decrease in functional decline. The relative risk of immunosuppression and the actuarial risk of each complication must be carefully measured in further research studies (Hoppe & Strober, 1992).

*Radiation Therapy Oncology Group

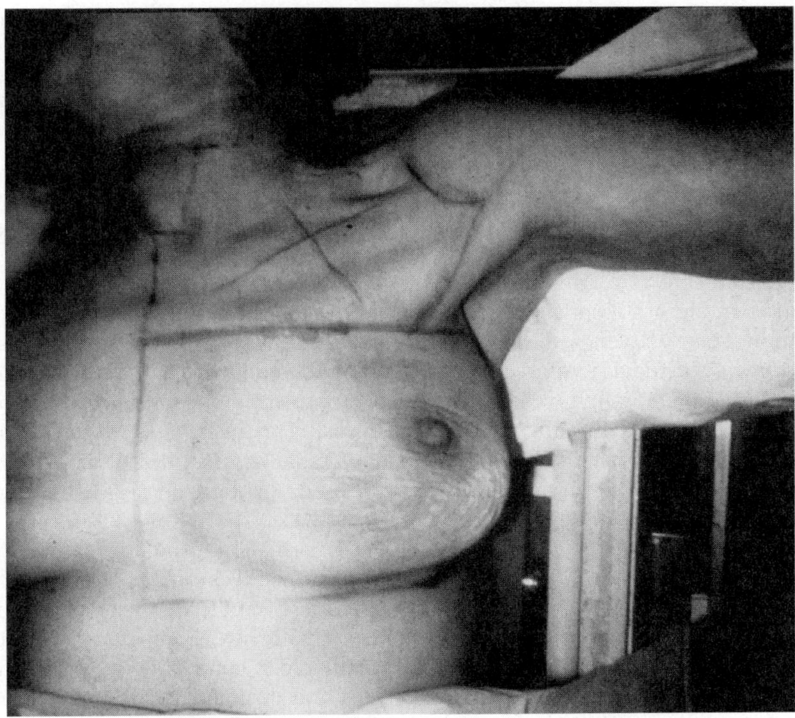

Fig. 4-3 Treatment setup for breast cancer.

THE TREATMENT PROCESS

Radiation therapy may be delivered in several ways. Most commonly patients receive external beam therapy using a linear accelerator. The treatment planning process begins with an initial consultation. In most settings, the radiation oncologist is not a primary care provider and is consulted after a cancer diagnosis has been made. Increasingly, the initial consultation may be done in the framework of an oncology clinic where a multidisciplinary approach is used to plan the patient's treatment. It is advantageous to discuss the treatment plan before any therapy is given to allow the patient to have input into the decision-making process. Radiation therapy is often given in combination with other modalities. How different modalities should be combined is the subject of intense study and debate. There are advantages and disadvantages to each approach that must be described and evaluated before a plan of care is developed. Ongoing Phase III clinical trials are exploring optimal treatment schedules (Purdy et al., 1992).

Radiation Therapy and Surgery

Radiation may be delivered either preoperatively or postoperatively in an attempt to improve local control. Preoperative radiation therapy has the advantage of increasing the tumor's resectability, eliminating potential seeding of tumor, destroying cells beyond the tumor margin, treating a well-oxygenated field, and allowing for a smaller field as the operative bed has not been contaminated. Disadvantages of preoperative radiation include delay in treatment, inability to tailor radiation to high-risk sites identified at the time of surgery, delay in wound healing, limitation of radiation dose because of surgery, and the pathologic down staging of a tumor (Sause, 1994).

Postoperative radiation therapy may be viewed as advantageous because the extent of disease is known, and treatment can be planned using that information. The surgical wound will be intact, and operative margins may be identified more easily. Difficult surgical procedures such as ileal conduits and tenuous anastomoses can be done in a nonirradiated field. Disadvantages of postoperative radiation include delay of treatment by poor wound healing or surgical complications, poor oxygen supply to the tumor because of the surgical intervention, increase in the volume of tissue that must be irradiated as the entire operative bed is included in the treatment field, and a potential for increased injury in tissues such as small bowel that may be fixed after surgery. Clearly, clinical trials are necessary to determine the optimal sequence of surgery and radiation therapy for different types of cancers (Sause, 1994).

Radiation Therapy and Chemotherapy

The timing and sequence of multimodal therapy consist of three approaches: sequential therapy, concurrent therapy, or alternating therapy. In sequential therapy, when chemotherapy is followed by radiation therapy, the smaller volume of tumor allows for a smaller treatment field thereby protecting more of the normal tissue. When radiation therapy precedes chemotherapy, the proliferating component of the tumor is destroyed and quiescent tumor cells may be recruited into cycle, making them more sensitive to the subsequent chemotherapy (Turrisi, 1994). Concurrent therapy allows the simultaneous action of each modality. An enhancement of the tumor's response implies that chemotherapy can make radiation therapy more effective or that irradiation can make cells more responsive to chemotherapy. Simultaneous therapy allows for local and metastatic sites to be treated at the same time. The toxic effects of simultaneous therapy require careful consideration especially if similar normal tissue toxicities are anticipated. The goal is to combine drugs with a variety of side effects that are not identical to those effects expected with radiation therapy. Even with this type of planning, concurrent therapy is a difficult journey for the patient (Turrisi, 1994). Alternating therapy involves the use of radiation therapy and chemotherapy in alternating cycles. This approach allows for the timely delivery of radiation and chemotherapy, reduced treatment toxicities, and improved adherence.

Treatment Planning

During the initial consultation, the physician assesses the patient's clinical condition. The stage and extent of disease are evaluated, and additional diagnostic tests are scheduled if needed. Physical examination evaluates the patient's condition before initiation of therapy. The nurse participates in this evaluation to ascertain what resources will be needed to assist patients to tolerate the proposed therapy. If patients require nutritional support, it is best to begin the therapy before radiation treatments start (Perez & Brady, 1992).

The initial step in the treatment planning process is the simulation. The treatment prescription is based on an evaluation of the full extent of the tumor, a knowledge of the patterns of spread of the cancer, a definition of the goals of therapy (i.e., curative or palliative), the selection of the modalities to be used, and an ongoing evaluation of the patient (Bomford et al., 1993; Purdy et al., 1992).

At the time of the simulation, a film is taken to identify the treatment volume (Fig. 4-4). Sensitive structures within the treatment field are identified. The goal of the simulation is to determine a set-up that can be reproduced on a daily basis. Treatment aids such as shielding blocks, molds, masks, and immobilization devices are used to maintain the desired position and protect normal structures (Bomford et al., 1993).

Information from the simulation including tumor volume, sensitive critical structures, and patient contact are used to compute the beams that will be used for the radiation treatments. Computed tomography (CT) scans are often available to contribute to the treatment planning. The physicist and dosimetrist will develop alternate treatment plans. The physician will select the plan that achieves the goal of delivering an adequate dose to the target volume and an acceptable dose to critical structures (Bomford et al., 1993; Purdy et al., 1992).

The patient will have a film taken on the treatment unit before the delivery of the first dose of radiation (Fig. 4-5). This portal film ensures that the treatment is being given as planned. These films are repeated at least weekly during treatment. Physicians examine patients who are receiving

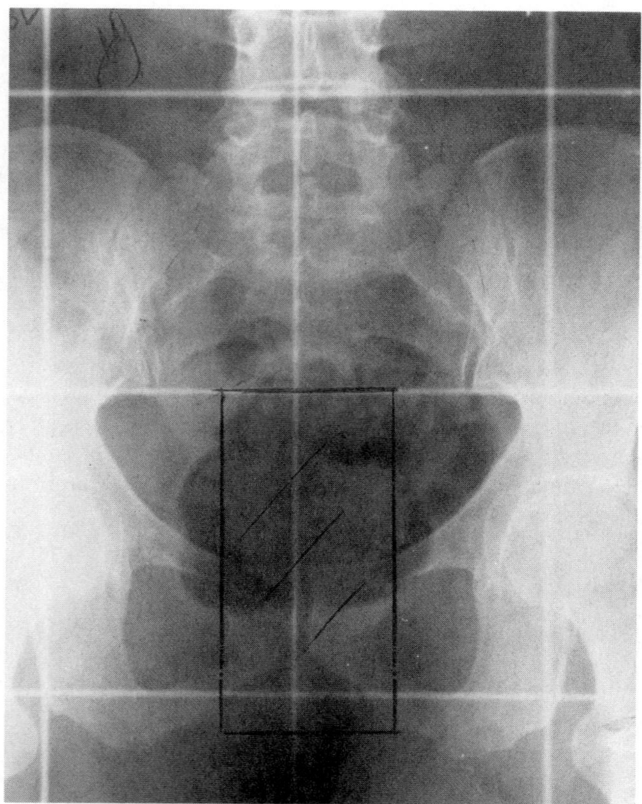

Fig. 4-4 Simulation film.

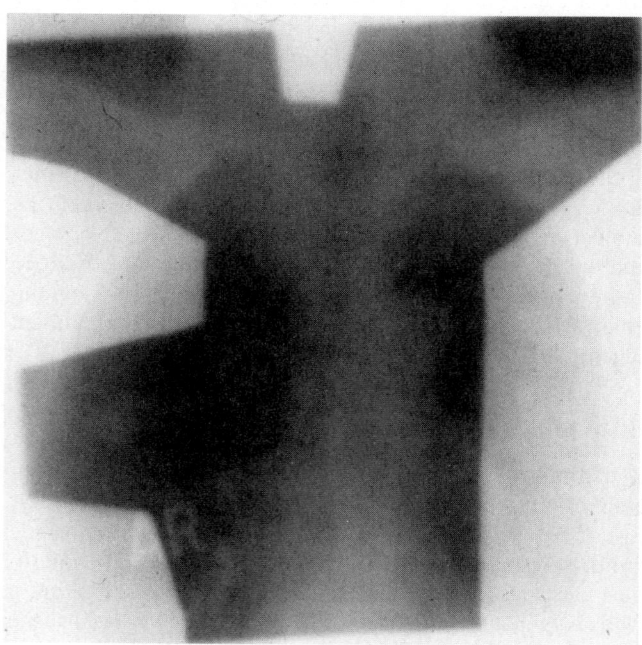

Fig. 4-5 Portal film.

treatment weekly to assess the response of the tumor and the response of normal tissues. At the completion of therapy, patients are given a follow-up appointment to return usually in 2 to 4 weeks. As radiation continues to work even after therapy is completed, it is usually not until the first follow-up visit that repeated scans are planned (Bomford et al., 1993; Purdy et al., 1992).

Nursing Management of Patients Receiving External Beam Radiation Therapy

The nurse meets the patient at the time of initial consultation. The initial nursing assessment is an opportunity to meet with the patient and family and/or significant other and prepare them for the journey through treatment. Information about the disease, prognosis, and treatment plan is clarified. What is the treatment plan? Do the family members and the patient understand the goals of treatment? Patients and families may view any therapy as curative, and, although it is critical to offer a focus of hope, the aims of treatment must be clarified. What has the family's cancer experience been like? Do they know anyone who received radiation therapy? The personal experience with cancer is a powerful teacher. If the experience was difficult, patients may be skeptical when they are given positive views or assured that symptoms can be managed. Radiotherapy is a difficult modality for the public to understand, and considerable time should be spent explaining the treatment.

Once treatment begins, the nurse assesses the patient at least once a week. If patients have had surgery before radiation therapy, they may need to be seen daily to assess their surgical wound. Individuals with new tracheostomies require suctioning before and after daily therapy as well as repeated instructions in suctioning techniques. Most patients are anxious when approaching the start of therapy. Anxiety that does not abate after a week or so of therapy, may require intervention by a social worker or psychiatrist. Patients are often depressed at the time of diagnosis, and the nurse should assess for depressive symptoms that require intervention. Each week, the nurse should assess for the side effects of radiation therapy and prepare the patient for the reactions that may occur during the next week. Teaching the patient and their family members about the treatment is an ongoing process. Patients may need encouragement to continue therapy as the side effects escalate. As most radiation therapy departments function as outpatient clinics, it is imperative that patients and family members know how to access care in the evenings and on weekends. Home care referrals are a critical part of the treatment plan to assist patients to manage ongoing symptoms. Individuals receiving combined modality treatments are monitored closely, as side effects may occur earlier and are usually more severe. Persons with malignancies related to acquired immunodeficiency syndrome (AIDS) should be assessed daily, as reactions occur earlier than anticipated and are often quite severe (Hughes-Davies, Young, & Spittle, 1991). The very young and the very old need special attention because side effects can occur earlier and may be more debilitating to them.

Helping parents prepare children for radiation treatment is a challenging nursing role. The necessary confinement in a treatment device and the fact that parents cannot be in the room with the child makes this experience extremely difficult. Children learn that the treatment does not hurt and is over quickly. Sedation may be necessary, but in our experience, casting and support by child life therapists have limited its use. Using behavior modification techniques and rewarding children with tokens such as stickers may assist them to cope better with the therapy. Parents may talk to the child during treatment, and a favorite toy may be brought into the treatment room. It has been our experience that children who initially feared the cast often want to take it home with them to show their family members and friends at the completion of therapy (Bucholtz, 1994).

As treatment ends, the nurse meets with the patient and family members to discuss follow-up care. The role of additional therapy is described. Late effects are reviewed. The concept that radiation damage occurs as cells divide and therefore continues after treatment ends is discussed. Patients often interpret this explanation as meaning that the "radiation is still in me." Fears of radioactivity often are voiced at this visit. Signs and symptoms that should be brought to the attention of the health care team are reviewed.

Follow-Up Care

The nurse will continue to see patients during follow-up care. Side effects are monitored on an ongoing basis. Coping with having cancer and having received radiation is an ongoing process for patients. Individuals treated as children continue to cope with the changes that radiation therapy may have caused as they develop and grow. Issues, such as infertility, that were not important at age 9 become a significant issue in adolescence and young adulthood. The nurse must be sensitive to the issues of survivorship and provide an ongoing opportunity for patients and family members to discuss their concerns.

If patients develop recurrent disease, the nurse helps patients and family members understand the goals of the proposed palliative care. In an academic setting, the nurse may be the consistent care provider and patients and family members often seek solace in an individual they have known, in some cases, for many years. The nurse plays a role in helping the other members of the health care team, especially the therapists, cope with the retreatment of a patient they have known.

Throughout the experience of receiving radiation therapy, the nurse helps patients understand the treatment and anticipate the reactions that will occur. Knowing what to expect and how to manage the sequelae of treatment as they evolve may help patients to decrease the anxiety and fear of receiving radiation therapy.

Brachytherapy

In addition to external beam treatment, brachytherapy, or close therapy is a delivery system that provides high doses of radiation to a limited volume of tissue. The goal of brachytherapy is to maximize the dose of radiation delivered to the tumor while sparing normal tissue by using radioactive material that only penetrates a short distance (Glasgow & Perez, 1992; Perez, Garcia, Grigsby, & Williamson, 1992).

Brachytherapy began in 1901 when Pierre Curie loaned a physician a small quantity of radium that was used in surface applicators to treat skin lesions. Reguad concluded that this type of therapy, extended over several days with low intensity sources, was an effective regimen for the treatment of cervical cancer (Perez et al., 1992).

Computers have enhanced the ability of clinicians to precisely calculate dose distributions. The most common use of brachytherapy is in conjunction with external beam treatment. External beam therapy encompasses a larger volume of tissue including the tumor and the draining lymph nodes. Application of brachytherapy allows for further administration of radiation to a small treatment volume and spares the previously treated normal tissue. It is useful in those cancers where a high local dose is needed but cannot be tolerated by the surrounding normal structures such as in cancers of the cervix, endometrium, and head and neck regions (Bomford et al., 1993; Perez et al., 1992) (Fig. 4-6).

Brachytherapy uses sealed sources of radioactive material. Patients are radioactive during the time that the source is within them. Because the source is sealed, their *body fluids are not radioactive.* Sources may be temporary or permanent. Permanent sources are used for prostate implants (Figs. 4-7 and 4-8). The permanent source is one with a short half-life, usually iodine-125, whose half-life is 60 days. The fact that the half-life is short and that the seeds are implanted in the deeply seated prostate tissues limits concern for exposure. Temporary sources vary in their half-life. The original source, radium-226, has a half-life of 1640 years. Radium was an energetic source that made protection difficult, and it has largely been replaced by cesium-137. It has a lower photon energy that requires less protection (Bomford et al., 1993; Perez et al., 1992).

The process used today to deliver temporary brachytherapy is a technique known as *afterloading.* The patient is sent to the operating room and, under anesthesia, has a device implanted that holds the radioactive material. After simulation, at which time films are taken to verify the accuracy of device placement, the patient returns to her room where the source is loaded. This procedure eliminates exposure of personnel in the operating room, recovery room, and radiation therapy department. It also provides a safety measure, allowing removal of the source if the patient's condition deteriorates to the point where staff feel uncomfortable with the amount of time they are spending in the room. After the source is removed, the patient is no longer radioactive. If the patient's condition improves, the source can be reinserted (Bomford et al., 1993; Perez et al., 1992).

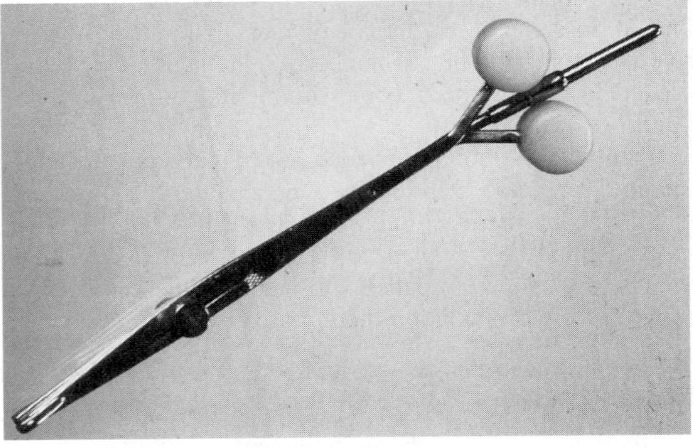

Fig. 4-6 Fletcher-suit brachytherapy device.

Low-dose brachytherapy is usually administered over 2 to 3 days. For head and neck cancers, hollow-tubes are inserted for a single application. In gynecologic cancers, two to three implants are planned. Permanent seeds are most commonly used in prostate cancer. These seeds are placed under ultrasound guidance using a template to assist in the placement of the seeds. The ultrasound verification allows the physician to ensure that an adequate volume of tissue has been implanted (Bomford et al., 1993.)

Another method to deliver implant therapy is the use of a remote control afterloading technique (Fig. 4-9). With this technique, the radioactive material is contained in a separate unit. The patient has an applicator or catheter inserted and simulation films are taken. The patient is then placed in a room and connected to a high-dose rate machine, and a radioactive source travels from the machine into the patient, remains for a period of time, and is returned to the treatment unit. Therefore, the patient is only radioactive when the source is within him. Applicators may be removed after each treatment for weekly therapy. In patients with soft tissue sarcomas, catheters are left in place between treatments. Safety precautions are not necessary, as the patient is not radioactive when returning to their hospital room (Perez et al., 1992.)

Nursing Management of Patients Receiving Brachytherapy

The patient receiving brachytherapy is often frightened by the thought of being radioactive. The necessary confinement and isolation further mystify this procedure. All of the nurses involved in the care of these patients must be knowledgeable about the procedure and related safety issues. Patients must be reassured that they can and will receive skilled and competent care. In this era of agency nurses and unlicensed personnel, the nurse in the radiation therapy department plays a critical role in providing ongoing education to the nurses who will care for implant patients. The radiation therapy nurse also has a role in supporting the decision of inpatient nurses to request source removal if a patient's condition warrants. Careful selection of patients for implants eliminates most of the difficulties encountered during treatment. Nurses and physicians should discuss concurrent medical problems that may contribute to difficulties during brachytherapy. Patients who are confused may not be candidates for brachytherapy unless the treatment can be given safely.

Radioisotopes

With isotope therapy, unsealed sources of radiation are given to the patient. Because the sources are unsealed, body fluids become contaminated. If necessary, patients are hospitalized during the time of greatest activity. Sources with short half-lives are used. The most commonly used source is iodine-131. As iodine is selectively concentrated in the thyroid, it is useful in the management of primary and metastatic thyroid cancer. Iodine-131 had a half-life of 8.06 days. Recently, strontium-89 (half-life, 50.5 days) has been administered for the palliation of bone pain related to metastatic prostate and breast cancer. Phosphorous-32 with a half-life of 14.3 days has been used intravenously in the management of polycythemia vera and intraperitoneally in the management of ovarian cancer (Perez & Brady, 1992).

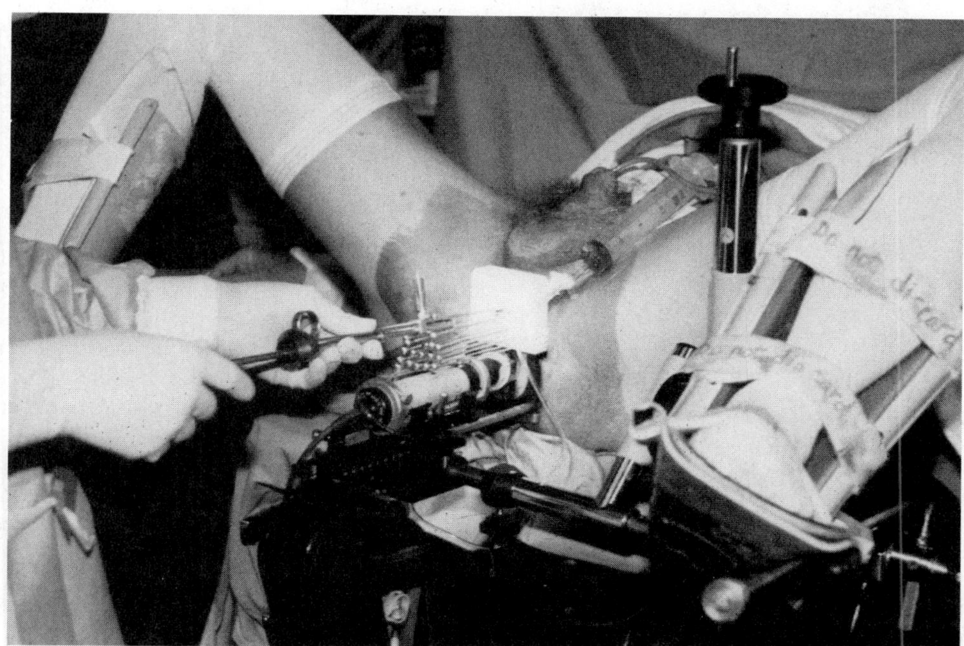

Fig. 4-7 Prostate implant.

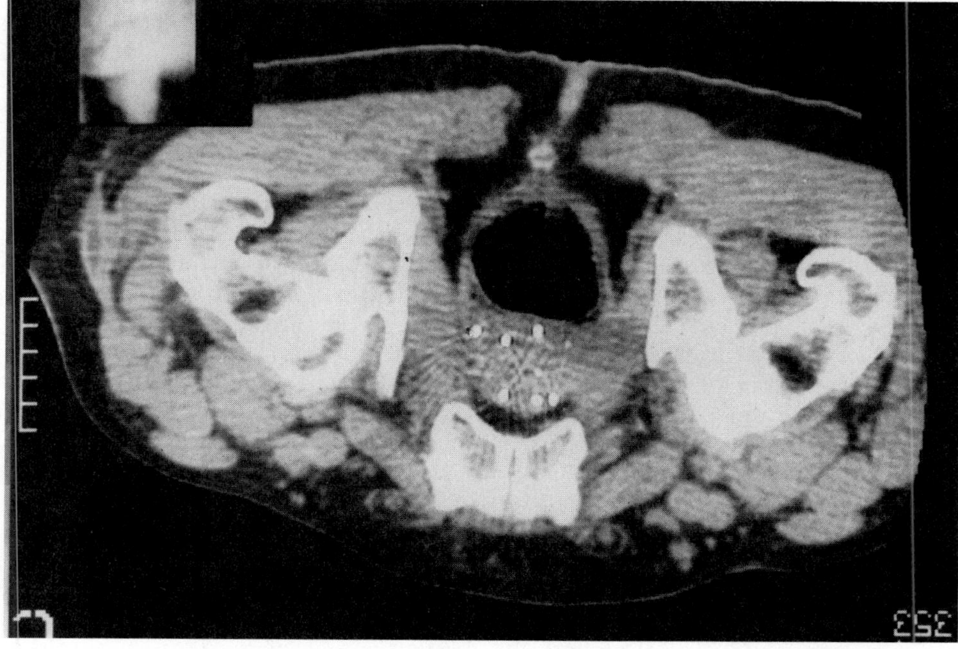

Fig. 4-8 Prostate implant.

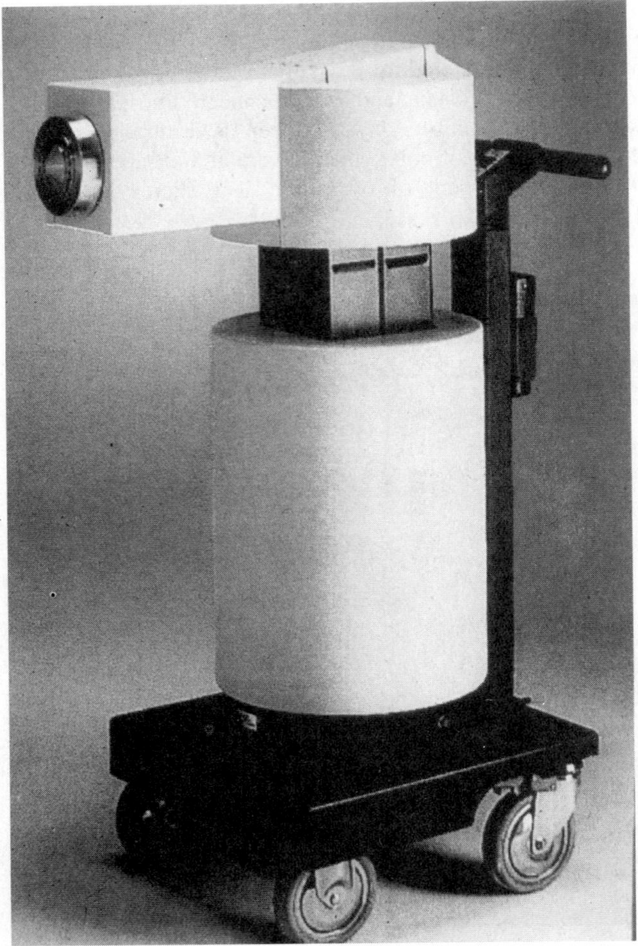

Fig. 4-9 High-dose remote applicator.

Radiation Safety

The nurse caring for a patient receiving brachytherapy needs to be knowledgeable about the type of implant and the source being used. Knowing if the source is sealed or not sealed is essential because this factor determines whether the patient's body fluids are radioactive. The key principle is to safeguard the personnel caring for the patient while providing quality care. Patients must never feel that they are abandoned or so dangerous to be near that care will not be available.

Every institution has a Radiation Safety officer who monitors radioactive substances and their use. This individual collects and distributes film badges that are used to monitor staff exposure. Concerns about the safety of caring for a brachytherapy patient can be addressed to this individual as well as to the radiation oncology nurse and physician. The three components of nursing care that provide protection are time, distance, and shielding.

Time. The total exposure received is related to the amount of time spent at specific distances from the source. Nurses need to determine what care is to be given so that, once in the room, care can be delivered efficiently. The time spent closest to the source should be limited. During this time, nurses should refrain from lengthy discussions about the patient's cancer experience. A sign on the door indicates the amount of time a person can spend at designated distances from the source. Implants are generally kept in place for 2 to 3 days. Patients should come to the experience prepared for the fact that staff will not be spending excessive amounts of time in the room.

Distance. The amount of exposure decreases as the distance from the source increases. Care should be given from a place as far from the source as possible. If the source is on one side (e.g., head and neck implants or breast implants), any intravenous infusions or monitors should be placed on the opposite side of the patient. Exposure decreases according to the inverse square law. Going from 2 feet from the source to 4 feet decreases the exposure by 25% (2 times the distance squared = 4, the inverse is ¼ or 25%) (Hilderly, 1993).

Shielding. Placing a shield made of absorbing material between the source and the caregiver also decreases exposure. If shielding is available, care that can be given from behind the shield should be delivered in that manner. One can talk to a patient from behind a shield. Direct care is usually not easily given from that vantage point. Careful patient selection eliminates most of the crises that occur during brachytherapy procedures. Unstable, confused, and combative patients must have appropriate evaluations by medical and psychiatric consults to assess whether any concomitant conditions can be managed during the implant. High-dose–rate remote therapy may be a useful alternative approach if clinically feasible. The nurse plays a critical role in patient assessment and must be comfortable expressing any concerns or reservations about the appropriateness of the proposed therapy.

ACUTE COMPLICATIONS ASSOCIATED WITH RADIATION TREATMENT

As radiation is a local treatment, the anticipated side effects are related to the site treated and the total dose given to the patient. The most common acute complications associated with radiation therapy are listed in Box 4-2.

Fatigue

Fatigue is a significant systemic effect associated with radiation therapy. In one study, 93% of patients with lung cancer, 68% of patients with head and neck cancer, 65% of patients with prostate cancer, and 72% of patients with gynecologic cancer reported fatigue (King, Nail, Kreamer, Strohl, & Johnson, 1985). Numerous factors can contribute to the development of fatigue in patients with cancer. Tumor burden, stress of treatment, hospitalization, psychosocial factors, nutritional changes, and side effects of therapy all contribute to fatigue (Nail & Winningham, 1993).

Oral Cavity Problems

The mucous membranes of the upper aerodigestive tract are sensitive to radiation. The fact that most cancers of the oral cavity are squamous cell carcinomas requiring a significant dose of radiation creates an environment in which side effects are anticipated (Fig. 4-10). In the setting of T3 and T4

Box 4-2
Common Acute Complications Associated With Radiation Therapy

Fatigue

Oral Cavity Problems
- Mucositis
- Dental caries
- Taste alterations
- Alterations in saliva
- Pain

Skin Problems
- Dry desquamation
- Wet desquamation
- Alopecia

Cardiac Problems
- Acute pericarditis

Pulmonary Problems
- Pneumonitis

Esophageal Problems
- Esophagitis
- Dysphagia

Stomach and Small Intestine Problems
- Gastritis
- Nausea
- Vomiting
- Diarrhea
- Enteritis

Colon and Rectal Problems
- Proctitis
- Rectal structure
- Diarrhea

Liver Problems
- Hepatitis

Kidney Problems
- Nephropathy

Bladder Problems
- Urinary frequency
- Urge incontinence

Testicular Problems
- Reduction in sperm count
- Azoospermia

Ovarian Problems
- Amenorrhea

Bone Marrow Problems
- Neutropenia
- Thrombocytopenia
- Anemia

disease where, increasingly, chemotherapy is added to the treatment plan, debilitating side effects can occur.

Meticulous daily assessments and early intervention are critical. All patients who have the oral cavity in the treatment field are referred to dentistry before initiation of treatment. Any necessary extractions are performed if teeth are decayed. A week to 10 days of healing is needed before the start of treatment. Patients are taught oral care and how to use fluoride trays during the course of treatment to prevent radiation cavities (Parson, 1994). Mucositis develops within 2 weeks of the initiation of treatment with 200 cGy fractions. The mucositis consists of fibrin, polymorphonuclear leukocytes, and dead surface epithelial cells. A sore throat is reported at about 3 weeks into therapy. It is important to note that certain populations of individuals may exhibit earlier and more severe reactions. Concomitant administration of chemotherapy contributes to the earlier development of and more severe mucositis. Individuals with AIDS often manifest mucositis during the first week of therapy. Combined modality treatment in the elderly results in earlier and more severe reactions (Parson, 1994; Hughes-Davies et al., 1991).

Mucositis develops throughout the treatment area on the soft palate, tonsillar pillars, buccal mucosa, lateral borders of the tongue, and portions of the larynx; but it is absent on the hard palate, gingival ridge, and the true vocal cords. After the completion of radiation therapy, the membranes usually heal within 2½ to 3 weeks. However, in individuals who are receiving chemotherapy, healing of the oral mucosa takes longer. After 1 month, the oral mucosa is healed in 90% to 95% of patients, and complaints of a sore throat are minimal.

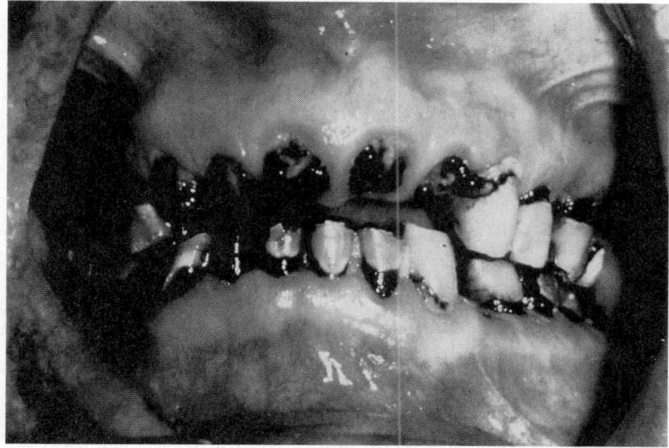

Fig. 4-10 Oral complications.

Changes in the salivary glands contribute to the development of mucositis. If they are included in the field, treatment results in a decrease in salivary flow. The serous component of saliva is most readily affected, leaving the mucous component and a tenacious, ropy saliva. The loss of saliva contributes to a loss of taste, as substances must be dissolved in saliva to initiate the taste response. Radiation therapy also damages the microvilli of the taste cells. Taste loss begins about 1 week into therapy and progresses as doses reach 4000 cGy. Activity is diminished significantly by the end of treatment. Recovery of taste generally improves within 20 to 60 days after the treatment is finished and is usually complete by 120 days. Some patients who have had the major salivary glands treated with high doses report a permanent sense of dryness with associated taste loss (Moss, 1994; Parson, 1994).

Nutritional management of persons receiving radiation therapy for head and neck cancer requires a multidisciplinary plan. Pain and sore throat are managed with good oral hygiene and analgesics if necessary. Rinsing and gargling with a solution of salt and baking soda (i.e., 1 teaspoon of salt and 1 teaspoon of baking soda in 1 quart of water) loosen thick saliva and decrease pain. Viscous lidocaine and other topical analgesics have also been used to decrease pain. However, it is essential that these substances be rinsed and not allowed to cake onto the oral mucosa. Patients receiving concomitant chemotherapy are at particular risk for the development of oral candidiasis. A topical broad-spectrum antimicrobial such as cholheyidine (i.e., 15 mL swish and gargle) may prevent development of oral candidias. Again, it is essential to carefully monitor the elderly and those patients with human immunodeficiency disease for the development of oral infections. All patients receiving radiation therapy for head and neck cancers should be weighed daily (Copeland & Ellis, 1994; Parson, 1994).

Percutaneous endoscopic gastrostomy tubes may be necessary to maintain nutritional intake. The family is placed in the unenviable position of encouraging food and fluid intake. If the patient cannot eat, a pattern of repeated admissions for weakness and dehydration ensues with the undesirable result of treatment breaks. Enteral nutrition, although sometimes seen as a burden for patients and families, often eliminates episodes of dehydration and contributes to maintaining a patient's quality of life. The nurse and dietitian working collaboratively can help the patient and family determine the best method to ensure adequate intake of food and fluids. It is clear that individuals who are able to maintain nutritional intake are better able to tolerate therapy. It has been determined that excessive treatment breaks alter outcomes in patients with head and neck cancer, so every attempt must be made to manage symptoms (Copeland & Ellis, 1994; Peters et al., 1992).

Skin Problems

The skin in the treatment field will react to the radiation therapy. Modern treatment equipment delivers the maximum radiation dose beneath the surface of the skin and has an effect known as *skin-sparing*. The severity of reactions seen today is much less than that observed in the early history of radiation therapy when the orthovoltage units delivered a significant dose of radiation to the skin. Nevertheless, a continuing fear of patients is that they will be "burned" by the radiation. This image of the effect of radiation must be addressed before therapy begins. Once skin reactions occur, patients are encouraged to view this problem in a positive framework (e.g., as evidence that something actually is happening when they are under this mysterious beam of energy) (Shimm & Cassady, 1994).

The skin consists of three layers: the epidermis, the dermis, and the subcutaneous tissues. The avascular epidermis is 0.05 to 0.15 mm thick. The dermis is 1 to 2 mm thick and is composed of blood vessels and lymphatics in a connective tissue stroma. The subcutaneous tissues underlie the dermis, are composed of areas of fat storage, and are a supportive structure for blood vessels and nerves (Archambeau, Pezner, & Wasserman, 1995; Shimm & Cassady, 1994).

A faint and transient erythema of the skin may be noted during the first week of radiation treatment. Dry desquamation of the skin occurs at 2 to 3 weeks and is the result of the killing of the basal cells in the epidermis (Fig. 4-11). Scaling of the skin occurs as a result of the caking of dead cells. These scales are often dark as radiation stimulates the melanocytes that are located between the epidermis and dermis. Patients report sensitivity to touch and itching and drawing of the skin (Archambeau et al., 1995; Shimm & Cassady, 1994).

With increasing doses of radiation, at 4 weeks, epidermal sloughing and oozing of serum from the denuded area occur. This problem is called *moist desquamation* (Fig. 4-12). Moist desquamation occurs as the capacity for the basal cell to repopulate the epidermis is exceeded by the rate at which cells are lost. Healing occurs spontaneously within 2 to 4 weeks. Re-epithelialization occurs from the periphery and from surviving cells within the field.

Skin adnexal structures such as hair follicles are also affected. In high-dose areas, hair loss may be permanent (Archambeau et al., 1995; Shimm & Cassady, 1994).

Treatment of acute skin reactions requires more research. Practices are based on conventional wisdom rather than em-

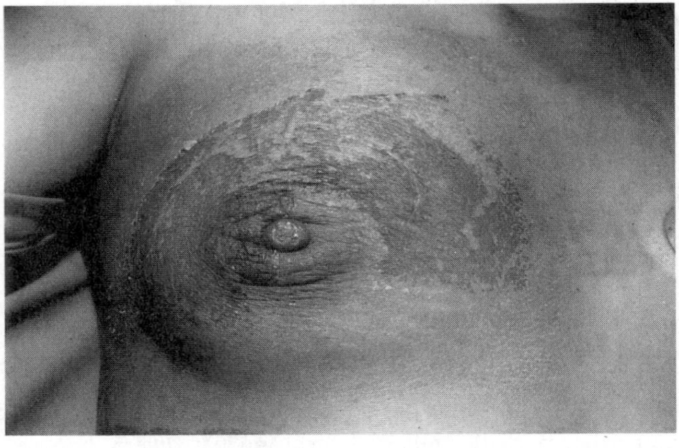

Fig. 4-11 Dry desquamation.

piric evidence. The main components of any skin care regimen are to promote healing, alleviate discomfort, and protect the skin from further damage. The skin should be protected from sun exposure and extremes of temperature. Harsh soaps and chemicals should not be used. Traditionally, treatment has been driven by a fear of infection, although it is difficult to find many individuals who can recall even a single case of an infection developing during a skin reaction. Traditional agents to treat skin reactions included astringents and antiseptics such as peroxide, hypochlorite (i.e., Dakin's solution), or iodine. Research findings suggest that these agents do not promote wound healing, as they produce an environment that does not support fibroblast migration and epithelial proliferation. Recently, agents that are hydrogels of the type used in the management of decubitus ulcers were found to promote faster healing and often allow radiation treatments to continue without interruption (Shimm & Cassady, 1994).

Cardiac Problems

The heart, in varying amounts, is included in the radiation field during the treatment of the mediastinum in several cancers (e.g., lung, esophagus, lymphomas, breast, and seminoma). The walls of the heart are composed of three layers: the epicardium, the myocardium, and the endocardium. Radiation-induced injuries of the heart trigger a dose-related thickening of the heart wall. The epicardium and pericardium provide a thin layer of avascular tissue that serves to minimize friction. These layers are particularly vulnerable to damage by radiation. The response of cardiac tissue is similar to that produced by an infection, the result being an acute pericarditis that appears a few weeks to several years after treatment. Pericarditis is manifested by fever, tachycardia, substernal pain, and a pericardial friction rub. This reaction is not a common complication of radiation therapy. Most symptomatic patients will have had at least 4000 cGy in 4 weeks to a major portion of the heart. It is postulated that tumor-related alteration in venous and lymphatic drainage from the heart may contribute to the accumulation of pericardial fluid.

Treatment planning that limits the dose of radiation to the heart prevents acute and chronic cardiac damage. Patients who have received combined modality therapy, with radiation to the mediastinum and cardiotoxic chemotherapeutic agents, will require long-term follow-up to assess cardiac damage (Byhardt & Moss, 1994; Stewart, Fajardo, Gillete, & Constine, 1995).

Pulmonary Problems

The lung is sensitive to radiation. The early reactions in the lung are considered a degenerative or pneumonitis phase. Type II pneumocytes in the lung, which are the cells that release surfactant, appear to be the foci for radiation damage. Surfactant is a phospholipid detergent-like substance that increases surface tension in the alveoli and prevents alveolar collapse. Initially, during radiation therapy, there is an increase in surfactant release followed by a steady decline (Komaki & Ox, 1994; McDonald, Rubin, Phillips, & Marks, 1995).

Patients may be asymptomatic, but some report fever and night sweats, as well as dyspnea and a cough with thick white sputum. Symptoms subside within 2 to 3 months. If a large volume of lung is treated above 2500 to 3000 cGy, signs and symptoms of radiation pneumonitis may appear at 3 to 6 weeks. The most common signs and symptoms are dyspnea, cyanosis, and fever. Frequently, the only clinical

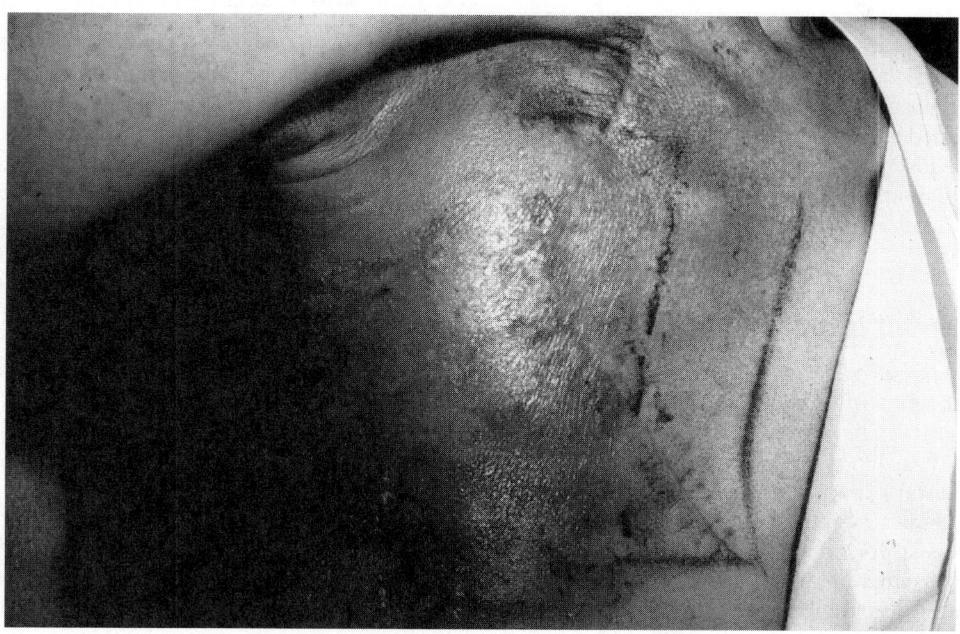

Fig. 4-12 Moist desquamation.

manifestations of pneumonitis are radiographic changes with an infiltrate seen on the chest film that conforms to the treatment field (Komaki & Ox, 1994; McDonald et al., 1995).

Pulmonary function studies are routinely obtained before the initiation of radiation therapy. Care is taken to treat as little volume of the lung as possible. Most patients remain asymptomatic. The RTOG reports a 10% grade 2 and 4.6% grade 3 incidence of pneumonitis. Corticosteroids may reverse symptoms, but they do not prevent or reverse fibrosis. Supportive care with bronchodilators, expectorants, bed rest, and oxygen may be indicated (Komaki & Ox, 1994; McDonald et al., 1995).

Dyspnea is a terrifying symptom for the patient and family members. The patient with lung cancer may present with significant shortness of breath and cough. Initially, treatment may cause these symptoms to increase, making patients believe they are getting worse. Patients with dyspnea are extremely anxious, making teaching difficult and sometimes futile. Patients may be so dyspneic that the first few radiation treatments must be given with the patient sitting up. Once the tumor has regressed and the dyspnea improves, teaching needs to be reinforced. Home care referrals may be needed if oxygen use is required. Patients who are receiving radiation therapy for lung cancer often present with late-stage disease. If therapy is palliative, the nurse plays a role in helping patients and family members make decisions to support comfort measures.

Esophageal Problems

The esophagus is lined with nonkeratinizing squamous epithelium similar to the cells of the oral cavity. The entire esophageal wall is less than 5 mm thick. The external muscle layer consists of striated fibers in the superior portion and smooth muscle in the inferior portion of the esophagus. Epithelial cell loss, associated with moderate to severe dysphagia, occurs during treatment. Patients often state that they feel as though food gets "stuck" here and point to an area in their chest. If dysphagia is severe, enteral feeding may be needed at the start of therapy. Antacids may help to alleviate the discomfort. Protocols combining radiation therapy and chemotherapy place the patient at risk for nutritional compromise, and early intervention is essential (Coia, 1994).

Stomach and Small Intestine Problems

The mucosal cells of the stomach are sensitive to radiation. The mucosal cells of the gastric pit are renewed every 2 to 6 days. Radiation alters gastric secretions by causing direct injury to mucosal cells and by altering the blood-borne and neural stimuli that regulate gastric secretions. Radiation gastritis begins about a week into treatment and may persist for a month or more. Radiation gastritis is usually asymptomatic and consists of edema, hyperemia, exudate formation, and microscopic hemorrhage. Regeneration of glandular cells begins 3 weeks after initiation of therapy. The gastric glands vary in their response to radiation. The pepsin-secreting cells appear to be more easily destroyed than the parietal and acid-producing cells, although both hydrochloric acid and pepsin secretion decrease with radiation treatment (Stevens, 1994a). Destructive changes are patchy throughout the stomach. Secretions remain depressed for a few weeks to several years after treatment. Then patients with Hodgkin's disease may develop ulcers related to the doses delivered to extended mantle fields.

The small intestine is one of the most radiosensitive tissues in the body. The mucosal cells turn over rapidly with a renewal time of 3 to 6 days. Mucosal cells are lost by denudation as the mitotically active crypt cells are destroyed. Attempts to treat the whole abdomen with radiation therapy have been limited by small bowel effects. Acute nausea, vomiting, and diarrhea result from radiation damage to the small intestine. Radiation enteritis results in a malabsorption of fat, carbohydrates, and protein. Excessive bile salts reach the colon instead of being reabsorbed and contribute to the development of diarrhea. Antiemetics, antispasmodics, and antidiarrheals are prescribed to treat the symptoms. Diets low in fat, milk, protein, and lactose have been advocated, although research about these approaches has shown variable results. As the mucosal cells of the small intestine begin to divide, rapid recovery begins as well. In animal studies, with single doses of radiation, re-epithelialization was extensive within 96 hours after treatment. Minimizing the dose delivered to and the volume of the small intestine in the treatment fields is one approach that can be used to decrease acute and late effects. Patients are instructed to drink fluids before treatment, as being treated with a full bladder pushes the intestine out of the treatment field (Stevens, 1994a).

Colon and Rectal Problems

The rectum and rectosigmoid colon tolerate higher doses of radiation than does the small intestine. Prostate cancer therapy results in a 2% incidence of severe proctitis and a 2% incidence of moderate rectal stricture. Diarrhea is the most significant side effect associated with radiation to the colon or rectal area. In most cases, diarrhea begins at about 3 weeks of therapy and resolves within 2 to 3 weeks after completion of treatment. Patients with hemorrhoids may experience an increase in discomfort during radiation therapy. Rectal cancer in persons with AIDS requires meticulous assessment, as the immunosuppressed patient is at risk for the development of systemic infections from any breaks in skin integrity (Stevens, 1994b).

Liver Problems

The entire liver tolerates about 3000 cGy, and 75% of patients who receive more than 4000 cGy develop liver dysfunction. Acute abnormalities occur primarily in the centrolobular region and include sinusoidal congestion, hyperemia or hemorrhage, dilation of central veins, and atrophy of central hepatic cells. Radiation hepatitis apparently occurs as a result of fibrinous deposits that trap erythrocytes in the liver and lead to collagen formation and venous obstruction. Chemotherapy influences the tolerance of the liver to radiation. Lower doses of radiation produce liver dysfunction in patients receiving chemotherapy. Chemotherapy potentiates the effects of radiation, lowering the tolerance of the liver to 2000-2500 cGy after high-dose chemotherapy. Treatment planning around unit doses and combined modality therapy reduces the risk of liver damage (Stevens, 1994c).

Kidney Problems

Radiation nephropathy is a slowly progressive disease that develops depending on the dose and volume of radiation delivered, the age of the patient, the presence of associated conditions such as hypertension and diabetes, and whether the patient receives chemotherapy. The pathogenesis of acute damage appears to be related to swelling of the capillary endothelium and the proximal tubular cells. After 30 to 60 days, capillary endothelium and proximal tubular cells exhibit patchy degeneration, separation from the basement membrane, and vocuolation. Acute radiation nephritis is characterized by hypertension, edema, proteinuria, anemia, and uremia and typically occurs 6 to 12 months after radiation. Segmental glomerular sclerosis and cellular proliferation mimic malignant hypertension. Doses of 2300 cGy in 5 weeks produce this picture in about 50% of patients and recovery is variable. Treatment planning identifies where the kidneys are within the treatment field. If the kidneys are within the treatment field and do not require treatment, attempts are made to block as much of the kidney as possible. If concerns about kidney function are warranted, function should be assessed frequently during treatment (Pearse, 1994a).

Bladder Problems

Early and late effects of radiation to the bladder can be readily observed clinically. The bladder is unavoidably treated during therapy for cervical and prostate cancer. Transient mucosal erythema occurs within 24 hours of treatment. Edema and a mild mucosal reaction occur at 3000 cGy given over 3 to 4 weeks. Submucosal petechiae appear and bladder capacity may be slightly diminished. At higher doses, bladder capacity is further reduced with increased mucositis. Most patients develop acute urinary symptoms within 4 to 5 weeks after the initiation of therapy. The most common problems are urinary frequency and urge incontinence. Cystoscopic examination of the bladder mucosa reveals acute inflammation with engorged capillaries, round cell infiltrates, and edema. Symptoms resolve within 3 to 4 weeks after therapy is completed. Management of acute bladder reactions includes the use of anticholinergics and antibiotics as indicated. Regeneration of the epithelium occurs rapidly after treatment ends. The severity of reactions is increased if chemotherapy agents, such as cyclophosphamide, are given during bladder irradiation (Pearse, 1994b).

Testicular Problems

The sensitivity of the germ cells of the testes to radiation therapy is related to their stage of development at the time they are irradiated. The type B spermatogonia are the most sensitive type of cells. The type A spermatogonia are somewhat sensitive, and primary and secondary spermatocytes and spermatids are much less sensitive than the germ cells. Except for the fact that type B spermatogonia are more sensitive than type A, radiosensitivity decreases along the maturation pathway. Primitive, type A, pale spermatogonia are more resistant than type B because they have a long (16-day) cell cycle and are therefore believed to be the cells that survive to repopulate the seminiferous tubules and reestablish fertility (Hussey, 1994).

Spermatogenesis appears to be more sensitive to fractionated irradiation than to single doses. The seemingly paradoxical observation has been seen in animal studies as well. The rationale for the increased cell kill with divided doses is related to the long cell cycle time of the primitive stem cells. The proportion of radioresistant cells is affected by fractions of treatment, as the cells are given time between doses to progress to a more sensitive phase of the cell cycle (Hussey, 1994).

Doses in the range of 15 to 30 cGy produce a temporary reduction of sperm count. Doses of 35 to 230 cGy produce a transient azoospermia. The time to recovery is also dose dependent. Recovery occurs within 21 to 41 weeks with doses of 60 cGy or less and within 47 to 88 weeks with doses of 60 to 140 cGy. Azoospermia may be permanent with doses of 140 to 300 cGy, and if recovery does occur, it may take as long as 3 to 13 years (Hussey, 1994).

Testicular shields should be used whenever possible to minimize the dose of radiation to the testes during pelvic radiation. Patients should be informed about the expected effects of radiation treatment on fertility. The contribution of chemotherapy also needs to be considered, as well as other causes of infertility in persons with cancer. For example, 50% of patients with seminoma have some degree of impairment in spermatogenesis at the time of presentation (Hussey, 1994). Infertility may not be the issue of greatest concern at the time of the cancer diagnosis. This issue often becomes more important as the patient enters adulthood and faces the consequences of cancer and cancer treatment. Ongoing involvement in the follow-up care of patients with cancer places the nurse in an ideal role to initiate discussions and referrals as they are indicated.

Ovarian Problems

The ovaries contain about 300,000 primordial follicles at puberty. When the ovaries become depleted of follicles, there is a cessation of ovulation and the production of estradiol and progesterone. The oocyte in the primitive follicle is more sensitive to radiation damage than is the ovum of the mature follicle. In the graafian follicle, the oocyte may be more radiosensitive than the ovum. The radiation dose necessary to induce ovarian failure is age dependent. Permanent cessation of menses occurs in 95% of women under 40 years of age who receive doses of 500 to 1000 cGy. In contrast, a lower minimum dose of 375 cGy achieved almost 100% amenorrhea in women over 40 years of age. Doses of 12.5 to 5.0 cGy produced permanent amenorrhea in 58% of younger women, whereas 1.25 to 3.75 cGy produced amenorrhea in 78% of women over 40. In young women, oogenesis is not quite as sensitive to internal scatter radiation as is spermatogenesis in males. In addition, function can be preserved by shielding the ovaries. Hormonal replacement therapy is indicated in young women (Thomas & Dembo, 1994). Infertility is a significant issue for young women. The nurse plays a significant role in helping patients understand their risks and options in terms of infertility.

Bone Marrow Problems

The bone marrow is extremely radiosensitive. After 3000 to 4000 cGy to large volumes of bone marrow, neutropenia occurs in 1 week; thrombocytopenia in 2 to 3 weeks; and anemia in 2 to 3 months. When small fields are irradiated, the unexposed bone marrow increases its population of progenitor cells, meeting the demands for hematopoiesis. When radiation is given alone, in conventional fields and with conventional doses, it is unusual to see a dramatic drop in blood counts. Larger field treatment and concomitant therapy produce a decrease in blood counts. Infection and bleeding are rarely seen with radiation alone. Because of the important role of oxygen in the effectiveness of radiation, patients may be transfused when hemoglobin levels fall below 9 g/dl (Mauch et al., 1995).

LATE COMPLICATIONS ASSOCIATED WITH RADIATION TREATMENT

The mitotic link of radiation effects means that cells continue to die for months to years after radiation is given. Late cellular death occurs in cell lines that are not mitotically active. Radiation effects on the vasculature appear to be a major contributor to late effects. Extracapillary fibrosis occurs in vessels in the treatment field. Vessel occlusion decreases the number of small vessels and inhibits capillary sprouting and vascular remodeling. The intima of blood vessels are swollen with a proliferation of endothelial cells and lipid deposits. These deposits resemble atheromatous plaques, except that they occur in the small arteries where plaques develop infrequently. The sequelae of vascular compromise vary from organ to organ. The skin can tolerate extensive damage before necrosis is seen, whereas small defects in the vasculature result in significant damage to the brain, myocardium, kidney, and lung. Late effects in specific sites are described in subsequent sections of this chapter (Box 4-3). There does not appear to be any correlation between the severity of acute reactions and late reactions.

Box 4-3
Late Complications Associated with Radiation Therapy

Central Nervous System Problems
- Myelopathy
- Leukoencephalopathy

Neuroendocrine Problems
- Growth hormone deficiency
- Gonadotropin deficiency
- Thyrotropin deficiency
- Adrenocorticotropin deficiency

Head and Neck Problems
- Soft tissue necrosis
- Xerostomia
- Radiation caries
- Osteoradionecrosis

Skin Problems
- Atrophy
- Subcutaneous fibrosis
- Necrosis

Lung Problems
- Pulmonary fibrosis
- Radiation pneumonitis

Cardiac Problems
- Cardiomyopathy
- Coronary artery disease

Gastrointestinal Tract Problems
- Esophageal stricture
- Ulceration in the pylorus
- Intestinal fibrosis
- Chronic proctitis

Liver Problems
- Fibrosis of hepatic tissue
- Hepatitis

Kidney Problems
- Nephropathy

Bone Marrow Problems
- Anemia

Skeletal Problems
- Skeletal growth arrest

In addition, early warning signs associated with late effects may not occur. Treatment planning that limits the normal tissue dose of radiation is the most important factor in limiting both acute and late effects. Unfortunately, individuals treated before computerized planning have provided evidence of the late effects of radiation therapy. As populations of individuals who received combined modality therapy begin to survive, late effects of combined modality therapy may appear. Chemotherapeutic agents often damage normal cells that are different from the cells damaged by radiation; therefore additive damage may occur. Agents that allow for the administration of increasing doses of chemotherapy, such as those that provide cardiac protection and increase blood counts, create a population of individuals who will need careful follow-up to identify the possible late effects of high doses of drug often given in combination with radiation therapy. The nurse plays a critical role in collecting these data and assisting patients and family members to cope with the unknown (Rubin, Constine, & Nelson, 1992).

Central Nervous System Problems

Proliferative and degenerative changes occur in astrocytes, oligodendrocytes, and other glial elements as a result of radiation therapy. Endothelial cell loss, capillary occlusion, and hemorrhagic exudates are seen with a resulting loss of the blood-brain barrier with increased vascular permeability. The late reaction is clinically manifested by focal neurologic deficits, including encephalopathy or neuropsychological dysfunction. Fraction size appears to be a dominant factor in the development of posttreatment necrosis. Brain tolerance is reported at 5200 cGy with 200 cGy daily fractions. At this dose, the incidence of necrosis is 0.04% to 4%. Tolerance is influenced by age and is 10% to 20% lower in children under 2 years of age, as their cells are mitotically more active because of ongoing myelination and neuronal replication (Schultheiss, Kun, Ang, & Stephens, 1995).

In children with acute lymphocytic leukemia (ALL) who receive combined modality treatment and in adults who receive cranial radiation for small cell lung cancer, leukoencephalopathy is a reported late effect that usually occurs 4 to 12 months after combined modality treatment. This demyelinating necrotizing reaction can progress to dementia, seizures, ataxia, and death. Discontinuing the intrathecal or intraventricular administration of chemotherapy allows for recovery, although there are often permanent neurologic deficits (Schultheiss et al., 1995.) Decline in intellectual functioning associated with neurocognitive changes correlates with the administration of cranial radiation to children who are 2 years of age or younger. This problem led to an alteration in the treatment of leukemia in children, with the elimination of prophylactic cranial radiation (Schultheiss et al., 1955).

Myelopathies are unusual late complications of radiation treatment. The initial symptoms may be subtle and include sensory deficits such as unilateral or bilateral leg weakness and diminished proprioception. Lhermitte syndrome, a sensation of a shock when the neck is flexed, may precede permanent myelopathy. Objective signs and symptoms include foot drop, spasticity, weakness, and hemiparesis with hyperreflexia and Babinski signs on examination. The severity of symptoms is usually progressive but may stabilize. Myelopathy occurs at doses greater than 5000 cGy and has a latency period of at least 6 months after treatment.

Because of the morbidity associated with radiation myelopathy, spinal cord doses are always calculated and considered, and doses are usually prescribed in the 4500 cGy to 5000 cGy dose range and administered in 22 to 25 fractions. It has been reported that 4500 cGy in 22 to 25 fractions yields an incidence of myelopathy of ≤0.2%. As the length of survival of patients increases, the question of retreating previously irradiated tissue, particularly the spinal cord, remains a dilemma. Up to 25% of patients with head and neck cancers develop a second primary close to or within a previously treated field. Animal studies suggest that the spinal cord does recover from occult injury. However, the severity of spinal cord sequelae is unknown at the present time (Schultheiss et al., 1995).

Neuroendocrine Problems

Abnormalities of the hypothalamic pituitary axis are seen as a result of radiation to the central nervous system, nasopharynx, or face. Abnormalities are related to the dose of radiation administered and are time-dependent, with the incidence increasing over time. Younger patients are more vulnerable to abnormalities than are adults. The hypothalamus is more radiosensitive than the pituitary gland and is commonly the site of damage at doses of 4000-5000 cGy (Sklar & Constine, 1995).

Growth hormone deficiency is the most common pituitary problem seen after cranial irradiation. In the growing child, this problem results in a reduction in growth velocity inappropriate for the age and stage of puberty, leading to short stature. A slowing of growth may not occur until 2 years after therapy. Nearly all children treated with doses in excess of 3500 cGy develop growth hormone deficiencies, generally occurring within 5 years of treatment.

Gonadotropin deficiency in a young child results in a failure to enter puberty and in primary amenorrhea. Milder forms lead to slow or arrested puberty, menstrual irregularities, and secondary amenorrhea. In adults, infertility and decreased libido occur. Doses of 5000 cGy or more result in gonadotropin deficiencies in 20% to 50% of patients. Early sexual maturation with precocious puberty, particularly in females, is also reported with gonadotropin and growth hormone deficiencies. This problem is reported with cranial radiation given in doses of 1800 to 2400 cGy for the treatment of leukemia.

Thyrotropin deficiency is generally subclinical, but may cause weight gain, lethargy, poor linear growth, and delayed puberty. It is rare with doses under 4000 cGy (Sklar & Constine, 1995). Decreased stamina, lethargy, and fasting hypoglycemia are associated with adrenocorticotropin hormone (ACTH) deficiency. At doses greater than 5000 cGy, the incidence of ACTH deficiency ranges from 18% to 35% after 5 to 15 years. Hyperprolactinemia is most common in adult women and can cause pubertal delay or arrest in children, galactorrhea and/or amenorrhea in women, or decreased libido and importance in men. Mild increases in prolactin are common after doses greater than 5000 cGy, and the incidence of hyperprolactinemia varies from 20% to 50%. Management of neuroendocrine effects is through the use of replacement hormones and is usually managed by a pediatric endocrinologist in children. The emotional sequelae of neuroendocrine effects need to be considered, and children may require ongoing support and counseling as they develop and grow into adults who must cope with treatment effects (Sklar & Constine, 1995).

Head and Neck Problems

Late effects of radiation on the mucosal linings of the oral cavity are characterized by paleness and thinning of the epithelium with loss of mucosal pliability, submucosal induration, and occasionally chronic ulceration and necrosis with exposure of bone and soft tissues. After surgery and radiation therapy, constricting fibrosis with loss of elasticity occurs. Soft tissue necrosis is related to the dose, time, and volume of tissue treated and is usually seen after interstitial implants (Cooper, Fu, Marks, & Silverman, 1995).

Mucosal changes usually do not require intervention. Soft tissue necrosis may be painful and requires topical treatments, such as, viscous xylocaine, Benadryl, and Mylanta. Meticulous oral hygiene is imperative. Pentoxifylline is being investigated for its ability to improve perfusion to ischemic tissues by increasing the deformity of red blood cells, inhibiting platelet aggregation, and stimulating fibrinolytic activity (Cooper et al., 1995). Long-term fibrosis can be minimized by teaching patients self-care exercises before treatment begins. Patients may be instructed to stretch the area 10 to 20 times in a row, several times per day. Inserting increasing numbers of stacked tongue blades into the oral cavity may be recommended to minimize or prevent trismus (Cooper et al., 1995).

The xerostomia that occurs after treatment may persist for several months to years and may or may not ever recover, depending on the volume of tissue treated and the dose administered. Xerostomia impedes talking, swallowing, and chewing. Increasing fluids is effective. Pilocarpine hydrochloride has been approved for posttreatment xerostomia. It has been shown to provide temporary relief of xerostomia in patients who have residual salivary function. Commercially prepared water and glycerin (i.e., artificial saliva), is available, although many patients find carrying a thermos of water to be as effective (Cooper et al., 1995).

The teeth and mandible can exhibit late effects of treatment. Prophylactic dental care with meticulous oral hygiene and fluoride treatments prevents many negative sequelae in the teeth and mandible. Radiation caries occur along the gum line and are related to changes in the composition and the amount of saliva. The mandible has a poor blood supply and is at risk for the development of osteoradionecrosis. This problem begins as an erythematous change in the overlying mucosa that ulcerates to reveal necrotic bone. Lytic destruction and periosteal thickening are seen and fractures can occur. Doses of greater than 6000 cGy to the entire mandible contribute to the risk of developing osteoradionecrosis. Other risk factors for osteoradionecrosis include dentulous patients, high-dose treatments to the bone, and tooth extractions after radiation therapy begins. Patients with head and neck cancers are seen routinely by a dentist before therapy begins. Any decayed or damaged teeth are removed before initiation of treatment, with a delay of 7 to 10 days to allow for wound healing. Studies exploring the preventive and therapeutic use of antibiotics and hyperbaric oxygen for osteoradionecrosis are ongoing. Prevention is the key, and the nurse plays a pivotal role in helping patients understand how critical oral hygiene measures are in the prevention of this devastating late effect (Cooper et al., 1995; Parson, 1994).

Skin Problems

Late effects in the skin include atrophy, subcutaneous fibrosis, and necrosis. Telangiectasias develop in an atrophic dermis with a reddish discoloration related to multiple, prominent, thin-walled, dilated vessels. Fibrosis is characterized by induration, edema, and thickening of the dermis and subcutaneous tissues. With skin-sparing equipment, subcutaneous fibrosis is more common. These chronic changes are generally painless. The skin in the field feels smoother and may have a permanent loss of sweat glands and hair. The area may react differently to the sun and should be protected. Although not symptomatic, these skin changes serve as a reminder of radiation therapy (Archambeau et al., 1995).

Lung Problems

Pulmonary fibrosis develops insidiously in a previously radiated field and stabilizes after 1 to 2 years. Most patients with radiation fibrosis are asymptomatic. The clinical symptoms relate to the extent of lung parenchyma involved and preexisting pulmonary function. With fibrosis limited to less than 50% of the lung, symptoms are minimal. Symptoms may include dyspnea, reduced exercise tolerance, cyanosis, finger clubbing, progressive cor pulmonale, and right heart failure. Chest radiographs show linear streaking that extends beyond the irradiated area with regional contraction, pleural thickening, and tenting of the diaphragm. These changes are seen 12 months to 2 years after therapy (McDonald et al., 1995) (Fig. 4-13).

Late lung injury consists of fibrosis of the alveolar septa associated with collapse and obliteration of alveoli by connective tissue. Mild deterioration in pulmonary function may occur with a reduction in maximum breathing capacity and tidal volume. When small volumes of lung are radiated, functional compensation of adjacent lung regions results in little change in pulmonary functions. The addition of chemotherapeutic agents to radiation therapy may potentiate lung damage. Bleomycin causes interstitial pneumonitis leading to fibrosis. Methotrexate can cause desquamative, interstitial pneumonitis. Doxorubicin and actinomycin do not cause pulmonary toxicity but do potentiate radiation pneumonitis. Careful follow-up is essential for individuals

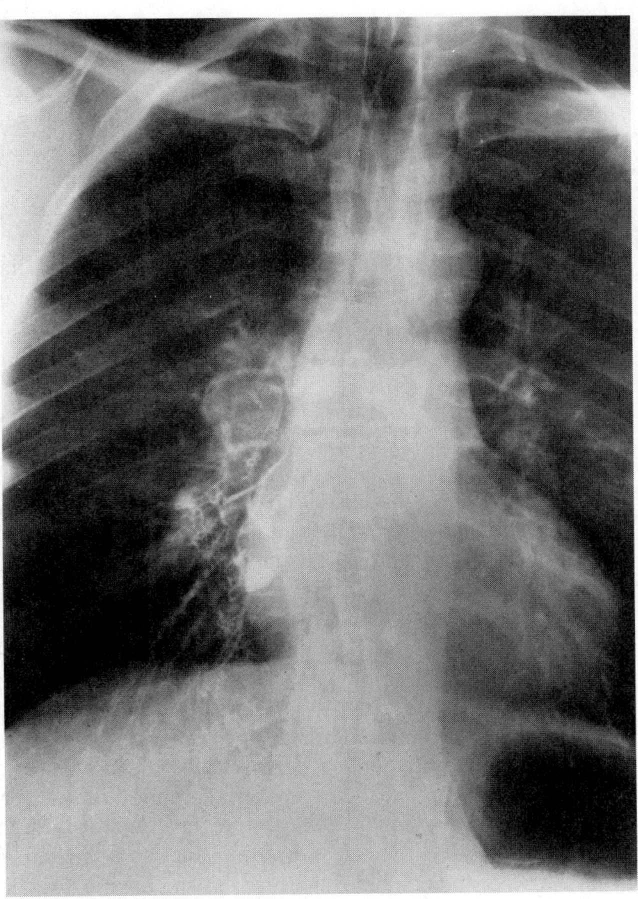

Fig. 4-13 Radiation fibrosis.

who receive combined modality treatment (McDonald et al., 1995).

Cardiac Problems

In patients treated with radiation alone, cardiomyopathy presents with signs and symptoms of pericardial disease with constriction and heart failure. The parietal pericardium develops variable degrees of fibrosis that replace the outer adipose tissue. Although pericardial fibrosis may progress to constriction, fibrous adhesions are not evident. The mechanism of pericardial fibrosis has not been determined, but may occur as a result of damage to blood vessels and subsequent ischemia. Radiation cardiomyopathy is aggravated by simultaneous or sequential chemotherapy with anthracyclines (Stewart et al., 1995).

Coronary artery disease is an important late effect of radiation therapy, particularly in children, and is related to the previously described vascular effects of radiation. Sudden cardiac deaths have been reported in young adults who received doxorubicin and radiation. Clearly, individuals who receive combined modality therapy require lifelong monitoring for evidence of late cardiac complications. Limiting the dose of radiation is the most effective preventive strategy (Stewart et al., 1995).

Gastrointestinal Tract Problems

Late effects in the esophagus are related to damage of the esophageal wall. Benign stricture is the most frequent complication, occurring at a rate of 2% at doses of 5000 cGy or less and increasing to a rate of 15% at doses of 6000 cGy. Stricture formation is not seen until 3 months after radiation, with a medium time of 6 months. Esophageal dilation is the management of choice (Coia, Myerson, & Tepper, 1995).

Ulceration in the pylorus is the most common late effect of radiation to the stomach. In most cases, these lesions heal spontaneously, although perforation can occur. Ulceration rarely occurs at doses under 4500 cGy, with higher doses per fraction predisposing an individual to ulcer formation. Patients may also develop dyspepsia 6 months to 4 years after treatment. Gastritis, arising 1 to 12 months after therapy, is related to spasm or stenosis of the antrum from mucosal atrophy and fibrosis of submucosal tissue. Agents used to treat ulcers have been effective. Studies have focused on testing the effects of agents such as sucralfate that form an ulcer-adherent complex (Coia et al., 1995).

Late injury in the intestine develops at a median time of 8 to 12 months. The most common symptom is frequent and urgent stools. Blood, rectal urgency, lower abdominal cramping, rectal pain, and chronic proctitis can occur. Fibrosis and ischemia with thickened folds, ulceration, and narrowing of segments of the intestine are seen. Dose of radiation and volume of tissue radiated are important determinants of risk, as are prior abdominal surgery and a history of pelvic inflammatory disease.

Management of gastrointestinal problems includes the use of low-residue diets. For diarrhea associated with small bowel injury, cholestyramine helps by reducing bile salts. Significant proctitis can be managed with sodium pentosanpolysulfate. This drug is a synthetic polysaccharide that improves mucosal integrity. Bowel obstruction can be managed by rest and decompression, but may require surgical intervention. Limiting the total dose of radiation delivered to the bowel is an essential component of treatment planning (Coia et al., 1995).

Liver Problems

In most instances, the liver heals after acute radiation injury. Late lesions may be seen and are usually asymptomatic. These lesions include distortion of lobular architecture, collapse of lobules, and concentric fibrosis of portal spaces. Radiation-induced hepatitis occurs 2 weeks to 4 months after hepatic irradiation and is characterized by anicteric ascites. Treatment is with diuretics; steroids are given in severe cases. Symptoms usually resolve in 1 to 2 months (Lawrence, Robertson, Anscher, Jirtle, Ensminger, & Fajardo, 1995).

Kidney Problems

Chronic radiation nephropathy with benign or malignant hypertension becomes evident at about 12 to 18 months after treatment. Symptoms include edema, dyspnea, hypertension, headache, nocturia, and lassitude. Signs include anemia, proteinuria, hypertension, and cardiac enlargement. Bed rest, low-protein diet, and fluids and salt restrictions reduce the workload of the kidney. Peripheral and pulmonary edema, as well as anemia, must be managed. Biologic response modifiers such as erythropoietin, along with transfusions, are indicated to manage anemia. Hypertension is managed medically. Tubular function does appear to recover. Dialysis and transplantation are treatments that have improved the survival of patients experiencing radiation-induced nephropathy. Treatment planning to reduce renal effects remains the standard of care (Cassady, 1995).

Bone Marrow Problems

Permanent ablation of bone marrow occurs in small treatment fields. The capacity of unexposed bone marrow to compensate by accelerating its rate of hematopoiesis obviates the need for repair. When larger areas of the bone marrow are irradiated, hematopoietic activity increases in unexposed segments followed by extension of functional marrow into previously quiescent areas such as femora and humeri. Hyperactivity in nonirradiated bone is seen as long as 8 to 13 years after treatment. In-field marrow regeneration occurs at doses of 3500 to 4000 cGy. Count recovery occurs within 1 to 2 months after therapy, whereas in 90% of patients, bone marrow regeneration takes longer. Management requires that counts be monitored. Growth factors are undergoing investigation but have not been used routinely in radiation therapy (Mauch et al., 1995).

Skeletal Problems

The effect of radiation on epiphyseal bone growth is a significant late effect. The growth plate includes rapidly proliferating cells that are sensitive to radiation. The severity of treatment-related damage depends on total dose administered, fractionation schedule, beam energy, treatment volume, and age of the patient. Probert and Parker (1975) were the first to describe and quantitate axial skeletal growth arrest in children who were treated with radiation to the entire spine. Heights of children were compared with the mean for a comparable group of children. They documented a disproportionate alteration in sitting as compared with standing height at doses greater than 3500 cGy. Disproportion was most severe in children treated under 6 years of age or for those treated between 11 and 13 years of age. The study did not include long-term follow-up and did not monitor younger children during the pubertal growth spurt.

In another study, Willman, Cox, and Donaldson (1994) found that children irradiated before puberty had more significant shortening than children radiated after puberty. During the orthovoltage era, scoliosis was noted in children treated for Wilms' tumor. This problem was a result of partial irradiation and inhomogeneous irradiation of the vertebral bodies. The portion of the vertebral body irradiated did not achieve normal height, but the nonirradiated portion did; thus, causing an unequal weighting and resulting in scoliosis. Soft tissue asymmetry from surgery and flank irradiation and rib hypoplasia also contributed to these effects. Children with Wilms' tumor no longer receive prophylactic radiation to the renal bed, and only those in high-risk groups receive radiation. Homogeneous distribution is planned, which may result in shortening but does not cause scoliosis. Abnormalities of craniofacial growth can cause significant cosmetic deformity in young children treated in the facial region for leukemia or tumors such as rhabdomyosarcomas (Eifel, Donaldson, & Thomas, 1995).

In most cases, careful planning with attention to the anatomy and location of the epiphyseal growth plate can minimize late effects. Actively growing epiphyseal cartilage is always excluded from the treatment field if possible. If a portion of the plate must be treated, the entire plate is included in the field to eliminate unequal growth. Parents must understand which bone effects are unavoidable. Pediatric oncologists, radiation oncologists, orthopedic surgeons, and occupational and physical therapists are challenged to develop a treatment plan to assess and minimize any deformities. Ongoing counseling may be required for the patient and family members. As children mature and come to terms with the deformities associated with radiation therapy they cannot remember, they may express anger toward their parents. Children treated today with the goal of limiting the use of radiation in pediatric protocols and, when necessary, having sophisticated treatment planning systems available should not suffer the same consequences as seen in the past (Eifel et al., 1995).

ETHICAL ISSUES

As the individual who provides continuity of care, patients and family members come to know the nurse. Questions about continuing therapy are presented to the nurse: *Is this therapy going to help? Should I stop treatment?* These types of issues can be difficult when a minor approaches the nurse with a desire to stop treatment. Ensuring that patients and family members are able to discuss their desires and goals is an essential part of treatment. In some clinical situations, the decision to stop treatment seems indicated, and the nurse may serve willingly as a patient advocate. A more difficult dilemma is to be an advocate for a patient who is informed and is making a decision that the nurse does not believe serves the patient's best interest. Ethical consultation is increasingly available in clinical areas and should be sought when difficult issues arise.

RESEARCH ISSUES

It is beyond the scope of this chapter to identify all of the ongoing clinical research in radiation therapy. Trials are ongoing to determine the optimal doses and combinations of radiation therapy, chemotherapy, and surgery for all of the major cancers.

FUTURE TRENDS

Altered Fractions

Modifications of fractionation have evolved in an attempt to address clinical situations in which responses to treatment have been inadequate. Delivering treatment over a shorter period has as its aim minimizing the potential for tumor growth or regeneration during therapy. Multiple standard fractions per day have been given in a continuous course, lasting less than 2 weeks, with good local control, but with a high frequency of complications. Lowering the fractions has yielded improved local control without an increase in late effects. Twice daily fractions (3 to 8 hours apart) of 110 to 120 cGy are being evaluated in the treatment of head and neck cancers. Studies are also ongoing in brainstem gliomas, lung, and bladder cancers. Acute effects are enhanced and may occur earlier than predicted. The disruption to the patient/family system is considerable and requires attention (Peters et al., 1992).

Chemical Modifiers

The biochemical effects of radiation are dependent on cellular physiology that may be modified through biochemical additives such as sensitizers and protectors. Following the limited success of the clinical trials with hyperbaric oxygen, an effort was made to study compounds that could modify the initial radiochemical event. These agents would mimic the ability of oxygen to sensitize hypoxic cells. Misonidazde was the first compound tested and proved to be too toxic to normal tissues (e.g., severe nausea and vomiting and the development of peripheral neuropathies). New nitromidizide analogs are under development. Chemical sensitization, through incorporation of pyrimidine analogs into DNA in rapidly dividing tumors, interferes with the repair of certain radiation injuries. Pyrimidine analogs, such as BUdR and LudR, are undergoing cooperative group trials. Alkylating chemotherapeutic agents have been studied for their sensitizing effects. As the chemical events associated with radiation therapy occur in a time sequence, sensitizers must be given in a timely fashion to be active when radiation is delivered. The goals of this research are to develop nontoxic chemicals that are selectively taken up by hypoxic tumor cells to increase their response to radiation, while not influencing normal tissue reactions (Wasserman & Kligerman, 1992).

Another strategy to increase the effectiveness of irradiation is to use radioprotector compounds that are absorbed by normal cells and reduce their response to radiation without reducing cytotic effects in tumor cells. One protector is 5-hydroxytryptamine (serotonin), which inhibits corticosteroid production, reducing sensitivity to ionizing radiation. Vitamins E and C, and β-carotene protect cellular membrane lipids from the action of free radicals by scavenging these radicals. The scavenging of the free hydroxyl radicals by compounds known as *aminothiols* and *thiourea* is undergoing clinical trials (Wasserman & Kligerman, 1992).

Sulfhydryl compounds protect cells from radiation damage by scavenging the products of irradiated water. The agent that has received the most study is WR2721 (S-2-C3 aminopropylamine-ethylphos-phorothioic acid). It is given 15 to 30 minutes before radiation therapy. Ongoing clinical trials are being designed to evaluate the effectiveness of these nontoxic agents that can selectively protect normal cells from radiation damage (Wasserman & Kligerman, 1992).

Intraoperative Radiation

Intraoperative radiation is a technique through which a single fraction of radiation is given during surgery. It is possible with intraoperative radiation to shield normal tissues or to move them out of the treatment field. The tumor can be visualized directly. Most intraoperative installations are done in the radiation therapy department. This procedure requires that patients and anesthesia services be moved from the operating room to the radiotherapy department so that the patient can receive treatment. The nurse should be involved in the complex planning involving patient transport. After the initial surgical procedure, hemostasis is obtained, the incision is loosely closed, and the patient under anesthesia is moved to the radiation therapy department. The incision is opened in the radiation therapy department, and a cylinder is placed over the tumor volume. The cylinder is attached to the treatment machine and therapy is given. During abdominal or pelvic treatments, a suction catheter may be needed in the operative site to prevent a buildup of blood. Typical doses are 1000 to 2000 cGy in a single dose, yielding a significant biologic effect (Tepper & Calvo, 1992).

Wound healing does not appear to be compromised after intraoperative radiation therapy. A pelvic pain syndrome has been reported and may be secondary to nerve entrapment in patients who have had extensive surgery and intraoperative radiation for recurrent tumors. Intraoperative radiation provides the benefits of being able to visualize tumors and being able to move or shield sensitive, normal tissues. Local control of tumor growth may be enhanced. Gynecologic and bladder cancers may adhere to the pelvic side wall, and intraoperative radiation therapy may be of benefit. Research with this technique is ongoing (Tepper & Calvo, 1992).

Stereotactic External Beam Therapy

Radiosurgery is a term that has been used to describe a variety of techniques that aim to deliver a large single fraction of radiation, with great accuracy, to a small intracranial target. Modified cobalt or linear accelerator and γ-knife units are used. The intracranial target is treated through a large number of small stationary portals by using a stereotactic frame and moving a collimator and x-ray tube circumferentially along the frame. The γ-knife produces multiple intersecting cobalt beams. Initial use of these units was for nonmalignant conditions such as arteriovenous malformations. Clinical trials are exploring the use of this therapy for primary and metastatic brain tumors (Karlsson et al., 1992).

NURSING RESEARCH

Symptom management strategies used in radiation therapy are not research based. Research on the management of all of the major symptoms that occur during and after radiation therapy is needed as the basis for practice. Management of skin reactions and mucositis and dietary modifications for pelvic radiation are important areas for nursing research. Randomized clinical trials are essential for the development of theory and practice related to the side effects associated with radiation therapy.

REFERENCES

Archambeau, J. O., Pezner, R., & Wasserman, T. (1995). Pathophysiology of irradiated skin and breast. *International Journal of Radiation Oncology, Biology, Physics, 31,* 1171-1187.

Bomford, C. K., Kunkler, I. H., & Sherriff, S. B. (1993). *Walter and Miller's textbook of radiotherapy* (5th ed.). New York: Churchill Livingston.

Bucholtz, J. D. (1994). Comforting children during radiotherapy. *Oncology Nursing Forum, 21,* 987-994.

Byhardt, R., & Moss, W. (1994). The heart and blood vessels. In J. Cox (Ed.), *Moss' radiation oncology: Rationale, technique, results* (7th ed.). St. Louis: Mosby.

Cassady, J. R. (1995). Clinical radiation nephropathy. *International Journal of Radiation Oncology, Biology, Physics, 31,* 1249-1257.

Coia, L. (1994). The esophagus. In J. Cox (Ed.), *Moss' radiation oncology: Rationale technique, results* (7th ed.). St. Louis: Mosby.

Coia, L., Myerson, R. J., & Tepper, J. E. (1995). Late effects of radiation therapy on the gastrointestinal tract. *International Journal of Radiation Oncology, Biology, Physics, 31,* 123-1237.

Cooper, J., Fu, K., Marks, J., & Silverman, S. (1995). Late effects of radiation therapy in the head and neck region. *International Journal of Radiation Oncology, Biology, Physics, 31,* 1141-1165.

Copeland, E., & Ellis, L. (1994). Nutritional management in patients with head and neck malignancies. In R. Million & N. Cassisi (Eds.), *Management of head and neck cancer: A multidisciplinary approach* (2nd ed.). Philadelphia: J. B. Lippincott.

Eifel, P., Donaldson, S., & Thomas, P. (1995). Response of growing bone to irradiation: a proposed late effects scoring system. *International Journal of Radiation Oncology, Biology, Physics, 31,* 1301-1309.

Fajardo, L. F. (1994). Morphology of radiation effects on normal tissues. In C. Perez & L. Brady (Eds.), *Principles and practice of radiation oncology* (2nd ed.). Philadelphia: J. B. Lippincott.

Glasgow, G., & Perez, C. (1992). Physics of brachytherapy. In C. Perez & L. Brady (Eds.), *Principles and practice of radiation oncology* (2nd ed.). Philadelphia: J. B. Lippincott.

Hall, E., & Cox, J. (1994). Physical and biologic basis of radiation therapy. In J. Cox (Ed.), *Moss' radiation oncology: rationale, technique, results* (7th ed.). St. Louis: Mosby.

Hanks, G. (1994). The prostate. In J. Cox (Ed.), *Moss' radiation oncology: rationale, technique, results* (7th ed.). St. Louis: Mosby.

Hilderly, L. (1993). Radiotherapy. In S. Groenwald, M. Frogge, M. Goodman, & C. Yarbro (Eds.), *Cancer nursing: Principles and practice* (2nd ed.). Boston: Jones and Bartlett.

Hoppe, R., & Strober, S. (1992). Tobil-lymphoid irradiation in the management of autoimmune disease and organ transplantation. In C. Perez & L. Brady (Eds.), *Principles and practice of radiation oncology* (2nd ed.). Philadelphia: J. B. Lippincott.

Hughes-Davies, L., Young, T., & Spittle, M. (1991): Radiosensitivity in AIDS patients. *Lancet, 337,* 1616.

Hussey, D. (1994). The testicle. In J. Cox (Ed.), *Moss' radiation oncology: rationale, technique, results* (7th ed.). St. Louis: Mosby.

Karlsson, V., Leibel, S., Wallner, K., Davis, L., Brady, L., Larson, D., Wasserman, T., Drzymala, R., & Simpson, J. (1992). Brain. In C. Perez & L. Brady (Eds.), *Principles and practice of radiation oncology* (2nd ed.). Philadelphia: J. B. Lippincott.

King, C., Nail, L., Kreamer, K., Strohl, R., & Johnson, J. (1985). Patients' descriptions of the experience of receiving radiation therapy. *Oncology Nursing Forum, 12,* 55-61.

Komaki, R., & Ox, J. (1994). The lung and thymus. In J. Cox (Ed.), *Moss' radiation oncology: rationale, technique, results* (7th ed.). St. Louis: Mosby.

Lawrence, T., Robertson, J., Anscher, M., Jirtle, R., Ensminger, W., & Fajardo, L. (1995). Hepatic toxicity resulting from cancer treatment. *International Journal of Radiation Oncology Biology, Physics 31,* 1237-1249.

Mauch, P., Constine, L., Greenberger, W., Knospe, J., Sullivan, J., Liesveld, J., & Deeg, H. (1995). Hematopoietic stem cell compartment: acute and late effects of radiation therapy and chemotherapy. *International Journal of Radiation Oncology, Biology, Physics, 31,* 1319-1341.

McDonald, S., Rubin, P., Phillips, T., & Marks, L. (1995). Injury to the lung from cancer therapy: Clinical syndromes, measurable endpoints and potential scoring systems. *International Journal of Radiation Oncology, Biology, Physics, 31,* 1187-1205.

Monyak, D., & Levitt, S. (1992). Breast: locally advanced (T_3 and T_4) and recurrent tumors. In C. Perez & L. Brady (Ed.), *Principles and practice of radiation oncology* (2nd ed.). Philadelphia: J. B. Lippincott.

Moss, W. (1994). The salivary glands. In J. Cox, (Ed.), *Moss' radiation oncology: rationale, technique, results* (7th ed.). St. Louis: Mosby.

Nail, L., & Winningham, M. (1993). Fatigue. In S. Groenwald, M. Frogge, M. Goodman, & C. Yarbro (Eds.), *Cancer nursing: Principles and practice* (2nd ed.). Boston: Jones and Bartlett.

Parson, J. (1994). The effect of radiation on normal tissues of the head and neck. In R. Million & N. Cassisi (Eds.), *Management of head and neck cancer: A multidisciplinary approach* (2nd ed.). Philadelphia: J. B. Lippincott.

Pearse, H. (1994a). The kidney. In J. Cox (Ed.), *Moss' radiation oncology: Rationale technique, results* (7th ed.). St. Louis: Mosby.

Pearse, H. (1994b). The urinary bladder. In J. Cox (Ed.), *Moss' radiation: Oncology rationale, technique, results* (7th ed.). St. Louis: Mosby.

Perez, C. (1992). Prostate. In C. Perez & L. Brady (Eds.). *Principles and practice of radiation oncology* (2nd ed.). Philadelphia: J. B. Lippincott.

Perez, C., & Brady, L. (1992). Overview. In C. Perez & L. Brady (Eds.), *Principles and practice of radiation oncology* (2nd ed.). Philadelphia: J. B. Lippincott.

Perez, C., Garcia, D., Grigsby, P., & Williamson, J. (1992). Clinical applications of brachytherapy. In C. Perez & L. Brady (Eds.), *Principles and practice of radiation oncology* (2nd ed.). Philadelphia: J. B. Lippincott.

Perez, C., Garcia, D., Kuske, R., & Levitt, S. (1992). Breast: stage T_1 and T_2 tumors. In C. Perez & L. Brady (Eds.), *Principles and practice of radiation oncology* (2nd ed.), Philadelphia: J. B. Lippincott.

Peters, L., Ang, K., & Thames, H. (1992). Altered fractionation schedules. In C. Perez & L. Brady (Eds.), *Principles and practice of radiation oncology* (2nd ed.). Philadelphia: J. B Lippincott.

Probert, J. C., & Parker, B. R. (1975). The effects of radiation therapy on bone growth. *Radiology, 114,* 155-162.

Purdy, J., Glasgow, G., & Lightfoot, D. (1992). Principles of radiologic physics, dosimetry, and treatment planning. In C. Perez & L. Brady (Eds.), *Principles and practice of radiation oncology* (2nd ed.). Philadelphia: J. B. Lippincott.

Rubin, P., Constine, L., & Nelson, D. (1992). Late effects of cancer treatment: Radiation and drug toxicity. In C. Perez & L. Brady (Eds.), *Principles and practice of radiation oncology* (2nd ed.). Philadelphia: J. B. Lippincott.

Sause, W. (1994). Principles of combining radiation therapy and surgery . In J. Cox (Ed.), *Moss' radiation oncology: Rationale, technique, results* (7th ed.). St. Louis: Mosby.

Sause, W., & Turrisi, A. (1996). Principles and application of preoperative and standard radiotherapy for regionally advanced non-small cell lung cancer. In H. Pass, J. Mitchell, D. Johnson, & A. Turrisi (Eds.), *Lung cancer: Principles and practice.* Philadelphia: Lippincott-Raven.

Schultheiss, T., Kun, L., Ang, K., & Stephens, L. (1995). Radiation response of the central nervous system. *International Journal of Radiation Oncology, Biology, Physics, 31,* 1093-1113.

Shimm, D., & Cassady, J. (1994). The skin. In J. Cox (Ed.), *Moss' radiation oncology: Rationale, techniques, results* (7th ed.). St. Louis: Mosby.

Sklar, C., & Constine, L. (1995). Chronic neuroendocrinological sequelae of radiation therapy. *International Journal of Radiation Oncology, Biology, Physics, 31,* 1113-1123.

Solan, M., Brady, L., Binnick, S., & Fitzpatrick, P. (1992). Skin. In C. Perez & L. Brady (Eds.), *Principles and practice of radiation oncology* (2nd ed.). Philadelphia: J. B. Lippincott.

Stevens, K. (1994a). The stomach and small intestines. In J. Cox (Ed.), *Moss' radiation oncology: rationale, technique, results* (7th ed.). St. Louis: Mosby.

Stevens, K. (1994b). The colon and rectum. In J. Cox (Ed.), *Moss' radiation: oncology rationale, technique, results* (7th ed.). St. Louis: Mosby.

Stevens, K. (1994c). The liver and biliary system. In J. Cox (Ed.), *Moss' radiation: oncology rationale, technique, results* (7th ed.). St. Louis: Mosby.

Stewart, J. R., Fajardo, L. F., Gillete, S. M., & Constine, L. S. (1995). Radiation injury to the heart. *International Journal of Radiation Oncology, Biology, Physics, 31,* 1205-1213.

Tepper, J., & Calvo, F. (1992). Intraoperative radiation therapy. In C. Perez & L. Brady (Eds.), *Principles and practice of radiation oncology* (2nd ed.). Philadelphia: J. B. Lippincott.

Thomas, G., & Dembo, A. (1994). The ovary. In J. Cox (Ed.), *Moss' radiation oncology: rationale, technique, results* (7th ed.). St. Louis: Mosby.

Turrisi, A. (1994). Principles of combined radiation therapy and chemotherapy. In J. Cox (Ed.), *Moss' radiation oncology: rationale, technique, results* (7th ed.). St. Louis: Mosby.

Wasserman, T., & Kligerman, M. (1992). Chemical modifiers of radiation. In C. Perez & L. Brady (Eds.), *Principles and practice of radiation oncology* (2nd ed.). Philadelphia: J. B. Lippincott.

Willman, K. Y., Cox, R. S., & Donaldson, S. S. (1994). Radiation-induced height impairment in pediatric Hodgkin's disease. *International Journal of Radiation Oncology, Biology, Physics, 28,* 85-92.

Withers, H. R. (1992). Biologic basis of radiation therapy. In C. Perez & L. Brady (Eds.), *Principles and practice of radiation oncology* (2nd ed.). Philadelphia: J. B. Lippincott.

Cancer Chemotherapy

Christine Miaskowski, RN, PhD, FAAN
Carol Viele, RN, MS

INTRODUCTION

This chapter provides an historical perspective on the use of chemotherapy in oncology patients and describes the major mechanisms of action of the drugs used in the treatment of cancer. In addition, the clinical aspects of cancer chemotherapy, including patient and family preparation, safe handling of chemotherapy drugs, and administration of these agents, are reviewed.

HISTORICAL PERSPECTIVE

The use of chemotherapy in the management of cancer dates back to the 1500s when heavy metals were used systemically to treat a variety of cancers. However, these agents were not effective in treating the disease and produced significant toxicity. The modern era of chemotherapy was launched during World War I when sulfur mustard gas was used in chemical warfare. Sailors who were exposed to the nitrogen mustard gas developed bone marrow suppression and lymphoid hyperplasia. These observations led investigators to speculate that if this agent had such profound effects on tissues that normally proliferate rapidly, they might be useful in eradicating cancer cells that also proliferate rapidly.

During World War II, the alkylating agents were recognized as having an antineoplastic effect. In addition, thioguanine and mercaptopurine were developed. The National Cancer Institute, established by an act of Congress in 1937, began specific research programs to develop and test new chemotherapeutic agents. In the 1950s, the antitumor antibiotics were discovered and tested on a variety of tumors.

Throughout the 1960s and early 1970s, work began on the development of platinum compounds. In addition, the first combination chemotherapy regimen (i.e., nitrogen mustard, oncovin, procarbazine, prednisone—or MOPP) was administered and found to be curative in patients with Hodgkin's disease.

With the advent of combination chemotherapy, significant toxicities were associated with the administration of these agents. Therefore the 1980s ushered in an era where a focus was placed on the development of strategies to alleviate the dose-limiting toxicities of chemotherapy (i.e., neutropenia, thrombocytopenia, nausea, and vomiting). Of note, during the 1980s and early 1990s, advances were made in the management of chemotherapy-induced nausea and vomiting with the release of drugs that antagonized dopamine or serotonin receptors. In addition, in 1992, the first granulocyte colony stimulating factor (G-CSF) was approved for use by the Food and Drug Administration (FDA). The development of these products allowed for an increase in the use of multimodal therapy regimens and made possible the development of high-dose chemotherapy regimens (Burke, 1997; Powell, 1996).

The 1990s saw the development of new drugs based on a better understanding of the genetic basis for cancer. Undoubtedly, combination regimens will continue to develop that will include not only multiple chemotherapy drugs, but additional therapies such as biologic response modifiers, monoclonal antibodies, potentiators, and gene therapy. In addition, as researchers gain a better understanding of the molecular biology of tumor growth and cell kinetics, approaches will be developed to overcome multidrug resistance to chemotherapy in patients with recurrent cancers.

BIOLOGIC AND PHARMACOLOGIC BASIS FOR CANCER CHEMOTHERAPY

Cancer is a disease of the cell that is characterized by abnormal growth and spread of affected cells. The purpose of treating cancer cells with chemotherapy is to prevent these cells from multiplying, invading, and metastasizing to distant sites. Unlike surgery or radiation therapy, cancer chemotherapy is a systemic treatment that enables drugs to reach the site of the tumor as well as distant sites.

The biologic basis of cancer chemotherapy rests on our understanding of the cell cycle. The cell cycle of cancer cells is qualitatively the same as that of normal cells (Skeel, 1991). As illustrated in Fig. 5-1, the cell cycle is the sequence of steps that both normal and cancer cells use to grow and replicate. This process of cell growth and replication involves five phases that are designated G_0, G_1, S, G_2, and M.

Cells begin their growth during a postmitotic phase called G_1. During G_1, the cells synthesize ribonucleic acid (RNA), various proteins, and the enzymes necessary for deoxyribonucleic acid (DNA) production. G_1 is highly variable in length. The variance in the length of time a cell spends in G_1 is mostly the result of another phase, called G_0, in which the cell is not actively committed to division (also termed the *resting phase* or *nonproliferative phase* of the cell cycle). When stimulated, the cell moves from G_0 into G_1 and begins the process of proliferation. G_1 is followed by a period of DNA synthesis, hence the name S phase. The S phase lasts approximately 10 to 20 hours. When DNA synthesis is complete, the cell enters a premitotic period called G_2. During G_2, DNA synthesis stops, but RNA and protein synthesis occurs. The G_2 phase of the cell cycle lasts approximately 2 to 10 hours. The G_2 phase is followed immediately by mitosis (M phase). During the M phase, the final steps in chromosome replication and segregation occur, and the cell undergoes cell division and produces two daughter cells. The M phase lasts about 30 minutes to 1 hour. During this time, the rate of RNA and protein synthesis slows as the genetic material is transferred into the daughter cells (Buick, 1994; Burke, 1997; Fischer, Knobf, & Durivage, 1993; Skeel, 1991).

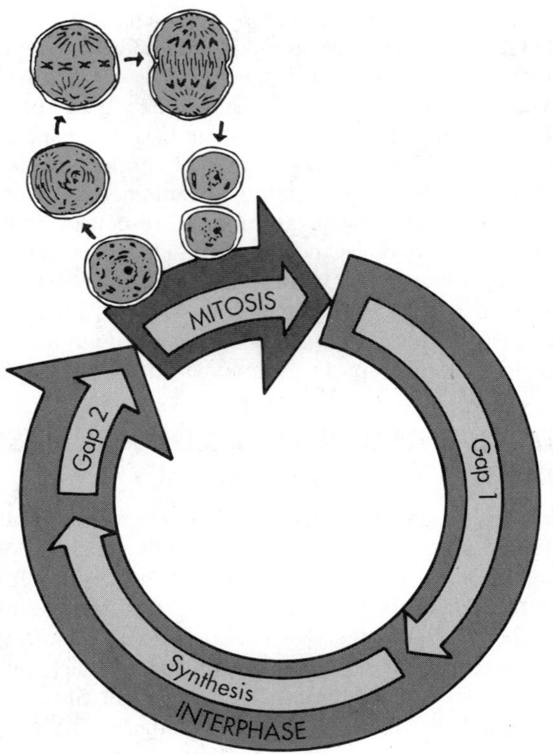

Fig. 5-1 Phases of the cell cycle. (From McCance, K., & Huether, S. [1998]. *Pathophysiology: The biologic basis for disease in adults and children* [3rd ed.]. St. Louis: Mosby.)

Most chemotherapeutic drugs can be grouped based on whether they exert their cytotoxic effects during a specific phase of the cell cycle (i.e., cell cycle phase–specific drugs). Cell cycle phase–specific drugs are usually not effective when cancer cells are predominantly in the dormant phase (i.e., G_0). In contrast, cell cycle–nonspecific drugs theoretically are more likely to be effective against cancer cells that are not in a state of rapid cell division.

Cell Cycle Specificity and Chemotherapy

Cell cycle phase–specific drugs are agents that are most active against cells that are in a specific phase of the cell cycle (Table 5-1). It is important to note that with cell cycle phase-specific agents there is a limit to the number of cells that can be killed with a single, short exposure to the drug, because only those tumor cells that are in the appropriate phase of the cell cycle will be killed. Because all of the cells in a given tumor do not cycle at the same time, one way to increase the number of tumor cells that are killed when they are exposed to a cell cycle phase–specific drug is to increase the time that the cancer cells are exposed to the drug or to administer repeated doses of the drug.

Cell cycle–specific drugs that are effective when cancer cells are actively in cycle but are not dependent on the cell being in a specific phase of the cell cycle are called *cell*

TABLE 5-1 Cell Cycle–Specific and Cell Cycle–Nonspecific Chemotherapeutic Agents

Cell Cycle Phase Specific Chemotherapeutic Agents	
G_1 Phase	**G_2 Phase**
Bleomycin	Bleomycin
Corticosteroids	Etoposide
Hormones	Taxol
L-asparaginase	Vinorelbine
S Phase	**M Phase**
Cytarabine	Vinblastine
5-Fluorouracil	Vincristine
Hydroxyurea	Vindesine
Methotrexate	Vinorelbine
Thioguanine	
Cell Cycle–Specific (Phase Nonspecific) Chemotherapeutic Agents	
Busulfan	Dactinomycin
Carboplatin	Daunorubicin
Chlorambucil	Doxorubicin
Cisplatin	Idarubicin
Cyclophosphamide	Melphalan
Dacarbazine	Liposomal doxorubicin
Cell Cycle–Nonspecific Chemotherapeutic Agents	
Carmustine	Mechlorethamine
Lomustine	Semustine

cycle–specific drugs (phase–nonspecific). This group includes most of the alkylating agents, antitumor antibiotics, and some miscellaneous agents. Many of these agents appear to have some activity in cells that are not in cycle, although not as much activity as when the cells are rapidly dividing. A third group of chemotherapeutic drugs appears to be effective whether cancer cells are in cycle or are resting. These agents are called *cell cycle-nonspecific drugs* (Table 5-1) (Skeel, 1991).

MECHANISM OF ACTION OF CHEMOTHERAPEUTIC DRUGS

Chemotherapeutic drugs are classified based on their mechanism of action (Fig. 5-2). The major classifications for the various chemotherapeutic drugs are listed in Box 5-1. With the exception of the hormones (see Chapter 6), the mechanism of action of each class of chemotherapeutic drugs is described here. In addition, summaries of the specific drugs in each class are provided in a tabular format.

Covalent DNA-Binding Drugs

Covalent DNA-binding drugs or alkylating agents form covalent bonds with DNA, RNA, and protein molecules. Alkylation of DNA produces a number of biochemical and cellular consequences, including DNA mutations, cross-linking of DNA, and strand breakage. These consequences interfere with the cellular replication of DNA, the transcription of RNA, and the translation of messenger RNA (m-RNA) into protein products. However, the precise mechanism by which alkylating agents produce DNA lesions that disrupt critical cellular processes are poorly understood. Tumor cell resistance to this class of chemotherapeutic drugs appears to be mediated by efficient glutathione conjugation or by enhanced enzymatic DNA repair processes (Grochow, 1996; McGovren, 1994).

All of the alkylating agents share the same dose-related toxicity of myelosuppression. These drugs exhibit a steep dose response curve that does not appear to plateau in terms of the drugs' cytotoxic effects. These properties make this class of drugs particularly suitable for the dose-intense preparative regimens used in bone marrow transplantation (Grochow, 1996). The various alkylating agents (Table 5-2) are subdivided according to their chemical structures and mechanisms of covalent bonding.

Box 5-1
Major Classification of Chemotherapeutic Drugs

Covalent DNA-Binding Drugs
Antimetabolites
Antitumor Antibiotics
Microtubule-Targeting Drugs
DNA Topoisomerase Inhibitors
Hormones
Enzymes

DNA, Deoxyribonucleic acid.

Antimetabolites

The antimetabolites are similar in structure to naturally occurring metabolites that are required for the normal functioning of the cell. These drugs interfere with the normal synthesis of nucleic acids by falsely substituting for biosynthetic precursors or other intermediates in metabolic pathways. Ultimately, the antimetabolites inhibit the replication or repair of DNA. This inhibition occurs because of either the direct inhibition of the enzymes needed for DNA replication or repair or because of the incorporation of the antimetabolite into the structure of the DNA molecule. The antimetabolites exert their major cytotoxic activity during the S phase of the cell cycle. Therefore, tumors with a high percentage of cells in the S phase, or with a high growth fraction, would be most sensitive to the action of the antimetabolites. Normal cells, with high growth fractions (e.g., gastrointestinal tract, bone marrow) are also sensitive to the action of the antimetabolites. Therefore gastrointestinal side effects and bone marrow suppression are the most common toxicities associated with this class of drugs. This class of chemotherapeutic agents is more effective when given as a prolonged infusion. Table 5-3 provides a list of the most common groups of antimetabolites (Gutheil & Kearns, 1996; McGovren, 1994).

Antitumor Antibiotics

All of the antitumor antibiotics share the same feature of being natural products of microbial metabolism. Efforts to improve the antiproliferative effects of the antitumor antibiotics and decrease their associated toxicities have resulted in the development of analog compounds. A variety of fungal organisms are the source of the antitumor antibiotics. These naturally occurring antibiotics are generated to protect the organism by interfering with the growth or proliferation of competing life forms. This property is what makes the antitumor antibiotics useful as chemotherapeutic agents (Riggs, 1996).

The antitumor antibiotics produce their cytotoxic effects by a variety of drug-specific mechanisms (Table 5-4). The most common antitumor antibiotics are listed in Table 5-5.

Microtubule-Targeting Drugs

Most of the microtubule-targeting drugs are plant alkaloids. These drugs appear to act by binding to specific sites on tubulin, a protein that polymerizes to form cellular microtubules. Microtubules are critical structural units that are involved in a number of cellular activities. One of these activities is the formation of the mitotic spindle (McGovren, 1994; Rowinsky & Donehower, 1996).

Currently, two classes of microtubule-targeting drugs are used in the treatment of cancer, the vinca alkaloids and the taxanes (Table 5-6). These two classes of microtubule-

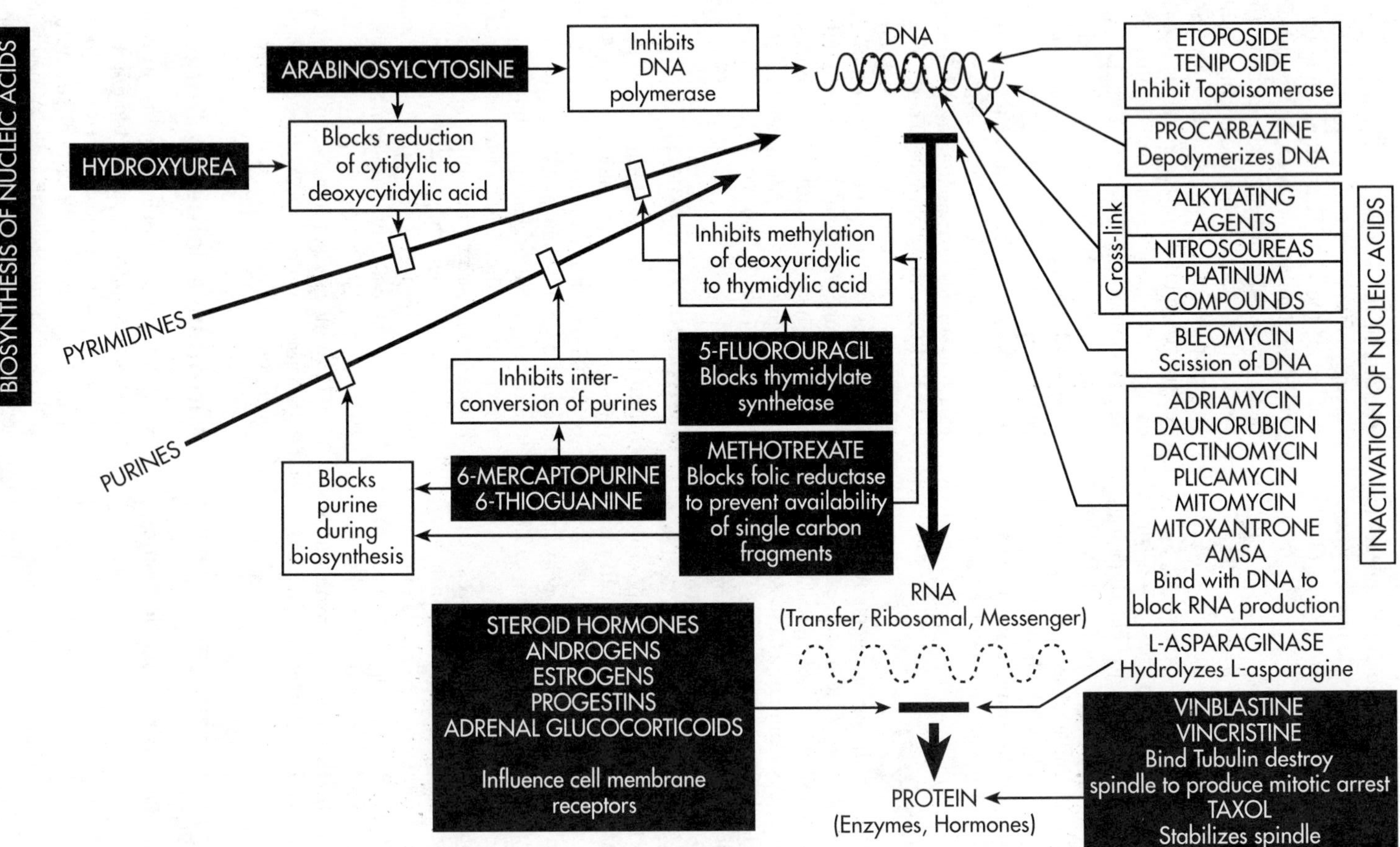

Fig. 5-2 Mechanism of action of chemotherapeutic agents. (From Krakoff I. [1991]. Cancer chemotherapeutic and biologic agents. *CA-Cancer Journal of Clinicians, 41*[5], 264-278.)

TABLE 5-2 Covalent DNA-Binding Drugs

Drug Name	Therapeutic Use	Side Effects/Toxicities
Nitrogen Mustards		
Mechlorethamine	Hodgkin's disease, NHL	Amenorrhea, drowsiness, fever, granulocytopenia, hyperpyrexia, nausea and vomiting, maculopapular rash, thrombocytopenia, thrombophlebitis, thrombosis, weakness
Chlorambucil	Breast, choriocarcinoma, CCL, Hodgkin's disease, NHL, ovarian	Amenorrhea, azoospermia, coma, drug fever, hepatitis, lymphocytopenia, nausea and vomiting, neutropenia, periorbital edema, pulmonary fibrosis, secondary malignancy, seizures, skin rash, thrombocytopenia
Melphalan	Breast, multiple myeloma, ovarian, rhabdomyosarcoma, sarcomas, testicular	Alopecia, dermatitis, hypersensitivity reactions, leukopenia, pulmonary fibrosis, stomatitis, thrombocytopenia
Cyclophosphamide	Acute leukemia, bladder, bone marrow transplant, breast, Burkitt's lymphoma, endometrial, multiple myeloma, neuroblastoma, non-Hodgkin's lymphomas, ovarian, sarcoma, small cell lung (oat cell) cancer, stem cell transplant, testicular, Wilms' tumor	Alopecia, amenorrhea, anorexia, bladder cancer, cardiotoxicity (high doses), hemorrhagic cystitis, hepatotoxicity, hyponatremia, leukopenia, nausea and vomiting, pneumonitis, SIADH, testicular atrophy, thrombocytopenia
Ifosfamide	Acute leukemia, breast, bronchogenic carcinoma, chronic leukemia, germ-cell testicular, Hodgkin's disease, non-small cell lung, ovarian, soft tissue sarcoma, stem cell transplant	Alopecia, ataxia, confusion, dysuria, hemorrhagic cystitis, hepatotoxicity, lethargy, leukopenia, nausea and vomiting, nephrotoxicity, pancytopenia, seizures, sterile phlebitis, stupor, urinary frequency, weakness
Aziridines		
Thiotepa	Bladder, breast, Hodgkin's disease, leukemia, lymphoma, lymphosarcoma, ovarian, stem cell transplant	Allergic reaction, anemia, dizziness, headache, leukopenia, nausea and vomiting, paresthesias, thrombocytopenia
Altretamine	Breast, bronchogenic carcinoma, cervical, childhood leukemias, lymphomas, NHL, ovarian	Agitation, abdominal cramps, anorexia, ataxia, confusion, depression, diarrhea, hallucinations, leukopenia, loss of deep tendon reflexes, nausea, paresthesias, Parkinson-like symptoms, peripheral neuropathy, petit mal-type seizures, skin rash, thrombocytopenia, vomiting
Mitomycin	Bladder, breast, cervical, CML, colon, gallbladder, gastric head and neck, non-small cell lung, ovarian, pancreatic, uterine	Alopecia, anemia, anorexia, confusion, drowsiness, extravasation, fatigue, interstitial pneumonia, leukopenia, nausea and vomiting, nephrotoxicity, purple-colored nail beds, stomatitis, thrombocytopenia, venoocclusive disease of the liver
Alkane Sulfonates		
Busulfan	Bone marrow transplant, CML, stem cell transplant	Adrenal insufficiency, amenorrhea, aplastic anemia, diarrhea, gynecomastia, hyperpigmentation, hyperuricemia, interstitial pulmonary fibrosis, leukopenia, ovarian suppression, secondary malignancies, thrombocytopenia
Carmustine	Bone marrow transplant, cutaneous T-cell lymphoma, glioblastoma, Hodgkin's disease, malignant melanoma, multiple myeloma	Burning sensation in extremity, facial flushing, gynecomastia, hepatotoxicity, hyperpigmentation, leukopenia, nausea and vomiting, optic neuroretinitis, pain at intravenous site, pulmonary fibrosis, renal toxicity, thrombocytopenia
Lomustine	Brain tumors, gastric cancer, Hodgkin's disease, multiple myeloma, non-small cell lung, prostate cancer	Alopecia, anorexia, ataxia, confusion, diarrhea, hepatotoxicity, lethargy, leukopenia, nausea and vomiting, nephrotoxicity, stomatitis, thrombocytopenia
Streptozocin	Beta pancreatic islet cell tumors, gallbladder, Hodgkin's disease, non-beta pancreatic islet cell tumors, non-small cell lung, oral cavity, synovial sarcoma, Zollinger-Ellison tumors	Altered glucose metabolism, burning sensation at injection site, duodenal ulcers, hepatotoxicity, nausea and vomiting, nephrotoxicity

CLL, Chronic lymphocytic leukemia; *CML*, Chronic myelogenous leukemia; *NHL*, Non-Hodgkin's lymphoma; SIADH, Syndrome of inappropriate antidiuretic hormone secretion

Continued

TABLE 5-2 Covalent DNA-Binding Drugs—cont'd

Drug Name	Therapeutic Use	Side Effects/Toxicities
Platinum Compounds		
Cisplatin	Bladder, bone marrow transplant, breast, colorectal, gastric, head and neck, non-small cell lung, osteosarcoma, ovarian, penile, pediatric brain tumors, small cell lung	Anaphylaxis, anemia, atrial fibrillation, bundle branch block, cellulitis at injection site, hepatotoxicity, hypomagnesemia, nausea and vomiting, nephrotoxicity, ototoxicity, peripheral neuropathy, SIADH, ST- and T-wave abnormalities
Carboplatin	Bladder, bone marrow transplant, endometrial, head and neck, non-small cell lung, ovarian, relapsed/refractory acute leukemia, testicular	Anemia, diarrhea, hematuria, hepatoxocity, leukopenia, nausea and vomiting, nephrotoxicity, thrombocytopenia
Methylating Agents		
Dacarbazine	Hodgkin's disease, malignant melanoma, soft tissue sarcomas	Alopecia, anemia, hepatotoxicity, extravasation, facial flushing, facial paresthesias, flulike syndrome, leukopenia, photosensitivity, nausea and vomiting, thrombocytopenia
Procarbazine	Brain tumor, bronchogenic carcinoma, Hodgkin's disease, malignant melanoma, multiple melanoma, NHL	Alopecia, amenorrhea, anemia, anorexia, ataxia, azoospermia, diarrhea, diplopia, dizziness, flulike syndrome, headache, nausea and vomiting, neuropathies, nystagmus, papilledema, paresthesias, photophobia, pruritus, retinal hemorrhage, thrombocytopenia

CLL, Chronic lymphocytic leukemia; *CML,* Chronic myelogenous leukemia; *NHL,* Non-Hodgkin's lymphoma; SIADH, Syndrome of inappropriate antidiuretic hormone secretion.

targeting drugs have different mechanisms of action. The vinca alkaloids (i.e., vincristine, vinblastine, vinorelbine, vindesine) exert their antitumor effects by disrupting the microtubules that comprise the mitotic spindle. The end result of this disruption is the arrest of mitosis. This group of drugs not only affects the M phase of the cell cycle but also has activity during the S phase of the cell cycle. Additional biochemical effects of the vinca alkaloids include the inhibition of DNA and RNA synthesis. In contrast, the taxanes exert their cytotoxic effects by blocking cells in mitosis by overstabilizing microtubule rather than by inhibiting microtubule assembly.

DNA-Topoisomerase Inhibitors

One of the major characteristics of DNA is its double helix structure. Scientists have wondered how these two supercoiled strands separate during replication. It is known that the dynamic three-dimensional arrangement of the DNA molecule is due to its topologic state, that is, its highly ordered twisting and winding of the double-strand molecule around itself. In the early 1970s, Wang (1969, 1971) found that cell extracts from *Escherichia coli* were capable of inducing coiling and relaxation of DNA. This protein, initially named the *omega protein,* was named 8 years later as *E. coli*-DNA topoisomerase I (Wang & Liu, 1979). Later a similar product was identified in mouse cell extracts (Champoux & Dulbecco, 1972). Then in 1976, Gellert, Mizuuchi, O'Dea, & Nash (1976) identified another enzyme from *E. coli* with effects exactly opposite to that of *E. coli*-DNA topoisomerase I. Therefore, the topoisomerases are classified as topoisomerase I or topoisomerase II based on their ability to cleave one or two strands of DNA, respectively. Both enzymes are found in the nucleus of the cell and are responsible for controlling, maintaining, and modifying the structure and function of DNA. To perform these activities, the topoisomerases induce transient breaks in one or both strands of DNA and then rejoin the nicked strand to the intact DNA. Therefore these enzymes play a critical role in the regulation of DNA replication and transcription (Berg, 1997; Donehower & Rowinsky, 1996; McGovren, 1994; Shahab & Perry, 1996).

The chemotherapeutic drugs that affect the topoisomerase enzymes are classified as DNA topoisomerase I inhibitors and DNA topoisomerase II inhibitors. It is believed that the formation of drug-topoisomerase-DNA complexes block critical functions within the cell such as DNA replication or serve to trigger as yet unknown mechanisms that mediate cell death.

The camptothecins are classified as DNA topoisomerase I inhibitors. Camptothecin is a plant alkaloid that exists in the wood, bark, leaves, and fruit of an Oriental tree called *Camptotheca acuminata.* This product has been used in traditional Chinese medicine to treat a variety of illnesses including cancer. The National Cancer Institute has tested an extract of *C. acuminata* and established its antitumor activity. In the 1980s, the target for camptothecin's activity, namely the enzyme topoisomerase I was identified. It was noted that topoisomerase I was overexpressed in human colon cancer and other malignancies. These findings led to the

TABLE 5-3 Antimetabolites

Drug Name	Therapeutic Use	Side Effects/Toxicities
Folate Antagonists		
Methotrexate	ALL, AML, breast, Burkitt's lymphoma, chorioadenoma, choriocarcinoma, chorioepithelioma, epidermoid cancer of the head and neck, hydatidiform mole, lung, NHL, osteogenic sarcoma, ovarian	Alopecia, anemia, anorexia, blurred vision, depigmentation, diarrhea, dizziness, erythematous rashes, folliculitis, gingivitis, glossitis, hepatotoxicity, hyperpigmentation, leukopenia, malaise, nausea and vomiting, nephrotoxicity, pharyngitis, photosensitivity, pruritus, stomatitis, thrombocytopenia, ulcerative stomatitis, urticaria, vasculitis
Trimetrexate	Bladder, colorectal, malignant mesothelioma	Alopecia, hyperpigmentation, maculopapular rash, mucositis, myelosuppression, vomiting
Pyrimidine Antagonists		
5-Fluorouracil	Basal cell, bladder, breast, colon, head and neck, pancreas, prostate, rectal, renal cell, squamous cell of the esophagus, stomach	Acute cerebellar syndrome, alopecia, diarrhea, esophagitis, headache, hyperpigmentation of the nail beds, leukopenia, maculopapular rash, MI, nausea and vomiting, palmar-plantar erythrodysesthesias, photosensitivity, visual disturbances, proctitis, stomatitis, thrombocytopenia
Fluorodeoxyuridine	Biliary tract, colon, GI tract adenocarcinoma, liver, oral cavity	Abdominal cramps, abdominal pain, alopecia, anemia, anorexia, biliary cirrhosis, blurred vision, depression, diarrhea, edema, gastric ulceration, hepatotoxicity, hyperpigmentation of veins, lethargy, leukopenia, mucositis, nausea and vomiting, nystagmus, pruritus, rash, thrombocytopenia, vertigo
Azacytidine	ANLL, myelodysplastic syndrome	Alopecia, azotemia, diarrhea, leukopenia, muscle weakness, myalgias, nausea and vomiting
Purine Antagonists		
6-Mercaptopurine	ALL, CML, NHL	Anemia, anorexia, drug fever, dry scaling rash, eosinophilia, hematuria, hepatotoxicity, leukopenia, mucositis, nausea and vomiting, thrombocytopenia
6-Thioguanine	ALL, AML, CML	Anemia, anorexia, diarrhea, hepatotoxicity, hyperuricemia, leukopenia, nausea and vomiting, stomatitis, thrombocytopenia, unsteady gait
Chlorodeoxy-adenosine	Hairy cell leukemia, AML	Anemia, fever, neutropenia, peripheral neuropathy, thrombocytopenia, transient blindness
Pentostatin	ALL, adult T-cell leukemia, CLL, hairy cell leukemia, mycosis fungoides	Dry skin, fatigue, granulocytopenia, hepatotoxicity, keratoconjunctivitis, lethargy, nausea and vomiting, nephrotoxicity
Sugar-Modified Analogues		
Cytarabine	ANLL, CML, CNS leukemia, Hodgkin's disease, NHL	Acral erythema (palms and soles), anorexia, cerebellar toxicity, diarrhea, flulike syndrome, GI ulceration, hepatotoxicity, leukopenia, nausea and vomiting, pain at injection site, rash, stomatitis, thrombocytopenia, thrombophlebitis, urinary retention
Fludarabine	ALL, ANLL, CLL, gliomas, low-grade lymphomas, mycosis fungoides	Anemia, CNS toxicity, diarrhea, granulocytopenia, interstitial pneumonitis, lymphocytopenia, nausea and vomiting, skin rash, somnolence, thrombocytopenia, tumor lysis syndrome
Ribonucleotide Reductase Inhibitors		
Hydroxyurea	CML, head and neck, malignant melanoma, refractory ovarian	Acral erythema, anemia, constipation, convulsions, diarrhea, dizziness, dysuria, facial erythema, fever, hallucinations, headache, leukopenia, maculopapular rash, nausea and vomiting, radiation "recall," stomatitis, thrombocytopenia

ALL, Acute lymphocytic leukemia; *ANLL,* Acute nonlymphocytic leukemia; *CLL,* Chronic lymphocytic leukemia; *CML,* Chronic myelogenous leukemia; *CNS,* Central nervous system; *GI,* Gastrointestinal; *MI,* Myocardial infarction; *NHL,* Non-Hodgkin's lymphoma.

TABLE 5-4 Mechanism of Action of Antitumor Antibiotics

Drug Name	Identified Mechanisms Producing Cytotoxicity
Doxorubicin	Intercalation into DNA and RNA
Daunorubicin	Inhibition of DNA and RNA polymerases
Idarubicin	Generation of oxygen-free radicals
Mitoxantrone	Single- and double-strand DNA breaks
	Peroxidation of cell membrane and mitochondrial lipids
	Cell surface cytotoxic action
	Inhibition of glutathione synthesis
Dactinomycin	Intercalation into DNA (G-C base pairs)
	Inhibition of DNA-directed RNA synthesis
Bleomycin	Generation of oxygen-free radicals
	Intercalation into DNA
	Single- and double-strand DNA breaks
Mitomycin C	Generation of oxygen-free radicals
	Alkylation of DNA
	Crosslinking of DNA strands
	Single-strand DNA breaks
Plicamycin	Binding to DNA requires a divalent cation
	Inhibition of RNA synthesis
	Single-strand DNA breaks
	Inhibition of adenosine deaminase

DNA, Deoxyribonucleic acid; *RNA,* Ribonucleic acid.
Reprinted with permission from Riggs, C.E. (1996). Antitumor antibiotics and related compounds. In M.C. Perry (Ed.), *The cancer chemotherapy sourcebook* (2nd ed). Baltimore: Williams & Wilkins.

development of two semisynthetic topoisomerase I inhibitors, topotecan and irinotecan (Table 5-7). Both of these drugs have a superior therapeutic index than that of camptothecin (Berg, 1997; Shahab & Perry, 1996).

The epipodophyllotoxins are classified as DNA topoisomerase II inhibitors. The epipodophyllotoxins are extracted from the roots and rhizomes of the May apple or mandrake plant, *Podophyllum peltatum.* These extracts have been used as cathartics, antiemetics, and antihelminthics and for the treatment of condylomata acuminata. Two derivatives of epipodophyllotoxin, etoposide and teniposide, are being used in the treatment of cancer (Donehower & Rowinsky, 1996) (Table 5-7).

Enzymes

In 1953, it was appreciated that guinea pig serum had antitumor activity particularly for acute lymphocytic leukemia (ALL). It was shown that this antitumor activity resides in the enzyme L-asparaginase. Most normal cells possess the ability to synthesize the amino acid asparagine, which is necessary for protein synthesis. Some tumor cells, especially ALL, do not possess this ability and require exogenous asparagine. The enzyme asparaginase converts asparagine to nonfunctional aspartic acid and deprives the cancer cells of a crucial amino acid. Therefore treatment of sensitive cancer cells with L-asparaginase results in the rapid inhibition of protein synthesis and delayed inhibition of DNA and RNA synthesis (Lyss, 1996; McGovren, 1994). The profile of L-asparaginase is found in Table 5-8.

DEVELOPMENT OF DRUG RESISTANCE

Resistance to antineoplastic chemotherapy is a combined characteristic of a specific drug, a specific tumor, and a specific host whereby the drug is ineffective in controlling the tumor without excessive toxicity (Skeel, 1991). Drug resistance is the opposite of sensitivity of a specific chemotherapeutic agent for a particular cancer. The ability of a specific cancer to develop resistance to a chemotherapeutic drug or drugs is similar to infectious organisms developing resistance to antimicrobial therapy. The ability of a tumor to develop resistance to cancer chemotherapy is a serious problem and one of the major limitations to achieving a cure for individuals with cancer.

Resistance to chemotherapeutic drugs can be either natural or acquired. *Natural resistance* refers to the initial unresponsiveness of a cancer to a given drug. *Acquired resistance* refers to the unresponsiveness of a cancer that emerges after initially successful treatment with chemotherapy.

The biologic basis for chemotherapeutic drug resistance appears to be related to genetic mechanisms. In tissue culture, drug-resistant cancer cells are generated at a frequency that is consistent with known rates of genetic mutation. In addition, mutagenic agents added to tissue culture increase the frequency of generation of drug-resistant cells. This finding may have significant clinical implications because most chemotherapeutic drugs are mutagenic. Furthermore, there is evidence that one can transfer drug-resistant phenotypes to cancer cells that are drug sensitive by transferring DNA in vitro (Buick, 1994).

Genetic changes underlying drug resistance may include point mutations or gene amplification. Much of the available evidence suggests that resistance to antineoplastic drugs occurs through gene amplification (e.g., by overproduction of P-glycoprotein; see later discussion). There are three basic categories of resistance to chemotherapy: kinetic, pharmacologic, and biochemical.

Drug Resistance Due to Cell Kinetic Phenomenon

Drug resistance based on cell kinetic phenomenon involves tumor growth fractions and cell cycle specificity and phase specificity. In other words, if a patient receives a chemotherapeutic agent that acts at the S phase of the cell life cycle, that patient's tumor will be resistant to the effects of chemotherapy if the tumor cells do not pass through the S phase of the cell life cycle during the time of drug exposure. In addition, if the tumor has reached a plateau growth phase with a small growth fraction, the tumor may be resistant or insensitive to many classes of chemotherapeutic agents (Goldie, 1996; Skeel, 1991). Strategies to overcome resistance resulting from cellular kinetics include (1) reduc-

TABLE 5-5 Antitumor Antibiotics

Drug Name	Therapeutic Use	Side Effects/Toxicities
Doxorubicin	ALL, ANLL, breast, bladder, Ewing's sarcoma, hepatocellular, Hodgkin's disease, neuroblastoma, NHL, non-small cell lung cancer, ovarian, small cell lung cancer, thyroid, Wilms' tumor	Alopecia, anemia, congestive heart failure, conjunctivitis, extravasation, hyperpigmentation, leukopenia, mucositis, nausea and vomiting, phlebosclerosis, radiation recall, thrombocytopenia
Daunorubicin	ALL, ANLL	Alopecia, congestive heart failure, contact dermatitis, extravasation, fever and chills, hepatotoxicity, hyperpigmentation of the nail beds, hyperuricemia, leukopenia, nausea and vomiting, nephrotoxicity, stomatitis, thrombocytopenia, urticaria
Dactinomycin	Embryonal carcinoma of the testis, Ewing's sarcoma, gestational choriocarcinoma, KS, melanoma, rhabdomyosarcoma, testicular, Wilms' tumor	Acne, alopecia, anemia, erythema, hepatotoxicity, hyperpigmentation, leukopenia, nausea and vomiting, radiation "recall" skin reactions, thrombocytopenia
Bleomycin	Anus, cervix, head and neck, Hodgkin's lymphoma, lung, NHL, penis, rectum, skin, testicular, vulva	Acute pulmonary edema, alopecia, desquamation, fever, headache, hyperpigmentation, lethargy, myelosuppression, nausea and vomiting, pain at injection site, pneumonitis, renal failure, stomatitis
Mitomycin C	Bladder, breast, cervical, CML, colon, gallbladder, gastric, head and neck, non-small cell lung, ovarian, pancreas, uterine	Alopecia, anemia, anorexia, confusion, drowsiness, extravasation, fatigue, interstitial pneumonia, leukopenia, nausea and vomiting, nephrotoxicity, purple-colored nail beds, stomatitis, thrombocytopenia, venoocclusive disease of the liver
Plicamycin	Disseminated embryonal cell carcinoma of the testis, germ cell tumor, hypercalcemia of malignancy	Anorexia, diarrhea, epistaxis, facial flushing, hemorrhage, hepatotoxicity, hypocalcemia, metallic taste, nausea and vomiting, nephrotoxicity, thrombocytopenia
Idarubicin	ALL, ANLL, CML	Alopecia, cardiotoxicity, diarrhea, extravasation, hepatotoxicity, leukopenia, mucositis, nausea and vomiting, rash, thrombocytopenia, urticaria
Mitoxantrone	ANLL, breast, ovarian	Alopecia, anemia, cardiac toxicity, leukopenia, nausea and vomiting, stomatitis, thrombocytopenia

ALL, Acute lymphocytic leukemia; *ANLL,* Acute nonlymphocytic leukemia; *CML,* Chronic myelogenous leukemia; *KS,* Kaposis' sarcoma; NHL, Non-Hodgkin's lymphoma.

ing tumor bulk with radiation therapy or surgery, (2) using combinations of chemotherapeutic agents such as drugs that are cell cycle phase–specific and cell cycle–nonspecific, and (3) scheduling chemotherapy administration to prevent phase escape or to synchronize cell populations and increase tumor cell kill (Skeel, 1991).

Pharmacologic Causes of Resistance

True pharmacologic resistance is caused by the poor transport of chemotherapeutic drugs into certain body tissues and tumor cells. For example, the central nervous system is a site where most drugs fail to reach effective concentrations (Skeel, 1991).

Biochemical Mechanisms of Drug Resistance

The major biochemical mechanisms involved in the development of resistance to chemotherapeutic drugs are listed in Box 5-2. The more that is known about the mechanism of action of a chemotherapeutic drug at a molecular level, the easier it will be to discern the mechanisms underlying the development of drug resistance. However, as noted by Goldie (1996), the general principle is that for a drug to have some lethal effect on the cell, it must first be transported across the cell membrane; it may require some form of intracellular activation; and then it may bind with an intracellular target. Whether the damage to the cell is lethal depends in part on the capacity of the cell to repair or circumvent the biochemical lesion induced by the chemotherapeutic drug.

Drug-resistant states can arise from modification of any or all of the processes indicated previously. Highly drug-resistant phenotypes may exhibit several changes that result in the drug's inability to produce a cytotoxic effect.

Impaired Transport of the Chemotherapeutic Drug Across the Cell Membrane. Two types of impaired drug transport can occur in chemotherapy-resistant tumor cells. Many chemotherapeutic agents enter the cell through some type of facilitated transport mechanism. In

TABLE 5-6 Microtubule-Targeting Drugs

Drug Name	Therapeutic Use	Side Effects/Toxicities
Vinca Alkaloids		
Vincristine	ALL, breast, Ewing's sarcoma, Hodgkin's disease, neuroblastoma, NHL, rhabdomyosarcoma, Wilms' tumor	Anorexia, constipation, fatigue, fever, extravasation, jaw pain, loss of deep tendon reflexes, paralytic ileus, SIADH
Vinblastine	Bladder, breast, choriocarcinoma, CML, histiocytosis X, Hodgkin's disease, NHL, renal cell carcinoma, testicular	Abdominal pain, adynamic ileus, alopecia, constipation, corneal irritation, depression, headache, jaw pain, leukopenia, malaise, muscle pain, nausea and vomiting, orthostatic hypotension, paresthesias, peripheral neuropathy, photosensitivity, rash, Raynaud's phenomenon, seizures, stomatitis, tachycardia, urine retention
Vindesine	ALL, breast, CML (blast crisis), colorectal, esophageal, Hodgkin's disease, lung, malignant glioma, melanoma, NHL	Abdominal cramping, alopecia, cellulitis, cortical blindness, distal paresthesias, interstitial pneumonitis, loss of deep tendon reflexes, maculopapular rash, nausea and vomiting, neutropenia, paralytic ileus, phlebitis, proximal muscle weakness, stomatitis, thrombocytopenia
Vinorelbine	Breast, non-small cell lung	Alopecia, constipation, diarrhea, dyspnea, extravasation, fatigue, granulocytopenia, injection site reactions, nausea and vomiting, peripheral neuropathy
Taxanes		
Paclitaxel	Breast, malignant melanoma, ovarian	Alopecia, bradycardia, diarrhea, dysgeusia, flulike symptoms, granulocytopenia, hypersensitivity reactions, mucositis, nausea and vomiting, peripheral neuropathy, phlebitis, rash
Docetaxel	Metastatic breast cancer, non-small cell lung, ovarian	Alopecia, fatigue, fluid retention syndrome, hypersensitivity reactions, maculopapular rash, mucositis, nausea, neutropenia, onychodystrophy, peripheral neuropathy, vomiting
Estramustine	Metastatic prostate cancer	Gynecomastia, hepatotoxicity, nausea and vomiting, rash, thrombocytopenia, thrombophlebitis (IV use)

ALL, Acute lymphocytic leukemia; *CML,* Chronic myelogenous leukemia; *IV,* Intravenous; *NHL,* Non–Hodgkin's lymphoma; *SIADH,* Syndrome of inappropriate antidiuretic hormone secretion.

TABLE 5-7 DNA Topoisomerase Inhibitors

Drug Name	Therapeutic Use	Side Effects/Toxicities
DNA Topoisomerase I Inhibitors		
Topotecan	Advanced ovarian epithelial cancers, leukemia, small cell lung cancer	Alopecia, myelosuppression, nausea and vomiting, paresthesias, peripheral neuropathy
Irinotecan	Advanced colorectal cancer	Alopecia, diarrhea (profound), myelosuppression, nausea and vomiting
DNA Topoisomerase II Inhibitors		
Etoposide	ALL, ANLL, Hodgkin's disease, lymphoma, lymphosarcoma, reticulum cell sarcoma, small cell bronchogenic carcinoma, small cell lung, testicular	Allergic reactions, alopecia, anorexia, bronchospasm, chemical phlebitis, fatigue, fever, headache, hypotension, leukopenia, nausea and vomiting, somnolence, stomatitis, thrombocytopenia
Teniposide	ALL, neuroblastoma, NHL	Chemical phlebitis, hemolytic anemia, hypersensitivity reaction hypertension, hypotension, leukopenia, thrombocytopenia

ALL, Acute lymphocytic leukemia; *ANLL,* Acute nonlymphocytic leukemia; *NHL,* Non-Hodgkin's lymphoma.

TABLE 5-8 Enzymes

Drug Name	Therapeutic Use	Side Effects/Toxicities
L-asparaginase	ALL	Acute pancreatitis, anaphylaxis, anemia, anorexia, depression, disorientation, hallucinations, hepatotoxicity, hypersensitivity reactions, lethargy, malaise, nausea and vomiting, somnolence, recent memory loss

ALL, Acute lymphocytic leukemia.

Box 5-2
Biochemical Mechanisms Involved in Drug Resistance

- Impaired transport of the chemotherapeutic drug across the cell membrane
- Decreased intracellular activation of the chemotherapeutic drug
- Altered or increased amounts of the intracellular target for the chemotherapeutic drug
- Increased intracellular detoxification of the chemotherapeutic drug
- Increased efficiency of DNA repair of cellular damage caused by the chemotherapeutic drug
- The development of the multidrug resistant (MDR) phenotype

many cases, this process involves the binding of the chemotherapeutic drug to a receptor protein on the cell membrane. Then the protein receptor-drug complex is translocated across the cell membrane, with release of drug into the cell where it exerts its cytotoxic effects. Some tumor cells become resistant to cancer chemotherapy by altering the structure of the protein receptor or by reducing the amount of receptor on the cell membrane. The net result is a decrease in the intracellular concentration of the chemotherapeutic drug to below cytotoxic concentrations. Two chemotherapeutic drugs that can exhibit this type of drug resistance are methotrexate and nitrogen mustard (Goldenberg & Begleiter, 1980; Goldie, 1996; Goldman, 1971).

The second type of transport alteration that can occur is an increase in cellular mechanisms that results in the extrusion of the drug after it has been transported into the cell. This process also reduces intracellular concentrations of the drug below cytotoxic levels (Gerlach, Kartner, Bell, & Ling, 1986; Goldie, 1996).

Decreased Intracellular Activation of the Chemotherapeutic Drug. Most of the purine and pyrimidine analogs (see Table 5-3) must be converted to an appropriate nucleoside or nucleotide within the cell to produce a cytotoxic effect. The conversion of the chemotherapeutic drug to a cytotoxic metabolite requires an enzyme. One biochemical change that can occur within cancer cells, which results in drug resistance, is the loss of one or another of these conversion enzymes. Examples of chemotherapeutic agents affected by this mechanism include 6-mercaptopurine, 6-thioguanine, cytosine arabinoside, and 5-fluorouracil (Goldie, 1996).

Altered or Increased Amounts of the Intracellular Target for the Chemotherapeutic Drug. Many chemotherapeutic drugs appear to exert their cytotoxic effects by binding to a normal cellular enzyme and rendering the enzyme nonfunctional. An example of this type of activity involves the chemotherapeutic drug, methotrexate. Methotrexate exerts its effect by binding to dihydrofolate reductase and blocking its effects. The result of the interaction between methotrexate and dihydrofolate reductase is a disruption in thymidine and purine biosynthesis and subsequent disruption in DNA synthesis. Tumor cells that are resistant to methotrexate may show increased amounts of dihydrofolate reductase or may produce a variant dihydrofolate reductase that is no longer inhibited by methotrexate (Bertino, Donahue, & Simmons, 1963; Flintooff & Asessani, 1980; Goldie, 1996; Williams, Duggleby, Cutler, & Morrison, 1980).

Increased Intracellular Detoxification of the Chemotherapeutic Drug. The glutathione-S-transferase (GST) system consists of a number of isoenzymes that are able to conjugate glutathione to a variety of xenobiotic substances. Such conjugation may significantly reduce the cytotoxic effects of a chemotherapeutic drug. This mechanism appears to play a role in the development of resistance to a number of the alkylating agents (Goldie, 1996; Moscow & Dixon, 1994).

Increased Efficiency of DNA Repair Mechanisms. Many of the chemotherapeutic drugs exert their effects by directly damaging the structural integrity of cellular DNA. Some tumor cells have evolved complex and highly effective mechanisms for repairing damaged DNA segments. These repair mechanisms may involve actually excising the segment of damaged DNA and replacing it with newly synthesized nucleotides that repair the areas of the drug-induced lesions (Goldie, 1996; Lawley & Brookes, 1968; Roberts, Brent, & Crathorn, 1971).

One specific example of increased efficiency in DNA repair mechanisms is observed with tumor cells that are resistant to alkylating agents. This resistance to alkylating agents is associated with a high methyl transferase repair capacity. Tumor cells that have a high methyl transferase repair capacity are designated as Mer^+. Cells with diminished activity of this enzyme are designated Mer^-, and they are particularly vulnerable to damage by nitrosourea-type alkylating agents (Lindahl, 1982; Yarosh, Foote, Mitra, & Day, 1983). It has been suggested that measuring the methyl transferase activity in tumor cells might permit identification of individual patients who would be particularly responsive to treatment with nitrosoureas (Goldie, 1996).

Development of the Multidrug-Resistant Phenotype. An important mechanism of general biochemical drug resistance has been identified. In the 1970s, a number of investigators (Biedler & Riehm, 1970; Ling & Thompson, 1974) showed that tumor cells that were rendered resistant to one class of chemotherapeutic drugs (e.g., vinca alkaloids) would demonstrate resistance to a number of other classes of chemotherapeutic drugs (e.g., anthracyclines). This phenomenon was called *pleiotropic drug resistance,* and in 1976, Juliano and Ling showed that pleiotropic drug resistance was mediated by a 170-kilodalton cell surface membrane glycoprotein called *P-glycoprotein,* which is widely distributed in nature and functions as an extracellular pump for extruding toxic molecules from inside the cell to the extracellular environment.

The substances that can bind and be extruded by the P-glycoprotein pump mechanism tend to be large heterocyclic compounds that are derived from the natural environment (e.g., plant alkaloids and antibiotics). This finding suggests a physiologic role for this drug-resistance marker and suggests why it is capable of mediating resistance to a broad range of chemotherapy drugs.

The P-glycoprotein associated with multidrug resistance (MDR) is coded by the gene *mdr-1.* It is one of a large family of transport glycoproteins that have significant degrees of homology with each other. These proteins are called *ATP-binding cassette (ABC) proteins,* and some of them mediate broad degrees of drug resistance. A recently described protein in this class is multidrug resistance protein (MRP), which is related to P-glycoprotein, and can confer multidrug resistance through the efflux of chemotherapeutic drugs (Goldie, 1996).

The terminology now used to describe the various multidrug resistance phenotypes is confusing. *Classic* MDR refers to the P-glycoprotein transporter described by Juliano and Ling (1976). *Nonclassical* or *atypical* MDR can refer to an ever-expanding list of cellular phenotypes that are characterized by their capacity to display MDR (Goldie, 1996).

The expression of P-glycoprotein can be measured in tumor cells. Studies indicate that there is an association between the expression of P-glycoprotein and prognosis. For example, patients with neuroblastomas or lymphomas, who had a high proportion of P-glycoprotein cells, had a significantly poorer prognosis (Chan et al., 1991; Gascoyne, Tolcher, Van Iderstine, & Connors, 1993). It should be noted that the relationship between P-glycoprotein expression and prognosis is extremely complex. The overexpression of P-glycoprotein may be associated with other markers of drug resistance or other biologic changes (e.g., mutations in the p53 gene) that may confer a poorer prognosis (Goldie, 1996).

Overcoming Multidrug Resistance

Theoretically, it would seem that once one understood the mechanisms underlying MDR, it would be relatively simple to develop and test strategies to overcome this phenomenon. Although many of the approaches to overcome MDR have been effective in the laboratory, none have been useful clinically. The most likely reason for the failure of these strategies in clinical practice is that the mechanisms underlying clinical drug resistance are multifactorial.

Several methods currently under investigation to overcome MDR are the use of drugs that inhibit calcium influx (e.g., verapamil), the use of drugs that inhibit the calcium-binding protein calmodulin, and the use of other drugs that tend to stabilize membranes (e.g., quinidine). Until these methods have undergone clinical trials, several clinical strategies are being used to circumvent MDR. These strategies include giving combination chemotherapy; initiating treatment at the earliest time feasible (i.e., adjuvant chemotherapy), and when available using unique new compounds against drug-refractory tumors. Another strategy used to circumvent MDR is to increase the dose of chemotherapy in order to increase the cellular concentration of the drug to the point that it will overcome the resistance. Administering these high concentrations of drugs will undoubtedly require the use of bone marrow rescue techniques.

CLINICAL USE OF CANCER CHEMOTHERAPY

More than 50 chemotherapeutic drugs are in use today to treat a wide variety of cancers. Depending on the type of cancer, these drugs are used as the primary modality of treatment or as adjuvant or neoadjuvant treatment (Box 5-3). These drugs can be given as single agents or as combination chemotherapy.

Principles of Combination Chemotherapy

Combination chemotherapy involves the use of combinations of drugs to treat a specific cancer. The concept of combination chemotherapy developed between 1960 and 1975 as the mechanisms of tumor cell growth began to be understood more clearly. The reasons that combination chemotherapy regimens may be more effective than the use of single agents in treating cancer and producing a cure are listed in Box 5-4. First, the use of combination chemotherapy regimens may prevent the development of resistant clones of cancer cells. The use of multidrugs with independent mechanisms of action should reduce the development of resistant clones and increase the likelihood of remission and cure. In addition, because most tumors are made up of heterogenous groups of cells, they require several drugs with different mechanisms of action to produce maximal cell kill.

The use of combination regimens that contain cell cycle–specific and cell cycle–nonspecific chemotherapeutic drugs results in the death of tumor cells that are slowly dividing, as well as the death of those cells that are dividing rapidly. The use of cell cycle–nonspecific drugs can also help recruit cells into a more actively dividing state, which results in their being more sensitive to the action of cell cycle–specific drugs (Friedland, 1996; Skeel, 1991).

The use of different combinations of chemotherapeutic agents, with different mechanisms of action, may enhance each other's activities through synergistic interactions (i.e.,

Box 5-3
Terminology Used in Describing Cancer Chemotherapy

1. *Induction:* High-dose, usually combination, chemotherapy given with the intent of inducing complete remission when initiating a curative regimen. The term is usually applied to hematologic malignancies but is applicable to solid tumors.
2. *Consolidation:* Repetition of the induction regimen in a patient who has achieved a complete remission after induction, with the intent of increasing the cure rate or the remission duration.
3. *Intensification:* Chemotherapy after complete remission with higher doses of the same agents used for induction or with different agents at high doses, with the intent of increasing the cure rate or the remission duration.
4. *Maintenance:* Long-term, low-dose, single or combination chemotherapy in a patient who has achieved a complete remission, with the intent of delaying the regrowth of residual tumor cells.
5. *Adjuvant:* A short course of high-dose, usually combination, chemotherapy in a patient with no evidence of residual cancer after surgery or radiotherapy, given with the intent of destroying a small number of residual tumor cells.
6. *Neoadjuvant:* Adjuvant chemotherapy given in the preoperative or perioperative period.
7. *Primary chemotherapy:* Sometimes used as a synonym for neoadjuvant chemotherapy, but also applied to chemotherapy given in the absence of intended surgery or radiotherapy.
8. *Palliative:* Chemotherapy given to control symptoms or prolong life in a patient in whom cure is unlikely.
9. *Salvage:* A potentially curative, high-dose, usually combination, regimen given in a patient who has failed or recurred following a different curative regimen.

Reprinted with permission from Yarbro, J. W. (1996). The scientific basis of chemotherapy. In M. C. Perry (Ed.), *The cancer chemotherapy sourcebook* (2nd ed.). Baltimore: Williams & Wilkins.

these chemotherapeutic agents interfere with different metabolic pathways or act at different sites in the same pathway). The concept of synergy suggests that these chemotherapeutic agents might be used to block the formation of essential cellular components that results in tumor cell death (Sartorelli, 1969).

Finally, the use of combination chemotherapy may decrease the rate at which mutations and therefore resistance develop because the combination regimens create a more hostile environment for tumor cell growth through the use of higher drug concentrations. Multiple drug regimens decrease the possibility that cells in the tumor will be resistant to all of the drugs simultaneously, thus tending to reduce the number of cells within the tumor that are capable of developing drug resistance (Friedland, 1996).

Principles of Selecting Agents for Combination Chemotherapy Regimens. Several principles guide the selection of agents for combination chemotherapy regimens. First, only individually active agents should be used in a combination regimen. An inactive agent should not be added to a combination regimen unless there is a clear and specific biologic or pharmacologic reason to do so (e.g., the use of high-dose methotrexate with leucovorin rescue [i.e., the inactive agent]). A second overriding principle that needs to be followed when selecting drugs for combination regimens is that one should choose drugs, when possible, that have different dose-limiting toxicities. Although adhering to this principle is extremely desirable, it is not always possible. When new combination regimens are developed, expected and unexpected side effects and toxicities must be evaluated carefully (Skeel, 1991).

Box 5-4
Rationale for Using Combination Chemotherapy

- May prevent the development of resistant clones of tumor cells
- Uses drugs with different mechanisms of action to maximize cell kill
- Provides the opportunity to use drugs that act at different phases of the cell cycle to maximize cell kill
- May result in synergistic interactions
- Creates a more "hostile environment" for tumor cell growth

The biologic or pharmacologic rationale for placing different drugs within a combination regimen should be described and tested in the appropriate tumor model. Tests in this model system should demonstrate that the combination regimen produces greater cell kill than any of the agents used alone.

Effectiveness of Combination Chemotherapy Regimens. The use of combination chemotherapy regimens has shown clear benefits in some, but not all, forms of human cancer. The benefits of combination chemotherapy, compared with the same drugs used sequentially, have been seen in such cancers as ALL, Hodgkin's disease, breast cancer, ovarian cancer, small cell and non-small cell cancer of the lung, testicular cancer, bladder cancer, head and neck cancers, and esophageal cancer (Friedland, 1996; Skeel, 1991).

Principles of Adjuvant Chemotherapy

Adjuvant chemotherapy involves a short course of high-dose, usually combination, chemotherapy in a patient who has no evidence of residual cancer after surgery or radiotherapy, given with the intent of destroying a small number of residual cells (Yarbro, 1996). The use of adjuvant chemotherapy is based on data from the 1950s and 1960s that showed that there was an inverse relationship between responses to chemotherapy and the number of tumor cells. In other words, the smaller the number of tumor cells, the better the response to chemotherapy and therefore the possibility of improved survival (Gilewski & Bitran, 1996; Goldin, Venditti, Humphreys, & Mantel, 1956; Martin & Fugmann, 1960; Shapiro & Fugmann, 1957).

According to Gilewski and Bitran (1996), several factors determine the effectiveness of adjuvant chemotherapy. These factors include tumor burden, dose and schedule of the administered chemotherapeutic agent, the use of combination chemotherapy, and the development of drug resistance. As noted earlier with regard to tumor burden, an inverse relationship was found in terms of the absolute number of tumor cells and an individual's response to adjuvant chemotherapy. Patients' responses to adjuvant chemotherapy are improved when their tumor burden is reduced with surgery or radiation therapy before the administration of the drugs. In addition, improvements in response rates are most dramatic when the maximum doses of adjuvant chemotherapy are administered to patients (Gilewski & Bitran, 1996).

Research has demonstrated that the use of combination chemotherapy in the adjuvant setting is beneficial. In addition, information from animal models indicate that the timing of drug administration may have an impact on the therapeutic outcome. However, in human trials, the best time to initiate adjuvant chemotherapy remains to be determined. Most adjuvant chemotherapy regimens begin 4 to 6 weeks after surgery. However, chemotherapy has also been administered in the perioperative (i.e., immediately postoperative) or preoperative (i.e, primary/neoadjuvant) setting. One final factor that may influence a tumor's response to adjuvant chemotherapy is whether the tumor cells that remain after the primary treatment have developed resistance to various chemotherapeutic drugs. One of the strategies used to overcome drug resistance tumors is to administer combination chemotherapy regimens in the adjuvant setting (Gilewski & Bitran, 1996).

Use of Investigational Protocols and Clinical Trials

The discovery of new drugs for use in cancer treatment occurs at a number of different levels. The National Cancer Institute, the pharmaceutical industry, and individual researchers all contribute to the development of new anticancer drugs. More than 10,000 new potential anticancer drugs are screened for antitumor activity each year. However, only a small fraction of these agents ever progress to clinical use (Conley & Van Echo, 1996).

New anticancer drugs proceed through in vitro screening procedures. After testing in cell cultures of human tumor cell lines, the most promising agents progress to animal studies. Pharmacologic and toxicologic studies are performed in animals either simultaneously with an evaluation of in vivo efficacy, or after a drug shows promise in vitro and in vivo. Ideally, the results from the animal studies are used to determine the logical schedule of administration and the initial dose for humans.

New anticancer drugs that demonstrate promising activity and acceptable toxicity in preclinical trials progress to clinical trials. Clinical trials occur in four phases (Table 5-9). The major purpose of a Phase I study is to determine drug toxicities relative to the dose of drug administered. Through a Phase I study, the maximum tolerated dose is determined for a particular drug administration schedule. Patients recruited for Phase I studies have cancers that are no longer responsive to standard therapy for those particular tumors.

The purpose of a Phase II trial is to determine the tumor types for which the new anticancer drug has some activity and to estimate the magnitude of the drug's activity. In addition, Phase II clinical trials attempt to refine the toxicity profile of the new anticancer drug and refine the drug's dosing parameters. Patients entered into Phase II clinical trials must have measurable disease. This criterion usually means that the tumor(s) can be measured accurately in at least two dimensions. Activity of the new anticancer drug is defined as a complete response, a partial response, or progression of disease after a defined period of time. A complete response requires the disappearance of all evidence of disease and no new appearance of disease for a specified interval, usually four weeks. A partial response requires a reduction of at least 50% in the sum of the products of the two longest diameters of all lesions, maintained for at least one course of therapy, and no new appearance of disease. Progression refers to the growth of disease while receiving chemotherapy (Conley & Van Echo, 1996).

Phase III studies of new anticancer drugs are performed with agents that demonstrate significant activity in Phase II studies. The purpose of a Phase III study is to compare the new drug to standard therapy for a particular cancer using a randomized controlled trial. Phase III studies also require patients with measureable disease and may require large numbers of patients, depending on the effectiveness of the new anticancer drug.

Phase IV studies are usually postmarketing studies that are done to define new uses for the drug, new dosing schedules, or additional information about the drug.

TABLE 5-9 Clinical Trials of New Anticancer Drugs

Study Phase	Major Outcomes
Phase I	• Determine the maximum tolerated dose (MTD) • Determine the major drug toxicities in relationship to the dose of drug administered
Phase II	• Determine the tumor types for which the drug has some activity, and estimate the magnitude of the drug's activity • Refine the toxicity profile of the drug • Refine the dosing regimen
Phase III	• Evaluate the effectiveness of the new drug compared with standard treatment
Phase IV	• Define new uses for the new drug, new dosing schedules, or additional information about the drug

Oncology nurses play a critical role in recruiting patients into clinical trials. Many of the Phase I and II clinical trials are conducted in large, comprehensive cancer centers. However, Phase III clinical trials, which require larger numbers of patients, are often conducted through large cooperative groups. Therefore, oncology nurses who work in a variety of settings can be involved in the recruitment of patients for clinical trials.

Oncology nurses need to serve as patient advocates and assist patients in the decision-making process regarding enrollment in a clinical trial. Patients and their family members require education about the goals of the clinical trial and the potential risks and benefits of the treatment regimen. Oncology nurses need to evaluate the patients' level of understanding about the trial within the context of the informed consent process.

PATIENT AND FAMILY PREPARATION FOR CHEMOTHERAPY ADMINISTRATION

The patient and family members need to be prepared for the administration of cancer chemotherapy. This preparation usually involves a prechemotherapy assessment and patient and family education.

Patient Assessment

The nurse who will be administering the patient's chemotherapy should conduct a pretreatment assessment of the patient using the guideline listed in Box 5-5. The assessment data should assist the nurse in developing a management plan and an educational program for the patient and the family members.

Box 5-5
Guidelines for the Pretreatment Assessment of the Chemotherapy Patient

Obtain a Complete Patient and Family History

1. Recent treatment, including surgery, prior chemotherapy, radiation therapy, biotherapy, or hormone therapy
2. Previous and concurrent medical illnesses
3. Previous and concurrent surgical problems
4. Laboratory data
   - Complete blood cell count with differential
   - *Liver function tests:* bilirubin, alkaline phosphatase, alamine aminotransferase
   - *Renal function tests:* serum creatinine, creatinine clearance, uric acid level

Obtain a Psychosocial Assessment of the Patient and the Family Members

1. Reactions to the diagnosis of cancer
2. Previous experience with chemotherapy
3. Coping styles
4. Interpersonal resources
5. Financial resources

Patient and Family Education

The education of patients and family members is an ongoing process that should begin before the administration of chemotherapy. The nurse should use the principles of adult learning to prepare the patient for the chemotherapy treatments. The nurse needs to ascertain the patient and family members' level of understanding of the proposed treatment regimen.

As part of formulating the teaching plan, the nurse should assess the patient and family members' primary language and level of understanding, ability to read, readiness to learn, anxiety levels, and any other potential barriers to learning (Miaskowski, 1997; Powell, 1996). The nurse should review the topics outlined in Box 5-6 and provide written materials to reinforce the verbal instructions.

SAFE HANDLING OF CHEMOTHERAPEUTIC DRUGS

The appropriate methods to ensure the safe handling of chemotherapeutic drugs have been the subject of intense discussion and scientific investigation. Exposure to cytotoxic drugs was recognized as a potential health hazard in the early 1970s (Baker & Connor, 1996; Bingham, 1985; McDiarmid, 1990; Powers et al., 1990; Stoikes, Carlson, Farris, & Walker, 1987). Falck and co-workers (1979) were one of the first groups to demonstrate the potential risks to nurses handling cytotoxic drugs by studying the mutagenicity of urine samples. Subsequent examinations of the workplace documented detectable levels of cytotoxic drugs in airborne samples and on work surfaces (Baker & Connor, 1996). These findings confirmed that exposure is possible even in the absence of obvious direct contact with the cytotoxic drugs.

No long-term adverse effects of exposure to cytotoxic drugs have been demonstrated conclusively. However, the potential risk has been deemed serious enough to warrant the publication of safe handling guidelines for cytotoxic drugs by several organizations and agencies, including the Occupational Safety and Health Administration (OSHA),

Box 5-6
Patient Education Regarding Chemotherapy

1. Review the treatment plan and protocol.
   - Names and actions of the drugs to be administered by the nurse
   - Names and actions of the drugs to be taken by the patient at home
   - Schedule of drug administration
   - Length of the treatment plan
2. Review the purpose or the goals (i.e., cure or palliation) of the chemotherapeutic treatment.
3. Review the potential side effects of chemotherapy and self-care activities to prevent or treat the side effects.
4. Review the schedule and rationale for diagnostic tests.
5. Provide the patient and family members with information on when and how to contact the nurse or the physician.

the American Society of Hospital Pharmacists, the Council on Scientific Affairs of the American Medical Association, the National Study Commission on Cytotoxic Exposure, and the Oncology Nursing Society. In addition, many hospitals and clinics have adapted these guidelines to their specific circumstances.

This section reviews some of the basic principles surrounding the safe handling of chemotherapeutic drugs. Nurses should refer to the guidelines provided by OSHA (Office of Occupational Medicine, Occupational Safety, and Health Administration, 1986; Instruction TED 1.15, 1995) and the Oncology Nursing Society (Powell, 1996) for more detailed information on this subject and for detailed recommendations to guide the development of institutional policies and procedures. Additional recommendations for policies, procedures, and safety materials for handling hazardous drugs were made by the American Society of Hospital Pharmacists (ASHP, 1990). The four major goals of these recommendations are listed in Table 5-10. In addition, practical clinical guidelines for the nurse and pharmacist to follow regarding the preparation and administration of chemotherapeutic drugs are summarized in Table 5-11.

Preparation, Storage, and Transport of Cancer Chemotherapy

Recommendations for the preparation, storage, and transport of cancer chemotherapy are outlined in the Cancer Chemotherapy Guidelines developed by the Oncology Nursing Society (Powell, 1996). The use of appropriate drug preparation, storage, and transport techniques reduces the health care professional's risk of exposure to chemotherapeutic drugs. The main routes of exposure include absorption through the skin, inhalation, and ingestion through contaminated food.

Drug Preparation. All personnel who prepare chemotherapeutic drugs require special training to perform these procedures safely. Chemotherapeutic drugs should be prepared under a Class II, biologic safety cabinet with vertical laminar airflow. Ideally, the hood should be vented to the outside with a blower operating continuously.

The person mixing the chemotherapeutic drugs should follow the manufacturer's recommendations for reconstitution. This individual should wear a long-sleeve, nonabsorbent gown with elastic at the wrists and back closure; the individual should use eye protection, as well as a mask and

TABLE 5-10 Goals, Criteria, and Recommendations for the Safe Handling of Chemotherapeutic Drugs

Goals	Criteria and Recommendations
Goal I Accidental contamination of health care environment, resulting in exposure of personnel, patients, visitors, and family members to hazardous substances, is prevented by maintaining the physical integrity and security of packages of hazardous drugs.	• Limited access to authorized staff • Hazardous drug identification • Policies for transporting hazardous drugs • Storage facilities designed to prevent breakage and limit exposure from leakage
Goal II The preparation of hazardous drugs does not result in contamination of the health care work environment or excessive exposure of personnel, patients, or family members to hazardous drug powders, dusts, liquids, or mists.	• Written policies for drug preparation • Orientation of personnel • Established method of evaluation of staff adherence to policies and procedures • Policies for protective apparel • Proper manipulative technique for drug mixture • Biologic safety cabinet • Procedures established for noninjectable dosage forms • Procedures for accidental exposure • Labeling for hazardous drug handling
Goal III Procedures for administering hazardous drugs prevent the accidental exposure of patients and staff and contamination of the work environment.	• Training programs for personnel • Standards for safe administration • Readily available protective materials
Goal IV The health care setting, its staff, patients, contract workers, visitors, and the outside environment are not exposed to or contaminated with hazardous drug waste materials produced in the course of using these drugs.	• Written policies established and maintained • Identification, containment, and segregation of hazardous drug waste materials • Protocols and materials available to clean up spills • Disposal in accordance with state, federal, and local regulations

Reprinted with permission from Fisher, D. S., Knobf, M. T., & Durivage, H. J. (1993). *The cancer chemotherapy handbook.* St. Louis: Mosby.

TABLE 5-11 Clinical Guidelines for the Preparation and Administration of Chemotherapeutic Drugs

Guideline	Comment
Drug Preparation	
Wash hands thoroughly before and after; wear protective gloves	Powder-free, of good quality; permeability has been demonstrated to be time dependent, and gloves should be changed every 30 min (Stoikes et al., 1987); double gloving is recommended as the safest procedure but does not appear to be common practice (Powers et al., 1990)
Wear disposable closed-front, long-sleeved, cuffed-wrist gowns; do not wear protective clothing out of the drug area	Gloves and a class II hood are perceived as adequate protection from exposure by many; gowns provide an additional barrier to potential skin contact (direct or aerosol), yet, in everyday practice, use of gowns may vary; factors cited are cost, employee adherence, individual technique, and level of benefit
Do not drink, eat, or smoke in the drug preparation area	Protects against ingestion exposure
Prepare drugs in a class II biologic safety cabinet (type B preferred)	The blower of the hood of the cabinet should be left on 24 hours a day, 7 days a week (ASHP, 1990; Powers et al., 1990)
Place absorbent plastic-backed pad on work surface; have a spill kit available in the drug preparation area; use aseptic techniques in drug preparation; use Luer lock fittings whenever possible	Should be changed every shift (hospital) or daily (ambulatory)
Wipe ampule with alcohol, and wrap a sterile gauze around the ampule when breaking; if diluent is added, inject slowly down the side wall of the ampule	Prevents cuts, aerosolization, and skin contamination
Examine vials for any cracks; avoid injecting positive pressure into the vial—slowly add diluent and allow displaced air to escape into the syringe periodically; venting devices may be used by experienced personnel	Venting reduces the pressure but it is not recommended unless a class II hood or hydrophobic filter needle is used; improper use of devices may increase risk of exposure; prevents aerolization
Wrap sterile gauze around the needle and vial when withdrawing solution, maintaining negative pressure; label all drugs; clean cabinet daily and decontaminate weekly (surface area cleansing with high-pH agents, followed by water)	
Administration	
Wash hands thoroughly before and after; wear protective gloves and a disposable gown; discard gloves after each use	Single pair of latex gloves recommended; in practice, adherence to the use of gowns for administration of drugs is much more variable and controversial than for admixture
Use Luer lock fittings for IV sets and syringes; use sterile gauze or alcohol pad for priming IV sets and for injecting and withdrawing the needle during drug administration	Prevents drug leakage and skin contact risk; for priming infusion sets and pumps, a plastic-backed absorbent pad can be used, and the line should be primed into a gauze inside a plastic bag
Do not clip needles, recap needles, or break syringes	Prevents possible contamination from needle sticks or aerosolization; in ambulatory care settings, disposal containers must be readily accessible to mediate the risk of walking with an uncapped needle vs. the risk of a needle stick from recapping at the site of the patient interaction; attention to individual technique is critical
Place all equipment in a puncture-resistant, leakproof container marked as hazardous waste or toxic material for incineration; dispose of protective materials according to institutional policy	Isolates and contains contaminated equipment
Spills	
Immediately remove protective clothing if contaminated; wash affected skin with soap and water; if eye exposure has occurred, flush with water or isotonic eyewash for 5 minutes; seek prompt medical attention	Reduces absorption exposure risk

Reprinted with permission from Fisher, D. S., Knobf, M. T., & Durivage, H. J. (1993). *The cancer chemotherapy handbook.* St. Louis: Mosby.

Continued

TABLE 5-11 Clinical Guidelines for the Preparation and Administration of Chemotherapy Drugs—cont'd

Guideline	Comment
Spills—cont'd	
Clean up spills dressed with disposable gown, eye protection, and double surgical latex gloves; wipe spills with absorbent pads, and cleanse the area 3 times with detergent solution, followed by water; dispose all materials for spill clean up immediately, according to institutional policy; Spill Kits, containing all the necessary equipment, are commercially available	
Personnel Policies and Surveillance	
Maintain a registry of staff who routinely handle antineoplastic drugs	Keep available a file on employees at potential risk for drug exposure and data for long-term follow-up (McDiarmid, 1990)
Offer continuing education for employees on occupational risk, policies, and procedures to reduce exposure; routine monitoring of protective measures and assessment of effectiveness	Required for employee occupational health protection
Pregnant or breast-feeding staff members should be offered alternative responsibilities to avoid drug contact, if desired	The data on reproductive risks are inconclusive, and action should not be to exclude potentially fertile or pregnant women from such tasks but to provide a safe work environment for all women (Bingham, 1985)

Reprinted with permission from Fisher, D. S., Knobf, M. T., & Durivage, H. J. (1993). *The cancer chemotherapy handbook.* St. Louis: Mosby.

powder-free latex gloves that are at least 0.007 inches thick. The chemotherapeutic drug should be reconstituted under the hood and then labeled with the patient's name, identification number, medication name and dose, route, diluent fluid, volume, and expiration date.

Drug Storage. All chemotherapeutic drugs should be stored at the temperature recommended by the manufacturer. The storage area should be labeled appropriately as to the hazardous nature of the drugs in the container and what an individual should do in case of accidental exposure. Spill kits (Table 5-12) should be readily available in areas where chemotherapeutic drugs are stored. Chemotherapeutic drugs stored in the home should be placed in containers that provide adequate protection from puncture or breakage.

Drug Transport. Syringes containing prepared chemotherapeutic drugs should be transported in sealed containers with the ends capped off. Syringes should *not* be transported with needles in place. All syringes should be transported in a leak-proof and sealable bag. If one is transporting chemotherapeutic drugs outside a health care agency (e.g., to a patient's home), additional impervious packing material or a leak-proof storage container should be used to prevent the contents from jostling or puncturing the leak-proof and sealable bag. All containers should be labeled to identify the hazardous nature of the contents (Powell, 1996).

Administration of Cancer Chemotherapy

The administration of chemotherapy requires specialized education and training regarding the mechanism of action of the various chemotherapeutic drugs; the procedures to be followed to ensure safe handling of these drugs; and the procedures to be followed to ensure the safe administration of these drugs to the patient. As with the administration of any other drug, the oncology nurse should compare the written orders to a formal drug protocol or reference book to determine the correctness of the prescription and the route of administration. The nurse should recalculate the drug dose and check the dose against the physician's prescription.

Most chemotherapeutic drug doses are calculated on the basis of body surface area (BSA) and are expressed in milligrams per square meter of body surface area (mg/m^2). BSA is generally calculated from the patient's height and weight using a BSA calculator (Box 5-7) or a nomogram (Fig. 5-3). After the patient's BSA is determined, the nurse should calculate the dose of chemotherapy to be administered by multiplying the patient's BSA by the dose of chemotherapy that was ordered in mg/m^2.

It should be noted that controversy exists about whether to use the patient's actual (i.e., current) or ideal body weight when calculating BSA. This question has significant clinical implications, particularly for obese patients or patients with amputations, (Table 5-13) because one could give the patient an overdose of the drug.

On the basis of an analysis of doses (actual compared with ideal weight) in a study of 3732 protocol patients, Gelman and colleagues (1987) suggested that actual body weight be used to calculate chemotherapy doses, with two exceptions: in clinical trials using very high doses (i.e., bone morrow transplantation) and in clinically obese patients de-

TABLE 5-12 Contents of a Chemotherapy Spill Kit

Number	Item
1	Gowns with cuffs and back closure (made of water nonpermeable fabric)
1 pair	Shoe covers
2 pair	Gloves
1 pair	Utility gloves
1 pair	Chemical splash goggles
1	Rebreather mask (National Institute of Occupational Safety and Health approved)
1	Disposable dust pan (to collect any broken glass)
1	Plastic scraper (to scoop materials into dust pan)
2	Plastic-backed or absorbable towels
1 each	250-ml and 1-L spill control pillows
2	Disposable sponges (one to clean up spill, one to clean up floor after removal of spill)
1	"Sharps" container
2	Large, heavy-duty waste disposal bags
1	Container of 70% alcohol for cleaning soiled area

From Occupational Safety and Health Administration. *Controlling occupational exposure to hazardous drugs,* 1994, OSHA Instruction CPL2-2.20B (pp. 21-1 to 21-34), 1994. Washington, DC: Author. Copyright 1995 by OSHA.

TABLE 5-13 Calculation of Body Surface Area in Adult Amputees*

Body Parts	Women (%)	Men (%)
Hand plus fingers	2.65	2.83
Lower part of arm	3.80	4.04
Upper part of arm	5.65	5.94
Foot	2.94	3.15
Lower part of leg	6.27	5.99
Thigh	12.55	11.80

*BSA (M^2) = BSA − [(BSA) × (%BSA_{part})], where BSA = body surface area; M^2 = meters squared; BSA_{part} = body surface area of amputated body part.

NOTE: Dose reductions may not be necessary in all amputee patients. Metabolism and clearance of a drug does not necessarily change in amputee patients. Use professional judgment when deciding to reduce drug doses.

From Colangelo, P. M., Welch, D. W., Rich, D. S., & Jeffrey, L. P. (1984). Two methods for estimating body surface area in adult amputees. *American Journal of Hospital Pharmacy, 41,* 2650-2655.

Box 5-7
Calculation of Body Surface Area*

Mostellar†

$$\text{BSA (m}^2) = \sqrt{\frac{\text{height} \times \text{weight}}{3600}}$$

DuBois and Du Bois‡

$$\text{BSA(m}^2) = (\text{wt}^{0.425}) \times (\text{ht}^{0.725}) \times 71.84$$

Haycock et al.§

$$\text{BSA(m}^2) = (\text{wt}^{0.5378}) \times (\text{ht}^{0.3964}) \times 0.024265$$

**BSA,* body surface area; m^2, meters squared; *ht,* height in centimeters; *wt,* weight in kilograms.

†From Mostellar, R. D. (1987). Simplified calculation of body-surface area. *New England Journal of Medicine, 317,* 1098.

‡From Du Bois, D., & Du Bois, E. F. (1916). A formula to estimate the approximate surface area if height and weight be known. *Archives of Internal Medicine, 17,* 863-871.

§From Haycock, G. G., Schwartz, G. J., & Wisotsky, D. H. (1978). Geometric method for measuring body surface area: A height-weight formula validated in infants, children, and adults. *Journal of Pediatrics, 93,* 62-66.

fined as those individuals weighing more than 30% of ideal body weight (Table 5-14). If actual weight had been used for dose calculations, 48% of the patients would have had a 10% increase in drug dose, and only 8% would have received a 25% increase (Gelman et al., 1987). In addition, dose reductions may be needed for patients with preexisting liver disease or impaired renal function, or for patients with an impaired performance status, toxicity related to prior chemotherapy administration, or other comorbid conditions (Powell, 1996). The nurse should follow the procedures outlined in Table 5-11 when administering chemotherapeutic drugs.

ROUTES OF CHEMOTHERAPY ADMINISTRATION

Chemotherapeutic drugs are administered by multiple routes to achieve systemic or regional delivery of the agents. The goal of systemic therapy is to attain a drug concentration that is sufficient to achieve a therapeutic toxic effect in presumed or proven metastatic disease without causing excessive toxicity to normal tissues. Regional chemotherapy is directed toward the goal of delivering the drug(s) directly into the blood vessel supplying the tumor or the cavity in which the tumor is isolated. Regional administration of chemotherapy often allows for higher concentrations of the drug to be delivered to the area of the tumor with fewer systemic side effects (Holmes, 1994). The major routes used for systemic and regional administration of chemotherapeutic drugs are listed in Table 5-15.

Oral Route

The oral route is the most convenient way to administer any medication. When considering the administration of chemotherapy through the oral route, several factors need to be evaluated: (1) the availability of the drug in an oral formulation; (2) the functioning of the gastrointestinal tract; (3) the presence of nausea, vomiting, or dysphagia; (4) the patient's level of consciousness; and (5) the patient's willingness and ability to adhere with the dosing schedule (Holmes, 1994).

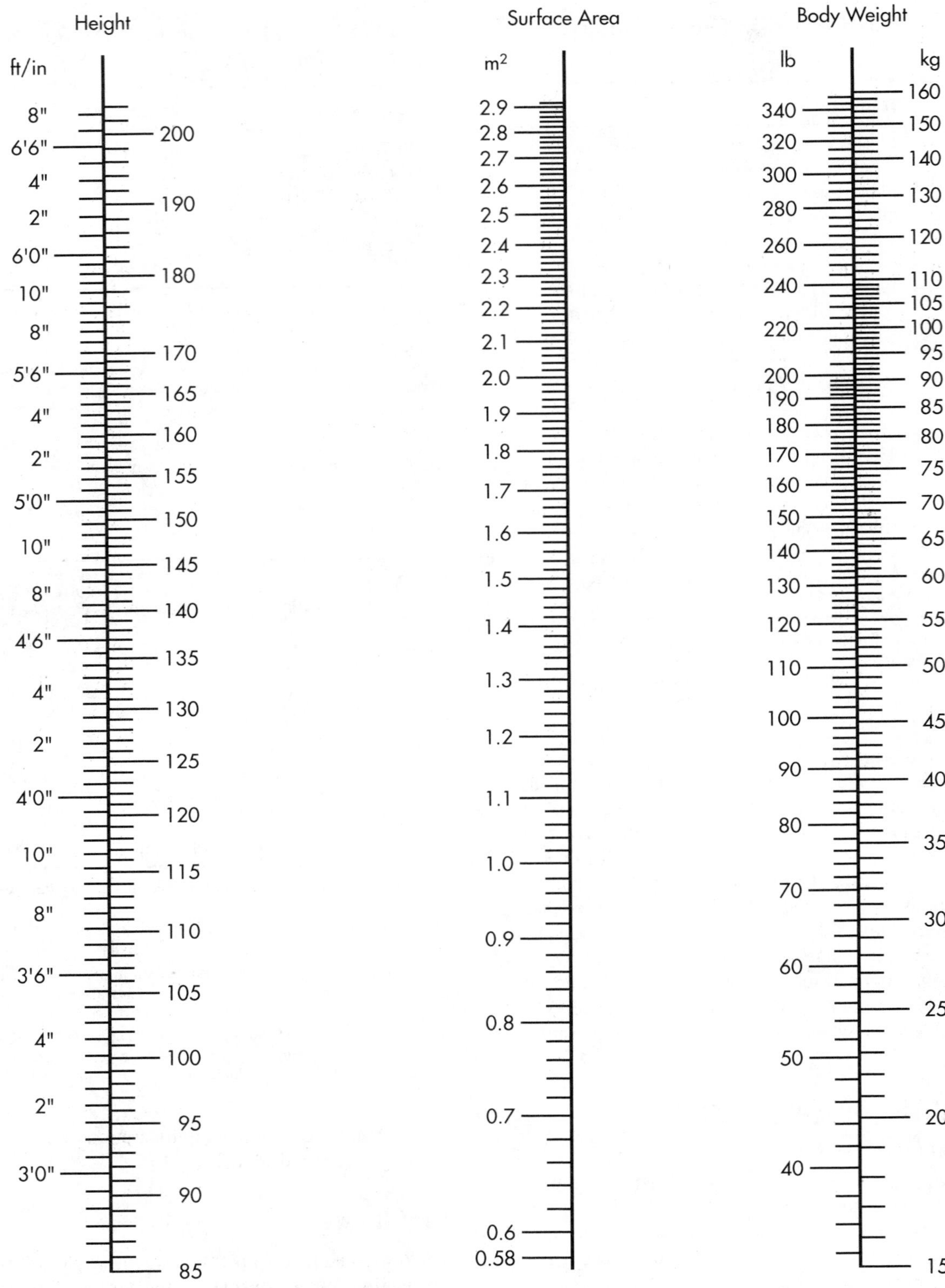

Fig. 5-3 Estimation of surface area from height and weight. An estimate of a patient's surface area can be obtained by marking the patient's height and weight and drawing a line between these two points; the point at which this line intersects the middle scale represents the patient's surface area.

TABLE 5-14 Ideal Body Weight*

Height (cm)	Weight (kg)	Height (cm)	Weight (kg)	Height (cm)	Weight (kg)
Males					
145	51.9	159	59.9	173	68.7
146	52.4	160	60.5	174	69.4
147	52.9	161	61.1	175	70.1
148	53.6	162	61.7	176	70.8
149	54.0	163	62.3	177	71.6
150	54.5	164	62.9	178	72.4
151	55.0	165	63.5	179	73.3
152	55.8	166	64.0	180	74.2
153	56.1	167	64.6	181	75.0
154	56.6	168	65.2	182	75.6
155	57.2	169	65.9	183	76.5
156	57.9	170	66.6	184	77.3
157	58.6	171	67.3	185	78.1
158	59.3	172	68.0	186	78.9
Females					
140	44.9	150	50.4	160	56.2
141	45.4	151	51.0	161	56.9
142	45.9	152	51.5	162	57.6
143	46.4	153	52.0	163	58.3
144	47.0	154	52.5	164	58.9
145	47.5	155	53.1	165	59.5
146	48.0	156	53.7	166	60.1
147	48.6	157	54.3	167	60.7
148	49.2	158	54.9	168	61.4
149	49.8	159	55.5	169	62.1

*Ideal body weight for height. This table corrects the 1960 Metropolitan Standards to nude weight without shoe heels.
From Fisher, D. S., Knobf, M. T., & Durivage, H. J. (1993). *The cancer chemotherapy handbook.* St. Louis: Mosby.

TABLE 5-15 Major Routes for Administration of Chemotherapy

Systemic Administration	Regional Administration
• Oral • Intravenous • Subcutaneous • Intramuscular	• Intrathecal • Intraarterial • Intracavitary

Patients and family members require extensive education to ensure adherence with the therapeutic regimen. At a minimum, patients and family members should receive verbal and written instructions that include the name of the chemotherapeutic drug, the dose of the drug, the times the drug should be taken, side effects associated with the medication, and when to call the physician or nurse. An assessment as to whether the patient will need nursing follow-up in the home care setting is necessary to ensure adherence with the administration schedule. Patients may benefit from using a pillbox and keeping a daily diary of chemotherapy administration. The nurse can review the diary during the next outpatient visit.

Intravenous Route

The intravenous (IV) route is the most common route used for the administration of cancer chemotherapy. Antineoplastic drugs may be given intravenously by several methods: (1) IV push (direct push method, two syringe technique), (2) IV sidearm (IV side port, IV Y-site), (3) mini-infusion (IV piggyback), or (4) IV infusion. The choice of intravenous method of administration depends on several factors, including the vesicant properties of the drugs, the potential for vein irritation by the drugs, the potential for immediate or delayed complications associated with drug administration (e.g., anaphylaxis, hypotension), and the specific logistics of the treatment protocol (Holmes, 1994).

Numerous controversies exist regarding the IV administration of vesicant drugs. The controversial issues and arguments for and against various vesicant chemotherapy administration practices are summarized in Table 5-16. Short-term infusions (30 minutes to 6 hours) are indicated when the chemotherapeutic drugs produce complications or

TABLE 5-16 Controversial Issues and Arguments For and Against Vesicant Chemotherapy Administration Practices

Controversial Practices	For	Against
Vesicant first	Vascular integrity decreases over time. Initially, practitioner's assessment skills more accurate. Patient may become more sedated from antiemetic and less able to report burning, pain at infusion site (Otto, 1991).	Vesicant is irritating, compromising integrity of vein. Nonvesicants are less irritating to veins. Venous spasm may occur early during injection, altering assessment of patency (Otto, 1991).
Side arm administration	Free-running IV lines allow for maximal dilution of drugs that could be potentially irritating.	
Direct push administration	Integrity of vein can be assessed more easily, and the early signs of extravasation can be noted more easily.	
Use of antecubital fossa	Larger veins permit more rapid infusion/administration of drug. Larger veins permit potentially irritating chemotherapeutic agents to reach the general circulation sooner with less irritation to small veins.	Arm mobility is restricted with a needle in place. The risk of extravasation is increased due to patient mobility (e.g., coughing, vomiting). Infiltration could require extensive reconstruction efforts with limited arm use during the healing process, resulting in increased morbidity and decreased function. Because of the subcutaneous tissues, early infiltration is more difficult to assess.
Large-gauge needles (e.g., #19 and #21 scalp vein needles)	Potentially irritating chemotherapeutic agents can reach the general circulation sooner, with reduced irritation to the peripheral veins. Drug administration time is decreased, which reduces the patient's exposure to a potentially stressful environment.	
Small-gauge needles (e.g., #23 and #25 scalp vein needles)	Smaller gauge needles are less likely to puncture the wall of a small vein. Scar tissue may be formed with needle insertion; small gauge needles cause less scar tissue formation. The patient may experience less pain during the insertion of a smaller needle. Increased blood flow around a smaller bore needle increases dilution of the chemotherapeutic agent. Mechanical phlebitis may be minimized with a smaller bore needle. Potential episodes of nausea and vomiting may be decreased by slow infusion of the chemotherapeutic agents.	

Reprinted with permission from Powell, L. L. (1996). *Cancer chemotherapy guidelines and recommendations for practice.* Pittsburgh: Oncology Nursing Press.

undesirable side effects when given by IV push. Long-term infusions (longer than 8 hours) are being used more often as knowledge regarding the benefits of this method of administration continue to increase. Several advantages of continuous infusions of chemotherapeutic drugs are summarized in Box 5-8 (Holmes, 1994).

Intrathecal Route

The intrathecal route of administration is used to treat meningeal metastases as a result of breast cancer, gastrointestinal cancer, brain tumors, leukemia, or lymphoma. Chemotherapy drugs must be administered through the intrathecal route because when these drugs are administered systemi-

Box 5-8
Advantages of Continuous Infusions of Chemotherapeutic Drugs

- Has the ability to overcome cytokinetic resistance mechanisms
- Maximizes the intracellular levels of the drugs by prolonging the tumor cells, exposure to low extracellular concentrations of the drugs
- Enhances the transport mechanisms of the cell membrane through saturation
- Avoids peak plasma levels, which minimizes the toxic effects of the drug

cally they do not cross the blood-brain barrier. Therefore chemotherapeutic drugs administered systemically have no effect on tumor cells located within the central nervous system.

Intrathecal administration of chemotherapy is accomplished through a lumbar puncture or through the placement of an Ommaya or Rickham reservoir (i.e., an indwelling subcutaneous cerebrospinal fluid reservoir). An Ommaya reservoir may be used instead of repeated lumbar punctures because administration of chemotherapy through a lumbar puncture does not ensure that the drug will reach the cerebral ventricles (Holmes, 1994).

Intra-Arterial Route

Intra-arterial administration of chemotherapy is most commonly used to treat an isolated organ. The chemotherapeutic drugs are administered through a catheter inserted into an artery that supplies the tumor. Intra-arterial chemotherapy has been used to treat primary hepatoma, metastatic disease of the liver, bladder cancer, head and neck cancer, melanoma, and osteogenic sarcoma (Holmes, 1994).

Intracavitary Route

The intracavitary route has been used to administer chemotherapy into the peritoneal cavity (i.e., intraperitoneal administration) and into the bladder (i.e., intravesical administration). Both forms of administration allow for the delivery of a higher concentration of the drug at the tumor site.

REFERENCES

American Society of Hospital Pharmacy (1990). Technical assistance bulletin on handling cytotoxic and hazardous drugs. *American Journal of Hospital Pharmacy, 47,* 1033-1049.

Baker, E. S., & Connor, T. H. (1996). Monitoring occupational exposure to cancer chemotherapy drugs. *American Journal of Health Systems Pharmacists, 53,* 2713-2723.

Berg, D. T. (1997). New chemotherapy treatment options and implications for nursing care. *Oncology Nursing Forum, 24*(Suppl. 1), 5-12.

Bertino, J. R., Donahue, D. R., & Simmons, B. (1963). Induction of dihydrofolate reductase activity in leukocytes and erythrocytes in patients treated with methopterin. *Journal of Clinical Investigation, 42,* 466-475.

Biedler, J. L., & Riehm, H. (1970). Cellular resistance to actinomycin D in Chinese hamster cells in vitro: Cross resistance autoradiographic and cytogenetic studies. *Cancer Research, 30,* 1174-1179.

Bingham, E. (1985). Hazards to health workers from antineoplastic drugs. *New England Journal of Medicine, 313,* 1220-1221.

Buick, R. N. (1994). Cellular basis of chemotherapy. In R. T. Dorr & D. D. Von Hoff (Eds.), *Cancer chemotherapy handbook* (2nd ed.). Norwalk, Connecticut: Appleton & Lange.

Burke, M. B. (1997). Cancer chemotherapy. In C. Varricchio (Ed.), *A cancer source book for nurses* (7th ed.). Atlanta: The American Cancer Society, Inc.

Champoux, J. J., & Dulbecco, R. (1972). Activity from mammalian cells that untwists superhelical DNA: Possible swivel for DNA replication. *Proceedings of the National Academy of Sciences, USA, 69,* 143-146.

Chan, H. S., Haddad, G., Thorner, P. S., DeBoer, G., Lin, Y. P., Ondrusek, N., Yeger, H., & Ling, V. (1991). P-glycoprotein expression as a predictor of outcome of therapy for neuroblastoma. *New England Journal of Medicine, 325,* 1608-1614.

Colangelo, P. M., Welch, D. W., Rich, D. S., & Jeffrey, L. P. (1984). Two methods for estimating body surface area in adult amputees. *American Journal of Hospital Pharmacy, 41,* 2650-2655.

Conley, B. A., & Van Echo, D. A. (1996). Antineoplastic drug development. In M. C. Perry (Ed.), *The cancer chemotherapy sourcebook* (2nd ed.). Baltimore: Williams & Wilkins.

Donehower, R., & Rowinsky, E. (1996). DNA topoisomerase II inhibitors. In M. C. Perry (Ed.), *The cancer chemotherapy sourcebook* (2nd ed.). Baltimore: Williams & Wilkins.

Falck, K., Gröhn, P., Sorsa, M., Vainio, H., Heinonen, E., & Holsti, L. R. (1979). Mutagenicity in urine of nurses handling cytostatic drugs. *Lancet, 1,* 1250-1251.

Fischer, D. S., Knobf, M. T., & Durivage, H. J. (1993). *The cancer chemotherapy handbook* (4th ed.). St. Louis: Mosby.

Flintooff, W. F., & Asessani, K. (1980). Methotrexate resistant Chinese hamster ovary cells contain a dihydrofolate reductase with an altered affinity for methotrexate. *Biochemistry, 19,* 4321-4327.

Friedland, M. L. (1996). Combination chemotherapy. In M. C. Perry (Ed.), *The cancer chemotherapy sourcebook* (2nd ed.). Baltimore: Williams & Wilkins.

Gascoyne, R. D., Tolcher, A., Van Iderstine, E., & Connors, J. M. (1993). The prognostic significance of P-glycoprotein expression in malignant lymphoma. *Modern Pathology, 6*(1A), 5-18.

Gellert, M., Mizuuchi, K., O'Dea, M. H., & Nash, H. A. (1976). An enzyme that induces superficial turns into DNA. *Proceedings of the National Academy of Sciences, USA, 73,* 3872-3876.

Gelman, R. S., Tormey, D., Betensky, R., Mansour, E. G., Galkson, H. C., Falkson, G., Creech, R. H., & Haller, D. G. (1987). Actual versus ideal weight in the calculation of surface area effects on dose of 11 chemotherapy agents. *Cancer Treatment Reports, 71,* 907-911.

Gerlach, J. H., Kartner, N., Bell, D. R., & Ling, V. (1986). Multidrug resistance. *Cancer Surveys, 5,* 25-46.

Gilewski, T., & Bitran, J. D. (1996). Adjuvant chemotherapy. In M. C. Perry (Ed.), *The cancer chemotherapy sourcebook* (2nd ed.). Baltimore: Williams & Wilkins.

Goldenberg, G. J., & Begleiter, B. (1980). Membrane transported alkylating agents. *Pharmacology and Therapeutics, 8,* 237-274.

Goldie, J. H. (1996). Drug resistance. In M. C. Perry (Ed.), *The cancer chemotherapy sourcebook* (2nd ed.). Baltimore: Williams & Wilkins.

Goldin, A., Venditti, J. M. Humphreys, S. R., & Mantel, N. (1956). Influence of the concentration of leukemic inoculum on the effectiveness of treatment. *Science, 123,* 840.

Goldman, I. D. (1971). The characteristics of the membrane transport of amethopterin and the naturally occurring folates. *Annals of the New York Academy of Sciences, 186,* 400-422.

Grochow, L. B. (1996). Covalent DNA-binding drugs. In M. C. Perry (Ed.), *The chemotherapy sourcebook* (2nd ed.). Baltimore: Wilkins & Wilkins.

Gutheil, J., & Kearns, C. M. (1996). Antimetabolites. In M. C. Perry (Ed.), *The cancer chemotherapy sourcebook* (2nd ed.). Baltimore: Williams & Wilkins.

Haycock, G. G., Schwartz, G. J., & Wisotsky, D. H. (1978). Geometric method for measuring body surface area: A height-weight formula validated in infants, children, and adults. *Journal of Pediatrics, 93,* 62-66.

Holmes, B. C. (1994). Administration of cancer chemotherapy agents. In R. T. Dorr & D. D. Von Hoff (Eds.), *Cancer chemotherapy handbook* (2nd ed.). Norwalk, Connecticut: Appleton & Lange.

Instruction TED 1.15. Directorate of Technical Support, Occupational Safety and Health Administration. (1995). *Controlling occupational exposure to hazardous drugs.* (Instruction TED 1.15, Section V, Ch. 3) Washington, D. C.: U.S. Department of Labor.

Juliano, R. L., & Ling, V. (1976). A surface glycoprotein modulating drug permeability in Chinese hamster ovary cell mutants. *Biochimica et Biophysica Acta, 455,* 152-159.

Krakoff, I. (1991). Cancer chemotherapeutic and biologic agents. *CA-Cancer Journal for Clinicians, 41*(5), 264-278.

Lawley, P. D., & Brookes, P. (1968). Cytotoxicity of alkylating agents toward sensitive and resistant strains of *E. coli* in relation to extent and mode of alkylation of cellular macromolecules and repair of alkylation lesions in deoxyribonucleic acid. *Biochemistry Journal, 109,* 433-447.

Lindahl, T. (1982). DNA repair enzymes. *Annual Review of Biochemistry, 51,* 61-92.

Ling, V., & Thompson, L. H. (1974). Reduced permeability in CHO cells as a mechanism of resistance to cultrasine. *Journal of Cell Physiology, 83,* 103-110.

Lyss, A. P. 91996). L-Asparaginase. In M. C. Perry (Ed.), *The cancer chemotherapy sourcebook* (2nd ed.). Baltimore: Williams & Wilkins.

Martin, D. S., & Fugmann, R. A. (1960). Clinical implications of the interrelationship of tumor size and chemotherapeutic response. *Annals of Surgery, 151,* 97-100.

McCance, K., & Huether, S. (1998). *Pathophysiology: The biologic basis for disease in adults and children* (3rd ed.). St. Louis: Mosby.

McDiarmid, M. A. (1990). Medical surveillance for antineoplastic-drug handlers. *American Journal of Hospital Pharmacy, 47,* 1061-1066.

McGovren, J. P. (1994). Pharmacologic principles. In R. T. Dorr, & D. D. Von Hoff (Eds.), *Cancer chemotherapy handbook* (2nd ed.). Norwalk, Connecticut: Appleton & Lange.

Miaskowski, C. (1997). *Oncology nursing: An essential guide for patient care.* Philadelphia: W. B. Saunders Company.

Moscow, J. A., & Dixon, K. H. (1994). Glutathione-related enzymes, flutathione, and multi-drug resistance. In M. Clynes (Ed.), *Multiple drug resistance in cancer.* Norwell, MA: Kluver Academic.

Office of Occupational Medicine, Occupational Safety and Health Administration. (1986). Guidelines for cytotoxic (antineoplastic) drugs. (Instructional publication 8-1.1). Washington, DC: U.S. Department of Labor.

OSHA. (1994). *OSHA INstruction CPL2-2.* Washington, DC: Occupational Safety and Health Administration. Copyright 1995 by OSHA.

Otto, S. (1991). *Oncology nursing.* St. Louis: Mosby.

Powell, L. L. (Ed.). (1996). *Cancer chemotherapy guidelines and recommendations for practice.* Pittsburgh: Oncology Nursing Press, Inc.

Powers, L. A., Anderson, R. W., Cortopassi, R., Gera, J. R., & Lewis, R. M., Jr. (1990). Update on safe handling of hazardous drugs: The advice of experts. *American Journal of Hospital Pharmacy, 47,* 1050-1060.

Riggs, C. E. (1996). Antitumor antibiotics and related compounds. In M. C. Perry (Ed.), *The cancer chemotherapy sourcebook* (2nd ed.). Baltimore: Williams & Wilkins.

Roberts, J. J., Brent, T. P., & Crathorn, A. R. (1971). Evidence for the inactivation and repair of mammalian DNA template after alkylation by mustard gas and half mustard gas. *European Journal of Cancer, 7,* 515-521.

Rowinsky, E. K., & Donehower, R. C. (1996). Microtubule-targeting drugs. In M. C. Perry (Ed.). *The cancer chemotherapy sourcebook* (2nd ed.). Baltimore: Williams & Wilkins.

Sartorelli, A. C. (1969). Some approaches to the therapeutic exploitation of metabolic sites of vulnerability of neoplastic cells. *Cancer Research, 29,* 2292-2299.

Shahab, N., & Perry, M. C. (1996). DNA topoisomerase I inhibitors. In M. C. Perry (Ed.), *The cancer chemotherapy sourcebook* (2nd ed.). Baltimore: Williams & Wilkins.

Shapiro, D. M., & Fugmann, R. A. (1957). The role of chemotherapy as an adjunct to surgery. *Cancer Research, 28,* 1098-1101.

Skeel, R. T. (1991). Biologic and pharmacologic basis of cancer chemotherapy. In R. T. Skeel (Ed.), *Handbook of cancer chemotherapy* (3rd ed.). Boston: Little, Brown and Company.

Stoikes, M. E., Carlson, J. D., Farris, F. F., & Walker, P. R. (1987). Permeability of latex and polyvinyl chloride gloves to fluorouracil and methotrexate. *American Journal of Hospital Pharmacy, 44,* 1341-1346.

Wang, J. C. (1969). Degree of superhelicity of covalently closed cyclic DNAs from *Escherichia coli. Journal of Molecular Biology, 43,* 263-272.

Wang, J. C. (1971). Interaction between DNA and *Escherichia coli* protein omega. *Journal of Molecular Biology, 55,* 523-533.

Wang, J. C., & Liu, L. F. (1979). DNA topoisomerases: Enzymes that catalyze the concreted breaking and rejoining of DNA back bone bonds. *Molecular genetics, Part III.* New York: Academic Press.

Williams, J. W., Duggleby, R. G., Cutler, R., & Morrison, J. F. (1980). The inhibition of dihydrofolate reductase by folate analogues: Structural requirements for slow and tight binding inhibitors. *Biochemistry and Pharmacology, 29,* 589-595.

Yarbro, J. W. (1996). The scientific basis of cancer chemotherapy. In M. C. Perry (Ed.), *The cancer chemotherapy sourcebook* (2nd ed.). Baltimore: Williams & Wilkins.

Yarosh, D. B., Foote, R. S., Mitra, S., & Day, R. S. (1983). Repair of 0 (6)-methylguanine in DNA by demethylation is lacking in MER minus human tumor cell strains. *Carcinogenesis, 4,* 199-205.

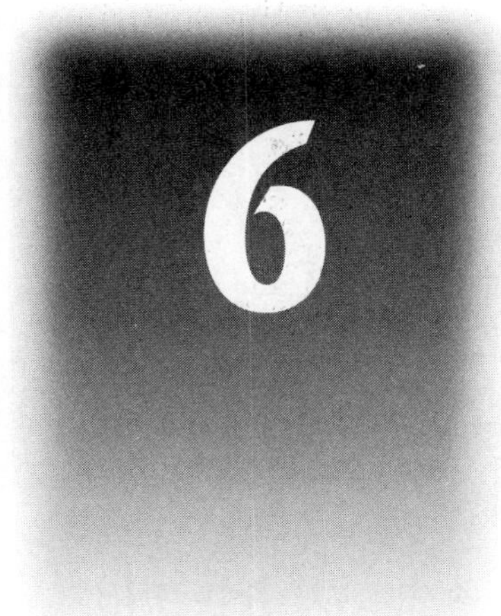

Hormonal Therapy

Christine Miaskowski, RN, PhD, FAAN
Carol S. Viele, RN, MS

Hormonal therapy may be an effective way to treat many "hormonally responsive" tumors such as breast cancer, prostate cancer, or endometrial cancer. In the past these cancers would have been treated with an ablative surgical procedure (e.g., castration, hypophysectomy, adrenalectomy). However, current approaches to treatment may include the use of hormonal agonists or antagonists, depending on the nature of the disease process. In addition, adrenocorticoids may be administered as part of the treatment regimen for lymphoid leukemias, Hodgkin's disease, non-Hodgkin's lymphoma, myeloma, and other lymphoproliferative disorders. Some hormonal therapies may be used in the treatment of ovarian cancer, renal cancer, and melanoma. Finally, hormonal therapy may be used as palliative or supportive therapy (e.g., steroids as antiemetics or adjuvant analgesics, androgens as anabolic agents, progestins as appetite stimulants) (Aisner, Fram, Eisenberger, & Fontana, 1996). The major classes of hormonal agents are listed in Box 6-1.

ADRENOCORTICOIDS

The adrenocorticoids are synthesized in the adrenal cortex and regulated through the action of adrenocorticotropic hormone (ACTH) which is produced in the anterior pituitary. The regulation of ACTH release depends on a precise balance between negative feedback from the level of adrenocorticoids in the blood and positive stimulation from the nervous system. Both of these effects are mediated through the hypothalamus. The main physiologic roles for the adrenocorticoids or glucocorticoids are control of glucose metabolism, gluconeogenesis, and regulation of the immune system. The major human forms of the hormone are cortisol and corticosterone (Aisner et al., 1996; McGovern, 1994; Schwartzman & Cidlowski, 1997).

Mechanism of Action of the Adrenocorticoids

The mechanism of action of the adrenocorticoids is illustrated in Fig. 6-1. The biologic effects of the adrenocorticoids are mediated through a specific intracellular protein receptor called the *glucocorticoid receptor.* This receptor is found in all tissues that are targets for the action of glucocorticoids (Burnstein & Cidlowski, 1989). The current model of glucocorticoid action suggests that the hormone diffuses passively through the cell membrane and enters the cytoplasm, where it binds with the glucocorticoid receptor. This binding causes a conformational change in the receptor that unmasks the portion of the receptor that can bind to deoxyribonucleic acid (DNA). The hormone-receptor complex translocates to the nucleus, where it binds to specific DNA sequences and alters the rate of gene transcription. This change in the rate of gene transcription leads to changes in the amount of messenger ribonucleic acid (m-RNA) that is produced and ultimately the amount of protein that the cell produces. The protein produced by a specific cell results in a specific cellular function (Schwartzman & Cidlowski, 1997).

Uses for Adrenocorticoids in Cancer Treatment

The corticosteroids used commonly in clinical practice are listed in Box 6-2. Tissue culture studies demonstrated that lymphoid cells were the most sensitive to glucocorticoids and that treatment with glucocorticoids resulted in decreases in DNA, RNA, and protein synthesis (Baxter et al., 1989). In addition, studies of proliferating human lymphocytes demonstrated that glucocorticoids had lymphocytolytic effects (Ernst & Killman, 1970). The mechanism of action by which the glucocorticoids inhibit the proliferation of lymphocytes is apoptosis (Cohen, 1989).

On the basis of these findings, the glucocorticoids are used in the management of acute lymphoblastic leukemia, chronic lymphocytic leukemia, Hodgkin's disease, non-Hodgkin's lymphoma, and multiple myeloma. In addition, glucocorticoids may be used to reduce edema in patients with primary or metastatic central nervous system tumors, to prevent allergic reaction, as part of the treatment regimen for hypercalcemia, as an appetite stimulant or to increase a patient's sense of well being during the terminal phases of the illness, or as an adjuvant analgesic for the pain associ-

Box 6-1
Major Classes of Hormonal Agents

- Adrenocorticoids
- Estrogens
- Progestins
- Antiestrogens
- Aromatase inhibitors
- Androgens
- Antiandrogens
- Lutenizing Hormone-Releasing Hormone (LHRH) agonists
- LHRH Antagonists

ated with bone metastasis (Schwartzman & Cidlowski, 1997).

Side Effects Associated With Adrenocorticoids

The adrenocorticoids are usually well tolerated. They often produce a feeling of euphoria and can act as an appetite stimulant. The long-term complications associated with the use of glucocorticoids include the appearance of Cushing's syndrome, hypertension, diabetes mellitus, and osteoporosis. In addition, these drugs can produce profound immunosuppression with the subsequent development of life-threatening infections. An additional problem associated with the chronic use of steroids is peptic ulcer disease. Finally, patients can develop a "steroid psychosis" while on or discontinuing high-dose therapy (McGovern, 1994). Oncology patients who are receiving glucocorticoids as part of their treatment regimen require ongoing assessments for these potentially life-threatening side effects.

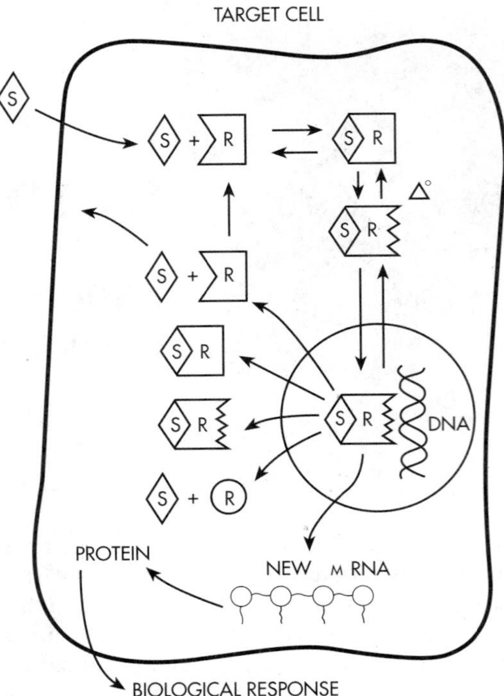

Fig. 6-1 Mechanism of action of adrenocorticords. (From Schwartzman, R. A., & Cidlowski, J. A. [1997]. Corticosteroids. In J. F. Holland, R. C. Bast, Jr., K. S. Morton, E. Frei, III, D. W. Kufe, & P. R. Weichselbaum [Eds.], *Cancer medicine* [4th ed]. Ontario, Canada: B. C. Decker.)

ESTROGENS

Estrogens are used in the management of patients with advanced prostate cancer. The effects of estrogen are mediated by a direct action on prostatic tissue and through a suppression of luteinizing hormone (LH) secretion from the adrenal glands. In addition, estrogens may be beneficial in the management of a small number of women with advanced-stage breast cancer. However, the exact mechanisms underlying the therapeutic benefit of estrogen therapy in advanced breast cancer remain to be elucidated (McGovern, 1994).

Use of Estrogens in Prostate Cancer

The dependence of prostate tumors on testosterone for growth has been recognized for many years since the description by Huggins and Hodges in 1941 of major clinical benefits associated with surgical castration or with the administration of pharmacologic doses of estrogens (Huggins & Hodges, 1941). However, orchiectomy is a procedure that some patients refuse to undergo.

An effective nonsurgical approach for suppressing testosterone levels is the administration of exogenous estrogen. Estrogen produces its effects by blocking the release of LH from the pituitary. The blockage of LH release results in the ablation of the production of testosterone by the Leydig cells in the testes (Vogelzang & Kennealey, 1992).

One of the most commonly used estrogens in the management of prostate cancer is diethylstilbestrol (DES). The administration of a daily oral dose of 3 mg or more of DES produces castration levels of testosterone within 7 to 21 days (Shearer, Hendry, Sommerville, & Fergusson, 1973).

Extensive studies of the safety and efficacy of DES in advanced prostate cancer have been carried out by the Veterans Administration Cooperative Urological Research Group (VACURG). One study (Byar, 1973) indicated that doses of 1 and 5 mg of DES were equivalent in efficacy and that the incidence of cardiovascular side effects was significantly less with the lower dose. However, although patients with stage C or D prostate cancer who received DES had a slightly lower mortality rate from progressive prostate cancer than the control group, the death rate from cardiovascular disease was increased in the DES-treated patients. The increased mortality associated with DES-induced cardiovascular disease virtually negated any of the survival benefits of estrogen treatment (Blackard, Byar, & Jordan, 1973; The Veterans Administration Cooperative Urological Research Group, 1967). Due to its side effect profile, DES is no longer used for the treatment of prostate cancer.

Side Effects Associated With the Use of Estrogens for Prostate Cancer. The acute side effects associated with the use of estrogen include nausea, vomiting, fluid retention, and headache. Long-term administration of

Box 6-2
Corticosteroids Commonly Used in Clinical Practice

Cortisone acetate
Hydrocortisone
Prednisone
Prednisolone
Methylprednisolone
Dexamethasone

estrogen can produce gynecomastia (which may be prevented by low-dose radiation therapy to the breasts), loss of libido, azoospermia, and impotence. The most serious adverse effects are an increased risk of cardiovascular complications (e.g., myocardial infarction, cerebrovascular accident, congestive heart failure, and arteriosclerotic heart disease), and thromboembolism (McGovern, 1994; Vogelzang & Kennealey, 1992).

Use of Estrogens in Breast Cancer

In general, the use of synthetic high-dose estrogens in the treatment of advanced breast cancer has been replaced by tamoxifen. However, selected patients may benefit from the use of estrogens (Teller & Jordan, 1995). The use of estrogens in advanced breast cancer is generally limited to postmenopausal women (Kennedy, 1962). The mechanism of action of estrogen in advanced breast cancer is not clear. However, the administration of the drug may cause a down-regulation of estrogen receptors (ERs) in malignant tissue (Kiang & Kennedy, 1976).

DES is the most frequently used estrogen. The drug is started at doses of 5 to 10 mg per day and escalated to doses of 15 to 25 mg per day based on the woman's level of tolerance. In some cases conjugated estrogen (Premarin, 7.5 mg/day) or ethinyl estradiol (3 mg/day) are used. Typical responses tend to occur slowly, and a prolonged trial of therapy (8 to 12 weeks) is usually indicated in the absence of progressive disease (Aisner et al., 1996).

Side Effects Associated With the Use of Estrogens for Advanced Breast Cancer. Administration of estrogen can result in nausea, vomiting, fluid retention, anorexia, enlargement and tenderness of breast tissue, softening of the skin, breakthrough bleeding, headaches, and pigmentation of the skin folds and areola. The fluid retention can exacerbate existing congestive heart failure (Aisner et al., 1996; McGovern, 1994; Teller & Jordan, 1995).

In some cases the administration of estrogen in patients with bone metastasis can result in an exacerbation of severe bone pain, often called a *flare* of the disease (Clarysse, 1985; Eisenberger, O'Dwyer, & Friedman, 1986). This early exacerbation of pain is frequently followed by a decrease in symptoms with the continuation of therapy and a disappearance after 2 to 3 weeks of treatment. In addition, hypercalcemia may occur during the early phase of therapy and resolve with subsequent treatment (Clarysse, 1985; Eisenberger et al., 1986; Henderson, 1987).

PROGESTINS

Progestins are compounds related to the steroid hormone progesterone. The most common progestins used in the management of cancer include: medroxyprogesterone acetate (e.g., Cycrin, Depo-Provera, Provera), hydroxyprogesterone caproate (e.g., Delalutin, Hydroxon, Pro-Depo), and megestrol acetate (Megace). The progestins are used in the management of breast and endometrial cancer. Megestrol acetate is also used in the management of ovarian cancer, and medroxyprogesterone acetate is used in the treatment of prostate cancer. In addition, they are used in the management of cachexia associated with cancer or acquired immunodeficiency syndrome (AIDS) (Aisner et al., 1996; Lonning & Lien, 1995; McCarty & McCarty, 1997; McGovern, 1994; Teller & Jordan, 1995).

Mechanism of Action of Progestins

Under normal physiologic conditions, progesterone is involved in the differentiation of a broad spectrum of tissues. For example, progesterone produces profound changes in the breast and uterus during the menstrual cycle. Progesterone is also required for the maintenance of pregnancy (McCarty & McCarty, 1997). However, the specific effect of progesterone appears to depend on the type of tissue.

Progestins have an indirect effect on tissue growth through their action on the hypothalamic-pituitary axis, which results in the inhibition of gonadotropin-releasing hormone. In addition, the progestins appear to have a direct effect on cellular proliferation, resulting in either inhibition or growth, depending on the growth conditions (Aisner et al., 1996; Alkhalaf & Murphy, 1992; VanderBurg, Kalkhoven, Isbrucher, & deLaat, 1992). The cellular effects of progestins appear to be mediated through the progesterone receptor located in the nucleus of the cell. The binding of progesterone to the receptor, with the formation of a progesterone-receptor complex, modulates the transcription of genes and results in the formation of various protein products. Recent studies have shown that the progesterone receptor has distinct agonist and antagonist binding sites (Tsai & O'Malley, 1994). In addition, estrogen is required for the activation of the progesterone receptor gene (Aisner et al., 1996; Horowitz & McGuire, 1978).

Use of Progestins in Breast Cancer

Progestins are used as second-line therapy, following tamoxifen, in the management of metastatic breast cancer (McCarty & McCarty, 1997). Both medroxyprogesterone and megestrol acetate have been used in the management of metastatic breast cancer. The response of metastatic breast cancer to therapy with progestins is predicted by the presence of estrogen receptors and/or progesterone receptors, but it is best predicted by the observation of an objective response to previous hormonal therapy (Robertson, Williams, Todd, Nicholson, Morgan, & Blamey, 1989).

Phase II trials demonstrated that the response rate of advanced breast cancer in postmenopausal women to medroxyprogesterone and megestrol acetate is approximately 30% (Alexieva-Figush, Blankestein, & Jop, 1984; Ansfield,

Kallas, & Singson, 1982; Canetta, Florentine, Hunter, & Lenaz, 1983). Of clinical importance is the finding that progestin therapy exhibits a dose-response increase in efficacy. Patients who have relapsed or progressed on conventional doses of medroxyprogesterone (100 to 200 mg/day) or megestrol (30 mg/day) may show an additional response with an increased dose (i.e., up to 2000 mg/day for medroxyprogesterone or 160 mg/day for megerstrol). Patients receiving progestins at these high doses seem to achieve an objective response rate comparable to that of tamoxifen or aminoglutethimide (Canney et al., 1988; Ingle et al., 1982; Lundgren et al., 1989; Morgan, 1985; Muss et al., 1985; Sedlacek & Horwitz, 1984; Van Veelen, Willemse, Tjabbes, Schwertzer, & Sleijfer, 1986; Wander et al., 1987; Willemse, van der Ploeg, Sleijfer, Tjabbes, & van Veelen, 1990).

Use of Progestins in Endometrial Cancer

Progestins are used in the management of recurrent endometrial cancer. The response rate is approximately 30% with minimal side effects (Bonte, Decoster, Ide, & Billiet, 1978; Geisler, 1973; Karlstedt, 1971; Malkasian, Decker, Mussey, & Johnson, 1971; Wait, 1973).

Side Effects of Progestins

The most common side effects associated with the administration of progestins include weight gain (18% to 50%), amenorrhea (37%), fluid retention (5% to 19%), skin abscesses (17%), sweating (17%), tremors (16%), muscle cramps (16%), and Cushingoid features (12%). Side effects that occurred in less than 10% of patients include hot flashes, constipation, hypercalcemia, nausea, vomiting, vaginal bleeding, and thrombophlebitis (Teller & Jordan, 1995).

ANTIESTROGENS

The role of estrogen in the pathophysiology of breast cancer unfolded through a series of clinical observations. For example, in the early 1900s it became known that approximately one third of premenopausal women with advanced breast cancer would respond to oophorectomy (Boyd, 1990; Jordan, 1997). In addition, some postmenopausal women with breast cancer responded to hypophysectomy (Pearson, Ray, & Harold, 1956) and adrenalectomy (Huggins & Bergenstad, 1952), whereas others in a somewhat paradoxical fashion responded to high doses of synthetic estrogens (e.g., DES) (Dodds, Lawson, & Nobel, 1938) or tripanisylchlorethylene (Thompson & Werner, 1951). However, it was not until the discovery of the estrogen receptor (Jensen & Jacobson, 1962; Toft & Gorski, 1966) that possible mechanisms of action for estrogen on various target tissues (i.e., breast, uterus, pituitary gland) and its role in the pathophysiology of breast cancer could be determined (Jordan, 1997).

An understanding of the basic mechanisms of action of estrogen on various target tissues, as well as malignant tissues, has led to the development of various synthetic estrogens and antiestrogens. In fact, as early as 1936, Lacassagne predicted that a drug might be found that could block the stimulatory effects of estrogen on breast tissue (Lacassagne, 1936). The first nonsteroidal antiestrogen to be developed was MER 25 (Lerner, Holthaus, & Thompson, 1958). However, trials with MER 25 were stopped because of toxic side effects.

However, because of the belief that antiestrogens would be useful in the management of breast cancer, several other compounds were developed and tested. Only one of these agents has been approved for clinical use (i.e., tamoxifen). However, several other nonsteroidal and pure antiestrogens are undergoing clinical trials (Box 6-3).

Box 6-3
Antiestrogens

Nonsteroidal Antiestrogens
Tamoxifen
Toremifene
Droloxifene

Pure Antiestrogens
ICI 182,780
ICI 164,384

Nonsteroidal Antiestrogens

The therapeutic use and side effects and toxicities associated with the nonsteroidal antiestrogens are summarized in Table 6-1.

Tamoxifen. Tamoxifen is a nonsteroidal antiestrogen that was developed in the late 1960s and entered clinical trials in 1971 (Cole, Jones, & Todd, 1971; Ward, 1973). Tamoxifen exhibits the properties of a partial estrogen agonist/antagonist in rats and women. It is these properties that contribute to its diverse effects in women.

In breast cancer, tamoxifen inhibits the binding of estradiol to the ER (Jordan, 1984). The binding of tamoxifen to the ER inhibits the growth of ER-positive breast cancer cells (Jordan, 1997). However, this cannot be the only mechanism of action of tamoxifen because up to 10% of patients whose tumors are ER negative respond to tamoxifen treatment (Rose & Mourisden, 1984). Although the specific mechanisms of action of tamoxifen have not been elucidated completely, administration of the drug is known to decrease DNA synthesis and lower levels of insulin growth factor (IGF)-II (Osborne et al., 1989, Yee et al., 1988), transforming growth factor (TGF)-α (Bates et al., 1988), and other mitogens that enhance the growth of breast cancer cells.

Tamoxifen is the endocrine treatment of choice for metastatic breast cancer in postmenopausal women (Furr & Jordan, 1984; Jordan, 1997). A summary of the phase II trials of tamoxifen treatment in postmenopausal women is found in Table 6-2. The response rate in these trials ranges from 15% to 53% in unselected patients, with a median duration

TABLE 6-1 Nonsteroidal Antiestrogens

Generic Name	Trade Name	Therapeutic Use	Side Effects/Toxicities
Tamoxifen	Nolvadex®	Breast cancer, endometrial cancer, melanoma, prostate cancer (stage D), renal cell cancer	Bone pain, cataracts, depression, dizziness, headache, hot flashes, leg cramps, lethargy, menstrual irregularities, nausea, peripheral edema, retinal hemorrhage, skin rash, vaginal bleeding
Toremifene	—	Breast cancer	Anorexia, hot flashes, nausea, sweating
Droloxifene	—	Breast cancer	Hot flashes, nausea

TABLE 6-2 Phase II Trials of Tamoxifen in Postmenopausal Women

Study	Number of Patients	Tamoxifen Dose (mg/day)	Response rates (%) (CR + PR)
Bratherton et al., 1984	116	20	34
	121	40	31
Hoogstraten et al., 1982	39	20	46
Kiang et al., 1977	59	40	39
Lerner et al., 1976	30	20	53
	44	15 mg/m^2	43
Morgan et al., 1976	72	40	33
Tormey et al.,	52	12 $\geq$ 32 mg/m^2	29
Ward, 1973	33	20	15
	35	40	20

CR, complete response; *PR,* partial response.
Reprinted with permission from Teller, C., & Jordan, V. C. (1995). Hormonal treatment of advanced breast cancer. *Surgical Oncology Clinics of North America, 4*(4), 751-777.

of response of 20 months (Teller & Jordan, 1995). However, patients with ER-positive tumors are more likely to benefit from tamoxifen therapy. Correlation of clinical response with ER status indicates that 48% of patients (159/333) with ER-positive disease had partial or complete responses, whereas only 13% (17/129) of ER-negative patients had responses (Jordan, 1997).

Tamoxifen is approved for the treatment of advanced breast cancer in premenopausal women with ER-positive disease. Phase II trials of tamoxifen have reported response rates of approximately 30% in premenopausal women not selected for hormone status (Planting, Alexieva-Figush, Blonk-vander Wijst, & van Patten, 1985; Pritchard, Meaken, & Sawka, 1985; Pritchard et al., 1980; Sunderland & Osborne, 1991). Responses appear to occur more frequently in soft tissue and bony lesions compared to visceral disease. For premenopausal patients with positive estrogen and progesterone receptors, the response rates range from 45% to 75% (Sawka et al., 1986).

Side Effects of Tamoxifen. The side effects associated with the administration of tamoxifen are summarized in Table 6-3. The most common side effects are fatigue, insomnia, hot flashes, headaches, nausea, vomiting, weight gain, and vaginal bleeding. In premenopausal women with

TABLE 6-3 Side Effects of Tamoxifen Treatment

Side Effect	Incidence (%)
Fatigue	5-70
Vasomotor instability	17-67
Insomnia	0-54
Headache	9-37
Depression	1-33
Altered menses	1-31
Fluid retention	2-25
Nausea	3-21
Anorexia	1-16
Emesis	1-12
Diarrhea	8-10
Constipation	2-4
Weight gain	4

Reprinted with permission from Teller, C., & Jordan, V. C. (1995). Hormonal treatment of advanced breast cancer. *Surgical Oncology Clinics of North America, 4*(4), 751-777.

ovarian cycles, the administration of tamoxifen causes ovarian stimulation (Litherland & Jackson, 1988). Women need to be advised about the use of barrier contraception while taking tamoxifen (Teller & Jordan, 1995).

In postmenopausal women tamoxifen exhibits weak estrogen-like properties that result in a decrease in levels of LH and follicle-stimulating hormone (FSH), an increase in sex hormone-binding globulin levels, a decrease in antithrombin III, changes in vaginal cytology, and hyperplasia of the endometrium (Jordan, 1997). These effects have resulted in investigations of the potential toxic effects of long-term tamoxifen use in postmenopausal women.

Estrogen is an important hormone in the maintenance of bone, and hormone replacement therapy is recommended for postmenopausal women to prevent osteoporosis. Therefore it is possible that the long-term administration of an antiestrogen such as tamoxifen could result in osteoporosis. However, clinical studies show that a 2-year period of adjuvant therapy with tamoxifen does not decrease bone density (Fentimen, Caleffi, & Rodin, 1989; Love et al., 1988; Powles et al., 1989; Turken et al., 1989). In addition, there is evidence that suggests that tamoxifen is beneficial and maintains bone in the lumbar spine and neck of the femur (Kristensen et al., 1994; Love et al., 1992; Ward, Morgan, Dalley, & Kelly, 1993).

Another beneficial effect of estrogen is that the hormone lowers the levels of low-density lipoprotein (LDL) cholesterol and that this change in lipid profile protects against myocardial infarction in premenopausal women. Again, the long-term use of an antiestrogen might lead to the risk of premature coronary artery disease. However, tamoxifen appears to have estrogenic effects that result in the lowering of cholesterol levels in female patients (Bagdade, Wolter, Subbaiah, & Ryan, 1990; Bertelli et al., 1988; Bruning et al., 1988; Caleffi et al., 1988; Love et al., 1990; Love, Wielbe, Newcomb, & Chappell, 1994; Love et al., 1991; Rossner & Wallgren, 1984). In fact, an analysis of the Scottish clinical trial of 5 years of adjuvant tamoxifen showed a significant decrease in fatal myocardial infarction (McDonald & Stewart, 1991).

Although the estrogenic effects of tamoxifen on bone and cholesterol levels appear to be beneficial to women, the estrogenic effects of tamoxifen on levels of antithrombin III and on the uterus may produce deleterious consequences. Tamoxifen decreases the levels of antithrombin III and, as a result, may place women at an increased risk for thromboembolic disorders. However, a study from Sweden showed no significant increase in thromboembolic disorders in women who were on long-term tamoxifen therapy (Rutqvist & Mattson, 1993). Nevertheless, women with a known history of thromboembolic disorders should be evaluated carefully before being placed on tamoxifen (Jordan, 1997).

Suggestions have been made that long-term use of tamoxifen may increase a woman's risk for developing endometrial cancer. In fact, the Stockholm (Fornander et al., 1989) and National Surgical Adjuvant Breast and Bowel Project (NSABP) (Fisher et al., 1994) noted an increase in endometrial cancer in the women on tamoxifen compared to women in the control arm. All cases of persistent vaginal bleeding in women on tamoxifen should be followed up with a gynecologic examination and endometrial biopsy.

Toremifene. Toremifene is a structural derivative of tamoxifen that was developed in 1979, and human studies began in 1982 (Kangas, 1990). Toremifene was found to have direct cytotoxic effects on tamoxifen-resistant estrogen receptor negative tumors (Kangas et al., 1986), but unlike tamoxifen the drug does not produce liver tumors in rats (Hirsimaki, Hirsimaki, Nieminen, Payne, 1993).

Phase I studies demonstrated that toremifene had activity against breast cancer and was well tolerated (Kivinen & Maenpaa, 1986). However, toremifene is less potent than tamoxifen and clinical studies are using a higher dose than tamoxifen. Phase II trials comparing toremifene to tamoxifen in metastatic breast cancer produced comparable results to tamoxifen with response rates ranging from 38% to 51% (Teller & Jordan, 1995; Valavaara, Tuominen, & Johansson, 1990). The drug appears to be well tolerated with 80% of patients reporting no side effects, only 12% reporting sweating, and 4% reporting nausea, depression, or dizziness (Kivinen & Maenpaa, 1986).

Droloxifene. Droloxifene is an antiestrogen with higher binding affinity for the ER than tamoxifen (Pritchard, 1991; Roos, Deze, & Loser, 1983). Droloxifene has been shown to have activity in the management of breast cancer. The major side effects reported by 20% of patients were hot flashes and nausea. In addition, two cases of pulmonary emboli were documented (Rauschning & Pritchard, 1994).

Pure Antiestrogens

The pure antiestrogens were developed with the goal of producing compounds that would have no estrogen-like activity. The potential advantages of pure antiestrogens compared with tamoxifen are summarized in Box 6-4. ICI 164, 384 and ICI 182,780 are two pure antiestrogens. The mechanism of action of these compounds remains unexplained. However, it is known that these drugs bind to the ER. In addition, the antiestrogens prevent the "shuttling" of newly synthesized ERs to the cell nucleus. These receptors are rapidly destroyed (Dauvois, Danielian, White, & Parker, 1992).

A preliminary clinical study of ICI 182,780 in patients with early stage breast cancer demonstrated a decrease in tumor Ki 67 proliferation index, a decrease in progesterone receptor content, and a disappearance of estrogen receptors (DeFriend et al., 1994).

AROMATASE INHIBITORS

Antiestrogens are the first line of endocrine therapy for women with hormonally responsive advanced breast cancer. However, second-line hormonal therapies are needed for women who initially respond to antiestrogens but whose disease relapses. Therefore work has progressed on the development of potent aromatase inhibitors for the management of postmenopausal women with hormone-sensitive breast cancer (Harvey & Manni, 1997).

Box 6-4
Potential Advantages of Pure Antiestrogens Compared With Tamoxifen

1. Higher affinity for the estrogen receptor
2. Better antiestrogenic — estrogenic ratio
   - Higher antitumor efficacy (?)
   - More effective in bone (?)
3. Inhibition of tamoxifen-stimulated growth of MCF-7 tumor cell lines in vitro and endometrial tumors grown in athymic mice
4. Effective in a significant number of patients who failed with tamoxifen
5. Effective in other estrogen-receptor negative experimental tumors (?)
6. Good tolerance at high doses
7. Less hepatocarcinogenicity in rats
8. Lower risk of endometrial cancer during long-term therapy (?)
9. Less tumor flare (?)
10. Reversal of multidrug resistance at high doses (?)

From Klijn, J. G. M., Setyono-Han, B., Bontenal, M., Seynaeve, C., & Foekens, J. (1996). Novel endocrine therapies in breast cancer. *Acta Oncologica, 35* (Suppl. 5), 30-37.

Rationale for the Use of Aromatase Inhibitors

In the postmenopausal or castrated woman, the major source of estrogen is not derived from the ovaries but from the adrenal glands. Androstenedione is produced in the adrenal glands and is converted to estrone by the peripheral cytochrome P450 enzyme system. This process of conversion is called *aromatisation.* This enzymatic conversion occurs at extra-adrenal or peripheral sites such as fat, liver, and muscles and is catalyzed by the aromatase enzyme complex. Some breast cancer tissues also contain the enzyme aromatase (Harvey & Manni, 1997). In premenopausal women, the synthesis of estrogen by the ovaries is under the control of pituitary gonadotrophins. Any interruption in estrogen synthesis results in a reflex increase in pituitary gonadotrophins. Therefore aromatase inhibitors are not able to cause significant decreases in estrogen levels in premenopausal women (Santen, 1981; Teller & Jordan, 1995).

Mechanism of Action of the Aromatase Inhibitors

The aromatase inhibitors are divided into two classes, namely mechanism-based or "suicide" inhibitors, or competitive inhibitors. The mechanism-based or "suicide" inhibitors initially compete with androstenedione for binding to the active site of the aromatase enzyme. The enzyme then acts on the inhibitor to yield reactive compounds which form covalent bonds at or near the site of the enzyme. Through this mechanism, the enzyme is *irreversibly* inactivated. On the other hand, competitive inhibitors bind *reversibly* to the active site of the enzyme and prevent the formation of estrogen for as long as the aromatase inhibitor occupies the active site (Harvey & Manni, 1997). The aromatase inhibitors that are in use or are being evaluated in clinical trials are listed in Table 6-4.

Prototype Aromatase Inhibitor

Aminoglutethimide was the prototype aromatase inhibitor. This drug prevents the synthesis of estrogen by two mechanisms: the inhibition of cholesterol metabolism in the adrenal glands, and the inhibition of the peripheral aromatase enzyme system. The first mechanism of action also reduces the production of glucocorticoids in the adrenal gland, which causes an increase in the levels of adrenocorticotropin hormone (ACTH) from the pituitary gland. This increase in ACTH reverses the effects of aminoglutethimide. Therefore hydrocortisone needs to be administered with aminoglutethimide to prevent an increase in ACTH (Teller & Jordan, 1995).

An evaluation of the overall responses of women with breast cancer to aminoglutethimide with hydrocortisone reveals results similar to responses to other forms of endocrine therapy. Approximately 33% of women experience a complete or partial response. However, women with ER-positive tumors experience a response rate of 54%. The mean duration of response is 13 months and mean survival is approximately 20 months (Santen, Lipton, & Kendall, 1974).

More specifically, when compared with tamoxifen, aminoglutethimide with hydrocortisone produced comparable response rates of the same duration (Petree & Schmahl, 1987). In addition, comparable response rates without the surgical morbidity were seen when aminoglutethimide was compared with adrenalectomy (Santen et al., 1981) and transphenoidal hypophysectomy (Harvey et al., 1979). The major side effects associated with the administration of aminoglutethimide are lethargy, skin rash, pruritus, orthostatic symptoms, and in rare cases, pancytopenia (Teller & Jordan, 1995).

Mechanism-Based or "Suicide" Aromatase Inhibitors

Formestane (1-hydroxyandrostenedione) is a structural analog of androstenedione and is more potent than aminoglutethimide (Brodie, Wing, Goss, Dowsett, & Coombes, 1986). The drug has been tested in several clinical trials of patients with advanced breast cancer, with response rates ranging from 14% to 29% (Goss et al., 1986; Hoffken et al., 1990; Pickels, Perry, & Murray, 1990). The major side effects associated with the administration of formestane are hot flashes, lethargy, rash, transient leukopenia, facial swelling, and anaphylaxis (Teller & Jordan, 1995).

Competitive Aromatase Inhibitors

Fadrozole. Fadrozole is a nonsteroidal competitive inhibitor of the aromatase enzyme system. In vitro studies demonstrated that fadrozole is 200 to 400 times more potent than aminoglutethimide (Steele, Mellor, Sawyer, Wasvary,

TABLE 6-4 Aromatase Inhibitors for Breast Cancer

Drug	Mechanism of Action	Dose Used in Clinical Studies
Aminoglutethimide	Prototype aromatase inhibitor	1000 mg/day with 40 mg of hydrocortisone
Formestane	Mechanism-based	250, 500 mg IM every 2 wk
Fadrozole	Competitive inhibitor	1 mg BID
Letrozole	Competitive inhibitor	0.5, 2.5 mg per day
Vorozole	Competitive inhibitor	2.5 mg per day
Arimidex	Competitive inhibitor	1, 10 mg per day

& Browne, 1987). In phase II studies, daily oral doses of 1 to 2 mg of fadrozole in postmenopausal women with advanced breast cancer showed an overall response rate of 23% and a median survival of 22.6 months. The most common side effects reported were hot flashes, nausea, and vomiting (Rauschning & Pritchard, 1994).

Letrozole. Letrozole appears to be more potent than fadrozole and exhibits increased sensitivity for the aromatase enzyme system (Goss & Gwyn, 1994). A phase I study that evaluated three different daily doses (i.e., 0.1, 0.5, and 2.5 mg) in postmenopausal patients demonstrated a 33% response rate. No adverse effects were reported (Demers et al., 1993).

Vorozole. Vorozole is another highly potent and specific aromatase inhibitor that has demonstrated little toxicity in animals (Wouters et al., 1989). Phase II studies of the dextroanantiomer of vorozole (i.e., R83842) in doses of 1 to 5 mg per day resulted in response rates ranging from 30% to 33% in previously treated women with advanced breast cancer (Goss, Clark, & Ambers, 1994; Johnston et al., 1994). The major side effects were hot flashes, headaches, and nausea that were each reported by 8% of the patients.

Arimidex. Arimidex is the first aromatase inhibitor approved for the treatment of advanced breast cancer in postmenopausal women who have disease progression following treatment with tamoxifen. Two large, phase III trials demonstrated that Arimidex (in doses of 1 mg or 10 mg once a day) is similar to megestrol acetate (40 mg 4 times a day) in efficacy but causes less weight gain and fewer thromboembolic side effects (Harvey & Manni, 1997). The most common side effects associated with the administration of Arimidex are fatigue, nausea, headache, hot flashes, and back pain.

ANDROGENS

Androgens are the major sex steroid hormones in males. Testosterone, the principal male hormone secreted by the testes is found in the plasma either bound to sex hormone binding globulin (SHBG) or albumin or in an unbound form (i.e., only 2% of testosterone is unbound). When unbound testosterone diffuses across a target cell (e.g., prostate gland), it is converted immediately to dihydrotestosterone by the enzyme 5α-reductase. Dihydrotestosterone binds to an androgen-receptive protein in the cytoplasm and is translocated into the nucleus of the cell, where it exerts its biologic effects (Bruchovsky, 1997).

Box 6-5
Antiandrogens

Cyproterone acetate
Flutamide
Nilutamide
Bicalutamide

The use of androgens in the management of breast cancer has been replaced by the use of tamoxifen or other hormonal agents. From the outset, the use of androgens in the treatment of breast cancer was associated with significant and distressing side effects (e.g., deepening of the voice, clitoral hypertrophy, alopecia) (Bruchovsky, 1997). In addition, androgens do not have a role in the management of prostate cancer.

ANTIANDROGENS

Antiandrogens bind to androgen receptors on target tissues and prevent the stimulatory effects of exogenous or endogenous androgens. In the treatment of prostate cancer, antiandrogens block the effects of testosterone on cell growth (Vogelzang & Kennealey, 1992). Specific antiandrogens are listed in Box 6-5 and Table 6-5.

Cyproterone Acetate

The first antiandrogen, developed in the early 1960s was cyproterone acetate. This drug is a synthetic steroidal antiandrogen. Although it was claimed to be as effective as orchiectomy or estrogen in the treatment of prostate cancer, cyproterone offered no survival advantage, and its steroidal side effects made it a less desirable drug (Vogelzang & Kennealey, 1992). The major side effects associated with cyproterone acetate are loss of libido, impotence, fatigue, weakness, nipple tenderness, breast swelling, shortness of breath, and thrombosis (Bruchovsky, 1997).

Flutamide

Flutamide is a nonsteroidal antiandrogen that inhibits the translocation of androgen receptor from the cytoplasm to the nucleus in both the prostate and the hypothalamus. Flutamide blocks the negative feedback loop to the hypothalamus, which results in increased secretion of lutenizing

TABLE 6-5 Antiandrogens

Generic Name	Trade Name	Therapeutic Use	Side Effects/Toxicities
Cyproterone acetate	—	Prostate cancer	Breast swelling, fatigue, impotence, loss of libido, nipple tenderness, shortness of breath, thrombosis, weakness
Flutamide	Eulexin	Prostate cancer	Anorexia, diarrhea, edema, gynecomastia, hot flashes, hypertension, impotence, loss of libido, nausea and vomiting, photosensitivity

hormone–releasing hormone (LHRH) and LH. The increased secretion of LHRH and LH causes the testes to increase the production of testosterone. In patients who receive flutamide, plasma concentrations of testosterone increase slowly to a peak of about 50% above the mean normal value after six months of treatment. A gradual decline in testosterone levels follows, such that after 12 months of therapy a normal baseline value is achieved (Bruchovsky, 1997). In clinical practice, an LHRH agonist (e.g., leuprolide, goserelin) is combined with flutamide to prevent the rise in plasma testosterone levels. The side effects associated with the administration of flutamide include gynecomastia, diarrhea, nausea, vomiting, hepatotoxicity, and neutropenia (Bruchovsky, 1997).

Bicalutamide

Bicalutamide is an extremely potent and pure antiandrogen. It is a nonsteroidal antiandrogen that has a long half-life of 6 days, compared with 5 hours for flutamide. The most frequent side effects associated with bicalutamide are gynecomastia and breast tenderness.

LHRH AGONISTS

Release of LHRH from the hypothalamus results in the secretion of LH and FSH from the pituitary, which in turn causes the secretion of estrogen from the ovaries and testosterone from the testes. The administration of an exogenous LHRH agonist results in the inhibition of LH and FSH secretion and subsequent inhibition of ovarian and testicular function (Bruchovsky, 1997; Teller & Jordan, 1995). The most common LHRH agonists are listed in Box 6-6.

Box 6-6
Lutenizing Hormone–Releasing Hormone Agonists

Leuprolide
Goserelin
Buserelin
Nafarelin
Typtorelin

The LHRH agonists have been used in the treatment of premenopausal and postmenopausal women with advanced breast cancer. The most common side effects observed in women include nausea and depression (Teller & Jordan, 1995). The LHRH agonists are usually administered in combination with an antiandrogen in the management of prostate cancer. The side effects observed when LHRH agonists are administered to males include a transient flare reaction and prostate enlargement (Bruchovsky, 1997).

LHRH ANTAGONISTS

LHRH antagonists may be useful in the management of hormone-dependent cancers. These antagonists act on the same receptor sites as LHRH and cause the immediate inhibition of release of gonadotropins (LH, FSH) and sex steroid hormones. Several drug formulations are undergoing clinical trials. This class of hormones may prove useful in the management of some cases of breast and prostate cancer (Schally & Comaru-Schally, 1997).

REFERENCES

Aisner, J., Fram, R. J., Eisenberger, M., & Fontana, J. A. (1996). Hormonal agents. In M. C. Perry (Ed.), *The chemotherapy sourcebook* (2nd ed.). Baltimore: Williams & Wilkins.

Alexieva-Figush, J., Blandestein, M. A., & Jop, W. C. J. (1984). Treatment of metastatic breast cancer patients with different doses of megestrol acetate, dose relations, metabolic and endocrine effects. *European Journal of Cancer and Clinical Oncology, 20,* 33-40.

Alkhalaf, M., & Murphy, L. C. (1992). Regulation of C-Jun and Jun-B by progestins in T47D human breast cancer cells. *Molecular Endocrinology, 6,* 1625-1633.

Ansfield, F. J., Kallas, G. J., & Singson, J. P. (1982). Clinical results with megestrol acetate in patients with advanced carcinoma of the breast. *Surgery, Gynecology, and Obstetrics, 155,* 888-890.

Bagdade, J. D., Wolter, J., Subbaiah, P. V., & Ryan, W. (1990). Effect of tamoxifen treatment on plasma lipids and lipoproteins lipid composition. *Journal of Clinical Endocrinology and Metabolism, 70,* 1132-1135.

Bates, S. E., Davidson, N. E., Volverius, E. M., Freter, C. E., Dickson, R. B., Tam, J. P., Kudlow, J. E., Lippmann, M. E., & Salomon, D. S. (1988). Expression of transforming growth factor alpha and its ribonucleic and in human breast cancer: Its regulation by estrogen and its function. *Molecular Endocrinology, 2,* 543-555.

Baxter, G. D., Collins, R. G., Harmon, B. V., Kumar, S., Prentice, R. L., Smith, P. J., & Lavin, M. F. (1989). Cell death by apoptosis in acute leukemia. *Journal of Pathology, 158,* 123-129.

Bertelli, G., Pronzato, P., Amoroso, D., Cusimano, M. P., Conte, P. F., Montagma, G., Bertolini, S., & Rosso, R. (1988). Adjuvant tamoxifen in primary breast cancer: Influence on plasma lipids and antithrombin III levels. *Breast Cancer Research and Treatment, 12,* 307-310.

Blackard, C. E., Byar, D. P., & Jordan, W. P. (1973). Veterans Administration Cooperative Urological Research Group: Orchiectomy for advanced prostatic cancer: A reevaluation. *Urology, 1,* 553-560.

Bonte, J., Decoster, M. J., Ide, P., & Billiet, G. (1978). Hormonoprophylaxis and hormonotherapy in the treatment of endometrial adenocarcinoma by means of medroxyprogesterone acetate. *Gynecologic Oncology, 6,* 60-75.

Boyd, S. (1990). On oophorectomy in cancer of the breast. *British Medical Journal, 2,* 1161-1167.

Bratherton, D. G., Brown, C. H., Buchanan, R., Hall, V., Kingsley Pillers, E. M., Wheeler, T. K., & Williams, C. J. (1984). A comparison of two doses of tamoxifen (Nolvadex) in postmenopausal women with advanced breast cancer. *British Journal of Cancer, 50,* 199-205.

Brodie, A. M. H., Wing, L. Y., Goss, P., Dowsett, M., & Coombes, R. C. (1986). Aromatase inhibitors and the treatment of breast cancer. *Journal of Steroid Biochemistry, 24,* 91-97.

Bruchovsky, N. (1997). Androgen and antiandrogens. In J. F. Holland, R. C. Bast, Jr., D. L. Morton, E. Frei, III, D. W. Kufe, & P. R. Weichselbaum (Eds.), *Cancer Medicine* (4th ed.). Baltimore: Williams & Wilkins.

Bruning, P. F., Foufer, J. M. G., Hart, A. A. M., de Jorg-Bakker, M., Linders, D., Van Loor, J., & Nooyen, W. J. (1988). Tamoxifen, serum lipoproteins and cardiovascular risk. *British Journal of Cancer, 58,* 497-499.

Burnstein, K. L., & Cidlowski, J. A. (1989). Regulation of gene expression by glucocorticoids. *Annual Review of Physiology, 51,* 683-699.

Byar, D. P. (1973). The Veterans Administration Cooperative Urological Research Group's studies of cancer of the prostate. *Cancer, 32(5),* 1126-1130.

Caleffi, M., Fentiman, I. S., Clark, G. M., Wang, D. Y., Needham, J., Clark, K., La Ville, A., & Lewis, B. (1988). Effect of tamoxifen on estrogen binding, lipid and lipoprotein concentrations and blood clotting parameters in premenopausal women with breast pain. *Journal of Endocrinology, 119,* 335-339.

Canetta, R., Florentine, S., Hunter, H., & Lenaz, L. (1983). Megestrol acetate. *Cancer Treatment Reviews, 10,* 141-157.

Canney, P. A., Priestman, T. J., Griffiths, T., Latief, T. N., Mould, J. J., & Spooner, D. (1988). Randomized trial comparing aminoglutethimide with high-dose medroxyprogesterone acetate in therapy for advanced breast carcinoma. *Journal of the National Cancer Institute, 80,* 1147-1151.

Clarysse, A. (1985). Hormone-induced tumor flare. *European Journal of Clinical Oncology, 21,* 545-548.

Cohen, J. J. (1989). Lymphocyte cell death induced by glucocorticoids. In R. P. Schleimer, H. N. Claman, & A. L. Dronsky (Eds.), *Anti-inflammatory steroid action: Basic and clinical aspects* (pp. 110-121). San Diego: Academic Press.

Cole, M. P., Jones, C. T. A., & Todd, I. D. H. (1971). A new antiestrogenic agent in late breast cancer: An early clinical appraisal of ICI 46474. *British Journal of Cancer, 25,* 270-275.

Dauvois, S., Danielian, P. S., White, R., & Parker, M. G. (1992). Antiestrogen ICI 164, 384 reduces cellular estrogen receptor by increasing its turnover. *Proceedings of the National Academy of Sciences, USA, 89,* 4037-4041.

DeFriend, D. J., Howell, A., Nicholson, R. I., Anderson, E., Dowsett, M., Mansel, R. E., Blamey, R. W., Bundred, N. J., Robertson, J. F., Saunders, C., Baum, G., Walton, P., Sutcliff, F., & Wakeling, A. E. (1994). Investigation of a new pure antiestrogen (ICI 182, 780) in women with primary breast cancer. *Cancer Research, 54,* 408-414.

Demers, L. M., Lipton, A., Harvey, H. A., Kambie, K. B., Grossberg, H., Brady, C., & Santen, R. J. (1993). The efficacy of CGS 20267 in suppressing estrogen biosynthesis in patients with advanced-stage breast cancer. *Journal of Steroid Biochemistry and Molecular Biology, 44,* 687-691.

Dodds, E. C., Lawson, W., & Noble, R. L. (1938). Biological effects of the synthetic oestrogenic substance 4:4′-dihydroxy-$\alpha \rightarrow \beta$ diethylstilbene. *Lancet, 1,* 1389-1391.

Eisenberger, M., O'Dwyer, P.F., & Friedman, M. (1986). Gonadotropin hormone–releasing hormone: A new therapeutic approach for the treatment of prostate cancer. *Journal of Clinical Oncology, 4,* 414-424.

Ernst, P., & Killman, S. (1970). Perturbation of generation of human leukemic blast cells by cytostatic therapy in vivo: Effects of corticosteroids. *Blood, 36,* 689-705.

Fentiman, I. S., Caleffi, M., & Rodin, A. (1989). Bone mineral content of women receiving tamoxifen for mastalgia. *British Journal of Cancer, 60,* 262-264.

Fisher, B., Constantino, J. P., Redmond, C. K., Fisher, E. R., Wickerman, D. L., Cronin, W. M., & other NSABP contributors. (1994). Endometrial cancer in tamoxifen treated breast cancer patients: Findings from the National Surgical Adjuvant Breast and Bowel Project (NSABP) B-14. *Journal of the National Cancer Institute, 80,* 527-534.

Fornander, T., Rutqvist, L. E., Cedermark, B. V., Glas, U., Mattson, A., Silversward, J. D., Skoog, L., Somell, A., Theve, T., Wilking, N., Askergren, J., & Hjolmar, M. C. (1989). Adjuvant tamoxifen in early breast cancer: Occurrence of new primary cancers. *Lancet, 1,* 117-120.

Furr, B. J. A., & Jordan, V. C. (1984). The pharmacology and clinical uses of tamoxifen. *Pharmacologic Therapies, 25,* 127-205.

Geisler, H. E. (1973). The use of megestrol acetate in the treatment of advanced malignant lesions of the endometrium. *Gynecologic Oncology, 1,* 340-344.

Goss, P. E., Clark, R., & Ambers, U. (1994). Phase II report of vorozale (R83842), a new aromatase inhibitor in postmenopausal women with breast cancer. *ASCO Proceedings, A156,* 88.

Goss, P. E., & Gwyn, K. M. E. H. (1994). Current perspectives on aromatase inhibitors in breast cancer. *Journal of Clinical Oncology, 12,* 2460-2470.

Goss, P. E., Powles, T. J., Dowsett, M., Hutchinson, G., Brodie, A. M., Gazet, J. C., & Coombes, R. C. (1986). Treatment of advanced postmenopausal breast cancer with an aromatase inhibitor, 4-hydroxy androstendione phase II report. *Cancer Research, 46,* 4823-4826.

Harvey, H. A., & Manni, A. (1997). Clinical use of aromatase inhibitors in breast carcinoma. In J. F. Holland, R. C. Bast, Jr., D. L. Morton, E. Frei, III, D. W. Kufe, & R. R. Weichselbaum (Eds.), *Cancer medicine* (4th ed., pp. 1113-1124). Baltimore: Williams & Wilkins.

Harvey, H. A., Santen, R. J., Osterman, J., Samojlik, E., White, D., & Lipton, A. (1979). A comparative trial of transsphenoidal hypophysectomy and estrogen suppression with aminoglutethimide in advanced breast cancer. *Cancer, 43,* 2207-2214.

Henderson, I. C. (1987). Treatment of metastases. In J. R. Harris, S. Hellman, I. C. Henderson, & D. W. Kinne (Eds.), *Breast diseases* (pp. 398-428). Philadelphia: J. B. Lippincott.

Hirsimaki, P., Hirsimaki, Y., Nieminen, A. L., & Payne, B. J. (1993). Tamoxifen induces hepatocellular carcinoma in rat liver: A 1-year study of 2 antiestrogens. *Archives of Toxicology, 67,* 49-59.

Hoffken, K., Jonat, W., Possinger, K., Kölbel, M., Kunz, T., Wagner, H., Becher, R., Callies, R., Friederich, P., & Willmanno, W. (1990). Aromatase inhibitor with 4-hydroxyandrostendione in the treatment of postmenopausal patients with advanced breast cancer: A phase II study. *Journal of Clinical Oncology, 8,* 875-880.

Hoogstraten, B., Fletcher, W. S., Gad-ei-Mawla, N., Maloney, T., Altman, S. J., Vaughn, C. B., & Foulkes, M. A. (1982). Tamoxifen and oophorectomy in the treatment of recurrent breast cancer. *Cancer Research, 42,* 4788-4791.

Horowitz, K. B., & McGuire, W. L. (1978). Estrogen control of progesterone receptor in human breast cancer: Correlation with nuclear processing of estrogen receptor. *Journal of Biological Chemistry, 253,* 2223-2228.

Huggins, C., & Bergenstad, D. M. (1952). Inhibition of human mammary and prostate cancers by adrenalectomy. *Cancer Research, 12,* 134-141.

Huggins, C., & Hodges, C. V. (1941). Studies in prostatic cancer. I. The effect of castration estrogens and androgen injections on serum phosphates in metastatic carcinoma of the prostate. *Cancer Research, 1,* 293-297.

Ingle, J. N., Ahmann, D. L., Green, S. J., Edmonson, J. H., Creagan, E. T., Hahn, R. G., & Rubin, J. (1982). Randomized clinical trial of megestrol acetate versus tamoxifen in paramenopausal or castrated women with advanced breast cancer. *American Journal of Clinical Oncology, 5,* 155-160.

Jensen, E. V., & Jacobson, H. I. (1962). Basic guidelines on the mechanism of estrogen action. *Recent Progress in Hormone Research, 18,* 387-414.

Johnston, S. R. D., Smith, I. E., Doody, D., Jacobs, S., Robertshaw, H., & Dowsett, M. (1994). Clinical and endocrine effects of the oral aromatase inhibitor vorozole in postmenopausal patients with advanced breast cancer. *Cancer Research, 54,* 5475-5881.

Jordan, V. C. (1984). Biochemical pharmacology of antiestrogen action. *Pharmacological Reviews, 36,* 245-276.

Jordan, V. C. (1997). Estrogens and antiestrogens. In J. F. Holland, R. C. Bast, Jr., D. L. Morton, E. Frei, III, D. W. Kufe, & R. R. Weichselbaum (Eds.), *Cancer medicine* (4th ed., pp. 1103-1111). Baltimore: Williams & Wilkins.

Kangas, L. (1990). Review of the pharmacologic properties of toremifene. *Journal of Steroid Biochemistry, 36,* 919-195.

Kangas, L., Nieminen, A. L., Blanco, G., Grānroos, M., Kallio, S., Karjalainen, A., Perilä, M., Södervall, M., & Toivola, R. (1986). A new triphenylethylene compound Fc-1157a. II Antitumor effects. *Cancer Chemotherapy and Pharmacology, 17,* 109-113.

Karlstedt, K. (1971). Progesterone treatment for local recurrence and metastases in carcinoma corpus uteri. *Acta Radiologica: Therapy, Physics, Biology, 10,* 187-192.

Kennedy, B. J. (1962). Massive estrogen administration in premenopausal women with metastatic breast cancer. *Cancer, 15,* 641-648.

Kiang, D. T., & Kennedy, B. J. (1976). "Intranuclear" castration effect of high-dose estrogen. *Proceedings of the American Association of Cancer Research, 17,* 194.

Kiang, D. T., & Kennedy, B. J. (1977). Tamoxifen therapy in advanced breast cancer. *Annals of Internal Medicine, 87,* 687-690.

Kivinen, S., & Maenpaa, J. U. (1986). *Effect of toremifene on clinical hematological and hormonal parameters in different dose levels: Phase I study* (Abstract 2994, p. 778) International Cancer Congress, Budapest.

Klijn, J. G. M., Setyono-Han, B., Bontenal, M., Seynaeve, C., & Foekens, J. (1996). Novel endocrine therapies in breast cancer. *Acta Oncologica, 35* (Suppl. 5), 30-37.

Kristensen, B., Ejlersten, B., Dalgaard, P., Larsen, L., Holmegaard, S. N., Transbol, I., & Mouridsen, H. T. (1994). Tamoxifen and bone metabolism in postmenopausal low-risk breast cancer patients: A randomized study. *Journal of Clinical Oncology, 12,* 992-997.

Lacassagne, A. (1936). Hormonal pathogenesis of adenocarcinoma of the breast. *American Journal of Cancer, 27,* 217-225.

Lerner, H. J., Band, P. R., Israel, L., & Leung, B. S. (1976). Phase II study of tamoxifen. Report of 74 patients with stage IV breast cancer. *Cancer Treatment Reports, 60,* 1431-1435.

Lerner, L. J., Holthaus, F. J., Jr., & Thompson, C. R. (1958). A nonsteroidal estrogen antagonist 1-(p-2-diethylaminoethoxy phenyl)-1-methoxyphenylethanol. *Endocrinology, 63,* 295-318.

Litherland, S., & Jackson, I. M. (1988). Antiestrogens in the management of hormone-dependent cancer. *Cancer Treatment Reviews, 15,* 183-194.

Lonning, P. E., & Lien, E. A. (1995). Mechanism of action of endocrine treatment in breast cancer. *Critical Reviews in Oncology/Hematology, 21,* 158-193.

Love, R. R., Mazess, R. B., Barder, H. S., Epstein, S., Newcomb, P. A. Jordan, V. C., Carbone, P. P., & De Mets, D. L. (1992). Effects of tamoxifen on bone marrow density in postmenopausal women with breast cancer. *New England Journal of Medicine, 326,* 852-856.

Love, R. R., Mazess, R. B., Tormey, D. C., Barden, H. S., Newcomb, P. A., & Jordan, V. C. (1988). Bone mineral density in women with breast cancer treated for at least two years with tamoxifen. *Breast Cancer Research and Treatment, 12,* 297-302.

Love, R. R., Newcomb, P. A., Wiebe, D. A., Surawicz, T. S., Jordan, V. C., Carbone, P. P., & De Mets, D. L. (1990). Lipid and lipoprotein effects of tamoxifen therapy in postmenopausal patients with node negative breast cancer. *Journal of the National Cancer Institute, 82,* 1327-1339.

Love, R. R., Wielbe, D. A., Newcomb, P. A., Cameron, H., Leventhal, H., Jordan, V. C., Feyzi, J., & De Mets, D. L. (1991). Effects of tamoxifen on cardiovascular risk factors in postmenopausal women. *Annals of Internal Medicine, 115,* 860-864.

Love, R. R., Wielbe, D. A., Newcomb, P. A., & Chappell, R. J. (1994). Effects of tamoxifen on cardiovascular risk factors in postmenopausal women after five years of treatment. *Journal of the National Cancer Institute, 86,* 1534-1539.

Lundgren, S., Gunderson, S., Klepp, R., Lonning, P. E., Lund, E., & Kvinnsland, S. (1989). Megestrol accetate versus aminoglutethimide for metastatic breast cancer. *Breast Cancer Research Treatment, 14,* 201-206.

Malkasian, G. D., Jr., Decker, D. G., Mussey, E., & Johnson, C. E. (1971). Progesterone treatment of recurrent endometrial carcinoma. *American Journal of Obstetrics and Gynecology, 110,* 15-21.

McCarty, K. S., Jr., & McCarty, K. S., Sr. (1997). Progestins. In J. F. Holland, R. C. Bast, Jr., D. L. Morton, E. Frei, III, D. W. Kufe, & P. R. Weichselbaum (Eds.), *Cancer medicine* (4th ed., pp. 1087-1102). Baltimore: Williams & Wilkins.

McDonald, C. C., & Stewart, H. J. (1991). Fatal myocardial infarction in the Scottish adjuvant tamoxifen trial. *British Medical Journal, 303,* 435-437.

McGovern, J. P. (1994). Pharmacologic principles. In R. T. Dorr, & D. D. Von Hoff (Eds.). *Cancer chemotherapy handbook* (2nd ed., pp. 15-34). Norwalk, CT: Appleton & Lange.

Morgan, L. R. (1985). Megestrol acetate versus tamoxifen in advanced breast cancer in postmenopausal patients. *Seminars in Oncology, 12,* 43-47.

Morgan, L. R., Schein, P. S., Wolley, P. V., Hoth, D., Macdonald, S., Lippmann, M., Posey, L. E., & Beazley, R. W. (1976). Therapeutic use of tamoxifen in advanced breast cancer: Correlation with biochemical parameters. *Cancer Treatment Reports, 60,* 1437-1443.

Muss, H. B., Paschold, E. H., Black, W. R., Cooper, M. R., Capizzi, R. L., Christian, R., Cruz, J. M., Jackson, D. V., Stuart, J. J., & Richards, F. (1985). Megestrol acetate versus tamoxifen in advanced breast cancer: A phase III trial of the Piedmont Oncology Association (POA). *Seminars in Oncology, 12,* 55-61.

Osborne, C. K., Coronado, E. B., Kilten, L. J., Arteaga, C. I., Fuqua, S. A., Ramasharma, K., Marshall, M., & Li, C. H. (1989). Insulin-like growth factor II (IGF II): A potential autocrine/paracrine growth factor for human breast cancer acting via the IGF I receptor. *Molecular Endocrinology, 3,* 1701-1709.

Pearson, O. H., Ray, B. S., & Harold, C. C. (1956). Hypophysectomy in the treatment of advanced cancer. *Journal of the American Medical Association, 161,* 17-21.

Petree, E., & Schmahl, D. (1987). On the role of additive hormone monotherapy with tamoxifen, medroxyprogesterone acetate, and aminogluthethimide in advanced breast cancer. *Klinische Wochenschrift, 65,* 959-966.

Pickels, T., Perry, L., & Murray, P. (1990). 4-hydroxyandrostenedione: Further clinical and extended endocrine observations. *British Journal of Cancer, 62,* 309-313.

Planting, A. S. T., Alexieva-Figush, J., Blonk-vander Wijst, L., & van Patten, W. L. (1985). Tamoxifen therapy in premenopausal women with metastatic breast cancer. *Cancer Treatment Reports, 69,* 363.

Powles, T. J., Hardy, J. R., Ashley, S. E., Farrington, G. M., Cosgrove, D., Davey, J. B., Dowsett, M., McKinna, J. A., Nash, A. G., Sinnett, H. D., Tilyer, C. R., & Treleven, J. G. (1989). A pilot trial to evaluate the acute toxicity and feasibility of tamoxifen for prevention of breast cancer. *British Journal of Cancer, 60,* 126-131.

Pritchard, K., Meaken, J. W., & Sawka, C. (1985). The role and mechanism of action of tamoxifen in premenopausal women with metastatic carcinoma of the breast. An update. *Proceedings of the American Society of Clinical Oncology, 4,* 54.

Pritchard, K. I. (1991). Droloxifene summary. *American Journal of Clinical Oncology, 14* (Suppl. 2), 562-563.

Pritchard, K. I., Thompson, D. B., Myers, R. E., Sutherland, D. J., Mobbs, B. G., & Meaken, J. W. (1980). Tamoxifen therapy in premonopausal patients with metastatic breast cancer. *Cancer Treatment Reports, 64,* 787-796.

Rauschning, W., & Pritchard, K. I. (1994). Droloxifene, a new antiestrogen: Its role in metastatic breast cancer. *Breast Cancer Research and Treatment, 31,* 83-94.

Robertson, J. R. R., Williams, M. R., Todd, J., Nicholson, R. I., Morgan, D. A. I., & Blamey, R. W. (1989). Factors predicting the response of patients with advanced breast cancer to endocrine (Megace) therapy. *European Journal of Cancer and Clinical Oncology, 25,* 469-475.

Roos, W. K., Deze, L., & Loser, R. (1983). Antiestrogen action of 3-hydroxy-tamoxifen in human breast cancer cell line MCF-7. *Journal of the National Cancer Institute, 71,* 55-59.

Rose, C., & Mourisden, H. T. (1984). Treatment of advanced breast cancer with tamoxifen. *Recent Results in Cancer Research, 91,* 230-242.

Rossner, S., & Wallgren, A. (1984). Serum lipoproteins after breast cancer surgery and effects of tamoxifen. *Atherosclerosis, 53,* 339-346.

Rutqvist, L. E., & Mattson, A. (1993). Cardiac and thromboembolic morbidity among postmenopausal women with early-stage breast cancer in a randomized trial of adjuvant tamoxifen. *Journal of the National Cancer Institute, 85,* 1398-1406.

Santen, R. J. (1981). Suppression of estrogen with aminoglutethimide and hydrocortisone (medical adrenalectomy) as treatment of advanced breast carcinoma. A review. *Breast Cancer Research and Treatment, 1,* 183-202.

Santen, R. J., Lipton, A., & Kendall, J. (1974). Successful medical adrenalectomy with aminoglutethimide. Role of altered drug metabolism. *Journal of the American Medical Association, 230,* 1661-1665.

Santen, R. J., Worgul, T. J., Samojlik, E., Interante, A., Boucher, A. E., Lipton, A., Harvey, H. A., White, D. S., Smart, E., Cox, C., & Wells, S. A. (1981). A randomized trial comparing surgical adrenalectomy with aminoglutethimide plus hydrocortisone in women with advanced breast cancer. *New England Journal of Medicine, 305,* 545-551.

Sawka, C. A., Pritchard, K. I., Paterson, A. H. G., Sutherland, D. J., Thomson, D. B., Shelley, W. E., Myers, R. E., Mobbs, B. G., Malkin, A., & Meakin, J. W. (1986). Role and mechanism of action of tamoxifen in premenopausal women with metastatic breast carcinoma. *Cancer Research, 46,* 3152-3156.

Schally, A. V., & Comaru-Schally, A. M. (1997). Hypothalamic and other peptide hormones. In J. F. Holland, R. C. Bast, Jr., D. L. Morton, E. Frei, III, D. W. Kufe, & P. R. Weichselbaum (Eds.), *Cancer medicine* (4th ed.). Baltimore: Williams & Wilkins.

Schwartzman, R. A., & Cidlowski, J. A. (1997). Corticosteroids. In J. F. Holland, R. C. Bast, Jr., D. L. Morton, E., Frei, III, D. W. Kufe, & P. R. Weichselbaum (Eds.), *Cancer medicine* (4th ed., pp. 1087-1102). Baltimore: Williams & Wilkins.

Sedlacek, S. M., & Horwitz, K. B. (1984). The role of progestins and progesterone receptors in the treatment of breast cancer. *Steroids, 44,* 467-484.

Shearer, R. J., Hendry, W. F., Sommerville, H. F., & Fergusson, J. D. (1973). Plasma testosterone: An accurate monitor of hormone treatment of prostate cancer. *British Journal of Urology, 45,* 668-677.

Steele, R. E., Mellor, L. B., Sawyer, W. K., Wasvary, J. M., & Browne, L. T. (1987). In vitro and in vivo studies demonstrating patient and selective estrogen inhibition with the nonsteroidal aromatase inhibitor, CGS 16949A. *Steroids, 50,* 147-161.

Sunderland, M. S., & Osborne, C. K. (1991). Tamoxifen in premenopausal women with metastatic breast cancer: A review. *Journal of Clinical Oncology, 9,* 1283-1297.

Teller, C., & Jordan, V. C. (1995). Hormonal treatment of advanced breast cancer. *Surgical Oncology Clinics of North America, 4*(4), 751-777.

The Veterans Administration Cooperative Urological Research Group. (1967). Treatment and survival of patients with cancer of the prostate. *Surgery, Gynecology, and Obstetrics, 124,* 1011-1017.

Thompson, C. R., & Werner, H. S. (1951). Studies of estrogen tri-p-anisylchlorethylene. *Proceedings of the Society of Experimental Biology and Medicine, 77,* 494-497.

Toft, D., & Gorski, J. (1966). A receptor molecule for estrogens: Isolation from the rat uterus and preliminary characterization. *Proceedings of the National Academy of Science, USA, 55,* 1574-1581.

Tormey, D. C., Lippmann, M. E., Edwards, B. K., & Cassidy, J. G. (1983). Evaluation of tamoxifen doses with and without fluoxymesterone in advanced breast cancer. *Annals of Internal Medicine, 98,* 139-144.

Tsai, M. J., & O'Malley, R. W. (1994). Molecular mechanisms of action of steroid/thyroid superfamily members. *Annual Review of Biochemistry, 63,* 451-486.

Turken, S., Siris, E., Seldin, E., Seldin, D., Flaster, E., Hyman, G., & Lindsay, R. (1989). Effects of tamoxifen on spinal bone density in women with breast cancer. *Journal of the National Cancer Institute, 81,* 1086-1088.

Valavaara, R., Tuominen, J., & Johansson, R. (1990). Predictive value of tumor estrogen and progesterone receptor levels in postmenopausal women with advanced breast cancer treated with toremifene. *Cancer, 66,* 2264-2269.

VanderBurg, B., Kalkhoven, E., Isbrucher, L., & deLaat, S. W. (1992). Effects of progestins on the proliferation of estrogen-dependent human breast cancer cells under growth-defined conditions. *Journal of Steroid Biochemistry and Molecular Biology, 42,* 457-465.

Van Veelen, H., Willemse, P. H. B., Tjabbes, T., Schwertzer, M. J., Sleijfer, D. T. (1986). Oral high-dose medroxyprogesterone acetate versus tamoxifen: A randomized crossover trial in postmenopausal patients with advanced breast cancer. *Cancer, 58,* 7-19.

Vogelzang, N. J., & Kennealey, G. T. (1992). Recent developments in endocrine treatment of prostate cancer. *Cancer, 70*(4), 966-976.

Wait, R. B. (1973). Megestrol acetate in the management of advanced endometrial carcinoma. *Obstetrics and Gynecology, 41,* 129-136.

Wander, H. E., Kleeberg, U. R., Gärtner, E., Hartlapp, J., Scherpe, A., Bönische, E., & Nagel, G. A. (1987). Megestrol acetate versus medroxyprogesterone acetate in the treatment of metastasizing carcinoma of the breast. *Onkologie, 10,* 104-106.

Ward, H. W. C. (1973). Antioestrogen therapy for breast cancer: A trial of tamoxifen at two dose levels. *British Medical Journal, 1,* 13-14.

Ward, R. L., Morgan, G., Dalley, D., & Kelly, P. J. (1993). Tamoxifen reduces bone turnover and prevents lumbar spine and proximal femoral bone loss in early post menopausal women. *Bone and Minerals, 22,* 87-94.

Willemse, P. H. B., van der Ploeg, E., Sleijfer, D. T., Tjabbes, T., & van Veelen, H. (1990). A randomized comparison of megestrol acetate (MA) and medroxyprogesterone acetate (MPA) in patients with advanced breast cancer. *European Journal of Cancer, 26,* 337-343.

Wouters, W., DeCoster, R., Krekels, M., Van Dun, J., Beirens, D., Haelterman, C., Raeymaekers, A., Freyne, E., Van Gelder, J., Venet, M., & Janssen, P. A. J. (1989). R76713. A new specific nonsteroidal aromatase inhibitor. *Journal of Steroid Biochemistry, 32,* 781-788.

Yee, D., Cullen, K., Paik, S., Perdue, J. F., Hampton, B., Schwartz, A., Lippmann, M. E., & Rosen, N. (1988). Insulin-like growth factor II MRNA expression in human breast cancer. *Cancer Research, 48,* 4491-6696.

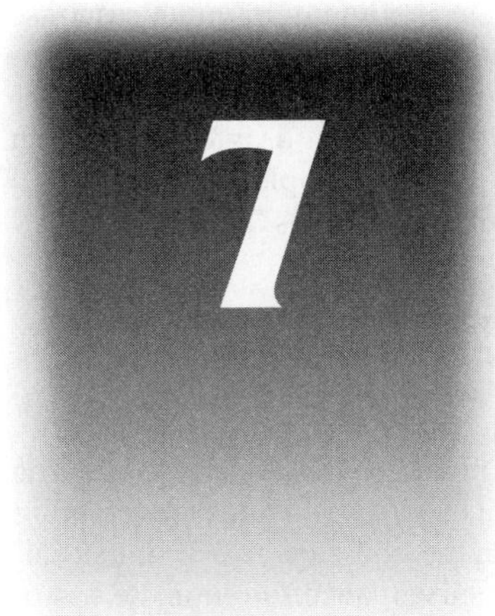

Biotherapy

Elaine DeMeyer, RN, MSN, OCN
Betsy A. Stein, BA, CCRN

INTRODUCTION

Historically, the term *immunotherapy* was used to describe modulation of the immune response. The term *biotherapy* or *biologic therapy* is now used instead to describe this treatment modality (Jassak, 1995). Biotherapy is generally used as a global term to describe the use of biologic agents to activate the immune system and treat cancer, as well as biologic approaches that manipulate the immune system, such as gene therapy and donor lymphocyte infusions (Tomaszewski, DeLa Pena, Molenda, Gantz, Bernato, and Folitz, 1995). The Food and Drug Administration (FDA) defines *biotherapy* as "the use of living organisms or products derived from living organisms to produce, modify, or improve a plant or animal for a specific purpose" (Wujick, 1993).

Biologic agents are substances that are extracted or produced from biologic material. Biologic agents used in biotherapy are called *biologic response modifiers* (BRMs). BRMs are naturally occurring substances produced in small amounts in the body that help regulate normal cellular function. In 1983 the National Cancer Institute's Division of Cancer Treatment Subcommittee on Biologic Response Modifiers defined BRMs as "agents or approaches that will modify the relationship between tumor and host by modifying the host's biologic response to tumor cells, with resultant therapeutic benefit" (Mihich & Fefer, 1983).

Along with surgery, radiotherapy, and chemotherapy, biotherapy is a primary treatment modality in cancer care. Biotherapy is considered the fourth treatment modality for patients with cancer. Many cancer patients receive some form of biotherapy during the course of their disease. Biologic agents can be used for diagnostic, therapeutic, or supportive therapy. They can also be used to assist with the diagnosis of cancer through radioimmune detection of the disease or to establish a differential diagnosis by assisting with tumor identification under the microscope or recognition of cell-surface markers. Therapeutic use of biologic agents (i.e., BRMs) can be implemented as primary or adjuvant therapy to cure, control, or stabilize the disease, or to maintain or enhance quality of life. Biologic agents can also be given in a supportive role to decrease the severity of toxicities associated with other treatment modalities (i.e., hematopoietic growth factors [HGFs]) to enhance neutrophil recovery (Conrad & Horrell, 1995).

Biotherapy is a treatment modality that has many more agents in development than are currently approved. Clinical trials are ongoing to determine the effectiveness and optimal use of BRMs, as single agents, in combination with other BRMs, or in conjunction with other cancer therapies. Future studies will decide how best to integrate BRMs with other treatment modalities to prolong disease-free survival and to improve the patient's quality of life by decreasing treatment-related toxicities.

Oncology nurses must become knowledgeable about this therapeutic modality so that they can provide quality care. With many of the BRMs in investigational stages, nurses are challenged to expand their knowledge base to keep pace with technology. Many principles of symptom management used in caring for patients who are receiving radiation therapy or chemotherapy can be applied to patients who are receiving biotherapy. However, the side effects differ, requiring new knowledge for successful symptom management. Oncology nurses have a crucial role in promoting patient self-care in medication administration and management of side effects, educating patients and families, and assisting with reimbursement issues within the changing health care system. There are numerous opportunities for oncology nurses in biotherapy research, since most of biotherapy is investigational.

HISTORICAL PERSPECTIVES

The theory of biotherapy arose from two types of observations occurring before the nineteenth century: (1) observations of unexplained spontaneous tumor regression, and (2) instances where patients lived longer than expected based on clinical experience or statistical chance. The actual use of biologic agents in the treatment of cancer can be traced back to the nineteenth century (Oettgen & Old, 1991). The development of cytokines, a form of biotherapy, resulted from Dr.

William Coley's work with cancer patients in the early 1900s. Coley, a surgeon at New York's Memorial Hospital from 1891 until 1936, noted that some patients experienced spontaneous tumor regression, where the tumor either decreased in size or disappeared entirely, whereas other patients quickly relapsed after surgery. Many of the patients who remained tumor-free had developed septicemia after surgery. Based on this observation, Coley developed toxins, attenuated or weakened forms of bacteria, to induce an infection assuming that the resulting immune response would destroy both the infection and the cancer. Coley's toxins continued to be used until 1975 and provided the background for the development of cytokine therapy.

Modern immunology emerged in the late 1950s with the recognition of histocompatibility antigens, the identification of antibody structure, and the study of the immune mechanisms that cause disease (Farrell, 1996). During this period, many clinical trials of bacterial agents used as cancer treatment in a variety of tumors were initiated, including *bacillus Calmette-Guérin* (BCG), *Corynebacterium parvum,* and levamisole. These early agents induced a nonspecific effect on the immune system, which resulted in poor clinical outcomes. These outcomes, as a result of the use of impure agents and variability in experimental procedures, led to a negative impression of the promise of immunotherapy in the next two decades (Jassak, 1995). Other biologic agents discovered during this time were interferon (IFN) and tumor necrosis factor (TNF). Both of these biologic agents exhibit antitumor activity. In 1975 the FDA approved IFN as the first biologic agent for use as a cancer therapy.

Key scientific and technologic advances in the 1980s led to a renewed interest in biotherapy including (1) increased understanding of the immune system, (2) genetic engineering, (3) molecular biology, and (4) computer technology. Improved techniques in identifying, isolating, producing, and using biologic agents to improve tumor responses led to further clinical research. As a result, a number of BRMs, including the BCG vaccine, erythropoietin, filgrastim, interleukin-2 (IL-2), levamisole, and sargramostim, were approved by the FDA.

In 1987 the FDA established the Center for Biologics Evaluation and Research (CBER). The mission of CBER is "to protect and enhance the public health through regulation of biological and related products including blood, vaccines, and biological therapeutics according to statutory authorities. The regulation of these products is founded on science and law to ensure their purity, potency, safety, efficacy, and availability" (CBER, 1997). With the establishment of an independent agency overseeing the development and approval of biotherapy, CBER enabled biotherapy to emerge as the fourth treatment modality of cancer.

CONCEPTS AND PRINCIPLES

BRMs may affect the host/tumor in three major ways: (1) by regulating the host's immune response to the tumor; (2) by providing direct antitumor activity to suppress or kill the tumor; or (3) by altering other biologic activities that have an effect on the tumor (Farrell, 1996). Examples of agents that restore, enhance, or modulate the host's immune response include the hematopoietic growth factors. The effect of interleukins (ILs) on the tumor is indirect via immunomodulation. IFNs are examples of BRMs that provide both direct and indirect antitumor activity. An example of an agent that has other biologic effects on the tumor is TNF.

Rationale for Biotherapy

The rationale for biotherapy as a treatment modality is based on the immune surveillance theory, originally proposed by Burnet in the 1970s and modified by Herberman (1992). The theory of immune surveillance proposes that cancer cells are constantly being produced in the body and that an intact immune system is in constant surveillance to eliminate tumor cells. This theory implies that tumors have antigens that, under normal circumstances, can be identified by the immune system, thus enabling the immune system to recognize and destroy tumors. Patients who have deficiencies of the immune system (e.g., acquired immunodeficiency syndrome [AIDS] or congenital deficiencies of the immune system) often develop neoplastic diseases, implying that the immune system may play a role in immune surveillance. Theoretically, when a tumor is diagnosed, it may be a result of a compromised immune system that allowed the tumor to evade the immune surveillance system (Gallucci & McCarthy, 1995). The immune system can be described as a watchdog, continuously searching for cancerous cells and destroying them before they grow numerous enough to become tumors (Rumsey & Rieger, 1992). Suggested mechanisms of how tumors escape immune surveillance are as follows:

- An immune system that is nonfunctioning, overwhelmed, and/or immature
- A reduction or absence of expressed tumor surface antigens, which allows the tumor cells to proliferate without stimulating an immune response
- A defective host antigen-processing (antigenic modulation) that reduces the host's ability to recognize the presence of tumor cells
- A suppression of the immune response due to secretion of substances (e.g., prostaglandins) from tumor cells

Biotherapy uses the body's own biologic agents to stimulate or "rev up" an immune response so that the tumor cells no longer escape the body's immune surveillance system. Not only can BRMs modulate the host's immune response to cancer, but they can have direct effects on the cancer by interfering with its ability to grow, invade, and metastasize (Tomaszewski et al., 1995).

Overview of the Immune System

To understand how BRMs work, as well as the basic principles of biotherapy, it is necessary to review the structure and function of the immune system. This chapter does not attempt to review the complex anatomy and physiology of the immune system. However, some basic principles as they apply to biotherapy are worth mentioning. The immune system is an elaborate, dynamic system with three major functions—defense, homeostasis, and surveillance. The immune system protects the body against bacterial, viral, fungal, and protozoan invasion or other cells that are capable of causing harm (defense); removes damaged cells, worn out cells, and debris from the body (homeostasis); and detects and removes nonself and mutated cells (surveillance) (Rumsey & Rieger, 1992).

The immune system is different from other organ systems of the body because the cells of the immune system are not in constant contact with each other—they circulate freely in and out of the circulatory and lymphatic systems. Immune system function occurs through the integrated interaction of lymphocytes, monocytes, macrophages, basophils, eosinophils, dendritic cells, endothelial cells, and many other cells throughout the body. Although these cells have specific functions, they interact with each other to regulate each other's activities (Rosenberg, 1993). BRMs use the host's immune cells to produce an antitumor effect.

TREATMENT APPLICATIONS

Traditionally, oncology care has primarily focused on surgery, radiotherapy, and chemotherapy. These treatment modalities have effects that are not limited to cancer tissue, including a suppressive effect on the immune system. BRMs act to stimulate rather than suppress antitumor immune mechanisms. Clinical applications for BRMs are expanding while new agents are being studied in clinical trials and approved by the FDA. The biotherapy agents and the indications for which they are currently approved by the FDA are listed in Table 7-1.

BRMs are used clinically to treat a variety of hematologic malignancies such as chronic myelogenous leukemia (CML), hairy cell leukemia, acute promyelocytic leukemia, non-Hodgkin's lymphoma, AIDS-related Kaposi's sarcoma, and myeloma. BRMs are also used to treat a number of solid tumor malignancies including renal cell carcinoma, melanoma, lung cancer, soft tissue sarcoma, and superficial blad-

TABLE 7-1 FDA-Approved Biologic Response Modifiers

Generic Name	Trade Name	FDA-Approved Indications
All-*trans*-retinoic acid, Tretinoin	Vesanoid	Acute promyelocytic leukemia remission induction
Bacillus Calmette-Guerin	TICE BCG	Primary and relapsed carcinoma in situ of the urinary bladder; immunization against tuberculosis
Erythropoietin	Epogen; Procrit	Anemia associated with chronic renal failure; AZT-induced anemia; cancer patients with disease-related or treatment-related anemia
Filgrastim (G-CSF)	Neupogen	Decrease febrile neutropenia in patients with nonmyeloid malignancies receiving myelosuppressive therapy; patients with nonmyeloid malignancies receiving BMT therapy; severe chronic neutropenia; mobilization of hematopoietic progenitor cells into the blood for collection by leukapheresis
Interferon α-2A	Roferon-A	Hairy cell leukemia; Kaposi's sarcoma of AIDS; chronic phase, Philadelphia chromosome positive chronic myelogenous leukemia
Interferon α-2b	Intron-A	Hairy cell leukemia; Kaposi's sarcoma of AIDS; condylomata acuminata; non-A, non-B hepatitis; adjuvant treatment to surgery for malignant melanoma in patients who are free of disease but at high risk for systemic recurrence
Interferon α-N3	Alferon	Condylomata acuminata
Interferon β-1a	Avonex	Multiple sclerosis
Interferon β-1b	Betaseron	Multiple sclerosis
Interferon γ-1b	Actimmune	Infection associated with chronic granulomatous disease
Interleukin-2, Aldesleukin	Proleukin	Metastatic renal cell carcinoma
Levamisole	Ergamisol	Adjuvant therapy with fluorouracil after surgical resection for Duke's Stage C colon cancer
Muromonab-CD3	Orthoclone OKT-3	Acute allograft rejection in renal transplant patients; steroid resistant acute allograft rejection in cardiac and hepatic transplant patients
Sargramostim (GM-CSF)	Leukine, Prokine	Following induction chemotherapy in acute myelogenous leukemia; mobilization and following transplantation of autologous blood cells; myeloid reconstitution after autologous marrow transplantation; myeloid reconstitution after allogeneic marrow transplantation; marrow transplantation failure or engraftment delay
Satumomab pendetide	OncoScint CR/OV	Diagnostic imaging for colon and ovarian cancer

FDA, Food and Drug Administration; *G-CSF,* granulocyte colony-stimulating factor; *BMT,* bone marrow transplantation; *AIDS,* acquired immunodeficiency syndrome; *GM-CSF,* granulocyte-macrophage colony-stimulating factor.
Physicians Desk Reference. (1997). Montvale, NJ: Medical Economics Company.

der cancer. Two diseases, CML and renal cell carcinoma, treated with biotherapy were chosen to illustrate the role of biologic agents in the treatment of hematologic malignancies and the treatment of solid tumor malignancies.

Chronic Myelogenous Leukemia

CML is a hematologic malignancy characterized by a cytogenetic abnormality, specifically a reciprocal translocation between chromosomes 9 and 22, known as the *Philadelphia chromosome.* The three phases of the disease are chronic phase, accelerated phase, and blastic crisis. Blastic crisis precedes the transformation to acute leukemia and is uniformly fatal (Kantarjian, Deisseroth, & Kurzrock, 1993). Therapeutic agents such as hydroxyurea and busulfan are successful in temporarily controlling the elevated white blood counts and splenomegaly but do not provide long-term disease control. The disease progresses to blastic crisis, despite treatment efforts, and patients eventually die. Allogeneic marrow transplantation is used in selected patients to treat CML.

Talpaz and colleagues (1986) first reported the use of a biologic agent, IFN-α, for the treatment of CML. With the use of IFN-α, the Philadelphia chromosome was seen in fewer cells and often completely eliminated. The clinical significance of eliminating the Philadelphia chromosome remains unclear. IFN-α-2a was approved by the FDA in 1995 for the treatment of CML. Although the use of IFN-α has been shown to alter the natural course of the disease, whether patients have an extended chronic phase, delayed onset of blastic crisis, or prolonged survival is still under investigation (see Chapter 57).

Renal Cell Carcinoma

The most common malignancy of the kidney is renal cell carcinoma. More than one third of patients present with metastatic disease at the time of diagnosis. Curative results with surgery are marginal with only 50% of patients with local disease cured, and patients with metastatic disease have a median survival of approximately 10 months (Moldawer & Figlin, 1995). Other treatment modalities such as chemotherapy or radiation therapy have not made an impact on the natural course of the disease.

The agent found to be effective in the treatment of metastatic renal cell carcinoma is IL-2, which was approved by the FDA in 1992 for this indication. The approval was based on a trial by Rosenberg and colleagues (1989) that involved high doses of IL-2 in 255 patients. The side effects of the doses of IL-2 used in the study were considerable, with some patients requiring intensive care support. Many of the current studies for renal cell carcinoma involve different doses, schedules, and combination regimens that are better tolerated while maintaining or improving efficacy. Table 7-2 shows a comparison of IL-2 treatment regimens in renal cell carcinoma patients based on dose level.

TABLE 7-2 Comparison of Interleukin-2 Treatment Regimens in Patients With Renal Cell Carcinoma Based on Dose Level

Type of Therapy/Care Setting	Dose and Schedule	Comparitive Dose*	Response Rate†	Major Toxic Effects
High dose Inpatient care with ICU support (Rosenberg, 1994)	600,000 or 720,000 IU/kg every 8 hours IV bolus for 15 doses and 2 cycles as tolerated	139-167 MID/d	19% (53/283)	Fever, chills, malaise, hypotension, weight gain, oliguria, dyspnea, nausea, vomiting, diarrhea, CNS changes, cardiac arrhythmias
Intermediate dose Inpatient care (Von der Maase, 1991)	18 MIU/m^2/d CIV for 15 days with two induction and four maintenance cycles	36 MID/d	16% (8/51)	Fatigue, hypotension, dyspnea, increased creatinine, weight gain, central and peripheral neurotoxicity
Intermediate dose Inpatient care (Yang, 1994)	72,000 IU/kg every 8 hours IV bolus for 15 doses and 2 cycles	16.7 MID/d	15% (9/60)	Fatigue, chills, naiaise, oliguria, nausea, vomiting, diarrhea, infection
Low dose Ambulatory care (Sleijfer, 1992)	9-18 MIU SC every day for 5 d/wk over 6 weeks	9-18 MID/d	23% (6/26)	Fever, chills, nausea, skin desquamation, SC site inflammation

ICU, intensive care unit; *IU,* international units; *IV,* intravenous; *MID,*minimal inhibitory dose; *CNS,* central nervous system; *MIU,* milli-International unit; *CIV,* continuous intravenous infusion; *SC,* subcutaneous.

*Dose based on a patient with the following dimensions: 77.3 kg (170 lbs); height, 6 ft; body surface area, 2.0 m. All doses have been translated into MIU.

†Response rate is the percentage of complete responders and partial responders of the total number of study patients.

From Wheeler, V.S. (1996). Interleukins: The search for an anticancer therapy. *Seminars in Oncology Nursing, 12*(2), 106-114.

Combination cytokine therapy is also being studied, especially the combination of IL-2 and IFN-α. These studies have shown mixed results. Most have demonstrated response rates comparable to IL-2 alone but with more side effects (fatigue and neurotoxicity) (Atkins, Trehu, & Mier, 1995; Wheeler, 1996). More information on renal cell carcinoma is available in Chapter 49.

CLASSIFICATION OF AGENTS

Classifying BRMs based on their mechanism of action is difficult since the function of many agents is still not completely understood and many agents have more than one antitumor mechanism (Rumsey & Rieger, 1992). Due to the multiple biologic actions and number of agents currently under investigation, no one classification system exists for biologic agents.

In general, BRMs can be classified by their effects on the immune system or their ability to alter and/or affect growth or function of cells (Conrad & Horrell, 1995). Two classification systems have been described based on the biologic actions of BRMs. First, Clark and Longo (1986) classify biologic agents by their primary function into three major categories:

1. Agents that augment, modulate, or restore the host's immune response
2. Agents that have a direct cytotoxic or antitumor activity
3. Agents that produce other biologic effects (e.g., differentiation or maturation of cells, or interference with tumor cell metastasis or transformation).

Second, Mitchell (1992, 1993) uses another approach to classify biologic agents into five broad categories based on their effect on the immune system, as described in Box 7-1.

Biotherapy can also be described as either an active or passive approach (Mitchell, 1992, 1993). An active approach refers to immunization of the tumor-bearing host with materials designed to elicit an immune response capable of retarding or eliminating tumor growth. The active approach can be subdivided into nonspecific or specific. A nonspecific active stimulation of the immune system involves a nonspecific increase in immune activity that could lead to an increase in immune reaction to a tumor. Much of the early attempts at biotherapy of cancer involved nonspecific active approaches with agents such as BCG (Rosenberg, 1993). To elicit a specific active immune response against a specific cancer, many attempts have been made at developing a cancer "vaccine."

The passive approach, also called *adoptive approach,* is the transfer or administration of sensitized immune products. Monoclonal antibodies are an example of a passive approach by mediating a complement-dependent cytotoxicity or antibody-dependent cellular cytotoxicity. The use of lymphocyte-activated killer cells (LAKs) and tumor-infiltrating lymphocytes (TILs) are other examples of passive biotherapy (Tomaszewski et al., 1995).

In addition to categorization, BRMs can also be placed into the four major groups: (1) IFNs, (2) ILs, (3) HGFs, and (4) monoclonal antibodies (MoAbs). Some literature describes a fifth major group of BRMs—other biologic agents—such as levamisole, TNF, or vaccines (Tomaszewski et al., 1995). IFNs and ILs can be combined into a broad class of BRMs called *cytokines.*

Cytokines are proteins that are released from activated immune system cells that affect the behavior of other cells (Jassak, 1990). Cytokines produced by lymphocytes are called *lymphokines,* and cytokines produced by monocytes are called *monokines.* Cytokines are pleiotropic, meaning they are capable of inducing multiple biologic activities in a variety of target cells. Production or administration of one cytokine influences production of or response to other cytokines (Jassak, 1995). The main function of cytokines is to affect the growth and differentiation of white blood cells (WBCs), as well as to regulate immune and inflammatory responses. Cytokines may also be responsible for communication between the neuroendocrine and immune systems. For example, fever can be induced by certain cytokines that act on the temperature-regulating center of the hypothalamus. Some cytokines may play an important role in integrating the immune system with the rest of the body (Gallucci & McCarthy, 1995).

All the major groups of BRMs—IFNs, ILs, HGFs, MoAbs, and "other biologic agents"—have now received regulatory approval for at least one indication (Rieger, 1996). Each of these five major categories is now discussed further.

Box 7-1

Mitchell Classification Scheme of Biologic Agents

Active: Directly stimulates the host's immune function

- *Specific:* Use of vaccines to augment or induce a host response to tumor cells or tumor-associated antigens
- *Nonspecific:* Use of microbial or chemical preparations to enhance overall immunity

Adoptive: Transfer to the host of immune cells with anti-tumor properties

Restorative: Replacement or restoration of deficient immune responses or cells

Passive: Transfer of antibodies or short-lived antitumor factors

Cytomodulatory: Increases recognition of tumor-associated antigens or human leukocyte antigens on the surface of tumor cells

From Mitchell, M. (1992, April). Chemotherapy in combination with biomodulation: A 5-year experience with cyclophosphamide and interleukin-2. *Seminars in Oncology 19*(2) [Suppl. 4], 80-87.

Interferons

Introduction. The IFNs are naturally occurring polypeptides belonging to the family of cytokines that are produced by a variety of immune cells and virally infected cells (Rumsey & Rieger, 1992). The term *interferon* comes from the original premise that it had the ability to "interfere" with viruses. IFNs have a potent antiviral effect, often acting as the first line of defense against many viruses. Since IFN was the first BRM to be discovered and FDA-approved for the treatment of cancer, it is considered the "prototype" of the BRMs.

History. IFN was identified in 1957 by British researchers Isaacs and Lindemann who named this protein *alpha interferon* because of its ability to "interfere" with viral replication (Isaacs & Lindemann, 1957). Other studies indicated that IFN did not directly attack or interfere with viruses but stimulated other cells to produce proteins that prevented reproduction and function of the invading virus. Further research showed that this protein enhances the ability of natural killer (NK) cells to destroy tumor cells, blocks or enhances antibody production by B lymphocytes, and enhances macrophages. Unfortunately, because of the slow and costly production of IFN, it was only used for in vitro studies (Gantz, Tomaszewski, DeLa Pena, Molenda, Bernato, & Kryk, 1995).

With the development of recombinant deoxyribonucleic acid (rDNA) technology in the 1980s, IFN was produced in sufficient quantities for large-scale clinical trials of various diseases, including cancer. In 1986, IFN was approved for the treatment of hairy cell leukemia. Today, IFN-α is also approved for the treatment of AIDS-related Kaposi's sarcoma, condyloma acuminatum, non-A/non-B hepatitis, melanoma at high risk of recurrence, and CML in the chronic phase. IFN-β is indicated for the treatment of multiple sclerosis and IFN-γ for the treatment of chronic granulomatous disease (Skalla, 1996). The role of IFN, alone or in combination with other BRMs or chemotherapy, remains under investigation in the management of other diseases such as non–Hodgkin's lymphoma, chronic lymphocytic leukemia, multiple myeloma, colon cancer, renal cell carcinoma, and other indications for the treatment of melanoma.

Classification. IFNs are classified based on their different amino acid sequence structure. They also differ in the cell receptors used to bind to cells and the signal transduction pathways for transmitting messages within the cell. Several IFNs have been identified: IFN-α, IFN-β, IFN-γ, IFN-ω, and IFN-τ (Gantz, et al., 1995). The following recombinant IFNs are approved: IFN-α-2a and -2b, IFN-α-n3, IFN-β, and IFN-γ-1b (Skalla, 1996).

Biologic Actions. IFNs are proteins that are produced by a variety of cells (B lymphocytes, T lymphocytes, null cells, macrophages, or fibroblasts) when a cell is activated by a stimulus such as a virus, foreign cell, or tumor cell. Once produced, IFNs bind to a specific cell receptor and are then internalized into the nucleus of the cell where they attach to a region of genes that regulates cellular function. As a result the rate at which transcription occurs is altered and cellular activity is modulated. Three major biologic actions of IFNs have been identified—antiviral, antiproliferative, and immunomodulatory (Box 7-2).

Both ribonucleic acid (RNA) and DNA viral replication can be inhibited by IFNs. IFNs have both direct and indirect antiproliferative effects against certain malignant tumor cells. The direct antiproliferative effect of IFNs is thought to be the major role of IFNs in killing tumors (Rosenberg, 1993). Immunomodulation occurs when IFNs stimulate or inhibit the activation of immune cells, such as NK cells or macrophages, or the secretion of other cytokines. Another

Box 7-2
The Biologic Effects of Interferon

Antiviral effect: When a cell is infected with a virus, it synthesizes and releases interferon into the extracellular space. The interferon then binds to receptors on other cells, causing a complex chain of reactions that results in the production of other proteins that interfere with viral replications

Antiproliferative effects: Interferon slows down the replications of some malignant tumor cells and reduces the rate at which the tumor grows.

Immunomodulatory effect: Interferon increases the killing potential of natural killer cells. In addition, interferon induces immune cells and tumor cells to express high levels of human lymphocyte antigens.

Modified from Yasko, J., M, Kearney, B., & Conrad, K. (1997). *Biotherapy in cancer.* Richmond, CA: Berlex Laboratories.

immunomodulatory effect of IFNs occurs when IFNs enhance the expression of tumor-associated antigens or oncogene expression (Moldawer & Figlin, 1995; Skalla, 1996; Gantz et al., 1995).

All IFNs have these three major biologic properties; however, the effects differ among the different subtypes of IFN. Some functions are specific to a particular IFN. For example, IFN-γ is a quantitatively potent immunostimulator (Bonnem & Oldham, 1987). Other functions seem to overlap, such as the potent antiviral effects of IFN-α, -β, and -γ. The therapeutic effectiveness, pharmacokinetics, and severity of side effects also differ between the different subtypes of IFNs. Because of these differences, one IFN cannot be substituted for another (Gantz et al., 1995).

Interleukins

Introduction. ILs are also naturally occurring proteins of the immune system under the broad category of cytokines. The term *interleukin* describes the communicating function of these proteins as "inter," meaning *between,* and "leukin," meaning *leukocytes* or *white blood cells* (Sharp, 1995). Cytokines can be thought of as the "telephone" of the immune system, because they assist with regulation of the immune system by communicating messages between cells and signaling cells to alter their function.

History. The first interleukin, IL-1, was originally known by three different names—endogenous pyrogen, lymphocyte activator, and B lymphocyte activator (Gery, Gershon, & Waksman, 1972a/1972b; DeLaPena, Tomaszewski, & Bernato 1996). To date, 17 ILs have been reported (Farrell, 1996). In 1992 the FDA approved recombinant IL-2, or aldesleukin, under the trade name Proleukin (Chiron Corp, Emeryville, CA) for the treatment of metastatic renal cell carcinoma. Aldesleukin is made through genetic engineering by inserting the human IL-2 gene into *Escherichia coli* bacteria (Wheeler, 1996). Other ILs are in various phases of clinical investigation.

Classification. ILs were first classified and named according to their function. When scientists discovered that ILs have pleiotropic functions, meaning they are capable of inducing multiple biologic activities in various cells, they realized that many of the ILs identified had several different names that described their different functions. This identification of ILs led to confusion as researchers thought they had discovered new ILs when in fact, they were describing a different function of one previously identified (Rosenberg, 1993). In an effort to standardize classification, a nomenclature was introduced in which each IL is named in the order that it was discovered (e.g., IL-1, IL-2, IL-3, etc.) rather than on the basis of function.

Biologic Actions. ILs provide communication between cells by binding to receptor sites on the cell-surface membranes of the target cell. Once bound, the cell receives a signal to alter its level of activity or function. Limited information is available about most cytokine receptors, with the exception of IL-2 (Rosenberg, 1993). IL binding and activation of cells can be described as autocrine action, paracrine action, or endocrine action. *Autocrine action* ("auto," meaning self) is known as the binding and activation of the IL to the same cell that produced the IL. *Paracrine action* refers to binding and activation of nearby cells, and when distant cells are bound and activated, it is called *endocrine action.* Paracrine action is the most common action of ILs.

There are three major biologic properties of ILs—immunomodulation, immunoregulation, and hematopoiesis. ILs exhibit an indirect antitumor effect through immunomodulation by stimulating other cells that have antitumor effects, such as monocytes, T lymphocytes, and NK cells. Immunomodulation also includes the secretion of other cytokines that may have antitumor effects. Immunoregulation is the regulation of the immune system by augmenting, restoring or suppressing immune functional activity (DeLaPena et al., 1996). ILs can either directly or indirectly stimulate hematopoiesis. For example, direct stimulation occurs when IL-4 stimulates B lymphocytes to grow and differentiate. An example of indirect stimulation is when ILs induce production of HGFs, such as granulocyte-macrophage colony-stimulating factor (GM-CSF) (Sharp, 1995) (Table 7-3).

Hematopoietic Growth Factors

Introduction. HGFs are a large group of naturally occurring glycoproteins that are responsible for the regulation of blood cell formation and function of many of the mature blood cells. The Greek term *hematopoietic* describes the role of these proteins as "haima," referring to *blood* and "poiein," meaning *to make.* (DeLaPena et al., 1996). The HGFs regulate cell production as part of the normal body processes or in response to a stimuli such as an infection or decrease in oxygen.

History. HGFs were originally discovered in the 1950s. However, like IFN, the production of HGFs was limited until the discovery of rDNA technology, which allowed HGFs to be cloned and reproduced in large quantities for clinical trials. HGFs were first identified through colony assays, where WBCs are grown in petri dishes when nutrients and marrow stem cells are combined and incubated. Hence the term *colony-stimulating factors* (CSFs) was coined to describe these factors that form specific colonies of cells. Today, CSFs are a subcategory of the broader category of HGFs. Three recombinant HGFs are currently approved by the FDA. They include erythropoietin (EPO) (Epogen, epoetin-alfa; Amgen Inc., Thousand Oaks, CA; Procrit, epoetin-alfa; Ortho Biotech, Raritan, NJ), granulocyte colony-stimulating factor (G-CSF) (Neupogen, filgrastim; Amgen Inc., Thousand Oaks, CA), and GM-CSF (Leukine, sargramostim; Immunex Corp., Seattle, WA).

In 1989, EPO was the first HGF to be approved for use with patients with chronic renal failure receiving dialysis. Other approved indications for EPO include the treatment of anemia in patients with human immunodeficiency virus (HIV) infection receiving zidovudine and chemotherapy-induced anemia in patients with nonmyeloid malignancies (Rieger & Haeuber, 1995). G-CSF, initially approved by the FDA in 1991, is approved for four indications (*Physicians Drug Reference* [PDR], 1997):

1. To decrease the incidence of infections in patients with nonmyeloid malignancies receiving myelosuppressive chemotherapy
2. To enhance myeloid recovery and decrease the incidence of infection after bone marrow transplantation for nonmyeloid malignancies
3. To manage severe chronic neutropenia
4. To initiate mobilization of hematopoietic progenitor cells into the blood for collection by leukapheresis

Also initially FDA-approved in 1991, GM-CSF is approved to enhance myeloid recovery in patients (PDR, 1997):

1. Receiving induction chemotherapy for acute myelogenous leukemia
2. With nonmyeloid malignancies undergoing autologous bone marrow transplantation
3. After human leukocyte antigen-related allogeneic bone marrow transplantation
4. After peripheral blood stem cell transplantation
5. Marrow transplantation failure or engraftment delay

GM-CSF is also approved for use in mobilization of hematopoietic progenitor cells into peripheral blood for collection by leukapheresis.

Although approved for specific uses, both G-CSF and GM-CSF are used clinically for patients with various malignancies and treatment-induced toxicities. These factors have significantly altered the care of many oncology patients by decreasing the period of neutropenia so that patients are less susceptible to opportunistic infection and enabling chemotherapy agents to be given according to schedule without delay. The field of blood and marrow transplantation has been significantly affected as a result of these factors. Higher doses of chemotherapy, with and without stem cell rescue, can be administered as a result of HGFs. Other HGFs are currently in various phases of clinical investigation, including those agents that stimulate platelet production.

Classification. HGFs are classified according to the cell line that is stimulated in the hematopoietic cascade (Fig. 7-1). Class I HGFs are multilineage, meaning they stimulate

Table 7-3 Biologic Activities of Interleukins

Type	Source	Main Functions
Interleukins (IL)		
IL-1 (α and β)	Predominantly macrophages	↑ Immune response; inflammatory mediator; activates T cells; activates phagocytes; ↑ prostaglandin production; induces a fever
IL-2 (T cell growth factor [TCGF])	Predominantly helper T lymphocytes; NK cells	↑ T lymphocytes and NK cells; ↑ growth and ↑ T cells
IL-3 (multiple colony-stimulation factor [CSF])	T lymphocytes, mast cells, NK cells	Hematopoietic growth factor for immature hematopoietic precursor cells, ↑ NK cells
IL-4 (B cell growth factor [BCGF])	T lymphocytes, mast cell	Growth factor for T cells, activated B cells, and mast cells; macrophage-activating factor, ↑ IgE reactions
IL-5	T lymphocytes, macrophages	↑ Growth and proliferation of activated B cells, ↑ eosinophils, ↑ T cell production
IL-6	Monocytes, T and B lymphocytes, fibroblasts, endothelial cells	B cell stimulatory and differentiation factor; ↑ hematopoiesis, ↑ inflammatory response, fever
IL-7	Bone marrow, thymus	↑ Lymphoid cells
IL-8 (monocyte-derived neutrophil chemotactic factor)	Macrophages, monocytes, endothelial cells	Triggers chemotactic activity of neutrophils and lymphocytes
IL-9	Helper T cells	T cell and mast cell growth factor; maturation of erythroid progenitors
IL-10	Helper T cells	↓ Proliferation of helper T cells; ↑ cytotoxic T cell differentiation; induces MHC antigen expression, ↓ cytokines
IL-11	Fibroblasts	↑ Monocyte and B cell function, ↓ some inflammatory cytokines
IL-12	Macrophages	↑ Helper T cells and production of other lymphocytes and cytokines
IL-13	Activated T cells	↑ Gene expression in nerve and intestinal cells, ↑ osteoclasts, ↑ progenitor cells in bone marrow
IL-14	T cells	B cell growth factor
IL-15	Macrophages	Activity identical to that of IL-2
IL-16	CD8+ T cells	Chemotactic factor and growth factor for CD4+ T cells, chemotactic for eosinophils
IL-17	Helper T cells	↑ IL-6 and IL-8
Interferon (IFN)		
IFN-α	T and B lymphocytes, macrophages	Provides antiviral protection; ↓ B cell proliferation; ↓ IL-8, ↓ tumor growth, ↑ NK cell
IFN-β	Fibroblasts, macrophages, epithelial cells	Provides antiviral protection; ↑ IL-6, ↓ IL-8
IFN-γ	T lymphocytes, NK cells	Activates macrophages; ↑ B cell differentiation and NK cell activity, ↓ tumor growth
Tumor Necrosis Factor (TNF)		
TNF-α	Macrophages, lymphocytes, fibroblasts, endothelial cells	↑ Cytokines, ↑ inflammatory and immune responses
TNF-β	T cells	Cytotoxic to tumor cells, ↑ phagocytosis by macrophage and neutrophil, ↑ macrophages, ↑ B cell proliferation
Colony-Stimulating Factors (CSF)		
G-CSF	Monocytes, fibroblasts	Myeloid growth factor
GM-CSF	T cells, fibroblasts, monocytes, endothelial cells	Myelocytic growth factor
M-CSF	Monocytes, lymphocytes, fibroblasts, endothelial and epithelial cells	Macrophage growth factor
Transforming Growth Factor (TGF-β)		
	Lymphocytes, macrophages, platelets, bone	Chemotactic for macrophages, ↑ IL-1 production; stimulates fibroblasts for wound healing; inhibits immune response; potentially inhibits mitotic division in other cells

↑, Increased; ↓, decreased; see text for other abbreviations.

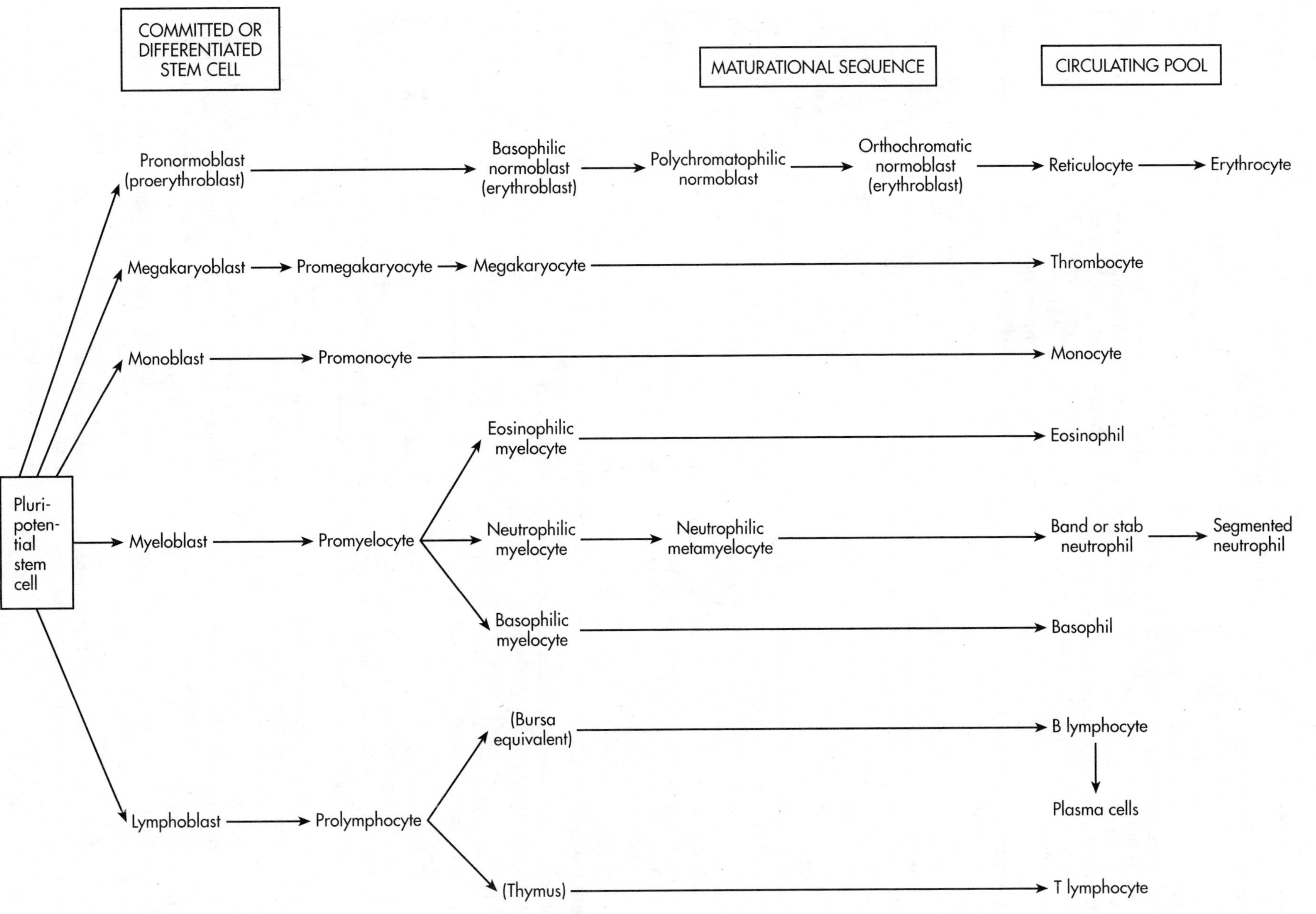

Fig. 7-1 Hematopoietic growth chart depicting proliferation, differentiation, and maturation of the various cell lineages. (From Amgen Inc., Thousand Oaks, CA.)

more than one cell line. For example, GM-CSF stimulates the production of granulocytes, monocytes, macrophages, and erythrocytes (Pitler, 1996). Lineage-specific HGFs stimulate one specific cell lineage. G-CSF is an example of a lineage-specific HGF because it primarily stimulates neutrophil production. Fusion molecules of growth factors can be engineered using molecular techniques. For example, IL-3 and GM-CSF have been fused together to create a molecule, PIXY321. Whether fusion molecules have greater biologic effects than either single agent alone remains unclear. Fusion molecules, like PIXY321, create a new breed of HGFs with potential differences in toxicities than either individual factor.

Biologic Actions. HGFs are produced by a variety of cells, including activated T lymphocytes, fibroblasts, endothelial cells, and macrophages (Wujick, 1995). HGFs can act directly or indirectly on cells to regulate blood cell proliferation, differentiation, maturation, and function. Similar to IFNs and ILs, HGFs act directly on cells by binding to receptor sites on the cell-surface membranes of the target cell and internalizing themselves into the cell, directing it to divide or mature (Wujick, 1995). Since both immature and mature cells contain receptors, HGFs also enhance the function of mature cells. Cells may express several receptors for more than one type of HGF, resulting in overlapping function and synergistic enhancement of the HGFs. Indirectly, HGFs can initiate a secondary cytokine cascade by stimulating other cytokines that interact with a different target cell (Pitler, 1996). For example, GM-CSF causes the release of TNF, which induces fever by affecting the temperature-regulating center in the hypothalamus.

Monoclonal Antibodies

Introduction. Antibodies, also called *immunoglobulins,* are naturally occurring proteins produced by B lymphocytes to protect the body from foreign antigens. The term *monoclonal antibodies* (MoAbs) arises from the fact that these antibodies are a clone of a single cell that reacts to a specific antigen. The term *magic bullet* was used by the media to describe MoAbs because of their ability to carry tumorcidal agents to cancer cells. Clearly, MoAbs have demonstrated effectiveness in the treatment of certain malignancies, but they are not the "magic bullet" cure that was touted by the media.

History. In 1975, Nobel prize winners Kohler and Milstein developed a technique called *hybridoma,* which allowed production of large quantities of pure antibodies against a target antigen. Mice were injected with a particular antigen, which resulted in the mouse's B lymphocytes recognizing the antigen as foreign and developing antibodies against the target antigen. The lymphocytes producing these antibodies were then fused with malignant mouse cells to form a new cell known as a *hybridoma.*

Chemotherapeutic drugs, toxins, radionuclides, and other BRMs are examples of some of the agents that have been conjugated with MoAbs (Baquiran, Dantis, & McKerrow, 1996). MoAbs can aid with diagnosis of cancer by assisting the pathologist in the histopathologic classification of cancer or by enhancing tumor imaging. They may be used for treatment of cancer by targeting therapy such as chemotherapy, biotherapy, or radiotherapy. Some MoAbs exhibit direct tumor kill by inducing cell membrane lysis (Rieger, 1992). Other clinical applications of MoAbs include the following:

- Assisting medical laboratories to improve understanding of cell differentiation and cancer biology
- Purging autologous bone marrow for the removal of cancer cells or to remove T lymphocytes that are responsible for graft versus host disease (GVHD) in allogeneic transplantation
- Treating allograft rejection in solid organ transplantation

MoAbs have also been used to manage GVHD after allogeneic marrow transplantation. Although numerous MoAbs have been studied, only two MoAbs have received FDA approval, muromonab-CD3 (Orthoclone OKT-3; OrthoBiotech, New Brunswick, NJ) and satumomab pendetide (OncoScint CR/OV; Cytogen, Princeton, NJ). By targeting the CD3 surface antigen of human T lymphocytes, muromonab-CD3 is indicated for the treatment of acute allograft rejection in renal transplant patients and steroid-resistant acute allograft rejection in cardiac and hepatic transplant patients. Satumonab pendetide is approved for diagnostic imaging for the detection of colorectal and ovarian cancers (PDR, 1997).

Classification. MoAbs can be placed into two broad categories, unconjugated or conjugated. Unconjugated MoAbs are considered "native" MoAbs because they are used alone. An example of an unconjugated MoAb is L6, which has strong reactivity with colon, ovarian, breast, and lung cancer. Conjugated MoAbs are developed by coupling the MoAbs with various agents such as drugs, toxins, radionuclides, or BRMs. Often the name of MoAbs consists of only numbers and letters that refer to the antigen for which it is targeted, the specific clone from which it originated, or the corporation that developed it. For example, OKT-3 is named after its target—CD3 receptors on T lymphocytes.

Biologic Actions. MoAbs function based on the passive antibody theory that states that the immune system is able to develop antibodies against any antigens encountered by the host. In general, when the B lymphocyte recognizes an antigen, the immunoglobulins on their cell surface act as receptors for the antigen, eventually forming an antigen/antibody complex. This complex binds to a helper T lymphocyte, which secretes cytokines that stimulate the B lymphocytes to transform into plasma cells that actively secrete antibodies. The complex can be eliminated by activation of complement or by the liver and spleen (Gallucci & McCarthy, 1995).

With the discovery of the hybridoma technique, researchers can now develop antibodies to any antigen they choose. The majority of MoAbs in use are made from the subgroup of immunoglobulin G (Bacquiran et al., 1996). Although MoAbs can be made for various antigens, several obstacles exist with their use. Tumor characteristics such as the size of the tumor, vascularity, removal of cell surface antigens by antigenic modulation, and interstitial pressure, can affect the efficiency of the targeting MoAb (Farrell, 1996; DiJulio & Liles, 1995). Another limitation with MoAb therapy has been the development of human antimurine antibodies (HAMA), which is a human antibody response against any antigens in the preparation of the murine MoAb (DiJulio & Liles, 1995).

Other Biologic Agents

Other biologic agents besides the four major categories of biologic agents (i.e., IFNs, ILs, HGFs, and MoAbs) have been used in cancer care. BRMs that do not fall under the previously mentioned categories include BCG, retinoids, levamisole, TNF, and effector (activated) cells such as LAK cells and TILs. Many biologic agents remain in the investigational stage and have yet to be categorized.

MANAGEMENT OF PATIENTS RECEIVING BIOTHERAPY

With the increasing use of biotherapy as the fourth treatment modality, both the novice and the experienced oncology nurse need to be knowledgeable about this treatment in order to provide quality patient care. Oncology nurses who have learned how to manage side effects of chemotherapy and radiation therapy will be able to apply that knowledge and skill in the management of the patient receiving biotherapy. However, some symptom management considerations of biotherapy require creative approaches, particularly when helping patients/families deal with the chronic effects of biotherapy, such as fatigue and flu-like symptoms (Table 7-4). Nurses must be knowledgeable about the side effects common to many of the BRMs and toxicities specific to the particular agent the patient is scheduled to receive. Nurses caring for patients receiving biotherapy must have a basic understanding of the immune system and how BRMs work in relation to the immune system. The Oncology Nursing Society (ONS) has published a biotherapy manual that contains an overview of the general concepts of biotherapy and recommendations for education and clinical practicum (Conrad & Horrell, 1995). The field of biotherapy is changing and evolving so rapidly that the oncology nurse is challenged to keep abreast of which BRMs remain in clinical trials and which BRMs have been FDA-approved for specific diseases and conditions. Since many patients receive biologic agents that are still under investigation, the nurse must also be familiar with the clinical trial and informed consent process (Farrell, 1996).

The Physician's Role

After deciding that a patient is a candidate for receiving biotherapy, either an approved or investigational agent, the physician advises the patient and family of the treatment plan. The physician discusses the purpose of therapy, treatment course, adverse reactions to treatment, and any alternative treatment options. The physician may use practice guidelines, in the form of standards or algorithms, to guide the care of patients receiving biotherapy with specific diseases or symptoms. The American Society of Clinical Oncology (ASCO) published guidelines or recommendations for the use of G-CSF and GM-CSF for patients not enrolled in clinical trials (ASCO, 1994). The ASCO guidelines are not intended to replace medical judgment or medical practice decisions but rather are meant to serve as a tool to provide recommendations for practice (Pitler, 1996).

Physicians conducting clinical trials are required to obtain Institutional Review Board approval and to follow Good Clinical Practice Guidelines as defined by the FDA. If the biologic agent is investigational, it is the responsibility of the physician to obtain a signed statement of informed consent from each patient. The nurse can assist in the informed consent process by reinforcing, clarifying, or providing additional information; assisting the patient and family in formulating questions and communicating concerns to the physician; and communicating to the physician any patient misunderstandings of the benefits and risks of therapy, as well as alternative therapy (Conrad & Horrell, 1995). Any patient questions or concerns should be conveyed to the physician for clarification before initiation of therapy.

Ambulatory or Home Care Considerations

Patients receiving biotherapy are often treated in the ambulatory or home care setting. Many of the biologic agents are given by the subcutaneous route and can be safely administered outside of an acute care setting. This shift in care from the acute care setting to the ambulatory care setting creates a unique set of challenges for patients and their families. Oncology nurses are in a key position to coordinate patient care with the multidisciplinary team as patients move from one health care setting to another. Continuity of care throughout the health care system must be provided by the oncology nurse in order to achieve optimal patient care.

When biotherapy is initiated in the outpatient setting, the first dose is typically given in a setting where the patient can be closely monitored. The type and length of monitoring depends on the specific agents being administered and the anticipated side effects. Emergency drugs, including diphenhydramine, epinephrine, and solumedrol, should be immediately available, particularly when administering biotherapy agents such as MoAbs, which can cause a hypersensitivity reaction. Quick response to these adverse reactions is important to prevent a negative patient outcome (Baquiran et al., 1996). Symptom report forms or nursing care flow sheets may be helpful to document the most common side effects experienced by patients, symptom management interventions, and patient response to intervention (White, 1992). Patient diaries or logbooks may also be useful for patients receiving biotherapy as an outpatient or in the home (Brophy & Sharp, 1991). An example of a patient diary for patients receiving IL-2 is provided in Fig. 7-2.

The Nurse's Role

Components of nursing practice pertinent to providing quality patient care to patients receiving biotherapy include side

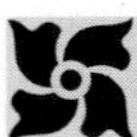

TABLE 7-4 Standard of Care for the Patient Undergoing Biotherapy

Patient Problem and Outcomes	Nursing Interventions and Rationales	Patient Education Instructions
Fatigue	1. Assess patient's level of fatigue using 0-5 verbal rating scale with 0 being no fatigue. 2. Assess patient's ability to perform activities of daily living. 3. Control other symptoms that may exacerbate fatigue (e.g., nausea, vomiting, diarrhea, anemia). 4. Assess the effects of fatigue on patient's sexuality. 5. Monitor the impact of fatigue on patient's perceived quality of life. 6. Offer resources for counseling or consult other members of the multidisciplinary team. 7. Suggest manipulation of treatment dose or schedule to the physician. 8. Encourage adequate nutrition and hydration.	1. Provide patient with information about the likelihood of experiencing fatigue. 2. Encourage patients to keep a diary or log of patterns of fatigue and activities that increase or decrease fatigue. 3. Instruct patient on interventions to decrease fatigue: • Balance periods of activity with periods of rest • Plan ahead; schedule activities when energy levels are highest • Realize limitations, prioritize activities, and delegate unimportant activities • Keep active—exercise when possible 4. Educate patient and family about the negative effect of prolonged bedrest and too much inactivity. 5. Provide patient with information on patient diary.
Flu-like syndrome	1. Assess patient for signs and symptoms associated with flu-like syndrome (e.g., fever, chills/rigors, myalgias, headache, malaise, bone pain). 2. Assess factors that may exacerbate symptoms (e.g., age, performance status, hydration status). 3. Obtain baseline temperature and vital signs. Continue to monitor vitals as needed. 4. Administer pharmacologic agents to decrease symptoms (e.g., antipyretics, antiemetics, antidiarrheals). 5. Request and administer premedications with subsequent doses. 6. Administer medications to control chills and rigors. 7. Provide comfort measures such as warm blankets, increase room temperature, sponge baths, ice packs, or hypothermia blankets. 8. Consider guided imagery or relaxation techniques to decrease chilling and anxiety.	1. Provide patient with information about the likelihood of experiencing flu-like symptoms. 2. Encourage patients to keep a diary or log of fever patterns. 3. Educate patient about when to notify health care team (e.g,. high fevers, uncontrollable symptoms). 4. Instruct patient to drink at least 8 to10 glasses of fluid per day. 5. Teach patient relaxation and guided imagery techniques.

effect management, patient education, assistance with economic issues, and psychosocial support (Tomaszewski et al., 1995). Fig. 7-3 provides a conceptual model for understanding the special needs of patients receiving biotherapy. Nurses must apply the nursing process to assess patient needs and to plan and implement interventions that assist patients and families (Farrell, 1996). In caring for patients undergoing biotherapy, the nurse should assess the following areas: the type of therapy and treatment plan; the goal of the therapy (e.g., diagnostic, therapeutic, or supportive); patient tolerance during therapy; patient and family understanding of therapy; and patient and family educational and resource needs (Sandstrom, 1996). An ongoing evaluation of patient tolerance to therapy and the effectiveness of interventions is critical to avoid patient early withdrawal from treatment and to assist patients in their quality of life.

Managing Physical Needs. Although some side effects are common to most BRMs, side effects of biotherapy often depend on the specific BRM with its own distinct biologic and chemical properties. Toxicities also depend on the dose, route of administration, and schedule, as well as concomitant therapy. Most biotherapy toxicity is dose related, meaning the intensity and often frequency of effects increase as the dose increases. Unlike chemotherapy, with biotherapy there are typically no cumulative dose-toxic effects. Furthermore, some side effects associated with biotherapy are immediately reversible once therapy is discontinued. Side effects from biotherapy can be acute or chronic. Acute complications such as hypotension occur early in therapy. Hypotension is a common dose-dependent effect of high-dose IL-2 that reverses once the drug is discontinued. Since many of the agents are given over a long period, many

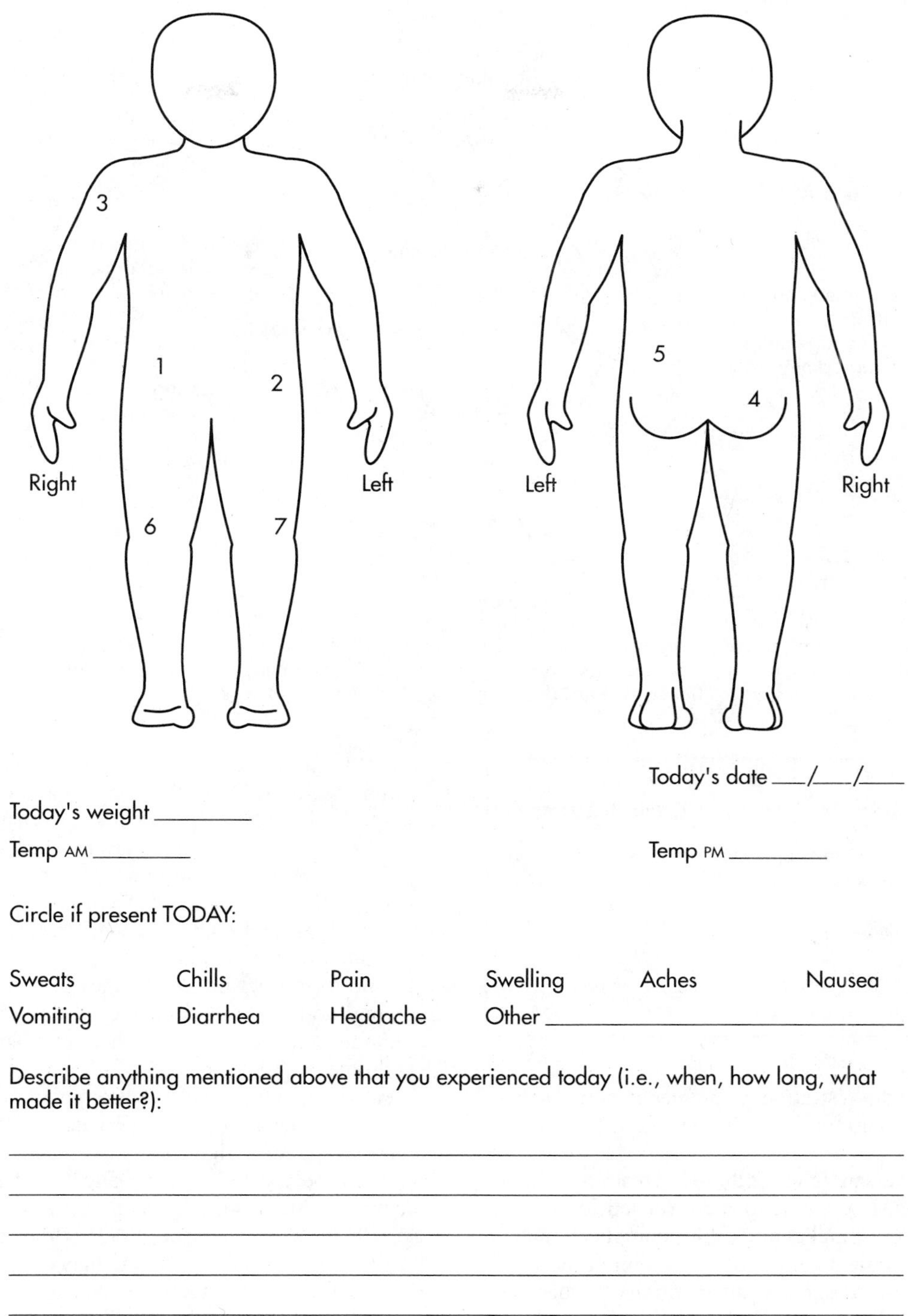

Fig. 7-2 **A,** Schematic for rotating injections of biologic agents. **1,** Monday; **2,** Tuesday; **3,** Wednesday; **4,** Thursday; **5,** Friday; **6,** Saturday; **7,** Sunday. **B,** A patient diary for patient's receiving IL-2. (From Aimee Lanier, Baylor University Medical Center, Dallas, TX.)

of the side effects are considered chronic complications (e.g., fatigue) (Sandstrom, 1996). The timing of biotherapy complications may differ significantly from the timing of chemotherapy side effects. Although most side effects are not life threatening, they often have a significant impact on the patient's quality of life (Rieger, 1995b). Nurses must be aware of potential toxicities with approved agents, as well as the research protocol parameters for acceptable toxicities of investigational agents. With this knowledge, nurses can predict potential complications to be proactive when caring for patients receiving BRMs. For example, with the knowledge that BRMs can cause flu-like symptoms, nurses can

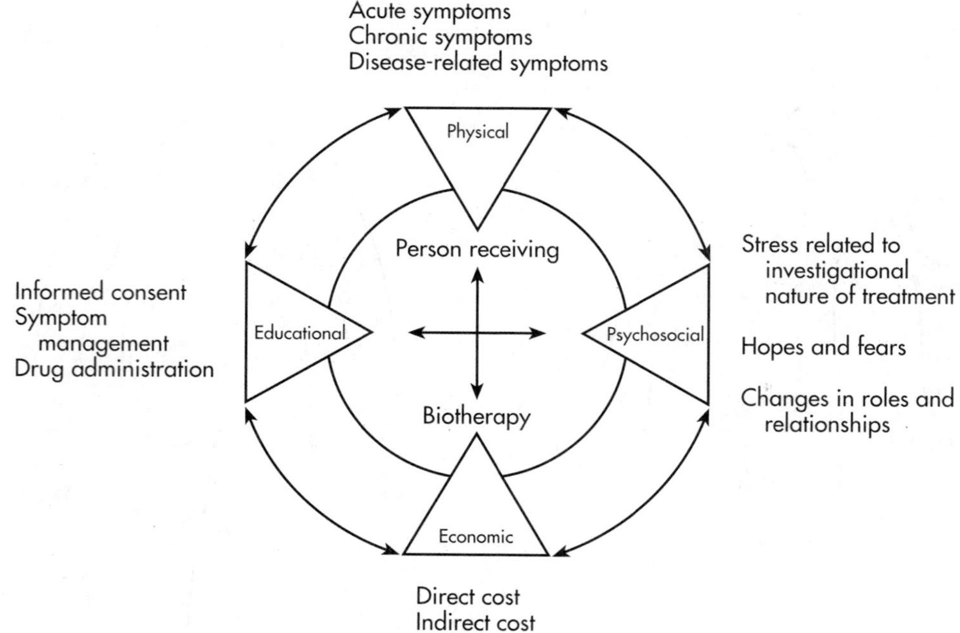

Fig. 7-3 Needs of biotherapy patients: a conceptual model. (From Tsevat, J., & Lacasse, C. [1992]. Understanding the special needs of patients receiving biotherapy: A conceptual model. In R. Carroll-Johnson [Ed.], *The biotherapy of Cancer-V.* Pittsburgh: Oncology Nursing Press.)

Box 7-3

Interventions to Decrease Site Complications

- Warm the agent to room temperature before administration.
- Rotate injection sites (select the abdomen whenever possible).
- Do not aspirate before injection.
- Use 27 G needle.
- Inject slowly (15-30 seconds) at a 90-degree angle.
- Apply gauze to the injection site.

advocate for the administration of premedications such as acetaminophen to help alleviate discomfort (Tomaszewski et al., 1995).

Biologic agents can have both local reactions and/or systemic toxicities. Local reactions are related to subcutaneous injection site complications. Site complications can include erythema, inflammation, and irritation at the injection sites. Box 7-3 describes interventions to decrease local or site complications (Comley, 1996; DeLaPena et al., 1996).

Since BRMs are naturally occurring proteins, it was initially thought that they would have minimal toxic effects. However, these agents have a toxicity profile that is unique when compared with other cancer treatment modalities (Sandstrom, 1996). Fig. 7-4 outlines some of the common systemic toxicities associated with BRMs. Systemic toxicities commonly associated with biotherapy include constitutional or flu-like symptoms, fatigue, anorexia, weight loss or gain, mental status changes, integumentary changes, hypotension, and hematologic changes. Other systemic toxicities of BRMs are limited to a particular agent or more prevalent with a specific BRM (Table 7-5). For example, HGFs have minimal side effects, whereas IL-2 affects nearly all systems (Sandstrom, 1996). Complications such as capillary leak syndrome and renal insufficiency are most commonly associated with IL-2. Rieger (1995a) uses a systems approach to thoroughly describe management strategies for side effects associated with biotherapy. The reader is referred to Rieger (1995a) for further information about care of the patient receiving biotherapy. This chapter discusses two of the most common side effects of biotherapy—fatigue and flu-like syndrome.

Fatigue is one of the most commonly occurring side effects of biotherapy (Skalla & Rieger, 1995). The incidence and severity of fatigue among patients receiving BRMs seems to be greater than in patients receiving other treatment modalities, such as chemotherapy, radiation, or surgery (Robinson & Posner, 1992). Other toxicities such as flu-like symptoms and anorexia may exacerbate the fatigue. Fatigue is so severe that it becomes a dose-limiting toxicity of biotherapy. Fatigue becomes a critically important issue when it begins to affect the person's well-being, daily activities, lifestyle, social and work-related activities, familial and sexual relations, and compliance with therapy. Patients may withdraw early from treatment when the fatigue outweighs the perceived benefit of biotherapy. Nurses play a key role in developing strategies to assist the patient to deal with fatigue. The goal of nursing care for the patient who is receiving biotherapy and experiencing fatigue is to facilitate adaptation, thereby minimizing it, and maintaining or enhancing quality of life. Winningham (1994) has identified four strategies for nurses to help patients manage fatigue.

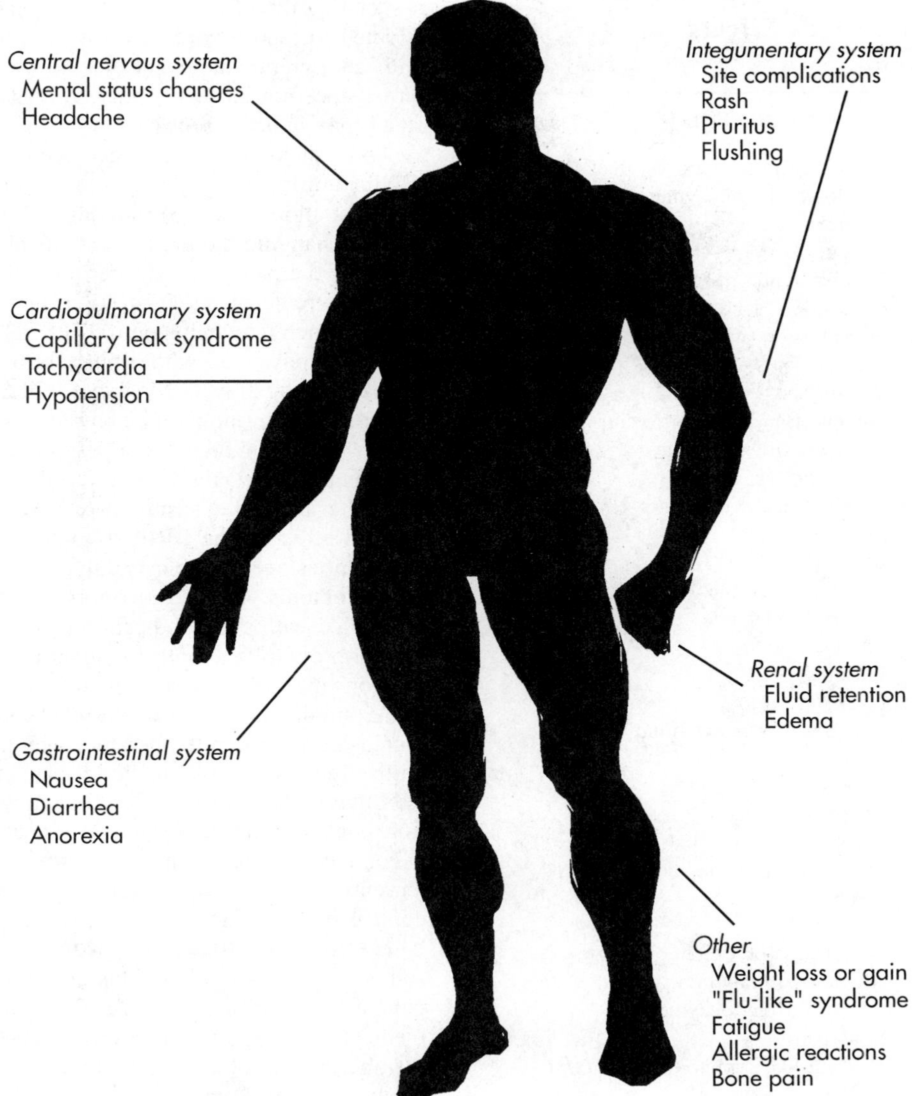

Fig. 7-4 Systemic toxicities associated with biotherapy.

These strategies could also be used by patients to help decrease fatigue:

1. *Activity-rest interventions.* Develop a schedule of activity and rest periods, and adhere to the schedule. Short naps followed by periods of activity, or a nap before a planned activity may increase energy levels.
2. *Plan ahead.* Plan ahead when stressful events can be anticipated, such as physician visits. More rest may be needed the day before and the day after a stressful event. If possible, schedule the event when energy levels are at their peak.
3. *Realizing limitations.* Conserve energy for more important activities. Activities may need to be ranked so that energy is spent on activities that are important. Delegate nonessential activities to family or friends whenever possible. Request assistance from family and friends with interventions that help reduce fatigue, such as assisting with household chores.
4. *Keep active.* Exercise daily. Too much rest can have a negative impact on energy production and may actually increase fatigue. Even short periods of activity or exercise are helpful in the management of fatigue.

Fatigue experienced by patients receiving biotherapy is subjective. Fatigue has different meanings for different individuals. Self-care interventions and interventions by others that decrease fatigue are also an individual matter. What one patient may find useful, may be of no help to another. Interestingly, in a research study by Robinson and Posner (1992), patients mentioned "encouraging activity" as an intervention by others that resulted in both reducing and increasing fatigue. Nurses need to explore with each patient what interventions are helpful in alleviating fatigue and develop a specific plan for that patient.

TABLE 7-5 Common Side Effects of Biologic Agents

Agent	Common Side Effects
Interferon	Alteration in laboratory values (hematologic, liver enzymes) Anorexia Fatigue Flu-like syndrome: chills, fever, myalgias, headache Hypotension (with IFN-γ) Mental status changes Weight loss
Interleukin-2	Alteration in laboratory values (hematologic, liver enzymes) Anorexia Capillary leak syndrome Diarrhea Fatigue Flu-like syndrome: chills, fever, myalgias, headache Fluid retention Flushing Hypotension Inflammatory reaction/induration at injection sites Nausea Periphral edema Pruritus Skin rash, erythema, and desquamation Tachycardia Weight loss or weight gain
Hematopoietic growth factors	Alteration in laboratory values (hematologic, liver enzymes) Bone pain Mild flu-like symptoms (with GM-CSF)
Monoclonal antibodies	Potential allergic reaction: hives, pruritis, anaphylactic reactions, hypotension

IFN, interferon; *GM-CSF,* granulocyte-macrophage colony-stimulating factor.

Another commonly occurring side effect of biotherapy is flu-like syndrome (FLS). FLS can be defined as a combination of signs and symptoms including fever, chills, rigors, myalgias, headache, malaise, respiratory symptoms (cough and nasal congestion), gastrointestinal symptoms (anorexia, nausea, vomiting, and diarrhea), and bone and joint pain. Fever, chills, rigors, myalgias, and headache are the most common side effects associated with the FLS (Haeuber, 1995). Similar to fatigue, FLS can affect a patient's ability to carry out activities of daily living (ADLs) and can significantly affect the patient's quality of life. FLS may be severe enough that patients consider discontinuing therapy.

Education about FLS is paramount to allay fears and give the patient and family a sense of control. Some patients may associate FLS with a worsening of their illness instead of associating the FLS with treatment. Patients need to be instructed to report extremely elevated fevers not controlled with antipyretics or fevers that do not follow normal patterns, since not all fevers may be related to therapy but instead may indicate sepsis.

Three main approaches have been identified in the management of FLS: (1) treatment manipulation, (2) medication administration, and (3) nursing interventions (Haeuber, 1989). Changing the dose or treatment time may not be an option if the patient is enrolled in a clinical trial. At times the dose, route of administration, or schedule may be adjusted, which may help control FLS. The nurse can give input to the physician who ultimately makes the decision to manipulate treatment. Most mild FLS symptoms can be controlled with antipyretics, antiemetics, and antidiarrheal agents. Many clinicians routinely prescribe premedications such as acetaminophen. Other clinicians avoid medication use either to help determine toxic effects or to achieve the optimal effect of the BRM (Haeuber, 1995). Occasionally, medications need to be scheduled around the clock to control symptoms. Chills and rigors related to BRMs can be controlled with a premedication of meperidine or a dose at the onset of chills. Finally, nonpharmacologic nursing interventions may help alleviate symptoms associated with FLS. For example, the use of warm blankets, warmer clothes, or increasing the room temperature may help patients tolerate chills. Tepid sponge baths, ice packs, or hypothermia blankets may help reduce fever. Encouraging adequate hydration is also an important nursing measure as patients may become dehydrated with a fever (Rieger, 1992). Nursing interventions such as relaxation or guided imagery may help control shivering and reduce anxiety.

Managing Educational Needs. Self-care skills and self-assessment of side effects are two important areas for patient teaching (Gantz et al., 1995). Self-administration of medications requires a highly motivated patient or family member who has the capacity to learn about the therapy. To safely self-administer medications in the home, patients or family members need to learn all the details of medication administration such as how to store, handle, and reconstitute the drug; inject the medication; and dispose of the syringe, needle, and medication vials (Tomaszewski et al., 1995). Patients should be provided with needle disposal containers with specific instructions according to institutional guidelines and Occupational Safety Health Administration (OSHA) guidelines (Sandstrom, 1996). An educational card for disposal of equipment at home is available from the U.S. Environmental Protection Agency (1990).

Another safety issue regarding biologic agents is the issue of radiation safety with radioactive MoAbs. Safety precautions for these agents are the same as safety guidelines for patients receiving other forms of radioactive isotopes used for cancer therapy. Patients and their families, as well as all medical personnel caring for these patients, need to be educated about the radiation safety principles of time, distance, and shielding. The institutional safety officer can assist with educational in-services, monitoring of patient radioactivity, proper waste disposal, and any patient precautions after discharge (Baquiran et al., 1996). Patients may be fearful about being close to family members or having an intimate relationship after receiving radioactive biotherapy. Nurses need to provide proper discharge education to allay these fears.

Since biotherapy is given in the home, patients must be able to self-assess side effects. It is the responsibility of the nurse to teach the patient anticipated side effects and measures to manage complications. For example, the first signs of central nervous system toxicity may involve subtle changes, such as slowed thinking, decreased concentration, or memory loss, that are often first recognized by family members. Additionally, patients and their families must be taught when to notify the health care professional, particularly if side effects are no longer manageable. If patients are enrolled in a clinical trial, they must also be aware of any special toxicity reporting or any special requirements for the purposes of the study, such as laboratory and diagnostic tests, specific monitoring, and inpatient admissions (Rumsey & Rieger, 1992). It may be helpful for patients to record side effects and interventions helpful in alleviating side effects. A journal or diary of recorded information may assist in planning further intervention or simply serve as a reminder to patients of the frequency of side effects, particularly when experiencing chronic effects such as fatigue or FLS (Gantz et al., 1995).

Numerous patient education materials are available for patients receiving biotherapy. Pamphlets, booklets, injection charts, self-injection video tapes, self-injection practice pads, and diaries are just a few examples of patient education materials that are available from pharmaceutical companies, national organizations, and individual cancer centers (Straw & Conrad, 1994). Information is also available on the World Wide Web.

Managing Economic Needs. Nurses must be aware of the economic issues surrounding biotherapy. Clearly, the cost of oncology care has been affected by biotherapy. As the use of cytokines is applied to broader clinical applications, the concerns about controlling cost pushes leading professional organizations such as the ASCO and private practice groups to develop practice guidelines for the use of cytokines. Obtaining reimbursement may require physicians, nurses, and pharmacists to define standards of practice that differentiate between state-of-the art and investigational therapy.

The reimbursement issues related to biotherapy have had a significant impact on oncology nursing practice. Nurses and/or patient service representatives may need to assist patients in obtaining information on reimbursement for biotherapy. Patients should review their insurance policies and coverage to determine the type of reimbursement for biotherapy. The coverage also depends on whether the care is delivered in the inpatient setting or outpatient clinic, or is self-administered in the home setting and whether the biotherapy agent is being used for an approved indication, "off-label" use, or investigational use in a clinical trial. Unfortunately, reimbursement issues are affecting patient participation in clinical trials. Yet clinical trials are critical in learning more about how to maximize the efficacy of biotherapy. Even if the biotherapy agent is being provided at no cost in a clinical trial, the payor may refuse to pay for associated costs such as clinic visits and clinical laboratory tests. Many payors do not have clearly defined standards for the coverage of biotherapy, so physicians and nurses can work with payors by providing scientific data in the form of manuscripts and abstracts to justify treatment.

A number of pharmaceutical companies have customer service programs available to assist with obtaining financial coverage for biotherapy. Oncology nurses are challenged with providing low-cost, quality patient care and achieving the highest reimbursement for their employer. This can create a conflict since many biotherapy agents are self-administered by patients in the home setting. As mentioned previously, patients must be educated on proper drug storage and preparation, subcutaneous injection techniques, and the injection sites to be used for frequent injections. Often there is no reimbursement for this time spent educating patients and for time spent following up with patients via phone calls. Oncology nurses play a pivotal role in identifying strategies for obtaining reimbursement of biotherapy.

Managing Psychosocial Needs. Finally, nurses need to be aware of the psychosocial needs of the patient receiving biotherapy that may affect the patient's quality of life. Limited publication and nursing research has been conducted on the numerous psychosocial difficulties of the patient receiving biotherapy. Nursing interventions and strategies used with other cancer patients undergoing other treatments should be able to be applied to the patient undergoing biotherapy. However, when compared with other treatment modalities, unique to biotherapy is the fact that agents are usually given in the home and often for several weeks to several years. Thus the burden of care is placed on the patient and family. Patients and family members may exhaust all resources to deal with the chronic effects of treatment. Nurses may need to explore novel approaches to assist patients and families with the management of chronic effects of biotherapy.

Many of the symptoms of biotherapy, such as fatigue, FLS, anorexia, and mental status changes, can interfere with ADLs and ultimately affect the patient's quality of life. Nurses can implement interventions to assist the patient with ADLs, which are no different than interventions used for individuals with other chronic illnesses (Gantz et al., 1995). Certainly, if the patient is experiencing fatigue, FLS, dry mucous membranes, or changes in body image, his or her sexuality may be altered as well. Counseling, education, and other nursing interventions used with other cancer patients with sexual concerns can be applied to the patient receiving biotherapy.

Biotherapy may be considered as a treatment option when all other treatment options have been exhausted. Patients may have unrealistic hope about what the treatment can offer and may become devastated if the treatment fails. The nurse should conduct a thorough psychosocial history including the patient's response to illness, current emotional status, ability to perform self-care, and support systems. The nurse also needs to assess the patient's understanding of the goal of therapy and feelings about the treatment. Misunderstandings should be conveyed to the physician before the start of therapy. The nurse plays a key role in making appropriate referrals and communicating patient concerns to the multidisciplinary team members.

Nurses caring for patients receiving biotherapy may deal with chronic stress. Stress may be related to the fact that the nurse may administer the agents or teach self-administration of agents that cause distressing side effects that may greatly affect the patient's quality of life. Personal values of the nurse may conflict with the patient's decision to continue therapy. Furthermore, the nurse may experience feelings of personal failure if the treatment is unsuccessful. To provide quality nursing care, some type of psychological support is needed for staff who routinely care for patients receiving biotherapy.

ETHICAL ISSUES

The ethical issues involving biotherapy center around the numerous agents being used in clinical trials and the frequency of "off-label" use. *Off-label use* can be defined as the use of drugs and biotherapy agents for nonapproved indications. IL-2, given postautologous transplantation as an immunomodulatory agent, is an example of an off-label use of a biotherapy agent. Although obtaining informed consent from patients participating in clinical trials is standard, it is unclear what extent of informed consent is needed for patients receiving biotherapy for off-label indications.

A controversial issue involves the use of cytokines in normal donors and certainly could be considered an ethical issue. For example, in allogeneic blood cell transplantation, normal donors are given HGFs before the collection of blood stem cells or donor lymphocytes. Since the long-term effects of donors receiving cytokines remains unknown, this practice could potentially have a negative effect on an otherwise healthy individual.

RESEARCH ISSUES

Clinical research in biotherapy involves both the study of biologic approaches and biologic agents. More biologic agents are in development than are currently approved for use in the United States. Agents in development are in a variety of phases of clinical research and are being evaluated in many disease types and treatment applications. Due to the volume of clinical research in biotherapy, six topics were chosen to be discussed: (1) donor lymphocyte infusions after allogeneic blood cell or marrow transplantation, (2) gene therapy, (3) chemokines, (4) immunomodulatory therapy after blood cell and bone marrow transplantation (BMT), (5) dendritic cells in the treatment of cancer, and (6) novel HGFs.

Donor Lymphocyte Infusions Post–Allogeneic Blood Cell or Bone Marrow Transplantation

Introduction. One novel approach of biotherapy that does not include the use of biotherapy agents but instead modifies the host's response to tumor cells is donor lymphocyte infusions (DLI). DLI is currently used after allogeneic blood cell and BMT in an attempt to reinduce remissions in patients who have relapsed. DLI is also being investigated in high-risk patients after allogeneic transplantation to prevent disease recurrence.

History. Abundant laboratory and clinical data have shown a powerful immune-mediated antitumor effect of allogeneic BMT. Clinical observations have suggested that this effect, termed *graft-versus-leukemia* (GVL) or *graft-versus-tumor* (GVT), is very potent and may account for at least half of the curative potential of BMT in certain diseases (Collins, 1996). Observations in humans have strongly suggested the existence of a GVL effect in allogeneic BMT, which includes relapse rates of identical twin BMT recipients that are higher than in allogeneic, nontwin BMT recipients; allogeneic BMT recipients who do not develop GVHD have a higher relapse rate than allogeneic BMT recipients who develop GVHD; and recipients of T lymphocyte–depleted BMT relapse more often than recipients of non-T lymphocyte–depleted BMT (Weiden, Sullivan, Flournoy, Storb, & Thomas, 1981; Gale & Champlin, 1984; Horowitz, Gale, Sondel, Goldman, Kersey, Kolb et al., 1990). In addition, complete remissions have been observed in patients with relapsed disease after allogeneic BMT in association with flares of GVHD (Odom, August, Githen et al., 1978; Higano, Brixey, Bryant, Durnam, Doney, Sullivan 1990; Collins, Rogers, Bennett, Kumar, Nikein, & Fay, 1990).

Numerous clinical trials have been conducted based on the apparent power of the GVL effect and its presumed mediation by donor lymphocytes (T lymphocytes and/or NK cells). Kolb and colleagues (1990) first described the activity of DLI in BMT recipients. Lymphocytes obtained from the original bone marrow donor have been infused into patients with relapsed malignancy after allogeneic BMT to induce GVT, hence the *donor lymphocyte infusions.*

Clinical Applications. The DLI approach typically involves histocompatible marrow donors who are apheresed for one to three sessions. Lymphocytes are then infused into the recipients, generally in the outpatient setting, to induce a GVT effect. The recipients do not take immunosuppressive medications and are observed closely for disease response and for the development of complications, including GVHD and pancytopenia. The clinical applications of DLI include the treatment of relapse after allogeneic BMT and the prevention of disease recurrence in high-risk allograft patients. In a complete analysis of 140 patients treated with DLI at 25 transplant centers in North America, 76% of patients with relapsed CML achieved a complete response that has lasted as long as 3 years after DLI (Collins, 1996).

Nursing Implications. During the infusion, nurses need to assess patients for signs and symptoms of a reaction not unlike those associated with allogeneic blood cell or marrow infusions. After the infusion, nurses have a key role in assessing patients for acute and chronic GVHD. Patient and family education includes the purpose of therapy, as well as the signs and symptoms to report to the health care team (e.g., rash, palmar erythema, diarrhea, petechiae, and bleeding). Patients receiving DLI often need psychosocial support since they are often devastated by a recurrence after transplant and they may have exhausted all other treatment options. The nurse should assess for psychosocial concerns and make referrals to appropriate multidisciplinary team members for any psychosocial difficulties.

Future Trends. The exact role of DLI is being investigated. Through a collaborative effort of more than 55 transplant centers, some of the following questions about DLI are being addressed: mechanism of action of DLI, role of DLI to treat hematologic diseases other than leukemia, safety and efficacy of DLI in unrelated donor transplants, the use of salvage chemotherapy before DLI in patients with advanced disease, and the role of hematopoietic progenitor cells in eliminating pancytopenia (Collins, 1996).

Gene Therapy

Another example of a type of biologic therapy in which the host's response to tumor cells is modified is gene therapy. *Gene therapy* is defined as "the alteration of an individual's genetic material to fight or prevent disease" (National Cancer Institute, 1993). This technology allows for the therapeutic transfer of genes to cells to restore lost function, to add function to cells, and to do cell marking. Technologic advances in molecular biology, cell biology, and immunology have moved the use of gene therapy from the laboratory into clinical trials. The first clinical attempts to use gene therapy to control cancer have been made in the past several years. Gene therapy is an investigational therapy and is therefore available only through carefully controlled clinical research trials. Gene therapy is covered in detail in Chapter 10.

Chemokines

Introduction. Basic science and clinical research have shown that cytokines exhibit a stimulatory effect on hematopoietic precursors. Chemokines are another group of small molecular weight proteins that exhibit inhibitory actions and suppress hematopoietic stem cell proliferation. Therefore instead of accelerating cell growth and differentiation like HGFs, chemokines slow down the growth of selected cells. Chemokines are also known as *stem cell protectors,* because by slowing down the cell cycle they may be able to protect the stem cell from the effects of chemotherapy. Chemokines are divided into two subfamilies, alpha and beta, based on sequence, function, and chromosomal location (Clore & Gronenborn, 1995). Examples of alpha chemokines are platelet factor 4 (PF4), interleukin-8 (IL-8), and neutrophil activating peptide 2 (NAP-2). Examples of beta chemokines are macrophage inflammatory protein-1 alpha (MIP-1-α), macrophage inflammatory protein-1 beta (MIP-1-β), and macrophage chemotactic and activating factor (MCAF).

History. Chemokines are a relatively new subclass of cytokines with the majority of reports in the literature starting in the early 1990s. National scientific conferences, where the latest basic science and therapeutic developments of chemokines are presented, have been held annually for the past 4 years. MIP-1-α is an example of a chemokine under investigation in a randomized trial that involved three varying schedules of administration—before, during, and after the administration of dose-intensive chemotherapy. The study objective was to determine if this chemokine could protect the stem cells from the effects of the chemotherapy as demonstrated by a reduction in the days of pancytopenia. Theoretically, other nonhematologic side effects may possibly be lessened with chemokine administration (e.g., mucositis and alopecia). The results of this novel study are pending publication. No chemokines are approved for clinical use by the FDA.

Clinical Applications. The potential clinical applications of chemokines include:

- Reduce incidence and severity of thrombocytopenia post intensive chemotherapy
- Reduce the myelosuppressive effects of chemotherapy
- Novel therapeutic targets of acute and chronic inflammatory diseases (e.g., treatment of acute respiratory distress syndrome [ARDS])
- Lessen nonhematologic side effects of chemotherapy (e.g., mucositis)

Immunomodulatory Therapy Post-Blood Cell and Marrow Transplantation

Introduction. Although the morbidity and mortality rate is significantly higher in allogeneic BMT, disease-free survival appears to be comparable or superior to autologous blood cell or marrow transplantation for diseases such as acute myelogenous leukemia, acute lymphocytic leukemia, and non–Hodgkin's lymphoma. The comparable results are due to a decreased risk of relapse after allogeneic BMT (Thomas, 1983). This decrease is partially a result of an immunologic effect known as *GVT* (Horowitz et al., 1990; Jones et al., 1991). The cellular mechanisms of GVT are not entirely known, but they appear to be similar to those that cause GVHD. Although the relapse rates are lower in allogeneic BMT patients who develop GVHD, they have higher toxicity associated. Allogeneic donor T lymphocytes appear to be in part responsible for the development of GVHD. In studies where the donor T lymphocytes were removed from the allogeneic marrow, the results showed higher relapse rates due to lack of GVT effect (Mitsuyasu, Champlin, Gale, Ho, Lenarsky, Winston et al., 1986).

Many patients do not have the option of having an allogeneic BMT primarily due to donor availability, age, and co-morbid disease, so autologous blood cell or BMT is pursued. In the autologous setting, there is no GVT because allogeneic T lymphocytes are not present. In addition the autologous cells may be contaminated with tumors, which may contribute to the higher relapse rates in patients who receive autologous transplant with preparative regimens similar to those used in allogeneic BMT. Nevertheless, autologous transplantation can be a curative treatment for relapsed malignancies. New therapies may be able to produce an immunologic effect similar to GVT after autologous transplantation, which may improve disease-free survival. This approach, where the immune system can be modulated to provide antitumor effects similar to GVT, is called *immunomodulatory therapy.*

History. Clinical application of immunomodulatory therapy postautologous transplantation began in the late

1980s. Examples of biologic agents used include IL-2 and quinoline-3-carboxamide (Linomide). IL-2 is approved by the FDA only for the treatment of metastatic renal cell carcinoma, so the use of IL-2 for this clinical application is not an FDA-approved indication. The use of Linomide as an immunomodulatory agent is still under investigation.

Clinical Applications. The use of IL-2 posttransplant to produce an immunomodulatory effect is still under investigation at both the scientific and clinical levels. Recent studies have shown that IL-2 can be safely administered posttransplant, which results in a rise in NK cell numbers and cytotoxicity. NK cells are large lymphocytes (non–B or T) that destroy a range of tumor cell targets without antigen specificity. Since the numbers of NK cells are decreased after intensive chemotherapy, it is being studied whether agents such as IL-2 can stimulate the production of NK cells and make them more functional. Posttransplant, when the tumor burden may be lowest, the NK cells may be able to destroy the residual tumor cells, leading to improved clinical outcomes. Other immunologic effects of IL-2 are also being studied. Since immunomodulatory agents are well tolerated and can be given in the outpatient setting, their clinical application to decrease disease recurrence posttransplant will continue to be explored.

Dendritic Cells in the Treatment of Cancer

Introduction. Dendritic cells are the most efficient antigen-presenting cells (APCs) that function to initiate an immune response such as the activation of naïve T lymphocytes, the rejection of organ transplants, and the formation of T lymphocyte–dependent antibodies (Steinman, 1991). APCs process peptides from foreign antigens and present these peptides bound to products of the major histocompatibility complex (MHC). The T lymphocyte receptor then recognizes the MHC-peptide complexes to initiate an immune response (Banchereau & Steinman, In press). Dendritic cells are found in many nonlymphoid tissues, such as the skin, mucosa, liver, and heart, but can migrate to the T lymphocyte-dependent areas of lymphoid organs via the lymph system or blood stream. Culture systems were designed in the early 1990s that permit the in vitro growth of large numbers of dendritic cells, allowing for an expansion of research opportunities.

History. Dendritic cells were identified in 1973 by Steinman and Cohn (Steinman, 1991). Through the late 1980s, there was considerable debate about the existence of dendritic cells as a specific cell lineage with unique functions. Now, dendritic cells are recognized as an integral part of the hematopoietic system and function to initiate immune responses.

Clinical Applications. The study of dendritic cells is currently limited to basic science research and early Phase I clinical trials in humans (Engleman, 1996). The clinical application of therapies using dendritic cells will likely require cells to be generated in vitro from progenitor cells because of the relatively small numbers of dendritic cells in the blood and tissue. Several cytokines such as IL-4, stem cell factor (SCF), IL-13, GM-CSF, TNF-α, and Flt-3 ligand protein stimulate the growth and differentiation of dendritic cells from hematopoietic cells and monocytes. Further investigation will be required to determine clinical applications of these cytokines. The diseases that might benefit from dendritic cell immunotherapy are cancer and infectious disease by the induction of immunity and autoimmunity, transplantation, and possibly allergy by the induction of tolerance. Early scientific results indicate that this treatment approach may prove useful in the treatment of a variety of tumors.

Novel Hematopoietic Growth Factors

Introduction. In an effort to decrease the hematologic toxicities associated with dose-intensive chemotherapy, researchers continue to develop and study novel HGFs for improved clinical applications. There are three categories of investigational HGFs: lineage-restricted HGFs, multilineage HGFs, and combination HGFs. Examples of lineage-restricted HGFs include thrombopoietin (TPO), IL-6, and IL-11. SCF, C-kit ligand, mast-cell growth factor, IL-1, and IL-3 are examples of multilineage HGFs. Combination HGFs involve concurrent or sequential administration of two or more HGFs. Combinations of HGFs may involve approved HGFs and/or novel HGFs.

History. Many of these novel HGFs have been studied in clinical trials since the early 1990s or are currently being investigated. None of the lineage restricted or multilineage HGFs referenced above have an FDA-approved indication.

Clinical Applications. Potential clinical applications of novel HGFs include chemotherapy, blood cell and BMT, blood cell mobilization, and prevention and treatment of infection. An example of the use of novel HGFs in chemotherapy is the use of single or combination agent HGFs for "priming." HGFs such as IL-3 and G-CSF are administered before and after intensive chemotherapy to increase the patient's WBC count; then chemotherapy is given with HGFs postchemotherapy. The objective is to reduce the period of neutropenia associated with intensive chemotherapy. Thrombopoietin is an example of a novel HGF being studied in blood cell and marrow transplantation to accelerate megakaryocyte maturation and increase the platelet count. Blood cells are typically mobilized with G-CSF or GM-CSF, and adequate cells are collected after an average of three apheresis procedures. One potential future application of novel HGFs is to use new single agents or combinations to enhance blood cell mobilization and decrease the number of collections required to achieve optimal cell counts in the blood cell product. An example of novel HGFs to treat infections is the off-label use of GM-CSF to prevent invasive fungal infections in allogeneic BMT patients with GVHD.

FUTURE TRENDS

Biotherapy is a treatment modality that holds great promise in the management of patients with neoplastic diseases. Sci-

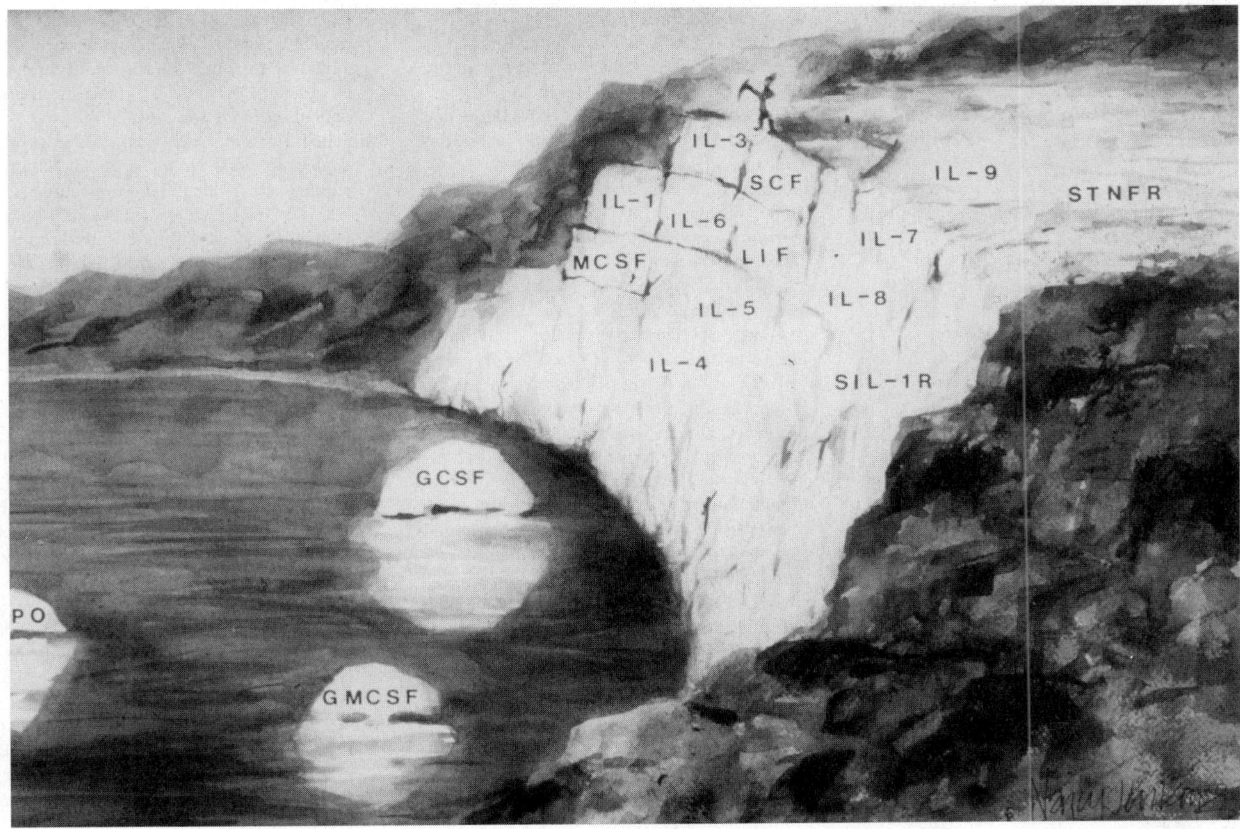

Fig. 7-5 Biotherapy at the tip of the iceberg. (From John Nemunaitis, M. D., Baylor University Medical Center and Texas Oncology Physicians Association, Dallas, TX.)

entists have just reached the "tip of the iceberg" in biotherapy (Fig. 7-5). Only a small number of biologic agents have clinical utility, and the vast majority of them await the results of ongoing clinical research. It is possible that biotherapy agents used in combinations for the optimal "cytokine cocktail" will result in improved outcomes. Combination therapy, however, may increase the complexity of patient management. For the majority of biotherapeutic agents, the optimal dose, route, and schedule administration remain unknown. Oncology nurses must have expertise in biotherapy and must play an active role in the development of biotherapeutic intervention.

NURSING RESEARCH

Since biotherapy is such a new field, numerous opportunities exist for nursing research. Nursing research related to fatigue associated with different types of therapy is rapidly emerging since the introduction of the Fatigue Initiative through Education and Research (FIRE) initiative in 1995. Since fatigue is one of the most common symptoms associated with biotherapy, further research is needed to better manage patients' fatigue.

Biotherapy has been used in standard clinical practice for a limited number of diagnoses or conditions only since the late 1980s. With more long-term cancer survivors who may have received biotherapy for several months to several years, further research is needed to explore the long-term issues such as long-term physical complications, economic impact of biotherapy, and quality-of-life issues. Quality-of-life studies related to biotherapy are beginning to appear in the literature. Both quality-of-life and pharmacoeconomic studies are being conducted during Phase III trials for many of the biotherapy agents now in development.

Opportunities also exist for collaborative research to develop effective symptom management strategies for novel biologic agents and biologic approaches. The financial impact of biotherapy on patient care and nursing practice also requires further investigation. Advanced practice nurses conducting research and oncology nurses experienced in biotherapy must disseminate new concepts in biotherapy to improve patient outcomes through research, presentations, and publications.

REFERENCES

American Society of Clinical Oncology. (1994). Recommendations for the use of hematopoietic colony-stimulating factors: evidence based, clinical practice guidelines. *Journal of Clinical Oncology, 12,* 2317-2508.

Atkins, M. B., Trehu, E. G., & Mier, J. W. (1995). Combination cytokine therapy. In V. T. DeVita, S. Hellman, & S. A. Rosenberg (Eds.), *Biologic therapy of cancer: Principles and practice* (2nd ed.). Philadelphia: J. B. Lippincott.

Banchereau, J., & Steinman, R. M. (In press). Antigen presentation in vivo and in disease states: functions of dendritic cells. *Nature.*

Baquiran, D. C., Dantis, L., & McKerrow, J. (1996). Monoclonal antibodies: Innovations in diagnosis and therapy. *Seminars in Oncology Nursing, 12*(2), 130-141.

Bonnem, E. M., & Oldham, R. K. (1987). Gamma-interferon: Physiology and speculation on its role in medicine. *Journal of Biological Response Modifiers, 6,* 275-301.

Brophy, L., & Sharp, E. (1991). Physical symptoms of combination biotherapy: A quality-of-life issue. *Oncology Nursing Forum, 18* (suppl 1), 25-30.

Burnet, F. M. (1970). The concept of immunologic surveillance. *Progress Experimental Tumor Research, 13,* 1-27.

Center for Biologics Evaluation and Research. (1997). *[Resource on the World-Wide-Web]* URL: http://www.octma@a1.cber.fda.gov: The Author.

Clark, J., & Longo, D. (1986). Biological response modifiers. *Mediguide Oncology, 6*(2), 1-4.

Clore, G.M., & Gronenborn, A.M. (1995). Three dimensional structures of alpha and beta chemokines. *FASEB-J, 9*(1), 57-62.

Collins, R. H. (1996). Donor leukocyte infusions for post-BMT relapse. *Transplantation Update: Baylor Institute for Transplantation Services, 1*(2), 1.

Collins, R. H., Rogers Z. R., Bennett, M., Kumar, V., Nikein, A., & Fay, J. W. (1990). Hematologic relapse of chronic myelogenous leukemia following allogeneic bone marrow transplantation: apparent graft-versus-leukemia effect following abrupt discontinuation of immunosuppression. *Bone Marrow Transplantation, 10,* 391-395.

Conley, A., & DeMeyer, E. (In press). Effect of subcutaneous GCSF injectable volume on drug efficancy: Site complications and client comfort. *Oncology Nursing Forum.*

Conrad, K. J., & Horrell, C. J. (Eds). (1995). *Biotherapy: Recommendations for nursing course content and clinical practicum.* Pittsburgh: Oncology Nursing Press.

DeLaPena, L., Tomaszewski, J. G., Bernato, D. L., Kryk, J. A., Molend, A. J., & Gantz, S. (1996). Programmed instruction: Biotherapy module IV: interleukins. *Cancer Nursing, 19*(1), 60-75.

DiJulio, J. E., & Liles, T. M. (1995). Monoclonal antibodies. In P.T. Rieger (Ed). *Biotherapy: A comprehensive overview.* Boston: Jones and Bartlett.

Engleman, E. G. (1996). Dendritic cells in the treatment of cancer. *Blood, 2,* 115-117.

Farrell, M. M. (1996). Biotherapy and the oncology nurse. *Seminars in Oncology Nursing, 12,* 82-88.

Gale, R. P., & Champlin, R. E. (1984). How does bone marrow transplantation cure leukaemia? *Lancet, 2,* 28-30.

Gallucci, B. B., & McCarthy, D. (1995). The immune system. In P. T. Rieger (Ed.), *Biotherapy: A comprehensive overview.* Boston: Jones and Bartlett.

Gantz, S., Tomaszewski, J. G., DeLaPena, L., Molenda J., Bernato D. L., & Kryk J. (1995). Programmed instruction: Biotherapy module II: interferons. *Cancer Nursing, 18*(5), 479-493.

Gery, I., Gershon, R., & Waksman, B. (1972a). Potentiation of the T-lymphocyte response to mitogens, I. The responding cell. *Journal of Experimental Medicine, 136*(1), 128-142.

Gery, I., Gershon, R., & Waksman, B. (1972b). Potentiation of the T-lymphocyte response to mitogens, II. The cellular source of potentiating mediators. *Journal of Experimental Medicine, 136*(1), 143-155.

Haeuber, D. (1989). Recent advances in the management of biotherapy-related side effects: Flu-like syndrome. *Oncology Nursing Forum, 16* (Suppl.), 35-41.

Haeuber, D. (1995). The flu-like syndrome. In P. T. Rieger (Ed.), *Biotherapy: A comprehensive overview.* Boston: Jones and Bartlett.

Herberman, R. (1992). Tumor immunology. *Journal of the American Medical Association, 268,* 2935-2939.

Higano, C. S., Brixey, M., Bryant, E. M., Durnam, D. M., Doney, C., Sullivan, K. M., & Singer, J. (1990). Durable complete remission of acute nonlymphocytic leukemia associated with discontinuation of immunosuppression following relapse after allogeneic bone marrow transplantation. A case report of probable graft-versus-leukemia effect. *Transplantation, 50,* 175-177.

Horowitz, M. M., Gale, R. P., Sondel, P. M., Goldman, J. M., Kersey, J., Koib, H.B., Rimm, A. A., Ringeden, O., & Rozman, C. (1990). Graft-versus-leukemia reactions after bone marrow transplantation. *Blood, 75,* 555-562.

Isaacs, A., & Lindemann, J. (1957). Virus interference. I. The interferon. *Proceeding from the Royal Society Service, B147,* 258-267.

Jassak, P. (1990). Biotherapy. In S. L. Groenwald, M. Frogge Hanse, M. Goodman, & C. H. Yarbro (Eds.), *Cancer nursing: Principles and practice.* Boston: Jones and Bartlett.

Jassak, P. (1995). An overview of biotherapy. In P. T. Rieger (Ed.), *Biotherapy: A comprehensive overview.* Boston: Jones and Bartlett.

Jones, R. J., Ambinder, R. F., Piantadosi, S., Santos G. W. (1991). Evidence of a graft-versus-leukemia effect associated with allogeneic bone marrow transplantation. *Blood, 77*(3), 649-653.

Kantarjian, H., Deisseroth, A., & Kurzrock, R. (1993). Chronic myelogenous leukemia: a concise update. *Blood, 82*(3), 691-703.

Kolb, H. J., Mittermuller, J, Clemm, C. H., Holler E., Ledderose G., Brehm G., Heim M., & Wilmanns W. (1990). Donor lymphocyte transfusions for treatment of recurrent chronic myelogenous leukemia in marrow transplant patients. *Blood, 76,* 2462-2465.

Mihich, E., & Fefer, A. (Eds.). (1983). *National Cancer Institute Monograph, 63.* National Institutes of Health: NIH Publication No. 83-2606, 3-31. U.S. Department of Health and Human Services, Public Health Service.

Mitchell, M. S. (1992). Chemotherapy in combination with biomodulation: A 5-year experience with cyclophosphamide and interleukin-2. *Seminars in Oncology, 19*(2) [Suppl. 4], 80-87.

Mitchell, M. S. (1993). *Biological approaches to cancer treatment—Biomodulation.* New York: McGraw-Hill.

Mitsuyasu, R. T., Champlin, R. E., Gale, R. P., Ho, W. G., Lenarsky, C., Winston, D., Selch, M., Elashofe, R., & Giorg, J. W. (1986). Treatment of donor bone marrow with monoclonal anti-T cell antibody and complement for the prevention of graft-versus-host disease. *Annals of Internal Medicine, 105,* 20.

Moldawer, N. P., & Figlin, R. A. (1995). The interferons. In P. T. Rieger (Ed.), *Biotherapy: A comprehensive overview.* Boston: Jones and Bartlett.

Mullen, C. A., & Blaese, R. M. (1994). Gene therapy of cancer. In H. M. Pinedo, D. L. Longo, & B. A. Chabner (Eds.), *Cancer chemotherapy and biological response modifiers annual 15.* New York: Elsevier.

National Cancer Institute. (1993). *Cancer facts: Questions and answers about gene therapy.* Washington, DC: Author.

Odom, L. F., August, C. S., Githen, J. H., et al. (1978). Remission of relapsed leukaemia during graft-versus-host reaction. *Lancet, ii,* 537-540.

Oettgen, H., & Old, L. (1991). The history of cancer immunotherapy. In V. T. DeVita, S. Hellman, & S. A. Rosenberg (Eds.), *Principles of cancer biotherapy* (2nd ed.). New York: Marcel Dekker.

Physicians Desk Reference. (1997). Montvale, NJ: Medical Economics Company.

Pitler, L. (1996). Hematopoietic growth factors in clinical practice. *Seminars in Oncology Nursing, 12*(2), 115-129.

Reiger, P. T. (1992). Biological response modifiers. In K. Rumsey & P. T. Rieger (Eds.), *Biological response modifiers: A self-instruction manual for professionals.* Chicago: Precept Press.

Reiger, P.T. (1995a). Dosing and scheduling of biological response modifiers. In P. T. Rieger (Ed.). *Biotherapy: A comprehensive overview.* Boston: Jones and Bartlett.

Reiger, P. T. (1995b). Patient management. In P. T. Rieger (Ed.). *Biotherapy: A comprehensive overview.* Boston: Jones and Bartlett.

Reiger, P. T. (1996). Future projections in biotherapy. *Seminars in Oncology Nursing, 12*(2), 163-171.

Reiger, P. T., & Haeuber, D. (1995). A new approach to managing chemotherapy-related anemia: Nursing implications of epoetin alfa. *Oncology Nursing Forum, 22,* 71-81.

Robinson, K. D. & Posner, J. D. (1992). Patterns of self-care needs and interventions related to biological response modifier therapy: Fatigue as a model. *Seminars in Oncology Nursing, 8*(4), 17-22.

Rosenberg, S. A. (1993). Principles and applications of biologic therapy. In V. T. DeVita, S. Hellman, S. A. Rosenberg (Eds.), *Cancer principles and practice of oncology,* (4th ed.). Philadelphia: J. B. Lippincott.

Rosenberg, S. A., Lotze, M. T., Yang, J. C., Aebersold, P. M., Lineham, W. M., Seipp, C. A., & White, D. E. (1989). Experience with the use of high-dose interleukin-2 in the treatment of 652 cancer patients. *Annals of Surgery, 316,* 898-905.

Rosenberg, S. A., Yang, J. C., & Topalian, S. L. (1994). Treatment of 283 consecutive patients with metastatic melanoma or renal cell cancer using high-dose bolus interleukin 2. *Journal of the American Medical Association, 271,* 907-913.

Rumsey, K., & Rieger, P. T. (Eds.). (1992). *Biological response modifiers: A self-instruction manual for professionals.* Chicago: Precept Press.

Sandstrom, S. K. (1996). Nursing management of patients receiving biotherapy. *Seminars in Oncology Nursing, 12*(2), 152-162.

Schlom, J. (1991). Antibodies in cancer therapy: Basic principles of monoclonal antibodies. In V. T. DeVita, S. Hellman, & S. A. Rosenberg (Eds), *Biologic therapy of cancer.* Philadelphia: J. B. Lippincott.

Sharp, E. (1995). The interleukins. In P. T. Rieger (Ed.), *Biotherapy: A comprehensive overview.* Boston: Jones and Bartlett.

Skalla, K. (1996). The interferons. *Seminars in Oncology Nursing, 12*(2), 97-105.

Skalla, K., & Reiger, P. T. (1995). Fatigue. In P. T. Rieger (Ed.), *Biotherapy: A comprehensive overview.* Boston: Jones and Bartlett.

Sleijfer, D. T., Janssen R. A., Buter, J., de Vries, E. G., Willemse, P. H., & Mulder, N. H. (1992). Phase II study of subcutaneous interleukin-2 in unselected patients with advanced renal cell cancer on an outpatient basis. *Journal of Clinical Oncology, 10,* 1119-1123.

Steinman, R. M. (1991). The dendritic cell system and its role in immunogenicity. *Annual Review of Immunology, 9,* 271-296.

Straw, L. J., & Conrad, K. J. (1994). Patient education resources related to biotherapy and the immune system. *Oncology Nursing Forum, 21*(7), 1223-1228.

Talpaz, M., McCredie, K. B., Maulight, G. M., Trujillo, J. M., Keating, J., & Gutterman, J. U. (1983). Leukocyte interferon induced myeloid cytoreduction in chronic myelogenous leukemia. *Blood, 62,* 689-692.

Talpaz, M., Kantarjian, H., McCredie, K., & Gutterman, J. U. (1986). Hematologic remission and cytogenetic improvement induced by recombinant human interferon alpha in chronic myelogenous leukemia. *New England Journal of Medicine, 314*(17), 1065-1069.

Thomas, E. D. (1983). Marrow transplantation for malignant disease. *Journal of Clinical Oncology, 9,* 517.

Tomaszewski, J. G., DeLaPena, L., Molenda, J., Gantz S., Bernato, D. L., & Foltz, S. (1995). Programmed instruction: Biotherapy module II: Overview of biotherapy. *Cancer Nursing, 18*(5), 397-414.

Tsevat, J., & Lacasse, C. (1992). Understanding the special needs of patients receiving biotherapy: A conceptual model. In R. Carroll-Johnson (Ed.), *The biotherapy of Cancer-V.* Pittsburgh: Oncology Nursing Press.

U. S. Environmental Protection Agency. (1990). *Disposal tips for home health care.* Washington, DC: Office of Solid Waste, United States Environmental Protection Agency.

von der Masse, J., Geertsen, P., Thatcher, N., Jasmin, C., Mercatello, A., Fosså, S. D., Symann, M., Stoler, G., Nagel, G., Israel, L., Oskam, R., Palmer, P., & Franks, C. R. (1991). Recombinant interleukin-2 in metastatic renal cell carcinoma: A European multicentre phase II study. *European Journal of Cancer, 27,* 1583-1589.

Weiden, P. L., Sullivan, K. M., Flournoy, N., Storb, R., & Thomas, E. D. The Seattle Marrow Transplant Team. (1981). Antileukemic effect of chronic graft-versus-host disease. Contribution to improved survival after allogeneic marrow transplantation. *New England Journal of Medicine, 304,* 1529-2533.

Wheeler, V. S. (1996). Interleukins: The search for an anticancer therapy. *Seminars in Oncology Nursing, 12*(2), 106-114.

White, C. (1992). Symptom assessment and management of outpatients receiving biotherapy: The application of a symptom report form. *Seminars in Oncology Nursing, 8*(4), suppl 1, 23-28.

Winningham, M. (1994). New concepts in the nursing care of fatigue. *Fighting fatigue: Resolving issues for the cancer patient.* Beachwood, OH: PreEd Communications.

Wujick, D. (1993). An odyssey into biologic therapy. *Oncology Nursing Forum, 20,* 879-887.

Wujick, D. (1995). Hematopoietic growth factors. In P.T. Rieger (Ed.), *Biotherapy: A comprehensive overview.* Boston: Jones and Bartlett.

Yang, J. C., Topalian, S. L., Parkinson, D. R., et al. (1994). Randomized comparison of high-dose and low-dose intravenous IL-2 for the therapy of metastatic renal cell carcinoma: An interim report. *Journal of Clinical Oncology, 12,* 1572-1576.

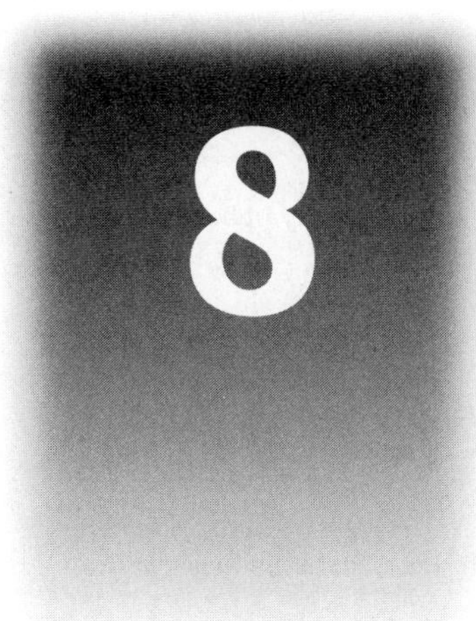

Bone Marrow Transplantation

Patricia C. Buchsel, RN, MSN

INTRODUCTION

Bone marrow transplantation (BMT) was introduced as an experimental therapy for end-stage cancer patients 40 years ago. Now this therapy is acknowledged as a recognized treatment, as witnessed by the twenty-fifth anniversary of the International Bone Marrow Transplant Registry (IBMTR). Treatment advances, successful recruitment of unrelated volunteer donors, and wider treatment and disease applications now offer this therapy to thousands who would otherwise die of the disease (Bortin, Horowitz, Rowlings, Rimm, Zhang, & Gale, 1993). One of the major impediments of successful BMT is relapse, and collaborate international trials using large numbers of recipients are investigating this problem. Renewed interest in T-lymphocyte depletion to reduce the incidence and severity of graft versus host disease (GVHD) without associated graft failure or relapse is the subject of collaborate trials. New questions challenging old practices, such as the value of skin and lip biopsies in predicating chronic GVHD with screening studies after allogeneic BMT are under scrutiny. Perhaps the most provocative query is when marrow will cease to be the most common source of hematopoietic stem cells. Many researchers believe this shift will evolve by the next millennium. Until stem cells derived from allogeneic donors, umbilical cord, and fetal cells are perfected, marrow will remain an important therapy. Nurses entering into the profession should learn basic BMT concepts, and those practicing in this field should keep abreast of new techniques and practice environments. As an increasing number of BMTs are offered in regional and community settings more general oncology nurses and some general nurses will give a large portion of the care of these recipients.

HISTORICAL PERSPECTIVES

The history of BMT has been reported to date back to the ancient Egyptians (Thomas, Storb, Clift, Fefer, Johnson, Neiman, & Lerner et al., 1988). Not until a late nineteenth-century article in the *New England Journal of Medicine* is BMT noted as a possible treatment for blood diseases. Table 8-1 notes a history of major events in BMT.

THE TENETS OF BONE MARROW TRANSPLANTATION

The concept of replacing diseased marrow for the purpose of care, quality of life, or years gained is as follows:

1. The dose intensity of most chemotherapeutic agents administered to cure a patient's disease is limited by subsequent dose-related marrow toxicity.
2. The availability of hematopoietic stem cells in the marrow allows the infused stem cells to reconstitute the hematopoietic and immunologic system.
3. Resulting complications occur secondary to the effects of dose-intensive conditioning regimens, GVHD, supportive medications, or treatment failure.
4. Supportive care techniques sustain the recipient until stabilized engraftment.

TYPES OF BONE MARROW TRANSPLANTATION

Successful BMT is dependent on an available and appropriate donor source. Donor sources include matched siblings, mismatched family members, matched volunteer donors, and autologous donation (self). If the recipient's donor is a relative or unrelated donor, the transplant is an allogeneic transplant. An autologous transplant is one in which the patient uses his or her own marrow. A syngeneic marrow transplant is one in which the donor is an identical twin (who by definition is a perfect histocompatible leukocyte antigen [HLA] match) (Box 8-1). Cadaveric donors have been the subject of period research but remain rare or unsuccessful (Blazer, Lasky, Perentesis, Watson, Steinberg, Filipoich, & Orr et al., 1986; Kapelushnick, Aker, Paggatsch, Samuel, & Slavin, 1998).

The IBMTR organizes and facilitates data collaboration

TABLE 8-1 Milestones in Bone Marrow Transplantation

1837	Bone marrow administered intramuscularly and intramedullary.
1891	First published record of the possibility of marrow as rescue therapy.
1892	The earliest BMT in humans administered by mouth to patients with pernicious anemia and lymphadenoma, reported by Brown-Sequard.
1893	Favorable results increase overuse of marrow for treatment of leukemias.
1894	Enthusiastic reports gain acceptance relative to marrow use in numerous anemias.
World War II (1940-1944)	Studies of radiation-induced bone marrow failure led to treatments using infusions of bone marrow in aplastic anemia and patients with radiation-induced bone marrow failure. Blood banking available in many U.S. hospitals.
1949 and 1951	Irradiation protection effect proven by infusion of syngeneic marrow. Murine and canine models showed that animals given lethal doses of irradiation survive after parenteral infusion of bone marrow.
1955	Graft versus host disease (GVHD), or "runt" disease, noted in animals.
1956	Cytogenetic techniques indicated that irradiation protection in animals was due to the transfer and survival of hematopoietic donor cells.
1956	The term *chimera* used for the first time to describe animals lethally irradiated and given a BMT from another animal.
1957	French and Yugoslav physicians work with workers exposed to radiation during the Vinca nuclear reactor accident.
1958	First human autologous BMT unsuccessful, and BMT largely abandoned until 1960. Learned that methotrexate mediates GVHD.
1960	Histocompatible leukocyte antigen (HLA) typing established to identify suitable sibling donors and successful human allogeneic transplants performed. Whole blood is divided into components. Platelet transfusion technology perfected. Antibiotics came of age.
1963	GVHD noted in allogeneic BMT.
1966	Recognition of the association between infection and low neutrophil counts.
1968	First BMT from a matched sibling for an infant with immunologic deficiency disease.
1969	Successful BMTs performed at Fred Hutchinson Cancer Research Center.
1970	Review of reported human BMTs published. Routine use of neutrophil transfusions abandoned due to concern of cytomegalovirus (CMV) exposure. Standard technique for marrow harvest described by Thomas et al., 1988.
1973	First unrelated donor transplant at Memorial Sloan Kettering Medical Center.
1975	Success of BMT established in acute leukemia and severe aplastic anemia recipient. Protective environments, including laminar airflow rooms (LAFs) high-efficiency particulate air filters, sterile diets, and topical and oral antibiotics were developed.
1975	Modern BMT comes of age. *New England Journal of Medicine* reported experimental background and the early clinical successes and problems reviewed.

From Ezzone S. A. & Fliedner, M. (1998). Transplant networks and standards of care: International perspectives. In M. B. Whedon & D. W. Wujick (Eds.), *Blood and marrow stem cell transplantation: Principles, practice, and nursing insights* (2nd ed.). Sudbury, MA: Jones and Bartlett; Whedon, M. B. (1995). Bone marrow transplantation nursing: Into the twenty-first century. In P. C. Buchsel & M. B. Whedon (Eds.), *Bone marrow transplantation: Administrative strategies and clinical concerns.* Sudbury, MA: Jones & Bartlett; Wingard, J. R. (1994). Bone marrow to blood stem cells: Past, present, future. In M. B. Whedon, & D. W. Wujick (Eds.), *Blood and marrow stem cell transplantation: Principles, practice, and nursing insights* (2nd ed.). Sudbury, MA: Jones and Bartlett.

with more than 47 countries. In 1997, 5500 allogeneic marrow/stem cell and 10,000 autologous stem cell transplants were performed (IBMTR, 1998).

DISEASES TREATED WITH AUTOLOGOUS BONE MARROW TRANSPLANTATION

Autologous

Autologous transplants are used most often to treat breast cancer, Hodgkin's disease, non–Hodgkin's lymphoma, acute leukemias, multiple myeloma, and neuroblastoma, as well as ovarian, testicular, brain, lung, and bone sarcomas (Table 8-2). With the exception of leukemia, diseases treated by autologous BMT usually are not disorders that begin in or involve the bone marrow.

Allogeneic Bone Marrow Transplantation

Until recently the number of allogeneic BMTs outnumbered autologous transplants. A successful allogeneic marrow transplant depends on the availability of a matched donor. GVHD, a phenomenon in which the donor graft rejects the host, is the major hurdle to successful marrow grafting.

Diseases Treated with Bone Marrow Transplantation

Allogeneic transplants are performed for acute and chronic leukemia, lymphomas, multiple myeloma, severe aplastic anemia, genetic disease, immunologic deficiencies, and inborn errors of metabolism. Children with genetic diseases such as thalassemia or Franklin's anemia are also candidates for allogeneic BMT. BMT for sickle cell anemia is being re-

TABLE 8-1 Milestones in Bone Marrow Transplantation—cont'd

1979	Graft versus leukemic effect noted. Hickman double-lumen catheter perfected.
1980	First nursing articles in BMT published. Cyclosporine introduced for GVHD management.
1981	T-cell depletion of donor bone marrow inhibits human GVHD.
1983	First nursing Bone Marrow Transplant Consortium formed.
	First collection of nursing BMT articles in *Nursing Clinics of North America.*
1978-1980	Psychological aspects of BMT explored.
1984	Minimal risks and problems with marrow harvesting in normal donors noted. Comprehensive review of the long-term complications of bone recipients.
1985	Capability to cryopreserve hematopoietic progenitor cells (HPCs) was developed. Plasma exchange perfected for ABO incompatible BMTs.
Late 1980	Cyclosporine in combination with methotrexate was largely abandoned, and standard prophylaxis for GVHD currently is cyclosporine with corticosteroids. Autologous peripheral stem cell transplantation (PSCT) recognized as a possible hematopoietic source.
	Improvements in pretransplant conditioning regimens, prophylaxis, and treatments of infectious diseases lead to decreased transplant-related morbidity and mortality. First unrelated allogeneic BMT.
1986	More than 200 centers performed almost 2000 BMTs. Development of the National Unrelated Donor Registry. Blood products screened for prevention of CMV. Granulocyte-macrophage colony-stimulating factor enhances white cell counts after BMT, decreasing infections and antibiotic use.
1988	Acyclovir for viral infection emerged. Quality of Life nursing article published.
1988-1990	Fractionated (vs single-dose total-body irradiation (TBI) and antileukemic drugs such as high-dose etoposide and high-dose cytosine arabinoside, with TBI increase markedly. The increased use of busulfan and cyclophosphamide without TBI for pretransplant conditioning is another important trend.
	T-lymphocyte marrow depletion to reduce the risk of GVHD largely abandoned because of significantly high relapse rates and graft failure in recipients of T-lymphocyte–depleted marrow infusions.
	Cyclosporine emerged as an important treatment with corticosteroids to prevent GVHD. By mid-decade, research demonstrated cyclosporine with or without corticosteroids was a more effective treatment than other regimens. Treatment of choice for chronic GVHD treatment is combination of steroids plus cyclosporine.
	Studies conducted on quality of life in the BMT recipient.
1993	Experiences of the first 493 unrelated marrow donors in the National Marrow Donor Program noted.
1994	Foundation for the Accreditation of Hematopoietic Cell Therapy established.
1998	Twenty-fifth anniversary of International Bone Marrow Transplant Registry.

Box 8-1

Types of Bone Marrow Transplantation

Syngeneic: The donor is an identical twin (who by definition is a perfect match).

Allogeneic: The donor is a matched sibling or family donor or an unrelated donor.

Autologous: The donor is one's own marrow after treatment for the disease

ported with increasing frequency but remains controversial in spite of encouraging results. A report of 50 patients by a European group indicated Kaplan-Meier estimates of overall survival (93%), even-free survival (82%), and disease-free survival (85%) (Vermylen, Cornu, Ferster, Brichard, Ninane, & Ferrant et al., 1998) The concerns raised by opponents to this treatment for sickle-cell anemia are the acute and long-term complications, morbidity, and costs compared with traditional therapy of disease (Beutler & Sullivan, 1994).

Immunologic deficiencies such as congenital immunodeficiency diseases, including severe combined immunodeficiency disease syndrome (SCIDS), Wiskott-Aldrich syndrome, and some rare inherited disorders are the treatment of choice only in the presence of an HLA-matched sibling. The first successful human gene therapy transplants were conducted in children with adenosine deaminase (ADA) in 1990 (Blaese, Culver, Miller, Carter, Fleisher, Clerici, & Shearer et al., 1995). Other gene therapy trials under review include treatment of Gaucher's disease, Fanconi's anemia, selected acute and chronic leukemias, multiple myeloma, breast cancer, Hodgkin's disease, and lymphoid malignancies. Gene therapy using marrow and stem cells alone or in combination are under way. However, efficacy, as well as ethical, economic, and technical concerns, are of major importance as this therapy advances (Jenkins, 1998). Chapter 10 offers a complete discussion of gene therapy.

Allogeneic BMT has been used successfully to treat diseases of inborn errors of metabolism, such as Gaucher's disease, chronic granulomatosis disease, osteoporosis, mucopolysaccharidosis (Hurler's syndrome), Sanfilipp B disease, and Maroteaux-Lamy syndrome. Lipidosis diseases include adrenoleukodystrophy (ADL) and metachromatic leukodystrophy (MLD). Treatment of these diseases has been limited to those patients with a histocompatible sibling. However, as increasing numbers of volunteer donors become available, more unrelated donor searches may be initiated (Armitage, 1994). Diseases currently being treated with allogeneic BMT are depicted in Fig. 8-1 and Table 8-3 illustrates estimated 5-year survival rates.

TABLE 8-2 Distribution Of Autotransplants Performed Between 1989 and 1995 and Registered With the Autologous Blood and Marrow Transplant Registry (ABMTR) by 220 Teams in North and South America

Disease	No. of Transplants	Percent (%)
Breast cancer	10,556	35
Non–Hodgkin's lymphoma	7653	25
Hodgkin's lymphoma	3593	12
Acute myelogenous leukemia (AML)	2330	8
Acute lymphoblastic leukemia (ALL)	590	2
Chronic myelogenous leukemia (CML)	271	1
Multiple myeloma	1715	6
Neuroblastoma	735	2
Ovarian cancer	695	2
Testicular cancer	452	1
Brain cancer	370	>1
Lung cancer	128	>1
Bone sarcoma	118	>1
Other cancer	1189	4
TOTAL	30,395	

From Armitage, J. O. (1996). New ABMTR studies evaluate growing use of autologous transplantation. *ABMTR Newsletter, 3*(1):2.

DONOR ISSUES

Tissue Typing

The crux of allogeneic BMT is the presence of a compatible and healthy donor. Matching patients and donors is accomplished by examining the HLA tissue typing of each person. The major histocompatibility complex in humans is composed of a series of closely linked genetic loci or antigens on chromosome 6 and are referred to as *HLA-A, -B, -C, -DR,* or *-DQ, -DP* antigens. The HLA-A and -B antigens, referred to as *Class I antigens,* are readily identified on the surface of most nucleated cells, especially leukocytes. At the time of conception, the fetus inherits a set of antigens from the mother and one from the father. The HLA-DR and -DP antigens, known as *Class II* antigens are most commonly found on B lymphocytes. HLA-A, HLA-B, and HLA-C antigens have been historically defined serologically, but deoxyribonucleic acid (DNA)–based technologies now offer more accuracy. Those antigens at the HLA-DR, -DQ, and -DP loci (Class II) are identified most often. DNA technology that uses oligonucleotide probes is replacing the older, more inaccurate mixed leukocyte culture (MLC) serologic test. Several exciting methods to rapidly determine the most optimal marrow donor now exist. A new method is identification of HLA allelic polymorphism directed at the DNA level by hybridization with sequence-specific oligonucleotide probes (HLA oligotyping) after identification of DNA by polymerase chain reaction (PCR). PCR is a simple, rapid, inexpensive method of producing large quantities of a specific gene (DNA) from minute and/or poor-quality material. With the use of PCR techniques, additional HLA alleles, formerly unrecognized now allow more precise tissue typing, allowing for more matches and less morbidity and mortality.

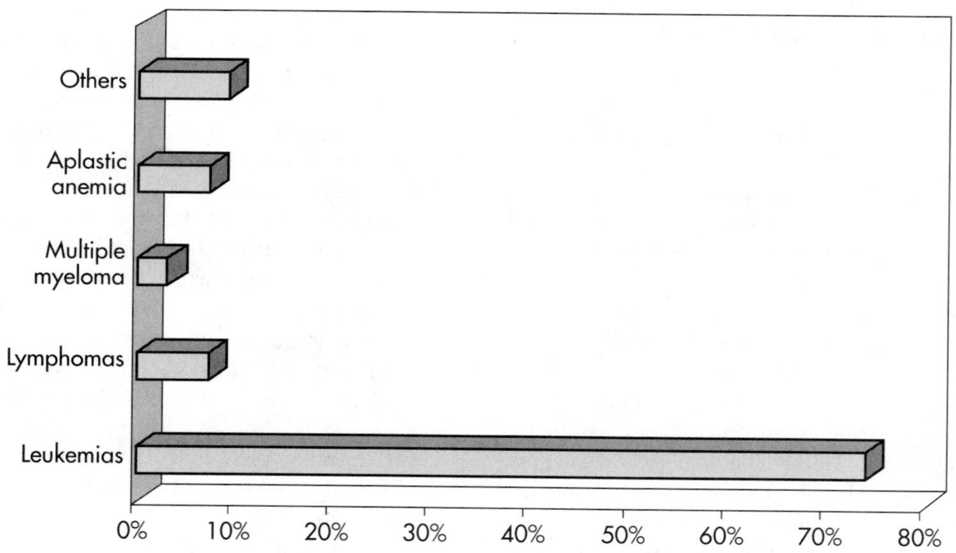

Fig. 8-1 Percentages of diseases treated with allogeneic bone marrow transplantation.

Most transplant clinicians require that five of six possible antigens match between patients and donors. Because only approximately 25% of patients have an HLA match with a family member, 75% of patients who could be potentially cured with allogeneic BMT are left untreated (Perkins & Hansen, 1994). The importance of recruiting unrelated donors from international and national donor pools, especially those of mixed diversity, is imperative to offer BMT to thousands who would otherwise die of the disease.

ABO Incompatibility. Major or minor ABO-incompatibility between patient and donor occurs in 20% to 30% of all allogeneic marrow grafting. However, BMT can be performed without significant hemolytic transfusion reactions (Bensinger, Buckner, & Thomas, 1982). Red blood cell (RBC) depletion is performed for any clinically significant incompatibility between the RBCs of the donor and the recipient. RBCs are depleted by hydroxyethyl (Hetastarch) sedimentation in two states, and produce two separate bags of RBC-depleted marrow for infusion. Hetastarch depletion results in a reduction of the red cell volume by 90% to 95%. If unmanipulated, incompatible ABO marrow is transfused, and it, like any incompatible blood product transfusion can cause a major hemolytic transfusion reaction, which can result in death. Blood transfusions after BMT are of the recipient's ABO blood type. After sustained engraftment occurs, the patient's ABO type converts to that of the marrow donor (Klingemann, 1992).

Allogeneic donors, in addition to being HLA matched, must be able to undergo general or spinal anesthesia, give informed consent, and, in some cases, be available for platelet donation. Marrow donation in adults involves giving voluntary informed consent to an operative procedure that may cause morbidity and the risk of death without any benefit to the donors. In rare cases, donors may be reluctant because of estranged family relations, financial issues, confidentiality concerns (i.e., a potential donor with acquired immunodeficiency syndrome [AIDS] who does not wish to reveal this illness). Recent attention to several families who have conceived children in hopes of obtaining an HLA match for a family member needing a BMT has come under scrutiny. Few have found fault with this practice. However, with the ability to perform HLA tissue typing on fetusus, parents could elect to abort a fetus until a successful HLA tissue-typed fetus is conceived. As more research and interests emerge in the use of fetal livers as a stem cell source, ethical issues are arising regarding fetal parts obtained through abortions.

Donor age at the time of marrow harvest has been a limiting factor for eligibility for allogeneic marrow donation, but as an aging healthy population increases, donor age is increasing. Currently unrelated volunteer age is limited to age 60.

TABLE 8-3 Estimated 5-Year Survival for Disease-Free Response Rates After Bone Marrow Transplantation

Disease	Stage	Allogeneic (%)	Autologous (%)
Aplastic anemia		50-80	
AML	First CR	45-65	30-50
	Second CR	20-45	20-40
ALL	First CR	40-70	30-50
	Second CR	25-45	15-25
Myelodysplastic syndrome	Combined	45	
CML	Chronic phase	60-75	0-5
	Accelerated phase	30-40	0-5
	Blast crisis	10-20	0-5
Non–Hodgkin's lymphoma	First relapse, second CR	40-60	40-60
	Advanced	10-25	10-25
Hodgkin's disease	First relapse, second CR	40-60	40-60
	Advanced	10-25	10-25
Multiple myeloma	Combined	30	0-5
Neuroblastoma	Stage IV	25-50	25-50
Thalassemia		70-80	NA
Breast cancer	Stage IV	ND	10-20
	Stage V		70
Lung cancer	Limited stage	ND	57 (2-year)
	Extensive stage		35 (2-year)
Testicular cancer	Recurrent	ND	20
Ovarian	ND	ND	ND

From Applebaum, F. R. (1996). The use of bone marrow and peripheral blood stem cell transplantation. *CA: A Cancer Journal for Clinicians, 46*(3), 142-164.
CR, complete remission; *NA*, not applicable; *ND*, not determined.

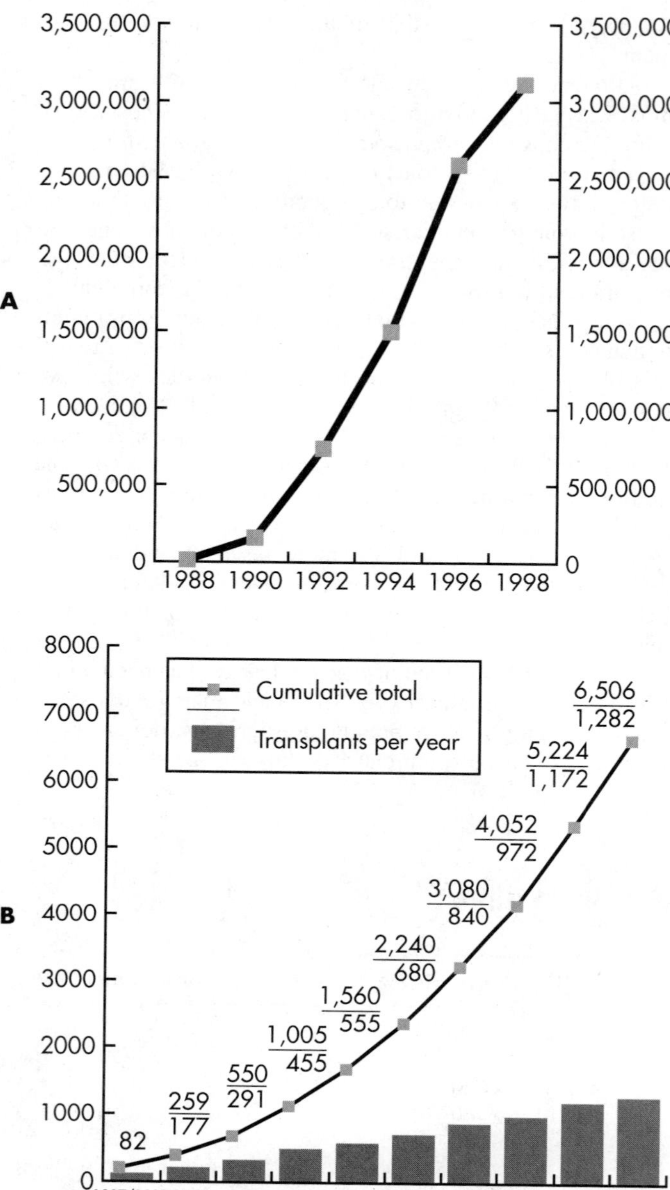

Fig. 8-2 **A,** Total number of unrelated marrow donors in the National Marrow Donor Program (NMDP). **B,** Number of unrelated bone marrow transplantations as facilitated through the NMDP as of November 1998.

Ethical Issues. Family marrow donors must consider issues of informed consent and confidentiality. Donors who are minors present certain legal and ethical concerns, and states vary on laws pertaining to this subject. For example, all minor donors in Washington are made wards of the court, legal guardians are appointed, and court approval obtained for marrow harvest. (Buckner, Peterson, & Bolonesi, 1994). In another incidence, the Illinois Supreme Court recently ruled that half siblings cannot be required to undergo tissue-typing for a stepbrother in need of BMT (Curran & Hyg, 1992).

Unrelated Donors. The National Marrow Donor Program (NMDP) is the largest unrelated donor registry worldwide and has a potential volunteer donor base of over 3.2 million (Fig. 8-2). The current number of unrelated transplants facilitated by the NMDP is more than 7000, 75% of which were for leukemic patients. This organization has cooperative relations between the United States and Puerto Rico, the Netherlands, Israel, Germany, Norway, and Sweden. Collaborative relationships with national registries were aimed at coordinating donor searches and marrow transport for unrelated donors from Australia, Austria, Canada, England, France, Spain, Singapore, Taiwan, Japan, Switzerland, Italy, and Ireland. The mission of the NMDP is to facilitate successful transplants of hematopoietic cells from volunteer unrelated donors for patients of all ethnic and socioeconomic backgrounds. Fig. 8-3 illustrates the cultural diversity growth over the past decade. Over 500 events per month are sponsored by religious groups, college sororities and fraternities, community groups, corporations and other groups to advance the benefits and decrease the myths of marrow donation (NMDP, 1998). As the success of allogeneic peripheral stem cell and umbilical stem cell transplants grows, the NMDP will be positioned to assist an increasing number of transplants. Volunteer donor safety is foremost in the minds of researchers and clinicians, and international and national standards now provide for optimal donor care. HLA typing remains the key factor to more successful unrelated allogeneic BMT. Simplistically, the more mismatched the patient is to the donor, the less successful the transplant. Thus more precise HLA-matching techniques employing high-resolution DNA typing is the subject of ongoing investigations. Successful efforts in this field will decrease historical and current problems such as infection, GVHD, graft failure, and relapse (Madrigal & Alejandro, 1998). Other investigations under way are refining T-lymphocyte manipulations to prevent graft failure and severe GVHD while persevering the graft versus leukemia benefit (Gajewski & Champlin, 1996). The phenomenon of graft versus leukemia is discussed in this chapter.

Leaders of a consensus conference have addressed the current problems of the unrelated BMT. Panel members included an expert in BMT, a general hematologist, a pediatrician, a patient advocate, and a medical journalist. The panel was asked to identify current indications for such transplants in adults and children, to consider appropriate donor care, and to identify studies that might contribute to improved evaluation of the procedure. Box 8-2 notes the heart of the consensus statement; however, some researchers took exception to some statements discussed below (A consensus statement, 1997).

One researcher reported that a National Marrow Donor Program comparing approximately 1400 unrelated and 700 related donor transplants showed that those chronic myelogenous leukemia (CML) recipients of unrelated donors had significant adverse disease-free survival. Another exception raised was the consensus that unrelated BMT for patients with CML is the optimal treatment. He argues that this point of view does not take into account patient characteristics such as older age, which represent poor prognostic indica-

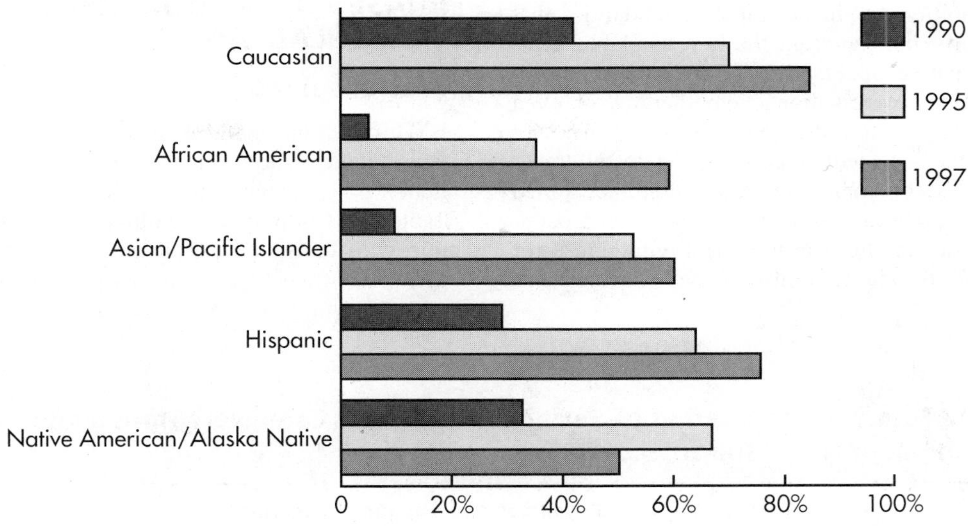

Fig. 8-3 Cultural diversity of unrelated bone marrow transplantations. (National Marrow Donor Registry [1998]. *About the National Marrow Donor Program.* www.marrow.org/WHATSNEW/FACTS/GUIDE.html.)

Box 8-2

Concensus on Unrelated Donor Bone Marrow Transplantation

Efficacy

Unrelated BMT for some types of leukemia produces prolonged quiescence and, in some cases cure.

Serologic HLA-A, -B, and -DR tissue typing may indicate appropriate matching, but new molecular typing may indicate less matching compared with serologic typing.

Toxicity

Increasing age and degree of mismatching each increase the probability of transplant-related mortality and morbidity.

In patients less than 20 years of age, the mortality of the procedure is 15%, then rises in older patients (45 years) to 30% or more.

Unrelated matched donor marrow has a high toxicity compared with matched marrow and cannot be equated with sibling transplants.

Quality-of-life studies in unrelated BMT recipients are needed. Data collected with well-validated standardized instruments are necessary.

Indications

Patients with chronic myelogenous leukemia (CML) in chronic phase or accelerated phase who do not have a matched sibling donor should be considered for the best available treatment. CML patients in blast crisis have a 10% survival rate or less.

Patients with acute myeloid leukemia (AML) in first remission should not be considered for unrelated BMT but should be considered in second complete remission.

Subgroups of patients with initial refractory disease, secondary AML, and high-risk myelodysplastic syndromes are candidates for unrelated BMT.

Children and adults with high-risk acute lymphocytic leukemia (ALL) in first remission and those in second remission sustaining bone marrow relapse may have a survival rate improved over those undergoing conventional chemotherapy. However, data are limited in the adult population.

Information for Decision Making

Unrelated BMT should be performed only in those centers having the ability to understand the patient's disease.

Patients having diseases for which there is no evidence and for whom there is some doubt about the benefits of unrelated BMT vs conventional treatment should be entered into randomized trials.

Donors

Uncertainties accompany short- and long-term complications with the administration of colony-stimulating factors (CSFs). Long-term studies are warranted.

Anonymity between donor and patient in the face of some problems should continue until long-term studies are performed.

Further research addressing complex ethical and psychosocial issues is required.

From A consensus statement on unrelated donor bone marrow transplantation from the Consensus Panel chaired by E. C. Gordon-Smith. (1997). *Bone Marrow Transplantation, 19,* 959-962.

tors or the availability of other therapeutic modalities that may not be curative but represent the best available treatment. These alternatives include interferon therapy, autologous transplantation, combination chemotherapy, or even conventional therapy with hydroxyurea (Hydrea). Another researcher found the statement on peripheral stem cell transplantation (PSCT) to be ambiguous. Careful studies aimed at evaluating the safety and efficacy of PSCT need occur before offering it as an alternate treatment. Guidelines for patient and donor education are also needed (A consensus statement, 1997).

PHASES OF BONE MARROW TRANSPLANTATION

Pretransplant

BMT, once considered as treatment when all other therapies have failed, is now often discussed at the time of the patient's initial diagnosis. The phases of BMT are shown in Table 8-4. Community oncologists often work in collaboration with transplant physicians to set the course of treatment. This trajectory is especially true in the case of patients who may store their undesired marrow in the event that tra-

TABLE 8-4 Key Points of Preparation of Recipients and Their Caregivers Throughout the Phases of Bone Marrow Transplantation

Phase of BMT	Resources and Support Mechanisms
Prearrival	
Patient and family will have knowledge of the following: 1. Daily living resources 2. Philosophy of health care provider 3. Members of health care team	1. Family has determined affordable housing arrangement, furnishings, lending closets, transportation availability, laundry facilities, banking, post office, shopping, mail systems, parking, child care, schools, grocery stores, ethnic food availability, medical care for family members, and recreational opportunities such as museums, movie theaters, and sporting events 2. Clinical mission statement, benefits and risks of research, confidentiality, and informed consent issue 3. Physician, physician assistant, nurse, pastor, social worker, dietitians, pharmacists, behavioral health therapist, physical therapist, and volunteers
Arrival/Transplantation Preparation	
Patient and family caregivers will demonstrate knowledge of anticipated responsibilities and expectations throughout BMT.	1. Prepare family caregivers to be patient advocates by gathering information, assisting with decision-making and financial issues, giving emotional support, and providing physical care. 2. Provide resource information of social worker, psychologist, volunteer services, chaplain, support groups, community support, and respite care for the family caregivers. 3. Support patient through informed consent procedure. 4. Provide transportation to and from appointments at hospital, clinics, and emergency care facility. 5. Provide formal classes that include: a. Transplant rationale, process, and expectations b. Protective isolation rationale and policies, LAF rooms, high-efficiency particulate air (HEPA) filtration rooms, protective isolation, masks and gowns, and effective handwashing techniques c. Common complications during transplantation and their management d. Orientation to health care team e. Written guidelines for all transplant phases f. Obtaining emergency and after-hour care g. Acquiring and maintaining medical supplies h. Taking and recording temperatures i. Assisting patient with central catheter management j. Assisting patient with blood draws from catheter and delivery to appropriate locations k. Identifying emotional self-care
Marrow Harvest	
Patient, donor, and family caregivers will understand responsibilities surrounding marrow harvest.	Provide classes for: 1. Principles of marrow harvest 2. Donor issues of marrow harvest, risks of general anesthesia, and autostorage of blood

ditional treatment fails. Another example is the appropriate timing and treatment of chronic myelogenous leukemia (CML). For example, a common treatment for CML is interferon-alpha. Recent research indicates that 60% of CML recipients who had undergone 6 months or less of interferon treatment before BMT survived more than 5 years. That result compared with a 43% 5-year survival rate for patients with CML who had transplants after 6 months or more of interferon. Of those who died, most succumbed to unresponsive GVHD between 100 and 300 days after transplantation. Furthermore, the researchers identified five criteria indicating favorable outcome for CML recipients (Box 8-3) (Morton, Gooley, Hansen, Appelbaum, Bruemmer, Bjerke & Clift et al., 1998).

Preparing for BMT. Historically, most BMTs were performed far from the patient's home, causing considerable isolation, anxiety, and out-of-pocket expenses. Research centers continue to investigate new disease applications, techniques, supportive care measures, and transplant for high-risk patients. As BMT moves from research centers to the community and as third-party payors select regional centers for the insured, some patients are able to remain near

TABLE 8-4 Key Points of Preparation of Recipients and Their Caregivers Throughout the Phases of Bone Marrow Transplantation—cont'd

Phase of BMT	Resources and Support Mechanisms
Marrow Harvest—cont'd	
	3. Managing postoperative complications (e.g., fever, pain, infection, nausea and vomiting, fatigue) 4. Symptoms to report to transplant team
Conditioning Regimens	
Patient and family caregivers will be knowledgeable about the type and effects of conditioning regimens for BMT.	Provide information for: 1. Type of chemotherapy, preparation for TBI, expected symptoms of conditioning regimens (e.g., nausea, vomiting, diarrhea, pain, mucositis, anemia, neutropenia, thrombocytopenia, anorexia, and anxiety) 2. Assure patient about medical supportive, comfort, and self-care measures (e.g., guided imagery, deep breathing)
Marrow Infusion	
Patient and family caregivers will be prepared for marrow infusions.	Explain to allogeneic recipient and family caregivers: 1. Possible adverse effects such as fever are similar to those of a red blood cell (RBC) transfusion. 2. Prepare recipient and family caregivers of autologous BMT of possible effects of dimethosulfate (chilling, fever, cough, hypotension). 3. Monitor patient compliance in self-administration of oral and intravenous (IV) medications.
Waiting for Engraftment	
Patient and family caregivers will be aware of possible complications and their management. Patient and family caregivers will be knowledgeable about expectations for hospital discharge.	Reinforce teaching about the complications following BMT, GVHD, failure to engraft RBC and platelet infusions, veno-occlusive disease, immobility, and fatigue. 1. Instruct patient and family: a. About diet b. Maintaining home environment, cleaning c. IV pump administration d. Recognition of common symptoms; symptom management e. Anticipating, recognizing, and directing emergencies; reporting symptoms 2. Initiate preparation for return home to primary care physician.
Engraftment and Recovery	
Patient and family caregivers will be aware of issues of recovery.	Classes for recognizing: 1. Common problems and symptoms: fatigue, weight loss, sexual dysfunction, cataracts 2. Chronic GVHD: skin, eyes, mouth, sinusitis 3. Infection: herpes zoster virus, depression, isolation, fatigue, and malaise 4. Survivorship issues reentry into community setting, insurance concerns 5. Availability of community support groups 6. Names and numbers of BMT long-term support group

their homes. An increasing number of written and electronic resources have emerged to prepare patients and families before and after BMT. Pharmaceutical companies and the National Institutes of Health (NIH) provide written and computer online material that explains the BMT process. Long-term survivors of BMT are participating with increasing frequency in advocacy and community support groups as more recipients recover from marrow and stem cell transplants.

Box 8-3
Ideal Criteria for Unrelated Bone Marrow Transplantation for Chronic Myelogenous Leukemia

- A matched donor
- Years of age or less
- Receipt of preventive fungal therapy after BMT
- Receipt of ganciclovir for CMV after BMT
- Less than 110% of ideal weight

Box 8-4
Pretransplantation Evaluation for Bone Marrow Transplantation Candidates

Complete medical history
Current medications
Performance status
Full discussion of BMT and its rationale, risks, and benefits.
Bone marrow aspiration and biopsy
Tumor-staging studies for malignant diseases
Immunization history
Complete blood count (CBC) with differential
Human immunodeficiency virus (HIV) titers
Hepatic-liver function studies, hepatitis screen
Renal urinalysis, serum creatinine, creatinine clearance
Pulmonary-arterial blood gases, pulmonary function studies, diffusing capacity of carbon monoxide
Chest x-ray
Cardiac-left ventricular function evaluation
Toxoplasma titers
Andrology for sperm banking
Human chorionic gonadotropin (HCG) titers
Follicle-stimulating hormone levels
Histocompatibility testing for allogeneic and syngeneic BMT
Restrictive fragment length
Serologic typing on patient and nuclear or extended family
Mixed leukocytes culture testing on the patient and prospective donor
Deoxyribonucleic acid (DNA) molecular studies
ABO typing
CMV status, hepatitis B and C
Nutritional evaluation
Dental consultation
Social support: 24-hour committed caregiver
Sperm or oocyte banking, if appropriate
Autologous whole blood storage for allogeneic donors
Financial screening and evaluation

BMT is a toxic procedure that is associated with considerable morbidity and mortality. Consequently, candidates require comprehensive evaluations to determine that there is no comorbid disease that will compromise a patient's ability to sustain the procedure (Box 8-4).

Concomitant with the evaluation, third-party payor coverage, or direct payment from patient is ensured by the financial offices within the institution. Once approved, a patient and family conference is held to obtain informed consent. Although the long-term complications of BMT are in the informed consent, patients rarely concentrate on problems that may occur months or years after BMT. Sterility, resulting from high-dose dose-conditioning regimens, is usually addressed, and for those patients who may already be sterile from prior treatment, several options exist. Sperm banking in boys and men with adequate sperm counts is an option, or fertilized ova storage for women may apply. Survival statistics presented may be stark, but at this point in the process, patients are usually hopeful but realistic. All patients have multilumen indwelling central catheters inserted before treatment begins.

Hospital lengths of stay for BMT are decreasing and patients and caregivers are becoming responsible for complex self-care. Classes focusing on central lumen catheter management, intravenous (IV) administration, infection control, emergency care, and nutrition are critical to outpatient management. Formalized instruction for the patient and family caregiver using educational classes particular to each stage of transplant has been shown to be an effective method of supporting patients. Most BMT centers provide written information about the center, including maps, important telephone numbers, activities, and a glossary of BMT terms.

The Donor. Although risks are minimal, donors need to be comprehensively evaluated before surgery, especially for the ability to tolerate general or spinal anesthesia (Buckner, Clift, Sanders, Stewart, Bensinger & Doney et al., 1984). Box 8-5 lists common tests for donor evaluation.

To minimize the risks of blood transfusion, donors weighing more than 50 kg donate a unit of autologous whole blood to be reinfused intraoperatively at the time of marrow harvest. Little documentation exists about the long-term consequences of marrow harvest on family members. More research is needed in this area. Several factors influence the amount of counseling and education a donor needs

Box 8-5
Pretransplantation Evaluation for Bone Marrow Transplantation Donors

Complete history and physical
Chest x-ray
12-lead electrocardiogram
CBC with differential
Serum chemistries
Urinalysis
HIV titer
Hepatitis B and C
CMV status
HCG titers

before donation. Older literature suggests that the relationship between the donor, the patient, and the family, as well as the donor's own life responsibilities significantly affect donor physiologic outcome (Ruggerio, 1988). Long-term sequelae, including mood changes, lack of self-esteem, altered relationships, and guilt, can occur depending on the donor's perception of the success or failure of the BMT (Paternaude, Szymanski, & Rappeport, 1979). Although research is forthcoming relative to the physiologic and psychological consequences of the unrelated donor, a gap exists in the related donor research.

The Unrelated Donor. In the case of unrelated volunteer donors, few psychological pressures are involved and most individuals donate out of altruism. Direct contact between unrelated marrow donors and recipients is prohibited by the National Marrow Donor Program in the United States. There is debate on this issue, and some centers allow written contact before transplantation and shortly thereafter. Some donors and marrow recipients have formed long-term relationships (Buckner, Peterson, & Bolonesi, 1994). Several significant studies assessing the effects of unrelated marrow donation have emerged. Butterworth, Simmons, and Bartsch (1993) noted the psychosocial effects of 493 donors from the National Marrow Donor Program. The majority (88%) reported a positive experience and that they would donate a second time. Stroncek, Holland, and Bartsch (1995) studied the same group for physiologic effects and found that fatigue (74.8%), pain at the collection site (67.8%), and lower back pain (51.6%) were reported.

MARROW COLLECTION

Donor marrow is harvested in the operating room under sterile conditions, with the donor anesthetized under general or spinal anesthesia. The marrow is obtained from the posterior iliac crests in 2-ml aspirates, up to a total of 10 to 15 mg/kg recipient body weight. If necessary, the anterior iliac crests and the sternum can be used. Although 150 to 200 aspirates are necessary to obtain sufficient marrow, only 6 to 10 skin punctures are made, with the aspiration needles redirected to different sites under the skin. The heparinized marrow is screened through a series of progressively finer mesh screens to filter out bone particles and fat. Marrow is then placed in blood administration bags and infused into the patient within 2 to 4 hours (Buchsel, 1997).

Marrow Purging

When bone marrow or peripheral stem cells are transplanted, the patient usually does not receive an infusion of a pure population of hematopoietic cells. Depending on the processing methods, a varying number of RBCs, granulocytes, and other cells also accompany the hematopoietic stem cells into the recipient's circulation. In an allogeneic BMT, RBCs can cause an ABO incompatible reaction, and donor T-lymphocytes can cause GVHD. In autologous transplants, tumor cells may contaminate the marrow or peripheral stem cells collected from autologous donors. To minimize this risk, marrow is usually collected from patients in remission. However, hidden tumor cells (occult) can be inadvertently infused with the marrow or stem cells during the transplant. The ultimate goal of any collection method is to remove as many of the undesired cells from the marrow as possible while conserving the greatest possible number of functional hematopoietic progenitor cells (HPCs). Therefore several techniques have been developed for purging the undesirable cells before infusion. *Negative selection* refers to removing undesirable cells from the marrow product by removing harmful cells. Almost all autologous purging involves combinations of positive and negative selection techniques in which contaminating cells are removed from the graft (negative), and the most desirable cells are selected (positive) for transplantation

Negative Purging Techniques. Pharmacologic purging techniques use 4-hydroperoxychchophosphamide (4HC) to remove undesirable cells while sparing some uncommitted HPCs. The cells are mixed with 4HC, incubated, washed, and cryopreserved until use. This type of purging is nonspecific and can lethally damage committed progenitor cells.

Antibody Purging. Certain cell surface markers have been identified that appear exclusively or predominately on certain tumor cells. Techniques have been developed that use monoclonal antibodies (MoAbs) against these antigens. An efficient technique for removal of cells that do not adversely affect HPCs involves the use of plastic polymer microspheres (beads) bound to one or more MoAbs. The antibody-coated beads attach to the cells of interest during an incubation period, after which the cell suspension is exposed to a strong magnet. The magnet holds the cells that have bound to the beads, allowing the unbound cells to be removed from the suspension.

Positive Selection Techniques. Immature HPCs have surface markers that gradually diminish as the cells differentiate and mature. If the patient's tumor cells are negative for this CD+ antigen, a more efficient method of tumor cell removal may be to isolate and infuse only those cells that bear this marker.

T-Lymphocyte Depletion. A major limiting factor of allogeneic BMT is GVHD and ex vivo T lymphocyte depletion of donor marrow has proven to be the most successful method to prevent this common complication. This technique has been largely abandoned because of associated graft failure and relapse. Renewed interest has arisen because more sophisticated T lymphocyte depletion techniques have been developed. Because aggressive studies continue in this area, it is important for oncology nurses to have some understanding of the T lymphocyte depletion process with complement alone or in combination with magnetic immunobeads to lysis the T cells while preserving progenitor cells. Finally, combinations of physical and MoAb techniques or soybean agglutination plus MoAbs are used (Ezzone & Camp-Sorrel, 1994)

Complications of Marrow Harvesting

Assessments of adverse effects associated with outpatient marrow harvesting revealed that donors harvested in outpatient areas had no adverse postoperative sequelae. In a large study of 211 unrelated marrow donors, participants were asked to describe the side effects of outpatient marrow donation. Of the 65% who responded, the most common side effects were pain at the donation site (90%), low-back pain (60%), nausea (43%), vomiting (31%), sore throat (43%), fever (8%), and bleeding at the donation site (6%). Similar complications are noted in marrow donors admitted for longer periods (Stroncek, Hollang, & Bartch 1995). Physical and psychological follow-up care for the donor is essential.

THE BONE MARROW TRANSPLANT

Hospital Admission

Once patients have been evaluated for BMT, they are admitted to the hospital and usually placed in a protective isolation room. Several isolation methods exist. Laminar airflow (LAF) rooms were extensively used during the past two decades to decrease infection-related morbidity and mortality but have largely fallen into disuse. Economic considerations, the advent of colony-stimulating factors (CSFs), and lack of convincing data to support installing and maintaining LAF rooms are responsible for this trend. Early studies showed that only patients with aplastic anemia admitted to LAF rooms survived longer when compared with patients not placed in LAF rooms (Buckner, Clift, & Sanders, 1978). Russell, Poon, and Jones (1992) argued that patients cared for in LAF rooms have no higher survival rates than patients placed in conventional hospital rooms where reverse isolation, gloves, face masks, or filtered air are used. In the face of mixed reports, little consistency in infection prophylaxis measures exists (Poe, Larson, McGuire & Krumm, 1994). Most recently, an impressive study determining how the use of high-efficiency particulate air (HEPA) filtration rooms and/or LAF rooms affect transplant-related mortality or survival in the first years after allogeneic transplantation was reported. Over 5000 recipients with leukemia receiving BMTs from an HLA identical sibling (N = 3982) or unrelated transplants (N = 1083) were included in the study. Patients were cared for in either (1) conventional protective isolation in a single-patient room, with any combination of handwashing, gloves, masks, and gowns; or (2) HEPA and/or LAF rooms. Decreased risks of TRM and death in the first 100 days posttransplant resulted in significantly high 1-year survival rates in patients treated in HEPA/LAF rooms compared with those in conventional isolation units. The study is limited because the researchers could not compare HEPA with LAF (Passweg, Rowlings, Atkinson, Barrett, Gale, Gratwohl, & Jacobsen et al., 1998). Decontamination of gastrointestinal tracts, skin, and body cavities with antibiotic solutions and applications of antibiotic powders in body cavities, as well as bathing with sterile water and antibacterial soap have been abandoned due to the lack of convincing survival data. For those centers performing autologous BMT, these expensive units may not be necessary because of the lower incidence of infection among these recipients compared with allogeneic recipients. Handwashing, scrupulous hygiene, and protective isolation may be the most cost-effective and meaningful conventions for infection control. The importance of handwashing protection of the immunocompromised patient was recently underscored by the findings that health care workers caring for low-birth-weight infants introduced *Mycobacterium pachydermatous* in a hospital nursery after being colonized from pets at home. Although this particular infection is not reported in the BMT population, the study makes a compelling statement in nosocomial infection from health care worker's hands (Chang, Miller, Watkins, Arduino, Ashford, & Aguero et al., 1998).

Pretransplant Conditioning Regimens

Recipients of marrow transplants usually are admitted to the hospital 1 day before the start of their conditioning regimen. The methods used to prepare patients for grafting differ according to the underlying disease. Patients receive high-dose chemotherapy alone or with supralethal doses of irradiation. This serves to eradicate malignant cells and to prevent graft rejection by the patient's own immune system.

The array of drugs for high-dose chemotherapy in preparation for marrow transplantation is limited secondary to major organ toxicity. For example, doxorubicin can cause cardiac toxicity, placing the patient at significant risk to succumb during or immediately after transplantation. Historically, cyclophosphamide (CY) in combination with total-body irradiation (TBI) has been the standard treatment used in BMT preparative regimens. CY is the most common chemotherapeutic agent because it provides tumor cell kill, as well as immune ablation. Other agents sometimes used in combination with TBI include cytosine arabinoside and etoposide. The use of busulfan and cyclophosphamide without TBI has increased markedly during the last decade, in an effort to avoid the long-term effects of irradiation, especially on children (Bortin, Horowitz, & Rimm, 1992).

TBI is delivered in varying doses from cobalt or linear accelerator units. TBI offers optimal tumor cell kill because of its ability to penetrate the central nervous system (CNS) and other privileged sites. Lung shielding sometimes is used in an effort to reduce life-threatening pulmonary complications. TBI can be delivered in single or fractionated doses, but prevailing practice favors fractionated doses to reduce toxicities. Pretransplant "booster" radiotherapy to previous tumor sites may be used in patients with bulky disease to reduce the chances of relapse.

Marrow Infusion

The day of marrow infusion is "day 0," with subsequent days numbered from this time. The actual marrow infusion is a procedure similar to a blood transfusion. The marrow is infused through a central lumen catheter over the course of several hours. Marrow cells pass through the lung and home to the marrow cavity. Complications are dependent on the type of cells infused, marrow preservatives, or allergic reactions. For example, dimethylsulfoxide (DMSO) or MoAbs may cause fever, dyspnea, nausea, and vomiting or hematuria. Volume overload and pulmonary abnormalities from fat emboli may also occur. Symptoms similar to blood transfu-

TABLE 8-5 Cause of Symptoms and Nursing Interventions Related to Autologous Blood Cell Infusion

Cause	Symptoms	Interventions
Dimethylsulfoxide toxicity	• Nausea, vomiting, diarrhea, severe hemolysis, anaphylactic reaction, occasional bronchospasm, renal failure, diastolic and systolic hypertension, bradycardia, rare pulmonary edema, or cardiac arrest • Garliclike taste and breath; garliclike odor from urine and stool • Facial flushing	• Administer prophylactic premedications (diphenhydramine, corticosteroids, acetaminophen, antiemetics, mild sedatives, diuretics, mannitol) and hydration; continue during stem cell infusion to prevent or manage nephrotoxicity; administer dexamethasone, ondansetron, lorazepam. • Closely observe patient for somnolence. • Monitor vital signs every 15 minutes. • Offer hard candy or citrus fruits. • Offer cool cloths.
Stem cell product contamination	• Hematuria, increased bilirubin or creatinine	• Draw and monitor serum bilirubin and creatinine levels, monitor thought daily and for 2-3 days after infusion.
Allergies	• Chills, fever, dyspnea, nausea, vomiting	• Premedications as above.

sion reactions can occur (i.e., chills, urticaria, and fever) and should be treated with antihistamines or antipyretics or by decreasing the rate of infusion Table 8-5 lists potential complications for autologous marrow or stem cell infusion.

EARLY COMPLICATIONS OF BONE MARROW TRANSPLANTATION

Acute and chronic complications can complicate the course of allogeneic BMT. Complications are the result of (1) high-dose chemotherapy and irradiation for conditioning regimens, (2) GVHD, (3) problems associated with the original disease and the adverse effects of medications used in the process. The major complications following autologous BMT are similar, except for GVHD. Acute complications declare themselves several days after BMT and compromise almost all organ systems. Because pretransplantation chemoradiotherapy ablates all cell lines thereby causing pancytopenia, complications are most severe until early engraftment. The type, duration, and severity of acute complications depend on the type of preparative regimens, the degree of histocompatibility and GVHD prophylaxis, and the occurrence of GVHD. Patients who have chemotherapy alone typically demonstrate less severe complications than those who receive combination chemotherapy with TBI. Other risk factors are patient age, disease status, and co-morbid condition before BMT complications.

Gastrointestinal Complications

The gastrointestinal tract is a major target of the direct consequences of high-dose chemotherapy, TBI preparative conditioning, infection, preexisting conditions of active periodontal disease, and dental caries. Inflammation of the oral and pharyngeal tissues may occur 2 to 3 days after marrow infusion and persist to approximately 21 days after BMT (Buckely & Syrjala, 1995). Patients can develop pharyngitis or sore throat, have difficulty swallowing, and have bleeding ulcerations from trauma on the sides of the tongue or buccal mucosa (Lloid, 1995). Endotracheal intubation may be required. Herpes simplex lesions, or local or systemic secondary infections with severe thrombocytopenia can further compromise the oral mucosa. In the face of these problems, nutrition concerns arise because of the patient's inability to tolerate most foods (Stern & Lensen, 1995). Airway management, symptom management for pain and anorexia, and antimicrobials are critical to the survival and comfort of the patient (Lloid, 1995). Mucosal coating agents such as antacids, sucralfate, sodium alginate, and cellulose film may increase comfort and promote healing. Benzydamine hydrochloride rinses aid in the reduction of oral mucositis (Epstein, Stevenson-Moor, & Jackson, 1988). Although these topical anesthetics may decrease pain, most patients require parenteral analgesics. Patient-controlled analgesia has been reported to offer optimal pain control in comparison to control in those receiving continuous infusion analgesics (Hill, Chapman, Kornell, Sullivan, Saegar, & Beneditti, 1990). Mouth care using toothbrushes, flossing, and saline sodium rinses are helpful to prevent some discomfort and infection, but the use of these tools is dependent on the patient's tolerance. Lanolin creams and lip balms can smooth lips, but petroleum jelly should be avoided when lips have sores or bleed. Dry mouth can be alleviated with saliva substitutes, sugarless candies, and gum.

Nausea and Vomiting. Nausea and vomiting following chemotherapy and TBI is a consistent problem. Protracted nausea and vomiting also may be caused by GVHD, CMV esophagitis, or gastrointestinal infections. In these cases, a differential diagnosis must be made and may include endoscopy with duodenal biopsy.

Diarrhea. Diarrhea occurs in approximately 50% to 70% of BMT recipients, is multifactorial, can be a life-threatening toxicity, and can result in prolonged hospitalization. Mucosal injuries associated with watery diarrhea result in dehydration, electrolyte disorders, and possible sepsis. (Wasserman, Hidalog, Hornedo, & Corotes-Funes, 1997). The most common causal factors of diarrhea are acute GVHD (48%) and infection (13%) resulting from viral (astrovirus and adenovirus) and bacterial *(Clostridium difficile)* infection. Diarrhea with no clear cause can be present in up to 40% of the patients with these disturbing symptoms, but oral magnesium and nonabsorbable antibiotics (vancomycin, tobramycin, and nystatin) can cause mild diarrhea. (Cox Matsui, Lo, Hinds, Bowden, & Hackman et al., 1995). Classic management of chemotherapy-induced diarrhea includes bowel rest, IV hydration with electrolyte replacement, use of opioid agents (loperamide or diphenoxylate), and total parenteral nutrition. Recently octreotide acetate, a synthetic polypeptide analog of somatostatin, has been found to be safe and effective in the control of diarrhea resulting from high-dose chemotherapy and GVHD (Lamberts, Van Derhely, & DeHerder, 1996).

Hematologic Complications

Transplant recipients are at high risk for pancytopenia and must be supported with blood component therapy and, in some cases with CSFs, until the donor marrow becomes fully engrafted and functional. The use of alpha-erythropoietin has been studied in clinical trials to reduce RBC transfusions but was found to be of little benefit in increasing return of the RBC line or decreasing RBC transfusions (Chao, Tierney, Bloom, Long, Barr & Stallbaum, 1992). Prevention of uterine bleeding after BMT remains a problem. Interest in addressing this problem with the use of leuprorelin acetate at 3.75 mg administered subcutaneously at least 30 days before the conditioning regimen and then 28 days after the first dose has been successful in women with hematologic malignancies or lymphoma. After transplantation, patients required hormone replacement with estroprogestinics or estrogens alone when indicated. Long-term studies are needed to evaluate for possible complications (Chiusolo, Salutari, Sica, Scirpa, Laurenti, & Picirillo et al., 1998). Blood products must be irradiated to destroy T lymphocytes that can cause GVHD in the marrow recipient. Patients whose platelets become refractory to random platelet transfusions can receive HLA-matched platelets from family or community donors, and platelets that have undergone plasmapheresis from marrow donors yield optimal increments. Alloimmunization and platelet refractoriness contribute to a 1% case fatality rate from hemorrhagic complications (Deeg, 1994). Bleeding can occur from all body orifices and requires immediate intervention.

Hemorrhagic Cystitis

Almost 70% of marrow recipients receiving cyclophosphamide in conditioning regimens develop hemorrhagic cystitis. Acroleic metabolite in cyclophosphamide causes ulceration of bladder mucosal tissue resulting in significant bleeding. Recently papovavirus and adenovirus infection have been found to contribute to this problem. Hemorrhagic cystitis has a sudden onset, may be delayed, or may manifest itself months after BMT. Preventive techniques with continuous bladder irrigation and/or aggressive IV therapy to flush cyclophosphamide metabolites from the bladder are common supportive care measures. Debate continues on the effectiveness of IV drug therapies (2-mercaptoethane sulfonate sodium), especially in today's health care economic climate. Nursing management includes management of continuous IV hydration and administration diuretics.

Pulmonary Complications

Life-threatening pulmonary complications occur in up to 40% to 60% of recipients. Causative factors are chemoradiotherapy toxicity or bacterial, viral, or fungal infection in severely immunosuppressed patients. The pathophysiology is characterized by alveolar capillary injury, leakage of plasma into the pulmonary interstitium, and reduced pulmonary compliance. Pulmonary edema syndromes caused by sodium excess and cardiomyopathy, myocarditis, and volume overload from veno-occlusive disease (VOD) can occur immediately after transplant. Interstitial pneumonia presents symptoms similar to those of adult respiratory distress syndrome (ARDS) and occurs early (before day 100) or late (after day 100) transplantation (Crawford, 1994).

Common symptoms associated with pneumonia may include rapid onset of nonproductive cough, dyspnea, hypoxemia, and fever. Chest radiographs can show interstitial infiltrates whereas arterial blood gas levels may indicate hypoxia. Diagnosis using open lung biopsies have been replaced by bronchoalveolar lavage and centrifugation culture techniques to identify causative organisms and treatment.

Interstitial Pneumonia. Interstitial pneumonia, a process that occurs in the interstitial spaces of the lungs, can be manifested in approximately 35% of allogeneic marrow recipients. This troublesome complication remains the most frequent cause of death during the first 100 days after transplant, carrying a mortality rate of approximately 20% in allogeneic recipients receiving transplants for advanced hematologic malignancy (Crawford, 1994).

Cytomegalovirus Pneumonia. CMV pneumonia, occurring in 20% of allogeneic recipients, continues to be the leading cause of infectious pneumonia. Onset of early CMV pneumonia is greatest between 5 and 13 weeks after transplantation. Allogeneic marrow recipients have a mortality rate of up to 85% (Crawford, 1994). It is thought that the incidence of CMV pneumonia in the allogeneic recipient exceeds the incidence in autologous graft recipients because of immunosuppressive medications given to prevent GVHD. Patients at risk are those older than 30 years of age with advanced disease who receive TBI. Severe GVHD and CMV seropositivity further compromise recipients (Goodrich, Boeckh, & Bowden, 1994). The most effective prophylaxis against CMV pneumonia is the avoidance of viral infection by infusing only CMV-negative blood products in cases in which both donor and patient demonstrated CMV seronegativity before BMT. Patients who receive screened blood products must continue to do so through day 100 after BMT. A seminal 5-year randomized study showed that recipients receiving blood component therapy via a mechanical device (experimental group) vs CMV blood screened at a blood bank (control) had a 2.4% probability of developing CMV infection, compared with those who received screened products. This percentage is within the acceptable rate of less than or equal to a 5% infection rate. This finding has changed practice guidelines and many BMT units use blood filtered to reduce the costs of transplantation without compromising patient care (Bowden, Slichter, Sayers, Weisdorg, Kays, & Banaji et al., 1995).

Medical Management

Patients who are seropositive for CMV whose donors are also seropositive may be managed with antiviral agents such as acyclovir or immunoglobulin. Recently, more than five studies using prophalatic ganciclovir have shown a reduction in CMV infection but without a reduction in transplant mortality. Treatments employing combination ganciclovir and IV CMV immunoglobulin have shown a 40% to 50% survival rate in marrow recipients whose diagnosis occurred during the initial episode of CMV pneumonia (Zaia, 1994).

Other Pneumonia. Idiopathic pneumonia is diagnosed when no specific organism is recovered in bronchial lavage washings or lung tissue biopsy (Crawford, 1994). Idiopathic pneumonia accounts for 30% of all interstitial pneumonias in marrow recipients. It is believed to be a result of high-dose irradiation. Other pneumonias that occur may be caused by a virus (e.g., adenovirus, herpes simplex, or varicella zoster), bacteria, or fungus. These account for 15% of pneumonia in marrow recipients and may be successfully treated (Crawford, 1994).

Community-acquired infections such as respiratory syncytial virus (RSV), influenza, parainfluenza rhinoviruses, adenoviruses, and coronaviruses are not well understood in the marrow transplant recipient. A recent study examining nasal and throat specimens in leukemia and transplant patients presenting with respiratory symptoms demonstrated community respiratory viruses in 27% of those cultured. Viral prevalence in this study mirrored that in the community except that RSV was more common than anticipated. RSV was, in fact, the most common respiratory virus isolate. RSV infections occurred primarily occurring in the winter and early spring. Strategies for preventing morbidity and mortality from community respiratory viruses require better understanding of their nosocomial transmission, immunization, and early diagnosis and treatment. Several studies demonstrate that respiratory viruses are often transmitted nosocomially, often from people with only mild symptoms of illness. Strict adherence to infection control measures that include contact isolation and prevention of exposure to people with even mild respiratory illnesses can decrease nosocomial risk. Immunization is available only for the influenza virus; passive immunization with immune globulin may be helpful for some viruses, including RSV. Effective antivirals are available for influenza A (amantadine, rimantadine) and ribavirin. However, successful treatment requires early diagnosis and intervention, as well as awareness of the prevalence of these viruses in the community, and appropriate investigation of respiratory symptoms.

Although it is well recognized that community-acquired respiratory virus can cause severe pulmonary infection and death in transplant recipients, their overall contribution to mortality after blood and marrow transplantation is still unclear. Most studies are limited by small numbers and inadequate sampling, and are restricted to patients with severe respiratory symptoms. A goal of the IBMTR and American Bone Marrow Transplant Registry (ABMTR) is to study seasonal incidence of fatal and nonfatal respiratory infections (Whimbey, Champlain, & Couch, 1996). *Pneumocystis carinii* pneumonia, discussed elsewhere in this chapter, caused significant mortality in the early years of BMT but has been successfully prevented by the use of prophylactic trimethoprim-sulfamethoxazole (TMP-SMX) (Sullivan, 1994).

Nursing Management

The median time of onset for interstitial pneumonias is 60 to 70 days after BMT. Typically, patients have been discharged from the acute care setting and are being followed up in a clinic or a physician's office. Classic symptoms are related to the patient's inability to engage in daily activities and may manifest as fatigue, malaise, and/or dyspnea. Patients must undergo routine chest x-rays and thorough physical examinations, including chest auscultation and determination of arterial blood gases (ABGs) in cases of suspected interstitial pneumonia. Readmission to the hospital is usually necessary, and patients may need respiratory support with mechanical ventilation (Wilke, 1991).

Renal Complications

Renal complications after BMT occur in more than 50% of marrow recipients and can be the result of one event or a combination of events (Ballard, 1991). Multiple nephrotoxic drugs used for prevention and treatment of transplantation-related problems (e.g., amphotericin B, cyclosporine, methotrexate, aminoglycosides) are implicated in renal toxicities. These toxicities, superimposed on patients with prerenal dysfunction, septic shock, volume depletion, VOD, or tumor necrosis syndrome act in concert to exacerbate renal hemodynamic complications further.

Patients at risk for renal failure are those with a pretransplant history of hypertension, diabetes mellitus, or vascular disease. Clinical manifestations of renal complications include the abrupt onset of anuria, heralding an early indication of acute tubular necrosis or acute renal failure. Acute tubular necrosis compromises renal flow, subsequent inability to effectively eliminate fluid, electrolytes, and metabolic wastes (Wujcik, Ballard, & Camp-Sorrel, 1994). Anuria is typically caused by postrenal obstruction resulting from hemorrhagic cystitis secondary to cyclophosphamide administration. *Renal failure,* defined as a doubling of baseline creatinine, stems from tumor lysis resulting from high-dose chemotherapy. Early symptoms of renal failure include anuria and acid-base imbalances from the lack of elimination of nitrogenous wastes, water, electrolytes, and acids. Renal dysfunction in marrow transplant recipients usually is mild, and patients can be managed by eliminating nephrotoxic agents, monitoring fluids and electrolytes, possible dopamine infusion to reduce renal perfusion or renal dialysis. After allogeneic transplantation, however, 5% to 10% of patients will require renal dialysis, and mortality is 85% in this group (Ballard, 1988).

Nursing assessment includes monitoring patients for confusion or complaints of thirst, as well as taking vital signs with postural blood pressures, measurements of urine specific gravity, urine electrolytes, and accurate intake and output of bodily fluids (Ballard, 1991). Assessing for distended neck veins or peripheral edema, coupled with accurate measurement of abdominal girth and daily weights, are also imperative to distinguish between prerenal and intrarenal conditions.

Veno-occlusive Disease of the Liver

VOD is almost exclusive to BMT and is the most common nonrelapse life-threatening complication of preparative-regimen–related toxicity for BMT. Peak onset is 21 weeks after transplant. The diagnosis of VOD often is clouded by overlapping BMT-related symptoms. Risk factors for developing VOD include (1) patients with hepatitis and infections before BMT, (2) those that receive repeated doses of chemotherapy before transplant in addition to high-dose irradiation in pretransplant conditioning regimens, (3) the use of antimicrobial therapy with acyclovir, amphotericin, or vancomycin, (4) and mismatched or unrelated allogeneic marrow grafts.

Liver damage caused by chemoradiotherapy involves two histopathologic processes: (1) venule occlusion and/or veno-occlusive process involving terminal hepatic venules and sublobular veins and (2) hepatocyte necrosis. Clinical symptoms, which occur in the first weeks after transplantation, include rapid fluid retention, sudden weight gain, abdominal distention, pain in the right upper quadrant of the abdomen, jaundice, hepatomegaly, icteric skin and sclerae, encephalopathy, possible bleeding, and elevated serum bilirubin levels (Ballard, 1991). These symptoms are the result of significant obstruction and intrasinusoidal hypertension, and morbidity ranges from 21% to 50% (McDonald, Sharma, Matthews, Shulman, & Thomas, 1984).

Currently, there is no prevention or treatment for VOD, although mild cases may respond spontaneously and treatment is mainly one of supportive care. Researchers are exploring the use of prostaglandins, tumor necrosis factor (TNF), and ursodeoxcycholic acid and recombinant tissue plasminogen activator, but these measures remain questionable. Treatment consists of fluid management, with diuresis and restriction of water. Hematocrit levels should be kept above 35% to maintain intravascular volume and renal perfusion. Supportive care must include the respiratory system as well because of fluid overload (Bearman, 1995).

Continuous and careful monitoring of the fluid status of the patient is a nursing responsibility. This includes weighing the patient twice a day, obtaining daily abdominal girth measurements, monitoring for signs of bleeding, monitoring postural blood pressures, and administering and monitoring the effectiveness of diuretics and colloids (Ballard, 1991).

Neurologic Complications

Acute manifestations of neurologic and neuromuscular compromise occur in 60% to 70% of marrow recipients, with a resulting 6% fatality rate (Openshaw & Slatkin, 1994). The underlying causes are pretransplant chemoradiotherapy (busulfan, cytarabine, cyclophosphamide, L-asparaginase), CNS infection, and immunosuppressive agents, such as cyclosporine, steroids, and intrathecal methotrexate. These problems occur from time of conditioning to weeks after transplantation. Neuropathy and somnolence occur earliest (13 to −8 days before BMT) whereas confusion or disorientation peak around 12 days after transplantation. Neurologic complications from hemorrhage are rare because of the administration of prophylactic platelet transfusions to prevent bleeding. Recurrence of malignancy after BMT may occur in the CNS in up to 38% of the recipients who receive no post-transplant intrathecal prophylaxis (Furlong, 1993).

Leukoencephalopathy

Leukoencephalopathy has been reported in a small number of marrow transplant recipients who have had prior cranial irradiation and intrathecal methotrexate (Thompson, Flournoy, Buckner, & Sanders, 1986). Signs and symptoms include lethargy, somnolence, dementia, coma, and personality changes. Patients who receive cyclosporine for post-transplantation immunosuppression have documented hypomagnesemia, which can result in seizure activity.

Cardiac Complications

Serious cardiac complications, although rare (5% to 10%) can occur several days after high-dose cyclophosphamide administration. Mortality rates are less than 1%. Other problems such as cardiomegaly, congestive heart failure (CHF), and fluid retention are more common and can be managed with fluid balance measures (Peterson, & Bearman, 1994). Recipients at risk are those with a history of receiving cardiotoxic drugs (e.g., doxorubicin).

Infection

Infections in BMT recipients result from neutropenia, depressed T- and B-lymphocyte function, and disruption of anatomic barriers (e.g., mucositis, central venous catheters) and immunosuppressive agents used to manage GVHD. The nature of GVHD is immunosuppressive, but, in a seemingly paradoxical approach, this complication must be managed with immunosuppressive agents. Thus the autologous recipient, once periods of neutropenia are resolved, is usually less susceptible to life-threatening infection. The most common sites of infection are the gastrointestinal tract, oropharynx, lung, skin, and indwelling catheter sites (Wingard, 1990). The temporal sequence of high-risk periods for bacterial, viral, fungal, and protozoal complications are classically divided into three periods: early (0 to 30 days); intermediate (30 to 100 days); and late (>100 days) (Bowden et al., 1995; Wingard, 1994; Zaia, 1994).

In general, the most common infections (90%) during the

first month after BMT are gram-negative and gram-positive bacterial, fungal, and herpes simplex virus (HSV) infections. During the second and third months CMV, fungal, gram-positive bacteria, and *P. carinii* are the dominant infections for patients. For those surviving more than 100 days after BMT, infections arising from encapsulated bacteria, varicella-zoster, and *P. carinii* (Wingard, 1990) are in evidence.

Early Infections

Bacterial infections caused by gram-positive organisms *(Staphylococcus epidermis, Streptoccus)* and gram-negative organisms *(Pseudomonas aeruginosa, Klebsiella pneumoniae)* place patients at risk for significant morbidity and mortality during the first week after BMT. A classic management approach is the use of semisynthetic penicillin, plus an aminoglycoside administered empirically at the first sign of fever during neutropenia. The use of the fluoroquinolones (e.g., norfloxacin, ciprofloxacin) and development of effective regimens that do not include aminoglycosides has improved the control and treatment of gram-negative infections.

HSV types I and II, Epstein-Barr virus, and CMV are the major viruses that occur during the early phase of BMT. Oral ulceration is the common clinical manifestation of HSV type I infection, and genital ulcerations are caused by HSV type II reactivation. Clinical features are painful vesicles, usually several millimeters in diameter. Standard treatment for HSV is acyclovir, but new strains of acyclovir-resistant herpes are emerging. Foscarnet may be employed in acyclovir-resistant disease (Bowden et al., 1995, Wingard, 1994; Zaia, 1994).

Local and systemic candidal infections commonly occur during periods of neutropenia. The most common fungal pathogens seen in the BMT recipient are *Candida* species and *Aspergillus* species. Colonization of cutaneous and mucosal surfaces such as those in the oropharynx, gastrointestinal tract, and vagina act as a portal of entry for broad-spectrum antibiotics. Treatments with topical antifungals include clotrimazole troches, nystatin suspension and tablets, and chlorhexadine oral rinses. Significant esophageal disease may require systemic antifungal therapy. Fluconazole, amphotericin B, and liposomal-encapsulated amphotericin B are recognized systemic agents. The advantages of fluconazole are that it can be administered either orally or intravenously, and one daily dose may be sufficient. Aspergillus is a major infectious problem during days 0 to 30 after BMT. The portal of entry for aspergillus infection is the respiratory tract, and the risk for aspergillus infection increases with the duration and degree of neutropenia. Diagnosis from blood cultures is difficult, and percutaneous-needle, bronchoscopic, or open-lung biopsy may be used.

CMV infection is the most significant infection during this phase, accounts for a 15% to 20% mortality rate in marrow recipients, and is discussed elsewhere in this chapter. Bacterial infections are less frequent from day 30 to day 90 following marrow transplantation. PCP accounts for 10% of interstitial pneumonitis during this period (Sullivan, 1994). TMP-SMX is the gold standard as a preventative and therapeutic agent, and daspone or IV pentamidine is an alternative therapy for those patients who report true allergies to TMP-SMX.

Medical Management. Infection prophylaxis is the first line of defense for the immunosuppressed marrow recipient. Prevention techniques vary among institutions, but generally involve handwashing, meticulous oral hygiene, prophylactic antibiotics, and protective isolation. Treatment of infection focuses on identifying the invasive organism and treating the accompanying infection with appropriate antibiotics. Immunoglobulin (IG) therapy is generally recommended for allogeneic BMT recipients to decrease bacterial sepsis and interstitial pneumonia, and modulate GVHD (Sullivan, Kopecky, & Jocom, 1990). Results of studies indicate that IG given before and at 100 days after transplantation reduced the incidence of CMV pneumonia, but no gain was realized in those receiving IgG after that time (Sullivan, 1994).

Acute Graft Versus Host Disease

GVHD occurs because T cells in the donor marrow recognize the patients as foreign and, similar to automimmune diseases, attempt to reject the host (patient). This phenomenon is in direct contrast to solid-organ transplant when the patient's antigens mount an immunologic effort to reject the transplanted organ. The key factors necessary for GVHD are (1) immunologically competent donor T lymphocytes, (2) histoincompatibility between donor and host, and (3) inability of the host to reject donor lymphocytes. Risk factors are (1) patient and donor age greater than 8 years of age, (2) donor alloimmunization through transfusion or pregnancy, (3) mismatched-gender BMTs, (4) CMV negativity in patient and donor, and (6) type of GVHD prophylaxis. (Chao et al., 1992; Sullivan, 1994).

GVHD exists in two forms, the acute and the chronic. The acute phase manifests itself between 70 to 90 days after allogeneic BMT, whereas the chronic form declares itself approximately 100 days after allogeneic BMT. Chronic GVHD is discussed later in this chapter. Acute GVHD occurs in 30% to 50% of HLA-identical recipients and up to 75% of unrelated donor transplants (Sullivan, 1994). Acute GVHD targets the skin, liver, and gut. Those recipients receiving unrelated donor BMT demonstrate a higher incidence compared with an HLA identical sibling transplant but no more than in mismatched family BMTs (Sullivan, 1994).

The clinical presentation of acute GVHD usually begin with a maculopapular rash typically beginning at the time of white blood cell (WBC) engraftment. The early stages may be pruritic, confined to 25% of the body, and appearing at the nape of the neck, ears, shoulder, palms of the hands or soles of the feet. Disease progression includes a confluent rash that involves the entire integument. In severe cases, bullous lesions, desquamation, and blistering similar to second-degree burns can occur. This syndrome may appear similar to other skin problems, but skin biopsies will declare a differential diagnosis.

The second most common organ involved in acute GVHD is the liver, which is almost always affected in conjunction with acute GVHD of the skin. The primary sign is a rise in conjugated bilirubin, alkaline phosphatase, and transaminase. Jaundice indicates progressive liver involvement. Diagnoses may be clouded by the appearance of VOD, CMV, HSV hepatitis, and drug toxicity, most notably cyclosporine or methotrexate. Liver biopsy by percutaneous methods or the transjugular route can confirm liver GVHD, but most recipients manifest thrombocytopenia at this time, thereby placing the patient at risk for life-threatening bleeding.

The third organ system involved with acute GVHD is the gastrointestinal tract, and it is characterized by nausea, vomiting, anorexia, abdominal cramping, pain, and diarrhea. Green, watery diarrhea may exceed 2 L per day, causing serious fluid and electrolyte losses and a portal of entry for infections. Severe ileus has also been noted in some patients.

Medical Management. The much sought-after quest in BMT is GHVD prevention, which has proven illusive and frustrating for investigators. Although T-lymphocyte–depleted marrow transplants can significantly reduce this problem, relapse and graft failure limit its utility. The three most common immunosuppressive medications are aimed at removing or inactivating T cells that attack target organs. Cyclosporine and methotrexate continue to be the first-line approach to treating GVHD, whereas adding corticosteroids (1 to 60 mg/kg) to the treatment regimen is the second line of therapy. Polyvalent IV immunoglobulin (IVIG) at a dose of 400 to 500 mg administered from day of transplant until 120 days afterward has been reported to reduce the frequency of acute GVHD. Other medications used to prevent and modify acute GVHD are antithymocyte globulin (ATG) and monoclonal antibodies. Tacrolimus, a macrolide lactone with potent immunosuppressive activity, is demonstrating significant efficacy in prevention and treatment of related and unrelated donor transplantations. Three multicenter randomized studies comparing tacrolimus with cyclosporine are now completed. All three studies show a significantly lower incident of acute GVHD in patients receiving this agent, but toxicities associated with its use are substantial. The adverse effects include nephrotoxicity, neurotoxicity, hyperglycemia, and hypertension. Future studies using tacrolimus in combination with other immunosuppressants and its use in patients with advanced malignancy is warranted.

Grading Acute Graft Versus Host Disease

Universally used grading systems to measure acute GVHD severity were established on an analysis of only 61 patients. Consequently, the categories do not clearly relate to current treatments and mortality. Recently, the IBMTR reevaluated the GVHD grading system and sought to reclassify GVHD relative to mortality risk and specific organ involvement. The new grading schema is more user friendly and correlates directly with mortality risk. The new schema, however, requires validation, and a prospective analysis comparing the Glucksbery and IBMTR grading system is under way.

Common Nursing Problems and Their Management

Nursing care for patients with acute GVHD demands an understanding of its tempo and symptoms so that timely assessments and symptom management be instituted. Knowledge of drugs administered in concert for other BMT-related drugs may confound the patient's clinical course (e.g., amphotericin). Nursing care includes management of burn-like wounds, abdominal pain, and voluminous diarrhea. Frequent clinical reassessment is required to monitor fluid replacement, hyperalimentation, transfusions, and antibiotic therapy.

Hospital Discharge

The amount of time recipients remain hospitalized depends on the institution's philosophy, the clinical course of the patient, the ability to offer BMT-trained staff on a 24-hour basis, and committed family caregivers. Discharge criteria will differ accordingly. The character of newly discharged marrow recipients has changed dramatically with patients and families responsible for the administration of multiple antibiotics and complex symptom management support. Patients are typically assessed daily to weekly, and blood products and IV therapy can be delivered either in the clinic or home care setting. Significant teaching is required, and patients are taught to prevent infections by avoiding crowds, school, and work for 1 year after BMT.

GVHD in Return to Community Oncologist

Typically, allogeneic marrow recipients remain with the BMT team until 100 days after BMT, or until stabilized immune recovery occurs and GVHD is controlled. Autologous recipients, because they are generally immunocompetent, usually return home as early as 50 days after BMT. Once an evaluation to assess the patient's clinical status is completed, patients often make this transition with mixed emotions. Fear of leaving the secure environment of specialized care often overrides the excitement of returning home. Once home, physician assessments occur weekly and then at monthly intervals, depending on the patients' clinical status. Communication between community-based oncologists and long-term follow-up is essential.

Annual Assessments

Patients typically return to the BMT center for annual evaluations for up to 3 years after BMT to evaluate engraftment and assess for possible adverse effects such as growth and development problems in children, resistant GVHD, or treatment failure.

LATE COMPLICATIONS OF BONE MARROW TRANSPLANTATION

Similar to the acute BMT complications, late complications (day 100 and after) arise from the results of high-dose conditioning regimens, GVHD and its long-term immunosuppressive management, and treatment failure. Table 8-6 lists the complications of chronic GVHD, and Table 8-7 lists the late effects of BMT and medical management. Table 8-8 discusses nursing care of the patient with late effects of BMT.

Chronic Graft Versus Host Disease (Allogeneic Bone Marrow Transplantation)

Chronic GVHD is the single major determinant of long-term outcome and quality of life in allogeneic BMT recipients. Once restricted to appearance 100 days after BMT, it is now thought this problem can occur as early as 50 days after allogeneic BMT but is often confounded by other complications. Numerous risk factors have been associated with chronic GVHD, such as mismatched donors, female-to-male transplants, positive HSV and CMV age over 8 years, prior grade 2 to 3 acute GVHD, and CML recipients who received methotrexate and cyclosporine as chronic GVHD prophylaxis. The primary risk factor is for those having had acute GVHD treated with steroids (Wagner, Flowers, Longton, Storb, & Schubert, 1998). Risk factors are cumulative, and those recipients having larger numbers of these threats have higher probabilities of extensive chronic GHVD. Chronic GVHD is noted in 33% of HLA-identical transplants, 49% of HLA-mismatched family members, and 65% of unrelated donor BMTs. Mismatched recipients have also been shown to manifest this problem earlier than matched sibling transplants (201 days vs 159 days). (Sullivan, 1994). Chronic GVHD is a multisystem disorder of the skin, mouth, eyes, sinuses, liver, gut, vaginal mucosa, and serosal surfaces, as well as pulmonary, nervous, urologic, hematopoietic, lymphoid, and endocrine systems.

Traditionally, chronic GVHD has been classified as progressive, quiescent, or *de novo.* Progressive onset that is an extension of acute GVHD has the poorest prognosis. Quiescent onset develops after primary acute GVHD has resolved and has fair prognosis. New onsets *(de novo)* in those with no prior acute disease present with the best prognosis. Historically, chronic GVHD has been graded according to a schema that divides this syndrome into limited or extensive categories. Limited disease targets only the skin and liver and has a favorable course if untreated, whereas extensive disease affects numerous organ systems and can be fatal if not treated. (Sullivan, 1994). New scoring is under investigation that may provide an analysis of the precise impact of chronic GVHD on an affected organ system (e.g., gastrointestinal, hepatic, integumentary, or pulmonary) (IBMTR, 1998).

Text continued on p. 174

TABLE 8-6 Complications of Chronic Graft Versus Host Disease

Site and Incidence	Signs and Symptoms	Medical Management
Skin, 70%	Dyspigmentation, erythema, hyperkeratosis, desquamation, facial butterfly rash, patchy hyperpigmentation, reticular mottling, perifollicular papules, and pruritus Hidebound skin texture, joint contracture, and guttate lesions (stretch marks) Ulcerations with serous drainage and concomitant infection Alopecia, nail ridging, and premature graying Loss of sweat gland function	Clinical examination and 3-mm skin biopsy Immunosuppressive therapy: Cyclosporine, corticosteroids, thalidomide, rapamycin, tacrolimus, psoralen, and ultraviolet irradiation Diphenhydramine and topical steroids for itching Burn treatment measures with silver sulfadiazine ointment, whirlpool débridement, and skin allografts
Mouth, 70%	Erythema, tissue atrophy, and lichenoid changes Hyperkeratotic striae, plaques, papules, and patches Pseudomembranous ulcerations of buccal mucosa and lateral tongue Infection Pain, burning, xerostomia, and loss of taste Sensitivity to spices, acidic foods, and temperature Difficulty opening mouth Dental caries	Immunosuppressive therapy Lip biopsy Salivary analysis for proteins and antibodies Culture and sensitivity for bacteria, fungus, and virus Pilocarpine and anetholetrithione for xerostomia Analgesics as needed Fluoride gels and mouthwashes
Esophagus, 10%	Difficulty swallowing Retrosternal pain Weight loss Esophageal web formation and stricture	Endoscopy and x-rays for diagnosis Esophageal dilation

From Buchsel, P. C., Wroblewski, E. L., & Randolph, S. R. (1996). Delayed complications of bone marrow transplantation: An update. *Oncology Nursing Forum, 23*(8), 1267-1291.

Continued

TABLE 8-6 Complications of Chronic Graft Versus Host Disease—cont'd

Site and Incidence	Signs and Symptoms	Medical Management
Gastrointestinal tract, rare	Anorexia, nausea, and vomiting Diarrhea and malabsorption Weight loss	X-rays for diagnosis Stool culture and sensitivity Total parenteral nutrition Immunosuppressive therapy
Liver, 30%	Jaundice Elevated bilirubin, SGOT, and alkaline phosphatase Increased prothrombin time and partial thromboplastin time Abdominal pain in the upper right quadrant	Immunosuppressive therapy Rule out viral and fungal infection, hepatotoxic drug reactions, gallstones, and neoplastic disease. Biopsy for diagnosis Liver function tests Prothrombin time, partial thromboplastin time, and fibrin split products Ursodeoxycholic acid
Eyes, 80%	Sicca syndrome Pain, burning, and itching Photophobia Corneal ulceration or scarring Cataracts Infection Positive Schirmer's tear test (less than 10 mm wetness)	Immunosuppressive therapy Ophthalmology consult Slit-lamp microscopy examination Lacriset plugs and punctural ligation Keratoplasty and tarsorrhaphies Ocular lens replacement
Lungs/bronchiolitis obliterans, 10%	Persistent cough, dyspnea, and wheezing Decreased forced expiratory volume and vital capacity Decreased serum immunoglobulin gamma and IgA levels	Immunosuppressive therapy Chest x-ray Pulmonary function tests Arterial blood gases and pulse oximetry
Vagina, incidence unknown	Vaginal stenosis and atrophy Decreased libido Fatigue Painful intercourse Obstruction of menstrual flow (swollen abdomen, pain, bloating)	Immunosuppressive therapy Gynecology consult Vaginal biopsy and Pap test Vaginal dilation and vaginal lubricants Sexual counseling
Myofascial, 10%	Muscle pain, aches, and cramping Arthralgia Synovial effusion Tendonitis and arthritis Limited range of motion	Immunosuppressive therapy Muscle biopsy and x-rays for diagnosis Analgesics as needed Physical therapy consult
Peripheral nervous system, extremely rare	Myasthenia gravis: Eyelid ptosis, extraocular weakness, and proximal limb and facial muscle weakness Polymyositis: Proximal muscle weakness and tenderness, dysphagia, and cardiac muscle involvement Demyelinating polyneuropathy: Difficulty chewing, swallowing, and speaking; progressive quadriplegia	Neurology consult Electromyography and nerve conduction studies Sural nerve biopsy Cholinesterase inhibitors (e.g., diphenhydramine, prochlorperazine) Immunosuppressive therapy Plasmapheresis Immunoglobulins Physical therapy consult
Immune system, 20% to 40%	Leukopenia, lymphopenia, and granulocytopenia Eosinophilia and thrombocytopenia Infection Anemia and bleeding Fatigue and malaise	Physical examination and health history Bone marrow aspiration and bone biopsy CBC and immunoglobulin levels Prophylactic antibiotics Immunoglobulins Granulocyte and granulocyte-macrophage colony-stimulating factors and epoetin-alfa Irradiated packed RBC and platelet transfusions Surveillance cultures of urine and central venous catheter site Sepsis work-up: Blood, urine, stool, sputum, catheter exit site, culture and sensitivity Chest x-rays Antibiotics

From Buchsel, P. C., Wroblewski, E. L., & Randolph, S. R. (1996). Delayed complications of bone marrow transplantation: An update. *Oncology Nursing Forum, 23*(8), 1267-1291.
SGOT, serum gluatamic oxalacetic transaminase.

TABLE 8-7 Late Effects of Bone Marrow Transplantation

Late Effect	Incidence*	Causes	Typical Onset Posttransplant	Signs and Symptoms	Medical Management
Pulmonary Complications					
	50% with chronic GVHD 21% without chronic GVHD 2% autologous BMT	Cytotoxic agents Irradiation Structural and functional damage Impaired immunity from chronic GVHD Infectious pathogens	100 days or until immune reconstitution	Fever, shaking chills, malaise, cough, dyspnea, wheezing, bronchospasm, bilateral interstitial infiltrates, and abnormal PFTs	Chest x-ray PFTs and ABGs Open lung biopsy Antibiotic therapy
Interstitial pneumonitis	10% to 15% allogeneic BMT	Irradiation Cytotoxic agents Impaired immunity Infectious pathogens	80 to 150 days	Nonproductive cough, fever, wheezing, dyspnea, bronchospasm, hypoxia, and reduced expiratory flow	Chest x-ray ABGs BAL Steroid and antibiotic therapy
Restrictive disease	20%	Irradiation Cytotoxic agents Chronic GVHD	365 days	Cough, dyspnea upon exertion, abnormal PFTs, mean loss in total lung capacity, reduced vital capacity, and impaired diffusion capacity May be asymptomatic	Respiratory therapy Bronchodilators
Obstructive disease	10% to 15%	Irradiation Cytotoxic agents Chronic GVHD	100 to 400 days	Dyspnea, cough, hypoxia, shortness of breath, reduced forced expiratory volume, and reduced IgG and IgA levels	Chest x-ray ABGs, pulse oximetry, and PFTs Lung biopsy Oxygen therapy and mechanical ventilation Immunosuppressive therapy

*Figures are intended as general guidelines. Incidence will vary/be uncertain depending on the number of patients, diseases, and transplant variables.

ABGs, arterial blood gases; *BAL,* broncho alveolar lavage; *BMT,* bone marrow transplant; *BUN,* blood urea nitrogen; *CBC,* complete blood count; *CMV,* cytomegalovirus; *CNS,* central nervous system; *CT,* computed tomography; *FSH,* follicle-stimulating hormone; *GI,* gastrointestinal; *GVHD,* graft vs host disease; *HLA,* human lymphocyte antigen; *IgA,* immunoglobulin alpha; *IgG,* immunoglobulin gamma; *IVIG,* intravenous immunoglobulin; *LH,* luteinizing hormone; *MRI,* magnetic resonance imaging; *MUD,* multiple unmatched donors; *PFT,* pulmonary function test; *SMX,* sulfamethoxazole; *TBI,* total body irradiation; *TMP,* trimethoprim; *TSH,* thyroid-stimulating hormone; *VZV,* varicella-zoster virus

From Buchsel, P. C., Wroblewski, E. L., & Randolph, S. R. (1996). Delayed complications of bone marrow transplantation: An update. *Oncology Nursing Forum, 23*(8), 1267-1291.

Continued

Table 8-7 Late Effects of Bone Marrow Transplantation—cont'd

Late Effect	Incidence*	Causes	Typical Onset Posttransplant	Signs and Symptoms	Medical Management
Infectious Complications					
Bacterial Organisms: Blood and Sinopulmonary Sites					
• Encapsulated bacteria • *Streptococcus pneumoniae* • *Hemophilus influenzae*	38% MUD BMT 22% HLA-matched BMT Rare with autologous BMT	Immunodeficiency caused by chronic GVHD, HLA disparity, and hypogammaglobulinemia	100 to 365 days	*General:* Fever, sepsis, shaking chills, malaise, hypotension, changes in mental status, and headache. *Site specific:* Ear pain, sore throat, sensation of pressure/pain in frontal or maxillary sinuses, postnasal drip, cough, shortness of breath, abdominal pain/cramping, diarrhea, nausea, and vomiting	Appropriate cultures (e.g., blood, nasal, sputum, urine) Chest and sinus x-rays CBC with differential and immunoglobulin levels; PFTs Antibiotics and IVIG
Fungal Organisms: Oral, Esophageal, and Sinopulmonary Sites					
• *Aspergillus* • *Mucomycosis*	50%	Immunodeficiency GVHD HLA disparity	100 to 365 days	Positive blood culture, sore throat, difficulty swallowing, mucositis, and pulmonary infiltrates	Appropriate cultures (e.g., blood, nasal, sputum, urine); x-rays; CBC with differential and IgG levels; PFTs; and antifungal prophylaxis or IVIG therapy
Viral Organisms					
• CMV pneumonia	10% to 15% allogeneic BMT 2% to 3% autologous BMT	Immunodeficiency CMV-seropositive patient and donor GVHD	100 to 365 days	Rapid onset with fulminate respiratory failure in days or slow onset with nonproductive cough, prolonged fever, dyspnea, or lethargy May be asymptomatic	Rule out bacterial infection. Shell viral cultures Chest x-rays ABGs, PFTs, bronchoscopy, and BAL IgG and IgA levels Prophylaxis with ganciclovir, foscarnet, and acyclovir Surveillance cultures of blood, urine, and pharyngeal secretions Leukocyte-depleted blood products, CMV-negative blood products, and IVIG or CMV/IVIG with ganciclovir

• VZV, integument	>50% with chronic GVHD 33% to 50% without chronic GVHD	Immunodeficiency GVHD CMV-seropositive patient and donor Immunosuppression	180 to 365 days	Prodromal symptoms: Headache, irritability, malaise, pain, itching, burning along affected nerve tract, fever, chills, and vesicular lesions localized or disseminated along dermatones Neurologic manifestations: Facial palsy and hearing loss	VZV cultures Acyclovir IV 500 mg/m^2 q8h × 10 days Strict isolation until lesions are crusted Calamine lotion and antihistamines for pruritus Pain management as needed
• Visceral VZV dissemination	16%	Immunodeficiency GVHD CMV-seropositive donor and recipient Immunosuppression	180 to 365 days	Midepigastric or periumbilical pain, with or without nausea, vomiting, or fever	Monitor for possible complications: pancreatitis, hepatitis, GI hemorrhage, and disseminated intravascular coagulation Acyclovir IV 500 mg/m^2 q8h × 10 days
Protozoal Organisms					
• *Pneumocystis carinii* pneumonia	8% with chronic GVHD	Immunosuppression Chronic GVHD	100 to 200 days	Fever, nonproductive cough, dyspnea, tachypnea, hypoxia, reduced midexpiratory airflow, and progressive airflow obstruction	Chest x-ray Lung biopsy Oxygen therapy and mechanical ventilation Pulse oximetry and ABGs Prophylactic TMP-SMX
Central Nervous System Complications					
Neurologic sequelae	59% to 70%	CNS radiation Intrathecal methotrexate Immunosuppressive agents (e.g., steroids, cyclosporine) Drug withdrawal	Variable	Tremors, seizures, musculoskeletal changes, visual disturbances, peripheral neuropathy, and encephalopathy Depression, mood swings, nervousness, sleep disturbances, agitation Myopathy	Head CAT and MRI scan to rule out organic disease Drug dose adjustment Psychiatric, neurologic, and neuropsychiatric consultation
Leukoencephalopathy	7%	Prior CNS radiation Intrathecal methotrexate Conditioning regimens	30 to 150 days	Lethargy, confusion, somnolence, coma, and irritability Ataxia, tremors, and seizures Personality changes, impaired memory, and shortened attention span Ventricular dilation, calcification of brain tissue, and white-matter hypodensity	Head CT and MRI scan Neurologic and psychiatric consultations: Psychometric evaluation, symptom management, and periodic screening Occupational counseling Vocational rehabilitation Special education

From Buchsel, P. C., Wroblewski, E. L., & Randolph, S. R. (1996). Delayed complications of bone marrow transplantation: An update. *Oncology Nursing Forum, 23*(8), 1267-1291.

Continued

Table 8-7 Late Effects of Bone Marrow Transplantation—cont'd

Late Effect	Incidence*	Causes	Typical Onset Posttransplant	Signs and Symptoms	Medical Management
Central Nervous System Complications—cont'd					
Cognitive disabilities	Preliminary anecdotal reports	Prior CNS radiation Intrathecal methotrexate Systemic treatment	90 days to years	Short-term memory loss and shortened attention span Visual-motor coordination, abstract thinking, spatial processing, and behavioral and language processing deficits	(See Leukoencephalopathy above.)
Ocular Complications					
Cataracts	>50% with single-dose TBI <50% with fractionated dose TBI	TBI Steroids	1.5 to 5 years	Poor (cloudy) vision	Ophthalmology consultation and slit-lamp microscopy Surgical removal and intraocular lens replacement
Endocrine Complications					
Thyroid dysfunction	15%-25% with fractionated dose TBI 30%-50% with single-dose TBI	TBI	Immediate to years	Increased TSH and reduced thyroxine levels Lethargy, sluggishness, depression, sleep disturbances, weight gain, sparse/thinning hair, and dry skin	Endocrine consultation: Thyroid scan and thyroid replacement therapy
Growth and Development Alterations					
	100% Not yet known in children age 9 or younger 100% in children older than age 9	Cranial irradiation, TBI Glucocorticosteroids GVHD Busulfan and cyclophosphamide together (cyclophosphamide alone will not cause these problems)	At puberty	Delayed development/absence of secondary sexual characteristics, primary gonadal failure, reduced growth velocity curves, abnormal bone age, reduced growth hormone level, increased gonadotropin levels, reduced estradiol levels (females), azoospermia, reduced testicular volume (males), and reduced T_4 levels	Pediatric endocrine consultation Health history, physical examination, and monitoring of growth Tanner staging Menstrual history Semen analysis Growth hormone replacement (testosterone/estrogen) Sexual and reproductive counseling

Gonadal Complications					
Ovarian and testicular dysfunction	100% but varies with age and treatment; with TBI or combination chemotherapy (busulfan plus cyclophosphamide) or in women older than age 26, effects generally are permanent and irreversible With cyclophosphamide alone or in women younger than age 26, effects usually are transient	TBI Chemotherapy	Immediate Transient effects last 3-24 months	*Females:* Menstrual irregularities (scanty flow/amenorrhea), sterility, night sweats, hot flashes, vaginal atrophy, vaginal adhesions, osteoporosis, decreased libido, palpitations, dyspareunia, depression, altered self-esteem, elevated LH and FSH, and decreased estradiol *Males:* Sterility, azoospermia, elevated LH and FSH, premature ejaculation, and altered self-esteem	*Females:* Care by gynecologist familiar with BMT Monitor gonadotropin and hormone levels. Cyclic hormone therapy, water-soluble vaginal lubricants, and topical estrogen creams Vaginal stents and dilation Sexual counseling *Males:* Urology consultation Monitor gonadotropin and hormone levels. Semen analysis and sperm banking before transplant Sexual counseling
Dental/Oral Complications					
Retarded dental and facial bone development in children	Unknown Preliminary/anecdotal reports	Cranial irradiation and TBI	Months to years	Asymmetric face (e.g., reduced lengths of mandible and maxilla, reduced vertical growth of upper face) Abnormal tooth/root development, delayed tooth eruption, and disproportion between tooth and jaw size Pain and difficulty chewing	Cephalometric measurements and facial bone x-rays Annual orthodontia consultation and interventions
Dental caries	Common	TBI GVHD Immunosuppression Reduced IgA and IgG levels in saliva	90 days to 1 year	Tooth decay, pain, and sensitivity	Regular dental examinations: Panorex films, fluoride gels and rinses, and oral hygiene instruction
Temporomandibular joint dysfunction	Not known Anecdotal reports	Not known	Not known	Toothache and facial pain Dizziness, ringing in the ears, and headache	Rule out CNS disease, infection, and dental or periodontal disease. Dental consultation Treat underlying pathology. Occlusal splints, physical therapy, tricyclic antidepressants, and muscle relaxants

From Buchsel, P. C., Wroblewski, E. L., & Randolph, S. R. (1996). Delayed complications of bone marrow transplantation: An update. *Oncology Nursing Forum, 23*(8), 1267-1291.

Continued

Table 8-7 Late Effects of Bone Marrow Transplantation—cont'd

Late Effect	Incidence*	Causes	Typical Onset Posttransplant	Signs and Symptoms	Medical Management
Skeletal Complications					
Avascular Necrosis	10%	Glucocorticoid therapy GVHD	90 days to 1 year	Pain, discomfort, inflammation in femoral or humeral heads, limited range of motion in leg/hip or shoulder joints, and contractures	Pain management Antimicrobial therapy Femoral head replacement and physical therapy
Genitourinary Complications					
Chronic renal failure	Not known Anecdotal reports	Radiation injury to renal system/kidneys Chemotherapy regimens Antimicrobial and cyclosporine toxicity	4.5 to 26 months	Hematuria, proteinuria, increased serum creatinine levels, decreased glomerular filtration rate, fluid and electrolyte imbalances, anemia, and hypertension	Nephrology consultation, urinalysis, 24-hour creatinine clearance, and intravenous pyelogram Monitor BUN, serum creatinine, and electrolytes. Antihypertensive medications, epoetin-alfa, dialysis, and renal transplantation
Late hemorrhagic cystitis	Not known	Cyclophospamide Ifosfamide Adenovirus	>100 days	Microscopic or gross hematuria, dysuria, vague abdominal pain, anemia, bladder wall scarring, urinary musculature atrophy, and infection	Nephrology consultation, urinalysis, cystoscopy, and hydration Analgesics and antimicrobial therapy Urinary diversion CBC and viral cultures
Hemolytic uremic syndrome	Usually associated with renal failure	Possibly high-dose chemotherapy regimens Infection Cyclosporine	30 to 875 days	Microangiopathic hemolytic anemia, renal insufficiency, thrombocytopenia, hematuria, increased creatine levels, reduced creatinine clearance, fluid retention, and fatigue	Nephrology consultation, urinalysis, 24-hour creatinine clearance, BUN, serum creatinine, electrolytes, and irradiated packed RBC and platelet transfusions Hemodialysis

Graft Failure/Marrow Dysfunction					
	1% HLA-matched sibling donors 2% HLA 1-antigen-mismatched related donors 5%-40% T-cell-depleted marrow 20% autologous transplant	HLA disparity, chronic GVHD, T-lymphocyte–depleted marrow, disease status at time of transplant, insufficient stem cells in the donor graft, disease reoccurrence, infection, drug-related marrow suppression (e.g., TMP, ganciclovir), and damaged or insufficient stem cells	Weeks to months	Pancytopenia, hypocellular bone marrow, infection, bleeding, and anemia	CBC, bone marrow aspiration and bone biopsy, and cytogenetic studies Identification of underlying cause Interferon-alpha and hematopoietic growth factors Second BMT Supportive care interventions and hospice care
Secondary Malignancy					
Lymphoproliferative disorders (e.g., Hodgkin's and non-Hodgkin lymphomas, acute or chronic leukemia) Basal cell and squamous cell carcinoma	2% to 22%	Associated with TBI, Epstein-Barr virus, antithymocyte globulin, anti-CD-3 monoclonal antibody, immunosuppression, chronic immune stimulation, T-lymphocyte–depleted grafts, and HLA disparity	1 to 14 years	Fever, fatigue, swollen glands, abnormal CBC, night sweats, and pain	Periodic follow-up examination and screening Health history CBC, bone marrow aspiration, and bone biopsy CAT scans Biopsy suspicious lesions Health teaching
Psychosocial Complications					
	5% to 10%	Neuropsychological deficits, body image changes, malaise, sexual dysfunction, altered functional status, ineffective coping skills, and posttraumatic stress disorder	Months to years	Depression; feelings of loss, sadness, and helplessness; disruptive anxiety; inability to concentrate or make decisions; social isolation; altered interpersonal relationships; suicidal ideation; pathologic regression; and delirium	Rule out organic disease with psychometric tests (e.g., Beck's Depression Scale, Haberman's Demands of BMT Recovery). Head CAT and MRI scans Psychiatric evaluation and psychotherapy Antidepressants and antianxiety medications

From Buchsel, P. C., Wroblewski, E. L., & Randolph, S. R. (1996). Delayed complications of bone marrow transplantation: An update. *Oncology Nursing Forum, 23*(8), 1267-1291.

Continued

Table 8-7 Late Effects of Bone Marrow Transplantation—cont'd

Late Effect	Incidence*	Causes	Typical Onset Posttransplant	Signs and Symptoms	Medical Management
Quality-of-Life Disruption					
	Probably 100%	*Physical:* Decreased strength and stamina, altered level of function, visual disturbances/cataracts, recurrent infections, infertility, effects of chronic GVHD, and inadequate nutritional intake *Psychological:* Increased anxiety, fear of recurrence, depression, cognitive deficits, and altered role function *Social:* Difficulty in resuming intimate or sexual relationships, inability to return to former vocation or employment, increased anxiety regarding caregiver, and financial burden	Immediate to years	Per patient and family self-report	Symptom management according to physical findings Appropriate referrals (e.g., social worker, psychologist, financial counselor, vocational counselor) Physical therapy BMT support groups Antidepressants and antianxiety medication

From Buchsel, P. C., Wroblewski, E. L., & Randolph, S. R. (1996). Delayed complications of bone marrow transplantation: An update. *Oncology Nursing Forum, 23*(8), 1267-1291.

TABLE 8-8 Nursing Care of the Late Effects of Bone Marrow Transplantation

Nursing Diagnosis	Nursing Interventions
Knowledge deficit regarding late effects of BMT	Instruct patient/caregiver about potential late complications. Teach reportable signs and symptoms. Emphasize the importance of follow-up and medication compliance. Set mutual, realistic goals for return to school or work. Provide written instructions regarding medication schedule, central lumen catheter care, diet, activities of daily living (ADLs), and personal hygiene measures. Identify activity restrictions necessary until immune reconstitution. • Avoid crowds, infectious people, and construction areas. • Refrain from gardening. • Refrain from changing animal litter boxes. Monitor compliance with instructions. Communicate with primary physician and home care and interdisciplinary team members about patient status and treatment plan. Provide 24-hour emergency number. Refer patient to community support services such as support groups, the American Cancer Society, and the National Coalition of Cancer Survivors.
Knowledge deficit regarding clinical manifestations of chronic GVHD	Assess patient's and caregiver's understanding of chronic GVHD. Provide information about chronic GVHD and symptom management. Teach adverse effects of immunosuppressive medications. • Cyclosporine: Hypertension, seizures, magnesium wasting, and hirsutism • Steroids: Hypertension, fluid retention, aseptic necrosis of bone, and mood swings • Thalidomide: Drowsiness and constipation Document teaching plan and patient and family level of understanding. Monitor medication compliance.
Impaired skin integrity related to chronic GVHD and infection	Assess skin for signs and symptoms of altered integrity. • Texture: Scaling and dermatosclerosis • Color: Hypo/hyperpigmentation and erythema • Ulceration: Desquamation • Infection: Redness, drainage, and tenderness Clean skin with nonirritating soap. Apply creams such as Eucerin® and Aquaphor® (Beiersdorph Inc., Norwalk, CT) moisturizing lotion. Avoid direct sunlight, and apply sunscreen. Administer medications (e.g., immunosuppressive therapy, antibiotics, topical steroids, antihistamines), and monitor for desired effects. Promote range-of-motion exercises to prevent contractures. Provide consultation with a dermatologist familiar with BMT recipients.
Altered body image related to chronic GVHD and side effects of medication	Instruct patient about alterations in skin color and texture and other skin-related side effects of medications such as weight gain, hirsutism, alopecia, muscle wasting, and gingival hyperplasia. Reassure patient that appearance will improve with effective treatment. Offer counseling regarding cosmetic aids, make-up, wigs, hats, and scarves. Provide emotional support. Refer patient to a support group.
Altered oral mucous membranes related to chronic GVHD, sicca syndrome, and infection	Assess oral cavity for pain; xerostomia; striae on mucous membranes lining cheeks, lips, and palate; erythema progressing to ulceration; burning; loss of taste; and dental caries. Monitor immunosuppressive therapies. Culture suspicious lesions for bacteria, virus, and fungus. Instruct patient in oral hygiene regimen. • Use a soft toothbrush, and floss daily. • Rinse regularly with saline or water. • Avoid commercial mouthwashes. • Use artificial saliva. Provide salivary gland stimulants such as sugarless mints, gum, and hard candy. Encourage patient to eat a soft, bland diet. Avoid spices, acidic foods, and foods served at extreme temperatures. Refer patient to a nutritionist. Monitor response to topical anesthetics and parenteral analgesics.

From Buchsel, P. C., Wrobleski, E. L., & Randolph, S. R. (1996). Delayed complications of bone marrow transplantation: An update. *Oncology Nursing Forum, 23*(8), 1267-1291

Continued

TABLE 8-8 Nursing Care of the Late Effects of Bone Marrow Transplantation—cont'd

Nursing Diagnosis	Nursing Interventions
Altered nutrition (less than body requirements) related to chronic GVHD, infection, and medications	Assess signs and symptoms of esophageal dysfunction, such as difficulty swallowing, retrosternal pain, and esophageal stricture. Assess nutritional status, including monitoring weight, calorie count, and tissue turgor. Provide a low-bacterial diet. Administer antibiotic therapy as ordered. Record anthropometric measurements. Refer patient to a nutritionist, if necessary. Assess signs and symptoms, including anorexia, nausea, vomiting, diarrhea, malabsorption, and weight loss. Provide nutritional supplements, enteral feeding, and TPN as ordered. Culture suspicious sites. Determine whether esophageal dilation is necessary. Monitor serum albumin, ferritin, and electrolytes. Administer analgesics, antiemetics, antidiarrheal agents, fluids, and electrolyte replacements as ordered; monitor for desired effects.
Altered metabolic processes (impaired hepatic function) related to chronic GVHD, infection, and medications	Assess and monitor hepatic function, including liver function tests (SGOT, SGPT, gamma-glutamyl transferase, bilirubin, alkaline phosphatase), impaired hepatic function, hepatitis antigen and antibody levels, right upper quadrant pain, hepatomegaly, and ascites. Obtain medication and transfusion history. Assess current medication profile. Monitor abdominal girth. Monitor for signs and symptoms of infection. Observe for changes in level of consciousness. Assess coagulation profile (e.g., prothrombin time, partial thromboplastin time, fibrin split products). Observe sclera and skin for jaundice.
Altered metabolic processes (thyroid dysfunction) related to TBI	Instruct patient about signs and symptoms of hypothyroidism such as sluggishness, depression, lethargy, sleep disturbances, weight gain, sparse or thinning hair, and dry skin. Assess TSH and thyroxine levels. Monitor and instruct patient regarding thyroid replacement therapy compliance. Provide symptom management interventions. Discuss changes in functional capacity and ability to perform ADL. Reassure patient that thyroid replacement therapy will restore adequate thyroid function. Refer patient to an endocrinologist.
Altered growth and development related to cranial or TBI, GVHD, and glucocorticosteroids	Discuss growth and development effects with patient and family before BMT. • Delayed development of or difficulty in performing cognitive skills • Delayed development or absence of secondary sexual characteristics • Delayed or altered growth velocity Assess and monitor growth and development, including physical assessment; Tanner staging; neuropsychological evaluation; LH and FSH levels; semen analysis (males); and menstrual history (females). Refer patient to a pediatric endocrinologist. Monitor compliance with sex and growth hormone replacement. Monitor school performance history. Collaborate with school officials regarding development of social and cognitive skills. Refer for appropriate counseling (e.g., reproductive, educational, vocational).
Altered growth and development (retarded dental and facial bone development) related to cranial or TBI	Assess cephalometric measurements and dental development, including abnormal tooth/root development, delayed tooth eruption, disproportion between tooth and jaw dimensions, pain, and difficulty chewing. Refer for orthodontic consultation.

From Buchsel, P. C., Wrobleski, E. L., & Randolph, S. R. (1996). Delayed complications of bone marrow transplantation: An update. *Oncology Nursing Forum, 23*(8), 1267-1291

TABLE 8-8 Nursing Care of the Late Effects of Bone Marrow Transplantation—cont'd

Nursing Diagnosis	Nursing Interventions
Altered ovarian function (in women over age 26) related to TBI and cyclophosphamide	Assess signs and symptoms of ovarian failure such as sterility, premature menopause, amenorrhea, hot flashes, vaginal atrophy and dryness, heart palpitations, and osteoporosis. Monitor LH and FSH and estradiol levels. Assess for alterations in sexual response, including painful intercourse and decreased libido. Assess psychological status, including depression, poor self-esteem, and performance anxiety. Refer patient to a gynecologist who is familiar with BMT recipients. Recommend water-soluble vaginal creams and topical estrogen creams. Discuss/explain vaginal stents and dilation. Monitor patient response to hormone replacement therapy. Refer for sexual counseling as appropriate.
Impaired testicular function related to TBI	Discuss sperm banking before transplant. Assess for signs and symptoms of testicular dysfunction such as sterility, azoospermia, increased LH and FSH and premature ejaculation. Refer patient to a urologist.
Sexual dysfunction related to testicular/ovarian failure, chronic GVHD, fatigue, and impaired self-esteem	Establish a therapeutic relationship. Implement PLISSIT model interventions (i.e., *P* = permission, *LI* = limited fatigue and impaired self-information, *SS* = specific instructions, and *IT* = intensive treatment). Encourage communication between patient and partner. Assess etiology of sexual dysfunction, including altered body structure or function (e.g., vaginal dryness, stenosis, impotence, premature ejaculation), low self-esteem, altered body image, and anxiety/depression. Provide information about sexual aids, lubricants, vaginal dilator, and relaxation techniques. Recommend American Cancer Society publications *Sexuality and Cancer for the Man Who Has Cancer and His Partner* and *Sexuality and Cancer for the Woman Who Has Cancer and Her Partner* (Schover, 1988). Refer for sexual counseling as appropriate.
Altered visual sensory perception related to chronic GVHD, ocular sicca, infection, and plugged lacrimal ducts	Assess ability to perform ADL and changes in functional capacity. Assess/monitor for signs and symptoms of ocular alterations such as dry eyes/itching, corneal ulceration, photophobia, and pain/discomfort. Recommend artificial tears. Instruct patient about wearing sunglasses. Monitor for signs and symptoms of infection.
Altered visual sensory perception related to cataracts	Assess risk for cataract development, including transplant conditioning regimen, corticosteroids, and chronic GVHD. Assess for visual changes such as cloudy or blurred vision and opaque cornea. Refer patient to an ophthalmologist. Help explain surgical options. Reassure patient that vision will return with cataract removal or lens replacement.
Activity intolerance related to chronic GVHD, anemia, and infection; musculoskeletal, peripheral nervous system, or psychological late effects; and aseptic bone necrosis	Assess functional capacity (e.g., Karnofsky performance status, World Health Organization performance scale). Monitor signs and symptoms of physiologic and psychological peripheral dysfunction, including reports of weakness and fatigue, abnormal heart rate or blood pressure; dyspnea; pain; muscle weakness and wasting; limited range of motion; neuropathy; depression; social isolation; stress; and inability to complete ADL. Identify underlying etiology and contributing factors, and collaborate with interdisciplinary team to treat underlying causes. Promote balanced activity rest patterns. Teach stress management. Establish mutual and realistic goals.

Continued

TABLE 8-8 Nursing Care of the Late Effects of Bone Marrow Transplantation—cont'd

Nursing Diagnosis	Nursing Interventions
Impaired gas exchange, ineffective breathing pattern related to chronic GVHD, infection, restrictive/obstructive airway disease, and bronchiolitis obliterans	Assess for decreased activity tolerance and fatigue. Monitor for altered respiratory function, including abnormal or absent breath sounds; quality and rate of respiration; dusky or cyanotic color; dyspnea, shortness of breath on exertion, or wheezing; bronchospasm; and productive or nonproductive cough. Perform chest auscultation and percussion with each clinic or home visit. Assess vital signs and pulse oximeter regularly. Monitor PFTs, ABGs, CBC, IgG, and blood and sputum cultures. Prepare patient for bronchial lavage procedure and lung biopsy. Discuss potential for hospitalization with respiratory support, including mechanical ventilation. Administer supportive therapies, as ordered, such as ganciclovir, TMP-SMX pentamidine, amphotericin B, and broad-spectrum antibiotics; bronchodilators; immunosuppressive therapy; and immunoglobulins.
Risk for infection related to chronic GVHD, immunosuppression, and graft failure	Assess and monitor for signs and symptoms of infection, such as fever, chills, and hypotension; cough and dyspnea; painful urination, difficult urination, and foul-smelling urine; diarrhea, vomiting, and abdominal pain; redness, swelling, tenderness, and drainage; and malaise/arthralgia. Monitor CBC, IgG and IgA levels. Instruct patient regarding infection precautions. • Wash hands meticulously. • Avoid crowds and infectious individuals. • Avoid live vaccines. • Avoid trauma and invasive procedures. • Eat a low-bacterial diet. Monitor compliance with prophylactic medications such as TMP-SMX, ciprofloxin, nystatin/fluconozole, and acyclovir.
Risk of second malignancy related to chronic immune suppression, T-lymphocyte–depleted graft, TBI, alkylating chemotherapy, antithymocyte globulin, CD-3 monoclonal antibodies, and Epstein-Barr virus	Assess risk factors for development of a secondary malignancy. Discuss possibilities with patient and family. Instruct patient to report possible warning signs such as fever, fatigue/malaise, abnormal bleeding, night sweats, pain, and appearance of a painless lump. Emphasize the need for health screening and periodic check-ups.

From Buchsel, P. C., Wrobleski, E. L., & Randolph, S. R. (1996). Delayed complications of bone marrow transplantation: An update. *Oncology Nursing Forum, 23*(8), 1267-1291

Screening Studies

Screening tests to predict chronic GVHD have been performed for decades and included skin and lip biopsy, oral examination, Schiemer's test, serum alkaline phosphatase, aspartate transaminase, and immunoglobulin level and platelet count. The value of these tests has been studied in a retrospective trial at a major northwestern BMT center. Data strongly suggest that these tests may not, as previously thought, have predictive value. The strongest predictors of chronic GVHD were in those with a history of acute GVHD being treated with corticosteroids. New approaches for the prevention of extensive clinical chronic GVHD require study in prospective, controlled clinical trials (Wagner, Flowers, Longton, Storb, & Schubert, 1998)

Integumentary. Chronic GVHD affects more than 70% to 80% of patients diagnosed with chronic GVHD. The onset of skin involvement may be manifested as a generalized erythema or, more dramatically, hyperpigmentation or hypopigmentation, hide-bound skin and joint contractures, and skin ulcerations with poor wound healing. Lesser manifestations are alopecia and nail ridging. Sweat gland function can be decreased, leading to hyperthermia. Some patients have a sudden onset of erythema that can be activated by exposure to the sun. Skin biopsies may be required for differential diagnosis of chronic GVHD (Sullivan, 1994). The classic features of untreated skin in chronic GVHD is bronze-colored, hide-bound skins and pressure-point ulceration accompanied by joint contractures. However, these are rare today because of improved treatment protocols and long term follow-up.

Oral. Oral mucosal chronic GVHD can develop in approximately 70% of patients with extensive chronic GVHD. Xerostomia, including decreased or absent salivary lubrication and IgA secretion are common sequelae. Lichenoid lesions can be confused with candidiasis (Sullivan, 1994). Decreased saliva production affects oral integrity and nutritional intake and contributes to the development of dental caries. Early subtle signs are complaints of changes in food tastes and burning after brushing of the teeth. HSV often occurs in concert with chronic GVHD, and serial viral cultures may be needed to make a differential diagnosis of chronic GVHD (Lloid, 1995).

Ocular. The eye is involved in 50% of patients with extensive chronic GVHD. Common symptoms include burning, irritation, itching, pain, foreign body sensation, blurring of vision, photophobia, and excessive tearing. Supportive measures with artificial tears and ointments are recommended for comfort and cornea protection to prevent permanent blindness. Use of viscous eye drops such as Celluvisc® and Lacriserts® can decrease multiple daily dosing. Punctal ligation, (closure of tear draining ducts) may be necessary for those with severe eye involvement. Wearing glasses, avoiding dry and windy environments, and application of eye drops can prevent keratitis sicca, which can lead to corneal erosion, perforation, or scarring. Punctal ligation usually results in symptom relief, but eye drops may continue to be required. Early recognition with periodic ophthalmologic screening including Schirmer's tear test and slit lamp examination (Flowers, 1998).

Sinusal. Sinusitis is common in patients with chronic GVHD and is caused by a combination of sicca syndrome involving the sinuses and the predisposition to gram-positive bacterial infections. The most common causative organisms are *Streptococcus pneumoniae* and *Haemophilus influenzae*. Typical symptoms are fever and headache.

Gastrointestinal. Upper and lower intestinal involvement can occur in chronic GVHD. Symptoms include diarrhea and abdominal pain. Malabsorption and submucosal fibrosis also have been documented in advanced cases. Esophageal abnormalities, once a common complication in advanced cases of chronic GVHD, occur less often because of advances made in management of this disorder. Symptoms include dysphasia, painful swallowing, and retrosternal pain caused by esophageal thinning. Patients may need to be readmitted to inpatient care for management of nutritional problems and pain (Sullivan, 1994).

Hepatic. Liver disorders are observed in about 50% of patients with chronic GVHD. Alkaline phosphatase, serum glutamic oxaloacetic transaminase (SGOT), and bilirubin levels are elevated. With treatment, bilirubin values return to normal within several weeks, but elevated alkaline phosphatase and SGOT may persist for months (Sullivan, 1994).

Vaginal. Significant vaginal dryness and stricture formation have been documented in women with chronic GVHD; these symptoms manifest 1 to 3 years after transplantation. Stricture formation may be severe, requiring surgery to relieve menstrual obstruction. Treatment measures include vaginal dilation in conjunction with immunosuppressive therapies for chronic GVHD. It is not surprising that long-term survivors of BMT consistently list sexual problems as one of the major areas of dissatisfaction.

Musculoskeletal. The musculoskeletal system can be affected in a manner similar to rheumatoid arthritis, arthralgia, seral effusions, joint contracture, hemorrhagic cystitis, and polymyositis. Muscle biopsies reveal inflammation and necrotic muscle fibers. Tendinitis and arthritis accompanied by muscle aches, cramping, and carpal spasms have also been identified as long-term complications. Dyspnea may be a manifestation of bronchiolitis obliterans (Buchsel, Wroblewski, & Randolph, 1996).

Medical Management

Prevention of chronic GVHD has proven to be unsuccessful. Classic treatment of chronic GVHD is administration of cyclosporine and steroids. These medications, particularly steroids, cause distressing adverse effects of emotional lability, avascular necrosis, secondary malignancies, and increased susceptibility to infections (Russell, Blahey, Stuart, & Card, 1989; Witherspoon, Fisher, Sachet, Martin, Sullivan, & Sanders et al., 1992). Psoralen and ultraviolet (PUVA) therapy has shown some effectiveness for chronic GVHD of the mouth and skin (Vogelsang, Hess, & Santos, 1988). Clinical trials using thalidomide, an immunosuppressive agent, for prevention and treatment of chronic GVHD are underway and appear promising. This agent caused thousands of babies to be born with birth defects in the 1950s but was recently approved for use in the United States for immunosuppressed patients with AIDS and autoimmune disease. The drug is monitored under strict regulations, and health professionals prescribing and dispensing the drug are required to register with Clegen, the drug's manufacturer. The drug costs an average of $12 a day, and it is not clear if third-party payors will cover its use (Stolberg, 1998). Etretinate, a retinoid often used in the treatment of psoriatic patients, is being tested for efficacy and safety in the transplant recipient with chronic skin GVHD. Major adverse effects include teratogenetic effects, corneal erosion, hypertriglyceridemia, and hypercholesterolemia. Supportive care measures for patients with GVHD are prophylactic antibiotics, physical therapy, careful oral hygiene, and sunscreen.

Avascular Necrosis

Avascular necrosis of the bone, particularly of the humerus or femur head, has long been known to be an adverse effect from glucocorticoid therapy. Hence allogeneic recipients receiving long-term steroid treatment have an incidence rate of as high as 10%. Median time of onset is 545 (range: 249 to 731) days after BMT. Patients can present with complaints of pain and limited range of motion. Treatment often includes an interdisciplinary approach to provide symptom management for pain, physical therapy to maintain mobility, antimicrobial therapy, and femur head replacement (Buchsel, Wroblewski, & Randolph; Sullivan, 1996).

Graft Versus Leukemic Effect

The graft versus leukemic (GVL) effect is a curious phenomenon that has been known in vitro since the early 1950s. The GVL effect was first observed in twins receiving syngeneic marrow transplantations. It was noted that syngeneic marrow transplant patients had a twofold higher relapse rate than allogeneic marrow patients who developed GVHD. Studies of marrow recipients transplanted for leukemia suggest that GVHD is accompanied by a graft versus leukemic effect noted by a lower rate of relapse in patients with GVHD. Although not well understood, there is a significant interest in maintaining some GVHD in allogeneic recipients and inducing GVHD in the autologous recipient in an effort to decrease relapse rates A technique under investigation is manipulated donor T lymphocytes and donor lymphocyte infusions. Refer to section on Relapse, p. 179, for a further discussion (Buchsel, Wroblewski, & Randolph, 1996).

Late Infectious Complications

As the immune system recovers, infectious complications generally decline. However, marrow recipients with persistent acute GVHD or those who develop chronic GVHD remain at considerable risk for infection as a result of immune dysfunction (Sullivan, 1994; Wingard, 1994). Long-term survivors without chronic GVHD are remarkably free of infections after 1 year. In contrast, patients in whom chronic GVHD develops remain at high risk for bacterial pneumonia, septicemia, and sinusitis, because their donor-derived immune systems have not yet matured and cannot adequately protect against invasive organisms. The tempo and type of microbial infections follow a predicted path.

Varicella-Zoster Virus

Seropositive marrow recipients are at substantial risk for *varicella-zoster* virus (VZV) infection, and nearly one third to one half of long-term BMT survivors develop recurrent VZV. Peak time of onset is 6 to 9 months after BMT. Risk factors established from a study of more than 1100 marrow recipients are as follows (Chang, Miller, Watkins, Arduino, Ashford, & Midgley et al., 1998):

- Those greater than 10 years of age
- Those receiving TBI
- Those having seropostive VZV titers before transplantation
- There was no difference in incidence of HZV between allogeneic and autologous grafts

Reactivation occurs most often in marrow recipients with chronic GVHD; however, autologous BMT patients also are at risk. Patients may report the prodromal symptoms of burning, pain, and pruritus that may be accompanied by fever and chills. Dermatomal zoster represents 50% to 70% of post-BMT VZV with significant infections and complications in 20% to 30% of cases. As the infection progresses, vesicular lesions erupt and can be localized or disseminated over several dermatomes. Bacterial superinfection with subsequent scarring can be an additional problem if VZV is not treated promptly. Cutaneous infection can predispose BMT recipients to visceral VZV dissemination The lung, liver, and CNS are other common sites for VZV visceral dissemination, resulting in pneumonia, hepatitis, disseminated intravascular coagulopathy (DIC), and encephalitis. Aggressive antiviral therapy with IV acyclovir at 500 mg/kg every 8 hours for 7 to 10 days is the standard therapy (Nader & Arvin, 1994). Caution must be used in administering high-dose oral acyclovir (800 mg 5 times daily) because peak serum concentrations often are lower than the concentrations required to inhibit VZV in vitro. For seronegative marrow recipients exposed to VZV, early administration of VZV immunoglobulin may reduce the risk for infection. Patients with nonspecific suppressor cells and chronic GVHD may be at greater risk for VZV as a result of prolonged immunosuppression.

Encapsulated Bacteria. All marrow recipients with chronic GVHD are at risk for infection from encapsulated bacteria. The common cause is sinopulmonary infection caused by *S. pneumoniae, Neisseria meningitidis,* and *H. influenzae* (Hib). Resulting occult sinusitis and overwhelming sepsis can occur. All patients with chronic GVHD should receive antibiotic prophylaxis with penicillin or TMP-SMX. Marrow recipients with IgG subclass 2 deficiency and recurrent sinopulmonary infection may benefit from IV immunoglobulin supplementation. Current research is focusing on the cost-benefit ratio of this therapy.

A major concern after a BMT patient is discharged is infection. Historically, transplantation teams recommend that patients wear surgical masks for at least 6 months after transplant to reduce the risk of infections caused by microorganisms, fungal spores, and pollen. Because of a lack of convincing evidence that surgical masks prevent infection in combination with cost issues, mask wearing has been largely abandoned. Scrupulous handwashing, personal hygiene, and antibiotic and immunosuppressive agents continue to be the touchstone of prevention and treatment of infectious complications. Immunizations against a number of infectious diseases play an important role in these patients. Practices may differ among institutions. Some allogeneic recipients free of GVHD develop sufficient amounts of tetanus, diphtheria, and measles antibody virus from their donor marrow; however, standard practice is to reimmunize recipients so that antibody titers reflect normal laboratory values. For those patients free of chronic GVHD, booster immunizations with diphtheria, pertussis tetanus (DPT), Hib conjungae, inactivated Salk poliovirus and influenza and pneumococcal vaccines are advised. Live attenuated vaccines, such as for mumps, measles, and rubella should be given in the second year after BMT but only to those patients without chronic GVHD. Family members of BMT recipients should not be given the Sabin oral polio vaccine during the first years after BMT because of possible virus shedding with subsequent infection in the recipient. If the vaccine is given, the patient needs to be isolated from that family member for 8 to 12 weeks.

Pulmonary Complications

Restrictive pulmonary abnormalities are rarely observed in long-term survivors and are associated with chemoirradiation and recurrent pneumonia (Deeg, 1994). The incidence of restrictive disease peaks at 1 year. Obstructive pulmonary disease, which occurs in approximately 15% of long-term survivors with chronic GVHD, presents clinical and pathologic features of obliterative bronchiolitis. Late interstitial pneumonia occurs in 10% to 20% of long-term survivors with chronic GVHD and carries a 50% mortality rate. Studies have identified specific pneumonias as idiopathic, CMV, VSV, and *Pneumocystis carinii.*

Twenty percent of patients with chronic GVHD will have restrictive lung disease, 10% will have obstructive lung disease, and 10% will be at risk for bronchiolitis obliterans (Sullivan, 1994; Deeg, 1994). Complete nursing assessments of long-term survivors require careful histories and physical examinations. Specifically, inquire about changes in activities of daily living, perform chest auscultation and percussion, and monitor pulmonary capacities and volumes.

Gonadal Dysfunction

TBI used in conditioning regimens will render most recipients sterile and with significant gonadal dysfunction. Young women (under age 26) receiving single-agent chemotherapy alone will likely have restored gonadal function and some may successfully have children. The majority of those women who are older will likely not bear children and experience early menopause. Girls and boys receiving chemotherapy who are prepubertal at the time of BMT develop normally. Men usually return to normal gonadotropin levels and low to normal sperm counts, and can father children (Sanders, 1991). Initial data reviewing high-dose chemotherapy regimens containing combination therapy using cyclophosphamide and busulfan suggest that gonadal dysfunction is similar to that of regimens containing TBI.

Total Body Irradiation. Almost all female recipients conditioned with TBI have gonadal dysfunction, including sterility and early menopause. A few accounts exist about live births from women receiving such conditioning. Cyclic oral or transdermal hormone replacement therapy is commonly used to reduce symptoms of premature menopause and to prevent long-term disorders such as osteoporosis, or vulvar or vaginal atrophic changes. New questions arise about hormonal treatment for women receiving BMT for breast cancer. Box 8-6 lists nonhormonal strategies for women who are advised against hormonal therapy. In vitro fertilization in donors and artificial insemination are being reported with successful births (Rio, Letur-Konirsch, Ajchenbaum-Cymbalista, Bauduer, DeZiegler, & Pelissier et al., 1994).

Most men conditioned with TBI preserve Leydig cell function and testosterone, as well as luteinizing hormone (LH) production, but spermatogenesis usually is absent. A recently published study of gonadal function and psychosexual adjustment in male patients receiving autologous and allogeneic BMT noted that 50% (N = 29) were dissatisfied with their sexual life. None of these patients had a history of GVHD, and there was no difference between men who had received TBI and those who received chemotherapy—only in sexual concerns. The predominant problems reported were impotence/erectile difficulties (37.9%), low sexual desire (37.9%), and altered body image (20.7%) (Molassiotis Akker, van den Milligan, & Boughton, 1995).

Box 8-6
Nonhormonal Strategies for Menopausal BMT Recipients

- Identify situations that may trigger symptomatology (e.g., strong emotions, caffeine, alcohol, cayenne or other spices, occlusive clothing, heat).
- Exercise regularly. Walk, swim, dance, bike, or row 20 to 30 minutes a day.
- Consider daily mediation, tai chi, or yoga.
- Eat soy foods (e.g., tofu [80 g], tempeh, soy milk [400 ml]), papayas, yams, lentils, and beans.
- Join a support group.
- Drink 8 to 10 glasses of water daily.
- Practice relaxation techniques such as deep breathing.
- Sleep in a cool, well-ventilated room.
- Use fans during the day.
- Wear clothing made of breathable fabrics (e.g., cottons or clothes that wick away moisture).
- Dress in layers so that outer clothes can be discarded.

Modified from Schubert, M. (1998). *Nonhormonal strategies for menopausal BMT recipients.* Kirkland, WA: Evergreen Women's Care.

Most prepubertal girls who receive TBI have primary ovarian failure, do not achieve menarche, and do not develop secondary sexual characteristics. A few prepubertal boys conditioned with TBI develop secondary sexual characteristics, but most have delayed onset of puberty. The children most profoundly affected are prepubertal boys who receive testicular irradiation before marrow conditioning. Testosterone therapy may be effective, but longer follow-up is needed. Sexual counseling before BMT is important for all marrow transplant candidates.

Growth and Development Concerns

High-dose cyclophosphamide administered in BMT conditioning does not affect normal growth and development, but those receiving cyclophosphamide and busulfan are at risk for significant growth and development problems. Glucocorticoid treatment can suppress growth hormone, and those children treated with these agents for GVHD will also be at further risk. TBI used in conditioning regimens causes decreased production of growth hormone. Administration of growth hormone may improve the growth rates, but less so than seen with growth hormone deficiencies of other origins. In part, this is due to the fact that multiple factors, including thyroid dysfunction, also contribute to growth development in children. The availability of recombinant growth now paves the way for large studies, but primary care physicians should be alerted to the need for periodic growth and development follow-up in these children. Radiation can interfere with dental and facial bone development and is particularly harmful to pediatric patients, particularly those having prior cranial irradiation. TBI results in significantly reduced lengths of both the maxilla and the mandible, and reduction in vertical growth of the upper face, especially in children less than 6 years of age. Facial and dental bone development are compromised, resulting in poor calcification, root blunting, apical closure, and mandibular hypoplasia (Sanders, 1994). A recent study of dental health in 27 children receiving BMT demonstrated soft deposits in 77.7%, serious gingivitis in 59.2%, and paradental involvement in 3.7% of patients, whereas 62.9% had tooth abnormalities or agenesis. Nine out of 27 patients (33%) had root hypoplasia (Uderzo, Fraschini, Balduzzi, Galimberti, Arrigo, & Biagi et al., 1997). This study emphasizes the need for long-term dental evaluation after BMT. Correction of these problems may require years of dental surgery and orthodontist care.

Establishing parental awareness of the potential late effects of irradiation is an important nursing function and should be addressed before and at regular intervals after transplant. The administration of hormones may be necessary to ensure appropriate sexual maturity. As the pediatric BMT survivor approaches adolescence and young adulthood, sexual and reproductive counseling should be part of routine long-term follow-up care. Adversely affected children should be referred to endocrinologists for evaluation and intervention. Careful long-term follow-up through puberty will be necessary. Growth hormone and appropriate sex hormone therapy may be indicated. Growth patterns should be evaluated annually, and those who demonstrate a decreased growth rate should be referred to a pediatric endocrinologist. Tanner staging, a pubertal developmental staging tool, serum LH, and estradiol levels should be obtained in females at age 12 if the development of secondary sexual characteristics is not apparent. In addition to Tanner staging, assessment parameters for testicular dysfunction in adolescent males should include testicular volume, semen analysis, serum LH and follicle-stimulating hormone (FSH) if secondary sexual characteristics are not apparent by age 14. Education and counseling are key management and nursing considerations. It is essential that oncology nurses assess and evaluate growth and development patterns in children and young adults. Nurses should be mindful of pretransplant cranial radiation or TBI, as well as a history of chronic GVHD.

Thyroid Dysfunction

Thyroid dysfunction occurs in 40% to 50% of patients prepared with a regimen including single-dose TBI (Sanders, 1994). The most common clinical presentations compensated hypothyroidism with elevated TSH and normal T_4.

Ophthalmologic Effects

The late ophthalmologic effects of BMT are chronic GVHD of the eye and posterior capsular cataracts from TBI (Deeg, 1994; Tichelli, Gratwohl, Thomas, Roth, Prunte, & Nissen et al., 1994). Cataract formation peak onset is 3 years after BMT with a range of 1.5 to 5 years post-BMT and is caused by TBI and long-term steroid therapy for GVHD. Cataract formation was evaluated in 197 patients treated at a major international transplant center. Of patients studied, 36% (N = 197) developed cataracts, with 23% needing surgical repair. All recipients receiving single-dose TBI developed cataracts, whereas 86% of those treated with fractionated TBI had the probability of developing cataracts 6 years after BMT (Tichelli et al., 1994). For patients receiving TBI, lens shielding should be considered as a preventive measure. Keratoconjunctivitis sicca, or dry eye syndrome, also is noted as an ocular complication. Intraocular lens replacement is the treatment of choice for those with cataracts.

Dental Effects

Pretransplant conditioning regimens and GVHD have a deleterious effect on the oral cavity. A dry mouth, or sicca syndrome, constitutes an environment that contributes to oral caries and infection such as candida, HSV, and CMV. Brush-on fluoride gels or rinses can reduce these risks. Alteration in taste has a dramatic effect on nutrition, often leading to anorexia and substantial weight loss. Sensitivity to the taste of sweet and salty foods may also interfere with adequate nutrition, with hypersensitivity to cold further complicating this problem. Temporomandibular joint disorders manifested by patient complaints of toothache, facial pain, ear problems, and headache have been documented. Applications of hot or cold packs, physical therapy, and tricyclic antidepressants or muscle relaxants alleviate these symptoms (Lloid, 1995).

Genitourinary Effects

BMT recipients may develop chronic renal failure resulting from radiation injury, the chemotherapeutic process, or drug toxicity secondary to antimicrobial or immunosuppressive therapy (e.g., cyclosporine). Renal insufficiency is manifested by increased serum creatinine, decreased glomerular filtration rate, anemia, hypertension, and proteinuria. Chronic urinary infections, accompanied by abdominal pain, microscopic or gross hematuria, and anemia, are also an emerging problem in this patient population (Wujick, Ballard, & Camp-Sorrel, 1994).

Renal Complications

Radiation Nephritis. Radiation nephritis from radiation damage has recently been described and occurs approximately 5 months post-BMT, but it is a rare complication. Acute radiation nephritis declares itself 6 to 12 days after BMT (Juckett, Perry, Daniels, & Weisdorf, 1991). Hemolytic uremic syndrome (HUS) associated with renal failure is also a delayed and fatal complication after BMT. The etiologic factors are unclear, and some studies suggest HUS is related to high-dose conditioning regimens, infection, and cyclosporine (Wujick et al., 1994). Patients present with the triad of microangiopathic hemolytic anemia, renal insufficiency, and thrombocytopenia 30 to 875 days after BMT. Treatment consists of supportive care with administration of packed RBCs and platelets until HUS resolution (Juckett, Perry, Daniels, & Weisdorf, 1991). Prevention with vigorous pretransplant hydration and bladder irrigations may minimize these problems, but long-term studies are needed to document the true incident of these conditions.

Neurologic Complications

Neurologic complications in the BMT recipient are associated with intrathecal methotrexate, CNS irradiation, and immunosuppressive agents. The incidence of neurologic sequelae has been reported to be as high as 60% to 70% at various intervals along the transplantation continuum (Furlong, 1993). Many complications are reversible on drug withdrawal or dose reduction. However, leukoencephalopathy and irreversible CNS toxicity occur between 1 and 5 months after BMT in about 7% of patients transplanted for leukemia. Symptoms include impaired memory, shortened attention spans, and impaired verbal skills and may not appear for months or even years after transplantation. Learning disabilities in children and adults after BMT have been reported, but studies show conflicting data. A recent prospective, longitudinal study evaluated 65 pediatric BMT recipients with standardized measures of global intelligence and academic achievement and selected tests of neuropsychological function. Tests were administered pre-BMT and 12 to 16 months after BMT. Cognitive and neuropsychological function remained stable during the study periods. Declines were noted in social competence, self-esteem, and general emotional well-being. Surprisingly, and in contrast to other studies, BMT conditioning regimens were not associated with significant neuropsychologic impairment. Kramer and colleagues studied, prospectively and longitudinally, the intellectual and adaptive function of children receiving BMTs. Intelligent deficients compared with pretransplant baseline were found at 1 year after treatment, but no further changes were evident at the 3-year follow up (Kramer, Crittenden, DeSantes, & Cowan, 1997). Clinical signs and symptoms may be subtle and may require careful observation of the behavior of the pediatric patient. Meyers and colleagues (1994) studied 61 marrow recipients to evaluate cognitive and emotional functioning subsequent to BMT, at 2 weeks after BMT, at hospital discharge, and at 8 months after BMT. Baseline scores before BMT showed that 20% of the patients had mild cognitive dysfunction, and nearly 40% had significant anxiety. Although few patients developed problems with cognition or mood during the study, short-term memory deficits nearly doubled at follow-up compared with baseline. Anxiety decreased significantly during hospitalization and remained unchanged at follow-up evaluations. Oncology nurses assessing BMT survivors must be mindful of possible neurologic and developmental dysfunction and perform CNS assessments as part of follow-up care. Referral to rehabilitative programs is important.

Engraftment Problems

Graft Failure. Graft failure is a rare occurrence in HLA-matched marrow transplantation, but does manifest itself in HLA-mismatched or T-lymphocyte–depleted grafts. Graft failure can be a primary graft failure or transient engraftment. *Primary graft failure* is the failure of granulocyte counts to reach 0.2×10^9/L between 21 to 28 days after BMT. *Transient engraftment* is defined as complete or partial recovery of hematopoiesis in the absence of moderate to severe GVHD, followed by recurrent pancytopenia. The causes for graft failure include immunologic rejection at the donor, minor histocompatible antigens, and infection. Disease status at the time of transplantation, the degree of HLA compatibility, pretransplant treatment, preconditioning regimens, T-lymphocyte marrow depletion, and immunosuppressive therapy for GVHD also place recipients at risk. Diagnosis is usually determined by the presence of host T-lymphocytes. Booster grafts and administration of hematopoietic growth factors have been used as treatment measures but with limited success (Deeg, 1994).

Second Malignancy. As long-term survival improves, there is a growing concern about secondary malignancies resulting from TBI and high-dose chemotherapy used for pretransplant conditioning regimens and from compromised immune dysfunction. Only a few studies have emerged in this area. In 1992, Witherspoon and colleagues studied 1926 combined allogeneic and autologous marrow recipients transplanted for hematologic diseases and reported 35 secondary malignancies. The onset of *de novo* malignancy ranges from 2 to 4 years after BMT. More recently, an international team investigating solid tumors as a possible long-term BMT treatment sequelae, reported similar data. In over 20,000 allogeneic BMT recipients treated for leukemia (73%), 82 new invasive solid cancers were observed compared with 32 expected in the general population. The overall cancer risk rose steeply with increasing time of follow-up to reach eightfold among 10 or more survivors. The secondary cancers reported were cancers of the buccal cavity, liver, brain and other CNS locations, bone, connective tissue, along with melanoma (Curtis, Rowlings, Deeg, Shriner, Socie, & Travis et al., 1997). These studies indicate the vigilance that primary care providers need to assert in lifetime follow-up of these patients. Early detection of cancer and precursor lesions such as dysplastic nevi, actinic keratosis, and oral leukoplakia in combination of avoidance of carcinogenic exposures (e.g., tobacco) is essential in minimizing these deleterious effects.

Relapse. Relapse after BMT is a major impediment to long-term, disease-free survival or cure. Contributing factors include inadequate BMT conditioning regimens, disease T-lymphocyte–depleted marrow grafts, and GVHD (Deeg, 1994). Until recently, patients relapsing after BMT were referred for traditional chemotherapy, irradiation, surgery, second transplant. A number of investigational approaches are being employed to diminish recurrent disease. Posttransplant immunotherapy using active immunization is one approach that might eliminate tumor cells. Interferon-alpha administered to patients transplanted for CML may achieve or maintain complete hematologic and cytogenetic remissions. Other options for treatment of recurrent disease include salvage chemotherapy, second transplants, withdrawal of immunosuppressive medications (allogeneic), cytokine therapy, and therapy donor leukocyte infusions (DLIs). DLI, using buffy coat infusion or donor

T-lymphocytes to mediate a GVL effect, was first studied in clinical trials during the 1970s but was not widely accepted. In this process, donor leukocytes undergo leukopheresis in one or more sessions (cell dose varies) and administered to the recipient similar to a platelet transfusion. Results of DLI have been most striking among patients with CML who relapsed after a BMT. Of relapsed patients, 70% to 75% in chronic-stage CML have achieved a complete remission after DLI therapy. Most remissions are durable, and some survivors are alive and well more than 10 years after DLI therapy. Patients with more advanced disease (i.e., CML in the accelerated phase or blast crisis) have not responded as well to DLI therapy. DLI has been less effective in treating diseases other than CML. Approximately 15% of patients with acute myeloid leukemia have responded to DLI, and small numbers of patients with acute lymphocytic leukemia, myelodysplasia, multiple myeloma, and Fanconi's anemia have also responded. In most cases, patients with these diseases achieved remissions after DLI that were shorter than those seen in patients with CML, although some long-term remissions have been reported as well.

Most patients who respond to DLI therapy develop mild or moderate GVHD that is controlled on immunosuppressive medication, but approximately 5% of patients have died from GVHD-related complications. Although significant, these mortality rates still compare favorably with mortality rates after a second BMT for CML, which can be 40% or greater. Approximately 19% of patients treated with DLI have developed pancytopenia, which in most cases was short-term and was resolved without treatment or with administration of growth factors.

The success of DLI in treating relapsed patients with CML has encouraged investigators to minimize the toxic side effects. Some investigators have reported a lower incidence of GVHD in cases when specific T lymphocytes are removed from donor marrow before transplantation, without the loss of the beneficial GVL effect. Studies are under way to determine whether similar results can be achieved when these T lymphocytes are removed from donor leukocytes. It may be possible to treat these patients with lower doses of donor leukocytes when disease is minimal and reduce the incidence of GVHD. Studies are under way at a number of institutions to determine whether this approach will be efficacious and tolerable for the patient. Still others are investigating whether co-administering IL-2 with DLI can maximize its effect. Other investigators have hoped that DLI without hematologic transplantation can mediate the GVL effect, thereby avoiding the toxicities of radiation and chemotherapy. Success in this area would broaden its role, making it a standard component of allogeneic BMTs and potentially, an anti-cancer therapy outside the context of BMT (Collins, Shpilberg, Drobyski, Porter, Champlin, & Godman et al., 1997)

Consolidation therapy to decrease risks of relapse include DLIs. Involved-field irradiation given in addition to TBI to patients with lymphoma may reduce relapse rates and irradiation toxicity. The extra irradiation may be given before or after BMT and is being investigated in hopes of increasing tumor cell kill and lessening irradiation toxicities. Phases I and II trials in patients with recurrent leukemia using Iodine 131-labeled anti-CD45 antibody in combination with cyclophosphamide and TBI have demonstrated that delivery of 2000 cGY of radiation is possible without undue toxicity.

PSYCHOSOCIAL ISSUES

Patients

Rich research on the psychosocial issues unique to the BMT recipient is appearing with increasing regularity. Haberman (1988), in a seminal article, noted that patients have consistently identified specific stresses associated with each phase of the BMT process; each phase is eclipsed by particular concerns and provides a framework for nurses who care for these patients to offer appropriate support through patient preparation and teaching. More recently, Andrykowski and colleagues (1994) has advanced areas of psychosocial concerns of the marrow recipient into more succinct compartments with research recommendations for each phase. Nurses practicing in all areas of transplantation will find this latter article to be a helpful guide in planning research in this area.

Despite the continued research in psychological complications in the BMT recipient, few long-term problems have been identified. Once discharged from the hospital, marrow recipients often experience a normal reactive depression because of neuropsychological deficits, body image changes, malaise, sexual dysfunction, and a slower than anticipated return to normal activities. In contrast, in a recent study, Gaston-Johnsson and Foxall (1996) found that autologous recipients studied 2 days before BMT and 5 and 20 days after BMT were less depressed at 20 days. These symptoms might progress to clinical depression if not recognized and treated promptly. Recently, a small study of 20 families with children who underwent BMT documented that parents may develop posttraumatic stress disorder (PTSD). Parents considered the BMT process a traumatic occurrence and reexperienced the event through intrusive thoughts and a variety of emotional and cognitive responses. The investigators concluded that family preparation before BMT may decrease anxiety related to relocation to a BMT center and the BMT process. Little research has been done on the pretransplantation psychological and social status to determine their effects on morbidity and mortality after BMT. Syrjala and colleagues (1993) identified in a prospective study of allogeneic BMT recipients that emotional distress at 1 year after BMT was predicted by pretransplant family conflict, nonmarried status, and development of moderate chronic GVHD. Impaired physical recovery at 1 year after BMT was predicted by severe chronic GVHD, pretransplant physical impairment and family conflict.

Unusual psychological reactions include suicidal ideation, depression greater than expected from the normal grief reaction, disruptive anxiety, pathologic regression, and organic delirium. These cases represent a small but significant percentage of BMT recipients. Individual psychological counseling and antidepressant therapy may be required. Important consideration are early psychiatric intervention, ruling out organic factors, and identifying a consistent team to interact with these patients (Wellsich & Wolcott, 1994). Nurses can anticipate these normal reactions and direct patients and their families to supportive resources that include hospital- or community-based support groups, national survivorship organizations, and programs offered by the American Cancer Society. An Internet support group for BMT recipients meets weekly on America Online. As the cyberspace technologies advance, survivors will have rapid access to support systems in their own homes. Currently the Internet offers the *Bone Marrow Transplant Newsletter* and a home page for information exchange.

Donors

Donors experience a variety of psychological reactions before and after their marrow donation. Donor-related stresses have been identified and were reviewed earlier in this chapter. Family caregivers experience considerable psychological, emotional, and social problems before and after BMT. For example, transplant centers often are located far from familiar support systems, and relocation requires dramatic changes in every aspect of family dynamics. These changes include significant economic issues and medical consequences of BMT. Families need to confront the long-term issues of caring for a recovering family member until the physical sequelae of treatment have vanished. Strong social work teams are beneficial in transplant settings to prepare families for this experience and to identify community resources. This intervention lessens the likelihood of developing family-related dysfunctions. Studies examining the burden on the caregivers of BMT patients are needed to identify the nature and timing of stressors and caregiver burdens that can be alleviated through nursing interventions.

Staff

Psychological support for staff caring for patients undergoing marrow transplantation is essential to the quality of nursing care provided to marrow recipients and their families. Assisting staff in understanding family dynamics can alleviate the chronic stress of those continually caring for patients at considerable risk for morbidity and mortality. Winters, Miller, and Marachich (1995) characterized the nature of patient-nurse relations into five core concepts: (1) discovering the patient and families interpretation of the BMT experience, (2) intuitive awareness of the group relation, (3) undocumented and informal interactions between the nurse and patient, (4) direct and indirect interactions, and (5) monitoring family interactions in relation to the patient. The findings of this study can assist administrators in creating a framework for supporting staff in these environments. As the economics of health care increasingly influence practice by soaring work loads, former successful efforts to effect retention are rapidly disappearing. Perhaps some of the major impediments to staff satisfaction and subsequent retention of experienced nursing staff are administrative budgetary constraints, reducing or eliminating professional education, required travel, and subscription to professional nursing journals.

Quality of Life

The Karnofsky Performance Scale has been the most common physical function assessment of BMT recipients. More recently, researchers have assessed quality of life in four domains: physical, social, psychological, and spiritual (Ferrell, Grant, Schmidt, Whitehead, Fonbuena, & Forman, 1992). The numbers of quality-of-life studies are increasing, but few use prospective data with baseline data collected before BMT. Three notable studies are exceptions. Andrykowski and colleagues (1994) studied the physical and psychosocial status of 28 adult BMT recipients before BMT and at 12 to 16 months after BMT. Analysis of group means showed few significant differences between pre- and post-BMT assessments, but residual change scores suggested that physical and psychosocial status improved after BMT for women and younger recipients, whereas men and older recipients did less well. The second study showed that severe chronic GVHD coupled with pretransplant family conflict predicted subsequent impaired physical and emotional recovery. Patients with previous GVHD were least satisfied with major life domains (Syrjala et al., 1993). Eighty patients reported return of normal function with few physical problems. Few studies exist on pediatric quality-of-life issues, but anecdotal evidence from patients often praises the improved family life of disease-free survivors. Recently, a quality-of-life study was conducted to compare the health status of BMT survivors with age-adjusted population norms. Of 251 recipients studied, most survivors reported some diminished quality of life compared with the general population. Time after BMT was found to be a correlate with quality of life. Those patients transplanted for less than 3 years were experiencing considerable impairment, whereas those surviving beyond this point were indistinguishable from the normal population in most domains and fared significantly better in certain psychosocial aspects of health (Sutherland, Fyles, Adams, Hao, Lipton, & Minden, et al., 1997). More prospective studies using meaningful and reliable instruments specific to the recovering recipients over longer periods are needed. Instruments should be easy to use and not burdensome to a tool used in the easily fatigued or compromised recipient.

ETHICAL ISSUES

BMT is a useful metaphor for all that ails our current health care system. BMT is an expensive procedure carrying considerable morbidity and mortality. Cure rates have remained almost unchanged in several decades, and long-term complications persist. Questions of the allocation of resources are being examined. Concerns relative to the possible long-term effects of colony-stimulating factors used in normal stem cell and T-lymphocyte donors continue to be investigated. Worldwide banking of placental blood for transplant raises questions of (1) tissue ownership, (2) informed consent, (3) infectious disease and genetic information, (4) privacy and confidentiality, and (5) the need for fair and equitable access to placental blood. Gene manipulation will further challenge ethicists and researchers as alternative stem cell sources become available.

ECONOMIC ISSUES

Current health care mandates to reduce costs of BMT have led to economic studies of BMT, which, until now, have not been a concern to researchers. The first comprehensive study to examine the costs of BMT determined that allogeneic BMT for patients with AML was less than traditional treatment and provided patients with improved quality of life (Walsh & Larson, 1989). Since that time, various studies have been launched, but most used several methodologies and made numerous differing assumptions regarding costs and clinical practice. Variables such as data collection, length of time of study, type of transplant, use of direct or indirect costs, and charges were not consistent, and study results, with an exception of a few, were confusing. Few studies estimate the costs, life expectancy, and quality of life of marrow recipients. These early attempts at arriving at the costs and benefits of BMT reflect the infancy of this type of research, and those who have thus far contributed are to be applauded. Informed consent, especially for children and birth mothers donating placental blood for future use of unknown persons, effectiveness in medical models might serve as a model for future studies. Current challenges for researchers are to publish conducted studies in a timely fashion (Waters, Bennett, Pajeaü, Sobocinski, Rowlings, & Horowitz, 1998)

NEW SUPPORTIVE AGENTS

Supportive care agents are being investigated to prevent or reduce the incidences of serious and fatal infection, mucositis, and mortality among cancer patients receiving high-dose radiation and/or chemotherapy. Although recombinant colony-stimulating factors have decreased infections, they have been limited in preventing life-threatening infections such as those associated with the gastrointestinal tract. New agents such as lysoffline may protect the gastrointestinal epithelial cell lining and form an important physical barrier that separates the infectious pathogens from the sterile bloodstream. Initial trials in patients with AML showed promise, but recent studies in BMT recipients were disappointing. Amifostine is a new pancytoprotectant that holds promise for reducing nephrotoxic, neurotoxic, and hematologic complications resulting from chemotherapy and irradiation. The agent produces numerous side effects but tolerates the side effects of nausea and vomiting, hypotension, somnolence, hypocalcemia, sneezing, and warm, flushed feelings (Viele & Holmes, 1998).

FUTURE TRENDS

Bone marrow as a stem cell source is likely to give way to alternative stem sources such as blood, umbilical tissue, dendritic cells, and fetal cells. Chapter 9 discusses these options in detail. Diseases traditionally treated with marrow transplant will continue, but wider applications to autoimmune diseases are currently in clinical trials. The rational of treating autoimmune diseases with stem cells is that these diseases are the result of an altered immune response leading to an attack by the immune system against host antigens. Because all cells of the immune system are derived from the hematopoietic stem cell, replacing the immune system with healthy stem cells may lead to a cure. For example, rheumatoid arthritis, a persistent autoimmune inflammatory disease that attacks the joints, affects about 1% of the population in the United States. Although most live with sporadic symptoms and supportive care for pain, weakness, and other symptoms, others suffer rapidly progressing disease that confines them to a bed or wheelchair. Other disorders such as systemic lupus erythematosus, cerebral palsy, sickle cell anemia, cystic fibrosis, and multiple sclerosis affect millions of persons who may benefit from this therapy (Tyndall & Gratwohl, 1997). Only ongoing clinical trials will establish stem cell transplantation as a safe and cost-effective therapy compared with current supportive care measures.

Treatment failure or relapse remains one of the major impediments to successful allografting. Research on techniques for separation of hematopoietic stem cells include studies of sedimentation techniques, MoAbs, and immunoabsorption columns. Fetal liver stem cell transplants have been reported in treatment of selected patients with severe combined immunodeficiency disease (SCID). Successful allogeneic stem cell transplants for children and adults using umbilical cord blood are now being reported. Early fears that GVHD would be an insurmountable problem have not materialized. The ability to use cord blood has generated cord blood banks to store this tissue for possible autologous use and for unrelated ethically diverse transplants. Cord blood may be an optimal vehicle for gene therapy and treatment of metabolic diseases such as thalassemia and Fanconi's anemia (Gale, 1994).

Gene Transfer

Gene transfer holds dramatic promise for future applications of BMT and other genetic diseases. This involves replacement of defective genetic material with healthy genes in marrow transplantation candidates with genetic diseases (Kohn, Krall, Chalita, Skelnot, & Nolta, 1995). Adenosine deaminase deficiency is the first disease to be treated with gene transfer therapy, but other genetic disorders of lymphohematopoietic cells, including hemoglobinopathies, immune deficiencies, and storage diseases, are being studied in preclinical trials. Substantial preclinical improvements in transfer efficiency are required before wider clinical studies can be conducted.

CONCLUSION

Marrow will remain, for the time being, an important source for hematopoietic transplant, particularly for those requiring unrelated donor transplantation. However, alternative sources now dominate researchers' efforts. Because BMT is moving from an academic setting, community-based regional centers are rapidly becoming the most common site of marrow transplantation. Standards established by the Foundation for the Accreditation of Hematopoietic Cell Therapy, in hopes of facilitating consistent standards of care and outcomes, will unite and shape future research. General oncology nurses and general practice nurses will provide a large portion of transplant care. Advance practice nurses are contributing to the care of the marrow recipient, particularly in symptom management that ultimately affects the quality of life in these recipients. Nurse-managed outpatient clinics are being established with increasing frequency. Nursing case managers will continue to interact with corporate case managers to influence the quality of care of patients and their families. Earlier discharge of patients from hospital settings has more than likely flattened, but community oncologists and primary care physicians will play an even greater role in the long-term follow-up of recipient. Nurses will become more visible in educating advocacy and support groups for patients and family caregivers. More emphasis on the long-term complications of BMT, such as cognitive impairment and secondary malignancies, are critical to the continued success of this important treatment. Future nursing literature will not separate the concepts and care of marrow and stem cell recipients as one stem cell source gives way to more economical and efficient stem cell transplants. Growth of the unrelated donor pool will continue to increase, especially for those of cultural diversity. This shift will require that health care professionals working with these patients be sensitive to new belief systems and economic groups. Nursing administrators, because of economic restrains, now incorporate minimally trained caregivers to deliver complex care to highly symptomatic recipients. Staff retention in concert with optimal care in this milieu calls for creative and visionary leaders, especially in the face of an impending nursing shortage. Lastly, oncology nurse leaders will need to learn new negotiating and conflict management skills to gain influence in shaping the care of the marrow recipient and his or her family.

REFERENCES

A consensus statement on unrelated donor bone marrow transplantation from the Consensus Panel chaired by E. C. Gordon-Smith. (1997). *Bone Marrow Transplantation, 19,* 959-962.

Andrykowski, M. A., Bruehl, S., Brady, M, J., & Henslee-Downey (1994). Physical and psychosocial status of adults 1 year after bone marrow transplantation: A prospective study. *Bone Marrow Transplantation, 15,* 837-844.

Appelbaum F. R., Matthew, D. C., Eary, J. F. et al. The use of radiolabeled anti-CD33 antibody to augment marrow irradiation prior to marrow transplantation for acute myelogenous leukemia. *Transplantation 54*(5) 829-833, 1992.

Appelbaum, F. R. (1996). The use of bone marrow and peripheral blood stem cell transplantation in the treatment of cancer. *CA: A Cancer Journal for Clinicians, 46*(3), 142-164.

Armitage, J. O. (1994). Bone marrow transplantation. *New England Journal of Medicine, 330,* 827-838.

Armitage, J. O. (1996). New ABMTR studies evaluate growing use of autologous transplantation. *ABMTR Newsletter, 3*(1):2.

Baker, F., Wingard, J., Curbow, B., Zabora, Jodrey, D., Fogarty, L., & Legro, M. (1994). Quality of life of bone marrow transplant long-term survivors. *Bone Marrow Transplantation, 13,* 589-596.

Ballard, B. (1991). Renal and hepatic complications. In M. B. Whedon (Eds.), *Bone marrow transplantation: Principles, practice, and nursing insights.* Sudbury, MA: Jones and Bartlett.

Barnes, D. W. H., Corp, M. J., & Loutit, J. L. (1956). Treatment of murine leukæmia with x-rays and homologous bone marrow. *British Medical Journal, ii,* 96-99.

Bearman, S. I. (1995). The syndrome of hepatic veno-occlusive disease after marrow transplantation. *Blood, 85,* 3005-3020.

Bensinger, W. I., Buckner, C. D, & Thomas, E. D. (1982). ABO-incompatible marrow transplants. *Transplantation, 33,* 427-429.

Beutler, E., & Sullivan, K. (1994). Marrow transplantation in sickle cell disease. In S. J. Forman, K. Blume & E. D. Thomas (Eds.), *Bone marrow transplantation.* Cambridge, MA: Blackwell Scientific.

Blaese, R. M., Culver, K. W., Miller, A. D., Carter, C. S., Fleisher, T., Clerici, M., Shearer, G., Chang, L., Chiang, Y., & Tolstoshev, P. (1995). T lymphocyte-directed gene therapy for ADA-SCID: initial trial results after 4 years. *Science, 270,* 475-80.

Blazer, B. R., Lasky, L. C., Perentesis, J. P., Watson, K. V., Steinberg, S. E., Filipovich, A. H., Orr, H. T., & Ramsay, N. K. (1986). Successful donor cell engraftment in a recipient of bone marrow from a cadaveric donor. *Blood, 67,* 1655-1660, 1986.

Bortin, M. M., Horowitz, M. M., & Rimm, A. A. (1992). Progress report from the international bone marrow transplant registry. *Bone Marrow Transplantation, 10,* 113-122.

Bortin, M. M., Horowitz, M. M., Rowlings, P. A., Rimm, K. A., Zhang, M. J., & Gale, R. P. (1993). 1993 progress report from the international bone marrow transplant registry. *Bone Marrow Transplantation, 12,* 97-104.

Bortin, M. M., Bach, F. H., van Bekkumm, D. W., Good, R. A., & van Rood, (1994). Twenty-fifth anniversary of the first successful allogeneic bone marrow transplants. *Bone Marrow Transplantation 14* (2), 211-212.

Bowden, R. A., Slichter, S. J., Sayers, M., Weisdorg, D., Kays, M., Banaji, M., Haake, R., Welk, K., & Fisher, L. (1995). A comparison of filtered leukocyte-reduced and cytomegalovirus (CMV) seronegative blood products for the prevention of transfusion-associated CMV infection after marrow transplant. *Blood, 86,* 3599-3603.

Brandwine, J. M., Callum, J., Rubinger, M. (1989). An evaluation of outpatient bone marrow harvesting. *Journal of Clinical Oncology, 7,* 648-650.

Buchsel, P. C. (1991). Ambulatory care: Before and after BMT. In M. B. Whedon (Ed.), *Blood and marrow stem cell transplantation: Principles, practice, and nursing insights.* Sudbury, MA: Jones and Bartlett.

Buchsel, P. C., Wroblewski, E. L., & Randolph, S. R. (1996). Delayed complications of bone marrow transplantation: an update. *Oncology Nursing Forum, 23(8),* 1267-1291.

Buchsel, P. C. (1997). Bone Marrow Transplantation. S. L. Groenwald, M. H. Frogge, M. Goodman, & C. H. Yarbro. (Eds.), *Cancer nursing: Principles and practice.* (4th ed.). Sudbury, MA: Jones and Bartlett.

Buchsel, P. & Kapustay, P. (1998). New models of care for blood and marrow transplantation. In M. B. Whedon & D. Wujcik (Eds.), *Blood and marrow stem cell transplantation: Principles, practices, and nursing insights.* (2nd ed.). Sudbury, MA: Jones and Bartlett.

Buckley, F. P., & Syrjala, K. L. (1995). Pain management. In P. C. Buchsel & M. B. Whedon (Eds.). *Bone marrow transplantation: Administrative strategies and clinical concerns.* Sudbury, MA: Jones & Bartlett.

Buckner, C. D., Petersen, F. B., & Bolonesi, B. A. (1994). Bone marrow donors. In S. Foreman, K. Blume, & E. D. Thomas (Eds.), *Bone marrow transplantation.* Cambridge, MA: Blackwell Scientific.

Buckner, C. D., Clift, R. A., Sanders, J. E. Stewart, P., Bensinger, W. I., Doney, K. C., Sullivan, K. M., Witherspoon, R., Appelbaum, F. R., Storb, R., & Thomas, E. D. (1978). Protective environment for marrow transplant patients: A prospective study. *Annals of Internal Medicine, 89,* 893-901.

Burt, R. K., Deeg, H. J., Lothian, S. T., & Santos, G. W. (1996). *On call in bone marrow transplantation.* Austin, TX: R. G. Landes.

Butterworth, V. A., Simmons, R. G., & Bartsch V. (1993). Psychosocial effects of unrelated bone marrow donation: Experiences of the national marrow donor program. *Blood, 81* 947-1959.

Chang, H. J., Miller, H. L., Watkins, N., Arduino, M. J., Ashford, D. A., Midgley, G., Aguero, S. M., Pinto-Powell, R., Fordham von Reyn, C., Edwards, W., McNeil, M. M., & Jarvis, W. R. (1998). An epidemic of *malassezia pachydermatis* in an intensive care nursery associated with colonization of health care workers' pet dogs. *New England Journal of Medicine, 338,* 706-711.

Chao, N., Tierney, D., Bloom, J., Long, G., Barr, T., & Stallbaum, B. (1992). Dynamic assessment of quality of life after bone marrow transplantation. *Blood, 80,* 825-830.

Chiusolo, P., Salutari, P., Sica, S., Scirpa, P., Laurenti, L., Picirillo, N., & Leone, G. (1998). Luteinizing hormone-releasing hormone analogue: Leuprorelin acetate for the prevention of menstrual bleeding in premenopausal women undergoing stem cell transplantation. *Bone Marrow Transplantation, 21,* 821-823.

Collins, R. H., Shpilberg, O., Drobyski, W. R., Porter, D. L., Giralt, S., Champlin, R., Goodman, S. A., Wolff, S. N., Hu, W., Verfaillie, C., List, A., Dalton, W., Ognoskie, N., Chetrit, A., Antin, J. H., & Nemunaitis, J. (1997). Donor leukocyte infusions in 140 patients with relapsed malignancy after allogeneic bone marrow transplantation. *Journal of Clinical Oncology, 15*(2), 433-444.

Cox, G. J., Matsui, S. M., Lo, R. S., Hinds, M., Bowden, R., Hackman, R., Meyer, W. G., Mori, M., Tarr, P. I., Oshiro, L. S., Ludert, J. E., Meyers, J. D., & McDonald, G. B. (1995). Etiology and outcome of diarrhea after marrow transplantation: A prospective study. *Gastroenterology, 107,* 1398-1407.

Crawford, S. W. (1994). Critical care and respiratory failure. In S. Forman, K. Blume, & E. D. Thomas (Eds.), *Bone marrow transplantation.* Boston: Blackwell Scientific.

Crawford, W. (1988). Decision making in critically ill patients with hematologic malignancy. *Western Journal Medicine, 115,* 488-493.

Curran, W. J. & Hyg, S. M. (1992). Beyond the best interests of a child: Bone marrow transplantation among half-siblings. *New England Journal of Medicine, 324,* 881-889.

Curtis, D. J., Smale, A., Thien, F., Schwarer, A. P., & Szer, J. (1995). Chronic airflow obstruction in long-term survivors of allogeneic bone marrow transplantation. *Bone Marrow Transplantation, 16,* 169-173.

Curtis, R. E., Rowlings P. A., Deeg, H. J., Shriner, D. A., Socie, G., Travis, L., Horowitz, M. M., Witherspoon, R. P., Hoover, R. N., Sobocinski, K. A., Schoch, G. H., Travis, W., Sale, G. E., Kolb, H. J., Storb, R., Gale, R. P., Passweg, J. R., Fraumeni, J. F., & Boice, J. D. (1997). Solid cancers after bone marrow transplantation. *New England Journal of Medicine, 336,* 897-904.

Deeg, J. H. (1994). Graft failure. In R. K. Burt, J. H. Deeg, S. T. Lothian, & G. W. Santos (Eds), *Bone marrow transplantation.* Austin: Chapman & Hall.

Epstein, J. B., Stevenson-Moore, P., Jackson, S. (1989). Prevention of oral mucositis in radiation therapy. A contrasted study of benzydamine hydrochloride rinse. *International Journal of Radiation of Oncology and Biological Physics,* 16, 1571-1575.

Ezzone S. A., & Fliedner, M. (1998). Transplant networks and standards of care; international perspectives. M. B. Whedon, & D. Wujcik (Eds), *Blood and marrow stem cell transplantation: Principles, practice, and nursing insights* (2nd ed.). Sudbury, MA: Jones and Bartlett.

Ezzone, S. & Camp-Sorrell, D. (1994). *Oncology Nursing Society manual for bone marrow transplant nursing: Recommendations for practice and education.* Pittsburgh: Oncology Nursing Society.

Ferrell, B., Grant, M., Schmidt, G., Whitehead, C., Fonbuena, P., & Forman, S. (1992). The meaning of quality of life for BMT survivors. Part 2: Improving quality of life for BMT survivors. *Cancer Nursing, 15,* 247-253.

Flowers, M. (1998). Ask the doctor. *Blood and marrow transplant newsletter, 9,* 6.

Ford, R. & Eisenberg, S: (1990). Bone marrow transplant: Recent advances and nursing implications. *Nursing Clinics of North America, 25,* 405-422.

Freedman, S., Hainsfield, M. E., & McQuire, D. B. (1990) Nursing considerations in the administration of blood component therapy. *Seminars in Oncology Nursing, 6,* 155-162.

Furlong, T. (1993). Neurologic complications of immunosuppressive cancer therapy. *Oncology Nursing Forum, 20,* 1337-1352.

Gajewski, J. & Champlin, R. (1996). Bone marrow transplantation from alternate donors. In R. D. Burt, H. J. Deeg, S. T. Lothian, & G. W. Santos (Eds.), *On call in bone marrow transplantation.* Austin: R. G. Landes.

Gale, R. P. (1994). Cord blood stem cell transplantation: A real sleeper? *New England Journal of Medicine, 332,* 367-369.

Gaston-Johnson, F. & Foxall, M. F. (1996). Psychological correlates of quality of life. Cancer Nursing, 19, 170-178.

Giralt, S. A. & Champlin, R. E. (1994). Leukemic relapse after bone marrow transplantation: A review. *Blood, 84,* 3603-3612.

Goldman, J. M. (1994). A special report: Bone marrow transplantation using volunteer donors—recommendations and requirement for a standardized practice throughout the world—1994 update. *Blood 84,* 2833-2838.

Goodrich, J., Boeckh, M., & Bowden, R. (1994). Strategies for the prevention of cytomegalovirus disease after marrow transplantation. *Clinical Infectious Diseases, 19,* 624-629.

Haberman, M., Bush, N., Young, K., & Sullivan, K. (1993). Quality of life of adult long-term survivors: A qualitative analysis of narrative data. *Oncology Nursing Forum, 20,* 1545-1553.

Haberman, M. R. (1988). Psychosocial aspects of bone marrow transplantation. *Seminars in Oncology Nursing, 4,* 55-59.

Han, C. S., Miller, W., Haake, R., & Weisdorf, D. (1994). Varicella zoster infection after bone marrow transplantation: Incidence, risk factors and complications. *Bone Marrow Transplantation, 13,* 277-283.

Hill, H. H., Chapman, R. C., Kornell, J. A., Sullivan, K. M., Saegar, L. C., & Beneditti, C. (1990). Self-administration of morphine in bone marrow transplant patients reduces drug requirement. *Pain, 40,* 121-129, 1990.

International Bone Marrow Transplant Registry (1998). *Personal communication.*

Jenkins, J., Wheeler, V., & Albright, L. (1994). Gene therapy for cancer. *Cancer Nursing, 17,* 447-456.

Jenkins, J. (1998). Genetics and gene therapy. In M. B. Whedon & D. Wujcik (Eds.), *Blood and marrow stem cell transplantation: Principles, practice, and nursing insights.* (2nd ed.). Sudbury, MA: Jones and Bartlett.

Juckett, M., Perry, E., Daniels, B., & Weisdorf, D. (1991). Hemolytic uremia syndrome following bone marrow transplantation. *Bone Marrow Transplantation, 7,* (5) 405-411.

Kapelushnick, M., Aker, M., Paggatsch, T., Samuel, S., & Slavin, S. (1998). Bone marrow transplantation from a cadaveric donor. *Bone Marrow Transplantation, 21,* 857-859.

Kennedy, M., Vogelsang, G., Beveridge, R., Farmer, E., Altomonte, V., Huelskamp, A., & Davidson, N. (1993). Phase I trial of intravenous cyclosporine to induce graft-versus-host disease in women undergoing autologous bone marrow transplantation. *Journal of Clinical Oncology,* 11, 478-484.

Klingemann, H. G. (1992). A guide to bone marrow transplantation. In H. J. Deeg, H. G. Klingemann, & G. L. Phillips (Eds.), *A guide to bone marrow transplantation.* (2nd ed.). New York: Springer-Verlag.

Kohn, D. B., Krall, W., & Chalita, H. Skelnot, D, & Nolta, J. A. (1995). Gene therapy for congenital hematologic and immune disorders. *Bone Marrow Transplantation, 15* (Suppl. 1), 291-296.

Kramer, J. H., Crittenden, M. R., DeSantes, K., & Cowan, M. J. (1997). Cognitive and adaptive behavior 1 and 3 years after bone marrow transplantation. *Bone Marrow Transplantation, 19,* 607-613.

Lamberts, S. W., van der Lely, A. J., de Herder, W. W., & Hofland, L. J. (1996). Octreotide. *New England Journal of Medicine, 334*(4), 246-254.

Ljungman, P., Bock, R. D., Cordonnier, C., Einsele, H., Engelhard, D., Grundy, J., Locasciulli, A., Reusser, P. (1993) Practices for cytomegalovirus diagnosis, prophylaxis and treatment in allogeneic bone marrow transplant recipients. A report from the working party for infectious diseases of the EBMT. *Bone marrow transplantation, 12,* 399-403.

Lloid, M. (1995). Oral complications in the bone marrow transplant recipient. In P. Buchsel & M. Whedon (Eds.), *Bone marrow transplantation: Administrative strategies and clinical concerns.* Boston: Jones & Bartlett.

Madrigal, J. A. (1998). Bone marrow transplantation using unrelated donors. *Bone Marrow Transplantation, 21* (Suppl 2), 2-3.

McDonald, G. B., Sharma, P., Matthews, D. E., Shulman, H. M., Thomas, E. D. (1984). Venocclusive disease of the liver after bone marrow transplantation: Diagnosis, incidence, and predisposing factors. *Hepatology, 4*(1), 116-122.

McNeil, C. (1995). A new generation of monoclonal antibodies arrives at the clinic. *Journal of the National Cancer Institute 87*(22).

Meyers, C. A., Weitzner, M., Bryne, K., Valentine, A., Champlin, R. E., & Przepiorka, D. (1994) Evaluation of the neurobehavioral functioning of patients before, during, and after bone marrow transplantation. *Journal of Clinical Oncology, 12,* 820-826.

Meyers, C. A., Weitzner, M. A., Valentine, A. D., & Levin, V. A. (1998). Methylphenidate therapy improves cognition, mood, and function of brain tumor patients. *Journal of Clinical Oncology, 16*(7), 2522-2527.

Molassiotis, A, Akker, O. B. A., van den Milligan, D. W., & Boughton, B. J. (1995). Gonadal function and psychosexual adjustment in male long-term survivors of bone marrow transplantation. *Bone Marrow Transplantation, 16,* (2), 253-259.

Morton, A. J., Gooley, T., Hansen, J. A., Appelbaum, F. R., Bruemmer, B., Bjerke, J. W., Clift, R., Martin, P. J., Petersdorf, E. W., Sanders, J. E., Storb, R., Sullivan, K. M., Woolfrey, A., & Anasetti, C. (1998). Association between pretransplant interferon-alpha and outcome after unrelated donor marrow transplantation for chronic myelogenous leukemia in chronic phase. *Blood, 92*(2), 394-401.

Nader, S. & Arvin, A. (1994). Varicella zoster virus infections. In S. Foreman, K. Blume, & E. D. Thomas (Eds.), *Bone marrow transplantation,* Cambridge, MA: Blackwell Scientific. National Marrow Donor Registry (1998). *About the National Marrow Donor Program.* www.marrow.org/WHATSNEW/FACTS/GUIDE.html.

Oncology Nursing Society Manual For Bone Marrow Transplantation. (1994). Recommendations for Practice and Education. Pittsburgh: Oncology Nursing Press.

Openshaw H., & Slatkin, N. E. (1994). Varicella zoster virus infections. In S. Foreman, K. Blume, & E. D. Thomas (Eds.), *Bone marrow transplantation.* Boston: Blackwell Scientific.

Passweg, J. R., Hoffmann, T., Tichelli, A., Favre, G., Rohner, F., & Gratwohl, A. (1998). Double allogeneic peripheral stem cell transplants for patients at high risk of relapse. *Bone Marrow Transplant, 22*(4), 321-324.

Passweg, J. R., Rowlings, P. A., Atkinson, K. A., Barett, A. J., Gale, R. P., Gratwohl, A., Jacobsen, N., Klein, J. P., Ljungman, P., Russell, J. A., Schaefer, U. W., Sobocinski, K. A., Vossen, J. M., Zhang, M. J., & Horowitz, M. M. (1998). Influence of protective isolation on outcome of allogeneic bone marrow transplantation for leukemia. *Bone Marrow Transplantation, 21*(12), 1231-1238.

Paternaude, A. F., Szymanski, L., & Rappeport, J. (1979). Psychological costs of bone marrow transplantation in children, *American Journal of Orthopsychiatry, 49*(3), 409-422.

Perkins, H. A. & Hansen, J. A. (1994). The U.S. National Marrow Donor Program. *American Journal of Hematology and Oncology, 16* (1):30-34.

Peterson, F. B. & Bearman, S. J. (1994). Preparative regimens and their toxicity. In S. Forman, K. Blume, & E. D. Thomas (Eds.), *Bone marrow transplantation.* Boston: Blackwell Scientific.

Phipps S., Brenner, M., Heslop, H., Krance, R., Jayawardene, D., & Mulhern (1995). Psychological effects of bone marrow transplantation on children and adolescents: Preliminary report of a longitudinal study. *Bone Marrow Transplantation, 15,* 829-835.

Poe, S. S., Larson, E., & McGuire, D. (1994). A national survey of infection prevention practices on bone marrow transplantation units. *Oncology Nursing Forum 21,* 1687-1694.

Quine, W. E. (1896). The remedial application of bone marrow. *Journal of the American Medical Association, 26,* 1012 1013.

Rio, B., Letur-Konirsch, H., Ajchenbaum-Cymbalista, F., Bauduer, F., DeZiegler, D., Pelissier, C., Bernadou, A., Fryman, R., & Zittoun, R. (1994). Full-term pregnancy with embryos from donated oocytes in a 36-year-old woman allografted for chronic myeloid leukemia. *Bone Marrow Transplantation, 13,* 487-488.

Roncarolo, M. G., Bachetta, R., & Touraine, J. L. (1992). SCID patients reconstituted by fetal liver stem cell. *Journal of Cellular Biochemistry, 16a* (Abst. 180), 22.

Rowe, J., Ciobanu, N., Ascensao, J., Stadmauer, E., Weiner, R., Schenkein, D., McGlave, P. & Lazarus, H. (1994). Recommended guidelines for the management of autologous and allogeneic bone marrow transplantation. *Annals of Internal Medicine, 120,* 143-158.

Ruggiero, M. R. (1988). The donor in bone marrow transplantation. *Seminars in Oncology Nursing, 4,* 914, 1988.

Russell, J. A., Blahey, W. A., Stuart, T. A. & Card, R. T. (1989). Avascular necrosis of bone in bone marrow transplant patients. *Medical Pediatrics of Oncology, 17,* 1140-143.

Russell, J. A., Poon, M. C., Jones, A. R., et al: (1992). Allogeneic bone-marrow transplantation without protective isolation in adults with malignant disease. *Lancet, 339,* 38-40.

Sanders, J. (1991). Endocrine problems in children after bone marrow transplant for hematologic malignancies. *Bone Marrow Transplantation, 8,* 2-4.

Sanders, J. (1994). Growth and development after bone marrow transplantation. In S. Forman, K. Blume, & E. D. Thomas (Eds.), *Bone marrow transplantation.* Boston: Blackwell Scientific.

Sanders, J. E., Pritchard, S., Mahoney, P., Amos, D., Buckner, C. E., Witherspoon, R. P., Deeg, H. J., Doney, K. C., Sullivan, K. D., Appelbaum, F. R., Storb, R., & Thomas E. D. (1988). Growth and development following marrow transplantation for leukemia. *Journal Title,* 68(5), 1129-1135.

Santos, G. W. (1983). History of bone marrow transplantation. *Clinics of Hæmatology,* 12: 611-639.

Schover, L. (1988). *Sexuality and cancer.* Atlanta: American Cancer Society.

Schubert, M. (1998). *Nonhormonal strategies for menopausal BMT recipients.* Kirkland, WA: Evergreen Women's Care.

Serota, F. T., O'Shea, A., T., & Woodward, W. T., et al. (1981). Role of a child advocate in the selection of donors for pediatric bone marrow transplantation. *Journal of Pediatrics, 98,* 847-850.

Stern, J. M. & Lenssen, P. (1995). Food and nutrition services for the BMT patient. In P. Buchsel & M. Whedon (Eds.), *Bone marrow transplantation: Administrative strategies and clinical concerns.* Boston: Jones & Bartlett.

Stolberg, S. G. (1998 July). Thalidomide wins FDA approval. *The New York Times,* p. 1.

Storb, R., Deeg, H. J., & Whitehead, J. (1986). Methotrexate and cyclosporine compared with cyclosporine alone for prophylaxis of acute graft-versus-host disease after marrow transplantation for leukemia. *New England Journal of Medicine, 314,* 729-735.

Stroncek, D. F., Holland, P., Bartch, V. (1995). Experiences of the first 493 unrelated marrow donors in the national marrowdonor program. *Blood, 81* 1940-1946.

Sugarman, J., Reisner, E. G., & Kurtzberg, J. (1988) Ethical aspects of banking placental blood for transplantation. *Journal of American Medical Association, 274,* 1783-1785.

Sullivan K. & Witherspoon, R. (1995). Ask the doctor. *Bone Marrow Transplantation Newsletter. 6,*(4) 5.

Sullivan K. (1994). Graft-versus-host disease. In S. Forman, K. Blume, & E. D. Thomas Thomas (Eds.), *Bone marrow transplantation.* Boston: Blackwell Scientific.

Sullivan, K. M., Kopecky, K. J., Jocom, J., (1990). Immunomodulatory and antimicrobial efficacy of intravenous immunoglobulin in bone marrow transplantation. *New England Journal of Medicine, 323,* 705-712.

Sullivan, K. M., Moinpouir, C., Chapko, M., Buchsel, P., & Applebaum, F. (1995). *Reducing the costs of blood and marrow transplantation: A randomized study of early hospital discharge and the results of revised standard practice guidelines.* (Abstract). Nashville: American Society of Hematology.

Sutherland, H. J., Fyles, G. M., Adams, G., Hao, Y., Lipton, J. H., Minden, M. D., Meharchand, J. M., Atkins, H., Tejpar, I., & Messner, H. A. (1997). Quality of life following bone marrow transplantation: a comparison of patients reports with population norms. *Bone Marrow Transplantation, 19,* 1129-1136.

Syrjala, K. L., Chapko, M., Vitaliano, P., Cummings, C., & Sullivan, K. (1993). Recovery after graft-vs-host disease and other late complications of bone marrow transplantation, allogeneic marrow transplantation: Prospective study of predictors of long-term physical and psychosocial function. *Bone Marrow Transplantation, 11,* 319-327.

Syrjala K. (1995). Meeting the psychological needs of recipients and families. In P. C. Buchsel & M. B. Whedon (Eds.), *Bone marrow transplantation: Administrative strategies and clinical concerns.* Sudbury, MA: Jones and Bartlett.

Thomas E. D., Storb, R., Clift, R. A., Fefer, A., Johnson, L., Neiman, P. E. Lerner, K. G., Glucksberg, H., and Buckner, C. B. (1988), Bone-marrow transplantation. *New England Journal of Medicine, 292,* 832-843, 895-902.

Thompson, C., Flournoy, N., Buckner, D, & Sanders J. (1986) The risk of central nervous system relapse and leukoencephalopathy in patients receiving marrow transplants for acute leukemia. *Blood, 67* (1) 195-199.

Thomas, E. D. & Storb, R. (1970). Technique for human marrow grafting. *Blood, 36,* 507-515.

Thompson, C. B.,, June, C. H., Sullivan, K. M., & Thomas, E. D. (1984). Association between cyclosporine neurotoxicity and hypomagnesemia. *Lancet, 2,* 1116-1120.

Tichelli, A., Gratwohl, A., Thomas, E., Roth, J., Prunte, A., Nissen, C., & Speck, B. (1994). Cataract formation after BMT. *Annals of Internal Medicine, 119,* 1175-1180.

Tiercy, J. M., Morel, C., & Freidel, A. C. (1988). Selection of unrelated donors for bone marrow transplantation is improved by HLA class II genotyping with oligonucleotide hybridization. *Program of National Academic Sciences, 88,* 7121-7125.

Turkeri, L. N., Lum, L. G., Uberti, & J. P., Abella, E., Momin, F., Karanes, C., Sensenbrenner, L. L., Haas, G. P. (1995). Prevention of hemorrhagic cystitis following allogeneic bone marrow transplant preparative regimens with cyclophosphamide and busulfan: role of continuous bladder irrigation. *Journal of Urology, 153,* 637-640.

Tyndall A. & Gratwohl, A. (1997). Blood and marrow stem cell transplants in auto-immune disease: A consensus report written on behalf of the European League against rheumatis (EULAR) and the European groups for blood and marrow transplantation (EBMT). *Bone Marrow Transplantation, 19,* 643-645.

Tyndall, A. G. (1996). Options for bone marrow transplantation in severe arthritis. Blood cell and bone marrow transplants (Abstract 15) *Proceedings,* 28.

Tzakis, A., Abu-Elmaagd, K., & Fung, J. (1991). FK 506 rescue in chronic graft-versus-host disease after bone marrow transplantation. *Transplant Proceedings, 23,* 3225-3227.

Uderzo, C., Fraschini, D., Balduzzi, A., Galimberti, S., Arrigo, C., Biagi, E., Pignanelli, Nicolin, B., & Rovelli, A. (1997). Long term effects of bone marrow transplantation on dental status in children with leukæmia. *Bone Marrow Transplantation, 20,* 865-869.

Vermylen, C., Cornu, G., Ferster, A., Brichard, B., Ninane, J., Ferrant, A., Zenebergh, A., Maes, P., Dhooge, C., Benoit, Y., Dresse, M. F., & Sariban, E. (1998). Hematopoietic stem cell transplantation for sickle cell anaemia: The first 50 patients transplanted in Belgium. *Bone Marrow Transplantation, 22*(1), 1-6.

Viele, C. S. & Holmes, B. C. (1998). Amifostine: drug profile and nursing implications of the first pancytoprotectant. *Oncology Nursing Forum, 25,* 515-526.

Vogelsang, G., Farmer, E., & Hess, A. (1992). Thalidomide therapy of chronic graft-versus host disease. *New England Journal of Medicine, 326,* 1055-1058.

Vogelsang, G. B., Hess, A. D., & Santos, G. W. (1988). Thalidomide for treatment of graft vs host disease. *Bone Marrow Transplantation, 3,* 393-398.

Wagner, J. L., Flowers, M. E. D., Longton, G., Storb, R., & Schubert, M. (1998). The development of chronic graft-versus host disease: an analysis of screening studies and the impact of corticosteroid use at 100 days after transplantation. Bone Marrow Transplantation, 22, 139-146.

Walsh, G. & Larson, E. (1989). Cost-effectiveness of bone marrow transplantation in acute nonlymphocytic leukemia. *New England Journal of Medicine, 32,* 807-812.

Wasserman, E., Hidalgo, M., Hornedo, J., & Cortes-Funes, H. (1997). Octreotide (SMS 201-995) for hematopoietic support-dependent high-dose chemotherapy (HSD-HDC)-related diarrhoea: Dose-finding study and evaluation of efficacy. *Bone Marrow Transplant 20*(9):711-714.

Waters, T. M., Bennett, C. L., Pajeaü, T. S., Sobocinski, K. A. K. J. P., Rowlings, P. A., & Horowitz, M. M. (1998). Economic analyses of bone marrow and blood stem cell transplantation for leukemias and lymphoma: What do we know? *Bone Marrow Transplantation, 21,* 641-650.

Weinberg, P. (1988) The human leukocyte antigen (HLA) system, the search for a matching donor, national marrow donor program development, and marrow donor issues. In M. B. Whedon (Ed.), *Blood and marrow stem cell transplantation: Principles, practice, and nursing insights* Sudbury, MA: Jones and Bartlett.

Welch, H. G. & Larsen, E. B. (1989). Cost effectiveness of bone marrow transplantation. *New England Journal of Medicine,* B1, 807-811.

Wellisch, D., & Wolcott, D. (1994). Psychological issues in bone marrow transplantation. In S. Forman, K. Blume, & E. D. Thomas (Eds.), *Bone marrow transplantation.* Boston: Blackwell Scientific.

Whedon, M. B. (1995). Bone marrow transplantation nursing: into the twenty-first century. P. Buchsel & M. Whedon (Eds), *Bone marrow transplantation: Administrative strategies and clinical concerns.* Sudbury, MA: Jones and Bartlett.

Whimbey, E., Champlain, R. E., & Couch, R. B. (1996). Community respiratory virus infections among hospitalized adult bone marrow transplant recipients. *Clinics of Infectious Disease, 22,* 778-782.

Wilke, T. J. (1991). Pulmonary and cardiac complications of bone marrow transplantation. In M. B. Whedon (Ed.). *Blood and marrow stem cell transplantation: Principles, practice, and nursing insights.* Sudbury, MA: Jones and Bartlett.

Wingard, J. R. (1997). Bone marrow to blood stem cells: Past, present, future. In W. B. Whedon, & D. Wujcik. *Blood and marrow stem cell transplantation: Principles, practice, and nursing insights.* (2nd ed.). Sudbury, MA: Jones and Bartlett.

Wingard, J. R. (1994). Prevention and treatment of bacterial and fungal infections. In S. Forman, K. Blume, & E. D. Thomas (Eds.), *Bone marrow transplantation.* Boston: Blackwell Scientific.

Wingard, J. R. (1990). Management of infectious complications of bone marrow transplantation. *Oncology, 2,* 69-76.

Wingard, J., Curbow, B., Baker, F., & Piantadosi, S. (1991). Health, functional status, and employment of adult survivors of bone marrow transplantation. *Annals of Internal Medicine,* 114, 113-118.

Wingard, J., Curbow, B., Baker, F., Zabora, J., & Piantadosi, S. (1992). Sexual satisfaction in survivors of bone marrow transplantation. *Bone Marrow Transplantation, 9,* 185-190.

Wingard, J. R., Plotnick, L. P., Freemer, C. S., Zahurak, M., Piantadosi, S., Miller, D. F., Vriesendorp, H. M., Yeager, A. M., & Santos, G. W. (1992). Growth in children after bone marrow transplantation: Busulfan plus cyclophosphamide versus cyclophosphamide plus total body irradiation. *Blood, 79,* 1068-1073.

Winters, G., Miller C., Marachich, L. (1995). Provisional practice: The nature of psychological bone marrow transplant nursing. *Oncology Nursing Forum, 21,* 1147-1154.

Witherspoon, R. (1991). Chronic graft-versus-host disease and other late complications of bone marrow transplantation. *Seminars in Hematology, 28,* 250-259.

Witherspoon, R., Fisher, L., Sachet, G., Martin, P., Sullivan, K., Sanders, J., Deeg, H., Downy, K., Thomas, D., Storb, R., & Thomas, E. D. (1992). Secondary cancers after bone marrow transplantation for leukemia or aplastic anemia. *New England Journal of Medicine, 321,* 784-798.

Wujcik, D., Ballard, B., & Camp-Sorrel, D. (1994). Selected complications of allogeneic bone marrow transplantation *Seminars in Oncology Nursing, 10,* 28-41.

Zaia, J. (1994). Cytomegalovirus infection. In S. Foreman, K. Blume, & E. D. Thomas (Eds.), *Bone marrow transplantation.* Boston: Blackwell Scientific.

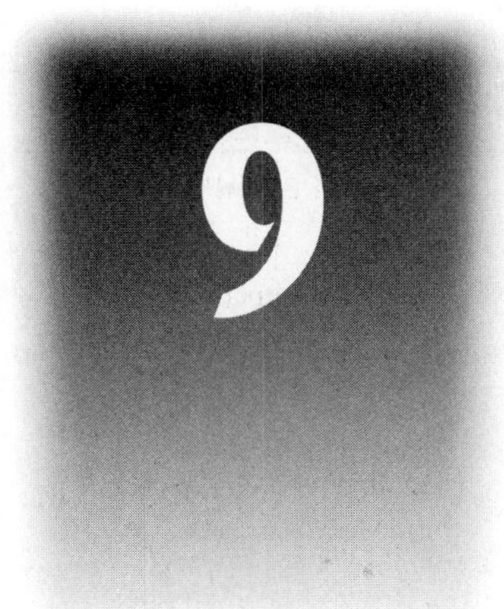

Peripheral Stem Cell Transplantation

Patricia C. Buchsel, RN, MSN
Pamela Kapustay, RN, MS

INTRODUCTION

The shift from marrow to peripheral and umbilical cord blood as a viable stem cell source has been one of the most rapid changes in transplantation medicine. Remarkably, this evolution occurred during this decade. Autologous bone marrow transplantations (BMTs) have given way to peripheral stem cell transplantations (PSCTs), and more than 80% of all autologous transplantations are performed using peripheral stem cells (Figs. 9-1 and 9-2). It is estimated that more than 2500 allogeneic PSCTs have been performed worldwide. Most were human leukocyte antigen (HLA) sibling grafts, but some were from unrelated doors. More than 600 umbilical cord blood transplantations have been documented. Interest in other stem cell sources such as fetal liver for cure of genetic diseases is being studied. Other stem cell applications are the use of dendritic cells to stimulate the immune systems of stem cell recipients and donor T lymphocytes to achieve the graft versus leukemic (GVL) effect. Novel stem cell growth factors to ensure purified products with minimal collection are the subject of laboratory study (Gratwohl, Hermans, & Baldomero, 1996).

Despite documented success in PSCT, unresolved questions prevail. The issues relate to donor type and source, mobilization techniques, graft versus host disease (GVHD), durable engraftment, graft engineering, and disease-free survival. Prospective comparative trials are ongoing. When results are published, in combination with large, carefully designed retrospective analyses, guidance for future research will be forthcoming (Gratwold, 1998). Table 9-1 compares the advantages of allogeneic peripheral stem cell to bone marrow transplantation.

This chapter addresses the common premises of the clinical practice of PSCT. See Chapter 10 for common complications shared on marrow and PSCT recipients. The issues, problems, and concerns of alternate stem cell sources (e.g., umbilical, fetal) are addressed later in the chapter.

HISTORICAL PERSPECTIVE

The evolution of PSCT from BMT has occurred over the last 100 years. As early as 1909, it was postulated that small cells circulating in the blood were capable of not only traveling to all organs but also self-generating from a primitive stem cell (Maximov, 1909). This discovery was debated until the mid 1950s when a greater understanding of the nature and characterization of the stem cells was improved through research (Korbling, 1995). Studies in the 1950s and 1960s reported the existence of stem cells in the peripheral blood of rates, mice, guinea pigs, and dogs. Goodman and Hodgson (1962), using the term *blood stem cell,* were the first to record evidence that circulating stem cells are capable of restoring hematopoiesis after marrow ablation. Successful animal transplantation with peripheral stem cells soon led to the conviction that human blood cell transplantation (BCT) was a possibility. New understandings and improvements in leukopheresis and cryopreservation techniques followed these findings. The development of the continuous flow stem cell separator in 1965 gave birth to the first clinical BCT, but findings were not published until 1971.

The modern age of PSCT began in the early 1980s. The first significant studies were reported in 1986 from four centers using BCT for patients with chronic myelogenous leukemia in accelerated phase. Although patients were returned to their chronic disease phase after treatment, they retained the Philadelphia + chromosome. Another limiting factor was the need for multiple collection to attain sufficient numbers of stem cells to successfully repopulate the marrow after ablating therapy. Administering cyclophosphamide and cytokines to mobilize stem cells was determined in the late 1980s to contribute to earlier engraftment, fewer infections, less antibiotic use, and shorter hospital stays when compared with BMT.

The first published report of an allogeneic PSCT was in a patient with acute lymphoblastic leukemia. The investigators reported rapid marrow engraftment using peripheral stem cells; however, nine aphereses were required to obtain sufficient cells. Paralleling this event, Dreger and colleagues (1994) noted successful PSCT in a marrow recipient after

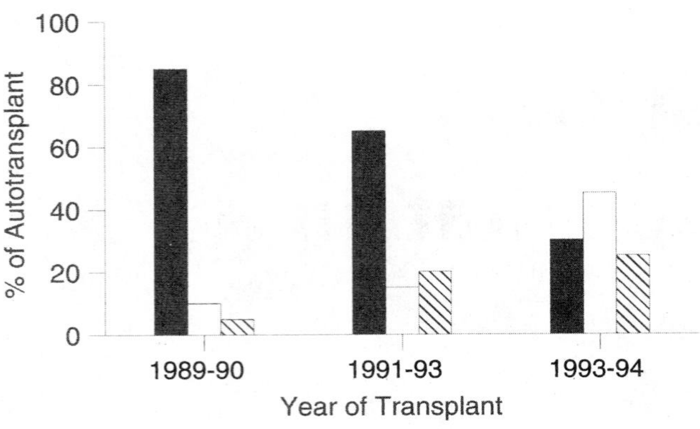

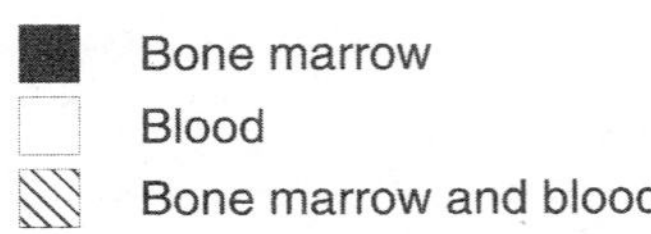

Fig. 9-1 Stem cell source for autotransplants. The most common source of cell used for hematopoietic recovery in autotransplants has shifted from bone marrow to blood. (From International Bone Marrow Transplant Registry. [1995].

TABLE 9-1 Advantages and Disadvantages of Allogeneic Peripheral Blood Transplantation.

Marrow	Peripheral Blood
General anesthesia for marrow harvest	Stem cells collected by apheresis in an outpatient setting, avoiding risks of general anesthesia and postoperative discomforts of pain, anemia, nausea, and fatigue.
No mobilization for harvest, therefore avoiding unknown risks of long-term complications of colony-stimulating factors	Cost-effective harvest compared with marrow
	Donor may require multiple vena punctures and a temporary central catheter for multiple leukopheresis, placing donor at risk for infection, discomfort, and decreased in activities of daily living
Slower engraftment	More rapid engraftment, reducing transplant-related morbidity and mortality
Graft versus leukemic effect present	Graft versus leukemic effect may be enhanced compared with marrow because of the larger number of lymphocytes collected and infused
	Graft versus host disease may be greater than marrow because of the larger number of lymphocytes collected and infused
	Possible cost savings because of ability to perform a significant part of care in ambulatory care models
Lower yield of CD34+ cells and colony-forming units	Higher yield of CD34+ cells and colony-forming units

Modified from Buchsel, P.C., & Kapustay, P.M. (1995). Peripheral stem cell transplantation. *Oncology Nursing: Patient Treatment and Support, 2*(2), 1-24.

marrow rejection. Initial studies using placenta blood for transplantation occurred in France in 1988. In utero transplantations first studied in the animal model were in humans by 1986 (Linch, Rodeck, Nicolaldes, Jones, & Brent, 1986). Since then, this method has increased dramatically.

TENETS OF PERIPHERAL STEM CELL TRANSPLANTATION

The concept of using stem cells collected from peripheral blood to be transfused into a patient for purposes of a cure or quality life years gained is as follows:

- The dose-intensity of most chemotherapeutic agents administered to cure a patient's disease is limited by subsequent dose-related marrow toxicity.
- The availability of hematopoietic stem cells collected from the peripheral blood allows infused stem cells to reconstitute the patient's hematopoietic and immunologic system after high-dose chemotherapy or total-body irradiation given alone or in combination.
- Resulting complications occur secondary to the effects of dose-intensive conditioning regimens, GVHD (allogeneic) supportive medications (amphotericin), or treatment failure (relapse).
- Supportive care techniques sustain the recipient until stabilized engraftment (Buchsel & Kapustay, 1995).

Hematopoiesis

One of the pivotal premises of BCT is new understanding of the hematopoietic process. Hematopoiesis is the process by which circulating blood cells are produced in adequate numbers, under normal conditions and in times of increased demand (i.e., in response to infection, after chemotherapy) (Messner & McCulloch, 1994). The origin of all blood cells is derived from the pluripotent stem cell found primarily in the bone marrow (Fig. 9-3). The important characteristics of pluripotent stem cells are their unlimited ability to replicate repeatedly and differentiate to either myeloid or lymphoid stem cells. Only a small population is required to accomplish this process. Once a cell begins to differentiate, it is known as a *progenitor cell.* These cells further differentiate and become committed to a specific cell lineage, resulting in

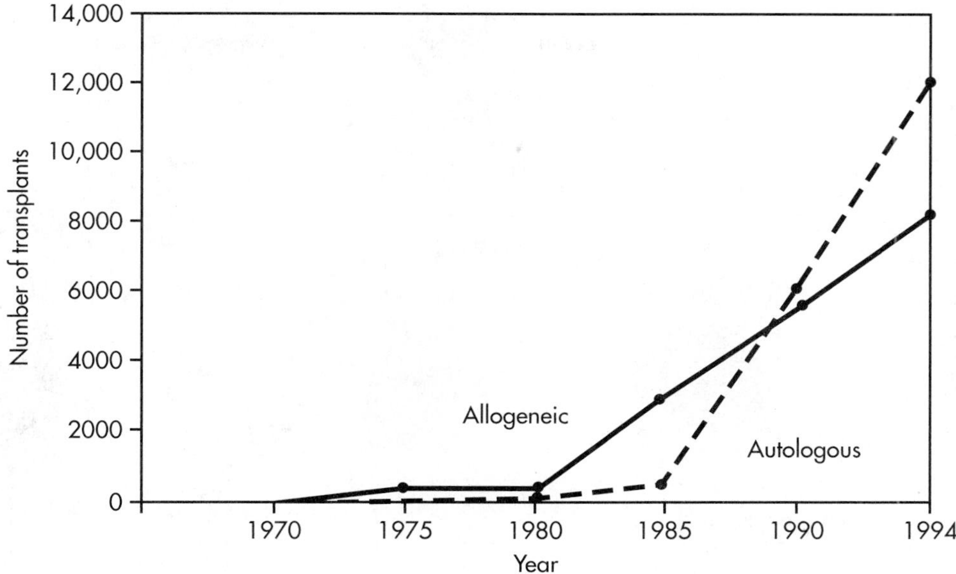

Fig. 9-2 Annual number of transplantations worldwide, 1970-1994. (From International Bone Marrow Transplant Registry [1995].

the various mature blood and lymphocyte cells (Vescio, Hong, & Cao, 1994).

Stem Cell Expression and Isolation

Identifying the number of CD34+ cells in the harvested product is a more timely method to determine hematopoietic capability. In 1984, a monoclonal antibody (MoAb), known as Civin's antibody, was isolated and found to be useful in identifying stem cells. This antibody reacts with a cell protein marker or antigen, known as CD34, which is present on all committed hematopoietic progenitor cells and pluripotent stem cells (Vescio, Hong, & Cao, 1994; Golde, 1991). CD34+ cells can now be readily identified and isolated from the masses of other cells in the circulation by using flow cytometry and MoAbs. During the normal maturation of blood cells, the expression of the CD34 antigen on the cell surface diminishes; therefore they are no longer identified as progenitor cells (Vescio, Hong, & Cao, 1994). Because the CD34+ cell count can be determined within hours of an apheresis, the need for excessive collections can be eliminated. Identification of a stem cell and/or progenitor cell is essential to ensure that sufficient numbers are collected to enable marrow engraftment after BCT. The higher the yield the more likely that a rapid, sustained marrow engraftment after myeloablative therapy will occur. A total stem cell harvest with a CD34+ cell count of 5×10^6/kg is considered sufficient to provide for rapid engraftment and marrow recovery after myeloablative chemotherapy (Bensinger, Applebaum, Rowley, Storb, Sanders, & Lilleby, 1995; Szilvassy & Hoffman, 1995).

The number of granulocyte-macrophage colony-stimulating factors (GM-CSFs) or CD34+ cells infused during PSCT is directly related to the rate of recovery for neutrophils and platelets (To, 1995). For this reason, it is vital to collect the optimal number of stem cells to ensure a rapid and enduring marrow engraftment. The data collected are inconclusive as to the accuracy of one cell measurement assay over the other (Bensinger et al., 1995). Both are somewhat variable, and the need to standardize them is crucial to ensure accurate measurements of stem and progenitor cells (Juttner, Fibbe, & Neumunaitis, 1994).

TYPES AND DONOR SOURCES

Autologous

In an autologous PSCT, selected patients with malignant disease have their own healthy stem cells reinfused after dose-intensive chemotherapy and possible irradiation to cure them of their disease. Diseases currently under evaluation treated with autologous PSCT are those of solid tumors such as breast, multiple myeloma, Hodgkin's disease (HD) and non–Hodgkin's lymphoma (NHL), small cell carcinoma of the lung, and acute nonlymphoblastic leukemia.

Allogeneic

An allogeneic PSCT is similar to an autologous PSCT but is dependent on the availability of an HLA donor. Diseases for which this modality are now being used are acute myelogenous leukemia (AML), acute lymphoblastic leukemia (ALL) in first and second complete remission, and chronic myelogenous leukemia in first chronic and accelerated phase. Advantages are identical to those of autologous BMT, such as accelerated engraftment and avoidance of general anesthesia for the donor. Some studies have been published, but they are limited in size. Pavletic and

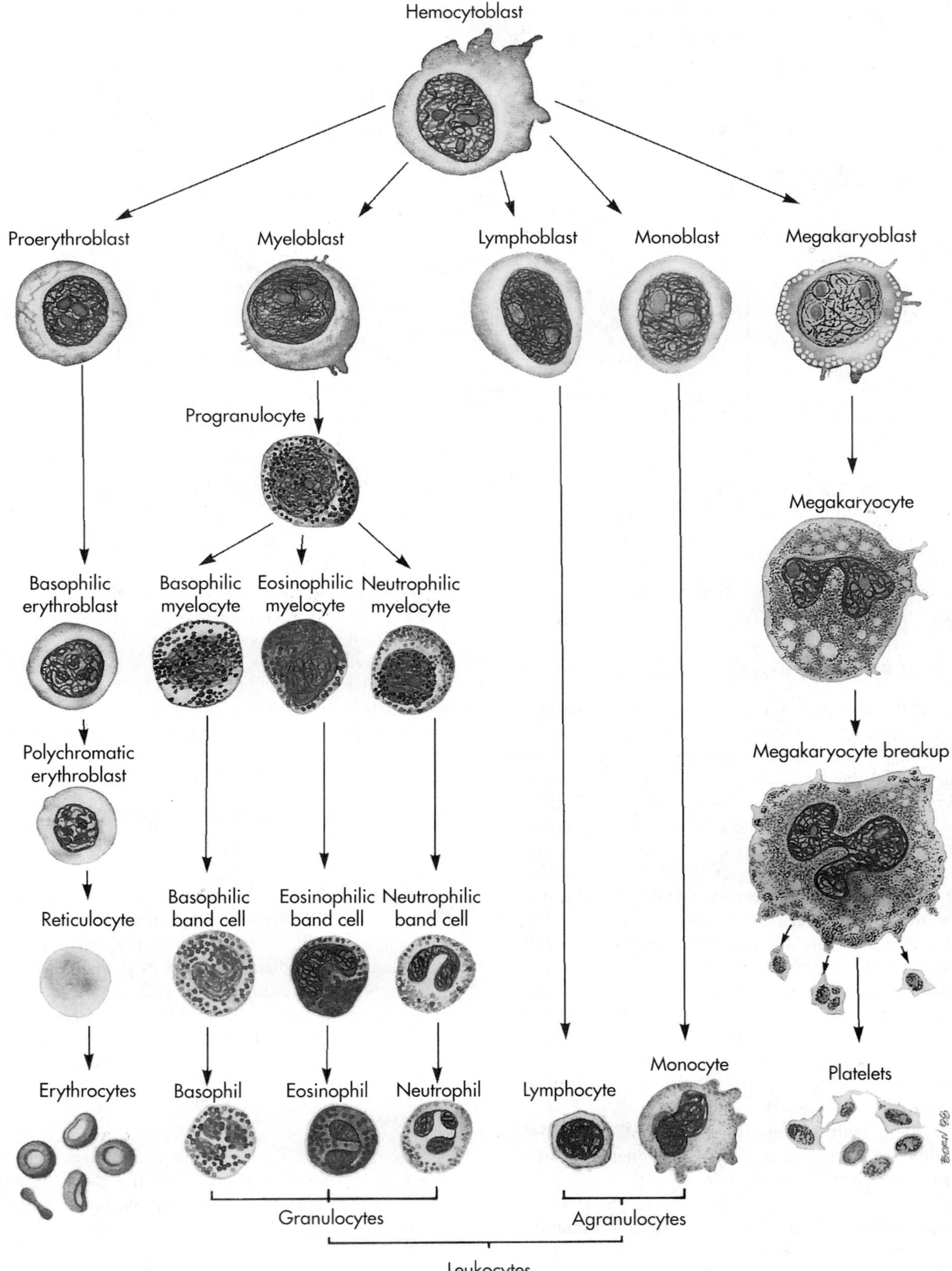

Fig. 9-3 Hematopoiesis. (Thibodeau, G., & Patton, K. T. [1996]. *Anatomy and physiology.* [3rd ed.]. St. Louis: Mosby.)

colleagues studied hematopoietic recovery after allogeneic blood stem cell transplantation to compare hematopoietic recovery, duration of hospitalization, and 100-day survival in recipients who received eight allogeneic blood or marrow transplantations (Pavletic, Bishop, Tarantolo, Martin-Algarra, Bierman, & Vose, 1997). Blood stem cell transplantation resulted in faster hematopoietic recovery, shorter hospital stays, and similar survival time. Many issues related to efficacy, adverse effects, and safety remain to be addressed.

Because only data gathered from large randomized clinical trials indicate the superiority of marrow over peripheral blood stem cells, the International Bone Marrow Transplant Registry (IBMTR) and the European Bone Marrow Transplant Registry (EBMT) have entered a joint project. The purpose of the project is to establish a large database of allogeneic peripheral stem cell transplantations with detailed patient, disease, and transplantation-related information to be used to address issues of safety and efficacy. Outcomes to be measured are (1) time to hematopoietic recovery, (2) grade and severity of acute and chronic GVHD, (3) transplant-related mortality and disease recurrence, (4) optimal methods of stem cell collection and CD34+ selection, and (5) T-cell depletion. Comparison of these data with those of marrow GVHD caused by donor T cells is a major complication after allogeneic BMT. Stem cell infusion has a larger ratio of T cells compared with marrow cells, and GVHD may be an even greater problem in PSCT. Other questions relate to the role of the donor.

Early toxicities arising from autologous and allogenic PSCT are reported to be less than those associated with BMT, but because the number of long-term survivors is small because of the infancy of PSCT, morbidity and mortality for these recipients are as yet undertermined.

DISEASES TREATED WITH PERIPHERAL STEM CELL TRANSPLANTATION

Multiple Myeloma

Achieving a complete response in the bone marrow of patients with multiple myeloma using conventional dose chemotherapy is difficult. Median survival generally ranges from 2 to 3 years.

Many questions remain regarding myeloma tumor cell contamination in the peripheral stem cell collection and the relationship of these cells to relapse. The use of various immunologic or pharmacologic purging methods has not been sufficiently investigated, but reports of studies using various methods are beginning to appear in the literature.

Lymphoma

Patients recently diagnosed with intermediate or high-grade NHL or HD have a 40% to 70% cure rate when treated with conventional chemotherapy or radiotherapy. Patients who do not achieve a complete remission or who experience relapse, for the most part, cannot be cured with conventional salvage therapies.

Non–Hodgkin's Lymphoma

Most patients with NHL have developed relapse or refractory disease at the time of PSCT, when the risks associated with the procedure were justified in light of the potential for cure. However, some patients with poor-risk disease received high-dose therapy as consolidation after achieving a complete remission with conventional therapy. A primary issue concerning the use of PSCT in NHL is the timing of the transplantation. Although there are few data regarding long-term outcomes, it appears that long-term responses to high-dose chemotherapy and PSCT are similar to those obtained after marrow infusion, although fewer toxicities, shorter lengths of hospitalization, and reduced costs have been reported.

Hodgkin's Disease

The number of patients with Hodgkin's disease who experience relapse after treatment with high-dose therapy and PSCT is increasing. The vast majority of these patients received this therapy because they had an underlying marrow abnormality that precluded a traditional bone marrow harvest. The ability to harvest the necessary quantity of autologous bone marrow may be limited in these patients because of fibrosis, prior pelvic irradiation, or hypocellularity resulting from extensive chemotherapy.

Questions regarding the superiority of PSCT over autologous BMT are the subject of much research and debate. The Working Party of the European Group for Blood and Marrow Transplantation addressed the question of short-term and long-term advantages of PSCT over autologous BMT. The group reviewed data from 3214 recipients treated for lymphoma; 2859 had marrow transplantations, and 355 had PSCTs. The overall disease-free survival was superior for marrow vs PSCTs, transplant-related mortality was lower but significant, and hematologic recovery occurred more rapidly. However, the study failed to show superiority in the long term. These data reaffirm the need for randomized clinical trials (Majolino, Pearce, Taghipour, & Goldstone).

Leukemia

Initial interest in PSCT for the treatment of acute myelogenous leukemia was based on the premise that there might be less malignant contamination of stem cells than in bone marrow. The additional benefit of rapid hematopoietic reconstitution also was quickly recognized. Future research in PSCT for leukemia should address whether there is a correlation between cell dose and the risk of relapse. Preliminary conclusions that can be drawn are that PSCT offers no advantage in leukemia-free survival over conventional BMT. However, many critical questions about the overall benefit of BCT in acute leukemia have yet to be answered (Yoder, 1997).

Chronic Myelogenous Leukemia

Chronic myelogenous leukemia (CML) cannot be cured with conventional chemotherapy, and there is little evidence to support prolongation of life with high doses of chemotherapy in the chronic phase of disease. Interferon-alpha-2a (IFN-α-2a) allows approximately 70% of patients to achieve a complete hematologic response, and 20% to 40% will achieve a level of cytogenic reversion. Refer to Chapter 8 for a critical discussion of the possible disadvantages of prior IFN treatment to the success of marrow and stem cell transplantation in this patient population.

Epithelial Ovarian Cancer

Seventy-five percent to 80% of women with ovarian cancer have advanced disease (stage III/IV) at the time of diagnosis. The 5-year survival for all cases combined is less than 40%, and ovarian cancer is fifth among causes of cancer death in women. For a less chemosensitive tumor, such as ovarian cancer, multiple cycles of high-dose chemotherapy with repetitive cytoreduction may be needed to produce a cure. The increasing use of stem cells has made such an approach technically possible, and clinical trials evaluating this protocol are underway at several transplantation centers.

Breast Cancer

Various stages (II, IIIa, IIIb, and IV) of breast cancer have been treated with PSCT, using multiple treatment regimens, but the effectiveness of this therapy for metastatic breast cancer has yet to be proven in randomized clinical trials. Two large randomized National Cancer Institute trials are expected to finish patient accrual in 1998, but results will not be available for several years. Few studies of women with stage IV breast cancer have reported disease-free survival rates of more than 3 years. Even in this selected subset of patients with metastatic breast cancer, at best, 30% to 40% will maintain a complete remission beyond 2 years.

Multiple Sclerosis

Multiple sclerosis (MS) is a demyelinating disease of the central nervous system. The disease manifests itself in characteristic relapses, remissions, and primary and secondary progressive stages. Acute MS plaques are notable by their infiltration with lymphocytes and macrophages. Because these cells arise from bone marrow progenitor cells, destruction of the immune system followed by reinfusion of hematopoietic progenitor CD34+ cells may be beneficial for some patients. Only long-term observation can determine if stem cell transplantation can induce durable stabilization of the disease course and prevent further neurologic deterioration, consistent with the arrest of progressive MS (Burt et al., 1998). (Wagner & Quinones, 1998).

THE PROCESS OF PERIPHERAL STEM CELL TRANSPLANTATION

There are numerous phases in a typical PSCT. For the purposes of this chapter they are delineated into five steps: (1) evaluation, (2) stem cell mobilization, (3) apheresis and cryopreservation, (4) dose-intensive therapy and reinfusion, (5) total body irradiation, and (6) engraftment and recovery.

Evaluation

The PSCT process involves an initial clinical evaluation to determine appropriate patients, mobilization of stem cells collecting progenitor stem cells through apheresis cryopreserving or freezing the cells, administering dose-intensive chemotherapy/irradiation and reinfusion, and engraftment and recovery.

Eligibility criteria for PSCT depend on the patient's disease and its status, prior treatment, treatment protocol, age, economic resources, and the presence of a committed family member. Box 9-1 illustrates common tests for patient evaluation.

Patients presenting for PSCT require central venous access for stem cell collection and reinfusion, administration of medications, and drawing blood specimens. A large-bore, permanent or temporary double-lumen catheter such as the Perm Cath (Quinton Instrument Company, Bothell, Wash.)

Box 9-1
Patient Eligibility Characteristics for Peripheral Stem Cell Transplantation

Disease and status treatable with PSCT
Appropriate age, usually not over 65 years
Third-party coverage or ability to pay for PSCT
A family or friend caregiver
History and physical examination to determine organ function
Performance status
Tests usually include:
- Complete blood count, reticulocyte
- Type and cross match, ABO type
- Diagnostic bone marrow aspirate and biopsy
- HLA testing for allogeneic PSCT transplantation
- Urinalysis and creatinine clearance
- Serum or urine pregnancy test
- BUN, creatinine
- SGOT or SGPT, LDH, alkaline phosphate, total/direct bilirubin
- Chest x-ray study
- Pulmonary function tests, DLCO, spirometry
- Arterial blood gases
- Herpes simplex, CMV, varicella-zoster, titers
- HIV antibodies
- Hepatitis B and C surface antigens/antibodies
- Tumor markers
- ECG
- Muga scan
- Bone scan, CT, MRI scans
- Allergy testing (if indicated)
- Dental consult
- Psychosocial consult
- Fertility counseling

HLA, human leukocyte antigen; *BUN,* blood urea nitrogen; *SGOT,* serum glutamic-oxaloacetic transaminase; *SGPT,* serum glutamic-pyruvic transaminase; *LDH,* lactate dehydrogenase; *DLCO,* diffusing capacity of the lung for carbon dioxide; *CMV,* cytomegalovirus; *ECG,* electrocardiogram; *CT* computed tomography; *MRI,* magnetic resonance imaging.

is inserted for stem cell collection to accommodate large and fluctuating circulating blood volumes. Adverse events such a perforation to the venous wall, pneumothorax, and/or hemothorax, although rare, can result during placement. Patients should be monitored closely for signs and symptoms of hypotension, shortness of breath, decreased breath sounds, and/or tracheal shift during the immediate postoperative period. Those presenting with risks for these complications, such as women who have had a mastectomy for breast cancer, may require evaluation for catheter placement in the femoral vein. Patient discomfort, potential risk of contamination, and subsequent infection in this site may necessitate catheter removal after completion of apheresis. After harvest is completed, some clinicians replace the apheresis catheter with temporary or small lumen catheters or with peripherally inserted catheters.

Nursing care of the patient with a central venous catheter includes monitoring patient compliance and patient education in aseptic dressing changes, flushing techniques, and reportable signs and symptoms of infection. Local bleeding may occur and may be prevented or alleviated through the application of ice packs or sandbags at the catheter insertion site. In some instances, substantial amounts of heparin (e.g., 5000 U/ml) may be required to maintain the patency of these large-bore catheters. In these cases, heparin must be removed before accessing the catheter to avoid the coagulopathies consistent with heparin therapy. The patient is then prepared for the next steps: mobilization, stem cell collection, and cryopreservation.

During peripheral stem cell collection, for normal donors it is common practice to use the antecubital vein with an angiocatheter rather than a central catheter. Avoiding catheter-related problems such as infection, catheter maintenance, and general inconvenience is imperative for donor safety and minimizing discomfort. If the donor has adequate venous access, stem cells are collected through a large-bore angiocatheter inserted in the antecubital fossa. Long-term, indwelling catheters are avoided to prevent risks of infection, pneumothorax, and the inconvenience of a catheter. BCTs are obtained based on the recipient's size. If an ABO incompatibility exists between the patient and donor, the cells are processed to accommodate ABO incompatibility (see Chapter 8).

Stem Cell Mobilization

Mobilization is a method to stimulate progenitor marrow cells to the peripheral circulation to be collected, or aphere-sed, and subsequently reinfused. After a sufficient amount of cells are harvested, the cells are mixed with anticoagulants, possibly purged for tumor cells, and cryopreserved until the time for reinfusion. In the case of allogeneic PSCT, stem cells may be collected, processed, and immediately infused into the patient.

Stem cell mobilization is achieved with administration of chemotherapy and recombinant growth factors either alone or in combination in autologous recipients. Allogenic donors receive colony-stimulating factor only (Table 9-2). Current belief is that a combination of these agents provides an optimal stem cell yield with the potential to ensure durable engraftment and disease-free survival. Chemotherapy offers the additional benefit of decreasing tumor burden; but immunosuppression, mucositis, hemorrhagic cystitis, and other dose-related complications can occur. Depending on the dose and duration of therapy, prophylactic antimicrobial agents such as ciprofloxacin and fluconazole may be ordered.

Nursing Management. Nursing management of the patient receiving chemotherapy for mobilization centers around patient preparation, assessment, and management of particular symptoms expected from various agents. Chemotherapy-related complications depend on the agent, dose, and duration of administration. Some complications and management are similar to those manifested during and immediately after high-dose conditioning therapy. Patients with neutropenia require patient teaching in neutropenic precautions, signs and symptoms of infection, and the possibility of hospitalization for septic events. In the event of febrile episodes, patients require cultures of blood, urine, stool, throat, and central venous catheter exit sites. Uroprotectant therapy using mesna (Mesnex, Bristol Myers, Princeton, NJ), bladder irrigation, and forced diuresis are all methods used to prevent hemorrhagic cystitis associated with cyclophosphamide and other alkylating agents. Daily weights are required to determine nutritional status and fluid retention. Obtaining and monitoring complete blood counts, serum electrolytes, and creatinine levels are necessary. Table 9-3 lists common complications and clinical and nursing interventions. Colony-stimulating factors are administered subcutaneously rather than intravenously because of ease of administration and decreased costs compared with intravenous administration. Both patients and caregivers require information on obtaining, reconstituting, administering, and storing the drug, as well as disposal of biohazard wastes. Compliance requires attention, and patients and caregivers benefit from medication diaries to record their doses and sites of injection (King, 1995).

Patients receiving colony-stimulating factors report bone pain, headaches, fevers, nausea, diarrhea, rash, and malaise; but they are usually able to tolerate these side effects. Nursing assessments include identification of bone pain, fever, chills, rigors, fatigue, cough, or nasal congestion. Allergic reactions such as rash, erythema, dry skin, parities, dyspnea, or hypotension are rare, but may occur. Monitoring blood counts and CD34+ cell assays are necessary to determine the effects of colony-stimulating factors on stem cell production.

Stem cells are collected or harvested on an outpatient basis through an apheresis process using the patient's central venous access device and blood cell separators programmed to collect either lymphocytes or low-density leukocytes (Fig. 9-4). The apheresis process takes approximately 2 to 4 hours and requires between three and eight collections over 3 to 5 days to obtain sufficient progenitor cells. The collections are monitored by the total cumulative number of collected nucleated cells, colony-forming unit–granulocyte macrophage (CFU_{GM}), or CD34+ cells. The minimal number of cells needed for successful engraftment is approximately 3 to 5 $\times$ 10^6 CD34+ cells/kg of recipient body weight.

TABLE 9-2 Allogeneic Peripheral Stem Donor Clinical Management

Nursing Diagnosis	Donor Education
Knowledge deficit regarding donor responsibilities and risks	Explain process of obtaining HLA tissue typing. Be available before, during, and after informed consent to answer questions the donor may have. Reassure donor that although there is no data on long-term effects of colony-stimulating factors, few long-term adverse effects have been noted.
Risk of injury related to vascular access and complications secondary to insertion and maintenance of access device	If donor has central venous access, teach management of central catheter relative to patency and infection prevention.
Knowledge deficit regarding mobilization techniques and apheresis procedure	Provide donor with rationale of colony-stimulating factor use to mobilize and collects stem cells. Teach donor reconstitution, self-injection, and hazardous waste methods.
Complications related to colony-stimulating factors	Emphasize possible "flu-like syndrome" effects of colony stimulating factors, such as fever, fatigue, chilling, and bone pain, and their management. Acetaminophen (extra strength) as needed; avoid aspirin products that may cause platelet dysfunction; provide donor with physician access information if discomfort is unrelieved.
Risk for hypocalcemia related to citrate toxicity	Instruct donor to increase calcium intake (dairy products, calcium supplements, calcium-based antacids before and during apheresis
Risk for injury related to thrombocytopenia secondary to apheresis procedure	Explain rationale for routine complete blood counts; teach patient to report petechiae, gum oozing, or nose bleeds.

From Kapustay, P.M. (1997). Peripheral stem cell transplantation program development using the foundation for the accreditation of hematopoietic therapy standards. In P. C. Buchsel (Ed.), *Advance concepts in peripheral stem cell transplantation.* Pittsburgh: Oncology Nursing Press; Buchsel, P., & Kapustay, P. (1995). Blood cell transplantation. *Patient Treatment and Support, 2*(2), 1-14; Wagner, N., & Quinones, V.W. (1998). Allogeneic peripheral blood stem cell transplantation. *Oncology Nursing Forum, 25*(6), 1049-1054.

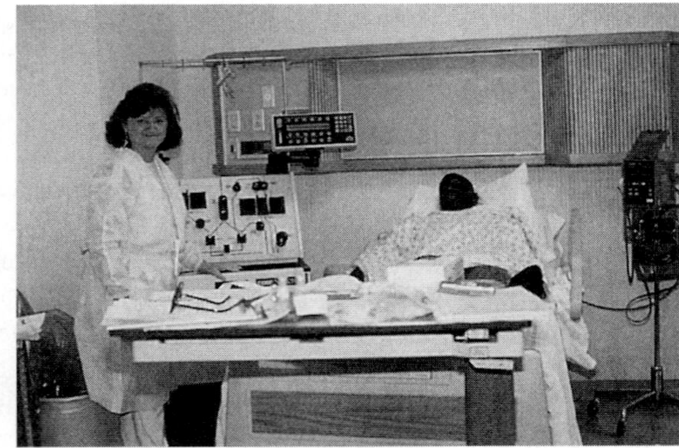

Fig. 9-4 Donor undergoing stem cell collection using the COBE BCT Spectra. (From Gee, A. P. [1988]. Collection and processing of peripheral blood hematopoietic progenitor cells. In J. Reiffers, J. M. Goldman, & J. Armitage [Eds.], *Blood stem cell transplantation.* St. Louis: Martin Dunitz.)

Allogeneic donors receive colony-stimulating factors only for stem cell mobilization. Dosages of up 10 μg/kg/day show a consistent dose-response relationship with the mobilization and collection of CD34+ precursor cells, and this dose is acceptable for routine clinical use. Higher dosages are feared to cause leukocytosis (arbitrarily defined as a leukocyte count of more 70 × 10/9/l). The most commonly reported symptoms by mobilized donors are bone pain, headache, fatigue, and nausea. Other side effects, such as noncardiac chest pain, insomnia, night sweats, low-grade fever, fluid retention, and dizziness, have been reported less frequently. A recent study of donors by a major transplantation center showed that of 280 donors, 53% experienced moderate to severe filgrastim-related toxicities. Of those, 71% took oral analgesics. Despite these problems, less than 2% of donors refused to complete stem cell mobilization and collection. Donors who experience thrombocytopenia (platelet count <80 to 100 × 10/9/l usually remain asymptomatic, but for those who demonstrate bleeding symptoms, reinfusion of autologous platelet-rich plasma may be considered. The total blood volume processed per apheresis for donors is usually 1.5 to 3 times the donor's total blood volume; however, large-volume collections of up to six times the donor's total volume have been reported (Anderlini, Przepiorka, Korbling, & Champlin, 1998).

Apheresis and Cryopreservation

Complications. Morbidity associated with stem cell apheresis is minimal. Complications are usually the result of problems with the central venous catheter, citrate toxicities, and thrombocytopenia. Catheter occlusions are common

TABLE 9-3 Complications of Peripheral Stem Cell Mobilization and Harvest and High-Dose Conditioning Therapy

Complications	Time of Onset	Symptoms	Cause	Clinical Management	Nursing Management
Central Venous Catheter					
Exit site infection	Duration of catheter placement	Fever, skin breakdown, local erythema, pain, tenderness at catheter insertion site, possible purulent drainage, sepsis	Neutropenia secondary to high-dose conditioning regimens, poor catheter management techniques, commonly gram-positive organisms	Vancomycin 1 g IV every 2 h or vancomycin 15 mg/kg IV every 12 h for gram-positive organisms, ceftriazone sodium 1-2g IV every 24 hr	Blood and exit site cultures, administration of antibiotics if indicated. Teach aseptic technique in dressing changes and catheter flushing, signs and symptoms of infection, and emergency instructions
Tunnel infection	As above	Erythema, induration, tenderness along subcutaneous track of catheter, possible purulent exudate	As above	Vancomycin 15 mg/kg every 12 hr for gram+ organisms, ceftriazone sodium 1-2 g IV every 24 hr, possible catheter removal	Blood cultures, culture exudate if present, administer appropriate antibiotics
Line infections	As above	Cellulitis	As above Colonization of infecting organisms, (i.e., *Staphylococcus epidermis, Staphylococcus aureus*)	As above	As above
Catheter occlusion	As above, particularly during apheresis procedure	Inability to aspirate from, or flush catheter, arm swelling, pain may be asymptomatic	G-CSF, GM-CSF Thrombus, technical or mechanical problems, blood clotting, drug precipitate	Venogram, doppler study, dye study, chest x-ray. Urokinase 5,000 IU/mL (urokinase not effective on drug precipitate)	Gentle catheter flushing with heparin, reposition patient, possible catheter removal. Instill urokinase 5000 IU/ml into lumen of catheter and let stand for 5 min Attempt to aspirate every 5 min × 30 min Wait 30-60 min and attempt to aspirate again
Catheter-related venous thrombus	Duration of catheter placement, particularly during mobilization and stem cell collection	Arm swelling, pain may be asymptomatic. Venous congestion in neck on side of catheter	Venous collateral circulation	Venogram, Doppler study, dye study, chest x-ray. Urokinase 5000 IU/ml	Reposition patient, gentle catheter flushing, possible catheter removal, monitor daily prothrombin time/partial prothrombin time

IV, intravenous; *GI,* gastrointestinal; *G-CSF,* granulocyte colony-stimulating factor; *GM-CSF,* granulocyte-macrophage colony-stimulating factor; *GU,* genitourinary; *I & O,* intake and output.

Continued

TABLE 9-3 Complications of Peripheral Stem Cell Mobilization and Harvest and High-Dose Conditioning Therapy—cont'd

Complications	Time of Onset	Symptoms	Cause	Clinical Management	Nursing Management
Central Venous Catheter—cont'd					
Catheter rupture	As above	Pain, shortness of breath, air and blood emboli, leakage from catheter, inability to aspirate catheter	Frequent catheter manipulation, forceful flushing against resistance	Replace catheter	Turn patient on left side and call MD, clean and secure catheter, repair or exchange if possible, possible catheter removal
Phlebitis	0-7 days after insertion	Inflamed area in proximal upper extremity	Peripherally inserted central catheters	Heparin therapy	Apply warm compresses to affected area; may necessitate catheter removal
Infection	Chemotherapy-induced mobilization, high-dose conditioning regimens	Fever, shaking, chills, hypotension	Chemotherapy, *S. aureus*	Prophylactic antimicrobials	Teach neutropenic precautions, monitor prophylactic medications; acyclovir, ciprofloxacin, fluconazole
Skin toxicity	Mobilization, high-dose conditioning regimens	Indurated skin, rash	GM-CSF, G-CSF	Topical cortisones	Assess injection site daily
Hemorrhagic cystis	Mobilization, high dose cyclophosphamide	Hematuria, blood clots	Exposure of bladder lining to cyclophosphamide metabolites, adenovirus	Mesna, aggressive hydration, bladder irrigation may be necessary	Strict I & O, administer mesna and IV fluids
Thrombocytopenia					
Most frequent sites of bleeding: mucous membranes, skin, GI, respiratory and GU systems, intracranial	Chemotherapy induced mobilization, apheresis, high-dose conditioning regimens	Shortness of breath, headache, blurred vision Petechiae, ecchymosis, frank bleeding or oozing from any orifice or injection site	Loss of platelets during stem cell collection Toxic effects of chemotherapy induced mobilization	Monitor platelet count before apheresis Vital signs before and during apheresis Platelet and/or red blood cell transfusion Administer anovulatory therapy for menstruating females. (Begin 1 week before starting chemotherapy, continue until recovery of platelets)	Hematest urine, stool for occult blood, avoid invasive procedures, discontinue drugs that interfere with platelets, institute bleeding precautions, maintain integrity of the skin and mucous membranes Avoid increased intracranial pressure, administer blood products as indicated

Citrate toxicity	Apheresis	Perioral tingling, numbness/tingling in hands and feet, paresthesias, and muscle and/or abdominal cramps	Mixing of blood and anticoagulant (ACD) in apheresis machine resulting in hypocalcemia (free-floating calcium in the blood binds to citrate molecule)	Calcium gluconate 1 g IV every 1 hr as needed throughout duration of procedure	Administer calcium gluconate (Tums) at least 6 tabs/day for 3-4 days before apheresis. Continue throughout the apheresis procedure as needed, monitor vital signs
Flu-like syndrome	Mobilization	Fever, chills, arthralgias, myalgias, chills, headache, malaise	CSFs G-CSF GM-CSF	Acetaminophen 500 mg orally every 4 hr	Administer analgesics, reassure patient that symptoms will resolve after medication is stopped
Mucositis	Mobilization, high-dose conditioning regimens	Pain, facial and throat swelling, airway occlusion, anorexia, difficulty swallowing & talking, divided mucosal lining	Cyclophosphamide Bulsulfan	Opioids, topical anesthetics, infection prophylactic measures Nystatin Bleeding (GI) prophylaxis: carafate	Frequent mouth care with use of toothbrush/floss/toothette, bland rinses with 0.9 saline or saline/sodium bicarbonate. Mucosal coating agents, antacids, sodium alginate, cellulose film, ice bag applications. Assess mouth for signs and symptoms of herpes simplex and candidiasis. Teach patient to avoid irritants such as alcohol and tobacco, monitor nutritional status, avoid mouthwash containing alcohol
Nausea, vomiting	Chemotherapy-induced mobilization, high-dose conditioning regimens	Myriad of symptoms resulting from a complex neurophysiologic phenomenon	Conditioning regimens: bulsulfan, melphalan, thiopeta. Constipation/GI obstruction, infection, medications, anxiety	Ondansetron/decadron, granisetron hydrochloride, lorazepam, diphenhydramine hydrochloride, stool softener, Milk of Magnesia for constipation with ondansetron	Cold, small, bland, frequent liquid meals, decrease external stimuli, hard mints, sour candy. Sour foods are sometimes tolerated. Administer medication as ordered
VOD	High-dose conditioning regimens	Ascites, weight gain, confusion, jaundice	High-dose conditioning	Supportive care, diuretics	Weigh patient 2 times/day, measure abdominal girth

IV, intravenous; *GI,* gastrointestinal; *G-CSF,* granulocyte colony-stimulating factor; *GM-CSF,* granulocyte-macrophage colony-stimulating factor; *GU,* genitourinary; *I & O,* intake and output.

and usually caused from a thrombus or malpositioned catheter secondary to the fluctuating flow rates in the apheresis machine, as well as from the use of recombinant growth factors. Nursing interventions to alleviate decreased blood flow include repositioning the patient, flushing the catheter with mild force, or instilling urokinase to dissolve the clot. A venogram may be indicated to identify catheter obstruction.

Complications can arise as a result of anticoagulant citrate dextrose used to prevent the patient's blood from clotting during apheresis and can be defined as citrate toxicities. Clinical manifestations include circumoral numbness or tingling and cramping in the hands and legs, paresthesis, and muscle and/or abdominal cramps. Administration of oral calcium supplements or intravenous calcium gluconate may be necessary to manage persistent hypocalcemia. Hypovolemia caused by alterations in extracorporeal volume can result in light-headedness, vertigo, tachycardia, hypotension, and arrhythmias. These side effects can be minimized by reducing flow rates or administering blood products. Table 9-3 illustrates nursing management of the patient throughout stem cell collection.

After the stem cells are collected, they are removed from the blood cell separator, isolated using a density gradient or other apheresis procedure to reduce contaminating red and white cells and other cellular debris inadvertently collected. To ensure their viability, the cells are mixed with cryopreservatives until time of reinfusion (Figs. 9-5 and 9-6). Manipulation of cells for tumor reduction may be accomplished through purging techniques; pharmacologic (e.g., mafosfamide), immunologic (e.g. monoclonal antibodies), or physical methods (e.g. density separation) can be used. The cells and their cryopreservatives, often referred to as the *cell product*, are taken to the cryopreservation laboratory and placed in liquid nitrogen. The patient then proceeds to the preparative or conditioning regimen.

Dose-Intensive Chemotherapy and Reinfusion

The doses of chemotherapeutic agents used alone or in combination with radiation therapy are substantially higher than conventional therapy and vary according to the underlying disease or the clinical trial. Most protocols involve 3 to 7 days of conditioning. The conditioning regimen can take place in various care settings, including inpatient and outpatient ambulatory care settings, with supportive care provided in the hospital, local housing facilities, or in the home. Decisions regarding the location of therapy are based on availability of supportive care and types of conditioning regimens.

Busulfan (Myleran), an alkylating agent, is frequently administered in BCT conditioning regimens. Because the medication is taken orally, it is attractive for outpatient administration. Major disadvantages are the administration of a large number of pills and its highly emetic- and seizure-producing properties. Patients require detailed teaching and preparation to manage the protocol as an outpatient. Patients are taught to record the dose and time of swallowing the pills and any resulting emesis. The emesis must be examined for pills, and if any are vomited, the dose must be repeated. Box 9-2 presents a teaching guide for patients receiving busulfan (Myleran).

BCT or stem cell reinfusion occurs several days after high-dose therapy. The day of BCT is referred to as day "0" and following days as Day +1. The cryopreserved stem cells are transported to the patient's room in ice and thawed one at a time in a 98.6° F to 104° F (37° C to 40° C) water bath to prevent cell damage caused by premature thawing and to ensure a continuous infusion of cells. Some protocols require that the thawed stem cells be washed to remove dimethyl sulfoxide and cell lysis products before infusion to minimize side effects. Aggressive hydration is initiated before the infusion and for several hours after to prevent nephrotoxicity associated with the large amount of stem cells reinfused. In addition, premedications such as diphen-

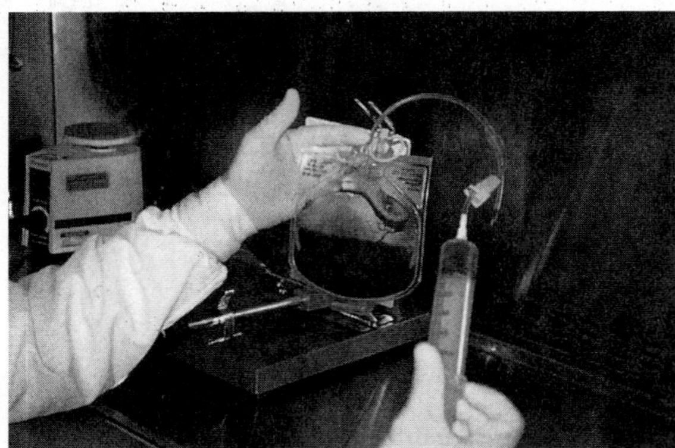

Fig. 9-5 Adding of cryopreservation medium to a stem cell product. Freezing medium is added slowly with mixing to the stem cell products. (From Gee, A. P. [1988]. Collection and processing of peripheral blood hematopoietic progenitor cells. In J. Reiffers, J. M. Goldman, & J. Armitage [Eds.], *Blood stem cell transplantation.* St Louis: Martin Dunitz.)

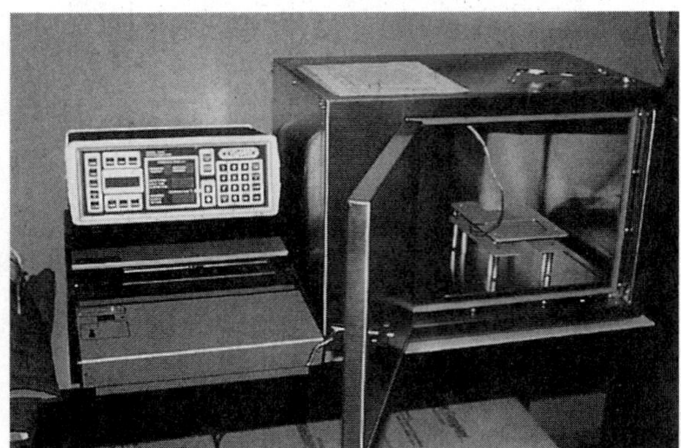

Fig. 9-6 Programmable freezer. The canisters containing the product are stacked horizontally in the freezing chamber *(right).* Liquid nitrogen is pumped into the chamber to achieve the preprogrammed temperature stored in the control device *(upper left).* The temperature of the chamber and a "dummy" product during cryopreservation are printed out by the chart recorder *(lower left).*

hydramine, corticosteroids, acetaminophen, ondansetron, lorazepam, diuretics, or mannitol may be given before reinfusion.

Unirradiated, unfiltered stem cells are infused intravenously piggybacked over 15 to 20 minutes by gravity drip or through a large-bore (60 ml) syringe into the patient's central venous catheter. The infusion is often accompanied by a normal saline infusion to prime the tubing and to clear remaining stem cells from the IV tubing. It is important not to insert medications into the infusion line, because of possible hemolytic reactions.

Complications. Complications usually occur immediately and resolve in 24 to 48 hours. Common adverse effects include nausea, vomiting, facial flushing, hypertension, hypotension, bradycardia, tachycardia, cardiac arrhythmias, tachypnea, cough, chest tightness, fever, chills, and abdominal cramping. Table 9-4 lists common complications, their causes, and nursing management.

Box 9-2

Patient Instruction for High-Dose Myleran Conditioning Regimen for Home Administration

Antiseizure Medication

Phenytoin (Dilantin) is taken to prevent rare seizures that may be caused by busulfan (Myleran). Take Dilantin 12 hours before your first dose of busulfan. This first dose is referred to as *a loading dose* and is a higher dose than doses on the following days. You will need to take this dose in divided doses only on the first day. The following days you will take only one dose a day until 2 days after your last busulfan dose. It is important that you do not drive because the medication can make you drowsy.

Antinausea Medication

Busulfan causes nausea and vomiting. You must take antinausea medication to prevent vomiting before you take your dose of busulfan.

Chemotherapy

Busulfan is a chemotherapy agent that destroys cancer cells. It is usually given 4 times a day until your entire dose is completed. This drug is made only in small doses, but the dose required for you is high. You will need to take about 25 to 30 pills for each of your doses. The pills are placed in a gelatin capsules by the pharmacist to make it easier for you to swallow.

Take busulfan capsules 1 hour before or 1 hour after you eat to reduce nausea.

Take the busulfan with fat-free liquids.

Eat your regular meals between busulfan doses.

If you vomit, examine the vomit for the presence of whole pills only. Retake the same number of whole pills with the replacement dose the pharmacist has given you. Readminister the busulfan from the extra supply the pharmacists has given you.

Record the dose, time, and any replacement medication you take. Bring the medication record to your clinic visit each day.

Medication Record

Patient Name
Date
Dose #1

Medication	Time	Comments
Dilantin	8 AM 2 PM	
Antinausea medication Type ____ Dose ____	____ AM ____ PM	
Myleran	8 AM	Replacement dose No □ Yes □ Number of pills ____
	2 PM	Replacement dose No □ Yes □ Number of pills ____
	8 PM	Replacement dose No □ Yes □ Number of pills ____
	2 PM	Replacement dose No □ Yes □ Number of pills ____

TABLE 9-4 Complications, Symptoms, and Nursing Interventions for Autologous Peripheral Stem Cell Infusion

Cause	Symptoms	Interventions
DMSO toxicity	Nausea, vomiting, diarrhea, severe hemolysis, anaphylactic reaction, occasional bronchospasm, renal failure, diastolic and systolic hypertension, bradycardia, rare pulmonary edema or cardiac arrest	Administer prophylactic premedications (diphenhydramine, corticosteroids, acetaminophen, antiemetics, mild sedative, diuretics, mannitol, and hydration; continue during stem cell infusion to prevent or manage nephrotoxicity; dexamethasone, ondansetron, lorazepam, closely observe patient for somnolence; monitor vital signs every 15 minutes
	Garliclike taste and breath; garliclike odor from urine and stool	Offer hard candy or citrus fruits
	Facial flushing	Offer cool cloths
Stem cell product contamination	Hematuria, increased bilirubin or creatinine	Draw and monitor serum bilirubin and creatinine levels, monitor throughout and daily for 2-3 days after infusion
Allergies	Chills, fever dyspnea, nausea, vomiting	Premedications as above

DMSO, dimethyl sulfoxide.

Although it is tempting to superimpose the long-term complications of BMT onto BCT, one must carefully review the BMT literature to identify those complications related to total-body irradiation (TBI) before assigning these problems to BCT recipients who receive only chemotherapy. For example, in describing cataract development in BMT recipients, researchers found that complications depended on single dose vs fractionated TBI, GVHD, and steroid treatment. Similarly, growth and development problems were linked to the child's age at time of transplantation; prior cranial irradiation; and type, dose, and duration of high-dose therapy. Children who received cyclophosphamide only in conditioning regimens had normal growth rates, whereas children receiving TBI demonstrated decreased growth rates. Consequently, cataract formation after PSCT or growth and development problems in children may be less apparent for recipients who do not receive TBI. However, combinations of cyclosporine and busulfan have altered growth rates in children.

Long-Term Complications. The long-term effects of PSCT will be forthcoming as more PSCT recipients become long-term survivors. Prolonged abnormalities in humoral and cell-mediated immunity have been reported after PSCT, and secondary complications such as varicella-zoster infection and cytomegalovirus infection are not uncommon. Delayed engraftment and graft failure have also been documented.

Total Body Irradiation

Few protocols for peripheral blood cell transplantation use total body irradiation (TBI) in conditioning regimens. Several investigators have reported safe and cost-effective administration of TBI in outpatient settings. Toxicities and their management are discussed in Chapter 8.

Complications. Complications following PSCT depend on the type, dose, and duration of the agents used in the conditioning regimens; supportive medications; graft failure; relapse; and in the allogeneic recipient, GVHD. Other factors that may contribute to the incidence of side effects include age, performance status, and infectious disease profile. Most complications are related to pancytopenia and are similar to those encountered during the mobilization phase and pre-engraftment. (See Chapter 8 for a complete discussion of complications, their causes, supportive care, and nursing management).

Engraftment and Recovery

Care and management of the PSCT recipient do not end with successful engraftment and resolution of all complications. As with PSCT, the outcome of transplantation is not always successful. For patients with disease recurrence, there are numerous physical, psychological, quality of life, family caregiver burden, and economic issues to address.

Discharge criteria for the PSCT recipient, either from the hospital or for return to their referring physician, are highly variable and depend on the condition of the recipient, 24-hour availability of the transplant team, geographic proximity to the transplant facility, availability of transportation to outpatient and emergency facilities, and availability of a competent caregiver. Typically, patients must be free of overwhelming clinical problems, be afebrile, and have a strong family caregiver to manage their care.

ALLOGENEIC BLOOD CELL TRANSPLANTATION

The process of an allogeneic BCT is similar to an allogeneic BMT in patient and donor eligibility.

Allogeneic BCT recipients receive prophylaxis and treatment for GVHD with cyclosporine and corticosteroids. Ini-

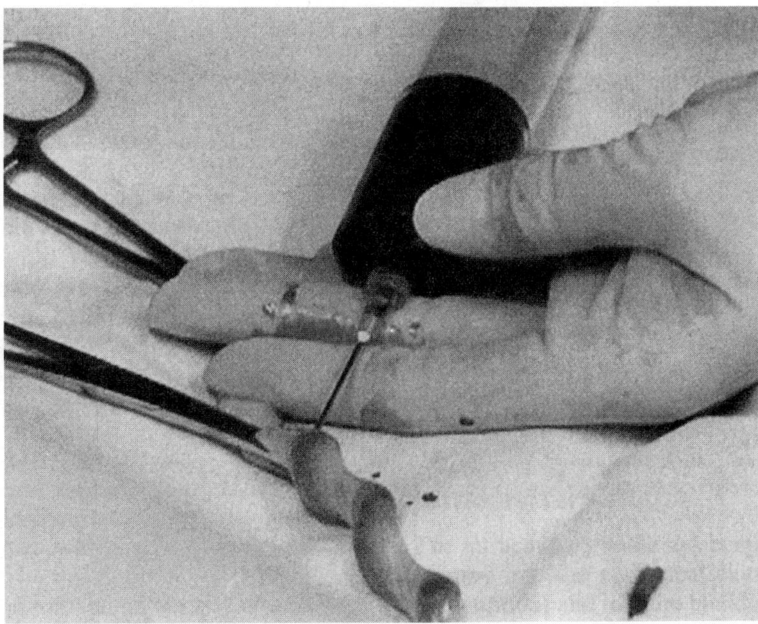

Fig. 9-7 About 25 ml of umbilical blood is drawn from the clamped and cut umbilical cord. (Courtesy Cord Blood Registry, San Bruno, California.)

tial data indicate that the incidence and severity of acute GHVD after allogeneic BCT are not significantly different from those after marrow transplantation. In a small cohort of 73 patients receiving HLA-identical BCT and GVHD prophylaxis, 56% of 23 evaluable patients developed some form of chronic GVHD. Manifestation of chronic GVHD in allogeneic BCT recipients is being studied closely. Initial fears that chronic GVHD would present with even greater morbidity and mortality than in BMT recipients was based on the knowledge that peripheral blood contains approximately 20 times the number of T cells compared with marrow. Because donor T cells cause GVHD, it is postulated that chronic GVHD would be a major limitation to successful BCT.

Although it is believed that BCT is less expensive, less toxic, and as beneficial as BMT, more research is needed to document these potential advantages. Transplantation researchers predict that BCT will replace BMT within the next 5 years, but much research is needed before these predictions become a reality. Currently several randomized clinical trials are comparing PSCT and BMT.

ALTERNATIVE HEMATOPOIETIC SOURCES

Umbilical Cord Blood Transplantations

There is a growing enthusiasm for umbilical cord blood as an alternative for marrow or stem cell transplantation. The advantages of cord blood use are the abundance of the product, possible decreased GVHD compared with marrow and blood, increased number of donors, especially for patients not having a matched donor, and elimination of TBI in conditioning regimens. Another advantage of umbilical blood transplantations is that only a small number of stem cells are collected (Fig. 9-7). Kurtzberg (1996) reported that cord blood transplantations from unrelated donors were successfully engrafted in more than half of a group of high-risk patients, most of them children. Despite the HLA incompatibility, GVHD was mild, which may be expected because most recipients were children who typically demonstrate milder GVHD than adults. One important finding in this study is that placental-blood transplants that differed from the recipients' blood by as many as three HLA antigens or alleles engrafted and produced a trilineage graft and no clinically significant GVHD. Further investigations are warranted to achieve the desired GVHD effect and to determine the incidence and severity of GVHD. Other considerations are the establishment of the GVL benefit for patients not having GVHD (Kurtzberg, 1996)

A subject of major debate is whether placental blood contains sufficient stem cells to repopulate the hematopoietic systems of adults. The controversy is based on the absence of reliable assays to measure cell counts. Also described is the successful engraftment of placental blood from an unrelated donor in a 26-year-old woman with CML weighing more than 50 kg. Similar reports have been submitted by Kurtzberg (1996). These studies suggest that long-term engraftment of placental hematopoietic stem cells is possible in adults who receive relatively small amounts of placental blood.

Umbilical/Placenta Stem Cell Banking

Concomitant with the success of umbilical cord blood transplants is the feasibility of placental blood banks to expedite large-scale placental blood transplantation. These banks could offer quality control of collection, processing, and storage. Universal standards, recently established by the Foundation for Accreditation of Hematopoietic Cell Therapy (FAHCT), may allow for such a model. Issues of consent and testing for infectious diseases (e.g., human immunodeficiency virus [HIV], hepatitis B and C viruses, human T-cell lymphotropic virus types I and II) and genetic disorders (e.g., sickle cell anemia, congenital immunodeficiency disease) remain a serious concern for confidentiality and follow-up care. Questions concerning abnormal genetic results beg the question of what information, if any, should be communicated to the family even though there is no cure or treatment. Such questions pose difficult and interesting challenges to government agencies such as the Food and Drug Administration, ethicists, and transplant physicians.

The number of placental blood transplantations is increasing because the National Heart, Lung, and Blood Institute is supporting a network of placental blood banks. The short-term goal is to produce documentation of the safely and efficacy of this type of transplantation. Future development may include the ex vivo expansion of placental blood stem cell progenitor cells. Other novel approaches include the feasibility of transient placental blood stem cells for gene therapy. As this therapy grows, comparisons with blood and marrow stem cells sources for transplantation warrant study.

Costs of Banking. The cost of storing and collecting placenta blood is usually not covered by third-party payors, but most charges are reasonable. Approximate costs are $25 for a collection kit used by the obstetrician, $25 to collect the blood after delivery, $25 for the storage process, and a $40 a year storage fee.

Ethical Issues

Ethical issues are associated with banking umbilical cord blood. Consensus on these issues was recently published, which represented the work of experts experienced in anthropology, blood banking, stem cell transplantation, ethics, obstetrics, pediatrics, law, and social sciences. The group maintained that (1) although umbilical cord blood technology is promising, much more investigation is needed; (2) secure linkage of the stored cells to the donor must be maintained throughout the investigational stage; (3) umbilical cord blood banking for autologous use is associated with even greater uncertainty than banking for allogeneic use; (4) marketing practices for umbilical banking in the private sector require close attention; (5) more data are needed to ensure the recruitment for banking and use of umbilical cord blood are equitable; and (6) the process of obtaining informed consent for collection should begin before labor and delivery (Sugarman, Kaalund, Kodish, Mashall, Reisher, & Nilfond, 1977).

In Utero Transplantations

In utero transplantation of hematopoietic cells is a novel therapeutic option that may hold promise for families with increased risk of having a child with an inherited disorder. Genetic diseases collectively occur in tens of thousands of births per year, making this treatment option an exciting and hopeful investigational challenge. One of the first marrow transplantations in a fetus was performed to eliminate severe combined immunodeficiency disease (SCID) in 1997. The recipient was the second son of a woman who carried a mutant gene for SCID. Her first son died of the disease at age 7 months. After genetic testing during the second pregnancy determined genetic disease, the father's bone marrow was collected and injected into the abdomen of the fetus in three aliquots administered 1 week apart. This unique approach is based on the knowledge that (1) the immunologic naiveté of the fetus prevents rejection of the donor stem cells and (2) hematopoietic cells expand rapidly in the first trimester (Flake & Zanjani, 1997).

Another option is the use of fetal liver stem cells harvested from aborted fetuses or ectopic pregnancies for in utero transplantation for immunodeficiency disorders such as SCID, hemoglobinopathies, B thalassemia, and sickle cell disease. Ethical imperatives about the use of such sources are the subject of considerable debate. Under the Bush administration, all fetal tissue research was banned, but this decision was subsequently reversed by President Clinton. Although it is now recognized that fetal tissue can be used to understand human development and provide therapeutic strategies, concerns remain that medical gains should not be made thorough the use of fetal tissue because this would legitimize pregnancy termination (Jones, Miles, Warner, Colwell, Bryant, & Warner, 1996). Much research is needed in this area to determine the mode or timing of in utero transplantation, the ideal source and dose of donor cells, estimation of maternal and fetal risk, appropriate candidate diseases, and important ethical issues (Jones, Bui, Ek, Liu, Ringden, & Westgren, 1996). Maternal risks include procedural complications such as infection and bleeding, and fetal risks include infectious disease and GVHD.

Dendritic Cells

Dendritic cells are being studied to enhance patients' immune systems to ward off infectious disease or cancers. Dendritic cells were first identified by Steinman and Cohn in 1973, but modern collection technology was not yet available to implement their use. Dendritic cells are located in the lymphoid and nonlymphoid tissue such as the dermis and epidermis. When a foreign antigen enters the skin, an immune response is initiated in which the antigen-presenting dendritic cell travels through the lymphic system to the T cell–containing lymph nodes. Dendritic cells can be collected from patients and treated with CD34+ cells, treated with cytokines such as interleukin (IL)-4, stem cell factor, IL-13, tumor necrosis factor-alpha, and flt-3 ligand protein to stimulate the growth and differentiation of dendritic cells. Phase II clinical trials are now in progress because large numbers of dendritic cells grown from CD34+ cells collected from patients or volunteer donors can be collected and infused into patients. Dendritic cells travel directly to the spleen when given intravenously, whereas subcutaneous administration allows them to journey through lymphoid tissue. Researchers have treated patients with B cell lymphoma by collecting patient CD34+ cells, loading them with the B-cell tumor-associated antigen, and administering the cells intravenously. All patients tolerated the procedure without significant adverse effects, and they subsequently developed a cellular response (Engelman, 1996). Further areas of research include (1) the optimal culture medium in which to grow these cells, (2) loading antigens, (3) determining the number of dendritic cells required, and (4) treatment efficacy (DeMeyer, 1997).

ADOPTIVE IMMUNOTHERAPY

Donor Leukocyte Infusions

Recipients of stem cell transplantation for hematologic malignancies are at considerable risk for treatment failure or relapse because dose-limiting toxicities in conditioning regimens are barriers to sufficient tumor kill. Patients relapsing after allogeneic BMT have few treatment options. New approaches to eliminate this problem include administration of donor lymphocyte infusions for allogeneic recipients and GVHD induction for autologous recipients. Both techniques are based on inducing the GVL effect.

The GVL effect has been recognized for decades and is discussed at length in Chapter 8. Early studies demonstrated that recipients of allogeneic BMT with chronic GVHD had a lower relapse rate than those with no GVHD (identical twin donors) or those receiving T-cell–depleted marrow. These observations led researchers to suggest a GVL, mediated in part by donor T cells. Donor lymphocytes, mobilized with CSFs, adhered and subsequently infused into the patient (donor lymphocyte infusion) is being used to prevent or reverse transplant relapse. The most striking evidence in support of this effect is that 70% of patients with CML who experience relapse can achieve remission with donor lymphocyte infusions. The toxicity associated with donor lymphocyte infusion may be significant if severe GVHD or marrow toxicity from lymphocyte infusion occurs (Collins, Shpilberg, Drobyski, Porter, Giralt, & Champlin, 1997). GM-CSF modified donor lymphocyte infusions, raising the perennial question of the possible long-term effects of CSF in healthy donors.

Autologous Graft Versus Host Disease

Autologous marrow recipients experience fewer regimen-related toxicities than allogenic recipients because of GVHD. As stated previously, GVHD does confer some benefit relative to reducing relapse rates. The challenge is to induce sufficient GVHD without causing GVHD severe enough to harm the patient. Current studies in breast cancer, lymphoma, leukemia, and myeloma are underway in this effort. Autologous GVHD is induced by administering low-dose cyclosporine after transplantation. The clinical syndrome of autologous GVHD is characterized by a mild skin rash, but other organ involvement such as the gastrointestinal tract and liver is rarely demonstrated. Other antitumor strategies are to induce autologous GVHD using a combination of cyclosporine, IL-2, and interferon-alpha. Adverse effects include possible nephrotoxicity secondary to cyclosporine administration and flu-like syndrome from interferon-alpha.

Graft Failure in Allogeneic Stem Cell Transplantation

Patients with engraftment failure after allogeneic BMT also have been treated with allogeneic stem cells from the donor. From clinical use in two patients, Arseniev and colleagues concluded that CD34+ cells immunoselected from the stem cells of an HLA-identical sibling donor are appropriate for the treatment of bone marrow graft failure. However, the risk of severe GVHD prompted by such an infusion is still unknown. To determine whether allogeneic T-cell–depleted immunoselected CD34+ or unmanipulated stem cells produce full hematopoietic recovery requires clinical trials with larger numbers of patients.

HOME CARE ISSUES

With the institution of PSCT transplantations and their decreased toxicities compared with BMT, most institutions are offering and marketing "new models of care" for patients and their families. Candidates and their family caregivers are usually given the opportunity to receive part or all of their care in an outpatient area, provided they are clinically stable. Although appearing to be "new" models, most research centers have offered this type of care for many years. For institutions requiring certification by the FAHCT, however, critical staffing and geographic criteria must be met (Table 9-5). Residential living facilities located within walking distance of the clinic and designed for the immunosuppressed and debilitated patient require careful planning. This model has been described elsewhere (Buchsel & Kapustay, 1995). Although several transplantation centers offer "outpatient" transplantations, few, if any, actually administer conditioning regimens in the outpatient area. Typical outpatient regimens admit patients to the hospital for conditioning and resolution of mucositis or other acute complications and then discharge patients to the outpatient setting for 24-hour follow-up. Recipients are readmitted to the hospital for fevers, organ dysfunction, and GVHD, if necessary.

Costs

Successful models can reduce the overall number of hospital days, thereby decreasing costs. Although published studies are emerging relative to cost reduction of outpatient models, few cost analysis studies have captured the direct and indirect costs associated with this type of care. For example, one of the earliest studies assessing the feasibility of outpatient transplantation selected patients receiving the condition regimen combinations cyclophosphamide/

TABLE 9-5 Minimal Criteria for a Blood Cell Transplant Program

Components	Criteria
The Clinical Program	Integrated medical team housed in geographically contiguous space with a Program Director, common training programs, protocols, and quality assessment systems
	Access to accredited collection and process laboratory that meet the standards for the Foundation for the Accreditation of Hematopoietic Cell Therapy (FAHCT) and American Blood and Marrow Transplant Registry
Allogeneic BCT units	Access to blood bank providing 24-hour service for CMV-blood products; HLA testing laboratory accredited by the American Society of Histocompatibility and Immunogenetics; and the capability of performing deoxyribonucleic acid-based HLA typing
Accreditation criteria	Minimum of 10 transplantations performed year before application for program accreditation
	Perform minimum of 10 BCTs per year of each type (allogeneic or autologous) for which the program is accredited
Institutional Review Board	Formal review of investigational treatment protocols and patient consent forms approved by the Office for Protection from Research
Blood Cell Transplant Team	
Program Transplant Director	Responsible for administrative and medical operations of the clinical transplantation program, including compliance with standards. Licensed to practice medicine in the United States or Canada and board certified (or non-Untied States/Canadian equivalent) in one or a combination of: hematology, medical oncology, immunology, and/or pediatrics
Attending physicians	Demonstrate a minimum 1-year experience in management of transplant recipients in both inpatient and outpatient settings
	Understand indications for BCT
	Ability to perform evaluation and selection for BCT
	Management of high-dose chemotherapy and irradiation, growth factors, neutropenic fever, bacterial, viral, and fungal infection, veno-occlusive disease, thrombocytopenia, hemorrhagic cystitis, nausea and vomiting, pain, posttransplant immunodeficiencies, acute and chronic GVHD and terminal care
	Blood cell infusion management
	Allogeneic PSCT considerations
	Identify and select appropriate blood cell sources for BCT, including donor registries
	Demonstrate knowledge of human leukocyte antigen typing, ABO-incompatible hematopoietic progenitor cell components
Consulting physicians	Board certified in surgery, pulmonary intensive care, gastroenterology, nephrology, infectious disease, cardiology, pathology, psychiatry, and radiation therapy
Collection Medical Director	Ensures compliance with all medical aspects of the cell processing facilities (i.e., donor care)
Laboratory Medical Director	Responsible for all administrative operations of the cell processing facility, including all medical aspects of the activities of the cell processing facility
Laboratory Director	Responsible for administrative operations of cell processing facility, including compliance with FAHCT standards
	Possess PhD in appropriate discipline
Nursing	
Nursing supervisor	Formally trained and experienced in the management of patients receiving BCTs care
Nursing staff	Training in hematology/oncology patient care, ability to perform pediatric and outpatient care when appropriate, administration of high-dose therapy, growth factors, blood component therapy, management of infectious complications
	Nurse:patient ratios satisfactory to cover the severity of patient clinical status
Pharmacy	Ensure appropriate use and management of pharmaceuticals
Dietary	Provide dietary consultations regarding patients' nutritional status, including total parenteral nutrition
Other	Social services and physical therapy
	Staff to provide efficient pretransplant patient evaluation and coordinate treatment and post-transplant follow-up care
Clinical Unit	
Inpatient	Written policies for all procedures, including prevention and infection control and administration of high-dose therapy, immunosuppressive agents, and blood component therapy
	Create designated inpatient unit that minimizes airborne microbial contamination

Modified from Foundation for the Accreditation of Hematopoietic Cell Therapy (FAHCT). *CMV,* cytomegalovirus; *HLA,* histocompatibility locus antigen; *BCT,* blood cell transplantation.

TABLE 9-5 Minimal Criteria for a Blood Cell Transplant Program—cont'd

Components	Criteria
Clinical Unit—cont'd	
Outpatient care	Create patient care area reasonably free of infectious agents Provide administration of long-term infusions and blood products
Emergency care	Prompt 24-hour evaluation and treatment by an attending transplant physician
Other Departments	
Data management	Complete and accurate patient records required by the International Bone Marrow Transplant Registry (IBMTR) or Autologous Bone Marrow Transplant Registry (ABMTR).
Quality management plan	Responsible for review and approval of policies and procedures that document compliance with regulatory requirements and standards Provide documentation of research protocols Ensure Institutional Review Board protocol approval Document implementation of new drugs or devices with any adverse outcomes Develop system for detection, evaluation, documenting and reports errors, accidents, and adverse reactions

cisplatin/carmustine because of the limited amount of mucositis associated with these agents compared with regimens containing TBI or high-dose melphalan or thiotepa. The investigators showed that the regimen was well tolerated, allowing 95% of eligible patients to be discharged soon after chemotherapy and followed up by outpatient care. Of those, 70% required no or brief hospitalization of 1 to 4 days (Peters, Ross, Vredenburg, Husseinn, Rubin, & Dukelow et al., 1994).

A Canadian team reported its experience with 51 consecutive patients treated for metastatic breast cancer who were managed in outpatient settings. Strategies used were symptom management with once daily prophylactic oral antibiotics, GM-CSF, ketoconazole, acyclovir, and instructions in scrupulous hygiene (Clever & Goldman, 1998).

The Community Setting

A landmark study documented the feasibility of offering PSCT in the community setting. Weaver and colleagues described 100-day treatment mortality of the first 1000 consecutive patients receiving high-dose myeloablative chemotherapy within a multicentered community-based clinical trials program (Weaver, Schwartzberg, Hainsworth, Greco, Li, & Bucker, 1997). Thirty-four patients experienced treatment-related mortality, 15 patients died from infection, and 19 died from regimen-related toxicities. Increasing age and lower numbers of CD34+ cells per kilogram were associated with an increased risk of 100-day mortality. Patient age, the type of preparative regimen, and the number of CD34+ cells infused were important determinants of morbidity. These data documented no apparent increase in treatment-related mortality compared with published reports of similar regimens.

Family Caregivers

Family caregiver burden is inherent for those caring for transplant recipients. Although clinical observations and anecdotal accounts report significant caregiver burden in marrow transplant recipients, few published reports exist regarding peripheral stem cell recipients. Much information, however, can be extrapolated from the BMT literature. One must be cautious and look at the severity of the clinical status of the recipient, rather than the stem cell source, to assess for caregiver burden. Eliers studied baselines scores of 81 family caregivers in the BMT population. Baseline data indicated that family members enter transplant at varying levels of family function. Family stressors, family strains, family distress, social support, and relative and friend support instruments showed scores higher than established norms; and family hardiness and social support scores were lower than established norms. Rivera (1997) noted the pivotal role that family and friends play in maintaining quality of life in recounting her personal story as a wife/oncology nurse caring for her husband who received a stem cell transplant. In her own studies in this area, Rivera (1997) noted the role of family and friends in maintaining quality of life in BMT survivors. A total of 465 questionnaires were mailed to BMT recipients requesting them to identify a personal exemplar of the impact of family and friends during their treatment. A total of 296 surveys were returned (64%). The findings of the study stressed the need to (1) sensitize oncology nurses to the importance of providing psychological support for family and friends of transplant recipients, (2) educate family and friends about the important role that they play in maintaining quality of life for transplant recipients, and (3) encourage ongoing research to describe the impact of cancer and its treatment on family and friends (Rivera & Grant, 1997).

As nonhospitalized patients and family caregivers participate in increasingly complex self-care management and coping strategies, there is a more critical need for collaborative nursing research studies to identify methods to decrease stressors associated with these new care environments. Family caregivers require special attention and education to prepare them for the responsibilities in managing the patient throughout the transplant trajectory. Stetz and

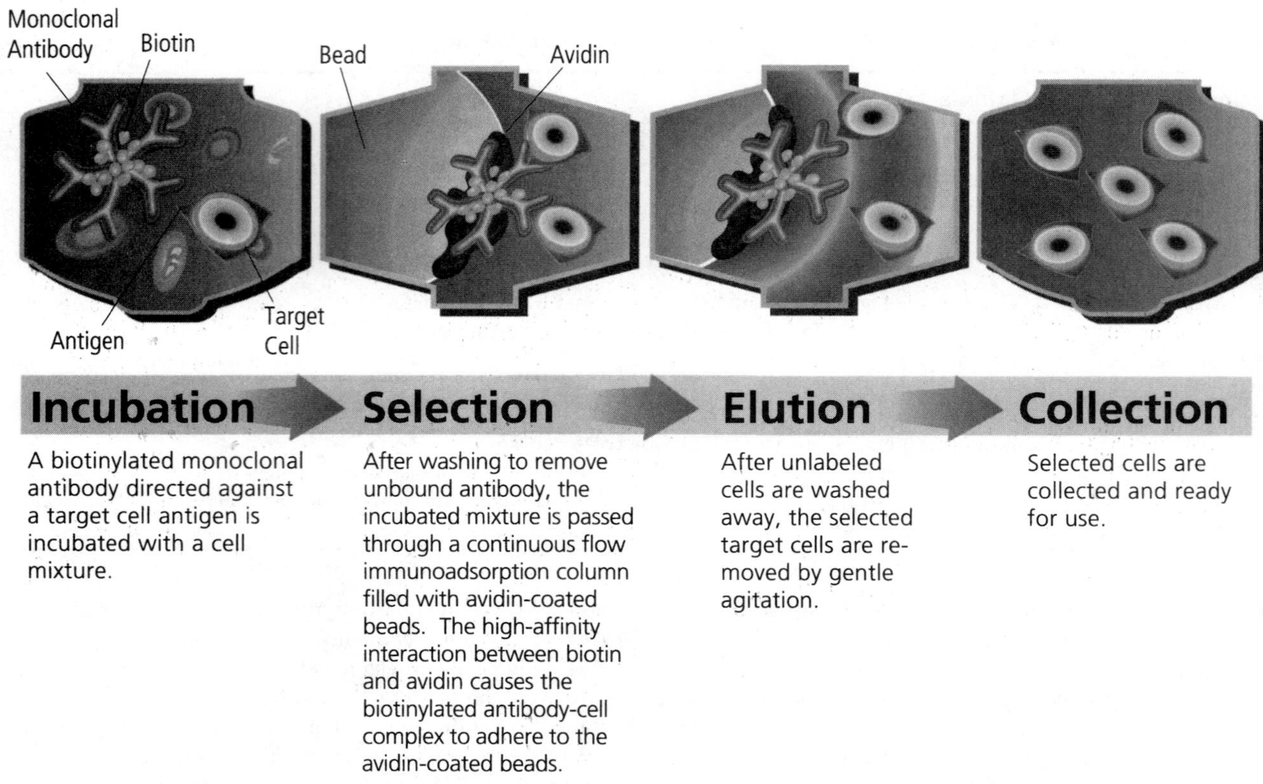

Fig. 9-8 A schematic of a stem cell purging process using Cell Pro.

colleagues (1996) recently identified family caregiver needs so that transplantation teams may provide optimal support to them. Families identified the following needs: assistance in selecting the most qualified transplant center, assistance in obtaining accurate information about the patient's diagnosis and treatment, strategies to manage patient care in the home, and opportunities for them to obtain support. Thus educational and supportive programs to provide family caregivers with knowledge and respite care will allow family members to share in the care of the BCT recipient. Institutions implementing support systems that offer caregivers respite have been shown to diminish caregiver stress (Compton, McDonald, & Stetz, 1996). Not all patients have willing family caregivers. In these cases, some centers have created a bank of approved "lay" people capable of assisting patients with some aspects of their outpatient management.

FOUNDATION FOR ACCREDITATION OF HEMATOPOIETIC CELL THERAPY STANDARDS

The major objective of the FAHCT is to promote quality medical and laboratory practice in hematopoietic progenitor cell transplantation. Facilities accredited by FAHCT are required to meet, at a minimum, criteria for centers performing blood and marrow transplantation as outlined in Table 9-5. The standards apply to all sources of hematopoietic progenitor cells and all phases of collection, processing, and administration of bone marrow, peripheral blood, or placental/umbilical cord blood (FAHCT Standards, 1996; Kapustay, 1997)

The standards were initially developed by the Regulatory Affairs Committee of the International Society for Hematotherapy and Graft Engineering (ISHAGE) and a subcommittee of the Clinical Affairs Committee of the American Society of Blood and Marrow Transplantation (ASBMT). In December 1994, the ISHAGE laboratory standards and the ASBMT clinical standards were merged into a single document, and FAHCT was established to develop and implement the accreditation program. Accreditation is determined by evaluation of the written information provided by the applicant facility and by on-site inspection. Site inspections are performed every 3 years by persons expert in hematopoietic cell therapy. Institutions currently performing transplantations and who wish to be accredited are assessing or revising their current guidelines to prepare for FAHCT accreditation. The financial impact of creating administrative and clinical positions may appear to increase the cost of care, but because of the growing number of transplantations for stem cell sources such as allogeneic and umbilical cord quality must be assured.

FUTURE TRENDS

PBCT and umbilical stem cell transplantations are likely to replace BMT. In utero transplantations for genetic diseases will continue to be the subject of considerable investigation,

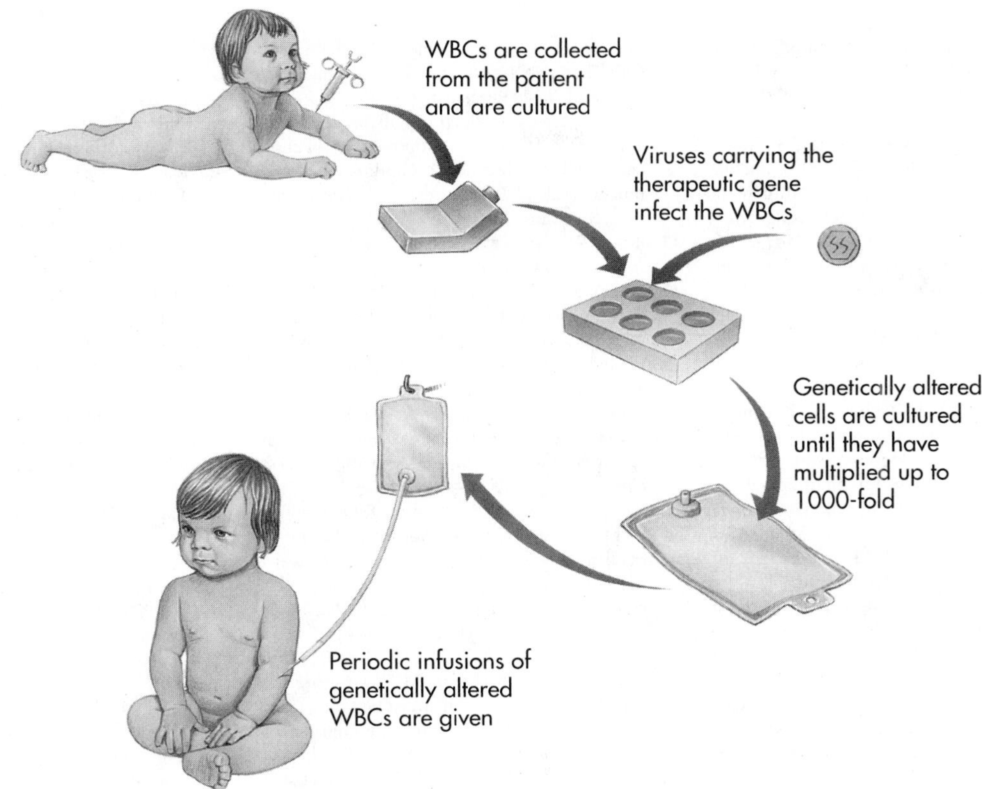

Fig. 9-9 Ex vivo expansion.

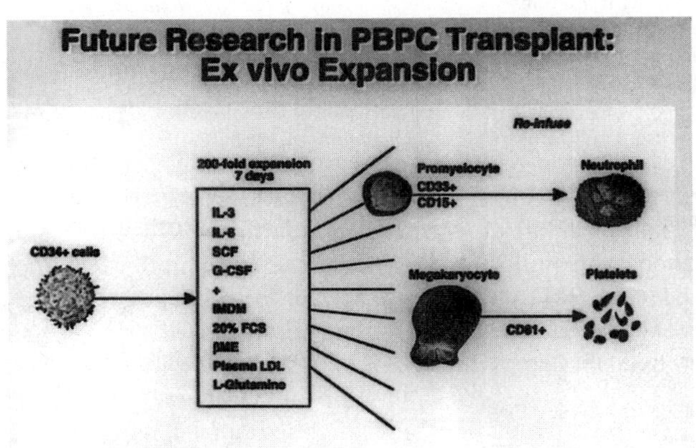

Fig. 9-10 Gene therapy. (Thibodeau, G., & Patton, K. T. [1996]. *Anatomy and physiology.* [3rd ed.]. St. Louis: Mosby.)

but ethical issues may prevail. Diseases traditionally treated by PSCT can be expanded to autoimmune diseases such as rheumatoid arthritis, multiple sclerosis, and scleroderma, possibly offering cure to hundreds of thousands of patients. The rationale of treating autoimmune diseases with stem cells is that these diseases are the result of an altered immune response leading to an attack by the immune system against host antigens. Only ongoing clinical trials can establish stem cell transplantation as a safe and cost-effective therapy compared with current supportive care measures.

Treatment failure or relapse remains one of the major impediments to successful allografting. Research on techniques for separation of hematopoietic stem cells include studies of sedimentation techniques, monoclonal antibodies, and immunoabsorption columns (Fig. 9-8). Fetal liver stem cell transplantations have been reported in treatment of selected patients with SCID. Successful allogeneic stem cell transplants for children and adults using umbilical cord blood are now being reported. Early fears that GVHD would be an insurmountable problem have not materialized. The ability to use cord blood has generated cord blood banks to store this tissue for possible autologous use and for unrelated ethical diverse transplantations. Cord blood may be an optimal vehicle for gene therapy and treatment of metabolic diseases such as thalassemia and Fanconi's anemia (Fig. 9-9).

Gene transfer holds dramatic promise for future applications of BMT and other genetic diseases. This involves replacement of defective genetic material with healthy genes in marrow transplantation candidates with genetic diseases. Use of dendritic cells to mount immune-mediated responses to cancer and other diseases may negate the need for transplantation itself. The use of ex vivo expansion in concert with cytokine cocktails may make it possible for donors to give only a few milliliters of blood to be expanded and administered to patients after they have received chemotherapy (Fig. 9-10). This phenomenon would enhance the recruitment of unrelated donors, as predicted by Thomas (1989).

REFERENCES

Anderlini, K., Przepiorka, D., Korbling, M., & Champlin, R. (1998). Blood stem cell procurement: Donor safety issues. *Bone Marrow Transplantation, 21,* S35-S39.

Bensinger, W., Appelbaum, F., Rowley, S., Storb, R., Sanders, J., & Lilleby, K. (1995). Factors that influence collection and engraftment of autologous peripheral-blood stem cells. *Journal of Clinical Oncology, 13*(10), 2547-2555.

Buchsel, P., & Kapustay, P. (1995). Blood cell transplantation. *Patient Treatment and Support, 2*(2), 1-14.

Buchsel, P.C., & Whedon, M.B. (1995). (Eds.), *Bone marrow transplantation: Issues and clinical strategies.* Boston: Jones & Bartlett.

Burt, R. K., Traynor, A. E., Cohen, B., Karlin, K. H., Davis, F. A., & Steforeski, D. (1998). T-cell depleted autologous hematopoietic stem cell transplantation for multiple sclerosis: Report on the first three patients. *Bone Marrow Transplantation, 21,* 537-541.

Clever, S. A., & Goldman, J. M. (1998). Use of G-CSF to mobilize PBSC in normal healthy donors—an international study. *Bone Marrow Transplantation, 21,* Supplement 3, S29-31.

Coiffier, B., Phillip, T., Burnett, A. K,. & Symann, M. L. (1994). Consensus conference on intensive chemotherapy plus hematopoietic stem-cell transplantation in malignancies. Lyon France, June 4-6, 1993. *Journal of Clinical Oncology, 12,* 226-231.

Collins, R. H., Jr., Shpilberg, O., Drobyski, W. R., Porter, D. L., Giralt, S., & Champlin, R. (1997). Donor leukocyte infusions in 140 patients with relapsed malignancy after allogeneic bone marrow transplantation. *Journal of Clinical Oncology, 15*(2), 433-444.

Compton, K., McDonald, J. C., & Stetz, K. M. (1996). Understanding the caring relationship during marrow transplantation: Family caregivers and healthcare professionals. *Oncology Nursing Forum, 23,* 1428-1432.

DeMeyer, E. (1997). Advanced concepts in peripheral stem cell transplantation. In P. B. Buchsel (Ed.), *Advanced concepts in peripheral stem cell transplantation.* Pittsburgh: Oncology Nursing Press.

Dreger, Haferlach, Eckstein, Jacobs, Suttarp, Happler, Mueler-Ruchholtz, & Schmitz (1994).

Eliers, J. (1997). Stressors, strains, distress, resources and supports: Longitudinal study of families of adult BMT recipients. *Oncology Nursing Forum, 24,* 323 (Abstract 147).

Engelman, E. C. (1996). Dentritic cells in the treatment of cancer. *Biology of Blood and Marrow Transplantation, 2,* 115-117.

Faucher, C., Le Corroller, A. G., Blaise, D., Novakovitch, G., Manonni, P., & Moatti, J. P. (1994). Comparison of G-CSF-primed peripheral blood progenitor cells and bone marrow auto transplantation: Clinical assessment and cost-effectiveness. *Bone Marrow Transplant, 14,* 895-901.

Flake, G. W., & Zanjani, E. D. (1997). *In utero* hematopoietic stem cell transplantation. *Journal of the American Medical Association, 278,* 932-937.

Fliedner, T. M., Calvo, W., Korbling, M., & et al. (1978). Hematopoietic stem cells in blood: Characteristics and potentials. In D. W. Gold, et al. (Eds.), *Hematopoietic cell differentiation, ICN-UCLA Symposia on Molecular Biology, Vol X.* New York: Academic Press.

Foundation for Accreditation of Hematopoietic Cell Therapy. (1996). Standards of care. Location published: Publisher.

Gee, A. P. (1998). Collection and processing of peripheral blood hematopoietic progenitor cells. In J. Reiffers, J. M. Goldman, & J. Armitage (Eds.), *Blood stem cell transplantation.* St. Louis: Mosby.

Golde, D.W. (1991). The stem cell. *Scientific American, December,* 86-93.

Goodman, J. W. & Hodgson, C. S. (1962). Evidence for stem cues in the peripheral blood of mice. *Blood, 19,* 702-714.

Gratwohl A. (1998). Forward. *Bone Marrow Transplant,* (21), S.

Gratwohl, A., Hermans, J., & Baldomero, H. (1996). Indications for hemopoietic precursor cell transplants in Europe. *British Journal of Haematology, 92,* 35-43.

Jones, A. C., Miles, E. A., Warner, J. O., Colwell, B. M., Bryant, T. N., & Warner, J. A. (1996). Fetal peripheral blood mononuclear cell proliferative responses to mitogenic and allergenic stimuli during gestation. *Pediatric Allergy and Immunology, 7*(3), 109-116.

Jones, D. R. E., Bui, T.-H., Ek, S., Liu, T. D. Y., Ringden, O., & Westgren, M. (1996). *In utero* hematopoietic stem cell transplantation: Current perspectives and future potentials. *Bone Marrow Transplantation, 18,* 831-837.

Juttner, C.A., Fibbe, W.E., & Neumunaitis, J. (1994). Blood cell transplantation: Report form an international consensus meeting. *Bone Marrow Transplantation, 14,* 689-693.

Kapustay, P. M. (1997). Peripheral stem cell transplantation program development using the foundation for the accreditation of hematopoietic cell therapy standards. In P. C. Buchsel (Ed.), *Advanced concepts in peripheral stem cell transplantation.* Pittsburgh: Oncology Nursing Press.

King, C. R. (1995). Peripheral stem cell transplantation: Past, present, and future. In P. C. Buchsel, & M. B. Whedon (Eds.), *Bone marrow transplantation.* Boston: Jones & Bartlett.

Korbling, M., & Fliedner, T. M. (1996). The evolution of clinical peripheral blood stem cell transplantation. *Bone Marrow Transplantation, 17,* S4-S11.

Kurtzberg. (1996). Placental blood as a source of hematopoietic stem cells for transplantation into unrelated recipients. *New England Journal of Medicine, 335,* 157-166.

Linch, D.C., Rodeck, C.H., Nicolaldes, K., Jones, H.M., & Brent, L. (1986). Attempted bone-marrow transplantation in a 17-week fetus. [Letter] *Lancet, 2,* 1453.

Majolino, I., Pearce, R., Taghipour, G., & Goldstone, A. H. (1997). Peripheral-blood stem-cell transplantation versus autologous bone marrow transplantation in Hodgkin's and non-Hodgkin's lymphomas: A new matched-pair analysis of the European Group for blood and marrow transplantation registry data. *Journal of Clinical Oncology, 15,* 509-517.

Maximov, A. (1909). Der Lymphozyt als gemeinsame Stammzelle Der verschideneen Blutelemente in der embryonalen Entwicklung und im postfetalen Leben der Saugetiere. *Folia Haemat, 8,* 125-141.

Messner, H.A., & McCulloch, E.A. (1994). Mechanisms of human hematopoiesis. In S. J. Formon, K. G. Blume, & E. D. Thomas (Eds.), *Bone marrow transplantation.* Boston: Blackwell Scientific Publishers.

Pavletic, Z. S., Bishop, M. R., Tarantolo, S. R., Martin-Algarra, S., Bierman, P. J., & Vose, J. M. (1997). Hematopoietic recovery after allogeneic blood stem-cell transplantation compared with bone marrow transplantation in patients with hematologic malignancies. *Journal of Clinical Oncology 15,* 1608-1616.

Peters, W. P., Ross, M., Vredenburg, J. J., Husseinn, A., Rubin, P., Dukelow, K., Cavanaugh, C., Beauvais, R., & Kasprzak, S. (1994). The use of intensive clinic support to permit outpatient autologous bone marrow transplantation for breast cancer. *Seminars in Oncology, 21,* 25-31.

Rivera, L. M. (1997). Blood cell transplantation: The impact on one family. *Seminars in Oncology Nursing, 13,* 194-199.

Rivera, L. M. & Grant, M. (1997). The role of family and friends in maintaining quality of life in bone marrow transplantation survivors. *Oncology Nursing Forum, 24,* 323 (Abstract 146).

Stetz, K. M., McDonald, J. C., & Compton, K. (1996). Needs and experiences of family caregivers during marrow transplantation. *Oncology Nursing Forum 23* (9), 1422.

Sugarman, J., Kaalund, V., Kodish, E., Marshall, M. F., Reisner, E. G., & Wilfond, B. S. (1997). Ethical issues in umbilical cord blood banking. *Journal of the American Medical Association, 278,* 938-943.

Szilvassy, S.F., & Hoffman, R. (1995). Enriched hematopoietic stem cells: Basic biology and clinical utility. *Biology of Bone Marrow Transplantation, 1,* 3-17.

Thomas, E. D. (1995). History, current results, and research in marrow transplantation. *Perspectives in Biology and Medicine, 38*(2), 230-237.

Thomas, E. D. (1989). The future of marrow transplantation. *Seminars in Oncology Nursing, 4,* 74-78.

To, L. B. (1995). Mobilizing and collecting blood stem cells. In R. P. Gale, C. A. Juttner, & P. Henon (Eds.), *Blood stem cell transplants.* New York: New York Press Syndicate of the University of Cambridge.

Vescio, R. A., Hong, C. H., & Cao (1994). The hematopoietic stem cell antigen, CD34, is not expressed on the malignant cells in multiple myeloma. *Blood, 84,* 3283-3290.

Wagner, N., & Quinones, V. W. (1998). Allogeneic peripheral blood stem cell transplantation. *Oncology Nursing Forum, 25*(6), 1049-1054.

Weaver, C. H., Schwartzberg, L. S., Hainsworth, F. A., Greco, F. A., Li, W., & Bucker, C. D. (1997). Treatment-related mortality in 1000 consecutive patients receiving high-dose chemotherapy and peripheral blood progenitor cell transplantation in community cancer centers. *Bone Marrow Transplantation, 19,* 671-678.

Yoder, L. (1997). Diseases treated with blood cell transplantation. *Seminars in Oncology Nursing, 13,* 164-171.

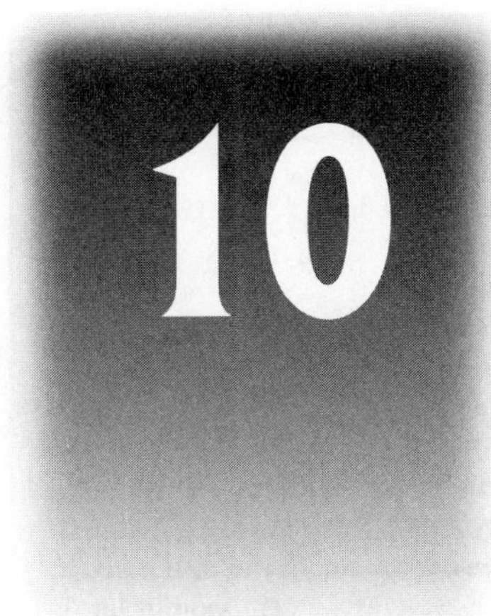

Gene Therapy

Christine Miaskowski, RN, PhD, FAAN

INTRODUCTION

Gene therapy is a therapeutic technique in which a functioning gene is inserted into a cell to correct a metabolic abnormality or to introduce a new function (Hwu & Rosenberg, 1997). This therapy should be useful in the treatment of cancer because cancers are the result of genetic mutations or the loss of genetic material. Therefore it seems reasonable to assume that, if the genetic abnormality were corrected, the cancer cell would no longer express the malignant phenotype.

The idea of gene therapy is not a new concept. In fact, Runnebaum (1997) points out that "the basic concept of human gene therapy has a history of more than twenty years," citing the reference by Friedmann and Roblin (1972).

Gene therapy represents an attempt to take lessons learned in the basic science laboratory (e.g., oncogenes; see Chapter 1) and apply them to the treatment of human cancers (Fine & Kufe, 1997). This form of cancer therapy has generated a great deal of interest and has been the subject of a large number of review articles (Bank, 1996; Barnes, Deshane, Rosenfield, Siegal, Curiel, & Alvarez, 1997; Forbes & Hodgson, 1997; Hall, Chen, & Woo, 1997; Hussein, 1996; Jenkins, Wheeler, & Albright, 1994; Lea, 1997; Lebkowski, Philip, & Okarma, 1997; Mastrangelo, Berd, Nathan, & Lattime, 1996; Peters, Dimond, & Jenkins, 1997; Weichselbaum & Kufe, 1997). However, as noted by Melcher, Garcia-Ribas, & Vile (1997), "gene therapy has not fulfilled its early promise." The authors are quick to point out that gene therapy has failed to live up to expectations so far because these expectations have not been realistic. They argue that studies of gene therapy should not be abandoned prematurely because the trials fail to produce a cure. Rather, clinicians and basic scientists need to collaborate to develop different approaches to more effectively use gene therapy to treat cancer.

Purposes of Gene Therapy

In general, two forms of gene therapy exist: gene correction and gene addition. Gene correction is the most straightforward form of therapy. It appears to be the most effective and desirable approach to correcting a deoxyribonucleic acid (DNA) defect associated with a disease when the genetic defect is known. Gene correction involves replacing a defective gene with its corresponding normal DNA sequence (Fig. 10-1). This exchange of DNA sequences can be accomplished by the process of homologous recombination, which involves the precise excision of DNA sequences and the replacement of the excised sequences with other homologous pieces of DNA (Bank, 1996).

Homologous recombination occurs normally in many organisms. It functions as a repair mechanism and as a means for organisms to increase their genetic diversity (Forbes & Hodgson, 1997). Homologous recombination has been accomplished with embryonic stem cells of mice to create transgenic mice with specific genetic characteristics (Capecchi, 1989; Thomas & Capecchi, 1987).

Gene addition or augmentation (Fig. 10-1) is used to overcome a genetic defect or to add a new function to cells by either increasing new gene expression or preventing the expression of unwanted genes. New genes or their complementary DNAs (cDNAs) can be used to express new cellular functions or to increase the level of already functioning genes. An alternative approach would be to add antisense DNA or ribonucleic acid (RNA) molecules that block the expression of specific unwanted or harmful genes. Gene addition has the advantage of delivering genes to cells much more efficiently than gene correction. The great disadvantage of gene addition over homologous recombination (i.e., gene correction) is that the added genes are not integrated or are integrated randomly and not in a site-specific manner into the host cell's chromosomal DNA (Bank, 1996).

Categories of Gene Therapy

Gene transfer is generally divided into two categories: in vitro and in vivo. In vitro gene therapy occurs when genes are transferred (or transduced) into target cells outside the host (i.e., ex vivo) and those cells are then placed back into the animal or the patient. In vivo gene therapy occurs when

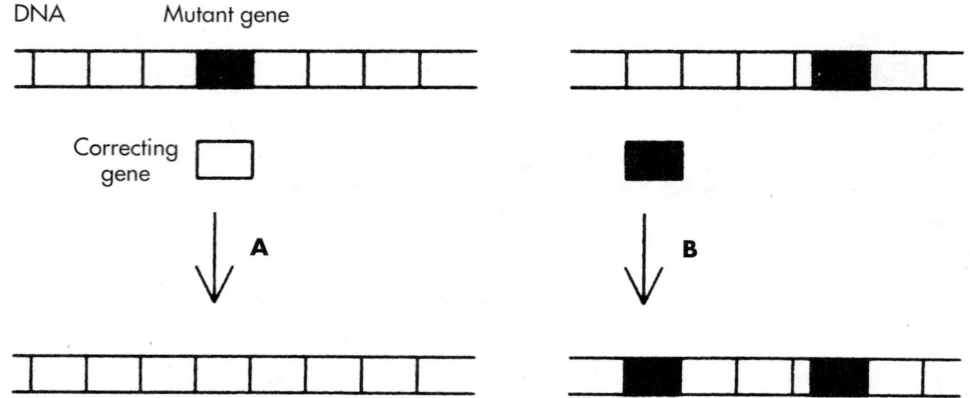

Fig. 10-1 In homologous recombination **(A)** the abnormal gene is replaced with a correcting gene of similar homology. In gene augmentation **(B)** the correcting gene inserts randomly, leaving the abnormal gene within the chromosome. (From Forbes, S. J., & Hodgson, H. J. F. [1997]. Review article: Gene therapy in gastroenterology and hepatology. *Alimentary Pharmacology and Therapy, 11,* 823-836.)

the gene is transduced directly into target cells within the host (Fine & Kufe, 1997).

METHODS OF GENE TRANSFER

The success of gene therapy depends on two distinct but interrelated components: the gene itself and the delivery system used to move the gene into the cell. Several factors listed in Box 10-1 must be considered when selecting an appropriate therapeutic gene. The second component of gene transfer involves the delivery of the therapeutic gene to the intended target cell that expresses or will express the gene that is transfected (Fine & Kufe, 1997).

A variety of gene delivery systems exist (Table 10-1). In general, these delivery systems can be divided into two major categories: viral-based and non–viral-based vectors. At the present time, viral vectors are more efficient than non–viral-based vectors. A great deal of research is ongoing to develop more efficient viral vectors.

Box 10-1
Factors to Consider When Selecting a Therapeutic Gene

- Mechanism of action of the gene product
- Size of the gene
- Need for stability of gene expression
- Expected effect of the gene on the transduced cell and the host

Box 10-2
Common Viral Vectors for Gene Therapy

- Retroviral vectors
- Adenoviral vectors
- Adeno-associated virus vectors
- Pox vectors
- Herpes simplex virus–based vectors

Viral Vectors

The basic premise underlying the use of viral-based vectors is the attempt to use the inherent ability of the virus to carry foreign genetic material into cells and exploit the innate abilities of the cells to encode the new genes and produce protein products. The viral vectors used in gene therapy are listed in Box 10-2.

Retroviral Vectors. The most common vectors currently in use for gene therapy are retroviral vectors (Fine & Kufe, 1997) (Box 10-3). Retroviruses are RNA viruses that are capable of stably integrating DNA within the host cell genome. The replication cycle of a retrovirus begins with the attachment of the virus to a cell through a specific receptor (Fig. 10-2). The RNA virus enters the cell and is transcribed into DNA by the enzyme reverse transcriptase. The viral DNA is then transported to the nucleus of the cell, where it is integrated into the DNA of the host cell. The viral DNA is transcribed and then translated into specific viral proteins. Some of the viral transcripts are packaged into newly formed viral particles and released by budding (Hwu & Rosenberg, 1997).

Retroviral RNA contains three genes that are required to form intact retroviral particles: *gag,* which is needed to encode viral core proteins; *pol,* which encodes the enzyme reverse transcriptase; and *env,* which encodes the protein envelope of the virus. In addition, a packaging signal sequence (Ψ) is needed to package the mature virus so that it is able to infect target cells (Fig. 10-3, *A*).

Retroviral vectors for gene therapy are constructed by substituting the gene of interest in place of the viral protein coding regions (Danos & Mulligan, 1988). The most frequently used retroviruses are murine viruses, usually the Moloney murine leukemia virus (MoMULV). When creating retroviral vectors, one of the major dangers, which has

TABLE 10-1 Comparison of Gene Transfer Methods

	Gene Transfer Method					
Profile	**Retrovirus**	**Adenovirus**	**AAV**	**Vaccinia**	**Fowlpox**	**Nonviral**
Efficiency of gene transfer*	Moderate	High	Moderate	High	High	Low
Stable vs transient	Stable	Transient	Stable	Transient	Transient	Transient
Gene expression	Variable†	Variable†	Variable†	High	High	Variable†
Immunogenicity‡	Low	Moderate	Low	High	High	Low
In vitro toxicity	Low	Low	Low	High	Low	Low
Titer	Low	High	See comments	High	High	N/A
Comments	Requires replicating cells	New vector design should lead to decreased immunogenicity	High-titer preparations difficult to produce; production requires replication competent adenovirus	Most infected cells die within 24 hours; replication competent	Easy to produce clinical-grade material; fewer safety issues compared with viral methods	

From Hwu, P., & Rosenberg, S. A. (1997). Gene therapy of cancer. In V. T. DeVita, Jr., S. Hillman, & S. A. Rosenberg (Eds.), *Cancer: Principles and practice of oncology* (5th ed.). Philadelphia: Lippincott-Raven.
*Can be variable, depending on cell type.
†Gene expression depends on specific promoter and cell type.
‡Immunogenicity from expression of normal viral proteins.

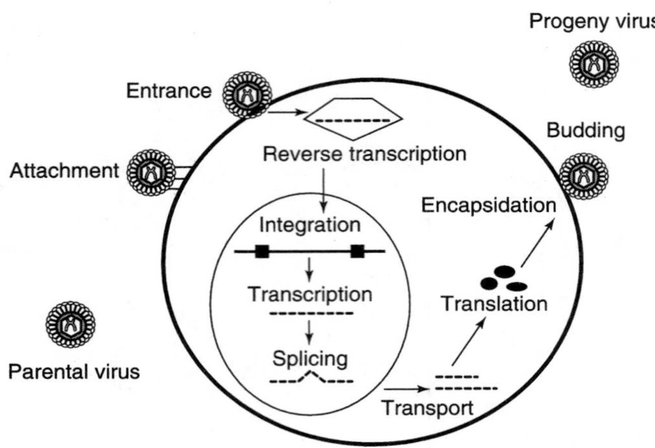

Fig. 10-2 Retrovirus replication cycle. The retrovirus uses envelope glycoproteins to bind to specific receptors on the cell surface. Viral RNA then enters the cell and is reverse transcribed to DNA. The viral DNA is transported to the nucleus, where it integrates in the host chromosome and directs transcription of the provirus, using the viral long terminal repeat. Viral transcripts are translated by the infected cell to form viral structural proteins. Some of the unspliced viral transcripts are packaged into the newly formed viral particles and released by budding. (From: Hwu, P., & Rosenberg, S. A. [1997]. Gene therapy of cancer. In V. T. DeVita, Jr., S. Hillman, & S. A. Rosenberg [Eds.], *Cancer: Principles and practice of oncology* [5th ed.]. Philadelphia: Lippincott-Raven.)

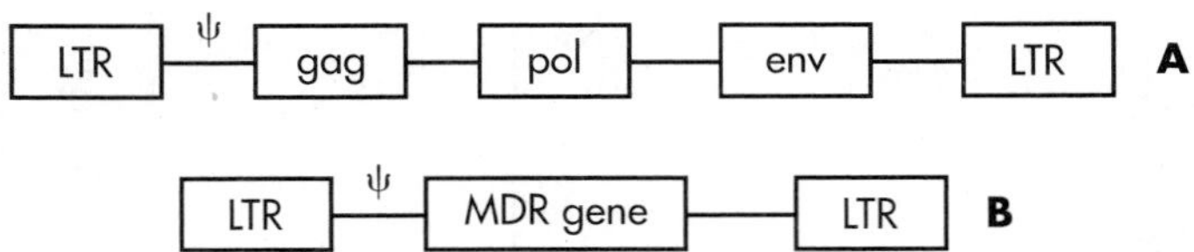

Fig 10-3 **A,** Schematic diagram of retrovirus genome. **B,** Example of a retroviral vector. *MDR,* multidrug-resistant gene; *LTR,* long terminal repeat; *ψ,* packaging signal sequence; *gag,* encodes viral proteins; *pol,* encodes the enzyme reverse transcriptase; *env,* encodes the protein envelope of the virus.

Box 10-3
Advantages and Disadvantages of Retroviral-Based Vectors

Advantages

A high degree of infection and gene expression can be achieved
A single copy of the desired gene can be integrated into the DNA of the recipient cell
Retroviral infection does not confer any harmful effects on the infected cell

Disadvantages

The virus may be pathogenic in humans
The retrovirus only infects replicating cells

been overcome, is the possibility of generating growth of the virus within the host.

To avoid the possibility of producing a retroviral infection in the host, the creation of a retroviral vector and gene transfer requires several manipulations of the retroviral genome to ensure its safe use. To accomplish these manipulations, so-called *safe packaging* or *helper cell lines* are used (Danos & Mulligan, 1988; Eglitis & Anderson, 1988; Markowitz, Goff, & Bank, 1988a,b; Miller & Buttimore, 1986). As illustrated in Fig. 10-4, the process of safe packaging involves the use of specific cell lines that stably express structural genes of different retroviruses (i.e., *gag, pol, env*) but do not express the packagable RNA transcripts. An example of such a cell line is the NIH 3T3 cells. These are mouse fibroblast cells that are transfected with plasmids that permit the production of *gag, pol,* and *env* retroviral proteins but do not allow the packaging of the RNA containing the retroviral functions into retroviral particles. These cells that contain the viral plasmids are called *packaging cells.* They are then transfected with the vector plasmid that contains the desired gene, at which point they are called *producer cells.* Only the vector plasmid with the desired gene has an intact Ψ sequence. Therefore producer cells are able to produce the retroviral vector, with the desired gene, that is able to infect cells. However, a competent retrovirus that can cause an infection cannot be reproduced (Bank, 1996; Fine & Kufe, 1997; Hwu & Rosenberg, 1997).

Retroviral vectors have advantages. Their relative simplicity makes construction of a variety of vectors relatively simple. In addition, these vectors are able to stably integrate into the DNA of a cell, and they do not express viral proteins, which reduces the risk of developing significant antiviral immune responses. Disadvantages include their low levels of gene transfer efficiency and low level of activity because of complement-mediated inactivation of the gene (Challita & Kohn, 1994). In addition, these vectors can only infect and integrate into actively dividing cells. This property has important therapeutic implications in the use of these vectors to treat cancer because most solid tumors have relatively low growth fractions in vivo (i.e., less than 20% of tumor cells are actively dividing at any one time). This low growth fraction makes it highly unlikely that retroviral vectors would be capable of transducing a significant portion of the tumor. Finally, two potential safety concerns with the creation of retroviral vectors are (1) the possible replication of a competent virus that is capable of producing an infection, and (2) the potential of producing an insertional mutation that could result in a malignant transformation because of the random integration of the provirus into the host genome. Although this second possibility seems unlikely and no murine retrovirus has been demonstrated to be pathogenic in humans, a recent study in nonhuman primates (Donahue, Kessler, Bodine, McDonagh, Dunbar, Goodman et al., 1992) demonstrated the development of leukemias/lymphomas in three of eight monkeys following treatment with high doses of retroviral vectors that were contaminated with helper viruses. For many of these reasons, retroviruses appear to be best suited for in vitro transduction (Bank, 1996; Fine & Kufe, 1997; Hwu & Rosenberg, 1997).

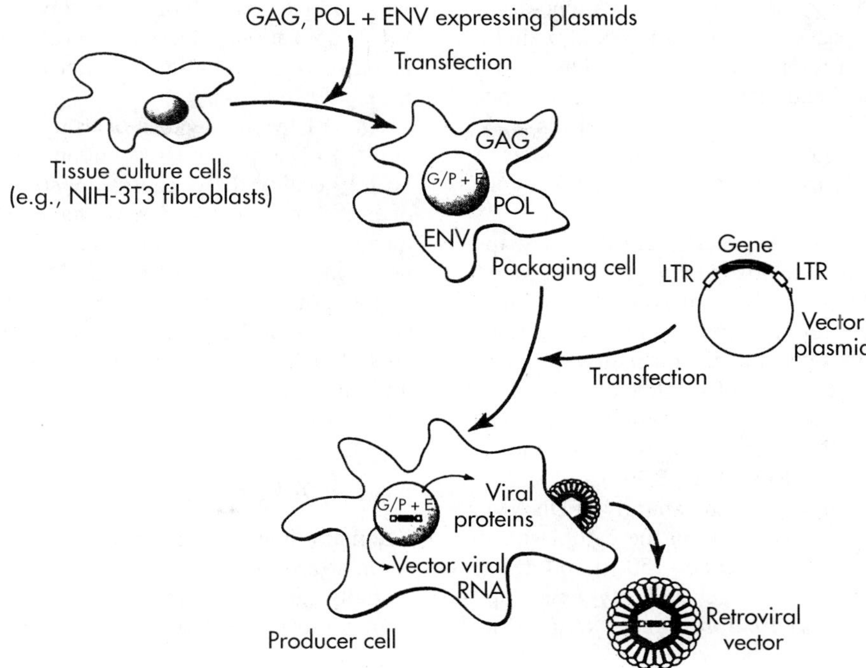

Fig. 10-4 Production of retroviral vectors with packaging cells. The gene of interest is cloned into a retroviral vector and then is transfected into a helper cell line, which provides the retroviral structural genes in trans. The retroviral structural genes cannot be packaged because of the absence of a packaging sequence (ψ), whereas the retroviral vector can be packaged, thereby producing a replication incompetent retrovirus. (From Hwu, P., & Rosenberg, S. A. [1997]. Gene therapy of cancer. In V. T. DeVita, Jr., S. Hillman, & S. A. Rosenberg [Eds.], *Cancer: Principles and practice of oncology* [5th ed.]. Philadelphia: Lippincott-Raven)

Adenoviral Vectors. Adenoviruses contain double-stranded DNA complexed with core proteins and surrounded by capsid proteins (Fine & Kufe, 1997). The genome of the adenovirus is divided into two regions: the early gene region (i.e., E1 to E4) and the late gene region. The early gene region is involved in viral replication, whereas the late gene region encodes structural proteins. Of particular interest in gene therapy is the E1 gene, whose products are expressed first and are responsible for activating other genes that begin a cascade of events that lead to viral replication. Removal of the E1 region results in an adenovirus particle that is not able to replicate (Fine & Kufe, 1997, Hwu & Rosenberg, 1997).

Adenoviral vectors have been produced by removing the E1 region and cloning the gene of interest into the deleted E1 region (Berkner, 1992). The recombinant adenovirus must be produced using cell lines that provide the E1 products in trans (e.g., 293 cells).

The major advantages of adenoviral vectors over retroviral vectors are: (1) they can infect most human cells with a high level of efficiency, (2) they can infect both dividing and nondividing cells, (3) they can be concentrated and frozen for use at later times, and (4) they are less likely to cause an insertional mutation (Berkner, 1992; Quantin, Perricaudet, Tajbakhsh, & Mandell, 1992; Rosenfeld, Yoshimura, Trapnell, Yoneyama, Rosenthal, Dalemans et al., 1992). The major disadvantage of adenoviral vectors is that they provoke a significant immune response in the host (Yang, Nunes, Berencsi, Furth, Gonczol, & Wilson, 1994).

Herpes Simplex Virus–Based Vectors. Herpes simplex virus (HSV)–based vectors were originally developed for gene transfer into the central nervous system (Manthorpe et al., 1993). However, this vector may prove useful in gene therapy for cancer. HSV is a large virus of double-stranded DNA that naturally infects nerves and many types of epithelial cells. The HSV-based vectors are made in a manner similar to the way that the adenoviral vectors are constructed. The theoretical advantages of HSV-based vectors include (1) the ability to accommodate at least 30 kilobases (kb) of foreign DNA, (2) the ability to infect cells with a high level of efficiency, and (3) the possibility that these vectors may be able to establish latency with long-term expression of the gene.

The development of HSV-based vectors will require a great deal of research before these vectors are available for widespread clinical use. One of the major problems with the development of this type of vector is the complexity of the HSV genome and an incomplete knowledge of the functions of all of the genes. In some cases, expression of ill-defined genes in replication-incompetent HSV vectors has resulted in cytotoxic effects in a number of cells. In addition, the HSV-based vectors can produce an immune response and, because of the propensity of the virus for neural tissue, may produce neurotoxic effects (Fine & Kufe, 1997).

Adeno-Associated Virus Vectors. Adeno-associated virus (AAV) is a parvovirus that consists of a single strand of DNA made up of approximately 5000 base-pairs. The AAV genome is small and theoretically can be manipulated relatively easily. The major characteristic of the AAV is that it requires a helper virus (e.g., adenovirus) in order to replicate (Siegl, Bates, Berns, Carter, Kelly, Kurstak, et al., 1985).

The major advantages of AAV vectors are that they appear to stably integrate into the host genome (with a special predilection for a small region of chromosome 19) and that they are capable of integrating into nondividing cells. However, in practical terms these vectors are difficult to produce in sufficient quantities that are free of viable helper virus. In addition, because of the vector's size, it is constrained in terms of the amount of DNA that can be packaged into it (Fine & Kufe, 1997; Hwu & Rosenberg, 1997).

Pox Vectors. The pox viruses are a family of DNA viruses that have the ability to replicate in the cytoplasm of infected cells. The pox genome encodes 150 to 200 genes that are divided into early and late genes. Early genes (approximately 100) are expressed before viral DNA replication, and late genes (approximately 100) are expressed after DNA replication. Infection of a cell with a pox virus results in cell lysis within 48 hours after infection (Hwu & Rosenberg, 1997).

One of the advantages of using pox virus vectors is the ability to incorporate large amounts of foreign DNA into the vector because these viruses are so large. In addition, large quantities of gene expression have been observed because the gene expression is entirely cytoplasmic and does not depend on the regulatory mechanisms of the host cell. The major disadvantages of pox virus vectors are (1) the transient nature of the gene expression, (2) the cell lysis that occurs after infection, and (3) the ability of the virus to produce an immune response (Hwu & Rosenberg, 1997; Moss, 1992a, b).

Nonviral Vectors

The major nonviral vectors or methods for gene transfer are summarized in Table 10-2. These nonviral methods are potentially safer than viral vectors and should not produce an immune response. However, most current methods of non-

TABLE 10-2 Nonviral Vectors for Gene Therapy

Method	Characteristics
Calcium phosphate precipitation (Graham & van der Eb, 1973)	Oldest method to deliver foreign genes to cells DNA is complexed to calcium phosphate crystals, and the complex enters the cell through the cell membrane Results in a low percentage of cells being transfected
Electroporation	Common laboratory technique for gene transfer Involves the passage of an electric current across cells that destabilizes the cell membrane and opens undefined channels that facilitate the entry of DNA into the cell Results in a low percentage of cells being transfected
Injection of naked DNA (Wolff & Lederberg, 1994)	Simplest method of gene transfer In vitro procedure that uses microinjection techniques to introduce DNA into individual cells Tedious process that allows the transduction of only a limited number of cells Useful for the transduction of highly selected cells (e.g., oocytes, embryonic cells)
Gene gun (Wolff, Malone, Williams, Chong, Acsadi, Jani, et al., 1990)	Naked DNA is coated onto micropellets and injected into target tissue by means of a burst of air Improves gene expression by allowing DNA to be injected with greater force May be useful for vaccine gene therapy strategies
Liposomes (Nicolau, LePape, Soriano, Fargette, & Juhel, 1983)	Widely used method of gene transfer Liposomes are bilipid membranes that surround an aqueous core; hydrophilic substances can be maintained in the aqueous core until the liposome membrane fuses with a cell membrane Liposomal DNA gene transfer is more efficient than calcium phosphate transfection or electroporation in vitro Major limitation is that liposomes lack target specificity
DNA-polypeptide ligand complexes (Wu, Wilson, Shalaby, Grossman, Shafritz, & Wu, 1991)	Development of a complex with plasmid DNA and specific polypeptide ligands This approach exploits receptor-mediated endocytic pathways

viral gene transfer result in transient gene expression, and the efficiency of gene transfer is lower when compared with viral vectors. Until better nonviral vectors are developed, most gene therapy research will continue to be done using viral vectors.

GENE THERAPY APPROACHES FOR CANCER

The use of gene therapy approaches to treat human cancers is theoretically possible. However, several limitations associated with the delivery of gene therapy will need to be overcome before it can be used more widely as adjuvant treatment for malignant disease. For example, a significant limitation of the current vectors is their inability to transfer therapeutic genes uniformly into all tumor cells in situ. To increase cell kill within tumors and make metastatic disease more manageable, new methods will be needed to deliver therapeutic genes systemically or to induce systemic antitumor responses following local therapy (Hall, Chen, & Woo, 1997).

A simple categorization of the approaches that are being evaluated that use gene therapy for the treatment of cancer are listed in Box 10-4. In general, gene therapy can be used (1) to produce direct antitumor effects, (2) to decrease the toxic effects of chemotherapy, and (3) to modify the response of the immune system to cancer. Each of these approaches is discussed in more detail in subsequent sections of this chapter.

Gene Therapy for Direct Antitumor Effects

In general, three approaches are being used to produce direct antitumor effects by adding genes that (1) are tumor suppressors, (2) encode antisense or ribozyme molecules to inhibit the expression of oncogenes, or (3) act as suicide genes within the tumor.

Box 10-4
Gene Therapy Approaches for the Treatment of Cancer

- Use gene therapy to produce direct antitumor effects
  - Use of tumor suppressor genes
  - Use of antisense oligodeoxynucleotide or ribozyme molecules
  - Use of suicide genes
- Use gene therapy to decrease the toxic effects of chemotherapy
  - Use of drug-resistance genes
- Use gene therapy to modify the immune system's response to cancer
  - Active immunization
    - Use genes to enhance the immunogenicity of tumor cells
    - Immunize with genes that encode tumor-specific antigens
  - Use gene therapy to modify immune effector cells
    - Use genes to enhance the survival of immune cells
    - Use genes to increase the ability of immune cells to recognize tumor cells
    - Use genes to increase the ability of immune cells to produce an antitumor response
    - Use gene therapy to decrease the toxicity of effector cells

Tumor Suppressor Gene Therapy. Normal cells contain genes whose primary purpose is to regulate cell growth and proliferation. These genes are called *tumor suppressor genes.* Many human cancers exhibit mutations in a tumor suppressor gene. For example, normal p53 genes (i.e., a tumor suppressor gene) are required for the maintenance of the normal cell cycle and regulated cell growth. These regulatory functions are disrupted by p53 mutations in cancer cells. Because p53 is the most commonly mutated gene in human cancer, it has received the most interest as a target for tumor suppressor gene therapy (Bank, 1996; Hall et al., 1997).

The overall goals of tumor suppressor gene therapy are the replacement of the defective gene with a correct copy and the reversal of the malignant phenotype. Additional effects associated with tumor suppressor gene therapy include the death of malignant cells, changes in tumor growth patterns, changes in the behavior of the tumor, and changes in the ability of the tumor to invade or metastasize.

Experiments have been conducted in which the transduction of cancer cells with the p53 gene significantly inhibited growth and angiogenesis or induced apoptosis (i.e., cell-death) in mutant p53 cells in several tumor models, including lung and breast cancer (Fujiwara, Cai, Georges, Mukhopadhyay, Grimm, & Roth, 1994; Lesoon-Wood, Kim, Kleinman, Weintraub, & Mixson, 1995; Xu, Kumar, Srinivas, Detolla, Yu, & Stass et al., 1997). Enthusiasm has continued for the idea of tumor suppressor gene therapy after a phase I clinical trial in which injection of lung tumors with a p53 retrovirus was nontoxic and suppressed tumor growth in six of nine patients (Roth, Jguyen, Lawrence, Kemp, Carrasco, & Ferson et al., 1996).

One of the major limitations of tumor suppressor gene therapy is the lack of appropriate vectors that are capable of efficiently delivering the gene therapy to all tumor cells within the body. However, research will continue to develop this approach into an effective clinical strategy.

Use of Antisense and Ribozyme Molecules. The use of antisense oligodeoxynucleotides as gene therapy has been tested in cell culture and mouse models. The rationale for this approach is that in certain tumors, cellular protooncogenes that are normally silent in cells become activated and this activation results in abnormal cell growth. For example, mutations in the *ras* gene are associated with human cancers. One way to interfere with these genes is to use antisense oligodeoxynucleotides or ribozymes. Antisense oligodeoxynucleotides are short sequences of RNA that are complementary to a target messenger RNA (mRNA) and act to inhibit the translation of the RNA transcript into a protein product (Calabretta, 1991; Mercola & Cohen, 1995).

Gene therapy using antisense molecules has been shown to reduce tumor cell growth in vitro when antisense oligonucleotides were directed against Bcl-2 in leukemic cells (Reed et al., 1990), BCR-ABL in chronic myelogenous leukemia cells (Szczylik, Skorski, Nicolaides, Manzella, Malaguarnera, Venturelli, et al., 1991), MYC in lymphoma cell lines (McManaway, Neckers, Loke, al-Nassar, Redner, & Shiramizu et al., 1990), and MYB in adenocarcinoma and leukemia cell lines (Anfossi, Gerwitz, & Calabretta, 1989; Melani, Rivoltini, Parmiani, Calabretta, & Colombo, 1991). In addition, several studies have been done in mice demonstrating in vivo efficacy of antisense oligonucleotides against tumors (Higgins, Perez, Colemann, Dorshkind, McComas, & Sarmiento et al., 1993; Ratajczak, Kant, Luger, Hijiya, Zhang, & Zo et al., 1992). A current limitation of this approach is the inability to successfully deliver the antisense genes to tumor cells in vivo with adequate efficiency. In addition, antisense studies must be interpreted carefully because of the possibility of nonspecific effects (Hwu & Rosenberg, 1997).

Another potential gene therapy approach to target-activated oncogenes is through the use of ribozymes. These are mRNA molecules that have catalytic activity. Some ribozymes are being used to cleave mRNA from activated oncogenes, which results in a disruption of the creation of a protein product (Poeschla & Wong-Staal, 1994). However, at the present time there are no adequate in vivo systems to deliver ribozymes to target cancer cells.

Use of Suicide Genes. Suicide gene therapy is defined as the transduction of a gene into a cell that converts a prodrug into a toxic substance. The gene product and the prodrug are nontoxic (Hall et al., 1997). Two suicide gene systems have been investigated: the *Escherichia coli* cytosine deaminase (CD) gene with the prodrug 5-fluorocytosine (5-FC) and the herpes simplex virus thymidine kinase gene (HSV-tk) with the prodrug ganciclovir (GCV).

The CD gene converts 5-FC into the chemotherapeutic agent 5-fluorouracil (5-FU) (Huber, Austin, Good, Knick, Tobbels, & Richards, 1993). This form of suicide gene therapy has been tested as a treatment for hepatic metastasis from gastrointestinal tumors, for which 5-FU is commonly used. Systemic administration of 5-FC to animals with CD-transduced tumors resulted in the suppression of tumor growth, whereas little suppression was achieved with systemic administration of high doses of 5-FU (Huber et al., 1993).

Another example of suicide gene therapy is the HSV-tk gene with GCV. The HSV-tk gene acts by phosphorylating GCV into a nucleoside analog that inhibits DNA synthesis (Moolten, 1986). This approach was first used to treat patients with brain tumors (Barba, Hardin, Sadelin, & Gage, 1994; Chen, Shine, Goodman, Grossman, & Woo, 1994; Culver, Ram, Wallbridge, Ishii, Oldfield, & Blaese, 1992). In these studies the HSV-tk gene is transferred by direct injection of retroviral producer cells into multiple areas of the tumor under stereotactic monitoring. Dividing tumor cells integrate the virus and produce the enzyme herpes simplex thymidine kinase. Following the gene therapy injections, the patients receive GCV systemically. The HSV-tk-expressing transduced tumor cells are killed by the phosphorylated GCV. Preliminary results suggest a modest anti-tumor effect (Bank, 1996).

An interesting phenomenon associated with suicide gene therapy is termed the "bystander effect." This effect is reported with CD and HSV-tk gene therapy. The bystander effect is the term applied to the observation that although only a small percentage of tumor cells are in cycle (i.e., dividing) and are transduced with the suicide gene, the death of a greater number of tumor cells is sometimes observed. The exact mechanisms underlying the bystander effect remain to be elucidated. However, several mechanisms have been proposed, including the following: gap junctions transport nondiffusable phosphorylated GCV to the nontransduced cells; nontransduced cells endocytose debris containing phosphorylated GCV from dying cells; and an induced immune response leads to tumor cell killing (Elshami, Saavedra, Zhang, Kucharczuk, Spray, & Fishman et al., 1996; Hamel, Magnelli, Chiarugi, & Israel, 1996; Mesnil, Piccoli, Tirabi, Willecke, & Yamasaki, 1996; Vile, Nelson, Castleden, Chong, & Hart, 1994).

Additional studies using the HSV-tk gene and GCV are being conducted in patients with mesotheliomas (Elshami, Kucharczuk, Zhang, Smythe, Hwang, & Liteky 1996), liver metastasis (Caruso, Panis, Gagandeep, Houssin, Salzmann, & Klatzmann, 1993), and peritoneal-based metastases (Tong, Block, Chen, Contant, Agoulnik, & Blankberg et al., 1996, Yee, McGuire, Brunner, Kozelsky, Allred, & Chen et al., 1996). However, the use of suicide gene therapy is not a panacea. A number of inadequacies exist with this therapy, including the need to have localized disease because the suicide genes need to be injected directly into the tumor, the variability of the bystander effect, the lack of a tissue-specific systemic vector to deliver the gene therapy, and the possibility of treatment-related toxicities.

Gene Therapy to Decrease Toxicity of Chemotherapy

Gene therapy may be used to protect hematopoietic stem cells from the toxic effects of chemotherapy and allow higher doses of these drugs to be administered to enhance the ability of the drugs to kill tumor cells. The human multidrug resistance (MDR) gene is one of the genes that is involved in this application of gene therapy. The protein product of the MDR gene is a transmembrane *p*-glycoprotein that normally pumps toxic natural substances out of cells (Pastan & Gottesman, 1991). These substances include certain classes of widely used chemotherapy drugs: anthracycline antibiotics, vinca alkaloids, podophyllins, and taxol and its derivatives. When this gene is expressed in cancer cells, it is associated with tumor resistance to chemotherapy drugs.

Bone marrow cells normally express low levels of MDR and thus are especially sensitive to the toxic effects of chemotherapy drugs (Bank, 1996). In a mouse model, investigators have been able to transfer the human MDR gene into bone marrow cells. The transfer and expression of the MDR gene in the mouse bone marrow cells were shown to protect mice from the leukopenic effects of taxol and anthracycline antibiotics (Podda, Ward, Himelstein, Richardson, de la Flor-Weiss, & Smith et al., 1992; Richardson, Ward, & Bank, 1995; Richardson, Ward, Podda, & Bank, 1994; Sorrentino, Brandt, Bodine, Gottesman, Pastan, & Cline et al., 1992).

The transfection of the MDR gene into human hematopoietic stem cells will most likely be done using peripheral blood stem cells. These peripheral blood stem cells can be transduced efficiently with a MDR retrovirus (Ward, 1996). Phase I clinical trials are underway using safe and efficient MDR retroviral supernatants to test the feasibility of MDR gene transfer in humans (Hesdorffer, Antiman, Bank, Fetell, & Mears, 1994).

Gene Therapy to Modify the Immune Response

Efforts are being made to use gene therapy to modulate the response of the immune system to tumor cells. Two assumptions underlie this approach to gene therapy: (1) tumor-specific antigens exist, and (2) the immune system of the host is potentially capable of recognizing these tumor antigens and destroying the tumor cells (Fine & Kufe, 1997). A variety of gene therapy approaches are being developed that seek to modify the response of the immune system to tumor cells (see Box 10-4).

Active Immunization. One approach to modifying the immune system using gene therapy is active immunization. Two types of active immunization are being investigated. In one type, tumor cells are modified with genes that enhance the immunogenicity of the tumor by producing a variety of cytokines (e.g., interleukin-2 [IL-2], granulocyte-macrophage colony-stimulating factor, tumor necrosis factor [TNF]). The introduction of genes encoding cytokines into the tumor can result in the production of very high levels of cytokines in the tumor microenvironment. This increase in cytokine concentration enhances the immune response of the host to the tumor cells (Hwu & Rosenberg, 1997).

Another type of gene therapy that uses the principles of active immunization is the development of recombinant vaccines. This research has been supported by the cloning of several melanoma antigens that are recognized by T lymphocytes. Recent studies in mice have shown that antigens expressed at high levels in recombinant adenoviral, fowl pox, and vaccinia vector systems can induce a significant immune response against tumors that contain the same antigen (Hwu & Rosenberg, 1997).

Genetic Modification of Immune Effector Cells

Several genetic approaches are being designed to modify immune effector cells. One approach focuses on using gene therapy to enhance the survival of immune cells. More specifically, T cells grow in response to stimulation by IL-2. By inserting the gene for IL-2, T cells may be able to stimulate themselves and enhance their immunogenicity. Another strategy to enhance in vivo survival of immune effector cells would be to insert receptor genes that bind cytokines into these cells; they could then be administered to patients in large amounts with minimal toxicities.

Another approach to enhancing the effector function of immune cells would be to use novel receptor genes (e.g., for antibodies) to allow lymphocytes to recognize new targets on tumor cells. Yet another gene therapy approach is to transduce tumor infiltrating lymphocytes (TILs) with the TNF gene. TNF has potent antitumor activity against large tumor burdens in mouse models. However, humans cannot tolerate large doses of TNF because of profound hypotension. Thus the ability to transduce TILs with the TNF gene may allow for high concentrations of TNF to be delivered locally to the tumor without systemic side effects (Hwu, Yannelli, Kriegler, Anderson, Perez, & Chiang et al., 1993). This approach has been tested in patients in a phase I trial; no safety or toxicity problems were detected. Despite the achievement of a fivefold increase in TNF production, this amount does not appear to be clinically effective (Hwu & Rosenberg, 1997).

NURSING IMPLICATIONS OF GENE THERAPY

Two review articles (Jenkins, Wheeler, & Albright, 1994; Lea, 1997) provide an excellent overview of the nursing implications of gene therapy. These issues can be broadly divided into education, safety, and clinical practice issues.

Education Issues

Oncology nurses will need a tremendous amount of education concerning genetics and gene therapy. Nursing curriculums need to be developed around the areas of basic genetics, genetic diseases, principles of gene therapy, and methods used in gene therapy. Simple methods for teaching these concepts must be made available to oncology nurses who will need to educate patients and their family members.

Safety Issues

Potential safety issues include both the immediate and long-term complications of gene therapy for both the patient and the health care provider. In the limited number of clinical studies done to date, gene therapy does not appear to produce severe toxicities. However, no data are available on the long-term consequences of this therapy. Long-term follow-up care needs to be built into gene therapy protocols.

With regard to health care workers' safety, clinicians should use universal precautions when administering gene therapy. An expressed concern associated with gene therapy is the possibility of infectious transmission of altered genes, especially when viral vectors are used. Infectious spread of viruses as a result of viral vectors has not been observed with the present generation of retroviral vectors. Thus the risk of this problem occurring appears to be remote (Jenkins, Wheeler, & Albright, 1994; Lea, 1997).

Practice Issues

The ethical issues to be considered surrounding gene therapy are enormous. In 1980 the World Council of Churches wrote a letter to President Carter expressing concern about potentially dangerous consequences of genetic engineering and the lack of governmental review. This action prompted a Presidential Commission and congressional hearings on the subject. Guidelines were developed to assist investigators and reviewers of human gene therapy protocols (Jenkins, Wheeler, & Albright, 1994).

In the United States the National Institutes of Health Recombinant DNA Advisory Committee (RAC), the Food and Drug Administration, and the institutional review boards are required to evaluate proposed gene therapy clinical studies that will use federal funding or be conducted at an institution that receives federal funding. The role of the RAC is to promote broad public discussion of this new technology, with special attention to social and ethical concerns (Jenkins, Wheeler, & Albright, 1994).

A tremendous amount of patient and public education regarding the risks and benefits of gene therapy needs to be done to provide consumers with realistic expectations of this approach to cancer treatment. The news media tend to sensationalize any advances in cancer treatment and make the public think that these approaches are available to all patients. Patients and the public need realistic information about what to expect from gene therapy. This approach may be the therapy of the future, but it is not an effective approach or mainstay of cancer treatment at the present time.

REFERENCES

Anfossi, G., Gerwitz, A. M., & Calabretta, A. (1989). An oligomer complementary to c-myb-encoded mRNA inhibits proliferation of human myeloid leukemia cell lines. *Proceedings of the National Academy of Sciences, USA, 86,* 3379-3383.

Bank, A. (1996). Human somatic cell gene therapy. *Bio Essays, 18*(12), 999-1007.

Barnes, M. N., Deshane, J. S., Rosenfeld, M., Siegal, G. P., Curiel, D. T., & Alvarez, R. D. (1997). Gene therapy and ovarian cancer. *Obstetrics and Gynecology, 89*(1), 145-155.

Barba, D., Hardin, J., Sadelin, M., & Gage, F. H. (1994). Development of antitumor immunity following thymidine kinase-based killing of experimental brain tumors. *Proceedings of the National Academy of Sciences, USA, 91,* 4348-4352.

Berkner, K. L. (1992). Expression of heterologous sequences in adenoviral vectors. *Current Topics in Microbiology and Immunology, 158,* 39-66.

Calabretta, B. (1991). Inhibition of protooncogene expression by antisense oligodeoxynucleotides: Biologic and therapeutic implications. *Cancer Research, 51,* 4505-4510.

Capecchi, M. R. (1989). Altering the genome by homologous recombination. *Science, 244,* 1288-1292.

Caruso, M., Panis, Y., Gagandeep, S., Houssin, D., Salzmann, J. L., & Klatzmann, D. (1993). Regression of established macroscopic liver metastases after in situ transduction of a suicide gene. *Proceedings of the National Academy of Sciences, USA, 90*(15), 7024-7028.

Challita, P. M., & Kohn, D. B. (1994). Lack of expression from a retroviral vector after transduction of murine hematopoietic stem cells is associated with methylation in vivo. *Proceedings of the National Academy of Sciences, USA, 91,* 2567-2571.

Chen, S. H., Shine, H. D., Goodman, J. C., Grossman, R. G., & Woo, S. L. C. (1994). Gene therapy for brain tumors: Regression of experimental gliomas by adenovirus-mediated gene transfer in vivo. *Proceedings of the National Academy of Sciences, USA, 91,* 3054-3057.

Culver, K. W., Ram, Z., Wallbridge, S., Ishii, H., Oldfield, E. H., & Blaese, R. M. (1992). In vivo gene transfer with retroviral vector-producer cells for treatment of experimental brain tumors. *Science, 256,* 1550-1552.

Danos, O., & Mulligan, R. C. (1988). Safe and efficient generation of recombinant retroviruses with amphotropic and ectotropic host ranges. *Proceedings of the National Academy of Sciences, USA, 85,* 6460-6464.

Donahue, R. E., Kessler, S. W., Bodine, D., McDonagh, K., Dunbar, C., Goodman, S., Agricola, B., Byrne, E., Raffeld, M., Moen, R., Backer, J., Zsebo, K. M., & Nienhuis, A. W. (1992). Helper virus induced T-cell lymphoma in nonhuman primates after retroviral mediated gene transfer. *Journal of Experimental Medicine, 176,* 1125-1135.

Eglitis, M. A., & Anderson, W. F. (1988). Retroviral vectors for introduction of genes into mammalian cells. *Biotechniques, 6,* 608-614.

Elshami, A. A., Kucharczuk, J. C., Zhang, H. B., Smythe, W. R., Hwang, H. C., Litzky, L. A., & Kaiser, L. R. (1996). Treatment of pleural mesothelioma in an immunocompetent rat model utilizing adenoviral transfer of herpes simplex virus thymidine kinase gene. *Human Gene Therapy, 7,* 141-148.

Elshami, A. A., Saavedra, A., Zhang, H., Kucharczuk, J. C., Spray, D. C., Fishman, G. I., & Amin, K. M. (1996). Gap junctions play a role in the "bystander effect" of the herpes simplex virus thymidine kinase/ganciclovir system in vitro. *Gene Therapy, 3,* 85-92.

Fine, H. A. & Kufe, D. W. (1997). Cancer gene therapy. In J. F. Holland, R. C. Bast, Jr., D. L. Marton, E. Frei, D. W. Kufe, & R. R. Weichselbaum (Eds.), *Cancer medicine* (4th ed., 1265-1275). Baltimore: Williams & Wilkins.

Forbes, S. J., & Hodgson, H. J. F. (1997). Review article: Gene therapy in gastroenterology and hepatology. *Alimentary Pharmacology and Therapy, 11,* 823-836.

Friedmann, T., & Roblin, R. (1972). Gene therapy for human genetic disease? *Science, 175,* 949-955.

Fujiwara, T., Cai, D. W., Georges, R. N., Mukhopadhyay, T., Grimm, E. A., & Roth, J. A. (1994). therapeutic effect of a retroviral wild type p53 expression vector in an orthotopic lung cancer model. *Journal of the National Cancer Institute, 86,* 1458-1462.

Graham, F. L., & van der Eb, A. J. (1973). A new technique for the assay of infectivity of human adenovirus 5. *Virology, 52,* 456-462.

Hall, S. J., Chen, S. H., & Woo, S. L. C. (1997). Gene therapy '97: The promise and reality of cancer gene therapy. *American Journal of Human Genetics, 61,* 785-789.

Hamel, W., Magnelli, L., Chiarugi, V. P., & Israel, M. A. (1996). Herpes simplex virus thymidine kinase/ganciclovir-mediated apoptotic death of bystander cells. *Cancer Research, 56,* 2697-2702.

Hesdorffer, C., Antiman, K., Bank, A., Fetell, M., & Mears, G. (1994). Clinical protocol: Human MDR gene transfer in patients with advanced cancer. *Human Gene Therapy, 5,* 1151-1160.

Higgins, K. A., Perez, J. R., Colemann, T. A., Dorshkind, K., McComas, W. A., Sarmiento, U. M., Rosen, C. A., & Narayanan, R. (1993). Antisense inhibition of the p65 subunit of NF-kappa B blocks tumorigenicity and causes tumor regression. *Proceedings of National Academy of Sciences, USA, 90,* 9901-9905.

Huber, B. E., Austin, E. A., Good, S. S., Knick, V. C., Tobbels, S., & Richards, C. A. (1993). In vivo antitumor activity of 5-fluorocytosine on human colorectal carcinoma cells genetically modified to express cytosine deaminase. *Cancer Research, 53,* 4619-4626.

Hussein, A. M. (1996). The potential applications of gene transfer to the treatment of patients with cancer: A concise review. *Cancer Investigation, 14*(4), 343-352.

Hwu, P., & Rosenberg, S. A. (1997). Gene therapy of cancer. In V. T. DeVita, Jr., S. Hellman, & S. A. Rosenberg (Eds.), *Cancer: Principles and practice of oncology* (5th ed.). Philadelphia: Lippincott-Raven Publishers.

Hwu, P., Yannelli, J., Kriegler, M., Anderson, W. F., Perez, C., Chiang, Y., Schwarz, C., Cowherd, R., Delgado, C., & Mulé, J. (1993). Functional and molecular characteristics of TIL transduced with TNFα cDNA for gene therapy of cancer in man. *Journal of Immunology, 150,* 4104-4115.

Jenkins, J., Wheeler, V., & Albright, L. (1994). Gene therapy for cancer. *Cancer Nursing, 17*(6), 447-456.

Lea, D. H. (1997). Gene therapy: current and future implications for oncology nursing practice. *Seminars in Oncology Nursing, 13*(2), 115-122.

Lebkowski, J. S., Philip, R., & Okarma, T. B. (1997). Breast cancer: Cell and gene therapy. *Cancer Investigation, 15*(6), 568-576.

Lesoon-Wood, L. A., Kim, W. H., Kleinman, H. K., Weintraub, B. D., & Mixson, A. J. (1995). Systemic gene therapy with p53 reduces growth and metastases of a malignant human breast cancer in nude mice. *Human Gene Therapy, 6,* 395-405.

Manthorpe, M., Cornefert-Jensen, F. J., Hartikka, J., Felgner, J., Rundell, A., Margalith, M., & Dworki, V. (1993). Gene therapy by intramuscular injection of plasmid DNA: Studies of firefly luciferase gene expression in mice. *Human Gene Therapy, 4,* 419-431.

Markowitz, D., Goff, S., & Bank, A. (1988a). A safe packaging line for gene transfer: Separating viral genes on two different plasmids. *Journal of Virology, 62,* 1120-1125.

Markowitz, D., Goff, S., & Bank, A. (1988b). Construction and use of safe and efficient amphotropic packaging cell line. *Virology, 167,* 400-405.

Mastrangelo, M. J., Berd, D., Nathan, F. E., & Lattime, E. C. (1996). Gene therapy for human cancer: An essay for clinicians. *Seminars in Oncology, 23*(1), 4-21.

McManaway, M. E., Neckers, L. M., Loke, S. L., al-Nasser, A. A., Redner, R. L., Shiramizu, B. T., Goldschmidts, W. L., Huber, B. E., Dhatai, K., & Magrath, I. T. (1990). Tumour-specific inhibition of lymphoma growth by an antisense oligodeoxynucleotide. *Lancet, 335,* 808-811.

Melani, C., Rivoltini, L., Parmiani, G., Calabretta, B., & Colombo, M. P. (1991). Inhibition of proliferation by c-myb antisense oligodeoxynucleotides in colon adenocarcinoma cell lines that express c-myb. *Cancer Research, 51,* 2897-2901.

Melcher, A. A., Garcia-Ribas, I., & Vile, R. G. (1997). Gene therapy for cancer-managing expectations. *British Medical Journal, 315,* 1604-1607.

Mercola, D., & Cohen, J. S. (1995). Antisense approaches to cancer gene therapy. *Cancer Gene Therapy, 2,* 47-59.

Mesnil, M., Piccoli, C., Tirabi, G., Willecke, K., & Yamasaki, H. (1996). Bystander killing of cancer cells by herpes simplex virus thymidine kinase gene is mediated by connexins. *Proceedings of the National Academy of Sciences, USA, 93,* 1831-1835.

Miller, A. D., & Buttimore, C. (1986). Redesign of retrovirus packaging cell lines to avoid recombination leading to helper virus production. *Molecular and Cell Biology 6*(8), 2895-2902.

Moolten, F. L. (1986). Tumor chemosensitivity conferred by inserted herpes thymidine kinase genes: Paradigm for a prospective cancer control strategy. *Cancer Research, 46,* 5276-5281.

Moss, B. (1992a). Vaccinia virus vectors. *Biotechnology, 20,* 345-362.

Moss, B. (1992b). Poxvirus expression vectors. *Current topics in microbiology and immunology, 158,* 25-38.

Nicolau, C., LePape, A., Soriano, P., Fargette, F., & Juhel, M. F. (1983). In vivo expression of rat insulin after intravenous administration of the liposome-entrapped gene for rat insulin 1. *Proceedings of the National Academy of Sciences, 80,* 1068-1072.

Pastan, I., & Gottesman, M. M. (1991). Multidrug resistance. *Annual Review of Medicine, 41,* 277-286.

Peters, J., Dimond, E., & Jenkins, J. (1997). Clinical applications of genetic technologies to cancer care. *Cancer Nursing, 20*(5), 359-377.

Podda, S., Ward, M., Himelstein, A., Richardson, C., de la Flor-Weiss, E., Smith, L., Gottesman, M., Pastan, I., & Bank, A. (1992). Transfer and expression of the human multiple drug resistance gene into live mice. *Proceedings of the National Academy of Sciences, USA, 89,* 9676-9680.

Poeschla, E., & Wong-Staal, F. (1994). Antiviral and anticancer ribozymes. *Current Opinion in Oncology, 6,* 601-606.

Quantin, B., Perricaudet, L. D., Tajbakhsh, S., & Mandell, J. L. (1992). Adenovirus as an expression vector in muscle cells in vivo. *Proceedings of the National Academy of Sciences, 89,* 2581-2584.

Ratajczak, M. A., Kant, J. A., Luger, S. M., Hijiya, N., Zhang, J., Zon, G., & Gerwitz, A. M. (1992). In vivo treatment of human leukemia in a scid mouse model with c-myb antisense oligodeoxynucleotides. *Proceedings of the National Academy of Sciences, USA, 89,* 11823-11827.

Reed, J. C., Stein, C., Subasinghe, C., Haldar, S., Croce, C. M., Yum, S., & Cohen, J. (1990). Anti-sense mediated inhibition of BCL-2 protooncogene expression and leukemic cell growth and survival: Comparisons of phosphodiester and phosphorothioate oligodeoxynucleotides. *Cancer Research, 50,* 6565-6570.

Richardson, C., Ward, M., & Bank, A. (1995). MDR gene transfer into live mice. *Journal of Molecular Medicine, 73,* 189-195.

Richardson, C., Ward, M., Podda, S., & Bank, A. (1994). Mouse fetal liver cells lack functional amphotropic retroviral receptors. *Blood, 84,* 433-439.

Rosenfeld, M. A., Yoshimura, K., Trapnell, B. C., Yoneyama, K., Rosenthal, E. R., Dalemans, W., Fukayami, M., Bargon, J., Stier, L. E., & Stratford-Perricaudet, L. (1992). In vivo transfer of human cystic fibrosis transmembrane conductance regulator gene into the airway epithelium. *Cell, 68,* 143-155.

Roth, J. A., Jguyen, D., Lawrence, D. D., Kemp, B. L., Carrasco, C. H., Ferson, D. Z., & Hong, W. K. (1996). Retrovirus-mediated wild type p53 gene transfer to tumors of patients with lung cancer. *Nature Medicine, 2,* 985-991.

Runnebaum, I. B. (1997). Basics of cancer gene therapy. *Anticancer Research, 17,* 2887-2890.

Siegl, G., Bates, R. C., Berns, K. I., Carter, B. J., Kelly, D. C., Kurstak, E., & Tattersall, P. (1985). Characteristics and taxonomy of Parvoviradae. *Intervirology, 23,* 61-73.

Sorrentino, B. P., Brandt, S. J., Bodine, D., Gottesman, M., Pastan, I., Cline, A., & Nienhuis, A. W. (1992). Selection of drug-resistant bone marrow cells in vivo after retroviral transfer of human MDR1. *Science, 257,* 99-103.

Szczylik, C., Skorski, T., Nicolaides, N. C., Manzella, L., Malaguarnera, L., Venturelli, D., Gerwitz, A. M., & Calabretta, B. (1991). Selective inhibition of leukemia cell proliferation by BCR-ABL antisense oligodeoxynucleotides. *Science, 253,* 562-565.

Thomas, K. R., & Capecchi, M. R. (1987). Site-directed mutagenesis by gene targeting in mouse embryo-derived stem cells. *Cell, 51,* 503-512.

Tong, X. W., Block, A., Chen, S-H., Contant, C. F., Agoulnik, I., Blankberg, K., & Kaufman, R. H. (1996). In vivo gene therapy of ovarian cancer by adenovirus-mediated thymidine binase gene transduction and ganciclovir administration. *Gynecological Oncology, 61,* 175-179.

Vile, R. G., Nelson, J. A., Castleden, S., Chong, H., & Hart, I. R. (1994). Systemic gene therapy of murine melanoma using tissue specific expression of the HSV-tk gene involves an immune component. *Cancer Research, 54,* 6226-6234.

Ward, M. (1996). Transfer and expression of the human MDR gene in peripheral blood progenitor cells. *Clinical Cancer Research, 2,* 873-876.

Weichselbaum, R. R., & Kufe, D. (1997). Gene therapy of cancer. *Lancet, 349*(Suppl. 11), 10-12.

Wolff, J. A., & Lederberg, J. (1994). An early history of gene transfer and therapy. *Human Gene Therapy, 5,* 469-480.

Wolff, J. A., Malone, R. W., Williams, P., Chong, W., Acsadi, G., Jani, A., & Felgner, P. L. (1990). Direct gene transfer into mouse muscle in vivo. *Science, 247,* 1465-1468.

Wu, G. Y., Wilson, J. M., Shalaby, F., Grossman, M., Shafritz, D. A., & Wu, C. H. (1991). Receptor-mediated gene delivery in vivo. *Journal of Biological Chemistry, 266,* 14338-14342.

Xu, M., Kumar, D., Srinivas, S., Detolla, L. J., Yu, S. F., Stass, S. A., & Mixson, A. J. (1997). Parenteral gene therapy with p53 inhibits human breast tumors in vivo through a bystander mechanism without evidence of toxicity. *Human Gene Therapy, 8,* 177-185.

Yang, Y., Nunes, F. A., Berencsi, K., Furth, E. E., Gonczol, E., & Wilson, J. M. (1994). Cellular immunity to viral antigens limits E-1 deleted adenoviruses for gene therapy. *Proceedings of the National Academy of Sciences, 91,* 4407-4411.

Yee, D., McGuire, S. E., Brunner, N., Kozelsky, T. W., Allred, D. C., Chen, S. H., & Woo, S. L. C. (1996). Adenovirus-mediated gene transfer of herpes simplex virus thymidine kinase in an ascites model of human breast cancer. *Human Gene Therapy, 7,* 1251-1257.

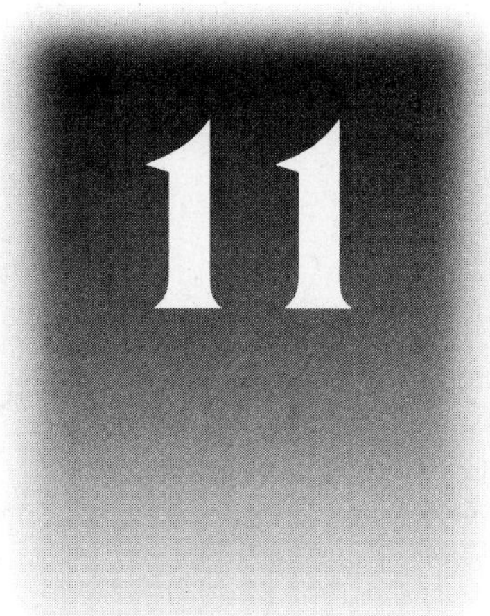

Oncologic Emergencies

Christine Miaskowski, RN, PhD, FAAN

INTRODUCTION

Cancer is becoming a chronic illness. Therefore patients are living longer with the disease and have a greater chance of developing an oncologic emergency associated with their disease or treatment. Oncology nurses are experts at assessing and monitoring patients during and after the completion of cancer therapy. One of the most important principles in the accurate diagnosis of an oncologic emergency is to maintain a high index of suspicion. The morbidity associated with an oncologic emergency may be significantly reduced with prompt recognition and the initiation of appropriate therapy.

A complete review of all of the oncologic emergencies experienced by oncology patients is beyond the scope of this book. A summary of the pathophysiologic mechanisms underlying some of the most common oncologic emergencies is presented. In addition, an approach to assessing the patient for a specific oncologic emergency and a standard of care for each emergency are included in this chapter.

DISSEMINATED INTRAVASCULAR COAGULATION

Pathophysiology

The condition of disseminated intravascular coagulation (DIC) can be described as a process where clotting suddenly occurs throughout the vascular system. DIC represents a two-stage process of an acceleration of the normal clotting process and a decrease in the amount of circulating clotting factors. The pathophysiologic processes involved in DIC are illustrated in Fig. 11-1.

Normally a balance exists and equilibrium is maintained between the clotting mechanisms and the process of fibrinolysis. With the occurrence of DIC, an overwhelming thrombogenic stimulus triggers the process of DIC. As the process continues, coagulation occurs at the same time as fibrinolysis. The diffuse intravascular coagulation results in fibrin deposits in the microcirculation. The development of microvascular thrombi results in ischemic tissue injury in major organs, including the heart, lungs, kidneys, liver, central nervous system, and skin. In addition, red blood cell (RBC) damage and hemolysis occurs as RBCs attempt to pass through the capillaries that contain microthrombi. Ischemic tissue injury and subsequent end organ failure can potentiate the development of shock. It should be noted that the intravascular coagulation process results in the consumption of platelets and clotting factors. These substances are consumed faster than they can be replaced. The end result is that the patient has the tendency to bleed (Bailes, 1992; Bick, 1994).

The mechanisms by which tumors activate the hemostatic system with the subsequent development of DIC are extremely complex. Tumors have been shown to produce procoagulants (e.g., tissue factor, cancer procoagulant) that activate the clotting cascade. In addition, tumor cells have been shown to activate platelets and promote platelet aggregation (Bick, 1994). The cancers most commonly associated with the development of DIC, as well as other conditions that can contribute to the development of DIC in oncology patients, are listed in Box 11-1.

Assessment

The key to accurate assessment of the patient for DIC is to maintain a high index of suspicion. Patients with DIC tend to bleed from at least three unrelated sites simultaneously. Patients with fulminating DIC can progress rapidly to a shocklike state with associated end organ dysfunction (e.g., renal failure, pulmonary failure) (Table 11-1).

Medical Management

The medical management of DIC involves removing the trigger of the disorder. In oncology patients who are experiencing DIC, this approach may not always be feasible. Additional approaches to treatment include stopping the intravascular clotting process, administering blood component therapy as indicated, and inhibiting residual fibrinolysis. All treatment approaches must be individualized.

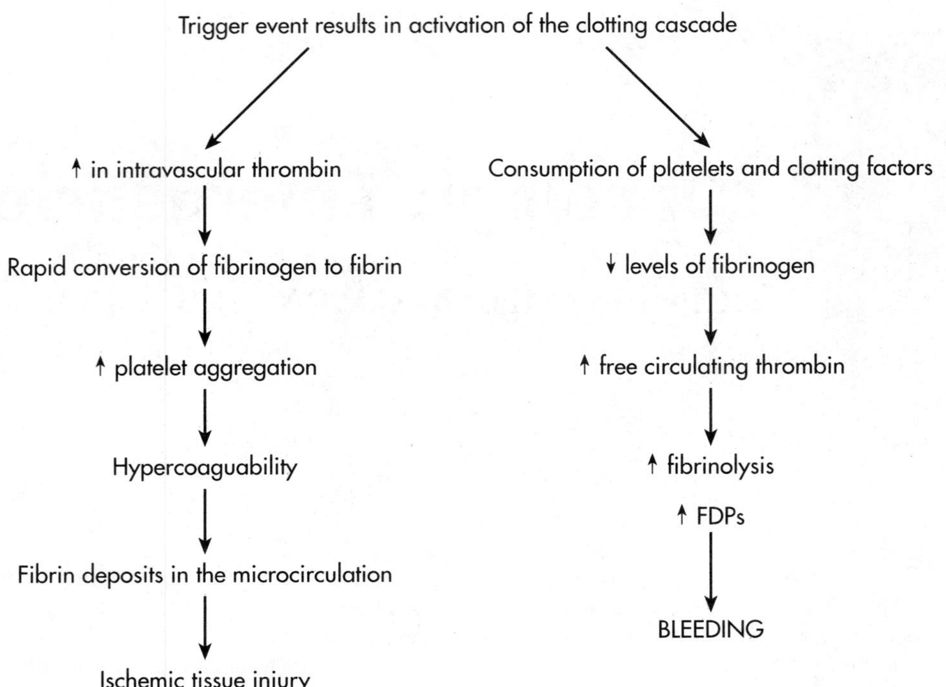

Fig. 11-1 The pathophysiology of disseminated intravascular coagulation.

Box 11-1
Cancers and Conditions Associated With Disseminated Intravascular Coagulation

Cancers Associated With DIC
Acute promyelocytic leukemia
Acute myelomonocytic leukemia
Acute myeloblastic leukemia
Immunoblastic lymphomas
Hodgkin's disease
Biliary cancer
Breast cancer
Colon cancer
Gastric cancer
Lung cancer
Malignant melanoma
Ovarian cancer
Prostate cancer

Other Conditions Associated With DIC
Sepsis
Massive tissue injury (e.g., major surgery)
Placement of an intraperitoneal shunt
Transfusion reaction

The major intervention to decrease thrombin formation and intravascular clotting is the administration of heparin. In most instances, heparin is administered as a low-dose continuous infusion (e.g., 5 to 10 units per kg/hour) (Williams & Mosher, 1995). Additional therapy may include the administration of antithrombin concentrates. Antithrombin is a coagulation factor that inhibits the competitive action of thrombin during heparin therapy.

Approximately 75% of patients with DIC respond to the first two steps in the treatment plan—removing the trigger and initiating therapy to stop the intravascular clotting process. If patients continue to bleed, the most probable cause is the depletion of blood components. These patients may require the administration of blood components (e.g., washed, packed RBCs; platelet concentrates; nonclotting, protein-containing volume expanders). The general rule, if the patient requires blood component therapy, is to administer concentrates and components that are devoid of fibrinogen.

In a small percentage of cases, patients require fibrinolytic therapy. This therapy is directed at preventing or controlling additional bleeding. The agent most commonly used is epsilon-aminocaproic acid. Another antifibrinolytic agent that may be used is tranexamic acid (Bailes, 1992; Bick, 1994).

Nursing Management

The nursing management of the patient with DIC centers on monitoring the patient for excessive bleeding or clotting, allaying the patient's anxiety, and providing reassurance that the medical management helps reverse the disease process (Collins, 1995; Dangel, 1991; Murphy-Ende, 1998).

Particular attention should be paid to the prevention of injury. A fall or any other type of injury could result in a fatal hemorrhage. The nursing care of the patient with DIC is summarized in Table 11-2.

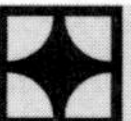

TABLE 11-1 Assessment of the Patient for Disseminated Intravascular Coagulation

	Assessment Parameters	Typical Abnormal Findings
History	A. Cancer diagnosis	A. Cancers associated with the development of DIC are listed in Box 11-1.
	B. Concurrent conditions	B. Concurrent conditions associated with the development of DIC are listed in Box 11-1.
Physical Examination	A. Evaluate the patient for evidence of bleeding.	A. Evidence of bleeding 1. Predominant signs of DIC a. Petechiae b. Ecchymosis c. Prolonged bleeding from injection sites 2. Additional signs of bleeding include: a. Epistaxis b. Oozing from old injection sites c. Bleeding from incision sites d. Intestinal bleeding
	B. Evaluate for major internal hemorrhage.	B. Signs and symptoms of a major internal hemorrhage include hypotension, tachycardia, decreased hematocrit, decreased urine output.
	C. Assess the patient for evidence of clotting.	C. Evidence of clotting may include: 1. *Renal system:* hematuria, renal failure 2. *Central nervous system:* mental status changes 3. *Integumentary system:* presence of acrocyanosis (i.e., generalized sweating with cold, mottled fingers and toes)
Diagnostic Tests	A. General comments regarding laboratory tests	A. The laboratory diagnosis of DIC is complex. Most laboratory tests that are abnormal in DIC are abnormal only in the fulminant form of DIC. In subacute or low grade DIC associated with cancer, many laboratory tests of hemostasis may be difficult to interpret or are within normal limits.
	B. Prothrombin time (PT)	B. Usually prolonged
	C. Activated partial thromboplastin time (aPTT)	C. May be prolonged
	D. Thrombin time (TT)	D. Usually prolonged
	E. Fibrinogen level	E. Usually decreased
	F. Fibrin degradation products (FDPs)	F. Elevated
	G. D-dimer assay	G. Elevated
	H. Platelet count	H. Usually decreased

HYPERCALCEMIA

Pathophysiology

Calcium is the fifth most abundant cation in the body and exists in insoluble (99%) and soluble forms (1%). The soluble or freely exchangeable calcium exists in three forms: (1) ionized or free calcium (40% to 50%); (2) calcium bound to plasma proteins (40% to 45%); and (3) calcium combined with anions such as citrate or phosphate (5% to 10%). Only the ionized calcium is physiologically active and is one of the most precisely controlled constituents of body fluids.

Normal serum calcium levels range from 9 to 11 mg/dl. If ionized calcium levels are not available (normal value ranges from 1.16 to 1.32 mmol/L), then serum calcium levels must be evaluated in relationship to the patient's serum albumin level. If the serum albumin is reduced, which is likely to occur in oncology patients, then less calcium is bound to protein. Because serum calcium is often reported and measured as total serum calcium, it should be noted that a decrease in serum albumin results in an elevation of unbound or ionized calcium. Clinicians need to measure either ionized calcium levels or correct the serum calcium level in relationship to serum albumin using the formula found in Table 11-3.

Calcium is involved in numerous physiologic functions, including the clotting cascade, neuromuscular activity, muscular depolarization, secretion of hormones and neurotransmitters, and neutrophil chemotaxis. Normal levels of calcium are maintained through a complex feedback loop involving parathyroid hormone, calcitonin, and 1,25 dihydroxy vitamin D_3. The overall schema for regulation of serum calcium level is shown in Fig. 11-2.

A decrease in serum calcium level causes a release of parathyroid hormone (PTH) from the parathyroid gland. The release of PTH causes the kidney to release the enzyme

TABLE 11-2 Standard of Care for the Patient With Disseminated Intravascular Coagulation

Patient Problems and Outcomes	Nursing Interventions and Rationales	Patient Education Instructions
Alteration in Tissue Perfusion		
Patient will:		
• Maintain adequate tissue perfusion	1. Assess skin for signs of thrombosis (i.e., acrocyanosis). 2. Assess for signs and symptoms of thrombosis, vascular occlusion, and organ ischemia: a. *Neurologic:* syncope, change in level of consciousness, paresthesias b. *Renal:* progressive oliguria c. *Gastrointestinal:* bowel necrosis 3. Monitor laboratory values (see Table 11-1). 4. Administer heparin as prescribed. 5. Administer fibrinolytic agents as prescribed.	1. Explain the rationale for the interventions. 2. Provide information and reasons for maintaining a safe environment to protect the patient from injury or falls.
Anxiety		
Patient will:		
• Experience a tolerable level of anxiety	1. Assess concerns regarding the problem and the medical management of the problem. 2. Assess usual coping strategies. 3. Administer sedative medications as needed.	1. Provide an explanation of DIC. 2. Explain the rationale for the therapeutic interventions. 3. Teach relaxation exercises.

25-hydroxycalciferol-1-hydroxylase. This enzyme converts a circulating metabolite of vitamin D_3– called *25 hydroxycholecalciferol (25-OH-D_3)* into an active metabolite called *1,25 dihydroxy vitamin D_3 (1,25 diOHD_3)*. The active metabolite, 1,25 diOHD_3, is one of the most potent substances known to raise serum calcium levels. This metabolite causes increased absorption of calcium and phosphate from the intestine and increases the activity of osteoclasts in bone. Osteoclast activity results in the release of calcium from storage in bone into the serum.

In addition, PTH acts directly on the ascending limb of the loops of Henle, distal tubules, and collecting ducts of the kidney to increase the renal absorption of calcium. Taken together, these mechanisms result in an increase in serum calcium levels. An increase in serum calcium levels results in the secretion of calcitonin from the thyroid gland. Calcitonin has several mechanisms of action. The hormone activates an enzyme, which converts 1,25 diOHD_3 to an inactive metabolite (e.g., 24,25 diOHD_3) excreted by the kidneys. In addition, calcitonin acts on the osteoblasts of the bone to increase the uptake serum calcium into the bone. This feedback system maintains the levels of serum calcium under tight control.

Hypercalcemia associated with cancer occurs as a result of a number of different mechanisms. Current evidence suggests that hypercalcemia of malignancy is a complex metabolic complication in which the primary defect is an increase in bone resorption of calcium that exceeds both bone formation and the kidney's ability to excrete serum calcium (Adami & Rossini, 1992; Goni & Tolis, 1993). The cancers most commonly associated with hypercalcemia are listed in Box 11-2. Hypercalcemia is associated with a 50% mortality rate if not properly treated.

TABLE 11-3 Formula to Correct Serum Calcium Level in a Patient With a Decreased Level of Serum Albumin

$$\frac{\textit{Corrected calcium}}{(\textit{mg/dL})} = \frac{\textit{measured calcium}}{(\textit{mg/dL})} \quad \frac{\textit{albumin}}{(\textit{g/dL})} + 4.0$$

EXAMPLE: Cancer patient has a calcium level of 11.5 mg/dL and a serum albumin of 1.5 g/dL.
Corrected calcium = 11.5 − 1.5 + 4
Corrected calcium = 14

Box 11-2

Cancers Associated With the Development of Hypercalcemia

- Squamous cell carcinoma of the lung
- Squamous cell carcinoma of the head and neck
- Breast cancer
- Multiple myeloma
- T-cell lymphoma
- Renal cancer
- Ovarian cancer
- Prostate cancer
- Bladder cancer
- Ewing's sarcoma
- Thyroid cancer

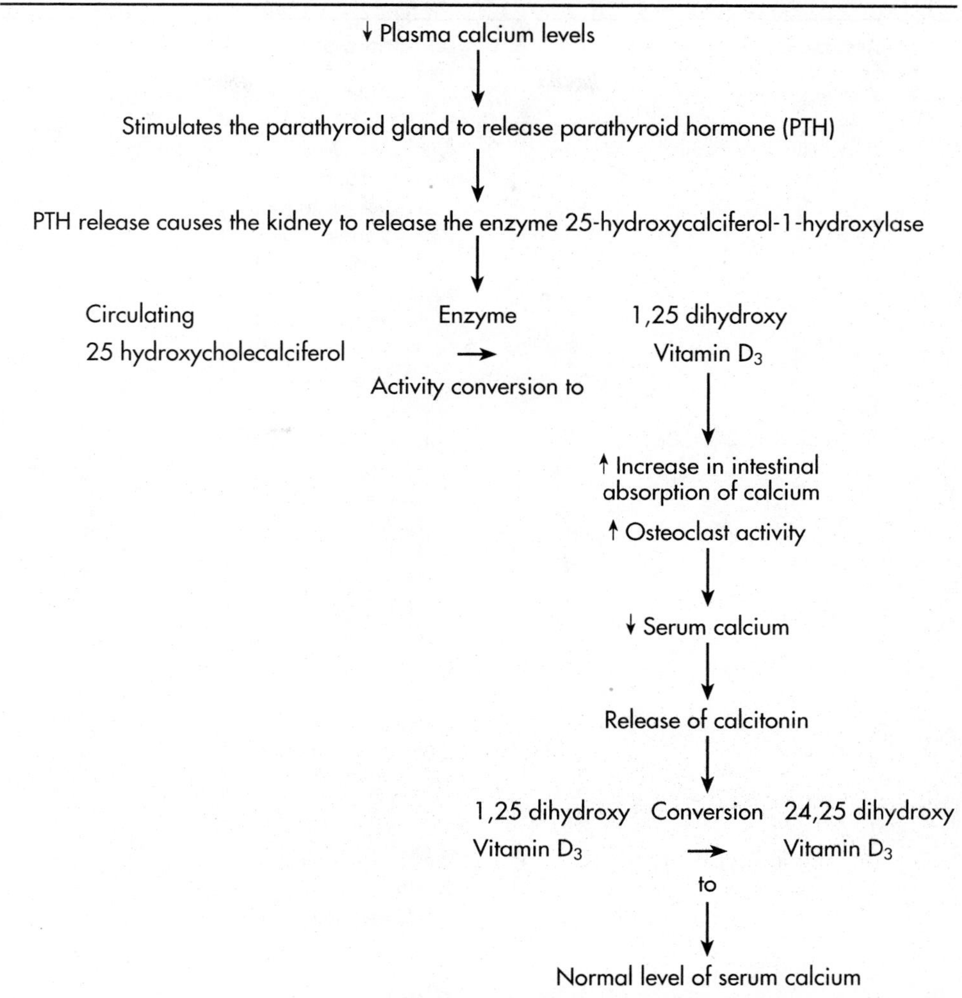

Fig. 11-2 Control of serum calcium levels.

Several mechanisms may be involved in the development of hypercalcemia associated with malignant disease. First of all, hypercalcemia of malignancy is thought to occur because certain tumors produce a parathyroid hormone-related protein (PTH-rP). This PTH-rP has been isolated from a variety of tumor cells and is known to have significant sequence homology with the NH_2-terminal region of PTH. Since the NH_2-terminal region of PTH is responsible for the hormone's biologic activity, PTH-rP mimics the effects of PTH by binding to the PTH-receptor. The increased levels of PTH-rP result in increased osteoclast bone resorption of calcium and increased renal absorption of calcium that results in hypercalcemia. The PTH-rP has been identified in the following tumor types: squamous cell cancer of the lung, squamous cell cancer of the head and neck, T-cell lymphoma, breast cancer, and renal cancer (Adami & Rossini, 1992; Goni & Tolis, 1993).

A second mechanism involved in the development of hypercalcemia of malignancy is the production of prostaglandins of the E series by certain tumors. Prostaglandins of the E series have complex effects on bone, including the stimulation of osteoclast resorption of bone. The third mechanism involved in the hypercalcemia of malignancy is the production of osteoclast activating factors by certain tumors. A number of cytokines (e.g., transforming growth factor-alpha, lymphotoxin, tumor necrosis factor [TNF], or interleukin-1 [IL-1]) stimulate osteoclast resorption of bone. The increased resorption of calcium from bone results in an elevation in serum calcium levels (Adami & Rossini, 1992; Goni & Tolis, 1993).

Assessment

Patients with hypercalcemia exhibit a variety of signs and symptoms because calcium is involved in the regulation of numerous physiologic processes. Signs and symptoms vary depending on the rapidity with which hypercalcemia develops (Table 11-4).

TABLE 11-4 Assessment of the Patient for Hypercalcemia

	Assessment Parameters	Typical Abnormal Findings
History	A. Cancer diagnosis	A. Cancers associated with the development of hypercalcemia are listed in Box 11-3.
	B. Concurrent medical conditions	B. Patients should be evaluated for the following concurrent medical conditions: 1. Hyperparathyroidism 2. Sarcoidosis 3. Immobility 4. Dehydration 5. Renal dysfunction 6. Malnutrition 7. Skeletal fractures 8. Acute osteoporosis
Physical Examination	A. Neuromuscular effects	A. Signs and symptoms include: 1. Apathy 2. Depression 3. Malaise 4. Fatigue 5. Profound muscle weakness 6. Hyporeflexia 7. Occasionally, anxiety or agitation 8. Rarely, psychotic behavior 9. Hypercalcemic crisis would present with mental obtundation 10. Bone pain
	B. Renal effects	B. Signs and symptoms include: 1. Polyuria 2. Nocturia 3. Dehydration
	C. Gastrointestinal effects	C. Signs and symptoms include: 1. Anorexia 2. Nausea and vomiting 3. Abdominal pain 4. Constipation 5. Ileus
Diagnostic Tests	A. Serum calcium level	A. Elevated serum calcium >11 mg/dl
	B. Serum phosphorus	B. Decreased serum phosphorus <2.5 mg/dl
	C. Blood urea nitrogen (BUN)	C. Elevated BUN >18 mg/dl
	D. Serum creatinine	D. Elevated serum creatinine >1.2 mg/dl
	E. Electrocardiogram	E. Changes indicative of hypercalcemia include: 1. Shortening QT-interval 2. Prolongation of PR-interval 3. Dysrhythmias.

Medical Management

As with other oncologic emergencies, treatment of the underlying cause of the hypercalcemia is the most effective approach to the problem. However, in some cases this approach may not be possible, and symptomatic relief becomes the priority. Medical interventions focus on increasing the renal excretion of calcium, decreasing the gastrointestinal absorption of calcium, and decreasing the renal absorption of calcium. With mild hypercalcemia (less than 13 mg/dl) the patient may be asymptomatic. Treatment with oral hydration (3 to 4 L/day) and an increase in the patient's level of mobility may be sufficient to reduce serum calcium levels.

Patients with serum calcium levels between 13 and 15 mg/dl are usually moderately symptomatic and require more aggressive treatment. Intravenous (IV) hydration with normal saline (4-6 L in 24 hours) is required to replenish intravascular volume and restore the glomerular filtration rate. After intravascular volume is restored, a calciuric diuretic (e.g., furosemide 40-100 mg every 12 to 24 hours) can be administered.

With serum calcium levels greater than 15 mg/dl, more aggressive hydration is required. In addition, agents that inhibit bone resorption of calcium are administered. These agents include calcitonin, plicamycin, gallium nitrate, the bisphosphonates (etidronate, pamidronate, clodronate) or

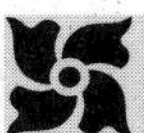

TABLE 11-5 Standard of Care for the Patient With Hypercalcemia

Patient Problems and Outcomes	Nursing Interventions and Rationales	Patient Education Instructions
Dehydration Patient will: • Maintain an adequate fluid volume	1. Monitor intake and output. 2. Weigh patient daily. 3. Assess skin integrity and skin turgor. 4. Monitor vital signs for hypovolemia. 5. Monitor serum electrolytes, level of blood urea nitrogen, and serum creatinine. 6. Administer intravenous hydration with normal saline.	1. Teach patient to use comfort measures for dehydration: a. Moisturize lips and skin b. Perform frequent oral hygiene c. Apply ointment or drops to eyes 2. Teach patient the importance of drinking 3 to 4 liters of fluid per day. Suggest that patient divide fluid intake over the course of the day to maximize fluid intake.
High Risk for Injury Patient will: • Remain free of bodily injury	1. Modify and maintain a safe environment. 2. Assess mental status and determine risk for falls. 3. Assist patient to perform activities of daily living. 4. Assist patient to increase mobility or to perform range-of-motion exercises if on bedrest.	1. Teach patient to evaluate his home environment for potential hazards and to remove these hazards.
Fatigue Patient will: • Maintain optimal activity level	1. Perform a fatigue assessment. 2. Assess patient's daily schedule of activities and his level of endurance.	1. Teach patient to prioritize activities to conserve energy. 2. Explore and provide opportunities that are restful and restorative of energy.

the oral phosphates. In addition, strategies should be employed to increase the mobility of patients with hypercalcemia. Additional benefits may be derived from reducing the dietary intake of calcium (Chisholm, Mulloy, & Taylor, 1996).

Nursing Management

The patient with hypercalcemia requires intensive nursing care. The changes in mental status that occur with hypercalcemia can result in increased risk for injury. In addition, severe hypercalcemia can result in fatal dysrhythmias and renal failure. Depending on the patient's overall prognosis, a decision may need to be made regarding the use of hemodialysis (Calafato & Jessup, 1991; Cockburn, 1995; Meriney & Reeder, 1998) (Table 11-5).

NEOPLASTIC CARDIAC TAMPONADE

Pathophysiology

Cardiac tamponade is an acute compression of the heart by fluid (usually blood) in the pericardial sac. In oncology patients, cardiac tamponade can develop suddenly or insidiously. This oncologic emergency can go unrecognized! The normal mortality rate for cardiac tamponade is 25%. However, if cardiac tamponade goes unrecognized, the mortality rate rises to 65% (Ameli & Shah, 1991; Kralstein & Frishman, 1987).

The pericardium is a double-walled sac that surrounds the heart and the roots of the great vessels. The visceral layer of the pericardium adheres directly to the surface of the heart. The parietal layer is the outer, fibrous layer that can move freely. Between the visceral and the parietal layer is the pericardial sac. The sac contains approximately 25 to 30 ml of straw-colored serous fluid that has the composition of lymph. The pericardium provides a frictionless sac for the heart's contractions. It serves as a restraining force against cardiac overdistention and supports the heart in a stable position.

Fig. 11-3 shows the pathophysiologic processes involved in cardiac tamponade. The basic mechanism underlying cardiac tamponade is an increase in intrapericardial pressure that results from fluid filling the pericardial sac. The increase in pressure causes a decrease in cardiac filling with subsequent decreases in cardiac output. The pericardial wall is made of stiff membranous material that makes it resistant to stretching. Normally, the pericardial sac holds approximately 50 ml of fluid. A sudden increase of as little as 100 ml of fluid in the pericardial sac can precipitate severe car-

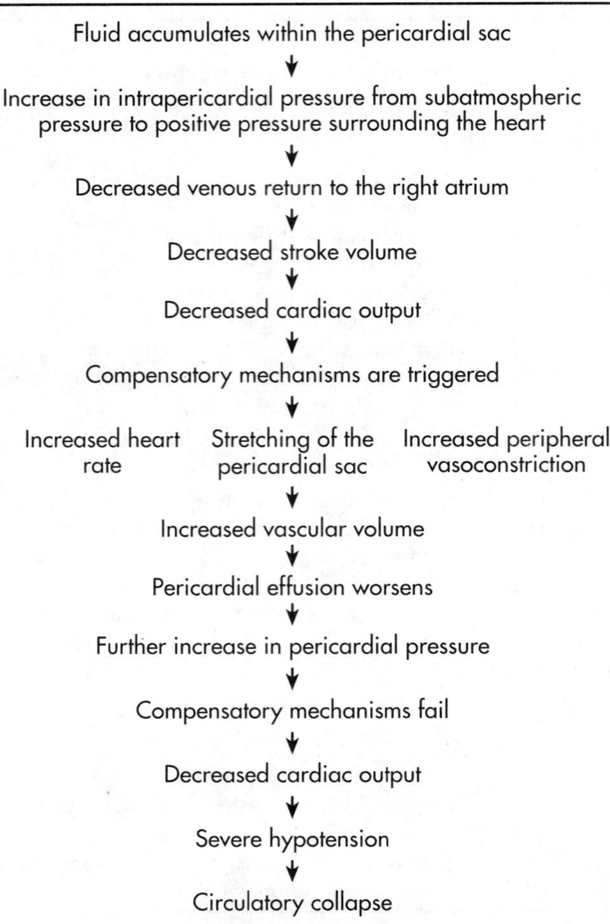

Fig. 11-3 Pathophysiologic processes in cardiac tamponade.

diovascular compromise and a shock state. However, if the pericardial effusion develops slowly, as much as 2 L of fluid can accumulate because the pericardial wall stretches over time.

The major causes of neoplastic cardiac tamponade are listed in Box 11-3. The most common cause of a malignant pericardial effusion is metastases from lung cancer, breast cancer, leukemia, Hodgkin's or non–Hodgkin's lymphoma, or melanoma. Radiation-induced pericarditis can occur when the heart receives 4000 or more cGys. Pericarditis can develop during the course of radiation therapy or within weeks or months after completing radiation therapy, as with acute pericarditis, or it can develop within a few months or up to 20 years after treatment, as with chronic pericarditis (Ameli & Shah, 1991; Kralstein & Frishman, 1987).

Assessment

The signs and symptoms that the patient exhibits are extremely variable depending on whether the effusion develops suddenly or insidiously (Table 11-6).

Box 11-3
Causes of Neoplastic Cardiac Tamponade

- Malignant pericardial effusion—most common cause
- Tumor directly encases the heart—rare cause
- Combination of pressure and constriction from a tumor mass and fluid
- Postirradiation pericarditis

Medical Management

The medical management of this oncologic emergency involves a pericardiocentesis. This procedure involves the insertion of a needle in the left lateral xiphoid insertion site between the xiphoid process and the left costal margin. The insertion of a needle into the pericardial sac allows for the removal of fluid, which reduces intrapericardial pressure. This decrease in pericardial pressure results in significant improvement in the patient's cardiac output and often a dramatic improvement in the patient's symptoms. During and following the emergency pericardiocentesis, the patient may require supportive therapy, including fluids and oxygen.

Chronic treatment of neoplastic cardiac tamponade can take the form of a pericardial window, pericardectomy, or a pericardioperitoneal shunt. Other treatment options include the administration of chemotherapy to treat the underlying cancer or the use of radiation therapy if the tumor is radiosensitive. The choice of treatment depends on the patient's underlying disease, as well as his or her physical condition (Ameli & Shah, 1991; Kralstein & Frishman, 1987).

Nursing Management

Nursing management of the patient with neoplastic cardiac tamponade centers on relieving anxiety and fear and making the patient as comfortable as possible during the acute phase of treatment. Attention must be paid to maintaining an adequate cardiac output to ensure adequate oxygenation and perfusion of major organ systems (Davies, 1995; Dragonette, 1998; Hydzik, 1991). Table 11-7 describes the nursing management of the patient with neoplastic cardiac tamponade.

SEPSIS

Pathophysiology

Sepsis is one of the most challenging problems faced by clinicians who care for oncology patients. In 1991 a new nomenclature was developed by members of the Society of Critical Care Medicine and the American College of Chest Physicians that defined sepsis as a type of systemic inflammatory response syndrome (SIRS) that occurs in response to infection. The specific response criteria for sepsis are listed in Box 11-4 (Ackerman, 1994).

In sepsis, a substance in the microbial cell wall, usually an endotoxin initiates the activation of the complement and clotting cascades. The consequences of activation of the

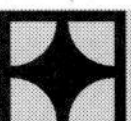

TABLE 11-6 Assessment of the Patient for Neoplastic Cardiac Tamponade

	Assessment Parameters	Typical Abnormal Findings
History	A. Cancer diagnosis	A. Patients are at risk for the development of neoplastic cardiac tamponade with any of the following cancer diagnoses: 1. Metastatic disease from: a. Lung cancer b. Breast cancer c. Leukemia d. Hodgkin's disease e. Non-Hodgkin's lymphoma f. Melanoma
	B. History of radiation to the thorax including the heart	B. Patients who have received 4,000 or more cGys to the heart
Physical Examination	A. Initial signs and symptoms	A. Patient may present with: 1. Weakness 2. Fatigue 3. Anxiety, apprehension
	B. Progressive signs and symptoms	B. As the effusion enlarges, patients experience: 1. Dyspnea and tachypnea 2. Precordial oppressive feeling 3. Perfuse perspiration 4. Tachycardia 5. Pulsus paradoxus 6. Decreased systolic blood pressure
	C. Additional signs and symptoms	C. Additional signs and symptoms that can occur depending on the extent of the effusion and the structures that are impinged on by the effusion include the following: 1. Cough 2. Dysphagia 3. Hoarseness 4. Hiccups 5. Nausea and vomiting 6. Abdominal pain 7. Seizures 8. Jugular venous distention 9. Ascites 10. Distant or muffled heart sounds
Diagnostic Tests	A. Chest x-ray	A. The cardiac silhouette may be enlarged with a water bottle appearance or globular shape
	B. Electrocardiogram	B. Sinus tachycardia; widespread ST-segment elevations; PR-segment depression; T-wave inversion; electrical alternans
	C. Echocardiogram	C. Pericardial effusion appears as an echo-free space between the pericardium and the heart
	D. Cardiac catheterization	D. Can determine the size and exact location of the effusion
	E. Computerized tomography or magnetic resonance imaging	E. Can distinguish between a pericardial effusion and pericardial thickening caused by radiation fibrosis

complement and clotting cascades include increased capillary permeability, vasodilation, and coagulopathies. In addition, phagocytic cells are activated that produce TNF and IL-1.

TNF is a cytokine produced by the monocyte/macrophage family of white blood cells (WBCs). This cytokine plays a role in the immediate inflammatory response and induces the release of other mediators that are part of the inflammatory response. The pathophysiologic effects of TNF include hypotension, tachycardia, tachypnea, hyperglycemia, metabolic acidosis, and alveolar thickening.

IL-1 is another cytokine that is released by macrophages and other cells during the process of inflammation. The effects of IL-1 include leukocytosis, fever, and metabolic changes. The effects of TNF and IL-1 appear to be synergistic.

The initial systemic inflammatory response to an infection results in an increase in cardiac output because of gen-

TABLE 11-7 Standard of Care for the Patient With Neoplastic Cardiac Tamponade

Patient Problems and Outcomes	Nursing Interventions and Rationales	Patient Education Instructions
Decreased Cardiac Output Patient will: • Maintain an adequate cardiac output	1. Monitor vital signs. 2. Maintain an intravenous line for administration of emergency medication. 3. Prepare patient for emergency pericardiocentesis or transfer to the operating room.	1. Inform patient of the purpose of all procedures and the reason for frequent monitoring of vital signs. 2. Explain the purpose of the pericardiocentesis as well as the steps of the procedure. 3. Try to allay patient's anxiety by providing simple explanation. 4. Allow patient to discuss concerns.
Altered Peripheral, Cerebral, and Renal Tissue Perfusion Patient will: • Maintain adequate peripheral, cerebral, and renal tissue perfusion	1. Assess skin color, temperature, moisture, and capillary refill time (should be less than 3 seconds). 2. Assess for changes in level of consciousness. 3. Monitor intake and output. 4. Monitor arterial blood gases.	1. Explain to patient the reason for the frequent monitoring.

eralized peripheral vasodilation and reflex tachycardia. As the SIRS continues, there is an increase in capillary permeability and microvascular clotting occurs. These changes lead to a maldistribution of circulating blood volume, an imbalance in oxygen supply and demand in vital organs, and alterations in metabolism. These processes are manifested as profound hypotension and multiple organ dysfunction (Ackerman, 1994).

Sepsis is the most significant complication of cancer treatment. The numerous factors that contribute to infectious complications in oncology patients are listed in Box 11-5.

Assessment

Clinicians need to maintain a high index of suspicion for sepsis when evaluating oncology patients who are immunosuppressed (Emmanouilides & Glaspy, 1996; Rubin & Ferraro, 1993). In addition to the risk factors listed in Box 11-6, very young and elderly patients are at increased risk for the development of sepsis because of the decreased production of T lymphocytes and a limited ability to mount an inflammatory response (Table 11-8).

Medical Management

The medical management of sepsis focuses on identifying the infectious organism and selecting the most appropriate empiric antibiotic therapy (Freifeld, 1993). Patients who are experiencing sepsis and who are progressing to septic shock require fluid resuscitation usually with normal saline or lactated Ringer's solution (150 to 500 ml/hour). If hypotension continues after fluid resuscitation, the patient will be started on vasoactive therapy (e.g., dopamine with or without dobutamine to maintain a mean arterial pressure of more than 60 mm Hg).

Nursing Management

Patients with cancer are at extremely high risk for developing sepsis. Since sepsis is associated with significant mor-

Box 11-4
Criteria for Sepsis

Sepsis is a systemic response to infection. This systemic response is manifested by two or more of the following conditions as a result of an infection:

- Temperature >100.4° F (38° C) or <96.8° F(36° C)
- Heart rate >90 beats/minute
- Respiratory rate >20 breaths/minute or $Paco_2$ <32 torr
- White blood cell count >12,000 cells/mm^3, <4,000 cells/mm^3, or >10% immature (band) forms

Box 11-5
Factors That Contribute to Infectious Complications in Oncology Patients

- Neutropenia
- Any break in the integrity of the skin or gastrointestinal tract
- Disease or drug-induced immunosuppression
- Decreased nutritional status
- Presence of a foreign body (e.g., intravascular catheter)

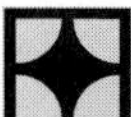

TABLE 11-8 Assessment of the Patient for Sepsis

	Assessment Parameters	Typical Abnormal Findings
History	A. Appraisal for risk factors	A. The risk factors that predispose an oncology patient to develop sepsis are listed in Box 11-6.
	B. High risk cancer diagnoses	B. The high risk cancer diagnoses for the development of sepsis include the following: 1. Acute leukemia 2. Lymphoma 3. Hodgkin's disease 4. Chronic leukemia 5. Multiple myeloma 6. Gastric cancer 7. Esophageal cancer 8. Colon cancer 9. Ovarian cancer 10. Lung cancer 11. Melanoma
Physical Examination	A. Cardiovascular system	A. Signs and symptoms: 1. Hypotension 2. Tachycardia
	B. Respiratory system	B. Signs and symptoms: 1. Tachypnea and dyspnea 2. Respiratory alkalosis → respiratory acidosis 3. Hypoxemia 4. Crackles
	C. Renal system	C. Signs and symptoms: 1. Decreased urine output
	D. Neurologic system	D. Signs and symptoms: 1. Decreased level of consciousness
	E. Hematologic system	E. Signs and symptoms: 1. Petechiae 2. Ecchymosis
	F. Changes in metabolism	F. Signs and symptoms include the following: 1. Hyper/hypothermia 2. Hyperglycemia → hypoglycemia
Diagnostic Tests	A. Cultures of blood and body fluids	A. Positive for an infectious organism
	B. Coagulation profile	B. Decreased platelet count, decreased clotting factors, decreased fibrinogen level, and increased fibrin degradation products
	C. Chest x-ray	C. May diagnose a pulmonary infection or acute respiratory distress syndrome

bidity and mortality, sepsis should be prevented or detected in the early stages whenever possible. Nursing interventions and patient education can help reduce the risk of sepsis or allow for prompt identification of the problem with the subsequent initiation of appropriate treatment (Peterson, 1998; Rostad, 1995) (Table 11-9).

SPINAL CORD COMPRESSION

Pathophysiology

Spinal cord compression (SCC) occurs in approximately 10% to 15% of patients with cancer. The most common error in the management of the patient with SCC is failure to consider the diagnosis in an oncology patient who complains of back pain. This problem represents a clinical emergency that requires prompt diagnosis, evaluation, and treatment if permanent neurologic deficits are to be prevented.

SCC results from one of two mechanisms. Tumors can cause SCC through direct extension from the paravertebral nodes to the spinal cord or through metastatic involvement of the vertebral column. Approximately 70% of all SCCs occur in the thoracic area, 20% occur in the lumbosacral area, and 10% occur in the cervical area. The most common cancers causing SCC in each of these areas are listed in Box 11-6. The pathophysiologic response to SCC includes edema of the spinal cord, diminished blood supply at the cord, and mechanical distortion of neural tissue that can lead to paresis or paralysis (Dyck, 1991; Forster, 1998).

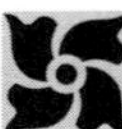

Table 11-9 Standard of Care for the Patient with Sepsis

Patient Problems and Outcomes	Nursing Interventions and Rationales	Patient Education Instructions
Infection Patient will: • Be free of infection or the signs and symptoms of infection will be recognized as early as possible	1. Assess for changes in vital signs that are indicative of the development of sepsis: • Hypotension • Tachycardia • Changes in level of consciousness • Decreased urine output 2. Evaluate catheter sites for redness, drainage, or tenderness 3. Evaluate specific sites for signs and symptoms of infection: • Wounds • Perirectal area • Oral mucosa • Skin 4. Monitor the patient for fever or hypothermia 5. Administer antibiotics on a strict administration schedule 6. Administer antipyretics or apply fever-reduction strategies	1. Explain to patient the need for protective isolation and the need to restrict the number of visitors. 2. Emphasize the importance of handwashing for the patient, visitors, and staff. 3. Teach the patient to wear a mask when he is out of his room. 4. Teach patient the rationale for and importance of: • Good oral care • Good hygiene practices 5. Teach patient to use a cooked food diet.
Fluid Volume Deficit Patient will: • Maintain a normal fluid balance and adequate circulatory volume	1. Assess the patient's circulatory status: • Dependent or peripheral edema • Tachycardia • Hypotension 2. Measure and record urine output and urine-specific gravity 3. Weigh patient daily 4. Administer intravenous fluids and/or colloids as prescribed 5. Monitor laboratory values of hydration status: • Hematocrit • Blood urea nitrogen • Serum creatinine	1. Explain to patient the reason for the frequent vital signs.
High Risk for Injury Patient will: • Prevent or avoid injury	1. Evaluate the patient for signs of bleeding including: • Bleeding from mucous membranes • Oozing of blood from wounds or intravenous sites • Presence of petechiae, purpura, or hematomas 2. Monitor laboratory values including: • Coagulation profile • Hemoglobin and hematocrit 3. Perform neurologic assessment	1. Teach patients to remove unwanted clutter from their environment to prevent falls.

Box 11-6
Common Cancers Causing Spinal Cord Compression (SCC)

Thoracic area (70% of SCCs)
- Lung cancer
- Breast cancer
- Renal cancer
- Prostate cancer
- Lymphoma
- Multiple myeloma
- Melanoma
- Gastrointestinal cancers

Lumbosacral Area (20% of SCCs)
- Gastrointestinal cancers
- Melanoma
- Lymphoma
- Multiple myeloma
- Renal cancer
- Prostate cancer
- Breast cancer
- Lung cancer

Cervical area (10% of SCCs)
- Lung cancer
- Breast cancer
- Melanoma
- Lymphoma
- Renal cancer
- Multiple myeloma

Assessment

The initial symptom of SCC is pain. The characteristics of the pain depend on the location of the tumor. The usual sequelae of symptoms in SCC are pain, motor weakness, sensory deficits, and autonomic dysfunction. The rapidity with which symptoms develop usually depends on the growth rate of the tumor (Boogerd & van der Sande, 1993; Portenoy, Lipton, & Foley, 1987) (Table 11-10).

Medical Management

Numerous factors interrelate and influence the patient's treatment plan for SCC, including the patient's primary tumor, level of SCC, rapidity of onset of symptoms, degree and duration of the blockage, and patient's general condition. The major interventions for SCC can include surgery, chemotherapy, radiation therapy, and medications.

Surgery is warranted in patients with rapidly progressing symptoms or with acutely severe neurologic deficits. Laminectomy may also be performed if the tumor is resistant to radiation therapy. Spinal fusion may be done to stabilize the spine. Usually after a laminectomy, patients receive radiation therapy.

Radiation therapy can be used to treat patients who have slowly progressing symptoms or who have an incomplete spinal cord blockage. Generally, chemotherapy is used as adjuvant therapy in the management of SCC. Patients with SCC usually receive corticosteroids (e.g., methylprednisolone sodium or dexamethasone) to decrease spinal cord edema.

SCC requires prompt recognition and treatment. There is a positive correlation between preoperative motor status and posttreatment outcome. In other words, if patients are ambulatory at the time of diagnosis of SCC, most likely they will continue to remain ambulatory after treatment for SCC (Boogerd & van der Sande, 1993).

Nursing Management

The nursing management of the patient with SCC involves extensive assessments of the neurologic and musculoskeletal systems to detect early changes in sensory and motor function. Depending on the outcomes of the medical and surgical management of SCC, patients may have extensive needs for rehabilitative consultation and services (Forster, 1998; Gentzch, 1991; Reese, 1995) (Table 11-11).

SUPERIOR VENA CAVA SYNDROME

Pathophysiology

Superior vena cava (SVC) syndrome describes the compression of the SVC and its tributaries with subsequent engorgement of the vessels of the upper trunk. The most common cause of SVC syndrome is malignant disease.

The SVC is a thin-walled, low-pressure vessel that lies within the anterior mediastinum. In the adult the SVC measures 6 to 8 cm in length and is approximately 1.5 to 2 cm in diameter. The SVC receives blood from the head and neck, upper extremities, thoracic wall, and through the azygos venous system from the back. The SVC is surrounded by other vital structures within the mediastinum, including the vertebral column, trachea, esophagus, right mainstem bronchus, aorta, and pulmonary artery. The SVC is also surrounded by lymph nodes and loose connective tissue. Because the SVC is a thin-walled, low-pressure vessel, it is easily collapsed by external pressure. Since the mediastinum is a rigid anatomical structure with little ability to expand and accommodate the growth of neoplastic tissue, malignant neoplasms in the mediastinum cause displacement and compression of major organs and blood vessels, including the SVC.

The major mechanisms underlying the development of SVC syndrome include (1) eternal compression of the SVC by an extrinsic mass, (2) occlusion of the SVC by invasion of a tumor into the wall of the vessel, (3) intraluminal thrombosis due to a neoplastic thrombus, and (4) intravascular thrombosis related to the presence of an intravascular catheter in a major vessel of the upper thorax (Stewart, 1996). The clinical picture of SVC syndrome is due to venous hypertension in areas normally drained by the SVC and its tributaries.

Malignant diseases account for 80% to 90% of the reported cases of SVC syndrome. The major malignant and nonmalignant causes of SVC syndrome are listed in Box

TABLE 11-10 Assessment of the Patient for Spinal Cord Compression

	Assessment Parameters	Typical Abnormal Findings
History	A. Cancer diagnosis	A. Cancer diagnoses associated with the development of SCC are listed in Box 11-7.
	B. Detailed pain assessment 1. General evaluation of the pain complaint includes: a. Description b. Location and radiation c. Severity d. Aggravating and relieving factors e. Previous treatment modalities and effectiveness	
	C. Characteristics of pain associated with SCC	C. Common characteristics of the pain associated with SCC include: 1. Pain is the most frequent initial symptom of SCC. 2. Pain is usually localized to the involved spinal segment. 3. Localized pain usually increases with: a. Movement b. Coughing c. Sneezing d. Valsalva maneuver 4. Pain is often radicular in nature. 5. Vertebral tenderness is usually present over the site of SCC. 6. Pain associated with SCC in the thoracic area is often described as a tight band around the patient's chest.
Physical Examination	A. Neurologic examination	
	1. Evaluate muscle strength	1. Decrease in muscle strength occurs with SCC.
	2. Evaluate muscle tone	2. Damage to the corticospinal tracts results in spasticity. Damage to lower motor neurons results in hypotonicity.
	3. Evaluate motor coordination	3. Loss of motor coordination may occur with SCC.
	4. Evaluate for weakness and gait abnormalities	4. Weakness and ataxia may occur with SCC.
	5. Inspect muscles of the arms and legs for: a. Atrophy b. Fasciculations c. Involuntary movements d. Abnormal positioning of the extremities	
	6. Test all reflexes	6. Damage to the corticospinal tracts results in hyperreflexia. Damage to the lower motor neurons results in hyporeflexia.
	B. Sensory examination 1. Light touch 2. Temperature 3. Pain 4. Position 5. Vibration	B. Sensory deficits result from pressure on the spinothalamic tracts. Involvement of the anterior spinothalamic tract causes loss of light touch. Involvement of the lateral spinothalamic tract results in loss of pain followed by the loss of temperature. The posterior columns (i.e., proprioception) are usually involved late in SCC.
	C. Evaluate for autonomic dysfunction	C. Late-sign of SCC
	1. Bowel dysfunction	1. Bowel dysfunction includes: rectal anesthesia, constipation, obstipation, encopresis.
	2. Bladder dysfunction	2. Bladder dysfunction includes: bladder anesthesia, enuresis.

Continued

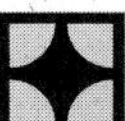

TABLE 11-10 Assessment of the Patient for Spinal Cord Compression—cont'd

	Assessment Parameters	Typical Abnormal Findings
Diagnostic Tests	A. X-ray of the vertebral column	A. X-rays can reveal vertebral abnormalities, including bone lesions and areas of vertebral collapse.
	B. Bone pain	B. Bone scan can reveal multiple lesions.
	C. Computed tomography (CT) scan	C. CT scan can provide information on the vertebral column as well as on the paravertebral structures.
	D. Magnetic resonance imaging (MRI)	D. MRI can reveal the extent of SCC, the type of injury, and the condition of the soft tissues over the spinal cord.
	E. Myelogram	E. Myelogram reveals the area of SCC and an outline of the spinal cord and nerve roots.

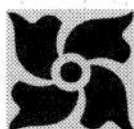

TABLE 11-11 Standard of Care for the Patient With a Spinal Cord Compression

Patient Problems and Outcomes	Nursing Interventions and Rationales	Patient Education Instructions
Pain Patient will: • Experience adequate pain control	1. Perform a pain assessment a. Description b. Location and radiation c. Severity d. Aggravating and relieving factors e. Previous treatment and effectiveness f. Associated symptoms 2. Administer opioid analgesics on a regular schedule. 3. Administer short-acting analgesics for breakthrough pain. 4. Administer steroid medications.	1. Explain the rationale for taking analgesics on a regular schedule. 2. Explain the differences between physical dependence, tolerance, and psychological addition to opioid analgesics. 3. Use nonpharmacologic interventions for pain management: a. Relaxation exercises b. Hypnosis
Impaired Physical Mobility Patient will: • Maintain optimal level of physical mobility	1. Assess mobility status, including: a. Gait and coordination b. Range of motion of extremities c. Muscle strength and tone d. Deep tendon reflexes 2. Obtain a physical therapy consult.	1. Explain to patient the importance of notifying a health care professional of any changes in mobility. 2. Assist patient to develop an exercise program to maintain optimal level of functioning.
Constipation Patient will: • Maintain a normal bowel pattern	1. Assess usual bowel pattern for frequency, size, shape, consistency, and color of stools. 2. Auscultate the abdomen. 3. Evaluate medication regimen. 4. Institute a bowel regimen with a stool softener and a stimulant.	1. Teach patient the following measures to promote elimination: a. Respond immediately to the urge to defecate. b. Obtain privacy to defecate. c. Facilitate a proper position for defecation. 2. Teach patient to maintain a high fiber diet and adequate fluid intake.

Box 11-7
Causes of Superior Vena Cava Syndrome

Malignant Etiologies

- Bronchiogenic carcinoma
- Lymphoma
- Thymoma
- Germ cell tumor
- Kaposi's sarcoma
- Metastatic disease associated with esophageal, colon, breast, or testicular cancers

Nonmalignant Etiologies

- Aortic aneurysm
- Infectious agents
- Substernal thyroid
- Central venous catheter

11-7. The malignancy that is most commonly associated with the development of SVC syndrome is bronchiogenic carcinoma, or small cell carcinoma of the lung. These tumors account for approximately 75% of the cases of SVC syndrome. The second most common cause of SVC syndrome is lymphoma, which accounts for approximately 15% of the cases (Stewart, 1996; Yellin, Rosen, Reichart, & Lieberman, 1990).

Assessment

The severity of the patient's symptoms depends on the rapidity, degree, and location of the obstruction, as well as on the development and adequacy of collateral circulation. If the onset of the SVC syndrome is gradual, then collateral circulation has time to develop and compensate for the obstructed blood flow within the SVC. In general, a slowly developing obstruction is generally well tolerated. A rapidly occurring obstruction usually produces more acute symptoms. The assessment of the patient for SVC syndrome is described in Table 11-12.

Medical Management

The medical management of SVC syndrome depends on whether the onset of the syndrome is acute or insidious. With an acute onset of symptoms, interventions are directed at preventing life-threatening complications by maintaining a patent airway and cardiac output. If the onset of the SVC syndrome is more gradual, initial interventions are directed at symptom management and determining the underlying cause of the disorder.

In many cases, patients are treated with radiation therapy as first-line therapy, particularly for an acute onset of SVC. The total dose of radiation therapy depends on the underlying histology of the tumor and the patient's general condition. The usual dosing schedule for adults is high-dose fractions (300-400 cGy) for the first two to four doses followed by conventional fractions (150-200 cGy) over 3 to 6 weeks (with a total dose of radiation of 300-500 cGy). Subjective relief of symptoms is usually reported within 3 to 4 days. Objective responses (i.e., decreased edema, decreased venous distention) are usually observed within 1 to 2 weeks after the initiation of treatment (Loney, 1998).

The use of chemotherapy to treat SVC syndrome depends on the cause of the syndrome. The specific chemotherapy agents used depend on the type of tumor being treated.

Supportive medical therapy includes the use of strategies to maintain a patent airway and relieve airway obstruction. Oxygen therapy should be used with patients who are hypoxic. Diuretics may be used to reduce edema. However, these agents should be used cautiously because they may produce a decrease in venous return to the heart and cause dehydration and thrombosis.

If the SVC syndrome is a result of thrombosis, IV heparin may be administered. Urokinase can be used to resolve a thrombosis that fails to respond to heparin therapy.

A recent development in the management of SVC syndrome is the use of expandable wire stents that are placed into the obstructed or stenosed portion of the SVC. Patients need to be placed on anticoagulants after stent placement. Complications associated with stent placement include hematoma formation, perforation of the SVC, infection, and transient renal insufficiency (Loney, 1998).

Nursing Management

The nursing management of the patient with SVC syndrome centers on maintaining the patient's cardiac output and maintaining an effective breathing pattern until the medical interventions are effective in shrinking the tumor or the obstruction is relieved. Measures to decrease anxiety and fear are often warranted, as well as comfort measures (Cawley, 1991; Gates, 1995; Loney, 1998) (Table 11-13).

SYNDROME OF INAPPROPRIATE ANTIDIURETIC HORMONE SECRETION

Pathophysiology

The syndrome of inappropriate antidiuretic hormone secretion (SIADH) is a condition in which an excessive amount of antidiuretic hormone (ADH) is secreted or produced, resulting in an increase in body water and relative or dilutional decrease in body sodium. To understand the clinical manifestations of SIADH, one needs to have an understanding of the role of ADH in regulating normal fluid balance.

Water balance is regulated through a negative feedback loop (Fig. 11-4). ADH is an octapeptide produced in the supraoptic nucleus of the hypothalamus and stored in the posterior pituitary. The major stimulus for the release of ADH is an increase in serum osmolality (normal = 275-295 mOsm) and/or a decrease in blood volume. As shown in Fig. 11-4, an increase in serum osmolality is associated with a decrease in extracellular fluid concentration. The major extracellular cation is sodium, which is the primary determinant of extracellular fluid concentration. The increase in solute in the extracellular fluid causes water to shift from the intracellular fluid space to the extracellular fluid space.

Water, leaving specialized cells, called *osmoreceptors,* within the hypothalamus, causes these cells to decrease in

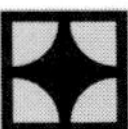

TABLE 11-12 Assessment of the Patient for Superior Vena Cava Syndrome

	Assessment Parameters	Typical Abnormal Findings
History	A. Cancer diagnoses	A. Cancers associated with the development of superior vena cava (SVC) syndrome include the following: 1. Bronchiogenic carcinoma 2. Lymphoma 3. Thymoma 4. Germ cell tumor 5. Kaposi's sarcoma 6. Metastatic disease (see Box 11-8)
	B. Concurrent medical illness or conditions	B. Concurrent medical illnesses or conditions associated with the development of SVC include the following: 1. Aortic aneurysm 2. Infectious agents 3. Substernal thyroid 4. Central venous catheter
Physical Examination	A. Initial signs/symptoms	A. Initial signs/symptoms: 1. Usually occur in early morning 2. Early morning signs and symptoms include the following: a. Periorbital edema b. Conjunctival edema c. Facial swelling d. Stoke's sign-tightness of a shirt collar
	B. Evolutionary signs/symptoms	B. Evolutionary signs and symptoms include the following: 1. Fullness of the arms 2. Swelling of the fingers and hands 3. Difficulty in putting on and removing rings 4. Erythema of the face, neck, and upper trunk 5. Epistaxis
	C. Late signs/symptoms	C. Late signs and symptoms include the following: 1. Distention of the veins in thorax and upper extremities 2. Painless dysphagia 3. Throat tightness 4. Cough 5. Dyspnea 6. Tachypnea 7. Anxiety 8. Cyanosis 9. Hoarseness 10. Chest pain 11. Headache 12. Irritability 13. Lethargy 14. Blurred vision 15. Impaired memory
Diagnostic Tests	A. Thoracotomy and biopsy	A. Major surgical procedure, will establish a definitive tissue diagnosis
	B. Mediastinoscopy and biopsy	B. Can be used to establish a tissue diagnosis
	C. Ultrasound-guided transthoracic needle aspiration biopsy	C. Determines tissue diagnosis of cancer, pattern of collateral circulation in and around tissue mass
	D. Bronchoscopy and biopsy	D. Determines tissue diagnosis of cancer
	E. Lymph node biopsy	E. Determines tissue diagnosis of cancer
	F. Sputum cytology	F. Determines tissue diagnosis of cancer
	G. Chest x-ray	G. Mass located in the superior mediastinum (75% of lesions are on the right side); pulmonary lesions, hilar adenopathy
	H. Computerized tomography of the chest	H. Can visualize a mediastinal mass and thoracic anatomy, determine the extent of occlusion and existence of collateral circulation, determine presence and degree of thrombus formation
	I. Venography of the SVC	I. Determine site and degree of obstruction and the presence of collateral circulation
	J. Radionuclide scan of the SVC	J. Can determine the source of the obstruction and the pattern of collateral circulation
	K. Magnetic resonance imaging	K. Detailed imaging of the SVC and the source of the obstruction

TABLE 11-13 Standard of Care for the Patient With Superior Vena Cava Syndrome

Patient Problems and Outcomes	Nursing Interventions and Rationales	Patient Education Instructions
Decreased Cardiac Output Patient will: • Maintain an adequate cardiac output	1. Perform a cardiovascular assessment to determine decreases in cardiac output including: a. Heart rate b. Blood pressure c. Respiratory rate d. Pulsus paradoxus 2. Assess for central and peripheral cyanosis 3. Maintain bedrest and elevate the head of the bed to 60° 4. Maintain an intravenous line	1. Teach patient to keep the head of the bed elevated to improve his level of comfort.
Ineffective Breathing Pattern Patient will: • Maintain an adequate level of oxygenation	1. Perform a respiratory assessment 2. Evaluate arterial blood gases for respiratory acidosis and hypoxemia 3. Administer oxygen, as needed 4. Administer corticosteroids and diuretics, as prescribed	1. Encourage patient to verbalize his concerns and fears. 2. Teach patient to limit activities based on level of pulmonary dysfunction.
Altered Cerebral Tissue Perfusion Patient will: • Maintain adequate cerebral perfusion pressure	1. Assess level of consciousness and orientation to time, place, and person 2. Orient patient to time, place, person, and environment	1. Instruct patient to avoid maneuvers that increase intracranial pressure: a. Valsalva maneuver b. Bending forward c. Lifting from the waist
Anxiety Patient will: • Remain calm and will be able to attend to instructions	1. Medicate patient for pain or anxiety as needed	1. Inform the patient that dyspnea is a time-limited symptom and will decrease within 3-4 days. 2. Instruct patient to decrease activity, which will improve his shortness of breath. 3. Teach patient relaxation techniques that do not focus on rhythmic breathing. 4. Explain the benefits of all interventions and procedures.
Impaired Skin Integrity Skin surface will remain intact	1. Examine skin surfaces in the radiation treatment field for erythema and breakdown 2. Elevate upper extremities if swollen	1. Teach patient to clean skin gently in the radiation treatment field with a mild soap. 2. Teach patient to avoid tight or abrasive clothing.
Esophagitis Patient will: • Maintain adequate dietary intake	1. Obtain a dietary consult 2. Administer systemic analgesics, as needed	1. Teach patient to avoid trauma to the mucous membranes: a. Avoid extreme temperatures in foods b. Avoid spicy foods c. Avoid the use of alcohol and tobacco

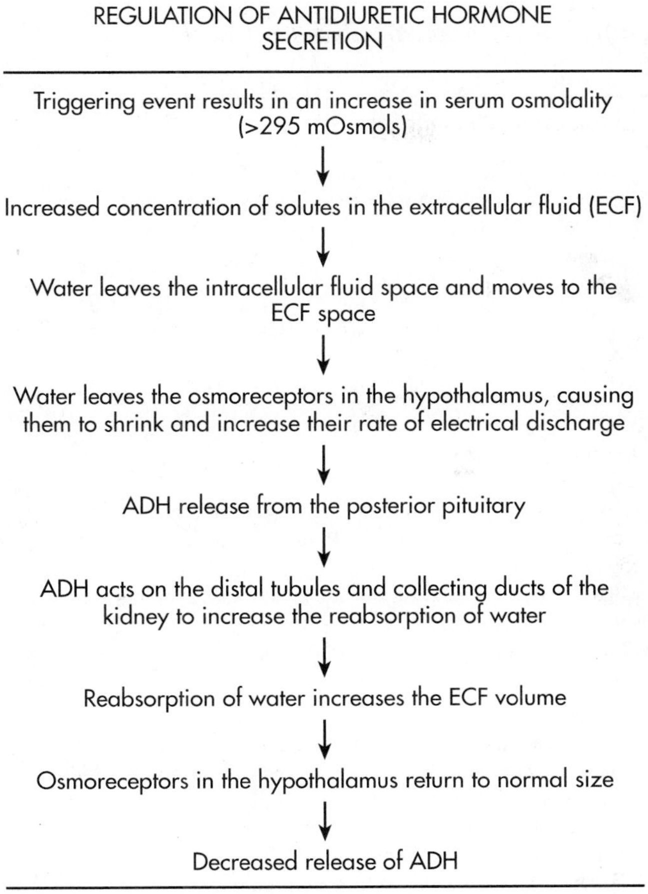

REGULATION OF ANTIDIURETIC HORMONE SECRETION

Triggering event results in an increase in serum osmolality (>295 mOsmols)

↓

Increased concentration of solutes in the extracellular fluid (ECF)

↓

Water leaves the intracellular fluid space and moves to the ECF space

↓

Water leaves the osmoreceptors in the hypothalamus, causing them to shrink and increase their rate of electrical discharge

↓

ADH release from the posterior pituitary

↓

ADH acts on the distal tubules and collecting ducts of the kidney to increase the reabsorption of water

↓

Reabsorption of water increases the ECF volume

↓

Osmoreceptors in the hypothalamus return to normal size

↓

Decreased release of ADH

Fig. 11-4 Regulation of antidiuretic hormone (ADH) secretion.

size and increase their rate of electrical discharge. This stimulation results in the release of ADH from the posterior pituitary. Circulating ADH acts on the distal tubules and the collecting ducts of the kidney to increase the reabsorption of water. The reabsorption of water results in an increase in extracellular volume and a dilution of the solutes. Cells in the hypothalamus return to normal size, and the release of ADH decreases. Conditions that can cause an increase in serum osmolality and an associated increase in the release of ADH include dehydration, vomiting, diarrhea, hyperthermia, stress, pain, hemorrhage, and certain medications (e.g., morphine, barbiturates, diuretics, cytoxan, vincristine).

The major causes of SIADH are listed in Box 11-8. The primary cause of SIADH is malignant disease. The most common cancer associated with the development of SIADH is small cell carcinoma of the lung (SCLC). Approximately 80% of patients with SCLC have evidence of impaired ability to excrete water. Research has demonstrated that the malignant cells from patients with SCLC are capable of synthesizing, storing, and releasing ADH (i.e., ectopic production of ADH). The amount of ADH produced by the tumor cells is released independent of normal physiologic controls (Kinzie, 1987; Poe & Taylor, 1989; Sørensen, Andersen, & Hansen, 1995).

Box 11-8

Causes of the Syndrome of Inappropriate Antidiuretic Hormone Secretion

Cancer

- Small cell carcinoma of the lung
- Pancreatic cancer
- Duodenal cancer
- Bladder cancer
- Lymphosarcoma
- Thymoma
- Reticulum cell sarcoma
- Ewing's sarcoma
- Hodgkin's disease
- Malignant histiocytosis

Central Nervous System Disorders

- Skull fractures
- Subdural hematoma
- Subarachnoid hemorrhage
- Cerebral atrophy
- Cerebral vascular thrombosis

Infectious and Inflammatory Central Nervous System Disorders

- Encephalitis
- Meningitis
- Guillain-Barré syndrome
- Systemic lupus erythematosus
- Acute intermittent porphyria

Pulmonary Disorders

- Tuberculosis
- Lung abscesses
- Status asthmaticus
- Pneumonia

Medications

- Opioids
- Barbiturates
- Anesthetics
- Thiazide diuretics
- Tricyclic antidepressants
- Chlorpropamide
- Clofibrate
- Carbamazepine

Cancer Chemotherapy

- Vincristine
- Vinblastine
- Cyclophosphamide
- Cisplatin
- Melphalan

The development of SIADH has been associated with a variety of other cancers (see Box 11-8). In addition, central nervous system (CNS) trauma and infectious and inflammatory disorders of the CNS are associated with the development of SIADH. The SIADH secretion can be precipi-

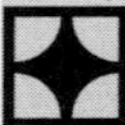

TABLE 11–14 Assessment of the Patient for Syndrome of Inappropriate Antidiuretic Hormone Secretion

	Assessment Parameters	Typical Abnormal Findings
History	A. Cancer diagnosis	A. Patients are at risk for the development of SIADH with any of the following cancer diagnoses: 1. Small cell carcinoma of the lung 2. Pancreatic cancer 3. Duodenal cancer 4. Bladder cancer 5. Lymphosarcoma 6. Thymoma 7. Reticulum cell sarcoma 8. Ewing's sarcoma 9. Hodgkin's disease 10. Malignant histiocytosis
	B. Concomitant medical conditions	B. Evaluate patient for central nervous system trauma, inflammatory or infectious disorders of the CNS, and pulmonary disorders (refer to Box 11-9).
	C. Chemotherapy administration	C. Evaluate for administration of vinca alkaloids, cyclophosphamide, cisplatin, or melphalan.
	D. Medication history	D. Evaluate for medications listed in Box 11-9.
Physical Examination	A. For patients with serum sodium of <130 mEq/L	
	1. Neurologic	1. Headache, mental confusion, lethargy, disorientation, sleepiness, weakness, personality changes, sluggish deep tendon reflexes
	2. Gastrointestinal	2. Anorexia, abdominal cramps, diarrhea, nausea and vomiting
	3. Musculoskeletal	3. Muscle cramps, weakness
	4. Renal	4. Edema is rarely seen, mild weight gain
	5. Cardiovascular	5. Increased heart rate, increased blood pressure
	B. For patient with a serum sodium <110 mEq/L	
	1. Neurologic	1. Seizures, coma
	2. Gastrointestinal	2. Anorexia, nausea and vomiting
	3. Musculoskeletal	3. Weakness
	4. Renal	4. Weight gain, oliguria
	5. Cardiovascular	5. Increased heart rate, increased blood pressure
Diagnostic Tests	A. Laboratory tests for patients with a serum sodium of <130 mEq/L	
	1. Serum osmolality	1. Decreased <280 mOsm/kg
	2. Urine osmolality	2. Increased >300 mOsm/kg
	3. Urine sodium	3. Increased >20 mEq/L
	4. Blood urea nitrogen (BUN)	4. Normal
	5. Serum creatinine	5. Normal
	6. Serum potassium	6. Normal
	7. Serum calcium	7. Normal
	B. Laboratory tests for patients with a serum sodium of <110 mEq/L	
	1. Serum osmolality	1. Decreased <280 mOsm/kg
	2. Urine osmolality	2. Increased >500 mOsm/kg
	3. Urine sodium	3. Increased >20 mEq/L
	4. BUN	4. Decreased
	5. Serum creatinine	5. Decreased
	6. Serum potassium	6. Decreased (probably dilutional)
	7. Serum calcium	7. Decreased (probably dilutional)

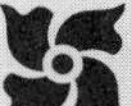

Table 11-15 Standard of Care for the Patient With the Syndrome of Inappropriate Antidiuretic Hormone Secretion

Patient Problems and Outcomes	Nursing Interventions and Rationales	Patient Education Instructions
Fluid Volume Excess		
Patient's serum sodium and serum osmolality levels will return to normal.	1. Monitor laboratory tests: a. Serum sodium b. Serum osmolality c. Urine osmolality d. Urine sodium e. BUN f. Creatinine 2. Maintain strict intake and output 3. Weigh patient daily 4. Initiate fluid restriction a. For serum sodium between 125 to 134 mEq/L, give 800 to 1,000 milliliters/day b. For serum sodium <125 mEq/L, give 500 milliliters/day 5. Administer oral hygiene every 2-4 hours. 6. Administer demeclocycline hydrochloride as prescribed.	1. Explain to patient the rationale for the frequent laboratory tests to monitor serum sodium levels. 2. Teach patient how to allocate fluids over the course of the day to maintain the fluid restriction. 3. Teach patient measures to control thirst, including avoidance of salty foods and mouthwashes containing alcohol, and to use a saline mouth rinse on a regular basis. 4. Inform patient of the need to avoid sun exposure while on demeclocycline hydrochloride, as well as the other side effects of the medication (e.g., nausea, urinary tract infections).
Risk for Injury Patient will:		
• Remain free from injury	1. Provide safety measures for confused and disoriented patients, including: a. Orientation b. Use of soft restraints when necessary c. Assistance with ambulation 2. Institute seizure precautions if serum sodium level falls below 110 mEq/L.	1. Teach patient to examine home environment and remove hazards.

tated by several chemotherapeutic drugs. The vinca alkaloids (e.g., vincristine and vinblastine) produce SIADH by directly stimulating the release of ADH. The administration of cyclophosphamide may produce SIADH by decreasing the renal excretion of the free water. Administration of cisplatin is associated with the development of SIADH. Although the exact mechanism by which cisplatin produces SIADH is unknown, it is hypothesized that cisplatin may have a central effect on ADH secretion, as well as a direct effect on the functioning of the renal tubules.

Assessment

A careful history, physical examination, and diagnostic tests all contribute to making an accurate diagnosis of SIADH. This syndrome is characterized by water retention that progresses to water intoxication. The signs and symptoms that are observed in the patient often depend on the patient's serum sodium level (Table 11-14).

Medical Management

The medical management of SIADH depends on the severity of the hyponatremia, the patient's clinical condition, and the underlying cause of the syndrome. The ideal initial treatment for SIADH is to eliminate the underlying cause of the syndrome. Since this approach is not always possible for patients with cancer, treatment of SIADH is directed at managing the patient's symptoms and preventing life-threatening complications.

The mainstay of medical management of SIADH is to restrict patients' fluid intake (i.e., for serum sodium of 125-134 mEq/L, give 800-1000 mL/day; for serum sodium of less than 120 mEq/L, give 500 mL/day). Any medications that can induce SIADH (see Box 11-8) must be discontinued and substitutions prescribed. Chronic treatment of SIADH may be initiated with demeclocycline hydrochloride, a tetracycline derivative. This drug inhibits the action of ADH at the renal tubule. Patients may be started on an initial dose of 1200 mg/day. The dose is reduced to the lowest effective dose (usually 300-900 mg/day). Patients may be able to increase their fluid intake while on this medication. Side effects of demeclocycline hydrochloride include polyuria, nephrotoxicity, photosensitivity, and urinary tract infections. Severe hyponatremia (less than 110 mEq/L) requires aggressive treatment with hypertonic saline.

Nursing Management

The nursing care of patients with SIADH centers on reversing the hyponatremia and protecting patients from injury due to changes in their mental status (Hawthorne Maxson, 1998; Kratcha-Sveningson, 1991; Miaskowski, 1995). Nursing management and education of patients with SIADH are summarized in Table 11-15.

REFERENCES

Ackerman, M. H. (1994). The systemic inflammatory response, sepsis, and multiple organ dysfunction. *Critical Care Nursing Clinics of North America, 6*(2), 243-250.

Adami, S., & Rossini, M. (1992). Hypercalcemia of malignancy: Pathophysiology and treatment. *Bone, 13,* 551-555.

Ameli, S., & Shah, P. K. (1991). Cardiac tamponade: Pathophysiology, diagnosis, and management. *Cardiology Clinics, 9*(4), 665-674.

Bailes, B. K. (1992). Disseminated intravascular coagulation. *AORN Journal, 55*(2), 517-529.

Bick, R. L. (1994). Disseminated intravascular coagulation - Objective laboratory diagnostic criteria and guidelines for management. *Clinics in Laboratory Medicine, 14*(4), 729-768.

Boogerd, W., & van der Sande, J. J. (1993). Diagnosis and treatment of spinal cord compression in malignant disease. *Cancer Treatment Reviews, 19,* 129-150.

Calafato, A., & Jessup, A. L. (1991). Body fluid composition, alteration in: Hypercalcemia. In J. C. McNally, E. T. Somerville, C. Miaskowski, & M. Rostad (Eds.), *Guidelines for oncology nursing practice.* Philadelphia: W. B. Saunders.

Cawley, M. M. (1991). Alteration in cardiac output, decreased: Related to superior vena cava syndrome. In J. C. McNally, E. T. Somerville, C. Miaskowski, & M. Rostad (Eds.), *Guidelines for oncology nursing practice.* Philadelphia: W. B. Saunders.

Chrisholm, M. A., Muloy, A. L., & Taylor, A. T. (1996). Acute management of cancer-related hypercalcemia. *The Annals of Pharmacotherapy, 30,* 507-513.

Cockburn, D. (1995). Hypercalcemia. In C. Miaskowski (Ed.), *Plans of care for specialty practice-Oncology nursing.* Albany, New York: Delmar Publications.

Collins, P. (1995). Disseminated intravascular coagulation. In C. Miaskowski (Ed.), *Plans of care for specialty practice-Oncology nursing.* Albany, New York: Delmar Publishers.

Dangel, R. H. (1991). Injury, potential for, related to disseminated intravascular coagulopathy (DIC). In J. C. McNally, E. T. Somerville, C. Miaskowski, & M. Rostad (Eds.), *Guidelines for oncology nursing practice.* Philadelphia: W. B. Saunders.

Davies, P. S. (1995). Neoplastic cardiac tamponade. In C. Miaskowski (Ed.), *Plans of care for specialty practice-Oncology nursing.* Albany, New York: Delmar Publishers.

Dragonette, P. (1998). Malignant pericardial effusion and cardiac tamponade. In C. C. Chernecky & B. J. Berger (Eds.), *Advanced and critical care oncology nursing-Managing primary complications.* Philadelphia: W. B. Saunders.

Dyck, S. (1991). Surgical instrumentation as a palliative treatment for spinal cord compression. *Oncology Nursing Forum, 18*(3), 515-521.

Emmanouilides, C., & Glaspy, J. (1996). Opportunistic infections in cancer patients. *Hematology/Oncology Clinics of North America, 10*(4), 841-860.

Forster, D. A. (1998). Spinal cord compression. In C. C. Chernecky & B. J. Berger (Eds.), *Advanced and critical care oncology nursing-Managing primary complications.* Philadelphia: W. B. Saunders.

Freifeld, A. G. (1993). The antimicrobial armamentarium. *Hematology/Oncology Clinics of North America, 7*(4), 813-839.

Gates, M. L. (1995). Superior vena cava syndrome. In C. Miaskowski (Ed.), *Plans of care for specialty practice - Oncology nursing.* Albany, New York: Delmar Publishers.

Gentzch, P. (1991). Mobility, impaired physical, related to spinal cord compression. In J. C. McNally, E. T. Somerville, C. Miaskowski, & M. Rostad (Eds.), *Guidelines for oncology nursing practice.* Philadelphia: W. B. Saunders.

Goni, M. H., & Tolis, G. (1993). Hypercalcemia of cancer: An update. *Anticancer Research, 13,* 1155-1160.

Hawthorne Maxson, J. L. (1998). Syndrome of inappropriate antidiuretic hormone secretion. In C. C. Chernecky & B. J. Berger (Eds.), *Advanced and critical care oncology nursing-Managing primary complications.* Philadelphia: W. B. Saunders.

Hydzik, C. A. (1991). Alteration in cardiac output, decreased: Related to cardiac tamponade. In J. C. McNally, E. T. Somerville, C. Miaskowski, & M. Rostad (Eds.), *Guidelines for oncology nursing practice.* Philadelphia: W. B. Saunders.

Kinzie, B. J. (1987). Management of the syndrome of inappropriate secretion of antidiuretic hormone. *Therapy Reviews, 6,* 625-633.

Kralstein, J., & Frishman, W. (1987). Malignant pericardial diseases: Diagnosis and treatment. *American Heart Journal, 113*(3), 785-790.

Kratcha-Sveningson, L. (1991). Body fluid composition, alteration in: Syndrome of inappropriate antidiuretic hormone (SIADH). In J. C. McNally, E. T. Somerville, C. Miaskowski, & M. Rostad (Ed.), *Guidelines for oncology nursing practice.* Philadelphia: W. B. Saunders.

Loney, M. (1998). Superior vena cava syndrome. In C. C. Chernecky & B. J. Berger (Eds.), *Advanced and critical care oncology nursing-Managing primary complications.* Philadelphia: W. B. Saunders.

Meriney, D. K., & Reeder, S. J. (1998). Hypercalcemia. In C. C. Chernecky & B. J. Berger (Eds.), *Advanced and critical care oncology nursing-Managing primary complications.* Philadelphia: W. B. Saunders.

Miaskowski, C. (1995). Syndrome of inappropriate secretion of antidiuretic hormone. In C. Miaskowski (Ed.), *Plans of care for specialty practice-Oncology nursing.* Albany, New York: Delmar Publishers.

Murphy-Ende, K. (1998). Disseminated intravascular coagulation. In C. C. Chernecky & B. J. Berger (Eds.), *Advanced and critical care oncology nursing-Managing primary complications.* Philadelphia: W. B. Saunders.

Peterson, P. G. (1998). Sepsis and septic shock. In C. C. Chernecky & B. J. Berger (Eds), *Advanced and critical care oncology nursing-Managing primary complications.* Philadelphia: W. B. Saunders.

Poe, C., & Taylor, L. (1989). Syndrome of inappropriate antidiuretic hormone: Assessment and nursing implications. *Oncology Nursing Forum, 16*(3), 373-381.

Portenoy, R. K., Lipton, R. B., & Foley, K. M. (1987). Back pain in the cancer patient: An algorithm for evaluation and management. *Neurology, 37,* 134-138.

Reese, K. (1995). Spinal cord compression. In C. Miaskowski (Ed.), *Plans of care for specialty practice-Oncology nursing.* Albany: New York: Delmar Publishers.

Rostad, M. E. (1995). Sepsis. In C. Miaskowski (Ed.), *Plans of care for specialty practice-Oncology nursing.* Albany, New York: Delmar Publishers.

Rubin, R. H., & Ferraro, M. J. (1993). Understanding and diagnosing infectious complications in the immunocompromised host: Current issues and trends. *Hematology/Oncology Clinics of North America, 7*(4), 795-812.

Sørensen, J. B., Andersen, M. K., & Hansen, H. H. (1995). Syndrome of inappropriate secretion of antidiuretic hormone (SIADH) in malignant disease. *Journal of Internal Medicine, 238,* 97-110.

Stewart, I. E. (1996). Superior vena cava syndrome: An oncologic complication. *Seminars in Oncology Nursing, 12*(4), 312-317.

Williams, E. C., & Mosher, D. F. (1995). Disseminated intravascular coagulation. In R. Hoffman, D. J. Benz, S. J. Shattil, B. Furie, H. J. Cohen, & L. E. Silberstein (Eds.), *Hematology: Basic principles and practice.* New York: Churchill-Livingstone.

Yellin, A., Rosen, A., Reichert, N., & Lieberman, Y. (1990). Superior vena cava syndrome-The myth-The facts. *American Review of Respiratory Diseases, 141,* 1114-1118.

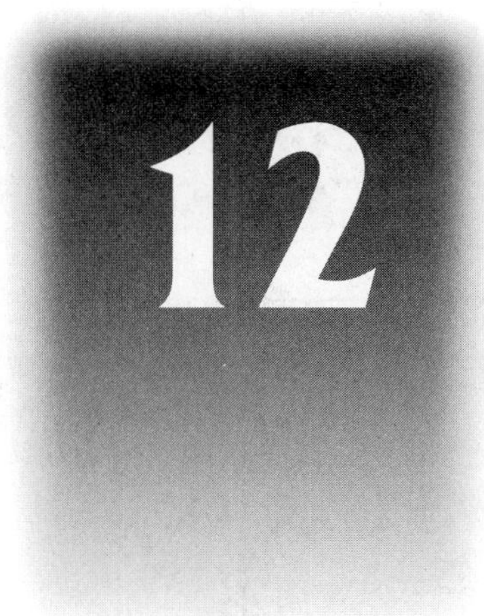

Genetic Counseling in Cancer Care

Susan T. Tinley, RN, MS, CGC
Amy Strauss Tranin, RN, MS, OCN

INTRODUCTION

The pathogenesis of cancer involves a multifactorial process. This progressive process arises from a single cell that has accumulated a series of changes that cause its growth pattern to become progressively more abnormal. Genetic alterations are at the very center of cancer development so that, at the cellular level, cancer is a genetic disorder (Ruddon, 1995). Nevertheless, most cancer is the result of a complex interplay of multiple genetic and environmental factors.

Cancer can result from lifestyle factors such as smoking or exposure to other specific physical, chemical, and infectious agents that are etiologically linked to cancer. In addition to these external factors, cancer can result from endogenous factors, many of which are genetic in origin. These genetic elements influence the relative susceptibility of the individual target tissue to developing particular cancers, as well as the manner in which the organism metabolizes a specific carcinogen (Lowy, 1996). Genetic differences in metabolism can profoundly influence the rate of carcinogenesis.

Genetic mechanisms that control cellular growth and proliferation can become abnormal and lead to the development of cancer. These genetic abnormalities (mutations) are usually acquired over time, but in some families with a hereditary predisposition to cancer, they can be passed on from generation to generation.

Cancer-prone families are uncommon, comprising approximately 15% or less of all cancers, but these families are incredibly important to study. High-risk families are those who may benefit most from early intervention such as targeted cancer surveillance or chemoprevention. The examination of cancer-prone families has also uncovered specific genes that serve as catalysts in initiating the process of carcinogenesis. The mechanisms of cancer causation gleaned from these families will help to identify the mechanisms involved in the more commonly caused sporadic cancers.

Recent progress in understanding changes in cell behavior that lead to cancer has been extraordinary. Revolutionary approaches to the prevention, early detection, and treatment of cancer are now underway. Therapies targeted at the molecular alterations in cells will become standard. These advances are changing the way cancer care is practiced. The genetic revolution impacts the specialty of oncology nursing because cancer is a genetic disease.

Oncology nurses have tremendous opportunities to participate in the exciting scientific changes taking place in cancer treatment and research. However, for their efforts to be successful, oncology nurses need to have a strong foundation in cancer genetics. Most oncology nurses will not become so specialized in cancer genetics as to provide cancer genetic counseling. However all nurses at all levels of practice need a basic level of understanding of genetics to provide any level of oncology care. Taking a family history after all involves a basic understanding of genetics. This chapter is written to provide oncology nurses with a basic overview of not only cancer genetics, but also the practice of genetic counseling in cancer care.

The first part of this chapter focuses on basic genetic principles and the intrinsic genetic factors that influence the development of cancer. Selected inherited cancer-predisposing syndromes in adults are also described and explored. The nurse's role in genetic counseling encompasses the remaining sections of this chapter.

FUNDAMENTALS OF GENETICS

Chromosomes and DNA

Deoxyribonucleic acid (DNA) is the blueprint of life and provides the code for the structural and enzymatic proteins that make up every cell in the human body. DNA is tightly packaged into units called *chromosomes.* In humans, the normal chromosome number in every cell except the mature egg and sperm is 46, or 23 pairs. Just as there are pairs of chromosomes, the genes that make up the chromosomes are in pairs called *alleles.* The mature egg and sperm have only one set of 23 chromosomes. If the chromosomes in a single

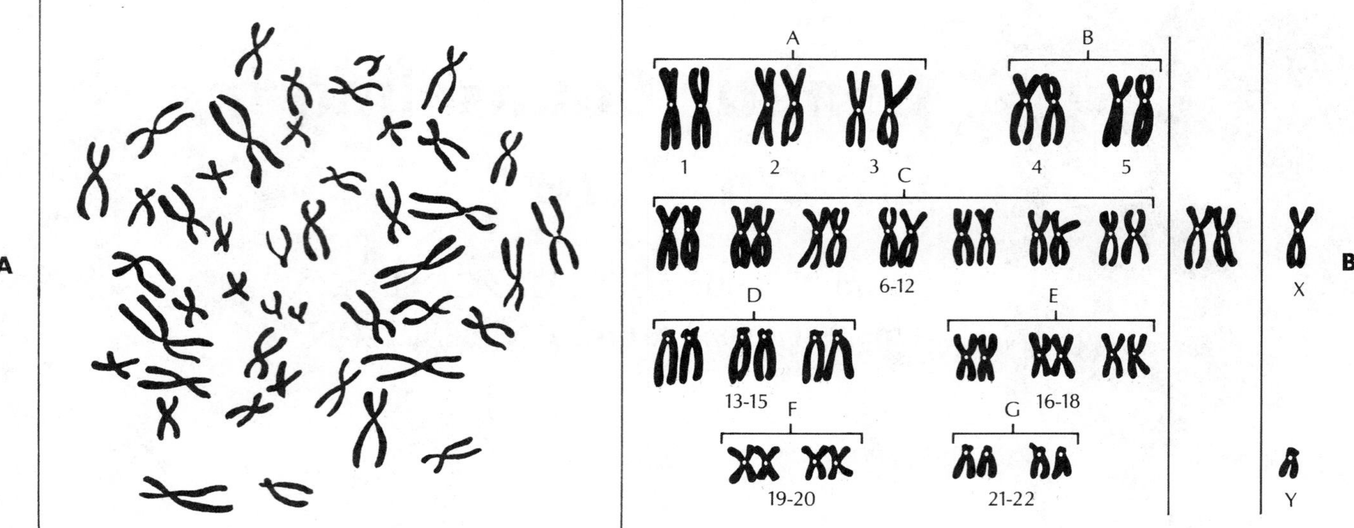

Fig. 12-1 Chromosomes during cell division. **A,** Example of photomicrograph. **B,** Chromosomes arranged in karotype; female and male sex-determining chromosomes. (From Bobak, I.M. [1995]. *Maternity nursing.* (4th ed.). St. Louis: Mosby.)

cell were stretched out and laid end to end, the DNA would be more than 5 feet long.

Chromosomes vary in size and shape. The pairs of autosomal chromosomes are arranged from the largest, 1, to the smallest, 22 (Fig. 12-1). The sex chromosomes are found to the right of chromosome 22 and are labeled XX (female) or XY (male). Chromosomes are divided by the centromere into a short arm (called *p* for *petite*) and a long arm (called *q*). Each chromosome can be identified by light microscopy with staining techniques that give a characteristic pattern of alternating light and dark bands. Banding patterns are distinct and consistent for each chromosome and assist in identifying specific chromosomes. The bands are individually numbered so that a specific location on a chromosome may be stated as 17q21, which refers to band number 21 on the long arm of chromosome 17.

A DNA molecule consists of two strands that wrap around each other to resemble a twisted ladder. The sides of the ladder are made of sugar and phosphate molecules, and the rungs of the ladder are nitrogen-containing chemicals called *bases* (Fig. 12-2). Four different bases are present in DNA—adenine (A), thymine (T), cytosine (C), and guanine (G). The sequence of bases specifies the exact genetic instructions required to create a particular organism with its own unique traits.

The two strands of DNA are held together by bonds between the bases on each strand, forming base pairs (bp). Gene size is usually stated as the total number of base pairs. The entire human gene sequence is thought to contain roughly 3 billion base pairs. The smallest human chromosome, the Y chromosome, contains 50 million base pairs, and the largest human chromosome, chromosome 1, contains 250 million base pairs.

Each time a cell divides into two daughter cells, its full genetic sequence is duplicated. Cell division in somatic cells (mitosis) results in the creation of two daughter cells with the same number of chromosomes as the original cell, a total of 46 chromosomes. Each new daughter cell contains the exact same genetic information as the parent cell. Germ cells, ovum, and sperm are formed through meiosis, a two-stage process of reduction and division, resulting in one chromosome from each pair in every germ cell. This reduction in the number of chromosomes is important so that the original number of 46 chromosomes is restored after fertilization of the egg by the sperm. Without the reduction, each generation would double the number of chromosomes and hence double the genetic information.

During cell division the DNA molecule unwinds and the bonds between the base pairs break, allowing the strands to separate (Fig. 12-3). Strict base-pairing rules are adhered to—adenine will pair only with thymine, and cytosine will pair only with guanine. Each strand directs the synthesis of a complementary new strand, with free nucleotides matching up with their complementary bases on each of the separated strands. Adherence to the base-pairing rules ensures that the new strand is an exact copy of the old pair so that each daughter chromosome receives one old and one new DNA strand.

Genes

Each DNA molecule and therefore each chromosome contains many genes that reside in the cell nucleus. Genes are the units of inheritance and the source of heritable biologic variation. A gene is a specific sequence of nucleotide bases that provides the information required for the produc-

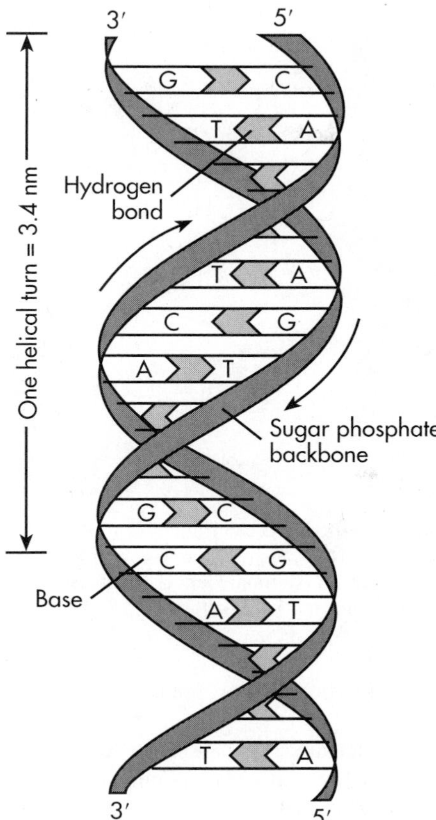

Fig. 12-2 Structure of the double helix that forms the DNA molecule. Sugar-phosphate bonds are the backbones of the two polynucleotide chains. The nitrogenous bases are in the center of the molecule and correspond to the "rungs" in the usual schematic representations of DNA. (From McCance, K. L., & Huether, S. E. [1994]. *Pathophysiology: The biologic basis for disease in adults and children.* (2nd ed.). St. Louis: Mosby.)

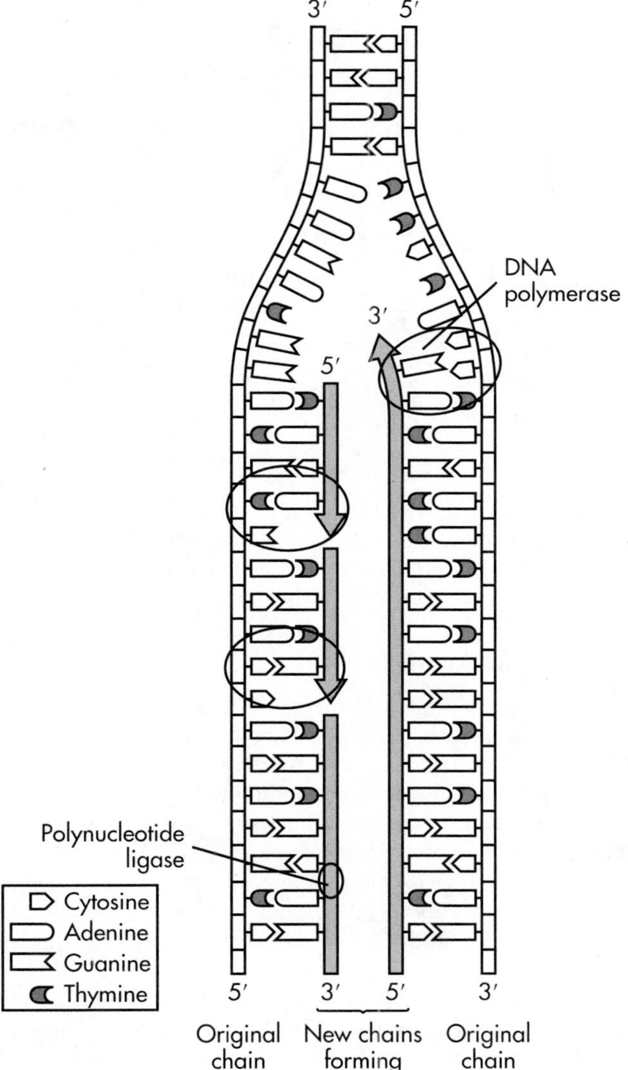

Fig. 12-3 Replication of DNA. The two chains of the double helix separate, and each chain serves as the template for a new complementary chain. (From McCance K. L. & Huether, S. E. [1994]. *Pathophysiology: The biologic basis for disease in adults and children.* (2nd ed.). St. Louis: Mosby.)

tion of a functional product. This product is a protein that provides the structural components of cells and tissues, as well as enzymes for essential biochemical reactions. The human genome, which is the complete DNA sequence in human cells, is estimated to contain approximately 100,000 genes.

The coding instructions of the genes are transmitted from the cell nucleus to the cytoplasm indirectly through messenger ribonucleic acid (mRNA), which is a transient intermediary molecule similar to a single strand of DNA. For the information within a gene to be expressed, a complementary RNA strand is produced through a process called *transcription from the DNA template.* In the cytoplasm, protein is produced by the translation of the mRNA into a string of amino acids, which make up the specific protein (Fig. 12-4).

The coding region of the gene, which is the part of the gene that determines the final amino acid sequence, is only part of a gene's features. The portions of the DNA sequence that code for the protein are called *exons.* The exons are separated by noncoding regions called *introns,* which are excised during RNA processing. The beginning and end of a gene, known as the *flanking region,* determines when, where, and how much of the gene product will be produced. The initial RNA product contains copies of exons and introns, but the mRNA has been processed to remove introns before translation into the protein.

Different forms of a gene are called *alleles.* If a pair of alleles are alike, the individual is said to be homozygous; if the pair of alleles is different, the individual is heterozygous. The genotype of a person is the individual's genetic constitution or genome. The phenotype is the observable expression of a genotype as a morphological, biochemical, or molecular trait.

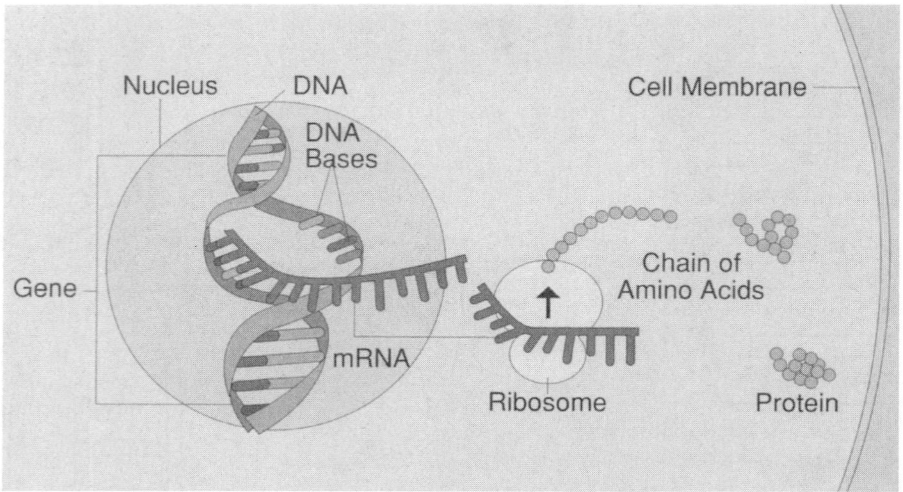

Fig. 12-4 Gene expression. The coding instructions of genes are transmitted from the cell nucleus to the cytoplasm through messenger RNA (mRNA). In the cytoplasm, protein is produced by the translation of the mRNA into a string of amino acids that make up the specific protein. (From National Cancer Institute. [1995]. *Understanding gene testing* [NIH Publication No. 96-3905]. Washington, DC: Author.)

Genetic Mutations

Since the DNA sequence directs protein production, it follows that changes in the DNA sequence (mutations) may result in altered characteristics of an organism. A mutation in a gene may lead to the formation of a variant protein, which may have altered properties as a result of its changed structure. Mutation is an essential feature of heredity because it increases genetic variation. However, some DNA changes may have no phenotypic effect because the changes do not alter the protein product. These types of changes are known as *polymorphisms.*

Mutations can occur anywhere along the length of the gene, affecting introns, exons, or the immediate flanking regions. These mutations can affect the function or amount of protein that is produced. Mutations can occur in any cell and can either be inherited from a parent or acquired during a person's lifetime. An inherited mutation, or germ line mutation, is a mutation that is present in the DNA of all cells in the body. Since the genetic mutation is present in a reproductive cell (germ cell), it can be passed from generation to generation. Acquired mutations, also known as somatic mutations, are changes in DNA that occur throughout an individual's life. In contrast to germ line mutations, somatic mutations arise in the DNA of individual cells and the genetic errors are passed only to the offspring of that cell line, not to all cells in the body.

Mechanisms of Inheritance

A single gene disorder is one that is determined by a mutated allele at a single spot (locus) on one or both members of a chromosome pair. Single gene disorders are characterized by their patterns of transmission in families. The pattern in families is dependent on two factors: (1) the chromosomal location of the gene locus, which can be autosomal (chromosomes 1-22) or X-linked (located on the X chromosome); and (2) whether the phenotype is dominant or recessive.

Dominant inheritance is observed when one gene is enough to establish a trait or individual characteristic. For a recessive trait to be observed, however, two recessive alleles must be present. If a cell contains at least one dominant allele, the presence of the recessive allele will be masked. When a cell has two recessive alleles, then the recessive trait will be expressed. Many of the cancer susceptibility genes function as autosomal dominant genes at the phenotypic level, but at the molecular level, they have recessive characteristics. This observation is elaborated on below with a description of Knudson's two-hit hypothesis.

Traits that are a result of the combined effects of multiple genes are polygenic. When environmental factors also play a role in the development of a trait, the term *multifactorial* is used to refer to the additive effects of many genetic and environmental factors. Most cancers do not arise from a single gene disorder, but are multifactorial. Multifactorial conditions tend to run in families, but the pattern of inheritance is not as predictable as with single gene disorders. The degree of risk of a multifactorial disorder occurring in relatives is related to the number of genes they share in common.

TYPES OF GENETIC ALTERATIONS IN CANCER CELLS

All cancer cells have some alteration of gene expression. These alterations include chromosomal duplications or losses of whole chromosomes, translocations, inversions, deletions, amplifications, and single gene mutations. Until recently, most of the information about genetic alterations in cancer came from studies of leukemias and lymphomas because of the ease in obtaining single-cell populations of cells from peripheral blood or bone marrow. However, a significant amount of information has now been obtained about genetic alterations in solid tumors. Different patterns of gene alteration can produce common changes in cells that lead to improperly regulated cell proliferation, invasion, and metastasis. The more subtle changes in the genome—point mutations, gene deletions, and gene rearrangements—may be associated with the initiation of the malignant transformation process, whereas gross changes in the number of chromosomes usually occur as tumors progress in malignancy.

Aneuploidy

Abnormal chromosome number is referred to as *aneuploidy.* Changes in ploidy are associated with a variety of tumor types in their advanced stages and may be random in their pattern of occurrence. The frequency of aneuploidy increases with progressive stages of disease and may have prognostic value.

Loss of Chromosomal Material

The most common defects observed in solid tumors are chromosomal deletions including loss of specific gene sequences, sometimes observed as loss of heterozygosity of a specific genetic allele. This loss of chromosome material can result in the loss of function of a tumor suppressor gene.

Translocations and Inversions

Translocations are typical in leukemias and lymphomas. However, they can occur in any malignancy. The multiplicity of translocation events in various cancers suggests that they have a causal relationship in inducing malignancy (Ruddon, 1995). Some translocations may be primary events and many may be secondary events. The first genetic alteration described in cancer was the Philadelphia chromosome seen in chronic myelocytic leukemia (Nowell & Hungerford, 1960). The Philadelphia chromosome is a translocation of a piece of chromosome 22 to chromosome 9. More than 90% of patients with chronic myelocytic leukemia have the Philadelphia chromosome in their leukemic cells. This translocation involves a breakpoint near the *abl* proto-oncogene, which provides evidence for the involvement of proto-oncogenes in the malignant process, particularly in leukemias and lymphomas (Ruddon, 1995). Because of the chromosomal translocation, the oncogene is activated. The Philadelphia chromosome is just one example of many such translocations that lead to malignant cell transformation in all types of tumors.

Gene Amplification

A gene that is normally present in a single copy may be duplicated or may undergo a small increase in copy number. Genes can also be amplified when whole chromosomes are duplicated as in trisomy or polyploidy. Gain of chromosomal material might promote cell proliferation by amplification of an oncogene or interfere with normal cell development. Amplifications of genes observed in human cancers include amplification of the N-*myc* gene in advanced neuroblastoma or of the epidermal growth factor receptor-regulated gene her-*2/neu* that proves to be a prognostic marker in advanced breast and ovarian cancer (Fearon, 1996).

Single Gene Mutations

A variety of mutations can alter the coding sequence of a single gene, resulting in the predisposition to cancer. A point mutation, which is a single base-pair substitution, may not alter the ultimate protein product, or it can result in premature termination of the product. Deletions or insertions of a multiple of three base-pairs can result in the deletion or insertion of one or more amino acids, which can result in a significant alteration in the protein product. If a deletion or insertion is not a multiple of three base-pairs, all the following amino acid sequences will be altered. If this type of mutation occurs at the end of the gene sequence, it may not result in a significant functional change, but earlier in the gene sequence, it may result in a string of amino acids with no functional purpose.

Mutations in the regulatory regions, known as *promoter* or *enhancer mutations,* can alter the rate of protein production. Splice site mutations occur at the boundaries of exons and introns, where the introns are cut out in the production of mRNA. As a result, the splice may occur in the middle of the exon or may not occur until the next exon, causing a complimentary change in the protein product.

The phenotypic expression of a single gene mutation on the ultimate gene product is not only dependent on the original normal gene instruction, but also on the position and type of mutation within the gene. As an example, the phenotypic expression of one mutation in a gene associated with breast cancer may include an increased risk for ovarian cancer, whereas another mutation of a different type or in a different position in the gene may not increase the risk of ovarian cancer. There is ongoing study of the phenotypes associated with specific mutations in cancer-related genes (Eng, 1996; Gayther et al., 1997). It is hoped that such studies eventually will provide a family with risk information specific to the mutation they carry.

Knudson's Two-Hit Hypothesis

Retinoblastoma is described as the prototype disease caused by a genetic mutation. It is a rare childhood malignant tumor of the retina. In the hereditary form of retinoblastoma, a parent is likely to be affected, whereas in the sporadic form, neither parent is affected. Inherited retinoblastoma has an earlier age of onset and is usually bilateral, but sporadic retinoblastoma usually involves only a single tumor of one retina.

By studying families with inherited retinoblastoma, Knudson realized that the inherited dominant mutation is not in itself sufficient to ensure that a retinal cell bearing the mutated gene will become a cancer cell. Knudson's hypothesis says that two mutational events must occur before a retinoblastoma will occur (Knudson, 1971). In inherited cancer, the first mutation is a germ-line mutation (inherited from one of the parent's germ cells) and a second somatic mutation must occur for the tumor to actually develop. In nongenetically linked tumors, the retinoblastoma arises as a result of two somatic mutations.

Knudson's two-hit theory of carcinogenesis in retinoblastoma became the paradigm model to describe how inheritance of an altered gene predisposes to cancer (Jorde, Carey, & White, 1995). Genes that are associated with cancer syndromes are the same genes that can cause cancers by somatic mutation. The more that is understood about the inherited mutant genes, the more the somatic pathway to cancer will be understood.

GENES THAT PREDISPOSE TO MALIGNANCY

The three main classes of genes known to predispose to malignancy are oncogenes, tumor suppressor genes, and genes involved in DNA repair. These gene classes constitute only a small proportion of the full genetic set. However, they play major roles in triggering cancer. For a malignancy to develop, mutations must occur in numerous growth-controlling genes. Altered forms of other classes of genes may also participate in the malignant process by specifically enabling a proliferating cell to become invasive or capable of metastasis. Only the three classes of genes that predispose to malignancy will be discussed here.

Oncogenes

Proto-oncogenes are genes that regulate and encourage cell growth and differentiation. A proto-oncogene may become activated by a genetic mutation to become an oncogene, which sends a message to the cells to divide in an uncontrolled manner. Mutations in proto-oncogenes result in altered, enhanced, or inappropriate expression of the gene product leading to neoplasia. Proto-oncogenes may be activated by point mutations, gene amplifications, or chromosomal translocations. Table 12-1 lists some examples of known oncogenes, their genetic alterations, and the tumors that may result from activation of these genes. Oncogenes act in a dominant fashion in tumor cells in that mutation in one copy of the gene is sufficient to cause neoplasia. The activation of an oncogene typically occurs at the somatic level, causing sporadic cancers. However, a notable exception is the germ-line mutation in the *ret* oncogene responsible for multiple endocrine neoplasia type 2A, explained in detail later in this chapter.

TABLE 12-1 Oncogenes and Human Tumors

Oncogene	Neoplasm	Genetic Alteration
abl	Chronic myelogenous leukemia	Translocation
erb B-2 (neu)	Adenocarcinoma of breast, ovary, and stomach	Amplification
myc	Burkitt's lymphoma	Translocation
	Carcinoma of lung, breast, and cervix	Amplification
H-ras	Acute myelogenous and lymphoblastic leukemia, carcinoma of the thyroid, melanoma	Point mutation
N-ras	Carcinoma of genitourinary tract and thyroid, melanoma	Point mutation
ret	Carcinoma of the thyroid	Rearrangement

From Bishop, J. M. (1995). Molecular themes in oncogenesis. *Cell, 64,* 235.

TABLE 12-2 Tumor Suppressor Genes, Sporadic Tumors, and Hereditary Cancer Syndromes

Tumor Suppressor Gene	Sporadic Tumor	Hereditary Cancer Syndrome
APC	Colon cancer	Familial adenomatous polyposis
DCC	Colon cancer	—
NF1	Neurofibromas	Neurofibromatosis type 1
p53	Colon cancer; many other epithelial malignancies	Li-Fraumeni syndrome
RB	Retinoblastoma	Retinoblastoma
VHL	Kidney cancer	von Hippel-Lindau syndrome

From Mars. (1993). Learning to suppress cancer. *Science, 261,* 1385.

Tumor Suppressor Genes

The presence of genes to inhibit uncontrolled cell proliferation helps to explain why cancer does not occur in all human beings. Tumor suppressor genes play a central role as regulators of cell growth as growth suppressors. When inactivated by a mutation, tumor suppressor genes allow cells to grow and divide uncontrollably. The loss of tumor suppressor genetic information is a common event in human malignant disease. At the cellular level, tumor suppressor genes act in a recessive fashion, since loss of activity of both copies of the gene is required for malignancy to develop. Tumor suppressor gene inactivation occurs in both sporadic and hereditary cancers. Table 12-2 lists some examples of known tumor suppressor genes and the cancers that may occur if mutations occur in these genes.

The first tumor suppressor gene that was cloned was the *RB* gene, which is the defective gene in retinoblastoma

(Friend et al., 1986). This germ-line mutation, uncovered by the loss of heterozygosity, substantiated Knudson's two-hit hypothesis. The most commonly altered gene in human cancer is the p53 tumor suppressor gene, which occurs in approximately 70% of all malignancies (Kingston, 1994).

DNA Repair Genes

Each time a cell divides, the DNA bases must be replicated. DNA replication remains surprisingly accurate, considering the exposure to mutations that the cell may encounter. This accuracy is a result of the process of DNA repair, which takes place in all normal cells. DNA repair genes correct DNA errors generated during cell division. DNA repair genes specify the code for repair enzymes that recognize an altered base, excise it by cutting the DNA strand, replace it with the correct base (determined by the complementary strand), and reseal the DNA. If the DNA repair system fails, the damaged DNA becomes a permanent mutation in one of the cell's genes and in all the descendants of that cell. Hereditary nonpolyposis colorectal cancer (HNPCC), described later in the chapter, is a result of defects in DNA mismatch repair genes.

HEREDITARY CANCER SYNDROMES

Breast and Ovarian Cancers

In 1998, more than 180,000 new cases of invasive breast cancer are estimated to be diagnosed in women, with about 1600 new cases occurring in men (Landis, Murray, Bolden, & Wingo, 1998). The lifetime risk for a woman to develop breast cancer is approximately 1 in 8. Ovarian cancer accounts for 4% of all cancers among women and an estimated 25,000 new cases are estimated to be diagnosed in 1998 (Landis et al., 1998). Ovarian cancer causes more deaths than any other cancer of the female reproductive system.

Hereditary breast and ovarian cancers account for approximately 5% to 10% of all breast and ovarian cancers (Ford & Easton, 1995). The existence of a hereditary influence on the occurrence of breast and ovarian cancers at a higher rate of cancer than expected in certain families has now been confirmed with the discovery of the BRCA1 and BRCA2 genes. These genes predispose women to both breast and ovarian cancers. Familial breast and ovarian cancer syndromes are usually divided into five groups: (1) site-specific breast cancer, (2) site-specific ovarian cancer, (3) breast-ovarian cancer syndrome, (4) Li-Fraumini syndrome (LFS), and (5) HNPCC. The BRCA1 and BRCA2 genes are implicated in the first three groups, with distinctly different genes causing the LFS and HNPCC syndromes that are discussed elsewhere in this chapter.

Since breast cancer is a common cancer, it is important to differentiate sporadic from inherited cases. The total number of individuals affected with breast and/or ovarian cancer in the family is the most important measure used in making a diagnosis of hereditary breast or ovarian cancer (Narod, 1994). Hereditary breast cancer is usually considered when several early onset breast cancer cases occur in a family in at least two generations. Early onset breast cancer occurs at age 45 or younger. The occurrence of ovarian cancer at any age is significant when there are also multiple cases of breast cancer in the family.

Site-specific ovarian cancer is rare, if indeed it really occurs. Usually, when site-specific ovarian cancer families are followed over time, they are found to contain cases of breast cancer or colon and endometrial cancers as in HNPCC. In fact, the clinical distinction between the breast-ovarian cancer syndrome and site-specific ovarian cancer is not supported in the literature (Narod, 1996). Until genotype/phenotype correlations can be made with specific BRCA1 or BRCA2 mutations, all women who carry BRCA1 and BRCA2 mutations are at risk for not only breast cancer, but also ovarian cancer, regardless of what cancers have occurred in the family.

BRCA1. In 1990, Mary-Claire King's research team (Hall et al., 1990) published the landmark paper identifying linkage of a breast cancer susceptibility gene to the long arm of chromosome 17 (17q21). They called the gene the BRCA1 gene for the first breast cancer gene identified. The gene was fully cloned in 1994 (Miki et al., 1994). BRCA1 is a tumor suppressor gene important in regulating the growth of breast epithelial cells.

BRCA1 is thought to be responsible for the majority of families with multiple cases of early onset breast and ovarian cancer, as well as site-specific ovarian cancer and for a minority of families with site-specific breast cancer (Couch et al., 1997; Narod et al., 1995; Steichen-Gersdorf et al., 1994). However, newer data may prove otherwise.

In a recent study of more than 200 women with breast cancer, Couch and colleagues (1997) found that only 16% of women with breast cancer, and a family history of breast or ovarian cancer or both, had detectable BRCA1 mutations. This percentage is far lower than previous studies, which estimated that 45% of hereditary breast cancer and 80% to 90% of hereditary breast and ovarian cancer are caused by BRCA1 mutations (Easton, Ford, Bishop, & Breast Cancer Linkage Consortium, 1995). Couch (1997) attributes this difference to the study population. The 45% risk estimate is derived from large research families with multiple cases of breast and ovarian cancer. Couch's population is more representative of families seen in a referral clinic for the evaluation of breast cancer risk. Couch goes on to estimate that BRCA1 and BRCA2 mutations together account for only 40% to 50% of the hereditary cases of breast cancer, not 90%, which had been reported previously (Wooster et al., 1994).

The BRCA1 gene is a large gene with approximately 100,000 base pairs. More than 300 mutations have been identified scattered throughout the gene (Calzone, 1997). The majority of BRCA1 mutations interrupt the genetic coding sequence and result in a shortened protein, which is thought to be nonfunctional (Narod, 1996). Mutations in noncoding regions of the gene could account for up to 20% of BRCA1 mutations (Couch et al., 1997). These noncoding region mutations would not be detectable by current commercial testing technology.

BRCA2. The BRCA2 gene is located on the long arm of chromosome 13 and was identified in 1995 (Wooster et al., 1995). BRCA2 is a very large gene, even larger than BRCA1, consisting of more than 10,000 nucleotides encoded by 26 exons. The majority of exons are relatively small, although exon 10 and 11 account for 60% of the entire coding region of the gene (Gayther et al., 1997).

Almost all BRCA2 mutations cause premature termination of the protein that is encoded by the normal BRCA2 gene. The effect of a BRCA2 mutation on protein function may depend on where the mutation shortens the protein (Krainer et al., 1997). Mutations that truncate the protein toward the end of the gene may affect protein function minimally and therefore have little effect on the development of breast cancer.

Risk of Cancer Associated With BRCA1 and BRCA2 Mutations. Initial estimates of risk of breast cancer in a woman with a BRCA1 or BRCA2 mutation who is from a family with multiple cases of breast or ovarian cancer, or both, range from 76% to 87% (Struewing et al., 1997). Risk estimates of ovarian cancer in a woman with the same type of family history range from 40% to 60% for BRCA1 carriers (Ford et al., 1994) but are considerably lower for BRCA2 mutation carriers in the range of 20% or less. A male with a BRCA2 mutation has a 6% lifetime risk for breast cancer. Women who have had breast cancer are estimated to have a 64% lifetime risk of a contralateral breast cancer (Easton et al., 1995). There may also be an increased risk for colon and prostate cancer with BRCA1 and BRCA2 mutations and for pancreatic and intraocular cancer with BRCA2 mutations. These risk figures are thought to be as high as the risk estimates will range because they are derived from research studies of high-risk families and may not apply to all carriers of BRCA1 or BRCA2 mutations. Risk estimates should be used cautiously and judiciously, since they are likely to represent a sample biased toward increased risk and may overestimate the cancer risk associated with BRCA1 and BRCA2 mutations (Burke et al., 1997a).

BRCA1 and BRCA2 Mutations in the Ashkenazi Jewish Population. Two specific mutations in BRCA1 (185delAG and 5382insC) and one in BRCA2 (6174delT) occur with a relatively high frequency in the Ashkenazi Jewish population, a genetically distinct population of Jewish people whose ancestors lived in central and eastern Europe (Struewing et al., 1997). The combined frequency of these three mutations exceeds 2% in this population. Like in the general population, these three mutations are associated with an increased risk of breast, ovarian, and prostate cancers in the Ashkenazi Jewish population. However, the cancer risk in this specific population is higher than for individuals without the alterations but is lower than risk estimates stated previously. Struewing and colleagues (1997) estimate, in the Ashkenazi Jewish population, that the lifetime risk for breast cancer among carriers of one of these three mutations is 56% compared with 85% in the carrier population at large. The estimated lifetime risk for ovarian cancer is 16% compared with a 20% to 60% risk.

It is important to recognize that although these mutations are more prevalent in the Ashkenazi Jewish population, only about 7% of the breast cancer in Jewish women is due to these alterations. Another significant finding from the Struewing study that is supported by other studies is that the risk of beast cancer is not uniformly high for all women who carry a BRCA1 or BRCA2 mutation. Research still must answer the questions of which mutations carry what risk and what are the modifying factors that alter the risk among families and individuals.

Screening for BRCA1 and BRCA2 Mutation Carriers. The optimal cancer risk management strategies for BRCA1 and BRCA2 mutation carriers are not known at this time. Counseling regarding screening recommendations should take into account the efficacy of the cancer surveillance strategies and the uncertainties in risk estimates (Burke et al., 1997a). Decision making about the timing and surveillance methods that should be used should be a joint effort between the high-risk individual and the health care provider. Table 12-3 provides surveillance options that should be discussed with mutation carriers. It should be noted that the efficacy of breast cancer surveillance is more widely established than surveillance for ovarian cancer. In

TABLE 12-3 Surveillance Options for BRCA1 and BRCA2 Mutation Carriers

Method	Recommendation
Breast Cancer	
Breast self-examination	Education regarding monthly self-examination beginning at age 18
Clinical breast examination	Annually or semi-annually beginning at age 25-35 years
Mammography	Annually beginning at age 25-35 years
Ovarian Cancer	
Transvaginal ultrasound with color Doppler and CA-125 tumor marker	Annually or semi-annually beginning at age 25-35 years
Prostate Cancer	
Prostate cancer surveillance	Education regarding options for screening utilizing digital rectal exam and prostate-specific antigen level annually beginning at age 50 years
Colon Cancer	
Colon cancer surveillance	Fecal occult blood test annually and flexible sigmoidoscopy every 3-5 years, beginning at age 50 years

From: Burke, W., Daly, M., Garber, J., Botkin, J., Kahn, M. J. E., & Lynch, P., et al., for the Cancer Genetics Studies Consortium. (1997a). Recommendations for follow-up care of individuals with an inherited predisposition to cancer II: BRCA1 and BRCA2. *Journal of the American Medical Association, 277,* 997-1003.

fact, ovarian cancer screening is not recommended for the general population at any age and is controversial in high-risk women (National Institutes of Health, 1994).

In addition to the increased cancer surveillance methods listed in Table 12-3, all high-risk individuals should be educated about risk avoidance and maintenance of a healthy lifestyle. This approach includes not smoking or chewing tobacco; eating a low-fat, high-fiber diet; regular exercise; and maintaining a healthy weight.

Prophylactic surgery is another option that female carriers of the BRCA1 and BRCA2 genes are often given. Prophylactic mastectomy and/or oophorectomy as a measure of reducing breast and ovarian cancer risk can be used. However, there is insufficient evidence to recommend for or against either surgical procedure (Burke et al., 1997a). Women need to be informed that cancer has been documented after these surgeries have been performed.

Colon Cancer

It is estimated that in 1998 there will be approximately 131,600 new cases of colorectal cancer with 56,500 deaths from the disease. The lifetime probability of colon cancer for the general population is 1 in 17 (Landis et al., 1998). However, for a member of a family with hereditary colon cancer, the probability is much higher and may approach 85% to 100% for a carrier of a hereditary colon cancer–causing mutation. Hereditary colon cancer includes the polyposis syndromes and hereditary nonpolyposis colorectal cancers that are listed in Table 12-4. Each year, the polyposis syndromes account for approximately 1% of colon cancers and the nonpolyposis syndromes account for 5% to 10% of colon cancers (Rustgi, 1994).

Adenomatous Polyposis Syndromes. Familial adenomatous polyposis (FAP) has an autosomal dominant mode of inheritance and is the most common of the polyp-

TABLE 12-4 Hereditary Forms of Colorectal Cancer

Syndrome	Chromosome Inheritance	Colon Cancer Risk	Colonic Phenotype	Extracolonic Phenotype
Familial adenomatous polyposis	5 q AD	High	Adenomas (100 to >1000; colorectal cancer)	Periampullary adenoma and carcinoma; periampullary carcinoma most common cancers of stomach, small bowel, pancreas, thyroid (papillary histology), sarcomas, brain tumors Desmoid tumors, particularly intraabdominal; congenital hypertrophy of retinal pigment epithelium
AFAP	5q AD	High	Flat adenomas (1 to >100); right side > left; ordinary adenomas	Fundic gland polyps; adenomas of stomach and periampullary region; periampullary carcinoma
Hereditary nonpolyposis colorectal cancer	2p,3p AD	High	Occasional adenomas; may be larger, high-grade dysplasia	Carcinomas of endometrium, ovary, stomach, small bowel, pancreas, and transitional cell carcinoma of ureter and renal pelvis
Juvenile polyposis	Slight controversial	Juvenile polyps	Occasional juvenile polyps in small bowel and stomach; rare gastric carcinoma	
Peutz-Jeghers syndrome	? AD	Slight	Hamartomatous polyps; small intestine > stomach, colon	Mucocutaneous melanin deposits; hamartomatous polyps (Peutz-Jeghers polyps) in stomach, small bowel, colon; carcinoma of duodenum; there may be an excess of cancer of other sites, but more research required

AD, autosomal dominant; *AFAP*, attenuated familial adenomatous polyposis.

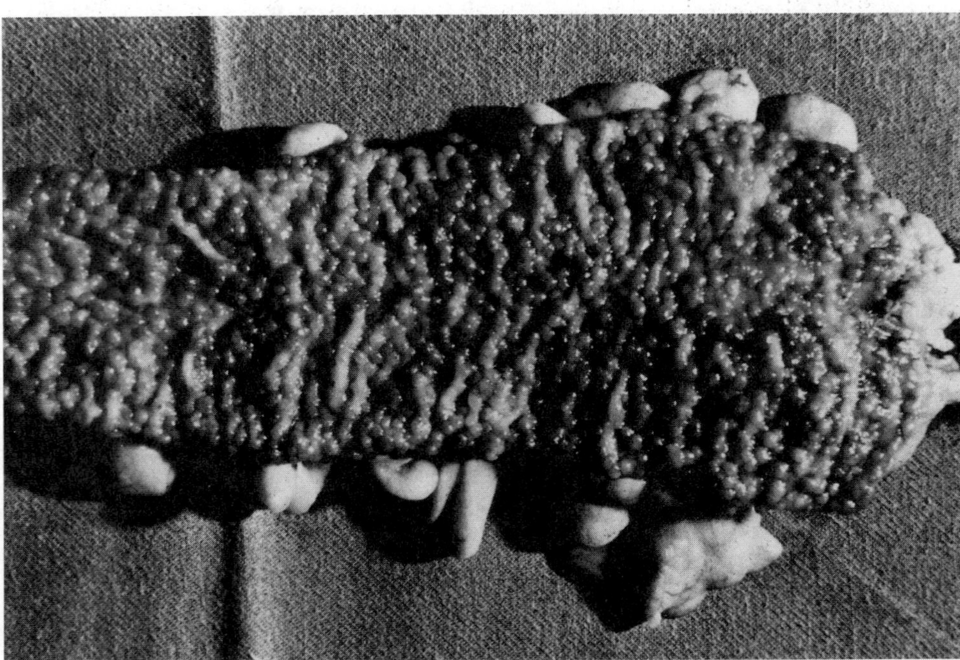

Fig. 12-5 Colon specimen blanketed with polyps.

osis syndromes. It is caused by a germ-line mutation in the *APC* gene, which is located on the long arm of chromosome 5. As illustrated in Fig. 12-5, patients with FAP develop hundreds to thousands of colorectal adenomatous polyps. Although these tumors are benign, it is almost certain that some will progress to cancer. The progression from adenoma to carcinoma in this syndrome is dependent on a somatic mutation in the normal *APC* gene of a colonic epithelial cell (Kinzler & Vogelstein, 1996). The average age at the onset of polyps is 15. If left untreated, the risk for colon cancer is virtually 100% usually by the fourth decade of life but has been reported at as early as 9 years of age. Annual screening with sigmoidoscopy is usually initiated by about 10 years of age, and prophylactic colectomy is performed after the teen years or earlier if polyps become too numerous to remove at endoscopy. There is an increased risk for upper gastrointestinal (GI) cancers, so periodic upper endoscopy is indicated for these patients even after colectomy.

In addition to the colon polyps, individuals with FAP may have a variety of other clinical finding, including osteomas: congenital hypertrophy of the retinal pigment epithelium, which is a benign finding in the retina; epidermoid cysts; and desmoid tumors. In the past, polyposis with these additional findings was thought to represent a separate syndrome called *Gardner syndrome.* It has been determined that Gardner syndrome is associated with a mutation in the *APC* gene. With careful examination, most individuals with FAP have some of these additional findings. Of all of the extracolonic findings, desmoids and extracolonic cancers are the only ones that result in increased morbidity and mortality. Desmoid tumors are fibrous masses that often have aggressive growth patterns that cause pain from pressure on other structures, small bowel obstruction, ureteric compression, and respiratory failure. In fact, desmoids are the second most common cause of death among those with FAP, and for those who have had prophylactic colectomy, they are the most common cause of death (Clark & Phillips, 1996).

An attenuated phenotype of FAP (AFAP) has been identified and associated with specific mutations in the APC gene. AFAP is associated with a later age of onset and a much smaller number of polyps ranging from 100 to 0 in affected family members. Because of the lower incidence of colon cancer in this form of FAP, prophylactic colectomy is not recommended for all mutation carriers (Lynch, Smyrk, & Lynch, 1995). Another rare form of intestinal polyposis, familial juvenile polyposis (FJP), is not linked to the APC gene (Leggett et al., 1993). Juvenile polyps are characterized by a distinctive histologic appearance and occur most commonly as single lesions in children. Familial juvenile polyposis is characterized by the existence of multiple juvenile polyps throughout the colon and may not appear until the adult years. The lifetime risk of colon cancer has been estimated to be 50%, and prophylactic colon resection is recommended for affected family members. The risk for gastric cancer is also elevated, but it is not known to what degree (Scott-Connor et al., 1995). Peutz-Jeghers syndrome consists of GI polyposis and a greenish black-to-brown pigmentation of the mucous membranes and skin around the nose, lips, hands, and feet. As with the other polyposis syndromes, it is autosomal dominant. However, the gene has not been identified yet. Approximately 50% of the affected family members develop cancer, which is most common in the GI tract but can also be of the breast, pancreas, and gallbladder (Rustgi, 1994).

Hereditary Nonpolyposis Colorectal Cancer. Hereditary nonpolyposis colorectal cancer (HNPCC) is the most common of the hereditary colon cancers, accounting for up to 5% of all colon cancers. Patients with HNPCC have a mutation in one of four genes that are responsible for the repair of DNA mismatches. Mutations in MLH1 are the most common, accounting for 33% of the cases of HNPCC. In addition, mutations in MSH2 account for 31%, whereas PMS1 and PMS2 account for 2% and 4% of the cases, respectively (Lynch & Smyrk, 1996). Cells that are heterozygous for one of these mismatch repair genes have normal DNA repair mechanisms, but a loss or mutation of the normal gene results in an accumulation of mutations at a rapid rate.

Recent data indicate that the risk for colorectal cancer in HNPCC may be higher in males than in females up to the age of 70 (74% vs 30%), and the female risk for endometrial cancer of 42% exceeds the colorectal risk (Dunlop et al., 1997). Other estimates for extracolonic cancer risks include a 14%-to-20% risk for transitional cell carcinoma of the ureter and renal pelvis; a 5% risk for cancers of the hepatobiliary tract; and increased risk for the development of cancers of the pancreas, small bowel, and stomach (Lynch & Smyrk, 1996).

Management of HNPCC family members with colon cancer should include subtotal colectomy because of the high incidence of second colonic primaries as the entire colonic mucosa is vulnerable to malignant transformation. Total abdominal hysterectomy and bilateral oophorectomy should be considered for women at the time of colectomy for colon cancer, especially if the woman has completed childbearing (Lynch & Smyrk, 1996).

Due to the early age of cancer onset, the proximal location of 70% of colon cancers, the problem of missed cancers, and accelerated carcinogenesis, colonoscopy is recommended for gene carriers or those at 50% risk between the ages of 20 and 25. It should be repeated at least every other year until age 30 and annually thereafter. Women should have endometrial aspiration, CA125 levels, and transvaginal ultrasound annually.

Prophylactic surgery, which is offered as an option to screening, includes subtotal colectomy, total abdominal hysterectomy, and salpingo-oophorectomy for women who have completed childbearing or reached menopause. Women need to be informed of the remaining risk for peritoneal cystadenocarcinoma consistent with ovarian origin even after removal of histologically normal ovaries (Lynch, Smyrk, & Lynch, 1996). After subtotal colectomy is performed prophylactically or for cancer, there is still a risk for rectal cancer, so endoscopic surveillance of the rectum is still required.

Muir-Torre syndrome is a subset of HNPCC which includes the classical features of HNPCC, as well as sebaceous adenomas, sebaceous carcinomas, and keratocanthomas. Muir-Torre syndrome has been shown to be associated with the same mutations that predispose to HNPCC (Lynch & Smyrk, 1996).

Familial Colorectal Cancer. Preliminary evidence indicates that a familial form of colorectal cancer may be caused by a specific mutation (I1307K) in the *APC* gene (Laken et al., 1997). This mutation is different from the *APC* gene mutations that cause the FAP phenotype. The I1307K mutation is estimated to occur in 1 in 16 Ashkenazi Jewish people. The lifetime risk for colon cancer associated with the mutation is in the range of 18% to 30%. Further study is required to determine the frequency of this mutation in other populations and to further delineate its phenotypic expression.

Familial Atypical Multiple Mole Melanoma

It is commonly known that individuals with fair skin who react to sunlight exposure by burning instead of tanning are more likely to develop melanoma. However, the greatest risk for melanoma is among those with a large number of moles (nevi) and/or atypical or dysplastic nevi (Easton, 1996). Melanoma, in association with a large number of nevi and dysplastic nevi clusters, indicates an inherited component. This autosomal dominant predisposition to melanoma is called *familial atypical multiple mole melanoma* (FAMMM). A gene responsible for FAMMM, p16, is located on the short arm of chromosome 9 (Cannon-Albright et al., 1992).

Recent evidence supports the view that p16 is a general tumor suppressor gene, and mutations may predispose not only to cutaneous and ocular melanoma, but also to other malignancies (Gruis, Sandkuijl, van der Velden, Bergman, & Frants, 1995). There is evidence that at least some p16 mutations increase the risk for pancreatic cancer (Bergman, Watson, de Jong, Lynch, & Fusaro, 1990), and further studies are required to determine the full spectrum of risks associated with the gene.

Screening of at-risk family members includes careful dermatologic and ophthalmologic examinations annually, as well as monthly self-skin examinations, starting in the teenage years. Nevi can occur in such unlikely areas as between the toes, on the labia, and in the perianal area so these areas need to be included in the examination. Any dysplastic nevi should be biopsied. Family members need to be taught that they are looking for any changes in nevi and the difference between normal and dysplastic nevi.

Li-Fraumeni Syndrome

Li-Fraumeni syndrome (LFS) is a rare autosomal, dominantly inherited cancer syndrome caused by a germ-line mutation in the p53 gene located on chromosome 17. Multiple cancers are associated with LFS (Li et al., 1988) with the most commonly associated cancers listed in Box 12-1. Individuals with LFS appear to have a 50% risk of developing cancer by age 30 and a risk to age 70 of approximately 90% (Malkin et al., 1990). The diverse tumor types in family members characteristically develop at unusually early ages, and multiple primary tumors are a frequent occurrence.

Direct DNA analysis is available for families suspected of having a germ-line p53 mutation that causes the Li-Fraumeni syndrome. However, the sensitivity and specificity of testing is not well established (Calzone, 1997). Once a mutation is confirmed in a family, predisposition testing can be useful to identify those in the family who are not at high risk for the development of various cancers.

Multiple Endocrine Neoplasia

Multiple endocrine neoplasia (MEN) represents another familial group of diseases that are subdivided into four different types: MEN1, MEN2A, MEN2B, and familial medullary thyroid cancer (FMTC). Table 12-5 outlines the disease characteristics of each of the four types of MEN syndromes.

Multiple Endocrine Neoplasia Type 1. Multiple endocrine neoplasia type 1 (MEN1) is an autosomal dominant condition characterized by the development of tumors of the parathyroid glands, anterior pituitary, pancreatic islet cells, adrenal glands, and thyroid glands. Duodenal gastrinomas, carcinoid tumors, and multiple lipomas are also described in this syndrome (Hodgson & Maher, 1993). Hypercalcemia is the most common manifestation of the disorder secondary to hyperparathyroidism. This disease is 94% penetrant by the age of 50 (Chandrasekharappa et al., 1997). Presenting symptoms are variable, depending on the tumor's prevalence. Except for gastrinomas, most of the tumors in MEN1 are nonmetastasizing.

Box 12-1
Li-Fraumeni Syndrome

Commonly Associated Cancers

Breast
Leukemia
Osteosarcoma
Brain
Soft tissue sarcomas
Adrenal cell carcinomas
Lung
Laryngeal

Genetics of MEN1. Chandrasekharappa and colleagues (1997) reported the cloning of the MEN1 gene in 1997. The gene is thought to be a tumor suppressor gene located on the long arm of chromosome 11. The protein product of the MEN1 gene is proposed by these researchers to be called *menin.* The function of the protein is unknown.

Screening of MEN1. Screening of at-risk individuals should start at age 10 and continue at 5-year intervals (Hodgson & Maher, 1993). Screening usually involves symptom inquiry; complete physical examination; measurement of serum calcium levels; and parathyroid, pituitary, and pancreatic hormone level assays. Currently, linkage analysis is available in families where two affected family members are willing to be tested. Since the gene for MEN1 has now been identified, direct DNA analysis will be available in the future. Linkage or direct DNA analysis will clarify the risks to relatives of clinically diagnosed individuals, allowing a modification of screening protocols to those who test negative.

Multiple Endocrine Neoplasia Type 2A. Multiple endocrine neoplasia type 2A (MEN2A) is an autosomal dominant syndrome that includes medullary thyroid carcinoma (MTC), pheochromocytoma, and parathyroid hyperplasia. The hereditary type of MTC, which accounts for about 25% of the cases, is characterized by C-cell hyperplasia, a precursor lesion for the tumor (Hodgson & Maher, 1993). Most hereditary MTC tumors are bilateral and multifocal and develop in the 20-to-40-year-old age group. Pheochromocytomas are also bilateral and occur in about one half of affected individuals. Approximately 10% of the pheochromocytomas become malignant.

Multiple Endocrine Neoplasia Type 2B. Multiple endocrine neoplasia type 2B (MEN2B) is a variant of MEN2A and comprises individuals with MTC, with or without pheochromocytoma in association with a characteristic phenotype. The phenotype includes multiple mucosal neuromas, intestinal ganglioneuromatosis, neurological abnormalities, joint laxity, kyphoscoliosis, enlarged and nodular lips, and Marfanoid build (Hodgson & Maher, 1993). The medullary thyroid carcinomas in MEN2B are more ag-

Table 12-5 Disease Characteristics of Multiple Endocrine Neoplasia Syndromes

MEN1	MEN2A	MEN2B	FMTC
Parathyroid hyperplasia or adenoma	Parathyroid hyperplasia or adenoma		
Anterior pituitary hyperplasia	Pheocromocytoma	Pheocromocytoma	
Pancreatic islet cell hyperplasia, adenoma or cancer			
Adrenal hyperplasia or adenoma			
Thyroid hyperplasia or adenoma	Medullary thyroid cancer	Medullary thyroid cancer	Medullary thyroid cancer
Duodenal gastrinomas, carcinoid tumors, multiple lipomas		Mucosal neuromas, intestinal ganglioneuromatosis	
		Joint laxity, kyphoscoliosis, Marfanoid habitus, enlarged and nodular lips	

gressive and develop earlier than in MEN2A, with a mean age at diagnosis of 20 years. Virtually all patients affected with MEN2B will develop MTC, with about one quarter developing pheochromocytoma. Parathyroid disease is rare in MEN2B.

Familial Medullary Thyroid Carcinoma. FMTC encompasses families in which there is a minimum of four individuals affected with MTC but no evidence of pheochromocytoma or parathyroid disease (Hodgson & Maher, 1994).

Genetics of MEN2A, MEN2B, and FMTC. Mutations in the RET receptor tyrosine kinase gene are associated with MEN2A, MEN2B, and FMTC. The RET gene was cloned in 1985 (Takahashi, Ritz, & Cooper, 1985) and is located on chromosome 10. Activating mutations in this proto-oncogene have been identified in approximately 95% of MEN2A and 90% of FMTC families (Eng, 1996).

Screening and Treatment for MEN2A, MEN2B, and FMTC. Prospective screening and early treatment of manifestations of MEN2 and FMTC can prevent metastasis of medullary thyroid carcinoma and the morbidity and mortality of pheochromocytoma (Gagel et al, 1988). Before genetic screening was available, the following was indicated (Calmettes, Ponder, Fischer, Raue, & members of the European community Concerted Action Medullary Thyroid Carcinoma, 1992):

- Beginning at age 3, screening by the pentagastrin stimulation test
- Annual screening for pheochromocytoma by measurement of urinary excretion of catecholamines
- Annual screening for hyperparathyroidism by serum calcium determination

Currently, biochemical screening can be reserved for gene carriers only. Genetic screening is now considered a standard of care for MEN2 families (Wells et al., 1994). Curative treatment for MTC is total thyroidectomy by age 5.

Neurofibromatosis

Neurofibromatosis-Type 1. Neurofibromatosis-type 1 (NF-1) is one of the most common of all human neurogenetic disorders with a frequency of 1 in 3000. It is a disorder of hyperplasia, dysmorphology, and oncology and does not discriminate among racial, ethnic, and national groups, or geographic locations. Neurofibromatosis is an autosomal dominant disorder characterized by café-au-lait spots and neurofibromatous tumors of the skin.

Neurofibromatosis-type 1 varies from one family to another, from each individual within a family, and even from one body part to another for any given individual (Riccardi, 1994). Nearly half of all cases are new mutations, which means the mutation originated in the presenting individual and no family history will be detectable (Stephens et al., 1992). Individuals with NF-1 do not manifest all of the disorder's features, and many characteristics of NF-1 are age-related. Characteristic clinical features of NF-1 are listed in Box 12-2. Most individuals with the NF-1 gene mutation develop six or more café-au-lait spots and Lisch nodules by age 5 (Riccardi, 1992). Individuals affected with NF-1 are at increased risk for a variety of neoplastic lesions that are also listed in Box 12-2 (Hodgson & Maher, 1993).

Genetics of NF-1. The location of the NF-1 gene on the long arm of chromosome 17, near the centromere, was reported in 1989 (Goldgar, Green, Parry, & Mulvihill, 1989), and the complete cloning of the coding region of the gene occurred in 1991 (Marchuk et al., 1991). The NF-1 gene appears to be a tumor suppressor gene (Legius, Marchuk, Collins, & Glover, 1993) with its protein product, called *neurofibromin,* functioning to downregulate the RAS oncogene (Basu et al, 1992). Diagnosis of NF-1 is usually a clinical diagnosis and does not require or necessitate DNA testing. However, DNA testing may be useful in the presymptomatic and prenatal setting, if a mutation is already identified in the family.

Neurofibromatosis-Type 2. Neurofibromatosis-type 2 (NF-2) is an autosomal dominant disorder that is distinct from NF-1 and is characterized by bilateral vestibular schwannomas (acoustic neuromas), schwannomas of other central and peripheral nerves, cranial meningiomas, and ependymomas (Parry et al., 1994). The incidence of NF-2 is approximately 1 in 35,000, and the disorder is recognized for its clinical heterogeneity. Peripheral neurofibromas may occur in NF-2, although they are rarely as numerous as is usually seen in NF-1. Diagnostic criteria for NF-2, established by an National Institutes of Health (NIH) Consensus Development Conference (1988), are outlined in Box 12-3.

Generally, NF-2 does not become clinically evident until after puberty or well into adulthood. Vestibular schwannomas are benign, slow-growing tumors located on the vestibular branch of the eighth cranial nerve. The clinical course may include severe to profound deafness.

The tumors of NF-2 are histologically benign, but their anatomic locations make treatment challenging. Early surgical intervention can produce dramatic results by preventing long-term disability. The single most important factor in the treatment of NF-2 is early detection. A program of presymptomatic testing of individuals at risk, including both

Box 12-2
Clinical Features of Neurofibromatosis Type 1

Neurofibromas
Café-au-lait spots
Axillary freckling
Lisch nodules
Short attention span, hyperactivity, learning disabilities
Macrocephaly
Kyphoscoliosis
Pseudoarthrosis
Renal artery stenosis
Optic glioma
Astrocytoma
Neurofibrosarcoma
Leukemia
Pheochromocytoma
Carcinoid

Box 12-3
Diagnostic Criteria for Neurofibromatosis Type-2

Bilateral eighth nerve masses

OR

First-degree relative with NF - 2

AND

Either unilateral eighth nerve mass OR two of the following:

- Neurofibroma
- Meningioma
- Glioma
- Schwannoma
- Juvenile posterior subcapsular lenticular opacity

Neurofibromatosis: *NIH Consensus Statement 1987 Jul 13-15,* 6(12), 1-19.

Table 12-6 Screening Recommendations for Families With Von Hippel-Lindau Syndrome

Medical Procedure	Age for Initiation	Frequency
H&P	Infancy	Annual
Ophthalmoscopy	Infancy	Annual
24-hour urinary catecholamines	2 years	Every 1-2 years
MRI of brain and spine	11 years	Every 2 years
Abdominal CT scan with contrast	20 years	Annual
MRI or CT internal auditory canals	20 years	To evaluate symptoms

magnetic resonance imaging (MRI) and audiologic evaluations, is usually recommended (MacCollin et al., 1993).

Genetics of NF-2. In 1993 the NF-2 gene was cloned and characterized as a tumor suppressor gene located on the long arm of chromosome 22 (Rouleau et al., 1993; Trofatter et al., 1993). The cloning of the NF-2 gene allows for identification of mutation carriers in high-risk families. Using DNA testing technology for risk assessment should result in a greatly reduced number of individuals who require periodic screening. Therefore presymptomatic and prenatal diagnosis is feasible in families in which a mutation has been identified.

Von Hippel-Lindau Syndrome

Von Hippel-Lindau (VHL) syndrome is a rare multiple-tumor syndrome with an estimated frequency of 1 in 36,000 (Maher et al., 1991). The VHL gene is a tumor suppressor gene on the short arm of chromosome 3. Mutations in the VHL gene can result in a retinal angioma, central nervous system (CNS) hemangioblastoma, clear cell renal carcinoma, pheochromocytoma, and cysts in the pancreas and epididymis (Humphrey, Klausner, & Linehan, 1996). Symptomatic patients with VHL are diagnosed at a mean age of 26. The most frequent initial manifestation is retinal angioma or cerebellar hemangioblastoma. Approximately 28% of patients develop clear cell renal carcinoma, which is almost invariably bilateral. Identification of mutation carriers by DNA testing can be essential for targeting the extensive surveillance in VHL families as seen in Table 12-6.

CASE IDENTIFICATION

The primary purpose of cancer risk assessment and counseling is to reduce the morbidity and mortality of cancer for individuals and families that are at an increased risk for cancer due to their genetic make-up, lifestyle, and/or environmental exposures. Cancer risk assessment enables the development of management plans, including surveillance recommendations, lifestyle modifications and options for DNA testing, prophylactic surgeries, and chemoprevention, as appropriate. Cancer risk counseling provides the opportunity to educate family members, to assist the individual in making the best decisions for himself or herself, and to promote optimal adaptation to the risk and occurrence of cancer within the family.

Identification of Individuals at Increased Risk

One of the primary nursing roles in cancer genetics is the identification of individuals and families at increased risk for cancer, based on their family history. As the nurse is collecting historical data as part of the assessment of a new patient, the family history, including any history of cancer, should always be recorded. Explaining the rationale for taking a family history may decrease the reluctance of some patients to share information about other family members. Issues such as nonpaternity, consanguinity, or suicide need to be acknowledged with sensitivity (Bennett et al., 1995).

The family history should include all first-degree (i.e., parents, siblings, and children) and second-degree (i.e., grandparents, aunts, uncles, nieces, nephews, and grandchildren) relatives. Inquiry about each individual's history reduces the chance of the patient forgetting about someone who has a history of something pertinent. Patient recall can also be augmented by inquiring, during the review of systems, if anyone in the family has a history of cancer of the respective anatomic sites. Young people are less likely to be aware of their family history and may need to discuss it with other members of the family. There is often an unofficial historian in the family who is aware of the history of previous generations, or it may be recorded in a Holy Bible or other genealogy records.

Keeping in mind that cancer is a common occurrence, the nurse's next step is to determine if the family history is one that should lead to a referral for further evaluation. Factors to be considered in this determination are listed in Box 12-4.

Even in the presence of a rather insignificant family history, some individuals may have intense concern about their risks or that of their offspring. In an English study, it was found that many women over age 50 with breast cancer and

Box 12-4
Characteristics of Hereditary Cancer

Age of cancer onset; on average 10-20 years earlier than in sporadic cancers
Two or more first-degree relatives with the same cancer site
Cancer occurrences in more than one generation
More than one primary cancer in one individual
A pattern of different cancers, which is consistent with a hereditary cancer syndrome

no other risk factors overestimated the breast cancer risk for their daughters (Luker, Leinster, Owens, Beaver, & Degner, 1994). The patient's level of anxiety and concerns related to cancer risks associated with the family history of cancer should be assessed. The concern may be related to witnessing a relative or friend experience cancer, or it may be due to misinformation or a misunderstanding of information about risks. Identification of the source of concern can facilitate the nurse's attempt to allay the anxiety, but if unsuccessful, a referral for a formal cancer risk assessment may be indicated.

Identification of Providers

Cancer risk assessment and genetic counseling services are provided by a variety of professionals, including advanced practice nurses, genetic counselors, oncologists, and geneticists. Some centers have a team of professionals providing services and in other centers; it may be one individual providing the service with other professionals consulted on an as-needed basis. For the purpose of this chapter, the provider of cancer risk assessment and counseling is referred to as the *counselor.* The National Cancer Institute's Cancer Information Service maintains a listing of cancer genetic services for the United States. This resource can be accessed on the Internet at http://cancernet.nci.nih.gov/wwwprot/genetic/genesrch.html or by calling 1-800-4CANCER.

Preparation for Comprehensive Evaluation

At the time of referral, the nurse's role includes conveying information to both the counselor and the patient. Communicating the nurse's assessment of the family history and the patient's questions and concerns about cancer, as well as any other pertinent data to the counselor, can facilitate continuity of care for the patient. Likewise, the patient should be informed of what to expect from a comprehensive cancer genetic evaluation.

The patient is asked to assume a partnership role in the evaluation of the significance of the family history. The patient collects additional information about all first-degree, second-degree, and at least some third-degree relatives such as great-grandparents and first cousins. The information to be gathered on each family member includes name, date of birth or current age, date of or age at death, cause of death, all primary cancer sites with age at diagnosis, and any other significant health problems. The ethnic backgrounds or nationalities of those in the earliest generation should be identified.

If there is suspicion of a cancer syndrome that includes specific physical findings, the patient should be asked to inquire among relatives about the existence of those findings, such as multiple atypical moles in FAMMM. Likewise the patient should be informed to collect information about specific health problems if the recommendations or options for medical management might be affected by a familial risk for those problems. As an example, heart disease or osteoporosis in a family suspected of having hereditary breast and ovarian cancer (HBOC) may affect recommendations for hormone replacement after prophylactic oophorectomy or menopause.

Some individuals may be able to access little information about the health history of other family members. Families and individual members vary in their openness about sharing medical information. The patient should be encouraged to try to gather as much family history information as possible without damaging family relationships.

Ideally, the cancer occurrences in the family should be documented with medical and pathology records. There may be confusion within a family related to cancer; in some families, surgical removal of any type of tumor may equate with malignancy. Even when cancer has occurred, the site reported may be the metastatic site rather than the primary site. Nurses can help families with obtaining medical records by explaining the necessity for accurate information and assuring that the release of information forms are completed by the individual with a history of cancer or the nearest surviving relative. Pathology reports are the preferred source of documentation of the site of cancer and the age of diagnosis, and are most easily obtained from the hospital where the diagnosis was made. Medical records related to treatment can be an additional source of documentation. If all records have been destroyed, the death certificate may be an additional source for documentation. It is important to note that death certificates may be fraught with errors in diagnosis and should be used only as a secondary source of information. These records can be obtained from the health department of the state in which the individual died.

The patient should be encouraged to bring a spouse, family member, or friend to the evaluation. The presence of a significant other can provide support when the information that is shared during the evaluation and counseling has strong emotional overtones. Some individuals choose to bring several family members who share the concern about their risk so that they all receive the information at the same time. Each may ask questions or remember information that was shared that others did not consider or remember.

CANCER RISK ASSESSMENT

Construction of the Pedigree

At the time of the evaluation, the counselor reviews the family history with the patient(s) and constructs a pedigree (Fig. 12-6). The purpose of the pedigree is to facilitate visualiza-

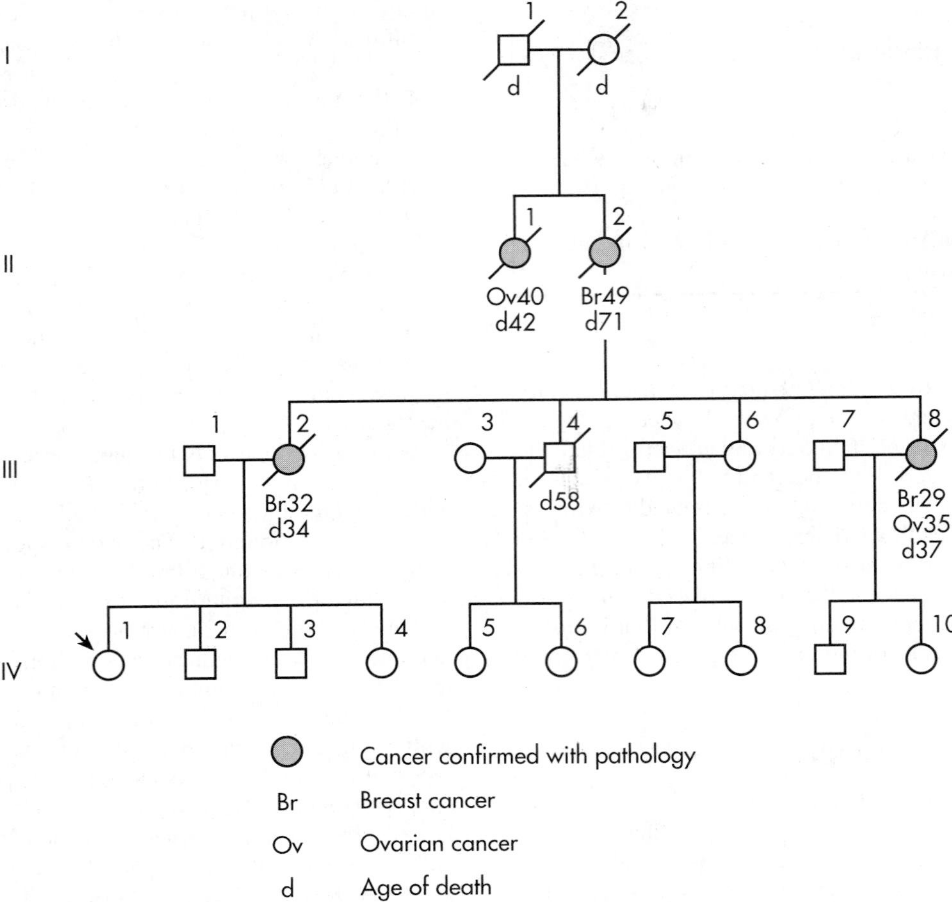

Fig. 12-6 Family pedigree indicative of hereditary breast and ovarian cancer.

tion of all of the history and discernment of any pattern to the cancer occurrences. Circles represent females, and squares represent males. A horizontal line drawn from the middle of one symbol to the middle of another represents a marriage or a procreative union. A vertical line represents the relationship between parents and children. The symbols for siblings are joined by a horizontal line. The current age or age at death is usually recorded below the symbol along with the individual's name. A diagonal line is drawn through the symbol for an individual who is deceased. Pedigrees for publication do not have names, but numbers are assigned for each generation and each individual within a generation. These pedigrees are generally encrypted to preserve the privacy of the family without destroying the scientific significance of the report. The cancer site(s) with age of onset are recorded for each affected individual. Shading of symbols can be used to identify other pertinent diagnoses or to indicate the level of documentation of the cancer occurrences. Notations of a significant surgical history are also made. Legends are provided to define the abbreviations of cancer sites and the representations of the shaded symbols. In Fig. 12-6, it is easy to see from the pattern of the breast and ovarian cancers in multiple generations, the early age of onset, and the multiple primary tumors that this is a high-risk family. In Fig. 12-7 the abbreviations are used to indicate the clinical findings in addition to colon cancer that are associated with FAP.

Medical History and Physical Examination

A complete medical history is obtained from the patient. Special attention is paid to environmental exposures and lifestyle issues that may contribute to the risk of cancer, surgeries or biopsies, cancer screening practices, and other significant physical findings or conditions that may relate to the diagnosis or have an impact on medical management. Some centers also provide a physical examination as part of the evaluation, while others do not.

Psychosocial Assessment

While the family and medical history are being reviewed, the counselor assesses the psychosocial impact of the cancer occurrences and threat of cancer for the individual and the family. This assessment may require little or no prompting if it is the first time that the patient has had an opportunity to tell the story of the personal and family impact of multiple cancer occurrences and early deaths.

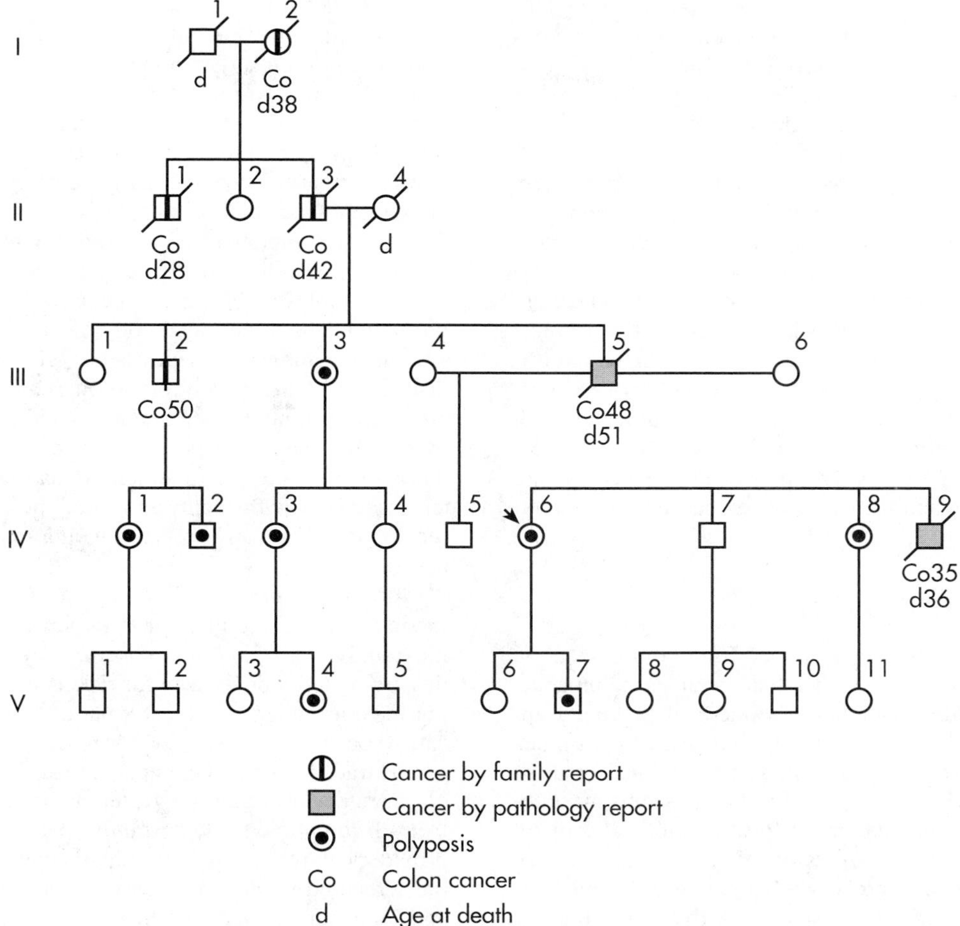

Fig. 12-7 Family pedigree indicative of familial adenomatous polyposis.

In Fig. 12-6 (IV-1), the consultant related the experience of witnessing her mother's (III-2) battle and death with ovarian cancer when IV-1 was 13 years of age, followed 5 years later by the death of her aunt (III-8) who had assumed the maternal role for her and her siblings. The consultant has assumed the maternal role among her siblings, and there is a tight bond among them. However, the consultant also has an intense underlying fear of "losing" her sister to a similar fate.

In Fig. 12-7 (IV-6), the consultant also fears for the life of her siblings, but the "story" in her family is somewhat different. In his 20s, the consultant's father reportedly received a recommendation for a colectomy because of multiple colonic polyps, which he chose to ignore. In his 30s, he abandoned his family. The family lost all contact with him until shortly before his death. The consultant and her full siblings were raised by their mother who was unaware of their father's family history. When the father (III-5) re-established contact with his children, he informed them of the family's diagnosis of FAP and their own risk. Several years later when the consultant sought a cancer risk assessment, she could provide history for her grandparents, parents, full siblings, and their children. With some help from one of her paternal aunts (III-3), the rest of the family history was taken. The family has been dysfunctional for several generations; there is bitterness and anger among family members, and some do not talk with each other. The response to the threat of colon cancer within this family varies from a rather matter-of-fact acceptance to complete denial.

The family experience with cancer can have a profound impact on individual members' beliefs about cancer treatment and survival. The risk of cancer is often equated with the risk of dying (Kelly, 1992). As many as 50% of first-degree relatives (FDRs) of breast cancer patients have reported the experience of traumatic stress symptoms related to their cancer risk, including sleep disturbances, as well as intrusive thoughts and feelings that interfere with daily activities (Lerman et al., 1993). Compassionate, understanding, sympathetic attention to the individual's response to the family cancer experience may also provide some relief in and of itself.

Identification of physical traits of affected members with the risk of cancer is a common myth in families that affects risk perception (e.g., identifying the children who resemble the affected parent as more likely to develop cancer). A woman with breast cancer said she was sure that her older daughter would have breast cancer because that daughter has dark hair and eyes like her side of the family, whereas her other daughter would not have it because she has blond hair and blue eyes. In other families, there may be a belief in an association between inheritance of cancer risk and a certain personality characteristic.

The counselor also assesses the individual's support systems within and outside of the family. As with the family in Fig. 12-6, some families are supportive of each other, and others are more like the family in Fig. 12-7. Spouses and close friends are an important source of support, especially if an individual needs a more objective perspective or feels that the family is currently overwhelmed with its experience. Support from a relationship with God, a formal religion, or clergy carries some individuals or families through many painful experiences. Some individuals turn to professionals or support groups when their needs for support are not being met or when they are concerned about overloading the family system.

GENERAL COUNSELING

Genetic counseling has been defined as a communication process about a genetic disorder that includes helping the individual or family understand the medical facts and appreciate the contribution of heredity and risk of recurrence in specified relatives; understanding their options for dealing with the risk; choosing the option(s) that seems most appropriate for them; and making the best possible adjustment to the disorder or the risk of its occurrence (Fraser, 1974). The genetic counseling process is an active, dynamic process for all the individuals involved, with each counselor and patient learning from the other. The ultimate goal of cancer risk counseling is the prevention of cancer or, at the least, the early identification and successful treatment of cancer. Although this type of genetic counseling at times may have a more directive approach than traditional genetic counseling, respect is maintained for the patient's right to make autonomous informed decisions. The counselor's role is not limited to providing information and care, but he or she is also involved in empowering the patient to take an active role in decision making about genetic testing and cancer risk management, and in developing or reinforcing healthy coping behaviors.

Cancer risk counseling may be provided to an individual or to a small group of family members as determined by the patient. Individual counseling provides an opportunity to focus on the informational and psychological needs of the patient. Group counseling provides an opportunity for several family members to contribute to the family history, to hear the same information at the same time, and to derive support from each other.

Medical and Genetic Facts

The medical and genetic facts provided in the counseling session include the diagnosis, treatment, prognosis, contribution of heredity, and genetic and cancer risks. The psychosocial assessment performed during the evaluation phase is used to determine the counselor's approach to conveying the information. The individual's knowledge and educational level should determine the complexity of the information that will be provided and the amount of explanation that will be required. The emotional and cognitive aspects of faulty beliefs and family myths need to be dispelled so that new information can be integrated into the individual's knowledge base and belief system.

Drawings, pictures, and other visual materials are used to assist in providing understandable information about the complex topics of cancer and genetics. A description of the normal anatomy and physiology of the predominant cancer sites in the family provides a background for subsequent discussion of medical information. The medical facts that are explained include the diagnosis and the associated findings such as any cancers at other sites for which there is an increased risk; current treatment modalities and the prognosis associated with them; and the appropriate surveillance recommendations and prevention options with their benefits and limitations.

Sporadic Cancer. Because cancer is so frequent, affecting one in three individuals at some time in their lives, most individuals have some history of cancer in their families. Some individuals seen for risk assessment and counseling have a family history of what are most likely sporadic cancer occurrences. These occurrences may be cancers that can be traced to environmental exposures, have an older age of onset, occur at multiple different sites, or affect relatives from different sides of the family. Often, the primary care provider can relieve the individual's concerns during an initial screening by phone; however, others require evaluation and counseling. Afterward, these individuals can be told that they have only a slightly increased risk for specific cancers. The American Cancer Society screening recommendations for the general population are discussed with them. If their cancer anxiety is still at a level that interferes with quality of life, they are referred for psychological counseling.

Familial Cancer. *Familial cancer* is defined as the occurrence of cancer at the same site in more than one relative, usually at an older age, and without the presence of other cancers or of a pattern to the occurrences that would be associated with a hereditary syndrome. Empiric models have been developed for estimating breast cancer risk based on large population studies. Frequently used models include the Claus and the Gail models. The Claus model (Claus, Risch, & Thompson, 1991) was derived specifically for women who have a family history of breast cancer and takes into consideration the age of onset of the cancer for various combinations of first- and second-degree relatives. The Gail model calculates risk based on the individuals' current age, age at menarche, age at first live birth, number of previous biopsies, and number of FDRs with breast cancer (Gail et al., 1989). The most appropriate use of the Gail model is with women undergoing annual mammography and without a strong family history of breast cancer (Spiegelman, Colditz, Hunter, & Hertzmark, 1994). Both models calculate cumulative risks for specific points in the life span, and underestimates the risk for some and overestimates the risk for others. Whatever method is used for familial cancer risk assessment, the patient needs to be informed of the limitations associated with risk calculations derived from epidemiologic studies.

There are no studies that show benefit to a specific surveillance program for individuals with a familial risk for cancer. Therefore surveillance recommendations are a matter of clinical judgment. Many clinicians recommend instituting the appropriate surveillance measures somewhat earlier than in the general population. The patient should also be informed of the availability of any chemoprevention trials that may be available.

Hereditary Cancer. When a hereditary cancer syndrome is diagnosed, the mode of inheritance should be explained adequately to assist the individual with understanding the role heredity plays in the syndrome. The concepts of variable expression, gene penetrance, and heterogeneity are explained if the syndrome is autosomal dominant. If the syndrome is autosomal recessive, the carrier state needs to be adequately defined. The patient should be informed of the increased chance of mating with a carrier of the same ethnic background, if from a high-risk population or in a consanguineous union.

The genetic risk is defined for the patient and selected others in the family based on their positions in the pedigree. Some people understand risk information better if it is provided as chance (e.g., 1 in 4), whereas others better understand the percentage of likelihood (e.g., 25% risk). Generally, it is helpful to present the risk both ways and to balance the chance of an event happening with the chance that it will not happen.

The risk of cancer at the various sites needs to be differentiated from the risk of inheriting a mutation. Transmission of the gene in a syndrome with a gender-limited cancer site such as breast cancer is no different than in syndromes in which both genders are equally likely to be affected with cancer. This fact can be quite surprising to individuals who have assumed that transmission of the breast cancer gene is only from mother to daughter based on their observations within their own family.

Psychosocial Counseling

The psychosocial aspect of cancer risk counseling may be centered primarily on the individual, but it always includes a focus on the family as a whole. The goal of the psychosocial component of genetic counseling is the empowerment of the individual to be able to integrate factual information provided; to make informed decisions related to testing issues and medical management; to make an optimal adaptation to the family history of cancer occurrences and personal risk status; and to realistically, and with a sense of hope and purpose, plan for the future. Achievement of these goals takes time and patience, keeping in mind that many of these family members have been dealing with their cancer legacy for most of their lives.

The individual's anxieties, fears, and perception of the risk for cancer, as well as his or her beliefs about cancer treatment and survival, can have a profound impact on the acceptance and integration of information that is provided during counseling. In a randomized trial, Lerman and colleagues (1995) found that two thirds of women who received individualized breast cancer risk counseling continued to extremely overestimate their risks. Since these were the women who were the most preoccupied with their cancer risk, it was hypothesized that their anxieties interfered with their attention to and comprehension of new risk information.

Some of the common emotional themes related to multiple cancer occurrences in a family and the risk of future occurrences include grief, anxiety, guilt, and depression. The manner in which individuals and families deal with these emotions has as many permutations as the cancer-causing genes have mutations. The role of the counselor or the nurse is to support healthy coping mechanisms, and in the event of ineffective or destructive coping, to suggest or teach alternatives. The first step in supporting healthy coping is listening with acceptance and acknowledgment of feelings while seeking clarification of the personal meaning of the individual's experience.

The death of a family member may be the motivating force for seeking a cancer risk assessment. In this situation the individual may be immersed in the grieving process and may be unable to integrate new information until some of the grief is dealt with. The individual who is grieving has three tasks: (1) to experience the feelings associated with the loss; (2) to review the history of the attachment; and (3) to confront the task of moving on (Cassem, 1978). The role of the nurse or counselor is to allow the expression of feeling and to help the individual understand the grieving process as a normal reaction. It is also important to encourage family members to share memories and experiences with each other, to recall and utilize past strengths and successful coping strategies, and to return to activity.

Guilt is witnessed in a variety of situations within families with hereditary cancer. There is the guilt experienced by the individual with cancer over being sick and unable to perform their usual roles, the guilt of a parent for passing on a cancer-causing mutation to their children, or the survivor guilt of a family member for being fortunate enough to avoid the cancer-causing mutation. Although guilt is a common human experience, in these instances, it is destructive, since it is due to events out of the individual's control. After encouraging the expression of guilty feelings, the individual can be assisted to develop a more constructive attitude by acknowledging that as part of the human condition, everyone has deleterious genes with no control over the genes that are received nor over the ones that are passed on.

The experience of being at significantly increased risk for the development of cancer is bound to be associated with a certain degree of anxiety. A high level of anxiety about developing cancer may interfere with the ability of an individual to carry out daily activities or to comply with the recommended cancer surveillance strategies. The effectiveness of coping mechanisms that are being used can be assessed with the individual. In the event of ineffective coping, strategies successfully used in the past may be explored as alternatives, or new strategies may be suggested. Some individuals find activity to be a mechanism for working out the excessive energy they experience with strong emotions. Others may deal with that energy with intense expression of their feelings, such as crying, yelling, or laughing. Others cope by using quiet contemplation, whether it be in prayer, meditation, relaxation techniques, or thinking things through.

The supportive roles within a family change with the development of cancer or death and even with the discovery of the genetic status of family members. Family members may need help finding an alternative source of support within or outside of the family. Just as the supportive roles within the family may change with the occurrence of cancer or death, genetic test results may alter other family roles, as well as family functioning and communication patterns. Families may need some help in adapting to these changes and exploring alternative strategies. The perceptions and experiences of family members have a strong influence on each other. If a family member's perceptions are unrealistic, eliciting the perceptions of other family members may be supportive of more realistic coping by the family as a whole.

GENETIC TESTING AND INFORMED CONSENT

Guidelines for Providers

Genetic testing is available for a number of hereditary cancer syndromes, and this procedure increases as more genes associated with an increased risk for cancer are identified. However, there is concern and controversy over when, how, to whom, and by whom these tests should be offered. Position statements and guidelines have been established for predictive testing by several professional and lay organizations, including the American Society of Clinical Oncology (1996), American Society of Human Genetics (1994), National Action Plan on Breast Cancer (1996), National Breast Cancer Coalition (1995), National Advisory Council for Human Genome Research (1994), and Oncology Nursing Society (1997).

Some concerns leading to attempts at limiting the availability of genetic testing include the following:

- Inadequate knowledge about the frequency of the various gene mutations and the risks of cancer associated with each mutation
- Insufficient professionals who are prepared to provide the education and counseling for the informed consent and beneficial integration of this powerful information into the lives of consumers
- Incomplete understanding of laboratory issues such as frequencies of false-positive and false-negative results
- Lack of proven effectiveness of the interventions to decrease the morbidity and mortality of cancer in high-risk individuals
- The potential for financially devastating discrimination by insurers and employers.

Despite the positions of these organizations, the fact is that DNA testing for hereditary cancer syndromes is commercially available from a growing number of laboratories, not all of which share these views. Nurses need to be prepared to act as advocates for their patients to ensure they receive appropriate services and complete information.

There has also been concern about the potential for an overwhelming consumer demand for DNA testing. Studies of interest among the general population in genetic testing for colon cancer susceptibility (Croyle & Lerman, 1993) revealed interest in 83% of the respondents. As the potential for refining an individual's cancer risk through DNA testing was approaching a reality, several studies were performed to determine the level of interest in testing among FDRs of patients with colon, breast, or ovarian cancer. In each of these studies, more than 80% to 95% of the subjects indicated they would or probably would want to obtain a genetic test for susceptibility to the cancer of their FDR (Lerman, Daly, Masny, & Balshem, 1994; Lerman, Marshall, Audrain, & Gomez-Caminero, 1996; Lerman, Seay, Balshem, & Audrain, 1995). Based on psychological measures, those who would elect to be tested tended to be more pessimistic about outcome and to have more mood disturbance. Common motivations for seeking testing were to determine what cancer screening should be performed, to identify their children's risk for cancer, and to be reassured. These studies were performed with FDRs of individuals with cancer, regardless of whether the cancers were sporadic, familial, or hereditary. They were also lacking discussion of any of the risks or limitations of DNA testing, resulting in a gross overestimation of the demand for testing. When BRCA1 test results were offered to a cohort of HBOC family members who had participated in DNA research studies, only 43% chose to receive their results after genetic counseling (Lerman, Narod, et al., 1996).

Due to all of the aforementioned concerns, many have advocated for testing to be limited to well-controlled situations such as within research programs with protocols approved by the Institutional Review Board (IRB). Others have felt the limitation to a research protocol restricts access to testing and its potential benefits by too many high-risk individuals and that clinical testing with the same safeguards can be provided when the family history is consistent with a hereditary cancer syndrome.

One area of consensus is the need for informed consent and genetic counseling to be an integral part of the testing process. Another area of consensus is that until more is known about the polymorphisms and mutations of the various genes, testing needs to be initiated with a member who has a history of a syndrome cancer to identify the cancer-causing mutation in the family. A negative test result for an at-risk member of a family in which the family mutation has not yet been identified cannot be interpreted. The individual may not have the mutation in the family, or there may be a mutation present that the test could not identify. Lacking awareness of this limitation, almost 32% of requesting physicians misinterpreted negative test results for the *APC* gene during the first year the test was commercially available (Giardello et al., 1997). Therefore testing has to be initiated with an affected family member to identify the mutation. If a mutation is not identified in the affected individual, testing is not offered to unaffected family members.

Although the collection of the specimen may be as routine as drawing a blood sample, DNA testing cannot be equated with other laboratory tests. Its unique nature resides in the information that is obtained. Genetic information is permanent, has implications for others in the family, can affect relationships within the family, may have implications for reproductive decision making or choice of a partner, may be a source of pressure for one to take a course of action opposed to one's desires or values, may alter one's perception of his or her health status, may result in one being stereotyped, or may be used as a source of discrimination (Scanlon & Fibison, 1995).

Before giving consent for DNA testing, the individual needs to be informed about the test(s) to be performed, the cost, the implications of both positive and negative results, and the likelihood of not receiving informative results. Patients need to know that they can decline testing and employ surveillance and/or prevention strategies based on family history alone. Assistance should be provided in making a comparison between the potential outcomes of having and of not having the test performed. Ideally, there should be a time interval, between the delivery of information and the consent, for the individual to absorb the information and consider the consequences of each alternative for oneself, one's family, and significant others. The nurse's role during the informed consent process includes protection of the individual's autonomy, provision or reinforcement of information, assurance of the individual's comprehension of the facts, and assistance with making a decision that is in the individual's best interest (Lessick & Williams, 1994).

Testing of Minors

The generally accepted practice of parents providing the consent for their children's medical tests and treatments is not considered appropriate for predisposition testing for hereditary cancer syndromes. Children may experience heightened anxiety about their future health or a loss of self-esteem. Parents may lower their expectations or be overprotective of the child who is found to be at high risk for cancer. The unaffected siblings may feel left out or experience survivor guilt. Another reason for not testing minors is to preserve the child's right as an adult to make an informed decision about the course of action that is best for him or her (Ackerman, 1996).

If the welfare of the child outweighs the preceding considerations, testing of minors is acceptable. Predictive tests (e.g., *RET* gene testing for retinoblastoma) for syndromes with childhood onset of cancer offer the potential for substantial therapeutic benefit for a child. Genetic testing may also exclude a child from expensive and invasive medical surveillance such as colonoscopies for children who are negative for the *APC* gene. There have also been some arguments in favor of testing adolescents if substantial psychosocial benefit is to be obtained. This last situation could occur if the adolescent is found to be competent, provides voluntary consent, and has adequate understanding of the necessary information (American Board of Medical Genetics & American College of Medical Genetics Board of Directors, 1995).

Benefits of Testing

At this time, there are no proven methods of preventing the occurrence of most of the hereditary cancers, although a number of chemoprevention trials are in progress. There also are no unique treatment modalities for hereditary cancers once they occur, but there is the hope of gene therapy at some time in the future. In the meantime, the only interventions available for reducing morbidity and mortality are intensive targeted surveillance for early detection and treatment and the option of prophylactic surgeries to remove organs at high risk for syndrome cancers. The effectiveness of these interventions is promising but not proven.

For many individuals, relief from the uncertainty about their future is the primary benefit. People tend to cope with uncertainty in two ways: some prefer to retain the uncertainty so that they do not have to deal with the bad news until it is inescapable, whereas others try to resolve the uncertainty so that they can proceed with their lives accordingly. For the latter group, knowing their true genetic status may provide relief to many years of anxiety related to the uncertainty of their future.

The knowledge of one's genetic status also may provide benefit to others in the family. The first member of the family to be tested frequently has altruistic motives, since that individual, by current practice, already has a personal history of cancer. By undergoing testing to identify the cancer-causing mutation, they make it possible for others in the family to learn their genetic status. Unaffected parents such as males in families with HBOC may choose to undergo testing for the benefit of their offspring, since their result will clarify their children's risk. Among families with HBOC (Lynch et al., 1997), the most frequent reason for seeking genetic test results was to clarify the risk status for the individual's offspring.

DNA test results can also be helpful in making life decisions. They may influence an individual's career or family planning decisions. This has been witnessed with individuals who previously chose not to have children because of their high risk of cancer, but on receiving a negative result, have declared an intent to have children (H. T. Lynch, personal communication, January 20, 1997).

Risks of Testing

Psychological Risks. A positive result to DNA testing for hereditary cancer carries with it a risk for an adverse psychological impact such as depression, anxiety, anger, or hopelessness related to an increased risk of developing cancer. Clearly, the individual's past experiences and discernment of the effectiveness of cancer treatment and survivability, as well as individual personality characteristics, influence the psychological response. Those who have children are likely to experience concern and worry about their genetic status. Although they had no control over what genes they passed on to their children, there is often a sense of guilt related to the possibility of passing on the cancer-causing mutation. These psychological repercussions may be of such an extent as to impair the individual's performance of daily activities.

The individual who receives the good news of a negative result may also experience a negative impact. Many have described a kind of survivor guilt in which the family member with a negative result feels that he or she should not be relieved of the cancer burden that others in the family have to carry. He or she may feel unworthy of being spared what others in the family have experienced, or may possibly feel in a better position than a sibling to deal with a positive result.

Alterations in Family Relationships. The emotional relations among family members and expectations for the roles that each member is to play may be altered as individuals are trying to deal with their own results, as well as the results of others in the family. One young woman who was the only one of four sisters in her family to receive a negative result described a sense of alienation when her sisters looked to each other for support in coping with their cancer or risk for cancer.

Individuals who undergo genetic testing frequently are encouraged to inform other family members who may benefit from the knowledge of the results. Some individuals may experience anxiety about how this information may be received by their relatives who may not want to know of their increased risks. There is the potential for private information previously unknown in the family to be revealed, such as an adoption or paternity being other than what was thought. This possibility should always be discussed as part of the informed consent process to provide the individual an opportunity to avoid such a situation.

Insurance and Employment Discrimination. The issue that currently is receiving the greatest amount of attention by family members, cancer genetic professionals, the media, and now legislators relates to use of genetic information by insurers and employers. There is significant concern that genetic information will be used to discriminate against members of families with hereditary cancer. A 1992 survey of genetics professionals uncovered 41 examples of insurance discrimination, almost all by insurers or employers (Billings et al., 1992). Due to the uncertainty about the potential of losing their insurance or employment, and the possibility of being locked into a job so as to safeguard insurance or having to pay excessively high premiums, many patients have chosen to forego genetic testing for hereditary cancer.

Employer discrimination refers to the possibility that an employer may choose to not employ or to terminate employment of a hereditary cancer mutation carrier rather than risk the expense of that individual requiring a long period(s) of employee sick leave. If the employer offers a self-funded insurance policy for employees, the potential expense of the individual's cancer treatment may also be a factor. In 1995 the U.S. Equal Employment Opportunity Commission (EEOC) officially interpreted the Americans with Disabilities Act as protective of employment for individuals who carry a disease susceptibility gene. However, attorneys caution that this interpretation has not been tested in the courts.

Life and disability insurers regularly screen potential patients for the existence or risk of disease as part of their underwriting practices. It has been determined by one insurance company that females with a BRCA1 mutation would qualify for life insurance on an affordable basis, and someone who is being followed carefully because of a hereditary predisposition for colon cancer may qualify as a relatively normal risk (Chambers, 1997). However, discrimination by health insurers, if it occurs, is likely to be in the form of denying coverage at all or at least for the cancer for which there is such a high risk. Some states have enacted legislation against genetic discrimination in health insurance. However, approximately one third of the privately insured population receives coverage through self-funded plans, and these plans are not regulated by state insurance laws (Hudson et al., 1995). At the Federal level, the Kassebaum-Kennedy Health Insurance Portability and Accountability Act (Pub. L 104-191) was enacted in July 1997. This law provides a guarantee of the portability of health insurance when a person moves from one group plan to another, and it prohibits denial of coverage for a preexisting condition, including genetic information. Since this legislation is at a federal level, self-insured plans are included in its jurisdiction. However, it is just a start because it fails to provide any safeguards for those with private health insurance plans and those without insurance who want to obtain it at a later date (Genome Action Coalition, 1996). It also does not prohibit an insurer from raising the premiums charged to entire group plans.

Obtaining coverage for surveillance or prophylactic surgeries outside of what is recommended for the general population has long been a problem for members of families with hereditary cancer. Many health insurance plans do not cover mammography screening until the age of 40, yet women with a mutation or at 50% risk for HBOC are urged to initiate screening between the ages of 25 and 35. Revealing the individual's genetic risk may result in a company covering the surveillance procedures, but a future change in insurers may result in a denial of all coverage or prohibitive rates.

Prophylactic surgeries have been denied as part of preventive medicine and therefore are not a part of the usual health care plan. One woman took her insurance provider to court after its refusal to cover a prophylactic oophorectomy. The woman was part of an HBOC family, but the insurance company reasoned that she was healthy at the time of her surgery so they did not need to cover it. The district court upheld the denial of benefits, but on appeal, the state supreme court overruled the district court's decision (Lynch et al., 1995). In another state a woman experienced a similar denial of benefits, so she revealed her BRCA1 positive results in hopes of explaining the need for her oophorectomy. The insurance company again denied her claim, the second time on the basis of her having a preexisting condition. It is extremely frustrating for family members to realize there are medical options for managing their high risk, only to be thwarted with every attempt they make to preserve their health and lives.

Individuals who are considering DNA testing may wish to discuss issues of confidentiality with their primary care providers before making a final decision. Some providers agree to keep no written record of the test result to prevent inadvertent copying and sharing of results with the rest of the patient record, which could result in discrimination. Others keep results in a locked, confidential file separate from the routine medical records. Confidentiality of genetic information is imperative because of the potential for discrimination. These test results should never be released without a written consent that specifically identifies their inclusion.

Cost of Testing. The cost of clinical DNA testing varies from laboratory to laboratory and within laboratories from test to test. Due to the labor-intensive nature of the original test to identify the mutation in a family, the cost of that test may be as high as between $2000 and $3000. Once the mutation is identified, testing for anyone else in the family generally costs several hundred dollars. The cost of testing will likely decrease as new technologies make the testing process less labor-intensive.

Limitations of DNA Testing

Although the advent of DNA testing has provided many new capabilities, there are limitations to the information that can be provided. With current testing technologies, not all possible mutations within a gene are identifiable. It has been estimated that using the current clinical testing method, a mutation cannot be identified in 40% to 50% of families with HNPCC (Kinzler & Vogelstein, 1996). It is known that there is at least one additional gene associated with hereditary breast cancer beyond the BRCA1 and BRCA2, although it has not yet been identified. This means that the first individual in the family to be tested could incur the expense of testing and have no more information than what was possessed before testing.

The risks for cancer at specified sites have been identified for the genes for which testing is available. However, this risk may be inflated or deflated for a specific family. There is evidence that the risks may vary for the different mutations within a given gene. Investigations are underway to determine the risks associated with specific mutations within each gene, but these can only be calculated for the more common mutations. Even with more exact risk calculations, identification as a mutation carrier cannot tell an individual when or with any certainty if cancer will occur.

Anticipatory Guidance in the Decision-Making Process

It is not sufficient for the counselor to provide the individual with all of the factual information along with a discussion of risks, benefits, and limitations. Generally, health care providers respond with concern and support to those individuals with a high level of distress and try to assist them during the decision-making process. However, the results of one study indicate that a low level of distress may indicate greater denial and avoidance behaviors and poor anticipation of DNA test outcomes (DudokdeWit et al., 1997). This problem can be addressed in pretest counseling by encouraging the individual to anticipate the outcome of various options. This approach can be accomplished by asking questions such as those in Box 12-5. These same questions should be framed for a decision in favor of testing with potential positive results and potential negative results. The counselor should also point out common responses that the individual may not anticipate on his or her own, such as survivor guilt over a negative result.

Box 12-5 Decision-Making Regarding Genetic Testing

1. Why do you want to have this genetic test?
2. What will you do with the information if the test is positive?
3. What will you do with the information if the test is negative?
4. Do you plan to involve other members of your family in the decision-making process about whether or not to be tested?
5. Do you plan to tell any members of your family about the results of the genetic testing?
6. What do you anticipate will be the reactions of your family members if the test is positive?
7. What do you anticipate will be the reactions of your family members if the test is negative?

Support in Decision Making

For an unaffected family member, the decision about whether to undergo DNA testing is often a difficult one to make. Some individuals agonize over the risks and benefits of their options. Older family members who are accustomed to a paternalistic attitude from health care providers may find the decision especially difficult. The nurse can be an important and impartial support for individuals going through this process.

The decision related to DNA testing should not only be informed, it should be totally voluntary. However, in some families, there is a great deal of pressure for one decision or another. Sometimes, parents feel that they know what is best for their offspring and bring a great deal of pressure to bear on an adult child's decision. The nurse may need to assume an advocacy role, reminding the parent that because of the potential repercussions, the decision rightfully belongs to the individual.

In some situations, family members may have conflicting interests that affect each other's decisions. In one situation, a young adult wanted to be tested for the mutation known to exist in her family. This woman's mother had no history of cancer, had not been tested, and did not want to know what her status was. It was pointed out to the young woman that a negative result for her would not reveal anything about her mother, but a positive result would reveal that her mother was also a carrier of the mutation. A week later, the mother called the counselor to ask how she was supposed to deal with the dilemma of her daughter wanting to be tested when she did not want to know her own status. The counselor explored the options and possible outcomes, and the two women were encouraged to work this conflict out between themselves. The mother did decide that she would proceed with testing, thinking it would be better for her to find out that way if she were a mutation carrier, than through a positive result for her daughter. If the mother was negative for the mutation, the daughter could avoid testing entirely.

CLINICAL MANAGEMENT

Surveillance

The information obtained during the assessment phase of an individual's cancer risk evaluation is invaluable for the counseling related to medical management. It is essential to dispel myths and misinformed beliefs about the cause of cancer in the family, as well as any associations made between cancer risk and family characteristics, so that recommendations for screening can be integrated into the individual's lifestyle. The individual's current surveillance practices should be discussed to identify the source of inappropriate methods, frequency, and practices.

In a study of the impact of family history of breast cancer, it was found that only 27% of the high-risk women were performing breast self-examinations on a regular basis, and 10% were not performing breast self-examinations at all. Noncompliance was most closely associated with emotional distress, anxiety, and fear of findings (Rosenthal, Kash, & Diemer, 1995). Not performing breast self-examinations gives some women, especially those who lack confidence in their ability to detect a lump, a sense of control over their feelings of anxiety and fear (Chalmers & Luker, 1996).

As was reported by Lerman, Kash, and Stefanek (1994), psychological distress can be associated not only with infrequent self-examinations for some, but also with excessive examinations by others. Similarly, it has been found that some women deal with their acute anxieties with hypervigilance by performing breast self-examinations weekly or daily. One woman even reported that she checked her breasts several times a day, feeling that this approach provided her with a sense of control over what she perceived as the inevitability of breast cancer. She needed support in exploring her fears and anxiety, as well assistance in the development of more effective coping behaviors, so that she could incorporate the information that her hypervigilant behavior could fail to detect an incipient change in breast tissue.

When screening recommendations include a self-assessment such as breast self-examination, the most effective technique needs to be taught with a return demonstration by the patient to help assure confident practice of the technique. Tactile models can be used to help an individual develop confidence about being able to distinguish between normal breast tissue and a source of concern. Before high-risk women can integrate monthly breast self-examination, as a part of their routine care, they will need an opportunity to discuss their previous experiences with cancer and express their fears and perceptions about breast cancer detection, treatment, and survivability. This discussion can then be followed by reassurance that most unusual lumps are not cancer, and reinforcement of the need for professional evaluation of any change to ensure early detection and treatment if a cancer is present.

FDRs of ovarian cancer patients were found to be more likely to undergo CA 125 screening and abdominal ultrasound (Schwartz et al., 1995). However, this positive correlation held only for FDRs with only one affected relative. FDRs with more affected relatives, and therefore probably with a higher risk, were less likely to demonstrate the same positive correlation between level of worry and surveillance activities. The investigators suggested that worry is a motivation only when screening is likely to be negative. They called for improved education and management of anxiety to reduce unnecessary use of surveillance among low-risk women and to increase use among high-risk women.

Prophylactic Surgeries

One of the most controversial procedures for preventing breast cancer in high-risk women is prophylactic mastectomy. Although controversial and frequently discussed, there have been few studies addressing the issues. Houn, Helzlsouer, Friedman, and Stefanek (1995) found that 85% of the plastic surgeons, 47% of the general surgeons, and 38% of the gynecologists that they surveyed agreed that prophylactic mastectomy does have a role in the care of women at high risk for breast cancer. In another study, one third of oncologists would recommend prophylactic surgery for women with a 35% to 40% risk for breast cancer, one third would recommend close follow-up, and one third would present both options and leave the decision to the patient (Belanger, Moore, & Tannock, 1991). Patients' perceptions about prophylactic mastectomy have been studied even less. FDRs of breast cancer patients were asked before their cancer risk assessment whether they would be interested in prophylactic mastectomy. Fourteen who expressed interest in surgery proceeded to have it performed, and at least 6 months postoperatively they were satisfied with their decision and with the surgery. Ninety-two women who were interested before the risk assessment decided against the procedure, and 58 did not express interest before or after the risk assessment (Stefanek, Helzlsouer, Wilcox, & Houn, 1995).

There is a lack of data for or against the effectiveness of prophylactic surgeries in HNPCC (Burke et al., 1997a) and HBOC (Burke et al., 1997b). However, preliminary findings from one study suggest that prophylactic mastectomy significantly reduces the risk of breast cancer even in women with a positive family history (Hartmann, Jenkins, Schaid, & Yang, 1997). Until there are data to show substantial benefits to be secured by such surgeries, prophylactic surgery will remain an option to be discussed with high-risk individuals, especially if their fear of cancer interferes with their ability to conduct their daily activities or undergo the recommended surveillance program. These discussions need to include information that prophylactic surgery does not provide 100% protection from the cancers they are intended to prevent. Also, the psychological impact of such surgery is important to explore. Although there is a lack of literature on the latter for prophylactic surgeries, findings from studies that deal with the psychological impact of surgeries for therapeutic reasons may provide some insight into what can be anticipated (Bellerose & Binik, 1993; Northouse, Cracchiolo-Caraway, & Appel, 1991; Schover et al., 1995; Walsh, Grunert, Telford, & Otterson, 1995; Weinryb & Rossel, 1986).

Chemoprevention

There are clinical trials of the effectiveness of chemoprevention agents such as tamoxifen for those at high risk for breast cancer and nonsteroidal antiinflammatory drug (NSAID) trials to prevent colon cancer among those with FAP or HNPCC. The discussion of the risks, benefits, and limitations associated with the chemoprevention trials belongs with those who are working with the trials. However, nurses share in the responsibility of informing family members of their existence and helping those who want more information to get it.

FOLLOW-UP CARE

Reinforcement of Counseling

The amount of information that is discussed in the process of cancer risk assessment and counseling is overwhelming and too much for anyone to be expected to retain. Therefore it is customary to send the patient a letter summarizing everything that has been discussed. Typically this letter includes a review of the family history as it was presented so that corrections can be made if new information is obtained. The diagnosis and the associated medical and genetic facts are explained. Recommendations for surveillance and potential options for chemoprevention or prophylactic surgery are reviewed. The letter serves not only as a reminder to the patient, but also as an aid in sharing information with primary care providers or other family members if he or she so chooses. Patients are encouraged to call if questions arise, and most cancer risk counselors make follow-up contacts to assess how their patients are adapting.

Promotion of Compliance

One of the major concerns about DNA testing for cancer risk has been the potential for a level of anxiety that is so acute as to interfere with an individual's compliance with medical recommendations. Kash and colleagues (1992), Lerman, Kash, and Stefanek (1994), and Chalmers and Luker (1996) have stressed the need for psychological interventions to reduce stress to increase compliance with surveillance recommendations. Nurses can carry out an important role in helping family members gain a sense of control over their feelings of risk by including, in the education about surveillance recommendations, a psychological component of addressing their relatives' experiences with cancer and their own fears of developing cancer. By addressing the past experiences and fears for the future, family members may be able to develop a greater sense of hope for having some control over their risks.

Support Needs

The support needs of individuals who discover they did not inherit the mutation in their family may easily be overlooked. It is natural to assume that negative results decrease anxiety and increase freedom from concern. These individuals need to be reassured that guilty feelings about survival are relatively common and are a normal reaction. They also need to know that if they feel somewhat displaced or alienated from their family, there are others in a similar situation with whom they can talk.

Those who opt not to have testing may also need continued support from primary providers. They remain in a situation of not having their status clarified. If this is a choice made from an awareness of their best coping style, they will probably do quite well. However, if this is a decision forced by fears of discrimination or due to a lack of access to testing, there may be an ongoing need for support in coping with uncertainty.

Referrals

In a study of the impact of having a family history of breast cancer, more than 23% of high-risk women had a level of psychological distress consistent with a need for psychological counseling. These women were more likely to report fewer social supports, greater perceived risk and more barriers to screening. Psychotherapists need to be identified who can help these women deal with and reduce their psychological distress (Rosenthal et al., 1995).

The extended family, which has been the traditional source of support for many with hereditary cancer, is often eroded in a highly mobile society. Even when the family unit is intact and supportive, there are times and circumstances when a family member needs to turn to someone outside of the family. Support groups have been formed for individuals with some forms of hereditary cancer. It is the commonality of experience and emotion that makes it possible for members of such groups to provide comfort, support, and strength to each other. By promoting healthy coping, support groups have the potential to improve the quality of life and thus prolong lives by increasing compliance with surveillance.

Some support groups also provide a mechanism through which family members are able to become part of larger advocacy movements to eliminate discrimination and improve access to medical management. Newsletters and annual meetings provide education and up-to-date information about progress in research. Support groups for hereditary cancer can help family members deal with the unique issues of their own risk and the passing on of that heritage to their offspring.

Notification of Relatives

Individuals in hereditary cancer families are encouraged to inform appropriate relatives of their potential risk so that their relatives can make decisions about seeking genetic counseling and testing. Some individuals may be reluctant to provide this information to their relatives for a variety of reasons. This situation presents a dilemma for the counselor and other health care providers who might be involved. The counselor has an obligation to maintain the confidentiality of the patient, but it has been questioned if there is not an equal obligation to warn others in the family of their potential risk. Some attorneys say that U.S. case law raises the possibility that such a duty to disclose does exist, whereas others have said that the issue is not established. Obviously, the solution that is favored is for the counselor to convince the patient of the need to share the information with his or her relatives.

CONCLUSION

The advances in cancer genetics have been incredibly rapid in the last few years, and there is every reason to believe that this pace will continue as new discoveries are made. However, for families with hereditary forms of cancer, the advances in identifying effective preventive measures and the legal safeguards to their privacy are not coming quickly enough. Nurses play an important role as advocates for these individuals as they try to make decisions based on uncertain benefits of testing and management. To fulfill this role, nurses need to increase their knowledge of cancer genetics by obtaining current and accurate information from local cancer risk assessment programs, by taking part in educational programs, and through print or electronic exchange of information, such as web sites sponsored by professional genetic and oncology organizations. Cancer risk assessment and counseling is also a dynamic, gratifying arena for nursing role expansion.

REFERENCES

Ackerman, T. F. (1996). Genetic testing of children for cancer susceptibility. *Journal of Pediatric Oncology Nursing, 13,* 46-49.

American Board of Medical Genetics & American College of Medical Genetics Board of Directors. (1995). Points to consider: Ethical, legal and psychosocial implications of genetic testing in children and adolescents. *American Journal of Human Genetics, 57,* 1233-1241.

American Society of Clinical Oncology. (1996). Statement of the American Society of Clinical Oncology: Genetic testing for cancer susceptibility. *Journal of Clinical Oncology, 14,* 1730-1736.

American Society of Human Genetics. (1994). Statement of the American Society of Human Genetics on genetic testing for breast and ovarian cancer predisposition. *American Journal of Human Genetics, 55,* i-iv.

Basu, T. N., Gutmann, D. H., Fletcher, J. A., Glover, T. W., Collins, F. S., & Downward, J. (1992). Aberrant regulation of ras proteins in malignant tumor cells from type 1 neurofibromatosis patients. *Nature, 356,* 713-715.

Belanger, D., Moore, M., & Tannock, I. (1991). How American oncologists treat breast cancer: An assessment of the influence of clinical trials. *Journal of Clinical Oncology, 9,* 7-16.

Bellerose, S. B., & Binik, Y. M. (1993). Body image and sexuality in oophorectomized women. *Archives of Sexual Behavior 22,* 435-459.

Bennett, R. L., Steinhaus, K. A., Uhrich, S. B., O'Sullivan, C. K., Resta, R. G., Lochner-Doyle, D., Markel, D. S., Vincent, V., & Hamanishi, J. (1995). Recommendations for standardized human pedigree nomenclature. *Journal of Genetic Counseling, 4,* 267-279.

Bergman, W., Watson, P., deJong, J., Lynch, H. T., & Fusaro, R. M. (1990). Systemic cancer and the FAMMM syndrome. *British Journal of Cancer, 81,* 932-936.

Billings, P. R., Kohn, M. A., deCuevas, M., Beckwith, J., Alper, J. S., & Natowicx, M. R. (1992). Discrimination as a consequence of genetic testing. *American Journal of Human Genetics, 50,* 476-482.

Burke, W., Daly, M., Garber, J., Botkin, J., Kahn, M. J. E., Lynch, P., McTiernan, A., Offit, K., Perlman, J., Petersen, G., Thomson, E., & Varricchio, C., for the Cancer Genetics Studies Consortium. (1997a). Recommendations for follow-up care of individuals with an inherited predisposition to cancer II: BRCA1 and BRCA2. *Journal of the American Medical Association, 277,* 997-1003.

Burke, W., Peterson, G., Lynch, P., Botkin, J., Daly, M., Garber, J., Kahn, M. J. E., McTiernan, A., Offit, K., Thomson, E., & Varricchio, C., for the Cancer Genetics Studies Consortium. (1997b). Recommendations for follow-up care of individuals with an inherited predisposition to cancer I: Hereditary nonpolyposis colon cancer. *Journal of the American Medical Association, 277,* 915-919.

Calmettes, C., Ponder, B. A. J., Fischer, J. A., & Raue, F., the members of the European Community Concerted Action Medullary Thyroid Carcinoma. (1992). Early diagnosis of the multiple endocrine neoplasia type 2 syndrome: Consensus statement. *European Journal of Clinical Investigation, 22,* 755-760.

Calzone, K. A. (1997). Predisposition testing for breast and ovarian cancer susceptibility. *Seminars in Oncology Nursing, 13,* 82-90.

Cannon-Albright, L. A., Goldgar, D. E., Meyer, I. J., Lewis, C. M., Anderson, D. E., Fountain, J. W., Hegi, M. E., Wiseman, R. W., Petty, E. M., Bale, A. E., Olopade, O. I., Diaz, M. O., Kwiatkowski, D. J., Piepkorn, M. W., Zone, J. J., & Skolnick, M. H. (1992). Assignment of a locus for familial melanoma. *Science, 258,* 1148-1152.

Cassem, N. (1978). Treating the person confronting death. In A. M. Nicoli Jr. (Ed.), *The Harvard guide to modern psychiatry.* Cambridge, MA: Harvard University Press.

Chalmers, K. I., & Luker, K. A. (1996). Breast self-care practices in women with primary relatives with breast cancer. *Journal of Advanced Nursing, 23,* 1212-1220.

Chambers, D. (1997). Ethical issues in genetic testing. *Medical Resource, 9*(1), 5-6.

Chandrasekharappa, S. C., Guru, S. C., Manickam, P., Olufemi, S. E., Collins, F. S., Emmert-Buck, M. R., Debelenko, L. V., Zhuang, Z., Lubensky, I. A., Liotta, L. A., Crabtree, J. S., Wang, Y., Roe, B. A., Weisemann, J., Boguski, M. S., Agarwal, S.K ., Kester, M. B., Kim,Y. S., Heppner, C., Dong, Q., Spiegel, A. M., Burns, A. L., & Marx, S. J. (1997). Positional cloning of the gene for multiple endocrine neoplasia-type 1. *Science, 276,* 404-406.

Clark, S. E. & Phillips, R. K. S. (1996). Desmoids in familial adenomatous polyposis. *British Journal of Medicine, 83,* 1494-1504.

Claus E. B., Risch N., & Thompson W. D. (1991). Genetic analysis of breast cancer in the cancer and steroid hormone study. *American Journal of Human Genetics, 48,* 232-242.

Couch, F. J., DeShano, M. L., Blackwood, A., Calzone, K, Stopfer, J., Campeau, L., Ganguly, A., Rebbeck, T., & Weber, B.L. (1997). BRCA1 mutations in women attending clinics that evaluate the risk of breast cancer. *New England Journal of Medicine, 336,* 1409-1415.

Croyle, R. T., & Lerman, C. (1993). Interest in genetic testing for colon cancer susceptibility: Cognitive and emotional correlates. *Preventive Medicine, 22,* 284-292.

DudokdeWit, A. C., Tibben, A., Duivenvoorden, H. J., Frets, P. G., Zoeteweij, M. W., Losekoot, M., van Haeringen, A., Niermeijer, M. F., & Passchier, J. (1997). Psychological distress in applicants for predictive testing for autosomal dominant, heritable, late onset disorders. *Journal of Medical Genetics, 34,* 382-390.

Dunlop, M. G., Farrington, S. M., Carothers, A. D., Wyllie, A. H., Sharp, L., Burn, J., Liu, B., Kinzler, K. W., & Vogelstein, B. (1997). Cancer risk associated with germline DNA mismatch repair gene mutations. *Human Molecular Genetics, 6,* 105-110.

Easton, D. (1996). The role of atypical mole syndrome and cutaneous nevi in the development of melanoma. *Cancer Surveys, 26,* 237-249.

Easton, D. F., Ford, D., Bishop, D. T., & the Breast Cancer Linkage Consortium. (1995). Breast and ovarian cancer incidence in BRCA1-mutation carriers. *American Journal of Human Genetics, 56,* 265-271.

Eng, C. (1996). The RET proto-oncogene in multiple endocrine neoplasia type 2 and Hirschsprung's disease. *New England Journal of Medicine, 335,* 943-951.

Fearon, E. R. (1996). Genetic lesions in human cancer. In J. M. Bishop, & R. A. Weinberg (Eds.), *Molecular oncology.* New York: Scientific American.

Ford, D., & Easton, D. F. (1995). The genetics of breast and ovarian cancer. *British Journal of Cancer, 72,* 805-812.

Ford, D., Easton, D. F., Bishop, D. T., Narod, S. A., Goldgar, D. E., & the Breast Cancer Linkage Consortium. (1994). Risk of cancer in BRCA-1 mutation carriers. *Lancet, 343,* 692-695.

Fraser, F. C. (1974). Genetic counseling. *American Journal of Human Genetics, 26,* 284-292.

Friend, S. H., Bernards, R., Rogelj, S., Weinberg, R. A., Papaport, J. M., Albert, D. M., & Dryja, T. P. (1986). A human DNA segment with properties of the gene that predisposes to retinoblastoma and osteosarcoma. *Nature, 323,* 643-646.

Gagel, R. F., Tashjian, A. H., Cummings, T., Papathanasopoulos, N., Kaplan, M. M., DeLellis, R. A., Wolfe, H. J., & Reichlin, S. (1988). The clinical outcome of prospective screening for multiple endocrine neoplasia type 2a: An 18-year experience. *New England Journal of Medicine, 318,* 478-484.

Gail, M. H., Brinton, L. A., Byar, D. P., Corle, D. K., Green, S. B., Schairer, C., & Mulvihill, J. J. (1989). Projecting individualized probabilities of developing breast cancer for white females who are being examined annually. *Journal of the National Cancer Institute, 81,* 1879-1886.

Gayther, S. A., Mangion, J., Russell, P., Seal, S., Barfoot, R., Ponder, B. A. J., Stratton, M. R., & Easton, D. (1997). Variation of risks of breast and ovarian cancer associated with different germline mutations of the BRCA2 gene. *Nature Genetics, 15,* 103-105.

Giardello, F. M., Brensinger, J. D., Peterson, G. M., Luce, M. C., Hylind, L. M., Bacon, J. A., Booker, S. V., Parker, R. D., & Hamilton, S. R. (1997). The use and interpretation of commercial APC gene testing for familial adenomatous polyposis. *New England Journal of Medicine, 336,* 823-827.

Goldgar, D. E., Green, P., Parry, D. M., & Mulvihill, J. J. (1989). Multipoint linkage analysis in neurofibromatosis type 1: An international collaboration. *American Journal of Human Genetics, 44,* 6-12.

Gruis, N. A., Sandkuijl, L. A., van der Velden, P. A., Bergman, W., & Frants, R. R. (1995). CDKN2 explains part of the clinical phenotype in Dutch familial atypical multiple-mole melanoma FAMMM syndrome families. *Melanoma Research, 5,* 169-177.

Hall, J. M., Lee, M. K., Newman, B., Morrow, J., Anderson, L. A., Huey, B., & King, M. C. (1990). Linkage of early onset breast cancer to chromosome 17q21. *Science, 250,* 1684-1689.

Hartmann, L., Jenkins, R., Schaid, D., & Yang, P. (1997). Prophylactic mastectomy (PM): Preliminary retrospective cohort analysis [Abstract]. *Proceedings of the American Association of Cancer Research, 38,* 168.

Hodgson, S. V., & Maher, E. R. (1993). *A practical guide to human cancer genetics.* New York: Cambridge University Press.

Houn, F., Helzlsouer, K. J., Friedman, N. B., & Stefanek, M. E. (1995). The practice of prophylactic mastectomy: A survey of Maryland surgeons. *American Journal of Public Health, 85,* 801-805.

Hudson, K. L., Rothenberg, K. H., Andrews, L. B., Ellis Kahn, M. J., & Collins, F. S. (1995). Genetic discrimination and health insurance: An urgent need for reform. *Science, 270,* 391-393.

Humphrey, J. S., Klausner, R. D., & Linehan, W. M. (1996). Von Hippel Lindau syndrome: Hereditary cancer arising from inherited mutations of the VHL tumor suppressor gene. In H. J. Pienta (Ed.), *Diagnostic advances: The use of molecular medicine in the diagnosis and prognosis of genitourinary malignancies.* Boston: Kluwer Academic Publishers.

Jorde, L. B., Carey, J. C., & White, R. L. (1995). *Medical genetics.* St. Louis: Mosby.

Kash, K. M., Holland, J. C., Halper, M. S., & Miller, D. G. (1992). Psychological distress and surveillance behaviors of women with a family history of breast cancer. *Journal of the National Cancer Institute, 84,* 27-30.

Kelly, P. T. (1992). Breast cancer risk analysis: A genetic epidemiology service for families. *Journal of Genetic Counseling, 1,* 155-168.

Kingston, H. M. (1994). *ABC of clinical genetics* (2nd ed.). London: BMJ Publishing Group.

Kinzler, K. W., & Vogelstein, B. (1996). Lessons from hereditary colon cancer. *Cell, 87,* 159-170.

Knudson, A. G. (1971). Mutation and cancer: Statistical study of retinoblastoma. *Proceedings of the National Academy of Science, 68,* 820-823.

Krainer, M., Silva-Arrieta, S., FitzGerald, M. G., Shimada, A., Ishioka, C., Kanamaru, R., MacDonald, D. J., Unsal, H., Finkelstein, D. M., Bowcock, A., Isselbacher, K. J., & Haber, D. A. (1997). Differential contributions of BRCA1 and BRCA2 to early-onset breast cancer. *New England Journal of Medicine, 336,* 1416-1421.

Laken, S. J., Peterson, G. M., Oddouz, C., Ostrer, H., Giardello, F. M., Hamilton, S. R., Hampel, H., Markowitz, A., Klimstra, D., Jhanwar, S., Winawar, S., Offit, K., Luce, M. C., Kinzler, K. W., & Vogelstein, B. (1997). Familial colorectal cancer in Ashkenazim due to a hypermutable trait in APC. *Nature Genetics, 17,* 79-83.

Landis, S. H., Murray, T., Bolden, S., & Wingo, P. A. (1998). Cancer statistics, 1998. *CA: A Cancer Journal for Clinicians, 48*(1), 6-29.

Leggett, B. A., Thomas, L. R., Knight, N., Healey, S., Chenevix-Trench, G., & Searle, J. (1993). Exclusion of APC and MCC as the gene defect in one family with familial juvenile polyposis. *Gastroenterology, 105,* 1313-16.

Legius, E., Marchuk, D. A., Collins, F. S., & Glover, T. W. (1993). Somatic deletion of the neurofibromatosis type 1 gene in a neurofibrosarcoma supports a tumour suppressor gene hypothesis. *Nature Genetics, 3,* 122-125.

Lerman, C., Daly, M., Masny, A., & Balshem, A. (1994). Attitudes about genetic testing for breast-ovarian cancer susceptibility. *Journal Clinical Oncology, 12,* 843-850.

Lerman, C., Daly, M., Sands, C., Balshem, A., Lustbader, E., Heggan, T., James, J., Goldstein, L., & Engstrom, P. (1993). Psychological distress interferes with breast cancer screening in high risk women. *Journal National Cancer Institute, 85,* 1074-1080.

Lerman, C., Kash, K. M., & Stefanek, M. (1994). Younger women at increased risk for breast cancer: Perceived risk, psychological well-being, and surveillance. *Monographs National Cancer Institute, 16,* 171-176.

Lerman, C., Lustbader, E., Rimer, B., Daly, M., Miller, S., Sands, C., & Balshem, A. (1995). Effects of individualized breast cancer risk counseling: A randomized trial. *Journal National Cancer Institute, 87,* 286-292.

Lerman, C., Marshall, J., Audrain, J., & Gomez-Caminero, A. (1996). Genetic testing for colon cancer susceptibility: Anticipated reactions of patients and challenges to providers. *International Journal Cancer, 69,* 58-61.

Lerman, C., Narod, S., Schulman, K., Hughes, C., Gomez-Caminero, A., Bonney, G., Gold, K., Trock, B., Main, D., Lynch, J., Fulmore, C., Snyder, C., Lemon, S. J., Conway, T., Tonin, R., Lenoir, G., & Lynch, H. T. (1996). BRCA1 testing in families with hereditary breast-ovarian cancer: A prospective study of patient decision making and outcome. *Journal Americam Medical Association, 275,* 1885-1892.

Lerman, C., Schwartz, M. D., Lin, T. H., Hughes, C., Narod, S., & Lynch, H.T. (1997). The inflence of psychological distress on use of genetic testing for cancer risk. *Journal Consulting and Clinical Psychology, 65,* 414-420.

Lerman, C., Seay, J., Balshem, A., & Audrain, J (1995). Interest in genetic testing among first degree relatives of breast cancer patients. *American Journal Human Genetics, 57,* 385-392.

Lessick, M., & Williams, J. (1994). The human genome project: Implications for nursing. *Medsurg Nursing, 3,* 49-58.

Li, F. P., Fraumeni, J. F., Mulvihill, J. J., Blattner, W. A., Dreyfus, M. G., Tucker, M. A., & Miller, R. W. (1988). A cancer family syndrome in twenty-four kindreds. *Cancer Research, 48,* 5358.

Lowy, D. R. (1996). The causes of cancer. In J. M. Bishop & R. A. Weinberg (Eds.), *Molecular oncology.* New York: Scientific American.

Luker, K. A., Leinster, S., Owens, G., Beaver, K., & Degner, L. (1994). Preferences for information and decision-making in women with breast cancer: A follow-up study. *Research Report.* London: Cancer Macmillan Fund.

Lynch, H. T., Lemon, S. J., Durham, C., Tinley, S. T., Connolly, C., Lynch, J., Surdam, J., Orinion, E., Slominski-Caster, S., Watson, P., Lerman, C., Tonin, P., Serova, O., Lenoir, G., & Narod, S. (1997). A descriptive study of BRCA1 testing and reactions to disclosure of test results. *Cancer, 79,* 2219-2228.

Lynch, H. T., Severin, M. J., Mooney, M. J., & Lynch, J. (1995). Insurance adjudication favoring prophylactic surgery in hereditary breast-ovarian cancer syndrome. *Gynecologic Oncology, 57,* 23-26.

Lynch, H. T., & Smyrk, T. (1996). Hereditary nonpolyposis colorectal cancer (Lynch syndrome): An updated review. *Cancer, 78,* 1149-1167.

Lynch, H. T., Smyrk, T., & Lynch, J. (1996). Overview of the natural history, pathology, molecular genetics and management of HNPCC (Lynch syndrome). *International Journal Cancer, 69,* 38-43.

Lynch, H. T., Smyrk, T., & Lynch, J. (1997). Genetics and cancer of the gastrointestinal tract. In H. J. Wanebo (Ed.), *Surgery for gastrointestinal cancer: A mutidisciplinary approach.* Philadelphia: Lippincott-Raven Publishers.

Lynch, H. T., Smyrck, T., McGinn, T., Lanspa, S., Cavalieri, J., Lynch, J., Slowminski-Castor, S., Cayouette, M. C., Priluck, I., & Luce, M. C. (1995). Attenuated familial adenomatous polyposis (AFAP). *Cancer, 76,* 2427-2433.

MacCollin, M., Mohney, T., Trofatter, J., Wertelecki, W., Ramesh, V., & Gusella, J. (1993). DNA diagnosis of neurofibromatosis 2: Altered coding sequence of the *merlin* tumor suppressor in an extended pedigree. *Journal of the American Medical Association, 270,* 2316-2320.

Maher, E. R., Iselius, L., Yates, J. R., Littler, M., Benjamin, C., Harris, R., Sampson, J., Williams, J., Ferguson-Smith, M. A., & Morton, N. (1991). Von Hippel Lindau disease: A genetic study. *Journal Medical Genetics, 28,* 443-447.

Malkin, D., Li, F. P., Strong, L. C., Fraumeni, J. F., Nelson, C. E., Kim, D. H., Kassel, J., Gryka, M. A., Bischoff, F. Z., Tainsky, M. A., & Friend, S. H. (1990). Germ line p53 mutations in a familial syndrome of breast cancer, sarcomas, and other neoplasms. *Science, 250,* 1233-1238.

Marchuk, D. A., Saulino, A. M., Tavakkol, R., Swaroop, M., Wallace, M. R., Andersen, L. B., Mitchell, A. L., Gutmann, D. H., Boguski, M., & Collins, F. S. (1991). cDNA cloning of the type 1 neurofibromatosis gene: Complete sequence of the NF1 gene product. *Genomics, 11,* 931-940.

Miki, Y., Swansen, J., Shattuck-Eidens, D., Futreal, F. A., Harshman, K., Tavrigan, S., Lui, Q., Cochran, C., Brennen, L. M., Ding, W., Bell, R., Rosenthal, J., Hussey, C., Tran, T., McClure, M., Frye, C., Harder, T., Phelps, R., Haugen-Strano, A., Katcher, H., Yakumo, K., Gholarni, Z., Shaffer, D., Stone, S., Bayer, S., Wray, C., Bogden, R., Dayanath, P., Ward, J., Tonin, P., Narod, S.A., Bristow, P. K., Norris, F. H., Helvering, L., Morrison, P., Rosteck, P., Lai, M., Barrett, J. C., Lewis, C., Neuhausen, S., Cannon-Albright, L., Goldgar, D., Wiseman, R., Kamb, A., & Skolnick, M. H. (1994). A strong candidate for the breast and ovarian cancer susceptibility gene BRCA1. *Science, 266,* 66-71.

Narod, S. A. (1994). Genetics of breast and ovarian cancer. *British Medical Bulletin, 50,* 656-676.

Narod, S. A. (1996). Families with cancer at multiple sites. In W. Weber, J. J. Mulvihill, & S. A. Narod (Eds.), *Familial cancer management.* New York: CRC Press.

Narod, S. A., Ford, D., Devilee, P., Barkardottir, R., Lynch, H. T., Smith, S. A., Ponder, B. A. J., Weber, B. L., Garber, J., Birch, J. M., Cornelis, R. S., Kelsell, D. P., Spurr, N., Smyth, E., Haites, N., Sobol, H., Bignon, Y. J., Claude-Chang, J., Hamann, U., Lindblom, A., Borg, A., Piver, M. S., Gallion, H. H., Struewing, J., Whittemore, A., Tonin, P., Goldgar, D., & Easton, D. F., and the Breast Cancer Linkage Consortium. (1995). An evaluation of genetic heterogeneity in 145 breast-ovarian cancer families. *American Journal of Human Genetics, 56,* 254-264.

National Action Plan on Breast Cancer. (1996, March). *Position paper: Hereditary susceptibility testing for breast cancer.* Washington, DC: US PHS Office on Women's Health.

National Breast Cancer Coalition. (1995, September 28). *Presymptomatic genetic testing for heritable breast cancer risk.* Press Release. Washington, DC: Author.

National Institutes of Health Consensus Development Conference. (1988). Neurofibromatosis: Conference statement. *Archives in Neurology, 45,* 475-578.

National Institutes of Health. (1994). *Ovarian cancer: Screening, treatment, and followup.* (NIH Consensus Statement, 12[3], April 5-7). Washington, DC: Author.

Northouse, L. L., Cracchiolo-Caraway, A., & Appel, C. P. (1991). Psychologic consequences of breast cancer on partner and family. *Seminars Oncology Nursing, 7,* 216-223.

Nowell, P. C., & Hungerford, D. A. (1960). Chromosome studies on normal and leukemic human leukocytes. *Journal of the National Cancer Institute, 25,* 85-109.

Oncology Nursing Society. (1997, September). *ONS Position Statement: Cancer genetic testing and risk assessment counseling.* Pittsburgh, PA: Author.

Parry, D. M., Eldridge, R., Kaiser-Kupfer, M. I., Bouzas, E. A., Pikus, A., & Patronas, N. (1994). Neurofibromatosis 2 (NF2): Clinical characteristics of 63 affected individuals and clinical evidence for heterogeneity. *American Journal of Medical Genetics, 52,* 450-461.

Riccardi, V. M. (1992). Type 1 neurofibromatosis and the pediatric patient. *Current Problems in Pediatrics, 22,* 66-106.

Riccardi, V. M. (1994). The neurofibromatoses. *Hematology/Oncology Annals, 2,* 119-128.

Rosenthal, G., Kash, K., & Diemer, K. (1995). The Strang National High Risk Registry: A program for delivery of cancer risk information and a resource for research. *Annals of New York Academy of Sciences, 768,* 317-322.

Rouleau, G. A., Merel, P., Lutchman, M., Sanson, M., Zucman, J., Marineau, C., Hoang-Xuan, K., Demczuk, S., Desmaze, C., Plougastel, B., Pulst, S. M., Lenoir, G., Bijlsma, E., Fashold, R., Dumanski, J., de Jong, P., Parry, D., Eldrige, R., Aurias, A., Delattre, O., & Thomas, G. (1993). Alteration in a new gene encoding a putative membrane-organizing protein causes neuro-fibromatosis type 2. *Nature, 363,* 515-521.

Ruddon, R. W. (1995). *Cancer biology* (3rd ed.). New York: Oxford University Press.

Rustgi, A. K. (1994). Hereditary gastrointestinal polyposis and nonpolyposis syndromes. *New England Journal Medicine, 331,* 1694-1702.

Scanlon, C., & Fibison, W. (1995). *Managing genetic information: Implications for nursing practice.* Washington, DC: American Nurses Association Publishing.

Schover, L. R., Yetman, R. J., Tuason, L. J., Meisler, E., Esselstyn, C. B., Hermann, R. E., Grundfest-Broniatowski, S., & Dowden, R. V. (1995). Partial mastectomy and breast reconstruction. A comparison of their effects on psychosocial adjustment, body image, and sexuality. *Cancer, 75,* 54-64.

Schwartz, M., Lerman, C., Daly, M., Audraiu, J., Masny, A., & Griffith, K. (1995). *Cancer Epidemiology, Biomarkers & Prevention, 4,* 269-273.

Scott-Connor, C. E. H., Hausmann, M., Hall, Skelton, D. S., Anglin, B. L., & Subramony, C. (1995). Familial juvenile polyposis: Patterns of recurrence and implications for surgical management. *Journal American College Surgery, 181,* 407-413.

Spiegelman, D., Colditz, G. A., Hunter, D., & Hertzmark, E. (1994). Validation of the Gail et al. model for predicting individual breast cancer risk. *Journal of National Cancer Institute, 86,* 600-607.

Stefanek, M. E., Helzlsouer, K. J., Wilcox, P. M., & Houn, F. (1995). Predictors of and satisfaction with bilateral prophylactic mastectomy. *Preventive Medicine, 24,* 412-419.

Steichen-Gersdorf, E., Gallion, H. H., Ford, D., Girodet, C., Easton, D. F., DiCioccio, R. A., Evans, G., Ponder, M. A., Pye, C., Mazoyer, S., Noguchi, T., Karengueven, F., Sobol, H., Hardouin, A., Bignon, Y. J., Piver, M. S., Smith, S. A., & Ponder, B. A. J. (1994). Familial site-specific ovarian cancer is linked to BRCA1 on 17q12-21. *American Journal of Human Genetics, 55,* 870-875.

Stephens, K., Kayes, L., Riccardi, V. M., Rising, M., Sybert, V. P., & Pagon, R. M. (1992). Preferential mutation of the neurofibromaosis type 1 gene in paternally derived chromosomes. *Human Genetics, 88,* 279-282.

Struewing, J. P., Hartge, P., Wacholder, S., Baker, S. M., Berlin, M., McAdams, M., Timmerman, M. M., Brody, L. C., & Tucker, M. A. (1997). The risk of cancer associated with specific mutations of BRCA1 and BRCA2 among Ashkenazi Jews. *New England Journal of Medicine, 336,* 1401-1408.

Takahashi, M., Ritz, J., & Cooper, G. M. (1985). Activation of a novel human transforming gene, ret, by DNA rearrangement. *Cell, 42,* 581-588.

Trofatter, J. A., MacCollin, M. M., Rutter, J. L., Murrell, J. R., Duyao, M. P., Parry, D. M., Eldridge, R., Kley, N., Menon, A. G., Pulaski, K., Haase, V. H., Ambrose, C. M., Munroe, D., Bove, C., Haines, J. L., Martuza, R. L., MacDonald, M. E., Seizinger, B. R., Short, M. P., Buckler, A. J., & Gusella, J. F. (1993). A novel moesin-, ezrin-, radixin-like gene is a candidate for the neurofibromatosis 2 tumor suppressor. *Cell, 72,* 791-800.

U. S. Equal Employment Opportunity Commission. (March 14, 1995). *Directives Transmittal Number 915.002.* Washington, DC: Author.

Walsh, B. A., Grunert, B. K., Telford,G. L., & Otterson, M. F. (1995). Multidisciplinary management of altered body image in the patient with an ostomy. *Journal Wound and Ostomy Care Nursing, 22,* 227-236.

Weinryb, R., & Rossel, R. (1986). Personality traits that can affect adaptation after colectomy: A study of 10 patients treated for ulcerative colitis either with proctocolectomy and ileostomy or with colectomy, proctomucosectomy, ileal pouch and ileoanal anastomosis. *Psychotherapy and Psychosomatics, 45,* 57-65.

Wells., S. J., Chi, D. D., Toshima, K., Dehne, L. P., Coffin, C. M., Dowton, B., Ivanovich, J. L., DeBenedetti, M. K., Dilley, W. G., Moley, J. F., Norton, J. A., & Donis-Keller, H. (1994). Predictive DNA testing and prophylactic thyroidectomy in patients at risk for MEN type 2a. *Annals of Surgery, 220,* 237-250.

Wooster, R., Neuhausen, S. L., Mangion, J., Quirk, Y., Ford, D., Collins, N., Nguyen, K., Seal, S., Tran, T., Averill, D., Fields, P., Marshall, G., Narod, S. A., Lenoir, G. M., Lynch, H. T., Devilee, P., Cornelisse, C. J., Menko, F. H., Daly, P. A., Ormiston, W., McManus, R., Pye, C., Cannon-Albright, L., Peto, J., Ponder, B. A. J., Skolnick, M., Easton, D. E., Goldgar, D. E., & Stratton, M. R. (1994). Localization of a breast cancer susceptibility gene, BRCA2, to chromosome 13q12-13 by genetic linkage analysis. *Science, 265,* 2088-2090.

Wooster, R., Bignell, G., Lancaster, J., Swift, S., Seal, S., Mangion, J., Collins, N., Gregory, S., Gumbs, C., Micklem, G., Barfoot, R., Hamoudi, R., Patel, S., Rice, C., Biggs, P., Hashim, Y., Smith, A., Connor, F., Arason, A., Gudmundsson, J., Ficenec, D., Keisell, D., Ford, D., Tonin, P., Bishop, D. T., Spurr, N. K., Ponder, B. A. J., Eeles, R., Peto, J., Devilee, P., Cornelisse, C., Lynch, H., Narod, S., Lenoir, G., Egilsson, V., Barkadottir, R. B., Easton, D. F., Bentley, D. R., Futreal, P. A., Ashworth, A., & Stratton, M. R. (1995). Identification of the breast cancer susceptibility gene BRCA2. *Nature, 378,* 789-792.

13 Symptom Management

Judith A. Paice, PhD, RN, FAAN

INTRODUCTION

Importance of Symptom Identification and Management

The identification and management of symptoms associated with cancer and its treatment are critical to the patient's quality of life. Severe pain, fatigue, nausea, and other complications reduce mobility, impair ability to interact with loved ones, and diminish capacity to enjoy life. Several studies have explored the prevalence of diverse symptoms in cancer patients. The majority of patients experience at least one, usually several, symptoms, either as a presenting sign, during diagnosis and treatment, while surviving cancer, or at the end of life. The clinical utility of such investigations is to make clinicians aware of the spectrum of symptoms associated with cancer so that they might more aggressively assess for and manage these complications at all phases of care. In addition, these studies provide clues for needed prevention strategies and treatment approaches.

Nurses play a critical role in the management of symptoms associated with cancer and its treatment. At all stages of the cancer experience, nurses prevent, assess, detect, and manage these symptoms. As oncology nurses are aware, it is inadequate and unacceptable merely to deliver cancer treatment without also anticipating and treating the complications of this disease and associated therapies. Symptom control is the essence of oncology nursing.

Prevalence

It is generally believed that cancer-related symptoms are common. However, few studies systematically evaluate the prevalence of these symptoms. One of the barriers to conducting these studies has been the lack of comprehensive tools to systematically measure the symptoms associated with cancer. Most tools currently in use evaluate a single symptom or include small aspects of symptom evaluation within the context of the larger quality of life assessment. Examples of single-symptom assessment tools include the Brief Pain Inventory (BPI) (Daut, Cleeland, & Flanery, 1983) used to evaluate pain and the Constipation Assessment Scale (CAS) (McMillan & Williams, 1989), which measures bowel function. Quality of life tools include the Functional Assessment of Cancer Therapy (FACT) (Cella, Tulsky, Gray, Sarafian, Linn, & Bonomi et al., 1993) and the Ferrans and Powers Quality of Life Index (QLI) (Ferrans & Powers, 1985). Few comprehensive symptom assessment tools have been developed and validated.

One of the few comprehensive, valid tools is the Memorial Symptom Assessment Scale (MSAS) (Fig. 13-1). Validated in cancer patients, the MSAS is a patient-rated tool that assesses the prevalence, characteristics, and distress associated with 33 symptoms common to cancer (Portenoy, Thaler, Kornblith, McCarthy Lepore, Friedlander-Klar, & Kiyasu et al., 1994). Portenoy and colleagues studied 297 randomly selected cancer patients at Memorial Sloan Kettering Cancer Center with a wide range of tumors and disease severity. The most common symptoms were lack of energy (73.4%), worrying (72.4%), feeling sad (67.4%), and pain (63.1%). Thus, in a sample of general oncology patients, most suffered physical and emotional responses to their disease or its treatment. Additional multicenter studies are needed to support the validity and utility of this tool.

More commonly, symptom prevalence studies are conducted at the end of life. As disease progresses and the end of life approaches, it is generally believed that symptoms also increase. Patients and their loved ones fear that the final days will be filled with pain and suffering, and the results of many of these studies do little to allay these fears. Coyle and colleagues (1990) evaluated terminally ill cancer patients during the last 4 weeks of life. They recorded only those symptoms voluntarily described by the patient. Fatigue (58%), pain (54%), and generalized weakness (43%) were the most commonly reported symptoms (Table 13-1). At 4 weeks before death, 71% reported three or more symptoms. By 1 week before death, 73% of patients reported three or more symptoms, with 27% describing five or more.

Brescia and colleagues (1990) evaluated the prevalence of symptoms in 1103 admissions to a hospital specializing

NAME:	DATE:

SECTION 1:

INSTRUCTIONS: We have listed 24 symptoms below. Read each one carefully. If you have had the symptom during this past week, let us know how OFTEN you had it, how SEVERE it was usually and how much it DISTRESSED OR BOTHERED you by circling the appropriate number. If you DID NOT HAVE the symptom, make an "X" in the box marked "DID NOT HAVE."

DURING THE PAST WEEK Did you have any of the following symptoms?	DID NOT HAVE	IF YES, How OFTEN did you have it?				IF YES, How SEVERE was it usually?				IF YES, How much did it DISTRESS or BOTHER you?				
		Rarely	Occasionally	Frequently	Almost constantly	Slight	Moderate	Severe	Very severe	Not at all	A little bit	Somewhat	Quite a bit	Very much
Difficulty concentrating		1	2	3	4	1	2	3	4	0	1	2	3	4
Pain		1	2	3	4	1	2	3	4	0	1	2	3	4
Lack of energy		1	2	3	4	1	2	3	4	0	1	2	3	4
Cough		1	2	3	4	1	2	3	4	0	1	2	3	4
Feeling nervous		1	2	3	4	1	2	3	4	0	1	2	3	4
Dry mouth		1	2	3	4	1	2	3	4	0	1	2	3	4
Nausea		1	2	3	4	1	2	3	4	0	1	2	3	4
Feeling drowsy		1	2	3	4	1	2	3	4	0	1	2	3	4
Numbness/tingling in hands/feet		1	2	3	4	1	2	3	4	0	1	2	3	4
Difficulty sleeping		1	2	3	4	1	2	3	4	0	1	2	3	4
Feeling bloated		1	2	3	4	1	2	3	4	0	1	2	3	4
Problems with urination		1	2	3	4	1	2	3	4	0	1	2	3	4

DURING THE PAST WEEK Did you have any of the following symptoms?	DID NOT HAVE	IF YES, How OFTEN did you have it?				IF YES, How SEVERE was it usually?				IF YES, How much did it DISTRESS or BOTHER you?				
		Rarely	Occasionally	Frequently	Almost constantly	Slight	Moderate	Severe	Very severe	Not at all	A little bit	Somewhat	Quite a bit	Very much
Vomiting		1	2	3	4	1	2	3	4	0	1	2	3	4
Shortness of breath		1	2	3	4	1	2	3	4	0	1	2	3	4
Diarrhea		1	2	3	4	1	2	3	4	0	1	2	3	4
Feeling sad		1	2	3	4	1	2	3	4	0	1	2	3	4
Sweats		1	2	3	4	1	2	3	4	0	1	2	3	4
Worrying		1	2	3	4	1	2	3	4	0	1	2	3	4
Problems with sexual interest or activity		1	2	3	4	1	2	3	4	0	1	2	3	4
Itching		1	2	3	4	1	2	3	4	0	1	2	3	4
Lack of appetite		1	2	3	4	1	2	3	4	0	1	2	3	4
Dizziness		1	2	3	4	1	2	3	4	0	1	2	3	4
Difficulty swallowing		1	2	3	4	1	2	3	4	0	1	2	3	4
Feeling irritable		1	2	3	4	1	2	3	4	0	1	2	3	4

Fig. 13-1 Memorial Symptom Assessment Scale. (Reprinted with permission from Portenoy, R. K., et al. [1994]. The Memorial Symptom Assessment Scale: An instrument for the evaluation of symptom prevalence, characteristics and distress. *European Journal of Cancer, 30A,* 1326-1336.)

TABLE 13-1 Prevalence of Symptoms in Cancer Patients

	Coyle et al., 1990	Brescia et al., 1990	Vainio et al., 1996
Study Design	Prospective, telephone and office visits	Chart review	Prospective, 40 international palliative care centers
Patients	90 advanced cancer patients enrolled in Supportive Care Program at Memorial Sloan Kettering Cancer Center	1013 inpatients admitted to Calvary Hospital	1640 patients with advanced or terminal cancer
Prevalence of Symptoms	At 4 weeks before death: Fatigue (58%) Pain (54%) Weakness (43%) Sleepiness (24%) Confusion (24%) Anxiety (21%) Leg weakness (18%) Shortness of breath (17%) Nausea (12%)	Severe pain (38%) Confusion (33%) Anorexia (31%) Shortness of breath (27%) Dysphagia (22%) Nausea (19%)	Pain (51%) Weakness (51%) Weight loss (39%) Anorexia (30%) Constipation (23%) Nausea (21%) Dyspnea (19%) Insomnia (9%) Confusion (8%)

From Brescia, F. J., Adler, D., Gray, G., Ryan, M. A., Cimino, J., & Mamtani, R. (1990). Hospitalized advanced cancer patients: A profile. *Journal of Pain and Symptom Management, 5,* 221-227; Coyle, N., Adelhardt, J., Foley, K. M., & Portenoy, R. K. (1990). Character of terminal illness in the advanced cancer patient: Pain and other symptoms during the last four weeks of life. *Journal of Pain and Symptom Management, 5,* 83-93; Vainio, A., Auvinen, A., with Members of the Symptom Prevalence Group. (1996). Prevalence of symptoms among patients with advanced cancer: An international collaborative study. *Journal of Pain and Symptom Management, 12,* 3-10.

in the care of patients with advanced cancer. Severe pain was the most common symptom (38%), followed by confusion (33%) and anorexia (31%). There were statistically significant, age-related differences in the prevalence of certain symptoms. Higher percentages of patients under 65 years of age had pain (47% vs 33%). As one might expect, confusion was significantly more common in patients over 65 years of age (35% vs 29%).

Vainio, Auvinen, and Members of the Symptom Prevalence Group (1996) investigated the prevalence of eight symptoms associated with cancer in a recent international study of 40 palliative care centers. This prospective study of 1640 patients with advanced or terminal cancer revealed that pain and weakness were the most common symptoms, each occurring in 51% of the patient population. The prevalence of other symptoms were weight loss (39%), anorexia (30%), constipation (23%), nausea (21%), dyspnea (19%), insomnia (9%), and confusion (8%).

It is apparent from these and other studies that symptom prevalence increases during aggressive treatment, as the disease progresses, and as the end of life approaches. Furthermore, recent studies have documented that symptoms persist in long-term cancer survivors, altering quality of life (Ferrell & Dow, 1997). Oncology nurses must consider the potential for each symptom throughout the disease trajectory. This approach begins with a careful study of each of the most common symptoms experienced by patients with cancer.

CANCER PAIN

Of the many symptoms associated with cancer, pain is the most feared. Unfortunately this fear is warranted for many, even though most cancer patients can obtain sufficient relief from available therapies (Jacox, Carr, & Payne, 1994). Barriers to good relief are numerous, including myths regarding the beneficial properties of pain, attitudes associated with the use of opioids, and the lack of knowledge concerning methods for assessing and treating pain. These barriers were comprehensively analyzed and documented in Box 13-1 (Jacox, Carr, & Payne, 1994).

Epidemiology

Many studies have investigated the prevalence of pain in subpopulations of cancer patients. In a randomly selected sample of postoperative oncology patients, 70.6% were in pain at the time of interview, and 91.2% reported pain during the previous 24 hours (Paice, Mahon, & Faut-Callahan, 1991). Ambulatory cancer patients cared for at Eastern Cooperative Oncology Group (ECOG)-affiliated research centers were evaluated for pain (Cleeland, Gonin, Hatfield, Edmonson, Blum, & Stewart et al., 1994). More than two thirds had pain during the previous week, and more than one third of these patients felt pain significant enough to impair function. In a study of advanced cancer patients, Coyle and colleagues (1990) found that pain occurred in 54% of those in their last 4 weeks of life. Pain was the second most common symptom after fatigue.

Fewer studies have examined the prevalence of pain in children with cancer. In a study of children and young adults at the time of cancer diagnosis, Miser and colleagues (1987a, b) found that 78% reported pain, which lasted a median duration of 74 days. Moderate to severe pain was experienced by 18% of children treated in an outpatient clinic (McGrath, Hsu, & Cappelli, 1990). These studies

Box 13-1
Barriers to Cancer Pain Management

Problems Related to Health Care Professionals

Inadequate knowledge of pain management.
Poor assessment of pain.
Concern about regulation of controlled substances.
Fear of patient addiction.
Concern about side effects of analgesics.
Concern about patients becoming tolerant to analgesics.

Problems Related to Patients

Reluctance to report pain
- Concern about distracting physicians from treatment of underlying disease.
- Fear that pain means disease is worse.
- Concern about not being a "good" patient.

Reluctance to take pain medications.
- Fear of addiction or of being thought of as an addict.
- Worries about unmanageable side effects.
- Concern about becoming tolerant to pain medications.

Problems Related to the Health Care System

Low priority given to cancer pain treatment.
Inadequate reimbursement.
Restrictive regulation of controlled substances.
Problems of availability of treatment or access to it.

From Jacox, A. et al. (1994). *Management of cancer pain.* Clinical practice guideline No. 9. AHCPR Publication No. 94-0592. Rockville, MD: Agency for Health Care Policy and Research, U.S. Department of Health and Human Services, Public Health Service, March, 1994.

support the widely held belief that a diagnosis of cancer is often associated with pain. An examination of risk factors assists clinicians in identifying groups in danger of being undertreated.

Risk Factors

Among ambulatory oncology patients, unrelieved pain was more prevalent among minority patients, the elderly, and females (Cleeland et al., 1994). These findings may be related to assumptions about pain perception, pain expression, and concerns about addiction in these populations. In an international study conducted by Vainio et al. (1996), more than half of breast and lung cancer patients had at least moderate pain. Moderate to severe pain was most common in patients with gynecologic or head and neck cancers. Severe pain was most common in patients with prostate cancer. Thus, primary cancer sites may be correlated with varying risks of increased pain intensity.

Ward and colleagues (1993) examined patient-related barriers to cancer pain relief using the Barriers Questionnaire (BQ). This self-report tool evaluates eight areas of concern often associated with pain and its treatment, including fear of addiction and concern about side effects of pain medication. High levels of concern were correlated with higher levels of pain intensity. Therefore, patients' fears act as risk factors for unrelieved pain. This finding was supported in a quality improvement study evaluating cancer inpatients and outpatients (Paice, Toy, & Shott, in press). Factors associated with higher pain intensity included inpatient setting, presence of metastatic disease, hesitancy to bother the nurse, and concerns regarding tolerance and addiction. Although concerns about addiction and tolerance correlated strongly in this study, fear of tolerance seemed to increase pain intensity scores more than did fear of addiction.

These and other studies suggest that risk factors for unrelieved pain are often related to biases and attitudes held by patients and health care professionals. Professional and lay education aimed at correcting these biases would assist in relieving much of the pain seen in those with cancer. Other efforts should include standardizing pain practice through the development of institutional programs. Policies, procedures, pathways, and algorithms provide structure for those not familiar with pain assessment and treatment. Finally, regulatory barriers must be overcome so that opioids can be available for those in need.

Prevention

As much as is possible, pain prevention is crucial. Preemptive analgesia for postoperative and procedural pain is rapidly gaining acceptance. Although difficult to design, numerous studies have documented the advantages of preoperative or intraoperative medication to relieve postoperative pain (Richmond, Bromley, & Woolf, 1993). Potential benefits of preemptive analgesia are reduced postoperative opioid requirements, accelerated recovery, and reduced morbidity. Specific agents used include nonsteroidal anti-inflammatory drugs (NSAIDs), opioids, local anesthetics, and other adjuvant analgesics (Dahl & Kehlet, 1993).

Within the setting of chronic cancer pain, prevention of pain recurrence includes use of around-the-clock administration of medication (Jacox et al., 1994). This approach prevents the recurrence of pain by providing stable plasma levels of drug. Immediate release products should also be available for breakthrough pain (see Pharmacologic Therapies).

Pathophysiology

Understanding the pathophysiology of pain assists clinicians in making educated decisions regarding treatment. Four basic processes are involved in the pathophysiology of pain: transduction, transmission, perception, and modulation (Fig. 13-2) (Fields, 1987). Pain is relayed through the peripheral and central nervous systems to higher centers in a process that begins with transduction. Tissue damage, such as mechanical trauma induced by pressure from a metastatic tumor, elicits changes in substrates at the site of injury. The release of these substances, including prostaglandin, bradykinin, histamine, serotonin, substance P, and others, evokes an inflammatory response. This response includes erythema, edema, and pain. Anti-inflammatory drugs, such as the NSAIDs, block prostaglandin synthesis and inhibit transduction.

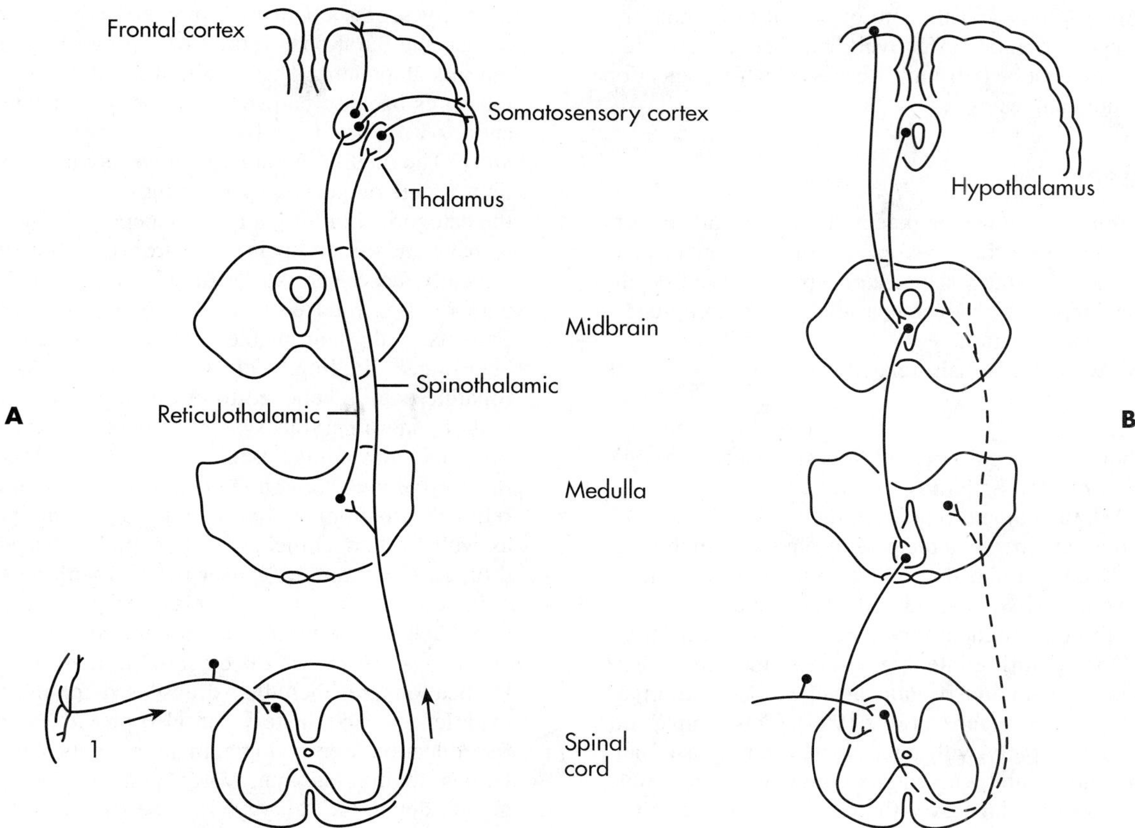

Fig. 13-2 Pathophysiology of pain. **A,** Transmission; **B,** modulation. (Reprinted with permission from Fields, H. L. [1987] *Pain.* New York: McGraw-Hill.)

The inflammatory response results in the stimulation of nociceptors, sensory neurons distributed throughout the periphery (Rang, Bevan, & Dray, 1994). Nociceptors include C fibers, associated with dull, aching, and diffuse sensations, and A fibers, identified with more localized, sharp, and acute episodes of pain. Extending from the periphery to the dorsal horn of the spinal cord, these neurons continue transmission to the central nervous system. The stimulation of these fibers is called *transmission*. Local anesthetics and anticonvulsants block pain transmission along the axon of the neuron (Tanelian & MacIver, 1991).

Within the dorsal horn, neurotransmitters are released from primary afferent terminals that bind to receptors on ascending nociceptive spinal neurons. Thus, pain signals are communicated by chemical means across the synapse between afferent fibers and dorsal horn neurons. Substances released in the dorsal horn include adenosine triphosphate, aspartate, calcitonin gene-related peptide, cholecystokinin, glutamate, neurokinins, neuropeptide Y, substance P, vasoactive intestinal polypeptide, and others (Dray, Urban, & Dickenson, 1994).

Other substances within the dorsal horn serve as inhibitory mediators. Opioids, including endogenous substances such as enkephalin, as well as exogenously administered opioids such as morphine, block the release of specific neurotransmitters, suppressing the transmission of pain within the region of the dorsal horn. This mechanism provides the rationale for using morphine and other opioids to treat cancer pain.

Ascending fibers, originating from nociceptive neurons in the spinal cord, terminate in numerous areas of the brain stem and thalamus. From the thalamus, neurons project widely throughout the cerebral cortex, where several areas process nociceptive information. These areas include the primary somatosensory cortex (SI), located in the parietal lobe, and the secondary, or association, somatosensory cortex (SII) (Talbot, Marrett, Evans, Meyer, Bushnell, & Duncan, 1991). It is believed that perception of the pain occurs at these sites and within other regions in higher centers of the brain, although the precise location of pain perception remains elusive.

In addition to the ascending pain systems, descending pathways originating in the brain stem modify pain (Besson & Chaouch, 1987). Many substances, including endogenous opioids, as well as serotonin and norepinephrine, released by these descending neurons inhibit pain. This process is referred to as *modulation*, the final of the four processes. Tricyclic antidepressants block the reuptake of serotonin and norepinephrine. This blockade allows more of these substances to be available for binding, which enhances the pain modulatory system.

Clinicians must understand these basic mechanisms of

pain pathophysiology and the site of action of commonly-used analgesics to more effectively manage cancer pain. However, pain must be thoroughly assessed before selection of appropriate analgesics.

Assessment

Clinicians must recognize the potential for pain and perform an assessment before the development of a treatment plan. Pain assessment includes a thorough history, based on the patient's self-report whenever possible, and a comprehensive physical examination.

Pain History. The pain-related history consists of the following:

Onset: When did the pain begin? Was the onset accompanied by associated activities?

Location: Ask the patient to point to the site(s) of pain. Use a figure diagram in which the patient can shade in the sites of pain. Keep in mind that many patients have multiple sites of pain, some associated with cancer and others associated with nonmalignant conditions, such as arthritis.

Intensity: For measuring intensity, use a rating scale where 0 indicates no pain and 10 indicates the worst pain imaginable (Fig. 13-3) (Jacox et al., 1994). This simple tool can be used verbally with patients who have visual and motor handicaps and who cannot complete written tools, and it allows for triage over the telephone (Paice & Cohen, 1997). Determine intensity scores before and after a new analgesic or treatment is administered. These intensity scores provide information regarding the degree of response; a weak response warrants a dose increase. Pain intensity scores obtained at predetermined intervals establish the duration of effect of a drug or therapy in an individual patient. These pain intensity scores are key measures because patients' responses to analgesic medications vary significantly.

Quality: The quality of pain, obtained spontaneously by patient report or guided by offering descriptors, assists in the categorization of pain as nociceptive (which includes somatic and visceral pain) or neuropathic. Somatic pain is typically described as "aching," "throbbing"; visceral pain is often referred to as "squeezing" or "cramping." Patients with neuropathic pain describe their pain as "burning," "tingling," "electrical," or "shocklike." Neuropathic pain is believed to occur in response to peripheral or central nervous system damage, and the treatment often includes adjuvant analgesics.

Exacerbating and alleviating factors: Factors that worsen or relieve the pain may provide clues regarding its etiology, as well as alert clinicians to potentially dangerous syndromes. For example, cancer patients with metastases to the spine who complain of elevated pain during cough may have an impending spinal cord compression.

Pain treatment history: It is essential to ask about previous medication use, including drugs used for previous pain experiences. This history can also provide opportunities for education. For example, many patients may report allergies to opioids, but, when patients are queried in greater detail, the "allergy" may be nausea and vomiting, a known adverse effect of opioids. At this time, it is useful to ask patients about their beliefs regarding morphine and other opioids, offering the opportunity to correct ungrounded fears regarding tolerance and addiction.

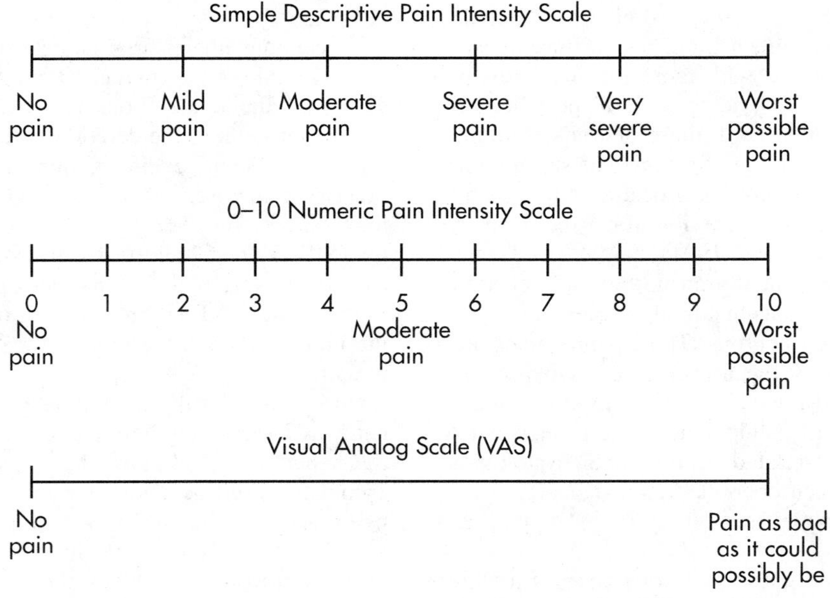

Fig. 13-3 Pain intensity scales. (Reprinted from Jacox, A., Carr, D. B, Payne, R., et al. [1994]. *Management of cancer pain.* Clinical practice guideline No. 9. AHCPR Publication No. 94-0592. Rockville, MD: Agency for Health Care Policy and Research, U.S. Department of Health and Human Services, Public Health Service.)

Medication use: Patients should be questioned with regard to both the medications for pain that have been prescribed and the medications they are actually taking. For a variety of reasons, patients may not take the medication ordered by their physician or may take reduced amounts of the drug. This lack of adherence may be due to fears of tolerance (wanting to "save" the drug for later), concerns regarding addiction, or cost barriers. Ask patients about over-the-counter medicines, with particular attention to the total daily amount of acetaminophen intake. Opioids such as codeine, hydrocodone, or oxycodone often contain admixtures with acetaminophen. Patients who take these drugs can easily exceed the maximum recommended daily intake of acetaminophen, approximately 4000 mg, particularly when they use supplemental "non-aspirin" pain relievers or other products. Finally, assess patients' use of recreational drugs, as this may affect the dose of opioid required to relieve pain.

In addition to a complete pain history, patients should be queried with regard to their medical history, and records should be examined for information regarding extent of disease and past cancer therapy. For example, concurrent medical problems, such as narrow angle glaucoma or cardiac arrhythmia, might preclude prescribing some tricyclic antidepressants for pain. Past treatment with radiotherapy may not absolutely preclude current use to reduce tumor bulk, and thereby reduce pain.

It can be useful to understand the patient's previous pain experiences, the meaning of these experiences, as well as the meaning of the current pain to both the patient and family members. Ask about information regarding past and present social and psychological functioning and the level of medical and social support, which will assist when developing a plan of care. Finally, evidence of patient and family fatigue warrants contact with support services.

Physical Examination. A thorough physical examination is essential, with particular attention given to the neurologic examination. This examination can reveal sources of pain such as infection, which may require additional treatment, or etiologies that might respond to antitumor therapies, including radiation therapy. Radiographic procedures may be necessary to document the cause of the pain when the etiology is unclear. For example, opioid-induced confusion can be differentiated from hypercalcemia through laboratory tests. The data obtained from the history and physical examination are then applied to develop a plan of care.

Staging

Pain staging systems were developed to standardize various pain syndromes cited within the literature, provide more accurate sharing of information, and allow clinicians to use available treatments more logically. One of the earliest classifications of cancer pain was described by Foley (1985). In this system, pain is related to the cancer, treatment, or nonmalignant causes. Another method of classifying cancer pain is based on the quality of the pain. This system broadly categorizes pain as nociceptive or neuropathic. Within nociceptive pain, there are two subtypes: somatic and visceral. Neuropathic pain is generally believed to be related to neuronal damage, either within the peripheral (e.g., postherpetic neuropathy) or central nervous system (e.g., thalamic pain after stroke).

The International Association for the Study of Pain developed a classification system for coding chronic pain diagnoses (Merskey & Bogduk, 1994). Pain is coded by region (e.g., abdominal region), system (e.g., gastrointestinal), temporal characteristics (e.g., continuous), intensity and time since onset (e.g., severe lasting 1 to 6 months), and etiology (e.g., neoplasm).

The Edmonton staging system was developed to be more useful for clinicians by predicting prognosis for pain relief (Bruera, Macmillan, Hanson, & MacDonald, 1989). This tool is based on the mechanism of pain, pain characteristics, previous opioid exposure, cognitive function, psychological distress, tolerance, and a past history of drug addiction or severe alcoholism. Three stages were originally proposed: stage I (good prognosis), stage II (intermediate prognosis), and stage III (poor prognosis). Subsequent validation studies have led the investigators to collapse the stages into I (good prognosis) and II (poor prognosis) (Bruera, Schoeller, Wenk, MacEachern, Marcelino, & Hanson et al., 1995). All current cancer pain staging systems must be refined, simplified, and disseminated for their use to become more widespread.

Medical Management

Pain treatments consist of two broad categories: pharmacologic and nonpharmacologic. Clinicians select the appropriate treatment or treatments based on the patient's history and physical examination. Other factors that aid selection of treatment include availability of care, physical or cognitive limitations that affect ability to participate in the treatment plan, and financial concerns.

Pharmacologic Therapies. Analgesic drug categories include nonopioids, opioids, and adjuvant agents. Each category produces analgesia by a different mechanism of action and therefore are indicated in different types of pain syndromes.

Nonopioids. Nonopioids include NSAIDs and acetaminophen. The rationale for the clinical use of NSAIDs pertains to the role of prostaglandins in pain. The phospholipid bilayer of the cellular membrane of traumatized cells is metabolized into arachidonic acid, which is further broken down into prostaglandins by the enzyme, cyclooxygenase. Prostaglandins are rich in the periosteum of the bone and in the uterus and are believed to be involved in bone pain and dysmenorrhea. NSAIDs, such as aspirin, block cyclooxygenase and thereby inhibit the conversion of arachidonic acid into prostaglandins (Insel, 1991). These agents have demonstrated efficacy in a variety of pain syndromes, including pain associated with cancer.

The most common adverse effects associated with NSAID use include gastrointestinal ulceration, bleeding, and renal dysfunction. The etiology and treatment of these effects are included in Table 13-2. Many NSAIDs are avail-

TABLE 13-2 Management of Adverse Effects Associated with NSAIDS

Adverse Effect	Mechanism	Prevention/Management
Gastrointestinal erosion	Prostaglandins are responsible for generating the mucous coating that protects the lining of the stomach from exposure to enzymes and other caustic substances responsible for digesting food. Inhibition of prostaglandins to relieve pain also results in breakdown of this mucous coating.	*Prevention:* Prophylactic use of prostaglandin analogs (e.g., misoprostol) prevents loss of the mucous coating. Avoid concomitant use with other drugs that cause erosion (e.g., corticosteroids). *Management:* Discontinue NSAID. Restore hemostasis if bleeding occurs.
Bleeding	Prolonged bleeding times occur due to inhibition of prostaglandin synthetase. This is reversible and lasts as long as the drug remains in the plasma (except for aspirin, which has an irreversible effect on platelets).	*Prevention:* Discontinue NSAID one to two days before planned invasive procedures (discontinue aspirin approximately 7 days before procedure). Avoid NSAID use in thrombocytopenic patients or those receiving anticoagulants. Monitor bleeding times (platelet numbers are not predictive of risk). *Management:* Discontinue NSAID and restore hemostasis.
Renal dysfunction	Inhibition of renal vasodilatory prostaglandins	*Prevention:* Keep patient hydrated. Avoid use of NSAIDS in those with chronic renal disease, and those receiving diuretics. *Management:* Assess for oliguria and sodium and water retention. Stop the NSAID.

NSAID, Nonsteroidal anti-inflammatory drug.

able (Table 13-3), some without a physician's prescription. If there is no relief with one agent, or if side effects occur, another NSAID from a different category may be of use. Patients should be cautioned that, unlike most opioids, there are maximum recommended doses of NSAIDs, so that orders regarding dose and frequency must be strictly followed.

Opioids. Opioids provide the foundation for cancer pain treatment (Levy, 1996; Cherny & Portenoy, 1995). Opioids bind to receptors in the spinal cord to prevent the release of neurotransmitters involved in pain transmission. Pure opioid agonists bind primarily to the μ-opioid receptor, and include agents such as morphine, codeine, fentanyl, hydromorphone, methadone, and others. Some opioids, particularly codeine, hydrocodone, and propoxyphene, are compounded with acetaminophen or aspirin. The acetaminophen content limits dose escalation. For example, most hydrocodone preparations contain 500 mg of acetaminophen. Because the maximum recommended daily dose of acetaminophen is approximately 4000 mg, patients are limited to approximately eight tablets of the hydrocodone preparations. However, this dose limitation assumes that they are not taking any other compounds containing acetaminophen. In addition, propoxyphene (Darvon) is not recommended for routine use because of its long half-life and the risk of accumulation of norpropoxyphene, a metabolite toxic to the central nervous system.

Tramadol (Ultram) has weak opioid binding as well as inhibition of serotonin and norepinephrine reuptake (Sunshine, 1994; Wilder-Smith, Schimke, Osterwalder, & Senn, 1994; Portenoy, 1996). The usual starting dose is 50 to 100 mg and can be given at 4- to 6-hour intervals, not to exceed 400 mg/day. It is unique in that it does not contain acetaminophen or aspirin. Side effects include sedation, nausea, and vomiting.

Single-entity pure opioid agonists have no ceiling effect or maximum dose. These drugs include morphine, fentanyl, hydromorphone, levorphanol, methadone, and oxycodone. These opioids can be administered by parenteral, oral, transdermal, transmucosal, rectal, stomal, vaginal, inhaled, nasal, and spinal routes (Table 13-4). As a general guideline, oral, rectal, and transdermal routes are preferred over parenteral or spinal routes (Jacox et al., 1994). Other opioid formulations include controlled- or sustained-release delivery and transmucosal administration. Factors to consider when selecting the opioid, the dose, and the route of administration include the severity of the pain, previous adverse or favorable responses to a specific opioid, age, preexisting renal and hepatic function, skill of the patient and caregiver in drug administration, and cost (Hammack & Loprinzi, 1994).

Partial agonists and mixed agonist-antagonists either block or remain neutral at μ-opioid receptors while activating κ-opioid receptors (Drug Facts and Comparisons, 1997). These agents are not appropriate choices in the treatment of cancer pain for several reasons. Partial agonists (e.g., butorphanol, dezocine, and pentazocine) have limited analgesic effects, are associated with greater cognitive effects, and are primarily available in parenteral formulations. In addition, they may precipitate withdrawal symptoms in patients currently taking pure opioid agonists (Jacox et al., 1994).

Another opioid analgesic, meperidine hydrochloride (Demerol), is not appropriate for long-term use in cancer patients because it has a short duration of action and it metabolizes to normeperidine. Normally excreted by the kidney, normeperidine accumulates in patients with renal dysfunction, causing central nervous system toxicity, including tremulousness and seizures (Drug Facts and Comparisons, 1997; Jacox et al., 1994). Therefore meperidine may be use-

TABLE 13-3 Nonopioid Analgesics Used to Treat Cancer Pain

Chemical Class	Generic Name	Half-life (h)	Starting Dose (mg)	Maximum Recommended Dose (mg/day)	Comments
Nonacidic					
p-Aminophenol	Acetaminophen	3-4	750 every 4 h	6000	Available OTC derivatives
Acidic					
Salicylates	Aspirin	3-12	650 every 4-6 h	6000	Available OTC
	Diflunisal	8-12	500 every 12 h	1500	Less GI toxicity than aspirin
	Choline Magnesium Trisalicylate	8-12	1000 every 12 h	4000	Minimal GI toxicity No effect on platelet function at usual doses
	Salsalate	8-12	1000 every 12 h	4000	Minimal GI toxicity. No effect on platelet function at usual doses
Propionic acids	Ibuprofen	3-4	400 every 6 h	4200	Available OTC
	Naproxen	1-3	250 every 12 h	1000	Available OTC
	Fenoprofen	2-3	200 every 6 h	3200	
	Ketoprofen	2-3	25 every 8 h	200	
	Oxaprozin	40	600 every 24 h	1800	
	Flurbiprofen	5-6	100 every 12 h	300	
Acetic acids	Indomethacin	4-5	25 every 12 h	200	Sustained-release and rectal preparations
	Sulindac	14	150 every 12 h	400	
	Diclofenac	2	25 every 8 h	200	
	Ketorolac	4-7	30x1: then 15 mg every 6 h or 10 mg every 6 h by mouth	90	Oral or parenteral preparation
	Tolmetin	1	200 every 8 h	2000	
Oxicams	Piroxicam	45	20 every 24 h	40	
Fenamates	Mefenamic acid		250 every 6 h	1000	
Pyranocarboxylic acids	Etodolac	7	1000 every 24 h	2000	
Naphthylalkalones	Nabumetone	24	1000 every 24 h	2000	

Reprinted with permission from Cherny, N. I., & Portenoy, R. K. (1995). Systemic drugs for cancer pain. *Pain Digest, 5,* 235-263.
GI, Gastrointestinal; *OTC,* over the counter; *PO,* parenteral.

ful only for brief courses over a few days to treat acute pain or rigors.

Opioid antagonists, including naloxone (Narcan) and naltrexone (ReVia), are used clinically for reversal of opioids when untoward side effects such as respiratory depression occur. The only acceptable use of opioid antagonists in cancer patients is the rare episode of opioid overdose resulting in respiratory depression. Naloxone is not an innocuous drug and, therefore, should not be used indiscriminately. Standard doses of naloxone have been associated with acute hypertensive reactions (Tanaka, 1974), pulmonary edema (Flacke, Flacke, & Williams, 1977; Prough, Roy, Bumgarner & Shannon, 1984), ventricular tachycardia and fibrillation (Michaelis, Hickey, Clark, & Dixon, 1974), and sudden death (Andree, 1980). Additionally, the half-life of naloxone is much shorter than that of morphine, with a duration of effect of approximately 30 to 60 minutes, so patients must be carefully monitored for possible recurrence of respiratory depression after this time.

Adjuvants. Adjuvant analgesics are indicated primarily for other purposes, but they also produce significant analgesic effects. These include tricyclic antidepressants, local anesthetics, anticonvulsants, corticosteroids, and others (Table 13-5).

The analgesic effect of tricyclic antidepressants is believed to be due to their ability to block the reuptake of serotonin and norepinephrine. These substances are released endogenously in response to painful stimuli. Blocking their reuptake theoretically allows more of these agents to be available for binding in the spinal cord, which produces an-

TABLE 13-4 Formulations and Routes of Administration of Opioids

Formulation	Drug	Frequency of Administration	Trade Name	Doses
Inhaled (nebulized)	Morphine	As needed	No commercially available preparations; safety and efficacy not studied	
Nasal	Butorphanol (mixed agonist-antagonist, not recommended in cancer pain)	As needed	Stadol	
Rectal (can also be used in stomas and vagina)	Morphine	As needed	MS/S RMS suppositories Roxanol suppositories	5, 10, 20, 30 mg 10, 20, 30 mg
	Hydromorphone	As needed	Dilaudid rectal suppositories	3 mg
Spinal delivery	Preservative-free morphine	Continuous infusion or bolus administration	AstramorphPH Duramorph Infumorph	0.5 and 1 mg/mL 0.5 and 1 mg/mL 10 mg/mL 25 mg/mL
Sustained-release oral opioids	Morphine	Twice daily	MS Contin, Oramorph	15, 30, 60, 100, and 200 mg tablets
	Morphine	Daily	Kadian	20, 50, and 100 mg capsules
	Oxycodone	Twice daily	OxyContin	10, 20, and 40 mg tablets
Transdermal delivery	Fentanyl	Every 3 days	Duragesic	25, 50, 75, and 100 μm patches
Transmucosal delivery	Fentanyl	As needed	Oralet (approved for use in surgical settings, shown to be safe and effective in cancer pain)	200, 300, or 400 μm lozenges attached to a plastic holder; to be available in higher doses soon

algesia. Tricyclic antidepressants are indicated in neuropathic pain, producing analgesic effects distinct from their antidepressant outcome. Because they sedate the patient, these drugs are often given at night to also enhance sleep. Starting doses typically are low to avoid excessive sedation and a "hung over" feeling; doses are increased gradually every 3 to 4 days. Contraindications include narrow angle glaucoma, symptomatic prostatic hypertrophy, and significant cardiovascular disease.

Clinicians disagree about the analgesic effects of newer, selective serotonin reuptake inhibitors (SSRIs). There are currently little data to support the use of SSRIs in relieving pain. In one exception, a controlled trial of paroxetine (Paxil) for diabetic neuropathy pain suggested that this agent may provide relief.

Local anesthetics and anticonvulsants inhibit sodium channels in sensory neurons, which reduces ectopic impulses generated by damage to peripheral nerves. These agents are of particular use in treating trigeminal neuralgia and neuropathic pain. Local anesthetics have been limited by the lack of an oral formulation. Topical application of lidocaine or other anesthetics is useful before invasive procedures, but only for a short duration. Epidural anesthetics, alone or in combination with an opioid, have proven successful; however, few patients are candidates for long-term epidural administration. Oral local anesthetics such as mexiletine can relieve continuous, lancinating neuropathic cancer-related pain apparently by stabilizing neuronal membranes (Dejgard, Petersen, & Kastrup, 1988). The starting dose of mexiletine is 150 mg orally at bedtime for 7 days and, if tolerated, is increased to 150 mg three times a day. If the relief is inadequate, the dose can be slowly escalated every 5 to 7 days to a maximum of 1200 mg/day. Side effects include arrhythmias, syncope, hypotension, ataxia, tremors, nervousness, upper gastrointestinal distress, dizziness, hepatotoxicity, skin rash, visual changes, fever, and chills (Mohamed, Mohamed, & Borsook, 1996).

Anticonvulsants include carbamazepine (Tegretol), phenytoin (Dilantin), and valproic acid (Depakene). Each has a distinct side effect profile that must be carefully weighed when considering these drugs. Anecdotal reports suggest a newer anticonvulsant, gabapentin (Neurontin), provides relief of neuropathic pain syndromes. The mechanism of this effect is unknown. Although its name suggests

TABLE 13-5 Adjuvant Analgesics

Drug	Approximate Adult Daily Dose Range	Route of Administration	Type of Pain
Corticosteroids			
Dexamethasone	16-96 mg	PO, IV	Pain associated with brain metastases and epidural spinal cord compression
Prednisone	40-100 mg	PO	
Anticonvulsants			
Carbamazepine	200-1,600 mg	PO	Neuropathic pain
Phenytoin	300-500 mg	PO	
Antidepressants			
Amitriptyline	25-15 mg	PO	Neuropathic pain
Doxepin	25-150 mg	PO	
Imipramine	20-100 mg	PO	
Trazodone	75-225 mg	PO	
Neuroleptics			
Methotrimeprazine	40-80 mg	IM	Analgesia; sedation; antiemetic
Antihistamines			
Hydroxyzine	300-450 mg	IM	Adjuvant to opioids in postoperative and other types of pain; relief of complicating symptoms including anxiety, insomnia, nausea
Local Anesthetics/Antiarrhythmics			
Lidocaine	5 mg/kg	IV/SC	Neuropathic pain
Mexiletine	450-600 mg	PO	
Tocainide	20 mg/kg	PO	
Psychostimulants			
Dextroamphetamine	5-10 mg	PO	Improve opioid analgesia, decrease sedation
Methylphenidate	10-15 mg	PO	

PO, By mouth; *IV,* intravenous; *IM,* intramuscular; *SC,* subcutaneous.
Reprinted from Jacox, A. et al. (1994). *Management of cancer pain.* Clinical practice guideline No. 9. AHCPR Publication No. 94-0592. Rockville, MD: Agency for Health Care Policy and Research, U.S. Department of Health and Human Services, Public Health Service, March, 1994.

γ-aminobutyric acid (GABA) activity, gabapentin does not bind significantly to GABA receptors. Case reports suggest the drug is useful in neuropathic pain at doses that range from 900 to 2400 mg/day (Mellick & Mellick, 1995). Case reports of lamotrigine (Lamictal) in the treatment of diabetic neuropathy are also promising, although controlled clinical trials are needed to establish the safety and analgesic efficacy of these agents in cancer pain.

Corticosteroids such as prednisone (40 to 100 mg/day) or dexamethasone (16 to 24 mg/day) are used to treat various cancer pain syndromes, including bone pain, neuropathic pain, headache associated with intracranial tumors, and pain resulting from tumor growth within the liver leading to expansion of the capsule. Pain relief may be due in part to reduction of edema surrounding the tumor. Improved mood and appetite and reduced nausea are additional benefits of corticosteroid therapy. Adverse effects (including hyperglycemia, dysphoria, and myopathy) are more prevalent with prolonged use. High-dose intravenous dexamethasone has been suggested for the treatment of severe, progressive neuropathic or bone pain that does not respond to opioids. A bolus dose of 100 mg is followed by 96 mg daily in divided doses.

Another adjuvant analgesic is capsaicin, an active ingredient in red chilies, which relies on the release of substance P from sensory nerve terminals. Capsaicin causes the release and depletion of substance P when applied topically. Substance P release initially causes a burning pain, but depletion is believed to reduce pain. Capsaicin is effective in the relief of postherpetic neuropathy, rheumatoid and osteoarthritis, and postmastectomy and postthoracotomy incisional pain syndromes.

Epidural clonidine, an α_2-adrenergic agonist, produces analgesia by mimicking the body's modulatory system. Now available commercially, epidural clonidine has been effective when given to postoperative and cancer patients; however, significant orthostatic hypotension can occur (Eisenach, DuPen, Dubois, Miguel, Allin & the Epidural Clonidine Study Group, 1995). Alternative α_2-adrenergic agonists that may produce fewer adverse effects are currently under investigation.

New agents are constantly being studied for safety and efficacy. Oncology nurses aware of new developments can provide optimal care to their patients.

Nonpharmacologic Therapies. Nonpharmacologic therapies to relieve pain include invasive procedures such as nerve blocks or surgical procedures, cognitive-behavioral strategies, and physical modalities. Examples of nerve blocks include injection of local anesthetics or lytic substances in the dorsal root ganglion (Raj, 1993). These procedures are effective for selected, usually well-localized pain problems. For example, a celiac plexus block is effective in the relief of pain in up to 90% of patients diagnosed with pancreatic cancer. Cognitive-behavioral strategies include relaxation exercises and hypnosis to reduce both the sensory and affective components of pain. Physical modalities include the use of heat, cold, vibration, massage, counterstimulation, and bracing to relieve pain (Spross & Burke, 1995). These nonpharmacologic measures are useful adjuncts to drug therapies and are rarely used alone in the relief of cancer-related pain.

Principles of Treatment. When developing a plan of care using the preceding pharmacologic and nonpharmacologic interventions, the World Health Organization three step ladder is a useful guide (Fig. 13-4) (World Health Organization, 1990). Other principles of pain management guide the use of these therapies (Box 13-2).

Nursing Management

In the management of pain, the role of the nurse is diverse and vital. Nurses are active participants in the entire clinical process of pain control. This process includes assessment, planning, actually administering the treatment in most cases, and evaluating the efficacy of pain therapies. The nurse works proactively to prevent and treat adverse effects associated with analgesics. The nurse documents the patient's pain and responses to treatment. In the treatment of pain, nurses often collaborate with physicians and other health care professionals and serve as advocates when patients' complaints of pain are not taken seriously.

Nurses are uniquely prepared to educate patients about biases toward pain medications, particularly fears of addiction and tolerance. In fact, merely providing permission to discuss these concerns can allay fears. Other essential nursing roles related to pain management include developing health care policies and conducting research.

Home Care Issues

Most pain management in cancer care is provided at home by the patient and family or support persons. This care often creates excess burden for support persons, with feelings of guilt, inadequacy, and frustration when pain is not well-managed (Johnston-Taylor, Ferrell, Grant, & Cheyney,

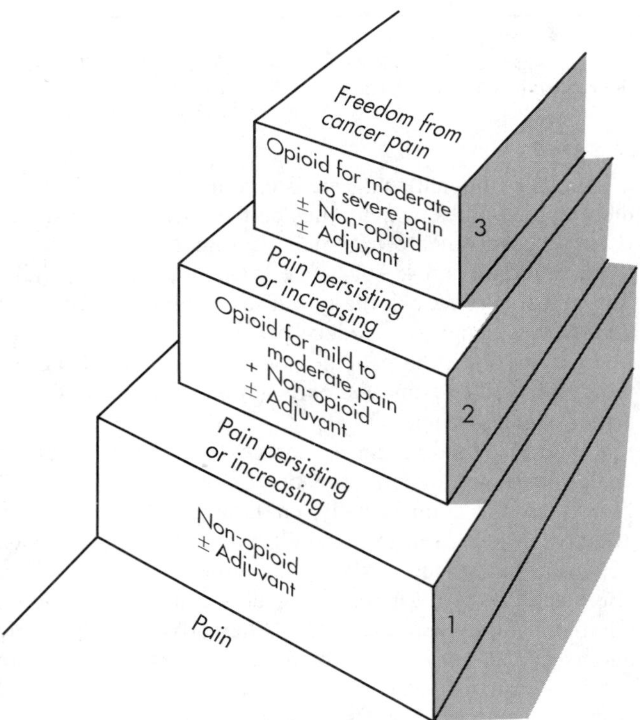

Fig. 13-4 World Health Organization three-step ladder. (Reprinted with permission from World Health Organization. [1990]. *Cancer pain relief and palliative care.* Geneva: World Health Organization.)

Box 13-2
Principles of Opioid Use

- Individualize the regimen to the patient.
- Use the simplest dosing schedules, and the least invasive and safest routes of opioid administration whenever possible, including oral, rectal and transdermal delivery.
- Avoid the intramuscular route of administration because this route is painful and absorption is unreliable.
- Avoid meperidine if continued opioid use is anticipated.
- Beginning doses for opioid naive patients in severe pain should be equal to 5 to 10 mg intramuscular morphine.
- Administer analgesics on an "around-the-clock" or fixed schedule to provide more stable plasma levels of drug.
- Rescue doses of an opioid, on an "as needed" basis, should be available to all patients for breakthrough pain. The rescue dose should equal approximately 5% to 15% of the 24-hour fixed schedule opioid dose.
- Switching routes, when necessary, should be performed gradually over a 2- to 3-day period.
- When converting from one opioid to another in patients with good pain control but significant side effects, reduce the dose to 50% to 75% of the equianalgesic dose.
- When converting from one opioid to another in patients with poor pain control and significant side effects, use 75% to 100% of the equianalgesic dose.
- When pain persists, opioid doses can be safely escalated in increments of 30% to 50% of the daily dose.
- Most patients taking opioids for pain relief should be given a stool softener and laxative regimen to prevent constipation and these doses should be increased as the opioid dose is increased.
- Placebos should not be used in cancer pain management.

From Cherny, N. I., & Portenoy, R. K. (1995). Systemic drugs for cancer pain. *Pain Digest, 5,* 235-263; Jacox, A. et al. (1994). *Management of cancer pain.* Clinical practice guideline No. 9. AHCPR Publication No. 94-0592. Rockville, MD: Agency for Health Care Policy and Research, U.S. Department of Health and Human Services, Public Health Service, March, 1994.

1993). Family members fear that they will cause their loved one to become addicted or that the medication will cause respiratory depression. These fears result in undermedication. Ill health or advanced age of caregivers is not uncommon, compounding these difficulties.

Professional support within the home is vital. The home care nurse can assess whether the analgesic regimen is being followed and whether fears present obstacles to good relief. Home care nurses can educate all caregivers and determine what other supports might be necessary, such as respite care or assistive devices. All members of the treatment team, including home care nurses, physicians, and others, must investigate the patient's and family members' goals and understanding of the disease. Only then can the health care professionals develop a treatment plan that includes competent pain control.

Evaluation of the Quality of Care

Nurses and other health care professionals should formally evaluate pain management practices including patient satisfaction with pain control. The American Pain Society published Quality Improvement (QI) Guidelines on Acute and Cancer-Related Pain (American Pain Society Quality of Care Committee, 1995). These standards require that patient satisfaction be measured; a recently updated tool has been released.

One of the difficulties in measuring patient satisfaction with pain management has been the incongruity between high satisfaction ratings and high pain intensity scores. In a survey of 72 hospitalized medical-surgical patients, the majority reported satisfaction with their pain treatment, although they also reported moderate to severe pain (Miaskowski, Nichols, Brody, & Synold, 1994). Ward and Gordon (1994) reported similar findings in a survey of 248 hospitalized patients. Mean pain intensity scores were high, but so was patient satisfaction with the pain management provided by clinicians. A 2-year follow-up study conducted by these investigators revealed similar findings: pain intensity ratings remained high, yet many patients were either satisfied or highly satisfied (Ward & Gordon, 1996). The reasons for these discrepancies are not clear, although a contributing factor may be low patient expectations.

Other aspects of quality pain management include evidence of patient education, documentation regarding assessment, response to therapy and other indicators, and adherence to treatment protocols.

Research Issues

There are many opportunities for research related to cancer pain. The mechanisms of pain are complex; their elucidation leads to more effective prevention and treatment. Further identification of the prevalence of cancer pain, as well as risk factors, is critical. New drugs and other treatments are currently under exploration, and this pursuit must be continued. As active participants in the research process, nurses can contribute to our understanding of cancer pain and its treatment.

FATIGUE

Fatigue is now recognized as a symptom of major importance in cancer. Patients complain of an overwhelming lack of energy that severely limits daily activities. Until recently, fatigue was poorly understood and health care professionals had little to offer to treat fatigue. Presently, more is known about fatigue, although much remains to be discovered.

Epidemiology and Risk Factors

Few studies have systematically evaluated the prevalence of fatigue in cancer patients. Blesch and colleagues (1991) found that 99% of a convenience sample of patients with breast and lung cancer complained of some degree of fatigue. In this study, fatigue was highly correlated with pain. Other studies have confirmed these findings. Risk factors associated with fatigue are also poorly defined. Physical risk factors include decreased hemoglobin, dehydration, electrolyte imbalances, and cancer treatment (e.g., surgery, chemotherapy, radiation therapy, and biotherapy). Psychosocial risk factors for fatigue are depression and anxiety. The patient's role within the family may place them at risk for fatigue, particularly single parents or others trying to work while undergoing therapy.

Ferrell, Grant, Dean, Funk, and Ly (1996) conducted an exploratory study using surveys, interviews, and focus groups of 910 cancer patients and survivors. Fatigue affected all aspects of quality of life, including physical, psychological, social, and spiritual well-being. Patients had difficulty differentiating fatigue related to disease from that associated with aging. In this study, pain increased fatigue and fatigue often lowered tolerance to pain. Patients often expressed frustration that fatigue was not taken seriously by health care professionals.

Prevention

Few studies examine the efficacy of interventions designed to prevent fatigue. Good sleep patterns, including regular times for sleep and rising, probably prevent fatigue. However, too much bed rest and sleep result in worsening fatigue and decreased functional status (Winningham, 1994). Exercise, rest, naps, adequate nutrition, and hydration may be helpful. A recent study confirms the role of moderate exercise in preventing fatigue associated with radiation therapy for breast cancer. Mock, Dow, Meares, Grimm, and Dienemann (1997) conducted an investigation of a moderate, self-paced walking program using two groups. The 46 female patients were randomly assigned to the walking program or usual care. Patients in the exercise group demonstrated physical and psychosocial benefits, including reduced fatigue, anxiety, depression, and improved sleep. Additional research is needed in the area of fatigue prevention.

Pathophysiology

The underlying pathophysiology of fatigue is complex and poorly understood. Abnormalities that produce altered nutrition, hydration, oxygenation, and biochemical markers may lead to fatigue. Multiple factors, rather than one single factor, probably contribute to fatigue in persons with cancer. Nutrients and electrolytes are altered by nausea, vomiting, diarrhea, and anorexia. Dehydration can also result from these syndromes, leading to fatigue. Oxygen intake is diminished in dyspnea and other respiratory syndromes, and decreased hemoglobin results in reduced oxygen delivery to the tissues. Biochemical factors include increases in tumor necrosis factor and interleukin-1, believed to contribute to fatigue. Although these factors may be elevated, there is no one biochemical marker for fatigue.

Assessment

Several tools have been developed to measure fatigue in research settings. These tools include the Functional Assessment of Cancer Therapy-Fatigue (FACT-F) (Yellen, Cella, Webster, Blendowski, & Kaplan, 1997), the Multidimensional Fatigue Inventory (Smets, Garssen, Bonke, & deHaes, 1995), the Piper Fatigue Scale (PFS) (Piper, 1993), and the Rhoton Fatigue Scale (Rhoten, 1982). Furthermore, several comprehensive tools include fatigue subscales such as the Profile of Mood States (POMS) (Shachman, 1983). A few of these tools may be of value in quantifying fatigue in the clinical setting. One major limitation of many of these tools for widespread clinical use is their excessive length, which could lead to respondent fatigue. An equally important limitation is that several of these tools rely on observations of the patient's behavior by health care professionals. Like pain, fatigue is a subjective phenomenon; therefore, self-report is the most valid measure. Similar to pain, a simple 0 to 10 scale is useful in measuring the intensity of fatigue, where 0 indicates no fatigue and 10 indicates the worst fatigue imaginable.

For a more comprehensive clinical tool, Winningham (1996) has developed a clinical assessment guide (Box 13-3) that also incorporates functional ability. The guide can be used by the oncology nurse to assess symptom distress associated with fatigue in persons with cancer.

Medical Management

Although universal and usually mild in persons without cancer (most oncology nurses would respond affirmatively if queried regarding the presence of fatigue), fatigue owing to malignancy or its treatment is not a trivial symptom. Fatigue may cause delays in cancer treatment; therefore, identification and management are critical. Management includes correction of metabolic abnormalities by administering supplemental potassium or magnesium, replacement of hemoglobin with infusion of blood products, and restoration of fluids through hydration. Recombinant human erythropoietin has also been administered to stimulate the production of red blood cells, reducing the need for transfusions (Case, Bukowski, Carey, Fishkin, Henry, Jacobson et al., 1993). Exercise plans incorporating low intensity activities such as walking can enhance energy (Winningham, 1996). Management of other symptoms, including pain, nausea, vomiting, anorexia, and depression, will reduce fatigue in most patients. Acknowledging the relationship between fatigue and depression mandates that depressed patients be treated with antidepressants and psychotherapy if fatigue is to be relieved.

Nursing Management

Nursing care of fatigued patients begins with assessment. The nurse should assess the physiologic and psychological aspects of fatigue, as well as social factors that may affect fatigue. Of particular concern is an assessment of the patient's home environment, daily responsibilities, and accessibility of support persons. After determining potential causes of fatigue, the nurse should develop a treatment plan in concert with other health care professionals, including physicians, physical and occupational therapists, psychologists, and others.

Education is critical. Nurses should explain the known causes of fatigue, the treatment plan, and the dangers of excessive bed rest. As with other symptoms, reassessment is also critical. As disease progresses or treatment changes, the intensity of fatigue may also change, necessitating modifications in the treatment plan. Coordination with professional and lay caregivers in the home is essential.

Home Care Issues

Nurses should assess the physical layout of the patient's home, as well as the need for assistive devices and support persons. Creative strategies must be developed to overcome obstacles such as stair climbing and the availability of bathrooms on floors not easily accessed by patients. Unsteady gait can be supported with assistive devices such as canes, walkers, bars in the bathroom, raised toilets, and braces. Family members may be recruited to assist in tasks, but this is difficult with today's geographic diversity of families and the limited time available to working mothers and fathers. Unskilled personnel may be hired to care for household tasks usually conducted by the patient. Unfortunately, few third-party payers cover these expenses.

Nurses need to maintain constant vigilance in the home regarding other symptoms that may enhance fatigue, including anorexia, nausea, and pain, and incorporate interventions for these symptoms into the treatment plan. Finally, psychological factors may become more apparent to nurses in the home. Education informs patients regarding the underlying causes of fatigue and possible treatment. However, fatigue brings deep meaning to many patients and family members. Inability to perform previously simple tasks is a potent reminder to the patient and caregivers of the cancer and all of its limitations on their lives. Cognitive reappraisal can assist in redefining the meaning of fatigue for the patient and family members.

Evaluation of the Quality of Care

Few quality improvement tools include assessment of fatigue or patient satisfaction with its treatment. This deficit highlights the lack of attention given this prevalent symptom

Box 13-3
Clinical Assessment Guide for Fatigue and Functioning

Background

Brief history of individual
1. Age
2. Gender
3. Cultural/lifestyle orientation
4. Role expectations
   - Occupation
   - Home
   - Social
   - Economic (insurance coverage)
   - Breadwinner?
   - Living with? Responsible for?
5. Normal activity patterns
6. Normal sleep patterns
7. Preexisting conditions
8. Diagnosis
9. Treatment regimen

Functional Work Output

Focus on changes
1. Are routine tasks getting harder?
2. Have you slowed down?
3. Have you stopped doing some things because of fatigue or any other symptom?

Changes in everyday activities
1. Are you capable of complete self-care?
2. Have you changed your bedtime? How much time do you spend in bed, resting, napping?
3. Are your activity-rest patterns changing?
4. Are you able to participate in family activities?
5. Are you making occupation-related changes?
6. Have you changed your social activities?
7. Have you changed your eating habits? Drinking habits?
8. Do you have any other health problems? Anything that affects your activity? (Consider need for referrals.)

Impairment/Pathophysiology

Diagnostic and laboratory tests
1. Decreased hemoglobin?
2. Hydration status?
3. Electrolyte imbalance? (potassium and magnesium!)

Preexisting conditions or disabilities?

Physical assessment—look for changes in:
1. Alertness and focus? Confusion, irritability, or short attention span?
2. Posture (slumped or erect)?
3. Gait, coordination, and balance (shuffle? steady pace? moving slowly and deliberately?)
4. Ability to arise from seated position?
   - Needs to use hands?
   - Able to rise rapidly from seated to standing position and keep balance?

Feelings Related to Fatigue

Describe sensation of fatigue
1. Ask specifically about no energy, tiredness, or exhaustion.
2. Ask about other symptoms (weakness, depression, dyspnea, pain, etc.).

Establish symptom burden
1. Check intensity of fatigue and related symptoms (get rating on fatigue and other prominent symptoms such as dyspnea, depression, weakness, pain).

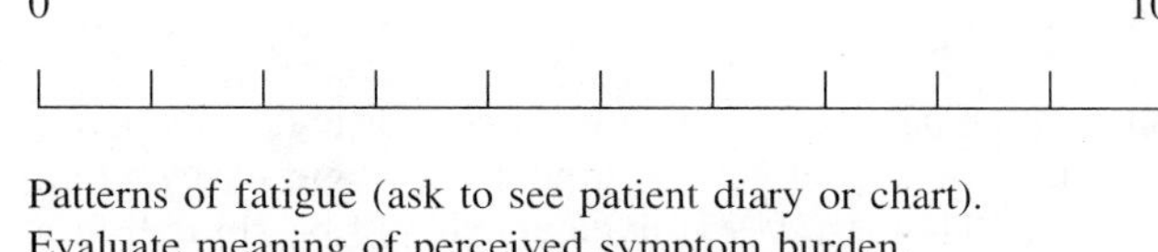

Patterns of fatigue (ask to see patient diary or chart).
Evaluate meaning of perceived symptom burden.
How do any of the above affect your quality of life?

From Winningham, M. L. (1996). Fatigue. In S. L. Groenwald, M. Goodman, M. H. Frogge, & C. H. Yarbro (Eds.), *Cancer symptom management*. Boston: Jones and Bartlett Publishers.

by health care professionals. Documentation of fatigue intensity alerts clinicians to the prevalence and severity of this syndrome, a first step toward changing practice. Intensity and satisfaction scales can be borrowed from the pain field, using a 0 to 10 scale to measure fatigue intensity and a 6-item Lickert scale to measure satisfaction with the treatment of fatigue (e.g., very satisfied, moderately satisfied, satisfied, dissatisfied, moderately dissatisfied, very dissatisfied).

Research Issues

Much research is needed to identify the underlying mechanisms of fatigue. Factors associated with fatigue should be defined, including laboratory values that might be predictors of fatigue. A better definition of fatigue is warranted and would assist clinicians in the differential diagnosis. Delineating fatigue from depression would ensure appropriate treatment of each of these syndromes. Finally, better methods for treating this prevalent problem are essential to good cancer care.

CONSTIPATION

Constipation is a frequent outcome of cancer and its treatment. Left untreated, reduced motility and constipation can lead to a serious bowel obstruction, nausea and vomiting, urinary retention, and cognitive impairment. Like pain, fatigue, and other symptoms, one difficulty in the identification of constipation is the lack of agreement on a definition of the problem. Normal bowel function varies greatly; therefore, abnormal conditions may be difficult to quantify. Constipation is generally defined as the passage of hard, dry stools, requiring straining and force, occurring with decreased frequency.

Epidemiology

The reported prevalence of constipation in cancer patients ranges from 23% to 45% (although the prevalence is probably closer to 100%); not surprising given the frequency of this syndrome in healthy individuals (Sykes, 1994; Vainio et al., 1996). This problem is apparent when viewing the laxative section within any retail pharmacy. Numerous commercial products and many more home remedies are used daily to treat constipation. Given the prevalence of this syndrome in the general population, it is surprising that constipation prevention and assessment are often overlooked within the health care system. Yet constipation can result in pain, nausea, vomiting, reduced food intake, trauma to the mucosa of the rectum and anus, and lethargy. In severe cases, constipation can lead to obstruction. Thus, good cancer care includes prevention and management of constipation.

Risk Factors

Constipation can be related to the cancer or can be iatrogenically induced. Constriction of the bowel by tumor, compression, or damage to the spinal cord at the T8-L3 level, hypercalcemia, hypokalemia, and hypothyroidism can all lead to constipation (Sykes, 1994). Iatrogenic causes include the administration of opioids, anticholinergic agents, tricyclic antidepressants, and some chemotherapeutic agents (such as vincristine). Box 13-4 lists many factors that lead to constipation.

Prevention

Constipation can usually be prevented, particularly when it is due to cancer treatment or a pharmacologic intervention (Wright & Thomas, 1995). Patients should be started on a bowel regimen consisting of laxatives and stool softeners whenever drugs known to cause constipation are administered. If practical, an exercise program can be instituted, as mild exercise is known to stimulate peristalsis. One can use glycerin suppositories or other lubricants to ease defecation and provide comfortable commodes and privacy whenever possible. Unfortunately, although causing great distress to patients, constipation is often overlooked and prophylactic treatment is rarely implemented (Sykes, 1994).

Box 13-4

Factors Leading to Constipation in the Cancer Patient

Dietary Changes

Low fiber
Reduced fluid intake

Pharmacologic Therapies

Antacids containing aluminum or calcium
Anticonvulsants
Antiemetics (5-HT_3 receptor antagonists)
Antihypertensives
Calcium supplements
Chemotherapeutics (e.g., vincristine, vinblastine, vinorelbine)
Diuretics
Iron supplements
Opioids
Phenothiazines
Tricyclic antidepressants

Complications of Cancer or Cancer Therapy

Ascites
Hypercalcemia
Hypokalemia
Obstruction of bowel by tumor
Spinal cord compression

Hospitalization

Lack of privacy within hospital
Altered timing in bowel routine
Use of bedpans
Reduced mobility and exercise

Related Conditions

Addison's disease
Confusion
Cushing's syndrome
Diabetes mellitus
Hemorrhoids, fissures
Hypothyroidism
Lead poisoning
Preexisting laxative dependence

Pathophysiology

Pathophysiologic mechanisms of constipation include altered strength of contractions within the intestines, poor muscle tone within the colon, and sensory changes within the rectum and anus, which make the individual unaware of the fecal mass. Weak propulsive contractions do not sufficiently push fecal material through the colon to the rectum. Conversely, strong contractions clamp down and block the flow of stool. Poor muscle tone inhibits sufficiently strong contractions to move stool toward the rectum. Finally, sensory changes in the anorectal area can occur from damage in the nervous system serving this area (Levy, 1991). Damage may be due to surgery, presence of tumor, fissures, or prolonged desensitization of nerves that occurs when individuals override the urge to defecate. If patients are not aware of rectal fullness and distension, they may not assist in the muscle movements necessary for defecation to take place (Sykes, 1994).

Assessment

Assessment for constipation begins with a thorough history of the patient's usual and current bowel habits (Box 13-5). The CAS is one tool that may assist in the clinical assessment of cancer-related constipation (McMillan & Williams, 1989). After the history is obtained, a physical examination should be conducted, including palpation of the abdomen, auscultation for bowel sounds, and digital examination of the rectum. The rectal examination includes exploration of

Box 13-5
Assessment of Constipation in the Cancer Patient

Past History

Past frequency of bowel movements
Character of the stool (soft, formed, inspissated)
Volume of stool
Chronic use of laxatives or softeners
Other measures used to enhance bowel function

Present History

Date of last bowel movement
Whether patient had to strain or use suppositories or enemas to defecate
Character of stool (soft, formed, inspissated)
Presence of abdominal fullness and gas
Volume of stool eliminated

Physical Examination

Abdominal palpation
Rectal examination

Radiographic Evaluation

Flat plate of abdomen

the rectum for the presence of stool as well as determination of the muscle tone of the anal sphincter. During the rectal examination, observe the anus for fissures, hemorrhoids, and other lesions that may cause painful defecation or alter sphincter function. Bruera and colleagues (1994) suggest obtaining an abdominal radiograph in terminally ill patients to allow faster diagnosis of constipation, because the accuracy of present history and diagnostic techniques is inadequate.

Medical Management

Constipation can be prevented in most cases. Because prevention is often overlooked, treatment of constipation is often necessary. This treatment includes pharmacologic therapies, physical measures, and dietary changes.

Pharmacologic Therapies. The pharmacologic agents used to treat constipation are listed in Table 13-6, and a protocol for treatment is depicted in Fig. 13-5. Few studies have been conducted that compared the efficacy of one treatment with another. In general, the caliber of the stool dictates the type of agents to be used. Soft stool that is difficult to expel demands a laxative. Frequent, firm stools would benefit from a softening agent. Most patients, particularly those experiencing opioid-induced constipation, have both inspissated and infrequent stools that require a combination of laxatives and stool softeners.

When constipation occurs owing to opioids and all other standard therapies have been ineffective, naloxone can be administered orally. Orally administered naloxone has low systemic bioavailability and is believed to relieve constipation by binding to opioid receptors within the enteric wall. This binding antagonizes the constipating effects of opioids. Two studies report beginning oral naloxone doses at 0.4 or 0.5 mg, respectively, with upward titration as needed (Sykes, 1996; Culpepper-Morgan, Intarrisi, Portenoy, Foley, Houde, Marsh et al., 1992). Sykes (1996) observed withdrawal symptoms in two patients at doses of 5 mg. Culpepper-Morgan and colleagues (1992) recommended a maximum dose of 12 mg administered no more than every 6 hours to prevent withdrawal. Therefore oral naloxone should be reserved only for patients who do not respond to laxatives, suppositories, and enemas, because of cost and the possibility that opioid withdrawal symptoms may occur.

Several agents have little role in relieving cancer-related constipation. Bulk laxatives, often containing psyllium or methylcellulose, increase the weight of the stool. This therapy requires a significant increase in fluid intake, however, and is more useful in treating mild constipation. Chronic use of oral mineral oil also should be avoided, as it coats the lining of the gastrointestinal tract and prevents absorption of vitamins, particularly the fat-soluble vitamins. Furthermore, mineral oil may cause anal leakage or incontinence of stool, particularly in the weak and elderly. Finally, mineral oil should not be administered to weak patients who are recumbent, or to anyone who is at risk for aspiration, as lipoid pneumonia may result (Levy, 1991).

Nonpharmacologic Therapies

Physical Measures. Physical measures include enemas and disimpaction. Because these procedures can be extremely painful, they should be used only when pharmacologic interventions are ineffective. When necessary, efforts should be made to reduce the pain and discomfort, including the use of lubricants and analgesics. Soap suds enemas, a therapy in favor several decades ago, is no longer recommended owing to the potential for local irritation and electrolyte imbalance.

Dietary Changes. Dietary changes may help prevent mild constipation, but are of questionable value in treating severe cases. Increased fiber intake is often recommended, but fluid intake must also be increased for fiber to be effective. Furthermore, high fiber foods may not be well tolerated by very ill patients. Several home preparations have been advocated. These generally consist of prunes, bran, senna, and other compounds; most of these recipes have not been adequately tested for their ability to prevent or relieve constipation. One pilot study of a bran-based pudding in 16 homebound elderly patients with varying diagnoses revealed an increase in the number of weekly bowel movements (Neal, 1995) (Box 13-6).

Nursing Management

Nursing care consists of prevention whenever possible, as well as comfort measures while patients undergo treatment for constipation. Nurses determine risk factors and assess for the existence of constipation. Nurses also educate patients regarding risks, prevention, and treatment strategies. Nurses can also provide the appropriate environment, including privacy, commodes, and other positioning measures, to assist defecation.

TABLE 13-6 Management of Constipation in the Cancer Patient

Category	Mechanisms of Action	Example	Onset of Action	Comments
Bulk forming	Absorbs water; increases bulk, thereby stimulating peristalsis	Metamucil, Perdiem, Konsyl, Hydrocil	Usually within 24 hr	Contraindicated in patients with abdominal pain, nausea, and vomiting and in patients suspected of having appendicitis, biliary tract obstruction, or acute hepatitis; needs to be taken with fluids
Stimulants	Increase peristalsis by irritating colon wall and stimulating enteric nerves	Antraquinone drugs Cascara sagrada, senna Phenolphthalein drugs Ex-Lax, Correctol, Feen-a-Mint, Bisacodyl, Dulcolax	Usually within 12 hr	Cause melanosis coli (brown or black pigmentation of colon), are most widely abused laxatives; should not be used in patients with impaction or obstipation
Stool softeners and lubricants	Lubricate intestinal tract and soften feces, making hard stools easier to pass; do not affect peristalsis	Mineral oil, dioctyl sodium, sulfosuccinate, Colace, Peri-Colace, Doxidan	Softeners up to 72 hr, lubricants up to 8 hr	Can block absorption of fat-soluble vitamins such as vitamin K, which may increase risk of bleeding in patients on anticoagulants
Saline and osmotic solutions	Cause retention of fluid in intestinal lumen caused by osmotic effect	Magnesium salts Magnesium citrate, Milk of Magnesia Sodium phosphates Fleets enema, Phospho-soda Lactulose Polyethylene glycol-saline solutions Go-Lytely, Colyte	15 min to 3 hr	Magnesium-containing products may cause hypermagnesemia in patients with renal insufficiency

From Lewis, S. (1996). *Medical-surgical nursing.* St Louis: Mosby.

Comfort measures during painful bowel movements, enemas, or disimpactions are essential. Glycerin suppositories or water-soluble jellies lubricate the rectum and anus, preventing fissures or tears. Topical anesthetics may be applied to reduce pain. Systemic opioids may be administered to relieve pain, and benzodiazepines may help relax and alleviate cramping (Curtiss, 1996). Abdominal cramping also may be reduced by heat or massage. In fact, massage in a clockwise motion following the ascending, transverse, and descending colon may be useful in stimulating peristalsis. Skin care after defecation is essential. Fecal material should be completely removed to prevent excoriation, and lotions, creams, or barriers applied to reduce exposure of the skin to stool.

Home Care Issues

Prevention of constipation is even more important in the home care setting, as many of the treatments used to relieve constipation may prove difficult for caregivers. For example, very weak or elderly patients may be too immobile to place a suppository and their elderly caregivers may also be unable to physically position the patient for suppository placement or administration of an enema. Bedside commodes, elevated toilet seats, and other assistive devices may provide greater comfort and safety. Hospital beds may be of benefit to nonambulatory patients, as they are not as low as most beds in the home; caregivers would not have to bend as deeply to provide care. Education in the home is imperative, including the importance of prevention and strategies for relief.

Evaluation of the Quality of Care

Constipation is often neglected in quality improvement tools. Inpatient records and outpatient charts should demonstrate evidence of patient teaching regarding prevention and

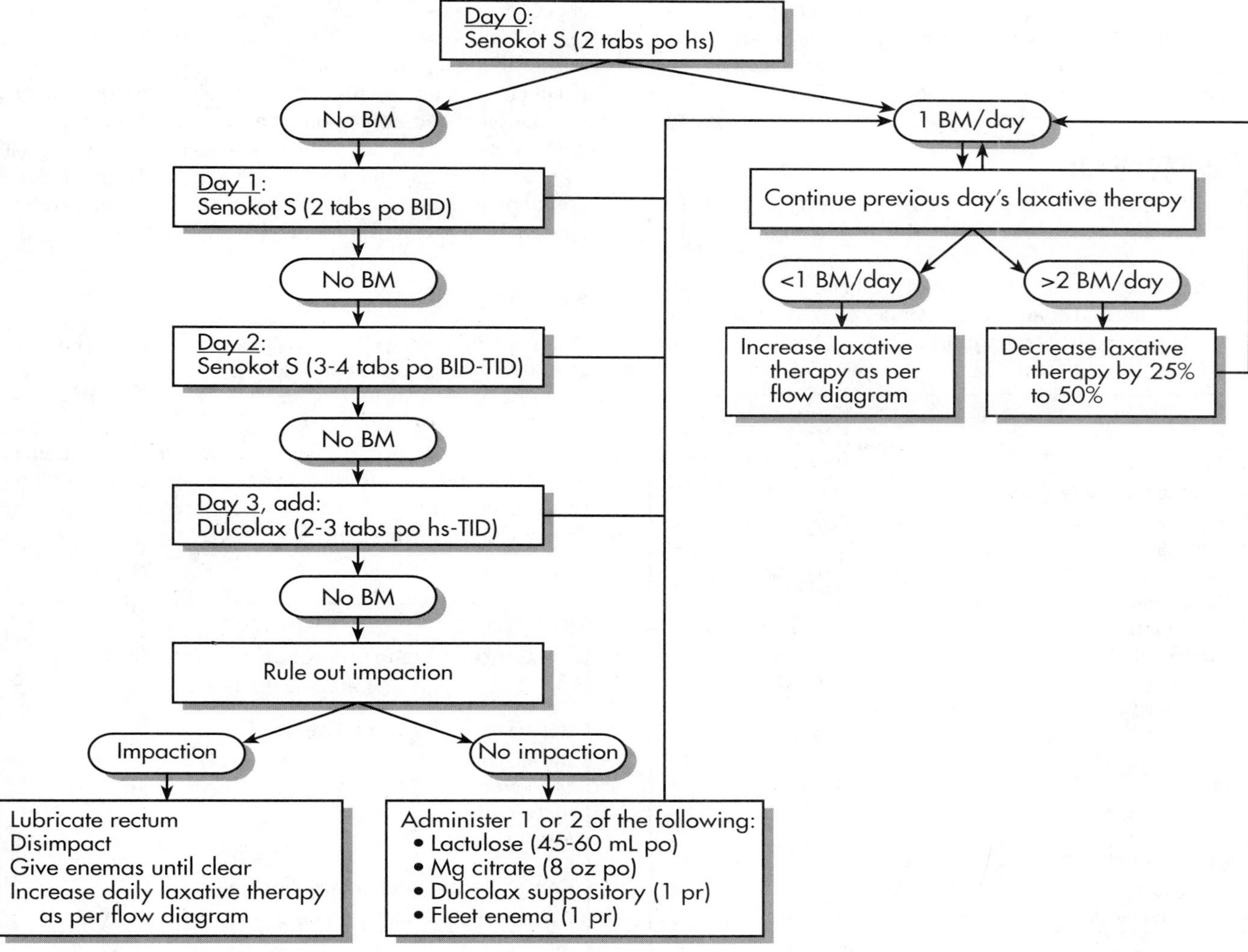

Fig. 13-5 Protocol for the treatment of cancer-related constipation. NOTE: *Tabs,* tablets; *po,* per os; *hs,* bedtime; *BM,* bowel movement; *BID,* twice a day; *TID,* three times a day; *Mg,* magnesium; *pr,* per rectum. (Reprinted with permission from Levy, M. H. (1991). Constipation and diarrhea in cancer patients. *Cancer Bulletin, 43,* 412-422.)

treatment of constipation. Protocols designed to treat pain should include the administration of a bowel regimen whenever opioids are ordered. Finally, patients should be queried regarding their satisfaction with constipation prevention and management in the same manner that the quality of pain management is evaluated.

Research Issues

Future research should compare the most effective agents and protocols in the prevention and treatment of constipation. The efficacy of nonpharmacologic treatments should also be evaluated, including diet, massage, and complementary treatments.

Box 13-6
Recipe for "Power Pudding" for Relief of Constipation

½ cup prune juice (if needed to blend only)
½ cup applesauce*
½ cup wheat bran flakes
½ cup whipped topping*
½ cup canned stewed prunes
Blend ingredients, cover, and refrigerate, and keep as long as 1 week. Take ¼ cup portions of recipe with breakfast.

*Diabetics may use "no added sugar" applesauce and "light" whipped topping.

From Neal, L. J. (1995). "Power pudding": natural laxative therapy for the elderly who are homebound. *Home Healthcare Nurs, 13,* 66-71.

DYSPNEA

Dyspnea is an unpleasant sensation of breathlessness or awareness of breathing. It is an extremely distressing symptom to both patients and their caregivers. Dyspnea can occur during all phases of cancer care, but is most frequent during the end of life. Treatment entails pharmacologic and nonpharmacologic interventions.

Epidemiology

Studies of dyspnea in cancer have primarily evaluated its prevalence in later stages of the disease. In an investigation of patients presenting to an emergency department in a large cancer hospital, the prevalence of dyspnea was 11.1% (Escalante, Martin, Elting, Cantor, Harle, & Price et al., 1996). In a study of patients with prostate, colon, breast, or ovarian cancer, shortness of breath occurred in 22.9% (Portenoy et al., 1994). Conversely, in a study of 1500 cancer patients during the last 6 weeks of life, 70% experienced dyspnea (Reuben & Mor, 1986). As one might expect, 90% of a population of end-stage, non-small-cell lung cancer patients complained of dyspnea (Muers & Round, 1993). As with pain and other symptoms, dyspnea is probably underreported by patients and frequently missed by health care professionals (Roberts, Thorne, & Pearson, 1993).

Risk Factors

Patients with primary or metastatic disease to the lungs are at significant risk for the development of dyspnea, followed by those with a history of cardiac or pulmonary disease (Dudgeon & Rosenthal, 1996). Escalante and colleagues (1996) found that 37% of persons presenting to the emergency department with dyspnea had lung cancer, 30% had breast cancer, and 34% had other cancers. In patients with breast cancer, pleural effusions were the most common

Box 13-7
Causes of Dyspnea

Dyspnea Directly Due to Cancer

Pulmonary parenchymal involvement (primary or metastatic)
Lymphangitic carcinomatosis
Intrinsic or extrinsic airways obstruction by tumor
Pleural tumor
Pleural effusion
Pericardial effusion
Ascites
Hepatomegaly
Phrenic nerve paralysis
Multiple tumor microemboli
Pulmonary leukostasis
Superior vena cava syndrome

Dyspnea Indirectly Due to Cancer

Cachexia
Electrolyte abnormalities
Anemia
Pneumonia
Pulmonary aspiration
Pulmonary emboli
Neurologic paraneoplastic syndromes

Dyspnea Due to Cancer Treatment

Surgery
Radiation therapy
Chemotherapy-induced pulmonary disease
Chemotherapy-induced cardiomyopathy

Dyspnea Unrelated to Cancer

Chronic obstructive pulmonary disease
Asthma
Congestive heart failure
Interstitial lung disease
Pneumothorax
Anxiety
Chest wall deformity
Obesity
Neuromuscular disorders
Pulmonary vascular disease

From Dudgeon, D. J., & Rosenthal, S. (1996). Management of dyspnea and cough in patients with cancer. *Hematology/Oncology Clinics of North America, 10,* 157-171.

Box 13-8
Cancer Chemotherapeutic Agents That May Cause Dyspnea

Hypersensitivity Lung Disease

Bleomycin
Methotrexate
Procarbazine
Mitomycin

Noncardiogenic Pulmonary Edema

Cytosine arabinoside
Methotrexate
Teniposide
Ifosfamide
Cyclophosphamide

Chronic Pneumonitis/Pulmonary Fibrosis

Bleomycin
Methotrexate
Busulfan
Cyclophosphamide
Carmustine (BCNU)
Mitomycin
Ifosfamide
Fludarabine

Congestive Heart Failure

Doxorubicin
Daunorubicin
Mitoxantrone
Amsacrine
Estrogens
Progestins
Androgens

From Dudgeon, D. J., & Rosenthal, S. (1996). Management of dyspnea and cough in patients with cancer. *Hematology/Oncology Clinics of North America, 10,* 157-171.

cause (31%) of dyspnea. Causes of dyspnea have been classified as those directly due to tumor, those related to treatment, and those indirectly associated with cancer (Box 13-7). In addition to the obstructive effect of tumors, cancer chemotherapeutic agents can produce dyspnea (Box 13-8). In an investigation of the seriously ill, many of whom had cancer, dyspnea occurred in 48.6% of those studied. In this study, nausea and dyspnea were related to pain intensity, although the causal relationship between these three symptoms is not clear (Desbiens, Mueller-Rizner, Connors, & Wenger, 1997).

Prevention

Because there are many associated factors, it is unlikely that dyspnea can be completely prevented at this time. However, early detection and treatment can prevent the worsening of symptoms. Additionally, aggressive management of pain, nausea, and other symptoms may delay the onset of dyspnea or reduce its severity.

Pathophysiology

Breathing is regulated through the interaction of the respiratory center in the brain stem, central respiratory receptors in the medulla, peripheral respiratory receptors in the carotid and aortic bodies, and the respiratory muscles (Ripamonti & Bruera, 1997) (Fig. 13-6). Three pathophysiologic mechanisms for dyspnea have been proposed: (1) respiratory effort increases to overcome obstruction, effusion, or restrictive lung disease; (2) a greater proportion of respiratory muscle is required to preserve normal function; and (3) ventilatory requirements increase owing to hypoxemia, acidosis, anemia, and other factors (Ripamonti & Bruera, 1997). One or more of these mechanisms may contribute to the dyspnea seen in patients with cancer.

Assessment

A complete assessment of dyspnea is critical, as some causes are potentially reversible (Box 13-9). The assessment of dyspnea begins with a thorough history, although this may present a challenge if patients are in extreme distress. Family members and caregivers may be of assistance at this time; however, there may be errors in their report owing to the subjective nature of this symptom. Factors to consider include the onset of dyspnea (acute or chronic), words used to describe the sensation (e.g., tight, heavy, suffocating), precipitating events, and associated symptoms. Past history should consist of the details associated with cancer, any past or concurrent medical diseases (particularly cardiac and pulmonary disorders), and smoking history. A confused, agitated mental status may denote dyspnea that is significant enough to lead to cerebral anoxia.

As with all other symptoms, the most reliable measure of dyspnea is the patient's self-report. The magnitude of dyspnea can be rated using a 0 to 10 or 0 to 100 scale. Other scales have been used, but are probably more useful in measuring chronic dyspnea or for research settings (Ripamonti & Bruera, 1997; van der Molen, 1995). Regardless of the availability of these tools, no one scale measures all of the essential components of dyspnea in patients with cancer.

After a thorough history, the physical examination is essential. This examination includes a general review of systems, with attention given to the patient's general condition. Weak, cachectic patients are at risk for developing dys-

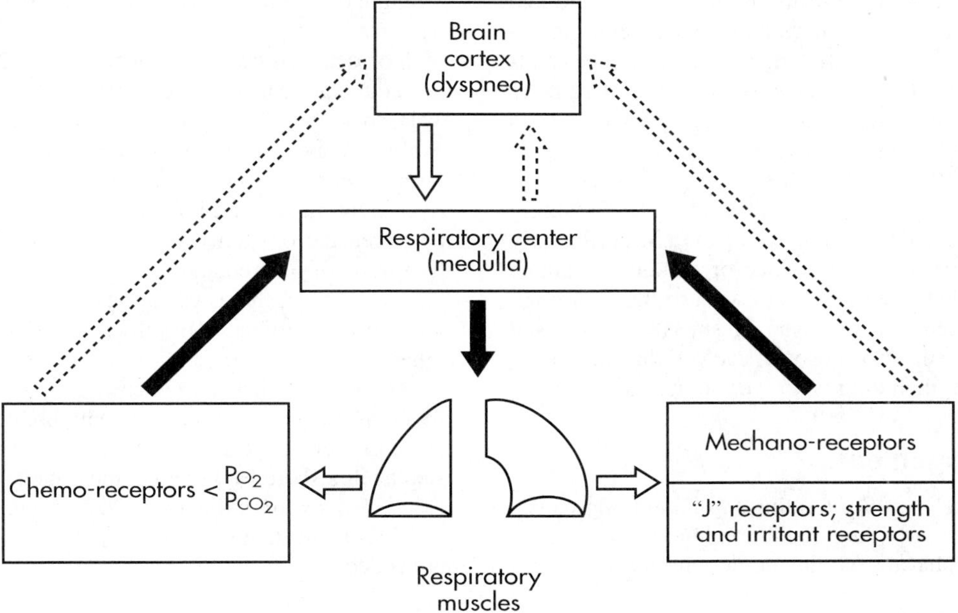

Fig. 13-6 Mechanisms of normal respiration. (Drawing adapted from original by Gail Wilkes. Reprinted with permission from Ripamonti, C., & Bruera, E. [1997]. Dyspnea: pathophysiology and assessment. *Journal of Pain and Symptom Management, 13,* 220-232.)

Box 13-9
Assessment of Dyspnea

Mental status
- Clear?
- Confused?
- Panicked?

Cyanosis?
- (Blood gases)

Cardiovascular status
- Hypotensive?
- Peripheral vasoconstriction?
- Ambulatory?
- Edema?

Pulmonary status
- Secretory/airway problems
- Air movement
- Rales
  - Segmented
  - Generalized
- Wheezes/bronchospasm
- (Chest x-ray)

Environment
- Receiving oxygen?
- Climbing stairs?
- Distance to toilet
- Temperature
- Air quality
  - Humidity
  - Irritants
- Medication compliance
- Caregiver stress

pnea. Moderate to severe dyspnea is associated with tachypnea and tachycardia. Observe the thorax for the rate and rhythm of respiration, as well as skin and mucous membranes for cyanosis. Auscultate lungs for the presence of effusions, bronchoconstriction, rales, or wheezing. Chest radiographs, pulse oximetry, and pulmonary function tests may reveal possible causes of dyspnea.

Assessment of the home is critical, including environmental and psychosocial factors that might alter breathing (Storey, 1994). Consider the quality of the air, particularly the degree of humidity and presence of irritants. Evaluate the temperature, distance required to walk to the bathroom, and whether oxygen is being used (if so, is it being used correctly?). Weigh the psychosocial factors that may contribute to dyspnea, including caregiver anxiety and fatigue.

Medical Management

Dyspnea can be relieved by treating the underlying cause, when possible, or providing palliation. Palliation can be achieved through pharmacologic and nonpharmacologic interventions.

Pharmacologic Therapies. Opioids are the most effective treatment for dyspnea in the patient with cancer. Bruera and colleagues (1990) systematically studied the effects of subcutaneous morphine on dyspnea in terminally ill cancer patients. In this open-labeled clinical trial, 95% of patients reported improvement in dyspnea with no significant decrease in respiratory function, including respiratory rate, effort, oxygen saturation, or respiratory carbon dioxide. A later, controlled trial supported the beneficial effects of subcutaneous morphine without respiratory depression (Bruera, MacEachern, Ripamonti, & Hanson, 1993).

Suggested opioid doses start at 2.5 to 5 mg of morphine for opioid naive patients (Bruera, Macmillan, Pither, MacDonald, Pither, & MacDonald, 1990). Dose increases for non-naïve patients range from 30% to 50% every 12 to 24 hours (Storey, 1994) or to increase the usual dose by 2.5 times (Bruera et al., 1990). Patients who are dyspneic may be unable to swallow pills or tablets; alternative routes, such as liquids, transdermal, or parenteral delivery can ease administration of the drug. Anecdotal reports suggest that nebulized morphine is an effective method for reducing dyspnea (Famcombe & Chater, 1993), although controlled clinical trials comparing nebulized with systemic morphine are needed.

Other pharmacologic therapies include corticosteroids, adrenergic antagonists, and benzodiazepines. Corticosteroids may limit airway obstruction by reducing edema and inflammation around the tumor. These are useful second line agents that can be administered as adjuncts to opioids. Although some individuals recommend bronchodilators or adrenergic agonists, these agents can also produce an elevated heart rate and tremors that worsen the patient's condition. Benzodiazepines do not reduce dyspnea directly; rather these drugs decrease the anxiety that so often accompanies dyspnea. Short-acting benzodiazepines such as lorazepam are preferred. Lorazepam can be given orally or by the sublingual route if the patient is unable or too weak to swallow (Storey, 1994). Midazolam, given subcutaneously or intravenously, has been added to the opioid to reduce the terminal agitation and anxiety that is frequently associated with dyspnea.

Nonpharmacologic Therapies. The use of oxygen in reducing dyspnea is controversial. Bruera, de Stoutz, Velasco-Leiva, Schoeller, and Hanson (1993) prospectively evaluated the effects of supplemental oxygen compared with air in a crossover study. Both oxygen and air were delivered by mask in a blinded fashion. Twelve of 14 patients preferred the oxygen. Conversely, a single-blind, prospective study of oxygen and air revealed that although both reduced dyspnea, there was no statistically significant difference in their efficacy (Booth, Kelly, Cox, Adams, & Guz, 1996).

Acupuncture has also been reported to reduce dyspnea. In an open study of 20 patients with breathlessness, 70% reported relief of symptoms, there was a reduction in the visual analog score for breathlessness, and respiratory rate decreased for approximately 90 minutes after treatment (Filshie, Penn, Ashley, & Davis, 1996). Additional research is needed.

Nursing Management

Several nursing measures can provide comfort to the person experiencing dyspnea. Position the patient upright on the edge of the bed, or sit the patient up with arms resting on an overbed table. A fan directed toward the patient's face is often comforting, reducing the sensation of breathlessness (Kerr, 1989). Deep or pursed lip breathing slows respirations, making breathing more efficient and less tiring. Relaxation techniques and a calm, soothing environment may also be effective in reducing anxiety. A recent randomized study of lung cancer patients with breathlessness revealed that a nurse-run clinic providing relaxation, coping strategies, and other rehabilitation techniques significantly reduced breathlessness (Comer, Plant, Hem, & Bailey, 1996).

Home Care Issues

As discussed earlier, thorough assessment of dyspnea demands evaluation of psychosocial and environmental factors in the home. Home care nurses are uniquely prepared to assess and plan for those factors that can be modified. Safety concerns must be addressed when educating patients and their caregivers regarding the use of oxygen in the home. Observing dyspnea in a loved one is extremely distressing; therefore, family support is critical. This support may include respite care and more frequent visits by support staff.

Research Issues

Much research is needed to clarify the most effective pharmacologic and nonpharmacologic treatments in the relief of dyspnea. Randomized, controlled clinical trials are difficult to initiate in patients with dyspnea; however, it is only by comparing treatments that optimal therapies can be identified.

NAUSEA AND VOMITING

As with the previous symptoms, nausea and vomiting can be related directly to the cancer, to cancer treatment, or to causes unrelated to cancer. These symptoms can be physically and emotionally devastating to patients and their family and, as a result, demand prompt recognition and treatment.

Epidemiology and Risk Factors

Studies have demonstrated the prevalence of nausea and/or vomiting. Of course, if treated with certain chemotherapeutic regimen without antiemetic pretreatment, almost 100% of patients would experience nausea and vomiting. Fortunately, effective antiemetics can prevent or manage nausea and vomiting in the majority of these patients. The emetogenic potential of various chemotherapeutic agents is listed in Table 13-7.

Nausea and vomiting that occur immediately after chemotherapy administration is described as acute. Delayed nausea and vomiting can occur with several chemotherapeutic agents; this is typically defined as nausea and vomiting occurring 24 hours after drug administration. In a recent study of 327 patients receiving diverse chemotherapeutic regimens, 33% reported delayed nausea, and 26% experienced delayed vomiting (Morrow, Hickok, Burish, & Rosenthal, 1996). Anticipatory nausea and vomiting generally occur after several cycles of chemotherapy. Patients begin to feel nauseated and may vomit before actually receiving the chemotherapeutic agent. Patients at risk for anticipatory nausea and vomiting include female patients, patients under 40 years of age, those receiving high doses of cisplatin, and individuals with a prior susceptibility to nausea and vomiting, such as motion sickness.

Many other cancer therapies and conditions are associated with nausea and vomiting. Radiotherapy to the upper abdomen may produce nausea and vomiting as can antibiotics given for sepsis. The prevalence rates for nausea and vomiting in general cancer populations vary widely. Portenoy and colleagues discovered that 44.7% of 218 cancer patients experienced nausea, whereas 21.1% experienced vomiting (Portenoy, 1996). Nineteen percent of a sample of hospitalized advanced cancer patients experienced nausea, with ovarian cancer patients having the greatest prevalence at 56% (Brescia, Adler, Gray, Ryan, Cimino, & Mamtani, 1990). In patients admitted to a palliative care unit, 32% had nausea that required treatment, whereas nausea was the primary reason for admission in 2% (Bruera, Seifert, Watanabe, Babul, Darke, Harsanyi et al., 1996). Furthermore, during their stay in the palliative care unit, 98% of patients developed nausea that required treatment. Etiologies often include obstruction of the intestinal lumen by tumor or administration of opioids and other agents that may produce nausea and vomiting.

Prevention

Nausea and vomiting should be prevented whenever feasible. Examples of prevention include administering antiemetics before chemotherapy known to be emetogenic. The patient who has a prior history of nausea and vomiting after receiving an opioid should be given antiemetics before the next dose of an opioid and for the next several days. The antiemetic dose can then be tapered to determine if the patient has developed tolerance to the emetic effect of the opioid.

Pathophysiology

Many mechanisms are responsible for nausea and vomiting (Fig. 13-7). The chemoreceptor trigger zone (CTZ) in the area postrema is activated by substances within the blood and cerebrospinal fluid. Emetic stimuli acting on dopamine receptors within the CTZ include drugs (such as chemotherapeutic agents, opioids, hormones), hypercalcemia, and toxins from tumor breakdown products or infectious organisms. Visceral activation occurs when tumor compresses or obstructs the gastrointestinal tract or other abdominal organs. Distension, constipation, and obstruction can also produce visceral disturbances that cause nausea and vomiting. Vestibular effects include motion-induced nausea and vomiting, tumors affecting the vestibular system (intracranial lesions and acoustic neuroma), and certain drugs such as aspirin and opioids. Finally, other factors can result in nausea and vomiting, including severe pain, infection, and emotional responses.

Table 13-7 Emetogenic Potential of Cancer Chemotherapeutic Agents

Emetic Potential	Agent/Dose (mg/m^2)	Onset (Latency: Hours)	Reported Duration (Hours)
Very High: >90%	Cisplatin ≥75mg	1-6	48-72+
	Nitrogen mustard	0.5-2	6-24
	Streptozotocin	1-6	12-24
	Dacarbazine ≥500 mg	0.5-6	6-24
	Cyclophosphamide >1 g	4-12	12-24+
	Cytarabine >500-1000 mg	1-4	12-24
	Carmustine ≥200 mg	2-6	4-24
	Melphalan, high dose	0.3-6	6-12
	Lomustine ≥60 mg	4-6	12-24
High: 60%-90%	Cisplatin <75 mg	1-6	48-72
	Dacarbazine <500 mg	1-6	6-24
	Cyclophosphamide <1 g	4-12	12-24+
	Cytarabine 250-500 mg	2-4	12-24
	Carmustine <200 mg	2-6	4-24
	Lomustine <60 mg	4-6	12-24
	Doxorubicin ≥75 mg	4-6	6-24+
	Methotrexate ≥200 mg	4-12	3-24+days
	Procarbazine	24-72	variable
	Etoposide, high dose	4-6	12-24
	Ifosfamide	—	—
	Carboplatin	4-9	12-48
Moderate: 30%-60%	Cyclophosphamide <750 mg	4-12	12-24+
	Fluorouracil ≥1000 mg	3-6	24+
	Doxorubicin	4-6	6-24+
	Daunorubicin	2-6	24
	Asparaginase	—	—
	Cytarabine 20-200 mg	2-4	12-24
	Methotrexate >100 mg	4-6	6+
	Mitoxantrone	1-4	48-72
	Mitomycin	1-6	2-12
	Teniposide	—	—
Moderately Low: 10%-30%	Fluorouracil <1000 mg	—	—
	Doxorubicin ≤20 mg	—	—
	Cytarabine ≤20 mg	3-12	—
	Etoposide	3-8	6-12
	Melphalan	6-12	—
	Vinblastine	4-8	—
	Hydroxyurea	—	—
	Bleomycin	3-6	—
	Melphalan	6-12	—
	Mercaptopurine	4-8	—
	Methotrexate <100 mg	4-12	3-12
	Paclitaxel	—	—
Low: <10%	Vincristine	4-8	—
	Busulfan	—	—
	Chlorambucil	4-12	—
	Thioguanine	—	—
	Cyclophosphamide (oral)	—	—
	Thiotepa	—	—
	Hormones	—	—
	Steroids	—	—

From Wickham, R. (1996). Nausea and vomiting. In S. L. Groenwald, M. Goodman, M. H. Frogge, & C. H. Yarbro (Eds.), *Cancer symptom management.* Boston: Jones and Bartlett Publishers.

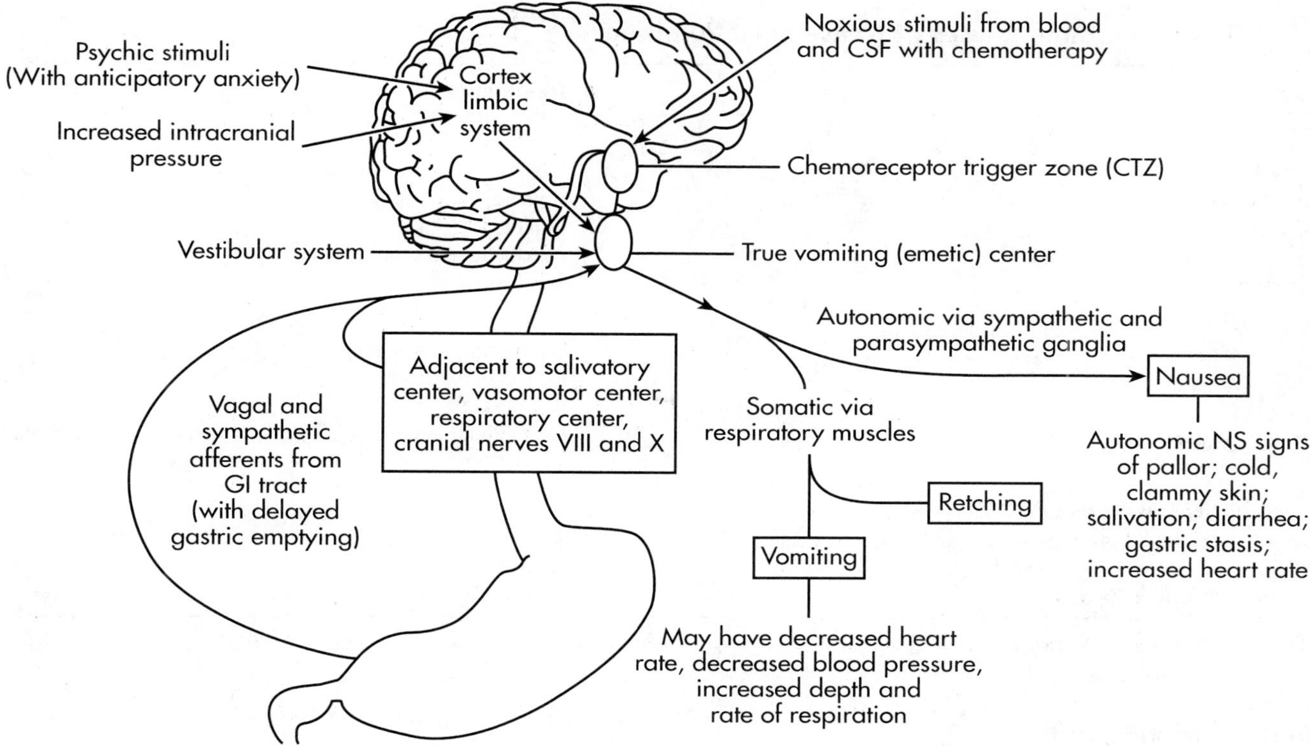

Fig. 13-7 Mechanisms of cancer-related nausea and vomiting. (Reprinted with permission from Wilkes, G. M., Ingwersen, K., & Burke, M. B. [1997]. *1997-1998 Oncology nursing drug handbook.* Boston: Jones and Bartlett Publishers.)

TABLE 13-8 Opioid-Induced Nausea and Vomiting

Inferred Mechanism	Clinical Features	Antiemetic Drugs of Choice
Stimulation of the medullary chemoreceptor trigger zone	Nausea or vomiting or both shortly after opioid administration	Metoclopramide, prochlorperazine, chlorpromazine, haloperidol, corticosteroids, or lorazepam
Enhanced vestibular sensitivity	Prominent movement-induced nausea and vomiting or vertigo	Scopolamine, meclizine or lorazepam
Increased gastric antral tone	Early satiety, postprandial bloating, or vomiting	Metoclopramide or cisapride
Constipation	Passage of small, hard infrequent stool, with difficulty	Proactive bowel regimen

From Coyle, N., Cherny, N., Portenoy, R. K. (1996). Pharmacologic management of cancer pain. In D. B. McGuire, C. H. Yarbro, & B. R. Ferrell (Eds.), *Cancer pain management (2nd ed.).* Boston: Jones and Bartlett.

Assessment

Assessment incorporates a complete history and thorough physical examination. All systems should be assessed during the physical examination, including the patient's general appearance. Skin turgor and integrity of mucous membranes may reveal signs of dehydration. Palpation, auscultation, and percussion of the bowel can identify obstruction or the presence of constipation. Rectal examination determines the presence of stool or the absence of tone in the rectum or anal sphincter (Lichter, 1996). Examination of the vomitus may reveal new or old blood, warranting an extensive evaluation for gastrointestinal bleeding. Intake and output should be measured to rule out dehydration. Radiographic evaluation should be conducted to rule out bowel obstruction.

Assessment is essential even when the underlying cause of nausea and vomiting is known. For example, although opioids are known to produce nausea and vomiting, multiple mechanisms can lead to these symptoms. Clear delineation of the symptoms through accurate assessment can assist in determining therapy (Table 13-8).

Table 13-9 Treatable Causes of Nausea and Vomiting

Causes	Treatments
Gastrointestinal Tract	
Constipation	Laxative, enema, manual disimpaction
Gastric irritation	Antacid, H_2 receptor blocker, misoprostol
Gastric stasis	Prokinetic
Squashed stomach syndrome	Prokinetic and antiflatulent
Intestinal obstruction	Surgical relief
Metabolic	
Hypercalcemia	Hydration, biphosphonate
Uremia	Relieve obstruction
Sepsis	Antibiotic
Drug-induced	Discontinue nonessential drugs; switch to alternative drug
Central Nervous System	
Raised intracranial pressure—brain and meningeal cancer	Steroid; possible radiotherapy
Pain	Analgesics
Emotional factors, anxiety	Counseling; anxiolytic

From Lichter, I. (1996). Nausea and vomiting in patients with cancer. *Hematology/Oncology Clinics of North America, 10,* 207-220.

Medical Management

Many causes of nausea and vomiting can be corrected, such as gastric irritation or hypercalcemia (Table 13-9). Pharmacologic intervention is the primary treatment for cancer-related nausea and vomiting.

Pharmacologic Therapies. Three major categories of antiemetics are used to treat nausea and vomiting associated with cancer: serotonin antagonists, dopamine antagonists, and corticosteroids. Miscellaneous antiemetic agents include benzodiazepines, cannabinoids, antihistamines, and anticholinergics. Box 13-10 lists these agents, as well as the effective doses and indications.

Combination therapy may be required when administering highly emetogenic chemotherapies. One study evaluated the efficacy of dexamethasone added to ondansetron, a serotonin antagonist. Patients treated with the combination therapy of ondansetron and dexamethasone received better relief with cisplatin-induced delayed nausea and vomiting when compared with ondansetron therapy alone (Olver, Paska, Depierre, Seitz, Stewart, Goedhals et al., 1996).

Although the oral route is preferred, the very nature of nausea and vomiting may limit this route of administration. Alternate routes of administration of antiemetics include rectal, vaginal, and parenteral (Wickham, 1996). Novel formulations of antiemetics may also be useful. Controlled-release metoclopramide has been shown by Bruera, MacEachern, and colleagues (1994) to be safe and effective in relieving chronic cancer-related nausea.

Nonpharmacologic Therapies. Nonpharmacologic interventions to control nausea and vomiting are frequently recommended and anecdotally reported to be effective. Unfortunately, few of these interventions, including exercise, cognitive-behavioral techniques, and dietary changes, have undergone rigorous study. Oncology nurses should be aware of the research findings, ever cognizant of the limitations of these studies, but the lack of data should not prevent patients from using these treatments. If a particular intervention seems appealing to the patient or it has been effective in the past, it should be incorporated into the treatment plan as an adjunct to pharmacologic therapy.

In a controlled study of exercise conducted in 42 patients with breast cancer, those patients in the experimental group (aerobic exercise three times a week for 10 weeks) reported significant decreases in nausea (Winningham & MacVicar, 1988). A meta-analysis of literature related to the effects of exercise on physical and psychological outcomes in cancer patients revealed that breast cancer patients participating in an exercise intervention had reduced nausea and fatigue (Friendenreich & Coumeya, 1996). This analysis was based on only a few studies, however; more research is needed to identify the potential beneficial effects of exercise in patients with cancer.

The role of cognitive-behavioral therapies in reducing nausea and vomiting is uncertain. Group psychotherapy (90 minute sessions held weekly for 10 sessions) during radiotherapy has been shown to reduce emotional and physical symptoms, including nausea and vomiting (Forester, Kornfeld, Fleiss, & Thompson, 1993). However, no differences in nausea and vomiting were seen in patients taught to use guided imagery (Troesch, Rodehaver, Delaney, & Yanes, 1993). Progressive muscle relaxation was more effective than listening to relaxing music or no intervention in decreasing vomiting immediately after chemotherapy (Cotanch & Strum, 1987).

Acupressure and acupuncture have been reported as useful in relieving nausea and vomiting associated with motion sickness, pregnancy, and chemotherapy. The pressure point is located on the inner wrist, and elastic wristbands with projecting rounded tips are commercially available. As

Box 13-10
Antiemetics

Belladonna alkaloids	**Prokinetics**
Scopolamine	Metaclopramide
Phenothiazines	Domperidone
Prochiorperazine	Cisapride
Chlorpromazine	**Cytoprotectant**
Antihistamines (H_1)	Sucralfate
Cyclizine	**Anxiolytic**
Meclizine	Lorazepam
Antihistamines (H_2)	**Glucocorticoid**
Cimetidine	Dexamethasone
Ranitidine	**5-HT$_3$ Antagonists**
Famotidine	Ondansetron
	Granisetron

From Fessele, K. S. (1996). Managing the multiple causes of nausea and vomiting in the patient with cancer. *Oncology Nursing Forum, 23,* 1409-1415.

Box 13-11
Nursing Measures in the Relief of Nausea and Vomiting

Maintain a calm, reassuring environment
Provide fresh air
Avoid foods known to precipitate nausea, (e.g., sweet, fatty, highly salted, spicy foods, dairy products)
Rinse mouth with weak lemon juice
Suggested bland foods (e.g., mashed potatoes, dry biscuits, toast, cottage cheese, sherbet)
Offer sour foods (e.g., lemons)
Minimize unpleasant odors
Avoid exposure to perfumes
Provide distraction, including talk, music, television, and radio

From Lichter, I. (1996). Nausea and vomiting in patients with cancer. *Hematology/Oncology Clinics of North America, 10,* 207-220; Wickham, R. (1996). Nausea and vomiting. In S. L. Groenwald, M. Goodman, M. H. Frogge, & C. H. Yarbro (Eds.), *Cancer symptom management.* Boston: Jones and Bartlett.

complementary approaches gain greater acceptance, these techniques are likely to be used more frequently. More research is needed to establish their efficacy.

Dietary changes are often recommended, although there are few studies evaluating their efficacy. Furthermore, wide variability exists in patient food preference; therefore, a dietary plan should be highly individualized. A small pilot study found reduced nausea and vomiting, as well as improved food intake, in patients given colorless and odorless foods while receiving cisplatin (Menashian, Flam, Douglas-Paxton, & Raymond, 1992). In general, recommendations include the avoidance of hot foods (which may have a more pronounced odor) and the addition of clear liquids.

Nursing Management

Nursing care of the patient at risk for, or already experiencing, nausea and vomiting includes obtaining a thorough assessment, including treatments that have been effective in the past. With their physician colleagues, nurses then develop a plan of care incorporating the preceding pharmacologic and nonpharmacologic approaches. Many nursing measures have been recommended in the relief of nausea and vomiting, although few have undergone any systematic evaluation. These measures are listed in Box 13-11.

Home Care Issues

Patients and family members must be given adequate instruction regarding the causes and treatment of nausea and vomiting to be able to continue the therapeutic regimen at home. Assessment of the kitchen and food storage is useful, as is determination of the patient's ability to prepare food. If the patient is unable to do so, identify other options, including caregivers who might cook meals or social services that might deliver prepared foods. Obtain custodial services that might fix meals, as well as clean up after meals. This approach limits the patient's contact with food and food odors outside of the meal time.

Research Issues

Now that more effective antiemetics are available, much research is being directed toward performing cost analyses. This research is particularly relevant given the high costs of some of these effective antiemetics in an environment of reduced resources. Grunberg (1995) questions the use of standard cost-effectiveness analyses and recommends cost-utility (which considers quality adjusted life years rather than increased years of survival) when calculating the advantages of effective antiemetics. This methodology has undergone pilot testing in 30 cancer patients who received chemotherapy. Patients were asked to determine quality of life while undergoing the current cycle of chemotherapy with hypothetical presence or absence of nausea and vomiting. The mean quality of life score was significantly higher for patients without nausea and vomiting (Grunberg, Goutin, Ireland, Miner, Silveira, & Ashikaga, 1996). Additional research validating this and other methods is needed.

CONCLUSION

Symptom management is the essence of oncology nursing. This chapter addressed several of the more common symptoms that occur in people with cancer. Many other symptoms may also occur, including alopecia, anorexia, anxiety, cachexia, cough, depression, diarrhea, hormonal changes, mucositis, pruritus, and others. To provide optimal care to all persons with cancer, oncology nurses must be constantly vigilant for the presence of these symptoms, regardless of stage of disease. Careful, thorough assessment contributes to a comprehensive treatment plan, including both pharmacologic and nonpharmacologic interventions. Effective, timely treatment enhances comfort, allows delivery of potentially curative antitumor therapies, prevents the onset of related symptoms, and overall, enhances the quality of the patient's life.

REFERENCES

American Pain Society Quality of Care Committee. (1995). Quality improvement guidelines for the treatment of acute pain and cancer pain. *Journal of the American Medical Association, 274,* 1874-1880.

Andree, R. A. (1980). Sudden death following naloxone administration. *Anesthesia & Analgesia, 59,* 782-784.

Besson, J. M., & Chaouch, A. (1987). Peripheral and spinal mechanisms of nociception. *Physiological Reviews, 67,* 67-186.

Blesch, K. S., Paice, J. A., Wickham, R., Harte, N., Schnoor, D. K., Purl, S., Rehwalt, M., Kopp, P. L., Manson, S., Coveny, S. B., McHale, M., & Cahill, M. (1991). Correlates of fatigue in people with breast or lung cancer. *Oncology Nursing Forum, 18,* 81-87.

Booth, S., Kelly, M. J., Cox, N. P., Adams, L., & Guz, A. (I 996). Does oxygen help dyspnea in patients with cancer? *American Journal of Respiratory & Critical Care Medicine, 153,* 1515-1518.

Brescia, F. J., Adler, D., Gray, G., Ryan, M. A., Cimino, J., & Mamtani, R. (1990). Hospitalized advanced cancer patients: A profile. *Journal of Pain and Symptom Management, 5,* 221-227.

Bruera, E., de Stoutz, N., Velasco-Leiva, A., Schoeller, T., & Hanson, J. (1993). Effects of oxygen on dyspnoea in hypoxaemic terminal-cancer patients. *Lancet, 342,* 13-14.

Bruera, E., MacEachern, T., Ripamonti, C., & Hanson, J. (1993). Subcutaneous morphine for dyspnea in cancer patients. *Annals of Internal Medicine, 119,* 906-907.

Bruera, E., MacEachern, T. J., Spachynski, K. A., LeGatt, D. F., MacDonald, R. N., Babul, N., Harsanyi, Z., & Darke, A. C. (1994). Comparison of the efficacy, safety, and pharmacokinetics of controlled release and immediate release metoclopramide for the management of chronic nausea in patients with advanced cancer. *Cancer, 74,* 3204-3211.

Bruera, E., Macmillan, K., Hanson, J., & MacDonald, R. N. (1989). The Edmonton staging system for cancer pain: preliminary report. *Pain, 37,* 203-209.

Bruera, E., Macmillan, K., Pither, J., & MacDonald, K., Pither, J., & MacDonald, R. N. (1990). Effects of morphine on the dyspnea of terminal cancer patients. *Journal of Pain and Symptom Management, 5,* 341-344.

Bruera, E., Schoeller, T., Wenk, R., MacEachern, T., Marcelino, S., Hanson, J., & Suarez-Almazor, M. (1995). A prospective multicenter assessment of the Edmonton system for cancer care. *Journal of Pain and Symptom Management, 10,* 348-355.

Bruera, E., Seifert, L., Watanabe, S., Babul, N., Darke, A., Harsanyi, Z., & Suarez-Almazor, M. (1996). Chronic nausea in advanced cancer patients: A retrospective assessment of metoclopramide-based antiemetic regimen. *Journal of Pain and Symptom Management, 11,* 147-153.

Bruera, E., Suarez-Almazor, M., Velasco, A., Bertolino, M., MacDonald, S. M., & Hanson, J. (1994). The assessment of constipation in terminal care patients admitted to a palliative care unit: a retrospective review. *Journal of Pain and Symptom Management, 9,* 515-519.

Case, Jr., D. C., Bukowski, R. M., Carey, R. W., Fishkin, E. H., Henry, D. H., Jacobson, R. J., Jones, S. E., Keller, A. M., Kugler, J. W., & Nichols, C. R. (1993). Recombinant human erythropoietin therapy for anemic cancer patients on combination chemotherapy. *Journal of the National Cancer Institute, 85,* 801-806.

Cella, D. F., Tulsky, D. J., Gray, G., Sarafian, B., Linn, E., Bonomi, A., Silberman, M., Yellen, S. B., Winicour, P., & Brannon, J. (1993). The Functional Assessment of Cancer Therapy Scale: Development and validation of the general measure. *Journal of Clinical Oncology, 11,* 570-579.

Cherny, N. I., & Portenoy, R. K. (1995). Systemic drugs for cancer pain. *Pain Digest, 5,* 235-263.

Cleeland, C. S., Gonin, R., Hatfield, A. K., Edmonson, J. H., Blum, R. H., Stewart, J. S., & Pandya, K. J. (1994). Pain and its treatment in outpatients with metastatic cancer. *New England Journal of Medicine, 330,* 592-596.

Comer, J., Plant, H., Hem, R. A., & Bailey, C. (1996). Non-pharmacological intervention for breathlessness in lung cancer. *Palliative Medicine, 10,* 299-305.

Cotanch, P. H., & Strum, S. (1987). Progressive muscle relaxation as antiemetic therapy for cancer patients. *Oncology Nursing Forum, 14,* 33-37.

Coyle, N., Adelhardt, J., Foley, K. M., & Portenoy, R. K. (1990). Character of terminal illness in the advanced cancer patient: Pain and other symptoms during the last four weeks of life. *Journal of Pain and Symptom Management, 5,* 83-93.

Coyle, N., Cherny, N, & Portenoy, R. K. (1996). Pharmacologic management of cancer pain. In D. B. McGuire, C. H. Yarbro, & B. R. Ferrell (Eds.), *Cancer pain management* (2nd ed.). Boston: Jones and Bartlett.

Culpepper-Morgan, J. A., Inturrisi, C. E., Portenoy, R. K., Foley, K., Houde, R. W., Marsh, F., & Kreek, M. J. (1992). Treatment of opioid-induced constipation with oral naloxone: A pilot study. *Clinical Pharmacology and Therapeutics, 52,* 90-95.

Curtiss, C. P. (1996). Constipation. In S. L. Groenwald, M. Goodman, M. H. Frogge, & C. H. Yarbro (Eds.), *Cancer symptom management.* Boston: Jones and Bartlett.

Dahl, J. B., & Kehlet, H. (1993). The value of pre-emptive analgesia in the treatment of postoperative pain. *British Journal of Anaesthesia, 70,* 434-439.

Daut, R. L., Cleeland, C. S., & Flanery, R. C. (1983). Development of the Wisconsin Brief Pain Questionnaire to assess pain in cancer and other diseases. *Pain, 17,* 197-210.

Dejgard, A., Petersen, P., Kastrup, J. (1988). Mexiletine for treatment of chronic painful diabetic neuropathy. *Lancet, 1,* 9-11.

Desbiens, N. A., Mueller-Rizner, N., Connors, A. F., & Wenger, N. S. (1997). The relationship of nausea and dyspnea to pain in seriously ill patients. *Pain, 71,* 149-156.

Dray, A., Urban, L., & Dickenson, A. (1994). Pharmacology of chronic pain. *Trends in Pharmacological Sciences, 15,* 190-197.

Drug facts and comparisons (1997). Author.

Dudgeon, D. J., & Rosenthal, S. (1996). Management of dyspnea and cough in patients with cancer. *Hematology/Oncology Clinics of North America, 10,* 157-171.

Eisenach, J. C., DuPen, S., Dubois, M., Miguel, R., Allin, D., & the Epidural Clonidine Study Group. (1995). Epidural clonidine analgesia for intractable cancer pain. *Pain, 61,* 391-399.

Escalante, C. P., Martin, C. G., Elting, L. S., Cantor, S. B., Harle, T. S., Price, K. J., Kish, S. K., Manzullo, E. F., Rubenstein, E. B. (1996). Dyspnea in cancer patients. Etiology, resource utilization, and survival-implications in a managed care world. *Cancer, 78,* 1314-1319.

Famcombe, M., & Chater, S. (1993). Case studies outlining use of nebulized morphine for patients with end-stage chronic lung and cardiac disease. *Journal of Pain and Symptom Management, 8,* 221-225.

Ferrans, C. E., & Powers, M. J. (1985). Quality of life index: Development of psychometric properties. *Advances in Nursing Science, 8,* 15-24.

Ferrell, B. R., & Dow, K. H. (1997). Quality of life among long-term cancer survivors. *Oncology, 11,* 565-571.

Ferrell, B. R., Grant, M., Dean, G. E., Funk, B., & Ly, J. (1996). "Bone tired": The experience of fatigue and its impact on quality of life. *Oncology Nursing Forum, 23,* 1539-1547.

Fessele, K. S. (1996). Managing the multiple causes of nausea and vomiting in the patient with cancer. *Oncology Nursing Forum, 23,* 1409-1415.

Fields, H. L. (1987). *Pain.* New York: McGraw-Hill.

Filshie, J., Penn, K., Ashley, S., & Davis, C. L. (1996). Acupuncture for the relief of cancer-related breathlessness. *Palliative Medicine, 10,* 145-150.

Flacke, J. W., Flacke, W. E., & Williams, G. D. (1977). Acute pulmonary edema following naloxone reversal of high-dose morphine anesthesia. *Anesthesiology, 47,* 376-378.

Foley, K. M. (1985). The treatment of cancer pain. *New England Journal of Medicine, 313,* 84-95.

Forester, B., Kornfeld, K., Fleiss, J. L., & Thompson, S. (1993). Group psychotherapy during radiotherapy: effects on emotional and physical distress. *American Journal of Psychiatry, 150,* 1700-1706.

Friendenreich, C. M., & Coumeya, K. S. (1996). Exercise as rehabilitation for cancer patients. *Clinical Journal of Sports Medicine 6,* 237-244.

Grunberg, S. M. (1995). Economic impact of antiemesis. *Oncology, 9,* 155-160.

Grunberg, S. M., Goutin, N., Ireland, A., Miner, S., Silveira, J., & Ashikaga, T. (1996). Impact of nausea/vomiting on quality of life as a visual analogue scale-derived utility score. *Supportive Care in Cancer, 4,* 435-439.

Hammack, J. E., & Loprinzi, C. L. (1994). Use of orally administered opioids for cancer related pain. *Mayo Clinical Proceedings, 69,* 384-390.

Insel, P. A. (1991). Analgesic-antipyretics and anti-inflammatory agents: Drugs employed in the treatment of rheumatoid arthritis and gout. In A. G. Gilman, T. W. Rall, A. S. Nies, & P. Taylor (Eds.), *Goodman and Gilman's the pharmacological basis of therapeutics* (8th ed.). New York, NY: Pergamon Press.

Jacox, A., Carr, D. B., & Payne, R. (1994). *Management of cancer pain.* Clinical Practice Guideline No. 9. AHCPR Publication No. 94-0592. Rockville, MD: Agency for Health Care Policy and Research, U.S. Department of Health and Human Services, Public Health Service, March, 1994.

Johnston-Taylor, E., Ferrell, B. R., Grant, M., & Cheyney, L. (1993). Managing cancer pain at home: The decisions and ethical conflicts of patients, family caregivers, and homecare nurses. *Oncology Nursing Forum, 20,* 919-927.

Kerr, D. (1989). A bedside fan for terminal dyspnea. *The American Journal of Hospice Care, 6,* 22.

Levy, M. H. (1991). Constipation and diarrhea in cancer patients. *Cancer Bulletin, 43,* 412-422.

Levy, M. H. (I 996). Pharmacologic treatment of cancer pain. *New England Journal of Medicine, 335,* 1124-1132.

Lichter, I. (1996). Nausea and vomiting in patients with cancer. *Hematology/Oncology Clinics of North America, 10,* 207-220.

McGrath, P. J., Hsu, E., & Cappelli, M. (1990). Pain from pediatric cancer: A survey of an outpatient oncology clinic. *Journal of Psychosocial Oncology, 8,* 109-124.

McMillan, S. C., & Williams, F. A. (1989). Validity and reliability of the Constipation Assessment Scale. *Cancer Nursing, 12,* 183-188.

Mellick, G. A., & Mellick, L. B. (1995). Gabapentin in the management of reflex sympathetic dystrophy. *Journal of Pain and Symptom Management, 10,* 265-266.

Menashian, L., Flam, M., Douglas-Paxton, D., & Raymond, J. (1992). Improved food intake and reduced nausea and vomiting in patients given a restricted diet while receiving cisplatin chemotherapy. *Journal of the American Dietetic Association. 92,* 58-61.

Merskey, H., & Bogduk, N. (Eds.). (1994). *Classification of chronic pain: Descriptions of chronic pain syndromes and definitions of pain terms* (2nd ed.). Seattle: IASP Press.

Miaskowski, C., Nichols, R., Brody, R., & Synold, T. (1994). Assessment of patient satisfaction utilizing the American Pain Society's Quality Assurance Standards on Acute and Cancer-Related Pain. *Journal of Pain and Symptom Management, 9,* 5-11.

Michaelis, L. L., Hickey, P. R., Clark, T. A., & Dixon, W. M. (1974). Ventricular irritability associated with the use of naloxone hydrochloride. *Annals of Thoracic Surgery, 18,* 608-614.

Miser, A. W., Dothage, J. A., Wesley, R. A., & Miser, J. S. (1987). The prevalence of pain in a pediatric and young adult cancer population. *Pain, 29,* 73-83.

Miser, A. W., McCall, J., Dothage, J. A., Wesley, M., & Miser, J. S. (1987). Pain as a presenting symptom in children and young adults with newly diagnosed malignancy. *Pain, 29,* 85-90.

Mock, V., Dow, K. H., Meares, C. J., Grimm, P. M., Dienemann, J. A., Haisfield-Wolfe, M. E., Quitasol, W., Mitchell, S., Chacravarthy, A., & Gage, I. (1997). Effects of exercise on fatigue, physical functioning, and emotional distress during radiation therapy for breast cancer. *Oncology Nursing Forum, 24,* 991-1000.

Mohamed, S. A., Mohamed, K., & Borsook, D. (1996). Pharmacotherapeutic approach: Non-opioid and adjuvant analgesics. In D. Borsook, A. LeBel, & B. McPeek (Eds.), *The Massachusetts General Hospital handbook of pain management.* Boston: Little, Brown.

Morrow, G. R., Hickok, J. T., Burish, T. G., & Rosenthal, S. N. (1996). Frequency and clinical implications of delayed nausea and delayed emesis. *American Journal of Clinical Oncology, 19,* 199-203.

Muers, M. F., & Round, C. E. (1993). Palliation of symptoms in non-small cell lung cancer: a study by the Yorkshire Regional Cancer Organisation Thoracic Group. *Thorax, 48,* 339-343.

Neal, L. J. (1995). "Power pudding": Natural laxative therapy for the elderly who are homebound. *Home Healthcare Nurse, 13,* 66-71.

Olver, I., Paska, W., Depierre, A., Seitz, J. F., Stewart, D. J., Goedhals, L, McQuade, B., McRae, J., & Wilkinson, J. R. (1996). A multicentre, double-blind study comparing placebo, ondansetron, and ondansetron plus dexamethasone for the control of cisplatin-induced delayed emesis. *Annals of Oncology, 7,* 945-952.

Paice, J. A., & Cohen, F. L. (1997). Validity of a verbally administered numeric rating scale to measure cancer pain intensity. *Cancer Nursing, 20,* 88-93.

Paice, J. A., Mahon, S. M., & Faut-Callahan, M. (1991). Factors associated with adequate pain control in hospitalized postsurgical patients diagnosed with cancer. *Cancer Nursing, 14,* 298-305.

Paice, J. A., Toy, C., & Shott, S. (in press). Barriers to cancer pain relief: fear of tolerance and addiction. *Journal of Pain and Symptom Management.*

Piper, B. F. (1993). Fatigue. In V. Carrieri-Kohlman, A. M. Lindsey, & C. M. West (Eds.), *Pathophysiological phenomena in nursing: Human responses to illness* (2nd ed.). Philadelphia: W. B. Saunders.

Portenoy, R. K. (1996). Cancer pain. In M. Lefkowitz & A. H. Lebovitis (Eds.), *A practical approach to pain management.* Boston: Little, Brown.

Portenoy, R. K., Thaler, H. T., Kornblith, A. B., McCarthy Lepore, J., Friedlander-Klar, H., Kiyasu, E., Sobel, K., Coyle, N., Kemeny, N., Norton, L., & Scher, H. (1994). The Memorial Symptom Assessment Scale: An instrument for the evaluation of symptom prevalence, characteristics and distress. *European Journal of Cancer, 30A,* 1326-1336.

Prough, D. S., Roy, R., Bumgarner, J., & Shannon, G. (1984). Acute pulmonary edema in healthy teenagers following conservative doses of intravenous naloxone. *Anesthesiology, 60,* 485-486.

Raj, P. P. (1993). Local anesthetic blocks. In R. B. Patt (Ed.), *Cancer pain.* Philadelphia: J. B. Lippincott.

Rang, H. P., Bevan, S., & Dray, A. (1994). Nociceptive peripheral neurons: Cellular properties. In P. D. Wall, & R. Melzack (Eds.), *Textbook of pain* (3rd ed.). Edinburgh: Churchill Livingstone.

Reuben, D. B., & Mor, V. (1986). Dyspnea in terminally ill cancer patients. *Chest, 89,* 234-236.

Rhoten, D. (1982). Fatigue and the postsurgical patient. In D. M. Norris (Ed.). *Concept clarification in nursing.* Rockville, MD: Aspen.

Richmond, C. E., Bromley, L. M., & Woolf, C. J. (1993). Preoperative morphine preempts postoperative pain. *Lancet, 342,* 73-75.

Ripamonti, C., & Bruera, E. (1997). Dyspnea: pathophysiology and assessment. *Journal of Pain and Symptom Management, 13,* 220-232.

Roberts, D. K., Thorne, S. E., & Pearson, C. (1993). The experience of dyspnea in late-stage cancer. Patients' and nurses' perspectives. *Cancer Nursing, 16,* 310-320.

Shacham, S. (1983). A shortened version of the Profile of Mood States. *Journal of Personality Assessment, 47,* 305-306.

Smets, E. M., Garssen, B., Bonke, G., & deHaes, J. C. (1995). The Multidimensional Fatigue Inventory (MFI): psychometric qualities of an instrument to assess fatigue. *Journal of Psychosomatic Research, 39,* 315-325.

Spross, J. A., & Burke, M. W. (1995). Nonpharmacological management of cancer pain. In D. B. McGuire, C. H. Yarbro, & B. R. Ferrell (Eds.), *Cancer pain* (2nd ed.). Boston: Jones and Bartlett.

Storey, P. (1994). Symptom control in advanced cancer. *Seminars in Oncology, 21,* 748-753.

Sunshine, A. (1994). New clinical experience with tramadol. *Drugs, 47*(Suppl. 1), 8-18.

Sykes, N. P. (1994). Current approaches to the management of constipation. *Palliative Medicine, 21,* 137-146.

Sykes, N. P. (1996). An investigation of the ability of oral naloxone to correct opioid-related constipation in patients with advanced cancer. *Palliative Medicine, 10,* 135-144.

Talbot, J. D., Marrett, S., Evans, A. C., Meyer, E., Bushnell, M. C., & Duncan, G. H. (1991). Multiple representations of pain in human cerebral cortex. *Science, 251,* 1355-1358.

Tanaka, G. Y. (1974). Hypertensive reaction to naloxone. *Journal of the American Medical Association, 228,* 25-26.

Tanelian, D. L., & MacIver, M. B. (1991). Analgesic concentrations of lidocaine suppress tonic A-delta and C-fiber discharges produced by acute injury. *Anesthesia, 74,* 934-936.

Troesch, L. M., Rodehaver, C. B., Delaney, E. A., & Yanes, B. (1993). The influence of guided imagery on chemotherapy-related nausea and vomiting. *Oncology Nursing Forum, 20,* 1179-1185.

Vainio, A., Auvinen, A., with Members of the Symptom Prevalence Group. (1996). Prevalence of symptoms among patients with advanced cancer: An international collaborative study. *Journal of Pain and Symptom Management, 12,* 3-10.

van der Molen, B. (1995). Dyspnoea: a study of measurement instruments for the assessment of dyspnoea and their application for patients with advanced cancer. *Journal of Advanced Nursing, 22,* 948-956.

Ward, S. E., Goldberg, N., Miller-McCauley, V., Mueller, C., Nolan, A., Pawlik-Plank, D., Robbins, A., Stormoen, D., & Weissman, D. E. (1993). Patient-related barriers to management of cancer pain. *Pain 52,* 319-324.

Ward, S. E., & Gordon, D. (1994). Application of the American Pain Society quality assurance standards. *Pain, 56,* 299-306.

Ward, S. E., & Gordon, D. (1996). Patient satisfaction and pain severity as outcomes in pain management: a longitudinal view of one setting's experience. *Journal of Pain and Symptom Management, 11,* 242-251.

Wickham, R. (1996). Nausea and vomiting. In S. L. Groenwald, M. Goodman, M. H. Frogge, & C. H. Yarbro (Eds.), *Cancer symptom management.* Boston: Jones and Bartlett Publishers.

Wilder-Smith, C. H., Schimke, J., Osterwalder, B., Senn, H. J. (1994). Oral tramadol, a mu-opioid agonist and monoamine reuptake-blocker, and morphine for strong cancer-related pain. *Annals of Oncology, 5,* 141-146.

Wilkes, G. M., Ingwersen, K., & Burke, M. B. (1997). *1997-1998 Oncology nursing drug handbook.* Boston: Jones and Bartlett.

Winningham, M. L. (1994). Exercise and cancer. In L. Goldberg, D. L. Elliot, (Eds.), *Exercise for prevention and treatment of illness.* Philadelphia: F. A. Davis.

Winningham, M. L. (1996). Fatigue. In S. L. Groenwald, M. Goodman, M. H. Frogge, & C. H. Yarbro (Eds.), *Cancer symptom management.* Boston: Jones and Bartlett.

Winningham, M. L., & MacVicar, M. G. (1988). The effect of aerobic exercise on patient reports of nausea. *Oncology Nursing Forum, 15,* 447-450.

World Health Organization. (1990). *Cancer pain relief and palliative care.* Geneva: World Health Organization.

Wright, P. S., & Thomas, S. L. (1995). Constipation and diarrhea: The neglected symptoms. *Seminars in Oncology Nursing, 11,* 289-297.

Yellen, S. B., Cella, D. F., Webster, K., Blendowski, C., & Kaplan, E. (1997). Measuring fatigue and other anemia-related symptoms with the Functional Assessment of Cancer Therapy (FACT) measurement system. *Journal of Pain and Symptom Management, 13,* 63-74.

14 Psychosocial Issues In Cancer Care

Myra Glajchen, DSW, ACSW, MSW, BSW

INTRODUCTION

A diagnosis of cancer presents a series of both medical and psychosocial crises to patients and their family members. To some extent, all cancer patients must overcome a common set of illness-related issues. At the same time, variation in background characteristics such as symptomatology, age, personality factors, and availability of social support results in individual reactions and styles of coping. Patients fear that they will die from the illness. In addition, they dread disfigurement, painful medical procedures, rigorous treatment schedules, high costs, stigma, and abandonment (Spiegel, 1997). Therefore, it is important to investigate the individual meaning of the illness for each patient, because the impact of the disease can be understood only when viewed within the context of the patient's goals, values, needs, and lifestyle (Anderson, 1989).

Weisman (1979) viewed each phase of cancer as having a unique constellation of predictable adjustment tasks. Although emotional distress is a normal reaction to catastrophic illness, each patient's reaction will be unique, as will be his or her ability to cope with the adaptational tasks that are necessary at different stages of the disease process. The pattern of living with illness changes over time. Therefore, coping strategies have to be revised to meet each new set of challenges, with concomitant alterations in lifestyle (Anderson, 1989). This chapter identifies various psychosocial reactions to each stage of the disease process for both the patient and their family members.

HISTORICAL PERSPECTIVES

Interest in the psychosocial and behavioral aspects of cancer has increased steadily over the last 40 years. Initially, researchers focused on the search for variables that might predict a predisposition to develop cancer. Anger, depression, and exposure to environmental carcinogens were originally studied but were never shown to definitively cause cancer (Holland, 1991). During the 1960s, cancer treatment improved survival time dramatically, and the rise of the consumer movement saw increased attention to the rights of patients and the need for informed consent. With new diagnostic and treatment modalities, many people with cancer were able to enjoy longer periods of remission, improved quality of life, and more frequent cure than in previous decades (Glajchen & Moul, 1996). The transformation of cancer from an inevitably fatal disease to a chronic illness of uncertain duration increased the relevance of patients' psychosocial and rehabilitation needs and made these increasingly long-term concerns.

The 1970s saw an upsurge in psychosocial and behavioral research into a host of new issues. Care of the terminally ill, pain management, ethical concerns in clinical trials, quality of life, and valid measurement of cancer symptomatology became legitimate concerns in the field of oncology (Holland, 1991). The last 10 years have seen increasing precision in research and clinical treatment, with our ability to measure endocrine and immune function in cancer, with the recognition that the definitions of medical outcomes must include functional status (Holland, 1991), and with a greater understanding of the role that genetics and family variables play in predisposing individuals to developing cancer.

The role of psychosocial factors in promoting effective coping strategies and prolonging survival has achieved recognition and respect through several landmark studies. In 1981, Spiegel and his colleagues (Spiegel, Bloom, & Yalom, 1981) demonstrated a survival effect for women with breast cancer who had participated in group therapy. In this study, 50 women were assigned randomly to a weekly support group that emphasized group cohesion, emotional expression, direct confrontation of death and dying, relationships with family members and friends, communication skills, problem-solving skills, and self-hypnosis for pain control. At the 10-year follow-up, group participants had an average of 18 months longer survival time.

A similarly positive relationship between psychotherapy and disease progression has been shown in at least two other studies. Richardson and colleagues (Richardson, Shelton, Krailo, & Levine, 1990) randomized patients with lymphoma and leukemia to an intervention that consisted of a combination of counseling and home visiting. Patients in the experimental group lived significantly longer than those in the control group. Fawzy and colleagues (Fawzy, Kemeny, Fawzy, Elashoff, Morton, & Cousins, 1990; Fawzy, Fawzy, Hyun, Elashoff, Guthrie, & Fahey, 1993) found that patients with malignant melanoma who participated in a series of six structured psychoeducational groups had significantly lower rates of disease recurrence after 6 months. In seeking an explanation for this survival effect, researchers have postulated that adherence to treatment regimens and changes in endocrine or immune functioning may serve as the underlying mechanisms that influence survival (Spiegel, 1997).

PSYCHOSOCIAL ADJUSTMENT TO CANCER

Researchers have studied a number of variables that predict psychosocial adjustment to cancer (Gordon, Friedenbergs, Diller, Hibbard, Wolf, & Levine, 1980). Identification of vulnerable individuals at risk for poor coping is useful because it can facilitate earlier intervention by health care professionals. The general consensus among psycho-oncologists is that psychological, social, and medical variables combine to influence adjustment and coping.

Psychological, Social, and Medical Factors That Influence Adjustment to Cancer

Psychological characteristics of importance include prior psychiatric history, previous experience with illness, history of a recent loss or a stressful life event, low ego strength, fewer coping strategies, pessimism, and anxiety. Social risk factors include lower socioeconomic status, poor social support, social isolation, marital or relationship strain, lower religiosity, work instability, and financial strain. Medical factors are also significant, given the fact that cancer comprises a constellation of diagnoses that vary in symptomatology, staging, treatment, and prognosis. Degree of illness, level of symptomatology, prognosis, and the doctor-patient relationship have been identified as critical stressors that have an impact on adjustment to and coping with cancer (Fawzy, Fawzy, Arndt, & Pasnau, 1995; Holland, 1989a; Spiegel, 1997).

Psychosocial support affects adjustment to cancer by encouraging adherence to the treatment regimen, mobilizing strategies for coping, promoting hope, and reducing anxiety and distress (Iacovino & Reesor, 1997). Such support can be made available to the patient in a formal manner through education, behavioral training, individual counseling, or group psychotherapy (Fawzy et al., 1995), or informally, through a social support network of family members, friends, and colleagues. As described in the next sections, several studies have demonstrated the beneficial effects of psychosocial interventions for cancer patients with different diagnoses, demographic backgrounds, and stages of disease.

Education

Adaptation to cancer necessitates the acquisition of new information and coping skills (Glajchen & Moul, 1996). Patient education reduces anxiety, decreases helplessness, and normalizes experiences. New information can help patients use medical care more effectively by improving adherence to medical regimens, strengthening recall of instructions, and facilitating the amelioration of side effects. Knowledge about cancer, its treatment, and anticipated medical and psychosocial consequences can reduce unpredictability and uncertainty while encouraging participation by keeping patients apprised of new and ongoing developments in their care (Fawzy et al., 1995).

Wells and associates (Wells, McQuellon, Hinkle, & Cruz, 1995) demonstrated that even a simple orientation program for newly diagnosed cancer patients was effective in reducing anxiety and overall distress. Patients were provided with a clinic tour, general information, and a question-and-answer session with a counselor. The actual information, the vicarious experience of visiting the practice setting, and the acquisition of resources and support services combined to lower distress and foster adaptation. These results have been borne out by other programs such as the Sunday Admissions Program at Memorial Sloan-Kettering Cancer Center. Group sessions before admission orient patients and their family members to the hospital system, restoring a sense of control and helping to contain acute anxiety (Christ, 1991).

Education is a useful tool for helping patients and their families understand the disease process, symptoms, side effects, and treatment options. Such education should include technical, disease-specific information, which can facilitate participation in and control over physical care. Information about normal coping strategies and common emotional reactions to serious illness encourage open communication and efforts to seek social support. Education can take many forms, including one-on-one discussion, videotapes, use of the Internet, and written materials (Fawzy et al., 1995; Glajchen, Blum, & Calder, 1995). Practical information related to resources and entitlements gives patients additional guidance in negotiating the maze of medical and social services.

Opportunities for education at each disease stage are highlighted throughout this chapter, with special attention given to the role of the oncology nurse in facilitating this education.

Behavioral Training

Behavioral training involves the use of such techniques as relaxation, hypnosis, visualization, imagery, meditation, biofeedback, and cognitive therapy to teach patients to control physical and psychological symptoms. Behavioral interventions can help patients control aversive reactions to medical procedures, radiation therapy, and chemotherapy. After these techniques have been learned, the patient can draw on them at any time, independent of outside professional help.

Edgar, Rosberger, and Nowlis (1992) studied 133 patients with a variety of cancers who were assigned randomly to one of two intervention groups. A five-session intervention was designed to increase knowledge about cancer, enhance personal control, strengthen coping mechanisms, and reduce emotional distress. One group of patients received the intervention immediately after their diagnosis, the other group, 6 months after their diagnosis. At the 8- and 12-month follow-up examinations, the group that participated 6 months after diagnosis reported less depression, anxiety, and illness-related concerns. These findings suggest that the timing of the intervention, as well as its content, influences adjustment to cancer.

Behavioral techniques are useful at every stage of the disease process, but particularly during active medical treatment. Behavioral interventions are effective for controlling physical pain and associated anxiety and can be used as an adjunct to other forms of psychosocial intervention.

Individual Counseling

Individual counseling can be provided to offer patients support, compassion, and empathy in an effort to bolster ego strength during the acute distress that accompanies cancer. At every stage of the disease, the patient may need counseling to help him or her make difficult decisions, express intense emotions, explore personal feelings of hopelessness and helplessness, and still maintain effective channels of communication with family members, friends, and coworkers (Blum, 1993). Psychotherapy involves three fundamental approaches: emotional expression, social support, and cognitive symptom management skills (Spiegel, 1995).

Greer, Moorey, and Baruch (1991) studied 44 patients with various types of cancer who received weekly counseling aimed at cognitive restructuring. Sessions were geared toward reducing emotional distress and inducing a "fighting spirit." Significant reductions in anxiety, depression, helplessness, and fatalism, as well as significant increases in fighting spirit, were observed in patients who participated in individual counseling. Such therapy can help patients retain a sense of individuality and humanity during a time when they may feel devoid of both.

Group Counseling

Group counseling can relieve tension and depression, decrease isolation, and enhance coping skills through education, sharing of feelings, emotional support, and the promotion of problem-solving behaviors (Lorenz, 1998). Group counseling can take place using a variety of formats. In psychoeducational groups, where education and support are provided simultaneously, patients have demonstrated improved attitudes toward treatment, as well as enhanced coping skills (Fawzy et al., 1993; Feldman, 1993; Glajchen & Magen, 1995). Self-help groups improve self-reported quality of life (Cella, Sarafin, Snider, Yellen, & Cruz, 1993). Data from supportive-expressive groups indicate that they lower tension, fatigue, and confusion among patients while increasing their vigor (Spiegel, 1997). In addition, researchers have postulated that the opportunity for structured emotional expression and frank discussion about death frees patients' problem-solving abilities, lowers pain and other symptoms, and strengthens their relationships with caregivers (Cain, Kohorn, Quinlan, & Latimer, 1986; Ferlic, Goldman, & Kennedy, 1979; Spiegel, 1997; Spiegel & Bloom, 1983; Spiegel & Glafkides, 1983).

Many cancer centers provide group counseling through their departments of social work, psychiatry, or psychology. Support groups are also available in community locations, as well as through toll-free lines, the Internet, and the American Cancer Society. Ideally, information about such groups should become a routine part of psychosocial care that is offered to all patients and family members as an additional resource for consideration during the treatment process.

Family Functioning

Family functioning can be an important resource to the cancer patient and have a powerful influence on adjustment and coping (Fobair & Zabora, 1995). Cancer involves the entire family system. During the cancer workup and treatment, family members are expected to support the patient while concurrently meeting their own developmental needs, as well as assume caretaking roles and responsibilities (Woods, Lewis & Ellison, 1989). Functional families can act as a buffer against the problems faced by the patient through four types of support: informational, emotional, instrumental, and affiliational. Advice and information can lessen the burden of decision making for the patient. Expressions of love and encouragement can reduce distress and affirm positive appraisal during the acute stress of the illness. The provision of tangible support and material aid can lessen the concrete needs of the cancer patient. In addition, affiliational support can help to reduce isolation and meet the patient's needs for socialization (Blanchard, Albrecht, Ruckdeschel, Grant, & Hemmick, 1995). Social support is not necessarily restricted to family support, although the family members are by far the most intimate sources of social support. Social friendships and work outside the home are also associated with better adjustment to cancer (Blanchard et al., 1995).

On the other hand, family problems can undermine the patient's ability to use medical or psychosocial services effectively, impair adherence to the treatment regimen, and complicate discharge planning, as well as impinge on the efforts of the health care team to help the patient. Zabora and colleagues (Zabora, Smith, & Baker, 1992) identified six family behaviors that create problems for the medical staff. These behaviors are listed in Box 14-1. Working with such families is a challenge requiring the collaboration of an interdisciplinary team.

Box 14-1

Family Member Behaviors That Create Problems for the Medical Staff

- Interfering directly with treatment
- Making excessive demands on staff time
- Refusing to comply with medical unit guidelines
- Forming alliances with other family members against the staff
- Using the staff inappropriately
- Being unavailable to provide support to the patient

Kristjanson and Ashcroft (1994) reviewed the literature on the family cancer experience and identified four major dimensions for consideration: developmental stage of the family, cancer illness trajectory, family members' responses to cancer, and the behaviors of health care providers. These variables are useful in assessing the needs and strengths of each patient-family unit and in implementing specific interventions to facilitate coping.

Each family will experience the illness in a distinct manner depending on its developmental stage and the role of the patient within the family (Woods et al., 1989). Families with preexisting strains or recent losses may have fewer emotional resources to deal with a newly diagnosed cancer in another family member. Adult children trying to coordinate medical care for older parents in a remote location will have more complex resource and service needs than will children who live close by. Younger families facing breast or prostate cancer will have to deal with loss of fertility and loss of potential for procreation, whereas older patients may feel cheated if diagnosed with cancer in their "golden years." Whatever the developmental stage of the family, these factors must be taken into account during the period of initial assessment so that needs can be anticipated and areas of vulnerability identified as early as possible.

The illness trajectory is another aspect of the family's cancer experience. This dimension will change in accordance with the course of the patient's disease and treatment (Kristjanson & Ashcroft, 1994). For example, spouses have been shown to demonstrate levels of distress equal to or above those of the patient during the time of the initial surgery and hospitalization (Spiegel, 1997). The speed with which the illness advances will also affect the family's experience. A sudden, downward slope in the health status of the patient will challenge family members' capabilities to integrate new information, adapt to the necessary changes, and prepare for the patient's death. Conversely, if patients take longer than expected to die, family members may withdraw prematurely and begin a watch until death. In the terminal phase of the illness, the quality and setting of the patient's death will influence grief work in the bereavement period. Therefore, the shape and speed of the disease trajectory must be taken into account when working with family members.

Family members' responses to cancer include demands placed on the family members, role changes necessitated by the illness, communication challenges, and coping responses (Kristjanson & Ashcroft, 1994). Such variables as family cohesion (emotional bonding), adaptability (ability to change roles and rules in response to outside demands), communication (expressiveness, degree of conflict and problem solving), and environment (relationships, resources) are important influences on patients' adjustments and ability to interact effectively with the health care team (Fobair & Zabora, 1995).

Kristjanson and Ashcroft (1994) identified health care provider behaviors perceived as helpful to family members. In the studies they reviewed, provision of comfort and high-quality medical care to the patient, followed by provision of information and supportive communication, were the professional behaviors most highly rated by family members. Support from health care professionals is an important source of effective coping for the individual patient as well. Several researchers have suggested that a strong doctor-patient relationship is a prerequisite for patients undergoing chemotherapy (Holland & Lesko, 1989; Spiegel, 1997). Given that chemotherapy treatment can last for months, with physical and emotional side effects accumulating over time, patient adherence to the therapeutic regimen may hinge on physician commitment and encouragement. Quality of communication, collaboration in decision making, and perception of physician caring have been linked to patients' level of distress, trust in the medical treatment, adjustment to treatment outcomes, and satisfaction (Roberts, Cox, Reintgen, Baile, & Gilbertini, 1994). For less assertive patients who have difficulty asking questions, expressing feelings, or comprehending medical information, the oncology nurse can play an important role in facilitating doctor-patient communication.

Common psychosocial reactions to cancer are discussed within the context of the major crisis points during cancer: diagnosis, primary treatment, rehabilitation, long-term survival, recurrence, and the terminal phase of the illness. Within each treatment phase, the patient's psychosocial adjustment tasks, the family members' adaptive challenges, and the role of the oncology nurse are discussed.

DIAGNOSIS OF CANCER

Patient's Adaptational Tasks

The major adaptational tasks for the patient at the time of diagnosis are listed in Box 14-2.

Receiving a diagnosis of cancer is a universally catastrophic event that patients can recall with immediacy and precision for the rest of their lives. The initial diagnosis of cancer follows a period of uncertainty, multiple medical tests, and emotional upheaval. Inevitable time lags during diagnostic testing tend to escalate anxiety as patients and their loved ones wait in limbo for a definitive answer. The inherent ambiguity of this phase hinders the use of psychosocial interventions, but provision of information and education related to the tests can be enormously helpful. Once the diagnosis of cancer is confirmed, opportunities for psychosocial intervention become more apparent.

Whatever the type of cancer and its treatment course, the life-threatening nature of the disease disrupts the continuity of the patient's life, challenges existential beliefs, undermines the basic sense of personal control over life, and

Box 14-2
Adaptational Tasks for the Patient at the Time of Diagnosis

- Integrate the cancer diagnosis
- Mobilize coping strategies
- Mount psychological defense mechanisms
- Acquire medical information

threatens hope for the future. Patients tend to be emotionally overwhelmed when diagnosed with cancer, which hinders their ability to integrate new information and make informed treatment decisions. According to Holland (1989a), shock, numbness, denial, dysphoria, anxiety, depression, and anger are all common at this initial stage. In addition, guilt related to the etiology of the disease and helplessness in the wake of an uncontrolled illness may surface.

The individual must attempt simultaneously to integrate the reality of cancer into his or her self-concept, mobilize coping strategies such as information-seeking and locating a cancer specialist, and mount psychological defense mechanisms to avoid total devastation. Yet, in the face of increased anxiety and distress, patients may be unable to use their normal coping styles (Fawzy et al., 1995). This period of acute distress generally dissipates within 2 weeks, as a constructive plan of action is developed. However, longer-term adaptation generally takes months (Holland, 1991).

Role of the Physician in Breaking Bad News

How the diagnosis and treatment plan are presented has a major impact on the patient's well-being, willingness to adhere to the treatment plan, and subsequent adjustment. Ideally, the physician should present a realistic explanation of the type of cancer and staging, along with a treatment plan that includes medical and psychological management. Simultaneously, the task of giving the diagnosis must be moderated with sensitivity to the patient's reactions and a solid commitment to the patient's ongoing care (Holland, 1989a).

Before the 1960s, there was much debate among health care professionals about whether to reveal or conceal the diagnosis of cancer from patients and their loved ones. Societal demands for informed consent, patient autonomy, and patients' rights resulted in a groundswell of support for honest communication and involvement of patients in treatment decision making (Holland, 1991). Unfortunately, the responsibility for breaking this news falls to physicians with little training. In addition, environmental barriers may preclude the sharing of the diagnosis under optimal conditions. These problems can lead to the appearance of insensitivity and tactlessness on the part of physicians who give the cancer diagnosis over the telephone, in public places, or without the presence of relatives and friends. In reality, the patient and family members may need to hear the information about the diagnosis and treatment plan in a variety of settings and formats until their anxiety has decreased to a level that enables them to integrate this new knowledge.

Family Members' Reactions to the Diagnosis of Cancer

Once the diagnosis of cancer is made, the patient and family members enter into a new relationship with the health care system. They must learn to negotiate new treatment settings, unfamiliar terminology, new personnel, and frightening procedures. Current research confirms that family members also experience a complex array of powerful emotions during the initial crisis of diagnosis (Sales, 1991). They express many parallel emotions to the person with cancer, including a strong need to trust and depend on the members of the health care team. Those family members who conceal their feelings in an effort to protect the patient may feel isolated, unsupported, and excluded from the focus of care. Therefore, it is essential that family members be included as active participants in the patient's treatment from the onset.

Role of the Oncology Nurse

The oncology nurse's role during the initial period of diagnosis and treatment planning is that of educator, counselor, and coordinator. The nurse can reinforce and repeat the new medical information for patients and family members, provide reassurance and hope about the treatment plan, and directly address the patient's concerns as they arise. The nurse can also begin to play a coordinator role by anticipating concrete and psychosocial needs that may arise and by helping the patient plan for the upcoming phase of primary treatment.

PRIMARY TREATMENT

Patient's Adaptational Tasks

The major adaptational tasks for the patient during the time he or she undergoes the primary treatment for cancer are listed in Box 14-3.

Primary treatment for cancer today is generally multimodal, consisting of surgery, radiation therapy, and/or chemotherapy, each of which carries its own set of stressors. Before treatment begins, patients need specific information about treatment options to participate actively in the decision-making process. Although making decisions can be burdensome for patients, most are relieved to "finally do something" active to treat their disease (Christ, 1991). Patients gain a sense of mastery and competency by integrating new medical information, participating actively in making treatment decisions, and identifying resources to help them cope with their illness.

The period of initial hospitalization is one of acute stress for cancer patients and their family members. With the introduction of surgery, radiation therapy, or chemotherapy, the cancer diagnosis becomes more tangible and frightening for the patient. Loss of control and personal identity are highlighted by accepting hospital attire, undergoing preoperative preparation, and placing one's trust in the medical team (Jacobsen & Holland, 1989).

Box 14-3
Adaptational Tasks for the Patient During the Primary Phase of Treatment

- Participate in treatment decision making
- Adjust daily routines
- Accommodate the treatment schedule
- Accept the sick role
- Manage treatment-related side effects

Role of Family Members

The importance of family members in promoting adjustment to cancer is increasingly well understood. Family members typically have to manage multiple and conflicting roles during this initial period. They are expected to provide emotional and tangible support to the patient in the hospital while assuming the patient's role responsibilities outside of the medical system. They must develop collaborative working relationships with the medical staff, but also advocate for the patient and ensure the best possible medical treatment. On a practical level, the demands of transportation, hospital visits, financial strain, and the need to deal with insurers can be physically and emotionally exhausting. Understandably, the focus must be on the patient's well-being, but if family members neglect their health, sleep, diet, or well-being, physical and psychological problems may result, and the patient will lose a major source of social support. Therefore, the patient and family members must be seen as the unit of care from the onset.

Role of the Oncology Nurse

The oncology nurse plays a vital role during primary cancer treatment by helping the patient and family members integrate new medical information, anticipate and treat side effects as they occur, and make adjustments to changes in their functional status during treatment. The nurse can address common concerns associated with the onset of treatment, provide reassurance about the expected course of that treatment, and help facilitate the adjustment to a new environment and medical team. The oncology nurse can reduce the patient's level of distress and maximize his or her level of coping through education, counseling, and the use of cognitive-behavioral techniques such as relaxation and imagery. In addition, the nurse can play a role in helping the family members adapt to the demands of treatment, offer support to the patient, and continue to involve the patient in family life and decision making (Christ, 1991). The nurse can serve as a resource person for information about alternative therapies for cancer.

In general, a combination of psychotherapeutic, pharmacologic, and behavioral interventions can be used to reduce the distressing consequences of surgery, radiation therapy, and chemotherapy and help patients to endure primary treatment as a whole (Holland & Lesko, 1989).

Surgery

Surgery carries with it universal fears of mortality, disfigurement, and pain. Loss of control while under anesthesia is another common concern. There is evidence that psychological preparation for surgery promotes postoperative adjustment and recovery, reduces postsurgical pain, and increases satisfaction with care (Devine, 1992; Jacobsen & Holland, 1989). Helpful interventions include a rehearsal of the activities and procedures involved in the surgery, informed consent accompanied by a thorough explanation of the likely benefits and risks of the surgical procedure, and emotional support.

After surgery, depression is a common reaction, especially if the diagnosis of cancer is confirmed and accompanied by a poor prognosis. In addition, different psychological reactions can be expected according to surgical site and associated functional loss. For example, head and neck surgery may be associated with fears of stigma and social revulsion in the wake of visible disfigurement. Recovery from mastectomy or prostatectomy is likely to evoke concerns about gender identity and loss of fertility or sexuality. Such reactions should be anticipated and appropriate interventions planned accordingly.

With shorter hospital stays and the shift to outpatient treatment for cancer, most patients will need a period of convalescence at home. This approach necessitates the need for home care (e.g., wound care, pain management), which is generally provided by home care nurses, physical therapists, and family members. Given the complexity of cancer surgery, recovery, and rehabilitation, a collaborative interdisciplinary approach is needed to provide optimal care. The surgeon, oncology nurse, physical therapist, home care nurse, and mental health professional each have specific expertise that can facilitate the postoperative course and subsequent adaptation. A key principle to consider during this phase is that early emotional support and education about surgery will have an impact on subsequent adjustment and coping. Understanding normal reactions can help the oncology nurse identify aberrant responses early on and intervene accordingly.

During cancer surgery, the nurse is in an ideal position to provide patient education related to preoperative preparation, orient patients and family members to the operating room procedures, and teach them about the management of postoperative side effects. In their role as counselors, nurses can allow patients to express concerns, provide emotional support, and reassure the patient and family members through the waiting period. The nurse can also act as the liaison between the surgeon and the patient and family members, maintaining open lines of communication and ensuring that the informational needs of the patient are met.

Radiation Therapy

Radiation therapy is associated with primitive fears of confinement, loss of privacy, and frightening x-ray beams given in specially shielded rooms. Fears about the harmful effects of radiation are widely held and must be systematically dispelled through accurate education. Additionally, the typical radiation therapy regimen is given five times a week for an average of 6 weeks, and the patient is soon faced with the practical difficulties related to the regimen itself. Even as patients are encouraged to maintain daily routines and a sense of normalcy in their lives, other parts of their lives must be suspended to accommodate the rigorous treatment schedule. The onset of radiation therapy also means that the patient must develop a working relationship with a new physician, nurses, and other members of the health care team.

The simulation procedure allows for realistic medical and psychosocial preparation of the patient for the radiation treatments. Once the treatments begin, the patient is able to establish a familiar and comforting routine by seeing the same patients and radiation staff each day. During radiation treatments, some patients find it difficult to lie still and remain isolated in a protected room. Most will experience side effects such as nausea, vomiting, fatigue, malaise, and possibly sore throat or diarrhea. Lengthy waits and patient groupings of less ill with seriously ill patients can heighten anxiety and anger among patients undergoing radiation therapy.

When radiation treatment ends, the patient moves on to the next treatment phase. Continuity of care and emotional support can be engendered by identifying a point person among staff members to maintain contact with the patient during the transition period. The oncology nurse is ideally situated to undertake this coordination role (Holland, 1989b). In fact, the oncology nurse can play a pivotal role in the patient's care throughout this period by preparing the patient and family members for the treatment regimen before treatment commences and by providing a detailed explanation about anticipated side effects. The nurse can decrease uncertainty and anxiety by giving advice about skin care, mouth care, and diet while encouraging adherence to the treatment regimen and problem solving in the wake of distressing symptoms. Verbal instructions may be supplemented with written educational materials and videotapes. Finally, the nurse can make appropriate referrals to a social worker or psychiatrist for counseling, for information about resources, and for the management of acute symptoms, such as anxiety and depression.

Chemotherapy

Chemotherapy may result in medical complications and a host of side effects that impair quality of life and escalate distress among the patient and family members. Usually, it is chemotherapy that forces the transition from feeling and appearing healthy to becoming visibly sick. Hair loss, nausea and vomiting, loss of appetite, weight loss, diarrhea, sexual problems, weakness, and fatigue are common side effects associated with chemotherapy. However, serious and even toxic side effects must be tolerated to achieve the desired effect on the disease process. Patients generally understand the relationship between full chemotherapy doses and survival. This insight can be highly distressing for patients who must delay treatment or accept a lower dose owing to myelotoxicity. If the goal of treatment is curative, patients are more willing to tolerate distressing symptoms. When chemotherapy is given for palliative reasons, quality of life and comfort concerns should be more important (Holland & Lesko, 1989).

In addition to the physical strain of undergoing chemotherapy, the patient must cope with the disruption of daily routines necessitated by the rigorous treatment schedule. The strain of waiting for appointments, arranging transportation, traveling to and from treatment, and trying to meet work and family obligations combine to exact a high toll on the person with cancer. The nurse's attention to the discomforts of chemotherapy and suggestions for dealing with nausea, vomiting, hair loss, and other symptoms indicate concern for the patient as a person. The nurse's role as a resource for organizing transportation, home care, and administration of medication at home gives family members a sense of continuity and confidence throughout this difficult stage of treatment.

Alternative/Complementary Therapies

Alternative medicine has become increasingly popular with the public and more integrated into the major institutions of mainstream medicine (Cassileth & Chapman, 1996), culminating in the inauguration of the Office of Alternative Medicine (OAM) established by the United States Congress in 1992. According to the OAM, alternative therapies fall into seven major categories: diet and nutrition, mind-body techniques, bioelectromagnetics, alternative systems of medical (folk remedy) practice, pharmacologic and biologic treatments, manual healing methods, and herbal medicine. The percentage of Americans using alternative medicine has been estimated at approximately 34% (Cassileth & Chapman, 1996) and as high as 76% among cancer patients in Canada (Montbriand, 1994). Careful assessment and understanding of the alternative therapies used by patients are essential to help patients make informed health care choices while avoiding some of the pitfalls characteristic of these approaches.

Factors contributing to growing acceptance of complementary cancer therapies by the public are noteworthy because they highlight shortcomings in conventional cancer treatment. First, quality and quantity of life have become increasingly important to people with chronic and life-threatening illnesses. Second, there is widespread dissatisfaction and distrust with traditional medicine, including its impersonal nature and lack of sensitivity to patients' psychosocial and spiritual concerns (Cassileth & Chapman, 1996). Patients with cancer may be drawn toward alternative medicine because of dissatisfaction with conventional treatment, treatment ineffectiveness, the need for control over health care decisions, and the desire for a more holistic treatment approach that embodies spiritual beliefs (Astin, 1998). In addition, they may be drawn to the more egalitarian and less paternalistic relationship with a physician and captivated by overly optimistic promises of complete cure (Montbriand, 1994).

Variables predictive of alternative health care use by cancer patients include higher education, poorer health status, a holistic health orientation, interest in spirituality and personal growth, and anxiety (Astin, 1998). Because the majority of patients may choose not to tell their physicians about alternative health care practices, it is essential that the oncology nurse remain neutral and establish a trusting relationship so that she or he can encourage full disclosure of these practices by patients.

Careful assessment of alternative health care practices is essential for monitoring the safety of these treatments and ensuring patient adherence to conventional treatment. Toxic side effects of some alternative therapies include poisoning, irreversible neuropathy, organ failure, bleeding, emaciation, electrolyte imbalance, and death (Montbriand, 1994). Unfortunately, desperate patients may make erroneous decisions based on biased information from the lay press. If the oncology nurse becomes knowledgeable about the risks and benefits of alternative therapies, the nurse can communicate accurate, nonbiased information, ensure informed decision making, and monitor the patient's vital signs as indicated. In addition, the nurse should try to achieve this type of education and care without destroying the patient's hope or creating division among family members.

REHABILITATION

Patient's Adaptational Tasks

The major adaptational tasks for the patient during the rehabilitation phase of the illness are listed in Box 14-4.

Rehabilitation for the person with cancer involves restoration to normal functioning in the physical, psychosocial, vocational, and economic realms of life (Ganz, 1990). Physical rehabilitation strategies should be tailored to the type of cancer, its treatment sequelae, and the performance status of the patient at every stage of treatment. Wherever established physical therapy regimens exist for surgical treatments, they should be offered to patients before the surgical procedure. Physical therapy can also be used to maintain function and mobility, improve stamina, and retain independence in activities of daily living (Ganz, 1990).

In the realm of psychosocial functioning, the challenge facing the patient is to make a cognitive shift from adjusting to the idea of death to resuming life-oriented modes of thinking (Christ, 1991). Both patients and family members need information about psychosocial recovery, which may lag behind physical convalescence. If patients have not been educated to expect the intermittent mood shifts that characterize this stage, they may consider their reactions abnormal. On a more existential level, patients must successfully integrate a changed body image, damaged sense of future health, and overriding fear of recurrence into a functioning personality. The powerful impact of living with uncertainty in the wake of a life-threatening illness can create a sense of discontinuity that persists for many years.

Sexuality and problems with intimacy often surface during this stage of the illness, after the acute stress of diagnosis and treatment have somewhat abated. Decline in sexual desire may occur as a result of a physical etiology (e.g., fatigue from treatment, tumor progression, pain, nerve damage) or psychosocial factors (e.g., poor body image, feelings of unattractiveness, anxiety, depression). Couple counseling and education about reversible versus long-term consequences can help patients make a successful adaptation and regain sexual functioning after treatment.

Box 14-4

Adaptational Tasks for the Patient During the Rehabilitation Phase of Treatment

- Shift to life-oriented thinking
- Resume obligations at home and work
- Integrate a changed body image

Patients face a return to their responsibilities in the workplace and resumption of their normal family roles and functions, but often with lingering side effects and treatment sequelae (Holland, 1989a). The establishment of advocacy groups such as the National Coalition for Cancer Survivorship has done much to highlight the barriers of societal stigma and workplace and insurance discrimination for cancer survivors. When they return to work, many cancer survivors find that knowledge about their illness is an "open secret." They may encounter hostility from co-workers who have carried an extra workload for a period of time; employers may be resentful if insurance premiums rise following the patient's treatment course; and they may experience expectations of low productivity, high absenteeism, or favoritism (Glajchen, 1994). Because health insurance is linked to employment in the United States, many cancer survivors face "job lock," the inability to change jobs because of difficulty attaining insurance coverage because of a "preexisting condition." These problems can conspire to block successful re-entry into the workplace for cancer survivors. Yet this transition is essential to restoration of confidence and self-esteem (Clark, 1995).

Family Members' Reactions

When the patient is discharged from the hospital, family members must adapt their preexisting lifestyle to the patient's new needs. For patients whose treatment is followed by rehabilitation, long-term survival, and cure, the family members may revert to normal levels of functioning within a short period. A positive prognosis and lack of permanent debilitation and disfigurement are associated with better adjustment (Sales, 1991).

Treatment cessation can be a paradoxical time for the patient. On one hand, this important milestone is met with a sense of relief and accomplishment. At the same time, the patient may experience anxiety about decreased contact with the medical staff and the loss of the treatment's protective shield. For patients who reorganize their lives around the treatment schedule, the end of treatment can signify the loss of an important goal that gave their life meaning and purpose. Reactions to the end of treatment vary according to the reasons for treatment cessation. The patient who has achieved a successful treatment outcome and hope of cure will react differently from the patient for whom treatment was unsuccessful or was stopped prematurely owing to toxicity (Christ, 1991).

As disease-free intervals increase, confidence builds, coupled with hope that the patient will return to previous levels of functioning and coping. Most family members are able to reintegrate the recovering patient into their preexisting lifestyles, although short-term tentativeness and lack of future planning are common. It is also noteworthy that as direct caregiving tasks subside, family members attempt to re-establish their own equilibrium, and they are often more able and willing to acknowledge their own emotions (Sales, 1991). Typically, family members report that the medical and social support characteristic of earlier illness phases greatly diminishes during the posttreatment period.

Role of the Oncology Nurse

The oncology nurse can play a helpful role in the cancer patient's rehabilitation by focusing on preventive interventions to decrease functional impairment and maximize quality of life (Ganz, 1990). Pretreatment discussion about anticipated changes in physical functioning, including sexuality, can diminish anxiety and help locate medical and social services to help ease the patient back into the community. Psychosocial support, counseling, and referral to community resources can help patients re-establish a sense of self-worth as a cancer survivor. Counseling may also be necessary for patients who lose their jobs or are unable to return to work after treatment. Finally, the oncology nurse can involve the patient's social support network in accomplishing rehabilitation goals and refer family members for their own counseling when this approach is appropriate.

LONG-TERM SURVIVAL

Patient's Adaptational Tasks

The major adaptational tasks for the oncology patient during the period of survivorship are listed in Box 14-5. Early studies of cancer survivors looked exclusively at the delayed physical sequelae of cancer treatment and considered survival a one-time event that occurred once the patient had been free of disease for 5 years or longer. In 1985, Mullan (Mullan, 1985) challenged the field by introducing his conceptualization of "seasons of survival," suggesting that long-term survival is a process that unfolds over time. Mullan identified three distinct stages of cancer survivorship: surviving the period of diagnosis and treatment; extended survival, which is dominated by fear of recurrence; and permanent survival, during which the patient is no longer defined by the cancer. This schema is useful and has been expanded by others (Dow, 1990; Fredette, 1995).

During the acute distress of diagnosis and treatment for cancer, many patients describe being on "automatic pilot" and "just getting through treatment." Realistically, there is little time for existential reflection or integration of the diagnosis into the patient's self-concept. During the period of extended survival, fear of recurrence generally predominates, as patients begin to grapple with the meaning of the disease to their lives. Acute uncertainty about future health can persist for years after the end of cancer therapy. Fear of recurrence is generally activated by the anniversary of the cancer diagnosis, check-up visits, the appearance of new symptoms, diagnosis of cancer in others, and hospital visits to family members and friends. Survivors describe conflicting feelings of joy at having survived and regret for their lost potential (Christ, 1991). Oversimplifying survivorship as treatment success and cure does a great disservice to patients confronting interruption of commitments, postponed goals, or altered relationships (Dow, 1990; Quigley, 1989).

Finally, the patient moves into the stage of permanent survival, which requires acquisition of a new set of skills so that the person can return to a healthy status, decrease vigilance over health, and allow fear of recurrence to recede into the background. In fact, controlling the fear of recurrence and reducing associated anxiety are essential for making the transition to being a survivor and helping patients re-establish their quality of life (Mahon, Cella, & Donovan, 1990).

It is important to understand that survivorship, like rehabilitation, embodies physical, social, and psychological components. Physical vulnerability, increased health concerns, fatigue, loss of energy, infertility, decreased mobility, and irritability can persist for years after treatment (Fredette, 1995; Spiegel, 1997). Social re-entry requires that the survivor make the leap from an ill patient with special status to a healthy person with full expectations for meeting previous obligations. Social stigma and fears of contagion persist to this day; and many survivors endure inconsistent, destructive, and inaccurate advice from well-meaning friends and colleagues. Employment and insurance discrimination can maintain survivors in the sick role long after they are ready to move ahead with their lives. Denial of promotion, loss of a job, denial of benefits, hostility in the workplace, and difficulty obtaining health and life insurance are unwelcome reminders of the survivor's former status (Clark, 1995).

Tross and Holland (1989) list a host of psychological adjustment tasks confronted by survivors: greater sense of vulnerability and uncertainty about the future, sense of personal inadequacy, fear of social rejection, diminished sense of control, anxiety, and depression. Others have highlighted the sense of isolation and loneliness that can surface during the transition to survivorship (Fredette, 1995). Cancer treatment fosters disconnection from social contacts for a period of time; restoring those connections takes time and energy. Intimacy and sexual relationships may suffer in the wake of physical and emotional changes after cancer treatment, a further source of loneliness for the survivor. Finally, fear of self-disclosure, which may lead to rejection, can leave the patient lacking the needed support and closeness.

Box 14-5
Adaptational Tasks for the Survivor of Cancer

- Maintain functional level of hope
- Maintain healthy denial of recurrence
- Live with uncertainty
- Re-enter social circle as a survivor
- Resume normal work and functioning

Finding Meaning After Cancer

For patients who are able to find meaning in their cancer experience, optimism and a heightened appreciation of life are associated with resumption of normal work and social functioning. Successful adaptation includes making sense of the event, finding ways to re-exert control, and maintaining a positive self-image (Thompson & Pitts, 1993). Many patients experience disruption in goals related to external achievements: income accumulation, career advancement, and reproduction. A shift in perspective and the development of attainable, internal goals, such as living life one day at a time, acquiring self-knowledge, and spending quality time with family members and friends, are associated with finding meaning in life after cancer (Thompson & Pitts, 1993).

Role of the Oncology Nurse

The oncology nurse plays a pivotal role in helping the cancer patient make the transition away from the hospital setting back to the community. First, the nurse may provide patients with an action list of interventions for disease monitoring and prevention (Dow, 1990). Behaviors such as eating, exercise, dental care, self-examination, and management of side effects are useful in restoring a semblance of mastery and control to patients. Making referrals to primary health care providers and ambulatory community settings can provide cancer survivors with continuity of care at a time of heightened anxiety. Links to advocacy organizations, such as the National Coalition for Cancer Survivorship, Y-Me for breast cancer survivors, and Us Too for prostate cancer survivors, can give recovered patients healthy role models and peer group support to facilitate adaptation. Third, the nurse can suggest new coping skills based on methods that have worked for others. Patient education courses and materials should be made accessible to patients who are willing and able to use them. Finally, the oncology nurse can educate the patient and family members to anticipate a long-term period of readjustment to survivorship, reassuring them that the members of the health care team will always be available and committed to their health and welfare.

RECURRENCE OF CANCER

Patient's Adaptational Tasks

The major adaptational tasks for the patient whose cancer has recurred are listed in Box 14-6.

Recurrence presents both a medical and psychosocial crisis to the patient, forcing a return to active medical management of the disease. Patients may become immobilized when faced with new treatment decisions, expressing doubt and remorse for past treatment choices. The immediate tasks at hand are adjusting to the changed medical status, accepting functional limitations and impaired quality of life, and adjusting to a new prognosis. The acute emotional turmoil characteristic of diagnosis generally recurs but with intensified existential fears, depression, anger, disappointment, and hope (Holland, 1989a). In fact, some research has suggested that patients with recurrent cancer demonstrate poorer psychological adjustment than newly diagnosed patients (Mahon et al., 1990). Treatment and personal goals have to be redefined, goals of care may shift from curative to palliative or from first-line to experimental therapy, and patients have to re-enter treatment with full comprehension about the difficulties that lie ahead (Montbriand & Casperson, 1995).

Box 14-6

Adaptational Tasks for the Patient Experiencing a Recurrence

- Adjust to changed medical status
- Accept functional limitations
- Adjust to altered prognosis
- Maintain quality of life

Mahon et al. (1990) studied 40 patients recently diagnosed with recurrent cancer. A majority of patients (78%) reported that recurrence was more upsetting than the initial diagnosis because the threat of death was "more real," treatment decisions were more weighty, side effects and pain were more severe, and they were more fatigued and preoccupied with anxiety about the illness. The authors concluded that patients with recurrent cancer have concerns and fears that are different from those experienced at the time of the initial diagnosis.

The chronicity of the patient's illness can take its toll on such personality characteristics as optimism and self-esteem. Functional limitations that increase dependence on others, inability to work, and difficulty maintaining family roles are painful reminders of increasing illness severity (Munkres, Oberst, & Hughes, 1992). Poor physical status and increased severity of symptoms are associated with pessimism, less denial, and depressed mood (Holland, 1989a).

The financial burden of cancer in general, and recurrence in particular, cannot be underestimated. Patients are expected to meet innumerable out-of-pocket medical expenses related to diagnostic tests, hospitalization, insurance copayments, and medications. In addition, patients may lose income due to loss of wages, travel expenses, housing near the hospital, parking fees, home care, and child care. Given that cancer treatment is highly specialized and expensive, the expense of a recurrence may place patients and family members in adversarial relationships with insurers, the hospital, or the physician's office. If patients are forced to use savings or investments to meet their medical expenses, other life goals, such as taking a vacation, going to college, or buying a home, might have to be sacrificed. This situation can lead to anxiety and hopelessness about the future (Houts et al., 1988).

Family Members' Reactions to Recurrence

Recurrence may engender a sense of hopelessness about achieving a cure in physically and emotionally depleted family members. Optimism and faith in the medical establishment tend to be eroded with the diagnosis of recurrent disease (Sales, 1991). Family members may re-experience the acute distress of the initial diagnostic period and may have substantial difficulty mustering the energy necessary to deal with new treatments, new side effects, and the renewal of time demands linked to hospital visits and home responsibilities. If treatment is prolonged, the capacity of family caregivers to meet the daily needs of patients is severely strained. Most family members report a decrease in formal and informal social support at the time of recurrence. However, mastery of the previous stages of the illness and the development of new coping skills will have strengthened the family members' ability to meet this new challenge. Family members can be reassured that they coped effectively with the previous treatment course and should be encouraged to participate actively in the new phase of treatment planning.

Role of the Oncology Nurse

The oncology nurse continues to play a critical role as educator, counselor, and coordinator during the period of recurrence. The nurse can help alleviate acute anxiety, restore hope no matter what the goals of care, foster problem-solving skills, and promote new coping behaviors (Anderson, 1989). Although it may be difficult to treat each recurrence as a new episode worthy of education regarding the treatment regimen, side effect management, and social support resources all over again, patients express the need for these interventions.

When Mahon and Casperson (1995) studied the needs of patients with recurrent cancer, they learned that patients perceived the health care team as less concerned and involved than they had been at the time of initial diagnosis. Yet patients expressed difficulty making treatment decisions, communicating with health care professionals, and initiating discussions about their needs and concerns. The nurse can help the patient and family members redefine their goals and develop a plan for the management of side effects, pain, and other symptoms. Such individualized treatment planning can do much to reassure patients facing recurrence that their care is being carefully monitored by a committed and involved health care team (Mahon & Casperson, 1995; Mahon et al., 1990).

TERMINAL PHASE

Patient's Adaptational Tasks

The major adaptational tasks for the patient during the terminal phases of the illness are listed in Box 14-7.

During the terminal phase of the illness, the cancer patient must integrate the reality that the goals of care have changed from curative to palliative. This stage of the illness is a time when intense emotions are evoked. The patient has to cope with a deteriorating physical condition, relevant existential and spiritual issues, and planning for a future without his or her presence. The patient may require additional help to compensate for loss of function and maintain quality of life for whatever time remains.

Box 14-7
Adaptational Tasks for the Patient During the Terminal Phase of the Illness

- Shift from curative to palliative treatment
- Confront existential and spiritual issues
- Complete advanced directives
- Deal with impending loss and separation
- Achieve resolution and fulfillment

Discussion of advance directives should begin as early as possible because even the sickest cancer patients can gain a sense of control over how and where they die. Frank interchanges about resuscitation orders, artificial nutrition, hydration, and life support, as well as arranging personal affairs, help the patient prepare psychologically for death. Existential soul searching about the meaning of the patient's life helps patients establish a legacy of their contribution to family members, friends, and society at large. Regret about lost opportunities, guilt for risky behaviors, and sadness about the future are also normal. The work involved in resolving these issues gives the patient the sense of completion and resolution necessary to deal with the impending sense of loss and separation (Christ, 1991).

Demands on Family Members

The physical and emotional demands on family members reach their peak as the disease progresses to the terminal phase (Sales, 1991; Vachon, Kristjanson, & Higginson, 1995). Physical fatigue, mental exhaustion, sleep disorders, depression, anxiety, and chronic health problems among family members are well documented in the literature (Holland, 1989a; Spiegel, 1997). In addition to assuming many of the patient's prior domestic responsibilities, family caregivers may be increasingly called on to function as nursing assistants. Surprisingly, family members express unmet concrete needs to a much greater extent than they do emotional needs during the terminal phase. Home care, transportation, dealing with medical staff, filling prescriptions, dealing with finances, and insurance were cited as the most pressing needs for 433 caregivers of terminal cancer patients (Houts et al., 1988). Those family caregivers who care for the patient at home may also forego social activities and work duties, resulting in social isolation and job instability. Role overload and exhaustion are common.

Role of the Oncology Nurse

During the terminal phase of the illness, patients need aggressive symptom management, an understanding of existential distress, and participation in effective decision making. The oncology nurse can help with these tasks. In addition, dying patients report that they need someone to listen to their concerns and give them hope, give them control over their environment, and provide comfort measures to alleviate pain and spiritual distress (Waltman, 1990). The psychosocial concerns of patients and family members during the terminal phase are discussed more fully in Chapter 18.

CONCLUSION

An understanding of individual variation in psychosocial adaptation and coping is helpful in guiding the cancer patient and family members through the upheaval of diagnosis, treatment, and treatment outcome. Early recognition of the psychological vulnerability of patients and family members can guide the oncology nurse in the assessment, education, counseling, and coordination of services for these individuals. In addition, the ability to recognize vulnerability will help the nurse integrate a variety of strategies with specific stages of the disease and treatment process. Specific nursing interventions can then be implemented to promote adaptive coping, relieve acute anxiety, encourage problem solving, and maintain hope (Anderson, 1989). A thorough understanding of patients' major adaptational tasks in the areas of psychological, social, and medical functioning can result in more targeted interventions, better allocation of limited resources, and, ultimately, improved quality of life.

REFERENCES

Anderson, J. L. (1989). The nurse's role in cancer rehabilitation: A review of the literature. *Cancer Nursing, 12,* 85-94.

Astin, J. A. (1998). Why patients use alternative medicine: Results of a national study. *Journal of the American Medical Association, 279,* 1548-1553.

Blanchard, C. G., Albrecht, T. L., Ruckdeschel, J. D., Grant, C. H., & Hemmick, R. M. (1995). The role of social support in adaptation to cancer and to survival. *Journal of Psychosocial Oncology, 13,* 75-95.

Blum, D. (1993). Social work services for adult cancer patients and their families. In N. Stearns, M. Lauria, J. Hermann, & P. Fogelberg (Eds.), *Oncology social work: A clinician's guide.* New York: American Cancer Society.

Cain, E. N., Kohorn, E. I., Quinlan, D. M., & Latimer, K. (1986). Psychosocial benefits of a cancer support group. *Cancer, 57,* 183-189.

Cassileth, B. R., & Chapman, C. C. (1996). Alternative and complementary cancer therapies. *Cancer, 77,* 1026-1034.

Cella, D. F., Sarafin, B., Snider, P. R., Yellen, S. B., & Cruz, J. M. (1993). Evaluation of a community-based cancer support group. *Psychooncology, 2,* 123-132.

Christ, G. (1991). Principles of oncology social work. In A. I. Holleb, D. J. Fink, & G. R. Murphy (Eds.), *American Cancer Society textbook of clinical oncology.* Atlanta: ACS.

Clark, E. J. (1995). *You have the right to be hopeful.* Maryland: National Coalition for Cancer Survivorship.

Devine, E. C. (1992). Effects of psychoeducational care for adult surgical patients: A meta-analysis of 191 studies. *Patient Education and Counseling, 19,* 129-142.

Dow, K. H. (1990). The enduring seasons in survival. *Oncology Nursing Forum, 17,* 511-517.

Edgar, L., Rosberger, Z., & Nowlis, D. (1992). Coping with cancer during the first year after diagnosis: Assessment and intervention. *Cancer, 69,* 817-828.

Fawzy, F. I., Fawzy, N. W., Arndt, L. A., & Pasnau, R. O. (1995). Clinical review of social interventions in cancer care. *Archives of General Psychiatry, 52,* 100-113.

Fawzy, F. I., Fawzy, N. W., Hyun, C. S., Elashoff, R., Guthrie, D., Fahey, J. L., & Morton, D. L. (1993). Malignant melanoma: Effects of an early structured psychiatric intervention, coping, and affective state on recurrence and survival six years later. *Archives of General Psychiatry, 50,* 681-689.

Fawzy, F. I., Kemeny, M. E., Fawzy, N. W., Elashoff, R., Morton, D., Cousins, N., & Fahey, J. L. (1990). A structured psychiatric intervention for cancer patients: Changes over time in methods of coping and affective disturbance. *Archives of General Psychiatry, 47,* 720-725.

Feldman, J. S. (1993). An alternative approach: Using multidisciplinary expertise to support patients with prostate cancer and their families. *Journal of Psychosocial Oncology, 11,* 83-93.

Ferlic, M., Goldman, A., & Kennedy, B. J. (1979). Group counseling in adult patients with advanced cancer. *Cancer, 44,* 760-766.

Fobair, P. A., & Zabora, J. R. (1995). Family functioning as a resource variable in psychosocial cancer research: Issues and measures. *Journal of Psychosocial Oncology, 13,* 97-114.

Fredette, S. L. (1995). Breast cancer survivors: Concerns and coping. *Cancer Nursing, 18,* 35-46.

Ganz, P. A. (1990). Current issues in cancer rehabilitation. *Cancer, 65,* 742-751.

Glajchen, M. (1994). Psychosocial consequences of inadequate health insurance for patients with cancer. *Cancer Practice, 2,* 115-120.

Glachen, M., Blum, D., & Calder, K. (1995). Cancer pain management and the role of social work: Barriers and interventions. *Health and Social Work, 20,* 200-206.

Glajchen, M., & Magen, R. (1995). Evaluating process, outcome, and satisfaction in community-based cancer support groups. *Social Work with Groups, 18,* 27-40.

Glajchen, M., & Moul, J. (1996). Teleconferencing as a method of educating men about managing advanced prostate cancer and pain. *Journal of Psychosocial Oncology, 14,* 73-87.

Gordon, W. A., Freidenbergs, I., Diller, L., Hibbard, M., Wolf, C., Levine, L., Lipkins, R., Ezrachi, O., & Lucido, D. (1980). Efficacy of psychosocial intervention with cancer patients. *Journal of Consulting and Clinical Psychology, 48,* 743-759.

Greer, S., Moorey, S., & Baruch, J. (1991). Evaluation of adjuvant psychological therapy for clinically referred cancer patients. *British Journal of Cancer, 63,* 257-260.

Holland, J. C. (1989a). Clinical course of cancer. In J. C. Holland & J. H. Rowland (Eds.), *Handbook of Psychooncology.* New York: Oxford University Press.

Holland, J. C. (1989b). Radiotherapy. In J. C. Holland & J. H. Rowland (Eds.), *Handbook of psychooncology.* New York: Oxford University Press.

Holland, J. C. (1991). Progress and challenges in psychosocial and behavioral research in cancer in the twentieth century. *Cancer, 67*(3 Suppl.), 767-773.

Holland, J. C., & Lesko, L. M. (1989). Chemotherapy, endocrine therapy and immunotherapy. In J. C. Holland & J. H. Rowland (Eds.), *Handbook of psychooncology.* New York, Oxford University Press.

Houts, P., Yasko, J., Harvey, H., Kahn, S. B., Hartz, A. J., Hermann, J. F., Schelzel, G. W., & Bartholomew, M. J. (1988). Unmet needs of persons with cancer in Pennsylvania during the period of terminal care. *Cancer, 62,* 627-634.

Iacovino, V., & Reesor, K. (1997). Literature on interventions to address cancer patients' psychological needs: What does it tell us? *Journal of Psychosocial Oncology, 15,* 47-71.

Jacobsen, P., & Holland, J. C. (1989). Psychological reactions to cancer surgery. In J. C. Holland & J. H. Rowland (Eds.), *Handbook of psychooncology.* New York: Oxford University Press.

Kristjanson, L. J., & Ashcroft, T. (1994). The family's cancer journey: A literature review. *Cancer Nursing, 17,* 1-17.

Lorenz, L. (1998). Selecting and implementing cancer support groups for bereaved adults. *Cancer Practice, 6,* 161-166.

Mahon, S. M., & Casperson, D. S. (1995). Psychosocial concerns associated with recurrent cancer. *Cancer Practice, 3,* 372-380.

Mahon, S. M., Cella, D. F., & Donovan, M. I. (1990). Psychosocial adjustment to recurrent cancer. *Oncology Nursing Forum, 17*(Suppl.), 47-54.

Montbriand, M. J. (1994). An overview of alternate therapies chosen by patients with cancer. *Oncology Nursing Forum, 21,* 1547-1554.

Montbriand, S. M., & Casperson, D. S. (1995). Psychosocial concerns associated with recurrent cancer. *Cancer Practice, 3,* 372-380.

Mullan, F. (1985). Seasons of survival: Reflections of a physician with cancer. *New England Journal of Medicine, 313,* 270-273.

Munkres, A., Oberst, M. T., & Hughes, S. H. (1992). Appraisal of illness, symptom distress, self-care burden and mood states in patients receiving chemotherapy for initial and recurrent cancer. *Oncology Nursing Forum, 19,* 201-209.

Quigley, K. M. (1989). The adult cancer survivor: Psychosocial consequences of care. *Seminars in Nursing Oncology, 5,* 63-69.

Richardson, J. L., Shelton, D. R., Krailo, M., & Levine, A. M. (1990). The effect of compliance with treatment on survival among patients with hematologic malignancies. *Journal of Clinical Oncology, 8,* 356-364.

Roberts, C. S., Cox, C. E., Reintgen, D., Baile, W. F., & Gilbertini, M. (1994). Influence of physician communication on newly diagnosed breast cancer patients' psychological adjustment and decision-making. *Cancer, 74,* 336-341.

Sales, E. (1991). Psychosocial impact of the phase of cancer on the family: An updated review. *Journal of Psychosocial Oncology, 9,* 1-18.

Spiegel, D. (1995). Essentials of psychotherapy for cancer patients. *Supportive Care in Cancer, 34,* 252-256.

Spiegel, D. (1997). Psychosocial aspects of breast cancer treatment. *Seminars in Oncology, 24*(Suppl. 1), 36-47.

Spiegel, D., & Bloom, J. R. (1983). Group therapy and hypnosis reduce metastatic breast carcinoma pain. *Psychosomatic Medicine, 45,* 333-339.

Spiegel, D., Bloom, J. R., & Yalom, I. (1981). Group support for patients with metastatic cancer: A randomized outcome study. *Archives of General Psychiatry, 38,* 527-533.

Spiegel, D., & Glafkides, M. C. (1983). Effects of group confrontation with death and dying. *International Journal of Group Psychotherapy, 33,* 433-474

Thompson, S. C., & Pitts, J. (1993). Factors relating to a person's ability to find meaning after a diagnosis of cancer. *Journal of Psychosocial Oncology, 11,* 1-21.

Tross, S., & Holland, J. (1989). Psychological sequelae in cancer survivors. In J. C. Holland, & J. H. Roland (Eds.), *Handbook of psychooncology.* New York: Oxford University Press.

Vachon, M. L. S., Kristjanson, L., & Higginson, I. (1995). Psychosocial issues in palliative care: The patient, the family, and the process and outcome of care. *Journal of Pain and Symptom Management, 10,* 142-150.

Waltman, N. L. (1990). Attitudes, subjective norms, and behavioral intentions of nurses toward dying patients and their families. *Oncology Nursing Forum, 17*(Suppl.), 55-62.

Weisman, A. D. (1979). *Coping with cancer.* New York: McGraw-Hill.

Wells, M. E., McQuellon, R. P., Hinkle, J. S., & Cruz, J. M. (1995). Reducing anxiety in newly diagnosed cancer patients: A pilot program. *Cancer Practice, 3,* 100-104.

Woods, N. F., Lewis, F. M., & Ellison, F. S. (1989). Living with cancer: Family experiences. *Cancer Nursing, 12,* 28-33.

Zabora, J. R., Smith, E. D., & Baker, (1992). The family: The other side of bone marrow transplantation. *Journal of Psychosocial Oncology, 10,* 35-46.

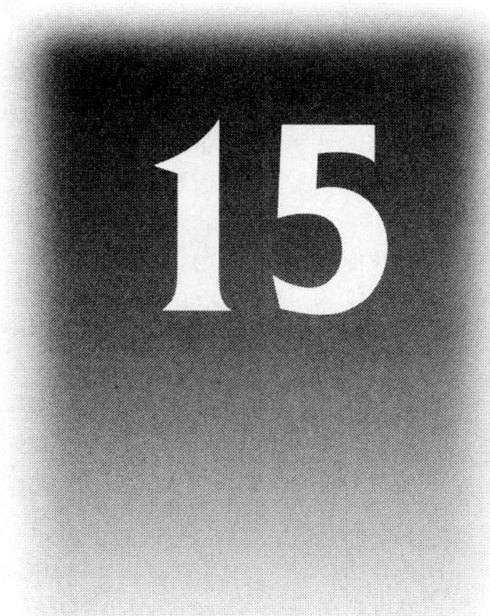

Family Issues in Cancer Care*

Frances Marcus Lewis, RN, MN, PhD, FAAN

INTRODUCTION

In addition to the patient, the family also experiences the impact and ongoing demands of a cancer diagnosis in a member. The work for the family is to integrate the cancer diagnosis and treatment into its everyday lives while still maintaining the family's life. During the family's work, the objective reality of the disease is interpreted and worked through at the levels of the individual members, dyads, total household, and the extended family and friendship network. Working through the illness is more than a cognitive-emotional process; it involves the development and refinement of often complex new behaviors of family members, including the development of new ways of working and interacting with each other. Each new piece of work adds its own challenges to the individual and family, as they attempt to integrate the cancer in ways that are least disruptive to their ongoing lifestyles while still assisting the diagnosed member.

This chapter has three purposes: to offer a theoretical framework within which nurses can understand cancer as a family-level experience, to identify implications for clinical services and programs for families with a member with cancer, and to identify areas for future needed family-level research.

Unshackling Our Assumptions and Myths

Personal views about the family experiencing cancer is colored by individual experiences with families, including family of origin. Although professional education teaches nurses to appreciate the importance of families adjusting to chronic medical illness like cancer (Lewis, 1990; Lewis & Bloom, 1979), nurses carry their own biases and assumptions about families. Among these assumptions are what is believed to be a "good" family, what is a "high functioning" family, and how families' reactions are manifested when they have a member diagnosed with cancer.

Full engagement with the family experiencing cancer requires that nurses unshackle themselves from their assumptions and past experiences. Stated in another way, beliefs about how an "ideal" family operates need to be abandoned. Full interaction with the family requires that prior assumptions be placed in abeyance (Lewis & Zahlis, 1997). Before reading this chapter, review Table 15-1. Answers to these questions will help clarify your personal beliefs about families functioning with cancer. The questionnaire is readdressed at the end of the chapter.

HISTORICAL PERSPECTIVES

In the last 10 years, there has been an accentuated awareness of cancer as a family experience, as contrasted with viewing cancer as an individual patient's personal diagnosis. This perspective was heralded in early theoretical papers by Barckley (1967), Litman (1974), Litman and Venters, (1979), and Parkes (1975).

Only recently, however, has family-level research in cancer come to empirical fruition in the research programs of a group of scientists: Armsden & Lewis, 1993, 1994; Compas et al., 1994; Compas, Worsham, Ey, & Howell, 1996; Germino, 1984; Given & Given, 1992; Gotay, 1984; Hilton, 1989, 1993, 1996; Issel, Ersek, & Lewis, 1990; Lewis & Hammond, 1996; Lewis, Hammond, & Woods, 1993; Lewis, Woods, Hough, & Bensley, 1989; Lewis, Zahlis, Shands, Sinsheimer, & Hammond, 1996; Northouse, 1988, 1992; Northouse & Peters-Golden, 1993; Northouse & Swain, 1987; Welch, Wadsworth, & compas, 1996; Wellisch, 1979, 1981; Wellisch, Gritz, Schain, Wang, & Siau, 1991, 1992; Yates, Bensley, Lalonde, Lewis, & Woods, 1995. This chapter excludes literature on the child as the di-

*This chapter derives in part from completed research that was supported by grants R01-NR-01000 from the Center for Nursing Research and R01-CA-55347 from the National Cancer Institute, National Institutes of Health, from the Oncology Nursing Foundation and ONS/Sigma Theta Tau Award, and an American Cancer Society Oncology Nursing Professorship. The author acknowledges the contributions of Lisa E. Hales in the preparation of this manuscript, and all members of the teams in the Family Functioning Research Program.

TABLE 15-1 The Family's Functioning with Cancer: Clarifying Assumptions and Beliefs

Instructions: Please choose the answer for each sentence below that best represents your beliefs.

1.	The person most severely affected by the cancer is the diagnosed patient.	True	False
2.	The children do well if they are told the facts about the cancer.	True	False
3.	The family does best when they don't try to dwell on the cancer.	True	False
4.	Thinking positive thoughts is the best way to heal from the cancer.	True	False
5.	A close marriage or partnership means that the woman and her mate think about the cancer in similar ways.	True	False
6.	Adolescents are hardly affected by a parent's cancer.	True	False
7.	Girls, more than boys, have the most difficult time when the mother is diagnosed with cancer.	True	False
8.	The diagnosed parent, more than the non-ill parent, has the key role to play in helping the family cope with cancer.	True	False
9.	If negative feelings and thoughts are put aside, families manage better with the cancer.	True	False
10.	A healthy family is able to manage the impact of the cancer without experiencing conflict.	True	False
11.	It is best not to give the child additional thoughts about the cancer; it only frightens the child.	True	False
12.	Families use their social support as a source of assistance for the cancer.	True	False
13.	Depressed mood in the diagnosed or non-ill parent has negative consequences for the children.	True	False
14.	Families do best when they focus on their family life more than on their life related to the cancer.	True	False
15.	Perceived illness-related demands are less important than is the severity of the cancer in terms of staging and treatment.	True	False
16.	The family member's negative feelings about the cancer will give way to positive feelings.	True	False
17.	Family members view the use of outside resources as a positive behavior.	True	False

Iagnosed cancer patient, caregiver research, and research with persons with late-stage disease. These areas of research and practice have extensive literatures and are deserving of their own analyses.

Family-level research in cancer evolved through four discernible phases (Lewis & Hammond, 1992). The first phase of research was represented by clinical papers written primarily by physicians. These papers raised concerns about the potential psychosocial morbidity in the patient and its potential ramifications for family members. These included recommendations from physicians about ways to minimize distress for the couple (Ervin, 1973); the value of including the partner in the preoperative phase of treatment for breast cancer (Kent, 1975); and the importance of encouraging the partner's participation in decisions about cancer treatment (Ervin, 1973; Wellisch, Jamison, & Pasnau, 1978). Although these initial papers were important conscience-raising papers, they lacked a database on which the clinical recommendations were made. Wisdom instead of data was the basis for the recommendations.

A second phase of research studies emerged in the 1970s and 1980s that went beyond the anecdotal information reflected in the early clinical papers. These database studies documented the impact of cancer on individual family members, including the partner. Breast cancer was the clinical prototype that received the greatest amount of attention. Research by Wellisch and Northouse were exemplary within this second phase (Northouse, 1988; Northouse & Swain, 1987; Wellisch et al., 1978). Both Northouse and Swain (1987) and Oberst and James (1985) were among the first to reveal a pattern of responses that further heightened our awareness of the partner's dilemma. The impact on the partner was not only a function of the impact on the patient, but often the partner's distress increased over time even as the patient's concerns decreased. Baider and De-Nour (1984) were the first to follow partners of women with breast cancer for more than a few months and documented that the partners had higher levels of distress over time and lower levels of adjustment than did the diagnosed women. Furthermore, this disturbance existed up to 3 years postsurgically (Baider & De-Nour, 1984).

Zahlis and Shands (1991) found that the spouses/partners of women with breast cancer experienced substantial concerns and difficulties in dealing with physicians, obtaining adequate information for making informed treatment decisions, adapting lifestyles to meet the pressures of the illness, and being sensitive to the diagnosed woman's emotional and physical needs. The partners also talked about the uncertainty of the future, their fear of disease recurrence, and the difficulties they experienced in their relationship with the women, including their struggles to communicate as couples about what was happening because of the breast cancer.

The third phase of studies (Lewis & Hammond, 1996; Lewis et al., 1989; Lewis et al., 1993; Woods & Lewis, 1995) identified the complexity of family life; considered multiple variables affecting the family; specified the mediating variables that potentially explained differential outcome in families (Moyer & Salovay, 1996); focused family members' behavior to function with the cancer; and included multiple outcomes of the household family's adjustment. The following discussion was derived from lessons learned from these empirical studies and is offered as a framework for oncology nursing practice.

THE RELATIONAL MODEL OF THE FAMILY FUNCTIONING WITH CANCER

To understand the family's work in functioning with cancer is to see the family as a relational, interacting system trying to be responsive to the illness-related demands and moderating the cancer's intrusion into the family's life. In the process of moderating cancer's intrusion and maintaining the household, the family is engaged in cancer-related work as a family (Box 15-1).

This model depicts cancer as a psychosocial transition in which a family attempts to balance its ongoing life as a family and its life with cancer. The following seven concepts form the basis for this model: (1) the family members' perceived illness-related demands, (2) the child's frame of reference for understanding the cancer, (3) the parent's depressive mood, (4) parenting quality, (5) social support available to the family, (6) marital adjustment, and (7) family member coping and management strategies. Each of these concepts are elaborated on in the following discussion. Within this model, cancer is viewed as a psychosocial transition, and the family is viewed as balancing two lives.

CANCER AS A PSYCHOSOCIAL TRANSITION

Cancer constitutes a psychosocial transition, not just a crisis event. Psychosocial transitions are characterized by deep personal reflection, cognitive-emotional searching, and existential questions such as "Why me? Why now? Why this? Why us?" It is through these reflective and search processes that family members attempt to maintain some sense of control and predictability over what is happening to them. Even when things are not under the control of the family members, the hope is that things are *in* control (Lewis, 1987; Lewis & Daltroy, 1990).

Psychosocial transitions cause a profound threat to the family member's entire assumptive world during which values, orientation, and self-formulation are reevaluated (Feldman, 1974; Strauss, 1959). For example, cancer can threaten a child's view of the parent as invincible and ever-present; the adolescent's life plan; the partner's sense of future and stability in the relationship, as well as vision of a shared future with the patient; and the patient's deepest sense of self. Viewing the cancer-related transitions as normal is part of the work of the family.

Box 15-1
The Work of the Family Experiencing Cancer

The ongoing tasks of the family experiencing cancer are:

- Viewing the psychosocial transitions caused by the cancer as normal processes
- Focusing on the *perceived* illness-related demands of the diagnosed person and their partner
- Being responsive to the child and adolescent's *perceived* illness-related concerns and related distress
- Attending to the child and adolescent's understanding and cognitive-behavioral management of the cancer
- Establishing boundaries around the parent's depressive mood so that the negativity does not diffuse into other relationships in the household (e.g., to the child-parent relationship or to the patient-partner dyad)
- Providing attentive and accessible parenting
- Accessing and utilizing social support in ways that are healing and not further burdensome to family members
- Working out ways to manage the tension in the family members' relationships that is caused by the cancer, including the marital dyad and the parent-child dyad
- Attending to and reciprocating the concerns and distress of the family members
- Self-monitoring and self-correcting behavioral management strategies that deal with both the cancer and its impact on the family relationships and activities

FAMILIES AS THE BALANCING OF TWO LIVES

A family is assumed to consist of intimate, interacting, and interdependent members. It has the potential to be an active manager of its own resources, ways of working and interacting with each other, and negotiations with the community. Illness in a parent requires that the family operate to maintain both stability in its routine internal arrangements and activities, as well as restructure its interactions and activities to manage the ongoing demands of cancer (Broderick & Smith, 1979; Buckley, 1967; Hough, Lewis & Woods, 1991; Lewis et al., 1989).

Families experiencing cancer must balance two lives—ongoing life as a family and life linked to the cancer. The ongoing life of the family involves maintaining the household's and other members' non–illness-related routines, activities, interactions, rituals, fun, and nurturing. Successful family functioning involves rearranging routines and daily responsibilities in ways that accommodate the demands of the illness while still maintaining time and energy for non–illness-related family life (Fig. 15-1).

The family's life regarding cancer involves reconfiguring life around the patient in ways that assist in the healing of that member. Problems occur for members of the household when there is an insufficient balance between these two lives. If the cancer consumes the family's life, there will be tension and problems. If the family fails to attend to the illness-related demands of the cancer, there will also be tension and problems.

The actual processes of the family adjusting to the cancer involve the work of both destructuring and restructuring

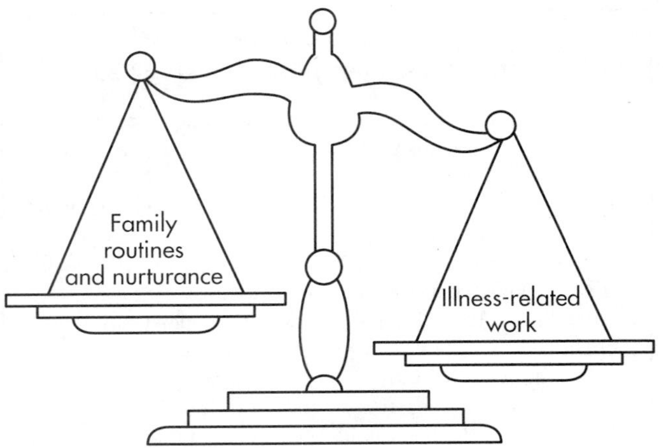

Fig. 15-1 The family's balancing of two lives.

(Hill, 1972). The challenge for family members is to give away old ways of thinking, doing, or interacting as a family, and to rebuild themselves around a new way; in a real sense the family evolves a new self-identity as a result of this cancer-related work (Feldman, 1974). Successful resolution of the destructuring and restructuring processes involves the family relinquishing past ways of functioning and working that are resistant or nonresponsive to the patient. Successful resolution also maintains the essential or core functions of the household. New ways of functioning that evolve from the family members have the potential to help them be the most effective managers of the cancer's intrusion into the family's life. Holding onto old ways of working or interacting that are nonresponsive to the illness-related demands create difficulties for the household. The successful family learns to "put the illness on the table, not under it" (Lewis et al., 1989).

Problems arise when destructuring is not balanced with restructuring. This occurs when the family's non–illness functioning is underemphasized or when individual members' affect and emotional needs are not considered. Balancing their lives as a family also means that the household does not overly dwell on the cancer. If most or all of the family's resources (i.e., time, sense of family identity, energy, commitments, and interactions) focus on the cancer, there will be problems for the household. In such a household, the cancer becomes dominant, not a part of the household's life. Imbalance is commonly reflected when clinicians say things such as, "This family can't get past its cancer," "They're consumed by the cancer," or "These family members have lost their sense of themselves as a family." Although these statements are overly general, they carry the connotation that the family is out of balance in what its doing to move ahead with both family life and life as a family working to manage the cancer.

Family Members' Perceived Illness-Related Demands

Family members are directly and indirectly affected by the cancer. Illness-related pressures or demands are subjective events (Haberman, Woods, & Packard, 1990). It is the perception of the family member, not the objective characteristics of some aspect of the cancer (Compas et al., 1994; Lewis et al., 1989; Lewis & Hammond, 1993, 1996), that affects how the family member responds and is affected by the cancer. The family is affected by the emotional pressures caused by the diagnosis. There are also interruptions or changes in life plans, priorities, and goals (Stetz, Lewis, & Houck, 1994; Stetz, Lewis, & Primomo, 1986). Cancer causes pressures on family members because they are affected by the negative mood, symptom state, and diminished activity level of the patient. In related studies with both recent and long-term diagnoses, these illness-related demands have deleterious consequences for the quality of the marital relationship. Heightened tension in the marital relationship, brought on or accentuated by the cancer's illness-related demands, has documented deleterious consequences for the household family (Box 15-2).

Parents' Illness-Related Demands

For a woman and her partner, cancer is associated with fears of death, recurrence, uncertainty, disruptions in lifestyle, and distress and mood disturbances (Bloom et al., 1987; Chekryn, 1984; Gotay, 1984; Hilton, 1989; Loveys & Klaich, 1991; Northouse, 1992; Northouse & Swain, 1987; Oberst & James, 1985; Packard, Haberman, Woods, & Yates, 1991; Wellisch et al., 1978; Zahlis & Shands, 1991). In both cross-sectional and longitudinal descriptive studies, the diagnosed woman's depressive mood is known to exceed those of referent samples. Furthermore, evidence shows this depressive mood remains significantly higher than the level in normative samples for an estimated 25% of women up to 1 year after diagnosis (Maguire et al., 1978). When anxiety and disturbance in self-image are also considered, 25% to 33% of diagnosed women also experience elevated levels in these additional areas (Maguire et al., 1978; Morris, Greer & White, 1977).

A significant amount of documentation suggests that partners of women diagnosed with breast cancer have demands that they attribute to the breast cancer and its contingencies (Northouse & Swain, 1987; Peters-Golden, 1982; Sabo, Brown & Smith, 1986; Zahlis & Shands, 1991, 1993). Illness-related demands pile up as treatment-related issues increase, the diagnosed woman becomes more symptomatic (fatigue, depressive mood, nausea and vomiting), and family routines are disrupted. These subjective or perceived illness pressures consistently predict family members' functioning with cancer (Lewis & Hammond, 1996; Lewis et al., 1989; Woods & Lewis, 1995).

Family members each have their own perception of the illness pressures that are affecting them; there is no core or consistent shared view of these pressures (Lewis, 1993). One of the fallacies of early family-level research was that family members, especially the diagnosed patient and the partner, would hold similar views or concerns about the cancer. This fallacy was even reinforced by researchers who claimed there was a singular most valid reporter of the family's experience. Over time, with different research methods and study samples, this fallacy was exposed (Gotay, 1984; Lewis & Hammond, 1996; Lewis et al., 1993). The fallacy

Box 15-2
Abstracts of Selected Studies from the Family Functioning Research Program

Lewis, F. M., & Hammond, M. A. (1992). Psychosocial adjustment of the family to breast cancer: A longitudinal analysis. *Journal of the American Women's Association, 47*(5), 194-200.

Data were obtained from 111 child-rearing mothers with breast cancer on three occasions at 4-month intervals using standardized measures of psychosocial adjustment. Results revealed that over time, the families experienced significantly lower levels of illness-related demands, and the marriages became better adjusted. Levels of depressive mood in the women, however, remained stable. This negative mood negatively affected the quality of the marriage, which, in turn, caused the family to cope less frequently with its problems and to function less well. Results strongly suggest the importance of formally assessing the woman's level of depressed mood and channeling women with stable depressive mood and their families into more intensive support services than those typically provided. Evidence from the current study is that, when not attended to, this depressive mood has sustained, deleterious effects on how well the family does during rehabilitation.

Lewis, F.M., & Hammond, M.A. (1996). The father's, mother's and adolescent's functioning with breast cancer. *Family Relations, 45,* 456-465.

The current study used path analysis to examine the impact of early stage breast cancer on the functioning of families with adolescents. Results revealed that the illness-related demands that the mothers and fathers saw impinging on their family predicted higher levels of maternal depressive mood, poorer marital adjustment, or lower parenting quality. When parenting quality was lower, the adolescent scored lower on self-esteem. Family professionals can help couples gain cognitive behavioral control over their perceived illness-related demands, help husbands avoid transferring illness-related tension onto their appraisal of the marriage, and help adolescents appropriately interpret parenting behavior.

Lewis, F. M., Hammond, M. A., & Woods, N. F. (1993). The family's functioning with newly diagnosed breast cancer in the mother: The development of an explanatory model. *Journal of Behavioral Medicine, 16*(4), 351-370.

The current study tested an explanatory model of family functioning with breast cancer based on data obtained from standardized questionnaires from 80 diagnosed mothers and partners with young school-aged children. Path analysis results for data obtained from both the mothers and the partners revealed a similar pattern. More frequently experienced illness demands were associated with higher levels of parental depressed mood which negatively affected the marriage. When the marriage was less well adjusted, it negatively affected the family's coping behavior. Household functioning was positively affected by heightened coping activity and by higher levels of marital adjustment. Children functioned better when the nonill parent more frequently interacted with them and their families coped more frequently with their problems.

Lewis, F. M., Woods, N. F., Hough, E. E., & Bensley, L. S. (1989). The family's functioning with chronic illness in the mother: The spouse's perspective. *Social Science in Medicine, 29*(11), 1261-1269.

The purpose of the current exploratory study was to test a set of interrelated hypotheses about family functioning with the mother's chronic illness from the spouse's perspective. Data were obtained from standardized questionnaires from 48 fathers with young school-aged children whose wife had either breast cancer, diabetes, or fibrocystic disease. Results of a path analysis revealed that the number of illness demands the father experienced was a significant predictor of his level of depression. More demands resulted in higher depression scores. Marital adjustment was significantly affected by both the father's level of depression and his wife's type of disease. Spouses of women with breast cancer had significantly higher levels of marital adjustment than did partners of the other women. More depressed spouses had lower levels of marital adjustment. Both illness demands and level of marital adjustment significantly predicted the type of coping behavior the family used. More frequent illness demands and higher levels of marital adjustment were associated with familial introspection, that is, coping behavior characterized by frequent feedback, reflection, and discussion in the family. The quality of the father-child relationship was significantly affected by this type of coping behavior. Families characterized as introspective had fathers who reported more frequent interchange with their children. This frequent exchange, as well as higher levels of marital adjustment, significantly affected the child's level of psychosocial functioning. Finally, higher levels of marital adjustment and more frequent exchange between the father and child positively affected the family's level of psychosocial functioning.

Woods, N. F., & Lewis, F. M. (1995). Women with chronic illness: Their views of their families' adaptation. *Health Care for Women International, 16,* 135-148.

Data were obtained from standardized questionnaires from 48 women who resided with an adult partner and one or more school aged children and had breast cancer, diabetes, or fibrocystic breast disease. Path analysis indicated that the women experienced more demands associated with their illness as the time since their initial diagnosis lengthened. The number of demands associated with the illness in turn produced problems with marital adjustment. Introspective coping behaviors were used more frequently by families in which the woman experienced high marital adjustment but depressed mood than by families in which the woman was not depressed but experienced marital difficulties. Women's relationships with their children were positively influenced by better marital adjustment, and women who had positive relationships with their children described their children's relationships with their peers as positive. Family functioning was optimum when the family frequently engaged in introspective coping behavior, when the woman had a low level of depressed mood, and when marital adjustment was positive.

of a consistent or similar view of the illness needs to give way to appreciating the multiple and often nonconvergent views individual family members hold of the illness. Research even suggests that family members often have discordant or nonconvergent views of the illness-related pressures (Germino, 1984; Gotay, 1984; Oberst & James, 1985). Each family member's perception of the illness is unique and deserving of its own attention (Lewis, 1993). Focusing on the perceived illness-related demands of the diagnosed person and the partner is part of the work of the family experiencing cancer.

Children's Perceived Illness Demands

There is beginning documentation that the school-age, adolescent, and adult children of individuals with cancer experience illness-related pressures when a parent is diagnosed with cancer (Armsden & Lewis, 1994; Compas et al., 1994;

Germino, 1984; Issel et al., 1990; Welch et al., 1996). To what extent these illness-related pressures have long-range, deleterious consequences for the child or adolescent is unknown. Also unexplained are the reasons that a large proportion of school-age and adolescent children experience cancer in a parent but demonstrate no short- or long-term impact; they appear to be unscathed by the experience, judging by their scores on batteries of standardized measures of adjustment (Lewis, 1996a). In recent research, a large percentage of the school-age and adolescent children scored out-of-range of normal on standardized measures of psychosocial functioning, but the majority of children (approximately 68% or more) scored within the normal range of scores on standardized measures of psychosocial adjustment (Lewis, 1996a). Recently Compas et al also reported similar variability on the proportion of children scoring in the clinical range (Compas et al., 1994). However, the proportion of children and adolescents who do score out of range of normative samples raises a host of research questions about this special group of young persons. Furthermore, the absence of psychosocial morbidity does not address the possible level of undocumented distress, sorrow, unanswered questions, concerns, or disenfranchised grief the children and adolescents may be experiencing, all of which are essentially undocumented in the existing research literature (Lewis, 1996a).

Within the relational model of functioning with cancer, child and adolescent functioning is hypothesized to be related to six major factors: (1) the child's frame for understanding and managing the cancer cognitively and behaviorally, (2) the quality of the child's past, (3) current parenting, (4) marital tension, (5) the depressive mood of the parent(s), and (6) the resources available to assist the child. These factors are summarized in Fig. 15-2. The discussion that follows relates to children ages 6 through 19. Although the child's past experiences, including the quality of past parenting, are important factors that affect the child's response to the cancer, we assume, for purposes of this chapter, that the child has a parenting history characterized by attentiveness, accessibility, and nurturance. Being responsive to the child's and adolescent's perceived illness-related demands is part of the work of the family experiencing cancer.

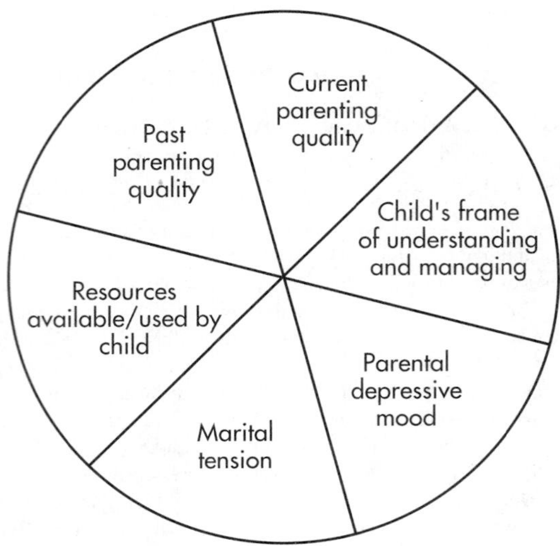

Fig. 15-2 Factors affecting child and adolescent's functioning with parental cancer.

THE CHILD AND ADOLESCENT FRAME OF REFERENCE FOR UNDERSTANDING AND MANAGING CANCER

Parental cancer poses some degree of threat to the psychologic security of the child (Armsden & Lewis, 1993). Even with older children and adolescents, cancer has the potential to cause attachment anxiety (Kobak & Sceery, 1988; Kobak, Sudler & Gamble, 1991; Morgan, Sanford & Johnson, 1992).

Children generate a frame of reference for understanding the cancer and for dealing with its impact (Armsden & Lewis, 1993). This occurs even in the absence of information from outside sources such as siblings or parents. When a child, for example, sees that his mother is vomiting or fatigued, the child will generate an explanation for this. Many times, particularly for the young child, the line between reality and fantasy is very thin (Armsden & Lewis, 1993). In the absence of information, the child may even generate explanations that are *more* frightening or *more* distressing than the reality of the situation.

Analytically we claim that the frame of reference of the child or adolescent has three components: a cognitive or intellectual component, a behavioral component, and an emotional or affective component. There is only a beginning research base that documents the child's response to cancer within each of these components; more descriptive research is needed to elaborate this frame of reference in both the school-aged and adolescent child.

Cancer is not an affect-free phenomenon; it is fraught with emotion. This is true for both children and adolescents (Compas et al., 1994; Grandstaff, 1976; Wellisch et al., 1978; Wellisch, 1981). Few research studies, however, enable us to know the level of emotions and distress that the diagnosis of cancer in a parent causes in the child or adolescent (Armsden & Lewis, 1993). Available data suggest enormous variability in the child and adolescent's affective response to cancer in a parent, including their level of distress or concern (Compas et al., 1994). Furthermore, there is evidence that this variability can be a function of the research methods used to measure the child's functioning. For example, the child or adolescent may have thoughts or fears that are never made visible to an outsider and are never reflected in the observable behavior of the child or adolescent (Armsden & Lewis, 1994). A quiet child or adolescent does not indicate or should not be interpreted as an "adjusted" or a "happy" child. His or her internal world of understanding, concerns, fears, and worries is not always visible, even when experiencing substantial distress (Armsden & Lewis, 1993, 1994; Buehler, Krishnakumar, Anthony, Tittsworth, &

Stone, 1994; Lewis, 1986; Lewis, 1996a). This affective response can include a stable, self-deprecating view (Armsden & Lewis, 1994). To what extent this occurs is essentially unknown and deserves further study.

School-age children have a sense of both personal agency and the importance of doing things to help with the cancer, including doing things that take away the pressures of the cancer on the parent. Unknown is to what extent the child or adolescent's engagement in cancer-related tasks and activities assists their sense of personal agency, sense of belonging, or positive self-worth (Brody, Moore, & Glei, 1994).

Adolescents are known to be active agents in co-constructing instead of passively accepting their experiences (Buehler et al., 1994; Maccoby, 1992). Little is known, however, about the models that adolescents have constructed about the parent's cancer. Merely tacking on the research labels of an adult's management or cognitive frame of reference is likely to be uninformed if not misinformed. Phrases such as "coping with the cancer" may be little understood by the child or adolescent (Issel et al., 1990). Interpretive research is clearly indicated as scientists and clinicians try to assess the understanding of children and adolescents. Attending to the child and adolescent understanding and cognitive-behavioral management of the cancer is part of the work of the family experiencing cancer.

Depressive Mood in Parents

Depressive mood in the patient or partner can produce problems in the marriage, in the quality with which they each parent the children, and in the tension and functioning of the household (Cancer Care, 1977; Forehand, McCombs, & Brody, 1987; Goodman, & Brumley, 1990; Hirsch, Moos, & Reischl, 1985; Lewis & Hammond, 1996; Orvaschel, 1983; Panaccione & Wahler, 1986; Tronick & Field, 1986; Kobak & Sceery, 1988).

Frank depression in a parent, particularly the mother, is known (from prior research in both clinical and nonclinical samples) to deleteriously affect the continued quality of parenting (Orvaschel, 1983). Less clear, however, is the effect of parental depressive mood on the parenting behavior during the family's cancer experience. The conditions under which parental depressed mood does *not* affect parenting quality in a household experiencing cancer is an important area that needs further examination. Unknown are the mechanisms that protect the child or adolescent from depressive parental mood caused by the parent's cancer. Little known, too, are the processes by which family members interact with the child or adolescent in ways that buffer the impact of parental depressed mood on them.

Results from research suggest that parents experiencing cancer and depressive mood are capable of maintaining solid parenting practices despite the cancer; their depressive mood does not always spill over into the ways in which they parent their child (see Table 15-1). Establishing boundaries around the parent's depressive mood so that the negativity does not diffuse to other relationships in the household (e.g., to the child-parent relationship) is part of the work of the family experiencing cancer (Lewis & Zahlis, 1997).

Quality of Parenting

The quality of parenting is a consistent and significant predictor of both the school-age and adolescent children's functioning a family member's cancer. The relative absence of nurturing and attentive parenting is a hypothesized risk factor for potential difficulty for both the school-age and adolescent child. See evidence for this claim in Lewis and Hammond (1996), Lewis, Hammond and Woods (1993), and Lewis et al., (1989). Current parenting practices do indeed matter to the child's adjustment. What may be difficult is stabilizing quality parenting while still attending to the cancer-related issues in the ill parent. Even as adolescents developmentally struggle with their own evolving independence, there is evidence that these same emerging adults benefit from parental attentiveness during the parent's cancer (Lewis & Hammond, 1996). The provision of attentive, accessible, and nurturant parenting is part of the work of the family experiencing cancer.

Resources Available to Children and Adolescents

Social support can be a valued resource for families who are experiencing cancer (Funch & Mettlin, 1982; Lindsey, Norbeck, Carrieri, & Perry, 1981). Social support is known from prior research to act in one of two ways: to affect the parents' appraisal of the illness or to make available tangible resources for family members to manage the illness (Bloom, 1982; Cohen & Wills, 1985; Northouse, 1988; Stewart, 1989; Thoits, 1982; Wortman, 1984). Prior research has documented significant positive associations between perceived social support and psychosocial adjustment levels in male partners of women with breast cancer at 3 and 30 days postoperatively (Northouse, 1988). These support variables accounted for more variance in the partner's adjustment than did medical variables (e.g., type of surgery, type of treatment or extent of disease) or demographic variables (e.g., age, education, length of marriage) (Northouse, 1988).

Results from research program have yielded inconsistent associations between social support and the household family's level of functioning (Primomo, Yates, & Woods, 1990). Our evidence is that some families may have difficulty accessing or successfully using social support, even when support is available. It may be that support, when available, is unable to respond in ways in which families find it helpful (Lewis et al., 1996). The reality is that many families work through and on the cancer in the absence of resources from their network. Results from some research suggest that some or many of the partners manage the cancer in relative isolation of existing support, and some patients are only burdened by support that is available to them (Lewis & Hammond, 1996). The provision of social support to assist the family needs more research; Samarel's intervention study will be helpful in this regard (Samarel & Fawcett, 1992; Samarel, Fawcett, & Tulman, 1993). The conditions are unknown under which family members fail to successfully use support, even when it exists. Also unknown are the forms with which nurses can best offer sources of support that assist families to normalize the use of such support. It may be, for example, that a prescription for healing is needed in which the use of social support is made normative, much like physical therapy is prescribed and used for persons with a broken leg (Lewis, 1996b). The family's access and utilization of social support in ways that are healing and not further burdensome to family members is part of the family's work with the cancer.

Marital Tension

The presence of heightened marital tension in a couple experiencing cancer should be expected. It is not a matter of whether it will occur but when it will occur, at what intensity it will occur, and what will reduce it. Heightened marital tension need not be interpreted as a failure in the marriage but as an opportunity for the couple to surface the sources of their tension and to manage the tension. In prior research with other clinical populations, spouses of persons with chronic illness have attributed marital problems to either the patient's illness or to its related treatments (Brown et al., 1978; Molumphy & Sporakowski, 1984; Peterson, 1979). Prior research has also raised the importance of marital tension as a factor affecting the adjustment of the child or adolescent (Emery, 1982; Emery & O'Leary, 1982; Fauber, Forehand, Thomas, & Wierson, 1990; Gable, Belsky, & Crnic, 1992; Porter & O'Leary, 1980). The real challenge for the couple is to work out ways to manage the tension rather than to let it go unattended. Working out ways to manage the tension caused by the cancer is part of the couples' work with the cancer.

Although an individual family members has his or her own journey through the cancer experience, this journey is not carried out in isolation of others. Rather, it is punctuated by interactions with other family members. When the feelings, affect, concerns, distress, or behavioral responses to the cancer experience are not attended to and reciprocated by the other person, there is heightened tension and distress in the relationship. Both attending and reciprocating are important components of interpersonal sensitivity in a family experiencing cancer. Attending to and reciprocating the concerns and distress of each family member is an essential activity of the family experiencing cancer.

Attending and reciprocating mean two separate things: (1) the *attending* behavior (family members deeply listen and give recognition to the importance of the concern or issue that the other family member is sharing, even when it is not their own concern); and (2) the *reciprocated* behavior (family members give or demonstrate the behavior to the other family member that is expected or desired by that family member because of their concern). In reciprocating, the other family member delivers the response or behavior that is expected by the family member expressing concern.

Sometimes family members have difficulty both attending to and reciprocating the expressed concerns of others. Not uncommonly, partners want the patient to carry a positive attitude, to "be up" in his or her thinking, and to not talk or cry about the cancer. When the patient is a woman and she wants to express sad, bad, or negative thoughts, it may be difficult for her male partner to attend to such talk and reciprocate it by listening without judgment and offering the deserved behavioral response. This is not because these partners are uncaring or insensitive. Such labels prematurely dismiss their behavior. Rather, male partners may have difficulty engaging in, attending to, and reciprocating the behavior because of a myriad of reasons, all of which are motivated by a deep caring for the female patient (Samms, 1996; Zunkel, 1996). In another example, the female patient may be concerned about her own vulnerability and ability to deal effectively with the demands of the medical treatment for the cancer. When the partner is concurrently concerned with how the children and house will be managed while she is symptomatic from the treatments, the female patient may find it difficult to attend to her partner's concerns. Furthermore, she may not view her partner's situation as difficult or as pressing as her own situation and may have difficulty delivering the behavioral response her partner expects. Attending and reciprocating are part of the family's work in dealing with the cancer.

FAMILY MEMBER COPING AND MANAGEMENT STRATEGIES

Higher functioning families actively modify what, when, and how they manage their daily lives to include the cancer-related contingencies. They not only focus on what they need to do to deal with the regular, daily issues of family life; they also talk about how well they dealt with their concerns and how they could better deal with the challenges in future situations. They provide strokes and feedback to each other about how they handled the problems and challenges (Stetz, Lewis, & Primomo, 1986). In this form of interacting, the family members self-reflect and self-correct their behavior as needed.

Families whose coping behavior is self-reflective, goal-focused, self-correcting, and punctuated by feedback to its members have demonstrated higher levels of household functioning and higher quality parenting (Lewis & Hammond, 1996; Lewis et al., 1989; Lewis et al., 1993). Self-monitoring and self-correcting behavior that manages the cancer and its impact on the household is part of the work of the family experiencing cancer.

Clinical Implications and Services for Families

Despite both the documented levels of distress in family members and the declared importance of family-level nursing services in cancer care, there is an extremely limited set of services that systematically assist the family with its experience with cancer. Most interventions and services focus on the adjustment of the patient, partner, and children (Lewis, 1983 , 1990, 1993, 1996a). Johnson and Norby's (1981) *We Can Week-End* program is a noted exception. When services are available for the family, they may have poor attendance, they often are short-term, or they may emphasize treatment or medical information, not cognitive-emotional-behavioral management by the family. Still needed are programs and services that focus on the family as a family. The reality is that families are primarily on their own to manage the transitions and contingencies related to parental cancer. A self-diagnosis is in order. In your own practice and in your place of employment, what family-level services exist? Box 15-3 summarizes five levels of services. To what extent and at what level is your agency offering family-level services and programs? It is not a matter of caring about families; it is a matter of developing services that deliver concrete, specific family-focused care. In the absence of family-focused services, family care in oncology is only an ideology, not a reality.

Evidence from our own program of research is that such family-focused services and programs should consider six potential targets: (1) the individual family member's perceptions of his or her illness-related demands, (2) the household family's coping and management of its experience, (3) the parent's depressive mood, (4) tension in the marriage that escalated because of the cancer, (5) the quality of the parenting during the illness, and (6) the utilization of support by the paient's parents.

Illness-Related Demands

Programs need to be developed that invite the family members to report of their illness-related pressures. Without disclosure, these illness-related demands have the potential to cause negative mood and consequences for the family. Although multiple methods could be used to assist family members to describe and cognitively and emotionally process these demands, the reality is that few opportunities, if any, are provided for family members to talk about their concerns. During the course of gaining clarity on the family member's concerns, the nurse will have opportunities to help decrease the threat of the demands. Attentive listening, grief counseling, and additional strategies can potentially assist family members (Lewis & Daltroy, 1990; Lewis &

Box 15-3
Family Focused Oncology Nursing: Five Levels of Services

Level 1: Courtesy Level

- Nurse introduces self to family member as a resource person to family.
- Nurse advocates for family in assisting them clarify treatment/care information from agency or physician.
- Nurse introduces family member to physical layout of unit/agency; structure of existing services.

Level 2: Engagement Level

- Nurse explicitly identifies family member who will act as family representative and spokesperson to family about patient's status/condition.
- Nurse actively invites and encourages family members to ask questions/clarify issues with nurse about patient's condition/treatment.

Level 3: Family Instructional Level

- Nurse operationalizes specific plan for teaching families about patient conditions and services.
- Nurse develops explicit goal-directed educational plan for triaged families.
- Nurse directs family members to explicit sources of printed, audio, or audiovisual materials for better understanding or managing the patient's condition.

Level 4: Family Psychoeducational Services

- Agency develops specific operational plans for eliciting and responding to the needs of the family members as direct clients in need of supportive services.
- Agency develops a file system of printed educational and support materials for check-out or distribution to the family.
- Agency updates regularly the file system of materials for family members.
- Agency systematically and regularly schedules face-to-face meetings with family members in need of support or assistance.
- Agency develops and implements group-level services for families sharing common issues, concerns, or challenges.
- Agency develops and regularly updates a clearinghouse of information on services and resources available to the family.
- Agency invites and engages multiple family members, as appropriate, in the family's solution and self-care.
- Reporting mechanisms between professionals include assessed family-level services.

Level 5: Agency Level Institutionalized Services

- Printed and highly visible philosophy of oncology nursing practice explicitly addresses the family as a highly valued client.
- Nursing *protocols* are developed and used for commonly encountered family problems or challenges.
- Record-keeping forms are explicitly developed for family focus, including: documented concerns addressed and followed up with family; family-level teaching plans; stationary with a family logo.
- Quality Assurance Committee reviews documented family-level services.
- Nurse job descriptions include family focused nursing services.
- Physical space is allocated for family conferences and counseling, and teaching meetings
- Physical space is allocated for family-focused printed materials.
- Systematized release mechanisms are allocated for "being with" a family.
- Merit raise and promotion criteria include special recognition of family-level services.
- Dedicated phone line exists for family members' calls.
- Trained volunteers assist with selected aspects of family-level services under the guidance of professional nursing staff.

Zahlis, 1997). Families can potentially benefit from having a forum in which to reflect on and augment, as necessary, the particular strategies the family members use to manage the impact of the cancer on their lives. By putting the illness "on the table" and working on it, the family's agency is enhanced, and there is the potential to advance the family's self-care and self-management skills. Face-to-face or phone interviews with the family members can be used to offer problem-focused management counseling with their expressed concerns (Roberts et al., 1995). Emphasis in such contacts should include both an emotive and a behavioral management focus. Assisting the family to express their concerns through empathic listening is important, but it does nothing to assist the family members' cognitive or behavioral management of the concern. Both are needed.

Depressive Mood in the Parent(s)

Family professionals need to assess depressive mood in both the diagnosed parent and the non-ill parent. The person with the depressive mood is not the problem; rather, the causes of the depressive mood are the problem. Nurses need to develop formal ability to assess the presence of signs and symptoms of depressive mood and to triage into referral those family members manifesting signs of clinical depression. In addition, the causes of this depressive mood are directly linked in our research program with the illness-related demands the family members are reporting. By assisting in the management of these illness-related demands, the nurse is potentially helping family members remove or reduce a major source of their depressive mood.

Marital Tension

Oncology nurses are not marital counselors or therapists, but they do have the potential to reduce tension caused by or accentuated by the cancer. Current research program experience shows that this tension is commonly generated when an illness-related concern of the couple is not clearly identified and dealt with by the couple (Lewis & Zahlis, 1997; Shands, Sinsheimer, & Lewis, 1997). In face-to-face interactions, it may be helpful to assist the couple to share with each other, in the presence of a skilled and objective listener, concerns or issues related to the cancer with which they as a couple want to work through. Skills are needed to facilitate such interaction, as well as the couple's enhancement of self-management of cancer-related concerns. More than 25 standardized protocols have been developed for assisting couples to work through their sources of tension from the cancer, including renegotiating sexual intimacy, dealing with emotions caused by the cancer, and interpreting the cancer for the children. Future research should include the development and evaluation of programs and services that assist couples to work through the cancer-related sources of their tension. Such services are not therapy; rather they focus on the couple's self-management and self-care.

Quality of Parenting

Nurses need to support the importance of quality parenting for the child or adolescent, even if the children are erroneously perceived as independent and not needing attention when the parent has cancer. Research evidence documents that the quality of parenting makes a significant impact on the success with which the children and adolescents respond to cancer in a parent.

Reinforcing the importance of parental responsiveness is a delicate matter in families experiencing cancer because the parents are already taxed by illness-related issues. The form of inviting the parent's reflection on their parenting needs to be concrete, nonthreatening, and nondemanding.

Some nurses might work directly with the child or adolescent whose parent has cancer (Heiney & Lesesne, 1997). A first step in any program or interaction is to determine the child and adolescent's perception of how they view the parent's cancer and how, if at all, the child or adolescent thinks the cancer is affecting them. Both young and school-age children and adolescents may need assistance from the nurse in interpreting alterations in parenting as illness-related. It is the illness, not the child, that is causing changes in parenting. In the absence of such interpretive assistance, research shows that some children and adolescents may be at risk for perceiving themselves as unworthy or devalued (Armsden & Lewis, 1994; Lewis et al., 1993, 1996).

Utilization of Social Support

The challenge for the nurse is to assist the family to more effectively use existing resources. Without such assistance, it is possible, if not probable, that many families will attempt to manage the cancer on their own. When there are no existing resources to which the family is able to turn, the nurse needs to assist the family to generate resources.

The use and access to resources needs to be normalized so that utilization is not interpreted by the family members as failure or weakness. Nurses need to directly recommend the use of resources for the families in much the same way that an orthopedic surgeon would recommend the use of physical therapy after surgery for repair of a broken bone. By framing these resources as part of a natural healing process, resource utilization is normalized and the family members are not stigmatized as failing or as being less competent. Research is needed on ways to normalize the referral to and utilization of social support by the family.

THE CHILD AND ADOLESCENT MODEL FOR UNDERSTANDING AND MANAGING CANCER

Few resources are available to either nurses or family members to help a child or adolescent deal with the impact of cancer in a parent (Lewis, 1996a). The small number of pamphlets or booklets that are available, although potentially helpful, may not go far enough in assisting children to deal with a parent's cancer. The development of multiple programs, services, and materials is clearly needed. The materials that do exist deserve to be rigorously evaluated either alone or in combination with other program components (e.g., with a support group for the child or the parent[s]). Unclear is what is needed; what is effective; or what can be done to improve the effectiveness of programs, materials, and services to help the children. In truth, we have treated the children and adolescents of parents with cancer with benign neglect (Lewis, 1996a).

CONCLUSION

The majority of studies with families experiencing cancer in a parent have been conducted in middle class, predominately highly educated white families. Essentially unknown is the experience of other family members from other socioeconomic, ethnic, or cultural groups (Tharp, 1991). Additional descriptive research is needed to develop culturally sensitive and informed programs and services (Lewis, 1996a).

This chapter has implicitly defined the *household family* in terms of two or more adult members living in the house, including those with one or more dependent children. There are other types of family constellations, including male-male families, female-female families, grandparent families, and others. To the authors' knowledge, none of these types of families have been studied, even though they are also experiencing cancer. Additional family constellations, including singles, deserve particular attention.

There is more than suggestive evidence that single women are experiencing greater levels of distress and disruption in their daily lives and households than are women with partners (Lewis et al., 1996). Additional research is needed with single parents and other special populations including couples experiencing cancer recurrence (Lewis & Deal, 1995).

The Family's Functioning With Cancer: Myth and Reality

This chapter began by asking questions about your beliefs about the family's functioning with cancer. These questions are now revisited. All of the items in Table 15-1 are *false.* If you hold beliefs and assumptions that caused you to select "true" for any of the items, return to your initial answers to see what changes you may want to consider making. Although assumptions and beliefs are personal, they affect how we work with and orient ourselves toward families experiencing cancer. In reflecting on your own assumptions about how families function with cancer, you add to your own practice expertise.

REFERENCES

Armsden, G.C., & Lewis, F.M. (1993). The child's adaptation to the mother's illness: Theory and clinical implications. *Patient Education and Counseling, 22,* 153-165.

Armsden, G. C., & Lewis, F. M. (1994). Behavioral adjustment and self-esteem among school-age children of mothers with breast cancer. *Oncology Nursing Forum, 21,* 39-45.

Baider, L., & De-Nour, A. K. (1984). Couples' reactions and adjustment to mastectomy: A preliminary report. *International Journal of Psychiatry in Medicine, 14,* 265-276.

Barckley, V. (1967). The crisis in cancer. *American Journal of Nursing Research, 67*(2), 278-280.

Bloom, J. R. (1982). Social support systems and cancer: A conceptual view. In J. Cohen, J. W. Cullen, & L. R. Martin, (Eds.), *Psychosocial aspects of cancer.* New York: Raven Press.

Bloom, J. R., Cook, M., Fotopoulis, S., Flamer, D., Gates, C., & Holland, J. C. (1987). Psychological response to mastectomy: A prospective comparison study. *Cancer, 59,* 189-196.

Broderick, C., & Smith, J. (1979). The general systems approach to the family. In W.R. Burr, R. Hill, F. I. Nye, & I. L. Reiss (Eds.), *Contemporary theories about the family.* New York: The Free Press.

Brody, G. H, Moore K., & Glei D. (1994). Family processes during adolescent development as predictors of parent-young adult attitudes similarity: A six-year longitudinal analysis. *Family Relations, 43,* 369.

Brown, D.J., Craick, C.C., Davies, S.E., Johnson, M.L., Dawborn, J.K., & Heale, W.F. (1978). Physical, emotional and social adjustments to home dialysis. *Medical Journal of Australia, 1,* 245-247.

Buckley, W. F. (1967). *Sociology and modern systems theory.* Englewood Cliffs, NJ: Prentice-Hall.

Buehler, C., Krishnakumar, A., Anthony, C., Tittsworth, C., & Stone, G. (1994). Hostile interparental conflict and youth maladjustment. *Family Relations, 43,* 409-416.

Cancer Care, Inc., & National Cancer Foundation, Inc. (1977). *Listen to the children! A study of the impact on the mental health of children of a parent's catastrophic illness.* New York: Authors.

Chekryn, J. (1984). Cancer recurrence: Personal meaning, communication, and marital adjustment. *Cancer Nursing, 7,* 491-498.

Cohen, S., & Wills, T. A. (1985). Stress, social support, and the buffering hypothesis. *Psychological Bulletin, 98,* 310-357.

Compas, B.E., Worsham, N.L., Epping-Jordan, J. E., Grant, K.E., Mireault, G., & Howell, D.C. (1994). When Mom or Dad has cancer: Markers of psychological distress in cancer patients, spouses, and children. *Health Psychology, 13*(6), 507-515.

Compas, B.E., Worsham, N.L., Ey, S., & Howell, D.C. (1996). When Mom or Dad has cancer: II. Coping, cognitive appraisals, and psychological distress in children of cancer patients. *Health Psychology, 15*(3), 167-175.

Emery, R. E. (1982). Interparental conflict and the children of discord and divorce. *Psychological Bulletin, 92,* 310-330.

Emery, R. E., & O'Leary, K. D. (1982). Children's perceptions of marital discord and behavior problems of boys and girls. *Journal of Abnormal Child Psychology, 10,* 11-24.

Ervin Jr., C. (1973). Psychologic adjustment to mastectomy. *Medical Aspects in Human Sexuality, 7,* 42-65.

Fauber, R., Forehand, R., Thomas, A. M., & Wierson, M. (1990). A mediational model of the impact of marital conflict on adolescent adjustment in intact and divorced families: The role of disrupted parenting. *Child Development, 61,* 1112-1123.

Feldman, D.J. (1974). Chronic disabling illness: A holistic view. *Journal of Chronic Disease, 27,* 287-291.

Forehand, R., McCombs, A., & Brody, G. H. (1987). The relationship between parental depressive mood states and child functioning. *Advances in Behavior Research and Therapy, 9,* 1-20.

Funch, D. P., & Mettlin, C. (1982). The role of support in relation to recovery from breast surgery. *Social Science and Medicine, 16,* 91-98.

Gable, S., Belsky, J., & Crnic, K. (1992). Marriage, parenting and child development: Progress and prospects. Special issue: Diversity in contemporary family psychology. *Journal of Family Psychology, 5,* 276-294.

Germino, B.B. (1984). *Family members' concerns after cancer diagnosis.* Unpublished doctoral dissertation, University of Washington.

Given, B., & Given, C.W. (1992). Patient and family caregiver reaction to new and recurrent cancer. *Journal of The American Medical Women's Association, 47*(5), 201-206.

Goodman, S., & Brumley, H. (1990). Schizophrenic and depressed mothers: Relational deficits in parenting. *Developmental Psychology, 26,* 31-39.

Gotay, C. C. (1984). The experience of cancer during early and advanced stages: The views of patients and their mates. *Social Science and Medicine, 18,* 605-613.

Grandstaff, N. W. (1976). The impact of breast cancer on the family. *Frontiers of Radiation Therapy and Oncology, 11,* 146-156.

Haberman, M.R., Woods, N.F., & Packard, N.J. (1990). Demands of chronic illness: Reliability and validity assessment of a demands of illness inventory. *Holistic Nursing Practice, 5*(1), 25-35.

Heiney, S.P., & Lesesne, C.A. (1997). *Quest: An intervention program for children whose parent or grandparent has cancer.* Manuscript submitted for publication.

Hill, R. (1972). Modern systems theory and the family: A confrontation. *Social Science and Information, 10,* 7-26.

Hilton, B. A. (1989). The relationship of uncertainty, control, commitment, and threat of recurrence to coping strategies used by women diagnosed with breast cancer. *Journal of Behavioral Medicine, 12,* 39-54.

Hilton, B.A. (1993). Issues, problems, and challenges for families coping with breast cancer. *Seminars in Oncology Nursing, 9*(2), 88-100.

Hilton, B.A. (1996). Getting back to normal: The family experience during early stage breast cancer. *Oncology Nursing Forum, 23*(4), 605-614.

Hirsch, B.J., Moos, R.H., & Reischl, T.M. (1985). Psychosocial adjustment of adolescent children of a depressed, arthritic, or normal parent. *Journal of Abnormal Psychology, 94,* 154-164.

Hough, E.E., Lewis, F.M., & Woods, N.F. (1991). Family response to mother's chronic illness: Case studies of well- and poorly-adjusted families. *Western Journal of Nursing Research, 13*(5), 568-596.

Issel, L.J., Ersek, M., & Lewis, F.M. (1990). How children cope with mother's breast cancer. *Oncology Nursing Forum, 17*(3), 5-13.

Johnson, J.L., & Norby, P.A. (1981). We can weekend: A program for cancer families. *Cancer Nursing, February,* 23-28.

Kent, S. (1975). Coping with sexual identity crises after mastectomy. *Geriatrics, 30,* 145-146.

Kobak, R. R., & Sceery, A. M. (1988). Attachment in late adolescence: Working models, affect regulation, and representations of self and others. *Child Development, 59,* 135-146.

Kobak, R. R., Sudler, N., & Gamble, W. (1991). Attachment and depressive symptoms during adolescence: A developmental pathways analysis. *Development and Psychopathology, 3,* 461-474.

Lewis, F.M. (1983). Family-level services for the cancer patient: Critical distinctions, fallacies, and assessment. *Cancer Nursing, 6*(3), 193-200.

Lewis, F. M. (1986). The impact of cancer on the family: A critical analysis of the research literature. *Patient Education and Counseling, 8,* 269-289.

Lewis, F. M. (1987). The concept of control: A typology and health-related variables. *Advances in Health Education and Promotion, 2,* 277-309.

Lewis, F. M. (1990). Strengthening family supports: Cancer and the family. *Cancer, 65,* 158-165.

Lewis, F.M. (1993). Psychosocial transitions and the family's work in adjusting to cancer. *Seminars in Oncology Nursing, 9*(2), 127-129.

Lewis, F. M. (1996a). The impact of breast cancer on the family: Lessons learned from the children and adolescents. In L. Baider & C.L. Cooper (Eds.), *Cancer and the family.* Sussex: John Wiley & Sons.

Lewis, F.M. (1996b). The Single Woman's Journey: Listening to and Learning From Her Story. Y-ME National Breast Cancer Conference. Chicago, August 1-2.

Lewis, F.M., & Bloom, J.R.. (1979). Psychosocial adjustment to breast cancer: A review of selected literature. *International Journal of Psychiatry in Medicine, 9*(1), 1-17.

Lewis, F. M., & Daltroy, L. (1990). How causal explanations influence health behavior: Attribution theory. In K. Glanz, F.M. Lewis, & B. Rimer (Eds.), *Health behavior and health education: Theory, research and practice.* San Francisco: Jossey-Bass.

Lewis, F. M., & Deal, L. (1995). Balancing our lives: A study of the married couple's experience with breast cancer recurrence. *Oncology Nursing Forum, 22*(6), 943-953.

Lewis, F. M., & Hammond, M. A. (1992). Psychosocial adjustment of the family to breast cancer: A longitudinal analysis. *Journal of the American Medical Women's Association, 47,* 194-200.

Lewis, F. M., & Hammond, M. A. (1996). The father's, mother's and adolescent's adjustment to a mother's breast cancer. *Family Relations, 45,* 456-465.

Lewis, F.M., & Zahlis, E.H. (1997). *The nurse as coach: A conceptual analysis for clinical practice.* Manuscript submitted for publication.

Lewis, F. M., Hammond, M. A., & Woods, N. F. (1993). The family's functioning with newly diagnosed breast cancer in the mother: The development of an explanatory model. *Journal of Behavioral Medicine, 16,* 351-370.

Lewis, F. M., Woods, N. F., Hough, E. E., & Bensley, L. S. (1989). The family's functioning with chronic illness in the mother: The spouse's perspective. *Social Science and Medicine, 29,* 1261-1269.

Lewis, F.M., Zahlis, E.H., Shands, M.E., Sinsheimer, J.A., & Hammond, M.A. (1996). The functioning of single women with breast cancer and their school-aged children. *Cancer Practice, 4*(1), 15-24.

Lindsey, A. M., Norbeck, J. S., Carrieri, V. L., & Perry, E. (1981). Social support and health outcomes in post-mastectomy women: A review. *Cancer Nursing, 4,* 377-384.

Litman, T.J. (1974). The family as a basic unit in health and medical care: A social-behavioral overview. *Social Science Medicine, 8,* 495-519.

Litman, T.J., & Venters, M. (1979). Research on health care and the family: A methodological overview. *Social Science Medicine, 13A,* 379-385.

Loveys, B. J., & Klaich, K. (1991). Breast cancer: Demands of illness. *Oncology Nursing Forum, 18,* 75-80.

Maccoby, E.E. (1992). The role of parents in the socialization of children: An historical overview. *Developmental Psychology, 28,* 1006-1017.

Maguire, G. P., Lee, E. G., Bevington, D. J., Kuchemann, C. S., Crabtree, R. J., & Cornell, C.E. (1978). Psychiatric problems in the first year after mastectomy. *British Medical Journal, 1,* 963-965.

Molumphy, S.D., & Sporakowski, M.J. (1984). The family stress of hemodialysis. *Family Relations 33,* 33-39.

Morgan, J., Sanford, M., & Johnson, C. (1992). The impact of a physically ill parent on adolescents: Cross-sectional findings from a clinic population. *Canadian Journal of Psychiatry, 37,* 423-427.

Morris, T., Greer, S., & White, P. (1977). Psychological and social adjustment to mastectomy: A two-year follow-up study. *Cancer, 40,* 2381-2387.

Moyer, A., & Salovay, P. (1996). Psychosocial sequelae of breast cancer and its treatment. *Annals of Behavioral Medicine, 18*(2), 110-125.

Northouse, L. L. (1988). Social support in patients' and husbands' adjustment to breast cancer. *Nursing Research, 37,* 91-95.

Northouse, L. L. (1992). Psychological impact of the diagnosis of breast cancer on the patient and her family. *Journal of the American Medical Women's Association, 47,* 161-164.

Northouse, L. L., & Peters-Golden, H. (1993). Cancer and the family: Strategies to assist spouses. *Seminars in Oncology Nursing, 9,* 74-82.

Northouse, L., & Swain, M. A. (1987). Adjustment of patients and husbands to the initial impact of breast cancer. *Nursing Research, 36,* 221-225.

Oberst, M. T., & James, R. H. (1985). Going home: Patient and spouse adjustment following cancer surgery. *Topics in Clinical Nursing, 7,* 46-57.

Orvaschel, H. (1983). Maternal depression and child dysfunction. In B. B. Lahey & A.E. Kazdin (Eds.), *Advances in child clinical psychology* (Vol. 6). New York: Plenum.

Packard, N. J., Haberman, M. R., Woods, N. F., & Yates, B. C. (1991). Demands of illness among chronically ill woman. *Western Journal of Nursing Research, 13,* 434-457.

Panaccione, V. F., & Wahler, R. G. (1986). Child behavior, maternal depression, and social coercion as factors in the quality of child care. *Journal of Abnormal Child Psychology, 14,* 263-278.

Parkes, C.M. (1975). The emotional impact of cancer on patients and their families. *Journal of Laryngology and Otolaryngology, 89,* 1271-1279.

Peters-Golden, H. (1982). Breast cancer: Varied perceptions of social support in the illness experience. *Social Science and Medicine, 16,* 483-491.

Peterson, Y. (1979). The impact of physical disability on marital adjustment: A literature review. *Family Coordinator, 28,* 47-51.

Porter, B., & O'Leary, D. (1980). Marital discord and childhood behavior problems. *Journal of Abnormal Child Psychology, 8,* 287-295.

Primomo, J., Yates, B., & Woods, N.F. (1990). Social support for women during chronic illness. Sources, types and outcome. *Research in Nursing and Health, 13,* 153-161.

Roberts, J., Browne, G.B., Streiner, D., Gafni, A., Pallister, R., & Hoxby, H. (1995). Problem-solving counseling or phone-call support for outpatients with chronic illness: Effective for whom? *Canadian Journal of Nursing Research, 27*(3), 111-136.

Sabo, D., Brown, J., & Smith, C. (1986). The male role and mastectomy: Support groups and men's adjustment. *Journal of Psychosocial Oncology, 4,* 19-31.

Samarel, N., & Fawcett, J. (1992). Enhancing adaptation to breast cancer: The addition of coaching to support groups. *Oncology Nursing Forum, 19,* 591-596.

Samarel, N., Fawcett, J., & Tulman, L. (1993). The effects of coaching in breast cancer support groups: A pilot study. *Oncology Nursing Forum, 20*(5), 795-798.

Samms, M. (1996). *The husband's unheard story of sustaining his wife with breast cancer.* Unpublished master's thesis, University of Washington, Seattle.

Shands, M.E., Sinsheimer, J., & Lewis, F.M. (1997). *Coaching couples experiencing early stage breast cancer: An analysis of their concerns.* Manuscript in preparation.

Stetz, K. M., Lewis, F. M., & Houck, G. M. (1994). Family goals as indicants of adaptation during chronic illness. *Public Health Nursing, 11,* 385-391.

Stetz, K., Lewis, F. M., & Primomo, J. (1986). Family coping strategies and chronic illness in the mother. *Family Relations, 35,* 515-522.

Stewart, M. J. (1989). Social support: Diverse theoretical perspectives. *Social Science and Medicine, 28,* 1275-1282.

Strauss, A.L. (1959). *Mirrors and masks: The search for identity.* Glencoe, IL, Free Press.

Tharp, R. G. (1991). Cultural diversity and treatment of children. *Journal of Consulting and Clinical Psychology, 59*(6), 799-812.

Thoits, P. A. (1982). Conceptual, methodological, and theoretical problems in studying social support as a buffer against life stress. *Journal of Health and Social Behavior, 23,* 145-159.

Tronick, E.Z., & Field, T. (Eds.). (1986). *Maternal depression and infant disturbance.* San Francisco: Jossey-Bass.

Welch, A., Wadsworth, M., & Compas, B. 1996. Adjustment of children and adolescents to parental cancer: Parents' and children's perspectives. *Cancer, 77*(7): 1409-1418.

Wellisch, D. K. (1979). Adolescent acting-out when a parent has cancer. *International Journal of Family Therapy, 1,* 230-241.

Wellisch, D. K. (1981). Family relationships of the mastectomy patient: Interactions with the spouse and children. *Israel Journal of Medical Sciences, 17,* 993-996.

Wellisch, D. K., Gritz, E. R., Schain, W., Wang, H. J., & Siau, J. (1991). Psychological functioning of daughters of breast cancer patients. Part I: Daughters and comparison subjects. *Psychosomatics, 32,* 324-336.

Wellisch, D. K., Gritz, E. R., Schain, W., Wang, H-J., & Siau, J. (1992). Psychological functioning of daughters of breast cancer patients. Part II: Characterizing the distressed daughter of the breast cancer patient. *Psychosomatics, 33,* 171-179.

Wellisch, D. K., Jamison, K. R., & Pasnau, R. O. (1978). Psychosocial aspects of mastectomy II: The man's perspective. *American Journal of Psychiatry, 135,* 543-546.

Woods, N. F., & Lewis, F. M. (1995). Living with chronic illness: Women's perspectives on their families' adaptation. *Health Care for Women International, 16,* 135-148.

Wortman, C. B. (1984). Social support and the cancer patient: Conceptual and methodological issues. *Cancer, 53,* 2339-2359.

Yates, B.C., Bensley, L.S., Lalonde, B., Lewis, F.M., & Woods, N.F. (1995). The impact of marital status and quality on family functioning in maternal chronic illness. *Health Care for Women International, 16*(5), 437-449.

Zahlis, E. H., & Shands, M. E. (1991). Breast cancer: Demands of illness on the patient's partner. *Journal of Psychosocial Oncology, 9,* 75-93.

Zahlis, E. H., & Shands, M. E. (1993). The impact of breast cancer on the partner 18 months after diagnosis. *Seminars in Oncology Nursing, 9,* 83-87.

Zunkel, G. (1996). *Women with breast cancer: Couple processes as a context for recovery.* Unpublished doctoral dissertation. University of Washington, Seattle.

The Cancer Patient and Psychoneuroimmunology

Kathryn Ann Caudell, PhD, RN, AOCN

INTRODUCTION

The neuroendocrine and immune systems have the ability to receive input from the environment and respond accordingly. It was long thought that these systems functioned independently of each other in a Cartesian dualistic manner. However, in the last 25 years, researchers have identified communication networks that exist between these systems. In an effort to further explore and communicate these mind-body relationships, the field of psychoneuroimmunology developed.

The idea that the body responds to stressful events in the environment is not new. In 1914 Cannon proposed a psychophysiologic model of the fight-or-flight response during which acute responses to stress were characterized (Cannon, 1914). He proposed that the sympathetic nervous system was responsible for a person's defense against stress, whereas the parasympathetic nervous system controlled functions such as digestion. Selye (1936, 1956) further delineated the body's response to acute and chronic stressors in his general adaptation syndrome (GAS). He proposed that two neuroendocrine axes became activated during the body's response to stress: the hypothalamic-pituitary-adrenal-cortical and the sympathoadrenal-medullary axes. He also characterized the GAS as having three stages of response: the acute phase, or the alarm reaction; the second phase, the stage of resistance; and the third phase, the stage of exhaustion.

Research in the area of mind-body interactions continued, and in 1964 Solomon and Moos published a paper that theoretically integrated the relationships between stress, immunologic dysfunction, and psychological disturbances. They extensively investigated the areas of personality and emotional factors, focusing specifically on the failure of psychologic defenses in the development and course of rheumatoid arthritis. These findings, in addition to data that suggested that autoimmune diseases were associated with immunoincompetence and that immunosuppressive adrenocortical hormones become elevated during periods of stress, motivated the development of a psychoimmunology laboratory in 1965 at the Palo Alto Veterans Administration Hospital.

Another important area of investigation that provides strong support for the mind-body interaction involves conditioned immunosuppression. In the early 1970s Ader and Cohen discovered that rodents given saccharin-flavored water before administration of cyclophosphamide, a potent immunosuppressant antineoplastic agent, exhibited immunosuppression when administered subsequent saccharin-flavored water without cyclophosphamide. Several other groups repeated this murine protocol and found similar results (Rogers, Reich, Strom, & Carpenter, 1976; Wayner, Flannery, & Singer, 1978).

More recently, Giang, Goodman, Schiffer, Mattson, Petrie, Cohen, et al. (1996), using a human model, administered intravenous (IV) cyclophosphamide paired with anise-flavored water to a group of 10 people with multiple sclerosis. During the subsequent two monthly treatments, the subjects alternately received either a considerably lower nonimmunosuppressive dose of IV cyclophosphamide with the flavored water or the full-strength cyclophosphamide (1100 to 1800 mg). Eighty percent of the subjects who received the nonimmunosuppressive dose exhibited immunosuppression. These studies suggest that in both animals and humans the immune response can be conditioned and that the immune system can be controlled by the nervous system.

Research in the area of psychoneuroimmunology is currently becoming more sophisticated. Investigations into bidirectional communication networks between lymphoid tissue, hormones, and cells of the immune system are greatly expanding our knowledge of the mind-body connection. An increasing number of interdisciplinary research teams are also improving the development of sound, research protocols based on well thought out models that control for confounding variables. Protocols frequently include immune measurements of absolute numbers of cell types, functional assays such as the chromium release assay, and activation assays that monitor the appearance of specific membrane-bound proteins. Many investigators have evaluated responses in a number of clinical populations, which has led to the identification of potential immunologic markers for various disorders. Research continues in an attempt to elucidate the mechanisms involved between immune down-regulation and the development of disease. Other research examines the effects of behavioral interventions in reducing the maladaptive responses to stress and improving immunocompetence in various populations.

This chapter provides an overview of several critical components included in psychoneuroimmunology, focusing primarily on the neuroendocrine and immune responses to stress, bidirectional communication networks between the neuroendocrine and immune systems, and factors that mediate the responses. Finally, interventions that have been found to reduce maladaptive neuroendocrine and immune responses are discussed.

STRESS AND NEUROENDOCRINE RESPONSES

In reviewing the stress literature, it is apparent that the concept of stress means many things to many people. For example, stress can be viewed as the initiating event, the response, or the interactional process experienced. It can be acute or chronic in nature, both of which yield different physiologic responses. Stress can also be caused by external psychological or physiologic stimuli such as examination stress or extreme physical exercise or by internal factors such as an infection. It has also become apparent that a person's response is strongly associated with his or her appraisal of the event.

Generally, when a person is exposed to a stressful event, afferent stimuli enter the neocortex and travel to the limbic system, which consists of the cingulate gyrus, the amygdala, the hippocampus, and other related structures. In the limbic system the stimuli are processed and evaluated. The limbic system is extensively interconnected with the hypothalamus. Both maintain homeostasis by regulating endocrine secretion, the autonomic nervous system, emotion, and motivation. Excitatory impulses received by the hypothalamus cause neurons to release corticotropin-releasing hormone (CRF). CRF is secreted into the portal hypophyseal vascular network between the hypothalamus and the anterior pituitary gland and travels to the anterior pituitary, where cells

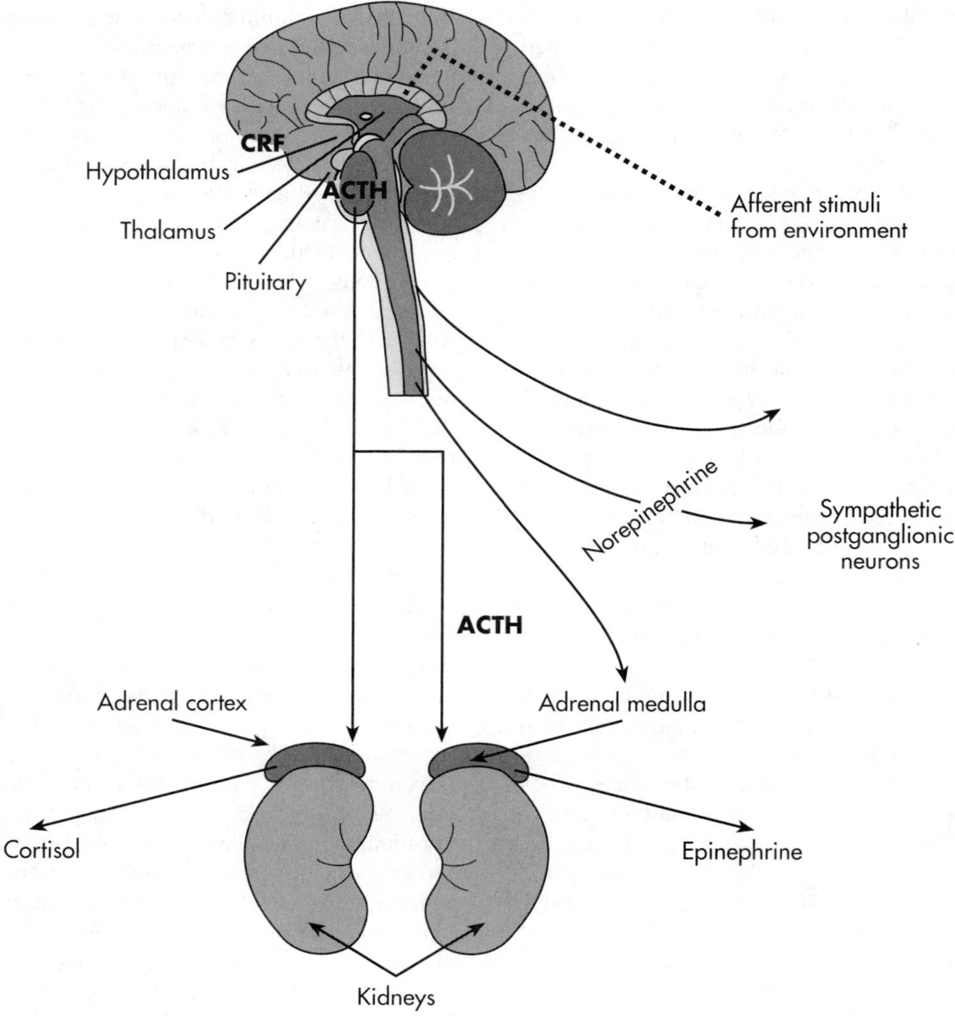

Fig. 16-1 Activation of the hypothalamic-pituitary-adrenal-cortical and the sympathoadrenal-medullary axes in response to stressful stimuli.

are stimulated to release adrenocorticotropic hormone (ACTH) into the circulation. ACTH ultimately activates corticotrophs in the adrenal cortex to secrete the glucocorticoid hormone cortisol. Concurrent with the activation of the hypothalamic-pituitary adrenal axis, the sympathoadrenal medullary axis is activated, during which hypothalamic efferent neurons stimulate the adrenal medulla to secrete both epinephrine and norepinephrine (in smaller amounts) and the sympathetic postganglionic neurons to secrete norepinephrine (Fig. 16-1).

Many studies use acute stress paradigms to examine the physiologic responses of persons experiencing them. Realistically, however, many people are exposed to stressors over an extended period. Chronic stress has been defined as "demands, threats, perceived harm or loss, or responses that persist for long periods of time" (Baum, 1990). This definition suggests that the perceived loss or harm can continue to elicit responses in animals or humans long after the specific event has terminated.

Responses to chronic stressors have been observed to vary. For example, some investigators propose that persons exposed to prolonged stressors tend to respond in a more subdued manner. Pulse rates and blood pressure tend to be lower. The person eventually habituates to the stressor and adapts by suppressing his or her responses. Habituation is defined as the "learned suppression of the response to a repeated stimulus" (Kandel, 1991).

Other investigators suggest that the physiologic response does not adapt during periods of prolonged stress and may remain elevated for a prolonged time (Davidson & Baum, 1986). A study examining the effects of a novel stressor on a group of chronically stressed rats and a group of nonstressed rats revealed that mean arterial pressures, heart rates, and epinephrine and norepinephrine levels did not differ considerably between groups before the novel stressor. However, when both groups were exposed to the new stressor, the chronically stressed rats exhibited significant increases in both epinephrine and norepinephrine, as well as mean arterial pressure and heart rate. The authors suggested that the sympathetic adrenal-medullary activation in the chronically stressed rodents became sensitized such that a heightened physiologic response occurred when the animal was then exposed to a novel stressor (Konarska, Stewart, & McCarty, 1989) (Fig. 16-2). Like habituation, sensitization is a form of nonassociative learning that helps an animal learn to strengthen its defensive reflexes when withdrawal and escape are required (Kandel, 1991).

Individuals living near the Three Mile Island nuclear plant in 1979 during the destruction of its nuclear core experienced a number of stressors over an extended period. Radioactive gas and water were released periodically, potentially exposing residents who resided in close proximity to the plant. Mismanagement of information provided to the residents, loss of privacy as a result of increased news media coverage, and evacuation of pregnant women and small children added to the threat of the incident (Baum, 1990). Residents that lived within 5 miles of the plant exhibited higher levels of urinary epinephrine and immunosuppression and reported more symptoms than matched controls living 80 miles away. Data continued to be collected on the residents throughout the early 1980s. A significant number of residents continued to experience elevated catecholamine levels and higher blood pressure, report more health problems, and purchase more prescriptions than people living a distance away (Baum, Gatchel, & Schaeffer, 1983). Data from these two studies in both animals and humans support the suggestion that exposure to chronic stress can induce long-term responses.

NEUROENDOCRINE AND IMMUNE COMMUNICATION

In recent years an increasing number of communication mechanisms have been discovered between the neuroendocrine and immune systems. Cell membrane receptors for a

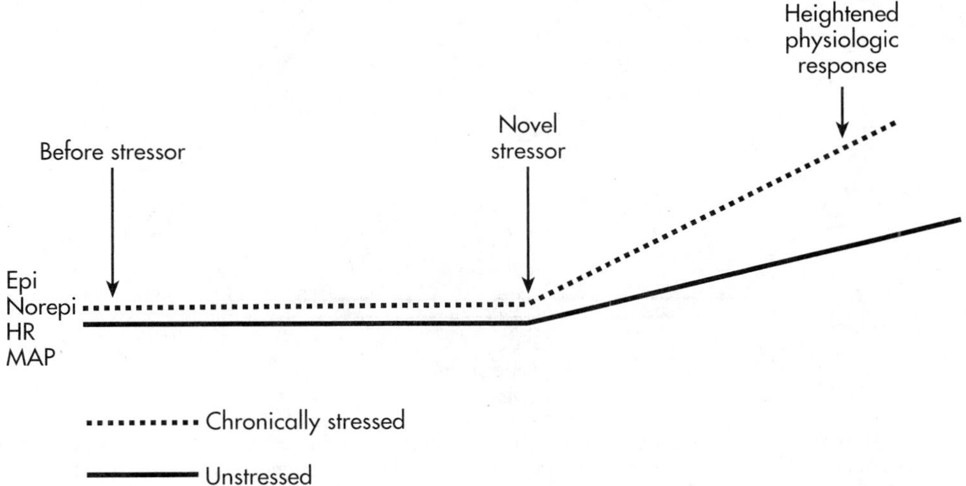

Fig 16-2 Heightened physiologic reactivity in chronically stressed animals. *Epi,* Epinephrine; *Norepi,* norepinephrine; *HR,* heart rate; *MAP,* mean arterial pressure.

number of hormones, including epinephrine, norepinephrine, vasoactive intestinal peptide, growth hormone, and prolactin, are found on the cell surface of several lymphocytes. The hormones that are secreted in response to emotion appear to control the distribution and migration of monocytes. These monocytes, in turn, communicate with B-cells and thymocytes and interact with the entire immune system to protect the body against foreign antigens.

White blood cells have been observed to produce peptides that were originally thought to be produced only by endocrine glands. For example, during viral or bacterial infections, leukocytes synthesize ACTH molecules. After a thorough examination of the molecular weights, amino acid sequences, reactivity with monospecific antibodies, and biologic function, it was determined that the peptides produced by leukocytes were basically identical to the peptides produced by the anterior pituitary gland. Similar findings have been observed for thyrotropin, chorionic gonadotropin, growth hormone, prolactin, and others (Carr & Blalock, 1991).

A number of peptides have been found to modulate immune function. For example, α-endorphin suppresses antigen specific T-lymphocyte helper factor. Luteinizing hormone suppresses natural killer cell activity. Immunoglobulin and interferon-gamma synthesis is suppressed by ACTH. Conversely, various cytokines produced by leukocytes modulate hormonal functions. For example, interferon-alpha leads to elevated levels of plasma cortisol (Carr & Blalock, 1991). Furthermore, lymphoid tissues have also been shown to be innervated by nerve fibers.

These data strongly suggest that anatomic, biochemical, and molecular communication pathways exist between the immune and neuroendocrine systems (Fig. 16-3). The cellular components of the immune system are producing chemicals that were historically thought to control mood. Thus there is increasing evidence that the relationship between stressors and immune function is influenced by the neuroendocrine system, which is directly responsive to psychosocial factors.

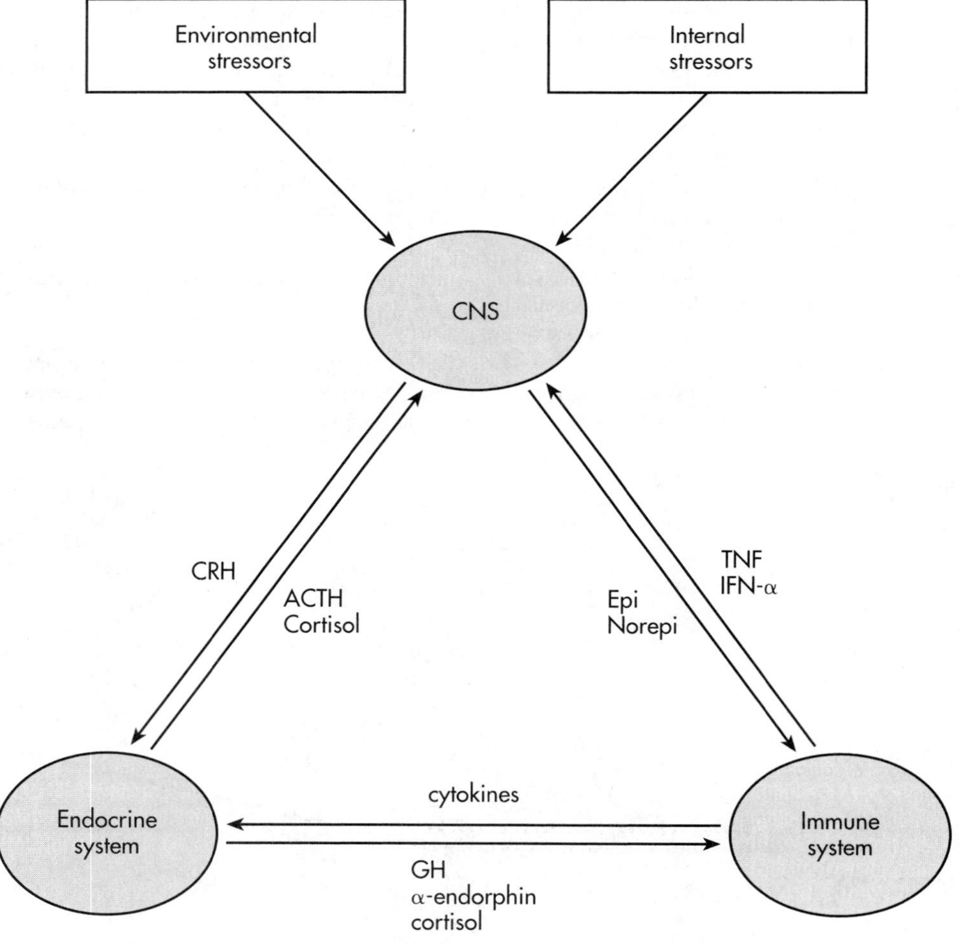

Fig. 16-3 Complex psychoneuro-endocrine-immune interactions in response to environmental and internal stressors. *CRH,* Corticotropin-releasing hormone; *ACTH,* adrenocorticotropic hormone; *Epi,* epinephrine; *Norepi,* norepinephrine; *TNF,* tumor necrosis factor; *IFN-α*, interferon-alpha; *GH,* growth hormone.

PSYCHOLOGICAL FACTORS THAT MEDIATE THE PSYCHONEUROIMMUNOLOGIC RESPONSE

Appraisal, coping, social support, mood, and personality factors all influence the way in which individuals respond to stressors (Table 16-1). The type of stressor, the duration and intensity of the event, and the individual's perception determine the way in which the individual responds. If the stressor is perceived as a threat, there is likely to be a more pronounced neuroendocrine response than if it is thought be insignificant to the individual's well-being.

The way in which individuals cope with the stressor also determines how they respond. For example, Laudenslager, Ryan, Drugan, Hyson, & Maier (1983) monitored the proliferation ability of lymphocytes from rodents who were able to control electric shock vs those who could not control the shock. Lymphocytes taken from the two groups of rats were exposed to tritiated thymidine, a growth factor. In normal circumstances the lymphocyte should proliferate when exposed to this substance. The rats that could not control their exposure to the shock demonstrated greater suppression of lymphocyte proliferation (Laudenslager et al, 1983). Other electric shock studies on rodents have found that those without the ability to turn off the shock exhibit lower natural killer cell cytotoxicity (Millar, Thomas, Pacheco, & Rollwagen, 1993).

Turner, Clancy, & Vitaliano (1987) observed that individuals' appraisals of their pain levels were significantly associated with the way in which they coped with the pain. If individuals accepted the pain and did not think that the pain would restrict their activities, they were more likely to use problem-focused coping. These data may suggest that an individual's initial appraisal affects not only his or her physiologic response, but also the coping strategies used.

Early studies using animal models found that behavioral subtypes demonstrated different physiologic responses (Ingram & Corfman, 1980). Investigators have more recently examined the effects of stressors such as examinations on individuals categorized as high stress and low stress (Workman and LaVia, 1987). The high-stress students who also had high scores on stress intrusion exhibited a greater reduction in lymphocyte proliferation to the mitogen phytohemagglutinin when compared with other stressed students. These "high-stress intrusion" students also acquired more viral upper respiratory infections after experiencing stressful situations.

Personality factors and mood disturbances have also been implicated in the development of cancer. In 1926 Evans reported that the loss of an important personal relationship frequently occurred before the development of cancer. Similar connections have subsequently been made in the areas of cardiovascular disease, low-birth-weight children, and several other types of malignancies, including gastric carcinoma, lung and breast cancers, and pediatric cancers.

Several investigators have examined personality factors in women undergoing diagnostic breast biopsies. These studies found that women who were diagnosed with breast cancer reported elevated feelings of anger and loss of control during anger episodes (Morris, Greer, Pettingale, & Watson, 1981); had problems in expressing anger, tended to avoid conflict, were more aloof, and reported being more self-sufficient (Wirsching, Stierlin, Hoffman, Weber, & Wirsching, 1982); and exhibited lower aggression scores but higher depression scores (Jansen & Muenz, 1984)

TABLE 16-1 Psychosocial Variables and Observed Outcomes

Psychosocial Variable	Outcome
Appraisal	May directly affect initial neuroendocrine activation
	Influences mood (Caudell, Gallucci, & Betrus, 1996)
	Major determinant of coping styles (Bush, 1998)
Coping	Influences affect, symptom perceptions, reasons to seek medical care, neuroendocrine-immune responses (Stone & Porter, 1995)
	Helps people find meaning in life (i.e., life goals reprioritized, value changes, increased appreciation for life (Bush, 1998)
Social support	Lessens anxiety
	Facilitates more adaptive coping
	Facilitates reinterpreting significance of stressor
	Improves quality of life (Post-White, 1998)
	Lengthens survival (Spiegel, Bloom, Kraemer, & Gottheil, 1998)
	Fewer health consequences (Kennedy, Kiecolt- Glaser, & Glaser, 1988)
	Enhanced immune function (Fawzy & Fawzy, 1994)
Personality	Influences speed of recovery from illness (Greenfield, Roessler, Corsley, 1959)
	Reduces illness during stressful life events (Johnson & Sarason, 1978; Kobasa, Maddi, & Courington, 1981)
Mood	Depression mediates high cortisol levels and lowers helper T-cell numbers and natural killer cell cytotoxicity
	Humor potentially immunoenhancing (Martin & Dobbin, 1988)

Social support has also been found to be significantly associated with survival in cancer patients. Individuals who report satisfaction with their support networks also tend to exhibit fewer health consequences when exposed to stressful events compared with those with inadequate social networks.

Uchino and colleagues (1992) examined the effects of social support as a potential buffer to stress in family caregivers of people with Alzheimer's disease. The family members who reported high levels of social support demonstrated normal age-related decreases in heart rate. Those who reported low levels of support exhibited elevations in heart rate reactivity and blood pressure. The data suggest that autonomic reactivity in people experiencing chronic stress may be moderated by social support. Kiecolt-Glaser, Dura, Speicher, Trask, & Glaser (1991) found in a similar population that caregivers of Alzheimer's patients experience declines in immune function and that those with the lowest levels of support show the largest declines.

A seminal study by Speigel and colleagues (1989) discovered that women with advanced breast cancer who attended weekly support groups as part of a multicomponent intervention survived on the average of 36 months, whereas women who did not participate in a support group lived for 18.9 months. Fawzy & Fawzy (1994) developed a 6-week psychoeducational intervention for patients with malignant melanoma that included stress management, coping information, and psychologic support. Forty patients were randomized to participate in the intervention, and another 40 were assigned to the control group. Those who participated in the intervention were found to use more active behavioral coping techniques, exhibit less psychologic distress, and have a significant increase in the number and cytotoxicity of natural killer cells. Of the 37 subjects who completed the entire 5-year study, three died and six developed recurrence of their disease. On the other hand, 12 of the control group died and three developed recurrence. These data suggest that a multicomponent intervention that includes stress management and support and teaches affective coping strategies is useful in reducing distressing psychophysiologic responses and may be of some benefit in lengthening survival.

These studies represent a sampling of the literature on the effects of psychosocial factors that mediate the neuroendocrine and immune responses to stressors. Although it is premature to assume that these factors play direct roles in the development of disease, there have been statistically significant associations between these variables and psychophysiologic responses to stress.

Nonpsychosocial factors also mediate neuroendocrine and immune function. These can be categorized as constitutional, such as a person's age, gender, genetics, and the circadian rhythms that modulate physiologic and cellular activity, or they can pertain to behaviors that have either beneficial or detrimental effects. Aging individuals normally experience a decline in cell-mediated immunity, a change that places older individuals at risk for developing diseases such as cancer and autoimmune diseases (Haddy, 1987). Men and women exhibit different responses to stressful events and perceive the same events differently. Women have been found to secrete lower levels of epinephrine than men in response to stress (Ziegler, 1989).

Studies of adopted children also demonstrate that they are at higher risks for dying from certain illnesses if their biologic parents died from the illness, a finding that suggests that nature, or a person's genetic predisposition, may have a stronger influence on outcomes than nurture, or one's environment (Sørenson, Nielsen, Anderson, 1988). Several neuroendocrine peptides have been found to be secreted in a circadian pattern. Lymphocytes also tend to exhibit patterns throughout the day with decreased activity, with lower levels of absolute numbers occurring approximately around 10 AM. (Dammacco, Campobasso, Altomare, & Iodice, 1984).

Poor health behaviors such as sleep deprivation, nutritional deficits, and smoking or activities such as intensive exercise have been found to alter immunocompetence. For example, sleep deprivation suppresses the function of several white blood cells, including proliferation in response to mitogens and phagocytosis (Palmblad, Petrini, Wasserman & Akerstedt, 1979). Individuals with both calorie and protein deficits exhibit suppression of cell-mediated immunity (Chandra, 1980).

Both cigarette smoking and exercise have stimulating and suppressive effects on immune function. Smoking depresses lymphocyte responses but has been found to increase proliferation of cytotoxic T lymphocytes (Petersen, Steimel, & Callaghan, 1983; Holmen, Karlsson, Bratt, & Hogstedt, 1995). The effects of exercise on immune function depend on its intensity and duration. Exercise causes temporary increases in catecholamines, glucocorticoids, and β-endorphins (Howlett, Tomlin, Hgahfoong, Rees, Bullen, & Skrinar, et al., 1984). Glucocorticoids are immunosuppressive, whereas catecholamines tend to induce the distribution of leukocytes from the bone marrow to the peripheral circulation (Shinkai, Shore, Shek, & Shephard, 1992). Many behavioral activities that have detrimental effects on immunocompetence can be changed, unlike the constitutional factors.

Clinicians developing behavioral interventions aimed at reducing psychological distress during diagnosis, treatment, and follow-up of cancer patients should incorporate components that address the psychosocial factors. Furthermore, educational programs should be offered to patients, which include ways to change detrimental behaviors to ones that improve immunocompetence when diagnosis and treatment stress may affect immune function.

MIND-BODY INTERVENTIONS

A number of complimentary interventions are demonstrating promising results in reducing both psychologic and physiologic distress. Individuals can do several of these at their convenience and their location of choice after instruction, whereas other interventions require the presence of a trained practitioner.

Relaxation is defined as a state of decreased cognitive, physiologic, and/or behavioral arousal. During the relaxation process, muscle fibers become elongated, neural impulses to the brain are reduced, and overall activity of the body is reduced. The relaxation response is characterized by decreased heart rate, respiratory rate, blood pressure, perspiration rate, and oxygen consumption and increased alpha brain activity and skin temperature. The relaxation response may be achieved through a variety of techniques that involve a repetitive mental focus and adoption of a calm, peaceful attitude (Mandle, Jacobs, Arcaro, & Domar, 1996).

There are two types of relaxation strategies. During passive relaxation, individuals are taught to focus on internal sensory processes such as breathing while relaxing various muscle groups. No energy expenditure is required. This form of relaxation is ideal for individuals who have minimal energy reserves. Active relaxation, on the other hand involves tightening specific muscle groups at varying degrees followed by relaxing the muscle. This helps the individual learn to recognize variations in muscle tension so that relaxation techniques may be instituted while the muscle tension is still at a manageable level (McGuigan, 1993). The type of relaxation intervention, whether it be active or passive, should be determined according to the individual's functional status, the energy expenditure required by the technique, and the motivation of the individual for frequent practice. A critical outcome of relaxation is the acquisition of cognitive skills that people develop during relaxation training that help them reduce detrimental responses to stressful events within their environment.

Individuals with chronic pain who experience elevated muscular tension and emotional distress have been found to exhibit a lowered pain tolerance and increased exacerbations of pain and distress. Relaxation training combined with pleasing imagery has been found to decrease pain intensity and distress (Ferrell, Dean, & Funk, 1996). Similar relaxation interventions have also produced beneficial effects by reducing anticipatory nausea and vomiting in a variety of cancer patients (Burish, Snyder, Krozely, & Greco, 1987; Carey & Burish, 1987; Burish, Snyder, & Jenkins, 1991).

Imagery is another strategy frequently used in combination with relaxation therapy. Imagery can be self-directed, in which the individual creates his or her own mental images, or guided, during which a practitioner leads the individual through a particular scenario. In guided imagery a practitioner describes a pleasing environment into which the individual visualizes being immersed. The use of various senses is encouraged to make the environment to seem more realistic. For example, a person may be encouraged to visualize walking through a flowered meadow through which a babbling brook is running. The person is encouraged to feel the warmth of the sun on his or her arms, to hear the birds singing and the relaxing sound of running water, and to see and smell the wild flowers surrounding him or her.

Self-directed imagery is characterized by instructing the person to visualize his or her own special place. This strategy is frequently used by persons who are more experienced in practicing relaxation because it gives them, rather than the practitioner, the opportunity to choose a place they prefer. As in guided imagery, the practitioner encourages the use of senses and quietly reminds them to feel the warmth entering with each inspiration, the warmth spreading throughout their body, and the tension being released with each expiration.

Imagery has applications in a number of patient populations. It has been used by cancer patients to visualize cancer cells being destroyed by cells of the immune system, to control pain, and to achieve an overall feeling of well-being. It was also found to increase the cytotoxic ability of lymphokine-activated killer cells in a group of patients with solid tumor cancer (Post-White, 1991).

Prayer or meditation is used frequently by persons diagnosed with cancer. The diagnosis leads to increased fear, uncertainty, and anxiety about the future. Frequently the highest levels of psychologic distress occur at the completion of treatment during survivorship, rather than at the beginning (Levenson & Lesko, 1990). Throughout the cancer continuum, patients are searching for answers to existential questions related to death and what will happen after death. It is not surprising that cancer patients use an increased number of spiritual coping strategies (Fleming, Scanlon, & D'Agostino, 1987). Prayer has also been associated with improved health outcomes in other patient populations. For example, prayer was found to reduce the number of cardiac arrests, the amount of diuretics used, and the need for ventilatory assistance in cardiac patients (Byrd, 1988).

Prayer represents one method of meeting spiritual needs of persons with serious illnesses. Meditation is another technique that helps to focus an individual by directing attention to a single unchanging or repetitive stimulus (Carrington, 1993). Meditation can be easily learned, does not require memorization or particular procedures, and requires less self-discipline than most other behavioral therapies. Meditation induces a deeply restful state, reduces oxygen consumption, decreases respiratory and heart rates, and reduces anxiety.

Therapeutic touch; reiki; massage; acupuncture; and aroma, art, music, and pet therapies are being used with increasing frequency in efforts to decrease distress and improve quality of life. The decision as to which intervention is the best for specific individuals depends on the person's motivation and interest, philosophic and religious perspectives, and functional status, as well as the availability of trained practitioners. Therefore a highly individualized approach with input from the patient is needed to select the most appropriate behavioral intervention. This is particularly important, given that the major tenet of behavioral interventions is based on the individual's participation in the therapy.

CONCLUSION

The increased interest by basic scientists, clinicians in interdisciplinary fields, and health care consumers in psychoneuroimmunology suggests that a major shift in our thinking and approach to health care is occurring. Although advances are rapidly being made in psychoneuroimmunologic research, many questions remain. For example, the health implications of short-term immunosuppression have not been determined. The mechanisms that lead to enhanced versus suppressed immune function during exposure to stress are unclear. The complex interactions and interdependence of psychosocial variables, neuroendocrine hormones, and immune cells and products contribute to the difficulty in determining causal relationships between stress and disease.

Given the enormous variety in the way people perceive, cope with, and respond to stress, it is not surprising that PNI research is difficult. When multiple psychological, hormonal, and immune variables are included in studies, large numbers of subjects are needed to obtain the power necessary to observe significant findings. Functional immune, flow cytometric, and biochemical assays are expensive, and skilled laboratory technicians are needed for reliable and valid assays to be performed.

Despite the complexity of psychoneuroimmunology, researchers and clinicians maintain interest in assessing the efficacy of behavioral interventions that influence the mind-body connection. Multicomponent programs are useful for patients undergoing difficult diagnoses and treatments. However, the ability to ascertain which component had the greatest effect is difficult unless large numbers of subjects are randomized into the various components. Nonetheless, programs that can help people learn to reduce detrimental responses to stress and improve a sense of well-being are critical.

REFERENCES

Ader, R., & Cohen, N. (1975). Behaviorally conditioned immunosuppression. *Psychosomatic Medicine, 37,* 333-340.

Baum, A. (1990). Stress, intrusive imagery, and chronic distress. *Health Psychology, 9,* 653-675.

Baum, A., Gatchel, R. J., & Schaeffer, M. A. (1983). Emotional, behavioral, and physiological effects of chronic stress at Three Mile Island. *Journal of Consulting and Clinical Psychology, 51,* 565-572.

Burish, T. G., Snyder, S. L., Krozely, M. G., & Greco, F. A. (1987). Conditioned side effects induced by cancer chemotherapy: Prevention through behavioral treatment. *Journal of Consulting and Clinical Psychology, 55,* 42-48.

Burish, T. G., Snyder, S. L., & Jenkins, R. A. (1991). Preparing patients for cancer chemotherapy: Effect of coping preparation and relaxation interventions. *Journal of Consulting and Clinical Psychology, 59,* 518-525.

Bush, N. J. (1998). Coping and adaptation. In R. M. Carroll-Johnson, L. M. Horman, N. J. Bush (Eds.), *Psychosocial nursing care: Along the cancer continuum.* Pittsburgh: Oncology Nursing Press.

Byrd, R. C. (1988). Positive therapeutic effects of intercessory prayer in a coronary care unit population. *Southern Medical Journal, 81,* 826-829.

Cannon, W. B. (1914). The emergency function of the adrenal medulla in pain and the major emotions. *American Journal of Physiology, 33,* 356-372.

Carey, M. P. & Burish, T. G. (1987). Providing relaxation training to cancer chemotherapy patients: A comparison of three delivery techniques. *Journal of Consulting and Clinical Psychology, 55,* 732-737.

Carr, D. J. J., & Blalock, J. E. (1991). Neuropeptide hormones and receptors common to the immune and neuroendocrine systems: Bidirectional pathway of intersystem communication. In R. Ader, D. L. Felten, & N. Cohen (Eds.), *Psychoneuroimmunology.* (2nd ed.). San Diego: Academic Press.

Carrington P. (1993). Modern forms of meditation. In Lehrer P. M. and Woolfolk R. L. (Eds.), *Principles and practice of stress management,* (2nd ed.). New York: Guilford Press.

Caudell, K. A., Gallucci, B. B., & Betrus, P. (1996). A psychoneuroimmunological perspective of resistance. Implications for clinical practice. *Mind/Body Medicine, 1,* 192-202.

Chandra, R. (1980). Cell-medicated immunity in nutritional imbalance. *Federal Proceedings, 39,* 3088-3092.

Dammacco, F., Campobasso, N., Altomare, E., & Iodice, G. (1984). Analogues in immunology. *LaRicerca Clinical Lab, 14,* 137-147.

Davidson, L. M., Baum, A. (1986). Chronic stress and posttraumatic stress disorder. *Journal of Consulting and Clinical Psychology, 54,* 303-308.

Evans, E. (1926). *A psychological study of cancer.* New York: Dodd-Mead.

Fawzy, F., & Fawzy, N. W. (1994). Psychoducational interventions and health outcomes. In R. Glaser, & J. Kiecolt-Glaser J., (Eds.), *Handbook of human stress and immunity* (365-402). San Diego: Academic Press.

Ferrel, B. R., Dean, G. E., & Funk, B. (1996). Nondrug pain interventions. In R. McCorkle, M. Grant, M. Frank-Stromberg, & S. B. Baird (Eds.), *Cancer nursing: A comprehensive textbook.* (2nd ed.). Philadelphia: W. B. Saunders.

Fleming, C., Scanlon, C., & D'Agostino, N. S. (1987). A study of the comfort needs of patients with advanced cancer. *Cancer Nursing, 10,* 237-243.

Giang, D. W., Goodman, A. D., Schiffer, R. B., Mattson, D. H., Petrie, M., Cohen, N., & Ader, R. (1996). Conditioning of cyclophosphamide-induced leukopenia in humans. *Journal of Neuropsychiatry and Clinical Neurosciences, 8,* 194-201.

Greenfield, N. S., Roessler, R. & Corseley, A.P. (1959), Ego strength and length of recovery from infectious mononucleosis. *Journal of Nervous and Mental Disease,* 128, 125-128.

Haddy, R. I. (1987). Aging, infections and the immune system. *Journal of Family Practice, 27,* 409-413.

Holmen, A., Karlsson, A., Bratt, I., & Hogstedt, B. (1995). Increased frequencies of micronuclei in T8 lymphocytes of smokers. *Mutation Research, 334,* 205-208.

Howlett T. A., Tomlin S., Ngahfoong, L., Rees, L. H., Bullen, B. A., Skrinar, G. S., & McArthur, J. W. (1984). Release of β-endorphin and met-enkephalin during exercise in normal women: Response to training. *British Medical Journal, 288,* 1950-1952.

Ingram, D. K. & Corfman, T. P. (1980). An overview of neurobiological comparisons in mouse strains. *Neuroscience and Biobehavioral Reviews, 4,* 421-435.

Jansen, M. A., & Muenz, L. R. (1984). A retrospective study of personality variables associated with fibrocystic disease and breast cancer. *Journal of Psychosomatic Research, 28,* 35.

Johnson, J. H. & Sarason, I. G. (1978). Life stress, depression and anxiety: Internal-external control as a moderator variable. *Journal of Psychosomatic Research, 22,* 205-208.

Kandel, E. R. (1991). Cellular mechanisms of learning and the biological basis of individuality. In E. R. Kandel, J. H. Schwartz, & T. M. Jessel (Eds.), *Principles of neural science.* (3rd ed.). New York: Elsevier.

Kennedy, S., Kiecolt-Glaser, J. K., & Glaser, R. (1988). Immunological consequences of acute and chronic stressors: Mediating role of interpersonal relationships. *British Journal of Medical Psychology, 61,* 77-85.

Kiecolt-Glaser, J. K., Dura, J. K., Speicher, C. E., Trask, & Glaser, R. (1991). Spousal caregivers of dementia victims: Longitudinal changes in immunity and health. *Psychosomatic Medicine, 53,* 345-362.

Kiecolt-Glaser, J. K., Ricker, D., George, J., Mexxick, G., Speicher, C. E., Garner, W., & Glaser, R. (1984). Urinary cortisol levels, cellular immunocompetency, and loneliness in psychiatric inpatients. *Psychosomatic Medicine, 46,* 15-21.

Kobasa, S. C., Maddi, S. R., & Courington, S. (1981). Personality and constitution as mediators in the stress-illness relationship. *Journal of Health and Social Behavior, 22,* 368-378.

Konarska M., Stewart, R.E., & McCarty, R. (1989). Sensitization of sympathetic-adrenal medullary responses to a novel stressor in chronically stressed laboratory rats. *Physiological Behavior, 46*(2), 129-135.

Laudenslager, M. L., Ryan, S. M., Drugan, R. C., Hyson, R. L., and Maier, S. F. (1983). Coping and immunosuppression: inescapable but not escapable shock suppresses lymphocyte proliferation. *Science, 221,* 568.

Levenson, J. A., & Lesko, L. M. (1990). Psychiatric aspects of adult leukemia. *Seminars in Oncology Nursing, 6,* 76-83.

Mandle, C. L., Jacobs, S. C., Arcaro, P.M., & Domar, A. D. (1996). The efficacy of relaxation response interventions with adult patients: a review of the literature. *Journal of Cardiovascular Nursing, 10,* 4-26.

Martin, R. A., & Dobbin, J. P. (1988). Sense of humor, hassles, and immunoglobulin A: Evidence for a stress-modulating effect of humor. *International Journal of Psychiatry Medicine, 18,* 93-105.

McGuigan, F. J. (1993). Progressive relaxation: Origins, principles, and clinical applications. In P. Lehrer & R. L. Woolfolk (Eds.). *Principles and practice of stress management* (2nd ed.). New York: Guilford Press.

Millar, D. B., Thomas, J. R., Pacheco, N. D., & Rollwagen, F. M. (1993). Natural killer cell cytotoxicity and T-cell proliferation is enhanced by avoidance behavior. *Brain, Behavior, & Immunity, 7,* 144-153.

Morris, T., Greer, S., Pettingale, K. W., & Watson, M. (1981). Patterns of expression of anger and their psychological correlates in women with breast cancer. *Journal of Psychosomatic Research, 25,* 111-117.

Palmblad, J., Petrini, B., Wasserman, J., & Akerstedt, T. (1979). Lymphocyte and granulocyte reactions during sleep deprivation. *Psychosomatic Medicine, 41,* 273-278.

Petersen, B. H., Steimel, L. F., & Callaghan, J. T. (1983). Suppression of mitogen-induced lymphocyte transformation in cigarette smokers. *Clinical Immunology and Immunopathology, 27,* 135-140.

Post-White, J. (1991). The effects of mental imagery on emotions, immune function, and cancer outcome. (Doctoral dissertation, University of Minnesota. Dissertation Abstracts International, 52, 12B (University Microfilms No. 92-5462).

Post-White, J. (1998). Psychoneuroimmunology: The mind-body connection. In R. M. Carroll-Johnson, L. M. Horman, & N. J. Bush (Eds.), *Psychosocial nursing care: Along the cancer continuum.* Pittsburgh: Oncology Nursing Press.

Rogers, M. P., Reich, P., Strom T. B., & Carpenter, C. B. (1976). Behaviorally conditioned immunosuppression: replication of a recent study. *Psychosomatic Medicine, 38,* 447-452.

Selye, H. (1936). Thymus and adrenals in the response of the organism to injuries and intoxications. *British Journal of Experimental Pathology, 17,* 234-248.

Selye, H. (1956). *The stress of life.* New York: McGraw-Hill.

Shinkai, S., Shore, S., Shek, P. N., & Shephard, R. J. (1992). Acute exercise and immune function. *International Journal of Sports Medicine, 13,* 452.

Solomon, G. F., & Moos, R. H. (1964). Emotions, immunity and disease: A speculative theoretical integration. *Archives of General Psychiatry, 11,* 657-674.

Sørensen, T. I. A., Nielsen, G. G., Anderson, P. K., & Teasdale, T. W. (1988). Genetic and environmental influences on premature death in adult adoptees. *New England Journal of Medicine, 318,* 727-732.

Spiegel, D., Bloom, J. R., Kraemer, H. C., & Gottheil, E. (1989). Effect of psychosocial treatment on survival of patients with metastatic breast cancer. *Lancet, 2,* 888-891.

Stone A. A. & Porter L. S. (1995). Psychological coping: Its importance for treating medical problems. *Mind/Body Medicine, 1,* 46-54.

Turner, J. A., Clancy, S., & Vitaliano, P. P. (1987). Relationships of stress, appraisal, and coping to chronic low back pain. *Behavior, Research, & Therapy, 25,* 281-288.

Uchino, B. N., Kiecolt-Glaser, J. K., & Caioppo, J. T. (1992). Age-related changes in cardiovascular response as a function of a chronic stressor. *Journal of Personality and Social Psychology, 63,* 839-846.

Wayner, E. R., Flannery, G. R., & Singer, G. (1978). Effects of taste aversion conditioning on the primary antibody response to sheep red blood cells and *Brucella abortus* in the albino rat. *Physiological Behavior, 21,* 995-1000.

Wirshing, M., Stierlin, H., Hoffman, F., Weber, G., & Wirsching, B. (1982). Psychological identifications of breast cancer before biopsy. *Journal of Psychosomatic Research, 26,* 1-10.

Workman, E. A., & LaVia, M. F. (1987). T lymphocyte polyclonal proliferation: effects of stress and stress response style on medical students taking national board examinations. *Clinical Immunology and Immunopathology, 43,* 303-313.

Ziegler, B. G. (1989). Catecholamine measurement in behavioral research. In N. Schneiderman, S. M. Weiss, P. B. Kaufmann (Eds.), *Handbook of research methods in cardiovascular behavioral medicine.* New York: Plenum Press.

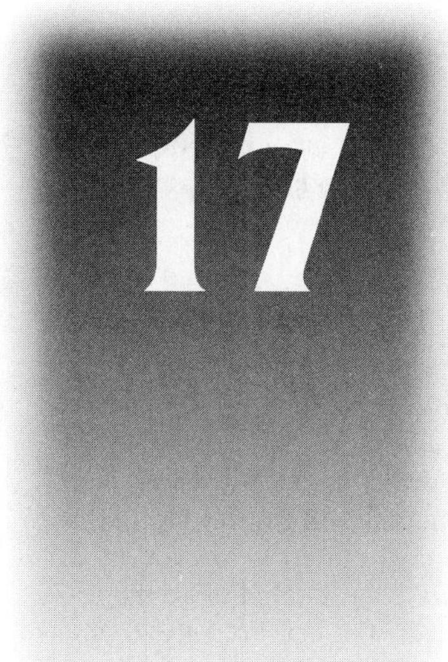

Nursing Management Across the Continuum of Care

Patricia C. Buchsel, RN, MSN
Brenda Nevidjon, RN, MSN
Tricia Corbett, MSPH

THE CURRENT HEALTH CARE ENVIRONMENT

The health care environment often poses unprecedented challenges to nurses practicing at all levels and settings across the trajectory of cancer care. The cumulative events of rising health care costs spurred by sophisticated technology, an aging population of survivors subject to long-term sequelae, a generation of aging baby boomers with political clout, and economic restraints have created a dynamic synthesis that demands creative solutions to meet the needs of oncology patients. A nursing shortage, particularly in the specialty areas, looms ahead, threatening the quality of care oncology patients will receive. Departures from traditional systems include emphasis on disease prevention with use of screening clinics, outpatient vs inpatient care, physician's managed groups, managed care conglomerates, and advocacy groups. These forces, in turn, direct the influence, scope, and practice of oncology nursing. The current influences affecting health care delivery are as follows:

- Managed care
- Aging baby boomers
- The elderly
- Technology

Almost all oncology care has moved from traditional settings in a rapidly paced transition through various health care settings from physicians' office to hospice care. The purpose of this chapter is to review the changing influences and issues that affect health care, the shifting foci of health care delivery, and the current roles and opportunities for oncology nurses across the continuum of care. This chapter does not discuss specific clinical and administrative issues respective to the traditional sites of care, but rather critical, global concerns related to components of care. The reader is referred to specific administrative and clinical management resources relative to inpatient, ambulatory, and home care for oncology patients and family members and caregivers. Chapter 18 discusses death and dying issues and Chapter 19 describes cultural concerns.

NURSING FRAMEWORK

To meet health care demands now and into the next millennium, oncology nurses can rely on the rich and consistent tradition of nursing leaders from the past to guide them through the medical maze confronting all health care professionals. Many outstanding nursing theorists and leaders have contributed to the shape of the nursing profession; however, Florence Nightingale's basic and authoritative principles of preventing disease and maintaining health remain a constant and consistent theme in today's oncology nursing practice. She changed nineteenth-century nursing into the profession it is today by encouraging what nursing "ought to be" (Nightingale, 1969). Her emphasis on disease prevention was the basis of reducing the death rate of the British army during the Crimean War from 42% to 2% within 6 months. Her treatment, or "reparative process" for cure, in addition to administration of medications, was "the use of fresh air, light, warmth, cleanliness, quiet, and the proper use and administration of diet." As an educator she founded the first training school for nurses at St. Thomas' Hospital in 1860. As a researcher she used statistical analysis to convince the English government to improve medical care at military and civilian hospitals. Nightingale's administrative acuity and vision of the scope of nursing practice was further underscored by nursing curriculum development that extended nursing care from the hospital to the home to teach patients and families about the preservation and maintenance of health (Nightingale, 1969). Her enormous efforts to shape the professional nurse to be a clinician, educator, researcher, and consultant serve as the basis for the direction and commitment of oncology nurses today.

CHANGES IN CARE VENUES

The care setting in which oncology patients are treated has changed dramatically over the past decade, and the tenets of excellence in delivering and receiving care are not always consistent across care settings. Issues once specific to a particular care location (mastectomy) no longer are the concern of a particular location (inpatient). In today's marketplace, standards of care leading to positive clinical outcomes remain a benchmark for excellence. Safety concerns are paramount as more high-risk procedures and techniques are delivered in the nonacute setting. Often patient safety is compromised by the inappropriate use of unlicensed personnel with limited experience. The Oncology Nursing Society (ONS) has outlined minimal standards for delivery of oncology services (Box 17-1).

Box 17-1
Oncology Nursing Society Position on Medical Services in the Nonacute Medical Oncology

- Regardless of setting, patient safety is the priority in planning and providing cancer care.
- Cancer care for patients is best accomplished by registered nurses educated and certified in oncology.
- During all hours of operation, nonacute services must ensure that personnel treat antineoplastic medications in accordance with ONS and Occupational Safety and Health Administration guidelines.
- Emergency services are available during the administration of blood products or any medications associated with severe adverse reactions, and response must incorporate.
- Care providers should include Advanced Cardiac Life Support (ACLS)–trained personnel or a physician who directs emergency medication administration, and a certified clinical staff of direct-care providers certified in cardiopulmonary resuscitation.
- Emergency medications (e.g., epinephrine, atropine, diphenhydramine) are stocked and available within the facility.
- Guidelines appropriate to the risk potential of regimens and procedures being used in the facility are written and followed for cardiac/respiratory arrest, anaphylactic reaction, fluid overload, hypertension and hypotension, seizures, extravasations, chemical spills, and other emergency situations.
- Before infusion of medications in the home setting, patients are assessed for their ability to identify and report untoward or adverse effects and provide self-care and for their willingness to follow directions by a registered nurse who has been educated and certified in the specialty of oncology.
- Patients receiving continuous infusion therapy in the home setting and having a central vascular access catheter are under the care or supervision of a home infusion service that follows these guidelines or have a 24-hour ambulatory office or professional staff available to them.
- Patients and caregivers are provided with written and verbal information for self-care.
- The patient/staff mix is consistent with a hazard-free, safe, and therapeutic environment. When conscious sedation is used, written guidelines and policies are followed, state regulations enforced, and oxygen and reversal medications (e.g., naloxone) are stocked and available for use. When state regulations have not been developed to guide staff mix, ACLS certification designates the preferred level of emergency.

Modified from the Oncology Nursing Society (1998) and American Society of Clinical Oncology (1997). Criteria for facilities and personnel for the administration of parenteral system antineoplastic therapy. *Journal of Clinical Oncology, 15,* 3416-3417.

Prevention

During the past decade, health promotion, prevention, and early detection of illnesses have gained increasing attention in the field of health. The volume of research and literature in these specific areas continues to grow. A new focus on the economic bottom line in health care reform has brought the realization that it is far more cost effective to prevent disease than to treat it. Cancer care costs totaled more than $96 billion in 1985 (Schuette, Tucker, Brown, Potosky, & Samuel, 1995). Money spent on prevention is money well spent.

In 1991 the Department of Health and Human Services published a landmark document entitled *Healthy People 2000: National Health Promotion and Disease Prevention Objectives* (U. S. Public Health Service, 1991a). Many states have used this document to tailor objectives to the specific characteristics and needs of their populations. Cancer is targeted as a major focus for prevention, and many of the national and state objectives deal specifically with cancer prevention and control.

Research has demonstrated that many cancers can be prevented and others cured if detected and treated in early stages. In addition, the potential for reducing cancer incidence and mortality is great. Cigarette smoking is responsible for 30% of all cancer deaths. Thirty-five percent of all cancer deaths may be related to diet, particularly those high in certain fats and low in fiber (Eddy, 1986). High alcohol consumption has been implicated in cancers of the buccal cavity, pharynx, larynx, esophagus, liver, large bowel, breast, and head and neck (National Cancer Institute, 1986). Occupational and environmental exposure to identified carcinogens such as asbestos, benzene, radon, and ionizing radiation have been associated with specific cancers. Strides in preventing such illnesses as hepatitis B human immunodeficiency virus infections may well reduce the incidence of liver cancer, Kaposi's sarcoma, and related cancers (U.S. Public Health Service, 1991a).

Research and clinical trials have also found screening procedures for early detection of some cancers such as breast, gynecologic, prostate, colorectal, and skin to be effective in reducing the morbidity and mortality associated with these cancers, as well as cost effective. Additional prevention and early detection measures are being evaluated currently in ongoing studies and clinical trials.

In the *Healthy People 2000* document, 16 national objectives specific to cancer have been identified with clearly stated outcome targets. For example, the first objective is to reverse the rise in cancer deaths to achieve a rate of no more than 130 per 100,000 people* (U. S. Public Health Service, 1991b). In addition, the means for accomplishing each ob-

*Age-adjusted baseline: 133 per 100,000 in 1987.

jective are discussed in a detailed summary, complete with references for each objective.

The remaining objectives relate to reducing rates of lung, breast, cervical, and colorectal cancers and targeting these areas for improvement: cigarette smoking; dietary fat intake; daily intake of vegetables, fruits, and grain products; actions to reduce sun exposure; tobacco, diet, and cancer screening counseling by clinicians; breast examinations; mammograms and mammography quality; Papanicolaou (Pap) tests and test quality; fecal occult blood tests; proctosigmoidoscopy; oral, skin, and digital rectal examinations.

The U.S. Public Health Service is in the process of evaluating the achievement of the *Healthy People 2000* objectives and identifying new objectives for the coming decade. These will be published within the next few years.

In the development and provision of prevention and early detection services, special consideration should be given to two population groups with disproportionate cancer-related mortality rates: minorities, especially African Americans (particularly males), whose rate of 5-year survival is 37% compared with 50% for whites; and the elderly, the only age group for whom cancer mortality rates continue to rise (U.S. Public Health Service, 1991b).

In recognition of the disproportionately high mortality rates for African Americans, the ONS offers a series of 2-day intensive workshops for nurse educators. The purpose of these workshops is to provide the information and resources needed "to introduce issues, trends, and concepts related to cancer prevention and early detection among African Americans within nursing curricula" (*ONS News,* 1998). Implementation issues surrounding ethnicity and culture, which may influence the accessibility and acceptability of these services, are also covered, as are the knowledge and skills required for undertaking cancer risk appraisal and health assessment. Chapter 19 discusses issues in cultural diversity.

Nurses are in an ideal position to provide health education and cancer screening, as well as initial patient referrals for cancer care. This is particularly true for nurse oncologists who work in or have contact with primary care settings. Prevention and early detection have the greatest potential for reducing the burden of cancer in our society.

Surgery

One of the key issues emerging in the wake of health system restructuring is the increased pressure for and use of short-stay/ambulatory surgery. For example, many breast cancer–related surgeries, including mastectomy, lumpectomy, axillary node sampling, and dissection, are now performed in the ambulatory setting. Although short-stay procedures do significantly reduce the costs of care, the quality of care may well be jeopardized in the process. It is of critical impor-

Box 17-2

The Oncology Nursing Society Position on Short-Stay Surgery for Cancer Patients

- A comprehensive preoperative assessment of the patient, including preexisting conditions, medications, social situation, and support systems, is essential.
- Complete preoperative education of patient and family (caretaker), including presurgery preparation, the procedure, postoperative care, and availability of appropriate resources, is mandatory. Referrals are implemented at this time.
- The patient and caretaker must have contact information for preoperative and postoperative questions or problems. Optimally, the patient or caretaker should be contacted the night before and the day after the procedure to ensure that questions are answered and or to promptly intervene should complications occur.
- An interdisciplinary approach to care must be used and should include nursing, medicine, pharmacy, respiratory therapy, physical therapy, rehabilitation, and home health.
- Readiness for discharge will be carefully assessed to include evaluation of symptomatology, including pain; nausea and vomiting; preexisting complicating health conditions; postoperative complications; and support system, including caretakers' abilities at home. If deemed medically necessary, a patient must be admitted to the hospital for ongoing postoperative recovery without delay.

Modified from Oncology Nursing Society Online (1998). *Regarding the use of short-stay surgery for patients with cancer.* Available at http://www.ons.org/ons/main/journals.

Box 17-3

The Oncology Nursing Society Position on Short-Stay Surgery for Breast Cancer

- Length-of-stay decisions must be made solely between the health care provider and the patient (and family), without influence of financial incentives.
- Decisions about length of stay must be based on individual patient variables (including co-morbid conditions, age, anesthetic risk, and attitudes toward short stay); type of surgery; health care provider evaluation; and caretaker support, burden, and resources.
- An interdisciplinary team must be used to ensure comprehensive presurgical assessment and patient/caregiver education and preparation for self-care at home; evaluate readiness for discharge; and ensure appropriate communication, physical care, symptom management, follow-up evaluation, and continuity of care in recovery and rehabilitation phases.
- Issues to be addressed with patents and caregivers must include physical care (e.g., wound care, drain care, minimization of infection, postsurgical arm exercises), symptom management (e.g., pain, nausea, vomiting), and the social (e.g., resources, transportation), psychological (e.g., alterations in body image, femininity, sexuality), and emotional (e.g., depression, anxiety) impact of breast cancer and its treatment.
- Patients and caregivers must be physically and psychologically prepared to manage self-care or caregiving in the home.
- Appropriate referrals, including referrals for social services and home care and to programs such as Reach to Recovery, must be made before discharge and evaluated for efficacy in the immediate recovery phase.
- Policies that mandate outpatient mastectomies must be eliminated.

Modified from Oncology Nursing Society Online (1998). *Short-stay surgery for breast cancer.* Available at http://www.ons.org/ons/main/journals.

tance to monitor this financial/quality relationship to determine the consequences of this strategy. The ONS has addressed the issue of short-stay surgery and written guidelines for making length-of-stay decisions. Guidelines call for both a preoperative assessment and a careful evaluation of readiness for postoperative discharge as the basis for such decisions (Boxes 17-2 and 17-3).

The preoperative assessment must include patient variables such as preexisting or co-morbid conditions, age, type of surgery, anesthetic risk, and attitudes toward short stay. It must also assess family (caregiver) variables regarding willingness and ability (physical, emotional, and financial) to provide appropriate postoperative care and follow-up. A readiness for discharge evaluation must include symptomatology, including pain, nausea and vomiting; preexisting complicating health conditions; postoperative complications; and support systems, including caretaker's abilities at home.

If a decision for ambulatory surgery is made, education for the patient and family (caregiver) in preparation for the home care role is imperative, and availability of required resources is mandatory. The patient and caregiver must be able to provide adequate postoperative care (e.g., wound care) and management of symptoms (e.g., pain, nausea), as well as address the social, psychological, and emotional impact of cancer and its treatment. The patient and caregiver must also have a specific contact for information if questions or problems arise, as well as coordination of follow-up and continuum of care requirements. A list of appropriate community service and support referrals should also be provided. Chapter 3 gives a complete discussion of further issues surrounding surgical oncology nursing.

Chemotherapy

The major issue in chemotherapy, as in other treatment modalities, is staying abreast of the rapid advances in cancer treatment required for the provision of optimal patient care. Continuing competency of nurse oncologists is addressed through required continuing education and certification courses. Thus many resources are available for keeping up with important advances.

Most professional associations monitor advances in the field and maintain continually updated standards of practice. The ONS recently published *Cancer Chemotherapy Guidelines and Recommendations for Practice* (1996). This document identifies the didactic content and clinical experience needed to provide quality care for patients during the continuum of care and in different settings (Box 17-4).

Periodic review of pertinent literature, particularly reports of ongoing drug and treatment clinical trials, is most helpful in staying abreast of advances. Updated reading lists and summaries of various oncologic topics can be obtained through a regional medical (health sciences) library or on websites, including the Institute of Medicine and Oncology Nursing Society Online. In addition, of the total number of MEDLINE searches, 30% are by the general public. An increasing number of cancer patients now search websites for the latest in treatments and/or the "miracle" drug to cure their cancer (see Chapter 5).

Box 17-4

ONS Position Statement on the Preparation of the Professional Registered Nurse Who Administers and Cares for the Individual Receiving Chemotherapy

The Oncology Nursing Society takes the position that the utilization of the following course contents will provide the information necessary to prepare the professional registered nurse to practice at a safe and competent level.

Basic didactic content and clinical experiences necessary for the preparation of the professional registered nurse to care for individuals during the treatment continuum and in different settings are as follows:

- Drug development
- Principles of cancer chemotherapy
- Chemotherapy preparation, storage, and transport
- Nursing assessment
- Chemotherapy administration
- Safety precautions during chemotherapy administration
- Disposal, accidental exposure, and spills
- Institutional considerations

Modified from Oncology Nursing Society (1998). *Regarding the preparation of the professional nurse who administers and cares for the individual receiving chemotherapy.* Available at http://www.ons.org/ons/main/journals.

Radiation Oncology

Radiation oncology has traditionally been the domain of radiologist technicians, in part because nurses are not solidly educated in the academic setting for the technical aspects of radiation biology and equipment. Rather, this specialty area is learned in the clinical setting. Much of the role of radiation oncology nurses is focused on the traditional nursing role of patient teaching, coordinating procedures, symptom management, and follow-up care after therapy (Hillary, 1997). However, radiation oncology, similar to other venues, has been affected by the changes in health care delivery relative to the use of new technology delivered as outpatient procedures. Examples are the increasing use of stereotactic radiosurgery for brain tumors and radiation seeding for prostate cancer. Stereotactic radiosurgery is a knifeless procedure used to deliver a single high dose of radiation to limited intracranial lesions while avoiding adjacent critical structures in the brain. This procedure is usually performed on an outpatient basis or with an overnight hospitalization and requires expert nursing care and support (Morgan, 1998). Similarly, increasing numbers of prostate cancer patients are electing iodine-125 radioactive seed implants in lieu of traditional prostate cancer irradiation therapy. As successful prostate cancer screening increases early detection, this treatment, if proven to have long-term benefits, will have a twofold impact on oncology nurses practicing in this area. Although these patients require considerable counseling about the risks and benefits of either treatment, the overall workload and revenues of this department are diminished and placed nursing positions at risk (Iwamoto, 1998). Alternatively, as novel techniques such as the use of proton or heavy-particle beams, photodynamic therapy, and radiodynamic therapy move from the research to the community setting, complex patient care will be required in the clinical setting. As in other care settings, the nursing care of these patients has been provided by advanced nurse practitioners or certified oncology nurses. However, economic constraints may further compromise the ability to offer professional nursing support to these patients. Chapter 4 addresses further issues in this area. The reader is also referred to other sources (Bruner, Bucholtz, Iwamoto, & Strohl, 1998).

Bone Marrow Transplantation

The trend to perform a large part of bone marrow transplantation in outpatient settings has increased over the past 5 years, especially with the advent of peripheral stem cell transplantations. Although numerous transplant care settings market "outpatient transplants," few, indeed, have the capability to offer high-dose chemotherapy and total body irradiation in outpatient settings. Rarely are recipients sufficiently clinically stable to be outpatients during the conditioning regimen or early engraftment period. Chapters 8 and 9 discuss the process of each therapy, its complications, and recovery issues. Investigators of new supportive care therapies such as antiemetics and colony-stimulating factors have shortened hospital stays and the length of time to discharge to a referring oncologist, but most recipients are inpatients for several weeks after transplantation. Specialized nursing care is required to monitor and care for patients throughout this process. As the number of trained bone marrow and stem cell transplant nurses decrease, general nurses are increasingly caring for these patients (Buchsel & Kapustay, 1997).

SPECIAL SETTINGS

Survivors

Scientific and medical advances have altered the course of cancer care in this country. Currently there are approximately 10 million cancer survivors in the United States, 7 million of whom have survived for at least 5 years. By the year 2000 there will be approximately 200,000 survivors of childhood cancer who will have access to 30 specialty survivor clinics nationwide (National Cancer Institute, 1997). Conversely, millions of adult long-term survivors have no specialized follow-up care. Recovering patients and their families require continued access to psychosocial support via individual or family counseling, support groups, information and referral services, and vocational counseling. Few guidelines for long-term care by primary care physicians now exist. Long-term support for patients who will need to address the known and unknown long-term consequences of cancer therapy is a growing need; medical centers, community cancer centers, and advocacy groups are providing multifaceted support services for recovering patients and their families in significant numbers.

As patients live longer after treatment, they must become increasingly aware of the possibility of long-term complications. Organ damage and failure can result from chemotherapy, radiotherapy, and biologic response modifiers; compromised immune systems place patients at risk for infection, and damaged endocrine systems lead to thyroid dysfunction. Hypothalamic-pituitary dysfunction, premature menopause, and reproductive problems or sexual dysfunction are also potential risks. Recurrence and secondary malignancies are increasingly noted as therapies become more intense and patients live longer. Related functional problems and psychosocial issues also occur. As more research priorities addressing the long-term consequences of cancer therapy come to fruition, oncology nurses will play a pivotal role in identifying, treating, and supporting patients at risk for these problems.

Community Outreach Programs

A number of outreach programs offered by medical centers to communities are gaining impetus across the country. Cancer prevention programs staffed by volunteers from cancer specialty centers such as breast self-examination, smoking cessation, nutrition guidance, and weight management support groups offer mutually beneficial adjuncts to the missions of participating organizations. An example is Project CHOICE (Choosing Healthy Options in Cancer Education) located in Seattle, Wash. This program is a comprehensive K to 12 curriculum designed to be offered in a 2-week time frame and offers health, science, and language arts instruction. Through the assistance of the community hospital, programs such as this provide successful hospital-school partnerships that enrich the community by developing habits in children that will assist them in preventing and understanding the risk factors associated with an unhealthy lifestyle (Miller, 1993). Large tertiary and metropolitan medical centers can extend their networks into rural and smaller communities where hospitals may not have a cancer committee, continuing medical education conferences, tumor registry, and multidisciplinary consultation.

Telemedicine is a method of telecommunications that brings physicians and/or patients in multiple areas together by means of two-way interactive video conferencing, using computers and fiberoptic transmission. This technique has been shown to be successful as a means of access to high-quality health care for an increased number of rural residents. Rural cancer centers in particular enjoy numerous benefits such as improved access to high-quality patient health care, patient retention, physician and midlevel practitioner retention, and cost reduction. Distance learning, often referred to as "college without walls," allows oncology nurses and other clinicians to obtain continuing education credits and decrease their sense of isolation by being connected to the larger medical community. Limitations with this technology do exist. Telemedicine needs to be supported by an infrastructure for it to survive. Acceptance levels among the oncology practitioners vary, and managers' sensitivity to doubts and skepticism are inherent in their acceptance of new technology. Legal issues such as patient confidentiality will also need to be addressed. In spite of these hurdles, telemedicine will play an important part in bringing state-of-the-art health care services to many (Dawson, 1995). Oncology nurses can be champions of úse of this technology in their communities.

Rural Cancer Care

The number of people living in rural America has increased; almost one quarter of the American population live in rural areas. Of these, eight million are over the age of 65 (U.S. Bureau of the Census, 1987). Cantril & Haylock (1996) studied the characteristics of rural nurses compared with those of urban nurses and found that rural nurses generally are older, practice solely in one area for many years, serve a larger patient population, lack the anonymity common to urban nurses, have higher visibility, are more autonomous, and are skilled generalists. The patients for whom these nurses serve have world views on health care that differ from their city counterparts. Their major focus is on a strong work ethic, and they are less concerned about their physical health and often reject the sick role. The elderly optimize their health status by measures of absence of fatigue or pain, and women desire adaptation and coping in defining their health care needs. Other hallmarks of the rural community are that these residents have higher rates of unemployment and chronic or serious illness. It is not unusual for families to travel hundreds of miles for health care, and often health care providers provide large parking areas where families can live in motor homes for the duration of their treatment. In this challenging milieu, health care programs that are effective in urban areas often fail in this setting, and nurses specializing in highly technical fields usually are not accepted by the rural population, nor do they find job satisfaction.

To identify and overcome barriers in this setting, the ONS held a "think tank" to link rural nursing theory with the conceptualized vision of oncology nursing practice. Twenty nurses from 13 states identified the urgent need to provide "seamless" cancer care that was anchored in knowledge, equipment, and technologic assistance for optimal symptom management of the cancer patient. In addition to primary care, the scope of services would include prevention, long-term care, and survivorship and bereavement support. Nursing researchers are challenged to continue to define the characteristics of the cancer patient in the rural area and assist nurses working in this area to collaborate with urban and rural teams to bring optimal health care to this understudied and underserved group.

Cancer and Aging

Senior citizens 65 years and older currently comprise 13% (approximately 24 million) of the U.S. population. By 2030 they will account for an estimated 22% of the population (U.S. Public Health Service, 1991a). The elderly have unique cancer-specific needs and problems, and the fact that they are the fastest growing segment of our population presents special challenges for the provision of oncologic services. (The current issues in cancer and aging are covered in some detail in this section because it is a topic of major importance not addressed elsewhere in this book.)

The risk of cancer rises exponentially with age (Yancik & Ries, 1989). Over 57% of all cancers occur in people over the age of 65, and cancer is the second leading cause of death in this age group. The increased risk for and incidence of cancer is likely caused by prolonged exposure to carcinogens, coupled with a decreased ability of the body to repair deoxyribonucleic acid and an often inefficient immune system as a result of bodily changes (and morbidity) that accompany aging (Cohen, 1990).

Cancer in the elderly tends to be diagnosed at a more advanced state, and mortality rates are disproportionately high, especially among the socioeconomically disadvantaged (Baranovsky & Myers, 1986). In addition, studies have shown that the elderly more often receive substandard care and less rigorous pursuit of primary and adjuvant cancer treatment therapies.

A variety of age-related factors no doubt contribute to this inequity in cancer-related outcomes. A recent article has demonstrated that the elderly patient is often undertreated for pain. Those particularly at risk are individuals in nursing homes (SAGE Study Group, 1998). Senior citizens often have diminished access and increased barriers to prevention, screening, and primary care. Existing morbidity related to aging; the tendency of many toward loneliness, depression, and dementia; and decreasing familial and community support networks complicate the effectiveness of cancer diagnosis and treatment and recovery. In addition, an age bias often precludes the elderly from the more aggressive treatment modalities and clinical trials available to younger and healthier patients (Derby, 1991).

Gerontologic oncology is one of the fastest growing and least studied areas of cancer care. That aging influences the availability, accessibility, and quality of care and alters the provision of care throughout the continuum is clear. But how these aging and cancer care factors interplay is not as clear and is a topic in great need of basic and clinical research. The aged account for over half of all cancer victims, and yet we know little of the aging-related sequelae of cancer and its management in the elderly.

An ONS task force recently studied the issue of aging and cancer and determined that "oncology nurses have a clear mandate to establish a formal framework within which nursing care can be augmented or modified to meet the unique cancer-specific needs of the elderly." The resulting position paper entitled *Oncology Nursing Society Position Paper on Cancer and Aging: The Mandate for Oncology Nursing* (1996), identifies ten "imperatives" for oncology nurses (Boyle, Engelking, Bliesch, Dodge, Sarna, & Weinrich, 1992). These include prevention and screening services, "appropriate diagnosis, treatment, and rehabilitation for cancer and its associated conditions, research . . ., and promotion of public health policies that will support the programs, services, and care required for older adults" (Boyle et al., 1992). This paper should be perused by all oncology nurses providing care to the elderly. The following paragraphs briefly mention important issues in cancer care of the elderly.

Four sites account for the vast majority of cancers in those over 65. These are breast, prostate, colon, and lung; and it is likely that the incidence of lung cancer will increase in a lag response to increased rates of smoking during the earlier years of both men and women in (and approaching) this age group (Anisimov, 1989). All of these cancers are amenable to prevention and/or early detection strategies. If detected early in their course, colon, breast, and prostate cancers can be cured; and morbidity associated with treatment can be reduced (Satariano, Ragheb & Dupuis, 1989). Unfortunately, the elderly have limited access to prevention and particularly screening programs (Weinrich, 1990).

The availability of and easy accessibility to prevention and screening services for the elderly are clearly important. Recent studies have shown that older smokers who quit increase their life expectancy, reduce their risk of cancer and heart disease, and improve respiratory function and circulation (Office on Smoking and Health, 1989). Screening programs for prostate, cervical, skin, colon, and breast cancer at the very least should be available. Mammography and clinical breast examinations are estimated to reduce mortality in women over 50 by about 30% (Shapiro, Venet, Strax, & Roeser, 1985).

Age-related physiologic and psychosocial changes can complicate the diagnosis, choices of treatment, and management of the clinical manifestations of cancer and cancer therapies. Such changes in the elderly are not always caused by aging; thus the possibility that they are age related must be taken into account but never assumed. Aged-induced impairments include compromised hematologic and immune status, altered skin and mucous membrane integrity, and impaired neurosensory/perceptual acuity (Boyle et al., 1992).

Diagnosis and treatment management are particularly influenced by these physiologic changes. The ONS position paper on this subject identifies six conditions seen in the aged that may have either malignant or nonmalignant origins. These include (1) high risk for injury and trauma (Perry, 1982; Nickens, 1985; Jenkins, Reynolds, & Seviech, 1986); (2) altered thought processes/acute confusion/dementia (Foreman, 1986); (3) altered nutrition; (4) altered patterns of bowel and bladder elimination (Boyle et al., 1992; Dodge, Bachman, & Silverman, 1988); (5) impaired skin, tissue, and mucous membrane integrity (Fitzsimons, 1983; Frantz, Kinney, & Dowing, 1986); and (6) sleep pattern disturbances (Colling 1983; Hayter, 1983).

Conditions related to aging also influence the options for treatment. The majority of older people have multiple, concurrent chronic illnesses (Mandelblatt, Wheat, Monane, Moshief, Hollenberg, & Tang, 1992), which can diminish cardiac, pulmonary, renal, and liver function and for which they may be taking numerous medications. These problems often limit involvement in clinical trials and reduce available treatment options. Concurrently they may also increase the risk of adverse reactions to treatment. However, age alone is a poor predictor of side effects in cancer treatment.

Many older adults can safely undergo cancer surgery. The risk increases not with age but rather with co-morbid conditions. Obesity, compromised cardiac and vascular statuses, lung disease, and impaired immune function increase surgical risk. Radiation therapy side effects/toxicity may be enhanced by decreased bone marrow reserves and coexisting disease at the irradiated site. Reduced nutritional status also can complicate the need for increased caloric intake during treatment.

Little data are available on age-related drug-induced toxicity or other side effects or chemotherapy in the elderly. However, age-related changes may influence how drugs are absorbed, distributed, metabolized, and excreted. In addition, many older adults are on multiple drugs to treat co-morbid conditions. Multiple-drug therapy can lead to problems with drug interactions and enhanced side effects. Currently, little is known about problems related to concurrent medical treatment of preexisting conditions and cancer.

Psychosocial changes related to aging may also compromise the ability and desire of the patient to comply with treatment and recovery regimens. Social isolation caused by a lack of a familial/community support system for the elderly is a very real problem. Nearly one third of those over 65 live alone; of these, 27% have no children (Boyle et al., 1992). In addition, as older adults age, the loss of spouses, family, and close friends increases, further isolating these individuals and often leading to a profound bereavement.

Depression and discouragement are common outcomes of age-related changes that can have significant impact on cancer care. These conditions can be treated but are often overlooked by both the family and health care professionals or are considered a natural result of aging and/or the least of the patient's problems. Depression is a major risk factor for suicide, the highest rate of which occurs in men 65 to 74 years of age. Symptoms of depression in the elderly include bereavement, loneliness, and low self-esteem. Great care should be taken to recognize and treat depression and discouragement in this age-group.

A comprehensive gerontologic assessment (physical, psychological [cognitive and affective], social, economic, functional, and environmental) aimed at differentiating normal age-related changes, co-morbid illnesses, and specific cancer-related problems and needs is critical to the provision of quality of care along the cancer care continuum.

The goal of such an assessment is to improve "diagnostic accuracy, selection of appropriate interventions, identification of the optimal environment for care, prediction of outcomes, and the monitoring of change(s) over time. Identification of rehabilitation needs is also aided by such an assessment (Boyle et al., 1992).

Basic and clinical research relating to all aspects of cancer care for the aged must become a major priority if cancer care for the elderly is to be improved and morbidity and mortality rates for cancer reduced.

The nurse oncologist is in an ideal position to coordinate care and ensure the quality of care along the continuum of cancer-related services for the elderly, as well as act as an advocate for the availability of needed support services in the community and the patient's ability to access these services.

NEW ROLES AND DIRECTIONS

Nursing Administration

Consistent with the shifts in the current health care system, transformation of the traditional nurse manager roles has been rapid, dynamic, and in constant flux. In fact, today's nursing leader has few role models and is most often in the position of using vision enhanced by creativity in providing leadership to a shifting health care system. Changes in roles from manager to leader, from director to coach, from participatory management to self-governance, and from control to partnerships are a few of the profound shifts demanded of this generation of nursing leaders.

Nurse Practitioners

History and Current Status. The role of the nurse practitioner was first noted almost 30 years ago and had a focus on primary care; it has expanded dramatically. Some notable pioneers who helped develop and secure this role deserve mentioning. Brooten, Kumar, & Brown (1986), in a seminal study, determined that low-birth-weight neonates, discharged with early discharge criteria (1500 g) and cared for by home care advanced practice nurses, demonstrated no greater morbidity or mortality compared with a similar group who remained hospitalized until reaching traditional criteria (2200 g). Furthermore, the study showed reduced costs of the early discharge group compared to the traditional group. The vast majority of nurse practitioners have a master's degree, and a smaller number have received training in certificate programs that require up to 2 years of additional training beyond the master's degree in nursing. McCorkle, Benoliel, Donaldson, Georgiadou, Moinpour, & Goodell (1989) studied the effectiveness of follow-up home care by oncology advanced nurse practitioners for patients with progressive lung cancer. One hundred and sixty-six patients were randomly assigned to one of three groups. One group received care from advanced practice oncology home care nurses. A standard home care group received care from generalist home care nurses, whereas the physician group received no home care. Patients cared for by oncology advanced nurse practitioners had fewer complications and fewer hospital readmissions. No cost analysis was performed in this study, but the investigators clearly supported the important role of advanced practitioners.

Recently a study in New York City found that patients covered by an Oxford health care plan chose nurse practitioners instead of physicians as their principle primary care provider. Simultaneously, another northeastern hospital found that 66% of visits during 1994 could have been performed by a nurse practitioner rather than physicians. Both studies encouraged the PEW Health Professions Commission to double the number of nurse practitioner graduates by the year 2000 to counter the shortage of primary physicians in major metropolitan inner cities and rural areas (PEW Health Professions Commission, 1994).

Compensation. In 1997 nurse practitioners nationally earned an average salary of $52,532, ranging from averages of $43,386 in college health clinics to $58,515 in health maintenance organizations, $59,285 in private practice, $60,050 in emergency room departments, and $60,000 in surgical facilities (Leccese, 1998).

Cost Effectiveness. Education for an oncology nurse practitioner costs four to five times less and can be completed at least 4 years sooner than that for oncologists and hematologists, strongly supporting the cost benefit of placing nurse practitioners on staff in oncology settings. It is estimated that the underuse of nurse practitioners because of practice restrictions costs the United States approximately $9 billion annually. In addition a meta analysis of nurse practitioners and nurse midwives in primary care determined that, compared with physicians, nurse practitioners scored high on patient satisfaction in areas of hypertension and diabetes. The patients surveyed were also found to be more compliant in keeping appointments, taking medications, and following lifestyle changes compared with a similar group being followed by physicians. The U.S. Congressional Office of Technology (OTA) Assessment, examining studies reporting the roles of nurse practitioners, found that up to 80% of health services and 90% of pediatric services can be provided by nurse practitioners at equal or better quality and less cost than those provided by primary care physicians. In the 12 reviewed studies the OTA concluded that quality of care surpassed that delivered by physicians and included communication with patients, prevention strategies, and symptom management. In a separate study it was determined that nurse practitioners are more likely than physicians to suggest counseling, relaxation programs, and diet changes rather than medications, suggesting a reduced cost of care.

Scope of Practice. With increasing managed care control of the health care market and decreasing inpatient volumes, more cancer health care providers are employing the nurse practitioner to meet the escalating need for accessible high-quality health care. A growing number of cancer nurse practitioners are providing services ranging from preventive and screening services to services in acute inpatient settings, outpatient areas, and rural care settings. In 1996 more than 53,000 registered nurses (RNs) were nationally certified as nurse practitioners or held state recognition as nurse practitioners or advanced practice nurses (Moses, 1997). Except for Georgia and Illinois, every state and the District of Columbia have granted nurse practitioners authority to write and prescribe medications independent of the physician. In 25 states and the District of Columbia, nurse practitioners can practice independently without physician collaboration or supervision (Pearson, 1998).

According to the American Association of Colleges of Nursing, 0.6% of nurse practitioner students enrolled in 1997 were in oncology tracks (Moses, 1997). In general, nurse practitioners perform physical examinations; diagnose and treat common acute illness and injuries; provide immunizations; manage hypertension, diabetes, and other chronic problems; order and interpret x-rays and other laboratory tests; and counsel patients on disease prevention and health care options. In addition, nurse practitioners perform invasive procedures such as inserting and removing central venous and pulmonary artery catheters and practice in roles once reserved for interns and fellows. Several symptom management clinics directed by nurse practitioners are well established and respected within the health care institutions, and often these nurses are able to bill directly for their services.

The oncology nurse practitioner is a relatively new advanced practice nursing specialty that is expanding nationwide. According to the ONS, 549 nurses identified them-

Table 17-1 Percent of Respondents Who Examine Specific Case Types Without Physician Supervision

Case Type	N	%
Long-term follow-up (disease-free)	60	52
Patients receiving chemotherapy or biologic response modifiers	71	61
Symptom management	89	77
Newly diagnosed patients	25	22
Reevaluation or restaging	30	26
Patients on a clinical trial	68	59
Cancer screening and early detection	43	37

From Kinney, A. Y., Hawkins, R., & Hudman, K. S. (1997). A discipline study of the role of the oncology nurse practitioner, *Oncology Nursing Forum, 24,* 811-820.

Table 17-2 Respondents' Perceptions of Role

	$\bar{X}$*	SD
Satisfaction with role	3.99	0.85
Physician's acceptance and support of role	4.31	0.86
Other nurses' acceptance and support of role	4.02	0.90
Nursing administration's acceptance of role	3.79	1.04
Administrative support of role	3.66	1.06
Patients' acceptance of role	4.67	0.55
Satisfaction with current salary	3.62	1.08

*Possible range: 1 (not very satisfied) to 5 (very satisfied).
SD, Standard deviation.

selves as nurse practitioners. Accordingly, the membership of the nurse practitioner special interest group grew from 29 in 1991 to 300 in 1998 (*ONS News,* 1998). The number of oncology nurse graduate programs grew from two in 1990 to an estimated 23 today. Kinney, Hawkins, & Hudman (1997) delineated the characteristics and practices of oncology nurse specialists. The most frequently cited employment settings were university-affiliated hospitals (33%), comprehensive cancer centers (26%), and ambulatory care centers (23%). Other work settings cited were cancer detection and prevention clinics, children's hospitals, hospitals with radiation facilities, medical schools, nursing homes, and community cancer centers. Table 17-1 lists the percent of respondents who examine patients independent of a physician, and Table 17-2 describes the respondents' perceptions of their roles. The role of oncology nurse practitioner brings credibility to the nursing profession by enhancing the level of care to cancer patients across all settings.

Advanced Practice Nursing

The ONS has endorsed the title "Advanced Practice Nurse" to designate clinical nurse specialist and nurse practitioner roles in oncology nursing. The advanced nurse is prepared at a minimum with a master's degree in nursing, with specialty education and clinical experience in oncology. This individual coordinates and/or provides direct and indirect care to cancer patients. Components of responsibility include making differential diagnoses, having prescriptive authority, and treating various conditions in cancer patients throughout the care trajectory. The ONS has issued strategies to promote and enhance this role. These strategies include developing a model core curriculum for advanced practice nursing in oncology graduate programs, supporting funding and access for postgraduate education, providing opportunities for continuing education at the ONS offerings, including the role of advanced practice nurses in health care policy-making arenas, establishing advanced practice nursing outcomes as research priorities, providing information to practice in case management and cancer genetic counseling, supporting mechanisms to obtain reimbursement for services, and facilitating avenues of communication among other nursing disciplines (*ONS News,* 1998).

Genetics

As the Human Genome Project nears completion, anticipated ethical, social, and legal consequences are emerging that will affect oncology nurses' daily practice. Surveys show that nurses have little or insufficient preparation in basic sciences to be able to integrate this new information into clinical care. It is not surprising that, when the ONS surveyed their membership to evaluate the need to offer educational programs in basic science, 96% replied affirmatively. Because of the far-reaching impact of genetic testing, ONS has developed positions related to the role of oncology nurses in cancer genetics counseling, as well as to risk assessment and counseling needs associated with cancer genetics testing (Box 17-5 and Table 17-3). In addition, ONS Online (www.ons.org) recently launched a cancer genetics area to aid members in understanding clinical genetics and its relevance to cancer nursing. Jenkins (1998) has outlined the areas in which oncology nurses will have the greatest responsibilities and impact.

As it is more widely recognized that genetics has implications for all nurses, organizations such as the ONS are assessing the knowledge and skills needed by members to assimilate this new technology. Oncology nurses have new opportunities to become genetic counselors who have expertise in counseling about family risk for cancer and testing for genetic susceptibility. Individuals who are considering genetic testing for cancer susceptibility require support in understanding the appropriateness and implications of these tests. Two organizations have created guidance to help professional health care workers in this critical process. The National Cancer Institute, using Cancernet, offers a direc-

Box 17-5
The Role of the Oncology Nurse in Cancer Genetic Counseling

It is the Position of the Oncology Nursing Society That . . .

The rapid integration of advances in cancer genetics will require increased numbers of individuals educated in genetics and cancer care:

- Oncology nurses possess the skills and are well-suited to assume expanded roles in cancer genetics and genetic counseling.
- Oncology nurses at both the general and advanced practice levels must have a foundation in genetics knowledge.
- Cancer genetics content must be incorporated into all levels of nursing curricula and be provided through continuing education and specialized cancer genetics programs.
- Nurses providing cancer genetic counseling must be advanced practice oncology nurses with specialized education in genetics.
- Partnering with specialty organizations with a focus in genetics is essential for providing comprehensive care to high-risk individuals.

Oncology Nursing Practice Related to Cancer Genetics

Includes three levels of practice:

- The general oncology nurse
- The advanced practice oncology nurse, basic level
- The advanced practice oncology nurse with specialty training in cancer genetics

Will vary according to practice level, but will include activities related to assessment, diagnosis, planning/implementation, and evaluation:

- Must be consistent with guidelines defined by an individual's state nurse practice act
- Must be consistent with the nurse's educational preparation and the role, scope, and standards of oncology nursing practice

Modified from Oncology Nursing Society Online (1998). *The role of the oncology nurse in cancer counseling.* Available at http://www.ons.org/main/journals.

Table 17-3 Requirements for Genetics Assessment and Counseling

Health Care Service	Responsibility
Risk assessment	Include family histories in nursing assessments and refer high-risk individuals for counseling.
Referral	Become familiar with referral sources (e.g., www.ons.org [Clinical Practice]; http://cancernet.nci.nih.gov/wwwprot/genetic/genesrch.html).
Access to services	Advocate for equal access to reliable genetics services.
Informed consent	Elements should include pretest and posttest counseling by qualified individuals.
Stored tissue sample and databanks	Involvement is ethical decision making about the use of stored genetic material for research.
Management of genetics information	Maintain confidentiality of genetics testing.
Family implications	Provide psychological support and counseling for families having a member predisposed to cancer.
Implications for children	Predictive testing for children is not recommended for adults, children, and adolescents.
Screening recommendations	Assist in decisions about screening protocols and recommendation for individuals predisposed to cancer.
Treatment recommendations	Interact on research teams to determine optimal treatment for those predisposed to cancer.

Modified from Jenkins, J. (1998). Common questions about the implications of integrating genetics information. Fact Sheet: Common Concerns in Cancer Care. *Oncology Nursing Society, March,* 1-4.

tory of genetic counselors for persons who have a family history of cancer or other risk factors that may indicate inheritable cancers. More than 200 health care professionals are currently listed in the directory (http://cancernet.nci.nih.gov/wwwprot/genetic/genesrch.html). As genetic testing and therapies become available, nurses will be assuming education and counseling responsibilities to help consumers make choices about obtaining genetic testing and the appropriate use of that information in making health care choices. Genetic counseling is discussed in Chapter 12.

The Case Manager

Another emerging and dynamic role is that of the nurse case manager. This role has arisen out of the managed care environment to ensure a designated overseer of a patient as he or she progresses through the maze of our current health care system. The American Nurses Association (ANA) urges that nurses practicing in these roles acquire a minimum of a baccalaureate degree in nursing, followed by 3 years of clinical nursing. In these changing times the case manager may have diverse responsibilities, depending on the organization in which he or she is practicing. But many health care providers insist that nurse case managers be advanced nurse practitioners because of the intensity of patient care needs from time of diagnosis through treatment and follow-up care. Galassi (1997) emphasizes the essential components of the role to be that of coordinating comprehensive cost-effective care for the oncology patients. Others have broadened the definition as a process of identifying, coordinating, and monitoring the implementation of services needed to achieve desired patient care outcomes within a specified period. The framework from which case managers practice is (1) collaboration with all health care team members, (2) use of clinical pathways, (3) continuous quality improvement, and (4) promotion of professional practice.

To meet the needs of the oncology case manager, the ONS recently held a national conference to educate and direct the efforts of these important care coordinators. A recent collection of articles contains an excellent multifaceted discussion of use of the case manager in cross-functional practice (Baird, 1996).

Nurse Entrepreneurs

Numerous oncology nurses have lost their positions through the effects of downsizing, and many more will do so in the near future. Projections indicate that over one half of the nation's inpatient beds will become unavailable because of hospital closures within 5 years and 9 million hospital-based nurses will be displaced. As of 1996 most nurses leaving the hospital setting were successful in finding ambulatory care positions (Buerhause & Staiger, 1996). Other dissatisfied nurses or those who were unable to find satisfying employment within their community have become specialists in various creative roles. A recent nursing newsletter interviewed oncology nurses who took charge of their future and sought new avenues to use their skills to implement and enhance patient care. New careers discussed were patient counseling; wound care, incontinence, and patient education consultants; web page designers and editors; and lymphedema clinicians. Many nurses also work for oncologic pharmaceutic firms for which they design, implement, and market educational programs; assist in writing research studies; and collect and analyze data (Sanoshy, 1998). These new roles call for self-direction, business acumen, efficiency, ego strengths, and flexibility. Oncology nurses practicing in these roles offer a new dimension to the delivery of quality care to the cancer patient and his or her family.

Nurse Educators

Ongoing nursing education is a critical component in delivering optimal patient care. The American Association of Colleges of Nursing (AACN) has recently characterized the nature of nursing education in the face of dramatic health care shifts. A recent position statement stressed the need for nurse educators to analyze health care trends and create flexible curricula that provide students with the skills and knowledge required for diverse settings. Education must be directed at computer and technical skills and the ability to practice within ethically charged settings such as rationing of heath care and research advances such as the Human Genome Project. Universities and colleges that extend oncology nursing tracks and who adopt the directions of the AACN need to prepare faculty and students for practicing among end-of-life issues, rationed care, more complex clinical trials, access to clinical trials, and caregiver burden.

Box 17-6
The Oncology Nursing Position on the Identification of Registered Nurses in the Workplace

- The registered nurse should, at all times when on duty, wear an insignia that identifies him/her as a registered nurse (RN).
- The RN should verbally inform health care consumers of *who* he or she is and about his or her role in providing care.
- Health care facilities should never prohibit personnel from wearing an insignia that identifies credentials.
- Health care consumers should be informed of the caregiver's demonstrated specialized knowledge in oncology nursing through identification of the credentials "OCN" and "AOCN," earned by the RN through the Oncology Nursing Certification Corporation examinations.
- Advanced practice nurses should identify themselves as such (e.g., as clinical nurse specialists or nurse practitioners).
- In the event that a facility (including private offices, ambulatory clinics, and home care agencies) prohibits or discourages identification of staff credentials, staff members and consumers should submit written protest to facility administrators, the state's nurses association, the state's board of nursing, and the Joint Commission on Accreditation of Healthcare Organizations (JCAHO).

Every RN should advocate that his or her state nurse practice act mandate identification of professional title and credentials.

Modified from The Oncology Nursing Society Online (1998). *Position on the identification of registered nurses in the workplace.* Available at http://www.ons.org/ons/main/journals.

Another important direction from the AACN is to acknowledge the importance of lifelong learning for the professional nurse. Attention should be paid to the lifelong experiences that matriculated students bring to nursing programs, and nursing skills should be built on these talents. Programs using creative and flexible approaches may attract students who would otherwise be deterred from entering traditional programs. The executive summary is a vision of baccalaureate undergraduate nursing (AACN, 1998).

Titles in Oncology Nursing

One of the most common means of decreasing the cost of health care has been to replace the professional nurse with less skilled workers, often referred to as "assistive personnel." Often consumers and their family caregivers are not aware of the qualifications of their direct caregiver, and some institutions have mandated that nurses not display professional or academic accreditation. Joint Commission Accreditation Standards stipulate that "staff members inform patients of the identity and professional status of individuals responsible for or authorizing and performing treatments and or procedures." Oncology nurses are encouraged to wear an insignia identifying their credentials and roles relative to their care. Nurses practicing in facilities discouraging this practice need to report this practice to their nursing state board and the Joint Commission on Accreditation of Healthcare Organizations (Box 17-6).

Future Trends

There are predictions that an imminent nursing shortage threatens the quality of care for oncology patients. The issue is one of improper distribution, with emphasis on unmet needs for specialized nursing such as emergency room, operating room, and intensive care nurses. Two major factors in the general nursing shortage are an aging nurse population and an aging America. The average age of professional nurses is 44, approximately 50% of nurses are entering their 50s, and many will retire shortly. Only 9% of the nursing population in the United States is under age 30. Other contributing concerns are decreased quality of patient care, poor working conditions, and increased need for education to meet growing complex technology (Stewart, 1998). The ANA recently addressed issues of RN staffing relative to rising record-breaking profits, due in part to the use of unlicensed nursing personnel. In a statement released in January 1998, the ANA called for the Patient Safety Act that demands that health care institutions make public specific information on nurse staffing levels, staff mix, and patient outcome (Carswell, 1998).

These dismal statistics are particularly disturbing for the oncology nurse and patient. The foreseeable shortfalls in the profession of nursing lie in the specialty areas of practice. To avoid a worsening scenario, undergraduate enrollments need to increase and the image of an abundance of nurses flooding the marketplace must vanish. Organizations such as the ONS and the ANA will continue to play a major role in the education, recruitment, and retention of qualified oncology nurses.

EVALUATION OF THE QUALITY OF CARE

Profound shifts during the past 2 decades have forced health care providers to define, deliver, and measure the type, duration, intensity, and place of health care. In addition, providers dictate to the insured the time and place at which they can receive that care. Thus the nation struggles to provide a benchmark for assessment of quality of care to measure positive outcomes in an economical manner.

To meet this challenge, the ONS has issued a position paper to characterize components of quality of care (Mooney, 1997). The major goals of the statement are to (1) offer nurses and others a framework within which to design and implement holistic and programmatic approaches to quality cancer care, (2) stress the important role of the RN or certified nurse, and (3) give patients a definition to select services consistent with their needs and expectations (Haylock, 1997). The position paper outlines eight statements about quality care. The ONS believes that quality cancer care, a right of all citizens, entails timely access and reimbursement across the trajectory of care, including prevention, early detection, treatment, supportive care, long-term follow-up, and end-of-life care. A summary of the position paper can be found in Box 17-7. Concomitantly, a Patients' Bill of Rights was issued (Box 17-8).

Box 17-7

Components of Quality of Care for Cancer Patients and Their Families

Quality cancer care:

- Is a right of all citizens.
- Is culturally competent, ethical, and cost effective.
- Entails timely access to and reimbursement for a coordinated, comprehensive approach to care provided by a multidisciplinary team throughout the cancer trajectory that includes prevention, early detection, treatment, supportive care, long-term follow-up, and end-of-life care.
- Incorporates the individual with cancer (and the patient's family) as fully informed partners and decision makers.
- Is best accomplished by registered nurses who have been educated and certified in the oncology specialty.
- Is coordinated and delivered by competent cancer care providers.
- Oncology advanced practice nurses should be used in all cancer care delivery systems.
- Oncology nursing must be included in the planning and implementation of cancer care services with equal parity to that of medicine and other disciplines.

Mooney, K.H. (1997). Oncology Nursing Society position paper on quality cancer care. *Oncology Nursing Forum, 24,* 951-953.

THE INFORMATION AGE

One of the greatest impacts of the electronic age is the use of the Internet for medical information not only for the professional, but also for the lay public. MEDLINE for the National Library of Medicine for the National Institutes of Health alone totaled 7 million in 1997 but exceeded 7 million for the month of March, 1998 alone (Fig. 17-1). A total of 70 (million) searches are expected this year, and 30% of the users are the general public (*Gratefully Yours*, 1998). For the first time, consumer health publications whose primary audience is the lay public will be indexed in MEDLINE and available on both Internet Grateful Med and PubMed. The goal is to provide affordable, secure information that will enhance public information, advanced telemedicine conferences, digital libraries, and distance learning.

In a similar action, the ONS Online is now available to other health care providers and consumers. The public accesses the service over 80,000 times a month, and this number grows exponentially (Gomez, 1998). Oncology nurses are now, more than ever, in a position of staying current by familiarizing themselves with Internet access, interpreting information that patients access, and guiding patients to reliable electronic resources.

RESEARCH AND CLINICAL TRIALS

Advances in cancer care come primarily from basic and clinical research and from clinical trials that test the efficacy of research findings in the clinical setting. Basic research provides a better understanding of the molecular

Box 17-8

Patients' Bill of Rights for Quality Cancer Care

- Availability and access to education about cancer risks and lifestyle changes that influence the incidence of cancer, including educational activities that are effective and appropriate for diverse populations
- Reimbursement for screening activities that facilitate the early detection of cancer when there is a greater potential for cure; these screening activities should be tailored to individual risk, including family history, age, race, gender, and socioeconomic status
- Timely access to the appropriate spectrum of treatment options provided in the most appropriate setting for the management of the specific cancer and symptoms; these options include but are not limited to surgery, radiotherapy, chemotherapy, hormonal therapies, biologic therapies, marrow or blood stem cell transplant, complementary therapies, and rehabilitative therapies
- Administration of cancer care by qualified practitioners who have oncology knowledge and who successfully complete ongoing programs that prove their competency
- Access to adequate health plan coverage for supportive therapies that help to decrease the side effects from cancer treatments
- Access to scientifically sound and culturally relevant clinical trials that provide necessary information to advance the implementation of effective screening, diagnostic, and treatment modalities
- Access to long-term follow-up by oncology specialists that focuses on health promotion, prompt detection of cancer recurrence, and the evaluation and identification of physical and psychosocial effects of cancer and its treatment
- Availability of palliative care modalities that improve quality at the end of life, with the focus on symptom management, psychosocial support for patients and families, hospice care, and bereavement counseling; this care must be provided in a manner that respects the individual's cultural, spiritual, and ethical needs.
- Access to culturally competent care provided by culturally competent caregivers.

Modified from Mooney, K.H. (1997). Oncology Nursing Society position paper on quality cancer care. *Oncology Nursing Forum, 24,* 951-953.

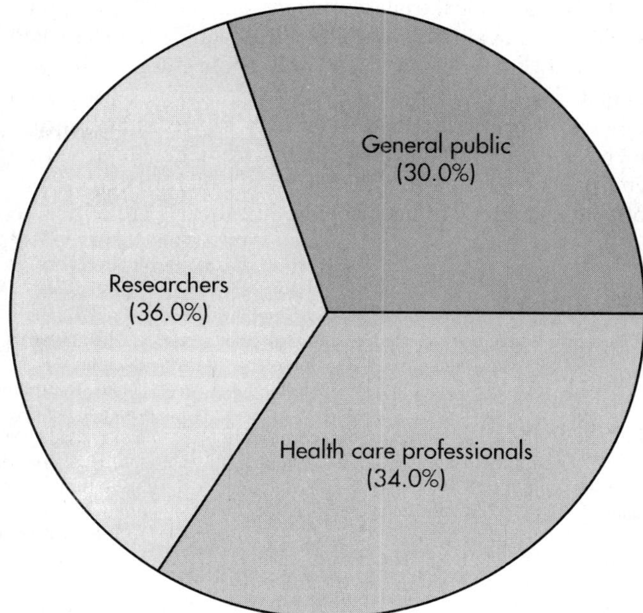

Fig. 17-1 Populations accessing MEDLINE. (From *Gratefully yours* [1998]. March-April, 5.)

and genetic bases of cancer, the pharmacology of potential cancer drugs, and the bases for developments of other technology-dependent therapies. Clinical research helps determine the effectiveness of the translation of basic knowledge to clinical practice. Clinical trials provide the setting for the application and refinement of all aspects of cancer care from prevention and early screening to enhancement of quality of life for patients and survivors.

Advances from basic research are emerging at a startling pace. Although improved funding levels would be most helpful, the real challenge is in keeping pace with these advances in effective translation to clinical practice. Clinical trials are the key to this process. However, they are plagued by a lack of sufficient funds, problems with the design and implementation of trials, and a very low rate of potential subject (patient) participation.

Participation in clinical trials is very costly for health care delivery institutions and organizations, as is the design and implementation of investigatively sound study protocols. Study outcomes can be influenced by a myriad of factors or variables. These variables include patient characteristics, patient environmental factors, cancer-related factors such as stage and prior treatment, treatment provision, data collection, and health/study provider variables. Great care must be taken to see that members of the study cohort (patients) are comparable in terms such as relevant individual characteristics and severity of illness. In addition, other variables such as clinical setting, provision of treatment, study personnel behavior, and the collection and analysis of data must be carefully controlled if one is to be confident that the outcomes of the trial are due to the variable being investigated (e.g., different drugs, different doses) and not some other factor. Unintentional (or intentional) bias introduced into a study design or implementation can compromise the validity of trial results and complicate the required duplication of the study by others. This, unfortunately, is not an uncommon occurrence.

The availability of subjects for clinical trials is also an important problem. The more rare the cancer, the more difficult it is to find sufficient subjects for a statistically relevant outcome. Consortia of clinical sites with adequate numbers of pooled patients are now being used for clinical trials related to these cancers.

For most clinical trials, sufficient numbers of appropriate subjects are available for study. However, of the estimated 12% to 44% eligible subjects, only about 3% actually participate in studies (Morrow, Hickok, & Burish, 1994). Such low enrollment is caused by barriers to access and enrollment on the part of the health care system, health providers, and patients. Increasing awareness of, altering perceptions of, and changing attitudes about clinical trials are critical to overcoming these barriers to enrollment (ONS Online, 1998).

The nurse oncologist can play an important role in identifying subjects and facilitating their enrollment in clinical trials. In addition, those involved in clinical trials can take special care to see that protocols are implemented as designed and study results incorporated into state of the art clinical cancer care.

REFERENCES

American Association of Colleges of Nursing. (1998). Executive summary: A vision of baccalaureate and graduate nursing. Washington, D.C.: The Association.

Anisimov, V. N. (1989). Age-related mechanisms of suseptibility to carcinogenesis. *Seminars in Oncology, 15,* 10-19.

Baird, S. B. (1997). Cross-functional practice. *Innovations in Breast Cancer Care, 3*(2), 43-46.

Baird, S. B. (1996). Rural cancer care: A nursing challenge. *Innovations in Breast Cancer Care 1,* 45.

Baranovsky, A. & Myers, M. H. (1986). Cancer incidence and survival in patients 65 years of age and older. *Cancer, 36,* 26-41.

Bernreuter, M. & Cardona, S. (1997). Survey and critique of studies related to unlicensed assistive personal from 1975 to 1997: Part I. *Journal of Nursing Administration, 27*(6), 24-29.

Bernreuter, M. & Cardona, S. (1997). Survey and critique of studies related to unlicensed assistive personal from 1975 to 1997: Part II. *Journal of Nursing Administration, 27*(6), 49-55.

Boyle, D.M., Engelking, C., Blesch, K.S., Dodge, J., Sarna, L., & Weinrich, S. (1992). Oncology Nursing Society position paper on cancer and aging: The mandate for oncology nursing. *Oncology Nursing Forum, 19,* 913-932.

Brooten, D., Kumar S., & Brown, L. P. (1986). A randomized clinical trial of early hospital discharge and home follow-up of very-low-birthweight infants. *New England Journal of Medicine, 315,* 934-939.

Bruner, D. W., Bucholtz, J. D., Iwamoto, R., & Strohl, R.(Eds). (1998). *Manual for radiation oncology nursing practice and education.* Pittsburgh: Oncology Nursing Society Press.

Buchsel, P. C. & Kapustay, P. M. (1997). In M. B. Whedon & D. Wujick (Eds.), *Blood and marrow stem cell transplantation: Principles, practice, and nursing insights* (2nd ed.). Sudbury, MA: Jones and Bartlett.

Buerhause, P. I. & Staiger, D. O. (1996). Managed care and the nursing workforce. *Journal of the American Medical Association, 276*(18): 1487-1493.

Colling, J. (1983). Sleep disturbances in aging: A theoretic and empiric analysis. *Advances in Nursing Science, 6,* 36-44.

Cantril, C. A. & Haylock, P. J. (1996). Cancer care in rural settings. *Innovations in Breast Cancer Care, 1*(3), 46-49.

Carswell, A. (1998). ANA reacts to release of data on U. S. Hospitals. *The Pennsylvania Nurse, March,* 11.

Cohen, H. J. (1990). Oncology and aging: general principles of cancer in the elderly. In W.R. Hazard, R. Andres, & E. L. Bierman (Eds.), *Principles of geriatric medicine and gerontology.* (2nd ed.). New York: McGraw-Hill.

Dawson, L. J. (1995). Telemedicine and its benefits to rural communities. *The Journal of Oncology Management,* March/April.

Derby, S. E. (1991). Ageism in cancer care of the elderly. *Oncology Nursing Forum, 18,* 921-926.

Dodge, J., Backman, C., & Silverman, H. (1988). Fecal incontinence in elderly patients. *Postgraduate Medicine, 83,* 258-270.

Eddy, D. M. (1986). Setting priorities for cancer control programs. *Journal of the National Cancer Institute, 76,* 187-199.

Fitzsimons, V. M. (1983). The aging integument: A sensitive and complex system. *Topics of Clinical Nursing, 5*(2), 32-38.

Foreman, M. D. (1986). Acute confusional starts in hospitalized elderly: A research dillemma. *Nursing Research, 35,* 34-87.

Frantz, R. A. & Kinney, X. (1986). Variables associated with skin dryness in the elderly. *Nursing Research, 35,* 98-110.

Galassi, A. (1997). Role of the oncology advanced practice nurse. In S. L. Groenwald, M. H. Frogge, M. Goodman, & C. H. Yarbro (Eds.). *Cancer nursing: Principles and practice* (4th ed). Sudbury: Jones and Bartlett Publishing.

Gomez, L. (1998). ONS online redesign offers improved functionality, expanded content, and increased access. *ONS News, 13*(4), 11.

Gratefully yours (1998), http://www.nlm.gov, *March-April,* 5.

Haylock, P. J. (1997). Improving the quality of cancer care. *Oncology Nursing Forum, 24,* 924.

Hillary, L. J. (1997). Radiotherapy. In S. L. Groenwald, M. H. Frogge, M. Goodman, & C. H. Yarbro (Eds.), *Cancer nursing: Principles and practice* (4th ed), Sudbury: Jones and Bartlett.

Iwamoto, R. (1998). *Personal communication.*

Jenkins, J. (1998). Common questions about the implications of integrating genetics information. Fact sheet: Common concerns in cancer care. *Oncology Nursing Society, March,* 1-4.

Jenkins, J. K., Reynolds, B., Seviech, K. (1986). Patient falls in the acute care setting: Identifying risk factors. *Nursing Research, 35,* 34-37.

King, C. R., Forth, D., Ayette, M., & Harrington, A. (1997). Planning, implementing, and evaluating a patient-centered care model for oncology patients. *Innovations in Breast Cancer Care, 3*(2)22:27.

Kinney, A. Y., Hawkins, R. H., & Hudman, K. S. (1997). A descriptive study of the role of the oncology nurse practitioner. *Oncology Nursing Forum, 24,* 811-820.

Leccese, C. (1998). Who's making what and where: The ADVANCE salary survey. *Advanced Nurse Practitioner, 6*(1), 30-5.

Mandelblatt, J. S., Wheat, M. E., Monane, M., Moshief, R. D., Hollenberg, J. P., & Tang, J. (1992). Breast cancer screening for elderly women with and without comorbid conditions. A decision analysis model. *Annals of Internal Medicine, 116*(9), 722-730.

McCorkle, R., Benoliel, J. A., Donaldson, G., Georgiadou, F., Moinpour, C., & Goodell, B. (1987). A randomized clinical trial of home nursing care for lung cancer patients. *Cancer, 64,* 1375-1382.

Miller, S. (1993). Hospital-school partnerships: Linking vital community institutions. *The Journal of Oncology Management, July/August,* 35-42.

Mooney, K. H. (1997). Oncology nursing society position paper on quality cancer care. *Oncology Nursing Forum, 24,* 951-953.

Morgan, R. H. (1998). Stereotactic radiosurgery: Procedures and nursing care. *Supportive Cancer Care, 1,* 88-91.

Morrow, G., Hickok, J., & Burish, T. (1994). Behavioral aspects of clinical trials. *Cancer, 74,* 2676-2682.

Moses, E. B. (1997). The registered nurse population: March 1996. Washington, D. C.: U. S. Department of Health and Human Services, Division of Nursing.

National Cancer Institute (1997). The cancer journey: Issues for survivors. A training program for health professions. Bethesda, MD: U. S. Department of Health and Human Services.

National Cancer Institute (1986). Cancer control objectives for the nation: 1985-2000. National Cancer Institute Monographs 2 (1986). Pub. No. 86-2880. Bethesda, MD: U. S. Department of Health and Human Services.

Nickens, H. (1985). Intrinsic factors in falling among the elderly. *Archives of Internal Medicine, 145,* 1089-1093.

Nightingale, F. (1969). *Notes on nursing: What it is and what it is not.* New York: Dover.

Office on Smoking and Health (1989). Reducing the health consequences of smoking: 25 years of progress. A report of the Surgeon General. DHHS Publication No. (CDC) 89-8411. Washington, D.C.: U.S. Department of Health and Human Services.

Oncology Nursing Society (1998) and American Society of Clinical Oncology (1997). Criteria for facilities and personnel for the administration of parenteral system antineoplastic therapy. *Journal of Clinical Oncology, 15,* 3416-3417.

Oncology Nursing Society (1996). Position paper on cancer and aging: The mandate for oncology nursing. *ONS Online,* http://www.ons.org.

Oncology Nursing Society News (1998). NP SIG promotes high standards for advanced practice RNS. *ONS News, 13*(10), 6.

Oncology Nursing Society Online (1998). *Various articles.* Available at http://www.ons.org/ons/main/journals.

Oncology Nursing Society Online (1996). *Cancer chemotherapy guidelines and recommendations for practice.* Available at http://www.ons.org/ons/main/journals.

Pearson, L. J. (1998). Annual update of how each state stands on legislative issues affecting advanced nursing practice. *Nurse Practitioner, 23*(1), 14.

Perry, B. C. (1982). Falls among the elderly: A review of the methods and conclusions of epidemiologic studies. *Journal of American Gerontology Society, 30,* 367-371.

PEW Health Professions Commission (1994).

SAGE Study Group. (1998). Management of pain in elderly patients with cancer. *Journal of the American Medical Association, 279*(23), 1877-1914.

Sanoshy, J. (1998) Nurse entrepreneurship: An alternative career choice worth considering. *ONS News 13*(7), 1-6.

Satariano, W. A., Ragheb, N. E., & Dupuis, M. H. (1989). Co-morbidity in older women with breast cancer: An epidemiologic approach. In R. Yancek & J. W. Yales (Eds.), *Cancer in the elderly: Approaches to early detection and treatment.* New York: Springer.

Schuette, H. L., Tucker, T. C., Brown, M. L., Potosky, A. L., & Samuel, T. (1995). The costs of cancer care in the United States: Implications for action. *Oncology, 9*(11 Suppl.), 19-22.

Shapiro, S., Venet, W., Strax, L., & Roeser, R., (1985). Selection, follow-up, and analysis in the Health Insurance Plan Study: A randomized trial with breast cancer screening. *NCI Monographs, 67,* 65-74.

Stewart, M. (1998). New nursing shortage hits; causes complex. *The American Nurse, March/April,* 32.

U. S. Bureau of the Census (1987). Statistical abstract of the United States (108th ed.). Washington Printing Office.

U.S. Public Health Service. (1991a). *Healthy People 2000: National health promotion and disease prevention objectives,* Pub. No. (PHS) 91-50212. Washington D.C.: U. S. Department of Health and Human Services.

U.S. Public Health Service. (1991). *Healthy People 2000: National health promotion and disease prevention objectives.* Pub. No. 91-50213. Washington D.C.: U.S. Department of Health and Human Services.

Waltman, N. L., Bergstrom, N., Armstrong, N., Norvell, K., & Braden, B. (1991). Nutritional status, pressure sores, and mortality, in elderly patients with cancer. *Oncology Nursing Forum, 18*(5), 867-874.

Weinrich, S. P. (1990). Predictors of older adults' participation in fecal occult blood screening. *Oncology Nursing Forum, 17*(15), 715-720.

Whedon, M. B. & Wujcik, D. (1997). *Blood and marrow stem cell transplantation: Principles, practices, and nursing insights* (2nd ed.). Sudbury, MA: Jones and Bartlett.

Yancik, R. & Ries, L. G. (1989). Epidemiologic features of cancer in the elderly. In T. V. Zinser & R. M. Coe (Eds.), *Cancer and aging.* New York: Springer.

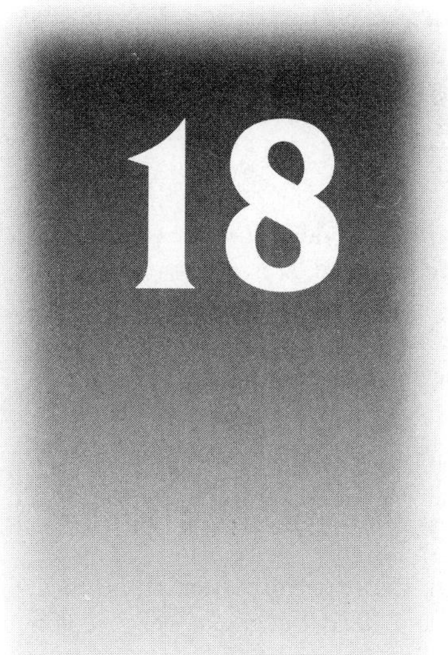

Care of the Terminal Patient's Physical and Psychosocial Needs

Nessa Coyle, RN, MS, FAAN
Jane Ingham, MD
Theresa Altilio, MSW

INTRODUCTION

Palliative care has been defined as "the active total care of patients whose disease is not responsive to curative treatment" (World Health Organization [WHO], 1990). More encompassing definitions consider that palliative care should be delivered in conjunction with therapies aimed at cure or life prolongation to all patients living with life-threatening illness. Regardless of whether illness is "life-threatening" with the retained hope for cure, or unresponsive to cure, the goal of palliative care is the achievement of the best possible quality of life for patients and their families. For the purpose of this chapter, *family* is defined as the primary supports identified by the patient, regardless of blood or legal ties. In this context, aggressive attention to symptom control is considered an imperative with concurrent and ongoing attention to the psychological and spiritual concerns of the individual and his or her family. Although such an approach to care is certainly applicable at any stage of illness, it is especially important, and frequently becomes the primary focus of care at the end of life (Cassem, 1991; Corr, Morgan, & Wass, 1993; Twycross & Lichter, 1993).

At the core of palliative care is attention to symptom management. Such management must always be viewed in the light of the patient's priorities. Much fear can be alleviated if the patient and family can be assured that priorities will be established for symptom management and distress aggressively treated by attentive and knowledgeable caregivers (Cherny, Coyle, & Foley, 1996). To achieve these goals, nurses and physicians must be well versed in symptom management strategies and attentive to patients' subjective reports. To facilitate both effective symptom management and optimal care at the end of life, it is also important for patients to understand the relevance of advanced directives, including living wills and health care proxies. Such directives reflect an attempt to ensure that the patient's wishes surrounding end-of-life care are known, and preferences regarding life-sustaining treatments and "do not resuscitate orders" are clear (Grant, 1992; Latimer & Dawson, 1993; Virmani, Schneiderman, & Kaplan, 1994).

The role of the nurse throughout illness is vital but especially so at the end of life (American Nurses Association, 1991). To optimize care, nurses work in close liaison with others such as physicians, social workers, and pastoral care personnel, so that the skills of a "team" can be brought to the patient and family. By becoming knowledgeable about the principles and practice of palliative care, the oncology nurse will often be in a position to help educate other team members. This chapter provides an overview of the principles of palliative care, describes some programmatic approaches to the delivery of this care, and addresses some of the tasks that are an integral part of the practice of palliative care. Because symptom control is addressed in an earlier chapter, this chapter focuses on the aspects of symptom control that are particular to the time near the end of life.

DEFINITIONS OF PALLIATIVE CARE AND ELIGIBILITY

Although palliative care has been defined as "the active total care of patients whose disease is not responsive to curative treatment" (WHO, 1990), recently, there has been recognition that many aspects of palliative care can be applied throughout the course of any life-threatening disease. Those who are at the end of life, a time that health care professionals and patients alike often find difficult to recognize and accept, should not be the only population who receive care with an intensive focus on symptom management and psychosocial and spiritual support. Further, those patients who elect life-sustaining therapies and/or experimental therapies should not suffer as a consequence of having limited, or no, access to palliative care expertise.

The Canadian Palliative Care Association has been an exponent of this concept and defines palliative care in this broader sense as "the combination of active and compassionate therapies intended to comfort and support individuals and families who are living with life-threatening illness" (Ferris & Cummings, 1995). Within this definition is a recognition that the concerns of patients who are living with incurable, life-threatening illness are similar to those experiencing life-threatening but potentially curable illness. An acceptance of this broader definition allows all those with life-threatening illness to receive, and benefit from, palliative care.

MODELS FOR PROVIDING PALLIATIVE CARE

As indicated previously, to address the needs of all cancer patients comprehensively, and given the difficulty of precisely defining the end of life, it is generally accepted that a palliative care model that is integrated throughout the course of illness is ideal so as to ensure quality and continuity. Institutions caring for cancer patients, and for others with life-threatening illness, must address integrating palliative care throughout the care delivery system in a manner that addresses the needs of *all* patients, specifically the needs of both inpatients and outpatients. This approach applies to institutions and organizations providing acute and chronic care and to those involved in the delivery of care to patients who reside in their homes. The ideal model for each institution or organization varies.

At the time of writing, palliative care in the United States is a rapidly evolving field, and new models for care delivery are being developed. For example, some cancer centers are developing palliative care programs and are including palliative and end-of-life care into disease management pathways. In other countries and parts of the world, for example Canada, Australia, and Europe, models of palliative care have been functioning for many years. Regardless of which model is selected as the optimal mechanism for the delivery of palliative care, the common theme for *all* models is one of an interdisciplinary team approach to care, with the patient and family at the center of care. The key components of palliative care are listed in Box 18-1.

Box 18-1
Components of Palliative Care

Palliative Care

- Is provided by an interdisciplinary team
- Affirms life and regards dying as a normal process
- Provides relief from pain and other distressing symptoms
- Integrates the psychological and spiritual aspects of care
- Seeks to ensure that a support system is available to help the patient cope throughout life-threatening illness
- Seeks to ensure a support system is available to help the family cope during the family member's illness and in their own bereavement

Palliative Therapies

- Are never administered with the intent of hastening death
- Do not, of themselves, postpone death but can be delivered in conjunction with life-sustaining therapies

Adapted from World Health Organization (1990). *Cancer pain relief and palliative care.* Report of a WHO Expert Committee on Cancer Pain Relief and Palliative Care. Geneva: World Health Organization.

Hospice Care

In the United States the most commonly delivered and well-known model for specialized end-of-life care is hospice care. The first American Hospice opened in New Haven, Connecticut, in 1974. The National Hospice Organization, founded in 1977, defines a *hospice program* as a "centrally administered program of palliative and supportive services which provides physical, psychological, and spiritual care for dying persons and their families" (National Hospice Organization, 1989). In 1983, after evaluation of government-sponsored demonstration projects on the efficacy and cost of hospice care, hospice services became a Medicare benefit (Mor, Greer, & Kaastenbaum, 1988; Mor & Masterson-Allen, 1987). Hospice programs are now run by both for-profit and not-for-profit organizations and are becoming part of the standard of care offered to patients nearing the end of life.

Unfortunately, the Medicare hospice benefit, which mandates a 6-month prognosis criterion for eligibility for hospice, has come to be viewed as hospice. However, hospice is not a government-defined benefit, but rather a philosophy of care that essentially is identical to the philosophy of palliative care, but specifically focuses on optimizing quality of life in those not seeking, and unlikely to benefit from, life-sustaining treatments (Saunders, 1990). As a consequence, hospice care generally provides palliative care at the very end of life. Hospice benefits are now available to many patients, but most insurance programs and the Medicare program continue to restrict the delivery of hospice care to those patients who have a prognosis of less than 6 months. These criteria, along with various financial constraints and an approach that focuses only on comfort for the most part, prevent hospice programs from offering palliative care throughout the full spectrum of cancer care. Most hospice programs do not offer care to patients who are nearing the end of life but still seek life-sustaining treatments.

In the United States, hospice programs offer palliative care to patients and families through a medically supervised interdisciplinary team approach to care. Teams include nursing, medical, social work, chaplaincy, and volunteer personnel. For the most part, hospice teams work with the patient's own physician. Medicare-certified hospices must also have a medical director whose role is to supervise the overall program, to act as a resource for hospice staff and primary attending physicians, and more rarely, to provide direct care for hospice patients. Although hospice care is available on both an inpatient and outpatient basis, the focus is on home care, with brief periods of hospitalization for symptom control or to provide respite for the caregivers. A major advantage to patients and families is the availability of regular home visits by the hospice nurse and 24-hour emergency support from skilled hospice nurses with back up from the hospice medical staff. Because of the variety of models of hospice programs, levels of sophistication, and depth of services offered, the needs of the patient and the services offered through the program should be evaluated before referral of a patient (Coyle, Loscalzo, & Bailey, 1989). For example, although most hospice programs have changed their policy toward the use of technology in end-of-life care, in contrast to an earlier "no high-tech" approach, severe restrictions on the financial reimbursement for programs may limit their ability to deliver care to patients seeking or requiring such treatment approaches.

The hospice model has the potential to, and frequently does, provide optimal palliative care for patients who meet eligibility criteria. Unfortunately, many eligible patients are not offered hospice care or are referred only in the last days of their illness. In the past this referral pattern may have been influenced by the need for patients to have a "Do Not Resuscitate" (DNR) status. This requirement has changed, and a DNR status is not required for admission to a hospice program (National Hospice Organization, 1992). However, some inpatient facilities question the role of inpatient hospice care for an ill patient seeking life-sustaining therapies. Such patient's needs may be better met in an acute hospital setting.

Individuals involved in providing oncologic care should familiarize themselves with hospice services in their area and seek to establish a relationship with a particular program. Given that the hospital nursing staff and physicians may become geographically distanced from the patient who elects hospice home care, a good working relationship with the hospice nursing staff will help facilitate continuity and reassure patients and families of ongoing communication between staff in both settings. Further, if there is mutual respect for the expertise of team members in both settings, the development of relationships among oncology and hospice nurses can facilitate the sharing of knowledge and expertise (Coyle, 1987).

Palliative Care and Supportive Care Programs

To address the gap in the delivery of specialized palliative care services that has existed in cancer centers and other hospitals, some institutions develop in-house palliative care and supportive care programs that link with community resources such as home nursing agencies and hospice programs. Indeed, sometimes the needs of the dying patient and their family are best served by a joint effort between a cancer center or hospital and community services and programs (Coyle, 1987; Ingham & Coyle, 1997).

There are a variety of models of in-house palliative care programs, ranging from a one-time consultative model, with the primary service continuing to have overall responsibility for the patient's care, to models in which the palliative care service both consults at times, and at other times assumes primary responsibility for the patient's care, to still other models in which the palliative care service sometimes consults and at other times assumes primary responsibility for the ongoing care of the patient and family. Although the concept of a "program" in an institution may seem to imply that many personnel are involved in a specialized team, these programs often consist of a dedicated physician, nurse, or both, who aim to complement the existing expertise within an institution while, at the same time, reach out to community resources. However, some programs have a large number of staff and offer a comprehensive range of services (Kellar, Martinez, Finis, Bolger, & Von Gunten, 1996; Von Gunten, Neely, & Martinez, 1996; Walsh, 1990). Their services may include a hospice program, a link with a hospital-based home nursing service, and inpatient and home care for patients who are not enrolled in the hospice program but are in need of palliative care interventions while still pursuing life-sustaining therapies. Examples of such highly developed programs are the palliative care programs at the Cleveland Clinic in Ohio and at Northwestern University in Chicago (Von Gunten et al., 1996; Walsh, 1990).

An example of a long-running program that provides palliative care with a small number of personnel is the Supportive Care Program (SCP), a part of the Pain and Palliative Care Service at Memorial Sloan-Kettering Cancer Center (MSKCC) in New York City (Coyle, 1987). This program utilizes institutional and community resources to optimize care for patients who are in need of palliative care but may have goals that still focus on the prolongation of life. The program is a patient and family-centered, nurse-coordinated program that provides 24-hour access to palliative care nurse specialists, daily telephone contact (or more often if indicated), ongoing monitoring and treatment of symptoms, psychological support, and liaison and coordination among the physicians, nurses, and social workers involved in care of the patient in the hospital and at home. The nurse clinical specialists who coordinate this program have access to the pain service palliative care physicians and social worker as well as to the broader resources within the institution.

All of these programs emphasize continuity of care, home management, education, and support for those providing care in the community. Further, each recognizes the need to bridge the gap between hospital and community. It is important to note that hospital or cancer-center-based palliative care programs are relatively new to the United States. Although insurance providers and the Health Care Financing Administration recognize the need to reimburse most hospice programs, they are only just beginning to explore reimbursement mechanisms for hospital programs, many of which are seeded in and/or gain their ongoing support through philanthropic funds.

The reasons for referral to a palliative care or supportive care program may be diverse. Some programs, for example the Supportive Care Program of MSKCC, provide care for a limited number of select patients and families who are at high risk for complex and difficult symptom-related or psychological and spiritual-related distress, with concomitant family burden. Other programs may encourage early referrals for all patients with a particular diagnosis where there is a high prevalence of distressing symptoms such as pancreatic cancer. Most programs see patients for evaluation of evolving or poorly controlled symptoms, multiple symptoms, progressive functional decline, and increasing nursing requirements.

Other Models for Delivery of Palliative Care

Just as in the hospital system, there are gaps in availability and delivery of palliative care. These gaps also exist in the home environment for patients seeking life-sustaining or highly technical care. To address this need, some home nursing agencies are beginning to develop programs that may facilitate the delivery of palliative care. Traditionally, these agencies deliver highly technical or skilled nursing services to patients in the home. Recently many are beginning to link with, or develop, home care programs to deliver prehospice care. In doing this, agencies frequently use the services of the same nursing staff from their home care programs to provide prehospice and hospice home care. Through this system, the patient and family can benefit from continuity of care in the setting of changing goals of care.

It is important to note that, for the most part, these agencies *do not* provide a model for palliative care delivery, as they generally provide nursing care alone and do not offer specialized medical, social work, and other personnel to assist in care. These agencies generally rely on the system that referred the patient to them to provide such personnel and to provide emergency support for the patient and family. Nonetheless, when the referring system is responsive and *does* address these other needs of their patients, these programs can greatly assist in the delivery of palliative care, particularly to those patients who are seeking life-sustaining treatments toward the end of life.

ROLE OF THE HEALTH CARE TEAM IN END-OF-LIFE PALLIATIVE CARE

Throughout the course of illness and particularly at the end of life, the multidimensional nature of disease and the diverse manifestations of distress suggest that care is best provided using a team approach. Each of the models for palliative care reviewed previously utilizes this team concept, with care delivered by nurses, physicians, social workers, chaplains, volunteers, and others. Diverse skills and training frequently are required to help the patient and family best deal with the physical, psychosocial, and spiritual issues that are so common toward the end of life. Delivery of optimal end-of-life care, therefore, requires incorporation of the concepts of team and continuity.

A *team* can be defined as a group of individuals with a common purpose working together (Ajemian, 1993). The common purpose should be understood by the individual members who come together to share knowledge and information and then plan for future action. Each individual brings particular expertise and training to the team and within the team is responsible for making individual decisions within his or her area of responsibility. The most common version of a team in health care systems is the collaborative multidisciplinary group. In this type of team, the individuals are known first by their professional identities and only secondarily by their team affiliation. They share information using the vehicle of the medical record, and the leader is the highest ranking member. The multidisciplinary team approach is the usual approach taken in the early phase of illness. As an illness becomes more complex both physically and socially, and as goals of care shift, it is likely that care will be best provided by an interdisciplinary team. In this type of team, the identity of the team itself supersedes the individual professional identities. Members share information and work together to develop goals, and leadership is shared among team members depending on the task at hand. Because the team is the vehicle of action, the communication process is vital to success. Good communication and mutual respect among disciplines, for example, nurses, physicians, social workers, and chaplains, are essential (Ingham & Coyle, 1997; Saunders, 1990).

The composition of the team caring for the dying patient will vary, depending on the goals of the institution and the available resources. In most instances, regardless of whether a hospice program, cancer center, or other service is providing care, most teams consist of at least a nurse and a physician. As discussed previously, a hospice team is more defined and has a number of team members with differing skills and expertise. The patient and family are always considered central to the care structure and are encouraged to have a central role in decision making. It is important for health care providers to be aware that family members have a unique role in the home care setting and often need ongoing support, education, and advice from the health care team. Family members need concrete information and education with regard to providing physical care for the patient. In addition, they need acknowledgment, validation, and support for the care they are giving, as well as the distress and grieving they are experiencing. Although nurses and physicians can accomplish much in providing such care for patients and families, social workers and chaplains also play a vital role in the team, particularly in the area of supportive counseling.

Regardless of the components of the team, the nurse is the primary liaison, the coordinating figure in the care of the dying, and the individual who brings the team plan to the bedside whether at home or in the hospital. Because of the close proximity of the nurse to the patient and family through day-to-day observation and care, there is often a shift in the balance of decision making at the end of life from the physician to the nurse. If and when this shift does occur, it should always happen within the broad construct of goals of care arrived at by the team, and with a recognition of the nurse's need for ongoing support and advice. The coordinating figure must recognize the often increasing difficulty that patient and families have with their own care-coordination as illness becomes more burdensome and demands more complex. A nurse who is cognizant of this burden can assist patients and families by a proactive approach to problems, both physical and social. A great burden can be lifted if the nurse, for example, considers calling a patient to ascertain how things are going rather than waiting for a crisis to occur; assists with coordination of appointments; refers when appropriate to social work services; suggests pastoral intervention; or calls to explain the patient's condition to a new health care provider, such as another home care nurse or physician.

Continued involvement of the patient's physician in end-of-life care should be fostered and encouraged. That a physician needs to be less involved with the patient when the goal of care changes from cure to comfort is a myth. At no time does the patient and family need the physician more than at the end of life when fears of abandonment are often a major source of worry for the dying patient and family.

PALLIATIVE CARE IN THE CONTEXT OF A MULTICULTURAL SOCIETY

To deliver optimum palliative care, health care professionals need an understanding of, and sensitivity to, the cultural factors relevant to individuals receiving care. Respect for patient dignity and self-determination involves acknowledgment of these cultural differences.

Awareness of Culture in Palliative Care

Kagawa-Singer (1996) described culture as the "core element within which the cancer experience is constructed." She goes on to say that culture is "the milieu in which all human life occurs and it affects every aspect of the cancer experience for patient, family, and nurse." It is beyond the scope of this book to review fully the many cultural approaches to, and views of, end of life. Excellent texts are available that provide information specific to a range of cultures (Lipson, Dibble, & Minarik, 1996; Waxler-Morrison, Anderson, & Richardson, 1990).

Health care providers must be sensitive to the many ways that culture can affect significant aspects of the patient-family/health care providers interface and show respect for cultural diversity. For example, privacy, touch, space, time, communication, and spirituality are culturally informed aspects of living. Culture and often religion are major factors that guide the approaches of individuals, families, and societies to role expectations, family lifestyles, child rearing, authority patterns, and dietary practices (Tripp-Reimer & Brink, 1985). Cultural variables affect beliefs and behaviors, some of which relate to pain, suffering, decision making, death, and grief (Kagawa-Singer, 1996). If not recognized and understood, cultural practices and beliefs may put the patient and family in conflict with an institutional or other medical culture.

When discussions about health are initiated or health care decisions are being considered, it is important to recognize that the culture of consumerism, individuality, and positive thinking often encountered within the North American health care system is not an approach embraced by all patients and families. The North American approach to care, with its focus on respect for individual autonomy, self-determination, and informed consent, may well conflict with cultures in which either a community, family, or paternalistic approach to health care decisions is the norm. For example, some cultures place family needs and decision making above the needs of the individual; some protect their family members from knowing a diagnosis of cancer and a terminal prognosis; some believe that a discussion of death might hasten death and interfere with divine will; and some do not involve elderly relatives in decision making in the belief that they have earned the right to be protected from such tasks (Klessig, 1992).

Being sensitive to cultural diversity means being aware that individuals may respond to similar situations in dissimilar ways. For example, whereas some cultures value privacy and hence appreciate a private room, others would consider the offer of a single room a sign of abandonment (Kagawa-Singer, 1996). Cultural differences may be present even in those who do not "appear" to be "different" from the health care provider. Differences may also exist within a family and within health care teams.

Sensitivity to cultural issues at the end of life solidifies the patient-family/health care provider relationship and can prevent or reduce conflicts at a time of crises. Lack of sensitivity can lead to conflict. Given the extraordinary cultural diversity that is encountered in health care delivery today, it is clearly not feasible for the nurse to have an awareness of all cultures. When caring for someone of an unfamiliar culture, it may be appropriate to ask patients and family members about their cultural values and beliefs and about the way issues are managed in their family. This approach can be an important symbol of a willingness to understand and respect the individual's experience and beliefs. Such an approach can also mobilize the strengths and supports that often come from cultural identity (Irish, 1994; Lipson et al., 1996; Pagli & Abramovitch, 1984; Waxler-Morrison et al., 1990).

Awareness of Spirituality in Palliative Care

Through their work of coordinating overall care at the end of life, nurses can be instrumental in initiating discussions on the spiritual aspects of the patient and family's life. Patients and families are often involved in a structured religion and adhere to a set of beliefs. Even those who do not participate in organized religion may have a spiritual belief system that can provide comfort and support. It is not necessary to share similar beliefs or to have the "answers" to create an environment that enhances discussion of issues of meaning (Doyle, 1992).

The discussion of issues of meaning can sometimes help to lessen isolation and create avenues for intervention. Questions such as "Why does God allow me to suffer?" offer an opportunity to explore fears, doubts, and despair. Encouraging referrals to chaplains and other community spiritual resources provides a fundamental source of support for patients and families throughout the illness and into the bereavement period. In addition, the role of the chaplain can be vital in concrete ways. For example, patients and families may struggle with decision making within the context of their belief system. Often difficult decisions, such as those involving the withdrawal of a ventilator, the cessation of total parenteral nutrition, or a DNR directive, can be made less burdensome for the patient or family by this suggestion: "This is something that patients/families often struggle with, and many find that talking this over with their chaplain is helpful." Finally, religious communities can often be sources of practical help by providing meals, drivers for patients to attend appointments, or volunteers to visit and provide respite for family members.

COMMUNICATION IN PALLIATIVE CARE

Central to the shared experience of patients, family members, and caregivers at the end of life is communication: speaking through use of, and listening to, verbal and nonverbal language. Communication in health care may be spontaneous and informal, as in the case of an interaction between a nurse and patient at the bedside or in the hallway. More formal communication usually is initiated by the patient, family member, or a member of the health care team with a specific goal or purpose in mind. That goal or purpose will determine the setting and the participants. The following section reviews some general principles involved in communication in palliative care.

Sensitivity to the Use of Language

By paying careful attention to the words and phrases used when caring for patients, health care professionals can provide support and reassurance despite being in situations in which they must communicate what may be viewed as "bad news." The words that are chosen convey powerful messages. Certain phrases and words may help patients and families understand and cope with illness, whereas others can create a confusing vocabulary that can exacerbate distress and suffering. For example, it is not uncommon for patients to be told that they "have failed treatment," that "there is no hope," that they are "terminal." By describing a dying patient as having "failed therapy" or as "giving up," the nursing and medical professions may convey a message of failure that implies blame and choice. The phrase "there is nothing more I can do for you" can greatly increase patient and family fears of abandonment and helplessness. In reality, there is nearly always something that can be done to improve a patient's quality of life, including symptom control, family support, and assistance in helping them address a variety of existential issues. In addition, by exploring the interpretation, by patient and family, of words that have been used by staff and others, the nurse can do much to maximize mutual understanding and minimize distress.

Sensitivity to Issues Relating to How Much and Whom to Tell

The use of language in health care is particularly relevant with regard to sharing information about prognosis and outcome. In general, although not always, information is likely to aid patients in adjusting to illness and may decrease uncertainty and unrealistic fears. Further, it may help a patient and family members to prepare and make decisions on the basis of the best available information. In some cultures, this approach may be considered overly harsh and abnormal. In many settings, discussion of the reality of life-threatening illness may increase anxiety in the short term, but ultimately maximizes patients' ability to cope with and to make decisions that will allow them to use their time in a meaningful way (Spiegel, Bloom, & Yalom, 1981). All discussions should reinforce the commitment of staff to help, to be available when needed, and to arrange care for the patient and family.

Age, cultural and religious influences, and education are some variables that influence preferences for information (Cassileth, Zupkis, Sutton-Smith, & March, 1980). The medical and legal bias in the United States toward autonomy and individual self-determination is sometimes at variance with patient and family preferences. Open discussion about how a patient wishes to handle this part of the care preserves autonomy and reinforces respect for personal and cultural differences. Although autonomy must be respected, this may reasonably involve the patient's right not to know or his or her right to delegate decision making to others. Simple questions can convey a tone of collaboration, respect, and acceptance: "How would you like me to deal with information that might come up about your illness and perhaps even require some difficult decisions?" "Who within your family should I be speaking with about your illness?" "How are decisions made within your family?" "Who is the spokesperson for your family?" The stress of severe illness may interfere with the ability of patients and families to integrate and retain distressing information. Ill patients often report that it is beneficial to have family members and a nurse present when complex decisions are being discussed or bad news is being broken. If they are not present at such meetings, inaccurate information can be received by family members who rely on distressed and ill patients to interpret and report medical data. Especially in the setting of far advanced illness, but only with the patient's consent, a proactive approach on the part of health care professionals to communicating with the family is optimal. Often, however, stressed family members need encouragement to establish direct contact with staff. A sensitive nurse can be the bridge for such family members.

Sensitivity to the Setting for Communication

Creating conditions that maximize successful communication and respect the patient's wishes and need for privacy supports individual dignity and diminishes unnecessary distress for patients, family members, and staff. Simple techniques can add a great deal to the patient's sense of comfort. These approaches may include drawing a curtain, sitting at eye level, or returning at a time when it is more convenient for the patient and the family. Although ensuring that the patient is included in the conversation, even if he or she is not able to respond verbally, demonstrates both respect for the individual and recognition that he or she exists, there are also times when it is more appropriate to discuss certain issues away from the bedside of the patient.

Family Meetings

From the health care professional's perspective, family meetings can be a useful approach to facilitate the provision of information, to reassess practical and emotional needs and resources, to review goals of care, and to validate family efforts and stresses. Family members can view meetings as useful times to be updated, obtain information, consolidate plans, gain support, and/or resolve conflicts. Such meetings can be concrete representations of the health care team's alliance and support and can decrease feelings of isolation for the family. A family meeting may or may not include the patient; this will depend on the individual patient, the family, and the goals of the meeting. Broadly speaking, the purpose and outcomes of such meetings can be categorized under three general headings: clarification of goals, problem solving, and counseling (Walsh, 1990).

The counseling potential within a family meeting is based in the hearing and validation of individual feelings. Inviting the discussion and expression of differing opinions and views can provide an opportunity to clarify misconceptions and normalize ambivalent and painful decisions. Counseling can be centered around any one of numerous issues that may be related to the illness or may have existed before the illness. For example, patients and families often need permission to maintain some normalcy and aspects of their original roles. Being a patient does not mean that other roles are necessarily lost, and being a caregiver does not preclude continuing as spouse, lover, child, or parent. Examples of highly charged decision-making areas are those around resuscitation and hydration (Ellershaw, Sutcliffe, & Saunders, 1995; Fainsinger & Bruera, 1994). These areas often evoke strong emotions in staff who need to recognize and acknowledge their reactions and to separate their own responses from the feelings and decision-making process of the family. Family members may ask the nurse what he or she would do in the same situation. This question provides an opportunity for the nurse to reinforce that there is no right or wrong decision, but rather a decision based on the particular person's needs, goals, culture, and belief system (Figs. 18-1 and 18-2).

APPROACHING THE EMOTIONS AND RESPONSES TO ILLNESS THAT OCCUR NEAR THE END OF LIFE

Psychosocial concerns at the end of life are best understood in the context of multiple factors that interact to create a unique patient and family dynamic. Patients and family members bring their individual and collective life stories, as well as their hopes, goals, and fears, to situations. When delivering care, it is important to individualize the needs of the dying patient and family members and to recommend interventions that are responsive to the uniqueness of the patient and family experience.

Many have attempted to explore the response of individuals to life-threatening illness and impending death. For example, Kubler-Ross (1969) describes five stages in coping with the knowledge of terminal illness: denial, anger, bargaining, depression, and acceptance. The delineation of these stages provides a useful framework for nurses working with the dying. They should not, however, be viewed as goals or expected responses. A person's dying is a unique, fluid process, a time of loss and transition, and an experience to be shared within the context of family, culture, and spiritual belief system. It should not be viewed as a symptom to be fixed or cured. The task of the nurse and others on

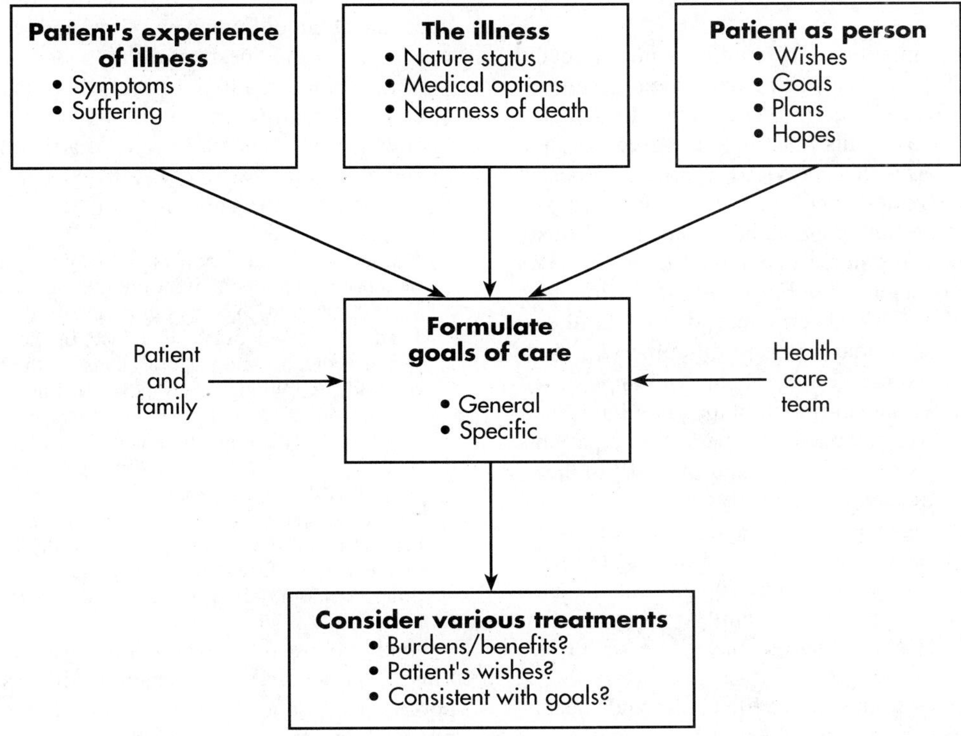

Fig. 18-1 Potential paths to care.

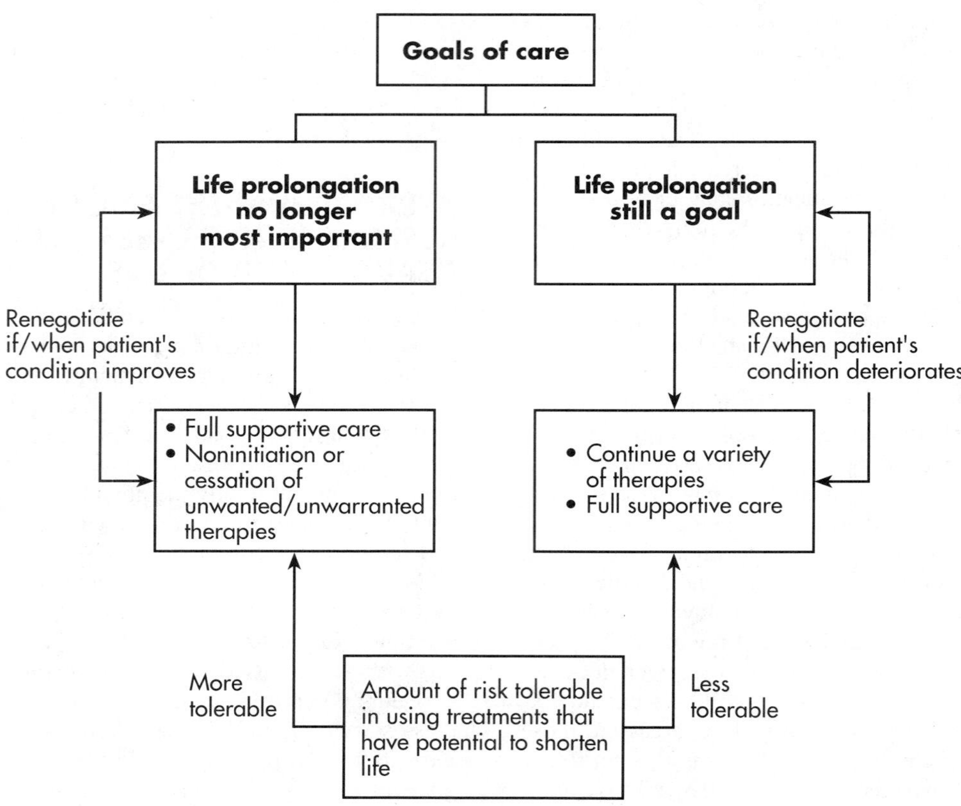

Fig. 18-2 Medical decision making with dying patients.

the team is to accompany the patient and family through the experience, to provide expertise in the relief of physical and psychosocial distress, and to provide guidance and support.

An individual's adaptation to impending death is affected by current physical, functional, and psychosocial issues, as well as by variables that directly relate to previous illness experiences. Thus assessments must include an exploration of the present illness as well as previous significant illnesses experienced by the patient and their close relatives and friends. Understanding how patients have coped previously with illness may help the nurse understand their approach to the end phase of their life. For example, individuals who have focused on empowerment, positive attitudes, and fighting their disease may come to this time with feelings of blame and personal failure. Those who approached illness in a controlling manner may find the potential loss of control ahead more frightening than others. Some patients may find value and purpose in the limited time left to them, but others may not (Bernardin, 1997; Byock, 1997; Groopman, 1997). By creating an environment that encourages patients and families to share their beliefs, thoughts, and worries, avenues for intervention may open that have a profound impact on the patient and family's experience of the illness (Byock, 1997). Isolation may be lessened and fear diminished.

Emotional reactions to the end of life can include acceptance, a sense of peace, joy, anger, anxiety, denial, relief, terror, sadness, fear, irritability, despair, or guilt. It is common for seemingly opposite responses to coexist in the one individual. Those living with life-threatening illness experience the gamut of human emotions and fears. Some describe experiencing the "best" and the "worst" (Coyle, 1995).

The Roman Catholic Archbishop of Chicago, Joseph Cardinal Bernardin, in a book written in the months before his death from pancreatic cancer, articulated some aspects of his experience with advanced cancer. His words reflect this flood of contrasting emotion:

> I experienced in a very personal way the chaos that serious illness brings into one's life. Initially, I felt as though floodwaters were threatening to overwhelm me. For the first time in my life I had to truly look death in the face. In one short moment all my personal dreams and pastoral plans for the future had to be put on hold. Everything in my personal life and pastoral ministry had to be re-evaluated from a new perspective. My initial experience was of disorientation, isolation, a feeling of not being "at home" anymore . . . Blessedly, a peace of mind and heart and soul quietly flooded through my entire being, a kind of peace I had never known before. Nevertheless, during my convalescence I found the nights to be especially long, a time for various fears to surface. I sometimes found myself weeping, something I seldom did before (Bernardin, 1997).

Such contrasting expressions are not uncommon for those experiencing life-threatening illness and provide opportunities for nursing interventions that respond to both the physical and existential suffering.

Specific Emotions and Psychological Responses Experienced by Patients and Families

A number of emotional and psychological responses are common in those with advanced illness who are approaching death. The emotions and psychological responses discussed in this section are not listed in any particular order, nor is the list all inclusive. The review aims to provide some insights for nurses who are likely to encounter patients and families experiencing these reactions.

Distinguishing Between Psychological Symptoms and Psychiatric Disorders. The prevalence of individual psychological symptoms in cancer patients has rarely been addressed. However, individual symptoms or complexes of symptoms may occur in the absence of specific psychiatric disorders. One recent survey demonstrated that the prevalence of "worrying," "feeling sad," and "feeling nervous" (71%, 65%, and 61%, respectively) far exceeded the prevalence of any psychiatric diagnoses (Portenoy et al., 1994a). A number of surveys have nonetheless documented a high prevalence of psychiatric diagnoses (Derogatis et al., 1983; Levine, Silberfarb, & Lipowski, 1978; Massie, Holland, & Glass, 1983). For example, in a survey of 215 hospitalized and ambulatory patients at three cancer centers, 47% met the criteria for a psychiatric disorder. Of these, 69% had an adjustment disorder with anxious or depressed mood, and 13% had a major depression (Derogatis et al., 1983). In psychiatry, just as in internal medicine, it is the nature of the symptoms (including but not only their severity and temporal patterns) and the other symptoms with which they are associated that facilitates the formulation of a diagnosis. The formulation of a diagnosis facilitates the implementation of appropriate treatment strategies.

The diagnosis of a particular psychiatric illness requires that the patient meet published criteria as outlined by the American Psychiatric Association (American Psychiatric Association, 1994). Many patients present with symptoms that are too transitory or mild to meet criteria for any diagnosis. It is important to understand that symptoms are indeed symptoms and are of themselves not likely to be specific for any psychiatric diagnosis. For example, sadness or anxiety may be transient and normal expressions in response to a particular situation, and may not be the manifestation of an adjustment disorder, a delirious state, or a major depression. Only when symptoms and symptom complexes are fully assessed can a diagnosis be made and appropriate treatment initiated. The observations and assessment of nurses are an important source of information to clarify any diagnosis.

Anxiety and Fear. Anxiety and fear are common in the setting of life-threatening illness and may be a reaction to physical factors or to existential and psychological distress. Anxiety is a feeling of apprehension caused by anticipation of danger that may be internal or external (Kaplan & Sadock, 1991; Tomb, 1988). It can occur in isolation or be a manifestation of an underlying psychiatric condition such as delirium. Anxiety differs from fear in that fear is more directed. In fear, the threat is recognizable; in anxiety "it is difficult to identify the cause of the feeling" (Rando, 1984). Both anxiety and fear are extremely common in the medically ill near the end of life. Assessment of the patient to define the source and severity of these symptoms is essential. Just as their etiology needs to be explored through the assessment so must their impact be defined (Roth & Breitbart, 1996).

As indicated previously, any assessment must include a careful mental status examination to clarify the role of delirium and other reversible medical factors in the etiology of these symptoms. Anxiety and fear can be associated with, or compounded by, medical problems including pain, medication use, metabolic states, and drug withdrawal states. Accompanying physical symptoms such as palpitations, shortness of breath, and diaphoresis may further exacerbate feelings of fear, loss of control, and helplessness. Inquiring about the physical, emotional, and cognitive aspects of the experience can in itself diminish anxiety, allowing an opportunity to correct misconceptions and to problem solve. It is also important to assess environmental factors including family, caregiver, and staff behaviors that may cause or exacerbate patient anxiety (Rando, 1984). Examples of such behaviors include whispered conversations in hallways and visible medical disagreements in front of patients.

Appropriate treatment of anxiety and fear includes specific treatment of any underlying and reversible conditions, for example, delirium or hypoxia. Psychological support, anxiolytics, and/or behavioral interventions may be indicated to reduce symptoms to a manageable level (Roth & Breitbart, 1996). Simple behavioral techniques such as focused breathing can affect the physiologic response of fight or flight that exacerbates the physical symptoms and distress that accompany anxiety. These interventions can be integrated into the nursing relationship with patients and thereby promote cognitive control. Such behavioral techniques may also be useful for family members and staff in managing their own anxiety and distress (Loscalzo & Jacobson, 1990).

Just as some may find a sense of meaning and value in this final period of their life and appear to harbor few fears of death, others may be overwhelmed by fear. Whereas anxiety may represent apprehension in the absence of a specific danger and be nondirected, fear is focused on a recognizable, tangible concern (Rando, 1984). The intensity of private worries and fears about, for example, uncontrolled pain, dying alone, or punishment in an afterlife can be diminished by the provision of an opportunity to share and address these aspects of suffering (Buckman, 1993). It is important to explore patient and family fears in a considerate manner that does not engender new fears. For example, a fear of suffocation that may accompany acute shortness of breath requires the nurse to respond immediately in a calm, confident manner so as not to increase the patient's fear and anxiety. The nurse may also feel somewhat anxious and fearful when encountering such a clinical situation, but must focus attention and skill on the patient in need and the task at hand. Although in some instances, aspects of fear may be best explored by others on the team, the nurse is in the best position to address many fears. Practical, supportive, and reassuring nursing input can do much to alleviate fear. Some patients may respond to broad reassurances, whereas others may need some specific details to feel comforted and safe. The approach is determined by the patient's coping style and needs.

Much can be learned from the patient's emotional state, manner, and the words chosen to articulate concerns. For example, a frightened patient who is openly acknowledging death might be asked, "What aspects of dying do you fear most?" In other instances, when it is unclear as to what the patient understands or chooses to know about his or her prognosis, a beginning inquiry might be, "What has your doctor told you about your illness?" or "Are there things about the future that are worrying you?" The nature of the patient's worries and the nature of the patient's relationship with team members help determine the most appropriate team member to handle individual concerns. Fears and concerns are not always solvable, but the expression and sharing of them can diminish isolation and reinforce the team's availability and commitment.

Sadness and Depression. Given the many losses associated with dying, it is expected that sadness will be part of this process. Most patients use established coping mechanisms to handle these feelings. Nonetheless, it can be helpful to acknowledge and to allow the patient to express sadness. It is also important for nurses to be aware that, although severe clinical depression is not expected, it may occur. It is most important to differentiate between syndromes that require psychiatric intervention and an expected emotional response. When the pervading mood is one of hopelessness, morbid guilt, and persistent low self-esteem, and when the patient expresses that he or she feels "depressed most days," a major depression is likely (Bukberg et al., 1984; Endicott, 1983; Massie & Holland, 1990; Roth & Breitbart, 1996). A patient who is tearful and emotionally labile with evidence of cognitive impairment may be experiencing delirium. The prevalence of delirium is high toward the end of life, indeed in the last days of life it occurs in most patients (Bruera et al., 1992; Massie et al., 1983). The importance of examining the mental state in full, as opposed to assuming that depression is normal in this setting, cannot be overstated.

The reported incidence of depression in cancer patients has varied significantly depending on the diagnostic criteria that have been used and the population of cancer patients surveyed (Chochinov, Wilson, Enns, & Lander, 1994). For example, Bukberg and colleagues (1984) studied 62 oncology inpatients applying DSM-III diagnostic criteria, patient self-report, and interview report rating scales and found that 42% met criteria for nonbipolar major depression (24% with severe and 18% with moderately severe symptoms), 14% had depressive symptoms that did not meet criteria for a major depression, and 42% had no depressed effect. As reviewed earlier, Derogatis found, in 215 hospitalized and ambulatory patients, that 69% had an adjustment disorder with anxious or depressed mood and 13% had a major depression (Derogatis et al., 1983).

Patients in the advanced stages of cancer report fatigue, pain, anxiety, insomnia, and anorexia, with prevalence rates often greater than 50% (Brescia et al., 1990; Coyle, Adelhardt, Foley, & Portenoy, 1990; Curtis, Krech, & Walsh, 1991; Dunlop, 1989; Dunphy & Amesbury, 1990; Fainsinger, Miller, Bruera, Hanson, & MacEachern, 1991; Grosvenor, Bulcavage, & Chlebowski, 1989; Portenoy et al., 1994; Rueben, Mor, & Hiris, 1988; Ventafridda, DeConno, Ripamonti, Gamba, & Tamburini, 1990). In the physically healthy, the diagnosis of a major depression depends heavily on the presence of these somatic symptoms. The high prevalence of somatic symptoms in cancer patients reduces their utility as diagnostic criteria for psychiatric disorders (Bukberg et al., 1984; Plumb & Holland, 1977, 1981). Although it could be postulated that these symptoms may be more severe in cancer patients who have concurrent depression, a study that investigated the relationship between physical and nonphysical symptoms of depression in patients with advanced cancer found no correlation between anorexia or weight loss and the nonphysical symptoms of depression (Holland, Rowland, & Plumb, 1977; Plumb & Holland, 1977). In these studies, anorexia was associated with physical symptoms, such as insomnia and fatigability, but not with feelings of guilt, worthlessness, or hopelessness. These data suggest that an etiology other than depression should be considered in cancer patients with anorexia and weight loss. In summary, given these findings, psychological symptoms, including persistent low self-esteem, morbid guilt, hopelessness, and suicidal ideation, are better indicators of clinical depression in the cancer patient (Bukberg et al., 1984; Endicott, 1983; Massie & Holland, 1990).

Although it is beyond the scope of this chapter to fully review depression in the cancer patient, this condition is optimally managed with supportive therapy, antidepressant medication, and cognitive behavioral techniques (Massie & Holland, 1990). Antidepressants with a prompt onset of action and occasionally stimulants should be considered in those nearing the end of life. Psychiatric input by a practitioner skilled in this aspect of psychiatry is often invaluable for the management of patients who have difficult symptoms.

Suicidal thoughts may occur at any time throughout illness. In a study of 200 terminally ill inpatients, desire for death and major and minor depressive episodes were evaluated (Chochinov et al., 1995). Although occasional wishes that death would come soon were common (reported by 44.5% of the patients), only 17 (8.5%) of these individuals acknowledged a serious and pervasive desire to die. Although their desire for death was correlated with ratings of pain and low perceived family support, it was most significantly correlated with measures of depression. The prevalence of diagnosed depressive syndromes was 58.8% among patients with a desire to die and 7.7% among patients without such a desire. The authors concluded that the desire for death in terminally ill patients is closely associated with clinical depression, a potentially treatable condition, and also concluded, based on follow-up interviews, that this desire is commonly transient and can decrease over time.

Many factors contribute to these transient desires, but given that the incidence of depression is high, its contributing role must be assessed in every case.

In cancer patients, serious depression and delirium are treatable and common entities that must be addressed. Neurologic complications of cancer such as cerebral metastases may also change mood, and investigation of these problems may need to be considered (Patchell & Posner, 1989). Personal and emotional factors that increase vulnerability to suicide include: prior history of suicide (personal or family), prior psychiatric disorder, alcohol or drug use, depression, recent bereavement, and poor social support (Roth & Breitbart, 1996). Medical risk factors include pain, delirium with poor impulse control, advanced illness, debilitation, and exhaustion or fatigue (Breitbart, 1989; Chochinov et al., 1995; Holland, 1993; Tomb, 1988).

Although few patients commit suicide, by contemplating the option some do retain a sense of control and avoid feeling overwhelmed. Nonetheless, suicidal ideation and related statements always need to be taken seriously (Box 18-2).

Psychiatric assessment and appropriate pharmacologic and psychotherapeutic interventions are essential. Twenty-four-hour companions should be used when a patient is actively suicidal. The approach to the suicidal patient should both reassure and minimize risk (Roth & Breitbart, 1996). Developing and maintaining a supportive relationship while helping the patient focus on remaining areas of control are an integral part of care. It is important that nursing staff and others convey a sense of confidence and honesty with regard to their ability to improve the patient's quality of life and to effectively treat symptoms. Family counseling is almost always required. The family, whose support often needs to be mobilized for the patient, is frequently distressed and in need of support themselves.

Box 18-2

Requests for Euthanasia and Assisted-Suicide: Nursing Management Principles

Establish a rapport with the patient.

Assess mental status:

- Issues for the individual patient:
  - Inadequate symptom control
  - Depression, hopelessness, spiritual despair
  - Being a burden on the family
  - Altered quality of life and unacceptable limitation
  - Has lived a full life and wants to die while still in control
- Suicide vulnerability factors
- Family status and adequacy of support resources

Address the reversible issues (e.g., symptom control); acknowledge other issues:

- The involvement of colleagues from other disciplines, do not act independently

Know the law.

From Coyle, N. (1992). The euthanasia and physician-assisted suicide debate: issues for nursing. *Oncology Nursing Forum, 19,* 41-46.

Awareness and Denial. Awareness and denial sometimes seem to coexist in cancer patients and their families, running parallel to each other, with one or the other taking prominence at different times. Sometimes patients and family members may be described as "in denial" when, in fact, they have not been offered the opportunity to discuss the seriousness of the illness with either their close family members and/or medical team. At other times caregivers may make the assumption that an individual is denying the serious nature of the illness when the individual has made the choice to discuss dying with certain people to the exclusion of others.

Denial is an unconscious process aimed against a threat that is perceived as intolerable. It can be a phase in the process of integrating a threatening reality (Vachon, 1993). Therefore, staff need to be supportive of the patient and to provide information, as requested, in an empathic manner. Decisions to confront denial should be driven by patient needs and based on the team's assessment that denial is preventing the patient from receiving support, maintaining emotional stability, and/or participating in necessary medical treatment. It is important that denial is distinguished from avoidance. Avoidance is a conscious process that protects patients from bringing stressful aspects of their reality to the forefront (Vachon, 1993). Patients who acknowledge that they are dying, but do not wish to discuss it, are using avoidance. This approach may be their chosen way of coping.

Loss. Life-threatening illness can be demoralizing for many patients. It may involve losses at multiple levels, including loss of bodily function, independence, decision-making capabilities, and sometimes, loss of the meaning of life itself. Individual approaches to loss are shaped to a significant degree by life experience, family support, and spiritual or philosophical approaches to life and death.

The support and respect of the nurse and other members of the health care team are critical to fostering dignity and respect for the individual in the setting of physical decline and dependency. Dignity is viewed in its broadest context and is not limited to the function of a body but is expressed through respect for the essence of a life lived and through the behavior and attitudes of those caring for that life. The patient's physical environment can support dignity and be enriched by personalizing the space with pictures, mementos, and symbols of the individual and his or her life history. Simple behaviors that enhance dignity include ensuring that needed items are within reach, knocking before entering a patient's room, and changing soiled linen promptly and without fuss. Such behaviors send a message of respect. Although the process of dying involves relinquishing many aspects of control, this process does not always have to be accompanied by feelings of powerlessness and hopelessness. Advanced directives, legacy and financial planning, and being kept informed about everyday family life all contribute to a feeling of personal worth.

Anger. Some patients and family members come to the end of life with histories of difficult family relationships and ongoing conflicts. These conflicts may be exacerbated by the impending death of a family member. "Unfinished business" is not always resolved, and anger can continue to pervade the dying patient and family member interactions. In other situations, patients may be enraged as they recognize that cancer will deprive them of the future they had planned. Many patients express anger and rage at those closest to them, those whom they feel can be counted on not to abandon them. It is often difficult and stressful for staff to maintain an attentive and caring attitude towards angry patients. Avoidance of such patients, however, exacerbates their anger and increases their fears. Helping patients and family members to identify thoughts and feelings that may underlie their anger can offer an opportunity to deepen communication and resolve conflicts. Limit setting and structure can be helpful for some patients and family members when tension and crises have challenged their own limit-setting ability (Rando, 1984).

Guilt. Guilt, in the setting of life-threatening illness, may originate from various sources. Whereas some patients feel guilty for "past transgressions," others are concerned about causing suffering in people they love or for being sick. Some feel guilty consequent to unexpressed feelings of resentment and anger toward others, and others for not having been able to cure their illness or conquer their disease. Guilt often arises when people feel they have fallen short of their own standards, and this threatens self-image and self-esteem. In seeking a reason for illness, some patients may see their illness and suffering as retribution and atonement for past offenses. Thus the illness and related guilt can have symbolic significance and possible redeeming value in the patient's eye. This symbolic meaning needs to be recognized and understood by the nurse if interventions are to be helpful. Interventions to alleviate guilt depend on its etiology and range from normalizing such feelings to encouraging self-forgiveness and completing unfinished business (Rando, 1994).

Hope. Having focused on many of the emotional responses that may in some way be viewed as difficult and challenging, and perhaps by some as "negative," we now turn to hope. Hope often confounds caretakers, as well as patients and family members. When death is the likely outcome, it is frequently stated that there is "no hope"; yet many can find hope without "cure." According to Byock (1997):

> In the midst of profound suffering, not only comfort, but also triumph and exhilaration, are possible. The separation between suffering and the sense of growth and transformation is but a membrane. The clinical skills required to help a person explore the boundaries of his unique suffering and pierce that membrane can be delicate, sophisticated and sometimes subtle. But they are not mystical, and they can be taught.

Within the fields of nursing and medicine, nursing has led the way in recognizing and studying the clinical significance of hope in medical illness, with the result that there is an emerging literature to guide interventions. The approach and language used in encounters with patients and families can have enormous impact in this area. Questions such as "can you tell me something about your hope?" or "in addition to hoping for a cure, are there other things you hope for during the time ahead?" may widen the patient's and family's view of hope to new possibilities of meaning (Callan, 1989). Broadly speaking, exploring hope involves exploring the thoughts, feelings, beliefs, and actions that provide new areas of meaning and possibility. Hope is a unique, personal, and energizing force that adjusts as reality changes (Herth, 1990).

Pastoral interventions are frequently paramount in fostering hope (Herth, 1990; Jones, 1993; Verwoerdt, 1966). These interventions were touched on by Bernardin (1997), who wrote:

> Even if they are not committed to a specific religion, men and women everywhere have a deep desire to come in contact with the transcendent. Members of the clergy can facilitate this through the simple goodness they show in being with their people. The things people are naturally attracted to and remember most are small acts of concern and thoughtfulness . . . *that* is what they tell you about their priests and other clergy.

This is also what patients and family members tell you about the staff who care for them.

Finally, hope is frequently sustained by reflections on the continuity of life; past, present, and future. For the dying person and family members, reminiscences and life reviews can validate and give meaning to the life lived (Herth, 1990; Jones, 1993; Verwoerdt, 1966). By expressing interest in unique aspects of the patient's experience and by listening to their narrative, nurses may assist patients in their struggle to find hope and to validate feelings of worth and self-esteem.

Bereavement

The circumstances of both illness and death influence the process of bereavement (Chochinov & Holland, 1989). It is important, therefore, that the nurse recognize that interventions along the continuum of illness have the potential to affect a family's bereavement. Ultimately, the experience of the death of a family member will become part of the narrative of the whole family and be integrated into the family myth. The experience of the death becomes in a sense, "part" of the family (Coyle, 1995).

Although before death the patient and family often share a period of anticipating loss and separation, family members who intellectually prepare for the death may still react with shock and disbelief when death occurs. Even though the process of preparation is ongoing, when the final stages of illness are approaching, the family members, often exhausted, may become overwhelmed with the feeling of responsibility for the decisions that are made and the events that have occurred throughout the illness. Frequently expressions of "what if" are verbalized (Coyle et al., 1989). By addressing these "what ifs" concretely before the death (and often repeatedly), the bereavement process may be made easier for family members.

Family members are likely to focus on the time of death and the events that occur immediately around that time. For example, final words may be given special meaning, and if these words are not heard, or the primary care provider is not there at the moment of death, there may be a sense of loss or inadequacy. Alternatively the actual moment of death, so long anticipated and feared, may be anticlimactic, with the family members feeling "Is that all there is?" Although the manner of death and potential symptom constellation can be predicted for many patients, for some it cannot. With the provision of good palliative care, unanticipated distress should be dealt with swiftly and effectively. It is important for staff to be aware of the significance of this time and to be considerate and proactive of the family members' needs and wishes.

For example, in an anticipated death, staff should consider notifying the relevant family members that the time of death may be close. If family members were not present, it is important to inform at least the spokesperson for the family of the circumstances of the death. Family members are often greatly reassured to know that someone was with the person when they died, that he or she died peacefully, or that he or she did not suffer for a long period. The care that is given to the body after death, and to the patient's possessions, can leave a lasting impression on the survivors. The loss, for example, of small personal possessions in the hospital at the time of death may symbolize a lack of respect and diminish the positive impact of care that may have been provided earlier. Support of patient dignity extends to the rituals and care that are provided both during *and* after the death. The nurse can contribute greatly in this area. After the death, family members are likely to feel an intense void and loneliness. This feeling may be expressed as a sense of loss of purpose. A focus of energy and caring is gone, family roles must realign, and the staff are less of a presence in the life of the family. For some, the most important work they have ever done has been taken from them. Work and everyday life pale in comparison to the intensity of the recent experience. The "what ifs" may become "if onlys," and it is not uncommon for a sense of guilt to surface (Coyle et al., 1989).

Family members may express thoughts such as these: "What if I lacked sensitivity?" "Maybe I thought too much about myself;" "Did I do everything I could have done?" Guilt may also be expressed in relation to the feeling of relief and freedom after death has occurred: "I didn't think I could live without him and yet I am doing so." Another fear often expressed is the possibility of forgetting the deceased loved one, or that the family will only recall the last days of the illness, and not the earlier, happier times. Discussion of the psychological, cognitive, and physical symptoms of grief can sometimes be helpful in preparing families for a wide range of possible feelings and behaviors (Rando, 1984). The nurse and other members of the health care team in their review and debriefing after a death must decide which team member is most appropriate to handle bereavement follow-up or seek appropriate counseling resources either through hospice programs or churches.

Emotions and Responses of Professional Caregivers

Nurses and other caregivers in oncology are involved in a constant process of attachment and loss occurring in the context of their own personal histories and the setting in which they work. Staff reactions to caring for patients at the end of life are highly individual. These reactions are influenced by specific patient and family situations, as well as by the staff members' own skills, history of loss, experiences, and resources (Chochinov & Holland, 1989; Mount, 1986; Vachon, 1993; Vincent, 1982).

Diverse issues may trigger stress in those providing care for individuals and families who are nearing the end of life. For example, feelings of ambivalence, guilt, and failure over the inability to cure, and worry about being overwhelmed by multiple losses may present difficulties for staff (McEvoy, 1990). Ongoing, unresolved stress can trigger burnout, the features of which may include shifts from a caring approach to apathy, involvement to distancing, openness to self-protection, trust to suspicion, enthusiasm to disillusionment or cynicism, and self-esteem to personal devaluation (Vincent, 1982).

Given the perception that expression of emotion is incongruous with being a "professional," the emotional aspects of loss may go unacknowledged and unsupported in institutional settings. Just as bereavement is a most important issue for families, the impact of loss on staff can also be significant in a setting where close and valued relationships have developed with patients and family members over a long time (Chochinov & Holland, 1989). The experience of repeated losses without an opportunity for mourning, replenishment, and support can also create symptoms of "burnout." The stresses that can be triggered by work in this field can be expressed in the physical, cognitive, emotional, personal, and work-related realms. Responsibility for preventing and recognizing such stresses lies with the individual, the team of caregivers, and the institution involved in the provision of care. Nurses in the field need to watch out for each other.

From the perspective of the individual, the ability to continue to care for others presupposes a responsibility and commitment to care for self. In the setting of choosing to care for patients at the end of life, it is clear that death is the expected outcome and that the work of helping patients and family members live through to that end is enormously valuable. Setting priorities and limits, establishing attainable goals, and celebrating the achievement of such goals are antidotes to burnout. Increasing knowledge adds to competence and can be a source of replenishment for many. Awareness of feelings, energy levels, and thoughts are important in creating the kind of self-knowledge that alerts nurses and other health care professional to mounting stress. Thoughts that serve to increase distress and feelings of failure need to be identified and expressed either to colleagues or confidants (Larson, 1993).

In addition, the use of a journal, which allows for written expression and externalization, provides a vehicle to validate and sort out feelings and thoughts. Such a journal may also be a tool for stress reduction and provides a continuing narrative of events and people that have been meaningful to the writer. Exercise and relaxation can counter stress as can exposure to people and activities that are life affirming. Relaxation and meditative techniques, often taught to patients, may also be useful additions to the staff's coping techniques and can be integrated into the work environment.

Although many aspects of caring for patients who are nearing the end of life can be stressful, it is clear that systems, team interactions, and institutions also have the potential to cause considerable stress. These issues often are the most stressful aspect of working in this field (Vachon, 1993). Team communication may be challenging because of overlapping or unclear roles, issues of control, and competitive strivings. Within the team of caregivers, it is important to develop open and clear lines of communication, with common goals and role expectations. This approach, along with an ability to acknowledge and respect differences, can minimize team-related stresses (Mount, 1986; Vachon, 1993). In addition to interteam stressors, external stressors are imposed on the team through the increasing challenges and demands of the larger health care system. It is important for staff to have mechanisms to ventilate, address, and potentially resolve these concerns. Mechanisms to achieve these goals can include staff meetings and support groups, as well as an occasional event or activity that fosters staff interaction in a "social" setting. Committed, available, and understanding leadership of the team is essential.

APPROACHING THE PHYSICAL CONCERNS AND SYMPTOMS THAT OCCUR NEAR THE END OF LIFE

Despite growing interest in quality-of-life outcomes, the nursing and oncology literature in general contain little information about the nature of the dying process and the discomfort or distress associated with each different cancer. The nurse, who aims to provide optimal care for the dying, needs to develop an understanding of the dying process. Only a small number of studies have described the experience of the last days or hours of patients with cancer and, for the most part, these studies have been undertaken in the hospice or palliative care setting. Because a large proportion of the deaths that occur in developed countries occur in the hospital setting, the absence of data on this group represents a significant gap in both nursing and medical knowledge. Other sections in this textbook have focused on symptom management. This section addresses symptom prevalence; awareness, consciousness and delirium; and the ethics of symptom management at the end of life.

Prevalence and Impact of Symptoms

The spectrum of symptoms experienced by cancer patients at various points during the course of advanced disease has been assessed in a number of studies that focus on the time of admission to a hospice or palliative care unit (Brescia, 1990; Brescia et al., 1990; Curtis et al., 1991; Donnelly & Walsh, 1995; McCarthy, 1990; Wilkes, 1974). Several investigations, including those summarized in Table 18-1, have focused specifically on the dying process or the last weeks of life (Bedard, Dionne, & Dionne 1991; Brock, Holmes, Foley, & Holmes, 1992; Coyle et al., 1990; Exton-Smith, 1961; Fainsinger & Bruera, 1994; Fainsinger et al., 1994; Hinton, 1963; Hockley, Dunlop, & Davies, 1988; Ingham et al., 1994; Lichter & Hunt, 1990; Morris, Suissa, Sherwood, Wright, & Greer, 1986; Reuben et al., 1988; Saunders, 1984; Ventafridda, Ripamonti, De Conno, Tamburini, & Cassileth, 1990; Ward, 1974; Witzel, 1975). Some studies have explored the prevalence and impact of particular symptoms in the setting of advanced malignant disease (Bukberg et al., 1984; Dunlop, 1989; Goldberg, Mor, Weimann, Greer, & Hiris, 1986; Grosvenor et al., 1989; Heyse-Moore & Baines, 1984; Heyse-Moore, 1991; Higginson & McCarthy, 1989; Kane, Wales, Bernstein, Leibowitz, & Kaplan. 1984; Levine et al., 1978; McKegney, Bailey, & Yates, 1981; Morris, Mor, et al., 1986; Morris, Suisa, et al., 1986; Plumb & Holland, 1977, 1981; Portenoy et al., 1994; Reuben & Mor, 1986a, b; Twycross, 1975; Ventafridda et al., 1990). Others have highlighted other aspects of the dying process by characterizing the differences in the quality of care provided by inpatient and homecare services (Dunphy & Amesbury, 1990; Greer et al., 1986; Kane, Wales, Berstein, Leibowitz, & Kaplan, 1984; Searle, 1991; Ventafridda et al., 1989; Vinciguerra, Degnan, Sciortino, O'Connell, Moore, & Brody, 1986).

The most commonly reported symptoms experienced by patients with far-advanced cancer are fatigue, pain, anxiety, and anorexia. Each of these symptoms has been reported to have a prevalence rate of greater than 50% (Brescia et al., 1990; Coyle et al., 1990; Curtis et al., 1991; Dunlop, 1989; Dunphy & Amesbury, 1990; Fainsinger et al., 1991; Grosvenor et al., 1989; Portenoy et al., 1994; Reuben et al., 1988; Ventafridda et al., 1990). In addition, most patients with advanced cancer experience multiple symptoms (Curtis et al., 1991; Coyle et al., 1990; Portenoy et al., 1994). Although the commonly reported symptoms are generally considered to be "physical" (e.g., pain, fatigue, or nausea), these findings most likely reflect a survey methodology that often does not address psychological symptomatology. When measures to assess psychological distress are incorporated into survey methodology, high prevalence rates for psychological symptoms, including depressed mood and anxiety, have been reported (Bukberg et al., 1984; Holland et al., 1977; McCarthy, 1990; Plumb & Holland, 1977, 1981; Portenoy et al., 1994).

Although fatigue, pain, anxiety, and anorexia are commonly reported symptoms during the course of advanced cancer, the shifts that may occur in symptom prevalence during the last week of life are poorly documented. However, some shifts have been demonstrated, particularly with regard to pain and dyspnea. In a study of 1754 cancer patients, The National Hospice Study documented that pain became more prevalent during the last weeks of life (Morris, Mor, et al., 1986). More recent information has been provided by the investigators of the Support Study (Lynn et

TABLE 18-1 Symptom Prevalence in the Last Week of Life in Patients With Cancer

Symptoms (%)	Bedard N = 952[1,5]	Coyle N = 90[3,5]	Fainsinger N = 100[1,5,7]	Hinton N = 82[2,4]	Lichter N = 200[1,5]	Saunders N = 200[1,5]	Ward N = 200[2,7]
Pain	12-30	34	99	71	51	23	62
Dyspnea	9	28	46	4-20	22	21	52
Nausea	16	13	71	12-17	14	3	
Vomiting	16			12-17	14	7	38
Sleepiness	5	57				46	
Congestion		6			56	53	
Confusion	4	28	39		9	12	39
Restlessness		7			42	31	
Anorexia	14	6					61
Fatigue		52					
Urinary incontinence	4	6			32		28

NOTE: Symptoms are recorded if any two surveys demonstrated a prevalence of greater than 25% or if any one survey demonstrated a prevalence of 50% or more for a specific symptom.

[1]Hospice or palliative care inpatients only.
[2]General patients, type of care not specified.
[3]Cancer center in- and outpatients.
[4]Data provided directly by patient.
[5]Data provided by patient or primary care.
[6]Data provided by carer.
[7]Indicators of overall distress included, as well as prevalence.

al., 1997; SUPPORT, 1995). The data from the Support Study were combined with those from another survey to clarify the perceptions of family members who observed the dying experiences of 3357 patients, of whom approximately 12% had lung cancer and 5% had colon cancer. In the groups with cancer, 40% to 46% of patients were judged by their relatives to have moderate to severe pain for more than half of the time during the last 3 days of life.

Toward the end of life, the prevalence of cancer-related dyspnea is high, in the range 20% to 78% (Heyse-Moore, 1991; Higginson & McCarthy, 1989; Hockley et al., 1988; Reuben & Mor, 1986b). It is likely that this wide variation reflects variability in the definitions for dyspnea, the methods used for eliciting the symptom, and patient selection criteria. In the National Hospice Study, dyspnea was seen in 70% of 1754 patients during the final 6 weeks of life, and this prevalence increased as death approached (Reuben & Mor, 1986b). Higginson and McCarthy (1989) studied a group of 86 cancer patients and noted that dyspnea was a severe and often uncontrollable symptom near death. In the SUPPORT study, dyspnea was reported to be moderate to severe for the last few days of life in 30% of colon cancer patients and almost 70% of the patients with lung cancer.

It is difficult to draw conclusions concerning the factors that contribute to the prevalence and severity of pain and dyspnea before death. Most studies do not include detailed discussions of pain syndromes and treatments. Moreover, when the reports are provided by staff or family members, they must be interpreted with caution, as numerous studies have demonstrated that observer and patient assessments are not highly correlated (Clipp & George, 1992; Grossman, Sheidler, Swedeen, Mucenski, & Piantadosi, 1991; Higginson, Priest, & McCarthy, 1994; Kahn, Houts, & Harding, 1992; Slevin, Plant, & Lynch, 1988). Consequently, it is not possible to ascertain whether the reported high incidence rates for pain and dyspnea before death reflect perceived distress, worsening pathology, undertreatment, or all three.

Despite some uncertainty about the factors contributing to the high prevalence of potentially distressing symptoms, undertreatment of pain is a significant and common problem (Cleeland et al., 1994; VonRoenn, Cleeland, Gonin, Hatfield, & Pandya, 1993). A survey of 1308 oncology outpatients being treated by the physician members of the Eastern Cooperative Oncology Group documented that 67% had reported recent pain, with 36% describing pain severe enough to impair function (Cleeland et al., 1994). Forty-two percent of the patients who reported pain were not given adequate analgesia (VonRoenn et al., 1993). Poor pain assessment was rated by 76% of the physicians in this survey as the single most important barrier to adequate pain management, and 61% of these physicians indicated that physician reluctance to prescribe opioids was also a barrier to adequate pain management.

Although significant gaps in knowledge exist, the studies that have been undertaken highlight the spectrum of symptoms experienced by cancer patients nearing the end of life. The available information also highlights the investigations that will be necessary if we are to adequately characterize the dying process and the distress associated with this process.

Awareness, Consciousness, and Delirium Near the End of Life

The level of consciousness during the time near an individual's death is influenced by many factors, including the nature of the specific illness, rapidity of physical deterioration, coexisting organ failure, and medication use. Although for cancer patients, the level of consciousness and ability to interact before death have been explored peripherally in several studies, specific diagnoses or conditions, such as delirium and cognitive impairment, have been less commonly studied.

Lynn and colleagues (1997) combined SUPPORT data with data from another group of 4622 elderly patients to evaluate patients' level of consciousness before death. Eighty percent of the lung cancer patients in this population and almost 70% of the colon cancer patients were reported to be conscious 3 days before death; 55% and 40% of these groups, respectively, were also able to communicate effectively at this time. At St. Christopher's Hospice in the United Kingdom, a survey of 100 cancer patients found that 10% were alert, 67% drowsy or semiconscious, and 23% unarousable or unconscious during the 24 hours before death (Saunders, 1984). Finally, a recent survey of inpatient and home care cancer deaths found that one third of the patients were able to interact 24 hours before death; this decreased to one fifth at 12 hours before death, and one tenth in the hour before death (Ingham et al., 1994).

Although the preceding surveys suggest that the ability to interact frequently is maintained until close to death in cancer patients, several small studies explored specifically the mental disturbances that occur before death and demonstrated that cognition during this time is frequently impaired. In one of the first studies of delirium in cancer patients, Massie and colleagues (1983) found, in a small series of 13 terminally ill cancer patients, that 11 (85%) developed delirium before death. The authors also noted that the early symptoms of delirium were frequently misdiagnosed anxiety, anger, depression, or psychosis (Massie et al., 1983). Bruera and colleagues (1992) studied 66 episodes of cognitive failure in 39 patients admitted to a palliative care service and cited drugs, sepsis, and brain metastasis as the most frequently detected etiologic factors. These authors also demonstrated the benefits of an active approach to the diagnosis and treatment of cognitive decline. Careful assessment and adjustment of medications and treatments in this population were undertaken, and 22 of the episodes (33%) of cognitive failure improved, 10 spontaneously and 12 as a result of treatment.

Given the high prevalence of impaired cognitive functioning and the possibility of improvement with intervention, it is important to consider and explore the reversible etiologies of delirium and impaired cognition. Although the goals of care and life expectancy may limit the investigations that are undertaken, it is important to consider the range of strategies that may improve the patient's quality of life. Potential etiologic factors for delirium and impaired cognition in cancer patients may be divided into direct effects related to tumor involvement and indirect effects (Posner, 1979). The latter category includes drugs, electrolyte imbalance, cranial irradiation, organ failure, nutritional deficiencies, vascular complications, paraneoplastic syndromes, and many other factors (Barbato, 1994; Meyers & Abbruzzese, 1992; Oxman & Silberfarb, 1980; Patchell & Posner, 1989; Posner, 1979; Silberfarb, Philibert, & Levine, 1980; Silberfarb, 1983). A survey of 94 cancer patients referred initially for a neurology consultation demonstrated a multifactorial etiology to impaired cognitive functioning in most patients (Tuma & DeAngelis, 1992). In this survey, metabolic causes, drugs, and central nervous system metastases were the most common identifiable etiologic factors.

Broadly, the treatment of delirium and impaired cognition should involve a search for reversible etiologic factors, behavioral and environmental management, and pharmacologic therapy. Regardless of the cause, treatment of the patient who is perplexed, confused, restless, or agitated should include the manipulation of the environment to provide a safe, quiet, and reorienting milieu, with the availability of support and reassurance for both the patient and family. The implementation of measures aimed at increasing structure and familiarity, and reducing anxiety and disorientation should be considered. For example, the family may be encouraged to sit with the patient while avoiding intense and complex conversation. The patient may be best nursed in a quiet, well-lit room with familiar personnel and the use of orienting devices, such as clocks, calendars, and familiar objects. The safety of the patient with delirium must be ensured, and one-to-one nursing observation may be necessary. Family members will likely need the condition repeatedly explained to them. It is often reassuring for them to know that the patient, although confused, can still often understand the presence of family members and may be more peaceful in the presence of familiar and comforting family members. Pharmacologic symptomatic treatment of delirium is often, but not always, necessary. Although treatment is being instituted for specific etiologic factors, it is important to alleviate immediate distress. Except in the case of delirium tremens, for which a benzodiazepine is the first-line drug, a neuroleptic is the most appropriate drug for the initial management of delirium (Breitbart, Bruera, Chochinov, & Lynch, 1995; Fainsinger & Bruera, 1992; Fleishman, Lesko, & Breitbart, 1993).

Ethics of Symptom Management Near the End of Life

Ethical concerns are frequent in the care of symptomatic advanced cancer patients. Often such concerns surface when opioids or sedative-type drugs are escalated to control refractory pain or shortness of breath. The result may be inadequate symptom control for the patient and/or a sense of guilt on the part of family and staff. A process for the resolution of these ethical concerns by the nurse and other team members includes establishing and clarifying the extent of disease and treatment options; establishing goals of care; exploring, defining, and discussing ethical concerns; defining the plan of care and clarifying it within an ethical framework; and establishing routine mechanisms for assessment of ongoing concerns and exploration of conflicts.

The ethical principles underpinning symptom management near the end of life are autonomy, nonmaleficience, beneficence, justice, and the principle of double effect. The nurse, acting as a patient advocate, must be aware of the clinical implications of these principles at the bedside. Tacit assumptions (values) from which these ethical principles governing nursing practice are derived include alleviation of suffering, preservation of human dignity, existence of meaningfulness, sanctity of life, and compassion (Table 18-2).

Autonomy. Autonomy recognizes an individual's rights to make decisions according to beliefs, values, and a life plan. Respect for autonomy relies on truth-telling, the conveying of accurate information, and the determination that a patient or surrogate decision maker understands the facts of the situations and implications of the decisions. Respect for autonomy requires the nurse to enter into a dialogue with the patient, listening to patient priorities, transmitting information to enable informative decision making, respecting the patient's choice to limit exposure to information, and exploring patient and family decisions to ensure that they are not based on misconceptions or coercion. Respect for autonomy implies respect for the person and protects the rights of the individual with diminished capacity through honoring advanced directives. However, the exercise of autonomy does not imply an obligation on others to act. This is an important construct for nurses, especially at a time when society is grappling with issues surrounding the legalization of physician-assisted suicide and euthanasia (Mendelson, 1996; Velleman, 1992). For example, increasing an opioid dose in a dying patient to manage pain or shortness of breath is good palliative care, but increasing the opioid with the intent of hastening a death believed to be too prolonged is not.

Nonmaleficence. This principle is embodied in the concept "one ought not to inflict evil or harm." Implicit in this principle is the recognition of the vulnerability of the dying, and it mandates a strong commitment that the patient will come to no harm through the care provided to him or her. This ethical principle requires a high level of nursing vigilance and awareness of the needs, desires, and sensitivities of a particular patient. Continued aggressive, life-prolonging, or cure-oriented treatment that is not suited to the patient's needs or wishes is a violation of nonmaleficence. Unnecessary and unwanted sedation or premature, unrequested, or uninformed withdrawal of treatment is another. History taking, physical examinations, and conveying of information in an insensitive manner are less obvious examples of violation of the principle of nonmaleficence.

Beneficence. This concept states that "one ought to prevent or remove evil or harm, and promote good." Beneficence implies positive acts and includes all the strategies that nurses and other health care professionals use to support patients and families and reduce suffering. Included here are the effective treatment of pain and other symptoms. In addition, proposed treatments and in some instances the active withdrawal of other treatments should be evaluated in terms of their potential to relieve suffering and thereby promote good. Treatment plans that are concordant with the patient's goals of care and advanced directives would, for example, convey beneficence.

Justice. Justice deals with the concept of fairness. Justice demands that dying patients have access to care equal to others. However, the concept of justice may limit autonomy for the individual, as what the individual wishes, chooses, or feels entitled to may not be allowable in the context of the greater good. This is a complex ethical concept, often requiring the weighing of competing claims. (Nurses may be caught in this dilemma when caring for the dying in an acute care setting.) Decisions and actions that may seem morally compelling and appropriate for a particular person may not be allowable because of the wider risk they are seen to present to the greater society. The current debate on legalization of physician-assisted suicide and euthanasia is an example of this conflict (Coyle, 1992; Emanuel, 1988; Hendin & Klerman, 1993; Young, Volker, Riegler, & Thorpe, 1993).

The Principle of Double Effect. This principle distinguishes between the compelling primary therapeutic intent (to relieve suffering) and unavoidable untoward consequences (such as the likely diminution of interactional function and the potential for accelerating death) (Latimer, 1991). The principle of double effect is most commonly evoked in the use of high-dose opioid analgesics or induced sedation in the management of otherwise refractory pain or shortness of breath (Cavanaugh, 1996; Cherny & Portenoy, 1994). The principle of double effect is predicated on the

TABLE 18-2 Tacit Assumptions (Values) From Which Ethical Principles Governing Nursing Practice Are Derived and their Associated Obligations

Value	Obligation
Alleviation of suffering	To seek to relieve suffering and not to cause suffering
Preservation of human dignity	To seek to preserve and respect dignity, and not to act in such a way as to impair dignity
Existence of meaningfulness	To act to preserve and enhance the meaningfulness of life, and to act in such a way as not to remove or destroy the meaningfulness of any human life
Sanctity of life	To act to preserve human life
Compassion	To perform all compassionate deeds and not to refuse to perform compassionate deeds, unless contrary to law or conscience

Adapted from Coyle, N. (1992). The euthanasia and physician-assisted suicide debate: issues for nursing. *Oncology Nursing Forum, 19,* 41-46.

axioms that intent is a critical ethical concern, and that the distinction between foreseeing and intending an unavoidable maleficent outcome is ethically significant (Latimer, 1991). When caring for dying patients with intractable symptoms, invocation of this principle allows suffering to be relieved and symptoms to be controlled (Box 18-3). In the absence of this ethical principle, some patients would likely suffer a consequence of catastrophic symptoms.

FAMILY SUPPORT AND EDUCATION

Although in palliative care the patient and family members are both to be considered the unit of care, the needs of the patient take primary focus. A focus on the physical and emotional well-being of the family, however, implies respect for the patient's life that extends beyond the illness experience. The nurse has an opportunity to maximize the family members' ability to cope with the death in a way that positively affects their future life and adjustment. Although caring for a dying patient will change the balance within a family, this time of crisis can be influenced positively by nursing expertise, support, and intervention.

Family support begins with the nurse and other members of the team developing an understanding of who the key family members are, who speaks for the family, and the cultural milieu in which family members define themselves. Many aspects of family support have been discussed in earlier sections of this chapter. One extremely important aspect of the family role to be reiterated is that of direct caregiver. In many instances, especially with shorter hospital stays, family members have roles as an extension of the health care team.

Communication between the health care team and the family remains the moral and human imperative that it has always been, but now has also become an imperative to optimize care. Nursing staff frequently play the key role in this aspect of care. Many of the skills that represent the most basic and important aspects of nursing, those that involve the physical care of the ill person, must be taught to family members. In essence, it is important to recognize that family members who often provide physical and emotional care to the patient are in need of emotional support and care themselves. Those involved in the health care team must be cognizant of this delicate balance and the stresses to the family that can come with this combined role.

Box 18-3
What Does *Not* Constitute Euthanasia

- Giving a patient who is dying, hypotensive, and in pain sufficient opioid to control pain (Principle of Double Effect)
- Giving a patient who is dying and dyspneic sufficient morphine to control symptoms (Principle of Double Effect)
- Withholding nutrition or hydration at the request of the patient who is dying (Principle of Autonomy)

Modified from Coyle, N. (1992). The euthanasia and physician-assisted suicide debate: issues for nursing. *Oncology Nursing Forum, 19,* 41-46.

ADVANCED CARE PLANNING

Frequently an individual's first real encounter with the prospect of death comes at the time of diagnosis of a serious medical illness in self or in a family member. Although it is common for the initial focus of treatment to be on cure, fears surrounding end-of-life scenarios are often present. By addressing concerns early in the illness and in an ongoing forthright manner, and by facilitating advanced care planning, the quality of end-of-life care is likely to be improved. The aim of advanced care planning is to facilitate continuity of care and respect for an individual's wishes as an illness progresses. Unfortunately, discussions about end-of-life care are often not initiated until death is imminent. The failure of the medical team to assist patients and families in planning for end-of-life care earlier may result in patients proceeding with treatments that are burdensome and ineffective and that have a negative impact on the patient's overall quality of life. However, it must be recognized that individuals may change their wishes and goals as transitions occur in illness. These periods of transition are highly stressful, and the team can expect confusion, ambivalence, and conflicting opinions as the process of transition evolves.

The use of advanced directives such as living wills, health care proxies, and "do not resuscitate orders" helps to articulate the patient's values and ensure that their wishes surrounding end-of-life care are known. Many, when assisted in an appropriate manner, come to view completion of an advanced directive as a positive tool of empowerment rather than a negative or frightening process. In addition, knowledge by an individual that he or she has the right to have care directed solely towards quality of life can do much to alleviate both his or her fears and those of his or her family. Frequently the notion of the appropriateness of foregoing life-sustaining treatments must be discussed repeatedly and at some length, as some patients and families view this as "giving up." In these discussions, it can be helpful to introduce the concept of "optimal medical treatment" in the setting of incurable illness. Such care has been defined as depending "upon the careful determination of appropriate and realistic goals of medical treatment and implementing appropriate treatment measures designed to achieve those goals" (American Academy of Neurology, 1996).

Many factors, ranging from social to religious, influence a patient's or a family member's perception of "optimal" care at the end of life. An exploration of these factors may assist the health care team in ascertaining the patient and family member goals, as well as providing information to aid the patient or family in decision making. For example, a family member who feels hesitant about withdrawal of a ventilator may be expressing hesitancy based on a fear that he or she will be responsible for ending life and that such an action is against a personal code of ethics and/or against the will of God. Another family member in the same scenario may be concerned primarily as to how the person will die and whether the person will be breathless and distressed.

Discussions around advanced directives need to be ongoing, concrete, proactive, and specific. It is often important to address both broad and specific issues. For example, although patients and families with life-threatening illness need to be informed that they have the right to discontinue life-sustaining treatments at any time and may focus on care directed solely toward quality of life, discussions around specific interventions such as ventilatory support or hydration and nutrition are also often needed. Patients and family members need assistance to move from the generic concept of withdrawal of treatment to "shifting the focus" from ineffective treatments to those that will benefit the patient. When discussing "withdrawing treatment," it is important to specify the treatment that will be withdrawn and why, and the aspects of care that will be continued or initiated. Members of the health care team should also be understanding of the patient and family motives and goals in seeking specific treatments, and should assist them in understanding what is possible and what is not possible to achieve from such treatments.

End-of-life discussions around advanced directives are frequently difficult for staff as well as patients and families. A variety of actions by team members may give the appearance of conflict within the health care team and can make difficult decisions even more difficult. For example, a physician may continue to focus on life-sustaining treatments, whereas a nurse is encouraging the patient and family members to withdraw from such treatments. In most cases, it is more helpful to the patient if the team can present consistent advice having resolved its own conflicts elsewhere. It is key that information regarding the discussion process and final decisions is accessible to all involved in the continuum of care. In summary, patients can be assisted greatly with advanced planning if the health care team is in agreement, proactive, compassionate, and attentive to the patient and family priorities, and is knowledgeable about end-of-life care.

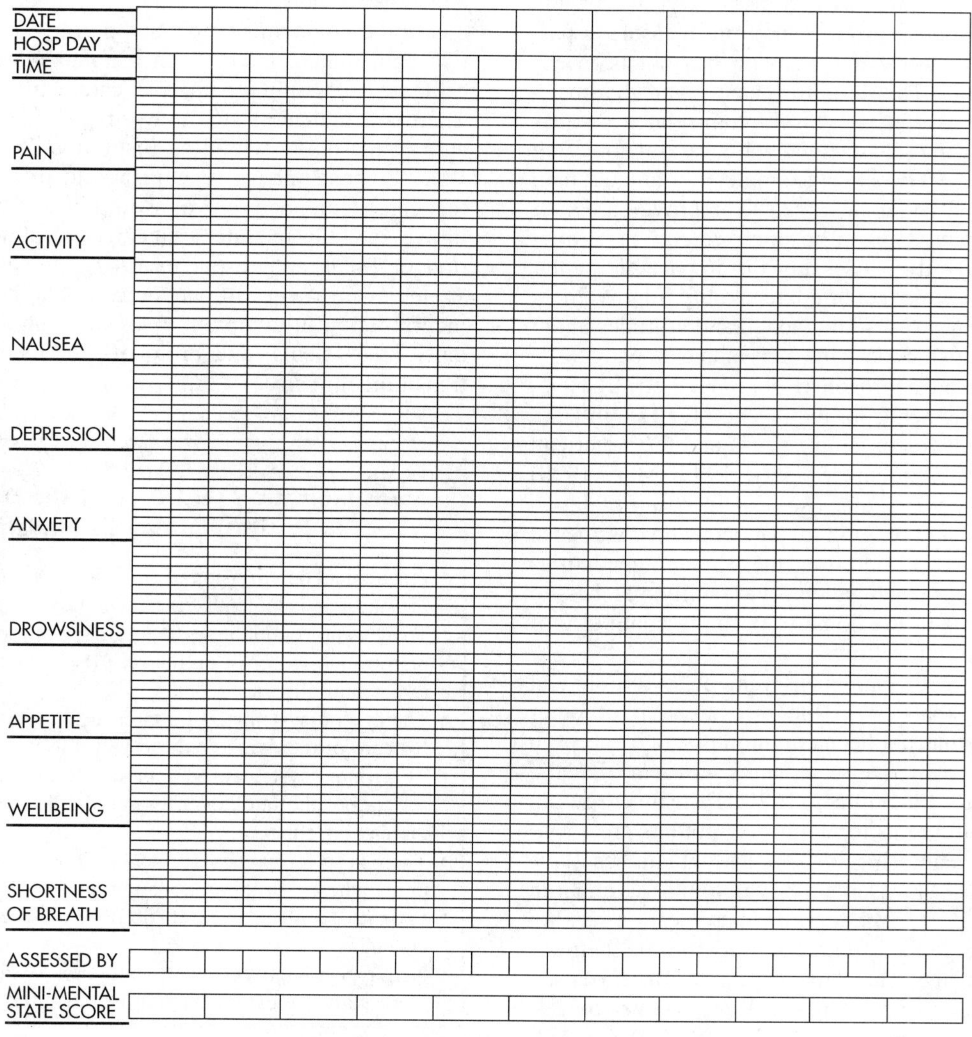

Fig. 18-3 Symptom assessment graph.

Ongoing dialogue and clear, specific documentation are core elements of such care.

MONITORING THE EFFECTIVENESS OF END-OF-LIFE CARE AND IMPLEMENTING INSTITUTIONAL CHANGE

For palliative care to be effective, its delivery must be optimized at the bedside and in the outpatient setting by nurses, physicians, social workers, and other team members; and it must be supported and encouraged at an institutional level. This chapter has focused on a practical approach to delivering front-line palliative care. Monitoring the effectiveness of such care is a complex area, and a full review is beyond the scope of this chapter. Outcomes measures in palliative care rarely have been implemented, and only recently have such measures been considered within institutions. As a consequence, although a number of investigators are developing methods of approaching this matter, much work is needed in this field, and the ideal instruments have not yet been developed.

At the bedside and patient level, an array of instruments exist for monitoring symptoms and distress. However, the routine clinical application of symptom measures, particularly for symptoms other than pain, has not been explored systematically. This is unfortunate given the possibility of increased awareness of symptom-related distress and improved outcomes associated with careful, ongoing monitoring (Foley, 1995). For example, systematic pain measurement has been demonstrated to improve caregiver understanding of pain status in hospitalized patients (Au et al., 1994), and early data assessing the impact of regular pain measurement within a continuous quality improvement strategy suggest that nurse's knowledge and attitudes about pain and patient satisfaction with pain management can be improved by such an approach (Bookbinder et al., 1995, 1996). Recent guidelines from the Agency for Health Care Policy and Research (Jacox et al., 1994) and the American Pain Society (American Pain Society, 1995; Max, 1990) have recommended the regular use of pain rating scales to assess pain severity and relief in all patients who commence or change treatments. In addition, these recommendations suggest that clinicians teach patients and family members to use assessment tools in the home to promote continuity of pain management in all settings.

The experience with pain measurement in the clinical setting could be expanded to the measurement of other symptoms, but this has not been common practice except in some specialized palliative care units (Bruera, Kuehn, Miller, Selmser, & Macmillan, 1991; Fainsinger et al., 1991), where specific tools to monitor symptoms are a routine part of such care (Fig. 18-3). Recent studies have yielded new validated measures for symptom assessment in the research setting and, although their application has not been explored outside the research setting, in time their use may prove beneficial in the clinical setting (Bruera et al., 1991; de Haes, Raatgever, van der Burg, Hamersma, & Neijt, 1987; de Haes, van Kippenberg, & Neijt, 1990; McCorkle & Young, 1978; McCorkle & Quint-Benoliel, 1983; Portenoy et al., 1994). In addition to focusing staff attention on symptom assessment, such measures may be used as a means of reviewing the quality of patient care and ascertaining situation-specific barriers to symptom control (Bruera et al., 1991; Bruera, Hanson, & MacDonald, 1990; Fainsinger et al., 1991; Stiefel, Fainsinger, & Bruera, 1992).

It is generally accepted that to optimize palliative care within an institution, there must be a strong commitment to the provision of such care, and that this will generally require institutional change. Some institutions are beginning to include palliative care and end-of-life care in disease management pathways, and in such endeavors the principles of quality improvement can be extremely effective. A useful template for institutional change can be taken from work relating to the implementation of a pain management improvement initiative by Bookbinder and colleagues (1995). The interventions in this initiative include developing a structured pain management program, regular education for professionals, and an institutional emphasis on the processes of pain management through continuous quality improvement (CQI) training and unit-based CQI teams. Outcome measures were directed toward both patients and professionals. For patients, these outcomes focused on satisfaction and adequacy of pain relief; and for professionals, on attitudes, documentation, and perceived barriers to effective pain management. Such a template is directly applicable to integrating palliative care within an institution. There are indicators that may suggest inadequacies in the care of the dying within an institution. These are listed in Box 18-4 and may give guidance to immediate problems that can be attended to. An institutional commitment to palliative care can include a statement of philosophy; dedication of funds and resources to the process, systematized strategies for review of care delivered at the end of life, the incorporation of symptom assessment and monitoring into daily assessments, and protocols for the management of transitions in care.

Box 18-4

Signs Indicating That Care of the Dying Within an Institution May Be Inadequate

- A statement on provision of end-of-life care is not included in the mission statement of the institution.
- There is no routine assessment of symptoms, family, social, or spiritual concerns, on the records of those with life-threatening illness.
- There is no systematized approach to monitoring outcomes for care of the dying or those with life-threatening illness.
- There is no systematized approach to monitoring outcomes for care of the families of those who die or experience life-threatening illness.
- There is no formal bereavement follow-up for families of patients who die within the institution.
- Patients, families, and staff do not have access to trained chaplains.
- No support is provided for health care professionals who work with dying patients and their families.

Adapted from Super, A., & Plutko, L. A. (1996). Danger signs: Coalition points to causes and consequences of inadequate care of the dying. *Health Progress, 77,* 50-54.

CONCLUSION

Clearly palliative care involves far more than symptom management, and as a consequence, both its implementation and assessment of its delivery are complex. In addition, integrating palliative care into the mainstream of oncology practice is in its infancy. However, nurses are in an excellent position to highlight the need for such care and the instrumental in its development.

REFERENCES

Ajemian, I. (1993). The interdisciplinary team. In D. Doyle, G. W. C., & N. MacDonald (Eds.), *Oxford textbook of palliative medicine.* Oxford: Oxford University Press.

American Academy of Neurology Ethics and Humanities Subcommittee. (1996). Palliative Care in Neurology. *Neurology, 46,* 870-872.

American Nurses Association. (1991). *Position statement on promotion of comfort and relief of pain in dying patients.* Kansas City: American Nurses Association.

American Pain Society Consensus Statement. (1995). Quality improvement guidelines for the treatment of acute pain and cancer pain. *Journal of the American Medical Association, 274,* 1872-1880.

American Psychiatric Association. (1994). *Diagnostic and statistical manual of mental disorders* (4th ed.) Washington, DC: American Psychiatric Association.

Au, E., Loprinzi, C. L., Dhodapkar, M., Nelson, T., Novotny, P., & Hammack, J. (1994). Regular use of a verbal pain scale improves the understanding of oncology impatient intensity. *Journal of Clinical Oncology, 12,* 2751-2755.

Barbato, M. (1994). Thiamine deficiency in patients admitted to a palliative care unit. *Palliative Medicine, 8,* 320-324.

Bedard, J., Dionne, A., & Dionne, L. T. (1991). The experience of La Maison Michel Sarrazin (1985-1990): Profile analysis of 952 terminal cancer patients. *Journal of Palliative Care, 7,* 48-53.

Bernardin, J. L. (1997). *The gift of peace: Personal reflections by Joseph Cardinal Bernardin.* Chicago: Loyola Press.

Bookbinder, M., Coyle, N., Kiss, M., Layman-Goldstein, M., Holritz, K., Thaler, H., Gianella, A., Derby, S., Brown, M., Racolin, A., Nah Ho, M., & Portenoy, R. K. (1996) Implementing national standards for cancer pain management: Program model and evaluation. *Journal of Pain and Symptom Management, 12,* 334-347.

Bookbinder, M., Kiss, M., Coyle, N.; Brown, M. H., Gianella, A., & Thaler, H. T. (1995). Improving pain management practices. In. D. B. McGuire, C. H. Yarbo, & B. R. Ferrell (Eds.), *Cancer pain management* (2nd ed.). Boston: Jones and Bartlett.

Breitbart, W. (1989). Psychiatric management of cancer pain. *Cancer, 63,* 2334-2342.

Breitbart, W., Bruera, E., Chochinov, H., & Lynch, M. (1995). Neuropsychiatric syndromes and psychological symptoms in patients with advanced cancer. *Journal of Pain and Symptom Management, 10,* 131-141.

Brescia, F. (1990). Approaches to palliative care: Notes of a deathwatcher. In K. M. Foley, J. J. Bonica, & V. Ventafridda (Eds.), *Advances in pain research and therapy: Second International Congress on Cancer Pain* (Vol. 16). New York: Raven Press.

Brescia, F. J., Adler, D., Gray, G., Ryan, M. A., Cimino, J., & Mamtani, R. (1990). Hospitalized advanced cancer patients: A profile. *Journal of Pain and Symptom Management, 5,* 221-227.

Brock, D. B., Holmes, M. B., Foley, D. J., & Holmes, D. (1992). Methodological issues in a survey of the last days of life. In R. B. Wallace & R. F. Woolson (Eds.), *The epidemiologic study of the elderly.* New York: Oxford University Press.

Bruera, E., Hanson, J., & MacDonald, N. (1990). Palliative care in a cancer center: Results in 1984 versus 1987. *Journal of Pain and Symptom Management, 5,* 1-5.

Bruera, E., Kuehn, N., Miller, M. J., Selmser, P., & Macmillan, K. (1991). The Edmonton Symptom Assessment System (ESAS): A simple method for the assessment of palliative care patients. *Journal of Palliative Care, 7,* 6-9.

Bruera, E., Miller, L., McCallion, J., Macmillan, K., Krefting, L., & Hanson, J. (1992). Cognitive failure in patients with terminal cancer: A prospective study. *Journal of Pain and Symptom Management, 7,* 192-195.

Buckman, R. (1993). Communication in palliative care. In D. Doyle, G. W. C. Hanks, & N. MacDonald (Eds.), *Oxford textbook of palliative medicine.* New York: Oxford University Press.

Bukberg, J., Penman, D., & Holland, J. C. (1984). Depression in hospitalized cancer patients. *Psychosomatic Medicine, 46,* 199-212.

Byock, I. (1997). *Dying well: The prospect for growth at the end of life.* New York: Riverhead Books.

Callan, D. (1989). Hope as a clinical issue in oncology social work. *Journal of Psychosocial Oncology, 7,* 31-46.

Cassem, N. H. (1991). The dying patient. In N. H. Cassem (Ed.), *Massachusetts General Hospital handbook of general hospital psychiatry.* St Louis: Mosby.

Cassileth, B. R., Zupkis, R. V., Sutton-Smith, K., & March, V. (1980). Information and participation preferences among cancer patients. *Annals of Internal Medicine, 92,* 832-836.

Cavanaugh, T. A. (1996). The ethics of death: Hastening or death-causing palliative analgesic administration to the terminally ill. *Journal of Pain and Symptom Management, 12,* 248-254.

Cherny, N., Coyle, N., & Foley, K. M. (1996). Guidelines in the care of the dying cancer patient. *Hematology Oncology Clinics of North America, 10,* 261-286.

Cherny, N. I. & Portenoy, R. K. (1994). Sedation in the management of refractory symptoms: Guidelines for evaluation and treatment. *Journal of Palliative Care, 10,* 31-38.

Chochinov, H. & Holland, J. C. (1989). Bereavement: a special issue on oncology. In J. C. Holland & J. E. Rowland (Eds.), *Handbook of psychooncology.* New York: Oxford University Press.

Chochinov, H. M., Wilson, K. G., Enns, M., & Lander, S. (1994). Prevalence of depression in the terminally ill: Effects of diagnostic criteria and symptom threshold judgments. *American Journal of Psychiatry, 151,* 537-540.

Chochinov, H., Wilson, K. G., Enns, M., Mowchun, N., Lander, S., & Levitt, M. (1995). Desire for death in the terminally ill. *American Journal of Psychiatry, 152,* 1185-1191.

Cleeland, C. S., Gonin, R. Hatfield, A. K., Edmonson, J. H., Blum, R. H., & Stewart, J. A. (1994). Pain and its treatment in outpatients with metastatic cancer. *New England Journal of Medicine, 330,* 592-596.

Clipp, E. C. & George, L. K. (1992). Patients with cancer and their spouse caregivers. Perceptions of the illness experience. *Cancer, 69,* 1074-1079.

Corr, C. A., Morgan, J. D., & Wass, H. (Eds.). (1993). *International work group on death and dying and bereavement: Statements on death, dying and bereavement.* Ontario, Canada: Canadian Palliative Care Association.

Coyle, N. (1987). A model of continuity of care. *Medical Clinics of North America, 71,* 259-270.

Coyle, N. (1992). The euthanasia and physician-assisted suicide debate: issues for nursing. *Oncology Nursing Forum, 19,* 41-46.

Coyle, N. (1995). Suffering in the first person. In B. R. Ferrell (Ed.), *Suffering.* Boston: Jones and Bartlett.

Coyle, N., Adelhardt, J., Foley, K. M., & Portenoy, R. K. (1990). Character of terminal illness in the advanced cancer patient: pain and other symptoms during the last four weeks of life. *Journal of Pain and Symptom Management, 5,* 83-93.

Coyle, N., Loscalzo, M., & Bailey, L. (1989). Supportive home care for the advanced cancer patient and family. In J. C. Holland & J. H. Rowland (Eds.), *Handbook of psychooncology.* New York: Oxford University Press.

Curtis, E. B., Krech, R., & Walsh, T. D. (1991). Common symptoms in patients with advanced cancer. *Journal of Palliative Care, 7,* 25-29.

de Haes, J. C. J. M., Raatgever, J. W., van der Burg, M. E. L., Hamersma, E., & Neijt, J. P. (1987). Evaluation of the quality of life of patients with advanced ovarian cancer treated with combination chemotherapy. In N. K. Aaronson & J. Beckman (Eds.), *The quality of life of cancer patients.* New York: Raven Press.

de Haes, J. C. J. M., van Kippenberg, F. C. E., & Neijt, J. P. (1990). Measuring psychological and physical distress in cancer patients: Structure and application of the Rotterdam Symptom Checklist. *British Journal of Cancer, 62,* 1034-1038.

Derogatis, L. R., Morrow, G. R., Fetting, J., Penman, D., Piasetsky, S., & Schmale, A. M. (1983). The prevalence of psychiatric disorders among cancer patients. *Journal of the American Medical Association, 249,* 751-757.

Donnelly, S., & Walsh, D., (1995). The symptoms of advanced cancer. *Seminars in Oncology, 22*(2, Suppl. 3), 67-72.

Doyle, D. (1992). Have we looked beyond the physical and the psychosocial? *Journal of Pain and Symptom Management, 7,* 302-311.

Dunlop, G. M. (1989). A study of the relative frequency and importance of gastrointestinal symptoms and weakness in patients with far advanced cancer. *Palliative Medicine, 4,* 37-43.

Dunphy, K. P. & Amesbury, B. D. W. (1990). A comparison of hospice and homecare patients: patterns of referral, patient characteristics and predictors on place of death. *Palliative Medicine, 4,* 105-111.

Ellershaw, J. E., Sutcliffe, J. M., & Saunders, C. M. (1995). Dehydration in the dying patient. *Journal of Pain and Symptom Management, 10,* 192-197.

Emanuel, E. J. (1988). A review of the ethical and legal aspects of terminating medical care. *American Journal of Medicine, 84,* 291-301.

Emanuel, E. J. (1994). Euthanasia: historical, ethical, and empirical perspectives. *Archives of Internal Medicine, 154,* 1890-1901.

Endicott, J. (1983). Measurement of depression in patients with cancer. *Cancer, 53,* 2243-2248.

Exton-Smith, A. N. (1961) Terminal illness in the aged. *Lancet, 2,* 305-308.

Fainsinger, R. & Bruera, E. (1992). Treatment of delirium in the terminally ill patient. *Journal of Pain and Symptom Management, 7,* 54-56.

Fainsinger, R. & Bruera, E. (1994). The management of dehydration in terminally ill patients. *Journal of Palliative Care, 10,* 55-59.

Fainsinger, R., MacEachern, T., Miller, M. J., Bruera, E. Spachynski, K., Kuehn, N., & Hanson, J. (1994). The use of hypodermoclysis for rehydration in terminally ill cancer patients. *Journal of Pain and Symptom Management, 9,* 298-302.

Fainsinger, R., Miller, M. J., Bruera, E., Hanson, J., & MacEachern, T. (1991), Symptom control during the last week of life on a palliative care unit. *Journal of Palliative Care, 7,* 5-11.

Ferris, F. & Cummings. (1995). *Palliative care: towards a consensus in standardized practice.* Ontario, Canada: Canadian Palliative Care Association.

Fleishman, S. B., Lesko, L. M., & Breitbart, W. (1993). Treatment of organic mental disorders in cancer patients. In W. Breitbart & J. C. Holland (Eds.), *Psychiatric aspects of symptom management in cancer patients.* Washington, DC: American Psychiatric Press, Inc.

Foley, K. M. (1995). Pain relief into practice: Rhetoric without reform. *Journal of Clinical Oncology, 13,* 2149-2151.

Goldberg, R. J., Mor, V., Weimann, M., Greer, D. S., & Hiris, J. (1986). Analgesic use in terminal cancer patients: Report from the National Hospice Study. *Journal of Chronic Disease, 39,* 37-45.

Grant, K. D. (1992). The Patient Self-Determination Act: Implications for physicians. *Hospital Practice, 27,* 44-48.

Greer, D. S., Mor, V., Morris, J. N., Sherwood, S., Kidder, D., & Birnbaum, H. (1986). An alternative in terminal care: results of the National Hospice Study. *Journal of Chronic Disease, 39,* 9-26.

Groopman, J. (1997). The last deal. *New Yorker Magazine,* (September 8), 62-74.

Grossman, S. A., Sheidler, V. R., Swedeen, K. Mucenski, J., & Piantadosi, S. (1991). Correlation of patient and caregiver ratings of cancer pain. *Journal of Pain and Symptom Management, 6,* 53-57.

Grosvenor, M., Bulcavage, L., & Chlebowski, R. T. (1989). Symptoms potentially influencing weight loss in a cancer population. Correlations with primary site, nutritional status, and chemotherapy administration. *Cancer, 63,* 330-334.

Hendin, H. & Klerman, G. (1993). Physician-assisted suicide: The dangers of legalization. *American Journal of Psychiatry, 150,* 143-145.

Herth, K. (1990). Fostering hope in terminally ill patients. *Journal of Advanced Nursing, 15,* 1250-1259.

Heyse-Moore, L. H. (1991). How much of a problem is dyspnea in advanced cancer? *Palliative Medicine, 5,* 20-26.

Heyse-Moore, L. & Baines, M. J. (1984). Control of other symptoms. In C. Saunders (Ed.), *The management of terminal malignant disease.* London: Edward Arnold.

Higginson, I. & McCarthy, M. (1989). Measuring symptoms in terminal cancer: Are pain and dyspnoea controlled? *Journal of the Royal Society of Medicine, 82,* 264-267.

Higginson, I., Priest, P., & McCarthy, M. (1994). Are bereaved family members a valid proxy for a patient's assessment of dying? *Social Science Medicine, 38,* 553-557.

Hinton, J. M. (1963) The physical and mental distress of the dying. *Quarterly Journal of Medicine, 32,* 1-21.

Hockley, J. M., Dunlop, R., & Davies, R. J. (1988). Survey of distressing symptoms in dying patients and their families in hospital and the response to a symptom control team. *British Medical Journal (Clinical Research Edition), 296,* 1715-1717.

Holland, J. (1993). Letter to the task force on life and the law. *When death is sought: Assisted suicide and euthanasia in the medical context.* Albany, NY: New York State Task Force on Life and the Law.

Holland, J. C., Rowland, J., & Plumb, M. (1977). Psychological aspects of anorexia in cancer patients. *Cancer Research, 37,* 2425-2428.

Ingham, J. & Coyle, N. (1997). A practical approach for the provision of end-of-life care: A nurse-physician perspective. In D. Clark, S. Ahmedzai, & J. Hockley (Eds.), *New themes in palliative care.* London: Open University Press.

Ingham, J. M., Layman-Goldstein, M., Derby, S., Coyle, N., Adelhardt, J., & Hawke, W. (1994). Pain and distress in cancer patients during the dying process. *American Pain Society Abstracts,* No. 94623.

Irish, P. B. (1994). *Ethnic variations on dying.* Bristol, PA: Taylor & Francis Publishing.

Jacox, A., Carr, D. B., Payne, R., et al. (1994). *Management of cancer pain. Clinical Practice Guideline. No. 9.* Bethesda, MD: U. S. Department of Health and Human Services, Public Health Service, Agency for Health Care Policy and Research.

Jones, S. A. (1993). Personal unity in dying: Alternative conceptions in the meaning of health. *Journal of Advanced Nursing, 18,* 88-94.

Kagawa-Singer, M. (1996). Cultural systems. In R. McCorkle, M. Grant, M. Frank-Stromborg, & S. Baird (Eds.), *Cancer nursing: A comprehensive textbook.* Philadelphia: W. B. Saunders.

Kahn, S. B., Houts, P. S., & Harding, S. P. (1992). Quality of life and patients with cancer: A comparative study of patient versus physician perceptions and its implications for cancer education. *Journal of Cancer Education, 7,* 241-249.

Kane, R. L., Wales, J. Bernstein, L., Leibowitz, A., & Kaplan, S. (1984). A randomised controlled trial of hospice care. *Lancet, 1,* 890-894.

Kaplan, H. I. & Sadock, B. J. (1991). *Synopsis of psychiatry behavioral sciences clinical psychiatry* (6th ed.). Baltimore: Williams & Wilkins.

Kellar, N., Martinez, J., Finis, N., Bolger, A., & VonGunten, C. F. (1996). Characterization of an acute inpatient palliative care unit in a U.S. teaching hospital. *Journal of Nursing Administration, 26,* 16-20.

Klessig, J. (1992). The effect of values and culture on life support. *Western Journal of Medicine, 157,* 316-322.

Kubler-Ross, E. (1969). *On death and dying.* New York: MacMillan.

Larson, D. G. (1993). Self-concealment: implications for stress and empathy in oncology care. *Journal of Psychosocial Oncology, 11,* 1-16.

Latimer, E. J. (1991). Ethical decision-making in the care of the dying and its application to clinical practice. *Journal of Pain and Symptom Management, 6,* 329-336.

Latimer, E. J. & Dawson, H. R. (1993). Palliative care, principles and practice. *Ontario Medical Association Journal, 148,* 933-936.

Levine, P. M., Silberfarb, P. M., & Lipowski, Z. J. (1978). Mental disorders in cancer patients: A study of 100 psychiatric referrals. *Cancer, 42,* 1385-1391.

Lichter, I. & Hunt, E. (1990). The last 48 hours of life. *Journal of Palliative Care, 6,* 7-15.

Lipson, J. G., Dibble, S. L., & Minarik, P. A. (Eds.). (1996). *Culture and nursing care: A pocket guide.* San Francisco, CA: University of California, School of Nursing Press.

Loscalzo, M. & Jacobson, P. (1990). Practical behavioral approaches to the effective management of pain and distress. *Journal of Psychosocial Oncology, 8,* 134-169.

Lynn, J., Teno, J. M., Phillips, R. S., Wu, A. W., Desbiens, N., & Harrold, J. (1997). Perceptions by family members of the dying experience of older and seriously ill patients. *Annals of Internal Medicine, 126,* 97-106.

Massie, M. J. & Holland, J. C. (1990). Depression and the cancer patient. *Journal of Clinical Psychiatry, 51,* 12-17.

Massie, M. J., Holland, J., & Glass, E. (1983). Delirium in terminally ill cancer patients. *American Journal of Psychiatry, 14,* 1048-1050.

Max, M. (1990). American Pain Society quality assurance standards for relief of acute pain and cancer pain. In M. R. Bond, J. E. Charlton, & C. J. Woolf (Eds.), *Proceedings VI World Congress on Pain.* Amsterdam: Elsevier Press.

McCarthy, M. (1990). Hospice patients: A pilot study in 12 services. *Palliative Medicine, 4,* 93-104.

McCorkle, R. & Quint-Benoliel, J. (1983). Symptom distress, current concerns and mood disturbance after diagnosis of a life-threatening disease. *Social Science Medicine, 17,* 431-438.

McCorkle, R. & Young, K. (1978). Development of a symptom distress scale. *Cancer Nursing, 1,* 373-378.

McEvoy, M. D. (1990). When your dying becomes my dying: Aspects of caregivers' grief. *Communicating with cancer patients and their families.* Philadelphia: The Charles Press.

McKegney, F. P., Bailey, L. R., & Yates, J. W. (1981). Prediction and management of pain in patients with advanced cancer. *General Hospital Psychiatry, 3,* 95-101.

Mendelson, D. (1996). Historical evolution and modern implications of concepts of consent to, and refusal of, medical treatment in the law of trespass. *The Journal of Legal Medicine, 17,* 1-71.

Meyers, C. A. & Abbruzzese, J. L. (1992). Cognitive functioning in cancer patients: Effect of previous treatment. *Neurology, 42,* 434-436.

Mor, V., Greer, D. S., & Kaastenbaum, R. (1988). *The hospice experiment.* Baltimore: Johns Hopkins University Press.

Mor, V. & Masterson-Allen, S., (1987). *Hospice care system: Structure, process, costs, and outcome.* New York: Springer Publishing Company.

Morris, J. N., Mor, V., Goldberg, R. J., Sherwood, S., Greer, D. S., & Hiris, J. (1986). The effect of treatment setting and patient characteristics on pain in terminal cancer patients: A report from the National Hospice Study. *Journal of Chronic Disease, 39,* 27-35.

Morris, J. N., Suissa, S., Sherwood, S., Wright, S. M., & Greer, D. (1986) Last days: A study of the quality of life of terminally ill cancer patients. *Journal of Chronic Disease, 39,* 47-62.

Mount, B. M. (1986). Dealing with our losses. *Journal of Clinical Oncology, 4,* 1127-1134.

National Hospice Organization. (1989). *Hospice surveyor operation manual.* Arlington, VA: Author.

National Hospice Organization (1992). *Do not resuscitate (DNR): Decisions in the context of hospice care.* Arlington, VA: Author.

Oxman, T. E. & Silberfarb, P. M. (1980). Serial cognitive testing in cancer patients receiving chemotherapy. *American Journal of Psychiatry, 137,* 1263-1265.

Pagli, P. & Abramovitch, H. (1984). Death: A cross cultural perspective. *Annual Review of Anthropology, 13,* 385-417.

Patchell, R. A., & Posner, J. B. (1989). Cancer and the nervous system. In J. C. Holland & H. Rowland (Eds.), *Handbook of psychooncology.* New York: Oxford University Press.

Plumb, M. M. & Holland, J. (1977). Comparative studies of psychological function in patients with advanced cancer. I. Self-reported depressive symptoms. *Psychosomatic Medicine, 39,* 264-276.

Plumb, M. & Holland, J. (1981). Comparative studies of psychological function in patients with advanced cancer. II. Interviewer-rated current and past psychological symptoms. *Psychosomatic Medicine,* 43, 243-254.

Portenoy, R. K., Thaler, H. T., Kornblith, A. B., Lepore, J. M., Friedlander, K. H., & Coyle, N. (1994a). Symptom prevalence, characteristics and distress in a cancer population. *Quality of Life Research, 3,* 183-189.

Portenoy, R. K., Thaler, H. T., Kornblith, A. B., Lepore, J. M., Friedlander, K. H., & Kiyasu, E. (1994b). The Memorial Symptom Assessment Scale: An instrument for the evaluation of symptom prevalence, characteristics and distress. *European Journal of Cancer, 30A,* 1326-1336.

Posner, J. B. (1979). Neurologic complications of systemic cancer. *Disease-a-Month, 25,* 1-60.

Rando, T. A. (1984). *Grief, dying and death: Clinical interventions for caregivers.* Chicago: Research Press.

Reuben, D. B. & Mor, V. (1986a). Nausea and vomiting in terminal cancer patients. *Archives of Internal Medicine, 146,* 2021-2023.

Reuben, D. B. & Mor, V. (1986b). Dyspnea in terminally ill cancer patients. *Chest, 89,* 234-236.

Reuben, D. B., Mor, V., & Hiris, J. (1988). Clinical symptoms and length of survival in patients with terminal cancer. *Archives of Internal Medicine, 148,* 1586-1591.

Roth, A. & Breibart, W. (1996): Psychiatric emergencies in terminally ill cancer patients. *Hematology/Oncology Clinics of North America, 10,* 235-259.

Saunders, C. (1984). Pain and impending death. In P. Wall & R. Melzack (Eds.), *Textbook of Pain.* New York: Churchill Livingstone.

Saunders, C. (1990). *Hospice and palliative care: An interdisciplinary approach.* London: Edward Arnold.

Searle, C. (1991). A comparison of hospice and conventional care. *Social Science Medicine, 32,* 147-152.

Silberfarb, P. M. (1983). Chemotherapy and cognitive defects in cancer patients. *Annual Review Medicine, 34,* 35-46.

Silberfarb, P. M., Philibert, D., & Levine, P. M. (1980). Psychosocial aspects of neoplastic disease: II. Affective and cognitive effects of chemotherapy in cancer patients. *American Journal of Psychiatry, 137,* 597-601.

Slevin, M. L., Plant, H., & Lynch, D. (1988). Who should measure quality of life, the doctor or the patient. *British Journal of Cancer, 57,* 109-112.

Spiegel, D., Bloom, J., & Yalom, G. (1981). Group support for patients with metastatic cancer. *Archives of General Psychiatry, 38,* 527-533.

Stiefel, F., Fainsinger, R., & Bruera, E. (1992). Acute confusional states in patients with advanced cancer. *Journal of Pain and Symptom Management, 7,* 94-98.

Super, A., & Plutko, L. A. (1996). Danger signs: coalition points to causes and consequences of inadequate care of the dying. *Health Progress, 72,* 50-54.

SUPPORT. (1995). A controlled trial to improve care for seriously ill hospitalized patients: *Journal of the American Medical Association, 274,* 1591-1598.

Tomb, D. A. (1988). *Psychiatry for the house officer.* Baltimore: William and Wilkins.

Tripp-Reimer, T., & Brink, P. (1985). Culture brokerage. In G. Bulechek & J. McCloskey (Eds.), *Nursing interventions and treatments for nursing diagnosis.* Philadelphia: W. B. Saunders Company.

Tuma, R. & DeAngelis, L. (1992). Acute encephalopathy in patients with systemic cancer. *Annals of Neurology, 32,* 288-290.

Twycross, R. G. (1975). The use of narcotic analgesics in terminal illness. *Journal of Medical Ethics, 1,* 10-17.

Twycross, R. G. & Lichter, I. (1993). The terminal phase. In D. Doyle, G. W. Hanks, & N. MacDonald (Eds.), *Oxford textbook of palliative medicine.* Oxford: Oxford University Press.

Vachon, M. L. S. (1993). Emotional problems in palliative medicine: Patient, family, and professional. In D. Doyle, G. W. C. Hanks, & N. MacDonald (Eds.), *Oxford textbook of palliative medicine.* Oxford: Oxford University Press.

Velleman, J. D. (1992). Against the right to die. *Journal of Medical Philosophy, 17,* 665-681.

Ventafridda, V., DeConno, F., Ripamonti, C., Gamba, A., & Tamburini, M. (1990). Quality-of-life assessment during a palliative care programme, *Annals of Oncology, 1,* 415-420.

Ventafridda, V., De Conno, F., Vigano, A., Ripamonti, C., Gallucci, M., & Gamba, A. (1989). Comparison of home and hospital care of advanced cancer patients. *Tumori, 75,* 619-625.

Ventafridda, V., Ripamonti, C., De Conno, F., Tamburini, M., & Cassileth, B. R. (1990). Symptom prevalence and control during cancer patients' last days of life. *Journal of Palliative Care, 6,* 7-11.

Verwoerdt, A. (1966). *Communication with the fatally ill.* Springfield, IL: Charles C. Thomas.

Vincent, M. O. (1982). The doctors own wholeness: "Burned out or refueled." *Canadian Medical Association Meeting.* Saskatoon, Saskatchewan.

Vinciguerra, V., Degnan, T. J., Sciortino, A., O'Connell, M., Moore, T., & Brody, R. (1986). A comparative assessment of home versus hospital comprehensive treatment for advanced cancer patients. *Journal Clinical Oncology, 4,* 1521-1528.

Virmani, J., Schneiderman, L. J., & Kaplan, R. M. (1994). Relationship of advance directives to physician-patient communication. *Archives of Internal Medicine, 154,* 909-913.

Von Gunten, C. F., Neely, K. J., & Martinez, J. (1996). Hospice and palliative care: Program needs and academic issues. *Oncology, 10,* 1070-1074.

VonRoenn, J. H., Cleeland, C. S., Gonin, R., Hatfield, A. K., & Pandya, K. J. (1993). Physician attitudes and practice in cancer pain management: A survey from the Eastern Cooperative Oncology Group. *Annals of Internal Medicine, 119,* 121-126.

Walsh, D. (1990). Continuing care in a medical center: the Cleveland Clinic Foundation Palliative Care Service. *Journal of Pain and Symptom Management, 5,* 273-278.

Ward, A. W. M. (1974). Terminal care in malignant disease. *Social Science Medicine, 8,* 413-420.

Waxler-Morrison, N., Anderson, J. M., & Richardson, E. (Eds.). (1990). *Cross Cultural caring: A handbook for health professionals in Western Canada,* British Columbia: University of BC Press.

Wilkes, E. (1974). Some problems in cancer management. *Proceedings Royal Society of Medicine, 67,* 1001-1005.

Witzel, L. (1975). Behavior of the dying patient. *British Medical Journal, 2,* 81-82.

World Health Organization. (1990). *Cancer pain relief and palliative care.* Report of a WHO Expert Committee on Cancer Pain Relief and Palliative Care. Geneva: World Health Organization.

Young, A., Volker, D., Riegler, P. T., & Thorpe, D. M. (1993). Oncology nurses attitudes regarding voluntary, physician-assisted dying for competent, terminally ill patients. *Oncology Nursing Forum, 20,* 445-451.

Cultural Issues in Cancer Care

Lisa Karlin Schulmeister, RN, MS, CS, OCN

INTRODUCTION

Every individual has a cultural heritage, which provides a framework for viewing the world. The lens through which the world is viewed is a product of values, beliefs, customs, and practices shared by a group of people and passed down from one generation to the next (Helman, 1990). Values and beliefs are expressed through language, dress, dietary choices, role behaviors, perceptions of health and illness, and health-related behaviors (Spector, 1991).

Socioeconomic influences also affect health care perceptions and behaviors. Several research studies that have included socioeconomic factors as a variable have shown that differences commonly ascribed to cultural heritage are often social in origin and reflect the key role of social conditions (Sheldon & Parker, 1992). Social conditions that affect health care practices include inadequate housing, malnutrition, unemployment or underemployment, racial discrimination, violence, and poverty. These social conditions transcend culture and are observed in nations throughout the world (Sowell, 1994).

Health care providers therefore must consider health care delivery in a sociocultural framework (Culley, 1996). However, the task of identifying a person's cultural heritage and socioeconomic influences is often not a simple, straightforward process. Viewing a person's culture as a uniform body of practices to which all members of the given group conform does not allow consideration of individual variation within the group, which is often the norm and not the exception. A person may also modify cultural beliefs and actions because of migration to another culture and may begin to acquire some of the new culture's values and practices. Lastly, a person's heritage may be mixed, resulting in a blurring of cultural identity. Perhaps the most relevant approach is to conceptualize the sociocultural framework in a model of reality. From this standpoint, a person's experiences of health and illness can be understood as an effort to model reality in terms of a socially shared system of meaning that he or she has assimilated as a member of a human society (Donnelly, 1995).

HISTORICAL PERSPECTIVES

Exploration of sociocultural concepts in health care delivery is relatively new. The field of transcultural nursing, which emphasizes cultural sensitivity in providing appropriate, individualized care, was founded in the mid-1960s by Madeleine Leininger. The Transcultural Nursing Society has promoted transcultural nursing since 1974, and certification in transcultural nursing became available in 1988. International conferences, international journals, and nursing research on patient approaches in culturally diverse situations are proliferating as nurses recognize the influence and importance of sociocultural concepts on health care delivery (Giger & Davidhizar, 1995). Approximately 22 books, 70 book chapters, and 900 articles on transcultural nursing have been published, and four graduate programs in transcultural nursing currently exist. These accomplishments are significant, especially when considering that the concept of transcultural nursing came into existence only in 1960 (Leininger, 1994).

Leininger (1996) contends that transcultural nursing research findings are gradually transforming nursing practice by providing a paradigm shift from a traditional unicultural model of practice to a multicultural model. This increased emphasis on cultural considerations in providing care is evident in the curriculums of nursing education programs. An increased emphasis on cultural considerations is also seen in the delivery of patient-centered nursing care. Incorporation of cultural concepts in all facets of nursing care delivery has come to be viewed as essential if nursing care is to be delivered sensitively and effectively.

The need for transcultural nursing knowledge is, in part, based on changing demographics. The United States is rapidly becoming a multicultural, pluralistic society. In 1990, 75% of the U.S. population was of white European decent. It is projected that by the year 2020, only 53% of the U.S. population will be white or of European decent. The number of Asian Americans and Hispanic Americans is expected to triple, and the number of African Americans will double (U.S. Department of Commerce, 1992). Nurses must be aware of changing demographics so that they can address the future nursing care needs of a changing population.

Shifting economics and social trends are also occurring. Between 1963 and 1991, high-paying manufacturing jobs, as a percentage of total jobs in the United States, fell by 43.3%. Service jobs increased, but many are low-paying, low-production jobs, the so-called "McJobs." The majority of these jobs are held by minorities and women and are often part-time positions with few benefits such as health insurance coverage (Schmidt, 1994). As the older population swells, millions of older women are predicted to experience economic stressors because women over age 65 receive an average of less than 60% of what men average in annual social security income. Female-headed families in the United States are four times as likely to be poor as male-headed or couple-headed families. At the present rate, by the year 2000, the poor will be made up almost entirely of women and children. The National Organization for Women refers to this phenomenon as the "feminization of poverty" (National Organization for Women, 1996).

Trends in the health care marketplace have placed care for the catastrophically ill and uninsured at risk. In 1995, approximately 39.4 million people in the United States did not have health insurance of any kind (Berk, Schur, & Cantor, 1995). The numbers of uninsured are growing, and safety net providers, such as public hospitals and community health centers, are feeling the financial strain. A recent estimate by the American Hospital Association places the cost of uncompensated care for acute care hospitals at more than $16 billion a year (Weissman, 1996). Without health care reform, the ranks of the uninsured and underinsured are anticipated to grow.

Because most workers obtain health insurance through their place of employment, loss of a job often triggers loss of health insurance coverage. Maintaining employment after a diagnosis of cancer and even during therapy is a major challenge; the majority of people with cancer who have attempted to return to the workplace have confronted a variety of issues and barriers (Berry, 1993; Berry & Catanzaro, 1992; Herbst, 1995). Work-related problems, loss of jobs, and lack of opportunities for education and professional training are occurring with greater frequency (Brown & Tai-Seale, 1992). Although the Consolidated Omnibus Budget Reconciliation Act (COBRA) provisions permit continuation of health coverage following loss of a job, such an option is often not financially feasible for economically stressed families. Only an estimated 20% of eligible people participate (Davis, 1996).

Historically, individuals who have experienced chronic illness, or a catastrophic illness such as cancer, have had few options in terms of employment mobility or insurability. Preexisting conditions often prevented or affected an individual's access to health insurance. The Kennedy-Kasseam bill signed into law in 1996 provides firmer health insurance portability and coverage to the 25 million Americans who wish to change jobs and/or have a preexisting medical condition. The Health Insurance Portability and Accountability Act guarantees access to continued health insurance when workers leave or lose their jobs, limits exclusions for preexisting conditions to 12 months, and mandates that health plans cover all employees in a group, not just healthy members (Murata, 1996; Neus, 1996). Estimates of how many Americans might be able to take advantage of the new portability provisions have ranged from 400,000 to 25 million. Although the act guarantees portability, there is no provision that ensures affordable health insurance premiums (McIlrath, 1996).

Another trend in health care is the growth in managed care. In 1996, 44% of Americans were enrolled in managed care plans, 41% had indemnity/fee-for-service plans, and 15% were uninsured (Meyer, 1996; Davis, 1996). Health maintenance organizations have been cited for denying access to care for patients with cancer seeking experimental or nonstandard therapies. Several landmark cases have occurred, including one in which a health maintenance organization in California denied a bone marrow transplant to a woman with metastatic breast cancer. An arbitration panel ruled that the transplant should have been approved and awarded the woman's family $1 million, plus $300,000 for court costs and attorney fees (Rice, 1996).

In 1996, mastectomies for breast cancer were considered an outpatient procedure by many managed care plans. Consequently, the media began referring to "drive-through" mastectomies and noted that although insurance companies were managing costs, families were expected to manage care at home after the procedure. A federal bill was introduced to protect mastectomy patients, and several state bills were proposed to require allowing a 2-day stay after a mastectomy (Roukema, 1997). Ross (1996) noted that the solution to the length of stay dilemma is not to legislate minimal hospital coverage for every medical procedure, but rather to have Congress mandate that managed care companies cannot interfere in decisions made between physician and patient. The federal bill also included a provision mandating that reconstructive surgery following a mastectomy must be covered by insurance and not considered a noncovered cosmetic procedure. Other parts of the legislation would require insurers to cover second opinions, including those by specialists not specifically covered by the insurance plan, for all cancer diagnoses (Skorneck, 1997).

Cost controls imposed by managed care delivery systems have prompted the consolidation and integration of hospitals with other health service providers. Hospitals have merged, consolidated, and sometimes closed. Hospitals are no longer the dominant setting for health care; outpatient clinics, the home, and long-term care facilities have become the norm (Bocchino, 1993). Historically, outpatient oncology care has been commonplace; the trend that has most affected patients with cancer is consolidation. Specialized oncology services, such as radiation therapy facilities, are increasingly being consolidated and offered at a few locations in a community. Large corporate mergers and acquisitions have mandated the downsizing of costly specialized services.

Socioeconomic influences on cancer-related practices and outcomes are profound, and recent trends in health care delivery are affecting the delivery of cancer-related services. Distinguishing between effects of cultural influences and socioeconomic factors is hampered methodologically, as well as conceptually. Both factors are closely related; disproportionate numbers of ethnic groups are in the lower socioeconomic category. Because definitive ethnic identifiers have only recently been used in the collection of cancer-related data, comparisons among ethnic groups are limited (Kagawa-Singer, 1995).

The complex interaction between culture and socioeconomic influences on the cancer experience requires that the nurse possess sensitivity and knowledge about transcultural theory. Because culture is the larger milieu in which the interaction between the patient and nurse occurs, knowledge about cultural differences and similarities facilitates more accurate communication, and interventions have a greater potential for success.

CONCEPTS AND PRINCIPLES OF TRANSCULTURAL CARE

Culture is a term used to describe the patterned behavioral response that develops over time as a result of imprinting the mind through social and religious structures and intellectual and artistic manifestations. Culture is shaped by values, beliefs, norms, and practices that are shared by members of the same cultural group. Transcultural nursing is viewed as a culturally competent practice field that is client centered and research focused (Giger & Davidhizar, 1995).

Oncology nurses must consider their own cultural beliefs and values and recognize that they may influence the care they provide. Sometimes inherent biases or inaccurate perceptions exist without the nurse being aware of them. Situations can arise that may cause the nurse to consider or reevaluate personal beliefs; confronting these biases and perceptions often leads to growth and understanding on the part of the nurse. However, at the other extreme, nurses may allow their perceptions or biases to affect the care they deliver. To deliver culturally sensitive care, nurses must be guided by acquired knowledge in the assessment, diagnosis, planning, implementation, and evaluation of a patient's needs based on culturally relevant information. Nurses must also remember that there may be as much cultural diversity within a group as across cultural groups. Regardless of educational preparation or experience, every nurse who provides care must try to deliver culturally sensitive care that is free of inherent bias.

Culturally Diverse Care

Culturally diverse nursing care refers to the variability in nursing approaches needed to provide culturally appropriate, competent care. In the twenty-first century, nurses will need to use transcultural knowledge to provide care to a rapidly changing, heterogeneous patient population. Culturally diverse care considers six cultural phenomena that vary with use, yet are evident in all cultural groups: communication, space, social organization, time, environmental control, and biologic variations (Giger & Davidhizar, 1995; Griffen, 1994).

Communication. As the matrix for thought and relationships among people, communication provides the means by which people connect. It establishes a sense of commonality with others and permits the sharing of information, signals, or messages in the form of ideas and feelings. Communication may occur through use of language or nonverbally, through touch, expressions, or movement (Giger & Davidhizar, 1995; Nance, 1995).

Oncology nurses often use touch as a method of communication. Bottorff (1993) reviewed the use and meaning of touch in caring for patients with cancer. Five types of touch were identified: comforting, connecting, working, orienting, and social. These types of touch were comparable to the two major kinds of touch previously identified in the literature: task-related touch and affective touch.

Therapeutic touch has been used in oncology as a routine part of care (Porter, 1996), as an adjuvant therapy for cancer pain (Gehlhaart, 1995), and to assist in reducing chemotherapy-induced nausea (Peters, Smith, Horrigan, & Mills, 1994). Little information is available on the use of therapeutic touch in specific ethnic groups. Morales (1994) explored the meaning of touch to eight Puerto Rican patients with cancer. Two types of touch, procedural and affective, were identified, and the predominant theme about perception of the nurse's touch was that of conveying confidence. Although nonverbal, touch was viewed as an integral communication method.

Space. The phenomenon of space is best understood as a component of the sensory system. Spatial behavior encompasses a variety of behaviors, including proximity to others, objects in the environment, and movement. Although spatial requirements vary among individuals, people in the same cultural group tend to act similarly. The nurse's responsiveness to the patient's spatial requirements is an important factor in the patient's emotional comfort.

In oncology, the concept of space is often linked to privacy (Glen & Jownally, 1995). Many oncology units have been designed to have single bedrooms, often with a foldout chair or additional bed for family use. When cancer treatment is long, as in the case of bone marrow transplantation, issues related to personal space become significant. The patient's desire to be surrounded by personal items may not be feasible, and frequent staff visits may be perceived as intrusive.

Other nursing care settings, such as outpatient treatment facilities and private practice office settings, also have space and privacy needs. A treatment area that accommodates several patients simultaneously may prevent patients from asking questions or talking about personal matters. The proximity of each treatment chair or bed should also be considered. When the chairs or beds are placed close together, patients may perceive an invasion of their personal space. Lack of privacy can also occur when there is no mechanism for creating a personal space. For instance, curtain dividers or room dividers are helpful in creating an area that patients can identify as theirs. Recognizing the patient's needs with regard to space considerations, especially the need for privacy, is crucial.

Social Organization. Cultural behavior, or how a person acts in certain situations, is socially acquired and not genetically inherited. Patterns of cultural behavior are learned through a process called *acculturation* or *socialization,* which involves acquiring knowledge and internalizing values. Because people learn a specific culture as they grow from infancy to adulthood, they live within a certain reality. This existence is sometimes termed *culture-bound.* Most people, therefore, have learned ways to interpret their world that are understandable to those who share the same frame of reference, a phenomenon often called *ethnocentrism.* People who are not members of the cultural group may not share these interpretations (Giger & Davidhizar, 1995).

Ethnicity is a term often used to mean race, but the term encompasses more than biologic identification. Ethnicity has a broader definition that refers to group identification based on a shared social and cultural tradition. Examples of shared traditions include language, place of birth, kinship patterns, and observable characteristics influenced by environment and genetics (Tripp-Reimer & Lively, 1988).

In any society, cultural groups can be arranged in a hierarchical power structure. Dominant groups are considered powerful, whereas those in minority groups are considered inferior and lacking in power. Although the term *minority* actually refers to "less than a numerical majority of the population" (Hautman & Bomar, 1995), the term has been interpreted and used in a variety of ways, most often to represent inequalities. In a number of cancer-related articles and publications, the term *minority* has been used to refer to people of color; however, the newer, more appropriate term of *underserved population* is being increasingly used.

Social organizations view groups as systems; they are in a steady state that is maintained even as the group changes. These groups include family, religious, ethnic, racial, tribal, kinship, clan, and other special interest groups. Most groups form, grow, and reach a state of maturity. In the course of development of the group, a pattern of behavior and set of norms, beliefs, and values evolve (Giger & Davidhizar, 1995).

Time. *Environmental control* refers to the ability of an individual or group of individuals from a particular cultural group to plan activities and control nature. Environmental control also refers to the individual's perception of the ability to direct factors in the environment. Environmental influences, along with sociocultural forces such as economics, politics, and the health care delivery system, affect a person's health care practices.

Health care practices include the Western medical system of diagnoses and scientific explanations for illness; religious systems that dictate social, moral, and dietary practices; and unconventional methods. A patient's world view largely determines beliefs about disease and appropriate treatment interventions. Culture therefore influences choices made by patients regarding their health care practices (Griffin, 1994).

In addition to receiving traditional Western medical treatment, a significant number of patients with cancer use or seriously consider using unconventional methods (Fletcher, 1992; Montbriand, 1995; Morrison, 1996). These unconventional methods include folk remedies (Cronsberry, 1996; Skinn, 1994) and the use of traditional healers (Nwoga, 1994). The appeal of unconventional methods may be related to the unpredictable and prevalent nature of cancer, the patient and family's needs to reduce anxiety, and spiritual and cultural beliefs (Fletcher, 1992). Montbriand (1995) noted that alternate health care practices are a way in which patients with cancer can be in control of their illness situation.

Use of traditional vs nontraditional health care practices is determined, in part, by the person's locus of control. People who subscribe to an internal locus of control have internal feelings of control and thus act to influence future behaviors and situations. People with an external locus of control view the future as the result of fate or chance and are less likely to take action to change the future (Figer & Davidhizar, 1995).

The locus of control construct is influenced by culture. Cancer fatalism is a phenomenon observed among African Americans; it has been suggested that African Americans perceive that there is no escape from the inevitability of death if cancer occurs (Powe, 1995). In the Latino population, specific beliefs about cancer reflect the moral framework within which they interpret disease. Latinos often believe that cancer is God's punishment for improper or immoral behavior (Perez-Stable, Sabogal, Otero-Sabogal, Hiatt, & McPhee, 1992).

Biologic Variations. Although culture differences are clearly evident in communication, spatial relationships, and social organizations, less recognized and understood are the biologic differences among people in various racial groups. Knowledge regarding biologic variations can aid the nurse in providing culturally competent care.

A direct relationship exists between race and body structure, skin color and other visible physical characteristics, enzymatic and genetic variations, nutritional preferences and deficiencies, electrocardiographic patterns, and susceptibility to disease. Body structure, which includes body shape and size, differs among racial groups. Bone density also differs among adults. The prevalence of osteoporosis is reported to be substantially lower in African-American women than in white American women (Pollitzer & Anderson, 1990). Bone mineral density has been shown to predict the risk of breast cancer in older nonblack women. Cauley, et al. (1996) conducted a prospective cohort study of 6854 nonblack women in four clinical sites. They found that the risk of breast cancer in women with bone mineral density above the 25th percentile was increased 2.0 to 2.5 times compared with women below the 25th percentile.

Early age at menarche and late menopause have been identified as risk factors in the development of breast cancer. Epidemiologic studies worldwide support this finding within and between cultural groups. Recent genetic research has identified markers within families for predisposition to breast, colon, and skin cancers, as well as genetic mutations that have been linked to the development of ovarian, colorectal, breast, and skin cancers (Boente et al., 1996; Box & Watne, 1995; Foulkes et al., 1996; Garrett, Liscia, Nasim, & Ferreira-Gonzalez, 1995; Gapstur, Duppuis, Gann, Collila, Winchester, 1996; Lancaster et al., 1996; Modan, 1996; Robinson, Rademaker, Goolsby, Traczyk, & Zoladzc, 1996).

No association between bladder cancer and ethnicity was found among Hispanic, white, and Pacific Islander ethnic groups. Differences were attributed to smoking and occupational exposures rather than genetic or biologic factors (Anton-Culver, Lee-Feldstein, & Taylor, 1993). Similarly, in examining survival from prostate cancer, the stage and grade of the cancer, as well as the patient's age, affected survival, but race did not (Optenberg et al., 1995).

Reactions to drugs vary by race. Caffeine, a component of many drugs, as well as coffee, tea, and colas, appears to be metabolized and excreted faster by whites than Asians. It is suggested that differences in caffeine metabolism are correlated with liver-enzyme differences (Kudzma, 1992). Nutritional preferences, which include habits and patterns, are developed during childhood as a result of family lifestyle and ethnic or cultural, social, religious, geographic, economic, and psychological influences. Food also has a symbolic meaning in many cultures. It may be symbolic in a religious context or other contexts, such as the use of food as a reward (Giger & Davidhizar, 1995; Otero-Sabogal, Sabogal, Perez-Stable, & Hiatt, 1995; Sekhon, 1996).

The cultural phenomena that are seen in all cultural groups vary in application across cultures. Therefore individualized assessment of each of these areas is necessary when working with patients from diverse cultural groups.

CULTURAL ASSESSMENT

Since its introduction in 1991, the Giger and Davidhizar Transcultural Assessment Model (Box 19-1) has been applied to the care of a variety of patients in a variety of clinical specialists (Giger & Davidhizar, 1995). The comprehensive model elicits information about key assessment areas, including information about the culturally unique individual, communication, space, social organization, time, environmental control, and biologic variations.

CULTURAL INFLUENCES ON CANCER PREVENTION, SCREENING, AND DETECTION

Health beliefs and behaviors of cancer prevention, screening, and detection are influenced by sociocultural factors. A person's desire to participate or not participate in cancer prevention and detection activities may be attributed to a variety of sociocultural factors. In addition, major risk factors for cancer (e.g., smoking; a high-fat, low-fiber diet; and occupational exposures to carcinogens) appear to be more prevalent among the economically disadvantaged.

Pfeffer and Moynihan (1996) noted that assessing ethnicity and health beliefs with respect to cancer is difficult. They assert that what people say in response to questions about health beliefs and ethnicity depends on the time and place that the questions are asked, and the identity, purpose, and method of approach that is used by the person posing the question. In addition to these methodologic issues, Zahm and Fraumeni (1995) noted that research has historically been hampered by vague classifications of ethnicity.

A person's health beliefs and the way in which a cancer screening program is presented also influence the desire to participate. Culturally sensitive programs such as outreach efforts targeted to a specific ethnic group are being implemented in many communities. Research is also being conducted on perceived barriers to cancer screening. In one study, Kelly et al. (1996) used a focus group composed of Cambodian women to identify their perceived barriers to cancer screening in an effort to design culturally sensitive programs. Thirteen barriers were identified, including the basic barrier of lack of understanding of the purpose of cancer screening and distorted beliefs about cancer. Fear, shyness, lack of transportation, expense, and discomfort were also identified as barriers. Fear and shyness are common among the Cambodian culture. Other barriers, such as the lack of transportation and costs associated with cancer screening, are not culture-specific.

Socioeconomic Influences

Ethnicity must be understood as a marker of behaviors and beliefs within a social context and not as a risk factor in and of itself. The separate effects of ethnicity and social status on attitudes and health-promoting behaviors cannot be extricated from one another. The two together interact with the environment in which the individual lives (Kagawa-Singer, 1995).

Gorey and Vena (1994) noted that epidemiologic evidence supports the interrelationship of race, socioeconomic status, and cancer in the United States. They reviewed 10 independent studies published between 1992 and 1996 and found that one of every three occurrences of stomach cancer and one out of every seven occurrences of lung or cervical cancer were related to low socioeconomic status. Other studies have supported the link between low socioeconomic status and low utilization of cancer screening programs. After accounting for socioeconomic factors, a study comparing Latinos and Anglos found Latino ethnicity to be a minor predictor of use of cancer screening tests. Increasing the availability of universal health coverage was thought to be an important priority to promote the use of cancer screening by Latinos (Perez-Stable, Sabogal, & Otero-Sabogal, 1995).

The most serious effect of low socioeconomic status is the delay of early detection, resulting in the diagnosis of disease at advanced stages. Mandelblatt, Andrews, Kerner, Zauber, and Burnett (1991) found that, in New York City, older African-American, lower-class women in public hospitals were 3.75 times more likely to have late-stage breast cancer and 2.54 times more likely to have late-stage cervical cancer than were younger, white, higher social class women in nonpublic hospitals. Racial differences were also observed in cervical cancer mortality in a study conducted by Samelson, Speers, Ferguson, and Bennett (1994). Age-adjusted mortality in African-American women was twice the rate found in white American women. These racial differences are particularly significant, as cervical cancer is curable when detected early, and breast cancer is most effectively treated when detected early.

When patients are poor, they often seek orthodox health care for cancer symptoms only after those symptoms have

Box 19-1

Transcultural Assessment Model

Culturally Unique Individual

1. Place of birth
2. Cultural definition: What is . . .
3. Race: What is . .
4. Length of time in country (if appropriate)

Communication

1. Voice quality
   - Strong, resonant
   - Soft
   - Average
   - Shrill
2. Pronunciation and enunciation
   - Clear
   - Slurred
   - Dialect (geographic)
3. Use of silence
   - Infrequent
   - Often
   - Length: brief, moderate, long, not observed
4. Use of nonverbal
   - Hand movement
   - Eye movement
   - Entire body movement
   - Kinesics (gestures, expression, or stances)
5. Touch
   - Startles or withdraws when touched
   - Accepts touch without difficulty
   - Touches other without difficulty
6. Ask these and similar questions:
   - How do you get your point across to others?
   - Do you like communicating with friends, family, and acquaintances?
   - When asked a question, do you usually respond (in words or body movement, or both?)
   - If you have something important to discuss with your family, how would you approach them?

Space

1. Degree of comfort
   - Moves when space invaded
   - Does not move when space invaded
2. Distance in conversations
   - 0 to 18 inches
   - 18 inches to 3 feet
   - 3 feet or more
3. Definition of space
   - Describe degree of comfort with closeness when talking with or standing near others
   - How do objects (e.g., furniture) in the environment affect your sense of space?
4. Ask these and similar questions:
   - When you talk with family members, how close do you stand?
   - When you communicate with coworkers and other acquaintances, how close do you stand?
   - If a stranger touches you, how do you react or feel?
   - If a loved one touches you, how do you react or feel?
   - Are you comfortable with the distance between us now?

Social Organization

1. Normal state of health
   - Poor
   - Fair
   - Good
   - Excellent
2. Marital status
3. Number of children
4. Parents living or deceased?
5. Ask these and similar questions:
   - How do you define social activities?
   - What are some activities that you enjoy?
   - What are your hobbies, or what do you do when you have free time?
   - Do you believe in a Supreme Being?
   - How do you worship that Supreme Being?
   - What is your function (what do you do) in your family unit/system?
   - What is your role in your family unit/system (father, mother, child, advisor)?
   - When you were a child, what or who influenced you most?
   - What is/was your relationship with your siblings and parents?
   - What does work mean to you?
   - Describe your past, present, and future jobs.
   - What are your political views?
   - How have your political views influenced your attitude toward health and illness?

Time

1. Orientation to time
   - Past-oriented
   - Present-oriented
   - Future-oriented
2. View of time
   - Social time
   - Clock-oriented
3. Physiochemical reaction to time
   - Sleeps at least 8 hours a night
   - Goes to sleep and wakes on consistent schedule
   - Understands the importance of taking medication and other treatments on schedule
4. Ask these and similar questions:
   - What kind of timepiece do you wear daily?
   - If you have an appointment at 2 PM, what time is acceptable to arrive?
   - If a nurse tells you that you will receive a medication in "about a half hour," realistically, how much time will you allow before calling the nurses' station?

From Giger, J. N. & Davidhizar, R. E. (1995). *Transcultural nursing: Assessment and intervention* (2nd ed.). St. Louis: Mosby.

Box 19-1
Transcultural Assessment Model—cont'd

Environmental Control

1. Locus of control
   - Internal locus of control (believes that the power to affect change lies within)
   - External locus of control (believes that fate, luck, and chance have a great deal to do with how things turn out)
2. Value orientation
   - Believes in supernatural forces
   - Relies on magic, witchcraft, and prayer to affect change
   - Does not believe in supernatural forces
   - Does not rely on magic, witchcraft, or prayer to affect change
3. Ask these and similar questions:
   - How often do you have visitors at your home?
   - Is it acceptable to you for visitors to drop in unexpectedly?
   - Name some ways your parents or other persons treated your illnesses when you were a child.
   - Have you or someone else in your immediate surroundings ever used a home remedy that made you sick?
   - What home remedies have you used that worked? Will you use them in the future?
   - What is your definition of "good health"?
   - What is your definition of "poor health"?

Biologic Variations

1. Conduct a complete physical assessment noting:
   - Body structure (small, medium, or large frame)
   - Skin color
   - Unusual skin discolorations
   - Hair color and distribution
   - Other visible physical characteristics (e.g., keloids, chloasma)
   - Weight
   - Height
   - Check laboratory work for variances in hemoglobin, hematocrit, and sickle phenomena if black or of Mediterranean descent
2. Ask these and similar questions:
   - What diseases or illnesses are common in your family?
   - Describe your family's typical behavior when a family member is ill.
   - How do you respond when you are angry?
   - Who (or what) usually helps you to cope during a difficult time?
   - What foods do you and your family like to eat?
   - Have you ever had any unusual cravings for:
     -White or red clay dirt?
     -Laundry starch?
   - When you were a child what types of foods did you eat?
   - What foods are family favorites or are considered traditional?

Nursing Assessment

1. Note whether the client has become culturally assimilated or observes own cultural practices.
2. Incorporate data into plan of nursing care:
   - Encourage the client to discuss cultural differences; people from diverse cultures who hold different world views can enlighten nurses.
   - Make efforts to accept and understand methods of communication.
   - Respect the individual's personal need for space.
   - Respect the rights of clients to honor and worship the Supreme Being of their choice.
   - Identify a clerical or spiritual person to contact.
   - Determine whether spiritual practices have implications for health, life, and well-being (e.g., Jehovah's Witnesses may refuse blood and blood derivatives; an Orthodox Jewish person may eat only kosher food high in sodium and may not drink milk when meat is served).
   - Identify hobbies, especially when devising interventions for a short or extended convalescence or for rehabilitation.
   - Honor time and value orientations and differences in these areas. Allay anxiety and apprehension if adherence to time is necessary.
   - Provide privacy according to personal need and health status of the client (NOTE: perception and reaction to pain may be culturally related).
   - Note cultural health practices:
     -Identify and encourage efficacious practices.
     -Identify and discourage dysfunctional practices.
     -Identify and determine whether neutral practices will have a long-term ill effect.
   - Note food preferences:
     -Make as many adjustments in diet as health status and long-term benefits will allow and that dietary department can provide.
     -Note dietary practices that may have serious implications for the client.

become severe and sometimes unbearable. Explanations for this phenomenon include feelings of pessimism, fatalism, and low self-esteem in addition to faith in a belief system that does not regard the physician as the person to whom one goes for disease prevention. Inaccessibility of facilities, high-risk behavior, and inability to pay are also associated with delay in seeking health care. The culture of poverty transcends ethnicity (Parham & Hicks, 1995).

In addition to low income, impact of low literacy level and knowledge and attitudes toward mammography were assessed by Davis et al. (1996). A lack of accurate information about mammography was prevalent among low-level readers in the sample of 445 women. Although the average highest grade completed in school was the tenth grade, 77% of the sample could not read above a seventh to eighth grade level. In certain areas, it may be necessary to screen the population for literacy level, instead of considering the highest grade in school completed, before offering information in written form.

Low income was also a strong predictor of underuse of

mammography in a study of 12,252 women conducted by Calle, Flanders, Thun, and Martin (1993). Other predictors of underuse of mammography included Hispanic ethnicity, low levels of education, age over 65, and residence in a rural area. In the same study, Pap smear use was examined. Women of all races and all income levels were found to underuse Pap smear screening, and underuse was most prevalent among older African-American women.

In a similar study, women with low levels of education, who had incomes below 200% of the poverty level, who had no health insurance, who were 80 years of age or older, and who resided in Appalachian West Virginia, as well as Hispanic women in urban Texas communities, had the lowest rates of breast and cervical cancer screening in a sample of 6648 women in three geographic target areas (National Cancer Institute Cancer Screening Consortium for Underserved Women, 1995). Older age appears to be a factor in underuse and cancer screening.

Caplan, Wells, and Haynes (1992) found several barriers to early detection of breast cancer among older minorities, including inaccurate knowledge, virtually no data on knowledge and attitudes for a number of minority groups, low awareness of the necessity of early detection, lack of health insurance to cover screening programs, and lack of reimbursement to health care providers for clinical breast examinations. The older minority woman therefore is at high risk for delayed diagnosis of cancer.

To overcome the inequality in terms of both the increased incidence and mortality from cancer that the poor encounter, health care reform is essential. Additional attention must be given to ensure that cancer prevention, screening, and treatment services for the poor overcome language barriers, geographic barriers, knowledge deficits, and literacy and linguistic hurdles. In addition, simply making health care services available is not sufficient. Health promotion of the poor will require societal changes that ensure safe, healthy living conditions, including a nutritious diet, exercise, safety, and an environment free of tobacco, alcohol, and other harmful substances (Wilkes, Freeman, & Prout, 1994).

Cultural Factors

Degree of acculturation has been recognized as a factor in utilization of cancer screening programs. Suarez (1994) measured acculturation by using five scales to assess English language proficiency, English language use, value placed on culture, traditional family attitudes, and social interaction. When an individual integrates into a new culture, he or she acquires and assimilates the values and beliefs of the new culture. The extent to which the individual adopts and integrates the new culture's practices reflects the individual's degree of acculturation.

Geographics is another cultural factor influencing utilization of cancer prevention and detection programs. Individuals living in rural areas, and particularly the rural poor, are often in great need of cancer detection services, yet have little or no local access to them. Rural hospitals typically lack state-of-the-art equipment and are unable to provide a full range of specialized oncology services. Because rural areas have higher proportions of older people, cancer risk is high in these areas. Rural dwellers often are less educated and do not practice prevention or early detection behaviors that could identify cancer at an early stage (Given, Given, & Harlan, 1994).

Box 19-2

Cultural Factors Affecting Cancer Prevention, Screening, and Early Detection Beliefs and Practices

Ethnic or racial identity
Level of acculturation
Religious beliefs
Socioeconomic level
Age
Education
Literacy level
Locus of control
Social support
Area of residence

Cultural factors influencing cancer screening and early detection behaviors therefore are diverse and often act as barriers to cancer control activities. Box 19-2 lists sociocultural factors that influence cancer prevention, screening, and detection beliefs and practices. Although many of these factors can be applied to most populations, culturally diverse populations with varying degrees of acculturation and assimilation are primarily affected by language preference, education or literacy level, ethnicity, religion, and support systems (Palos, 1994).

In a review by Olsen and Frank-Stromborg (1993), cancer rates, risks, knowledge, and screening practices in five ethnically diverse populations in the United States were examined (Table 19- 1). African Americans, the largest minority group, experienced some of the highest cancer incidence and mortality rates, and their 5-year cancer survival rate was 30% lower than that for white Americans. More is known about the cancer beliefs and practices of African Americans than any other minority group.

The Hispanic subgroup, composed of Mexican, Puerto Rican, Cuban, and other Hispanics, makes up the second largest minority group and is rapidly growing. By the year 2000, Hispanic Americans are projected to outnumber African Americans. Carpenter and Colwell (1995) found that the majority of 112 Hispanic women surveyed had significant misconceptions about cancer causation, symptoms, and treatment. They expressed feelings of little control over prevention, suggesting an external locus of control that is common among the Latino culture.

The third largest minority group in the United States, the Asian-American group, is highly diverse, and cancer rates vary among subgroups within this culture. Native-American Alaska Natives have the lowest overall cancer incidence and mortality rates of all minority groups, but there is significant disparity in cancer rates among tribes. Native Hawaiians rank first or second in the United States for cancers of the esophagus, lung, stomach, breast, uterus, and ovary

TABLE 19-1 Racial/Ethnic Populations Cancer Profile

Ethnic Group	Cancer Problems	Lifestyle Risk Factors	Barriers to Prevention	Possible Approaches
African American	Highest overall cancer incidence rate Highest overall cancer mortality rate Survival 30% lower than for whites Prostate cancer Breast cancer Lung cancer Colorectal cancer Pancreatic cancer Esophageal cancer	Poverty Diet Smoking Hazardous occupational exposures Obesity Alcohol consumption Urban living	Low education and literacy levels Lack of credible messengers with whom community can identify For the poor, survival, not prevention, is priority Decreased access to health care and prevention	Use African-American professional for health care and as speakers Church-based information and speakers Forums at public housing sites Smoking-cessation efforts directed to unique smoking habits of this group
Hispanic	Gallbladder cancer among New Mexico Hispanics of Native American ancestry Liver cancer among Mexican Americans	Genetic tendency Possibly diet	Low literacy, even in Spanish Fear of cancer General belief that cancer is God's will and only God can cure	Public service advertisements, Hispanic media Speakers bureau of Hispanic health professionals Outreach through neighborhood stores, restaurants Spanish videotapes Footonovelas Use Hispanic professionals for health care Use of comadres and copadres as role models Advocate use of 1-800-4CANCER number for Spanish translation and counseling
	Cervical cancer among women from Central and South America	Young age of first sexual encounter	Modesty and sexuality issues associated with gynecologic exams	
	Pancreatic cancer among Mexican Americans	Poverty and possibly associated alcohol use	Lack of Spanish-speaking caregivers Male reluctance to have exams	
	Prostate cancer	Dietary changes with associated acculturation	Decreased access to health care and prevention Decreased awareness of cancer warning signs and screening tests	
Asian/Pacific Islander *Chinese*	Nasopharyngeal cancer	Epstein-Barr virus Salt fish consumption Genetic predisposition	Low education and literacy in native languages "Prevention model" nonexistent Lack of trust in Western health care Leaders lack health knowledge Decreased access to health care	Include screening examinations and prevention education crisis care visits Outreach with messages through stores Tie in with English as second language classes Integrate traditional healers, herbs, and practices
	Liver cancer	Hepatitis B		
	Esophageal cancer	Consumption of salted foods, hot tea, silica fiber, and contaminated grain Smoking		
	Lung cancer	Indoor pollutants Smoking and passive smoke exposure Vitamin A deficiency		
	Stomach cancer	Loss of gastric acidity Salted food consumption Family history of gastric cancer		

Modified from Olsen, S. J., & Frank-Stromberg, M. (1993). Cancer prevention and early detection in ethnically diverse populations. *Seminars in Oncology Nursing, 9*(3), 198-209.

Continued

TABLE 19-1 Racial/Ethnic Populations Cancer Profile—cont'd

Ethnic Group	Cancer Problems	Lifestyle Risk Factors	Barriers to Prevention	Possible Approaches
Asian/Pacific Islander—cont'd				
Japanese	Stomach cancer	Age over 65 years Salted food consumption Low vitamin C intake Family history of gastric cancer Loss of gastric acidity		
	Esophageal cancer	Consumption of rice gruel cooked in hot tea Chronic esophagitis		
	Liver cancer	Hepatitis B Low vitamin C intake		
	Gallbladder cancer	Gallstones High-fat diet		
Korean	Liver cancer	Hepatitis B		
	Biliary cancer	History of gallstones High-fat diet		
	Lymphoma cancer	Unknown		
	Thyroid cancer	Unknown		
Filipino	Liver cancer	Hepatitis B		
	Biliary cancer	History of gallstones High-fat diet		
	Lymphoma cancer	Unknown		
Native American	Lowest overall cancer incidence and mortality of all U.S. populations Survival rates are uniformly low Tribal cancer rate differences are important		Inhospitable health care environment and insensitive personnel Lack of transportation to health clinic Low education and literacy levels Underfunded and overburdened health care system	Integrate cultural beliefs and practices Enlist support of key tribal leaders and organizations Perform examinations with strict attention and concern for modesty, tribal customs, gender and dress differences
Ogalala women	Lung cancer Cervical cancer Stomach cancer	Smoking Lack of services	Generalized lack of financial resources	Integrate prevention and screening into other health care visits
Ogalala, Alaska, Oklahoma, Northern Plains tribes	Lung cancer	Cigarette smoking	Lack of integration of traditional practices with western health care practice	
Oklahoma tribes and Alaska natives	Stomach cancer Colon cancer	Lack of dietary fiber		
Oklahoma, Navajo, and Aberdeen tribes	Breast cancer	Obesity		

Modified from Olsen, S. J., & Frank-Stromberg, M. (1993). Cancer prevention and early detection in ethnically diverse populations. *Seminars in Oncology Nursing, 9*(3), 198-209.

TABLE 19-1 Racial/Ethnic Populations Cancer Profile—cont'd

Ethnic Group	Cancer Problems	Lifestyle Risk Factors	Barriers to Prevention	Possible Approaches
Native American—cont'd				
Tribes of Rosebud Sioux Reservation, Ft. McDowell community, North Carolina	Cervical cancer	Lack of adequate nutrition		
Alaska natives	Liver cancer Nasopharyngeal cancer	Hepatitis B Epstein-Barr virus Cigarette smoking Salted fish consumption		
Southwestern and Oklahoma tribes	Gallbladder cancer	Diet Genetic factors		
Navajo men	Lung cancer	Uranium mining		
Western Washington tribes	Gallbladder cancer Cervical cancer	Diet Possibly genetics Access to care issues		

(Nomura, 1994). Lifestyle factors of this group include a high-fat diet, smoking, heavy alcohol consumption, obesity, and lack of exercise (Olsen & Frank-Stromberg, 1993).

Specific cancer screening practices of other ethnic groups have received little attention. Not much is known about cancer detection knowledge and practices for Chinese women either living in their homeland or worldwide, yet China is the most populated continent. Hoeman, Ku, and Ohl (1996) found that early detection of cancer was not a clear concept for the 23 Chinese women they interviewed; 80% believed performing breast examinations and 70% believed having Pap smears would prevent cancer.

Another understudied ethnic group is the Vietnamese. Yi (1994a) surveyed 141 Vietnamese women and found that their use of Pap tests was lower than Pap test utilization for the U.S. female population in general; 50% of the Vietnamese migrant respondents reported having had a Pap smear compared with 88% of the general population in 1987. Pham and McPhee (1992) found that Vietnamese women indicated that just over half believed they could do little to prevent cancer, and 54% had never had a Pap smear. In a study of breast cancer screening practices, Yi (1994b) found that half of 141 Vietnamese women surveyed had never had a clinical breast examination, and only 65 had ever had a mammogram.

It is believed that Asian Americans, including individuals from Southeast Asia, do not participate in cancer screening and education programs because of their traditional health beliefs and standards of modesty, misconceptions and fears about cancer, lack of knowledge about the U.S. health care system and how to access it, and inability to pay for care. As a result, the cancer screening rates for this population are low (Jackson, 1994).

Culturally Sensitive Cancer Screening

A variety of cancer screening programs addressing the needs of a culturally diverse population have been studied. In examining life span and ethnicity issues in breast cancer screening, Rimer (1994) noted that interventions to increase mammography utilization include individual-directed, system-directed, social network, and multistrategy interventions. Both individual interventions and multistrategy interventions increased the use of mammography among African-American women over the age of 50. Brown and Williams (1994) asserted that culturally sensitive breast screening programs need to be developed for older black women. Increased screening could be accomplished if the cost of mammography and clinical breast examinations were reduced, accessibility and availability were increased, educational programs were provided, and the community became involved. Furthermore, assessing specific health beliefs about cancer (Jennings, 1996) and educating African Americans about cancer prevention and detection (Lowe, Barg, & Bernstein, 1995) may reduce the high incidence of cancer mortality and morbidity in the African-American population.

In the Hispanic population, Carpenter and Colwell (1995) determined that increased knowledge is associated with increased self-efficacy for cancer screening. Russell and McCammon (1995) advocated using a multidisciplinary approach to improve access to health care for Latinos. Lack of bilingual providers, lack of health materials written in Spanish, and costs were identified as significant health care barriers for the Latino population.

To increase breast and cervical cancer screening for Cambodian women, Kelly et al. (1996) examined an intervention of providing informational programs in the Cambodian language, making group screening appointments, providing transportation, and using female physicians and interpreters in an informal clinic setting. The female physicians and group appointments were used in response to the women expressing feelings of fear and shyness when examined. After the intervention, community screening rates for Cambodians were almost five times higher than at baseline.

Lovejoy (1996) reviewed multinational approaches to cervical cancer screening and found that cohort screening policies, as well as provider attitudes, absence of public health campaigns, and lack of organized follow-up, tended to deter older, low-income women from obtaining adequate prevention care. Providing small monetary rewards or transportation incentives, making invitational phone calls, providing mailing lists of nonadherers to providers, creating clinic education programs, and sending letters of invitation were suggested as cost-effective methods for promoting cervical cancer screening adherence rates.

Although considerable attention has focused on ethnicity in relation to screening for cancer in women, little attention has been given to ethnicity in relation to screening for cancer in men. Prostate cancer is the most common cancer among American men and is now the second leading cause of cancer death in men (American Cancer Society, 1997). Since 1990, the reported number of new cases of prostate cancer has doubled from fewer than 100,000 annually to an estimated 184,500 in 1997 (Hanks & Scardino, 1996; Landis, Murray, Bolden, & Wingo, 1998). This increase has been attributed mostly to greater utilization of prostate cancer screening tests and, to a small extent, to the aging of the U.S. population. A major risk factor for prostate cancer is race; the incidence of prostate cancer is 66% higher for African-American men than for white American men. In fact, African-American men have the highest rate of prostate cancer in the world (American Cancer Society, 1998).

In addition to race, large population studies suggest that prostate cancer risk is significantly higher among men with a history of prostate cancer in a first-degree relative (Hayes et al., 1995; Whittemore et al., 1995). Familial risk of prostate cancer is also more pronounced in younger patients. Coffey (1993) estimates that 43% of prostate cancer deaths in men less than age 55 years old occur in men with a familial risk of the disease. In an early detection program targeted at African Americans, four prostate cancers were detected among 169 high-risk men, and all four reported having a positive family history of prostate cancer (Sartor, 1996).

Few strategies for addressing the screening needs of the rural population have been published. A community-based education program that included onsite mammography and colposcopy improved compliance and tracking in rural West Virginia. Recognizing local culture, geography, educational level, and economics for the target area is believed to be a critical consideration in designing a program to address the needs of rural dwellers (Walker, Lucas, & Crespo, 1994). Butterfoss, Goodman, and Wandersman (1993) advocate using community coalitions for prevention and health promotion, which may enhance health promotion activities, such as cancer screening, in underpopulated areas.

Olsen and Frank-Stromberg (1993) identified generic recommendations for interacting with different ethnic groups to conduct culturally sensitive cancer screening. Proceeding slowly and respectfully with great attention to dignity and modesty, and clearly explaining what will occur and why it is important are critical. Preferably, intimate examinations should be provided by clinicians of the same gender as the individual being screened. It is important to provide permission to ask questions and express discomfort. It is also necessary to obtain permission to touch the individual's body and learn to recognize clinical signs that may indicate the individual's use of traditional healers, such as medicine bundles or bracelets and religious articles.

ETHNOSENSITIVE CANCER CARE

The body of knowledge of the cultural issues that affect oncology care delivery is growing. Because the United States has such a sophisticated health care delivery system, patients from other countries often travel to the United States for treatment. Provision of effective oncology care is contingent on an accurate assessment of the patient's health care needs, which often differ from those of the dominant U.S. culture. For instance, Crom (1995) examined the experiences of South-American mothers who traveled to the United States to have their children treated for cancer. Emerging themes from interviews with the mothers included their belief that no sacrifice was too great to save their children's lives, the overwhelming impact of a cancer diagnosis, and economic and cultural hardship. The greatest challenges identified were difficulties associated with language and communication.

When patients with cancer travel to the United States for treatment, or conversely when Americans travel to other countries seeking cancer treatment, exposure to another culture occurs. This exposure may be brief or long. Patients must adapt to the new culture and cope with cancer and its treatment in an unfamiliar environment, which may be difficult, since few patients are able to bring all of their resource and support persons with them. For instance, patients may not have the same religious support they had in their native country, or they may find that their other methods of treatment, such as folk medicine, are not available. Patients coming to or leaving the United States for cancer treatment may encounter culture shock if they are not prepared for the new culture (Montbriand, 1993).

Pain and Culture

It is estimated that between 30% and 50% of patients with cancer either experience pain or are being treated for pain. The way in which pain is experienced and the way it is described and treated vary among cultures, and are often related to the degree of pain management resources available. When resources for pain management are lacking, pain control is often inadequate (Banoub-Baddour & Laryea, 1992; Kodiath & Kodiath, 1995). It has also been suggested that the pain management needs of ethnic minorities may be neglected by palliative care providers (O'Neill, 1994). The ability to assess pain across diverse cultures is important for understanding the universal aspects of this symptom and expediting nursing interventions. The McGill Pain Questionnaire is the most valid and reliable single multidimensional pain instrument available for measuring pain, and it has been translated into several languages. Translated tools such as the McGill Pain Questionnaire in the Norwegian language have been found to be reliable, sensitive, and culturally acceptable (Kim, Schwartz-Barcott, Holter, & Lorensen, 1995).

Ethnicity and Cancer Survival

Differences in cancer survival among ethnic groups have only recently received attention. One reason for the lack of attention to ethnicity in reviewing survival statistics is the lack of uniformity in defining ethnic group membership (Greenwald, Polissar, & Dayal, 1996).

In a study to determine whether ethnicity is an independent prognostic factor for survival, Perkins, Cooksley, and Cox (1996) reviewed 3382 patients treated over 30 years at a comprehensive cancer center. Survival differences were significant; African-American females had a 1.63 times higher risk of mortality at 5 years compared with white Americans, with ethnicity a strong predictor of survival. However, when stage and treatment were controlled, ethnicity was no longer a strong predictor of survival.

Ethnic variation in prostate cancer survival in New Mexico was assessed by Gilliland, Hunt, and Key (1996). American Indians and African Americans had the lowest 5-year survival rate. Poor survival may be explained by delayed detection and differences in treatment. Ethnicity and cure rates for children in Texas with acute lymphoid leukemia were reviewed by Hord, Smith, Culbert, Frankel, and Pinkel (1996). Although event-free survival and cure rates were lower for children of Mexican descent when compared with American children of European descent, the differences were not statistically significant. Earlier studies showed that children of African, Polynesian, Native American, and Mexican ancestry had a less favorable outcome than children of European ancestry when treated in a similar manner by the same physicians and nurses.

The association of Hispanic ethnicity and poverty with general survival in 14,896 patients with breast cancer was examined by Delgado, Lin, and Coffey (1995). Poverty and Hispanic race were significant predictors for reduced general survival time.

With improved methods of defining various ethnic groups, data on cancer survival in relation to ethnicity can be obtained. In addition, research using methodologies to discern whether survival is related to ethnicity or low socioeconomic status is needed to better clarify the role of ethnicity in cancer survival.

Death and Dying

Two concepts that transcend all cultural boundaries are loss and grief. Although expressions of loss and grief vary among members of diverse cultures, understanding the culture of the person experiencing loss assists in designing culturally appropriate nursing care. Culture brokerage, or the act of translation in which messages, instructions, and belief systems are exchanged between cultural groups, has potential for increasing understanding between oncology nurses and patients from diverse cultural backgrounds (Pickett, 1993). One of the keys to effective culture brokering is for the nurse to be aware of his or her own beliefs about death and dying, and to be aware of inherent biases.

Many times it is assumed that because a family has a shared cultural background, that each member experiences the loss and grieves in the same way. However, this assumption is not true (Nishimoto, 1996). Coping with death and dying is a process as unique as each person experiencing it. Although the person's culture often provides a framework for this process, each person experiences loss and grieves in his or her own way. Individual assessment of beliefs about death and dying is therefore crucial.

Only recently, research examining loss and grief experienced by specific ethnic groups has been conducted. Papadatou, Yeantopoulos, and Kosmidis (1996) explored the experiences of Greek mothers who cared for a child dying of cancer at home or in the hospital. The decision to remain at home or go to the hospital was based on the child's expressed wish and parental preference. Death in the hospital was believed to be as culturally acceptable as death at home.

Death at home is preferred in many cultures. Whereas a century ago virtually everyone died at home, more than three fourths of Americans now spend their final days in acute care hospitals (McCue, 1993). Death is still viewed as a natural and expected milestone of human existence by many ethnic groups (Morrison & Meier, 1995); for example, African Americans prefer to care for a dying relative in their home environment. The immediate and extended family typically mobilizes to coordinate care, and the goal of care is for the patient to remain at home whenever possible.

Asian-American women also feel culturally obligated to provide care for elders; however, as Asian women culturally assimilate, family and cultural obligations often conflict with employment (Jones, 1996). The traditional role of woman as caregiver may not be possible in a changing society in which women compose a significant portion of the work force.

In a study of Japanese families who have lost children to cancer, the main caregiver was consistently the mother, and the mother was viewed as the family leader (Saiki, Martinson, & Inano, 1994). Nurses should identify who the family looks to as its leader and be aware that, in some cultures, women rather than men are perceived as the family leader.

Funeral rites and religious rituals also vary among cultural groups. Being knowledgeable about culturally specific death-related rituals and beliefs could both prepare nurses for what they may encounter and increase their understanding of the responses of patients and their relatives. Nurses should ask direct questions about levels of religious observance and inquire about cultural death rites (Katz, 1996). For instance, in the Taiwanese culture, rituals include caring for the body, making funeral arrangements, wearing mourning clothes, spreading ashes, using spirit tablets, and visiting the grave (Gudmundsdottir, Martinson, & Martinson, 1996). Strong communication skills and an openness to accept cultural differences are essential qualities if nurses are to respond appropriately to reduce bereavement distress experienced by people from other cultures.

RECRUITING ETHNICALLY DIVERSE RESEARCH PARTICIPANTS

Evidence indicates that certain groups, such as women, ethnic minorities, the elderly, and the poor, may be underrepresented in clinical research. Larson (1994) conducted a review of 754 approved research protocols at a teriary care center over 2 years to examine demographic characteristics of subjects and found that exclusions for which a justification was least frequently given were age (44.9%), socioeconomic status (42.9%), and race (38.1%). When certain subgroups are underrepresented in clinical research, inappropriate and inaccurate inferences from the results may be made.

In oncology, clinical trials have been federally supported since 1995 as a program of cooperative clinical study directed toward better methods of treating malignant disease. Early clinical trials were successful in general accrual efforts, but minority and economically disadvantaged patient participation was lacking. In 1989, the National Cancer Institute established a specific initiative to meet the needs of minority patients with cancer and individuals at risk for cancer (McCabe, Varricchio, & Padberg, 1994). Recognition of the need to include minority and economically disadvantaged patients and their actual inclusion in clinical trials is a great challenge that requires awareness of recruitment factors.

McCabe et al. (1994) identified four major factors that affect access to care and therefore recruitment to clinical trials: availability, affordability, accessibility, and acceptability. These factors may be more critical to successful recruitment efforts in prevention trials than in treatment trials. Barriers to participation in clinical trials include fear and distrust, perceptions of costs, difficulty accessing the clinical site, recruitment information and informed consent in a language not used by the patient, lack of valid and culturally appropriate sampling tools or questionnaires, and lack of protocols available for the disease and stage of presentation. Suggestions for increasing recruitment to clinical trials include identifying barriers for the targeted population, determining and using key decision makers in the targeted group, contacting potential subjects through community events, advertising clinical trials where potential subjects will see it, offering tours of the clinical site to prospective subjects, making recruitment and retention a top priority, publicizing eligibility requirements, and providing cultural- and language-appropriate information materials.

Interactional Recruitment Model

Hautman and Bomar (1995) developed an interactional model for recruiting ethnically diverse research participants (Fig. 19-1). The model consists of four key players: the re-

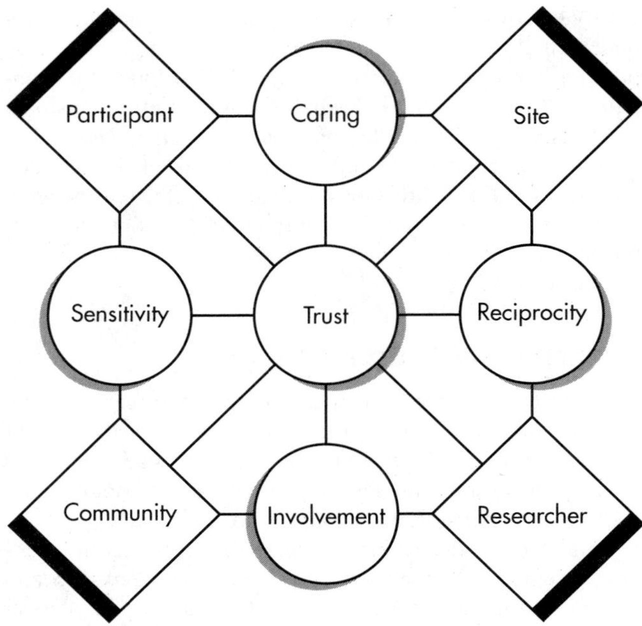

Fig. 19-1 The International Recruitment Model. (From Hartman, M. A. & Bomar, P. [1995]. International model for recruiting ethnically diverse research participants. *Journal of Multicultural Nursing & Health, 1*[4], 8-15, 27.)

searcher, the participant, the site, and the community. Underlying assumptions include caring, reciprocity, trust, sensitivity, and involvement. The model is open and interactive, thus allowing for creative and meaningful interactions. Success in recruiting and maintaining participants in research is often related to the assumptions on which the interaction model is based. Specific strategies to recruit ethnically diverse research participants are outlined in Table 19-2.

PROVIDING CULTURALLY DIVERSE ONCOLOGY NURSING CARE

Understanding cultural differences among people of different cultural backgrounds has considerable relevance in the cancer setting. Entering a hospital, losing a relative, undergoing a physical examination, experiencing a chronic illness, or accepting a permanent physical disability means different things to different people. Although an in-depth cultural assessment of all patients is recommended, constraints often limit the extent of the cultural assessment that can be conducted. Trill and Holland (1993) identified major cultural areas that should be considered essential when assessing the patient with cancer. They include family function, gender roles, language, disclosure of information, pain, attitudes toward illness and practices, immigration, religion, autonomy/dependency, death, and bereavement. Factors such as the level of involvement of family members in a patient's care, the degree of dependency among them, and their expectations of each other during the course of the disease are all highly influenced by sociocultural values and are important determinants of decision making and treatment planning. Culturally defined gender roles may affect a

Table 19-2 Recruitment Strategies for Ethnically Diverse Research Participants

Source	Group	Strategy
Affonso et al (1993)	Filipino, Chinese, Japanese, Hawaiian, Part Hawaiian	• Use of focus group as a safe to share and receive support. • Story telling in groups is a form of communication among members of these ethnic groups.
Bomar & Hautman (1990)	African-American	• Contact ministers. • Provide services such as health education and screening in the community.
El-Sadr & Capps (1992)	African-American	• Development of trust. • Close to home or transportation. • Provide a warm meal • Provide child care. • Education about research process. • Use culturally sensitive materials.
Frye & D'Avanzo (1994)	Cambodian refugee woman	• Use of consistent translator/culture broker known to the study population.
Hooks et al (1988)	Multiethnic families	• Begin with newspapers/posters, then use take-home information. • Home visits. • Telephone calls. • Clergy commenting on project during service enhances trust.
Howard et al (1983)	Hispanics	• Telephone interviewing more helpful than mailed questionnaires. • Spanish language with older persons.
Huttinger & Drevdahl (1994)	Navajo and Hopi	• Focused on preparing Navajo and Hopi students for careers in research, thereby increasing minority participation.
Lipson (1992)	Iranian Immigrants	• Persian-speaking research associate. • Face-to-face interviews preferred to written survey (only 38 of 200 surveys completed).
Marin and Marin (1991)	Hispanic	• Become familiar with the community demographics through available statistical information. • Obtain an initial "windshield" assessment of the community to identify and contact key community meetings. • Attend community meetings. • Locate key informants and be aware of rivalries.
Muecke (1992)	Refugees	• Negotiate with refugee leader to assume role of intermediary. • Language facility. • Educate community about the research process. • Consideration of refugees as "vulnerable population."
Munet-Vilaro (1988)	Not specified	• Identify formal and informal gatekeepers. • Personal contacts. • Personal interviews. • Work with the group before starting research.
Murdaugh (1990)	Multiethnic	In order of usefulness: • Recruitment coordinator. • Community support. • Visible and accessible site. • Telephone recruiting. • Newspaper ad. • Incentives.
Rosenbaum (1991)	Greek-Canadian women	• Become involved in participants' daily lives. • Participate in church, school, and community activities. • Assist with child care and mental preparation.
Saint-Germain, Bassford & Montano (1993)	Hispanic	For focus groups: • Person-to-person contacts rather than printed information. • Hold focus group in familiar community facility. • Homogenous groups in terms of neighborhood, church attendance, shared friends, or kin. • Moderator from same ethnic group and with community ties.
Shin (1993)	Korean	• Need for personal contact—not responsive to unknown persons or agencies.

Modified from Hautman, M. A. & Bomar, P. (1995). Interactional model for recruiting ethnically diverse research participants. *Journal of Multicultural Nursing and Health, 1*(4), 8-15, 27.

patient's ability to cope, and language barriers impose an additional burden on the patient facing a life-threatening disease. In the disclosure of information revealed to the patient, it is critical that the health care provider be responsive to the patient's wishes as to how much information is revealed and the meaning it has for the patient.

To study differences in the attitudes of elderly subjects from different ethnic groups toward disclosure of the diagnosis and prognosis of a terminal illness, Blackhall, Murphy, Frank, Michel, and Azen (1995) surveyed 200 subjects in each of four ethnic groups (African American, European American, Korean American, and Mexican American). Korean Americans and Mexican Americans were significantly less likely than African Americans or European Americans to be told the diagnosis of metastatic cancer. Korean and Mexican Americans believed that the family should make decisions about life support and end-of-life decision making. Ethnicity was a primary factor related to attitudes; Korean and Mexican Americans held a family-centered model of decision making, whereas African Americans and European Americans favored a patient autonomy model.

An increasing number of patients with cancer have a blurred or mixed cultural identity. Interfaith or interracial marriage or cohabitation, assimilation into a new culture, or a myriad of other reasons may cause a person to have a cultural identity that is a composite of two or more cultures. Receiving a diagnosis of cancer can compound cultural identity conflicts. Religion is yet another factor that determines a patient's acceptance of a cancer diagnosis, and it influences a patient's perceptions of death and the process of dying. The need for autonomy or dependency is culturally influenced and has important implications for the patient in assuming, or not assuming, a participative role in nursing care.

Although there is a trend toward increasing cultural sensitivity in health care settings, there is also the danger of cultural stereotyping. Generic culturally sensitive care plans may not be applicable to all patients of particular ethnicity. Health care providers must relate to each patient as an individual and accommodate the patient's cultural preferences as much as possible.

Educational programs should emphasize the impact of a family's cultural values and beliefs because culturally embedded meanings are attached to illness. For patient teaching to be successful, cultural influences must first be explored (Boston, 1993). Miano, Rojas, and Trujillo (1996) developed the "Platicas Y Merienda" program for the Hispanic population after realizing that the traditional support group model used in many oncology settings had not been effective in reaching this population. The program used education with social and peer support to expand health knowledge.

Mark and Roberts (1994) advocated using ethnosensitive techniques during each patient encounter. Use of this approach ensures that each ethnic group receives the same level of service without having to conform to an arbitrary norm. For example, Hasidic Jewish individuals, members of ultraorthodox sects, represent a cultural subgroup found predominantly in large urban areas. As a result of cultural and religious differences, both Hasidic Jewish groups and health care providers must confront a set of unique issues related to the way in which Hasidim approach a cancer diagnosis. Key variables influencing the patient's response include his or her cultural view of cancer, understanding the role of medicine, theologic world view, issues related to Holocaust survivorship, and sense of identity as expressed in ritual practice.

FUTURE TRENDS

A multicultural approach to health care and cultural awareness education will become important components of future health care delivery systems. Nursing education programs need to fully integrate transcultural nursing in curricula for nurses to be sensitive, knowledgeable, and competent in transcultural nursing. Kulwicki and Bolonik (1996) documented the inadequacy of our current nursing education curriculum; senior baccalaureate nursing students reported little self-confidence in their abilities to deliver care across five major ethnic groups. Rooda (1993) examined knowledge and attitudes of registered nurses toward patients from culturally different backgrounds and found that the nurses in the study knew more about Asian Americans than Hispanic Americans or African Americans, yet the number of African Americans and Hispanic Americans far exceeds the Asian-American population. It was recommended that nurse educators examine the differences in objectives, content, and learning experiences related to cultural diversity that might account for the differences in the nurses' knowledge. Such an examination is essential to prepare nurses to practice in a global society.

Oncology nurses will be practicing in a new era, defined by demographic changes and multicultural challenges. These challenges will be influenced by trends in health care delivery, such as the transformation from traditional health care delivery models to integrated systems. Nurses must be committed to teach and practice holistic health care that is grounded in diverse social structure and cultural and economic realities (Leininger, 1995).

Advances in science and technology will continue to extend life expectancy, alter age distribution in society, and provide new modalities for living and dying. Expanding world economies will enhance opportunities for sharing health information internationally. Burgeoning information systems and communication networks will bridge world distances (Parse, 1995).

CONCLUSION

Although the concepts of cultural diversity and transcultural nursing are fairly new, they have great relevance for patients with cancer. Patients with cancer, in confronting a potentially life-threatening diagnosis, look to their families, friends, and cultural heritage for guidance and support. The patient's cultural heritage influences the patient's perceptions about cancer and its treatment, perceptions about their degree of control over the situation, and beliefs about death and dying.

Nurses' awareness of cultural influences on all aspects of oncology care is needed to effectively provide comprehensive and sensitive nursing care. Nurses must also be aware of their own cultural beliefs and biases and be knowledgeable of how they influence the care they deliver. Although great strides have been made in recognizing cultural influences on health care delivery, embracing cultural diversity and fully integrating transcultural nursing care theory into practice have yet to occur.

REFERENCES

American Cancer Society (1997). *re the key statistics about prostate cancer?* Available URL: http://www.cancer.org.

Anton-Culver, H., Lee-Feldstein, A., & Taylor, T. H. (1993). The association of bladder cancer risk with ethnicity, gender, and smoking. *Annals of Epidemiology, 3,* 429-433.

Banoub-Baddour, S., & Laryea, M. (1992). Culture brokering: The essence of nursing care for preschool children suffering from cancer-related pain. *Canadian Oncology Nursing Journal, 2* (4), 132-136.

Berk, M. L., Schur, C. L., & Cantor, J. C. (1995). Ability to obtain health care: Recent estimates from the Robert Wood Johnson Foundation National Access to Care Survey. *Health Affairs, 14,* 139-146.

Berry, D. L. (1993). Return-to-work experiences of people with cancer. *Oncology Nursing Forum, 20,* 905-911.

Berry D. L., & Catanzaro, M. (1992). Persons with cancer and their return to the workplace. *Cancer Nursing, 15* (1), 40-46.

Blackhall, L. J., Murphy, S. T., Frank, G., Michel, V., & Azen, S. (1995). Ethnicity and attitudes toward patient autonomy. *Journal of the American Medical Association, 274,* 820-825.

Bocchino, C. A. (1996). A new accountability in health care: Providers, insurers, and patients. *Nursing Economics, 11* (1), 44, 51.

Boente, M. P., Hamilton, T. C., Godwin, A. K., Buetow, K., Kohler, M. F., Hogan, W. M., Berchuck, A., & Young, R. C. (1996). Early ovarian cancer: A review of its genetic and biologic factors, detection, and treatment. *Current Problems in Cancer, 20* (2), 83-137.

Boston, P. (1993). Culture and cancer: The relevance of cultural orientation within cancer education programmes. *European Journal of Cancer Care, 3* (2) 72-76.

Bottorff, J. L. (1993). The use and meaning of touch in caring for patients with cancer. *Oncology Nursing Forum, 20,* 1531-1538.

Box, J. C., & Watne, A. L. (1995). Inherited syndromes of colon polyps. *Seminars in Surgical Oncology, 11,* 394-398.

Brown, H. G., & Tai-Seale, M. (1992). Vocational rehabilitation of cancer patients. *Seminars in Oncology Nursing, 8* (3), 202-211.

Brown, L. W., & Williams, R. D. (1994). Culturally sensitive breast cancer screening programs for older Black women. *Nurse Practitioner: American Journal of Primary Health Care, 19* (3), 21, 25-26, 31.

Butterfoss, F. D., Goodman, R. M., & Wandersman, A. (1993). Community coalitions for prevention and health promotion. *Health Education Research, 8,* 315-330.

Calle, E. E., Flanders, W. D., Thun, M. J., & Martin, L. M. (1993). Demographic predictors of mammography and Pap smear screening in U.S. women. *American Journal of Public Health, 83* (1), 53-60.

Caplan, L. S., Wells, B. L., & Haynes, S. (1992). Breast cancer screening among older racial/ethnic minorities and whites: Barriers to early detection. *Journal of Gerontology, 47,* 101-110.

Carpenter, V., & Colwell, B. (1995). Cancer knowledge, self-efficacy, and cancer screening behaviors among Mexican-American women. *Journal of Cancer Education, 10* (4), 217-222.

Cauley, J. A., Lucas, F. L., Kuller, L. H., Vogt, M. T., Browner, W. S., & Cummings, S. R. (1996). Bone mineral density and risk of breast cancer in older women: The study of osteoporotic fractures. Study of Osteoporotic Fractures Research Group. *Journal of the American Medical Association, 276,* 1404-1408.

Chalanda, M. (1995). Brokerage in multicultural nursing. *International Nursing Review, 42* (1), 19-22, 26.

Coffey, D. S. (1993). Prostate cancer: An overview of an increasing dilemma. *Cancer, 71,* 880-886.

Crom, D. B. (1995). The experience of South American mothers who have a child being treated for malignancy in the United States. *Journal of Pediatric Oncology Nursing, 12* (3), 104-114.

Cronsberry, T. (1996). Alternative cancer therapies. *Canadian Nurse, 92* (4), 35-38.

Culley, L. (1996). A critique of multiculturalism in health are: The challenge for nurse education. *Journal of Advanced Nursing, 23,* 564-570.

Davis, K. (1996). Incremental coverage of the uninsured. *Journal of the American Medical Association, 276,* 831-832.

Davis, T. C., Arnold, C., Berkel, H. J., Nandy, I., Jackson, R. H., & Glass, J. (1996). Knowledge and attitude on screening mammography among low-literate, low-income women. *Cancer, 78,* 1912-1920.

Delgado, D. J., Lin, W. Y., & Coffey, M. (1995). The role of Hispanic race/ethnicity and poverty in breast cancer survival. *Puerto Rico Health Sciences Journal, 14* (2), 103-116.

Donnelly, E. (1995). Culture and the meanings of cancer. *Seminars in Oncology Nursing, 11* (1), 3-8.

Fletcher, D. M. (1992). Unconventional cancer treatments: Professional, legal, and ethical issues. *Oncology Nursing Forum, 19,* 1351-1354.

Foulkes, W. D., Bolduc, N., Lambert, D., Ginsburg, O., Olien, L., Yandell, D. W., Tonin, P. N., & Narod, S. A. (1996). The increased incidence of cancer in first degree relatives of women with double primary carcinomas of the breast and colon. *Journal of Medical Genetics, 35,* 534-539.

Gapstur, S. M., Dupuis, J., Gann, P., Collila, S., & Winchester, D. P. (1996). Hormone receptor status of breast tumors in black, Hispanic, and non-Hispanic white women. An analysis of 13,239 cases. *Cancer, 77,* 1465-1471.

Garrett, C. T., Liscia, D. S., Nasim, S., & Ferreira-Gonzalez, A. (1995). Genetics of colorectal and breast cancer. *Clinical Laboratory Medicine, 15,* 957-971.

Gehlhaart, C. (1995). Therapeutic touch as adjuvant therapy for cancer pain. *Cancer Pain Update, 36,* 5-6.

Giger, J. N., & Davidhizar, R. E. (1995). *Transcultural nursing: Assessment and intervention* (2nd ed.). St. Louis: Mosby.

Gilliland, F. D., Hunt, W. C., & Key, C. R. (1996). Ethnics variation in prostate cancer survival in New Mexico. *Cancer Epidemiology, Biomarkers, and Prevention, 5,* (4), 247-251.

Given, B. A., Given, C. W., & Harlan, A. N. (1994). Strategies to meet the needs of the rural poor. *Seminars in Oncology Nursing, 10,* (2), 114-122.

Glen, S., & Jownally, S. (1995). Privacy: A key nursing concept. *British Journal of Nursing, 4* (2), 69-72.

Gorey, K. M., & Vena, J. E. (1994). Cancer differentials among U. S. blacks and whites: Quantitative estimates of socioeconomic-related risks. *Journal of the National Medical Association, 86* (3), 209-215.

Greenwald, H. P., Polissar, N. L., & Dayal, H. H. (1996). Race, socioeconomic status and survival in three female cancers. *Ethnicity and Health, 1* (1), 65-75.

Griffin, F. N. U. (1994). The health care system: Factoring in the ethnicity, cultural, and health care needs of women and children of color. *ABNF Journal, 5* (5), 130-133.

Gudmundsdottir, M., Martinson, P. V., & Martinson, I. M. (1996). Funeral rituals following the death of child in Taiwan. *Journal of Palliative Care, 12* (1), 31-37.

Hanks, G. E., & Scardino, P. T. (1996). Does screening for prostate cancer make sense? *Scientific American, 275* (3), 114-115.

Hautman, M. A., & Bomar, P. (1995). Interactional model for recruiting ethnically diverse research participants. *Journal of Multicultural Nursing & Health, 1* (4), 8-15, 27.

Hayes, R. B., Liff, J. M., Pottern, L. M., Greenberg, R. S., Schoenberg, J. B., Schwartz, A. G., Swanson, G. M., Silverman, D. T., Brown, L. M., Hoover, R. N., & Fraumeni, J. F. (1995). Prostate cancer risk in U. S. blacks and whites with a family history of cancer. *International Journal of Cancer, 60,* 361-364.

Helman, C. G. (1990). *Culture, health, and illness* (2nd ed.). Oxford: Butterworth-Heinemann.

Herbst, S. (1995). Survivorship: Redefining the cancer experience. The economics of long-term survival. *Oncology Nursing Forum, 22,* 527-532.

Hoeman, S. P., Ku, Y. L., & Ohl, D. R. (1996). Health beliefs and early detection among Chinese women. *Western Journal of Nursing Research, 18,* 518-533.

Hord, M. H., Smith, T. L., Culbert, S. J., Frankel, L. S., & Pinkel, D. P. (1996). Ethnicity and cure rates of Texas children with acute lymphoid leukemia. *Cancer, 77,* 563-569.

Jackson, L. (1994). Cancer education and screening for Asian-Americans. *Journal of the American Academy of Physician Assistants, 7,* 693-699.

Jennings, K. (1996). Getting black women to screen for cancer: Incorporating health beliefs into practice. *Journal of the American Academy of Nursing Practitioners, 8,* (2), 53-59.

Jones, P. S. (1996). Asian American women caring for elderly patients. *Journal of Family Nursing, 2* (1), 56-75.

Kagawa-Singer, M. (1995). Socioeconomic and cultural influences on cancer care of women. *Seminars in Oncology Nursing, 11* (2), 109-119.

Katz, J. S. (1996). Caring for dying Jewish people in a multicultural/religious society. *International Journal of Palliative Nursing, 2* (1), 43-47.

Kelly, A. W., Fores Chacori, M. D. M., Wollan, P. C., Trapp, M. A., Weaver, A. L., Barrier, P. A. Franz, W. B., & Kottke, T. E. (1996). A program to increase breast and cervical cancer screening for Cambodian women in a midwestern community. *Mayo Clinic Proceedings, 71,* 437-444.

Kim, H. S., Schwartz-Barcott, D., Holter, I. M., & Lorensen, M. (1995). Developing a translation of the Mcgill pain questionnaire for cross-cultural comparison: An example from Norway. *Journal of Advanced Nursing, 21,* 421-426.

Kodiath, M. F., & Kodiath, A. (1995). A comparative study of patients who experience chronic malignant pain in India and the United States. *Cancer Nursing, 18,* 189-196.

Kudzma, E. C. (1992). Drug response: All bodies are not created equal. *American Journal of Nursing, 92* (12), 48-50.

Kulwicki, A., & Bolonik, B. J. (1996). Assessment of level of comfort in providing multicultural nursing care by baccalaureate nursing students. *Journal of Cultural Diversity, 3* (2), 40-45.

Lancaster, J. M., Wooster, R., Mangion, J., Phelan, C. M., Cochran, C., Gumbs, C., Seal, S., Barfoot, R., Collins, N., & Bignell, G. (1996). BRCA2 mutations in primary breast and ovarian cancers. *Nature Genetics, 13* (2), 238-240.

Landis, S. H., Murray, T., Bolden, S., Wingo, P. A. (1998). Cancer statistics, 1998. *CA: A Cancer Journal for Clinicians, 48*(1) 6-29.

Larson, E. (1994). Exlusion of certain groups from clinical research. *Image: Journal of Nursing Scholarship, 26* (3), 185-190.

Leininger, M. (1996). Culture care theory, research, and practice. *Nursing Science Quarterly, 9* (2), 71-78.

Leininger, M. (1995). Teaching transcultural nursing to transform nursing for the 21st century. *Journal of Transcultural Nursing, 6* (2), 2-3.

Leininger, M. (1994). Time to celebrate and reflect on progress with transcultural nursing. *Journal of Transcultural Nursing, 6* (91), 2-3.

Lovejoy, N. C. (1996). Multinational approaches to cervical cancer screening: A review. *Cancer Nursing, 19* (2), 126-134.

Lowe, J. I., Barg, F. K., & Bernstein, M. W. (1995). Educating African Americans about cancer prevention and detection: A review of the literature. *Social Work in Health Care, 21* (4), 17-36.

Mandelblatt, J., Andrews, H., Kerner, J., Zauber, A., & Burnett, W. (1991). Determinants of late stage diagnosis of breast and cervical cancer: The impact of age, race, social class, and hospital type. *American Journal of Public Health, 81,* 646-649.

Mark, N., & Roberts, L. (1994). Ethnosensitive techniques in the treatment of the Hasidic patient with cancer. *Cancer Practice: A Multidisciplinary Journal of Cancer Care, 2* (3), 202-208.

McCabe, M. S., Varricchio, C. G., & Padberg, R. M. (1994). Efforts to recruit the economically disadvantaged to national clinical trials. *Seminars in Oncology Nursing, 10* (2), 123-129.

McCue, J. D. (1993). The naturalness of dying. *Journal of the American Medical Association, 273,* 1039-1043.

McIlrath, S. (1996). Leave job, keep insurance. *American Medical News, 39* (31), 1, 38.

Meyer, H. (1996, August 12). Indemnity insurance: Down but not out. *Medical Economics, 73* (16), 209-215, 219, 220.

Miano, L. Y., Rojas, M. S., & Trujillo, M. (1996). "Platicas y merienda": Reaching Spanish-speaking patients in an oncology setting. *Cancer Practice: A Multidisciplinary Journal of Cancer Care, 4* (4), 199-203.

Modan, B. (1996). Carrying a genetic passport for ovarian cancer. *Lancet, 348,* 1328.

Mokuau, N., & Fong, R. (1994). Assessing the responsiveness of health services to ethnic minorities of color. *Social work in health care, 20* (2), 23-34.

Montbriand, M. J. (1995). Alternative therapies as control behaviours used by cancer patients. *Journal of Advanced Nursing, 22,* 646-454.

Montbriand, M. J. (1993). Freedom of choice: An issue concerning alternative therapies chosen by patients with cancer. *Oncology Nursing Forum, 20,* 1195-1201.

Morales, E. (1994). Meaning of touch to hospitalized Puerto Ricans with cancer. *Cancer Nursing, 17,* 464-469.

Morrison, C. (1996). Determining crucial correlates of breast self-examination in older women with low incomes. *Oncology Nursing Forum, 23,* 83-93.

Morrison, R. S., & Meier, D. E. (1995). Managed are at the end of life. *Trends in Health Care, Law, & Ethics, 10* (1 and 2), 91-96.

Murata, S. (1996, September 23). At last, a presidential signature on a health bill. *Medical Economics, 73* (18), 8-9.

Nance, T. A. (1995). Intercultural communication: Finding common ground. *JOGNN: Journal of Obstetric, Gynecologic, and Neonatal Nursing, 24* (3), 249-255.

National Cancer Institute Cancer Screening Consortium for Underserved Women (1995). Breast and cervical cancer screening among underserved women. *Archives of Family Medicine, 5,* 617-624.

National Organization for Women (1996) *[Online].* Available URL.: http://www.now.org.

Neus, E. (1996, August 22). Health care reform: Who it helps, how it works. *USA Today,* p. A4.

Nishimoto, P. (1996). Venturing into the unknown: Cultural beliefs about death and dying. *Oncology Nursing Forum, 23,* 889-894.

Nomura, A. M., Goodman, M. T., Kolonel, L. N., & Fu, T. (1994). The rise of cancer among the elderly in Hawaii. *Hawaii Medical Journal, 53* (7), 188-193, 200.

Nwoga, I. A. (1994). Traditional healers and perceptions of the causes and treatment of cancer. *Cancer Nursing, 17,* 470-478.

Olsen, S. J., & Frank-Stromberg, M. (1993). Cancer prevention and early detection in ethnically diverse populations. *Seminars in Oncology Nursing, 9* (3), 198-209.

O'Neill, J. (1994). Ethnic minorities neglected by palliative care providers? *Journal of Cancer Care, 3* (4), 215-220.

Optenberg, S. A., Thompson, I. M., Friedrichs, P., Wojcik, B., Stein, C. R., & Kramer, B. (1995). Race, treatment, and long-term survival from prostate cancer in an equal-access medical care deliver system. *Journal of the American Medical Association, 274,* 1599-1605.

Otero-Sabogal, R., Sabogal, F., Perez-Stable, E. J., & Hiatt, R. A. (1995). Dietary practices, alcohol consumption, and smoking behavior: Ethnic, sex, and acculturation differences. *Journal of the National Cancer Institute, 18* (Monograph), 73-82.

Palos, G. (1994). Cultural heritage: Cancer screening and early detection. *Seminars in Oncology Nursing, 10* (2), 104-113.

Papadatou, D., Yeantopoulos, J., & Kosmidis, K. V. (1996). Death of a child at home or in hospital: Experiences of Greek mothers. *Death Studies, 20* (3), 215-235.

Parham, G. P., & Hicks, M. L. (1995). Gynecologic cancer among the socioeconomically disadvantaged. *Cancer, 76* (Suppl 10), 2176-2180.

Parse, R. R. (1995). Nursing knowledge for the 21st century: An international commitment. *Nursing Science Quarterly, 5* (1), 8-12.

Perez-Stable, E. J., Sabogal, F., & Otero-Sabogal, R. (1995). Use of cancer-screening tests in the San Francisco Bay area: comparison of Latinos and Anglos. *Journal of the National Cancer Institute, 18* (Monograph), 147-153.

Perez-Stable, E. J., Sabogal, F., Otero-Sabogal, R., Hiatt, R. A., & McPhee, S. J. (1992). Misconceptions about cancer among Latinos and Anglos. *Journal of the American Medical Association, 268,* 3219-3223.

Perkins, P., Cooksley, C. D., & Cox, J. D. (1996). Breast cancer. Is ethnicity an independent prognostic factor for survival? *Cancer, 78,* 1241-1247.

Peters, D., Smith, J., Horrigan, C., & Mills, S. (1994). Chemotherapy-induced nausea, *Complementary Therapies in Medicine, 2* (4), 193-194.

Pfeffer, N., & Moynihan, C. (1996). Ethnicity and health beliefs with respect to cancer: A critical review of methodology. *British Journal of Cancer, 29* (Suppl.), 66-72.

Pham, C. T., & McPhee, S. J. (1992). Knowledge, attitudes, and practices of breast and cervical cancer screening among Vietnamese women. *Journal of Cancer Education, 7,* 305-310.

Pickett, M. (1993). Cultural awareness in the context of terminal illness. *Cancer Nursing, 16* (2), 102-106.

Pollitzer, W., & Anderson, J. (1990). Ethnic and genetic differences in bone mass: A review with a hereditary and environmental perspective. *American Journal of Clinical Nutrition, 52,* 181.

Porter, H. (1996). In profile. Therapeutic touch in part of Windsor's cancer care. *Canadian Oncology Nursing Journal, 6* (3), 157-160.

Powe, B. D. (1995). Cancer fatalism among elderly Caucasians and African Americans. *Oncology Nursing Forum, 22,* 1355-1359.

Rice, B. (1996, August 12). Look who's on the malpractice hot seat now. *Medical Economics, 73* (13), 193-205.

Rimer, B. K. (1994). Interventions to increase breast screening. Lifespan and ethnicity issues. *Cancer, 74* (Suppl. 1), 323-328.

Robinson, J. K., Rademaker, A. W., Goolsby, C., Traczyk, T. N., & Zoladzc, C. (1996). DNA ploidy in nonmelanoma skin cancer. *Cancer, 77,* 284-291.

Rooda, L. A. (1993). Knowledge and attitudes of nurses toward culturally different patients: Implications for nursing education. *Journal of Nursing Education, 32,* 209-213.

Ross, B. M. (1996, November 19). Drive-through mastectomies the next target. *USA Today,* p. 13A.

Roukema, M. (1997, February 14). Quit putting profits first. *USA Today,* p. 13A.

Russell, K. M., & McCammon, A. O. (1995). Health are barriers for Latinos: An assessment for advocacy. *Journal of Multicultural Nursing & Health, 1* (3), 8-16.

Saiki, S. C., Martinson, I. M., & Inano, M. (1994). Japanese families who have lost children to cancer: A primary study. *Journal of Pediatric Nursing: Nursing Care of Children and Families, 9,* 239-250.

Samelson, E. J., Speers, M. A., Ferguson, R., & Bennett, C. (1994). Racial differences in cervical cancer mortality in Chicago. *American Journal of Public Health, 84,* 1007-1009.

Sartor, O. (1996). Early detection of prostate cancer in African American men with an increased familial risk of disease. *Journal of the Louisiana State Medical Society, 148,* 179-185.

Schmidt, R. H. (1994, December 18). Services: A future of low productivity growth? *The Washington Times,* p. A2.

Sekhon, S. K. (1996). Insights into South Asian culture: Food and nutrition values. *Topics in Clinical Nutrition, 11* (4), 47-56.

Shanahan, M., & Brayshaw, D. L. (1995). Are nurses aware of the differing health care needs of Vietnamese patients? *Journal of Advanced Nursing 22,* 456-464.

Sheldon, T., & Parker, H. (1992). The use of 'ethnicity' and 'race' in health research: A cautionary note. In W. I. U. Ahmad (Ed.), *The politics of race and health.* Bradford, England: University of Bradford Press.

Skinn, B. (1994). The relationship of belief in control and purpose in life to adult lung cancer patients' inclination to use unproven cancer therapies. *Canadian Oncology Nursing Journal, 4* (2), 66-71.

Skorneck, C. (1997, January 30). Mastectomy reconstruction coverage urged. *The Times-Picayune,* p. A9.

Sowell, T. (1994). *Race and culture: A world view.* New York: Basic Books.

Spector, R. (1991). *Cultural diversity in health and illness* (3rd ed.). Norwalk, CT: Appleton & Lange.

Suarez, L. (1994). Pap smear and mammogram screening in Mexican-American women: The effects of acculturation. *American Journal of Public Health, 84,* 742-746.

Trill, M. D., & Holland, J. (1993). Cross-cultural differences in the care of patients with cancer: A review. *General Hospital Psychiatry, 15,* 21-30.

Tripp-Reimer, T., & Lively, S. (1988). Cultural considerations in therapy. In C. K. Beck, R. P. Rawlins, & S. Williams (Eds.), *Mental health and psychiatric nursing.* St. Louis: Mosby.

U. S. Department of Commerce, Bureau of Census (1992). *Population projections of the Untied States by age, sex, and Hispanic origins: 1990 to 2050.* Washington, DC: U. S. Government Printing Office.

Walker, R., Lucas, W., & Crespo, R. (1994). The West Virginia rural cancer prevention project. *Cancer Practice: A Multidisciplinary Journal of Cancer Care, 2,* 421-426.

Weissman, J. (1996). Uncompensated hospital care: Will it be there when we need it? *Journal of the American Medical Association, 276,* 823-828.

Whittemore, A. S., Wu, A. H., Kolonel, L. N., John, E. M., Gallagher, R. P., Howe, G. R., West, D. W., Teh, C. Z., & Stamey, T. (1995). Family history and prostate cancer risk for black, whites and Asian men in the United States and Canada. *American Journal of Epidemiology, 141,* 732-740.

Wilkes, G., Freeman, H., & Prout, M. (1994). Cancer and poverty: Breaking the cycle. *Seminars in Oncology Nursing, 10* (2), 79-88.

Yi, J. K. (1994a). Factors associated with cervical cancer screening behavior among Vietnamese women. *Journal of Community Health, 19,* 189-200.

Yi, J. K. (1994b). Breast cancer screening practices by Vietnamese women. *Journal of Women's Health, 3* (3), 205-213.

Zahm, S. H., & Fraumeni, J. F. (1995). Racial, ethnic, and gender variations in cancer risk: Considerations for future epidemiologic research: *Environmental Health Perspectives, 103* (Suppl.), 283-286.

Practice of Oncology Nursing

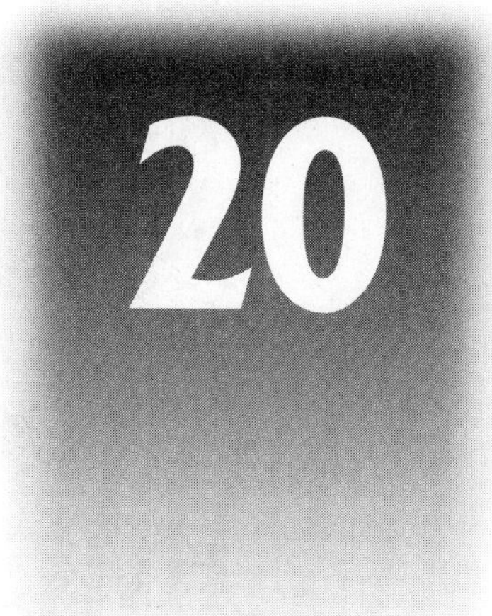

Breast Cancer-In Situ Disease

Noreen Facione, RN, PhD
Deborah Hamolsky, RN, MS

EPIDEMIOLOGY

According to American Cancer Society's (ACS's) estimates of cancer prevalence, in 1998, 180,300 women will be newly diagnosed with breast cancer (Landis, Murray, Bolden, & Wingo, 1998). An estimated 12% of the cases will be women with carcinoma in situ (Hankey, Brinton, Kessler, & Abrams, 1993; Surveillance, Epidemiology and End Results [SEER], 1995).

Carcinoma in situ (CIS) is defined as a malignant cellular proliferation that has not extended through the basement membrane into the surrounding tissue. Lobular carcinoma in situ (LCIS) can be present in lobules or ducts, as can ductal carcinoma in situ (DCIS). The exact diagnosis is made based on pathologic interpretation of the structure and cellular elements of the tumor, not on the location of the abnormal cellular proliferation (Barth, Brenner, & Giuliano, 1995; Carty, Royle, Carter, & Johnson, 1995; Connolly & Nixon, 1996; Hetelekidis, Schnitt, Morrow, & Harris, 1995; Wood, 1996).

Data from the National Cancer Institute's (NCI's) SEER program demonstrate a 213% increase in the incidence of breast cancer in white women and 153% increase in black women from 1983 to 1989. Since the 1973 baseline statistics, the overall increase in the incidence of DCIS is 557%, with 15.8 American women per 100,000 developing DCIS in 1992 (Ernster, Barclay, Kerlikowske, Grady, & Henderson, 1996). In the early 1980s, DCIS accounted for only 0.8% to 3.2% of all breast cancers. By 1990, DCIS accounted for 13% of all breast cancers and 20% to 30% of breast cancers detected by mammography (Barth et al., 1995; Ernster et al., 1996). This large increase is believed to be the result of an increase in the use of screening mammography in the United States. From 1983 to 1992 the overall incidence of DCIS has increased by more than 300% for women over age 40 (SEER, 1995). It has been estimated, that by the year 2005, the proportion of breast cancers that are diagnosed as DCIS will approach 33% (Cady et al., 1996). Figs. 20-1 and 20-2 display the incidence of carcinoma in situ in white and black women reported in the National Cancer Institute's SEER data.

Although most breast cancer is discovered by women themselves, CIS is most often first identified by screening mammography and only a minority of the cases are found by clinical breast examination (Weiss et al., 1996). DCIS is most typically identified as visible, suspicious microcalcifications on mammography. When the disease presents as a palpable mass, it is usually subsequently diagnosed as comedo-type DCIS. The diagnosis of LCIS is often an incidental finding that is made based on pathologic examination of the tissue obtained during a biopsy or surgery. Lobular carcinoma in situ is a pathologic diagnosis that is distinct from lobular hyperplasia and atypical lobular hyperplasia.

LCIS and DCIS share a common characteristic—their lack of metastatic potential. However, these two in situ breast cancers differ in terms of biologic behavior, prognosis, treatment, and follow-up care. Table 20-1 lists the features of DCIS and LCIS. With the increased incidence of both of these noninvasive or preinvasive tumors, there is clinical controversy and changing recommendations regarding surveillance and treatment, particularly for DCIS.

The most provocative question surrounding this disease is the exact relationship between CIS of the breast and other more typically invasive forms of breast cancer. Approximately 15% to 20% of women with LCIS go on to develop breast cancer in the same breast. An additional 10% to 15% of these women develop breast cancer in the contralateral breast. Based on these findings, LCIS is generally believed to represent a potential precursor of invasive disease (Kerlikowske, Barclay, Grady, Sickles, & Ernster, 1997). Some investigators have estimated that the proportion of CIS tumors that develop into invasive forms of breast cancer may be as high as 50% (Weiss et al., 1996). The evidence for this progression of disease was strengthened by the recent demonstration that a tumor suppressor gene on chromosome 11 is mutated or missing in both in situ and invasive breast cancers (Holzman, 1995).

A diagnosis of LCIS places an individual at an increased risk for developing invasive breast cancer in the future. Invasive breast cancer can develop in one or both breasts. In those women who do develop invasive lobular breast can-

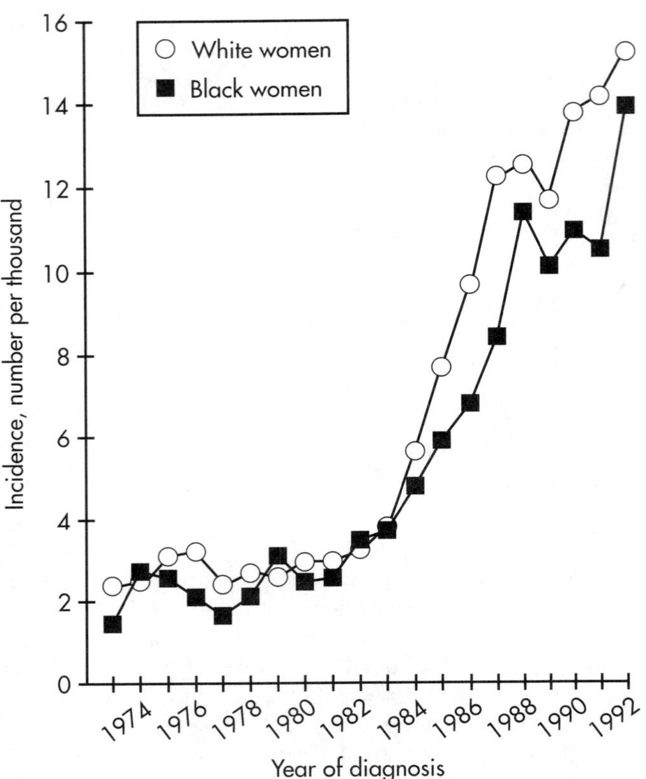

Fig. 20-1 Age-adjusted incidence rates for ductal carcinoma in situ of the breast from 1973 to 1992 for white and black women in the United States. (From DiSaia, P. J. [1997]. *Clinical gynecologic oncology.* [5th ed.]. St. Louis: Mosby.)

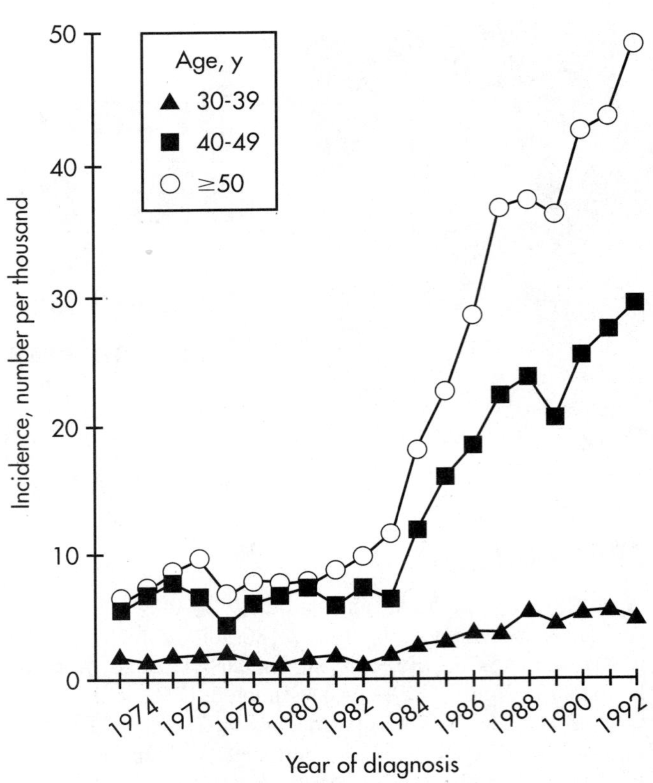

Fig. 20-2 Age-adjusted incidence rates in the United States for ductal carcinoma in situ (DCIS) of the breast from 1973 to 1992, all races combined. (From DiSaia, P. J. [1997]. *Clinical gynecologic oncology.* [5th ed.]. St. Louis: Mosby.)

TABLE 20-1 Features of Ductal and Lobular Carcinoma In Situ

	Ductal Carcinoma	Lobular Carcinoma
Average age	Late 50s	Late 40s
Menopausal status	70% postmenopausal	70% premenopausal
Clinical signs	Breast mass, Paget's disease, nipple discharge	None
Mammographic signs	Microcalcification	None
Risk of subsequent carcinoma	30%-50% at 10-18 years	25%-30% at 15-20 years
Site of subsequent carcinoma:		
Same breast	99%	50%-60%
Other breast	1%	40%-50%

Adapted from Page, D. L., Steel, C. M., & Dixon, J. M. (1995). Carcinoma in situ and patients at high risk of breast cancer. *British Medical Journal, 310,* 39-42.

cer, the average time from the diagnosis of LCIS to the development of invasive cancer is 10 to 15 years. This risk is higher than in the general population, and most patients who develop invasive breast cancer are diagnosed with ductal carcinoma (Morrow & Schnitt, 1996).

At the present time, women begin their menses many years earlier; have many more menstrual cycles, fewer pregnancies, and later menopause; and give birth to their first child on average at an older age than women in the past. In addition, they have exogenous oral contraceptive hormones available to them for pregnancy prevention, and women may use perimenopausal and postmenopausal hormone replacement therapy, extending the years that estrogen and progesterone are active on their breast tissue. Many researchers and clinicians are wondering if the current increase in the incidence of in situ breast cancer is attributable to these changes in women's lifestyle.

RISK FACTORS

Risk factors describe characteristics and behaviors that are associated with an increased likelihood of developing a dis-

TABLE 20-2 Risk Factors for Ductal Carcinoma In Situ (DCIS)

Risk Factors	Association with DCIS
Age	Older women have an increasing incidence of DCIS
Family history of breast cancer	Increased incidence DCIS in women with familial history of infiltrating breast carcinoma
Previous breast surgery or a history of benign breast disease	Mixed reports of an increased incidence of DCIS
Later age at birth of first child or nulliparity	Mixed reports of an increased incidence of DCIS
Early menarche or late menopause	Mixed reports of an increased incidence of DCIS
Alcohol consumption	No relationship reported

ease compared with the likelihood of the population as a whole developing the same disease. Not everyone who shares the characteristic or behavior pattern will actually develop the disease. In time, causal explanations connecting various risk factors to the development of breast cancer may become available. At the present time, however, the task of explaining why each of the identified risk factors is associated with an increased likelihood of developing breast cancer remains to be determined.

Researchers are working to determine specific risk factors associated with the development of CIS. Several studies have noted a number of shared risk factors with invasive breast cancer, namely increasing age and a positive family history of breast cancer (i.e., first-degree relative with breast cancer) (Kerlikowske et al., 1997; Weiss et al., 1996). Most investigators have observed a relationship between nulliparity, early menarche, later age at first child birth, and previous breast surgery and an increased incidence of DCIS (Kerlikowske et al., 1997; Weiss et al., 1996).

In a study of nearly 40,000 women, 30 years of age and older, who were undergoing screening mammography, Kerlikowske and colleagues (1997) reported that an increased incidence of DCIS was associated with nulliparity, early menarche, later age at first child birth, and previous breast surgery in women who were 50 years of age or older, but not in women between the ages of 30 and 49. These investigators noted that among women 50 years of age and older, a palpable mass was associated with an increased incidence of invasive cancer but not with an increased risk for DCIS. In addition, an apparent decreased risk of DCIS was noted for younger women who had a body mass index greater than or equal to 25 kg/m^2. As of January 1998, no studies have been reported linking alcohol consumption, the use of oral contraceptives, or the use of hormone replacement therapy with in situ disease in the breast. Table 20-2 lists the risk factors for DCIS of the breast.

CHEMOPREVENTION

Chemoprevention is defined as the use of specific natural and synthetic chemical agents to reverse or suppress carcinogenesis and prevent the development of invasive cancer. Carcinogenesis is a multistep process including a premalignant phase that does not always proceed to malignancy. Therefore certain compounds may be capable of reversing premalignant changes or preventing the formation of second primary tumors. The principles of chemoprevention are to identify agents that have the capability to inactivate oncogenes or activate tumor suppressor genes. Chemoprevention activities in breast cancer target women at increased risk for cancer development and uses systemic drugs and nutrient therapies.

Women with breast cancer who are at highest risk for the development of a secondary tumor and women with a known genetic predisposition to develop breast cancer (e.g., Li Fraumeni syndrome; BRCA1 families; and individuals at risk for hereditary breast, ovarian, or colon cancer) are considered candidates for chemoprevention. Chemopreventive agents are believed to work in several ways, including (1) changing the pathway of cells from proliferation to differentiation; (2) binding with carcinogens present in the body and/or enhancing the metabolic breakdown of these carcinogens, making them inactive agents; or (3) inducing the death of the aberrant (i.e., premalignant or malignant) cell.

Currently, two agents are under investigation for the chemoprevention of breast cancer—tamoxifen and retinoid compounds. Tamoxifen has been shown in large clinical trials of women with breast cancer to decrease the incidence of contralateral (opposite side) breast cancer and to increase patients' disease-free interval and overall survival (Cook et al., 1995; Early Breast Cancer Trialists' Collaborative Group, 1992). In addition, tamoxifen has been shown to prevent the development of mammary cancer in animal models. However, long-term use of tamoxifen has been reported to increase women's risk of endometrial cancer and, particularly in premenopausal women, to increase women's risk of developing ovarian cancer (Cook et al., 1995).

Retinoid compounds (e.g., vitamin A compounds) have been shown to control abnormal proliferation of the epithelium. In animal models a decrease in mammary tumors has been demonstrated. A major clinical hurdle that needs to be overcome before vitamin A can be used as a chemopreventive agent is the liver toxicity associated with the compound. An open clinical trial of fenretinide, a retinoid less toxic to the liver, is under way in Italy to examine the impact of the drug on breast cancer prevention (NSABBP, 1994; Veronesi, DePalo, Costa, Fornelli, & Decensi, 1996; Veronesi, Salvadori et al., 1996). In addition, a trial was opened recently in the United States to test the effectiveness of beta carotene as a chemopreventive agent for breast cancer in postmenopausal women (Hunter & Willett, 1996).

Chemoprevention trials use biomarkers as indicators of

the advancement or reversal of the process of carcinogenesis as a result of the treatment under study. Currently, two of the most commonly studied biomarkers are indicators of genetic mutations within the cells: the presence of micronuclei and the presence of abnormal cellular proliferation. Using biomarkers as an intermediate indicator of the effects of a treatment on carcinogenesis has provided an improvement over awaiting evidence of the occurrence of a malignancy, but to date, the identification of biomarkers for breast carcinogenesis lacks the specificity needed (i.e., the presence of known biomarkers does not guarantee that carcinogenesis will occur) to warrant the launching of an intervention trial to identify women at risk for developing breast cancer (Hong & Lippman, 1995).

A chemoprevention trial is in process at the M. D. Anderson Cancer Center in Houston, Texas to develop biomarkers for tamoxifen and 4-hydroxyphenylretinamide (4-HPR: fenretinide). One or both of these drugs are being given to women with DCIS or small invasive breast lesions in the interval between the initial diagnostic core biopsy and definitive surgery. These researchers will track excessive cell proliferation, alterations in nuclear morphology, and angiogenesis, as well as oncogenes and tumor suppressor genes regulated by the proposed chemopreventive agents (Dhingra, 1995).

PATHOPHYSIOLOGY

Normal Anatomy and Physiology of the Female Breast

The female breasts lie on the ventral surface of the thorax within the superficial facia of the chest wall. The breasts begin at the second rib and extend vertically to the sixth or seventh intercostal space and laterally from the sternum to the midaxillary line. An important consideration, particularly in relationship to breast cancer, is that breast tissue extends into the axilla. This area should be included in an examination of the breast.

As illustrated in Fig. 20-3, the female breast is composed of 15 to 20 pyramid-shaped lobes that are separated and supported by Cooper ligaments. Each lobe contains approximately 20 to 40 lobules or alveoli that subdivide into numerous functional units called *acini.* Each acinus is lined with a layer of epithelial cells capable of secreting milk and a layer of subepithelial cells capable of contracting to squeeze milk from the acinus. The acini empty into a network of collecting and ejecting ducts that reach the nipple pores. The lobules are surrounded by muscle strands and fatty connective tissue.

The nipple is a pigmented, cylindrical structure usually located in the fourth or fifth intercostal space. On its surface

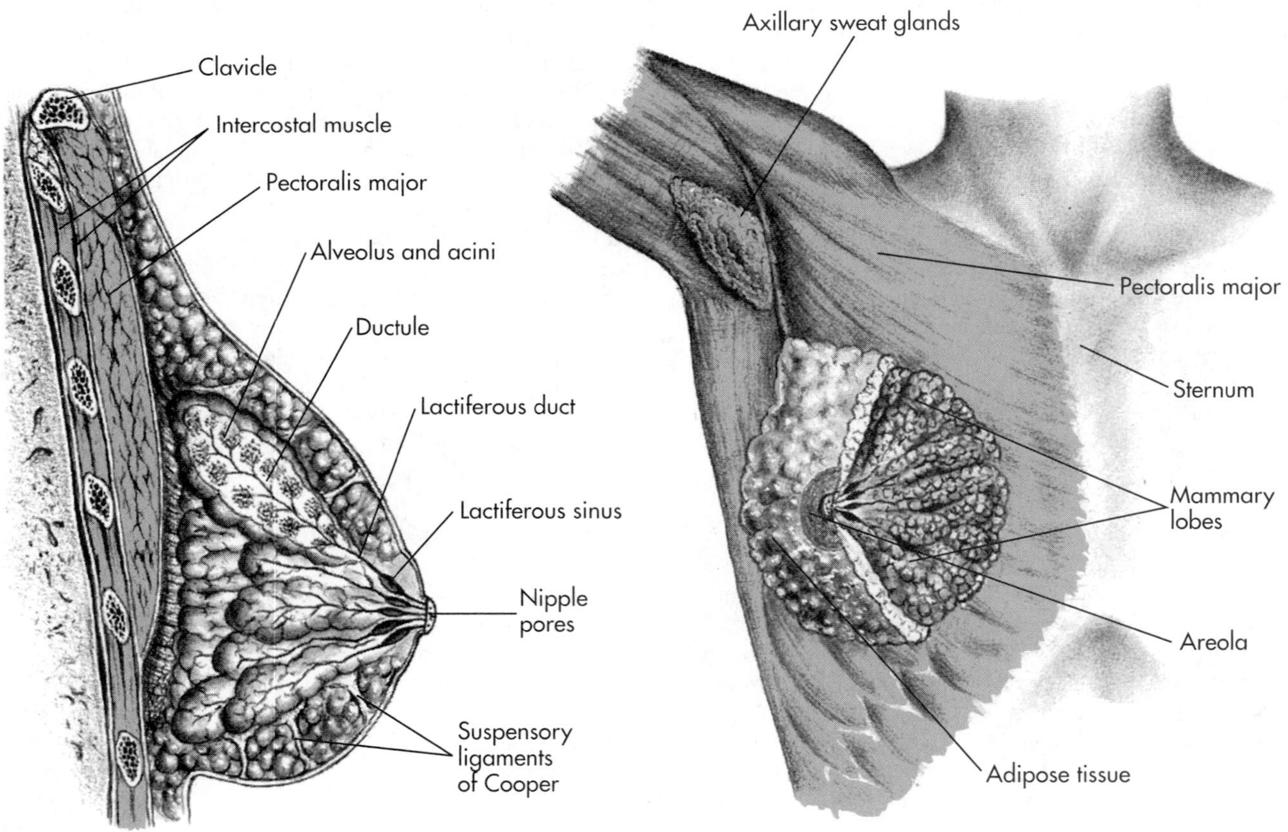

Fig. 20-3 The female breast. (From Thompson, J. M., McFarland, G. K., Hirsch, J. E., & Tucker, S. M. [1997]. *Mosby's clinical nursing.* [4th ed.]. St. Louis: Mosby.)

lie multiple openings, one from each lobule. The areola is the pigmented, circular area around the nipple and may be 15 to 60 mm in diameter. The nipple and areola contain smooth muscles that are innervated by the sympathetic nervous system.

The breast contains an extensive capillary network that is supplied by the internal and lateral thoracic arteries. The venous system empties into the superior vena cava. The breast receives sensory innervation from branches of the second and sixth intercostal nerves and from the cervical plexus. As illustrated in Fig. 20-4, the lymphatic drainage of the breast occurs largely through the axillary nodes. However, approximately 25% of lymphatic drainage of the breast occurs through the transpectoral and internal mammary routes.

Breast development occurs at the onset of puberty. Estrogen secretion stimulates the growth of breast tissue. Full differentiation and development of breast tissue are mediated by several hormones, including estrogen, progesterone, prolactin, growth hormone, thyroid hormone, insulin, and cortisol. The major function of the female breast is to provide a source of nutrition for the newborn. The breasts are also a source of sexual pleasure and in some cultures are associated with female sexuality (Robinson & Huether, 1996).

The Process of Carcinogenesis

CIS represents a histologically heterogeneous group of breast lesions characterized by the proliferation of neoplastic epithelial cells that are confined to the ducts or the lobules of the breasts. Carcinoma in situ can be divided histologically into groupings of cells in the lobules with varying degrees of atypia (LCIS) or more commonly, neoplastic cell clusters in the ducts (DCIS). The histopathologic diagnosis of DCIS is difficult. DCIS is a pathologic abnormality arising out of the terminal duct of the lobule. It is sometimes difficult to differentiate DCIS from atypical ductal hyperplasia in more low-grade lesions and from microinvasion or invasion with higher-grade lesions (Hetelekidis et al., 1995). There is no universal agreement among pathologists regarding the diagnosis of DCIS, as witnessed by the upgrading or downgrading of lesions when they are reviewed by another pathologist (Morrow, 1995a, 1996).

No universally accepted classification system for DCIS exists, but many pathologists divide the disease into comedo and noncomedo (e.g., papillary, micropapillary, cribriform, solid) types. Comedo-type DCIS is characterized by an outer ring of malignant cells and intraluminal necrosis. The tumor often shows a higher nuclear grade, aneuploidy, and a higher proliferation rate and is considered more aggressive than the noncomedo types (Barth et al., 1995).

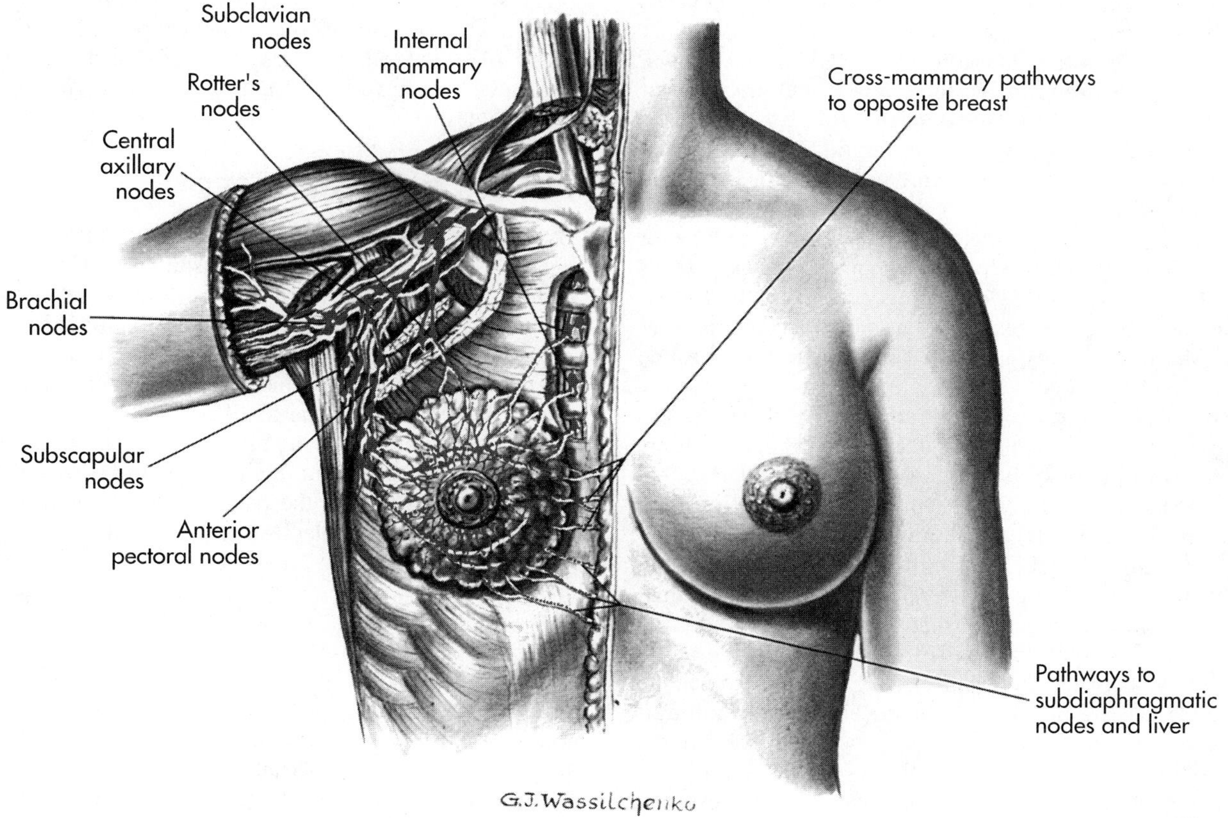

Fig. 20-4 Lymphatic drainage of the female breast. (From Bobak, I. M. [1993]. *Maternity and gynecologic care: The nurse and the family.* [4th ed.]. St. Louis: Mosby.)

Some in situ lesions exhibit features of both LCIS and DCIS. Women who are diagnosed through screening mammography may have localized or widespread microcalcifications. These microcalcifications typically show a branching pattern of varying density. Patients with symptomatic DCIS generally seek a provider evaluation because of a self-discovered breast mass, nipple discharge, or Paget's disease.

In a study that examined 96 patients from several studies whose DCIS was initially misdiagnosed (Frykberg, Ames, & Bland, 1991; Page, Dupont, Rogers, Jensen, & Schuyler, 1995), 30 patients (31%) went on to develop invasive carcinoma within the next 24 years, and most frequently within the next 10 years. These lesions were not discovered on the basis of screening mammography. However, these findings suggest the need for follow-up care of women with low-grade DCIS lesions, particularly when women are younger at the time of diagnosis of DCIS.

Many authors suggest that future research will assist them in differentiating higher-risk cases. Markers of the invasive potential of tumors such as proliferation rate, aneuploidy of the tumor cells, c-erB-2 (also HER2-neu) overexpression, or the absence of Nm23 gene expression (i.e., a suppressor gene of metastasis) are useful in identifying women at high risk (Barth et al., 1995; Carty et al., 1995). Work in this area is limited at the present time because in the past most women with DCIS were treated with mastectomy, and our estimates of the natural history of DCIS are based largely on retrospective data.

Although the exact natural history of CIS is not known, currently DCIS is considered to be a potential precursor of invasive disease and to the extent that this is so, it shares the same pathophysiology as infiltrating breast cancer. Breast cancer is the result of carcinogenic processes in a breast cell. The development of a breast tumor depends on the ratio of the rate of cell proliferation to the rate of genetically determined cell death (apoptosis). This ratio is dependent on the process of angiogenesis (i.e., the formation of new blood vessels that can support cell proliferation). Measures of apoptosis and angiogenesis determine tumor doubling time.

The development of an infiltrating breast cancer is believed to involve complex interactions between multiple factors. Most tumors arise from a single cell mutation that leads to uncontrolled cell growth. Specific genetic mutations have been identified that are associated with the relatively rare cases of inherited infiltrating breast cancer. The mechanisms underlying the development of CIS are less clear. Currently, geneticists using such techniques as fluorescence in situ hybridization (FISH) are attempting to establish links between the occurrence of CIS and the genetic mutations that are linked with the development of infiltrating breast cancer. Additional work focuses on performing a deoxyribonucleic acid (DNA) analysis of breast biopsies to evaluate for other genetic mutations that may be present in the tissues of women with DCIS and LCIS.

Many investigators are concluding that there is a very high concordance between genetic alterations in invasive carcinoma and genetic alterations in DCIS. This finding leads them to hypothesize that a continuum exists between the development of DCIS and invasive carcinoma, with the major genetic events in carcinogenesis already established at the time of preinvasive disease (Ottesen et al., 1995). Millikan, Dressler, Geradts, and Graham (1995) have argued that studying CIS may reveal more clearly the risk factors for infiltrating carcinoma because epidemiologic studies of precursor lesions are conducted closer in time to the exposures suspected to be causes of the cancer and may reduce recall bias and other errors. Box 20-1 lists the genetic anomalies that have been identified in DCIS and LCIS tissue samples.

Box 20-1
Genetic Findings Reported in DCIS and LCIS Tissue Samples

Ductal Carcinoma in Situ (DCIS)

- Alterations of chromosome 1 (Munn, Walker, & Varley, 1995)
- Alterations of chromosome 17 (Munn et al., 1996; Murphy et al., 1995; Visscher et al., 1996)
- Multiple sites of loss of heterozygosity (LOH) that is the loss of one allele (Radford et al., 1995; Zhuang et al., 1995)
- ERBB2 gene amplification (Murphy et al., 1995)
- Histologic necrosis (apoptotic death; Bodis et al., 1996)

Lobular Carcinoma in Situ (LCIS)

- Chromosome 17 abnormalities (Visscher et al., 1996)

ROUTES OF METASTASES

By definition, metastasis is not associated with CIS. However, CIS is treated based on the assumption that the natural history of CIS includes progression to invasive carcinoma of the breast. In nine studies that evaluated for axillary node metastases in patients with DCIS (Silverstein et al., 1991), the incidence of positive nodal involvement was 0. In a more recent review of the SEER data from 1973 to 1987, Berg and Hutter (1995) reported that the incidence of regional nodal involvement in patients with DCIS was 1% or less, with almost all of the patients (98%) cured by local-regional therapy regardless of the size of the tumor.

ASSESSMENT

History

Clinical evaluation of the patient involves a detailed history that is inclusive of all relevant history about physical symptoms and a full psychosocial history, a complete physical examination, and a variety of diagnostic tests (Table 20-3). The signs and symptoms depend on the stage of the disease at the time of diagnosis. To establish a definitive diagnosis, a tissue biopsy is performed.

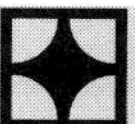

TABLE 20-3 Assessment of the Patient for In Situ Breast Cancer

	Assessment Parameters	Typical Abnormal Findings
History	A. Personal and Social History 1. Age 2. Family history 3. History of benign breast disease or breast surgery 4. Nulliparity 5. Age of menarche/menopause B. Breast Symptoms	A. Personal and Social Risk Factors 1. Increased incidence in older women 2. Increased incidence of ductal carcinoma in situ (DCIS) in women with a familial history of infiltrating breast cancer 3. Potential risk factor 4. Potential risk factor 5. Early menarche and late menopause may be a risk factor B. Usually asymptomatic disease that is detected on routine mammogram.
Physical Examination	A. Clinical Breast Examination (CBE)	A. Before the widespread use of screening mammography, patients presented with a palpable mass and nipple discharge. Patients may still present with a palpable mass.
Diagnostic Tests	A. Mammography B. Stereotactic Core Biopsy C. Needle Localization Biopsy D. Fine Needle Aspirate Biopsy	A. On mammography, DCIS exhibits a diffuse and often linear and extensive pattern of pleomorphic calcifications. B. Stereotactic core biopsy is the preferred procedure for suspected DCIS. C. Obtain a biopsy specimen for pathologic diagnosis. D. Not routinely used to establish a diagnosis of carcinoma in situ.

Physical Examination

Clinical Breast Examination. Breasts are glandular tissue that develop in the female to supply milk to infant offspring. The breasts are composed of lobules where milk is made and a tubule and duct system several inches long that conduct the milk to the nipple. Fat and connective tissue surround these structures in a sac that extends outward toward the axilla in the upper outer quadrant of each breast. The lymphatic system of the breast is composed of the axillary node chain. These are the lymph nodes where breast cancer cells are believed to immediately metastasize. Ten percent of breast cancers are identified primarily through observation and palpation during a clinical breast examination (CBE) (Farwell, Foster, & Costanza, 1993). Box 20-2 lists considerations that should be kept in mind when performing a CBE to decrease the chance of missing an early breast cancer.

Mammographic screening and CBE remain the most promising methods for early detection of breast cancer. As illustrated in Fig. 20-5, DCIS may be visible on a mammogram as microcalcifications (Foschini, Fornelli, Peterse, Mignani, & Eusebi, 1996; Walt, 1995). In the last few years, many dollars have been spent to educate women to have screening mammograms. Several large scale studies have attempted to demonstrate the potential benefit associated with screening mammography (Leitch, 1995; Miller, Baines, To, & Wall, 1992; Smart, Hendrix, Rutledge, & Smith, 1995). Because the relationship between CIS and infiltrating breast cancer still requires clarification, the definitive assessment of the benefit derived from screening mammography remains to be determined.

Box 20-2
Considerations for Clinicians Performing a Clinical Breast Examination

1. Perform a standardized examination, being mindful of the woman's life history. This examination includes an observation of the motion of the breast as the woman changes position.
2. Do not allow demographic statistics to influence conclusions drawn about any individual breast examination findings. An individual woman is not adequately represented by the aggregate profile of breast cancer.
3. Do not use risk factor status to influence conclusions drawn about any individual breast examination findings. Most breast cancers occur in women with no known risk factors, and in the absence of a known high risk genetic mutation, even women who are otherwise high risk have a low probability of breast cancer on any given examination throughout life.
4. A negative mammogram is not a reason to delay a biopsy of a suspicious breast abnormality found on clinical breast examination. In patients with observable/palpable breast abnormalities, the purpose of mammography is to further define the clinical findings and to rule out the presence of unexpected nonpalpable abnormalities in the ipsilateral or contralateral breast.
5. Take a careful history. The history-taking allows the clinician to know the concerns of the woman and to hear the character and duration of any abnormalities she may have noted on self-examination. It also provides the basis for future counseling and education.

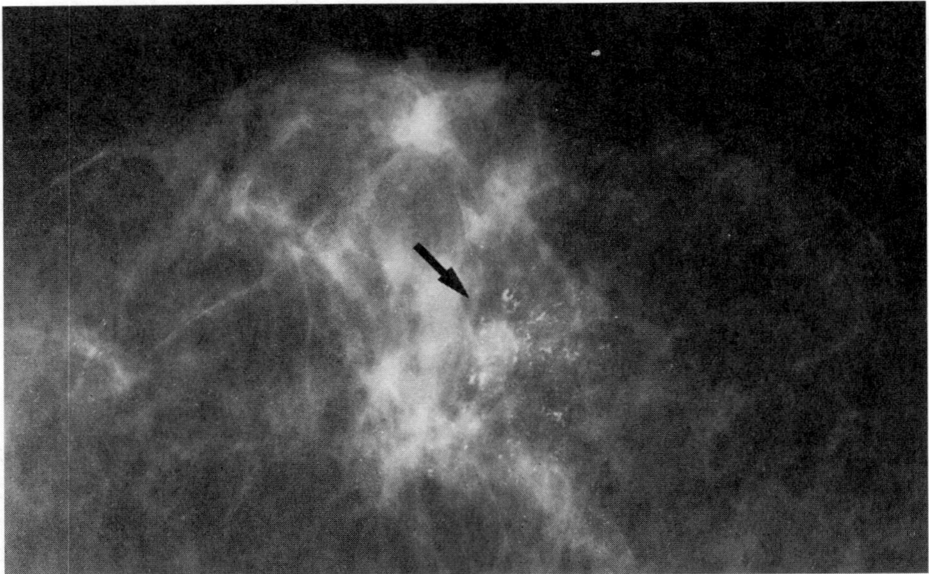

Fig. 20-5 A group of irregular microcalcifications *(arrow)* without associated mass or tissue density proved to be DCIS. (From Walt, A. J. [1995]. Screening for breast cancer. In J. L. Cameron [Ed.], *Current surgical therapy* [5th ed.]. St. Louis: Mosby.)

A useful quick reference guide for clinicians regarding mammography referral and follow-up recommendations is available through the U.S. Department of Health and Human Services (Bassett et al., 1994; Linver, Osuch, Brenner, & Smith, 1995). Despite these guidelines, women's participation in mammographic screening is suboptimal. The reasons for nonparticipation include disinterest, comorbid medical problems, fear of radiation associated with the procedure, and the lack of either medical insurance or available financial assets for either health promotion or the treatment of the disease if a breast cancer is discovered (Facione & Facione, 1997; Lidbrink, Frisell, Brandberg, Rosendahl, & Rutqvist, 1995).

Clinical Presentation of DCIS. Before the widespread use of screening mammography, most patients with DCIS had palpable breast masses or nipple discharge, or were seen in association with Paget's disease. In a study by Kerlikowske and colleagues (1997), palpable DCIS lesions were distributed in proportions similar to those observed with invasive tumors. Eleven percent were found in the upper quadrant and 47% in the upper outer quadrant, whereas approximately 10% of DCIS tumors were found in the retroareolar area. In the same study (Kerlikowske et al., 1997), infiltrating breast cancers were found in the upper (10%), upper-outer (43%), and retroareolar (14%) areas in a similar distribution.

Careful history-taking of a symptomatic woman may help differentiate DCIS from other types of breast disease. For example, lesions of the nipple that do not heal within 2 weeks should be regarded as suspicious of Paget's disease and not dismissed as topical skin irritations requiring little or no treatment. Discharge from the nipple, although most commonly associated with benign breast disease, should be evaluated as a possible indication of DCIS, particularly if the discharge is clear or bloody rather than milky (Ibanez, Giannotti-Filho, & Da Silva Neto, 1993).

Diagnostic Tests

Although presentation of DCIS as a palpable mass or its diagnosis as an incidental finding on a biopsy of an otherwise benign lesion still occurs, most DCIS is detected through a routine mammogram as microcalcifications (Fig. 20-5). The microcalcifications appear as white dots on the mammogram and are better visualized on spot magnification views (e.g., diagnostic mammograms with targeted magnified views of suspicious areas). These microcalcifications are thought to be secondary byproducts of cellular debris from cellular necrosis within the ducts involved with DCIS. Calcifications are classified as benign, indeterminate, or suspicious. Suspicious calcifications are further classified as being of low, moderate, or high suspicion. It is generally recommended to biopsy indeterminate or suspicious microcalcifications unless there is long-term stability in biopsy-proven benign microcalcifications. Not all microcalcifications, even those in characteristically suspicious or linear clusters with a coarse granular appearance, prove to be DCIS. Thus a biopsy (e.g., stereotactic core biopsy or needle localization) is required to make the definitive diagnosis (Foster, 1996).

Today, 60% to 65% of in situ cancer is diagnosed through mammography (Weiss et al., 1996). Currently, DCIS makes up about 17% to 35% of the breast cancers detected through mammography (Kerlikowske et al., 1997; Page, Steele, & Dixon, 1995). By comparison, LCIS is rare, making up only 1% of breast cancers detected by mammography screening (Page, Steele, & Dixon, 1995).

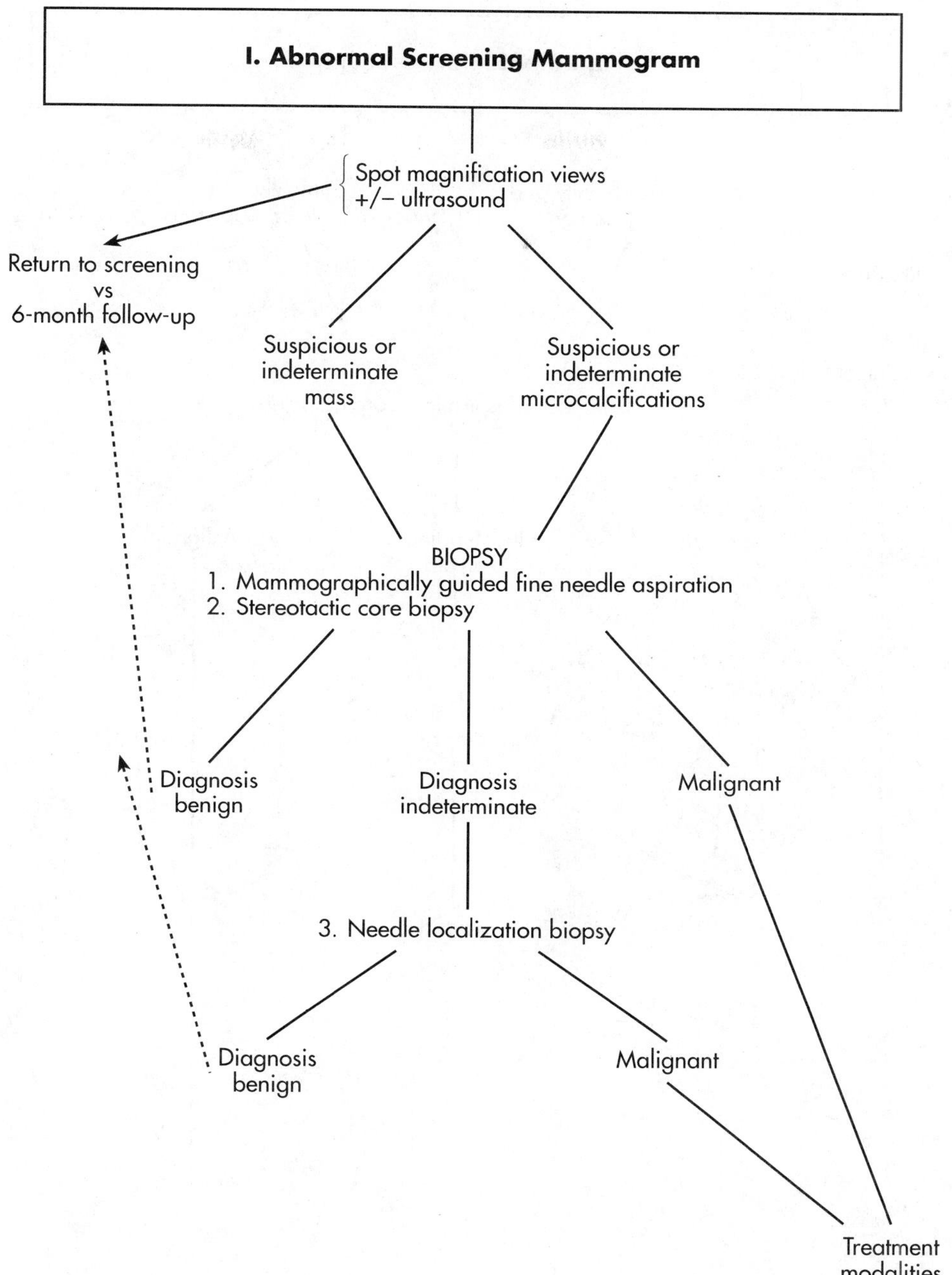

Fig. 20-6 Diagnostic workup: I. Abnormal screening mammogram.

Making or Ruling Out a Breast Cancer Diagnosis. Figs. 20-6 and 20-7 describe two pathways that can be used to guide the diagnostic workup for a breast abnormality, depending on the clinical presentation of the abnormality (e.g., abnormal mammogram, palpable breast lump, or palpable abnormal density). For a mammographic abnormality, radiologic or complementary radiologic and surgical procedures are used to obtain biopsy tissue. The radiologist recommends the appropriate biopsy procedure based on the size and position of the abnormality. All biopsies can be done under local anesthesia, with or without sedation, and on an outpatient basis. The number of breast biopsies performed in the United States each year has been estimated to be near 1 million (Hall, Storella, Silverstone, & Wyshak, 1988). Today, 4% of all breast biopsies are performed for CIS (Cady et al., 1996).

Stereotactic Core Biopsy. Stereotactic core biopsy has been advocated increasingly as an alternative to open excisional biopsy and is the preferred procedure for suspected DCIS. However, it is not recommended in women who are unable to tolerate lying on their abdomens. Table 20-4 describes the stereotactic core biopsy procedure. The postprocedure symptoms include breast soreness and possible bruising. There is no scar on the breast, and no notice-

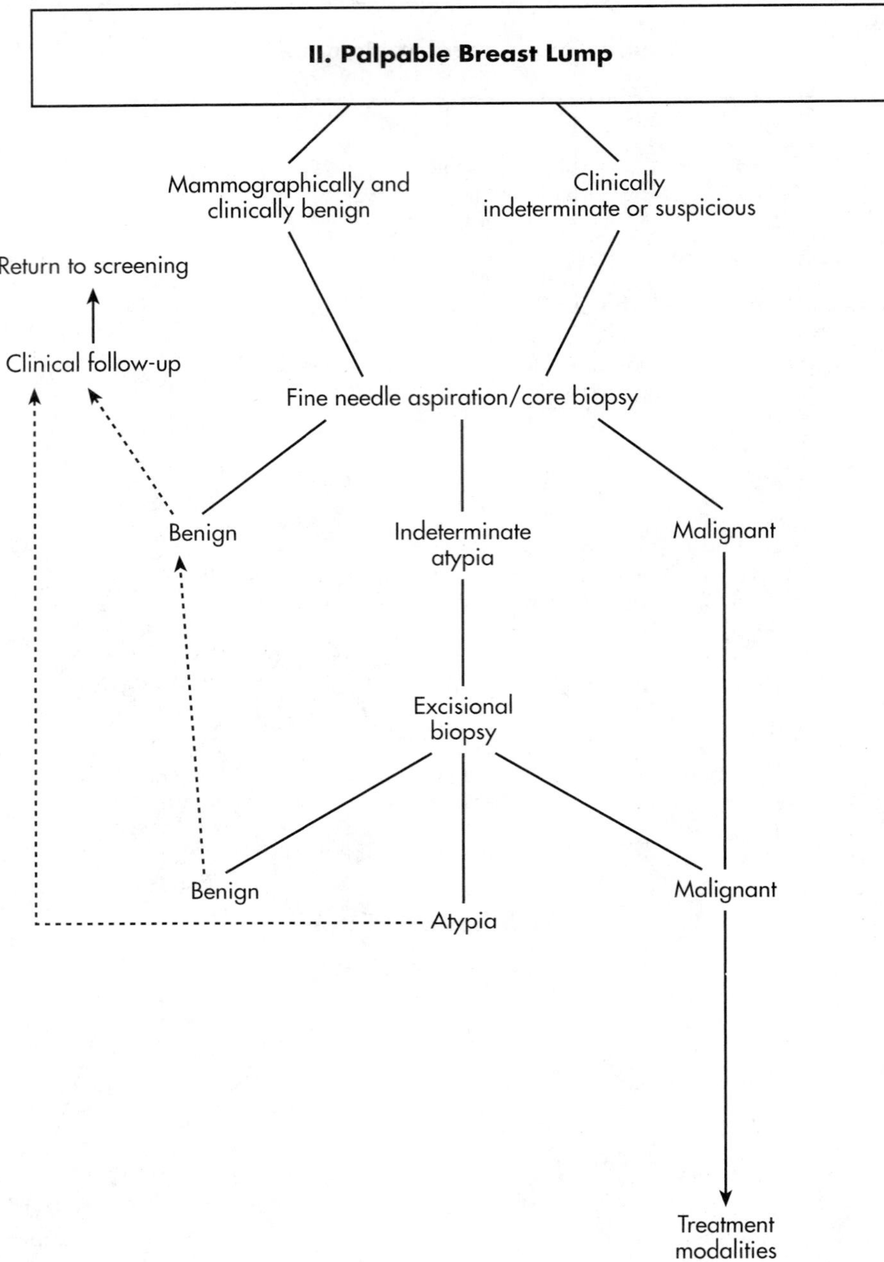

Fig. 20-7 Diagnostic workup: II. Palpable breast lump.

able scar tissue is evident on future mammograms. The advantages of stereotactic core biopsy include lower cost and less trauma to the patient, and when the lesions are benign, the absence of cosmetic deformity and breast scarring on follow-up mammograms. The stereotactic core biopsy, where there is a definitive diagnosis, allows for pretreatment planning and fewer steps in the diagnostic pathway.

A recent review of 431 core needle biopsies done at the University of California Los Angeles (UCLA) demonstrated a definitive outcome in 96% of the biopsies with 6 to 38 months of follow-up. Among the biopsies, 179 were malignant, 13 demonstrated atypia, and 239 were benign. A false-negative rate of 1.7% was reported. These data corroborate the safety and efficacy of stereotactic core biopsy in the hands of experienced providers (Nguyen et al., 1996). Even with this technique, there is still a small miss rate, usually owing to movement of the tissue after the breast has been removed from compression (Morrow, 1995b).

Needle Localization Biopsy. If the diagnosis following a stereotactic core biopsy is not definitive or if stereotactic core biopsy is not recommended clinically, a needle localization biopsy is performed. This procedure is done on an outpatient basis and is accomplished in two steps. Step 1 occurs in the radiology department, where a

TABLE 20-4 Patient Preparation for Stereotactic Core Biopsy

Procedural Considerations:

1. Position the woman on her stomach on the specially designed table (hole at breast level) with the breast positioned in the opening.
2. Elevate the table and place the breast in the plastic compression device.
3. Obtain mammographic images to visualize and position the abnormality.
4. Inject local anesthetic and make a small incision to accommodate the biopsy needle. A standard 14-gauge needle is used. In some cases, smaller needles are used.
5. Guided by computer visualization, obtain core biopsy samples from designated areas. These biopsies are obtained at the center of the visualized abnormality and usually in the areas that correspond with 12, 3, 6, and 9 o'clock on a watch face. The device makes a gunlike noise when it injects the needle through the skin.
6. Apply pressure to the site and a dry, sterile dressing.
7. If the workup is for a finding of abnormal calcifications on mammography, obtain a radiograph of the biopsy specimen to verify the presence of calcifications in the specimen before the specimen is taken to the pathology lab.
8. Discharge the patient home.

thin wire is placed into or around the abnormality with mammographic guidance. Step 2 occurs in the operating room, where the surgeon removes the abnormality using the wire to locate its exact position. The surgeon, with the patient under either local anesthesia alone or with local anesthesia and sedation, performs an excisional biopsy, and then a specimen radiograph is done to verify that the abnormality is in the specimen. The incision is sutured and a dressing is applied. The woman is discharged home after recovery from sedation, if it was used. Postprocedural symptoms may include breast pain or discomfort, bruising, bleeding, infection, or wound dehiscence. The woman will have a scar on the breast and architectural distortion evident on future mammograms. Many women report awareness of sensations in the area of the biopsy for months or years after the procedure (Kelly & Winslow, 1996).

Concern has been raised about whether there are major histologic discrepancies between stereotactic core biopsies and the more extensive needle localization biopsies, particularly in relation to differentiating between infiltrating carcinomas and DCIS (Morrow, 1995b). Neither biopsy method is without error, and additional studies are needed to determine which procedure results in the more accurate differential diagnosis of breast cancer.

Previously, excisional biopsies were performed as the initial procedure in a one-step approach to breast cancer surgery. Histologic analyses were performed on frozen sections of the breast biopsy tissue, and if the frozen sections were positive, the definitive surgical procedure was performed at the same time. Today most excisional biopsies are performed on an outpatient basis, usually under local anesthesia. Open biopsies for smaller tumors are intended to remove the entire observable lesion with clear margins. The lesion is classified histologically by using permanent sections of the tissue specimen, and the borders of the biopsy specimen are carefully examined for the presence of cancer. When the tumors are larger, a small portion of the tumor may be removed initially to determine its histologic classification and to perform receptor assays to determine the optimal treatment approach. Women with positive biopsies are provided with counseling regarding their treatment options and the advisability of a second surgical procedure, re-excision mastectomy, or lumpectomy. A part of the two-step surgical procedure, the mastectomy or partial mastectomy procedure is performed with the patient under general anesthesia.

Fine Needle Aspiration Biopsy. A fine needle aspiration biopsy (FNAB) is not performed routinely for the diagnosis of CIS because of the difficulty in obtaining accurate results. Occasionally, this procedure is used to diagnosis CIS when the patient's presenting symptom is a palpable mass and the diagnosis of DCIS is not suspected (Grant, Groellner, Welsh, & Martin, 1986).

STAGING

Staging is a method of describing the extent of a tumor at the time of diagnosis and is used as a prognostic indicator and to determine treatment options. Staging is determined based on the size of the tumor, presence of and number of positive lymph nodes, margins of the tumor resection, tumor histology (structure of the breast cancer cells), hormonal receptor status of the tumor, tumor grade, and other individually relevant prognostic factors. The American Joint Committee on Cancer's (AJCC, 1988) TNM classification system is used to stage breast cancer. The TNM system considers the primary tumor (T), lymph node involvement (N), and the presence or absence of metastatic spread (M). By definition, CIS lesions are staged as Tis lesions (carcinoma in situ or Paget's disease of the nipple).

MEDICAL MANAGEMENT

DCIS is believed to be a clinical entity requiring intervention at the time of diagnosis, as corroborated by studies that demonstrated progression of DCIS to invasive breast cancer in patients who refused the recommended therapy. Traditionally, symptomatic DCIS was treated with mastectomy. However, considerable controversy exists as to the most appropriate treatment options. The panel, who made recommendations about breast cancer treatment at the Fifth International Conference on Adjuvant Therapy of Primary Cancer, agreed that the population of patients having a lower than 10% mortality rate at 10 years should not be candidates for routine systemic adjuvant therapy (Goldhirch, Wood, Senn, Glick, & Gelber, 1995). Carty and colleagues (1995) argued that although local excision with or without radiation therapy is associated with a significant risk of local recurrence of DCIS or invasive cancer, salvage surgery is usually successful; they warn that clinicians may be overtreating small lesions discovered on screening mammography.

Table 20-5 displays the NCI's Patient Data Query (PDQ) State-of-the-Art Treatment Summary for CIS (1995). Updates are available to providers and clinicians by calling 1-800-4 CANCER or on the World Wide Web at http://www.icic.nci.nih.gov. Treatment for LCIS consists of observation with annual bilateral mammography or bilateral mastectomy.

Medical Management of LCIS

Definitive recommendations for treatment await results of randomized clinical trials and future genetic research. Although a diagnosis of LCIS indicates an increased risk for the development of invasive breast cancer, as of yet, there are no clear criteria to divide women with this diagnosis into subsets with different degrees of risk to match those who are at greatest risk with increased surveillance and earlier clinical interventions. It is possible that chemopreventive agents (e.g., tamoxifen and retinoids) may alter the natural history of LCIS.

Some patients inquire about, and some clinicians may favor, bilateral prophylactic mastectomy. However, this procedure is not recommended generally because most women with LCIS never develop invasive breast cancer, and even those who do are diagnosed 10 to 15 years later. In the future, women who test positive for BRCA1, BRCA2, and other genetic markers may be asked to consider prophylactic mastectomy or the use of chemopreventive agents or prevention strategies to reduce their risk of developing invasive breast cancer. However, at the present time, there is consensus to recommend and develop financial systems to support the use of long-term regular CBEs every 6 months and mammography every year. The mammographer and all clinicians who perform CBEs need to be informed if a woman has a history of LCIS in order to make appropriate decisions when subtle changes are noted during either or both of these procedures (Wood, 1996).

Table 20-5 State-of-the-Art Treatment Recommendations

Stage	Treatment
Stage 0 in situ (ductal)	1. Mastectomy with excision of lymph nodes around the axillary tail without a formal level I dissection of axillary lymph nodes 2. Lumpectomy or partial or segmental mastectomy with radiotherapy
in situ (lobular) Not considered breast cancer	1. No treatment after biopsy with careful follow-up examinations and mammograms 2. Bilateral prophylactic mastectomies 3. Tamoxifen (which is in clinical trials) after biopsy to help prevent development of invasive cancer

From National Cancer Institute PDQ State-of-the-Art Cancer Treatment Summary. (1995). *Breast Cancer, 1,* 39.

Medical Management of DCIS

A great deal remains to be learned about the natural history of DCIS. Progress in this area is limited by prior treatment practices and the number of studies of DCIS cases that compare, unlike presentations. Before widespread screening mammography, DCIS presented as a palpable mass, and the standard treatment was mastectomy. Now this population of patients can only be evaluated for the development of contralateral breast cancer or the occurrence of infiltrating breast cancer with metastatic disease. A small number of patients who refused treatment for their disease were followed, but in the comparison group who were treated, local excision with clear margins was not done consistently, making comparisons with the untreated patients problematic (Page, Dupont, Rogers, Jensen, & Schuyler, 1995).

A second group of studies (Wood, 1996) monitored patients who were treated for DCIS for recurrence after their initial treatment. Most of these studies now have 5 to 10 years of clinical follow-up; it is from these studies that the mean time from diagnosis of DCIS to the development of invasive breast cancer has been estimated at about 10 years (Wood, 1996).

A third group of studies consists of larger randomized clinical trials with better control of pathologic evaluation and tumor margins. These studies compared the efficacy of various treatment options (i.e., mastectomy, excision alone, excision with radiation alone, and excision with radiation followed by chemoprevention) for the treatment of DCIS (Fisher et al., 1993; National Surgical Adjuvant Breast and Bowel Project [NSABBP], 1994). Protocol B-06 from the NSABBP is one of the prospective, randomized trials trying to determine the efficacy of various treatment options for DCIS (NSABBP, 1994). Although Protocol B-06 was designed to compare mastectomy, lumpectomy alone, and lumpectomy with radiation therapy in patients with infiltrating carcinoma of the breast, 78 of the patients in this study were found to have only DCIS. Of these 78 patients, 28 had a mastectomy, and one died of metastatic disease without a local recurrence. An additional 27 patients were treated with lumpectomy and radiation therapy and two had local recurrences. Twenty-one patients with DCIS were treated with lumpectomy alone, and nine had a local recurrence. There was no difference in survival between the three treatment groups in this study, but larger studies are needed to definitively examine the value of these treatment approaches.

In a second NSABBP Protocol (B-17), 818 women with DCIS were assigned randomly to one or two treatment arms, namely lumpectomy or both lumpectomy and radiation therapy. The attainment of negative margins was required for all women in the study. There were fewer recurrences (7% vs 28%) and a decreased incidence of invasive breast cancer (2.9% vs 10.5%) in the group treated with lumpectomy and radiation therapy compared with the group treated with lumpectomy alone (Fisher et al., 1993).

Later, NSABBP Protocol B-24 was designed to measure the benefit of adding tamoxifen as a chemopreventive agent for patients treated with lumpectomy and radiation therapy. Patients were randomized to one of two treatment arms: 5 years of tamoxifen or a placebo. The definitive interpretation of this study's findings is limited by the lack of clear tumor margins and the incomplete removal of all microcalcifications in all of the study cases (NSABBP, 1994).

Currently, a number of European trials are evaluating the role of radiation therapy with excision in the treatment of DCIS (Wood, 1996). The controversy about treatment approaches for DCIS will continue until more is learned about the natural history of DCIS and the impact of various treatment modalities on the disease process, as well as on survival. To obtain definitive answers about the effectiveness of various treatment options, DCIS must be better defined pathologically and clinically. Precisely because DCIS has an unknown, but believed to be long trajectory or natural history, the development, implementation, and evaluation of clinical trials to resolve the existing controversies are likely to take years to accomplish.

Until then, an individual patient diagnosed with DCIS can choose from three treatment modalities: (1) mastectomy with or without reconstruction (immediate or delayed); (2) excision of the DCIS with the goal of obtaining clear margins, possibly followed by a re-excision to meet that goal; or (3) excision followed by radiation therapy. Careful pathologic evaluation, including a possible second opinion, should classify the DCIS by type (comedo vs noncomedo) and grade (low- vs high-grade). A thorough history should be done to determine the presence of other risk factors for the development of infiltrating breast cancer. Previous mammograms should be reviewed carefully, including spot magnification views, before the biopsy procedure and after the surgical excision to exclude the presence of other suspicious or indeterminate microcalcifications.

Careful collaborative reviews among the various specialties (e.g., surgery, pathology, radiology, radiation therapy), despite all of the debate it may engender, is essential to the development of an optimal treatment plan. Treatment recommendations can then be made with an honest description of what is and what is not known, and with a rationale for the subsequent recommendations that are tailored as much as possible to the individual patient. These interdisciplinary discussions must include input from the patient regarding her needs for risk aversion; the meanings she gives to her breast and its loss; her feelings and thoughts about radiation therapy; and her willingness to participate in randomized clinical trials. In an arena of controversy, with the possibility that a patient who seeks second and third opinions may hear two or three different opinions or differences in emphasis, medical uncertainty adds a great deal of stress to the diagnosis of DCIS for both women and their clinicians. It is important to attempt to incoporate patients into clinical trials, when relevant, so that more informed decisions about treatment options can be made.

Surgical Excision. The goal of surgical intervention is to remove all known DCIS from the breast. Mammography is used to define areas of suspicious calcifications for biopsy, localize the abnormality for biopsy and/or excision, supply intraoperative radiographs to confirm the location of microcalcifications in the specimen, verify that no other suspicious microcalcifications remain in the breast postoperatively, and provide a new postsurgical baseline. The pathologist delineates the surgical margins and describes the type, grade, and size of the DCIS in the specimen.

To define the margins accurately, the specimen must be removed as a single piece, the margins must be inked, and the sutures or some other mutually agreed on system must be used by the surgeon to orient the specimen. Because definitive pathologic examination requires time, a second surgery (re-excision) may be necessary to achieve clear margins. As with lumpectomy for invasive breast cancer, patients should be informed before surgery that there is a chance that a re-excision may be necessary. When fully informed of this possibility, some patients opt for a single surgery with mastectomy rather than face an uncertain outcome with a breast-conserving surgical excision.

No clear consensus standard exists for the attainment of adequate surgical margins, although the visualization of normal duct epithelium in the margin of tissue that is excised is the desired result. Wood (1996) suggests 5-mm margins for low-grade lesions and 8- to 10-mm margins for higher-grade and larger lesions.

Radiation Therapy. The next clinical decision that needs to be made, after completion of the excision with clear margins and a confirmatory postoperative mammogram, is whether the patient should receive radiation therapy. Adjuvant radiation therapy of the breast consists of 4500 to 5000 cGy, 5 days a week for 5 to 6 weeks of therapy. Controversy exists about whether and under what conditions to boost (treat with a concentrated dose) the prior tumor bed with additional radiation therapy (1500 to 2000 cGy). The decision-making process includes an evaluation of the risk of local recurrence as determined by type of DCIS, margins, size, location of known DCIS, and any other factors that influence a patient's risk.

Research findings, consisting mainly of small studies conducted under varying conditions, do not provide definitive information to guide decision making for an individual patient, but rather provide preliminary data about the differences between various treatment options. An examination of eight studies of excision alone for DCIS (311 patients) demonstrated a local failure rate of 2% to 54% (mean: 20%). Eleven studies of both excision and radiation therapy (525 patients) had a local failure rate ranging from 5% to 21% (average 9%). Overall, follow-up was longer for the excision-only studies, limiting comparison of the study findings. Approximately half the recurrences were DCIS and half were invasive breast cancer, regardleess of whether radiation therapy was used (Barth et al., 1995; Carty et al., 1995; Wood, 1996). Fig. 20-8 illustrates the development of noninfiltrating and infiltrating carcinoma in patients treated with and without radiation therapy.

Mastectomy. The final treatment option for DCIS is mastectomy with or without immediate or delayed reconstruction. Until recently, this classic approach was the only option used for DCIS. In six studies, involving 495 patients,

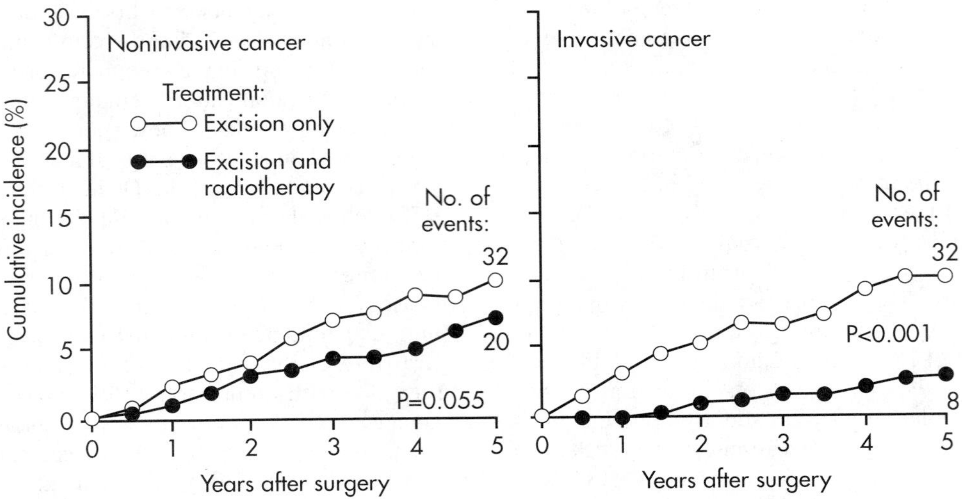

Fig. 20-8 Rate of development of noninvasive and invasive carcinoma after treatment of DCIS by wide excision alone or wide excision and radiotherapy. (All sizes and types of lesions of DCIS were included in this study.) (From Page, D. L., Steel, C. M., & Dixon, J. M. [1995]. Carcinoma in situ and patients at high risk of breast cancer. *British Medical Journal, 310,* 39-42.)

with most of the studies reporting 3- to 20-year follow-up, there is up to a 4% incidence of local failure (mean: 0.8%). Intuitively, both to patients and clinicians, it made little sense to offer more aggressive therapy for in situ disease than for invasive breast cancer. Currently, a mastectomy is recommended for the following:

- Extensive or multifocal disease that would prohibit excision and satisfactory cosmesis of the breast
- DCIS that is difficult or impossible to follow mammographically
- High-grade lesions
- Women who experience persistent worry over the years that is a serious detriment to their quality of life

ONCOLOGIC EMERGENCIES

Oncologic emergencies are not expected in patients with in situ breast cancer. However, clinicians are obligated to anticipate all possible intraoperative and perioperative complications in these patients.

NURSING MANAGEMENT

The perioperative treatment period is replete with informational needs, severe stress regarding a potential life threat, the need to make choices between treatment options, alterations in personal identity in terms of health and life potential, the need for support during adaptation to changes in family and sexual relationships, and reassurance that normal healing is occurring. Although some researchers have attempted to predict informational needs by demographic descriptors such as age (Bilodeau & Degner, 1996), such work is not intended to preclude the need to assess individual needs for breast cancer–related teaching (see Table 20-6 for a standard of care to assist patients with the decision-making process).

Careful attention to effective perioperative teaching for women undergoing surgery for breast cancer is more necessary than ever as hospital stays become increasingly brief. A complete educational program should include at least the following: information about breast and lymph node anatomy; the type and extent of the woman's breast cancer; the surgical procedure the woman will undergo or has undergone; what to expect in the immediate postoperative period in terms of wound care and the care of drains, pain management, and therapy for arm movement; numbness or other sensory sequelae; the availability of financial, sexual, and/or family counseling; all relevant information about treatment options; and information about managing symptoms associated with all treatments that the women will undergo subsequently.

Physical Aspects of Care

Women with LCIS are confronted with the choice of bilateral prophylactic mastectomies or with ongoing monitoring that includes CBEs every 6 months and annual bilateral mammographies. Women who undergo bilateral mastectomies need extensive physical and emotional care (see Chapter 19). Women monitored on an ongoing basis need extensive education that stresses the importance of adhering to the schedule of regular CBEs and mammograms.

Women with DCIS most likely undergo a surgical excision with or without radiation therapy. They require education about how to care for the surgical incision and postoperative pain management.

Side effects associated with radiation most commonly include fatigue and local skin reactions. A comprehensive guide for the management of side effects related to these

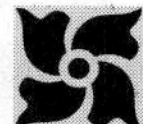

TABLE 20-6 Standard of Care: Decision Making in Breast Cancer

Patient Problem and Outcome	Nursing Interventions and Rationales	Patient Education Instructions
Undecided about treatment Patient will: • Feel comfortable with her decision and not experience regret	1. Determine the patient's decision-making style by asking: a. Does the patient have an independent, collaborative, or passive style of decision making? b. How is the current breast cancer diagnosis affecting the patient's ability to make decisions? c. What cultural or religious ideas may affect the patient's decision-making style? 2. Provide information to inform choices. 3. Provide emotional support to enable thinking, coping, and help for the psychological component of decision making. 4. Recommend (if feasible) that a support person be present during conversations with providers about treatment-related decisions. 5. Recommend taping provider education, particularly conversations with material designed to inform treatment decisions. 6. Review decisions once made to be sure that there is comprehension, agreement, and informed consent. 7. Access translation services or match caregivers fluent in the patient's native language (not family members or friends) for monolinguals not fluent in English.	1. Assess learning style and ask what if any materials will support the patient's ability to learn. 2. Provide appropriate educational materials (e.g., correct level of literacy, correct language) that will help the patient to make decisions about her treatment. 3. Offer books, pamphlets, videos, audiotapes, and consultations with providers or opportunities to meet with survivors. 4. Teach family members along with the patient. This approach involves the family members, and two or three people may remember the information provided more effectively. 5. Ask questions and engage in conversation to evaluate the patient's level of comprehension.

From Bilodeau, B. A., & Degner, L. F. (1996). Information needs, sources of information, and decisional roles in women with breast cancer. *Oncology Nursing Forum, 23*(4), 691-696.
Street, R. L., Jr., Voigt, B., Geyer, C., Jr., Manning, T., & Swanson, G. P. (1995). Increasing patient involvement in choosing treatment for early breast cancer. *Cancer, 76*(11), 2275-2285.
Beaver, K., Luker, K. A., Owens, R. G., Leinster, S. J., Degner, L. F., & Sloan, J. A. (1996). Treatment decision making in women newly diagnosed with breast cancer. *Cancer Nursing, 19*(1), 8-19.

therapies can be found in Dodd's *Managing the Side Effects of Chemotherapy and Radiation Therapy: A Guide for Patients and their Families* (1996).

Psychosocial and Cultural Concerns in the Management of CIS

Although the biologic threat associated with CIS is not comparable to that of infiltrating carcinoma of the breast, the diagnosis of CIS raises the specter of a cancer threat, and most patients diagnosed with CIS experience many of the emotional concerns faced by other breast cancer patients. These concerns include, for example, the potential threat related to a CIS diagnosis, coping with others' reactions to cancer, fear, anxiety, balancing the stressors of obtaining information while making treatment decisions, and all of the distress associated with treatment. It should be noted that there are many philosophic, theologic, and psychologically reflective writings, as well as a large body of research, that focuses on the psychosocial needs of women with breast cancer.

Specifically, we know less about the emotional responses to CIS. Much of the psychological research focuses on the use of therapeutic interventions to decrease distress and enhance coping and wellness (Fetting, 1991; Hilton, 1996; Lavery & Clarke, 1996; Tross et al., 1996; Walker, Nail, Larsen, Magill, & Schwartz, 1996). The focus areas for the research include sexuality and body image, fear of mortality, disclosure, social support and the impact of the disease on relationships (i.e., significant other, family, children, friends), as well as work, money, and insurance issues. Responses to breast cancer are affected by age (life cycle–specific issues); the amount and content of the disruption that a diagnosis and treatment of breast cancer has on one's life; prediagnosis personality, coping style, and crisis experience; and prior experience with breast cancer in women who come from high-incidence breast cancer families with early deaths (Rowland & Massie, 1996).

Underlying the differences between breast cancer and other cancers is the fact that the breast (and the loss of the breast) has distinct emotional and cultural meanings. The breast is associated with feeding one's child, and the threat to the breast magnifies fertility and childbearing issues in many premenopausal women. Stimulation of the breast and nipples is often part of sexual expression, and a threat to the breast may be intertwined with one's sexual identity, self-image, and how one imagines being perceived by an intimate. A woman may like or dislike her breasts and have complicated feelings related to the loss of or change in a healthy breast.

In addition to individual differences in reaction to the loss of a breast, a large amount of information has been reported on differences in the meaning of breast loss across the life span and across cultures. People of white Northern American and European cultures tend to focus on the breast as a seat of beauty. This interpretation may not reflect the impressions in many other cultures, and it certainly does not hold true for every woman in any one culture.

Kagawa-Singer (1996) delineated the ways in which Asian-American and Pacific-American women have distinct differences from American and European women regarding body image and sexuality (e.g., the breast has less sexual and more functional meaning). In addition, she described some specific differences among Asian cultures (e.g., what is beautiful is different in the Chinese culture [rounded vs squared shoulders], in the Korean culture [beauty being read in the shape of the heel of the foot], and in the Japanese culture [the nape of the neck and lightness of the skin]). Essential to sensitivity to cultural differences is the understanding of marked diversity among individuals within a culture and the wide differences in cultural adherence behaviors.

Brant (1996) reported on some of the responses of Native-American women to breast cancer. For example, some Native-American women may ask to save the postsurgical breast to bury it, some believe that their body must be intact for the next life, some believe that postoperative pain will be less, and some believe that the burial ceremony will help to heal the grief of the loss of the breast.

Phillips (1996) explored issues, primarily as they relate to screening and early detection, in African-American women. She focused on the need to thread empowerment strategies within the provision of education and emotional support. Additionally, she stressed the impact of the historical (and continued) lack of trust in health care providers' interventions based on documented breaches in the ethics of research (e.g., the Tuskegee Syphilis Study from 1932-1970 in which 400 African-American men, without their consent and after the discovery of therapy, were observed with untreated syphilis [Jones, 1981]).

It is difficult to establish therapeutic relationships, which are key to the provision of emotional support, without trust. The key health care issues for lesbians, who come from diverse cultural backgrounds, are dealing with homophobia (hatred and fear of people with same-sex intimate relationships); assumptions of heterosexuality by providers or other survivors; visitation and acknowledgment of a partner as family and significant other; disclosure of lesbian identification to providers, friends, and family members; and lack of knowledge about risk factors, the incidence of breast cancer, and emotional responses to diagnosis, treatment, and recovery (Denenberg, 1995; O'Hanlan, 1995; Rankow, 1995).

Emotional needs and effective interventions are also different for elderly women with breast cancer. Elderly women may have diminished social support mechanisms; have likely experienced more prior losses; have limited financial resources when they are on fixed incomes and limited health care coverage; come from a generation with less tendency to discuss breast cancer, their breasts, and sexuality; and may be less likely to perform breast self-examination and may be more uncomfortable with CBE (Cohen, 1996).

In addition to a commitment to learning about and respecting cultural diversity and the impact of culture on patients with breast cancer, it is vitally important that our programs, from screening through treatment for metastatic breast cancer, include the lived experience and knowledge of bicultural caregivers from diverse cultures. In addition, psychosocial resources must be made available to nonnative English speakers in their own language.

Psychological Interventions

Psychological assistance for patients with breast cancer is provided through individual or peer group support; professional support from various disciplines; and individual psychological consultation with psychologists, social workers, or psychiatrists. Counseling is often provided in concert with genetic testing, for a new diagnosis, or during a diagnostic crisis (e.g., metastatic disease or recurrence).

Although all of the benefits from participating in a breast cancer support group are not clear, the benefits are believed to be related to those derived from social support. As with all treatment recommendations and despite some data reporting their benefit, support groups are not perceived as beneficial for all women. Many women choose not to participate and others participate for a period and then choose not to continue. Some women report feeling overly affected by the difficult medical treatment and/or life experience stories of the other women. Some women with CIS may not feel "ill enough" to be in a breast cancer support group that includes women with more advanced disease. Others are not comfortable with the disclosure of feelings either in a group or to people they do not know. In addition, some women may not participate because of language or cultural barriers. In larger, urban areas or in areas where a specific population is well represented, culture- and language-specific support groups may be available to these women.

HOME CARE ISSUES

Much of a patient's postoperative nursing care must be delivered in the context of home care, given the current trend toward early discharge for mastectomy patients and for lumpectomies to be done on an outpatient basis. Referrals for in-home nursing care need to be considered for the following patients: women with functional limitations; elderly women; women without support from family and friends; and women with a prior history of severe co-morbid conditions, dementia, or mental illness.

TABLE 20-7 The Van Nuys Prognostic Index Scoring System

Score	1	2	3
Size (mm)	≤15	16-40	≥41
Margin width (mm)	≥10	1-9	<1
Pathologic classification	Nonhigh grade without necrosis	Nonhigh grade with necrosis	High grade with or without necrosis

One to three points are awarded for each of three different predictors of local breast recurrence (size, margin width, and pathologic classification). Scores for each of the predictors are totaled to yield a Van Nuys Prognostic Index score ranging from a low of 3 to a high of 9.

Modified from Silverstein, M. J., Lagios, M. D., Craig, P. H., Waisman, J. R., Lewinsky, B. S., Colburn, W. J., & Poller, D. N. (1996). A prognostic index for ductal carcinoma in situ of the breast. *Cancer, 77,* 2267-2274.

PROGNOSIS

As reported in the 1973 to 1987 SEER data (Berg & Hutter, 1995), the relative survival rate for all forms of CIS was approximately 100%. Breast-conserving surgery is used increasingly for localized CIS. At least one published study showed no difference in 8-year local recurrence rates, regardless of whether the patient had postoperative radiation therapy (Silverstein et al., 1996). In the only prospective randomized clinical trial, the NSABBP, the 5-year recurrence rate was 10% for patients treated with tumor excision and radiation and 21% for patients treated with tumor excision alone. These findings suggest that there may be a subset of women who could be managed with tumor excision alone, but few subset analyses were done to help clinicians decide who these women were likely to be (Fisher et al., 1993).

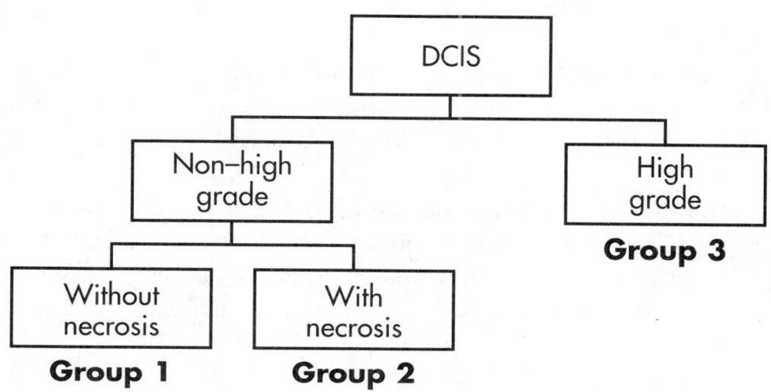

Fig. 20-9 Van Nuys DCIS classification. (From Silverstein, M. J., Lagios, M. D., Craig, P. H., Waisman, J. R., Lewinsky, B. S., Colburn, W. J., & Poller, D. N. [1996]. A prognostic index for ductal carcinoma in situ of the breast. *Cancer, 77,* 2267-2274.)

Prognostic Classification of DCIS

One of the striking features of the studies on DCIS is that the majority of them group all of the different types of DCIS into a single entity with presumed similar biologic behavior. However, DCIS is believed to be a spectrum of diseases, with different pathologic features proposed to be linked to different rates of recurrence. No single, adequately studied prognostic index can be used in clinical practice to match pathologic grade and disease characteristics with recommendations for an appropriate treatment modality.

However, one prognostic index has been studied in a series of 333 patients that offers an example of a rational system for differentiating DCIS and testing whether the recommended treatment proves to be appropriate and safe over time. The Van Nuys Prognostic Index (VNPI) developed by Melvin Silverstein (Silverstein et al., 1995, 1996) combines three predictors of local recurrence: tumor size, margin width, and pathologic classification. Scores of 1 (most favorable for prognosis) to 3 (least favorable for prognosis) are given to each predictor, and then all three predictor ratings are totaled to a prognostic index score (between 3 and 9). Table 20-7 displays the categories for the size, margin width, and pathologic classification for the VNPI.

The pathologic classification score, undoubtedly the most difficult criterion to standardize, depends on nuclear grade and comedo necrosis. Fig. 20-9 depicts the relationship between the three ratings on these criteria. Based on their observations of whether patients with differing VNPI ratings showed a local disease-free survival benefit from breast irradiation, Silverstein and colleagues (1995, 1996) suggested the VNPI ratings could be used as one indicator to determine treatment recommendations. Scores of 3 to 4 indicate the need for excision only, scores of 5 to 7 indicate the need for excision and radiation therapy, and scores of 8 to 9 indicate the need for mastectomy.

There are still concerns about the use of the VNPI in terms of ensuring consistency in the application of the scoring criteria, particularly the pathologic classification score (Schnitt, Harris, & Smith, 1996; Silverstein et al., 1996). The validation sample of 333 patients may be insufficient to assess whether this system's predictive value will be sustained over time. However, it represents an improvement over grouping all of the patients with DCIS into one category with three possible treatment outcomes.

EVALUATION OF THE QUALITY OF CARE

An assessment of what women know and are being taught about CIS as they are going through the diagnostic process is critical to providing quality care. This assessment would

TABLE 20-8 Quality of Care Evaluation of Treatment Decision Making Support in Breast Cancer

Disciplines participating in the quality of care evaluation:
□Surgery □Nursing □Medical Oncology □Radiation Oncology
□Social Work □Psychology/Psychiatry
Data from: □Mailed Questionnaire
□Patient Interview

Criteria	Yes	No
1. Were you told that you have choices regarding your breast cancer treatment?	□	□
2. Were those treatment choices explained to you?	□	□
3. Were you given information to help you decide what treatment to have?	□	□
4. Do you regret any of the decisions you made?	□	□
5. Who helped you to decide what treatment to do? You may check more than one. ___ Doctor ___ Nurse ___ Social Worker ___ Therapist ___ Family ___ Friends ___ Women with breast cancer ___ Other ___________	□	□
6. What kind of information helped you to make your decision? ___ Conversation with doctor(s) ___ Conversation with nurse(s) ___ Videotape ___ Conversation with women with breast cancer ___ Written patient education material ___ Professional medical literature ___Other ___________	□	□
7. Please feel free to add comments		

ideally include an evaluation of the informed consent process and support for treatment decision making. Table 20-8 is a tool developed by Hamolsky for assessing the quality of the process used to support patients with their decision making around treatment options. Clinical follow-up is essential to determine how oncology nurses should design systems to support follow-up care. Patient teaching should focus on anticipatory guidance for treatment-related side effects, clarification of recurrence rates, and the need for long-term follow-up. Particular attention should be given to helping women understand how their diagnosis of CIS differs from a diagnosis of infiltrating carcinoma. This approach assists them in correctly interpreting future reports of genetic studies and treatment-related research as it applies to themselves and to their families.

RESEARCH ISSUES

Many questions remain about improving clinical management and aiding decision making for women diagnosed with CIS. For example, what is the relationship between DCIS and LCIS lesions and invasive breast cancer? What is the etiology of DCIS and LCIS, and are there underlying causes that can be avoided?

Patients with DCIS or LCIS are confronted with numerous decisions that cause severe stress to women and their families and require supportive intervention. Research is needed to determine how to best help women with treatment decisions and how nurses can ensure that all women receive adequate support during treatment planning and follow-up care.

REFERENCES

American Joint Committee on Cancer. (1988). *Manual for staging of cancer* (3rd ed.). Philadelphia: J. B. Lippincott.

Barth, A., Brenner, R. J., & Giuliano, A. E. (1995). Current management of ductal carcinoma in situ. *Western Journal of Medicine, 163,* 360-366.

Bassett, L. W., Hendrick, R. E., Bassford, T. L., et al. (1994). *Quality determinants of mammography.* Clinical Practice Guideline No. 13 (AHCPR Publication No. 95-0632). Rockville, MD: Agency for Health Care Policy and Research, Pubic Health Service, U. S. Department of Health and Human Services.

Beaver, K., Luker, K. A., Owens, R. G., Leinster, S. J. Degner, L. F., & Sloan, J. A. (1996) Treatment decision making in women newly diagnosed with breast cancer. *Cancer Nursing, 19*(1), 8-19.

Berg, J. W., & Hutter, R. V. P. (1995). Breast cancer. *Cancer, 75,* 257-269.

Bilodeau, B. A., & Degner, L. F. (1996). Information needs, sources of information, and decisional roles in women with breast cancer. *Oncology Nursing Forum, 23*(4), 691-696.

Bodis, S., Siziopikou, K. P., Schnitt, S. J., Harris, J. R., & Fisher, D. E. (1996). Extensive apoptosis in ductal carcinoma in situ of the breast. *Cancer, 77*(9), 1851-1855.

Brant, J. M. (1996). Breast cancer challenges in Native American women. In K. Hasey Dow (Ed.), *Contemporary issues in breast cancer.* Boston: Jones and Bartlett.

Cady, B., Stione, M. D., Schuler, J. G., Thakur, R., Wanner, M. A., & Lavin, P. T. (1996). The new era in breast cancer. *Archives of Surgery, 131,* 302-308.

Carty, N. J., Royle, G. T., Carter, C., & Johnson, C. D. (1995). Management of ductal carcinoma in situ of the breast. *Annals of the Royal College of Surgery England, 77,* 163-167.

Cohen, H. J. (1996). Breast cancer screening in elder women: The geriatrician/internist perspective. *Journal of Gerontology, 47,* 134-136.

Connolly, J., & Nixon, A. (1996). Ductal carcinoma in situ of the breast: Histologic subtyping and clinical significance. Updates: Principles and practice of oncology 10. In V. DeVita, S. Hellman, & S. Rosenberg (Eds.), *Cancer principles and practice of oncology* (5th ed.). Philadelphia: Lippincott-Raven.

Cook, L. S., Weiss, N. S., Schwartz, S. M., White, E., McKnight, B., Moore, D. E., & Daling, J. R. (1995). Population-based study of Tamoxifen therapy and subsequent ovarian, endometrial, and breast cancers. *Journal of the National Cancer Institute, 87*(18), 1359-1364.

Denenberg, R. (1995). Invisible women: Lesbians and health care. *Health PAC Bulletin,* Spring 1992.

Dhingra, K. (1995). A phase II chemoprevention trial design to identify surrogate endpoint biomarkers in breast cancer. *Journal of Cellular Biochemistry, 3*(Suppl.), 19-24.

Dodd, M. J. (1996). *Managing the side effects of chemotherapy and radiation therapy: A guide for patients and their families.* San Francisco: University of California Press.

Early Breast Cancer Trialists' Collaborative Group (EBCTCB). (1992). Systemic treatment of early breast cancer by hormonal, cytotoxic, or immune therapy. 133 randomized trials involving 31,000 recurrences and 24,000 deaths among 75,000 women. *Lancet, 339,* 1-15, 71-85.

Ernster, V. L., Barclay, J., Kerlikowske, K., Grady, D., & Henderson, C. (1996). Incidence of and treatment for ductal carcinoma in situ of the breast. *Journal of the American Medical Association, 275,* 913-918.

Facione, N. C., & Facione, P. A. (1997). Equitable access to cancer services in the 21st century. *Nursing Outlook, 5*(4), 220-227.

Farwell, M. F., Foster, R. S., & Costanza, M. C. (1993). Breast cancer and earlier detection efforts—Realized and unrealized impact on stage. *Archives of Surgery, 128,* 510-514.

Fetting, J. (1991). Psychosocial aspects of breast cancer. *Current Science ISSN 1040-8746,* 1014-1018.

Fisher, B., Constantino, J., Redmond, C., Fisher, E. R., Margolese, R., Dimitrov, N., Wolmark, N., Wickerman, D. L., Deutsch, M., & Ore, L. (1993). Lumpectomy compared with radiation therapy for the treatment of intraductal breast cancer. *New England Journal of Medicine, 328,* 1581-1586.

Foschini, M. P., Fornelli, A., Peterse, J. L., Mignani, S., & Eusebi, V. (1996). Micro calcifications in ductal carcinoma in situ of the breast: Histochemical and immunohistochemical study. *Human Pathology, 27*(2), 178-183.

Foster, R. (1996). Techniques for diagnosis of palpable breast masses. In J. Harris, M. Lippman, M. Morrow, & S. Hellman (Eds.), *Diseases of the breast.* Philadelphia: Lippincott-Raven.

Frykberg, E. R., Ames, F. C., & Bland, K. L. (1991). Current concepts for management of early (in situ and occult invasive) breast carcinoma. In K. L. Bland & E. M. Copeland (Eds.), *Diseases of the breast* (4th ed.). Philadelphia: W. B. Saunders.

Goldhirch, A., Wood, W. C., Senn, H. J., Glick, J. H., & Gelber, R. D. (1995). Meeting highlights: International consensus panel on the treatment of primary breast cancer. *Journal of the National Cancer Institute, 87*(19), 1441-1445.

Grant, C. S., Groellner, J. R., Welsh, J. S., & Martin, J. K. (1986). Fine needle aspiration of the breast. *Mayo Clinic Proceedings, 61,* 377-381.

Hall, F. M., Storella, J. M., Silverstone, D. Z., & Wyshak, G. (1988). Nonpalpable breast lesions: Recommendations for biopsy based on suspicion of carcinoma at mammography. *Radiology, 167,* 353-358.

Hankey, B. F., Brinton, L. A., Kessler, L. G., & Abrams, J. (1993). Breast cancer. In B. A. Miller, L. A. G. Ries, B. F. Hankey, C. L. Kosary, A. Harras, S. S. Devesa, & B. J. Edwards (Eds.), *SEER Cancer Statistics Review 1973-1990.* U.S. National Institutes of Health Publication No. 93-2789. Washington, DC: National Cancer Institute.

Hetelekidis, S., Schnitt, S., Morrow, M., & Harris, J. (1995). Management of ductal carcinoma in situ. *CA: A Cancer Journal for Clinicians, 45*(4), 244-253.

Hilton, B. A. (1996). Getting back to normal: The family experience during early stage breast cancer. *Oncology Nursing Forum, 23*(4), 605-614.

Holzman, D. (1995). *News: Journal of the National Cancer Institute, 87,* 710-711.

Hong, W. K., & Lippman, S. M. (1995). Cancer chemoprevention. *Journal of the National Cancer Institute Monographs, 17,* 49-53.

Hunter, D., & Willett, W. (1996). Dietary factors. In J. Harris, M. Lippman, M. Morrow, & S. Hellman (Eds.), *Diseases of the breast.* Philadelphia: Lippincott-Raven.

Ibanez, J. A., Giannotti-Filho, O., & Da Silva Neto, J. B. (1993). Nipple discharge: Study on 100 patients. *Revista Paulista de Medicina, 111*(1), 305-308.

Jones, J. H. (1981). *Bad blood: The Tuskegee syphilis experiment.* New York: The Free Press.

Kagawa-Singer, M. (1996). Issues affecting Asian American and Pacific American women. In K. Hassey Dow (Ed.), *Contemporary issues in breast cancer.* Boston: Jones and Bartlett.

Kelly, P., & Winslow, E. H. (1996). Needle wire localization for nonpalpable breast lesions: Sensations, anxiety levels, and informational needs. *Oncology Nursing Forum, 23*(4), 639-645.

Kerlikowske, K., Barclay, J., Grady, D., Sickles, E. A., & Ernster, V. (1997). Comparison of risk factors for ductal carcinoma in situ and invasive breast cancer. *Journal of the National Cancer Institute, 89*(1), 76-82.

Landis, S. H., Murray, T., Bolden, S., & Wingo, P. A. (1998). Cancer statistics, 1998. *CA: A Cancer Journal for Clinicians 48*(1), 6-29.

Lavery, J., & Clarke, V. (1996). Causal attributions, coping strategies and adjustment to breast cancer. *Cancer Nursing, 19*(1), 20-28.

Leitch, A. (1995). Controversies in breast cancer screening. *Cancer, 76,* 2064-2069.

Lidbrink, E., Frisell, J., Brandberg, Y., Rosendahl, I., & Rutqvist, L. E. (1995). Nonattendance in the Stockholm mammography screening trial: Relative mortality and reasons for nonattendance. *Breast Cancer Research and Treatment, 35,* 267-275.

Linver, M. N., Osuch, J. R., Brenner, R. J., & Smith, R. A. (1995). The mammography audit: A primer for the mammography quality standards act (MQSA). *American Journal of Roentgenology, 165*(1), 15-19.

Miller, A. B., Baines, C. J., To, T., & Wall, C. (1992). Canadian National Breast Screening Study: Breast cancer detection and death rates among women ages 40-49. *Canadian Medical Association Journal, 147,* 1459-1476.

Millikan, R., Dressler, L., Geradts, J., & Graham, M. (1995). The need for epidemiologic studies of in-situ carcinoma of the breast. *Breast Cancer Research and Treatment.* The Netherlands: Kluer Academic Publishers.

Morrow, M. (1995a). The natural history of ductal carcinoma in situ. *Cancer, 76*(7), 1113-1115.

Morrow, M. (1995b). When can stereotactic core biopsy replace excisional biopsy? A clinical perspective. *Breast Cancer Research and Treatment, 36,* 1-9.

Morrow, M. (1996). Ductal carcinoma in situ. In J. Harris, M. Lippman, M. Morrow, & S. Hellman (Eds.), *Diseases of the breast.* Philadelphia: Lippincott-Raven.

Morrow, M., & Schnitt, S. (1996). Lobular carcinoma in situ. In J. Harris, M. Lippman, M. Morrow, & S. Hellman (Eds.), *Diseases of the breast.* Philadelphia: Lippincott-Raven.

Munn, K. E., Walker, R. A., Menasce, L., & Varley, J. M. (1996). Mutation of the TP_{53} gene and allelic imbalance at chromosome 17p13 in ductal carcinoma in situ. *British Journal of Cancer, 74*(10), 1578-1585.

Munn, K. E., Walker, R. A., & Varley, J. M. (1995). Frequent alterations of chromosome 1 in ductal carcinoma in situ of the breast. *Oncogene, 10*(8), 1653-1657.

Murphy, D. S., Hoare, S. F., Going, J. J., Mallon, E. E., George, W. D., Kaye, S. B., Brown, R., Black, D. M., & Keith, W. N. (1995). Characterization of extensive genetic alterations in ductal carcinoma in situ by fluorescence in situ hybridization and molecular analysis. *Journal of the National Cancer Institute, 87*(22), 1694-1704.

National Surgical Adjuvant Breast and Bowel Project (NSABBP). (1994). 4-HPR (fenretinide)—Stage 1:NSABP. *Journal of the National Cancer Institute, 86,* 527-537.

Nguyen, M., McCombs, M. M., Ghandehari, S., Kim, A., Wang, H., Barsky, S. H., Love, S., & Bassett, L. W. (1996). An update on core needle biopsy for radiologically detected breast lesions. *Cancer, 78,* 2340-2345.

O'Hanlan, K. (1995). Lesbians in health research. *Recruitment and retention of women in clinical studies.* Publication No. 95-3756. Bethesda, MD: Public Health Service, National Institutes of Health.

Ottesen, G. L., Christensen, I. J., Larsen, J. K., Christiansen, J., Hansen, B., & Andersen, J. A. (1995). DNA analysis of in situ ductal carcinoma of the breast via flow cytometry. *Cytometry, 22*(3), 168-176.

Page, D. L., Dupont, W. D., Rogers, L. W., Jensen, R. A., & Schuyler, P. A. (1995). Continued local recurrence of carcinoma 15-25 years after a diagnosis of low grade ductal carcinoma in situ of the breast treated only by biopsy. *Cancer, 76,* 1197-1200.

Page, D. L., Steel, C. M., & Dixon, J. M. (1995). Carcinoma in situ and patients at high risk of breast cancer. *British Medical Journal, 310,* 39-42.

Phillips, J. (1996). Breast cancer and African American Women. In K. Hassey Dow (Ed.), *Contemporary issues in breast cancer.* Boston: Jones and Bartlett.

Radford, D. M., Phillips, N. J., Fair, K. L., Ritter, J. H., Holt, M., & Donis-Keller, H. (1995). Allelic loss and the progression of breast cancer. *Cancer Research, 55*(22), 5180-5183.

Rankow, E. (1995). Lesbian health issues for the primary care provider. *Journal of Family Practice, 48*(5), 486-496.

Robinson, K. M., & Huether, S. E. (1996). Structure and function of the reproductive systems. In S. E. Huether & K. L. McCance (Eds.), *Understanding pathophysiology.* St. Louis: Mosby.

Rowland, J., & Massie, M. (1996). Psychologic reactions to breast cancer diagnosis, treatment and survival. In J. Harris, M. Lippman, M. Morrow, & S. Hellman (Eds.), *Diseases of the breast.* Philadelphia: Lippincott Raven.

Schnitt, S., Harris, J., & Smith, B. (1996). Developing a prognostic index for ductal carcinoma in situ of the breast: Are we there yet? *Cancer, 77*(11), 2189-2192.

Silverstein, M. J., Gierson, E. D., Colburn, W. J., Rosser, R. J., Waisman, J. R., & Gamagami, P. (1991). Axillary lymphadenopathy for intraductal carcinoma of the breast. *Surgery, Gynecology and Obstetrics, 172,* 211-214.

Silverstein, M. J., Lagios, M. D., Craig, P. H., Waisman, J. R., Lewinsky, B. S., Colburn, W. J., & Poller, D. N. (1996). A prognostic index for ductal carcinoma in situ of the breast. *Cancer, 77,* 2267-2274.

Silverstein, M., Poller, D., Waisman, J., Colburn, W., Barth, A., Gierson, E., Lewinsky, B., Gamagami, P., & Slamon, D. (1995). Prognostic classification of breast ductal carcinoma in situ. *The Lancet, 345*(May), 1154-1157.

Smart, C. R., Hendrix, R. E., Rutledge, J. H., & Smith, R. (1995). Benefits of mammography screening in women ages 40-49. *Cancer, 75,* 1619-1626.

Street, R. L., Jr., Voigt, B., Geyer, C., Jr., Manning, T., & Swanson, G. P. (1995). Increasing patient involvement in choosing treatment for early breast cancer. *Cancer, 76*(11), 2275-2285.

Surveillance, Epidemiology, and End Results (SEER) Program Public Use [CD-ROM] (1973-1992). Bethesda: National Cancer Institute, DCPC, Surveillance Program, Cancer Statistics Branch: July 1995.

Tross, S., Herndon, J., Korzun, A., Kornblith, A. B., Cella, D. F., Holland, J. F., Raich, P., Johnson, A., Kiang, D. T., Perloff, M., Norton, L., Wood, W., & Holland, J. C. (1996). Psychological symptoms and disease-free survival in women with Stage II breast cancer. *Journal of the National Cancer Institute, 88*(10), 631-661.

Veronesi, U., DePalo, G., Costa, A., Fornelli, F., & Decensi, A. (1996). Chemoprevention of breast cancer with fenretinide. *IARC Scientific Publications, 136,* 87-94.

Veronesi, U., Salvadori, B., Luini, A., Banfi, A., Zucali, R., & Del Vecchio, M. (1996). Conservative approaches for the management of stage I/II carcinoma of the breast: Milan Cancer Institute trials. *World Journal of Surgery, 18,* 70-75.

Visscher, D. W., Wallis, T. L., & Crissman, J. D. (1996). Evaluation of chromosome aneuploidy in tissue sections of preinvasive breast carcinomas using interphase cytogenetics. *Cancer, 77*(2), 315-320.

Walker, B. L., Nail, L., Larsen, L., Magill, J., & Schwartz, A. (1996). Concerns, affect, and cognitive disruption following completion of radiation treatment for localized breast cancer or prostate cancer. *Oncology Nursing Forum, 23*(8), 1181-1187.

Walt, A. J. (1995). Screening for breast cancer. In J. L. Cameron (Ed.), *Current surgical therapy* (5th ed.). St. Louis: Mosby.

Weiss, H. A., Brinton, L. A., Brogan, D., Coates, R. J., Gammon, M. D., Malone, K. E., Schoenberg, J. B., & Swanson, C. A. (1996). Epidemiology of in situ and invasive breast cancer in women aged under 45. *British Journal of Medicine, 73,* 1298-1305.

Wood, W. (1996). Management of lobular carcinoma in situ and ductal carcinoma in situ of the breast. *Seminars in Oncology, 23*(4), 446-452.

Zhuang, Z., Merino, M. J., Chuaqui, R., Liotta, L. A., & Emmert-Buck, M. R. (1995). Identical allelic loss on chromosome 11q13 in microdissected in situ and invasive human breast cancer. *Cancer Research, 55*(3), 467-471.

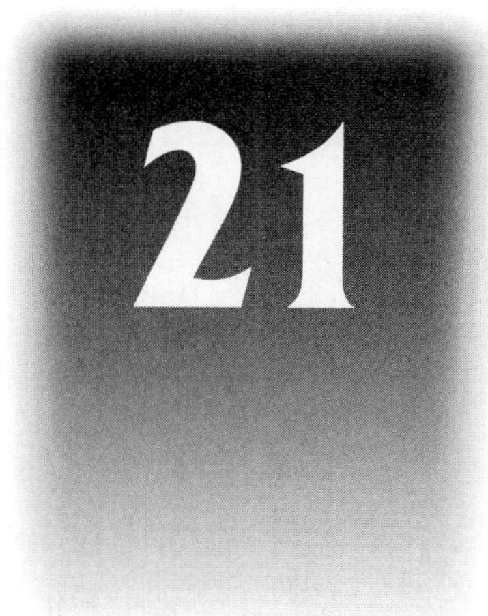

Infiltrating Breast Cancer

Deborah Hamolsky, RN, MS
Noreen Facione, RN, PhD

EPIDEMIOLOGY

In the United States, breast cancer is the leading cause of death for women between the ages of 40 and 55 years. In 1998, this disease will claim the lives of 43,500 mothers, partners, daughters, wives, or closest companions (Landis, Murray, Bolden, & Wingo, 1998). The biologic processes that give rise to the development of breast cancer are being described, but specific recommendations to prevent new cases remain elusive. Recent statistics demonstrate much larger increases in the incidence of breast cancer (4% per year) throughout the 1980s. Much of the rise is attributable to an increasing life expectancy and aging of the population, as well as to the earlier detection of many cases of breast cancer through the routine use of mammography screening. Taking these three factors into account, since the 1930s when accurate statistics began to be recorded, there has been an increase in the incidence of breast cancer cases of roughly 1% per year.

Some evidence exists that supports the beneficial effects of early detection. Since 1980 the number of women with newly diagnosed breast tumors measuring 2 cm or more has remained relatively stable, whereas the number of women with new tumors measuring less than 2 cm has increased (Miller, Feuer, & Hanky, 1991). If this trend of finding smaller-size tumors at the time of diagnosis continues, it has been estimated that by the year 2005, the median maximum diameter of an invasive carcinoma could approach as small as 1 cm (Cady et al., 1996). Even this level of early detection will leave room for improvement, as many breast tumors are visible as an area of density on a mammogram when the tumor reaches approximately 0.3 cm in diameter.

The majority of breast cancers are adenocarcinomas (arising from glandular tissue) and are classified on the basis of their microscopic appearance as either ductal (i.e., arising from the lactiferous ducts) or lobular (i.e., arising from the breast lobes). Infiltrating ductal carcinoma is the most commonly diagnosed female breast cancer, accounting for 67% to 75% of new cases. Less common types of breast cancer include infiltrating lobular carcinoma (5% to 10%), medullary carcinoma (5% to 7%), mucinous carcinoma (3%), tubular carcinoma (approximately 1% to 2%), and secretory carcinoma, which are seen rarely in children and adolescents (Berg & Hutter, 1995).

Invasive lobular carcinoma is believed to be more extensively infiltrative than ductal carcinoma. The disease presents with indistinct margins and is associated with a higher incidence rate (20% to 30%) of being present bilaterally (Yeatman, 1995). Other nonadenocarcinomas of the breast include metaplastic cancer, squamous cell cancer, apocrine cancer, and adenoid cystic carcinoma. Sarcomas (phyllodes tumors) in the breast are rare, and most are localized and treated by local surgical therapy. Less specific data and therefore less specific knowledge about the biologic behavior of the less common histologic types of breast cancer exist. However, routine treatment protocols for all types of breast cancer require consideration of both local and systemic therapies. Local therapy includes surgery and radiation; systemic therapy includes chemotherapy and hormone therapy.

There are differences in the incidence rates for breast cancer by race, with white women having an approximately 20% higher overall incidence of the disease than women of other racial or ethnic heritages (American Cancer Society [ACS], 1997). However, in women under 45 years of age, African-American women's incidence rates are higher than those of white women. At least a portion of this difference by race appears to be explained by differences in socioeconomic status, with the incidence of breast cancer in poorer women being *lower* across ethnic groups. Generally, women in developing nations are reported to have higher rates of breast cancer than women in less developed nations.

Breast cancer is exceedingly more prevalent in women than in men. Only 1600 cases of breast cancer are expected to occur in males in the United States in 1998 compared with 178,700 cases in females (Landis et al., 1998). Aside from the lower incidence, the clinical presentation, pathology, and natural history of breast cancer in men is remarkably similar to breast cancer in women. Stage and axillary node status are strong prognostic indicators in both women and men. Less gender-specific research is available, but

5-year disease-free survival rates in men are reported as high as 47%, similar to the rates reported for women (Williams, Powers, & Wagman, 1996). Men are generally older at the time of diagnosis and are diagnosed proportionally at a more advanced stage. The tumors are located most often beneath the nipple and are more often responsive to hormonal therapy than breast cancers in women (Donegan & Redlich, 1996). The treatment approach for male breast cancer is modified radical mastectomy with systemic adjuvant therapy when lymph nodes are involved.

RISK FACTORS

The National Institutes of Health (NIH) estimate that women have a 1 in 8 lifetime risk for developing breast cancer. This statistic is puzzling and misleading for many women. An individual woman's risk may be considerably lower or much higher given her particular circumstances. Therefore helping women make realistic appraisals of their personal risks for breast cancer is an important role for nurses involved in breast health education.

Risk factors for breast cancer are not *causes* of breast cancer. Risk factors describe characteristics and behaviors that have been associated with an increased likelihood of developing a disease compared with the likelihood of the population as a whole developing the same disease (e.g., age, use of oral contraceptives). Not everyone who shares the characteristic or behavior pattern will actually develop the disease. In time, causal explanations connecting these risk factors to the development of breast cancer may become available. However, the task of explaining why each of the identified risk factors is associated with an increased likelihood of developing breast cancer remains to be determined through extensive research studies.

Studies of men with breast cancer offer little reliable information about breast cancer risk factors in men, but a number of risk factors associated with the development of breast cancer in women have been identified. Increasing age is the single most important risk factor. The median age of women diagnosed with breast cancer today is 61 years of age (Simon & Severson, 1996). Table 21-1 displays the age-specific probabilities of developing infiltrating breast cancer.

Table 21-2 displays other risk factors that researchers have linked with the development of breast cancer. Relative risk expresses the odds relationship between the incidence of breast cancer among persons possessing the characteristic, divided by the incidence among otherwise similar persons without the characteristic (odds ratio: OR). For example, the relative risk of a woman with a history of the risk factor "atypical hyperplasia" to develop breast cancer is calculated by dividing the incidence of breast cancer in women with a history of atypical hyperplasia (presence of the risk factor) by the known incidence of breast cancer in women without atypical hyperplasia (comparison group). This ratio is about 4:1, and thus the relative risk associated with a history of atypical hyperplasia is 4.0.

Because many of the studies that support these characteristics as risk factors were carried out in samples of white women, the relevance of these risk factors for women in other ethnic and racial groups remains to be tested. Similarly, there are many unanswered questions about how differences in women's lifestyles may affect their individual breast cancer risk. Research that describes breast cancer rates and risk factors in lesbian women has yet to be reported. However, some have speculated that lesbians and celibate women may have increased relative risks because of lifestyle choices related to limited or absence of childbearing, and oral contraceptive use (Denenberg, 1995; O'Hanlan, 1995; Rankow, 1995).

TABLE 21-1 Age-Specific Probabilities of Developing Breast Cancer

Age	Probability of Developing Breast Cancer in the Next 10 Years	Odds Ratio
20	0.04%	1 in 2500
30	0.43%	1 in 233
40	1.55%	1 in 65
50	2.44%	1 in 41
60	3.44%	1 in 29

Data from American Cancer Society (1997). *Cancer facts and figures 1997*, Atlanta: The Society; Reis, L. A. G., Miller, B. A., Hankey, B. F., Kosary, C. L., Harras, A., & Edwards, B. K. *Surveillance and Epidemiologic End Results cancer statistics review, 1973-1991.* U.S. National Institutes of Health Publication No. 94-2789. National Cancer Institute.

Research to determine epidemiologic links between the incidence of breast cancer and personal and environmental risk factors is also hampered by inaccuracies in describing and recording cultural behavior and life events, particularly in countries where a cancer diagnosis remains a stigmatized condition. Further complicating this picture is the observation that women in industrialized and developed countries around the world are reported to have lower incidence rates for breast cancer than women in the United States, yet their rates approach our own when they immigrate to this country.

Fat composition in the diet has been studied as a breast cancer risk factor with inconclusive results. This research is based on an ecologic relationship between the higher rates of breast cancer in nations where there is high consumption of animal fats vs lower rates in countries where there is a prevalence of vegetable and fish oil consumption (Glanz, 1994; Hunter & Willett, 1996). Reeves and colleagues (1996) reported that obesity was associated with an increased stage of breast cancer at the time of diagnosis and a poorer survival prognosis in women who detected their own breast cancer but not for those cases detected by mammography.

Women who have both atypical hyperplasia and a family history of breast cancer have an absolute risk of 20% to 30% of developing breast cancer within the next 15 to 20 years. At the present time, women begin their menses many years

TABLE 21-2 Breast Cancer Risk Factors

Risk Factors Other Than Age	Comparison Group		Odds Ratio
Family history of breast cancer (Henderson et al., 1995)	No first-degree relatives	2 first-degree relatives:	4-6.0
Personal history of breast cancer (Plotkin, 1995)	Never diagnosed with breast cancer	30 years later risk of dying of breast cancer:	16.0
History of benign breast disease (Willett et al., 1987; Hunter, 1986; Dupont & Page, 1985)	Any biopsy or aspiration	Any benign disease:	1.5
		Proliferation:	2.0
		Atypical hyperplasia:	4.0
Age at birth of first child (White, 1987)	<20 years old	20-24 years:	1.3
		25-29 years:	1.6
		>29 years:	1.9
Oral contraceptives	Never used	Current use:	1.4
		Past use:	1.0
Hormone replacement (Colditz et al., 1995; Romieu et al., 1989)	Never used	Current use, all ages:	1.4
		Age 50-59 years	1.5
		Age >59 years	2.1
Age at menopause	45-54 years old	Age >54 years	1.5
		Age <45 years	0.7
		Oophorectomy <35 years	0.4

earlier, have many more menstrual cycles, fewer pregnancies, a later menopause, and give birth to their first child on average at an older age than women in the past. They also have exogenous oral contraceptive hormones available to them for pregnancy prevention and may use perimenopausal and postmenopausal hormone replacement therapy, extending the years when estrogen and progesterone are active on their breast tissue. Many scientists are wondering if the current increase of in situ breast cancer being detected on mammography represents more than simply an early detection phenomenon but rather a true increase in the number of new in situ cases that may be attributable to changing lifestyle in relationship to the use of reproductive hormones.

CHEMOPREVENTION

Chemoprevention is defined as the use of specific natural and synthetic chemical agents to reverse or suppress carcinogenesis and prevent the development of invasive cancer. Carcinogenesis is a multistep process including a premalignant phase that does not always proceed to malignancy, and certain compounds may be capable of reversing premalignant changes or preventing the formation of second primary tumors. The principles of chemoprevention are to identify agents that have the capability to inactivate oncogenes or activate tumor suppressor genes. Chemoprevention in breast cancer targets women at increased risk for the development of cancer through systemic drug and nutrient therapies.

Women with breast cancer who are at highest risk for the development of a secondary tumor and women with a known genetic predisposition for developing breast cancer (e.g., Li Fraumeni syndrome; BRCA1 families; and individuals at risk for hereditary breast, ovarian, or colon cancer) are considered candidates for chemoprevention. Chemopreventive agents are believed to work in several ways, including: (1) changing the pathway of cells from proliferation to differentiation, (2) binding with carcinogens present in the body and/or enhancing the metabolic breakdown of these carcinogens making them inactive agents, or (3) inducing the death of the aberrant (premalignant or malignant) cell.

Currently, two agents are under investigation for the chemoprevention of breast cancer, tamoxifen and retinoid compounds. Tamoxifen has been shown in large clinical trials to decrease the incidence of contralateral (opposite side) breast cancer in addition to having an impact on an individual's disease-free interval and overall survival (Cook et al., 1995; Early Breast Cancer Trialists' Collaborative Group, 1992). In addition, tamoxifen was shown to prevent the development of mammary cancers in animals. However, long-term use of tamoxifen has been reported to increase a woman's risk of developing endometrial cancer and, particularly in premenopausal women, to increase their risk of developing ovarian cancer (Cook et al., 1995).

Retinoid compounds (i.e., vitamin A compounds) have been shown to control the abnormal proliferation of epithelial cells. In animal models, a decrease in mammary tumors has been demonstrated using retinoid compounds. A major clinical hurdle is the liver toxicity associated with vitamin A therapy. An open clinical trial of fenretinide, a less liver-toxic retinoid, is underway in Italy to examine its impact on the prevention of breast cancer (National Surgical Adjuvant Breast and Bowel Project [NSABBP], 1994; Veronesi, DePalo, Costa, Fornelli, & Decensi, 1996; Veronesi, Salvadori, et al., 1996). In addition, a trial is open in the United States to test the effect of beta-carotene on the development of breast cancer in postmenopausal women (Hunter & Willett, 1996).

Chemoprevention trials use biomarkers as indicators of the advancement or reversal of the process of carcinogenesis as a result of the treatment under study. Two of the most commonly studied biomarkers are indicators of genetic mutations within cells; namely, the presence of micronuclei and the presence of abnormal cell proliferation. Using biomarkers as an intermediate indicator of the effects of a treatment on carcinogenesis has provided an improvement over awaiting evidence of the occurrence of the disease. However, to date, the identification of biomarkers for breast carcinogenesis lacks the specificity needed (the presence of known biomarkers does not guarantee that carcinogenesis will occur) to warrant the launching of an intervention trial to identify women at risk for developing breast cancer (Hong & Lippman, 1995).

PATHOPHYSIOLOGY

Normal Anatomy and Physiology of the Female Breast

Refer to Chapter 20 for a review of the normal anatomy and physiology of the female breast.

The Process of Carcinogenesis

Breast cancer is not one disease but rather a cluster of diseases that results when breast cells undergo a process of carcinogenesis. The development of a breast tumor depends on the ratio of the rate of cell proliferation to the rate of genetically determined cell death (apoptosis). This ratio is dependent on the process of angiogenesis (the formation of new blood vessels that can support cell proliferation). Inhibition of angiogenesis appears to lead to increased apoptosis and decreased tumor growth. Measures of apoptosis and angiogenesis determine tumor doubling time, another important biomarker that is a strong prognostic indicator and also useful for determining the response to primary and adjuvant chemotherapy agents (Heimann et al., 1996). The threat to survival from breast cancer is the ability of most invasive breast cancers to metastasize and carry the disease throughout a woman's body.

Once the tumor has metastasized, the implications for a woman's survival is highly influenced by the tumor's doubling time. Aggressive tumors have doubling times of less than 60 days, whereas others double over a period as long as 300 days and are considered very indolent. Tumor doubling time can be roughly estimated by the S-phase fraction that is derived from deoxyribonucleic acid (DNA) flow cytometry. In this test procedure, a small amount of the tumor is prepared and the nuclei of the cells are stained. The cells are then expressed in a fine spray, and the nuclei are visualized with a laser beam. Computer scans of these cells record the number of cells that are dividing, and from this count, the doubling time of the tumor can be estimated. However, it should be noted that after reviewing what is currently known about the relationship between S-phase and ploidy, the American Society of Clinical Oncology (ASCO) does not at this time recommend using these test measures (i.e., S-phase, ploidy) to estimate women's survival potential (ASCO, 1996).

The etiology of a breast cancer involves complex interactions between multiple factors, one of which is the genetic alterations in the chromosomes that can influence breast cells. Approximately 5% to 10% of breast cancers follow a familial pattern; that is, the genetic abnormality triggering the cancer is inherited from one generation to another (King, Rowell, & Love, 1993; Weber, 1996). The remainder of the breast cancers occur as sporadic events, most likely due to a genetic alteration in a single mature breast cell or because of a series of events in a group of susceptible cells (Brock, 1993). Most breast cancers are believed to arise from a single cell mutation that results in uncontrolled cellular growth.

Two types of genes that contribute to the process of carcinogenesis are oncogenes and tumor suppressor genes. Oncogenes are instrumental in the malignant transformation of the affected breast cell. The *c-erbB2* and *myc* are protooncogenes (i.e., normal genes that can undergo a mutation and become an oncogene) that have been identified as active in malignant breast cell proliferation. Tumor suppressor genes are genes that restrain cell proliferation. A mutation in a tumor suppressor gene leads to unrestrained proliferation, usually of an already specialized cell type. Tumor suppressor genes have been identified in several breast cancers. Persons with Li Fraumeni syndrome, a rare inheritable cancer accounting for about 1% of breast cancer cases (Evans et al., 1994), have been shown to have genetic mutations on one small area of the p53 gene (Brock, 1993).

Patients with breast/ovarian cancer syndrome appear predisposed to cancer because of the presence of a BCRA1 gene located on chromosome 17. Genetic alterations of BCRA1 are thought to be responsible for half of all inherited breast cancers in women younger than 45 years of age, and in 90% of families with breast and ovarian cancer syndrome (Easton, Bishop, Ford, & Crockford, 1993; Hoskins et al., 1995). Members of these families have a 50% chance of inheriting BCRA1 mutations. Female carriers of this mutation are estimated to have about an 87% risk of developing breast cancer by age 70, and those who develop one cancer also have an additional higher risk of developing second cancers (Ford et al., 1994). The deletion of two nucleotides, adenine and guanine (AG), at position 185 on the BCRA1 gene, is present in 1% of Ashkenazi Jewish women and in 20% of these women who develop breast cancer by 40 years of age (Weber, 1996). The risk for developing breast cancer associated with the presence of a BRCA1 mutation is estimated to be 87% by 80 years of age (Easton et al., 1993).

A second, more recently identified genetic mutation, BCRA2, occurs on chromosome 13. This mutated gene appears to predispose carriers to breast cancer but less so to ovarian cancer. Lifetime risk for breast cancer in BCRA2 mutation carriers is also high, estimated at 85% for women and 6% for men (Wooster et al., 1994). Much remains to be learned about tumorigenesis, which in most cases is much more complex than simply the occurrence of a tumor suppressor gene mutation or an oncogene mutation.

The role of hormonal factors, oncogenes, and growth factors in the development of breast cancer will remain an active area of research for years. Efforts to predict patterns of and reasons for tumor metastases continue. Estrogen and progesterone receptor status are relatively weak predictors of long-term relapse and breast cancer mortality rates (ASCO, 1996). The majority of studies show an increased survival potential associated with negative node status and a positive estrogen receptor status.

Tumor suppressor genes, particularly p53, are being studied aggressively. Mutations in this gene were demonstrated in the earliest phase of breast neoplasia and were shown to be maintained throughout a tumor's progression to an infiltrating carcinoma (Davidoff, Kerns, Inglehart, & Marks, 1991). Two potential markers for metastases in breast cancer are nm23-H1 and Cathepsin-D (CD). In a variety of animal models and in one in vitro human study, nm23-H1 was seen in tumors less likely to metastasize (Leone et al., 1991). CD has been proposed to facilitate invasion of tumors into neighboring tissues through its proteolytic enzyme activity. In one study, increased levels of CD were associated with an increase in tumor recurrence in node-positive and node-negative women and in women who were both premenopausal and postmenopausal (Seshadri et al., 1994).

Recently, researchers engineered an immunoliposome (i.e., a fat molecule attached to an antibody and a chemotherapy drug) and used it in animal studies to eradicate the *c-erbB2* oncogene's protein product that interacts with cell growth factors (News JNCI, 1996a). Over expression of the c-erbB2 gene is seen in 20% of breast cancers and is known to be associated with a poorer prognosis. This study represents the beginning of gene therapy treatment for breast cancer. However, in its most recent statement, ASCO found insufficient evidence to recommend the routine use of these tumor markers, oncogenes, and hormonal factors for most screening, diagnosis, staging, or intervention decisions (ASCO, 1996).

A controversial preventive measure in women at high risk for breast cancer is prophylactic mastectomy. Most investigators and clinicians are reluctant to recommend a more drastic intervention to prevent breast cancer than would be recommended for the treatment of many invasive breast cancers. There are limited data on the effectiveness of prophylactic mastectomy in ensuring prevention of systemic disease in patients who have this local therapy before the occurrence of any disease. However, questions regarding the benefits of prophylactic mastectomy will become more important with the advent of genetic screening and with the ability to more accurately determine future risk for the disease (Bilimoria & Morrow, 1995).

Women with a genetic predisposition for breast cancer and the members of their families require compassionate and ethical treatment by their health care providers, as well as by all of the researchers involved in the Human Genome Project. Nurses with expertise in genetic counseling will play important roles in guiding the decision-making processes regarding the advisability of genetics testing, ensuring comprehension and completeness of the informed consent process, facilitating social support for women newly diagnosed with hereditary breast cancer and their family members, serving as a source of much-needed information, and providing appropriate referrals for these individuals (Lerman, Schwartz, Miller, Daly, & Sands, 1996; Vandegriff & Williams, 1996).

The Oncology Nursing Society (ONS), a 25,000 member specialty organization, is active in supporting ethical and clinically relevant genetics counseling and care. Box 21-1 summarizes the basic elements of informed consent for germline DNA testing that have been proposed by ASCO (1996).

Box 21-1
Informed Consent for Genetics Testing: Essential Elements

1. Provide information on the specific test that will be done.
2. Fully describe the implications of both a positive and a negative test result.
3. Provide full information on the probability that the test will not prove informative.
4. Describe alternative options for risk estimation if genetics testing is not performed.
5. Explain the probable risk of passing the suspected mutation on to offspring.
6. Describe the technical accuracy of the test.
7. Describe the complete fees involved in testing and counseling.
8. Describe the risks of psychological distress.
9. Describe the risks of health/life insurance or employer discrimination.
10. Discuss the issue of confidentiality.
11. Describe the options and limitations of follow-up and additional screening after testing.

ROUTES OF METASTASES

Breast cancers spread locally, regionally, and systemically. Although metastases can occur in any organ, the most common sites of metastases are lymph nodes (76%), bone (71%), lung (69%), liver (65%), pleura (51%), adrenals (49%), and skin (30%). Locally, tumors infiltrate and spread along the mammary ducts or spread through the lymphatic system within the breast. In addition, lymphatic spread carries the cancer regionally to axillary lymph nodes and from these regional nodes to the other lymphatic chains (Fig. 21-1). Nearly 50% of women undergoing surgery for infiltrating carcinoma of the breast have axillary node involvement (Engleking, 1989). Fig. 21-2 illustrates the major sites of breast cancer metastases at the time of first recurrence and at autopsy.

ASSESSMENT

History and Physical Examination

The assessment of a patient for infiltrating breast cancer is summarized in Table 21-3. Clinical evaluation of the patient involves a detailed history that is inclusive of all of the relevant history about physical symptoms and a complete psy-

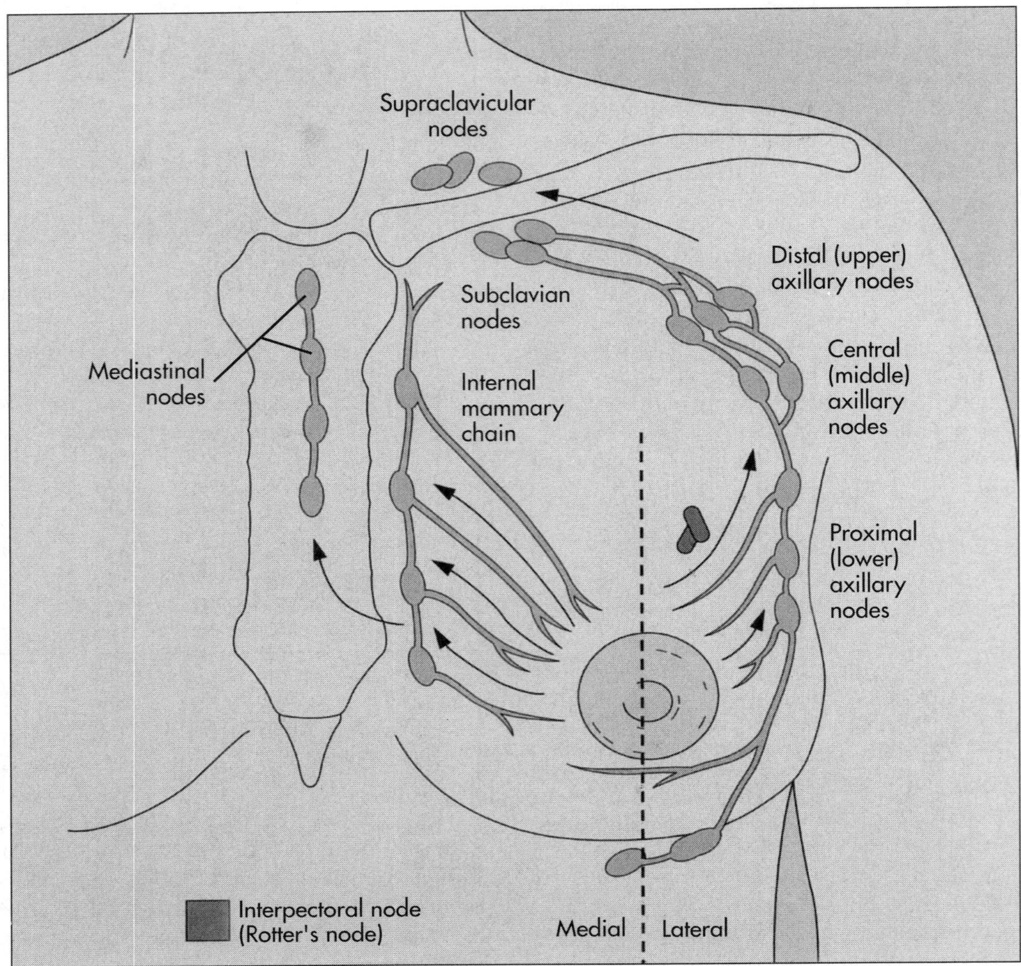

Fig. 21-1 Lymphatic spread of breast cancer. Lymph node metastases are present at the time of diagnosis in 60% of cases. In general, lateral lesions in the breast metastasize to the axillary and supraclavicular nodes, whereas medial tumors tend to metastasize to the internal mammary and mediastinal lymph nodes, as well as the supraclavicular nodes. However, lymph involvement is merely a marker for the probability that the cancer has spread from the breast. A positive finding implies that microdeposits of breast cancer will likely be present in other areas as well. (From Hayes, D. F. [1996]. Breast cancer. In A. T. Skarin [Ed.], *Atlas of diagnostic oncology* [2nd ed.]. London: Mosby-Wolfe.)

chosocial history, a complete physical examination, and a variety of diagnostic tests. The signs and symptoms that the patient presents with depend on the stage of the disease at the time of diagnosis. A biopsy is done to establish a definitive diagnosis.

Clinical Breast Examination and Mammography

Breasts are glandular tissue that develop in the female to supply milk to infant offspring. They are comprised of lobules where milk is made and a tubule and duct system several inches long that conducts milk to the nipple. Fat and connective tissue surround these structures in a sac that extends outward toward the axilla in the upper outer quadrant of each breast. The primary lymphatic system of the breast is the axillary node chain. These are the lymph nodes where breast cancer cells are believed to metastasize immediately (see Fig. 21-1). In addition, the internal mammary lymph nodes provide primary lymphatic drainage from the breast. It has been estimated that in about 9% of patients with breast cancer, the internal mammary lymph nodes contain metastatic disease when no positive axillary lymph nodes are present (Veronesi et al., 1985). The presence of disease in the supraclavicular nodes usually implies extensive metastases to the axillary chain, but can occur in the absence of axillary involvement. Ten percent of breast cancers are identified primarily through observation and palpation during a clinical breast examination (CBE) (Farwell, Foster, & Costanza, 1993).

Mammographic screening and CBE remain the most promising means for the early detection of breast cancer. Some breast cancers cannot be seen on mammography in their early stages, but often mammography is able to visualize breast tumors earlier than they can be detected by CBE or self-examination. Women with implants need to in-

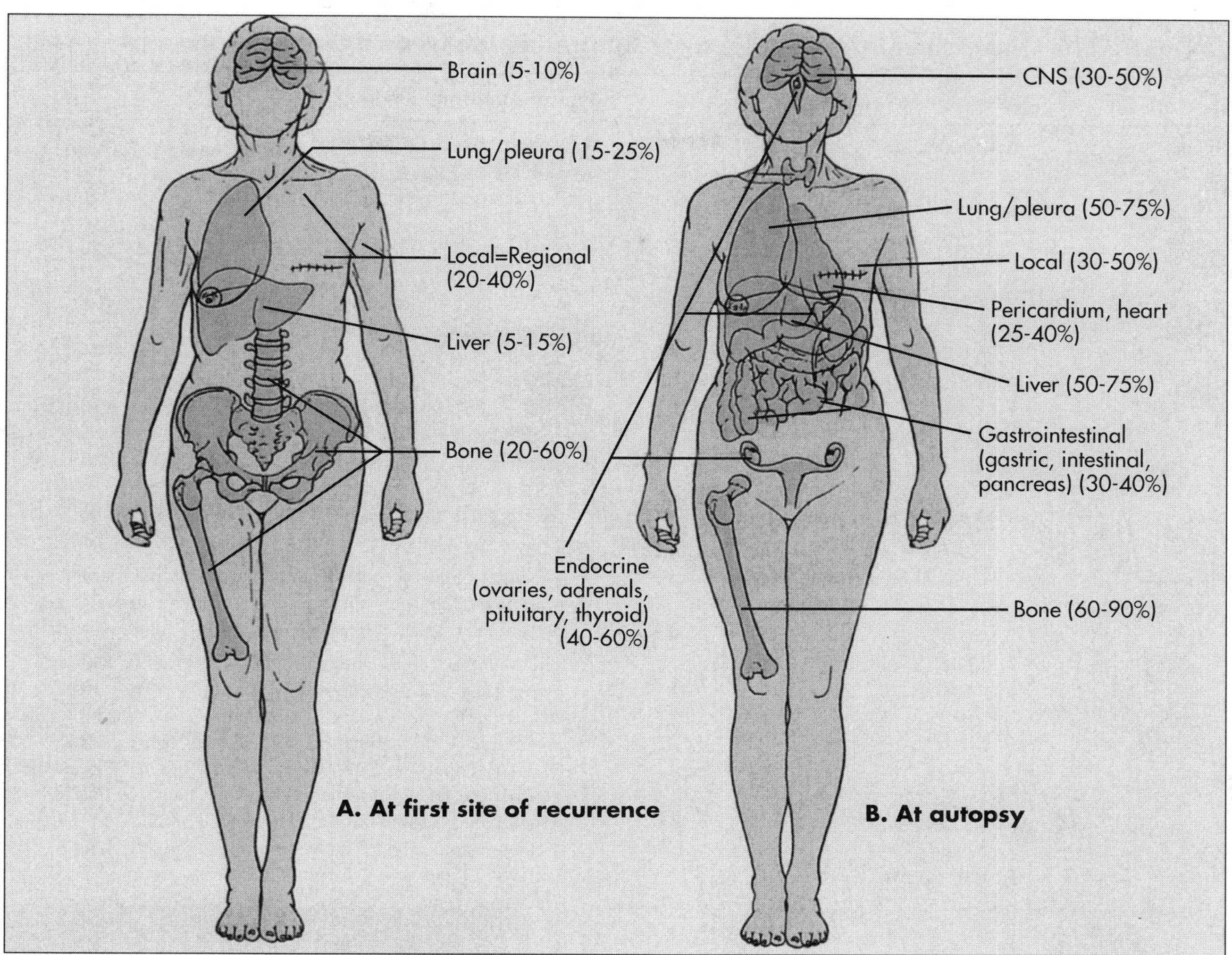

Fig. 21-2 Frequency of breast cancer metastases. The most common first sites of recurrent breast cancer are the chest wall, the regional lymph nodes, and/or bone. Liver, lung, and central nervous system (CNS) are less common sites of recurrence. In patients with well-advanced disease, breast cancer can be found in almost any organ. Autopsy studies show that metastases are most commonly found in the chest wall and in the surrounding lymph nodes, as well as in the bones, liver, lung, pleura, and CNS (brain, spinal cord, meninges). Metastases may also occur in gastrointestinal organs (pancreas, stomach, large and small intestine), endocrine organs (ovaries, adrenals, pituitary, thyroid), and in the cardiovascular system (pericardium, endocardium, myocardium). (From Hayes, D. F. [1996]. Breast cancer. In A. T. Skarin [Ed.], *Atlas of diagnostic oncology* [2nd ed.]. London: Mosby-Wolfe.)

form the mammographer of the presence of an implant so that displacement views (i.e., Ecklund views) may be performed.

In the last few years, many educational dollars have been spent to teach women the importance of screening mammograms. Several large-scale studies are attempting to show whether there is a survival advantage associated with screening mammography. The initial trials included the Health Insurance Plan of Greater New York (HIP) and the Kopparberg Swedish study. Each trial found a definite, albeit small, survival advantage in women who were 50 years of age and older who had obtained a mammogram over and above any lead-time bias (an apparent lengthening of survival related to earlier discovery of the tumor). Three subsequent trials have not confirmed these results, the most notable of them being the Canadian trial (Leitch, 1995; Miller, Baines, To, & Wall, 1992; Smart, Hendrix, Rutledge, & Smith, 1995).

Individuals who favor mammographic screening dismiss the negative results, believing that they occurred because the time frame for observation of survival was too short or because the sample sizes were inadequate. Others who doubt the benefits of screening mammography claim that the initial studies reporting a beneficial effect on survival were flawed by lead-time, length, and selection biases. For example, if a cancer is discovered earlier and treatment is ineffective, a woman may appear to live longer, but in fact her actual survival may be unaffected by the early detection of the tumor (i.e., lead-time bias). Cancers detected between mammograms (interim tumors) tend to be fast growing,

TABLE 21-3 Assessment of the Patient for Infiltrating Breast Cancer

	Assessment Parameters	Typical Abnormal Findings
History	A. Personal and social history	A. Personal and social risk factors
	1. Age	1. Increased incidence in older women
	2. Family history of breast cancer	2. Increased incidence in women with a positive family history
	3. Personal history of breast cancer	3. Increased incidence in women with a personal history of breast cancer
	4. History of benign breast disease	4. Increased incidence in women with a history of benign breast disease
	5. Age at birth of first child	5. Increased incidence in women who have their first child at an older age
	6. Age at menopause	6. Increased incidence in women who experience menopause at an older age
	B. Breast symptoms	
	1. Breast mass	1. Usually a painless mass or lump in the breast
	2. Changes in nipple or areola	2. Persistent dermatitis may be present over the nipple or areola. Serous or bloody nipple discharge may be reported.
Physical Examination	A. Clinical breast examination	A. A painless mass or lump in the breast requires mammographic evaluation. Nipple discharge may or may not be present. The axilla should be palpated for masses or lumps.
Diagnnostic Tests	A. Mammography	A. The mammographic abnormality having the highest rate of malignancy is a mass density on radiograph with associated calcifications. An associated calcification increases the rate of positivity for malignancy from 13% with density alone to 29% for density containing microcalcifications. The calcification pattern most characteristic of malignancy is one in which calcifications are typically linear, small (< 1 mm) in diameter, nonuniform in size, and clustered.
	B. Ultrasound	B. Ultrasound can be used to obtain a cross-sectional image of the breast. Ultrasonography is very accurate in the diagnosis of breast cysts (>95%).
	C. Computerized axial tomography scan	C. Computed tomography (CT) may be used as a supplement to mammography in evaluating dense breast tissue.
	D. Fine needle aspiration biopsy (FNAB)	D. Limited to determining whether or not a palpable breast lump is cancer.
	E. Stereotactic core biopsy	E. Used to establish a diagnosis of breast cancer.
	F. Needle localization biopsy	F. Used to establish a diagnosis of breast cancer.
	G. Hormone receptor assays of tissue specimen	G. Estrogen, >3 fmol/mg protein; progesterone, >3 fmol/mg protein.
	H. Liver function tests	H. May be elevated in patients with liver metastases.
	I. Bone scan	I. Bone scans are performed routinely in patients suspected of having advanced disease.
	J. CT scans of chest and abdomen	J. CT scans of the chest and abdomen are ordered in patients with early stage tumors only when the patient has elevated liver function tests.

more aggressive, detected by women themselves rather than found on mammographic screening. This fact tends to favor mammography as benefiting survival in studies that compare women's survival from breast cancers discovered by mammography with those discovered by palpation (i.e., length bias). The most important factor in any of these comparison studies is that the study populations be comparable to one another. Women who regularly obtain mammograms and those who participate in scientific experiments tend to be more affluent and more highly educated and thus may not be comparable to women in the general population (i.e., selection bias).

Screening mammograms are problematic in terms of both their sensitivity (i.e., whether the test truly determines the presence or absence of a breast tumor) and specificity (i.e., whether the mammogram correctly discriminates between breast cancer and other abnormalities). Mammograms that lack sensitivity (false-negative mammograms) were shown to be associated with provider delays in the diagnosis of breast cancer (Lannin, Harris, Swanson, & Pories, 1993). Mammograms that lack specificity (false-positive mammograms), estimated at 60% to 80% of the positive mammograms (Harris, Lippman, Veronesi, & Willett, 1992; Ziegler, 1996), result in women undergoing diagnostic procedures that are both emotionally and economically costly for themselves and their families. Studies that attempt to make the ultimate determination of whether women are benefiting adequately from screening mammography need to consider whether a significant proportion of tumors are being detected earlier, whether this earlier detection is translated into improved survival, and whether the cost is justifiable given the number of women benefited and harmed by the screening process.

Several researchers have published cost-benefit analyses for mammographic screening. Harris and Leininger (1995) estimated that the screening of 10,000 women between the ages of 50 and 60 will benefit only two to six of them a year. In another study, Eddy (1989) estimated that if 25% of the women in the United States between the ages of 40 and 75 were screened by both mammography and CBE, 4000 deaths per year would be avoided and the annual cost to the nation would be approximately $1.3 billion, or approximately $325,000 per woman benefited.

The useful *Quick Reference Guide for Clinicians* regarding mammography referral and follow-up recommendations is available through the U.S. Department of Health and Human Services (Bassett, Hendrick, Bassford, et al., 1994; Linver, Osuch, Brenner, & Smith, 1995). Despite these guidelines, women's participation in mammographic screening is suboptimal. The reasons for nonparticipation have been reported as disinterest, co-morbid medical problems, fear of radiation associated with the procedure, and the lack of either medical insurance or available financial assets for either health promotion or the treatment of a breast cancer illness if a tumor should be discovered (Facione & Facione, 1997; Lidbrink, Frisell, Brandberg; Rosendahl & Rutqvist, 1995).

Other Diagnostic Tests

Ultrasound (high-frequency sound waves) can be used to obtain a cross-sectional image of the breast and is reported to be as accurate as mammography in distinguishing between cystic and solid masses in the vast majority of cases. Ultrasound is generally ineffective in detecting small, nonpalpable cancers or in distinguishing between benign and malignant solid tumors.

Computed tomography (CT) scanning has a reported accuracy of 94% in distinguishing between benign and malignant lesions. It is useful as a supplement to mammography in evaluating dense breast tissue or to search for a primary tumor when mammogram scans are negative, but axillary lymph node biopsy is positive. The disadvantages of CT scans include radiation exposure to the thorax, a higher cost than mammography, the need for an intravenous (IV) contrast material, and the length of time required to perform the procedure.

Standard magnetic resonance imaging (MRI) uses the interaction between magnetism and radio waves to produce cross-sectional images of the breast. The adjustment of MRI to better evaluate microcalcifications seen on standard mammography appears to have the potential for diminishing false-positive rates and decreasing the number of unnecessary biopsy procedures (Ziegler, 1996). Also the application of satellite technologies to improve sensitivity and specificity in the early detection of breast cancer promises improved possibilities.

Until these and other modalities are developed to better detect breast cancers, the NIH continues to recommend that women obtain regular screening mammograms after the age of 50. The ACS continues to recommend that women between the ages of 40 and 50 obtain screening mammograms at least every 2 years (ACS, 1997). Some have suggested that the age for baseline mammogram should be as young as 35 years in African-American women because these women develop breast cancer on average at an earlier age. The availability of genetic screening for breast cancer vulnerability may lead to a refinement of these guidelines in the near future. The U.S. Preventive Task Force recommendations regarding routine breast cancer screening currently limits the use of mammography alone or mammography with annual CBE to women age 50 to 69, finding that there is currently insufficient evidence to recommend for or against routine mammography or CBE for women age 40 to 49 or age 70 and older (NEWS, Journal of the National Cancer Institute, 1996b). This limitation excludes women determined to be at high risk, who they recommend should have a screening mammography. They found insufficient evidence (i.e., the quality of the research data were inadequate) to recommend either CBE alone without accompanying mammography or breast self-examination (BSE) as proven methods for the earlier detection of breast cancer.

Making or Ruling Out a Diagnosis of Breast Cancer

A diagnostic workup to make or rule out a cancer diagnosis follows two pathways dependent on the presentation of the abnormality: abnormal mammogram or palpable breast lump or palpable abnormal density. Figs. 20-6 and 20-7 describe the pathways for making or ruling out a breast cancer diagnosis in women with an abnormal screening mammogram and a palpable breast lump.

For a mammographic abnormality, radiology alone or radiology/surgery complementary procedures are used to obtain a sample of breast tissue. Mammographic abnormalities include nonpalpable masses; suspicious architectural distortion (i.e., distortion of the normal structures of the breast tissue); or microcalcifications. Calcifications, seen as white flecks on a mammogram, are classified as benign, indeterminate, or suspicious. Suspicious calcifications are further classified to be of low, moderate, or high suspicion. It is generally recommended to biopsy indeterminate or suspicious microcalcifications unless there is long-term stability in biopsy proven benign microcalcifications.

A definitive diagnosis entails both a biopsy and histopathologic determination of the tissue sample. Indications for biopsy include any discrete, palpable mass in the breast regardless of mobility, negative mammogram, length of time the mass has been present, or benign nature of previous biopsies. Generally, it is recommended to biopsy indeterminate and suspicious microcalcifications. The radiologist will recommend the appropriate biopsy procedure based on the size and position of the abnormality and relevant clinical issues. All biopsies can be done under local anesthesia, with or without sedation, on an outpatient basis. The number of breast biopsies performed in the United States each year has been estimated as near 1 million (Hall, Storella, Silverstone, & Wyshak, 1988).

Biopsy Procedures Used to Establish a Diagnosis of Breast Cancer

Fine Needle Aspiration Biopsy. With a palpable breast mass, an in-office fine needle aspiration biopsy (FNAB) can be performed (Grant, Groellner, Welsh, & Martin, 1986). The technique involves palpating and holding the mass steady with one hand while inserting a small needle (22 to 25 gauge), generally held on a needle holder, and pulling the needle in and out of the lump while remaining in the breast to obtain tissue. This procedure is usually repeated (often for a total of two times, sometimes three) until the provider, usually a surgeon or a cytopathologist, is satisfied that there appears to be a sufficient sample of breast tissue. Some practitioners use injectable lidocaine to anesthetize the area. Applying firm pressure until bleeding or oozing has stopped will decrease bleeding and bruising after the procedure. The needle insertion site will heal, and no scar will be evident.

Patients experience a range of discomfort during the procedure, somewhat in relationship to location of the lump, baseline breast sensations, density of their breast tissue, time in the menstrual cycle, general pain sensitivity, prior experience, and level of anxiety. If feasible, it is useful to have a support person present during the procedure. In addition, some patients may benefit from the use of relaxation techniques, distraction, or humor. The patient will benefit from having a description of what to expect during the FNAB *before* the procedure and being shown the needle holder (which otherwise makes the small needle look frightening). Postprocedure teaching should include recommendations for use of ice, the use of acetaminophen or a nonsteroidal anti-inflammatory drug (NSAID) if needed, and a brief review of unusual complications (e.g., infection, bleeding, swelling).

The advantage of an FNAB is the availability of a fairly rapid tissue analysis without surgery. The general standard for diagnostic accuracy is triple diagnosis, that is, the use of three tests (i.e., CBE, mammogram, and FNAB). The FNAB procedure has been used more widely in Europe and in the Scandinavian countries but is gaining more acceptance in the United States. The false-positive rate is low (about 0.17% [Foster, 1996]) so a diagnosis of breast cancer from an FNAB allows for expeditious treatment planning. The false-negative rate has a wider range (0.4% to 35%) and is thought to be largely operator dependent (Foster, 1996). A patient with a benign result with sufficient tissue that matches CBE findings and is corroborated by a negative mammogram can be monitored safely in the clinic at 3- to 6-month intervals. Patients should be taught to do BSE and to report any changes in breast tissue to their health care provider.

An FNAB with insufficient tissue is comparable to no FNAB and should either be repeated or followed by an excisional biopsy. An FNAB with atypical or equivocal findings warrants follow-up with an excisional biopsy. A mammogram should be performed before the FNAB, as post-FNAB mammogram results can be obscured by bleeding and swelling. If an FNAB is done inadvertently before the mammogram, one should wait 4 to 6 weeks before the mammogram is done.

An FNAB is limited to determining whether a palpable lump is cancer. It is not a reliable determinant of tumor type or tumor biology, although tissue specially prepared from an FNAB can be used to test for estrogen and progesterone receptors. Some practitioners validate the malignant FNAB findings with frozen section tissue intraoperatively; others do not. Some clinicians do so only if the cytopathologist recommends confirmation.

Stereotactic Core Biopsy. Stereotactic core biopsy has been advocated increasingly as an alternative to open excisional biopsy. Some women are not candidates for this option because of dyspnea and/or obesity, or in some cases they may not be able to lie on their abdomen on the stereotactic core biopsy table. Patient Preparation Table 20-4 describes this procedure. Postprocedure symptoms include breast soreness and possible bruising. There is no scar on the breast and no noticeable scar tissue is evident on future mammograms. The advantages of stereotactic core biopsy include lower cost and less trauma to the patient and, in cases where the lesions are benign, the absence of cosmetic deformity and breast scarring on follow-up mammograms. When a definitive diagnosis is made using stereotactic core biopsy, this allows for pretreatment planning and fewer steps in the diagnostic pathway.

A recent review of 431 core needle biopsies, done at the University of California Los Angeles (UCLA), demonstrated a definitive outcome in 96% of the biopsies with 6 to 38 months of follow-up. Of the 431 biopsies, 179 were malignant, 13 demonstrated atypia, and 239 were benign. A false-negative rate of 1.7% was reported. These data corroborate the safety and efficacy of core biopsy in the hands of experienced providers (Nguyen et al., 1996). Even with this technique there is still a small miss rate, usually due to movement of the tissue after the breast has been removed from compression.

Needle Localization Biopsy. If the diagnosis following a stereotactic core biopsy is not definitive or if a stereotactic biopsy is not recommended clinically or is technically not feasible, a needle localization biopsy will be performed. This outpatient procedure is accomplished in two-steps. Step 1 occurs in the radiology department where a thin wire is placed into or around the abnormality with mammographic guidance. Step 2 occurs in surgery where the surgeon removes the abnormality using the wire to locate its exact position. The surgeon, with the patient under

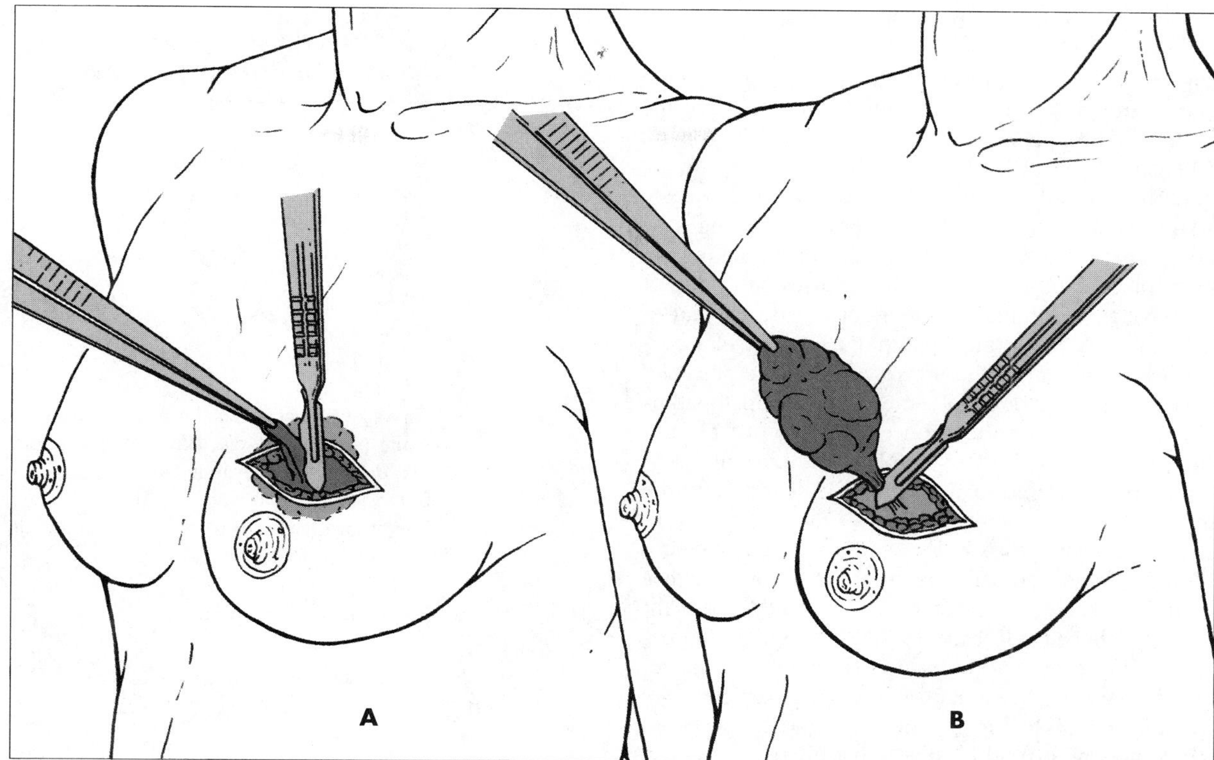

Fig. 21-3 **A,** An incisional biopsy allows for a definitive diagnosis. **B,** Excisional biopsies, although diagnostic, can also be therapeutic by eliminating the need for further breast surgery when radiation therapy is performed. (From Hayes, D. F. [1996]. Breast cancer. In A. T. Skarin [Ed.], *Atlas of diagnostic oncology* [2nd ed.]. London: Mosby-Wolfe.)

either local anesthesia alone or with local anesthesia and sedation, performs an excisional biopsy, and then a specimen radiograph is done to verify that the abnormality is in the specimen. The incision is sutured and a dressing is applied. The woman is discharged home after recovering from the sedation, if any was used. Postprocedure signs and symptoms may include breast pain or discomfort, bruising or bleeding, infection, or wound dehiscence. The woman will have a scar on the breast and architectural distortion evident on future mammograms. Many women report awareness of sensations in the area of a biopsy for months or years after the procedure.

Summary of Biopsy Procedures. Previously, excisional biopsies were performed as the initial procedure in one-step breast cancer surgery. Histologic analyses were preformed from frozen sections of the breast biopsy tissue, and if the frozen section was positive, the definitive surgery was performed during the same surgical procedure. Today, most excisional biopsies are performed on an outpatient basis, usually under local anesthesia. Open biopsies for smaller tumors endeavor to remove the entire observable lesion with clear margins. The histologic type of the lesion is determined from permanent sections of the tissue specimen and the borders of the specimen are carefully examined (Fig. 21-3).

In the case of larger tumors, a small portion of the tumor may be removed first to perform histologic and receptor assay examinations to determine the optimal approach to treatment. Women with positive biopsies are provided with counseling regarding their treatment options and the advisability of a second surgical procedure (i.e., re-excision mastectomy or lumpectomy) to complete the primary surgery. As the second step in breast cancer surgery, mastectomy or lumpectomy procedures usually are performed with the patient under general anesthesia, as they almost always include a lymph node dissection.

Improved tolerance for these procedures and decreased levels of anxiety are reported to occur when women are given sensory information before the biopsy procedure, including brochures and pictures of the procedure (Kelly & Winslow, 1996). Women undergoing an FNAB report moderate anxiety levels and sensations of pressure, stinging, and pain almost always rated to be in the moderate intensity range.

STAGING

Staging is a method of describing the extent of a tumor at the time of diagnosis. Staging is used as a prognostic indicator and to determine optimal treatment options. Staging is determined by considering the size of the tumor, presence of and number of positive lymph nodes, margins of the resected tumor, histology of the tumor (structure of the breast cancer cells), hormonal receptor status of the tumor,

tumor grade, and other individually relevant prognostic factors.

A general staging system used to standardize a portion of this determination is the American Joint Committee on Cancer's (AJCC, 1988) TNM classification system. The TNM system considers the characteristics of the primary tumor (T), lymph node involvement (N), and the presence or absence of metastatic spread (M). Standardized staging systems help guide treatment and provide uniform tracking information for research. Clinical staging uses information from the physical examination, laboratory tests, and radiographic findings. A postsurgical pathologic staging of a cancer describes the extent of the primary tumor; the presence or absence of lymph node involvement; and the histopathologic diagnosis based on a careful examination of the excised breast tissue. Table 21-4 displays the current TNM classification system used to stage breast cancer at the time of diagnosis.

Stage at diagnosis differs by race/ethnicity, age, and economic status. Usually, older women are diagnosed with a more advanced stage of breast cancer (Mandalblatt, Andrews, Kao, Wallace, & Kerner, 1995). The association between increasing stage and older age is believed to be related to a decrease in breast cancer screening participation; a decrease in access to breast cancer diagnostic services; and higher rates of co-morbid illness that distract providers from attention to breast cancer risk in this patient population. Several studies have shown that older women with breast cancer undergo fewer treatment modalities than younger women (Goodwin & Samet, 1994; Merchant, McCormick, Yahalom, & Borgen, 1996; Newschaffer, Penberthy, Desch, Retchin, & Whittemore, 1996). The claim that older women are offered fewer treatment modalities because of co-morbidity issues was refuted by Newschaffer and colleagues (1996). The most important issue is whether older women have lower survival rates if they fail to receive the same level of aggressive treatment. This issue remains unresolved at the present time. Some researchers have reported that older women have poorer treatment outcomes as a result of less aggressive treatment approaches (Goodwin & Samet, 1994), whereas others have observed no differences in 5- or 10-year survival rates when pathologic staging is controlled for in the statistical analyses (Merchant et al., 1996).

African-American women are more likely to present with regional or distant disease (45%) than white women (37%) (Simon & Severson, 1996). Table 21-5 displays differences in stage of breast cancer at the time of diagnosis between whites and African-American women (Reis et al., 1994). In recent years, the proportion of white women with more advanced cancer at the time of diagnosis has been decreasing, a gain not demonstrated in the African-American population. Reports from the National Cancer Institute (NCI)/Surveillance, Epidemiology and End Results (SEER) data documented larger tumor diameters and increased numbers of positive axillary nodes in African-American women when compared with whites (Boring, Squires, Tong, & Montgomery, 1994). Separating the effects of racial heritage (genetics) from social and behavioral variables (ideas, values, and the circumstances of women's lives) on the development of breast cancer have been difficult (Facione & Dodd, 1995). Some studies have suggested a difference in tumor biology by ethnicity or race (Ownby et al., 1985; Richardson et al., 1992), whereas others have shown no differ-

TABLE 21-4 The TNM Four-Stage System: Clinical Evaluation of Primary Breast Cancer

Tumor (T)	
To	No evidence of tumor
Tis	Carcinoma in situ or Paget's disease of nipple with no tumor
T1	2 cm
T1a	0.5 cm
T1b	>0.5 cm-1 cm
T1c	>1cm-2 cm
T2	>2cm-5 cm
T3	>5 cm
T4	Any size: direct extension to chest wall (excluding pectoral muscle, skin infiltration, peau d'orange, satelite nodules)
T4a	Extension to chest wall
T4b	Edema or ulceration of skin or presence of satellite nodules
T4c	Both T4a and T4b
T4d	Inflammatory carcinoma
Nodes (N)	
No	No regional lymph node metastases
N1	Metastasis to movable ipsilateral axillary lymph node(s)
N2	Metastasis to ipsilateral axillary lymph node or nodes fixed to one another or to other structures
N3	Metastasis to ipsilateral internal mammary node or nodes
Metastasis (M)	
Mo	No distant metastasis
M1	Distant metastasis, including metastasis to ipsilateral supraclavicular lymph node or nodes

AJCC Classification for breast cancer based on TNM Criteria

Stage	Tumor	Nodes	Metastases
0	Tis	N0	M0
I	T1	N0	M0
IIA	T0,1	N1	M0
	T2	N0	M0
IIB	T2	N1	M0
	T3	N0	M0
IIIA	T0,1,2	N2	M0
	T3	N1,2	M0
IIIB	T4	N1,2	M0
	Any T	N3	M0
IV	Any T	Any N	M1

American Joint Committee on Cancer (AJCC). (1988). *Manual for staging of cancer* (3rd ed.). Philadelphia: J. B. Lippincott.

TABLE 21-5 Percentage Distribution of Breast Cancer Cases by Race and Stage at Diagnosis

Stage	African Americans	Whites
Localized	48	60
Regional	37	31
Distant	9	6
Missing Data	6	3

National Cancer Institute Surveillence and Epidemiologic End Results Data 1986-1992.

ences in stage of disease at the time of diagnosis when access to care is not an issue (Zaloznik, 1995).

An early survey report of why cancer stage was significantly more advanced in African-American women focused on a lack of knowledge of cancer-related symptoms (EVAXX, Inc., 1980). More recent studies have added to this understanding, delineating the relative lack of access to breast cancer diagnosis and detection services and the inability for many African-American and other poor Americans to pay for cancer early detection and treatment services as contributing to women's decision to delay the evaluation of breast symptoms that later prove to be signals of breast cancer (Simon and Severson, 1996; Weiss et al., 1995). Other researchers have examined differences in the beliefs of women about the likelihood of curability of breast cancer and social role constraints women experience in relationship to seeking a diagnosis or treatment of their breast cancer symptoms (Facione & Dodd, 1995; Facione, Dodd, Holzemer, & Meleis, 1997).

MEDICAL MANAGEMENT

The major treatment options for infiltrating breast cancer are shown in Fig. 21-4.

Surgical Management

Surgery is most often the first treatment modality used in the management of breast cancer regardless of whether the invasive breast cancer is infiltrating ductal, infiltrating lobular, or one of the less common types of breast cancer. The classic exception to this rule is metastatic disease or inflammatory breast cancer because of its poorer prognosis. In addition, in some settings, large breast cancers may be treated initially with chemotherapy. Initial treatment with chemotherapy does not preclude the subsequent use of surgery for local control. However, at the present time, if a patient experiences a good response to a course of presurgical chemotherapy, there are no definitive outcome data to guide decision making regarding subsequent treatment with breast conservation surgery or the advisability of radiation therapy for these women. The standard approach has been to recommend mastectomy after chemotherapy for large (i.e., >5 cm) tumors (Bonadonna, Valgussa, Zucali, & Salvadori, 1995; Harris & Swain, 1996; Hortobagyi et al., 1995).

Once the diagnosis of invasive breast cancer has been made, treatment options for local and systemic control of the disease must be addressed immediately. Women with early stage disease are offered the choice of breast-conserving surgery followed by radiation therapy to the breast or mastectomy. Although local reoccurrence rates differ between the two choices, survival outcomes continue to be borne out as equivalent between the two treatment approaches (Veronesi & Salvadori, 1996). In 1990, the use of breast-conserving surgery was supported by an NCI expert panel, for most women with stage I and II breast cancers. The acceptance of this approach continues to grow. The medical criteria that need to be evaluated before recommending lumpectomy (partial mastectomy) and breast irradiation or a modified radical mastectomy include (1) tumor size; (2) skin involvement, edema, erythema (inflammatory breast cancer); (3) presence or absence of multifocal disease; (4) extent of intraductal disease, if it is also present; (5) whether the position of the cancer and the size of the woman's breast allow for cosmetically acceptable conservative surgery; and (6) whether there are reasons why the patient could not receive radiation therapy. In addition, it is important for the patient to understand that a lumpectomy is successful only if there are clear surgical margins and that in a percentage of cases, a re-excision, or more rarely if a complication occurs, a mastectomy may be recommended that was not foreseen earlier.

The key components that affect a woman's decisions regarding a specific surgical treatment option vary widely and are highly personal. Decisions are influenced by the full diversity of cultural, ethnic, religious, regional, and generational factors. The major factors that influence a woman's decision about breast cancer treatment include the following: how a woman (and her perception of how significant other[s]) feels about her breast and her body; her degree of worry about local recurrence; and her and her family's and friends' previous encounters with illness, medicine, and breast cancer. Women express a wide spectrum of responses when confronted with the need to make choices about the options regarding breast cancer surgery. These range from a woman feeling that she would lose her sense of self and could not tolerate losing a breast, to feeling that her breast is a threat to her life and therefore she wants "it" removed. The difficulties surrounding decision making are compounded by the lack of definitive medical knowledge, conflicting opinions, and the emotional crisis precipitated by the cancer diagnosis.

Surgical Procedures for Breast Cancer. A modified radical mastectomy (MRM) is removal of the breast, dissection of the axillary nodes, and preservation of the pectoral muscles. An MRM is sufficient for local control unless the tumor is close to or invading the underlying muscle. A lumpectomy (partial mastectomy) is removal of the tumor resected widely enough to obtain clear margins. A quadrantectomy is the removal of a quadrant of the breast, removing more ductal tissue in line with the nipple than what is removed in a lumpectomy. A separate incision is also made to do an ipsilateral axillary lymph node dissection. There has been a recent shift in practice from a former attempt to

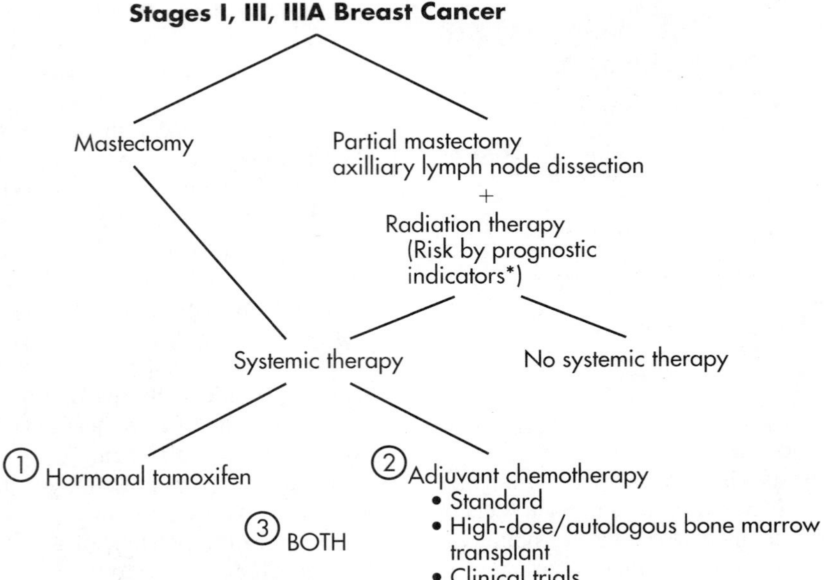

Fig. 21-4 Treatment options: invasive breast cancer. (*Age, lymph nodes, estrogen, progesterone receptors, tumor size, tumor rate of growth, differentiation.)

dissect all level I, II, and III lymph nodes to matching the clinical presentation of the disease with the warranted level of aggressiveness in an attempt to better control procedure-related morbidity. In general, level I and II lymph nodes are dissected along with tissue that appears to contain disease at the time of the dissection (Mackarem, Barbarisi, & Hughes, 1992). Table 21-6 lists some of the common sequelae associated with mastectomy or axillary node dissection.

Currently, studies are emerging that identify and biopsy the sentinel lymph node (SLN), then compare that pathologic data to standard level I and II dissection. Albertini and colleagues (1996), in a study of 62 patients, first identified the SLN by injection of a blue dye and a technetium-labeled sulfur colloid. The SLN was excised and the axillary lymph node dissected. The SLN was correctly identified in 92% of the patients in the study. All women with regional disease had positive SLNs, and in 67% of the women with regional disease, the SLN was the only positive lymph node. If these types of studies continue to produce similar results, the advantages of using SLN biopsies as indicators of the need for a full axillary dissection will include decreased patient morbidity (by potentially eliminating the need for further lymph node dissection in women with negative SLNs) and a potential for an improvement in pathologic assessment because fewer nodes will need to be examined.

The timing of the primary surgery has been the topic of a number of studies. Results from some studies suggest that surgery during the luteal phase of the menstrual cycle (mid cycle, day 7 to 20) may be associated with a better prognosis than surgery on or near the follicular phase (perimenstrually: day 0 to 6 or day 21 to 36). Davidoff and Abeloff (1993) reviewed six studies that found a relationship between timing of surgery and survival and nine studies that did not demonstrate the same relationship. At the present time, it appears that there are insufficient data to link timing of surgery to survival outcome.

Reconstructive Surgery. Choices regarding reconstruction range from doing it at all to not having the procedure, the timing of the procedure, and the type of procedure. A presurgical consultation with a plastic surgeon before surgery is recommended when the patient is considering having reconstructive surgery. Some practitioners do not recommend immediate reconstruction, and others offer it as an option. The two major types of breast reconstructive surgery are an implant or a flap procedure using autologous muscle to reshape muscle from a donor site into a breast mound. The timing of a consultation with a plastic surgeon may vary depending on variations in the decision-making process. However, when a patient is considering breast reconstruction, consultation with the plastic surgeon is a key element of pretreatment planning.

Reconstruction with an Implant. In 1963, the silicone implant was developed for breast augmentation. Since 1965, silicone gel implants were used in reconstructive surgery following mastectomy. In response to a reported or suspected relationship between silicone implants and the development of connective tissue disease, the Food and Drug Administration (FDA) conducted hearings and currently has prospective trials underway to study the physiologic effects of silicone implants. To date, the FDA has not established a link between connective tissue disorders and silicone implants. However, saline implants are currently being used widely for breast reconstruction.

The approach used to surgically place an implant depends on the amount and condition of the skin overlying the chest wall after mastectomy. If there is an adequate amount of tissue, direct implantation of a saline prosthesis can be accomplished relatively easily. With the most com-

Table 21-6 Common Sequelae of Mastectomy, Axillary Dissection, or Both

Sequelae	Patients Affected (%)
Pain or Discomfort	
Incisional	90-100
Paresthesia of the arm	90-100
Hypesthesia of the arm	90-100
Cords	40-50
Pectoralis spasm	20-30
Chest wall	25-35
Trigger point	<10
Edema	
One arm, transient	<50
Arm requiring Jobst sleeve (increase >2 cm)	18
Breast	90-100
Neurapraxia	
Serratus anterior	15
Others	15
Limitation in range of motion	Initially, 100; after 9 mo, 2

Gerber, L. (1996). Rehabilitation management for women with breast cancer: Maximizing functional outcomes. In J. Harris, M. Lippman, M. Morrow, & S. Hellman (Eds.), *Diseases of the breast.* Philadelphia: Lippincott Raven.

mon procedure, an expander is implanted under the pectoralis muscle (Fig. 21-5). This procedure allows for implant reconstruction without the use of an imported skin flap and results in improved cosmesis (Fig. 21-6).

Several different tissue expanders are on the market, but most of them are attached to filling valves that are injected percutaneously with normal saline over time (usually 6 to 8 weeks) until full inflation is achieved. The initial inflation begins after adequate postoperative healing has occurred and generally involves the injection of 100 to 150 ml of normal saline, one to two times per week, until an average total of 600 to 800 ml has been injected. Variations in these procedures are influenced by preoperative breast size, the condition and amount of skin involved at the site of the implant, and whether the patient smokes cigarettes. The implant is overinflated to promote more natural shaping of the breast and softer tissue. Women are often concerned at this point about the size and lack of a match to the contralateral breast. This concern may be alleviated by re-education about the entire process of breast reconstruction. When skin expansion is accomplished, a second surgical procedure is done to remove the expander and replace it with the implant.

The most common complications that may occur with tissue expanders are mechanical failure of the device, contracture, or deflation. With mechanical failure or deflation, surgical replacement is necessary. If a contracture produces symptoms of pain or impaired range of motion or if the cosmetic result is unacceptable to the patient, a surgical capsulotomy is indicated. Women with implants need to inform

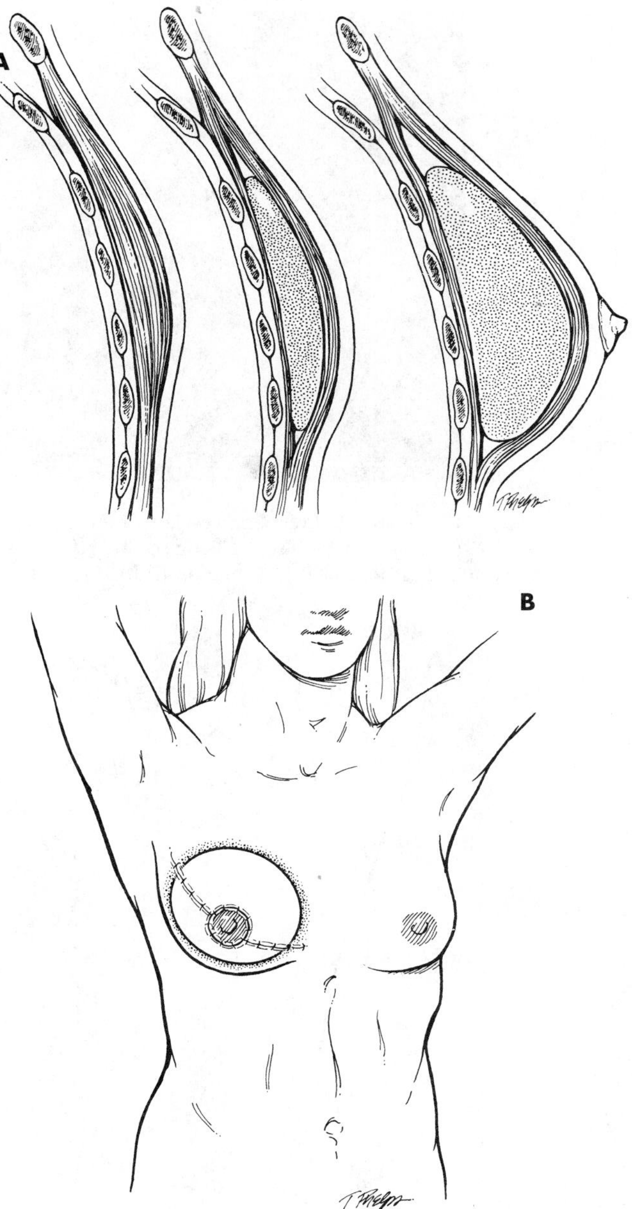

Fig. 21-5 **A,** Placement of tissue expander beneath the pectoralis major muscle and skin with serial expansion. **B,** Permanent saline implant in place. (From Chang, B. W. [1995]. Reconstruction following mastectomy: Timing, indications, and results. In J. L. Cameron [Ed.], *Current surgical therapy* [5th ed.]. St. Louis: Mosby.)

the mammographer of the presence of the implant so that displacement views (i.e., Ecklund views) can be performed.

Reconstruction of the Breast with Autologous Tissue and Skin. A transverse rectus abdominis myocutaneous (TRAM) flap is the most frequently performed autologous reconstruction procedure (Figs. 21-7 and 21-8 pp. 442-443). A good candidate for this surgery is a woman who has adequate abdominal skin and underlying tissue and who chooses this procedure with a good understanding of the realities of the surgery. This surgery takes 2 to 6 hours and requires a 3- to 7-day hospitalization. A large ellipse of

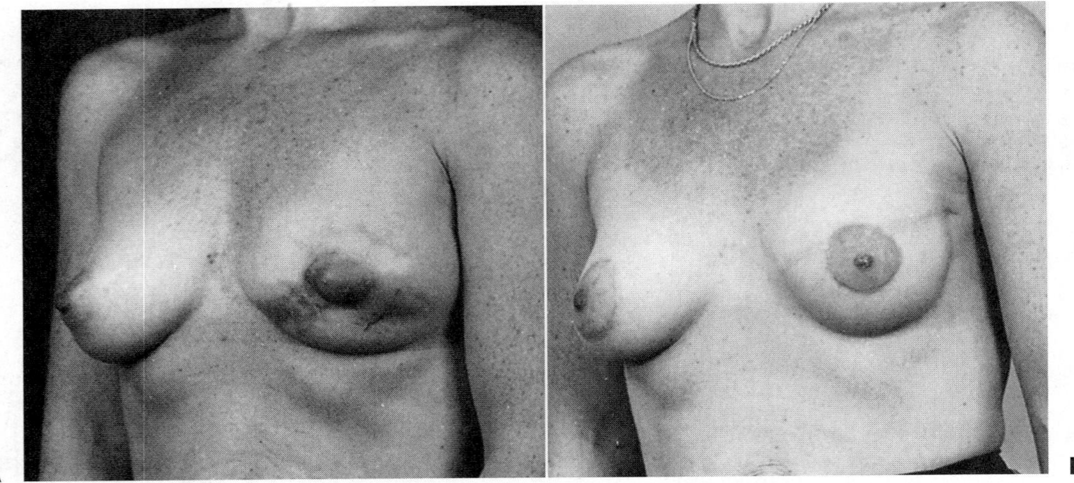

Fig. 21-6 **A,** Preoperative view of a patient before expander/implant reconstruction. **B,** Results 8 months after operation. (From Chang, B. W. [1995]. Reconstruction following mastectomy: Timing, indications, and results. In J. L. Cameron [Ed.], *Current surgical therapy* [5th ed.]. St. Louis: Mosby.)

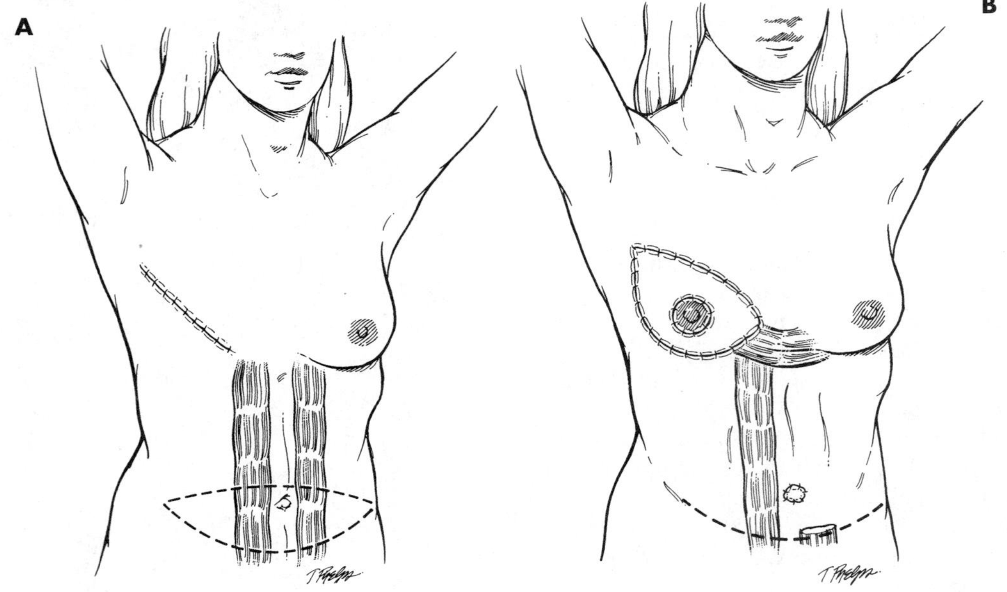

Fig. 21-7 **A,** Outline of a transverse rectus abdominis myocutaneous (TRAM) flap donor site. **B,** Inset of a contralateral-pedicle TRAM flap breast reconstruction. (From Chang, B. W. [1995]. Reconstruction following mastectomy: Timing, indications, and results. In J. L. Cameron [Ed.], *Current surgical therapy* [5th ed.]. St. Louis: Mosby.)

skin and subcutaneous tissue is harvested from the abdomen and transferred to the chest wall to create a breast mound. The tissue remains attached to one or both rectus muscles so that the epigastric artery and vein maintain tissue viability. In addition to the creation of the breast mound, this procedure results in a transverse scar on the lower abdomen and a change in contour of the abdomen resulting from removal of skin, fat, and muscle.

Free flap reconstruction is microsurgery involving the resection of a mass of tissue comprised of skin, fat, and muscle with its key vessel attached and transferring this tissue to the chest wall where it is reattached to a blood supply and fashioned to match the contralateral breast. The common donor sites include the lower abdomen (TRAM free flap) or gluteal tissue (gluteus maximus musculocutaneous flap). The latissimus dorsi musculocutaneous flap is performed by moving back tissue (skin and muscle) to the chest wall to create a breast mound.

Complications encountered with autologous reconstruction include a weakening of the abdominal wall because of loss of the rectus abdominis muscle, possibly resulting in a hernia, although the incidence is reported at less than 5%

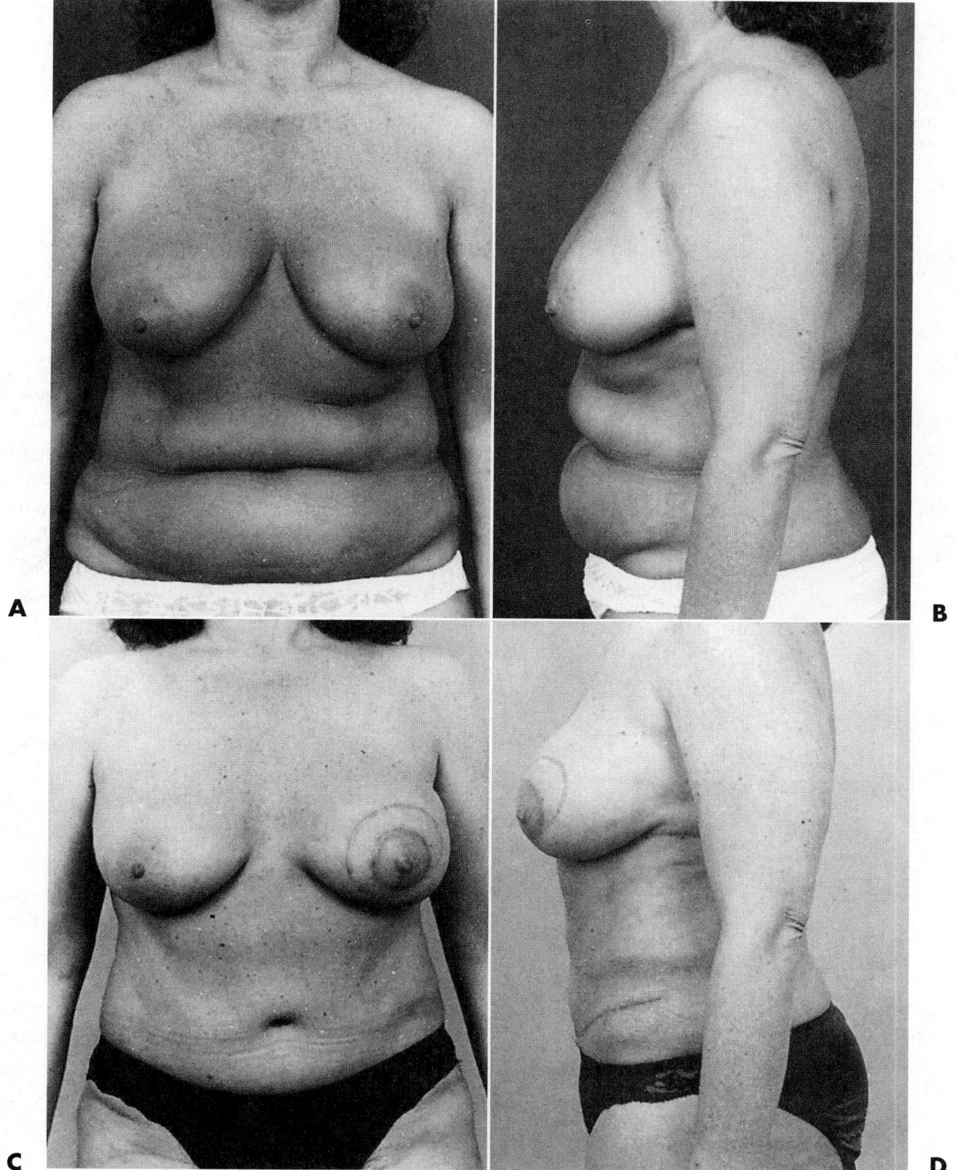

Fig. 21-8 **A,** Preoperative view of a patient before mastectomy and immediate reconstruction with a single-pedicle TRAM flap. **B,** Preoperative lateral view. **C,** Results 8 months after operation. **D,** Postoperative lateral view. (From Chang, B. W. [1995]. Reconstruction following mastectomy: Timing, indications, and results. In J. L. Cameron [Ed.], *Current surgical therapy* [5th ed.]. St. Louis: Mosby.)

(Handel, 1991). Complications at the donor site include infection, hematoma, and fat necrosis. Fat and skin necrosis can develop in the reconstructed breast that may require débridement. The most serious complication following a free flap involves a loss of tissue viability of the flap. The immediate postoperative period is the time of greatest risk. Other complications include infection, bleeding, seroma formation, and difficulties with wound healing. Complications involving viability of the flap are more common in women with compromised circulation resulting from smoking, morbid obesity, diabetes mellitus, or hypertension. Other complications include infection, hematomas, and seromas (Mackay & Bostwick, 1996).

Reconstruction of the Nipple Areola. Generally, this part of the breast reconstruction is done as an outpatient procedure, after complete healing from prior reconstructive surgery. The tissue used is most often from the skin and subcutaneous tissue of the breast or from a small portion of the opposite nipple (Figs. 21-9 and 21-10). Tattooing can be used to create the areola with a more natural skin tone, eliminating the need for more surgery (Bostwick, 1995; Mackay & Bostwick, 1996).

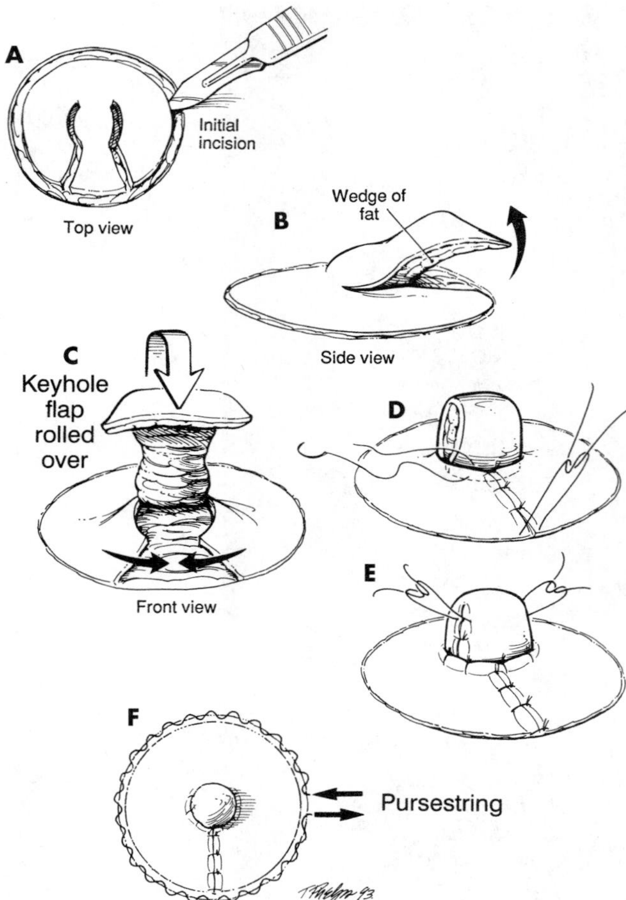

Fig. 21-9. Circumscribed keyhole nipple-areola reconstruction. **A,** Initial incisions. **B,** Keyhole flap elevated. **C,** Keyhole flap rolled over and areola flaps mobilized. **D** and **E,** Incisions closed. **F,** Areola diameter adjusted with a pursestring suture. (From Chang, B. W. [1995]. Reconstruction following mastectomy: Timing, indications, and results. In J. L. Cameron [Ed.], *Current surgical therapy* [5th ed.]. St. Louis: Mosby.)

Radiation Therapy

Radiation therapy to the breast is a primary therapy done for local control of disease or as palliative treatment for metastatic disease. According to a report that evaluated studies of women who underwent lumpectomy (Fisher et al., 1995), radiation therapy following lumpectomy decreases the risk of local or regional recurrence from 5% to 10%. Ideally, the patient who is considering breast-conserving surgery should meet with the radiation oncologist and the surgeon before the surgical procedure so that there is collaborative professional agreement that the choice of surgery followed by radiation therapy is feasible and safe. There are patients whose risk for local recurrence is high, and the risks should be made clear to the patient. High-risk patients include those with extensive intraductal carcinoma; those who have tumors with multiple microcalcifications, especially if these lesions are shown to be associated with invasive or in situ disease; and those who have a tumor with a subareolar location.

After adequate wound healing from breast-conserving surgery (i.e., wide local excision, segmental or partial mastectomy, or quadrantectomy), the breast is irradiated. The whole breast, underlying chest wall, and a small area of the lung are included in the treatment field. The breast is irradiated with lateral and medial tangential portals. In most cases, the total dose of radiation therapy is 4500-5000 cGy given over 5 to 6 weeks to the whole breast followed by a boost (concentrated dose) of an additional 1500 to 2000 cGy to the portion of the breast that contained the primary tumor. The dose of external beam radiation is delivered by a linear accelerator.

The boost dose is given because the majority of local recurrences occur near the site of the primary tumor. A boost dose may not be judged clinically necessary in defined subsets of patients (e.g., stage I tumors, wide surgical margins, quadrantectomy, low-grade tumors), but it is done for most patients. It is possible, and at one time it was more common, to use interstitial implants for the boost dose. However, the use of an interstitial implant appears to have no additional clinical benefit, and because it requires an inpatient hospitalization, its use has become rare.

At the time of treatment planning and simulation, wedges or compensating filters are designed or placed to allow for uniform dosing across the breast. Clinical consideration, depending on the stage and presentation of the disease, may also be given to radiating the axillary, supraclavicular, and rarely, the internal mammary lymph nodes. Radiation therapy to the axillary lymph nodes increases morbidity because of the increased incidence of lymphedema. Chest wall irradiation after a modified radical mastectomy may be considered for large tumors (i.e., >5 cm); in patients with numerous positive lymph nodes; or when the tumor is at or near the margin or the invading muscle is excised incompletely by the surgeon.

Common side effects from primary breast irradiation include fatigue that appears to be cumulative, local breast edema, breast tenderness or pain, and skin reactions. The spectrum of responses varies widely from women who continue their full-time lives with little accommodation to women (rarely) who are unable to work or perform their accustomed activities of daily life. Women with fair skin are at higher risk to develop skin reactions from radiation therapy. It is rare to see "skin burns," yet some care providers and the population as a whole still carry that fear (O'Rourke & Robinson, 1996). Table 21-7 lists the side effects of radiation therapy to the breast and chest wall and provides suggested interventions (O'Rourke & Robinson, 1996).

Chemotherapy

The rationale for systemic therapy is based on work done in the 1960s and 1970s. The fact that micrometastases may exist in some women at the time of diagnosis forms the basis for the use of systemic therapy. Therefore systemic therapies (i.e., chemotherapy and hormonal therapy) are consid-

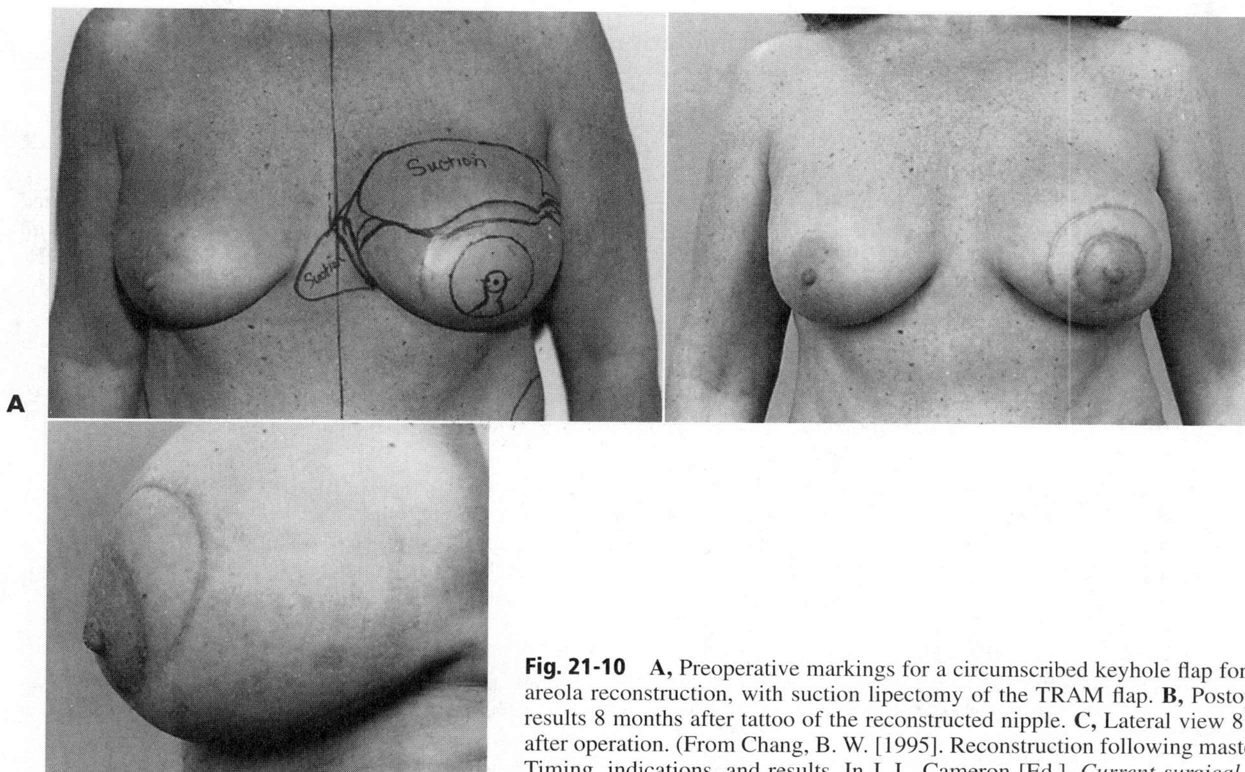

Fig. 21-10 **A,** Preoperative markings for a circumscribed keyhole flap for nipple-areola reconstruction, with suction lipectomy of the TRAM flap. **B,** Postoperative results 8 months after tattoo of the reconstructed nipple. **C,** Lateral view 8 months after operation. (From Chang, B. W. [1995]. Reconstruction following mastectomy: Timing, indications, and results. In J. L. Cameron [Ed.], *Current surgical therapy* [5th ed.]. St. Louis: Mosby.)

ered in addition to local and regional therapeutic modalities for the management of breast cancer. There are numerous controversies and unanswered research questions regarding the use of chemotherapy in the management of infiltrating breast cancer: Which regimens? At what doses? Over what time interval? What is the correct sequencing of chemotherapy with local regional therapy? How does one compute the percentage of benefit for a specific patient? The decision to receive chemotherapy is difficult for the patient who may receive conflicting treatment recommendations. In addition, she may qualify for one or more clinical trials and will need to factor participation in a clinical trial into her decision-making processes.

Establishing prognostic indicators for the use of chemotherapy is an attempt to describe the biology and predict the behavior of breast cancer for the purpose of matching appropriate treatment recommendations to subsets of patients and ultimately to individual patients. Prognostic factors that have been evaluated include the duration and rate of tumor growth, degree of invasiveness of the tumor, and metastatic potential of the tumor. Prognostic indicators that are used currently include numbers of pathologically positive axillary lymph nodes; measurement of estrogen and progesterone responsiveness; growth rate measurement by flow cytometry calculating the percentage of cells in S-phase; DNA ploidy; demonstration of the occurrence of oncogene amplification by measuring over expression of the *c-erbB2* gene product (i.e., *Her-2/neu*) and measurement of CD levels (Simpson & Page, 1996). As a marker of drug resistance, *c-erbB2* has been associated with resistance to cyclophosphamide, methotrexate, 5-fluorouracil (CMF) combination chemotherapy (Gusterson et al., 1992), and increased sensitivity to doxorubicin (Muss et al., 1994).

Currently, the best, but an imperfect, prognostic indicator for the use of chemotherapy is lymph node status. The numbers of lymph nodes are used for pathologic staging, matching patients to treatment recommendations for systemic therapy, and assigning patients to clinical trials (Dhingra & Hortobagyi, 1996; Simpson & Page, 1996).

Primary (Neoadjuvant) Chemotherapy. Chemotherapy given before surgery (up front) is primary or neoadjuvant chemotherapy. The hypotheses guiding trials of primary chemotherapy are that systemic therapy might eliminate or reduce microscopic disease; that the tumor in the breast, if responsive, would decrease in size and allow for breast conserving surgery; and that tumor responsiveness to systemic therapy might be gauged at the onset of therapy, before surgery. The bulk of clinical experience with primary chemotherapy has been in preoperative chemotherapy of stage III breast cancer with larger tumors. Objective response rates of up to 90%, with complete response rates of 50%, have been observed (Veronesi & Salvadori, 1996). However, an overall improved survival benefit

TABLE 21-7 Potential Acute Side Effects of Radiation Therapy to Breast/Chest Wall

Side Effect	Average Onset	Usual Duration	Appearance/ Presentation	Intervention
Intermittent aches and pains in breast	May occur approximately 1 week after start of radiation	Can persist for months after radiation finishes although usually with decreased frequency.	Patient often describes pain as intermittent sharp twinge in the breast.	Reassurance that this is a normal occurrence and may be alleviated with use of a nonsteroidal antiinflammatory drug (NSAID).
Breast edema	As above	Can persist for months after radiation therapy.	Slight to moderate swelling of the treated breast. Breast may feel full or heavy.	As above. Wearing a supportive bra may improve comfort.
Hair loss in the treatment portal (fine hair of breast, nipple, and possibly small amount of axillary hair)	Usually starts 3-4 weeks at doses of 30-35 Gy.	Variable. May take 1-6 months for hair to grow back.	Typically not very noticeable or bothersome to patients except when associated with folliculitis or itching.	Follow interventions for itching/folliculitis.
Dry desquamation	Approximately 3 weeks after starting radiation.	Usually resolves within 2 weeks of finishing radiation treatments.	Dry flaking or peeling of skin frequently associated with erythema or hyperpigmentation of skin.	Use of highly moisturizing hydrophilic creams such as Aquaphor and Eucerin.
Moist desquamation	4-5 weeks after start of radiation therapy.	Usually completely healed within 2-3 weeks after end of radiation treatments.	Moist peeling of the skin with associated erythema. Area may ooze or weep. May be associated with mild to moderate discomfort depending on severity of reaction. Increased reaction is possible if patient is receiving concurrent chemotherapy. Often occurs in areas with increased shearing friction such as intramammary fold and axilla.	Gentle rinsing with drying antibacterial solutions such as chlorhexidine gluconate or ¼-½ strength H_2O_2. Pat dry with soft clean towel 2-3 times a day. Above can be followed by application of unscented hydrophilic cream such as Aquaphor, followed by nonadherent dressing such as Aquaphor gauze, covered with a soft abdominal pad and held in place by a bra or large-size body netting. Moist soaks can be used such as aluminum acetate solutions: Bluboro and Domeboro for 20 minutes 3 times a day. Moisture vapor permeable dressing may be used such as Op-Site, although it can be difficult to adhere in skin folds. Avoid use of tape on irritated skin.

O'Rourke, N., & Robinson, L. (1996). Breast cancer and the role of radiation therapy. In K. Hassey-Dow (Ed.), *Contemporary issues in breast cancer,* Sudbury, MA: Jones and Bartlett.

TABLE 21-7 Potential Acute Side Effects of Radiation Therapy to Breast/Chest Wall—cont'd

Side Effect	Average Onset	Usual Duration	Appearance/ Presentation	Intervention
				Patient can use gentle lukewarm shower spray to help debride the skin. Allow area to be open to air, whenever possible. If pain is moderate or severe, use of NSAID, or mild narcotic may be indicated.
Skin erythema	Approximately 2 weeks after start of treatment	Resolution usually within 10 days to 2 weeks after end of treatment.	Variable. Mild redness to brisk or bright redness. Mild to moderate discomfort.	Apply unscented hydrophilic creams such as Aquaphor, Eucerin, Lubriderm Unscented, 99%-100% pure aloe vera gel (no added perfumes, colors). Avoid tight bras; underwire bras.
Hyperpigmentation	Approximately 2 weeks after start of treatment. May be more pronounced in darker pigmented women.	Resolves slowly after end of treatments. Mild hyperpigmentation may last for months.	Presents as mild to deep tanning of the skin. May be associated with mild discomfort.	As above.
Itching/folliculitis (irritation of hair follicles)	Approximately 10 days to 2 weeks after start of treatment.	Variable—may start to resolve at end of treatment course to entire breast (before start of boost treatment) usually much improved by end of treatment course.	Itchy skin appears slightly red and dry. Folliculitis appears as small red dots often in sternal, infraclavicular, and supraclavicular area. Occasionally found on back below the clavicle. May cause mild discomfort and itching.	Oatmeal colloidal-based soaps (such as Aveeno). Make paste and apply to affected area, let dry for 3-5 minutes and rinse off with cool water. Oatmeal colloidal based bath products may be added to tub bath. Use 99-100% pure aloe vera gel (no added dyes or perfumes). Use unscented hydrophilic creams such as those listed above for erythema. Diphenhydramine—25 mg may be taken at night for severe itching.
Fatigue	Highly variable approximately 2-3 weeks after start of treatment. May be an increased effect with previous or concurrent chemotherapy.	Fatigue may last up to 2-3 weeks after finishing radiation treatments. Average is 10 days to 2 weeks. May be more prolonged if patient is receiving chemotherapy.	Increased tiredness late afternoon or early evening. Most women are able to continue their usual routines.	Earlier bedtime, late afternoon, or early evening rest period. Good nutrition—avoid dieting during course of treatment. Conserve energy by having family and friends help as needed. Moderate exercise such as walking has been found to help energy levels.

has not been demonstrated using primary or neoadjuvant chemotherapy.

The Early Breast Cancer Trialists' Collaborative Group (EBCTCG, 1992) does periodic meta-analyses that combine clinical trial data to increase the power to analyze for statistical differences among therapies (Hortobagyi & Buzdar, 1995). The EBCTCG meta-analysis from 1990 demonstrated that chemotherapy compared with no chemotherapy in all patients studied resulted in an overall reduction of 21% in recurrence rates and an 11% reduction in mortality. For women under 50 years of age, the rate of recurrence was reduced by 28% and the mortality rate was reduced by 17%. In women over 50 years of age, the percentages were 17% and 9%, respectively.

The goals of primary chemotherapy are to achieve both local and systemic control of the disease. Although there are insufficient data to prove that primary chemotherapy results in better survival than adjuvant chemotherapy, important findings from several studies (Bonadonna et al., 1995) clarify many issues and provide evidence for the benefits associated with primary chemotherapy. There is a hypothesis, as of yet not disproven, that early eradication of micrometastases results in longer disease-free intervals. Breast conservation can be completed successfully in more women with larger tumors who received primary chemotherapy. If a tumor does not respond to primary chemotherapy, clinically or mammographically, this early indicator of drug resistance may prompt an earlier trial of newer agents or strategies. There is some preliminary discussion (Bonadonna et al., 1995; Harris & Swain, 1996) about the use of prognostic indicators from tissue obtained by FNAB that would tailor pretreatment planning. Currently, FNAB is most often performed to diagnose cancer or to rule it out. As our knowledge of the various indicators becomes more predictive (e.g., Does the overexpression of the *c-erbB2* oncogene predict anthracycline resistance, and if so, would it be more effective to start with the Taxanes?), the use of FNAB will provide the information that is now obtained from primary surgical pathology. In addition, research needs to determine whether it is beneficial to treat the disease systematically before tumor disruption by surgery.

Adjuvant Chemotherapy. Adjuvant chemotherapy is chemotherapy treatment, most often a multidrug regimen, given to treat presumed micrometastasis. Adjuvant therapy is most useful in the treatment of patients who meet two conditions: (1) they have micrometastasis at the time of diagnosis or surgery or (2) their tumor cells are not resistant to chemotherapy. However, clinical trials measure the benefit to all women who are treated with adjuvant chemotherapy. There is no way to differentiate between women with micrometastasis and those who are cured by local therapy or those with drug-resistant tumors (Hortobagyi & Buzdar, 1995). Patients at higher risk for recurrence and death obtain the greatest benefit from adjuvant chemotherapy.

Establishing that degree of risk, using tumor stage and grade, estrogen and progesterone receptor status, age, premenopausal or postmenopausal status, the presence or absence of lymph nodes, and the number of positive lymph nodes, is an essential part of making treatment recommendations. Patients need to know the percentage of risk for recurrence and death with and without adjuvant chemotherapy. These discussions need to take place in the context of statistics that represent large groups of patients with the limited ability to predict the risk of recurrence for a single individual. It is useful to express survival benefit in terms of years of life prolongation so that the physician and patient can subtract the costs (e.g., side effects of therapy, financial cost, impact on quality of life) from the expected projected gain in survival (Henderson, 1995). Table 21-8 lists randomized trials of adjuvant therapy that were begun before 1985 for early stage breast cancer. Table 21-9 explains the mechanism of action of the common endocrine therapies used in the management of breast cancer.

Clinical trials that evaluated the effectiveness of adjuvant chemotherapy began in the 1970s. Meta-analyses of many trials conclude that there is an improvement in disease-free survival and overall survival in women treated with adjuvant chemotherapy, tamoxifen (hormone therapy), and ovarian ablation. The EBCTCG (1992) concluded that there was an overall increase of 20% in survival rates in treated patients compared with untreated patients. The questions that remain regarding the use of adjuvant chemotherapy include the following: Who should be treated? Which drugs and drug combinations and dosages are best for which groups of patients? When and for how long should patients be treated? What is the optimal sequencing of radiation therapy with adjuvant chemotherapy?

A meta-analysis done in 1990 concluded that chemotherapy was more efficacious in women younger than 50 years of age and that tamoxifen was more effective in women 50 years of age or older (EBCTCG, 1992). In the first (1988) and second (1992) reports of these meta-analyses, most trials were of single agent antineoplastics or combination drug protocols, for instance the combination of CMF. Fewer data were available from these early meta-analyses on anthracycline-based regimens (e.g., adriamycin).

Clinical trials have demonstrated that combination chemotherapy regimens result in improved outcomes over a single agent (EBCTCG, 1988, 1992). Six cycles of CMF were shown to be more than or equally beneficial when compared with other chemotherapy regimens. Therefore in subsequent clinical trials, CMF is considered to be the "gold standard" adjuvant chemotherapy regimen against which other treatment regimens are compared. Four cycles of adriamycin and cytoxan (AC) demonstrated similar efficacy with a trend toward recommending adriamycin for patients who were at a higher risk for recurrence. Studies that have addressed the question of the duration of therapy and its impact on relapse and survival have shortened the average time frame for adjuvant chemotherapy from 1 to 2 years to 4 to 6 months (Hortobagyi et al., 1995). However, when the International Study Group studied the use of CMF for only three cycles, a survival rate of 53% was reported as compared with a survival rate of 58% with a six-cycle program.

TABLE 21-8 Randomized Trials That Began Before 1984 of Systemic Adjuvant Therapy for Early Breast Cancer: Numbers Available and Approximate Numbers Not Yet Available

	Available for Analysis				Not Yet Available	
Treatment Comparison	**Trials**	**Women**	**Deaths**	**Recurrences**	**Trials**	**No. of Women (%)**
Tamoxifen vs same without tamoxifen*	40	29,892	8219	11,055	4	700 (2)
• Mean scheduled duration ≥5 yr	4	4551	667	1030	0	—
• Mean scheduled duration 3 yr	3	1847	371	536	0	—
• Mean scheduled duration 2 yr	23	15284	4196	5698	3	500 (3)
• Mean scheduled duration ≥1 yr	12	8210	2985	3791	1	200 (2)
Longer vs shorter tamoxifen	5	2319	317	492	0	
Ovarian ablation vs same without ablation	10	3072	1658	1817	2	878 (22)
Other hormonal therapy vs same without hormonal therapy†	12	3014	1138	1464	2	41 (1)
Cytotoxic chemotherapy vs same without cytotoxic*	44	18,403	6582	8320	14	4500 (20)
• Pre/perioperative only	6	4985	1610	2028	3	920 (16)
• Prolonged single agent	11	2744	1,526	1703	2	1120 (29)
• Prolonged polychemotherapy (PPC)	31	11041	3640	4818	9	2500 (19)
Cytotoxic vs other cytotoxic*	46	19,260	6048	8207	13	3300 (15)
• PPC vs pre/perioperative only	3	1223	403	603	0	—
• PPC vs prolonged single agent	13	3462	1683	1988	2	400 (10)
• PPC vs shorter PPC	6	2485	1084	1316	0	—
• Other cytotoxic comparison†	28	15,292	3022	4518	11	2900 (16)
Immunotherapy vs same without immunotherapy	24	6300	2527	3210	5	550 (8)
TOTAL: All systemic trials*	133	74,652	23,956	31,299	35	9400 (11)

NOTE: A detailed list of these trials is available on request from the secretariat.
*Reduced to avoid "double counting" of trials that contribute to more than one therapeutic comparison. (Numbers of women include those randomized before or after January 1, 1985).
†These comparisons do not contribute to the present analyses. If they are excluded, leaving only the currently relevant treatment comparisons, then in the total the proportion available is increased from 89% to 90%.
Early Breast Cancer Trialists' Collaborative Group (EBCTCG). (1992). Systemic treatment of early breast cancer by hormonal, cytotoxic, or immune therapy. 133 randomized trials involving 31,000 recurrences and 24,000 deaths among 75,000 women. *Lancet, 339,* 1-15 and 71-85.

Commonly used adjuvant chemotherapy regimens for infiltrating breast cancer are shown in Table 21-10.

Side Effects of Chemotherapy. The side effects that breast cancer patients experience are not specific to breast cancer, but to the drugs that they receive. The common breast cancer adjuvant chemotherapy regimens (CMF; cyclophosphamide, adriamycin 5-fluorouracil [CAF]; AC) produce the following side effects: nausea and vomiting (generally well controlled with antiemetics); alopecia; weight gain; fatigue; premature menopause (particularly in women over 40), with its attendant long-term increased risk for osteoporosis and cardiovascular disease; second malignancies (leukemias are rare, except with melphalan, but increase with radiation to the chest wall and lymph nodes);

TABLE 21-9 Mechanisms of Treatment Effects of Endocrine Therapies

Treatments	Effects on Estrogen	Remarks and Additional Mechanisms
Oophorectomy (in premenopausal women)	Eliminates ovarian estrogens	Reduces TGF-α, IGF-i, PDGF, Cathepsin D, all of which are stimulated by estrogens
Adrenalectomy	Reduces androgens (thus estrogens)	
Hypophysectomy	Reduces ACTH, FSH and LH levels (thus adrenal androgens and ovarian sex steroids)	
Estrogens (in postmenopausal women)	Occupies estrogen receptors (thus reducing estrogen effects)	Probably also directly cytotoxic
Androgens (in postmenopausal women)	Suppresses FSH and LH levels (thus reducing estrogens) Occupies androgen receptors (subsequent reduction of estrogen receptors limiting the effects of estrogens)	
Tamoxifen	Occupies estrogen receptors	Metabolites with estrogenic and antiestrogenic effects might explain effectiveness and resistance. Estrogenic effects also explain protection of bone and beneficial effects on the cardiovascular system Slowing of cell cycling; reduced IGF-1; increased TGF-β
Tamoxifen withdrawal	Hypothesized change in estrogenic effects of tamoxifen metabolites	
Other antiestrogens	"Total blockade" of estrogen action for "pure" antiestrogens	
Progestins	Occupy progesterone receptors (reducing ER and estrogen action)	Glucocorticoid effects with effects on the hypothalamic pituitary axis Direct inhibition of breast cancer cells Androgen receptor-mediated effect is postulated
Aromatase inhibitors (in postmenopausal women)	Interferes with aromatase which converts androstenedione to estrone and then to estradiol (reducing estrogen levels)	*Type I:* steroidal agents bind irreversibly to the catalytic site of the aromatase cytochrome P-450 causing loss of aromatase activity *Type II:* nonsteroidal agents which interact with the cytochrome P-450 moiety of the flavor protein of the super family of enzymes, causing more or less extensive interference with the synthesis of cortisol and aldosterone
GnRH analogs (mainly in premenopausal women)	Inhibitors of gonadotrophin release from the pituitary (reduced estrogen levels)	LH and FSH levels are first stimulated then almost completely inhibited: reduces testosterone, progesterone, and estradiol to castration levels
Antiprogestins	Occupy nuclear progesterone receptor (reduced progesterone action)	Mifepristone also binds glucocorticoid receptors Cell cycle arrest in G_0 or G_1 phase with subsequent terminal differentiation of the cells and increased cell death
Antiandrogens	Occupy androgen receptors (thus inhibit the conversion of testosterone into a more active dihydrotestosterone and reduced synthesis of adrenal precursors of active androgens)	Postulated to have direct cytotoxicity

TGF-α, transforming growth factor alpha; *IGF-I,* insulin-like growth factor I; *PDGF,* platelet-derived growth factor; *ACTH,* adrenocorticotrophic hormone; *FSH,* follicle-stimulating hormone; *LH,* luteinizing hormone; *ER,* estrogen receptor.
From Goldhirsch, A., & Gelber, R. D. (1996). Endocrine therapies of breast cancer. *Seminars in Oncology, 23*(4), 496.

TABLE 21-10 Popular Chemotherapy Regimens Useful in the Adjuvant Treatment of Breast Cancer

Regimen	Dose and Schedule	Cycle Interval	Cycles
CMF (Standard)			
Cyclophosphamide	100 mg/m^2/d PO × 14 days	28 days	6
Methotrexate			
5-Fluorouracil			
CMF (IV; Tested in Node-Negative Patients Only)			
Cyclophosphamide	600 mg/m^2 IV	21 days	12
Methotrexate	40 mg/m^2 IV	21 days	12
5-Fluorouracil	600 mg/m^2 IV	21 days	12
CMFVP			
Cyclophosphamide	60 mg/m^2/d PO	Daily	1 year
5-Fluorouracil	400 mg/m^2 IV	Weekly	1 year
Methotrexate	15 mg/m^2	Weekly	1 year
Vincristine	0.625 mg/m^2	Weekly × 10	
Prednisone	30 mg/m^2 tapering over 10 weeks	—	
CAF			
Cyclophosphamide	100 mg/m^2/d PO × 14 days	28 days	6
Doxorubicin	30 mg/m^2 IV day 1 & day 8	28 days	6
5-Fluorouracil	500 mg/m^2 IV day 1 & day 8	28 days	6
CAF			
Cyclophosphamide	600 mg/m^2 IV day 1	21-28 days	4-6
Doxorubicin	60 mg/m^2 IV day 1	21-28 days	4-6
5-Fluorouracil	600 mg/m^2 IV day 1 & day 8	21-28 days	4-6
AC			
Doxorubicin	60 mg/m^2 IV day 1	21 days	4
Cyclophosphamide	600 mg/m^2 IV day 1	21 days	4
A → CMF (Tested in Node-Positive Patients Only)			
Doxorubicin	75 mg/m^2 IV day 1	21 days	4
Cyclophosphamide	600 mg/m^2 IV	21 days	8 (cycles 5-12)
Methotrexate	40 mg/m^2 IV	21 days	8 (cycles 5-12)
5-Fluorouracil	600 mg/m^2 IV	21 days	8 (cycles 5-12)

From Osborne, C. K., Clark, G., & Ravdin, P. (1996). Adjuvant systemic therapy of breast cancer. In J. Harris, M. Lippman, M. Morrow, & S. Hellman. *Diseases of the breast.* Philadelphia: Lippincott Raven.

cardiac toxicity with anthracycline-containing regimens; and febrile neutropenia (uncommon with standard dose regimens, more common with high-dose regimens).

Weight gain while on adjuvant chemotherapy is a unique problem for women with breast cancer. Dow (1996) and Barnicle (1996) reported that 50% to 90% of women with breast cancer who are on adjuvant chemotherapy regimens gain weight. The cause of the weight gain is not clear, and there is no convincing data to substantiate the impact of hormonal changes, depression, increased food intake, or decreased activity level (particularly when associated with fatigue) on the increase in the patient's weight. Regular exercise, decreased fat intake, and a range of stress management and emotional support strategies are recommended to help women manage the weight gain. Women commonly report that weight gain compounds the other difficult changes in body image, such as alopecia, or the loss of or change in the breast after surgery and radiation therapy.

High-Dose Adjuvant Chemotherapy. There is a trend suggesting improved outcomes with high-dose adjuvant chemotherapy (Gradishar, Tallman, & Abrams, 1996). Preliminary results of trials of high-dose therapies (e.g., using accelerated doses of standard agents with growth factors and/or autologous stem cell support and/or autologous bone marrow transplant) have demonstrated some benefit in patients with 10 or more positive lymph nodes (Osborne, Clark, & Radvin, 1996). However, the use of this type of therapy is extremely controversial. Many patients are treated in community settings and are not enrolled in clinical trials. As a result, clinicians have learned a great deal about how patients tolerate therapy, but the questions of efficacy and outcome remain unanswered for this costly and toxic therapy.

Currently, three NCI trials are comparing standard chemotherapy with high-dose chemotherapy. Peters and colleagues (1993) studied 85 patients who received standard CAF followed by high-dose chemotherapy. They also received chest wall irradiation and 5 years of tamoxifen. At 6 years, the event-free survival was 64% and the overall survival was 75%. This study was not a randomized prospective trial comparing the use of high-dose chemotherapy to standard chemotherapy, but rather a comparison was made to historical controls with event-free survival of 30% to 35% and overall survival of 37% to 48% (Peters et al., 1993, 1995). Thus although the differences are encouraging, critics raise the issues of different study entry criteria between the high-dose chemotherapy protocol and the historical controls. Patients were disqualified from the high-dose chemotherapy studies if they had metastatic disease. However, the historical controls were not as carefully screened for the presence of metastatic disease.

Biologic therapies, immunotoxins, antibodies, and gene therapy for breast cancer remain to be tested in clinical trials. These approaches involve explorations of growth factors and angiogenesis factors and will be aimed initially at patients with advanced disease. Table 21-11 displays the NCI/Physician Data Query (PDQ) State-of-the-Art Cancer Treatment Summary for infiltrating breast cancer (1995).

TABLE 21-11 State-of-the-Art Treatment Recommendations

Stage	Treatment
Stage 0 In situ (ductal)	1. Mastectomy with excision of lymph nodes around the axillary tail without a formal level I dissection of axillary lymph nodes 2. Lumpectomy or partial or segmental mastectomy with radiotherapy
In situ (lobular) Not considered breast cancer	1. No treatment after biopsy with careful follow-up examinations and mammograms 2. Bilateral prophylactic mastectomies 3. Tamoxifen (which is in clinical trials) after biopsy to help prevent development of invasive cancer
Stage I	Treatment based on tumor size, location, appearance on mammogram, and breast size 1. Lumpectomy—removal of cancer and some surrounding breast tissue followed by radiation 2. Partial or segmental mastectomy, followed by radiation 3. Modified radical mastectomy with reconstruction. All procedures should include axillary node dissection. 4. Clinical trials continue on adjuvant therapy, chemotherapy, hormonal therapy (tamoxifen to determine if trials will improve disease-free and overall survival rates)
Stage II Positive nodes	1. Lumpectomy and axillary node dissection followed by radiation 2. Modified radical mastectomy with lymph node dissection and reconstruction 3. Adjuvant therapy • Combination chemotherapy—not to exceed 1 year • Hormone therapy—tamoxifen for 2 years • Clinical trial of chemotherapy before surgery • Clinical trial of chemotherapy and/or hormone therapy after surgery • Clinical trial of no additional therapy after surgery
Stage IIA Negative nodes	1. Lumpectomy/segmental mastectomy with axillary node dissection and radiotherapy 2. Modified radical mastectomy with axillary dissection. Radical mastectomy only to accomplish complete humor resection 3. Clinical trials studying adjuvant therapy with chemotherapy or hormonal therapy
Stage IIIA Operable	1. Modified radical mastectomy and lymph node dissection 2. Radiation therapy both before and after surgery 3. Chemotherapy with or without hormone therapy in conjunction with surgery and radiation 4. Clinical trials testing new chemotherapeutic drugs with or without hormonal drugs. Clinical trials testing chemotherapy before surgery.
Stage IIIB Inoperable	1. Radiotherapy to control local and regional disease 2. Systemic chemotherapy recommended to control occult metastatic disease 3. Surgery may be limited to diagnostic biopsy and receptor protein assay, or to remove tumor following other therapy 4. Ongoing clinical trials studying use of combination chemotherapy initially, followed by surgery and/or radiotherapy, and maintenance chemotherapy 5. Phase 2 studies are evaluating new chemotherapeutic or biologic agents when local disease
Stage IV Cancer has metastasized to other parts of the body	1. Surgery to determine histology and estrogen- and progesterone-receptor levels 2. Disease control through surgery, radiotherapy, hormonal therapy, chemotherapy 3. Clinical trials—studying role of bisphosphonates in reducing skeletal morbidity in women with metastases to the bone

From National Cancer Institute Physician Data Query State of the Art Cancer Treatment Summary. (1995). *Breast Cancer, 1*, 39.

ONCOLOGIC EMERGENCIES

Although patients being treated with surgery, radiation therapy, chemotherapy, and hormonal therapies experience complications of treatment, the major oncologic emergencies in breast cancer are associated with metastatic disease. Symptoms associated with various oncologic emergencies (e.g., cardiac tamponade, hypercalcemia, pulmonary embolism, pleural effusion, superior vena cava syndrome, spinal cord compression) should precipitate a workup for metastatic disease.

NURSING MANAGEMENT

General Considerations

The perioperative treatment period is replete with informational needs, severe stress regarding the diagnosis of a life-threatening illness, the need to make choices among various treatment options, alterations in personal identity in terms of health and life potential, the need for support during adaptation to changes in family and sexual relationships, and reassurance that normal healing is occurring. Although some researchers have attempted to predict informational needs by demographic characteristics such as age (Bilodeau & Degner, 1996), such work is not intended to preclude the need to assess individual patients for their specific needs related to breast cancer teaching.

Careful attention to effective perioperative teaching for women undergoing surgery for breast cancer is more necessary than ever as hospital stays become increasingly brief. An educational program should include the following: information about breast and lymph node anatomy; the type and extent of the woman's breast cancer; the surgical procedure she will undergo or has undergone; what to expect in the immediate postoperative period in terms of wound care and the care of drains, pain management, and rehabilitation therapy for arm movement; appropriate postoperative care of the arm to prevent pressure damage or infection; the possibility of experiencing acute or long-term lymphedema, numbness, or other sensory sequelae; the availability of financial, sexual, and/or family counseling; all relevant information about treatment options; and information about managing symptoms associated with all treatments she will undergo following the postoperative recovery period. Table 21-12 provides a surgical standard of care for the patient with infiltrating breast cancer.

Physical Care

Immediate Postoperative Management. Women with mastectomies and less frequently, those with lumpectomies are discharged with a Jackson-Pratt drain in place. They require teaching regarding the emptying, measuring, and recording of output from the drain. Most drains remain in place until the output is 30 ml or less per 24 hours, which generally occurs within 4 to 10 days. Postoperative care is aimed at healing the surgical wound and achieving the functional recovery of the arm and shoulder. Limited exercise (e.g., squeeze ball and wrist flexion) is encouraged for the first 24 hours after surgery. Range of motion exercises are begun thereafter. Precautions that need to be taught to women who have had an axillary node dissection include protecting the extremity from trauma and monitoring for signs and symptoms of infection and lymphedema. If a seroma occurs, it is managed with aspiration if it does not reabsorb spontaneously. Usually, hematomas resolve spontaneously, unless there is a continuing bleed that necessitates surgical revision.

Management of Lymphedema. Secondary or acquired lymphedema is an accumulation of protein-rich fluid in the subcutaneous tissue of the skin resulting from blocked or damaged lymphatic vessels. Postmastectomy lymphedema has been reported to occur in 10% to 63% of patients. This wide variance in occurrence attests to the variability in the type and extent of the surgical procedures, the expertise of the surgeon, co-morbidity associated with radiation therapy, age and health status of the patient, and the patient's use of self-care behaviors. Lymphedema can result in pain, compromised mobility, infection, impaired cosmesis, psychological distress, and decreased quality of life. It has a wide range of onset from weeks to years from the date of the lymph node dissection. The three-stage system for classifying lymphedema is found in Table 21-13.

The range of conventional treatments for lymphedema can include the use of a compression sleeve or stocking, or a single-cell pump, or a sequential gradient pump. Daily treatment is required at a substantial cost that may or may not be reimbursed by third-party payers. In addition, the success of these compression procedures and devices on reducing lymphedema is highly variable. Complete or complex decongestive physiotherapy (CDP) includes four therapeutic steps: (1) skin and nail care and treatment of infection, (2) manual lymph drainage (MLD), (3) compression bandaging after MLD by applying bandages from the fingers to the axilla, and (4) while bandaged, doing a series of exercises to increase lymph flow. Manual lymph drainage is mild, rhythmic massage designed to stimulate the lymphatics of the contralateral normal quadrant, decongest the ipsilateral quadrant, and evacuate lymph from the hand, fingers, and upper arm. Patients can be taught to do CDP, and many can maintain the benefits realized by regular exercises and practice of MLD (Petrek & Lerner, 1996).

An elastic sleeve garment measured for the patient from her wrist to her axilla and including the hand, if swollen, should be ordered to achieve the appropriate amount of compression for the degree of lymphedema. Diuretics, while often prescribed, should not be used, as this drug therapy may result in increased fluid retention in the extremity when increased protein in the interstitial space results in the reaccumulation of fluid. There is some evidence that the benzopyrones, including bioflavonoids and the coumarins, may decrease the symptoms of chronic lymphedema by increasing proteolysis and decreasing the osmotic pressure in the extremity, resulting in less edema. FDA approval is still pending for the use of benzopyrones for the treatment of breast cancer–related lymphedema.

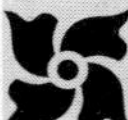

TABLE 21-12 Standard of Care for the Patient Undergoing Modified Radical Mastectomy or Lumpectomy

Patient Problems and Outcomes	Nursing Interventions and Rationales	Patient Education Instructions
Knowledge Deficit: Patient will be able to: • Verbalize understanding of surgical procedure • Verbalize understanding of postoperative pain, signs and symptoms of infection, numbness, mobility deficits and increased infection risk to affected arm	1. Assess patient's level of understanding of surgical procedure 2. Provide pre-, peri-, and postoperative teaching 3. Verify patient's level of comfort with and understanding of procedure a. Refer to physician if conflict with plan of care b. Refer for psychosocial support if anxiety, fear, and other responses require intervention	1. Demonstrate with diagram of anatomy of breast, axillary lymph nodes and part of breast to be removed. 2. Teach general preoperative instructions re coughing and deep breathing. 3. Introduce patient to postoperative range of motion exercises. Instruct patient to begin limited exercise 24 hours after surgery. 4. Demonstrate drain care if drain will be left in. Obtain return demonstration. 5. Explain postoperative procedures: a. Pain management b. Range of motion exercises c. Reporting of bleeding, signs and symptoms of infection, nonfunctioning drain d. Drain care and documentation e. Dressing care f. Who and how to call for problems 6. Make postoperative appointment.
Pain Patient will: • Experience optimal pain relief with minimal side effects • Be able to perform postoperative exercises and recover range of motion	1. Provide postoperative pain medications with instructions for use 2. Inform patients to call if inadequate relief 3. Assess pain intensity on a 0-10 scale. Assess type of pain by descriptors (persistent pain is often neuropathic from axillary lymph node dissection). Assess pain medications and effectiveness. 4. Determine the correct medications from opioids, nonsteroidal anti-inflammatories and antidepressants for neuropathic pain. Re-evaluate for effectiveness after trial use.	1. Teach 0-10 assessment for pain intensity; teach patient to describe pain. 2. Inform patient about pain medications, side effects and dosing intervals. 3. Teach patient to take appropriate pain medication 20-30 minutes before exercise.
Postoperative Swelling Excess fluid will reabsorb into tissue	1. With a Jackson Pratt drain left in: a. Assess function of drain b. Examine for signs and symptoms of infection Drains are usually removed when drainage is less than 30 cc in 24 hours. 2. Without a drain: a. Assess for swelling that increases b. Aspiration of fluid from site of swelling; if continues to reaccumulate, drain may be placed.	1. Teach patient to strip and empty drain and document output BID. 2. Teach patient signs and symptoms of infection and what to report. 3. Teach patient to report malfunction of drain, excess bleeding, swelling that increases.

TABLE 21-12 Standard of Care for the Patient Undergoing Modified Radical Mastectomy or Lumpectomy—cont'd

Patient Problems and Outcomes	Nursing Interventions and Rationales	Patient Education Instructions
Infection		
Prevent infection or treat it early	1. Observe incision for signs and symptoms of infection 2. Take temperature 3. Share strategies for infection prevention from axillary lymph node dissection 4. Maintain dressing	1. Teach patient signs and symptoms of infection and parameters for reporting. 2. Teach patient infection prevention behaviors: a. Avoid cuts (use gardening gloves, oven mitts, thimble, electric razor) b. No injections; no IV in the affected arm c. Use sunscreen; limit sun exposure d. Avoid constricting the circulation of the arm by jewelry, watch, tight sleeves e. If a cut occurs, wash with soap and water; observe closely for signs and symptoms of infection and report 3. Postoperatively, steri strips and a dressing cover the incision a. Leave dressing in place until postoperative visit or remove outside dressing as instructed. Do not remove steri strips b. Patient may bathe or take sponge bath; instruct patient not to get dressing wet 4. Instruct patient not to use deodorant until incision heals.
Limited range of motion from axillary lymph node dissection		
Patient will: • Achieve baseline range of motion • "Frozen shoulder' will be prevented	1. Provide rehabilitation exercises and monitor progress until full range of motion is achieved. 2. Refer to/consult physical therapy if range of motion is compromised and is not responding to exercises. 3. Evaluate inadequate pain control as a barrier to exercise compliance.	1. Teach the patient to begin limited exercise 24 hours after surgery. a. Flex fingers b. Squeeze ball c. Move wrist and elbow; do not keep arm in fixed position d. Brush hair and teeth 2. Teach patient restrictions a. No heavy lifting b. No aerobic exercises until drain removed or wound healed (4-10 days) 3. Demonstrate (with return demonstration) range of motion exercises for shoulder and arm. a. Begin exercises 2-3 times per day b. Continue at least once per day for 4-6 months or until other exercises resumed (swimming, dance) 4. Demonstrate massage to axilla and underarm to soften scar tissue.
Cosmesis		
Patient will: • Have access to short- and long-term resources for cosmesis • Receive emotional support for alteration in body image	1. Provide preoperative discussion of potential changes in operative breast for lumpectomy; refer to plastic surgeon if immediate reconstruction is an option with mastectomy.	1. Encourage patients to begin to state their preferences for cosmesis preoperatively. 2. Show sample prostheses to patients. 3. Share with patients the range of feelings women experience.

Continued

TABLE 21-12 Standard of Care for the Patient Undergoing Modified Radical Mastectomy or Lumpectomy—cont'd

Patient Problems and Outcomes	Nursing Interventions and Rationales	Patient Education Instructions
Cosmesis—cont'd		
	2. Identify emotional issues of concern re alteration in body image. 3. For mastectomy without immediate reconstruction: a. Have temporary prosthesis postoperatively before prosthesis can be fitted b. At postoperative visit, supply prescription for prosthesis and updated community resources for prosthesis and bras. 3. Mastectomy with immediate reconstruction: a. Describe changes in appearance in reconstructed breast from expander to permanent implant b. Autologous flap (e.g., Tram) requires healing; changes in body appearance in reconstructed breast and donor site. 4. Address cosmesis issues related to systemic chemotherapy: alopecia, skin changes, nail bed changes, weight gain Encourage patient to address issues of changes in appearance with staff, in support groups with other women with breast cancer.	4. Teach patient that immediate cosmetic result is not permanent result. 5. Give healing timeline based on procedure. 6. Prepare patient for expected occurrence and timing of alopecia based on drug regimen. 7. Give patient relevant community resources for wigs, scarves, turbans, make-up.

TABLE 21-13 Staging System for Lymphedema

Stage I	Pitting edema, soft tissue, spontaneously reversible
Stage II	Firmer skin, nonpitting edema, possible inflammation, spontaneously irreversible
Stage III	Elephantiasis, hardening of the skin, overproduction of connective tissue, severe swelling

Management of the Side Effects of Chemotherapy and Radiation Therapy. Radiation and chemotherapy produce an array of side effects that are specific to the treatment regimen. A comprehensive guide for the management of side effects associated with these therapies can be found in Dodd's *Managing the Side Effects of Chemotherapy and Radiation Therapy: A Guide for Patients and their Families* (1996).

Table 21-14 lists symptoms associated with the use of tamoxifen as adjuvant therapy (Ganz, Day, Ware, Redmond, & Fisher, 1995). The women in this study reported an average of 8.9 distinct symptoms over 4 weeks. A decline in sexual activity has also been reported with the use of tamoxifen (Ganz et al., 1995) and was more marked in older than in younger women. Declines in sexual activity have also been reported in women who were receiving chemotherapy. Young-McCaughan (1996) reported that, controlling for endocrine therapy, women who were receiving chemotherapy for breast cancer were more likely to report vaginal dryness (OR $= 5.7$, $P < .01$), decreased libido (OR $= 3.0$, $P < .04$), dyspareunia (OR $=5.5$, $P < .01$), and difficulty achieving orgasm (OR $=7.1$, $P < .01$). A standard of care for the management of menopausal symptoms in women receiving treatment for infiltrating breast cancer is found in Table 21-15.

Psychosocial and Cultural Concerns of Patients with Breast Cancer

Many of the emotional concerns faced by breast cancer patients share common themes with patients diagnosed with other cancers. For example, the range of responses to life-threatening illness, coping with others' reactions to "cancer," fear, anxiety, balancing the stressors of obtaining information while making treatment decisions, and all of the distress associated with subsequent treatments are experienced by most patients with a diagnosis of cancer. However, many philosophic, theologic, and psychological reflective writings, as well as a large body of research, focus on the psychosocial needs of women with breast cancer.

Work by Speigel and colleagues (1989) attempts to explore the effect of psychological health or distress of women with breast cancer on disease-free survival and overall sur-

TABLE 21-14 Frequency of Symptoms Associated With Tamoxifen Therapy by Percent

Symptom	Overall %	Age		
		35-49	50-59	>60
Unhappy with appearance of body	58.7	59.8	60.8	53.2
Headaches	56.5	67.0	57.4	41.6
Joint pains	49.3	38.6	52.4	60.3
General aches and pains	48.9	43.5	53.3	51.5
Muscle stiffness	41.8	34.6	45.3	47.8
Breast sensitivity	40.9	58.3	35.3	23.8
Early awakening	39.1	31.4	42.8	45.3
Forgetfulness	38.2	29.9	53.6	47.5
Hot flashes	34.6	26.0	53.6	26.4
Swelling of hands and feet	28.6	26.8	29.7	29.8

From Ganz, P. A., Day, R., Ware, J. E., Redmond, C., & Fisher, B. (1995). Base-line quality-of-life assessment in the National Surgical Adjuvant Breast and Bowel Project Cancer Prevention Trial. *Journal of the National Cancer Institute, 87,* 1372-1382. Oxford University Press: Oxford, England.

vival. Much of the psychological research with breast cancer patients focuses on therapeutic interventions to decrease distress and enhance coping and wellness (Fetting, 1991; Hilton, 1996; Lavery & Clark, 1996; Tross et al., 1996; Walker, Nail, Larsen, Magill, & Schwartz, 1996). The areas of focus include sexuality and body image, fear and threat to mortality, disclosure, social support and its impact on relationships (e.g., significant other, family, children, friends), work, money, and insurance issues.

Responses to breast cancer are believed to be influenced by age (life cycle–specific issues), the amount and content of the disruption breast cancer has on one's life; an individual's prediagnosis personality, coping style, and prior crisis experience; and an individual's prior experience with breast cancer in women who come from high-incidence breast cancer families with early deaths (Rowland & Massie, 1996). One of the underlying differences between breast cancer and other cancers is the fact that the breast (and the loss of breast) has distinct emotional and cultural meanings. The breast is associated with feeding one's child. The threat to the breast magnifies fertility and childbearing issues for many premenopausal women. Stimulation of the breasts and nipples is often part of sexual expression. Therefore a threat to the breast may be intertwined with one's sexual identity or self-image, as well as with how one imagines being perceived by an intimate. A woman may like or dislike her breasts and have complicated feelings related to the loss or change of the healthy breast.

In addition to the individual differences in reaction to the loss of a breast, a wide spectrum of meanings associated with the breast is found across the life span and cultures. Persons of white North-American and European cultures tend to focus on the breast as a seat of beauty. This idea may not be reflective of views held by many other cultures, and it certainly does not hold true for every woman in any culture. Kagawa-Singer (1996) delineated the ways in which Asian-American and Pacific American women have distinct differences from North-American and European women with respect to body image and sexuality (e.g., the breast has less sexual and more functional meaning). Kagawa-Singer describes some specific differences among Asian cultures (e.g., what is beautiful is different in the Chinese culture [rounded vs squared shoulders], in the Korean culture [beauty read in the shape of the heel of the foot], and in the Japanese culture [the nape of the neck and lightness of skin]). Essential to the consciousness of cultural differences is an understanding of the marked diversity in cultural adherence behaviors among individuals within a culture and the wide differences, especially in the United States, within the generations of immigrants from every world culture.

Brant (1996) explored some of the responses of Native-American women to breast cancer. She noted how some Native-American women asked to save the postsurgical breast to bury it, believing that their body must be intact for the next life; how some women believed that postoperative pain would be less if the breast was buried; and how some women believed that the burial ceremony would help to heal the grief of the loss of the breast. Colomeda (1996) interviewed women in Alaska and Northern Canada regarding their experiences with breast cancer and how their illness influenced their family life.

Phillips (1996) explored issues, primarily as they relate to screening and early detection behaviors, in African-American women. She stressed the need to thread empowerment strategies throughout the provision of education and emotional support. Additionally, she discussed the impact of history and the continued lack of trust in interventions recommended by health care providers, based on documented breaches in the ethics of research. Many African-American women still recall the Tuskegee Syphilis Study in which 400 African-American men were observed with untreated syphilis, without their consent, and after the discovery of therapy (Jones, 1981).

It is difficult to establish therapeutic relationships, the key to the provision of emotional support, without trust. The key issues for lesbians, who come from diverse cultures when they enter the health care system, are dealing with homophobia (i.e., hatred and fear of people with same sex in-

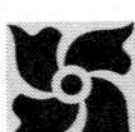

TABLE 21-15 Standard of Care for the Management of Selected Menopausal Symptoms

Patient Problems and Outcomes	Nursing Interventions and Rationales	Patient Education Instructions
Potential for Menopausal Symptoms Patient will: • Expect symptoms and learns how to manage symptoms most effectively	1. Warn patient of potential for menopausal symptoms secondary to stopping hormone replacement therapy (HRT); with the use of hormonal therapies; or with the use of chemotherapy.	1. Teach patient the spectrum of potential side effects: hot flashes, night sweats, vaginal dryness, headaches, mood changes, cognitive changes/memory, changes in libido, sleep deprivation.
Hot Flashes and Nightsweats Patient will: • Experience a decreased incidence of hot flashes and nightsweats	1. Trial the following interventions: a. Avoid hot drinks and food, hot weather, alcohol, caffeine b. Low-dose clonidine (0.1 mg/day) orally or patch, titrate the dose to effect Monitor blood pressure; warn of α-adrenergic agonist effects of clonidine (dizziness, dry mouth, nausea, headache) c. Progestins (side effects of breast pain, mood changes, abdominal bloating) • Medroxyprogesterone acetate (Provera) • Low dose Megace (20 mg) d. Benadryl at bedtime (decreases insomnia, decreases awareness) e. Vitamin E 200-800 mg/day Do not use in women with diabetes, hypertension, cardiac disease without medical supervision 2. Encourage patient to report the use of complementary medicine interventions (e.g., herbs, homeopathy).	1. Teach patients the use and side effects of each intervention. 2. Have patients report trial benefits and side effects to decide to pursue interventions.
Vaginal Dryness Patient will: • Experience a decrease in vaginal dryness, discomfort, and painful sexual intercourse	1. Encourage patient to report vaginal dryness and related discomforts. 2. Trial the following interventions: a. Use topical lubricants (e.g., Replens, Astroglide) regularly and before sexual activity; use water soluble lubricants only b. Use low-dose topical testosterone 3. Teach patient to avoid products that dry or irritate the vagina. 4. Encourage the use of loose fitting clothing.	1. Teach patient the interventions and potential problems. 2. Encourage patient to report effectiveness or problems with the various interventions. 3. Teach patient to avoid soaps, bath gels or bubbles, powders or vaginal deodorants that contain perfumes or alcohol. 4. Teach patient to wear cotton underwear and avoid silk, polyester, nylon fabrics.

timate relationships); assumptions of heterosexuality by providers or other survivors; visitation and acknowledgment of partner as family and significant other; disclosure of lesbian identification to providers, friends, and family; and lack of knowledge about risk factors, incidence of breast cancer, and emotional responses to diagnosis, treatment, and recovery (Denenberg, 1995; O'Hanlan, 1995; Rankow, 1995).

Emotional needs and effective interventions will undoubtedly be different for elderly women with breast cancer. Elderly women may have diminished social support; will likely have experienced more prior losses; will have limited financial resources because they are on fixed incomes and have limited health care coverage; come from a generation with less of a tendency to discuss breast cancer, their breasts, or sexuality; be less likely to perform BSE; and be more uncomfortable with clinical breast examinations (Caplan, Wells, & Haynes, 1992; Champion, 1992).

In addition to a commitment to learning about and respecting the impact that culture may have on the reactions and behaviors of women with breast cancer, it is vitally important that our programs, from screening through treatment of metastatic breast cancer, include the lived experience and knowledge of bicultural caregivers from diverse cultures. In addition, psychosocial resources must be available to non-English speakers in their own native language.

Rowland and Massie (1996) have compiled a review of 12 controlled studies that compare the emotional responses of women to mastectomy and breast-conserving surgery. The studies were compared using the following criteria: satisfaction with body image, marital adjustment, satisfaction with sexual functioning, psychological adjustment, and fear of recurrence. For the measures of marital adjustment and fear of recurrence, no differences were found between the two surgical groups. Women who had breast-conserving surgery reported consistently more positive feelings about their body image than did women who had a mastectomy. Satisfaction with sexual functioning was found to be equal in five studies and less problematic after breast-conserving surgery in five studies. Two of the studies did not evaluate satisfaction with sexual functioning. Psychological adjustment was equal in five studies, better with breast-conserving surgery in five studies, better with mastectomy in one study, and not measured in one study. The timing of measurement, although potentially relevant, was not consistent across the 12 studies that were evaluated. Clinicians have wondered whether the higher incidence of distress from mastectomy may be an earlier phenomenon, with delayed distress accompanying breast-conserving surgery. Understanding the timing of various surgical interventions for breast cancer and their psychological sequelae is an important area for study. For example, it would be useful to compare the psychological impact of immediate vs delayed reconstruction following mastectomy.

Psychological Interventions for Women with Infiltrating Breast Cancer. Psychological help for patients with breast cancer is provided by individual and peer group support, through professional support from members of various health care disciplines, as well as through individual consultations with psychologists, social workers, or psychiatrists. Psychological help is often provided in concert with genetic counseling; at the time of diagnosis, or at the time of a diagnostic crisis (e.g., diagnosis of metastatic disease or recurrence).

Breast cancer support groups are an active part of many comprehensive breast cancer treatment programs. Speigel and colleagues (1989) studied the effect of participation in a breast cancer support group on the survival of women with metastatic breast cancer. Eighty-six women participated in the study (50 in the intervention group and 36 in the control group). Survival time was significantly longer for women who participated in the support group. In addition, the interval of time from first metastasis to death was longer for women who participated in the support group.

Although all of the benefits of participating in a breast cancer support group are not clear, it is believed that the benefits are derived from social support. As with all treatment recommendations and despite some data reporting their benefit, support groups are not perceived as beneficial by all women. Many women choose not to participate, and others give participation a trial and then choose not to continue. Some women report feeling overly affected by the difficult medical treatment and/or life experiences of the other women. Others are not comfortable with the disclosure of feelings either in a group or to individuals they do not know. In addition, for some women, language or cultural barriers may inhibit participation. In larger, urban areas or in areas where a specific population is well represented, culturally specific or language-specific support groups may be available for these women. Box 21-2 provides information

Box 21-2

Common Breast Cancer Support Group Themes

1. Alteration in body image: loss of breast, change in breast, weight gain, hair loss, stories about prosthetics and wigs, reconstruction issues, feeling different in one's body, concern regarding ohers' response to changes (spouse, partner, child)
2. Coping with medical decision making and treatment issues
3. Hypervigilance to symptoms and fear of their meaning, fear of reoccurrence, generalized fear and anxiety
4. Fear of death, threat to mortality, coping with those fears in loved ones (particularly difficult with parent/child)
5. Reassessment of meaning in life: What and who matters when one is not working or care-giving or doing? What mark does one wish to leave on the world?
6. Sharing coping strategies, comparing experiences
7. Using the group as a safe place to trial run honest expression of feelings, encouragement (homework) to be more honest in relationships outside the group
8. Learning from, struggling with the recurrences and deaths of group members. Learning to talk about the feelings about one's own death, fears, survivor guilt when doing well, or guilt when too defended to feel at all
9. Sexuality: feeling sexual, wanting to feel sexual, a spouse or partner wanting to be sexual, how to be sexual with fatigue, vaginal dryness, and hot flashes

Box 21-3
Words of Women Living with Breast Cancer

One restless night just after being diagnosed with breast cancer, I picked up a pencil and a piece of paper and tried to sketch the fear that was stirring inside of me. At the time all I could think of was the hourglass in the movie *Wizard of Oz* where Dorothy is trapped in dark chambers of the Wicked Witch's castle. Time was running out. . . I have no idea how much sand remains in the upper half of my hourglass; however, I remain hopeful that new methods of diagnosis and treatment will prolong my life and the lives of many others.

Kathleen Gardner

Gardner, K. (1998). Personal communication.

on some common themes identified by women who participate in breast cancer support groups.

At the University of California San Francisco Mount Zion Medical Center, there is an Art for Recovery program directed by Cindi Perlis (begun in 1987). One of the projects of this program is the creation of beautiful quilts composed of quilt squares made by women living with breast cancer. The quilt project is inspirational and healing for the women who choose to participate. It is a concrete way for women to give voice to many thoughts and feelings and to be honored. For family members, friends, and health care professionals, the quilt project is an educational and moving experience. Along with the making of the quilt square, women are invited to write words to accompany their squares. Box 21-3 is an example of women's voices of their lived experience of breast cancer.

HOME CARE ISSUES

Much of the postoperative nursing care following breast cancer surgery is delivered in the home as a result of the current trend of early discharge after mastectomy patients and the performance of lumpectomies on an outpatient basis. A standard of care that can be used when caring for a patient in the home is found in Table 21-11. Referrals to home care agencies need to be considered for the following patients: women with functional limitations, elderly women, women without the support of family and friends, and women with a prior history of severe co-morbid conditions or mental illness.

Little data are available on the prevalence and incidence of pain associated with breast cancer and its treatments. Postmastectomy pain (PMP) syndrome occurs after any breast surgery that includes axillary lymph node dissection. It is thought that PMP syndrome occurs primarily after injury to the intercostobrachial nerve. Patients with a PMP syndrome describe "nerve pain," as well as aching, burning, and numbness in the affected upper arm and chest wall or breast. The pain may be chronic and often does not respond well to opioid analgesics. It is generally believed that the prevalence of PMP syndrome is low, but this issue is not well studied, and reports have varied widely. In an early study, Daut and Cleeland (1982) reported a prevalence rate for pain of 68% in a mixed inpatient and outpatient sample of patients with breast cancer. Foley (1987) reported an incidence rate of 4% to 6%. Four other studies of pain in patients with cancer have been reported (Ahles, Ruckdeschel, & Blanchard, 1984; Bressler, Hange, & McGuire, 1986; Miaskowski & Dibble, 1995; Peteet, Tay, Cohen, & MacIntyre, 1986) but none have been specifically examined pain in patients with cancer of the breast.

Stevens, Dibble, and Miaskowski (1995) reviewed a subset of 97 patients with breast cancer from a larger study of 435 cancer patients. The prevalence of the PMP syndrome in the patients with breast cancer was 20% (19 of 97 women). Of these 19 women with PMP syndrome, approximately half had intermittent pain and half had continuous pain. Their PMP was characterized by inadequate pain control and exacerbation of the pain with movement, and the pain was described as interfering with daily functioning. Stevens and colleagues (1995) point out that the reported proportion of patients in this sample with PMP syndrome may be underestimated, as it was not possible to determine whether any of the additional 14 women with advanced breast cancer in the sample also had PMP syndrome.

Ongoing research is needed to better understand the prevalence of breast cancer–related pain during all phases of the breast cancer experience. In addition, studies need to be done to determine how best to manage the different types of pain associated with breast cancer. Clinical practice must become more informed by the continued assessment and evaluation of pain and the development of effective strategies for pain management. Nurses should be challenged by the general perception that breast cancer pain is a rarity except with metastatic disease.

Another pain syndrome associated with breast cancer is characterized by pain in the axilla, arm, and/or elbow accompanied by cordlike material that can be palpated. The "cords" are thought to be sclerosed lymphatic structures. These cords cause tightness, pain, and impaired mobility; and the associated symptoms are often responsive to massage and stretching. The discomfort decreases or stops after spontaneous or massaged rupture of the cordlike structures.

A decrease in shoulder mobility, accompanied by pain, can be a consequence of axillary lymph node dissection or radiation therapy. Shoulder pain may be caused or exacerbated by edema, bleeding, or scarring. Range of motion exercises may prevent and can decrease mobility limitations and pain (Gerber, 1996).

In addition to the PMP syndrome, pain associated with breast cancer includes pain from bone metastases as well as acute pain associated with surgery for local recurrence. Frequently, bone metastases presents as pain that is described as dull, continuous rather than intermittent, and worsening gradually unless there is a fracture. Radiation therapy is an effective local palliative pain control therapy, particularly for a single lesion. Systemic therapy may provide effective pain control if it is successful in shrinking tumor size (Aaron, Jennings, & Springfield, 1996). In most cases, opioid analgesics are required for pain control, often in concert with NSAIDs.

Pain is usually the presenting symptom of brachial plex-

TABLE 21-16 Prognostic Indicators Used to Predict Tumor Recurrence and Survival from Breast Cancer

Prognostic Indicator	Favorable Value	Unfavorable Value
Axillary lymph nodes	No metastases	Metastasis in nodes
Number of positive axillary nodes	1-3 (0 most favorable)	4+ (>10 least favorable)
Internal mammary lymph nodes	No metastases	Metastases in nodes
Tumor size	Small (≤1 cm)	Large (>1 cm)
Histologic grade	I (Well differentiated)	III (Poorly differentiated)
Nuclear grade	I (Well differentiated)	III (Poorly differentiated)
Estrogen receptor	Present at ≥10 fmol/mg	<10 fmol/mg protein
Progesterone receptor	Present at ≥10 fmol/mg	<10 fmol/mg protein
p52 protein	High (>11ng/mg)	Low (<11ng/mg)
S-phase fraction	Low	High
Ploidy	Diploid	Aneuploid
Her-2/neu (c-erbB2)	Absent	Present
p53	Absent	Present
Cathepsin-D	Low	High
uPA	Low	High

uPA, urokinase plasminogen activato

opathy (invasion of the tumor into the brachial plexus). Brachial plexopathy can also be caused by surgical trauma to the brachial plexus, radiation-induced injury, lymphedema, or a new primary breast cancer. In addition to pain in the brachial plexus, other symptoms of brachial plexopathy include paresthesias, arm pain, heaviness, muscle weakness, and edema. Arm pain can also be caused by carpal tunnel syndrome. Radiation therapy may be used to treat brachial plexopathy if the skin in the treatment field has not received the maximum tolerated dose. Systemic therapies (chemotherapy, hormonal therapy) are variably effective in cases of tumor recurrence or new primary tumors. Effective dosing of analgesics for pain management often requires the use of a combination of analgesics, including opioids, NSAIDs, antidepressants, and/or anticonvulsants (Cherney & Foley, 1996).

PROGNOSIS

Prognostic Indicators

Prognostic indicators for recurrence and survival from infiltrating carcinoma include the following: lymph node status, tumor size, hormone receptor status, nuclear grade, histologic type, proliferative rate, and certain genetic markers. Features of tumors that are being explored for their ability to predict metastasis, tumor recurrence, and survival have increased considerably in recent years. Table 21-16 lists a variety of prognostic indicators and the characteristics that make them favorable or unfavorable. It is hoped that refinement of our understanding of carcinogenesis in relationship to these indicators will assist in identifying patients most at risk for recurrence so that they can receive adjuvant therapy, and that those not at risk for recurrence can be spared the morbidity associated with adjuvant therapy.

The SEER statistics for women diagnosed from 1989 to 1991 and followed up in 1993 report 5-year relative survival rates by stage at diagnosis to be 97% for tumors that exhibit only local extension at diagnosis, 76% for tumors with regional extension, and 20% for women with distant metastases at the time of diagnosis (ACS, 1997). When all prognostic factors are considered together, using multivariate analyses, the presence or absence of metastases to the axillary lymph nodes is the single most influential predictor of recurrence and mortality rates. However, the presence or absence of diseased lymph nodes is an imperfect indicator when taken alone because approximately 25% of patients without axillary node metastases are not cured by local regional therapy alone, and some patients with metastases are alive and well for many years (at 10 years: 30% overall, and 17% with 4 or more positive nodes) (Gardner & Feldman, 1993).

The presence of metastases in the internal mammary nodes is second only to the presence of metastases in axillary nodes as a predictor of recurrence or higher mortality (Noguchi et al., 1991). Long-term survival for patients with supraclavicular node involvement is considered to be equal to patients with stage IV disease, although 5-year survival rates (30% to 34%) are often better than in patients who present with metastases to distant organ systems (18%) (Kiricuta et al., 1994).

Several histologic types are associated with a reduced risk of invasive cancer: pure mucinous, pure tubular, pure medullary, and pure capillary carcinoma. However, these tumors make up less than 6% of invasive carcinomas and are usually diagnosed while still localized. The 5-year relative survival rate for patients with these pure histologic types of breast cancers is 95% (Berg & Hutter, 1995). Five-year survival rates for infiltrating tumors with less well-differentiated histology are overall (83%), ductal carcinoma

(79%), lobular carcinoma (84%), and medullary carcinoma (82%) (Berg & Hutter, 1995).

Histologic grade is based on the degree of tubule formation, the number of mitoses, and nuclear pleomorphism seen in routine tissue sections. These parameters are combined as the Scarff-Bloom-Richardson (SBR) grade. Well-differentiated tumors (grade 1) are relatively rare, and histologic grade usually increases with tumor size and stage. Both histologic and nuclear grades are predictors of mortality, but they provide no additional benefit as prognostic indicators once tumor size, node status, nipple involvement, and estrogen receptor status are considered (Fisher, Constantino, Fisher, & Redmond, 1993).

Increased numbers of microvessels (i.e., veins and arteries) in the invasive carcinomas were reported originally to be a predictor of nodal disease and distant metastases (Weidener et al., 1991); however, other investigators have failed to replicate this finding. In one blinded study of 220 cases of invasive carcinoma, there was considerable variation in the number of microvessels in different parts of the same tumor. At this time, there is no strong evidence that an increase in the number of microvessels is associated with increased risk of metastases or decreased survival.

The presence of estrogen or progesterone receptors in the tumor is associated with a better prognosis because the tumor may be responsive to hormone therapy. It has been estimated that between 50% and 85% of breast cancers contain measurable amounts of estrogen receptor (ER) (Donegan, 1997). ER-positive tumors are more common in older patients and are most common in postmenopausal women. The presence of ERs in the tumor indicates that normal cellular mechanisms for processing estrogen still exist despite the malignant process. The presence of progesterone receptors suggests that the same system is functioning and as a result offers little additional prognostic information.

About 50% to 60% of patients with ERs are observed to respond favorably to hormone or endocrine therapies, with the actual percentage that respond being correlated with the level of ERs present in the tumor. ER-positive patients have prolonged disease-free survival after primary treatment, superior overall survival rates, and longer survival after recurrence than patients with ER-negative tumors (Donegan, 1997). Limitations on the value of this prognostic indicator arise because ER-positive tumors tend also to be low in histologic and nuclear grade, and have a low S-phase fraction. Therefore the use of this indicator alone or in combination with node status has not been found to be a reliable indicator for which patients should be given adjuvant therapy. The importance of ER-positive status is most beneficial in the selection of hormone treatment.

Additional indicators are being sought to identify which patients with ER-positive tumors may have a particularly favorable outlook. One such indicator is the pS2 protein whose actual function is not yet well understood but is believed to be associated with a more intact cellular estrogen-processing mechanism.

Ploidy is another marker being studied for its ability to predict patients more likely to have recurrence or poorer survival potential. Diploid cells are in the resting phase (termed the *G phase*) or in the first phase of the cell cycle (termed G_1), whereas cells with twice the number of normal DNA content are in the mitotic phase (termed *M* phase). Cells with intermediate amounts of DNA are in the synthesis *(S)* phase. When a high proportion of the breast cells in a tissue sample are observed to be in the S-phase (i.e., S-phase fraction is high), prognosis is poorer. The process for calculation of the S-phase fraction is not standardized at this time, making the study of its value as a prognostic indicator more problematic. To date, this indicator has not been found to contribute additional predictive information about recurrence and mortality after tumor size and node status is taken into account.

CD is an estrogen-dependent lysosomal protease that is synthesized by normal tissues and is overexpressed and secreted by some breast cancers. As a result, CD has been suspected as facilitating the metastatic process. This hypothesis is supported by reports of increased levels of CD in patients with nodal metastases (Donegan, 1997). The overexpression of CD is associated with higher levels of recurrence and lower survival rates (Gasparini et al., 1991; Seshadri et al., 1994). However, the presence of CD has not provided additional prognostic information in node-positive patients once tumor size is considered. The situation surrounding the overexpression of CD in patients with node-negative tumors is more puzzling. Findings have been conflicting in these patients, with initial studies reporting a poorer prognosis in patients with overexpression of CD (Isola et al., 1993; Tandon et al., 1990). However, a later, larger study failed to replicate this finding (Ravdin et al., 1994).

Urokinase plasminogen activator (uPA) is a protease that has been implicated in the metastatic process. In animals, the activation of this protease has been shown to lead to the metastatic growth of tumors. In addition, high levels of uPA in human breast tumors have been correlated with a shorter disease-free interval and poorer survival rates. More important, this indicator appears to be independent of tumor size and node status (Duffy et al., 1994). This work shows promise as being able to provide additional information about patterns of recurrence and survival potential, but the findings await replication in future reports.

c-erbB2 (also called *Her-2/neu,* or *erbB2*) is a protooncogene. It is believed that when this and other protooncogenes undergo mutation, they promote neoplastic transformation. The overexpression of c-erbB2 has been observed to be associated with a poorer prognosis, but this association appears to be confined almost entirely to node-positive patients (Marks et al., 1994).

p53 is a tumor suppressor gene that is believed to function by blocking cells in G_1 or by programming cell death. The expression of mutant p53 is the most commonly observed genetic defect found in human cancers. It can be demonstrated in 14% to 26% of in situ and invasive cancers depending on which criteria are used to determine its presence (Isola, Visakorpi, Holli, & Kallioniemi, 1992; Thor et al., 1992). Mutant p53 is more common in familial cases of breast cancer and has been found in up to 52% of cases of breast and ovarian cancer syndrome and in all cases of Li

Fraumeni syndrome (Thor et al., 1992). The expression of p53 is associated with an overall decrease in survival, as well as in time to recurrence.

Race and Cultural Considerations in Terms of Prognosis

In a recent analysis of all white female breast cancer cases in the United States, decreasing trends in breast cancer mortality of approximately 2% per year from 1989 to 1993 were reported across all age ranges (Chu et al., 1996). The researchers concluded that both the onset of mammographic screening in the 1980s and the availability of new treatments account for these gains in breast cancer survival. This improvement appears to be most demonstrable in white women (Chu et al., 1996).

Improving breast cancer survival may be more complicated than simply decreasing the overall stage of breast cancer at the time of diagnosis. Even when the stage of breast cancer is taken into account, African-American women still have lower survival rates. Five-year survival rates for breast cancer patients differ by race, with 1986 to 1991 SEER data showing African-American women having lower overall survival rates (70%) than white women (85%) (ACS, 1997; Phillips, 1996). Table 21-17 lists the 5-year mortality rates by stage for white American and African-American women as calculated from the 1986 to 1992 SEER data (ACS, 1997).

Hispanics with breast cancer of similar socioeconomic status to African-American women have survival rates closer to those of whites. This finding suggests that biologic differences may account for some of these differences in survival rates by race. Initial studies have suggested that a higher proportion of ER-negative tumors and alterations in relationship to the p53 gene (Shiao et al., 1995) predispose African-American women to poorer survival. Other recent studies, controlling for the effects of age, tumor size, histology, estrogen and progesterone receptor levels, ploidy status, S-phase, Her-2/neu expression, and tumor grade have failed to demonstrate biologic differences by race (Gapstur, Dupuis, Gann, Collila, & Winchester, 1996; Weiss et al., 1996). The effects of poverty and genetics have been difficult to separate, even in large national data sets.

TABLE 21-17 Percentage 5-Year Relative Survival Rates by Race and Stage at Diagnosis

Stage	African American	Caucasian American
All stages combined	70	85
Localized	89	97
Regional	61	77
Distant	16	21

National Cancer Institute Surveillance and Epidemiologic End Results Data 1986-1992.

Treatments for infiltrating breast cancer show improvements in the eradication of the primary tumor but little progress in preventing metastases. Little is known about when a breast tumor metastasizes to local, regional, and then distant tissues; as a result, systemic therapies have become the standard of care. In a study that analyzed 133 randomized clinical trials from around the world (Early Breast Cancer Trialists' Collaborative Group, 1992), women who underwent either chemotherapy or tamoxifen therapy after

TABLE 21-18 Quality of Care Evaluation for a Patient Undergoing Lumpectomy/Modified Radical Mastectomy and Lymph Node Dissection

Disciplines participating in the quality of care evaluation:
☐ Surgery ☐ Nursing ☐ Physical Therapy
☐ Psychological Services ☐ Discharge Planning
Data from:
☐ Medical Record Review ☐ Patient Interview
I. Postoperative Management Evaluation

Criteria	Yes	No
1. Patient given preoperative information about		
a. treatment choices	☐	☐
b. potential for lymphedema	☐	☐
2. Patient given postoperative information:		
a. If drain is present, how to empty drain	☐	☐
b. If drain is present, how to document drainage	☐	☐
c. How to prevent infection in ipsilateral arm	☐	☐
d. Mobility and range of motion exercises and when to start	☐	☐
e. Information re bra and /or prosthesis	☐	☐
3. Patient offered emotional support/referral	☐	☐
4. Patient experienced the following complications		
a. Postoperative seroma	☐	☐
b. Blood draw, blood pressure, IV start on ipsilateral arm (except emergency)	☐	☐
c. Unrelieved pain	☐	☐

II. Patient/Family Satisfaction

Criteria	Yes	No
1. On a scale of 0-10, with 0 being totally dissatisfied and 10 being totally satisfied, how satisfied were you with your pain control?	☐	☐
2. Were you taught not to have blood pressures, IVs, blood draws on the surgical side?	☐	☐
3. If you have a drain, were you shown how to take care of it?	☐	☐
4. Did you know who to call for a problem and at what telephone number?	☐	☐

TABLE 21-19 Quality of Care Evaluation for a Patient Undergoing Lumpectomy/Modified Radical Mastectomy Without a Lymph Node Dissection

Disciplines participating in the quality of care evaluation:
☐ Surgery ☐ Nursing ☐ Physical Therapy
☐ Psychological Services ☐ Discharge Planning
Data from:
☐ Medical Record Review ☐ Patient Interview
I. Postoperative Management Evaluation

Criteria	Yes	No
1. Patient given preoperative information about		
a. treatment choices	☐	☐
b. no lymph node dissection, therefore no lymphedema	☐	☐
2. Patient given postoperative information:		
a. Information about bra and /or prosthesis	☐	☐
b. Who/where to call with a problem	☐	☐
3. Patient offered some type of emotional support/referral	☐	☐
4. Patient experienced the following complications		
a. Postoperative infection	☐	☐
b. Postoperative bleeding	☐	☐

surgery had a 12% to 14% greater chance of surviving for 10 years than those who did not. Without chemotherapy or tamoxifen, women with breast cancer have a 55% chance of dying within 10 years. Once a woman is diagnosed with infiltrating breast cancer, she is always more likely to die of the disease than women in the general population; thus use of the word *cure* is always questionable when describing breast cancer survival.

EVALUATION OF THE QUALITY OF CARE

What needs to be evaluated and how can this be accomplished? Two main areas for evaluating the quality of breast cancer care include an assessment of (1) equity in access to breast cancer early detection and treatment services, and (2) the delivery of optimal treatment services to patients under care. Our national goals for cancer prevention, detection, and treatment services imply an equity of access to cancer services for populations at risk for the disease (Healthy People 2000, 1992). Our urban cancer centers still fall short in communicating and facilitating the availability of diagnostic and treatment services for the populations they serve. Few centers have evaluated their efforts to facilitate early detection for symptomatic individuals in local communities who are not yet patients.

Ensuring that clients are treated with dignity, that culturally competent cancer information is available to all, and that no segments of the population are systematically denied cancer care is the shared ethical responsibility of providers, policy-makers, and concerned citizens. This philosophy requires us, as providers, to advocate for those who have been poorly served or not served at all (Facione & Facione, 1997).

Suominen and colleagues (1995) have documented that nurses' opinions of how well care was delivered do not always agree with the opinions of cancer patients and their families. Nurses need to evaluate the quality of the care they deliver in the context of the health care setting, the percep-

Box 21-4
Research Issues in the Diagnosis and Treatment of Breast Cancer

Biologic

The relationship between in situ and infiltrating breast cancer
The role of oncogenes, growth factors, and hormonal factors
The relationship between tumor doubling time and cell differentiation and real survival improvements from any of our current treatment modalities
The timing, mechanism, and prevention of breast cancer metastatic spread
The association between hormone replacement therapy and the development of breast cancer
Efficacy of complementary medicine therapies
Impact of dietary changes (e.g., low fat) on prevention and recurrence of breast cancer

Hereditary Breast Cancer

The indications for prophylactic mastectomy
Use of chemopreventive agents
Guidelines for intensified screening
Ethical delivery of genetic screening and information to families
Effective prevention against insurance and job discrimination

Social and Behavioral Research Issues

The ethics and cultural considerations surrounding genetics testing
Ways to better evaluate cancer prevention, detection, and treatment services delivery
The impact on utilization of cost, provider relationships, and availability of services
Ethical/spiritual/political influences on early detection and treatment decisions for breast cancer

Treatment Issues

Effective preventative measures and treatment strategies for lymphedema
Improved pain management
Interventions that effectively decrease or enhance coping with symptoms: fatigue, cognitive changes, alopecia, psychological distress
Provider communication and teaching skills to support patient decision making
Treatment of menopausal symptoms without estrogen

Box 21-5
A Breast Cancer Agenda for Women in the Twenty-First Century

- Shall I consult my provider regarding an estimate of my personal risk of developing breast cancer in the next ten years?
- How frequently shall I undergo routine mammography and professional breast examination?
- Should I obtain more information regarding breast cancer symptoms and breast cancer treatments?
- Should I perform breast self-examination? Should I obtain training in breast self-examination?
- Shall I participate in prospective breast cancer prevention and screening studies (Tamoxifen, retinoids, mammography screening pilots, etc.)?
- Shall I participate in genetic screening as it becomes more widely available?
- Shall I expend personal financial resources for my own breast cancer screening?
- Shall I become an agent for family and friends in regard to breast cancer prevention and early detection?
- Shall I advocate the increased spending for the development of improved breast cancer screening modalities?
- Shall I advocate the use of communal resources for breast cancer screening for all women?

tion of needs from the perspective of the patient and/or the family, and the goals for breast cancer management held by the health care team. Ultimately, the judgments of the patient and/or the family members determine the major portion of the quality assessment of nursing interventions; as a result, input from these individuals needs to be included in any evaluation tools used to evaluate quality.

Tracking tools can be useful devices to document progress in teaching key information and communicating to staff the remaining educational needs in both inpatient and outpatient settings. When charts do not reliably follow patients to their postoperative outpatient appointments, women should be provided with copies of the educational program.

Merrouche and colleagues (1996) continued their evaluation of care through the terminal stages of illness by surveying the family members of terminal cancer patients 6 months after the death of the patient. They included an assessment of the quality of information given to patients and their families, estimates of the quality of pain control, nursing care services, psychological support, and the family members' opinions of the practical conditions at the time of the patient's death at home or in an institutional setting. Inadequate pain management was reported by 21% of their sample, and the majority (67%) of these families preferred death to occur in the hospital rather than in the home.

Tools for the collection of data developed by Hamolsky are shown in Tables 21-18 and 21-19. It can be used to begin to gather data to evaluate the quality of care for patients with breast cancer in relationship to perioperative nursing care. Another tool for evaluating nursing care of breast cancer patients has been developed by Sciartelli (1995).

RESEARCH ISSUES

The research issues surrounding breast cancer are complex and broad in domain, encompassing biologic, social, and behavioral issues; issues surrounding hereditary breast cancer; and issues surrounding specific treatment options. Box 21-4 provides a list of some of the future research questions. Box 21-5 lists a group of questions that frame the breast cancer early detection and treatment agenda for the twenty-first century. How we choose to answer these questions will influence the lives of women with breast cancer in the years to come.

REFERENCES

Aaron, A., Jennings, L., & Springfield, D. (1996). Local treatment of bone metastases. In J. Harris, M. Lippman, M. Morrow, & S. Hellman (Eds.), *Diseases of the breast.* Philadelphia: Lippincott Raven.

Ahles, T. A., Ruckdeschel, J. C., & Blanchard, E. B. (1984). Cancer related pain: Prevalence in an outpatient setting as a function of stage of disease and type of cancer. *Journal of Psychosomatic Research, 28,* 115-119.

Albertini, J. J., Lyman, G. H., Cox, C., Yeatman, T., Balducci, L., Ku, N., Shivers, S., Berman, C., Wells, K., Rapaport, D., Shons, A., Horton, J., Greenberg, H., Nicosia, S., Clark, R., Cantor, A., & Reintgen, D. S. (1996). Lymphatic mapping and sentinel mode biopsy in the patient with breast cancer. *Journal of the American Medical Association, 276*(22), 1818-1822.

American Cancer Society. (1997). *Cancer facts and figures 1997.* Atlanta: The Author.

American Joint Committee on Cancer. (1988). *Manual for staging of cancer* (3rd ed.). Philadelphia: J. B. Lippincott

American Society of Clinical Oncology. (1996). Statement of the American Society of Clinical Oncology. Genetic testing for cancer susceptibility. *Journal of Clinical Oncology, 14,* 1730-1736.

Barnicle, M. (1996). Managing symptoms related to chemotherapy. In K. Hassey-Dow (Ed.), *Contemporary issues in breast cancer.* Sudbury, MA: Jones and Bartlett.

Bassett, L. W., Hendrick, R. E., Bassford, T. L., et al. (1994). *Quality determinants of mammography. Clinical Practice Guideline No. 13* (AHCPR Publication No. 95-0632). Rockville, MD: Agency for Health Care Policy and Research, U. S. Department of Health and Human Services, Public Health Service.

Berg, J. W., & Hutter, R. V. P. (1995). Breast cancer. *Cancer, 75*(Suppl.), 257-269.

Bilimoria, M., & Morrow, M. (1995). The woman at increased risk for breast cancer: Evaluation and measurement strategies. *CA: A Cancer Journal for Clinicians, 45*(5), 263-278.

Bilodeau, B. A., & Degner, L. F. (1996). Information needs, sources of information, and decisional roles in women with breast cancer. *Oncology Nursing Forum, 23*(4), 691-696.

Bonadonna, G., Valgussa, P., Zucali, R., & Salvadori, B. (1995). Primary chemotherapy in surgically resectable breast cancer. *CA: A Cancer Journal for Clinicians, 45*(4), 227-243.

Boring, C. C., Squires, T. S., Tong, T., & Montgomery, S. (1994). Cancer statistics. *CA: A Cancer Journal for Clinicians, 44*(1), 7-26.

Bostwick, J. (1995). Breast reconstruction following mastectomy. *CA: A Cancer Journal for Clinicians, 45*(5), 289-304.

Brant, J. M. (1996). Breast cancer challenges in Native American women. In K. Hassey Dow (Ed.), *Contemporary issues in breast cancer.* Sudbury, MA: Jones and Bartlett.

Bressler, L. R., Hange, P.A., & McGuire, D. B. (1986). Characteristics of the pain experience in a sample of cancer outpatients. *Oncology Nursing Forum, 13*(6), 51-55.

Brock, D. J. H. (1993). *Molecular genetics for the clinician.* Cambridge, Great Britain: Cambridge University Press.

Cady, B., Stione, M. D., Schuler, J. G., Thakur, R., Wanner, M. A., & Lavin, P. T. (1996). The new era in breast cancer. *Archives of Surgery, 131,* 301-308.

Caplan, L. S., Wells, B., & Haynes, S. (1992). Breast cancer screening among older racial/ethnic minorities and whites: Barriers to early detection. *Journals of Gerontology, 47,* 101-110.

Champion, V. (1992). Breast self-examination in women 65 and older. *Journals of Gerontology, 47,* 75-79.

Chang, B. W. (1995). Reconstruction following mastectomy: Timing, indications, and results. In J. L. Cameron (Ed.), *Current surgical therapy* (5th ed.). St. Louis: Mosby.

Chereney, M., & Foley, K. M. (1996). Brachial plexopathy in patients with breast cancer. In J. Harris, M. Lippman, M. Morrow, & S. Hellman (Eds.), *Diseases of the breast.* Philadelphia: Lippincott Raven.

Chu, K. C., Tarone, R. E., Kessler, L. G., Ries, L. G. A., Hankey, B. F., Miller, B. A, & Edwards, B. K. (1996). Recent trends in U.S. breast cancer incidence, survival, and mortality rates. *Journal of the National Cancer Institute, 88*(21), 1571-1579.

Colomeda, L. A. L. (1996). *Through the looking glass: Breast cancer stories told by northern native women.* New York: NLN Press.

Cook, L. S., Weiss, N. S., Schwartz, S. M., White, E., McKnight, B., Moore, D. E., & Daling, J. R. (1995) Population-based study of tamoxifen therapy and subsequent ovarian, endometrial, and breast cancers. *Journal of the National Cancer Institute, 87*(18), 1359-1364.

Daut, R. L., & Cleeland, C. S. (1982). The prevalence and severity of pain in cancer. *Cancer, 50,* 1913-1918.

Davidoff, A. M., Kerns, B. Inglehart, J. D., & Marks, J. R. (1991). Maintenance of p53 alterations throughout breast cancer progression. *Cancer Research, 51,* 2605-2610.

Davidson, N. E., & Abeloff, D. W. (1993). Menstrual effects of surgical treatment for breast cancer. *Current Treatment Reviews, 19,* 105-112.

Denenberg, R. (1995). Invisible women: Lesbians and health care. *Health PAC Bulletin,* Spring, 1992.

Dhingra, K., & Hortobagyi, G. (1996). Critical evaluation of prognostic factors. *Seminars in Oncology, 23*(4), 436-445.

Dodd, M. J. (1996). *Managing the side effects of chemotherapy and radiation therapy: a guide for patients and their families.* San Francisco: University of California Press.

Donegan, W. L. (1997). Tumor-related prognostic factors for breast cancer. *CA: Cancer Journal for Clinicians, 47,* 28-51.

Donegan, W. L., & Redlich, P. N. (1996). Breast cancer in men. *Surgical Clinics in North America 76*(2), 343-363.

Dow, K. H. (1996). *Contemporary issues in breast cancer.* Sudbury, MA: Jones and Bartlett Publishers.

Duffy, M. J., Reilly, D., McDermott, E., O'Higgins, N., Fennelly, J. J., & Andreasen, P. A. (1994). Urokinase plasminogen activator as a prognostic marker in different subgroups of patients with breast cancer. *Cancer, 74,* 2276-2280.

Dupont, W. D., & Page, D. L. (1985). Risk factors for breast cancer in women with proliferative breast cancer. *New England Journal of Medicine, 312,* 146-151.

Early Breast Cancer Trialists' Collaborative Group, EBCTCG. (1988). Effects of adjuvant tamoxifen and of cytotoxic therapy on mortality in early breast cancer. An overview of 61 randomized trials among 28,896 women. *New England Journal of Medicine, 319*(26), 1681-1692.

Early Breast Cancer Trialists' Collaborative Group (1992). Systemic treatment of early breast cancer by hormonal, cytotoxic, or immune therapy. 133 randomized trials involving 31,000 recurrences and 24,000 deaths among 75,000 women. *Lancet, 339,* 1-15, 71-85.

Easton, D. F., Bishop, D. T., Ford, D., & Crockford, G. P. (1993). Genetic linkage analysis in familial breast and ovarian cancer: Results from 214 families. *American Journal of Human Genetics, 52,* 678-701.

Eddy, D. M. (1989). Screening for breast cancer. *Annals of Internal Medicine, 111,* 389-399.

Engelking, C. (1989). Recurrent breast cancer: Physical and psychosocial sequelae. *Innovations in Oncology Nursing, 3,* 2-6.

Evans, D. G. R., Fentiman, I. S., McPherson, K., Asbury, D., Ponder, B. A. J., & Howell, A. (1994). Familial breast cancer. *British Medical Journal, 308,* 183-187.

EVAXX, Inc. (1980). Black Americans' attitudes toward cancer and cancer tests. *Cancer, 31*(4), 212-218.

Facione, N. C., & Dodd, M. J. (1995). Women's narratives of help seeking for breast cancer. *Cancer Practice, 3*(4), 219-225.

Facione, N. C., Dodd, M. J., Holzemer, W., & Meleis, A. (1997). Helpseeking for self-discovered breast symptoms: Implications for cancer early detection. *Cancer Practice, 5*(4), 220-227.

Facione, N. C., & Facione, P.A. (1997). Equitable access to cancer services in the 21st century, *Nursing Outlook, 45*(3), 118-124.

Farwell, M. F., Foster, R. S., & Costanza, M. C. (1993). Breast cancer and earlier detection efforts: Realized and unrealized impact on stage. *Archives of Surgery, 128,* 510-514. Fetting, J. (1991). Psychosocial aspects of breast cancer. *Current Science ISSN 1040-8746,* 1014-1018.

Fisher, B., Andersen, S., Redmond, C. K., Wolmark, N., Wickerham, D. L., & Cronin, W. M. (1995). Re-analysis and results after 12 years of follow-up in a randomized clinical trial comparing total mastectomy with lumpectomy with or without irradiation in the treatment of breast cancer. *New England Journal of Medicine, 333*(22), 1456-1461.

Fisher, E. R., Constantino, J., Fisher, B., & Redmond, C. (1993). Pathologic findings from the National Surgical Adjuvant Breast Project (Protocol 4). *Cancer, 71,* 2141-2150.

Foley, K. M. (1987). Pain syndromes in patients with cancer. *Medical Clinics of North America, 71,* 169-184.

Ford, D., Easton, D. F., Bishop, D. T., Narod, S. A., Godgar, D. E., & the Breast Cancer Linkage Consortium. (1994). Risks of cancer in BRCA1 mutation carriers. *Lancet, 343,* 692-695.

Foster, R. (1996). Techniques for diagnosis of palpable breast masses. In I, J. Harris, M. Lippman, M. Morrow, & S. Hellman (Eds.), *Diseases of the breast.* Philadelphia: Lippincott Raven.

Ganz, P. A., Day, R., Ware, J. E., Redmond, C., & Fisher, B. (1995). Base-line quality-of-life assessment in the National Surgical Adjuvant Breast and Bowel Project Cancer Prevention Trial. *Journal of the National Cancer Institute, 87,* 1372-1382.

Gapstur, S. M., Dupuis, J., Gann, P., Collila, S., & Winchester, D. P. (1996). Hormone receptor status of breast tumors in black, Hispanic, and non-Hispanic white women. An analysis of 13,239 cases. *Cancer, 77*(8), 1465-1471.

Gardner, B., & Feldman, J. (1993). Are positive axillary nodes in breast cancer markers for incurable disease? *Annals of Surgery, 218,* 270-278.

Gasparini, G. Pozza, F., Meli, S., Reitano, M., Santini, G., & Bevilacqua, P. (1991). Breast cancer cell kinetics: Immunocytochemical determination of growth fractions by monoclonal antibody Ki-67 and correlation with flow cytometric S-phase and some features of tumor aggressiveness. *Anticancer Research, 11,* 2015-2021.

Gerber, L. (1996). Rehabilitation management for women with breast cancer: Maximizing functional outcomes. In J. Harris, M. Lippman, M. Morrow, & S. Hellman (Eds.), *Diseases of the breast.* Philadelphia: Lippincott Raven.

Glanz, K. (1994). Reducing breast cancer risk through changes in diet and alcohol intake: From clinic to community. *Annals of Behavioral Medicine, 16*(4), 334-336.

Goldhirsch, A., & Gelber, R. D. (1996). Endocrine therapies of breast cancer. *Seminars in Oncology, 23*(4), 496.

Goodwin, J. S., & Samet, J. M. (1994). Care received by older women diagnosed with breast cancer. *Cancer Control, 1,* 313-319.

Gradishar, W., Tallman, M., & Abrams, J. (1996). High-dose chemotherapy for breast cancer. *Annals of Internal Medicine, 120*(7), 599-604.

Grant, C. S., Groellner, J. R., Welsh, J. S., & Martin, J. K. (1986). Fine needle aspiration of the breast. *Mayo Clinic Proceedings, 61,* 377-381.

Gusterson, B. A., Gelber, R. D., Goldhirsch, A., Price, K. N., Säve-Söderborgh, J., Anbazhagan, R., Styles, J., Rudenstam, C. M., Golouh, R., & Reed, R. (1992). Prognostic importance of c-erb B-2 expression in breast cancer. *Journal of Clinical Oncology, 10,* 1049-1056.

Hall, F. M., Storella, J. M., Silverstone, D. Z., & Wyshak, G. (1988). Nonpalpable breast lesions: Recommendations for biopsy based on suspicion of carcinoma at mammography. *Radiology, 167,* 353-358.

Handel, N. (1991). Current status of breast reconstruction after mastectomy. *Oncology, 5*(11), 73-89.

Harris, R., & Leininger, L. (1995). Clinical strategies for breast cancer screening: Weighing and using the evidence. *Annals of Internal Medicine, 122*(7), 539-547.

Harris, J. R., Lippman, M. E., Veronesi, U., & Willett, W. (1992). Medical progress: Breast cancer. *New England Journal of Medicine, 327,* 319-328.

Harris, L., & Swain, S. (1996). The role of primary chemotherapy in early breast cancer. *Seminars in Oncology, 23*(1, Suppl. 2), 31-42.

Hayes, D. F. (1996). Breast cancer. In A. T. Skarin (Ed.), *Atlas of diagnostic oncology* (2nd ed.). London: Mosby-Wolfe.

Healthy people 2000: National health promotion and disease prevention objectives (1992). U. S. Dept. of Health & Human Services, Public Health Service. Boston: Jones & Bartlett.

Heimann, R., Ferguson, D., Powers, C., Recant, W. M., Weichselbaum, R. R., & Hellman, S. (1996). Angiogenesis as a predictor of long-term survival for patients with node-negative breast cancer. *Journal of the National Cancer Institute, 88*(23), 1764-1769.

Henderson, C. I. (1995). Breast cancer. In G. P. Murphy, W. L. Lawrence, & R. E. Lenhard (Eds.), *Clinical oncology.* Atlanta: American Cancer Society.

Hilton, B. A. (1996). Getting back to normal: The family experience during early stage breast cancer. *Oncology Nursing Forum, 23*(4), 605-614.

Hong, W. K., & Lippman, S. M. (1995). Cancer chemoprevention. *Journal of the National Cancer Institute Monographs, 17,* 49-53.

Hortobagyi, G. N., & Buzdar, A. U. (1995). Current status of adjuvant systemic therapy for primary breast cancer: Progress and controversy. *CA: A Cancer Journal for Clinicians, 45,* 199-226.

Hortobagyi, G. N., Buzdar, A. U., Strom, E. A., Ames, F. C., & Singletary, S. E. (1995). Primary chemotherapy for early and advanced breast cancer. *Cancer Letters, 90,* 103-109.

Hoskins, K. F., Stopfer, J. E., Calzone, K. A., Merajver, S. D., Rebbeck, T. R., Garber, J. E., & Weber, B. L. (1995). Assessment and counseling for women with a family history of breast cancer: A guide for clinicians. *Journal of the American Medical Association, 273,* 577-585.

Hunter, D., & Willett, W. (1996). Dietary factors. In J. Harris, M. Lippman, M. Morrow, & S. Hellman (Eds.), *Diseases of the breast.* Philadelphia: Lippincott Raven.

Hunter, R. V. P. (1986). Consensus meeting: Is "fibrocystic disease" of the breast precancerous? *Archives of Pathology and Laboratory Medicine, 110,* 171.

Isola, J., Visakorpi, T., Holli, K., & Kallioniemi, O. P. (1992). Association of overexpression of tumor suppressor protein p53 with rapid cell proliferation and poor prognosis in node-negative breast cancer patients. *Journal of the National Cancer Institute, 84,* 1109-1114.

Isola, J., Weitz, S., Visakorpi, T, Holli, K., Shea, R., Khabbaz, N., & Kallioniemi, O. P. (1993). Cathepsin D expression detected by immunohistochemistry has independent prognostic value in axillary node-negative breast cancer. *Journal of Clinical Oncology, 11,* 36-43.

Jones, J. H. (1981). *Bad blood: The Tuskegee syphilis experiment.* New York: The Free Press.

Kagawa-Singer, M. (1996). Issues affecting Asian American and Pacific American women. In K. Hassey Dow (Ed.), *Contemporary issues in breast cancer.* Sudbury, MA: Jones and Bartlett.

Kelly, P., & Winslow, E. H. (1996).Needle wire localization for nonpalpable breast lesions: Sensations, anxiety levels, and informational needs. *Oncology Nursing Forum, 23*(4), 639-645.

King, M. C., Rowell, S., & Love, S. (1993). Inherited breast and ovarian cancer: What are the risks? What are the choices? *Journal of the American Medical Association, 269,* 1975-1980.

Kiricuta, I. C., Willner, J., Kolbl, O., & Bohndorf, W. (1994). The prognostic significance of the supraclavicular lymph node metastases in breast cancer patients. *International Journal of Radiation Oncology, Biology, and Physics, 28,* 387-393.

Landis, S. H., Murray, T., Bolden, S., Wingo, P. A. (1998). Cancer statistics, 1998. *CA: A Cancer Journal for Clinicians, 48*(1), 6-30.

Lannin, D. R., Harris, R. P., Swanson, F. H., & Pories, W. J. (1993). Difficulties in diagnosis of carcinoma of the breast in patients less than 50 years old. *Surgery, Gynecology and Obstetrics, 177,* 457-462.

Lavery, J., & Clarke, V. (1996). Causal attributions, coping strategies and adjustment to breast cancer. *Cancer Nursing, 19*(1), 20-28.

Leitch, A. (1995). Controversies in breast cancer screening. *Cancer, 76,* 2064-2069.

Leone, A., Flatow, King, C. R., Sandeen, M. A., Marguiles, I. M. K., Liotta, L. A., & Steeg, P. S. (1991). Reduced tumor incidence, metastatic potential, and cytokinetic responsiveness of nm-23-transfected melanoma cells. *Cell, 65,* 25-35.

Lerman, C., Schwartz, M. D., Miller, S. M., Daly, M., & Sands, C. (1996). A randomized trial of breast cancer risk counseling: Interacting effects of counseling, emotional level and coping style. *Health Psychology, 15*(2), 75, 83.

Lidbrink E, Frisell J, Brandberg Y, Rosendahl I, & Rutqvist, L. E. (1995) Nonattendance in the Stockholm mammography screening trial: Relative mortality and reasons for nonattendance. *Breast Cancer Research and Treatment, 35,* 267-275.

Linver, M. N., Osuch, J. R., Brenner, R. J., & Smith, R. A. (1995). The mammography audit: A primer for the mammography quality standards act (MQSA). *American Journal of Roentgenology, 165*(1), 19-25.

Mackarem, G., Barbarisi, L., & Hughes, K. (1992). The role of axillary dissection in early stage breast cancer. *Cancer Investigation, 10*(5), 461-470.

Mackay, G., & Bostwick, J. (1996). Reconstructive breast surgery. In J. Harris, M. Lippman, M. Morrow, & S. Hellman (Eds.), *Diseases of the breast.* Philadelphia: Lippincott Raven.

Mandalblatt, J., Andrews, H., Kao, R., Wallace, R., & Kerner, J. (1995). Impact of access and social context on breast cancer stage at diagnosis. *Journal of Health Care for the Poor and Underserved, 6*(3), 342-351.

Marks, J. R., Humphrey, P. A., Wu, K., Berry, D., Bandarenko, N., Kerns, B. J., & Iglehart, J. D. (1994). Overexpression of p53 and HER-2/neu proteins as prognostic markers in early stage breast cancer. *Annals of Surgery, 219,* 332-341.

Merchant, T. E., McCormick, B., Yahalom, J., & Borgen, P. (1996). The influence of older age on breast cancer treatment decisions and outcome. *International Journal of Radiation Oncology Biology and Physics, 34*(3), 565-570.

Merrouche, Y., Freyer, G., Saltel, P., & Rebattu, P. (1996). Quality of final care for terminal patients in a comprehensive cancer centre from the point of view of patients' families. *Supportive Care in Cancer, 4*(3), 163-168.

Miaskowski, C., & Dibble, S. (1995). The problem of pain in outpatients with breast cancer. *Oncology Nursing Forum, 22*(5), 791-797.

Miller, A. B., Baines, C. J., To, T., & Wall, C. (1992). Canadian National Breast Screening Study: 1) Breast cancer detection and death rates among women ages 40-49. *Canadian Medical Association Journal, 147,* 1459-1476.

Miller, B. A., Feuer, E. J., & Hanky, B. F. (1991). The increasing incidence of breast cancer since 1982: Relevance of early detection. *Cancer Causes and Control, 2,* 67-74.

Muss, H. B., Thor, A. D., Berry, D. A., Kute, T., Liu, E. T., Koerner, F., Cirrincione, C. T., Budman, D. R., Wood, W. C., & Barcos, M. (1994). c-erbB-2 expression and response to adjuvant therapy in women with node-positive early breast cancer. *New England Journal of Medicine, 330,* 1260-1266.

National Cancer Institute PDQ State of the Art Cancer Treatment Summary. (1995). *Breast Cancer, 1,* 39.

National Surgical Adjuvant Breast and Bowel Project (NSABBP). (1994). 4-HPR (fenretinide) - Stage 1: NSABP. *Journal of the National Cancer Institute, 86,* 527-537.

Newschaffer, C. J., Penberthy, L., Desch, C. E., Retchin, S. M., & Whittemore, M. (1996). The effect of age and comorbidity in the treatment of elderly women with nonmetastatic breast cancer. *Archives of Internal Medicine, 156,* 85-90.

NEWS. (1996a). *Journal of the National Cancer Institute, 88*(23), 1710.

NEWS. (1996b). *Journal of the National Cancer Institute, 88*(2), 75.

Nguyen, M., McCombs, M. M., Ghandehari, S., Kim, A., Wang, H., Barsky, S. H., Love, S., & Bassett, L. W. (1996). An update on core needle biopsy for radiologically detected breast lesions. *Cancer, 78,* 2340-2345.

Noguchi, M., Ohta, N., Koyasaki, N., Taniya, T., Miyazaki, I., & Mizukami, Y. (1991). Reappraisal of internal mammary node metastases as a prognostic factor in patients with breast cancer. *Cancer, 68,* 1918-1925.

O'Hanlan, K. (1995). Lesbians in health research. *Recruitment and retention of women in clinical studies.* U. S. National Institutes of Health Publication No. 95-3756. Bethesda, MD: Public Health Service, National Institutes of Health.

O'Rourke, N., & Robinson, L. (1996). Breast cancer and the role of radiation therapy. In K. Hassey-Dow (Ed.), *Contemporary issues in breast cancer,* Sudbury, MA: Jones and Bartlett.

Osborne, C. K., Clark, G., & Ravdin, P. (1996). Adjuvant systemic therapy of breast cancer. In J. Harris, M. Lippman, M. Morrow, & S. Hellman (Eds.), *Diseases of the breast.* Philadelphia: Lippincott Raven.

Ownby, H. E., Frederick, J., Russo, J., Brooks, S. C., Swanson, G. M., Heppner, G. H., & Brennan, M. J. (1985). Racial differences in breast cancer patients. *Journal of the National Cancer Institute, 75,* 55-60.

Peteet, J., Tay, V., Cohen, G., & MacIntyre, J. (1986). Patient characteristics and treatment in an outpatient cancer population. *Cancer, 57,* 1259-1265.

Peters, W. P., Bernyi, D., Vredenburgh, J. J., & Hossein, A. (1995). Five year follow-up of high dose combination alkylating agents with autologous bone marrow transplant as consolidation after standard dose CAF for primary breast cancer involving 10 axillary lymph nodes (Duke University/ Protocol CALGB No. 8782) Abstract. *Association of the Society for Clinical Oncology, 14,* 317.

Peters, W. P., Ross, M., Vredenburgh, J. J., Hussein, A., Meisenberg, B., Gilbert, C., Petros, W. P., & Kutzberg, J. (1993). High dose chemotherapy and autologous bone marrow support as consolidation after standard dose adjuvant therapy for high risk primary breast cancer. *Journal of Clinical Oncology, 11,* 1132-1143.

Petrek, J., & Lerner, R. (1996). Lymphedema. In J. Harris, M. Lippman, M. Morrow, & S. Hellman (Eds.), *Diseases of the breast.* Philadelphia: Lippincott Raven.

Phillips, J. (1996). Breast cancer and African American Women. In K. Hassey Dow (Ed.), *Contemporary issues in breast cancer.* Sudbury, MA: Jones and Bartlett.

Rankow, E. (1995). Lesbian health issues for the primary care provider. *Journal of Family Practice, 48*(5), 486-496.

Ravdin, P. M., Tandon, A. K., Allred, D. C., Clark, G. M., Fuqua, S. A., Hilsenbeck, S. H., Chamness, G. C., & Osborne, C. K. (1994). Cathepsin-D by western blotting and immunohistochemistry: Failure to confirm correlations with prognosis in node negative breast cancer. *Journal of Clinical Oncology, 12,* 467-474.

Reeves, M. J., Newcomb, P. A., Remington, P. L., Marcus, P. M., & MacKenzie, W. R. (1996). Body mass and breast cancer. Relationship between method of detection and stage of disease. *Cancer, 77*(2), 301-307.

Reis, L. A. G., Miller, B. A., Hankey, B. F. Kosary, C. L., Harras, A., & Edwards, B. K. (1994). *Surveillance and Epidemiologic End Results: Cancer statistics review, 1973-1991.* U. S. National Institutes of Health Publication No. 94-2789. National Cancer Institute.

Richardson, J. L., Langholz, B., Bernstein, L., Burgiaga, C., Danley, K., & Ross, R. K. (1992). Stage and delay in breast cancer diagnosis by race, socioeconomic status, age, and year. *British Journal of Cancer, 65,* 922-926.

Romieu, I., Willett, W. C., Colditz, G. A., et al. (1989). Prospective study of oral contraceptive use and the risk of breast cancer in women. *Journal of the National Cancer Institute, 81,* 1313-1321.

Rowland, J., & Massey, M. (1996). Psychologic reactions to breast cancer diagnosis, treatment and survival. In J. Harris, M. Lippman, M. Morrow, & S. Hellman (Eds.), *Diseases of the breast.* Philadelphia: Lippincott Raven.

Sciartelli, C. H. (1995). Using a clinical pathway approach to document patient teaching for breast cancer surgical patients. *Oncology Nursing Forum, 22*(1), 131-137.

Seshadri, R., Horsfall, D. J., Firgaira, F., McCaul, K., Setlur, V., Chalmers, A. H., Yeo, R., Ingram, D., Dawkins, H., & Hahnel, R. (1994). The relative prognostic significance of total Cathepsin D and HER-2/neu oncogene amplification in breast cancer: The South Australian Breast Cancer Study Group. *International Journal of Cancer, 56,* 61-65.

Shiao, Y. H., Chen, V. W., Scheer, W. D., Wu, X. C., & Correa, P. (1995). Racial disparity in the association of p53 gene alterations with breast cancer survival. *Cancer Research, 55*(7), 1485-1490.

Simon, M. S., & Severson, R. K. (1996). Racial differences in survival of female breast cancer in Detroit metropolitan area. *Cancer 77*(2), 308-314.

Simpson, J., & Page, D. (1996). The role of pathology in premalignancy and as a guide for treatment and prognosis in breast cancer. *Seminars in Oncology, 23*(4), 428-435.

Smart, C. R., Hendrix, R. E., Rutledge, J. H., & Smith, R. (1995). Benefits of mammography screening in women ages 40-49. *Cancer,* 75, 1619-1626.

Souminen, T., Leino-Kilpi, H., & Laippala, P. (1995). Who provides support and how? *Cancer Nursing, 18*(4), 278-285.

Spiegel, D., Bloom, J., Kraemer, H., & Gottheil, E. (1989). Effect of psychosocial treatment on survival of patients with metastatic breast cancer. *The Lancet (October),* 888-891.

Stevens, P., Dibble, S., & Miaskowski, C. (1995). Prevalence, characteristics, and impact of postmastectomy pain syndrome: An investigation of women's experiences. *Pain, 61,* 61-68.

Tandon, A. K., Clark, G. M., Chamness, G. C., Chirgwin, J. M., & McGuire, W. L. (1990). Cathepson D and prognosis in breast cancer. *New England Journal of Medicine, 322,* 297-302.

Thor, A. D., Moore, D. H., Edgerton, S. M., Kawasaki, E. S., Reihaus, E., Lynch, H. T., Marcus, J. N., Schwartz, L., Chen, L. C., Mayall, B. H., et al. (1992). Accumulation of p53 tumor suppressor gene protein: An independent marker of prognosis in breast cancers. *Journal of the National Cancer Institute, 84,* 845-855.

Tross, S., Herndon, J., Korzun, A., Kornblith, A. B., Cella, D. F., Holland, J. F., Raich, P., Johnson, A., Kiang, D. T., Perloff, M., Norton, L., Wood, W., & Holland, J. C. (1996). Psychological symptoms and disease-free survival in women with Stage II breast cancer. *Journal of the National Cancer Institute, 88*(10), 661.

Veronesi, U., Cascinelli, N., Greco, M., Bufalino, R., Morabito, A., Galluzzo, D., Conti, R., De Lellis, R., Delle Donne, V., Piotti, P., et al. (1985). Prognosis of breast cancer patients after mastectomy and dissection of internal mammary nodes. *Annals of Surgery, 202*(6), 702-707.

Veronesi, U., DePalo, G., Costa, A., Fornelli, F., & Decensi, A. (1996). Chemoprevention of breast cancer with fenretinide. *Iarc Scientific Publications, 136,* 87-94.

Veronesi, U., & Salvadori, B. (1996). Breast conservation trials from the Milan National Cancer Institute. In J. Harris, M. Lippman, M. Morrow, & S. Hellman (Eds.), *Diseases of the breast.* Philadelphia: Lippincott Raven.

Veronesi, U., Salvadori, B., Luini, A., Banfi, A., Zucali, R., & Del Vecchio, M. (1996). Conservative approaches for the management of stage I/II carcinoma of the breast: Milan Cancer Institute trials. *World Journal of Surgery, 18,* 70-75.

Walker, B. L., Nail, L., Larsen, L., Magill, J., & Schwartz, A. (1996). Concerns, affect and cognitive disruption following completion of radiation treatment for localized breast cancer or prostate cancer. *Oncology Nursing Forum, 23*(8), 1181-1187.

Weber, B. (1996). Breast cancer susceptibility genes: Current challenges and future promises. *Annals of Internal Medicine, 124(12),* 1088-1090.

Weidner, N., Semple, J. P., Welch, W. R., & Folkman, J. (1991). Tumor angiogenesis and metastasis-correlation in invasive breast carcinoma. *New England Journal of Medicine, 324*(1), 1-8.

Weiss, H. A., Brinton, L. A., Brogan, D., Coates, R. J., Gammon, M. D., Malone, K. E., Schoenberg, J. B., & Swanson, C. A. (1996). Epidemiology of in situ and invasive breast cancer in women under 45. *British Journal of Cancer, 73*(10), 1298-1305.

Weiss, S. E., Tartter, P. I., Ahmed, S., Brower, S. T., Brusco, C., Bossolt, K., Amberson, J. B., & Bratton, J. (1995). Ethnic differences in risk and prognostic factors for breast cancer. *Cancer, 76*(2), 268-274.

White, E. (1987). Projected changes in breast cancer incidence due to the trend toward delayed childbearing. *American Journal of Public Health, 77,* 495-497.

Willett, W. C., Stampfer, M. J., Colditz, G. A., Rosner, B. A., Hennekens, C. H., & Speizer, F. E. (1987). Dietary fat and the risk of breast cancer. *New England Journal Medicine, 316,* 22-28.

Williams, W. L., Powers, M., & Wagman, L. D. (1996). Cancer of the male breast: A review. *Journal of the National Medical Association. 88*(7), 439-443.

Wooster, R., Neuhausen, S. L., Magion, J., Quirk, Y., Ford, D., Collins, N., Nguyen, K., Seal, S., Tran, T., Averill, D., et al. (1994). Localization of a breast cancer susceptibility gene, BCRA2, to chromosome 13q12-13. *Science, 265,* 2088-2090.

Yeatman, T. J. (1995). The natural history of locally advanced primary breast carcinoma and metastatic disease. *Surgical Oncology Clinics of North America, 4*(4), 569-589.

Young-McCaughan, S. (1996). Sexual functioning in women with breast cancer after treatment with adjuvant therapy. *Cancer Nursing, 19*(4), 308-319.

Zaloznik, A. L. (1995). Breast cancer stage at diagnosis: Caucasians versus Afro-Americans. *British Cancer Research and Treatment, 34,* 195-198.

Ziegler, J. (1996). New techniques promise improved breast imaging. *News: Journal of the National Cancer Institute, 88*(21), 1518-1521.

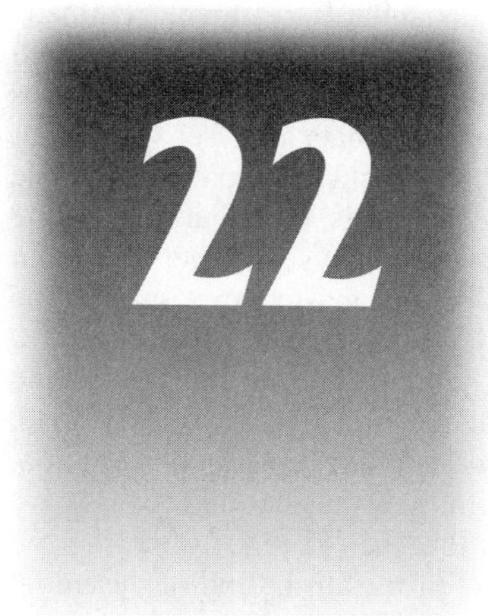

Metastatic Breast Cancer

Noreen Facione, RN, PhD
Deborah Hamolsky, RN, MS

EPIDEMIOLOGY

Although the overall breast cancer mortality rate has been declining since 1989, breast cancer remains the leading cause of cancer death for women between 15 and 55 years of age and claimed the lives of 43,500 women in the United States in 1998. This number represents 17% of all female cancer deaths (Landis et al, 1998). Approximately 10% of these women will be diagnosed with metastatic breast cancer. An additional 30% to 40% will develop metastatic breast cancer with recurrence of the disease after initial treatment (Engleking & Kalinowski, 1995).

The majority of breast cancers are adenocarcinomas (arising from glandular tissue) and are classified on the basis of their microscopic appearance as either ductal (arising from the lactiferous ducts) or lobular (arising from the breast lobes). Infiltrating ductal carcinoma is the most commonly diagnosed female breast cancer, representing 67% to 75% of the new cases. Less common types are infiltrating lobular carcinoma (5% to 10%), medullary carcinoma (5% to 7%), mucinous carcinoma (3%), tubular carcinoma (approximately 1% to 2%), and secretory carcinoma seen rarely in children and adolescents (Berg & Hutter, 1995).

Invasive lobular carcinoma is believed to be more extensively infiltrative than ductal carcinoma, often presenting with indistinct margins and having a higher incidence (20% to 30%) of being present bilaterally (Yeatman, 1995). Other nonadenocarcinomas of the breast include metaplastic cancer, squamous cell cancer, apocrine cancer, and adenoid cystic carcinoma. Sarcomas (i.e., phyllodes tumors) in the breast are very rare, and most are localized and treated by local surgical therapy. Less specific data and therefore less specific knowledge are available about the behavior of the less common histologic types of breast cancer, but routine treatment protocols for all types require consideration of both local and systemic therapies. Local therapies include surgery and radiation, whereas systemic therapies include chemotherapy and hormone therapy.

There are differences in breast cancer incidence by race, with white women having an approximately 20% higher overall incidence rate than women of other racial or ethnic heritages (ACS, 1996). However, in women 45 years of age, the rate of incidence is higher in African-American women than in white women. African-American women have higher rates of metastatic breast cancer at the time of diagnosis than do white American women. Table 21-5 displays differences by race in the stage of breast cancer at the time of diagnosis.

Metastatic breast cancer is not a disease of women exclusively. Aside from its lower incidence, breast cancer in men is remarkably similar to breast cancer in women with regard to the clinical presentation, pathology, and natural history. Stage and axillary node status are strong prognostic indicators in men as well. Less gender-specific research is available, but 5-year disease-free survival in men is reported to be as high as 47%, similar to that of women (Williams, Powers, & Wagman, 1996). Men are generally older at the time of diagnosis and proportionally are diagnosed with a more advanced stage of the disease. The tumors are located most often beneath the nipple and are more often responsive to hormonal therapy than breast cancers in women (Donegan & Redlich, 1996). The treatment approach for male breast cancer is modified radical mastectomy with systemic adjuvant therapy when lymph nodes are involved.

RISK FACTORS

Poverty has long been considered a risk factor for being diagnosed with a more advanced stage of breast cancer. This fact may account, to some degree, for the higher rates of metastatic disease, at the time of diagnosis, in African-American women and Latinas (Freeman & Wasfie, 1989; Richardson et al., 1992).

Reports from the National Cancer Institute's (NCI) Surveillance Epidemiology and End Results (SEER) data have documented larger tumor diameters and increased numbers of positive axillary nodes in African-American women compared with whites (Boring et al., 1994). Separating the effects of ethnic heritage (i.e., genetics) from social and behavioral variables (i.e., ideas, values, and the circumstances of women's lives) has been difficult. Some studies have demonstrated a possible difference in tumor biology by ethnicity or race (Ownby et al., 1985; Richardson et al., 1992), whereas others have shown no difference in the stage of disease at the time of diagnosis when access to care is not an issue (Zaloznik, 1995).

An early survey report of why cancer stage was significantly more advanced in the African-American population focused on a lack of knowledge of cancer-related symptoms (EVAXX, Inc., 1980). More recent studies have added to this understanding, delineating that the relative lack of access to breast cancer diagnosis and detection services and the inability for African Americans and other poor Americans to pay for cancer early detection and treatment services are factors that contribute to women's decisions to delay an evaluation of breast symptoms that later prove to be signals of breast cancer (Simon & Severson, 1996; Weiss et al., 1995).

Factors that have been suggested to have an impact on the timing of diagnosis in some ethnic populations, as well as in all women with advanced disease at the time of diagnosis, include conflicting role responsibilities that lead women to prioritize others' needs over their own health needs (Facione, 1993; Facione & Dodd, 1995; Facione, Dodd, Holzemer, & Meleis, 1997; Lierman, 1988), attributing the breast cancer symptom to a benign process (Facione & Dodd, 1995; Facione et al., 1997), and holding fatalistic beliefs about breast cancer and the likelihood of dying from the disease regardless of whether they seek treatment (Facione & Dodd, 1995; Facione et al., 1997; Lauver & Tak, 1995).

Older age itself has been associated with higher rates of metastatic breast cancer in some studies (Mandalblatt, Andrews, Kao, Wallace, & Kerner, 1995; Satariano, Belle, & Swanson, 1986), but not in others (Menon, Teh, & Chua, 1992; Rossi et al., 1990). Those who have observed a relationship between older age and a more advanced stage of disease at the time of diagnosis have suggested that this finding is due to decreased breast cancer screening participation, a decrease in strategic and economic access to breast cancer diagnosis services, and higher rates of co-morbid illness that distract providers from attention to breast cancer risk in the older age groups. Researchers have suggested that the existence of co-morbid conditions in older women may complicate the early diagnosis of breast cancer in some women (Mandalblatt et al., 1995; Satariano et al., 1986). The combination of older age, African-American ethnicity, and poverty was calculated to increase the risk of metastatic breast cancer at the time of diagnosis by a factor of 3.75 (Mandalblatt, Andrews, Kao, Wallace, & Kerner, 1991).

Several studies have shown that older women undergo fewer treatment modalities than younger women with breast cancer (Goodwin & Samet, 1994; Merchant, McCormick, Yahalom, & Borgen, 1996; Newschaffer, Penberthy, Desch, Retchin, & Whittemore, 1996). The claim that older women are advised about fewer treatment modalities because of co-morbidity issues was refuted by Newschaffer and colleagues (1996). The most important issue that needs to be addressed is whether women have poorer survival rates if they fail to receive the same level of aggressive treatment. This issue remains unresolved, as some researchers have reported that older women have poorer treatment outcomes as a result of changes in the standard treatment regimens (Goodwin & Samet, 1994), whereas others have observed no differences in 5- or 10-year survival rates when pathologic staging is controlled for in the data analyses (Merchant et al., 1996). Eighty percent of breast cancer patients relapse within 2 years of their initial diagnosis, but recurrence of the disease has been reported as late as 20 years after the initial diagnosis. Local recurrence in the mastectomy scar or the chest wall is usually a harbinger of metastatic disease.

Men are more at risk for being diagnosed with metastatic breast cancer at the time of the initial diagnosis. To date, there are no behavioral studies to explain this observation, but the mean age of men with breast cancer and the relative rarity of the disease suggest that the existence of co-morbid conditions and the likelihood of misattribution of the initial breast cancer symptoms may play a part in delaying the diagnosis.

Determining who is at risk for the development of metastatic breast cancer after the initial treatment of local disease is done through a consideration of a variety of prognostic indicators. Tumor histology helps to determine some of the risk for metastatic disease. Several histologic types of breast cancer pose a smaller risk for invasive cancer, including: pure mucinous, pure tubular, pure medullary, and pure capillary carcinomas. However, these tumor types account for less than 6% of invasive carcinomas and are usually diagnosed while they are still localized. The 5-year relative survival rate for patients with these pure histologic types of breast cancer is 95% (Berg & Hutter, 1995). Five-year survival rates for infiltrating tumors with less well-differentiated histology are overall (83%), ductal carcinoma (79%), lobular carcinoma (84%), and medullary carcinoma (82%) (Berg & Hutter, 1995).

Increased numbers of microvessels (veins and arteries) in the invasive carcinomas originally were reported to be a predictor of nodal disease and distant metastases (Weidener, Semple, Welsh, & Folkman, 1991); however, other investigators have failed to replicate this finding. In one blinded study of 220 cases of invasive carcinoma, there was considerable variation in the amount of microvessel counts in different parts of the same tumor. At this time, there is no strong evidence that an increase in microvessel counts is associated with increased risk of metastases or a decreased survival.

Tumor suppressor genes, particularly p53, are being studied aggressively for their potential to predict tumor metastasis. Mutations in this gene have been demonstrated in the earliest phase of breast neoplasia and shown to be maintained through the tumor's progression to an infiltrating carcinoma (Davidoff, Kerns, Inglehart, & Marks, 1991). Two potential markers of metastases in breast cancer are nm23 and Cathepsin-D (CD). In animal models and in one in vitro human study, the expression of nm23-H1 has been observed in tumors less likely to metastasize (Leone et al., 1991). CD is an estrogen-dependent, lysosomal protease that is synthesized by normal tissues and overexpressed and secreted by some breast cancers. As a result, CD has been suspected to be a protease that facilitates the metastatic process. This hypothesis is supported by reports of increased levels of CD in patients with nodal metastases (Donegan, 1997).

CHEMOPREVENTION

Adjuvant systemic therapy can be considered chemoprevention for metastatic disease because it is a treatment for micrometastases that may not be apparent at the time of the initial breast cancer diagnosis. Adjuvant chemotherapy is a chemotherapy program, most often a multidrug regimen, given to treat presumed micrometastasis. Adjuvant chemotherapy is most useful for patients who meet two clinical criteria: They have micrometastasis at the time of diagnosis or at surgery or their tumor cells are not resistant to chemotherapy. However, clinical trials measure the benefits to all women who are treated with a particular adjuvant chemotherapy regimen. Therefore there is no way to differentiate between women who have micrometastasis and those who are cured by local therapy or those who had drug-resistant tumors (Hortobagyi & Buzdar, 1995).

Patients at higher risk for recurrence and death obtain the greatest benefit from adjuvant chemotherapy. Establishing the degree of risk by evaluating tumor stage and grade, estrogen and progesterone receptor status, age, premenopausal or postmenopausal status, presence or absence of lymph nodes, and the number of positive lymph nodes is an essential component in the development of treatment recommendations. Patients need to know: "What is the percentage of risk to me of recurrence and death with and without adjuvant chemotherapy?" These discussions need to take place in the context of data that represent large groups of patients with limited ability to predict for a single individual. It is useful to express survival benefit in terms of prolongation of life so that the physician and the patient can subtract the costs (e.g., side effects of therapy, financial cost, impact on quality of life) from the expected projected gain in survival (Henderson, 1996). Table 21-8 lists randomized clinical trials of adjuvant chemotherapy that were begun before 1985 for early stage breast cancer. Table 21-9 explains the mechanism by which common endocrine therapies work in the management of breast cancer.

Tamoxifen (Hormone Therapy) and Ovarian Ablation

Clinical trials that evaluated the effects of adjuvant chemotherapy began in the 1970s. Meta-analyses of many trials generally conclude that there is improvement in disease-free survival and overall survival from the use of adjuvant chemotherapy. The Early Breast Cancer Trialists' Collaborative Groups (EBCTCG) concluded that there was an overall increase of 20% in survival rates in treated compared with untreated patients (1992). The questions, then, surrounding adjuvant chemotherapy include these: Who should be treated? Which drugs and drug combinations and dosages are best for which groups of patients? When and for how long should patients be treated? What is the optimal sequencing of drugs when chemotherapy is used in conjunction with radiation therapy?

The 1990 meta-analysis concluded that adjuvant chemotherapy was more efficacious in women younger than 50 years of age and that tamoxifen was more effective in women 50 years of age or older (EBCTCG, 1992). In these reports of the meta-analyses of the adjuvant chemotherapy clinical trials, most trials were of single-agent antineoplastics or combination drug protocols (e.g., cytoxan, methotrexate, 5-fluorouracil, also known by the drug combination acronym CMF). Less data were available from these early meta-analyses on anthracycline-based protocols (e.g., adriamycin). Clinical trials have demonstrated that multiple drug therapy results in improved outcomes over monodrug therapy (EBCTCG, 1988, 1992).

Six cycles of CMF were more than or equally beneficial compared with other protocols. Therefore this regimen is considered the "gold standard" adjuvant chemotherapy protocol against which other protocols are compared in clinical trials. Four cycles of adriamycin and cytoxan (AC) demonstrated similar efficacy with a trend towards recommending adriamycin in patients with a higher risk of recurrence. Studies that addressed the duration of therapy and its impact on relapse and survival have shortened the average time frame for the administration of adjuvant chemotherapy from 1 to 2 years to 4 to 6 months (Hortobagyi et al., 1995). However, when the International Study Group studied the use of CMF for three cycles, there was a 53% survival rate compared with the six-cycle program outcome of 58% (Hortobagyi, 1996). Commonly used adjuvant chemotherapy regimens are listed in Table 21-10.

PATHOPHYSIOLOGY

The threat to survival from breast cancer is the ability of invasive breast cancers to metastasize and carry the disease throughout a woman's body. Measures of apoptosis (i.e., the ratio of the rate of cell proliferation to the rate of genetically determined cell death) and angiogenesis (i.e., the formation of new blood vessels that can support cell proliferation) determine tumor doubling time. The time in which a tumor doubles in size is an important prognostic indicator for the development of metastatic breast cancer.

Once the tumor has metastasized, the implications for survival are highly influenced by the tumor's doubling time. Aggressive tumors have doubling times of less than 60 days, whereas others double in as long as 300 days and are considered very indolent. Tumor doubling time can be estimated roughly by the S-phase fraction, which is derived from deoxyribonucleic acid (DNA) flow cytometry. In this test procedure, a small amount of the tumor is prepared with staining of the cell nuclei. The cells are then expressed in a fine spray, and the nuclei are visualized with a laser beam. Computer scans of the cells record the number of cells that are dividing, and from this count one can estimate the tumor's doubling time. It should be noted that after reviewing what is currently known about the relationship between S-phase and ploidy, the American Society of Clinical Oncology (ASCO) does not recommend at this time using these measures to estimate women's survival potential (ASCO, 1996).

ROUTES OF METASTASES

Breast cancers spread locally into the tissue of the mammary ducts and skin, regionally to the lymphatics, and systemically through the bloodstream. Although metastases can occur in any organ, the most common sites of metastases are lymph nodes (76%), bone (67% to 71%), lung (>69%), liver (>65%), pleura (51%), adrenals (49%), and the brain and central nervous system (25%). Involvement of the skin (30%), as in inflammatory breast cancer, is a precursor to major organ involvement (Cook & Troutner, 1996). Nearly 50% of women undergoing surgery for infiltrating carcinoma of the breast have axillary node involvement (Engleking, 1989) (Table 22-1).

ASSESSMENT

Patients With Metastatic Breast Cancer at the Time of Initial Diagnosis

Most metastatic breast cancer is diagnosed after symptoms that precede a confirmatory diagnosis of metastatic breast cancer. The signs and symptoms depend on whether there are distant or only regional metastases at the time of diagnosis. The symptoms and physical findings associated with the major sites of metastatic breast cancer are listed in Table 22-1. Clinical evaluation of the patient involves a detailed history that includes all of the relevant history about physical symptoms, a full psychosocial history, a complete physical examination, and a variety of diagnostic tests (Table 22-2).

The lymphatic system of the breast, composed of the axillary node chain, is where breast cancer cells are believed to metastasize immediately. Approximately 10% of breast cancers are identified primarily through observation and palpation during a clinical breast examination. Many women are diagnosed with metastatic disease (Farwell, Foster, & Costanza, 1993).

A diagnostic workup to make or rule out a diagnosis of metastatic breast cancer occurs after the diagnosis of an invasive breast cancer. Once the tissue diagnosis of an invasive breast cancer has been confirmed, general screening procedures for metastatic disease include a chest radiograph, liver function tests, and, if indicated, a bone scan. Any additional symptoms should trigger a symptom-specific workup (e.g., severe headaches would warrant a magnetic resonance imaging [MRI] scan of the brain). The suspicion of a local or regional recurrence (e.g., chest wall nodule, palpable axillary lymph node) should be evaluated

TABLE 22-1 Major Sites of Breast Cancer Metastasis/Recurrence

Sites	Percentage	Symptoms
CNS	25%	Headache
		Unilateral sensory loss
		Focal muscular weakness
		Hemiparesis
		Incoordination (ataxia)
		Visual defects
		Speech disorders (aphasia)
		Impaired cognition (memory loss and concentration)
		Behavioral/mental changes
		Loss of sphincter control
		Papilledema
		Persistent nausea/vomiting
		Paresthesia in one or more extremities
		Progressive back pain (localized and radicular)
Liver	65%	Abdominal distention
		RLQ abdominal pain ± radiation to scapular region
		Nausea/vomiting, anorexia, weight loss
		Weakness/fatigue
		Hepatomegaly
		Jaundice
		Peripheral edema
		Elevated LFTs: alkaline phosphatase, total bilirubin
Lung	69%	Chest pain (pleuritic if inflammatory process present)
		Dyspnea on exertion, shortness of breath, tachypnea
		Nonproductive cough (unless pneumonia is present, then productive)
		With pleural effusion, adventitious breath sounds, dullness to percussion, and restricted chest wall expansion on affected side
Skeletal	67%	Localized pain of gradually increasing intensity, tendency to worsen at night and with positional change (percussion tenderness at involved sites)
		Anemia secondary to neoplastic marrow involvement

CNS, central nervous system; *RLQ,* right lower quadrant; *LFTs,* liver function tests

Cook, G.A., & Troutner, K. (1996). *Taxotere: An important advance in the treatment of metastatic breast cancer.* Pittsburgh: Oncology Nursing Society: Rhone-Poulenc Rorer.

by biopsy. A positive supraclavicular node is diagnostic of metastatic disease.

Biopsy Procedures to Diagnose Breast Cancer

The most common biopsy procedures to diagnose breast cancer are fine needle aspiration biopsy (FNAB), stereotactic core biopsy, and needle localization biopsy. These procedures are described in detail in Chapter 21.

Patients Diagnosed With Metastatic Cancer at a Breast Cancer Recurrence

A wide variety of diagnostic tests are done to screen for metastatic breast cancer. Two distinct philosophies guide the timing of these diagnostic screening decisions. One approach recommends screening for abnormalities. The other approach recommends a workup for a presenting problem when a patient becomes symptomatic. Because there is no definitive data to substantiate the practice of checking every potential recurrence site periodically, the current trend is to

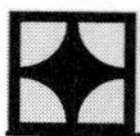

TABLE 22-2 Assessment of the Patient for Metastatic Breast Cancer

	Assessment Parameters	Typical Abnormal Findings
History	A. Personal and social history	A. Personal and social risk factors.
	1. Age	1. Increased incidence in older women
	2. Family history of breast cancer	2. Increased incidence in women with a positive family history
	3. Personal history of breast cancer	3. Increased incidence in women with a personal history of breast cancer
	4. History of benign breast disease	4. Increased incidence in women with a history of benign breast disease
	5. Age at birth of first child	5. Increased incidence in women who have their first child at an older age
	6. Age at menopause	6. Increased incidence in women who experience menopause at an older age
	B. Breast symptoms	
	1. Breast mass	1. Usually a painless mass or lump in the breast. Tumor may be >5 cm with mobile axillary nodes or tumor may be of any size with fixed axillary or clinically enlarged mammary nodes
	2. Other presentations	2. Tumor may exhibit direct extension to the chest wall and/or skin
	C. Symptoms associated with skeletal metastases	
	1. Pain	1. Localized pain of gradually increasing intensity that worsens at night and with positional changes
	2. Weakness	2. Weakness may result from anemia that occurs with bone marrow involvement
	D. Symptoms associated with liver metastases	
	1. Pain	1. Typically right lower quadrant pain with or without radiation to the scapular region
	2. Nausea and vomiting	
	3. Anorexia	
	4. Fatigue	
	E. Symptoms associated with central nervous system metastases	
	1. Pain	1. Headache or progressive back pain that is localized or radicular in nature
	2. Persistent nausea and vomiting	2. May be a sign of increased intracranial pressure.
	3. Paresthesias, numbness, tingling	3. May be indicative of nerve injury
	F. Symptoms associated with pulmonary metastases	
	1. Chest pain	1. Pleuritic chest pain will occur if an inflammatory process is present
	2. Pulmonary symptoms	2. Patient may exhibit dyspnea on exertion, shortness of breath, tachypnea, productive or nonproductive cough

Continued

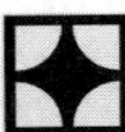

TABLE 22-2 Assessment of the Patient for Metastatic Breast Cancer—cont'd

	Assessment Parameters	Typical Abnormal Findings
Physical Examination	A. Clinical breast examination	A. A painless mass or lump in the breast requires a mammogram. Nipple discharge may or may not be present. The axilla should be palpated for masses or lumps.
	B. Evaluation for skeletal metastases	
	1. Bone scan	1. Bone scan may show evidence of single or multiple metastases sites
	2. Complete blood cell count	2. Evaluate for anemia that may be due to bone marrow involvement
	C. Evaluation for liver metastases	
	1. Abdominal examination	1. Abdominal distention, hepatomegaly, jaundice
	2. Liver function tests	2. Elevated liver function tests
	D. Evaluation for central nervous system metastases	
	1. Complete neurologic examination	1. Symptoms will depend on the site of the metastatic disease within the central nervous system and can include: unilateral sensory loss, focal muscle weakness, ataxia, visual defects, aphasia, memory loss, mental status changes, behavior changes
	E. Evaluation for pulmonary metastases	
	1. Complete respiratory examination	1. With a pleura effusion, there will be adventitious breath sounds, dullness to percussion and restricted chest wall expansion on the affected side
Diagnostic Tests	A. Mammography	A. The mammographic abnormality having the highest rate of malignancy is a mass density on radiograph with associated calcifications. An associated calcification increases the rate of positivity for malignancy from 13% with density alone to 29% for density containing microcalcifications. The calcification pattern most characteristic of malignancy is one in which calcifications are typically linear, small (<1 mm) in diameter, nonuniform in size, and clustered.
	B. Ultrasound	B. Ultrasound can be used to obtain a cross-sectional image of the breast. Ultrasonography is very accurate in the diagnosis of breast cysts (>95%).
	C. Computed tomography (CT) scan	C. CT may be used as a supplement to mammography in evaluating dense breast tissue.
	D. Fine needle aspiration biopsy (FNAB)	D. Limited to determining whether or not a palpable breast lump is cancer.
	E. Stereotactic core biopsy	E. Used to establish a diagnosis of breast cancer.
	F. Needle localization biopsy	F. Used to establish a diagnosis of breast cancer.
	G. Hormone receptor assays of tissue specimen	G. Estrogen, >3 fmol/mg protein; progesterone, >3 fmol/mg protein.
	H. Liver function tests	H. May be elevated in patients with liver metastases.
	I. Bone scan	I. Bone scans are performed routinely in patients suspected of having advanced disease.
	J. CT scans of chest and abdomen	J. CT scans of the chest and abdomen are ordered in patients with early stage tumors only when the patient has elevated liver function tests.

do fewer tests. As with any shift in practice, there is wide variation and controversy in this area of clinical practice. As a result, patients sharing treatment stories in support groups will wonder why they may have received more or fewer diagnostic tests than a woman with a seemingly similar story.

The diagnostic workup is tailored to the presenting symptoms. For example, abdominal pain, ascites, or jaundice would warrant a clinical examination and liver function tests. If these tests are abnormal, an abdominal computed tomography (CT) scan should be performed. The new onset of bone pain would trigger a bone scan and plain radiographic films targeted at a suspicious or indeterminate abnormality. Once a diagnosis of metastatic disease is made, effective clinical strategies, including symptom management (e.g., management of bone pain with radiation therapy and analgesics), local therapy (e.g., surgery to debulk the tumor or radiation therapy for bone metastases in a weight-bearing bone at risk for fracture), and then systemic therapy (chemotherapy or hormonal therapy), would be initiated. Systemic therapy, with hormonal interventions and/or chemotherapy, offers the best possibility for a clinical response. The anticipated and hoped for clinical response includes the control of symptoms and the extension of life.

STAGING

Staging is a method of describing the extent of a tumor at diagnosis and is used as a prognostic indicator and to determine optimal treatment strategies. Staging is determined by considering the size of the tumor, the presence and number of positive lymph nodes, margins of the tumor resection, tumor histology (structure of the breast cancer cell), hormone receptor status of the tumor, tumor grade, and other individually relevant prognostic factors. A general staging system used to standardize a portion of this determination is the American Joint Committee on Cancer's (AJCC, 1988) TNM classification system. The TNM system considers the primary tumor (T), lymph node involvement (N), and the presence of metastatic spread (M). Breast cancers that present with regional metastases to lymph nodes are staged as N_{1-3}, and those tumors that have advanced to more distant metastatic disease are all staged as M_1.

Staging guides treatment and provides uniform tracking information for research. Clinical staging includes information from the physical examination, as well as laboratory and radiographic tests. A postsurgical pathologic staging describes the extent of the primary tumor, lymph node involvement, and histopathologic information using data from the biopsy or surgical procedures and the examination of excised tissues. Table 21-4 displays the current TNM four-stage categorization used to stage breast cancers at the time of diagnosis.

MEDICAL MANAGEMENT

Surgical Management at the Time of Diagnosis

Once the diagnosis of metastatic breast cancer is made, treatment options for local and systemic control of the disease must be addressed immediately. Metastatic disease is the classic exception to the rule that surgery is the first treatment modality for breast cancer. With metastatic breast cancer, hormonal therapy or chemotherapy usually is given first. Giving these therapies first does not preclude subsequent surgery for local control. In patients who achieve a good response to a course of presurgical chemotherapy, there are no definitive outcome data that guide decision-making with respect to a recommendation for breast conservation surgery and the advisability of radiation therapy for these women. The standard practice has been to recommend mastectomy after chemotherapy for large tumors (i.e., >5 cm). (Bonadonna, Valgussa, Zucali, & Salvadori, 1995; Harris & Swain, 1996; Hortobagyi et al., 1995). Table 21-11 provides the NCI Physician Data Query State of the Art Treatment Recommendations for Stage III and IV (metastatic) breast cancer.

The key components that affect a woman's decisions regarding surgical treatment options are widely variable, personal, and influenced by the full diversity of cultural, ethnic, religious, regional, and generational factors. Principal influences include how a woman (and perception of how significant other[s]) feels about her breast and her body; her degree of worry about local recurrence; and both her and family and friends' previous encounters with illness, medicine, and breast cancer. There is a wide spectrum of responses to the need to make choices about breast cancer surgery. These range from women feeling that they would lose their sense of self and could not tolerate losing a breast to women feeling that their breast is a threat to their life and therefore they want "it" removed. The difficulties associated with decision making about treatment options are compounded by the lack of medical knowledge, conflicting opinions, and the emotional crisis precipitated by the cancer diagnosis.

Local treatment of metastatic breast cancer can control the disease and prevent pain, infection, and profound body image changes. A modified radical mastectomy (MRM) includes removal of the breast, dissection of the axilla, and preservation of the pectoral muscles. An MRM is sufficient for local control unless the tumor is close to or invading the underlying muscle. A lumpectomy (partial mastectomy) is removal of the tumor resected widely enough to obtain clear margins. A quadrantectomy is the removal of a quadrant of the breast removing more ductal tissue in line with the nipple than is removed in a lumpectomy. A separate incision is also made to do an ipsilateral axillary lymph node dissection. For metastatic disease, a decision must be made regarding whether to remove the lymph nodes. This decision is made by considering the level of aggressiveness of the tumor in an attempt to better control procedure-related morbidity. In general, all lymph nodes are dissected that appear to be involved with disease at the time of the surgical procedure (Mackarem, Barbarisi, & Hughes, 1992). Table 21-6 lists the common sequellae of mastectomy or axillary node dissection.

Reconstructive Surgery

Women face numerous choices regarding reconstructive surgery, ranging from whether to do the procedure to the timing and type of procedure. Most physicians would be reluctant to recommend reconstruction in women with metastatic disease. However, for some patients, it may be critically important to consider this option. The two major types of breast reconstructive surgery are an implant and a flap procedure that uses autologous muscle from a donor site that is reshaped into a breast mound. The timing of a consultation with a plastic surgeon may vary depending on variations in the decision-making process. However, with any patient who is considering the procedure, it is a key element of pretreatment planning.

Decision Making Regarding Treatment

Depending on the presenting symptoms, the extent and site(s) of disease, previous treatment and response, history, age, health status, and estrogen and progesterone status, various treatment options are outlined for the patient. As with a new diagnosis of local or regional disease, the resources for emotional support and decision-making support must be readily available to a patient at this juncture in her treatment. The factors that differentiate treatment decision making in the context of metastatic disease include the following: (1) the patient may be sicker and not as physically able to think clearly (e.g., cognitive impairment associated with brain metastasis or liver failure); (2) if experimental therapies are being considered, available financial resources may be a barrier to treatment; (3) if the metastatic disease presents emergently, there may not be the luxury of time for thought, research, and seeking second opinions; and (4) quality of life issues are generally more intense. It is considerably more difficult for a patient to evaluate the potential benefits of therapy against the toxicities and risks of therapy in the context of markedly worsened survival outcomes associated with metastatic disease. However, the imminent threat for some women embolden them to take major treatment risks and participate in experimental therapies. Many women may be saying, "What have I got to lose?"

The treatment profile for metastatic disease is influenced by measures of tumor biology and prior therapy. Women with estrogen and progesterone receptive tumors have the range of hormonal therapies available to them for systemic therapy. If there is a local or regional recurrence, it may be useful to repeat tests of this prognostic indicator, as this index of hormonal responsiveness does not always remain constant. Women who have had adjuvant chemotherapy respond less well to systemic chemotherapy than do women who have not been treated previously. However, two relatively new agents, paclitaxel (Taxol) and vinorelbine tartrate (Navelbine), are being evaluated in the treatment of metastatic breast cancer. In addition, a number of new agents in phase I and II clinical trials have broadened the choices for patients who have been treated previously. If autologous bone marrow transplant (BMT) was not done in the setting of high-dose adjuvant therapy, it might be considered in the range of experimental treatment options.

Clinical trials are attempting to discover more effective therapies for patients for whom standard therapies have failed, or for whom they are no longer effective. Phase I trials test new therapies on a small number of patients to determine the dose required to produce a biologic effect and to determine the major toxicities associated with the drug. Phase II trials test new therapies on a small number of patients with specific tumor types to test the responsiveness of these tumors to the drug and to continue to study toxicities and appropriate dose ranges. Phase III trials compare the new therapy with standard therapy in large, multisite studies. A new therapy may become a standard therapy with evidence of improved responsiveness or decreased toxicity (Dollinger, Rosenbaum, & Cable, 1992).

Hormonal Therapy

Hormonal therapy has long played a role in the management of breast cancer. The breast is stimulated by multiple endocrine pathways, offering many opportunities to block hormonal stimulation of breast cancer. Fig. 22-1 depicts these processes. As early as the late 1800s, bilateral oophorectomy was described as a treatment option for women with breast cancer. Adrenalectomy and hypophysectomy were utilized in the 1950s before medical ablation of the ovaries became possible. The technologic advances enabling the development of estrogen and progesterone receptor assays in the 1970s were critical elements in helping to match hormonal manipulations to women most likely to benefit from them. Approximately two thirds of postmenopausal women have tumors that are estrogen and/or progesterone receptor positive, which signals tumor growth in response to hormonal stimulation. The use of surgical or medical inhibition of estrogen production can be an effective strategy to inhibit tumor growth in hormonally responsive breast cancer. There are two approaches to blocking estrogen stimulation through the use of drugs: the use of antiestrogens that compete with estrogens on the surface of tumor cells (e.g., tamoxifen) or the use of drugs that inhibit the production of estrogen by inhibiting the enzyme aromatase required to synthesize estrogen (e.g., aminogluthethamide or anastrazole).

Approximately one third of all patients with metastatic disease respond to endocrine therapies (Harris, Lippman, Veronesi, & Willett, 1992). The mechanisms for blocking hormonal stimulation and therefore decreasing the growth of breast cancer include surgery and the administration of medications that are effective at a number of sites involved in the pathways for hormonal stimulation. In the premenopausal woman, the majority of estrogen is produced by the ovary. In the postmenopausal woman, estrogen production increases in the peripheral tissues and blocking estrogenic effects is better done systemically than by surgery (Brodie & Njar, 1996).

Tamoxifen, a complex medication with both estrogen agonist and antagonist features, is most effective in women with estrogen-responsive tumors. The EBCTCG meta-analysis (1992) reviewed clinical trials on the use of tamoxifen with 30,081 women. Tamoxifen reduced the annual odds of recurrence or death by 25% and the mortality rate by 17%. Because tamoxifen blocks the effects of estrogen, initially there was concern that its use would increase the incidence of cardiovascular disease and osteoporosis in women taking the medication. However, it is believed that the estrogen agonist features of tamoxifen result in an offsetting protective benefit with respect to osteoporosis.

In addition to its estrogen receptor blockade, tamoxifen has additional effects, including increasing natural killer cells, increasing sex hormone-binding globulin, increasing tumor suppressive growth factors, and decreasing tumor-stimulating growth factors (Vogel, 1996). The short-term side effects associated with tamoxifen include hot flashes, nausea, vaginal dryness, mood changes, and changes in libido. Two potential long-term complications associated

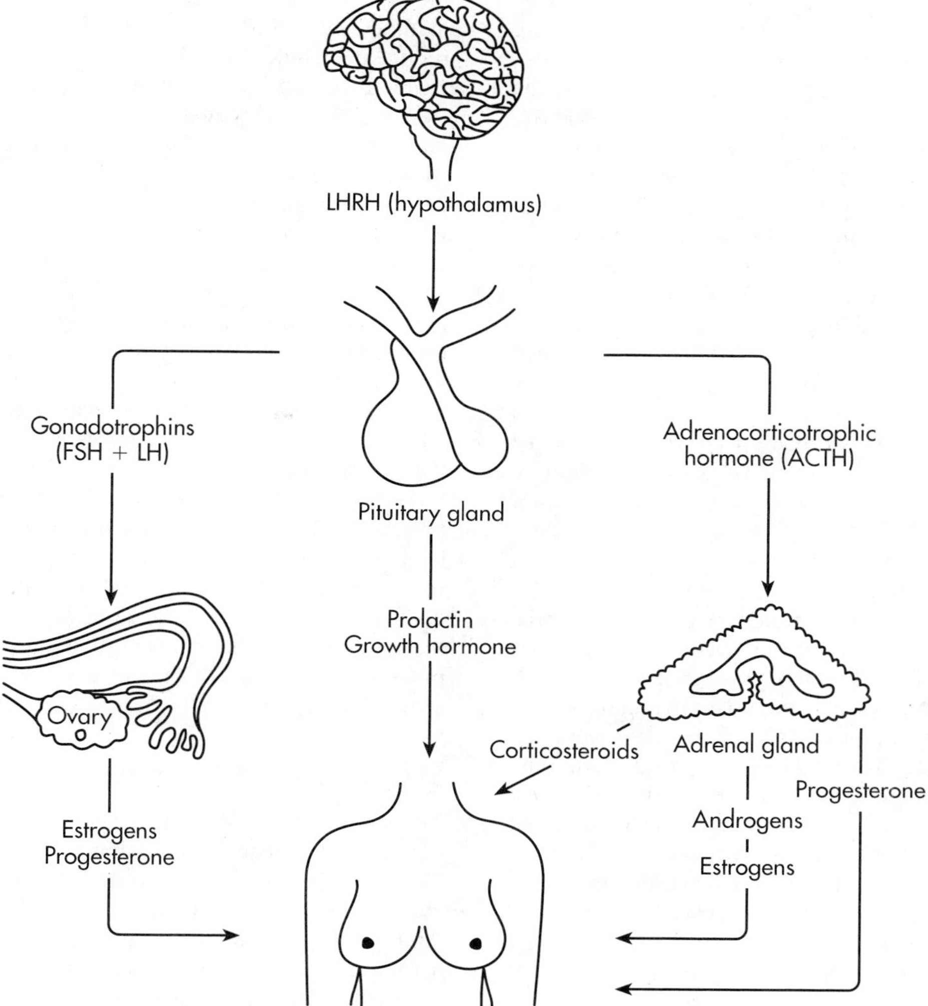

Fig. 22-1 Glands and hormones affecting the breast.

with tamoxifen use include an increase in endometrial cancer and liver toxicity. These rare, but significant complications, have shaped the recommendations for closer gynecologic follow-up.

Guidelines for the use of ultrasound to detect endometrial thickening and endometrial biopsies to assess the presence of endometrial cancer are not yet universally agreed upon or universally practiced. However, any woman on tamoxifen who experiences spotting or vaginal bleeding should be evaluated to rule out endometrial cancer. Data from six randomized tamoxifen trials indicate that of 3097 women taking tamoxifen, 3 in 1000 will develop uterine cancer (EBCTCG, 1992).

Two cases of hepatocellular cancer were reported in the 8034 women taking tamoxifen in seven clinical trials. Liver damage is indicated by increases in bilirubin and aminotransferase levels. The incidence of this complication is very rare. However, if symptoms of liver dysfunction occur in a woman taking tamoxifen, the drug should be considered as a causative factor along with a workup for metastatic disease to the liver.

Fueled by concerns about the carcinogenic effects of tamoxifen, other antiestrogens are being investigated. Toremifene, at a dose of 60 mg/day, appears to have less estrogenic effects and does not induce liver carcinogenesis in laboratory rats. Droloxifene has a shorter elimination time from the body and is less carcinogenic in animal models. It is postulated that droloxifene might be used in conjunction with chemotherapy because, with its shorter elimination time, it might interact less with the antineoplastic agents. Idoxifene is an antiestrogen currently in phase I trial, and its mechanism of action is not well understood (Goldhirsch & Gelber, 1996). ICI 182780 is a compound without estrogenic effects. In phase II trials, it has been shown to produce a good response in a small number of patients.

Because of its efficacy and the large body of evidence supporting its effectiveness, tamoxifen is used as the first-line hormonal therapy for metastatic disease in postmenopausal women. For premenopausal women, some would argue in favor of oophorectomy and the use of luteinizing hormone-releasing hormone (LH-RH) analogs (e.g., buserelin, luprelide, goserelin, triptorelin) to medically ablate the ovaries.

The second-line therapies are used when the response to a first-line therapy has ended; that is, when there is a recurrence or progression of disease. Second-line therapies include the use of the progestins and the aromatase inhibitors. The progestins (e.g., medroxyprogesterone acetate or megestrol acetate) generally are well tolerated. Their side effect profile includes weight gain and dyspnea. The aromatase inhibitors block the actions of the enzyme aromatase. Aromatase is an enzyme complex that propels the conversion of the adrenal androgen androstenedione and testosterone to estrone. This process is responsible for the production of circulating estrogens in postmenopausal or castrated women. Aromatase can be found in breast tumor epithelial cells and in the surrounding tissue (Harvey, 1996).

Original aromatase inhibitor drugs had severe side effect profiles including skin rash sometimes associated with fever, lethargy, orthostatic hypotension, ataxia, nausea, anorexia, and less commonly experienced but serious complications such as hypothyroidism, thrombocytopenia, agranulocytosis, pancytopenia, and systemic lupus erythematosus. The advantages of the newer aromatase inhibitors are specificity, potency, and decreased toxicity. There is no need to administer these drugs with corticosteroids. In addition they are nonestrogenic and noncarcinogenic and show no evidence of weight gain (Harvey, 1996). Anastrozole (Arimidex), administered once a day in a dose of 1 mg, has been shown in clinical trials to have similar efficacy to megestrol acetate and a less toxic side effect profile than the progestins. It is the first aromatase inhibitor to be approved for use in the United States for the treatment of advanced breast cancer in postmenopausal women who have not responded to tamoxifen.

Formestane, given intramuscularly in doses of 250 to 500 mg every 2 weeks, is commercially available, but not in the United States. Other aromatase inhibitors (e.g., exemestane, rogletimide, fadrozole, letrozole and vorozole) are in various stages of clinical trials. As a result, over the next decade, there will likely be a series of new hormonal interventions with decreased toxicity and increased specificity of action available for the treatment of metastatic breast cancer (Brodie & Njar, 1996; Buzdar, Plourde, & Hortobagyi, 1996; Goldhirsch & Gelber, 1996; Harvey, 1996; Smith & Henderson, 1996; Vogel, 1996).

Chemotherapy for Metastatic Disease

Hormonal therapy is often the preliminary therapy for patients with metastatic disease, particularly if the patient has positive estrogen and progesterone receptor status. Systemic chemotherapy is recommended for patients with receptor-negative breast cancer or for patients when hormonal therapy is no longer, or never was, effective (Winer, 1996).

Systemic chemotherapy for metastatic disease includes first-line chemotherapy regimens. First-line therapies include the following combinations: cyclophosphamide, methotrexate, CMF or doxorubicin, cyclophosphamide, and at times fluorouracil (AC +/− F). Less commonly used regimens include cyclophosphamide, novantrone, and fluorouracil (CNF); mitoxantrone, methotrexate, mitomycin (MMM); novantrone and 5-fluorouracil (NFL); and calcium leucovorin. Paclitaxel (Taxol) is now used for the treatment of metastatic breast cancer, particularly if there is a history of drug resistance or tumor progression while the patient is on active treatment with any of the standard first-line therapies.

Sometimes systemic therapies (e.g., chemotherapy and hormonal therapy) are used in conjunction with local and regional therapeutic modalities. There are controversies and unanswered research questions about the treatment of metastatic breast cancer: Which regimens? At what doses? Over what time interval? With what treatment toxicities? What is the correct sequencing with local regional therapy? How does one compute the percentage of benefit for a specific patient? Making decisions about the treatment options may be extremely difficult for the patient. She may receive conflicting treatment recommendations. In addition, she may qualify for one or more clinical trials and will need to factor those options into her decision-making process. Table 22-3 provides a summary of the current clinical trials for metastatic disease.

Side Effects of Chemotherapy

The side effects that breast cancer patients experience are not specific to breast cancer, but to the drugs they receive. The common breast cancer chemotherapy regimens (CMF; cyclophosphamide, adriamycin, and 5-fluororacil [CAF]; AC) result in side effect profiles that include the following: nausea and vomiting (generally well controlled with antiemetics), alopecia, weight gain, fatigue, premature menopause (particularly in women over 40 years of age) with its attendant long-term increased risk of osteoporosis and cardiovascular disease, second malignancies (leukemias are rare except with melphalan, but increase with radiation to the chest wall and lymph nodes), cardiac toxicity with anthracycline containing regimens, and febrile neutropenia (uncommon with standard doses, more common with high-dose regimens).

Weight gain is a problem for women with breast cancer while they are on chemotherapy and hormonal therapy. This side effect has been studied more in women who are receiving adjuvant chemotherapy (Barnicle, 1996; Dow, 1996). However, there are anecdotal reports of weight gain during treatment for metastatic disease. The cause of the weight gain is not clear. Possible factors that may be associated with weight gain include the impact of hormonal changes, depression, increased food intake, and decreased activity level. Regular exercise, decreased fat intake, and a range of stress management and emotional support strategies are recommended. Women report that weight gain compounds with the other changes in body image, such as alopecia or loss of or change in the breast from surgery and radiation therapy. Weight loss resulting from wasting is generally a late sign in breast cancer and signals advanced disease.

Table 22-3 Current Clinical Trials for Metastatic Breast Cancer

The following cytotoxic agents have been shown to have activity in metastatic breast cancer and are in clinical trials designed to test their efficacy and toxicity:

Drug Name	Dose	Trial Results
Ammonified	300 mg/m^2 qd × 5d	Modest response rate; tolerable side effects
Class: **New Anthracyclines**		
Theprubicin		No demonstrated increased efficacy over doxorubicin
Liposomal Doxorubicin	60-90 mg/m^2 q3w	Permits increased doxorubicin dosage without additional cardiotoxicity
Class: **Anthropyrazoles—Being Developed to Decrease Cardiotoxicity**		
Losoxantrone	55 mg/m^2 (maximum)	Active agent; less cardiotoxicity
Teloxantrone		Similar toxicity to Losantrone
Piroxantrone		No reports yet in breast cancer
Class: **Campothecin Analogs—Semisynthetic and Synthetic Analogs of Plant Alkaloid Found to Be Too Toxic for Use as Chemotherapeutic Drug in Its Natural Form**		
Topotecan	1.5 mg/m^2 qd × 5d q 3 wks	Demonstrating response Side effects: myelosuppression, alopecia, skin rashes
Irinotecan	350 mg/m^2 q 3 wks	Demonstrating some response Side effects: nausea, vomiting, diarrhea, abdominal cramps, alopecia, neutropenia, asthenia and hot flashes
Class: **Elliptinium Analogs—Plant Alkaloid Too Toxic; Semisynthetic and Synthetic Compounds**		
		Entering Phase I Trials
Class: **New Antifolates—Inhibition of the Enzyme Dihydrofolate Reductase**		
Edatrexate		Some partial and complete responses, unpredictable toxicity
Trimetrexate		Less successful than edatrexate, but demonstrates some activity
Class: **Pyridimine Antimetabolite**		
Gemcitabine	1,200 mg/m^2 qwk For 3 to 4 wk	Inhibits DNA synthesis Side effects: neutropenia, nausea, vomiting, liver toxicity, lethargy, alopecia
Milefosine	6% solution in aqueous glycol for dermal application to skin metastasis	Oral administration has multiple toxicities These are not seen with dermal application No current U.S. trial
Class: **Vinca Alkaloids—Includes Vincristine and Vinblastine Superior in Breast Cancer**		
Vindesine		Never approved, not better than Vinblastine
Vinorelbine (Navelbine)	20-25 mg/m^2 qwk	Promising effectiveness. Side effects: myelosuppression, minimal neurotoxicity
Class: **Taxanes—Being Studied Now in Combination with Other Cytotoxics, Side Effects; Hypersensitivity Reactions, Skin Toxicity, Fluid Retention**		
Paclitaxel (Taxol)	175 mg/m^2 over 3 hr Originally: 24h infusion-q21d	Tubulin-active, from bark of yew tree Shown to be effective, even in anthracycline resistant tumors
Docetaxel (Taxotere)	100 mg/m^2 over 1 hr q3wk	Approved by FDA for anthracycline resistant or metastatic breast cancer

From Hortobagyi, G. (1996). New cytotoxic agents from the treatment of breast cancer. *Oncology, 10*(6, Suppl.), 21-29; Ravdin, P. (1995). Taxoids: Effective agents in anthracycline-resistant breast cancer. *Seminars in Oncology, 22*(6, Suppl. 13), 29-34; Smith, G., & Henderson, C. (1996). New treatments in breast cancer. *Seminars in Oncology, 23*(4), 506-528.

High-Dose Adjuvant Chemotherapy

Improved outcomes are suggested with higher doses of adjuvant chemotherapy. Trials of high-dose therapies (i.e., accelerated doses of standard agents with growth factors and/or autologous stem cell support and/or autologous bone marrow transplant have demonstrated some benefit in patients with 10 or more positive lymph nodes (Osborne, Clark, & Ravdin, 1996). However, this arena of therapy is highly controversial. Many patients are treated in community settings and are not enrolled in clinical trials. Therefore clinicians have learned a great deal about how patients tolerate this therapy, but questions of efficacy and outcome remain unanswered for this costly and toxic therapy. Three NCI trials are currently comparing standard chemotherapy with high-dose chemotherapy.

Peters and colleagues (1993) studied 85 patients who received standard CAF followed by high-dose chemotherapy. They also received chest wall irradiation and 5 years of tamoxifen. At 6 years, the event-free survival rate was 64% and the overall survival rate was 75%. This study was not a randomized prospective trial comparing the high-dose group with standard chemotherapy, but the comparison was made with historical controls with event-free survival of 30% to 35% and overall survival of 37% to 48% (Peters et al., 1993; 1995). Thus although the percentage differences are encouraging, critics raise the issues of different study entry criteria between the high-dose chemotherapy protocol and the historical controls. Patients were disqualified from the high-dose chemotherapy studies for metastatic disease that was not as carefully screened for in the historical controls. Biologic therapies, immunotoxins, antibodies, and gene therapy have yet to enter full-fledged clinical trials. These approaches will involve explorations of growth factors and angiogenesis and will be aimed at patients with advanced disease.

Treatment for Patients with Recurrent Disease That Has Advanced to Regional or Distant Metastatic Disease

Any recurrence may signal systemic disease, but local therapies (e.g., mastectomy for recurrence in a breast treated with breast-conserving surgery, radiation to axillary lymph nodes or chest wall recurrence) are appropriate for local or regional recurrences. Local control of disease can decrease symptoms and overall tumor burden. It is essential to weigh the potential benefits against related morbidity.

Radiation Therapy

Radiation therapy for metastatic breast cancer is done as palliative. The sites most commonly treated are the bones and the brain. Bone metastases are common and are associated with side effects that negatively affect the quality of life of patients with metastatic breast cancer. More than 67% of patients with metastatic disease will develop evidence of bone metastasis, and this will be the first site of metastasis in 40% of the patients (Cook & Troutner, 1996). When bone metastasis is the only evidence of metastatic disease, survival may be prolonged for years. Bone metastasis is usually associated with pain and a 15% incidence of pathologic fractures. The goals of radiation therapy for the treatment of bone metastases are pain control, prevention of fractures, and improvement of function and quality of life. The radiation dose can be given as a single dose of 6 to 8 Gy or in fractionated doses over 10 treatments (3 Gy). If a relapse occurs, surgical stabilization of the bone may be required, particularly if the spinal cord is threatened (Aaron, Jennings, & Springfield, 1996).

In the treatment of intracranial metastases, whole brain irradiation therapy (WBXRT) is generally delivered in 200 cGy over five treatments, 4000 cGy in 20 treatments over 4 weeks, or 1500 cGy in two treatments within 3 days. Although patients may benefit from the reduction in symptoms; the prognosis is grave once intracranial metastases are present. Fewer than 10% of patients survive longer than 1 year. The side effects of WBXRT include headache, nausea, vomiting, fever, and potential brain stem herniation (Glass & Foley, 1996).

Palliative Chemotherapy and Drug Therapy for Metastatic Disease

Drug therapy includes analgesics to treat the pain and steroids to decrease edema. In addition, chemotherapy may be administered if the tumor is sensitive to antineoplastic agents. Treatment for metastatic breast cancer has the following goals: to control and contain the disease, to palliate symptoms, and to maintain the patient's quality and length of life.

Between 1974 and 1993, no new drugs for breast cancer treatment were approved by the Food and Drug Administration (FDA). Two new drugs, paclitaxel (Taxol) and docetaxel (Taxotere) were approved in 1995. A newly approved drug for breast and ovarian cancer is mitoxantrone (Novantrone), and an existing agent that demonstrates clinical efficacy in small cell lung disease but is not yet approved for use in breast cancer is vinorelbine (Navelbine) (Miaskowski, 1997). Table 22-3 displays current clinical trials testing pharmacologic agents.

Paclitaxel, with FDA approval, is currently a part of second-line treatment for metastatic breast cancer. Vinorelbine, without FDA approval for use in breast cancer, is also in current clinical use. Much is unknown about the use of chemotherapeutic agents, patient selection for treatment options, the timing of drug administration, combinations of agents, and long-term outcomes associated with the use of these antineoplastics. However, it is clear that the spectrum of choices for the treatment of metastatic breast cancer is widening and that the next decade of research will help to better delineate which combinations will benefit which subsets of patients (Henderson, 1996; Hortobagyi, 1996; Hortobagyi & Ibrahim, 1996; Ravdin, 1995; Smith & Henderson, 1996; Vogel, 1996; Winer, 1996).

Historically, in addition to local radiation therapy and pain management with opioid analgesics and nonsteroidal anti-inflammatory drugs (NSAIDs), the treatment of bone metastases has included systemic therapy with hormonal interventions and chemotherapy. Therapies are under investigation that hold promise for local treatment of osteoblastic lesions. Biphosphonates inhibit bone resorption and have been studied and used in the treatment of hypercalcemia. Two drugs, pamidronate, 60 to 90 mg intravenous (IV) every 4 weeks, and dichloromethylene biphosphonate (Clodronate), 1600 mg daily by mouth, have shown promise and efficacy in decreasing hypercalcemia, bone pain, and fractures and appear to be effective in healing osteolytic lesions. In one randomized clinical trial (Hortobagyi, Theriault, Porter, Blayney, Lipton, Sinoff, et al., 1996), 382 patients with metastases to the bone reported decreased bone pain, decreased time to skeletal complication, and less deterioration in performance status using pamidronate.

Strontium 89 (Metastron) is a radionuclide that is given as a single injection of 40 to 55 uCi/kg and has been demonstrated to provide pain relief in 81% of breast cancer patients studied. In addition, more than 50% of the patients reported decreased pain and improved quality of life for 3 to 6 months after treatment. The major toxicity of strontium 89 is bone marrow suppression that includes decreases in both platelets and white blood cell counts. In addition, a pain flare 48 hours after treatment has been reported in 10% to 20% of patients (Smith & Henderson, 1996).

Box 22-1
Hypercalcemia in Women with Metastatic Breast Cancer

Diagnostic Tests

Elevated serum and urine calcium levels, possible elevation of BUN and creatinine

Electrocardiogram: prolongation of the PR interval, shortened QT interval, changes in ST wave

Medical and Nursing Management

Ensure adequate hydration (3 L of normal saline per 24 hr. unless contraindicated)

Record fluid balance, diuretics prn (furosemide) to increase urine flow

Optimize mobilization (ambulation, isometric exercise)

Administer medications to inhibit bone resorption (mithramycin 25 μg/kg over 48 hours IV; side effect: thrombocytopenia) and to decrease calcium absorption from the gastrointestinal tract (oral phosphates; side effect: diarrhea)

Monitor the ECG and calcium, potassium, BUN and creatinine

Assess for confusion and weakness and anticipate safety precautions

BUN, blood nitrogen; *ECG*, electrocardiogram

Modified from Ziegfeld, C. R. (1992). *Core curriculum for oncology nursing*, Philadelphia: W. B. Saunders Company: Oncology Nursing Society.

ONCOLOGIC EMERGENCIES

Hypercalcemia

Hypercalcemia is defined as a serum calcium level of greater than 11 mg/100 ml and can be an oncologic emergency in women with infiltrating breast cancer who develop bone metastases. The incidence of hypercalcemia in women with metastatic breast cancer is between 40% and 50%. Metastatic disease and immobility result in the release of high levels of calcium from the bones. Signs and symptoms of hypercalcemia are primarily neurologic (e.g., fatigue, lethargy, irritability, weakness, depression, hyporeflexia), gastrointestinal (e.g., nausea, vomiting, anorexia, constipation), renal (e.g., polyuria, polydipsia, dehydration, occurrence of renal calculi), and ocular (e.g., white crystals may be visible on the cornea). Box 22-1 lists diagnostic tests and treatments for the management of hypercalcemia in patients with metastatic breast cancer.

Spinal Cord Compression

Spinal cord compression is a relatively uncommon but debilitating complication of metastatic breast cancer. Spinal cord compression is due to direct tumor invasion of the spinal canal or to the collapse of vertebrae due to bone metastases. The cord is damaged as a result of diminished blood supply or tumor invasion. Pain is the most common presenting symptom of spinal cord involvement. The pain may be localized to the back or may be referred to the abdomen, chest, or more rarely, the extremities. Eventually the pain, numbness, or tingling may give way to muscle weakness or paralysis.

The success of treatment depends on an accurate diagnosis and prompt initiation of therapy before the development of neurologic compromise. The effectiveness of radiotherapy alone depends on the presenting neurologic deficits, extent of disease, duration of symptoms, and overall clinical status of the patient (Janjan, 1996). In one study of surgical cord decompression, improved spinal stabilization and improved quality of life were reported in patients with long life expectancy and neurologic improvement and only pain relief in patients with short life expectancy (Shimizu, Shikata, Iida, Iwasaki, Yoshikawa, & Yamamuro, 1992).

Malignant Pleural Effusion

In women, breast cancer is the malignancy most commonly associated with pleural effusion. Median survival from the time of diagnosis of a pleural effusion matches that of metastatic breast cancer: (i.e., 1 to 2 years). Most patients present with symptoms including dyspnea, cough, and pain. Management includes treatment of the underlying malignancy with systemic therapies (i.e., chemotherapy and/or hormonal manipulation) and local treatment for the pleural effusion. Local treatment includes thoracentesis, first done to establish the diagnosis while providing symptomatic relief by draining fluid and then sometimes continued intermittently for symptom management. Because the benefits from systemic therapy occur slowly and intermittent thoracenteses are generally less effective, the approach of choice is often instillation of a sclerosing agent into the pleural space. Current effective sclerosing agents include doxycycline (formerly tetracycline), bleomycin, or talc. Any of these agents can be delivered through a chest tube after adequate drainage of the pleural space. Talc can be instilled, with very effective outcomes, with the patient under thoracoscopy using local anesthetic with sedation or under general anesthesia. Surgical thoracotomy and sclerosis are rarely used in clinical practice.

The goal of this procedure is to achieve a chemical irritation that will fuse the pleura to prevent future reaccumulation of fluid. If the pleural fluid is loculated (trapped in areas not drained by the chest tube), the pleural sclerosis will not be successful. Before the instillation of the sclerosing agent through a chest tube, premedication with an opioid analgesic is essential to control pain. In addition, a local anesthetic can be administered with the sclerosing agent. The provision of analgesics and local anesthetics will permit repositioning of the patient to allow maximum exposure of the sclerosing agent to the pleura (Shulman & Sugarbaker, 1996).

Cardiac Tamponade

Cardiac tamponade is a condition characterized by increased intrapericardial pressure caused by metastatic tumor invasion. This condition can also occur as a result of a thickening of the pericardium after radiation therapy (dose of 4000 Gy or more) to the thorax. The hemodynamic changes associated with cardiac tamponade include a decreased diastolic filling pressure and a subsequent decrease in cardiac stroke volume. Signs and symptoms of cardiac tamponade are directly related to decreased circulatory capacity and subsequent diminished oxygenation, and include dyspnea, cough, chest pain, anxiety and apprehension, signs of heart failure (jugular venous distention, cyanosis, edema, rales), pulsus paradoxus, muffled heart sounds, narrowed pulse pressure, and increased central venous pressure. Table 22-4 lists the diagnostic tests and procedures for the management of cardiac tamponade.

TABLE 22-4 Diagnostic Tests and Procedures for Cardiac Tamponade

Diagnostic Tests	Findings Associated with Cardiac Tamponade
Electrocardiogram	Low voltage, elevated ST segment, sinus tachycardia ventricular electrical alternans
Chest radiograph	May demonstrate cardiomegaly, or the tumor may be visualized
Echocardiogram	Two echos instead of one
Nursing Management	
Monitor ECG, vital signs and fluid balance, administer oxygen and pain medication, and prepare the patient for emergency medical management procedures listed below.	
Emergency Medical Management	
Emergency pericardiocentesis	The removal of 50-100 ml of fluid to provide temporary relief
Pericardial window	Performed for palliative purposes to allow pericardial fluids to drain into the pleural space
Chemotherapy or radiation therapy (2000-3000 rads)	To induce fibrosis of the pericardium stabilizing intrapericardial pressure
Total pericardectomy	Treatment when tamponade is sequela of radiation therapy

Modified from Ziegfeld, C. R. (1992). *Core curriculum for oncology nursing*. Philadelphia: W. B. Saunders, Oncology Nursing Society.

Superior Vena Cava Syndrome

Superior vena cava syndrome occurs when the superior vena cava is obstructed externally by the tumor itself or by enlarged metastatic lymph nodes or internally by the presence of a thrombus. The signs and symptoms are dramatic and are related to disturbances in circulation and to hypooxygenation. They include dyspnea; chest pain; cough; tachypnea; facial, trunk, and arm edema; thoracic and neck vein distention; hypotension; cyanosis; headache; and vision changes. Table 22-5 lists the diagnostic tests and management approaches for superior vena cava syndrome.

NURSING MANAGEMENT

The treatment period for metastatic breast cancer is replete with informational needs, severe stress associated with a life-threatening illness, the need to make choices among treatment options, alterations in personal identity in terms of health and life potential, the need for support during periods of adaptation to changes in family and sexual relationships, and the need for reassurance that normal healing is occurring. Although some researchers have attempted to predict informational needs by demographic descriptors such as age (Bilodeau & Degner, 1996), such work is not intended to preclude the need to assess for individual learning needs associated with the management of metastatic breast cancer. Table 20-6 provides a standard of care for decision-making about the various approaches used to manage metastatic breast cancer.

Careful attention to effective perioperative teaching for patients undergoing surgery for breast cancer is more necessary than ever as hospital stays become increasingly brief. A complete educational program should include at least the following: information about the type and extent of the patient's breast cancer; the surgical procedure that has occurred or will occur; what to expect in the immediate postoperative period in terms of wound care and the care of drains, pain management, and therapy for arm movement; care of the arm to prevent pressure damage or infection; the possibility of acute and long-term lymphedema, numbness, or other sensory sequelae; the availability of financial, sexual, and/or family counseling; all relevant information

TABLE 22-5 Diagnostic Tests and Procedures for Superior Vena Cava Syndrome

Diagnostic Tests	Potential Findings
Chest radiograph	May show the obstructing mass
NB: superior vena cavogram	*Contraindicated* due to increased venous pressure and the potential for internal bleeding
Nursing Management	
Monitor hydration and renal output, maintain airway and elevate upper body to promote gravity drainage of the upper torso, provide psychological supportive care for anxiety related to hypoxia	
Medical Management	**Focused on local control of the tumor**
Radiation therapy	Treatment of choice, expected response in 72 hours
Chemotherapy	Less effective in breast cancer patients
Mediation: diuretics and steroids	Reduce edema

Modified from Ziegfeld, C. R. (1992). *Core curriculum for oncology nursing.* Philadelphia: W. B. Saunders, Oncology Nursing Society.

about treatment options; and information about managing symptoms associated with all treatments the patient will undergo subsequently.

Physical Care

Immediate Postsurgical Care. Women with mastectomies are discharged with a Jackson-Pratt drain in place and require teaching regarding the emptying, measuring, and recording of the drain output. Most drains remain in place until the output is 30 ml or less per 24 hours, which generally occurs within 4 to 10 days. Directives for postoperative care are aimed at healing and functional recovery of the arm and shoulder. Limited exercise is encouraged for the first 24 hours (i.e., squeeze ball and wrist flexion). Range of motion exercises are begun thereafter. Precautions include watchfulness against trauma and monitoring for signs of infection and lymphedema after an axillary node dissection (see Table 21-12). If a seroma occurs, it may resolve spontaneously, or it may need to be aspirated. A hematoma usually resolves spontaneously, unless there is continuing bleeding that necessitates surgical revision.

Management of Lymphedema

Secondary or *acquired lymphedema* refers to the accumulation of protein-rich fluid in the subcutaneous tissue of the skin resulting from blocked or damaged lymphatic vessels. Postmastectomy lymphedema occurs in 10% to 63% of patients. This wide variance in outcome attests to the variability in the types and extent of the surgical procedure, surgical expertise, co-morbidity from radiation therapy, age and health status, and patient self-care behaviors. Lymphedema can result in pain, compromised mobility, infection, impaired cosmesis, psychological distress, and decreased quality of life. It has a wide range of onset from weeks to years from the date of lymph node dissection. A three-stage system is used to classify lymphedema:

1. *Stage I:* Pitting edema, soft tissue, spontaneously reversible
2. *Stage II:* Firmer skin, nonpitting edema, possible inflammation, spontaneously irreversible and
3. *Stage III:* Elephantiasis, hardening of the skin, overproduction of connective tissue, severe swelling.

The range of conventional treatments for lymphedema includes the use of a compression sleeve or stocking, a single cell pump, or a sequential gradient pump. Daily treatments are required for the remainder of the patient's life at high cost with variable payment by third-party payers and a range of clinical outcomes. Complete or complex decongestive physiotherapy (CDP) includes four therapeutic steps: (1) skin and nail care and the treatment of infection; (2) manual lymph drainage (MLD); (3) compression bandaging after MLD by applying bandages from the fingers to the axilla; and (4) while bandaged, doing a series of exercises to increase lymph flow. MLD is mild, rhythmic massage designed to stimulate the lymphatics of the contralateral normal quadrant, decongest the ipsilateral quadrant, and evacuate lymph from hands, fingers, and the upper arm. Patients can be taught to do CDP, and many can maintain the benefits realized by regular exercises and the use of MLD (Petrek & Lerner, 1996). A patient teaching guide for the management of lymphedema is found in Box 22-2.

An elastic sleeve garment measured for the patient from her wrist to her axilla and including the hand, if swollen, should be ordered to the appropriate compression as indicated by degree of lymphedema. In addition, medications are sometimes prescribed. Diuretics, although often prescribed, should not be, as this drug therapy might result in increased fluid retention in the extremity when increased protein in the interstitial space results in reaccumulation of edema. There is some evidence that the benzpyrenes, including bioflavonoids and the coumarins, may decrease the symptoms of chronic lymphedema by increasing proteolysis and decreasing the osmotic pressure in the extremity, resulting in less edema. FDA approval is still pending for the use of benzpyrenes for breast cancer–related lymphedema.

Management of Side Effects of Chemotherapy and Radiation Therapy

Radiation and chemotherapy each bring an array of side effects specific to the agent and dose. A comprehensive guide for the management of side effects related to these therapies can be found in Dodd's *Managing the Side Effects of Chemotherapy and Radiation Therapy: A Guide for Patients*

Box 22-2
Patient Instructions for the Management of Lymphedema

Lymphedema refers to swelling in an arm that may occur after lymph node surgery or if the lymph nodes become compressed or blocked with a tumor. Various strategies can be used to prevent lymphedema or to decrease lymphedema when it occurs.

1. You can help to prevent pressure on the lymphatic vessels by:
   - Wearing clothing that does not constrict the arm (e.g., avoid elastic sleeves, tight wrist bands)
   - Avoiding keeping the arm in a dependent position
   - Elevating the arm several times a day using a pillow or foam wedge
   - Preventing injury to the affected hand and arm
   - Applying skin lotion to the arm and hand on a daily basis
   - Performing hand and arm exercises on a daily basis
2. Obtain a prescription for a compression sleeve or stocking if lymphedema occurs. The sleeve should be fitted by a professional when the arm is not swollen.
3. Report any signs and symptoms of infection (i.e., redness, pain or soreness in the arm, swelling in the hand or arm) to your doctor or nurse.

and their Families (1996). Table 21-15 provides a standard of care for the management of postmenopausal symptoms associated with hormonal therapy.

Psychosocial and Cultural Concerns of Patients with Metastatic Breast Cancer

Many of the emotional concerns faced by patients with metastatic breast cancer share common themes with patients diagnosed with other cancers, for example, the range of responses to life-threatening illness, coping with others' reactions to "cancer," fear, anxiety, and balancing the stressors of obtaining information while making treatment decisions. However, there is a body of information, thought, and research that particularly focuses on the psychosocial needs of women with breast cancer. Confirmation of distant metastases or stage IV disease is both a medical and emotional crisis. For patients who are diagnosed with metastatic disease as their index (initial) breast cancer diagnosis there is the experience of a dual crisis, a new diagnosis of cancer and the reality of a life-threatening illness. For patients with recurrent and/or initial diagnosis of metastatic disease, it is the realization of the patient's worst nightmare. It is the advent of loss of a seemingly certain future, as well as the likely loss of self and loved ones.

Much of the focus of psychosocial research is to increase our knowledge base about those issues that, when identified, can allow for therapeutic interventions to decrease distress and enhance coping and wellness (Fetting, 1991; Hilton, 1996; Lavery & Clark, 1996; Tross et al., 1996; Walker, Nail, Larsen, Magill, & Schwartz, 1996). The areas of focus include sexuality and body image, fear and threat of mortality, disclosure, social support and the impact of the disease on relationships (significant other, family, children, friends), work, money, and insurance issues. Responses to metastatic breast cancer are believed to be affected by age (life cycle–specific issues), the amount and content of the disruption the disease has on one's life, prediagnosis personality, coping style and prior crisis experience, and prior experiences with breast cancer in family or friends (Rowland & Massie, 1996).

It is difficult to establish therapeutic relationships, key to the provision of emotional support, without trust. To support women through treatment and end-of-life decision making, it is essential that nurses understand the diverse cultural meanings associated with the breast, its loss, and the risk of impending death as a result of advanced disease. The key issues for lesbians, who come from diverse cultures of origin, are dealing with homophobia (hatred and fear of people with same sex intimate relationships); assumptions of heterosexuality by providers or other survivors; visitation and acknowledgment of partner as family and significant other; disclosure of lesbian identification to providers, friends, and family; and emotional responses to diagnosis, treatment, and recovery (Denenberg, 1995; O'Hanlan, 1995; Rankow, 1995). Emotional needs and effective interventions are also different for elderly women with metastatic breast cancer. Elderly women may have diminished social support, will likely have experienced more prior losses, have limited financial resources on fixed incomes and limited health care coverage, and come from a generation with less of a tendency to discuss breast cancer, their breasts, or sexuality (Caplan, Wells, & Haynes, 1992; Champion, 1992).

In addition to a commitment to learning more about and respecting the impact that culture may have on breast cancer patients, it is vitally important that our programs for the treatment of metastatic breast cancer include the lived experience and knowledge of bicultural caregivers from diverse cultures. In addition, psychosocial resources must be available to non-English speakers in their own native language.

Psychological Interventions

Psychological help for patients with breast cancer is provided by individuals and peer support groups, by professionals from a variety of disciplines, and through individual psychological consultations with psychologists, social workers, or psychiatrists. It is often provided for a new diagnosis or for a diagnostic crisis (e.g., metastatic disease or recurrence). Breast cancer support groups are an active part of the landscape of breast cancer treatment programs. Spiegel and colleagues (1989) studied the effect on survival of participation in a breast cancer support group for women with metastatic breast cancer. Eighty-six women participated: 50 in the intervention group and 36 in the control group. Survival time was significantly longer for patients in the treatment group, The interval of time from first metastasis to death was longer in the treatment group. Although all the components of benefit from participating in a breast cancer support group are not clear, it is believed to be related to the benefits derived from social support.

Box 22-3

1985 . . . 1995 . . . 10 years of living with breast cancer and the operative word is living. Those of us LIVING with breast cancer would certainly choose other methods to open our eyes to the beauty of life . . . This disease often has that kind of effect. I feel that it is my obligation to bring as much to the fight as I can, using my firm belief in the interconnectedness of mind and body. I have learned a great deal about death from the terrible vantage point of watching many women die of breast cancer. I'm learning to accept and embrace the idea of my own death, ironically strengthened and healed by a disease with no cure. I hope that newly diagnosed women, or those facing yet another round of treatment, find both education and inspiration from the fact that I have hung on for ten years, fought many battles, expanded my capacity for learning and compassion, and prepared myself for whatever lies ahead.

Susan Claymon

Claymon, C. (1998). *Personal communication.*

As with all treatment recommendations and despite some data reporting their benefit, support groups are not perceived as beneficial by all women. Many women choose not to participate, and others give participation a trial and then choose not to continue. Some women report feeling overly affected by the difficult medical treatment and/or life experience stories of the other women. Others are not comfortable with the disclosure of feelings either in a group or to people they do not know. There may also be language or cultural barriers for some women. In larger, urban areas or in areas where a specific population is well represented, culture- and language-specific support groups may be available.

At the University of California San Francisco and Mount Zion Medical Center, there is an Art for Recovery program directed by Cindi Perlis (begun in 1987). One of the projects of the program is the creation of beautiful quilts composed of quilt squares made by women living with breast cancer. The quilt project is inspirational and healing for the women participating. It is a concrete way to have women give voice to thoughts and feelings and be honored. For family, friends, professional caregivers, and the community, viewing the quilts is an educational and moving experience. Along with the making of the quilt squares, women are invited to write words to accompany their squares. Box 22-3 is an example of the lived experience of breast cancer.

HOME CARE ISSUES

Although issues of facing one's own mortality are present from the moment of the diagnosis of breast cancer, the diagnosis of recurrence of disease or metastatic breast cancer makes the threat of death an ever-present reality. On a practical level, there are increased needs for physical care. Referrals for home nursing care need to be considered more quickly for the following patients: those with functional limitations, frail elderly, persons without the support of family and friends, and those with a prior history of severe comorbid conditions or mental illness.

The decision-making focus shifts from therapy with curative intent to therapy with the intent to control the disease, and the focus may shift again to an emphasis on palliative care to control the symptoms. Decisions must be made about the nature of the care, decisions that are often influenced jointly by what third-party payers will pay for, as well as what the patient and family members prefer. Depending on the caregiving site(s) and the extent of metastatic disease, a patient with metastatic breast cancer may have an experience that ranges from a long life span living at home with limited care needs to a rapidly declining course requiring the urgent institution of inpatient or outpatient hospice services.

The timing of appropriate shifts in care goals and treatment is a learned skill, shifting with variations in the patient's disease trajectory and personality and preferences. For example, some patients initiate a hospice referral before their life expectancy would appear to be limited to 6 months, whereas others have been placed on home care services waiting for the moment, which may never come, when they will accept hospice services.

Pain in Breast Cancer

There are little data on the prevalence and incidence of breast cancer pain across the spectrum of illness. Postmastectomy pain syndrome (PMP) occurs after any breast surgery that includes axillary lymph node dissection. It is thought that PMP occurs primarily after injury to the intercostobrachial nerve. The PMP syndrome includes "nerve pain," aching and burning, and numbness in the affected upper arm and chest wall or breast. It may be chronic and is usually only poorly responsive to opioid analgesics. Generally, it is believed that the prevalence of PMP is low, but this issue is not well studied, and reports have varied widely. In an early study, Daut and Cleeland (1982) reported a 68% prevalence rate of pain in a mixed sample of inpatients and outpatients with breast cancer. Later, Foley (1987) reported an incidence rate of 4% to 6%. Four other studies of pain in patients with cancer have been reported (Ahles, Ruckdeschel, & Blanchard, 1984; Bressler, Hange, & McGuire, 1986; Miaskowski & Dibble, 1995; Peteet et al., 1986), but none specifically examined pain in patients with cancer of the breast.

Stevens, Dibble, and Miaskowski (1995) reviewed a subset of 97 breast cancer patients from a larger study of 435 cancer patients. They observed the prevalence of PMP syndrome in the breast cancer patients to be 20% (19 of 97 women). Of these 19 women with the PMP syndrome, approximately half had intermittent pain and half had continuous pain. Their PMP was characterized by inadequate pain control, exacerbations of the pain with movement, and pain experienced as interfering with daily functioning. There were no males with breast cancer in this study. Stevens and colleagues (1995) point out that the reported proportion of patients in this sample with PMP may be underestimated, as it was impossible to determine whether any of the additional 14 women with advanced breast cancer in the sample also had PMP.

There is continued need for nursing research to better understand the prevalence of breast cancer–related pain in all phases of the breast cancer experience, as well as how best to manage this pain for all patients with breast cancer. Clinical practice must become more informed by the continued assessment and evaluation of pain and develop effective strategies for pain management.

There is also a reported syndrome that includes pain in the axilla, arm, and/or elbow accompanied by cordlike material that can be palpated. The "cords" are thought to be sclerosed lymphatic structures. These cords cause tightness, pain, and impaired mobility. The associated symptoms are often responsive to massage and stretching. The discomfort decreases or stops after spontaneous or massaged rupture of the cordlike structures.

A decrease in shoulder mobility, accompanied by pain, can be a consequence of axillary lymph node dissection or radiation therapy. Shoulder pain may be caused or exacerbated by edema, bleeding, or scarring. Range of motion exercises may prevent and certainly can decrease mobility limitations and pain (Gerber, 1996).

In addition to PMP syndrome, breast cancer–related pain includes pain related to bone metastases and pain related to local surgical therapy, for recurrence. Bone metastases frequently present as pain often characterized as dull, continuous rather than intermittent, and worsening gradually unless there is a fracture. Radiation therapy is an effective local palliative pain control therapy, particularly for a single lesion. Systemic therapy can also provide effective pain palliation if successful in shrinking tumor size (Aaron, Jennings, & Springfield, 1996). Opioid analgesics are most often required for pain control, often in concert with NSAIDs.

Pain is usually the presenting symptom of brachial plexopathy (invasion of the tumor into the brachial plexus). Brachial plexopathy can also be caused by surgical trauma to the brachial plexus, radiation-induced injury, lymphedema, or a new primary breast cancer. In addition to brachial plexus pain, other symptoms of brachial plexopathy include paresthesias, arm pain, heaviness, muscle weakness, and edema. Arm pain can also be caused by carpal tunnel syndrome. Radiation therapy may be used if the skin in the treatment field has not been over exposed. Systemic therapies (chemotherapy, hormonal therapy) are variably effective in cases of tumor recurrence or new primary tumors. Effective dosing of analgesics for pain management often requires combination analgesia: opioids, NSAIDs, and antidepressant or anticonvulsant medications (Cherney & Foley, 1996).

PROGNOSIS

The SEER statistics for women diagnosed from 1989 to 1991 and followed through 1993 report 5-year relative survival rates by stage at diagnosis to be 97% for tumors that exhibit only local extension at diagnosis, 76% for tumors with regional extension, and 20% for women with distant metastases at the time of diagnosis (ACS, 1996). In women who have negative lymph nodes at the time of diagnosis (local disease), 20% to 30% will develop metastatic disease. Once a patient is diagnosed with metastatic disease, the 5-year survival rates range from 12% to 35% and the 10-year survival rates range from 5% to 22%. The range of survival time varies in relationship to the site of disease, with patients whose recurrence is limited to bone metastases having longer survival times. The overall mean survival time after recurrence with metastatic breast cancer disease is approximately 2 years (Cook & Troutner, 1996; Engleking & Kalinowski, 1995; Winer, 1996).

The 5-year survival rate in African-American women (70%) remains significantly lower than the rate for white American women (85%) in the NCI SEER program data from 1988 to 1993, although both rates have shown gains over the last 25 years (Parker et al., 1997). Perhaps more significant is the fact that 5-year survival rates are lower for African-American women even when stage at diagnosis is taken into account. Table 21-17 depicts 5-year survival rates by stage at diagnosis and race.

Prognostic indicators for recurrence and survival of infiltrating carcinoma include lymph node status, tumor size, hormone receptor status, nuclear grade, histologic type, proliferative rate, and certain genetic markers. When all prognostic factors are considered together (i.e., multivariate analyses), the presence or absence of metastases to axillary lymph nodes is the single most influential predictor of recurrence and mortality rates. However, they are an imperfect indicator taken alone, as approximately 25% of patients without axillary metastases are not cured by local regional therapy alone, and some patients with metastases are alive and well for many years (at 10 years, 30% overall and 17% with 4 or more positive nodes) (Gardner & Feldman, 1993).

The presence of metastases in the internal mammary nodes is second only to the presence of metastases in axillary nodes as a predictor of recurrence or higher mortality (Noguchi et al., 1991). Long-term survival for patients with supraclavicular node involvement is considered to be equal to patients with stage IV disease, although 5-year survival (30% to 34%) is often better than in patients who present with metastases to distant organ systems (18%) (Kiricuta et al., 1994).

Table 21-16 lists these prognostic indicators and the favorable and unfavorable values. It is hoped that refinement of our understanding of the process of carcinogenesis in relationship to these indicators will assist in identifying patients most at risk for recurrence so that they may be selected for adjuvant therapy, and so that those not at risk for recurrence can be spared the morbidity associated with adjuvant therapy.

Histologic grade is based on the degree of tubule formation, the number of mitoses, and nuclear pleomorphism seen in routine tissue sections. These factors are combined as the Scarff-Bloom-Richardson (SBR) grade. Well-differentiated tumors (grade 1) are relatively rare, and histologic grade usually increases with tumor size and stage. Both histologic and nuclear grade are predictors of mortality, but they provide no additional benefit as prognostic indicators once tumor size and node status, nipple involvement, and estrogen receptor status are considered (Fisher, Constantino, Fisher, & Redmond, 1993).

The presence of estrogen or progesterone receptors in the tumor is associated with a better prognosis as a result of the responsivity of the tumor to hormone therapy. It has been estimated that between 50% and 85% of breast cancers contain measurable amounts of estrogen receptor (ER) (Donegan, 1997). ER-positive tumors are more common in older patients and most common in postmenopausal women. The presence of ER in the tumor indicates that normal cellular mechanisms for processing estrogen still exist despite the malignant process. The presence of the progesterone receptor implies function of this same system and, as a result, offers little additional prognostic information.

About 50% to 60% of patients with ER have been observed to respond favorably to hormone or endocrine therapies; the actual percentage that responds is correlated with the level of ER present in the tumor. ER-positive patients have prolonged disease-free survival after primary treatment, superior overall survival rates, and longer survival rates after recurrence than patients with ER-negative tumors (Donegan, 1997). Limitations on the value of this prognostic indicator arise because ER-positive tumors tend also to be low in histologic and nuclear grade, and have a low S-phase fraction (see later); and use of this indicator alone or in combination with node status has not been found to be a reliable indicator of which patients should be given adjuvant therapy. The importance of ER-positive status is most influential in the selection of hormone treatment.

Additional indicators are being sought to identify which patients with ER-positive tumors may have a particularly favorable outlook. One such indicator is the pS2 protein whose actual function is not yet well understood but is believed to be associated with a more intact cellular estrogen-processing mechanism.

Ploidy is another marker being studied for its ability to predict patients more likely to have recurrence or poorer survival potential. Diploid cells are in the resting phase (termed the *G phase*) or in the first phase of the cell cycle (termed G_1), whereas cells with twice the number of normal DNA content are in the mitotic phase (termed *M*). Cells with intermediate amounts of DNA are in the synthesis (S) phase. When a high proportion of the breast cells in a tissue sample are observed to be in the S-phase (S-phase fraction is high), prognosis is poorer. The process for calculation of the S-phase is not standardized at this time, making the study of its value as a prognostic indicator more problematic. To date, this indicator has not been found to contribute significant additional predictive information about recurrence and mortality after tumor size and node status are considered.

The overexpression of CD is associated with higher levels of recurrence and lower survival rates (Gasparini et al., 1991; Seshadri et al., 1994), but once again the presence of CD has not provided additional prognostic information in node-positive patients once tumor size is considered. The situation surrounding the overexpression of CD in patients with node-negative tumors is more puzzling. Findings have been conflicting in these patients, with initial studies reporting a poorer prognosis in patients with an overexpression of CD (Isola, Visakorpii, Holli, & Kallioniemi et al., 1992; Tandon et al., 1990) but a later, larger study failing to replicate this relationship (Ravdin et al., 1994).

Urokinase plasminogen activator (uPA) is a protease that has been implicated in the metastatic process. In animal research, the activation of this protease has been shown to lead to metastases in animal tumors. In addition, high levels of uPA in human breast tumors are correlated with a shorter disease-free interval and poorer survival rates. More important, this indicator is claimed to be independent of tumor size and node status (Duffy et al., 1994). At the moment, this research holds promise for providing additional information about recurrence and survival potential, but the findings await replication in future reports.

ERBB2 (also *Her-2/neu, c-erbB2*) is a proto-oncogene. It is believed that when this and other proto-oncogenes are mutated, they promote neoplastic transformation. The overexpression of *c-erbB2* has been associated with a poorer prognosis, but this finding is confined almost entirely to node-positive patients (Marks et al., 1994). Recently, researchers have engineered an immunoliposome (i.e., a fat molecule attached to an antibody and a chemotherapy drug) and used it in animal studies to eradicate the c-erbB2 oncogene's protein product, which interacts with cell growth factors (NEWS, *Journal of the National Cancer Intstitute,* 1996). Overexpression of the c-erb B2 gene is seen in 20% of breast cancers and is associated with a poorer prognosis. This study represents the beginning of genetic breast cancer treatment modalities. However, in its most recent statement, the ASCO found insufficient evidence to recommend the routine use of these tumor markers, oncogenes, and hormonal factors for most screening, diagnosis, staging, or intervention decisions (ASCO, 1996).

p53 is a tumor suppressor gene that is believed to function by blocking cells in G_1 or by programming cell death. The expression of mutant p53 is the most commonly observed genetic defect found in human cancers. It can be demonstrated in 14% to 26% of in situ and invasive cancers depending on what criteria are used to determine its presence (Isola et al., 1992; Thor et al., 1992). Mutant p53 is more common in familial cases of breast cancer and has been found in up to 52% of cases of breast and ovarian syndrome and in all cases of Li Fraumeni syndrome (Thor et al., 1992). The expression of p53 is associated with an overall decrease in survival, as well as in the time to recurrence.

EVALUATION OF THE QUALITY OF CARE

Ensuring that clients are treated with dignity, that culturally competent cancer information is available to all, and that no segments of the population are systematically denied cancer care is the shared ethical responsibility of providers, policy makers, and concerned citizens. This philosophic approach requires us, as providers, to advocate for those who have been poorly served or not served at all (Facione & Facione, 1997).

Suominen and colleagues (1995) have documented that nurses' opinions of how well care was delivered do not always agree with the opinions of cancer patients and their families. Nurses need to evaluate the quality of the care they deliver in the context of the caregiving setting, the perception of needs from the perspective of the patient and the family, and the goals for breast cancer management held by

Table 22-6 Quality of Care Evaluation of Treatment of Pain in Breast Cancer

Disciplines participating in the quality of care evaluation:
☐ Surgery ☐ Nursing ☐ Medical Oncology
☐ Radiation Oncology ☐ Social Work
☐ Psychology/Psychiatry
Data from: ☐ Mailed Questionnaire
☐ Patient Interview

Criteria	Yes	No
1. Do you currently have pain?	☐	☐
2. Have you been asked by doctor(s) and/or nurse(s) about pain?	☐	☐
3. If you do have pain, is it being treated?	☐	☐
4. How good is your pain relief? (Circle one) Poor Fair Good Very good Excellent		
5. Describe your pain:		
a. Where is the pain?		
b. What does it feel like?		
c. How long have you had it?		
d. What helps?		
6. Comments:		

Box 22-4
Research Issues in the Diagnosis and Treatment of Metastatic Breast Cancer

Biologic

The timing, mechanism, and prevention of breast cancer metastatic spread
Efficacy of complementary medicine therapies

Social and Behavioral Research Issues

Effective prevention against insurance and job discrimination
Ways to better evaluate cancer detection and treatment services delivery
The impact on utilization of cost, provider relationships, and availability of services
Ethical/spiritual/political influences on treatment decisions for breast cancer

Treatment Issues

Effective preventive measures and treatment strategies for lymphedema
Improved pain management
Interventions that effectively decrease or enhance coping with symptoms: fatigue, cognitive changes, alopecia, psychologic distress
Provider communication and teaching skills to support patient decision making
Treatment of menopausal symptoms without estrogen

the health care team. Ultimately, the judgments of the patient and/or family determine the major portion of the quality assessment of nursing care interventions, and as a result, input from these individuals needs to be included in any evaluation tools that are used.

Tracking tools can be useful devices to document progress to date in teaching key information and communicating remaining educational needs to staff in both inpatient and outpatient settings. When charts do not reliably follow patients to their postoperative outpatient appointments, women should be provided with copies of the educational program.

Merrouche and colleagues (1996) continued their evaluation of care through terminal care by surveying the families of terminal cancer patients 6 months after the death of the patient. They included an assessment of the quality of information given to patients and their families, estimates of the quality of pain control, nursing care services, psychological support, and the families' opinions of the practical conditions at the time of the patient's death at home or in an institutional setting. Inadequate pain management was reported by 21% of their sample, and the majority (67%) of these families preferred death to occur in the hospital rather than the home.

Two tools that can be used for the collection of data to begin to evaluate the treatment of pain and the quality of decision-making support are shown in Tables 20-8 and 22-6.

RESEARCH ISSUES

Research issues are complex and broad in domain, encompassing biologic, social, and behavioral issues; issues surrounding hereditary breast cancer; and issues surrounding specific treatment options. Box 22-4 displays a list of some of the many future research questions applicable to the prevention and treatment of metastatic carcinoma.

REFERENCES

Aaron, A., Jennings, L., & Springfield, D. (1996). Local treatment of bone metastases. In J. Harris, M. Lippman, M. Morrow, & S. Hellman (Eds.), *Diseases of the breast.* Philadelphia: Lippincott Raven.

Ahles, T. A., Ruckdeschel, J. C., & Blanchard, E. B. (1984). Cancer related pain: Prevalence in an outpatient setting as a function of stage of disease and type of cancer. *Journal of Psychosomatic Research, 28,* 115-119.

American Cancer Society. (1996). *Cancer facts and figures 1996.* Atlanta: The Author.

American Joint Committee on Cancer (AJCC). (1988). *Manual for staging of cancer* (3rd ed.). Philadelphia: J. B. Lippincott.

American Society of Clinical Oncology (ASCO). (1996). Statement of the American Society of Clinical Oncology. Genetic testing for cancer susceptibility. *Journal of Clinical Oncology, 14,* 1730-1736.

Barnicle, M. (1996). Managing symptoms related to chemotherapy. In K. Hassey-Dow (Ed.), *Contemporary issues in breast cancer.* Sudbury, MA: Jones and Bartlett.

Berg, J. W., & Hutter, R. V. P. (1995). Breast cancer. *Cancer Supplement, 75,* 257-269.

Bilodeau, B. A., & Degner, L. F. (1996). Information needs, sources of information, and decisional roles in women with breast cancer. *Oncology Nursing Forum, 23*(4), 691-696.

Bonadonna, G., Valgussa, P., Zucali, R., & Salvadori, B. (1995). Primary chemotherapy in surgically resectable breast cancer. *CA: Cancer Journal for Clinicians, 45*(4), 227-243.

Boring, C. C., Squires, T. S., Tong, T., & Montgomery, S. (1994). Cancer statistics. *CA: A Cancer Journal for Clinicians, 44*(1), 7-26.

Bressler, L. R., Hange, P. A., & McGuire, D. B. (1986). Characteristics of the pain experience in a sample of cancer outpatients. *Oncology Nursing Forum, 13*(6), 51-55.

Brodie, A. M., & Njar, V. C. (1996). Aromatase inhibitors and breast cancer. *Seminars in Oncology, 23*(4, Suppl. 9), 10-20.

Buzdar, A. U., Plourde, P. V., & Hortobagyi, G. N. (1996). Aromatase inhibitors in metastatic breast cancer. *Seminars in Oncology, 23*(4, Suppl. 9), 28-32.

Caplan, L. S., Wells, B., & Haynes, S. (1992). Breast cancer screening among older racial/ethnic minorities and whites: Barriers to early detection. *Journals of Gerontology, 47,* 101-110.

Champion, V. (1992). Breast self-examination in women 65 and older. *Journals of Gerontology, 47,* 75-79.

Cherney, N., & Foley, K. (1996). Brachial plexopathy in patients with breast cancer. In J. Harris, M. Lippman, M. Morrow, & S. Hellman (Eds.), *Diseases of the breast.* Philadelphia: Lippincott Raven.

Cook, G. A., & Troutner, K. (1996). *Taxotere: An important advance in the treatment of metastatic breast cancer.* Pittsburgh: Oncology Nursing Society: Rhone-Poulenc Rorer.

Daut, R. L., & Cleeland, C. S. (1982). The prevalence and severity of pain in cancer. *Cancer, 50,* 1913-1918.

Davidoff, A. M., Kerns, B., Inglehart, J. D., & Marks, J. R. (1991). Maintenance of p53 alterations throughout breast cancer progression. *Cancer Research, 51,* 2605-2610.

Denenberg, R. (1995). Invisible women: Lesbians and health care. *Health PAC Bulletin,* Spring, 1992.

Dodd, M. J. (1996). *Managing the side effects of chemotherapy and radiation therapy: A guide for patients and their families.* San Francisco: University of California Press.

Dollinger, M. Rosenbaum, E., & Cable, G. (1992). Deciding on the appropriate treatment. *Everyone's guide to cancer therapy.* Toronto: Somerville House Publishing.

Donegan, W. L. (1997). Tumor-related prognostic factors for breast cancer. *CA: Cancer Journal for Clinicians, 47,* 28-51.

Donegan, W. L., & Redlich, P. N. (1996). Breast cancer in men. *Surgical Clinics in North America, 76*(2), 343-363.

Dow, K. H. (1996). *Contemporary issues in breast cancer.* Sudbury, MA: Jones and Bartlett Publishers.

Duffy, M. J., Reilly, D., McDermott, E., O'Higgins, N., Fennelly, J. J., & Andreasen, P. A. (1994). Urokinase plasminogen activator as a prognostic marker in different subgroups of patients with breast cancer. *Cancer, 74,* 2276-2280.

Early Breast Cancer Trialists' Collaborative Group (EBCTCG). (1988). Effects of adjuvant tamoxifen and of cytotoxic therapy on modality in early breast cancer. An overview of 61 randomized trials among 28,896 women. *New England Journal of Medicine, 319*(26), 1681-1692.

Early Breast Cancer Trialists' Collaborative Group (EBCTCG). (1992). Systemic treatment of early breast cancer by hormonal, cytotoxic, or immune therapy. 133 randomized trials involving 31,000 recurrences and 24,000 deaths among 75,000 women. *Lancet, 339, 3,* 1-15 and 71-85.

Engelking, C. (1989). Recurrent breast cancer: Physical and psychosocial sequellae. *Innovations in Oncology Nursing, 3,* 2-6.

Engleking, C., & Kalinowski, B. (1995). *A comprehensive guide to breast cancer treatment: Current issues and controversies.* New York: Triclinica Communications Inc.

EVAXX, Inc. (1980). Black Americans' attitudes toward cancer and cancer tests. *Cancer, 31*(4), 212-218.

Facione, N. C. (1993). Delay versus helpseeking for breast cancer symptoms: A critical review of the literature on patient and provider delay. *Social Science and Medicine, 36,* 1521-1548.

Facione, N. C., & Dodd, M. J. (1995). Women's narratives of helpseeking for breast cancer. *Cancer Practice, 3*(4), 219-225.

Facione, N. C., Dodd, M. J., Holzemer, W., & Meleis, A. (1997). Help-seeking for self-discovered breast symptoms: Implications for cancer early detection. *Cancer Practice, 5*(4), 220-227.

Facione, N. C., & Facione, P.A. (1997). Equitable access to cancer services in the 21st century. *Nursing Outlook, 45*(3), 118-124.

Farwell, M. F., Foster, R. S., & Costanza, M. C. (1993). Breast cancer and earlier detection efforts: Realized and unrealized impact on stage. *Archives of Surgery, 128,* 510-514.

Fetting, J. (1991). Psychosocial aspects of breast cancer. *Current Science ISSN 1040-8746,* 1014-1018.

Fisher, E. R., Constantino, J., Fisher, B., & Redmond, C. (1993). Pathologic findings from the National Surgical Adjuvant Breast Project (Protocol 4). *Cancer, 71,* 2141-2150.

Foley, K. M. (1987). Pain syndromes in patients with cancer. *Medical Clinics of North America, 71,* 169-184.

Freeman, H. P., & Wasfie, T. J. (1989). Cancer of the breast in poor black women. *Cancer, 63,* 2562-2568.

Gardner, B., & Feldman, J. (1993). Are positive axillary nodes in breast cancer markers for incurable disease? *Annals of Surgery, 218,* 270-278.

Gasparini, G., Pozza, F., Meli, S., Reitano, M., Santini, G., & Bevilacqua, P. (1991). Breast cancer cell kinetics: Immunocytochemical determination of growth fractions by monoclonal antibody Ki-67 and correlation with flow cytometric S-phase and some features of tumor aggressiveness. *Anticancer Research, 11,* 2015-2021.

Gerber, L. (1996). Rehabilitation management for women with breast cancer: Maximizing functional outcomes. In J. Harris, M. Lippman, M. Morrow, & S. Hellman (Eds.), *Diseases of the breast.* Philadelphia: Lippincott Raven.

Glass, P., & Foley, K. (1996). Brain metastases in patients with breast cancer. In J. Harris, M. Lippman, M. Morrow, & S. Hellman (Eds.), *Diseases of the breast.* Philadelphia: Lippincott Raven.

Goldhirsch, A., & Gelber, R. D. (1996). Endocrine therapies of breast cancer. *Seminars in Oncology, 23*(4), 496.

Goodwin, J. S., & Samet, J. M. (1994). Care received by older women diagnosed with breast cancer. *Cancer Control, 1,* 313-319.

Harris, J. R., Lippman, M. E., Veronesi, U., & Willett, W. (1992). Medical progress: Breast cancer. *New England Journal of Medicine, 327,* 319-328.

Harris, L., & Swain, S. (1996). The role of primary chemotherapy in early breast cancer. *Seminars in Oncology, 23*(1, Suppl. 2), 31-42.

Harvey, H. A. (1996). Aromatase inhibitors in clinical practice: Current status and a look to the future. *Seminars in Oncology, 23*(4 Suppl 9), 33-38.

Henderson, C. (1996). Recent advances in the treatment of refractory advanced breast cancer. *Oncology, 10*(6, Suppl.), 5-6.

Hilton, B. A. (1996). Getting back to normal: The family experience during early stage breast cancer. *Oncology Nursing Forum, 23*(4), 605-614.

Hortobagyi, G. (1996). New cytotoxic agents for the treatment of breast cancer. *Oncology, 10*(6, Suppl.), 21-29.

Hortobagyi, G. N., & Buzdar, A. U. (1995). Current status of adjuvant systemic therapy for primary breast cancer: Progress and controversy. *CA: A Cancer Journal for Clinicians, 45,* 199-226.

Hortobagyi, G. N., Buzdar, A. U., Strom, E. A., Ames, F. C., & Singletary, S. E. (1995). Primary chemotherapy for early and advanced breast cancer. *Cancer Letters, 90,* 103-109.

Hortobagyi, G., & Ibrahim, N. (1996). Combinations of new and old agents for breast cancer treatment: Future directions. *Oncology, 10*(6, Suppl.), 30-36.

Hortobagyi, G. N., Theriault, R. L., Porter, L., Blayney, D., Lipton, A., Sinoff, C., Wheeler, H., Simeone, J. F., Seaman, J., Knight, R. D., et al. (1996). Efficacy of pamidronate in reducing skeletal complications in patients with breast cancer and lytic bone metastases. Protocol 19 Aredia Breast Cancer Study Group. *New England Journal of Medicine, 335*(24), 1785-1791.

Isola, J., Visakorpi, T., Holli, K., & Kallioniemi, O. P. (1992). Association of over expression of tumor suppressor protein p53 with rapid cell proliferation and poor prognosis in node-negative breast cancer patients. *Journal of the National Cancer Institute, 84,* 1109-1114.

Janjan, N. A. (1996). Radiotherapeutic management of spinal metastases. *Journal of Pain and Symptom Management, 11*(1), 47-56.

Kiricuta, I. C., Willner, J., Kolbl, O., & Bohndorf, W. (1994). The prognostic significance of the supraclavicular lymph node metastases in breast cancer patients. *International Journal of Radiation Oncology, Biology, and Physics, 28,* 387-393.

Landis, S. H., Murray, T., Bolden, S., & Wingo, P. A. (1998). Cancer Statistics, 1998. *CA: A Cancer Journal for Clinicians, 48:* 6-29.

Lauver, D., & Tak, Y. (1995). Optimism and coping with a breast cancer symptom. *Nursing Research, 44,* 202-206.

Lavery, J., & Clarke, V. (1996). Causal attributions, coping strategies and adjustment to breast cancer. *Cancer Nursing, 19*(1), 20-28.

Leone, A., Flatow, King, C. R., Sandeen, M. A., Marguiles, I. M. K., Liotta, L. A., & Steeg, P. S. (1991). Reduced tumor incidence, metastatic potential, and cytokinetic responsiveness of nm-23-transfected melanoma cells. *Cell, 65,* 25-35.

Lierman, L. M. (1988). Discovery of breast changes. *Cancer Nursing, 11,* 352-358.

Mackarem, G., Barbarisi, L., & Hughes, K. (1992). The role of axillary dissection in early stage breast cancer. *Cancer Investigation, 10*(5), 461-470.

Mandalblatt, J., Andrews, H., Kao, R., Wallace, R., & Kerner, J. (1995). Impact of access and social context on breast cancer stage at diagnosis. *Journal of Health Care for the Poor and Underserved, 6*(3), 342-351.

Mandalblatt, J., Andrews, H., Kerner, J., Zauber, A., & Burnett, W. (1991). Determinants of late stage diagnosis of breast and cervical cancer: The impact of age, race, social class, and hospital type. *American Journal of Public Health, 81*(5), 646-649.

Marks, J. R., Humphrey, P. A., Wu, K., Berry, D., Bandarenko, N., Kerns, B. J., & Iglehart, J. D. (1994). Over expression of p53 and HER-2/neu proteins as prognostic markers in early stage breast cancer. *Annals of Surgery, 219,* 332-341.

Menon, M., Teh, C. H., & Chua, C. L. (1992). Clinical and social problems in young women with breast carcinoma. *Australian and New Zealand Journal of Surgery, 62,* 364-367.

Merchant, T. E., McCormick, B., Yahalom, J., & Borgen, P. (1996). The influence of older age on breast cancer treatment decisions and outcome. *International Journal of Radiation Oncology Biology and Physics, 34*(3), 565-570.

Merrouche, Y., Freyer, G., Saltel, P., & Rebattu, P. (1996). Quality of final care for terminal patients in a comprehensive cancer centre from the point of view of patients' families. *Supportive Care in Cancer, 4*(3), 163-168.

Miaskowski, C. (1997). *Oncology nursing: An essential guide for patient care.* Philadelphia: WB Saunders Co.

Miaskowski, C., & Dibble, S. (1995). The problem of pain in outpatients with breast cancer. *Oncology Nursing Forum, 22*(5), 791-797.

Newschaffer, C. J., Penberthy, L., Desch, C. E., Retchin, S. M., & Whittemore, M. (1996). The effect of age and comorbidity in the treatment of elderly women with nonmetastatic breast cancer. *Archives of Internal Medicine, 156,* 85-90.

NEWS (1996). *Journal of the National Cancer Institute, 88*(23), 1710.

Noguchi, M., Ohta, N., Koyasaki, N., Taniya, T., Miyazaki, I., & Mizukami, Y. (1991). Reappraisal of internal mammary node metastases as a prognostic factor in patients with breast cancer. *Cancer, 68,* 1918-1925.

O'Hanlan, K. (1995). Lesbians in health research. *Recruitment and Retention of Women in Clinical Studies.* Public Health Service. NIH Publication No. 95-3756, Department of Health and Human Services.

Osborne, C. K., Clark, G., & Ravdin, P. (1996). Adjuvant systemic therapy of breast cancer. In J. Harris, M. Lippman, M. Morrow, & S. Hellman (Eds.), *Diseases of the breast.* Philadelphia: Lippincott Raven.

Ownby, H. E., Frederick, J., Russo, J., Brooks, S. C., Swanson, G. M., Heppner, G. H., & Brennan, M. J. (1985). Racial differences in breast cancer patients. *Journal of the National Cancer Institute, 75,* 55-60.

Peteet, J., Tay, V., Cohen, G., & MacIntyre, J. (1986). Patient characteristics and treatment in an outpatient cancer population. *Cancer, 57,* 1259-1265.

Peters, W. P., Bernyi, D., Vredenburgh, J. J., & Hossein, A. (1995). Five year follow-up of high dose combination alkylating agents with autologous bone marrow transplant as consolidation after standard dose CAF for primary breast cancer involving 10 axillary lymph nodes (Duke University/ Protocol CALGB No. 8782) [Abstract]. *Association of the Society for Clinical Oncology, 14,* 317.

Peters, W. P., Ross, M., Vredenburgh, J., Hussein, A., Meisenberg, B., Gilbert, C., Petros, W. P., & Kurtzberg, J. (1993). High dose chemotherapy and autologous bone marrow support as consolidation after standard dose adjuvant therapy for high risk primary breast cancer. *Journal of Clinical Oncology, 11,* 1132-1143.

Petrek, J., & Lerner, R. (1996). Lymphedema. In J. Harris, M. Lippman, M. Morrow, & S. Hellman (Eds.), *Diseases of the breast.* Philadelphia: Lippincott Raven.

Rankow, E. (1995). Lesbian health issues for the primary care provider. *Journal of Family Practice, 48*(5), 486-496.

Ravdin, P. (1995). Taxoids: Effective agents in anthracycline-resistant breast cancer. *Seminars in Oncology, 22*(6, Suppl. 13), 29-34.

Ravdin, P. M., Tandon, A. K., Allred, D. C., Clark, G. M., Fuqua, S. A., Hilsenbeck, S. H., Charmness, G. C., & Osborne, C. K. (1994). Cathepsin-D by western blotting and immunohistochemistry: Failure to confirm correlations with prognosis in node negative breast cancer. *Journal of Clinical Oncology, 12,* 467-474.

Richardson, J. L., Langholz, B., Bernstein, L., Burgiaga, C., Danley, K., & Ross, R. K. (1992). Stage and delay in breast cancer diagnosis by race, socioeconomic status, age and year. *British Journal of Cancer, 65,* 922-926.

Rossi, S., Cinini, C., Di Pietro, C., Lombardi, C., Crucitti, A., Bellatone, R., & Crucitti, F. (1990). Diagnostic delay in breast cancer: Correlation with disease state and prognosis. *Tumori, 76,* 559-562.

Rowland, J., & Massie, M. (1996). Psychologic reactions to breast cancer diagnosis, treatment and survival. In J. Harris, M. Lippman, M. Morrow, & S. Hellman (Eds.), *Diseases of the breast.* Philadelphia: Lippincott Raven.

Satariano, W. A., Belle, S. H., & Swanson, G. M. (1986). The severity of breast cancer at diagnosis: A comparison of age and extent of disease in black and white women. *American Journal of Public Health, 76*(7), 779-782.

Seshadri, R., Horsfall, D. J., Firgaira, F., McCaul, K., Setlur, V., Chalmers, A. H., Yeo, R., Ingram, D., Dawkins, H., & Hahnel, R. (1994). The relative prognostic significance of total cathepsin D and HER-2/neu oncogene amplification in breast cancer: The South Australian Breast Cancer Study Group. *International Journal of Cancer, 56,* 61-65.

Shimizu, K., Shikata, J., Iida, H., Iwasaki, R., Yoshikawa, J., & Yamamuro, T. (1992). Posterior decompression and stabilization for multiple metastatic tumors of the spine. *Spine, 17*(11), 1400-1404.

Shulman, L., & Sugarbaker, D. (1996). Malignant effusions. In J. Harris, M. Lippman, M. Morrow, & S. Hellman (Eds.), *Diseases of the breast.* Philadelphia: Lippincott Raven.

Simon, M. S., & Severson, R. K. (1996). Racial differences in survival of female breast cancer in Detroit metropolitan area. *Cancer 77*(2), 308-314.

Smith, G., & Henderson, C. (1996). New treatments in breast cancer. *Seminars in Oncology, 23*(4), 506-528.

Spiegel, D., Bloom, J., Kraemer, H., & Gottheil, E. (1989). Effect of psychosocial treatment on survival of patients with metastatic breast cancer. *The Lancet, 2*(8668), 888-891.

Stevens, P., Dibble, S, & Miaskowski, C. (1995). Prevalence, characteristics, and impact of postmastectomy pain syndrome: An investigation of women's experiences. *Pain, 61,* 61-68.

Suominen, T., Leino-Kilpi, H., & Laippala, P. (1995). Who provides support and how? *Cancer Nursing, 18*(4), 278-285.

Tandon, A. K., Clark, G. M., Chamness, G. C., Chirgwin, J. M., & McGuire, W. L. (1990). Cathepsin D and prognosis in breast cancer. *New England Journal of Medicine, 322,* 297-302.

Thor, A. D., Moore, D. H., Edgerton, S. M, Kawasaki, E. S., Reihaus, E., Lynch, H. T., Marcus, J. N., Schwartz, L., Chen, L. C., Mayall, B. H., et al. (1992). Accumulation of p53 tumor suppressor gene protein: An independent marker of prognosis in breast cancers. *Journal of the National Cancer Institute, 84,* 845-855.

Tross, S., Herndon, J., Korzun, A., Kornblith, A.B., Cella, D. F., Holland, J. F., Raich, P., Johnson, A., Kiang, D.T., Perloff, M., Norton, L., Wood, W., & Holland, J. C. (1996). Psychological symptoms and disease-free survival in women with Stage II breast cancer. *Journal of the National Cancer Institute, 88*(10), 661.

Vogel, C. (1996). Current status of salvage chemotherapy for refractory advanced breast cancer. *Oncology, 10*(6, Suppl.), 7-15.

Walker, B. L., Nail, L., Larsen, L., Magill, J., & Schwartz, A. (1996). Concerns, affect and cognitive disruption following completion of radiation treatment for localized breast cancer or prostate cancer. *Oncology Nursing Forum, 23*(8), 1181-1187.

Weidner, N., Semple, J. P., Welsh, W. R., & Folkman, J. (1991). Tumor angiogenesis and metastasis: Correlation in invasive breast carcinoma. *New England Journal of Medicine, 324,* 1-8.

Weiss, S. E., Tartter, P. I., Ahmed, S., Brower, S. T., Brusco, C., Bossolt, K., Amberson, J. B., & Bratton, J. (1995). Ethnic differences in risk and prognostic factors for breast cancer. *Cancer, 76*(2), 268-274.

Williams, W. L., Powers, M., & Wagman, L. D. (1996). Cancer of the male breast: A review. *Journal of the National Medical Association. 88*(7), 439-443.

Winer, B. (1996). Treatment options for patients with refractory breast cancer. *Oncology, 10*(6, Suppl.), 16-20.

Yeatman, T. J. (1995). The natural history of locally advanced primary breast carcinoma and metastatic disease. *Surgical Oncology Clinics of North America, 4*(4), 569-589.

Zaloznik, A. L. (1995). Breast cancer stage at diagnosis: Caucasians versus Afro-Americans. *British Cancer Research and Treatment, 34,* 195-198.

Ziegfeld, C.R. (1992). *Core curriculum for oncology nursing.* Philadelphia: W. B. Saunders Company: Oncology Nursing Society.

Astrocytoma

Karen Belford, RN, MS
Ruth Gargon-Klinger, RN, MSN, ANP

EPIDEMIOLOGY

Primary central nervous system (CNS) cancers include tumors of the brain and spinal cord. They account for less than 2% of all cancers diagnosed in the United States and are a major source of morbidity and mortality. An estimated 34,422 new cases of primary benign and malignant CNS tumors were diagnosed in 1996 (Central Brain Tumor Registry of the United States [CBTRUS], 1997). Of these cases, 17,600 were malignant (Parker, Tong, Bolden, & Wingo, 1997). It is estimated that 17,400 new malignant CNS tumors will be diagnosed in 1998 (Landis, Murray, Bolden, & Wingo, 1998). Astrocytomas are the most common primary CNS tumor. Spinal cord tumors compose only 4% to 10% of CNS tumors (Constantini, Allen, & Epstein, 1997), and 20% are estimated to be malignant (McCormick & Stein, 1996). Spinal cord astrocytomas account for 6% to 8% of all spinal cord tumors. Approximately 13,300 deaths in 1996 were attributed to malignant CNS tumors (Central Brain Tumor Registry of the United States [CBTRUS], 1997), making them responsible for 2.4% of all cancer-related deaths (Parker et al., 1997). In women between the ages of 15 and 34, CNS tumors are now the fourth leading cause of cancer mortality (they had been the third). In men between the ages of 15 and 34, they are the third, and in men between 35 and 54 years, CNS cancers are the fourth leading cause of cancer-related mortality (Parker et al., 1997; Landis et al., 1998). The majority of these deaths result from high-grade astrocytomas (Levin, Leibel, & Gutin, 1997).

Low-grade astrocytomas (LGAs) represent approximately 10% of all CNS tumors, whereas the high-grade astrocytomas (anaplastic astrocytoma [AA] and glioblastoma multiforme [GBM]) account for 33% to 45% of these tumors (Bruner, 1994). Of these high-grade astrocytomas, 20% to 40% are the AAs (GBM is discussed in Chapter 25). LGAs are most prevalent in the 20 to 40 year age range and the AAs in the 30 to 50 year age range. AAs are slightly more prevalent in men than women and in whites than blacks, Latinos, and Asians (Radhakrishnan, Bohnen, & Kurland, 1994).

The incidence of primary malignant brain tumors may be increasing in the elderly (Riggs, 1995). However, controversy exists as to whether the reported increase is a true increase or the result of improved and increasingly available diagnostic methods. Other possible explanations include increased longevity, changing attitudes toward the care of the elderly, more physician awareness of the prevalence of the disease, and more informed medical consumerism (American Brain Tumor Association, 1996).

Historically, it has been difficult to estimate the true epidemiology of CNS tumors. Fifteen cell types can potentially give rise to CNS tumors (Levin et al., 1997), and many tumors consist of a combination of these cell types. Many classification systems are used to group these tumors, which may lead to inconsistency in data collection and interpretation. In the United States, data on the incidence of cancer are routinely collected by two organizations, the Surveillance, Epidemiology, and End Results (SEER) program of the National Cancer Institute (NCI) and the North American Association of Central Cancer Registries (NAACCR). Currently, these programs report only malignant CNS tumors in their standard incidence reports (CBTRUS, 1997). Therefore the true incidence of CNS tumors may be underreported because many benign tumors are excluded. Recently, the American Brain Tumor Association (ABTA) founded the CBTRUS to gather incidence information on all benign and malignant brain tumors. The registry is working toward including data from all tumor registries in the United States and is attempting to standardize the histologic classification of CNS tumors based on the World Health Organization's (WHO) system (CBTRUS, 1997).

RISK FACTORS

The majority of CNS cancers are sporadic and are not thought to be associated with specific risk factors. Many factors have been evaluated as possible etiologic agents, but much of the epidemiologic evidence is inadequate, inconclusive, or mostly negative (Bohnen, Radhakrishnan, O'Neill, & Kurland, 1997; Wrensch, Bondy, Wiencke, & Yost, 1993). As shown in Box 23-1, some of the potential risk factors that have been examined include heredity,

Box 23-1
Risk Factors for Astrocytomas

Previous radiation to the head and neck area
Genetic disorders
- Neurofibromatosis Type I (NF-1)
- Tuberous Sclerosis (Bourneville's Disease)
- Li-Fraumeni Syndrome
- Turcot Syndrome

Electromagnetic fields (? association)
Chemical and occupational exposure (? association)
Chromosomal alterations (? association)

chemicals, environment, ionizing radiation, and electromagnetic fields (EMFs).

Genetic Disorders

Only approximately 5% of all CNS tumors are associated with specific hereditary factors (American Brain Tumor Association, 1996). This group of tumors is the basis for the National Familial Brain Tumor Registry whose goals are to document that some brain tumors can occur as a familial disorder, to gain further insight into the etiologic factors of these tumors by evaluating affected families, and to serve as a resource for investigators interested in pursuing this area of study (Brem, Rozental, & Moskal, 1995). Persons with four autosomal dominant disorders (i.e., neurofibromatosis, Li-Fraumeni syndrome, tuberous sclerosis, and Turcot's syndrome) have a higher incidence of brain tumors than the general population (American Brain Tumor Association, 1996).

Neurofibromatosis type 1 (NF-1) has an incidence of 1 in 3000 (Watkins & Rouleau, 1994). Approximately 15% of patients with NF-1 have low-grade optic nerve gliomas, cerebellar astrocytomas, pilocytic astrocytomas, and high-grade astrocytomas (Bohnen et al., 1997). Neurofibromatosis type 2 (NF-2) occurs only about one-tenth as frequently as NF-1 and has been associated with LGAs and other tumor types (Bondy, Wiencke, Wrensch, & Kyritsis, 1994). The Li-Fraumeni syndrome has an increased incidence of a number of different types of cancer including gliomas. In a study by Li and colleagues (1988), this cancer family syndrome was described in 24 kindreds in whom 9% of the tumors were brain tumors. Tuberous sclerosis (Bourneville's disease) has a reported incidence of 1 in 10,000 to 1 in 50,000 people (Watkins & Rouleau, 1994). About one half of the patients who have this disorder develop subependymal giant cell astrocytomas (National Brain Tumor Foundation, 1994). Turcot syndrome, a syndrome of CNS tumors, occurs in 5% of patients with adenomatous polyposis coli (Watkins & Rouleau, 1994).

Previous Radiation Therapy

A history of therapeutic radiation to the head and neck is associated with the subsequent development of malignant astrocytomas. Brain tumors have occurred after radiation therapy (RT) in childhood for the treatment of acute lymphoblastic leukemia (Neglia et al., 1991; Shapiro & Mealey, 1989), after RT for the treatment of tinea capitis (Ron et al., 1988), and after RT for the treatment of pituitary adenomas in adults (Tsang et al., 1993). Hodges, Smith, and Garrett (1992) performed a retrospective review of 100 patients with malignant astrocytomas and reported that 17% had previously received therapeutic RT. However, a history of prior RT accounts for only a small percentage of the cases of astrocytomas.

Chemical and Occupational Exposure

Thomas and Waxweiler (1986) reviewed brain tumors and possible occupational risk factors. Although a variety of chemicals have been shown to induce brain tumors in experimental animals, the possible association between brain tumors and chemical exposure is limited to a few occupations. Occupational groups reported to have an elevated risk of astrocytomas and other brain tumors include those working with synthetic rubber production, petroleum refining and petrochemical production, polyvinyl chloride, formaldehyde, pesticides, herbicides, and precision metal work. At this time, no association with a specific occupational exposure and the increased risk of developing a brain tumor is recognized universally (Berleur & Cordier, 1995). The nature and strength of the role specific chemicals play in neuro-oncogenesis in human beings remain controversial (Wrensch, Bondy, Wiencke, & Yost, 1993) in part because of various methodologic limitations in the epidemiologic studies. In many instances, it is extremely difficult to isolate a particular chemical or exposure. Many workers have multiple types of exposures. Small numbers of cases make it difficult to reach statistical significance. Work histories and brain tumor confirmation are often difficult to ascertain, and an adequate means of assessing cumulative exposures is lacking.

Electromagnetic Fields

Controversy exists regarding the possible association between extremely low frequency electromagnetic fields (ELF-EMFs) and the development of brain tumors. Occupations likely to have higher than average levels of exposure to EMFs include electricians, railway workers, communications workers, and welders (Berleur & Cordier, 1995; Bohnen et al., 1997). However, occupational exposure may be just a fraction of the total EMF exposure (Floderus et al., 1993). Nonoccupational exposure to EMFs is extremely widespread in today's industrialized society; sources include residential heating and electrical appliances, electric power lines and transformers, hand-held radios, and cellular telephones.

The mechanism of the carcinogenic action of EMFs is not well understood. It has been suggested that EMFs may act as a cancer promoter. Although some positive correlations have been reported, the evidence is inconsistent. No definitive studies have linked exposure to EMFs with astrocytomas. Methodologic problems in some of the studies include small sample sizes, few studies conducted in adults, an inability to precisely measure the overall EMF exposure, incorrect classification of individuals as either exposed or unexposed, and lack of attention to the potential interactions between EMFs and other carcinogenic factors. Further studies of the possible association between residential, occupational, and recreational exposure of ELF-EMFs and brain tumors are required.

CHEMOPREVENTION

No chemoprevention, screening, or early detection activities are available for astrocytomas. However, individuals with specific hereditary syndromes that may suggest a predisposition to astrocytomas can be informed of their genetic risk.

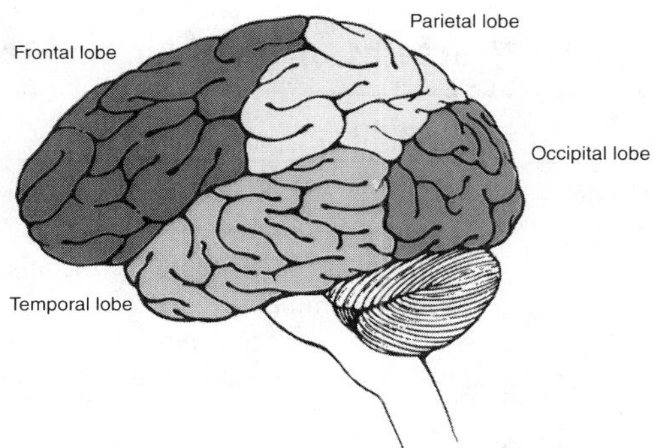

Fig. 23-1 Lobes of the cerebral hemispheres.

PATHOPHYSIOLOGY

The nervous system is composed of the peripheral nervous system and the CNS. The peripheral nervous system includes the cranial and spinal nerves; the CNS includes the brain and spinal cord. The autonomic nervous system, often considered separately, is part of both the central and peripheral nervous systems. The nervous system contains two types of cells: neurons and glial cells. Neurons are the basic functional unit of the nervous system. They respond to sensory and chemical stimuli, conduct impulses, and release chemical regulators (Hickey, 1992). The glial cells support, nourish, and protect the neurons. Six types of glial cells are found in the nervous system: astrocytes, oligodendrocytes, ependymal cells, Schwann cells, microglia, and satellite cells. The glial cells compose almost half the volume of the CNS and outnumber the neurons 10 to 1. Unlike neurons, glial cells in the adult nervous system retain their capacity to divide. Glial cells can undergo anaplasia and are the major source of primary tumors of the CNS.

The specific tumor type is derived from its glial cell of origin. For example, astrocytomas arise from the glial cell, the astrocyte. The astrocytes have a characteristic starlike appearance. These cells are commonly found between nerve tissue and blood vessels. Astrocytes form a structural support between capillaries and neurons; convey nutrients, gases, and wastes between neurons and blood vessels or between neurons and cerebrospinal fluid (CSF); and make repairs after damage caused by disease or trauma (Hickey, 1992). For the purposes of review and discussion, sections of this chapter have been divided into astrocytomas of the brain (intracranial) and astrocytomas of the spinal cord.

Normal Anatomy and Physiology of the Brain

The brain is divided into three main areas: the cerebrum, brain stem, and cerebellum. The cerebrum consists of the two cerebral hemispheres and the diencephalon. The two cerebral hemispheres are connected by a thick band of nerve fibers, the corpus callosum, which enables each portion of one hemisphere to connect with its corresponding portion in the other. It essentially allows communication between the two hemispheres (Leahy, 1990). The surface of the cerebral hemispheres contains folds or convolutions called *gyri,* which increase the surface area of the brain. Deeper grooves between the gyri are called *fissures* or *sulci.* The right hemisphere is separated from the left by the longitudinal fissure. Each cerebral hemisphere is anatomically divided into a frontal, parietal, temporal, and occipital lobe based on these fissures (Fig. 23-1). The central sulcus separates the frontal and parietal lobes. The lateral fissure, also called the *Sylvian fissure,* separates the frontal and temporal lobes. The parieto-occipital sulcus divides the parietal and occipital lobes. The separation between the occipital and temporal lobes is less obvious. Other structures located deep within the cerebral hemispheres are the basal ganglia, which are masses of gray matter.

The diencephalon consists of the thalamus, hypothalamus, epithalamus, and subthalamus. The midbrain, pons, and medulla form the brain stem. The cerebellum consists of two lobes or hemispheres and a midline portion called the *vermis.* The cerebellum is attached to the brain stem by cerebral peduncles. The functions of these structures are listed in Table 23-1.

The brain is a delicate structure requiring protection and support. It is encased by the rigid bony skull and surrounded by the CSF and meninges. The meninges are the three layers of connective tissue covering the brain and spinal cord. They are the dura mater, arachnoid, and pia mater (Fig. 23-2). The outermost meningeal layer, the dura mater, is a thick tough double-layered membrane. The outer dural layer adheres to the inner surface of the skull forming the periosteum of the cranial cavity. A potential space between the dura and the skull is the epidural space. The inner dural layer contains blood vessels and nerves and folds in on itself to create anatomic compartments. The falx cerebri, the tentorium cerebelli, and the falx cerebelli are three such folds (Belford, 1997). The falx cerebri extends vertically and separates the two cerebral hemispheres. The tentorium cerebelli lies between the occipital lobes of the cerebral hemispheres and the cerebellum, dividing the cranial cavity into the supratentorial and infratentorial compartments. Structures and tumors found above the tentorium cerebelli (cerebral hemispheres, diencephalon, and basal ganglia) are said to be in the supratentorial compartment. Those below the

Table 23-1 Structures of the Brain and Their Functions

Location	Function	Pathology
Frontal lobe	Motor/motor association (contralateral)	Hemiparesis, hemiplegia
	Personality features	Mood disturbances, affect
	Intellect, judgment (dominant frontal lobe)	Cognitive deficits
	Speech (dominant frontal lobe)	Dysphasia, Broca's aphasia, word-finding difficulty
	Secondary urinary control	Incontinence
Parietal lobe	Sensory modalities: touch, pain, vibration, pressure (contralateral)	Loss of sensation
	Ability to carry out and understand special constructs (e.g., math, reading)	Construction apraxia, astereognosis, finger agnosia, loss of right-left discrimination, agraphia, acalculi
	Visual	Visual loss in the inferior aspect of the contralateral visual field
Temporal lobe	Visual	Visual field loss in the superior quadrant of the contralateral field
	Speech (dominant temporal lobe)	Inability to understand simple or multistep commands, Wernicke's aphasia
	Short-term memory	Memory loss
Occipital lobe	Vision	Contralateral homonymous hemianopsia
		Visual hallucinations
Cerebellum	Reflex/involuntary fine tuning of muscle control	Ataxia, coordination abnormalities, nystagmus
	Gait and station	Wide-based gait
Brain stem	Corticospinal tracts (motor)	Motor abnormalities
	Spinothalamic tracts (sensory)	Sensory abnormalities
	Spinocerebella tracts	Coordination abnormalities
Midbrain	Voluntary gaze stimulated	Gaze abnormality
	Stimulus-induced involuntary gaze	Gaze abnormality
	Cranial nerves III, IV	Cranial nerve deficit, eye movement
Pons	Cranial nerves V, VI, VII, VIII	Facial sensation, eye movement, facial movement, and hearing
	Respiratory control	Abnormal respiratory patterns
Medulla	Reflex activities: heart rate, respiration, blood pressure, cough, sneezing, swallowing, vomiting	Abnormalities of reflex activities
	Cranial nerves IX-XII	Cranial nerve deficit, dysphagia
Thalamus	Major integrating center for sensory impulses to the cerebral cortex	Hyperesthesia, sensory abnormalities, contralateral impairment of peripheral sensation, astereognosis, hemiataxia
	Conscious awareness of pain	Spontaneous pain in the contralateral half of the body
Pineal gland	Secretory role related to growth and development—not well understood	?
Hypothalamus	Temperature control	Hypo/hyperthermia
	Water metabolism	Abnormalities in the reabsorption of free water
	Appetite control	Increase/decrease in appetite
	Autonomic nervous system control of visceral and somatic activities	Abnormalities in sweating, vasodilation, hypotonia, pulse
	Growth hormone	Growth abnormalities
	Regulation of part of the sleep/wake cycle	
	Control of affective behavior	Emotional liability
	Sexual behavior	
Basal ganglia	Fine motor control	Intention tremors, weakness or paralysis, parkinsonism

tentorium (brain stem and cerebellum) are in the infratentorial compartment, also known as the *posterior fossa.* The falx cerebelli separates the two lobes of the cerebellum. In addition, the dural layers separate and form large venous sinuses. These sinuses or endothelial-lined spaces occur along the attachment of dural folds and are part of the venous circulation of the brain.

The middle meningeal layer, the arachnoid, is a nonvascular membrane between the pia mater and dura mater. It loosely covers the brain, passing over the sulci without following their contours. The potential space between the dura and arachnoid is the subdural space, a common site of hematomas. The pia mater, the innermost meningeal layer, is a thin vascular translucent membrane that dips into all the

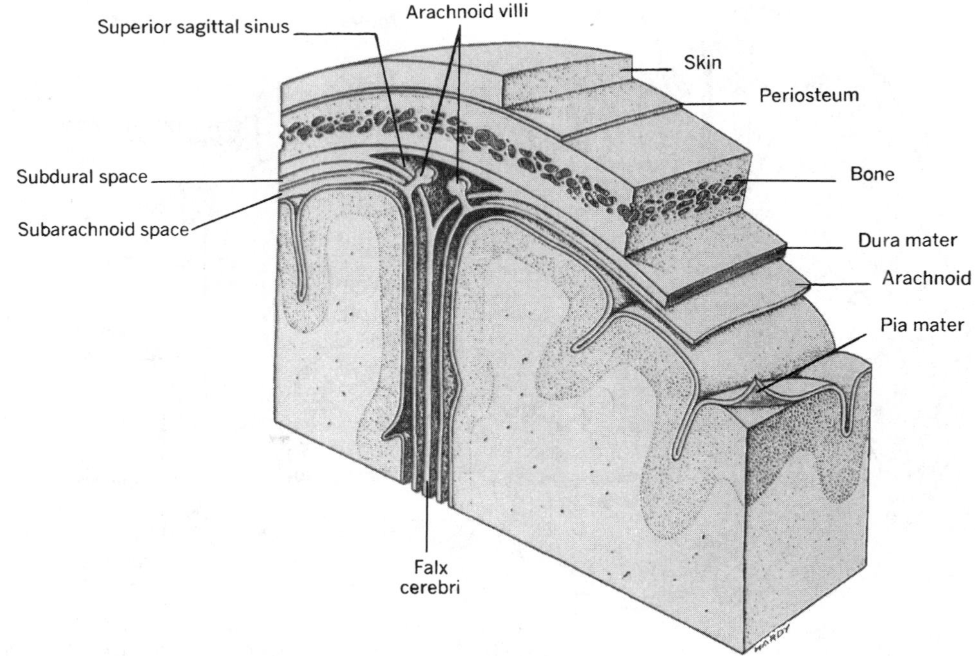

Fig. 23-2 The cranial meninges. (From Hickey, J. V. [1992]. *The clinical practice of neurological and neurosurgical nursing* [3rd ed.]. Philadelphia: J. B. Lippincott.)

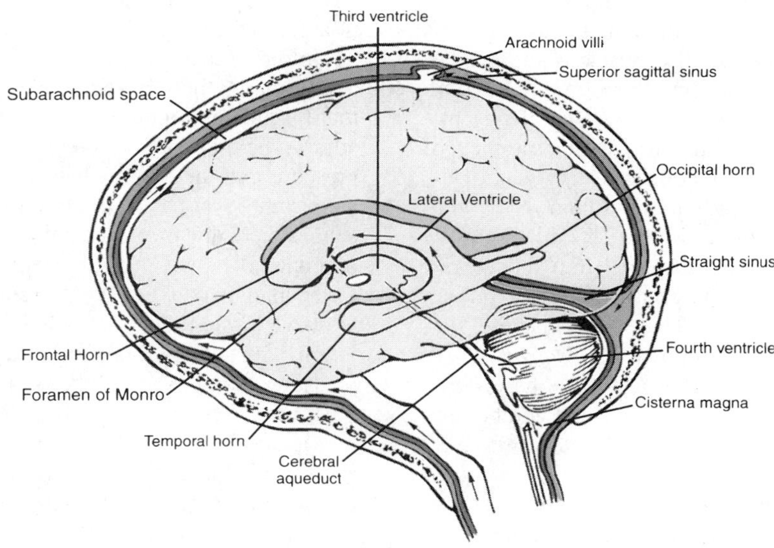

Fig. 23-3 The ventricular system.

fissures and sulci and adheres directly to the surface of the brain. The pia and the arachnoid layers together are referred to as the *leptomeninges.* The space between the arachnoid and the pia mater is the subarachnoid space, where CSF circulates.

The ventricular system (Fig. 23-3) consists of a series of interconnected chambers and pathways responsible for the production and circulation of CSF around the brain and spinal cord (Gilman & Newman, 1992). CSF is a clear, colorless fluid containing protein, glucose, electrolytes, and other substances. The CSF may allow for the exchange of nutrients and waste materials between the blood and cells of the CNS. It is formed by the choroid plexuses, the cauliflower-like structures located in the two lateral, third, and fourth ventricles. Approximately 20 ml of CSF are produced hourly. The lateral ventricles, located in the cerebral hemispheres, are divided into the frontal, temporal, and occipital horns. The lateral ventricles communicate with the third

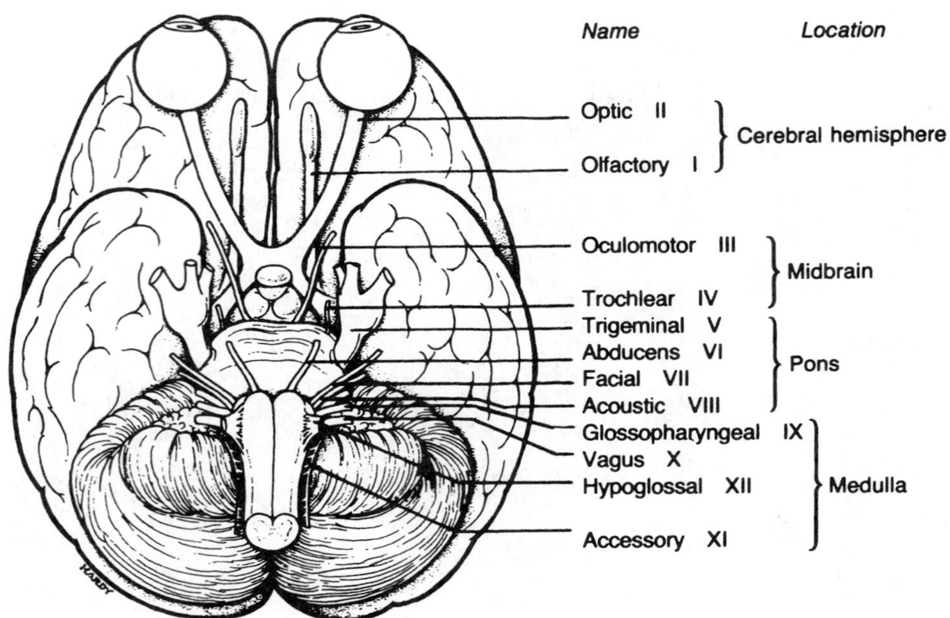

Fig. 23-4 The cranial nerves. (From Hickey, J. V. [1992]. *The clinical practice of neurological and neurosurgical nursing* [3rd ed.]. Philadelphia: J. B. Lippincott.)

ventricle through the foramina of Monro (intraventricular foramina). The third ventricle is located beneath the corpus callosum and surrounded by the thalamus. The third and fourth ventricles are connected by the aqueduct of Sylvius or the cerebral aqueduct. The fourth ventricle is situated between the two hemispheres of the cerebellum. The CSF leaves the fourth ventricle through the foramina of Luschka to circulate around the brain and through the foramen of Magendie to circulate around the spinal cord by way of the subarachnoid space. The volume of CSF found in the ventricular system at any one time is 125 to 150 ml. From the subarachnoid space, the CSF is absorbed into the venous circulation by the arachnoid villi, small fingerlike projections of the arachnoid membrane. There are expanded sections of the subarachnoid space known as *cisterns,* where CSF may be aspirated. Two major cisterns are the cisterna magnum, located between the medulla and the cerebellum, and the lumbar cistern, between vertebrae L2 and S2 (Hickey, 1992).

The 12 pairs of cranial nerves found in the brain are responsible for sensory and motor functions of the head and neck (Fig. 23-4). Each pair of cranial nerves is represented by a Roman numeral and can be classified as motor, sensory, motor and sensory, or autonomic. The cranial nerves and their functions are listed in Table 23-2.

The cerebral circulation is one of the body's most complex and metabolically active systems. The human brain constitutes only 2% of the total body weight; yet, it receives 15% to 20% of the body's cardiac output each minute. Approximately 20% of the oxygen consumed by the body is used for the oxidation of glucose to provide energy. The brain is totally dependent on glucose for its metabolism. An adequate cerebral blood flow (CBF) is necessary to deliver oxygen, glucose, and other nutrients and to remove carbon dioxide and other metabolic products. Because the CNS has little ability to store oxygen and glucose in its tissue, the CBF must remain relatively constant. Even a brief circulation failure can result in temporary or permanent loss of neurologic function.

Normally, the CBF is maintained at a relatively constant rate by the autoregulatory mechanism, which automatically adjusts the diameter of cerebral blood vessels in response to pressure and metabolic changes. The CBF is maintained at a constant level by the dilation or constriction of blood vessels. When the mean systemic arterial pressure (SAP) is maintained between 60 mm Hg and 140 mm Hg, there is little change in CBF and cerebral blood volume (CBV). However, when the SAP falls below 60 mm Hg, autoregulation fails and CBF begins to fall passively with the blood pressure. Conversely, if the SAP rises above 160 mm Hg, CBF increases.

Metabolic factors that influence autoregulation include $PaCO_2$, pH, and PaO_2. The autoregulation is most sensitive to $PaCO_2$. Increases in $PaCO_2$ cause vasodilation leading to an increase in CBF and conversely, a decrease in $PaCO_2$ results in vasoconstriction and a decrease in CBF. The cerebral blood vessels are less sensitive to changes in the PaO_2. Generally, vasodilation does not occur until the PaO_2 falls in the hypoxic range, leading to an increase in CBF.

The arterial blood supply of the brain is supplied by the two internal carotid and the two vertebral arteries. The internal carotid arteries form the anterior circulation and the vertebral arteries form the posterior circulation. An important subdivision of the internal carotid arteries is their bifurcation into the anterior and middle cerebral arteries. The anterior cerebral artery supplies the corpus callosum and the medial aspect of the anterior half of each cerebral hemisphere. The anterior cerebral artery also has subdivisions

TABLE 23-2 Assessment and Function of the Cranial Nerves

Cranial Nerve	Major Function	Method of Testing	Expected Response
I. Olfactory	Sense of smell	Have patient close eyes, occlude one nostril, and identify commonly recognized odors such as coffee, mint, lemon, etc. Repeat with other nostril. Avoid noxious substances such as alcohol or ammonia.	The patient will correctly identify substances with each nostril.
II. Optic	Vision	Have patient read Snellen chart with one eye covered to assess visual acuity. Repeat with the other eye.	The patient accurately reads the eye chart.
		To assess visual fields, have patient close one eye. The examiner closes the opposite eye and positions his finger off to the side and then brings his moving finger into the boundaries of the visual field. Repeat with the other eye.	The patient is able to see the moving finger within acceptable distance with both eyes.
		The optic disc is visualized with an ophthalmoscopic examination.	The appearance of the optic disc is normal.
III. Oculomotor	Lid elevation Pupil constriction and accommodation	Observe for ptosis of the eyelid. Assess pupillary response to light.	Eyes are symmetrical. Pupils react equally and briskly to light, have a consensual response, and accommodate.
	Movement of eyes in 4 of the 6 cardinal directions of gaze (inward, upward, downward, upward and outward)	Have patient follow examiner's finger with his eyes while not moving his head through the six cardinal directions of gaze.	The eye movements are equal in the cardinal directions of gaze. Diplopia and nystagmus are absent.
IV. Trochlear	Movement of eyes down and inward	Have patient follow examiner's finger with his eyes while not moving his head through the six cardinal directions of gaze.	The eye movements are equal. Diplopia and nystagmus are absent.
V. Trigeminal	Jaw movement	Have patient open his mouth and hold open tightly while examiner attempts to close it.	Jaw movement is strong and symmetrical.
	Facial sensation (scalp, face, and mouth)	Have patient close eyes and then have examiner touch various parts of face on both sides to assess touch, pain, and temperature.	Patient correctly identifies sensations.
	Corneal reflex	Examiner gently touches patient's cornea with a cotton wisp.	There is rapid blinking.
VI. Abducens	Lateral movement of the eyes	Have the patient follow examiner's finger with his eyes while not moving his head through the 6 cardinal directions of gaze.	The eye movements are equal. Diplopia and nystagmus are absent.

Continued

Table 23-2 Assessment and Function of the Cranial Nerves—cont'd

Cranial Nerve	Major Function	Method of Testing	Expected Response
VII. Facial	Facial muscles	Have patient smile, show teeth, frown, wrinkle brow, and close eyes tightly.	Movements are symmetrical.
	Taste to anterior 2/3 of tongue	Have patient taste sweet, sour, salty, and acidic flavors.	Patient correctly identifies flavors.
	Tearing Salivation		
VIII. Acoustic (Cochlear and Vestibular)	Hearing	Examiner assesses hearing ability using whispered words and tuning fork at varying distances from the ear.	Patient recognizes sound.
	Balance and equilibrium	Have patient stand on one foot with eyes closed. Switch feet.	Patient maintains balance.
IX. Glossopharyngeal (IX and X are assessed together because of overlapping innervation of the pharynx)	Gag and swallowing	Have patient say "Ah."	Soft palate and uvula elevate in the midline.
		Have patient protrude tongue. Examiner gently touches back of pharynx with tongue depressor.	Gag response is present.
		Have patient drink fluid.	No dysphagia present.
	Taste to posterior 1/3 of tongue	Have patient taste different flavors.	Patient correctly identifies flavors.
	Salivation		
X. Vagus	Gag and swallowing Articulation and phonation Heart rate, peristalsis (parasympathetic innervation to thoracic and abdominal viscera)	Have patient cough and speak.	Patient articulates clearly. No hoarseness is present.
XI. Accessory	Head and shoulder movement (Control of trapezius and sternocleido-mastoid muscles)	Have patient raise (shrug) shoulders and hold tightly while examiner applies pressure. Have patient turn his head to the side and resist the examiner's attempt to bring head back to midline.	Strength is equal bilaterally.
		Repeat on opposite side. Assess for muscle symmetry.	No atrophy is present.
XII. Hypoglossal	Tongue movement	Have patient protrude tongue and move from side to side and up and down.	Tongue is midline. No atrophy or tremors are present.

that supply the basal ganglia and other deep structures. The middle cerebral arteries supply the anterior two thirds of the temporal lobe and the lateral aspect of the frontal and parietal lobes. The middle cerebral artery also has small branches that supply deep structures including the basal ganglia.

The vertebral arteries run along the vertebral column and join to form the basilar artery at the pontomedullary junction (where the pons and medulla join). Branches of the vertebral arteries include the posterior inferior cerebellar arteries and the anterior and posterior spinal arteries. Along its course the basilar artery has further subdivisions, which include the anterior inferior cerebellar, the superior cerebellar, the posterior cerebral, and the pontine arteries. These vessels supply the occipital lobe, brain stem, and cerebellum. These major vessels are independent until they become interconnected at the circle of Willis.

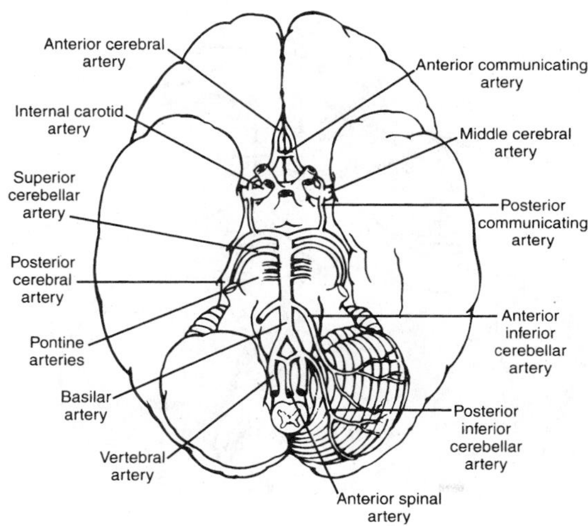

Fig. 23-5 The circle of Willis.

The circle of Willis (Fig. 23-5) is located at the base of the brain and is formed by the anterior and posterior communicating arteries and part of the anterior, middle, and posterior cerebral arteries. It can permit an adequate blood supply to all parts of the brain even when flow is impaired in one of the major vessels. However, collateral circulation through the circle depends on the presence and patency of all of its components. Significant anatomic variations are common, especially with the communicating arteries. Blood vessels in the meninges also help to ensure collateral circulation in the brain (Belford, 1997).

The cerebral venous circulation consists of veins located on the surface of the brain and dural venous sinuses deep within the brain. Dural sinuses are vascular channels located between the two dural layers. An important sinus is the superior sagittal sinus. It lies superior to the falx cerebri and drains the lateral and superior aspects of the hemispheres. In addition, this area is the major site of CSF reabsorption. Cerebral veins drain into the cerebral sinuses, empty into the jugular veins, and return blood to the heart. Obstruction of venous outflow can result in increased intracranial pressure (ICP).

Dynamics of ICP

A review of normal ICP dynamics is helpful in understanding the pathophysiology of brain tumors. *ICP* is defined as the pressure exerted within the skull and meninges by the brain tissue, CSF, and CBV. The brain tissue makes up 80%, the CSF 10%, and the blood volume 10% of this intracranial volume. The skull and meninges form a rigid compartment around the three components and are unyielding to any increase in volume. According to the Monro-Kellie doctrine, if one component increases in volume, a concomitant decrease in the volume of one or both of the remaining components must occur to maintain a normal ICP. If this reciprocal decrease does not occur, ICP begins to rise. The normal range of ICP is 0 to 15 mm Hg. The mechanism by which the body attempts to decrease the volume is called *compensation.*

Compensation can occur whenever an insult to the brain leads to an increase in brain, blood, or CSF volume (Andrus, 1991). Astrocytomas increase the brain mass, and the often accompanying edema further expands the volume. To maintain a normal ICP, the compensatory mechanisms begin to reduce the amount of CSF, blood volume, or both. The CSF in the cranial subarachnoid space is displaced to the spinal subarachnoid space, and the arachnoid villi increase the amount of CSF that is absorbed into the venous circulation. When increased ICP is sustained for prolonged periods, the choroid plexuses can decrease the amount of CSF they produce. The next mechanism decreases the CBV, and the venous blood is shunted away from the affected area into the venous sinuses (Barr & Kiernan, 1988).

Increases in volume made over long periods can be better accommodated than the same amount introduced within a much shorter interval. The compensatory mechanisms are usually more effective if the tumor is small or grows slowly. However, these mechanisms are finite and eventually become exhausted. Once they have been depleted, ICP rises. At this point, relatively small increases in volume will result in large increases in ICP.

Another important consideration associated with ICP is the cerebral venous system. The cerebral veins do not have valves as do other venous blood vessels in the body. Any condition that obstructs or compromises venous outflow can increase CBV because more blood backs up in the intracranial cavity (Hickey, 1992). Activities such as coughing, sneezing, straining at stool, or performing a Valsalva maneuver increase intrathoracic and intraabdominal pressures. Cerebral venous outflow by way of the jugular veins decreases, leading to increased ICP (Andrus, 1991). Extreme flexion or extension of the neck or sudden position changes may also obstruct venous outflow. Maintaining proper head alignment and elevating the head of the bed facilitate venous drainage. Hip flexion, lying on the abdomen, and positive end-expiratory pressure may also increase intrathoracic and intra-abdominal pressures, leading to increased ICP.

Normally, fluctuations in intracranial volume are constantly occurring in response to changes in systemic blood pressure, changes in arterial blood gas values, and alterations in intrathoracic and intra-abdominal pressures. However, these fluctuations are transient, and the autoregulatory and compensatory mechanisms function appropriately. The presence of a brain tumor can compromise these mechanisms and cause sustained elevations in ICP.

Normal Anatomy and Physiology of the Spinal Cord

The spinal cord is part of the CNS. It is an elongated cylindrical mass of nervous tissue encased in the bony structure of the vertebral column (Fig. 23-6). The spinal cord extends from the first cervical vertebra to the level of the intravertebral disk between the first and second lumbar vertebrae. The most inferior portion of the spinal cord, the conus medullaris, is usually found at the intravertebral level between

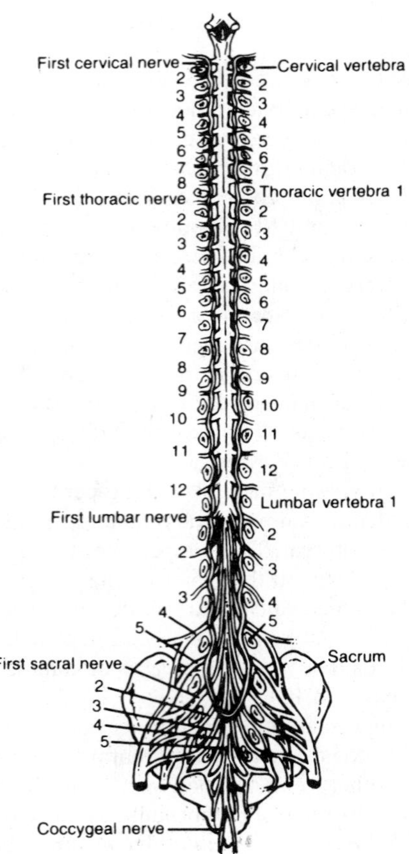

Fig. 23-6 The spinal cord lying within the vertebral column. The vertebrae are numbered on the right side and the spinal nerves are numbered on the left side.

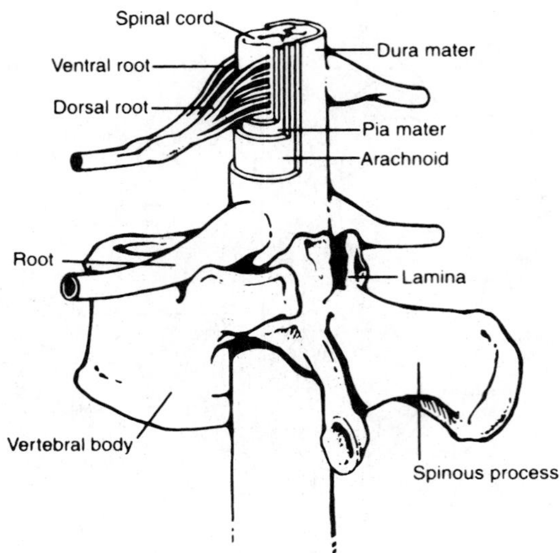

Fig. 23-7 The spinal meninges.

L1 and L2. The cauda equina, which consists of the lumbar and sacral nerve roots, begins at the level of the conus medullaris. Beyond the conus, the spinal cord itself continues as the filum terminale, a thin cord of connective tissue with no nervous elements.

The spinal cord is enclosed in the meninges (Fig. 23-7). The spinal dura mater, arachnoid, and pia mater are contiguous with the brain coverings. The outer layer, the dura mater, extends below the cauda equina, ending as a blind sac at the level of the second sacral vertebra. The dura covers the spinal nerve roots as they leave the cord and exit through the intervertebral foramina. The arachnoid forms the middle layer. The pia mater is the thin vascular membrane that adheres to the cord and ends as the filum terminale.

Thirty-one pairs of spinal nerves originate from the spinal cord: 8 cervical, 12 thoracic, 5 lumbar, 5 sacral, and 1 coccygeal nerve (Fig. 23-6). They innervate specific regions of the skin, muscle, and connective tissue with sensory and motor fibers. The posterior or dorsal root is the sensory portion and supplies impulses from the periphery to the cord. The spinal nerves are organized in a segmental fashion and are illustrated by the sensory dermatomes. A dermatome is a region of the skin supplied by individual sensory fibers. A chart of the dermatomes is a useful aid in the localization of spinal cord lesions (Fig. 23-8); however, some overlap exists between dermatomes. The anterior or ventral root is the motor portion and sends impulses to the periphery. A similar segmental organization is present with regard to motor innervation. Specific areas of muscle innervation are referred to as *myotomes* and are listed in Table 23-3.

The spinal cord is composed of two types of tissue: gray matter and white matter; the glial cells provide a supportive framework. Gray matter consists of nerve cells, dendrites, blood vessels, and a large number of neuroglial cells. A cross-section of the spinal cord shows the distribution of the gray matter within the central cord and the white matter forming the periphery. The pattern of gray and white matter viewed through a cross-section forms an H shape. This distribution of gray and white matter varies at different levels in the cord. The variations in the amount of gray matter at each segmental level relate to the number of nerve fibers. In the cervical and lumbar-sacral regions, the enlargement of the gray matter is responsible for limb innervation. The gray matter is divided into two ventral (anterior) horns, two dorsal (posterior) horns, and the intermediate gray region. In the thoracic and upper lumbar regions, a lateral horn is present. The neuronal cell bodies in the posterior horns are responsible for sensory input to the spinal cord. The anterior horns contain motor neurons responsible for motor functions. The lateral horn contains autonomic preganglionic motor neurons.

White matter forms the bulk of the spinal cord. It consists of a bundle of myelinated and nonmyelinated nerve fibers. Each half of the spinal cord is divided into funiculi (columns). The posterior, lateral, and anterior funiculi contain the long ascending and descending fiber tracts. The tracts are arranged according to their function, origin, and termination. The main tracts, their functions, and possible pathology are presented in Table 23-4.

The blood supply to the spinal cord is provided by the anterior spinal artery and the two posterior spinal arteries. The posterior spinal arteries descend along the posterior cord and receive additional blood supply from posterior radicular arteries. The anterior spinal artery supplies the anterior two thirds of the spinal cord. It arises from two small

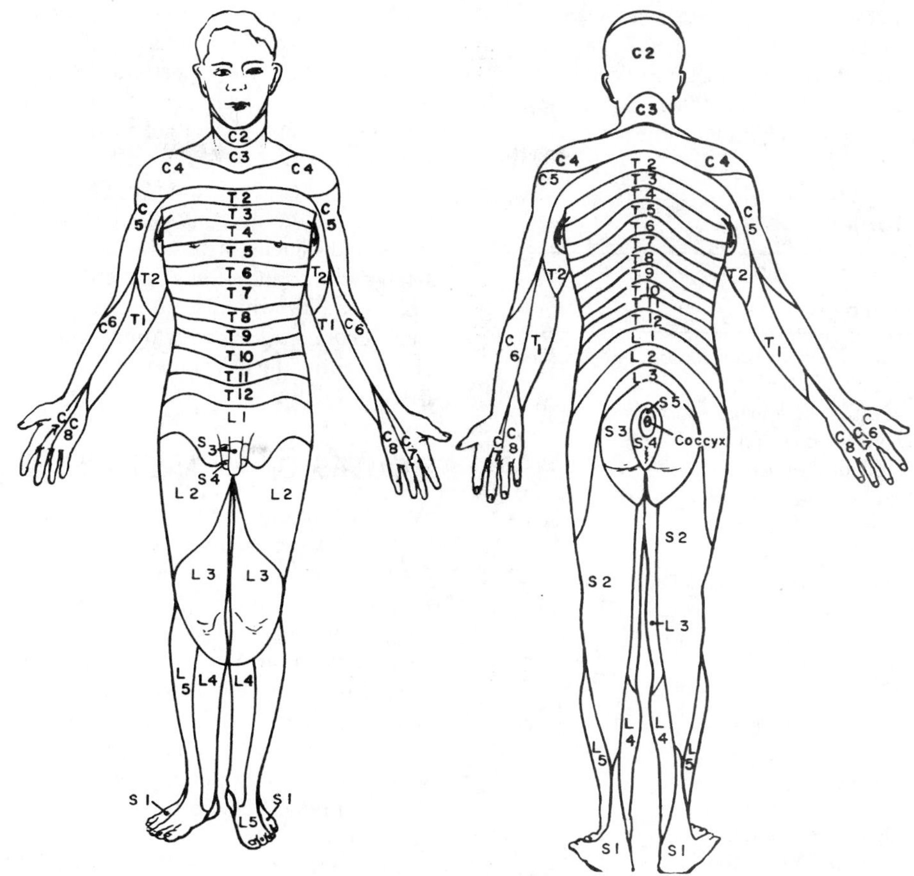

Fig. 23-8 Cutaneous distribution of the spinal nerves (dermatomes). (From Barr, M. L., & Kiernan, J. A. [1988]. *The human nervous system* [5th ed.]. Philadelphia: J. B. Lippincott.)

branches of the vertebral arteries. Additional blood supply comes from radicular arteries. The midthoracic region has the least number of radicular arteries and is at the greatest risk for ischemia. The most prominent feeding artery in this region is the artery of Adamkiewicz, which generally arises from a left radicular artery between T9 and L2.

The Process of Carcinogenesis

As with other cancers, the development of an astrocytoma appears to occur as a multistep process that ultimately leads to dysregulation of cell growth. The changes may be due to hereditary, environmental, and dietary factors; related to the aging process; or may be due to elements that remain to be identified. Current research is directed toward understanding cellular pathways involving growth factors, signal transduction, and deoxyribonucleic acid (DNA) transcription (Hubbard, Goodman, & Knobf, 1997). The molecular events that lead to the development of glial tumors involve at least two types of cellular genes, oncogenes and tumor suppressor genes. Proto-oncogenes are normal cellular genes that encode for proteins that stimulate cell growth, inhibit differentiation, or block apoptosis (i.e., programmed cell death). The conversion of a proto-oncogene to an oncogene is the result of some genetic alteration. Mutation or alteration of a proto-oncogene leads to oncogene activation and results in cell proliferation. Tumor suppressor genes normally function to prevent the continuous growth of cells by promoting differentiation and inducing apoptosis. Mutation or alteration of a tumor suppressor gene leads to loss of tumor suppressor function. The significance of genetic alterations in proto-oncogenes and tumor suppressor genes in the development of cancer has been well demonstrated in studies of families with hereditary cancer (Bondy et al., 1994).

The p53 tumor suppressor gene has been implicated in a number of human malignancies, and mutations of p53 are one of the most commonly detected genetic alterations found in gliomas. The p53 gene regulates phosphorylation of the Rb gene, which is critical for progression of the cell cycle (Kordek et al., 1995). Another function of wild-type p53 (i.e., normal p53) is its role in inhibiting angiogenesis. Angiogenesis is the development, growth, and production of new blood vessels. Loss of p53 protein function promotes the formation of a neovasculature critical for tumor growth. It has been postulated that the loss of wild-type p53 function may be important in the early pathogenesis of astrocytomas.

Another class of proteins that has been implicated in cell proliferation is growth factors. Mutation of growth factors or their receptors results in abnormal cell function, including increased proliferation, migration, and the ability of cells to invade surrounding tissues and metastasize. These growth factors include epidermal growth factor (EGF), transforming growth factors alpha and beta, platelet-derived growth factor, fibroblast growth factor, vascular endothelial growth factor, nerve growth factor, and brain-derived neurotropic factor (Levine & Schmidet, 1993). For example, mutations of the EGF receptor are found in at least 50% of GBMs, less than 10% of AAs, and rarely in LGAs, suggesting a role for this mutation in astrocytoma progression (Wong, Zoltick, & Moscatello, 1994). Additionally, glial tumors have increased expression of several growth factors and their receptors that act to stimulate angiogenesis, leading to increased tumor growth.

The mechanics of the process of oncogenesis in astrocytomas is not completely understood. It is clear that brain tumors and cancer in general are genetic diseases resulting from the accumulation of genetic alterations and mutations, only a few of which were noted previously. Understanding the genetics of astrocytoma formation and progression should allow the development of more specific and effective therapies.

TABLE 23-3 Myotomes

Spinal Cord Segment	Action
C1-C4	Flexion, extension, rotation, and lateral bending of neck
C3-C5	Elevation of upper thorax and scapula Diaphragm (inspiration)
C4-C6	Abduction of arm Lateral rotation of arm
C5-C7	Shoulder movement Flexion of elbow
C5 C6 C7 C8 T1	Adduction of arm from back to front
C6-C8	Extension of forearm and wrist
C6 C7 C8 T1	Index, middle, ring, and pinky fingers
C7 C8 T1	Flexion of hand Thumb
T1-T12	Control of thoracic, abdominal, and back muscles
L1-L3	Flexion of hip
L2-L4	Extension of leg Adduction of thigh
L4 L5 S1	Dorsal flexion of foot
L4 L5 S1 S2	Flexion of thigh (L4 L5) Rotation of thigh Abduction of thigh Extension, flexing, and spreading of toes Flexion of leg
L5 S1 S2	Plantar flexion of foot
S2-S4	Perineum and sphincters

ROUTES OF METASTASES

Astrocytomas grow by expansion, infiltration, or both. They invade locally, diffusely involving the surrounding normal CNS tissue. Astrocytomas have a tendency to grow in an octopus-like shape, with an actively proliferating front zone that advances into the surrounding normal brain tissue with extensions along the white matter tracts (Ceberg et al., 1995). Another characteristic of these tumors is the migration of malignant cells from the tumor into the surrounding brain. Most of these cells reside in the normal brain tissue within a few centimeters from the tumor border, but other cells can reach remote parts of the CNS. These tumor cells can spread to other areas in the CNS by way of the cerebral blood vessels and CSF, but they rarely metastasize to other parts of the body outside the CNS.

Metastases outside the CNS may occur when tumor cells are transferred to the scalp, cerebral blood vessels, or dural sinus during surgery (Willis, 1991). Once tumor cells invade the cerebral blood vessels, they can then enter the systemic circulation. The CNS does not contain lymphatic vessels (Freilich & DeAngelis, 1995; Posner, 1995), but when tu-

TABLE 23-4 Major Spinal Cord Tracts

Tract	Function	Pathology
Ascending Tracts (Sensory)		
1. Spinocerebellar	Reflexes, proprioception, smooth and coordinated movements	Loss of coordinated movements, lack of awareness of body position in relation to space
2. Dorsal columns Funiculus gracilis (lower extremities) Fasciculus cuneatus (upper extremities)	Vibration, proprioception, two-point discrimination	Loss of vibration sense, loss of two-point discrimination, lack of awareness of body position in relation to space, paresthesias
3. Spinothalamic	Touch, pressure, pain, temperature	Contralateral (opposite side) pain and loss of temperature
Descending Tracts (Motor)		
1. Corticospinal	Voluntary muscle activity	Weakness, spasticity, hyperactive reflexes
2. Extrapyramidal	Maintenance of balance, muscle tone, coordination, subconscious motor control, reflex movements of the head	Altered muscle tone and posture, loss of balance, loss or reflex response
3. Descending autonomic fibers	Bowel and bladder function	Loss of bowel and bladder function

mor cells have traveled outside the CNS, they can potentially spread through the lymphatic system. The spread of glial tumor cells through ventriculopleural and ventriculoperitoneal shunts has also been reported. A higher incidence of distant spread has been reported in high-grade spinal astrocytomas. This increased propensity for dissemination of spinal cord astrocytomas compared with intracranial astrocytomas is thought to result from the close proximity of tumor cells to the subarachnoid space and CSF pathways (Cohen, Wisoff, Allen, & Epstein, 1989).

ASSESSMENT

Signs and Symptoms of Intracranial Astrocytomas

The assessment of the patient with an astrocytoma is summarized in Table 23-5. The clinical evaluation of the patient involves a detailed history, a complete physical and neurologic examination, and a variety of diagnostic tests. The presenting signs and symptoms are primarily dependent on the size and location of the tumor and the rapidity with which it

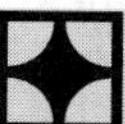

TABLE 23-5 Assessment of the Patient with an Astrocytoma

	Assessment Parameters	Typical Abnormal Findings
History	A. Personal and social history	A. Personal and social factors
	1. Age	1. Low-grade astrocytomas are most prevalent in the 20- to 40-year age range. Anaplastic astrocytomas are most prevalent in the 30- to 50-year age range.
	2. Ethnicity	2. Anaplastic astrocytomas are slightly more prevalent in men than women and in whites than Blacks, Latinos, and Asians.
	3. Family History	3. Positive family history may increase the risk. Specific hereditary syndromes may increase risk.
	4. Occupational history and environmental factors	4. Exposure to various chemical substances and industries or radiation sources may increase risk.
	5. Previous treatment with radiation therapy	5. Previous treatment with radiation to the head and neck increases the risk.
	B. A history of the presenting symptoms is obtained. A detailed review of systems is performed since the presenting symptoms are quite variable depending on the location of the tumor, the extent of its infiltration into and destruction of normal tissue, the rapidity at which it develops, and the amount of edema.	B. Common symptoms include altered mental status, impaired cognition, personality changes, impaired speech and comprehension, memory loss, motor and sensory impairment, gait disturbance, cranial nerve dysfunction, nausea/vomiting, headache, seizure, and bowel and bladder incontinence.
Physical Examination	A. A detailed physical is necessary to obtain information concerning the patient's general medical condition.	A. Patients may have pre-existing medical conditions such as cardiac, pulmonary, or endocrine that may affect treatment options.
Neurologic Examination	B. Comprehensive Examination	
	1. Mental Status Parameters Orientation and LOC Attention and ability to concentrate Memory Calculations General fund of knowledge Abstract thinking Language Ability to follow commands (Tools can be used to assess these functions [refer to Figs. 23-10 and 23-11], along with questions during the general interview.)	1. Depending on the location of the tumor, patients may present with problems such as disorientation, confusion, memory loss, impaired judgment, aphasia, and apraxia (inability to perform a skilled act, such as combing ones hair).
	2. Cranial Nerve Examination A detailed cranial nerve examination is presented in Table 23-2.	2. Abnormalities related to cranial nerves can be found in Table 23-2.

Continued

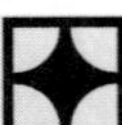

TABLE 23-5 Assessment of the Patient with an Astrocytoma—cont'd

	Assessment Parameters	Typical Abnormal Findings
	3. Motor Examination Evaluation of muscle tone, bulk, and strength are performed. Generally a grading scale is used to evaluate and document motor strength. 5 - normal muscle strength, full resistance 4 - some resistance, examiner can overcome muscle tone 3 - active movement against gravity 2 - movement of the limb is possible if gravity is removed 1 - weak palpable muscle contraction 0 - no movement	3. Depending on the location of the lesion, patients may exhibit hemiparesis, hemiplegia, flaccid or spastic extremities, muscle atrophy, ataxia, or incoordination. Patients with spinal cord lesions may present with paresis, quadriparesis, or quadriplegia, atrophy, spasticity, bladder and bowel dysfunction, and sexual dysfunction.
	4. Deep Tendon Reflexes These are graded according to a scale that evaluates the briskness of the response. 4+ - hyperactive 3+ - brisker than average 2+ - normal, average 1+ - diminished 0 - absent	4. Abnormalities may include hyperreflexia or absence of reflexes.
	5. Sensory Examination Light touch, pinprick (pain), temperature and position sense (vibration) are evaluated. In the evaluation of patients with spinal cord lesions it is important to identify and document a sensory level, if present. This helps to localize the level of the lesion and can be used as a monitor over time.	5. Depending on the location of the lesion, patients may present with paresthesia, loss of touch sensation, pinprick (pain), temperature, and position sense. The degree of loss can be partial to complete.
	6. Cerebellar Examination Coordination and the ability to perform rapid alternating movements are accessed.	6. Patients with involvement of the cerebellar hemispheres can present with dysmetria (inability to control accurately the range of movement in muscle action). In addition, abnormalities in balance and coordination can be present.
	7. Gait Evaluation of the manner of walking and posture is performed.	7. Patients may present with abnormal gait, including wide-based gait, ataxic gait, and spastic hemiparesis.
Diagnostic Tests A detailed description is included in the text.	A. Computerized Tomography Scan with iodinated contrast agents	A. Regions of contrast enhancement may exist where there is a disruption in the blood brain barrier or regions of low attenuation indicative of edema.
	B. Magnetic Resonance Imaging with paramagnetic contrast (gadolinium). This is the study of choice for lesions involving the brain and spinal cord.	B. The study generally provides clear anatomical images that can depict tumors in the structure of the brain and spinal cord.

develops. The pattern of the symptoms is often useful in localizing the site of the tumor. The signs and symptoms of intracranial astrocytomas can be divided into three main categories: general symptoms of increased ICP, focal effects related to tumor location, and herniation syndromes.

General Symptoms of Increased ICP. Increased ICP results from the enlarging tumor mass and development of vasogenic edema in the surrounding tissues. The increased permeability of the capillary endothelial cells and the leakage of plasma into the extracellular spaces result from the tumor's disruption of the blood brain barrier (BBB). As cerebral edema increases, the intracranial contents attempt to compensate. When the compensatory mechanisms are depleted, ICP rises and signs and symptoms occur. The presentation of symptoms depends on the rate of tumor growth and the development of edema. Symptoms may progress rapidly or slowly. LGAs that grow very slowly may not present with symptoms until the mass is quite large. More aggressive AAs may rapidly develop extensive edema with little time for the intracranial components to compensate or accommodate. The earliest generalized symptoms of astrocytomas may be vague and nonspecific.

Headaches are a frequent complaint experienced by 30% to 50% of patients with astrocytomas (Wen et al., 1995). The headaches are typically nonspecific; they can present as tension headaches. As ICP increases, the character of the headache may change, becoming bifrontal or bioccipital. Patients may experience early morning headaches that awaken them.

Personality changes or cognitive deficits, including difficulty concentrating, difficulty with memory, slowing of mental processes, impaired judgment, irritability, lack of initiative or loss of interest in things, and changes in mood and affect, are often described by patients and significant others. Approximately 20% to 40% of patients have some changes in cognitive function. Often families retrospectively describe behavioral changes that they thought were related to stress or other reasons. As ICP increases, confusion, lethargy, and somnolence may be evident.

Patients with lesions involving the posterior fossa may present with vomiting. Typically, vomiting is projectile in nature and patients do not experience nausea. Episodes of vomiting commonly occur in the early morning.

Focal Effects. Focal neurologic symptoms relate to the tumor's direct infiltration or compression of specific regions of the brain. Presenting signs and symptoms are directly related to the functions of these regions. For example, patients with tumors involving the frontal or parietal lobes of the brain may present with sensory or motor symptoms, whereas lesions of the occipital lobe cause visual symptomatology, and cerebellar astrocytomas result in balance and coordination difficulties. Table 23-1 provides a detailed summary of the regions of the brain, their functions, and possible pathology.

Herniation Syndromes. As mentioned previously, the brain is surrounded by the rigid skull and the dural layer of the meninges. The dura folds in on itself in the brain to create anatomic compartments. The faux cerebri separates the two cerebral hemispheres, and the tentorium cerebelli (located beneath the temporal and occipital lobes and above the cerebellum) separate the supratentorial and infratentorial compartments. Expanding tumors or other lesions, along with the accompanying cerebral edema, cause pressure to increase within the intracranial compartment. Initially, the brain's compensatory mechanisms attempt to accommodate for the increased pressure. However, these mechanisms quickly become exhausted, and nervous tissue is displaced from one compartment to another. The brain tissue shifts or herniates from the higher-pressure compartment into a lower-pressure compartment. The shifting brain tissue compresses other nervous tissue and structures, further increases cerebral edema, compresses blood vessels leading to ischemia, and may obstruct the CSF pathways causing hydrocephalus. Hydrocephalus is an enlargement of the ventricles and CSF spaces with an abnormal amount of CSF.

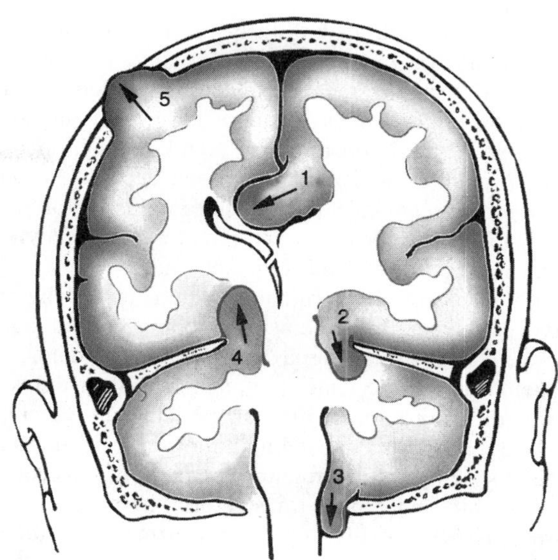

Fig. 23-9 The herniation syndromes. (1) Cingulate herniation. (2) Uncal herniation. (3) Cerebellar tonsillar (downward) herniation. (4) Upward herniation of the cerebellum. (5) Herniation through a cranial defect. (Central transtentorial herniation, unlabeled, may occur between numbers [2] and [4] and progress downward.)

These compressive, ischemic, and obstructive processes further contribute to the already increased ICP (Belford, 1997). This process is called *herniation* and is considered a life-threatening neurologic emergency. If untreated, the herniation syndromes can lead to coma, respiratory arrest, and death. There are several types of herniation syndromes. Supratentorial lesions can cause cingulate, uncal, or central transtentorial herniation. Tumors in the infratentorial compartment can cause an upward herniation of the cerebellum through the tentorium or a downward cerebellar herniation through the foramen magnum. Fig. 23-9 depicts the different herniation syndromes.

Cingulate herniation occurs when the cingulate gyrus (an area of the frontal lobe above the corpus callosum) is forced under the falx cerebri by the expanding tumor and edema in one hemisphere. The frontal lobes are compressed and the ipsilateral (same side) anterior cerebral artery may also be compressed, causing frontal lobe ischemia. The patient can present with an altered level of consciousness (LOC), hemiparesis or hemiplegia, and urinary incontinence.

Uncal herniation results from expanding tumors or lesions located in the temporal or frontal lobes. The uncus, the medial portion of the temporal lobe, is compressed and forced over the edge of the tentorium cerebelli. Structures compromised are the oculomotor nerve, the brain stem, and the posterior cerebral artery. The third cranial nerve (oculomotor) is compressed, leading to ipsilateral pupillary dilation. Eventually, the pupil does not respond to light and ptosis develops. The brain stem is displaced to the opposite side causing an ipsilateral hemiparesis, a false localizing sign. Patients exhibit a diminishing LOC and changes in their respiratory pattern. Irregular rhythm and depth of respirations are more meaningful than changes in respiratory rate. Compression of the posterior cerebral artery causes a visual field cut on the contralateral (opposite) side.

Central transtentorial herniation is the result of the progressive downward displacement of both cerebral hemispheres and the basal ganglia onto the diencephalon and brain stem through the tentorial notch. A shift of this kind occurs with lesions in the frontal, parietal, and occipital lobes. With unilaterally expanding tumors, a shift across the midline and cingulate herniation commonly precedes a downward shift and central transtentorial herniation (Plum & Posner, 1980). Initially, there is impairment in patients' LOC. Patients may become drowsy, inattentive, or agitated. They may sigh deeply or yawn with respirations. Their pupils become small but are still reactive. As the tumor continues to push tissue downward, there is a progressive loss of consciousness, and the patient becomes stuporous. Other signs at this time may include Cheyne-Stokes respirations that progress to hyperventilation, nonreactive pupils, dysconjugate (uncoordinated) eye movements, and decorticate posturing in response to noxious stimuli. In decorticate posturing, there is hyperflexion of the upper extremities and hyperextension of the lower extremities. Decorticate posturing soon deteriorates to decerebrate posturing. In decerebrate posturing, there is hyperextension of both upper and lower extremities. Oculocephalic and oculovestibular reflexes are lost, and patients become comatose.

Oculocephalic reflexes (doll's eyes) are tested by holding the comatose patient's eyelids open and briskly turning the head from side to side or by briskly flexing and extending the neck. The eyes normally should move to the opposite side conjugately. If the eyes remain fixed in the midline, the reflex is considered absent, and there is no brain stem function. Oculovestibular reflexes (i.e., ice water calorics) are tested by injecting ice water into the external auditory meatus of the comatose patient. Normally, the eyes deviate toward the stimulus. If brain stem function is lost, the eyes move away from the stimulus. These two tests are performed only in the comatose patient to assess the presence of brain stem function. Finally, medullary dysfunction occurs and there is ataxic breathing with periods of apnea leading to respiratory arrest.

In downward cerebellar herniation, the cerebellar tonsils are forced down through the foramen magnum, compressing the lower brain stem. Patients can present with signs of brain stem dysfunction such as lower cranial nerve palsies, abnormal respiratory pattern, fluctuating blood pressure, and cardiac dysrhythmias (Plum & Posner, 1980). When the compression is acute, it can cause sudden loss of consciousness followed by respiratory arrest (Posner, 1995). Downward cerebellar herniation may be precipitated by events causing sudden increases in ICP such as sneezing, coughing, or performing a Valsalva maneuver. Downward tonsillar cerebellar herniation may be the cause of sudden death that follows lumbar puncture in patients with brain tumors or meningitis (Plum & Posner, 1980).

In upward herniation, the cerebellum is displaced upward through the tentorium and the brain stem is compressed. Patients develop pupillary abnormalities and upward gaze paralysis. Other signs of brain stem compression may be coma, hyperventilation, vomiting, and decerebrate posturing. Hydrocephalus may also occur as a result of interference with the CSF pathways.

Signs and Symptoms of Spinal Astrocytomas

Patients with spinal cord astrocytomas typically present with pain. Pain syndromes associated with intramedullary (i.e., within the spinal cord) lesions depend on the specific nerve tracts involved. The pain is characterized as a deep, severe type of pain that can be worse at night and may have a radicular or radiating component (Kornblith, Walker, & Cassady, 1987). The local symptoms are specific to the tumor's location along the spinal cord. The symptoms generally present slowly, reflecting the slow growth of the majority of intramedullary tumors. The signs and symptoms of these lesions result from parenchymal destruction and lead to compression of adjacent areas. Compression of adjacent areas can compromise the vascular supply to the spinal cord. Intramedullary spinal cord astrocytomas that affect the gray matter can cause segmental sensory and motor changes.

Deficits below the level of the spinal cord tumor result from the involvement of the sensory and motor tracts. Characteristic signs and symptoms are motor deficits, sensory dysfunction, and bowel and bladder impairment. Motor deficits include unilateral or bilateral paresis, progressive spastic paraparesis, and muscle wasting. Sensory dysfunction usually begins distally, and the patient complains of numbness and tingling.

History

The patient should be evaluated for any of the risk factors associated with the development of an astrocytoma. In addition, a careful history of any of the aforementioned symptoms must be obtained. The description and duration of symptoms, when they occur, the presence of exacerbating or relieving factors, and the order of their appearance are important pieces of information (Belford, 1997). Mental status changes, for example, are a common symptom of intracranial astrocytomas and often go unnoticed by patients. For this reason, family members, significant others, or work colleagues often initially identify a problem. They can provide valuable information regarding the onset and progression of symptoms.

Physical Examination

The history is followed by a complete neurologic examination. A thorough initial examination is essential because it provides a baseline assessment of the patient's level of neurologic function. Future assessments are compared with this initial examination and facilitate the detection of changes or abnormalities. The neurologic examination includes an assessment of the patient's LOC and mental status, cranial nerve function, motor and sensory function, cerebellar function and gait, and reflexes.

Mental status is composed of LOC, mood, affect, attention span, language comprehension, memory, judgment, and insight. An evaluation of LOC includes both arousal and awareness. Arousal indicates wakefulness and reflects only brain stem function. A patient who is unarousable to any stimuli has brain stem dysfunction. Awareness, which refers to the functioning of the cerebral cortex, the thinking part of the brain, means that the patient can interact with and interpret his or her environment (Lower, 1992). A patient's level of orientation is always determined in three spheres: person, place, and time. A patient's LOC can be described as alert and oriented, confused, lethargic, restless, stuporous, semicomatose, or comatose. The individual whose LOC is impaired must be sufficiently stimulated to appropriately assess the degree of impairment. Many institutions use the Glasgow Coma Scale, a tool that assesses neurologic function in comatose patients or components of it as part of their neurologic assessment flow sheets. An example of such a tool is shown in Fig. 23-10.

Observations of the patient's actions, facial expressions, appearance, posture, and responses to the environment and conversation around him or her provide information about mood and affect. Language is evaluated for content, flow of speech, speech patterns, and comprehension. The presence of aphasia (i.e., the inability to understand or express one's own language), agnosia (i.e., the inability to recognize common objects through the senses of sight, touch, and sound), and apraxia (i.e., the inability to perform a skilled motor act in the absence of weakness or paralysis) is noted.

Aphasia can be expressive, receptive, or both. In expressive aphasia, the patient is unable to self-express verbally or in writing but has full comprehension. In receptive aphasia, the patient is unable to understand the spoken language and is unable to self-monitor language. However, many patients have a combination of expressive and receptive aphasia known as *global aphasia.* General knowledge and long- and short-term memory are assessed by eliciting information that can be validated easily. Attention span, abstract reasoning, insight, and judgment are also evaluated. An example of a tool used to assess mental status is the Mini Mental Status Examination (Fig. 23-11).

The focus of the neurologic examination in patients with spinal cord astrocytomas is a detailed assessment of motor, sensory, and autonomic function.

Diagnostic Tests

Computed Tomography. Computed tomography (CT) is often the first study performed in an individual with symptoms suggestive of a brain tumor. CT is an imaging technique that combines x-ray with computerized data analysis. The primary function of CT scanning is to define the structural anatomy and characteristics of tissue within the body. The acquisition of images is accomplished by passing a narrow x-ray beam through successive layers of an object. Energy is absorbed as the x-ray beam is rotated 180 degrees around the object. The amount of absorption is dependent on the density of the structure. The radiation that passes through the tissue is detected by the scanner. The computer system manipulates the data to produce images that represent the successive slices or sections of the object (McCullough & Coulam, 1976).

In imaging the brain, the bone absorbs the most radiation and air absorbs the least. The energy detected by the scanner is seen on the x-ray films as varying shades of black, gray, and white. Bone is most dense and appears white on CT, whereas air, being least dense, appears black. The density of the brain is in between and appears as various shades of gray. Areas that contain fluid such as CSF, cystic collections, and cerebral edema appear as various shades of black. The images are generally obtained in the axial plane. In this plane, the brain is cut horizontally, providing a downward view of the brain sections. The sectional images of the brain are evaluated for changes in tissue density, displacement of structures, evidence of bleeding, and abnormalities in the size and shape of structures (Hickey, 1992). The CT scan is routinely performed with and without contrast. Noncontrast images are performed first and are used to look for evidence of blood or calcium within the brain tissue. Contrast administration using an iodinated radiopaque material is then performed. Both CT and magnetic resonance imaging (MRI) contrast agents depend on the integrity of the BBB. Normally, only a few structures such as blood vessels are enhanced with contrast. The contrast agents extravasate into the extravascular space at sites of BBB disruption (Castillo, 1994). Density changes produced by contrast material in a tumor help to distinguish the lesion from the surrounding brain structure and can aid in biopsy, resection, and evaluation of treatment.

The advantages of CT in evaluating patients with suspected or known brain astrocytomas are as follows: it is a noninvasive inpatient/outpatient procedure, it provides rapid images that provide a great deal of information about the structure of the brain, and it is readily available at a reasonable cost. On the other hand, it provides less detail than MRI, and small lesions can be missed; radiation exposure is small but exists; and patients with iodine or shellfish allergies may be unable to receive the contrast agent.

In adults, LGAs are characteristically located in the cerebral white matter. They are hypodense in appearance, can lack evidence of a sharp margin, and display little or no enhancement with contrast agents. The amount of surrounding edema and shift is minimal and may not be detectable on CT images (Earnest et al., 1988).

Cerebellar astrocytomas typically have a large cystic component with a homogeneous, round, contrast-enhancing solid region. They can obstruct the fourth ventricle and produce hydrocephalus. Edema within the surrounding tissues is generally minimal. These tumors typically do not display evidence of hemorrhage or calcification (Barnes, Robertson, & Poussaint, 1997).

CONFIDENTIAL PATIENT INFORMATION - HANDLE ACCORDING TO HOSPITAL POLICY

Memorial Hospital for Cancer and Allied Diseases

Neurological Assessment

Patient Identification

Date		
Time		
Initial		
COMA SCALE — 1. Eyes Open (eyes closed by swelling = c)	Spontaneously	
	To Speech	
	To Touch	
	To Pain	
	None	
	Eyes closed by swelling	
2. Best verbal response	Oriented	
	Confused	
	Inappropriate	
	Incomprehensible	
	None	
3. Best Motor Response	Obeys commands	
	Localizes Pain	
	Withdraws	
	Decorticate (Flexion)	
	Decerebrate (Extension)	
	None	
4=Normal Strength	Arm Rt.	
3=Lifts and Holds	Leg Rt.	
2=Lifts and Falls Back	Arm Lt.	
1=Moves on Bed 0=No Movement	Leg Lt.	
PUPILS (2mm, 3mm, 4mm, 5mm, 6mm, 7mm, 8mm) N=Normal	Size Rt.	
S=Sluggish	Size Lt.	
F=Fixed	React. Rt.	
	React. Lt.	
CONSCIOUSNESS		
RESPIRATIONS		

CODES

COMA SCALE
CHECK (✓) APPROPRIATE BOX

ORIENTATION
3 ORIENTED X 3 SPHERES
2 ORIENTED X 2 SPHERES
1 ORIENTED X 1 SPHERE

CONSCIOUSNESS
4 ALERT
3 LETHARGIC
2 RESTLESS, AGITATED
1 STUPOROUS
0 COMATOSE

˅˄ **BLOOD PRESSURE**
• **PULSE**

200
190
180
170
160
150
140
130
120
110
100
90
80
70
60
50
40
30
20

56-08187 F16 CIMC Approval Date: 6/96 *Signatures Required on Back* /11.050

Fig. 23-10 Neurological Assessment Form. (Courtesy of Memorial Sloan-Kettering Cancer Center, Division of Nursing.)

Continued

CONFIDENTIAL PATIENT INFORMATION - HANDLE ACCORDING TO HOSPITAL POLICY

	Memorial Hospital for Cancer and Allied Diseases
Patient Identification	

INIT.	FULL SIGNATURE	TITLE	INIT.	FULL SIGNATURE	TITLE

56-08187 F16 CIMC Approval Date: 6/96 **/11.050**

Fig. 23-10, cont'd For legend see opposite page.

Neurological Examination:

Level of Alertness:

Mini-Mental Status Examination:

5 ( ) What is the (year) (season) (date) (month)?

5 ( ) Where are we: (state) (borough) (city) (hospital) (floor)?

Registration

3 ( ) Name 3 objects: 1 second to say each. Then ask the patient all 3 after you have said them. Give 1 point for each correct answer. then repeat them until he learns all 3. Count trials and record.
Trials ________. (Score 1st trial only.)

5 ( ) Serial 7's. 1 point for each correct. Stop after 5 answers. (93,86,79,72,65). Alternatively spell ''world'' backwards

Recall

3 ( ) Ask for the 3 objects repeated above. Give 1 point for each correct.

Language

9 ( ) Name a pencil and watch (2 points).
Repeat the following: ''No ifs, ands or buts''. (1 point)
Follow a 3 stage command: ''Take a paper in your right hand, fold it in half, and put it on the floor.'' (3 points)
Read and obey the following:

CLOSE YOUR EYES (1 point)

Write a sentence (1 point).

Copy design (1 point).

__________ Total Score

Fig. 23-11 Mini Mental Status Examination. (Courtesy of Memorial Sloan-Kettering Cancer Center, Department of Neurology.)

On CT, brain stem gliomas may have similar characteristics to LGAs and AAs of the cerebral hemispheres. The sensitivity of CT may not be adequate for distinguishing these tumors. For spinal cord intramedullary tumors, MRI is the imaging technique of choice. Evaluation of the spine and spinal cord with CT generally involves the use of myelography and the acquisition of images with contrast in the subarachnoid space. The images demonstrate widening of the cord at the level of the lesion but may provide no other information.

High-grade astrocytomas are best seen with contrast. The lesions typically have a heterogeneous quality and often have a central region with low density and irregularly enhancing borders. Although areas of calcifications are not seen, they may display an area of hemorrhage within the tumor. The degree of edema and mass effect can be extensive (Grossman, 1990).

Magnetic Resonance Imaging. MRI was developed in the 1980s. Today, MRI has replaced CT for the evaluation of the CNS. MRI uses a magnetic field and sequencing of radiofrequency pulses for the production of computerized images. This technique depends on the mobile hydrogen atom concentration in tissues. Hydrogen has magnetic nuclei and makes up two thirds of the atoms in living tissues (Oldendorf & Oldendorf, 1991). When the hydrogen ions in the body are placed within the magnetic field of the MRI, the ions align with the magnetic field. The frequency at which hydrogen ions oscillate in the magnetic field is termed the *resonant frequency.* Radiofrequency waves are used to stimulate the nucleus of the hydrogen ions in the body, which absorb energy and then re-emit energy in the form of radio waves that can be detected by the MRI scanner. In imaging of the brain, slices of the brain are isolated by stimulating the hydrogen ions in a plane and changing the gradient of the magnetic field.

The MRI scanner measures the total amount of hydrogen along a slice of tissue. By varying the sequence of the radiofrequency pulses, different types of information can be obtained. *T1* and *T2* refer to the relaxation times, as they define the rate that a signal fades after stimulation. T1 measures the rate of energy loss. T2 represents the dephasing or the hydrogen nuclei drifting out of phase with each other. These two components of relaxation time can be isolated to a greater or lesser degree. Pulse sequences cause the re-emitted signal to contain information about T1 and T2. T1-weighted scans demonstrate excellent gray/white differentiation and high spatial resolution (Oldendorf & Oldendorf, 1991). They look at the structure of the brain. T2 images better demonstrate pathologic brain lesions by evaluating water content (Oldendorf & Oldendorf. 1991). The tissues, fluid, and blood of the brain have different characteristics that can be evaluated by MRI.

Computer-generated images such as CT define tissues according to different levels of brightness from white to black. MRI uses a variety of sequences to produce the brain images. It produces high-resolution images in any plane without the loss of detail. MRI has the ability to demonstrate tumors as small as 3 to 5 mm. It has the ability to demonstrate brain edema before there are changes in the

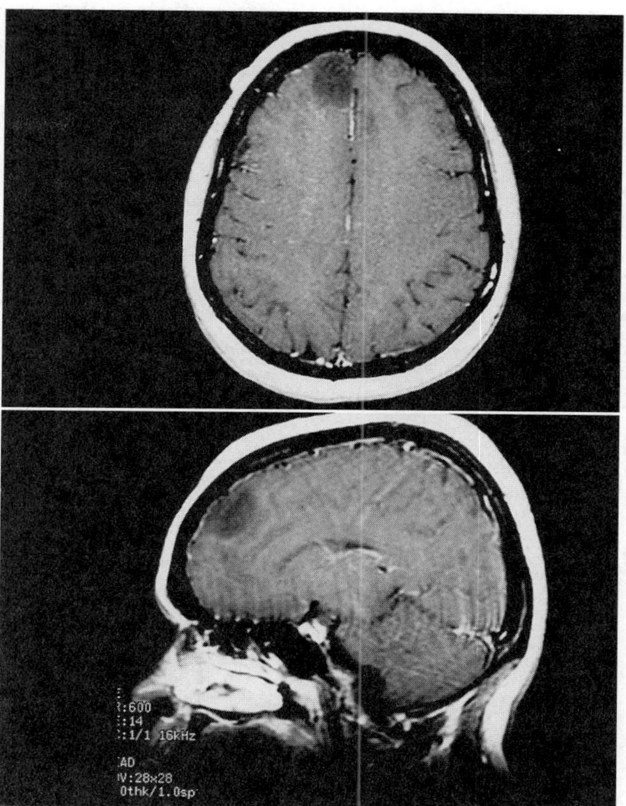

Fig. 23-12 MRIs of a low-grade astrocytoma in the right frontal lobe. (Courtesy of Memorial Sloan-Kettering Cancer Center, Department of Neuroradiology.)

BBB or compression related to mass effect (Levin et al., 1997). MRI provides better imaging of the posterior fossa compared with CT where bony artifact may obscure lesions. These lesions may or may not exhibit focal areas of contrast enhancement with gadolinium. The LGAs usually appear hypointense (blacker) or isointense (grayer like normal brain) on T1-weighted images and hyperintense (brighter or whiter) on T2-weighted images (Bentson, 1996). In Fig. 23-12, a LGA of the right frontal lobe in two views is depicted. High-grade astrocytomas evaluated by MRI have characteristics similar to CT images; they both enhance these tumors. Both T1 and T2 images have a heterogeneous appearance. When gadolinium is administered, the appearance of an irregular nodular border surrounding a cystic or low signal area can be demonstrated. Fig. 23-13 is an MRI of a right frontal lobe AA.

Spinal cord tumors appear hypointense on T1-weighted images. T2-weighted images are generally more sensitive to tumors but do not distinguish tumor, edema, or cyst formation. The appearance of spinal cord astrocytomas on T1 images with gadolinium demonstrates heterogeneous uptake with patchy, irregular margins that may extend over many vertebral segments (McCormick & Stein, 1996). The MRI in Fig. 23-14 is a T2-weighted image of an astrocytoma of the cervical spine.

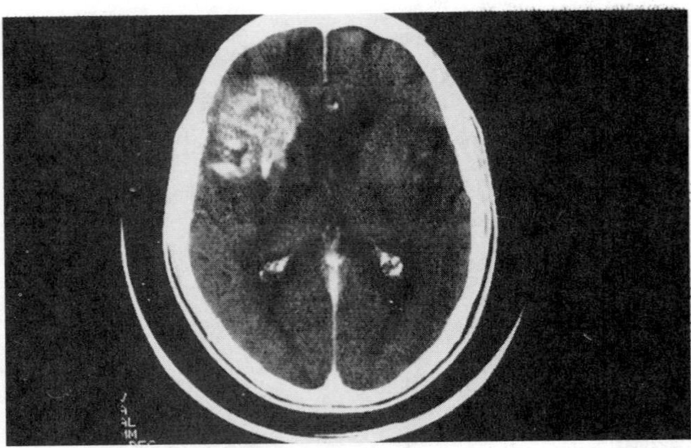

Fig. 23-13 MRI of an anaplastic astrocytoma in the right frontal lobe. (Courtesy of Memorial Sloan-Kettering Cancer Center, Department of Neuroradiology.)

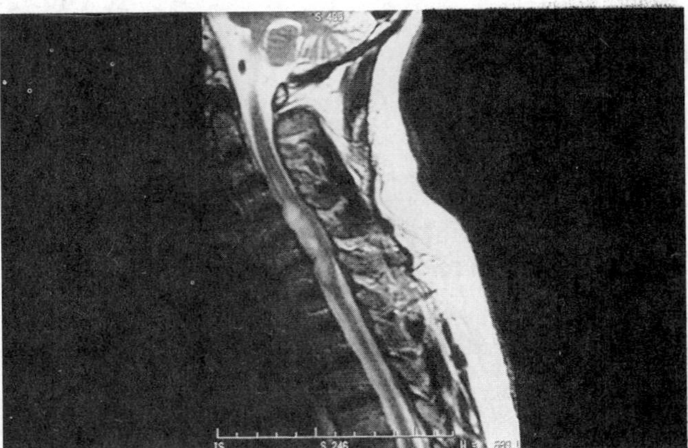

Fig. 23-14 T2-weighted image of an astrocytoma in the cervical spine. (Courtesy of Memorial Sloan-Kettering Cancer Center, Department of Neuroradiology.)

Three-dimensional reconstruction of the brain, tumor mass, and edema patterns is possible with MRI. MRI has become the modality of choice for treatment planning and evaluating residual tumor after surgery, radiation, and chemotherapy (Tice et al., 1993). It has many advantages in its ability to image the CNS. However, disadvantages to this technology include the following: It is more expensive than CT imaging; it is not as widely available as CT, although this is becoming less of an issue; it requires more time for data acquisition; patients must remain in a tight, claustrophobic tube for a prolonged time; and there is concern about the magnet and patient safety with regard to metallic implants. Close patient screening is necessary to detect for metal, including some types of clips, heart valves, pacemakers, eye implants, and inferior vena cava filters. Patients with nonferromagnetic metallic implants may need to wait several weeks for the implant to become firmly imbedded in the tissue before they are permitted in the scanner.

Angiogram. Cerebral angiography is used to define the vasculature of the brain. It involves the percutaneous puncture of the femoral artery with injection of a radiopaque medium to visualize the circle of Willis and the cerebral blood vessels by serial imaging of the transit of the contrast medium through the vessels (Leahy, 1990; Wegmann, 1993). Invasive angiography has largely been replaced with the introduction of CT and MRI, which define the structure and location of astrocytomas. The ability to look at flow characteristics with less invasive magnetic resonance angiography has also diminished the use of angiograms in the evaluation of astrocytomas.

Positron Emission Tomography. Positron emission tomography (PET) is a functional imaging technique used in patients with intracranial astrocytomas to evaluate brain tissue and tumor metabolism. A cyclotron produces radioactive isotopes from oxygen, carbon, nitrogen, and fluorine. These isotopes are then combined with a chosen brain metabolite and injected intravenously. The isotopes disintegrate spontaneously in the brain and eject a positively charged electron called a *positron* (Schwartz, 1995). As the positron moves through the tissue, it encounters a negatively charged electron. The resulting collision neutralizes the charges and produces electromagnetic energy in the form of two photons (gamma rays), which travel in opposite directions (Thiessen & Blasberg, 1996). A ring of collimators surrounding the patient's head records these events, computers calculate measurements, and an image of brain uptake is produced.

The most common radionucleotide used for PET studies in brain tumor patients is F-fluoro-deoxyglucose (FDG). The FDG is a glucose analog transported across the BBB by the same mechanism as glucose, but it does not undergo further metabolism (Roelcke, 1994). The amount of FDG uptake represents the metabolic activity of the tissue. High FDG uptake correlates with increased metabolic activity, and low FDG uptake is associated with decreased metabolic activity. In patients with astrocytomas, PET has been used to predict the degree of malignancy. High FDG uptake (hypermetabolic activity) generally correlates with high-grade tumors, and low FDG uptake (hypometabolic activity) correlates with low-grade tumors (Di Chiro et al., 1982).

Currently, FDG-PET is most widely used to distinguish between radiation necrosis and recurrent or residual tumor. The radiographic appearance of radiation necrosis and recurrent tumor is often indistinguishable on both CT and MRI. In the PET image, however, lesions caused by tumor are generally associated with moderate to high FDG uptake, whereas radiation necrosis has very low FDG uptake (Thiessen & Blasberg, 1996). However, many patients with high-grade astrocytomas have a mixture of necrosis and tumor. A biopsy may be necessary to confirm the diagnosis, especially when the area in question is at or near the original tumor site (Levin et al., 1997). PET has also been used to distinguish residual tumor from postoperative changes, study the response to therapy (chemotherapy, RT, and steroids), evaluate remote effects of the tumor itself on brain metabolism, localize areas of probable tumor for biopsy, and monitor patients with LGAs for transformation to high-grade tumors (Byrne, 1994).

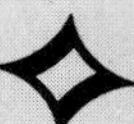

TABLE 23-6 Patient Preparation for Stereotactic Brain Biopsy

Description of the Procedure: A stereotactic brain biopsy is a computer-assisted technique that precisely locates an area of the brain using three dimensional coordinates. These coordinates are then used to guide a needle to that specific location to obtain brain tissue for histologic evaluation.

Patient Preparation: The patient will be instructed not to eat or drink past midnight the night before the procedure. The patient should not have taken aspirin, products containing aspirin, or anticoagulants for 7-10 days, or nonsteroidal anti-inflammatory drugs for 48 hours before the procedure. The stereotactic frame is placed on the patient's head before the procedure and should be described in detail to the patient.

Procedural Considerations: Informed consent is obtained. The patient is prepared for surgery. The base of the stereotactic head frame is placed on the patient while in a sitting position before undergoing an imaging study (CT or MRI). Often, an analgesic, anxiolytic, or both are administered before the frame placement. The patient is transported to CT or MRI where a localizing frame is attached to the base. This base is secured to the CT or MRI table to avoid movement that may distort the images. The imaging study is performed with and without a contrast agent (assess for iodine or shellfish allergies). The information from the study is then entered into a computer that plans the path of the biopsy needle and the depth it is to be inserted. The patient may be taken directly to the operating room from CT or MRI or he may be returned to his room to await the biopsy. The procedure is generally performed under monitored sedation. Once the procedure is completed, the patient recovers in the Postanesthesia Care Unit and then returns to his room. Neurologic assessments are performed every hour for 8-12 hours.

Although PET is not used to diagnose astrocytomas, it does supplement information obtained from CT and MRI. Unfortunately, PET is not yet widely available because of the high cost of obtaining and operating the equipment.

Single Photon Emission Computed Tomography. Single photon emission computed tomography (SPECT), a technique used for the imaging of the functional neuroanatomy, involves the intravenous (IV) administration of isotopes transported to the brain in proportion to the regional blood flow and their uptake by brain and tumor cells (Schwartz, 1997). Rotating gamma cameras and computer reconstruction techniques then produce high-resolution cross-sectional or three-dimensional brain images (Schwartz, 1995). SPECT has proven useful in predicting the presence of necrosis or recurrent tumor following RT, distinguishing infiltrating tumor from solid tumor or recurrence, and differentiating abscesses from tumor sites. Recent developments have allowed SPECT to overlap MRI data using computer processing techniques, so that it is possible to directly correlate anatomic and functional information (Schwartz, 1995). This important development allows biopsy sites to be selected on the basis of functional imaging data, thereby minimizing tissue sampling errors and increasing the yield of stereotactic biopsies (Schwartz, 1997). SPECT is more widely available than PET and is useful in complementing the information obtained from CT and MRI. Presently, it provides only an indirect measure of brain metabolism and is not generally used in the initial diagnosis of astrocytomas.

BOX 23-2
World Health Organization (WHO) Histologic Classification of Astrocytic Tumors

Astrocytic Tumors

Astrocytoma
  Variants: fibrillary, protoplasmic, gemistocytic
Pilocytic astrocytoma
Pleomorphic xanthoastrocytoma
Subependymal giant cell astrocytoma
Anaplastic (malignant) astrocytoma
Glioblastoma
  Variants: Giant cell glioblastoma, gliosarcoma

From Kleihues, P., Burger, P. C., & Scheithauer, B. W. (1993). *World Health Organization histological typing of tumours of the central nervous system* (2nd ed.). Berlin, Heidelberg: Springer-Verlag.

Stereotactic Brain Biopsy. Stereotactic biopsy is performed to obtain tissue for histology. It is a surgical procedure that can be considered the definitive test in the diagnosis of astrocytomas. The procedure and its indications are presented in the surgery section of this chapter. The preparation of a patient for a stereotactic biopsy is outlined in Table 23-6.

STAGING

Classification of brain and spinal cord tumors is based on the identification of the presumed cell of origin. In astrocytomas, the cell of origin is the astrocyte. Histologic grading also determines the grade or biologic aggressiveness of the tumor and is able to predict prognosis. Astrocytomas often represent a heterogeneous group of tumors. They are characterized by different degrees of cellularity, endothelial proliferation, pleomorphism, and necrosis. For this reason, several grading systems have been proposed that consist of either a three-tier or a four-tier grading of malignancy. Unfortunately, the development of multiple grading systems has led to difficulty in defining incidence, prognosis, treatment, and comparison among clinical studies. The WHO classification system was developed to provide an international classification system that would help standardize the histologic grading of these tumors. Specific criteria allow neuropathologists around the world to determine the type of tumor so that it is recognized as the same type by every specialist. A uniform basis is available for the evaluation of the effectiveness of various new therapies, and prognosis can be predicted more accurately. The WHO system, shown in Box 23-2, characterizes a tumor histologically by its cell of origin and then designates a grade based on its similarity to normal cells. The WHO system is a three-tier system that divides astrocytic tumors

Box 23-3
TNM Classification of Brain Tumors

Primary Tumor (T)

TX - Primary tumor cannot be assessed
TO - No evidence of primary tumor

Supratentorial Tumor

T1 - Tumor 5 cm or less in greatest dimension; limited to one side
T2 - Tumor more than 5 cm in greatest dimension; limited to one side
T3 - Tumor invades or encroaches upon the ventricular system
T4 - Tumor crosses the midline, invades the opposite hemisphere, or invades infratentorially

Infratentorial Tumor

T1 - Tumor 3 cm or less in greatest dimension; limited to one side
T2 - Tumor more than 3 cm in greatest dimension; limited to one side
T3 - Tumor invades or encroaches upon the ventricular system
T4 - Tumor crosses the midline, invades the opposite hemisphere, or invades supratentorially

Regional Lymph Nodes (N)

This category does not apply to this site.

Distant Metastasis (M)

MX - Presence of distant metastasis cannot be assessed
M0 - No distant metastasis
M1 - Distant metastasis

Histopathologic Grade (G)

GX - Grade cannot be assessed
G1 - Well-differentiated
G2 - Moderately well-differentiated
G3 - Poorly differentiated
G4 - Undifferentiated

Stage Grouping

Stage IA	G1	T1	M0
Stage IB	G1	T2	M0
	G1	T3	M0
Stage IIA	G2	T1	M0
Stage IIB	G2	T2	M0
	G2	T3	M0
Stage IIIA	G3	T1	M0
Stage IIIB	G3	T2	M0
	G3	T3	M0
Stage IV	G1,2,3	T4	M0
	G4	Any T	M0
	Any G	Any T	M1

From American Joint Committee on Cancer (AJCC®), Chicago. (1992). *AJCC® manual for staging of cancer* (4th ed.). Philadelphia: Lippincott-Raven.

into astrocytomas, anaplastic astrocytomas, and glioblastoma multiforme. In addition to the histologic grading of astrocytomas, the anatomic extent of disease can be defined by the TNM Classification of Brain Tumors. This system evaluates the extent of the primary tumor (T), involvement of regional lymph nodes (N), and the presence of distant metastasis (M). The TNM Classification of Brain Tumors is found in Box 23-3.

MEDICAL MANAGEMENT

The treatment of astrocytomas is extremely complicated and depends on many factors. Generally, a combination of surgery, RT, and chemotherapy is used for AAs. The management of LGAs remains controversial because large-scale prospective randomized studies are unavailable. Patients with LGAs are often observed, but treatment may include surgery, RT, or both.

Surgery

The initial approach for the majority of individuals with an astrocytoma is surgery. The two most common surgical procedures in the diagnosis and treatment of intracranial astrocytomas are stereotactic biopsy and craniotomy with resection of the tumor. The surgical approach used is dependent on many variables including the goal of surgery, the location and grade of the tumor, and the extent of the lesion. The principal goal of surgery is to obtain tissue for histology and grading. The histology of the lesion may make a difference in the intraoperative approach, medical management, and the overall prognosis of the patient. Patients with LGAs often present with seizures, but have no other localizing clinical symptoms. A small percentage of the lesions, which have the typical appearance of LGAs on CT and MRI, are high-grade tumors on histologic review (Kondziolka, Lundsford, & Martinez, 1993; Widen & Kelly, 1987). This disparity argues for biopsy of lesions presumed low-grade by radiographic criterion. Shaw et al. (1997) reviewed the surgical literature related to the extent of surgical resection of LGAs and survival. They concluded that a survival benefit is suggested with a gross total or a substantial subtotal surgical resection of these lesions. With LGAs, the goal may be to cure the tumor, although this is rarely achieved. The tumors often undergo malignant degeneration.

Beyond histology, surgical resection may be undertaken to relieve symptoms associated with increased ICP or direct compression of adjacent tissue. In patients with high-grade astrocytomas, surgical intervention alone is rarely curative. In most instances, the reduction of tumor bulk during craniotomy produces a decrease in local compression and ICP. Patients often experience a reduction in their symptoms. Surgery is believed to reduce the tumor burden and increase the effectiveness of adjuvant therapy. The alteration in cell kinetics that converts tumor cells not actively growing to an active cell cycle phase may render the cells more responsive to radiation and chemotherapy. Surgery also removes necrotic tissue, which is not responsive to adjuvant therapy and may be a nidus for increased cerebral edema. The decrease in tumor mass makes the reduction in the dosage of corticosteroids possible, thereby limiting the potential side effects of the medication.

The location of the tumor may limit the ability of the surgeon to perform an extensive resection. Planning an aggressive tumor resection must include an assessment of potential neurologic morbidity. A rapidly growing infiltrative astrocytoma that extends across the midline or into the eloquent motor cortex, sensory cortex, or speech cortex may not be completely excised and increases the risk of producing new neurologic deficits. Astrocytomas exhibit an infiltrative growth pattern between normal cells and are difficult to distinguish from normal nervous tissue. In these instances, a partial resection or biopsy may be the optimal approach. Lesions in the superficial, noneloquent cortex are more amenable to resection than deeper lesions.

Patient factors considered in the surgical approach include the patient's age, preexisting medical condition, and neurologic deficit. Whether this is a progressive or recurrent tumor and whether surgery will potentially improve the individual's quality of life are also important considerations.

Craniotomy. Craniotomy involves opening the skull. A bone flap is raised to provide access to the brain for tumor resection. The procedure is performed with the patient under general anesthesia except when intraoperative monitoring requires the patient to be awake. Technologic advances, including the development of pharmacologic agents for brain edema; neuroanesthesia; the operating microscope; microsurgical neuroanatomy; imaging systems (e.g., CT, MRI, and PET); the fusion of imaging systems with resection techniques; intraoperative monitoring of evoked responses; advanced stereotactic and ultrasound technology; and improved resection tools have led to improvements in surgical resection of both spine and brain tumors (Arbour, 1994; Black, 1991; Black et al., 1997; Epstein & Ozek, 1993).

The CT and MRI scans have made it possible to measure tumor volumes and evaluate the location of the tumor in relationship to critical brain structures. Iodine contrast and paramagnetic agents aid in defining tumor margins. Magnetic resonance angiography is a noninvasive technique useful in defining the vascular structure of the tumor. Functional MRI is being developed for preoperative planning. Although not readily available, it is capable of localizing critical structures. Techniques for functional mapping of language, visual, motor, and sensory areas utilizing MRI are being developed (Kim et al., 1993).

Tumors are localized intraoperatively using ultrasonography, stereotactic frames, and more recently, frameless image-guided interactive surgical systems. Intraoperative ultrasound technology is used to both localize and remove tumors. In addition, it aids intraoperatively in assessing the resection of the lesion. Intraoperative ultrasound assists in defining the borders of the tumor and its transition toward normal brain tissue and differentiating solid tumor from edema. The ultrasonic aspirator combines a vibrating head with suction to remove the tumor.

Interactive, image-guided, stereotactic systems allow for improved accuracy in the localization of a lesion, provide optimization of a safe surgical approach, and aid in defining tumor margins (Black, 1991; League, 1995). These systems use CT or MRI images acquired before surgery. Fiducials (markers) are applied to the patient's head at the time of the scan. The markers are visible on the scanned images. Some systems do not require markers to be placed, but instead use identified surface points on the patient's head. The data are loaded into a computer system and a three-dimensional reconstruction of the data is made. In the operating room, the patient's fiducials or coordinates are integrated by point-matching or surface-matching to the CT or MRI image. The registration process varies according to the specific system used. A pointing device communicates the surgical location to a computer system. Some systems use a mechanically linked arm; other systems communicate through sonic, optical, or magnetic digitizers (Chen & Apuzzo, 1997). The major limitation of this technology is the inability to take into account changes in anatomic structure, which occur during surgery. Changes in CSF, in cerebral edema, or related to the resection cannot be reflected in the images.

Intraoperative brain mapping techniques use either direct stimulation of the cerebral cortex or somatosensory-evoked potentials (SSEPs). Cortical mapping is used to localize the sensory, motor, or speech cortex. The technique requires the use of local anesthesia and a cooperative, informed patient, who may be required to perform repetitive tasks (Lehman, 1995). In direct cortical stimulation, electrical stimulation is applied to the cortex to elicit a response. This technique often allows a more extensive surgical resection to be performed with a decreased risk of permanent morbidity. In a study of 40 patients with dominant temporal lobe tumors, cortical mapping techniques helped maximize the extent of surgery with decreased permanent language deficits (Haglund, Berger, Shamseldin, Lettich, & Ojemann, 1994). Also, the distance of the surgical resection from the language site was significant in predicting postoperative language function and recovery. The procedure has disadvantages. Responses that occur with stimulation of the sensory cortex can be ambiguous. Failure to elicit a response from an area of the cortex does not mean that the resection will not result in deficits. The necessity of using conscious sedation rather than general anesthesia may eliminate this procedure as an option for some patients (Lehman, 1995; Sawaya, Rambo, Hammoud, & Lee Ligon, 1995).

Sensory-evoked potentials include SSEPs, brain stem auditory-evoked potentials, and visual-evoked potentials. They consist of recorded electrical potentials produced by repetitive stimulation of a sensory nerve. The technique permits mapping of the somatosensory, auditory, and visual cortex. In SSEPs, stimulation of a peripheral sensory nerve and recording of the electrical potentials along its entire course to the cortex are performed (Black & Cucchiara, 1993). Monitoring of SSEPs is often used in spine surgery and with tumors located near the motor cortex. The problem with the use of SSEPs is that it does not monitor motor function (Lehman, 1995).

The intraoperative microscope provides magnification and intense illumination within the operative field. Microsurgery has improved the approach to these lesions by providing the ability to make smaller cortical incisions and reach deep areas with less surgical retraction. This approach has led to a decrease in postoperative morbidity. The improved magnification allows more accurate determination of tissue borders, nerves, and vascular structures.

Stereotactic Biopsy. In many patients with known or suspected astrocytomas, the use of cytoreductive surgery may not be the appropriate treatment option. Stereotactic biopsy is indicated for patients whose lesions are located in functionally eloquent areas or in regions difficult to approach without an increased risk of neurologic deficit. Stereotactic biopsy is used to differentiate between radiation necrosis and tumor recurrence, or when tumor progression to a higher grade is suspected. Stereotactic surgery using CT or MRI guidance has permitted biopsy of virtually any abnormality evident on imaging (Apuzzo, Chandrasoma, Cohen, Zee, & Zelman, 1987). In addition, the technique can be used with patients who are unable to tolerate general anesthesia for craniotomy.

Stereotaxis uses three-dimensional coordinates to precisely locate lesions in the brain. The technique uses a stereotactic frame, such as the Brown-Roberts-Wells (BRW) or Leksell system that is secured with screw pins to the patient's head. Fig. 23-15 illustrates the BRW system. A localizing crown with horizontal and vertical rods is attached to the base ring. A CT scan or MRI scan is obtained. The rods are seen on each slice of the imaging study. The x and y coordinates of these points are obtained and transformed to three-dimensional space. In the operating room, an arc guidance system is attached to the base ring. The target lesion can be approached from any angle or point on the arc quadrant. A burr hole or small twist drill hole is made in the skull. The biopsy probe is guided to the tumor site using the x, y, and z coordinates.

The selection of the biopsy site in patients with a presumed astrocytoma is critical. The potential for a nondiagnostic biopsy, inaccurate diagnosis, or underestimation of

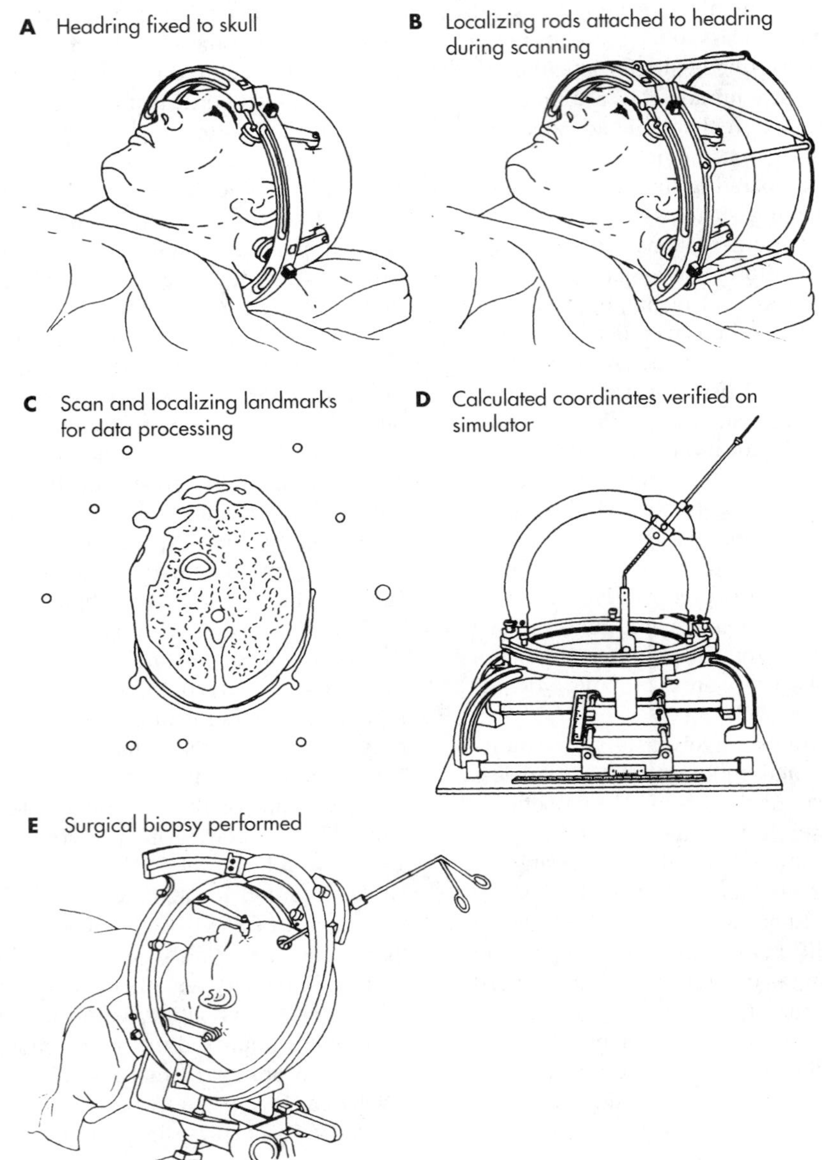

Fig. 23-15 The sequence of steps in stereotactic biopsy using the Brown-Roberts-Wells stereotaxic guidance system. (From Heilbrun, M. P., Roberts, T. S., Apuzzo, M. L. J., Wells, Jr., T. H. & Sabshin, J. K. [1983]. Preliminary experience with Brown-Roberts-Wells [BRW] computerized tomography stereotaxic guidance system. *Journal of Neurosurgery, 59,* 217-222.)

histologic grade exists with astrocytomas (Levivier et al., 1995), which are often histologically heterogeneous. Small tissue samples or inadequate localization may not provide tissue that is representative of the entire lesion. Recent studies using FDG-PET to define biopsy targets have been undertaken to evaluate whether this technique adds to the diagnostic yield. In a study by Greene, Hitchon, Schelper, Yult, and Dyste (1989), the greatest diagnostic yield based on CT data came from the contrast-enhancing tumor rim. The integration of FDG-PET data in the planning of intracranial procedures allows surgeons to biopsy abnormal metabolic regions of the tumors (Levivier et al., 1992, 1995). The procedure is not without risk. The primary surgical risk is hemorrhage at the biopsy site. After the procedure, patients often experience increased cerebral edema and increased neurologic deficits.

Kelly, Alker, and Goerss (1982) and Arbour (1993) described computer-assisted stereotactic resection. A laser is guided through a speculum that is placed using stereotactic guidance. The laser is used to vaporize the lesion. This technique may be beneficial for small, deep tumors.

Laminectomy. The surgical procedure used for spinal cord astrocytomas tumors is a laminectomy. Spinal cord astrocytomas are intramedullary lesions. A laminectomy involves removal of the spinous process and part of the lamina, which constitutes the posterior arch of the spinal canal. Depending on the location and extent of the tumor, multiple levels may require removal. Removal of the lamina provides exposure to the spinal cord. The dura covers the spinal cord and is opened in the midline. Before the dura is opened, intraoperative ultrasound may be used to define the length of the lesion and the presence of cysts. Ultrasonography facilitates the determination of the site for placement of a myelotomy (incision of the spinal cord) at the start of the resection and provides real time images that are useful in evaluating the completeness of the resection (Epstein, Farmer, & Schneider, 1991). The operating microscope is used to visualize the cord as a midline myelotomy is made. The development of the bipolar coagulating forceps, the operating microscope, and the Cavitron ultrasonic surgical aspirator has facilitated the removal of these tumors.

Removal of the tumor is determined by its size, the surgical objectives, and the gross and histologic characteristics of the lesion (McCormick & Stein, 1996). Histologic grade is the most important factor affecting the prognosis of the patient with intramedullary spinal cord astrocytomas. The traditional surgical approach to astrocytomas has been biopsy followed by RT. Epstein, Farmer, and Freed (1992) advocate an aggressive approach to the resection of low-grade tumors. There was minimal morbidity and mortality and good long-term prognosis in a series of adult patients with intramedullary LGAs who had a radical surgical resection performed before significant neurologic deterioration. Of the six adults with an AA at the time of surgery, four had further neurologic deficits, and two remained at their preoperative wheelchair-bound level. Five of the six died between 4 and 23 months postoperatively. These researchers no longer propose aggressive surgery in patients with AAs.

As with astrocytomas of the brain, a more aggressive surgical resection of spinal cord tumors reduces the risk of sampling error in the establishment of a diagnosis. Astrocytomas present with varying degrees of demarcation between the tumor and the spinal cord. Surgical removal alone may provide long-term tumor control or a cure for well-delineated astrocytomas, such as pilocytic astrocytomas and gangliogliomas.

Complications. Neurosurgical procedures are associated with many potential complications. The postoperative management of patients focuses on the early detection of neurologic deterioration. Timely interventions can prevent or reduce permanent neurologic dysfunction. A second goal of postoperative management is maintaining or reestablishing neurologic and systemic homeostasis.

The most common complications that occur following intracranial procedures include the development of a new neurologic deficit, deep venous thrombosis (DVT), pulmonary embolus, hematoma formation, wound infection, and pneumonia. Less commonly occurring complications include hyponatremia, diabetes insipidus, aseptic meningitis, urinary tract infection, sepsis, and drug reactions (Wilson, 1993). A new neurologic deficit or worsening of a preoperative deficit can result from direct injury to brain tissue, cerebral edema, hemorrhage, or metabolic abnormalities. The signs and symptoms commonly observed are alterations in LOC, including lethargy, somnolence, agitation, and confusion; signs of increasing ICP; and increasing focal neurologic deficits.

Cerebral edema, if not recognized and treated early, can be fatal. Postoperative cerebral edema may be exacerbated by the manipulation of brain tissue during surgery, excessive retraction, interference with venous drainage, and cerebral infarction. The maximum amount of cerebral edema occurs 48 to 72 hours postoperatively. Salcman (1993) reviewed complications of stereotactic biopsy in 357 patients and found that the major postoperative morbidities were related to cerebral edema and hemorrhage. Medical management can often reverse edema. High-dose steroids, diuretics (such as mannitol and furosemide), hyperventilation, and intraventricular spinal fluid drainage are the most frequent methods used to reduce cerebral edema.

Hematomas are the result of bleeding into the operative cavity or bleeding from tearing of bridging veins between the brain and dura (subdural hematoma) or the skull and the dura (epidural hematoma). Bleeding within the operative cavity is more common with incompletely resected malignant astrocytomas (Wilson, 1993). Stereotactic biopsy is a blind procedure with the potential risk of injuring vessels and producing bleeding within the tumor because there is no direct visualization of the area. Patients generally present with a new or an exacerbation of a preoperative deficit and CT confirms the region of the bleeding. Management is generally surgical with evacuation of the hematoma (Chin, Zee, & Apuzzo, 1993). Bleeding can extend into the ventricles, producing obstruction of CSF and the development of hydrocephalus. Management of this complication requires placement of a ventriculostomy for external drainage of the CSF. The patient may ultimately need a shunt placed when the CSF clears. Blood may enter the CSF and cause aseptic meningitis, an inflammation of the meninges, which is managed with steroids and symptomatic relief. Placement of an external ventricular or lumbar drain may be needed if signs of increased ICP develop.

Seizures may occur postoperatively and can be a source of increased neurologic injury. Seizures in the postoperative period could result from the tumor itself, the craniotomy, cerebral edema, hemorrhage, or metabolic abnormalities. The risk of seizures is greater with certain types of craniotomies. Anticonvulsants are often administered prophylactically following both craniotomies and stereotactic biopsies. Phenytoin is the most commonly used antiseizure medication. The incidence of postoperative seizures may be associated with subtherapeutic anticonvulsant levels. Levels should be obtained preoperatively and postoperatively to ensure appropriate dosage. Hyponatremia can decrease the seizure threshold, exacerbate cerebral edema, and worsen neurologic deficits. Hyponatremia generally responds to fluid restriction. It may be necessary in the immediate postoperative period to limit fluids to 1500 ml/day, although generally patients are kept euvolemic. Other common causes of seizures include low magnesium or calcium levels, hyperglycemia, hypoxemia, alcohol withdrawal, meningitis, hematoma, cerebral edema, or pneumocephalus. It is essential to determine the cause of the seizure so that the underlying cause can be treated appropriately (Kelly, 1994).

Postoperative DVT is often seen in patients with astrocytomas. The high incidence is caused by a number of factors including limited mobility, hemiparesis, and the release of factors that increase the coagulability of the blood. The use of compression boots in the perioperative period is helpful in reducing the incidence of clots. Early ambulation is encouraged whenever possible. The use of heparin prophylaxis remains controversial. Because pulmonary emboli can be a fatal complication of DVT, early recognition and treatment are vital. This complication can present early or late in the postoperative period.

Pneumonia is a concern in any surgical procedure that requires general anesthesia. Neurosurgical procedures are generally long, with the patient remaining in a fixed position. Patients must be evaluated for increased risk of pneumonia. Patients at higher risk are those with an altered LOC, cranial nerve deficits, impaired mobility, and those who have recently experienced seizures. Other general surgical complications encountered include wound infection, sepsis, myocardial infarction (MI), gastrointestinal (GI) hemorrhage, and drug reactions.

Short-term use of antibiotics during the perioperative period reduces the incidence of infection. Patients undergoing recurrent craniotomies who have also undergone prior treatment with RT are at greater risk for wound-healing difficulties and infection. Superficial wound infections are treated locally. More extensive infections may require removal of the bone flap and several weeks of IV antibiotics. Patients with reconstructed bone flaps are also at an increased risk for infection. Urinary tract infections are a risk because of the use of indwelling urinary catheters. These catheters should be removed as quickly as possible postoperatively.

Patients who are on high-dose steroids are at risk for the development of steroid-induced diabetes. Serum glucose levels should be evaluated. If they are elevated, blood glucose monitoring should be initiated. The use of high-dose steroids has been associated with GI bleeding, and many advocate the use of prophylactic treatment with antacids, H_2 blockers, or sucralfate.

Complications following biopsy or resection of intramedullary spinal cord lesions include the standard risks, such as infection, MI, hemorrhage, DVT, and pulmonary embolus. Complications specific to spinal surgery are bladder or bowel dysfunction, sexual dysfunction, CSF leakage, pseudomeningocele formation, and the onset of new neurologic deficits, such as proprioception deficits. It is common for patients to complain of sensory loss in the early postoperative period. The patient may experience difficulty with position sense, although this problem generally improves with time. The patient with significant or long-standing preoperative neurologic deficits is likely to have no improvement or even progression after surgery.

Radiation Therapy

Radiation therapy is an important adjuvant therapy in the treatment of AAs. Early large, randomized, multiinstitutional trials firmly established the role of external beam RT as standard postoperative therapy for patients with both AAs and other malignant gliomas (Walker, Strike, & Sheline, 1979). Patients with AAs who received postoperative RT had a significantly prolonged median survival time compared with those who received only postoperative supportive care. These studies were so convincing that almost all subsequent clinical trials evaluating adjuvant therapy for malignant astrocytomas have included some form of RT in all of the treatment arms (Fine, Dear, Loeffler, Black, & Canellos, 1993).

Conventional External Beam Radiation Therapy. Conventional external beam RT has traditionally been delivered to the whole brain (WBRT). However, many patients who survive for extended periods after WBRT develop significant treatment-related morbidity (Shapiro, 1986). Furthermore, neuroimaging studies have demonstrated that the majority of these tumors recur within 2 cm of their original location. Improved imaging techniques and the recognition that tumor recurrence is generally local, combined with the known deleterious side effects of RT to the normal brain, have led many cancer centers and cooperative groups to use limited field radiotherapy. The radiation is delivered to the tumor and a 2 to 3 cm margin of surrounding tissue (Laperriere & Bernstein, 1994). This method of partial brain irradiation has become a standard treatment approach for AAs and other brain tumors. It is generally agreed that the deleterious effects of radiation to the brain for long-term survivors with malignant astrocytomas occur less often with limited field irradiation, and that this has been achieved without any loss in treatment efficacy (Vick & Paleologos, 1995). WBRT is usually recommended for patients with multifocal tumors (Leibel, Scott, & Loeffler, 1994).

Conventional external beam cranial irradiation is given in divided doses (fractions) over an extended period. Generally, in patients with AA, a total dose of 60 Gy is administered in daily fractions of 1.8 to 2.0 Gy over 6 weeks. Many of these tumors have poorly defined borders and infiltrate into surrounding normal brain tissue. Therefore it is often necessary to irradiate a substantial amount of normal tissue within the target volume, and the tolerance of this normal tissue becomes the dose-limiting factor. Damage to normal brain tissue is related not only to a higher total dose of radiation, but also to the size of the fraction administered. The amount of fractionation is the predominant factor in determining the incidence of late toxicity in normal tissue (Jeremic, Grujicic, Antunovic, Djuric, & Shibamoto, 1995). Higher doses delivered in a conventional fashion have not improved the outcome and have resulted in increased toxicity. Approximately 50% of patients with AA show evidence of a response with conventional RT (Shrieve & Loeffler, 1995).

The role of RT in LGAs remains controversial. No prospective randomized clinical trials have compared surgery alone with surgery plus RT in the treatment of LGAs (Levin et al., 1997). Nor does any consensus exist with regard to the proper timing of postoperative RT for these tumors (National Comprehensive Cancer Network, 1997). The analysis of two randomized trials comparing immediate and delayed radiation in patients with LGA will provide more information on this subject. For some completely resected astrocytomas (cystic cerebellar astrocytoma and pilocytic astrocytoma), postoperative RT is not recommended, as complete surgical removal is often curative.

Many retrospective reviews suggest that postoperative RT is beneficial for incompletely resected low-grade tumors, and some medical professionals advocate that postoperative RT should be routinely given to these patients (Shaw, Scheithauer, & O'Fallon, 1993). The rationale for early intervention is based on the poor long-term survival of these patients, the likelihood that low-grade tumors will transform into high-grade tumors, and the advances in the delivery of modern RT (Shaw, 1990). Other physicians prefer to observe patients on anticonvulsants and defer RT until the tumor progresses or recurs. Proponents of the watchful, waiting approach base it on the lack of proven benefit or improved prognosis of early RT compared with delayed RT and the known potential long-term complications of RT. When radiation is given to patients with these tumors, it should be administered using limited field or conformal methods. WBRT results in more treatment-related neurotoxicity than localized RT, and these patients are often young and may survive for years (National Comprehensive Cancer Network, 1997). The standard radiation dose for LGAs is 54 Gy delivered over 6 weeks in fractions of 1.8 Gy (Shaw et al., 1993). The selection of 54 Gy as the standard dose is based on its relative safety when applied to a limited volume of the brain and the lack of evidence for increased efficacy with higher doses (National Comprehensive Cancer Network, 1997).

The side effects of cranial irradiation can be divided into acute, early-delayed, and late-delayed reactions. The acute reactions occur during the course of therapy, often after the first few treatments. They are believed to result from disruption of the BBB by ionizing radiation, causing increased cerebral edema and a rise in ICP (Posner, 1995). Patients may experience headache, nausea, vomiting, somnolence, and worsening neurologic symptoms. Many patients receive corticosteroids 24 to 72 hours before beginning treatment, especially if a large tumor is present, a large volume of brain is to be irradiated, or if symptoms of increased ICP already exist. Corticosteroids substantially diminish the disruption of the BBB and prevent or improve most clinical symptoms (Posner, 1995). The symptoms usually become less severe with subsequent treatments. Other acute effects are fatigue, anorexia, alopecia, and skin irritations.

The early-delayed reactions occur 1 to 4 months after treatment has been completed and may last for several months. These effects are thought to result from the temporary disruption of myelin formation or changes in capillary permeability. Symptoms include headache, somnolence, and an increase or worsening of neurologic deficits. Symptoms appearing within this time frame are generally anticipated and may not require treatment with corticosteroids. However, patients may be evaluated for possible disease progression.

Late-delayed effects of cranial irradiation are the most serious and usually occur 6 to 24 months after completion of treatment. These effects are irreversible and often progressive. They are believed to result from direct injury to brain cells and blood vessels. This reaction typically occurs after a large volume of or the whole brain is irradiated and presents as white matter changes or degeneration at the tumor site and surrounding irradiated brain. The clinical presentation ranges from seizure disorders, varying degrees of neuropsychological impairment, dementia, or death. The neuropsychological impairment most often is short-term memory loss and a decreased attention span. Elderly patients are more severely affected. The onset and progression of impairment are quite variable. Radiation necrosis, although more common after brachytherapy and radiosurgery, may also occur as a late-delayed effect of conventional external beam RT. Patients who develop radiation necrosis often present with localizing neurologic signs, symptoms of increased ICP, or both. The necrosis may mimic signs and symptoms of tumor occurrence. Corticosteroids may improve the neurologic symptoms associated with radiation necrosis. Patients often undergo reoperation of the necrotic tissue. Other long-term complications of RT are optic atrophy leading to visual loss, hypopituitarism, and secondary malignancies.

Although the role of radiotherapy in spinal cord astrocytomas has not been evaluated in prospective studies because of the rarity of these tumors (Jyothirmayi, Madhaven, Nair, & Rajan, 1997), the use of postoperative RT is generally recommended. In one review of patients with spinal cord astrocytomas (Minehan, Shaw, Scheithauer, Davis, & Onofrio, 1995), survival was improved in all patients who received RT despite different histologic subtypes. In another review (Jyothirmayi et al., 1997), patients with these tumors were treated with conservative surgery and RT, and 90% demonstrated improvement or stabilization of their neurologic status.

Radiation doses of 50 to 54 Gy are used to minimize the risk of radiation injury to the spinal cord (Levin et al., 1997). Radiation therapy to the spinal cord does not cause acute clinical syndromes. However, it can result in transient early-delayed or late-delayed radiation myelopathy. The transient early-delayed syndrome develops 3 to 5 months after treatment and generally resolves within 6 months. It is characterized by momentary paresthesias or electric shock-like sensations radiating from the neck down to the extremities upon flexion of the neck (Lhermitte's sign). Symptoms of late-delayed radiation myelopathy begin 12 to 50 months after RT has been completed. The first symptom may be Brown-Sequard syndrome with paresthesias and weakness in one leg and a loss of temperature and pain sensation in the other leg (Posner, 1995). The signs and symptoms are irreversible and often progressive. Some patients may develop only mild to moderate weakness and sensory loss, although others go on to lose, within several months, all motor, sensory, and autonomic function below the involved level of the spinal cord. Less commonly, radiation myelopathy is manifested by the acute onset of paraplegia or quadriplegia that evolves over several hours or a few days, resulting from infarction of the spinal cord.

Demyelination, white matter necrosis, and intramedullary microvascular injury each play a role in the development of radiation myelopathy (Levin et al., 1997), which can occur after RT has been administered for other malignant processes in the neck, chest, or abdominal region if the spinal cord is accidentally or unavoidably included in the RT port (DeAngelis, 1996). It is estimated that with conventionally fractionated RT (1.8 to 2.0 Gy per fraction, 5 fractions per week), the incidence of delayed myelopathy is 5% for doses in the range of 57 to 61 Gy (Schultheiss, 1990). A large retrospective study indicated that 50 Gy delivered in 25 daily fractions is associated with an approximate 1% incidence of late myelopathy (Wong, Van Dyk, Milosevic, & Laperriere, 1994).

A number of new radiotherapy approaches have been evaluated and continue to be evaluated in patients with astrocytomas in an attempt to improve on the unsatisfactory results obtained with conventional RT. These strategies include three-dimensional conformal RT (3D-CRT), alternative methods of fractionation, radiosensitizers, focal dose escalation with brachytherapy or radiosurgery, stereotactic radiotherapy, particle therapy, and boron neutron capture therapy (BNCT).

3D-CRT. 3D-CRT is a relatively new method of treatment planning that uses CT and MRI information and powerful computer technology to optimize the delivery of external beam RT. The radiation treatments shape the prescribed dose to conform to the anatomic boundaries of the tumor in its entire three-dimensional configuration (Leibel et al., 1994). Complete anatomic and dose information for the entire tumor volume and its surrounding tissues are provided so that the high radiation dose is limited to the tumor, and the dose to the surrounding normal tissue is minimized.

Thorton and colleagues (1991) compared conventional RT (two-dimensional) and three-dimensional treatment planning studies in brain tumor patients. When 3D-CRT was used, a 30% reduction in the volume of normal brain irradiated was noted. This method of highly precise RT should improve outcomes by reducing toxicity to the normal brain and subsequent long-term effects. It may also allow safe administration of higher doses than are possible using standard treatment planning techniques. Until recently, 3D-CRT was impractical and not widely available because of the highly complex software required for treatment planning and computer-controlled dose delivery.

Alternative Methods of Fractionation. Two alternative methods of fractionation that have been studied are hyperfractionation (HF) and accelerated fractionation. In HF, two or more treatments are given daily using smaller than the standard dose fractions of 1.8 to 2.0 Gy. The goal of HF is to administer a higher total dose in the same overall time without increasing toxicity. Normal glial and vascular cells limit the total amount of radiation that can be administered. If smaller sized fractions are administered (by HF) and the amount of normal tissue irradiated decreases (by high precision RT), a higher total dose may not cause increased damage or late sequelae. The interval between the twice daily dose fractions allows sufficient time for normal tissues to repair radiation damage. During the time between doses, the rapidly proliferating tumor cells may progress into more radiosensitive phases of the cell cycle, thus increasing the opportunity for tumor cell killing (Leibel et al., 1994). An example of an HF regimen is the delivery of 1.2 Gy twice daily over 6 weeks for a total dose of 72 Gy. The Radiation Therapy Oncology Group (RTOG) conducted dose escalation trials with HF and reported that 72 Gy delivered with HF was no more toxic that 60 Gy delivered with conventional RT (Nelson et al., 1993). However, a significant survival advantage with HFRT was not clearly demonstrated.

In accelerated fractionation, standard size fractions (1.8 to 2.0 Gy) are administered more than once a day to complete treatment in a shorter overall time. This approach may be appropriate for patients with poor prognostic factors and relatively short life expectancies such as the elderly (Leibel et al., 1994).

Radiosensitizers. Radiosensitizers are chemicals that potentially increase the lethal effects of radiation by preferentially sensitizing tumor cells to radiation. A number of agents administered during RT have been evaluated in patients with malignant astrocytomas, including metronidazole, misonidazole, etanidazole, hydroxyurea, and alkylating agents; but they have not demonstrated a significant increase in survival. The halogenated pyrimidines, particularly 5-bromodeoxyuridine (BUdR), have been under investigation. The radiosensitizer, BUdR, is similar to the normal DNA precursor, thymidine. The BUdR is incorporated into the DNA of cells undergoing DNA synthesis (Shrieve & Loeffler, 1995). The mitotically active tumor cells are much more likely to incorporate the BUdR than the slowly replicating normal glial cells (Laperriere & Bernstein, 1994). As a result of the substitution, the tumor cells are more sensitive to the DNA-damaging effects of radiation. In a study by Levin and colleagues (1995), patients with AA who received RT with BUdR and chemotherapy had a significantly prolonged median survival (272 weeks). In comparison, an earlier study (Levin et al., 1990) evaluated patients with AA who received nonsensitized RT and the same chemotherapeutic agents. Median survival in this group was 151 weeks. A randomized study comparing BUdR-sensitized RT with nonsensitized RT (followed by chemotherapy in both groups) is further evaluating the efficacy of this form of therapy in patients with AA.

Focal Dose Escalation. Interstitial brachytherapy, a method of focal irradiation, delivers a high dose of radiation to the tumor while decreasing the radiation exposure to the surrounding normal brain tissue. It involves the temporary implantation of radioactive sources directly into the tumor using CT- and MRI-guided stereotactic surgical techniques. The radiation sources most commonly used are iodine 125 (^{125}I) and iridium 192 (^{192}I), and they remain in place for several days to weeks. Because the sources are placed directly within the area to be irradiated, the tumor volume receives the highest radiation dose. The rapid fall-off in dose as the distance from the radiation source increases spares the surrounding normal brain tissue (Shrieve & Loeffler, 1995).

It has been estimated that less than one third of all patients with malignant astrocytomas are candidates for brachytherapy (Sneed, Larson, & Gutin, 1994). Patients with tumors that are large, multifocal, cross the midline, located in functionally vital areas, and have borders that are not reasonably well demarcated are not eligible for this form of therapy. Neither are patients whose performance status is low. Brachytherapy has been used in both patients with recurrent disease and those with newly diagnosed tumors. In newly diagnosed patients with AA who were treated with brachytherapy following external beam RT, median survival was 158 weeks, with a 51% 3-year survival, and in patients with recurrent disease, the median survival was 53 weeks, with a 23% 3-year survival (Sneed et al., 1994). The role of interstitial brachytherapy in the initial management of patients with AA remains to be determined. It does appear to benefit selected patients with recurrent disease (Laperriere & Bernstein, 1994).

Another form of focal irradiation is radiosurgery, which uses an imaging-compatible stereotactic device to precisely localize an intracranial target and deliver a high radiation dose in a single fraction without delivering a significant dose to the surrounding normal brain tissue (Leibel et al., 1994). Stereotaxy is necessary because such a high dose of radiation can be given without complications only if the normal brain is not included in the treatment field. The planning and accuracy of the treatment are critical (Krause, Lamb, Ham, Larson, & Gutin, 1991). Stereotactic radiosurgery is similar to stereotactic craniotomy in its use of modern neuroradiologic and computer technology to target the lesion in three-dimensional space (Ward-Smith, 1997). Radiosurgery is being used as a boost after external beam RT in patients with malignant astrocytomas. It may also be used to retreat patients with small previously irradiated lesions. Unfortunately, only 10% to 20% of patients with AAs are eligible for this method of therapy (Shrieve & Loeffler, 1995). Tumors must be small and well circumscribed.

The major complication of both interstitial brachytherapy and radiosurgery is the development of symptomatic radiation necrosis requiring the prolonged administration of steroids and reoperation. There has not yet been a randomized trial comparing radiosurgery and brachytherapy in the management of either newly diagnosed or recurrent patients with AA. Although the outcomes for brachytherapy and radiosurgery appear similar, radiosurgery offers several advantages over brachytherapy. Radiosurgery is noninvasive, thus avoiding the risks of hemorrhage, infection, and tumor seeding (Leibel et al., 1994) and is often done in an outpatient setting. Radiosurgery may be used on tumors located within regions of the brain that are unsuitable for brachytherapy. However, brachytherapy has the advantage of better contouring of dose distribution for large or irregularly shaped tumors (Flickinger, Loeffler, & Larson, 1994).

Stereotactic Radiotherapy. Stereotactic radiotherapy uses the planning technology of stereotactic radiosurgery but delivers the treatment using standard fractionation doses. Stereotactic hardware and head frames that can be relocalized daily in a nontraumatic and reproducible fashion are used (Leibel et al., 1994). Standard fractionation avoids the toxicities associated with large single doses, and tumors located near critical structures may be treated more successfully because of the precision of the stereotactic technique (Belford, 1997).

Particle Therapy. Particle therapy uses subatomic particles as opposed to photons as a form of radiation. These particles, which include neutrons, protons, helium ions, and pions, allow better dose localization to the tumor volume, thus decreasing damage to normal brain tissue. Particle beams also have a greater biologic effect than photons; that is, they are more effective in killing tumor cells (Laperriere & Bernstein, 1994). Research of this form of radiation will continue as additional facilities become available.

Boron Neutron Capture Therapy. Theoretically, boron neutron capture therapy (BNCT) could be a very effective form of RT in the treatment of malignant astrocytomas. The concept involves the systemic administration of a boron compound that has selective uptake in rapidly dividing tumor cells, followed by irradiation of the tumor with thermal neutrons (Ceberg et al., 1995). Neutron-capture reactions will then occur in the cell containing the boron, followed by a prompt emission of lithium and helium particles. These particles release sufficient energy to be cytotoxic to the individual cell in which the reaction takes place (Laperriere & Bernstein, 1994). The energy resulting from this reaction is lost in a very small diameter, so normal brain cells are not affected. Thus if a boron carrier with high tumor specificity can be found, BNCT could be an effective method of killing tumor cells with boron uptake while sparing the surrounding healthy tissue.

For BNCT to cure patients with astrocytomas, the injected boron compound must not only be taken up in the bulk of the tumor, but also must reach the nearby infiltrated areas and the migrating cells that have traveled to other parts of the CNS. Widespread use of this technique has been limited by the high cost, limited availability of nuclear reactors, and lack of suitable boron compounds that do not have harmful side effects (Belford, 1997). Furthermore, the boron uptake in the tumor is often quite inhomogeneous so that there is an insignificant concentration of the compound in infiltrating cells. However, interest in this form of therapy is growing.

Chemotherapy

The addition of chemotherapy to the treatment regimen of AAs has not greatly improved the survival of these patients. The nitrosoureas have been the most widely studied group of chemotherapeutic agents in patients with high-grade astrocytoma. These drugs are highly lipid soluble and readily cross the BBB. Early studies by the Brain Tumor Study Group (BTSG) found an improved 18-month survival with adjuvant carmustine (BCNU) and radiation as compared with radiation alone (Walker et al., 1978). Despite the large number of subsequent trials evaluating other single agents and combination chemotherapy, BCNU remains the single-most active nitrosourea for high-grade astrocytomas. Partial responses have been observed in up to 30% of patients (Moynihan & Grossman, 1994).

To clarify the value of adjuvant chemotherapy for malignant gliomas, Fine and colleagues (1993) reviewed 16 randomized studies investigating chemotherapy in high-grade astrocytomas conducted over a 15-year period. They concluded that adjuvant chemotherapy after surgery and RT in patients with high-grade astrocytomas increased survival by 10.1% at 1 year and 8.6% at 2 years. Although none are superior to BCNU (Conrad, Milosavljevic, & Yung, 1995; Nicholas, Prados, Larson, & Gutin, 1997), other agents that have demonstrated some activity against high-grade astrocytomas include procarbazine, carboplatin, etoposide, cisplatin, cyclophosphamide, dacarbazine, streptozocin, hydroxyurea, and tamoxifen.

Until recently, no other agent or combination of agents has been shown conclusively to be more effective against these tumors (Kaye & Laidlaw, 1992). In a reanalysis of a randomized prospective study (Levin et al., 1990), the combination of lomustine, procarbazine, and vincristine (PCV) significantly increased the median survival of patients with AA (151.1 weeks) compared with BCNU (82.1 weeks). The PCV regimen, as opposed to BCNU, is being used increasingly in many centers as standard adjuvant chemotherapy for patients with AA.

Many of these earlier studies evaluating the effectiveness of chemotherapeutic agents in astrocytomas show only marginally significant or conflicting results. These findings stem in part from several methodologic problems. Historically, it has been difficult to accrue large enough numbers of patients with these tumors into clinical studies. Many of the studies conducted included heterogeneous patient populations and failed to separate patients according to prognostically significant variables such as age, histology, and performance status. Patients with different tumor histologies were often included in these studies. The inconsistent use of a uniform histologic classification system and a lack of uniform response criteria have also contributed to the difficulty in interpreting the results of these chemotherapy trials. Most contemporary chemotherapy trials now control for these variables (Conrad et al., 1995).

A major barrier in delivering chemotherapy to primary brain tumors is the presence of the BBB. This barrier is comprised of a continuous lining of capillary endothelial cells that are connected by tight junctions. These tight junctions provide a selective mechanism that can exclude or allow the transport of substances depending on their physical characteristics. Large, hydrophilic compounds tend to be excluded from the brain by this poorly understood anatomic and physiologic barrier, whereas smaller, lipid-soluble agents pass through more rapidly into the brain (Moynihan & Grossman, 1994). The BBB exists to prevent harmful substances from reaching the brain. Unfortunately, many chemotherapeutic agents are unable to penetrate the BBB because of their physical characteristics. New approaches to chemotherapy administration are being investigated in an attempt to increase the delivery and efficacy of chemotherapeutic agents to astrocytomas. These approaches include continuous infusion chemotherapy, intra-arterial administration of chemotherapy, BBB disruption, high-dose chemotherapy with autologous bone marrow transplantation, and interstitial chemotherapy.

Continuous Infusion Chemotherapy. As previously mentioned, most chemotherapy regimens for astrocytomas have relied on lipid-soluble agents that pass through the BBB. However, most high-grade astrocytomas are characterized by some degree of BBB disruption. Contrast enhancement within these tumors on CT or MRI studies represents local BBB disruption. For this reason, treatment with water-soluble chemotherapeutic agents may be effective. Short-term infusions or boluses of water-soluble agents may reach the outer perimeter where the BBB is disrupted. When contrast is administered, the tumor rim initially enhances, but it may take several hours for the contrast to reach the center of the tumor. Water-soluble agents may be able to reach a wider area of the tumor over a longer time if sustained blood levels of the drug are maintained. Treatment of these diffusely infiltrating tumors with only water-soluble agents is of little value because these tumors extend beyond the regions of contrast enhancement on CT and MRI. A combination of a water-soluble agent and a lipid-soluble agent with nonoverlapping toxicities can provide chemotherapy to regions of the brain where the BBB is intact and where it is disrupted. Continuous 72-hour infusions of cisplatin and carmustine administered to patients with high-grade astrocytoma before RT have demonstrated a 40% response rate, with three patients alive at 5.2, 5.6, and 7.9 years after their diagnoses (Grossman et al., 1997). Additional studies are needed to determine if this type of regimen is superior to conventional therapy.

Intra-arterial Chemotherapy. The method of direct intra-arterial administration of chemotherapy has been used in an attempt to increase drug delivery to the tumor while limiting systemic exposure. Chemotherapy can be delivered into the internal carotid or vertebral arteries, which provide the arterial supply to intracranial astrocytomas (Lesser & Grossman, 1994). Cisplatin and BCNU are two agents that have been evaluated in this fashion. Overall, tumor responses with this technique have been variable with substantial toxicity (Armstrong & Gilbert, 1996). Shapiro and colleagues (1992) reported on a large BTSG study evaluating intra-arterial BCNU in one treatment arm that was discontinued because of toxicity. Ipsilateral visual loss occurred in 15% of the patients, and 10% developed severe neurotoxicity. Also, survival rates for those who received the intra-arterial chemotherapy were worse than those who received IV BCNU.

BBB Disruption. Disruption of the BBB is another method of chemotherapy administration that has been investigated for malignant astrocytomas in an attempt to improve the delivery of chemotherapy to the tumor. An osmotic agent such as mannitol is administered through the carotid or vertebral arteries on the side of the tumor just before administering intra-arterial or IV chemotherapy. This approach results in shrunken vascular endothelial cells with widened intercellular tight junctions, leading to an increased passage of previously restricted substances across the vascular endothelium. This disruption allows higher concentrations of the drug to reach the tumor. However, the normal brain tissue is also exposed to an increased amount of chemotherapy. This approach has resulted in substantial toxicities including seizures and increased neurologic deficits. The procedure is performed with the patient under general anesthesia, and the possibility of complications from anesthesia itself exists. Disruption of the BBB is transient and returns to normal within 4 hours after the hypertonic infusion (Lesser & Grossman, 1994).

High-dose Chemotherapy with Bone Marrow Rescue. High-dose chemotherapy, followed by autologous bone marrow rescue, has also been evaluated in patients with malignant astrocytomas in the hope that dose intensification might improve drug delivery into the brain and overcome drug resistance (Armstrong & Gilbert, 1996). These tumors rarely metastasize to the bone marrow, and patients often have a low total-body tumor burden after surgery, theoretically making this form of therapy an attractive option (Grossman & Norris, 1995). The chemotherapeutic agent most often used in the preparative regimen is carmustine. Carmustine has a steep dose-response curve, its dose-limiting toxicity is delayed, and it is an effective agent against malignant astrocytomas. These factors make it a good agent for dose intensification followed by bone marrow rescue (Lesser & Grossman, 1993). Other agents that have been used in this fashion include etoposide and thiotepa. Although longer survivals have been noted in some patients, significant systemic toxicities have been reported including pulmonary, hepatic, neurologic, and infectious complications (Grossman & Norris, 1995).

Interstitial Chemotherapy. Interstitial chemotherapy is another form of chemotherapy administration being investigated. It involves the use of biodegradable polymers impregnated with chemotherapy. The major goal of interstitial chemotherapy is to maximize the local cytotoxic effects of the administered drug while minimizing or eliminating its systemic toxicity (Lesser & Grossman, 1994). These polymers can be placed intraoperatively in the walls of the cavity left after surgical resection. They continuously release over several weeks high concentrations of the incorporated drug. Chemotherapy delivered in this fashion bypasses the variably disrupted BBB, results in high local drug concentrations, and minimizes systemic toxicities.

Brem and colleagues (1995) reported on a randomized Phase III trial in patients with recurrent malignant gliomas who underwent reoperation with implantation of polymer wafers containing carmustine into the tumor bed. Patients who received the carmustine wafers had a moderate but statistically significant improvement in survival with no untoward events. Future studies are planned to evaluate the effectiveness of higher doses of carmustine and the use of polymer implants as initial therapy for brain tumors. It may be possible to use this type of delivery system with other agents.

Chemotherapy in Low-grade Astrocytomas. Few randomized prospective studies have evaluated the role of chemotherapy in LGAs. Currently, there is no proven role for chemotherapy in the initial management of these tumors (Shaw, Scheithauer, & Dinapoli, 1997). Chemotherapy is generally reserved for patients with recurrent or progressive disease (Conrad et al., 1995). When chemotherapy is administered to these patients, the same agents are used as in patients with AAs. Prospective studies are in progress evaluating several chemotherapeutic regimens in patients with low-grade tumors.

Chemotherapy in Spinal Cord Astrocytomas. There are no reports of controlled clinical trials of chemotherapy for primary spinal cord astrocytomas. It is possible that chemotherapeutic agents active against intracranial astrocytomas may be equally efficacious against this same histology in the spinal cord (Levin et al., 1997). Anecdotal reports suggest that patients have been treated with nitrosourea-based chemotherapy regimens.

Biotherapy

The majority of available methods of biotherapy have not been successful in improving the survival of patients with astrocytomas when compared with conventional therapy (Jaeckle, 1994). Methods investigated include the use of cytokines (interferons, interleukins, and tumor necrosis factor), interleukin-stimulated lymphokine-activated killer cells, antigen-stimulated lymphocytes, and monoclonal antibodies. Research continues to grow in this area as more selective methods of administration are developed, newer agents are identified, and the use of biotherapy in combination with other treatment modalities is tested.

Gene Therapy

Gene therapy is a promising biologic therapy being investigated for malignant astrocytomas. There are two major components to gene therapy, the delivery system and the therapeutic gene. The most commonly used delivery system or vector is a virus. The three predominant vectors are retroviruses, adenoviruses, and herpes viruses. Retroviruses will insert their genes only into dividing cells, making them particularly useful in brain tumors. The viral vector infects the tumor cell with a previously incorporated therapeutic gene. As the cell divides, it produces other cells that are now genetically altered with the incorporated gene.

The most widely used therapeutic gene in brain tumor trials is one of the herpes simplex virus genes, thymidine kinase (TK). The TK gene is inserted into the brain tumor and is subsequently replicated. The tumor cells now carrying the gene are destroyed when the antiviral agent ganciclovir is administered (Randal, 1993). Although initial gene therapy trials are encouraging, the development of more efficient and selective vector systems is needed. This method of therapy is still in its infancy, and it remains to be seen what role gene therapy will play in the treatment of astrocytomas.

An additional area being investigated is antiangiogenesis. Tumor growth is dependent on the development of a new vascular supply. Endothelial proliferation is a uniformly accepted characteristic of malignant astrocytomas; the degree of neovascularization increases with the degree of malignancy (Fine, 1995). Antiangiogenesis, or the inhibition of new blood vessel growth, is believed to inhibit tumor growth. Studies are currently underway evaluating several antiangiogenesis inhibitors in the treatment of malignant astrocytomas.

Treatment of Recurrent Astrocytomas

Treatment of recurrent intracranial and spinal cord astrocytomas is greatly dependent on the same factors as had been evaluated at diagnosis plus the current neurologic condition of the patient and which previous therapies have been administered. In general, patients with recurrent AA are evaluated for surgery as a first therapeutic intervention. Reoperation often provides improvement in neurologic status and a decrease in symptoms. An alternative form of RT may be considered, such as stereotactic radiosurgery or brachytherapy. Patients who have received a full dose of external beam RT may not be reirradiated in this manner. Additional chemotherapeutic agents may be recommended, depending on which agents the patient received previously. Agents that may be used include carboplatin, procarbazine, and tamoxifen. Patients may also be referred for investigational therapies. A list of current clinical trials is available through the NCI.

Patients with recurrent LGAs are also evaluated for reoperation first. Many LGAs progress to a higher grade tumor, and a histologic diagnosis is necessary. Patients who have not received RT will usually receive some form of this therapy, either limited field RT or 3D-CRT. Chemotherapy may also be considered even though definitive clinical trials are not available to support that this approach is an effective treatment strategy. Chemotherapeutic agents that may be used in LGAs include BCNU, carboplatin, vincristine, and procarbazine.

Patients with spinal cord astrocytomas may receive further RT if the maximal dose has not been administered or if the lesion extends outside the originally treated field. Generally, surgical intervention is not recommended. Chemotherapy may be considered with the same agents that were described previously.

ONCOLOGIC EMERGENCIES

The major oncologic emergency associated with intracranial astrocytomas is increased ICP. Signs and symptoms of increased ICP are discussed extensively elsewhere in this chapter. The early recognition of signs and symptoms is essential to ensure the best possible neurologic outcome in these patients. Often, subtle changes in the LOC may be the first sign of ICP. Untreated increased ICP can lead to further neurologic deterioration, herniation syndromes, and death. Treatment of increased ICP and cerebral herniation consists of corticosteroids, careful fluid management, hyperosmolar agents, surgical decompression, and hyperventilation.

NURSING MANAGEMENT

Surgery

The nursing management of the astrocytoma patient undergoing surgery is summarized in Table 23-7. The nursing care varies depending on the surgical procedure performed and the extent of the neurologic deficits. Patients undergoing craniotomy are usually hospitalized for 3 to 5 days if there are no complications. Patients having a stereotactic biopsy require a 24- to 48-hour hospital stay. Patient education is the major focus of care for the preoperative outpatient. Patients require information on the type of procedure, the usual perioperative routine, common medications, and self-care activities. Fig. 23-16, pp. 531-532, is an example of a documentation tool for preoperative teaching for patients undergoing neurosurgery. Postoperative recovery practices vary among institutions. Some patients will be cared for in an intensive care setting or a postoperative stepdown unit for 24 to 48 hours. Others will not require intensive monitoring beyond the postanesthesia care unit environment. Patients must be instructed to refrain from taking aspirin or products containing aspirin for 10 days or nonsteroidal anti-inflammatory drugs (NSAIDs) for 48 hours. This restriction is essential to prevent bleeding complications.

The major focus of inpatient nursing care is on the early recognition of neurologic changes. Corticosteroids are administered to reduce postoperative cerebral edema. Maximal postoperative cerebral edema occurs 48 to 72 hours after surgery. Early recognition may be critical in the prevention of permanent or life-threatening deficits. In addition, the prevention of postoperative complications including DVT, pulmonary embolus, pneumonia, infection, and pressure ulcers is essential. Patients with astrocytomas often have neurologic deficits that include cognitive changes, motor and sensory deficits, language dysfunction, and difficulty with balance. The nurse must individualize the patient's plan of care depending on the specific neurologic deficits. Safety measures assume the utmost importance for all involved in the patient's care. Family members and primary caregivers may not be aware of the severity of the potential risks. The nursing care plan should reflect the high-risk activities, including impaired judgment, high risk for falls, and altered thought processes. The nursing standards of care present the management of these patient problems in detail.

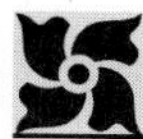

TABLE 23-7 Standard of Care for the Patient Undergoing a Neurologic Procedure

Patient Problem and Outcomes	Nursing Interventions and Rationales	Patient Education Instructions
Knowledge Deficit Patient will: • Verbalize understanding of the purpose, benefits, and risks of the planned surgical procedure. • Verbalize understanding of the planned diagnostic tests, consults, or procedures required before surgery. • Verbalize understanding of risk factors that can impact in the postoperative recovery.	1. Assess patient's level of knowledge about the disease, surgical procedure, and risks of the procedure. 2. Explain consults and diagnostic tests required preoperatively. 3. Encourage questions and allow time for discussion. 4. Make referrals as needed to obtain answers to questions (physician, anesthesiologist). 5. Instruct patient in self-care measures to prevent complications (leg exercises, coughing and deep-breathing exercises). 6. Document patient and family teaching.	1. Provide and review educational materials with patient and family, including booklets and pamphlets on the disease, procedure, and preoperative teaching. 2. Provide a list of drugs to avoid preoperatively such as aspirin and ibuprofen. 3. Patient will demonstrate self-care measures to prevent complications (leg exercises, coughing and deep-breathing exercises).
Anxiety Patient will: • Verbalize concerns and fears related to the surgery or diagnosis. • Verbalize coping strategies and available resources.	1. Assess patient's level of anxiety. 2. Encourage expression of feelings and concerns. 3. Assist patient in identification of coping strategies that have helped in the past. 4. Offer new techniques for coping (relaxation, visualization, therapeutic touch). 5. Explore cultural and religious aspects of responses to illness, loss, or death.	1. Teach strategies such as diversion techniques to minimize focusing on somatic or emotional response. 2. Provide information on hospital and community resources for emotional support.
High Risk for Seizures • Therapeutic anticonvulsant levels will be maintained. • Patient will remain free from injury in the event of a seizure.	1. Obtain seizure history if applicable (focal or generalized, duration, frequency, presence of an aura, precipitating factors). 2. Document history in patient chart. 3. Medicate with anticonvulsants as ordered. 4. Ensure patient safety (call bell within reach, bed in lowest position, functioning suction machine at bedside). 5. Do not stop the anticonvulsants without a physician's order. 6. Monitor anticonvulsant levels as ordered and notify physician if level is low or in toxic range. 7. Assess patient for signs of drug toxicity (ataxia, gait disturbances, lethargy, visual problems). 8. Be aware of potential drug interactions that may interfere with absorption of anticonvulsant (enteral feedings). 9. If a seizure occurs, remain with patient, call for help, notify physician, get patient to a safe position such as on the floor, protect patient's head, place patient on side to prevent aspiration, ensure IV access is available.	1. Teach patient and family member about the medication, dosage, frequency, side effects, and interactions with alcohol and sedatives. 2. Teach patient and family member not to abruptly stop the medication. If patient is unable to take oral medication, a physician is to be contacted. 3. Instruct patient and family member of the safety measures others should take if the patient has a seizure (lower patient to floor, turn patient's head to side to protect airway, do not hold patient down, loosen restrictive clothing, do not put anything in patient's mouth). 4. Inform patient and family member about medic alert bracelets and how to obtain one. 5. Instruct patient and family member about pertinent state law regarding driving and seizure history.

Continued

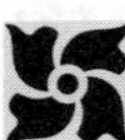

TABLE 23-7 Standard of Care for the Patient Undergoing a Neurologic Procedure—cont'd

Patient Problem and Outcomes	Nursing Interventions and Rationales	Patient Education Instructions
High Risk for Injury: Falls Patient and family will: • Identify risk factors for falls. • Verbalize measures to reduce the risk of falls in the hospital and at home.	1. Place bedside items, personal items, and call bell within patient's reach. 2. Keep side rails up at all times when patient is unsupervised. 3. Leave the bathroom light on at night. 4. Include patient and family in planning fall precautions. 5. Evaluate potential risk factors for falls in the home. 6. Refer to visiting nurse or home health agency for physical or occupational therapy evaluation of the home environment. 7. Evaluate patient for personnel response system if living alone.	1. Instruct patient on proper footwear (non-skid soles, laced or closed-back shoes). 2. Instruct patient and family in ambulation and transferring techniques. 3. Instruct family member to support weak side if appropriate.
Pain Patient will: • Report pain intensity and satisfaction with pain relief. • Experience optimal pain relief with minimal side effects. • Describe pain management regimen.	1. Assess patient's pain history including prior pain medications, dosage, and frequency. 2. Assess pain intensity using 0 to 10 scale (0 = no pain; 10 = most severe pain) every 3 to 4 hours postoperatively and prn. 3. Instruct patient on rationale and use of analgesics. 4. Administer prescribed analgesics and evaluate effectiveness following administration. 5. Consult physician if pain regimen is ineffective, if pain is rated 5 or more twice in a 24-hour period, or if patient is unable to participate in self-care activities because of pain. 6. Monitor for analgesic side effects and administer medications to prevent or treat the effects.	1. Teach patient and family member about the pain medication including dose and side effects. 2. Reinforce the importance of taking pain medication on a regular basis. 3. Instruct patient on non-pharmacologic methods of pain relief (relaxation techniques, breathing exercises, distraction, imagery).
Infection • Incision and drain site will be free from signs and symptoms of infection. • Patient and family member will demonstrate appropriate hygiene measures to minimize infection. • Patient and family member will demonstrate appropriate incision and drain site care.	1. Monitor patient's temperature as often as the patient's condition warrants. 2. Observe dressing for drainage and proper placement. Notify physician if drainage becomes excessive or its character changes. 3. Assess and empty drainage systems according to routine and prn; record amount and character of drainage; notify physician if amount is excessive. 4. Change dressing over incision site according to routine and prn. 5. Assess incision and drain site for signs of infection (redness, swelling, drainage). 6. Document all assessments and interventions. 7. Initiate visiting nurse referral if necessary.	1. Teach patient and family member hygiene measures to minimize infection. 2. Teach patient and family member signs and symptoms of infection and what steps to take if they develop. 3. Teach patient and family member care of the incision and drain site.

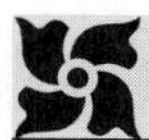

TABLE 23-7 Standard of Care for the Patient Undergoing a Neurologic Procedure—cont'd

Patient Problem and Outcomes	Nursing Interventions and Rationales	Patient Education Instructions
Constipation • Patient will have a bowel movement at least every 3 days. • Patient's abdomen will be soft and distended.	1. Identify patient's normal bowel pattern (character, frequency, and amount). Document last bowel movement. 2. Assess abdomen for bowel sounds, distension, and tenderness. 3. Identify prior interventions that were effective in the past. 4. Evaluate patient's diet. Increase intake of fiber, fruits, vegetables, whole grains, and bran. 5. Maintain adequate fluid intake of 30 cc/kilogram per day unless contraindicated. 6. Increase activity. 7. Establish a bowel regimen as ordered, especially if patient is thrombocytopenic, on steroids, vinca alkaloids, taking analgesics, or has spinal cord disease.	1. Teach patient to avoid constipation by regular use of diet, fluids, and activity. 2. Teach patient and family side effects of constipation and the indications to call physician (severe pain or blood with bowel movement, constipation not relieved with usual bowel regimen.
Impaired Physical Mobility Related to Muscle Weakness, Paralysis, Spasticity, or Pain		
Patient and family member will: • Identify measures to maintain range of motion (ROM) and optimize mobility. • Verbalize understanding of interventions to prevent injury caused by motor dysfunction. • Demonstrate ability to use assistive devices.	1. Evaluate motor function including tone and strength and notify physician of any change. 2. Evaluate the patient's ability to manage activities of daily living. 3. Perform ROM exercises every 4 hours and prn if indicated. 4. Perform position changes every 2 to 3 hours, maintaining proper body alignment using support devices. 5. Assess skin integrity as often as indicated. 6. Consult rehabilitation service. 7. Provide appropriate tools to assist patient with mobility (cane, walker, wheelchair). 8. Assess for thrombophlebitis and take measures to prevent its development (antiembolic stockings, compression boots). 9. Ambulate patient postoperatively as ordered, if appropriate.	1. Teach principles of ROM and position changes to patient and family member. 2. Teach ROM exercises to the patient and family to continue at home. 3. Teach transfer techniques with assistive devices. 4. Instruct the patient and family member on the potential injuries caused by decreased mobility (pressure ulcers, deep vein thromboses, contracture deformities).
Sensory/Perceptual Alteration The patient will: • Verbalize an understanding of the risks associated with sensory dysfunction. • Learn to compensate for the lost sensory modality.	1. Identify highest level of sensory function. 2. Develop specific interventions to compensate for deficits. 3. Obtain assistive devices as necessary (eating utensils, touch-tone phones, velcro straps). 4. Identify ability to ambulate secondary to sensory deficits (position sense, neglect). 5. Prevent injury to areas with decreased sensory innervation (burns, trauma, pressure ulcers).	1. Teach the patient to visually check the affected limbs. 2. Instruct patient and family to evaluate skin for evidence of trauma. 3. Instruct patient to compensate for sensory and perceptual deficits using special techniques and assistive devices.

Continued

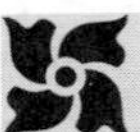

TABLE 23-7 Standard of Care for the Patient Undergoing a Neurologic Procedure—cont'd

Patient Problem and Outcomes	Nursing Interventions and Rationales	Patient Education Instructions
High Risk for Altered Cerebral Tissue Perfusion		
• The patient will maintain optimal cerebral perfusion. Neurologic changes will be identified promptly and definitive action taken to prevent neurologic compromise.	1. Perform neurologic assessments as often as indicated (every hour for the first 12 hours and then every 2 to 4 hours). 2. Elevate the head of the bed 30 degrees. 3. Administer steroids as ordered. 4. Avoid activities that may increase ICP (cumulative activities, suctioning, Valsalva maneuver, isometric exercises). 5. Administer anticonvulsants and antipyretics to reduce the occurrence of seizures and fevers. 6. Administer oral and intravenous fluids as ordered. Monitor intake and output.	1. Instruct patient and family member about steroids, including indication, dose, and side effects. 2. Teach patient and family importance of spacing activities. 3. Teach patient and family member stress reduction techniques. 4. Instruct patient to avoid Valsalva maneuver. 5. Instruct patient and family member on fluid restrictions, if appropriate. 6. Instruct patient and family member on early signs on increased ICP and to call physician if they occur.

Radiation Therapy

Nursing management of the astrocytoma patient receiving RT is summarized in Table 23-8. Nursing care varies depending on the method of irradiation used and the extent of the patient's neurologic deficits. The most common method, external beam RT, is often provided on an outpatient basis. Assistance may be required for transportation arrangements. However, some patients require hospitalization for part of or the entire course of RT because of their neurologic condition. The major problems associated with external beam RT are hair loss; dry, itchy scalp; changes in skin color; headache; lethargy; nausea; and fatigue. Patients must be told to avoid sun exposure and to use hats and sunscreen. Patients undergoing RT are usually receiving dexamethasone and need to be instructed on the possible side effects and dosage schedule. Nurses evaluate the patient on a consistent basis for any signs and symptoms of cerebral edema, and family members are instructed to report any increases in neurologic dysfunction. Patients receiving brachytherapy are hospitalized for several days. They require preoperative teaching, perioperative neurologic assessments, and instruction on pin site care. Radiosurgery is often provided on an outpatient basis. Coordination among the person(s) applying the stereotactic head frame, the CT or MRI personnel, and the radiation oncologist is essential.

Chemotherapy

Nursing management of the astrocytoma patient receiving chemotherapy is summarized in Table 23-9, pp. 534-535. Management is dependent on the specific chemotherapeutic agent(s) being used and the method of administration. Nursing care focuses on assessment and management of side effects, evaluation of toxicities, prevention of complications, patient and family teaching regarding treatment schedules, managing side effects at home, maximizing function, and maintaining quality of life. It is essential to provide written information and instructions for patients and their caregivers and to follow up with phone calls.

Many chemotherapeutic agents are administered in an outpatient setting. Some protocols require short hospitalizations because of the method of administration such as intraarterial chemotherapy with BBB disruption. The use of biodegradable wafers impregnated with chemotherapy requires a surgical procedure. In this case, patients require preoperative teaching, perioperative neurologic assessments, prevention of complications, possible pain management, instruction on incision care, and medications. Other methods, such as in high-dose chemotherapy with autologous bone marrow rescue, require prolonged hospitalization. These patients require treatment for prolonged myelosuppression including antibiotic support and blood product administration, possible treatment of mucositis and pain, nutritional support, careful monitoring for complications, and neurologic assessments. The most common chemotherapeutic agents administered to patients with astrocytomas and their side effects are listed in Table 23-10, p. 536.

HOME CARE ISSUES

Whether the patient with an astrocytoma is diagnosed in an outpatient or inpatient setting, issues related to home care are at the forefront. The initial presentation, clinical progression, course of treatment, and complications vary with the type of astrocytoma and its location. Depending on the treatment approaches used in the management of this disease process, patients and their family caregivers will be faced with several issues in the home care setting. Potentially, the most devastating issues are the psychologic impact of the diagnosis and the relatively poor prognosis associated with the disease. Communication and information are vital to patients and significant others. Information provides a means of having some control over a situation that is perceived as uncontrollable. Patients and significant others

CONFIDENTIAL PATIENT INFORMATION - HANDLE ACCORDING TO HOSPITAL POLICY

Memorial Hospital for Cancer and Allied Diseases

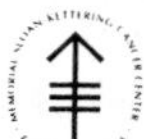

Patient Education Documentation Form

Patient Identification

LEARNING NEEDS ASSESSMENT

Date	Check any of the following that impact teaching/learning:
Initials	☐ Physical disability ☐ Religion ☐ Culture ☐ Emotional issues ☐ Language ☐ Cognitive changes ☐ Lack of agreement with learning objectives

TEACHING FOR NEUROSURGERY

Taught to: ☐ patient ☐ other ____________	Teaching Sessions				Outcome Achieved	
The Patient/Family is able to	Date	Initials	Date	Initials	Date	Initials
1. Describe the operative procedure to be performed.						
2. Describe any significant physical changes likely to result from surgery (i.e., incision, skull defect, motor/sensory loss, speech loss).						
3. State that aspirin or products containing aspirin must be discontinued 10 days before surgery.						
4. State that the physician should be notified if any new illness develops before surgery (i.e., cold, flu, fever, sore throat).						
5. State that he/she will be NPO after midnight.						
6. State that valuables (dentures, etc.) will be removed before he/she leaves the unit to go to the O.R.						
7. Demonstrate proper technique for coughing and deep breathing.						
8. Demonstrate proper use of the incentive spirometer.						
9. Demonstrate proper technique for leg exercises.						
10. State the reason for log rolling while on bedrest (laminectomy only).						
11. State the reason for the use of Venodyne® boots.						
12. State that he/she might remain in PACU overnight.						
13. State the reason for NICU stay and probable length of stay in NICU.						
14. Describe catheters/tubes that he/she may have upon return from surgery (i.e., Foley®, IV/arterial lines, Jackson Pratt®, chest tube, nasogastric tubes).						
15. Describe how and where family can obtain information on patient's status during surgery.						
16. State the importance of taking pain medication.						
17. State that pain medication will not be given automatically and describe how to obtain it.						
18. State the reason for not giving sleeping medication immediately after surgery.						
19. State that P.O. fluids will be restricted.						
20. State the reason that he/she will be awakened every hour for 12 hours and then every two hours through the first night after surgery.						

SEE BACK FOR COMMENTS / NOTES / SIGNATURES / RESOURCES

56-11330 Q98 CIMC Approval Date: 6/96 **B/02.050.72**

Fig. 23-16 Patient education documentation form for the patient undergoing neurosurgery. (Courtesy Memorial Sloan-Kettering Cancer Center, Division of Nursing). *Continued*

CONFIDENTIAL PATIENT INFORMATION - HANDLE ACCORDING TO HOSPITAL POLICY

Memorial Hospital for Cancer and Allied Diseases

Patient Education Documentation Form

Patient Identification

Initials	Signature/Title	Initials	Signature/Title

Educational Materials / Methods

Cancer
___ What Are Clinical Trials All About?
___ What You Need to Know About Cancer
___ Taking Time
___ When Cancer Recurs
___ Other ______________________________

Hematology
___ Blood Counts and Infections: A Guide For Patients with Cancer
___ Facts About Blood and Blood Cells
___ Guidelines for Patients with Low Platelet Count

Information
___ Disposal Tips for Home Health Care
___ Giving Blood: The Ultimate Gift
___ Medic Alert Forms
___ When Your Doctor Recommends A Transfusion

Neurology
___ Carcinomatous Meningitis
___ Ommaya Reservoir
___ Ventriculo-Peritoneal Shunt
___ What You Need to Know About Cancer of the Spinal Cord

Nutrition
___ Eating Hints: Recipes and Tips for Better Nutrition During Cancer Treatment

Pain
___ Coping With Pain

Pharmacology
___ Common Medicines Containing Aspirin and Ibuprofen
___ ______________________________
___ ______________________________
___ ______________________________

Procedures
___ Arteriogram
___ Lumbar Puncture
___ MRI Patient Information Card
___ Pneumoencephalogram

Radiation Therapy
___ Radiation Therapy and You: A Guide to Self-Help During Treatment.
___ Simulation

Self-Care
___ Care of Your Suture Line
___ ______________________________
___ ______________________________
___ ______________________________

Surgery
___ Before, During, and After Surgery: A Guide for Patients and Families
___ Getting Ready for Surgery

Date	Comments/Notes

56-11330 Q98 CIMC Approval Date: 6/96 **B/02.050.72**

Fig. 23-16, cont'd For legend see previous page.

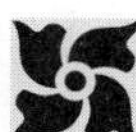

TABLE 23-8 Standard of Care for the Astrocytoma Patient Undergoing Radiation Therapy

Patient Problem and Outcomes	Nursing Interventions and Rationales	Patient Education Instructions
Nausea Patient will: • Verbalize absence of or a decrease in nausea and vomiting. • State plan for management of nausea at home. • Verbalize signs and symptoms of dehydration and electrolyte imbalance.	1. Administer antiemetics before radiation, meals, and prn. 2. Assess patient for nausea and vomiting. 3. Document frequency and characteristics of emesis. 4. Monitor effectiveness of treatment and document. 5. If nausea and vomiting persist, notify physician for possible adjustment in treatment plan. 6. If appropriate, consider hydration or alternative methods of nutrition.	1. Instruct patient and family on dietary modifications, if necessary (spicy or odiferous foods). 2. Instruct patient on antiemetics, including dosage and side effects.
High Risk for Impaired Cognition Patient will: • Experience minimal disorientation. • Not experience any physical injury.	1. Identify the existence and nature of the cognitive deficit. 2. Reorient patient as needed (post calendar and clock in patient's view). 3. Maintain safe environment (call bell within reach, side rails up, frequent checks). 4. Administer steroids as ordered during radiation. 5. Perform neurologic assessments as necessary. 6. Provide continuity of care as often as possible to minimize anxiety. 7. Provide instruction or direction to patient in simple, easily understood language. 8. Utilize alternative methods of communication if appropriate (letter board, pictures, magic slate). 9. Place patient in room close to the nurses' station, if appropriate.	1. Explain cause of cognitive impairment to patient and family member. 2. Discuss strategies to enhance communication with family member. 3. Instruct patient and family member on steroids (dose, side effects, tapering schedule if appropriate, never to discontinue the drug without consulting physician). 4. Educate family member on methods to maintain safe environment at home. 5. Instruct family member to notify physician for changes in mental status (lethargy, confusion), increased headaches, worsening neurologic deficits, or seizures.
Skin Integrity Patient will: • Verbalize acceptable level of discomfort. • Demonstrate skin care regimen. • Maintain intact skin.	1. Assess treatment field daily and document appearance. 2. Assess for signs and symptoms of infection. 3. Assess for itching or discomfort. 4. Moisturize prn only with approved creams, but not 4 hours prior to treatment. 5. If drainage or breakdown is present, apply appropriate type of dressing or protective agent.	1. Teach patient to cleanse skin with mild unscented soap. 2. Instruct patient to assess skin daily for redness, peeling, or signs and symptoms of infection. 3. Instruct patient on use of creams and moisturizers. Use only those approved by radiation oncologist and not 4 hours before treatment. 4. Instruct patient to avoid sources of irritation (tight-fitting clothing, scarves, or hats; application of extreme heat or cold; sun exposure without protective clothing or sun block).

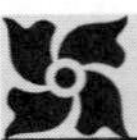

TABLE 23-9 Standard of Care for the Astrocytoma Patient Undergoing Chemotherapy

Patient Problem and Outcomes	Nursing Interventions and Rationales	Patient Education Instructions
Infection Patient will: • Remain free from infection. • Promptly report signs and symptoms of infection.	1. Monitor patient's complete blood count, including neutrophils. 2. Monitor patient's temperature every 4 hours when neutropenic or if chills occur. 3. Assess patient for signs and symptoms of infection. 4. Maintain strict aseptic technique when caring for catheters, tubes, etc. 5. Follow strict handwashing and infection control guidelines. 6. If febrile, obtain cultures and start antibiotics as ordered. 7. Administer neupogen if ordered.	1. Instruct patient and family on appropriate hygiene measures. 2. Demonstrate to patient and family proper handwashing techniques and have them give a return demonstration. 3. Instruct patient on signs and symptoms of infection. 4. Instruct patient and family on catheter care using aseptic or sterile technique if appropriate. 5. Instruct patient and family to avoid crowds and persons with colds, flu-like symptoms, or infections. 6. Instruct patient on method of obtaining accurate temperatures. 7. Instruct patient to keep a log of daily temperatures and related symptoms. 8. Instruct patient to notify physician if fever or signs of infection develop. 9. Instruct patient and family In neupogen administration techniques.
Bleeding Patient will: • Verbalize when risk of bleeding is highest. • Identify safety measures to reduce risk of bleeding. • Verbalize steps to take if a bleeding episode occurs.	1. Monitor patient's platelet count. 2. Assess for signs and symptoms of minor bleeding (petechiae, epistaxis, gum bleeding, ecchymoses, occult blood in urine and stool). 3. Assess for signs and symptoms of major bleeding (headache, changes in mentation, blurred vision, melena, tachycardia, dizziness, orthostatic blood pressure). 4. Maintain safe environment. 5. Maintain current type and crossmatch. 6. Place patient on bleeding precautions. 7. Administer platelet transfusions as ordered and evaluate response.	1. Review with patient and family etiology of thrombocytopenia and time frame to expect symptoms to occur. 2. Instruct patient and family on ways to prevent bleeding. 3. Instruct patient and family on signs and symptoms of bleeding. 4. Instruct patient and family on avoiding aspirin, products that contain aspirin, and nonsteroidal anti-inflammatory agents. 5. Provide list of common products that contain aspirin and nonsteroidal anti-inflammatory agents. 6. Inform patient and family of importance of contacting physician if episodes or symptoms of bleeding occur. 7. Instruct patient to avoid constipation. 8. Instruct patient to take steroids with food if appropriate.

should be encouraged to seek needed information including printed literature and personal discussions with physicians, nurses, other health care workers, and family members. National and community support groups can be of enormous assistance to patients and significant others (Box 23-4).

Discharge Planning

Discharge planning begins when the patient is admitted to the hospital. Assessment of the patient's functional limitations, cognitive ability, and home situation are performed and a tentative discharge plan is identified. Discharge planning will evolve during the hospitalization. Before discharge, it is essential that the patient and family caregiver understand who is the primary care physician, as well as the roles of other physicians. Specific written instructions concerning persons to call and their phone numbers should be provided at the time of discharge. If the patient is not receiving cancer treatment locally, a local physician who can provide emergency services and address other medical

TABLE 23-9 Standard of Care for the Astrocytoma Patient Undergoing Chemotherapy—cont'd

Patient Problem and Outcomes	Nursing Interventions and Rationales	Patient Education Instructions
Activity Intolerance/Anemia		
Patient will: • Verbalize strategies to avoid fatigue (spreading out activities during day, frequent rest periods). • Maintain normal activities of daily living.	1. Monitor patient's hemoglobin and hematocrit. 2. Assess patient's ability to perform activities of daily living. Provide assistance if needed. 3. Assess for signs and symptoms of anemia (fatigue, dyspnea, tachycardia, orthostatic hypotension, headache, dizziness). 4. Administer epogen as ordered. Instruct patient on the expected length of treatment time. 5. Transfuse patient with packed red blood cells as ordered and evaluate response. 6. Encourage dietary modifications (foods high in iron, protein). 7. Schedule frequent rest periods and space nursing activities.	1. Instruct patient and family member on strategies to minimize fatigue. 2. Review cause of fatigue and expected start and duration of symptoms. 3. Instruct a family member on epogen administration technique if appropriate. 4. Instruct patient on importance of adequate diet and sources of iron.

problems is needed. The local physician must be informed of the treatment plan and updated as treatment progresses. Nurses play a vital role in this coordination of care. Providing continuity of care reduces anxiety and fear for patients and their family caregivers.

Patients recovering from a surgical intervention will need to care for their surgical incision. They require instruction on how to cleanse the suture line, the frequency of the assessment, and how to evaluate the incision for signs and symptoms of infection. They need to be informed when the sutures or surgical staples are to be removed. The procedure for this may vary among institutions.

An important aspect of home care is the education of the patient and the family caregiver concerning medications. Patients will be placed on new medications at the time of surgery and during their course of treatment. As with any medication, teaching is critical to its safe and effective use. The majority of patients will be discharged on tapering doses of dexamethasone or another steroid medication. They should be taught the potential short- and long-term side effects, how to decrease the medication dose, and never to discontinue the drug abruptly. Written materials are often useful for the patient and family members.

Patients continue to take phenytoin (or another anticonvulsant) when they leave the hospital. Patients receive anticonvulsants because they often present with seizures at the time of diagnosis or are prophylactically placed on anticonvulsants before surgery. How the medication is given, side effects, drug/nutrient interactions, special points of emphasis, and when to call the physician should be included in the discharge instructions. Patients and caregivers should be encouraged to obtain a medical identification bracelet, especially if the patient has a seizure history. It should be stressed that another individual in addition to the patient be included in the teaching. Brain tumors often cause cognitive disabilities including short-term memory loss, poor concentration, and disruption in understanding written and spoken language. Anxiety alone may impair an individual's ability to retain new information.

At the time of discharge, an accurate assessment of the patient's neurologic deficits and functional limitations is needed to identify home care support. Patients with functional motor or sensory deficits will require physical therapy, occupational therapy, or both. The physical structure of the home may limit the patient's access to specific areas. The patient may require safety rails in the bathroom to facilitate a safe and functional environment. Rehabilitation services can assist in identifying changes needed in the home to maximize patient safety. Some patients may require speech therapy. This therapy can be provided in the home or at an outside facility depending on the patient's functional abilities. Other patients may not require any physical support or care, but cognitive deficits may make it unsafe for the patient to be left alone. A more intensive or inpatient rehabilitation program may be important for an individual with a primary spinal cord tumor because these individuals often have extended periods between recurrences or progression of disease. Vocational rehabilitation is sometimes required. A thorough assessment of health care benefits and family, community, and agency support is necessary.

The patient and significant others may find themselves dealing with increasing disability as the disease progresses. The progression of the disease and disabilities may be slow or may occur rapidly. One's coping ability is based largely on past experiences. Individuals have different styles and techniques. Coping mechanisms of patients and family caregivers should be assessed. Nurses facilitate coping by listening openly and attentively. Patients and significant others

Table 23-10 Common Chemotherapeutic Agents and Their Side Effects Used in Astrocytomas

Chemotherapeutic Agent	Side Effects
Carmustine (BCNU)	Pain and burning along IV site Facial flushing Delayed myelosuppression (4-6 weeks) Cumulative bone marrow toxicity Nausea, vomiting, and stomatitis Pulmonary fibrosis Brown skin discoloration (hyperpigmentation) Hepatotoxicity Nephrotoxicity Dizziness and ataxia
Procarbazine	Nausea, vomiting, anorexia, and stomatitis Myelosuppression Peripheral neuropathy Confusion, lethargy, and ataxia Interstitial pneumonitis Hypertensive crisis with foods containing tyramine (Chianti wine, cheeses, cola, tea, coffee, dark beer, bananas, and yogurt) Flu-like symptoms Skin rash, pruritus, and dermatitis Hyperpigmentation Hepatotoxicity Alopecia
Lomustine (CCNU)	Nausea and vomiting Diarrhea, stomatitis, and anorexia Delayed myelosuppression (4-6 weeks) Cumulative bone marrow toxicity Nephrotoxicity Hepatotoxicity Pulmonary fibrosis Confusion, lethargy, ataxia, and dysarthria Alopecia
Vincristine	Nausea, vomiting, and stomatitis Constipation (can lead to paralytic ileus) Peripheral neuropathy, motor weakness Extraocular muscle paralysis Can cause extravasation Myelosuppression Alopecia Acute bronchospasm and shortness of breath Syndrome of inappropriate antidiuretic hormone (SIADH)
Cisplatin	Severe and delayed nausea and vomiting Alterations in taste Ototoxicity Nephrotoxicity Peripheral neuropathy Hepatotoxicity Myelosuppression Hypokalemia Hypomagnesemia Hypocalcemia
Carboplatin	Nausea, vomiting, and alterations in taste Myelosuppression Ototoxicity Nephrotoxicity (less than cisplatin) Peripheral neuropathy Abnormal liver function (reversible) Skin rash, urticaria, pruritus Alopecia

Box 23-4
Patient Support and Advocacy Groups

American Brain Tumor Association
2720 River Road, Suite 146
Des Plaines, IL 60018
Phone: (800) 886-2282
Fax: (847) 827-9918
American Cancer Society
1599 Clifton Road, NE
Atlanta, GA 30329
Phone: (800) 227-2345 or (404) 320-3333
Fax: (404) 325-0230
Brain Tumor Foundation of Canada
111 Waterloo Street, Suite 600
London, Ontario N6B 2M4
Phone: (519) 642-7755
Brain Tumor Information Services
University of Chicago Hospitals
Box 405, Room J341
5841 S. Maryland Avenue
Chicago, IL 60637
Phone: (312) 684-1400
Cancer Care, Inc.
1180 Avenue of the Americas
New York, NY 10036
Phone: (800) 813-HOPE or (212) 302-2400
Fax: (212) 719-0263
Cancer Research Institute
681 Fifth Avenue
New York, NY 10022
Phone: (800) 99-CANCER or (212) 688-7515
Epilepsy Foundation of America
4351 Garden City Drive
Landover, MD 20785
Phone: (800) 332-1000
Families Against Cancer
P. O. Box 588
DeWitt, NY 13214
Phone: (315) 446-6385
Fax: (315) 446-5326
National Brain Tumor Foundation
785 Market Street, Suite 1600
San Francisco, CA 94103
Phone: (800) 934-CURE or (415) 284-0208
Fax: (415) 284-0209
National Cancer Institute
Cancer Information Service
National Cancer Institute Public Inquiries
9000 Rockville Pike
Building 31, Room 10A-19
Bethesda, MD 20892-3100
Phone: (800) 422-6237 or (301) 496-5583
Fax: (301) 402-5874
National Coalition for Cancer Survivorship
1010 Wayne Avenue, Suite 300
Silver Springs, MD 20910
Phone: (301) 585-2616
National Familial Brain Tumor Registry
The John Hopkins Oncology Center
600 N. Wolfe Street, Room 132
Baltimore, MD 20892-2540
Phone: (800) 352-9424
National Institute of Neurological Disorders and Stroke
31 Center Drive
Building 31, Room 8A06, MSC 2540
Bethesda, MD 20892-2540
Phone: (800) 352-9424
National Neurofibromatosis Foundation
95 Pine Street, 16th Floor
New York, NY 10005
Phone: (800) 323-7938
National Organization for Rare Disorders
P. O. Box 8923
New Fairfield, CT 06812-8923
Phone: (800) 942-6825
National Organization on Disability
910 Sixteenth Street, N. W.
Washington, DC 20006
Phone: (202) 293-5960
Neurofibromatosis, Inc.
8855 Annapolis Road, Suite 110
Lanham, MD 20706-2924
Phone: (800) 942-6825
National Tuberous Sclerosis Association
8181 Professional Place, Suite 110
Landover, MD 20785
Phone: (800) 225-6872
Physician's Data Query
9000 Rockville Pike
Bethesda, MD 20205
Phone: (301) 496-7403
South Florida Brain Tumor Association
P. O. Box 7770182
Coral Springs, FL 33077-0182
Phone: (954) 755-4307
The Brain Tumor Society
84 Seattle Street
Boston, MA 02134
Phone: (800) 770-8287
Fax: (617) 783-9712

are often grieving for their losses. For patients, this may mean a loss of motor strength, sensory dysfunction, endurance, memory, and autonomy. They may grieve and become angry at their inability to perform simple tasks. The patient's significant others may grieve the loss of the person they knew, and they may have to assume new responsibilities or roles that they feel ill-equipped to handle. These responsibilities may include issues related to employment, finances, or young children. Maintaining an open pattern of communication facilitates identification of perceived losses.

Actively and honestly discussing these issues helps them verbalize their sense of loss, identify what these changes mean to them, and explore ways to deal with them. Family caregivers often feel helpless in their inability to control the disease and focus their attention on patient comfort (Gargan-Klinger, 1988).

Astrocytomas of the CNS present a challenge to all involved. The patient requires a highly individualized plan of care. The neurologic symptoms and complications produced by these tumors are, unfortunately, profoundly disabling and impact severely on the patient's quality of life.

Quality of Life

There is scant literature about the quality of life of patients with astrocytomas. Although the objective of treatment for the majority of these patients is palliation, the goal is to maintain the patient's neurologic and general functional status at a level that is "meaningful" for them as long as possible. The effect of the treatment on the tumor is most often the main focus of the physician. Patients and significant others may be more concerned about the impact of the disease and therapy on their daily functioning and lifestyle (Aiken, 1994). The concept of "meaningful" varies among patients and family caregivers, and it is essential to understand this concept on an individual basis. In addition, what individuals perceive as "meaningful" at one phase of their illness may not reflect their concept at a later stage. Health care personnel, including physicians, nurses, social workers, and psychologists, agree that the effects of treatments on the cognitive functioning and quality of life of patients with brain tumors are important outcome measures. However, the majority of the treatment regimens continue to use the Karnofsky Performance Status (KPS) scale as the quality-of-life measure. The KPS scale is an inadequate assessment tool, since it looks only at the reviewer's perception of the patient's external performance status and not at the neurobehavioral or the more intrinsic and psychosocial concerns.

Two recent studies have used a more focused and systematic method of assessing the neuropsychologic function and impact on quality of life in the adult population. Archibald and colleagues (1994) evaluated concentration and short-term memory in patients who had received radiation and chemotherapy. All patients had some degree of cognitive impairment. A second study evaluated cognitive function in patients with low-grade gliomas who had received radiotherapy (Taphoorn et al., 1992). These investigators reported that patients had significantly more cognitive dysfunction and suffered from fatigue and depressed mood. The poor performance of the patients with brain tumors in tests of cognitive functioning and quality of life was not reflected in their neurologic examination or KPS scores. Available studies are limited by their small samples and the use of study-specific quality-of-life questionnaires that make cross-study comparisons difficult (Meyers & Weitzner, 1995).

Aaronson (1988) recommended that, for quality-of-life assessment, 10 factors should be measured in all populations of cancer patients: (1) pain and pain relief, (2) fatigue and malaise, (3) psychological distress, (4) nausea and side effects, (5) body image, (6) sexual function, (7) social functioning, (8) memory and concentration, (9) economic disruption, and (10) global quality of life. Mackworth, Fobair, and Prados (1992) devised a quality-of-life self-report tool and evaluated 200 patients with primary brain tumors. The components in the scale were depression, socialization, energy, symptoms, leisure, age, cognition, and memory. Results of the study indicated that elderly patients tend to have lower quality-of-life scores and a higher incidence of depression.

Quality of life has emerged as an important consideration in the treatment of patients with astrocytomas. New attempts are being made to include more specific and sensitive tools to measure quality of life in this patient population.

PROGNOSIS

The prognosis for patients with intracranial astrocytomas is quite variable. The most important prognostic factors are age at diagnosis, histologic grade of the tumor, and patient's performance status. Patients diagnosed with an LGA at a young age (less than 35 years old) with a high performance status have a more favorable prognosis than an older individual with an AA whose performance status is low. Other factors that have been suggested as favorably influencing prognosis include long duration of symptoms, seizures as a presenting symptom, absence of neurologic deficits, complete or gross total surgical resection, frontal or temporal tumor location in the nondominant hemisphere, and absence of enhancement on CT or MRI.

Median survival for patients with intracranial LGAs is approximately 5 years. Five-year survival rates range from 50% to 68% and 10-year rates from 20% to 39%. The majority of LGAs will transform to a higher grade tumor. Median survival for patients with AAs is approximately 3 years; the 3-year survival rate is 50%. Five-year survival rates for patients with low-grade spinal cord astrocytomas vary from 60% to 90% and the 10-year rates from 40% to 90%. The prognosis of patients with malignant astrocytomas of the spinal cord is much poorer; these patients generally survive less than 12 months (Levin et al., 1997).

EVALUATION OF THE QUALITY OF CARE

Accreditation organizations such as the Joint Commission for the Accreditation of Health Care Organizations require evaluation of the quality of care provided to patients. Because the care provided to patients with astrocytomas requires input from a multidisciplinary team, an evaluation of the quality of care provided to these patients should include aspects of care provided by various members of the team. Table 23-11 provides an example of a quality of care evaluation tool that can be initiated preoperatively in the outpatient setting, continued postoperatively in the inpatient setting, and completed after discharge in the outpatient setting.

RESEARCH ISSUES

Numerous research issues surrounding the diagnosis and management of astrocytomas require further investigation.

TABLE 23-11 Quality of Care Evaluation for a Patient with an Astrocytoma Undergoing a Neurosurgical Procedure

Disciplines participating in the quality of care evaluation:
☐ Nursing ☐ Surgery ☐ Dietary ☐ Respiratory ☐ Pharmacy
☐ Rehabilitation ☐ Social Work
Data from: ☐ Medical Record Review
☐ Patient/Family Interview

Criteria	Yes	No
1. Patient/Family provided with preoperative teaching, including:		
a. Diagnostic tests	☐	☐
b. Operative procedure	☐	☐
c. Potential complications	☐	☐
d. Use of aspirin, products containing aspirin, and nonsteroidal anti-inflammatory agents preoperatively	☐	☐
e. Perioperative routine	☐	☐
2. Prevention of complications:		
a. Patient can verbalize frequency of incentive spirometer use	☐	☐
b. Patient can correctly demonstrate use of incentive spirometer	☐	☐
c. Patient can verbalize rationale for external compression devices, antiembolic stockings, anticoagulation, isometric exercises or whichever combination is appropriate	☐	☐
d. Patient consistently receiving appropriately prescribed method of DVT prophylaxis	☐	☐
e. Fluid and electrolyte balance evaluated postoperatively	☐	☐
f. Neurologic assessments are performed and documented and reported according to the standard of care	☐	☐
g. Appropriate referrals are made according to the level of neurologic deficits	☐	☐
3. Patient experienced the following complications:		
a. Postoperative pneumonia	☐	☐
b. Deep-vein thrombosis	☐	☐
c. New neurologic deficit	☐	☐
4. Patient education regarding steroid therapy:		
a. The patient/family can verbalize the rationale for the steroids	☐	☐
b. The patient/family can verbalize correct dose of medication and administration schedule	☐	☐
c. The patient/family can verbalize at least three side effects of the medication	☐	☐
d. The patient/family can verbalize the importance of taking food with the medication and if applicable, avoiding certain foods (concentrated sweets)	☐	☐
e. The patient/family received instructions on how to taper the dose of medication	☐	☐
f. The patient/family can verbalize rationale and administration schedule for Bactrim,® if applicable	☐	☐

II. Patient/Family Satisfaction
Data from: ☐ Patient/Family Interview
☐ Patient/Family Satisfaction Survey

Criteria	Yes	No
1. On a scale of 0 to 10, with 0 being totally dissatisfied and 10 being totally satisfied, how satisfied were you with the pain management you received?	☐	☐
2. Were you instructed to call your nurse for specific needs or concerns?	☐	☐
3. Did you receive any type of written information regarding your diagnosis, surgical procedure, treatment, or medications?	☐	☐
4. Did you receive a follow-up phone call from a nurse after discharge?	☐	☐
5. Was a follow-up appointment or appropriate referral made for you before your discharge from the hospital?	☐	☐

Currently, the standard therapies following surgery are radiation techniques, chemotherapy, and biotherapy. However, these therapies are often only palliative in nature, and the adverse side effects from these treatments can be serious. Molecular and genetic therapies may potentially offer more specific and effective therapeutic options without the side effects. An understanding of the gene alterations specific to astrocytomas is needed. Current research demonstrates the presence of multiple genetic defects associated with astrocytomas. It may not be feasible to correct all of these alterations. Possible goals of gene therapy may be to block the expression of activated oncogenes and to increase the expression of tumor suppressor genes to prevent tumor development and progression. RT techniques have advanced, but are still limited by the deleterious effects on normal cells. Genetics may offer a means to protect normal tissues from the effects of radiation by manipulating the expression of antioxidants (Rosenfeld, 1996).

Continued research in the development of imaging technologies using noninvasive methods may lead to improvements in the diagnosis of these tumors. The ability to accurately differentiate radiation necrosis from a recurrent or progressive tumor could reduce the need for reoperation. The development of the operating room MRI can provide the neurosurgeon with real-time images and facilitate a gross total tumor resection with less morbidity. Further development of instrumentation that can be used in the environment of the magnet is critical.

Nursing research is vital to the supportive care of patients, caregivers, and significant others. Quality-of-life issues remain a vast area for nursing research directed at understanding the meaning of the disease and neurologic deficits to the patient. It can also provide information needed to develop more effective nursing strategies. The role of the family caregiver is critical in the management of patients with astrocytomas. The impact of the disease on the family caregivers needs to be evaluated as well so that they can continue to support the patient and maintain their own quality of life.

REFERENCES

Aaronson, N. K. (1988). Quality of life: What is it? How should it be measured? *Oncology, 2,* 69-76.

Aiken, R. D. (1994). Quality-of-life issues in patients with malignant gliomas. *Seminars in Oncology, 21,* 273-275.

American Brain Tumor Association (Ed.). (1996). *A primer of brain tumors.* (Available from the American Brain Tumor Association, 2720 River Road, Des Plaines, IL 60018-4110.)

Andrus, C. (1991). Intracranial pressure: Dynamics and nursing management. *Journal of Neuroscience Nursing, 23,* 85-92.

Apuzzo, M. L. J., Chandrasoma, P. T., Cohen, D., Zee, C. S., & Zelman, V. (1987). Computed imaging stereotaxy: Experience and prospective related to 500 procedures applied to brain masses. *Neurosurgery, 20,* 930-937.

Arbour, R. B. (1993). Stereotactic localization and resection of intracranial tumors. *Journal of Neuroscience Nursing, 25,* 14-21.

Arbour, R. (1994). Laser and ultrasound technology in aggressive management of central nervous system tumors. *Journal of Neuroscience Nursing, 26,* 30-35.

Archibald, Y. M., Lunn, D., Ruttan, L. A., Macdonald, D. R., Del Maestro, R. F., Barr, H. W. K., Pexman, J. H. W., Fischer, B. J., Gaspar, L. E., & Cairncross, J. G. (1994). Cognitive functioning in long-term survivors of high-grade glioma. *Journal of Neurosurgery, 80,* 247-253.

Armstrong, T. S., & Gilbert, M. R. (1996). Glial neoplasms: Classification, treatment, and pathways for the future. *Oncology Nursing Forum, 23,* 615-625.

Barnes, P. D., Robertson, R. L., & Poussaint, T. Y. (1997). Structural imaging of central nervous system tumors. In P. M. Black & J. S. Loeffler (Eds.), *Cancers of the nervous system.* Cambridge: Blackwell Science.

Barr, M. L., & Kiernan, J. A. (1988). *The human nervous system* (5th ed.). Philadelphia: J. B. Lippincott.

Behars, O. H., Henson, D. E., & Hutter, R. (1992). *Manual for staging of cancer* (4th ed.). Philadelphia: J. B. Lippincott.

Belford, K. (1997). Central nervous system cancers. In S. L. Groenwald, M. H. Frogge, M. Goodman, & C. H. Yarbro (Eds.), *Cancer nursing principles and practice.* Boston: Jones and Bartlett.

Bentson, J. R. (1996). Magnetic resonance imaging. In J. R. Youmans (Ed.), *Neurological surgery.* Philadelphia: W. B. Saunders.

Berleur, M. P., & Cordier, S. (1995). The role of chemical, physical, or viral exposures and health factors in neurocarcinogenesis: Implications for epidemiologic studies of brain tumors. *Cancer Causes and Control, 6,* 240-256.

Black, P. M. (1991). Brain tumors. *The New England Journal of Medicine, 324,* 1555-1564.

Black, P. M., Moriarty, A. E., Stieg, P., Woodard, E. J., Gleason, P. L., Martin, C. H., Kikinis, R., Schwartz, R. B., & Jolesz, F. A. (1997). Development and implementation of intraoperative magnetic resonance imaging and its neurosurgical applications. *Neurosurgery, 41,* 831-845.

Black, S., & Cucchiara, R. F. (1993). Anesthetic considerations. In M. L. J. Apuzzo (Ed.), *Brain surgery: Complication avoidance and management.* New York: Churchill Livingstone.

Bohnen, N. I., Radhakrishnan, K., O'Neill, B. P., & Kurland, L. T. (1997). Descriptive and analytic epidemiology of brain tumors. In P. M. Black & J. S. Loeffler (Eds.), *Cancer of the nervous system.* Cambridge: Blackwell Science.

Bondy, M., Wiencke, J., Wrensch, M., & Kyritsis, A. P. (1994). Genetics of primary brain tumors: A review. *Journal of Neuro-Oncology, 18,* 69-81.

Brem, H., Piantadosi, S., Burger, P. C.., Walker, M., Selker, R., Vick, N. A., Black, K., Sisti, M., Brem, S., Mohr, G., Muller, P., Morawetz, R., & Schold, S. C. (1995). Placebo-controlled trial of safety and efficacy of intraoperative controlled delivery by biodegradable polymers of chemotherapy for recurrent gliomas. *The Lancet, 345,* 1008-1012.

Brem, S., Rozental, J. M., & Moskal, J. R. (1995). What is the etiology of human brain tumors? *Cancer, 76,* 709-713.

Bruner, J. M. (1994). Neuropathology of malignant gliomas. *Seminars in Oncology, 21,* 126-138.

Byrne, T. N. (1994). Imaging of gliomas. *Seminars in Oncology, 21,* 162-171.

Castillo, M. (1994). Contrast enhancement in primary tumors of the brain and spinal cord. *Neuroimaging Clinics of North America, 4,* 63-80.

CBTRUS. (1997). *1996 Annual report.* The Central Brain Tumor Registry of the United States.

Ceberg, C. P., Persson, A., Brun, A., Huiskamp, R., Fyhr, A. S., Persson, B. R. R., & Salford, L. G. (1995). Performance of sulfhydryl boron hydride in patients with grade III and IV astrocytoma: A basis for boron neutron capture therapy. *Journal of Neurosurgery, 83,* 79-85.

Chen, T. C., & Apuzzo, M. L. J. (1997). Principles of stereotactic surgery. In P. M. Black & J. S. Loeffler (Eds.), *Cancer of the nervous system.* Boston: Blackwell Science.

Chin, L. S., Zee, C. S., & Apuzzo, M. L. J. (1993). Special considerations in point stereotactic procedures. In M. L. J. Apuzzo (Ed.), *Brain surgery: Complications avoidance and management.* New York: Churchill Livingstone.

Cohen, A. P., Wisoff, J. H., Allen, J. C., & Epstein, F. (1989). Malignant astrocytomas of the spinal cord. *Journal of Neurosurgery, 70,* 50-54.

Conrad, C. A., Milosavljevic, V. P., & Yung, W. K. A. (1995). Advances in chemotherapy for brain tumors. In P. Y. Wen & P. M. Black (Eds.), *Neurologic clinics: Brain tumors in adults.* Philadelphia: W. B. Saunders.

Constantini, S., Allen, J. C., & Epstein, F. (1997). Pediatric and adult spinal cord tumors. In P. M. Black & J. S. Loeffler (Eds.), *Cancer of the nervous system.* Cambridge: Blackwell Science.

DeAngelis, L. M. (1996, December). Neurologic complications of RT. In M. G. Malkin (Program Director), *Neuro-oncology VI: Recent advances in diagnosis and treatment.* New York: Postgraduate Course at Memorial Sloan-Kettering Cancer Center.

Di Chiro, G., DeLaPaz, R. L., Brooks, R. A., Sololoff, L., Kornblith, P. L., Smith, B. H., Patronas, N. J., Kufta, C. V., Kessler, R. M., Johnston, G. S., Manning, R. G., & Wold, A. P. (1982). Glucose utilization of cerebral gliomas measured by [18F]-fluorodeoxyglucose and positron emission tomography. *Neurology, 32,* 1323-1329.

Earnest, F., Kelly, P. J., Scheithauer, B. W., Kall, B. A., Cascino, T. L., Ehman, R. L., Forbes, G. S., & Axley, P. L. (1988). Cerebral astrocytomas: Histopathologic correlation of MR and CT contrast enhancement with stereotactic biopsy. *Radiology, 166,* 823-827.

Epstein, F. J., Farmer, J. P., & Freed, D. (1992). Adult intramedullary astrocytomas of the spinal cord. *Journal of Neurosurgery, 77,* 355-359.

Epstein, F. J., Farmer, J. P., & Schneider, S. J. (1991). Intraoperative ultrasonography: An important surgical adjunct for intramedullary tumors. *Journal of Neurosurgery, 74,* 729-733.

Epstein, F. J., & Ozek, M. (1993). The plated bayonet: A new instrument to facilitate surgery for intra-axial neoplasms of the spinal cord and brain stem. *Journal of Neurosurgery, 78,* 505-507.

Fine, H. A., Dear, K. B., Loeffler, J. S., Black, P. M., & Canellos, G. P. (1993). Meta-analysis of RT with and without adjuvant chemotherapy for malignant gliomas in adults. *Cancer, 71,* 2585-2597.

Fine, H. W. (1995). Novel biologic therapies for malignant gliomas. In P. Y. Wen & P. M. Black (Eds.), *Neurologic clinics: Brain tumors in adults.* Philadelphia: W. B. Saunders.

Flickinger, J. C., Loeffler, J. S., & Larson, D. A. (1994). Stereotactic radiosurgery for intracranial malignancies. *Oncology, 8,* 81-86.

Floderus, B., Persson, T., Stenlund, C., Wennberg, A., Ost, A., & Knave, B. (1993). Occupational exposure to electromagnetic fields in relation to leukemia and brain tumors: A case-control study in Sweden. *Cancer, Causes and Control, 4,* 465-476.

Freilich, R. J., & DeAngelis, L. M. (1995). Primary central nervous system lymphoma. In P. Y. Wen & P. M. Black (Eds.), *Neurologic clinics: Brain tumors in adults.* Philadelphia: W. B. Saunders.

Gargan-Klinger, R. (1988). *Family caregivers of patients with malignant brain tumors.* Unpublished Master's thesis, Garden City, NY: Adelphi University.

Gilman, S., & Newman, S. W. (1992). *Manter and Gatz's essentials of clinical neuroanatomy and neurophysiology* (8th ed.). Philadelphia: F. A. Davis.

Greene, G. M., Hitchon, P. W., Schelper, R. L., Yult, W., & Dyste, G. N. (1989). Diagnostic yield in CT-guided stereotactic biopsy of gliomas. *Journal of Neurosurgery, 71,* 494-497.

Grossman, C. B. (1990). *Magnetic resonance imaging and computer tomography of the head and spine.* Baltimore: Williams & Wilkins.

Grossman, S. A., & Norris, L. K. (1995). Adjuvant and neoadjuvant treatment for primary brain tumors in adults. *Seminars in Oncology, 6,* 530-539.

Grossman, S. A., Wharam, M., Sheidler, V., Kleinberg, L., Zeltzman, M., Yue, N., & Piantadosi, S. (1997). Phase II study of continuous infusion carmustine and cisplatin followed by cranial irradiation in adults with newly diagnosed high-grade astrocytoma. *Journal of Clinical Oncology, 15,* 2596-2603.

Haglund, M. M., Berger, M. S., Shamseldin, M., Lettich, E., & Ojemann, G. A. (1994). Cortical localization of temporal lobe language sites in patients with gliomas. *Neurosurgery, 18,* 33-39.

Heilbrun, M. P., Roberts, T. S., Apuzzo, M. L. J., Wells, Jr., T. H., & Sabshin, J. K. (1983). Preliminary experience with Brown-Roberts-Wells (BRW) computerized tomography stereotaxic guidance system. *Journal of Neurosurgery, 59,* 217-222.

Hickey, J. V. (1992). *The clinical practice of neurological and neurosurgical nursing* (3rd ed.). Philadelphia: J. B. Lippincott.

Hodges, L. C., Smith, J. L., & Garrett, A. (1992). Prevalence of glioblastoma multiforme in subjects with prior therapeutic radiation. *Journal of Neuroscience Nursing, 24,* 79-83.

Hubbard, S. M., Goodman, M., & Knobf, M. T. (1997). Cancer genetics for nurses: Part I. The genetic basis of cancer. *Oncology Nursing Updates, 4,* 1-11.

Jaeckle, K. A. (1994). Immunotherapy of malignant gliomas. *Seminars in Oncology, 21,* 249-259.

Jeremic, B., Grujicic, D., Antunovic, V., Djuric, L., & Shibamoto, Y. (1995). Accelerated hyperfractionated RT for malignant glioma. *American Journal of Clinical Oncology, 18,* 449-453.

Jyothirmayi, R., Madhaven, J., Nair, M. K., & Rajan, B. (1997). Conservative surgery and radiotherapy in the treatment of spinal cord astrocytoma. *Journal of Neuro-Oncology, 33,* 205-211.

Kaye, A. H., & Laidlaw, J. D. (1992). Chemotherapy of gliomas. *Current Opinions in Neurology and Neurosurgery, 5,* 526-533.

Kelly, D. F. (1994). Neurosurgical postoperative care. *Neurosurgery Clinics of North America, 5,* 789-810.

Kelly, P. J., Alker, G. J., & Goerss, S. (1982). Computer assisted stereotactic laser microsurgery for the treatment of intracranial neoplasm. *Neurosurgery, 10,* 324-331.

Kim, S. G., Ashe, J., Georgopoulos, A. P., Merkle, H., Ellermann, J. M., Menon, R. S., Ogawa, S., & Ugurbil, K. (1993). Functional imaging of human motor cortex at high magnetic field. *Journal of Neurophysiology, 69,* 297-302.

Kleihues, P. Burger, P. C., & Scheithauer, B. W. (1993). *The WHO histological typing of the central nervous system* (2nd ed.). Berlin, Heidelberg: Springer-Verlag.

Kondziolka, D., Lunsford, L. D., & Martinez, A. J. (1993). Unreliability of contemporary neurodiagnostic imaging in evaluating suspected adult supratentorial (low-grade) astrocytoma. *Journal of Neurosurgery, 79,* 533-536.

Kordek, R., Biernat, W., Alwasiak, J., Maculewicz, R., Yanagihara, R., & Liberski, P. P. (1995). P53 protein and epidermal growth factor receptor expression in human astrocytomas. *Journal of Neuro-Oncology, 26,* 11-16.

Kornblith, P., Walker, M. D., & Cassady, J. R. (1987). *Neurologic oncology.* Philadelphia: J. B. Lippincott.

Krause, E. A., Lamb, S., Ham, B., Larson, D. A., & Gutin, P. H. (1991). Radiosurgery: A nursing perspective. *Journal of Neuroscience Nursing, 23,* 24-28.

Landis, S. H., Murray, T., Bolden, S., & Wingo, P. A. (1998). Cancer statistics, 1998. *CA: A Cancer Journal for Clinicians, 48,* 6-29.

Laperriere, N. J., & Bernstein, M. (1994). Radiotherapy for brain tumors. *CA: A Cancer Journal for Clinicians, 44,* 96-108.

League, D. (1995). Interactive image-guided stereotactic neurosurgery systems. *American Operating Room Nurses' Journal, 61,* 360-370.

Leahy, N. M. (1990). *Quick reference to neurological critical care nursing.* Rockville, MD: Aspen.

Lehman, R. A. W. (1995). Intraoperative cortical stimulation and recording. In G. B. Russell & L. D. Rodichok (Eds.), *Primer of intraoperative neurophysiologic monitoring.* Boston: Butterworth-Heinemann.

Leibel, S. A., Scott, C. B., & Loeffler, J. S. (1994). Contemporary approaches to the treatment of malignant gliomas with RT. *Seminars in Oncology, 21,* 198-219.

Lesser, G. J., & Grossman, S. A. (1993). Tumor review: The chemotherapy of adult primary brain tumors. *Cancer Treatment Reviews, 19,* 261-281.

Lesser, G. J., & Grossman, S. A. (1994). The chemotherapy of high-grade astrocytomas. *Seminars in Oncology, 21,* 220-235.

Levin, V. A., Leibel, S. A., & Gutin, P. A. (1997). Neoplasms of the central nervous system. In V. T. DeVita, S. Hellman, & S. A. Rosenberg (Eds.), *Cancer principles and practice of oncology.* Philadelphia: J. B. Lippincott.

Levin, V. A., Prados, M. R., Wara, W. M., Davis, R. L., Gutin, P. H., Phillips, T. L., Lamborn, K., & Wilson, C. B. (1995). Radiation therapy and bromodeoxyuridine chemotherapy followed by procarbazine, lomustine, and vincristine for the treatment of anaplastic gliomas. *International Journal of Radiation Oncology, Biology, Physics, 32,* 75-83.

Levin, V. A., Silver, P., Hannigan, J., Wara, W. M., Gutin, P. H., Davis, R. L., & Wilson, C. B. (1990). Superiority of postradiotherapy adjuvant chemotherapy with CCNU, procarbazine, and vincristine (PCV) over BCNU for anaplastic gliomas: NCOG 6G61 final report. *International Journal of Radiation Oncology, Biology, Physics, 18,* 321-324.

Levine, A. J., & Schmidet, H. H. (1993). *Molecular genetics of nervous system tumors.* New York: John Wiley & Sons.

Levivier, M., Goldman, S., Bidaut, L. M., Luxen, A., Stanus, E., Przedborski, S., Baleriaux, D., Hildebrand, J., & Brotchi, J. (1992). *Neurosurgery, 31,* 792-797.

Levivier, M., Goldman, S. L., Pirotte, B., Brucher, J. M., Baleriaux, D., Luxen, A., Hildebrand, J., & Brotchi, J. (1995). Diagnostic yield of stereotactic brain biopsy guided by positron emission tomography with [18F] fluorodeoxyglucose. *Journal of Neurosurgery, 82,* 445-452.

Li, F. P., Fraumeni, J. F., Jr., Mulvihill, J. J., Blattner, W. A., Dreyfus, M. G., Tucker, M. A., & Miller, R. W. (1988). A cancer family syndrome in twenty-four kindreds. *Cancer Research, 48,* 5358-5362.

Lower, J. S. (1992). Rapid neuro. *American Journal of Nursing, 92,* 38-48.

Mackworth, N., Fobair, P., & Prados, M. D. (1992). Quality of life self-reports from 200 brain tumor patients: Comparisons with Karnofsky performance scores. *Journal of Neuro-Oncology, 14,* 243-253.

McCormick, P. C., & Stein, B. M. (1996). Spinal cord tumors in adults. In J. R. Youmans (Ed.), *Neurological surgery.* Philadelphia: W. B. Saunders.

McCullough, E. C., & Coulam, C. M. (1976). Physical and dosimetric aspects of diagnostic geometrical and computer-assisted tomographic procedures. *Radiologic Clinics of North America, 14,* 3-14.

Meyers, C. M., & Weitzner, M. A. (1995). Neurobehavioral functioning and quality of life in patients treated for cancer of the central nervous system. *Current Opinions in Oncology, 7,* 197-220.

Minehan, K. J., Shaw, E. G., Scheithauer, B. W., Davis, D. L., & Onofrio, B. M. (1995). Spinal cord astrocytoma: Pathological and treatment considerations. *Journal of Neurosurgery, 83,* 590-595.

Moynihan, T. J., & Grossman, S. A. (1994). The role of chemotherapy in the treatment of primary tumors of the central nervous system. *Cancer Investigation, 12,* 88-97.

National Brain Tumor Foundation. (Ed.). (1994). *Brain tumors: A guide.* (Available from the National Brain Tumor Foundation, 785 Market Street, Suite 1600, San Francisco, CA 94103.)

National Comprehensive Cancer Network. (1997). NCCN adult brain tumor practice guidelines. *Oncology, 11,* 237-277.

Neglia, J. P., Meadows, A. T., Robison, L. L., Kim, T. H., Newton, W. A., Ruymann, F. B., Sather, H. N., & Hammond, G. D. (1991). Second neoplasms after acute lymphoblastic leukemia in childhood. *New England Journal of Medicine,* 325, 1330-1336.

Nelson, D. F., Curran, W. J., Jr., Scott, C., Nelson, J. S., Weinstein, A. S., Ahmad, K., Constine, L. S., Murray, K., Powlis, W. D., Mohiuddin, M., & Fischbach, J. (1993). Hyperfractionated RT and bis-chlorethyl nitrosourea in the treatment of malignant glioma - possible advantage observed at 72 Gy on 1.2 Gy b.i.d. fractions: Report of the Radiation Therapy Oncology Group protocol 8302. *International Journal of Radiation Oncology, Biology, Physics, 25,* 193-207.

Nicholas, M. K., Prados, M. D., Larson, D. A., & Gutin, P. H. (1997). Malignant astrocytomas. In P. M. Black & J. S. Loeffler (Eds.), *Cancer of the nervous system.* Cambridge: Blackwell Science.

Oldendorf, W., & Oldendorf, Jr., W. (1991). *MRI primer.* New York: Raven Press.

Parker, S. L., Tong, T., Bolden, S., & Wingo, P. A. (1997). Cancer statistics, 1997. *CA: A Cancer Journal for Clinicians, 47,* 5-27.

Plum, F., & Posner, J. B. (1980). *Diagnosis of stupor and coma.* Philadelphia: F. A. Davis.

Posner, J. B. (1995). *Neurologic complications of cancer.* Philadelphia: F. A. Davis.

Radhakrishnan, K., Bohnen, N. I., & Kurland, L. T. (1994). Epidemiology of brain tumors. In R. A. Morantz & J. W. Walsh (Eds.), *Brain tumors.* New York: Marcel Dekker.

Randal, T. (1993). Gene therapy for brain tumors in trials, correction of inherited disorders a hope. *Journal of the American Medical Association, 269,* 2181-2182.

Riggs, J. E. (1995). Rising primary malignant brain tumor mortality in the elderly. *Archives in Neurology, 52,* 571-575.

Roelcke, U. (1994). PET: Brain tumor biochemistry. *Journal of Neuro-Oncology, 22,* 275-279.

Ron, E., Modan, B., Bolce, Jr., J. D., Alfandary, E., Stovall, M., Chetrit, A., & Katz, L. (1988). Tumors of the brain and nervous system after radiotherapy in childhood. *New England Journal of Medicine, 319,* 1033-1039

Rosenfeld, M. R. (1996, December). Oncogenes, tumor suppressor genes and gene therapy. In M. G. Malkin (Program Director), *Neuro-oncology VI: Recent advances in diagnosis and treatment.* New York: Postgraduate Course at Memorial Sloan-Kettering Cancer Center.

Salcman, M. (1993). Intrinsic cerebral glioma. In M. L. J. Apuzzo (Ed.), *Brain surgery: Complication avoidance and management.* New York: Churchill Livingstone.

Sawaya, R., Rambo, Jr., W. M., Hammoud, M. A., & Lee Ligon, B. (1995). Advances in surgery for brain tumors. In P. Y. Wen & P. M. Black (Eds.), *Neurologic clinics: Brain tumors in adults.* Philadelphia: W. B. Saunders.

Schultheiss, T. E. (1990). Spinal cord radiation "tolerance": Doctrine versus data. *International Journal of Radiation Oncology, Biology, Physics, 19,* 219-221.

Schwartz, R. B. (1997). Functional imaging of brain tumors. In P. M. Black & J. S. Loeffler (Eds.), *Cancer of the nervous system.* Cambridge: Blackwell Science.

Schwartz, R. B. (1995). Neuroradiology of brain tumors. In P. Y. Wen & P. M. Black (Eds.), *Neurologic clinics: Brain tumors in adults.* Philadelphia: W. B. Saunders.

Shapiro, S., & Mealey, Jr., J. (1989). Late anaplastic gliomas in children previously treated for acute lymphoblastic leukemia. *Pediatric Neuroscience, 15,* 176-180.

Shapiro, W. R. (1986). Therapy of adult malignant brain tumors: What have the clinical trials taught us? *Seminars in Oncology, 13,* 38-45.

Shapiro, W. R., Green, S. B., Burger, P. C., Selker, R. G., VanGilder, J. C., Robertson, J. T., & Mahaley, M. S. (1992). A randomized comparison of intra-arterial versus intravenous BCNU, with or without intravenous 5-fluorouracil for newly diagnosed patients with malignant glioma. *Journal of Neurosurgery, 76,* 772-781.

Shaw, E. G. (1990). Low grade gliomas—to treat or not to treat? The radiation oncologist's perspectives. *Archives of Neurology, 47,* 1138-1139.

Shaw, E. G., Scheithauer, B. W., & Dinapoli, R. P. (1997). Low-grade hemispheric astrocytomas. In P. M. Black & J. S. Loeffler (Eds.), *Cancer of the nervous system.* Boston: Blackwell Science.

Shaw, E. G., Scheithauer, B. W., & O'Fallon, J. R. (1993). Management of supratentorial low-grade gliomas. *Oncology, 7,* 97-111.

Shrieve, D. C., & Loeffler, J. S. (1995). Advances in RT for brain tumors. In P. Y. Wen & P. M. Black (Eds.), *Neurologic clinics: Brain tumors in adults.* Philadelphia: W. B. Saunders.

Sneed, P. K., Larson, D. A., & Gutin, P. H. (1994). Brachytherapy and hyperthermia for malignant astrocytomas. *Seminars in Oncology, 21,* 186-197.

Taphoorn, M. J. B., Heimans, J. J., Snoek, F. J., Lindeboom, J., Oosterink, B., Wolbers, J. G., & Karim, A. B. M. F. (1992). Assessment of quality of life in patients treated for low-grade glioma: A preliminary report. *Journal of Neurology, Neurosurgery, and Psychiatry, 55,* 372-376.

Thiessen, B., & Blasberg, R. B. (1996, December). The PET scanner: Research tool and diagnostic aid. In M. G. Malkin (Program Director), *Neuro-oncology VI: Recent advances in diagnosis and treatment.* Postgraduate Course at Memorial Sloan-Kettering Cancer Center, New York, New York.

Thomas, T. L., & Waxweiler, R. J. (1986). Brain tumors and occupational risk factors. *Scandinavian Journal of Work Environmental Health, 12,* 1-15.

Thorton, A. F., Jr., Hegarty, T. J., Haken, R. K. T., Yanke, B. R., LaVigne, M. L., Fraass, B. A., McShan, D. L., & Greenberg, H. S. (1991). Three-dimensional treatment planning of astrocytomas: A dosimetric study of cerebral irradiation. *International Journal of Radiation Oncology, Biology, Physics, 20,* 1309.

Tice, H. M., Jones, K. M., Mulkern, R. V., Schwartz, R. B., Kalina, P., Ahn, S., Barnes, P., & Jolesz, F. (1993). Fast spin-echo imaging of intracranial neoplasms. *Journal of Computer Assisted Tomography, 17,* 425-431.

Tsang, R. W., Laperriere, N. J., Simpson, W. J., Brierly, J., Panzarella, T., & Symth, H. S. (1993). Glioma arising after RT for pituitary adenoma. *Cancer, 72,* 2227-2233.

Vick, N. A., & Paleologos, N. A. (1995). External beam radiotherapy: Hard facts and painful realities. *Journal of Neuro-Oncology, 24,* 93-95.

Walker, M. D., Alexander, E., Jr., Hunt, W. E., MacCarty, C. S., Mahaley, M. S., Mealey, J., Jr., Norrell, H. A., Owens, G., Ransohoff, J., Wilson, C. B., Gehan, E. A., & Strike, T. A. (1978). Evaluation of BCNU and/or radiotherapy in the treatment of anaplastic gliomas. *Journal of Neurosurgery, 49,* 333-343.

Walker, M. D., Strike, T. A., & Sheline, G. E. (1979). An analysis of dose-effect relationship in radiotherapy of malignant gliomas. *International Journal of Radiation Oncology, Biology, Physics, 5,* 1725-1731.

Ward-Smith, P. (1997). Stereotactic radiosurgery for malignant brain tumors: The patient's perspective. *Journal of Neuroscience Nursing, 29,* 117-122.

Watkins, D., & Rouleau, G. A. (1994). Genetics, prognosis and therapy of central nervous system tumors. *Cancer Detection and Prevention, 18,* 139-144.

Wegmann, J. (1993). Central nervous system cancers. In S. L Groenwald, M. H. Frogge, M. Goodman, & C. H. Yarbro (Eds.), *Cancer nursing principles and practice.* Boston: Jones and Bartlett.

Wen, P. Y., Fine, H. A., Black, P. M., Shrieve, D. C., Alexander, E., & Loeffler, J. S. (1995). High-grade astrocytomas. In P. Y. Wen & P. M. Black (Eds.), *Neurologic clinics: Brain tumors in adults.* Philadelphia: W. B. Saunders.

Widen, J. N., & Kelly, P. J. (1987). CT computerized stereotactic biopsy of low density CT lesions presenting with epilepsy. *Journal of Neurology, Neurosurgery, and Psychiatry, 50,* 1302-1305.

Willis, D. (1991). Intracranial astrocytoma: Pathology, diagnosis and clinical presentation. *Journal of Neuroscience Nursing, 23,* 7-14.

Wilson, C. B. (1993). General considerations. In M. L. J. Apuzzo (Ed.), *Brain surgery: Complication avoidance and management.* New York: Churchill Livingstone.

Wong, A. J., Zoltick, P. W., & Moscatello, D. K. (1994). The molecular biology and molecular genetics of astrocytic neoplasms. *Seminars in Oncology, 21,* 139-148.

Wong, S. C., Van Dyk, J., Milosevic, M., & Laperriere, N. J. (1994). Radiation myelopathy following single courses of radiotherapy and retreatment. *International Journal of Radiation Oncology, Biology, Physics, 30,* 575-581.

Wrensch, M., Bondy, M. L., Wiencke, J., & Yost, M. (1993). Environmental risk factors for primary malignant brain tumors: A review. *Journal of Neuro-Oncology, 17,* 47-64.

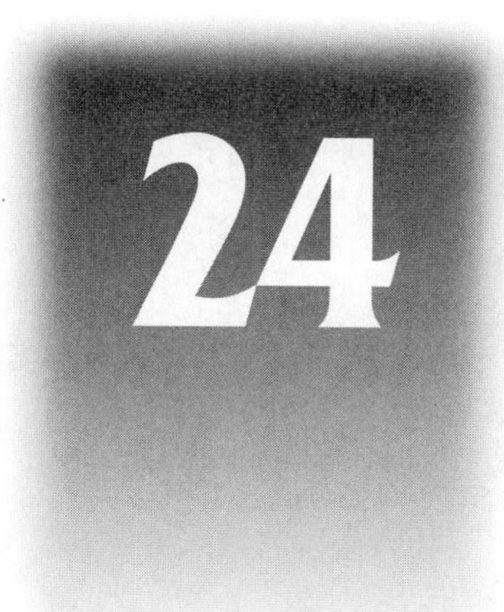

Primary Central Nervous System Lymphoma

Kathy Lilleby, RN

EPIDEMIOLOGY

Primary central nervous system lymphoma (PCNSL) is a rare tumor arising in the central nervous system (CNS). It has been called *microglioma, reticulum cell sarcoma,* or *periarticular sarcoma* (Taylor, Russell, Lukes, & Davis, 1978) and is usually associated with congenital, acquired, or iatrogenic immunodeficiency disease such as Wiskott-Aldrich syndrome, ataxia telangiectasia, severe combined immunosuppression, X-linked immunodeficiency, or renal transplantation (Rubinstein, 1972; Jellinger, Radaskiewicz, & Slowik, 1975; Zimmerman, 1975).

Because the origin of the B-cell lymphocyte is known, the question remains how a lymphoma can develop in an area that has no lymph nodes or lymphatic system. Circulating lymphocytes may be the source of the tumor. The rising incidence of T-cell CNS lymphoma may be due to newer immunohistochemical techniques. T-cell CNS lymphoma is more common in the leptomeninges. Studies suggest that the Epstein-Barr virus may contribute to its development (Adams, 1985).

The incidence of CNS lymphoma is 0.31 per 100,000 person-years in the United States (a 3-fold increase between 1973 and 1984) and a 10-fold increase in incidence has been seen in southeast England (Devesa & Fears, 1992). Primary CNS lymphoma affects all ages but is more common in the sixth and seventh decade of life and in younger immunocompromised patients (DeAngelis, Yahalom, Rosenblum, & Posner, 1987). There is a 3:2 male/female ratio in immunocompetent people, and more than 90% of acquired immune deficiency syndrome (AIDS) patients with CNS lymphoma are men (So et al., 1988).

RISK FACTORS

Patients with AIDS have the highest incidence of CNS lymphoma; about 3% will develop it. (Rosenblum et al., 1988; Welch et al., 1984). Other immunosuppressed patients such as transplant recipients and those with congenital immunodeficiencies are at most risk (Stein, 1985) (Box 24-1).

CHEMOPREVENTION

Chemoprevention refers to the use of drugs or certain foods to prevent malignancies from developing or progressing. Although many chemoprevention trials are currently being investigated, a review of the literature does not reveal any type of chemoprevention efforts for medulloblastoma.

PATHOPHYSIOLOGY

Normal Anatomy and Physiology of the CNS

The CNS is composed of the brain and spinal cord, which are enclosed within the cranium and bony spinal column. The brain can be divided into four regions: cerebrum, diencephalon, brain stem, and cerebellum (Fig. 24-1). The cerebrum makes up approximately 80% of the brain, is the second largest part, and includes the right and left hemispheres. The diencephalon, meaning "between brain," includes the thalamus and hypothalamus. At the base of the brain lies the cerebellum, which is responsible for coordination of movement. The brain stem, which is made up of the midbrain, pons, and medulla, connects the upper portion of the brain to the spinal cord. Brain tissue consists of gray matter, which is composed of nerve cell bodies, and white matter, which is composed of myelinated nerve fibers. The brain also contains four irregularly shaped spaces within the brain called *ventricles.* These four ventricles are interconnected and assist in the production and circulation of cerebrospinal fluid (CSF), which functions as a cushion and support to the brain and spinal cord. There are two lateral ventricles, one in each cerebral hemisphere; they contain a major portion of the choroid plexus, which produces the CSF. The third ventricle is located just posterior to the hypothalamus, and the fourth is located in the brain stem, anterior to the cerebellum.

The Lymphatic System: T- and B-Cell Origins

The lymphatic system consists of a network of vessels that branch throughout the body, with hundreds of small, bean-

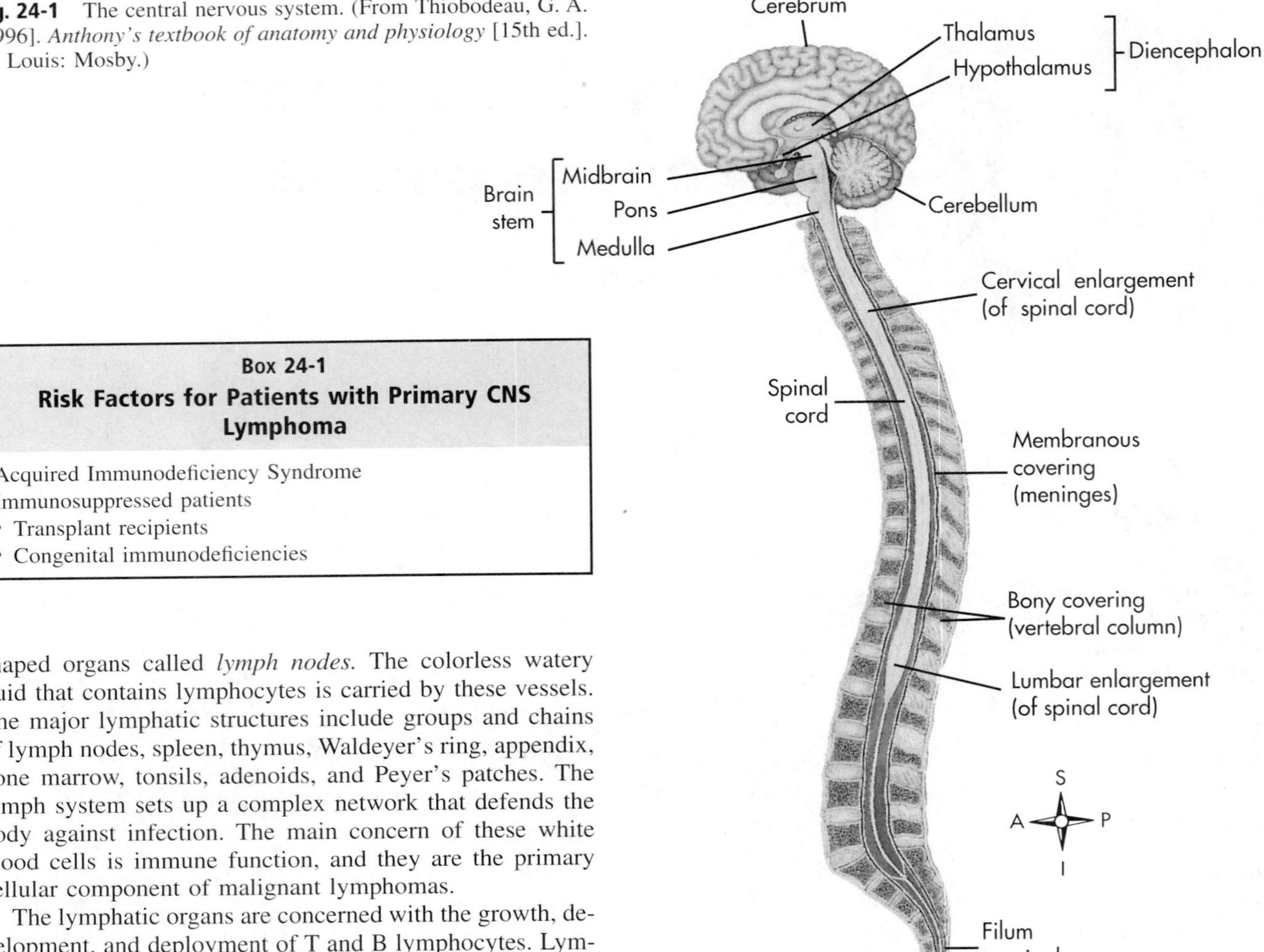

Fig. 24-1 The central nervous system. (From Thiobodeau, G. A. [1996]. *Anthony's textbook of anatomy and physiology* [15th ed.]. St. Louis: Mosby.)

Box 24-1
Risk Factors for Patients with Primary CNS Lymphoma

Acquired Immunodeficiency Syndrome
Immunosuppressed patients
- Transplant recipients
- Congenital immunodeficiencies

shaped organs called *lymph nodes.* The colorless watery fluid that contains lymphocytes is carried by these vessels. The major lymphatic structures include groups and chains of lymph nodes, spleen, thymus, Waldeyer's ring, appendix, bone marrow, tonsils, adenoids, and Peyer's patches. The lymph system sets up a complex network that defends the body against infection. The main concern of these white blood cells is immune function, and they are the primary cellular component of malignant lymphomas.

The lymphatic organs are concerned with the growth, development, and deployment of T and B lymphocytes. Lymphatic precursors arise from pluripotent stem cells in the marrow and are carried through the blood to the lymph nodes and spleen. They proliferate and differentiate on contact with antigens. T cells are memory cells and cells that regulate both antibody production by B cells and the cell-mediated effector responses of other T cells. B cells are memory and plasma cells, which are factories for the production of antibodies (Fig. 24-2).

PCNSL is an intermediate grade non-Hodgkin's lymphoma; however, AIDS-related PCNSL is usually high or intermediate grade. Histology is usually diffuse large-cell lymphoma or diffuse large-cell, immunoblastic lymphoma. The disease may arise in any part of the cerebrum, cerebellum, or brain stem. It may be either monofocal or multifocal (Scott, Hagan, Carter, Garin, Brieman, & Kurent, 1990).

The cells comprise a brownish space-occupying mass in the deep white matter of the CNS (Rubenstein, 1972). Sometimes, the corpus callosum is only thickened and not discolored; in other cases, the brain may appear normal but microscopic evidence of the malignancy is seen. The cells grow as sheets or in a characteristic vasocentric growth pattern with tumor infiltrating the brain parenchyma and adjacent blood vessels. Neither necrosis nor hemorrhage is common. On autopsy, tumor is found in many areas of the brain that have appeared normal on imaging studies. No unique tumor marker has been found to distinguish PCNSL from other systemic lymphomas (DeAngelis & Yahalom, 1997).

ROUTES OF METASTASES

PCNSL does not metastasize to visceral organs because, by definition, it is confined to the CNS. However, malignant cells may shed into the CSF by perivascular and meningeal spread (Scott et al., 1990).

ASSESSMENT

Patient History

Patients may present with symptoms of localized neurologic dysfunction, apathy, confusion, or personality changes. These symptoms can be classified into three categories: the effects of increased intracranial pressure, shifts of brain structure, and focal effects (Wegmann, 1993) (Table 24-1).

TABLE 24-1 Clinical Manifestations of Intracranial Tumors

Location	Function	Abnormality
Frontal lobes	Intellect	Intellectual deterioration
	Personality	Personality changes
	Judgment	Impaired judgment
	Abstract thinking	Bowel and bladder incontinence
	Mood and affect	Emotional lability
	Memory	Memory loss
	Motor activity (contralateral)	Muscle weakness or paralysis
		Babinski sign
	Expressive speech (left hemisphere)	Expressive aphasia
Parietal lobes	Sensory input (contralateral)	Decrease or loss of sensation (pain, temperature, pinprick, light touch, proprioception, vibration, two-point discrimination, double simultaneous stimulation, stereognosis, graphesthesia)
Occipital lobes	Sight	Visual field defects, hallucinations
	Visual identification of objects	Inability to identify objects or symbols
Temporal lobes	Hearing	Hearing changes, hallucinations
	Memory	Memory loss
	Receptive speech	Receptive aphasia
Cerebellum	Coordination	Ataxia, action tremor
		Nystagmus
	Balance (ipsilateral)	Loss of balance, wide-base gait
		Decreased deep tendon reflexes

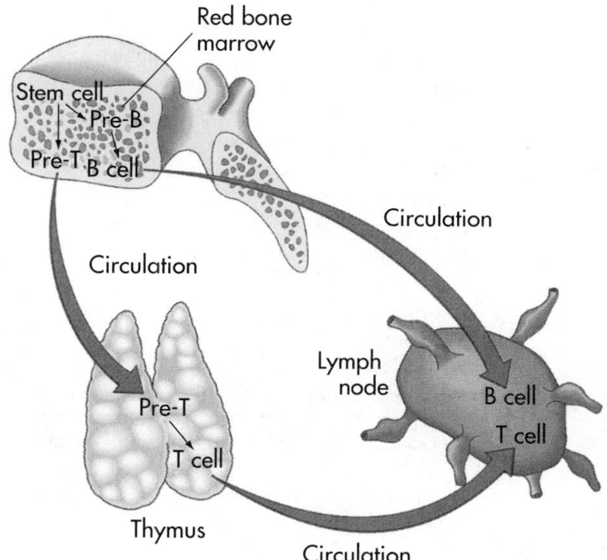

Fig. 24-2 Development of T and B cells of the immune system. (From Thibodeau, G. A. [1996]. *Anthony's textbook of anatomy and physiology* [15th ed.]. St. Louis: Mosby.)

See Table 24-2 for an assessment guide for patients with suspected CNS lymphoma.

Physical Examination

Brain. The patient may present with symptoms of an intracranial mass depending on the location of the tumor. The frontal lobe of the brain is frequently the site of tumor or tumors, so changes in personality or level of alertness and headaches are common. Seizures occur in only 10% of patients presenting with CNS lymphoma because the tumor involves deep brain structures rather than the seizure-prone cerebral cortex. Because PCNSL is a rapidly growing tumor, symptoms are seen for only weeks to a few months before the patient presents for diagnosis (Fig. 24-3) (DeAngelis & Yahalom, 1997).

CNS lymphoma is usually multifocal within the nervous system at diagnosis. The diagnosis can be confusing because 13% of the patients have a history of a prior malignancy (DeAngelis, 1991). These lesions can be microscopically connected to other tumors and not observed by magnetic resonance imaging (MRI). Periventricular lesions frequently infiltrate the CSF (Balmaceda, Gaynor, Sun, Gluck, & DeAngelis, 1995).

Eye. The eye, a direct extension of the brain, is a common site for CNS lymphoma. About 20% of CNS lymphoma patients have involvement of their eye at diagnosis (DeAngelis, 1995). Of patients in whom lymphoma originates in the eye, 50% to 80% develop cerebral lymphoma after several years. Ocular lymphoma involves the vitreous, retina, choroid, or optic nerve. Symptoms can include blurred vision or floaters, unilaterally or bilaterally, or there may be no symptoms (Char, Ljung, Miller, & Phillips, 1988).

Leptomeninges. Primary leptomeningeal lymphoma is found in only 7% of patients with CNS lymphoma. Presenting symptoms are progressive leg weakness, urinary incontinence or retention, cranial neuropathies, increased intracranial pressure, confusion, or a combination of these

Table 24-2 Assessment Guideline for Patients with CNS Lymphoma

Problem	Cause	Solution
Increased intracranial pressure (ICP)	Tumor size Cerebral edema Obstruction of CSF pathways	Corticosteroid administration
	Increased systemic arterial blood pressure	Avoid Valsalva maneuvers, isometric muscle contractions, coughing, emotional arousal
	Decreased cranial venous outflow	Elevate head of bed, avoid head rotation, neck flexation, and extension
	Increased intraabdominal and intrathoracic pressure	Avoid sneezing, coughing, straining Avoid hip flexion, prone position Monitor ICP level
Seizures	Disturbance of intracranial contents	Prophylactic anticonvulsants Safe environment Prevent harm during seizure activity Skin and oral hygiene following seizure activity
Personality changes	Frontal lobe involvement Cerebral edema	Maintain normal function Maintain orientation Acceptance of subtle change Avoid perilous behavior Encourage use of remaining cognitive functions Encourage social activities
Loss of sensation	Parietal, occipital, temporal lobe involvement	Monitor for visual disturbances Monitor for hearing loss Maintain orientation Safe environment, clothing
Disturbances in coordination	Cerebellum involvement	Ongoing assessment Intervention in physical surroundings Safety devices (bed rails, walker) Close off stairway Protect access to outdoors
Poor nutrition and hydration	Decreased activity GI effects of medications Overall deterioration	Frequent, small, attractive meals Dietary supplements Frequent oral fluids Use of alternative feeding routes, if necessary
Need for supportive care	Breakdown of patient/family social network	Assessment of: Priorities Environment Resources Roles and family functioning

From Wegmann, J. A. (1993). Central nervous system cancers. In S. Groenwald, M. H. Frogge, M. Goodman, & C. H. Yarbro (Eds.), *Cancer nursing: Principles and practice* (3rd ed). Boston: Jones & Bartlett.

symptoms. Patients usually have these symptoms for 2 to 3 months, but sometimes 1 to 2 years, before being diagnosed (Lachance et al., 1991). An examination of the CSF shows increased protein and lymphocyte values and a low glucose level (Taylor, Russell, Lukes, & Davis, 1978). An MRI of the head or spine shows meningeal enhancement and hydrocephalus, but no tumors in the brain or intradural nodules (DeAngelis & Yahalom, 1997).

Spinal Cord. Primary spinal cord lymphoma is less common than primary leptomeningeal lymphoma (Hochberg & Miller, 1988). Lymphoma in the spinal cord occurs alone or with brain lymphoma. Symptoms include painless bilateral leg weakness and sensory symptoms and may be recognized only after spinal cord decompression surgery. These signs may be in a radicular pattern, but eventually a sensory level is identified. The CSF may be normal or have a slightly elevated protein concentration with a few lymphocytes (DeAngelis & Yahalom, 1997).

Diagnostic Tests

Imaging (MRI) with Gadolinium. The cranial image of CNS lymphoma has a distinctive isointense signal before administration of the pregadolinium contrast. After the contrast, there is dense and diffuse enhancement. The lesions have indistinct borders with varying surrounding edema. Ring enhancement as seen with brain metastases or malignant gliomas is rare. Nonenhancing CNS lymphoma is

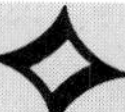

TABLE 24-3 Patient Preparation for a Lumbar Puncture

Description of the Procedure: A lumbar puncture is performed to withdraw a small amount of cerebral spinal fluid (CSF) from the spinal canal to measure readings and obtain CSF for laboratory examination. This is a safe procedure and requires about 15 minutes to perform. The health care provider performing the procedure, as well as an assistant, are present.

Patient Preparation: Patient may eat or drink before the procedure. Patient must empty the bladder before the procedure to avoid needing to do so during or immediately after the procedure.

Procedural Considerations

1. Obtain informed consent.
2. Patient should disrobe, wear a gown, and sit upright with head bent or lie sideways in a knee-chest position. Assuming these positions allow spaces in the spinal column to separate between the vertebrae and allow easy access to spinal fluid.
3. While in this position, the health care providers cleanse patient's skin with antiseptic solution to prevent bacteria from being introduced into the spinal spaces. A local anesthetic will be given through a small needle to inject medications to reduce your discomfort.
4. During the procedure, patient should remain still, should not cough or sneeze, and should continue to breathe slowly.
5. A small dressing such as an adhesive bandage is placed over the site. It can be removed in 12-24 hours.
6. On completion of the procedure, patient must lie still for a short period to prevent headaches. Headaches are a common side effect of the procedure.
7. At home, patient should lie down for several hours, consume plenty of fluids, and report any symptoms of headache or diziness to the health care provider.

Modified from Schenk, E. A. (1995). Assessment of the nervous system. In W. J. Phipps, V. L. Cassmeyer, J. K. Sands, and M. K. Lehman (Eds.), *Medical-surgical nursing: Concepts and clinical practice* (5th ed.). St. Louis: Mosby.

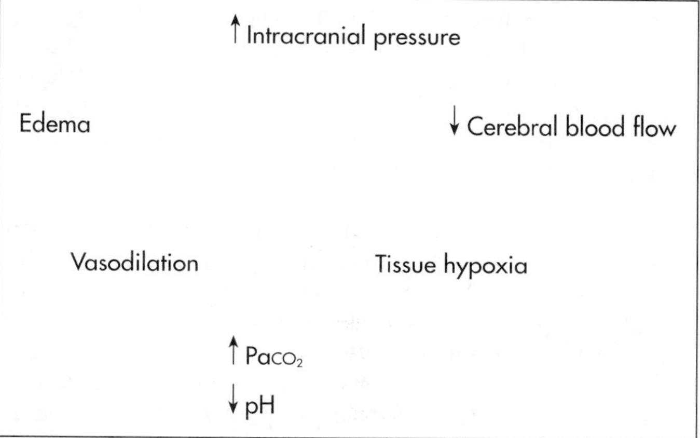

Fig. 24-3 Cycle of increased intracranial pressure.

important to recognize because it indicates tumor behind the blood-brain barrier. Spinal MRI with gadolinium should be done when appropriate (DeAngelis & Yahalom, 1997).

Lumbar Puncture. Lumbar puncture should be a standard diagnostic evaluation of every patient with CNS lymphoma. The protein concentration, glucose concentration, and lymphocyte count are the key values for diagnosis (Balmaceda et al., 1995). Elevated tumor markers such as beta-2 microglobulin, lactic acid dehydrogenase isoenzyme, and beta-glucuronidase give some evidence of leptomeningeal involvement (DeAngelis & Yahalom, 1997). See Table 24-3 for a lumbar puncture procedure.

Ophthalmologic Examination. Ophthalmologic examination with slit-lamp is required to detect a cellular infiltrate, as 20% of patients have ocular involvement at diagnosis (DeAngelis, Yahalom, Thaler, & Kher, 1992). Indirect ophthalmoscopy is used to detect choroidal or retinal lesions (Char et al., 1988). A vitrectomy specimen is sometimes needed for diagnosis, but a false-negative biopsy is possible when patients have too few vitreal lymphocytes or when they have been given corticosteroids to treat a presumed uveitis (Whitcup et al., 1993).

Box 24-2
Tests for Staging for CNS Lymphoma

Staging Examinations

Cranial magnetic resonance imaging (MRI) with gadolinium
Lumbar puncture
Ophthalmologic examination with slit-lamp
Spinal MRI with gadolinium (when appropriate)
Abdominal computerized tomograph scan
Bone marrow aspiration and biopsy
Chest radiograph

Abdominal Computerized Tomography Scan. An abdominal computerized tomography (CT) scan is used to establish a diagnosis of PCNSL. By definition, if lymphoma is found outside the CNS, the diagnosis is actually non-Hodgkin's lymphoma with metastasis to the nervous system.

Bone Marrow Aspiration and Chest Radiograph. Examination of the bone marrow by aspiration or biopsy also confirms that the lymphoma is not involved in areas outside of the CNS. A chest radiography or CT scan is also necessary to assess for lymphoma outside of the CNS.

STAGING

The clinical staging criteria for systemic lymphoma is used to stage CNS lymphoma. Stage IE is the stage for disease confined to a single extranodal site (DeAngelis & Yahalom, 1997) (Box 24-2).

MEDICAL MANAGEMENT OF CNS LYMPHOMA IN THE IMMUNOCOMPETENT PATIENT

Corticosteroids

CNS lymphoma is highly sensitive to corticosteroids. In 40% of patients, the tumor masses shrink significantly or disappear on MRI after administration of these medications. (DeAngelis, Yahalom, Heinemann, Cirricione, Thaler, & Krol, 1996). This seems to be due to the cytotoxic effects of corticosteroids because a biopsy of the mass after treatment shows normal, necrotic, or nondiagnositc tissue. In some patients, disappearance of the CNS lymphoma leads to clinical improvement that lasts for some time after the corticosteroids have been stopped. A few patients have been cured or have had prolonged survival after treatment with corticosteroids alone. However, in most patients, a steroid-induced remission is short and therefore not definitive treatment (Singh et al., 1982). This rapid disappearance of tumor, called *ghost tumor,* after administration of steroids is specific to PCNSL.

Surgery

Surgical resection is useful only in confirming the histologic diagnosis; it has no effect on survival. The mean survival of a patient after biopsy, resection only, and supportive care is 3.3 to 5 months (Henry, Heffner, Dillard, Earle, & Davis, 1974). Complete resection is difficult because the tumors are deep and multiple, and there is a high risk of severe physical deficits postoperatively (DeAngelis et. al., 1996). The diagnostic method of choice is stereotactic biopsy, which allows for a safer approach to the deep lesions. The other method of obtaining a biopsy specimen is a craniotomy, in which case an intraoperative frozen section can be obtained, a diagnosis made immediately, and the question of whether a resection is necessary answered (DeAngelis & Yahalom, 1997).

Radiotherapy

The conventional treatment for CNS lymphoma is whole brain radiotherapy with concurrent administration of corticosteroids. Retrospective studies have shown that doses of 4000 to 5000 Gy yielded better survival rates than lower doses. The median survival with this treatment is 12 to 18 months (DeAngelis, 1995). The Radiation Therapy Oncology Group reported, in their retrospective study of patients treated with 4000 Gy whole brain radiotherapy plus a 2000 Gy boost to the involved area, that the median survival was only 12.2 months and that most recurrences were in the boosted field (Nelson et al., 1992). The Memorial Sloan-Kettering Cancer Center has adopted the use of 4500 Gy whole brain radiotherapy without the boost, as the added therapy does not improve relapse rates and can cause late neurologic complications (DeAngelis et al., 1982).

The primary treatment of ocular disease is 3500 to 4500 Gy to the globe over 4 to 5 weeks. Both eyes should be irradiated whether one or both eyes are involved. Most patients have improved vision and vitreal clearing after treatment, but some have vitreal clearing without improvement of their vision. Other patients have no response to the treatment. Long-term side effects from ocular radiotherapy is unknown. Conjunctivitis, dry eyes, retinal atrophy, vitreous hemorrhage, and cataracts have all been reported in patients receiving ocular radiotherapy (Margolis, Fraser, Lichter, & Char, 1980).

Craniospinal irradiation has been suggested as additional therapy for CNS lymphoma owing to the high incidence of recurrence in the leptomeninges. It does, however, compromise the ability to give systemic chemotherapy at relapse because of the effect on hematologic toxicity in the large area of bone marrow irradiated (Rampen, van Andel, Sizoo, & van Unnik, 1980).

Chemotherapy

The combination of intrathecal chemotherapy plus radiotherapy has been studied in various institutions; even with small numbers in the trials, this treatment seems to be most effective (Shibamoto et al., 1990). The question of when to give the chemotherapy in relation to the radiotherapy has been studied. Researchers have concluded that giving chemotherapy before beginning radiotherapy is best for two reasons: (1) It allows for assessment of response of the tumor to chemotherapy, as most patients have a complete although short-lived response to radiotherapy, and (2) the risk of late neurologic toxicity by chemotherapy is reduced because the blood-brain barrier is not yet broken down by radiotherapy (DeAngelis & Yahalom, 1997).

The most commonly studied chemotherapeutic regimen is cyclophosphamide, doxorubicin, and vincristine with prednisone (CHOP) or dexamethasone. Patients who initially responded to CHOP quickly developed metastasis in a site distant from the original disease before chemotherapy was completed (Stewart et al., 1984). Other patients had longer survival rates with CHOP plus whole brain radiotherapy. Other researchers report poor outcome and high toxicity with this regimen (Liang et al., 1993).

Methotrexate, doxorubicin, cyclophosphamide, vincristine, prednisone, and bleomycin was given to a group of patients before radiotherapy, but the median survival was only 14 months (Brada, Dearnaley, Horwich, & Bloom, 1990). Methotrexate, procarbazine, cyclophosphamide, and doxorubicin have all been used in small groups of patients with success (Shibamoto et al., 1990). These agents should have activity against CNS lymphoma cells, but they are unable to cross the blood-brain barrier, so they can be effective only against bulky disease and not microscopic disease. Intraarterial chemotherapy has been studied after blood-brain barrier disruption, as well as intrathecal chemotherapy with varied results (DeAngelis & Yahalom, 1997).

High-dose cytarabine has been given for the treatment of ocular lymphoma with therapeutic levels documented in the aqueous and vitreous humor 90 minutes after the infusion was completed. Five of six patients responded (Strauchen, Dalton, & Friedman, 1989). The combination of high-dose

TABLE 24-4 Management of the Immunocompetent Patient

Surgery
Diagnosis biopsy
Resection should be avoided
Chemotherapy
Considered at diagnosis for every patient
Must penetrate the blood-brain barrier:
- Lipophilic (e.g., procarbazine)
- High-dose with CNS penetration (e.g., methotrexate)
- Antilymphoma activity
- Administered before radiotherapy

Radiotherapy
Whole brain, if used
4500 Gy boost not necessary
3600 Gy to eyes, if indicated
Deferred in some patients demonstrating complete remission after chemotherapy

From DeAngelis, L. M., & Yahalom, J. (1997). Primary central nervous system lymphoma. In V. T. DeVita, S. Hellman, & S. A. Rosenberg (Eds.), *Cancer, principles and practice of oncology* (5th ed., vol. 2). Philadelphia: Lippincott-Raven.

methotrexate and ocular radiotherapy has also been successful (DeAngelis & Yahalom, 1997).

The current regimen at Memorial Sloan Kettering Cancer Center combines methotrexate, vincristine, and procarbazine given intravenously on days 1, 3, and 5 along with methotrexate given through an Ommaya reservoir on days 2, 4, and 6. Whole brain irradiation begins on day 11 followed by intravenous high-dose cytarabine on days 16 and 20 (Freilich, Delattre, Monjour, & DeAngelis, 1996).

The scheme for disrupting the blood-brain barrier with chemotherapy includes intravenous cyclophosphamide and intra-arterial infusions of methotrexate on days 1 and 2. Leukovorin is given on days 2 through 7, and procarbazine and dexamethasone are given on days 3 through 7 and repeated on days 8 through 16. The dose of dexamethasone is then tapered beginning on day 17 (Dahlborg et al., 1996).

The Harvard regimen consists of methotrexate given intravenously on days 1, 11, and 21 followed by whole brain irradiation beginning on day 42 (Glass, Gruber, & Cher, Hochberg, 1994). Table 24-4 gives an overview of medical management of the immunocompetent patient.

MEDICAL MANAGEMENT OF CNS LYMPHOMA IN THE IMMUNOCOMPROMISED PATIENT

The difference in managing the immunocompromised patient must be considered at presentation. In patients with AIDS, CNS toxoplasmosis is the most common cause of an intracranial lesion that can be detected by MRI. In the non-AIDS immunocompromised patient, a stereotactic biopsy should be done (Ciricillo & Rosenblum, 1990).

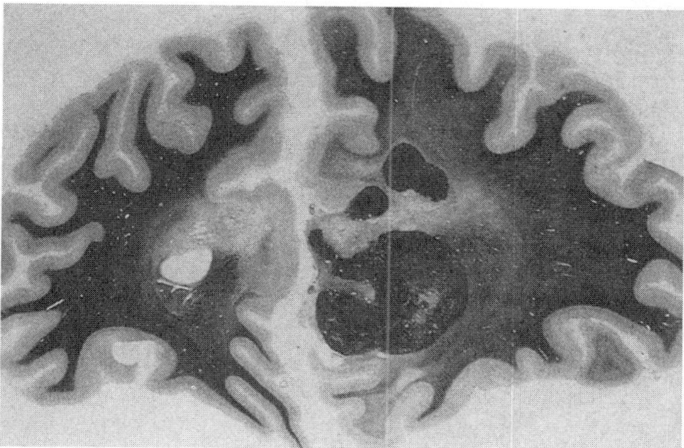

Fig. 24-4 Edema is represented in the pale areas surrounding the tumor nodules. (From Skarin, A. T. [1996], *Atlas of diagnostic oncology.* London: Mosby-Wolfe.)

Therapy

Corticosteroids and cranial irradiation are the treatment of choice for immunocompromised patients. However, care should be taken when administering corticosteroids to these patients, as they can contribute to their immunosuppression (Liang, Roach, Larson, & Wara, 1994; Matthews, Barba, & Fullerton, 1995).

Chemotherapy has not been used in this population, except for relapse after whole brain radiotherapy. Intrathecal methotrexate has been effective for leptomeningeal lymphoma, although the length of the response was short (DeAngelis & Yahalom, 1997).

NURSING MANAGEMENT

Supportive measures are the goal in caring for a patient with PCNSL because the prognosis is usually poor. However, several acute problems require special attention.

Increased Intracranial Pressure

Brain tumors increase intracranial pressure (ICP) by their size, cerebral edema, or obstruction of CSF flow (Fig. 24-4). Cerebral edema may be treated with a hyperosmolar agent such as mannitol given intravenously (IV) to cause fluid to be drawn across the semipermeable membrane and into the circulating bloodstream. Corticosteroids are given with the osmotherapy because they are believed to have an effect on vasogenic brain edema. Other IV and oral fluids are restricted to prevent intracellular edema (Wegmann, 1993).

Activities that may aggravate ICP are coughing, sneezing, Valsalva maneuvers, straining, isometric muscle contraction, and emotional arousal. Suctioning of the oropharynx reduces $PACO_2$, as does poor respiratory gas exchange. Positions that decrease venous outflow by compression of the jugular vein should be avoided. Care should be taken when turning a patient or doing range of motion exercises to

Table 24-5 Family Teaching and Home Care Guidelines for Patients with CNS Lymphoma

Problem	Care Guidelines
Physical injury due to unsteady gait	Call local American Cancer Society or other support organizations to obtain equipment (three-prong cane, walker, wheelchair, bedside commode, guard rail for bathroom, stool for shower) Do not use throw rugs to prevent tripping Wear nonskid shoes when out of bed Eliminate the need to walk up or down stairs Obtain assistance with physical care through home health aide and visiting nurse service
Decreased mobility due to physical disability	Obtain hospital bed to assist with care and change position Range of motion exercises four times daily Physical therapy consult Occupational therapy consult Change position in bed every 4 hours
Skin breakdown due to immobility and chronic steroid use	Bathe every 2-3 days using a nondeodorant soap Apply aloe-based cream or Eucerin cream daily, especially to pressure points Massage pressure points daily to stimulate blood flow Change position every 4 hours Keep perineum dry
Oral fungal infections due to chronic steroid use	Oral hygiene three times a day Inspect oral cavity for white plaque build-up Mycostatin mouth wash
Hyperglycemia due to steroid use	Medical management with sliding scale insulin administration Test blood sugar or urine sugar as directed Report sugar results to doctor or nurse Report unusual symptoms to your doctor such as: increased thirst, dry mouth, flushed skin, polyuria, nausea and vomiting
Stomach irritation and possible ulcer formation due to chronic steroid use	Eat small meals frequently Use antacids to minimize stomach upset Avoid caffeine Eat foods that are soft and easy to digest Soft feeding tube may be necessary to maintain nutrition
Fatigue, dizziness, muscle weakness and joint pain due to chronic steroid use and immobility	Conserve energy for activities patient enjoys Be out of bed as much as possible Walk out of doors daily as tolerated Nonsteroidal anti-inflammatory agent as needed for joint pain Vary activities to combat fatigue Avoid sleeping during the day Removable splinting may be used for weakened muscles Slide objects rather than lifting and carrying
Difficulty with dressing and personal hygiene due to decreased mobility and/or perception	Assess basic functional abilities to identify effective assistance devices Provide garments that are easy to put on, with large fasteners in accessible areas Nonskid shoes with Velcro closings Assess need for raised toilet seat, shower stool, tilted mirrors, and large faucets Lower closet rods Store frequently used items within easy reach, in consistent places
Memory impairment, perceptual deficits and cognitive processing impairments due to tumor growth or cerebral edema	Establish habitual use of safety devices and routines Provide compensatory cognitive devices: • Labels • Written instructions • Reminders and memory logs
Urinary incontinence due to confusion, loss of muscle control	Note patterns of incontinence Establish habit retraining based on time intervals Assess need for mechanical methods of urine collection Maintain positive attitude and recognize incontinence as a symptom, not a disease

From Wegmann, J. A. (1993). Central nervous system cancers. In S. Groenwald, M. H. Frogge, M. Goodman, & C. H. Yarbro (Eds.), *Cancer nursing: principles and practice* (3rd ed.). Boston: Jones and Bartlett.

TABLE 24-5 Family Teaching and Home Care Guidelines for Patients with CNS Lymphoma—cont'd

Problem	Care Guidelines
Impending death related to anticipated cardiopulmonary failure and advanced disease	Family teaching regarding: • Diminishing level of consciousness • Decreased oral fluid intake • Oliguria • Labored, irregular breathing • Bubbling in throat and chest • Progressive cyanotic mottling in lower extremities Encourage participation in home hospice program Determine unfinished business Encourage worship and prayer that are consistent with family beliefs

avoid positions or activities that increase ICP. Elevating the head of the bed promotes venous drainage and is recommended for increased ICP (Wegmann, 1993).

Use of Corticosteroids

Corticosteroids are used to treat PCNSL and to reduce cerebral edema. However, patients must be carefully monitored for side effects common to the use of this drug. The side effects can affect several body systems. First, acute adrenal insufficiency can cause fatigue, muscular weakness, joint pain, fever, anorexia, nausea, and orthostatic hypotension. Second, cardiovascular problems can include increased cardiac output and atrioventricular node conduction rate problems. Third, the kidneys may be affected by sodium retention. Fourth, gastrointestinal disturbances such as formation of peptic ulcers and melena with resulting anemia are seen. Fifth, metabolic problems may include hyperglycemia and glucosuria, polydypsia, and polyuria. Finally, the musculoskeletal system is affected by muscular atrophy and osteoporosis in patients who are immobile (Wegmann, 1993).

Discharge planning for patients who have been hospitalized should center on rehabilitation and home care. Table 24-5 contains teaching guidelines for home care. Hospice care may be necessary as the disease progresses (Wegmann, 1993).

HOME CARE ISSUES

Care of the patient with PCNSL centers around safety and mobility. An unsteady gait and decreased ability to walk due to weakness, confusion, or balance require assessment. Assistive devices such as canes, walkers, or wheelchairs, as well as nursing personnel or family members, may be necessary. Protective devices such as bed rails, hand rails, or cushions should be evaluated. Reality orientation devices such as clocks and calendars should be available (Wegmann, 1993).

EVALUATION OF THE QUALITY OF CARE

The quality of a patient's care should be monitored. Specific aspects of care can be evaluated through the use of a tool seen in Table 24-6.

TABLE 24-6 Quality of Care for a Patient with Primary CNS Lymphoma

Disciplines participating in the quality of care evaluation:
☐ Nursing ☐ Physician
☐ Physical Therapy ☐ Social Services
Data from:
☐ Medical Record Review ☐ Patient/Family Interview

Criteria	Yes	No
1. Patient provided with information about:		
a. Signs and symptoms of hyperglycemia	☐	☐
b. Safety measures to prevent falling at home	☐	☐
c. Signs and symptoms of a gastric ulcer	☐	☐
d. Signs and symptoms of increased intracranial pressure	☐	☐
2. The following assessments are made at each visit:		
a. Level of consciousness, personality changes	☐	☐
b. Blood glucose	☐	☐
c. Functional status and mobility	☐	☐
d. Skin integrity	☐	☐
3. Patient experienced the following complications:		
a. Ulcer formation	☐	☐
b. Joint pain or injury	☐	☐
c. Skin breakdown	☐	☐
d. Seizure	☐	☐

Patient/Family Satisfaction
Data from: ☐ Patient Interview ☐ Family Interview

Criteria	Yes	No
1. On a scale of 0 to 10, with 0 being totally dissatisfied and 10 being totally satisfied, how satisfied were you with the home care management guidelines you received? ______	☐	☐
2. Were you told to call the nurse if your blood sugar or urine sugar was not in the normal range you were taught?	☐	☐
3. Were you taught to eat frequent small meals of soft, easily digested food and to drink 8 glasses of liquid a day?	☐	☐

PROGNOSIS

The prognosis for CNS lymphoma is poor. Even though it is highly responsive to treatment, the median survival is only 12 to 18 months with cranial radiotherapy. The 5-year survival rate is 3% to 4% because of recurrence of disease. Relapse occurs primarily in the brain within the radiation port or in the leptomeninges or eye. Prognosis is poor for spinal cord lymphoma, with survival only a few months from onset of symptoms to death. Poor survival may be due to lack of diagnosis and treatment (DeAngelis, 1995).

RESEARCH ISSUES

Earlier detection and new treatments need to be developed because of the poor prognosis of the disease.

REFERENCES

Adams, R. D., & Victor, M. (1985). *Principles of Neurology* (3rd ed.). New York: McGraw Hill.

Balmaceda, C., Gaynor, J. J., Sun, M., Gluck, J.T., & DeAngelis, L. M. (1995). Leptomeningeal tumor in primary central nervous system lymphoma: recognition, significance, and implications. *Annals of Neurology, 38,* 202-209.

Brada, M., Dearnaley, D., Horwich, A., & Bloom, H. J. G. (1990). Management of primary cerebral lymphoma with initial chemotherapy: preliminary results and comparison with patients treated with radiotherapy alone. *International Journal of Radiation, Oncology, Biology, Physics, 18,* 787-792.

Char, D. H., Ljung, B. M., Miller, T., & Phillips, T. (1988). Primary intraocular lymphoma (ocular reticulum cell sarcoma) diagnosis and management. *Ophthalmology, 95,* 625-630.

Ciricillo, S. F., & Rosenblum, M. L. (1990). Use of CT and MR imaging to distinguish intracranial lesions and to define the need for biopsy in AIDS patients. *Journal of Neurosurgery, 73,* 720-724.

Dahlborg, S. A., Henner, W. D., Crossen, J. R., Tableman, M., Petrillo, A., Braziel, R., & Neuwelt, E. A. (1996). Non-AIDS primary CNS lymphoma. *Cancer Journal Science American, 2,* 166.

DeAnglis, L. M. (1991). Primary central nervous system lymphoma as a secondary malignancy. *Cancer, 67,* 1431-1435.

DeAngelis, L. M. (1995). Current management of primary central nervous system lymphoma. *Oncology, 9,* 63-71.

DeAngelis, L. M., & Yahalom, J. (1997). Primary central nervous system lymphoma. In V. T. DeVita, S. Hellman, & S. A. Rosenberg (Eds.), *Cancer, principles and practice of oncology* (5th ed., vol. 2). Philadelphia: Lippincott-Raven Publishers.

DeAngelis, L.M., Yahalom, J., Heinemann, M-H., Cirrincione, C., Thaler, H.T., & Krol, G. (1990). Primary CNS lymphoma: combined treatment with chemotherapy and radiotherapy. *Neurology, 40,* 80-86.

DeAngelis, L. M., Yahalom, J., Rosenblum, M., & Posner, J. B. (1987). Primary CNS lymphoma patients with spontaneous and AIDS-related disease. *Oncology, 1,* 52-62.

DeAngelis, L. M., Yahalom, J., Thaler, H.T., & Kher, U. (1992). Combined modality treatment for primary CNS lymphoma. *Journal of Clinical Oncology, 10,* 635-643.

Devesa, S. S., & Fears, T. (1992). Non-Hodgkin's lymphoma time trends: United States National Data. *Cancer Research, 52,* 5432s-5440s.

Freilich, R. J., Delattre, J.Y., Monjour, A., & DeAngelis, L.M. (1996). Chemotherapy without radiation therapy as initial treatment for primary central nervous system lymphoma in older patients. *Neurology, 46,* 435-439.

Glass, J., Gruber, M. I., Cher, I., & Hochberg, H.J. (1994). Preirradiation methotrexate chemotherapy of primary central nervous system lymphoma: long-term outcome. *Journal of Neurosurgery, 81,* 188-195.

Henry, J.M., Heffner, R. R., Dillard, S. H., Earle, K.M., & Davis, R.L. (1974). Primary malignant lymphomas of the central nervous system. *Cancer, 34,* 1293-1302.

Hochberg, F.H., & Miller, D.C. (1988). Primary central nervous system lymphoma. *Journal of Neurosurgery, 68,* 835-853.

Jellinger, K., Radaskiewicz, T.H., & Slowik, F. (1975). Primary malignant lymphomas of the central nervous system in man. *Acta Neuropatholgoica (Berlin), Suppl VI,* 95-102.

Lachance, D. H., O'Neill, B. P., MacDonald, D. R., Jaeckle, K.A., Witzig, T. E., Li, C.Y., & Posner, J.B., (1991). Primary leptomeningeal lymphoma: report of 9 cases, diagnosis with immunocytochemical analysis, and review of the literature. *Neurology, 41,* 95-100.

Liang, B. C., Grant, R., Junck, L., Sandler, H. M., Papadopoulous, S. M., Kaminski, M.S., & Greenberg, H. S. (1993). Primary central nervous system lymphoma: treatment with multiagent systemic and intrathecal chemotherapy with radiation therapy. *International Journal of Oncology, 3,* 1001-1004.

Ling, S.M., Roach, III, M., Larson, D.A., & Wara, W.M. (1994). Radiotherapy of primary central nervous system lymphoma in patients with and without human immunodeficiency virus. *Cancer, 73,* 2570-2582.

Margolis, L., Fraser, R., Lichter, A., & Char, D. H. (1980). The role of radiation therapy in the management of ocular reticulum cell sarcoma. *Cancer, 45,* 688-692.

Matthews, C., Barba, D., & Fullerton, S.C. (1995). Early biopsy versus empiric treatment with delayed biopsy of non-responders in suspected HIV-associated cerebral toxoplasmosis: a decision analysis. *AIDS, 9,* 1243-1248.

Nelson, D.F., Martz, K.L. Bonner, J., Nelson, J.S., Newall, J., Kerman, H. D., Thomson, J.W., & Murray, K.J. (1992). Non-Hodgkin's lymphomas of the brain: can high dose, large volume radiation therapy improve survival? Report on a prospective trial by the radiation therapy oncology group (RTOG): RTOG 8315. *International Journal of Radiation Oncology, Biology Physics, 23,* 9-17.

Rampen, F.H., van Andel, J.G., Sizoo, W., & van Unnik, J.A.M. (1980). Radiation therapy in primary non-Hodgkin's lymphomas of the CNS. *European Journal of Cancer, 16,* 177-184.

Rosenblum, M. I., Levy, R. M., Bredesen, D. E., So, Y. T., Wara, W., & Ziegler, J.L. (1988). Primary central nervous system lymphoma in patients with AIDS. *Annals of Neurology, 23,* 13-16.

Rubinstein, L.J. (1972). *Tumors of the central nervous system: atlas of tumor pathology; second series.* Fascicle 6, Washington, D.C.: Armed Forces Institute of Pathology.

Scott, T. F., Hogan, E. L., Carter, T. D., Garen, P. D., Brillman, J., & Kurent, J. E. (1990). Primary intercranial menengeal lymphoma, *American Journal of Medicine 89,* 536-545.

Shibamoto, Y., Tsutsui, K., Dodo, Y., Yamabe, H., Shima, N., & Abe, M. (1990). Improved survival rate in primary intracranial lymphoma treated by high-dose radiation and systemic vincristine-doxorubicin-cyclophosphamide-prednisone chemotherapy. *Cancer, 65,* 1907-1912.

Singh, A., Strobos, R. J., Singh, B. M., Rothballer, A. B., Reddy, V., Puljic, S., & Poon, T.P. (1982). Steroid-induced remissions in CNS lymphoma. *Neurology, 32,* 1267-1271.

Skarin, A. T. (1996). *Atlas of diagnostic oncology.* London: Mosby-Wolfe,

So, Y. T., Coucair, A., Davis, R. L., Wara, W. M., Ziegler, J. L., Sheline, G. E., & Beckstead, J. H. (1988). Neoplasms of the central nervous system: an immunodeficiency syndrome. In R. M. Rosenblum, & D. E. Bredesen (Eds.), *AIDS and the nervous system.* New York: Raven Press.

Stein, R. C. (1995). Hodgkin's disease and malignant lymphomas. In R. T. Skeel, & N. A. Lachant (Eds.), *Handbook of cancer chemotherapy.*

Stewart, D. J., Russell, N., Dennery, M., Richard, M., Atack, E., & Eapen, L. (1984). Cyclophosphamide, adriamycin, vincristine and dexamethasone in the treatment of bulk central nervous system lymphoma (Abstract). *Journal of Neuro-Oncology, 2,* 289.

Strauchen, S. A., Dalton, J., & Friedman, A.H. (1989). Chemotherapy in the management of intraocular lymphoma. *Cancer, 63,* 1918-1921.

Taylor, C.R., Russell, R., Lukes , R. J., & Davis, R. I. (1978). An immunohistological study of immunoglobulin content of primary central nervous system lymphomas. *Cancer, 41,* 2197-2205.

Thibodeau, G. A., & Patton K. T. (1996). *Anatomy & physiology* (3rd ed.). St. Louis: Mosby.

Wegmann, J. A. (1993). Central nervous system cancers. In S. Groenwald, M. H. Frogge, M. Goodman, & C. H. Yarbro (Eds.), *Cancer nursing: Principles and practice* (3rd ed.). Boston: Jones & Bartlett.

Welch, K., Finkbeiner, W., Alpers, C. E., Blumenfeld, W., Davis, R.L., Smuckler, E.A., & Beckstead, J. H. (1984). Autopsy findings in the acquired immunodeficiency syndrome. *Journal of the American Medical Association 252,* 1152-1159.

Whitcup, S.M., deSmet, M.D., Rubin, B. I., Palestine, A. G., Martin, D. F., Burnier, M, Jr., Can, C. C., & Nussenblatt, R. B. (1993). Intraocular lymphoma clinical and histopathologic diagnosis. *Ophthalmology, 100,* 1399-1406.

Zimmerman, H.M. (1975). Malignant lymphomas of the nervous system. *Acta Neuropathologica (Berlin) Suppl VI,* 69-74.

Glioblastoma

Mary P. Lovely, RN, PhD

EPIDEMIOLOGY

Malignant gliomas account for 2.5% of cancer deaths annually in the United States. Astrocytomas form the largest group among the primary gliomas (i.e., 75% to 90%) (Bruner, 1994). Other types of gliomas include oligodendrogliomas, ependymomas, and mixed gliomas. The most malignant type of glioma is glioblastoma multiforme, which may arise from any of the various types of glioma. Glioblastoma multiforme accounts for more than 50% of all malignant gliomas (Bruner, 1994; Central Brain Tumor Registry of the United States (CBTRUS), 1996).

Glioblastomas are found more often in men than in women. The average age for a patient with a glioblastoma is between 65 and 75 years (CBTRUS, 1996). Twenty years ago, the average age at time of diagnosis of a glioblastoma was within the fifth decade (Schoenberg, Christine, & Whisnant, 1976). Whites are more commonly diagnosed with glioblastoma than people of any other race.

Survival rates for patients with a glioblastoma are age dependent. However, the average length of life after diagnosis is about 10 months (Berens, Rutka, & Rosenblum, 1990). Five years after diagnosis, patients less than 21 years old have a 21% chance of survival, whereas patients older than 44 have a 2% chance of survival. Patients older than 65 years have a less than 1% chance of survival. (CBTRUS, 1996). Survival rates have increased for younger patients, but not for older patients.

RISK FACTORS

The main risk factors associated with the development of glioblastoma are increasing age, gender, and ethnicity. Other possible risk factors include occupational exposure and previous radiation therapy. The evidence supporting each of these risk factors is reviewed in the next section of this chapter (Box 25-1).

Age

Age is an important risk factor in the development of glioblastoma. Approximately two thirds of patients with a glioblastoma are diagnosed at age 65 and older (CBTRUS, 1996). The next largest age group to develop glioblastomas are patients between 55 and 64 years of age. One reason for increased number of diagnoses of glioblastoma at a late age may be that older people have imaging studies more often than younger people; thus more cases are found. Glioblastomas are seen in children, and the occurrence in this group has increased in the last decade (DeVesa et al., 1995).

Gender and Ethnicity

Glioblastoma occurs more frequently in males than in females (i.e., male/female ratio = 1.6:1) (CBTRUS, 1996). There is no apparent reason for the gender difference in occurrence rates. During the last decade, the incidence of malignant brain tumors has increased in white males (12.9%) and in white females (16.3%) (DeVesa, Blot, Stone, Miller, Tarone, & Fraumeni, 1995). Glioblastoma is diagnosed twice as often in whites as in African Americans (CBTRUS, 1996).

Occupational Exposure

Research indicates that occupational exposure to vinyl chloride increases the incidence of glioblastoma. Workers exposed to vinyl chloride, a substance found in rubber factories, developed a greater number of brain tumors, mostly glioblastomas, than the general population (Moss, 1985). The average time from exposure to vinyl chloride to the time of diagnosis was 21 years (Waxweiler et al., 1976).

The relationship between exposure to petrochemicals in large petroleum plants and the development of glioblastoma has been explored (Moss, 1985). There is a consistently elevated relative risk (1.0 to 2.9) for the development of brain cancer in this group of workers (Moss, 1985).

A question has arisen about whether exposure to pesticides, herbicides, and fertilizers increases the risk for glioblastoma. A large cohort study of Canadian farmers (156,242 farmers) revealed a statistically significant association between the risk of dying of glioblastomas and increased fuel/oil expenditures ($P = 0.03$, relative risk 2.11) (Morrison, Semenciw, Morison, Magwood, & Mao, 1992). Low income was associated with reduced risk of brain cancer mortality. The number of acres sprayed with herbicides did not show a relationship with an increased risk for brain cancer.

Prior Exposure to Therapeutic Radiation

One risk factor associated with the development of glioblastoma is previous radiation therapy for another disorder (Hodges, Smith, Garrett, & Tate, 1992). In a review of 100 patients, 17 had received previous radiation therapy. Four of the 17 patients fit established criteria for the development of glioblastoma. These criteria are as follows: (1) the tumor must arise in a previously irradiated field, (2) the tumor must differ histologically from the previous tumor, (3) the latency must be long enough that symptoms do not result from the original lesion, and (4) the neoplastic growth facilitating conditions such as neurofibromatosis are eliminated. Two of the patients had radiation for prolactinomas, one for pinealoma, and one for squamous cell cancer of the ethmoid sinus.

Electromagnetic Fields

Exposure to electromagnetic fields has been thought to lead to the development of brain tumors. Numerous studies have evaluated the effects of electromagnetic fields in residential areas and in specific occupations (Heath, 1996). The studies that evaluated a person's risk for developing a brain tumor if the individual lived in a residential area around power lines and electrical transformers remain inconclusive. One study showed a relative risk for developing a glioblastoma of 1.5 for people in jobs that are associated with possible exposure to electromagnetic fields (Tornquist, Knave, Ahlbom, & Persson, 1991).

In summary, the main risks associated with the development of a glioblastoma are older age, male gender, and white race. Except for the working around polyvinyl chloride, other occupations carry a low risk for developing glioblastomas. Although most risks are not preventable, there must be awareness that patients who present with neurologic signs and symptoms and risk factors related to glioblastoma must be thoroughly assessed for glioblastoma.

CHEMOPREVENTION

Although a large body of knowledge exists about the chromosomal changes associated with glioblastomas, there are no chemoprevention strategies to prevent their initiation or promotion.

Box 25-1
Risk Factors for Glioblastoma

- Age
- Ethnicity
- Gender
- Previous therapeutic radiation
- Occupation exposure:
  Vinyl chloride exposure
  Petrochemical exposure
  Electromagnetic fields (?)

PATHOPHYSIOLOGY

Normal Anatomy and Physiology

The brain is divided into the supratentorial and infratentorial areas. The supratentorial area contains the frontal lobe (responsible for higher mental functions, primary motor ability), the temporal lobe (responsible for speech, memory, hearing), the parietal lobe (responsible for primary sensory functions, visual spatial recognition, and association with other lobes), and the occipital lobe (responsible for primary vision functions) (Fig. 25-1). More centrally located in the supratentorial area is the basal ganglia (controls some motor coordination) and the thalamus (a large area that is a network of nerve fibers that connects the supratentorial area to the infratentorial area).

The infratentorial area of the brain includes the brain stem (responsible for control of vital functions such as respiratory and cardiac functions, and nerve fibers that carry impulses from the spinal cord to the brain.) The cerebellum (responsible for motor coordination) is also located in the infratentorial area.

In adults, glioblastoma occurs predominantly in the supratentorial areas of the brain. The frontal lobe is the most common site for the development of glioblastoma, followed by the temporal, parietal, and occipital lobes. Glioblastomas are rarely found in the ventricular area. Glioblastomas in children usually occur in the infratentorial area, namely, in the brain stem and cerebellum.

Common Forms of Gliomas

The most common forms of gliomas in adults are glioblastoma, astrocytoma, oligodendroglioma, and ependymoma (McKeran & Thomas, 1980). The astrocytoma originates from the astrocyte, a stellate cell that surrounds and

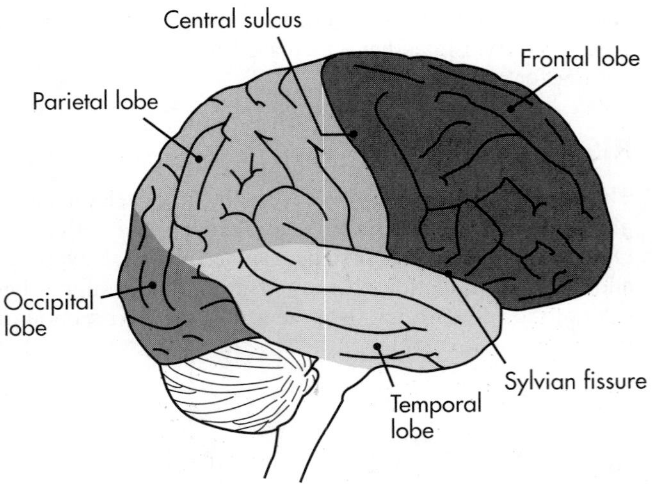

Fig. 25-1 The lobes of the supratentorial area of the brain.

supports neurons and blood vessels. The ependymoma develops from ependymal cells that line the ventricles of the brain and the central spinal cord. The oligodendroglioma derives from the oligodendrocyte, the cell that provides the myelin sheath in the cerebrum. The glioblastoma, a highly malignant and anaplastic tumor, represents more than 50% of all malignant gliomas. This tumor is an undifferentiated, invasive, aggressive neoplastic mass that can arise from any of the different types of gliomas. However, most glioblastomas are thought to develop from astrocytomas (Bruner, 1994).

The Process of Carcinogenesis

Changes in five specific chromosomes (i.e., 7, 22, 17, 10, and 9) have been seen in patients with gliomas. Chromosomes 7 and 22 are overrepresented in malignant gliomas (Kurpad, Wikstrand, & Bigner, 1994). The oncogenic, or abnormal growth, factor that is associated with chromosome 7 is epidermal growth factor.

Another chromosomal abnormality associated with glioblastomas is the loss of tumor suppressor genes. Tumor suppressor genes are located on different chromosomes, and deletion of these genes is associated with the progression of malignant gliomas. The most common deletion is the loss of the short arm of chromosome 17, which is found in astrocytomas and glioblastomas (Shapiro, Shapiro, & Walker, 1995). The loss of chromosome 9 appears to be an intermediate step in the development of a malignant astrocytoma (Shapiro et al., 1995). In glioblastoma, the most common defect is the loss of genetic material in chromosome 10. The deletions in chromosome 10 may permit the cells to evolve to a more malignant state (Kurpad et al., 1994).

Aberrations in the levels of cytokines and the number of growth factor receptors also occur in astrocytes. Transforming growth factor is seen throughout the astrocytoma and glioblastoma. Epidermal growth factor is secreted in large amounts during the development of a glioblastoma. In addition, epidermal growth factor receptors enlarge and are able to interact with epidermal growth factor as well as transforming growth factor. Activation of these cytokines and their receptors may play an important role in the process of tumor initiation (Shapiro et al., 1995).

In summary, both chromosomal abnormalities and cytokine and cytokine receptor abnormalities have been identified in patients with various types of gliomas. Further research is continuing to focus on how these abnormalities are involved in the initiation and promotion of malignant gliomas.

Pathophysiology of Increased Intracranial Pressure

A tumor growing in one part of the brain compresses and destroys brain tissue. Two pathophysiologic processes occur as a brain tumor develops. The first process involves an edema reaction in tissues surrounding the tumor, and the second process involves the distortion and displacement of brain tissue produced by mechanical forces (Zulch, 1986). Both of these processes can produce clinically significant signs and symptoms.

Extracellular, or vasogenic, edema is the initial reaction in the tissue surrounding the tumor (Adams & Victor, 1989; Zulch, 1986). Extracellular edema is a localized process that occurs as a result of increased permeability in capillary endothelial cells. Plasma enters the extracellular space, and the excess fluid begins to cause a compressive effect on the outflow of the surrounding veins. The edema begins to create a mass effect.

Localized compression resulting from edema and the tumor mass causes a distortion in the equilibrium of the three major elements in the cranial cavity: the brain, the cerebrospinal fluid (CSF), and blood. If an increase in one element occurs, a decrease in one or both of the other elements must occur to maintain a normal intracranial pressure of 5 to 15 mm Hg (Hickey, 1997). Fig. 25-2 illustrates the results of brain compression due to a tumor.

Clinical symptoms that may occur when intracranial pressure increases include headache, focal or generalized seizures, or decreases in motor, sensory, speech, or memory functions depending on the particular part of the brain that is affected (Zulch, 1986).

To accommodate a localized increase in mass in the brain, in this case by a brain tumor, initially CSF shifts into the ventricular system followed by displacement of arteries and veins. When the CSF can no longer shift, the brain begins to shift from one compartment into another. The direction of displacement is determined by the partitioning of the intracranial cavity, the attachments at the base, and the stresses and strains on fiber tracts. Frontal masses will shift the brain posteriorly, medially, or laterally. Parietal masses

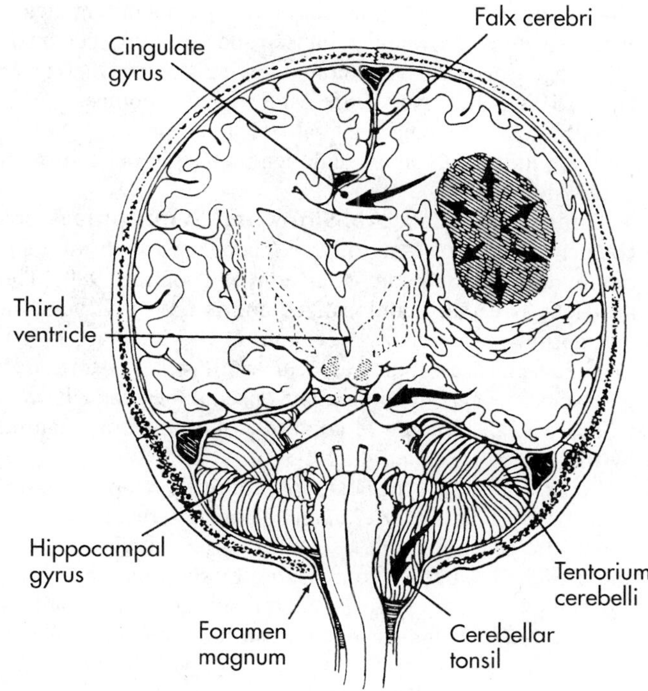

Fig. 25-2 Results of brain compression due to a tumor.

shift the brain toward the base of the skull, where there are large cisterns. Temporal masses shift the brain medially or laterally or toward the posterior fossa. Occipital masses shift the brain anteriorly into the parietal, frontal, and temporal lobes.

The shifting of brain substance from one area to another is known as *brain herniation.* The most clinically significant types of herniation are temporal lobe–tentorial and cerebellar–foramen magnum herniation. Temporal lobe-tentorial herniation occurs when the medial portion of the temporal lobe is displaced into the tentorial opening. The herniation is usually caused by a unilateral supratentorial lesion and results in pressure on the midbrain, thalamus, and vessels surrounding these structures. Cerebellar–foramen magnum herniation occurs when the inferior mesial cerebellum is forced through the foramen magnum. This type of herniation may be due to a cerebellar lesion or massive pressure from a supratentorial lesion. Unilateral or bilateral herniation may result.

Symptoms associated with transtentorial herniation include mydriasis and a sluggish pupillary response followed by a nonreactive pupil. Symptoms associated with cerebellar herniation include arching of the neck and back, respiratory disturbances, change in pulse rate, loss of consciousness, areflexia, cardiac arrhythmias, electrical shocks, and paresthesias (Zulch, 1986).

With either type of herniation, if the intracranial pressure continues to rise, the reticular formation and cranial nuclei or nerves controlling vital functions in the brain stem will be affected. Ultimately, herniation will lead to coma and respiratory arrest.

Signs and Symptoms of Glioblastoma

The most common signs and symptoms associated with glioblastomas are generalized in nature, including headaches, seizures, drowsiness, nausea and vomiting, personality changes, and/or psychomotor slowing (Levin, Sheline, & Gutin, 1993; Salcman, 1985; McKeran & Thomas, 1980). Box 25-2 lists the major generalized signs and symptoms as well as the focal signs and symptoms associated with glioblastomas.

Generalized Cerebral Signs and Symptoms Associated with Glioblastoma. Headache is the most commonly reported symptom (McKeran & Thomas, 1980). The headache is usually nonlocalized and is typically worse in the morning (Thomas & McKeran, 1990; Salcman, 1985). The headache is attributed to local swelling and distortion of pain-sensitive nerve endings. The onset of the headache correlates with the amount of compression in the brain caused by the tumor (Levin et al., 1993).

Seizure activity is the next most common symptom (Salcman, 1985). In the McKeran and Thomas series (1980), almost 40% of patients had seizures as an initial symptom, and 55% had experienced a seizure by the time of diagnosis. Half the seizures were generalized and manifested by tonic-clonic movements. In contrast, the remaining 50% of seizures were focal, reflecting the areas in the brain that were affected by the pressure of the tumor.

Focal Cerebral Signs and Symptoms Associated with Glioblastomas. Focal symptoms are related to the function of the specific brain structures that are affected by the tumor. The most common functional symptoms associated with glioblastomas in relationship to the anatomic location of the tumor are summarized in Box 25-2.

Frontal lobe symptoms vary markedly from patient to patient depending on the area, extent, and side of the frontal lobe involved (Levin et al., 1993). Personality changes may include marked mood elevation or loss of initiative. Other signs of frontal lobe disorders may include contralateral hemiplegia, dysphasia, and slowing of movements. Seizures may be manifested by contralateral motor movement of the face and limbs or by generalized tonic-clonic movements. Left frontal lobe syndromes cause a right hemiparesis, as well as nonfluent dysphasia with or without apraxia of the lips, tongue, or hands. Right frontal lobe syndromes include left hemiplegia, slight mood elevation, difficulty in adapting to new situations, loss of initiative, and occasionally primitive grasp and sucking reflexes.

Bifrontal glioblastoma disease involving the corpus callosum can occur with infiltrative glioblastomas (Levin et al., 1993; Thomas & McKeran, 1990). This syndrome causes a severe impairment of intellect, mood lability, and dementia associated with incontinence and prominent primitive grasping.

Box 25-2
Signs and Symptoms of Glioblastoma

Generalized Signs and Symptoms

Headache
Seizures

Focal Signs and Symptoms

Frontal lobe
- Personality changes
- Slowing movements

Temporal lobe
- Aggressive or irritable behavior
- Auditory hallucinations
- Memory disorders
- Impaired perception of verbal commands
- Spatial disorientation

Parietal lobe
- Decrease in sensory perception
- Receptive dysphasia
- Impairment in right-left discrimination
- Impairment in visual-spatial orientation

Occipital lobe
- Contralateral disturbances
- Cranial nerve palsies

Brain stem
- Gait disturbances
- Cranial nerve palsies

Cerebellum
- Headache and vomiting
- Gait ataxia
- Diplopia

Temporal lobe tumors, such as frontal lobe tumors, can produce subliminal to severe signs and symptoms (Levin et al., 1993). Superior quadrantanopia, auditory hallucinations, and even aggressive behavioral changes can occur. Medial temporal lobe tumors can lead to memory disorders and a more irritable personality. Seizures are relatively frequent in tumors affecting the temporal lobe (Thomas & McKeran, 1990). These seizures are manifested by gustatory hallucinations, feelings of fear or pleasure, and repetitive psychomotor movements. Tumors in the dominant temporal lobe can lead to inability to name objects and impaired perception of verbal commands. Nondominant lobe tumors can result in minor perceptual problems and spatial disorientation.

Parietal lobe syndromes affect sensory, perceptual, and speech functions. Glioblastomas in the sensory cortex of either parietal lobe can produce a decrease in perception of cortical stimuli such as a decrease in light touch, pressure, and two-point discrimination (Levin et al., 1993). Tumors in the dominant parietal lobe may cause a receptive dysphasia, whereas tumors in the nondominant parietal lobe cause impairment of right-left discrimination and visual-spacial orientation of the body (Thomas & McKeran, 1990). Seizures are a common feature, with sensory symptoms manifested by paresthesias of a limb or the face (Thomas & McKeran, 1990).

Occipital lobe glioblastomas are rare (Schoenberg et al., 1976). These tumors, if unilateral, can cause contralateral homonymous hemianopsia. Bilateral tumors can cause cortical blindness.

Third ventricle glioblastomas occur in the thalamus or the basal ganglia. The most common symptoms associated with these glioblastomas are contralateral motor and sensory changes (Thomas & McKeran, 1990). As the tumor progresses, the symptoms of increased intracranial pressure occur due to obstruction of the third ventricle. When the hypothalamus is affected, changes in growth, appetite, and temperature regulation may arise.

Brain stem glioblastomas are usually considered tumors of childhood, although these glioblastomas do occur in adults (Bruner, 1994). The symptoms are related to damage to the long tracts and to the cranial nerves. Gait disturbance is the most commonly seen problem, followed by inversion of the eyes (i.e., sixth nerve palsy) (O'Brien & Johnson, 1985). Symptoms of increased intracranial pressure are unusual, yet headaches may be reported (Thomas & McKeran, 1990). Long tract signs such as hemiparesis and hyperreflexia have been observed. In addition to the inversion of the eyes, cranial nerve dysfunction may cause motor or sensory changes and diplopia. Multiple symptoms often occur with brain stem glioblastomas because of the close proximity of various structures within the brain stem (Thomas & McKeran, 1990).

Cerebellar glioblastomas commonly manifest with an onset of headache and vomiting. Later signs include gait ataxia on the same side as the tumor and diplopia. In addition, head tilt and personality changes may occur (McLone, 1985).

McKeran and Thomas (1980) noted that tumor signs and symptoms can take a gradual, stepwise, or rapid decline. They evaluated 615 patients with gliomas and found that individuals with grade I (well-differentiated cells) to grade III (intermediate anaplastic changes) gliomas most commonly experienced a gradual decline in neurologic function. Grade II (intermediate anaplastic) to grade IV (glioblastoma) glioma patients commonly showed a stepwise progression, whereas 85% of the cases of rapid deterioration took place in patients with grades III and IV tumors. In all but one of the 615 cases, the tumor signs and symptoms were progressive.

The most common signs and symptoms of glioblastoma are headache and seizures. The headache is usually related to increased intracranial pressure caused by the mass and surrounding edema. Other signs and symptoms such as motor and sensory changes, speech disorders, and cranial nerve palsies are related to the anatomic site where the tumor is located and the extent of the mass.

ROUTES OF METASTASES

Most glioblastomas recur within 2 cm of the previous margins of the primary tumor site (Bruner, 1994). Glioblastomas are considered a regional disease because the tumor cells can migrate along nerve fibers, and a tumor can recur in another part of the central nervous system.

There is a 1% incidence of extraneural spread in glioblastoma (Kaplan, 1993). Extraneural spread can be to the bone (Chestnut, Abitbol, Chamberlain, & Marshall, 1993; LoRusso, Tapazogloa, Zarbo, Cullis, Austin, & Al-Sarral, 1988) or kidneys (Ruiz, Cotorruclo, Tudela, Ulate, Val-Bernal, & DeFrancisco et al., 1993).

ASSESSMENT

Assessment of a patient for a glioblastoma is summarized in Table 25-1. Clinical evaluation of the patient involves a detailed history, thorough physical examination, and diagnostic tests. The signs and symptoms may be generalized as a result of increased intracranial pressure, or focal, depending on the size and location of the tumor.

History

The patient should be identified for possible risk factors for glioblastoma. In addition, a careful history of neurologic status should be obtained from the patient and close family members if possible because the patient may have some mental compromise and be unaware of the progression of events. The patient may not be aware that subtle neurologic changes have been taking place. The generalized problems the patient may have encountered are seizures or headaches. Focal signs and symptoms may include personality changes, inability to think clearly, weakness in extremities, or changes in sensory patterns such as eyesight or feeling (Box 25-2). Usually these symptoms have been progressing over time.

Rarely, a patient with a glioblastoma may present in a state of somnolence or coma. In this event, a history from a family member or close friend will aid the nurse or doctor in understanding the previous events that led to the coma.

TABLE 25-1 Assessment of the Patient for Glioblastoma

	Assessment Parameters	Typical Abnormal Findings
History		
	A. Personal and social history 1. Age 2. Gender 3. Ethnicity	A. Personal and social history 1. Usually over 55 years old 2. More prevalent in men than women 3. More prevalent in whites than African Americans
	B. Evaluation of the central nervous system	B. Common signs and symptoms include seizures, headache, or changes in mental status such as personality, judgement, language, or ability to do calculations. Motor weakness or sensory changes in cranial nerves, upper or lower extremities. Signs and symptoms usually progress over time.
Physical Examination	A. Neurologic examination	A. On mental status testing: unusual affect, difficulty with understanding or expressing words, or difficulty with calculations. Asymmetrical motor weakness or sensory changes. Reflexes may show increased response. Some cases present with no neurologic signs or symptoms. Bradycardia, hypertension, or respiratory changes occur if brain stem is compromised. In cases of extreme compromise, the patient may be quite somnolent or comatose.
	B. Ophthalmoscopic examination	B. Papilledema
Diagnostic Tests		
	A. Magnetic resonance imaging (MRI)	A. MRI after gadolinium administration, will show a heterogenous mass
	B. Computed tomography (CT) scan	B. CT scan after intravenous contrast enhancement may show a hyperdense region, frequently ring-like, around a central lucent area.

Physical Examination

A neurologic examination provides information about the neurologic functioning of the patient. This examination involves an evaluation of the patient's mental status, cranial nerve function, motor and sensory function, and reflexes.

The mental status examination includes an evaluation of level of consciousness, attention, language, memory, calculations, and judgment. The cranial nerve examination includes testing the sensory and motor components of each cranial nerve (i.e., olfactory, optic, oculomotor, trochlear, trigeminal, abducens, facial, acoustic, glossopharyngeal and vagus nerves, the spinal accessory nerves, and the hypoglossal nerves). The functions of the cranial nerves are summarized in Table 25-2. The motor and sensory examination proceeds from the upper limbs to the neck and trunk, and then to the lower extremities. The symmetry of responses of each side of the body is compared for motor ability and sensation. Gait, coordination, and reflexes are evaluated. Abnormalities in any of these tests provide an indication of the presence and location of a tumor (Hickey, 1997).

Diagnostic Tests

Two most commonly used tests for the evaluation of glioblastoma are computed tomography (CT) and magnetic resonance imaging (MRI). These tests have revolutionized the diagnosis of brain disorders.

Computed Tomography. The CT scan provides a scan through radiation that has been digitized. The numbers are based on the density of the structure (Hickey, 1997). Bone, for example, is more dense than CSF. The CT scan is usually indicated if the patient is somnolent or in a coma, to evaluate the difference between a head injury or a stroke from a brain tumor.

CT is done initially without contrast medium to evaluate for changes in the status of blood in the brain (i.e., hemorrhage). The patient is usually skin tested to determine sensitivity to the contrast medium. If no reaction occurs, the patient is injected with the contrast medium, and another set of scans is obtained. The outline of a tumor is better visualized with a contrast medium.

Management of a patient during a CT scan includes en-

TABLE 25-2 Cranial Nerve Functions

Nerve	Function
I. Olfactory	Smell
II. Optic	Visual acuity, visual fields; examination of the fundi
III. Oculomotor	Pupillary reflex, external ocular muscles inducing upward, downward and medial movements; involvement will cause ptosis, dilation of pupils
IV. Trochlear	Ocular movements; involvement will cause inability to look downward and laterally; nystagmus
V. Trigeminal	Sensory function: corneal reflex, skin of face and forehead, mucosa of nose and mouth; motor function: maxillary "jaw" reflex
VI. Abducens	Ocular movements; involvement will cause inability to look downward and laterally, nystagmus
VII. Facial	Motor function of upper and lower face; involvement will cause asymmetry of face and paresis; sensory function is tested by taste
VIII. Acoustic	Cochlear nerve test: hearing, lateralization, air and bone conduction; involvement will cause tinnitus, decreased hearing, or deafness
IX. Glossopharyngeal X. Vagus	Motor function: pharyngeal gag reflex, swallowing; vocal cord assessment: speak clearly without any hoarseness
XI. Spinal accessory	Strength of trapezius and sternocleidomastoid muscle; involvement will cause inability to elevate shoulder
XII. Hypoglossal	Motor function of tongue; involvement will cause lateral deviation, atrophy, tremor, inability to extend or move tongue from side to side

From Tucker, S. M., Canobbio, M. M., Paquette, E. V., & Wells, M. F. (1996). *Patient care standards: Collaborative practice planning guides*. St. Louis: Mosby.

suring the patient has no metal clips in the hair. The patient should be told the machine produces a clacking sound. Patients need to be told to hold still for the procedure or the image will be blurred. See Table 25-3, which describes how to prepare a patient for a CT scan.

Magnetic Resonance Imaging. The MRI scanner uses magnetic fields and radiofrequency pulses to produce an image. Nuclei in the brain have a spin that generates a magnetic field. The magnet in the MRI scanner realigns these nuclei. A radiofrequency pulse is given that causes the hydrogen nuclei or protons to realign to the previous position. At the time of realignment, an image is taken (Arbour, 1993). The MRI scanner provides more detailed cross sections of living tissue and gives sharper anatomic information than the CT scan (Arbour, 1993).

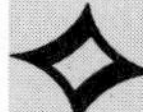

TABLE 25-3 Patient Preparation for Computerized Tomogram

Description of the Procedure: Computed tomography (CT) creates digital radiologic pictures that distinguish different densities in the brain.

Patient Preparation: If there is potential for feeling claustrophobic during the test, the patient may be given a sedative such as diazepam or lorazepam to take 1 hour before the procedure.

Procedural Considerations:

1. Obtain informed consent.
2. Patient does not need to disrobe.
3. Remove any metal hair clips or objects from hair.
4. Patient's skin is tested for reaction to iodine-based contrast medium.
5. Patient should be made aware of the clacking sound made by the machine during the test.
6. Patient must feel comfortable that although the staff are not in the room they will be available if needed.
7. Patient is monitored during and after the contrast medium injection for increased respirations and increased heart rate.

During the procedure, the patient is instructed to hold still because the images may become obscured with movement. An MRI scan will be taken initially without contrast. Another MRI scan will be taken after the patient has received a gadolinium-based contrast medium for better identification of a brain tumor.

Preparation of a patient who will have an MRI scan includes assessment for any metal objects in the patient's head such as hairpins, shrapnel in the eye, or metal aneurysm clips. The magnetic force of the MRI scan is so strong that the metal objects may be pulled out of the tissue. The metal may also obstruct the image by causing a glare. If the patient has any metal objects implanted in the head, these should be carefully evaluated before the MRI scan begins. See Table 25-4 for instructions on how to prepare a patient for a MRI scan.

STAGING

The glioblastoma is the most malignant stage of a glioma. Because most glioblastomas evolve from astrocytes, the grading system for astrocytomas is commonly used to determine the severity of a glioblastoma.

The most commonly used grading systems are usually four tiered, with the lowest grade (grade I) associated with

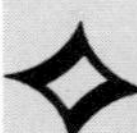

TABLE 25-4 Patient Preparation for Magnetic Resonance Imaging

Description of the Procedure: Magnetic resonance imaging (MRI) creates pictures of the brain using magnetic fields.

Patient Preparation: Patient may be given a sedative such as diazepam or lorazepam before the test to decrease feelings of claustrophobia.

Procedural Considerations:

1. Obtain informed consent.
2. Ask patient about any metal objects in the brain, scalp, or face such as metal aneurysm clips, shrapnel, or metal in eye or face from welding or other type of occupation since the magnetic force will try and pull out reactive metal.
3. Patient does not need to disrobe from the waist down.

the longest survival and the highest grade (grade IV, or glioblastoma) associated with the shortest survival period (Daumas-Duport, Scheithauer, O'Fallon, & Kelly, 1988). Grade I tumors contain well-differentiated astrocytes but with some changes in cytoplasmic processes (Bruner, 1994). Grade II tumors are considered moderately anaplastic, showing increased cellularity, microcytes, and nuclear and cellular pleomorphism. Grade III tumors are considered malignant astrocytomas, with even more diffuse cellular changes. Grade IV tumors (i.e., glioblastomas) contain undifferentiated cells and have the distinguishing characteristic of coagulative tumor necrosis (Bruner, 1994).

Some astrocytes progress through grades of malignancy with transformation from a low-grade tumor to anaplastic astrocytoma, to glioblastoma. Some glioblastomas seem to arise rapidly in otherwise healthy patients and are diagnosed at a small size. It is thought that this variety of glioblastoma may arise from malignant transformations of astrocytes and never pass through the lower grades of malignancy (Leibel, Scott, & Loeffler, 1994).

MEDICAL MANAGEMENT

Surgery

Surgery is the primary treatment modality because tumor bulk must be removed to reduce neurologic damage (Berger, 1994). The goals of glioblastoma surgery are to establish the diagnosis, remove as much of the tumor as possible, treat the signs and symptoms of cranial compression, and provide time to permit other therapy to work (Berger, 1994). When open craniotomy is not feasible, stereotaxic biopsies are done to obtain a definitive tissue diagnosis to guide further therapy (Levin et al., 1993).

Complications from surgery in the first 24 postoperative hours include anesthetic complications (0.2%), postoperative hemorrhage (<5%), wound infection (<2%), and increased neurologic deficit (<10%) (Mahaley, Mettlin, Machimuther, Laws, & Peace, 1990).

Before surgery the patient is placed on dexamethasone, a steroid that is used to decrease edema. The patient remains on this drug throughout surgery and may continue taking it throughout radiation therapy. If little or no edema is present and the patient has no neurologic symptoms, the patient is tapered off the dexamethasone over a period of a few weeks.

An antiepileptic drug, most commonly phenytoin, is prescribed before surgery to prevent seizure activity during and after surgery. The antiepileptic drug may be discontinued after surgery or may be continued if the patient has had seizures or is at high risk for seizures.

Radiation Therapy

In most cases of glioblastoma, the standard treatment involves surgical resection followed by radiation therapy (Leibel et al., 1994). Radiation therapy in conjunction with surgery has produced longer survival periods than surgery alone (Voets, Keyser, Lenders, & Meijer, 1987). Yet the ability to deliver curative doses of radiation to brain tumors is limited because the dose is dependent on the tolerance of normal brain tissue (Leibel & Sheline, 1990).

External Beam Radiation Therapy. Partial brain irradiation is considered the standard treatment for malignant gliomas. Most radiation is now done to include the tumor and the 3 cm margin of tissue surrounding the perimeter of the contrast-enhancing lesion on CT or MRI (Leibel et al., 1994). This treatment regimen is based on the observation that most glioblastomas are unifocal at the time of diagnosis. After initial treatment, most tumors recur within 1 to 2 cm of their original location (Gaspar, Fisher, MacDonald, LeBer, Halperin, & Schold, et al., 1992).

The standard dose, taking into consideration the risks of normal brain tissue, is a total of 60 Gy, with daily fractions of 1.7 to 2.0 Gy, for 5 consecutive days over 6 to 7 weeks (Leibel et al., 1994). It is expected that 25% of patients with glioblastoma will have a significant radiologic response, meaning that there will be a decrease in the size of the tumor area as seen on MRI or CT scan (Gaspa, Fisher, MacDonald, LeBer, Halperin, & Schold, et al., 1993).

Hyperfractionation is another dosing regimen that is used in the management of glioblastomas. This regimen is patterned so that the radiation is given in two daily fractions of about 1.2 Gy per fraction. The total amount of radiation given is 72.0 Gy over 4 weeks (Leibel et al., 1994). Smaller fractions of radiation at each treatment period should allow for less damage to normal tissue. A recent study ($N = 712$) compared standard external beam radiation followed by a chemotherapeutic agent (i.e., carmustine) to hyperfractionation followed by carmustine and found no survival benefit with hyperfractionation (Curran, Scott, Yung, Scarantino, Urtasun, & Movsas, et al., 1996). In fact, the standard treatment group had a slightly better survival rate in glioblastoma patients younger than 50 years of age (15.7 months for standard therapy vs 12.2 months for hyperfractionation). Hyperfraction is used when a shorter overall radiation time would seem more expedient (e.g., a patient with a larger tumor who is developing neurologic symptoms), because hyperfractionation takes 4 weeks and standard therapy takes 6 or 7 weeks to deliver. Hyperfractionation is used commonly in patients with brain stem gliomas because of the ability to give smaller doses in a confined area.

Radioenhancing drugs may be used to increase oxygen to tumor cells and provide a better opportunity for the radiation to kill the tumor cells. The most commonly used radioenhancing drug is hydroxyurea, an oral agent with few side effects. Hydroxyurea is started a few days before radiation therapy begins and is continued throughout the radiation treatments.

Neuropathologic Reactions to Radiation Therapy. Injury to the brain from radiation therapy falls into three categories: acute reactions, early delayed reactions, and late delayed reactions (Leibel et al., 1994; Rutten, 1991). Acute reactions occur during the course of therapy and are usually related to increased intracranial pressure causing intensification of preexisting neurologic signs and symptoms in addition to headaches, nausea, and vomiting (Rutten, 1991). Acute reactions are probably due to edema, as tumor cells exhibit an inflammatory response to radiation therapy (Sheline, 1986). Signs and symptoms associated with acute reactions decrease following steroid administration (Kramer, Hendrickson, Zelen, & Schotz, 1977. However, in one study (Kramer et al., 1977) patients who did not receive steroids for their acute symptoms improved to the same degree as patients who did receive them during a 4-week period. These data suggest that acute reactions to radiation therapy decrease with time, but that steroid therapy, if given early, may reduce the intensity and duration of the signs and symptoms associated with the acute reaction.

Early delayed reactions may develop a few weeks to a few months after radiation therapy. Patients experience a degree of somnolence and exacerbation of preexisting neurologic symptoms. Boldrey and Sheline (1966) described eight patients who developed signs and symptoms of malaise, increased seizures, paralysis, and increased symptoms related to the location of the tumor 1 week to 4 months after radiation therapy. These signs and symptoms resolved spontaneously approximately 6 weeks after they appeared. Hoffman, Levin, & Wilson (1979) reported on a series of patients who received radiation and chemotherapy; 49% (25 of 51) of the patients exhibited signs and symptoms of tumor progression such as weakness, increased number of seizures, and speech disorders within 18 weeks. However, 28% (7 of 25) of the patients with symptoms of progression improved spontaneously, suggesting that the signs and symptoms were the result of early delayed effects of radiation therapy.

Fatigue has been described in patients 6 weeks after radiation therapy (Faithfull, 1991). The patients described feeling exhausted and had difficulty initiating activity. Some patients described increased weakness and a return of their original symptoms about 3 weeks after radiation. The duration of the symptoms lasted about 11 days.

The timing of early delayed reactions are related to myelin turnover time and may be due to the occurrence of transient demyelination (Sheline, 1986). The effects of the transient demyelination should subside within 4 months after the completion of radiation therapy.

Late delayed reactions may develop several months to several years after radiation therapy. The level of responses to late reactions may vary from totally asymptomatic to a loss of function without changes in the patient's CT scan or MRI scan. On the other hand, tissue necrosis may be seen on CT or MRI scan. The late delayed reaction may be manifested as a secondary neoplasia (Leibel & Sheline, 1990).

Radiation necrosis is the outstanding pathologic feature of late delayed reactions. The necrotic lesion consists of a mass or area of discolored parenchyma of rubbery consistency that resembles a glial tumor. Microscopically, the tissues are characterized by hemorrhagic necrosis of the white matter, thrombosis of small vessels, endothelial proliferation of capillaries, and focal chronic inflammation (Rutten, 1991). Radiation necrosis is irreversible and potentially fatal. The prognosis may be favorable if the radiation necrosis is located in a single hemisphere and can be surgically removed.

Interstitial Brachytherapy. Interstitial brachytherapy is radiation therapy directly implanted in the periphery of the tumor bed to provide a very large dose of radiation to a specific area without damage to the surrounding brain tissue. Interstitial brachytherapy is considered adjuvant therapy because only a few patients with glioblastomas are eligible. Patients eligible for brachytherapy include those with a Karnofsky Performance Status (KPS) of at least 70 (i.e., able to care for themselves but unable to carry on normal activity or do active work) and those who have a unifocal, well-circumscribed, supratentorial tumor less than 5 or 6 cm in diameter (Sneed, Larson, & Gutin, 1994). Radiation seeds of iodine (^{125}I) are placed into the tumor bed through stereotaxic surgery (i.e., drilling a hole in the skull and placing the seeds through thin catheters into the tumor bed) and guided by the dimensions of the tumor seen on the CT or MRI scan. The radiation seeds remain in the patient's head for 5 to 7 days. During this time, the patient remains in the hospital. Because this radiation is done through stereotactic methods, radiation treatment for difficult to reach tumors through normal surgical procedures is possible.

Results of studies of patients with glioblastoma who have received conventional radiation therapy followed by interstitial brachytherapy are promising (Leibel et al., 1994). An improvement in survival of approximately 12 months has been observed in patients with glioblastoma when external beam radiation was combined with a boost of interstitial brachytherapy to cumulative doses of 11 to 120 Gy compared with patients who would have been eligible for implantation (Prados, Gutin, Phillips, Wara, Sneed, & Larson et al., 1992; Scharfen, Sneed, Wara, Larson, Phillips, & Prados et al., 1992). In addition, patients 18 to 29 years old had a 78% 3-year survival rate with the combination treatment (Sneed et al., 1995). Older patients with the same treatment had a 10% or less 3-year survival rate (Sneed et al., 1995).

Complications after interstitial brachytherapy are rare, but include increased neurologic impairment, infection, possible brain hemorrhage, and pulmonary embolus (Scharfen et al., 1992). As a result of the large amount of radiation given, radiation necrosis may develop about 6 months after the implant. Most patients require this surgery or neurologic symptoms develop that appear as a tumor recurrence.

Radiosurgery. Radiosurgery is another form of stereotactic radiation therapy used to augment the radiation dose for selected patients with glioblastoma. This radiation treatment includes a series of beams that, coordinated through a stereotactic coordinate system, intersect on a single intracranial target. This technique can deliver a high dose of radiation in a single session without damaging surrounding healthy tissue. This type of radiation is usually limited to lesions of 4 cm or less (Leibel et al., 1994).

Results of studies using external beam radiation therapy followed by a single dose of radiation through radiosurgery showed that the median survival of glioblastoma patients was 19.5 months (Flickinger, Loeffler, & Larson, 1994). One third of the patients required surgery approximately 6 months after radiosurgery for a mass due to radiation necrosis.

The advantage of radiosurgery over interstitial brachytherapy is that the patient does not undergo surgery. There is no invasion of the skin, so the patient is not susceptible to infection or hemorrhage at a wound site. The patient stays in the hospital only 1 day or overnight. In addition, the radiation exposure of personnel is reduced (Flickinger et al., 1994).

Chemotherapy

Chemotherapy as a treatment for glioblastoma has not been very successful, because most chemotherapeutic agents are unable to pass the blood-brain barrier. Whether to treat patients with chemotherapy remains controversial because the regimen may last about 6 months and the patient may have untoward side effects. Quality of life issues arise when the patient gains only a few months of survival in exchange for feeling ill during the course of chemotherapy. A common treatment pattern for the patient with glioblastoma is as follows: At the time of diagnosis, the patient undergoes surgery and radiation therapy; at recurrence, the patient is given chemotherapy. Chemotherapy may be given as adjuvant therapy after radiation to patients whose tumor is quickly progressing (Levin et al., 1993).

Three chemotherapeutic agents that have shown some effectiveness in the treatment of glioblastomas are carmustine (BCNU), procarbazine, and carboplatin (Levin et al., 1993). Carmustine and procarbazine have been used since the 1970s. Carboplatin is a newer drug that is being used to treat brain tumors. Carmustine remains the most effective drug for decreasing or stabilizing tumor growth in patients with glioblastomas (Levin et al., 1993). New drugs, such as interferon and phenylalanine drugs, are being evaluated in the management of glioblastomas. Combinations of drugs are also being tested.

Gene Therapy

Some studies have attempted to alter the genetic makeup of the tumor and to decrease its invasiveness by injecting the tumor with a virus. This type of therapy appears to be promising in animal models. Only a few patients have been entered into these trials, and there is insufficient data to determine whether gene therapy is beneficial to humans (Maskal, 1996).

ONCOLOGIC EMERGENCIES

Increased Intracranial Pressure

The main oncologic emergency related to glioblastoma is increased intracranial pressure resulting from edema, increased tumor growth, or the development of radiation necrosis from interstitial brachytherapy or radiosurgery. Increased intracranial pressure may cause an emergency situation because of somnolence, coma, or a change in respiratory rate or heart rate resulting from pressure on the brain stem.

First-line medical management of increased intracranial pressure includes intravenous administration of dexamethasone, a steroid that decreases edema in the brain. In addition, the patient may receive a bolus of mannitol, an osmotic diuretic, and/or an injection of furosemide to decrease swelling in the brain. An MRI or CT scan is done to identify the cause of the increased intracranial pressure. If there is a mass, further surgical debulking may be done if feasible.

Nursing care of the patient with life-threatening increased intracranial pressure includes vigilant monitoring of the patient's neurologic status and vital signs. The patient's intake is carefully monitored to prevent increased fluid in the brain. The patient's output is monitored to prevent fluid and electrolyte imbalances because of the strong diuretic effects of mannitol.

NURSING MANAGEMENT

Surgery

Preoperative teaching of the patient includes the need for the patient to understand the possible complications of surgery (e.g., changes in neurologic status, postoperative pain, and possible infection at the operative site). Analgesic medications are ordered for the patient directly after surgery and should be given as needed. The patients should be made aware that there will be a large head dressing that will stay in place for a few days. Fluid may accumulate in the subgaleal space around the face, which will decrease within 1 week. Optimally, a family caregiver should be included in the preoperative teaching session, because the patient may have difficulty remembering the information.

After surgery, the patient must be monitored continuously for changes in neurologic status. In addition to obtaining the patient's temperature, pulse, and blood pressure measurements, the nurse needs to evaluate the patient's level of consciousness and the size and equality of the patient's pupils. The patient is evaluated for movement of all extremities and checked to see whether strength is equal on both sides. A neurologic flow sheet is often used to document the vital signs during the first 24 to 48 hours postoperatively. Most patients do well after surgery. However, a wound infection is not uncommon, so monitoring the temperature and inspecting the site for drainage are important.

In addition, intake and output must be monitored, especially when surgery was performed near the hypothalamus or pituitary gland. Decreased production of antidiuretic hormone may result in a large urine output. The patient may need to be given antidiuretic hormone and have the hormone regulated for a period of time. In addition, the patient may require large amounts of diuretics, such as mannitol or furosemide, during surgery to manage brain swelling. Therefore, monitoring and management of intake and output in these patients are extremely important.

The patient may experience postoperative pain. Patients are usually given morphine for the first 72 hours after surgery, followed by oxycodone with acetaminophen or acetaminophen. If extreme pain continues, the patient is followed closely to manage pain and to decide whether the pain is indicative of infection or some other complication.

The patient's head dressing usually remains intact for 72 hours. The nurse needs to inspect the dressing for bleeding, CSF leakage, or other drainage from the wound. Any kind of drainage should be reported immediately. After 72 hours, the dressing is removed and the patient wears a stockinette cap for the next week to keep the head covered.

Patients are usually able to leave the hospital within 5 days after surgery. Patients may experience some difficulty with memory abilities and difficulty in processing new information (Armstrong, Ruffer, Corn, DeVries, & Mollman, 1995), so they need to be accompanied by an adult at this time.

To prevent cerebral edema, the patient is placed on dexamethasone, a steroid that specifically decreases edema in the brain. The patient is usually placed on a dose of 4 mg, 4 times per day. Side effects that the patient may experience include headaches, personality changes, and insomnia. If the patient does not have symptoms of edema, the dexamethasone is tapered to half the dose for 1 week and then the dose is decreased by half again. Some patients have difficulty with mood changes, headache, and insomnia during the tapering period. If this occurs, the dose of dexamethasone is increased and a taper initiated later. Dexamethasone can cause gastric distress. An antacid should be taken at the same time the steroid is administered.

Most patients with glioblastoma are placed on antiepileptic drugs before surgery and remain on the drug for approximately 6 months. The most common antiepileptic drug used is phenytoin. Phenytoin blood levels are monitored every 2 weeks when starting the drug to ensure that the patient's drug level is in the therapeutic range. Nurses must be alert for toxic side effects of phenytoin such as ataxia, nystagmus, and slurred speech (Table 25-5).

Care of the Patient Before and During Radiation Therapy

External beam radiation therapy occurs in three phases. The first phase is the simulation phase. A mask of the patient's face is made for consistent placement of the beam during treatments. While the mask is being made, the patient must be able to remain calm and still. The nurse needs to evaluate the patient's level of anxiety and to use pharmacologic or nonpharmacologic strategies to help the patient manage increased levels of anxiety.

The second phase of radiation therapy is the actual treatments. Most patients are given one or two treatments per day. A common side effect associated with external beam radiation is fatigue (King, Nail, Kreamer, Strohl, & Johnson, 1985). As the treatment progresses, patients become more fatigued. Measures to counteract fatigue include daily naps, limited daily exercise, and going to bed at the same time every night. As patients begin to understand the feelings of fatigue, they will begin to cut back on activities as the fatigue increases. Another side effect of radiation therapy is skin desquamation that leads to burning and itching at the external beam site. Several actions can be taken to alleviate the burning and itching such as lotions and compresses (Table 25-6).

The third phase of radiation therapy is the time after therapy. Patients may remain fatigued, develop seizures, or have an exacerbation of symptoms. The patients should be warned about the potential for fatigue to persist. If seizures or exacerbated symptoms develop, the patient or caregiver should immediately contact a health care provider. The patient may require an increase in dexamethasone because an inflammatory reaction may develop, causing edema in the brain. The patient's tumor may have increased in size, and the patient may require additional therapy.

Care of the Patient Receiving Chemotherapy

Nursing care of the patient undergoing chemotherapy requires knowledge of the drugs' toxicities including how to monitor and manage them. Table 25-7 lists the three chemotherapy drugs commonly used to manage glioblastoma, the side effects of these drugs, and specific nursing interventions. Patients require anticipatory counseling with regard to the toxicities so that they may be prepared in case these side effects occur.

HOME CARE ISSUES

Home care issues arise as the patient's disease progresses and the neurologic status deteriorates. Most of the problems relate to increased dependency.

Changes in Neurologic Status

The most common problem for the glioblastoma patient is impairment of mental status and an inability to make appropriate judgments (Armstrong et al., 1995). In addition, the patient may suffer changes in mobility, vision, and sensation. The patient needs rehabilitative services that may optimize the individual's ability to maintain independence at home (e.g., occupational therapist, physical therapist, visual impairment specialist, cognitive rehabilitation specialist).

Altered Role Performance

Because of the numerous mental and physical changes that occur, the patient may not be able to perform normal family activities and participate in normal social roles and functions. The changes usually require the patient to alter responsibilities at home and at work. Patients and family

TABLE 25-5 Standard of Care for the Patient Undergoing Surgery for a Glioblastoma

Patient Problem and Outcomes	Nursing Interventions and Rationales	Patient Education Instructions
Anxiety Patient will: • Verbalize an understanding of the surgical procedure • Express feelings of decreased anxiety • Identify strategies to cope with anxiety	1. Assess patient's level of understanding of the surgical procedure. 2. Give patient the opportunity to ask questions or verbalize concerns. 3. Determine which coping strategies the patient has used effectively in the past to decrease anxiety and reinforce the use of effective coping strategies.	1. Utilize diagram of the anatomy of the brain to explain the procedure. 2. Provide patient and family with information about the preoperative routine: a. Diagnostic tests b. Anesthesiology consult c. NPO after midnight 3. Teach the patient coughing and deep breathing exercises and obtain a return demonstration. 4. Provide patient with information about the postoperative plan of care: a. Monitoring neurologic vital signs b. Pain management c. Surgical incision care d. Intravenous hydration
Increased Intracranial Pressure Patient will be carefully monitored if changes in intracranial pressure occur	1. Assess baseline neurologic status before surgery. 2. Monitor vital signs and perform neurologic checks every 5 to 15 minutes, until stable. 3. Administer dexamethasone, if required. 4. Elevate head of bed 30 degrees for patients with supratentorial surgery.	1. Teach patient to inform the nurse immediately if a headache or motor or sensory changes occurs. 2. Teach patient about side effects of dexamethasone: headaches and insomnia.
Infection Patient will be free from infection	1. Monitor temperature. 2. Inspect head dressing for drainage. 3. Monitor patient for headache at the incision site.	1. Teach patient to inform the nurse of any wetness around dressing. 2. Teach patient to inform nurse if headache occurs around the incision site.
Pain Patient will not have pain after surgery	1. Assess the patient for pain using a 0 (no pain) to 10 (intolerable pain) scale. 2. Administer opioids for pain around the clock for the first 24 to 48 hours postoperatively. 3. Determine how pain is relieved through positioning. 4. Inform physician if pain persists because further surgical intervention may be required.	1. Teach patient to inform nurse if experiencing pain. 2. Teach patient the importance of taking pain medication on a regular basis to keep pain under control.
Fluid and Electrolyte Imbalance (Especially Hyponatremia) Patient will maintain an appropriate fluids and electrolyte balance	1. Monitor fluid and electrolytes for 72 hours after surgery. 2. Monitor changes in mental status that may be indicative of hyponatremia. 3. Restrict fluids until serum sodium levels return to normal.	1. Teach patient about the need to decrease fluid intake. 2. Inform the patient to drink only fluids that are specifically allocated. 3. Inform patient to measure urine output.
Seizures Patient will be seizure-free	1. Administer antiepileptic medication at prescribed intervals. 2. Maintain proper blood levels of antiepileptic medication. 3. Place patient on schedule for regular antiepileptic drug levels. 4. Assess for side effects or toxicity of antiepileptic drugs.	1. Teach patient to take antiepileptic medication as prescribed. 2. Teach patient side effects and toxicity of antiepileptic medication: • Ataxia • Nystagmus • Double vision • Skin rash

TABLE 25-6 Standard of Care for the Patient Receiving External Beam Radiation for Glioblastoma

Patient Problem and Outcomes	Nursing Interventions and Rationales	Patient Education Instructions
Knowledge Deficit Patient will verbalize an understanding of the purpose, benefits, and risks of radiation therapy	1. Assess patient's knowledge level about radiation therapy. 2. Assess patient's concerns and fears about radiation therapy.	1. Describe the routine procedures involved in radiation therapy: a. Consultation b. Simulation procedure c. Treatment procedures and routines 2. Describe the major side effects associated with radiation therapy, the importance of notifying the nurse should side effects occur, and self-care measures to manage side effects: a. Change in neurologic status b. Fatigue c. Skin redness
Fatigue Patient will be able to maintain normal activities throughout radiation therapy	1. Assess patient's present level of fatigue using a 0 (not at all tired, full of pep) to 10 (total exhaustion) rating scale. 2. Evaluate patient's sleep and activity pattern to teach patient ways to conserve energy.	1. Inform patient of the likelihood of fatigue toward the end of treatment and several weeks following treatment. 2. Teach patient energy conservation strategies: a. Take short naps during day b. Exercise in small amounts during the day c. Listen to body for cues that indicate a need to slow down
Change in Neurologic Status Patient or family caregiver will verbalize to nurse or doctor any neurologic changes seen in the patient during or following radiation therapy	1. Assess patient's present neurologic status. 2. Evaluate patient throughout the course of radiation therapy for changes that may occur due to edema or further tumor growth.	1. Teach the patient or family caregiver to call the doctor or nurse if the patient experiences changes in mental status or any other neurologic changes.
Skin Desquamation Patient will verbalize to nurse or doctor the skin friability at the radiation site	1. Assess the patient's skin around the area where external radiation will be given. 2. Check skin at entry site of the radiation beam and exit site for signs of irritation or injury.	1. Inform the patient that skin redness at the site may occur. 2. Bathe area with lukewarm water. 3. Do not use heat lamps or electric blankets around the area. 4. Do not use any lotions without instructions. 5. For itching, use a cool compress 3-4 times per day to itching site. 6. For dryness, use lanolin, eucerin, aquaphor, or natural care lotion. All care should be withheld within 2 hours of actual treatment. 7. For burning, cool compresses 3-4 times per day for 10 minutes. Apply refrigerated aloe vera gel (80%-90%) to irritated area 2-3 times per day. 8. If skin becomes moist, sticky, painful, or blistered, notify the nurse, doctor, or technician so that special skin care measures can be started.

Table 25-7 Commonly Used Chemotherapeutic Agents in Glioblastoma

Drug	Toxicities	Nursing Interventions
Carmustine (BCNU) Most commonly used chemotherapeutic agent Given intravenously Alkalating agent that inhibits a number of key enzymatic reactions involved in DNA synthesis	Burning sensation in the extremity	Explain to patient there may be a burning sensation.
	Nausea and vomiting 2 hours after the intravenous dose	Administer antiemetics before administration.
	Leukopenia and thrombocytopenia 3 to 5 weeks after administration Nadir white blood cell count recession occurs at 3 to 4 weeks	Obtain baseline bloodwork and followup bloodwork 3 weeks after initiation of drug.
	Rare toxic effects: • Liver and renal dysfunction (elevated blood serum gluatmic-oxalocetic transaminase, alkaline phosphatase, and bilirubin). Elevated blood urea nitrogen is common in about 10% of the patients with no harmful effects.	
	• Pulmonary fibrosis with long-term therapy	Obtain periodic chest x-ray if drug given over a long term.
Carboplatin Given intravenously Exact mechanism unknown: DNA is the predominant intracellular target	Nausea and vomiting that lasts less than 24 hours	Administer antiemetic.
	Bone marrow suppression; platelet nadir is 3 weeks and restored in 5 to 6 weeks	Obtain baseline bloodwork and monitor every 3 weeks and before cycle.
	Nephrotoxicity, elevated blood urea nitrogen Rare toxicities: alopecia, mucositis, skin rash, flu-like symptoms, hematuria, alterations in taste	Monitor possible side effects.
Procarbazine Given orally Exact mechanism of action unknown	Myelosuppression and thrombocytopenia at about 4 weeks	Obtain baseline bloodwork and followup bloodwork every 4 weeks and at beginning of cycle.
	Gastrointestinal toxicities: nausea, vomiting, diarrhea Tolerance to these symptoms develops in a few days. Flu-like symptoms: fever, chills, sweating Dermatologic reactions: alopecia, pruritus	Monitor gastric distress and flu-like symptoms.
	Central nervous system toxicities: paresthesias, neuropathy, dizziness, ataxia, headache, nightmares, depression, insomnia, nervousness, hallucinations. May limit ability to take this drug due to these effects.	Counsel patient about these side effects before treatment begins.
	Ophthalmic reactions: diplopia, nystagmus, papilledema, photophobia, retinal hemorrhages Rare pulmonary allergic response	Do ophthalmic check every cycle.
	No sperm and no menses with high-dose procarbazine. This effect may not be reversible.	Counsel patient about these side effects before treatment begins.

Modified from Hickey, J. V. (1997). *The clinical practice of neurological and neurosurgical nursing* (4th ed.). Philadelphia: J. B. Lippincott.

caregivers will experience increased stress as these transitions take place. Guidance is usually given to the patient and family to establish strong support systems. More than one person becomes involved with the patient. This approach allows the main caregiver some respite and a chance not to become overwhelmed while caring for the patient.

Resources that focus on enabling patients with glioblastoma to cope with their disease can be found through brain tumor organizations and other national resources. Local support groups, found in most communities, can help patients with glioblastoma and their families to feel less isolated and to learn more about the disease. These organizations provide information about institutions who are doing studies on the management of glioblastoma, the location of support groups, suggestions for rehabilitation resources, and

TABLE 25-8 Prognostic Variable Related to Glioblastoma

Age	Karnofsky Performance Status	Extent of Surgery	Mental Status	Median Survival (months)
<50	>90	>Partial resection	Able to work status	17.9
<50	<90	>Partial resection	Able to work status	11.1
>50	70-100			
>50	<70	>Partial resection or biopsy and radiation	Normal mental status	8.9 months
	70-100			
>50	<70	Biopsy only	Poor mental status	4.6 months
<50	70-100			

Modified from Leibel, S. A., Scott, B. B., & Loeffler, J. S. (1994). Contemporary approaches to the treatment of malignant glioma with radiation therapy. *Seminars in Oncology, 21*(2), 198-212.

BOX 25-3
National Brain Tumor Foundations

American Brain Tumor Association
2720 River Rd., Suite 146
Des Plaines, IL 60018
(847) 827-9910
(847) 827-9918 fax
(800) 886-2282
Brain Tumor Foundation for Children, Inc.
2231 Perimeter Park Drive, Suite 9
Atlanta, GA 30341
(770) 458-5554
(404) 458-5467 fax
Brain Tumor Society
84 Seattle St.
Boston, MA 02184
(617) 783-0340
(617) 730-8449 fax
(800) 770-8287
Children's Brain Tumor Foundation, Inc.
35 Alpine Lane
Chappaqua, NY 10514
(914) 747-0301
National Brain Tumor Foundation
785 Market Street Suite 1600
San Francisco, CA 94103
415 284-0208
(415) 284-0209 fax
(800) 934-2873

a network of other glioblastoma patients who are willing to share experiences (Box 25-3).

Care in the Advanced Stages of Glioblastoma

Patients usually remain stable for months after the diagnosis of glioblastoma. When tumor recurrence occurs, the family or caregivers may be the first to notice changes in neurologic function. An exacerbation of previous neurologic symptoms usually indicates a tumor recurrence. Anticipa-

TABLE 25-9 Quality of Care Evaluation for a Patient Undergoing Resection for Glioblastoma

Disciplines participating in the quality of care evaluation
☐ Nursing ☐ Surgery ☐ Social Work
☐ Physical Therapy

I. Postoperative Management Evaluation
Data from:
☐ Mailed Questionnaire ☐ Patient Interview

Criteria	Yes	No
1. Patient provided with pre-operative information about:		
a. Diagnostic tests	☐	☐
b. Pain management	☐	☐
2. Neurologic status evaluated postoperatively	☐	☐
3. Patient experienced the following complications:		
a. Infection	☐	☐
b. Hemorrhage	☐	☐
c. Further neurologic impairment	☐	☐

II. Patient/Family Satisfaction
Data from:
☐ Patient Interview ☐ Family Interview

Criteria	Yes	No
1. On a scale of 0 to 10, with 0 being totally satisfied, how satisfied were you with the pain management you received? ________		
2. Were you told to call the nurse if you experienced any changes in movement or sensation?	☐	☐
3. Were you told to have a family member or friend help you in the next few weeks in remembering important events?	☐	☐

tory guidance about the possible increase in symptoms and the potential for the occurrence of seizures is important at this time. Patients and families need to watch for symptoms and to contact a health care provider if these symptoms occur. The patient may require medication to decrease edema and may need another tumor resection. Because a decrease in function may occur, the patient will benefit from a visiting nurse service to evaluate new home care needs, such as aids or devices to facilitate living at home.

Patients who have entered the advanced stages of glioblastoma usually have extensive neurologic dysfunction and may become somnolent and comatose. This condition usually lasts a short time (Sachsenheimer, Piotrowski, & Bimmler, 1992). Hospice has become the standard of care for these patients and families. Hospice provides assistance with pain relief, symptom management, and overall care required by the patient and family caregivers.

PROGNOSIS

As previously stated, glioblastoma is a life-threatening disease with a median survival of about 8.8 months (Daumas-Duport et al., 1988). The factors that play a major role in length of survival are age, functional and neurologic status, and extent of surgery (Curran, Scott, Horton, Nelson, Weinstein, & Fischbach et al., 1993). In a series of 1578 patients, those less than 50 years of age with a KPS of 90 to 100 had a median survival of 17.9 months. Patients less than 50 years of age with a KPS of less than 90 had a median survival of 11.1 months. Patients 50 years of age or older, with a partial resection and a KPS of 70 to 100 had a median survival of 8.9 months. In contrast, older patients with a KPS of 70 to 100 and a biopsy had only a 4.6-month median survival. Refer to Table 25-8 for a summary of the median survival statistics for patients with glioblastoma.

Another study (Sachsenheimer et al., 1992) followed patients with high-grade tumors and noted that in most patients, their KPS usually remained stable for 7 to 9 months after diagnosis, then rapidly declined. The decline in KPS was associated with tumor recurrence.

EVALUATION OF THE QUALITY OF CARE

Accreditation organizations require evaluation of quality of care provided to patients. Care for glioblastoma patients is provided by a multidisciplinary team that includes nurses, physicians, rehabilitation staff, and social workers. Tables 25-9 and 25-10 provide evaluation tools that can be used in inpatient or outpatient settings.

TABLE 25-10 Quality of Care Evaluation for a Patient Receiving Radiation Therapy for Glioblastoma

Disciplines participating in the quality of care evaluation:
☐ Nursing ☐ Medicine ☐ Social Services
Data from:
☐ Medical Record ☐ Patient/Family Interview

Criteria	Yes	No
1. Did the doctor or nurse explain to you that you might experience some of these side effects from radiation?		
a. Fatigue	☐	☐
b. Redness of the skin at radiation site	☐	☐
2. Were you taught how to manage fatigue during and after radiation therapy?	☐	☐
3. Were you taught to report any new or changing neurologic symptoms to your doctor or nurse?	☐	☐

RESEARCH ISSUES

Gene therapy appears to be one of the most promising areas in glioblastoma research. This research focuses on increasing our understanding of the changes that occur in the cell during the process of neoplastic transformation. The research is focusing on interventions to stop the process of malignant transformation by interrupting the cellular growth processes that take place in the tumor cell.

New chemotherapeutic agents that will decrease tumor size or stabilize tumor growth need to be evaluated. The key factor to overcome when using chemotherapy is the inability of these agents to cross the blood-brain barrier.

Finally, there is very little information regarding how to manage symptoms associated with glioblastoma, particularly fatigue. Additional research needs to focus on the patterns of fatigue in this patient population and optimal strategies to manage fatigue.

REFERENCES

Adams, J., & Victor, P. (1989). *Principles of neurology.* New York: McGraw-Hill.

Arbour, R. B. (1993). Stereotactic localization and resection of intracranial tumors. *Journal of Neuroscience Nursing, 25*(1), 14-21.

Armstrong, C., Ruffer, J., Corn, B., DeVries, K., & Mollman, J. (1995). Biphasic patterns of memory deficits following moderate-dose partial-brain irradiation: Neuropsychologic outcome and proposed mechanisms. *Journal of Clinical Oncology, 12*(9), 2263-2271.

Berens, M. E., Rutka, J. T., & Rosenblum, M. L. (1990). Brain tumor epidemiology, growth and invasion. *Neurosurgery Clinics of North America, 1*(1), 1-18.

Berger, M. (1994). Malignant astrocytomas: Surgical aspects. *Seminars in Oncology. 21,* 172-185.

Boldrey E., & Sheline, G. E. (1966). Delayed transitory clinical manifestations after radiation treatment of intracranial tumors. *Acta Radiologica (Therapy, Biology, Physics), 5,* 5-10.

Bruner, J. M. (1994). Neuropathology of malignant gliomas. *Seminars in Oncology, 21*(2), 126-138.

Central Brain Tumor Registry of the United States First Annual Report. (1996). Chicago: Central Brain Tumor Registry of the United States Press.

Chestnut, R. M., Abitbol, J. J., Chamberlain, M., & Marshall, L. F. (1993). Vertebral collapse with quadraparesis due to metastatic glioblastoma multiforme: Case report and review of the literature. *Journal of Neuro-Oncology, 16,* 135-140.

Curran, W. J., Scott, C. B., Horton, J., Nelson, J. S., Weinstein, A. S., Fischbach, A. J., Chang, C. H., Rotman, M., Asbell, S. O., Krisch, R. E., & Nelson, D. F. (1993). Recursive partitioning analysis of prognostic factors in three radiation therapy oncology group malignant glioma trials. *Journal of the National Cancer Institute, 85,* 704-710.

Curran, W. J., Scott, C. B., Yung, W. K. A., Scarantino, C., Urtasun, R., Movsas, B., Jones, C., Simpson, J. R., Fischbach, A. J., Petito, C., & Nelson, J. (1996). No survival benefit of hyperfractionated radiotherapy (RT) to 72.0/Gy and carmustine versus standard RT and carmustine for malignant glioma patients: Preliminary results of RTOG 90-06. *Program/Proceedings of the American Society of Clinical Oncology, 15,* 154.

Daumas-Duport, C., Scheithauer, B., O'Fallon, J., & Kelly, P. (1988). Grading of astrocytomas, a simple and reproducible method. *Cancer 62*(10), 2151-2165.

DeVesa, S. S., Blot, W. J., Stone, B. J., Miller, B. A., Tarone, R. E., & Fraumeni, J. F. (1995). Recent cancer trends in the United States. *Journal of the National Cancer Institute, 87,* 175-181.

Faithfull, S. (1991). Patient's experience following cranial radiotherapy: A study of the somnolence syndrome. *Journal of Advanced Nursing 16,* 939-946.

Flickinger, J. C., Loeffler, J. S., & Larson, D. A.. (1994). Stereotactic radiosurgery for intracranial malignancies. *Oncology, 8,* 81-86.

Gaspar, L. E., Fisher, B. J., MacDonald, D. R., LeBer, R. T., Halperin, E. C., Schold, S. C., & Cairncross, J. G. (1993). Malignant glioma—timing of response to radiation therapy. *International Journal of Radiation, Biology, Physics, 25,* 877-879.

Gaspar, L. E., Fisher, B. J., MacDonald, D. R., LeBer, R. T., Halperin, E. C., Schold, S. C., & Cairncross, J. G. (1992). Supratentorial malignant glioma: Patterns of recurrence and implications for external beam local treatment. *International Journal of Radiation Oncology, Biology, Physics, 24,* 55-57.

Heath, C. W. (1996). Electromagnetic field exposure and cancer: A review of epidemiologic evidence. *CA: A Cancer Journal for Clinicians, 65,* 29-44.

Hickey, J. V. (1997). *The clinical practice of neurological and neurosurgical nursing* (4th ed.). Philadelphia: J. B. Lippincott.

Hodges, L. C., Smith, J. L., Garrett, A., & Tate, S. (1992). Prevalence of glioblastoma multiforme in subjects with prior therapeutic radiation. *Journal of Neuroscience Nursing, 24,* 2, 79-83.

Hoffman, W. F., Levin, V. A., & Wilson, C. B. (1979). Evaluation of malignant glioma patients during the postirradiation period. *Journal of Neurosurgery, 50,* 624-628.

Kaplan, R. S., (1993). Supratentorial malignant gliomas: Risk patterns and therapy. *Journal of the National Cancer Institute, 85*(9), 690-691.

King, K. B., Nail, L. M., Kreamer, K., Strohl, R. A., & Johnson, J. E. (1985). Patients' descriptions of the experience of receiving radiation therapy. *Oncology Nursing Forum, 12,* 55-61.

Kramer, S., Hendrickson, F., Zelen, M., & Schotz, W. (1977). Therapeutic trials in the management of metastatic brain tumors by different time/dose fractionation schemes of radiation therapy. *National Cancer Institute Monograph, 46,* 213-221.

Kurpad, S. N., Wikstrand, C. J., & Bigner, D. D. (1994). Immunobiology of malignant astrocytomas. *Seminars in Oncology, 21,* 149-161.

Leibel, S. A., Scott, B. B., & Loeffler, J. S. (1994). Contemporary approaches to the treatment of malignant glioma with radiation therapy. *Seminars in Oncology, 21*(2), 198-212.

Leibel, S. A., & Sheline, G. E. (1990). Radiotherapy in the treatment of cerebral astrocytomas. In D. G. T. Thomas (Ed.), *Neurooncology: primary malignant brain tumors.* Baltimore: Johns Hopkins University Press.

Levin, V. A., Sheline, G. E., & and Gutin, P. H. (1993). Neoplasms of the central nervous system. In V. T. DeVita, Jr., S. Hellmen, & S. Rosenberg (Eds.), *Cancer: Principles and practices of oncology: Vol. 2* (3rd ed.). Philadelphia: J. B. Lippincott Company.

LoRusso, P. M., Tapazogloa, E., Zarbo, R. T., Cullis, P. A., Austin, D., & Al-Sarral, M (1988). Intracranial astrocytoma with diffuse bone marrow metastasis: A case report and review of the literature. *Journal of Neuro-Oncology, 6,* 53-59.

Mahaley, M. S., Mettlin, C., Machimuther, N., Laws, E. R., & Peace, B. B., (1990). Analysis of patterns of care of brain tumor patients in the United States: A study of the brain tumor section of the AANS and the CNS and the commission on cancer of the ACS. *Clinical Neurosurgery, 36,* 347-352.

Maskal, J. R. (1996). New treatments for brain cancer. *Cope, 12,* 4-6.

McKeran R. O., & Thomas, D. G. T. (1980). The clinical study of gliomas. In D. G. T. Thomas & D. I. Graham (Eds.), *Brain tumors.* London: Butterworths.

McLone, D. G. (1985). Cerebellar astrocytomas. In R. H. Wilkins & S. S. Rengachary (Eds.) *Neurosurgery.* New York: McGraw-Hill.

Morrison, H. I., Semenciw, R. M., Morison, D., Magwood, S., & Mao, Y. (1992). Brain cancer and farming in western Canada. *Neuroepidemiology, 11,* 267-276.

Moss, A. R. (1985). Occupational exposure and brain tumors. *Journal of Toxicology, Environment and Health, 16,* 703-711.

O'Brien, M. S., & Johnson, M. M. (1985). Brain stem gliomas. In R. H. Wilkins & S. S. Rengachary (Eds.), *Neurosurgery.* New York: McGraw-Hill.

Prados, M. D., Gutin, P. H., Phillips, T. L., Wara, W. M., Sneed, P. K., Larson, D. A., Lamb, S. A., Ham, B., Malec, M. K., & Wilson, C. B. (1992). Interstitial brachytherapy for newly diagnosed patients with malignant gliomas: The UCSF experience. *International Journal of Radiation Oncology, Biology, Physics, 24,* 593-597.

Ruiz, J. C., Cotorruclo, J. G., Tudela, V., Ulate, P.G., Val-Bernal, M., De Francisco, A. L., Zublmend, J. A., Prieto, M., Canga, E., & Arias, M. (1993). Transmission of glioblastoma multiforma to two kidney transplant recipients from the same donor in the absence of ventricular shunt. *Transplantation, 55*(3), 682-683.

Rutten, E. H. J. M. (1991) Radiation injury to the brain. In A. B. M. F. Karim & E. R. Laws (Eds.), *Glioma.* Berlin, Germany: Springer-Verlag.

Sachsenheimer, W., Piotrowski, W., & Bimmler, T. (1992). Quality of life in patients with intracranial tumors on the basis of Karnofsky's performance status. *Journal of Neuro-Oncology, 13,* 177-181.

Salcman, M. (1985). Supratentorial gliomas: Clinical features and surgery. In R. H. Wilkins & S. S. Rengachary (Eds.), *Neurosurgery.* New York: McGraw-Hill.

Scharfen, C. O., Sneed, P. K., Wara, W. M., Larson, D. A., Phillips, T. L., Prados, M. D., Weaver, K. A., Malec, M., Acord, P., Lamborn, K., Lamb, S. A., Ham, B., & Gutin, P. H. (1992). High activity iodine 125 interstitial implant for gliomas. *International Journal of Radiation Oncology, Biology, Physics, 24,* 583-591.

Schoenberg, B. S., Christine, B. W., & Whisnant, J. P. (1976). The descriptive epidemiology of primary intracranial neoplasms: The Connecticut experience. *American Journal of Epidemiology, 104*(3), 499-510.

Shapiro, W. R., Shapiro, J. R., & Walker, R. W. (1995). Central nervous system. In M. D. Abeloff, J. O. Armitage, A. S. Lichter, J. E. Niederhuber (Eds.), *Clinical oncology.* New York: Churchill-Livingstone.

Sheline, G. E. (1986). Normal tissue tolerance and radiation therapy of gliomas of the adult brain. In N. M. Bleehen (Ed.), *Tumours of the brain.* Berlin: Springer-Verlag.

Sneed, P. K., Larson, D. A., & Gutin, P. H., (1994). Brachytherapy and hyperthermia for malignant astrocytomas. *Seminars in Oncology, 21*(2), 186-197.

Sneed, P. K., Prados, M. D., McDermott, M. W., Larson, D. A., Malec, M. K., Lamborn, K. R., Davis, R. L., Weaver, K. A., Wara, W. M., Phillips, T. L., & Gutin, P. H. (1995). Large effect of age on the survival of patients with glioblastoma treated with radiotherapy and brachytherapy boost. *Neurosurgery, 36,* 898-903.

Thomas, D. G. T., & McKeran, R. O. (1990). Clinical manifestations of brain tumors. In D. G. T. Thomas (Ed.), *Neuro-oncology: Primary malignant brain tumours.* Baltimore: The Johns Hopkins University Press.

Tornquist, S., Knave, B., Ahlbom, A., & Persson, T. (1991). Incidence of leukaemia and brain tumours in some electrical occupations. *British Journal of Medicine, 48,* 597-603.

Voets, A. J., Keyser, A., Lenders, M., & Meijer, E. (1987). High graded astrocytoma: Results of treatment. In M. Chatel & J. Pecker, (Eds.), *Brain oncology.* Dordrecht, Netherlands: Marinus Nijhoff Publishers.

Waxweiler, R. J., Stringer, W., Wagoner, J. K., Jones, J., Falk, H., & Carter, C. (1976). Neoplastic risk among workers exposed to vinyl chloride. *Annals of the New York Academy of Science, 271,* 40-48.

Zulch, K. (1986). *Brain tumors: Their biology and pathology.* New York: Springer-Verlag.

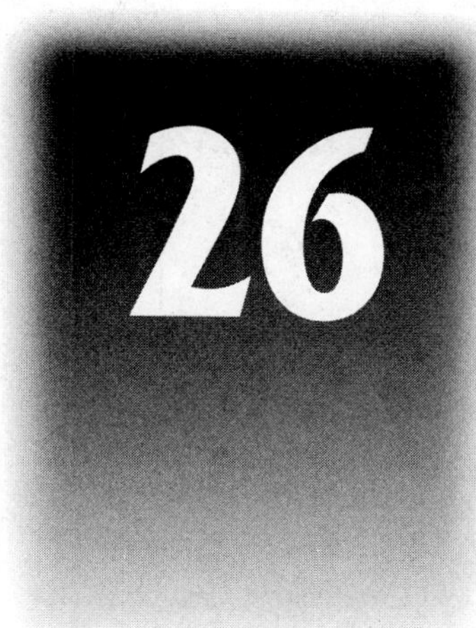

Glioma

Tricia Corbett, MSPH

INTRODUCTION

Central nervous system (CNS) tumors are masses of abnormal cells that grow in the brain or spinal cord. These tumors arise primarily from neuroectodermal and meningeal tissues (Alavi, 1995). Eighty-five percent occur in the cranium, or intracranially, and 15% in the spinal cord (McKee, 1996; Murphy, Morris, & Lange, 1997; Prados & Wilson, 1997).

Brain tumors may be *benign* or *malignant,* but these terms are used in a different context than when applied to most other tumors. Because brain tumors develop within a confined space, even a small, benign tumor can be life-threatening. These terms refer to *slow-growing* and *fast-growing* tumors and are used primarily for histologic grading of brain tumors for treatment purposes. Additional factors such as location must be also used to determine treatment and prognosis.

Brain tumors are either primary, those originating from cells within the brain, or metastatic, those arising from primary cancers elsewhere in the body that spread to the brain. Primary brain tumors arise from a diverse group of phenotypically distinct cells found in the brain. Metastatic tumors are more common than primary tumors of the brain. The most common tumors responsible for metastases to the brain are the lung, breast, colon, kidney, thyroid, and prostate. Metastatic meningeal tumors may arise from leukemias, lymphomas, small cell lung cancer, breast cancer, and some primary brain tumors such as ependymomas and medulloblastomas (ARC/NCI, 1998; Levin, Leibel, & Gutin, 1997). Approximately 35% of cancer victims have metastatic brain disease (Murphy, 1997).

Table 26-1 lists brain and spinal cord tumors by percentage, location, characteristics, and cell of origin. Primary tumors are typically divided into glial tumors, which arise from the cells that support and nourish the nerve cells, and nonglial tumors, which arise from brain cells other than the glial cells. Nonglial tumors include acoustic neuromas, arising in the acoustic nerve; craniopharyngiomas, emerging in structures near the pituitary gland; meningiomas, arising in the meninges; pineal parenchymal tumors, developing in the pineal gland; and primary lymphomas, arising in the lymph tissue of the CNS.

Tumors that originate in astrocytes, ependymocytes, or oligodendrocytes are termed *gliomas.* These tumors are known as *astrocytomas, ependymomas,* and *oligodendrogliomas.* Fig. 26-1 illustrates the most common location of many of these tumors. The fact that mixed glial tumors exist, such as oligoastrocytoma, oligoependymomas, or a combination of all three glial cells, suggests that these cells may originate from common stem or progenitor cells (Levin, Leibel, & Gutin, 1997). Several types and subtypes of glial cells exist, and various tumors can develop in each subtype.

- Astrocytomas are the most common of the glial tumors and are typically found in the cerebrum. The glioblastoma multiforme (GBM) is a fast-growing, highly malignant form of astrocytoma accounting for nearly half of all glial tumors.
- Oligodendrogliomas arise from the cells that provide a protective sheath (myelin) around nerves in the white matter. They are most commonly found in the frontal lobes of the cerebrum, usually in younger adults.
- Ependymomas originate from the cells that line the ventricles of the brain. They are most commonly found in the fourth ventricle and the region of the cauda equina. Ependymomas tend to spread to the spinal cord and meninges.
- Mixed gliomas arise from more than one type of glial cell and are usually oligoastrocytomas but may also be oligoependymomas or a mixture of all three glial cell types.
- Brain stem gliomas develop from glial cells in the brain stem, usually the astrocytes, and are most commonly located in the pons. These tumors are classified

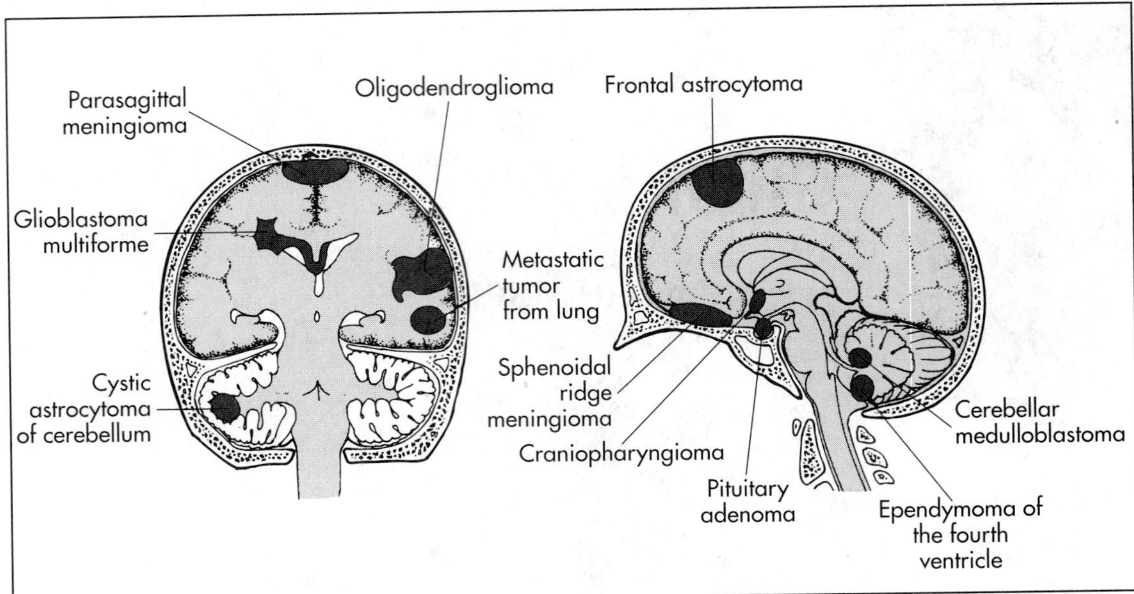

Fig. 26-1 Common sites of intracranial tumors. (From K. L. McCance & S. E. Huether [1994]. *Pathophysiology: The biologic basis for disease in adults and children* [2nd ed.] St. Louis: Mosby.)

TABLE 26-1 Brain and Spinal Cord Tumors

Neoplasm	Percentage of Tumors	Location	Characteristics	Cell of Origin
Gliomas				
Astrocytoma	20	Anywhere in brain or spinal cord	Grades I and II Slow growing, invasive	Supportive tissue, astrocytes, glial cells
Glioblastoma multiforme	30	Common in cerebral hemispheres	Grades III, IV Highly invasive and malignant	Thought to arise from mature astrocytes
Oligodendrocytoma	4	Common in frontal lobes deep in white matter; may arise in brain stem, cerebellum, and spinal cord	Avascular, tends to be encapsulated; more malignant form called *oligodendroblastoma*	Oligodendrites, glial cells
Ependymoma	5	Intramedullary; wall of ventricles; may arise in caudal tail of spinal cord	Common in children, variable growth rates; more malignant, invasive form called *ependymoblastoma;* may extend into ventricle or invade brain tissue	Ependymal cells
Neurilemoma	4	Cranial nerves (most often vestibular division of cranial nerve VIII)	Slow growing	Schwann cells
Neurofibroma		Extramedullary: spinal cord	Slow growing	Neurilemma, Schwann cells
Pituitary Tumors	8	Pituitary gland; may extend to or invade floor of third ventricle	Age linked, several types slow growing, macroadenomas and microadenomas may be secreting or nonsecreting	Pituitary cells, pituitary chromophobes, basophils, eosinophils

From Boss, B. J., Sunderland, P. M., & Heath, J. (1994). Alterations of neurological function. In K. L. McCance & S. E. Huether (Eds.), *Pathophysiology: The biologic basis for disease in adults and children.* St. Louis: Mosby; Murphy, M. E. (1997). Cancers of the brain and central nervous system. In S. E. Otto (Ed.), *Oncology nursing.* (3rd ed.) St. Louis: Mosby.

TABLE 26-1 Brain and Spinal Cord Tumors—cont'd

Neoplasm	Percentage of Tumors	Location	Characteristics	Cell of Origin
Pineal Region Tumors	1	Pineal region; pineal parenchyma, posterior or third ventricle	Several types (e.g., germinoma, pineocytoma, teratoma)	Several types with different cell origin
Blood Vessel Tumors				
Angioma	3	Predominantly in posterior cerebral hemispheres	Slow growing	Arising from congenitally malformed arteriovenous connections
Neuronal Cell Tumors				
Medulloblastoma	1	Posterior cerebellar vermis, roof of fourth ventricle	Well demarcated, rapid growing, fills fourth ventricle	Embryonic cells
Mesodermal Tissue Tumors				
Meningioma	20	Intradural, extramedullary; sylvian fissure region, superior parasagittal surface of frontal and parietal lobes, olfactory groove, wing of sphenoid bone, superior surface of cerebellum, cerebellopontine angle, spinal cord	Slow growing, circumscribed, encapsulated, sharply demarcated from normal tissues, compressive in nature	
Choroid Plexus Tumors				
Papilloma	1	Choroid plexus of ventricular system; lateral ventricle in children, fourth ventricle in adults	Usually benign; slow in expansion, inducing hemorrhage and hydrocephalus; malignant tumor is rare	Epithelial cells
Cranial Nerve and Spinal Nerve Root Tumors				
Hemangioblastoma	2	Arises from blood vessels, predominant in cerebellum	Benign, slow growing	Embryonic vascular tissue
Lymphoma	1	Cerebral hemispheres	Metastasis common	B cells
Metastatic Tumors	35 of all cancer patients	Cerebral cortex diencephalon	Malignant spread	From lung, breast, colon, kidney, thyroid, prostate

separately from cerebral gliomas because their location has a major impact on the clinical course and survival of patients. In addition, involvement of the cranial nerves associated with the brain stem leads to significant neural deficits in most patients. Brain stem gliomas are more commonly found in children than adults.

- Pilocytic astrocytomas develop in the cerebellum and the hypothalamus.
- Medulloblastomas occur in the developing nerve cells of the cerebellum and are most commonly found in children. Although this tumor is not a true glioma, it is often included with the gliomas.

This chapter is concerned primarily with the oligodendrogliomas, ependymomas, mixed gliomas, and adult brain stem gliomas. Although covered elsewhere, astrocytomas are included in this chapter in a cursory manner, since they account for the majority of brain stem gliomas. Astrocytomas are detailed in Chapter 23, glioblastoma multiformes in Chapter 25, medulloblastomas in Chapter 27, and childhood brain tumors in Chapter 70.

EPIDEMIOLOGY

Primary brain cancer accounts for 1% of all cancers and 2.5% of all cancer deaths in the United States annually. It is the second most common cancer (20% of total cases) and the most common solid tumor in children (Boss, Sunderland, & Heath, 1994; Fisher, Linggood, & Recht, 1995; Murphy, Morris, & Lange, 1997). These tumors are responsible for the highest number of cancer deaths in children less than 15 years of age (Mack, 1993; McKee, 1996). Primary brain tumors are the eighth most common cancer in adults (Murphy, Morris, & Lange, 1997).

The incidence rate for primary brain tumors for the U.S. population as a whole is 5:100,000. However the rate for children younger than 15 years of age is 6.5, and the elderly between 65 and 79 years of age have a rate approaching 19:100,000 (Alavi, 1995; McKee, 1996; Werner, Phuphanich, & Lyman, 1995). Peaks in the incidence rates occur between 0 and 4 years of age, 15 and 24 years, and 65 and 75 years. A gradual increase in rates begins at about 50 years of age and continues through the 70s (McKee, 1996; Murphy, Morris, & Lange, 1997). Tumors are more common in men than in women by a 3:2 ratio, except for meningiomas, which affect women more often than men (Mack, 1993). Ethnic differences have not been documented.

During the last decade the incidence of tumors has been rising at an alarming rate. Reported cases increased by nearly 50% from 12,800 in 1984 to 17,900 in 1996 (*Cancer Statistics,* 1997). Although some of these numbers reflect a very real increase in tumor rates of the elderly, primarily malignant gliomas and lymphomas (Werner, Phuphanich, & Lyman, 1995), the vast majority of the numbers are in the immune suppressed population, particularly patients with acquired immune deficiency syndrome (AIDS), who tend to have a high rate of brain lymphomas. Other possible explanations for this increase are an aging population and an improved ability to diagnose brain tumors. However, the rise in the incidence rate of tumors in the elderly is of major concern, and the causes are currently unknown. The American Cancer Society projected a total of 17,600 primary brain cancer diagnoses for 1997.

The location of tumors within the brain varies with age. The frequency of primary tumors by age is listed in Table 26-2. Ninety percent of adult tumors are supratentorial (anterior and middle fossae), most commonly in the cerebral hemispheres. Almost half of these tumors are gliomas; approximately 20% are meningiomas. Seventy percent of all childhood tumors are infratentorial (posterior fossa) and are usually medulloblastomas, ependymomas, or low-grade gliomas. Less than 20% are glioblastoma (Alavi, 1995; McKee, 1996; Chipps, Clanin, & Campbell, 1992). The incidence of CNS tumors after treatment for prior malignancies is very low (Levin, Leibel, & Gutin, 1997).

Oligodendrogliomas constitute about 4% of all CNS tumors, and between 5% and 19% of all gliomas (McKee, 1996). They tend to arise in the frontal lobes of the middle aged, with a peak incidence between ages 35 and 40 years. One third of these tumors are anaplastic (grade III). Progression to the glioblastoma (grade IV) stage is rare. Nearly one half of tumors classified as oligodendroglioma are actually oligoastrocytomas (mixed gliomas) (Boss, Sunderland, & Heath, 1994).

Ependymomas arise in the ventricles and may extend into adjacent brain tissue. They are not encapsulated. Ependymomas account for about 4% of all intracranial tumors. They compose between 5% of all intracranial gliomas in adults and 20% in children and adolescents. The majority (70%) occur in the fourth ventricle. Of those that arise in the

TABLE 26-2 Frequency of Intracranial Tumors as a Function of Age Range

	Patient Age (y)						
Histology	**0-9**	**10-19**	**20-29**	**30-39**	**40-49**	**50-59**	**60-74**
Astrocytoma	60.0	59.0	76.0	81.0	86.0	87.0	91.0
"Low-grade"	9.8	7.1	7.1	4.9	2.5	1.5	1.8
Astrocytoma and anaplastic	46.5	42.6	51.4	54.7	47.8	39.4	39.8
Glioblastoma	1.3	7.4	14.4	18.2	32.9	44.2	51.0
Mixed oligoastrocytoma	2.5	2.7	2.8	3.4	2.2	2.1	0.7
Oligodendroglioma	1.1	4.0	5.0	6.4	6.2	3.6	1.6
Ependymoma*	8.7	2.7	4.3	1.8	0.8	1.3	0.5
Medulloblastoma	21.0	10.0	5.5	2.3	1.0	0.1	0
Embryonal/teratoid†	1.0	1.3	0.3	0.3	0	0	0
Meningioma‡	0.2	0.4	1.2	1.7	1.2	2.0	2.4

From Levin, V. A., Leibel, S. A., & Gutin, P. H. (1997). Neoplasms of the central nervous system. In V. T. DeVita, S. Hellman, & S. A. Rosenberg (Eds.), *Cancer: The principles and practice of oncology.* (5th ed.). Philadelphia: J. B. Lippincott.
*Includes differentiated and anaplastic ependymoma.
†Includes germinoma, mixed embryonal pinealomas, and malignant teratomas.
‡Underestimate since SEER does not include many "benign" tumors in its registry; these are probably malignant meningiomas.
(Data based on unpublished SEER program search 1978-1984)

infratentorium, 40% occur in children younger than 10 years of age. Supratentorial ependymomas are equally distributed by age, but are the most common cerebral tumor in children (Boss, Sunderland, & Heath, 1994).

Brain stem gliomas are typically diffuse, fibrillary astrocytomas most commonly found in children. (Ependymomas related to the ventricular components of the brain stem also may be found.) The majority of these tumors occur in the pons. They tend toward early malignant transformation, and because of their deep location and infiltrating character, prognosis is usually poor.

ETIOLOGIC/RISK FACTORS

The cause of most brain cancers is unknown. However, factors associated with the risk of developing tumors continue to emerge (Box 26-1).

Environmental Factors

Several environmental factors show an association with tumor development (Mack, 1993). (It is important to note that "association" does not imply "causation.")

- Ionizing radiation is thought by some to play a role in inducing meningiomas, nerve sheath tumors (schwannomas), sarcomas, and, less commonly, astrocytomas.
- Concern regarding the role of electromagnetic fields in the development of certain tumors has been raised. However, the vast majority of studies undertaken in this area do not support this contention.
- Animal studies indicate that exposure to N-nitroso compounds, aromatic hydrocarbons, triazenes, and hydrazines increases risk for astrocytomas.

Box 26-1
Possible Risk Factors for Gliomas

Age:
  Children and the Elderly
Sex:
  Males (3:2 ratio)
Ethnicity:
  None documented
Prior Injury:
  None documented
Environmental/occupational exposure:
  X-ray exposure (especially for tinea capitis)
  Ionizing radiation
  Electromagnetic fields (?)
  N-nitroso compounds
  Aromatic hydrocarbons
  Friazenes
  Hydrazines
  Vinyl chloride
Precursor Morbidity:
  Epstein-Barr viral infections
  Compromised immune systems (AIDS, transplants)
Hereditary Conditions:
  von Hippel-Lindau
  Tuberous sclerosis
  Turcot's syndrome
  Neurofibromatosis I & II
  Nevoid basal cell carcinoma syndrome
  Li-Fraumini syndrome
  Osler-Weber-Rendu syndrome

Ethnicity

Risk factors related to ethnicity have not been documented.

Prior Injury

There appears to be no association between prior head trauma and the development of tumors.

Individuals at Risk

The following groups of individuals are at an increased risk of developing primary brain tumors:

- Age—children and the elderly
- Sex—men at a 3:2 ratio except for meningiomas (Mack, 1993; McKee, 1996; Murphy, Morris, & Lange, 1997)
- People exposed to x-rays, particularly those treated for scalp irradiation from tinea capitis, for meningioma (Levin, Leibel, & Gutin, 1997; McKee, 1996; Murphy, Morris, & Lange, 1997);
- People exposed at work to chemicals such as solvents, pesticides, petrochemicals, and rubber (e.g., anatomists, farm workers, and petrochemical workers) (McKee, 1996; Murphy, Morris, & Lange, 1997);
- People exposed to vinyl chloride for gliomas and astrocytomas (Mack, 1993; Murphy, Morris, & Lange, 1997);
- People with the Epstein-Barr virus for brain lymphomas (McKee, 1996; Murphy, Morris, & Lange, 1997);
- People with compromised immune systems, such as individuals with AIDS and transplant recipients, as well as those with CNS lymphoma but not gliomas (Levin, Leibel, & Gutin, 1997; Mack, 1993; McKee, 1996; Murphy, Morris, & Lange, 1997)
- People with certain hereditary conditions (Mack, 1993):
  - von Hippel-Lindau disease is a dominant disorder characterized by cerebellar hemangioblastomas
  - Tuberous sclerosis is a dominantly transmitted disorder associated with giant cell astrocytomas
  - Turcot's syndrome (familial intestinal polyposis) is associated with glioblastoma and medulloblastoma
  - Neurofibromatosis I is a dominantly inherited condition associated with intracranial astrocytomas, schwannomas, neurofibrosarcomas, and neural crest–derived tumors
  - Neurofibromatosis II is a condition of multiple schwannomas associated with ependymomas and meningiomas

- Nevoid basal cell carcinoma syndrome may be associated with medulloblastoma and meningioma
- Li-Fraumini syndrome is a syndrome of familial breast cancer, sarcomas, and primary brain tumors
- Osler-Weber-Rendu syndrome is a hereditary condition that affects the blood vessels, causing a tendency to hemorrhage; this syndrome is associated with angiomas

CHEMOPREVENTION AND SCREENING

Chemoprevention involves the use of drugs and certain foods as a means to prevent development of tumors. To date, nothing has emerged from a growing number of clinical trials as helpful in preventing brain tumors nor are there any other preventive measures of note. No screening tests for brain tumors currently exist.

PATHOPHYSIOLOGY

A good understanding of the structure and functions of the brain is fundamental to the diagnosis, grading, and selection of treatment options for primary brain tumors. The various components of the brain each have specialized functions, which, if interfered with, usually manifest as recognizable symptoms. For instance, a neurologic examination of the 12 cranial nerves, 10 of which originate in the brain stem, can help locate tumors in the infratentorium. The location of a tumor in the brain greatly influences the diagnostic and therapeutic procedures that may be used and thus the survival time of the patient.

Normal Anatomy and Physiology of the Brain

The brain is one of the most complex and least understood organs of the human body. Much is known about individual parts such as the neurons and which sections of the brain are associated with certain mental and bodily functions. However, the way the brain works as a whole, its many components in unison, is not fully understood.

The brain accounts for about 2% of the total body weight of an adult. It demands 20% of the cardiac output, uses 20% of the body's oxygen supply, and requires 400 kcal of energy a day. Its tissue is extremely fragile, and its need for oxygen and glucose via the blood supply is constant and critical. Hypoglycemia can cause damage to the brain cells, and an interruption of blood supply for only a few minutes can result in irreversible damage (Wilson & Hartwig, 1997). Although the brain initially has approximately 1 trillion neuron cells, these cells do not divide to form new cells. Neurons that die cannot be replaced by the brain.

Histology of the Neural Tissue

The brain consists of nerve cell bodies and their nerve fibers (neurons, axons, and dendrites) that evolve from the precursor neural crest cells to primitive nerve cells called *neuroblasts* to differentiated true nerve cells. These cells are enmeshed in a connective tissue unique to the CNS. This tissue is called *neuroglia.* Unlike other connective tissue that arises from the mesoderm, CNS connective tissue has its origins in the ectoderm (Levin, Leibel, & Gutin, 1997).

Neuroglia

Neuroglia are the supporting cells of the CNS. Approximately 10 glial cells exist for every one neuron. The glial cells compose about 40% of the total volume of the brain and spinal cord (Wilson & Hartwig, 1997). Four distinct types of glial cells exist: astroglia, oligodendroglia, ependymal cells, and microglia.

Astroglia are the "caretakers" of the neurons. They play a role in neuronal nutrition and maintenance of the proper bioelectrical environment needed for impulse conduction and synaptic transmission. Their cell bodies are star-shaped (astro) and have multiple processes extending from them, many of which are attached to blood vessels. When neurons die, astrocytes fill in the empty space (Wilson & Hartwig, 1997).

Oligodendroglia surround the neuronal processes (axons and dendrites) and produce a myelin sheath around them. This sheath protects the neurons and increases the rate at which a signal impulse can be transmitted along a neuronal network. Myelinated fibers in the brain are called *white matter.* Schwann cells myelinate the fibers in the spinal cord.

The ependymal cells line the ventricular system and its choroid plexi, which are responsible for producing, maintaining, and circulating the cerebrospinal fluid (CSF).

The microglia are the "janitors" of the brain. Because these cells are of mesodermal embryologic origin, they are not always classified as glial. Microglia enter the CNS through the vascular system and are responsible for disposing of the debris of damaged neural tissue, much like the macrophages elsewhere in the body. They also have a role in fighting infection.

The fragile biochemical environment of the brain is protected in part by two cellular barriers known as the *blood-brain barrier* and the *blood-cerebral spinal fluid barrier.* These barriers prevent harmful and disruptive macromolecular substances, such as proteins, some glucoses, free fatty acids, drugs, and toxins from entering the neural tissue or the CSF. The barriers appear to be formed by the tight junctures between the endothelial cells lining the capillaries (blood-brain), and the cuboidal epithelial cells forming the choroid plexus (blood-CSF). The barriers allow water, oxygen, carbon dioxide, glucose, and essential amino acids to pass freely, but regulate the movement of sodium (NA^+), chlorine (Cl^-), and potassium ions across the membrane (Wilson & Hartwig, 1997). Although these barriers play a very important role in maintaining a healthful environment for the brain, they greatly complicate the effective use of chemotherapy as a means of treating tumors.

Neurons. Neurons are the basic and the most important functional cell of the nervous system. Neurons consist of a cell body and one or more extensions, or processes, termed *nerve fibers.* These include the rather short fibers called *dendrites,* of which there may be many, and/or a single, longer fiber known as an *axon.* Neurons are classified according to the length of their axons. Golgi type I neurons have axons that may extend more than a meter long and are found in the peripheral nervous system. Golgi type II neurons have short axons terminating close to the cell body and are numerous in the brain and spinal column.

Typically, dendrites receive and convey signals to the cell body, and axons convey signals away from the cell body and send them on to adjoining dendrites across the gap, known as a *synapse,* which separates them. Although most synapses are between axons and dendrites, they may also be between axons and cell bodies, between axons, and between dendrites. The ability of the neurons "to receive, convey, and transmit neural messages is a result of the specialized neural cell membrane properties of excitability and electrical-chemical conductibility" (Wilson & Hartwig, 1997).

Neurons are categorized according to their directional flow of information. The three categories are the afferent, or sensory neurons (body to brain); the efferent, or motor neurons (brain to body); and the internuncal, or associative neurons.

Neurons normally communicate between the axon and dendrite synapses. Neurotransmitters, chemicals enzymatically produced in the neurons, are stored at the terminal ends of the axon and released when the "excitability" phase of transmission occurs. These chemicals change the permeability of the membranes, allowing the neurons to transmit the impulse from the axon of one to the dendrites of the other. The impulse is conducted electrically through the neuron, and chemically from the axon to the dendrites. Approximately 30 neurotransmitters are currently known or thought to exist. They include acetylcholine, dopamine, norepinephrine, serotonin, and glycine (Wilson & Hartwig, 1997). Depending on their location, neurons are of varying sizes with varying numbers of dendrites and have fibers anywhere from 1 mm to 1 m long.

Nerves

A nerve is a bundle of neuronal fibers that is found outside of the CNS. Neuronal fibers found inside the CNS are called *fiber tracks.*

Gross Anatomy of the Brain

The brain itself is grossly divided into at least three main regions: the cerebrum, the cerebellum, and the brain stem. The diencephalon, composed of the thalamus and hypothalamus, is sometimes added as a fourth region (Fig. 26-2).

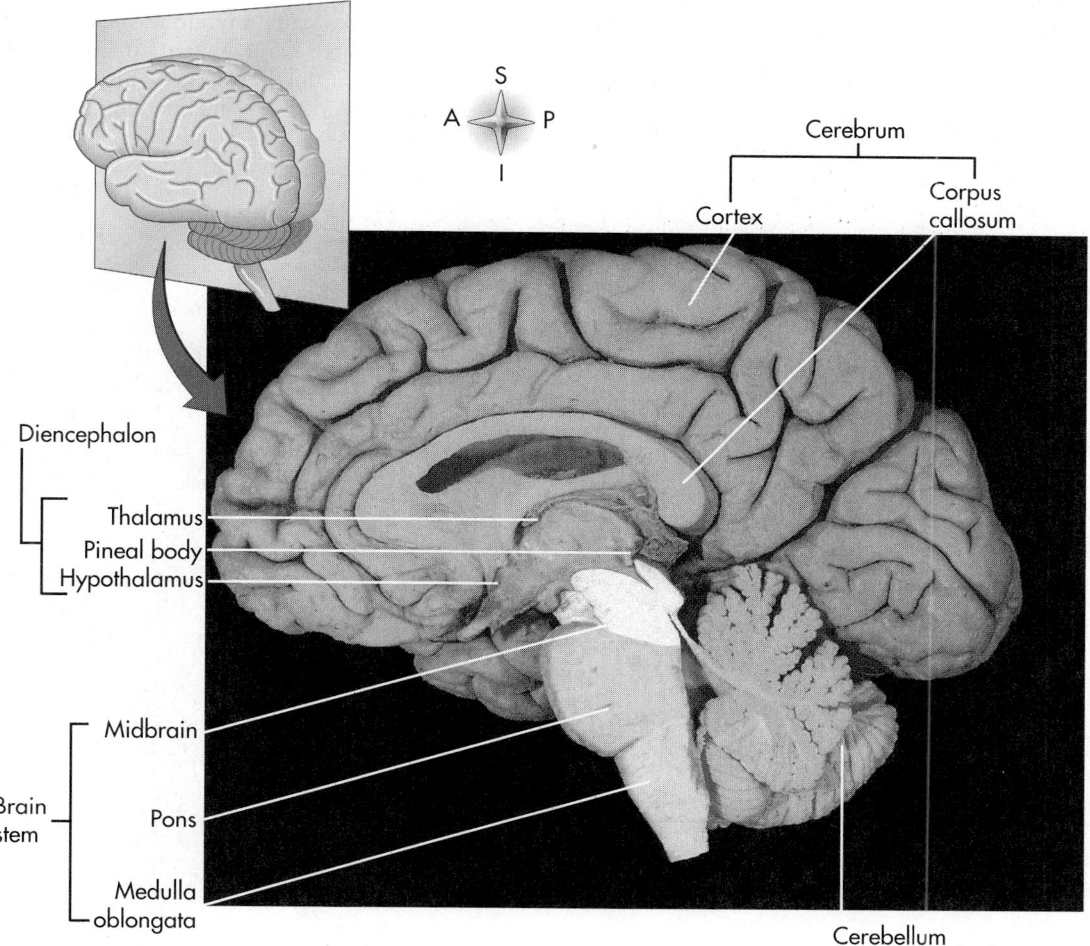

Fig. 26-2 Divisions of the brain. A midsagittal section of the brain reveals features of its major divisions. (From Thibodeau, G. A. [1999]. The central nervous system. In *Anatomy and physiology* [4th ed.], St. Louis, Mosby).

The cerebral region is often referred to as the *supratentorium,* and the cerebellum and the lower part of the brain stem as the *infratentorium.* They are separated by the tentorium cerebelli, thick-layered, shelflike projections of dura that lie in a transverse plain between the lower (distal) surfaces of the cerebral hemispheres and the upper (ventral) surfaces of the cerebellum, and roof of the posterior cranial fossa (Fig. 26-3). The tentorium does not form a continuous shelf but rather has a central oval aperture termed the *tentorial notch.* This notch is occupied in part by the upper end of the midbrain. The tentorium provides a convenient demarcation line for the location of tumors in the cerebrum vs the posterior fossa region of the brain. The foramen magnum is the opening in the base of the skull through which the spinal cord passes, becoming the brain stem.

The Cerebrum. The cerebrum accounts for about 80% of the brain mass. It is physically divided medially by the longitudinal cerebral fissure into nearly identical left and right hemispheres. One hemisphere is dominant over the other and typically is determined by handedness. Because each hemisphere controls the contralateral side of the body, right-handed individuals tend to have left hemisphere dominance. The dominant hemisphere controls performance of speech and understanding of language and is responsible for verbal and analytic skills. The nondominant hemisphere, usually the right, is responsible for creative arts and spatial reasoning (Fig. 26-4).

Each hemisphere has four functionally distinct lobes: frontal, parietal, occipital, and temporal (Fig. 26-5). The frontal lobe runs from the frontal pole of the brain to the central sulcus. Some distance behind the frontal pole is a fissure called the *lateral sulcus,* which runs backward and upward into the hemisphere. The area below this sulcus is the temporal lobe. The occipital lobe lies in the posterior end of the cerebral hemisphere and is continuous with the temporal lobe. The occipital lobe and the posterior part of the temporal lobe, the medial gyrus, rest on the tentorium cerebelli, which separate them from the posterior cranial fossa. The parietal lobe lies between the frontal, temporal, and occipital lobes, separated from the frontal by the central sulcus and the anterior portion of the temporal by the lateral sulcus. Although not visible from the lateral surface of the hemispheres, the boundaries between the parietal, temporal, and occipital lobes can actually be seen on the medial surface (Hollinshead, 1967).

Each of the cerebral lobes appears to be the center of specific mental and/or bodily functions peculiar to that lobe. These differing functions of the hemispheres and lobes of the cerebrum often provide important localizing symptoms for diagnosis of a tumor (Table 26-3).

The cerebrum is composed of thick outer walls of nerve fibers called *white matter.* The interior contains concentrations of nerve cells (gray matter), which are usually in close proximity to the ventricles and the CSF. However, some nerve cells migrate to the outer surface of the brain and cover the white matter with a layer of gray matter from 1 to 4 mm thick. This gray matter is called the *cerebral cortex.* A protective membrane, the meninges, covers

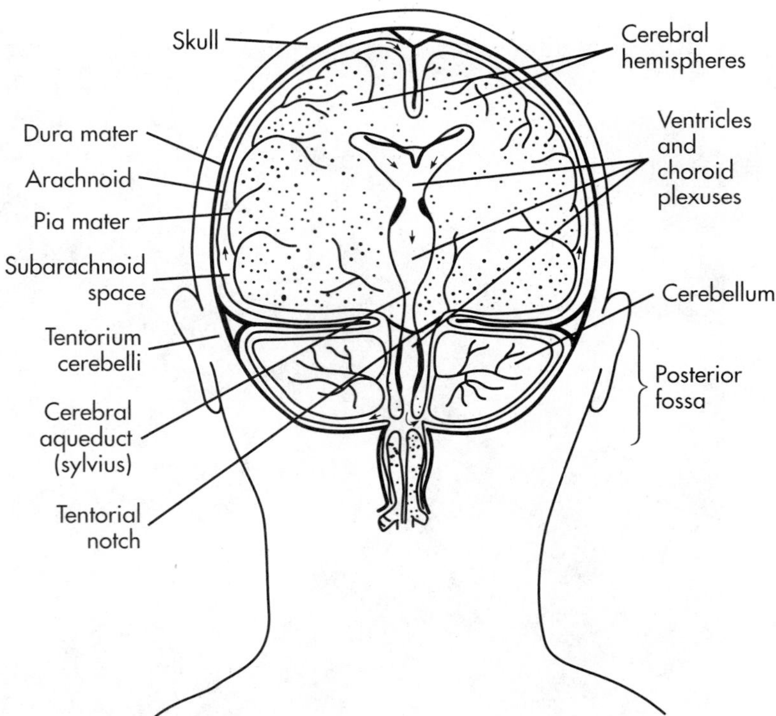

Fig. 26-3 View of the tentorium cerebelli and tentorial notch. (From Owens, B. [1992]. Neurological cancers. In J. C. Clark & R. F. McGee [Eds.], *Core curriculum for oncology nursing* [2nd ed.]. Philadelphia: W. B. Saunders.)

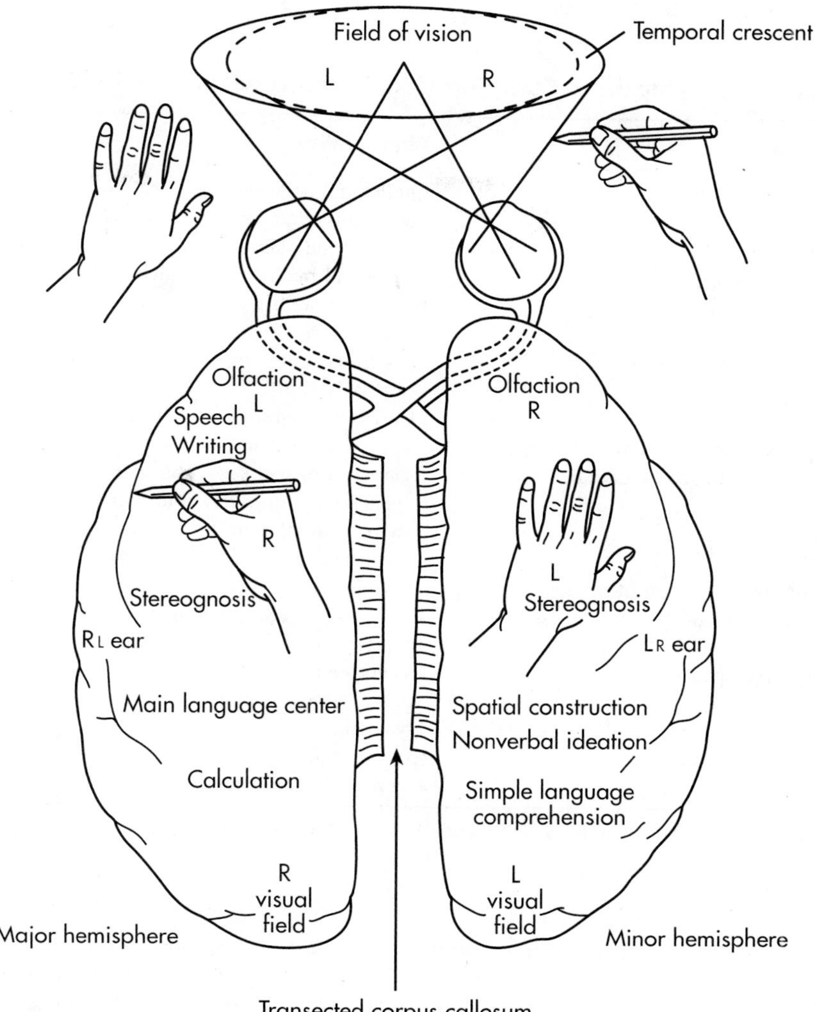

Fig. 26-4 Functions of the hemispheres. (From Wilson, L. M. & Hartwig, M. S. [1997]. Anatomy and physiology of the nervous system. In S. A. Price & L. M. Wilson [Eds.], *Pathophysiology: Clinical concepts of disease processes* [5th ed.] St. Louis: Mosby.)

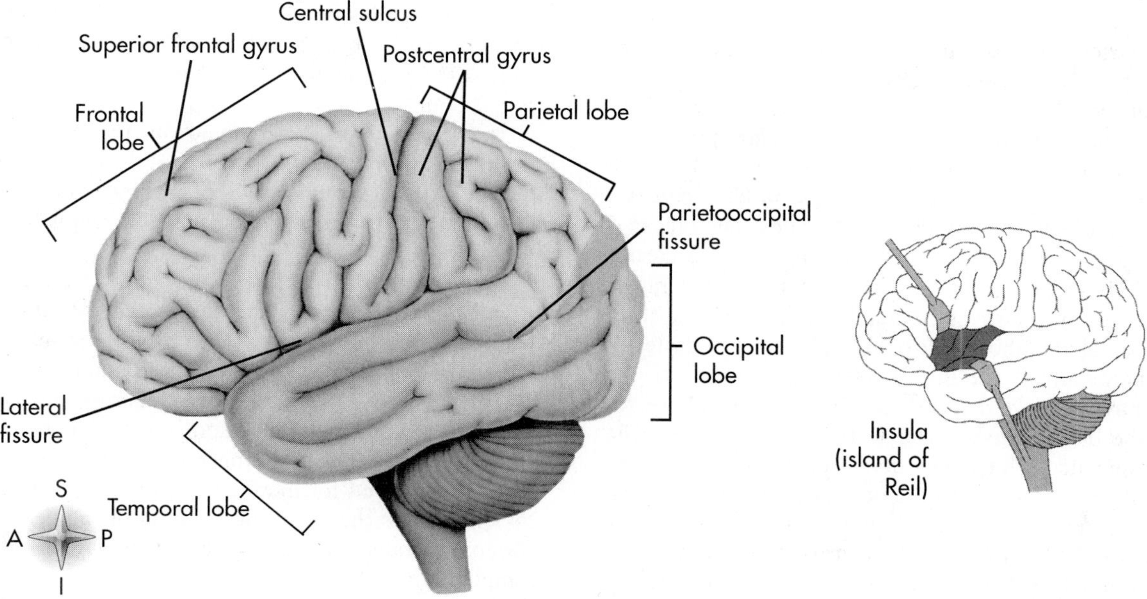

Fig. 26-5 Left hemisphere of cerebrum, lateral surface. (From Thibodeau, G. A. [1999]. The central nervous system. In *Anatomy and Physiology* [4th ed.], St. Louis: Mosby.)

TABLE 26-3 Functions and Symptoms Commonly Associated with Specific Cerebral Lobes

Location	Function	Abnormality
Frontal lobes	Intellect	Intellectual deterioration
	Personality	Personality changes
	Judgment	Impaired judgment
	Abstract thinking	Bowel and bladder incontinence
	Mood and affect	Emotional lability
	Memory	Memory loss
	Motor activity (contralateral)	Muscle weakness or paralysis
		Babinski's sign
		Decreased deep tendon reflexes
	Expressive speech (left hemisphere)	Expressive aphasia
Parietal lobes	Sensory input (contralateral)	Decreased or lost sensation (pain, temperature, pinprick, light touch, proprioception, vibration, two-point discrimination, double simultaneous stimulation, stereognosis, graphesthesia)
Occipital lobes	Sight	Visual field defects, hallucinations, inability to identify objects or symbols
	Visual identification of objects	
Temporal lobes	Hearing	Hearing changes, hallucinations
	Memory	Memory loss
	Receptive speech	Receptive aphasia
Cerebellum	Coordination	Ataxia, action tremor
		Nystagmus
	Balance (ipsilateral)	Loss of balance, wide-base gait
		Decreased deep tendon reflexes

Modified from Kerr, M. E. & Wallack, C. A. (1996). Intracranial problems. In S. M. Lewis, I. C. Collier, & M. M. Heitkemper [Eds.], *Medical surgical nursing assessment and management of clinical problems.* St. Louis, Mosby.

the entire cerebrum and is firmly attached to the cranium (Hollinshead, 1967).

The fibers in the walls of the hemispheres interconnect different parts of a hemisphere. These fibers also connect the cerebrum to the lower parts of the brain and the spinal cord. Some are ascending from the body to the brain, and others are descending from the brain to the body. The two hemispheres are connected with each other via the corpus collosum.

The ventricles are four irregularly shaped extensions of the neural tube that produce the CSF in the choroid plexus of each ventricle (Fig. 26-6). They also provide a circulation system for the CSF throughout the brain and spinal cord where the fluid acts as a cushion and support for the CNS. The two lateral ventricles are located one in each cerebral hemisphere and extend through all four lobes. They lie sagittally to each side of and extend the length of the corpus collosum. These two ventricles do not connect, but rather empty through the intraventricular foramina into the third ventricle, situated in the posterior cranial fossa just posterior to the hypothalamus. The third ventricle connects with the fourth ventricle, located in the pontine and medullary regions of the brain stem anterior to the cerebellum, via the cerebral aqueduct, which runs dorsal to the midbrain. The fourth ventricle extends into the central canal of the spinal column. The ventricles are also connected to the subarachnoid space of the meninges, which surrounds the brain and spinal column. The ventricular system supplies, maintains, and circulates about 150 ml of CSF at any given time (Hollinshead, 1967; Wilson & Hartwig, 1997).

The Cerebellum. The cerebellum lies below and is separated from the posterior portions of the cerebral hemisphere by the tentorium cerebelli. It is split laterally into paired cerebellar hemispheres. These are connected posteriorly and inferiorly by the much smaller vermis, which occupies a notch between them. The cerebellum is a solid structure, as it contains no ventricles. Although no cranial nerve emerges from or is attached to the cerebellum, cranial nerve VIII (vestibulocochlear) has intimate contact with it (Fig. 26-7).

The cerebellum is involved in the maintenance of balance, as well as helping to control the contraction of voluntary muscles, especially the timing and strength of the contractions for smooth and accurate movement (Hollinshead, 1967).

The Brain Stem. The 12 cranial nerves arise in the brain and exit the skull via openings called *foramina.* These nerves are commonly referred to by Roman numerals. The nuclei of 10 of the cranial nerves are found in the brain stem (III-XII). Because these nerves are identified throughout the description of the brain stem and can be important locational clues in diagnosing tumors, Fig. 26-7 and Table 26-4 are provided for the reader's review and referral. Fig. 26-7 illustrates the anatomic location of the nerves in relation to the brain. Table 26-4 lists the cranial nerves by nerve component and function.

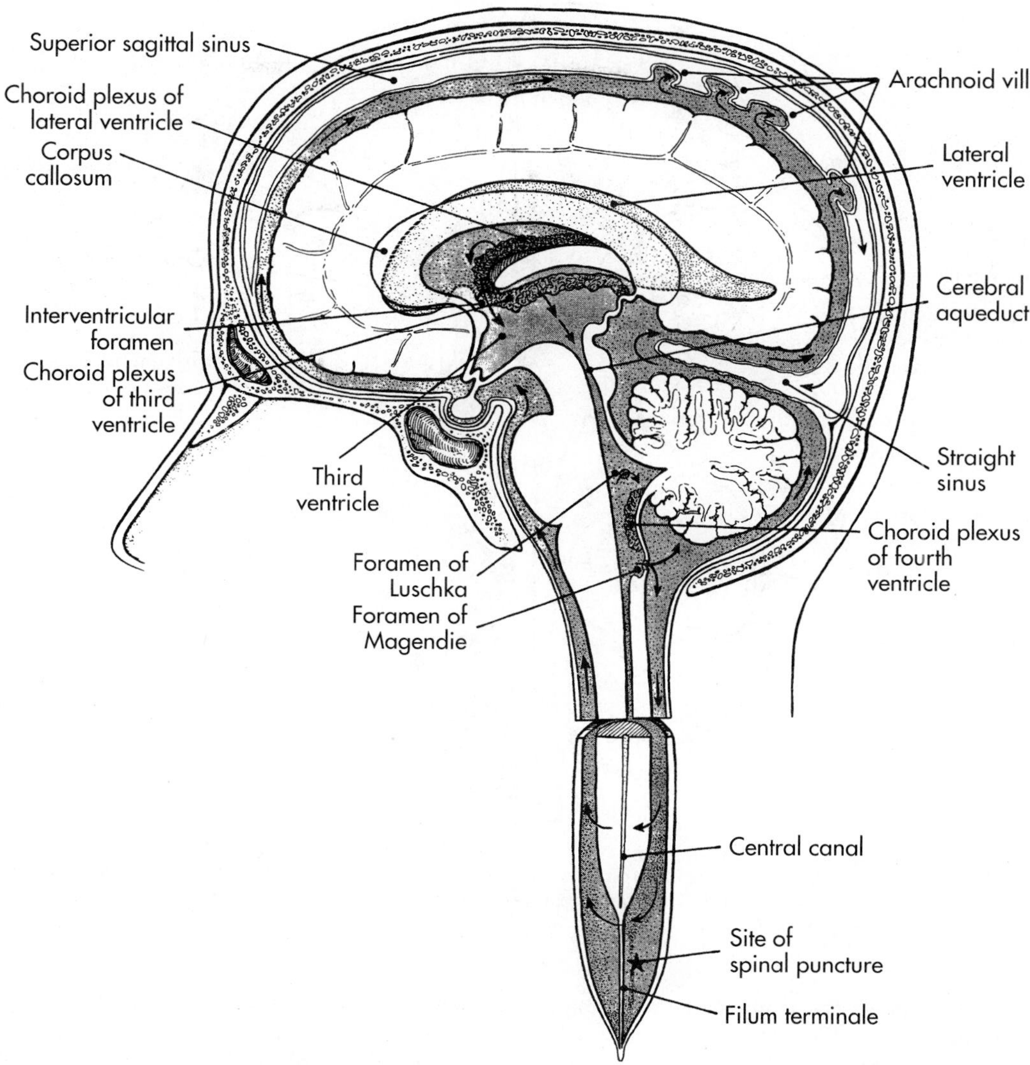

Fig. 26-6 Ventricular system and circulation of the cerebral spinal fluid. (From Wilson, L. M. & Hartwig, M. S. [1997]. Anatomy and physiology of the nervous system. In S. A. Price & L. M. Wilson [Eds.], *Pathophysiology: Clinical concepts of disease processes* [5th ed.]. St. Louis: Mosby.)

The brain stem is the upward continuation of the spinal cord. It resembles the spinal cord in general, but is more complex. Whereas the gray and white matter tend to be more intermixed than in the cerebral and cerebellar hemispheres, the white matter lies largely on the exterior and the gray matter is located more centrally, near the fourth and third ventricles and their connecting cerebral aqueduct. Ascending and descending nerve tracks run through the brain stem, making it an important relay and reflex center in the CNS.

The brain stem comprises, in ascending order, the medulla oblongata, the pons, and the midbrain. The medulla oblongata, or myelencephalon, begins at the root of the first spinal nerve and extends laterally, disappearing into the pons. The medulla plays an important role as a reflex center for cardiac, vasoconstrictor, respiratory, sneezing, coughing, swallowing, salivating, and vomiting reflexes (Wilson & Hartwig, 1997). Two anterior enlargements called the *pyramids* contain voluntary motor fibers. Posteriorly two swellings named the *fasciculi gracilis* and the *fasciculi cuneatus* are the dorsal column's ascending sensory tracts. The tracts carry pressure, conscious muscle proprioception, vibratory sensations, and two-point tactile discrimination (Wilson & Hartwig, 1997). The nuclei of the cranial nerves (CNs) IX, X, XI, and XII are in the medulla.

The pons, or metencephalon, is a transverse bundle of fibers that appears to connect the cerebral hemispheres (*pons* is Latin for "bridge"). However, each side of the pons is actually part of the connection between one cerebral hemisphere and its opposite cerebellar hemisphere. The lower portion of the pons is involved in respiratory regulation. The pons also connects the medulla

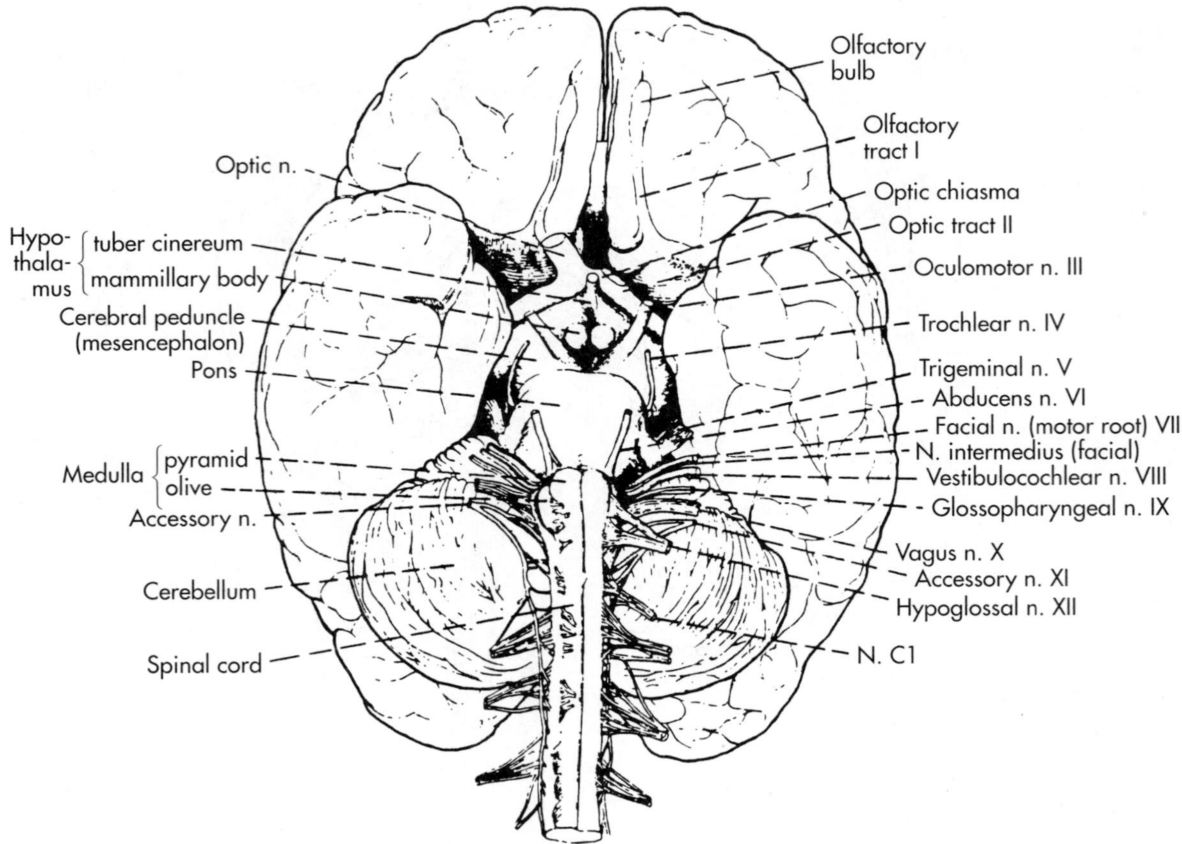

Fig. 26-7 View of the cranial nerves from the base of the brain and ventral surface of the brain stem. (From Hollinshead, W. H. [1967]. The cranial parts of the nervous system. In *Textbook of anatomy* [2nd ed.], New York: Harper & Row.)

below with the midbrain above and contains the upper part of the fourth ventricle. The nuclei of the cranial nerves V through VIII are located in the pons. The majority of brain stem gliomas arise in this structure (Hollinshead, 1967; Wilson & Hartwig, 1997).

The midbrain, or mesencephalon, is located above the pons. The midbrain lies at the junction of the posterior and middle cranial fossae, partly in both. The posterior portion of the midbrain, the tectum, contains the superior colliculi, involved with visual reflexes and tracking, and the inferior colliculi, involved with auditory reflexes and turning one's head toward a sound (Wilson & Hartwig, 1997).

The anterior portion of the midbrain contains the cerebral peduncles, which are bundles of descending motor fibers from the cerebrum. The CNs III and IV emerge from the midbrain. CN IV is the only cranial nerve that exits on the posterior surface of the brain stem and crosses around to the opposite side, putting this nerve at risk during any surgical procedure involving the midbrain (Hollinshead, 1967; Wilson & Hartwig, 1997).

The midbrain also contains the substantia nigra and the red nucleus, which are part of the involuntary motor pathways. The substantia nigra's neurotransmitter is dopamine. The red nucleus has a role in posture and righting reflexes dealing with the orientation of the head in space (Wilson & Hartwig, 1997).

The Diencephalon. The diencephalon is composed of the thalamus and the hypothalamus. It lies anterior to the tentorium cerebelli and below the cerebral hemispheres. The thalamus is the largest part of the diencephalon and is separated into right and left hemispheres by the third ventricle. Most of the dienchephalon is buried in the cerebral hemispheres.

The hypothalamus lies ventrally, above and posterior to the optic chiasm, where a prominent band of the optic nerve (II) is located. The two optic tracts run opposite each other through this chiasm. The hypothalamus provides a floor and part of the lower walls for the third ventricle. It controls many basic functions, including temperature regulation and appetite, and also controls the hypophysis (pituitary gland), the "master gland" of the endocrine system. The posterior-part of the hypophysis is an outgrowth from the floor of the hypothalamus (Hollinshead, 1967).

Blood Supply to the Brain. The blood supply to the brain arrives through the paired vertebral arteries and the paired inferior carotid arteries. The vertebral arteries supply the spinal cord, the posterior fossa structures, and the posterior portion of the cerebrum (temporal and occipital lobes)

TABLE 26-4 Summary of Cranial Nerve (CN) Functions

Cranial Nerve	Nerve Component	Function
I. Olfactory	Sensory	Smell
II. Optic	Sensory	Vision
III. Oculomotor	Motor	Elevation of upper lid Pupillary constriction Most extraocular movements
IV. Trochlear	Motor	Downward inward movement of eye
V. Abducens	Motor	Lateral deviation of eye
VI. Trigeminal	Motor	Temporal and masseter muscles (jaw clenching, chewing); lateral movement of the jaw
	Sensory	Skin of face and anterior two thirds of scalp; mucosa of eyes; mucosa of nasal and oral cavities, tongue, and teeth Corneal or blink reflex: sensory limb carried in CN V, motor response in CN VII
VII. Facial	Motor	Muscles of facial expression, including those of forehead and around eyes and mouth Lacrimation and salivation
	Sensory	Taste on anterior two thirds of tongue (sweet, sour, salty)
VIII. Vestibulocochlear		
Vestibular branch	Sensory	Equilibrium
Cochlear branch	Sensory	Hearing
IX. Glossopharyngeal	Motor	Pharynx: swallowing, gag reflex Parotid: salivation
	Sensory	Pharynx, posterior tongue, including taste (bitter)
X. Vagus	Motor	Pharynx, larynx: swallowing, gag reflex, phonation; abdominal viscera
	Sensory	Pharynx, larynx: gag reflex; neck, thoracic, and abdominal viscera
XI. Accessory	Motor	Sternocleidomastoid and upper portion of trapezius: head and shoulder movements
XII. Hypoglossal	Motor	Tongue movements

From Wilson, L. M., & Hartwig, M. S. (1997). Anatomy and physiology of the nervous system. In S. A. Price & L. M. Wilson (Eds.), *Pathophysiology: Clinical concepts of disease processes.* (5th ed.). St. Louis: Mosby.

(Fig. 26-8). The posterior portion of the cerebrum is fed by the posterior cerebral artery.

The internal carotid arteries supply the optic region, the meninges, the choroid plexus of the lateral ventricles, and the anterior and middle portions of the cerebrum. These portions of the cerebrum are fed by the anterior and middle cerebral arteries.

These two blood supplies interconnect via the communicating arteries in the hexagonal formation of blood vessels at the base of the brain called the *circle of Willis.* The two separate sides of each arterial supply also interconnect in the circle of Willis (Fig. 26-9). Venous drainage occurs via veins that enter a series of venous sinuses located in the dura mater throughout the brain (Fig. 26-10).

The Process of Carcinogenesis

A cancer cell originates when the genetic coding (deoxyribonucleic acid [DNA]) of a single cell is altered in such a way that the cell can no longer normally regulate cell division and differentiation. Eventually, the cell begins to multiply unchecked and no longer functions in its original role in the body.

A cell's transformation to a cancer cell involves the interaction of at least two classes of genes: oncogenes and tumor suppressor genes. The normal function of an oncogene is to enhance cell growth and development in a manner that balances cell proliferation and cell death. When abnormally expressed, oncogenes promote cell proliferation and the development of cancer growth. Tumor suppressor genes normally inhibit cell proliferation and growth. Alterations in this gene that lead to inactivation result in uncontrolled growth, and tumor formation and progression. Oncogene activation and tumor suppressor inactivation, combined with genetic alterations of other factors involved in the cell-cycle regulatory pathway, appear to be central to the current molecular understanding of human tumor formation (Louis & Cavenee, 1997; Volker, 1992).

The information emerging from ongoing molecular genetic studies indicates that carcinogenesis is a complex, multifactorial, multistep process that may have several different genetic pathways to the same malignant outcome. In addition, these pathways may differ among cell types.

The development of primary brain tumors, like other cancers, is thought to occur in a three-stage process of initiation, promotion, and tumor formation (progression) (Murphy, Morris, & Lange, 1997). In the initiation stage, a critical mutating event occurs, usually involving an oncogene, irreparably altering the DNA of a specific gene (or

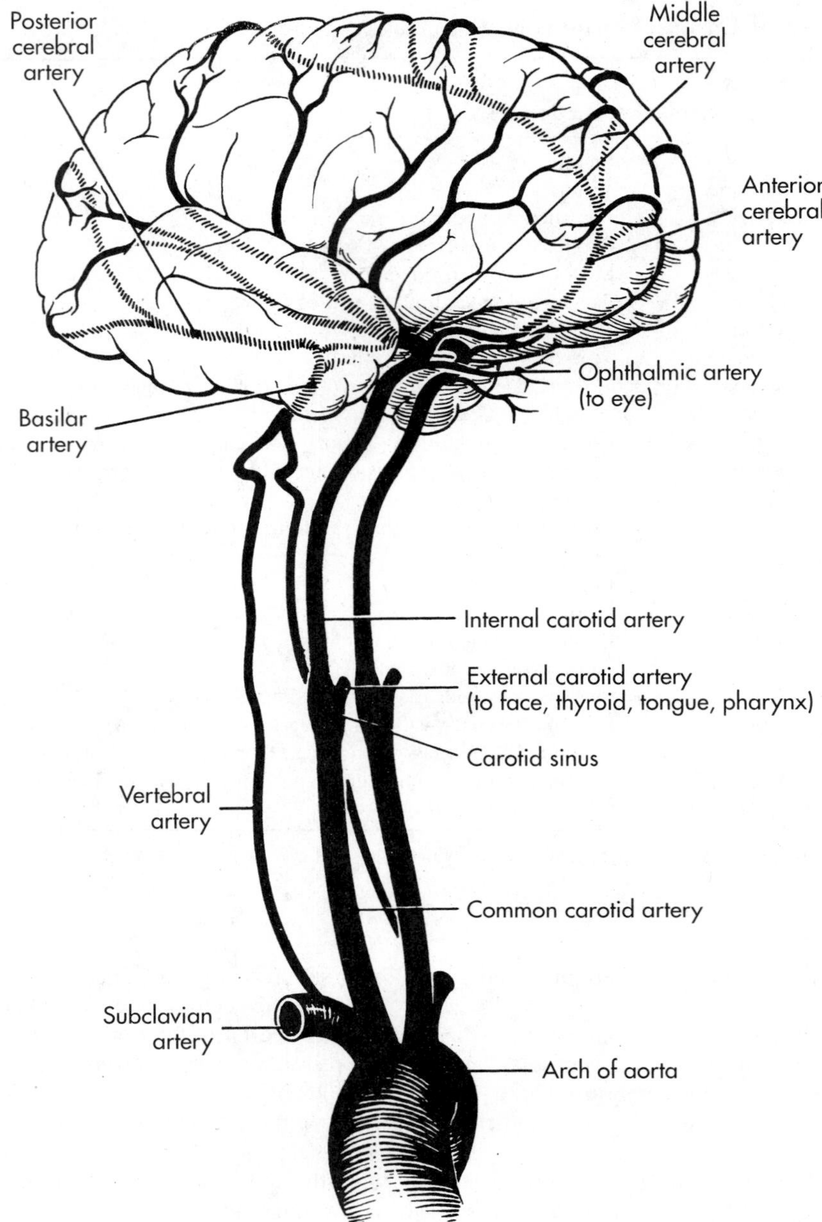

Fig. 26-8 Arterial blood supply to the brain. (From Wilson, L. M., & Hartwig, M. S. [1997]. Anatomy and physiology of the nervous system. In S. A. Price & L. M. Wilson [Eds.], *Pathophysiology: Clinical concepts of disease processes* [5th ed.]. St. Louis: Mosby.)

genes). The gene then lies latent for an unspecified period until a "promoter" activates the carcinogenic process.

The promotion stage occurs when a latent gene is exposed to a promoter carcinogen, one that promotes uncontrolled growth in an already "initiated" cell. Some carcinogens, such as many found in tobacco, are both initiators and promoters. Others, especially dietary factors such as fat, can act only as promoters. Some promoters are relatively weak, and others such as aflatoxin, a mold found particularly on peanuts, is very potent. Each of these promoter carcinogens appears to have a required threshold level of exposure below which carcinogenesis will not take place.

The progression stage is hallmarked by tumor invasion, metastasis, and heterogeneity (Volker, 1992). Proliferation of the cancerous cells reaches a point at which the increasing bulk and pressure result in local spread and invasion of surrounding structures.

Metastasis (the development of secondary tumors distant from the primary site) occurs when cancer cells spread either by seeding throughout a body cavity (e.g., the peritoneum) and/or disseminating via the lymphatic system or the blood capillaries and veins. Although metastatic tumors from other primary sites commonly arise in the brain, the spread of primary brain tumors outside of the CNS is extremely rare.

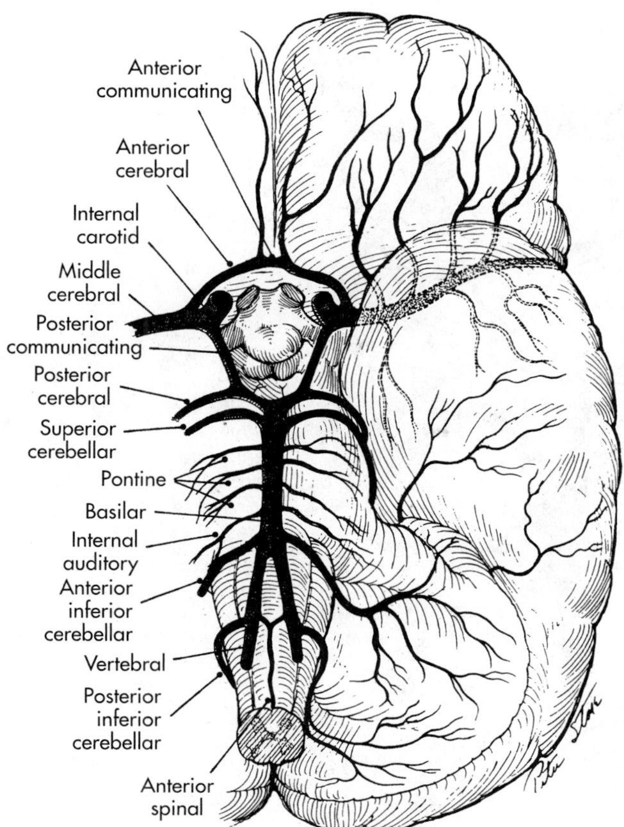

Fig. 26-9 The circle of Willis. (From Wilson, L. M., & Hartwig, M. S. [1997]. Anatomy and physiology of the nervous system. In S. A. Price & L. M. Wilson [Eds.], *Pathophysiology: Clinical concepts of disease processes* [5th ed.]. St. Louis: Mosby.)

Heterogeneity refers to the differences among individual cells in a tumor. As the tumor grows, differences increase as a result of random mutations during tumor growth. Differences in the individual cells can include genetic composition, invasiveness, growth rate, hormonal responsiveness, metastatic potential, and susceptibility to antineoplastic therapies. Heterogeneity often results in tumors highly resistant to any one form of therapy (Volker, 1992).

Although early neoplastic cells often resemble normal cells, more "mature" cells are usually easily identified as abnormal. Noncancerous and precancerous histologic changes include atrophy, hypertrophy, hyperplasia, metaplasia, and dysplasia. Dysplasia is considered to be precancerous because these cells display abnormal cytologic features and tissue organization. Anaplastic cells exhibit cytologic and positional disorganization. The degree of anaplasia varies with the level of cell differentiation: the more poorly differentiated the cell (those with a high degree of pleomorphic and bizarre cytologic features), the more malignant the neoplasm (Volker, 1992).

The time it takes a cancer to become clinically detectable varies by the particular tumor growth fraction (the ratio of total cells to proliferating cells) and the volume-doubling time of a given cancer. In many solid tumors, 2% to 8% of the cells are proliferating; the more malignant tumors have 20% to 30% proliferating cells. The average volume-doubling time for primary solid tumors is 2 to 3 months, with a range of 11 to 90 weeks. The smallest clinically detectable tumor is considered to be 1 g in weight and/or 1 cm^3 (10 billion to 100 billion cells), which requires approximately 30 tumor volume-doubling times (Volker, 1992).

Genetic and Molecular Basis for Primary Gliomas

Significant progress has been achieved in recent years in the identification of genetic factors and sites (translocations, deletions, additions, and fragile genetic sites) related to gliomas and to syndromes associated with these primary brain tumors. The molecular basis for malignant tumor progression is also becoming better understood (Seizinger, Klinger, Junien, Nakamura, Le Beau, & Cavanee, 1991).

Research in the field of molecular genetics is progressing rapidly, and significant new knowledge is emerging faster than it can be incorporated into oncologic practice. The following sections review the latest information on the molecular basis of primary gliomas. Astrocytomas are included in this review because the majority of brain stem gliomas are astrocytomas.

Diffuse Astrocytomas. Recent studies have uncovered the key molecular features of the genetic process underlying the malignant progression for grade II: diffuse, fibrillary astrocytoma through grade III: anaplastic astrocytoma to grade IV: GBM. Fig. 26-11 illustrates this progression.

The grade II astrocytomas are low-grade tumors that have a tendency to diffusely infiltrate surrounding tissue, complicating therapeutic attempts at local control. These tumors tend toward malignant progression.

The *p53* gene on chromosome *17p* plays a key role in the cellular processes of DNA repair, cell-cycle arrest, apoptosis, angiogenesis, and cell differentiation. This role is of such significance that the *p53* gene is commonly known as the *guardian of the genome.* The loss of *p53* results in genome instability and has been implicated in the early stages of astrocytoma tumorigenesis. It also appears to set the stage for malignant progression. Gene *p53* mutations are seen in about one third of all three grades of adult astrocytomas (Louis & Cavenee, 1997; Louis, 1994; Livingstone, White, Sprouse, Livanos, Jacks, & Tlsty, 1992).

Several growth factors and their receptors, including platelet-derived growth factor (PDGF), fibroblast growth factors (FGFs), and vascular endothelial growth factor (VEGF), are overexpressed in astrocytomas (Hermanson, Funa, Hartman, Claesson-Welsh, Heldin, & Westermark, 1992). Loss of the *p17* chromosome in the region of *p53* correlates highly with PDGF alpha-receptor overexpression (Hermanson, Funa, Koopman, Maintz, Waha, & Westermark, 1996). Such findings suggest that *p53* alterations may require PDGF overexpression to have a carcinogenic effect (Louis & Cavenee, 1997). These growth factors also stimulate cell migration, which may be why astrocytomas typically infiltrate the surrounding brain tissue (Pilkington, 1994).

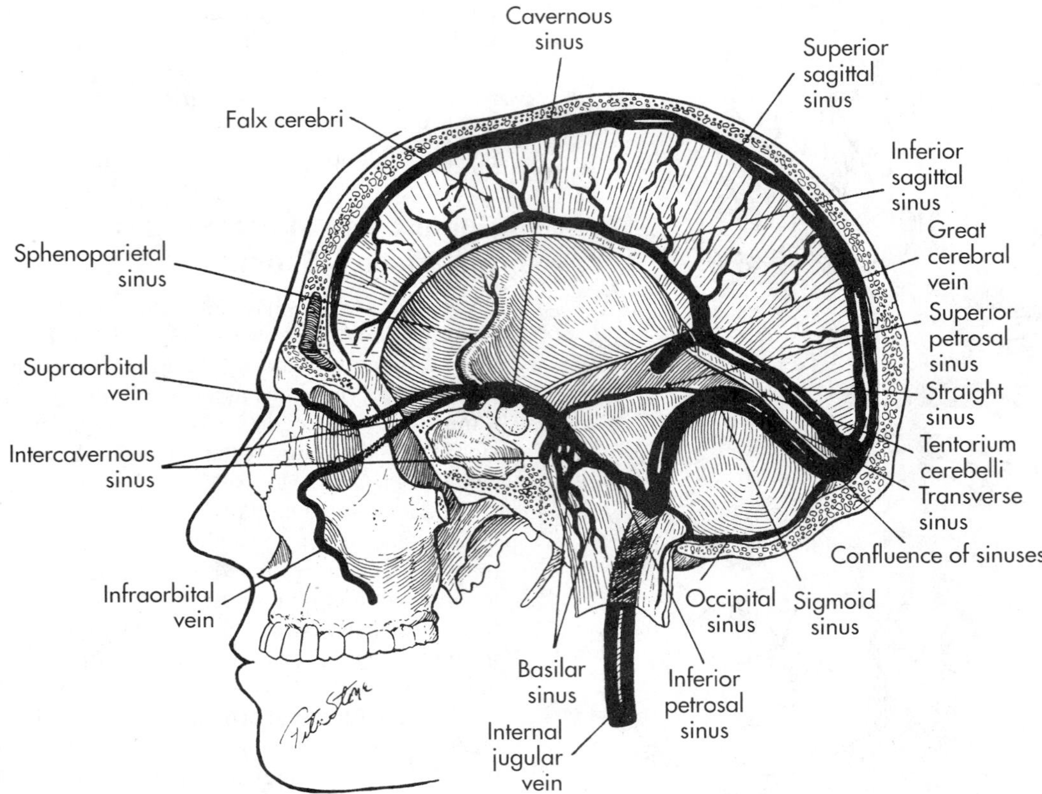

Fig. 26-10 Venous sinuses of the head. (From Wilson, L. M., & Hartwig, M. S. [1997]. Anatomy and physiology of the nervous system. In S. A. Price & L. M. Wilson [Eds.], *Pathophysiology: Clinical concepts of disease processes* [5th ed.]. St. Louis: Mosby.)

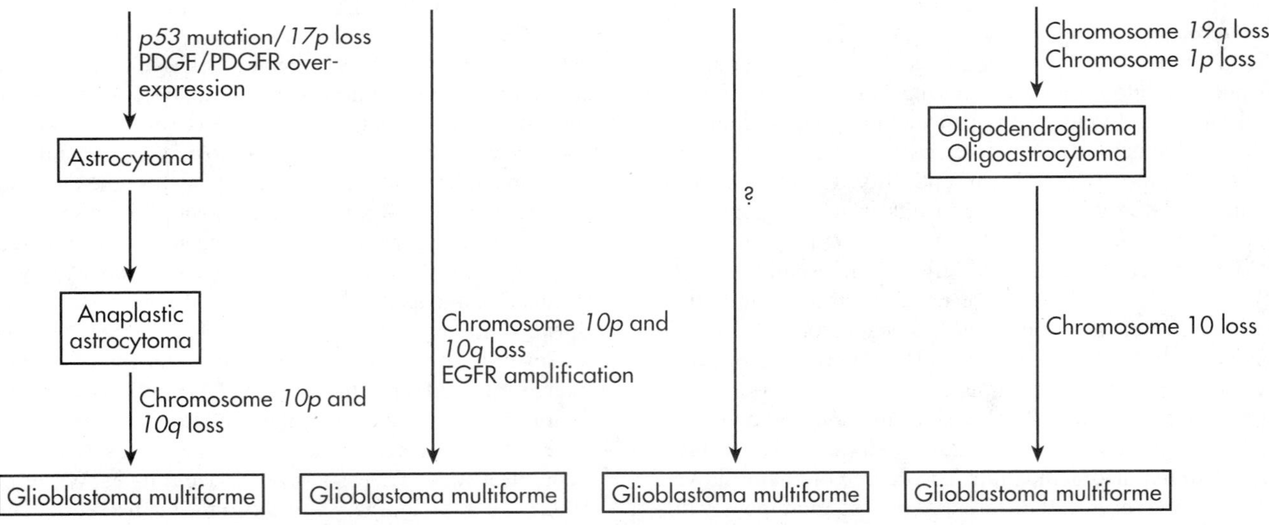

Fig. 26-11 Molecular genetic subsets of glioblastoma multiforme. (From Louis, D. N., & Cavenee, W. K. [1997]. Molecular biology of central nervous system neoplasms. In V. T. De Vita, S. Hellman, & S. A. Rosenberg [Eds.], *Cancer: The principles and practice of oncology* [5th ed.]. Philadelphia: J. B. Lippincott.)

Anaplastic Astrocytoma and Glioblastoma Multiforme. A higher level of cell proliferation activity is the histologic indicator of progression from grade II to grade III anaplastic astrocytoma. These tumors often show transformation to grade IV GBM.

A number of molecular abnormalities appear in anaplastic astrocytomas. The majority of these abnormalities involve one critical cell-cycle complex that includes *p16,* cyclin-dependent kinase 4 (cdk4), cyclin D1, and retinoblastoma (Rb) proteins. The Rb proteins maintain a brake on the cell cycle; the others ensure that the Rb proteins do so. Fifty percent of anaplastic astrocytomas and the majority of GBMs have abnormalities in this system. These tumors show a chromosome *9p* loss in the *p16* region. The frequency of 9p tumor suppressor loss increases as the tumor progresses to the higher grades III and IV. Primary GBMs almost always show deletions of *COKN2/p16* (Louis & Cavenee, 1997).

Loss of chromosome *13q* occurs in up to 50% of high-grade astrocytomas, implying that a tumor suppressor gene is located in that area. This gene is also involved in the cell-cycle pathway. Studies suggest that the Rb gene found on *13q* is inactive in about 20% of grade III and 35% of grade IV tumors (Henson, Schnitker, Correa, von Deimling, Fassbender, & Xu, 1994).

It appears that up to 50% of anaplastic astrocytomas and nearly all GBMs have mutations in at least one component of the critical cell-cycle regulatory pathway (Louis & Cavenee, 1997).

Allelic losses on *19q* have been found in 40% of the higher grade astrocytomas, indicating the presence of a progression-related tumor suppressor gene (von Deimling, Louis, von Ammon, Petersen, Wiestler, & Seizinger, 1992). This gene may be unique to glial tumors, since it is involved in all three diffuse cerebral gliomas (astrocytomas, oligodendrogliomas, and mixed gliomas). It has not yet been identified.

Brain Stem Gliomas. Brain stem gliomas are diffuse, fibrillary astrocytomas that usually follow a malignant course. Brain stem glioblastoma multiformes (GBM) show frequent *p53* gene and chromosome *17p* alterations without EGFR gene amplification (Louis, Rubio, Correa, Gusella, & von Deimling, 1993). Because these alterations are so similar in childhood and adult tumors, it appears that certain astrocytes can display differing responses at different ages to the same genetic mutations (Louis & Cavenee, 1997).

Oligodendrogliomas and Oligoastrocytomas. Oligodendrogliomas and oligoastrocytomas (mixed gliomas) are typically diffuse tumors most commonly found in the cerebrum, especially the frontal lobe. These tumors are biologically and clinically similar to the diffuse, fibrillary astrocytoma. They are far less common than astrocytomas, tend to be more chemosensitive, and generally have a better prognosis. The prognosis for oligoastrocytomas is somewhere between the same grade of astrocytomas and oligodendrogliomas.

Between 40% and 80% of oligodendrogliomas and oligoastrocytomas show allelic losses on chromosomes *1p* and *19q* (Kraus, Koopman, Kaskel, Maintz, Brandner, & Louis, 1995; Reifenberger, Reifenberger, Lui, James, Wechsler, & Collins, 1994; von Deimling et al., 1992). The tumor suppressor genes on these chromosomes are likely important in early tumorigenesis. The suspected gene on *19q* is probably the same gene that is implicated in astrocytomas, and indeed, the molecular changes in both cell types of the oligoastrocytoma appear to be identical (Kraus et al., 1995). Oligoastrocytomas may also have allelic losses on chromosome *17p* not associated with *p53* mutations. This suggests that a second glioma gene may reside on *17p.* Amplification of oncogenes is rarely identified in oligodendroglial tumors (Fuller & Bigner, 1992; Louis & Cavenee, 1997; Reifenberger et al., 1994).

Oligodendrogliomas and oligoastrocytomas may progress to grade III and grade IV (GBM) tumors, implying yet another genetic alteration pathway to glioblastomas. Anaplastic grades of these tumors sometimes show allelic losses of chromosomes *9p* and *10* (Reifenberger et al., 1994). Such losses on chromosome 10 may be a common finding in GBMs regardless of the cell of origin (James, Carlblom, Dumanski, Hansen, Nordenskjold, & Collins, 1988).

Ependymomas. Ependymomas are clinically diverse gliomas ranging from aggressive malignancies in children to benign spinal cord tumors in adults. Chromosome *22q* loss is common in ependymomas. Although the neurofibromatosis II (NF2) gene is on this chromosome and NF2 patients have a higher incidence of gliomas, particularly ependymomas, this gene does not appear to be the same as the yet unidentified ependymoma-related gene. The *p53* gene is not mutated in either the ependymoma or the anaplastic ependymoma. Progression to GBM is extremely rare and has not been studied (Ohgaki, Eibl, Wiestler, Yasargil, Newcomb, & Kleihaus, 1991).

There is some evidence that oncogenic viruses can cause human cancer. One study reported finding a viral sequence similar to the SV40 virus, an oncogenic virus that can deactivate the Rb and *p53* proteins, in ependymomas and choroid plexus papillomas. However, the SV40 viral sequence has not been seen in subsequent ependymoma studies. The role of these viruses, if there is one, has not been identified (Bersagel, Finnegold, Butel, Kupsy, & Garcea, 1992).

Genetic and molecular data for the various gliomas are incomplete. Once the genetic mutations and molecular pathways are better understood, new and more effective therapies may be developed to treat many of these tumors.

Neurologic Tumor Syndromes. The associations of certain neurologic syndromes with specific CNS tumors are listed in the section on Risk Factors in this chapter. The specific correlations between these syndromes and glial tumors, as well as the linked genetic site are indicated in Table 26-5.

ROUTES OF METASTASES

Primary brain tumors rarely, if ever, metastasize beyond the CNS. However, intracranial medulloblastomas and ependymomas may spread to the spinal cord. In addition, meningeal involvement, usually via the subarachnoid space, may be seen with medulloblastoma and, to a lesser degree, ependymomas. Nonglial tumors that may spread to the meninges include pinealoblastomas, germinomas, and primary lymphomas (Mack, 1993).

SIGNS AND SYMPTOMS

As tumor volume increases, progressive neurologic deficits and associated symptoms begin to emerge. The degree of severity of the deficits and symptoms is determined by tumor location, size, and degree of malignancy. Most symptoms manifest as either focal disturbances or increased intracranial pressure (ICP), or both. It is important to note that slow-growing tumors rarely cause focal deficits or increased ICP and are often difficult to diagnose.

TABLE 26-5 Correlations Among Neurologic Tumor Syndromes, Glial Tumors and Linked Genetic Alteration Sites

Syndrome/ Disease		Glioma Genetic Site
Neurofibromatosis I (NF1)	Optic nerve glioma astrocytoma	*17q*
Neurofibromatosis II (NF2)	Ependymoma astrocytoma	*22q*
Tuberous sclerosis	Subependymal giant cell astrocytoma	*9q, 16p*
Li-Fraumini syndrome	Various malignant gliomas	*17p (p53)*
Turcot's syndrome	Various malignant gliomas	*5q (ARC* gene)

Focal Disturbances

Focal disturbances are caused by compression of brain tissue due to mass effect, infiltration of the tumor into surrounding tissue, and/or direct invasion of the brain parenchyma with destruction of neural tissue and disruption of neural function. The pathologic process is one alteration of the blood supply resulting in tissue necrosis and acute loss of function. This process is often accompanied by peritumoral edema, which exerts pressure on neuronal elements (Lombardo, 1997).

General Symptoms

Classic symptoms include headache, nausea and vomiting, seizures, and papilledema. Other common symptoms include mental changes in such areas as personality, memory, concentration, and intellect; fatigue and drowsiness; and visual changes.

Headaches, caused by tumor pressure, are the most common symptom of glial tumors. They tend to be worse in the morning and are exacerbated by coughing, exercise, a change in body position, or any other action that normally raises ICP. Headaches can have localizing value in that one third overlie the tumor area and two thirds are near or above the tumor bed. Frontal headaches are associated with one third of supratentorial tumors. Headaches in the occipital region usually indicate a tumor in the posterior fossa (Lombardo, 1997; New hope for patients, 1997).

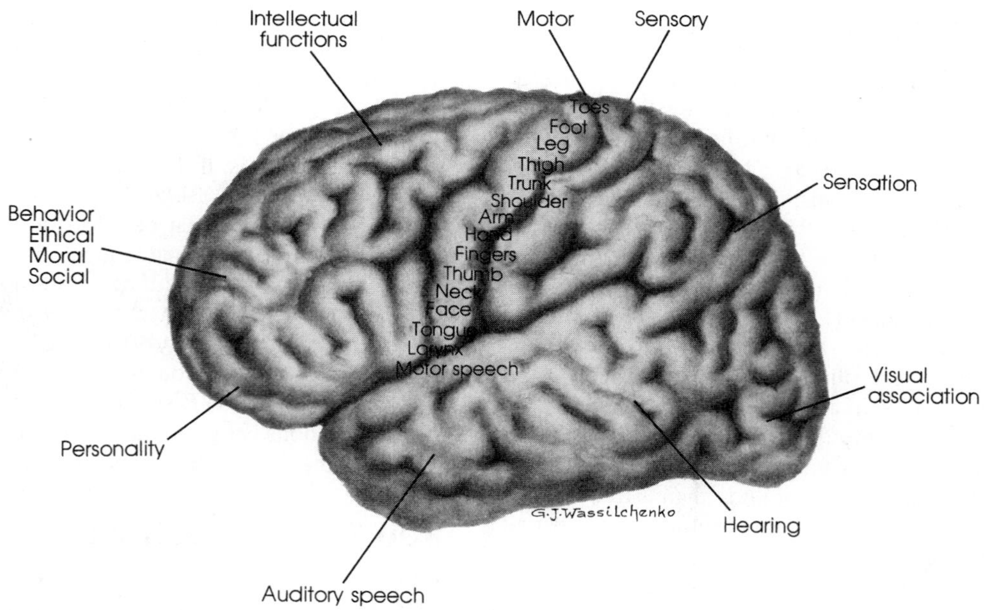

Fig. 26-12 Functional subdivisions of the cerebral hemisphere. (From Kerr, M. E. & Walleck, C. A. (1996). Intracranial problems. In S. M. Lewis, I. C. Collier, & M. M. Heitkemper. *Medical surgical* nursing. (4th ed.) St. Louis: Mosby.

Seizures are caused by altered neuronal excitability and may be accompanied by convulsions, tingling sensations, and loss of consciousness. Seizures are a symptom in 20% to 50% of all tumors, especially oligodendrogliomas, and tumors of the temporal and parietal lobes (Armstrong & Gilbert, 1996; Lombardo, 1997; New hope for patients, 1997).

Nausea and vomiting are caused by stimulation of the emetic center in the medulla. Vomiting may occur without nausea and may be projectile in children. These symptoms are most commonly associated with increased ICP, especially with brain stem displacement.

Papilledema is a result of venous stasis leading to engorgement and swelling of the optic disc. Fundoscopy is the usual means of identifying this sign, but the fundi of some people may not show papilledema. Disturbances of vision and an enlarged blind spot may also be associated with papilledema (Lombardo, 1997).

Localizing Symptoms

The location of a tumor determines the kind of neural dysfunction that emerges. Each component of the brain has specialized roles and functions whose disruption provides localizing clues for diagnosis. In the cerebrum, symptoms are related to lobular functions, and, very often, hemispheric dominance. Fig. 26-12 illustrates hemispheric functional differences. The functions unique to each of the four cerebral lobes are shown in Fig. 26-13, and symptoms commonly associated with the lobes in Table 26-3. Because the frontal lobe is the most common site of oligodendrogliomas, ependymomas originate in the ventricles, and brain stem gliomas arise in the brain stem, localizing signs and symptoms for each of these areas are discussed in detail in the following sections.

Frontal Lobe Symptoms. Oligodendrogliomas are almost exclusively found in the frontal lobes. These tumors cause symptoms nearly identical to astrocytomas, with the exception that the majority of individuals with oligodendrogliomas experience seizures before diagnosis. It is also not uncommon for these tumors to have been present for 7 to 8 years before diagnosis.

Frontal lobe tumors are often known as "silent" tumors because many frontal lobe tumors are slow growing, and symptoms are often difficult to recognize and assess. In particular, the kinds of dysfunction that can occur in the mental processes of the frontal lobe often make it difficult for the patient to recognize problems and/or accurately verbalize complaints. Tumor symptoms can present as dementia, confusion, anxiety, and depression, making it easy to misdiagnose these tumor symptoms. In such cases, input from the family can be a valuable source of diagnostic information.

Tumor-induced dysfunctions of the frontal lobe depend on the particular region of the frontal lobe affected. The prefrontal cortex is associated with personality, behavior, and the intellect. Functions of this cortex include complex intellectual activities, ideation, creative thought, judgment, foresight, some memory functions, and a sense of responsibility for socially acceptable behavior (Wilson & Hartwig, 1997). Tumors in this area affect higher-level reasoning and judgment skills, as well as memory. Subtle changes in personality, including depression, anxiety, confusion, and bizarre behavior, may occur. Difficulty in sequencing actions and lack of initiative are also common signs.

The primary motor area, located along the precentral gyrus and in front of the central sulcus, is responsible for voluntary movement. A tumor in this area can lead to jacksonian seizures, as well as contralateral motor weakness or hemiplegia. The premotor cortex, anterior to the primary motor area, controls learned skilled movement such as writing, driving, and typing. A lesion in the dominant hemisphere can lead to loss of writing ability (agraphia) (Wilson & Hartwig, 1997). Posterior precentral cortex tumors can cause weakness of the face, tongue, and larynx. Tumors of the paracentral lobule result in weakness in the foot and lower extremities (Lombardo, 1997).

The frontal eye field, located just anterior to the premotor cortex, is responsible in conjunction with the cortex for voluntary scanning movements of the eyes and conjugate

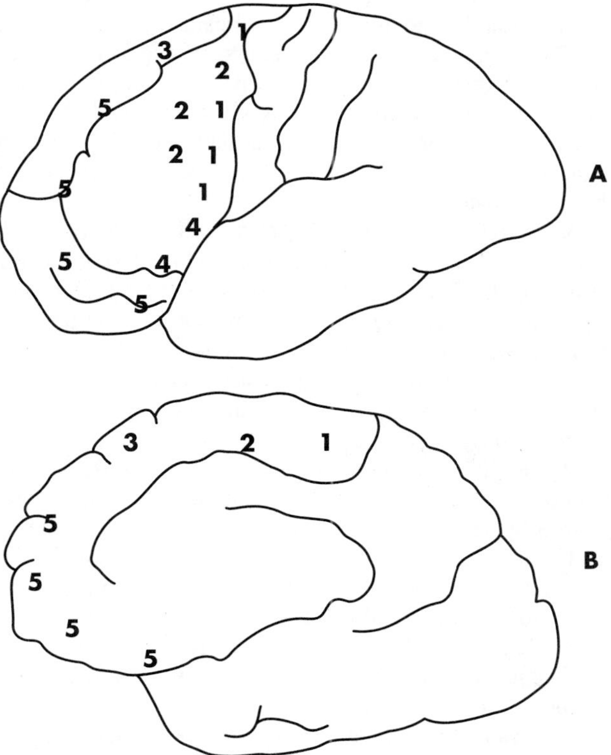

Fig. 26-13 Functions of the frontal lobe cerebral cortex. **A,** Lateral surface. **B,** Medial surface.

deviation of the eyes and the head. A tumor located in this field disrupts these visual abilities.

Broca's motor speech area, located adjacent to the prefrontal cortex along the lateral sulcus, is responsible for motor execution of speech. A lesion in this area in the dominant hemisphere causes expressive aphasia.

Brain Stem Glioma Symptoms. Gliomas of the brain stem almost always involve dysfunctions of the cranial nerves III through XII that arise in this area. The nuclei of the efferent (motor) fibers of these nerves are located in the brain stem and all emerge from the brain stem area. Thus a thorough examination of the cranial nerves is important for localizing brain stem gliomas.

Ninety percent of patients with brain stem gliomas have unilateral palsies of cranial nerves VI and VII. Long tract involvement usually follows with signs such as hemiplegia, unilateral limb ataxia, ataxia of gait, paraplegia, hemisensory syndromes, gaze disorders, and, sometimes, hiccups. Long tract signs may precede cranial nerve symptoms in confined central intrinsic tumors. Most of these tumors arise in the pons.

Tumors of the midbrain are usually well-differentiated or anaplastic astrocytomas, which often present with symptoms of hydrocephalus, vomiting, drowsiness, and cerebellar symptoms. Tumors in the anterior portion of the midbrain can result in muscle rigidity, fine motor tremors at rest, slow and shuffling gait, and masklike facies. Problems with posture and righting of the head can also occur.

Tumors of the medulla are usually glioblastomas. These tumors are rapidly progressive; symptoms include deficits in cranial nerves V, VII, IX, and X; dysarthria; personality changes; and head tilt. Whereas headache, vomiting, and papilledema occur early in the course of expansive posterior fossa tumors, these symptoms appear late in glioblastomas of the medulla (Levin, Leibel, & Gutin, 1997). Because the medulla is responsible for the cardiac, blood pressure, and respiratory reflexes, an increase of pressure in this area can be life-threatening.

Ventricle-Related Symptoms of Ependymomas. The ventricles (paired lateral, third, and fourth) produce and store the CSF and constitute the CSF circulation system with the subarachnoid space. Extraventricular supratentorial tumors cause focal neurologic deficits. Tumors in the ventricles or their communicating structures (interventricular foramina, cerebral aqueduct, and the lateral and median apertures) may occlude the flow of fluid, resulting in hydrocephalus, increased cranial pressure, and papilledema. Hydrocephalus symptoms include gait ataxia, vertigo, nausea, vomiting, headache, and ultimately a decrease in the level of consciousness. Specifically, invasive lesions of the third ventricle and hypothalamus result in somnolence, diabetes insipidus, obesity, and disturbances of temperature regulation. Tumors in the third ventricle present with a steady headache and papilledema with few localizing signs. Tumors in the fourth ventricle lead to rapid increase in cranial pressure with papilledema and cerebellar symptoms. Rapid increase in ICP, if left untreated, can result in central herniation.

Increased Intracranial Pressure. Increased ICP can be the result of an increase in mass within the confined space of the skull, peritumoral edema, hydrocephalus due to blockage of the CSF, and/or tumor-caused hemorrhage due to venous obstruction.

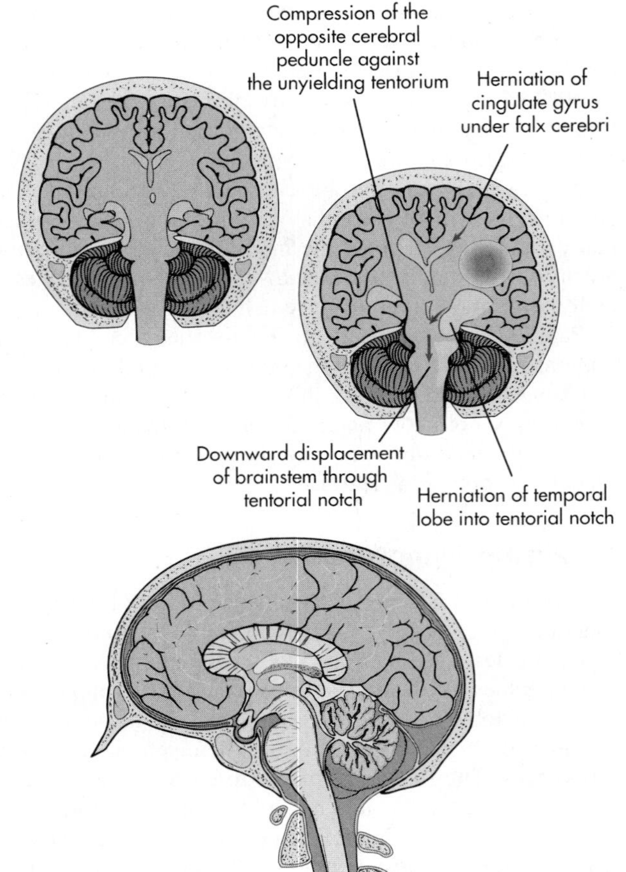

Fig. 26-14 Intracranial herniation. (From Lewis S. M. [1997]. *Medical-surgical nursing.* [4th ed.] St. Louis: Mosby.)

Acute and rapid onset of ICP is life-threatening and is considered a medical emergency, as it portends imminent herniation of the uncus or cerebellum, and ensuing death (Figs. 26-14 and 26-15). Herniation of the uncus occurs when the medial gyrus of the temporal lobe is displaced inferiorly through the tentorial notch by a mass in the supratentorium. The resulting pressure on the midbrain can cause a loss of consciousness and compression of cranial nerve III (Lombardo, 1997).

Cerebellar herniation occurs when the cerebellar tonsils are displaced downward through the foramen magnum by a mass in the posterior fossa. Compression of the medulla and respiratory arrest quickly follow. Other symptoms of rapid onset ICP include bradycardia, systemic hypertension with widening pulse pressure, and respiratory failure (Lombardo, 1997).

ASSESSMENT

A patient's presenting complaints fall into two categories: those related to neurologic dysfunction and those arising from depression, anxiety, or other psychosomatic symptoms

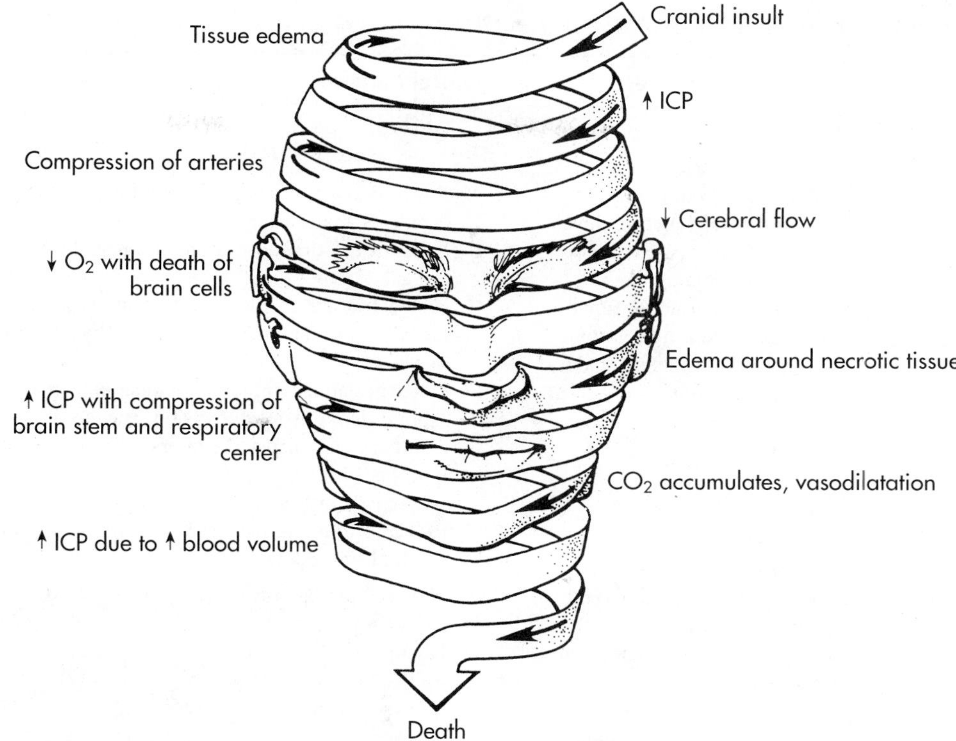

Fig. 26-15 Progression of increased intracranial pressure. (From Murphy, M. E. [1997]. Cancers of the brain and central nervous system. In S. E. Otto [Ed.], *Oncology nursing.* [3rd ed.] St. Louis: Mosby.)

related to a person's coping mechanisms. The second category can be as troublesome as the first and is an important component of nursing management for these patients and their families (Table 26-6).

Headaches and seizures are the most common presenting signs in patients with glial tumors. However, complaints such as nausea and vomiting, speech and vision problems, fatigue and drowsiness, muscle weakness, and often vague complaints of mental and behavioral problems are also often voiced (Armstrong & Gilbert, 1996; Lombardo, 1997; New hope for patients, 1997; Wilson & Hartwig, 1997).

Any patient with presenting symptoms that possibly indicate a tumor should undergo a careful neurologic evaluation, which should include a history, physical examination, neurologic assessment, and diagnostic procedures as indicated. The purpose of the evaluation is to systematically investigate the patient's complaints and symptoms. Such an evaluation can rule out other possible causes of signs and symptoms and provide a fairly accurate prediction of the location and extent of the tumor, even before radioimaging procedures are used (Armstrong & Gilbert, 1996).

History

A careful history should be taken and recorded in the patient's own words whenever possible. A good history and a subsequent interview with the patient's family can alert the clinician to important issues, direct the physical and neurologic examinations, and, most important, build a good rapport with the patient and his/her family that can ensure future cooperation during what likely may be a very difficult period in their lives.

The history should include past medical history, social history, genetic and family history, the onset and progression of presenting symptoms, and what additional problems have occurred in each major body system and parts. The patient should be queried about dizziness, headaches, visual disturbances, bowel or bladder problems, weakness, numbness, and pain. During the history taking, the clinician should carefully observe the patient's behavior, attitudes, personal appearance and grooming, ability to answer the questions appropriately, and ability to concentrate (Lombardo & Hartwig, 1997). For patients with suspected frontal lobe tumors, an interview with the family is of utmost importance, because it can provide both the verification of complaints that may be difficult for the patient to articulate and additional information that may be unrecognized by the patient.

Physical Examination

A complete physical examination and diagnostic procedures should be performed to rule out processes other than a tumor that could be responsible for the symptoms, and to assess the patient's general state of health. A differential diagnosis may include such possibilities as multiple sclerosis, sarcoid, stroke, vascular malformation, cerebral abscess, and other medical problems as indicated by the symptoms. If a tumor is suspected, the following diagnostic tests should

TABLE 26-6 Assessment of the Patient for Glioma

	Assessment Parameters	Typical Abnormal Findings
History	A. Personal and social history 1. Occupation	A. Personal and social risk factors 1. Exposure to ionizing radiation, vinyl chlorides
Physical examination	A. Neurologic examination to assess mental function, level of consciousness, cerebral functions, language and speech, cranial nerve function, motor function, muscle tone and strength, reflexes, and sensory function	A. Signs and symptoms are determined by the tumor location and decree of malignancy. B. Seizures are the most common presenting symptom in astrocytoma. C. Headaches are characterized by increased severity in the morning and may be accompanied by vomiting in the absence of nausea. D. Other possible symptoms include paralysis, personality changes, failing vision or loss of vision, speech difficulties, behavioral disorders, or sensory disorders, such as "smelling something burning." R/O depression, anxiety, psychologic disease as primary disorder E. R/O multiple sclerosis, sarcoid, stroke, vascular malformation, cerebral abscess
Diagnostic tests	A. Computed tomography (CT) of brain	A. Shows brain calcification but not brain stem anatomy well. May show early stage tumor.
	B. Computerized tomograph of chest, abdomen, pelvis, bone	B. Diagnostic of metastasis.
	C. Mammograms	C. Shows metastasis to breast.
	D. Magnetic resonance imaging (MRI) scan with gadolinium k	D. Shows more anatomic detail compared with computed tomography and better defines tumor.
	E. Stereotactic needle biopsy or open craniotomy with resection	E. Stereotactic surgery can safely sample deep regions of tumor.
	F. Positron emission tomograph (PET)	F. Allows uptake of patterns of deoxyglucose by brain cell, making it possible to determine tumor recurrence or necrosis from previous treatment with radiation or chemotherapy
	G. Posterior-anterior and lateral chest x-rays, mammogram, pelvic examination	G. R/O underlying system malignancy.
	H. Guaiac stool for occult blood	H. R/O metastasis.
	I. Complete blood count, renal and liver function tests, electrolytes, calcium, magnesium, glucose and thyroid tests	I. R/O metastasis.

From Armstrong, T. & Gilbert, M. (1996). Glial neoplasms: classification, treatment, and pathways to the future. *Oncology Nursing Forum, 23,* 615-625; Mack, E. E. (1995). Neurologic tumors. In D. A. Casciato & B. B. Lowitz (Eds.), *Manual of clinical oncology* (3rd ed.). Boston, Little, Brown.

be undertaken to rule out a systemic malignancy elsewhere in the body:

- Posteroanterior and lateral chest x-ray films
- Complete blood count, renal and liver function tests, electrolytes, calcium, magnesium, glucose, and thyroid function tests
- Mammogram and pelvic examination
- Stool guaiac for occult blood (Mack, 1993)

Neurologic Evaluation

A neurologic evaluation as part of the physical examination is fundamental to confirming and localizing a neurologic lesion. The suggested order for a neurologic evaluation is (1) mental status and function, (2) level of consciousness, (3) cerebral functions, (4) language and speech, (5) cranial nerve function (critical for the diagnosis of brain stem tumors), (6) motor function (coordination and gait, muscle tone and strength), (7) reflexes, and (8) sensory function. The evaluation is so organized because each segment builds on information previously gathered, leading to the localization of the disease process (Lombardo & Hartwig, 1997). Table 26-7 outlines the procedure for the examination of the cranial nerves.

Special Diagnostic Procedures

Neuroimaging. Radiographic imaging is required to confirm the presence of intracranial tumors. Two recent ra-

TABLE 26-7 Examination of Cranial Nerves

Cranial Nerve	Method of Testing	Desired Response
I. Olfactory	Inhalation of commonly recognized aromatic substance such as cloves; avoid the use of ammonia or alcohol because they stimulate the trigeminal nerve and evoke a pain response	Identification of the substance with each nostril
II. Optic	Direct ophthalmoscopy; use finger movement and eye charts to test visual acuity and fields	Note the appearance of the optic disk, macula, vessels, and retina; correct eye movement and chart identification with each eye separately
III. Oculomotor IV. Trochlear VI. Abducens	Individual follows the examiner's finger with the eyes to test eye movement; check pupil response to light; observe for ptosis of the eyelid, which indicates destruction of cranial nerve III	Movement of eyes should be equal in all six cardinal directions of gaze; pupils react to direct and consensual response to light: eyes are symmetric at rest and move conjugatively
V. Trigeminal	Individual clamps the jaw, opens the mouth against resistance, and masticates to check motor division of the nerve; touch both sides of the person's face, checking for pain, touch, and temperature response; gently touch the person's cornea with a cotton wisp to check the corneal reflex	Correct identification of sensations; rapid blinking
VII. Facial	Observe for facial symmetry and the person's ability to contract muscles to check motor division; individual tastes sweet, sour, salty, and acidic flavors	Person smiles and frowns with symmetry; correct identification of tastes
VIII. Acoustic	Test hearing ability with the use of whispered voice and tuning fork at various distances from the ear to check the cochlear nerve; check the vestibular nerve by having the person stand on one foot with eyes closed	Recognition of sound; maintains balance
IX. Glossopharyngeal	Check the gag reflex by touching the pharynx with a tongue depressor	Gag response
X. Vagus	Check the individual's swallowing ability; ask the person to cough and speak; glossopharyngeal and vagus nerves are easily examined together because of overlapping innervation of the pharynx	Speaks without hoarseness or weakness
XI. Spinal accessory	Ask the individual to elevate the shoulders, turn the head, and resist the examiner's attempts to pull the chin back to midline; check the symmetry of the trapezius and sternocleidomastoid muscles	Equal bilateral muscle strength; atrophy may indicate nerve dysfunction
XII. Hypoglossal	Ask the individual to protrude the tongue	Absence of deviations, atrophy, or tremors

From Owens, B. (1992). Neurological cancers. In J. C. Clark, & R. F. McGee (Eds.), *Core curriculum for oncology nursing* (2nd ed.). Philadelphia: W. B. Saunders.

diologic advances, computed tomography (CT) and magnetic resonance imaging (MRI), are ideally adapted for the brain and spinal cord, and initial evaluation always includes one or the other (Lombardo, 1997; Kaiser & Kralendonk, 1991). Both produce cross-sectional digital images, but the MRI appears to have distinct advantages as a diagnostic tool.

CT is based on a single parameter and the electron density of the tissue being studied, and it can be obtained only in the axial or half-axial planes. MRI creates images based on the interrelation of four parameters: proton density, T1 and T2 relaxation times, and blood flow. In addition, MRI data can be acquired in any plane with no compromise of spatial or contrast detail (Levin, Leibel, & Gutin, 1997). It is also more effective for evaluating edema, hydrocephalus, or hemorrhage (Brant-Zawadski, Badami, Mills, Norman, & Newton, 1984) and provides a superior visualization of the relation of the tumor to adjacent cranial structures. Another advantage of MRI is that the patient is not exposed to radiation. Contrast agents used with CT (iodinated) and MRI (gadolinium) scans greatly improve the ability to discern tumors from other pathologic entities, one tumor type from another, and lower- from higher-grade malignancies (Butler, Horii, Kricheff, Shannon, & Budzilovich, 1978; Levin, Leibel, & Gutin, 1997).

MRI is particularly effective in the diagnosis of oligodendrogliomas and mixed gliomas, ependymomas, and brain stem gliomas. Oligodendrogliomas and astrocytomas are often slow-growing tumors and difficult to differentiate from normal surrounding tissue. Nearly 50% of these do not enhance on CT scans, and many are not detected at all if the tumor is isodense with brain. These tumors show clearly on MRIs even without enhancement. In addition, oligodendrogliomas occasionally bleed, and the MRI can distinguish between acute and subacute hemorrhage (Levin, Leibel, & Gutin, 1997).

Because they arise in the ventricles many ependymomas obstruct the flow of CSF in the ventricular system, causing hydrocephalus. MRI is a superior means of identifying hydrocephalus and locating either intrinsic or extrinsic ventricular obstruction. By visualizing which parts of the system are dilated, locations of obstruction (usually downstream) can be determined.

Because the MRI can be obtained in the sagittal and coronal planes and lacks bone artifact, it is ideal for detecting and characterizing tumors in the posterior fossa, brain stem, and base of the skull. Intra-axial and extra-axial tumors are both easily visualized (Levin, Leibel, & Gutin, 1997).

MRI is also valuable for radiation therapy planning and follow-up evaluation. The sagittal plane image can be superimposed on radiographic simulation films for accurate location of the tumor in preparation for port design. In addition, the new technique of dynamic contrast–enhanced MRI can differentiate the slow uptake of radiation injury from the fast uptake of highly malignant primary tumors (Levin, Leibel, & Gutin, 1997). Until the advent of this technique, separating signs, symptoms, and even radiographic images of radiation damage from tumor growth or recurrence was impossible without tissue biopsy.

As a result, MRI is the imaging procedure of choice for neoplasms. If MRI technology is not available in a given community, a CT scan with administration of an iodinated contrast is an acceptable second choice. However, when using a CT with contrast it is important to take precautions for a possible allergic reaction.

Additional Diagnostic Tests

MRI is so effective in identifying lesions in the CNS that many of the older and/or more invasive diagnostic procedures are seldom used except for confirmation of a diagnosis. However, several additional diagnostic procedures are still occasionally used. For instance, myelography is sometimes required for staging of anaplastic ependymomas.

Cerebral angiography is an invasive procedure usually not required for the evaluation of tumors, but it may be obtained to verify that a lesion is a vascular malformation or an aneurysm as opposed to a tumor. Angiography is also used for evaluation of highly vascular tumors or tumors sharing a blood supply with other neural structures before surgery (Mack, 1993).

Pneumoencephalography is an invasive procedure used to improve imaging of the cavities of the brain by filling them with air. It is a risky and uncomfortable procedure. This procedure is rarely used since the advent of MRI and CT.

Lumbar puncture (LP) is useful for staging tumors such as medulloblastomas and ependymomas, which are known to spread along the neural axis, or for evaluating patients with evidence of meningeal seeding. However, its use before radiographic studies is contraindicated in any patient with a suspected CNS tumor. The LP creates an unacceptable risk for cerebellum–foramen magnum or temporal lobe–tentorial herniation, both of which are fatal. Once radiographic confirmation and location of a tumor are obtained, the examination of CSF may be justified for tumors such as ependymomas and medulloblastomas. The fluid can be examined for cytology (malignant cells), protein, glucose, and specific markers such as beta–human chorionic gonadotropin (HCG) and alpha fetoprotein (AFP), all of which are indicators of tumor presence (Levin, Leibel, & Gutin, 1997).

Electroencephalography is used primarily to diagnose seizure disorders and to determine whether neurologic deterioration may be due more to subclinical seizures than tumor growth (Levin, Leibel, & Gutin, 1997).

Tissue Biopsy

Biopsy of a tissue sample from the tumor is imperative for the definitive diagnosis and histologic staging of the tumor. The exception is deep-seated or inaccessible tumors, especially those for which radiographic and clinical findings are characteristic. The techniques currently in use for obtaining biopsies are diagnostic neurosurgery and resection, during which a tissue sample is obtained, or stereotactic needle biopsy.

Surgery should be the first treatment modality for any patient with a primary tumor, because total resection is the best opportunity for cure. Even if total resection is not possible, as is the case with most gliomas, aggressive tumor debulking and consequent decompression of the brain are important clinical goals, because they reduce intracranial pressure and alleviate symptoms (Levin, Leibel, & Gutin, 1997; Murphy, Morris, & Lange, 1997). A tumor tissue biopsy can be obtained as a by-product of complete tumor resection of surgically accessible primary tumors.

When open cranial surgery is not a viable option, a stereotactic needle biopsy should be used. This would be the case for patients who are a poor surgical risk and for tumors for which surgical resection is not practical. These tumors include intrinsic tumors of the deep midline (pontine or corpus callosum gliomas), deep tumors of the dominant hemisphere, or diffuse nonfocal tumors.

Stereotactic biopsy involves the use of a stereotactic frame and CT, MRI, or ultrasound guidance for accurate insertion of the needle into the tumor bed. CT-guided stereotaxy is considered to be the easiest method for needle biopsy (Levin et al., 1977). This biopsy technique has the advantage of a short hospital stay, usually 24 hours, a less than 3% occurrence of hemorrhage, low morbidity, and a low mortality of 1% (Salcman, 1990). However, the downside may be insufficient yield of specimen for biopsy (Murphy, 1997) or missing the tumor altogether.

GRADING/STAGING

Grading of a tumor refers to the histologic pathology of a tumor, and *staging* refers to the extent of spread or infiltration. The histopathologic analysis of biopsied tumor tissue is the key element in grading gliomas and the most important factor in determining outcome. Staging is based on histopathology, grade, tumor location, and microscopic evidence of the completeness of tumor resection and is classified in ascending grades of malignancy.

Because the distinction between benign and malignant tumors is of little use, and because brain tumors do not spread outside of the CNS, the staging system used for most cancers has limited application in the brain. From review of the literature, no one system is universally used in classifying primary brain tumors.

The Kernohan staging system is widely used (Kernohan, Moborn, & Svien, 1949; Zulch, 1979). This system is based on degree of malignancy and uses a I through IV staging, with IV being the most malignant grade (GBM). Unfortunately, it is of little prognostic value since the life expectancies for stages I and II are generally equivalent (5+ years), as are those for stages III and IV (Laws, Taylor, Clifton, & Ozaki, 1984).

The World Health Organization (WHO) system is a three-tier system also commonly used and tends to avoid the prognosis problem of the Kernohan system. The classification categories with median survival rates are the astrocytoma (grades I and II, 5 to 7 years), the anaplastic astrocytoma (grade III, 18 to 24 months), and GBM (grade IV, 8 to 10 months).

The TNM (tumor, node, metastases) classification system, although more complex because of additional variables, is also used. Table 26-8 details how this staging system is used. The American Joint Committee on Cancer has developed a new system based on signs and symptoms and the results of various diagnostic tests. It appears to be a streamlined version of the TNM classification (Murphy, Morris, & Lange, 1997). Levin and colleagues (1997) have deemed the three-tier system satisfactory for most purposes.

Unfortunately, the lack of a common system for tumor grading renders the comparability of cohorts among different studies, and thus the comparability and reliability of study results, difficult to judge.

TREATMENT MODALITIES

Surgery, radiotherapy, and chemotherapy, alone and in combination, are the three treatments most commonly used for gliomas. Although surgery with total gross resection remains the treatment of choice, the infiltrative nature of glio-

TABLE 26-8 TNM Classification of Brain Tumors

Primary Tumor (T)
TX Primary tumor cannot be assessed
T0 No evidence of primary tumor

Supratentorial Tumor
T1 Tumor 5 cm or less in greatest dimension; limited to one side
T2 Tumor more than 5 cm in greatest dimension; limited to one side
T3 Tumor invades or encroaches on ventricular system
T4 Tumor crosses midline, invades opposite hemisphere, or invades infratentorially

Infratentorial Tumor
T1 Tumor 3 cm or less in greatest dimension; limited to one side
T2 Tumor more than 3 cm in greatest dimension; limited to one side
T3 Tumor invades or encroaches on the ventricular system
T4 Tumor crosses midline, invades opposite hemisphere, or invades supratentorially

Regional Lymph Nodes (N)
This category does not apply to this site.

Distant Metastasis (M)
MX Presence of distant metastasis cannot be assessed
M0 No distant metastasis
M1 Distant metastasis

Histopathologic Grade (G)
GX Grade cannot be assessed
G1 Well differentiated
G2 Moderately well differentiated
G3 Poorly differentiated
G4 Undifferentiated

Stage Grouping

Stage IA	G1-T1-M0
Stage IIB	G1-T2-M0
	G1-T3-M0
Stage IIA	G2-T1-M0
Stage IIB	G2-T2-M0
	G2-T3-M0
Stage IIIA	G3-T1-M0
Stage IIIB	G3-T2-M0
	G3-T3-M0
Stage IV	G1, G2, G3-T4-M0
	G4-any T-M0
	Any G-any T-M1

From Beahrs, O. H., Henson, D. E., Hutter, R. V. P., & Kennedy, J. (1992). *Manual for staging of cancer* (4th ed.). Philadelphia: J. B. Lippincott; Murphy, M. E. (1997). Cancers of the brain and central nervous system. In S. E. Otto (Ed.), *Oncology nursing*. (3rd Ed.). St. Louis: Mosby.

mas and their resiliency make a cure difficult but not impossible to achieve. As a result, radiation therapy plays an important role in the treatment of gliomas, most often in combination with surgery. Chemotherapeutic applications have not been particularly effective, but this modality is currently used as a palliative measure and is usually reserved for the more highly malignant tumors and recurrent tumors, which do not have good prognoses. Chemotherapy is also plagued with delivery and toxicity problems. Other modalities are being investigated, such as brachytherapy and radiosensitizers in radiotherapy, regional infusion of chemotherapy, and bone marrow transplantation in conjunction with high doses of chemotherapy, hyperthermia, biotherapy, and photodynamic therapy. These and other new and experimental methods are reviewed later in this section.

Surgery

Gross total resection is the initial treatment goal for all primary glial tumors because it offers the best chance for a cure. Recent advances in surgery have made nearly every tumor accessible and the surgical procedures reasonably safe. However, surgery should not be attempted if tumor location presents too great a risk, multiple tumors exist, the patient is in poor medical condition, major neurologic deficits are not responsive to steroid therapy, or the tumor is rapidly spreading (Owens, 1992).

For tumors that cannot be totally removed, aggressive cytoreduction should be undertaken. With careful resection, using modern surgical technology, 90% of the typical astrocytoma or oligodendroglioma can be removed. In a review of retrospective studies, Armstrong and Gilbert (1996) cited several authors who reported significant improvement in patient outcomes with aggressive subtotal resection (Devaux, O'Fallon, & Kelly, 1993; Franklin, 1992; Nazarro & Neuwelt, 1990; Simpson, Horton, Scott, Curan, Rubin, & Fischbach, 1993; Vecht, Avezaat, van Putten, Eijkenboom & Stefanko, 1990). Evidence exists that radiotherapy and chemotherapy outcomes are enhanced by aggressive cytoreduction, or debulking, of the tumor mass (DeVita, 1983; Laws et al., 1984; Waller, Alexander, Hunt, McCarty, Mahaley, & Mealey, 1978; Salcman, 1990).

Several studies have shown an inverse correlation between the amount of residual tumor with positive outcomes such as patient survival time (Winger, MacDonald, & Cairncross, 1989; Wood, Green, & Shapiro, 1988) and quality of life as measured by the Karnofsky performance score (Andreou, George, Wise, deLeon, Kricheff, & Ransohoff, 1983). In addition, a direct relationship has been seen in the burden of postirradiation necrotic tissue in the tumor site and the level of resulting cerebral edema. Aggressive cytoreduction greatly reduces this dead cell mass (Gutin, Leibel, Wara, Choucair, Levin, & Philips, 1987; Kumar, Hoshino, Wheeler, Barker, & Wilson, 1974). Finally, DeVita (1983), following a review of the literature, cited three additional benefits of aggressive resection: (1) the number of separate cell populations in these heterogeneous tumors is reduced, thereby eliminating some already radioresistant or chemoresistant populations; (2) the probability of further mutation toward resistance is decreased by lowering the overall number of tumor cells; and (3) the number of cells in regions remote from blood vessels where chemotherapeutic agents cannot penetrate and where hypoxia can (theoretically) confer radioresistance is reduced.

Studies also indicate that surgical resection of recurrent tumors is a valuable treatment approach (Harsh, Levin, Gutin, Seager, Silver, & Wilson, 1987; Salcman, 1990; Young, Oldfield, Markesbery, Haack, Tibbs, & McCombs, 1981). Harsh and colleagues reported that reoperation significantly enhanced chemotherapy response in recurrent tumors. Resection of recurrent tumors appears to be of benefit regardless of patient age, tumor grade, performance status, or interval between initial treatment and recurrence (Salcman, 1990). However, because of tissue damage from previous treatments, the postoperative infection rates tend to be high.

The safe surgical approach and resection of a tumor are facilitated by an operating microscope. Most glial tumor margins are demarcated by glistening peritumoral white matter easily identified through the microscope. Because glial tumors are infiltrative, a 2-cm margin of microscopically confirmed healthy tissue is usually excised to increase the probability of total tumor removal.

The recently developed surgical technique of cortical mapping now allows the removal of tumors in functionally critical areas of the brain. The procedure uses intraoperative cortical stimulation to determine the safest routes through cortical tissue to underlying tumors, as well as optimal resection limits of tumors adjacent to these areas (Berger, Kincaid, Ojemann, & Lettich, 1989).

Stereotactic Surgery. Perhaps the most important current advancement in tumor treatment has been the introduction and continuing refinement of stereotatic surgery. Stereotactic surgery uses computerized guidance systems to locate tumors and conduct the process of surgery with unprecedented accuracy. This new system greatly improves accessibility and resectability of tumors previously thought to be inoperable. Because the extent of tumor removal is the most important indicator of patient outcome, stereotactic surgery is a major technologic advancement in the field (Sawaya, 1991).

Stereotactic surgery relies on high-quality radiologic images obtained by CT or MRI. These images allow for a three-dimensional depiction of the tumor and surrounding tissue and structures. Reference points (usually 6) around the tumor are selected and displayed on the images, which appear on a monitor. All of the information goes into a computer that is connected to a new device that has a movable arm that ends in a "wand" that the surgeon can move over the surface of the head to pinpoint the tumor and obtain precise information about tumor dimensions (NEWS, 1997).

With this new technology, surgeons can identify and have safe surgical access to small tumors, deep tumors, and tumors that arise in particularly complex or sensitive areas of the brain. In addition, resectability of these tumors is greatly improved since surgeons are able to determine when they have reached the margin of a tumor.

A recent and significant advancement has connected CT/MRI and a computer system to a surgical microscope, allowing surgeons to keep both hands free of stereotactic devices (NEWS, 1997). Refinements in this system continue to be made. New technology is in various stages of development and evaluation. Those considered imminent are discussed in the Research Issues section of this chapter.

Pharmaceutical agents normally given preoperatively and postoperatively are corticosteroids (usually dexamethasone) for control and reduction of edema and swelling in the brain, and antiseizure drugs (usually phenytoin). These drugs may be used indefinitely after surgery since they are also helpful for combatting some treatment complications and tumor progression symptoms.

Radiation Therapy

As is the case with surgery, radiation therapy is a localized treatment that targets only the tumor and surrounding tissue. Brain parenchyma is not particularly radiosensitive because of a relatively low vascularization of this tissue. However, it does tolerate radiation therapy fairly well.

Radiotherapy uses high-energy beams or radioactive isotopes as the source of radiation for treatment. The two types of radiotherapy used are the standard external beam radiation with the source outside the body, and brachytherapy, or internal therapy, in which a radioactive source is placed inside the body close to the tumor. Both types have standard and experimental applications in various phases of study.

Radiotherapy is used as adjuvant treatment with complete surgical resection to destroy any remaining stray tumor cells, as combined therapy with surgery in subtotal resection of tumors, and as a primary means of treating inoperable, high-grade and recurrent tumors (not previously treated with radiation). At times, adjuvant chemotherapy is given with the radiotherapy. The response rate of slow-growing tumors tends to be low, but medulloblastomas, glioblastomas, high-grade gliomas, and, to a lesser extent, oligodendrogliomas are particularly radiosensitive.

The benefit of postsurgical adjuvant irradiation for adults with complete tumor resection is currently under debate. Some advocate immediate radiotherapy (Shaw, Daumas-Duport, Scheithauer, Gilbertson, O'Fallon, & Earle, 1989; Shaw, Scheithauer, & O'Fallon, 1991), whereas others prefer to wait for signs of tumor progression before proceeding (Leibel, Sheline, Wara, Boldrey, & Nielsen, 1975; Morantz, 1987; Berger, Deliganis, Dobbins, & Keles, 1994).

For subtotal tumor resection, the radiotherapy question is not whether, but when. Irradiation is standard treatment for these tumors either immediately after surgery or at the first sign of progressive, nonresectable tumor (MacDonald, 1994; Van Glabbeke, Karim, Hamers, Harlevoll, Pierat, & Bartelink, 1995). This recommendation holds true for both low- and higher-grade gliomas. Patients who receive radiotherapy have a significant survival advantage over those who do not (Berger, Leibel, Bruner, Finlay, & Levin, 1996; MacDonald, 1994; Shaw, Scheithauer, & O'Fallon, 1991). For patients with high-grade or inoperable tumors, radiation therapy is the treatment of choice, often followed by chemotherapy (Urtasun, Kinsella, Farman, Del-Rowen, Lester, & Fulton, 1996).

The standard form of radiation treatment is external beam radiotherapy targeted at a field volume that includes the tumor and the surrounding edematous area, plus a 2-cm margin (Armstrong & Gilbert, 1996). The conventional total dosage is up to 60 Gy in 30 fractions (2 Gy per day) over 6 weeks. Dosage is limited by a brain tolerance threshold that appears to be at, or close to, this dosage. Sheline and associates have estimated threshold levels to be 35 Gy for 10 fractions, 60 Gy for 35 fractions, and 76 Gy for 60 fractions (Sheline, Wara, & Smith, 1980).

Another method of external radiation therapy, intraoperative radiation therapy (IORT), is delivered during surgery via external beam radiation equipment with a special adapter for intraoperative use. This technique allows for high-dose delivery of radiation directly to the tumor without harming healthy tissue that would otherwise be in the beam's path.

Stereotactic radiation therapy is a recently developed procedure currently only used to treat brain tumors. During the procedure, the head is immobilized by a surgically attached stereotactic frame, such as the one used for needle biopsy. Using an MRI or CT scan–generated map of the tumor and brain, a movable robotic arm of the radiotherapy machine is computer guided around the head, delivering hundreds of beams of radiation to the tumor site. The procedure typically lasts 40 minutes (Murphy, Morris, & Lange, 1997) (Table 26-9).

Brachytherapy involves the use of interstitial (Bernstein, Lapperriere, Leung, & McKenzie, 1990) or intraventricular (or spinal) implants of radioactive sources placed directly into or adjacent to the tumor bed during surgery (Florell, MacDonald, Irish, Bernstein, Leibel, & Gutin, 1991). Brachytherapy has most often been used as an adjunct to standard external beam radiation, particularly for recurrent tumors, but is currently being evaluated as an initial therapy (Murphy, Morris, & Lange, 1997). A recent randomized, comparative study showed a survival advantage for patients treated with both brachytherapy and standard external beam radiation over those with external beam only (Green, Shapiro, Burger, Selker, VanGilder, & Saris, 1994).

Interstitial implants placed during surgery are later "afterloaded" with ribbons of radioactive seeds smaller than grains of rice. The implant typically remains in the tumor bed for 3 to 5 days while the radioactive source decays and the necessary dose is delivered. In intraventricular implants, an applicator is placed in the ventricle and afterloaded with the radioactive source. The applicator is removed when the prescribed dosage has been achieved (Murphy, Morris, & Lange, 1997).

Two experimental therapies currently being evaluated are of particular note. The first is the use of drugs termed *radiosensitizers.* These drugs enhance the effects of radiation. Some drugs take the place of oxygen in hypotic cells (the more highly oxygenated the cell, the more effective is the radiotherapy outcome), some transport oxygen to the cells, and others are absorbed by the DNA inhibiting the ability of the cell to repair itself (Murphy, Morris, & Lange, 1997).

A recent study of an experimental treatment for patients with anaplastic gliomas using the radiosensitizer BrdU (5-

TABLE 26-9 Patient Preparation for Stereotactic Radiosurgery

Description of Procedure: Stereotactic radiosurgery is a nonsurgical procedure using focused beam of high-dose radiation to correct vascular malformations or treat brain tumors.

Patient Preparation

1. Wash your hair with the shampoo containing iodine given you at the clinic.
2. Do not eat or drink after midnight of the night before your procedure unless you are taking medications. In this case, take your medication with sips of water only. Be sure to check with your physician before taking the medications.
3. Bring your regular medications to the hospital with you.
4. Bring music to listen to after the procedure.
5. You may bring a family member.

Procedural Considerations:

1. You will sign an informed consent.
2. You will always have a physician or nurse with you during and after the procedure.
3. An IV is inserted into your arm and you will be given medication to help you relax.
4. A local anesthetic (2% lidocaine with epinephrine) will be given to your head to prepare you for the metal frame on your head.
5. The metal frame will then be placed on your head.
6. The frame will be attached in four places: two on your forehead and two on the back of your head.
7. You will then have computed tomography (CT), magnetic resonance imaging (MRI), or angiograph scans to locate the exact site to be treated.
8. Once the treatment is completed, the frame will be removed and bandages applied to your head.
9. After the treatment is completed, you will be placed on a radiation treatment table.
10. You will not be able to move your head, but you can move your arms and legs and; if you have not had an angiogram, you may walk around.
11. If you have had an angiogram, you may need to stay in bed for 8 to 12 hours.
12. Your pulse and blood pressure will be taken frequently.
13. You can be discharged from the treatment center when you feel well, which is usually the same day or the next morning.
14. You may rinse your scalp with warm water only after you return home.

Special Considerations

1. You may experience some side effects, but they are usually not serious.
   a. a dull headache easily controlled with medication
   b. nausea/vomiting related to headache or not eating
   c. swelling/bruising that can be managed with warm soaks
   d. seizures (patients with previous seizures are at higher risk)
   e. infection (rare), but can be managed with antibiotics
2. If you have any of these problems, call your physician.

From Morgan, R. H., Rines, T., D'Aquila, K., Merlo, M., & Benzil, D. L. (1997). Preparing for stereotactic radiosurgery. *Developments in Supportive Cancer Care, 1*(4), 101:102.

bromo-2′-deoxyuridine) plus radiotherapy (totally 60 Gy) followed by chemotherapy with procarbazine, lomustine, and vincristine (PCV) yielded a significantly improved progression-free survival than that of other therapies commonly used (Levin, Prados, Wara, Davis, Gutin, & Phillips, 1995). This regimen is currently being evaluated as a possible new standard of treatment.

The second experimental therapy currently being evaluated is hyperthermia. Tumor cells are known to be heat sensitive, and temperatures in the range of 105°F to 110°F (43°C) will either kill the cells outright or greatly enhance their radiosensitivity. In a recent study of stereotactic, MRI-guided thermal ablation using radiofrequency energy, the authors reported no disease progression in any of the 12 patients treated (Anzai, Lufkin, DeSalles, Hamilton, Farahani, & Black, 1995). This treatment method appears promising, but additional evaluation is necessary to corroborate its effectiveness.

Recent and ongoing radiotherapy investigations are generally focused on identifying methods for achieving more frequent exposure of mitotic tumor cells to radiation, increasing radiation dosage directly to the tumor tissue, and identifying means for increasing the radiosensitivity of tumor tissue.

Chemotherapy

Chemotherapy is currently used as a palliative measure, normally for inoperable, high-grade or recurrent tumors, in combination with surgery and/or radiotherapy. The goals of chemotherapy are to reduce edema and the size of the tumor mass so as to reduce neurologic deficits and prolong a useful and comfortable life. Unfortunately, response rates for chemotherapeutic agents remain low, usually 20% to 40%.

Several key factors are likely responsible for the low response rate of chemotherapy. The main problem most often cited is the blood-brain barrier. Most agents effective elsewhere in the body have restricted blood-brain barrier permeability (Levin, 1986). To pass the barrier, agents must be lipid soluble and/or of low molecular weight. The agents currently most active against parenchymal tumors, the nitrosoureas, readily cross the blood-brain barrier (Levin, 1985).

Neurotoxicity is almost equally as important a limiting factor as the blood-brain barrier for many chemotherapy agents due to the high doses required to be effective. Many of the infiltrating gliomas have cell populations that are remote from vasculature, particularly the larger tumors, limiting agent access to portions of the tumor. In addition, a large percentage of the cells in gliomas are in a resting state and relatively insensitive to cell-cycle agents. Another complicating factor is the tendency of these tumors to have a heterogeneous population of cells. To be effective, either an agent must be able to achieve cell kill in a variety of cells, or multiple agents, each targeted at specific cells, must be administered. Because of these efficacy-limiting factors, a paucity of drugs with demonstrable antitumoral activity has been identified for treatment of gliomas.

Nitrosoureas, such as carmustine (BCNU), semustine (PCNU), lomustine (CCNU), and nimustine (ACNU), are permeable to the blood-brain barrier and have been effective as single agents (Levin & Wilson, 1981). They typically are used concurrent with or after radiation therapy. Other single agents, such as diaziquone, cisplatin, and thioTEPA, have been used in adjuvant settings. Upchurch and colleagues initially reported a response rate of 30% to 40% for these agents, but a reanalysis of the data using new, more stringent response criteria yielded a response rate of 5% to 7% (Armstrong & Gilbert, 1996; Upchurch, Goodwin, Brown, Selby, Vogel, & Eyre, 1993).

Other agents used include the alkylating (nitrogen gas, cyclophosphamide) and antitumoral (bleomycin, mythramycin, doxorubicin) antibiotics, plant alkaloids (vincristine, etoposide), antimetabolics (methotrexate), and procarbazine, among others (Murphy, 1997). Procarbazine has been identified as an active agent and is commonly used (Kumar, Renaudin, Wilson, Boldrey, Enot, & Levin, 1974). Bleomycin, doxorubicin, cisplatin, vincristine (VCR), and mithramycin have shown no activity in adults but some show activity for primitive childhood and embryonal tumors (Levin, Leibel, & Gutin, 1997). All of these agents have side effects detailed in the upcoming section on Medical Management.

Alavi (1995) reported that for anaplastic astrocytomas and oligodendrogliomas adjuvant chemotherapy can prolong survival. The agents most often used are carmustine (BCNU) or the PCV regimen of procarbazine, lomustine, and vincristine. These agents are administered with or immediately after radiation and continued up to 1 year. Little evidence exists that adjuvant chemotherapy improves survival time for GBM. Another group has used intravenous carboplatin for recurrent malignant gliomas (Yung, Mechtler, & Gleason, 1991).

Regional drug delivery is far preferable to oral or systemic intravenous (IV) administration for optimal drug exposure to the tumor. Three methods are currently used: intra-CSF therapy, intra-arterial infusion, and intratumoral therapy.

Intra-CSF therapy is used primarily to treat meningeal neoplasia, and to a lesser extent, ventricular tumors. Drugs are administered usually by ventricular reservoir. This method has the advantages of high local drug levels, low system toxicity, and the ability to adjust frequency of treatments. However, it can be dangerous and tends to have a high morbidity rate.

Methotrexate, cytarabine, and thioTEPA are the drugs most commonly used in intra-CSF therapy, but all three have side effects ranging from fever to leukoencephalopathy and myelitis. The effectiveness of the drugs is limited by the size of the tumor and by any interruption of the CSF flow. In addition, the slow clearance of the drug from the CSF system, which is common, increases the neurotoxicity of the drug (Levin, Leibel, & Gutin, 1997).

Intra-arterial infusion of antitumor agents via the vertebral or interior carotid arteries has recently been under study. This method has the supposed advantage of increased uptake of the drug by the tumor tissue on the first pass through the tumor capillaries. However, it turns out that the amount of drug absorbed by the tumor is but a small fraction of the injected dose. Initial infusions were also administered just below the branch of the ophthalmic artery, resulting in significant retinal morbidity (Elsas, Watne, Fostad, & Hager, 1989; Feun, Wallace, Yung, Lee, Leavens, & Moser, 1984; Maiese, Walker, Gargan, & Victor, 1992).

Another difficulty with the intra-arterial method is the inability of the injected drugs to mix adequately with the pulsing arterial flow. The drugs tended to "stream," following along the wall of the artery until they reached a branch, where they veered off in high concentration into the brain tissue lying ahead. Severe neurotoxicity and tissue necrosis resulted (Armstrong & Gilbert, 1996). Because of these problems, intra-arterial infusion currently is not recommended as a delivery mechanism.

Intratumoral therapy is used primarily for cystic tumors with narrow rims of surrounding tumor. Initial applications of this method have been plagued by difficulties in maintaining sufficient cavity drug levels, diffusion distances to the outer margins of the tumor, biodegradation and binding of the drug, and the need for repeat treatments (Levin, Leibel, & Gutin, 1997). Clinical trials evaluating this delivery method have yet to be published.

Several experimental therapies aimed at improving drug dose delivery directly to the tumor are currently being evaluated. Several of these are of interest. The first involves the disruption of the blood-brain barrier. Mannitol is administered intra-arterially via the carotid artery located on the same side of the tumor. This drug provides a transient opening of the blood-brain barrier through which subsequently injected intra-arterial or IV chemotherapy can pass. Clinical trails demonstrated that normal brain tissue received a much greater concentration of the drug than did the tumor, and neurotoxicity was high. Seizures occurred in 56% of the patients, transient focal neurologic deficits in 58%, and permanent deficits in 8% (Neuwelt, Howieson, Frenkel, Specht, Weigel, & Buchan, 1986).

The second experimental therapy appears more promising. A bioerodable polymer wafer, saturated with a chemotherapy agent, is placed directly into the tumor cavity after surgical resection. Carmustine is the most commonly used agent and is incorporated into polyanhydride compounds, which slowly release the drug into the tumor cavity over 3 to 5 weeks. No system toxicity was found in phase I and II studies, and the mean survival from the time of wafer placement was 48 weeks (Brem, Mahaley, Vick, Black, Schold, & Burger, 1991). In a recently completed phase III blind study, the overall increase in survival between the group receiving the wafer and the group with the placebo was 8 weeks. The median time was 31 weeks compared with 23 weeks (Brem, Piantadosi, & Burger, 1994).

The third experimental therapy is continuous infusion of a chemotherapy agent(s) using prolonged IV administration. Armstrong and Gilbert (1996) report that results of a phase II pilot study of the continuous infusion of carmustine and cisplatin before radiation has shown dramatic response rates for newly diagnosed tumors (67% response, 17% remission) (Gilbert, Lunsford, Kondzsiolka, Flickinger, Matey, & Armstrong, 1993; Gilbert, Lunsford, Kondzsiolka, Flickinger, Shumaker, & Ziegler, 1993; Grossman, Sheidler, Ahn, Gilbert, Wharam, & Bucholtz, 1989). The response rate for patients treated at recurrence was 50%, with 15% showing complete remission (Gilbert, Matey, Minhas, Bozik, Armstrong, & Shumaker, 1994). A phase II trial is currently under way to further evaluate this promising treatment.

Another area of investigation, also reported by Armstrong and Gilbert, is focused on determining means to treat malignant gliomas that become refractory to chemotherapy. Acquired resistance to nitrosoureas is thought to be a result of increased intracellular concentration of the enzyme 06-AGAT (D'Incalci, Citti, Taverna, & Catapano, 1988). The experimental treatment is designed to inhibit this enzyme. Patients who originally failed carmustine therapy are treated with a combination of 6-mercaptopurine and streptozocin, which have been shown to inhibit 06-AGAT, followed by a continuous infusion of carmustine. The objective response rate was 29% (Gilbert et al., 1994). Newly identified inhibitors such as 06-benzylguanine are currently being evaluated in preclinical and phase I trials (Marathi, Kroes, Dolan, & Erickson, 1993).

Biotherapy

Biotherapy is an emerging field of treatment that is attracting great interest. Biotherapy stimulates the body's own immune system to recognize, attack, and destroy cancer cells. It is not, as yet, a frontline therapy (except for hairy cell leukemia, chronic myeloid leukemia, Kaposi's sarcoma, and kidney cancer) and is generally considered an experimental treatment. Biotherapy is currently likely to benefit only a very small percentage of cancer patients (2%).

The two basic categories of biotherapy are immunotherapy, both active and passive, and tumor cell modulation therapy (cytotoxic therapy). Immunotherapy works by triggering an immune response or by using immune cells to create a hostile environment for the cancer cells. Tumor cell modulation therapy uses proteins called *cytotoxins,* produced by the body's cells, to attack the cancer by destroying the cells or by inhibiting their ability to grow and reproduce. Table 26-10 lists agents currently under investigation in each category.

Active immunotherapy uses agents that trigger a general immune response activating a wide range of immune cells. Agents used for this purpose include interferon, interleukin-2 (IL-2), and the tuberculosis bacillus Calmette-Guerin (BCG). The immune response to tuberculosis has long been known to cause certain cancers to regress. The injection of these agents into the area where tumors are growing has met with some success but unfortunately not for parenchymal brain tumors.

As reported by Armstrong and Gilbert (1996), systemic administration of IL-2 and lymphokine-activated killer (LAK) cells resulted in severe neurologic damage with profound edema, and, in many cases, herniation (Yamasaki, Kikuchhi, Paine, Yamashita, Miyatake, & Iwasake, et al., 1989). In addition, local delivery of IL-2 and LAK cells into the tumor bed showed little effect (Merchant, Ellison, & Young, 1990; Merchant, McVicar, Merchant, & Young, 1992; Merchant, Merchant, Cook, McVicar, & Young, 1988). The use of beta-interferon and gamma-interferon showed little benefit over that of conventional treatment (Jaeckle, 1994).

Passive immunotherapy appears to have more potential as a treatment because components of the immune system are treated and activated in the laboratory and readministered to the patient. This approach is also known as *adoptive immunotherapy.* This technique uses genetic engineering technology and thus is expensive.

The agents most commonly used are tumor cell vaccines,

TABLE 26-10 Biologic Therapies for Glioma

Classification
Active immunotherapy
Nonspecific; immune-boosting substances (i.e., bacillus Calmette-Guerin [BCG])
Interferon
Interleukin-2
Passive immunotherapy
Specify; immunization with tumor cell vaccines
Antibodies
Monoclonal antibodies
Lymphokine-activated killer cells
Tumor-infiltrating lymphocytes (TIL)
Cytotoxic (tumor cell modulation)
Inhibition of tumor growth factors or angiogenic (blood vessel) factors

Modified from Murphy, G. P., Morris, L. B., & Lange, D. (1997). *Informed decisions: The complete book of cancer diagnosis, treatment, and recovery.* New York: Viking.

antibodies and monoclonal antibodies, LAK cells, and tumor-infiltrating lymphocytes (TIL). LAK cells have been found to be highly neurotoxic, and antiglioma antibody treatment outcome is no better than with conventional treatment (Jaeckle, 1994). The use of TIL is currently under investigation.

Tumor cell modulation therapy uses cytotoxins to change the cancer cell's biology to weaken and kill the cell. The best known cytotoxin is a growth factor called *tumor necrosis factor* (TNF), a toxin produced by macrophages that inhibits the blood supply to the cells. Other growth factors including granulocyte-macrophage colony-stimulating factor (GM-CSF), transforming growth factor-beta (interferes with tumor cells supporting structures and blood cells), thymic hormones (stimulates the immune system, used as a supporting therapy), and the use of vaccines are all cytotoxic therapies currently being studied. The use of bacterial derivatives and retinoids is also under investigation.

Although nothing of much value in the treatment of brain tumors has yet emerged, biotherapy is a rapidly growing field of cancer treatment, and a myriad of studies are underway. The results of these studies should be carefully monitored.

Bone Marrow Transplantation

High-dose chemotherapy (HDC) followed by autologous stem cell recovery (ASCR) and transplantation is a treatment currently being evaluated for brain tumors rarely cured by conventional therapies. Patients with high-grade gliomas such as anaplastic astrocytoma, anaplastic oligodendrogliomas and oligoastrocytomas, brain stem gliomas, and GBM, as well as those with recurrent gliomas, may benefit from this therapy. Because gliomas do not spread beyond the CNS, these patients are good candidates for marrow-related transplants.

The chemotherapy agents that are most active against gliomas are the alkylating agents such as carmustine. These agents have a steep dose-responsive curve in which higher doses may produce dramatic improvement. However, increased dosages also have a dramatic devastating effect on the bone marrow. HDC/ASCR therapy allows higher dosages to be used while still salvaging the marrow.

A combination of two or more drugs is used in high doses following the harvesting of the stem cells. These drugs include thiotepa, etoposide, BCNU (carmustine), carboplatin cyclophosphamide, and/or melphalon. Combinations are now used to limit the toxicity of single agents. After the administration of chemotherapy, the stem cells are transfused back into the patient. Blood and platelet transfusion are given until the stem cells have begun to produce an adequate supply of blood cells.

The August 1997 issue of *The Blood and Marrow Transplant Newsletter* reviewed the findings of the approximately 400 patients treated to date (New hope for patients with a brain tumor, 1997). HDC/ASCR has been found to benefit some patients with recurrent high-grade gliomas and medulloblastoma/PNET. However, for patients with brain stem gliomas and ependymomas, treatment was of little benefit. Successful treatment appears to be linked to the amount of postsurgery residual tumor. Those with at least 90% tumor removal seem to benefit the most.

Armstrong and Gilbert (1996) reported that initial studies using nitrosoureas found severe, irreversible systemic toxicity. When diaziquone and VP-16 were used, only modest results were noted (19% partial response) (Giannone & Wolf, 1987). In addition, nearly all of the tumors treated recurred, and the patients, because of depleted marrow reserves, could not continue to receive further cytotoxic chemotherapy. Subsequent studies using a combined high-dose treatment of thioTEPA and bone marrow transplantation appeared more promising (Ascensao, Ahmed, Feldman, Agoliti, Perchick, & Goldberg, 1989).

Research in the HDC/ASCR treatment is still in the early stages, and results are inconclusive. Studies are underway to determine which combination of chemotherapy drugs are most effective against which tumors, and to identify the optimal timing for HDC/ASCR therapy.

Photodynamic Therapy

Experimental research is underway to evaluate the effectiveness of intensive light treatment for brain tumors. Some feel photodynamic therapy (PDT) has the greatest potential for positive outcomes of any of the experimental treatment currently being studied.

PDT is an oxygen-dependent, photochemical oxidative process using photosensitive agents that are retained in cancer cells. These agents are activated by an illuminating source with resulting destruction of the tumor's neovasculation, leading to tumor necrosis. The most commonly used photosensitizing agent is hamatoporphyrin derivative (Photofrin). Photofrin is administered intravenously, through an artery, or directly into the tumor bed during surgery, and activated with outside lumination of the tumor bed. Currently PDT is limited to treating small tumors (<1 cm) because Photofrin is unable to reach the outer margins of the larger infiltrating gliomas (Murphy, 1997).

Gene Therapy

Gene therapy is a relatively new field with seemingly excellent potential for the treatment of neoplasms. The goals of gene therapy include replacing the damaged genes of tumor cells with healthy ones, halting the cells' uncontrolled growth, and introducing genetic material that alters the cell's metabolism, either causing it to self-destruct or making it more vulnerable to additional forms of treatment. Both of these strategies are currently under intensive investigation.

One area of experimental gene therapy being followed with great interest is the use of an altered cancer-specific "suicide" virus known as *GLI-328.* The treatment uses a genetically altered mouse leukemia virus containing a gene from the herpes simplex virus called *thymidine kinase-1* (herpes TK gene). The leukemia virus, genetically altered to self-destruct after invading a cancer cell, infects only dividing cells. Normal brain cells do not divide and thus are not invaded. Once infected, the tumor cells produce thymidine kinase, making them vulnerable to the antiviral drug ganciclovir. However, the results of several recent clinical studies, although encouraging, have been inconclusive.

A recent National Institutes of Health (NIH) pilot study used a herpes TK gene delivered directly to the tumor bed to treat 10 patients with recurrent glioblastoma (DeVroom, 1994). These patients received no additional treatment. The therapy appeared to reduce 4 of the 10 tumors, some as much as 50%, but produced no impact on overall survival, with the exception of one patient still alive 5 years after treatment (Goldberg, 1998). A Phase II study begun in 1994 used direct injection of an improved clone of the TK virus on 31 patients with recurrent glioblastomas concurrent with surgery to resect as much as possible of the tumor regrowth. Although average survival showed no improvement over repeat surgery and chemotherapy, 20% of the patients were still living 3 to 4 years after treatment. Whether those who survived did so solely as a result of the gene therapy is controversial. However, the director of the study stated that these 20% achieved a major benefit not seen with any other therapy (Goldberg, 1998).

A phase III study is currently underway at 44 university and other hospitals in the United States and nine other countries. A total of 250 patients with newly diagnosed glioblastomas are receiving treatment either with surgery, radiotherapy, and gene therapy; or with surgery and radiotherapy alone. This is the first large, randomized trial to evaluate any form of gene therapy. Results are pending.

More than 100 clinical trials for the treatment of a variety of illnesses have been undertaken with little uncontested evidence of therapeutic benefit. Regardless of these inconclusive results, however, the field of gene therapy is in its infancy. Many basic components of the therapy, such as the optimal techniques for and the best timing of gene delivery are still being determined. Whether gene therapy can achieve the results once thought to be so promising has yet to be determined.

TREATMENT OF SPECIFIC GLIOMAS

Because oligodendrogliomas, oligoastrocytomas, and ependymomas are fairly rare, accounting for only about 7% to 9% of primary brain tumors, information on the treatment of these tumors is limited compared with astrocytomas and glioblastomas. Brain stem gliomas are typically astrocytomas but tend to have a poor prognosis due to their location and the diffuse, infiltrative nature of these tumors. The information in this section on the suggested treatment regimens for each tumor type and the outcomes of studies evaluating standard and experimental treatment is taken primarily from two sources: the National Cancer Institute (NCI) CancerNet (1998) and the section on Neoplasms of the Central Nervous System by Levin, Leibel, and Gutin (1997). This latter source is an excellent review of the recent literature regarding treatment of these tumors. References to the original sources are noted in the text.

General Treatment Options

Surgical removal of the tumor to the greatest extent possible while preserving neurologic function is the first treatment option for all tumors. The exceptions are deep-seated tumors, such as pontine gliomas, which are diagnosed on clinical evidence and treated by radiation therapy without prior surgery about 50% of the time. However, stereotactic surgery can now be used for many such tumors that have been difficult to reach and resect in the past. Surgery is also the treatment of choice for recurrent tumors.

Radiation therapy has a major role in the treatment of many of these tumors and has been shown to increase the cure rate or prolong disease-free survival. Radiotherapy is also used to treat recurrent tumors not previously treated by radiation. Chemotherapy has had modest results in lengthening disease-free survival in patients with gliomas and medulloblastomas.

Patients with tumors that are deemed incurable should be considered for clinical trials that evaluate radiosensitizers, hyperthermia, or interstitial brachytherapy used with external-beam radiotherapy to control tumor progression. They should also be considered for studies evaluating new chemotherapy drugs and biologic response modifiers (BRMs) (NCI/CancerNet; Allen, Bloom, Ertel, Evans, Hammond, & Jones, 1986).

Adult Brain Stem Gliomas

Astrocytomas are the most prevalent of the brain stem gliomas, although oligodendrogliomas and ependymomas are occasionally seen. These tumors generally have a poor prognosis because they tend to be central, diffuse, and infiltrative and often involve both the cranial nerves and the afferent and efferent nerve tracks of the CNS. Tumors that are more focally infiltrative have a better prognosis.

Brain stem gliomas are most commonly found in the pons and are usually slow-growing astrocytomas. Tumors involving the midbrain tend to be well differentiated or anaplastic astrocytomas. Those involving the medulla are typically rapidly progressing glioblastomas found mostly in children.

The NCI recommends the following treatment options:

- Standard: Radiotherapy (Greenberger, Cassady, & Levene, 1977; Levin, Edwards, Wara, Allen, Ortega, & Vestnys, 1984). The best results have been attained with hyperfractionated doses (Shrieve, Wara, Edwards, Sneed, Prados, & Cogen, 1992).
- Under clinical evaluation: At recurrence, patients should be considered for clinical trials evaluating new drugs and BRMs (Rodriguez, Prados, Fulton, Edwards, Silver, & Levin, 1988).

The treatment options reviewed by Levin and associates (1997) are summarized below with augmentation as available.

Surgery. The location and critical functions of the brain stem generally preclude tumor resection as a therapeutic goal. The use of MRI for diagnosing brain stem gliomas now allows differentiation of gliomas from other lesions such as multiple sclerosis, brain stem abscesses, foramen magnum meningiomas, arteriovenous malformations, and clivus tumors; and biopsy is no longer critical for this purpose. Biopsies of gliomas on the lateral surface of the pons, or those accessible through the floor of the fourth ventricle, can be safely procured, and associated cysts drained. Complete resection should not be attempted (Levin, Leibel, Gutin, 1997).

Radiotherapy. Radiation therapy is the primary treatment of brain stem gliomas. Use of this therapy improves survival and, in the majority of cases, can stabilize or reverse neurologic dysfunction (Eifel, Cassady, & Belli, 1987; Kim, Chin, Pollan, Hazel, & Webster, 1980).

Gliomas are currently treated with doses of up to 50 to 60 Gy (1.8 Gy/fraction/day) through parallel opposed portals. Sagittal MRI use and the newer three-dimensional radiation therapy planning technology have improved targeting to the specific contours of the tumor. Usually, a margin of 2 cm of normal tissue is included in the irradiated volume.

The use of hyperfractionated irradiation designed to deliver higher tumor doses is under evaluation as a means of improving outcomes and better preventing the common recurrence of these tumors (Edwards, Wara, Urtasun, Rados, Levin, & Fulton, 1989; Freeman, Krischer, Sanford, Cohen, Burger, & Kun, 1991; Freeman, Krischer, Sanford, Cohen, Burger, & DelCaprio, 1993; Halperin, 1985; Packer, Allen, Goldwein, Newell, Zimmerman, & Priest, 1990; Packer, Boyett, Zimmerman, Rorke, Kaplan, Albright, 1993; Prados, Wara, Edwards, Larson, Lamborn, & Levin, 1995). The dosage recommended is 70.2 Gy (1 Gy twice daily). No increase in acute or delayed radiation-induced toxicity using this dose has yet been documented. Initial findings indicate a consistent, if modest, improvement in median survival for patients treated with hyperfractionated irradiation (Packer et al., 1990; Freeman et al., 1991). This dosage is currently being used in a POG randomized trial comparing hyperfractionated radiotherapy with 54-Gy conventional fractionation. Both groups of patients receive displatin during radiotherapy (Freeman et al., 1993). Results of this trial are not yet available.

In a more recent study, patients with anaplastic gliomas were given the radiosensitizer BrdU (5-Bromo-2'-deoxyuridine) plus radiotherapy (total of 60 Gy) followed by PCV chemotherapy. Results showed a better progression-free survival (4-year survival rate of 46%) than other therapies (Levin, Prados, Wara, Davis, Gutin, & Phillips, 1995). Pending the results of additional studies, this regimen could be a new standard of treatment.

Chemotherapy. The use of chemotherapy for brain stem gliomas is palliative. Nitrosoureas are the most commonly used agents. Chemotherapy as an adjunct to irradiation has been used infrequently. Studies comparing radiation therapy with radiation therapy followed by chemotherapy (CCNU, PCV and prednisone), and 5-fluouracil (5-FU) and CCNU before irradiation found no differences in the groups (Jenkin, 1983; Levin et al., 1984). However, as mentioned previously, results using the radiosensitizer BrdU plus radiotherapy followed by PCV were encouraging.

Few therapies have been evaluated for progressive or recurrent brain stem gliomas. One study showed some improvement in patients treated with 5-FU, CCNU, hydroxyurea, and 6-mercaptopurine. Although the group was small ($n = 13$) 69% had response or stabilization, with a relapse-free survival of 25 weeks (Rodriguez et al., 1988). A phase II study was undertaken in 5 patients with recurrent malignant glioma treated with a combination of BCNU and DFMO (difluoromethylornithine). Three of the five had continuing benefit of 1 to 3 years after treatment (Prados, Rodriguez, Chamberlain, Silver, & Levin, 1989).

Oligodendrogliomas

Treatment options for oligodendrogliomas are nearly identical to those for astrocytomas, although they tend to be more chemosensitive. Oligodendrogliomas most often arise in the frontal lobes of the cerebrum. However, they are occasionally found in the other cerebral lobes, the third or lateral ventricles, or protruding into a ventricle from the hypothalamus. About 10% spread through the CSF. These tumors are usually either differentiated or anaplastic. Progression to GBM is rare, although nearly two thirds of oligodendrogliomas that recur do so as an anaplastic astrocytoma or a glioblastoma. Nearly half of the oligodendrogliomas actually contain astrocytoma or ependymoma cells and are then referred to as mixed gliomas.

The NCI recommends the following treatment options for adult, well-differentiated oligodendrogliomas:

- Standard: Surgery plus radiation therapy; however, some controversy exists. Some physicians treat patients less than 45 years of age with surgery alone if the tumor is not contrast-enhanced on CT or MRI scan.
- Under clinical evaluation: Clinical trials are evaluating the effect of adding drugs to radiotherapy for tumors that are incompletely resected.

The cure rate for adult anaplastic oligodendroglioma is very low using standard local treatment (Kyritsis, Yung, Bruner, Gleason, & Levin, 1993). The NCI recommends the following treatment options:

- Standard: (1) Surgery plus radiotherapy. (Bullard, Rawlings, Phillips, Cox, Schold, & Burger, 1987; Burger, Rawlings, Cox, McLendon, Schold, & Bullard, 1987; Lindegaard, Mørk, Eide, Halvorsen, Hatlevoll, & Solgaard, 1987; Wallner, Gonzales, & Sheline, 1988) and (2) surgery plus radiotherapy plus chemotherapy (Cairncross & MacDonald, 1988; Cairncross, MacDonald, Ludwin, Lee, Cascino, & Buckner, 1994).
- Under clinical evaluation: Clinical trials are underway evaluating the use of interstitial brachytherapy, radiosensitizers, hyperthermia, and intraoperative radiotherapy in conjunction with external-beam radiotherapy.

Mixed gliomas (oligoastrocytomas, oligoependymomas, and oligoastroependymomas) have a prognosis somewhere between the anaplastic grade of each of the involved cells. The NCI recommends the following treatment options:

- Standard: (1) Surgery plus radiotherapy and (2) surgery plus radiotherapy plus chemotherapy (Kyritsis et al., 1993)
- Under clinical evaluation: The same trials are available as described for patients with anaplastic oligodendroglioma.

The treatment options reviewed by Levin and associates (1997) are summarized below with augmentation as available.

Surgery. Surgery, with the goal of total resection, is the first-line treatment for oligodendrogliomas and mixed gliomas. Unfortunately, although these tumors appear to have distinct margins, their infiltrative nature makes surgical cure the exception. However, as is the case with astrocytomas, subtotal resection, or debulking of the tumor mass, has benefits that far outweigh the risk of surgery.

Radiotherapy. Radiation therapy plays an important role in the treatment of oligodendrogliomas, but the typically long prediagnosis, and posttreatment natural history of these tumors renders the evaluation of the value of radiation treatment inconclusive and controversial. In addition, the lack of randomized trials makes firm recommendations for treatment difficult to determine.

Recent studies comparing subtotal resection with and without irradiation seem to point to the advantages of radiation as an adjunct treatment. Five- and 10-year survival rates for the irradiated cohorts ranged from 36% to 83% and 30% to 46%, respectively. Rates for the nonirradiated cohorts were 25% to 55% and 13% to 25% (Berger et al., 1996; Chin, Hazel, Kim, & Webster, 1980; Gannett, Wisbeck, Silbergeld, & Berger, 1994; Halperin, Kun, Constine, & Tarbell, 1989; Lindegaard et al., 1987; MacDonald, 1994; Shimizu, Tran, Mark, & Selch, 1983; Sun, Genka, Shitara, Akanuma, & Takakura, 1988; Wallner et al., 1988). A meta-analysis of reports from the current literature undertaken by Shimizu and colleagues indicates that postoperative irradiation conferred a 14% improvement in 5-year survival (Shimizu et al., 1993).

Most retrospective studies comparing surgery alone to surgery and radiation have flaws in the comparability of treatment groups, raising concerns about the validity of the study results. Many studies combined patients with differentiated and anaplastic oligodendrogliomas in the same study groups when such histologic differences have very different survival outcomes (9 years vs 2.2 years).

Many physicians currently recommend postoperative irradiation for all patients with subtotal resection of oligodendrogliomas. Others argue that only those with anaplastic tumors or mixed oligoastrocytomas should be treated (Halperin et al., 1989); still others contend that treatment should be delayed until evidence of tumor progression or recurrence appears (Mørk, Halvorsen, Lindegaard, & Eide, 1986).

Taken as a whole, the data suggest a benefit of irradiation to patients with large, symptomatic, unresectable or subtotally resected low-grade oligodendrogliomas. The radiation target field is recommended to include the tumor volume plus a 2- to 3-cm margin. Adult doses are recommended to be between 54 and 60 Gy (50 Gy for children).

Anaplastic oligodendrogliomas and mixed gliomas have a considerably poorer prognosis than the differentiated tumors, with the mixed gliomas having the worse prognosis of the two. Patients with these higher-grade tumors generally receive a radiation dose of 60 Gy (1.8 to 2.0 per day).

Chemotherapy. Prospective chemotherapy trials for the treatment of oligodendrogliomas are currently underway. Chemotherapy has been used for the primary treatment of highly anaplastic tumors adjuvant to surgery and radiation therapy, as well as for recurrent well-differentiated and moderately anaplastic tumors.

Treatment with chemotherapy included nitrosourea-based therapies, and the combination of PCV, procarbazine, DFMO-MGBG, and thioTEPA. Cairncross and Macdonald (1988, 1991, 1993) have used a combination of CCNU, procarbazine, and VCR for treatment of recurrent oligodendrogliomas. PCV therapy has been tried for recurrent anaplastic oligodendrogliomas with outcomes of a median survival of 1.2 years. Recurrent oligoastrocytomas treated with the same regimen showed a median relapse-free period of 1 to 1.2 years (Cairncross & MacDonald, 1991; Kyritsis et al., 1993).

Levin, Leibel, and Gutin (1997) reported that the efficacy of this regimen is currently being tested in newly diagnosed patients through a Radiation Therapy Oncology Group (RTOG) combined intergroup randomized trial comparing neoadjuvant intensive PCV chemotherapy followed by radiation therapy with radiation therapy alone. Results are not yet available.

Table 26-11 shows relapse-free survival and overall survival of the various treatments for initial and recurrent oligodendroglioma, mixed oligoastrocytoma, and anaplastic oligodendrogliomas.

Ependymomas

Ependymomas arise in the ependymal lining of the ventricles and the CSF pathways. They typically occur in the white matter adjacent to a ventricular surface. Sixty percent of these tumors are infratentorial, the majority of which are found in the fourth ventricle. Extension into the subarachnoid space occurs in nearly half of these cases. The remaining 40% are supratentorial, half of which are intraventricular and the other half parenchymal arising from ependymal rests. Seventy-five percent of the intraventricular tumors are in the lateral ventricles, with the remaining 25% in the third ventricle.

Ependymomas are usually of low grade and less likely to be anaplastic compared with other gliomas. However, they tend to spread through the CSF pathways. The well-differentiated ependymomas are often curable. The anaplastic ependymomas and ependymoblastomas are malignant with prognoses dependent on location and extent of disease. The ependymoblastoma is rare.

The NCI recommends the following treatment for well-differentiated adult ependymoma (Shaw, Evans, Scheit-

TABLE 26-11 Outcomes of Patients Treated for Oligodendroglioma, Oligoastrocytoma, and Anaplastic Oligodendroglioma Initially and at Recurrence

Oligodendroglioma	
Initial Treatment	
Surgery only (mean 8 studies)	43% 5-yr survival
Surgery + RT (mean 9 studies)	58% 5-yr survival ($P = 0.02$)
PCV + RT	
Treated at First Relapse	
Median time to first tumor recurrence ($n = 21$)†	2.4 yr
Median time from recurrence to death ($n = 12$)*†	1.4 yr
Median relapse-free survival for PCV ($n = 12$)	1.2 yr
Mixed Oligoastrocytoma	
Initial Treatment	
PCV + RT	80% 2-yr relapse-free survival
Treated at First Relapse	
Median time to first tumor recurrence ($n = 53$)†	1.8 yr
Median time from recurrence to death ($n = 20$)*†	1.6 yr
Median relapse-free survival for PCV ($n = 10$)	1.3 yr
Anaplastic Oligodendroglioma	
Initial Treatment	
RT only†	50% 3-yr survival
RT + chemotherapy*†	50% 3-yr survival
RT + PCV	57% 2-yr relapse-free survival
Treated at Recurrence	
Median relapse-free survival for mPCV, carmustine, diaziquone ($n = 8$)	1.2 yr
Median relapse-free survival for PCV ($n = 14$ therapies in 12)	1.0 yr

From Levin, V. A., Leibel, S. A., & Gutin, P. H. (1997). Neoplasms of the central nervous system. In V. T. DeVita, S. Hellman, & S. A. Rosenberg (Eds.), *Cancer: The principles and practice of oncology* (5th ed.). Philadelphia: J. B. Lippincott.
RT, Radiation therapy; *PCV*, Procarbazine, lomustine, and vincristine.
*Chemotherapy included nitrosourea-based therapies, the combination of PCV, procarbazine, DFMO-MGBG, and thioTEPA.
†V. A. Levin et al., unpublished observations 1987, 1995.

hauer, Ilstrup, & Earle, 1987; Wallner, Wara, Sheline, & Davis, 1986):

- Standard: (1) Surgery alone if totally resectable and (2) surgery followed by radiotherapy to known or residual tumor.
- Under clinical evaluation: At recurrence following surgery, patients should be considered for reoperation and radiotherapy if not previously used. Those who have already received radiotherapy could be candidates for nitrosourea-based chemotherapies and for clinical trials that evaluate new drugs and biological response modifiers.

For adult malignant ependymoma, the NCI recommends the following treatment options:

- Standard: Surgery plus radiotherapy.
- Under clinical evaluation: Adjuvant chemotherapy before, during, and after radiation are treatment options currently being evaluated. At recurrence, treatment is the same as that recommended for low-grade ependymomas.

The review and recommendations for treatment of ependymomas by Levin and associates (1997) follows.

Surgery. Supratentorial ependymomas are usually amenable to gross total resection, as they tend to be well circumscribed from surrounding brain tissue. They are also often cystic. A wide craniotomy is required for total resection, and the tumor is removed with the aid of an operating microscope. Minimal bleeding into the ventricle is key, and bleeding that does occur must be removed to avoid CSF pathway blockage and irritation to the brain tissue from bloody CSF.

Ependymomas arising in the floor of the fourth ventricle are approached through a wide bilateral suboccipital craniectomy and laminectomy of C1. The tumor is exposed by retracting the cerebellar tonsils laterally and splitting the inferior aspect of the vermis (Levin, Leibel, & Gutin, 1997). These tumors are typically attached to the floor of the ventricle and must be carefully exposed for evaluation. If the tumor is firmly attached to the floor and/or infiltration into the cranial nerves of the cerebropontine angle has occurred, total resection is contraindicated. Maximal resection should be undertaken when possible using the illumination and magnification of the operating microscope. An inverse correlation exists between the level of residual tumor and the efficacy of radiation therapy.

Radiotherapy. Patients with intracranial ependymomas clearly benefit from postsurgical irradiation. Doses of 45+ Gy are usually administered. Five-year survival rates range from 40% to 78% (Leibel & Sheline, 1987). However, the amount of normal tissue to be included in the target volume, and whether the prophylactic irradiation of the entire craniospinal axis should be undertaken, are currently controversial. Ironically, a recent review of the literature by Vanuytsel and Brada seemed to indicate a higher incidence of ependymal tumor seeding in those who received prophylactic craniospinal axis irradiation than in those treated with local radiation only (Vanuytsel & Brada, 1995). Other studies concluded that because tumor recurrence appears to be limited to the original site, the inclusion of anything other than a generous local field was unnecessary.

Low-grade supratentorial ependymomas are currently treated with a generous target volume to a dose of at least 54 Gy. The same recommendation is true for patients with low-grade infratentorial tumors. The craniospinal axis is included only if malignant cytology is found in the CSF or radiologic studies confirm tumor spread.

Radiation treatment for anaplastic ependymomas should include the entire craniospinal axis (Salazar, Castro-Vita, Van Houtte, Rubin, & Aygun, 1983; Vanuytsel, Bessell, Ashley, Bloom, & Brada, 1992; Wallner et al., 1986). The primary tumor site should receive a dose of 54 Gy with a 36-Gy dose given to the axis. If subsequent spread of the tumor is seen, the entire brain should receive 54 Gy; spinal irradiation is raised to 50 Gy. Given that ependymomas recur locally, spinal metastasis does not occur without local tumor recurrence, prophylactic treatment does not appear to prevent spinal seeding, and local field inclusion in the irradiated volume appears to be sufficient, many question whether use of spinal radiation or whole brain radiation results in improved survival.

The high rate of eventual treatment failure is primarily due to the current inability to eradicate the original tumor in both low- and high-grade ependymomas (Vanuytsel et al., 1992). More aggressive methods to achieve local control are currently being examined in clinical trials.

Chemotherapy. Because ependymomas are uncommon, few chemotherapeutic trials are underway. Table 26-12 provides published and unpublished data regarding chemotherapy for recurrent ependymomas. The best single agents appear to be carmustine (BCNU) and dibromodulcitol. Results from the use of these drugs are better than those achieved for anaplastic astrocytomas. TPDCV (6-thioguanine, procarbazine, dibromodulcitol, lomustine [CCNU], and vincristine [VCR]) has the best response among the drug combinations (Bertolone, Baum, Krivit, & Hammond, 1989; Gaynon, Ettinger, Baum, Siegel, Krailo, & Hammond, 1990; Ettinger, Ru, Krailo, Ruccione, Krivit, & Hammond, 1990; Goldwein, Leahy, Packer, Sutton, Curran, & Rorke, 1990; Levin, Edwards, Gutin, Vestnys, Fulton, & Seager, 1984).

TABLE 26-12 Chemotherapy for Recurrent Ependymoma and Anaplastic Ependymomas

Treatment	Number	Responding[a] (%)	Median Time to Progression (mo)
BCNU[b]	14	78	13
Dibromodulcitol[c]	12	75	16
AZQ[d]	12	42	10
Carboplatin[e]	14	28	14
Cisplatin[f]	8	75	3.8
VCR-CDDP-CCNU-PCB-VP16-IFSO[g]	16	22	9
6TG-PCB-DBD-CCNU-VCR[h]	11	82	21.6
Weighted mean			16

From Levin, V. A., Leibel, S. A., & Gutin, P. H. (1997). Neoplasms of the central nervous system. In V. T. DeVito, S. Hellman, & S. A. Rosenberg (Eds.), *Cancer: The principles and practice of oncology.* (5th Ed.). Philadelphia: J. B. Lippincott.

[a]Responding (%) = $\frac{\text{(response + stable patients)}}{\text{total patients}}$.

[b]V. A. Levin et al., unpublished observations, 1987.
[c]Levin, Edwards, Gutin, Vestnys, Fulton, & Staeger, 1984.
[d]Ettinger, Ru, Krailo, Ruccione, Krivit, & Hammond, 1990.
[e]Gaynon, Ettinger, Baum, Siegel, Krailo, & Hammond, 1990.
[f]Bertolone, Baum, Krivit, & Hammond, 1989.
[g]Goldwein, Leahy, Packer, Sutton, Curran, & Rorke, 1990.
[h]16 patients were treated on 37 different trials.

MEDICAL MANAGEMENT

Medical management of gliomas is required on two fronts: problems related to the tumor and complications resulting from treatment.

Tumor-Related Problems

The first priority of clinical intervention is to alleviate symptoms produced by the tumor. These symptoms are the result of mass effect (and increased intracranial pressure) due to the tumor and peritumoral edema, and/or by tumor infiltration and destruction of normal tissue. Patients must be monitored and treated, if necessary, for the following tumor-related problems: edema, hydrocephalus, hemorrhage, increased ICP, seizures, neurologic dysfunction, and impending herniation, which is a medical emergency.

Malignant gliomas often produce profound cerebral edema. The edema appears to result from the disruption of the blood-brain barrier and the endothelia of surrounding vasculature.

The degree of edema is directly associated with the increase in ICP. Cerebral edema leads to tissue hypoxia and acidosis. Symptoms include headaches and neurologic dysfunctions depending on the location of the edema. This condition is countered with corticosteroids, which is part of the presurgical protocol. Dexamethasone is the drug of choice, but methylprednisolone is also used. Side effects of these drugs include osteopenia, hyperglycemia, poor wound healing, proximal muscle weakness, and weight gain (Armstrong & Gilbert, 1996).

Intratumoral or peritumoral hemorrhage can occur and is usually associated with oligodendrogliomas and glioblastomas. (Hemorrhage can also be due to thrombocytopenia secondary to chemotherapy and to the use of the anticonvulsant drug valproate.) The use of osmotic agents and glucocorticoids may reduce signs and symptoms, but an extensive hemorrhage usually requires surgical decompression.

Hydrocephalus occurs when the CSF pathway is blocked by either a tumor in the ventricles, such as an ependymoma, or pressure from tumors in the brain stem. Hydrocephalus also contributes to increased ICP. Symptoms are headache, nausea, vomiting, gait ataxia, urinary incontinence, and lethargy. Conventional treatment is the placement of a ventriculoperitoneal shunt.

Increased ICP usually results from an increase in intracranial volume due to an expanding tumor and related edema. It is a potentially fatal complication and rapid onset of ICP is considered a medical emergency (ICP/herniation is discussed later in this section). Management includes surgical removal or debulking of the mass with subsequent diuretic and corticosteroid therapy.

Seizures occur in 20% to 40% of patients with brain tumor, and are particularly associated with oligodendrogliomas. They usually indicate neurologic deterioration and can lead to permanent neurologic dysfunction and medical complications such as aspirative pneumonia, and can be life threatening. Treatment either for the presence of seizures or prophylactically for the prevention of seizures is also part of the presurgical protocol. Patients typically remain on antiseizure medications for at least 1 year after surgery.

Most anticonvulsant drugs require the attainment and maintenance of therapeutic levels in the blood. This can be achieved either through a loading dose in emergent situations or through maintenance therapy given until a therapeutic level is reached. The most commonly used agent is phenytoin (Dilantin), which in adults requires a loading dose of 1 g/kg weight, and a maintenance dose of 300 mg/day for a therapeutic level of 10 to 20 μg/ml. Phenobarbital is most often used in an emergency setting, since it can be administered intravenously. The loading dose is 20 mg/kg with maintenance doses of 90 to 120 mg/day and a therapeutic level of 15 to 40 μg/ml. The only major side effect is sedation. Carbamazepine is often used in nonemergent treatment. It is available only in oral form. Maintenance levels must be attained slowly, because a loading dose is not tolerated. Doses range from 60 to 100 mg/day with a therapeutic level of 6 to 12 μg/ml. Valproate, also administered orally, is given at a dose of 15 mg/kg/day with a therapeutic level of 50 to 100 μg/ml. Table 26-13 lists the dose, therapeutic blood levels, and side effects of common anticonvulsant medications (Mack, 1993).

Thromboembolitic events are common in patients with gliomas, especially deep venous thrombosis. Armstrong and Gilbert (1996) report that studies have shown a 23% to 54% incidence of thromboembolism in patients with glial tumors at some point in the course of their disease (Altshuler, Moosa, Selker & Vertosick, 1990; Dhami, Bona, Calogero, & Hellman, 1993). These events appear to be related to the increased production of clotting factor by glial tumors (Sawaya et al., 1991).

Patients should be carefully monitored for onset of thromboembolitic symptoms, especially since corticosteroids tend to mask related inflammation. DVT presents with soreness in the calf, asymmetric leg swelling, and edema. Pulmonary emboli manifest with pleuritic chest pain, transient nonproductive cough, tachypnea, and hyponatremia. DVT can be confirmed with Doppler studies, and moderate

TABLE 26-13 Common Anticonvulsant Medications

Medication Barbituates	Dose	Therapeutic Blood Level (μg/ml)	Side Effects/Toxicities
Phenobarbital	60-400 mg/day	10-30	Drowsiness, mental dullness, nightmares, dizziness, fever, depression, irritability, rash, loss of libido, ataxia, anemia, nystagmus
Mephobarbital (Mebaral)	400-600 mg/day	25-50	Same as phenobarbital plus facial edema and possible hypersensitivity reactions
Primidone (Mysoline)	250-1500 mg/day	5-15	Same as phenobarbital plus diplopia, alopecia, impotence, lupus-like syndrome
Hydantoin			
Phenytoin (Dilantin)	300-600 mg/ml	10-20	Gastrointestinal upset, ataxia, diplopia, nystagmus, gingival hyperplasia, dermatitis, hirsutism, hypocalcemia, osteomalacia, agranulocytosis, leukopenia, megaloblastic anemia, insulin suppression, increased cholesterol, lupus-like syndrome, low bound thyroxin level
Others			
Carbamazepine (Tegretol)	600-1200 mg/day	2-8	Drowsiness, psychotic behavior, ataxia, dizziness, diplopia, nystagmus, dry mouth, skin eruptions, jaundice, edema, leukopenia, aplastic anemia, pancytopenia
Valproic acid (Depakene)	15-60 mg/kg/day	50-100	Drowsiness, ataxia, altered bleeding times, liver toxicity, transient hair loss, leukopenia, nausea and vomiting, depression, hallucinations, bone marrow depression
Clonazepam (Klonopin)	3-12 mg/day		Drowsiness, ataxia, dizziness, thick speech, hypotonia, hyperactivity, anorexia, rash, thrombocytopenia, palpitations, bradycardia, hirsutism, hysteria

Modified from Rudy, E. (1984). *Advanced neurological and neurosurgical nursing.* St. Louis: Mosby.
From Owens, B. (1992). Neurological cancers. In J. C. Clark & R. F. McGee (Eds.), *Core curriculum for oncology nursing* (2nd ed.). Philadelphia: W. B. Saunders.

hypoxia with a decreased PCO_2 indicates a pulmonary embolus (Armstrong & Gilbert, 1996). Both are life threatening, and the optimal treatment is insertion of a filter in the vena cava. Use of anticoagulants is risky immediately after surgery, but they may be used with careful monitoring if a filter cannot be placed (Mack, 1992). Some studies suggest the incidence of DVT can be reduced by the use of compression stockings and the administration of subcutaneous heparin during hospitalization (Cerrato, Ariano, & Fiaccjiono, 1978; Skillman, Collins, Coe, Goldstein, Shapiro, & Zervas, 1978).

Neurologic dysfunctions are related to tumor destruction of neuronal tissue, edema, hemorrhage in or around the tumor, and focal seizure activity. Usually, treatment of the tumor and the underlying edema significantly improve neurologic dysfunction. The effect of remaining deficits may be eased with rehabilitation services.

ONCOLOGIC EMERGENCIES

The major oncologic emergency associated with gliomas is the rapid onset of increased ICP with its impending brain herniation and death.

Increased ICP can be the result of an increase in mass within the cranium, peritumoral edema, hydrochephalus, and/or tumor-related hemorrhage. Rapid-onset ICP is a medical emergency. Immediate measures must be taken to prevent herniation of the brain and resulting death. Figure 26-15 illustrates the physiopathologic progression to death as a result of ICP. Accompanying symptoms include headache, vomiting, mental acuity changes, seizures, alterations in motor and sensory responses, changes in vital signs, ocular changes, wide pulse pressure, irregular respirations and bradycardia (Murphy, 1997).

Herniation of the uncus occurs when the medial gyrus of the temporal lobe is displaced inferiorly through the tentorial notch by a mass in the supratentorium. The resulting pressure on the midbrain can cause a loss of consciousness and compression of cranial nerve III (Lombardo, 1997). Table 26-14 lists the neurologic findings and related pathologic causes of uncal herniation.

Cerebellar herniation occurs when the cerebellar tonsils are displaced downward through the foramen magnum by a mass in the posterior fossa. Compression of the medulla and respiratory arrest quickly follow. Table 26-15 lists the neurologic findings and associated causes of cerebellar herniation. This herniation syndrome often results from obstructive hydrocephalus. In such cases, emergency removal of fluid from the ventricular system may be life saving. Ventriculoperitoneal shunting is often required as a follow-up measure.

Prompt intervention is necessary to prevent these herniation syndromes and impending death. Immediate IV administration of hyperosmotic agents such as mannitol at 50 to 100 g/kg in adults, and large doses of synthetic glucocorticoids such as dexamethasone (up to 100 mg) or methylprednisolone should be undertaken. The head of the bed should also be elevated and hyperventilation to a PCO_2 of about 30 mm Hg pursued.

TABLE 26-14 Temporal Lobe and Tentorial (Uncal) Herniation

Neurologic Findings	Pathologic Cause
Pupillary dilation and ptosis	Compression of ipsilateral oculomotor nerve between herniating tissue and petroclinoid ligament
Ipsilateral hemiplegia	Compression of contralateral cerebral peduncle against tentorium (Kernohan's notch)
Contralateral hemiplegia	Compression of ipsilateral cerebral peduncle; when associated with compression of contralateral peduncle, bilateral corticospinal tract signs will be present
Homonymous hemianopia	Compression of posterior cerebral artery against the tentorium can lead to occipital ischemia or infarction and contralateral homonymous hemianopia; occasionally bilateral field-cuts will occur.
Midbrain syndrome: Cheyne-Stokes respirations, stupor–coma, bipyramidal signs, decerebrate rigidity, dilated fixed pupils, gaze paresis, altered oculocephalic reflexes	Crushing of midbrain between herniating temporal lobe and leaf of tentorium associated with vascular occlusion and perivascular hemorrhage
Coma, rising blood pressure, and bradycardia	These late signs occur from rising intracranial pressure and hydrocephalus as the aqueduct is compressed and subarachnoid space compromised.

Modified from Adams, R. D. & Victor, M. (1977). *Principles of neurology.* New York: McGraw-Hill.
From Levin, V. A., Leibel, S. A., & Gutin, P. H. (1997). Neoplasms of the central nervous system. In V. T. DeVita, S. Hellman, & S. A. Rosenberg (Eds.), *Cancer: The principles and practice of oncology* (5th ed.). Philadelphia: J. B. Lippincott.

Therapy-Related Complications

Complications of Surgery. Potential complications of surgery include intracranial bleeding, cerebral edema, infection, thrombosis, hydrocephalus, and neuromotor deficits. Treatment for infection involves the use of antibiotics that can be undertaken prophylactically. Treatment for the remaining complications have been discussed previously.

TABLE 26-15 Cerebellar–Foramen Magnum Herniation

Neurologic Findings	Pathologic Cause
Head tilt, stiff neck, posturing of neck, or paresthesias over the neck	Downward displacement of inferior hemispheres through the foramen magnum; may be unilateral or bilateral
Tonic extensor spasms of limbs and body (cerebellar "fits") and later coma	Compressive effects of cerebellum or hydrocephalus on the upper brain stem
Respiratory arrest	Medullary compression

Modified from Adams, R. D., & Victor, M. (1977). *Principles of neurology.* New York: McGraw-Hill.
From Levin, V. A., Leibel, S. A., & Gutin, P. H. (1997). Neoplasms of the central nervous system. In V. T. DeVito, S. Hellman, & S. A. Rosenberg (Eds.), *Cancer: The principles and practice of oncology* (5th ed.). Philadelphia: J. B. Lippincott.

Therapeutic Efficacy Surveillance. A reliable means of monitoring the regression (response) or the continued progression of tumor (deterioration) is critical to the evaluation of the efficacy of the therapy in use. Contrast-enhanced MRI is used if possible; otherwise CT is used. However, tumor progression is extremely difficult to differentiate from radiation damage either by symptoms or conventional MRI/CT. Magnetic resonance spectroscopy, diffusion-perfusion algorithms, and dynamic contrast-enhanced MRI aid in this differentiation and should be used for postirradiation patients.

Tumor progression and peritumoral edema are the most common causes of neurologic deterioration during and after treatment. However, in the presence of deterioration without evidence of tumor progression, the following alternative causes should be considered (Levin, Leibel, & Gutin, 1997):

- Obstructive hydrocephalus
- Intratumoral and peritumoral hemorrhage
- Fluid imbalance, usually caused by excessive administration of parenteral dextrose in water solutions
- Hypertension, which can accentuate edema
- Reactive peritumoral edema due to radiotherapy
- Radiotherapy early-delayed syndrome
- Radiation necrosis (>6 months to 10 years)
- Seizures, even subclinical (may be indication tumor is progressing); electroencephalogram is diagnostic
- Infection and fever (may worsen neurologic signs and symptoms regardless of site of infection)
- Metabolic disorders, anemia, fatigue, and depression (are difficult to differentiate from tumor progression as none produce alteration of neuroimages)
- Increased need for corticosteroids (indicator of tumor progression) and the side effects of these drugs (Box 26-2).

Levin et al. (1997) stated that, from their experience, approximately 10% of patients responding to chemotherapy become significantly worse after the first course of treatment. They suggest the cause to be the initial increase in tumor bulk as a result of the effectiveness of therapy.

BOX 26-2
Steroid Therapy Side Effects

Hyperglycemia
Irritability
Insomnia
Psychotic reactions, mood swings
Hypokalemia
Hypernatremia
Depressed immune response
Elevated lipid and cholesterol levels
Fluid retention
Cataract formation
Osteoporosis
Thrombophlebitis
Steroid-induced gastric ulcers
Relocation of fat deposits (round face and thick trunk)
Cutaneous striae
Withdrawal symptoms (doses must be reduced from intravenous to oral and then in amount and frequency)

From Murphy, M. E. (1997). Cancers of the brain and central nervous system. In S. E. Otto (Ed.), *Oncology nursing* (3rd ed.). St. Louis: Mosby.

Because radiotherapy is used so extensively in the treatment of gliomas, and several of the potential causes of deterioration listed previously are due to radiotherapy, the following section discusses radiation side effects in detail.

Radiotherapy-Induced Brain Injury. The adult brain appears to have a general threshold level of radiation tolerance identified at 60 Gy in 2-Gy fractionated daily doses of 30 sessions over 6 weeks. The increase of total or fractionated doses beyond this threshold has a direct relationship to the probability of increasing injury to the brain (Leibel & Sheline, 1987; Marks, Baglan, Prassad, & Black, 1981).

The likelihood of brain damage also correlates with the total volume of tissue irradiated. Large-volume and whole-brain irradiation represent the greatest risk. In addition, some chemotherapeutic agents, given either concurrent with or after radiation therapy, appear to amplify radiation injury (DeAngelis & Shapiro, 1991). This is particularly the case with methotrexate, and attention to this discovery has greatly reduced the incidence of injury related to this agent (Bleyer & Griffin, 1980).

Clinical reactions to irradiation have differing causes and tend to appear on a continuum during the course of the illness. Reactions are temporally classified as acute reactions, which occur during or shortly after radiotherapy treatment; early-delayed reactions, which tend to appear between 2 weeks and 4 months posttreatment; and long-delayed injury which can manifest from several months to many years after treatment (Leibel & Sheline, 1991).

Acute reactions appear to be due to radiation-induced edema and may cause headache, nausea, vomiting, somnolence, fever, and worsening neurologic symptoms within hours of the first fractionated dose. These reactions are most commonly seen with large fractions (3.0 to 6.0 Gy) administered to a large volume of brain in patients with underlying tumor-related ICP. Such patients may be protected by corticosteroids administered 48 to 72 hours before the onset of treatment (Posner, 1995). Increased fractionated doses can lead to neurologic deterioration or death (Young, Posner, Chu, & Nisce, 1974). Typical adverse reactions to standard doses are mild headache and nausea lessening with subsequent doses.

Early-delayed reactions are thought to be caused by temporary demyelination of the oligodendroglial cells (Hoffman, Levin, & Wilson, 1979) or alteration of capillary permeability (Delattre, Rosenblum, Thaler, Mandell, Shapiro, & Posner, 1988). Symptoms may include transient neurologic deterioration, somnolence, and focal encephalopathy and are influenced by the presence of tumor, volume of field, and dosage (Leibel & Sheline, 1991). Corticosteroids and intensive medical support may be required to alleviate symptoms.

Late-delayed reactions are the most serious of radiation-induced injuries. The etiologic factors appear to be similar to those of early-delayed radiation damage. Complications range from asymptomatic focal or diffuse white matter injury to potentially fatal necrosis (Leibel & Sheline, 1991). Focal damage most often is associated with increased intracranial pressure. Diffuse white matter damage is typically due to large-volume or whole-brain irradiation and can present with seizure disorders, varied neuropsychological impairment, and, in the worst-case scenario, debilitating dementia. Cerebrocortical atrophy and enlarged central sulci and ventricles are seen in 17% to 39% of patients treated with whole-brain irradiation and chemotherapy for malignant gliomas (Posner, 1995). Vascular occlusion (Brant-Zawadzki, Anderson, De Armond, Conley, & Jahnke, 1980) and neoplasms secondary to irradiation are rare (Bernstein & Laperriere, 1991). Corticosteroids may improve or stabilize neurologic symptoms, and surgical resection has been beneficial for those with focal damage, especially those who become steroid dependent (Gutin, 1991).

Neuroendocrine sequelae are also a side effect of radiation therapy. Hypothalamic-pituitary dysfunction has been observed, and the degree of hormonal suppression appears to be dose related (Shalet, Beardwell, Pearson, & Jones, 1976). Deficiencies in growth hormones, gonadotropins, thyroid-stimulating hormone, adrenocorticotropins, and hyperprolactinemia have also been reported in patients treated with doses higher than 40 Gy (Sklar & Constine, 1995).

Additional long-term neurologic dysfunctions may include impaired intellect, recent memory loss, emotional lability, fatigue, and initiative and concentration problems, which make attending to tasks difficult (Hochberg & Slotnik, 1980; Maire, Coudin, Guerin, & Caudry, 1987; Corbett, personal communication, 1998). These symptoms can be devastating, or at the very least disruptive, and referral to such services as rehabilitation clinics, brain injury clinics, and individual and family counseling may be of benefit to both the patient and the family (Corbett, personal communication, 1998).

Until recently, the differentiation of radiotherapeutic injury from tumor activity on brain scans was nearly impossible. Today, the thallium-201 single-photon emission computed tomography, the F-18 fluorodeoxyglucose positron emission tomography, and dynamic-enhanced MRI can all clearly differentiate radiation damage from tumor progression or recurrence. However, because most patients have a mixture of necrotic and tumor cells, a biopsy may still be needed (Levin, Leibel, & Gutin, 1997).

Chemotherapy Complications

Complications associated with chemotherapy are almost always caused by dose-related neurotoxicity and the therapy's impact on other systems of the body, such as the bone marrow and the gastrointestinal tract. Most chemotherapeutic agents are administered in regimens and cycles that allow the body to recover as much as possible between treatments. Dosage of the agents and related side effects must be carefully monitored. Table 26-16 lists commonly used chemotherapy drugs and their side effects.

Biotherapy Complications

Complications commonly resulting from biotherapy relate to the specific agent, dosage, and the combined modalities used. The systemic administration of IL-2 and LAK is highly neurotoxic and leads to profound edema and herniation. The use of interferons has had little effect. The side effects of the most common biotherapy agents are listed in Box 26-3.

NURSING MANAGEMENT

The nursing management of patients with CNS tumors is focused on education that includes the family diad. The effects of malignancy, its treatment, and recovery represent devastating consequences to all domains of well-being—physical, spiritual, economic, and social functioning. Treatments are frightening and elicit anxiety that may surpass that of initial diagnosis. For those patients having craniotomies, intensive teaching and reassurance are required of the health care team to prepare and care for the patient throughout the trajectory of the treatment (Table 26-17). Safety issues are paramount because of impairments from tumors or treatment. For patients not having seizures as part of their presenting diagnosis, this terrifying sequelae may occur as a result of tissue damage and edema arising from surgery. Careful and calm instructions for both the patient and family are essential for optimal seizure management. Even as the early complications associated with treatment occupy the patient and health care team, overriding concerns about the possible permanent and longterm effects of the disease and multimodal therapy are omnipresent.

HOME CARE ISSUES

Even in the face of CNS treatment with its accompanying complex care, patients continue to be discharged early from

TABLE 26-16 Chemotherapy Drugs and Related Side Effects

Drug	Side Effects
BCNU	Bone marrow suppression
CCNU	Nausea, alopecia, pulmonary fibrosis
Cisplatin	Ototoxicity, renal dysfunction, bone marrow depression, anorexia, nausea/vomiting
Cyclophosphamide	Nausea/vomiting, diarrhea, alopecia, bone marrow suppression
Nitrogen mustard	Nausea/vomiting, anorexia, alopecia, diarrhea, bone marrow suppression, hepatic/neurologic dysfunction
Bleomycin	Nausea/vomiting, stomatitis, hepatic/ neurologic dysfunction, pulmonary fibrosis
Vincristine	Nausea/vomiting, anorexia, alopecia, neurologic dysfunction
Etoposide	Nausea/vomiting, anorexia, hypotension, bone marrow suppression
Methotrexate	Bone marrow suppression, renal tubular necrosis, stomatitis, diarrhea, hepatic dysfunction
Procarbazine	Nausea/vomiting, diarrhea, alopecia, myelosuppression, hepatic and neurologic dysfunction

From Murphy, M. E. (1997). Cancers of the brain and central nervous system. In S. E. Otto (Ed.), *Oncology nursing* (3rd ed.). St. Louis: Mosby.

BOX 26-3
Biotherapy Side Effects

Flu-like symptoms (headache, fever, chills, arthralgia, myalgia)
Nausea/vomiting (varies with individual and amount of dose)
Weight loss (amount depends on amount of side effects)
Altered neurologic functioning (decreased short-term memory concentration and attention)
Alopecia (partial)
Skin changes (erythema, rash, pruritus)
Fluid and electrolyte imbalances (hypocalcemia, hypomagnesemia)
Bone marrow suppression (pancytopenia)

From Murphy, M. E. (1997). Cancers of the brain and central nervous system. In S. E. Otto (Ed.), *Oncology nursing* (3rd ed.). St. Louis: Mosby.

hospitals (Table 26-18). Consequently, intense outpatient and home care support is vital for patient recovery. Table 26-19 details a standard of care plan that, although initiated in the hospital setting, requires consistent and careful adherence.

One of the critical components for ongoing care is long-term support. Leavitt, Lamb, & Voss (1996) have addressed the importance of expert nurse clinicians to organize and lead support groups as a therapeutic forum for patients with brain tumors and their families. The content can be aimed at the difficulties of survival and maintaining quality of life after treatment. In their own research with support groups, the investigators found five conceptual themes emerging from the support groups (Table 26-20). Recommendations to nurses practicing in this area are to provide support groups in which accurate information, realistic reassurances, and emotional and practical support prevail. The group itself can serve as a network and resource for information about conventional and unconventional care, symptom management, and family and caregiver issues.

Long-Term Cognitive Effect

Most patients with malignant glioma have behavioral, emotional, and intellectual difficulties that can compromise their ability to function independently. Cognitive impairment is a major impediment to achieving the quality of life enjoyed by patients before diagnosis. Stimulant treatment with methylphenidate has shown some improvement in those with psychomotor retardation, fatigue, and depression and is now under investigation to diminish this disturbing acute and chronic problem in glioma and other brain cancer patients. Investigators recently studied the use of methylphenidate in brain tumor patients and found that cognition, mood, and functional abilities were improved. Significant positive changes in improved gait, increased stamina, and motivation to perform activities were noted (Meyers, Weitzner, Valentine, & Levin, 1998). Numerous nationwide anecdotal accounts are emerging about the positive benefits experienced by patients with cognition deficiencies after cancer therapy. Much research is needed in generalized use of a CNS stimulant in this population, particularly regarding the long-term effects. However, for patients with possible terminal disease, short-term quality of life rather than long-term effects are the issue. This view must be respected.

PROGNOSIS

The prognosis for gliomas is based on histologic type, tumor grade, size and extent of tumor, location, patient's age, performance status, and residual tumor. For instance, younger neurologically intact patients tend to survive longer than the elderly. The most important prognosticators appear to be total resection vs partial (or none) resection, and the amount of tumor remaining.

Survival rates range from a cure to rapid deterioration and death. Grades I and II astrocytomas, oligodendrogliomas, and operable ependymomas can be cured with total resection. On occasion, a small amount of residual tumor treated with radiotherapy may be curable. Otherwise, life expectancy for patients with these low-grade tumors is measured in years (sometimes 10 years or more) (McCormack, Miller, Budzilovich, Voorhees, & Ransohoff, 1992). The prognosis for the malignant higher-grade (grades III and IV) tumors and brain stem tumors in general is poor, ranging from 1 to more than 2 years, usually depending on the amount of residual tumor. For patients with brain stem glio-

Text continued on p. 620

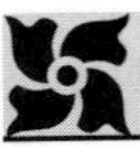

TABLE 26-17 Standard of Care for a Patient Having a Craniatomy

Patient Problem and Outcomes	Nursing Interventions and Rationales	Patient Education and Instruction
Anxiety Related to Impending Surgery and Perceived Negative Effects on Life-style.		
The patient will: 1. State the reason for surgery 2. Describe postoperative restrictions 3. Verbalize decreased anxiety related to impending surgery	1. Assess the patient's knowledge level to plan effective teaching strategies. 2. Information about what to expect can reduce anxiety associated with the unknown.	1. Teach patient about the surgical procedure using a sketch of the anatomy and physiology of the brain. 2. Teach the patient and family to inform the patient of past operative expectations in recovery room. 3. Prepare for possible loss of function. 4. Explain the specific postoperative experience, which may include the following: a. A large head dressing b. Swollen eyes c. Tracheostomy or endotracheal intubation 5. Discuss the possibility of cognitive and behavioral changes related to site of surgery: a. Frontal—lack of spontaneity and initiative, childlike impulsivity, decreased concentration and attention, loss of recent memory, or inability to plan/organize b. Temporal (1) Dysnomia (2) Aphasia (3) Test taking abilities (4) Impairments (5) Apathy (6) Placidity c. (7) Parietal (8) Cognitive deficits (9) Inattention (10) Language disorders (11) Astereognosis (12) Apraxia (13) Apathy d. Occipital (1) Visual agnosia (2) Alexis 6. Discuss the uncertainty of resolution of previous cognitive or behavior patterns. 7. Assess and document cognitive function preoperatively: a. Orientations (place, person, and time) b. Short-term memory (ask to repeat a set of words) c. Long-term memory (ask to identify name of high school) d. Affect (apathetic, hostile, or labile) e. General behavior (appropriate/inappropriate) f. Abstract reasoning (ask to relate the meaning of a proverb) g. Ability to calculate h. Attention (easily distracted or attentive) 8. Inform the client if an alternative form of communication to speech (e.g., note pad and pencil, or hand signals) will be necessary postoperatively.

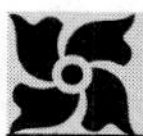

TABLE 26-17 Standard of Care for a Patient Having a Craniatomy—cont'd

Patient Problem and Outcomes	Nursing Interventions and Rationales	Patient Education and Instruction
Intracranial Pressure The patient will have minimized complications of increased intracranial pressure (ICP).	1. Monitoring ICP serves as an indicator of cerebral perfusion. a. Assess cortical auditory lack of response to evaluate patient's ability to integrate commands with conscious and involuntary movement function by evaluating eye opening and motor response. No response may indicate damage to the midbrain. b. Assess vital sign change for increasing ICP	1. Explain to the patient that coughing, sneezing, lifting heavy objects, straining during a bowel movement may cause increased ICP. 2. Teach patient to exhale during these activities to reduce pressure in head.
	(1) Pulse changes: slowing rate to 60 or below or increasing rate to 100 or above (2) Respiratory irregularities: slowing of rate with lengthening periods of apnea (3) Rising blood pressure or widening pulse pressure c. Assess pupillary response: (1) Inspect the pupils with a bright pinpoint light to evaluate size, configuration, and reaction to light. Compare both eyes for similarities and differences. (2) Evaluate gaze to determine whether it is conjugate (paired, working together) or if eye movements are abnormal. (3) Evaluate ability of the eyes to adduct and abduct. d. Note the presence of the following: (1) Vomiting (2) Headache (constant, increasing in intensity, or aggravated by movement or straining) (3) Subtle changes (e.g., lethargy, restlessness, forced breathing, purposeless movements, and changes in mentation) 2. Elevate the head of the bed 15 to 30 degrees unless contraindicated. Avoid changing position rapidly. 3. Avoid the following: a. Carotid massage b. Neck flexion or extreme rotation c. Digital anal stimulation d. Breath holding e. Straining f. Extreme flexion of hips and knees	3. Explain to patient that he/she will be asked 10 questions about pain and orientation to person, place, and time so that cortical function can be evaluated. 4. Explain to patient the need to obtain frequent vital signs to measure hemadynamic stability.
	4. Consult with the physician for stool softeners, if needed 5. Maintain a quiet, calm, softly lit environment. Plan activities to minimize interruptions.	5. Explain to patient that stool softeners prevent constipation and straining, which initiates Valsalva's maneuver.

Continued

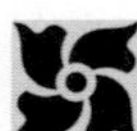

TABLE 26-17 Standard of Care for a Patient Having a Craniatomy—cont'd

Patient Problem and Outcomes	Nursing Interventions and Rationales	Patient Education and Instruction
Intracranial Pressure—cont'd		
	6. Assess cranial nerve function by evaluating the following: a. Pupillary responses b. Corneal reflex c. Gag reflex d. Cough e. Swallow f. Facial movements g. Tongue movements 7. Assess motor and sensory function by observing each extremity separately for strength and normalcy of movement, response to stimuli. 8. Assess cerebellar function by observing for the following: a. Ataxic movements b. Loss of equilibrium 9. Carefully monitor hydration status; evaluate fluid intake and output, serum osmolality, and urine specific gravity and osmolality. 10. Identify possible causes of hyposmolar state. a. Excess IV fluids b. Inappropriate antidiuretic c. Hormone secretion	
	11. Identify possible causes of hyperosmolar state. a. Fever b. Diarrhea c. Osmotic diuretic d. High-protein tube feeding e. Surgically induced diabetes insipidus f. Hyperglycemia 12. Monitor intake and administer necessary IV fluids via infusion pump. 13. Monitor for signs and symptoms of diabetes insipidus: a. Excessive urinary output b. Dilute urine 14. Monitor urinary output and urine specific gravity. 15. Monitor temperature 16. Monitor the would site for the following: a. Bleeding b. Bulging c. CSF leakage d. Infection	6. Explain to patient need for high-solute tube feeding to draw water from tissues by osmosis.

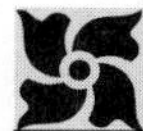

TABLE 26-17 Standard of Care for a Patient Having a Craniatomy—cont'd

Patient Problem and Outcomes	Nursing Interventions and Rationales	Patient Education and Instruction
Intracranial Pressure—cont'd		
	17. Consult with the physician if the client experiences seizure activity. 18. Avoid sequential performance of activities that increase ICP (e.g., coughing, suctioning, repositioning, and bathing) 19. Administer medication as indicated: a. Antihypertensives b. Peripheral vasodilators c. Anticoagulants d. Stool softeners e. Corticosteroids 20. Administer IV therapy as indicated: a. Fluid and electrolyte replacement 21. Collect specimens for laboratory studies: a. Complete blood count b. Blood chemistry profile c. Prothrombin time d. Urinalysis 22. Apply, if indicated: a. Antiembolism stockings b. Speech therapy	Teach the client to avoid the following: a. Coughing b. Neck hyperextension c. Neck hyperflexion d. Neck turning These measures help prevent hypercapnia, which can increase cerebral vasodilation and raise ICP and prevent cerebral ischemia
Pain		
The patient will report progressive pain reduction after pain relief measures.	1. Ascertain the location, nature and intensity of the pain. 2. If the pain is a headache, slightly raise the head of the bed, reduce bright lights and room noise, and loosen head dressings if constrictive. 3. Provide nonpharmacologic relief measures, as appropriate: a. Eye patches for eye edema b. Frequent immobility position changes and backrubs 4. Observe for a decrease in level of consciousness and respiratory rate after narcotic administration.	Teach the patient that mild headaches may persist, but will gradually diminish; to indicate pain on a scale of 1 to 10
Impaired Corneal Tissue Integrity		
The patient will demonstrate continued corneal integrity.	Assessment 1. Eyes: moisture, lid, closure, drainage, abrasions a. If eyelids do not close completely, use an eye shield or tape lids closed per protocol. b. Loosen any tight dressings over the eyes. c. Instill normal saline or hydroxethylcellulose (Artificial Tears), as necessary. d. Assess for irritation and drainage. e. Apply cool compresses to the eye area, if necessary.	1. Teach patient necessity of maintaining moisture in eyes

TABLE 26-18 Discharge Instructions for Craniotomy Patients

Incision care	Wear a cap or hat after bandages are removed to protect the surgical site. Shampoo hair after the sutures are removed, but avoid scrubbing near the incision. Pat the incision dry because vigorous rubbing can separate the wound edges. Do not use hair dryers or hot curlers until hair has regrown because direct heat can burn the unprotected surgical site.
Increased intracranial pressure	Do not hold your breath because this can activate the Valsalva maneuver, which impairs venous return to your head. Do not strain during a bowel movement, lift heavy objects, blow your nose hard, or cough or sneeze. Try to exhale during these events to reduce pressure in your head.
Cognitive function	You may have some concentration problems or be unable to do multiple tasks. You may be emotional at times and tire easily. Please feel free to discuss these changes with your health care provider.
Infection	Watch for drainage from the surgical site, nose, or ears and call your physician if this occurs. This may indicate an infection or increased intracranial pressure.

mas in particular, the 5-year survival rates range from 0% to 38%, with a median survival of less than a year (Petronio, Edwards, Prados, Freyberger, Rabbitt, & Silver, 1990; Rodriguez, Edwards, & Levin, 1990; Rosenstock, Packer, & Bilaniuk, Bruce, Radcliffe, & Savino, 1985). GBM and ependymoblastomas (classified as primitive neuroectodermal) have the worst expected survival of 6 to 12 months (Healy, Barnes, Kupsky, Scott, Salan, & Black, 1991; Ross & Rubinstein, 1989). Table 26-21 lists the gliomas by grade and expected survival.

EVALUATION OF THE QUALITY OF CARE

Measurement of the quality of care rendered to patients and their caregivers is mandated by a growing number of governmental agencies, regulatory bodies, and third-party payors (Table 26-22). Data collected from sources such as these can lead to improved outcomes.

RESEARCH ISSUES

The poorly understood etiologic and associated risk factors for CNS tumors warrant continuing intensive research as a means for identifying possible prevention strategies for these insidious diseases. Developing a means for screening for these cancers should also be a high priority considering most are well advanced by the time of diagnosis.

In terms of treatment, brain tumors have one clear advantage over most other tumors of the body: they rarely metastasize. If local control can be achieved, the chances for a cure are very good. Thus a focus on the development and refinement of treatment modalities, in particular complete surgical resection, which can accomplish local control, should be the highest priority for research in this area.

The recent advent and continuing refinements of stereotactic surgery are a major advancement in the ability to achieve local control, particularly for those tumors previously thought to be inoperable. Stereotactic surgery is also a valuable tool in achieving the highest rate of cytoreduction possible for those tumors, which currently cannot be totally resected. This "Star Wars–like" technology is literally on its way to virtual reality surgery. By using special goggles or helmets (currently under development), surgeons may be able to actually see inside the skull and visualize tumors and brain anatomy with unequaled precision.

For tumors that are still inoperable and those with residual tumor tissue after resection, including some thought to be totally resected, an effective means for destroying residual cancer cells must be found. This requires continuing research in the following area:

- A means for destroying potential residual periphery tumor cells in "total" resection of astrocytomas, oligodendrogliomas, and mixed gliomas
- Methods for achieving the highest rate of cytoreduction, particularly for brain stem gliomas and posterior fossa intraventricular tumors
- Methods for increasing radiation dosage to tumor tissue with optimal protection of surrounding healthy tissue
- Prevention and improved management of radiation damage and necrosis
- Methods to improve chemotherapeutic dosage to tumor tissue currently limited by the blood-brain barrier, toxicity, the poor vasculation of the brain tissue, and the infiltrative diffusion of most gliomas
- Improved chemotherapy methods for treating tumors that are slow-growing (low cell division rate) and contain heterogeneous populations requiring multiple agents
- Continuing research in gene therapy and other cell modulation strategies
- Continuing research in photodynamic therapy

One key component of the improvement in treating the more rare tumors, such as oligodendrogliomas, mixed gliomas, and ependymomas, is the ability to undertake trials with larger populations of patients. To have a large enough database for statistically significant findings, clinical consortia are now being formed to pool patients for larger, randomized studies with common selection and evaluation protocols to determine the efficacy of new and experimental treatments.

Regardless of the specific research undertaken, all of the studies must consider not only the efficacy of the treatment in improvement of patient survival but also the short- and long-term treatment-related deficits and the impact of the treatment on a patient's quality of life. Attention also should be paid to the cost of and potential for equal access to care for all patients who might benefit from the treatment.

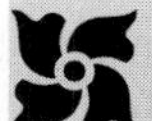

TABLE 26-19 Standard of Care for Home Care for the Glioma Patient Receiving Surgery and Radiation

Patient Problem and Outcomes	Nursing Interventions and Rationales	Patient Education Instructions
Cognition		
The patient will achieve optimal level of consciousness.	1. Assess patient for ability to be safe in his or her home care environment.	1. Teach patient and caregiver to create a safe environment by: a. Implementing visual clues such as clocks, calendars, colored labels, timers b. Encouraging social interactions with family and friends c. Providing patient with written instructions for tasks d. Assessing ability of patient to drive e. Inspecting home for slippery rugs or floors; move objects obstructing patient's path f. Inspect shower for safety 2. Teach patient and caregiver that steroids given for tissue inflammation (steroids) or anticonvulsants may cause cognitive dysfunction.
Seizures		
The patient or family caregiver will verbalize the seizure management.	1. Assess patient for risk of seizures. 2. Monitor patient compliance with medications and blood levels.	1. Teach patient that seizures are caused by irritation to the brain resulting from the tumor or surgery. Phenytoin and carbamazepine are the two most common drugs. Both drugs are taken for 7 to 10 days to reach a therapeutic blood level. Give clear instructions for patients to keep an accurate record of drug administration and not to double the dose if they should miss taking the medication. 2. Teach patient the most common side effects of phenytoin such as skin rash, drowsiness, or sleepiness. Major toxicities to be reported immediately are nystagmus, slurred speech, dysarthria, hypotension, and coma (rare).
Increased Intracranial Pressure		
The patient will verbalize management of intracranial pressure.	1. Identify the patient at risk for increased intracranial pressure, ie. those having a craniotomy.	1. Teach patients that tissue inflammation and swelling of the brain, particularly after surgery, cause increased intracranial pressure, leading to possible life-threatening problems. 2. Teach patient the rationale, dose, and administration. 3. Explain side effects: a. Short-term steroid use may produce mild side effects (i.e., mood swings; facial flushing; mild fluid retention; swelling of the hands, feet, or face; appetite increase) b. Long-term use includes body changes with swelling of the face, arms, legs, and abdomen; acne; mood swings; osteoporosis, diabetes, cataracts, immunosuppression with accompanying infections c. Gastrointestinal complications can be diminished by taking antacids d. Emphasize that medications should not be discontinued unless the physician directs the patient to do so.
Recovery		
The patient will achieve optimal recovery.	1. Assess patient emotional/ social, economic, medical, community, and spiritual needs.	1. Guide patient and caregivers to support groups such as the National Brain Tumor Foundation 800-934-CURE. 2. Direct patients to advocacy groups who can assist with financial, insurance, and employment issues. National Coalition for Cancer Survivorship 301-585-2616. Social Security Disability 800-772-1213. 3. Instruct patient on use of Physicians Data Query 301-496-7403. 4. Refer patient to American Cancer Society for transportation and home care equipment.

From *Brain tumors: A guide* (1992). San Francisco, National Brain Tumor Foundation; Belford, K (1997). Central nervous system cancers. In S. L. Groenwald, M. H. Frogge, M. Goodman, & C. H. Yarbro, (Eds.), *Cancer nursing: Principles and practice.* (4th ed). Sudsbury: Jones and Bartlett Publishers; Owens, B. Neurological cancers. (1992). In J. C. Clark & R. F. McGee (Eds.), *Core curriculum for oncology nursing.* Philadelphia: W. B. Saunders Company.

Table 26-20 Themes of Recovery of Brain Tumor Patients

Theme	Characteristics
1. Telling the story	1. Reliving the experience of coming to a diagnosis, warning signs, feeling alone and helpless, anger, shock, and confusion, adapting to a changed life, resolving to survive
2. Managing medical advice	2. Confusion in making choices in medical treatment, ie., is there a place for alternative treatment (herbal remedies versus clinical trials)? Traveling between treatment sites and health care providers seeking options.
3. Information seeking and exchange	3. Learning the pathophysiology of various brain tumors, survival data, elements of treatments and procedures, medications and adverse effects, and return to work. Understanding what "shadow" on magnetic resonance imaging indicates, reoccurrence, necrosis, spaces left after excision?
4. The long haul	4. Disillusionment and difficulties with continued and unexpected complications, disability, and search for quality of life. Experiencing diminishing professional health care support. "The doctor stops talking if I cry."
5. Family life changes	5. Family role changes such as adult children caring for parents, grandparents caring for grandchildren; personality changes, mood swings, aggressive or abusive behavior "I am losing my optimism."

From Leavitt, M., Lamb, S. A., & Voss, B. S. (1996). Brain tumor support group: Content themes and mechanisms of support. *Oncology Nursing Forum, 23,* 1247:1255.

Table 26-22 Quality of Care Evaluation of a Patient with Glioma

Disciplines participating in the quality of care evaluation:
Medical ☐ Nursing ☐ Dietary ☐ Pharmacy ☐

Data from: ☐ Medical Record Review
☐ Patient Family Interview

Criteria	Yes	No
Were you given information about how glioma is different from other brain cancers?	☐	☐
Were you given sufficient information to make an informed choice about your treatment options?	☐	☐
Did your family feel included in your treatment process?	☐	☐
Were you and your family adequately prepared for the tests you underwent for diagnosis of glioma?	☐	☐
If you were placed on a clinical trial, were you given information as to your right to withdraw from the trial at any time?	☐	☐
Were you told about the possible immediate symptoms related to your treatment, such as headaches, disorientation, infection, or bleeding?	☐	☐
Were you given instruction on how to take care of yourself at home?	☐	☐
Did the nurse provide you with education materials?	☐	☐
Were education materials helpful to you?	☐	☐
Did you receive information about after-hours care, the phone number to call, and what symptoms to report?	☐	☐
Were you given dietary information?	☐	☐
Did pharmacists fill your prescriptions promptly and give you medication instructions?	☐	☐
Were you given community and national support resources to contact such as the National Brain Tumor Foundation?	☐	☐
Were there things about the care you received that you did not like?	☐	☐

Table 26-21 Mean Survival Times for Patients with Gliomas by Grade

Tumor	Grade	Mean Survival*
Astrocytoma	I & II	Cure possible with total resection; years (10+)
Anaplastic astrocytoma	III	18-24 months
Glioblastoma multiforme	IV	9-12 months
Brain stem glioma		1-5 years mean: 12 months
Oligodendroglioma	I & II	Cure possible with total resection; years (5-10+)
Anaplastic oligodendroglioma	III & IV	Similar to high-grade astrocytoma
Ependymoma	I & II	Cure possible with total resection; years (5-10+)
Ependymoblastoma	III & IV	9-12 months

*With conventional treatment.

REFERENCES

Adams, R. D. & Victor, M. (1977). Principles of neurology. New York: McGraw-Hill.

Alavi, J. B. (1995). Primary and metastatic brain tumors. In R. T. Skeel & N. A. Lachant (Eds.), *Handbook of cancer chemotherapy* (4th ed.) Boston: Little, Brown.

Allen, J. C., Bloom, J., Ertel, I., Evans, A., Hammond, D., & Jones, H. (1986). Brain tumors in children: Current cooperative and institutional chemotherapy trials in newly diagnosed and recurrent disease. *Seminars in Oncology, 13,* 110-122.

Altshuler, E., Moosa, H., Selker, R. G., & Vertosick, F. (1990). The risk and efficacy of anticoagulant therapy in the treatment of thrombo-embolitic complications in patients with primary brain tumors. *Neurosurgery, 27,* 74-77.

Andreou, J., George, A. E., Wise, A., de Leon, M., Kricheff, I. I., & Ransohoff, J. (1983). CT prognostic criteria of survival after malignant glioma surgery. *American Journal of Neuroradiology, 4,* 488-490.

Anzai, Y., Lufkin, R., DeSalles, A., Hamilton, D. R., Farahani, K., & Black, K. L. (1995). Preliminary experience with MR-guided thermal ablation of brain tumors. *American Journal of Neuroradiology, 16,* 39-48.

Armstrong, T. S. & Gilbert, M. R. (1996). Glial neoplasms: Classification, treatment, and pathways for the future. *Oncology Nursing Forum, 23,* 615-627.

Ascensao, J., Ahmed, T., Feldman, E., Agoliti, G., Perchick, J., & Goldberg, R. (1989). High-dose thioTEPA with autologous bone marrow transplantation (ABMT) and localized radiotherapy (RT) for patients with astrocytoma grade III-IV (glioma): A promising approach [Abstract]. *Proceeding of the American Society of Clinical Oncology, 8,* A353.

Beahrs, O. H., Henson, D. E., Hutter, R. V. P., & Kennedy, J. (1992). *Manual for staging of cancer.* (4th ed). Philadelphia: J. B. Lippincott.

Belford, K. (1997). Central nervous system cancers. In S. L. Graenwald, M. H. Frugge, M. Goodman, & C. H. Yarbro (Eds.), *Cancer nursing: Principles and practice.* (4th ed). Sudsburg: Jones & Bartlett Publishers.

Berger, M. S., Deliganis, A. V., Dobbins, J., & Keles, G. E. (1994). The effect of extent of resection on recurrence in patients with low grade cerebral hemisphere gliomas. *Cancer, 74,* 1784-1791.

Berger, M. S., Kincaid, J., Ojemann, G. A., & Lettich, B. A. (1989). Brain mapping techniques to maximize resection, safety, and seizure control in children with brain tumors. *Neurosurgery, 25,* 786-792.

Berger, M. S., Leibel, S., Bruner, J. M., Finlay, J., & Levin, V. A. (1996). In V. A. Levin (Ed.), *Cancer in the nervous system.* New York: Churchill Livingstone.

Bernstein, M., Laperriere, N., Leung, P., & McKenzie, S. (1990). Interstitial brachytherapy for malignant brain tumors: Preliminary results. *Neurosurgery, 26,* 371-380.

Bernstein, M. & Laperriere, N. (1991). Radiation-induced tumors of the nervous system. In P. H. Gutin, S. A. Leibel, & G. E. Sheline (Eds.), *Radiation injury to the nervous system.* New York: Raven Press.

Bersagel, D. J., Finnegold, M. J., Butel, J. S., Kupsy, W. J., & Garcea, R. I. (1992). DNA sequences similar to those of simian virus 40 in ependymomas and choroid plexus tumors of childhood. *New England Journal of Medicine, 326,* 988-992.

Bertoloni, S. J., Baum, E. S., Krivit, W., & Hammond, G. D. (1989). A phase II study of cisplatin therapy in recurrent childhood brain tumors. *Journal of Neuro-oncology, 7,* 5-11.

Bleyer, W. A. & Griffin, T. W. (1980). White matter necrosis, mineralizing microangiopathy, and intellectual abilities in survivors of childhood leukemia. In H. A. Gilbert, & A. R. Kagan (Eds.), *Radiation damage to the nervous system.* New York: Raven Press.

Boss, B. J., Sunderland, P. M., & Heath, J. (1994). Alterations of neurological function. In K. L. McCance & S. E. Huether (Eds.), *Pathophysiology: The biologic basis for disease in adults and children.* St. Louis: Mosby.

Brant-Zawadski, M., Badami, J. P., Mills, C. M., Norman, D., & Newton, T. H. (1984). Primary intracranial tumor imaging: A comparison of magnetic resonance and CT. *Radiology, 150,* 435-440.

Brant-Zawadski, M., Anderson, M., De Armond, S. J., Conley, F. K., & Jahnke, R. W. (1980). Radiation-induced large intracranial vessel occlusive vasculopathy. *American Journal of Radiology, 134,* 51-55.

Brem, H., Mahaley, M. S., Jr., Vick, N. A., Black, K. L., Schold, S. C., Jr., & Burger, P. C. (1991). Interstitial chemotherapy with drug polymer implants for the treatment of recurrent gliomas. *Journal of Neurosurgery, 74,* 441-446.

Brem, H., Piantadosi, S., & Burger, P. C. (1994). Intraoperative chemotherapy using bioerodable polymers: Safety and effectiveness for recurrent glioma evaluated by prospective, multi-institutional placebo controlled clinical trial [Abstract]. *Proceedings of the American Society of Clinical Oncology, 13,* A487.

Bullard, D. E., Rawlings, C. E., Phillips, B., Cox, E. B., Schold, S. C., & Burger, P. (1987). Oligodendroglioma: An analysis of the value of radiation therapy. *Cancer, 60,* 2179-2188.

Burger, P. C., Rawlings, C. E., Cox, E. B., McLendon, R. B., Schold, S. C., & Bullard, D. E. (1987). Clinicopathologic correlations in the oligodendroglioma. *Cancer, 59,* 1345-1352.

Butler, A. R., Horii, S. C., Kricheff, I., Shannon, M. B., & Budzilovich, G. H. (1978). Computed tomography in astrocytomas: A statistical analysis of the parameters of malignancy and the positive contrast enhanced CT scan. *Radiology, 129,* 433-439.

Cairncross, J. G., MacDonald, D. R., Ludwin, S., Lee, D., Cascino, T., & Buckner, J. (1994). Chemotherapy for anaplastic oligodendroglioma. *Journal of Clinical Oncology, 12,* 2013-2021.

Cairncross, J. G. & MacDonald, D. R. (1991). Chemotherapy for oligodendrogliomas: Progress report. *Archives of Neurology, 48,* 225-227.

Cairncross, J. G. & MacDonald, D. R. (1988). Successful chemotherapy for recurrent malignant oligodendroglioma. *Annals of Neurology, 23,* 360-364.

Cancer Statistics 1997. *CA A Cancer Journal for Clinicians, 47,* 8-9.

Cerrato, C., Ariano, C., & Fiaccjiono, F. (1978). Deep vein thrombosis and low dose heparin prophylaxis in neurosurgical patients. *Journal of Neurosurgery, 49,* 378-381.

Chin, H. W., Hazel, J. J., Kim, T. H., & Webster, J. H. (1980). Oligodendromas, 1. A clinical study of cerebral oligodendrogliomas. *Cancer, 45,* 1458-1466.

Chipps, E., Clanin, N., & Campbell, V. (1992). *Neurologic disorders.* St. Louis: Mosby.

CNS consortia reshaping brain tumor research. (1997). *NEWS,* pg. 1661, issue 22, vol. 89. URL: http//www.out.co.uk/jnci/hdb/Volume__89/Issue__22/html/891661.html

Corbett, T. (1998). Personal communication.

D'Incalci, M., Citti, L., Taverna, P., & Catapano, C. V. (1988). Importance of the DNA repair enzyme 06-alkyl guanine alkyltransferase (AT) in cancer chemotherapy. *Cancer Treatment Reviews, 15,* 279-292.

Daumas-Duport, C., Scheithauer, B., O'Fallon, J., & Kelly, P. (1988). Grading of astrocytomas, a simple and reproducible method. *Cancer, 62,* 2152-2165.

DeAngelis, L. M. & Shapiro, W. R. (1991). Drug/radiation interactions and central nervous system injury. In P. H. Gutin, S. A. Leibel, & G. E. Sheline (Eds.), *Radiation injury to the nervous system.* New York: Raven Press.

Delattre, J. Y., Rosenblum, M. K., Thaler, H. T., Mandell, L., Shapiro, W. R., & Posner, J. B. (1988). A model of radiation myelopathy in the rat: Pathology, regional capillary permeability changes and treatment with dexamethasone. *Brain, 111,* 1319-1336.

Devaux, B. C., O'Fallon, J. R., & Kelley, P. J. (1993). Resection, biopsy, and survival in malignant glial neoplasms: A retrospective study of clinical parameters, therapy, and outcome. *Journal of Neurosurgery, 78,* 767-775.

DeVita, V. T., Jr. (1983). The relationship between tumor mass and resistance chemotherapy: Implication for surgical adjuvant treatment of cancer. *Cancer, 51,* 1209-1220.

DeVroom, H. (1994). Glioblastoma multiforme: Current trends in brain tumor treatment. *Oncology Nursing Forum, 21,* 1317-1320.

Dhami, M. S., Bona, R. D., Calogero, J. A., & Hellman, R. M. (1993). Venous thromboembolism and high grade gliomas. *Thrombosis and Haemostasis, 70,* 393-396.

Edwards, M. S. B., Wara, W. M., Urtasun, R. C., Rados, M., Levin, V. A., & Fulton, D. (1989). Hyperfractionated radiation therapy for brainstem gliomas: A phase I-II trial. *Journal of Neurosurgery, 70,* 691-700.

Eifel, P. J., Cassady, J. R., & Belli, J. A. (1987). Radiation therapy of tumors of the brainstem and midbrain in children: Experience of the Joint Center For Radiation Therapy and Children's Hospital Medical Center (1971-1981). *International Journal of Radiation Oncology, Biology, Physics, 13,* 847-852.

Elsas, T., Watne, K., Fostad, K., & Hager, B. (1989). Ocular complications after intracarotid BCNU for intracranial tumors. *Acta Ophthalmologica, 67,* 83-86.

Ettinger, L. J., Ru, N., Krailo, M., Ruccione, K. S., Krivit, W., & Hammond, G. D. (1990). A phase II study of diaziquone in children with recurrent or progressive primary brain tumors: A report from the Children's Cancer Study Group. *Journal of Neuro-oncology, 9,* 69-76.

Feun, L. G., Wallace, S., Yung, W. K., Lee, Y. Y., Leavens, M. E., & Moser, R. (1984). Phase I trial of intracarotid BCNU and cisplatin in patients with malignant intracerebral tumors. *Cancer Drug Delivery, 1,* 239-245.

Fisher, E. G., Linggood, R. M., & Recht, L. D. (1995). Cancers of the central nervous system. In *Cancer manual* (7th ed.). Boston: American Cancer Society.

Florell, R. C., MacDonald, D. R., Irish, W. D., Bernstein, M., Leibel, S. A., & Gutin, P. H. (1991). Selection bias, survival, and brachytherapy for glioma. *Journal of Neurosurgery, 76,* 179-183.

Franklin, C. I. (1992). Does the extent of surgery make a difference in high grade malignant astrocytoma? *Australasian Radiology, 36,* 44-47.

Freeman, C. R., Krischer, J., Sanford, R. A., Cohen, M. E., Burger, P. C., & Kun, L. (1991). Hyperfractionated radiation therapy for brainstem tumors: Results of treatment at the 7020 cGy dose level of Pediatric Oncology Group Study No. 8495. *Cancer, 68,* 474-481.

Freeman, C. R., Krischer, J., Sanford, R. A., Cohen, M. E., Burger, P. C., & DelCarpio, R. (1993). Final results of a study of escalating doses of hyperfractionated radiotherapy in brain stem tumors in children: A Pediatric Oncology Group Study. *International Journal of Radiation Oncology, Biology, Physics, 27,* 197-206.

Fuller, G. N. & Bigner, S. H. (1992). Amplified cellular oncogenes in neoplasms of the human central nervous system. *Mutation Research, 276,* 299-306.

Gannett, D. E., Wisbeck, W. M., Silbergeld, D. I., & Berger, M. S. (1994). The role of postoperative irradiation in the treatment of oligodendroglioma. *International Journal of Radiation Oncology, Biology, Physics, 30,* 567-573.

Gaynon, P. S., Ettinger, L. J., Baum, E. S., Siegel, S. E., Krailo, M. D., & Hammond, O. D. (1990). Carboplatin in childhood brain tumors: A Children's Cancer Study Group phase II trial. *Cancer, 66,* 2465-2469.

Giannone, L. & Wolff, S. N. (1987). Phase II treatment of central nervous system gliomas with high-dose etoposide and autologous bone marrow transplantation. *Cancer Treatment Reports, 71,* 759-761.

Gilbert, M. R., Lunsford, L. D., Kondziolka, D., Flickinger, J. C., Shumaker, E., & Ziegler, K. J. (1993). A phase II trial of continuous infusion chemotherapy, external beam radiotherapy and local boost radiotherapy for malignant gliomas [Abstract]. *Proceedings of the American Society of Clinical Oncology, 12,* 176.

Gilbert, M. R., Lunsford, L. D., Kondziolka, D., Flickinger, J. C., Matey, L., & Armstrong, T. S. (1993). Phase II trial of continuous infusion chemotherapy and boost radiation for recurrent malignant gliomas [Abstract]. *Proceedings of the American Neurological Association, 119,* 60.

Gilbert, M. R., Matey, L., Minhas, T., Bozik, M., Armstrong, T. S., & Shumaker, E. (1994). Dual modulation of BCNU resistance in patients with refractory or recurrent glial neoplasms [Abstract]. *Proceedings of the American Association for Cancer Research, 35,* 361.

Goldberg, J. (1998). A head full of hope. *Discover,* 19(4), *April,* 70-76.

Goldwein, J. W., Leahy, J. M., Packer, R. J., Sutton, L. N., Curran, W. J., & Rorke, B. (1990). Intracranial ependymomas in children. *International Journal of Radiation Oncology, Biology, Physics, 19,* 1497-1502.

Green, S. B., Shapiro, W. R., Burger, P. C., Selker, R. G., VanGilder, J. G., & Saris, S. (1994). A randomized trial of interstitial radiotherapy (RT) boost for newly diagnosed malignant glioma: Brain Tumor Cooperative Group (BTCG) trial 8701 [Abstract]. *Proceedings of the American Society of Clinical Oncology, 13,* A486.

Greenberger, J. S., Cassady, J. R., & Levene, M. B. (1977). Radiation therapy of thalamic, midbrain and brain stem gliomas. *Radiology, 122*(2), 463-468.

Grossman, S. A., Sheidler, V. R., Ahn, H., Gilbert, R. R., Wharam, M., & Bucholtz, J. (1989). Complete and partial response of newly diagnosed malignant astrocytomas (MA) following continuous infusion BCNU and cisplatin [Abstract]. *Proceedings of the American Society of Clinical Oncology, 8,* A344.

Gutin, P. H. (1991). Treatment of radiation necrosis of the brain. In P. H. Gutin, S. A. Leibel, & G. E. Sheline (Eds.), *Radiation injury to the nervous system.* New York: Raven Press.

Gutin, P. H., Leibel, S. A., Wara, W. M., Choucair, A., Levin, V. A., & Philips, T. L. (1987). Recurrent malignant gliomas: Improved survival following interstitial brachytherapy with high-activity iodine-125 sources. *Journal of Neurosurgery, 67,* 864-873.

Halperin, E. C. (1985). Pediatric brain stem tumors: Patterns of treatment failure and their implications for radiotherapy. *International Journal of Radiation Oncology, Biology, Physics, 11,* 1293-1298.

Halperin, E. C., Kun, L. E., Constine, L. S., & Tarbell, N. J. (1989). *Pediatric Radiation Oncology.* New York: Raven Press.

Harsh, G. R., IV, Levin, V. A., Gutin, P. H., Seager, M., Silver, P., & Wilson, C. B. (1987). Reoperation for recurrent glioblastoma and anaplastic astrocytoma. *Neurosurgery, 21,* 615-621.

Healy, E. A., Barnes, P. D., Kupsky, W. J., Scott, R. M., Sallan, S. E., & Black, R. M. (1991). The prognostic significance of post-operative residual tumor in ependymoma. *Neurosurgery, 28,* 666-672.

Henson, J. W., Schnitker, B. L., Correa, K. M., von Deimling, A., Fassbender, F., & Xu, H-J. (1994). The retinoblastoma susceptibility (Rb) gene is involved in the malignant progression of human astrocytomas. *Annals of Neurology, 36,* 714-721.

Hermanson, M., Funa, K., Hartman, M., Claesson-Welsh, L., Heldin, C.-H., & Westermark, B. (1992). Platelet-derived growth factor and its receptors in human glioma tissue: Expression of messenger RNA and protein suggests the presence of autocrine and paracrine loops. *Cancer, 52,* 3213-3219.

Hermanson, M., Funa, K., Koopman, J., Maintz, D., Waha, A., & Westermark, B. (1996). Association of loss of heterozygosity (LOH) on chromosome 17p with high platelet-derived growth factor (PDGF) alpha-receptor expression in human malignant gliomas. *Cancer Research, 56,* 164-171.

Hochberg, F. H. & Slotnick, B. (1980). Neuropsychologic impairment in astrocytoma survivors. *Neurology, 30,* 172-177.

Hoffman, W. F., Levin, V. A., & Wilson, C. B. (1979). Evaluation of malignant glioma patients during the postirradiation period. *Journal of Neurosurgery, 50,* 624-628.

Hollinshead, W. H. (1967). The cranial parts of the nervous system. In *Textbook of anatomy* (2nd ed.). New York: Harper & Row.

Jaeckle, K. A. (1994). Immunotherapy of malignant gliomas. *Seminars in Oncology, 21,* 249-259.

James, C. D., Carlblom, E., Dumanski, J. P., Hansen, M., Nordenskjold, M., & Collins, V. P. (1988). Clonal genomic alterations in glioma malignancy stages. *Cancer Research, 48,* 5546-5551.

Jenkin, D. (1983). Posterior fossa tumors in childhood: radiation treatment. *Clinical Neurosurgery,* 30, 203-208.

Kaiser, M. C. & Kralendonk, J. H. (1991). Modern imaging for cerebral gliomas: Breakthroughs and limitations. In A. B. M. F. Karim, & E. R. J. Laws (Eds.), *Glioma: Principles and practice in neuro-oncology.* New York: Springer-Verlag.

Kernohan, J. W., Moborn, R. F., & Svien, H. J. (1949). A simplified classification of gliomas. *Proceedings of Staff Meetings at Mayo Clinic, 24,* 71-75.

Kerr, M. E. & Walleck, C. A. (1996). Intracranial problems. In S. M. Lewis, I. C. Collier, & M. M. Heitkemper. *Medical surgical nursing.* (4th ed.). St. Louis: Mosby.

Kim, T. H., Chin, H. W., Pollan, S., Hazel, J. H., & Webster, J. H. (1980). Radiotherapy of primary brainstem tumors. *International Journal of Radiation Oncology, Biology, Physics, 6,* 51-57.

Kraus, J. A., Koopman, J., Kaskel, P., Maintz, D., Brandner, S., & Louis, D. N. (1995). Shared allelic losses on chromosome 1p and 19q suggests a common origin of oligodendroglioma and aligoastrocytoma. *Journal of Neuropathology and Experimental Neurology, 54,* 91-95.

Kumar, A. R. V., Hoshino, T., Wheeler, K. T., Barker, M., & Wilson, C. B. (1974). Comparative rates of dead tumor cell removal from brain, muscle, subcutaneous tissue, and peritoneal cavity. *Journal of the National Cancer Institute, 52,* 1751-1755.

Kumar, A. R. V., Renaudin, J., Wilson, C. B., Boldrey, E. B., Enot, K. J., & Levin, V. A. (1974). Procarbazine hydrochloride in the treatment of brain tumors. *Journal of Neurosurgery, 40,* 365-371.

Kyritsis, A. P., Yung, W. K. A., Bruner, J., Gleason, M. J., & Levin, V. A. (1993). The treatment of anaplastic oligodendrogliomas and mixed gliomas. *Neurosurgery, 32,* 365-371.

Laws, E. R., Taylor, W. F., Clifton, M. B., & Ozaki, H. (1984). Neurosurgical management of low-grade astrocytoma of the cerebral hemispheres. *Journal of Neurosurgery, 61,* 665-673.

Leavitt, M., Lamb, S. A., & Voss, B. S. (1996). *Oncology Nursing Forum,* 23, 1247-1256.

Leibel, S. A. & Sheline, G. E. (1991). Tolerance of the brain and spinal cord to conventional irradiation. In P. H. Gutin, S. A. Leibel, & G. E. Sheline (Eds.), *Radiation injury to the nervous system.* New York: Raven Press.

Leibel, S. A. & Sheline, G. E. (1987). Radiation therapy for neoplasms of the brain. *Journal of Neurosurgery, 66,* 1-22.

Leibel, S. A., Sheline, G. E., Wara, W. M., Boldrey, E. B., & Nielsen, S. L. (1975). The role of radiation therapy in the treatment of astrocytomas. *Cancer, 35,* 1551-1557.

Levin, V. A. (1986). Pharmacokinetics and CNS chemotherapy. In K. Hellmann & S. K. Carter (Eds.), *Fundamentals of cancer chemotherapy.* New York: McGraw-Hill.

Levin, V. A. (1985). Chemotherapy of primary brain tumors. *Neurology Clinics of North America, 3,* 855-866.

Levin, V. A., Edwards, M. S., Wara, W. M., Allen, J., Ortega, J., & Vestnys, P. (1984). 5-fluorouracil and CCNU followed by hydroxyurea, misonidazole and irradiation for brain stem gliomas: A pilot study of the Brain Tumor Research Center and the Children's Cancer Group. *Neurosurgery, 14,* 679-681.

Levin, V. A., Edwards, M. S., Gutin, P. H., Vestnys, P., Fulton, D., & Seager, M. (1984). Phase II evaluation of dibromodulcitol in the treatment of recurrent medulloblastoma, ependymoma, and malignant astrocytoma. *Journal of Neurosurgery, 61,* 1063-1068.

Levin, V. A., Leibel, S. A., & Gutin, P. H. (1997). Neoplasms of the central nervous system. In V. T. DeVito, S. Hellman, & S. A. Rosenberg (Eds.), *Cancer: The principles and practice of oncology* (5th ed.). Philadelphia: J. B. Lippincott.

Levin, V. A., Prados, M. R., Wara, W. M., Davis, R. L., Gutin, P. H., & Phillips, T. L. (1995). Radiation therapy and bromodeoxyuridine chemotherapy followed by procarbazine, lomustine, and vincristine for the treatment of anaplastic gliomas. *International Journal of Radiation Oncology, Biology, Physics, 32,* 75-83.

Levin, V. A. & Wilson, C. B. (1981). Clinical characteristics of cancer in the brain and spinal cord. In S. T. Crook, & A. Prestayko (Eds.), *Cancer and chemotherapy: Introduction to neoplasms and antineoplastic chemotherapy* (Vol. 2). New York: Academic Press.

Lindegaard, K.-F., Mørk, S. J., Eide, G. E., Halvorsen, T. B., Hatlevoll, R., & Solgaard, T. (1987). Statistical analysis of clinicopathological features, radiotherapy and survival in 170 cases of oligodendroglioma. *Journal of Neurosurgery, 67,* 224-230.

Livingstone, L. R., White, A., Sprouse, J., Livanos, E., Jacks, T., & Tlsty, T. D. (1992). Altered cell cycle arrest and gene amplification potential accompany loss of wild-type p53. *Cell, 70,* 923-935.

Lombardo, M. C. & Hartwig, M. S. (1997). Evaluation of the neurologic patient. In S. A. Price, & L. M. Wilson (Eds.), *Pathophysiology: Clinical concepts of disease processes* (5th ed.). St. Louis: Mosby.

Lombardo, M. C. (1997). Central nervous system tumors. In S. A. Price, & L. M. Wilson (Eds.), *Pathophysiology: Clinical concepts of disease processes* (5th ed.). St. Louis: Mosby.

Louis, D. N. & Cavenee, W. K. (1997). Molecular biology of central nervous system neoplasms. In V. T. DeVito, S. Hellman, & S. A. Rosenberg (Eds.), *Cancer: The principles and practice of oncology* (5th ed.). Philadelphia: J. B. Lippincott.

Louis, D. N. (1994). The p53 gene and protein in human brain tumors. *Journal of Neuropathology and Experimental Neurology, 53,* 11-21.

Louis, D. N., Rubio, M.-P., Correa, K., Gusella, J. F., & von Deimling, A. (1993). Molecular genetic alterations in pediatric brain stem gliomas. Application of PCR techniques to small and archival brain tumor specimens. *Journal of Neuropathology and Experimental Neurology, 52,* 507-515.

MacDonald, D. R. (1994). Low-grade gliomas, mixed gliomas, and oligodendrogliomas. *Seminars in Oncology, 21,* 236-248.

Mack, E. E. (1993). Neurologic tumors. In D. A. Casciato & B. B. Lowitz (Eds.), *Manual of clinical oncology* (5th ed.). Boston: Little, Brown, & Company.

Maiese, K., Walker, R. W., Gargan, R., & Victor, J. D. (1992). Intra-arterial cisplatin-associated optic and otic toxicity. *Archives of Neurology, 49,* 83-86.

Maire, J., Coudin, B., Guerin, H., & Caudry, M. (1987). Neuropsychologic impairment in adults with brain tumors. *American Journal of Clinical Oncology, 10,* 156-162.

Marathi, U. K., Kroes, R. A., Dolan, M. E., & Erickson, L. C. (1993). Prolonged depletion of 06-methylguanine DNA methyltransferase activity following exposure to 06-benzylguanine with or without streptozotocin enhances 1,3-bis(2-chloroethyl)-1-nitrosourea sensitivity *in vitro. Cancer Research, 53,* 4281-4286.

Marks, J. E., Baglan, R. J., Prassad, S. C., & Black, W. F. (1981). Cerebral radionecrosis: Incidence and risk in relation to dose, time, fractionation and volume. *International Journal of Radiation Oncology, Biology, Physics, 7,* 243-252.

McCormack, B. M., Miller, D. C., Budzilovich, G. N., Voorhees, G. J., & Ransohoff, J. (1992). Treatment and survival of low-grade astrocytoma in adults: 1977-1988. *Neurosurgery, 31,* 636-642.

McKee, A. C. (1996). Neoplasms of the central nervous system. In A. T. Skarin, (Ed.), *Atlas of diagnostic oncology* (2nd ed.). Barcelona: Mosby-Wolfe.

Merchant, R. E., Ellison, M. D., & Young, H. F. (1990). Immunotherapy for malignant glioma using human recombinant interleukin-2 and activated autologous lymphocytes: A review of preclinical and clinical investigations. *Journal of Neuro-oncology, 8,* 173-188.

Merchant, R. E., McVicar, D. W., Merchant, L. H., & Young, H. F. (1992). Treatment of recurrent malignant glioma by repeated intracerebral injections of human recombinant interleukin-2 alone or in combination with systemic interferon-alpha: Results of a phase I clinical trial. *Journal of Neuro-oncology, 12,* 75-83.

Merchant, R. E., Merchant, L. H., Cook, S. H., McVicar, D. W., & Young, H. F. (1988). Intralesional infusion of lymphokine-activated killer (LAK) cells and recombinant interleukin-2(rIL-2) for the treatment of patients with malignant brain tumor. *Neurosurgery, 23,* 725-732.

Morantz, R. A. (1987). Radiation therapy in the treatment of cerebral astrocytoma. *Neurosurgery, 20,* 975-982.

Morgan, R. H., Rines, T., D'Aquila, K., Marlo, M., & Benzil, D. L. (1977). Preparing for steriotactic radiosurgery. *Developments in Supportive Cancer Care,* 1(4), 101-102.

Mørk, S. J., Halvorsen, T. B., Lindegaard, K-F., & Eide, G. E. (1986). Oligodendroglioma. Histologic evaluation and prognosis. *Journal of Neuropathology and Experimental Neurology, 45,* 65-78.

Murphy, G. P., Morris, L. B., & Lange, D. (1997). *Informed decisions: The complete book of cancer diagnosis, treatment, and recovery.* New York: Viking.

Murphy, M. E. (1997). Cancers of the brain and central nervous system. In S. E. Otto (Ed.), *Oncology nursing* (3rd ed.). St. Louis: Mosby.

National Cancer Institute. (1998). http://www.cancernet.com. *Adult brain tumor for physicians.*

Nazzaro, J. M. & Neuwelt, E. A. (1990). The role of surgery in the management of supratentorial intermediate and high-grade astrocytomas in adults. *Journal of Neurosurgery, 73,* 331-344.

Neuwelt, E. A., Howieson, J., Frenkel, E. W., Specht, H. D., Weigel, R., & Buchan, C. G. (1986). Therapeutic efficacy of multiagent chemotherapy with drug delivery enhancement by blood-brain barrier modification in glioblastoma. *Neurosurgery, 19,* 573-582.

New hope for patients with a brain tumor. (1997). *Blood and Bone Marrow Transplant Newsletter, 8*(3), 1-2, 8.

NEWS, *See CNS consortia.*

Ohgaki, H., Eibl, R. H., Wiestler, O. D., Yasargil, M. G., Newcomb, E. W., & Kleihaus, P. (1991). p53 mutations in monastrocytic human brain tumors. *Cancer Research, 51,* 6202-6205.

Owens, B. (1992). Neurological cancers. In J. C. Clark & R. F. McGee (Eds.), *Core curriculum for oncology nursing* (2nd ed.). Philadelphia: W. B. Saunders.

Packer, R. J., Boyett, J. M., Zimmerman, R. A., Rorke, L. N., Kaplan, A. M., & Albright, A. L. (1993). Hyperfractionated radiotherapy (72 Gy) for children with brain stem gliomas: A Children's Cancer Group phase I-II trial. *Cancer, 72,* 1414-1421.

Packer, R. J., Allen, J. C., Goldwein, J. L., Newell, J., Zimmerman, R. A., & Priest, J. (1990). Hyperfractionated radiotherapy for children with brainstem gliomas: A pilot study using 7,200 cGy. *Annals of Neurology, 27,* 167-173.

Petronio, J., Edwards, M. S. B., Prados, M., Freyberger, S., Rabbitt, J., & Silver, P. (1990). Management of chiasma and hypothalamic gliomas of infancy and childhood with chemotherapy. *Journal of Neurosurgery, 74,* 701-708.

Pilkington, G. J. (1994). Tumor cell migration in the central nervous system. *Brain Pathology, 4,* 157-166.

Polednak, A. P. & Flannery, J. T. (1995). Brain, other central nervous system and eye cancer. *Cancer, 75,* 330-337.

Posner, J. B. (1995). Side effects of radiotherapy. In R. Wiley (Ed.), *Neurologic complications of cancer.* Philadelphia: F. A. Davis.

Prados, M., Rodriguez, L., Chamberlain, M., Silver, P., & Levin, V. A. (1989). Treatment of recurrent gliomas with 1,3-bis(2-chloroethyl)-1-nitrosourea and alpha-difluoromethylornithine. *Neurosurgery, 24,* 806-809.

Prados, M. D. & Wilson, C. B. (1997). Neoplasms of the central nervous system. In J. F. Holland, E. Frei, III, R. C. Blast, Jr., D. W. Kufe, D. L. Morton, & R. R. Weichselbaum (Eds.), *Cancer medicine* (4th ed.). Baltimore: Williams & Wilkins.

Prados, M. D., Wara, W. M., Edwards, M. S. B., Larson, D. A., Lamborn, K., & Levin, V. A. (1995). The treatment of brain stem and thalamic gliomas with 78 Gy of hyperfractionated radiation therapy. *International Journal of Radiation Oncology and Biological Physics, 32,* 85-91.

Reifenberger, J., Reifenberger, G., Lui, L., James, C. D., Wechsler, W., & Collins, V. P. (1994). Molecular genetic analysis of oligodendroglial tumors shows preferential allelic deletions on 19q and 1p. *American Journal of Pathology, 145,* 1175-1190.

Rodriguez, L. A., Edwards, M. S. B., & Levin, V. A. (1990). Management of hypothalamic glioma in children: An analysis of 33 cases. *Neurosurgery, 26,* 242-247.

Rodriguez, L. A., Prados, M., Fulton, D., Edwards, M. S. B., Silver, P., & Levin, V. A. (1988). Treatment of recurrent brain stem gliomas and other CNS tumors with 5-fluorouracil, CCNU, hydroxyurea and 6-mercaptopurine. *Neurosurgery, 22,* 691-693.

Rosenstock, J. G., Packer, R. J., Bilaniuk, L., Bruce, D. A., Radcliffe, J.-L., & Savino, P. (1985). Chiasmatic optic glioma treated with chemotherapy. *Journal of Neurosurgery, 63,* 862-866.

Ross, G. W. & Rubinstein, I. J. (1989). Lack of histopathological correlation of malignant ependymomas with postoperative survival. *Journal of Neurosurgery, 70,* 31-36.

Rudy, E. (1984). *Advanced neurological and neurosurgical nursing.* St Louis: Mosby.

Salazar, O. M., Castro-Vita, H., Van Houtte, P., Rubin, P., & Aygun, C. (1983). Improved survival in cases of intracranial ependymoma after radiation therapy: Late report and recommendations. *Journal of Neurosurgery, 59,* 652-659.

Salcman, M. (1990). Malignant glioma management. *Neurosurgery Clinics of North America, 1,* 49-63.

Sawaya, R., Juhani, R. O., Glas-Greenwalt, P., & Wu, S. (1991). Plasma fibrinolytic profile in patients with brain tumors. *Thrombosis and Haemostasis, 65,* 15-19.

Seizinger, B. R., Klinger, H. P., Junien, C., Nakamura, Y., Le Beau, M., & Cavenee, W. (1991). Report of the committee on chromosome and gene loss in human neoplasia. *Cytogenetics and Cell Genetics, 58,* 1080-1096.

Shalet, S. M., Beardwell, C. G., Pearson, D., Jones, P. H. (1976). The effect of varying doses of cerebral irradiation on GH production in childhood. *Clinical Endocrinology, 5,* 287-290.

Shaw, E. G., Daumas-Duport, C., Scheithauer, B. W., Gilbertson, D. T., O'Fallon, J. R., & Earle, J. D. (1989). Radiation therapy in the management of low-grade supratentorial astrocytomas. *Journal of Neurosurgery, 70,* 853-861.

Shaw, E. G., Evans, R. G., Scheithauer, B. W., Ilstrup, D. M., & Earle, J. D. (1987). Postoperative radiotherapy of intracranial ependymoma in pediatric and adult patients. *International Journal of Radiation Oncology, Biology, Physics, 13,* 1451-1462.

Shaw, E. G., Scheithauer, B. W., & O'Fallon, J. R. (1991). Management of supratentorial low-grade gliomas. *Seminars in Radiation Oncology, 1,* 23.

Sheline, G. E., Wara, W. M., & Smith, V. (1980). Therapeutic irradiation and brain injury. *International Journal of Radiation Oncology, Biology, Physics, 6,* 1215-1228.

Shimizu, K. Y., Tran, L. M., Mark, R. J., & Selch, M. T. (1993). Management of oligodendrogliomas. *Radiology, 186,* 569-572.

Shrieve, D. C., Wara, W. M., Edwards, M. S., Sneed, P. K., Prados, M. D., & Cogen, P. H. (1992). Hyperfractionated radiation therapy for gliomas of the brainstem in children and in adults. *International Journal of Radiation Oncology, Biology, Physics, 24,* 599-610.

Simpson, J. R., Horton, J., Scott, C., Curan, W. J., Rubin, P., & Fischbach, J. (1993). Influence of location and extent of surgical resection on survival of patients with glioblastoma multiforme: Results of three consecutive Radiation Therapy Oncology Group (RTOG) clinical trials. *International Journal of Radiation Oncology, Biology, Physics, 26,* 239-244.

Skillman, J. J., Collins, R. E. C., Coe, B. P., Goldstein, B., Shapiro, R., & Zervas, N. (1978). Prevention of deep vein thrombosis in neurosurgical patients: A controlled, randomized trial of external pneumatic compression boots. *Surgery, 83,* 354-358.

Sklar, C. A. & Constine, L. S. (1995). Chronic neuroendocrinological sequelae of radiation therapy. *International Journal of Radiation Oncology, Biology, Physics, 31,* 1113-1121.

Steriotatic surgery boosts accuracy when treating "hidden" brain tumors. (1997). *NEWS, 89*(9), 610. URL: http://www.out.co.uk/jnci/hdb/Volume__89/Issue__09/html/890610.html.

Sun, Z. M., Genka, S., Shitara, N., Akanuma, A., & Takakura, K. (1988). Factors possibly influencing the prognosis of oligodendroglioma. *Neurosurgery, 22,* 886-891.

Upchurch, C., Goodwin, W., Brown, T., Selby, G., Vogel, F. S., & Eyre, H. (1993). Assessment of response to new agents for CNS malignancies [Abstract]. *Proceedings of the American Society of Clinical Oncology, 12,* 176.

Urtasun, R. C., Kinsella, T. J., Farman, N., DelRowen, J. D., Lester, S. G., & Fulton, D. S. (1996). Survival improvement in anaplastic astrocytoma, combining external radiation with halogenated pyrimidines. Final report of RTOG 86-12, phase I-II study [Abstract]. *International Journal of Radiation Oncology, Biology, Physics, 36,* 1163-1167.

Van Glabbeke, M., Karim, A. B. M. F., Hamers, H., Harlevoll, R., Pierart, M., & Bartelink, H. (1995). No improvement in survival by increased radiation dose given postoperatively to patients with low grade brain tumors: An EORTC randomized phase III study [Abstract]. *Proceedings of the American Society of Clinical Oncology, 14,* A275.

Vanuytsel, L. & Brada, M. (1991). The role of prophylactic spinal irradiation in localized intracranial ependymoma. *International Journal of Radiation Oncology, Biology, Physics, 21,* 825-830.

Vanuytsel, L. J., Bessell, E. M., Ashley, S. E., Bloom, J. G., & Brada, M. (1992). Long-term results of a policy of surgery and radiotherapy. *International Journal of Radiation Oncology, Biology, Physics, 23,* 313-319.

Vecht, C. J., Avezaat, C. J., van Putten, W. L., Eijkenboom, W. M., & Stefanko, S. Z. (1990). The influence of the extent of surgery on the neurological function and survival in malignant glioma: A retrospective analysis in 243 patients. *Journal of Neurology, Neurosurgery and Psychiatry, 53,* 466-471.

Volker, D. B. (1992). Pathophysiology of cancer. In J. C. Clark & R. F. McGee (Eds.), *Core curriculum for oncology nursing* (2nd ed.). Philadelphia: W. B. Saunders Company.

von Deimling, A., Louis, D. N., von Ammon, K., Petersen, I., Wiestler, O. D., & Seizinger, B. R. (1992). Evidence for a tumor suppressor gene on chromosome *19q* associated with human astrocytomas, oligodendrogliomas and mixed gliomas. *Cancer Research, 52,* 4277-4279.

Waller, M. D., Alexander, E., Jr., Hunt, W. E., McCarty, C. S., Mahaley, M. S., & Mealey, J. (1978). Evaluation of BCNU and/or radiotherapy in the treatment of anaplastic gliomas: A cooperative clinical trial. *Journal of Neurosurgery, 49,* 333-343.

Wallner, K. E., Gonzales, M., & Sheline, G. E. (1988). Treatment of oligodendrogliomas with or without postoperative irradiation. *Journal of Neurosurgery, 68,* 684-688.

Wallner, K. E., Wara, W. M., Sheline, G. E., & Davis, R. L. (1986). Intracranial ependymomas: results of treatment with partial or whole brain irradiation without spinal irradiation. *International Journal of Radiation Oncology, Biology, Physics, 12,* 1937-1941.

Werner, M. H., Phuphanich, S., & Lyman, G. H. (1995). The increasing incidence of malignant gliomas and primary central nervous system lymphoma in the elderly. *Cancer, 76,* 1634-1642. As reviewed by J. V. Simone. In J. V. Simone, G. J. Bosl, A. M. Cohen, E. Glatstein, R. F. Ozols, & M. Tallman (Eds.), *1996 Yearbook of oncology.* St. Louis: Mosby.

Wilson, L. M. & Hartwig, M. S. (1997). Anatomy and physiology of the nervous system. In S. A. Price, & L. M. Wilson (Eds.), *Pathophysiology: Clinical concepts of disease processes* (5th ed.). St. Louis: Mosby.

Winger, M. J., MacDonald, D. R., & Cairncross, J. G. (1989). Supratentorial anaplastic gliomas in adults. *Journal of Neurosurgery, 71,* 487-493.

Wood, J. R., Green, S. B., & Shapiro, W. R. (1988). The prognostic importance of tumor size in malignant gliomas: A computed tomographic scan study by the Brain Tumor Cooperative Group. *Journal of Clinical Oncology, 6,* 338-343.

Yamasaki, T., Kikuchhi, H., Paine, J. T., Yamashita, J., Miyatake, S., & Iwasake, K., Kobayashi, H., Namba, Y., Hanaoka, M. (1989). Murine intracerebral interleukin-2 injection: Pathological and immunological effects. *Journal of Neurosurgery, 71,* 732-740.

Young, B., Oldfield, E. H., Markesbery, W. R., Haack, D., Tibbs, P. A., & McCombs, P. (1981). Reoperation for glioblastoma. *Journal of Neurosurgery, 55,* 917-921.

Young, D. F., Posner, J. B., Chu, F., & Nisce, L. (1974). Rapid-course radiation therapy of cerebral metastases: results and complications. *Cancer, 34,* 1069-1076.

Yung, W. K. A., Mechtler, L., & Gleason, M. J. (1991). Intravenous carboplatin for recurrent malignant gliomas: A phase II study. *Journal of Clinical Oncology, 9,* 860-864.

Zulch, K. J. (1979). *Histologic type of tumors of the central nervous system.* Geneva: World Health Organization.

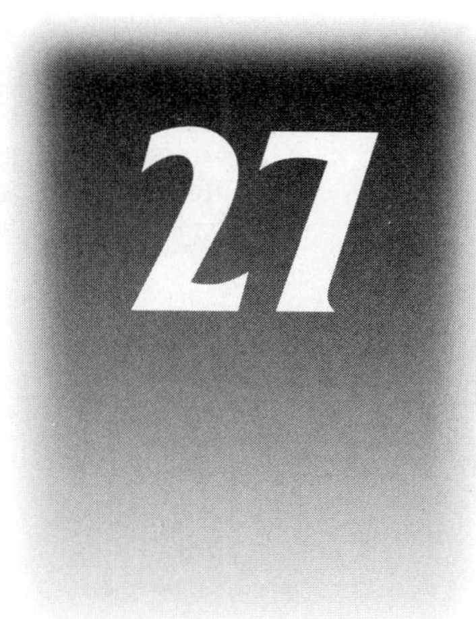

Medulloblastoma

Linda Worrall, RN, MSN, OCN

INTRODUCTION

Medulloblastoma is a primary central nervous system (CNS) tumor originally described more than 65 years ago and defined at that time as fatal despite the best of surgical efforts. Since then, evolution of therapeutic strategies has dramatically improved the prognosis for patients with medulloblastoma. These advances are a result of clinical trials that have attempted to improve the best available, accepted therapy. Medulloblastoma is rare in adults and is largely considered a pediatric disease (Albright, 1993).

EPIDEMIOLOGY

Medulloblastoma is one of the most common malignant brain tumors in children, accounting for approximately 20% of all childhood CNS neoplasms. The tumor demonstrates a bimodal incidence, showing a major early peak between 5 and 8 years of age, and a smaller peak between 20 and 30 years. Approximately 250 new pediatric cases of medulloblastoma are diagnosed in the United States each year (Prados & Wilson, 1997), and 20% of cases occur during late adolescence or early adulthood. In the adult population, medulloblastoma accounts for approximately 1% of all CNS neoplasms (Thaper, 1996).

The median age at diagnosis is 5 to 6 years, with approximately 20% of cases occurring in infants less than 2 years of age. Medulloblastoma is more common in boys than girls (2:1) (Halperin, Constine, Tarbell, & Kun, 1994). The 5-year survival rate for children diagnosed with medulloblastoma is approximately 50% (Packer, Sutton, Atkins, Radcliffe, Bunin, D'Angio, et al., 1989). Of interest, patients who receive treatment at large referral centers do better than those treated at smaller institutions (Boyett & Viehi, 1985; Cohen & Duffner, 1994).

RISK FACTORS

Risk factors associated with medulloblastoma are largely unknown. There has been some association with inherited syndromes, the most prominent of which are ataxia telangiectasia and Li-Fraumeni syndrome (Cohen & Duffner, 1994).

CHEMOPREVENTION

Chemoprevention refers to the use of drugs or certain foods to prevent malignancies from developing or progressing. Although many chemoprevention trials are currently in progress, review of the literature does not include any type of chemoprevention efforts for medulloblastoma.

PATHOPHYSIOLOGY

Normal Anatomy and Physiology of the CNS

The CNS is composed of the brain and spinal cord, which are enclosed within the cranium and bony spinal column. The brain can be divided into four regions: cerebrum, diencephalon, brain stem, and cerebellum (Fig. 27-1).

The cerebrum includes the right and left hemispheres and makes up approximately 80% of the brain. The diencephalon, meaning "between brain," includes the thalamus and hypothalamus. At the base of the brain lies the cerebellum, which is responsible for coordination of movement. The brain stem, which is made up of the midbrain, pons, and medulla, connects the upper portion of the brain to the spinal cord. Brain tissue consists of gray matter, which is composed of nerve cell bodies and white matter composed of myelinated nerve fibers. The brain also contains four irregularly shaped spaces within the brain called *ventricles.* These four ventricles are interconnected and assist in the production and circulation of cerebrospinal fluid (CSF), which functions as a cushion and support to the brain and the spinal cord. There are two lateral ventricles, one in each cerebral hemisphere; these contain a major portion of the choroid plexus, which produces the CSF. The third ventricle is located just posterior to the hypothalamus, and the fourth is located in the brain stem, anterior to the cerebellum. Approximately

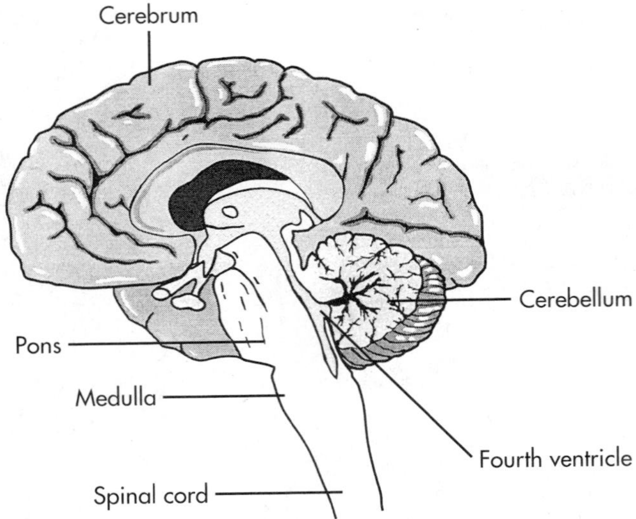

Fig. 27-1 Diagrammatic representation of the structures within the brain.

150 ml of CSF circulate through the CNS at any given time.

The Process of Carcinogenesis

Medulloblastoma is thought to arise from primitive neuroepithelial cells of the external granular layer of the cerebellum. Normally, these embryonal cells involute and disappear by 18 months of age. Their abnormal persistence, in the form of embryonal cells, rests the presumed basis for the development of these primitive tumors. Medulloblastoma usually originates in the midline cerebellar vermis. Initially, these tumors fill and expand the fourth ventricle, frequently infiltrating the ventricle walls and floor. Permeating along CSF pathways, the tumors ascend superiorly into the cerebral aqueduct, descend interiorly to the cisterna magna, and extend laterally via the foramina of Luschka into the cerebellopontine angle. By this point, CSF circulation has generally been blocked and an obstructive hydrocephalus results. The tumor may spread through the cerebellum, to the floor of the fourth ventricle, into the cervical spine or above the tentorium. In adolescents and adults, this disease occurs more frequently in the cerebellar hemisphere than within the fourth ventricle, where most childhood medulloblastomas present (Haplern et al., 1994; Louis & Cavenee, 1997).

Medulloblastoma is characterized by a highly cellular tissue that is well-demarcated (Cohen & Duffner, 1994). Medulloblastoma is a highly cellular tumor, believed to originate from primitive neuroepithelial cells with nonspecific differentiation. The term *primitive neuroepithelial tumor* (PNET) has been assigned to tumors that are histologically similar and occur in the cerebellum, cerebrum, and pineal region; medulloblastoma is among these (Prados, & Wilson, 1997). Current controversy exists about this nomenclature, and not all clinicians use this classification. PNET and medulloblastoma are frequently used interchangeably; however, this grouping of multiple CNS tumors into one category has made it difficult to compare clinical information related to the diagnosis.

Table 27-1 Sites of Relapse

Site	Percentage of Relapse/Site
Posterior fossa	50
Frontal lobe	20
Bone	10-15
Other cerebral and suprasellar regions	10-15

From Levin, V. A., Gutin, P. H., & Leibel, S. (1993). Neoplasms of the central nervous system. In V. T. DeVita, Jr., S. Hellman, & S. A. Rosenberg (Eds.), *Cancer: Principles & practice of oncology* (4th ed.). Philadelphia: J. B. Lippincott.

ROUTES OF METASTASES

At the time of diagnosis, 30% of patients have metastatic disease. The tumor spreads by seeding or direct extension of the tumor to the subarachnoid space intracranially and within the spinal canal. Medulloblastoma often spreads via CSF intracranially and/or into spinal cord or bones. Table 27-1 illustrates disease sites and percentages of relapse related to medulloblastoma.

ASSESSMENT

The clinical evaluation includes a thorough history, physical examination, and diagnostic evaluation (Table 27-2).

History and Physical Examination

A complete neurologic history for patients thought to have a CNS tumor is essential. Medulloblastoma presents with progressive features of an expanding posterior fossa mass associated with increased intracranial pressure (ICP) and resulting in vomiting, lethargy, and papilledema. Symptoms relating to hydrocephalus and elevated ICP frequently predominate, followed eventually by more specific posterior fossa symptoms of ataxia, morning headaches, and unsteadiness, as well as diplopia and nystagmus. Herniation or impaction of the cerebellar tonsils can cause neck stiffness and head tilting. (Albright, 1993). Obtaining a careful history from both the patient and family is mandatory. Observations by family members are particularly important because abnormalities unknown to the patient, especially children, may be noted.

A thorough neurologic physical examination, including the cranial nerves, cerebellar examination, motor strength, and the eye area, is essential to detect and document any abnormalities (Halpern et al., 1994). Cerebellar syndrome produces ataxia and problems with manual dexterity and is the result of interference with the function of an area of the cerebellum (Halperin et al., 1994).

TABLE 27-2 Assessment of the Patient with Medulloblastoma

	Assessment Parameters	Typical Abnormal Findings
History	A. Personal and social history 1. Age 2. Sex B. Evaluation of central nervous system	A. Personal and social history 1. Peak age 5 years 2. Males at greater risk than females B. Common symptoms include ataxic gait, headache, weakness, intention tremor, nausea and vomiting, papilledema, and diplopia; symptoms of increased intercranial pressure (ICP) appear early. Children less than 1 year of age may appear lethargic, have an increased head circumference, and have noted developmental delays.
Physical Examination	A. Neurologic assessment, including the cranial nerves, cerebellar examination, motor strength, and eye area	A. Essential to detect any abnormalities. Particular attention to gait alterations, impaired balance, loss of coordination and signs of increased ICP, all of which might indicate an alteration in the cerebellar area of the brain.
Diagnostic Tests	A. Magnetic resonance imaging (MRI) with gadolinium contrast B. Computed tomography (CT) C. Cerebrospinal fluid (CSF) cytology D. Bone scan	A. MRI is the scan of choice because it provides a greater resolution; therefore it is less likely to produce artifact, allowing a clearer image of the brain stem and cerebrum. B. CT without contrast provides tumor density, existence of hydrocephalus, and presence of calcification or hemorrhage. CT with contrast assists in identifying tumor margins and differentiating from vascular malformations. C. CSF measurements may detect the development of recurrence before they are detected on scans (Marton, Edwards, Levin, Lubich, & Wilson, 1981). D. Necessary to determine metastatic spread to bone.

Diagnostic Tests

Magnetic Resonance Imaging. Any patient suspected of having medulloblastoma should be evaluated with diagnostic imaging of the spinal cord and whole brain. The most sensitive method available for evaluating spinal cord subarachnoid metastasis is spinal magnetic resonance imaging (MRI) performed with gadolinium. If MRI is used, the entire spine must be imaged in at least two planes, with contiguous MRI slides performed after gadolinium enhancement. Because medulloblastoma occasionally metastasizes outside the CNS, especially to bone, a bone scan with plain film correlation as well as a bone marrow aspiration and biopsy may be useful in symptomatic patients or in those with abnormal blood cell counts. An MRI scan can provide information about the chemical makeup of tissues and can help distinguish between normal and cancerous tissue. The MRI is the scan of choice for medulloblastoma because it provides greater resolution and is less likely to produce artifact, allowing a clearer image of the brain stem and cerebrum. The MRI should encompass the cranium and spinal column. Unfortunately the MRI has difficulty distinguishing between tumor and surrounding edema and is not able to detect calcifications (Belford, 1997). During the MRI scan, the patient is required to lie completely still in a cylinder-shaped machine for the duration of the test. Patients often complain of claustrophobia and have difficulty remaining still, resulting in an incomplete examination. Table 27-3 outlines the patient preparation for an MRI. The MRI is useful not only in determining the extent of the disease upon diagnosis, but also in detecting the amount of disease present postoperatively, as well as disease recurrence (Grabenbauer, Beck, Erhardt, Seegenschmiedt, Seyer, & Thieraut et al., 1996).

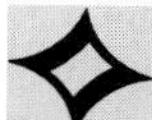

TABLE 27-3 Patient Preparation for MRI

Description of the Procedure: MRI uses a static magnetic field instead of radiation to visualize data.

Patient Preparation: Patient will be required to lie still in the scanner for an extended period. Children will require general anesthesia to complete the test, and some adult patients may require a sedative.

Procedural Considerations:

1. Jewelry and glasses are removed; patient wears a gown.
2. Administer sedation to patients unable to lie still.
3. Patient is placed inside scanner.
4. Scan is completed.
5. Patient is returned to room; if sedated, close monitoring of respiratory status and for safety is required.

Computed Tomography. A computed tomography (CT) scan provides radiologic images of the body including the densities of various structures. The addition of CT scanning without contrast provides tumor density, existence of hydrocephalus, and presence of calcification or hemorrhage.

CT with contrast assists in identifying tumor margins and differentiation from vascular malformations.

Cerebrospinal Fluid. An analysis of the CSF is rarely used for tumor staging or histologic diagnosis. The chemical tumor marker polyamines, specifically putrescine, are accurate markers for the recurrence of medulloblastoma (Yager, 1997) and may be found in the CSF. Putrescine is formed by bacterial action on the amino acid arginine. Serial polyamine measurement may detect the development of recurrence before they are detected on scans (Marton et al., 1981).

Bone Scan. It is not uncommon to have metastatic disease at diagnosis of medulloblastoma. Bone scans are used to determine if metastatic spread to bone has occurred.

STAGING

Staging of medulloblastoma is done after surgical resection is performed for initial treatment of this disease. Postoperative staging systems are now used based on surgical impression and postoperative imaging. Patients presenting with disseminated disease are at high risk for relapse. Box 27-1 outlines two subclassifications used for disease staging. The previous staging system proposed by Harisiadi and Chang was based on intraoperative staging and included size, extent, and the presence/absence of metastatic disease (Laurent, Chang, & Cohen, 1985).

MEDICAL MANAGEMENT

Management for medulloblastoma is based on the stage of disease at diagnosis and patient age. Treatment for medulloblastoma is multidimensional and can include surgery, radiation therapy, and/or chemotherapy.

Surgical Management

The goal of surgery is to remove the tumor completely without compromising neurologic function, decompress the cerebral ventricles, and relieve hydrocephalus (Albright, Wisoff, Zeltzer, Deutsch, Finlay, & Hammond, 1989; Park, Hoffman, Hendrick, Humphreys, & Becker, 1983). Surgery via the posterior fossa craniotomy with microsurgical resection has been documented to remove 90% or more of the tumor in about 80% of cases (Albright et al., 1989). At the time of this surgery, hydrocephalus may be treated with an external ventricular drain or a ventriculoperitoneal shunt (Dias & Albright, 1989). This drain may be maintained postoperatively up to 72 hours; however, controversy surrounds the use of shunting due to the possible spread of malignant cells (Cohen & Duffner, 1994).

Box 27-1
Staging Subclassifications

Average Risk (Low Stage)	Poor Risk (High Stage)
Child >3 years	Child <3 years
Posterior fossa tumor	Nonposterior fossa location
Tumor is totally or "near-totally" (<1.5 cm^3 of residual disease) resected	Subtotal tumor resection (>1.5 cm^3 of residual disease)
No dissemination	Metastatic disease

From Laurent, J.P., Chang, C.H., & Cohen, M. E. (1985). A classification system for primitive neuroectodermal tumors (medulloblastoma) of the posterior fossa. *Cancer, 56*(Suppl. 7), 1807-1809; Packer, R. J., Sutton, L. N., D'Angio, G., Evans, A. E., & Schut, L. (1985). Management of children with primitive neuroectodermal tumors of the posterior fossa/medulloblastoma. *Pediatric Neuroscience, 12,* 272-282.

Radiation Therapy

Medulloblastoma is relatively radiosensitive, and increasing the dose of radiation therapy to the posterior fossa, the site of most common relapse, has led to increased survival (Evans, 1994). The high incidence of CSF and meningeal seeding by the time of diagnosis is an indication for craniospinal radiation (Yager, 1997). Craniospinal radiation therapy is required in all patients at a dose of 36 to 40 Gy to the whole brain, 54 to 60 Gy to the posterior fossa, and 23 to 41 Gy to the spine (Albright, 1993; Evans, 1994; Graberbauer, Beck, Ehrhardt, Seegenschmiedt, Seyer, & Thieraut, 1996; Hughes, Shillito, Sallan, Loeffler, Cassady, & Tarbell, 1988). Radiation less than 50 Gy has been associated with increased recurrence and spinal metastasis.

One of the major negative effects of radiation therapy is the long-term intellectual deficits that result. This decrease in intellectual functioning has been shown to be more significant in children less than 3 years of age at treatment with radiation. Radiation therapy can cause leukoencephalopathy, vasculopathy, and radiation necrosis, which alters both cognitive development and function (Johnson, McCabe, Nicholson, Joseph, Getson, & Byrne et al., 1994; Kun, 1994). Intelligence quotient was less for children treated before the age of 3 years than those treated after that age (Johnson et al., 1994).

Radiation also affects the pituitary gland, resulting in a growth hormone deficiency. Supplemental growth hormone can be initiated in children requiring radiation therapy (Evans, 1994). Children less than 3 years have the greatest problem with intellectual functioning (Evans, 1994). Due to the extent of radiation required for medulloblastoma, it is impossible to avoid the thyroid gland during the spinal portion of craniospinal irradiation; the thyroid may receive up to 50% of delivered does. Hypothyroidism can be treated with daily thyroid replacement (Evans, 1994). The changes in the bone structure of vertebral bones is severe, resulting in a decrease in stature (Evans, 1994). Some deficits may develop over time; therefore, regular neuropsychological evaluations to assess the patient's abilities and to note any new deficits should be encouraged.

Chemotherapy

With the debilitating effects of radiation on growth and neurologic development in children, the use of chemotherapy to treat medulloblastoma has been incorporated into many treatment plans, thus allowing the delay of radiation and its negative sequelae. Di Rocco, Iannelli, La Marca, Tornesello, Mastrangelo, & Riccardi (1995) discussed the use of preoperative chemotherapy to reduce the size and extent of the medulloblastoma before surgery. Although this particular study involved only three patients, the investigators reported that the administration of carboplatin to children less than 3 years of age facilitated the surgical treatment by significantly reducing the tumor burden. Freeman (1994) lists the following reasons for preradiation chemotherapy:

- Cisplatin and methotrexate may be less toxic when administered before radiation.
- Microvascular changes and scarring after radiation may limit drug delivery to the tumor.
- Certain mechanisms of resistance may be shared by radiation and certain alkylating agents.
- Cisplatin may act as a radiosensitizer when administered before radiation.

Numerous other studies have all provided different chemotherapeutic regimens for treatment of medulloblastoma, with positive results achieved in the high-risk population (Duffner, Horowitz, Kirscher, Friedman, Burger, & Cohen et al., 1993; Evans, Jenkin, Sposto, Ortega, Wilson, & Wara et al., 1990; Horowitz, Kun, Mulhern, Kovnar, Sanford, & Hockenberger et al., 1988; Krischer, Ragab, Kun, Kim, Laurent, & Boyett et al., 1991; Packer, Sutton, Goldwein, Perilongo, Bunin, & Ryan, et al., 1991; Pendergrass, Milstein, Geyer, Mulne, Kosnik, & Morris et al., 1987; Tait, Thornton-Jones, Bloom, Lemerle, & Morris-Jones, 1990). Many different chemotherapeutic regimens have been described; carboplatin alone, cyclophosphamide, vincristine, lomustine and cisplatin in various combinations may increase survival for high-risk patients. A number of nitrosureas and platinum compounds, vinca alkaloids, and the epipodophylotoxins destroy recurrent medulloblastoma, including methotrexate, procarbazine,

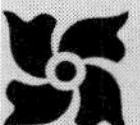

TABLE 27-4 Standard of Care for the Patient Undergoing Radiation Therapy for Medulloblastoma

Patient Problem and Outcomes	Nursing Interventions and Rationales	Patient Education Instructions
Knowledge Deficit Patient will: • Verbalize that radiation therapy is a major treatment for medulloblastoma • Discuss individual radiation treatment plan • State the purpose of "tattooing"	1. Assess current level of knowledge related to radiation therapy. 2. Assess level of understanding of radiation therapy related to disease process. 3. Provide time for questions. 4. Administer sedative as necessary to decrease anxiety before treatment, as ordered by physician.	1. Discuss the principles of radiation therapy as a treatment. 2. Provide patient with current literature related to radiation therapy. 3. Reassure patient/family that the patient is not radioactive. 4. Outline treatment schedule (include days, times, number of treatments). 5. Patient must lie still for entire treatment.
Alopecia Patient will: • Identify alopecia as a side effect to radiation treatments • List ways to manage hair loss	1. Assess patient's knowledge related to hair loss. 2. Assess patient's ability to cope with hair loss.	1. Instruct patient that hair loss is usually temporary and should return approximately 6 months after final treatment. 2. Caution not to wash off treatment guidelines. 3. Use wide tooth comb on hair, and avoid excessive brushing. 4. Encourage to purchase head covering (wig, turban, cap) before hair loss. 5. Avoid hair dyes or use of hot irons/rollers in hair during treatment.
Fatigue Patient will: • Identify fatigue as a side effect to radiation treatments • Verbalize the need for frequent rest periods while receiving radiation therapy	1. Assess patient's level of understanding related to fatigue being a major side effect of radiation therapy. 2. Assist the patient in recognizing the need to take rest periods.	1. Instruct patient that fatigue is a common side effect of radiation therapy and that it should be expected. 2. Encourage patient to plan rest periods throughout day. 3. Instruct patient that he/she may need to decrease normal activity during therapy.

and cyclophosphamide (Freeman, 1994). Newer treatments include using an 8-drugs-in-1-day regimen (vincristine, lomustine, procarbazine, hydroxyurea, cisplatin cytosine, arabinoside, methylprednisolone, and either cyclophosphamide or dacarbazine) to maximize toxicity by giving all the drugs in 12 hours (Krischer et al., 1991). Marrow ablative therapies are being initiated with follow-up bone marrow transplantation; results are better than with conventional chemotherapy. Albright (1993) recommends the following as follow-up for malignant tumors: "scans every 3 to 4 months for 2 years then at 2.5, 3, 4, 5, 7, and 10 years after diagnosis." Recurrence often takes place within 3 years of treatment.

ONCOLOGIC EMERGENCIES

The major oncologic emergency associated with medulloblastoma is the possibility of increased ICP. Radiation and/or recurrent disease also place patients at risk. The goals of each therapy—surgery, radiation, and chemotherapy—play a significant role in reducing ICP. Early signs of increasing ICP include headaches, especially early morning, nausea and vomiting, loss of appetite, blurred vision, and decreased visual fields. Late effects of increasing ICP could include bradycardia, shallow and slow respirations, decreased level of consciousness, seizures, and pupillary changes. Chapter 11 offers a complete discussion of oncologic emergencies.

NURSING MANAGEMENT

Nurses play a significant role in the care of the patient with medulloblastoma. Nursing care is required in all stages of the disease from diagnostic test preparation to support of potential long-term complications. During the diagnostic phase, it is not uncommon for children to require sedation to keep them still during MRI or CT scanning. Care must be taken during this period to maintain the respiratory status of the patient. In the adult population, it is not uncommon to administer an oral sedative before the scans to decrease anxiety. Care must be taken to ensure patient safety while sedated.

Patients with tumors in the cerebellar area are likely to have an altered gait, impaired balance, and loss of coordination, all of which will require safety precautions to prevent injury. Encouraging the patient not to ambulate unassisted, and keeping the call light within reach will assist in keeping the patient free of injury.

Nurses will be required to initiate a plan that will decrease ICP. In addition, observing for seizure activity is necessary, as well as initiating seizure precautions such as padding the side rails, having suction equipment available, and administering anticonvulsants as prescribed by the physician. The increased ICP may also cause nausea and vomiting, and the nurse may be required to administer antiemetics to help with this side effect.

Depending on the course of treatment planned for the patient, postoperative care may include the care of an intraventricular drain. Table 27-4 provides the nurse with a sample standard of care for the patient undergoing radiation therapy. Side effect management related to chemotherapy treatment will be specific to the agents used in the treatment plan.

HOME CARE ISSUES

Safety issues in the home are important to prevent injury to the patient. It is not uncommon for the patients to experience fatigue regardless of the type of treatment they receive for the medulloblastoma.

Nurses need to be aware of the many resources available to patients with medulloblastoma and their families. For example, the American Brain Tumor Association provides written materials for patients regarding their disease, its treatments, and treatment centers. It also offers listings of brain tumor support groups. The National Brain Tumor Foundation provides similar services. Cancer Information Service is available through the National Cancer Institute and can provide patient information to the health care professional.

PROGNOSIS

The prognosis for patients diagnosed with medulloblastoma varies. Five-year survival rates have been noted between

TABLE 27-5 Quality of Care Evaluation for a Child Receiving Radiation Therapy to the Head

Disciplines participating in the quality of care evaluation:
☐ Nursing ☐ Radiation Oncologist ☐ Radiation Technician

Data from:
☐ Mailed questionnaire ☐ Patient interview

Criteria	Yes	No
1. Did the doctor or nurse explain to you that your child may need to have an anesthetic before each radiation treatment in order for him/her to remain as still as possible during the treatment?	☐	☐
2. Did the doctor or nurse explain to you that your child would not be radioactive from receiving radiation treatment?	☐	☐
3. Did the doctor or nurse explain to you that you might notice the following side effects from radiation therapy to the head?		
a. Hair loss	☐	☐
b. Redness to the area	☐	☐
c. Nausea and vomiting	☐	☐
d. Drowsiness	☐	☐

40% and 75% (Yager, 1997). Age at diagnosis, location of tumor, degree of resection, and the absence or presence of metastatic disease on diagnosis all play an important role in long-term survival. Patients who are initially classified in the poor risk category (see Box 27-1) would be in the lower percentage, whereas patients initially classified in the average risk would be in the upper percentile of long-term survival.

EVALUATION OF THE QUALITY OF CARE

Quality patient care is a necessity in today's health care environment. Evaluation tools are an easy and efficient way to measure the quality of care administered to patients. Tools can be used by all disciplines coming into contact with the patient. Table 27-5 is an example of one type of tool that can be used to measure the quality of care in patients with medulloblastoma.

RESEARCH ISSUES

Research surrounding the treatment of medulloblastoma in the patient less than 3 years of age is critical. Radiation dosage needs additional research to provide patients with the maximum effective dose with the least amount of adverse effects. Unfortunately, a few studies have already demonstrated that decreasing the radiation dose leads to an increase in disease recurrence. Further research studies related to the varied chemotherapeutic regimens for this patient population is required. If adequate treatment can be obtained with chemotherapeutic agents, we may be able to eliminate high-dose radiation therapy and its sequelae.

REFERENCES

Albright, A. L. (1993). Pediatric brain tumors. *CA: A Cancer Journal for Clinicians, 43,* 272-288.

Albright, A. L., Wisoff, J. H., Zeltzer, P. M., Deutsch, M., Finlay, J., & Hammond, D. (1989). Current neurosurgical treatment of medulloblastomas in children: A report from the Children's Cancer Study Group. *Pediatric Neuroscience, 15,* 276-282.

Belford, K. (1997). Central nervous system tumors. In S. L. Groenwald, M. H. Frogge, M. Goodman, & C. H. Yarbro (Eds.), *Cancer nursing: Principles and practice* (4th ed.). pp. 980-1035, Sudsbury: Jones & Bartlett Publishing.

Boyett, J. M. & Viehi, T. J. (1985). Role of clinical trials and cooperative group studies in children. *Cancer, 56,* 1984-86.

Cohen, M. E. & Duffner, P. K. (1994). Medulloblastomas. In *Brain tumors in children: Principles of diagnosis and treatment* (2nd ed.). New York: Raven Press.

Di Rocco, C., Iannelli, A., La Marca, F., Tornesello, A., Mastrangelo, S., & Riccardi, R. (1995). Preoperative chemotherapy with carboplatin alone in high risk medulloblastoma. *Child's Nervous System, 11,* 574-578.

Dias, M. S. & Albright, A. L. (1989). Management of hydrocephalus complicating childhood posterior fossa tumors. *Pediatric Neuroscience, 15,* 283-289.

Duffner, P. K., Horowitz, M. E., Kirscher, J. P., Friedman, H. S., Burger, P. C., Cohen, M. E., Sanford, R. A., Mulhern, R. K., James, H. E., Freeman, C. R., Seidel, F. G., & Kun, L. E. (1993). Postoperative chemotherapy and delayed radiation in children less than three years of age with malignant brain tumors. *New England Journal of Medicine, 328,* 1725-1731.

Evans A. E., Jenkin, R. D., Sposto, R., Ortega, J. A., Wilson, C. B., Wara, W., Ertel, I. J., Dramer, S., Chang, C. H., & Leikin, S. L. (1990). The treatment of medulloblastoma: Results of a prospective randomized trial of radiation therapy with and without CCNU, vincristine, and prednisone. *Journal of Neurosurgery, 72,* 572-582.

Evans, R. G. (1994). The role of radiation therapy in the treatment of brain tumors in children. In R. A. Morantz & J. W. Walsch (Eds.), *Brain tumors: A comprehensive text.* New York: Marcel Dekker.

Freeman, A. I. (1994). Chemotherapy of pediatric brain tumors. In R. A. Morantz & J. W. Walsch (Eds.), *Brain tumors: A comprehensive text.* New York: Marcel Dekker.

Freeman, H. S., Oakes, W. J., Bigner, S. H., Wikstrand, C. J., & Bigner, D. D. (1991). Medulloblastoma: Tumor biological and clinical perspectives. *Journal of Neurooncology, 11,* 1-15.

Grabenbauer, G. G., Beck, J. D., Erhardt, J., Seegenschmiedt, M. H., Seyer, H., Thieraut, P., & Sauer, R. (1996). Postoperative radiation therapy of medulloblastoma: Impact of radiation quality on treatment outcome. *American Journal of Clinical Oncology, 19,* 73-77.

Halperin, E. C., Constine, L. S., Tarbell, N. J., & Kun, L. E. (Eds.). (1994). Tumors of the posterior fossa of the brain and the spinal canal. In *Pediatric radiation oncology* (2nd ed.). New York: Raven Press.

Horowitz, M. E., Kun, L. E., Mulhern, R. K., Kovnar, E. H., Sanford, R. A., Hockenberger, B. M., Greeson, F. L., Langston, J. W., Fairclough, D. L., & Jenkins, J. J., 3rd. (1988). Feasibility and efficacy of preirradiation chemotherapy for pediatric brain tumors. *Neurosurgery, 22,* 687-690.

Hughes, E. N., Shillito, J., Sallan, S. E., Loeffler, J. S., Cassady, J. R., & Tarbell, N. J. (1988). Medulloblastoma at the Joint Center for Radiation Therapy between 1968 and 1984. *Cancer, 61,* 1992-1998.

Johnson, D. L., McCabe, M. A., Nicholson, H. S., Joseph, A. L., Getson, P. R., Byrne, J., Brasseux, C., Packer, R. J., & Reaman, G. (1994). Quality of long-term survival in young children with medulloblastoma. *Journal of Neurosurgery, 80,* 1004-1010.

Krischer, J. P., Ragab, A. H., Kun, L., Kim, T. H., Laurent, J. P., Boyett, J. M., Cornell, C. J., Link, M., Luthy, A. R., & Camitta, B. (1991). Nitrogen mustard, vincristine, procarbazine, and prednisone as adjuvant chemotherapy in the treatment of medulloblastoma: A Pediatric Oncology Group study. *Journal of Neurosurgery, 74,* 905-909.

Kun, L. E. (1994), Principles of radiation therapy. In M. E. Cohen & P. K. Duffner (Eds.), *Brain tumors in children: Principles of diagnosis and treatment* (2nd ed.). New York: Raven Press.

Laurent, J. P., Chang, C. H., & Cohen, M. E. (1985). A classification system for primitive neuroectodermal tumors (medulloblastoma) of the posterior fossa. *Cancer, 56*(Suppl. 7), 1807-1809.

Levin, V. A., Gutin, P. H., & Leibel, S. (1994). Neoplasms of the central nervous system. In V. T. DeVita, Jr., S. Hellman, & S. A. Rosenberg (Eds.), *Cancer: Principles & practice of oncology* (4th ed.). Philadelphia: J.B. Lippincott Co.

Louis, D. & Cavenee, W. K. (1997). Neoplasms of the central nervous system. In V. T. DeVita, Jr., S. Hellman, & S. A. Rosenberg (Eds.), *Cancer: Principles & practice of oncology* (5th ed.). Philadelphia: Lippincott-Raven.

Marton, L. J., Edwards, M. S., Levin, V. A., Lubich, W. P., & Wilson, C. B. (1981). CSF polyamines: A new and important means of monitoring patients with medulloblastomas. *Cancer, 47,* 757-760.

Packer, R. J., Sutton, L. N., Atkins, T. E., Radcliffe, J., Bunin, G. R., D'Angio, G., Siegel, K. R., & Schut, L. (1989). A prospective study of cognitive function in children receiving whole brain radiation therapy and chemotherapy: 2-year results. *Journal of Neurosurgery,* 70, 707-713.

Packer, R. J., Sutton, L. N., D'Angio, G., Evans, A. E., & Schut, L. (1985). Management of children with primitive neuroectodermal tumors of the posterior fossa/medulloblastoma. *Pediatric Neuroscience, 12,* 272-282.

Packer, R. J., Sutton, L. N., Goldwein, J. W., Perilongo, G., Bunin, G., Ryan, J., Cohen, B. H., D'Angio, G., Kramer, E. D., & Zimmerman, R. A. (1991). Improved survival with the use of adjuvant chemotherapy in the treatment of medulloblastoma. *Journal of Neurosurgery, 74,* 433-440.

Prados, M. D. & Wilson, C. B. (1997). Neoplasms of the central nervous system. In J. F. Holland, E. Frei, III, R. C. Blast, Jr., D. W. Kufe, D. L. Morton, & R. R. Weichselbaum (Eds.), *Cancer medicine* (4th ed.). Baltimore: Williams & Wilkins.

Park, T. S., Hoffman, H. J., Hendrick, E. B., Humphreys, R. P., & Becker, L. E. (1983). Medulloblastoma, clinical presentation and management: Experience at the hospital for sick children, Toronto, 1950-1980. *Journal of Neurosurgery, 58,* 543-552.

Pendergrass, T. W., Milstein, J. M., Geyer, J. R., Mulne, A. F., Kosnik, E. J., Morris, J. D., Heideman, R. L., Ruymann, F. B., Stantz, J. T., & Bleyer, W. A. (1987). Eight drugs in one day chemotherapy for brain tumors: Experience of 107 children and rationale for preradiation chemotherapy. *Journal of Clinical Oncology, 5,* 1221-1231.

Rager, J. Y. & Vannucci, R. C. (1997). Brain tumors. In R. A. Hoekelman (Ed.), *Primary pediatric care* (3rd ed.). St. Louis: Mosby.

Tait, D. M., Thornton-Jones, H., Bloom, H. J. G., Lemerle, J., & Morris-Jones, P. (1990). Adjuvant chemotherapy for medulloblastoma: The first multi-centre control trial of the International Society of Paediatric Oncology (SIOP I). *European Journal of Cancer, 26,* 464-469.

Thaper K. & Laws, E. R. (1996). Tumors of the central nervous system. In G. P. Murphy, W. Lawrence, & R. E. Lenhard (Eds.), *Clinical oncology.* Atlanta: American Cancer Society.

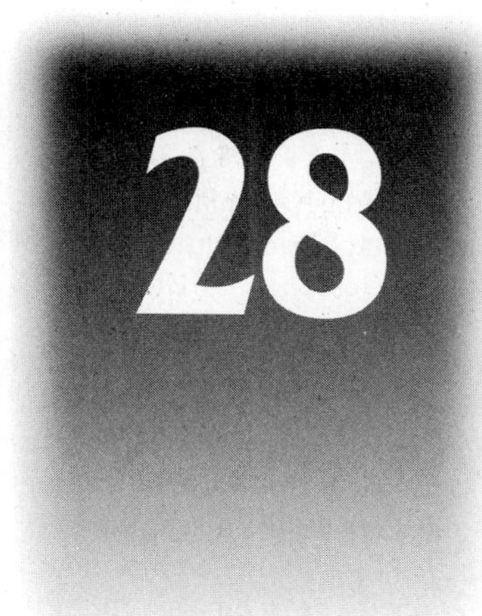

Neuroblastoma

Vivian Gates, RN, CS, MSN, AOCN

EPIDEMIOLOGY

Primary tumors of the central nervous system (CNS) are extremely rare, representing less than 2% of all reported malignancies. The estimated number of new brain and other CNS cancers in 1998 was less than 18,000. All CNS neoplasms will account for about 2% of all cancer-related deaths in 1999 (Landis, Murray, Bolden, & Wingo, 1998). Although primary brain tumors are found across the life span, they have two peak incidences. The first peak is in the first decade of life, and the second peak is in the fifth or sixth decade. Intracranial neoplasms are slightly more common in men (Keyser, 1993a). Some researchers have suggested that there has been an increasing incidence of primary brain tumors over the last few decades, but the reasons for this increase are not clear (Desmeules, Mikkelsen, & Mao, 1992; Grieg, Ries, & Yancik, 1990).

Primary cerebral neuroblastomas are extremely uncommon in adults. Two relatively large series demonstrate that most cerebral neuroblastomas occur in very young children (Bennet & Rubenstein, 1984; Horten & Rubenstein, 1976). However, those series and other smaller ones reported that cerebral neuroblastomas can occur at any time from adolescence to old age (Berger, Edwards, Wara, Levin, & Wilson, 1983; Davis, Wichman, Takei, & Hoffman, 1990; Louis, Swearingen, Linggood, Dickersin, Kretschmar, & Bhan et al., 1990; Nakagawa, Aoki, Sakata, Sasaki, Matsutani, & Akanuma, 1993; Ojeda, Stokes, Lee, Thomas, Papadimitriou & Cala et al., 1986). There does not seem to be a sex preference for the appearance of the tumor.

There is considerable controversy in the literature regarding the classification of cerebral neuroblastomas. They were first identified as a distinct clinical entity in 1976 (Horten & Rubenstein, 1976). Subsequent literature has demonstrated confusion concerning the diagnosis of cerebral neuroblastoma, differentiating it from an oligodendroglioma; a relatively benign tumor called *central neurocytoma;* and a group of tumors classed together as primitive neuroectodermal tumors (PNETs). Tumors traditionally classified as PNETs include medulloblastomas and, sometimes, pineoblastomas. (Kovnar, Kellie, Horowitz, Sanford, Langston, & Mulhern et al., 1990; Thomas, 1993). However, the most recent World Health Organization classification of brain tumors clearly delineates cerebral neuroblastomas as distinct from embryonal tumors, such as PNETs, and from both oligodendrogliomas and central neurocytomas. Mrak (1994) suggested that neuroblastomas fall at one end of a histologic continuum: Neurocytoma, with its relatively benign appearance and clinical course, is at one end, a variety of as yet unnamed tumors are in the middle of the continuum, and neuroblastomas mark the other, most malignant end of the continuum.

In addition, although there is clear and well-documented evidence that neurocytomas or, alternatively, central neurocytomas, occur almost exclusively in the intraventricular area (Hassoun, Soylemezoglu, Gambarelli, Figarella-Branger, von Amman, & Kleihues,1993; Maiuri, Spaziante, DeCaro, Cappabianca, Giamundo, & Iaconetta, 1995; Weprin, Hall, & Bergman, 1994), some authors have suggested that cerebral neuroblastomas may also occur in the periventricular area, as well as in the cerebral hemispheres (Davis et al., 1990; Rhodes, Cole, Takaoka, Roessman, Cotes, & Simon, 1994). Others maintain that "true" cerebral neuroblastomas occur only in the cerebral hemispheres themselves (Mrak, 1994). To add to the confusion, in some reports (Ferreol, Sawaya, & Courten-Myers, 1989), the terms *neuroblastoma* and *neurocytoma* are used interchangeably. In others, tumors once labeled as neuroblastomas would most likely be called *neurocytomas* today (Hassoun et al., 1993; Mrak, 1994).

Distinguishing among these varied types of tumors is critical, as treatment and especially prognosis vary considerably. However, because there is currently a lack of clarity regarding the histopathologic and clinical characteristics of cerebral neuroblastomas, confusion persists.

RISK FACTORS

As with most CNS tumors, no specific risk factors are associated with the development of cerebral neuroblastomas. Genetic links to many cancers are being explored with the goal of improved understanding of the etiology, progression, treatment, and prognosis of these tumors. There are documented clusters of CNS tumors in families. For instance, the Li-Fraumeni cancer family syndrome, linked with mutations of the p53 gene on chromosome 17, is associated with the development of many tumors, including gliomas and medulloblastomas. Neurofibromatosis (NF-1), or von Recklinghausen's disease, and neurofibromatosis type 2 (NF-2), which is more rare, are also linked to defects on chromosome 17. Both disorders are associated with the development of a variety of CNS and peripheral nervous system tumors, including optic gliomas, astrocytomas, ependymomas, acoustic neuromas, neurilemomas, meningiomas, neurofibromas, and schwannomas. In addition, Turcot syndrome, Gardner syndrome, and familial polyposis coli are all associated with medulloblastomas and glioblastomas. Von Hippel-Lindau disease is linked with the development of infratentorial hemangioblastomas. However, there is no documented genetic link with the development of cerebral neuroblastomas (Bondy, Wiencke, Wrensch, & Kyritsis, 1994; Frank-Stromborg, 1992; Martz, 1992; Thomas, 1993).

No demonstrable relationship has been established between exposure to chemical or environmental factors and the development of CNS tumors. Although some studies have suggested a link between exposure to herbicides, polyvinyl chlorides, petrochemicals, rubber, and organic solvents and the development of gliomas, no relationship to the development of cerebral neuroblastomas is suggested (Berleur & Cordier, 1995; Keyser, 1993a; Smith-Rooker, Garrett, Hodges, & Shue, 1992).

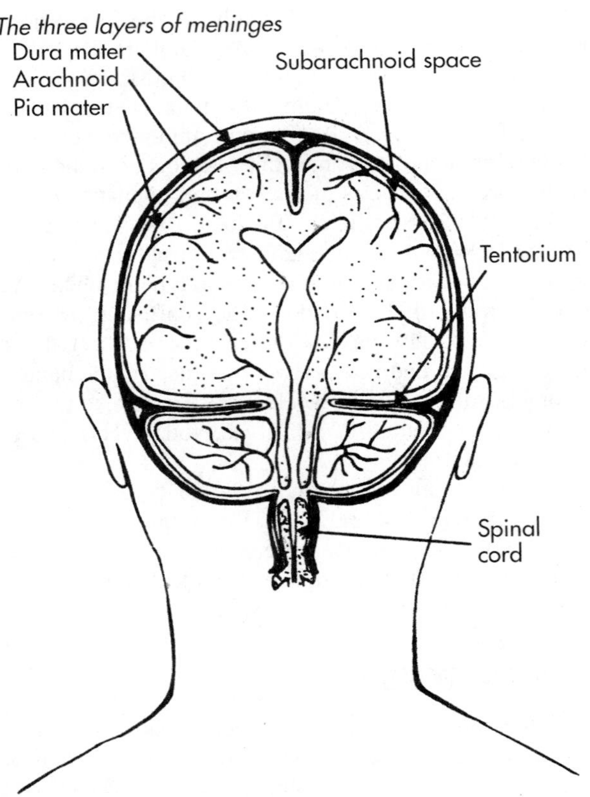

Fig. 28-1 The meninges.

Although there is some evidence to link the development of gliomas to a history of scalp or brain irradiation, there is none linking cerebral neuroblastomas to such a history (Keyser, 1993a). Some researchers have suggested a relationship between hormones, particularly female hormones, and the development of some primary brain tumors, but not with cerebral neuroblastomas (Schlehofer, Blettner, & Wahrendorf, 1992).

Overall, the rarity of this particular tumor (as well as that of all primary CNS tumors) and the dearth of epidemiologic information on such tumors make it difficult to establish the relative risk of intrinsic or extrinsic factors in the development of the tumor. Patients and families who seem to demonstrate a cluster of CNS tumors, including cerebral neuroblastomas, or have questions regarding their susceptibility to developing cerebral neuroblastoma should be encouraged to discuss their concerns with health care providers or should be referred to medical institutions with experience in cancer genetics and cancer risk counseling (Kelly, 1992).

PATHOPHYSIOLOGY

Anatomy and Physiology of the Brain

Microanatomy. The nervous system, containing at least 10 billion neurons, is among the first recognizable organ systems to develop in the embryo. Nerve tissue develops from the embryonic ectoderm. The ectoderm depresses along the midline of the embryo, forming the neural plate. The neural plate then deepens into the neural groove, and the edges grow toward each other, eventually fusing to form the neural tube. Extending from the head into the tail region, this structure gives rise to the entire CNS. Cells that are just lateral to the neural groove make up the neural crest. These cells give rise to most of the peripheral nervous system (PNS), as well as to other structures, including parts of the adrenal medulla, skin, meninges, and ganglia.

Nerve tissue itself consists of two types of cells: nerve cells, or neurons, which are the functional units of the

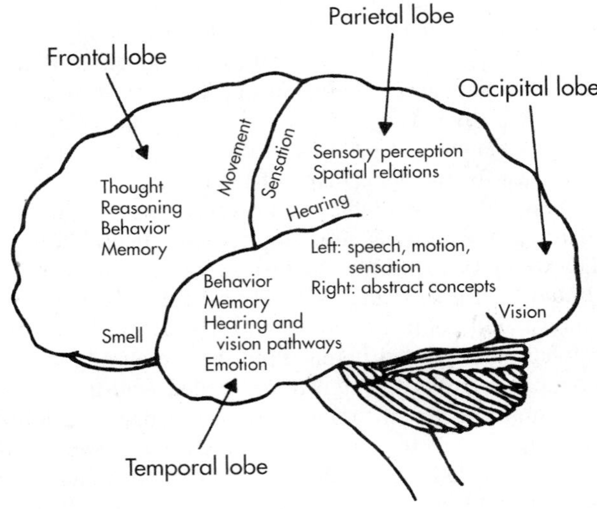

Fig. 28-2 Cerebral lobes. For right-handed individuals.

nervous system, and glial cells, or neuroglia, which support and protect the neurons. There are many more glial cells than neurons in the CNS, occurring in a ratio of 10 neuroglia to 1 neuron. There are four basic types of neuroglia: astrocytes, oligodendrocytes, microglia, and ependymal cells.

The neuroglia, from which most CNS tumors arise, play an essential role in the function of the nervous system, including maintaining the composition of fluids in the brain, assisting in the control of the chemical and electrical environment of the neuron, and forming the myelin sheath of axons (Junquerra, Caineiro, & Kelley, 1992).

Gross Anatomy. The nervous system is composed of the CNS and the PNS. The CNS is composed grossly of two parts: the brain and spinal cord. The components of the PNS include the 12 pairs of cranial nerves, the 31 pairs of spinal nerves, and the autonomic nervous system, which is further divided into the sympathetic and the parasympathetic nervous systems.

The brain is enclosed in a bony protective covering, the skull. It is further protected by the meninges, a triple-layered covering of the brain and spinal cord. The outermost layer, the dura mater, is a tough fibrous membrane that lines the skull's interior. The middle layer, the arachnoid, is named for its resemblance to a spider web. The innermost layer, the pia mater, is delicate and highly vascular. It adheres closely to the entire surface of the brain. The subarachnoid space, lying between the arachnoid and pia mater, is contiguous with the ventricles of the brain and is where the cerebrospinal fluid (CSF) flows (Fig. 28-1).

The brain itself is divided into three areas: the cerebrum, composed of the cerebral hemispheres, the thalamus, the hypothalamus and the basal ganglia; the brainstem, composed of the midbrain, pons, and medulla; and the cerebellum. The cerebral hemispheres are further divided into four areas or lobes: the frontal, parietal, temporal, and occipital lobes (Fig. 28-2). The major functions of all these areas are summarized in Table 28-1.

The Ventricles. The ventricular system is composed of the two lateral ventricles, as well as the third and the fourth ventricles (Fig. 28-3). The CSF is a clear, colorless fluid that is formed primarily by the choroid plexus, a collection of blood vessels covered by a thin layer of ependymal cells found in the ventricles. The CSF flows freely between the four ventricles and the subarachnoid space, cushioning the brain and spinal cord. Although about 500 ml of CSF is produced daily, only about 150 ml is contained in the adult ventricular system and subarachnoid space at any time. Thus, there is a fairly rapid turnover and reabsorption of CSF in the course of the day. Any disruption in the flow or reabsorption of CSF can result in overfilling of the ventricular system, resulting in hydrocephalus and increased intracranial pressure (ICP).

The Cranial Nerves. The cranial nerves, although part of the PNS, lie within the skull cavity. Assigned both a Roman numeral and a name, each cranial nerve exits in a systematic progression from the cerebral hemispheres (CNI), down to the lower portion of the medulla (CNXIII) (Fig. 28-4). Because of their location, functions of the cranial nerves can be affected by lesions in the brain. Lesions that occur in the brainstem or cerebellum can directly compress or invade these nerves. Lesions that occur further away in the cerebral hemispheres affect cranial nerve function indirectly through swelling and displacement of brain tissue.

TABLE 28-1 Areas of the Brain and Their Major Functions

Area of Brain	Major Functions
Cerebrum	
Frontal lobe	High-level cognitive functions, e.g., abstraction, concentration
	Memory
	Voluntary eye movements
	Somatic motor control of respiration, gastrointestinal activity, blood pressure
	Voluntary motor function (dominant side)
	Motor control of speech (dominant side)
Parietal lobe	Interpretation of sensory input
	Processing visual-spatial information (non-dominant side)
	Ideomotor praxis (dominant side)
Temporal lobe	Reception and interpretation of auditory stimuli
	Complex memory
	Emotional affect
Occipital lobe	Visual perception
	Visual reflexes and involuntary eye movements
Thalamus	Awareness of pain
	Maintenance of alertness
	Focusing attention
Hypothalamus	Regulation of body temperature
	Water metabolism
	Secretion of growth hormone, follicle-stimulating hormone
	Regulation of the sleep-wake cycle
	Appetite and satiety
	Sexual arousal
	Thirst
	Autonomic nervous system function
Basal ganglia	Fine motor control of the hands and lower extremities
Brain Stem	
Mid-brain	Relay station for cerebellar tracts
	Auditory, visual reflexes
	Origination of cranial nerves III and IV
Pons	Relay station for cerebellar, cerebral tracts
	Control of respiration
	Origination of cranial nerves V-VIII
Medulla	Coordination of head and eye movement
	Cardiac, vasomotor, respiratory centers
	Origination of cranial nerves IX-XII
Cerebellum	Fine motor control
	Coordination of muscle groups
	Balance

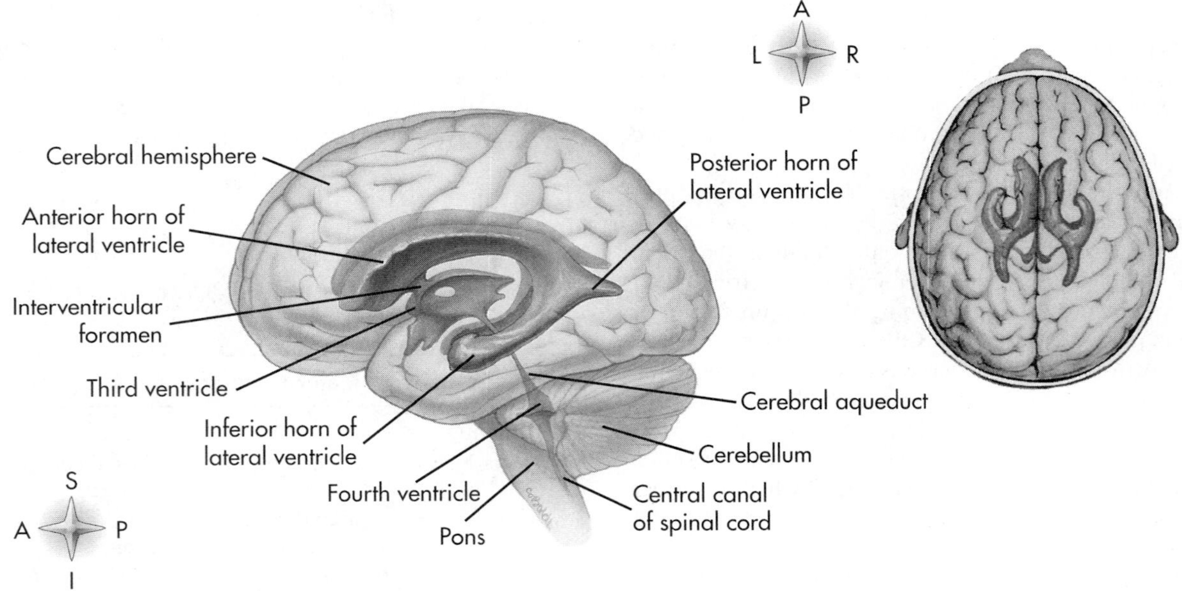

Fig. 28-3 The ventricles. (From Thibodeau, G. A. [1996]. *Anthony's textbook of anatomy and physiology* [15th ed.]. St. Louis: Mosby.)

Neurophysiology

Three concepts central to neuroanatomy and physiology are essential in understanding the signs, symptoms, and treatment of any CNS neoplasm. These concepts include the blood-brain barrier (BBB), cerebral dominance, and ICP.

Blood-Brain Barrier. Although homeostasis is critical for the function of the entire body, it is especially important in the nervous system. The passage of electrolytes through the nerve cell membrane helps maintain an environment that is essential for the generation and conduction of nerve impulses. In addition, the brain needs a constant nutrient supply of glucose and amino acids, as well as a means of eliminating waste products such as carbon dioxide. The brain also needs significant protection from chemical substances that could prove deleterious to its function.

Blood-brain barrier (BBB) is a term used to describe the process and structure of a system that maintains the homeostasis of the environment of brain cells and protects them as well. Structurally, the BBB is composed of the endothelial lining of capillaries in the brain and the tight junction between those endothelial cells and nearby astrocytes. Together, these structures filter the size and types of molecules that can diffuse across the capillaries into the neurons. In general, the BBB is permeable to water, oxygen, carbon dioxide and other gases, glucose, and lipophilic substances. Most drugs cannot cross the BBB (Hickey, 1997a). Although a body of evidence demonstrates that the BBB is disrupted in the area of a brain tumor, it remains a significant factor in determining the efficacy of chemotherapeutic agents in the treatment of brain tumors (Keyser, 1993b).

Intracranial Pressure. As discussed previously, the brain is encased in a rigid compartment composed of the bones of the skull. The contents of the skull include brain tissue itself, blood contained in the intravascular spaces, and the CSF found in the ventricles and subarachnoid space. As explicated by the Monroe-Kellie hypothesis, the relative volume of each of these three substances remains constant through a state of dynamic equilibrium that causes a decrease in one component in response to an increase in another component. The net effect is the maintenance of intracranial pressure (ICP) within acceptable parameters, allowing the brain to function normally.

Mechanisms such as shunting of CSF from the ventricles into the subarachnoid space and vasoconstriction of cerebral blood vessels can compensate for changes in the volume of intracranial contents for some time. In general, small volume changes can be compensated for much more readily than larger ones, especially over longer time intervals. Thus, slow-growing masses such as primary brain tumors can be accommodated for and achieve much larger sizes than faster-growing masses such as from a hemorrhage or metastatic tumor. However, at some point, compensatory mechanisms fail and ICP rises dramatically. This failure results in intracranial hypertension, or increased ICP.

Cerebral Dominance. In general, and especially in adults, most people demonstrate a high degree of specialization and development in one cerebral hemisphere over another. Functions of the various parts of the brain vary from one side of the brain to the other (Table 28-1). The most frequently observed pattern is that of left-hemisphere dominance, which occurs in most right-handed people, but also in some left-handed people. The consequence of this dominance is that the primary centers for language, motor skills, and sensory interpretation lie in one hemisphere, the dominant one. However, because pathways from the cerebral hemispheres cross over to the opposite side of the body as they descend through the brain stem and spinal cord, signs and symptoms from lesions in the cerebral hemispheres are seen on the opposite side of the body. Thus, a tumor in the left frontotemporal area will result in sensorimotor dysfunction on the right side of the body, along with language dysfunction.

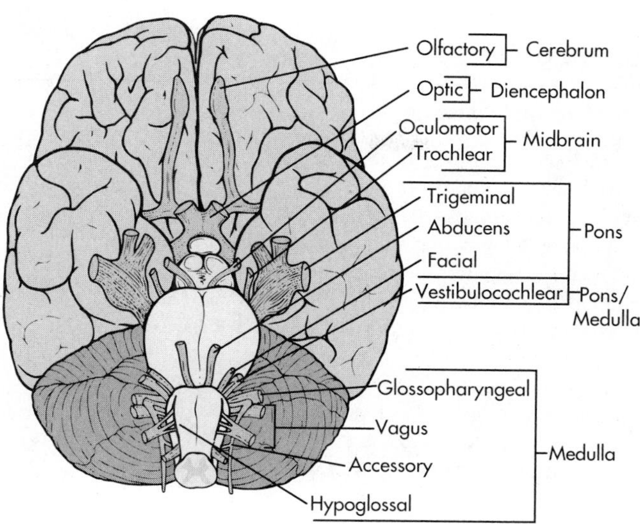

Fig. 28-4 Cranial nerves. (From Lewis, S. M. [1997]. *Medical-surgical nursing* [4th ed.]. St. Louis: Mosby.)

Box 28-1
Specific and Nonspecific Signs and Symptoms of Neuroblastomas

Specific signs and symptoms

- Hemiparesis
- Aphasia
- Papilledema
- Visual changes

Nonspecific signs and symptoms

- Headache
- Seizure
- Alterations in cognition
- Alterations in level of consciousness

ROUTES OF METASTASIS

The ability to spread to nonadjacent tissues is a characteristic of most malignancies. However, primary tumors of the CNS rarely metastasize outside the CNS. There is only one documented report of a cerebral neuroblastoma metastasizing outside of the CNS itself, to the T11 vertebral body (Louis et al., 1990). Tumors that arise in the ventricles, such as ependymomas and neurocytomas, or in periventricular areas may seed to the leptomeninges and CSF and may be found in any part of the neuroaxis (Cotran, Kumar, & Robbins, 1994; Meehan, 1994). Davis and colleagues (1990) suggested that cerebral neuroblastomas that appear to impinge on or invade the ventricles can seed into the ventricular system.

PATIENT ASSESSMENT

An essential part of the evaluation of the patient with a suspected cerebral neuroblastoma is the history and physical examination (Table 28-2). A careful and thorough neurologic examination often can pinpoint the location of a tumor, even in the absence of confirmatory diagnostic studies.

The history should begin with a detailed analysis of the presenting signs and symptoms, including temporal factors, precipitating and exacerbating events, and the sequence of their appearance. Because many of the cognitive and behavioral symptoms of brain tumors are subtle, it is important to include the patient's significant others when gathering this information. In general, the signs and symptoms associated with the presence of any brain tumor, including cerebral neuroblastomas, can be classified into two broad categories of specific and nonspecific signs and symptoms (Box 28-1).

Nonspecific Signs and Symptoms

Nonspecific signs and symptoms occur as a result of cerebral edema with its associated increase in ICP. Cerebral edema associated with brain tumors results from an increase in capillary permeability, which produces a breakdown of the BBB. This breakdown causes leakage of a protein-rich filtrate into the extracellular spaces. The overall increase in the bulk of the brain tissue produces pressure on the brain itself, causing generalized neurologic dysfunction.

Headache is a common presenting symptom of brain tumors (Jaeckle, 1993) and is described in patients with intraparenchymal cerebral neuroblastomas (Ojeda et al., 1986). Brain tissue itself does not have pain nerve endings. The pain associated with headache is thought to result from pressure on nerve endings in adjacent blood vessels. Headaches vary in severity, as well as in quality and location. Some patients with brain tumors complain of occipital headaches in the morning that subside with elevation of the head. Others may complain of more generalized head pain, especially in the frontal area (Fetell, 1995; Hickey & Armstrong, 1997; Levin, Leibel, & Gutin, 1997). A careful history and the specific characteristics of the headache are elicited as part of the neurologic examination.

Cognitive deficits, albeit quite subtle in some cases, are commonly found in patients with cerebral neoplasms and are described in patients with cerebral neuroblastoma (Berger et al., 1983). Other patients are described as demonstrating the signs and symptoms of increased ICP, which include changes in cognition (Bennet & Rubinstein, 1984, Berger et al., 1983). Cognitive deficits can vary widely and include changes in personality, mood, intellectual abilities, memory, and concentration. Changes in personality may include increased irritability, loss of social skills, and lack of initiative. Mood changes are demonstrated in emotional lability, flattened affect, and anhedonia. A history of having sought psychiatric help may be elicited in some patients experiencing these symptoms. Sometimes the patient is unaware of such symptoms, and family members seek help for the patient.

Alterations in intellectual abilities, including memory and concentration difficulties, overall slowing of thought processes, and difficulty in abstract thinking and problem solving are elicited during the mental status examination. Patients with highly technical or complex job requirements may be experiencing problems with job performance. Early

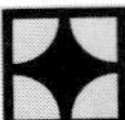

TABLE 28-2 Assessment of the Patient for a Neuroblastoma

	Assessment Parameters	Typical Abnormal Findings
History	A. Personal and Social History	A. Personal and social risk factors are not established for this tumor; such information would enhance current epidemiologic data that are available.
	B. History of Signs/Symptoms	B. Common symptoms may include those of generalized cerebral dysfunction. Seizures and headache are among the most common symptoms. Other symptoms may include lethargy, disorientation, sensory deficits, difficulty in concentration and slowed thinking, changes in customary behavior or personality. More specific signs and symptoms are related to the precise location of the tumor. These may include hemiparesis, hemisensory loss, visual changes, and speech difficulties, or inability to understand the written or spoken word.
Physical Examination	Neurologic Examination A. Mental Status 1. Lack of level of consciousness, orientation	A. 1. Family or significant others may report disruptions in sleep-wake cycle, increased sleepiness. Patient may present as lethargic (i.e., slowed responses, asleep in waiting area). Patient may exhibit confusion regarding the time of day, day of week, or date.
	2. Appearance and behavior	2. Previously well-groomed patients may present in a disheveled, unkempt manner. Subtle changes in behavior may only be obvious to family or significant others.
	3. Mood	3. Patients may present with a depressed or flattened affect.
	4. Speech pattern/language ability	4. Speech may be slowed or hesitant. Patient may exhibit difficulty in naming common objects. Patient's ability to follow commands may be impaired. Literate patients may have difficulty in writing or reading.
	5. Cognitive function a. Attention and concentration	a. Patients may exhibit difficulty in common tasks such as remembering a series of numbers, counting backward from 100 in decrements of 7, or spelling W-O-R-L-D backward.
	b. Memory	b. Patients may exhibit deficits in recent memory (e.g., what they had for breakfast) or in short-term memory, evaluated by asking them to recall three words given to them previously.
	c. Abstract thinking	c. Interpretation of a common proverb may demonstrate a concrete, literal response. A similar response may be given when asked to describe the similarities of two objects.
	B. Cranial Nerve Examination	B. Cerebral neuroblastomas appear to occur most often in the cerebral hemispheres, so much of the cranial nerve examination may be normal. However, papilledema, or blurring of the optic disk margin, is a relatively common finding found in examination of CN II. With increased intracranial pressure, CN III can be compressed, resulting in apoptosis, incomplete eyelid closure, and changes in the size, shape, and reaction to light of the affected pupil. Dysfunction of CN VI, resulting in inability to move the eye outward laterally, is also common.
	C. Motor Examination	C. Tumors affecting the motor cortex of the dominant frontal lobe will result in abnormal findings in the motor examination.
	1. Muscle size	1. Asymmetry in muscle size and wasting may be present if symptoms have persisted for some time.
	2. Muscle tone	2. Hypotonia (flaccidity) may be present in affected muscle groups or limbs.

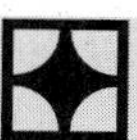

TABLE 28-2 Assessment of the Patient for a Neuroblastoma—cont'd

	Assessment Parameters	Typical Abnormal Findings
	3. Muscle strength	3. Changes in muscle strength, ranging from impaired movement when resisted to no contraction of the affected muscle(s), may be seen.
	4. Gait and posture	4. The patient may exhibit an unsteady or wide-based gait related to muscle weakness or sensory disturbance. There may be a tendency to "drift" to one side or the other while walking.
	D. Sensory Examination	D. Patients with lesions in the sensory cortex or parietal lobe may exhibit sensory loss (numbness) or loss of positive sense (inability to know the location of one's body in space).
Diagnostic Tests	A. Computed Tomography (CT) Scan	A. CT scan is likely to demonstrate a large intraparenchymal mass with heterogeneous contrast enhancement. Calcification intratumoral hemorrhage and cystic areas may be present. Mild peritumoral edema will be seen.
	B. Magnetic Resonance Imaging (MRI)	B. MRI may demonstrate an intraparenchymal mass with inhomogeneous enhancement patterns on T_1- and T_2-weighted studies. Contrast-enhanced MRI may demonstrate leptomeningeal seeding when tumor abuts or invades a ventricle.
	C. Cerebrospinal Fluid (CSF) Examination	C. In the presence of leptomeningeal seeding, elevations in CSF pressure, white blood cell count, and protein, as well as a decrease in CSF glucose, may be found.

signs of changes in level of consciousness are also subtle and may be limited to intermittent periods of confusion and an increased tendency to sleep or nap. Because many of these problems are commonly seen in other conditions, including anxiety disorders and depression, a fairly long history of such symptoms may be elicited.

Seizures are a common, nonspecific presenting sign of intracranial tumors including cerebral neuroblastomas (Bennet & Rubinstein, 1984; Davis et al., 1990; Louis et al., 1990). Cerebral edema and changes in the electrical activity of neurons result in abnormal electrical discharges, or seizures. The seizures may be generalized (resulting in loss of consciousness) or partial (associated with specific motor or sensory symptoms). The type of seizure and associated symptoms may help localize the tumor before other diagnostic studies are performed (Hickey & Armstrong, 1997). Vomiting, generally without accompanying nausea, is not as common as believed and occurs most often with lesions in the cerebellum.

Specific Signs and Symptoms

Discrete areas in the brain control specific functions (Table 28-1). Infiltration or destruction of these areas by tumors results in characteristic deficits. Cerebral neuroblastomas have been found in the frontal, temporal, parietal, and occipital lobes (Bennett & Rubinstein, 1984, Davis et al., 1990; Louis et al., 1990; Mrak, 1994; Ojeda et al., 1986). There are reports of cerebral neuroblastomas occurring in the cerebellum (Robey, Olson, Brem, & Epstein, 1988), but these are even more rare than reports of hemispheric lesions.

Frontal Lobe Signs and Symptoms. Tumors that arise in the frontal lobes cause a variety of signs and symptoms. Common behavioral symptoms include inappropriate behavior, personality changes, difficulty with thinking and concentration, emotional lability, and a flattened affect. In individuals with left hemisphere dominance, tumors in the posterior frontal lobe result in a right-sided spastic hemiparesis or hemiplegia and nonfluent (Broca's) aphasia (inability to express oneself). Agraphia (inability to express oneself in writing) may also be seen. Tumors occurring in the nondominant frontal lobe may not cause significant deficits. Bilateral frontal lobe tumors result in profound behavioral and cognitive changes.

Temporal Lobe Signs and Symptoms. Lesions in the temporal lobes may cause only subtle sensory-perceptual deficits that are elicited during a careful sensory examination. However, temporal lobe tumors may also result in aggressiveness, memory loss, and dementia. If the tumor occurs in the dominant (usually left side) temporal lobe, language dysfunction, especially fluent (Wernicke's) aphasia is found. Many patients with tumors in the frontotemporal area exhibit a mixed fluent and nonfluent aphasia, resulting in an inability to express oneself, as well as difficulty in comprehending the spoken word. In addition, gustatory, visual, olfactory, or auditory hallucinations are seen in temporal lobe disease.

Parietal Lobe Signs and Symptoms. Parietal lobe syndromes are characterized by sensory-perceptual losses. These losses may include a general loss of sensation, abnormal or painful sensations including tingling or burning, loss of position sense, or neglect (ignoring the affected side of one's body and environment). Other specific signs that occur with lesions in the dominant parietal lobe include left-right confusion, alexia (inability to understand the written word), acalculia (difficulty working with numbers), agraphia (inability to write in the absence of motor loss), and apraxia (inability to perform learned movements despite intact motor function).

Occipital Lobe Signs and Symptoms. Tumors are much less common in the occipital lobe. When present, they produce primarily visual symptoms, including contralateral homonymous hemianopsia (visual loss in half of each visual field, occurring on the opposite side of the tumor). Visual agnosia, or inability to interpret visual stimuli despite intact visual pathways, may also be seen.

Cerebellum Signs and Symptoms. Tumors in the cerebellum result in ataxia (incoordination of voluntary muscle action, especially muscles used for walking or reaching for objects), headache, and impaired articulation or dysarthria. Vomiting may also occur.

Cranial Nerve Signs and Symptoms. Because of their location relative to the CNS, some cranial nerves can be affected by cerebral tumors. Papilledema, blurring of the optic disc margin that is visualized in funduscopic examination of CN II, results from increased ICP. Papilledema is generally a late finding, occurring with marked increases in ICP.

CN III is easily compressed when mass lesions and edema in the cerebral hemispheres result in downward displacement of the brain. This compression results in changes in pupillary size and reactivity to light, initially on the ipsilateral (same) side as the tumor. If ICP continues to increase, bilateral dysfunction is seen. CN VI palsy, resulting in inability to move the eye laterally, may also be seen.

Obstruction of the Flow of CSF. Although cerebral neuroblastomas appear to occur most commonly in the cerebral hemispheres, there are reports that they can occur in the periventricular area. If the tumor invades the lateral ventricle, obstruction of CSF flow can occur, resulting in hydrocephalus or dilation of the ventricle. This obstruction, in turn, results in increased ICP and its associated symptoms.

Diagnostic Tests

Imaging techniques used to evaluate CNS tumors have improved dramatically in recent years. Neuroradiologists are able to determine quite accurately the size and location of tumors using a variety of imaging studies. In some cases, a differential diagnosis is possible based on evaluation of tumor characteristics, including peritumoral edema, intratumoral hemorrhage, calcifications, and cyst formation. Diagnostic imaging tests are also used to evaluate responses to therapy, as well as tumor progression or recurrence.

Computed Tomography. The most common and usually the first imaging technique used to evaluate CNS lesions is computed tomography (CT). CT produces an image in which tissues of different densities are assigned different shades of gray. It has the ability to differentiate among a wide variety of tissue types, including fat, soft tissue, and bone, as well as air. CT is also highly sensitive for evaluating the presence of blood in brain tissue and tumor.

Noncontrast CT is required to evaluate a tumor for the presence of hemorrhage and calcification. Contrast-enhanced CT assists in delineating tumor margins, as well as disruption of the BBB in the peritumoral area (Schwartz, 1995). A patient education tool that can be used to explain the CT scan procedure is found in Table 28-3.

Magnetic Resonance Imaging. Magnetic resonance imaging (MRI) allows for exquisitely detailed images of CNS tissue and structures. MRI produces three-dimensional images of the brain from a variety of perspectives, or planes. It may be used as an adjunct to CT scanning. Although it is more costly and not as widely available, MRI is the most accurate and therefore preferred technique for evaluating CNS neoplasms. In addition to providing superior images of brain structures, MRI is particularly useful in evaluating for the presence of edema, hemorrhage, and hydrocephalus. Use of a contrast agent, usually gadolinium-DTPA, results in superior imaging (Levin, Leibel, & Gutin, 1997; Schwartz, 1995).

Unlike CT, which uses x-ray technology, MRI uses

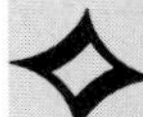

TABLE 28-3 Patient Preparation for Computed Tomography

Description of the procedure: A computed tomography (CT) scan is a special x-ray that makes pictures of the inside of your body.

How will the test help me? Your doctor can use the information from the CT scan to tell what is wrong with you. The doctor can also use it to see if your treatment is working.

Is there anything I need to do before the test? There are no special preparations for the test. Usually, you may eat and drink before the test and take your usual medication(s). However, if you will be getting dye with your CT scan, your doctor may ask you not to eat or drink before the test.

What will I feel? Having a CT scan does not hurt. You may have a needle put in a vein (an IV) so you can get dye for the test. Some people feel hot and flushed when they get the dye in their IV. This reaction is normal.
A technician will help you onto the CT scan table. Some people find lying still on the CT scan table uncomfortable. It is small and may feel hard. Your head will be strapped loosely to the table. This procedure helps make sure you will not move during the test. Moving can make the CT scan picture unclear, so try not to move.
Once you are comfortable, the table will slide into the machine. During the test, you will hear soft noises from the CT scan machine. Let the technician know if you need help during the test.

How long will the test take? A CT scan usually takes less than an hour.

What will happen after the test? The technician will help you off the table. You may leave as soon as you are ready. Your doctor will let you know the results of the CT scan as soon as they are ready.

powerful magnets and radiofrequency waves to produce images. Because of the magnets used, metal objects such as jewelry or glasses may not be worn during the scan. In addition, patients with certain metallic implants such as pacemakers or orthopedic prostheses may not be able to undergo MRI.

The most recently published data describing CT and MRI findings in cerebral neuroblastoma indicate that the tumors tend to be large (3 to 10 cm) intraparenchymal masses, some with calcifications and cystic components. As with other CNS neoplasms, intratumoral hemorrhage and peritumoral edema may be present. Unfortunately, none of these findings is considered pathognomonic, and histopathologic diagnosis is essential (Davis et al., 1990). An educational tool that can be used to prepare a patient for an MRI scan is found in Table 28-4.

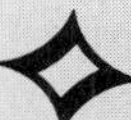

TABLE 28-4 Patient Preparation for Magnetic Resonance Imaging

What is an magnetic resonance imaging (MRI) scan? An MRI is a way to look inside your body. MRI is not an x-ray. MRI uses powerful magnets and radiowaves. A computer then makes a very detailed picture of parts of your body.

How will an MRI help me? Your doctor can use the information from the MRI to tell what is wrong with you. The doctor can also use it to see if your treatment is working.

Is there anything I need to do before the test? Because the MRI uses a magnet, you will be asked to remove any metal from yourself. This includes your glasses, jewelry, coins, keys, and so on. If you have a pacemaker or other medical device that may be made of metal, tell your doctor, since you may not be able to have an MRI. Ask your doctor if you can eat and drink before the test and take your usual medication(s).

What will I feel? Having an MRI does not hurt. You may have a needle put in a vein (an IV) so you can get dye for the test. Some people find lying still on the MRI table uncomfortable. Some people may not feel comfortable being inside the MRI machine. If you are worried about this, tell your doctor or nurse. You may be able to take medicine to help you feel more relaxed. A technician will help you onto the MRI table. It is small and may feel hard. Your head will be strapped loosely to the table. This procedure helps make sure you will not move during the test. Moving can make the MRI picture unclear, so try not to move. Once you are comfortable, the table will slide into the MRI machine. During the MRI, you will hear loud tapping and banging noises. The noises may stop and begin again. These sounds are normal. The technician(s) will be able to talk with you during the test. Let them know if you need help.

How long will the test take? An MRI usually lasts 30-60 minutes.

What will happen after the test? The technician will help you off the MRI table. You may leave as soon as you are ready. Your doctor will let you know the results of the MRI as soon as they are ready.

Other Diagnostic Imaging Modalities. Magnetic resonance angiography (MRA) has substantially replaced the need for invasive angiography procedures. MRA is used to differentiate tumors from vascular anomalies. It may also be used to evaluate the vascular supply of a tumor before surgery. Positron emission tomography (PET) and single photon emission computerized tomography (SPECT) are newer diagnostic modalities that are not used extensively in clinical settings. PET scan combines CT and radioisotope scanning to produce three-dimensional structural and functional images of brain tissue. It is particularly useful in differentiating tumor recurrence from radiation-induced necrosis. SPECT also uses radioisotopes in conjunction with rotating gamma cameras, primarily to image functional neuroanatomy. There are no published data evaluating the use of any of these techniques in the diagnosis of cerebral neuroblastomas (Schwartz, 1995).

CSF Examination. If cerebral neuroblastoma occurs or spreads to the ventricular area, there may be evidence of tumor seeding in the meninges, or meningeal carcinomatosis. In addition to characteristic changes on MRI, examination of the CSF, obtained through a lumbar puncture, may reveal elevated opening pressures, an increased white blood cell count and protein level, and a decreased glucose level. Cytologic examination of the fluid may not reveal malignant cells (Meehan, 1994; Posner, 1995).

STAGING

The current recommendation from the American Joint Committee on Cancer (AJCC) is that a formal classification and staging system of CNS tumors should not be attempted at this time (American Joint Committee on Cancer, 1997). This recommendation is based on factors that are peculiar to CNS tumors, including the fact that tumor size is not as important as tumor histology and location, and that primary CNS tumors generally do not metastasize outside the nervous system.

Some authors have suggested that neuroblastomas can be graded morphologically. In such a system, tumor cells are compared with normal cells of the same type and characterized according to degree of differentiation (Box 28-2). Using this system, neuroblastomas would be classified as grade III or grade IV neoplasms (poorly differentiated, undifferentiated). In contrast, central neurocytomas would be classed as grade I tumors (well differentiated) (Louis et al., 1990; Ojeda et al., 1986). The World Health Organization also

Box 28-2
Histopathologic Grading System

GX	Grade cannot be assessed
G1	Well differentiated
G2	Moderately differentiated
G3	Poorly differentiated
G4	Undifferentiated

From American Joint Commission on Cancer. (1997). *Cancer staging manual.* (5th ed.). Philadelphia: Lippincott-Raven.

classifies cerebral neuroblastomas as grade IV and notes that these tumors are generally associated with rapid progression (Kleihues, Burger, & Scheithauer,1993).

MEDICAL MANAGEMENT

Surgery

As with most CNS tumors, surgery is the mainstay of medical treatment for cerebral neuroblastomas. The goals of surgery are twofold. The first goal is to obtain tissue to make a histopathologic, definitive diagnosis. Because there are no pathognomonic characteristics associated with this tumor on standard imaging techniques, it is critical to obtain tissue to make the definitive diagnosis. The second goal is to remove (debulk) as much of the tumor as possible, both to relieve ICP and to improve symptoms. In addition, reduction of the tumor mass may improve the efficacy of radiation therapy and chemotherapy (Sawaya, Rambo, Hammond, & Ligon, 1995).

Unfortunately, subtotal resection through an open craniotomy may be the best surgical option (Berger et al., 1983; Davis et al., 1990; Louis et al., 1990; Mrak, 1994; Rhodes et al., 1994; Robey et al., 1988). Complete extirpation of the tumor is sometimes not possible, or ill-advised, when the tumor is relatively inaccessible or lies in, or adjacent to, an area that controls vital functions.

In some cases, for instance when the patient cannot tolerate a more complex procedure, biopsy alone may be the goal of the surgical intervention. Stereotactic biopsy is the most common method used. Stereotactic procedures are performed using a variety of devices. All devices allow for precise delivery of a probe using computer-generated, three-dimensional coordinates. The major risk associated with this type of procedure is hemorrhage at the biopsy site (Levin, Leibel, & Gutin, 1997).

Radiation Therapy

In general, most CNS neoplasms insidiously infiltrate normal tissue surrounding the tumor itself. Although such behavior is not described in the literature, it is reasonable to assume cerebral neuroblastomas share this characteristic, given their aggressive nature and propensity for local recurrence.

The intent of radiation therapy is to sterilize the tumor bed. Because of the infiltrative nature of CNS tumors, it is often necessary to irradiate a field that is somewhat larger than the actual dimensions of the resected area. When residual tumor remains after subtotal resection, radiation therapy is administered in the hope of ablating the tumor.

Cerebral neuroblastomas have been treated by either irradiating the whole brain (whole brain radiation therapy [WBRT]) or the tumor bed and surrounding area (Bennet & Rubenstein, 1984; Berger et al., 1983; Davis et al., 1990; Louis et al., 1990; Mrak, 1994; Ojeda et al., 1986; Robey et al., 1988). Data are too limited to evaluate the overall effectiveness of radiation therapy, or whether either method is preferred over the other. However, radiation therapy, when administered after resection, has shown a significant survival advantage for patients with other CNS neoplasms (Grossman & Norris, 1995; Shrieve & Loeffler, 1995).

With WBRT, both normal and malignant tissues are eradicated. WBRT can result in significant long-term morbidity, specifically leukoencephalopathy and cerebral atrophy, although this has not been documented for cerebral neuroblastomas. Clinically, patients present with varying degrees of dementia and functional deficits (Levin, Leibel, & Gutin, 1997). Even with focal or a more limited field of radiation, patients can still develop radiation necrosis. In this case, clinical signs and symptoms are related to the specific functional area that was radiated.

Doses of radiation therapy for cerebral neuroblastoma mimic those for other primary CNS malignancies. Documented doses range from 44 to 63 Gy. In one case, a cone-down of 9 Gy supplemented a 45 Gy dose to the whole brain was used. When tumor infiltration of the ventricles is suspected, spinal radiation therapy is also given (Berger et al., 1983; Louis et al., 1990; Ojeda et al., 1986; Robey et al., 1988).

New approaches to enhance the effectiveness of radiation therapy are being evaluated for many primary brain tumors. These approaches include the use of radiosensitizers, interstitial brachytherapy, radiosurgery techniques, varying hyperfractionation schedules, and conformational (three-dimensional) external beam radiation therapy. The use or effectiveness of any of these modalities is not documented for cerebral neuroblastomas (Shrieve & Loeffler, 1995).

Chemotherapy

Although effective for the treatment of other malignancies, chemotherapy has not been shown to play a major role in the treatment of primary CNS malignancies. Reasons for this ineffectiveness include the poor vascularization of central parts of many tumors and the heterogeneous cellular nature of most malignant CNS tumors. Although the BBB is disrupted in the peritumoral area, it is still considered a significant variable when evaluating the potential usefulness of many chemotherapeutic agents.

In addition, there is a problem entering patients into clinical trials because of the relative scarcity of these tumors. Fine (1994) suggested that a nihilistic attitude by the physician toward treatment of brain tumors contributes to the reluctance of some physicians to enter brain tumor patients into clinical trials.

Methodologic weaknesses also contribute to the difficulty in evaluating the role of chemotherapy for most brain tumors. Tumors of varying pathology are often evaluated together, and response criteria are not carefully spelled out (Conrad, Milosavljevic, & Yung, 1995).

In cerebral neuroblastomas, there are a few documented uses of chemotherapy (Bennet & Rubenstein, 1984; Berger et al., 1983; Louis et al., 1990). Because of the scarcity of literature documenting the use of chemotherapy in cerebral neuroblastomas, it is not possible to evaluate its efficacy.

The most commonly used drugs are the nitrosureas. Nitrosureas, which are lipid-soluble and thus more likely to penetrate the BBB, have been evaluated extensively in other primary brain tumors. Another agent used frequently is procarbazine. Procarbazine is known to cross the BBB and has shown activity in other CNS neoplasms. Intrathecal administration of chemotherapy is not documented in cerebral neuroblastomas. However, the drug used most often for meningeal tumor involvement is methotrexate (Alavi, 1995).

There are many clinical trials evaluating the use of new chemotherapeutic agents in patients with primary brain tumors, either alone or in combination with other drugs. There are also trials involving the use of monoclonal antibodies, biologic response modifiers, and hyperthermia. Although none are targeted specifically for cerebral neuroblastoma in adults, patients may be eligible for inclusion in some of these studies (National Cancer Institute, 1998).

ONCOLOGIC EMERGENCIES

The most common oncologic emergency likely to occur in patients with cerebral neuroblastoma is increased ICP. Some patients may present with the early signs and symptoms of increased ICP. Others may develop increased ICP during the course of their diagnosis and treatment.

Events likely to precipitate an increase in ICP include hemorrhage into the tumor, uncontrolled cerebral edema, initiation of radiation therapy, and obstruction of CSF flow. As discussed previously, mechanisms to maintain the dynamic equilibrium among the contents of the cranium (brain tissue, CSF, blood) are effective only to a certain point. When compensatory measures such as displacement, decreased production of CSF, and vasoconstriction fail, a dramatic increase in ICP occurs. As ICP rises, a cascade of events follows. There is a decrease in cerebral blood flow (CBF), which in turn results in a decrease in cerebral perfusion pressure (CPP), which is an estimate of the adequacy of cerebral circulation. As CPP falls, hypercapnia and hypoxia develop. Although ultimately self-defeating, vasodilation occurs in response to these changes, which only worsens the increase in ICP. Unless the vicious circle is interrupted, ischemia and infarction of cerebral tissue will result. Ultimately, cerebral herniation, or displacement of the brain, may occur.

The early signs and symptoms of increased ICP can be subtle and limited to a worsening of preexisting symptoms. Nursing staff and family members are often more likely to detect these changes, and interventions can be initiated before cerebral damage occurs.

A change in mental status or level of consciousness is often the earliest sign of increased ICP. Headache is also common. Changes in pupillary size and reactivity to light may occur, with the pupil on the ipsilateral side becoming dilated and sluggishly reactive to light. Palsies of the other cranial nerves may also occur. Hemiparesis (weakness) may develop or worsen to hemiplegia (paralysis). Increased ICP may precipitate seizure activity.

Without intervention, ICP continues to rise, and the late signs of increased ICP develop. Classic changes in vital signs (Cushing's triad) develop, consisting of an increase in blood pressure, with a widened pulse pressure; bradycardia; and changes in respiratory rate and pattern. The patient may vomit. Abnormal motor responses, such as decortication (hyperflexion of the upper extremities and hyperextension of the lower extremities) and decerebration (hyperextension of the upper and lower extremities) may be noted. The patient's level of consciousness will continue to deteriorate into coma.

Emergency management of the patient demonstrating the signs and symptoms of increased ICP is directed toward supporting the patient medically and reducing ICP by removing or alleviating the precipitating event. Patients may need to be admitted or transferred to critical care areas for closer observation and support. This move to a critical care unit can be frightening for both the patient and family members, and nursing support is critical. Common medical and nursing interventions to reduce ICP include respiratory support, cardiovascular support, and administration of diuretics and steroids.

Although mechanical ventilation may be needed to support the patient medically, it is also indicated for neurologic support. Hyperventilation to maintain hypocapnia (PCO_2 between 27 and 35 mm Hg) may be used to decrease cerebral edema, as CO_2 is a potent vasodilator. Although hypotension can result in cerebral ischemia, hypertension may develop in response to decreases in CBF. Management of the patient's blood pressure is complex and based on clinical judgment and patient response.

Osmotic diuretics, particularly mannitol (Osmitrol), are administered to reduce cerebral edema. Mannitol may be administered by bolus injection or as an infusion. Because the duration of action is limited, when mannitol is given by bolus, it may be necessary to repeat the dose based on the patient's response. Nursing management of the patient regarding fluid balance and electrolyte support is critical. Therapy with corticosteroids, usually dexamethasone (Decadron) is initiated or dosages increased. Doses in excess of 64 mg/day may be used (Levin, Leibel, & Gutin, 1997).

In addition, measures to control seizure activity by initiating or augmenting anticonvulsant use are instituted as necessary. If acute hydrocephalus is the precipitating cause of the increased ICP, emergency drainage of CSF, by insertion of a catheter through a burr hole into the lateral ventricle, may be performed. If time permits, or at a later point, a more permanent solution to CSF obstruction is obtained through placement of a ventriculoperitoneal catheter (Hickey, 1997b; McDonnell, 1994).

A medical crisis such as an acute increase in ICP can be extremely frightening to the patient and, perhaps more important, to family members. It is vital to keep the family members informed about the patient's condition and treatment. After the crisis resolves, the patient and family members need to know if and how such an emergency can be avoided in the future, or if this event signals progression of the disease.

NURSING MANAGEMENT

Diagnosis

The diagnosis of cerebral neuroblastoma profoundly and irrevocably changes the lives of patients and their family members. Because the common symptoms of a brain tumor can mimic those of many less serious disorders, patients and family members may be completely unprepared for the diagnosis. Additionally, little information is available on this tumor for clinicians and patients alike, and this can raise anxiety even more. As the patient undergoes diagnostic testing, nursing support is critical. Patient education assumes priority, as patients and their family members struggle to learn new and sometimes frightening information.

The symptoms the patient is experiencing, especially if they are cognitive, as well as anxiety about the diagnosis and future will impair the patient's ability to absorb and process information. Even simple facts may need to be repeated many times and reinforced with written materials when available and by other members of the health care team.

Most patients are started on a corticosteroid, usually dexamethasone (Decadron) to reduce cerebral edema. Because dexamethasone can cause serious side effects, including hyperglycemia, gastric irritation, ulcers, and mood swings, patients and their family members require considerable education to help them manage administration of the drug safely (Table 28-5). If the patient was diagnosed following a seizure, an anticonvulsant is prescribed. Most commonly, phenytoin (Dilantin) or carbamazepine (Tegretol) are the initial drugs of choice.

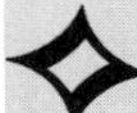

TABLE 28-5 Patient Preparation for the Use of Dexamethasone (Decadron)

What is dexamethasone? Dexamethasone is a steroid. It is used to decrease swelling.

Why am I taking dexamethasone? Dexamethasone is used to decrease swelling around your tumor or in the area where you had surgery.

How should I take my dexamethasone? Dexamethasone is a small pill. (Tape pill to paper here)
Your dexamethasone dose is ________ mg every ________ hours.
Dexamethasone can be irritating to your stomach, so take it with food or milk. Your doctor may prescribe medication to protect your stomach, too.
Take your dose exactly as prescribed. If you miss a dose, take it with your next dose. If you miss two doses, call your doctor or nurse.

What side effects should I know about? In addition to stomach irritation, Decadron can cause other side effects. These include the following:
- Hiccups
- Weight gain
- High blood sugar
- Mood swings (happy one minute, sad the next)
- Acne
- Muscle weakness

Let your doctor or nurse know **immediately** if you have any of the following problems:
- Fever
- Increased thirst; frequent urination
- Black bowel movements

Nursing Care in the Perioperative Phase

Preoperative Phase. Most patients with cerebral neuroblastoma undergo an operation to remove as much tumor as possible. Nursing research has demonstrated that patients anticipating craniotomy have specific and unique concerns. The most common concerns center on the potential loss of function and the return of function (Markin, 1986). These findings suggest that patients would benefit from a discussion of their current physical and functional status, as well as what temporary or permanent changes can be anticipated after surgery. Particular areas that should be addressed include hair loss, the location and appearance of the suture line, and the fact that symptoms may be worse initially because of swelling in the operative area.

In addition, patients need information regarding the surgical procedure itself, the sequence of events on the day of surgery, and measures such as deep breathing, leg exercises, and antiembolic devices that help prevent postoperative complications. It is also important to let patients know when and how often family members will be able to visit.

Postoperative Phase. Postoperatively, patients may require monitoring in an intensive care area. Close observation and careful nursing assessments are required to monitor for potential complications. These complications include an increase in cerebral edema, intracranial bleeding, and seizures.

Although cerebral edema is expected, close monitoring is necessary to prevent cerebral ischemia and infarction. Cerebral edema usually peaks around postoperative day 3 (Belford, 1997; Hickey, 1997c). Cerebral edema is managed by administering increasing doses of corticosteroids (Saba & Magolan, 1991).

Signs of intracranial bleeding, usually at the surgical site, are those of rapidly increasing ICP (Hickey, 1997c). Emergency interventions to control increases in ICP are required to prevent herniation and death.

Although most patients begin anticonvulsant drugs preoperatively for either therapeutic or prophylactic reasons, seizures are common in the postoperative period. Hyponatremia can precipitate seizure activity and should be avoided by close monitoring of serum sodium levels. Anticonvulsants must be given by alternative routes when patients are to receive nothing by mouth to maintain therapeutic serum levels. Phenytoin (Dilantin) is used most commonly. For status epilepticus, which is defined as continuous seizure activity that persists for 30 minutes or longer, or two or more seizures occurring sequentially without full recovery between each seizure, intravenous administration of lorazepam (Ativan) is recommended (Gilbert & Armstrong, 1995).

Other potential complications include respiratory compromise and, less commonly, wound infection and meningitis. Patients are at increased risk for the development of thrombophlebitis because of immobility and a hypercoagulable state secondary to the malignancy itself (Fowler, 1995; Sawaya et al., 1995). Constipation is also a common problem, secondary to immobility and dietary changes. Because straining at bowel movements can increase ICP, prophylactic use of stool softeners and laxatives is indicated.

Patients may complain of discomfort at the suture line or headache. The use of opioid analgesics is usually contraindicated because they can interfere with the neurologic examination. Acetaminophen or, if necessary, codeine may be prescribed and is usually effective.

Patients should be mobilized as soon as possible, both to avoid the complications of immobility and to promote self-care and self-esteem. Rehabilitation consults should be initiated early. Nurses can support and promote rehabilitation efforts by allowing the patient ample time to perform activities of daily living and by assisting the patient to incorporate newly gained skills into routine activities. Range-of-motion exercises should be performed on the affected side to maintain joint mobility. Family members often feel gratified to be able to assist their loved ones when assigned this task.

Swallowing may be impaired because of cranial nerve dysfunction or a depressed level of consciousness. Nutritional intake can be enhanced with supplements and careful dietary selection. Enteral tube feedings should be initiated if eating problems persist.

Aphasias, both fluent (receptive) and nonfluent (expressive), may result from surgery in the dominant frontotemporal region. Patients with nonfluent aphasia may feel frustrated and angry when attempts at communication fail. Patience and support, acknowledging the patient's frustration, are required by nurses and family members. Alternative means of communication such as pantomime or picture boards should be attempted and a referral for speech therapy initiated.

Patients with fluent aphasia often appear to be quite confused, as they have difficulty interpreting the spoken word. Their speech, although rhythmic, may contain many errors. Nurses should use visual cues to assist these patients to perform tasks. A mixed fluent and nonfluent aphasia leaves the patient profoundly impaired, with very little communication possible (Hickey, 1997d).

Nursing Care During Radiation Therapy

External beam radiation therapy is likely to be the most common treatment used postoperatively. Goals of nursing care during radiation therapy are centered on symptom control and patient support. A standard of care for the patient receiving external beam radiation to the brain is found in Table 28-6.

Patients receiving external beam radiation therapy experience complete alopecia in the irradiated area. Some patients have their entire head shaved preoperatively; for them, the prolongation of hair loss is not as traumatic as for patients who had only sections of their head shaved for surgery. Referrals to organizations and shops that can provide wigs, hairpieces, turbans, caps, and scarves help ameliorate the alterations in body image that occur with alopecia. Hair regrowth begins some time after radiation therapy stops, and the hair may regrow in a different shade and texture.

Irradiated skin will become erythematous and sensitive. Dry desquamation, with pruritus and flaking, may develop. General measures to avoid irritation should be instituted, including using only mild soaps and shampoos, avoiding tight or rough head coverings, and avoiding sunlight. If skin breakdown occurs, A&D or Aquaphor ointment may be prescribed (Hilderly, 1997).

Fatigue (see Home Care Issues) is also very common. Because radiation therapy often extends over 6 weeks, its effects on activities of daily living should not be underestimated or minimized.

Some patients may develop worsening of CNS symptoms when radiation therapy is initiated. This problem is due to a transient increase in cerebral edema and is usually treated with a temporary increase in corticosteroid dose.

Patients are usually maintained on corticosteroids throughout the course of radiation therapy. Patients and families need careful instructions when steroid doses are tapered after radiation therapy has ended, as over-rapid tapering can provoke adrenal insufficiency and increased cerebral edema (Table 28-5).

Because of the risk of developing *Pneumocystis carinii* pneumonia during a steroid taper, patients may receive prophylaxis for this complication, usually with oral trimethoprim/sulfamethoxazole (Bactrim). Therapy is continued for 1 month after discontinuation of radiation therapy (Belford, 1997; Slivka, Wen, Shea, & Loeffler, 1993).

Nursing Care During Chemotherapy

Although chemotherapy is not considered to have a major role in the treatment of many CNS neoplasms, some patients with cerebral neuroblastomas receive chemotherapy. The most common agents used include the nitrosureas, procarbazine, and methotrexate.

Nitrosureas. Nitrosureas, primarily BCNU (carmustine) and CCNU (lomustine), oral agents, are the mainstay of single-agent and combination chemotherapy protocols for many brain tumors, including cerebral neuroblastoma (Louis et al., 1990). Many patients experience nausea, perhaps with vomiting, although it is usually not severe. Nausea usually occurs 2 to 4 hours after administration of the chemotherapy. It responds well to standard antiemetic agents including granisetron (Kytril) or ondansetron (Zofran). Premedication with antiemetic drugs may be helpful.

Myelosuppression, which can be dose-limiting, occurs 4 to 5 weeks after treatment. Thrombocytopenia is common, as is leukopenia. Cumulative bone marrow toxicity can occur after repeated courses of treatment.

Renal toxicity, although not common, may occur with administration of high doses of CCNU. Irritation of the injection site and facial flushing is common with BCNU. Pulmonary toxicity from BCNU administration occurs with large cumulative doses and after prolonged administration, and can be fatal.

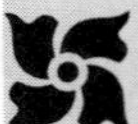

TABLE 28-6 Standard of Care for the Patient Receiving External Beam Radiation Therapy to the Brain

Patient Problems and Outcomes	Nursing Interventions and Rationales	Patient Education Instructions
Knowledge Deficit (Steroid Therapy)		
Patient will: • State indications for steroid use • List side effects that should be reported to MD/RN • Describe how to take dexamethasone safely	1. Assess patient/family knowledge of indications and side effects of steroid therapy. 2. Provide written materials to supplement verbal instruction. Reinforce as needed. 3. Assess for common side effects: • Hyperglycemia • Gastritis or gastrointestinal bleeding • Slowed wound healing • Sodium and fluid retention • Increased risk of infection	Teach patient to: 1. Take drug exactly as prescribed. 2. Not discontinue drug abruptly. 3. Take pills with food. 4. Report black stools. 5. Report fever over 100°F (38°C) 6. Report excessive thirst or urination 7. Expect mood swings, which are very common
Dry Desquamation (Scalp)		
Patient will: • Describe how to care for irradiated area	1. Assess irradiated skin for dryness, flaking, pruritus. 2. Apply A & D or other ointment (this may need to be removed prior to treatment).	Instruct patient to: 1. Use only mild soaps/shampoos. 2. Avoid washing off or "touching-up" radiation skin markings. 3. Avoid tight head coverings. 4. Avoid sun exposure. 5. Report areas of skin breakdown.
Knowledge deficit (external beam radiation therapy)		
Patient will: • Verbalize understanding of purpose and side effects of radiation therapy	1. Assess patient's understanding of purpose and side effects of radiation therapy. 2. Review anticipated schedule for receiving radiation therapy. Assist patient in prioritizing work and family responsibilities during extended course of treatment.	1. Teach patient expected side effects of radiation therapy: • Alopecia • Skin changes (dryness, erythema, pruritus) • Fatigue
Knowledge Deficit (surgery)		
Patient will: • State rationale for surgery • Discuss own symptoms in relation to location of tumor • Express general understanding of sequence of events on day of surgery • Return demonstrate deep breathing and leg exercises • Describe postoperative appearance (suture line, dressings, IV lines)	1. Assess understanding of rationale for surgery, procedure itself. 2. Include family members in discussion, as appropriate. 3. Provide ample time for repetition of information and questions.	1. Review relevant anatomy, focusing on functional anatomy. Avoid complex terms. 2. Tie anatomy to symptoms the patient is experiencing. 3. Discuss the surgical procedure, including rationale(s): • Obtain definitive diagnosis • Debulk tumor • Relieve pressure 4. Provide overview of sequence of events on day of surgery. 5. Give concrete information regarding the patient's appearance postoperatively. • Hair loss • Suture line • Dressing • IV lines • Catheter • Drains 6. Demonstrate deep breathing. 7. Demonstrate leg exercises.

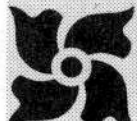

TABLE 28-6 Standard of Care for the Patient Receiving External Beam Radiation Therapy to the Brain—cont'd

Patient Problems and Outcomes	Nursing Interventions and Rationales	Patient Education Instructions
Anxiety Patient will: • Utilize effective coping mechanisms • Express feelings of decreased anxiety	1. Assess patient's level of anxiety. 2. Assess previous use of coping mechanisms in highly stressful situations. 3. Reinforce use of adaptive coping mechanisms. 4. Assist patient to identify specific areas of concern (loss of function, death, pain).	1. Teach patient relaxation techniques: • Guided imagery • Meditation • Focused breathing
Risk for Increased Intracranial Pressure (IICP) Patient will: • Not demonstrate signs of IICP	1. Monitor patient for signs and symptoms of increased intracranial pressure: • Deterioration in level of consciousness • Changes in motor/sensory function • Changes in pupil size and reaction • Headache • Seizures 2. Avoid clustering activities that are likely to increase ICP: • Arousal from sleep • Bathing • Turning • Suctioning • Isometric exercise 3. Maintain patient in neutral position: • HOB $\geq$ 30 • Avoid neck, hip, knee flexion 4. Administer stool softeners/laxatives to avoid straining at stool.	1. Instruct patient to avoid Valsalva maneuver, straining at stool.
Altered Thought Processes Patient will: • Return to baseline mental status, if possible	1. Assess neurological status, including alertness, orientation, memory and judgment. 2. Reorient patient regularly. Provide large clock and calendar at bedside, watch on wrist. 3. Assign consistent staff to care for patient. 4. Maintain consistent schedule if possible. 5. Implement appropriate safety measures.	Instruct family to: 1. Use familiar objects to re-orient patient. 2. Converse with patient about topics of interest to the patient, old hobbies, family events, etc.

Continued

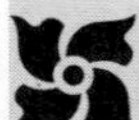

Table 28-6 Standard of Care for the Patient Receiving External Beam Radiation Therapy to the Brain—cont'd

Patient Problems and Outcomes	Nursing Interventions and Rationales	Patient Education Instructions
Nonfluent Aphasia Patient will: • Develop satisfactory method of expressing needs	1. Reassure patient that his/her needs will be met. 2. Allow patient to attempt speech. Do not interrupt. Do not rush patient. 3. Provide alternative means of communication. • Paper/pencil • Picture board 4. Initiate speech therapy referral.	1. Instruct patient to slow down. When stuck on a word, try another.
Self-Care Deficit: • Feeding • Bathing • Grooming • Toileting Patient will: • Demonstrate beginning skills in one-handed techniques for feeding, bathing, grooming, toileting	1. Assess degree of motor/sensory deficit postoperatively. 2. Initiate rehabilitation referral. 3. Maximize opportunities for patient to practice new skills learned in rehab. 4. Perform passive range of motion to affected extremities. 5. Avoid using terms such as *bad side* or *bad leg*. Use terms that are neutral, e.g., *affected* and *unaffected.*	1. Discuss with patient and family that severity of some symptoms may improve over time. 2. Teach family how to perform range-of-motion exercises.
Constipation Patient will: • Return to baseline bowel elimination patterns	1. Assess routine bowel habits and pattern of elimination. 2. Encourage as much activity as possible. 3. Alter diet to promote elimination. 4. Administer stool softeners and laxatives as prescribed. 5. Establish toileting schedule and adhere to it.	1. Teach patient/family how to increase fiber in diet. 2. Reinforce need for regular bowel elimination and early intervention for constipation. 3. Discuss effective ways to use laxatives and stool softeners.
Nausea Patient will: • Express tolerable relief of nausea associated with chemotherapy administration	1. Assess degree of nausea. 2. Assess response to anti-emetics. 3. Assess nutritional patterns: • Food intake • Taste changes • Weight loss	1. Teach patient relaxation techniques to help nausea. 2. Instruct patient to take anti-emetics as prescribed before and after treatment.
Risk for Bleeding Patient will: • Describe bleeding precautions	1. Assess for bleeding (gums, urine, stool, petechiae, headache). 2. Assess patient/family understanding of necessary precautions, reinforce as needed. 3. Monitor platelet count.	1. Instruct patient/family regarding bleeding precautions: • Soft toothbrush • Electric razor • Avoid falls
Risk for Infection Patient will: • Describe routine infection control practices	1. Assess patient/family understanding of risk(s) for infection and hygienic practices to follow.	1. Instruct patient to: • Maintain good general hygiene • Wash hands frequently • Avoid crowds • Notify nurse or doctor if temperature is elevated (≥100°F, 38°C)

TABLE 28-7 Resources for Adults with Neuroblastoma

American Brain Tumor Association	Provides excellent specific educational materials as well as listings of support groups for brain tumor patients. Also provides information on clinical trials for brain tumor patients. Sponsors a biennial symposium on current treatment for patients and family members.	(800) 886-2282
American Cancer Society	Provides educational materials on cancer and cancer treatment. Can provide information on the Look Good . . . . Feel Better program, which teaches cosmetic techniques to patients receiving chemotherapy and radiation therapy. May be able to provide medical equipment and rides to appointments and treatment.	(800) ACS-2345
Cancer Care	Provides one-on-one counseling, support groups, and educational programs for patients and family members. May be able to provide limited financial support for treatment-related expenses.	(800) 813 HOPE
National Brain Tumor Foundation	Provides brain tumor–specific educational materials, as well as a newsletter. Provides one-on-one counseling through a telephone network.	(800) 934 CURE
National Cancer Institute/ Cancer Information Service (CIS)	Provides accurate, up-to-date cancer information for patients and families. The CIS provides information on specific cancers in both English and Spanish, as well as information on clinical trials and how to obtain a second opinion.	(800) 4 CANCER

BCNU is also available as an implantable wafer, which can be placed in the tumor bed at the time of resection.

Procarbazine. Procarbazine is another oral agent used alone or in combination with the nitrosureas, as well as with other drugs. It is generally well tolerated. Patients may experience mild nausea throughout the treatment period. Because of potential food-drug interactions, patients should be instructed to avoid tyramine-containing foods, such as cheese and wine. Procarbazine can also precipitate a disulfiram-like reaction when ingested with alcohol. Myelosuppression occurs at 4 weeks and resolves slowly.

Methotrexate. If intrathecal (intraventricular) chemotherapy is indicated because of suspected or documented tumor seeding of the meninges or CSF, methotrexate is the agent used most often. It is injected into the CSF either through an Omaya reservoir (inserted into the lateral ventricle) or through a lumbar puncture. An acute chemical meningitis characterized by fever, headache, and nuchal rigidity may occur. Long-term intrathecal use is associated with leukoencephalopathy (Alavi, 1995).

HOME CARE ISSUES

Diagnosis of any cancer is a devastating event, but diagnosis of a primary brain tumor is particularly so. Repercussions reverberate throughout the patient's family system, related not only to the diagnosis and treatment of the tumor, but also to the impact of the tumor on the physical, social, and mental functioning of the patient. Alterations are likely to occur in all of these areas, especially as the tumor recurs or progresses. Singly and in combination, any of these areas of dysfunction places tremendous stressors on patients and their family members. These stressors are perhaps most apparent when the patient and family members are at home, attempting to regain a pattern in their daily lives. Preliminary nursing research demonstrates that a support group specifically for patients with brain tumors and their families can help provide information, guidance, and support, as well as enhance coping mechanisms and quality of life for the participants (Leavitt, Lamb, & Voss, 1996). Patients and family members should be assisted in searching for supportive resources (Table 28-7).

For patients coping with motor losses, the familiar environment of the home becomes a maze of difficulties. Nursing and occupational therapy assessments of the home before discharge from the hospital help family members make the physical adjustments necessary to accommodate the patient with hemiparesis, sensory or visual loss, and mental status changes. Such adjustments include rearranging furniture, adding grab bars and other safety features in the bathroom, rearranging supplies in the kitchen, and purchasing or altering clothing and footwear for ease in dressing.

A physical therapist can help prepare the patient for discharge by teaching stair climbing and safe ambulation and transfer techniques. It is essential to include family members in this preparation, as their knowledgeable support is vital. Rehabilitation should be addressed on an ongoing basis in the home, as the patient's level of functioning changes or deteriorates (Belford, 1997).

For patients receiving chemotherapy and especially radiation therapy, fatigue is an ever-present companion. It is important to ask about and acknowledge fatigue (Nail, 1997). Nurses can help patients and families set realistic goals, prioritize activities, and restructure activities of daily living to minimize frustration and fatigue and maximize productivity and feelings of satisfaction (Box 28-3).

PROGNOSIS

The ultimate prognosis is difficult to evaluate in a rare and relatively unstudied tumor such as cerebral neuroblastoma in adults. Published reports generally demonstrate an average life span after diagnosis of less than 5 years, with a range from less than 1 year to up to 64 months for intrapa-

Box 28-3
Managing Fatigue at Home

Many patients who are receiving treatments such as chemotherapy and radiation therapy experience fatigue. They feel "bone-tired" and "exhausted". You may feel that way, too. Although no one knows exactly why this happens, we do know that it is normal for you to feel tired or fatigued during treatment.

You may continue to feel tired for some time, even after your treatment ends. This feeling is normal, too.

Here are some tips to help you feel better while at home:

1. Get a bedtime routine and stick to it as much as possible. Some people find it helpful to have a warm drink before bedtime, such as warm milk or herbal tea. Avoid drinks with caffeine. Check with your doctor before drinking alcohol.
2. Try to arrange for your most important activities to occur early in the day, since you are more likely to feel rested then.
3. Decide what activities are most important to you and plan to do only them. Ask friends or family members to help with the rest of the activities.
4. Plan to rest or nap during the day. Avoid sleeping for long periods, though, since this will interrupt your nighttime rest. A one-hour nap can be refreshing!

renchymal tumors. In general, prognosis is poor, and, as with most primary CNS tumors, local recurrence can be expected (Bennet and Rubenstein, 1984; Berger et al., 1983; Davis et al., 1990; Horten & Rubenstein, 1976; Louis et al., 1990; Mrak, 1994; Ojeda et al., 1986).

QUALITY OF CARE EVALUATION

Inpatient and outpatient facilities are required to evaluate the quality of care provided to patients and their family members. Table 28-8 provides a tool to monitor the quality of care provided to a patient receiving external beam radiation to the brain.

Table 28-8 Quality of Care Evaluation for a Patient Receiving External Beam Radiation Therapy to the Brain

Discipline(s) participating in the quality of care evaluation:
☐ Nursing ☐ Medicine ☐ Social Services
Data From:
☐ Medical Record Review ☐ Patient/Family Interview

Criteria	Yes	No
1. Patient/family able to state rationale for radiation therapy	☐	☐
2. Patient/family able to identify expected side effects:		
a. Hair loss	☐	☐
b. Temporary worsening of symptoms	☐	☐
c. Fatigue	☐	☐
d. Scalp erythema, itching, dryness	☐	☐
3. Patient/family able to identify care priorities:		
a. Do not wash off markings	☐	☐
b. Use mild soap/shampoo	☐	☐
c. Avoid tight head coverings, rough fabrics	☐	☐
d. Notify MD/RN if skin is broken on scalp	☐	☐
e. Avoid sunlight	☐	☐
4. Patient/family able to state name/telephone number of resource person	☐	☐

RESEARCH ISSUES

Because there is relatively little information on cerebral neuroblastomas in adults, it is important for any patient diagnosed with the tumor to be reported in the literature. Case reports should highlight presenting signs and symptoms, characteristics of the tumor on imaging studies, histopathologic characteristics, detailed treatment protocols, and survival. An important area for nursing research is to evaluate the responses of patients and their family members to their diagnosis and treatment. A recent publication overviews instruments that can be used to measure quality of life in patients with CNS tumors ("Quality of Life," 1995). Issues specific to neuro-oncology patients have not been studied in detail, if at all. These issues include changes in body image and self-esteem in patients undergoing craniotomy, fatigue in patients receiving brain irradiation, role strain, caregiver stress and coping in family members of patients with brain tumors, and responses of patients and family members to being diagnosed with a rare tumor.

REFERENCES

Alavi, J. B. (1995). Primary and metastatic brain tumors. In R. T. Skeel & N. A. Lachant (Eds.), *Handbook of cancer chemotherapy* (4th ed.). Boston: Little, Brown and Company.

American Joint Commission on Cancer: *AJCC cancer staging manual.* (1997). (5th ed.). Philadelphia: Lippincott-Raven.

Belford, K. (1997). Central nervous system cancers. In S. Groenwald, M. H. Frogge, M. Goodman, & C. H. Yarbro (Eds.), *Cancer nursing: Principles and practice* (4th ed.). Sudbury, MA: Jones and Bartlett.

Bennet, J. P., Jr. & Rubenstein, L. J. (1984). The biological behavior of primary cerebral neuroblastomas: a reappraisal on the clinical course of 70 cases. *Annals of Neurology, 16,* 24-27.

Berger, M. S., Edwards, M. S. B., Wara, W., Levin, V. A., & Wilson, C. B. (1983). Primary cerebral neuroblastomas: Long term follow-up review and therapeutic guidelines. *Journal of Neurosurgery, 59,* 418-423.

Berleur, M. P. & Cordier, S. (1995). The role of chemical, physical or vial exposures and health factors in neurocarcinogenesis. Implications for epidemiologic studies of brain tumors. *Cancer Causes Control, 6,* 240-256.

Bondy, M., Wiencke, J., Wrensch, M., & Kyritsis, A. (1994). Genetics of primary brain tumors: a review. *Journal of Neuro-Oncology, 18,* 69-81.

Conrad, C., Milosavljevic, V. P., & Yung, W. K. A. (1995). Advances in chemotherapy for brain tumors. *Neurologic Clinics, 13,* 795-812.

Cotran, R. S., Kumar, V., & Robbins, S. L. (1994). *The central nervous system. Pathologic basis of disease* (5th ed.). Philadelphia: W. B. Saunders.

Davis, P. C., Wichman, R. D., Takei, Y., & Hoffman, J. C. (1990). Primary cerebral neuroblastoma: CT and MR findings in 12 cases. *American Journal of Radiology, 154,* 831-836.

Desmeules, M., Mikkelsen, T., & Mao, Y. (1992). Increasing incidence of primary malignant brain tumors: Influence of diagnostic methods. *Journal of the National Cancer Institute, 84,* 442-445.

Ferreol, E., Sawaya, R., & Courten-Myers, G. (1989). Primary cerebral neuroblastoma (neurocytoma) in adults. *Journal of Neuro-Oncology, 7,* 121-128.

Fetell, M. (1995). Tumors. In L. Rowland (Ed.), *Merritt's textbook of neurology* (9th ed.). Baltimore: Williams & Wilkins.

Fine, H. (1994). Brain tumor chemotherapy trials: Slow start, but quickly gaining (editorial). *Journal of Clinical Oncology, 12,* 2003-2004.

Fowler, S. B. (1995). Deep vein thrombosis and pulmonary emboli in neuroscience patients. *Journal of Neuroscience Nursing, 27,* 224-278.

Frank-Stromborg, M. (1992). Neurofibromatosis. *Seminars in Oncology Nursing, 8,* 265-271.

Gilbert, M. & Armstrong, T. S. (1995) Management of seizures in the adult patient with cancer. *Cancer Practice, 3,* 143-149.

Grieg, N. H., Ries, L. G., & Yancik, R. (1990). Increasing annual incidence of primary malignant brain tumors in the elderly. *Journal of the National Cancer Institute, 82,* 1621-1624.

Grossman, S. A. & Norris, L. K. (1995). Adjuvant and neoadjuvant treatment for primary brain tumors in adults. *Seminars in Oncology, 22*(6), 530-539.

Hassoun, J., Soylemezoglu, F., Gambarelli, D., Figarella-Branger, D., von Amman, K., & Kleihues, P. (1993). Central neurocytoma: A synopsis of clinical and histological features. *Brain Pathology, 3,* 297-306.

Hickey, J. V. (1997a). Overview of neuroanatomy and neurophysiology. In J. V. Hickey (Ed.) *The clinical practice of neurological and neurosurgical nursing* (4th ed.). Philadelphia: Lippincott.

Hickey, J. V. (1997b). Management of patients undergoing neurosurgical procedures. In J. V. Hickey (Ed.), *The clinical practice of neurological and neurosurgical nursing* (4th ed.). Philadelphia: Lippincott.

Hickey, J. V. (1997c). Intracranial pressure: Theory and management of increased intracranial pressure. In J. V. Hickey (Ed.), *The clinical practice of neurological and neurosurgical nursing* (4th ed.). Philadelphia: Lippincott.

Hickey, J. V. (1997d). Rehabilitation of neuroscience patients. In J. V. Hickey (Ed.), *The clinical practice of neurological and neurosurgical nursing* (4th ed.). Philadelphia: Lippincott.

Hickey, J. V. & Armstrong, T. (1997). Brain tumors. In J. V. Hickey (Ed.), *The clinical practice of neurological and neurosurgical nursing* (4th ed.). Philadelphia: Lippincott.

Hilderly, L. J. (1997). Radiotherapy. In S. Groenwald, M. H. Frogge, M. Goodman, & C. H. Yarbro (Eds.), *Cancer nursing: Principles and practice* (4th ed.). Sudbury, MA: Jones and Bartlett.

Horten, B. C. & Rubenstein, L. J. (1976). Primary cerebral neuroblastoma. *Brain, 99,* 735-756.

Jaeckle, K. A. (1993). Causes and management of headaches in cancer patients. *Oncology, 7,* 27-31.

Junquerra, L. C., Caineiro, J., & Kelley, R. O. (1992). Nerve tissue. *Basic histology* (7th ed.). Norwalk, CT: Appleton and Lange.

Kelly, P. T. (1992). Informational needs of families with hereditary cancers. *Seminars in Oncology Nursing, 8,* 288-292.

Keyser, A. (1993a). Epidemiology of neuro-oncological disease. In A. Twijnstra, A. Keyser, & B. W. Ongerboer DeVisser (Eds.), *Neuro-oncology: Primary tumors and neurological complications of cancer.* Amsterdam: Elsevier.

Keyser, A. (1993b). Current concepts on the interaction between nervous system and neuro-oncological processes. In A. Twvijnstra, A. Keyser, & B. W. Ongerboer DeVisser (Eds.), *Neuro-oncology: Primary tumors and neurological complications in cancer.* Amsterdam: Elsevier.

Kleihues, P., Burger, P. C., & Scheithauer, B. W. (1993). The new WHO classification of brain tumors. *Brain Pathology, 3,* 255-268.

Kovnar, R. H., Kellie, S. J., Horowitz, M. E., Sanford, R. A., Langston, J. W., Mulhern, R. K., Jenkins, J. J., Douglass, E. C., Etcubanas, E. E., Fairclough, D. L., & Kun, L. E. (1990). Pre-irradiation cisplatin and etoposide in the treatment of high risk medulloblastoma and other malignant embryonal tumors of the central nervous system. *Journal of Clinical Oncology, 8,* 330-336.

Landis, S. H., Murray, T., Bolden, S., & Wingo, P. A. (1998). Cancer statistics 1998. *CA: A Cancer Journal for Clinicians, 48,* 6-29.

Leavitt, M. B., Lamb, S. A., & Voss, B. S. (1996). Brain tumor support group: Content themes and mechanisms of support. *Oncology Nursing Forum, 23,* 1247-1255.

Levin, V., Leibel, S., & Gutin, P. (1997). Neoplasms of the central nervous system in cancer. In V. DeVita, S. Hellman, & S. Noremberg (Eds.), *Principles and practice of oncology* (5th ed.). Philadelphia: Lippincott.

Louis, D. V., Swearingen, B., Linggood, R. M., Dickersin, G. R., Kretschmar, C., Bhan, A. K., & Hedley-White, T. (1990). Central nervous system neurocytomas and neuroblastoma in adults: Report of eight cases. *Journal of Neuro-Oncology, 9,* 231-238.

Maiuri, F., Spaziante, R., DeCaro, M. L., Cappabianca, P., Giamundo, A., & Iaconetta, G. (1995). Central neurocytoma: Clinico-pathological study of 5 cases and review of the literature. *Clinical Neurology and Neurosurgery, 97,* 219-28.

Markin, D. M. (1986). Preoperative concerns of the patient undergoing craniotomy. *Journal of Neuroscience Nursing, 18,* 275-278.

Martz, C. M. (1992). Von Hippel-Lindau disease: A genetically transmitted multisystem neoplastic disorder. *Seminars in Oncology Nursing, 8,* 281-287.

McDonnell, K. K. (1994). Obstructive emergencies. In J. Gross & B. L. Johnson (Eds.), *Handbook of oncology nursing* (2nd ed.). Sudbury, MA: Jones and Bartlett.

Meehan, J. L. (1994). Mobility and neurological function. In J. Gross & B. L. Johnson (Eds.), *Handbook of oncology nursing* (2nd ed.). Sudbury, MA: Jones and Bartlett.

Mrak, R. E. (1994). Malignant neurocytic tumor. *Human Pathology, 25,* 747-752.

Nail, L. M. (1997). Fatigue. In S. Groenwald, M. H. Frogge, M. Goodman, & C. H. Yarbro (Eds.), *Cancer nursing: Principles and practice* (4th ed.). Sudbury, MA: Jones and Bartlett.

Nakagawa, K., Aoki, Y., Sakata, K., Sasaki, Y., Matsutani, M., & Akanuma, A. (1993). Radiation therapy of well-differentiated neuroblastoma and central neurocytoma. *Cancer, 72,* 1350-1355.

National Cancer Institute. (1998). *Current clinical trials in oncology.* New Jersey: Pyros Education Group.

Ojeda, V. J., Stokes, B. A. R., Lee, M. A., Thomas, G. W., Papadimitriou, J. M., Cala, L. A., Stevens, S. M. B., & O'Neill, P. (1986). Primary cerebral neuroblastomas: A clinicopathological study of one adolescent and five adult patients. *Pathology, 18,* 41-49.

Posner, J. B. (1995). *Neurologic complications of cancer.* Philadelphia: Davis.

Quality of life in the neuro-oncology patient: A symposium. (1995). *Journal of Neuroscience Nursing, 27,* 219-223.

Rhodes, R. H., Cole, M., Takaoka, Y., Roessman, U., Cotes, E. E., & Simon, J. (1994). Intraventricular cerebral neuroblastomas. *Archives in Pathology and Laboratory Medicine, 118,* 897-911.

Robey, S. S., Olson, J. L., Brem, H., & Epstein, J. (1988). Posterior fossa neuroblastoma occurring in an elderly man. *Human Pathology, 19,* 365-367.

Saba, M. & Magolan, J. (1991). Understanding cerebral edema: Implications for oncology nurses. *Oncology Nursing Forum, 18,* 499-505.

Sawaya, R., Rambo, W. M., Hammond, M. A., & Ligon, B. L. (1995). Advances in surgery for brain tumors. *Neurologic Clinics, 13,* 757-771.

Schlehofer, B., Blettner, M., & Wahrendorf, J. (1992). Association between brain tumors and menopausal status. *Journal of the National Cancer Institute, 84,* 1346-1349.

Schwartz, R. B. (1995). Neuroradiology of brain tumors. *Neurologic Clinics, 13,* 723-756.

Shrieve, D. & Loeffler, J. S. (1995). Advances in radiation therapy for brain tumors. *Neurologic Clinics, 13,* 773-793.

Slivka, A., Wen, P. Y., Shea, M., & Loeffler, J. S. (1993). *Pneumocystis carinii* pneumonia during steroid taper in patients with primary brain tumors. *The American Journal of Medicine, 94,* 216-219.

Smith-Rooker, J. L., Garrett, A., Hodges, L. C., & Shue, V. (1992). Prevalence of glioblastoma multiforme subjects with prior herbicide exposure. *Journal of Neuroscience Nursing 24*(5): 260-264.

Thomas, D. G. T. (1993). Primary tumors of the brain: genetic and chromosomal abnormalities. In A. Twijnstra, A. Keyser, & B. W. Ongerboer De Visser (Eds.), *Neuro-oncology: Primary tumors and neurological complications of cancer.* Amsterdam: Elsevier.

Weprin, B., Hall, W., & Bergman, T. (1994). Central neurocytoma: Diagnosis and treatment. *Minnesota Medicine, 77,* 43-46.

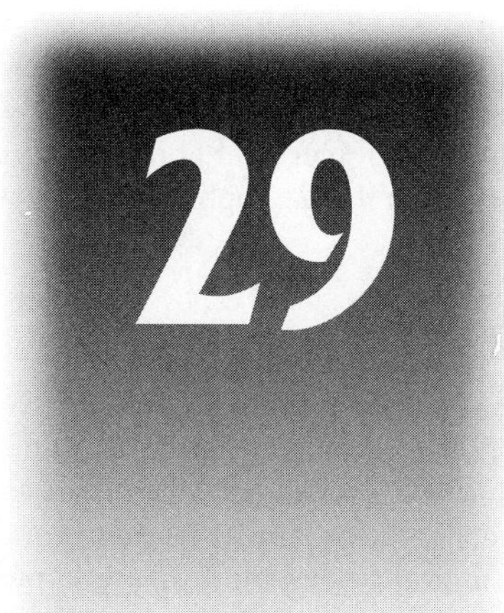

Cervical Cancer

Jeannine Brant, RN, MS, AOCN

EPIDEMIOLOGY

Cervical cancer represents the second most common cancer in women worldwide. The incidence varies geographically with rates in industrialized nations of 10 per 100,000 and in developing countries of 40 per 100,000. Approximately 80% of all new cases are diagnosed in developing nations of the world (Bosch et al., 1995).

In the United States, cervical cancer accounts for approximately 3% of all female cancers and 2% of female cancer deaths. It is the third most common of the female genital cancers. In 1998, it is estimated that 13,700 women will be diagnosed with invasive cervical cancer and 4,900 will die from the disease (Landis, Murray, Bolden, & Wingo, 1998). Carcinoma in situ of the cervix and other preinvasive forms of cervical abnormalities are not included in these statistics, and therefore the statistics are not representative of the actual problem.

Cervical cancer incidence and mortality within the United States is increased in women of color and in those with a low educational level and low socioeconomic status. This increased incidence is most likely related to the lack of screening and the practice of high-risk behaviors such as a smoking. The highest incidence occurs in Vietnamese-American women (43 : 100,000). Hispanic, Korean, and Native Alaskan women also have higher incidence rates of 15 : 100,000 or greater. These incidences are compared with 8.7 : 100,000 in white women (Fig. 29-1). Mortality rates, however, are highest among African-American women (6.7 : 100,000) compared with 2.5 : 100,000 among white women (Miller et al., 1996).

Of all female genital cancers, cervical carcinoma is the only one that can be detected and potentially prevented by regular screening activities. The morbidity and mortality of cervical cancer could be nearly eliminated if women participated in regular screening and evaluation. Approximately 35% of women who develop cervical cancer have never had a Papanicolaou (Pap) smear (Wain, Farnsworth, & Hacker, 1992).

The Breast and Cervical Cancer Early Detection Program, supported by the Centers for Disease Control and Prevention (CDC), is a national outreach education and screening program attempting to reach low-income, minority, and other underserved women. The program was started in 1991 in 12 states and expanded to all 50 states by 1996. As of May 1996, the program has provided 612,008 Pap smears, with 19,166 women found to have a precursor of cervical cancer. Invasive cervical cancer was diagnosed in 239 of these women (American Public Health Association, 1996).

Cervical cancer is a public health concern that challenges health care providers to seek new opportunities to educate and recruit underserved women for screening and early detection. When invasive cervical cancer is paramount, there are unique challenges related to diagnosis, treatment, and optimizing the quality of life of women with this cancer diagnosis.

RISK FACTORS

The etiologic factors for cervical cancer are multifactorial. The major risk factors associated with the development of cervical cancer are listed in Box 29-1. Many of the risk factors demonstrate a strong correlation with the development of cervical cancer, and yet the evidence supporting some proposed risk factors remains controversial and is discussed here.

Human Papilloma Virus

Human papilloma virus (HPV), a sexually transmitted agent, remains the single most important risk factor in the development of cervical cancer. More than 70 types of HPV have been identified, and about 20 types characteristically infect epithelial mucosa, usually of the genital tract (Birley, 1995). Two subtypes of HPV, 16 and 18, demonstrate the highest risk for the development of cervical cancer. Approximately 60% of squamous cell carcinomas (SCCs) of the cervix exhibit HPV 16, and 52% of adenocarcinomas of the cervix contain HPV 18 (Hording, Teglbjaerg, Visfeldt, & Bock, 1992; Lehtinen et al., 1996). It is important to note that HPV infection is one of several cofactors in the devel-

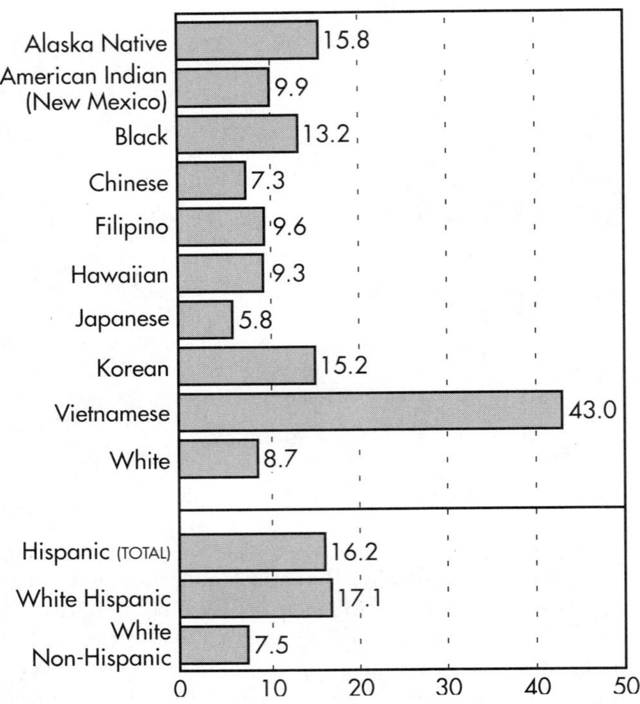

Fig. 29-1 The incidence of cervical cancer in minority women. (From Miller, B.A., Kolonel, L.N., Bernstein, L., Young, Jr. J.L., Swanson, G.M., West, D., Key, C.R., Liff, J.M., Glover, C.S., Alexander, G.A., et al. [eds]. [1996]. *Racial/ethnic patterns of cancer in the United States 1988-1992.* National Cancer Institute. NIH Pub. No. 96-4104. Bethesda, MD.)

Box 29-1
Risk Factors for Cervical Cancer

- Human papilloma virus
- Early sexarchy
- Multiple sexual partners
- Seminal chemicals (? association)
- Ethnicity (adenocarcinoma)
- In utero exposure to diethylstilbestrol (DES)
- Positive family history (? association)
- Tobacco use
- Oral contraceptives (? association)
- Retinoids (? association)
- Micronutrients (beta-carotene, folate, vitamin C, vitamin E - ? association)
- Immunosuppression (HIV Infection)
- Trichomonas vaginalis

opment of cervical cancer. HPV is not always present in cervical cancers or cervical intraepithelial neoplasia (CIN). A recent study evaluated for differences between HPV-positive and HPV-negative women with CIN. It was found that HPV-positive women were on average 2 years younger than HPV-negative women; had a median of four sex partners, compared with three in negative women; and 70.7% of HPV-positive women smoked, compared with 48.3% of HPV-negative women (Burger, Hollema, Pieters, Schroder, & Quint, 1996). HPV-negative cervical carcinomas also appear to have a worse prognosis than those that are HPV-positive (Herrington, 1995). The pathophysiology of HPV that is associated with conversion to cervical abnormalities and cervical cancer is discussed in the pathophysiology section of this chapter.

Trichomonas Vaginalis

Trichomonas vaginalis, a sexually transmitted pathogen of the male and female genital tracts may also play a role in the development of cervical cancer. Cervical cancer is the second most common fatal cancer in Chinese women, and trichomonas infection is common among the Chinese population. Women with trichomoniasis may exhibit a local production of nitrosamines by the vaginal microflora. It appears that women with *T. vaginalis* have an increased risk for cervical cancer (i.e., a relative risk of 3.3, compared with a relative risk of 0.9 in the general population [Zhang & Begg, 1994; Zhang et al., 1995]).

Herpes Simplex Virus-2/Cytomegalovirus

In vitro studies support an interaction between herpes simplex virus-2 (HSV-2) and HPV 16 and 18. It has also been suggested that cytomegalovirus (CMV) and HPV are cofactors in the development of cervical carcinoma. The exact independent role or associated role of these viruses with HPV is unknown at this time (Koffa, Koumantakis, Ergazaki, Tsatsanis, & Spandidos, 1995).

Early Sexarchy

Early sexarchy, or early initiation of sexual intercourse, is another significant risk factor in the development of cervical cancer, most likely due to the changes that occur within the transformation zone of the cervix during puberty. The transformation zone lies between the columnar epithelium of the endocervical canal and squamous epithelium of the exocervix and is comprised of squamous metaplasia. The squamous cells are replaced by basal reserve cells, and this high mitotic process peaks during puberty and pregnancy. The exotrophic zone during puberty and pregnancy renders itself susceptible to carcinogenic insults. The zone is also biologically immature during puberty, and biological immaturity may be extended by sexual activity. In addition, cervical mucous, a protective coat for the cervix, thins during puberty resulting in increased vulnerability to carcinogens (Lovejoy & Anastasi, 1994). Periods of active metaplasia may also coincide with rapid shedding of the HPV, resulting in cellular transformation.

Multiple Sexual Partners

The practice of having multiple sex partners is a considerable risk factor in the development of cervical cancer (Brinton et al., 1993). The data suggest that having various partners increases exposure to HPV and other sexually transmitted diseases such as human immunodeficiency virus (HIV) and HSV-2. It is also interesting to note that the risk of cervical cancer is increased in monogamous women whose husbands have extramarital partners. Women who are married to men with 15 or more partners have an increased relative risk of seven (Buckley, Harris, Doll, Vessey, & Williams, 1981).

Seminal Chemicals

Spermine and spermidine, two polyamines found in seminal fluid, have been found to accelerate cell proliferation and induce DNA changes in HPV 16-infected cervical cells. Bench pathology studies show that the chemicals may activate latent HPV infections by stimulating basal cell division, thus inducing squamous intraepithelial lesion (SIL) transformation (Fletcher, Neill, & Norval, 1990; Lovejoy, 1994).

Poor Hygiene

Assorted studies have examined the impact of poor genital and sexual hygiene on the development of cervical cancer. It has been suggested that penile cancer is a risk factor for cervical cancer. In men, penile cancer is associated with poor hygiene practices or is found in populations without public water and sewage systems (Franco, Filho, Billa, & Torloni, 1988). An increased risk for cervical cancer may also be associated with unsanitary conditions during the first coitus. One study found that women who experienced first coitus on the ground were more likely to develop invasive cervical cancer (Rotkin, 1967).

Genetic Predisposition

A few isolated case studies suggest that genetic predisposition may play a role in the development of SCC of the cervix. Two case histories in the literature report three sisters with SIL, and another study reports the presence of SIL in four daughters (Bender, 1976; Way, 1976). More recent studies are investigating the relationship between genes or antigens, and SCC of the cervix, specifically HLA-DQw3. Of the specimens examined, 88% contained the HLA-DQw3 antigen, whereas the expected value is 50% (Wank & Thomassen, 1991).

Ethnic Differences

Cervical cancer incidence rates vary throughout the world with the highest incidences in developing countries. It is unknown whether this increased incidence is a result of the lack of screening practices, thus more women have presenting symptoms of invasive cervical cancer, or whether there are true ethnic differences that place ethnic groups at increased risk for the development of cervical carcinoma.

It has also been speculated that there are variations worldwide of the types of HPV (e.g., HPV-16, 18, and other types). These variations could explain the pocket areas throughout the world with higher incidence rates for cervical cancer (Stewart et al., 1996). Further research is needed in this area.

An additional risk factor for cervical cancer is in utero exposure to diethylstilbestrol (DES) (McMullin, 1992). Pregnant women who took DES for pregnancy-induced nausea and vomiting in the mid-1900s have daughters who now have a higher incidence of cervical cancer.

Tobacco Use

Many studies indicate that tobacco use is directly correlated with the development of SIL and its progression to cervical carcinoma. Cigarette products, specifically cotinine and nicotine, are deposited in the cervical mucous. Passive smokers also experience elevations in cervical cotinine and nicotine. It is unknown whether the cigarette products exert a direct carcinogenic effect or localized immunosuppressive effects. It has also been noted that smoking cessation may trigger the acute shedding of occult HPV (Lovejoy & Anastasi, 1994). One proposed mechanism for the association between tobacco and cervical cancer is that there are reduced numbers of Langerhans cells in the cervical epithelium of smokers. This finding suggests that viral expression of HPV occurs as a result of reduced viral antigen presentation. Among women with HPV, the relative risk of invasive cancer is greater in smokers than in nonsmokers (Herrington, 1995; Yang, Jin, Nakao, Rahimtula, Pater, & Pater, 1996). However, smoking has also been shown to constitute a significant risk for cervical cancer in HPV-negative women (Kjaer et al., 1996).

Oral Contraceptives

The association between oral contraceptives and the risk for cervical cancer remains highly controversial. Most epidemiological studies have found a correlation between the risk of cervical cancer and oral contraceptives. However, other studies have not demonstrated an association. Long-term use of oral contraceptives (greater than 8 years) poses the highest risk, especially for the development of adenocarcinoma of the cervix. This finding suggests a hormonal link in the development of adenocarcinoma (Brinton, 1991; Kjaer & Brinton, 1993). A recent meta-analysis acknowledges an increased risk for the development of cervical cancer in women who have taken oral contraceptives for 8 years or more (Schlesselman, 1995). Another recent study revealed that the relative risk of cervical carcinoma in situ was estimated to be 1.3 in women who used oral contraceptives, compared with the lifetime risk of 0.9% in the general population. The greatest risk in this population was the use of oral contraceptives for greater than 60 months (Ye, Thomas, & Ray, 1995). Oral contraceptive use constitutes a significant risk factor in HPV-negative women (Kjaer et al., 1996).

Nutritional Deficiencies

The role of nutrition in the development of cervical cancer stems from the nutritional deficiencies observed among case patients in international epidemiological studies. The nutrients that spark the most interest include the retinoids, the micronutrients, and vitamin deficiencies.

Retinoids may play a role in epithelial cell development. Retinoic acid has been shown to reverse some preneoplastic

1. What is your age?

2. What is your marital status?

3. What is your race?
   __ White
   __ African American
   __ Hispanic
   __ Native American
   __ Other

4. What is your educational background?
   __ Less than high school
   __ High school
   __ Post high school

5. What is your current income?
   __ Less than $15,000
   __ $15,000-$30,000
   __ $30,000-$45,000
   __ More than $45,000
   __ Refused

6. Have you ever smoked?
   __ No
   __ Yes __ Pack years

7. Have you ever had condyloma (genital warts)?
   __ Yes
   __ No

8. Have you ever had gonorrhea?
   __ Yes
   __ No

9. How many sexual partners have you had in your lifetime?
   __ None
   __ 1
   __ 2-4
   __ 5-14
   __ 15+

10. How many sexual partners have you had in the past year?
    __ None
    __ 1
    __ 2-4
    __ 5-14
    __ 15+

11. How old were you when you first had intercourse?
    __ 15 or younger
    __ 16-19
    __ 20 or older

12. Have you ever used oral contraceptives (birth control pills)?
    __ Never
    __ Yes __ Years Total Use

Fig. 29-2 Risk assessment questionnaire for the development of cervical cancer. (Courtesy of Joyce Lavery, MFA, CMI, 1994, Reistertown, MD.)

cervical lesions and has been shown in vitro to reverse CIN III formation from HPV 16-immortalized endocervical cells. Beta-carotene deficiency has been correlated with CIN and cervical cancer. Beta-carotene is the most active and common carotenoid found in the diet (Sarma et al., 1996; Shindoh, Sun, Pater, & Pater, 1995). Folate deficiency has also been demonstrated in patients with CIN when compared with controls. Folic acid is involved in DNA synthesis, as well as cellular growth and proliferation. Erythrocytic folate levels below 660 nmol/L have been shown to enhance patient's susceptibility to HPV, which may predispose an individual to develop cervical carcinoma (Mitchell et al., 1995). Lower vitamin E and carotenoid levels are correlated with higher-grade cervical lesions (Potischman, 1993). However, higher levels of vitamin C have also been associated with a reduced risk for cervical cancer. Further epidemiological studies and chemoprevention studies are needed to determine whether strong correlations exist between various nutritional factors and the development of cervical cancer.

Immunosuppression

Immunosuppression is another risk factor associated with dysplasia of the uterine cervix, but it has not been shown to increase the incidence of cervical cancer. Patients with immunosuppressive disorders such as lupus, Hodgkin's and non-Hodgkin's lymphoma, sarcoidosis, and renal transplantation demonstrate increased rates in CIN (Mitchell, Sandella, & White, 1992). In addition, women with HIV are 7 to 10 times more likely to develop SIL than women of the general population (Lovejoy & Anastasi, 1994). HIV is also associated with enhanced replication of HPV, which may enhance cervical dysplasia and cervical cancer (Rabkin et al., 1993). Immunosuppressed patients are generally under close surveillance, and cases of CIN and SIL may be treated before invasive cervical cancer develops.

CHEMOPREVENTION

Chemoprevention is the use of chemical agents to delay or prevent the development of cancer in healthy populations. It may require 20 to 40 years for cancer to develop in humans. Chemoprevention encompasses populations of healthy individuals at normal risk for developing cancer, as well as those at intermediate and high risk for the development of cancer (Kelloff et al., 1996). The four factors pertinent to the development of chemoprevention trials include the following:

1. High-risk cohorts must be identified.
2. Suitable chemical agents must be identified.
3. Studies should include Phase I, II, and III designs.
4. Biomarkers must be used and identified to measure differences in high-risk and normal tissue.

Fig. 29-2 is an assessment tool for screening individuals at high risk for cervical cancer. The uterine cervix is well-suited for the development of chemoprevention trials. Clinicians can easily observe the organ over time, through the use of Pap smears and colposcopy. One can also observe the progression of dysplastic lesions to potentially invasive cancers. A summary of the numerous cervical cancer chemoprevention trials is presented below (Mitchell et al., 1995).

Retinoids

Retinoids are naturally occurring substances in the body. They include vitamin A and its natural and synthetic analogues. Retinoids have been shown to decrease the expression of HPV messenger ribonucleic acid (mRNA) and to increase the secretion of transforming growth factor-beta, the growth factor responsible for the promotion of HPV. Phase I, II, and III clinical trials are under way to investigate the use of topically applied retinoids to the uterine cervix in patients with CIN I-II. In one trial, retinyl acetate gel was applied to the cervix on 7 consecutive days for three sequential menstrual cycles. A 9-mg dose was established for the Phase III clinical trial currently in progress. A second trial involved the use of all-trans-retinoic acid delivered to the cervix with a cervical sponge and cap. The treatment duration was 4 days with a regression rate of 45% in patients receiving higher doses (Mitchell et al., 1995). The Phase III trial, with the 0.375% dose of topical all-trans-retinoic acid for patients with CIN II-III demonstrated a statistically significant regression in CIN II but not in CIN III (Meyskens et al., 1994).

An analog of vitamin A, N-4-hydroxyphenyl retinamide (4-HPR) is currently being investigated in a Phase II trial. The medication is given orally for 6 months to patients with CIN. Endpoint biomarkers include cell proliferation, regulation, and differentiation (Mitchell et al., 1995).

Micronutrients

Micronutrient studies involve the use of beta-carotene, vitamin C, and folate supplementation. These micronutrients have been observed as nutritional deficiencies in patients with CIN and cervical cancer. The micronutrients play a role in the normal growth, proliferation, and differentiation of cells.

A group of Phase II trials is currently under way to investigate supplementation with beta-carotene 30 mg/day in patients with CIN II-III. Approximately 200 patients are expected to participate in these trials (Current Clinical Trials Oncology, 1994; Southwest Oncology Group [SWOG], 1995). The combination of beta-carotene and vitamin C vs placebo is currently being investigated by SWOG in a Phase III trial (SWOG, 1995).

Folate supplementation is also being investigated in women with CIN and decreased erythrocytic folate levels. One Phase II trial compared folate 10 mg with vitamin C (placebo). Each drug was given for 90 days. Although patients treated with folate experienced a cytologic regression of their lesion(s), the difference was not statistically significant. Another trial compared folic acid 5 mg with placebo given over 6 months to women with cervical atypia and mild or moderate CIN. Although the folate levels increased considerably in treated patients, there were no significant differences in improvement in the treatment groups (Childers et al., 1995). Other trials using folate supplementation have yielded borderline statistical significance (Mitchell et al., 1995).

Folate supplementation for women taking oral contraceptives has also been investigated. One study showed that 10 mg of folic acid reversed megaloblastic features observed in Pap smears (Whitehead, Reyner, & Lindenbaum, 1973). Another study assessed folate concentrations in women who used oral contraceptives. The mean red blood cell folate concentration levels were lower in women taking oral contraceptives and even lower in women taking oral contraceptives with CIN. Women who received folic acid 10 mg orally for 3 months demonstrated improvement in CIN I-II (Butterworth et al., 1992).

Polyamine Amine Synthesis Inhibitors

Alpha-difluoromethylornithine (A-DFMO) is another agent under investigation for cervical cancer chemoprevention. DFMO is an agent that inhibits ornithine decarboxylase (ODC), a key enzyme of polyamine biosynthesis. Polyamines such as spermidine and spermine are found in seminal fluid and have been implicated as risk factors in the development of cervical cancer. These chemicals may be proto-oncogenes in cell growth and transformation. A-DFMO blocks endogenous ODC production in an attempt to inhibit cell transformation toward malignancy and to remove cells already transformed. Phase I and II trials are currently under way using oral A-DFMO at five-dose levels. Patients on the Phase I trial take A-DFMO for 1 month and are evaluated using a loop electrosurgical excision at the conclusion of the study. Patients enrolled on the Phase II trial take the dose determined in the Phase I trial for a 6-month period (Mitchell et al., 1995).

Chemoprevention studies present unique opportunities for the prevention and delay of cervical carcinoma. Further studies will clarify the usefulness of these agents.

PATHOPHYSIOLOGY

Normal Anatomy and Physiology of the Cervix

The cervix is an area of dense, connective tissue on the lower part of the uterus that extends from the isthmus into the vagina. The opening in the center of the cervix is called the *endocervical canal,* or the *endocervix.* The upper part of the opening is called the *internal os,* and the lower opening that opens into the vagina is called the *external os,* or *exocervix.* The endocervical canal is lined with columnar epithelial cells, whereas the exocervix is covered with squamous epithelial cells. The point where the columnar and squamous epithelial cells meet is called the *squamocolumnar junction* (Fig. 29-3).

The squamocolumnar junction is a dynamic area that changes in conjunction with a woman's fluctuating hormone levels. The junction is most exophytic (i.e., advances well out onto the exocervix) during neonatal life, menarche, and during the first pregnancy (Fig. 29-4). When the cervix is

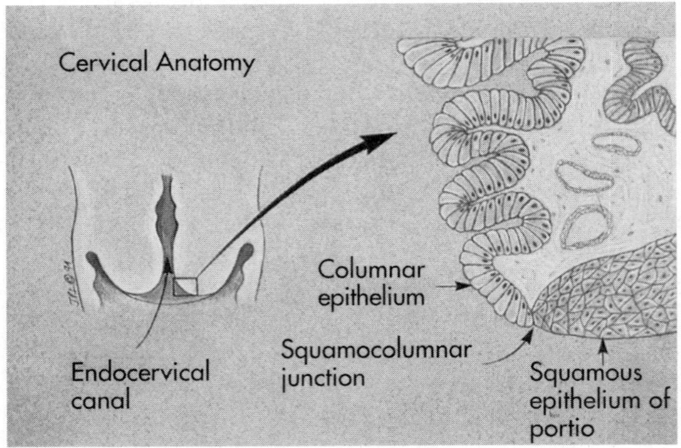

Fig. 29-3 Cervical anatomy. (Courtesy Joyce Lavery, MFA, CMI, 1994.)

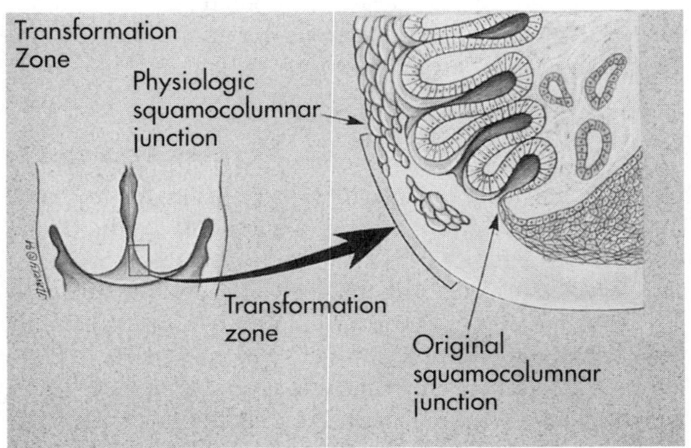

Fig. 29-5 The transformation zone of the cervix. (Courtesy Joyce Lavery, MFA, CMI, 1994, Reistertown, MD.)

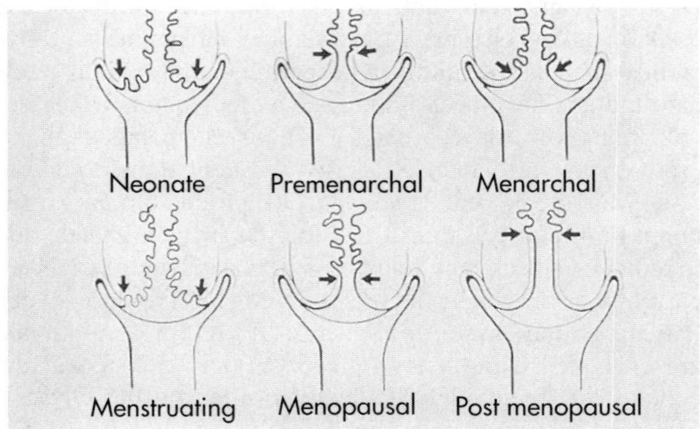

Fig. 29-4 Changes in the sqamocolumnar junction. (From Burke, L. [1991]. *Colposcopy text and atlas.* Norwalk, CT: Appleton & Lange.)

exophytic the columnar cells are exposed to the acidic pH of the vagina and are covered by squamous epithelium. This area of squamous metaplasia between the columnar and squamous epithelial cells of the endocervix and exocervix is called the *transformation zone.* It lies between the new original squamocolumnar junction and the physiologic squamocolumnar junction (Fig. 29-5) (American Medical Women's Association [AMWA], 1994). The zone is more susceptible to carcinogenic influences during exophytic phases. A larger transformation zone associated with biologic immaturity is also more susceptible to carcinogens (Lovejoy & Anastasi, 1994).

Normally, as the epithelial cells in the cervix mature, the keratinocytes flatten out and contain smaller nuclear-to-cytoplasmic ratios. These cells are ultimately sloughed off the surface and are replaced by the basal level of cells below the surface (Palefsky & Holly, 1995).

The cervical region contains several lymphatic chains that drain the area. The regional lymph nodes include the paracervical, parametrial, hypogastric, internal iliac, external iliac, common iliac, and presacral (Fig. 29-6). The major vascular network supplying blood to the cervix is the venous plexus and paracervical veins. These lymphatic and vascular networks play a major role in the metastatic spread of the disease (Perez, 1993a).

The Process of Carcinogenesis

The process of carcinogenesis in the cervix begins with cellular insult to the keratinocytes of the cervix and eventual DNA changes within the transformation zone. The carcinogenic insults are most likely multifactorial. However, HPV is presumed to play a major role in carcinogenesis.

The Role of HPV in Cervical Carcinogenesis. HPV infection occurs in the basal cell layer of the cervix that consists of the dividing level of the epithelium. Therefore the basal cells constitute a reservoir of HPV DNA, and the virus replicates in all daughter cells. HPVs, specifically types 16 and 18, may be responsible in part for the DNA transformation of the epithelial cells. The HPV contains two proteins, E6 and E7, that bind to and inhibit two key antioncogenes, p53 and the retinoblastoma protein. Only HPV 16 and 18 appear to have the binding affinity for these key antioncogenes. These proteins are necessary for full transformation of primary human keratinocytes. HPV may affect the keratinocyte in two ways: koilocytosis or dysplasia. Koilocytosis is presumed to be the direct effect of HPV and is characterized by irregular or enlarged nuclei. Dysplasia, however, is characterized by an increased nuclear-to-cytoplasmic ratio, an irregular-shaped nucleus, and chromatin abnormalities. The transformation period to cervical cancer is slow, estimated at 10 to 50 years (Birley, 1995; Cox, 1995; Fujii et al., 1995).

The Development of CIN. *CIN* is a term used to define epithelial cervical abnormalities. The classification system demonstrates the progression of the disease. CIN grade I is characterized by 20% to 25% replacement of the normal epithelium by immature cells with high cytoplasmic ratios. CIN grade II constitutes 50% replacement by immature cells, and CIN grade III reveals almost complete replacement by immature cells (Fig. 29-7). *Condyloma* is another

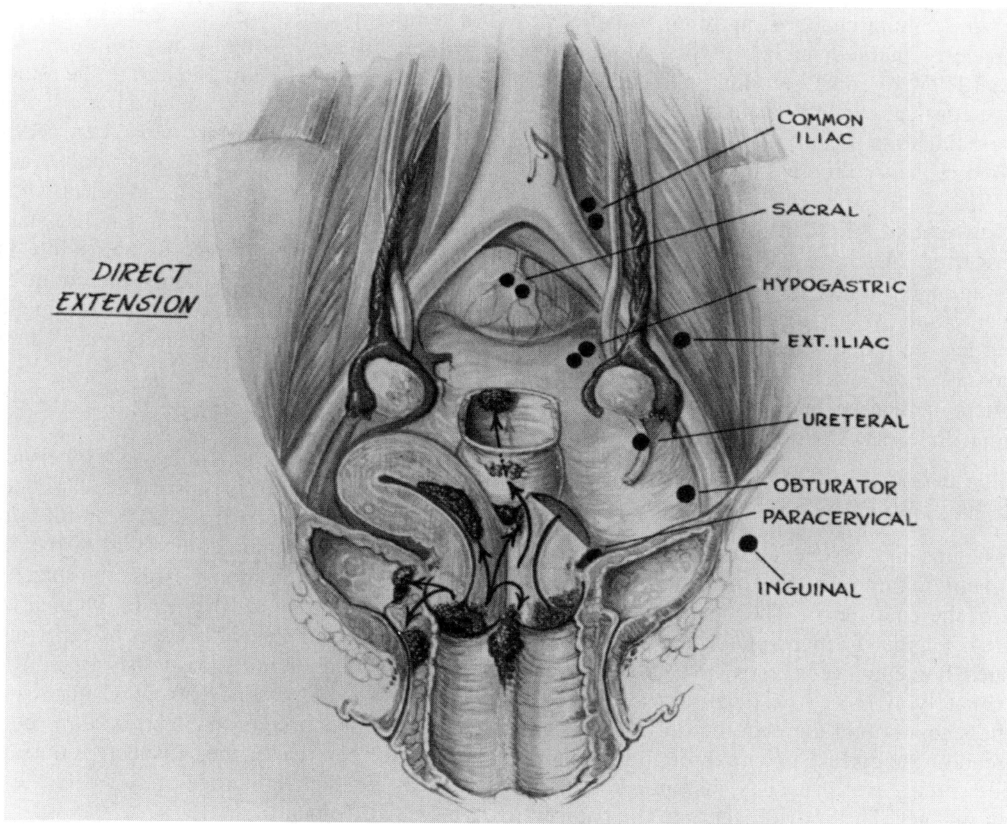

Fig. 29-6 Cervical regional lymph nodes. (From DiSaia, P.J. [1994]. Disorders of the uterine cervix. In J.R. Scott, P.J. DiSaia, C.B. Hammond, & W.N. Spellacy [Eds.], *Danforth's obstetrics and gynecology* [7th ed.]. Philadelphia: J.B. Lippincott.)

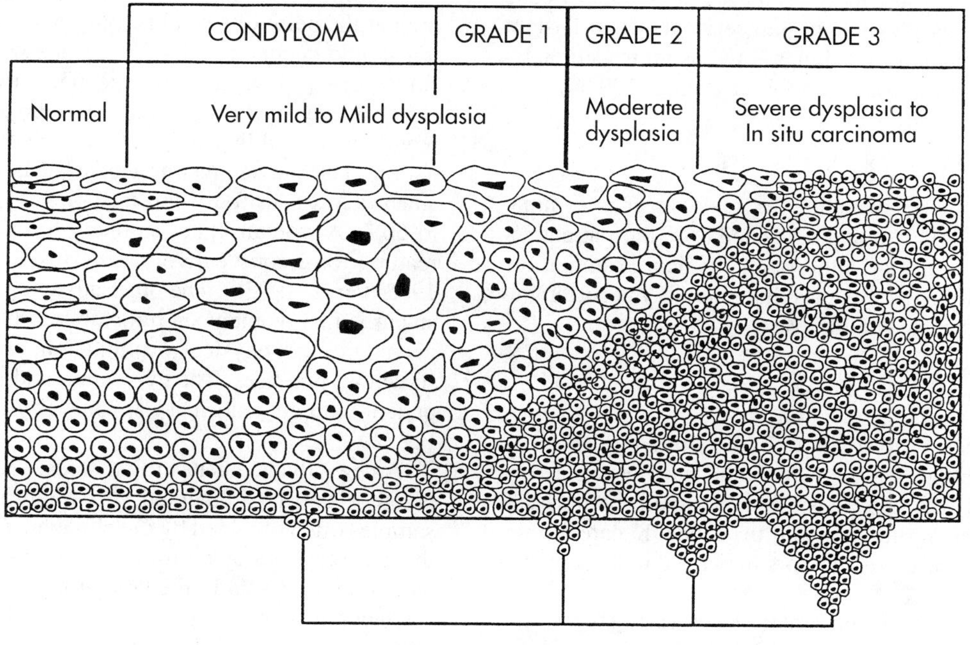

Fig. 29-7 The process of carcinoma intraepithelial neoplasia. (From Palefsky, J.M., & Holly, E.A. [1995]. Molecular virology and epidemiology of human papillomavirus and cervical cancer. *Cancer Epidemiology, Biomarkers, & Prevention, 4,* 415-428.)

term associated with cellular changes and refers to koilocytosis in the absence of marked nuclear atypia. Stong evidence suggest that HPV 16 and 18 are linked to high-grade CIN and invasive cervical cancer, whereas low-grade CIN and condyloma are linked to other types of HPV. Low-grade lesions are also more likely to regress (Cox, 1995; Palefsky & Holly, 1995).

The Development of Microinvasive and Invasive Cervical Carcinoma. Microinvasive cervical carcinoma occurs when the immature cells traverse or break through the basement membrane. Microinvasion occurs commonly with CIN III and less commonly with lower-grade lesions. Invasive carcinoma occurs when epithelial cells have traversed the basement membrane, and progress and invade the underlying stroma (Palefsky & Holly, 1995).

ROUTES OF METASTASIS

Cervical cancer begins as a superficial ulceration, or it may present as an exophytic tumor in the exocervix or as extensive infiltration of the endocervix. The cancer then spreads locally to adjacent vaginal fornices or to paracervical and parametrial tissues. It eventually invades the bladder and the rectum. Approximately 10% to 30% of all cases extend to the lower uterine segment and the endometrial cavity.

Regional spread of the disease occurs through lymphatic or hematogenous spread, and it usually disseminates in an orderly, adjacent manner. The spread occurs to the paracervical and parametrial lymphatics, a medial group of the external iliac nodes (obturator lymph nodes), other external iliac nodes, the hypogastric lymph nodes, and the common iliac or periaortic lymph nodes (see Fig. 29-6). Hematogenous spread occurs less often but is more common in advanced stages. This route involves the spread of cancer cells through the venous plexus and paracervical veins. Distant metastatic sites include the lungs, mediastinum, supraclavicular lymph nodes, bones, and liver (Perez, 1993a).

ASSESSMENT

The assessment of a patient for cervical cancer is summarized in Table 29-1. Clinical assessment of the patient includes a complete history, a thorough physical examination, and a number of diagnostic tests that may vary according to the suspected stage of the disease.

History

Whether a woman visits a clinic for a routine Pap smear or for another problem, the woman should have cervical cancer screening at that time. Risk factors should be assessed during a woman's routine visit to a health care clinic. Women with increased risk factors may need to be screened more often.

Cervical cancer is asymptomatic in its early stages, and most women do not have any complaints. Women with early invasive cancer may report vaginal discharge or vaginal bleeding, especially postcoitus. As the tumor progresses, vaginal bleeding becomes more extensive and persistent, and women may complain of continuous menstrual flow. Pain is a symptom of advanced cervical cancer. Chronic pelvic pain with a dull, aching quality may be associated with tumor invasion, necrosis, or inflammation. The tumor may also compress the lumbosacral spine and nerves, contributing to low back and leg pain. More advanced cervical cancer may cause genitourinary (GU) obstruction, as well as disturbances such as urinary frequency or urgency and hematuria. Gastrointestinal (GI) complaints in late stages include rectal tenesmus and rectal bleeding (Hoskins, Perez, & Young, 1993). The triad of symptoms, including back pain, edema of the lower extremities, and a nonfunctioning kidney, is evidence of an advanced carcinoma (Wharton, 1996).

Physical Examination

A general physical examination for cervical cancer begins with assessment of the supraclavicular nodes, abdominal assessment, and liver palpation. A careful bimanual pelvic examination is the main component of the physical examination. The clinician should assess the shape, consistency, and degree of mobility of the cervix. Vaginal or parametrial extension may be present in cases of cervical cancer (AMWA, 1994). The clinician should also assess for any pelvic tenderness or the presence of pelvic masses or abnormalities. Visual inspection of the cervix may be benign in early stages of cervical cancer. Inspection during late stages may reveal cervical inflammation, a visible lesion, or gross tumor involvement.

Diagnostic Tests

Papanicolaou Smear. The Pap smear is the most standard of all diagnostic tests. The American Cancer Society recommends that women undergo a Pap smear beginning at the point of sexual activity or at age 20. The screening should occur annually for 2 years with at least one Pap smear every 3 years until age 65. However, the American College of Obstetricians and Gynecologists recommends an annual Pap smear at the time of the annual examination. The annual recommendation is related to the Pap smear's low sensitivity and false-negative variability of 8% to 50%. A woman is not as likely to have a false-negative reading for 2 consecutive years (Hoskins, Perez, & Young, 1993; Perez, 1993a). The other advantage of the annual Pap smear is that women can remember to obtain an annual gynecologic and physical examination, which may increase screening practices. The evaluation and management of the patient with an abnormal Pap smear cytology is outlined in Fig. 29-8.

A new advancement in Pap smear technique, the monolayer or thin-layer method, may improve the insufficient samples often obtained by the clinician. Cells are taken from the cervix with a cytobrush and are rinsed in a preservative solution that is sent to the laboratory. A vacuum machine in the laboratory then deposits a uniform layer of cells on the slide to be stained and interpreted. The slide is much easier for the cytologist to read (AMWA, 1993) (Fig. 29-9). Unfortunately, the monolayer technique is much more expensive than the conventional Pap smear technique. The cytologist may potentially diagnose more CIN I Pap smears

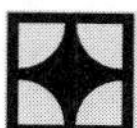

TABLE 29-1 Assessment of the Patient for Cervical Cancer

	Assessment Parameters	Typical Abnormal Findings
History	A. Personal and social history	A. Personal and social risk factors
	1. Sexual activity	1. Early sexarchy less than 18 years of age. Multiple sexual partners.
	2. Tobacco use	2. Increased risk in individuals who smoke.
	3. Immunosuppression	3. History of human immunodeficiency virus (HIV) infection, renal transplant, or other immunosuppressive disorder.
	B. Evaluation of the genitourinary system	B. Common symptoms include vaginal discharge or bleeding, vaginal spotting postcoitus. Advanced disease symptoms include urinary frequency or urgency, hematuria, and ureteral obstruction.
	C. Evaluation of the gastrointestinal (GI) system	C. Symptoms most likely to occur with advanced disease include rectal tenesmus, rectal bleeding, and obstruction.
	D. Evaluation for pain	D. Patients with metastatic disease may complain of lumbosacral back pain and unilateral or bilateral leg pain.
Physical Examination	A. Bimanual pelvic examination	A. The bimanual pelvic examination may be normal in patients with early stage disease. With advanced disease, the clinician may palpate a mass or lesion on the cervix or within the pelvis. The examination may also be uncomfortable for the patient.
	B. Weight	B. The patient may experience weight loss in advanced disease states.
	C. Lymph node evaluation	C. Patient may have palpable nodes in abdominal, femoral, or supraclavicular area.
Diagnostic Tests	A. Pap smear	A. May demonstrate abnormal cells within the cervix, including dysplasia and carcinoma. False-negative readings may be as high as 8%-50%.
	B. Colposcopy	B. Visually, the cervix may appear inflamed. Small lesions or gross tumor may be present.
	C. Cervical biopsy	C. Positive punch biopsies. If negative, cone biopsy may be necessary to demonstrate presence of cervical carcinoma.
	D. Endocervical and endometrial curettage	D. Endocervix and endometrium may contain malignant cells demonstrating upward extension of the carcinoma.
	E. Blood count and chemistries	E. Anemia present with heavy vaginal bleeding and metastatic disease. Increased blood urea nitrogen (BUN) and creatinine may indicate tumor involvement within the renal system. Increased liver enzymes are indicative of potential hepatic involvement of the tumor.
	F. Chest x-ray	F. Positive in patients with lung metastasis.
	G. Intravenous (IV) pyelogram	G. Complete or partial obstruction present in patients with renal involvement.
	H. Computed tomography (CT) or magnetic resonance imaging (MRI) scan	H. Enlarged lymph nodes may be present. Useful in diagnosis, staging, and treatment plan for cervical carcinoma.
	I. Cystoscopy or rectosigmoidoscopy, barium enema	I. Performed in patients with IIB, III, and IVA cervical cancer. Obstruction or tumor infiltration may be present in patients with GI or genitourinary (GU) involvement.

compared with CIN III; however, the treatment is the same for both, and it is questionable as to whether there is a therapeutic benefit in terms of patient outcomes. The cost-benefit ratio must also be considered.

There are three nomenclatures used to describe Pap smears. The Papanicolaou system was the initial system used; however, laboratories often interpret this system differently. The World Health Organization (WHO) system was established in 1973 in an attempt to standardize Pap smear terminology. The WHO system describes the degree of abnormal cells. The Bethesda system was developed in 1988 by a National Institutes of Health (NIH) consensus panel. In addition to providing a descriptive diagnosis, the Bethesda System estimates the adequacy of the smear and the characterization of the smear as normal or abnormal. The three systems are compared in Table 29-2.

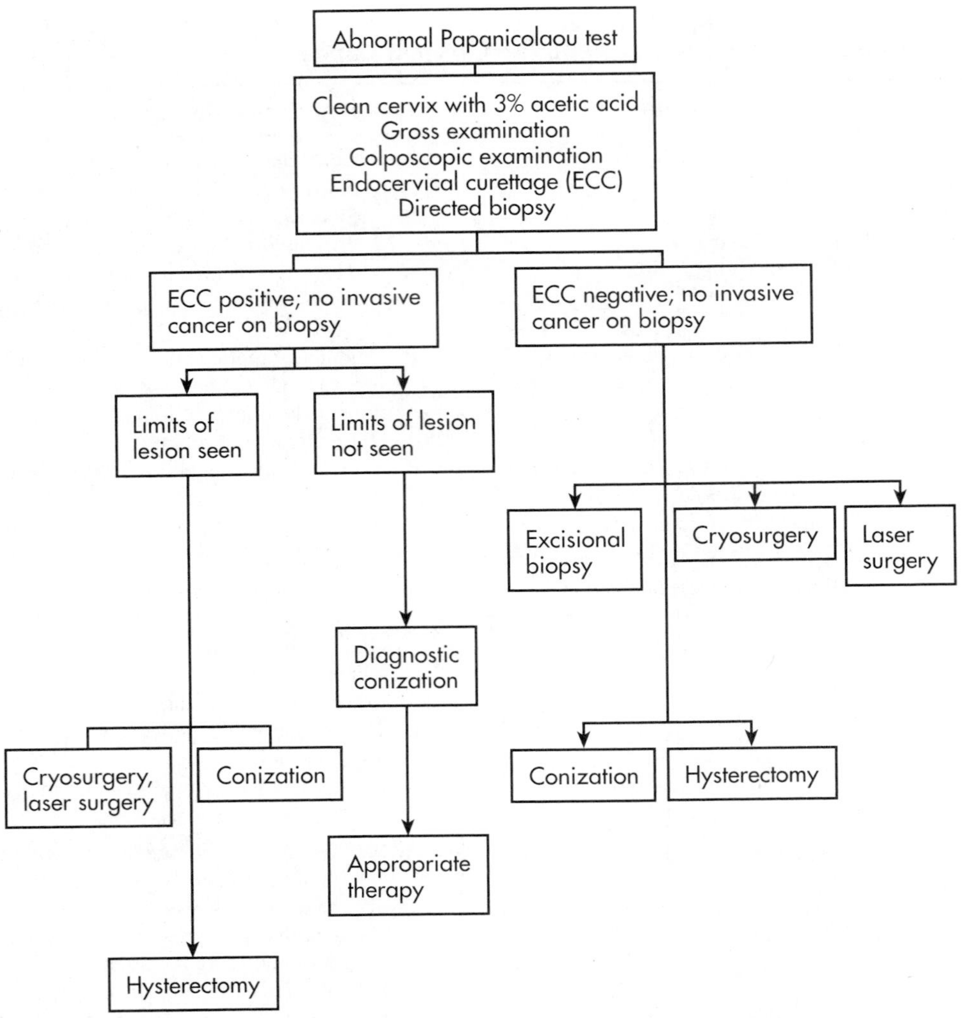

Fig. 29-8 Abormal pap smear: evaluation and management. (From DiSaia, P.J. [1994]. In J.R. Scott, P.J. DiSaia, C.B. Hammond, & W.N. Spellacy [Eds.], *Danforth's obstetrics and gynecology* [7th ed.]. Philadelphia: J.B. Lippincott.)

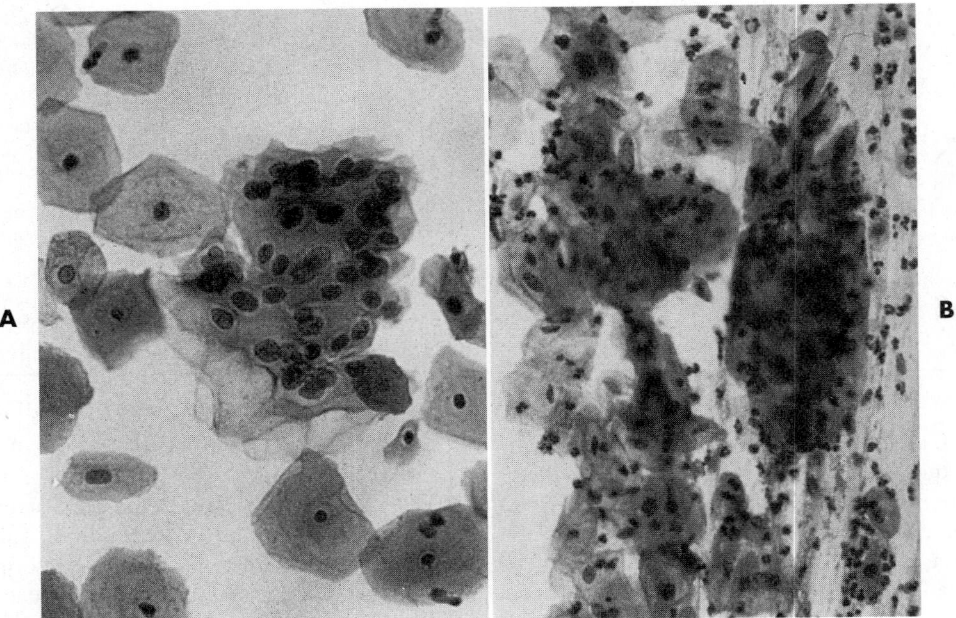

Fig. 29-9 **A,** Conventional Pap smear. **B,** Thin-layer preparation technique. (Courtesy Cytec Corporation.)

TABLE 29-2 Nomenclature in Cervical Cytology

Pap Smear	World Health Organization (WHO) System	Bethesda System
Class I	Normal	Within normal limits
Class II	Atypical	Reactive or reparative change
Class III	Dysplasia	Squamous epithelial cell abnormality; atypical squamous cells of undetermined significance; squamous intraepithelial lesion
	Mild dysplasia	Low grade (includes human papillomavirus [HPV])
	Moderate dysplasia	High grade
	Severe dysplasia	High grade
Class IV	Carcinoma in situ	High grade
Class V	Invasive squamous cell carcinoma	Squamous cell carcinoma
	Adenocarcinoma	Glandular cell abnormalities: adenocarcinoma or nonepithelial malignant neoplasm

From Wright, T. C., Richart, R. M. (1992). Preinvasive lesion of the lower genital tract. In W. J. Hoskins, C. A. Perez, R. C. Young (Eds.), *Principles and practice of gynecologic oncology*. Philadelphia: J. B. Lippincott.

Colposcopy. A colposcopy allows for enhanced visual inspection of the cervix when the Pap smear is abnormal. A bright light with a green filter and a 10-to-15 power magnification enhances the vascular patterns of the cervix and allows the clinician to identify suspicious areas for biopsy (Hoskins, Perez, & Young, 1993).

Biopsies. Visible gross tumors should be biopsied with a punch biopsy technique in all four quadrants of the cervix and from suspicious areas in the vagina. The clinician may also need to biopsy an inflammatory cervix that is suspicious. A cone biopsy is performed when a cervical punch biopsy fails to make the diagnosis of invasive cancer (Hoskins, Perez, & Young, 1993; Perez, 1993a).

Endocervical and Endometrial Curettage. An endocervical and endometrial curettage is recommended during the initial patient evaluation to assess for upper extension of the tumor. Upward extension of the tumor may modify the treatment plan (Perez, 1993a).

Blood Profile. A complete blood count (CBC) with hemoglobin and hematocrit indicates related blood loss and anemia from vaginal bleeding or invasive carcinoma. A biochemical evaluation includes renal and liver function tests that may be abnormal in late stages of the disease.

X-Rays. A chest x-ray is performed on all patients diagnosed with cervical carcinoma to rule out lung metastasis and to assess the lymph nodes located in the chest area. An intravenous pyelogram (IVP) to visualize potential renal involvement should also be obtained in all patients with a positive diagnosis (Perez, 1993a).

Lymphangiogram. Lymphangiograms may be useful if the evaluation is clearly positive. Unfortunately, false-negative rates may be as high as 20%. This diagnostic test is often replaced by more sophisticated examinations such as the computerized tomography (CT) scan.

Computerized Tomography With Contrast or Magnetic Resonance Imaging. The CT scan is being used extensively in the diagnosis of cervical cancer and may replace some of the other diagnostic tests such as the IVP and lymphangiogram. Although periaortic lymph nodes are easily detected on CT scan, histologically positive pelvic nodes may often be missed (Hoskins, Perez, & Young, 1993). There is increased interest in the use of magnetic resonance imaging (MRI). According to one study, MRI offered significant improvement in evaluation of the cervical cancer. One disadvantage of the MRI is the overestimation of the tumor size and the inability to differentiate between tissue edema and tumor invasion. In addition, lesions less than 1 cm cannot be differentiated from postbiopsy changes (Subak, Hricak, Powell, Azizi, & Stern, 1995). A comparison of the CT scan and MRI is found in Table 29-3.

Cystoscopy or Rectosigmoidoscopy. A cystoscopy or rectosigmoidoscopy should be performed on all patients with a complaint of urinary or lower GI tract disturbances. It is also routinely performed on patients with stages IIB, III, and IVA disease to assess potential GU or GI involvement of the tumor. A barium enema is also performed in this subgroup of patients (Perez, 1993a).

STAGING

The staging and classification of cervical cancer is based on the histopathological type of the tumor and clinical evaluation. The clinical staging of the tumor involves the use of two clinical staging systems (i.e., the 1992 TNM classification system or the Federation Internationale de Gynecologie et d'Obstetrique [FIGO] system). Examination of *t*umor extension, lymph *n*ode involvement, and the involvement of distant organs, or *m*etastases, is necessary for complete staging of cervical cancer. The staging is dependent on the results of the diagnostic tests and often times, the results of surgery—most generally a radical hysterectomy.

Laparoscopy is being investigated as a less invasive tool for staging ovarian cancer. A laparoscopy can be done to sample iliac and periaortic nodes and to obtain intraperitoneal washings. If the node status of the patient is clearly positive, the patient can be spared a radical hysterectomy. Laparoscopy has also been used successfully to stage patients with advanced disease before definitive radiation therapy (Childers & Surwit, 1993).

TABLE 29-3 Comparison of MRI and CT in the Diagnosis and Staging of Cervical Cancer

Diagnostic Criteria	MRI	CT
Tumor size	Within 5 cm of surgical sample (93% accuracy)	Could not be evaluated
Stromal invasion	88% accuracy	Could not be evaluated
Depth of invasion	78% accuracy	Only able to distinguish cancer from surrounding normal cervical tissue
Stage of disease	90% accuracy	65% accuracy
Parametrial invasion	94% accuracy	76% accuracy
Lymph node metastasis	86% accuracy	86% accuracy
Determining operative candidates (Stage I, minimal Stage IIA)	94% accuracy	76% accuracy

MRI, magnetic resonance imaging; *CT,* computed tomography.

Box 29-2
Histopathologic Types of Cervical Cancer

High grade squamous intraepithelial lesion
- Moderate dysplasia
- Severe dysplasia
- Cervical intraepithelial neoplasia grade III
- Squamous cell carcinoma in situ

Squamous cell carcinoma
- Keratinizing
- Nonkeratinizing
- Verrucous

Adenocarcinoma in situ
Adenocarcinoma, endocervical type
Endometrioid adenocarcinoma
Clear cell adenocarcinoma
Adenosquamous carcinoma
Adenoid cystic carcinoma
Small cell carcinoma
Undifferentiated carcinoma

Histologic Staging

Histologic staging of cervical cancer refers to the examination of the biopsy specimen(s) by a pathologist after punch biopsy, conization, or surgery. The histopathology of the tumor considers the tumor cell type and the grade of the tumor. SCC is the most common type of cervical cancer. However, the incidence of adenocarcinoma is increasing (Kjaer & Brinton, 1993). The various histopathologic types of cervical cancer are listed in Box 29-2. The histopathologic grade of the tumor cells is also part of the histological staging system. The *grade* refers to the maturity level (i.e., differentiation) of the tumor cells. The grade ranges from GX, when the grade cannot be assessed, to G1 (well-differentiated) and G4 (undifferentiated).

Clinical Staging

Two classification systems have been used for the clinical staging of cervical cancer: the 1992 TNM system and the FIGO system. The TNM staging system was developed by the American Joint Committee on Cancer (AJCC) and the International Union Against Cancer (UICC). The FIGO system was developed by the Federation Internationale de Gynecologie et d'Obstetrique (Beahrs, Henson, Hutter, & Kennedy, 1992). Both systems are commonly used in hospitals throughout the United States (Table 29-4). When there is a disagreement in the stage of the cancer, the earlier stage should be selected for statistical purposes (Perez, 1993a).

MEDICAL MANAGEMENT

The treatment of cervical cancer is most dependent on the stage of disease at the time of diagnosis. Table 29-5 provides a summary of the medical management options for cervical cancer, dependent on the stage of the disease. Other factors taken into consideration in determining the treatment plan are the patient's overall health status and age, the risk factors of the patient, the patient's desire to have children, the size of the tumor; and the histopathology of the tumor. When cervical cancer is diagnosed during pregnancy, the treatment can often be delayed depending on the stage of the cancer. The treatment of choice for early stage disease is surgery and/or radiation therapy. Patients with more advanced disease are generally treated with radiation therapy alone or in combination with chemotherapy. Controversies exist about the management of cervical cancer. Current clinical trials focus on developing conservative management strategies that achieve optimal quality-of-life outcomes and increased survival.

Surgical Management

Surgical treatment plays a vital role in the management of cervical cancer and other cervical abnormalities. Numerous surgical techniques are used at various stages of the disease, including cervical conization, laser therapy, hysterectomy, lymphadenectomy, and pelvic exenteration. Therapeutic laparoscopic surgery is also being investigated as a conservative surgical technique for a subset of this patient population (Hoskins, Perez, & Young, 1993).

TABLE 29-4 Classification Systems for Clinical Staging of Cervical Cancer

TNM and FIGO Systems

TNM* Category	FIGO† Stage	Definition
Tumor (T)		
pTX		Primary tumor cannot be assessed
pT0		No evidence of primary tumor
pTis		Carcinoma in situ
PT1	I	Cervical carcinoma confined to uterus (extension to corpus should be disregarded)
pT1a	IA	Preclinical invasive carcinoma, diagnosed by microscopy only
pT1a1	IA1	Minimal microscopic stromal invasion
pT1a2	IA2	Tumor with invasive component 5 mm or less in depth taken from the base of the epithelium, and 7 mm or less in horizontal spread
pT1b	IB	Tumor larger than T1a2
pT2	II	Cervical carcinoma invades beyond uterus, but not to pelvic wall or lower third of vagina
pT2a	IIA	Tumor without parametrial invasion
pT2b	IIB	Tumor with parametrial invasion
pT3	III	Cervical carcinoma extends to pelvic wall and/or involves lower third of vagina and/or causes hydronephrosis or nonfunctioning kidney
pT3a	IIIA	Tumor involves lower third of vagina, no extension to pelvic wall
pT3b	IIIB	Tumor extends to pelvic wall and/or causes hydronephrosis or nonfunctioning kidney
pT4	IVA	Tumor invades mucosa of bladder or rectum and/or extends beyond the pelvis
pM1	IVB	Distant metastasis
Lymph Nodes (N)		
NX		Regional lymph nodes cannot be assessed
N0		No regional lymph node metastasis
N1		Regional lymph node metastasis
Distant Metastasis (M)		
MX		Presence of distant metastasis cannot be assessed
M0		No distant metastasis
M1 IVb		Distant metastasis

AJCC/UICC/FIGO Staging System for Cervical Cancer

AJCC/UICC‡				FIGO
Stage 0	Tis	N0	M0	
Stage I	Ti	N0	M0	
Stage IA	T1a	N0	M0	IA
Stage IA1	T1a1	N0	M0	
Stage IA2	T1a2	N0	M0	
Stage IB	T1b	N0	M0	IB
Stage II	T2	N0	M0	
Stage IIA	T2a	N0	M0	IIA
Stage IIB	T2b	N0	M0	IIB
Stage IIIA	T3a	N0	M0	IIIA
Stage IIIB	T1	N1	M0	IIIB
	T2	N1	M0	
	T3a	N1	M0	
	T3b	Any N	M0	
Stage IVA	T4	Any N	M0	IVA
Stage IVB	Any T	Any N	M1	IVB

*Tumor, node, metastases
†Federation Internationale de Gynecologie et d'Obstetrique
‡American Joint Committee on Cancer/International Union Against Cancer

TABLE 29-5 Medical Management of Cervical Cancer Based on the Stage of the Disease

FIGO Stage	5-year Survival	Involvement	Therapeutic Options
Stage 0	100%	Carcinoma in situ	Conization Laser surgery Loop electrosurgical excision procedure (LEEP) Cryosurgery Hysterectomy
Stage I		Cervical carcinoma confined to uterus	
IA	100%	Preclinical invasive carcinoma	Total abdominal hysterectomy Conization Radical hysterectomy with lymphadenectomy for tumors deeper than 3 to 5 cm Intracavitary radiation therapy
IB	85%-90%	Tumor larger than 5 mm depth and 7 mm horizontal spread	Combined intracavitary and external beam radiation Radical hysterectomy and lymph node dissection with or without radiation therapy
Stage II		Cervical carcinoma invades beyond uterus, not to pelvic wall or lower third of vagina	
IIA	75%	Tumor without parametrial invasion	Combined intracavitary and external beam radiation Radical hysterectomy with lymphadenectomy followed by radiation therapy
IIB	60%-65%	Tumor with parametrial invasion	Combined intracavitary and external beam radiation Radiation therapy with or without chemotherapy
Stage III	25%-50%	Cervical carcinoma extends to pelvic wall and/or involves lower third of vagina and/or causes hydronephrosis or nonfunctioning kidney	Combined intracavitary and external beam radiation Intracavitary and external beam radiation combined with chemotherapy Lymphadenectomy followed by external beam radiation therapy
Stage IVA	10% or less for all stage IV	Tumor invades mucosa of bladder or rectum and/or extends beyond the true pelvis	Combined intracavitary and external beam radiation Pelvic exenteration External beam radiation plus chemotherapy Surgical staging plus external beam radiation therapy
IVB		Distant metastasis	Palliative external beam radiation Chemotherapy

Conization. Cervical conization is a surgical technique that removes a cone-shaped piece of tissue that includes most or all of the transformation zone. It may be used in both the diagnosis and treatment of microinvasive disease. Conization is the treatment of choice for patients with CIN-III. Patients may experience complications such as hemorrhage, cervical stenosis, and uterine perforation after the procedure (Hoskins, Perez, & Young, 1993).

Cryosurgery. Cryosurgery is used in the management of CIN. Cryotherapy causes local destruction of the abnormal cervical lesion(s) by the application of subfreezing temperatures to the tissue. The vagina is protected during the procedure. The patient may experience abdominal cramping and cervical scarring from the procedure (Mitchell, 1993).

Laser Therapy. Laser therapy is another treatment used in the management of CIN. A mixture of carbon dioxide, helium, and nitrogen forms an infrared laser beam that focuses on the abnormal lesion(s) of the cervix. High cure rates have been achieved with the use of laser therapy. Laser therapy also causes less cervical scarring than cryotherapy (Mitchell, 1993).

Loop Electrosurgical Excision Procedure. A loop electrosurgical excision procedure (LEEP) uses a thin wire loop with an electrical current to excise the abnormal cervical tissue. This procedure can be performed in the outpatient setting under local anesthesia. Like cervical conization, LEEP can be used in both the diagnosis and treatment of microinvasive cervical cancer. Complications of the procedure are intra- and postoperative bleeding with an incidence of about 7% (Ferenczy, Choukroun, & Arseneau, 1996). The procedure does not appear to have an adverse effect on subsequent pregnancies (Cruickshank, Flannelly, & Campbell, 1995). One problem with LEEP is overtreating the local area by removing excessive amounts of tissue. The depth of excision should be carefully controlled by colposcopy and loop electrodes of the appropriate size. Its use should be limited to cytologically and colposcopically unequivocal intraepithelial lesions. Additional reports are needed to define the role of LEEP in the management of cervical cancer (Ferenczy, Choukroun, & Arseneau, 1996).

Hysterectomy. Several hysterectomy techniques are employed to manage cervical cancer. The total abdominal hysterectomy that includes removal of the uterus and the cervix is indicated as the sole treatment for patient's with CIN-III and microinvasive cancer. A conservative hysterectomy may be adequate for patients with an early invasive cervical cancer when margins and depth of invasion are 3 mm or less, as established by conization (Jones, Mercer, Lewis, Rubin, & Hoskins, 1993). Hysterectomy may also be used after radiation therapy in early stage cervical cancer when there is endometrial involvement. The modified radical hysterectomy that removes a larger vaginal cuff and preserves the lateral attachments of the ureters is rarely used. However, some may recommend its use in microinvasive carcinoma of the cervix.

The radical hysterectomy, used for stages IB and IIA cervical carcinoma, includes complete dissection of the ureters from their tunnels and dissection of the bladder from the upper third of the vagina. This procedure allows complete removal of the parametrial, paracervical, and upper paravaginal tissues, the likely routes of cervical cancer metastasis. This surgery can also be combined with lymphadenectomy of the common and external iliac, hypogastric, obturator, presacral, and periaortic lymph nodes. A major complication of radical hysterectomy is blood loss, and patients often require transfusions postoperatively. Neurogenic bladder dysfunction is the most common complication with the incidence as high as 31.5%. Patients may require catheter drainage for up to 14 days postoperatively. Urinary tract fistulas can also occur, but the incidence is less than 2% (Hoskins, Perez, & Young, 1993).

Vaginal hysterectomy has also been used in the treatment of cervical carcinoma. One study demonstrated a 5-year survival of 81% in stage IB patients compared with 75% in patients treated with abdominal hysterectomy. Further studies are needed to determine and define the patient population most suited for a vaginal hysterectomy (Massi, Savino, & Susini, 1993).

Other potential complications of hysterectomy include thrombophlebitis, pulmonary embolism, lymphocysts, and intestinal obstruction (Nagell, DePriest, Higgins, & Powell, 1993). Psychosexual dysfunction is also a common problem. Both organic and psychogenic causes can be attributed to the problem. Diminished or disrupted sexual function occurs in 6% to 9% of patients after radical hysterectomy (Lamb, 1995).

Laparoscopy. Therapeutic laparoscopy is also being investigated in the treatment of cervical cancer. A pelvic lymphadenectomy is performed before radical hysterectomy to document nodal status. If negative, radical hysterectomy can be accomplished during the same intraoperative period. If the nodes are positive, the radical hysterectomy is aborted, and periaortic nodes are removed to define radiation fields. The use of therapeutic laparoscopy is also being explored in combination with radical vaginal hysterectomy for patients with small cervical lesions. The pelvic nodes are removed through laparoscopy followed by a vaginal hysterectomy, and the patient can be spared abdominal hysterectomy (Childers & Surwit, 1993).

Pelvic Exenteration. Pelvic exenteration is reserved for patients with advanced or recurrent disease. A total pelvic exenteration involves removal of the bladder, urethra, uterus, cervix, vagina, rectum, and lateral supporting tissues. The urinary tract is preserved in a posterior exenteration, and the rectum is preserved with an anterior exenteration (Hoskins, Perez, & Young, 1993). It is often difficult to determine if the tumor is resectable with current radiographic studies. The surgeon generally performs an exploratory laparotomy. However, aborted exenteration occurs in 28% to 56.5% of the cases. Laparoscopy is currently being explored to select patients for pelvic exenteration. This approach could prevent unnecessary laparotomies (Plante & Roy, 1995). The 5-year survival rate with pelvic exenteration ranges from 17% to 23%. Operative mortality is reported at approximately 9.8%. (Hoskins, Perez, & Young, 1993). Patients struggle with physical, psychosocial, and sexual morbidity after pelvic exenteration. Urinary and fecal diversions and loss of the vagina are common concerns. Vaginal reconstruction can be performed at the time of the surgery (Walczak & Klemm, 1993). The urologic complications resulting from the urinary conduit are higher in previously irradiated patients as a result of decreased pelvic vascularity and compromised healing (Magrina, 1993). Exenteration is used less often due to improved radiation therapy techniques.

Radiation Therapy

Intracavitary and external beam radiation therapy are both employed in the management of cervical carcinoma. The two types of radiotherapy can be used alone, in combination, or in conjunction with other treatment modalities. An example of the types and doses of radiotherapy in the treatment of different stages of cervical cancer is included in Table 29-6. Point A is the anatomical area that is 2 cm above and 2 cm lateral to the external os of the cervix (Perez, 1993a).

Patients who receive radiation therapy for cervical cancer may experience significant side effects, including GU, GI, and sexual dysfunction. Side effects are often dependent on the other types of treatment the patient has received and on the order of the treatment regimen. For example, patients who undergo radical hysterectomy for recurrence after pelvic irradiation experience an increased incidence of urologic complications. The urologic fistula rate is approximately 50%, and 45% of survivors have required urinary diversions and 23% have needed colostomies. This population is probably best managed with pelvic exenteration. Patients who

TABLE 29-6 Radiation Therapy as a Treatment Modality for Cervical Carcinoma

Carcinoma of the Uterine Cervix: Mallinckrodt Institute of Radiology Policies of Treatment with Irradiation

		External Irradiation (cGy)*		Brachytherapy		
Tumor Stage	**Tumor Extent**	**Whole Pelvis**	**Additional Parametrial Dose (Midline Shield)**	**Two Insertions (Milligram-Hours)†**	**Dose to Point A**	**Total Dose to Point A (cGy)**
IA		0	0	6500-8000	7000	6000-7000
IB (small)	Superficial ulceration; less than 2 cm in diameter or involving less than two quadrants	0	4500	8000	7000	7000
IB (2 to 4 cm)	Four quadrant involvement; no endocervical component or significant expansion	1000	4000	7000	6500-7000	7500-8000
IIA, IIB	Non-barrel shaped type	2000	3000	8000	7000	8500
IB-IIA (bulky),‡ IIB, IIIA	Barrel shaped cervix; parametrial extension	2000	3000	8000	7000	8500-9000
IIIB	Parametrial involvement	2000	4000	8000	7000	8500-9500
IIB, IIIB, IV	Poor pelvic anatomy; patients not readily treated with intracavitary insertions (barrel shaped cervix not regressing; inability to locate external os)	4000	2000	6500	6000	8500-9500

*180 cGy/d, five weekly fractions, using 15 MV or higher photon beams, two portals treated daily.
†60-80 cGy per hour at point A. In patients over age 65 or with history of previous pelvic inflammatory disease or pelvic surgery, reduce doses by 10%.
‡In stage IB and IIA, if complete regression is not obtained, do extrafascial conservative hysterectomy (reduce brachytherapy dose to 6,000 mgh).
Reprinted with permission from Perez, C. A. (1993a). Radiation therapy in the management of cancer of the cervix. *Oncology, 7*(2), 89-96.

receive radical hysterectomy plus pelvic irradiation experience a decrease in bladder compliance with greater problems occurring with higher doses of external beam radiotherapy. Urinary incontinence in this population has been reported at 63%, which is higher than radical hysterectomy alone (26%) or pelvic irradiation alone (23%). Patients receiving irradiation alone may report more problems with stress and urgency incontinence (Magrina, 1993). The risk of second malignancies is also prevalent among women treated with all modalities for cervical cancer (Werner-Wasik, Schmid, Bornstein, & Madoc-Jones, 1995). The balance of treatment that eradicates disease and yet preserves function is the most desirable modality.

External Beam Radiation Therapy. External beam irradiation is used in the management of patients with stage IB, IIA, IIB, III, or IVA disease. The goal is to treat the whole pelvis, which includes the parametria and the common iliac lymph nodes (Perez, 1993b). Patients treated with external beam radiotherapy may develop recurrence in the para-aortic nodes. Attempts have been made to extend the radiation field in tumors 4 cm or greater to reach para-aortic lymph nodes. The doses were 4000 to 5000 cGy. The 10-year survival rate in the pelvic-only arm was 44%, compared with 55% in the pelvic plus para-aortic irradiation arm. Unfortunately, disease-free survival was not different (Rotman et al., 1995). The volume of pelvis treated is dependent on the stage of disease. Patients with stage IB are treated with 15 cm x 15 cm portals, whereas patients with stage IIA, IIB, III, or IVA are treated with 18 cm x 15 cm portals. When there is vaginal involvement, the entire vagina is treated to the introitus. The spinal cord dose should be kept below 4500 cGy, and shields are typically used after 3800 to 4000 cGy have been delivered (Perez, 1993b).

A new technique combines external whole pelvic irradiation and an intravaginal cone boost of 2000 to 2600 cGy with an electron beam to the vaginal cuff. The goal of treatment is to decrease recurrence in the vaginal cuff area. The 5-year survival is reported at 89% for patients undergoing prophylactic treatment and 56% for patients undergoing treatment for recurrence. Complications may include vesicovaginal fistulas and rectal complications (Mitsuhashi et al., 1995).

Pelvic external beam irradiation can cause several adverse effects, including diarrhea, abdominal cramping, urinary changes, cystitis, rectal discomfort, bleeding bone marrow suppression, skin reactions, and fatigue (Dunne-Daly, 1994a). Pelvic irradiation can also cause vaginal thinning and narrowing, dryness, and stenosis that contribute to

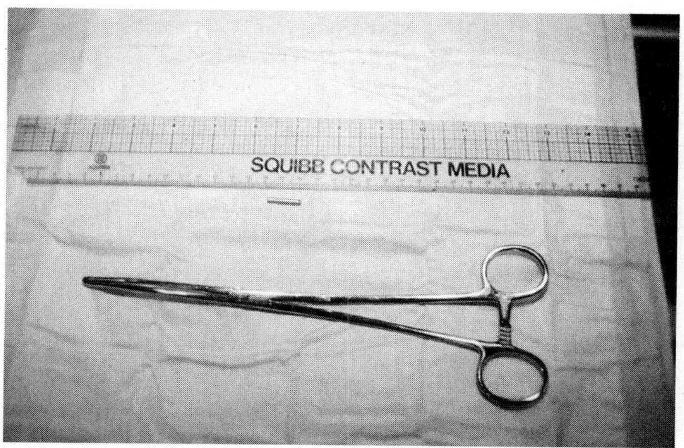

Fig. 29-10 Radioactive isotope for intracavitary irradiation.

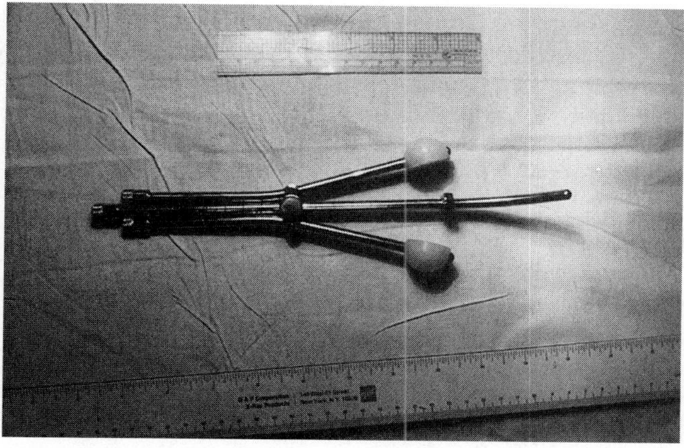

Fig. 29-11 Applicator for intracavitary irradiation for cervical cancer.

sexual dysfunction. The incidence is reported in up to 66% of patients (Cartwright-Alcarese, 1995; Lamb, 1995).

Intracavitary Radiation Therapy. Intracavitary radiation therapy involves implantation of a radioisotope into the cervical cavity. The most popular isotope is cesium (Cs); however, radium (Ra), cobalt (Co), and Iridium (Ir) have also been used. A picture of an isotope is found in Fig. 29-10. The isotopes are delivered using afterloading applicators that consist of an intrauterine tandem and vaginal colpostats. The tandem is the longest piece of the applicator, extending into the uterus. The two colpostats lie on each side of the tandem and lie within the vagina. Fig. 29-11 shows a picture of the applicator. The device is placed in the cervical and uterine area in the operating room or patient's room. The device is then "afterloaded" with the isotopes. The intrauterine tandem holds three to four isotopes within the uterus, and two colpostats are loaded with 20 mCiRa equivalent sources in the vaginal vault. The area is packed with iodoform gauze that is soaked in 40% iodinated contrast that can be identified on radiographic examination (Perez, 1993b). Fig. 29-12 depicts a radiographic picture of the intrauterine tandem and vaginal colpostats in place.

Afterloading reduces the radiation exposure to the health care workers. The afterloading technique can be manual or remote control. The remote control option further reduces the radiation exposure to the health care worker, lessens fear, improves control of isodose distributions, removes the possibility of misplacing or losing radiation sources, requires less source preparation for source curator, and allows for source loading, unloading, and automatic recording.

The adverse effects of intracavitary irradiation may be similar to those of external beam irradiation. An additional radiation effect is necrosis of the vaginal mucosa (Cartwright-Alcarese, 1995).

Combined External Beam and Intracavitary Radiation Therapy. External beam irradiation is used before intracavitary radiation with bulky cervical lesions, exophytic tumors, tumors with necrosis or infection, or when there is evidence of parametrial involvement. High-energy beams of 15 mV are used to help prevent damage to the surrounding peripheral tissues. Generally, the patient receives 1000 to 2000 cGy of external irradiation followed by an intracavitary dose. Approximately 1 to 2 weeks later, the patient receives 1000 to 2000 additional cGy of external irradiation followed by a second intracavitary dose (Perez, 1993b). The side effects from the combined irradiation techniques are minimal if the external beam dose is limited to 20 Gy, the dose at Point A to 70 Gy, and the dose to the bladder and rectum to 50 Gy (Magrina, 1993).

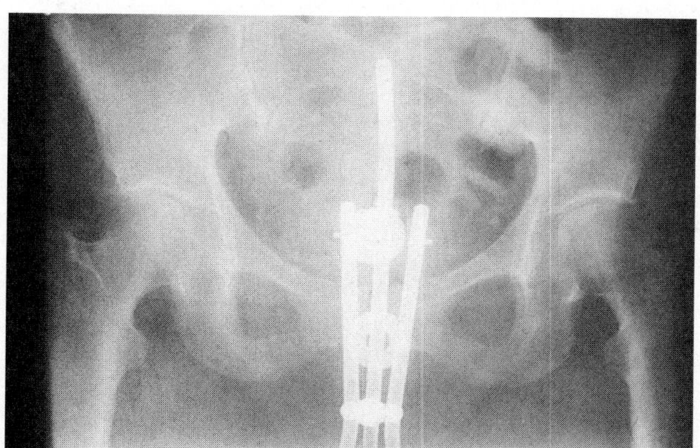

Fig. 29-12 Intrauterine tandem and vaginal colpostats in place.

Chemotherapy

The use of chemotherapy for cervical cancer is limited to patients with advanced or recurrent disease no longer amenable to control by surgery or radiotherapy or in a controlled clinical trial environment. Chemotherapy may also be used as a radiosensitizer. More than 38 chemotherapeutic agents have been tested in the management of cervical cancer. Cisplatin is the most effective agent used in the treatment of cervical cancer. As a single agent, it has a response rate of approximately 20% to 37% for both adenocarcinoma and SCC of the cervix. Many clinical trials compare combination regimens with cisplatin alone. It is most effective in patients who have not received prior chemotherapy, and complete responses (CRs) do occur in 6% to 10% of patients. Ifosfamide and dibromodulcitol both demonstrate a 22% response rate for SCC. Other responsive agents include epirubicin and vindesine. Advances in the use of chemotherapy for cervical cancer are discussed in a recent review article (Neijt, 1994).

Combination chemotherapy yields better results with response rates of about 40% to 60%. Cisplatin 100 mg/m^2 and cyclophosphamide 1000 mg/m^2 given every 3 weeks yields a 42% response rate, but the toxicity rate is fairly significant (Neijt, 1994; Park & Thigpen, 1993). A combination of ifosfamide 1.2 gm/m^2 with 300 mg/m^2 mesna, 5-fluorouracil (5-FU) 370 mg/m^2 for 5 days, and leucovorin 20 mg/m^2 was given every 28 days in patients with recurrent cervical cancer. Response rates were positive with 33% of patients demonstrating CRs and 20% of patients demonstrating partial responses (PRs). The dose-limiting toxicity was leukopenia, resulting in a dose reduction in 60% of the cases (Stornes, Mejlholm, & Jakobsen, 1994). A trial of cisplatin 90 mg/m^2, 5-FU 1500 mg/m^2, and ifosfamide 3 gm/m^2 with mesna was given over 3 days every 28 days. The response rate was 53% (with CRs in 17% of the patients and PRs in 36%). It is interesting to note that 78% of patients with adenocarcinoma responded (Fanning, Ladd, & Hilgers, 1995). A response rate of 60% (with CRs in 23% of the patients and PRs 37%) was obtained with the use of bleomycin 30 mg on day one, carboplatin 200 mg/m^2 on day one, and isfosfamide 2 g/m^2 plus mesna for 3 consecutive days. Toxicities included leukopenia, alopecia, and nausea and vomiting (Murad, Triginelli, & Ribalta, 1994). Although these combination trials demonstrate an improved response rate, overall survival was approximately 12 months in all trials.

Small cell cancer of the cervix is an aggressive disease, and few reports are found in the literature. Patients are treated with cisplatin-based therapy; however, the prognosis for this disease remains poor (Neijt, 1994).

Chemotherapy is also used as a radiosensitizer. The use of hydroxyurea with radiotherapy improved survival in patients with advanced cervical cancer from 49% without hydroxyurea to 68% with hydroxyurea. Other radiosensitizers have been investigated. Paclitaxel, administered approximately 48 hours before radiotherapy, has modest radiation-sensitizing effects in cervical cancer (Rodriguez et al., 1995).

Multimodal Therapy

Multimodal therapy involves the use of various treatment regimens to improve response rates and overall survival. The use of multimodal therapy in the management of cervical cancer is being investigated in patients with high risk for recurrent disease and in patients with inoperable tumors.

Neoadjuvant Chemotherapy Followed by Surgery. Neoadjuvant chemotherapy is the use of chemotherapy to reduce tumor bulk and diameter, decrease vascular space involvement, and lymph node involvement to allow surgical treatment in inoperable cases (Corn & Lanciano, 1994). The operability rate of stage I cervical cancer is approximately 70%, which leaves 30% of patients unresectable (Neijt, 1994). Patients who respond to adjuvant chemotherapy are eligible for radical surgery, and those ineligible are treated with radiotherapy. Chemoresponsiveness is the most predictive factor of cure in these scenarios (Benedetti-Panici et al., 1996). One clinical trial evaluated patients with stage IB cervical cancer. They were treated with cisplatin 50 mg/m^2 and vincristine 1 mg/m^2 at 10-day intervals for three courses. Patients then underwent a radical hysterectomy and pelvic lymphadenectomy. Survival after 24 months was 74% presumed disease-free, 12% died of their cancer, and 3% had developed recurrence (Eddy, Manetta, Alvarez, Williams, & Creasman, 1995). Another trial compared surgery alone with neoadjuvant vinblastine 4 mg/m^2, bleomycin 15 mg/m^2, and cisplatin 60 mg/m^2 (VBP) before radical surgery in patients with locally advanced stages IB, IIA, and IIB disease. The response rate for patients with SCC receiving VBP was 87% and 38% for patients with adenocarcinoma. The recurrence rate for patients treated with surgery was only 35.5%, compared with 18.5% treated with neoadjuvant chemotherapy and surgery, and the tumor-free survival rate was significant (Namkoong et al., 1995). The use of neoadjuvant chemotherapy plus surgery is promising for patients with locally advanced disease. However, more clinical trials are needed to demonstrate overall benefit.

Neoadjuvant Chemotherapy Followed by Radiation Therapy. Neoadjuvant chemotherapy before radiation therapy is another hopeful treatment combination. Patients in one clinical trial were given intraarterial (IA) cisplatin 120 mg/m^2 into the uterine artery for locally advanced cervical cancer. The IA chemotherapy was followed by external beam radiotherapy to the whole pelvis with or without intracavitary radiotherapy. A total of 76% of patients achieved CRs, and the 2- and 5-year survival rates were 64% and 55% respectively. The therapy was well-tolerated (Sueyama et al., 1995).

Concurrent Chemotherapy and Radiation Therapy Followed by Surgery. The use of concurrent chemoradiation followed by surgery has been used in patients with stages IB, IIB, III, and IVA disease. Two groups of patients were treated with cisplatin 40 or 60 mg/m^2 and 5-FU continuous infusion 400 or 600 mg/m^2/day over 96 hours on days 1 and 21. Radiotherapy (4500 cGy) was administered concurrently for 33 days through single-day administration or twice daily fractionation. A single intracavitary application with a parametrial boost was given to patients with disease reaching the pelvic wall. Next, patients were treated with hysterectomy and lymphadenectomy or with pelvic exenteration. Pelvic control was achieved in 81% of cases. The 2-year survival was 61% in patients with stages IB and IIB disease and 77% in patients with stages III and IVA disease. Complications included diarrhea, with some patients interrupting and discontinuing therapy; sepsis; and postexenteration complications. Toxicities were significant and must be weighed with the therapeutic benefit (Resbeut et al., 1994).

Patients with bulky stages I and II disease were also treated with radiation alone vs radiation with sequential or concurrent cisplatin 100 mg/m^2, and 5-FU 1000 mg/m^2 as a continuous infusion for 24 hours. Sequential chemotherapy was administered for two to three cycles and concurrent for one to six cycles. The 30-month survival was 79.5% in the radiotherapy alone arm, 89.5% in the sequential arm, and 100% in the concurrent therapy arm (Park et al., 1993).

ONCOLOGIC EMERGENCIES

The major oncologic emergencies associated with cervical cancer are septic shock and spinal cord compression (SCC). Septic shock is the result of neutropenia-induced infection after the administration of chemotherapy. Leukopenia and neutropenia are dose-limiting toxicities of many of the chemotherapy protocols used for cervical cancer. Treatment has resulted in septic deaths (Resbeut et al., 1994). Early detection and treatment of infection is paramount in managing this oncologic emergency.

Spinal cord compression in patients with cervical cancer may result from parametrial involvement of the tumor around the cord or bone metastasis that causes bone deterioration and compression onto the cord. The major complaint associated with SCC is back pain. The back pain is generally chronic and progresses with neurologic deficits such as weakness of the lower extremities, numbness, and bowel and bladder dysfunction. Patients with undiagnosed cervical cancer may also present at the time of diagnosis with SCC. This scenario is especially true in high-incidence populations where cervical screening is not a common practice. Back pain is not unusual in patients with cervical cancer, since it may be related to a pelvic tumor. However, the possibility of SCC should be investigated when a patient with cervical cancer complains of back pain. Rapid diagnosis and treatment are necessary to preserve function and maximize quality of life (Robinson & Muderspach, 1993).

Nursing care of the patient with an SCC includes educating the patient about the etiologic factors and treatment of the SCC, preventing further paralysis through proper body alignment and activity, protecting skin integrity, and alleviating pain. In addition, patients may experience difficulty in coping with the loss of normal functions and mobility (Held & Peahota, 1993).

NURSING MANAGEMENT

Nursing management of the patient with cervical cancer begins with cancer prevention, screening, and early detection. According to the Standards of Oncology Nursing Practice, oncology nurses serve an important role in the prevention and early detection of cancer (Brant, 1996). Advanced practice nurses often oversee cancer screening clinics where patients come to obtain a Pap smear for cervical cancer screening (Leslie, 1995). The nurses role is to inform the patient of the risk factors associated with cervical cancer and encourage prevention and regular screening for this disease. It is important to remind the patient that cervical cancer can usually be prevented when detected early. Women may not understand the reason or need for the Pap test and related diagnostic tests for cervical cancer. An educational visit before diagnostic tests may be beneficial (Tomaino-Brunner, Freda, & Runowicz, 1996). It is also important to provide culturally sensitive and educationally appropriate information to the patient. A list of culturally sensitive educational materials for cervical cancer is included in Table 29-7.

Nursing management continues through the diagnosis and treatment of the disease. The management is reflective of the stage of the disease process, the health status of the patient, and the treatment modalities employed. Each treatment modality exhibits its own side effects and complications. However, when treatment modalities are combined, the patient often experiences an exacerbation of the side effects. The patient with cervical cancer likely needs management in the inpatient, outpatient, and home settings. With care moving to the outpatient setting, nurses are challenged to educate patients and meet their needs in limited time frames.

Sexuality and Psychosocial Issues

Women diagnosed with cervical cancer often suffer psychological morbidity. Anxiety and depression occur with an increased frequency in women with cervical cancer compared with the general population, as well as when compared with other cancer survivors. One study assessed patients' concerns after surgery or radiotherapy for stage IB cervical cancer. Patients' concerns included fear of recurrence (91%), fear of general health (61%), self-blame about the cause of disease (39%), loss of self-control (37%), feeling old (29%), and feeling less attractive as a person (28%). Sexual concerns included pain with intercourse (60%), intercourse causing recurrence of the disease (37%), fear of their partner's attitude toward cancer (32%), blaming partner for the disease (29%), and feeling less sexually attractive (29%). Pain during intercourse is more common for patients who have received pelvic irradiation. Approximately 44% of women were unable to talk with their partner about their cancer, and greater than 50% needed additional information about the causes of cervical cancer and the risk for recurrence. Forty-nine percent of women would have preferred to have counseling (Cull et al., 1993). Nurses are instrumental in educating women about the potential causes, diagnosis, and management of cervical cancer. Counseling and education are necessary to decrease psychological and sexual morbidity. The nurse should encourage patients to talk about their feelings or concerns, plan periods of uninterrupted intimacy with their partners, and reinforce that pleasure and intimacy do not have to include intercourse, especially if this is uncomfortable for the patient (Cartwright-Alcarese, 1995; Cull et al., 1993; Lamb, 1995; McMullin, 1992). A sexual and psychosocial plan of care for the patient with cervical cancer is included in Table 29-8.

Surgery

Outpatient surgical procedures include cryosurgery, laser therapy, cervical biopsy, and conization. The patient may experience pain and cramping during the procedures that are

TABLE 29-7 Culturally Sensitive Cervical Cancer Resources

Population	Resources Available	Producer
Hispanic	1. *Hagase La Prueba Pap: Hagalo Hoy . . . Por Su Saludy Su Familia* brochure	1. National Cancer Institute
	2. *La Prueba Pap: Un Metodo Para Diagnosticar El Cancer Del Cuello Del Utero* booklet	2. National Cancer Institute
	3. *Women's Health Loteria* brochure	3. Norma Sheridan-Leos; San Antonio, Tex.
Native American	1. *Taking Control of Your Health: The Pap Test and Cervical Cancer* video	1. National Cancer Institute in conjunction with the Nebraska Department of Health
	2. *American Indian Women's Talking Circle* video	2. Center for American Indian Research and Education; Berkeley, Calif.
	3. *We Are the Circle of Life: Pass on the Gift of Health* poster	3. Native American Women and Wellness Project; St. Paul, Minn.
	4. *Health Risk Appraisal Project: Cervical Cancer* brochure	4. American Indian Health Care Association; Denver, Colo.
African American	1. *The Pap Test: It Can Save Your Life!* brochure	1. National Cancer Institute
Multicultural and Low-literacy	1. *Abnormal Pap Test Results: Understanding Your Diagnosis and Treatment* brochure	1. Krames Communications; San Bruno, Calif.
	2. *Having a Pelvic Examination and Pap Test* brochure	2. National Cancer Institute
	3. *The Pap Test: It Can Save Your Life* brochure	3. National Cancer Institute
	4. *Taking Control of Your Health: The Pap Test and Cervical Cancer* video	4. National Cancer Institute
	5. *Cervical Cancer: A Warning to Women* video	5. Films for the Humanities and Sciences; Princeton, NJ
	6. *Human Papilloma Virus* video	6. Milner-Fenwick, Inc.; Timonium, Md.

usually alleviated within 24 hours. Vaginal discharge and spotting is also common. The patient should be informed of the side effects of these procedures. Acetaminophen is usually sufficient to alleviate pain.

Hysterectomy is the most common surgical procedure done for the management of cervical cancer. The vaginal hysterectomy may be performed in the outpatient or inpatient surgical area. The patient arrives the morning of the procedure and is discharged that evening pending no complications. An abdominal hysterectomy, which requires a surgical incision, usually requires a 3-to-7-day stay in the inpatient setting. The major focus of inpatient nursing care is management of postoperative pain and potential complications such as bladder noncompliance, ureteral fistulas, rectovaginal fistulas, bowel obstruction, infection, and hemorrhage (Lui, 1993; Patterson & Carnago, 1996). Patients may also experience depression and may feel less attractive sexually. These feelings may be experienced by all patients undergoing hysterectomy regardless of the diagnosis of cancer (Cull et al., 1993).

Pelvic exenteration is a complex, radical surgery that requires extensive postoperative and ongoing nursing care. Postoperative problems include pulmonary embolism and edema, infection, hemorrhage, myocardial infarction, and small bowel obstruction (Walczak & Klemm, 1993). Long-term complications include urinary fistulas and obstruction, and infection. Depending on the extent of the exenteration, the patient may have a urinary diversion system or a colostomy that requires long-term management and prevention of infection and obstructive complications. Loss of the vagina is another traumatic aspect of the pelvic exenteration. Vaginal reconstruction should be offered at the time of the exenteration (Copeland, 1993; Nagell et al., 1993; Patterson & Carnago, 1996). Psychosocial and psychosexual support may assist the woman in adjusting to the vaginal reconstruction and urinary and fecal diversion devices. The nursing management of the patient undergoing hysterectomy and pelvic exenteration for cervical cancer is summarized in Table 29-9.

Radiation Therapy

Nursing management of the patient undergoing radiotherapy for cervical cancer is dependent on the type of therapy employed (external beam or intracavitary therapy) and whether the radiation therapy is combined with other treatment modalities. External beam therapy is administered in the outpatient setting. Intracavitary irradiation may be ad-

TABLE 29-8 Psychosocial and Psychosexual Standard of Care for the Patient With Cervical Cancer

Patient Problem and Outcomes	Nursing Interventions and Rationales	Patient Education Instructions
Knowledge Deficit Patient will: • Verbalize an understanding of the potential sexual complications associated with the treatment of cervical cancer	1. Assess patient's understanding of the potential sexual complications that can occur with cervical cancer treatment.	1. Describe the potential sexual complications that can occur with hysterectomy and/or pelvic exenteration: • Bladder noncompliance • Vaginal canal shortening • Vaginectomy
	2. Assess each patient's potential sexual complications in accordance with his or her individual treatment plan.	2. Describe the potential sexual complications that can occur with irradiation for cervical cancer: • Vaginal dryness • Vaginal stenosis • Painful intercourse
Anxiety Patient will: • Express feelings of anxiety • Identify strategies to cope with anxiety	1. Assess patient's fears and concerns about the diagnosis and treatment of cervical cancer.	1. Discuss the potential psychosocial difficulties that can occur with the diagnosis and treatment of cervical cancer: • Anxiety • Depression • Self-blame • Fear of recurrence
	2. Assess and encourage use of past effective coping strategies.	2. Review the potential causes of cervical cancer that potentiate self-blame (a woman may have had one or few sexual partners, yet is HPV-positive).
	3. Encourage patient to verbalize grief with loss of the uterus and loss of childbearing potential if applicable.	3. Offer a Cansurmount referral.
	4. Administer anxiolytic agents as needed to decrease anxiety.	4. Provide information about local support groups and individual counseling
Body Image Disturbance Patient will: • Be aware of treatment interventions that may interfere with body image such as ostomies and vaginal reconstruction • Express feelings about body image • Identify strategies that will assist to improve body image	1. Assess past perception of body image.	1. Use a diagram to describe anatomically, the changes that will occur with each individual patient's cancer treatment.
	2. Assess potential individual impact that cervical cancer treatment will have on body image disturbance: • Urinary diversion • Fecal diversion • Vaginectomy	2. Discuss vaginal reconstruction as necessary with patients undergoing complete vaginectomy.
	3. Encourage patient to verbalize concerns about body image changes.	3. Refer to an enterostomal therapist to provide information on means to manage diversion systems: • Regularity of stool • Odor management • Skin management under the devices • Hints to cover ostomy during intimacy
	4. Review the impact that diversion systems and vaginectomy can have on body image.	4. Provide information regarding ostomy support groups in the area.

Continued

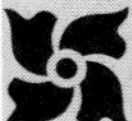

TABLE 29-8 Psychosocial and Psychosexual Standard of Care for the Patient With Cervical Cancer—cont'd

Patient Problem and Outcomes	Nursing Interventions and Rationales	Patient Education Instructions
Sexual Dysfunction Patient will: • Verbalize understanding of potential sexual dysfunction that occurs with treatment for cervical cancer • Identify strategies to minimize sexual dysfunction	1. Assess potential for sexual dysfunction that occurs with patient's individual treatment modality.	1. Teach patient about potential sexual changes that occur with hysterectomy: • Hormonal changes if ovaries are also removed: provide information about hormone replacement therapy • Temporary loss of vaginal sensation with vaginal hysterectomy: inform that longer period of stimulation may be necessary • Shortening of the vaginal canal: encourage patient to try alternative sexual positions to facilitate comfort
	2. Assess patient's level of sexual function prior to surgery.	2. Teach patient about the sexual changes that occur with vaginectomy and vaginal reconstruction for pelvic exenteration, especially change in sensation.
	3. Encourage patient to verbalize grief and concerns about potential loss of sexual functioning.	3. Teach patient that orgasm is still possible with the vaginectomy.
	4. Administer hormone replacement therapy as needed.	4. Teach patient about the potential sexual changes that occur from radiation therapy for cervical cancer: • Vaginal dryness: provide information on vaginal water-soluble lubricants • Vaginal stenosis: encourage sexual intercourse through radiation therapy to maintain vaginal elasticity and patency • Painful vaginal penetration: teach pelvic strengthening exercises, use vaginal lubricant • Vaginal burning: use vaginal lubricant, encourage male to use condom or ejaculation after withdrawal from the vagina

ministered in either the inpatient or the outpatient setting, depending on the dose of the intracavitary source. High-dose intracavitary irradiation (iridium) is given in the outpatient area, whereas low-dose intracavitary irradiation (cesium) is administered in the inpatient setting.

Radiation safety is a major responsibility of all health care workers (Dunne-Daly, 1994a). The radiation sources are kept in a safe until they are transported in a lead container to the patient's room for afterloading of the tandem and colpostats (Fig. 29-13). The patient is placed in a special room with lead walls and a lead door, and lead shields are also placed around the patient once the sources are implanted (Fig. 29-14). Radiation safety procedures for intracavitary irradiation are listed in Box 29-3.

The side effects of radiotherapy are similar for both external beam and intracavitary irradiation. Fatigue is the major complaint of all patients undergoing radiation therapy. Potential intestinal sequelae include proctitis, rectal ulcers, sigmoid stricture, diverticulitis, small bowel obstruction, small bowel perforation, and malabsorption. Urinary complications include chronic cystitis, bladder ulcer, vesicovaginal fistula, ureteral stricture, incontinence, and extensive cystocele. The GI and GU complications can occur during the treatment period or may be delayed. Delayed GI complications usually appear within the first 2 years of radiotherapy, whereas delayed GU complications occur more often 2 to 4 years after treatment. Other more common complications may include vault necrosis, vaginal stenosis, and arteriosclerosis. A greater incidence of complications occurs with higher doses of irradiation and irradiation of the periaortic lymph nodes (Dunne-Daly, 1994b; Perez, 1993b). The nursing management of the patient

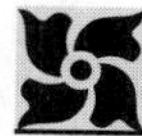

TABLE 29-9 Standard of Care For the Patient Undergoing Surgery For Cervical Cancer

Patient Problem and Outcomes	Nursing Interventions and Rationales	Patient Education Instructions
Anxiety Patient will: • Verbalize and understand the surgical procedure • Express concerns about the surgical procedure • Identify strategies to cope with anxiety and potential loss related to the surgical procedure	1. Assess patient's level of understanding of the surgical procedure. 2. Assess patient's concerns and questions related to the surgical procedure. 3. Assess ability to cope, and reinforce the use of past effective coping strategies. 4. Administer anxiolytic agents as necessary to decrease anxiety. 5. Offer a sleeping agent in the evenings prior to surgery and as needed thereafter. 6. Offer a Cansurmount referral.	1. Use visual diagrams to explain the type of surgical procedure employed: hysterectomy or various pelvic exenteration procedures. 2. Inform patient of preoperative routine: • Blood tests, ECG, chest x-ray • Bowel prep • Anesthesiology consult • Use of antiembolism stockings • NPO after midnight 3. Review postoperative plan with patient: • Coughing and deep-breathing exercises with use of an incentive spirometer • Pain management • Incision management • Drain and ostomy management • Use of indwelling catheter • Use of intravenous line(s) • Ambulation and activity postoperatively
Pain Patient will: • Verbalize an understanding of the postoperative pain management plan • Identify medical and self-care pain management interventions	1. Assess patient's location, intensity, quality, and temporality of pain at least every 4 hours around the clock. 2. Administer patient-controlled analgesia and supplemental opioids as needed. 3. Administer oral analgesics (when patient ready to be placed on oral), around the clock for the first week after surgery. 4. Administer additional or bolus opioids prior to ambulation or activity.	1. Teach patient about the use of patient-controlled analgesia. 2. Encourage patient to request additional pain medications or an increase in the PCA rate if uncomfortable. 3. Encourage patient to bolus self or request bolus medication prior to ambulation or activity such as bathing. 4. Provide patient with information about the use of oral analgesics when patient is ready.
Risk for Hemorrhage Patient will: • Maintain a normal hemoglobin and hematocrit • Maintain hemodynamic stability	1. Assess for bleeding: a. abdominal dressing with abdominal hysterectomy and pelvic exenteration b. sterile perineal pad with vaginal hysterectomy 2. Monitor hemoglobin and hematocrit postoperatively. 3. Monitor urinary output. 4. Monitor for hypotension.	1. Inform the patient to report any signs of bleeding: a. acute drainage on abdominal dressings b. increase in vaginal drainage 2. Teach the patient to avoid strenuous activity, which increases pelvic congestion, for 2 months after surgery: • Vacuuming • Dancing • Walking swiftly 3. Inform patient to avoid sexual intercourse for 4 to 6 weeks.

Continued

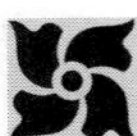

TABLE 29-9 Standard of Care for the Patient Undergoing Surgery for Cervical Cancer—cont'd

Patient Problem and Outcomes	Nursing Interventions and Rationales	Patient Education Instructions
Thrombophlebitis and Pulmonary Embolism Patient will: • Verbalize understanding of the risk for thrombophlebitis following surgery • Verbalize understanding of the risk for pulmonary embolism following pelvic exenteration • Identify strategies to prevent thrombophlebitis • Maintain normal arterial blood gases	1. Assess patient for individual risk of thrombophlebitis and embolism noting an increased risk in patients with: • Past history • Varicosities 2. Apply thromboembolitic stockings prior to surgery (may also use pneumatic compression stockings postoperatively). 3. Keep legs elevated postoperatively but avoid high Fowler's position. 4. Ambulate as soon as possible postoperatively. 5. Perform active range-of-motion exercises to prevent embolism. 6. Administer mini-dose heparin as ordered in patients undergoing pelvic exenteration.	1. Inform patient of potential risk of thromboembolism and pulmonary embolism with exenteration. 2. Teach patient to avoid pressure under the knees. 3. Teach patient to avoid high Fowler's position and demonstrate the position using the hospital bed. 4. Teach patient to perform leg exercises to promote circulation. 5. Teach patient about the use of thromboembolism stockings.
Incontinence Patient will: • Verbalize understanding of potential bladder noncompliance that occurs with hysterectomy • Identify strategies to strengthen bladder tone and manage incontinence	1. Assess for history of bladder noncompliance or incontinence. 2. Clamp urinary drainage system intermittently prior to removal to retrain bladder. 3. Assess for postoperative bladder noncompliance including stress incontinence.	1. Inform patient of the potential risk of bladder noncompliance following hysterectomy. 2. Teach patient pelvic strengthening exercises. 3. Provide information on methods to keep clothing dry.
Bowel Obstruction Patient will: • Verbalize understanding of risk of small bowel obstruction with pelvic exenteration	1. Assess bowel sounds every 4 hours following surgery. 2. Monitor output from fecal diversion system. 3. Maintain adequate intravenous hydration and nutrition postoperatively.	1. Teach patient to report any increased abdominal distention. 2. Teach patient to consume adequate fluids when oral intake resumes (3,000 fluids/day). 3. Teach patient dietary measures to regulate ostomy (i.e., adequate fiber intake). 4. Refer patient to an enterostomal therapist for ostomy management.

with cervical cancer undergoing irradiation is found in Table 29-10.

Chemotherapy

Cisplatin is the major chemotherapeutic agent used in the treatment of cervical cancer. Leukopenia is usually the dose-limiting toxicity, especially when combined with other agents. Other side effects include nausea and vomiting, alopecia, and renal toxicity. The nursing management for the patient undergoing chemotherapy for cervical cancer includes educating patients about potential sequelae and early detection of complications to decrease morbidity. Nursing management of the patient receiving chemotherapy is summarized within the Oncology Nursing Society's *Cancer Chemotherapy Guidelines and Recommendations for Practice* (Powel, 1996).

HOME CARE ISSUES

Home care issues are paramount for patients with cervical cancer. Psychosocial and sexual concerns are prevalent at all

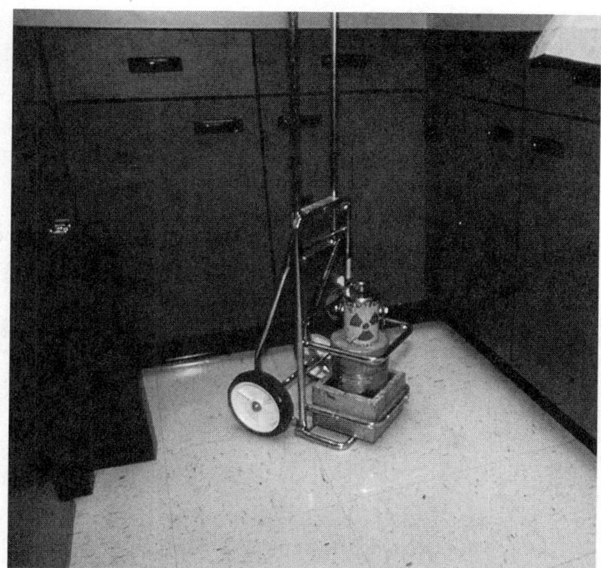

Fig. 29-13 Transporter of radioactive isotopes.

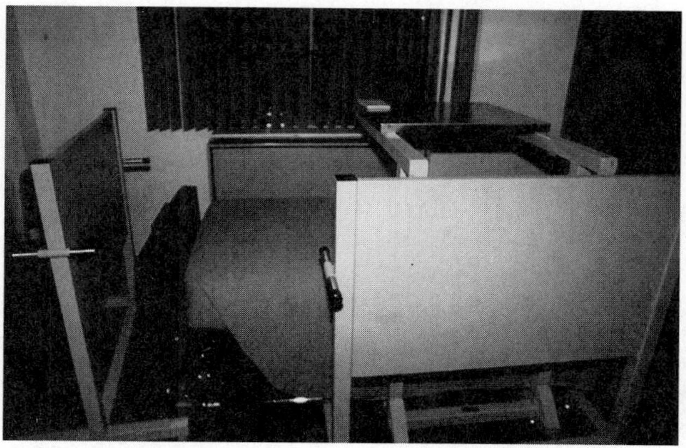

Fig. 29-14 Lead shields for the patient receiving intracavitary irradiation.

stages of the disease for both the patient and/or her significant other. Psychosocial and sexual issues should be addressed at the time of diagnosis and throughout treatment, and yet the issues are often lifelong. Physical problems are more diverse and are dependent on the treatment modalities employed, as well as the stage and prognosis of disease.

Psychosocial and Sexual Support

Regardless of the treatment modality employed, women with cervical cancer often suffer negative morbidity. The nursing management of the patient with sexual dysfunction is presented in Table 29-8. One home care intervention that can be recommended is pelvic muscle exercises for women who have undergone surgery and radiation treatment modalities. Pelvic muscle exercises strengthen the bladder after hysterectomy and external beam pelvic irradiation. In addition, they may help to relax the pelvis and minimize discomfort on vaginal penetration (Cartwright-Alcarese, 1995). A pelvic muscle exercise instruction sheet is included in Patient Preparation Table 29-11.

Box 29-3
Radiation Safety Procedures and Principles for Intracavitary Irradiation

All personnel should provide care using the principles of time, distance, and shielding:

1. Time: Minimize time spent in the patient's room.
2. Distance: Maximize distance between yourself and the patient.
3. Shielding: Stand behind the door or lead shielding whenever possible.

Visitation should be allowed within the following parameters:

1. Persons under 18 years of age and pregnant women should not be allowed in the room or in the adjacent rooms if indicated.
2. Other persons may visit patient for 15 minutes twice per day, unless otherwise ordered.
3. Visitors should stand behind the lead shields.

Ostomies and Urinary Diversion

Colostomies and urinary diversion systems require lifestyle changes and ongoing care. Diversion systems require a pouch that collects wastes outside of the body, and the patient and/or family needs education about the management of the system. Ostomies, which provide a route for elimination of stool from the body, are located in the ileus, or transverse, descending, or sigmoid colon. Ileostomies drain liquid stool. Transverse colostomies drain soft, mushy stool, whereas descending and sigmoid colostomies drain firmer stools. The most common type of urinary diversion is the ileal conduit. The ureters are attached to the small bowel, which is used as a conduit for the urine to exit at the skin surface. Diversion systems may also interfere with the patient's sexual functioning. The patient should be referred to the enterostomal therapist immediately after surgery. A home care guide for a urinary diversion is found in Box 29-4.

Community Resources

Several resources are available for patients diagnosed with cervical cancer. Cancer support groups are also available in most communities, and some larger metropolitan areas may offer cervical cancer–specific support groups. Support groups for persons with ostomies are also available. Persons with ostomies often gather to share information about living with the ostomy, and find support in meeting with one another.

Cansurmount, a program sponsored by the American Cancer Society, which links newly diagnosed cancer patients with cancer survivors, is another option. A woman who is a survivor of cervical cancer can meet with the newly diagnosed patient to share concerns about the diagnosis and

TABLE 29-10 Standard of Care for the Patient Undergoing Radiotherapy for Cervical Cancer

Patient Problem and Outcomes	Nursing Interventions and Rationales	Patient Education Instructions
Knowledge Deficit Patient will: • Verbalize an understanding of the radiation therapy procedures, including benefits and side effects • State when to call a health care provider when complications occur • Discuss strategies to manage complications	1. Assess patient's knowledge, fears, and misperceptions about radiation therapy. 2. Assess patient's individual therapy plan: intracavitary versus external beam therapy.	1. Describe the routine procedures involved with intracavitary irradiation: • Tandem/colpostat placement • Isotope placement • Radiation precautions 2. Describe the routine procedures involved with external beam irradiation: • Consultation • Simulation • Treatment 3. Provide information about the potential side effects and treatment complications of radiation therapy: • Fatigue • Diarrhea • Proctitis • Rectovaginal fistula • Small bowel obstruction • Cystitis • Vault necrosis • Vaginal stenosis
Fatigue Patient will: • Maintain activities of daily living and prioritize other activities that optimize her quality of life	1. Assess past activity level prior to radiation therapy and current level of activity. 2. Assess level of fatigue using a verbal numeric rating scale with 0 being not tired at all to 10 being exhausted.	1. Inform patient that the radiation therapy–induced fatigue is cumulative and extends beyond the course of treatment. 2. Teach patient methods to conserve energy: • Allowing a nap during the day • Maintaining a regular sleep schedule • Prioritizing activities by performing high priority or high quality-of-life activities first 3. Teach patient methods to enhance energy: • Exercise daily • Balance activity with rest
Diarrhea Patient will: • Maintain an adequate fluid and electrolyte balance • Identify self-care strategies to minimize and manage diarrhea	1. Assess elimination patterns including bowel frequency, quality, and quantity. 2. Provide a low-residue diet during therapy. 3. Administer antidiarrheal agents as needed such as immodium, lomotil, or tincture of opium. 4. Administer intravenous fluids as needed to maintain fluid and electrolyte balance. 5. Weigh daily.	1. Inform patient that diarrhea occurs after a couple of weeks of treatment, after approximately 2000 cGy have been given. 2. Provide patient with information about a low residue diet to control radiation-induced diarrhea: • Low fat • Avoid caffeine, which may stimulate bowel • Avoid fruits, except bananas and apples • Avoid vegetables, except for cooked squash, carrots, and green beans • Eat white bread and white starches (e.g., pasta) 3. Teach patient about the use of antidiarrheal agents to control diarrhea. 4. Encourage the patient to drink plenty of fluids (3000 cc/day).

TABLE 29-10 Standard of Care for the Patient Undergoing Radiotherapy for Cervical Cancer—cont'd

Patient Problem and Outcomes	Nursing Interventions and Rationales	Patient Education Instructions
Proctitis Patient will: • Maintain rectal comfort during radiotherapy • Identify self-care strategies to manage proctitis	1. Assess for rectal discomfort, itching, burning, or pain with bowel movements during the radiotherapy period. 2. Assess for skin breakdown that can occur with rectal irritation. 3. Administer steroidal antiinflammatory medications for discomfort such as Anusol HC suppository or ointment. 4. Administer aquaphor ointment for rectal irritation and itching.	1. Teach patient about the potential side effect of proctitis. 2. Teach patient pharmacologic and self-care strategies to enhance comfort: • Sitz baths • Epsom salts or Domeboro packets can be used in sitz baths • Anusol HC • Aquaphor 3. Teach patient to report any skin breakdown that may occur with proctitis.
Small Bowel Obstruction Patient will: • Maintain a patent GI tract • Verbalize understanding of the long-term risk of GI complications	1. Assess for bowel sounds during each visit. 2. Assess for GI disturbance such as bloating, nausea, vomiting, constipation, and diarrhea. 3. Administer antidiarrheal therapy appropriately to prevent constipation and obstruction.	1. Inform patient that GI complications can occur up to 2 years after radiation therapy. 2. Teach patient about the signs and symptoms of bowel obstruction: diarrhea, upper GI cramping, constipation. 3. Provide patient with a long-term follow-up schedule following radiotherapy.
Rectovaginal Fistula Patient will: • Maintain rectal and vaginal integrity	1. Assess vaginal drainage during radiotherapy: color, consistency, odor, correlation with bowel movements. 2. Monitor GI side effects of radiotherapy that may precede rectovaginal fistula.	1. Teach the patient about the potential radiotherapy side effect of rectovaginal fistula. 2. Teach the patient to report any signs or symptoms of rectovaginal fistula: • Vaginal drainage with fecal odor • Obvious stool evacuating vagina during bowel movements • Vaginal drainage that increases and is dark in color
Cystitis Patient will: • Identify signs and symptoms of cystitis • List self-care strategies to manage cystitis	1. Assess for signs of cystitis such as urinary burning or discomfort. 2. Administer Pyridium 200 mg three times per day when cystitis is present. 3. Administer antispasmodics as needed for discomfort (e.g., Oxybutin 5 mg, 2-3 times per day).	1. Teach the patient about the signs and symptoms of cystitis that can occur after approximately 3000 cGy of radiation. 2. Inform the patient to report signs and symptoms of cystitis. 3. Encourage the patient to drink plenty of fluids (3000 cc/day). 4. Inform the patient that Pyridium turns the urine an orange color. 5. Teach patient about the side effects of antispasmodics such as drowsiness, dry mouth, constipation, and urinary retention.
Vaginal Complications	See section on psychosexual standard of care	See section on psychosexual standard of care

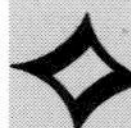

TABLE 29-11 Patient Preparation for Pelvic Muscle Exercises

Purpose of the Procedure: The purpose of pelvic muscle exercises is to strengthen the muscles of the pelvis to prevent unwanted leakage of urine and to learn to control muscles for more comfortable sexual intercourse.

Procedural Considerations:

1. Try to locate the muscles that surround the vagina and the urethra (the tube where urine leaves the body). Find these muscles by trying to stop the stream of urine midstream.
2. Get in a comfortable position. You can perform the exercises sitting or lying down.
3. Tighten the pelvic muscles and hold them tight for 10 seconds.
4. Relax now for 10 seconds.
5. Repeat the exercises 10 times.
6. Start out by performing these exercises 10 times per day. Try and increase this to 35 to 50 exercises (sets of 10) every other day.

Data from *Mosby's patient teaching guides.* (1996). St Louis: Mosby.

Box 29-4
Home Care Guide for Urinary Diversion

Purpose of the Procedure

The purpose of the procedure is to manage your urinary diversion system. A urinary diversion system is a system to pass urine to the skin's surface when the normal urinary system is no longer in place.

Steps to Follow

1. Wash around the stoma with soap and water. Make sure it is thoroughly dry before applying the ostomy appliance.
2. Apply a skin barrier or skin protectant before applying the ostomy pouch.
3. Obtain an ostomy pouch with an adhesive faceplate or backing.
4. Peel back the paper on the faceplate and press it around the stoma.
5. Compress the air from the bag, and clamp it at the bottom.
6. Change the ostomy pouch every 5 to 7 days.
7. Drink plenty of fluids, at least 8 glasses per day to maintain an acidic urine.
8. You may want to take a Vitamin C supplement, which will help maintain an acidic urine.

Data from *Mosby's patient teaching guides.* (1996). St. Louis: Mosby.

treatment of the cancer. Up to 37% of women in one study reported that they would have liked to talk with another woman with cervical cancer (Cull et al., 1993).

Sexual counseling and educational resources are other community services that should be recommended. The American Association of Sex Educators, Counselors, and Therapists provides names of sex therapists around the country. Cancer Care, Resolve, and the Wellness Community are other organizations that provide sexual and psychosocial assistance after a cancer diagnosis (Cartwright-Alcarese, 1995). Nursing's role is to provide patients and families with information about community resources and make referrals as needed.

PROGNOSIS

The prognosis of cervical cancer is greatly dependent on a number of host factors and the stage of the disease at the time of diagnosis. The stage of disease is the most significant prognostic variable. The 5-year survival rate for stage IA disease is close to 100%, whereas the 5-year survival rate for stage IV disease ranges from 18% to 30% (Hoskins, Perez, & Young, 1993). Individual tumor characteristics and behavior also share a role in the overall prognosis. The depth of invasion of the tumor is highly predictive of nodal spread or the progression-free interval (Zaino et al., 1992). Large bulky tumors larger than 4 cm have a poorer prognosis with a 5-year survival rate of 65% to 75%. Flow cytometry has also been used in attempts to monitor prognosis, and the findings from these studies are variable. There appears to be a greater number of relapses in patients with 20% or greater number of cells in the S-phase (Perez, 1993a). In addition, diploid tumors with a high proliferative phase have a significantly poorer prognosis with respect to stage, grade, nodal metastasis, and parametrial infiltration (Zanetta et al., 1992). Histologically, adenocarcinomas have a poorer prognosis than SCCs; however, statistically significant differences are only obvious for stage II disease (Shingleton et al., 1995). Small cell carcinoma of the cervix also has a very poor prognosis related to its high proliferative rate and propensity to spread to the lymphatics and distant sites (Perez, 1993a). A newly identified prognostic factor is the squamous cell carcinoma antigen (SCC-ag). A high SCC-ag level correlates with a poorer prognosis and a decreased disease-free survival (Duk et al., 1996). HPV-negative cervical carcinomas also appear to have a worse prognosis than those that are HPV-positive (Herrington, 1995).

Host factors associated with poorer prognosis include age less than 35 to 40 years, race, low socioeconomic status (SES), and a barrel-shaped cervix (Perez, 1993a). The low SES factors are attributed to the late detection of cervical cancer, thereby leading to increased mortality. There is poorer survival among women of color, which may be related to late detection or other potential genetic factors (National Cancer Institute, 1996). Clinical manifestations or symptoms that were possibly attributed to the cancer are also of prognostic value. Primary symptoms such as vaginal bleeding or discharge, systemic symptoms such as fatigue or nondeliberate weight loss, and metastatic symptoms such as profuse bleeding and/or nondeliberate weight loss of greater than 10 pounds were all associated with a poorer prognosis in patients with invasive cervical cancer. Five-year survival rates are increased in asymptomatic patients (Peipert, Wells, Schwartz, & Feinstein, 1994). Other clinical co-morbid

TABLE 29-12 Guidelines for Selecting a Pap Smear Lab

Criteria	Yes	No
1. Is the lab accredited by the College of American Pathologists?		
2. Are the Pap smear slides read on site?		
3. Does the lab read a minimum of 10,000 smears annually?		
4. Is a trained cytopathologist on staff?		
5. Is a pathologist readily available for consultation if needed?		
6. Are unsatisfactory and suboptimal slides identified?		
7. Is missing clinical information requested?		
8. Is the cost comparable to other facilities and not lower?		

If the answer to any of these questions is no, you may want to consult another facility for your annual Pap smear evaluation.

variables related to worse survival rates include anemia (<10-11 g/dL) and arterial hypertension (diastolic >110 mmHg), which are commonly associated with an increased number of pelvic recurrences. Fever is also associated with an increased incidence of distant metastasis (Perez, 1993a).

EVALUATION OF THE QUALITY OF CARE

Several organizations mandate the quality of care provided to patients with a diagnosis of cervical cancer. The Clinical Laboratory Improvement Amendments of 1988 (CLIA '88) monitors the quality of Pap smear techniques and cytologic reading of specimens. All College of American Pathologist laboratories must be CLIA '88–approved. Members of the health care team can provide women with information about quality indicators to be aware of when seeking cervical cancer screening. A quality tool reflecting where to obtain a Pap smear is included in Table 29-12 (Julian, 1993).

The Joint Commission for the Accreditation of Health Care Organizations (JCAHO) also evaluates quality care within the inpatient setting. The care of the patient with cervical cancer may be complex, and the care requires a multidisciplinary approach. The health care team should be involved in the delivery of care, as well as patient and family education. Table 29-13 provides an example of a quality-of-care evaluation tool that can be used for the patient with cervical cancer receiving intracavitary radiation therapy.

TABLE 29-13 Quality-of-Care Evaluation for a Patient Undergoing Intracavitary Radiotherapy

Disciplines participating in the quality-of-care evaluation:
☐ Nursing ☐ Surgery ☐ Radiology ☐ Social Services
Data from: ☐ Medical Record Review
☐ Patient/Family Interview

Criteria	Yes	No
1. Did the doctor or nurse explain the radiation safety procedures to you?	☐	☐
a. Health care workers would spend limited time in the hospital room	☐	☐
b. Visitor restrictions	☐	☐
c. Use of lead shields	☐	☐
2. Were you comfortable during the hospital stay?	☐	☐
a. Pelvic pain related to the implant	☐	☐
b. Comfort with position	☐	☐
3. Were you taught about the potential complications related to the radiation implant?	☐	☐
a. Vaginal dryness	☐	☐
b. Vaginal scarring	☐	☐
c. Possible pain with intercourse	☐	☐
4. Did the doctor or nurse provide you with materials and information about changes in sexuality?	☐	☐
5. Did the doctor or nurse offer a Cansurmount referral?	☐	☐

RESEARCH ISSUES

Many research opportunities exist for the diagnosis of cervical cancer. First, the use of HPV cervical smears is on the diagnostic horizon. Although current techniques can detect HPV DNA in more than 90% of preinvasive and invasive cervical lesions, HPV testing lacks specificity to be a universal screening test for all women. Second, automated cytology is also under investigation. An automated system could identify the most abnormal cells in the smear for review by the cytologist. This procedure could improve the false-negative readings. A third promising diagnostic technique is the use of cervicography. The cervix and upper vagina are visualized with a speculum, and the area is photographed using a special flash camera. The image can be magnified 16 times and projected on a large screen. Expert colposcopists can then interpret and evaluate the projection. Unfortunately, the high false-positive rates and technical problems currently make this technique unacceptable (AMWA, 1994).

Treatment issues are also being investigated. Intracavitary radiotherapy studies that compare the use of low-dose and high-dose administration of isotopes are currently in progress. Cesium-137 is the isotope used in low-dose therapy and delivers 0.5 cGy/minute or less. The patient is hospitalized for the duration of the therapy. The advantages of low-dose therapy include the following:

- Potentially better effects on the cell cycle and mitotic delay
- Decreased duration of therapy
- High doses delivered to the regions near the radiation sources
- Minimized irradiation to the normal tissue

Iridium-192, on the other hand, is used for high-dose therapy. The irradiation is delivered in fractionated doses of 200 to 300 cGy/minute. The therapy can be given in the outpatient setting. Advantages include the following:

- Potentially better survival rates
- Lower rates of serious complications
- Anesthesia-free, outpatient treatment

The disadvantage is that the patient receives fractionated doses. More investigation is needed to determine the exact role of these treatment modalities as they relate to overall survival and quality of life benefits (Brady, Micaily, Miyamoto, Heilmann, & Montemaggi, 1995).

Numerous chemotherapy clinical trials are also under way to improve the long-term survival of patients with locally advanced and advanced cervical cancer. More investigation in this area will better define the agents and the exact role of chemotherapy in the treatment of cervical cancer.

Finally, research and clinical experience is needed regarding cervical cancer screening and early detection. Because cervical cancer is a potentially preventable and curable type of cancer, it is important to investigate better strategies to recruit and follow women for cervical screening examinations, thus decreasing the overall morbidity and mortality of this disease.

REFERENCES

American Medical Women's Association. (1994). *Breast and cervical cancer education for primary care providers.* Alexandria, VA: American Medical Women's Association.

American Public Health Association. (1996). *The nation's health: The official newspaper of the American Public Health Association, 26*(10), 9. Washington, D.C.: American Public Health Association.

Beahrs, O. H., Henson, D. E., Hutter, R. V., & Kennedy, B. J. (1992). *Manual for staging of cancer.* Philadelphia: J. B. Lippincott.

Bender, S. (1976). Carcinoma in-situ of cervix in sisters. *British Medical Journal, 1,* 502.

Benedetti-Panici, P., Greggi, S., Scambia, G., Salerno, M.G., Amoroso, M., Maneschi, F., Cutillo, G., Caruso, A., Capelli, A., & Mancuso, S. (1996). Locally advanced cervical adenocarcinoma: Is there a place for chemosurgical treatment? *Gynecologic Oncology, 61,* 44-49.

Birley, H. D. L. (1995). Human papillomaviruses, cervical cancer and the developing world. *Annals of Tropical Medicine and Parasitology, 89*(5), 453-463.

Bosch, F. X., Manos, M. M., Munoz, N., Sherman, M., Jansen, A. M., Peto, J., Schiffman, M. H., Moreno, V., Kurman, R., & Shah, K.V. (1995). Prevalence of human papilloma virus in cervical cancer: A worldwide perspective. *Journal of the National Cancer Institute 87*(11), 796-802.

Brady, L. W., Micaily, B., Miyamoto, C. T., Heilmann, H. P., & Montemaggi, P. (1995). Innovations in brachytherapy in gynecologic oncology. *Cancer, 76,* 2143-2151.

Brant, J. (1996). *Statement on the scope and standards of oncology nursing practice.* Washington, D.C.: American Nurses' Association and Oncology Nursing Society.

Brinton, L. A. (1991). Oral contraceptives and cervical neoplasia. *Contraception, 43,* 581-596.

Brinton, L. A., Herrero, R., Reeves, W. C., De Britton, R. C., Gaitan, E., & Tenorio, F. (1993). Risk factors for cervical cancer by histology. *Gynecologic Oncology, 51,* 301-306.

Buckley, J. D., Harris, R. W. C., Doll, R., Vessey, M. P., & Williams, P. T. (1981). Case-control study of the husbands of women with dysplasia or carcinoma of the cervix uteri. *Lancet, 2,* 1010-1014.

Burger, M. P. M., Hollema, H., Pieters, W. J. L. M., Schroder, F. P., & Quint, W. G. V. (1996). Epidemiological evidence of cervical intraepithelial neoplasia without the presence of human papillomavirus. *British Journal of Cancer, 73,* 831-836.

Burke, L. (1991). *Colposcopy text and atlas.* Norwalk, CT: Appleton & Lange.

Butterworth, E. E., Hatch, K. D., Macaluso, M., Cole, P., Sauberlich, H. E., Soong, S. J., Borst, M., & Baker, V. V. (1992). Folate deficiency in cervical dysplasia. *Journal of the American Medical Association, 267,* 528-533.

Cartwright-Alcarese, F. (1995). Addressing sexual dysfunction following radiation therapy for a gynecologic malignancy. *Oncology Nursing Forum, 22*(8), 1229-1232.

Childers, J. M., Chu, J., Voigt, L. F., Feigl, P., Tamimi, H. K., Franklin, E. W., Alberts, D. S., & Meyskens, F. L. (1995). Chemoprevention of cervical cancer with folic acid: A Phase III Southwest Oncology Group intergroup study. *Cancer Epidemiology, Biomarkers, and Prevention, 4,* 155-159.

Childers, J. M. & Surwit, E. A. (1993). Current status of operative laparoscopy in gynecologic oncology. *Oncology, 7*(11), 47-51.

Copeland, L. J. (1993). Reconstructive surgery in gynecologic oncology. In D. M. Gershenson, A. H. DeCherney, & S. L. Curry (Eds.), *Operative Gynecology.* Philadelphia: W.B. Saunders.

Corn, B. W. & Lanciano, R. M. (1994). Combined modality treatment for carcinomas of the uterine cervix and vulva. *Current Opinion in Oncology, 6,* 524-530.

Cox, J. T. (1995). Epidemiology of cervical intraepithelial neoplasia: The role of human papillomavirus. *Bailliere's Clinical Obstetrics and Gynecology, 9*(1), 1-37.

Cruickshank, M. E., Flannelly, G., Campbell, D. M. (1995). Fertility and pregnancy outcome following large loop excision of the cervical transformation zone, *British Journal of Obstetrics and Gynaecology, 102,* 467-470.

Cull, A., Cowie, V. J., Farquharson, D. I. M., Livingstone, J. R. B., Smart, G. E., & Elton, R. A. (1993). Early stage cervical cancer: Psychosocial and sexual outcomes of treatment. *British Journal of Cancer, 68,* 1216-1220.

Current Clinical Trials Oncology. (1994). *Physician data query. National Cancer Institute, 1*(2) (protocol 09315, protocol 09088).

DiSaia, P. J. (1994). Disorders of the uterine cervix. In J. R. Scott, P. J. DiSaia, C. B. Hammond, & W. N. Spellacy (Eds.) *Danforth's obstetrics and gynecology* (7th ed.). Philadelphia: J.B. Lippincott.

Duk, J. M., Groenier, K. H., de Bruijn, H. W. A., Hollema, H., ten Hoor, K. A., van der Zee, A. G. J., Aalders, J. G. (1996). Pretreatment serum squamous cell carcinoma antigen: A newly identified prognostic factor in early-stage cervical carcinoma. *Journal of Clinical Oncology, 14,* 111-118.

Dunne-Daly, C. F. (1994a). Programmed instruction: Radiation therapy. Brachytherapy. *Cancer Nursing, 17*(4), 355-364.

Dunne-Daly, C. F. (1994b). Programmed instruction: Radiation therapy. Nursing care and adverse reactions of external radiation therapy: A self-learning module. *Cancer Nursing, 17*(3), 236-256.

Eddy, G. L., Manetta, A., Alvarez, R. D., Williams, L., & Creasman, W. T. (1995). Neoadjuvant chemotherapy with vincristine and cisplatin followed by radical hysterectomy and pelvic lymphadenectomy for FIGO stage IB bulky cervical cancer: A gynecologic oncology group pilot study. *Gynecologic Oncology, 57,* 412-416.

Fanning, J., Ladd, C., & Hilgers, R. D. (1995). Cisplatin, 5-fluorouracil, and ifosfamide in the treatment of recurrent or advanced cervical cancer. *Gynecologic Oncology, 56,* 235-238.

Ferenczy, A., Choukroun, D., & Arseneau, J. (1996). Loop electrosurgical excision procedure for squamous intraepithelial lesions of the cervix: Advantages and potential pitfalls. *Obstetrics and Gynecology, 87,* 332-337.

Fletcher, S., Neill, W. A., & Norval, M. (1990). Seminal polyamines as agents of cervical carcinoma. Production of aneuploidy in squamous epithelium. *Journal of Clinical Pathology, 44,* 410-415.

Franco, E. L., Filho, N. C., Villa, L. L., & Torloni, H. (1988). Correlation patterns of cancer relative frequencies with some socioeconomic and demographic indicators in Brazil: An ecologic study. *International Journal of Cancer, 41,* 24-29.

Fujii, T., Tsukasaki, K., Kiguchi, K., Kubushiro, K., Yajima, M., & Nozawa, S. (1995). The major E6/E7 transcript of HPV-16 in exfoliated cells from cervical neoplasia patients. *Gynecologic Oncology, 58,* 210-215.

Held, J. L. & Peahota, A. (1993). Nursing care of the patient with spinal cord compression. *Oncology Nursing Forum, 20*(10), 1507-1516.

Herrington, C. S. (1995). Human papillomaviruses (HPV) in gynaecological cytology: From molecular biology to clinical testing. *Cytopathology, 6,* 176-189.

Hording, U., Teglbjaerg, C. S., Visfeldt, J., & Bock, J. E. (1992). Human papilloma virus in type-16 and type-18 in adenocarcinoma of the uterine cervix. *Gynecologic Oncology, 46,* 313-316.

Hoskins, W. J., Perez, C. A., & Young, R. C. (Eds.). (1992). *Principles and practice of gynecologic oncology.* Philadelphia: J. B. Lippincott.

Hoskins, W. J., Perez, C. A., Young, R. C. (1993). Gynecologic tumors. In V. T. DeVita, Jr., S. Hellman, & S. A. Rosenberg (Eds.), *Cancer: Principles and practice of oncology* (4th ed.). Philadelphia: J. B. Lippincott.

Jones, W. B., Mercer, G. O., Lewis, J. L., Rubin, S. C., Hoskins, W. J. (1993). Early invasive carcinoma of the cervix. *Gynecologic Oncology, 51,* 26-32.

Julian, T. (1993). The minimally abnormal Pap smear and cervical cancer screening. *The Colposcopist, 25,* 1-6.

Kelloff, G. J., Hawk, E. T., Crowell, J. A., Boone, C. W., Nayfield, S. G., Perloff, M., Steele, V E., Lubet, R. A., Sigman, C. C. (1996). Strategies for identification and clinical evaluation of promising chemopreventive agents. *Oncology 10*(10), 1471-1480.

Kjaer, S. K. & Brinton, L. A. (1993). Adenocarcinomas of the uterine cervix: The epidemiology of an increasing problem. *Epidemiologic Reviews, 15*(2), 486-498.

Kjaer, S. K., VanDenBrule, A. J. C., Bock, J. E., Poll, P. A., Engholm, G., Sherman, M. E., Walboomers, J. M. M., & Meijer, C. J. L. M. (1996). Human papillomavirus: The most significant risk determinant of cervical intraepithelial neoplasia. *International Journal of Cancer 65,* 601-606.

Koffa, M., Koumantakis, E., Ergazaki, M., Tsatsanis, C., & Spandidos, D. A. (1995). Association of herpesvirus infection with the development of genital cancer. *International Journal of Cancer, 63,* 58-62.

Lamb, M. A. (1995). Effects of cancer on the sexuality and fertility of women. *Seminars in Oncology Nursing, 11*(2), 120-127.

Landis, S. H., Murray, T., Bolden, S., & Wingo, P. A. (1998). Cancer statistics 1998. *CA: A Cancer Journal for Clinicians, 48*(1): 6-29.

Lavery, J. (Consultant) (1997). *Personal communication.* Reistertown, MD.

Lehtinen, M., Dillner, J., Knekt, P., Luostarinen, T., Aromaa, A., Kirnbauer, R., Koskela, P., Paavonen, J., Peto, R., Schiller, J. T., & Hakama, M. (1996). Serologically diagnosed infection with human papillomavirus type 16 and risk for subsequent development of cervical carcinoma: Nested case-control study. *British Medical Journal, 312,* 537-539.

Leslie, N. S. (1995). Role of the nurse practitioner in breast and cervical cancer prevention. *Cancer Nursing, 18*(4), 251-257.

Lovejoy, N. C. (1994). Precancerous and cancerous cervical lesions: The multicultural "male" risk factor. *Oncology Nursing Forum, 21*(3), 497-504.

Lovejoy, N. C. & Anastasi, J. K. (1994). Squamous cell cervical lesions in women with and without AIDS. *Cancer Nursing, 17*(4), 294-307.

Lui, R. (1993). Abdominal and vaginal hysterectomy. In D. M. Gershenson, A. H. DeCherney, & S. L. Curry (Eds.), *Operative Gynecology.* Philadelphia: W. B. Saunders.

Magrina, J. F. (1993). Complications of irradiation and radical surgery for gynecologic malignancies. *Obstetrical and Gynecologic Survey, 48*(8), 571-575.

Massi, G., Savino, L., & Susini, T. (1993). Schauta-Amreich vaginal hysterectomy and Wertheim-Meigs abdominal hysterectomy in the treatment of cervical cancer: A retrospective analysis. *American Journal of Obstetrics and Gynecology, 168,* 928-934.

McMullin, M. (1992). Holistic care of the patient with cervical cancer. *Nursing Clinics of North America, 27*(4), 847-858.

Meyskens, F. L., Surwit, E. A., Moon, T. E., Childers, J. M., Davis, J. R., Dove, R. T., Johnson, C. S., & Alberts, D. S. (1994). Enhancement of regression of cervical intraepithelial neoplasia II (moderate dysplasia) with topically applied all-trans-retinoic acid: A randomized trial. *Journal of the National Cancer Institute, 86,* 539-548.

Miller, B. A., Kolonel, L. N., Bernstein, L., Young, J. L., Jr., Swanson, G. M., West, D., Key, C. R., Liff, J. M., Glover, C. S., & Alexander, G. A. (Eds.). (1996). *Racial/ethnic patterns of cancer in the United States 1988-1992.* National Cancer Institute. NIH Pub. No. 96-4104. Bethesda, MD.

Mitchell, M. F. (1993). Preinvasive diseases of the female lower genital tract. In D. M. Gershenson, A. H. DeCherney, & S. L. Curry, *Operative gynecology.* Philadelphia: W.B. Saunders.

Mitchell, M. F., Hittelman, W. K., Lotan, R., Nishioka, K., Luna, G. T., Kortum, R. R., Wharton, J. T., & Hong, W. K. (1995). Chemoprevention trials and surrogate end point biomarkers in the cervix. *Cancer, 76*(10), 1956-1972.

Mitchell, M. F., Sandella, J. A., & White, L. N. (1992). Cervical cancer: The role of the human papilloma virus. *Current Issues in Cancer Nursing Practice Updates, 1*(2), 1-9.

Mitsuhashi, N., Takahashi, M., Yamakawa, M., Nozaki, M., Takahashi, T., Sakurai, H., Maebayashi, K., Hayakawa, K., & Niibe, H. (1995). Results of postoperative radiation therapy for patients with carcinoma of the uterine cervix: Evaluation of intravaginal cone boost with an electron beam. *Gynecologic Oncology, 57,* 321-326.

Murad, A. M., Triginelli, S. A., & Ribalta, J. C. L. (1994). Phase II trial of bleomycin, ifosfamide, and carboplatin in metastatic cervical cancer. *Journal of Clinical Oncology, 12,* 55-59.

Nagell, J. R., DePriest, P. D., Higgins, R. V., & Powell, D. E. (1993). Surgical therapy for cervical cancer. In D. M. Gershenson, A. H. DeCherney, & S. L. Curry (Eds.), *Operative Gynecology.* Philadelphia: W.B. Saunders.

Namkoong, S. E., Park, J. S., Kim, J. W., Bae, S. N., Han, G. T., Lee, J. M., Jung, J. K., Kim, S. J. (1995). Comparative study of the patients with locally advanced stages I and II cervical cancer treated by radical surgery with and without preoperative adjuvant chemotherapy. *Gynecologic Oncology, 59,* 136-142.

National Cancer Institute. (1996). *Cancer rates and risks* (4th ed). Rockville, MD: National Institutes of Health.

Neijt, J. P. (1994). Advances in the chemotherapy of gynecologic cancer. *Current Opinion in Oncology, 6,* 531-538.

Palefsky, J. M. & Holly, E. A. (1995). Molecular virology and epidemiology of human papillomavirus and cervical cancer. *Cancer Epidemiology, Biomarkers, & Prevention, 4,* 415-428.

Park, R. C. & Thigpen, J. T. (1993). Chemotherapy in advanced and recurrent cervical cancer. *Cancer, 71,* 1446-1450.

Park, T. K., Lee, S. K., Kim, S. N., Hwang, T. S., Kim, G. E., Suh, C. O., & Loh, J. K. (1993). Combined chemotherapy and radiation for bulky stages I-II cervical cancer: Comparison of concurrent and sequential regimens. *Gynecologic Oncology, 50,* 196-201.

Patterson, K. A. & Carnago, L. (1996). Female reproductive problems. In S. M. Lewis, I. C. Collier, & M. M. Heitkemper (Eds.), *Medical-surgical nursing* (4th ed.). St. Louis: Mosby.

Peipert, J. F., Wells, C. K., Schwartz, P. E., & Feinstein, A. R. (1994). Prognostic value of clinical variables in invasive cervical cancer. *Obstetrics & Gynecology, 84,* 746-751.

Perez, C. A. (1993a). Radiation therapy in the management of cancer of the cervix. *Oncology, 7*(2), 89-96.

Perez, C. A. (1993b). Radiation therapy in the management of the cervix, part 2. *Oncology 7*(3), 61-70.

Plante, M. & Roy, M. (1995). The use of operative laparoscopy in determining eligibility for pelvic exenteration in patients with recurrent cervical cancer. *Gynecologic Oncology, 59,* 401-404.

Potischman, N. (1993). Nutritional epidemiology of cervical neoplasia. *Journal of Nutrition, 123,* 424-429.

Powel, L. (1996). *Cancer chemotherapy guidelines and recommendations for practice.* Pittsburgh, PA: Oncology Nursing Society.

Rabkin, C. S., Biggar, R. J., Baptiste, M. S., Abe, T., Kohler, B. A., & Nasca, P. C. (1993). Cancer incidence trends in women at high risk of human immunodeficiency virus (HIV) infection. *International Journal of Cancer, 55,* 208-212.

Resbeut, M., Cowen, D., Viens, P., Noirclerc, M., Perez, T., Gouvernet, J., Delpero, J. R., Gamerre, M., Boubli, L., Houvenaeghel, G. (1994). Concomitant chemoradiation prior to surgery in the treatment of advanced cervical carcinoma. *Gynecologic Oncology, 54,* 68-75.

Robinson, W. R. & Muderspach, L. I. (1993). Spinal cord compression in metastatic cervical cancer. *Gynecologic Oncology, 48,* 269-271.

Rodrigues, M., Sevin, B. U., Perras, J., Nguyen, G. N., Pham, C., Steren, A. J., Koechli, O. R., & Averette, H. E. (1995). Paclitaxel: A radiation sensitizer of human cervical cancer cells. *Gynecologic Oncology, 57,* 165-169.

Rotkin, I. D. (1967). Adolescent coitus and cervical cancer: Associations of related events with increased risk. *Cancer Research, 27,* 603-617.

Rotman, M., Pajak, T. F., Choi, K., Clery, M., Varcial, V., Grigsby, P. W., Cooper, J., & John, M. (1995). Prophylactic extended-field irradiation of para-aortic lymph nodes in stages II B and bulky IB and IIA cervical carcinomas. *Journal of the American Medical Association, 274,* 387-393.

Sarma, D., Yang, X., Jin, G., Shindoh, M., Pater, M. M., & Pater, A. (1996). Resistance to retinoic acid and altered cytokeratin expression of human papillomavirus type 16-immortalized endocervical cells after tumorigenesis. *International Journal of Cancer, 65,* 345-350.

Schlesselman, J. J. (1995). Net effect of oral contraceptive use on the risk of cancer in women in the United States. *Obstetrics and Gynecology, 85*(5), 793-801.

Shindoh, M., Sun, Q., Pater, A., & Pater, M. M. (1995). Prevention of carcinoma in situ in human papilloma type 16-immortalized human endocervical cells by retinoic acid in organotypic raft culture. *Obstetrics and Gynecology, 85*(5), 721-728.

Shingleton, H. M., Bell, M. C., Fremgen, A., Chmiel, J. S., Russell, A. H., Jones, W. B., Winchester, D. P., Clive, R. E. (1995). Is there really a difference in survival of women with squamous cell carcinoma, adenocarcinoma, and adenosquamous cell carcinoma of the cervix? *Cancer, 76,* 1948-1955.

Southwest Oncology Group (SWOG) Coordinating Center (1995). *Protocol SWOG - 9146.* San Antonio, TX.

Stewart, A. M., Eriksson, A. M., Manos, M. M., Munoz, N., Bosch, R. X., Peto, J., & Wheeler, C. M. (1996). Intratype variation in 12 human papillomavirus types: A worldwide perspective. *Journal of Virology, 70*(5), 3129-3136.

Stornes, I., Mejlholm, I., & Jakobsen, A. (1994). A phase II trial of ifosfamide, 5-fluorouracil, and leucovorin in recurrent uterine cervical cancer. *Gynecologic Oncology, 55,* 123-125.

Subak, L. L., Hricak, H., Powell, C.B., Azizi, L., & Stern, J. L. (1995). Cervical carcinoma: Computed tomography and magnetic resonance imaging for preoperative staging. *Obstetrics and Gynecology, 86*(1), 43-50.

Sueyama, H., Nakano, M., Sakumoto, K., Toita, T., Takizawa, Y., Moromizato, H., Kakihana, Y., Kushi, A., Moromizato, H., Higashi, M., Kanazawa, K. (1995). Intra-arterial chemotherapy with cisplatin followed by radical radiotherapy for locally advanced cervical cancer. *Gynecologic Oncology, 59,* 329-332.

Tomaino-Brunner, C., Freda, M. C., & Runowicz, C. D. (1996). "I hope I don't have cancer": Colposcopy and minority women. *Oncology Nursing Forum, 23*(1), 39-44.

Walczak, J. R. & Klemm, P. R. (1993). Gynecologic cancers. In S. L. Groenwald, M. H. Frogge, M. Goodman, & C. H. Yarbro (Eds.), *Cancer nursing: principles and practice* (3rd ed.). Boston: Jones & Bartlett.

Wain, G. V., Farnsworth, A., & Hacker, N. F. (1992). The Papanicolaou smear histories of 237 patients with cervical cancer. *Medical Journal of Australia, 157,* 14-16.

Wank, R. & Thomassen, C. (1991). High risk of squamous cell carcinoma of the cervix for women with HLA-DQw3. *Nature, 352,* 723-725.

Way, S. (1976). Carcinoma-in-situ of cervix in sisters. *British Medical Journal, 1,* 890.

Werner-Wasik, M., Schmid, C. H., Bornstein, L. E., & Madoc-Jones, H. (1995). Increased risk of second malignant neoplasms outside radiation fields in patients with cervical carcinoma. *Cancer, 75,* 2281-2285.

Wharton, J. T. (1996). Neoplasms of the cervix. In J. F. Holland, R. C. Bast, Jr, D. L. Morton, E. Frei, III, D. W. Kufe, & R. R. Weichselbaum (Eds.), *Cancer medicine* (4th ed.). Baltimore: Williams & Wilkins.

Whitehead, N., Reyner, F., & Lindenbaum, J. (1993). Megaloblastic changes in the cervical epithelium: Association with oral contraceptive therapy and reversal with folic acid. *Journal of the American Medical Association, 226,* 1421-1424.

Wright, T. C. & Richart, R. M. (1992). Preinvasive lesion of the lower genital tract. In W. J. Hoskins, C. A. Perez, & R. C. Young (Eds.), *Principles and practice of gynecologic oncology.* Philadelphia: JB Lippincott.

Yang, X., Jin, G., Nakao, Y., Rahimtula, M., Pater, M. M., & Pater, A. (1996). Malignant transformation of HPV 16-immortalized human endocervical cells by cigarette smoke condensate and characterization of multistage carcinogenesis. *International Journal of Cancer, 65,* 338-344.

Ye, Z., Thomas, D. B., & Ray, R. M. (1995). Combined oral contraceptives and risk of cervical carcinoma in situ. *International Journal of Epidemiology, 24*(1), 19-26.

Zaino, R. J., Ward, S., Delgado, G., Bundy, B., Gore, H., Fetter, G., Ganjei, P., & Frauenhoffer, E. (1992). Histopathologic predictors of the behavior of surgically treated stage IB squamous cell carcinoma of the cervix: A Gynecologic Oncology Group Study. *Cancer, 69,* 1750-1758.

Zanetta, G. M., Katzmann, J. A., Keeney, G. L., Kinney, W. K., Cha, S. S., Podratz, K. C. (1992). Flow cytometric DNA analysis of stages IB and 2A cervical cancer. *Gynecologic Oncology, 46,* 13-19.

Zhang, Z. F. & Begg, C. (1994). Is Trichomonas vaginalis a cause of cervical neoplasia? Results from a combined analysis of 24 studies. *International Journal of Epidemiology, 23,* 682-690.

Zhang, Z. F., Graham, S., Yu, S. Z., Marshall, J., Zielezny, M., Chen, Y. X., Sun, M., Tang, S. L., Liao, C. S., Xu, J. L., & Yang, X. Z. (1995). Trichomonas vaginalis and cervical cancer: A prospective study in China. *Annals in Epidemiology 5,* 325-332.

Endometrial Cancer

Catherine Hydzik, RN, MS
Margaret Cawley, RN, MS

EPIDEMIOLOGY

Endometrial cancer is the most prevalent and curable gynecologic malignancy in the United States. In 1998 the American Cancer Society estimated that 36,100 new cases were diagnosed and 6300 women died of the disease (Landis, Murray, Bolden, & Wingo, 1998). Early diagnosis, due to the occurrence of vaginal bleeding, is the major factor accounting for the low mortality rate (Creasman, 1994). Approximately 79% of all cases are diagnosed with the tumor confined within the uterus (Hubbard & Holcombe, 1990).

Ninety-seven percent of uterine cancers arise from the endometrial glands. The remaining 3% are sarcomas and are discussed in another chapter (Rose, 1996). Cancer of the endometrium is predominantly a disease of postmenopausal women; the median age at diagnosis is 63 years (Rose, 1996).

Presently there is a higher incidence of endometrial cancer in western societies compared with a low rate in eastern countries. Nutrition may be a causative factor because of the higher animal fat content in western diets (Park, Grigsby, Muss & Norris, 1992).

During the 1970s, the incidence of endometrial cancer rose to 39,000 cases. This eightfold increase was related to the use of unopposed estrogens for menopausal symptoms during the late 1960s and early 1970s. Since this practice has been discontinued and replaced with combined estrogen-progesterone preparations, the incidence of endometrial cancer has decreased (Rose, 1996). It is of interest to note that a worldwide increase in the incidence of endometrial cancer has been reported, even in countries where unopposed estrogen is not prescribed. This increase has been attributed in part to the increasing longevity of women (Rose, 1996).

RISK FACTORS

The major risk factors associated with the development of endometrial cancer are listed in Box 30-1. The evidence supporting each of these risk factors is reviewed and nursing implications for prevention and early detection are discussed. Approximately 50% of endometrial carcinomas occur in women with particular risk factors for the disease (Rose, 1996).

Unopposed Estrogen

That estrogen stimulates the endometrium when not opposed by progesterone has been recognized for a long time. Elevated levels of estrogen are directly related to the development of endometrial hyperplasia that may progress to a carcinoma. Sources of estrogen may be endogenous and exogenous.

Hormones such as estrogen influence the development of cancer by controlling the rate of cell division as well as cellular differentiation. Estrogen increases the mitotic rate of endometrial cells, whereas progestins oppose this effect by decreasing the number of estrogen receptors. The risk of cancer increases in proportion to the dose of estrogen and the duration of exposure to unopposed estrogen by progestins (Key, 1995).

It is thought that the decrease in estrogen levels associated with menopause may stimulate an increase in androstenedione, an estrogen precursor, in a negative feedback pathway. Androstenedione is converted to estrone, the most prevalent postmenopausal estrogen, which may lead to the development of endometrial hyperplasia (Martin & Braly, 1991).

Unopposed exogenous estrogens, as used for the treatment of menopausal symptoms in the late 1960s and early 1970s, resulted in an eightfold increase in endometrial cancer. The combined use of estrogen-progesterone preparations has decreased this incidence. However, endometrial cancer continues to be a problem in women treated with regimens that have less than the recommended 12 days of progesterone (Rose, 1996). Postmenopausal women on both estrogen and progestin replacement actually have a lower risk for endometrial cancer than untreated women (Muto & Friedman, 1995).

Box 30-1
Risk Factors for Endometrial Cancer

Unopposed estrogens
Obesity
Tamoxifen use
Early menarche, nulliparity, late menopause
Diabetes and hypertension

Obesity

In postmenopausal obese women, the increased risk may be related to the increase in production and bioavailability of endogenous estrogens. Adipose tissue is an excellent storage depot for estrogen, and the chronic release of estrogen from these cells may account for the increased risk. In addition, the secretion of serum sex hormone–binding globulin may be depressed in postmenopausal women, resulting in higher serum concentrations of free estradiol (Walczak & Klemm, 1993).

Twenty-five percent of the women who develop endometrial cancer are premenopausal; the majority of these women are obese. Premenopausal obese women often experience endocrine malfunction, such as polycystic ovarian disease, which causes chronic anovulation and irregular menses, resulting in reduced progesterone production and the inability to oppose the effects of estrogen on the endometrium (Walczak & Klemm, 1993; Rose, 1996).

The level of risk is directly related to the degree of obesity. Women who are 30 pounds over their ideal weight have a threefold increased risk of developing endometrial cancer. This risk increases tenfold if the women are 50 pounds or more over ideal weight (Park, Grigsby, Muss, & Norris, 1992).

Historically, hypertension, diabetes, and obesity have been referred to as a triad of disorders associated with endometrial cancer. However, studies appear to indicate a casual rather than a causal relationship. Hypertension and diabetes are altered physiologic states associated with endometrial cancer. Hypertension is prevalent in elderly, obese individuals but does not seem to be a significant factor in and of itself.

Tamoxifen Use

Since the mid 1970s, tamoxifen has been a mainstay in the treatment of breast cancer. Tamoxifen is a synthetic estrogen antagonist (antiestrogen) that acts by competing with estrogen for estrogen receptors. However, tamoxifen acts as a estrogenic agonist on the endometrium. A number of studies suggest an association between tamoxifen treatment and the development of endometrial cancer (Seoud, Johnson, & Weed, 1993). In a Swedish study of 1800 postmenopausal women (Abeler & Kjorstand, 1991), 12 new cases of endometrial cancer were found in women on tamoxifen compared with 2 in the control group. Data from the South Western Oncology Group identified that 4 of 966 women treated with tamoxifen developed endometrial cancer compared with none in the control group. Another study found that the relative risk of 2.6 for developing endometrial carcinoma with tamoxifen increased to 7.1 in women treated with tamoxifen and pelvic irradiation. Seoud, Johnson, & Weed (1993) concluded that tamoxifen is a safe and reliable treatment for breast cancer, but data suggest an association between tamoxifen and the development of endometrial cancer. These authors suggest that women on tamoxifen need to be monitored closely for endometrial cancer.

Early Menarche, Nulliparity, and Late Menopause

Epidemiologic data suggest that endometrial and breast cancers share similar risk factors, including early menarche, late menopause, and nulliparity. Early menarche and late menopause are factors that relate to the length of time that the endometrium is exposed to estrogen. Nulliparity is often associated with endocrine malfunction causing anovulatory cycles that result in failure of progesterone to oppose the continuous stimulation of estrogen on the endometrium. As mentioned previously, obesity is associated with endocrine malfunction in premenopausal women (Walczak & Klemm, 1993).

Protective Action of Oral Contraceptives

The use of oral contraceptives and the associated risk of endometrial cancer have changed with alterations in their formulations. Sequential contraceptives prescribed in the 1970s used unopposed estrogen and increased the risk of endometrial cancer by up to tenfold. Sequential oral contraceptives were removed from the American market in 1976 (Henderson, Ross, & Pike, 1993).

Presently, oral contraceptives have a lower dose of estrogen combined with progesterone, which provides a protective effect against endometrial cancer. The use of combined oral contraceptives for 1 year reduces the risk of endometrial cancer by approximately 20%, and their use for 4 years reduces the risk by 50% (Key, 1995). Epidemiologic studies confirm that protection lasts for at least 15 years after cessation of contraceptive use (Henderson, Ross, & Pike, 1993).

HEALTH PROMOTION

As the population ages, more women will be at risk for the development of endometrial cancer. Health promotion activities by oncology nurses directed toward a reduction in the prevalence of obesity will have several beneficial effects on women's health. Decreasing obesity in postmenopausal women will have a marked effect on the amount of endometrial exposure to unopposed estrogen, thereby decreasing the development of hyperplasia and the potential for progression to cancer.

Postmenopausal women need to be educated to report any vaginal bleeding that occurs 6 months after their menses stops. This abnormal symptom is often ignored and assumed to be related to menopausal changes. In addition,

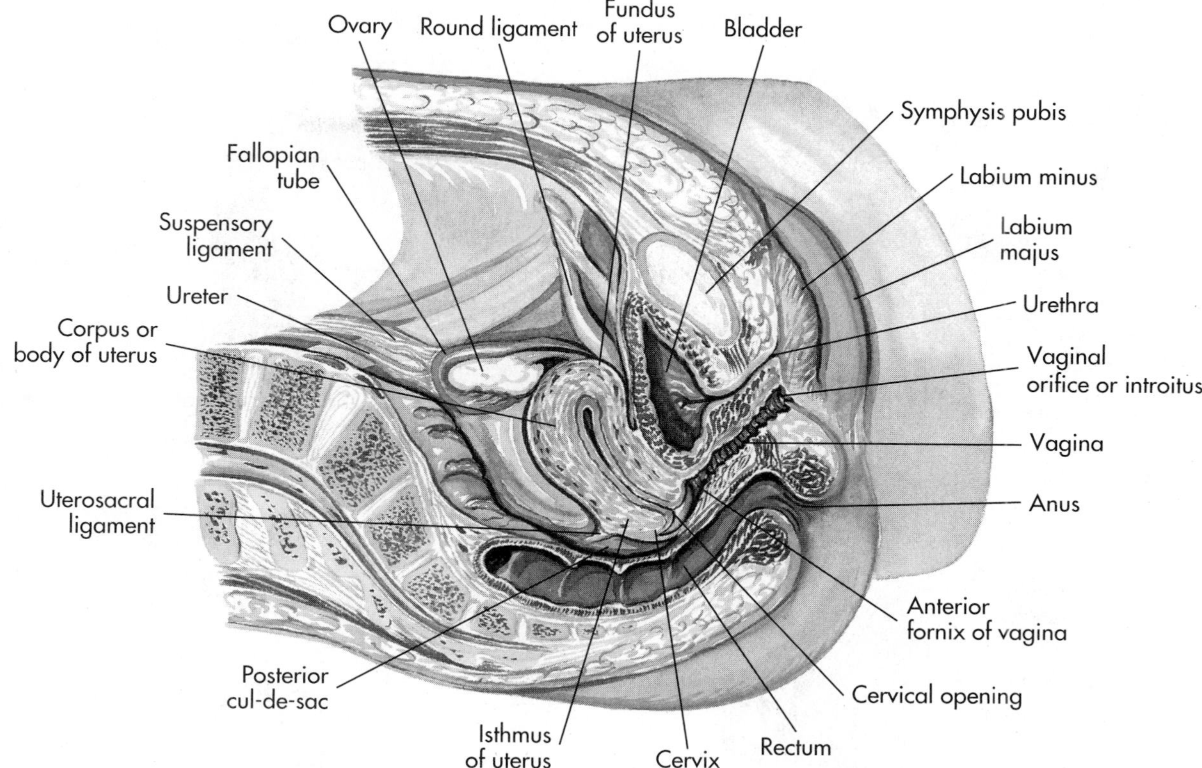

Fig. 30-1 Internal female genitalia and other pelvic organs. (From Bobak, I. M., Jensen, M. D., & Zalar, M. K. [1993]. *Maternity and gynecologic care: The nurse and the family.* [5th ed]. St. Louis: Mosby.)

women on tamoxifen for the treatment of breast cancer, as well as high-risk individuals receiving tamoxifen in clinical trials, need to be informed of the risks and benefits, as well as the potential adverse effects such as abnormal vaginal bleeding. It is essential that these women comply with annually scheduled gynecologic examinations, including a Pap smear. Premenopausal women need to be educated to report any abnormal vaginal bleeding to their health care team so an appropriate evaluation can be performed. An essential role for the oncology nurse is to educate women about early detection (Hall, Dewar, & Perchalski, 1992).

PREVENTION

Presently, there are no specific chemoprevention efforts in place to prevent the initiation or promotion of endometrial cancer. However, women diagnosed with atypical hyperplasia, the potential precursor to endometrial cancer, may be treated with hysterectomy or periodic use of progestins. Hysterectomy is the preferred treatment for postmenopausal women; premenopausal women with reproductive desires may be offered regimens of progestins (Park et al., 1992).

Premenopausal women who are amenorrheic or hypermenorrheic and who are experiencing fluctuating levels of estrogen should be treated periodically with progestins to create scheduled withdrawal bleeding, thereby preventing the development of hyperplasia and the potential progression to carcinoma (Park et al., 1992).

PATHOPHYSIOLOGY

Normal Anatomy and Physiology of the Uterus

The uterus is a hollow muscular organ located in the female pelvis (Fig. 30-1) between the bladder and rectum. It is divided structurally and functionally into two parts, the body (corpus) and the cervix, which are separated by a slight narrowing known as the *isthmus*. The cervix extends into the vagina.

The uterine corpus is attached to the surrounding pelvic structures by two pairs of ligaments, the broad and the round. Two other pairs of ligaments, the uterosacral and the cardinal, provide most of the support for the uterus and cervix.

The main blood supply to the uterus is from the uterine artery, which is a branch of the internal iliac artery. Lymphatic drainage begins in the retroperitoneal region through the obturator lymph nodes, then to the internal and external iliac nodes that then drain into the common and para-aortic nodes. The entire uterus is innervated by both motor and sensory neurons of the autonomic nervous system.

The uterine wall contains three layers: the perimetrium, the myometrium, and the endometrium (Fig. 30-2). An understanding of the layers is important because prognosis is related to the depth of invasion within the layers. The perimetrium is the outermost layer covering the uterus. The middle muscular layer, the myometrium, is thickest at

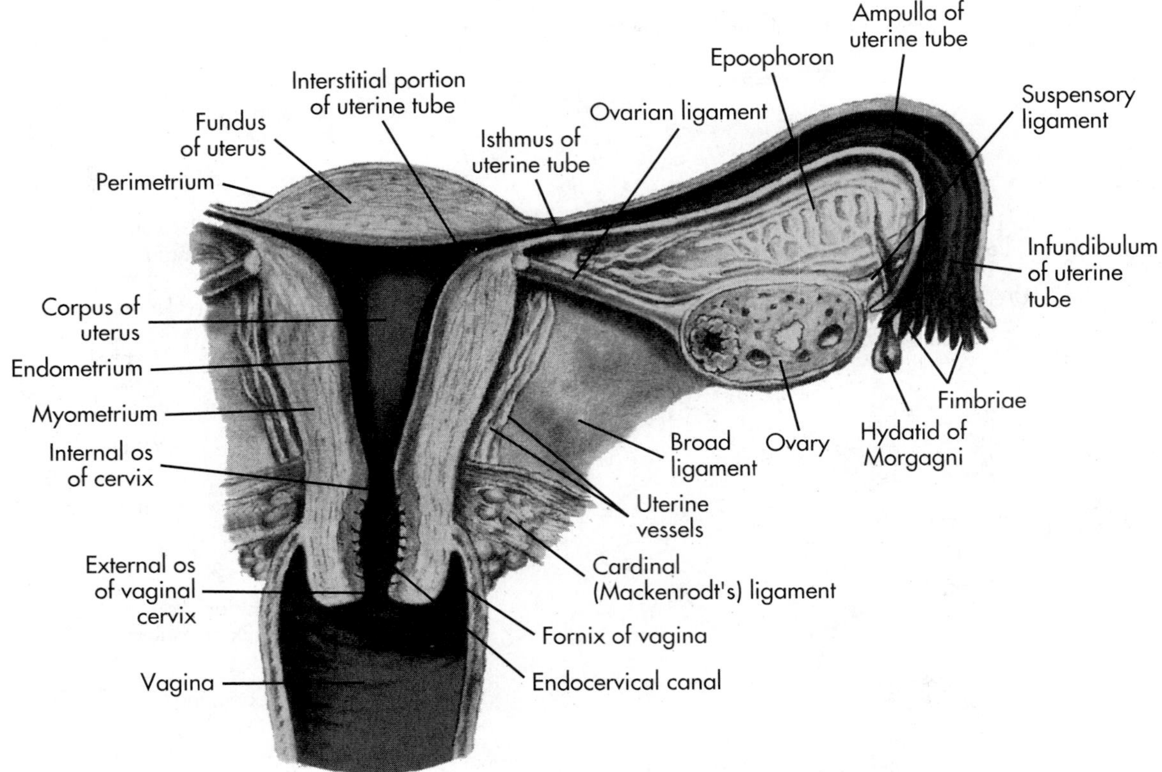

Fig. 30-2 Cross-section of the uterus, fallopian tube, and ovary. (From Lowdermilk, D. L., Perry, S. E., & Bobak, I. M. (1997). *Maternity and Women's Health Care* (6th ed.). St. Louis: Mosby.)

the fundus, facilitating the birthing process. The inner uterine layer that lines the uterus is composed of two layers: the functional layer that is responsive to sex hormones and the basal layer that is attached to the myometrium. Between puberty and menopause, the functional layer proliferates and sheds each month and is then regenerated by the basal layer (Robinson, McCance, & Gray, 1994).

At puberty, the uterus reaches adult size and descends from the abdomen into the lower pelvis. The uterus is approximately 9 cm long and 6.5 cm wide, with muscular walls 3.5 cm thick. In most women, the uterus is anteverted, or tipped forward, resting on the urinary bladder. Various degrees of flexion are within normal limits, and in some women their uterus may be retroverted.

The functions of the uterus include (1) anchoring and protecting the fertilized ovum, (2) providing an optimal environment while the ovum develops, and (3) expelling the fetus at the time of birth. In addition, the uterus plays an important role in sexual response and conception.

The uterus is an integral structure within the female reproductive system. Regulation between ovarian functions and endometrial changes are controlled by cyclic hormonal changes. Physiologic changes in the endometrium are initiated by the secretion of follicle-stimulating hormone and luteinizing hormone and involves the production of estrogens and progesterone from the ovaries.

During a normal menstrual cycle, the endometrium undergoes three specific phases: proliferative, secretory, and menstrual. During the proliferative phase, increased levels of estrogen contribute to the growth and thickening of the endometrium. After ovulation, the secretory phase occurs with an increase in the levels of progesterone. The endometrium continues to thicken and appears velvet-like. If implantation of the ovum does not take place, a sharp drop in estrogen and progesterone occurs. This drop in hormone levels results in ischemic changes in the arterioles, leading to sloughing of tissue, or menstrual bleeding.

The Process of Carcinogenesis

Just as with other cancers, the development of endometrial cancer appears to involve premalignant stages. Endometrial hyperplasia has long been regarded as a precursor of endometrial cancer. Hyperplasia of the endometrium is an abnormal increase in the number and size of proliferating glands in the endometrium. Hyperplasia may progress to the development of a carcinoma.

Simple hyperplasia is a benign proliferation of the endometrium with an increase in the number of cystically dilated glands that have outpouchings and invaginations that produce an irregular outline of the enlarged glands. In complex hyperplasia, the increased irregular glands are crowded back to back. Atypical hyperplasia is characterized by an increased number of cells with cytologic atypia. These atypical cells have an increased nuclear/cytoplasmic ratio. The enlarged nuclei are irregular in size and shape.

Simple and complex hyperplasias are proliferative responses to unopposed estrogenic stimulation and pose little risk of progression to a carcinoma. Conversely, nuclear atypia present in atypical hyperplasia is clearly associated with the subsequent development of carcinoma. It is the degree of cytologic atypia that determines the malignant potential of endometrial hyperplasia. Cytologic atypia progresses to adenocarcinoma 29% of the time (Muto & Friedman, 1995), whereas only 2% of cases of hyperplasia with atypia progress to carcinoma (Kurman, Zaino, & Norris, 1994).

Hyperplasia develops as a result of unopposed estrogen stimulation on the endometrium. Most women have a history of either persistent anovulation or exogenous unopposed estrogen use. In premenopausal women, an anovulatory state, such as polycystic ovarian syndrome, causes the nonproduction of progesterone by the corpus luteum, resulting in continuous estrogen levels and inducing endometrial proliferation. Women who are obese may have hyperplasia as a result of peripheral conversion of androstenedione to estrogen in adipose tissue.

Genetic Predisposition

A genetic predisposition for endometrial cancer has been suggested because of the results of several studies that correlate a high incidence of endometrial and breast cancer among sisters, mothers, and aunts of individuals with endometrial cancer (Kurman Zaino, & Norris, 1994).

Recently, two forms of inherited endometrial cancers have been proposed, namely a cancer family syndrome known as the *Lynch syndrome II* and a predisposition to endometrial carcinoma alone. In the Lynch syndrome II, females are at an increased risk of developing ovarian carcinoma, and 20% to 30% of affected women develop endometrial cancer. In addition, male and female family members are at an increased risk for developing colon cancers (Kurman, Zaino, & Norris, 1994).

Epidemiologic and clinicopathologic evidence supports the hypothesis that there may be two different genetic forms of endometrial carcinoma: an estrogen-dependent and a non–estrogen-related carcinoma. The estrogen-dependent form appears to occur in younger premenopausal and perimenopausal women with hyperplasia, tends to be low grade and well differentiated, has minimal myometrial invasion, and is associated with endometrial tumors. The non-estrogen-related tumors occur in postmenopausal women without hyperplasia, but with poorly differentiated high-grade tumors and deep myometrial invasion. In addition these tumors are associated in serous, clear cell, and adenosquamous endometrial carcinoma (Kurman, Zaino, & Norris, 1994).

ROUTES OF METASTASES

Cancer of the endometrium most often begins in the fundus and may spread throughout the entire endometrium. Through direct extension and infiltration, the cancer can spread to the myometrium, endocervix, cervix, vagina, fallopian tubes, and ovaries. Adnexal spread is not common; it is found in approximately 10% of women with stage I disease (Walczak & Klemm, 1993).

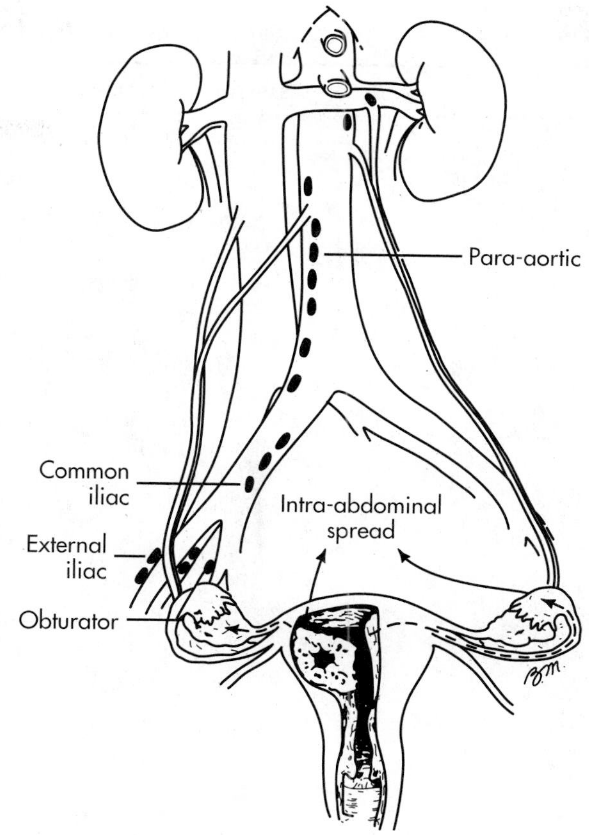

Fig. 30-3 Spread pattern of endometrial cancer. (From DiSaia P. J., & Creasman, W. T. [1993]. Adenocarcinoma of the uterus. In P. J. Di Saia & W. T. Creasman [Eds.], *Clinical gynecologic oncology.* St Louis: Mosby.)

Factors influencing metastatic spread include tumor differentiation, stage of the disease, and degree of myometrial invasion. Metastatic spread occurs through both lymphatic and hematogenous routes. Lymphatic spread begins in the pelvic lymph nodes and extends to the para-aortic lymph nodes (Fig. 30-3). The hematogenous route affects the lung, liver, bone, and brain (Walczak & Klemm, 1993).

ASSESSMENT

Clinical evaluation of the patient involves a detailed history, a thorough physical examination, and a variety of diagnostic tests (Table 30-1). The signs and symptoms present in the patient often depend on the stage of disease at the time of diagnosis.

History

The patient should be evaluated for all of the identified risk factors for endometrial cancer. In addition, a careful history of the patient's symptoms (e.g., vaginal bleeding) should be

Table 30-1 Assessment of the Patient for Endometrial Cancer

	Assessment Parameters	Typical Abnormal Findings
History	A. Personal and social history	A. Personal and social risk factors
	1. Age	1. Usually over age 50. Median age at time of diagnosis is 63 years.
	2. Ethnicity	2. The incidence among black women is significantly lower than among white women.
	3. Family history	3. Most common in women with the hereditary nonpolyposis colorectal cancer syndrome (Lynch syndrome II).
	4. Menstrual history a. Date of menarche/menopause b. Infertility	4. Early menarche and late menopause are factors that increase the length of estrogen exposure to the endometrium. Nulliparity is often associated with endocrine malfunction and failure of progesterone to oppose estrogen.
	5. Use of estrogen replacement therapy	5. Estrogen unopposed by progesterone stimulates the development of hyperplasia.
	6. Use of tamoxifen	6. Tamoxifen acts as an estrogenic agonist on the endometrium.
	7. Triad of medical disorders a. Diabetes b. Hypertension c. Obesity	7. This triad of disorders has been associated with endometrial cancer. However studies indicate a casual rather than a causal relationship.
	B. Evaluation of vaginal bleeding	B. Premenopausal women may report prolonged, heavy menstrual periods and intermenstrual spotting. Postmenopausal women may report abnormal vaginal bleeding and spotting.
	C. Evaluation of other signs/symptoms	C. Less frequent signs/symptoms include: yellow or serosanguineous vaginal discharge, pyometria, hematometria, and lumbosacral/pelvic pain.
	D. Evaluation for advanced disease	D. Presence of ascites, jaundice, bowel obstruction, respiratory distress, or hemorrhage may indicate advanced disease.
Physical Examination	A. Pelvic examination	A. Patient may have an enlarged uterus. Palpate the size and shape of the uterus.
	B. Rectal examination with stool guaiac test	B. Stool guaiac may be positive.
	C. Weight	C. Obesity is a risk factor.
Diagnostic Tests	A. Papanicolaou smear	A. About one third to one half of patients with adenocarcinoma of the endometrium have abnormal Pap smears. The reason is that the cells are not taken from the area of the lesion.
	B. Endometrial biopsy. Assess estrogen and progesterone receptors, ploidy, S-phase fraction, DNA index, proliferative index, p53 and *Her 2/neu* expression.	B. To diagnose and identify prognostic factors.
	C. Fractional dilation and curettage (D&C)	C. Provides histologic information regarding cell type and grade of tumor.
	D. Transvaginal ultrasound	D. To evaluate the depth of myometrial invasion. In women with cervical stenosis, the ultrasonography can be used to guide the performance of D&C.
	E. Blood tests Routine hematologic studies Clotting profiles Ca-125 Ca-15-3 or Ca-27-29	E. These markers may help to predict the risk and response to therapy.

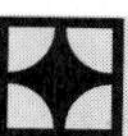

TABLE 30-1 Assessment of the Patient for Endometrial Cancer—cont'd

	Assessment Parameters	Typical Abnormal Findings
Diagnostic Tests—cont'd	F. Computerized tomography scan	F. To show extent of disease in the pelvis.
	G. Presurgical metastatic evaluation Chest x-ray Urogram	G. Changes on chest x-ray indicate metastatic disease. Positive urogram indicates spread of disease to the bladder.
	H. Palpable disease outside the uterus or symptoms related to bowel disease Sigmoidoscopy Barium enema	H. To assess extent of the disease if disease is suspected.
	I. Magnetic resonance imaging	I. To estimate the extent of myometrial invasion and identify possible nodal involvement. Frequently shows widening of the endometrial cavity or fluid.
	J. Peritoneal fluid obtained for cytologic analysis	J. To identify the presence of any suspicious cells.
	K. Surgical exploration	K. Peritoneal cytologic sampling, abdominal exploration, palpation, and biopsy of any suspicious lymph nodes or lesions.

obtained. The patient may less frequently report the following symptoms: yellow or serosanguineous vaginal discharge, pyometria, hematometria, or lumbosacral/pelvic pain. Patients with advanced disease may complain of ascites, jaundice, bowel obstruction, respiratory distress, or hemorrhage.

Physical Examination

A pelvic examination allows palpation of the uterus and noting of its size, shape, consistency, and mobility and enables the identification of any tenderness or masses. When performing a pelvic examination, particular attention to the vagina is important, as this is a frequent site of metastasis. The size of the uterus varies depending on the woman's age. The uterus usually starts to diminish in size after a woman reaches 40 years of age.

As part of the physical examination, other signs and symptoms must be assessed. The presence of vaginal bleeding, yellow or serosanguineous vaginal discharge, ascites, jaundice, bowel obstruction, respiratory distress, or hemorrhage should be determined.

Diagnostic Tests

Papanicolaou Smear. Detection of endometrial cancer by routine Papanicolaou (Pap) smear has been poor when compared with the efficacy of the Pap smear in diagnosing cervical cancer. Only one third to one half of patients with endometrial carcinoma have abnormal Pap smears. The poor detection rate is because the cells are not directly obtained from the lesion but from the cervix (DiSaia & Creasman, 1993).

Endometrial Biopsy, Hormone Receptor Status, and Tumor Ploidy. The presence of progesterone receptors is determined by an endometrial biopsy and is measured using competitive binding assays or by immunohistochemical techniques. A positive progesterone assay may predict the responsiveness of the tumor to progestational therapy and also indicates a survival advantage in patients with advanced endometrial cancer (Homesley & Zaino, 1994).

Using flow cytometry, the DNA in the biopsy specimen can be measured. This technique can distinguish if the malignant cells are diploid or aneuploid and can estimate the proportion of cells in different stages of the cell cycle.

Diploid tumors tend to be histologically well differentiated, whereas aneuploid tumors are poorly differentiated. Generally, women with poorly differentiated tumors are at high risk for extrauterine metastases and relapse (Homesley & Zaino, 1994).

Fractional Dilation and Curettage. Fractional dilation and curettage (D&C) provides the maximum amount of tissue from the endometrial cavity for diagnostic study. Tumor grade and histologic cell type are determined from the tissue sampling.

Transvaginal Ultrasound. Transvaginal ultrasonography provides an accurate measurement of the thickness of the endometrium. The thickness of normal and abnormal endometrium varies. Standard deviation measurements have been established for women with atrophic hyperplasia and those with carcinoma of the endometrium. According to Rose (1996), a cut-off value of 5 mm or more for abnormal endometrial thickness should result in few endometrial carcinomas being missed. A cut-off of 3 mm should be used for women of Asian descent (Rose, 1996). In women with cervical stenosis or abnormal anatomic features, ultrasonography can be used to guide the instrumentation of the dilation and curettage.

Blood Tests. In addition to routine hematologic studies (e.g., complete blood count, chemistries, and clotting profiles) required as a baseline and preoperatively, prognostic markers such as CA-125, CA-15-3, and CA-27-29 are analyzed to assist in determining the risk of extrauterine spread. Serum levels of CA-125 are elevated in most women with advanced or metastatic endometrial cancer. In addition, if the initial value of CA-125 is elevated with values exceeding 35 U/ml, responses to therapy may be evaluated if subsequent levels of CA-125 decrease.

Presurgical Metastatic Evaluation. Diagnostic tests performed to assist in the presurgical evaluation for metastatic disease include chest x-ray, pelvic computerized tomography scan, urogram, and barium enema. A cystoscopy and sigmoidoscopy may also be performed to determine metastatic spread to the mucosa of the bladder or rectum.

Magnetic Resonance Imaging. Magnetic resonance imaging can provide a preoperative estimate of myometrial invasion, as well as identify possible nodal involvement.

Cytologic Analysis of Peritoneal Fluid. Cytologic analysis of peritoneal fluids or washings is an important prognostic and staging test for pelvic malignancies. The presence of malignant cells in peritoneal fluid or washings in women with endometrial cancer is indicative of a poor prognosis. Women with positive cytologic washings may also have extrauterine disease that includes metastases to the pelvic or periaortic lymph nodes and intraperitoneal spread.

Surgical Exploration. At the time of surgery, pelvic and periaortic nodal sampling is performed, as indicated, for staging purposes. Peritoneal washings are obtained before the nodal sampling. As expected, women without lymph node metastases have a much better survival rate than those with lymph node metastases.

TABLE 30-2 Staging System for Endometrial Carcinoma

FIGO Classification of Endometrial Carcinoma

Stage Ia	G123 Tumor limited to endometrium
Ib G123	Invasion of less than half of the myometrium
Ic G123	Invasion of more than half of the myometrium
IIa G123	Endocervical glandular involvement only
IIb G123	Cervical stromal invasion
IIIa G123	Tumor invades serosa and/or adnexa and/or positive peritoneal cytology
IIIb G123	Vaginal metastases
IIIc G123	Metastases to pelvic and/or para-aortic lymph nodes
IVa G123	Tumor invasion of bladder and/or bowel mucosa
IVb	Distant metastases including intraabdominal and/or inguinal lymph node
Histopathology: Degrees of Differentiation	
Cases of carcinoma of the corpus should be grouped according to the degree of differentiation of the adenocarcinoma as follows:	
G1	5% or less of a nonsquamous or nonmorular solid growth pattern
G2	6% to 50% of a nonsquamous or nonmorular solid growth pattern
G3	More than 50% of a nonsquamous or nonmorular solid growth pattern

Modified from DiSaia, P. J. & Creasman, W. T. (1993). Adenocarcinoma of the uterus. In P. J. DiSaia & W. T. Creasman (Eds.), *Clinical gynecologic oncology.* St. Louis: Mosby.

STAGING

The staging of endometrial cancer involves the use of a surgical pathologic system adopted by the International Federation of Gynecology and Obstetrics (FIGO) in 1988. This staging system defines the extent of the patient's disease (Table 30-2). Classifications within this system consist of both surgical and histologic pathology.

Histologic Staging

Histologic staging refers to the examination of the biopsy specimen(s) by a pathologist after surgery. Surgical removal of the endometrial-curettage specimen, peritoneal cytologic sampling, and palpation and biopsy of any suspicious lymph nodes or lesions is required for complete histologic staging. The purpose of histologic staging is to determine the grade or biologic aggressiveness of the tumor.

The endometrial curettage specimen provides important information regarding the grade of the tumor (Table 30-2). The grade is a classification based on the tumor architecture and reflects the amount of non–gland-forming tumor. Grades 1, 2, and 3 indicate the percentage of tumor. The higher the grade, the greater the percentage of tumor. The grade of the tumor is highly predictive of the extent of disease, as well as an important predictor of survival. In addition, the endometrial curettage specimen identifies the histologic cell types of endometrial carcinoma (Box 30-2).

Surgical Staging

Surgical staging, performed at the time of treatment, involves an extensive evaluation of the abdominopelvic cavity and includes bimanual examination and palpation of all peritoneal surfaces, selective pelvic and para-aortic lymphadenectomy, total abdominal hysterectomy, bilateral salpingo-oophorectomy, and possible omentectomy and resection of tumor implants (Walczak & Klemm, 1993). On pathologic examination, the uterus is examined to identify the depth of myometrial invasion by the tumor. Myometrial invasion is a consistent indicator of tumor virulence. Metastatic disease appears directly related to the depth of myometrial invasion. Generally, the poorer the differentiation of the tumor, the greater is the myometrial invasion. This staging system allows patients to be treated by a primary surgical intervention that provides staging information and serves as a therapeutic intervention.

Box 30-2
Classification of Endometrial Carcinoma

Adenocarcinomas
Pure adenocarcinomas
Adenocanthoma
Adenosquamous
- Clear cell carcinoma
- Undifferentiated carcinoma
- Papillary carcinoma
- Endometroid
- Serous

Modified from Walczak, R. J. & Klemm, P. R. (1993). Gynecologic cancers. In S. L. Groenwald, M. H. Frogge, M. Goodman, & C. H. Yarbro (Eds.), *Cancer nursing principles and practice.* Boston: Jones and Bartlett Publishers.

MEDICAL MANAGEMENT

After the surgical procedure, the extent of the disease and various prognostic factors are determined so that a treatment plan can be developed for the patient. For those patients requiring additional interventions after surgery, the treatment plan may consist of radiation, hormonal agents, and/or chemotherapy. In addition, new approaches are being addressed in numerous randomized clinical trials by the Gynecologic Oncology Group (GOG).

The treatment of endometrial cancer depends on several factors, including the FIGO stage, the histologic type and grade of the tumor, the depth of myometrial penetration, and the medical condition of the patient. The medical management of endometrial cancer is summarized in Table 30-3. For most patients, surgery (hysterectomy) is the treatment of choice. Radiation therapy is used as adjuvant therapy with high-risk patients, in the management of advanced disease, and for patients who are medically inoperable. Hormonal therapy and chemotherapy are used for advanced, metastatic, or local recurrent disease.

Table 30-3 Treatment for Endometrial Cancer

Disease Stage	Treatment
Stage I, grades 1 and 2	Surgical staging
Stage I, grade 3	Surgical staging Radiotherapy of the whole pelvis (45-50 Gy)
Stage IC or IIA	Surgical staging Radiotherapy of the whole pelvis (45-50 Gy)
Stage II B	Surgical staging Radiotherapy of the whole pelvis (45-50 Gy) Intracavity radiotherapy
Stage III	Surgical staging Radiotherapy of the whole pelvis (45-50 Gy) Para-aortic radiotherapy (45 Gy) if para-aortic nodes are positive Possible pelvic and abdominal radiotherapy
Stage IV	Possible pelvic and abdominal radiotherapy Possible progestin therapy Possible chemotherapy

Modified from Rose, P. G. (1996). Endometrial cancer. *The New England Journal of Medicine, 335,* 640-649.

Surgical Management

Total Abdominal Hysterectomy and Bilateral Salpingo-Oophorectomy. The primary surgical management of endometrial cancer is summarized in Fig. 30-4. The most common surgical procedure for endometrial cancer is total abdominal hysterectomy and bilateral salpingo-oophorectomy for both therapeutic and staging purposes. Peritoneal fluid is obtained for cytologic analysis. Pelvic and periaortic nodal sampling should be considered in patients with suspicious adenopathy, high-grade tumors, or tumors of any grade invading into the middle third or greater of the myometrium or cervix. This surgical procedure requires removing the uterus, tubes, and ovaries; and an extrafascial hysterectomy is performed. A small vaginal cuff is usually excised and sampling of lymph nodes is performed. In Fig. 30-5, the schematic view of the operation is depicted. The immediate postoperative complications of this surgery include bleeding, thrombophlebitis, infection, and pulmonary emboli.

Presently, the GOG is evaluating the role of laparoscopic surgery for endometrial cancer. Operative laparoscopy and vaginal hysterectomy can both stage and treat endometrial cancer while avoiding an abdominal incision. The actual surgery takes longer than an abdominal approach. However, the hospital stay is significantly shorter for these patients. In the obese patient, laparoscopic surgery is not an option.

Pelvic Exenteration. Pelvic exenteration is used to treat central recurrence after radiation therapy. However, the utility of this surgery in endometrial cancer is limited (Hogan & Boente, 1993). This surgery combines the following three major procedures: radical hysterectomy with bilateral pelvic lymph node dissection and excision and bilateral salpingo-oophorectomy, total cystectomy, and combined abdominoperineal resection of the rectum. A pelvic exenteration is extensive surgery, and the patient must be prepared preoperatively, monitored postoperatively, and supported during the rehabilitation period (Hampton, 1986).

Medically Inoperable Patients. Approximately 10% of patients diagnosed with endometrial cancer are medically inoperable (Karasek & Faul, 1996). The primary treatment modality used for these patients is radiation therapy. Several reports suggest that the local control rates are inferior to the rates obtained with surgery. However, 5-year survival rates with the two modalities do not differ significantly, with both ranging between 45% and 88% (Karasek & Faul, 1996).

Brachytherapy can be used with patients who have clinical stage I disease of low grade. All other patients will re-

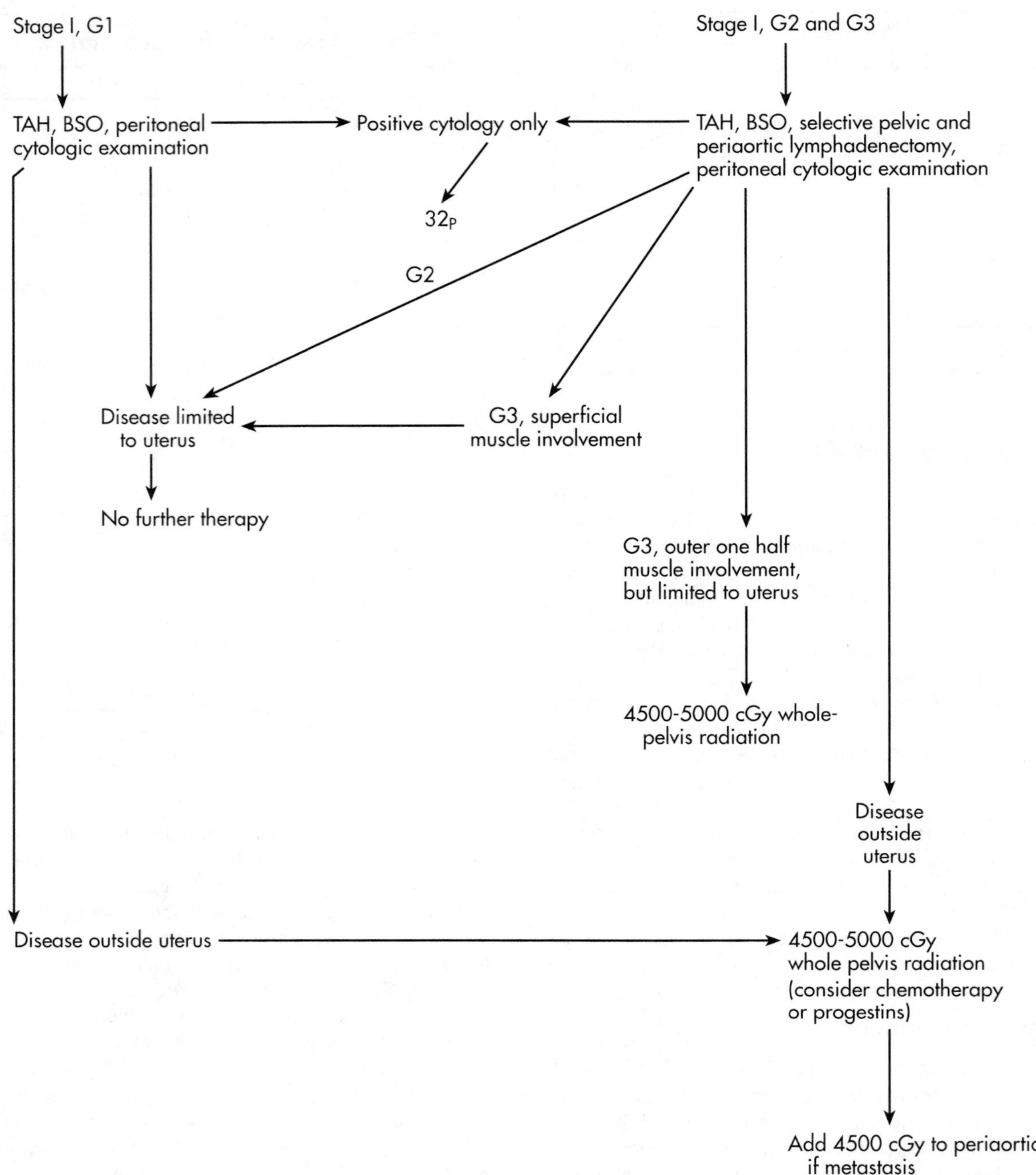

Fig. 30-4 Primary surgical management of endometrial cancer. (From DiSaia P. J, & Creasman, W. T. [1993]. *Clinical gynecologic oncology.* St. Louis: Mosby.)

quire radiation with external beam therapy and brachytherapy. Patients with local recurrences have been treated with additional therapy (Karasek & Faul, 1996).

Radiation Therapy

The role of radiation therapy has changed over the last decade. Radiation therapy has been given preoperatively followed by surgery; based on a postoperative assessment, some patients may be treated with additional external beam pelvic radiation. This approach is less popular today for the following reasons: It makes the pathologic evaluation of the uterus more difficult, women with less extensive disease may be overtreated, and women with more extensive disease may be undertreated. Primary radiation therapy is used for women who are medically inoperable, which accounts for approximately 10% of the women diagnosed with endometrial carcinoma (Karasek & Faul, 1996).

External Beam Radiation Therapy. Currently, women with endometrial cancer are staged surgically, and a

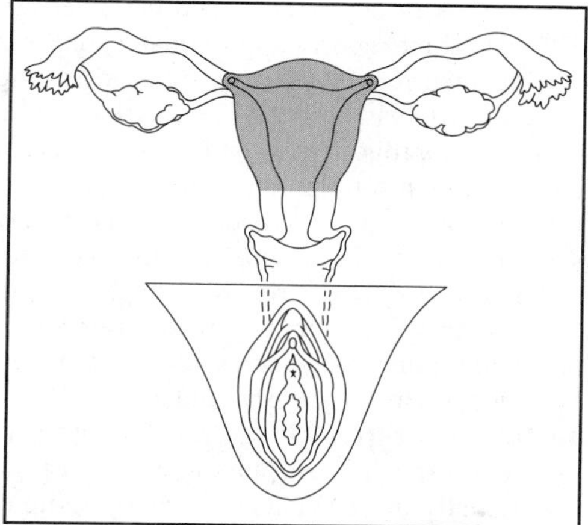

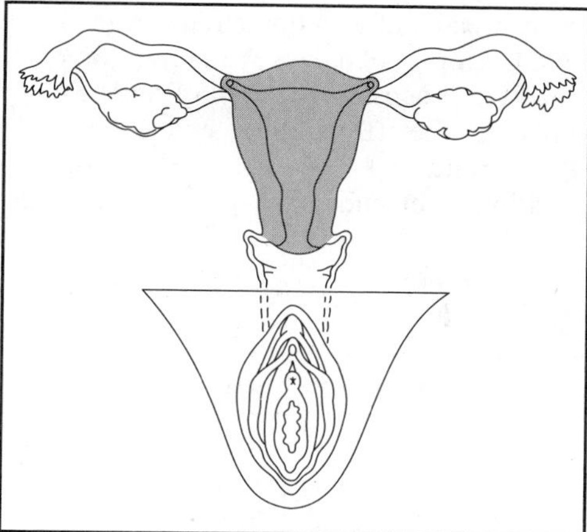

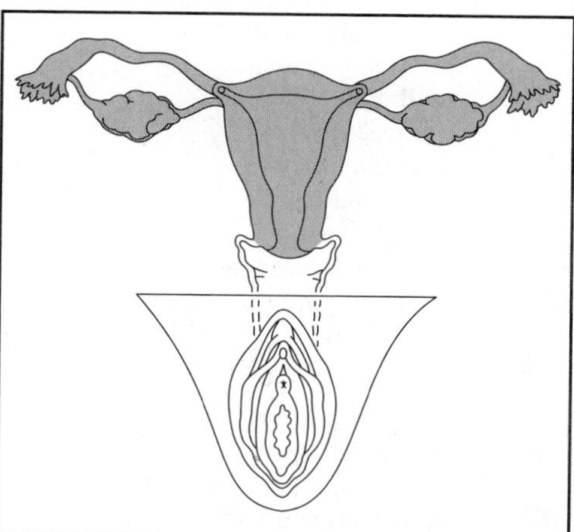

Fig. 30-5 Schematic view of a total abdominal hysterectomy and bilateral salpingo-ophorectomy. (From Butts, P. [1979]. Meeting the special needs of your hysterectomy patient. *Nursing, 79,* 41.)

decision to use external beam radiation is based on the patient's risk factors. In low-risk patients, adjuvant external beam radiation therapy is not necessary (Karasek & Faul, 1996). However, the use of adjuvant vaginal cuff irradiation alone is controversial because it has been difficult to demonstrate a significant clinical benefit (Carey & O'Connell, 1995; Elliot & Green, 1994).

Defining high-risk patients seems to be controversial. A majority of authors agree that high-risk patients are those with grade 3 tumors or those of any grade in which more than 50% of the myometrium is invaded with tumor (Karasek & Faul, 1996). It has been documented that adjuvant pelvic radiation has improved locoregional recurrence rates. Currently, the role of adjuvant radiation in surgically staged patients is being analyzed.

Patients with stage II endometrial cancer are usually treated like stage I patients. However, the use of adjuvant radiation therapy is based on prognostic factors. Patients with stage II disease are reported to have higher local recurrence rates when compared with stage I patients. Stage II patients tend to develop vaginal vault recurrences. This finding suggests a role for vaginal cuff irradiation after surgery (Morrow, Bundy, Kurman, Creasman, Heller, & Homesley, et al., 1991). Survival rates for clinical stage II disease range from 70% to 85% (Karasek & Faul, 1996).

The treatment options for patients with stage III disease include pelvic irradiation, extended-field radiation, or whole-abdominal radiation. In these patients treated with radiation alone, the 5-year survival rate ranges from 40% to 70% (Greven, Corn, & Lanciano, 1993). There is a need for improved strategies to manage these patients. Currently, combined chemoradiation and new chemotherapeutic regimens are being investigated.

Patients with stage IV endometrial cancer have a poor prognosis, with survival rates ranging from 5% to 15% (Karasek & Faul, 1996). If the tumor burden in the stage IV patient can be surgically debulked to less than 2 cm of residual disease, the use of whole abdomen radiation can be explored. This type of approach may result in improved patient outcomes.

Radiation therapy treatments are given 5 days a week, at doses of 45 to 50 Gy, for 5 to 6 weeks (total dose 4500 to 5000 Gy). The sites of radiation may include the pelvis, the entire abdomen, or the vaginal cuff. External beam radiation is generally well tolerated by the patient. Patients are assessed weekly during treatment, then monthly for about 3 months, and then every 6 months for 5 years. The acute problems associated with radiation therapy may include diarrhea, cystitis, alteration of vaginal membranes, and fatigue. Premenopausal women may experience menopause. The symptoms usually develop during the third week of treatment and resolve days to weeks after treatment is completed.

The occurrence of late complications of radiation therapy (i.e., complications that occur 6 or more months after the completion of treatment) is relatively rare. Possible late complications of external beam radiation include cystitis, vaginal changes, and chronic diarrhea.

Internal Radiation Therapy. Internal radiation therapy or brachytherapy may be considered a treatment option. Patients can receive high-dose brachytherapy as an outpatient, thereby avoiding an inpatient stay and the risk of complications associated with bed rest. At most centers, the treatment has been limited to the upper third of the vagina rather than the complete length. This change in treatment has reduced toxicities without decreasing results (Karasek & Faul, 1996).

Brachytherapy is used to give a high dose of radiation to a small area, minimizing the amount of radiation directed to the surrounding normal structures. Patients receive a total of three treatments, usually given every other week. The treatment is given by a hollow cylinder (applicator) attached by a catheter to a machine that contains the radioactive source. The patient should be prepared for the treatment, which includes putting on a hospital gown and having a pelvic examination performed. Then the patient receives treatment. There are no restrictions on the patient's activity level, and radiation precautions are not necessary. The patient may have a pinkish discharge after treatment and should be instructed that this is normal. Some patients report burning or pressure when urinating or pressure when having a bowel movement. These symptoms are expected, and if they do not improve after 2 days, the patient should be instructed to call her health care professional. Late effects might include vaginal dryness and vaginal tightening.

Hormone Therapy. Hormone therapy has been used for more than 20 years with documented objective responses in patients with recurrent or advanced endometrial cancer (Lentz, 1994). In some reports, approximately one third of all patients with recurrent disease responded to hormone therapy (DiSaia & Creasman, 1993; Karasek & Faul, 1996). Patients who have progesterone and estrogen receptors on their tumors and well-differentiated tumors are most apt to respond to hormone therapy (Rose, 1996). Disease-free interval is another factor that seems to influence response to hormone therapy (Hoskins, Perez, & Young, 1993). In addition, patients with vaginal or lung metastases and positive lymph nodes are more likely to respond than patients with pelvic recurrences (Hoskins, Perez, and Young, 1993).

Progestin Therapy. Progestin therapy involves agents that act on specific receptors in estrogen-primed target tissues. Usually these agents have an opposite effect to that of estrogen. The mechanism of action for progestin therapy in the treatment of endometrial cancers has not been determined. Examples of agents with progestational activity include medroxyprogesterone (Depo-Provera or Provera), hydroxyprogesterone (Delalutin), and megestrol acetate (Megace). Progestin is known to prevent clinical hyperplasia. In addition, premenopausal women taking combined

TABLE 30-4 Hormonal Therapy for Endometrial Cancer

Classification/Drug	Dosage Range	Cost*	Untoward Effects
Progestin			
Medroxyprogesterone acetate			• Nausea and vomiting • Edema
Depo-Provera (IM)	400-1000 mg weekly Average 400 mg/week	$400/month	• Weight gain • Fluid retention • Breast tenderness
Provera (Oral)	150-1000 mg Average 150 mg/day	$32/month	• Pruritus • Headache • Nervousness
Hydroxyprogesterone (Delalatin)	1-3 g IM weekly	$32-$96/month	• Hot flashes • Joint pain • Vaginal bleeding
Megestrol acetate (Megace)	40-320 mg/day Average 160 mg/day	$120/month	• Alteration in menstrual flow • Urticaria • Thrombophlebitis
Antiestrogen			
Tamoxifen (Nolvadex, Tam)	10-20 mg BID	$94-$198/month	• Hot flashes • Vaginal bleeding/discharge • Nausea and vomiting • Transient myelosuppression • Possible hyperkalemia • Tumor pain or flare • Light-headedness • Pruritus • Skin rash • Alopecia • Corneal changes, cataracts, retinopathy • Carpal tunnel syndrome • Can increase prothrombin time in patients taking coumadin

*Average wholesale price

oral contraceptives have a decreased risk for endometrial cancer. This research suggests a protective effect from progestin therapy. The use of progestin therapy in preventing recurrences has been disappointing and does not seem to prevent recurrence or affect survival (Lewis, Slack, Mortel, & Bross, 1974; DePalo, Spatti, Bandieramonte, & Luciani, 1983). Trials are ongoing to study the use of prophylactic progestational agents (Hoskins, Perez, & Young, 1993).

Antiestrogen Therapy. The use of antiestrogenic agents such as tamoxifen citrate (Nolvadex) in women with advanced endometrial cancer is being explored. Combining hormone therapies (e.g., medroxyprogesterone with tamoxifen) has not improved response rates compared with using a progesterone agent alone (Hoskins, Perez, & Young, 1993).

Summary. Hormone therapy is easy to administer with minimal side effects. The hormones used to treat endometrial cancer (including dosage, cost, and side effects) are summarized in Table 30-4. When administering hormone therapy, a few guidelines should be followed: patients should be on hormone agents for several weeks to months before discontinuing treatment, as there may be a delay in observing a clinical response. The side effects of hormone agents are generally tolerable. The patients should continue indefinitely on this therapy until there is a recurrence or distant metastases develop. Patients treated with progestin therapy have a median survival of 23 to 29 months compared with 6 months for patients who show no objective response (Kneale, 1986).

Chemotherapy

The role of chemotherapeutic agents in the treatment of advanced, metastatic, or recurrent disease is being investigated. A list of chemotherapeutic agents is provided in Table 30-5. The side effects and toxicities of these agents are summarized in Table 30-6.

Most patients seem to respond to chemotherapy and their symptoms improve (American Hospital Formulary Service, 1996; Levine, 1993). However, the duration of response to chemotherapy is usually short and has little to no effect on survival (Hoskins, Perez, & Young, 1993). The following factors seem to affect response rates: prior treatment, performance status, length of disease-free interval, and response criteria used for evaluation (Park et al., 1992).

The ideal chemotherapeutic agent(s) has not been found for the treatment of endometrial cancer. The agent most extensively evaluated for endometrial cancer is doxorubicin. The response rate for this agent ranges from 15% to 38%, with a median duration of response of 4 to 8 months (DiSaia & Creasman, 1993; Hoskins, Perez, & Young, 1993; Karasek & Faul, 1996; Rose, 1996). Doxorubicin is the standard drug with which new agents or combination therapy should be compared. The three most active agents in endometrial cancer are doxorubicin, cisplatin, and carboplatin.

The role of combination chemotherapy has not been studied extensively. Patients with advanced endometrial cancer should be considered for clinical trials. There is a need for large, well-controlled studies to explore the relationship between symptoms, quality of life, response rates, duration of response, and survival rate in patients with endometrial cancer who are treated with single versus combination chemotherapy and/or hormone therapy/radiation therapy. In one study (Thigpen, Blessing, DiSaia, Yordan, Carson, & Evers, 1994) comparing doxorubicin alone to cyclophosphamide and doxorubicin, there was slight advantage over doxorubicin alone in the treatment of endometrial cancer. However, the efficacy of this study requires careful evaluation, as there were heightened toxicities (i.e., myelosuppression and gastrointestinal) with the combination chemotherapy. Another randomized trial compared doxorubicin alone with doxorubicin and cisplatin (Thigpen, Vance, & Khansar, 1995). The response rate for cisplatin and doxorubicin was 66%, with a progression-free interval of 6.2 months compared with doxorubicin alone, which had a response rate of 35% and a progression-free interval of 3.9 months (Rose, 1996). The role of chemotherapy in the treatment of endometrial cancer continues to be investigated to develop better treatment approaches for this disease (Muggia & Gill, 1992; Muggia & Muderspach, 1994; Muss, 1994; Thigpen, Vance, & Khansar, 1995).

TABLE 30-5 Chemotherapeutic Agents Being Used or Studied in the Treatment for Endometrial Cancer

Classification	Agent
Alkylating agents	Carboplatin (Paraplatin) Cisplatin (Platinol, CIS-DDP) Cyclophosphamide (Cytoxan, CTX) Ifosfamide (Ifex)
Antimetabolites	5-Fluorouracil (Adrucil, 5-Fu)
Antitumor antibiotics	Doxorubicin hydrochloride (Adriamycin, Rubex, ADR)
Miscellaneous agent	Altretamine (Hexalen, hexamethymelamine)
Mitotic inhibitors	Paclitaxel (Taxol) Vincristine (Oncovin)

Estrogen Replacement Therapy

The use of estrogen therapy in the treatment of women with endometrial cancer is still controversial. Because endometrial cancer is an estrogen-dependent tumor, the risk of recurrence with estrogen replacement therapy remains to be determined. Retrospective studies of estrogen replacement therapy in low-risk women with stage I endometrial cancer have found no apparent increase in the risk of recurrence (Rose, 1996). In addition, these women are protected against the side effects and complication of estrogen deficiency. These data suggest that estrogen replacement therapy can be administered to women with stage I disease without increased risk of recurrence. The American College of Obstetrics and Gynecology recommends that an assessment of the risk of estrogen replacement therapy in relationship to the risk of recurrent disease be discussed by physi-

Table 30-6 Side Effects and Toxicities of Chemotherapy

Agents	Myelosuppression	Nausea and Vomiting	Stomatitis	Alopecia	Nephrotoxicity	Neurotoxicity	Vesicant	Cardiotoxicity	Photosensitivity	Constipation	Diarrhea	Darkening of Veins Used	Electrolyte Disturbances	Hypersensitivity Reaction	Hemorrhagic Cystitis	Altered Mental Status
Alkylating																
Carboplatin (Paraplatin)	X	X		X		X		X					X	X		
Cisplatin (Platinol, CIS-DDP)	X	X	X		X	X		Possible						X		
Cyclopsphamide (Cytoxan)	X	X		X				X							X	
Ifosfamide (Ifex)	X	X	X	X											X	X
Antimetabolites																
5-Fluorouracil (Adracil)	X	X	X						X		X	X				
Antitumor Antibiotics																
Doxorubicin hydrochloride (Adriamycin)	X	X	X	X			X	X	X					X		
Miscellaneous Agents																
Altretramine (Hexalen)	X	X		X		X										X
Mitotic Inhibitors																
Paclitaxel (Taxol)	X	X	X					X			X			X		X
Vincristine (Oncovin)	X			X		X	X			X				X		

X = Side effects.

cians and patients. Ultimately, the decision to use hormone replacement therapy should be the patient's choice.

ONCOLOGIC EMERGENCIES

The oncologic emergency associated with endometrial cancer is sepsis. Patients with cancer are at risk for developing sepsis. The cancer treatment, as well as the disease itself, places the patient at risk for infection. The early clinical signs and symptoms of sepsis may include chills, rigors, fever, subnormal temperature, malaise, tachycardia, tachypnea, and generalized complaints of discomfort. The late signs and symptoms of sepsis may include cool skin, hypotension, hyperventilation-respiratory failure, mental status changes/confusion, and oliguria-anuria. It is essential that the nurse determine whether the patient is at risk for sepsis, as prompt recognition and management of sepsis affect the mortality rate.

NURSING MANAGEMENT

The medical management of endometrial cancer is extremely complex and variable depending on the patient's age, clinical condition, and stage of disease at the time of diagnosis. The nursing management of patients with endometrial cancer is challenging, and these patients have numerous problems that require nursing interventions and patient education. Although a portion of the patient's care occurs in the inpatient setting, the majority of the care occurs in the outpatient and home care settings.

Early in the course of the patient's disease, the focus of nursing care may be on helping the patient understand and cope with the diagnosis and treatment plan. Patients need information about the different treatment modalities, as well as strategies for managing side effects associated with the disease or treatments. Because each major type of treatment for endometrial cancer (e.g., surgery, radiation therapy, hormonal therapy, chemotherapy) poses unique patient problems, the major issues associated with these treatments are discussed and five standards of care provided (Jansen, 1995; McNally, Somerville, Miaskowski, & Rostad, 1991).

The early diagnosis of endometrial cancer seems to affect survival. Health teaching is an essential nursing role. Patients being worked up for cancer are anxious, and the nurse plays a crucial role in assisting the women to cope by decreasing their anxiety level and providing necessary information. Patients should be encouraged to actively participate in their treatment decisions. The Patient Self-Determination Act requires hospitals to inform patients of their rights to make choices about their health care. Nursing can be instrumental in assisting patients in making treatment choices by actively listening and explaining the different options. The nursing management of the patient newly diagnosed with endometrial cancer is summarized in Table 30-7.

Surgery

The major focus of inpatient nursing care for patients undergoing total abdominal hysterectomy, bilateral salpingo-oophorectomy, and pelvic washing for cytology is on the prevention of postoperative complications, including bleeding, thrombophlebitis, infection, and pulmonary emboli. As hospital stays are shorter, education is essential for patients and family members. The patient should be instructed about postoperative care, including the need to report signs and symptoms of infection, how to perform wound care, the importance of fluid and food intake, activity levels, and the need for adequate rest periods. Follow-up care in the outpatient setting requires that nurses evaluate patients' level of functioning and their psychosocial adjustment to the surgical procedure.

The nursing management of the patient undergoing surgery for endometrial cancer is summarized in Table 30-8. The patient undergoing surgery may need information and education on the following topics: pain management, sexuality, and managing menopause. Box 30-3 provides information on various aspects of sexuality and the management of menopause and Table 30-9 offers a quick reference for managing menopausal symptoms.

Radiation Therapy

Patient problems vary depending on whether the patient is receiving external beam radiation therapy to treat the pelvis, the pelvic and para-aortic regions, the whole abdomen, or vaginal area, or high dose brachytherapy. External beam radiation therapy and high-dose brachytherapy are provided on an outpatient basis. The major problems associated with external beam radiation therapy include diarrhea, cystitis, alteration in vaginal mucous membranes, and fatigue. High-dose brachytherapy is done in the outpatient setting. Some institutions use low-dose brachytherapy in an inpatient setting. Patients and their significant other(s) require education to understand how radiation therapy works and how to manage the side effects associated with treatment. The nursing management of the patient with endometrial cancer receiving external beam radiation therapy is summarized in Table 30-10. A specific standard for knowledge deficit for patients receiving high-dose brachytherapy is provided in Table 30-11. Symptom management for patients receiving high-dose brachytherapy is similar to those patients treated with external beam therapy, which is summarized in Table 30-10 (Dow & Hilderley, 1992).

Hormone Therapy

Most patients receiving hormone therapy have advanced disease. In most cases, care is provided in the outpatient setting. Patients must be taught the rationale for therapy, as well as how to manage side effects. The major side effects (Table 30-4) associated with hormone therapy are vaginal bleeding, weight gain, edema, hot flashes, and tumor pain or flare. Patients report the most troublesome side effect is hot flashes (Clinical Handbook of Clinical preventive Services, 1995). The management plan for the patient with endometrial cancer who is receiving hormone therapy is summarized in Table 30-12.

Text continued on p. 713

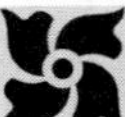

TABLE 30-7 Standard of Care for the Patient Newly Diagnosed with Endometrial Cancer

Patient Problem and Outcomes	Nursing Interventions and Rationales	Patient Education Instructions
Anxiety Related to New Diagnosis Patient will: • Be able to verbalize concerns, fears, and questions • Experience a decrease in anxiety as evidenced by a decrease in the signs and symptoms of anxiety	1. Assess for signs and symptoms of anxiety. 2. Establish a relationship with patient. 3. Assess effectiveness of coping skills. 4. Anticipate patient's needs. 5. Orient patient to environment. 6. Provide a calm, supportive, reassuring environment and reduce external stimuli. 7. Encourage verbalization of feelings and concerns. 8. Maintain a calm and tolerant manner. 9. Monitor changes in level of anxiety. 10. Administer antianxiety medications as prescribed, if necessary.	1. Provide patient with information about anxiety: a. Signs and symptoms b. Factors that lead to anxious feelings c. Alternatives to prevent anxiety d. Relaxation exercises e. Methods to reduce environmental stimuli
Knowledge Deficit Related to Early Detection and Diagnosis of Endometrial Cancer Patient will: • Be able to state the signs and symptoms of endometrial cancer • Keep regular appointments for gynecologic checkups	1. Assess past experience with the diagnosis of cancer and cancer treatment. 2. Determine present knowledge base and major concerns regarding diagnosis and treatment. 3. Assess readiness and ability to learn. 4. Assess risk factors. 5. Obtain history of signs and symptoms of bleeding.	1. Teach importance of proper nutrition and weight control. 2. Stress importance of regular checkups. 3. Teach signs and symptoms to report: a. Changes in bleeding patterns b. Breakthrough bleeding c. Irregular menses d. Bleeding occurring 6 months after cessation of menses in postmenopausal women 4. Teach patient the need for regular gynecologic checkups. 5. Instruct patient on American Cancer Society (ACS) guidelines: a. Pelvic examination every 3 years for woman 20-40 years old or older annually b. Endometrial tissue sampling at menopause in women at high risk

TABLE 30-7 Standard of Care for the Patient Newly Diagnosed with Endometrial Cancer—cont'd

Patient Problem and Outcomes	Nursing Interventions and Rationales	Patient Education Instructions
Knowledge Deficit Related to Early Detection and Diagnosis of Endometrial Cancer—cont'd		
	6. Assess gynecologic status.	6. Educate about pap smear and endometrial biopsy.
	7. Review ACS guidelines.	7. Discuss importance of follow-up for abnormal symptoms.
	8. Explain all tests and procedures.	8. Discuss modifications in lifestyle behaviors (i.e., diet, weight control, and exercise).
	9. Encourage verbalization of feelings and concerns.	9. Discuss treatment options when appropriate.
	10. Provide psychological and spiritual support.	
Grieving Patient will: • Identify areas of potential or real loss • Be able to recall past experiences with loss and use appropriate coping strategies • Identify roles and changes in relationships • Verbalize concerns	1. Assess patient's understanding of current health status and potential loss. 2. Teach patient about loss and grief to help her understand and identify feelings. In addition, providing accurate information may prevent misconceptions and decrease fear. 3. Give patient permission to grieve. 4. Discuss the reality of actual loss with patient. 5. Assess patient's response to loss. 6. Promote positive communication among family members. 7. Lead discussion of problems and solutions with patient and family members. 8. Facilitate patient's inquiry/discussion of implications of health care proxy, living will, and code status. 9. Encourage and maintain hope.	1. Instruct patient about the process of grieving and loss, including: a. Normal response to loss (include the stages of grief) b. Knowledge that individuals do not go through all the stages in sequence and may move back and forth c. Grieving is a normal response to a real or potential loss d. Grieving begins at time of diagnosis e. Grief response may be different for each person f. Importance of sharing information about diagnosis and role changes to foster mutual understanding and trust g. Importance of mutual acceptance and understanding of each other during the process h. The need for support i. The importance of maintaining health and welfare of the patient j. The importance of memories and the best way to preserve the memories

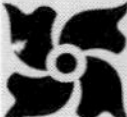

TABLE 30-8 Standard of Care for the Patient Undergoing Total Abdominal Hysterectomy and Bilateral Salpingo-Oophorectomy

Patient Problem and Outcomes	Nursing Interventions and Rationales	Patient Education Instructions
Knowledge Deficit Related to Surgery		
Patient will: • Verbalize an understanding of the surgical procedure: • Preoperative care • Postoperative care • Follow-up care after surgery	1. Assess past experience with surgery. 2. Determine present knowledge base and major concerns regarding surgery.	1. Use a diagram of the anatomy of the female genital tract to explain the procedure. 2. Provide patient with information about the preoperative routine: a. Diagnostic tests b. Bowel preparation c. Consent d. Anesthesiology consult e. Nothing by mouth (NPO) after midnight f. Skin preparation g. On call to operating room: (1) Hospital gown (2) Void on call (3) Preoperative medications h. Teach the patient to cough and deep breathe; use an incentive spirometer and perform foot and leg exercises i. Discuss pain and pain management
	3. Describe type of surgery and expected outcomes.	3. Provide patient with information about postoperative plan of care: a. Routine assessments b. Importance of pain management c. Need for leg exercises d. Use of thromboembolic stocking e. Use of incentive spirometers f. Teach coughing and deep breathing exercises g. Need to ambulate as soon as possible h. Explanation of equipment (e.g., Foley catheter, IV and nasogastric tubes, drains, and dressings)
	4. Assess patient's knowledge of potential sequelae, including loss of body organ and surgically induced menopause.	4. Instruct patient regarding postoperative care including: a. Avoiding tampons and douches b. Abstaining from intercourse for 4-6 weeks or as indicated by the physician c. Increasing activity gradually (i.e., limit stair climbing for 1-2 weeks, limit heavy housework and lifting of heavy objects for 6 weeks) d. Maintaining a high-protein diet and adequate fluid intake (2000 ml) e. Monitoring for signs and symptoms of infection f. Notifying physician if temperature is >100.5 °F (38 °C)

WBC, white blood cell.

TABLE 30-8 Standard of Care for the Patient Undergoing Total Abdominal Hysterectomy and Bilateral Salpingo-Oophorectomy—cont'd

Patient Problem and Outcomes	Nursing Interventions and Rationales	Patient Education Instructions
Knowledge Deficit Related to Surgery—cont'd		
		g. Taking pain medication as prescribed to control pain h. Avoiding constipation and straining i. Taking estrogen-progestin hormones as prescribed j. Keeping follow-up appointment
Pain		
Patient will: • Achieve satisfactory pain relief • Perform measures to manage pain	1. Assess pain intensity using a 0 to 10 pain rating scale, every 2-4 hours for the first 48 hours after surgery, then at least every 8 hours.	1. Teach patient to report pain to nurse.
	2. Administer opioid analgesics around the clock for the first 24-48 hours postoperatively.	2. Teach patient the importance of taking pain medication on a regular basis to keep pain under control.
	3. Monitor for analgesic side effects and use strategies to prevent or treat: a. Constipation b. Nausea c. Anxiety d. Depression e. Insomnia 4. Use nonpharmacologic pain control strategies.	3. Teach patient methods to minimize or reduce pain: a. Positioning b. Range of motion c. Gentle massage d. Cold or warm pack e. Distraction techniques f. Relaxation techniques g. Meditation or prayers h. Exercise or rest periods i. Transcutaneous electrical nerve stimulations (TENS)
High Risk for Infection		
Patient will: • Remain infection free • Verbalize signs and symptoms of infection	1. Perform a skin assessment 2. Perform a respiratory assessment 3. Perform nephrourologic assessment 4. Perform an oral assessment 5. Monitor for signs and symptoms of infection: a. Temperature <100.4 °F (38 °C) b. Shaking chills c. Tenderness, redness, heat, or pain d. Nonhealing, malodorous, or draining wound 6. Monitor vital signs. 7. Monitor WBC count and total neutrophil count. 8. Perform wound care and maintain a clean, dry incision. 9. Administer antipyretic or antibiotics as ordered.	1. Instruct patient/family members about preventing an infection: a. Signs and symptoms of infection b. Notify nurse/physician if the patient exhibits any symptoms c. Explain the rationale and importance of handwashing d. Explain the role of a balanced diet e. Explain the role of WBCs in preventing infection f. Strict aseptic technique should be used g. Teach perineal care h. Teach Foley care

Continued

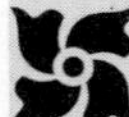

TABLE 30-8 Standard of Care for the Patient Undergoing Total Abdominal Hysterectomy and Bilateral Salpingo-Oophorectomy—cont'd

Patient Problem and Outcomes	Nursing Interventions and Rationales	Patient Education Instructions
Altered Sexuality Patterns Related to Diagnosis, Fear, Depression, and Treatment		
Patient will: • Demonstrate knowledge regarding potential alterations in sexual functioning • Maintain an optimal means of satisfaction with sexual expression or needs • Identify/demonstrate strategies to manage or correct alterations in sexual functioning	1. Establish a therapeutic relationship: a. Be nonjudgmental in your attitude b. Provide an atmosphere of acceptance c. Assure the patient that all discussions will be kept confidential d. Ensure privacy e. Start the discussion beginning with the least sensitive and progressing to the most sensitive issue f. Offer an opportunity for patient to ask questions and verbalize issues/concerns	1. Instruct patient and family members regarding the potential for an alteration in sexual functioning: a. Discuss impact of disease and treatment on sexuality b. Clarify terms, myths, and misconceptions as appropriate to ensure understanding c. Identify barriers to sexuality d. Identify strategies to a satisfying sexual function by managing side effects (e.g., pain, decreased libido, dyspareunia, and fatigue) e. Inform patient whether hormonal effects should be expected f. Prepare patient for anticipated menopausal symptoms
	2. Use Annon's PLISSIT model to guide your interventions: P = Permission LI = Limited Information SS = Specific Information IT = Intensive Therapy 3. Assess patient/family members' understanding of sexuality and physiology. 4. Obtain a sexual history including: a. Sexual activity b. Reproductive history c. Desire for children d. Use of contraceptives e. Attitudes about sex f. Impact of involved body part on sexuality g. Expectations 5. Allow patient to verbalize her perceptions of how the disease and treatment will affect sexuality and sexual function. 6. Elicit early identification of a specific problem, including: a. Nature b. Course of events c. Onset d. Duration e. Patient's perception of the problem 7. Encourage patient/family members to discuss concerns and/or problems. 8. Provide time for patient and family members to communicate privately.	2. Provide booklet entitled *Sexuality and Cancer For The Woman Who Has Cancer and Her Partner* by the American Cancer Society.

WBC, White blood cell.

Box 30-3

Regaining Sexual Confidence After Cancer

Having cancer can affect every aspect of your life, including your sexuality. Whether your treatment has entailed surgery, chemotherapy, radiotherapy, or any combination of the three, there will be adjustments to make as you recover. Remember that honest partner-to-partner communication is essential to maintaining a strong, supportive relationship. Be patient, be creative, and ask for advice when needed. The pleasure of sexual closeness enhances quality of life and can be adapted no matter what treatment has been used. After consulting your physician or nurse about specific restrictions, use the following suggestions to promote rehabilitation.

Before You Resume Sexual Activity

- Focus on your physical recovery first. Emphasize nutrition, rest, and progressive activity.
- Include your partner in all discussions about your care and treatment while you are still in the hospital.
- Be sure that your discharge instructions include advice about resuming sexual activity. If your nurse or doctor doesn't mention it, feel free to ask.
- Obtain a copy of the booklet, *Sexuality & Cancer,* a publication available from the American Cancer Society. (Your nurse can tell you how to contact this organization.) Separate booklets are published for men and women.
- Plan to use appropriate birth control measures, if indicated.
- Report any unusual bleeding, discharge, fever, or pain to your doctor or nurse.
- You've been through a lot, and it may take some time before your are interested in sex again. Be patient with yourself.

When You Feel Ready

- Remember that self-concept and sexuality are linked, so emphasize the positive aspects of your appearance and personality.
- Wear comfortable, attractive lounging clothes and perhaps perfume or cologne, not only to arouse your partner, but to feel good about yourself.
- Set the stage for sexual contact by choosing a time when both you and your partner are rested and free from distractions.
- A warm shower together allows partners to begin foreplay in a relaxed way.
- A glass of wine, candlelight, and music can add to a romantic mood.
- Mutual massage, not only of the genital area, but of the neck, chest, buttocks, and thighs, is stimulating to both partners.
- Use of erotic materials, such as books and movies, can help stimulate interest in sexual activity.
- Experiment with alternative positions until you find one that is most comfortable for you. If you are feeling fatigued, try positions that require minimal exertion.
- Use a water-soluble lubricant to increase vaginal moisture.
- Use prescribed pain medication or muscle relaxants, if necessary, to make sexual activity more comfortable.
- Conserve energy for sexual activity, perhaps by delegating certain household chores to others.
- Explore alternative ways of expressing physical love.

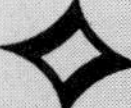

TABLE 30-9 Patient Preparation for the Management of Menopausal Symptoms

Women who undergo a hysterectomy with bilateral salpingo-oophorectomy will experience a surgically induced menopause. Each woman will react differently to menopause. Some of the symptoms and changes that women may experience include the following:

- Hot flashes and sweats
- Sleep disturbances
- Vaginal dryness
- Mood changes
- Changes in sexual desires

Several remedies, other than hormone replacement therapy, are used to manage menopausal symptoms. Most of these remedies have not been studied, but women report them to be helpful.

- For hot flashes and sweats—dressing in layers and natural fibers; reducing or avoiding alcohol intake
- Sleep disturbances—regular exercise; using stress reduction techniques; avoiding or reducing caffeine intake
- Vaginal dryness—using vaginal lubricants
- Mood changes—participating in a support group; regular exercise
- Changes in sexual desires—participating in a support group; encouraging sexual activities (e.g., fondling, kissing, hugging), which may increase desire

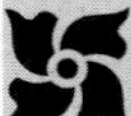

TABLE 30-10 Standard of Care for the Patient Receiving External Beam Radiation Therapy for Endometrial Cancer

Patient Problem and Outcomes	Nursing Interventions and Rationales	Patient Education Instructions
Knowledge Deficit Related to Radiation Therapy		
Patient will: • Demonstrate knowledge of radiation therapy, including purpose, benefits, and risks • Demonstrate knowledge related to treatment procedure and plan • Demonstrate knowledge related to managing side effects • Prevent/minimize fatigue • Promote adequate nutritional and fluid intake	1. Assess patient's knowledge of diagnosis and treatment plan. 2. Assess patient's physical and psychosocial status. 3. Assess patient's concerns and fears about radiation therapy.	1. Teach patient about: a. Principles of radiation therapy b. Treatment procedures: (1) Consultation (2) Simulation procedure (3) Treatment and routines c. Describe follow-up care d. Maintain adequate nutrition e. Describe side effects, stress the importance of notifying the health care member and self-care measures to manage the side effects of: (1) Diarrhea (2) Cystitis (3) Alteration in vaginal mucous membranes (4) Fatigue
Diarrhea		
Patient will: • Demonstrate knowledge related to side effect • Demonstrate strategies to prevent diarrhea • Achieves control or correction of diarrhea	1. Assess usual pattern of elimination, including use of laxatives. 2. Assess pattern of diarrhea including the onset, duration, character, amount, and frequency of stools. 3. Assess for the presence of associated symptoms such as flatus, cramping, abdominal distention, fatigue, rectal area excoriation, and the aggravation of hemorrhoids. 4. Assess nutritional status, including weight. 5. Encourage fluid intake of at least 2500 ml/day, unless contraindicated. 6. Maintain low-residue, bland, high-protein, high-carbohydrate, balanced diet 7. Monitor intake and output. 8. Increase foods high in potassium. 9. Try small, frequent meals. 10. Obtain a dietary consult if necessary. 11. Weigh weekly. 12. Provide Sitz bath as needed. 13. Administer antidiarrheal agent as prescribed.	1. Instruct patient to avoid liquids (e.g., orange juice, prune juice, lemonade, milk, caffeinated beverages) that may promote bowel movements. 2. Instruct patient to avoid extremes in food temperatures. 3. Teach patient to maintain low-residue diet, including foods to avoid, such as foods high in roughage, fried or highly seasoned foods, uncooked fruits or vegetables. 4. Teach patients to eat foods that are high in potassium (e.g., bananas, apricot and peach nectars, fish/meat and potatoes). 5. Teach patients to take antidiarrheal medications. Agents may include Lomotil 2.5 mg 1-2 tablets after each loose stool; or loperamide HCl (Imodium) 2 mg after each loose stool; or Tincture of Opium 0.5 to 1 ml q4h until diarrhea is controlled. 6. Instruct patient to: a. Monitor intake and output b. Follow diet restriction c. Take antidiarrheal agents d. Use Sitz bath e. Notify health care professional for excessive diarrhea

TABLE 30-10 Standard of Care for the Patient Receiving External Beam Radiation Therapy for Endometrial Cancer—cont'd

Patient Problem and Outcomes	Nursing Interventions and Rationales	Patient Education Instructions
Cystitis • Patient maintains urinary elimination within normal limits • Patient identifies strategies to prevent or minimize urotoxicity	1. Assess for signs and symptoms of urotoxicity, including dysuria, frequency, urgency, and burning. 2. Assess urine for the presence of urinary tract infection. 3. Initiate appropriate antibiotic therapy, if infection present. 4. Monitor intake and output. 5. Encourage oral intake. 6. Administer bladder antispasmodics/analgesics as prescribed.	1. Instruct patient to report symptoms and that symptoms may occur about 2 weeks into the treatment. 2. Instruct patient that phenazopyridine (Pyridium) will color urine orange-red.
Alteration in Vaginal Mucous Membranes Patient will: • Demonstrate knowledge of potential problem • Demonstrate absence of impairment	1. Assess for signs and symptoms of impaired vaginal membrane integrity, including pain, soreness, bleeding, discharge, pruritus, or dyspareunia. 2. Observe for signs of impaired vaginal membranes such as erythema, swelling, ulceration, decrease in vaginal size, muscle tone/lubrication and vaginal fibrosis/stenosis. 3. Instruct patient about preventive health practices. 4. Apply topical medications as prescribed. 5. Administer systemic medications as prescribed.	1. Teach patient to do the following: a. Gently pat dry skin after bathing b. Perform perineal care after defecation or urination c. Use cotton-lined underpants d. Use pantiliner e. Avoid tight-fitting slacks, jeans, or pantyhose f. Check with health care professional before douching 2. Teach patient how to take: a. Metronidazole (Flagyl) b. Estrogen creams 3. Teach patient strategies to decrease dyspareunia: a. Use of water-soluble lubricant b. Use of estrogen creams c. Female on top position for intercourse 4. Teach patient strategies to manage decreased vaginal size and tone: a. Use vaginal dilators b. Place a pillow under the women's hips for protection and control of penile thrusting c. Kegel exercises
Fatigue Patient will: • Be able to identify factors with the potential to cause fatigue • Maintain optimal function and comfort	1. Perform a fatigue assessment including pattern of fatigue, onset, duration, intensity, aggravating and alleviating factors, and impact of fatigue on the patient's activity level; assess for contributing factor(s) such as dyspnea, degree of anemia, infection, fever, anorexia, cachexia, and chronic pain.	1. Instruct patient to coordinate realistic daily activities. Teach patient to recognize fatigue and pace him- or herself. 2. Instruct patient to avoid doing too much too soon.

Continued

TABLE 30-10 Standard of Care for the Patient Receiving External Beam Radiation Therapy for Endometrial Cancer—cont'd

Patient Problem and Outcomes	Nursing Interventions and Rationales	Patient Education Instructions
Fatigue—cont'd	2. Encourage patient to set priorities and choose activities. 3. Plan intermittent rest periods as needed. 4. Assist the patient with activities as needed. 5. Provide emotional support. 6. Assess for the presence of anemia. 7. Administer packed red blood cells as prescribed. 8. Administer oxygen as prescribed. 9. Provide patient with feedback and encouragement in identifying abilities and limitations.	

TABLE 30-11 Standard of Care for the Patient Receiving High Dose Rate (HDR) Brachytherapy

Patient Problem and Outcomes	Nursing Interventions and Rationales	Patient Education Instructions
Knowledge Deficit Related to Brachytherapy Patient demonstrates knowledge of brachytherapy (internal radiation)	1. Assess patient's knowledge of diagnosis and treatment plan.	1. Teach patient about HDR, including: a. Explain the purpose b. Describe treatment procedure c. Describe routine including pelvic examination and measurement for cylinder d. No specific precautions

TABLE 30-12 Standard of Care for the Patient Receiving Hormonal Therapy for Advanced Endometrial Cancer

Patient Problem and Outcomes	Nursing Interventions and Rationales	Patient Education Instruction
Hot Flashes Patient will: • Experience a decrease in the number of hot flashes	1. Assess for hot flashes, including frequency. 2. Administer medications as ordered.	1. Teach patient to avoid situations that may trigger the hot flashes: a. Warm room b. Hot drinks c. Alcoholic drinks d. Caffeinated beverages 2. Instruct patient to dress in layers and natural fibers. 3. Have patient plan for regular exercise. 4. Have patient use stress reduction.

Chemotherapy

Most patients receiving chemotherapy have measurable disease either in the form of advanced-stage disease, metastatic disease, or recurrence of disease. In most cases, care is provided in the outpatient setting. The majority of these patients are refractory to hormone agents. Because the ideal regimen has not been identified, it is important that patients be offered an opportunity to participate in clinical trials (e.g., single- versus multiple-agent chemotherapy, chemotherapy versus radiation therapy, or chemotherapy plus radiation therapy). It is the responsibility of health care providers to obtain informed consent and explain the risks and benefits of participating in a clinical trial. By accruing patients into clinical trials, we will learn the best way to care for women with endometrial cancer. When administering chemotherapy, nurses must educate patients and their family members about the side effects associated with the drugs and self-care strategies to manage these side effects. The management plan for patients with endometrial cancer who are receiving chemotherapy is summarized in Table 30-13.

HOME CARE ISSUES

Depending on the treatment approaches used to manage endometrial cancer, patients and their family members will be faced with several issues in the home care setting. The focus in this setting is on symptom management. The nurse performs an assessment; identifies the problem(s); and plans, intervenes, and evaluates the plan. Areas for intervention may include changes in sexual functioning, the onset of menopause, psychosocial issues, and financial concerns.

The impact of the diagnosis and treatment of cancer has been recognized to affect sexual functioning. However, sexuality issues are not openly and readily discussed by health care professionals.

Sexual functioning has been documented to affect quality of life (Cartwright-Alcarese, 1995). Wilson and Williams (1988) documented that oncology nurses' attitudes toward sexuality may explain why little attention has been given to this issue. It is important for oncology nurses to examine their attitudes and feelings about sexuality (Hughes, 1996). Education to deal with sexual issues should include three domains: knowledge, skills, and attitudes. It is essential for the nurse to know what to ask about and then how to ask the question. Nurses with the knowledge and acquired skills need to incorporate sexual assessment into their practice. In addition, they must have an understanding of the effects of cancer and its treatment on sexual functioning.

The American Cancer Society (1996) has published a pamphlet, "Sexuality and Cancer for the Woman Who Has Cancer and Her Partner," that provides information about cancer and sexuality in understandable terms. The nurse could use this booklet to open a discussion with the patient and her partner regarding sexual functioning.

The oncology nurse is in a position to assist patients and their partners to cope with changes in sexual functioning that are related to the cancer diagnosis and its treatment. Annon's PLISSIT model (1976), provides a framework for sexual counseling. The four components of the model include permission, limited information, specific suggestions, and intensive therapy. It is thought that most sexual problems can be addressed by giving the patient permission to discuss sexual concerns.

For the cancer patient, education should include a discussion about sexuality and cancer therapy. The patient with endometrial cancer may be treated with surgery, radiation therapy, hormone agents, and chemotherapy. Other factors that influence sexual function include physical symptoms (e.g., pain, alopecia, fatigue, change in body image, anemia), menopausal symptoms, and changes in vaginal mucous membranes. An awareness and understanding of these sexual changes will enable the nurse to be a valuable resource and to have a positive impact on the patient's quality of life (Lamb, 1990, 1995; Lamb & Sheldon, 1994).

For patients who report a change in vaginal mucous membranes, a vaginal lubricant such as Astroglide or K-Y jelly may be used during intercourse to increase comfort. Patients may use a vaginal moisturizer such as Repens two to three times a weeks. Patients may have regular intercourse or use a dilator two to three times a week to prevent vaginal tightening. Strategies to enhance patients' sexual enjoyment may include trying new positions to increase comfort and instructing patients on the use of Kegel exercises to decrease pain and discomfort.

PROGNOSIS

The prognosis for patients with endometrial cancer varies depending on the stage of disease at the time of diagnosis. As shown in Table 30-14, endometrial cancer is a heterogeneous disease with a wide range in 5-year survival rates. Prognostic factors for endometrial cancer are listed in Box 30-4. The depth of myometrial invasion correlates directly with the incidence of extrauterine disease. The grade of the tumor is highly predictive of the extent of disease and pelvic nodal metastasis. Patients with high-grade tumors (i.e., grade 3) are more often associated with deep myometrial invasion and positive lymph nodes. The following histologic types are associated with a poorer prognosis: squamous component, clear cell, and papillary-serous (Kato, Ferry, Goodman, Sullinger, Scully, & Goff, et al., 1995). Lymph node metastasis has been identified as a negative prognostic factor and is associated with recurrence. A tumor size of greater than 2 cm is a negative prognostic factor. Hormone receptors for progesterone and estrogen are independent prognostic factors, but the presence of estrogen receptors not to the same degree as progesterone receptor-positive tumors. DNA ploidy may be a significant prognostic factor. Age may be a factor in prognosis; older age is associated with a poorer prognosis (Kosary, 1994). However, in some studies, after an adjustment is made for tumor grade, age is not an independent

Text continued on p. 721

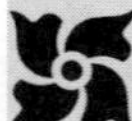

Table 30-13 Standard of Care for the Patient Receiving Chemotherapy for Endometrial Cancer

Patient Problem and Outcomes	Nursing Interventions and Rationales	Patient Education Instructions
Knowledge Deficit Related to Chemotherapy		
Patient will: • Verbalize an understanding of the purpose, benefits, and risks of chemotherapy	1. Assess patient's levels of knowledge about chemotherapy. 2. Assess patient's concerns and fears about chemotherapy.	1. Describe various aspects of chemotherapy treatments: a. Purpose of chemotherapy b. How chemotherapy affects cancer cells c. Name, dosage, route, and schedule of administration of the agents d. Side effects of chemotherapy e. Appropriate intervention to manage side effects including: (1) Nausea and vomiting (2) Alopecia (3) Anorexia (4) Mucositis (5) Infection (6) Fatigue f. Signs and symptoms to report to the health care team
High Risk for Injury Related to the Administration of Taxol		
Patient will: • Not experience a hypersensitivity reaction	1. Take patient's allergy history note if allergic to cremophor (polyoxyethylated castor oil). 2. Premedicate patient with the following: a. Decadron 20 mg PO 12 and 6 hours before Taxol administration b. Benadryl 50 mg PO or IV ½ hour before Taxol administration c. Cimetidine 300 mg IV ½ hour before Taxol administration 3. Monitor vital signs. 4. Observe for signs and symptoms of hypersensitivity reaction including: a. Hypotension b. Dyspnea c. Angioedema d. Urticaria e. Chest pain f. Flushing g. Skin reactions h. Tachycardia 5. Immediately stop the infusion if you suspect a reaction. Maintain intravenous access, notify physician, and administer emergency drugs as prescribed.	1. Teach the patient the importance of taking premedications.
Sensory-Perceptional Alteration Related to Peripheral Neuropathy Secondary to Chemotherapy		
Patient will: • Identify and report sensory-perceptual changes • Demonstrate measures to manage sensory-perceptual changes • Maintain optimal functioning	1. Assess baseline information regarding peripheral nervous system: a. Sensory responses b. Motor function c. Hearing test d. Vision test e. Deep tendon reflexes	1. Instruct patient regarding peripheral neuropathy: a. Definition b. Causes: (1) Name of chemotherapy agent (2) Dosage (3) Previous nerve condition

PO, Orally; *IV,* intravenously; *EMG,* electromyography; *CBC,* complete blood count; *BUN,* blood urea nitrogen; *TID,* 3 times a day; *ECG,* electrocardiogram; *MUGA,* multigated equilibrium heart scan.

TABLE 30-13 Standard of Care for the Patient Receiving Chemotherapy for Endometrial Cancer—cont'd

Patient Problem and Outcomes	Nursing Interventions and Rationales	Patient Education Instructions
Sensory-Perceptional Alteration Related to Peripheral Neuropathy Secondary to Chemotherapy—cont'd		
	f. Bowel function g. Bladder function h. Sexual function 2. Perform an ongoing assessment for peripheral neuropathy: a. Assess sensory function (1) Assess pain (2) Response to pain, touch, vibration, and sensation b. Assess motor function (1) Check Romberg's sign (2) Assess gait (3) Assess fine motor coordination c. Check deep-tendon reflexes d. History of falling 3. Evaluate patient's ability to perform activities of daily living. 4. Assist patient with activities of daily living as necessary. 5. Make referrals to physical therapy and occupational therapy. 6. Assess need for assistive devices. 7. Institute safety measures. 8. Evaluate bowel function and assess for signs and symptoms of intestinal obstruction.	c. Sign and symptoms of peripheral neuropathy d. Ongoing evaluation by physical examination or EMG e. Ways to promote safety: (1) Avoid extremes in temperature (2) Wear foot covering at all times (3) Use a pot holder in kitchen (4) Inspect skin for cuts, abrasions, or bruises (5) Maintain optimal functioning f. Maintain bladder/bowel functioning g. Tell patient that recovery may be complete or partial and is slow (months)
Anemia • Patient demonstrates adequate oxygen saturation of tissues: a. Laboratory values at satisfactory level b. Vital signs stable c. No evidence of obvious bleeding • Patient/significant other(s) demonstrates knowledge of relationship of red blood cells, hemoglobin, and availability of oxygen for normal function • Patient demonstrates knowledge of factors that contribute to anemia • Patient identifies measures to prevent anemia	1. Monitor CBC, including hemoglobin and hematocrit. 2. Assess for signs and symptoms of anemia including: a. Palpitations/chest pain upon exertion b. Dyspnea upon exertion c. Dizziness/syncope d. Fatigue/weakness e. Anorexia f. Headache g. Tinnitus h. Insomnia 3. Assess for signs of blood loss. 4. Monitor orthostatic vital signs. 5. Perform skin assessment. 6. Perform oral assessment. 7. Perform oral hygiene. 8. Perform cardiac assessment. 9. Assess patient's ability to perform activities of daily living. 10. Provide assistance for activities that cannot be performed independently. 11. Provide patient with rest periods.	1. Teach normal values for hemoglobin/hematocrit and relationship to overall health. 2. Teach signs and symptoms of anemia: a. Pallor b. Fatigue c. Shortness of breath d. Tachycardia on exertion e. Headache f. Dizziness g. Irritability h. Heart palpitations 3. Teach factors that cause anemia: a. Radiation b. Drugs (anticonvulsants, and chemotherapeutic agents) c. Alcohol d. Antibiotic therapy e. Bleeding 4. Refer to dietitian. 5. Encourage high-protein diet and vitamin and iron supplements. 6. Teach the importance of preventing infection.

Continued

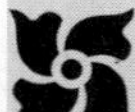

TABLE 30-13 Standard of Care for the Patient Receiving Chemotherapy for Endometrial Cancer—cont'd

Patient Problem and Outcomes	Nursing Interventions and Rationales	Patient Education Instructions
Anemia—cont'd	12. Increase activity level as tolerated by patient. 13. Provide diet high in protein, vitamins, and iron. 14. Consult dietitian if indicated. 15. Administer iron supplements as prescribed. 16. Administer erythropoietin as prescribed. 17. Administer blood products as prescribed. 18. Administer oxygen as prescribed.	7. Instruct patient to plan rest periods and adequate sleep time. 8. Explain treatment plan. 9. Instruct patient to maintain skin integrity: a. Turn and position b. Lubricate skin with cream or lotion after daily bath and as needed c. Avoid drying agents to the skin 10. Assess understanding of change in activity level and ability to perform activities.
Potential for Bleeding Related to Thrombocytopenia • Patient will not experience preventable bleeding • Patient will demonstrate knowledge of bleeding precautions and verbalize who to contact when signs and symptoms occur	1. Monitor CBC and platelet count. 2. Monitor for signs and symptoms of bleeding. 3. Monitor vital signs. 4. Institute thrombocytopenia protocol for a platelet count of 50,000/mm^3. 5. Institute safety standard. 6. Administer platelets as prescribed. 7. Avoid ASA-containing drugs and be aware of other drugs interfering with platelet function.	1. Explain the relationship between platelets and bleeding. 2. Teach patient about bleeding precautions. 3. Teach patient signs and symptoms of bleeding. 4. Instruct patient to notify health care professional if bleeding occurs. 5. Instruct patient on measures to manage bleeding.
Nausea and Vomiting Patient maintains adequate fluid balance as evidenced by: • Laboratory values within patient's baseline • Maintains stable weight • Decrease in nausea • Maintains adequate intake and output	1. Assess patient's pattern of nausea and vomiting including: a. Onset b. Frequency c. Duration d. Amount e. Color f. Character of the emesis g. Alleviating/exaggerating factors 2. Assess for signs and symptoms of fluid volume deficit including: a. Decreased skin turgor b. Thirst, parched tongue c. Warm, flushed skin d. Rapid, weak pulse e. Hypotension f. Lethargy g. Confusion, disorientation 3. Monitor patient for: a. Anorexia b. Altered taste c. Sore mouth d. Fatigue e. Pain f. Obstruction	1. Teach strategies to prevent nausea and vomiting: a. Small, frequent meals b. Rest period before and after meals c. Minimize stimuli d. Avoid sweet, highly seasoned, or greasy food e. Recommend foods with low potential to cause nausea (i.e., dry toast, crackers, ginger ale, cola, cold plates, boiled or baked potatoes) f. Experiment with sour foods g. Eat food cold or at room temperature h. Eat various kinds of candy (hard or soft mints and sour candy) i. Provide distraction

PO, Orally; *IV,* intravenously; *EMG,* electromyography; *CBC,* complete blood count; *BUN,* blood urea nitrogen; *TID,* three times a day; *ECG,* electrocardiogram; *MUGA,* multigated equilibrium heart scan.

TABLE 30-13 Standard of Care for the Patient Receiving Chemotherapy for Endometrial Cancer—cont'd

Patient Problem and Outcomes	Nursing Interventions and Rationales	Patient Education Instructions
Nausea and Vomiting—cont'd	4. Monitor intake and output. 5. Maintain fluid intake of at least 2500 ml/day, unless contraindicated. 6. Administer IV hydration as prescribed. 7. Inspect oral cavity to assess hydration status. 8. Perform oral care before/after meals and after emesis. 9. Administer antiemetic as prescribed and assess the effectiveness of antiemetic regimen. 10. Maintain patient in Fowler's position after eating. 11. Weigh weekly and report change in weight. 12. Refer for dietary consult. 13. Monitor lab values including: a. CBC b. electrolytes (K^+, Mg^{++}, Na^+) c. BUN/creatinine 14. Conduct a guaiac emesis. 15. Perform relaxation exercises.	
Oral Mucositis Related to: • Chemotherapy • Lack of oral intake • Immunosuppression and nutritional depletion Patient will: • Exhibit healing of oral mucosa • Maintain optimal level of comfort • Maintain sufficient oral intake • Identify factors that alter the integrity of the mucous membrane • Be able to perform an oral assessment and preventive measures • Identify signs and symptoms to report to health care team	1. Perform oral assessment including: a. Assessment of the lips, tongue, gums, and buccal mucosa for presence or absence of any of the following: (1) Change in color (2) Swelling (3) Pain (4) Bleeding/discharge (5) Lesions b. Assess the teeth for: (1) Missing teeth (2) Mobile teeth (3) Caps (4) Fractures (5) Pain/tenderness c. Assess for changes in taste d. Remove and assess denture fit (if applicable), amount and consistency of saliva, voice, and ability to swallow. e. Evaluate for evidence of infection 2. Provide oral hygiene care. 3. Apply lip lubricant. 4. Type of diet will depend on patient's condition. 5. Provide appropriate nutritional intake. 6. Refer for dietary consult.	1. Teach patient/others to perform an oral assessment: a. Wash hands b. Obtain a mirror and a light c. Observe for deviations from normal mucosa 2. Instruct patient to assess and report signs and symptoms of mucositis: a. Dry, rough lips b. Burning sensation/pain in the mouth or at mucocutaneous function c. Red, inflamed mucosa d. Small white or yellow patches e. Difficulty swallowing f. Red, swollen gums or tongue g. Coating, redness, ulceration h. Changes to sensation, appearance, or taste 3. Teach patient oral hygiene measures: a. Brush teeth with a soft nylon bristle toothbrush after meals and at bedtime b. Remove dentures/bridge cleanse and replace after oral hygiene care c. Keep dentures in water while out d. Remove dentures if evidence of alteration in oral mucosa

Continued

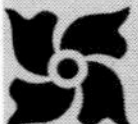

TABLE 30-13 Standard of Care for the Patient Receiving Chemotherapy for Endometrial Cancer—cont'd

Patient Problem and Outcomes	Nursing Interventions and Rationales	Patient Education Instructions
Oral Mucositis Related to:—cont'd		
	7. Encourage fluid intake (3000 ml of fluid daily unless contraindicated). 8. Monitor for signs and symptoms of infection. 9. Monitor vital signs. 10. Monitor WBC count and total neutrophil count. 11. Administer pain medication as prescribed. 12. Administer antimicrobial medication as prescribed. 13. Refer for dental consult.	4. Instruct patient to avoid irritants and irritation to mucosa: a. Commercial mouthwashes b. Alcohol c. Lemon-glycerin swab d. Tobacco e. Smoking f. Poorly fitted dentures g. Spicy foods h. Citrus fruit juices i. Extremes in food temperatures 5. Keep oral mucosa moist: a. Oral care at least TID and at bedtime b. Adequate fluid intake (3000 ml/day unless contraindicated) c. Artificial saliva d. Keep lips moist with K-Y jelly 6. Encourage patient to eat soft, moist food, avoiding dry, coarse food. 7. Instruct patient to administer prophylactic oral antifungal or antibacterial agents as prescribed.
Potential for Inadequate Nutrition Less than Body Requirements Related to:		
1. Inadequate intake: a. Decreased appetite b. Nausea/vomiting c. Mucositis d. Dysphagia 2. Increased excretion: a. Vomiting b. Diarrhea 3. Increased requirements: a. Fever b. Infection c. Stress Patient will: • Exhibit minimal signs and symptoms of malnutrition as evidenced by maintaining or increasing pretreatment body weight • Demonstrate knowledge about how to maintain adequate nutrition	1. Assess for nutritional deficits including: a. Lack of interest in food b. Problems or difficulties with eating: (1) Anorexia (2) Nausea and vomiting (3) Dysphagia (4) Early satiety (5) Mucositis 2. Monitor intake and output. 3. Measure height and weight on admission and weight weekly. 4. Evaluate dietary patterns: a. Obtain diet history, noting patterns in appetite and food preferences, aversions, and foods that are well tolerated b. Note best time to eat during the day 5. Obtain a dietary consult. 6. Monitor lab values: serum albumin, electrolytes, urinalysis, hemoglobin, hemocrit, serum total protein. 7. Observe for signs of dehydration: a. Decreased skin turgor b. Dry mouth and mucous membranes c. Thirst d. Scanty, concentrated urine	1. Instruct patient on eating hints and provide the booklet by the National Cancer Institute entitled *Eating Hints.*

PO, Orally; *IV,* intravenously; *EMG,* electromyography; *CBC,* complete blood count; *BUN,* blood urea nitrogen; *TID,* 3 times a day; *ECG,* electrocardiogram; *MUGA,* multigated equilibrium heart scan.

TABLE 30-13 Standard of Care for the Patient Receiving Chemotherapy for Endometrial Cancer—cont'd

Patient Problem and Outcomes	Nursing Interventions and Rationales	Patient Education Instructions
Potential for Inadequate Nutrition Less than Body Requirements Related to:—cont'd		
	8. Perform oral care before meals. 9. Administer antiemetic 30 minutes before meal as ordered. 10. Medicate with topical/systemic analgesics as ordered. 11. Position patient before meals for comfort. 12. Encourage patient to maintain a diet high in calories, protein, and vitamins. 13. Provide between-meals supplements. 14. Offer small, frequent meals. 15. Determine whether any other symptoms interfere with eating and utilize strategies to prevent the symptoms: a. Fatigue b. Pain c. Mucositis d. Diarrhea e. Anxiety f. Depression	
Alopecia Patient will: • Verbalize feelings related to hair loss • Utilize appropriate coping strategies to deal with alopecia	1. Inform the patient when hair loss is expected to begin and the anticipated degree and duration of the hair loss. 2. Inform patient that hair loss is temporary and that hair regrowth may differ in color and texture. 3. Assess the importance of hair to patient/significant other. 4. Encourage the patient to verbalize feelings about alopecia. 5. Identify possible measures to take during hair loss: a. Wig b. Scarf, hat, or turban c. Use make-up 6. Encourage patient to maintain self-image by: a. Socialization b. Wearing own clothes/pajamas 7. Instruct patient on interventions to minimize hair loss.	1. Teach the patient to utilize the following interventions: a. Use mild shampoo followed by a conditioner every 3-5 days b. Avoid excessive shampooing c. Minimize the use of electric hair dryer d. Discontinue the use of electric curlers and curling irons, hair clips, bobby pins, and barrettes e. Hair spray, hair dye, and bleach may increase the fragility of the hair and should be avoided f. Using a wide-tooth comb is preferred; avoid excessive brushing and combing of the hair. g. Use a satin pillowcase
Fatigue Patient will: • Be able to identify the factors with the potential to cause fatigue • Maintain optimal function and comfort	1. Perform a fatigue assessment including pattern of fatigue, onset, duration, intensity, aggravating and alleviating factors, and impact of fatigue on the patient's activity level and assess for contributing factor(s) such as dyspnea, degree of anemia, infection, fever, anorexia, cachexia and chronic pain.	1. Instruct patient to coordinate realistic daily activities. Teach patient to recognize fatigue and pace him- or herself. 2. Instruct patient to avoid doing too much too soon.

Continued

TABLE 30-13 Standard of Care for the Patient Receiving Chemotherapy for Endometrial Cancer—cont'd

Patient Problem and Outcomes	Nursing Interventions and Rationales	Patient Education Instructions
Fatigue—cont'd	2. Encourage patient to set priorities and choose activities. 3. Plan intermittent rest periods as needed. 4. Assist the patient with activities as needed. 5. Provide emotional support. 6. Assess for the presence of anemia. 7. Administer packed red blood cells as prescribed. 8. Administer oxygen as prescribed. 9. Provide patient with feedback and encouragement in identifying abilities and limitations.	
Potential Alteration in Renal Function Related to Nephrotoxic or Urotoxic Effects of Chemotherapy		
Patient will: • Maintain fluid intake of 2-3 L, unless contraindicated • Maintain urine output of 100 ml/hr or more	1. Encourage adequate fluid intake. 2. Monitor intake and output. 3. Administer fluids as prescribed. 4. Assess urine and report changes (i.e., color, sediment). 5. Monitor renal status.	
Constipation		
Patient will: • Demonstrate strategies to promote adequate bowel elimination • Demonstrate usual pattern of elimination	1. Assess the patient's usual patterns of elimination. 2. Encourage oral intake of at least 2500 ml/day, unless contraindicated. 3. Maintain high-fiber diet and avoid constipating foods. 4. Encourage physical activity as tolerated. 5. Administer stool softener and laxatives as needed. 6. Remind patient to respond immediately to the urge to defecate. 7. Administer prophylactic stool softeners and/or laxative as prescribed.	1. Teach signs and symptoms of constipation to report to the health care team. 2. Review foods that are high in fiber and those that are constipating. 3. Teach about modification of dietary habits (e.g., maintain oral intake, avoid constipating foods and increase fiber in diet).
Potential Alteration in Cardiac Output Related to Chemotherapy		
Patient maintains adequate cardiac output	1. Obtain baseline cardiac function studies as prescribed (e.g., ECG, MUGA scan). 2. Assess cardiac status: a. Vital signs b. Skin color c. Mental status	1. Explain test and procedures. 2. Instruct patient to report feelings of palpitations, irregular pulse, or fluttering in the chest.

TABLE 30-14 5-Year Survival for Endometrial Cancer by Stage

Stage	Population (%)	5-Year Survival Rates (%)
Stage I	81	83
Stage II	11	73
Stage III	6	52
Stage IV	2	27

From Abeler, V. M. & Kjorstad, K. E. (1991). Endometrial adenocarcinoma in Norway: A study of a total population. *Cancer, 67,* 3093-3103.

TABLE 30-15 Quality of Care Evaluation for a Patient Having Pain

Disciplines participating in the quality of care evaluation
☐ Nursing ☐ Medicine ☐ Rehabilitation
☐ Social Services ☐ Pharmacy ☐ Pain Service

Data from:
☐ Mailed Questionnaire ☐ Patient Interview

Criteria	Yes	No
1. Were you provided information on how to manage pain at home?	☐	☐
2. Were you given clear instructions about how to take your pain medication?	☐	☐
3. Were you instructed to report any change (increase) in pain or a new pain problem?	☐	☐
4. Were you satisfied with the way your health care provider managed you pain?	☐	☐

prognostic factor. Race is a prognostic factor. Nonwhite women have a poorer prognosis because these women are diagnosed with poorly differentiated endometrial cancer (Kosary, 1994).

In the literature, two groups of women have been described with endometrial cancer with different prognoses. Type I women have estrogen-related risk factors such as obesity, nulliparity, and unopposed estrogen therapy. The prognosis for these women with early-stage endometrial cancer is excellent. Women with type II endometrial cancer have poorly differentiated tumors with an adverse histologic type, deep myometrial invasion, and extrauterine disease. Type II women have a poorer prognosis, and the risk factors for these women have not yet been identified.

EVALUATION OF THE QUALITY OF CARE

Accreditation organizations, such as the Joint Commission for the Accreditation of Health Care Organizations, require that the quality of care provided to patients be evaluated. Because the care provided to patients with endometrial cancer requires input from a multidisciplinary team, an evaluation of the quality of care provided to these patients should include aspects of care provided by various members of the team. Tables 30-15 through 30-17 provide examples of quality of care evaluation tools that can be used in the inpatient and outpatient setting.

BOX 30-4
Prognostic Factors in Endometrial Cancer

Stage of disease
Depth of myometrial invasion
Tumor grade
Histologic type
Lymph node metastases
Tumor size
Hormonal receptors
DNA ploidy
Age
Race
Type I or II endometrial cancer

TABLE 30-16 Quality of Care Evaluation for a Patient Undergoing Total Abdominal Hysterectomy and Bilateral Salpingo-Oophorectomy

Disciplines participating in the quality of care evaluation
☐ Nursing ☐ Medicine
☐ Rehabilitation ☐ Social Services

Data from:
☐ Mailed Questionnaire ☐ Patient Interview

Criteria	Yes	No
1. Did the health care professional explain the type of surgery and expected outcomes?	☐	☐
2. Was the preoperative routine explained to you?	☐	☐
3. Were you taught to:		
a. Abstain from intercourse for 4-6 weeks or as indicated by the physician?	☐	☐
b. Report any signs and symptoms of infection?	☐	☐
c. Gradually increase activity?	☐	☐
4. Were you told to schedule a follow-up appointment?	☐	☐

RESEARCH ISSUES

Numerous research issues surrounding the management of endometrial cancer require further investigations. At the present time, cost-effective screening practices for endometrial cancer do not exist (Karasek & Faul, 1996). There is a need to develop cost-effective protocols to follow women who are identified to be at high risk for this disease. Currently, the Breast Cancer Prevention Trial is exploring the value of endometrial biopsy to screen women receiving tamoxifen therapy. Additional research is needed to determined the risks and benefits associated with hormone replacement therapy.

A major national research study (i.e., Women's Health Initiative) is being conducted to study postmenopausal women and their health. This study will explore the relationships among diet, hormone replacement therapy, calcium, and vitamin D, as well as the impact these factors have on heart disease, cancer, and bone fractures. The results of this study will have implications for women's health issues.

Numerous randomized clinical trails are needed to determine the most effective treatment for the various stages of endometrial cancer. Innovative strategies are needed for patients with advanced or recurrent disease. Additional research is warranted to determine the follow-up care for patients with endometrial cancer. There is a need to evaluate criteria for the purpose of developing guidelines for the management of follow-up care.

All of these research studies need to consider not only the effectiveness of the treatment in improving the patient's survival, but also the cost of the treatment modality, the associated treatment morbidities, and the impact of treatment on the patient's quality of life.

TABLE 30-17 Quality of Care Evaluation for a Patient Receiving Radiation Therapy

Disciplines participating in the quality of care evaluation
☐ Nursing ☐ Medicine ☐ Radiation Therapy

Data from:
☐ Mailed Questionnaire ☐ Patient Interview

Criteria	Yes	No
1. Did the health care professional explain the following:		
a. Purpose of radiation therapy?	☐	☐
b. Simulation procedure?	☐	☐
c. Treatment schedule?	☐	☐
2. Were you taught to minimize the side effects of		
a. Fatigue?	☐	☐
b. Cystitis?	☐	☐
c. Alteration of vaginal membranes?	☐	☐
3. Were you instructed on how to contact your health care professional?	☐	☐
4. Were you instructed when to call a health care professional about side effects?	☐	☐

REFERENCES

Abeler, V. M. & Kjorstad, K. E. (1991). Endometrial adenocarcinoma in Norway: A study of a total population. *Cancer, 67,* 3093-3103.

American Cancer Society. (1996). *Cancer facts and figures 1996.* Atlanta: American Cancer Society.

American Hospital Formulary Service. (1996). *Drug information.* Authority of the Board of Directors of the American Society of Health-System Pharmacists.

Annon, J. S. (1976). *Behavorial treatment of sexual problems: Brief therapy.* New York: Harper and Row.

Butts, P. (1979). Meeting the special needs of your hysterectomy patient. *Nursing, 79,* 40-47.

Carey, M. & O'Connell, G. (1995). Good outcome associated with a standardized treatment protocol using selective post-operative radiation with clinical stage I adenocarcinoma of the endometrium. *Gynecologic Oncology, 57,* 138-144.

Cartwright-Alcarese, F. (1995). Addressing sexual dysfunction following radiation therapy for a gynecologic malignancy. *Oncology Nursing Forum, 22,* 1227-1232.

Clinical Handbook of Clinical Preventive Services. (1995). Estrogen and progestin supplementation. *Nurse Practitioner, 20,* 63-64, 66.

Creasman, W. T. (1994). Limited disease role of surgery. *Seminar in Oncology, 21,* 79-83.

DePalo, G., Spatti, G. B., Bandieramonte, G., & Luciani, L. (1983). Pilot study with adjuvant hormone therapy in FIGO stage I endometrial carcinoma with myometrial invasion. *Tumori, 69,* 65-67.

DiSaia, P. J. & Creasman, W. T. (1993). Adenocarcinoma of the uterus. In P. J. DiSaia & W. T. Creasman (Eds.), *Clinical gynecologic oncology.* St. Louis: Mosby Company.

Dow, K. H. S. & Hilderley, L. J. (1992). *Nursing care in radiation oncology.* Philadelphia: W. B. Saunders Company.

Elliot, P. & Green, D. (1994). The efficacy of postoperative vaginal irradiation in preventing vaginal recurrence in endometrial cancer. *International Journal of Gynecologic Cancer, 4,* 84-93.

Greven K., Corn, B., & Lanciano, R. (1993). Pathologic stage III endometrial carcinoma: Prognostic factors and patterns of recurrence. *Cancer, 71,* 3697-3702.

Hall, K. L., Dewar, M. A, & Perchalski, J. (1992). Screening for gynecologic cancer. *Primary Care: Clinics in Office Practice, 19,* 607-619.

Hampton, B. G. (1986). Nursing management of a patient following pelvic exenteration. *Seminars in Oncology Nursing, 2,* 281-286.

Henderson, B. E., Ross, R. K., & Pike, M. C. (1993). Hormonal chemoprevention of cancer in women. *Science, 259,* 633-638.

Hogan, W. M. & Boente, M. P. (1993). The role of surgery in the management of recurrent gynecologic cancer. *Seminars in Oncology, 20,* 462-472.

Homesly, H. D. & Zaino, R. (1994). Endometrial cancer: Prognostic factors. *Seminars in Oncology, 21* 71-78.

Hoskins, W. J., Perez, C. A., & Young, R. C. (1993). Gynecologic tumors. In V. DeVita., S. Hellman, & S. A. Rosenberg (Eds.), *Cancer principles and practice of oncology.* Philadelphia: J. B. Lippincott Company.

Hubbard, J. L. & Holcombe, J. K. (1990). Cancer of the endometrium. *Seminars in Oncology Nursing, 6,* 206-213.

Hughes, M. K. (1996). Sexuality issues: Keeping your cool. *Oncology Nursing Forum, 23,* 1597-1600.

Jansen, C. (1995). Uterine cancer. In C. Miaskowski (Ed.), *Oncology nursing: Plans of care for specialty practice.* New York: Delmar.

Karasek, K. & Faul, C. (1996). Changing concepts in the management of endometrial cancer. *Oncology, 10,* 1099-1106.

Kato, D. T., Ferry, J. A., Goodman, A., Sullinger, J., Scully, E., Goff, B. A., Fuller, A. F., & Rice, L. W. (1995). Uterine papillary serous carcinoma. (UPSC): A clinicopathologic study of 30 cases. *Gynecology Oncology, 59,* 384-389.

Key, T. J. A. (1995). Hormones and cancer in humans. *Mutation Research, 333,* 59-67.

Kneale, B. L. (1986). Adjunctive and therapeutic progestins in endometrial cancer. *Clinical Obstetrics and Gynaecology, 13,* 789-809.

Kosary, C. L. (1994). FIGO stage, histology, histologic grade, age and race as prognostic factors in determining survival for cancers of the female gynecological system: An analysis of 1973-87 SEER cases of cancers of the endometrium, cervix, ovary, vulva and vagina. *Seminars In Surgical Oncology, 10,* 31-46.

Kurman, R. J., Zaino, R. J., & Norris, H. J. (1994). Endometrial carcinoma. In R. Kurman (Ed.), *Blaustein's pathology of the female genital tract.* New York: Springer-Verlag.

Lamb, M. A. (1995). Effects of cancer on the sexuality and fertility of women. *Seminars in Oncology Nursing, 11,* 120-127.

Lamb, M. A. (1990). Psychosexual issues: The woman with gynecologic cancer. *Seminars in Oncology Nursing, 6,* 237-243.

Lamb, M. A. & Sheldon, T. A. (1994). The sexual adaption of women treated for endometrial cancer. *Cancer Practice, 2,* 103-113.

Landis, S. H., Murray, T., Bolden, S., & Wingo, P. A. (1998). Cancer statistics, 1998. *CA: A Cancer Journal for Clinicians,* 48, 6-29.

Lentz, S. S. (1994). Advanced and recurrent endometrial carcinoma: Hormonal therapy. *Seminars in Oncology, 21,* 100-106.

Levine, G. N. (1993). *Pocket guide commonly prescribed drugs.* Connecticut: Appleton and Lange.

Lewis, G. J., Slack, N. H., Mortel, R., & Bross, I. D. (1974). Adjuvant progestogen therapy in the primary definitive treatment of endometrial cancer. *Gynecologic Oncology, 2,* 368-376.

Martin, L. K. & Braly, P. S. (1991). Gynecologic Cancers. In S. B. Baird, R. McCorkle, & M. Grant (Eds.), *Cancer Nursing: A comprehensive textbook.* Philadelphia: W. B. Saunders Company.

McCance, K. L. & Huether, S. E. (1998). *Pathophysiology: The biologic basis for disease in adults and children* (3rd ed.). St. Louis: Mosby Company.

McNally, J. C., Somerville, E. T., Miaskowski, C., & Rostad, M. (Eds.) (1991). *Guidelines for oncology nursing practice* (2nd ed.). Philadelphia: W. B. Saunders Company.

Morrow, C., Bundy, B., Kurman, R., Creasman, W. T., Heller, P., Homesley, H. D., & Graham, J. E. (1991). Relationship between surgical-pathological risk factors and outcomes in clinical stage I and II carcinoma of the endometrium. A Gynecologic Oncology Group Study. *Gynecologic Oncology, 40,* 55-61.

Muggia F. M. & Gill, I. (1992) Role of carboplatin in endometrial and cervical carcinomas. *Seminars in Oncology, 19,* 90-93.

Muggia, F. M. & Muderspach, L. (1994). Platinum compounds in cervical and endometrial cancers: Focus on carboplatin. *Seminars in Oncology, 21,* 35-41.

Muss, H. B. (1994). Chemotherapy of metastatic endometrial cancer. *Seminars in Oncology, 21,* 107-113.

Muto, M. G. & Friedman, A. J. (1995). The uterine corpus. In K. J. Ryan (Ed.), *Kistner's gynecology principle and practice.* St. Louis: Mosby Company

Park, R. C., Grigsby, P. W., Muss, H. B., & Norris, H. J. (1992). Corpus: Epithelial tumors. In W. J. Hoskin, C. A. Perez, & R. C. Young (Eds.), *Principle and practice of gynecologic oncology.* Philadelphia: J. B. Lippincott Company.

Robinson, K. M., McCance, K. L., & Gray D. P. (1994). Structures and functions of the reproductive systems. In K. L. McCance & S. E. Huether (Eds.), *Pathophysiology: The biologic bases for disease in adults and children.* St. Louis: Mosby Company.

Rose, P. G. (1996). Endometrial cancer. *The New England Journal of Medicine, 335,* 640-649.

Seoud, M A. F., Johnson, J., & Weed, J. C., Jr. (1993). Gynecologic tumor in tamoxifen treated women with breast cancer. *Obstetrical Gynecology, 82,* 165-169.

Thigpen, J. T., Blessing, J. A., DiSaia, P. J., Yordan, E., Carson, L. F., & Evers, C. (1994). A randomized comparison of doxorubicin alone versus doxorubicin plus cyclophosphamide in the management of advanced or recurrent endometrial carcinoma: A Gynecology Group Study. *Journal of Clinical Oncology, 12,* 1408-1414.

Thigpen, J. T., Vance, R. B., & Khansar, T. (1995). The platinum compounds and paclitaxel in the management of carcinomas of the endometrium, uterine and cervix. *Seminars in Oncology, 22,* 65-75.

Walczak, R. J. & Klemm, P. R. (1993). Gynecologic cancers. In S. L. Groenwald, M. H. Frogge, M. Goodman, & C. H. Yarbro (Eds.), *Cancer nursing principles and practice.* Boston: Jones and Bartlett Publishers.

Wilson, M. E. & Williams H. A. (1988). Oncology nurses' attitude and behavior related to sexuality of patients with cancer. *Oncology Nursing Forum, 15,* 49-53.

Epithelial Cancer of the Ovary

Catherine Jansen, RN, MS

EPIDEMIOLOGY

Ovarian cancer is the deadliest gynecologic malignancy in the United States, killing more women each year than cervical and endometrial cancers combined. Although ovarian cancer accounts for only approximately 4% of all female cancers, it is the fourth leading cause of cancer deaths in women. In 1998, the number of new cases of ovarian cancer in the United States was 25,400, and approximately 14,500 women died from this disease (Landis, Murray, Bolden, & Wingo, 1998). The most common type of ovarian cancers are epithelial, which encompass 85% to 90% of all tumors of the ovary. Epithelial ovarian tumors are rare in young women. They occur most commonly in postmenopausal women. Although available screening tools are more reliable in postmenopausal women than in young women, the variability in sensitivity, especially in earlier-stage tumors, and the lack of specificity negate the use of these tests in mass screening programs for the early detection of ovarian cancer.

Although the survival rate of women with early-stage disease is significantly higher than rates of women diagnosed with advanced-stage disease, this "silent killer" is rarely diagnosed in its early stages. Unfortunately, because of the vague nature or absence of symptoms and the lack of effective screening tools, more ovarian cancers are diagnosed with involvement at distant sites than localized and regional cancers combined. This pattern in diagnosis significantly affects treatment options and long-term survival. Despite aggressive operations and intensive chemotherapy, the overall 5-year survival rate for epithelial ovarian cancer remains less than 40%.

RISK FACTORS

The major risk factors associated with ovarian cancer are listed in Box 31-1. The evidence supporting each of these risk factors is reviewed and the nursing implications for prevention, and early detection activities are discussed in the next section of this chapter.

Increasing Age

Age is an important risk factor in the development of ovarian cancer. The risk of ovarian cancer increases with each decade of life until about age 75, when it reaches its peak, as reflected in Table 31-1. Eighty percent or more of the cases of epithelial ovarian cancer are diagnosed in postmenopausal women. The median age at the time of diagnosis is 62 years. Epithelial ovarian cancer is extremely rare in women younger than age 45. Various estimates have suggested only a 10% to 13% incidence of epithelial ovarian cancer in women younger than 40 years of age (Massi, Susini, Savino, Boddi, Amunni, & Maurizio, 1996; Yancik, 1993). Reports from the National Cancer Data Base estimate that the incidence of ovarian cancer in women under 45 years of age is 15.7 per 100,000 women and that the incidence increases to 54 per 100,000 in women between the ages of 75 and 79 years (Averette, Janicek, & Menck, 1995). In addition, older women usually have the most aggressive forms of ovarian cancer, present with advanced disease, and have a poorer prognosis (Merino & Jaffee, 1993). This risk factor has significant public health implications because of the increased longevity of women and the aging of the female population.

Ethnic Differences

As illustrated in Table 31-2, women who live in highly industrialized countries, with the exception of Japan, have the highest rates of ovarian cancer. In contrast, those who live in developing countries have a lower incidence of ovarian cancer. Whereas the incidence of ovarian cancer in industrialized countries has been constant, the incidence in developing countries has actually increased (Gershenson, Tortolero-Luna, Malpica, Baker, Whittaker, & Johnson et al., 1996). Several epidemiologic studies in the United States have shown ethnic differences, with Hawaiian and Caucasian women having the highest rates of ovarian cancer, followed by Hispanics, African Americans, Filipinos, Chinese, Japanese, and Native Americans with the lowest rates (Averette,

Box 31-1
Risk Factors for Epithelial Ovarian Cancer

- Age
- Ethnicity (whites > African Americans > Asians)
- Positive family history
- High-fat diet
- Talc (? association)
- Polycystic ovary syndrome (? association)
- Infertility
- Pelvic inflammatory disease

Janicek, & Menck, 1995; Devesa, 1995; Schiff, Becker, Smith, Gilliland, & Key, 1996).

Positive Family History

Recent evidence suggests a genetic risk for ovarian cancer, and three specific family types have been identified by pedigree studies. The most common type of positive family history is site-specific familial ovarian cancer syndrome. Women in this family type are at higher risk for the development of only ovarian cancers. Patients with a mother, sister, or daughter who has ovarian cancer are two to four times more likely to develop the disease than women without a positive family history (Gershenson et al., 1996). In addition, the risk for ovarian cancer increases as the affected number of first-degree relatives increases or second-degree relatives are added. This risk may be as high as 50% in women with two first-degree relatives who have ovarian cancer (Barber, 1993).

The second type of family history associated with ovarian cancer is breast-ovarian familial cancer syndrome. A mixture of epithelial ovarian and breast cancers are present in various first- and second-degree relatives. Similar to the first type of family history, women with this family history also have a twofold to fourfold increased risk for ovarian cancer and develop tumors at an earlier age. In the future, the presence of the BRCA-1 gene may be helpful in identifying women at risk for site-specific familial ovarian cancer and breast-ovarian familial cancer syndromes (Futreal, Liu, Shattuck-Eidens, Chochran, Harshman, & Tavtigian et al., 1994).

The third kind of family history associated with familial ovarian cancer is the Lynch II syndrome. This syndrome includes various adenocarcinomas, most commonly colorectal cancer, but has a high rate of breast, endometrial, and ovarian cancers as well. The risk of a woman developing ovarian cancer with this particular family history is variable and dependent on the number of first- and second-degree relatives with a cancer diagnosis.

A strong family history and the occurrence of these cancers at a significantly earlier age suggest an autosomal-dominant mode of inheritance. Women with any of these familial syndromes may benefit from prophylactic removal of both ovaries after they have completed childbearing. In addition, the Committee on Gynecologic Practice of the American College of Obstetricians and Gynecologists recommends periodic screening by transvaginal ultrasonography every 6 months and the use of oral contraceptives for women who wish to maintain fertility, until they have completed their families (Genetic risk, 1992). The Gilda Radner Familial Ovarian Cancer Registry recommends that women have a physical examination, serum CA-125 assay, and a sonogram every 6 months starting at the age of 20 until the age of 35, when prophylactic removal of the ovaries is recommended (Piver, Baker, Jishi, Sandecki, Tsukada, & Natarajan, et al., 1993). Although evidence exists for the role of family history, in actuality this risk factor may account for only 2% to 5% of all ovarian cancers (Gershenson et al., 1996; DiCioccio & Piver, 1996).

Table 31-1 Incidence of Ovarian Cancer in the United States Related to Age (1987-91)

Incidence per 100,000	Age
0.1	0-9 years
1.5	10-19
3.6	20-29
7.4	30-39
17.0	40-49
33.6	50-59
50.4	60-69
61.6	70-79
57.8	80+

From Ries, L.A.G., Miller, B.A., Hankey, B.F., Kosary, C.L., Harras, A., Edwards, B.K. (1994). *SEER cancer statistics review, 1973-1991: Tables and graphs, National Cancer Institute.* NIH Publication No. 94-2789. Bethesda, MD, 1994.

High-Fat Diet

Studies have reported a relationship between higher dietary fat intake and the development of ovarian cancer (Gershenson et al., 1996). For example, Japanese women who live in Japan have a low incidence of ovarian cancer. However, the higher rates of ovarian cancer in Japanese immigrants to the United States, especially in their descendants, suggests that the environment or diet may play a role in the development of ovarian cancer. Additionally, the rate of ovarian cancer in Japan actually doubled between 1958 and 1982, in concert with an increased daily consumption of fat in their diet from 10.6 g in 1950 to 84.5 g in 1986 (Wynder, Fujita, Harris, Hirayama, & Hiyama, 1991). Another study demonstrated a relationship between the consumption of dietary fat in milk and a higher risk for ovarian cancer (Mettlin & Piver, 1990). The actual mechanism by which dietary fat intake may increase the risk of ovarian cancer is unknown.

Talc

Previous studies suggested an increased risk for ovarian cancer in women who used talc powders for more than 3

TABLE 31-2 Age-Adjusted Incidence Rates of Ovarian Cancer in Selected Populations

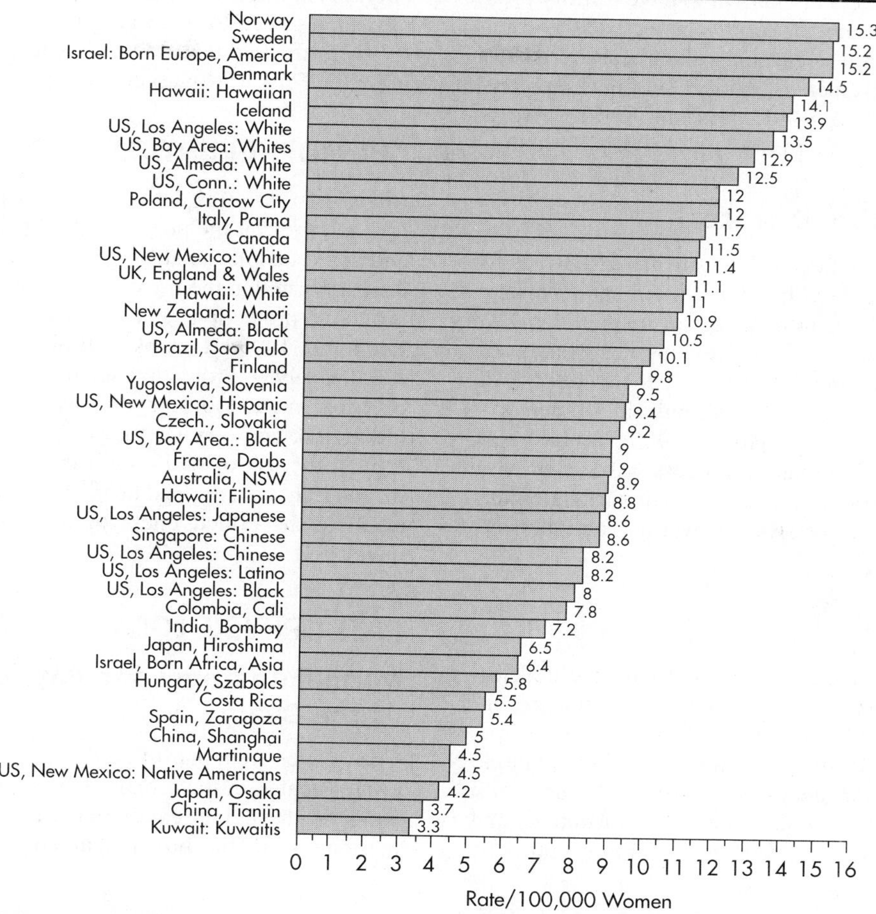

From Gershenson, D.M., Tortolero-Luna, G., Malpica, A., Baker, V.M., Whittaker, L., Johnson, E., & Mitchell, M.F. (1996). Ovarian intraepithelial neoplasia and ovarian cancer. *Obstetrics and Gynecology Clinics of North America, 23*(2), 475-543.

months (Harlow, Cramer, Bell, & Welch, 1992). It was thought that the powder could reach the ovaries after being absorbed through the cervix or vagina. Epidemiologic studies have been inconclusive, and because talc powders are no longer contaminated with asbestos, the possibility of risk is probably no longer important.

Infertility

Several studies have suggested an increased risk for ovarian cancer among nulliparous women and those with a history of infertility (DiCioccio & Piver, 1996). Individual case histories and findings from studies of infertile women who use fertility drugs suggest that these women have an increased risk for ovarian cancer compared with women without a history of infertility (Balasch & Barri, 1993; Bristow & Karlan, 1996; Goldberg & Runowicz, 1992; Karlan, Marrs, & Lagasse, 1994; Whittemore, Harris, Itnyre, Halpern, & The Collaborative Ovarian Cancer Group, 1992). In contrast, there is a decreased risk associated with increasing parity, such that women who have children may have a 45% decrease in risk compared with nulliparous women (Adami, Hsieh, Lambe, Trichopoulos, Leon, & Persson et al., 1994; Hankinson, Colditz, Hunter, Willett, Stampfer, & Rosner, et al., 1995; Piver & DiCioccio, 1996). Findings from some epidemiologic studies suggest a relationship between the use of oral contraceptives and a reduction in the risk for ovarian cancer by as much as 40%, especially with long-term users (Grimes, 1993; Grimes & Economy, 1995; DiCioccio & Piver, 1996; Rodriguez, Calle, Coates, Miracle-McMahill, Thun, & Heath, 1995). However, in other studies, a decreased risk was not as significant after controlling for other risk factors (Hankinson, Colditz, Hunter, Willett, Stampfer, & Rosner et al., 1995).

Polycystic Ovary Syndrome

Polycystic ovary syndrome (PCOS) is an endocrine disturbance characterized by abnormal patterns of hormone secretion, including luteinizing hormone (LH), androgens, and estrogen. This continual irregular stimulation results in the lack of consistent ovulation and the presence of multiple cysts on the ovaries, possibly leading to an increased risk of ovarian cancer. A study of women with PCOS revealed that the use of oral contraceptives was protective against ovarian cancer (Schildkraut, Schwingl, Bastos, Evanoff, & Hughes, 1996). Women with PCOS are known to have fertility problems and therefore are more likely to be exposed to drugs that stimulate the ovaries, causing an increased risk for ovarian cancer (Helzlsouer, Alberg, Gordon, Longcope, Bush, & Hoffman, et al., 1995; Rossing, Daling, Weiss, Moore, & Self, 1994; Whittemore et al., 1992).

Pelvic Inflammatory Disease

Some epidemiologic studies suggest an increased risk for ovarian cancer in women with pelvic inflammatory disease (PID). One study in Canada revealed an increased risk of greater than 30% in women with previous PID (Parazzini, La Vecchia, Negri, Moroni, dal Pino, & Fedele, 1996). Another study showed an increased risk only in women who had recurrent PID (Risch & Howe, 1995). It has been suggested that the inflammatory process associated with PID may stimulate proliferation of ovarian surface epithelium, thereby increasing the risk for ovarian carcinomas to develop.

Summary

Although several risk factors associated with the development of ovarian cancer (e.g., increasing age, ethnicity, and family history) cannot be modified, other risk factors may be reduced through lifestyle modifications. For example, women can reduce their dietary intake of fat through milk. In addition, the use of combination oral contraceptives may reduce the risk of ovarian cancer (see Chemoprevention for Ovarian Cancer). The use of tubal sterilization, especially for those with familial history types, may be useful in reducing risk (Gershenson et al., 1996; Grimes, 1993). Oncology nurses need to be aware of the potential risk factors to provide effective teaching to women concerned about their individual risk for ovarian cancer.

CHEMOPREVENTION

Chemoprevention is defined as the use of certain foods and drugs to prevent the progression of preneoplastic conditions and some neoplastic states (Thomas, 1993). Epidemiologic data confirm that the use of combination oral contraceptives provides protection against ovarian cancer (Grimes & Economy, 1995; Hankinson et al., 1995; Henderson, Ross, & Pike, 1993). Protection seems to occur after a minimum of 3 to 6 months of use, increases with extended length of utilization, and persists for years after discontinuation. Although the use of oral contraceptives for chemoprevention of ovarian cancer has been suggested, clinical trials to evaluate the effectiveness of these agents have not been developed.

PATHOPHYSIOLOGY

Normal Anatomy and Physiology of the Ovary

The ovaries are a pair of double glands (endocrine and exocrine) located in the female pelvis (Fig. 31-1) on the lateral walls of the pelvic cavity, each attached by a fold of the peritoneum to the broad ligament of the uterus on either

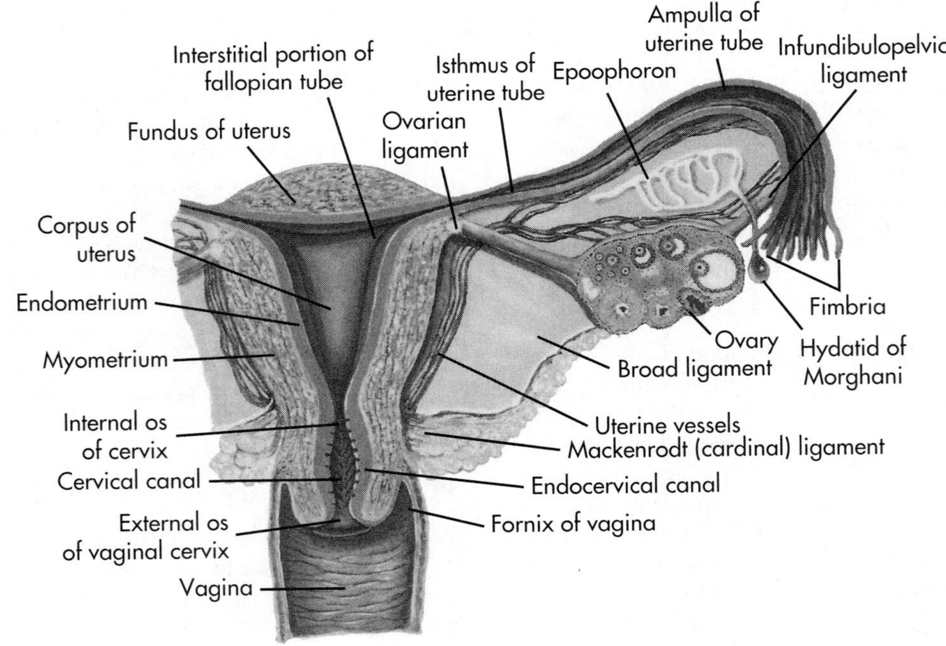

Fig. 31-1 Cross-sectional view of internal female organs. (From Seidel, H. M. [1995]. *Mosby's guide to physical examination* [3rd ed.]. St. Louis: Mosby.)

side. They are in close proximity to the fallopian tubes, which are connected to the uterus. The ovaries, fallopian tubes, uterus, cervix, and vagina constitute the internal genitalia. As displayed in Fig. 31-2, the diaphragm, ureters, colon, and bladder are in close proximity.

Ovary development is initiated by the mesodermal surface (i.e., primary germ layer) of the embryo, with the establishment of coelomic epithelium cells that form the ovaries, fallopian tubes, uterus, and cervix. Germ cells are then formed simultaneously with the proliferation of the coelomic epithelium and mesenchyme (i.e., diffuse network of cells forming connective tissue, blood, lymphatics). Finally, the ovary is divided into the cortex (outer portion) and the medulla (inner portion). The cortex is covered by a single layer of epithelium that functions as a protective layer. Its surface is smooth in early life and later becomes pitted as a result of atrophy. The cortex consists principally of follicles in various stages of development (i.e., primary, growing, and graafian, or mature). The medulla consists of a foundation of connective tissue encompassing nerves, smooth muscle, blood, and lymphatic tissues. The blood system is mainly derived from the ovarian artery, which arises from the abdominal aorta below the renal artery (Fig. 31-3). The lymphatics follow along the ovarian veins and drain into the para-aortic nodes at the level of the second lumbar vertebra (Fig. 31-4).

At birth the ovaries are approximately 3 mm wide and 10 mm long and almond-shaped. They contain up to 2 million ova (primitive female reproductive cells). During childhood, the ovarian ligaments form the outer ovarian layer of connective tissue, and only about 20% of the ova remain. Before puberty, all of the follicles present in the ovary are primary or primitive. Sexual maturity is characterized by the presence of growing follicles. At puberty, progressive development of the follicles is accompanied by growth and development of the ovaries, proliferation of follicles, and development of a connective tissue capsule from the surrounding stroma. Beginning with puberty and continuing through menopause (except during pregnancy), one graafian follicle develops approximately every 30 days. Each of these follicles contains a nearly mature ovum that, on rupture of the follicle through the cortex, is discharged from the ovary. This process is referred to as *ovulation.* The ovum then proceeds within 5 to 7 days through the fallopian tube, ending its journey in the uterus. If fertilization does not occur, menstruation takes place and another follicle goes through maturation. With the initiation of monthly ovulation, only a few hundredths of a percent of ova reach full maturity and even fewer remain at menopause. In an adult, the ovary is an egg-shaped body about 4 cm long, 2 cm wide, and 8 mm thick. The size of the ovaries decreases to 1 to 2 cm as their function decreases.

The functional activity and growth of these glands are primarily under the control of gonadotropins produced in the pituitary gland, in particular follicle-stimulating hor-

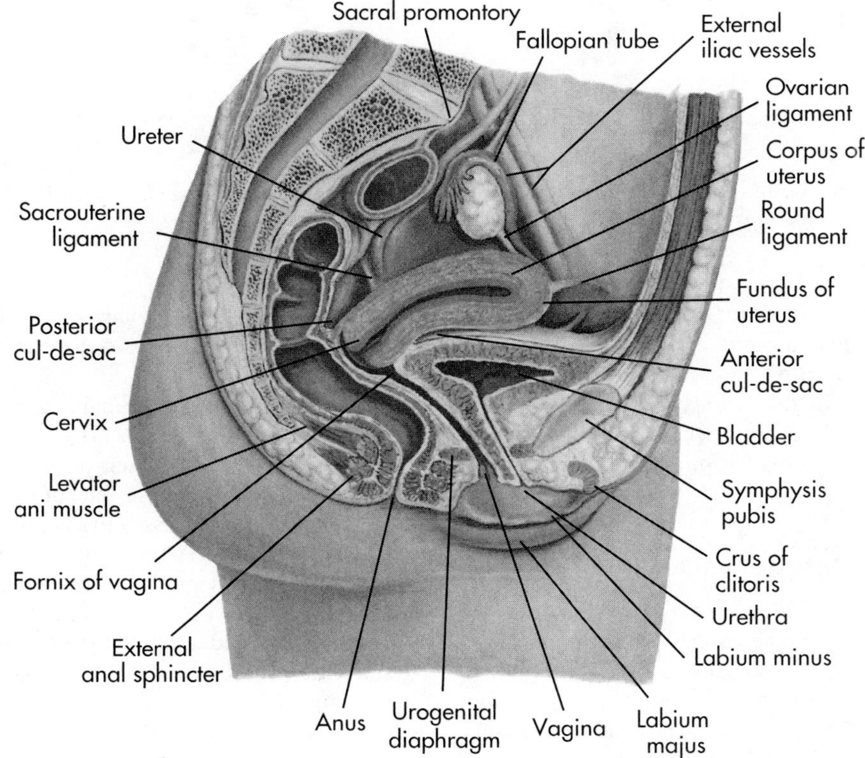

Fig. 31-2 Mid-sagittal view of female pelvic organs. (From Seidel, H. M. [1995]. *Mosby's guide to physical examination* [3rd ed.]. St. Louis: Mosby.)

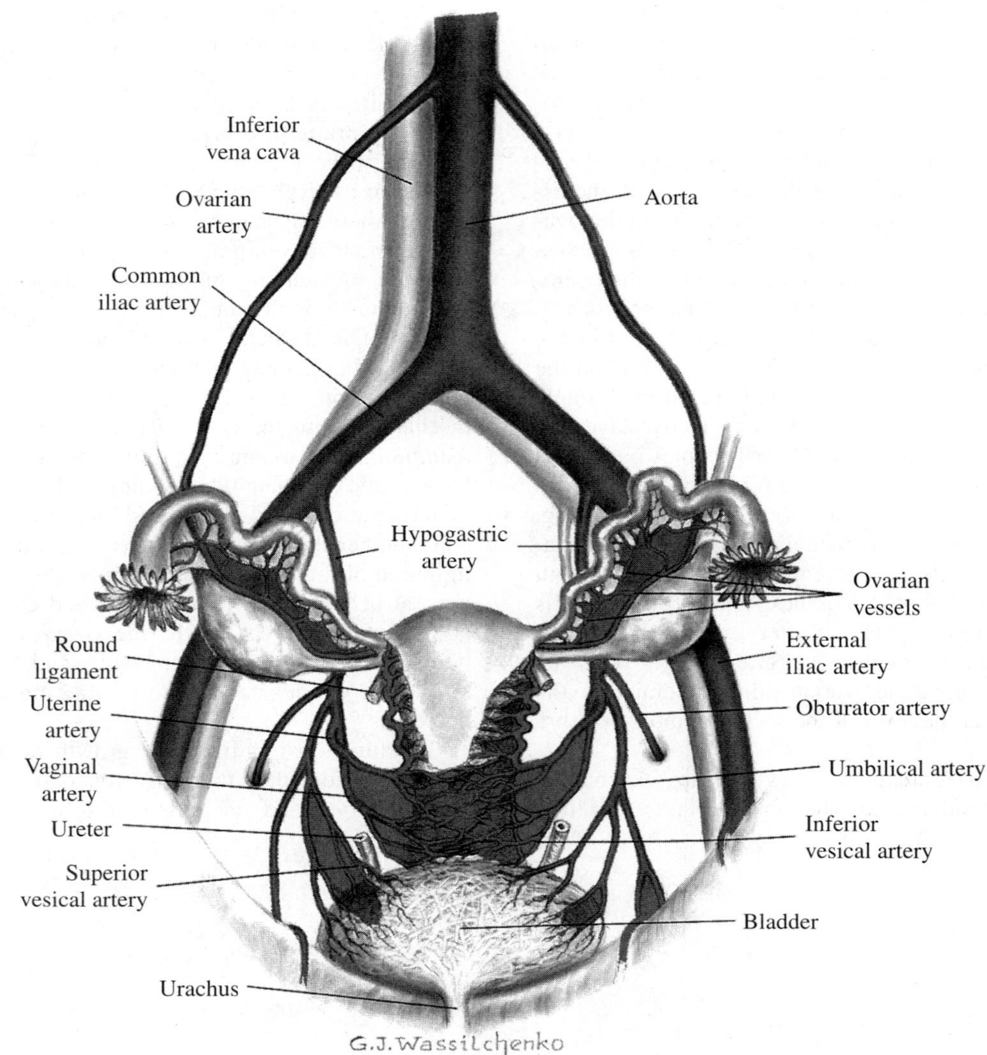

Fig. 31-3 Pelvic blood supply. (From Lowdermilk, D. L., Perry, S. E., & Bobak, I. M. [1993]. *Maternity and women's health care* [6th ed.]. St. Louis: Mosby.)

mone (FSH) and LH. The two major functions of the ovary are to produce and release ova (germ cells) regularly and to produce hormones. These hormones, mainly estrogen and progesterone, are secreted by the ovaries and are responsible for development and maintenance of secondary sexual characteristics, preparation of uterus for pregnancy, and development of the mammary gland.

The Process of Carcinogenesis

As with other cancers, development of ovarian cancer appears to occur as a multistage process including initiation, promotion, and progression. Because of this multistep process, the development of ovarian cancer may involve various premalignant stages. These premalignant lesions have been termed *ovarian intraepithelial neoplasia.* Studies reviewing potential premalignant lesions are limited and have focused on dysplasia of the epithelial tissue and inclusion cysts (Gershenson et al., 1996).

Two hypotheses have been proposed to explain the origin of ovarian cancer. Fathalla (1972) developed the incessant ovulation hypothesis, which proposes that repeated minor traumas to the epithelial surface of the ovary caused by continuous ovulation increases the opportunity for ovarian cancer. The hypothesis suggests that the epithelial lining of the ovaries might be sensitive to the constant trauma of ovulation and may act as a promoting factor in carcinogenesis. This theory would support the suppression of ovulation to reduce the risk of ovarian cancer. Another postulate, the gonadotropin hypothesis, proposes that the exposure of the ovary to continuous, high circulating levels of pituitary gonadotropins (LH and FSH) increases the risk of ovarian cancer (Whittemore et al., 1992). This theory would explain the

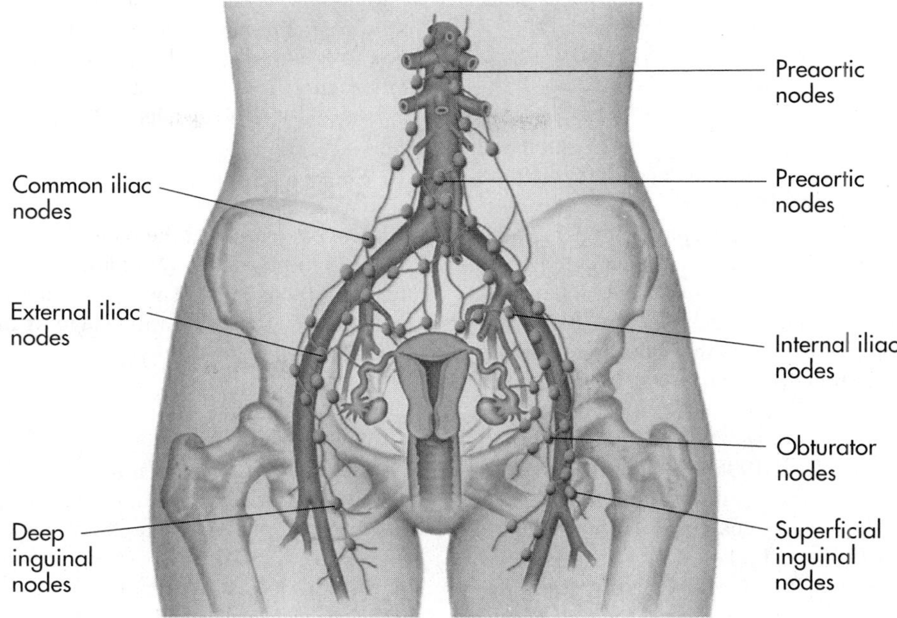

Fig. 31-4 Lymphatic drainage of the female genital tract. (From Seidel, H. M. [1999]. *Mosby's guide to physical examination* [4th ed.]. St. Louis: Mosby.)

protective effect observed with parity and oral contraceptive utilization.

Undoubtedly, changes at the molecular level are involved in the development and progression of ovarian cancer. With the use of sensitive molecular biology methods, the specific genetic (i.e., molecular) changes that occur during the process of carcinogenesis are being identified. As with other types of cancer, the molecular events that lead to the development of ovarian cancer occur in two types of cellular genes, oncogenes and tumor suppressor genes. Oncogenes normally function to enhance cell growth and development. The expression of these genes is tightly controlled, so that in normal adult tissues, a balance is maintained between cellular proliferation and cell death. Damage to a cellular oncogene can result in cellular proliferation and the development of ovarian cancer. One group of oncogenes that has been studied is the *ras* family of oncogenes (i.e., H, K, and N). A mutation of the Ki-*ras* oncogene may be involved in ovarian carcinogenesis and tumor progression of some epithelial cancers (Berchuck, Kohler, Boente, Rodriguez, Whitaker, & Bast, 1993; Cheung, 1996; Park, Kim, Han, Lee, Namkoong, & Kim, 1995; van Dam, Vergote, Lowe, Watson, van Damme, & van der Auwera et al., 1994). In contrast, Baker (1994) stipulates that Ki-*ras* amplification occurs too infrequently to play a role in tumor progression. Overexpression of oncogenes (i.e., epidermal growth factor receptor, c-erbβ-2) may be helpful in identifying which tumors are more aggressive (Cheung, 1996; Felip, Del Campo, Rubio, Vidal, Colomer, & Bermejo, 1995; van Haaften-Day, Russel, Boyer, Kerns, Wiener, & Jensen, 1996). Box 31-2 lists oncogenes that may be altered in ovarian tumors.

Box 31-2
Oncogenes Altered in Ovarian Tumors

BRCA1
c-*erb*β-2
c-*myb*
c-*myc*
EGF (epidermal growth factor)
FGF (fibroblast growth factor)
TGF-α (transforming growth factor-alpha)
Gi
Her-2/*neu*
K-*ras*
TGF-β (transforming growth factor-beta)

Tumor suppressor genes normally function to prevent the continuous growth of cells. A genetic mutation in a tumor suppressor gene could result in uncontrolled cellular proliferation. Several mutations in tumor suppressor genes may be involved in the progression of ovarian cancer from localized to metastatic disease. The most commonly studied tumor suppressor gene associated with ovarian cancer is p53. Mutations and overexpression of p53 have been observed in 50% of advanced ovarian cancers (Bast, Boyer, Jacobs, Xu, Wu, & Wiener et al., 1993). Prognosis tends to be poor in patients expressing high levels of p53 (Herod, Eliopoulos,

Warwick, Niedobitek, Young, & Kerr, 1996; Runnebaum, Kieback, Mobus, Tong, & Kreienberg, 1996).

ROUTES OF METASTASES

Epithelial cancers of the ovary spread by direct extension and seeding into the peritoneal cavity, by lymphatic dissemination, and by hematogenous spread affecting various organs (Fig. 31-5). Epithelial cancers grow through the surface of the gland, penetrating the tissue surrounding the ovary and invading the fallopian tubes and uterus. They may also invade the bladder, colon, and peritoneum. Peritoneal seeding into the abdominal cavity is the most frequent site of metastasis, and at the time of diagnosis as many as 85% of patients may have ascites. The presence of ascites results in a significantly poorer prognosis (Puls, Duniho, Hunter, Kryscio, Blackhurst, & Gallion, 1996). Seeding of the peritoneum facilitates spread of the ovarian cancer to the liver, diaphragm, bladder, spleen, and intestines following the circulatory path of the peritoneal fluid.

Lymphatic spread begins in the pelvic and para-aortic lymph nodes near the ovaries. It continues through the lymphatic channels of the diaphragm and retroperitoneal lymph nodes, upward to the supraclavicular lymph nodes. The incidence of lymph node metastases increases with advancement of clinical stage, 21% in stage I, 23% in stage II, 67% in stage III, and 75% in stage IV (Onda, Yoshikawa, Yokota, Yasugi, & Taketani, 1996).

Metastatic spread through the hematogenous route is uncommon but can affect the lungs and liver. Distant metastases related to ovarian cancer may include (in order of most commonly occurring): pleural effusion, lung, subcutaneous nodules, malignant pericardial effusion, central nervous system, and bone. Central nervous system involvement is rare and occurs in approximately 3% of patients with ovarian cancer (Geisler & Geisler, 1995).

ASSESSMENT

Clinical evaluation of the patient involves a detailed history, a thorough physical examination, and a variety of diagnostic tests (Table 31-3). The signs and symptoms present in the patient often depend on the stage of the disease at the time of diagnosis.

History

The patient should be evaluated for all of the identified risk factors for ovarian cancer. In addition, a careful history of the gynecologic and nearby systems should be obtained. When ovarian cancer is causing obstruction of the bladder, the patient typically reports urinary frequency, urgency, bladder discomfort, and/or distention. When the cancer is causing obstruction of the bowel, the patient may complain of rectal pressure, discomfort, or constipation.

Physical Examination

The bimanual pelvic examination (Fig. 31-6) allows for palpation of the vagina, uterus, and ovaries. The patient must empty the bowel and bladder before the examination and attempt to relax. The normal ovary is almond-shaped and

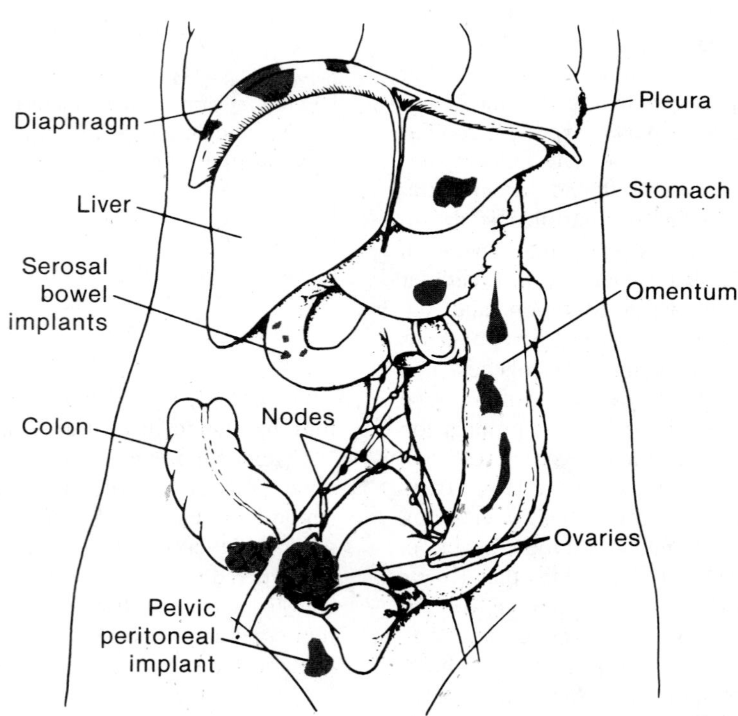

Fig. 31-5 Spread pattern for epithelial cancer of the ovary. (From DiSaia, P. J. [1997]. *Clinical gynecologic oncology* [5th ed.]. St. Louis: Mosby.)

measures approximately 4 × 2 cm. The presence of a normal-size ovary in a postmenopausal patient is cause for concern. The physical examination may reveal a mass in the ovarian area with relative immobility, irregularity, or a bilateral change. In asymptomatic patients, pelvic examinations probably reveal only 1 early-stage ovarian cancer for every 10,000 examinations. Despite the lack of sensitivity, repeat pelvic examinations every 6 months might be indicated in premenopausal women with abnormal findings, because most ovarian enlargements in this population are benign. The finding of weight loss and/or increased abdominal girth in a patient with suspected ovarian cancer is usually an indication of advanced disease.

Diagnostic Tests

Ultrasound. Ultrasound uses a transducer to create high-resolution images of the uterus, fallopian tubes, and ovaries. The procedure has the ability to detect lesions smaller than 4 cm in diameter. Initially, transabdominal ultrasound was used to evaluate the abdomen and had the advantage of visualizing the retroperitoneal structures within the pelvis. The technique is valuable in the diagnosis of ovarian cancer because it can be used to identify ovarian enlargement, distinguish between cystic and solid masses, and assess for the presence of ascites (NIH Consensus Panel, 1995). In transvaginal ultrasound, a vaginal probe is used that allows greater resolution of ovarian architectural detail and has replaced transabdominal ultrasound in some centers. Ultrasound is less specific in the premenopausal patient, because the ovary varies in size throughout the menstrual cycle. Because of this variability, the ultrasound should be performed a week after menses, and any ovary greater than 18 cm^3 should be evaluated further. In postmenopausal women, any ovary larger than 8 cm^3 in size should be evaluated. The observation of any complex or solid patterns should promote concern. A newer technique, transvaginal color Doppler ultrasonography, combines im-

TABLE 31-3 Assessment of the Patient for Ovarian Cancer

	Assessment Parameters	Typical Abnormal Findings
History	A. Personal and social history 1. Age 2. Ethnicity 3. Family history B. Evaluation of gynecologic and nearby systems: 1. Early signs/symptoms 2. Late signs/symptoms	A. Personal and social risk factors 1. Usually postmenopausal 2. More prevalent in whites than in African Americans or Asians 3. Positive family history increases risk B. Gynecologic and related system symptoms: 1. Early signs/symptoms may include: menstrual disturbances, urinary urgency or frequency; bladder discomfort or distention; lower abdominal pressure or discomfort; rectal pressure or discomfort 2. Late signs/symptoms may include: abdominal swelling or bloating (ascites); gastrointestinal disturbances (anorexia, indigestion, food intolerances, nausea and vomiting, constipation); abnormal bleeding (postmenopausal, irregular or excessive menses, precocious puberty); back pain
Physical Examination	A. Pelvic examination B. Weight	A. With early disease on pelvic examination, may palpate enlarged ovaries, especially in postmenopausal patient with advanced disease on pelvic examination, may palpate enlarged ovaries and involvement of other nearby organs (e.g., uterus) B. Weight loss is usually indicative of advanced disease
Diagnostic Tests	A. Transvaginal ultrasound B. Computed tomography (CT) C. Magnetic resonance imaging D. Chest x-ray E. Alpha fetoprotein F. Human chorionic gonadotropin G. Serum lactic dehydrogenase H. CA-125	A. Imaging reveals intraperitoneal masses, enlarged ovaries B. Imaging reveals enlarged ovaries and metastatic disease in the liver, retroperitoneum, and omentum C. Imaging reveals retroperitoneal nodes and masses (able to detect lesions smaller than seen on CT or ultrasound) D. Shows pleural effusions or other metastatic disease in the lungs E. Elevated $>$ 10 ng/ml in endodermal sinus tumors, immature teratomas, mixed germ cell tumors, and less commonly in dysgerminomas F. Elevated $>$ 5.0 mU/ml in choriocarcinomas, embryonal, polyembryonal, and mixed germ cell tumors G. Elevated $>$ 102 U/L in dysgerminomas H. Elevated $>$ 35 U/ml in 80% of postmenopausal patients with ovarian cancer

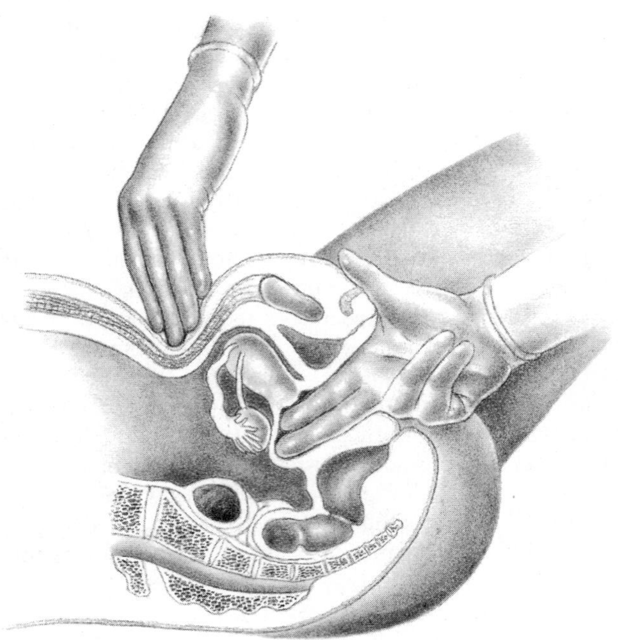

Fig. 31-6 Bimanual pelvic examination. (From Seidel, H. M. [1995]. *Mosby's guide to physical examination* [3rd ed.]. St. Louis: Mosby.)

proved anatomic resolution afforded by high-frequency transvaginal transducers with pathophysiologic evaluation of blood flow within the uterus and ovaries (Fleischer, Cullinan, Peery, & Jones, 1996). Although ultrasound may be helpful in identifying ovarian enlargement, it has not been useful in the screening and staging of ovarian cancer.

Computed Tomography. Computed tomography (CT) is a noninvasive scanning technique that uses a computer to produce three-dimensional images. It is highly acute in distinguishing between benign and malignant lesions. CT can image lesions 2 cm or greater and therefore may be helpful in determining disease volume and response to treatment. Although CT is not as reliable as ultrasound, it has the advantage of being able to detect possible metastatic disease in the liver, retroperitoneum, and omentum.

Magnetic Resonance Imaging. Magnetic resonance imaging (MRI) uses a magnetic field and radiofrequency energy to create multiplane and cross-sectional imaging of the pelvis and surrounding organs. It can depict abnormalities in the lymph nodes, peritoneum, pelvis, bone, and muscle. MRI is an expensive diagnostic tool that is not useful in screening, but may have a role in evaluating ovarian masses to determine the need for surgery (Outwater & Dunton, 1995). To alleviate anxiety, patients should be forewarned about confinement in the close quarters of the MRI equipment.

Barium Enema. A barium enema may be useful to rule out either a primary colon cancer or an ovarian cancer that has invaded the colon.

Chest X-ray. A chest x-ray may be done to determine if there is evidence of pleural effusions. It may also reveal metastatic spread to the lungs.

CA-125. CA-125 is an antigen produced by tissues derived from coelomic epithelium. Although CA-125 may be elevated (more than 35 U/ml) in 80% of epithelial ovarian tumors, most of these tumors present at advanced stages (Gershenson et al., 1996; Kramer, Gohagan, Prorok, & Smart, 1993). Only 50% of postmenopausal women have positive results in early stage I ovarian cancer; therefore its usefulness alone in picking up early cancers is limited (Tamakoshi, Kikkawea, Shibata, Tomoda, Obata, & Wakahara et al., 1996). It is even more unreliable for screening in premenopausal women. CA-125 is not specific to ovarian cancer and causes elevations in benign conditions such as ovarian cysts, endometriosis, pelvic adhesions, pelvic inflammatory disease, and pregnancy, or in other malignancies, such as breast, cervix, colon, endometrium, lung, and pancreas (Jacobs, Davies, Bridges, Stabile, Fay, & Lower et al., 1993; Teneriello & Park, 1995). Although CA-125 may not be helpful in screening, a decline in its level after surgery and during treatment can be correlated with tumor response (Buller, Vasilev, & DiSaia, 1996; Davelaar, Bonfrer, Verstraeten, ten Bokkel Huinink, & Kenemans, 1996; Frasci, Conforti, Zullo, Mastrantonio, Comella, & Comella et al., 1996; Rustin, Nelstrop, McClean, Brady, McGuire, & Hoskins et al., 1996).

Diagnosis. The diagnosis of ovarian cancer is suggested by an abnormal pelvic examination, an elevated CA-125, and abnormal findings on transvaginal ultrasound. However, all of these diagnostic tests have pitfalls. For example, only 80% of women with an abnormal pelvic examination will be found to have cancer. Although CA-125 may pick up some ovarian cancers in stage I, it is most useful for monitoring the effectiveness of treatment. No evidence is yet available that the current screening modalities of CA-125 and transvaginal ultrasonography can be used effectively for widespread screening to reduce mortality from ovarian cancer, or that their use will result in decreased rather than increased morbidity and mortality (NIH Consensus Panel, 1995). The diagnosis of an ovarian cancer requires an exploratory laparotomy.

STAGING

The staging of ovarian cancer involves the use of a histologic staging system (i.e., World Health Organization [WHO]) and one of two clinical staging systems (i.e., the 1992 TNM classification system or the 1985 International Federation of Gynecology and Obstetrics [FIGO] staging system).

Histologic Staging

Histologic staging refers to the examination of the biopsy specimen by a pathologist after surgery. Surgical removal of the ovarian tumor is required for complete histologic staging. In addition, if any free fluid is present in the peritoneum, it should be sampled; otherwise peritoneal washings should be performed and sent for cytologic evaluation. Finally, all intra-abdominal surfaces and viscera, the diaphragm, omentum, and pelvic and para-aortic lymph nodes

TABLE 31-4 Histologic Types of Epithelial Cancers

Type	Benign	Low Malignant Potential	Malignant
Serous	• Cystadenoma and papillary cystadenoma • Surface papilloma • Adenofibroma and cystadenofibroma	• Cystadenoma and papillary cystadenoma • Surface papilloma • Adenofibroma and cystadenofibroma	• Adenocarcinoma, papillary adenocarcinoma, and papillary cystadenocarcinoma • Surface papillary carcinoma • Malignant adenofibroma and cystadenocarcinoma
Mucinous	• Cystadenomas • Adenofibroma and cystadenofibroma	• Cystadenoma • Adenofibroma and cystadenofibroma	• Adenocarcinoma and cystadenocarcinoma • Malignant adenofibroma and cystadenofibroma
Endometrioid	• Adenoma and cystadenoma • Adenofibroma and cystadenofibroma	• Adenoma and cystadenoma • Adenofibroma and cystadenofibroma	• Carcinoma 1. Adenocarcinoma 2. Adenocanthoma 3. Malignant adenofibroma and cystadenofibroma • Endometrioid stromal sarcomas • Mesodermal [mullerian] mixed tumors, homologous and heterologous
Clear cell (mesonephroid)	• Adenofibroma	Carcinomas of low malignant potential	Carcinoma and adenocarcinoma
Brenner	• Benign	• Proliferating	• Malignant
Mixed epithelial	• Benign	• Of borderline malignancy	• Malignant
Undifferentiated carcinoma			

Box 31-3
Histopathologic Grade

GX	Grade cannot be assessed
G1	Well differentiated
G2	Moderately differentiated
G3-4	Poorly differentiated or undifferentiated

should be examined and biopsied if suspected. The purpose of histologic staging is to determine the grade or biologic aggressiveness of the tumor.

The WHO system classifies ovarian tumors by histologic types as outlined in Table 31-4. Each of these types is further defined as benign, borderline malignant (or low malignant potential), or malignant. Furthermore, a histopathologic grade is assigned to the tumor on a scale of 1 to 3. A higher score indicates a more aggressive disease (Box 31-3).

Clinical Staging

Two systems have been used for the clinical staging of ovarian cancer: the 1992 TNM classification system and the 1985 FIGO system. The TNM staging system was developed by the American Joint Committee on Cancer and the International Union Against Cancer. The two systems are displayed in Table 31-5. Since 1993, TNM staging is mandatory in all hospitals that are evaluated by the American Joint Commission on Cancer. However, the FIGO system is more commonly referred to when describing gynecologic tumors. The clinical staging system defines the extent of the patient's disease. The staging of ovarian cancer is depicted in Fig. 31-7.

MEDICAL MANAGEMENT

As summarized in Table 31-6, the treatment of ovarian cancer depends on several factors including the patient's age, the patient's general state of health, the tumor volume, the histologic grade of the tumor, and the stage of disease. In general, surgery with or without either radiation therapy or chemotherapy is used for localized disease. Surgery and chemotherapy are used for metastatic disease (Berek & Hacker, 1994).

Surgical Management

The most common surgical procedures for ovarian cancer are the initial staging laparotomy, interval debulking, and the second-look laparotomy. The amount of surgery required depends on the extent of disease.

Staging Laparotomy. Staging laparotomy is usually performed in patients who are in good health, less than 75 years of age, and without known metastatic disease outside

Table 31-5 TNM* and FIGO† Staging System for Epithelial Ovarian Cancer

TNM Staging System	
Primary Tumor (T)	
TX	Primary tumor cannot be assessed
T0	No evidence of primary tumor
T1	Tumor limited to ovaries (one or both)
T1a	Tumor limited to one ovary; capsule intact, no tumor on ovarian surface, no malignant cells in ascites or peritoneal washings
T1b	Tumor limited to both ovaries; capsules intact, no tumor on ovarian surface, no malignant cells in ascites or peritoneal washings
T1c	Tumor limited to one or both ovaries with any of the following: capsule ruptures, tumor on ovarian surface, malignant cells in ascites or peritoneal washings
T2	Tumor involves one or both ovaries with pelvic extension
T2a	Extension and/or implants on the uterus and/or tube(s); no malignant cells in ascites or peritoneal washings
T2b	Extension to other pelvic tissues; no malignant cells in ascites or peritoneal washings
T2c	Pelvic extension (2a or 2b) with malignant cells in ascites or peritoneal washings
T3	Tumor involves one or both ovaries with microscopically confirmed peritoneal metastasis outside the pelvis and/or regional lymph node metastasis
T3a	Microscopic peritoneal metastasis beyond the pelvis
T3b	Macroscopic peritoneal metastasis beyond the pelvis 2 cm or less in the greatest dimension
T3c	Peritoneal metastasis beyond the pelvis more than 2 cm in the greatest N1 dimension and/or regional lymph node metastasis
T4	Tumor involves distant metastasis in the liver parenchymal or pleural effusion with positive cytology
Node (N)	
NX	Regional lymph nodes cannot be assessed
N0	No regional lymph node metastasis
N1	Regional lymph node metastasis
Metastasis (M)	
MX	Presence of distant metastasis cannot be assessed
M0	No distant metastasis
M1	Distant metastasis (excludes peritoneal metastasis)
FIGO Staging System	
I	Growth limited to the ovaries
IA	Growth limited to one ovary; no malignant ascites. No tumor on the external surface; capsule intact
IB	Growth limited to both ovaries; no malignant ascites. No tumor on the external surface; capsule intact
IC	Either IA or IB but with tumor on the surface of one or both ovaries, or with capsule ruptured, or with malignant ascites, or positive peritoneal cytology
II	Growth involving one or both ovaries with pelvic extension
IIA	Extension and/or metastasis to the uterus and/or tubes
IIB	Extension to other pelvic tissues
IIC	Tumor either IA or IB but with tumor on the surface of one or both ovaries, or with capsule(s) ruptured, or with malignant ascites, or positive peritoneal cytology
III	Tumor involving one or both ovaries with peritoneal implants outside the pelvis and/or positive retroperitoneal or inguinal nodes. Superficial liver metastasis equals stage III. Tumor is limited to the true pelvis, but with histologically proven malignant extension to small bowel or omentum
IIIA	Tumor limited to the true pelvis with negative nodes but with histologically confirmed microscopic seeding of abdominal peritoneal surfaces
IIIB	Tumor of one or both ovaries with histologically confirmed implants of abdominal peritoneal surfaces, none exceeding 2 cm in diameter. Nodes negative
IIIC	Abdominal implants greater than 2 cm in diameter and/or positive retroperitoneal or inguinal nodes
Stage IV	Growth involving one or both ovaries with distant metastasis. If pleural effusion is present, there must be a positive cytology test to allot a case to stage IV. Parenchymal liver metastasis equals stage IV

Note: To evaluate the impact on prognosis of the different criteria for allotting cases to stage IC or IIC, it is of value to know if rupture of the capsule was spontaneous or caused by the surgeon, and if the source of the malignant cells detected was from peritoneal washings or ascites.

*Tumor, node, metastasis

†International Federation of Gynecology and Obstetrics

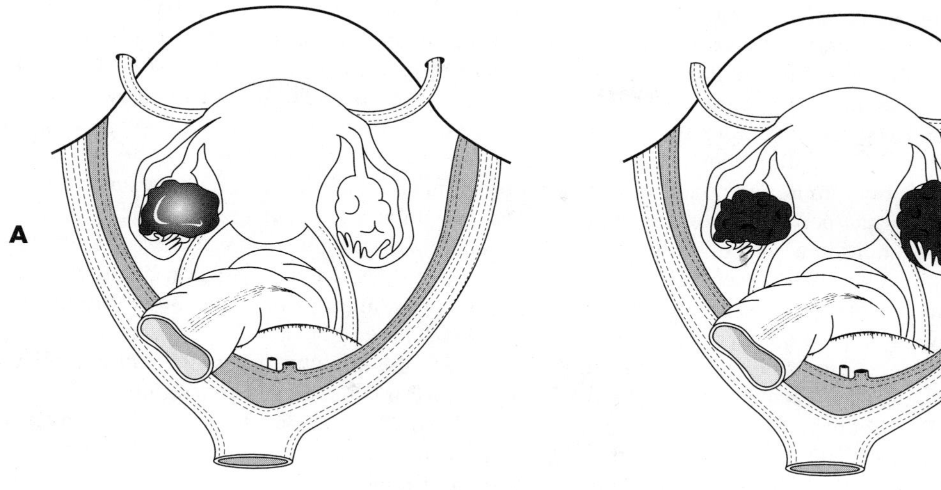

One ovary, capsule intact; no tumor on ovarian surface. Both ovaries, capsule intact; no tumor on ovarian surface.

Fig. 31-7 Carcinoma of the ovary by stage. (From DiSaia, P. J. [1997]. *Clinical gynecologic oncology* [5th ed.]. St. Louis: Mosby.)

TABLE 31-6 Medical Management of Ovarian Cancer

FIGO Stage	Involvement	Therapeutic Options
IA	Tumor limited to one ovary	• Total abdominal hysterectomy and bilateral salpingo-oophorectomy • If high grade would add
IB	Tumor limited to both ovaries	• Intraperitoneal radioactive colloidal phosphorus *or* • Chemotherapy
IC	Tumor limited to ovaries (one or both), with addition of ruptured capsule, malignant ascites or positive peritoneal cytology	• Total abdominal hysterectomy and bilateral salpingo-oophorectomy • Chemotherapy
IIA	Tumor involving one or both ovaries with extension or metastases involving the uterus and/or fallopian tubes	• Total abdominal hysterectomy and bilateral salpingo-oophorectomy • Intraperitoneal radioactive colloidal phosphorus *or*
IIB	Tumor involving one or both ovaries with extension into other pelvic tissues	• External radiation therapy *or* • Chemotherapy
IIC	Tumor involving one or both ovaries with pelvic extension and addition of ruptured capsule(s), malignant ascites or positive peritoneal cytology	• Total abdominal hysterectomy and bilateral salpingo-oophorectomy
IIIA	Tumor limited to pelvis, with microscopic seeding of abdominal peritoneum, but negative nodes	• Chemotherapy
IIIB	Tumor limited to pelvis with implants in the abdominal peritoneum (<2 cm), and negative nodes	• Total abdominal hysterectomy and bilateral salpingo-oophorectomy
IIIC	Abdominal implants >2 cm and/or positive nodes	• Chemotherapy including investigational drugs
IV	Distant metastases	

the abdomen. For older women who have completed childbearing, surgical management includes a minimum of a total abdominal hysterectomy (removal of the uterus), bilateral salpingo-oophorectomy (removal of the fallopian tubes and ovaries), and biopsies of the diaphragm, peritoneum, lymph nodes, omentum (covering of the peritoneum attached to the stomach), and peritoneal fluid. For younger women who wish to preserve childbearing capacity, a unilateral oophorectomy may be performed, if it is evident that only one ovary is involved.

The staging of ovarian cancer directs the overall treatment plan and depends on the extent and location of disease found at the initial laparotomy. A vertical midline incision provides excellent access to the pelvis and into the upper abdomen if needed. Both ovaries should be examined for the presence of tumor and removed intact. In addition, the uterus and fallopian tubes are also removed. Initial exploration must be thorough and starts with the collection of pelvic fluid for cytology. In the absence of pelvic fluid, peritoneal washings should be obtained. Exploration of all the intra-abdominal surfaces and organs, including the small and large intestines, kidneys, liver, gallbladder, and diaphragm is necessary to rule out common potential areas of metastases. Random biopsies of the peritoneal surfaces and diaphragm should be done, in addition to any suspicious areas. Staging should be completed with resection of the omentum and biopsies of pelvic, iliac, and para-aortic lymph nodes. Because pelvic and para-aortic lymph nodes are frequent sites of metastases, some studies recommend systematic pelvic and para-aortic lymphadenectomy to increase overall survival (Di Re, Baiocchi, Fontanelli, Grosso, Cobellis, & Raspagliesi et al., 1996). Others have found that the removal of macroscopic negative lymph nodes offers minimal benefit and therefore is unnecessary (Spirtos, Gross, Freddo, & Ballon, 1995). Accurate staging is essential, as it guides further treatment recommendations. Studies have shown that the size of residual tumor after primary surgery is a significant predictor of prognosis, and optimal debulking will leave 2 cm or less of residual disease (Hoskins, McGuire, Brady, Homesley, Creasman, & Berman et al., 1994; Makar, Baekelandt, Trope, & Kristensen, 1995).

The major complications of staging laparotomy are bleeding, prolonged ileus, wound infections, urinary tract infections, pulmonary complications, and bowel injury. Most patients present with advanced disease, necessitating the evaluation of whether nearby organs are involved, and lengthening the surgery. Blood loss is variable depending on the extent of surgery. Immediate postoperative complications may include bleeding, pulmonary emboli, urinary retention, and pain.

Interval Debulking. Residual tumor may be left behind after primary surgery in patients who present with bulky disease. The use of chemotherapy as adjuvant treatment is well accepted. Studies have shown that interval debulking after initial chemotherapy to resect small lesions significantly increases survival (Eisenkop, Nalick, Wang, & Teng, 1993; van der Burg, van Lent, Buyse, Kobierska, Colombo, & Favalli et al., 1995; Vaccarello, Rubin, Vlamis, Wong, Jones, & Lewis et al., 1995). Other studies have shown that despite optimal cytoreduction, patients with large metastases before resection had significantly poorer prognoses than patients with small lesions (Hoskins, Bundry, Thigpen, & Omura, 1992). Although debulking surgery may improve overall survival, it may be limited, as it does not provide a survival benefit equivalent to that of the presence of small-volume disease at the time of the staging laparotomy.

Second-Look Laparotomy. The second-look laparotomy is a surgical procedure that may be performed after treatment with staging laparotomy and chemotherapy to evaluate responsiveness to treatment. It is the most accurate method to rule out or confirm persistent disease that may not be evidenced by physical examination, imaging, or tumor markers. The technique is similar to the initial surgery and includes both a careful examination of the peritoneum, intra-abdominal surfaces, and organs and the performing of biopsies in areas of previous tumor. The odds of finding persistent disease is high in initially staged III and IV disease, and any gross residual disease found at this time should be resected. The use of second-look surgery is controversial, because recurrent ovarian cancer after negative findings is common, and therefore its effect on survival is questionable (Vaccarello et al., 1995).

The major complications of second-look laparotomy are prolonged ileus, wound infections, urinary tract infections, pulmonary complications, and bowel injury. Some studies suggest the use of laparoscopy for second-look operations to minimize the amount of surgery and complications (Abu-Rustum, Barakat, Siegel, Venkatraman, Curtin, & Hoskins 1996). Although laparoscopy is associated with fewer complications, it may provide inadequate visualization of residual tumor and therefore promote false-negative findings.

Radiation Therapy

Radiation therapy may be used to treat localized disease in patients after surgery. Radiation therapy treatments are administered through an external beam approach or by the placement of radioisotopes into the peritoneum.

External Beam Radiation Therapy. For patients with localized disease (stages I and II), radiation therapy after cytoreductive surgery may improve survival. Radiation treatments are given 5 days a week at doses of 100 to 150 Gy for 4 to 5 weeks to the entire abdomen and pelvis (total dose 2500 to 3000 Gy) (Fig. 31-8). Doses are restricted by neighboring organs (i.e., bone marrow, bowel, kidneys, and liver), and shields are used to protect the kidneys from the full dose. External beam radiation is not generally well tolerated by the patient, because the entire abdomen and pelvis are treated. The acute problems of anorexia, nausea and vomiting, diarrhea, vaginal discharge, bone marrow depression, dysuria, proctitis, and fatigue occur in most patients and may cause interruptions in therapy. Nausea and vomiting may occur within 1 or 2 hours after treatment. Although 67% of patients will have nausea, vomiting is infrequent and 75% of patients have mild diarrhea (Thomas & Dembo, 1993). Other side effects usually occur during the second or third week of treatment and resolve days to weeks after treatment is completed.

The occurrence of late complications associated with radiation therapy (i.e., complications that occur 6 or more months after the completion of treatment) are relatively common. Although small bowel obstruction is the most serious complication, it occurs infrequently. Other possible late complications of external beam radiation include cystitis, hematuria, radiation enteritis, chronic and recurrent diarrhea, and adhesive peritonitis. Limited field radiation therapy has been suggested for salvage therapy in localized recurrent ovarian cancer, as it is easier to tolerate with a decreased rate of bowel complications and because it has the potential to prolong symptom-free survival (Davidson, Rubin, Mychalczak, Saigo, Lewis, & Chapman et al., 1993). Effective treatment with radiation therapy is difficult

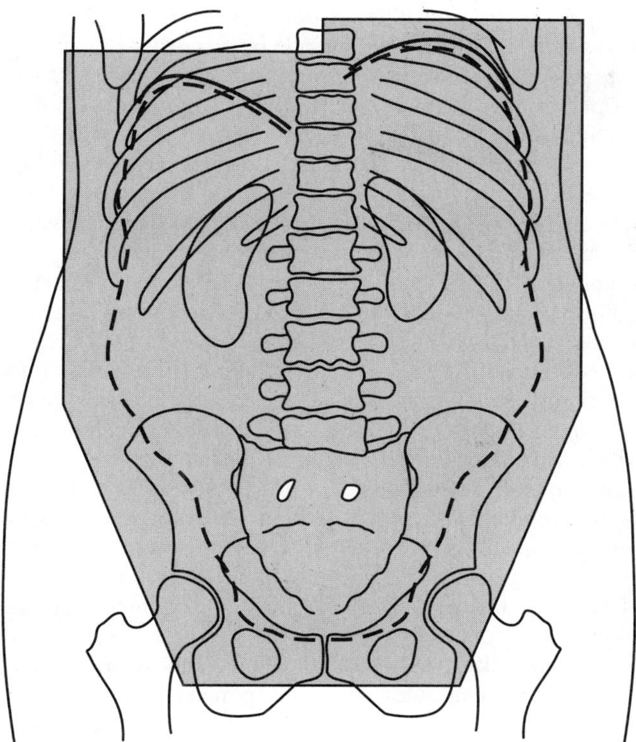

Fig. 31-8 Treatment portals for carcinoma of the ovary. (Redrawn from Berek, J. S. & Hacker, N. F. [1994]. *Practical gynecologic oncology.* Baltimore: Williams & Wilkins.)

because of the free mobility of tumor cells within the abdominal cavity and usually large tumor burden. Trials evaluating the use of chemotherapy alone versus chemotherapy followed by radiation therapy in patients with advanced ovarian cancer found no statistical differences in either survival or disease-free survival (Lambert, Rustin, Gregory, & Nelstrop, 1993). The use of radiation therapy has diminished over time with an increased use of chemotherapeutic agents. Radiation therapy may still play a palliative role in patients with brain or bone metastases.

Internal Radiation Therapy. The exact role for internal radiation therapy in the management of ovarian cancer has not been determined and may be limited to early-stage disease. Randomized trials comparing the use of radioactive isotopes and no treatment have not been done. Treatment involves the injection of a low-dose radioactive isotope into the peritoneum. After injection, the patient must be instructed to change her position frequently to ensure dispersion of the isotope in the peritoneum. The goal of intracavity radioisotopes is to achieve a predetermined dose of radiation that is effective enough to kill the tumor cells while keeping side effects at a minimum. Phosphorus-32 (P-32) is a radioactive colloidal that is injected into the peritoneum. The usual dose of P-32 is 15 to 20 mCi diluted in 1500 to 2000 ml of sterile saline. Low dose intraperitoneal treatments of P-32 may also be used in conjunction with platinum analog chemotherapy for the treatment of disseminated intraperitoneal ovarian cancer (Pattillo, Collier, Abdel-Dayem, Ozker, Wilson, & Ruckert et al., 1995). The potential side effects associated with radioactive isotopes are abdominal discomfort or pain, infection, and other small bowel complications. The procedure for administering a low-dose radioactive isotope into the peritoneum is outlined in Box 31-4.

Box 31-4
Administration of a Low-Dose Radioactive Isotope into the Peritoneal Cavity

- Phosphorus-32 (P-32), a beta emitter, is a colloid substance that can be instilled through an intraperitoneal catheter to treat microscopic disease in the peritoneum.
- The procedure to instill the P-32 is similar to a paracentesis and can be done on an outpatient basis.
  -Patient has an intraperitoneal catheter inserted and placement of the catheter is verified by x-ray.
  -P-32 is instilled through the patient's catheter with either a syringe or a closed intravenous pressurized system.
  -Once all the P-32 is instilled, the catheter is removed, and the patient is instructed to change positions to allow the P-32 to be distributed to the entire peritoneal cavity. Following this procedure, the patient is discharged home.

Chemotherapy

Chemotherapy is used most commonly as adjuvant treatment after surgery to treat residual or metastatic disease. It may also be used preoperatively for patients with bulky disease. Chemotherapy may be administered orally, intravenously, or intraperitoneally. Ovarian cancer has been shown to be highly sensitive to chemotherapy. Its use is most appropriate for patients with late-stage (III or IV) disease or early-stage (I or II) disease that is of high grade. Chemotherapy has been shown to be most effective when residual disease after surgery is less than 2 cm (Hoskins et al., 1992). A list of chemotherapy agents that have been used in ovarian cancer is summarized in Box 31-5.

Single-agent alkylator chemotherapy (i.e., melphalan, alkeran, or cyclophosphamide) was considered optimal treatment for ovarian cancer until the mid-1970s, when cisplatin was shown to have significant activity against ovarian cancer both as a single agent and in combination therapy. Trials comparing combination therapy, such as cyclophosphamide, hexamethylmelamine, doxorubicin, and cisplatin (CHAD), versus single-agent alkylators, such as melphalan, have revealed a higher complete response rate in the combination arm (Wadler, Yeap, Vogl, & Carbone, 1996). Since then, other drugs, such as paclitaxel, have been discovered, and the ideal combination continues to be under evaluation. Chemotherapy is used as initial adjuvant treatment. In addition, chemotherapy is given as salvage therapy because 75% to 85% of these patients experience relapse (Caldas, Morris, & McGuire, 1994).

Initial Chemotherapy. Platinum-containing regimens have resulted in 60% to 70% response rates, with median progression-free survival lasting 14 months, even in

Box 31-5
Chemotherapy Drugs Used in Ovarian Cancer

5-Fluorouracil (5-FU)
Carboplatin (Paraplatin)
Chlorambucil (Leukeran)
Cisplatin (Platinol)
Cyclophosphamide (Cyclophosphamide)
Doxorubicin (Adriamycin)
Epirubicin
Etoposide (VP-16)
Hexamethylmelamine (Hexalen)
Ifosfamide (Ifex)
Melphalan (Alkeran)
Methotrexate (MTX)
Mitomycin-C
Mitoxantrone
Paclitaxel (Taxol)

patients with large-volume residual disease (Thigpen, Blessing, Ball, Hummel, & Barrett, 1994). Cisplatin has been used in multiple combinations, including cisplatin and cyclophosphamide (PC); cisplatin, doxorubicin, and cyclophosphamide (PAC); and hexamethylmelamine, cyclophosphamide, doxorubidin, and cisplatin (CHAP). Major side effects associated with cisplatin include nausea and vomiting, myelosuppression, neurotoxicity, otoxicity, and renal toxicity. Dose intensification of cisplatin has resulted in greater toxicity (leukopenia, thrombocytopenia, neurotoxicity) without significant differences in efficacy or survival (Conte, Bruzzone, Carnino, Gadducci, Algeri, & Bellini et al., 1996; McGuire, Hoskins, Brady, Homesley, Creasman, & Berman et al., 1995).

Carboplatin has been substituted for cisplatin in many regimens due to its reduced incidence of nonhematologic toxicities. Although standard intravenous doses of carboplatin are equivalent to cisplatin in activity and less toxic, greater myelosuppression, in particular thrombocytopenia, has limited its use (Alberts, 1995; Calvert, Boddy, Bailey, Siddiqui, Humphreys, & Hughes et al., 1995; Lind, Ghazal-Aswad, Gumbrell, Fishwick, Craigs, & Millward et al., 1996). The use of carboplatin in combination with hexamethylmelamine and oral etoposide as first-line treatment has shown a promising 92% response rate with ovarian patients who have bulky disease (greater than 2 cm), but long-term survival data are still pending (Frasci, Comella, Comella, Conforti, Mastrantonio, & Zullo et al., 1995).

Paclitaxel, as first-line therapy, was shown to improve the duration of progression-free survival and of overall survival in women with incompletely resected stage III and stage IV ovarian cancer. Studies that compared paclitaxel plus cisplatin with cyclophosphamide plus cisplatin revealed a greater response to treatment (75% vs 60%), increased progression-free survival (18 months vs 13 months), and an overall increased survival rate (38 months vs 24 months) in the paclitaxel-containing arm (McGuire, Hoskins, Brady, Kucera, Partridge, & Look, et al., 1996; Thigpen, Vance, McGuire, Hoskins, & Brady, 1995). Toxicities related to paclitaxel include hypersensitivity, myelosuppression, nausea and vomiting, alopecia, arthralgias, and peripheral neuropathies (Ozols, 1995; Runowicz, Wiernik, Einzig, Goldberg, & Horwitz, 1993; ten Bokkel Huinink, Veenhof, Helmerhorst, Bierhorst, Dalesio, & Winograd et al., 1995). Peripheral neuropathy seems to be greater in both patients previously or simultaneously treated with cisplatin (Cavaletti, Bogliun, Marzorati, Zincone, Marzola, & Colombo et al., 1995; Connelly, Markman, Kennedy, Webster, Kulp, & Peterson et al., 1995). Studies have revealed comparable results when substituting carboplatin for cisplatin with paclitaxel. In addition, carboplatin has been shown to be less myelosuppressive when used in combinations with paclitaxel (Calvert et al., 1995). A pilot study of carboplatin with escalating doses of paclitaxel revealed an overall response rate of 81% (Bolis, 1995). Another study that escalated carboplatin doses with various infusion schedules of paclitaxel resulted in an overall response rate of 75% and median progression-free survival of 15 months (Bookman, McGuire, Kilpatrick, Keenan, Hogan, & Johnson et al., 1996).

Salvage Chemotherapy. Chemotherapy options are limited in patients with recurrent epithelial ovarian carcinoma who have been treated previously with platinum. Patients who relapse more than 6 months after completing first-line treatment are considered to have clinically platinum-sensitive disease. These patients have a significant response to a rechallenge with platinum-based therapy with response rates between 42% and 72% (Look, Muss, Blessing, & Morris, 1995). Patients who experience relapse within 6 months of platinum-based therapy are considered to have platinum-resistant disease. Only paclitaxel, ifosfamide, and hexamethylmelamine have yielded reproducible responses, which tend to be of short duration on the order of several months.

Paclitaxel has been found to be active in both drug-refractory (24%) and nonrefractory (40%) ovarian cancers (Runowicz, et al., 1993; Thigpen et al., 1994). It has been suggested that a more prolonged delivery of paclitaxel (more than 6 months) may potentially improve therapeutic outcome (Markman, Hakes, Barakat, Almadarones, & Hoskins, 1996a). Salvage ifosfamide in patients with refractory ovarian cancer has shown a 12% response rate (Markman, Iseminger, Hatch, Creasman, Barnes, & Dubeshter, 1996; Sorensen, Pfeiffer, & Bertelsen, 1995). Side effects of ifosfamide include myelosuppression, alopecia, and renal and neurologic toxicities. Hexamethylmelamine has produced a 12% to 14% overall response rate in cisplatin-resistant disease (Caldas, Morris, & McGuire, 1994). The most prevalent side effect of hexamethylmelamine is nausea and vomiting; other toxicities include myelosuppression and peripheral neuropathy.

In one study, oral etoposide produced a 26% response rate, with side effects of myelosuppression and mucositis. However, the response was of short duration (Hoskins & Swenerton, 1994). The use of 5-fluorouracil with leucovorin rescue has been disappointing, with only minimal activity in refractory ovarian cancer (Look et al., 1995; Morgan,

Speyer, Doroshow, Margolin, Raschoko, & Sorich et al., 1995; Prefontaine, Donovan, Powell, & Buley, 1996).

Response rates of 21%, with a median 7-month progression-free survival, have been observed with carboplatin as a single agent in patients refractory to a taxane with cisplatin (Kavanagh, Tresukosol, Edwards, Freedman, Gonzalez de Leon, & Fishman et al., 1995). Topotecan has also been studied as a single agent for cisplatin-refractory patients and produced a 14% response rate with a median duration of 8.9 months (Kudelka, Tresdukosol, Edwards, Freedman, Levenback, & Chantarawiroj et al., 1996).

Some new drugs currently being studied, including irinotecan, gemcitabine, and docetaxel, have shown reproducible activity after platinum failure. Irinotecan (CPT-11) has shown a 23% response rate (Runowicz, Fields, & Goldberg, 1995). Side effects include leukopenia, nausea and vomiting, diarrhea, and anorexia. Gemcitabine has produced some partial responses in previously treated patients with ovarian cancer (Hansen, Eisenhauer, Hansen, Neijt, Piccart, & Sessa et al., 1993; Qazi & McGuire, 1995).

Intraperitoneal Chemotherapy. The exact role for intraperitoneal chemotherapy in the management of ovarian cancer has not yet been determined. Treatment involves the placement of either a dialysis catheter, subcutaneous port, or single-use percutaneous catheter into the peritoneum. After access has been achieved, drug delivery to the intra-abdominal disease is dependent on positioning of the patient and gravitational flow. Additionally, the presence of intra-abdominal adhesions may limit drug delivery. The potential advantage of giving chemotherapy by this route is to deliver more drug to the tumor. Major complications associated with this route of delivery include catheter obstructions (i.e., due to the formation of a fibrin sheath), abdominal distention or pain, intestinal complications (i.e., small-bowel obstruction, ileus, or intestinal perforation), and infection (Schneider, 1994). Abdominal discomfort may be alleviated by warming the peritoneal fluid before infusion.

The same chemotherapy drugs that are used for initial or salvage treatment through the intravenous route have been studied using the intraperitoneal route. It has been suggested that cisplatin given intraperitoneally is actually superior to intravenous cisplatin when given with intravenous cyclophosphamide (Alberts, 1995). Intraperitoneal cisplatin in combination with 5-fluorouracil has shown a 66.7% response rate in patients previously sensitive to cisplatin (Braly, Berek, Blessing, Homesley, & Averette, 1995). Toxicities with this combination include neutropenia, thrombocytopenia, catheter-related complications, and gastrointestinal side effects. Paclitaxel appears to offer the greatest potential for intraperitoneal administration, and trials evaluating its use are in progress (Ozols, 1994). The toxicities of intraperitoneal paclitaxel include mild bone marrow suppression, nausea and vomiting, hypersensitivity reactions, and mild to moderate abdominal pain (Francis, Rowinsky, Schneider, Hakes, Hoskins, & Markman, 1995; Markman, Francis, Rowinsky, & Hoskins, 1995; Runowicz et al., 1993).

Other combinations have not been as easily tolerated, such as intraperitoneal high-dose carboplatin and etoposide with GM-CSF support. Although this combination elicited a 69% response rate, it was short lived. In addition, 78% of patients were removed from the study due to toxicities (McClay, Braly, Kirmani, Plaxe, Kim, & McClay et al., 1995).

Biologic Response Modifiers

Various biologic response modifiers, including α- and γ-interferons, have been studied for use in ovarian cancer. Biologic modifiers have had limited activity given intravenously, but have produced some responses when given intraperitoneally. In patients with minimal residual disease, α-interferon given intraperitoneally has produced response rates of up to 50% (Willemse, DeVries, Aalders, Bouma, & Sleijfer, 1990). Side effects may include fever, abdominal pain, and leukopenia. Intraperitoneal recombinant human interferon-γ, as second line treatment, has produced a 32% response rate with a median duration of 20 months. Additionally, patients younger than 60 with residual tumor less than 2 cm have higher response rates of 41% (Pujade-Lauraine, Guastalla, Colombo, Devillier, Francois, & Fumoleau et al., 1996) (see Chapter 7).

Hormonal Therapy

Hormonal therapy may be used to manage advanced-stage ovarian cancer that has not been responsive to chemotherapy. The ovaries produce estrogen and progesterone, so it is not surprising that ovarian cancers may be estrogen-receptor and/or progesterone-receptor positive, similar to breast cancer. Antiestrogen therapy has been useful for palliation of refractory ovarian cancer. Tamoxifen, in particular, has shown a 13% to 17% response rate (Ahlgren, Ellison, Gottlieb, Laluna, Lokich, & Sinclair et al., 1993; Markman et al., 1996b). Although the duration of response may be limited, tamoxifen is well tolerated. Other hormones, such as megestrol acetate and aminoglutethimide, have not shown similar responses. Side effects of hormonal therapy include hot flashes, vaginal dryness, emotional lability, and weight gain.

Bone Marrow Transplantation

Because the majority of patients with ovarian cancer are incurable with standard therapy, the use of high-dose chemotherapy with bone marrow or peripheral blood stem cell transplant rescue has been suggested as a potential solution. The chemotherapy drugs used in various trials have included carboplatin, cisplatin, cyclophosphamide, doxorubicin, etoposide, melphalan, mitoxantrone, and paclitaxel. Initial data are encouraging, with overall response rates of 80% to 100% in patients without previous chemotherapy after cytoreductive surgery (Benedetti-Panici, Greggi, Scambia, Salerno, Baiocchi, & Laurelli et al., 1995; Fennelly, Schneider, Spriggs, Bengala, Hakes, & Reich et al., 1995). Overall response rates in patients with relapsed ovarian cancer have been as high as 100% for patients with disease sensitive to cisplatin and 84% for patients with disease refractory to cisplatin (Samuels & Bitran, 1995; Stiff, McKenzie,

Alberts, Sosman, Dolan, & Rad et al., 1994; Stiff, Bayer, Camarda, Tan, Dolan, & Potkul et al., 1995). The major side effects seen are similar to those resulting from standard doses of these drugs and, although greater in intensity, seem to be well tolerated and may include myelosuppression, nausea and vomiting, diarrhea, mucositis, and peripheral neuropathy. Encouraging response rates, especially in patients with a poor prognosis, warrant further study of high-dose chemotherapy with bone marrow or peripheral stem cell support (see Chapter 8).

ONCOLOGIC EMERGENCIES

A major oncologic emergency associated with ovarian cancer treatment is anaphylaxis. Hypersensitivity is a potential side effect with the three most common chemotherapy drugs used for ovarian cancer: paclitaxel, carboplatin, and cisplatin. If a delayed hypersensitivity or anaphylactic reaction occurs when these drugs are given in combination, it may be difficult to determine which chemotherapy agent caused the reaction. Hypersensitivity and anaphylaxis with carboplatin have been observed even after several previous uncomplicated courses of treatment (Reed, Kohn, Sarosy, Dabhoka, Davis, & Jacob et al., 1995; Sood, Gelder, Huang, & Morgan, 1995; Weidmann, Mulleneisen, Bojko, & Niederle, 1994). An initial symptom of hypersensitivity may simply be facial flushing. Other signs and symptoms may include skin reactions, chest tightness, hypotension, tachycardia, and dyspnea. In the case of hypersensitivity reactions, one should immediately stop the chemotherapy infusion, notify the physician, maintain intravenous access, and administer oxygen and emergency drugs as needed.

Another major oncologic emergency associated with ovarian cancer and its treatment is disseminated intravascular coagulation (DIC). DIC may occur from chemotherapy, anaphylaxis, infection, massive tissue injury, or from the ovarian cancer itself. Symptoms of DIC may include bleeding from various sites, hypotension, abdominal pain, and confusion. In the case of DIC, one should immediately notify the physician, treat the underlying cause, maintain intravenous access (for heparin, blood products, and hydration), and administer oxygen as needed.

NURSING MANAGEMENT

The medical management of ovarian cancer is extremely complex and variable depending on the patient's age, clinical condition, and stage of her disease at the time of diagnosis. Patients with ovarian cancer have numerous problems that require nursing interventions and patient education. Although a portion of the patient's care will occur in the inpatient setting, the majority of the patient's care will occur in the outpatient and home care settings.

Early in the course of the patient's disease, the focus of nursing care may be on helping the patient understand the different treatment options. As the disease progresses, patients need information about the rationale for different types of pharmacologic interventions as well as strategies for managing the side effects associated with the disease or treatment. Because each major type of treatment for ovarian cancer (i.e., surgery, radiation therapy, chemotherapy, and hormonal therapy) poses unique patient problems, the major issues associated with these treatments are discussed below, and four standards of care are provided in this chapter.

Surgery

Patients undergoing a staging laparotomy are usually hospitalized for 5 days. Patients who present with extensive disease require more comprehensive surgery and possibly a longer stay. The major focus of inpatient nursing care is on the prevention of postoperative complications, including bleeding, thrombophlebitis, infection, and pulmonary emboli. Follow-up care in the outpatient setting may require that nurses evaluate patients for infection, wound care management, adequate nutritional intake, and ambulation. The nursing management of the patient undergoing surgery for ovarian cancer is summarized in Table 31-7.

Radiation Therapy

Patient problems vary depending on whether the patient is receiving external beam or internal radiation therapy. External beam therapy is provided on an outpatient basis. The major problems associated with external beam radiation therapy include myelosuppression, nausea and vomiting, diarrhea, and skin reactions. Internal radiation therapy is done in the inpatient setting. The patient requires a private room, and radiation precautions must be observed. Major problems associated with the use of radioisotopes include abdominal discomfort or pain, infection, ileus, and intestinal perforation. The nursing management of the patient with ovarian cancer who is receiving external beam radiation therapy is summarized in Table 31-8.

Chemotherapy

Most patients receiving chemotherapy have advanced disease. Care in most cases is provided in the outpatient setting. Patients must be taught the rationale for premedications, chemotherapy combinations, and any postchemotherapy directions. Additionally, patients and their families must be taught about potential side effects associated with different chemotherapy agents and their management. The nursing management of the patient with ovarian cancer who is receiving chemotherapy is summarized in Table 31-9.

Hormonal Therapy

Patients receiving hormonal therapy have advanced disease. Care is provided in the outpatient setting. Patients must be taught the rationale for hormonal treatment and potential side effects. The management plan for the ovarian cancer patient receiving hormonal therapy is summarized in Table 31-10.

Text continued on p. 748

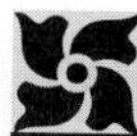

TABLE 31-7 Standard of Care for the Patient Undergoing Surgery for Ovarian Cancer

Patient Problem and Outcomes	Nursing Interventions and Rationales	Patient Education Instructions
Anxiety Patient will: • Verbalize an understanding of the surgical procedure • Express feelings of decreased anxiety • Identify strategies to cope with anxiety	1. Assess patient's level of understanding of the surgical procedure. 2. Review instruction with patient and allow time for questions and/or for patient to verbalize concerns. 3. Determine which coping strategies the patient has used effectively in the past to decrease anxiety and reinforce the use of these coping strategies. 4. Administer pharmacologic agents to decrease anxiety, if needed.	1. Utilize a diagram of the anatomy of the female reproductive system to explain the surgical procedure. 2. Provide patient with information about the preoperative routine: a. Diagnostic tests b. Bowel prep c. Anesthesiology consult d. Nothing by mouth after midnight 3. Teach patient coughing and deep breathing exercises; teach the use of an incentive spirometer and observe return demonstration. 4. Provide patient with information about the immediate postoperative routine: a. Routine assessments (including vital signs) b. Pain management c. Use of indwelling catheter d. Use of nasogastric tube e. Surgical incision, drains, and dressing f. Intravenous hydration g. Use of thromboembolic stockings and/or pneumoboots h. Ambulation 5. Provide patient with information about postdischarge instructions: a. Monitor for signs and symptoms of infection b. Notify physician if temperature is greater than 100.4° F (38° C) c. Take pain medications as needed to control pain d. Avoid constipation or straining e. Maintain adequate nutrition and fluid intake f. Increase ambulation and activity gradually g. Avoid tampons, douches, and intercourse for 4 to 6 weeks or as directed by physician h. Take hormones as prescribed i. Keep follow-up appointment
Pain Patient will experience optimal pain relief with minimal side effects	1. Assess pain intensity using a 0 to 10 verbal rating scale, every 2-4 hours for the first 48 hours after surgery, then at least once a shift. 2. Administer opioid analgesics around the clock for the first 24-48 hours postoperatively. 3. Monitor for analgesic side effects and administer medications to prevent or treat: a. Nausea b. Pruritus c. Constipation	1. Teach patient to inform the nurse if she is experiencing pain. 2. Describe the routine procedures for pain medication and explain how to use boluses if on a patient controlled analgesic pump. 3. Teach the patient the importance of taking pain medication on a regular basis to keep pain under control.

Continued

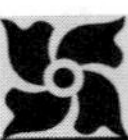

TABLE 31-7 Standard of Care for the Patient Undergoing Surgery for Ovarian Cancer—cont'd

Patient Problem and Outcomes	Nursing Interventions and Rationales	Patient Education Instructions
Dehydration Patient will maintain adequate fluid volume and electrolyte balance	1. Check CBC, electrolytes, blood urea nitrogen and creatinine. 2. Monitor intake and output. 3. Weigh patient daily. 4. Monitor vital signs. 5. Administer intravenous fluids as prescribed. 6. Assess patient for return of bowel sounds, flatulence. 7. Evaluate tolerance when patient resumes eating.	1. Teach the patient about the importance of maintaining adequate fluid intake. 2. Inform the patient of the need to measure all intake and output. 3. Teach patient to report persistent nausea and vomiting or decreased appetite after discharge.
Risk for Pulmonary Embolism	1. Apply antiembolic or compression stockings to both legs. 2. Ambulate as soon as possible. 3. Assess for leg pain and signs of thrombophlebitis. 4. Assess respiratory rate and rhythm.	1. Teach the patient the importance of wearing antiembolic or compression stockings and the rationale for ambulating as soon as possible.
High Risk for Urinary Retention Patient will be able to urinate without catheterization after surgery	1. Assess for bladder distention. 2. Monitor urinary output. 3. Assess for residual urine if needed.	1. Teach patient to report any change in bladder pattern (i.e., feeling of fullness, urinary frequency)
Risk for Bleeding Patient will maintain normal hemoglobin and hematocrit	1. Assess hemoglobin, hematocrit and platelet count. 2. Check surgical incision site, dressings and drains for excessive drainage.	1. Instruct patient to avoid strenuous exercise, tampons, and sexual intercourse for 4 to 6 weeks.
Infection Patient will remain free from infection	1. Assess incision site for redness, swelling, increased drainage, and approximation of surgical margins. 2. Monitor vital signs, especially temperature every 4 hours for first 48 hours. 3. Administer antibiotics as prescribed.	1. Teach patient the signs and symptoms of infection. 2. After discharge, instruct patient to call the doctor if presence of any symptoms of infection or temperature greater than 100.4° F (38° C).

CBC, Complete blood count.

TABLE 31-8 Standard of Care of the Patient Receiving External Beam Radiation Therapy for Ovarian Cancer

Patient Problem and Outcomes	Nursing Interventions and Rationales	Patient Education Instructions
Knowledge Deficit Patient will verbalize an understanding of the purpose, benefits and side effects of radiation therapy	1. Assess patient's level of understanding about radiation therapy. 2. Review instruction with patient and allow time for questions and/or for the patient to verbalize concerns.	1. Describe the purpose and routine procedures involved with radiation therapy: a. Local treatment for cure, control, or palliation b. Consultation c. Simulation procedure d. Treatment procedure and routine 2. Describe the major side effects associated with radiation therapy, the importance of notifying the nurse should side effects occur, and self-care measures to manage the side effects of: a. Skin reactions b. Nausea and vomiting c. Diarrhea d. Leukopenia e. Fatigue f. Cystitis
Skin Reactions Patient will be able to maintain intact, healthy skin	1. Assess skin in area of radiation field. 2. Notify physician if skin breakdown occurs. 3. Administer special skin products if needed.	1. Describe the appearance of skin reactions and inform the patient that skin reactions will usually occur during the second week of treatment, continue until approximately 7 days after the final treatment, and subside approximately 2 to 4 weeks later. 2. Teach patient to wash skin within radiation field with warm water only. 3. Teach patient to avoid restrictive clothing, extreme heat or cold, irritating substances on the skin (lotions, ointments, deodorants or substances containing zinc in the radiation field), sun exposure.
Nausea and Vomiting Patient will experience minimal or no nausea and vomiting	1. Assess for the presence of nausea and vomiting. 2. Administer antiemetics as needed. 3. Administer intravenous hydration if needed.	1. Teach patient to inform nurse if she is experiencing nausea and vomiting. Nausea and vomiting may occur 1 to 2 hours after treatment. This side effect may last until 1 week after treatment is completed. 2. Teach patient the importance of taking antiemetics as prescribed (usually 30 to 60 minutes before treatment). 3. Instruct patient to eat small snacks, drink fluids, avoid hot or greasy foods, and to rest after meals.

Continued

TABLE 31-8 Standard of Care of the Patient Receiving External Beam Radiation Therapy for Ovarian Cancer—cont'd

Patient Problem and Outcomes	Nursing Interventions and Rationales	Patient Education Instructions
Diarrhea Patient will maintain adequate fluid balance, weight, and energy level	1. Assess elimination patterns including frequency, quality, and quantity. 2. Initiate a low-residue diet at the start of treatment, including: a. Limit foods high in roughage b. Limit fried or highly seasoned foods c. Avoid alcohol 3. Refer for dietary consult. 4. Administer antidiarrheal medication as needed. 5. Monitor weight weekly.	1. Inform patient that diarrhea occurs within a few weeks of treatment. 2. Teach patient to maintain a low-residue diet until bowel patterns return to normal (usually a couple to few weeks after the radiation therapy treatments are completed). 3. Teach patient to keep track of number, quality, quantity and any patterns of diarrhea. 4. Instruct patient to drink three liters of fluid each day. 5. Instruct patient to cleanse affected skin with warm water and apply A & D ointment if sore.
Leukopenia Patient will be able to keep free of infections	1. Assess CBC with differential weekly 2. Hold treatment if patient becomes immunosuppressed.	1. Teach patient to call the doctor if she has a temperature greater than 100.4° F (38° C).
Fatigue Patient will be able to maintain normal activities	1. Assess patient's level of fatigue using a 0 (not at all tired) to 10 (total exhaustion) rating scale. 2. Evaluate patient's sleep and activity pattern to be able to teach patient ways to conserve energy.	1. Inform patient that she is likely to experience fatigue toward the end of treatment and for several weeks following treatment. 2. Teach patient how to pace herself and take rest periods as needed.
Cystitis Patient will experience relief of urinary symptoms	1. Assess for symptoms of urinary frequency, burning upon urination, urgency or blood in the urine. 2. Evaluate for the presence of a urinary tract infection and initiate appropriate antibiotic therapy if an infection is present.	1. Teach patient to notify the nurse if she has any symptoms of urinary frequency, burning upon urination, urgency, or blood in the urine. 2. Teach patient to drink three liters of fluid each day and avoid caffeine or alcohol.

CBC, Complete blood count.

TABLE 31-9 Standard of Care for the Patient Receiving Chemotherapy for Ovarian Cancer

Patient Problem and Outcomes	Nursing Interventions and Rationales	Patient Education Instructions
Knowledge Deficit		
Patient will verbalize an understanding of the purpose, benefits, and side effects of chemotherapy	1. Assess patient's level of understanding of chemotherapy. 2. Review instruction with patient and allow time for questions and/or for patient to verbalize concerns about chemotherapy.	1. Describe the purpose and routine procedures involved in chemotherapy: a. Systemic treatment, cure, control, and palliation b. Prechemotherapy lab assessments c. Premedications and antiemetics d. Hydration requirements 2. Describe the major side effects associated with chemotherapy, the importance of notifying the nurses should side effects occur, and self-care measures to manage the side effects of: a. Hypersensitivity b. Nausea and vomiting c. Peripheral neuropathy d. Diarrhea e. Myelosuppression f. Fatigue g. Myalgias h. Renal toxicity i. Ototoxicity
Acute Hypersensitivity Reaction		
Patient will be monitored and promptly treated if a hypersensitivity reaction occurs.	1. Review patient's drug history and any allergies. 2. Verify that patient took any premedications ordered prior to treatment. 3. Verify availability of emergency drugs 4. Give premedications prescribed. 5. Monitor vital signs prior to start of treatment, during, and after chemotherapy completed. 6. Assess for flushing, skin reactions, hypotension, dyspnea, urticaria, tachycardia, chest pain. 7. Stop infusion, maintain intravenous access, notify physician and administer emergency medications, oxygen, and intravenous fluids as prescribed, if reaction suspected.	1. Inform patient about possibility of allergic reaction and frequency of assessments. 2. Instruct patient to inform the nurse if she experiences lightheadedness, shortness of breath, or any unusual sensations.
Nausea and Vomiting		
Patient will experience minimal or no nausea and vomiting	1. Assess for the presence of nausea and vomiting (amount, frequency). 2. Administer antiemetics before chemotherapy. 3. Evaluate need for alternative or additional antiemetics. 4. Administer hydration as prescribed. 5. Monitor weight.	1. Teach patient about potential for nausea and vomiting. 2. Teach patient to inform the nurse if she is experiencing nausea. 3. Teach patient the importance of taking antiemetics as prescribed. 4. Instruct patient to avoid hot, spicy, and fatty foods and to try small, frequent feedings.

Continued

TABLE 31-9 Standard of Care for the Patient Receiving Chemotherapy for Ovarian Cancer—cont'd

Patient Problem and Outcomes	Nursing Interventions and Rationales	Patient Education Instructions
Peripheral Neuropathy Patient will: • Identify and report sensory changes • Maintain an optimal level of functioning	1. Assess baseline information about sensory functioning. 2. Evaluate patient's ability to perform activities of daily living. 3. Assess for numbness or tingling in hands or feet, decrease in fine and gross motor abilities, pain weakness, or constipation.	1. Instruct patient about safety measures: a. Avoid temperature extremes b. Wear shoes or slippers at all times c. Inspect skin for cuts, abrasions, or bruises 2. Teach patient to exercise the affected limb(s).
Diarrhea Patient will maintain adequate fluid balance, weight, and energy level	1. Assess elimination patterns including frequency, quality, and quantity. 2. Administer antidiarrheal medication as needed. 3. Administer intravenous hydration as needed.	1. Teach patient to inform the nurse if she is experiencing diarrhea. 2. Teach patient to cleanse rectal area with warm water. 3. Instruct patient to drink three liters of fluid each day.
Leukopenia Patient will be able to keep free of infections	1. Assess CBC with differential. 2. Hold chemotherapy if WBC < 3.0 or ANC < 1500. 3. Monitor vital signs, including temperature.	1. Teach patient about importance of blood work drawn prior to treatments and at nadir. 2. Inform patient to notify nurse if temperature greater than 100.4° F, especially at time of nadir.
Cystitis Patient will experience relief of urinary symptoms	1. Assess for symptoms of urinary frequency, burning upon urination, urgency or blood in the urine. 2. Evaluate for the presence of a urinary tract infection and initiate appropriate antibiotic therapy if an infection is present.	1. Teach patient to notify the nurse if any symptoms of urinary frequency, burning upon urination, urgency, blood in the urine, or low back pain occur. 2. Teach patient to drink three liters of fluid each day 3. Instruct patient to avoid urinary retention and void every two hours if able during chemotherapy.

CBC, Complete blood count; *ANC,* absolute neutrophil count.

HOME CARE ISSUES

Depending on the treatment approaches used to manage ovarian cancer, the patient and family caregivers will be faced with several issues in the home care setting. Symptoms associated with ovarian cancer and its treatment include fatigue, pain, numbness or tingling in hands or feet, nausea and vomiting, bloating, constipation, anorexia, diarrhea, edema, shortness of breath, and problems with urination (Portenoy, Kornblith, Wong, Vlamis, Lepore, & Loseth, et al., 1994). Patients who had extensive disease at presentation may have wound and/or colostomy care to perform at home. Many patients may have central lines placed for chemotherapy, antibiotics, total parenteral nutrition, and blood draws, which may require them to learn how to do flushes, dressing changes, and possibly infuse medication. Patients receiving chemotherapy may need to learn to manage delayed nausea and vomiting or give self-injections. Pain management both postoperatively and for advanced disease will be an issue for many patients and their family members.

Bowel Obstruction

Another problem patients may encounter while at home is bowel obstruction. *Malignant bowel obstruction* is defined as the cessation of normal progression of intraluminal contents (Labovich, 1994). Patients with ovarian cancer may have bowel obstruction from tumor involvement at diagnosis, surgical interventions, delayed side effects of radiation therapy or chemotherapy, or advancing disease.

TABLE 31-10 Standard of Care for the Patient Receiving Hormonal Therapy for Ovarian Cancer

Patient Problem and Outcomes	Nursing Interventions and Rationales	Patient Education Instructions
Knowledge Deficit		
Patient will verbalize an understanding of the purpose, benefits, and side effects of hormonal therapy	1. Assess patient's level of understanding of hormonal therapy. 2. Review instruction with patient and allow time for questions and/or for patient to verbalize concerns about hormonal therapy.	1. Describe the purpose and routine procedures involved in hormonal therapy: a. Systemic treatment, control, palliation b. Oral medication 2. Describe the major side effects associated with hormonal therapy, the importance of notifying the nurses should side effects occur, and self-care measures to manage the side effects of: a. Hot flashes b. Vaginal dryness c. Emotional lability d. Weight gain
Hot Flashes		
Patient will experience a reduction in the number of hot flashes	1. Assess for hot flashes.	1. Teach patient to avoid the following situations that may trigger her hot flashes: a. Warm room b. Hot drinks c. Alcohol
Weight Gain		
Patient will experience minimal weight gain	1. Monitor weight. 2. Assess ankles, feet, and hands for edema.	1. Instruct patient to restrict the amount of salt she eats. 2. Teach patient to weigh herself weekly and check her body for edema. 3. Instruct patient to elevate feet if edematous.
Vaginal Dryness		
Patient will experience minimal vaginal dryness	1. Assess patient for vaginal bleeding, discharge, pain, itching, soreness, redness, or swelling. 2. Administer estrogen cream or suppositories, as needed.	1. Instruct patient about signs and symptoms of vaginal dryness. 2. Teach patient to utilize a water-soluble lubricant to decrease dryness and cool compresses to the perineal area for comfort.

Patients with bowel obstruction may experience abdominal pain, nausea and vomiting, abdominal distention, dehydration, diarrhea, or constipation. Treatments may include the use of nasogastric tube, intravenous hydration, and possibly surgery. If surgery is not possible, patients and their caregivers may be required to learn how to care for a nasogastric tube with suction and the administration of intravenous hydration at home.

Ascites

Another problem patients may need to manage while at home is ascites. Malignant ascites is defined as the accumulation of fluid within the peritoneal cavity and is indicative of advanced disease (Labovich, 1994). Because the majority of patients with ovarian cancer have advanced disease at the time of their initial presentation, ascites may be present at diagnosis, or it may occur after treatment failure.

Patients may have several symptoms, including lack of appetite, feeling full, gastric reflux, inability to wear clothes, and difficulty with breathing. Treatment may include removal of the fluid by paracentesis and the use of diuretics. Patients should be given instructions about fluid and sodium restriction, diuretic use, positioning to aid breathing, monitoring weight, measurement of abdominal girth, and when to notify the physician of increasing symptoms (Table 31-11).

PROGNOSIS

The prognosis for patients with ovarian cancer varies depending on the stage of the disease at the time of diagnosis, the patient's age, and coexistent medical problems. Other factors that influence a patient's prognosis are the grade of the tumor, lymph node involvement, and presence or absence of ascites. Patients with disease confined to the ovary,

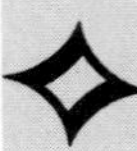

TABLE 31-11 Patient Preparation for the Monitoring and Management of Abdominal Ascites

Ascites is a problem that occurs when large amounts of fluid pool in the abdomen. This fluid can lead to feelings of fullness, loss of appetite, inability to wear clothes, and difficulty breathing. The doctor may do a procedure called a paracentesis to remove the fluid, or a shunt may be placed to drain the fluid from the abdomen into the bloodstream. The excess fluid in the blood can be removed by the kidneys into the urine.

Several actions may help to make you more comfortable:

1. Eat small, frequent meals that are high in protein and calories. The doctor may restrict your salt and fluid intake.
2. Measure the size of your abdomen (called *abdominal girth*) on a daily basis and record the measurement in a daily diary.
3. Perform as much activity as tolerated. Wear an abdominal binder while you are up to increase abdominal pressure and enhance fluid flow. Keep your legs and feet elevated when sitting.
4. Weigh yourself daily and keep a record of your weight.
5. Call your nurse or doctor if any of the following occurs:
    a. A weight gain or increase in abdominal girth so that your clothes do not fit
    b. Any difficulty breathing
    c. Nausea, vomiting, or abdominal pain

well- or moderately differentiated histology, an intact ovarian capsule, no adhesions or extracystic tumor, no ascites, and negative peritoneal washings have long-term survival rates greater than 90% without further treatment after surgery (Young, 1995). Patients with negative lymph nodes survive significantly longer than those with positive nodes at initial surgery, 46% versus 25% 5-year survival; median survival, 60 months vs 36 months (Di Re et al., 1996). When the initial surgery is able to cytoreduce the tumor to less than 1 cm, 5-year survival rates of 66% vs 85% may be achieved for patients with positive vs negative lymph nodes (Bolis, Villa, Guarnerio, Ferraris, Gavoni, & Giardina, et al., 1996). In addition, responsiveness of the tumor to chemotherapy and duration of that response affect survival. Primary postoperative radiation therapy to the abdomen and pelvis has resulted in a 68% 10-year relapse-free survival in patients with stages I and II disease (Morton & Thomas, 1994).

In general, when ovarian cancer is of early stage and low malignant potential, the disease may be curable. In fact, most patients with low-malignant-potential or borderline tumors have an extremely favorable prognosis, whether or not the disease is treated (Kennedy & Hart, 1996). Because only 23% of all ovarian cancers are detected at an early stage, only 76% of patients diagnosed with ovarian cancer will survive 1 year after diagnosis. Five-year survival rates are 91% for local disease, 49% for regional disease, and 23% for those who have distant metastases at the time of diagnosis (American Cancer Society, 1996).

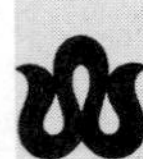

TABLE 31-12 Quality of Care Evaluation for a Patient Undergoing External Beam Radiation Therapy for Ovarian Cancer

Disciplines participating in the quality of care evaluation:
☐ Nursing ☐ Radiation Oncology

I. Outpatient Management Evaluation

Data from:
☐ Medical Record Review ☐ Patient/Family Interview

Criteria	Yes	No
1. Patient provided with information about:		
a. Purpose of the radiation therapy	☐	☐
b. Simulation procedure	☐	☐
c. Treatment procedures and routines	☐	☐
2. Complete blood cell count done weekly	☐	☐
3. Patient experienced the following side effects of external beam radiation therapy:		
a. Skin reaction	☐	☐
b. Nausea and vomiting	☐	☐
c. Diarrhea	☐	☐
d. Cystitis	☐	☐

II. Patient/Family Satisfaction

Data from:
☐ Patient Interview ☐ Family Interview

Criteria	Yes	No
1. On a scale of 0 to 10, with 0 being totally dissatisfied and 10 being totally satisfied, how satisfied were you with the information you received about the procedures and routines associated with your radiation treatments? ________	☐	☐
2. Were you told to call the physician if you had a temperature greater than 100.4° F (38° C)?	☐	☐
3. Were you taught to drink 3 liters of fluid each day?	☐	☐
4. Were you taught how to care for your skin while you were receiving radiation therapy?	☐	☐

EVALUATION OF THE QUALITY OF CARE

Accreditation organizations, such as the Joint Commission for the Accreditation of Health Care Organizations, require that the quality of care provided to patients be evaluated. Because the care provided to patients with ovarian cancer requires input from a multidisciplinary team, an evaluation of the quality of care provided to these patients should include aspects of care provided by various members of the team. Tables 31-12 and 31-13 provide examples of quality of care evaluation tools that can be used in the outpatient settings.

RESEARCH ISSUES

Numerous research issues surrounding the diagnosis and management of ovarian cancer require further investigations. The genetic basis for the disease, the risk factors associated with the development of ovarian cancer, and an optimal approach to early detection remain to be identified. At this time, guidelines or recommendations for early detection of ovarian cancer do not exist.

Numerous randomized, clinical trials are needed to determine the most effective treatments for the various stages of ovarian cancer. New chemotherapy drugs and combination regimens need to be studied and compared with current practice for responses, toxicities, and long-term survival. All of these research studies need to consider not only the effectiveness of the treatment in improving patient's survival, but also the costs of treatment, the morbidities associated with treatments, and the impact of treatments on the patient's quality of life.

TABLE 31-13 Quality of Care Evaluation for a Patient Receiving Hormone Therapy

Disciplines participating in the quality of care evaluation:
☐ Nursing ☐ Physician

Data from:
☐ Medical Record Review ☐ Patient/Family Interview

Criteria	Yes	No
1. Did the doctor or nurse explain to you that you might experience some of the following side effects from your hormonal therapy?		
a. Hot flashes	☐	☐
b. Vaginal dryness	☐	☐
c. Changes in your mood	☐	☐
d. Weight gain	☐	☐
2. Were you taught to avoid hot drinks and alcohol to reduce the number of hot flashes?	☐	☐
3. Were you taught to decrease your salt intake?	☐	☐

REFERENCES

Abu-Rustum, N. R., Barakat, R. R., Siegel, P. L., Venkatraman, E., Curtin, J. P., & Hoskins, W. J. (1996). Second-look operation for epithelial ovarian cancer: Laparoscopy or laparotomy? *Obstetrics and Gynecology, 88,* 549-553.

Adami, H. O., Hsieh, C. C., Lambe, M., Trichopoulos, D., Leon, D., Persson, I., Ekbom, A., & Janson, P. O. (1994). Parity, age at first childbirth, and risk of ovarian cancer. *Lancet, 344,* 1250-1254.

Ahlgren, J. D., Ellison, N. M., Gottlieb, R. J., Laluna, F., Lokich, J. J., Sinclair, P. R., Ueno, W., Wampler, G. L., Yeung, K. Y., Alt, D., & Fryer, J. G. (1993). Hormonal palliation of chemoresistant ovarian cancer: Three consecutive phase II trials of the mid-Atlantic oncology program. *Journal of Clinical Oncology, 11*(10),1957-1968.

Alberts, D. S. (1995). Carboplatin versus cisplatin in ovarian cancer. *Seminars in Oncology, 22*(5, Suppl. 12), 88-90.

American Cancer Society. (1996). *Cancer facts and figures—1996.* Atlanta: American Cancer Society.

Averette, H. E., Janicek, M. F., & Menck, H. R. (1995). The National Cancer Data Base report on ovarian cancer. *Cancer, 76*(6),1096-1103.

Baker, V. V. (1994). Molecular biology and genetics of epithelial ovarian cancer. *Obstetrics and Gynecology Clinics of North America, 21*(1), 25-38.

Balasch, J. & Barri, P. N. (1993). Follicular stimulation and ovarian cancer. *Human Reproduction, 8,* 990-996.

Barber, H. R. K. (1993). Prophylaxis in ovarian cancer. *Cancer, 71,* 1529-1533.

Bast, R. C., Jr., Boyer, C. M., Jacobs, I., Xu, F. J., Wu, S., Wiener, J., Kohler, M., & Berchuck, A. (1993). Cell growth regulation in epithelial ovarian cancer. *Cancer, 71,* 1597-1601.

Benedetti-Panici, P., Greggi, S., Scambia, G., Salerno, M. G., Baiocchi, G., Laurelli, G., Menichella, G., Pierelli, L., Roddai, M. L., Serafini, R., Bizzi, B., & Mancuso, S. (1995). Very high-dose chemotherapy with autologous peripheral stem cell support in advanced ovarian cancer. *European Journal of Cancer, 31A*(12), 1987-1992.

Berchuck, A., Kohler, M. F., Boente, M. P., Rodriguez, G. C., Whitaker, R. S., & Bast, R. C., Jr. (1993). Growth regulation and transformation of ovarian epithelium. *Cancer, 71,* 545-551.

Berek, J. S. & Hacker, N. F. (1994). *Practical gynecologic oncology.* Baltimore: Williams & Wilkins.

Bobak, L. M. & Jensen, M. D. (1993). *Maternity and gynecologic care: The nurse and the family* (3rd ed.). St. Louis: Mosby.

Bolis, G. (1995). Pilot study with fixed-dose carboplatin and escalating paclitaxel in advanced ovarian cancer. *Seminars in Oncology, 22*(6, Suppl. 14), 32-34.

Bolis, G., Villa, A., Guarnerio, P., Ferraris, C., Gavoni, N., Giardina, G., Melpignano, M., Scarfone, G., Zanaboni, F., & Parazzini, F. (1996). Survival of women with advanced ovarian cancer and complete pathologic response at second-look laparotomy. *Cancer, 77,* 128-131.

Bookman, M. A., McGuire, W. P., Kilpatrick, D., Keenan, E., Hogan, W. M., Johnson, S. W., O'Dwyer, P., Rowinsky, E., Gallion, H. H., & Ozols, R. F. (1996). Carboplatin and paclitaxel in ovarian carcinoma: A phase I study of the Gynecologic Oncology Group. *Journal of Clinical Oncology, 14*(6), 1895-1902.

Braly, P. S., Berek, J. S., Blessing, J. A., Homesley, H. D., & Averette, H. (1995). Intraperitoneal administration of cisplatin and 5-fluorouracil in residual ovarian cancer: A Phase II Gynecologic Oncology Group trial. *Gynecologic Oncology, 56*(2), 164-168.

Bristow, R. E. & Karlan, B. Y. (1996). The risk of ovarian cancer after treatment for infertility. *Current Opinion in Obstetrics and Gynecology, 8,* 32-37.

Buller, R. E., Vasilev, S., & DiSaia, P. J. (1996). CA 125 kinetics: A cost-effective clinical tool to evaluate clinical trial outcomes in the 1990s. *American Journal of Obstetrics and Gynecology, 174*(4), 1241-1254.

Caldas, C., Morris, L. E., & McGuire, W. P. (1994). Salvage therapy in epithelial ovarian cancer. *Obstetrics and Gynecology Clinics of North America, 21*(1), 179-191.

Calvert, A. H., Boddy, A., Bailey, N. P., Siddiqui, N., Humphreys, A., Hughes, A., Robson, L., Gumbrell, L., Thomas, H., Chapman, F., Proctor, M., Simmons, D., Oakey, A., Lind, M. J., Sinha, D. V., & Newell, D. R. (1995). Carboplatin in combination with paclitaxel I advanced ovarian cancer: Dose determination and pharmacokinetic and pharmacodynamic interactions. *Seminars in Oncology, 22*(5 Suppl. 12), 91-98.

Cavaletti, G., Bogliun, G., Marzorati, L., Zincone, A., Marzola, M., Colombo, N., & Tredici, G. (1995). Peripheral neurotoxicity of paciltaxel in patients previously treated with cisplatin. *Cancer, 75*(5), 1141-1150.

Cheung, A. N. Y. (1996). Oncogenes and other growth factors in gynaecological neoplasms. *Current Opinion in Obstetrics and Gynecology, 8,* 46-51.

Connelly, E., Markman, M., Kennedy, A., Webster, K., Kulp, B., Peterson, G., & Belinson, J. (1995). Paclitaxel delivered as a 3-hr infusion with cisplatin in patients with gynecologic cancers: Unexpected incidence of neurotoxicity. *Gynecologic Oncology, 62,* 166-168.

Conte, P. F., Bruzzone, M., Carnino, F., Gadducci, A., Algeri, R., Bellini, A., Boccardo, F., Brunetti, I., Catsafados, E., Chiara, S., Foglia, G., Gallo, L., Iskra, L., Mammoliti, S., Parodi, G., Ragni, N., Rosso, R., Rugiati, S., & Rubagotti, A. (1996). High-dose versus low-dose cisplatin in combination with cyclophosphamide and epidoxorubicin in suboptimal ovarian cancer: A randomized study of the Gruppo Oncologico Nord-Ovest. *Journal of Clinical Oncology, 14*(2), 351-356.

Davelaar, E. M., Bonfrer, J. M. G., Verstraeten, R. A., ten Bokkel Huinink, W. W., & Kenemans, P. (1996). CA 125 A valid marker in ovarian carcinoma patients treated with paclitaxel? *Cancer, 78*(1), 118-127.

Davidson, S. A., Rubin, S. C., Mychalczak, B., Saigo, P. E., Lewis, J. L., Jr., Chapman, D., & Hoskins, W. J. (1993). Limited-field radiotherapy as salvage treatment of localized persistent or recurrent epithelial ovarian cancer. *Gynecologic Oncology, 51,* 349-354.

Devesa, S. S. (1995). Cancer patterns among women in the United States. *Seminars in Oncology Nursing, 11*(2), 78-87.

DiCioccio, R. A. & Piver, M. S. (1996). A Polymorphism in intron 2 of the TPS3 gene. *Clinical Genetics, 50*(2), 108-109.

Di Re, F., Baiocchi, G., Fontanelli, R., Grosso, G., Cobellis, L., Raspagliesi, F., & Di Re, E. (1996). Systematic pelvic and paraaortic lymphadenectomy for advanced ovarian cancer: Prognostic significance of node metastases. *Gynecologic Oncology, 62,* 360-365.

DiSaia, P. J. (1997). *Clinical gynecologic oncology* (5th ed.). St. Louis: Mosby.

Eisenkop, S. M., Nalick, R. H., Wang, H. J., & Teng, N. N. (1993). Peritoneal implant elimination during cytoreductive surgery for ovarian cancer: Impact on survival. *Gynecologic Oncology, 51,* 224-229.

Fathalla, M. F. (1972). Factors in the causation and incidence of ovarian cancer. *Obstetrics and Gynecology Survey, 27,* 751-768.

Felip, E., Del Campo, J. M., Rubio, D., Vidal, M. T., Colomer, R., & Bermejo, B. (1995). Overexpression of c-erbB-2 in epithelial ovarian cancer. *Cancer, 75*(8), 2147-2152.

Fennelly, D., Schneider, J., Spriggs, D., Bengala, C., Hakes, T., Reich, L., Barakat, R., Curtin, J., Moore, M. A. S., Hoskins, W., Norton, L., & Crown, J. (1995). Dose escalation of paclitaxel with high-dose cyclophosphamide, with analysis of progenitor-cell mobilization and hematologic support of advanced ovarian cancer patients receiving rapidly sequenced high-dose carboplatin/cyclophosphamide courses. *Journal of Clinical Oncology, 13*(5), 1160-1166.

Fleischer, A. C., Cullinan, J. A., Peery, C. V., & Jones, H. W. (1996). Early detection of ovarian carcinoma with transvaginal color Doppler ultrasonography. *American Journal of Obstetrics and Gynecology, 174*(1, part 1), 101-106.

Francis, P., Rowinsky, E., Schneider, J., Hakes, T., Hoskins, W., & Markman, M. (1995). Phase I feasibility and pharmacologic study of weekly intraperitoneal paclitaxel: A Gynecologic Oncology Group pilot study. *Journal of Clinical Oncology, 13*(12), 2961-2967.

Frasci, G., Comella, G., Comella, P., Conforti, S., Mastrantonio, P., Zullo, F., & Persico, G. (1995). Carboplatin, hexamethylmelamine, oral etoposide first-line treatment of ovarian cancer patients with bulky disease: A phase II study. *Gynecologic Oncology, 58*(1), 68-73.

Frasci, G., Conforti, S., Zullo, F., Mastrantonio, P. Comella, G., Comella, P. Persico, G., & Iaffaioli, R. V. (1996). A risk model for ovarian carcinoma patients using CA 125: Time to normalization renders second-look laparotomy redundant. *Cancer, 77*(6), 1122-1130.

Futreal, P. A., Liu, Q., Shattuck-Eidens, D., Cochran, C., Harshman, K., Tavtigian, S., Bennett, L. M., Haugen-Strano, A., Swensen, J., Miki, Y., Eddington, K., McClure, M., Frye, C., Weaver-Feldhause, J., Ding, W., Gholami, Z., Soderkvist, P., Terry, L., Jhanwar, S., Berchuck, A., Iglehart, J. D., Marks, J., Ballinger, D. G., Barrett, J. C., Skolnick, M. H., Kamb, A., & Wiseman, R. (1994). BRCA1 mutations in primary breast and ovarian carcinomas. *Science, 266,* 120-122.

Geisler, J. P. & Geisler, H. E. (1995). Brain metastases in epithelial ovarian carcinoma. *Gynecologic Oncology, 57*(2), 246-249.

Genetic risk and screening techniques for epithelial ovarian cancer. (1992). *ACOG Committee Opinion,* 117.

Gershenson, D. M., Tortolero-Luna, G., Malpica, A., Baker, V. V., Whittaker, L., Johnson, E., & Mitchell, M. F. (1996). Ovarian intraepithelial neoplasia and ovarian cancer. *Obstetrics and Gynecology Clinics of North America, 23*(2), 475-543.

Golberg, G.L. & Runowicz, C. D. (1992). Ovarian carcinoma of low malignant potential, infertility, and induction of ovulation: Is there a link? *American Journal of Obstetrics and Gynecology, 166,* 853-854.

Grimes, D. A. (1993). Primary prevention of ovarian cancer. *Journal of the American Medical Association, 270*(23), 2855-2865.

Grimes, D. A. & Economy, K. E. (1995). Primary prevention of ovarian cancer. *American Journal of Obstetrics and Gynecology, 172*(1, part 1), 227-235.

Hankinson, S. E., Colditz, G. A., Hunter, D. J., Willett, W. C., Stampfer, M. J., Rosner, B., Hennekens, C. H., & Speizer, F. E. (1995). A prospective study of reproductive factors and risk of epithelial ovarian cancer. *Cancer, 76*(2), 284-90.

Hansen, H. H., Eisenhauer, E. A., Hansen, M., Neijt, J. P., Piccart, M. J., Sessa, C., & Thigpen, J. T. (1993). New cytostatic drugs in ovarian cancer. *Annals of Oncology, 7*(Suppl. 4), S63-S70.

Harlow, B. L., Cramer, D. W., Bell, D. A., & Welch, W. R. (1992). Perineal exposure to talc and ovarian cancer risk. *Obstetrics and Gynecology, 80*(1), 19-26.

Helzlsouer, K. J. Alberg, A. J., Gordon, G. B., Longcope, C., Bush, T. L., Hoffman, S. C., & Comstock, G. W. (1995). Serum gonadotropins and steroid hormones and the development of ovarian cancer. *Journal of the American Medical Association, 274*(24), 1926-1930.

Henderson, B. E., Ross, R. K., & Pike, M. C. (1993). Hormonal chemoprevention of cancer in women. *Science, 259,* 633-638.

Herod, J. J., Eliopoulos, A. G., Warwick, J., Niedobitek, G., Young, L. S., & Kerr, D. J. (1996). The prognostic significance of Bcl-2 and p53 expression in ovarian carcinoma. *Cancer Research, 56*(9), 2178-2184.

Hoskins, W. J. & Swenerton, K. D. (1994). Oral etoposide is active against platinum-resistant epithelial ovarian cancer. *Journal of Clinical Oncology, 12*(1), 60-63.

Hoskins, W. J., Bundry, B. N., Thigpen, J. T., & Omura, G. A. (1992). The influence of cytoreductive surgery on recurrence-free interval and survival in small-volume stage III epithelial ovarian cancer: A Gynecologic Oncology Group study. *Gynecologic Oncology, 47,* 159-166.

Hoskins, W. J., McGuire, W. P., Brady, M. F., Homesley, H. D., Creasman, W. T., Berman, M., Ball, H., & Berek, J. S. (1994). The effect of diameter of largest residual disease on survival after primary cytoreductive surgery in patients with suboptimal residual epithelial ovarian carcinoma. *American Journal of Obstetrics and Gynecology, 170,* 974-980.

Jacobs, I., Davies, A. P., Bridges, J., Stabile, I., Fay, T., Lower, A., Grudzinskas, J. G., & Oram, D. (1993). Prevalence screening for ovarian cancer in postmenopausal women by CA 125 measurement and ultrasonography. *British Medical Journal, 306,* 1030-1034.

Karlan, B. Y., Marrs, R., & Lagasse, L. D. (1994). Advanced-stage ovarian carcinoma presenting during infertility evaluation. *American Journal of Obstetrics and Gynecology, 171,* 1377-1378.

Kavanagh, J., Tresukosol, D., Edwards, C., Freedman, R., Gonzalez de Leon, C., Fishman, A., Mante, R., Hord, M., & Kudelka, A. (1995). Carboplatin reinduction after taxane in patients with platinum-refractory epithelial ovarian cancer. *Journal of Clinical Oncology, 13*(7), 1584-1588.

Kennedy, A. W., & Hart, W. R. (1996). Ovarian papillary serous tumors of low malignant potential (serous borderline tumors). *Cancer, 78,* 278-286.

Kramer, B. S., Gohagan, J., Prorok, P. C., & Smart, C. (1993). A National Cancer Institute sponsored screening trial for prostatic, lung, colorectal, and ovarian cancers. *Cancer, 71,* 589-593.

Kudelka, A. P., Tresdukosol, D., Edwards, C. L., Freedman, R. S., Levenback, C., Chantarawiroj, P., Gonzalez de Leon, C., Kim, E. E., Madden, T., Wallin, B., Hord, M., Verschraegen, C., Raber, M., & Kavanagh, J. J. (1996). Phase II study of intravenous topotecan as a 5-day infusion for refractory epithelial ovarian carcinoma. *Journal of Clinical Oncology, 14*(5), 1552-1557.

Labovich, T. M. (1994). Selected complications in the patient with cancer: Spinal cord compression, malignant bowel obstruction, malignant ascites, and gastrointestinal bleeding. *Seminars in Oncology Nursing, 10*(3), 189-197.

Lambert, H. E., Rustin, G. J. S., Gregory, W. M., & Nelstrop, A. E. (1993). A randomized trial comparing single-agent carboplatin with carboplatin followed by radiotherapy for advanced ovarian cancer: A North Thames Ovary Group study. *Journal of Clinical Oncology, 11,* 440-448.

Landis, S. H., Murray, T., Bolden, S., & Wingo, P. A. (1998). Cancer statistics, 1998. *CA: A Cancer Journal for Clinicians, 48,* 6-29.

Lind, M. J., Ghazal-Aswad, S., Gumbrell, L., Fishwick, K., Craigs, D., Millward, M. J., Bailey, N. P., Dore-Green, F., Chapman, F., Simmons, D., Proctor, M., Oakey, A., Robson, L., Middleton, I., McCann, E., Sinha, D., & Calvert, A. H. (1996). Phase I study of pharmacologically based dosing of carboplatin with filgrastim support in women with epithelial ovarian cancer. *Journal of Clinical Oncology, 14*(3), 800-805.

Look, K. Y., Muss, H. B., Blessing, J. A., & Morris, M. (1995). A phase II trial of 5-fluorouracil and high-dose leucovorin in recurrent epithelial ovarian carcinoma. A Gynecologic Oncology Group Study. *American Journal of Clinical Oncology, 18*(1), 19-22.

Makar, A. P., Baekelandt, M., Trope, C. G., & Kristensen, G. B. (1995). The prognostic significance of residual disease, FIGO substage, tumor histology, and grade in patients with FIGO stage III ovarian cancer. *Gynecologic Oncology, 56*(2), 175-180.

Markman, M., Francis, P., Rowinsky, E., & Hoskins, W. (1995). Intraperitoneal paclitaxel: A possible role in the management of ovarian cancer? *Seminars in Oncology, 22*(3, Suppl. 6), 84-87.

Markman, M., Hakes, T., Barakat, R., Curtin, J., Almadarones, L., & Hoskins, W. (1996). Follow-up of Memorial Sloan-Kettering Cancer Center patients treated on National Cancer Institute Treatment Referral Center protocol 9103: Paclitaxel in refractory ovarian cancer. *Journal of Clinical Oncology, 14*(3), 796-799.

Markman, M., Iseminger, K. A., Hatch, K. D., Creasman, W. T., Barnes, W., & Dubeshter, B. (1996). Tamoxifen in platinum-refractory ovarian cancer. A Gynecologic Oncology Group ancillary report. *Gynecologic Oncology, 62,* 4-6.

Massi, D., Susini, T., Savino, L. Boddi, V., Amunni, G., & Maurizio, C. (1996). Epithelial ovarian tumors in the reproductive age group. *Cancer, 77*(6), 1131-1136.

McClay, E. F., Braly, P. D., Kirmani, S., Plaxe, S. C., Kim, S., McClay, M. E., Wilgus, L., & Howell, S. B. (1995). A phase II trial of intraperitoneal high-dose carboplatin and etoposide with granulocyte macrophage-colony stimulating factor support in patients with ovarian carcinoma. *American Journal of Clinical Oncology, 18*(1), 23-26.

McGuire, W. P., Hoskins, W. J., Brady, M. F., Homesley, H. D., Creasman, W. T., Berman, M. L., Ball, H., Berek, J. S., & Woodward, J. (1995). Assessment of dose-intensive therapy in suboptimally debulked ovarian cancer: A Gynecologic Oncology Group study. *Journal of Clinical Oncology, 13*(7), 1589-1599.

McGuire, W. P., Hoskins, W. J., Brady, M. F., Kucera, P. R., Partridge, E. E., Look, K. Y., Clarke-Pearson, D. L., & Davidson, M. (1996). Cyclophosphamide and cisplatin compared with paclitaxel and cisplatin in patients with stage III and stage IV ovarian cancer. *New England Journal of Medicine, 334*(1), 1-6.

Merino, M. J. & Jaffe, G. (1993). Age contrast in ovarian pathology. *Cancer, 71,* 537-544.

Mettlin, C. & Piver, M. S. (1990). A case-control study of milk drinking and ovarian cancer risk. *American Journal of Epidemiology, 132,* 871-876.

Morgan, R. J., Jr., Speyer, J., Doroshow, J. H., Margolin, K., Raschko, J., Sorich, J., Akman, S., Leong, L., Somlo, G., Vasileve, S., Ahn, C., Johnson, D., & Beller, U. (1995). Modulation of 5-fluorouracil with high-dose leucovorin calcium: Activity in ovarian cancer and correlation with CA-125 levels. *Gynecologic Oncology, 58*(1), 79-85.

Morton, G., & Thomas, G. M. (1994). Role of radiotherapy in the treatment of cancer of the ovary. *Seminars in Surgical Oncology, 10,* 305-312.

NIH Consensus Panel. (1995). Ovarian cancer: Screening, treatment, and follow-up. *Journal of the American Medical Association, 273*(6), 491-497.

Onda, T., Yoshikawa, H., Yokota, H., Yasugi, T., & Taketani, Y. (1996). Assessment of metastases to aortic and pelvic lymph nodes in epithelial ovarian carcinoma. *Cancer, 78*(4), 803-808.

Outwater, E. & Dunton, C. J. (1995). Imaging of the ovary and adnexa: Clinical issues and applications of MR imaging. *Radiology, 194*(1), 1-18.

Ozols, R. F. (1994). Treatment of ovarian cancer: Current status. *Seminars in Oncology, 21*(2, Suppl. 2), 1-9.

Ozols, R. F. (1995). Carboplatin and paclitaxel in ovarian cancer. *Seminars in Oncology, 22*(3, Suppl. 6), 78-83.

Parazzini, F., La Vecchia, C., Negri, E., Moroni, S., dal Pino, D., & Fedele, L. (1996). Pelvic inflammatory disease and risk of ovarian cancer. *Cancer Epidemiology, Biomarkers and Prevention, 5,* 667-669.

Park, J. S., Kim, H. K., Han, S. K., Lee, J. M., Namkoong, S. E., & Kim, S. J. (1995). Detection of c-k-ras point mutation in ovarian cancer. *International Journal of Gynecologic Cancer, 5,* 107-111.

Pattillo, R. A., Collier, B. D., Abdel-Dayem, H., Ozker, K., Wilson, C., Ruckert, A. C., & Hamilton, K. (1995). Phosphorus-32-chromic phosphate for ovarian cancer: I. Fractionated low-dose intraperitoneal treatments in conjunction with platinum analog chemotherapy. *Journal of Nuclear Medicine, 36*(1), 29-36.

Piver, M. S., Baker, T. R., Jishi, M. F., Sandecki, A. M., Tsukada, Y., Natarajan, N., Mettlin, C. J., & Blake, C. A. (1993). Familial ovarian cancer: A report of 658 families from the Gilda Radner Familial Ovarian Cancer Registry 1981-1991. *Cancer, 71,* 582-588.

Portenoy, R. K., Kornblith, A. B., Wong, G., Vlamis, V., Lepore, J. M., Loseth, D. B., Hakes, T., Foley, K. M., & Hoskins, W. J. (1994). Pain in ovarian cancer patients. *Cancer, 74,* 907-915.

Prefontaine, M., Donovan, J. T., Powell, J. L., & Buley, L. (1996). Treatment of refractory ovarian cancer with 5-fluorouracil and leucovorin. *Gynecologic Oncology, 61*(2), 249-252.

Pujade-Lauraine, E., Guastalla, J. P., Colombo, N., Devillier, P., Francois, E., Fumoleau, P., Monnier, A., Nooy, M., Mignot, L., Bugat, R., Marques, C., Mousseau, M., Netter, G., Maloisel, F., Larbaoui, S., & Brandely, M. (1996). Intraperitoneal recombinant interferon gamma in ovarian cancer patients with residual disease at second-look laparotomy. *Journal of Clinical Oncology, 14*(2), 343-350.

Puls, L. E., Duniho, T., Hunter, J. E., Kryscio, R., Blackhurst, D., & Gallion, H. (1996). The Prognostic Implication of Ascites in Advanced-Stage Ovarian Cancer. *Gynecologic Oncology, 61,* 109-112.

Qazi, F. & McGuire, W. P. (1995). The treatment of epithelial ovarian cancer. *CA: A Cancer Journal for Clinicians, 45*(2), 88-101.

Reed, E., Kohn, E. C., Sarosy, G., Dabhokar, M., Davis, P., Jacob, J., & Maher, M. (1995). Paclitaxel, cisplatin, and cyclophosphamide in human ovarian cancer: Molecular rationale and early clinical results. *Seminars in Oncology, 22*(3, Suppl. 6), 90-96.

Ries, L. A. G., Miller, B. A., Hankey, B. F., Kosary, C. L., Harras, A., & Edwards, B. K. (1994). *SEER cancer statistics review, 1973-1991: Tables and graphs,* National Cancer Institute. NIH Publication No. 94-2789. Bethesda: National Cancer Institute.

Risch, H. A., & Howe, G. R. (1995). Pelvic inflammatory disease and the risk of epithelial ovarian cancer. *Cancer Epidemiology, Biomarkers and Prevention, 4,* 447-451.

Rodriguez, C., Calle, E. E., Coates, R. J., Miracle-McMahill, H. L., Thun, M. J., & Heath, C. W. Jr. (1995). Estrogen replacement therapy and fatal ovarian cancer. *American Journal of Epidemiology, 141*(9), 828-835.

Rossing, M. A., Daling, J. R., Weiss, N. S., Moore, D. E., & Self, S. G. (1994). Ovarian tumors in a cohort of infertile women. *New England Journal of Medicine, 331,* 771-776.

Runnebaum, I. B., Kieback, D. G., Mobus, V. J., Tong, X. W., & Kreienberg, R. (1996). Subcellular localization of accumulated p53 in ovarian cancer cells. *Gynecologic Oncology, 61*(2), 266-271.

Runowicz, C. D., Fields, A. L., & Goldberg, G. L. (1995). Promising new therapies in the treatment of advanced ovarian cancer. *Cancer, 76*(10), 2028-2033.

Runowicz, C. D., Wiernik, P. H., Einzig, A. I., Goldberg, G. L., & Horwitz, S. B. (1993). Paciltaxel in ovarian cancer. *Cancer, 71,* 1591-1596.

Rustin, G. J., Nelstrop, A. E., McClean, P., Brady, M. F., McGuire, W. P., Hoskins, W. J., Mitchell, H., & Lambert H. E. (1996). Defining response of ovarian carcinoma to initial chemotherapy according to serum CA 125. *Journal of Clinical Oncology, 14*(5), 1545-1551.

Samuels, B. L. & Bitran, J. D. (1995). High-dose intravenous melphalan: A review. *Journal of Clinical Oncology, 13*(7), 1786-1799.

Schiff, M., Becker, T. M., Smith, H. O., Gilliland, F. D., & Key, C. R. (1996). Ovarian cancer incidence and mortality in American Indian, Hispanic and non-Hispanic white women in New Mexico. *Cancer Epidemiology, Biomarkers and Prevention, 5,* 323-327.

Schildkraut, J. M., Schwingl, P. J., Bastos, E., Evanoff, A., & Hughes, C. (1996). Epithelial ovarian cancer risk among women with polycystic ovary syndrome. *Obstetrics and Gynecology, 88,* 554-559.

Schneider, J. G. (1994). Intraperitoneal chemotherapy. *Obstetrics and Gynecology Clinics of North America, 21*(1), 195-211.

Seidel, H. M. (1991). *Mosby's guide to physical examination* (3rd ed.). St. Louis: Mosby.

Sood, A. K., Gelder, M. S., Huang, S. W., & Morgan, L. S. (1995). Anaphylaxis to carboplatin following multiple previous uncomplicated courses. *Gynecologic Oncology, 57*(1), 131-132.

Sorensen, P., Pfeiffer, P., & Bertelsen, K. (1995). A phase 2 trial of ifosfamide/mesna as salvage therapy in patients with ovarian cancer refractory to or relapsing after prior platinum-containing chemotherapy. *Gynecologic Oncology, 56*(1), 75-78.

Spirtos, N. M., Gross, G. M., Freddo, J. L., & Ballon, S. C. (1995). Cytoreductive surgery in advanced epithelial cancer of the ovary: The impact of aortic and pelvic lymphadenectomy. *Gynecologic Oncology, 56*(3), 345-352.

Stiff, P., Bayer, R., Camarda, M., Tan, S., Dolan, J., Potkul, R., Loutifi, S., Kinch, L., Sosman, J., Peace, D., Rad, N., & McKenzie, R. S. (1995). A phase II trial of high-dose mitoxantrone, carboplatin, and cyclophosphamide with autologous bone marrow rescue for recurrent epithelial ovarian carcinoma: Analysis of risk factors for clinical outcome. *Gynecologic Oncology, 57*(3), 278-285.

Stiff, P. J., McKenzie, R. S., Alberts, D. S., Sosman, J. A., Dolan, J. R., Rad, N., & McCloskey, T. (1994). Phase I clinical and pharmacokinetic study of high-dose mitoxantrone combined with carboplatin, cyclophosphamide, and autologous bone marrow rescue: High response rate for refractory ovarian carcinoma. *Journal of Clinical Oncology, 12*(1), 176-183.

Tamakoshi, K., Kikkawea, F., Shibata, K., Tomoda, K., Obata, N. H., Wakahara, F., Tokuhashi, Y., Ishikawa, H., Kawai, M., & Tomoda, Y. (1996). Clinical value of CA 125, CA 19-9, CEA, CA 72-4, and TPA in borderline ovarian tumor. *Gynecologic Oncology, 62,* 67-72.

ten Bokkel Huinink, W., Veenhof, C., Helmerhorst, T., Bierhorst, F., Dalesio, O., Winograd, B., Depauw, L., & Pinedo, H. M. (1995). Paclitaxel plus carboplatin in the treatment of ovarian cancer. *Seminars in Oncology, 22*(3, Suppl. 6), 97-100.

Teneriello, M. G. & Park, R. C. (1995). Early detection of ovarian cancer. *CA: A Cancer Journal for Clinicians, 45*(2), 71-87.

Thigpen, J. T., Blessing, J. A., Ball, H., Hummel, S. J., & Barrett, R. J. (1994). Phase II trial of paclitaxel in patients with progressive ovarian carcinoma after platinum-based chemotherapy: A Gynecologic Oncology Group study. *Journal of Clinical Oncology, 12*(9), 1748-1753.

Thigpen, R., Vance, R. B., McGuire, W. P., Hoskins, W. J., & Brady, M. (1995). The role of paclitaxel in the management of coelomic epithelial carcinoma of the ovary: A review with emphasis on the Gynecologic Oncology Group experience. *Seminars in Oncology, 22*(6 Suppl. 14), 23-31.

Thomas, C. W. (1993). *Taber's cyclopedic medical dictionary.* Philadelphia: F. A. Davis Company.

Thomas, G. M. & Dembo, A. J. (1993). Integrating radiation therapy into the management of ovarian cancer. *Cancer, 71,* 1710-1718.

Vaccarello, L., Rubin, S. C., Vlamis, V., Wong, G., Jones, W. B., Lewis, J. L., & Hoskins, W. J. (1995). Cytoreductive surgery in ovarian carcinoma patients with a documented previously complete surgical response. *Gynecologic Oncology, 57*(1), 61-65.

van Dam, P. A., Vergote, I. B., Lowe, D. G., Watson, J. V., van Damme, P., van der Auwera, J. C., & Shepherd, J. H. (1994). Expression of c-erbB-2, c-myc, and c-ras oncoproteins, insulin-like growth factor receptor I, and epidermal growth factor receptor in ovarian cancer. *Journal of Clinical Pathology, 47,* 914-919.

van der Burg, M. E., van Lent, M., Buyse, M., Kobierska, A., Colombo, N., Favalli, G., Lacave, A. J., Nardi, M., Renard, J., & Pecorelli, S. (1995). The effect of debulking surgery after induction chemotherapy on the prognosis in advanced epithelial ovarian cancer. *The New England Journal of Medicine, 322*(10), 629-634.

van Haaften-Day, C., Russell, P., Boyer, C. M., Kerns, B. J. M., Wiener, J. R., Jensen, D. N., Bast, R. C. Jr., & Hacker, N. F. (1996). Expression of cell regulatory proteins in ovarian borderline tumors. *Cancer, 77*(10), 2092-2097.

Wadler, S., Yeap, B., Vogl, S., & Carbone, P. (1996). Randomized trial of initial therapy with melphalan versus cisplatin-based combination chemotherapy in patients with advanced ovarian carcinoma: Initial and long term results—Eastern Cooperative Oncology Group Study E2878. *Cancer, 77*(4), 733-742.

Weidmann, B., Mulleneisen, N., Bojko, P., & Niederle, N. (1994). Hypersensitivity reactions to carboplatin. *Cancer, 73,* 2218-2222.

Whittemore, A. S., Harris, R., Itnyre, J., Halpern, J., & The Collaborative Ovarian Cancer Group. (1992). Characteristics relating to ovarian cancer risk: Collaborative analysis of 12 US case-control studies. II. Invasive epithelial ovarian cancers in white women. *American Journal of Epidemiology, 136,* 1184-1203.

Willemse, P. H., DeVries, E. G., Aalders, J. G., Bouma, J., & Sleijfer, D. T. (1990) Intraperitoneal human recombinant interferon alpha-2b in minimal residual ovarian cancer. *European Journal of Cancer, 26,* 353-358.

Wynder, E. L., Fujita, Y., Harris, R. E., Hirayama, T., & Hiyama, T. (1991). Comparative epidemiology of cancer between the United States and Japan; A second look. *Cancer, 67,* 746-763.

Yancik, R. (1993). Ovarian cancer; Age contrasts in incidence, histology, disease stage at diagnosis, and mortality. *Cancer, 71,* 517-523.

Young, R. (1995). The treatment of early stage ovarian cancer. *Seminars in Oncology, 22*(5, Suppl. 12), 76-79.

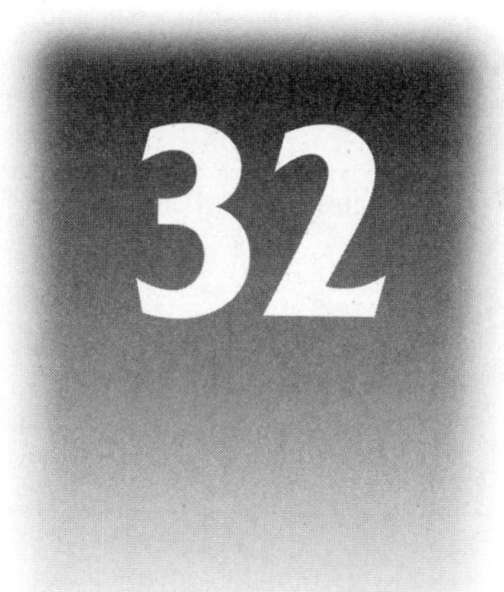

Stromal and Germ-Cell Cancer of the Ovary

Catherine Jansen, RN, MS

EPIDEMIOLOGY

Ovarian cancer is the deadliest gynecologic malignancy in the United States, killing more women each year than cervical and endometrial cancers combined. Although ovarian cancer accounts for only approximately 4% of all female cancers, it is the fourth leading cause of cancer deaths in women. In 1998 the number of new cases of ovarian cancer in the United States was 24,500, and approximately 14,500 women died from this disease (Landis, Murray, Bolden, & Wingo, 1998). The most common type of ovarian cancer is epithelial; these cancers encompass 85% to 90% of all tumors of the ovary. Germ-cell and sex-cord stromal cell tumors account for the other 10% to 15%. Germ-cell tumors tend to occur in adolescents and young adults, with a median age of 16 to 20 years. They are occasionally seen in infants and older women. In contrast, sex-cord stromal tumors may occur at any age and have a peak incidence in the postmenopausal years. Because these tumors are so rare and occur in multiple age groups, mass screening for early detection of nonepithelial ovarian cancer is not feasible.

The survival rate for women with early-stage disease is significantly higher than for those diagnosed with advanced-stage disease. Fortunately, unlike epithelial ovarian cancers, 60% to 70% of germ-cell tumors are diagnosed in stage I compared with 25% to 30% in stage III (Gershenson, Morris, Cangir, Kavanagh, Stringer, & Edwards et al., 1990; Schwartz, Chambers, Chambers, Kohorn, & McIntosh, 1992). Additionally, these tumors are sensitive to chemotherapy and radiation therapy. In contrast, sex-cord stromal tumors are not responsive to radiation therapy, and, although chemotherapy seems to be effective, experience is limited.

RISK FACTORS

The major risk factors associated with nonepithelial ovarian cancers are listed in Table 32-1. The evidence supporting each of these risk factors is reviewed, and the nursing implications for prevention and early detection activities are discussed.

Increasing Age

Age is an important risk factor in the development of ovarian cancer. The risk for ovarian cancer increases with each decade of life until about age 75 years, when it reaches its peak (see Table 31-1). Reports from the National Cancer Data Base estimate an incidence of ovarian cancer is 15.7 of 100,000 women under the age of 45 years, and this incidence increases to 54 of 100,000 women between the ages of 75 and 79 years (Averette, Janicek, & Menck, 1995). In addition, older women usually have the most aggressive forms of ovarian cancer, present with advanced disease, and have a poorer prognosis (Merino & Jaffee, 1993). The risk of increasing age is significant for sex-cord stromal ovarian tumors, which may occur at any age, although the age of peak incidence is in the postmenopausal years (Gershenson, 1994b). This risk factor is not shared with germ-cell tumors, in which the majority of malignancies occur in children or adolescents.

Ethnic Differences

Women who live in highly industrialized countries, with the exception of Japan, have the highest ovarian cancer rates. In contrast, those who live in developing countries have a lower incidence of ovarian cancer. Whereas the incidence of ovarian cancer in industrialized countries has been constant, the incidence in developing countries has actually increased (Gershenson, Tortolero-Luna, Malpica, Baker, Whittaker, & Johnson et al., 1996). Several epidemiologic studies in the United States have shown ethnic differences, with Hawaiian and white women having the highest rates of ovarian cancer, followed by Hispanic, African-American, Filipino, Chinese, Japanese, and Native-American women with the lowest rates (Averette, Janicek, & Menck., 1995; Schiff, Becker, Smith, Gilliland, & Key, 1996). Germ-cell tumors account for only approximately 10% of all ovarian neoplasms in Europe and North America, with a much greater incidence in Asia and Africa. Likewise, Japan has a higher incidence of germ-cell tumors owing to the decreased frequency of epi-

TABLE 32-1 Risk Factors for Sex-Cord Stromal and Germ-Cell Ovarian Cancer

Risk Factor	Sex-Cord Stromal	Germ-Cell
Age	Increasing age: highest incidence in post-menopausal years	Majority of tumors occur in children and adolescents
Ethnicity	Higher incidence in Hawaiian and white women	Higher incidence in Asia and Africa
Dysgenic gonad	Increased incidence of sex-cord stromal tumors	Increased incidence of germ-cell tumors
High-fat diet	Increased incidence	Increased incidence
Talc	? association	? association
Infertility	Use of oral contraceptives may have a protective effect	Weak negative association with parity

thelial tumors (Nakashima, Nagasaka, Fukata, Oiwa, Nara, & Fukatsu et al., 1990).

Dysgenetic Gonad

Dysgenetic gonad is a congenital endocrine disorder caused by failure of the ovaries to respond to pituitary hormone (gonadotropin) stimulation (Thomas, 1993). This anomaly is also known as *Turner's syndrome.* These patients have maldevelopment of their ovaries, chromosomal abnormalities, and a 20% to 25% chance of developing a gonadoblastoma and/or a germ-cell tumor (usually dysgerminoma) by age 20 (Lack, Young, & Scully, 1992). Gonadoblastomas are rare tumors that contain a combination of germ-cell and sex-cord stromal elements.

High-Fat Diet

Studies have reported a relationship between higher dietary fat intake and ovarian cancer (Gershenson et al., 1996b). For example, Japanese women who live in Japan have a low incidence of ovarian cancer. However, the higher rates of ovarian cancer in Japanese immigrants to the United States, especially in their descendants, suggests that the environment or diet might play a role in ovarian cancer risk. Additionally, the rate of ovarian cancer in Japan doubled between 1958 and 1982, in concert with an increased daily consumption of fat in the Japanese diet from 10.6 g in 1950 to 84.5 g in 1986 (Wynder, Fujita, Harris, Hirayama, & Hiyama, 1991). Another study demonstrated a relationship between the consumption of dietary fat in milk and a higher risk for ovarian cancer (Mettlin & Piver, 1990). The actual mechanism by which dietary fat intake may increase the risk of ovarian cancer is unknown.

Talc

Some studies have suggested an increased risk for ovarian cancer in women who used talc powders for more than 3 months (Harlow, Cramer, Bell, & Welch, 1992). It has been hypothesized that the powder could reach the ovaries after being absorbed through the cervix or vagina. Epidemiologic studies have been inconclusive and because talc powders are no longer contaminated with asbestos, the possibility of risk is probably no longer important.

Infertility

In epithelial ovarian cancers, there is a decrease in risk with increasing parity, such that women who have children may have a 45% decreased risk compared with nulliparous women (Adami, Hsieh, Lambe, Trichopoulos, Leon, & Persson et al., 1994). For germ-cell tumors, there appears to be a weak negative association with parity, but not a continual decrease in risk with increasing parity (Horn-Ross, Whittemore, Harris, & Itnyre, 1992). Some epidemiologic studies have suggested a relationship between the use of oral contraceptives and a reduction in risk for ovarian cancer by as high as 40%, especially with long-term users (Rodriguez, Calle, Coates, Miracle-McMahill, Thun, & Heath, 1995; Grimes, 1993; Grimes & Economy, 1995). Although the use of oral contraceptives seems to be protective for sex-cord stromal tumors, it may actually increase the risk for germ-cell tumors (Horn-Ross et al., 1992).

Summary

Although several risk factors associated with the development of nonepithelial ovarian cancer (i.e., increasing age, ethnicity, and dysgenetic gonads) cannot be modified, other risk factors may be reduced through lifestyle modifications. For example, women can reduce their dietary intake of fat through milk. In addition, the use of combination oral contraceptives may reduce the risk of sex-cord stromal ovarian cancer (see Chemoprevention below). Oncology nurses need to be aware of the potential risk factors to provide effective teaching for women concerned about their individual risk for ovarian cancer.

CHEMOPREVENTION

Chemoprevention is defined as the use of certain foods and drugs to prevent the progression of preneoplastic conditions and some neoplastic states (Thomas, 1993). Epidemiologic data confirm that the use of combination oral contraceptives provides protection against the development of ovarian cancer (Grimes & Economy, 1995; Henderson, Ross, & Pike, 1993). Protection seems to occur after a minimum of 3 to 6 months; increases with extended length of use, and persists for years after discontinuation. Although the use of oral contraceptives for chemoprevention has been suggested for ovarian cancer, trials evaluating their protective effects have not been developed.

PATHOPHYSIOLOGY

Normal Anatomy and Physiology of the Ovary

The ovaries are a pair of double glands (endocrine and exocrine) located in the female pelvis (see Fig. 31-1), on the lateral walls of the pelvic cavity, each attached by a fold of the peritoneum to the broad ligament of the uterus on either side, and are in close proximity to the fallopian tubes that are connected to the uterus. The ovaries, fallopian tubes, uterus, cervix, and vagina constitute the internal genitalia. The diaphragm, ureters, colon, and bladder are in close proximity (see Fig. 31-2).

Development of the ovary is initiated by the mesodermal surface of the embryo (i.e., primary germ layer), with the establishment of coelomic epithelium cells that form the ovaries, fallopian tubes, uterus, and cervix. Germ cells are then formed simultaneously with the proliferation of the coelomic epithelium and mesenchyme (i.e., a diffuse network of cells forming connective tissue, blood, lymphatics). Finally, the ovary is divided into the cortex (outer portion) and medulla (inner portion). The cortex is covered by a single layer of epithelium that functions as a protective layer. Its surface is smooth in early life and later becomes pitted as a result of atrophy. The cortex consists principally of follicles in various stages of development (primary, growing, and graafian or mature). The medulla consists of a foundation of connective tissue encompassing nerves, smooth muscle, blood, and lymphatic tissues. The blood system is mainly derived from the ovarian artery that arises from the abdominal aorta below the renal artery (see Fig. 31-3). The lymphatics follow along the ovarian veins and drain into the para-aortic nodes at the level of the second lumbar vertebra (see Fig. 31-4).

At birth, the ovaries are approximately 3 mm wide and 10 mm long, are almond-shaped, and contain up to 2 million ova (i.e., primitive female reproductive cells). During childhood, the ovarian ligaments form the outer ovarian layer of connective tissue, and only about 20% of the ova remain. Before puberty, all of the follicles present in the ovary are primary or primitive. Sexual maturity is characterized by the presence of growing follicles. At puberty, there is progressive development of the follicles, which is accompanied by growth and development of the ovaries, proliferation of follicles, and development of a connective tissue capsule from the surrounding stroma. Beginning with puberty and continuing through menopause (except during pregnancy), one graafian follicle develops approximately every 30 days. Each of these follicles contains a nearly mature ovum that, on rupture of the follicle through the cortex, is discharged from the ovary. This process is referred to as *ovulation.* The ovum then proceeds within 5 to 7 days through the fallopian tube, ending its journey in the uterus. If fertilization does not occur, then menstruation takes place and another follicle goes through maturation. With the initiation of monthly ovulation, only a few hundredths of a percent of ova reach full maturity, and even fewer remain at menopause. In an adult, the ovary is an egg-shaped body about 4 cm long, 2 cm wide, and 8 mm thick. The size of the ovaries decreases to 1 to 2 cm as their function decreases.

The functional activity and growth of these glands is primarily under the control of gonadoptropins produced in the pituitary gland, in particular the follicle-stimulating hormone and the luteinizing hormone. The two major functions of the ovary are to produce and release ova (germ cells) regularly and to produce hormones. These hormones, mainly estrogen and progesterone, are secreted by the ovaries and are responsible for the development and maintenance of secondary sex characteristics, the preparation of the uterus for pregnancy, and the development of the mammary glands.

The production of ova involves stimulation and development of the follicle to maturity, causing it to protrude through the ovarian surface (cortex), proceeding within 5 to 7 days through the fallopian tube and finally into the uterus. In the uterus, if fertilization does not occur, menstruation takes place and another follicle goes through maturation. Normally only one follicle matures each month.

The Process of Carcinogenesis

As with other cancers, the development of ovarian cancer appears to occur as a multistage process including initiation, promotion, and progression. Because of this multistep process, the development of ovarian cancer may involve various premalignant stages. Studies reviewing potential premalignant lesions are limited and have focused on dysplasia of the epithelial tissue and inclusion cysts (Gershenson et al., 1996b). Little is known about the carcinogenesis of germ cell and sex-cord stromal cell tumors. Dysgerminomas originate from primitive or undifferentiated germ cells of the embryonic gland that have lost their capacity to differentiate (Merino & Jaffe, 1993).

Undoubtedly, changes at the molecular level are involved in the development and progression of ovarian cancer. The specific genetic (i.e., molecular) changes that occur during the process of carcinogenesis are being identified with the use of sensitive molecular biology methods. As with other types of cancer, the molecular events that lead to the development of ovarian cancer occur in two types of cellular genes: oncogenes and tumor suppressor genes. Oncogenes are genes that normally function to enhance cell growth and development. The expression of these genes is tightly controlled, so that in normal adult tissues, a balance is maintained between cellular proliferation and cell death. Damage to a cellular oncogene can result in cellular proliferation and the development of ovarian cancer.

Tumor suppressor genes normally function to prevent the continuous growth of cells. A genetic mutation in a tumor suppressor gene could result in uncontrolled cellular proliferation. Several mutations in tumor suppressor genes may be involved in the progression of ovarian cancer from localized to metastatic disease.

ROUTES OF METASTASES

Nonepithelial cancers of the ovary spread by dissemination onto peritoneal surface, lymphatic dissemination, and by hematogenous spread that affects various organs. Germ-cell cancers usually spread unilaterally through the surface of the gland, penetrating the tissue surrounding the ovary and invading the adjoining fallopian tube. They tend to spread more commonly through the retroperitoneal or para-aortic nodes and hematogenously to the liver and lung. Sex-cord stromal cancers, such as granulosa tumors, tend to be slow growing and expand to fill the pelvis and abdomen (Segal, DePetrillo, & Thomas, 1995).

Lymphatic spread begins in the pelvic and para-aortic lymph nodes near the ovaries. It continues through the lymphatic channels of the diaphragm and retroperitoneal lymph nodes, upward to the supraclavicular lymph nodes.

Metastatic spread through the hematogenous route is uncommon. Distant metastases related to nonepithelial ovarian cancer may involve the bone, brain, liver, and lung.

ASSESSMENT

Clinical evaluation of the patient involves a detailed history, a thorough physical examination, and a variety of diagnostic tests (see Table 31-3). The signs and symptoms present in the patient often depend on the stage of the disease at the time of diagnosis.

History

The patient should be evaluated for all of the identified risk factors for nonepithelial ovarian cancer. In addition, a careful history of the gynecologic and nearby systems should be obtained. Abdominal pain, which may be accompanied by a palpable mass in approximately 85% of patients, is the most common symptom (Bonazzi, Peccatori, Colombo, Lucchin, Cantu, & Mangioni, 1994; De Palo, Zambetti, Pilotti, Rottoli, Spatti, Fontanelli, & Musumeci et al., 1992; Germa, Izquierdo, Segui, Climent, Ojeda, & Alonso et al., 1992; Pliskow, 1993; Williams, 1991). Ten percent of patients with germ-cell tumors will actually present with acute abdominal pain, caused by rupture, hemorrhage, or torsion of the ovarian tumor (Williams, 1994). Other less common presenting symptoms of germ-cell tumors are abdominal distention (35%), fever (10%) and vaginal bleeding (10%) (Williams, 1991).

When ovarian cancer causes obstruction of the bladder, the patient typically reports urinary frequency, urgency, bladder discomfort, and/or distention. When it causes obstruction of the bowel, the patient may complain of rectal pressure, discomfort, or constipation. It has been reported that 41% of patients with carcinoid tumors may have symptoms of pressure or pain with defecation, in the absence of bowel involvement (Davis, Hartmann, Keeney, & Shapiro, 1996). Granulosa cell tumors may cause precocious isosexual development in prepubertal females, menstrual irregularities in premenopausal patients, and postmenopausal bleeding in the older woman (Segal, DePetrillo, & Thomas, 1995).

Physical Examination

The bimanual pelvic examination (see Fig. 31-6) allows for palpation of the vagina, uterus, and ovaries. It is important that the patient empty the bowel and bladder before the examination and attempt to relax. The normal ovary is almond-shaped and approximately 4 × 2 cm in size. The presence of a normal-size ovary in a postmenopausal patient, or an adnexal mass measuring 2 cm or larger in a premenarchal girl, is cause for concern. The physical examination may reveal a mass in the ovarian area with relative immobility, irregularity, or a bilateral change. Nonepithelial ovarian tumors are usually unilateral and may be large at the time of diagnosis. In asymptomatic patients, pelvic examinations probably reveal only 1 early-stage ovarian cancer for every 10,000 examinations. Despite the lack of sensitivity, repeat pelvic examinations every 6 months might be indicated in premenopausal women with abnormal findings, as most ovarian enlargements in this population are benign. The finding of weight loss and/or increased abdominal girth in a patient with suspected ovarian cancer is usually an indication of advanced disease. As many as 20% of patients with malignant germ-cell tumors present with ascites.

Diagnostic Tests

Ultrasound. Ultrasound uses transducers to create high-resolution images of the uterus, fallopian tubes, and ovaries. The procedure has the ability to detect lesions smaller than 4 cm in diameter. Initially, transabdominal ultrasound was used to evaluate the abdomen and had the advantage of visualizing the retroperitoneal structures within the pelvis. The technique is valuable in the diagnosis of ovarian cancer because it can be used to identify ovarian enlargement, distinguish between cystic and solid masses, and assess for ascites (NIH Consensus Panel, 1995). Its main function with nonepithelial ovarian cancers may be to rule out benign cystic mature teratomas.

With a transvaginal ultrasound, a vaginal probe is used, which allows for greater resolution of the architectural detail of the ovaries. This procedure has replaced transabdominal ultrasound in some centers. Ultrasound is less specific in the premenopausal patient because the ovaries vary in size throughout the menstrual cycle. Because of this variability, the ultrasound should be performed a week after menses, and any ovary greater than 18 cm^3 should be evaluated further. In the postmenopausal woman, any ovary larger than 8 cm^3 should be evaluated. The observation of any complex or solid patterns should promote concern. A newer technique, transvaginal color Doppler ultrasonography, combines improved anatomic resolution afforded by high-frequency transvaginal transducers with pathophysiologic evaluation of blood flow within the uterus and ovaries (Fleischer, Cullinan, Peery, & Jones, 1996). Although ultrasound may be helpful in identifying ovarian enlargement, it has not been useful in the screening and staging of ovarian cancer. For an outline of a transvaginal ultrasound, see Table 32-2.

Computed Tomography. Computed tomography (CT) is a noninvasive scanning technique that uses a com-

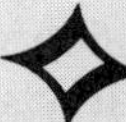

TABLE 32-2 Patient Preparation for Transvaginal Ultrasound

Description of the Procedure: Transvaginal ultrasound creates pictures of the structures and individual organs of the pelvic cavity from the echoes of high-frequency sound waves passing over the pelvic area. Unlike transabdominal ultrasound, a full bladder is not required for transvaginal ultrasound and therefore is better tolerated by the patient.

Patient Preparation: Patient should be instructed to fast from fluids for 4 hours before the procedure, and void just before the procedure.

Procedural Considerations:

1. Informed consent is not required.
2. Patient needs to disrobe below the waist or wear a gown.
3. Patient is assisted into a dorsal lithotomy position (i.e., lying on back with thighs flexed toward abdomen).
4. The probe is covered with an air-free, sterile, transparent condom, then lubricated and inserted slowly into the vagina.
5. After the probe is inserted, it is rotated to obtain multiple views of the pelvic organs.

Modified from Chernecky, C. C., Krech, R. L., & Berger, B. J. (1993). *Laboratory tests and diagnostic procedures.* Philadelphia: W. B. Saunders.

puter to produce three-dimensional images. It is highly accurate in distinguishing between benign and malignant lesions. CT is able to image lesions 2 cm or greater and therefore may be helpful in determining disease volume and response to treatment. Although CT is not as reliable as ultrasound, it can detect possible metastatic disease in the liver, retroperitoneum, and omentum. Table 32-3 contains patient preparation information for a CT of the pelvis.

Magnetic Resonance Imaging. Magnetic resonance imaging (MRI) uses a magnetic field and radiofrequency energy to create multiplane and cross-sectional imaging of the pelvis and surrounding tissues. It can depict abnormalities in the lymph nodes, peritoneum, pelvis, bone, and muscle. MRI is an expensive diagnostic tool that is not useful in screening, but may have a role in the evaluation of ovarian masses to determine the need for surgery (Outwater & Dunton, 1995). Patients should be forewarned about the confinement in the close quarters of the MRI equipment to alleviate anxiety.

Barium Enema and Chest Radiograph. A barium enema may be useful in the postmenopausal patient to rule out either a primary colon cancer or an ovarian cancer that has invaded the colon. A chest radiograph may be done to determine if there is evidence of metastatic disease in the lungs or mediastinum.

Alpha Fetoprotein. Alpha fetoprotein (AFP) is a globulin protein that is secreted by liver cells and is found in large amounts in fetal plasma. The normal AFP level in pregnant women varies from less than 75 to 450 ng/ml depending on the month of the pregnancy. In the nonpregnant female, the normal range of AFP is 0 to 10 ng/ml. AFP levels may be elevated in embryonal carcinomas, endodermal sinsus tumors, immature teratomas, mixed germ-cell tumors, and polyembryomas. In one study, AFP was positive in 100% of endodermal sinus tumors, 61.9% of immature teratomas, and 11.8% of dysgerminomas (Kawai, Kano, Furuhashi, Kano, Morikawa, & Oguchi et al., 1992). In one study, AFP was elevated above 1000 ng/ml in 93% of endodermal sinus tumors and mixed germ-cell tumors, regardless of stage (Kawai et al., 1990). AFP may be elevated in benign conditions such as ulcerative colitis, hepatitis, cirrhosis, and pregnancy, or in other malignancies such as pancreatic or gastric cancers with liver metastases (Chernecky, Krech, & Berger, 1993).

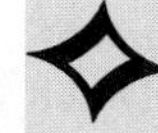

TABLE 32-3 Patient Preparation for Computed Tomography Scan of the Pelvis

Description of the Procedure: A computed tomography (CT) scan is an external examination that takes pictures of sections of the pelvis. The test you are scheduled for may involve the intravenous injection of an iodinated contrast agent. Although the contrast agent is very safe, some patients may experience a variety of side effects from this injection.

Patient Preparation: To reduce the side effects, you are asked to take the following medicines before your test: Atarax (hydroxyzine) 25 mg and Tagamet (cimetidine) 300 mg. *If you are allergic to Atarax (hydroxyzine) or Tagamet (cimetidine) or have asthma, multiple myeloma, sickle cell disease, or renal disease with elevated creatinine, pregnancy, or breastfeeding, please inform the pharmacist.*

Procedural Considerations: To ensure that you are properly prepared for the test, please carefully follow the instructions below:

1. Twelve (12) hours before your CT, take one (1) hydroxyzine (Atarax) and one (1) cimetidine (Tagamet).
2. At bedtime the night before your CT, drink one (1) full bottle (16 oz) of Prep-CAT.
3. Five (5) hours before your CT, do NOT eat or drink anything (except your Prep-CAT).
4. On the day of the exam drink eight (8) oz. of Prep-CAT at ________, and drink the remaining 8 oz. of Prep-CAT at ________.
5. Two (2) hours before your CT, take one (1) hydroxyzine one (1) cimetidine.

Human Chorionic Gondaotropin. Human chorionic gonadotropin (HCG) is a glycoprotein hormone that is normally produced by the developing placenta. The normal HCG level is less than 5.0 mU/ml. It is also produced by some germ-cell tumors such as choriocarcinoma, embryonal carcinoma, mixed germ-cell tumors, polyembryomas, and occasionally dysgerminomas. HCG may be elevated in benign conditions such as pregnancy, or in other malignancies including colon, hepatoma, lung, pancreas, and stomach cancers (Chernecky et al., 1993).

Serum Lactic Dehydrogenase. Lactic dehydrogenase (LDH) is an intracellular enzyme found in normal body tissues that is released in response to tissue damage. The normal LDH level in adults older than 60 years of age is 55 to 102 U/L; in younger adults the normal level is between 45 and 90 U/L. In one study, LDH was positive in 95% of dysgerminomas, and many values were greater than 1000 IU/L (Kawai et al., 1992).

LDH may be elevated in multiple benign conditions including alcoholism, anemia, burns, strokes, congestive heart failure, pneumonia, and ulcerative colitis, or in other malignancies such as liver cancer, leukemia, lymphoma, and renal cancers (Chernecky et al., 1993).

CA-125. CA-125 is an antigen produced by tissues derived from coelomic epithelium. CA-125 is not specific to ovarian cancer and can be elevated in benign conditions such as ovarian cysts, endometriosis, pelvic adhesions, pelvic inflammatory disease, and pregnancy, or in other malignancies such as breast, cervix, colon, endometrium, lung, and pancreas (Teneriello & Park, 1995). It may be positive in more than 50% of germ-cell tumors, except mature cystic teratomas, when it may be positive in approximately 24% of cases (Kawai et al., 1992). Although CA-125 may not be helpful in screening, a decline in its level after surgery and

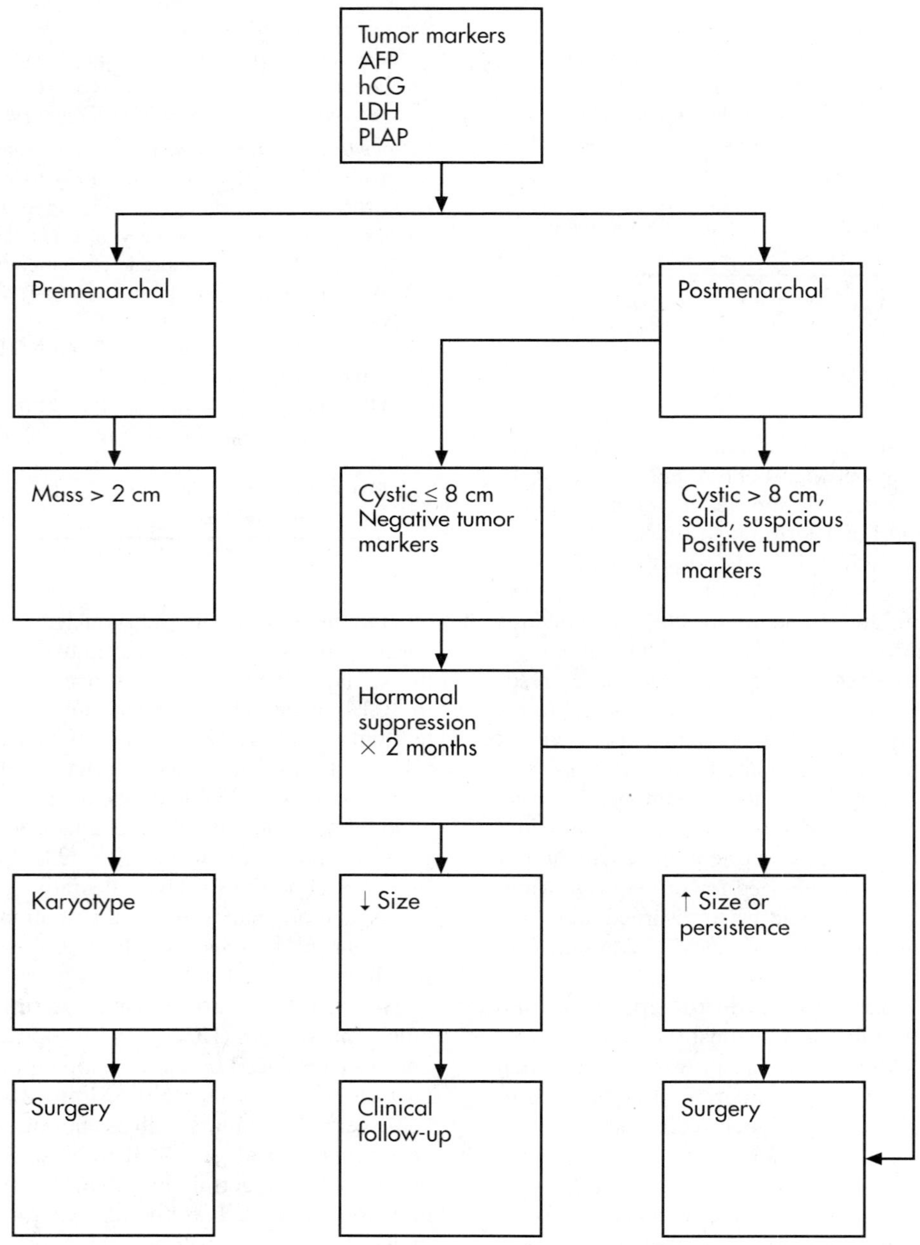

Fig. 32-1 Evaluation of pelvic mass in young female patients. (From Berek, J. S. & Hacker, N. F. (1994). *Practical gynecologic oncology.* Baltimore: Williams & Wilkins.)

during treatment may be correlated with tumor response (Rustin, Nelstrop, McClean, Brady, McGuire, & Hoskins et al., 1996).

Diagnosis. The diagnosis of ovarian cancer is suggested by an abnormal pelvic examination, elevated tumor markers, and abnormal findings on transvaginal ultrasound. However, all of these diagnostic tests have pitfalls. For example, only 80% of women with an abnormal pelvic examination are found to have cancer. Although tumor markers such as AFP and HCG may be helpful in identifying the presence of germ-cell tumors that are in an early stage, the incidence of germ-cell tumors does not warrant mass screening. These markers are most reliable for monitoring the effectiveness of treatment. No evidence suggests that available screening modalities (i.e., tumor markers and transvaginal ultrasonography) can be used effectively for widespread screening to reduce mortality from ovarian cancer, nor that their use will result in decreased rather than increased morbidity and mortality (NIH Consensus Panel, 1995). The diagnosis of an ovarian cancer requires an exploratory laparotomy. An algorithm depicting the evaluation of a pelvic mass in young female patients is displayed in Fig. 32-1.

STAGING

The staging of ovarian cancer involves the use of a histologic staging system (i.e., World Health Organization, [WHO]) and one of two clinical staging systems (i.e., the 1992 TNM classification system or the 1985 International Federation of Gynecology and Obstetrics [FIGO] staging system).

Histologic Staging

Histologic staging refers to the examination of the biopsy specimen by a pathologist after surgery. Surgical removal of an ovarian tumor is required for complete histologic staging. In addition, if any free fluid is present in the peritoneum, it should be sampled; otherwise peritoneal washings should be performed and sent for cytology. Finally, all intra-abdominal surfaces and viscera, the diaphragm, omentum, and pelvic and para-aortic lymph nodes should be examined and biopsied if suspect. The purpose of histologic staging is to determine the grade or biologic aggressiveness of the tumor.

The WHO system classifies nonepithelial ovarian tumors by histologic types according to the structure of the ovary from which the tumor is derived. This staging system is outlined in Box 32-1 for germ-cell tumors and Box 32-2 for sex-cord stromal tumors. Furthermore, a histopathologic grade is assigned to the tumor on a scale of 1 to 3. A higher score indicates more aggressive disease.

Clinical Staging

Two systems have been used for the clinical staging of ovarian cancer: the 1992 TNM classification system and the 1985 FIGO system. The TNM staging system was developed by the American Joint Committee on cancer (AJCC) and the International Union Against Cancer (UICC). The two systems are displayed in Table 31-5. Since 1993, TNM staging is mandatory in all hospitals that are evaluated by the American Joint Commission on Cancer. However, the FIGO system is more commonly referred to when describing gynecologic tumors. The clinical staging system defines the extent of the patient's disease. The staging of ovarian cancer is depicted in Fig. 31-7.

Box 32-1
Histologic Types of Germ-Cell Ovarian Cancers

Dysgerminomas
Endodermal sinus tumor
Embryonal carcinoma
Polyembryoma
Choriocarcinoma
Teratomas
1. Immature
2. Mature
    - Solid
    - Cystic: (1) *dermoid cyst* (mature cystic teratoma); (2) *dermoid cyst with malignant transformation*
3. Monodermal and highly specialized
    - Struma ovarii
    - Carcinoid
    - Struma ovarii and carcinoid
    - Others

Mixed forms

Box 32-2
Histologic Types of Sex-Cord Stromal Cell Ovarian Cancers

Granulosa-stromal cell tumor
1. Granulosa cell tumor
2. Tumors in the tecoma-fibroma group
    - Thecoma
    - Fibroma
    - Unclassified

Androblastomas; Sertoli-Leydig cell tumors
1. Well-differentiated
    - Tubular androblastoma; Sertoli cell tumor (tubular adenoma of Pick)
    - Tubular androblastoma with lipid storage; Sertoli cell tumor with lipid storage (folliculome lipidique of Lecene)
    - Sertoli-Leydig cell tumor (tubular adenoma with Leydig cells)
    - Leydig cell tumor; hilus cell tumor
2. Of intermediate differentiation
3. Poorly differentiated (sarcomatoid)
4. With heterologous elements

Gynandroblastoma
Unclassified

MEDICAL MANAGEMENT

The treatment of ovarian cancer depends on several factors including the patient's age, the patient's general state of health, tumor volume, histologic grade of the tumor, and the stage of the disease. In general, surgery with or without chemotherapy is used for localized disease. Radiation therapy may be used after surgery for patients with dysgerminoma. Surgery followed by chemotherapy is used for metastatic disease. An algorithm for the medical management of dysgerminoma of the ovary is displayed in Fig. 32-2.

Expectant Management

Seventy percent of simple cystic ovarian masses in premenopausal, asymptomatic women resolve without surgery (NIH Consensus Panel, 1995). Therefore, an option of watchful waiting may be appropriate in this population and should include repeated physical examinations and transvaginal ultrasound. Any changes during this time that suggest a malignancy should prompt a surgical intervention.

Expectant management has also been suggested for well-staged patients with stage IA dysgerminomas. Williams

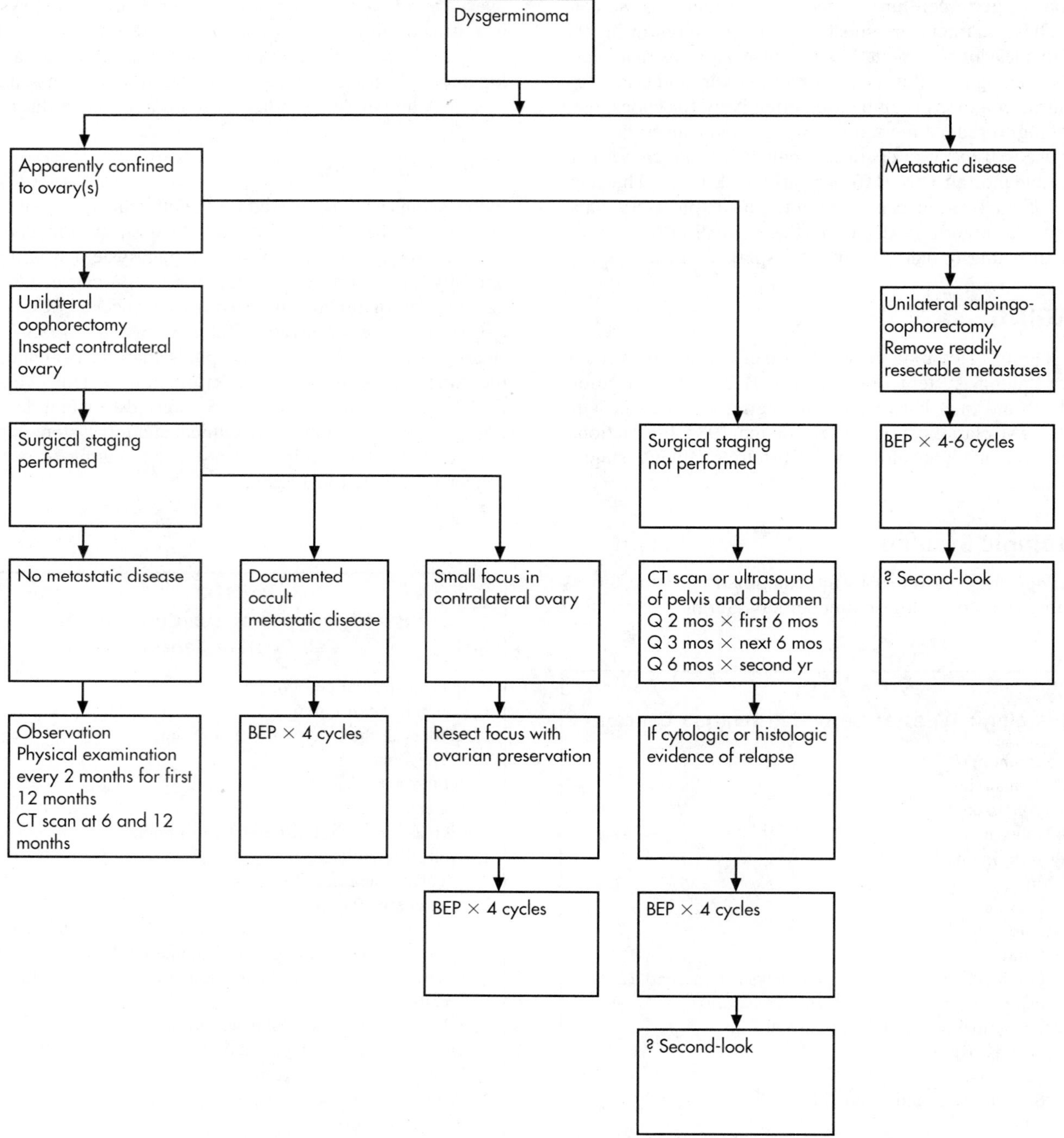

Fig. 32-2 Management of dysgerminoma of the ovary. (From Berek, J. S. & Hacker, N. F. (1994). *Practical gynecologic oncology.* Baltimore: Williams & Wilkins.)

(1994) advocated careful follow-up observation after unilateral salpingo-oophorectomy, regardless of the size of the tumor. These tumors are very sensitive to chemotherapy, which can be used in case of relapse.

Surgical Management

The most common surgical procedure for nonepithelial ovarian cancer is the initial staging laparotomy. The amount of surgery required depends on the extent of the disease. Surgery is used to establish a diagnosis, stage disease, and initiate treatment (Fishman & Schwartz, 1994). Cytoreductive surgery may be necessary for immature teratomas only. Second-look laparatomies may also be done, but their use is controversial in nonepithelial ovarian tumors.

Staging Laparotomy. Staging laparotomy is usually performed in patients who are in good health, less than 75 years of age, and without known metastatic disease outside the abdomen. Bilateral involvement is rare in most nonepithelial ovarian tumors and occurs in only 10% to 15% of pure dysgerminomas. A unilateral salpingo-oophorectomy (i.e., removal of the fallopian tube and ovary) can be performed for most cases, retaining the opposite ovary and the uterus for childbearing. Unless the contralateral ovary is grossly abnormal or enlarged, it should not be biospied. If the pathology on frozen section confirms dysgerminoma, a wedge biopsy of the other ovary should be performed (Piura, Dgani, Zalel, Nemet, Yanai-Inbar, & Cohen et al., 1995). The uterus can still be preserved for fertility if desired. Fertility-sparing surgery is warranted in all ovarian germ-cell tumors because it does not affect recurrence rates or survival (Peccatori, Bonazzi, Chiarai, Landoni, Colombo, & Mangioni, 1995). Preservation of fertility for young patients with germ-cell tumors of the ovary, regardless of stage, has been found to be safe in the absence of involvement of the contralateral ovary and uterus (Wu, Huang, Lang, Huang, Lian, & Tang, 1991).

For older women who have completed childbearing, surgical management may consist of a total abdominal hysterectomy (i.e., removal of the uterus), bilateral salpingo-oophorectomy, and biopsies of the diaphragm, peritoneum, lymph nodes, omentum (i.e., covering of peritoneum attached to the stomach), and peritoneal fluid.

Adequate surgical management of sex-cord stromal tumors of the ovary is similar to germ-cell tumors. When the findings of an exploratory laparotomy reveal a tumor confined to one ovary, a unilateral salpingo-oophorectomy may be performed. In the case of either a bilateral tumor or postmenopausal patient, a bilateral salpingo-oophorectomy, with or without hysterectomy, is indicated. Metastatic disease warrants aggressive cytoreductive surgery (Gershenson, 1994a). Fortunately, 95% of sex-cord stromal tumors are confined to only one of the ovaries (Gershenson, 1994b).

The staging of ovarian cancer directs the overall treatment plan and is dependent on the extent and location of disease found at the initial laparotomy. A vertical midline incision provides excellent access into the pelvis and upper abdomen, if needed. Both ovaries should be examined for the presence of tumor and removed intact. The uterus and fallopian tubes are also removed. Initial exploration must be thorough and starts with the collection of pelvic fluid for cytology. In the absence of pelvic fluid, peritoneal washings should be obtained. Exploration of all of the intra-abdominal surfaces and organs, including the small and large intestines, kidneys, liver, gallbladder, and diaphragm, is necessary to rule out common potential areas of metastases. The peritoneal surfaces and diaphragm should be biopsied randomly, in addition to any suspicious areas. Staging should be completed with resection of the omentum and biopsies of pelvic, iliac, and para-aortic lymph nodes. If metastatic disease is encountered during the initial surgery, the surgeon should attempt to resect as much tumor as possible (Gershenson, 1993). Accurate staging is essential, because it guides further treatment recommendations.

The major complications of staging laparotomy are bleeding, prolonged ileus, wound infections, urinary tract infections, pulmonary complications, and bowel injury. Most patients with nonepithelial ovarian cancer present with early-stage disease and require fewer surgical interventions. Blood loss is variable depending on the extent of the surgery. Immediate postoperative complications may include bleeding, pulmonary emboli, urinary retention, and pain.

Cytoreductive Surgery. Residual tumor may be left behind after primary surgery in patients who present with bulky disease. The use of chemotherapy as adjuvant treatment is well accepted. Secondary debulking or cytoreductive surgery may be beneficial for patients with immature teratoma or those whose tumors cannot be optimally debulked (Munkarah, Gershenson, Levenback, Silva, Messing, & Morris et al., 1994; Peccatori et al., 1995). Interval debulking may also be appropriate for symptom control and prolongation of survival in patients with granulosa cell tumors (Segal et al., 1995). The use of cytoreductive surgery is controversial, because it is not known whether patients who undergo salvage surgery followed by chemotherapy do better, or the same, as those treated with chemotherapy alone.

Second-Look Laparotomy. Second-look laparotomy is a surgical procedure that may be performed after treatment with staging laparotomy and chemotherapy to evaluate a patient's response to treatment. It is the most accurate method to rule out or confirm persistent disease that may not be evidenced by physical examination, imaging, or tumor markers. The technique is similar to the initial surgery and includes careful examination of the peritoneum, intra-abdominal surfaces, and organs, as well as performing biopsies in areas of previous tumor. The odds of finding persistent disease in patients with nonepithelial ovarian cancers without evidence of positive markers or imaging is low. The use of second-look surgery is controversial, because recurrent ovarian cancer after negative findings is common; therefore its effect on survival is questionable (Vaccarello, Rubin, Vlamis, Wong, Jones, & Lewis et al., 1995). Some studies have recommended second-look laparotomies for patients with a teratoma component in their primary tumor, persistent radiologic abnormalities, and normal tumor markers after chemotherapy (Culine, Lhomme, Michel, Leclere, Duvillard, & Droz, 1996; Marina, Rao, Etcubanans, Jenkins, Kun, & Thompson et al., 1991; Mayordomo, Paz-

Ares, Rivera, Lopez-Brea, Martin, & Mendiola et al., 1994; Williams, 1994). Others recommend it only for patients with advanced disease with initially negative markers (Gershenson, 1993; Gershenson, 1994b). Second-look laparotomy may uncover residual disease undetectable by tumor markers or clinical examination (Curtin, Morrow, D'Ablaing, & Schlaerth, 1994). However, many believe that second-look laparotomies are of limited value, preferring close follow-up and surveillance with serial imaging for patients with persistent masses after chemotherapy (Culine et al., 1996; Fishman & Schwartz, 1994; Segelov, Campbell, Ng, Tattersall, Rome, & Free et al., 1994).

The major complications of second-look laparotomy are prolonged ileus, wound infections, urinary tract infections, pulmonary complications, and bowel injury. Some studies have suggested the use of laparoscopy for second-look operations to minimize the amount of surgery and complications (Peccatori et al., 1995). Although laparoscopy is associated with fewer complications, it may provide inadequate visualization of residual tumor and therefore promote false-negative findings.

Radiation Therapy

Radiation therapy may be used to treat localized disease in patients after surgery. Radiation therapy treatments are administered through an external beam approach.

Dysgerminomas are very radiosensitive. For patients with localized disease (i.e., stages I and II), radiation therapy after cytoreductive surgery may improve survival. Radiation treatments are given 5 days a week at doses of 100 to 150 cGy for 4 to 5 weeks to the entire abdomen and pelvis (total dose 2500 to 3500 cGy). Doses are restricted by neighboring organs (e.g., bone marrow, bowel, kidneys, liver), and shields are used to protect the kidneys from the full dose of radiation. External beam radiation is not generally well tolerated by the patient, because the entire abdomen and pelvis are treated. Acute problems of anorexia, nausea and vomiting, diarrhea, vaginal discharge, bone marrow depression, dysuria, proctitis, and fatigue occur in most patients and may cause interruptions in therapy. Nausea and vomiting may occur within 1 to 2 hours after treatment. Although 67% of patients will experience nausea, vomiting is infrequent, and 75% of patients have mild diarrhea (Thomas & Dembo, 1993). Other side effects usually occur during the second or third week of treatment and resolve days to weeks after treatment is completed.

The occurrence of late complications of radiation therapy (i.e., complications that occur 6 or more months after the completion of treatment) are relatively common. Although small bowel obstruction is the most serious complication, it occurs infrequently. In one study (Mitchell, Gershenson, Soeters, Eifel, Delclos, & Wharton, 1991), 58% of patients continued to have multiple bowel movements each day, at least 3 years after receiving radiation therapy. Other possible late complications of external beam radiation include cystitis, hematuria, radiation enteritis, chronic and recurrent diarrhea, and adhesive peritonitis. Effective treatment with radiation therapy may be difficult because of the free mobility of tumor cells within the abdominal cavity and usually large tumor burden. In the younger patient, the loss of fertility after radiation therapy makes it a less attractive therapeutic option. Although radiation therapy has become less popular with the increased use of chemotherapeutic agents, it may be reserved for salvage therapy (Gershenson, 1994a). Radiation therapy may still play a palliative role in patients with brain or bone metastases. In addition, it has been shown to be effective for use in residual disease, localized pelvic recurrences, or for palliation with sex-cord stromal tumors (Segal et al., 1995).

Chemotherapy

Chemotherapy is used most commonly as adjuvant treatment after surgery to treat residual or metastatic disease. Germ cell ovarian cancers are highly sensitive to chemotherapy, even more so than epithelial tumors (Gershenson, 1993). Before the use of chemotherapy in germ-cell tumors, many of these tumors were fatal, with recurrences after surgery as high as 85% (Williams, 1994). Because germ-cell tumors grow rapidly, chemotherapy is often initiated within a week of surgery. Due to the aggressiveness of these tumors, granulocyte colony-stimulating factor (G-CSF) may be used to avoid any treatment delays (Motzer, Geller, & Bosl, 1990; Schwartz et al., 1992). An important consideration in the use of chemotherapy is that for most patients, normal menstrual function and fertility return after completion of therapy. A list of chemotherapy agents that have been utilized in nonepithelial ovarian cancer is summarized in Box 31-5.

Initial Chemotherapy. The first chemotherapy regimen found to be successful in treating germ-cell tumors was VAC (vincristine, dactinomycin, cyclophosphamide). Toxicities of this regimen include myelosuppression, myalgias, stomatitis, neurotoxicity, nausea, and vomiting (Schwartz et al., 1992). Unfortunately, less than 50% of patients with metastatic tumors have sustained remission rates after treatment with VAC (Gershenson, 1994a). Patients with nondysgerminomas, even with advanced and bulky disease, had high response rates to platinum-based chemotherapy regimens (Segelov et al., 1994). Therefore, subsequent regimens included cisplatin in their combination.

The use of PVB (cisplatin, vinblastine, bleomycin) resulted in response rates as high as 91.6% (Mayordomo et al., 1994). Side effects of this regimen may include leukopenia, peripheral neurotoxicity, nausea and vomiting, alopecia, and changes in skin pigmentation. Cure rates with PVB are 95% or better for patients with stage I or II disease, almost 80% for stage III, 60% for stage IV, and 40% for patients treated with recurrence (Gershenson, 1994b). Unfortunately, treatment fails for as many as 42% of patients with measurable disease (De Palo et al., 1992).

Etoposide has been substituted for vinblastine, reducing both bone marrow suppression and neuropathy (Schwartz et al., 1992). BEP (bleomycin, etoposide and cisplatin) has achieved sustained remission rates of more than 75% in patients with metastatic germ-cell tumors (Gershenson, 1994a). For patients with pure dysgerminomas, three cycles seem to be adequate therapy for patients with stage I disease, whereas a minimum of four cycles may be indicated for advanced or recurrent tumors. Patients with stage I nondysgerminomas generally receive four cycles, whereas four to six cycles are used for advanced or recurrent disease. A 100% response rates has been reported with this regimen (Mayordomo et al., 1994). Three cycles of BEP have produced 96% disease-free survival in patients with stage I, II, or III (Gershenson, 1994b). Toxicities includes leukopenia, alopecia, nausea and vomiting, mucositis, nephrotoxicity, and pulmonary toxicity (Gershenson et al., 1990). Carboplatin may be substituted for cisplatin in patients who experience severe nausea and vomiting, without affecting response rates (Cheung, Lau, Chan, Teng, Chan, & Ngan et al., 1994).

POMB/ACE (cisplatin, vincristine, methotrexate, bleomycin, actinomycin D, cyclophosphamide, and etoposide) has been used for patients newly diagnosed with metastatic ovarian germ-cell tumor with a 93% response rate (Bower, Fife, Holden, Paradinas, Rustin, & Newlands, 1996). Side effects of this regimen include leukopenia, alopecia, nausea, mucositis, peripheral neuropathy, nephrotoxicity, and pulmonary toxicity. If fertility-conserving surgery is done before chemotherapy, these patients are able to have children after completing treatment. The addition of cyclophosphamide, etoposide, doxorubicin, and vinblastine to create POMB/ACE/PAC has resulted in similar response rates of 95% in germ-cell tumors (Germa et al., 1992).

Other regimens for germ-cell tumors have had varying response rates and include PVeBV (high-dose cisplatin, vinblastine, bleomycin, and etoposide), AVAB (actinomycin D, cyclophosphamide, vincristine, doxorubicin, bleomycin), and VAB-6 (actinomycin D, cyclophosphamide, vinblastine, bleomycin, cisplatin). PVeBV has been used for malignant nondysgerminomas and may include toxicities such as leukopenia, thrombocytopenia, nausea and vomiting, alopecia, diarrhea, mucositis, and paresthesias (Culine, Kattan, Lhomme, Duvillard, Michel, & Castaigne et al., 1994a). VAB-6 has replaced AVAB, because of its greater response rates (86% vs 62.5%) and its milder profile of toxicities (Culine et al., 1994b).

Data regarding the use of chemotherapy for sex-cord stromal tumors are limited. Chemotherapy may be appropriate for sex-cord stromal patients with metastatic disease, and responses have been seen with PAC (cisplatin, doxorubicin, and cyclophosphamide), BEP (bleomycin, etoposide, and cisplatin), and paclitaxel (Gershenson, 1994a). Although BEP had response rates of 83% for patients with measurable disease, only 14% of patients had a durable response (Gershenson, Morris, Burke, Levenback, Matthews, & Wharton, 1996). Platinum-based chemotherapy, including PA (cisplatin and doxorubicin), BV-CAP (bleomycin, vinblastine, cyclophosphamide, doxorubicin, and cisplatin), PAC (cisplatin, doxorubicin, and cyclophosphamide), PVB (cisplatin, vinblastine, and bleomycin), and BEP, appears to be the most popular postoperative treatment for patients with sex-cord stromal tumors (Gershenson, 1994b), with response rates reported as high as 93% (Segal et al., 1995).

Salvage Chemotherapy. Chemotherapy options are limited in patients with recurrent ovarian carcinoma who have been previously treated with platinum. Patients who experience relapse more than 6 months after completing first-line treatment are considered to have clinically platinum-sensitive disease. Those who experience relapse within 6 months of platinum-based therapy are considered to have platinum-resistant disease.

EMA-CO (etoposide, methotrexate, dactinomycin, cyclophosphamide, vincristine) or vincristine, dactinomycin, and ifosfamide have been used for salvage therapy. For those with platinum-sensitive tumors, the most popular regimen includes ifosfamide, cisplatin, and either vinblastine or vincristine; for platinum-resistant treatment, options include either high-dose chemotherapy or phase II drugs. However, results have been variable (Gershenson, 1994a).

Hormonal Therapy

Hormonal therapy may be used to manage metastatic granulosa cell tumors that have not responded to chemotherapy. The ovaries produce estrogen and progesterone, so it is not surprising that ovarian cancers may be estrogen-receptor and/or progesterone-receptor positive, similar to breast cancer. Antiestrogen therapy is useful for palliation of refractory ovarian cancer. Progesterone treatment, tamoxifen, and leuprolide have been used with varying degrees of success (Gershenson, 1994a). Side effects of hormonal therapy may include hot flashes, vaginal dryness, emotional lability, and weight gain.

ONCOLOGIC EMERGENCIES

A major oncologic emergency associated with ovarian cancer and its treatment is disseminated intravascular coagulation (DIC). DIC may occur from chemotherapy, anaphylaxis, infection, massive tissue injury, or from the ovarian cancer itself. Symptoms of DIC may include bleeding from various sites, hypotension, abdominal pain, and confusion. When DIC occurs, one should notify the physician immediately, treat the underlying cause, maintain intravenous access (for heparin, blood products, and hydration), and administer oxygen as needed.

NURSING MANAGEMENT

The medical management of ovarian cancer is extremely complex and variable depending on the patient's age, clinical condition, and stage of disease at the time of diagnosis. Patients with ovarian cancer have numerous problems that require nursing interventions and patient education. Although a portion of the patient's care will occur in the inpatient setting, the majority of the patient's care will occur in the outpatient and home care settings.

Early in the course of the patient's disease, the focus of nursing care may be on helping the patient understand the different treatment options. As the disease progresses, patients need information about the rationale for different types of pharmacologic interventions, as well as strategies for managing the side effects associated with the disease or treatment. Because each major type of treatment for ovarian cancer (i.e., surgery, radiation therapy, and chemotherapy) poses unique patient problems, the major issues associated with these treatments are discussed, and three standards of care are provided.

Surgery

Patients undergoing a staging laparotomy are usually hospitalized for 5 days. Patients who present with extensive disease require more comprehensive surgery and possibly a longer stay. The major focus of inpatient nursing care is on the prevention of postoperative complications including bleeding, thrombophlebitis, infection, and pulmonary emboli. Follow-up care in the outpatient setting may require that nurses evaluate patients for infection, wound care management, adequate nutritional intake, and ambulation. The nursing management of the patient undergoing surgery for ovarian cancer is summarized in Table 31-7.

Radiation Therapy

External beam therapy is provided on an outpatient basis. The major problems associated with external beam radiation therapy include myelosuppression, nausea and vomiting, diarrhea, and skin reactions. The nursing management of the patient with ovarian cancer who is receiving external beam radiation therapy is summarized in Table 31-8.

Chemotherapy

Most patients receive chemotherapy in the outpatient setting. Patients must be taught the rationale for premedications, chemotherapy combinations, and any postchemotherapy directions. Additionally, patients and their families must be taught about potential side effects associated with different chemotherapy agents and their management. The nursing management of the patient with ovarian cancer who is receiving chemotherapy is summarized in Table 31-9.

HOME CARE ISSUES

Depending on the treatment approaches used to manage ovarian cancer, the patient and family caregivers will be faced with several issues in the home care setting. Symptoms associated with ovarian cancer and its treatment include fatigue, pain, numbness or tingling in hands or feet, nausea and vomiting, bloating, constipation, anorexia, diarrhea, edema, shortness of breath, and problems with urination (Portenoy, Kornblith, Wong, Vlamis, Lepore, & Loseth et al., 1994). Patients who had extensive disease at the time of presentation may have wound care to perform at home. Many patients may have central lines placed for chemotherapy, antibiotics, and/or total parenteral nutrition, which may require them to learn how to do flushes, dressing changes, and possibly infuse medication. Patients receiving chemotherapy may need to learn to manage delayed nausea and vomiting or give self-injections. Pain management, both postoperatively and for those with advanced disease, may be an issue for many patients and their family members.

Bowel Obstruction

Another problem patients may encounter while at home is bowel obstruction. *Malignant bowel obstruction* is defined as the cessation of normal progression of intraluminal contents (Labovich, 1994). Patients with ovarian cancer may experience a bowel obstruction from tumor involvement at the time of diagnosis, after surgical interventions, as a delayed complication of radiation therapy or chemotherapy, or associated with advancing disease.

Patients with bowel obstruction may experience abdominal pain, nausea and vomiting, abdominal distention, diarrhea, or constipation. Treatment may include use of nasogastric tube, intravenous hydration, and possibly surgery. If surgery is not possible, patients and their caregivers may be required to learn how to care for a nasogastric tube with suction and how to administer intravenous hydration at home.

Ascites

Another problem patients may need to manage while at home is ascites. *Malignant ascites* is defined as the accumulation of fluid within the peritoneal cavity and is indicative of advanced disease (Labovich, 1994). Ascites may be present at the time of diagnosis, or it may occur after treatment failure.

Patients may have several symptoms including lack of appetite, feeling full, gastric reflux, inability to wear clothes, and difficulty with breathing. Treatment may include removal of the fluid by paracentesis and the use of diuretics. Patients should be given instructions on fluid and sodium restriction, diuretic use, positioning to aid breathing, measurement of abdominal girth, and parameters on when to notify the physician of increasing symptoms.

PROGNOSIS

Prognosis varies depending on the stage of the disease at the time of diagnosis, the patient's age, and coexistent medical problems. Other factors that influence a patient's prognosis are the grade of the tumor, lymph node involvement, and presence or absence of ascites. The most powerful predictor for prognosis of patients with germ-cell tumors is histologic type. Survival rates are highest for dysgerminomas (78.5%), followed by immature teratomas (53.6%), mixed germ-cell tumors (33.3%), and endodermal sinus tumors (12%) (Ayhan, Tuncer, Yanik, Bukulmez, Yank, & Kucukali, 1995). Low-grade germ-cell tumors, such as immature teratomas, may be cured with fertility-sparing surgery alone (Bonazzi et al., 1994). In addition, responsiveness of the tumor to chemotherapy and duration of that response affect survival. Patients with endodermal sinus or mixed germ-cell tumors, stage I disease, and the absence of residual tumor and/or ascites have a significantly more favorable prognosis than pa-

TABLE 32-4 Quality of Care Evaluation for a Patient Undergoing Surgery for Ovarian Cancer

Disciplines participating in the quality of care evaluation:
☐ Nursing ☐ Surgery
☐ Physical Therapy ☐ Social Services

Data from:
☐ Medical Record Review ☐ Patient Interview

Criteria	Yes	No
1. Patient provided with preoperative information about:		
a. Diagnostic tests	☐	☐
b. Bowel preparation	☐	☐
c. Use of antiembolic stockings	☐	☐
d. Pain management	☐	☐
2. Hemoglobin and hematocrit evaluated postoperatively	☐	☐
3. Patient experienced the following complications:		
a. Infection	☐	☐

Patient/Family Satisfaction

Data from:
☐ Patient Interview ☐ Family Interview

Criteria	Yes	No
1. On a scale of 0 to 10, with 0 being totally dissatisfied and 10 being totally satisfied, how satisfied were you with the pain management you received?________		
2. Were you told to call the physician if you had a temperature greater than 100.4° F (38° C)?	☐	☐
3. Were you taught to avoid tampons, douches, intercourse, and strenuous exercise for 4 to 6 weeks after surgery?	☐	☐
4. Were you given a follow-up appointment before you left the hospital?	☐	☐

tients who present with stage II and IV disease and who have residual tumor and/or ascites (Kawai, Furuhashi, Kano, Nakashima, Hattori, & Okamoto et al., 1991). In general, when ovarian cancer is diagnosed at an early stage, the disease may be curable. Five-year survival rates are 91% for local disease, 49% for regional disease, and 23% when distant metastases are present at the time of diagnosis (American Cancer Society, 1996).

EVALUATION OF THE QUALITY OF CARE

Accreditation organizations, such as the Joint Commission for the Accreditation of Health Care Organizations, require evaluation of the quality of care provided to patients. Because the care provided to patients with ovarian cancer requires input from a multidisciplinary team, an evaluation of the quality of care provided to these patients should include aspects of care provided by various members of the team. See Tables 32-4 and 32-5 for evaluation tools that can be used in the inpatient and outpatient settings, respectively.

TABLE 32-5 Quality of Care Evaluation for a Patient Receiving Chemotherapy

Disciplines participating in the quality of care evaluation:
☐ Nursing ☐ Surgery
☐ Physical Therapy ☐ Social Services

Data from:
☐ Medical Record Review ☐ Patient Interview

Criteria	Yes	No
1. Did the doctor or nurse explain to you that you might experience some of the following side effects from your chemotherapy?		
a. Nausea and vomiting	☐	☐
b. Diarrhea	☐	☐
c. Low white blood cell count (bone marrow suppression)	☐	☐
d. Peripheral neuropathy	☐	☐
2. Were you given antinausea medications and instructions on their use?	☐	☐
3. Were you taught to call the doctor for temperature greater than 100.4° F (38° C)?	☐	☐

RESEARCH ISSUES

Numerous research issues surrounding the diagnosis and management of ovarian cancer require further investigations. The genetic basis for the disease and the risk factors associated with the development of ovarian cancer remain to be identified. An optimal approach to early detection still needs to be identified. At this time, guidelines or recommendations for early detection for ovarian cancer do not exist.

Numerous randomized, clinical trials are needed to determine the most effective treatments for the various stages of ovarian cancer. New chemotherapy drugs and combinations need to be studied and compared with current practice for response rates, optimal number of cycles, toxicities, and long-term survival. All of these research studies need to consider not only the effectiveness of the treatment in improving patient's survival, but the costs of treatment, the morbidities associated with the treatments, and the impact of the treatments on the patient's quality of life.

REFERENCES

Adami, H. O., Hsieh, C. C., Lambe, M., Trichopoulos, D., Leon, D., Persson, I., Ekbom, A., & Janson, P. O. (1994). Parity, age at first childbirth, and risk of ovarian cancer. *Lancet, 344,* 1250-1254.

American Cancer Society. (1996). *Cancer facts and figures-1996.* Atlanta: American Cancer Society.

Averette, H. E., Janicek, M. F., & Menck, H. R. (1995). The National Cancer Data Base report on ovarian cancer. *Cancer, 76*(6), 1096-1103.

Ayhan, A., Tuncer, Z. S., Yanik, F., Bukulmez, O., Yank, A., & Kucukali, T. (1995). Malignant germ-cell tumors of the ovary: Hacettepe hospital experience. *Acta Obstetricia et Gynecologica Scandinavica, 74,* 384-390.

Berek, J. S. & Hacker, N. F. (1994). *Practical gynecologic oncology.* Baltimore: Williams & Wilkins.

Bonazzi, C., Peccatori, F., Colombo, N., Lucchini, V., Cantu, M. G., & Mangioni, C. (1994). Pure ovarian immature teratoma, a unique and curable disease: 10 years experience of 32 prospectively treated patients. *Obstetrics and Gynecology, 84,* 598-604.

Bower, M., Fife, K., Holden, L., Paradinas, F. J., Rustin, G. J. S., & Newlands, E. S. (1996). Chemotherapy for ovarian germ-cell tumors. *European Journal of Cancer, 32A*(4), 593-597.

Chernecky, C. C., Krech, R. L., & Berger, B. J. (1993). *Laboratory tests and diagnostic procedures.* Philadelphia: W. B. Saunders.

Cheung, M. M., Lau, W. H., Chan, M., Teng, S. K., Chan, J. K. C., Ngan, R. K. C., Sin, V. C., & Tung, S. Y. (1994). Experience with the management of ovarian germ-cell tumors in Chinese patients. *Gynecologic Oncology, 52,* 306-312.

Culine, S., Kattan, J., Lhomme, C., Duvillard, P., Michel, G., Castaigne, D., Lechlere, J., Pico, J., & Droz, J. P. (1994a). A phase II study of high-dose cisplatin, vinblastine, bleomycin, and etoposide (PVeBV regimen) in malignant nondysgerminomatous germ-cell tumors of the ovary. *Gynecologic Oncology, 54,* 47-53.

Culine, S., Lhomme, C., Kattan, J., Duvillard, P., Michel, G., & Droz, J. P. (1994b). Long-term results of two VAB-like regimens (vinblastine + actinomycin-D + bleomycin + cyclophosphamide + cisplatin) in malignant germ-cell tumours of the ovary. *European Journal of Cancer, 30A*(9), 1239-1244.

Culine, S., Lhomme, C., Michel, G., Leclere, J., Duvillard, P., & Droz, J. P. (1996). Is there a role for second-look laparatomy in the management of malignant germ-cell tumors of the ovary? Experience at Institut Gustave Roussy. *Journal of Surgical Oncology, 62,* 40-45.

Curtin, P., Morrow, C. P., D'Ablaing, G., & Schlaerth, J. B. (1994). Malignant germ-cell tumors of the ovary: 20-year report of LAC-USC Women's Hospital. *International Journal of Gynecologic Cancer, 4,* 29-35.

Davis, K., Hartmann, L. K., Keeney, G. L., & Shapiro, H. (1996). Primary ovarian carcinoid tumors. *Gynecologic Oncology, 61,* 259-265.

De Palo, G., Zambetti, M., Pilotti, S., Rottoli, L., Spatti, G., Fontanelli, R., Musumeci, R., Kenda, R., Bombardieri, E., Stefanon, B., Escobedo, A., Del Vecchio, M., Di Donato, P., & Di Re, F. (1992). Nondysgerminomatous tumors of the ovary treated with cisplatin, vinblastine, and bleomycin: long-term results. *Gynecologic Oncology, 47,* 239-246.

Fishman, D. A. & Schwartz, P. E. (1994). Current approaches to diagnosis and treatment of ovarian germ cell malignancies. *Current Opinion in Obstetrics and Gynecology, 6,* 98-104.

Fleischer, A. C., Cullinan, J. A., Peery, C. V., & Jones, H. W. (1996). Early detection of ovarian carcinoma with transvaginal color Doppler ultrasonography. *American Journal of Obstetrics and Gynecology, 174*(1 part 1), 101-6.

Germa, J. R., Izquierdo, M. A., Segui, M. A., Climent, M. A., Ojeda, B., & Alonso, C. (1992). Malignant ovarian germ-cell tumors: The experience at the Hospital de la Santa Creu I Sant Pau. *Gynecologic Oncology, 45,* 153-159.

Gershenson, D. M. (1993). Update on malignant ovarian germ-cell tumors. *Cancer, 71,* 1581-1590.

Gershenson, D. M. (1994a). Chemotherapy of ovarian germ-cell tumors and sex cord stromal tumors. *Seminars in Surgical Oncology, 10,* 290-298.

Gershenson, D. M. (1994b). Management of early ovarian cancer: Germ-cell and sex cord-stromal tumors. *Gynecologic Oncology, 55,* S62-S72.

Gershenson, D. M., Morris, M., Burke, T. W., Levenback, C., Matthews, C. M., & Wharton, J. T. (1996). Treatment of poor-prognosis sex cord-stromal tumors of the ovary with the combination of bleomycin, etoposide, and cisplatin. *Obstetrics and Gynecology, 87,* 527-531.

Gershenson, D. M., Morris, M., Cangir, A., Kavanagh, J. J., Stringer, C. A., Edwards, C. L., Silva, E. G., & Wharton, J. T. (1990). Treatment of malignant germ-cell tumors of the ovary with the bleomycin, etoposide, and cisplatin. *Journal of Clinical Oncology, 8*(4), 715-720.

Gershenson, D. M., Tortolero-Luna, G., Malpica, A., Baker, V. V., Whittaker, L., Johnson, E., & Mitchell, M. F. (1996). Ovarian intraepithelial neoplasia and ovarian cancer. *Obstetrics and Gynecology Clinics of North America, 23*(2), 475-543.

Grimes, D. A. (1993). Primary prevention of ovarian cancer. *Journal of the American Medical Association, 270*(23), 2855-2865.

Grimes, D. A. & Economy, K. E. (1995). Primary prevention of ovarian cancer. *American Journal of Obstetrics and Gynecology, 172*(1 part 1), 227-235.

Harlow, B. L., Cramer, D. W., Bell, D. A., & Welch, W. R. (1992). Perineal exposure to talc and ovarian cancer risk. *Obstetrics and Gynecology, 80*(1), 19-26.

Henderson, B. E., Ross, R. K., & Pike, M. C. (1993). Hormonal chemoprevention of cancer in women. *Science, 259,* 633-638.

Horn-Ross, P. L., Whittemore, A. S., Harris, R., & Itnyre, J. (1992). Characteristics relating to ovarian cancer risk: Collaborative analysis of 12 U. S. case-control studies: VI. Nonepithelial cancers among adults. Collaborative Ovarian Cancer Group. *Epidemiology, 3*(6), 490-495.

Kawai, M., Furuhashi, Y., Kano, T., Misawa, T., Nakashima, N., Hattori, S., Okamoto, Y., Kobayashi, I., Ohta, M., Arii, Y., & Tomoda, Y. (1990). Alpha-fetoprotein in malignant germ-cell tumors of the ovary. *Gynecologic Oncology, 39,* 160-166.

Kawai, M., Kano, T., Furuhashi, Y., Mizuno, K., Nakashima, N., Hattori, S., Kazeto, S., Iida, S., Ohta, M., Arii, Y., & Tomoda, Y. (1991). Prognostic factors in yolk sac tumors of the ovary. *Cancer, 67,* 184-192.

Kawai, M., Kano, T., Furuhashi, Y., Kano, T., Morikawa, Y., Oguchi, H., Nakashima, N., Ishizuka, T., Kuzuya, K., Ohta, M., Arii, Y., & Tomoda, Y. (1992). Seven tumor markers in benign and malignant germ-cell tumors of the ovary. *Gynecologic Oncology, 45,* 248-253.

Labovich, T. M. (1994). Selected complications in the patient with cancer: Spinal cord compression, malignant bowel obstruction, malignant ascites, and gastrointestinal bleeding. *Seminars in Oncology Nursing, 10*(3), 189-197.

Lack, E. E., Young, R. H., & Scully, R. E. (1992). Pathology of ovarian neoplasms in childhood and adolescence. *Pathology Annual, 27*(2), 281-356.

Landis, S. H., Murray, T., Bolten, S., & Wingo, P. A. (1998). Cancer statistics: 1998. *CA: A Cancer Journal for Clinicians, 48,* 6-29.

Marina, N. M., Rao, B., Etcubanans, E., Jenkins, J. J., Kun, L., & Thompson, E. I. (1991). The role of second-look surgery in the management of advanced germ cell malignancies. *Cancer, 68,* 309-315.

Mayordomo, J. I., Paz-Ares, L., Rivera, F., Lopez-Brea, M., Martin, E. L., Mendiola, C., Diaz-Puente, M. T., Lianes, P., Garcia-Prats, M. D., & Cortes-Funes, H. (1994). Ovarian and extragonadal malignant germ-cell tumors in females: A single-institution experience with 43 patients. *Annals of Oncology, 4,* 225-231.

Merino, M. J. & Jaffe, G. (1993). Age contrast in ovarian pathology. *Cancer, 71,* 537-544.

Mettlin, C. & Piver, M. S. (1990). A case-control study of milk drinking and ovarian cancer risk. *American Journal of Epidemiology, 132,* 871-876.

Mitchell, M. F., Gershenson, D. M., Soeters, R. P., Eifel, P. J., Delclos, L., & Wharton, J. T. (1991). The long-term effects of radiation therapy on patients with ovarian dysgerminoma. *Cancer, 67,* 1084-1090.

Motzer, R. J., Geller, N. L., & Bosl, G. J. (1990). The effect of a 7 day delay in chemotherapy cycles on complete response and event-free survival in good risk disseminated germ-cell tumor patients. *Cancer, 66,* 857-861.

Munkarah, A., Gershenson, D. M., Levenback, C., Silva, E. G., Messing, M. J., Morris, M., & Burke, T. W. (1994). Salvage surgery for chemorefractory ovarian germ-cell tumors. *Gynecologic Oncology, 55,* 217-223.

NIH Consensus Panel. (1995). Ovarian cancer: screening, treatment, and follow-up. *Journal of the American Medical Association, 273*(6), 491-497.

Outwater, E. & Dunton, C. J. (1995). Imaging of the ovary and adnexa: Clinical issues and applications of MR imaging. *Radiology, 194*(1), 1-18.

Peccatori, F., Bonazzi, C., Chiarai, S., Landoni, F., Colombo, N., & Mangioni, C. (1995). Surgical management of malignant ovarian germ-cell tumors: 10 years' experience of 129 patients. *Obstetrics and Gynecology, 86,* 367-372.

Piura, B., Dgani, R., Zalel, Y., Nemet, D., Yanai-Inbar, I., Cohen, Y., & Gleerman, M. (1995). Malignant germ-cell tumors of the ovary: A study of 20 cases. *Journal of Surgical Oncology, 59,* 155-161.

Pliskow, S. (1993). Endodermal sinus tumor of the ovary: Review of 10 cases. *Southern Medical Journal, 86*(2), 187-189.

Portenoy, R. K., Kornblith, A. B., Wong, G., Vlamis, V., Lepore, J. M., Loseth, D. B., Hakes, T., Foley, K. M., & Hoskins, W. J. (1994). Pain in ovarian cancer patients. *Cancer, 74,* 907-915.

Rodriguez, C., Calle, E. E., Coates, R. J., Miracle-McMahill, H. L., Thun, M. J., & Heath, C. W., Jr. (1995). Estrogen replacement therapy and fatal ovarian cancer. *American Journal of Epidemiology, 141*(9), 828-835.

Rustin, G. J., Nelstrop, A. E., McClean, P., Brady, M. F., McGuire, W. P., Hoskins, W. J., Mitchell, H., & Lambert H. E. (1996). Defining response of ovarian carcinoma to initial chemotherapy according to serum CA 125. *Journal of Clinical Oncology, 14*(5), 1545-1551.

Schiff, M., Becker, T. M., Smith, H. O., Gilliland, F. D., & Key, C. R. (1996). Ovarian cancer incidence and mortality in American Indian, Hispanic and non-Hispanic white women in New Mexico. *Cancer Epidemiology, Biomarkers and Prevention, 5,* 323-327.

Schwartz, P. E., Chambers, S. K., Chambers, J. T., Kohorn, E., & McInosh, S. (1992). Ovarian germ cell malignancies: The Yale University experience. *Gynecologic Oncology, 45,* 26-31.

Segal, R., DePetrillo, A. D., & Thomas, G. (1995). Clinical review of adult granulosa cell tumors of the ovary. *Gynecologic Oncology, 56,* 338-344.

Segelov, E., Campbell, J., Ng, M., Tattersall, M., Rome, R., Free, K., Hacker, N., & Friedlander, M. L. (1994). Cisplatin-based chemotherapy for ovarian germ cell malignancies: the Australian experience. *Journal of Clinical Oncology, 12,* 278-384.

Teneriello, M. G. & Park, R. C. (1995). Early detection of ovarian cancer. *CA: A Cancer Journal for Clinicians, 45*(2), 71-87.

Thomas, C. W. (1993). *Taber's cyclopedic medical dictionary.* Philadelphia: F. A. Davis Company.

Thomas, G. M. & Dembo, A. J. (1993). Integrating radiation therapy into the management of ovarian cancer. *Cancer, 71,* 1710-1718.

Vaccarello, L., Rubin, S. C., Vlamis, V., Wong, G., Jones, W. B., Lewis, J. L., & Hoskins, W. J. (1995). Cytoreductive surgery in ovarian carcinoma patients with a documented previously complete surgical response. *Gynecologic Oncology, 57*(1), 61-65.

Williams, S. D. (1991). Chemotherapy of ovarian germ-cell tumors. *Hematology/Oncology Clinics of North America, 5*(6), 1261-1269.

Williams, S. (1994). Current management of ovarian germ-cell tumors. *Oncology, 8,* 53-67.

Wu, P. C., Huang, R. L., Lang, J. H., Huang, H. F., Lian, L. J., & Tang M. Y. (1991). Treatment of malignant ovarian germ-cell tumors with preservation of fertility: A report of 28 cases. *Gynecologic Oncology, 40,* 2-6.

Wynder, E. L., Fujita, Y., Harris, R. E., Hirayama, T., & Hiyama, T. (1991). Comparative epidemiology of cancer between the United States and Japan. A second look. *Cancer, 67,* 746-763.

Uterine Sarcoma

Frances Crighton, RN, PhD(c), OCN
Peggy J. Eldredge, RN, MS, AOCN
Amy Strauss Tranin, RN, MS, OCN

EPIDEMIOLOGY

Uterine sarcoma is a rare tumor accounting for approximately 1% to 3% of all gynecologic malignancies (DiSaia & Creasman, 1993). The overall annual incidence of uterine sarcoma is stable and only slightly higher than 1 in 100,000 women (Harlow, Weiss, & Lofton, 1986; Olah, Gee, Blunt, Dunn, Kelly, & Chan, 1991). Uterine sarcoma can generally be differentiated into three major histologic groups: leiomyosarcomas (LMS), mixed mesodermal tumors (MMT), and endometrial stromal sarcomas (ESS), with LMS and MMT accounting for approximately 85% of uterine sarcomas (Moskovic, MacSweeney, Law, & Price, 1993). The incidence of different histologies appear to be age-related, with the highest incidence of LMS occurring in women between 45 and 55 years of age, whereas MMT has a higher incidence between 65 and 75 years (Harlow, Weiss, & Lofton, 1986). Because of the rarity of these tumors, epidemiologic and treatment studies that have been reported include small samples or case reports. Although studies regarding risk factors are lacking, the literature presents evidence for potential risk factors.

RISK FACTORS

Epidemiologic studies that determined uterine cancer risks include results from the Surveillance, Epidemiology, and End Results (SEER) data (Harlow, Weiss, & Lofton, 1986; Schwartz & Weiss, 1990); a study of 167 newly diagnosed uterine sarcoma patients and 208 random control subjects (Schwartz, Weiss, Daling, Gammon, Liff, & Watt et al., 1996); a case-control study of 29 women with uterine sarcoma (Schwartz & Thomas, 1989); and retrospective analysis of 318 uterine sarcoma cases from a tumor registry (Olah et al., 1991).

The risk factors documented through this limited epidemiologic research are listed in Table 33-1. Except for obesity and nulliparity, the risk factors of endometrial carcinoma—obesity, diabetes, nulliparity, infertility, and hypertension—are not supported as risk factors among women with uterine sarcoma. Furthermore, in contrast to endometrial carcinoma, the one consistent risk factor for uterine sarcoma is ethnicity. The incidence of uterine sarcoma is approximately twice as high in African-American women (Harlow, Weiss, & Lofton, 1986). Other risk factors that have been suggested are menstrual and reproductive factors, marital status, prior pelvic irradiation, hormonal manipulation, and obesity. In addition, these reported risk factors vary with histologic types of uterine sarcomas, particularly when both sarcomatous and carcinomatous elements are present.

Menstrual and Reproductive Factors

From a retrospective study of 29 women diagnosed with uterine sarcoma, Schwartz and Thomas (1989) identified an increased risk for uterine sarcoma among women with short menstrual histories (i.e., menarche after age 13 and menopause before age 45). The same investigators found an increased risk for uterine sarcoma among nulliparous women and women who gave birth to their first child at 25 years of age or later. In contrast, a later study of 167 newly diagnosed women with uterine sarcoma found that these women were more likely to have had a prior live birth irrespective of age at first birth (Schwartz et al., 1996).

Marital Status

Schwartz and Weiss (1990) reviewed the SEER data for the incidence of uterine sarcoma and marital status. Risk for uterine sarcoma is 50% higher among women who have never married.

Pelvic Irradiation

Women previously treated with radiation therapy for malignant and benign conditions such as uterine bleeding, polyps, or fibroids are at increased risk for uterine sarcoma. Resnik, Chambers, Carcangiu, Kohorn, Schwartz, & Chambers (1995) reported an increased incidence of MMT after radiation therapy for benign lesions. Similarly, Olah et al. (1991)

discovered an increased incidence of MMT with prior history of pelvic irradiation for benign and malignant tumors. These findings support previous reports of pelvic irradiation as a risk factor for uterine sarcoma with unspecified histology (Clement & Scully, 1974; Meredith, Eisert, Kaka, Hodgson, Johnston, & Boutselis, 1986).

Hormonal Manipulation and Obesity

Unopposed estrogen may be a risk factor for MMT and LMS (Schwartz et al., 1996). One study of 167 women with uterine sarcoma examined risk factors including the use of oral contraceptives and the use of noncontraceptive estrogens. Oral contraceptive use was positively associated with an increased risk for leiomyosarcoma, and noncontraceptive estrogen use was associated with an increased risk for mixed mullerian tumors, both with long-term/recent use. As with findings from studies of endometrial carcinoma, these findings suggest a role for unopposed estrogen in the etiology of different histologic types of uterine sarcoma (Schwartz et al., 1996). The occurrence of LMS and MMT, as well as tumors of unspecified histology occurring in women after long-term use of tamoxifen, a nonsteroidal antiestrogen, have been cited in several case reports (Clarke, 1993; Fisher, Costantino, Redmond, Fisher, Wicherham, & Cronin, 1994; McCluggage, Varma, Weir, & Bharucha, 1996). Both Clarke (1993) and McCluggage, Varma, Weir, and Bharucha (1996) noted an increased incidence of uterine sarcoma in older postmenopausal women who received tamoxifen for 5 years or more. In addition, the occurrence of uterine sarcoma, as well as endometrial cancer, has been documented in women on tamoxifen for 5 years or more (Fisher et al., 1994).

Similar to women with endometrial cancer, obese women also may be at increased risk for uterine sarcoma. Schwartz and colleagues (1996) reported a higher incidence of obesity among a sample of 167 women with uterine sarcoma compared with 208 healthy control subjects. Obesity is a common risk for endometrial carcinoma as well.

TABLE 33-1 Reported Risk Factors for Uterine Sarcoma

Risk Factor	Histology
Ethnicity African American	All
Age < 54	LMS
Age > 55	MMT
Age of menarche > 13	All
Menopause < 45	All
Nulliparous	LMS, MMT
First birth > 25	All
Never married	All
History pelvic irradiation	MMT
>5-year history of tamoxifen	LMS, MMT
Tamoxifen	LMS, MMT
Unopposed estrogen	MMT
Obesity	All

LMS, Leiomyosarcoma; *MMT*, mixed mesodermal tumors.

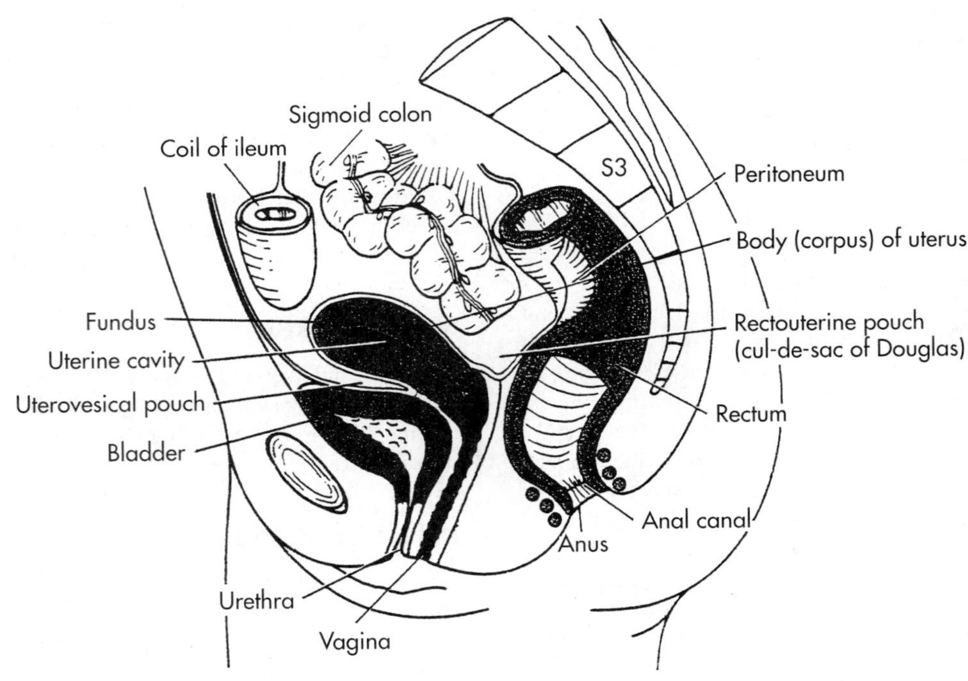

Fig. 33-1 Diagrammatic representation of the sagittal section of the uterus. (Modified from Snell, R. S. [1995]. The pelvis: The pelvis cavity [Part II]. In R. S. Snell [Ed.], *Clinical anatomy for medical students* [5th ed.]. Boston: Little Brown.)

PATHOPHYSIOLOGY

Normal Anatomy and Physiology of the Uterus

The uterus is a thick-walled, fibromuscular organ located in the pelvic cavity. It is hollow, pear-shaped, and positioned between the bladder anteriorly and the rectum posteriorly. In the adult the uterine corpus comprises the superior two thirds, and the cervix, the inferior one third of the uterus. The size of the normal uterus is quite variable, but generally is about 5.0 cm in height (length), 5.0 cm wide, and 2.5 cm in anteroposterior thickness, with a weight ranging from 40 to 100 g (Fig. 33-1).

The uterine cavity communicates with the fallopian tubes and the cervix. The uppermost portion of the uterus (above the level of communication with the tubes) is the fundus, which is the widest segment of the uterus. The lowermost portion, which joins with the cervix through the internal os, is the isthmus, or lower uterine segment. The rest of the organ is the body, or corpus (Silverberg & Kurman, 1992) (Fig. 33-2). The anterior and posterior surfaces of the uterus are covered by peritoneum or omentum, with the posterior (rectal) surface extending lower than the anterior (bladder) surface.

The anterior and posterior peritoneal coverings of the uterus join laterally and form the broad ligaments, which extend to the pelvic walls and include the fallopian tubes and the round and ovarian ligaments. The round ligaments help to maintain the uterus in its normal (anteverted) position, whereas the ovarian ligaments help maintain the position of the ovaries (Silverberg & Kurman, 1992) (Fig. 33-3).

The blood supply to the uterus is through the uterine arteries, which arise from the internal iliac arteries. The veins of the uterus drain to the uterovaginal venous plexus at the base of the broad ligament and then open into the internal iliac veins.

Lymphatic drainage is from a subserosal uterine plexus into the pelvic and para-aortic lymph nodes. Some lymphatics from the fundus accompany the round ligament of the uterus and drain into the superficial inguinal nodes. The myometrium has rich autonomic innervation that is primarily sympathetic. The function of this neural innervation is not known.

The Process of Carcinogenesis

The events leading to the development of uterine sarcoma are not clearly understood. Carcinomas arise from epithelial tissue, whereas sarcomas arise from connective tissue. Because uterine sarcomas may arise from muscle, cartilage, or bone (sarcoma) or endometrial tissue (carcinoma) *mixed* with sarcoma, the process may differ somewhat for the various histologic types. As with other cancers, it is most likely a multistage process (i.e., initiation, promotion, progression) resulting from genetic alterations and cellular transformation.

In a study of 14 patients with uterine sarcomas (LMS, ESS, and MMT), abnormalities of chromosomes 1, 7, and 11 were found. These chromosomal alterations may play a role in tumor initiation or progression of uterine sarcomas. Genomic alterations in the region of 11q22 suggest a relationship with malignant smooth muscle tumors of the uterus (Laxman, Currie, Kurman, Dudzinski, & Griffin, 1993). In addition, microsatellite instability (i.e., repetition of errors in nucleic acid sequences) observed in uterine sarcoma cell lines has been reported to be due to defective postreplication

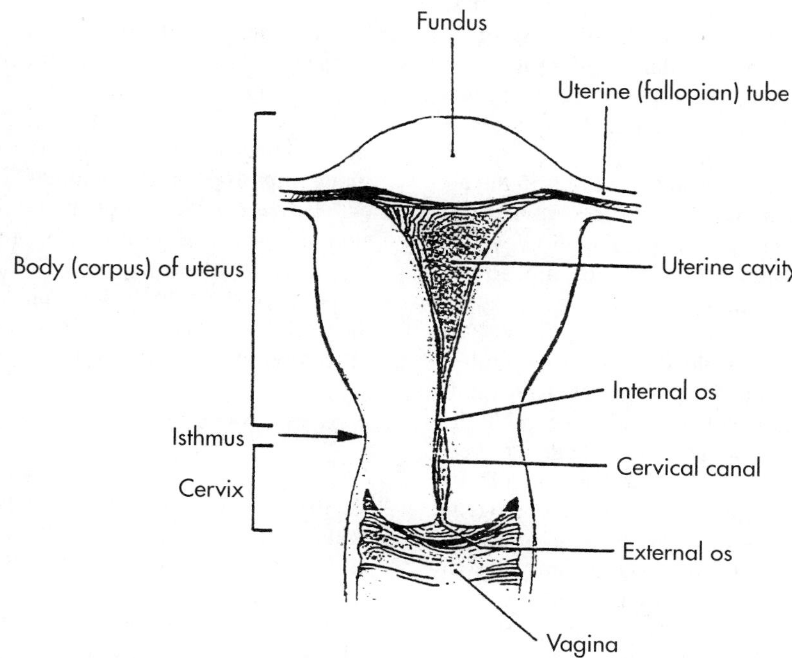

Fig. 33-2 Diagrammatic representation of the anterior view of the uterus. (Modified from Agur, A. M., & Lee, M. J. [1991]. Uterus and its adnexa. In A. M. R. Agur & M. J. Lee [Eds.], *Grant's atlas of anatomy* [9th ed.]. Baltimore: Williams & Wilkins.)

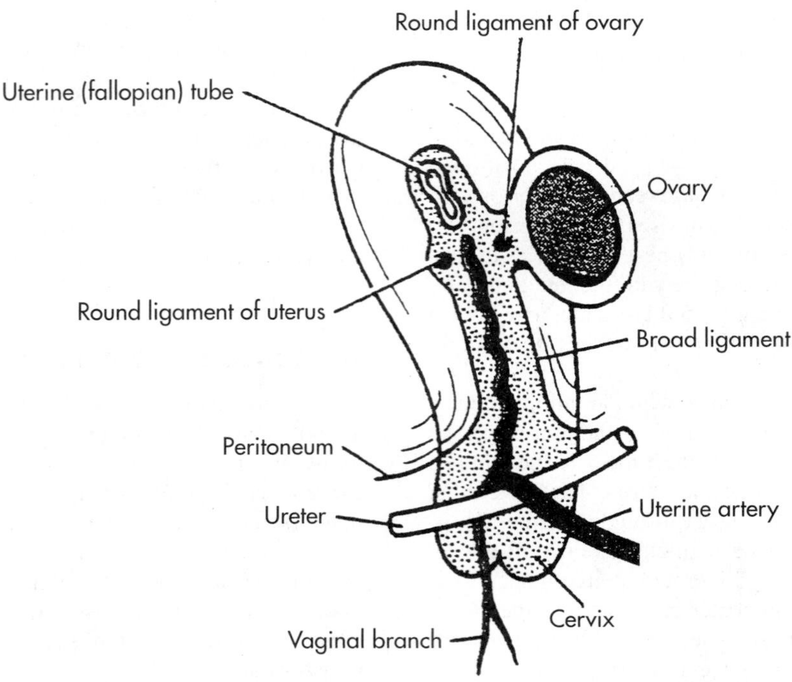

Fig, 33-3 Diagrammatic representation of the lateral view of the uterus. (Modified from Snell, R. S. [1995]. The pelvis: The pelvis cavity [Part II]. In R. S. Snell [Ed.], *Clinical anatomy for medical students* (5th ed.). Boston: Little Brown.)

mismatch repair (Risinger, Umar, Boyer, Evans, Berchuck, & Kunkel et al., 1995).

As with carcinomas, it appears that the molecular events leading to the development of sarcomas, or mixed tumors, also involve two types of cellular genes: oncogenes and tumor suppressor genes. Oncogenes promote the growth and development of cells. When functioning normally, these genes regulate cell proliferation and death. When an oncogene is defective, uncontrolled cellular proliferation may occur. Limited study of the relationship between oncogenes and uterine sarcoma suggests that there may be an association with the c-*myc* proto-oncogene (Jeffers, Richmond, & Macaulay, 1995). The role of c-*myc* abnormalities in the development of uterine sarcoma is not well understood.

The role of tumor suppressor gene mutation/overexpression has also been studied in relationship to the development of uterine sarcomas. As the name suggests, tumor suppressor genes normally function to prevent the unregulated growth of cells. A genetic mutation in a tumor suppressor gene could result in a loss of this tumor suppression and allow cancer cells to proliferate. Although p53, the first tumor suppressor gene identified, has been studied in relationship to uterine sarcomas, its clinical usefulness or its usefulness in elucidating the carcinogenic process has not been well established. It is reported that strong p53 overexpression in LMS is significantly associated with high-grade morphology and advanced-stage disease at the time of presentation (Niemann, Raab, Lenel, Rodgers, & Robinson, 1995). These findings might be useful in determining prognosis.

The role of hormonal stimulation in the pathogenesis of uterine sarcomas is unclear. Studies examining the relationship between hormonal milieu and the initiation and promotion of uterine sarcoma suggest potential harmful effects of contraceptive use, noncontraceptive estrogen supplementation, and tamoxifen therapy.

ROUTES OF METASTASES

Uterine sarcomas tend to be aggressive and commonly spread by direct extension into the peritoneal cavity and omentum at the time of diagnosis. Once it becomes extrauterine, uterine sarcoma is usually a systemic disease. Metastases may occur by both lymphatic and hematogenous routes. Involved sites are lung (52%), pelvic lymph nodes (41%), para-aortic lymph nodes (38%), and liver parenchyma (34%). Metastases to other distant sites include brain, heart, kidney, and bone (Rose, Piver, Tsukada, & Lau, 1989). Metastases to the lung and liver are best explained by the hematogenous route. Metastatic sites do not vary significantly by histologic type.

ASSESSMENT

The diagnosis of uterine sarcoma is formidable. Failure to identify populations at risk and a lack of adequate screening tools are major barriers. Furthermore, patients do not usually seek medical attention until symptoms are present.

Initial assessment involves a history and physical examination including a careful pelvic and rectal examination, laboratory tests to assess organ function, abdominal and pelvic computed tomography (CT), vaginal ultrasonography, and fractional dilation and curettage (D & C). Further x-ray films and scans are obtained to rule out metastatic dis-

TABLE 33-2 Assessment of the Patient for Uterine Sarcoma

Criteria	Assessment Parameters	Typical Abnormal Findings
History	A. Health history 1. Age 2. Ethnicity 3. Family history 4. Social history	A. Risk factors 1. Usually between age 45 and 75 2. More prevalent in African Americans
	B. Evaluation of gynecologic system	B. Menorrhagia, menstrual Irregularity, vaginal discharge, abdominal/pelvic pain, bowel symptoms, weight loss, infertility
	C. Menstrual status	C. Menarche >13 years and menopause < 45
Physical Examination	A. Abdominal examination	A. Abdomen 1. Ascites 2. Hepatomegaly 3. Abdominal mass 4. Increasing abdominal girth
	B. Weight	B. Weight loss
	C. Genitourinary	C. Obstructive urinary problems with advanced disease
	D. Pap smear	D. Abnormal in approximately 47% of diagnosed uterine sarcomas
	E. Pelvic/rectal examination	E. Palpable pelvic mass, enlarged uterus, broad-based or pedunculated lesion
Diagnostic Tests	A. Laboratory tests 1. CBC 2. Serum electrolytes 3. Blood glucose 4. BUN and creatinine 5. Hepatic function 6. CA-125	A. Usual Findings 1. Hemoglobin <12 2. Electrolyte imbalance with advanced disease 3. Within normal values 4. Abnormal with ureter obstruction 5. Increased with advanced disease 6. Slightly elevated or within normal limits
	B. Vaginal ultrasonography	B. Pelvic mass
	C. X-ray films and scans 1. Chest radiography/chest CT 2. Abdominal and pelvic CT/MRI	C. Findings 1. Abnormal in advanced disease 2. Enlarged uterus/abdominal mass, lymphadenopathy
	D. Fractional D & C/endometrial biopsy	D. Parametrial involvement (negative biopsy does not rule out presence of uterine sarcoma)

CBC, Complete blood count; *BUN,* blood urea nitrogen; *CT,* computed tomography; *MRI,* magnetic resonance imaging; *D & C,* dilation and curretage.

ease. Table 33-2 includes assessment criteria and abnormal diagnostic findings for a workup of uterine sarcoma

History

Patients with uterine sarcoma frequently present to their health care provider with a history of abnormal bleeding and abdominal/pelvic pain (Kunzel, Mills, Muderspach, & D'Ablaing, 1993; Murphy & Wallace, 1993; Olah et al., 1991; Parker, Fu, & Berek, 1994; Schwartz, Diamond, & Schwartz, 1993; Tinkler & Cowie, 1993). Uterine bleeding may present as menorrhagia or menstrual irregularity (Olah et al., 1991). Furthermore, it is not uncommon for premenopausal women to have a history of abnormal uterine bleeding for several months. Some report abnormal uterine bleeding as the only presenting symptom (Gerst, Levy, Swaminathan, Kshettry, & Albu, 1993; Schneider, Halperin, Segal, Maymon, & Bukovsky, 1995). Leiomyosarcoma arising in women suspected of having uterine fibroids has also been noted, particularly when "fibroids" are large. Less frequently, other presenting symptoms are noted. For example, urinary obstruction (Schwartz, Diamond, & Schwartz, 1993; Tinkler & Cowie, 1993), vaginal discharge, a self-detectable abdominal mass (To & Ngan, 1994), increasing abdominal girth (Kunzel, Mills, Muderspach, & D'Ablaing, 1993; Tinkler & Cowie, 1993), weight loss, bowel symptoms, and infertility (Olah et al., 1991) have been reported.

Physical Examination

The most common presenting sign on physical examination and at operation is uterine enlargement (Clement & Scully, 1974; Olah et al., 1991; Schneider et al., 1995). Abdominal palpation may reveal an abdominal mass (Schwartz, Diamond, & Schwartz, 1993), or a mass may be visible on speculum examination. Presence of a palpable pelvic mass other than the uterus, or lymphadenopathy, ascites, and/or hepatomegaly may also be noted (Olah et al., 1991). Less common physical findings include urinary obstruction and weight loss.

Diagnostic Tests

Laboratory tests, pathologic examination, vaginal ultrasonography, CT, and magnetic resonance imaging (MRI) are commonly used in the diagnosis of uterine sarcomas.

Laboratory Tests. Routine laboratory tests are conducted to define organ system involvement. Other abnormal laboratory findings may include decreased hemoglobin and hematocrit as a result of abnormal uterine bleeding.

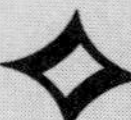

Table 33-3 Patient Preparation for Vaginal Ultrasonography

Description of the Procedure: Vaginal ultrasonography produces an image of the uterus from echoes recorded as they strike tissues of different densities.

Patient Preparation: No special preparation or procedure is required. Patient should void before the ultrasonography.

Procedural Considerations:

1. Obtain informed consent.
2. Patient needs to undress except for bra and put on gown.
3. Patient is assisted into lithotomy position.
4. Drape is applied to cover patient.
5. Transvaginal transducer is introduced into the vagina by the radiologist.
6. The transducer is introduced into the posterior vagina when the uterus is retroverted.
7. The transducer is introduced into the anterior vaginal fornix when the uterus is anteverted.
8. The uterus is scanned longitudinally and transversely.
9. The procedure lasts approximately 10 minutes.

There are no tumor markers with acceptable sensitivity or specificity for the detection of uterine sarcoma. Slight elevations in CA-125 at diagnosis that return to normal after treatment for uterine sarcoma have been reported (Kunzel et al., 1993; Gollard, Kosty, Bordin, Wax, & Lacey, 1995). Normal carcinoembryonic antigen and alpha-fetoprotein have been reported with MMT (Gollard et al., 1995). In contrast, Phillips, Scurry, and Toner (1996) reported possible efficacy in using alpha-fetoprotein for monitoring treatment response of MMT. Tumor-associated glycoprotein (TAG-72) is expressed by the majority of MMT of the uterus and may be helpful as a marker in the follow-up of affected patients (Hackett, Kaminski, Olt, Zaino, & Podczaski, 1994). Experimental studies are currently evaluating the usefulness of these and other tumor markers in the diagnosis and follow-up of patients with uterine sarcoma.

Surgical Pathology. The cervical cytopathology of MMT tumors demonstrates abnormal pathology in approximately 47% of patients (To & Ngan, 1994). Therefore, a biopsy is necessary to establish a definitive diagnosis. Furthermore, endometrial biopsy on frozen section is reported to detect less than one third of LMS (Schwartz, Diamond, & Schwartz, 1993). Leiomyosarcoma should be suspected when there is rapid growth of a fibroid tumor in the uterus (Olah et al., 1991). The occasional finding, on histologic examination, of malignant changes within fibroids underscores the need for an adequate inspection of the intra-abdominal contents at the time of total abdominal

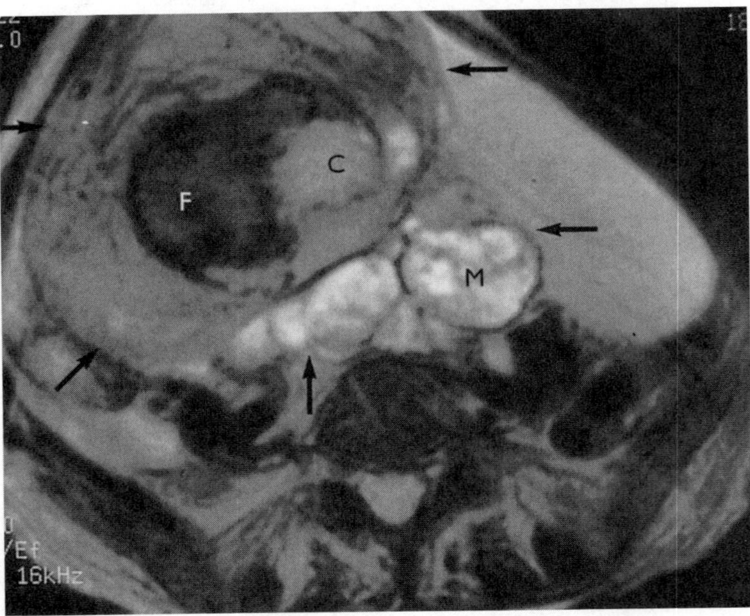

Fig. 33-4 Unresectable leiomyosarcoma. This MRI is from a 50-year-old woman who presented with abdominal swelling. The MRI shows a heterogeneous tumor *(arrows)* with areas of solid and cystic *(C)* tumor, mucin production *(M)*, and fibrosis *(F)*. CT scan can define a mass, whereas MRI can differentiate some tissue types within a tumor. (From Skarin, A. T. [1996]. *Atlas of diagnostic oncology* [2nd ed.]. St. Louis: Mosby-Wolfe.)

hysterectomy with bilateral salpingo-oophorectomy (TAH-BSO).

Vaginal Ultrasonography. Vaginal sonography is of limited benefit in the diagnosis of uterine sarcoma primarily because of the depth of the tumor. Nevertheless, in some patients, vaginal sonography is beneficial in assessing tumor location and size. Abdominal/pelvic sonography may be of benefit in staging disease or in assessing the presence or absence of ascites. Table 33-3 outlines instructions to prepare a patient for vaginal ultrasonography.

CT and MRI. CT and MRI are used to determine the extent of the tumor and tumor metastasis (Fig. 33-4). In addition, CT-guided biopsy of submucosal tissue with intraoperative frozen section has been successful in diagnosing LMS (Schwartz, Diamond, & Schwartz, 1993).

Sometimes uterine sarcoma is diagnosed from submucosal biopsy during D & C. However, it is not uncommon for a diagnosis of uterine sarcoma to be made after pathologic examination after a TAH-BSO (Schwartz, Diamond, & Schwartz, 1993; To & Ngan, 1994).

STAGING

Histologic examination of the tumor by a pathologist after surgery provides valuable information regarding the histologic type and the grade or biologic aggressiveness of the tumor. Uterine sarcomas are generally divided into three histologic types: LMS (40%), arising from smooth muscle; ESS (15%), arising from stroma; and MMT (30%), also referred to as *mixed mullerian tumors.* Mixed mesodermal tumors can have homologous or heterologous components, such as striated muscle, cartilage, and bone. Based on histologic criteria and distinct clinical behavior, ESS is comprised of two distinct entities (i.e., low grade and high grade), based on histologic criteria, but also with distinct clinical behavior (i.e., high grade). Other histopathologies make up the remaining 15% of uterine sarcomas and are rare.

No formal grading system is available for uterine sarcomas. This lack of uniformity among grading systems results in confusion and makes comparison of data difficult. However, tumor grading is similar to that for other sarcomas and takes into consideration the location and size of the tumor; the degree of differentiation (i.e., cellular pleomorphism); cellularity; the amount of stroma, necrosis, and vascularity; and the number of mitoses (Table 33-4). Other aspects of the histologic examination include tumor size, extent of tumor involvement, depth of myometrial invasion, and lymph nodal involvement.

Also suggested as prognostically important are ploidy status (the amount of DNA in the cells, aneuploid being an abnormal amount indicative of aggressive tumor growth), S-phase fraction (the percentage of cells in S phase, also indicative of aggressive tumor growth), and p53 mutation or overexpression (Nola, Babic, Ilic, Marusic, Uzarevic, & Petrovecki et al., 1996). However, the importance of these indicators in predicting survival has not been widely accepted.

Two systems have been used for the clinical staging of uterine sarcomas: the TNM classification system and the FIGO staging system. The TNM classification system was developed by the American Joint Committee on Cancer (AJCC) and the FIGO system by the Federation Internationale de Gynecologie et d'Obstetrique (Averette &Nguyen, 1995). The TNM system was developed for the grading of uterine carcinomas; therefore, it is of limited clinical usefulness in the classification of uterine sarcomas. The modified FIGO system is used most often in clinical practice (Table 33-5). Although clinical tumor stage is considered to be the strongest prognostic variable, the value of surgical staging laparotomy and tumor debulking remains controversial.

TABLE 33-4 Histologic Grading Guidelines for Uterine Sarcoma

Low Grade	High Grade
Well differentiated (minimal pleomorphism)	Poorly differentiated (much pleomorphism)
Hypocellular	Hypercellular
Much stroma	Little stroma
Hypovascular	Hypervascular
Minimal necrosis	Much necrosis
<5 mitoses per 10 HPF	>5 mitoses per 10 HPF

HPF, High-power field.
Modified from Averette, H. E. & Nguyen, H. (1995). Gynecologic cancer. In G. P. Murphy, W. Lawrence, & R. E. Lenhard (Eds.), *Texbook of clinical oncology* (2nd ed.). Atlanta: American Cancer Society.

MEDICAL MANAGEMENT

The primary treatment for uterine sarcomas is surgical. The TAH-BSO is the treatment of choice regardless of the histologic type or stage of the tumor, unless disease is known to be metastatic at the time of diagnosis. However, even with stage I-II disease, recurrence is likely and often occurs at distant sites. Adequate adjuvant treatment for uterine sarcomas is urgently needed. Radiation therapy may help locoregional control, but has not been shown to provide a survival benefit (Moskovic, MacSweeney, Law, & Price, 1993; Nickie-Psikuta & Gawrychowski, 1993,).

Although combination chemotherapy seems the only rea-

TABLE 33-5 FIGO* Staging System for Uterine Sarcoma

Stage	Description
I	Sarcoma confined to uterus
II	Extension to cervix
III	Extension to pelvic structures
IV	Extrapelvic metastases

*Federation Internationale de Gynecologie et d'Obstetrique
From Averette, H. E. & Nguyen, H. (1995). Gynecologic cancer. In G. P. Murphy, W. Lawrence, & R. E. Lenhard (Eds.), *Textbook of clinical oncology* (2nd ed.). Atlanta: American Cancer Society.

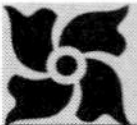

TABLE 33-6 Standard of Care for the Patient Undergoing TAH-BSO

Patient Problem and Outcomes	Nursing Interventions and Rationales	Patient Education Instructions
Potential Lack of Physiologic, Psychological, and Cognitive Readiness for Surgery		
Patient will verbalize an understanding and readiness for surgery	1. Assess patient's readiness to learn. 2. Give patient information about TAH-BSO. 3. Review side effects of surgery with patient. 4. Assess patient's understanding of impending surgery. 5. Witness informed consent. 6. Administer preoperative medication.	1. Describe surgical procedure to the patient. 2. Use diagram of pelvic anatomy to describe extent of surgery. 3. Describe preoperative procedure: a. Diagnostic tests b. Bowel prep c. Anesthesiology consult d. Use of antiembolism stockings e. Nothing by mouth after midnight 4. Instruct patient on potential complications of surgery: a. Hemorrhage b. Nausea and vomiting c. Wound infection d. Pneumonia e. Sexual dysfunction 5. Teach patient the plan for postoperative care: a. Turning, coughing, and deep breathing b. Pain management c. IV management d. Fluids and diet e. Surgical incision care
Altered Physiologic Status Related to the Immediate Postoperative Condition		
Patient's physiologic status will be hemoglobin 12 g/dl; hematocrit 37%; urinary output > 60 ml/hr; temperature <99° F (37.2° C	1. Assess vital signs every 15 min until stable and then as ordered. 2. Maintain IV. 3. Assess urinary output and report urinary output if <60 ml/hr. 4. Assess bowel sounds.	Teach patient to: 1. Report feelings of faintness. 2. Ask for assistance the first time she gets out of bed. 3. Report burning or pain at IV site. 4. Report when she passes flatus.
Patient will: • Maintain adequate fluid intake • Maintain adequate nutritional intake • Maintain an incision that is free of signs of infection	5. Assess incision for redness, tenderness, or drainage. 6. Offer clear fluids when bowel sounds are present.	5. Save urine to be measured when voiding. 6. Record fluids and dietary input. 7. Care for incision at home. 8. Sexual intercourse may be resumed when healing is complete, generally 1 month after surgery. 9. Management of menopausal symptoms if patient is premenopausal. 10. Use of vaginal lubricants such as K-Y jelly or Replens. 11. Vitamin E and clonidine may be ordered for hot flashes. 12. Dyspareunia may result with deep pelvic thrusting because of vaginal shorting.
Potential for Pulmonary Emboli		
Patient will: • Maintain breath sounds in all lung fields • Maintain respiratory rate between 12 and 20 respirations/min	1. Apply compression stockings to both legs. 2. Dangle patient's legs the evening of surgery. 3. Ambulate on day 1. 4. Assess breath sounds every shift. 5. Report shortness of breath. 6. Obtain chest x-ray as ordered.	Teach patient: 1. The importance of early ambulation. 2. To report shortness of breath, chest pain.

TAH-BSO, Total abdominal hysterectomy with bilateral salpingo-oophorectomy.

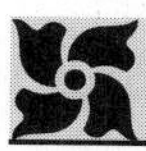

TABLE 33-6 Standard of Care for the Patient Undergoing TAH-BSO—cont'd

Patient Problem and Outcomes	Nursing Interventions and Rationales	Patient Education Instructions
Alteration in Comfort		
Patient will report on adequate comfort level	1. Assess patient's pain on a scale of 0 to 10, with 0 being no pain. 2. Administer pain medicine to keep patient's comfort at an acceptable level maintained at 0.	1. Teach patient the pain scale and to report pain to the nurse. 2. Teach patient protective body mechanics.
Potential Ineffective Coping Related to Hospitalization, Loss of Body Part, Altered Body Image, and Disease Prognosis		
Patient will verbalize/demonstrate effective coping skills	1. Assess patient's coping mechanisms, sources of support. 2. Have patient verbalize feelings about what the hysterectomy means to her. 3. Attempt to include significant other in discussion. 4. Allow patient and significant other to ventilate feelings regarding prognosis and need for further treatment. 5. Allow the patient to express feelings of anger and hurt. 6. Encourage the patient to express fear of cancer diagnosis.	1. Teach the patient effective coping strategies: a. Appropriate use of adaptive coping mechanisms b. Value of quiet time c. Use of distraction d. Appropriate use of anger e. Value of talking with significant other about the meaning of the hysterectomy

sonable treatment option, the search for an effective regimen has been unsuccessful. Chemotherapy regimens that have demonstrated at least some activity in one or more histologic type of uterine sarcomas are PAD (cisplatin, Adriamycin, and dacarbazine) (Baker, Piver, Caglar, & Piedmonte, 1991); VAC (vincristine, actinomycin-D, and cyclophosphamide) (Hannigan, Freedman, Elder, & Rutledge, 1983); etoposide, cisplatin, and doxorubicin (Resnik et al., 1995); hydroxyurea, dacarbazine, and etoposide (Currie, Blessing, Muss, Foweler, Berman, & Burke, 1996); and ifosfamide and doxorubicin (Sutton, Blessing, & Malfetano, 1996).

Biologic studies of the effect of estrogen and progesterone on uterine sarcomas suggest that a select group of tumors are sensitive to steroid hormones and may benefit from treatment with a progestational agent (Tseng, Tseng, Mann, Chumas, Stone, & Maxella et al., 1986). In general, low-grade ESS has high levels of steroid receptors and is hormonally sensitive to progestational agent treatment (Averette & Nguyen, 1995). However, estrogen and progesterone positivity does not necessarily predict hormone responsiveness.

ONCOLOGIC EMERGENCIES

There is no strong association of uterine sarcomas with any of the syndromes commonly thought of as oncologic emergencies. However, anecdotal reports describe an increased incidence of spontaneous/tension pneumothorax (Fenlon, Carney, & Breatnach, 1996; Moskovic et al., 1993), with the potential need for emergency chest tube placement and careful nursing assessment of the patient's pulmonary status.

NURSING MANAGEMENT

Nursing management focuses on three modalities of treatment: surgery, radiation therapy, and chemotherapy, as well as symptom management. Furthermore, nursing is instrumental in helping patients cope with the poor prognosis associated with this disease. Because many patients have metastatic disease at the time of diagnosis, patients need additional supportive care. Home care focuses on progressive symptoms such as anorexia and pain.

Surgery

Surgery is the primary method of treatment. The nurse plays an important role before surgery in explaining the treatment options to patients and providing necessary education, thereby facilitating treatment decisions. Leiomyosarcoma frequently affects women who are premenopausal; therefore, the decision to proceed with a hysterectomy may be especially difficult.

Postoperative nursing care focuses on patient monitoring and acute care interventions. Assessment criteria include physiologic status, patency of the airway, hemodynamic status, fluid volume, comfort, skin integrity, and coping. Nursing interventions are directed toward prevention of complications and early rehabilitation. Discharge teaching includes incision care and management of menopausal symptoms in premenopausal women. The patient is generally in the hospital for 3 to 5 days. For nursing management of the patient undergoing surgery for uterine sarcoma, see Table 33-6.

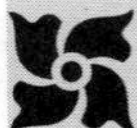

Table 33-7 Standard of Care for the Patient Receiving External Beam Radiation Therapy for Uterine Sarcoma

Patient Problem and Outcomes	Nursing Interventions and Rationales	Patient Education Instructions
Alteration in Skin Integrity Patient will: • Verbalize knowledge of skin care • Report skin integrity as dry and intact	1. Assess skin each visit. 2. Report signs of skin desquamation.	Teach patient: 1. Wash skin in treatment field with lukewarm water. 2. Use moisturizing soap. 3. Do not use a wash cloth. 4. Blot skin dry with a soft towel 5. Do not apply any ointment, lotions, or powder to the treatment area. 6. Do not remove the marks on the treatment field. 7. Do not use a heating pad on the treatment field. 8. Do not expose the treatment field to the sun. 9. Do not swim or use a hot tub. 10. Report skin changes in the treatment field such as dryness, redness, tanning or peeling. 11. If the skin in the treatment field becomes moist and sore, report it to the nurse.
Alteration in Bowel/Bladder Function Patient will: • Report normal bowel function for her • Report normal bladder function for her	1. Implement bowel management after barium study for treatment plan. 2. Assess preradiation bowel function. 3. Recommend magnesium citrate ½ bottle as needed for constipation. 4. Assess for diarrhea. 5. Assess for tenesmus. 6. Assess for urinary urgency. 7. Assess for urinary hesitancy. 8. Assess dysuria. 9. Assess if patient is following bladder filling technique.	Teach patient: 1. Drink 1 to 2 L of fluids a day after barium study. 2. Bowel movement will be white until barium is expelled. 3. Report if bowel movement does not return to normal color. 4. If constipated, take a mild laxative. 5. Report constipation if not relieved by laxative. 6. Purpose of the bladder filling technique is: a. Fill the bladder to help push the bowel up and out of the treatment field b. May swallow barium contrast during a latter portion of treatment to verify the procedure is working 7. Bladder filling technique a. Empty bladder 2 hours before treatment b. Drink 4 to 6 cups of fluids over 30 to 60 minutes after emptying bladder c. Abstain from voiding until after treatment
Fatigue Patient will: • Report understanding of fatigue process • Report management of activities of daily living without fatigue	1. Assess for fatigue. 2. Assess management of activities of daily living. 3. Assess dietary management. 4. Have patient rate fatigue on a scale of 0-10, with 0 being no fatigue. 5. Assess time of day fatigue is greatest for patient. 6. Assess degree fatigue interferes with activities of daily living. 7. Assess laboratory values. 8. Assess performance status.	1. Teach patient fatigue is normal and will be most severe toward the end of radiation therapy. 2. Teach patient energy conservation techniques: a. Make a list of activities b. Prioritize activities c. Plan rest periods to conserve energy for high priority events d. Group activities that can be done together e. Delegate activities that another member of the family can do 3. Eat high-energy foods. 4. Exercise daily.

Radiation Therapy

External beam radiation therapy is used occasionally as adjuvant therapy after surgery or for locoregional recurrent disease. Nursing care for patients receiving radiation therapy is adapted for patients with uterine sarcoma and includes prevention and treatment of side effects (Campbell & Pruitt, 1996; Holmes, 1996; Lowdermilk, 1995). The nurse assists in implementing bowel and bladder protection protocols. Radiation side effects are limited to skin desquamation and fatigue. For nursing care for a patient receiving radiation therapy, see Table 33-7.

Chemotherapy

Uterine sarcoma is frequently metastatic at the time of diagnosis, and recurrence is often at distant sites. Because of this pattern, a variety of chemotherapy regimens have been attempted in both primary and adjuvant settings. Tables 33-8 and 33-9 outline a specific standard of care for uterine sarcoma patients receiving the chemotherapy regimen outlined in the medical management section of this chapter.

Management of Metastatic Disease

Nursing management of metastatic disease focuses on supportive care and symptom management. Mahon and Casperson (1995) emphasized that patients have many psychosocial needs at the time of cancer recurrence. Symptom management is directed toward either local or distant disease spread and requires both acute and outpatient care. Acute care may include sclerotherapy for a pleural effusion (Goff, Mueller, Muntz, & Rice, 1993), management of respiratory failure, and postoperative care after surgical debulking procedures (Konski, Neisler, Phibbs, Bronn, & Dobelbower, 1993).

HOME CARE ISSUES

Patients with stage I and II disease require minimal home care; however, some follow-up during the immediate postoperative period may be needed (Lowdermilk, 1995). Home care primarily includes symptom management in patients with advanced-stage disease. Important quality of life issues include helping the patient adjust to a cancer recurrence, pain management, and control of weight loss and anorexia. In addition, nursing intervention for adjustment to body image changes, fatigue, and sexual function may be adapted for home care (Table 33-10).

PROGNOSIS

Clinical stage at the time of diagnosis is the most significant prognostic indicator. Patients with early-stage I and II

TABLE 33-8 Standard of Care for the Patient Receiving Chemotherapy Therapy for Uterine Sarcoma

Patient Problem and Outcomes	Nursing Interventions and Rationales	Patient Education Instructions
Infection Patient will: • Verbalize the signs and symptoms of infection: a. Temperature > 101° F (38.3° C) b. Productive cough c. Cough, shortness of breath d. Wound infection • Maintain temperature < 101° F (38.3° C) and be free of symptoms of infection	1. Assess vital signs each clinic visit or every 4 hr if patient is in the hospital. 2. Assess breath sounds each clinic visit or as needed if patient is in the hospital. 3. Assess wound or central line site. 4. Assess GU system. 5. Administer antibiotics as ordered. 6. Assess laboratory values.	Teach patient: 1. How to read thermometer 2. Signs of respiratory infection 3. To report redness, tenderness, or drainage at central line site 4. To report a cough or shortness of breath 5. To report burning or frequency of urination 6. To avoid crowded places or others with colds or influenza
Nausea and Vomiting Patient will maintain adequate nutrition	1. Assess emetic episodes. 2. Administer antiemetics as ordered. 3. Monitor nutritional intake. 4. Monitor intake and output. 5. Assess laboratory values.	Teach the patient: 1. To record number of emetic episodes 2. Restrict food before chemotherapy administration 3. Maintain a nutrition log 4. To self-administer oral antiemetic drugs as ordered for nausea 5. To report > 6 emetic episodes a day

Continued

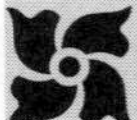

TABLE 33-8 Standard of Care for the Patient Receiving Chemotherapy Therapy for Uterine Sarcoma—cont'd

Patient Problem and Outcomes	Nursing Interventions and Rationales	Patient Education Instructions
Mucositis Patient will report oral integrity intact	1. Assess oral cavity. 2. Assess fluid intake. 3. Encourage mouth rinse of salt and soda. 4. Administer antifungal and antiviral agents as ordered.	Teach patient: 1. Importance of brushing and use of mouth rinse 2. To avoid mouth rinse with alcohol 3. To use soft-bristle tooth brush 4. To massage gums and tongue with soft-bristle tooth brush 5. To keep oral cavity moist with clear fluids or moisturizer 6. To use salt and soda dissolved in water for a mouth rinse 7. To check oral cavity daily for lesions 8. Importance of mouth care after any oral intake of food or beverage other than water 9. To report mouth sores
Body Image Resulting from Alopecia Patient will report adaptation to altered body image	1. Assess meaning of body image to patient. 2. Have patient get a snapshot showing usual hairstyle before treatment begins. 3. Have patient snip a swatch of hair before treatment begins. 4. Provide wig/turban resources. 5. Insurance will partially or totally reimburse for wigs with prescription for "hair prosthesis." 6. Assess patient's strengths.	Teach patient: 1. When to expect hair loss 2. How hair loss will occur 3. To protect scalp from sun or cold 4. To apply sunscreen to bare scalp if in sun 5. Encourage patient to obtain wigs or scarves before hair loss 6. To practice daily affirmations 7. To discuss meaning of altered body image with significant other
Thrombocytopenia Patient will report knowledge of care during thrombocytopenic episodes	1. Assess patient for bruising. 2. Assess laboratory values.	Teach patient: 1. To restrict activity to reduce chance of injury during nadir 2. Signs of abnormal bleeding such as nose bleeds, and blood in stool, urine, or bruising 3. To avoid aspirin or aspirin-containing drugs
Other Side Effects Patient will report knowledge of other side effects	1. Assess for neurotoxicity. 2. Assess for nephrotoxicity. 3. Assess renal function studies. 4. Assess for hematuria. 5. Assess mental status.	Teach patient: 1. Hands/fingers and feet may feel numb or lose sensation 2. To avoid going bare foot 3. To use caution when cooking 4. To drink 3 L of fluids daily unless contraindicated 5. To empty bladder before going to bed 6. To report pain in hands or loss of function 7. To report symptoms of hallucinations, depression, or somnolence

TABLE 33-9 Drug Regimens and Side Effects of Agents Used in Treatment of Uterine Sarcoma

Drug	Drug Regimen	Side Effects
Cisplatin	PAD or ECD	Slight to moderate myelosuppression, moderate to severe nausea and vomiting, irritant, nephrotoxicity, neurotoxicity, and ototoxicity
Doxorubicin (Adriamycin)	PAD or ID	Moderate to severe myelosuppression, slight mucositis, moderate nausea and vomiting, alopecia, vesicant, pulmonary toxicity, cardiomyopathy (cumulative dose dependent), radiation recall
Dacarbazine	PAD or HDE	Moderate myelosuppression, severe nausea and vomiting, alopecia, irritant, photosensitivity, flulike symptoms, hepatoxicity, diarrhea
Vincristine	VAC	Slight myelosuppression, mucositis, nausea/vomiting, alopecia, vesicant, moderate neurotoxicity, constipation
Actinomycin-D	VAC	Moderate to severe myelosuppression, slight to moderate mucositis, moderate to severe nausea and vomiting, alopecia, vesicant, pulmonary toxicity, hyperpigmentation (radiation recall), diarrhea
Cyclophosphamide	VAC	Moderate to severe myelosuppression, mucositis, nausea and vomiting, alopecia, irritant, pulmonary toxicity, nephrotoxicity, hyperpigmentation, hemorrhagic cystitis
Etoposide	ECD or HDE	Moderate myelosuppression, slight to moderate nausea and vomiting, alopecia, irritant, pulmonary toxicity, neurotoxicity, hypotension, anaphylaxis, headache
Hydroxyurea	HDE	Moderate myelosuppression, mucositis, slight to moderate nausea and vomiting, alopecia, neurotoxicity, diarrhea, anorexia
Ifosfamide	ID	Slight to moderate myelosuppression, moderate mucositis, moderate nausea and vomiting, alopecia, nephrotoxicity, mentation changes, hemorrhagic cystitis, and fatigue

NOTE: Key Drug Regimen: PAD (cisplatin, Adriamycin, dacarbazine); VAC (vincristine, actinomycin-D, cyclophosphamide); ECD (etoposide, cisplatin, doxorubicin); HDE (hydroxyurea, dacarbazine, etoposide); ID (ifosfamide, doxorubicin).
From Tenenbaum, L. (1994) Chemotherapeutic agents used in the treatment of cancer. In L. Tenenbaum (Ed.), *Cancer chemotherapy and biotherapy: A reference guide.* Philadelphia: W. B. Saunders.

TABLE 33-10 Home Care Management

Patient Problem	Focus of Nursing Intervention	Patient Problem	Focus of Nursing Intervention
Coping with cancer recurrence and advanced disease	Consideration of treatment options: • Chemotherapy • Radiation therapy • Surgery for debulking recurrent disease • Treatment of hydronephrosis • Treatment of pleural effusion Maintenance of feelings of control Promotion of self-efficacy Management of fatigue Coping with sexual dysfunction Maintenance of accurate expectations of disease Prognosis Refocusing of thoughts Finding hope and setting goals Referral to support groups and other community resources	Management of pain	Use of narcotic analgesia as needed for pain control Use of relaxation tapes Use of guided imagery Use of distraction techniques
		Management of anorexia	Meal planning and management: • High-calorie snacks • Frequent, small feedings • Limiting fluids before meals • Shakes with added protein supplement • Sampling a variety of foods • Making mealtime special • Maintenance of adequate fluid intake

TABLE 33-11 Factors Suggested to Influence Prognosis

Indicator	Favorable Prognostic Signs	Unfavorable Prognostic Signs
Size	Small	Large
Histologic grade	Low	High
Location	Confined to uterus	Extrauterine
Ploidy	Diploid	Aneuploid
S phase	Low	High
p53 mutation	Present	Absent
Clinical stage at diagnosis	I-II	III-IV

disease may have a chance of disease cure or control, whereas the goal of treatment for patients with advanced or recurrent disease is palliation. Dismal survival rates are frequently reported, with overall 5-year survival of only 34.5% to 37% (Malkasian, 1993; Nickie-Psikuta & Gawrychowski, 1993) and only 14.3% for MMT (To & Ngan, 1994). However, survival for low-grade stage I-II disease, such as LMS or ESS, may be significantly longer (Table 33-11). Death may be due to complications from local recurrence or distant metastasis.

EVALUATION OF THE QUALITY OF CARE

The Oncology Nursing Society has identified 11 standards for oncology nursing practice that serve as a guide in developing quality of care criteria for the evaluation of patient care. Tables 33-12 and 33-13 include examples of an inpatient and outpatient quality of care monitor adapted for patients with uterine sarcoma. The quality of care monitor includes indicators or standard of care assessed, threshold or desired outcome of compliance, data source, and criteria assessed. Because other disciplines such as dietary and social service are involved in care of patients with uterine sarcoma, the evaluation plan is multidisciplinary.

RESEARCH ISSUES

Both acute care and supportive care research is needed to advance the scientific knowledge of uterine sarcoma. Research exploring prognostic indicators for patients with uterine sarcoma to identify individuals who might benefit from adjuvant treatment for aggressive tumors must be carried out (Wolfson, Wolfson, Sittler, Breton, Markow, & Schwade et al., 1994). Other biologic factors deserving future consideration in predicting patients' prognosis include molecular markers, S-phase fraction, and estrogen and progesterone receptor status.

Oncology nurses rank symptom management first among the categories nurses need to research for improving the delivery of care to oncology patients (Stetz, Haberman, Holcombe, & Jones, 1995). Symptom management studies should include both qualitative and quantitative studies to determine appropriate nursing care to manage the distressing symptoms caused by uterine sarcoma. Because of the rarity of the disease, case report and qualitative studies are appropriate. Qualitative research questions might focus on body image changes, sexual dysfunction, coping with

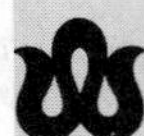

TABLE 33-12 Quality of Care Evaluation for a Patient Undergoing TAH-BSO*

Disciplines participating in the quality of care evaluation:
☐ Nursing ☐ Dietary
☐ Physical Therapy ☐ Social Services

Indicator: Preoperative Patient Care

Threshold expected to meet indicator: 95% indicated "yes"

Data from:
☐ Medical Record Review ☐ Patient/Family Interview

Criteria	Yes	No
1. Patient learning needs assessed		
a. Readiness to learn	☐	☐
b. Multiple methods of preoperative teaching offered	☐	☐
2. Preoperative plan of care for TAH-BSO		
a. Diagnostic tests	☐	☐
b. Bowel prep	☐	☐
c. Use of antiembolism stockings	☐	☐

Indicator: Postoperative Patient Care

Threshold expected to meet indicator: 90% indicated "yes"

Data From:
☐ Medical Record Review ☐ Patient/Family Interview

Criteria	Yes	No
1. Postoperative plan of care for TAH-BSO followed		
a. Dangled first evening	☐	☐
b. Ambulated day one	☐	☐
c. Discharged day five or before	☐	☐

Indicator: Patient/Family Satisfaction

Threshold expected to meet indicator: 95% indicated "yes"

Data from:
☐ Medical Record Review ☐ Patient/Family Interview

Criteria	Yes	No
1. Do you feel you were given enough information before surgery?	☐	☐
2. Were you given instruction on incisional care at home?	☐	☐
3. Were you informed or instructed on when you might resume sexual intercourse?	☐	☐

*Total abdominal hysterectomy with bilateral salpingo-oophorectomy.

TABLE 33-13 Quality of Care Evaluation for a Patient Coping with Metastatic Uterine Sarcoma at Home

Disciplines participating in the quality of care evaluation
☐ Nursing ☐ Dietary
☐ Physical Therapy ☐ Social Services

Indicator: Patient coping strategies
Threshold expected to meet indicator: 95% indicated "yes"

Data from:
☐ Medical Record Review ☐ Patient/Family Interview

Criteria	Yes	No
1. Did the nurse or social worker make referrals for:		
a. Support groups	☐	☐
b. Community agencies	☐	☐
2. Were the following coping strategies explained		
a. Setting short-term goals	☐	☐
b. Thought refocusing	☐	☐
c. Maintaining control	☐	☐
3. Were fatigue management steps taught?	☐	☐

chronic disease, and disruption in lifestyle as a result of the disease process.

Retrospective quantitative research of nursing care for uterine sarcoma can be conducted by assessing the tumor registrar data base to identify patients.

In addition, epidemiologic studies are needed to better identify the risk factors associated with uterine sarcoma. Although specific chemoprevention studies for uterine sarcoma are not currently available, nurses can focus on primary prevention measures including nutrition, exercise, and stress management, which can improve the quality of life for women of all ages at risk for cancer.

REFERENCES

Agur, A. M. & Lee, M. J. (1991). Uterus and its adnexa. In A. M. Agur & M. J. Lee (Eds.), *Grant's atlas of anatomy* (9th ed.). Baltimore: Williams & Wilkins.

Averette, H. E. & Nguyen, H. (1995). Gynecologic cancer. In G. P. Murphy, W. Lawrence, & R. E. Lenhard (Eds.), American Cancer Society: *Textbook of clinical oncology* (2nd ed.). Atlanta: American Cancer Society.

Baker, T. R., Piver, M. S., Caglar, H., & Piedmonte, M. (1991). Prospective trial of cisplatin, Adriamycin, and dacarbazine in metastatic mixed mesodermal sarcomas of the uterus and ovary. *American Journal of Clinical Oncology, 14,* 246-50.

Campbell, M. & Pruitt, J. (1996). Radiation therapy: Protecting your patient's skin. *RN, 59,* 46-47.

Clarke, M. R. (1993). Uterine malignant mixed mullerian tumor in a patient on long-term tamoxifen therapy for breast cancer [case report]. *Gynecologic Oncology, 51,* 411-415.

Clement, P. B. & Scully, R. E. (1974). Mullerian adenosarcoma of the uterus. *Cancer, 34,* 1138-1149.

Currie, J., Blessing, J.A., Muss, H. B., Fowler, J., Berman, M., & Burke, T. W. (1996). Combination chemotherapy with hydroxyurea, dacarbazine (DTIC), and etoposide in the treatment of uterine leiomyosarcoma: A Gynecologic Oncology Group study. *Gynecologic Oncology, 61,* 27-30.

DiSaia P. J. & Creasman, W. T. (1993). Sarcoma of the uterus. In P. J. DiSaia & W. T. Creasman. (Eds.), *Clinical Gynecologic Oncology* (4th ed.). St. Louis: Mosby.

Fenlon, H. M., Carney, D., & Breatnach, E. (1996). Bilateral recurrent tension pneumothorax complicating combination chemotherapy for soft tissue sarcoma, [case report]. *Clinical Radiology, 51,* 302-304.

Fisher, B., Costantino, J. P., Redmond, C. K., Fisher, E. R., Wicherham, L., & Cronin, W. M. (1994). Endometrial cancer in tamoxifen-treated breast cancer patients: Findings from the national surgical adjuvant breast and bowel project (NSABP) B-14. *Journal of the National Cancer Institute, 86,* 527-537.

Gerst, P. H., Levy, J., Swaminathan, K., Kshettry, V., & Albu, E. (1993). Metastatic leiomyosarcoma of the uterus: Unusual presentation of a case of late endobronchial and small bowel metastases, [case report]. *Gynecologic Oncology, 49,* 271-275.

Goff, B. A., Mueller, P. R., Muntz, H. G., & Rice, L. W. (1993). Small chest-tube drainage followed by bleomycin sclerosis for malignant pleural effusions. *Obstetrics & Gynecology, 81,* 993-996.

Gollard, R., Kosty, M., Bordin, G., Wax, A., & Lacey, C. (1995). Two unusual presentations of mullerian adenosarcoma: Literature review and treatment considerations, [case reports]. *Gynecologic Oncology, 59,* 412-422.

Hackett, T. E., Kaminski, P., Olt, G. J., Zaino, R., & Podczaski, E. (1994). Tissue distribution of TAG-72 in malignant mixed mullerian tumors of the uterus. *Gynecologic Oncology 52,* 165-171.

Hannigan, E. V., Freedman, R. S., Elder, K. W., & Rutledge, G. N. (1983). Treatment of advanced uterine sarcoma with vincristine, actinomycin D, and cyclophosphamide. *Gynecologic Oncology, 15,* 224-229.

Harlow, H. L., Weiss, N. S., & Lofton, S. (1986). The epidemiology of sarcomas of the uterus. *Journal of The National Cancer Institute, 76,* 399-402.

Holmes, S. (1996). Making sense of radiotherapy: Curative and palliative. *Nursing Times, 92,* 32-33.

Jeffers, M. D., Richmond, J. A., & Macaulay, E. M. (1995). Overexpression of the c-*myc* proto-oncogene occurs frequently in uterine sarcomas. *Modern Pathology, 8,* 701-704.

Konski, M. D., Neisler, J., Phibbs, G., Bronn, D., & Dobelbower, R. R. (1993). The use of intraoperative electron beam radiation therapy in the treatment of para-aortic metastases from gynecologic tumors. *American Journal of Clinical Oncology, 16,* 67-71.

Kunzel, K. E., Mills, N. Z., Muderspach, L. I., & D'Ablaing, G. (1993). Myxoid leiomyosarcoma of the uterus, [case report]. *Gynecologic Oncology, 48,* 277-280.

Laxman, R., Currie, J. L., Kurman, R. J., Dudzinski, M., & Griffin, C. A. (1993). Cytogenetic profile of uterine sarcomas. *Cancer, 71,* 1283-1288.

Lowdermilk, D. L. (1995) Home care of the patient with gynecologic cancer. *Journal of Obstetric Gynecologic Neonatal Nursing, 24,* 157-163.

Malkasian, G. D. (1993). Gynecologic sarcomas. In J. F. Holland, E. Frei, R. C. Bast, D. W. Kuse, D. L. Morton, & R. R. Weichselbaum (Eds.), *Cancer Medicine* (3rd ed., Vol. 2). Philadelphia: Lea & Febiger.

McCluggage, W. G., Varma, M., Weir, R., & Bharucha, H. (1996). Uterine leiomyosarcoma in patient receiving tamoxifen therapy. *Acta Obstetrica et Gynecology Scandinavica, 75,* 593-595.

Meredith, R. F., Eisert, D. R., Kaka, Z., Hodgson, S. E., Johnston, G. A., & Boutselis, J. G. (1986). An excess of uterine sarcomas after pelvic irradiation. *Cancer, 58,* 2003-2007.

Moskovic, E., MacSweeney, E., Law, M., & Price, A. (1993). Survival, patterns of spread and prognostic factors in uterine sarcoma: A study of 76 patients. *The British Journal of Radiology, 66,* 1009-1015.

Murphy, N. J. & Wallace, D. L. (1993). Gonadotropin releasing hormone (GnRH) agonist therapy for reduction of leiomyoma volume, [case report]. *Gynecologic Oncology, 49,* 266-267.

Nickie-Psikuta, M. & Gawrychowski, K. (1993). Different types and different prognosis—study of 310 uterine sarcomas. *European Journal of Gynaecological Oncology, 14* (Suppl.), 105-113.

Niemann, T. H., Raab, S. S., Lenel, J. C., Rodgers, J. R., & Robinson, R. A. (1995). p53 protein overexpression in smooth muscle tumors of the uterus. *Human Pathology, 26,* 375-379.

Nola, M., Babic, D., Ilic, J., Marusic, M., Uzarevic, B., Petrovecki, M., Sabioncello, A., Kovac, D., & Jukic, S. (1996). Prognostic parameters for survival of patients with malignant mesenchymal tumors of the uterus. *Cancer 78*(12), 2543-2550.

Olah, K. S., Gee, H., Blunt, S., Dunn, J. A., Kelly, K., & Chan, K. K. (1991). Retrospective analysis of 318 cases of uterine sarcoma. *Cancer, 27,* 1095-1099.

Parker, W. H., Fu, Y. S., & Berek, J. S. (1994). Uterine sarcoma in patients operated on for presumed leiomyoma and rapidly growing leiomyoma. *Obstetrics and Gynecology, 83,* 414-418.

Phillips, K. A., Scurry, J. P., & Toner, G. (1996). Alpha-fetoprotein production by a malignant mixed mullerian tumour of the uterus. *Journal of Clinical Pathology, 49,* 349-351.

Resnik, E., Chambers, S. K., Carcangiu, M. L., Kohorn, E. I., Schwartz, P. E., & Chambers, J. T. (1995). A phase II study of etoposide, cisplatin, and doxorubicin chemotherapy in mixed mullerian tumors (MMT) of the uterus. *Gynecologic Oncology, 56,* 370-375.

Risinger, J. I., Umar, A., Boyer, J. C., Evans, A. C., Berchuck, A., Kunkel, T. A., & Barrett, J. C. (1995). Microsatellite instability in gynecological sarcomas and in hMSH2 mutant uterine sarcoma cell lines defective in mismatch repair activity. *Cancer Research, 55,* 5664-5669.

Rose, P. G., Piver, M. S., & Tsukada, Y., & Lau, T. (1989). Patterns of metastasis in uterine sarcoma: An autopsy study. *Cancer, 63,* 935-938.

Schneider, D., Halperin, R., Segal, M., Maymon, R., & Bukovsky, I. (1995). Myxoid leiomyosarcoma of the uterus with unusual malignant histologic pattern, [case report]. *Gynecologic Oncology 59,* 156-158.

Schwartz, L. B., Diamond, M. P., & Schwartz, P. E. (1993). Leiomyosarcomas: Clinical presentation. *American Journal Obstetrics Gynecology, 168,* 180-183.

Schwartz, S. M. & Thomas, D. B. (1989). A case-control study of risk factors for sarcomas of the uterus. *Cancer, 64,* 2487-2492.

Schwartz, S. M. & Weiss, N. S. (1990). Marital status and the incidence of sarcomas of the uterus. *Cancer Research, 50,* 1886-1889.

Schwartz, S. M., Weiss, N. S., Daling, J. R., Gammon, M. D., Liff, J. M., Watt, J., Lynch, C. F., Newcomb, P. A., Armstrong, B. K., & Thompson, W. D. (1996) Exogenous sex hormone use, correlates of endogenous hormone levels, and the incidence of histologic types of sarcoma of the uterus. *Cancer, 77,* 716-724.

Silverberg, S. G. & Kurman, R. J. (1992). Tumors of the uterine corpus. In S. G. Silverberg & R. J. Kurman (Eds.), *Atlas of tumor pathology tumors of the uterine corpus and gestational trophoblastic disease.* Washington, D. C.: Armed Forces Institute of Pathology.

Snell, R. S. (1995). The pelvis: The pelvic cavity (Part II). In R. S. Snell (Ed.), *Clinical anatomy for medical students* (5th ed.). Boston: Little Brown.

Stetz, K. M., Haberman, M. R., Holcombe, J., & Jones, L. S. (1995). 1994 oncology nursing society research priorities survey. *Oncology Nursing Forum, 22,* 785-789.

Sutton, G. Blessing, J. A,, & Malfetano, J. H. (1996). Ifosfamide and doxorubicin in the treatment of advanced leiomyosarcoma of the uterus: A Gynecologic Oncology Group study. *Gynecology Oncology, 62,* 226-229.

Tenenbaum, L. (1994) Chemotherapeutic agents used in the treatment of cancer. In L. Tenenbaum (Ed.), *Cancer chemotherapy and biotherapy: A reference guide.* Philadelphia: W. B. Saunders.

Tinkler, S. D. & Cowie, V. J. (1993). Uterine sarcomas: A review of the Edinburgh experience from 1974 to 1992. *The British Journal of Radiology, 66,* 998-1001.

To, W. W. K. & Ngan, H. Y. S. (1994). Malignant mixed mullerian tumors of the uterus. *Gynecology and Obstetrics, 47,* 39-44.

Tseng, L., Tseng, J. K., Mann, W. J., Chumas, J. C., Stone, M. L., Maxella, J., Sun, B., Amalfitano, T. B., & Wallach, R. C. (1986). Endocrine aspects of human uterine sarcoma: A preliminary study. *American Journal of Obstetrical Gynecology, 155,* 95-101.

Wolfson, A. H., Wolfson, D. J., Sittler, S. Y., Breton, L., Markow, A. M., Schwade, J. G., Houdek, P. V., Averette, H. E., Sevin, B-U., Penalver, M., Duncan, R. C., & Ganjei, P. (1994). A multivariate analysis of clinicopathologic factors for predicting outcome in uterine sarcomas. *Gynecologic Oncology, 52,* 56-62.

Vaginal Cancer

Margaret Cawley, RN, MS
Catherine Hydzik, RN, MS

EPIDEMIOLOGY

Carcinoma of the vagina is the rarest of the female gynecologic cancers. Only 1% to 2% of malignant tumors originate in the vagina (Zaino, Robboy, Bentley, & Kurman, 1994). It occurs predominately in women 60 years of age or older. Squamous cell carcinoma represents 90% of the primary vaginal tumors. Other less common malignancies include melanoma, sarcoma, and clear cell adenocarcinoma (Zaino et al., 1994). Metastatic tumors from other genital sites such as the cervix or endometrium are more common than primary tumors of the vagina. The incidence rate for vaginal cancer is 0.42 cases per 100,000 in white women and 0.93 per 100,000 in black women (Zaino et al., 1994).

In utero exposure to diethylstilbestrol (DES) resulted in the development of clear cell vaginal carcinoma. From 1946 to 1970, 2 to 3 million women were prescribed nonsteroidal estrogens such as DES to prevent repeated spontaneous abortions. Although not all women exposed to DES in utero developed vaginal cancer, it occurred in approximately 1 in 1000 cases (Walczak & Klemm, 1993). Thus far, 520 cases have been reported. Nineteen is the average age at which clear cell carcinoma develops. The youngest case has been identified at 7 years of age and the oldest at 33. The incidence rises sharply at 14 years of age, with the peak at 19 years (Deppe & Lawrence, 1988).

In recent years, early detection with cervical cytology and rigid criteria that identify vaginal tumors as arising from other genital sites has resulted in a decrease in the incidence of primary vaginal cancers (Perez, Gersell, Hoskins, & McGuire, 1992).

RISK FACTORS

The major risk factors associated with the development of vaginal cancer are listed in Box 34-1. The evidence supporting each of these risk factors is reviewed, and the nursing implications for prevention and early detection activities are discussed.

With the exception of the casual relationship between in utero exposure to DES, the literature is sparse and conflicting with regard to the suggested risk factors predisposing women to vaginal carcinoma.

Chronic Irritation

Prolonged exposure of the vaginal mucosa to irritants is the premise underlying one theory of the etiology of vaginal squamous carcinoma. Because most tumors are located near the posterior fornix, a pooling effect has been suggested as a causative factor. However, there is no specific data to support the relationship between vaginal cancer and a chronic irritant such as pessaries. Although infrequent today, chronic or irritant vaginitis was commonly seen when pessaries were used therapeutically for uterine prolapse. The vaginal mucosa showed a thickening and inflammation, as well as metaplastic and dysplastic alterations, when pessaries were left in place for long periods (Merino, 1991).

Previous Hysterectomy for Benign Disease

Previous hysterectomy for benign disease may be a predisposing factor in primary vaginal cancer. One study (Bell, Bernd-uwe, Averette, & Nadji, 1984) reported a 36% incidence of vaginal carcinoma in 86 women who had a hysterectomy performed for benign disease. However, in a more recent study, the association between hysterectomy and vaginal cancer was not observed (Herman, Homesley, & Dignan, 1986). They compared 49 women with vaginal cancer with 49 control subjects matched for age, race, and a prior history of dysplasia or neoplasia. Findings from this study indicated that hysterectomy was associated with a very low risk for the development of vaginal cancer.

Irradiation for Cervical Disease

Irradiation for cervical cancer has been implicated as a risk factor for vaginal cancer. According to Merino (1991) many investigators support this concept. The amount of radiation that the vagina is exposed to, when the cervix is being radiated, may be sufficient to have a mutagenic effect. It is es-

Box 34-1
Risk Factors for Vaginal Cancer

Chronic irritation (e.g., pessaries)
Previous hysterectomy for benign disease
Irradiation for cervical disease
Immunosuppressive therapy
Viral infections (e.g., herpes simplex virus, human papilloma virus
DES exposure in utero

timated that 50% of women receiving cervical irradiation may develop dysplasias or in situ carcinomas (Merino, 1991). A study supporting this association was reported by Pride, Schultz, & Chuprevich (1979) who found that 5 of 43 women studied presented with invasive carcinoma of the vagina 7 years after radiation therapy for invasive cervical carcinoma. However, analysis of a 20-year follow-up of 1200 women failed to demonstrate the development of a second neoplasm following radiation therapy for cervical cancer (Lee, Perez, & Ettinger, 1982).

Immunosuppressive Therapy

Immunosuppressive therapy is another factor that may predispose women to vaginal cancer. Merino (1991) notes that in situ vaginal cancer has been found in organ recipients as well as in women with conditions such as chronic granulomatous disease. Vaginal tumors may present either as an isolated process or as part of a neoplastic syndrome of the lower genital tract. In addition, immunosuppression may increase the risk of certain viral infections associated with genital cancers.

Viral Infections

In recent years, viral infections such as herpes simplex virus (HSV) or human papillomavirus (HPV) have been implicated as an etiologic factor in the development of vaginal cancer. The infections follow the pattern of venereal disease and, except in rare cases, do not appear before the onset of sexual activity. Although there are more than 50 types of HPV, 12 are associated with lesions of the anogenital tract. Types 16 and 18 have been linked with squamous cell carcinomas (Merino, 1991). During malignant transformation, the virus becomes integrated into the human cells, with DNA abnormalities arising as the cells replicate.

Although it appears that infection with HPV contributes to the development of carcinoma, it has been proposed that HSV-2 infection may precede HPV infection and that the two may be essential to inducing squamous cell carcinoma (Merino, 1991).

DES Exposure In Utero

In utero exposure to DES and the subsequent development of clear cell adenocarcinoma of the vagina in young women has long been a well-recognized risk factor. Recently, the risk has been found to be higher for women whose mothers received DES before the twelfth week of gestation (Merino, 1991). The dose and duration of DES treatment of mothers of affected daughters have not been identified as a major factor (DiSaia & Creasman, 1993). However, factors such as a maternal history of prior miscarriage, birth in the fall, and prematurity may increase the risk for clear cell vaginal cancer in certain women exposed to DES in utero (Herbst, Anderson, & Hubby, 1986).

Melnick, Cole, Anderson, & Herbst (1987) postulated that DES is an incomplete carcinogen and other cofactors may be involved in the development of clear cell vaginal carcinoma. It appears that many DES daughters who develop clear cell vaginal adenocarcinoma are also infected with HPV. With the decreasing incidence of the malignancy in recent years, many unanswered questions remain as to the association of cofactors related to maternal complications (e.g., decreased birth weight), immunologic deficiencies, and the role of viruses in the development of clear cell adenocarcinoma.

DiSaia and Creasman (1993) note that the increased rate of prior spontaneous abortions and a history of vaginal bleeding during pregnancy among mothers whose daughters developed vaginal cancer raise the possibility that an inherited genetic predisposing factor may play a role in some cases.

Nursing Implications

Because the vaginal wall is highly distensible, it can accommodate the growth of a large tumor before the onset of symptoms. Unfortunately, many older women avoid medical care when symptoms develop, and diagnosis is delayed. Because vaginal cancer occurs in a clinically accessible site with the opportunity for earlier diagnosis and treatment, oncology nurses can play an important role in educating women about the signs, symptoms, and need for periodic examinations with their health care team.

Currently, there are no effective guidelines for the prevention and screening of women for vaginal cancer. However, nurses have the opportunity to play an important role in educating women who are sexually active or 18 years of age or older to have routine gynecologic examinations. In addition, nurses should educate women with predisposing factors (i.e., history of genital cancer, cervical dysplasia, HPV infection, previous irradiation for cervical cancer, or a hysterectomy for benign disease) to have vigilant follow-up by their health care team. Women with in utero DES exposure may have an increased risk of cervical neoplasia. As these women grow older and approach the age of peak incidence of invasive cancer, close follow-up will be required to exclude a higher risk (Bengtson, 1995).

PATHOPHYSIOLOGY

Normal Anatomy and Physiology of the Vagina

The vagina is an elastic fibromuscular canal 9 to 10 cm long that extends from the vestibule of the vulva to the uterine cervix, thereby interfacing with both the external and internal environment. The vagina is located posterior to the urinary bladder and anterior to the rectum (see Fig. 30-1, p. 691). The proximal third of the urethra is separated from the vagina by loose connective tissue and enters into the vaginal wall.

The mucous membrane lining of the vaginal wall consists of squamous epithelial cells. In response to hormones, such as estrogen, this lining thickens and thins. The vaginal wall consists of three layers: the mucosa, the muscularis, and the adventitia. The mucosal layer, which is arranged in transverse folds known as *rugae,* expands during childbirth. The middle layer consists of fibrous connective tissue containing numerous blood and lymph vessels. Smooth muscle constitutes the third layer.

Blood is supplied to the vagina by branches of the internal iliac artery, and a network of veins that surround the vagina drain into the interior iliac vein. The vagina is the passageway through which menstrual fluid passes from the uterus and through which the fetus is delivered; it is commonly referred to as the *birth canal.*

The Process of Carcinogenesis

As with other cancers, development of vaginal cancer may involve premalignant disease. Premalignant lesions of the vagina termed *vaginal intraepithelial neoplasia* (VAIN) have replaced older terminology of *dysplasia-carcinomas in situ.* The etiology of VAIN is unclear but may be related to an HPV infection (Deppe & Lawrence, 1988). The vaginal intraepithelium goes through a continuum of changes beginning with grade I (mild dysplasia) through grade II (moderate dysplasia) to grade III (severe dysplasia) or carcinoma in situ. The transit times for progression from a lesser degree of VAIN to invasive squamous cell carcinoma is poorly studied but appears to be slow (Deppe & Lawrence, 1988). Lesions may be single or multifocal and occur most frequently in the upper vagina. There is no certainty that these premalignant intraepithelial neoplasias will progress to vaginal cancer.

Most primary vaginal cancers are squamous cell in origin and may have different appearances on gross examination. Tumors may grow in a cauliflower-like fashion, or be infiltrative, nodular, or ulcerative (Merino, 1991). Histologically, squamous cell carcinomas of the vagina are similar to squamous cell tumors in other sites. Three histologic grades are recognized: well differentiated, moderately differentiated, and poorly differentiated. Although the grade assigned to a tumor is based on a combination of cytologic and histologic features, there is little correlation between tumor grade and survival (Perez, Gerse II, Hoskins, & McGuire et al., 1992). Primary vaginal squamous cell carcinomas most commonly arise from the posterior wall in the upper third of the vagina. The anterior wall of the lower third of the vagina is the next common site of origin (Deppe & Lawrence, 1988).

Much attention has been directed at the issue of iatrogenic carcinogenesis of clear cell carcinoma of the vagina associated with DES exposure in utero. In 1971, the Registry for Research on Hormonal Transplacental Carcinogenesis was established to study the clinical, epidemiologic, and pathologic aspects of this carcinoma.

Exposure to DES during the first 3 months of gestation inhibits the normal replacement of columnar epithelium by squamous epithelium in the vagina of the fetus. The columnar epithelium, which is not normally found in the vagina, may undergo malignant transformation.

Another structural abnormality of the genital tract that is prevalent in more than 90% of DES-exposed women is vaginal adenosis and is characterized by the presence of glandular-columnar epithelium and its mucinous secretary products. The strong association between adenosis and prenatal DES exposure suggests that the drug interferes with normal vaginal development (Bengtson, 1995). Vaginal adenosis is characterized by excessive vaginal secretions. White metaplastic changes may convert the columnar epithelium to the squamous type. The progression of adenosis to a carcinoma has not been identified (Bengtson, 1995).

ROUTES OF METASTASES

Cancers of the vagina spread by direct extension and through both lymphatic and hematogenous routes. Direct extension into the soft tissue of the pelvis or to the mucosa of the bladder or rectum occurs early because the vaginal wall is thin and separated from these organs by only a few millimeters of connective tissue (Zaino et al., 1994).

If the tumor occurs in the upper region of the vagina, lymphatic spread is through the obturator, iliac, and hypogastric lymph nodes. Tumors arising in the lower region of the vagina spread through inguinal nodes and then into the deep pelvic nodes (DiSaia & Creasman, 1993). Recurrent disease is usually local and occurs within 2 years, but metastasis may be discovered in the lung or supraclavicular nodes.

Squamous cell carcinoma, which composes 85% of vaginal cancers, initially spreads superficially within the vaginal wall, later invading the paravaginal tissue. Metastasis occurs most commonly in the lungs and liver.

ASSESSMENT

Clinical evaluation involves a detailed history, a thorough physical examination, and a variety of diagnostic tests (Table 34-1). The signs and symptoms often depend on the stage of disease at the time of diagnosis.

History

The patient should be evaluated for all the identified risk factors for vaginal cancer. In addition, a careful history of the genital, genitourinary, and gastrointestinal system should be obtained (Hall, Dewar, & Perchalski, 1992).

Tumors arising from the anterior vaginal wall may cause urinary symptoms, whereas posterior wall tumors may be associated with bowel symptoms. There is a relationship between the duration of symptoms and size and spread of tumor. Pain, if it occurs, depends on the location and size of the tumor and is often indicative of advanced disease.

Sexual History

A baseline history that includes sexual functioning, non–cancer-related dysfunction, and concerns related to treat-

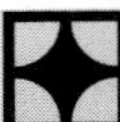

TABLE 34-1 Assessment of the Patient for Vaginal Cancer

	Assessment Parameters	Typical Abnormal Findings
History	A. Personal and social history	A. Personal and social risk factors
	1. Age	1. Usually over 60 for squamous cell carcinoma; peak age for clear cell carcinoma is 19 years of age
	2. Use of pessaries	2. Chronic irritation suggested as a causative factor
	3. Previous hysterectomy for benign disease	3. Considered a predisposing factor
	4. Irradiation for cervical disease	4. Suggested as having a mutagenic effect on the vaginal mucosa
	5. Immunosuppressive therapy	5. Considered to increase the risk of certain viral infections associated with genital cancer
	6. Viral infections Herpes simplex virus (HSV) Human papilloma virus (HPV)	6. Implicated as an etiologic factor
	7. Diethylstilbestrol (DES)	7. Recognized as a strong risk factor in young women
	B. Evaluation of systems:	B. Common symptoms include:
	1. Genital	1. Painless vaginal bleeding; spotting or discharge and/or dyspareunia
	2. Genitourinary	2. Dysuria, frequency and/or hematuria
	3. Gastrointestinal	3. Tenesmus; melena; pain
	C. Evaluation of pain	C. Symptom of advanced disease or infection. The nature of the pain depends on the location and size of the tumor
	D. Baseline sexual history 1. Frequency 2. Patterns of sexual activity 3. Attitudes about potential changes caused by treatment 4. Cultural and personal sexual preferences 5. Importance of sexuality in patient's relationship with a partner	
Physical Examination	A. Pelvic examination 1. Speculum examination of entire vagina and cervix 2. Palpation of both inguinal areas and pelvic organs	A. Identifies presence of tumor and extent of disease
Diagnostic Tests	A. Papanicolaou smear (Pap smear)	A. An abnormal Pap smear is usually the event that initiates the search for a definitive diagnosis since many lesions are asymptomatic
	B. Colposcopically directed biopsy	B. Confirms tumor type; determines size, location, and extent of disease
	C. Cystoscopy	C. Performed to assess for bladder invasion
	D. Sigmoidoscopy	D. Performed to rule out rectal invasion
	E. Intravenous pyelogram	E. Vaginal tumors may be in close proximity to the bladder neck and compress the urethra
	F. Barium enema	F. Performed to rule out rectal invasion
	G. Computerized tomography (CT) of pelvis and abdomen	G. Detects metastasis to pelvis and aortic lymph nodes
	H. Magnetic resonance imaging (MRI)	H. Shown to yield high positive values in identifying primary and metastatic disease
	I. Chest x-ray	I. Assess for metastatic disease

ment should be obtained. The patient's spouse or significant other should be present during the discussion.

According to Lamb (1990), nurses must be comfortable and knowledgeable regarding the topics of sexuality to assess, plan, and counsel patients and their partners. Some women may be uncomfortable revealing their sexual preferences, and nurses must communicate with an open, accepting attitude.

Different techniques can be used that may provide a comfortable environment for discussing sexual matters for both the nurse and patient. Lamb (1990) suggests a technique that involves moving from a less sensitive to a more sensitive topic so that abruptness and anxiety may be decreased. Assessing patients' activity patterns and attitudes about potential changes caused by treatment will assist the nurse in identifying potential body image disturbances (Cartwright-Alcarese, 1995).

Physical Examination

Many women report no symptoms, and the diagnosis is established by pelvic examination. Bleeding may occur only with intercourse or douching. All areas of the vagina and adjacent pelvic organs must be examined, including palpation of inguinal areas, to establish spread of the primary tumor or metastatic spread from tumors of the cervix, endometrium, vulva, bladder, or rectum. The presence of inguinal lymph nodes may indicate the presence of metastatic disease from either the primary vaginal cancer or spread from other genital cancers.

Diagnostic Tests

Papanicolaou Smear. The majority of vaginal cancers present in the upper third posterior portion of the vagina. Because of this presentation, the Papanicolaou (Pap) smear is an important diagnostic tool, especially in women with a prior history of hysterectomy (Chamorro, 1990). A cytologic specimen is usually obtained from the pooled secretions of the posterior vagina.

Colposcopic Directed Biopsy. Colposcopic examination of the vagina is difficult. The vaginal speculum must be repositioned several times to visualize the entire mucosal surface. An iodine stain, such as Schiller's solution, may be used to identify abnormal areas. Normal vaginal epithelial cells stain brown because of the high glycogen content. Dysplastic cells often contain less glycogen and therefore do not take up the dye (Bengtson, 1995).

Metastatic Workup. The metastatic workups for squamous cell carcinoma and clear cell adenocarcinoma are similar and include an evaluation of the pelvic and aortic lymph nodes preferably by computerized tomography (CT) scan. In addition, a cystoscopy and intravenous pyelogram should be performed to detect any bladder or ureter involvement. A sigmoidoscopy and barium enema are also necessary to rule out metastatic spread to the rectum. A chest x-ray is performed to assess for distant metastasis to the lung.

Diagnosis of Vaginal Cancer. The diagnosis of primary vaginal cancer requires that the cervix and vulva be intact and that no clinical evidence of the primary tumors exist (Merino, 1991). Because vaginal tumors resemble those in nearby structures, many authors do not accept a vaginal tumor as a primary tumor if it occurs in a woman with a history of cervical cancer. Generally, it is accepted as a primary tumor in women with a 5-year disease-free interval after treatment for invasive carcinoma and after a 2-year interval between a diagnosis of carcinoma in situ and the newly diagnosed vaginal tumor (Merino, 1991).

The diagnosis of squamous cell carcinoma is confirmed by biopsy of a visible, palpable vaginal lesion. Tumors may vary in appearance and may present as superficial plaques, ulcerative lesions, or exophytic growths (Bengston, 1995).

According to DiSaia and Creasman (1993), the diagnosis of squamous cell vaginal cancer is usually delayed, because many patients are elderly, sexually inactive, and unlikely to have periodic examinations. In addition, because these carcinomas are rare, physicians often fail to consider the possibility until the patient has symptoms of advanced disease. The diagnosis of clear cell adenocarcinoma most often can be accomplished with a digital examination and a Pap smear (Deppe & Lawrence, 1988).

STAGING

The staging of vaginal cancer as developed by the International Federation of Gynecology and Obstetrics (FIGO) is listed in Table 34-2 and is based on a clinical rather than a pathologic examination. In addition, a chest x-ray, intravenous pyelogram, cystoscopy, and proctosigmoidoscopy are performed to determine local and metastatic spread.

For a tumor to be considered a primary vaginal carcinoma, it must be located in the vagina without clinical or histologic evidence of involvement of the cervix or vulva. Squamous cell carcinomas of the vagina occurring within 5 years of cervical cancer are staged as recurrent cervical carcinomas.

TABLE 34-2 FIGO* Staging System for Primary Vaginal Cancer

Stage	Description
0	Carcinoma in situ, intraepithelial carcinoma
I	Carcinoma limited to the vaginal wall
II	Carcinoma involving the subvaginal tissue but not extending into the pelvic wall
III	Carcinoma extending into the pelvic wall
IV	Carcinoma extending beyond the true pelvis or involving the mucosa of the bladder or rectum (bullous edema, as such, does not permit a case to be allotted to stage IV)
IVA	Spread of the growth to adjacent organs and/or direct extension beyond the true pelvis
IVB	Spread to distant organs

*FIGO, International Federation of Gynecology and Obstetrics.

MEDICAL MANAGEMENT

Treatment of vaginal cancer depends on several factors including patient age, the patient's general state of health, the patient's desire for vaginal function, the patient's childbearing status, tumor volume and location, histologic grade of the tumor, and stage of the disease.

Radiation Therapy

Radiation therapy is the primary treatment for patients with squamous cell vaginal carcinoma, which accounts for about 90% of vaginal tumors. Radiation therapy is administered through an external beam approach and/or through internal implants.

External Beam Radiation Therapy. For patients with squamous cell carcinoma (bulky stage I, stage II, stage III, and stage IV with pelvic disease only), tumors are treated initially with external beam radiation (Table 34-3). A dose of 4000 to 5000 cGy is given over 5 to 6 weeks to shrink the neoplasm so that local radiation therapy will be more effective. In patients with stage III and IV tumors, the deep pelvic nodes are included in the treatment field, because large tumors have a higher incidence of regional metastasis (DiSaia & Creasman, 1993).

In clear cell adenocarcinoma of the vagina, external beam therapy to the whole pelvis is used after surgery for patients with tumors in the upper one third of the vagina (stage I) (Table 34-4) (DiSaia & Creasman, 1993).

Internal Radiation Therapy. Radiation delivered for local disease with an active radiation source is known as *brachytherapy*. The implantation techniques may be described as interstitial or intracavity. Interstitial brachytherapy occurs when small radioactive sources are surgically implanted directly into the target tissue. Intracavitary therapy uses tandem or colposot applicators with appropriate sources that are inserted into a body cavity in proximity to the target tissue. A catheter or applicator is placed intracavitary or near the tumor site, and the radiation source is placed through the catheter or applicator. Remote afterloading equipment (Fig. 34-1) is used to deliver high-dose radiation by automatically controlling the radioactive source. This treatment takes only 15 minutes.

The goal of interstitial or intracavity brachytherapy in the management of vaginal cancer is to deliver a predetermined dose of radiation that is effective enough to destroy the tumor cells while keeping side effects to a minimum (Philips, Dattatreyuda, & Peschel, 1990).

TABLE 34-3 Radiotherapy for Vaginal Cancer

Stage	External Irradiation	Vaginal Therapy
0	Surgical excision preferred for localized disease	7000 cGy surface doses
I (1-2 cm lesion)	Not indicated	Interstitial irradiation, 6000-7000 cGy
I (larger lesion)	4000-5000 cGy whole pelvis	Interstitial implant delivering 3000-4000 cGy
II	4000-5000 cGy whole pelvis	Same as above
III	5000 cGy whole pelvis (optional 1000-2000 cGy through reduced fields)	Interstitial implant, 2000-3000 cGy (if tumor regression is optimal)
IV (pelvis only)	Same as above	Same as above

From DiSaia, P. J. & Creasman, W. T. (1993). Invasive cancer of the vagina and urethra. In P. J. DiSaia & W. T. Creasman (Eds.), *Clinical gynecologic oncology*. St. Louis: Mosby.

TABLE 34-4 Suggested Management of Clear Cell Adenocarcinoma of the Vagina

Stage	Surgery	Radiation
I (upper one third of vagina)	Radical hysterectomy Bilateral pelvic lymphadenectomy Upper vaginectomy	5000 cGy WP in patients with positive lymph nodes
I (lower two thirds of vagina)	Radical hysterectomy Bilateral pelvic lymphadenectomy Total vaginectomy Vaginal reconstruction	5000 cGy WP vaginal application or interstitial implant
II	Consider pelvic exenteration for radiation failures	5000 cGy WP interstitial implant
III	Consider pelvic exenteration for radiation failures	6000 cGy interstitial implant
IV	Individualize	

WP, Whole pelvis.
From DiSaia, P. J. & Creasman, W. T. (1993). Invasive cancer of the vagina and urethra. In P. J. DiSaia & W. T. Creasman (Eds.), *Clinical gynecologic oncology*. St. Louis: Mosby.

Small squamous cell carcinoma of the vagina (stage 0) may be treated with interstitial radiation alone (not in combination with external beam radiation). A minimum of 6000 to 7000 cGy is delivered to the tumor in 5 to 7 days. Patients with larger neoplasms (stage I, stage II, stage III, and stage IV with only pelvic disease) require an interstitial implant with a treatment dose between 2000 and 3000 cGy. Interstitial implants are delivered by applicators such as Fletcher-Suit, Delclos, and Syed-Neblett. The Syed-Neblett applicator is illustrated in Fig. 34-2.

The short- and long-term sequelae associated with radiation to normal tissue, such as the bladder and rectum, depend mainly on the location of the tumor. During or shortly after therapy, as many as 35% of patients experience early side effects such as cystitis or proctitis. These symptoms usually resolve within a short time (DiSaia & Creasman, 1993).

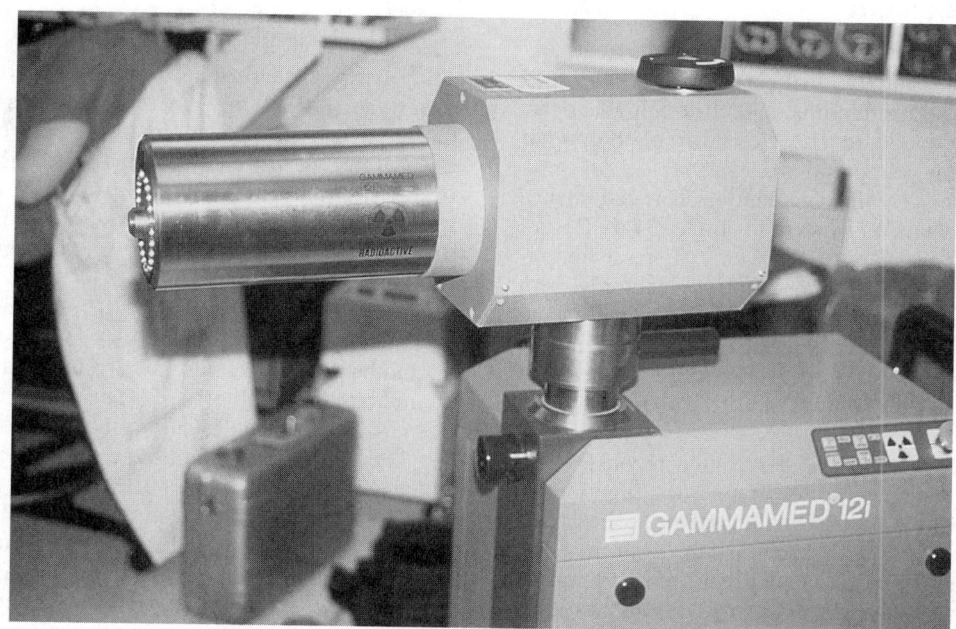

Fig. 34-1 Remote afterload machine. (Courtesy Dr. Borys Mychalczak, Radiation Oncology Department, Memorial Sloan-Kettering Cancer Center.)

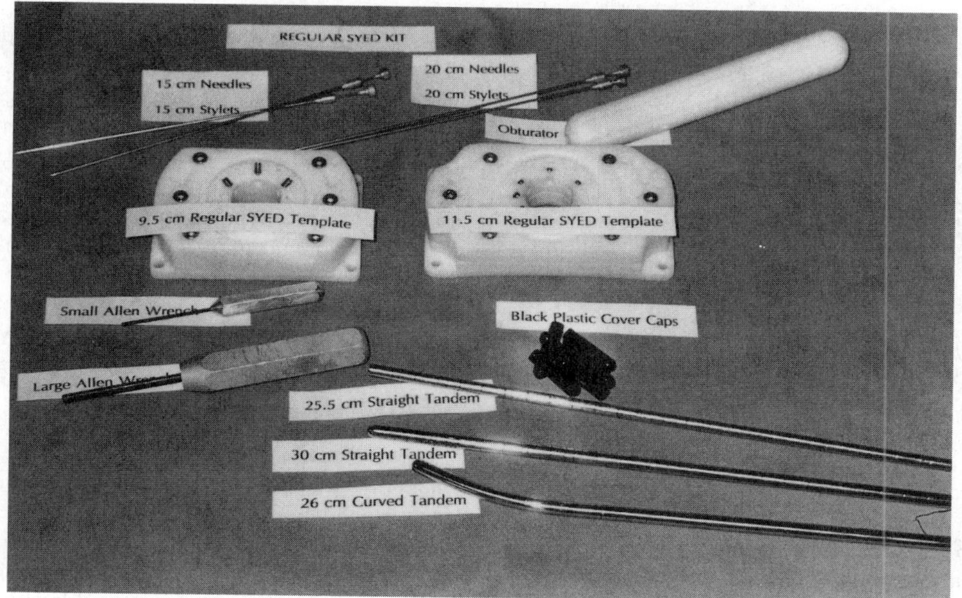

Fig. 34-2 The Syed-Neblett template. (Courtesy Dr. Borys Mychalczak, Radiation Oncology Department, Memorial Sloan-Kettering Cancer Center.)

Although the incidence of complications following radiation therapy is relatively low, serious complications occur in approximately 10% of patients and consist primarily of rectal stenosis, rectovaginal fistula, and severe rectal bleeding requiring diversion. In addition, a small number of patients experience extensive vaginal necrosis that usually resolves with prolonged conservative management (DiSaia & Creasman, 1993).

Surgical Management

Surgical excisions have been recommended as the treatment of choice for patients with vaginal carcinoma in situ, early invasive squamous cell carcinoma, and clear cell adenocarcinoma, as it may facilitate the preservation of optimal sexual functioning in young patients.

The suggested surgical management of clear cell adenocarcinoma of the vagina is listed in Table 34-4. Before radiation therapy, a radical hysterectomy, bilateral lymphadenectomy, and either partial or total vaginectomy with vaginal reconstruction are performed in patients with stage I disease. A radical hysterectomy consists of the removal of the uterus, cervix, adjacent supporting tissues, the uppermost part of the vagina, and the pelvic lymph nodes.

The patient may opt to have her vagina reconstructed. This procedure may or may not be done at the time of surgery. The best time for reconstruction seems to be at the time of surgery for the following reasons: the anatomy is restored, only one procedure is needed, and most important the woman's femininity is preserved. In addition the procedure helps fill the pelvic cavity, provides support for the intestines, introduces a source of vasculature, reduces exudate from the pelvic walls, and decreases the postoperative course.

Two techniques are used to reconstruct the vagina. In one type, the William procedure, a perineal pouch is formed by using labial skin and subcutaneous tissue. This procedure requires less operative time. However, the neovagina is hairy and may be displeasing. In addition, the angle of the neovagina makes sexual intercourse in any customary position difficult. A split-thickness graft using skin and muscle flaps resected from the gracilis muscle on the inner aspect of the thigh is used to construct the vagina. In the second technique, a tube is constructed that is inverted anteriorly into the pelvic cavity to replace the original vagina. Within 6 weeks sexual intercourse may be resumed, but it may take 6 months to 1 year for patients and their partners to attain satisfaction with vaginal function (Chamorro, 1990). The effect of vaginal reconstruction on women is not yet known. These procedures provide women with the opportunity to continue vaginal intercourse. The patient and her partner must receive education and support to adjust to the physical and psychological changes (Martello & Vasconez, 1995).

Surgery is also used for patients who develop recurrent local or persistent disease after radiation therapy. Ultraradical surgery referred to as *pelvic exenteration* encompasses removal of the uterus, bladder, and/or rectum and vagina (Barber, 1982). Little has been reported in the literature on this procedure for the management of vaginal cancers.

Chemotherapy

Chemotherapy with topical 5-fluorouracil (5-FU) is one of the modalities used for the treatment of carcinoma in situ. It offers the advantage of treating the entire vaginal mucosa, which has the potential to have multifocal lesions (Bengtson, 1995).

Chemotherapy for recurrent squamous cell and clear cell adenocarcinoma has been relatively ineffective. A phase II study using cisplatin had disappointing results (DiSaia & Creasman, 1993). Only isolated responses to individual cytotoxic agents have been noted. Several chemotherapeutic agents (e.g., doxorubicin [Adriamycin], 5-FU, methotrexate [MTX], mitomycin [mitomycin C], vincristine [Oncovin], cyclophosphamide [Cytoxan], and/or dactinomycin [actinomycin]) have been used with no total remissions observed (DiSaia & Creasman, 1993).

The role of chemotherapy is being investigated in the treatment of vaginal cancer. A list of most commonly used chemotherapeutic agents, side effects, and toxicities are summarized in Table 34-5. The ideal chemotherapeutic agent(s) has not been found for the treatment of vaginal cancer. There is a need for well-controlled studies to explore the efficacy of chemotherapy in the treatment of vaginal cancer. However, vaginal cancer is the rarest of the gynecologic cancers; therefore, sample sizes are limited. At present, there is limited use of chemotherapy in the treatment of vaginal cancer. In addition, no documented objective responses have been observed with the use of progestational agents.

ONCOLOGIC EMERGENCIES

The oncologic emergency associated with vaginal cancer is sepsis. Patients with cancer are at risk for developing sepsis. The cancer treatment as well as the disease itself place the patient at risk for infection. The early clinical signs and symptoms may include chills, rigors, fever, subnormal temperature, malaise, tachycardia, tachypnea, and generalized complaints of discomfort. Late signs and symptoms may include cool skin, hypotension, hyperventilation and respiratory failure, mental changes including confusion, and oliguria and anuria. It is essential that the nurse identify whether the patient is at risk for sepsis, as prompt recognition and management of sepsis affect the mortality rate.

NURSING MANAGEMENT

As illustrated in Tables 34-3 and 34-4, the medical management of vaginal cancer is extremely complex and individualized depending on the patient's age, desire for reproduction, sexual function, general clinical condition, and stage of disease at the time of diagnosis. Because of the rarity of this malignancy, there is a scarcity of publications on the nursing management of patients with vaginal cancer. Information addressing nursing management is often combined with other

Table 34-5 Side Effects and Toxicities of Chemotherapy

Agents	Myelosuppression	Nausea & Vomiting	Stomatitis	Alopecia	Nephrotoxicity	Neurotoxicity	Vesicant	Cardiotoxicity	Photosensitivity	Pulmonary Toxicity	Diarrhea	Darkening of Veins Used For Admin.	Hypersensitivity Reaction	HUS/Hemolytic Uremia Syndrome	Constipation	Hemorrhagic Cystitis
Alkylating																
Cisplatin (Platinol, CIS-DDP)	X	X	X		X	X		possible					X			
Cyclophosphamide (Cytoxan)	X	X		X				X								X
Antimetabolites																
5-Fluorouracil (Adracil)	X	X	X						X		X	X				
Antitumors Antibiotics																
Doxorubicin hydrochloride (Adriamycin)	X	X	X	X			X	X	X				X			
Mitomycin (Mutamycin, mitomycin C)	X	X	X	X	X		X			X	X					
Mitotic Inhibitors																
Vincristine (Oncovin)	X			X		X	X						X		X	

X, Side effects.

gynecologic cancer publications or chapters (Chamorro, 1990; Martin & Braly, 1991; Walczak & Klemm, 1993). Patients with vaginal cancer have numerous problems requiring nursing and patient education. Although a portion of patient care occurs in the inpatient setting, the majority of patient care occurs in the outpatient and home care settings.

Newly Diagnosed Patient

Early in the course of the patient's disease, nursing care should focus on assisting the patient in understanding the different treatment modalities. The nursing management of patients newly diagnosed with vaginal cancer is summarized in Table 34-6. During the treatment phase, the patient will require information about managing the side effects associated with the patient's specific treatments. Radiation and surgery are the two major treatment modalities, with each posing unique patient problems that are described in Tables 34-7 through 34-9 pp. 798-803. At the present time, chemotherapy has a limited role in the treatment of vaginal cancer. The nursing management is outlined in Table 34-10.

Radiation Therapy

Approximately 90% of patients with vaginal cancer have squamous cell carcinoma, which except for very small lesions, requires external beam therapy followed by interstitial brachytherapy. External beam therapy is provided on an outpatient basis. The major problems associated with external beam radiation therapy include fatigue, diarrhea, cystitis, and proctitis.

Interstitial brachytherapy is done in the inpatient or outpatient setting. The following side effects are associated with brachytherapy: proctitis, cystitis, fibrosis of the vagina, necrosis, and fistulae formation. Patients require a great deal of education to understand the precautions that must be instituted while they are receiving therapy (Tables 34-7 and 34-8). A specific standard for knowledge deficit for the patients receiving brachytherapy is provided in Table 34-8. Patients receiving brachytherapy should be instructed to receive nothing by mouth after midnight, and to take a Fleet enema and a vaginal douche. This is accomplished in the procedure room in 1 to 2 hours. An intravenous line is inserted, the patient's vital signs are monitored, and oxygen

Text continued on p. 800

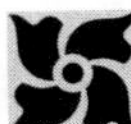 **TABLE 34-6 Standard of Care for the Patient Newly Diagnosed with Vaginal Cancer**

Patient Problem and Outcomes	Nursing Interventions and Rationales	Patient Education Instructions
Anxiety Related to New Diagnosis		
Patient will: • Be able to verbalize concerns, fears, and questions • Experience a decrease in anxiety as evidenced by a decrease in the signs and symptoms of anxiety	1. Assess for signs and symptoms of anxiety. 2. Establish a relationship with the patient. 3. Assess effectiveness of coping skills. 4. Anticipate patient's needs. 5. Orient patient to environment. 6. Provide a calm, supportive, reassuring environment and reduce external stimuli. 7. Encourage verbalization of feelings and concerns. 8. Maintain a calm and tolerant manner. 9. Monitor changes in level of anxiety. 10. Administer antianxiety medications as prescribed, if necessary. 11. Instruct patient about anxiety. Education reduces patient's anxiety level.	1. Provide patient with information about anxiety: a. Signs and symptoms b. Factors leading to anxious feelings c. Alternatives to prevent anxiety d. Relaxation exercises e. Reduction of stimuli
Knowledge Deficit Related to Early Detection and Diagnosis of Vaginal Cancer		
Patient will demonstrate knowledge related to early detection/ diagnosis of vaginal cancer	1. Assess past experience with the diagnosis of cancer and cancer treatment. 2. Determine present knowledge base and major concerns regarding diagnosis and treatment. 3. Assess readiness and ability to learn. 4. Assess risk factors. 5. Obtain history of signs and symptoms of bleeding. 6. Assess gynecologic status. 7. Review American Cancer Society (ACS) guidelines. 8. Explain all tests and procedures. 9. Encourage verbalization of feelings and concerns. 10. Provide psychological and spiritual support.	1. Patient education should include: a. Teach importance of proper nutrition and weight control. b. Stress importance of regular checkups. c. Teach signs and symptoms to report: (1) Changes in bleeding patterns (2) Breakthrough bleeding (3) Irregular menses (4) Bleeding occurring 6 months after cessation of menses in postmenopausal women 2. Teach patient the need for regular gynecologic check-ups: a. Instruct patient on ACS guidelines: pelvic examination every 3 years for woman 20-40 years old or older annually.

TABLE 34-6 Standard of Care for the Patient Newly Diagnosed with Vaginal Cancer—cont'd

Patient Problem and Outcomes	Nursing Interventions and Rationales	Patient Education Instructions
		b. Educate about Pap smear. c. Discuss importance of follow-up for abnormal symptoms. d. Discuss lifestyle behaviors (e.g., diet, weight control, and exercise). e. Discuss treatment options when appropriate.
Grieving Patient will: • Identify areas of potential or real loss • Be able to recall past experiences with loss and use appropriate coping strategies • Identify roles and changes in relationships • Verbalize concerns	1. Assess patient's understanding of current health status and potential loss. 2. Teach patient about loss and grief to help her understand and identify feelings. In addition, providing accurate information to prevent misconceptions and decrease fear. 3. Give patient permission to grieve. 4. Discuss the reality of actual loss with patient. 5. Assess patient's response to loss. 6. Promote positive communication among family members/significant others. 7. Lead discussion of problems and solutions with patient and significant others. 8. Facilitate patient's inquiry/discussion of implications of health care proxy, living will, and code status. 9. Encourage and maintain hope.	1. Instruct patient about the process of grieving and loss, including: a. Normal responses to loss (include the stages of grief) b. Knowledge that individuals do not go through all the stages in sequence and may move back and forth c. Grieving is a normal response to a real or potential loss d. Grieving begins at time of diagnosis e. Grief response may be different for each person f. Importance of sharing information about diagnosis and role changes to foster mutual understanding with trust g. Importance of mutual acceptance and understanding of each other during the process h. The need for support i. The importance of maintaining health and welfare of the patient j. The importance of memories and the best way to preserve the memories

TABLE 34-7 Standard of Care for the Patient Receiving External Beam Radiation Therapy for Vaginal Cancer

Patient Problem and Outcomes	Nursing Interventions and Rationales	Patient Education Instructions
Knowledge Deficit Related to Radiation Therapy		
Patient will: • Demonstrate knowledge of radiation therapy including purpose, benefits, and risk • Demonstrate knowledge related to treatment procedure and plan • Demonstrate knowledge related to managing side effects • Prevent/minimize/fatigue • Promote adequate nutritional and fluid intake	1. Assess patient's knowledge of diagnosis and treatment plan. 2. Assess patient's physical and psychosocial status. 3. Assess patient's concerns and fears about radiation therapy.	1. Teach patient about: a. Principles of radiation therapy b. Treatment procedures (i.e., consultation, simulation procedure, treatment and routine) c. Describe follow-up care d. Maintain adequate nutrition e. Describe side effects, stress the importance of notifying the health care member and self-care measures to manage the side effects of: (1) Diarrhea (2) Cystitis (3) Alteration in vaginal mucous membranes (4) Fatigue
Diarrhea		
Patient will: • Demonstrate strategies to prevent diarrhea • Achieve control or correction of diarrhea	1. Assess usual pattern of elimination including use of laxatives. 2. Assess pattern of diarrhea including the onset, duration, character, amount and frequency of the stools. 3. Assess for the presence of associated symptoms such as flatus, cramping, abdominal distention, fatigue, rectal area excoriation and the aggravation of hemorrhoids. 4. Assess nutritional status including weight. 5. Encourage fluid intake of at least 2500 ml/day, unless contraindicated. 6. Maintain low-residue, bland, high-protein, high-carbohydrate, balanced diet. 7. Monitor intake and output. 8. Increase foods high in potassium. 9. Try small frequent meals. 10. Obtain a dietary consult, if necessary. 11. Weight weekly. 12. Sitz bath as needed. 13. Administer antidiarrheal agent as prescribed.	1. Instruct patient to avoid certain liquids (e.g., orange juice, prune juice, lemonade, milk, caffeinated beverages) that will increase diarrhea. 2. Instruct patient to avoid extremes in food temperatures. 3. Teach patient to maintain low-residue diet and to avoid foods that are high in roughage, are fried, or highly seasoned, and cooked fruits or vegetables. 4. Suggest foods high in potassium (e.g., bananas, apricot and peach nectars, fish/meat, and potatoes) 5. Teach patients to use antidiarrheal medications. Agents may include Lomotil 2.5 mg 1-2 tablets after each loose stool or loperamide HCL (Imodium) 2 mg after each loose stool or tincture of opium 0.5 to 1 ml q4h until diarrhea is controlled. 6. Instruct patient to: • Monitor intake and output • Follow diet restriction • Take antidiarrheal agents • Use sitz bath • Notify health care professional

TABLE 34-7 Standard of Care for the Patient Receiving External Beam Radiation Therapy for Vaginal Cancer—cont'd

Patient Problem and Outcomes	Nursing Interventions and Rationales	Patient Education Instructions
Cystitis Patient will: • Maintain urinary elimination within normal limits • Identify/demonstrate strategies to prevent or minimize urotoxicity	1. Assess for signs and symptoms of urotoxicity including dysuria, frequency, urgency, and burning. 2. Assess urine for the presence of urinary tract infection and or blood. 3. If infection is present, initiate appropriate antibiotic therapy. 4. Monitor intake and output. 5. Encourage oral intake. 6. Administer bladder/antispasmodics or analgesics as prescribed.	1. Instruct patient to report symptoms that may occur about 2 weeks into the treatment. 2. Instruct patient that phenazopyridine (Pyridium) will color urine orange-red.
Alteration in Vaginal Mucous Membranes Patient will: • Demonstrate knowledge of potential problem • Demonstrate absence of impairment	1. Assess for signs and symptoms of impaired vaginal membrane integrity including pain, soreness, bleeding, discharge, pruritus, or dyspareunia. 2. Observe for signs of impaired vaginal membranes such as erythema, swelling, ulceration, decrease in vaginal size, muscle tone/lubrication and vaginal fibrosis/stenosis. 3. Apply topical medications, as prescribed. 4. Administer systemic medications as prescribed.	1. Instruct patient about preventive practices: a. Gently pat skin dry after bathing. b. After defecation or urination perform perineal care. c. Use cotton-lined underpants. d. Use pantiliner for discharge. e. Avoid tight-fitting slacks, jeans or pantyhose. f. Check with health care professional before douching. 2. Teach patient to use medications: a. Metronidazole (Flagyl) b. Water-soluble lubricant c. Estrogen creams 3. Teach patient strategies to decrease dyspareunia: a. Use of water-soluble lubricant b. Use of estrogen creams c. Female on top position for intercourse 4. Instruct patient how to manage decreased vaginal size and tone: a. Use of vaginal dilators b. Placing of a pillow under the woman's hips for projection and control of penile thrusting c. Kegel exercises

TABLE 34-7 Standard of Care for the Patient Receiving External Beam Radiation Therapy for Vaginal Cancer—cont'd

Patient Problem and Outcomes	Nursing Interventions and Rationales	Patient Education Instructions
Fatigue Patient will: • Be able to identify the factors that contribute to fatigue • Maintain optimal level of functioning and comfort	1. Perform a fatigue assessment including pattern of fatigue, onset, duration, intensity, aggravating and alleviating factors, impact on fatigue on the patient's activity level and assess for contributing factor(s) dyspnea, degree of anemia, infection, fever, anorexia, cachexia and chronic pain. 2. Encourage patient to set priorities and choose activities. 3. Plan intermittent rest periods as needed. 4. Assist the patient with activities as needed. 5. Provide emotional support. 6. Assess for the presence of anemia. 7. Administer packed red blood cells as prescribed. 8. Administer oxygen as prescribed. 9. Provide patient with feedback and encouragement in identifying abilities and limitations.	1. Instruct patient to coordinate realistic daily activities. Teach patient to recognize fatigue and pace themselves. 2. Instruct patient to avoid doing too much too soon.

TABLE 34-8 Standard of Care for the Patient Receiving High-Dose-Rate (HDR) Brachytherapy

Patient Problem and Outcomes	Nursing Interventions and Rationales	Patient Education Instructions
Knowledge Deficit Related to Brachytherapy		
Patient demonstrates knowledge of brachytherapy (internal radiation).	1. Assess patient's knowledge of diagnosis and treatment plan.	1. Teach patient about HDR: a. Explain the purpose of the procedure. b. Describe treatment procedure. c. Describe routine including pelvic examination and measurement for cylinder. d. No specific precautions are needed.

and medication are administered to relax the patient (Dow & Hilderley, 1992; Nail, 1993).

Surgery

Patients with vaginal cancer undergo a radical hysterectomy, with or without bilateral pelvic lymphadenectomy, and either partial or total vaginectomy. Patients are usually hospitalized for 6 to 7 days after a radical hysterectomy. The major focus of nursing care is to provide postoperative care (See Table 34-9). Psychosocial support is a priority, as problems with body image and sexual needs are prominent for these patients. It has been reported that women are able to maintain presurgical sexual functioning after a hysterectomy. Delayed bowel and bladder function is a temporary effect of a radical hysterectomy. Patients may be discharged with a Foley catheter.

According to Chamorro (1990), patients treated with radical surgery require intensive hemodynamic support. Bed rest and immobility are usual requisites and have the potential to increase postoperative complications. Deep vein thrombosis is recognized as the antecedent to a pulmonary embolus and occurs in nearly 20% of gynecologic malignancies. Half of all pulmonary emboli occur within the first 24 hours after surgery. External pneumatic calf compression stockings are effective in preventing vascular morbidity. Heparin may be administered to prevent this complication.

Wound care is a major concern postoperatively, as the skin flaps in the area of the pelvic lymphadenectomy are

Text continued on p. 809

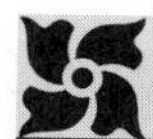

TABLE 34-9 Standard of Care for the Patient Undergoing Radical Hysterectomy

Patient Problem and Outcomes	Nursing Interventions and Rationales	Patient Education Instructions
Knowledge Deficit Related to Surgery		
Patient will verbalize an understanding of the surgical procedure: • Preoperative care • Postoperative care • Follow-up care after surgery	1. Assess past experience with surgery. 2. Determine present knowledge base and major concerns regarding surgery. Describe type of surgery and expected outcomes. 3. Assess patient's knowledge of potential sequelae, including loss of body organ and surgically induced menopause.	1. Describe type of surgery and expected outcomes. Use diagram of the anatomy of the female genital tract to explain the procedure. 2. Provide patient with information about the preoperative routine: a. Diagnostic tests b. Bowel preparation c. Consent d. Anesthesiology consult e. Nothing by mouth (NPO) after midnight f. Skin preparation g. On call to operating room: 1. hospital gown 2. void on call 3. preoperative medications h. Teach the patient to cough and deep breathe, use an incentive spirometer and perform foot and leg exercises. i. Discuss pain and pain management 3. Provide patient with information about postoperative plan of care: a. Routine assessment b. Importance of pain management c. Need for leg exercises d. Use of incentive spirometers e. Teach coughing and deep breathing exercises f. Need to ambulate as soon as possible g. Explanation of equipment (i.e., Foley catheter, IV and nasogastric tubes, drains and dressings) 4. Instruct patient regarding postoperative care including: a. Avoid tampons and douches. b. Abstain from intercourse for 4-6 weeks or as indicated by the physician. c. Increase activity gradually (i.e., limit stair climbing for 1-2 weeks, limit heavy housework and lifting of heavy objects for 6 weeks). d. Maintain a high-protein diet and adequate fluid intake (2000 ml). e. Monitor for signs and symptoms of infection. f. Notify physician if temperature is greater than 100.5° F (38° C). g. Take pain medication as prescribed to control pain. h. Avoid constipation and straining. i. Take estrogen-progestin hormones as prescribed. j. Keep follow-up appointment.

Continued

TABLE 34-9 Standard of Care for the Patient Undergoing Radical Hysterectomy—cont'd

Patient Problem and Outcomes	Nursing Interventions and Rationales	Patient Education Instructions
Pain Patient will: • Achieve satisfactory pain relief • Perform measures to manage pain	1. Assess pain intensity using a 0 to 10 pain rating scale, every 2-4 hours for the first 48 hours after surgery, then at least every 8 hours. 2. Administer opioid analgesics around the clock for the first 24-48 hours postoperatively. 3. Monitor for analgesic side effects and use strategies to prevent or treat: a. Constipation b. Nausea c. Anxiety d. Depression e. Insomnia 4. Use nonpharmacologic pain control strategies.	1. Teach patient to report pain to nurse. 2. Teach patient the importance of taking pain medication on a regular basis to keep pain under control. 3. Teach patient methods to minimize or reduce pain a. Positioning b. Range of motion c. Gentle massage d. Cold or warm pack e. Distraction techniques f. Relaxation techniques g. Meditation or prayers h. Exercise or rest periods i. Transcutaneous electrical nerve stimulations (TENS)
High Risk for Infection Patient will: • Remain infection free • Verbalize signs and symptoms of infection	1. Perform a skin assessment. 2. Perform a respiratory assessment. 3. Perform nephrourologic assessment. 4. Perform an oral assessment. 5. Monitor for signs and symptoms of infection: a. Temperature < 38° C b. Shaking chills c. Tenderness, redness, heat or pain d. Nonhealing, malodorous and or draining wound 6. Monitor vital signs. 7. Monitor white blood cell count and total neutrophil count. 8. Perform wound care and maintain a clean, dry incision. 9. Administer antipyretic or antibiotics as ordered. 10. Teach the patient to minimize anxiety, prepare the patient for discharge and allow the patient to be a partner in her care.	1. Instruct patient regarding preventing infection. a. Signs and symptoms of infection b. Notify nurse/MD if the patient exhibits any symptoms c. Explain the rationale and importance of handwashing d. Explain the role of balanced diet e. Explain the role of white blood cells in preventing infection f. Strict aseptic technique should be used g. Teach perineal care h. Teach Foley care

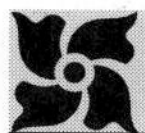

TABLE 34-9 Standard of Care for the Patient Undergoing Radical Hysterectomy—cont'd

Patient Problem and Outcomes	Nursing Interventions and Rationales	Patient Education Instructions
Altered Sexuality Patterns Related to Diagnosis, Fear, Depression, and Treatment		
Patient will: • Demonstrate knowledge regarding potential alterations in sexuality • Maintain an optimal means of satisfaction with sexual expression or needs • Identify/demonstrate strategies to manage or correct alteration in sexuality	1. Establish a therapeutic relationship a. Be nonjudgmental in your attitude b. Provide an atmosphere of acceptance c. Assure the patient that all discussions will be kept confidential d. Ensure privacy e. Start the discussion beginning with the least sensitive and progress to the most sensitive issue f. Offer an opportunity for patient to ask questions and verbalizes issues/concerns 2. Use Annon's Plisset model to guide your interventions: • P = Permission • LI = Limited Information • SS = Specific Information • IT = Intensive Therapy 3. Assess patient's/significant other(s) understanding of sexuality and physiology. 4. Perform a sexual history including: a. Sexual activity b. Reproductive history c. Desire for children d. Use of contraceptives e. Attitudes about sex f. Impact of involved body part on sexuality g. Expectations 5. Allow patient to verbalize her perceptions of how the disease/treatment will affect sexuality and sexual function. 6. Elicit early identification of a specific problem including: a. Nature b. Course of events c. Onset d. Duration e. Patient's perception of the problem 7. Encourage patient/significant other(s) to discuss concerns and or problems. 8. Provide time for patient and significant other to privately communicate.	1. Instruct patient and significant other regarding potential/alteration in sexuality: a. Discuss impact of disease and treatment on sexuality b. Clarify terms, myths and misconceptions as appropriate to ensure understanding c. Identify barriers to sexuality d. Identify strategies to a satisfying sexual function by managing side effects (i.e., pain, decreased libido, dyspareunia, and/or fatigue) e. Inform patient whether hormonal effects should be expected f. Prepared patient for anticipated menopausal symptoms 2. Provide booklet entitled *Sexuality and Cancer For The Woman Who Has Cancer and Her Partner* by the American Cancer Society

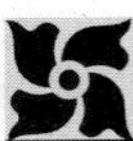

TABLE 34-10 Standard of Care for the Patient Receiving Chemotherapy for Vaginal Cancer

Patient Problem and Outcomes	Nursing Interventions and Rationales	Patient Education Instructions
Knowledge Deficit Related to Chemotherapy		
Patient will verbalize an understanding of the purpose, benefits and risks of chemotherapy.	1. Assess patient's levels of knowledge about chemotherapy. 2. Assess patient's concerns and fears about chemotherapy.	1. Describe the routine: a. Purpose of chemotherapy b. How chemotherapy affects cancer cells c. Name, dosage, route and schedule of administration of the agents d. Side effects of chemotherapy e. Appropriate intervention to manage side effects including: (1) Nausea and vomiting (2) Alopecia (3) Anorexia (4) Mucositis (5) Infection (6) Fatigue f. Signs and symptoms to report to the health care team
Anemia		
Patient will: • Demonstrate adequate oxygen saturation of tissues: 1. Laboratory values at satisfactory level for patient 2. Vital signs stable 3. No evidence of obvious bleeding • Demonstrate knowledge of relationship of red blood cells, hemoglobin and availability of oxygen for normal function. • Demonstrate knowledge of factors that contribute to anemia. • Along with significant other(s), identify/demonstrate measures to prevent anemia.	1. Monitor CBC including hemoglobin and hematocrit. 2. Assess for signs and symptoms of anemia including: a. Palpitations/chest pain on exertion b. Dyspnea on exertion c. Dizziness/syncope d. Fatigue/weakness e. Anorexia f. Headache g. Tinnitus h. Insomnia 3. Assess for signs of blood loss. 4. Monitor vital signs. 5. Monitor orthostatic vital signs. 6. Perform skin assessment. 7. Perform oral assessment. 8. Perform oral hygiene. 9. Perform cardiac assessment. 10. Assess patient's ability to perform ADL. 11. Provide assistance for activities that cannot be performed independently. 12. Provide patient with rest periods. 13. Increase activity level as tolerated by patient. 14. Provide diet high in protein, vitamins and iron. 15. Consult dietitian if indicated. 16. Administer iron supplements as prescribed. 17. Administer erythropoietin as prescribed. 18. Administer blood products as prescribed. 19. Administer oxygen as needed.	1. Teach normal values for hemoglobin/ hematocrit and relationship to overall health. 2. Teach signs and symptoms of anemia: a. Pallor b. Fatigue c. Shortness of breath d. Tachycardia on exertion e. Headache f. Dizziness g. Irritability h. Heart palpitations 3. Teach factors that cause anemia: a. Radiation b. Drugs (anticonvulsants and chemotherapeutic agents) c. Alcohol d. Antibiotic therapy e. Bleeding 4. Refer to dietitian. 5. Encourage a diet high in protein, vitamins, and iron. 6. Teach the importance of preventing infection. 7. Instruct patient to plan rest periods and adequate sleep time. 8. Explain treatment plan. 9. Instruct patient to maintain skin integrity: a. Turn and position b. Lubricate skin with cream or lotion after daily bath and as needed c. Avoid drying agents to the skin 10. Assess understanding of change in activity level and ability to perform activities.

CBC, Complete blood count; *ADL,* activities of daily living; *ASA,* acetylsalicylic acid; *hct,* hematocrit; *hgb,* hemoglobin; *BUN,* blood urea nitrogen.

TABLE 34-10 Standard of Care for the Patient Receiving Chemotherapy for Vaginal Cancer—cont'd

Patient Problem and Outcomes	Nursing Interventions and Rationales	Patient Education Instructions
High Risk for Injury: Bleeding, Related to Thrombocytopenia		
Patient will: • Not experience preventable bleeding • Demonstrate knowledge of bleeding precautions and verbalize who to contact when signs and symptoms occur	1. Monitor CBC and platelet count. 2. Monitor for signs and symptoms of bleeding. 3. Monitor vital signs. 4. Institute thrombocytopenia protocol for a platelet count of 50,000/ mm^3 or less. 5. Institute safety standard. 6. Administer platelets as prescribed. 7. Avoid ASA-containing drugs and be aware of other drugs interfering with platelet function.	1. Explain the relationship between platelets and bleeding. 2. Teach patient about bleeding precautions. 3. Teach patient signs and symptoms of bleeding. 4. Instruct patient to notify health care professional when/if bleeding occurs. 5. Instruct patient on measures to manage bleeding.
Fluid Volume Deficit Related to Nausea and Vomiting		
The patient maintains her status as evidenced by: 1. Laboratory values within patient's baseline 2. Maintains stable weight 3. Decrease in nausea 4. Maintains adequate intake and output	1. Assess patient's pattern of nausea and vomiting including: a. Onset b. Frequency c. Duration d. Amount e. Color f. Character of the emesis g. Alleviating/exaggerating factors 2. Assess for signs and symptoms of fluid volume deficit including: a. Decreased skin turgor b. Thirst, parched tongue c. Warm, flushed skin d. Rapid, weak pulse e. Hypotension f. Lethargy g. Confusion, disorientation 3. Monitor patient for: a. Anorexia b. Altered taste c. Sore mouth d. Fatigue e. Pain f. Obstruction 4. Monitor intake and output. 5. Maintain fluid intake of at least 2500 ml/day unless contraindicated. 6. Administer IV therapy as prescribed. 7. Inspect oral cavity to assess hydration status. 8. Perform oral care before/after meals and after emesis. 9. Administer antiemetic as prescribed and assess the effectiveness of antiemetic regimen. 10. Maintain patient in Fowler's position after eating. 11. Weigh and report change in weight. 12. Obtain dietary consult. 13. Monitor laboratory values including: a. CBC (hct/hgb) b. Electrolytes (K^+, Mg^{+2}, N^+) c. BUN/creatinine 14. Obtain guaiac of emesis. 15. Perform relaxation exercises.	1. Teach strategies to prevent nausea and vomiting: a. Small, frequent meals b. Rest period before and after meals c. Minimize stimuli d. Avoid sweet, highly seasoned or greasy foods e. Recommend foods with low potential to cause nausea (i.e., dry toast, crackers, ginger ale, cola, cold plates, boiled or baked potatoes). f. Experiment with sour foods g. Eat food cold or at room temperature h. Eat various kinds of candy (hard or soft mints and sour candy) i. Provide distraction technique

Continued

Table 34-10 Standard of Care for the Patient Receiving Chemotherapy for Vaginal Cancer—cont'd

Patient Problem and Outcomes	Nursing Interventions and Rationales	Patient Education Instructions
Oral Mucositis Related to Chemotherapy, Lack of Oral Intake, Immunosuppression, and Nutritional Depletion		
Patient will: • Exhibit healing of oral mucosa • Maintain optimal level of comfort. • Maintain sufficient oral intake. • Identify factors that alter the integrity of the mucous membrane. • Be able to perform an oral assessment and preventive measures. • Identify signs and symptoms to report to the health care team.	1. Perform oral assessment including: a. Assessment of the lips, tongue, gums, buccal mucosa for presence or absence of any of the following: (1) Change in color (2) Swelling (3) Pain (4) Bleeding/discharge (5) Lesions b. Assess the teeth for the following: (1) Missing teeth (2) Mobile teeth (3) Caps (4) Fractures (5) Pain/tenderness c. Assess for changes in taste. d. In addition remove dentures and assess denture fit (if applicable), amount and consistency of saliva, voice and ability to swallow e. Evaluate for evidence of infection 2. Provide oral hygiene care. 3. Instruct patient to administer mouthwash. 4. Apply lip lubricant. 5. Type of diet will depend on patient's condition. 6. Provide appropriate nutritional intake. 7. Refer for dietary consult 8. Monitor patient's hydration status. 9. Encourage fluid intake (3000 ml fluid daily unless contraindicated). 10. Monitor for signs and symptoms of infection. 11. Monitor vital signs. 12. Monitor WBC count and total neutrophil count. 13. Administer pain medication as prescribed. 14. Administer antimicrobial medication as prescribed. 15. Refer for a dental consult.	1. Teach patient to perform an oral assessment: a. Wash hands b. Obtain a mirror and a light c. Observe for deviations from normal mucosa 2. Instruct patient to assess and report signs and symptoms of mucositis: a. Dry, rough lips b. Burning sensation/pain in the mouth or at mucocutaneous junction c. Red, inflamed mucosa d. Small white or yellow patches e. Difficulty swallowing f. Red, swollen gums or tongue g. Coating, redness, ulceration h. Changes in sensation, appearance, or taste 3. Teach patient oral hygiene measures: a. Brush teeth with a soft nylon bristle toothbrush after meals and at bedtime b. Remove dentures/bridge, cleanse, and replace after oral hygiene care c. Keep dentures in water while out d. Remove dentures if evidence of alteration in oral mucosa. 4. Instruct patient to avoid irritants and irritation to mucosa: a. Commercial mouthwashes b. Alcohol c. Lemon-glycerin swab d. Tobacco e. Smoking f. Poorly fitted dentures g. Spicy foods h. Citrus fruit juices i. Extremes in food temperatures 5. Keep oral mucosa moist: a. Oral care at least 3 times a day and at bedtime b. Adequate fluid intake (3000 ml/day unless contraindicated) c. Artificial saliva d. K-Y jelly 6. Encourage patient to eat soft, moist food and to avoid dry, coarse food. 7. Instruct patient to administer prophylactic oral antifungal or antibacterial agents as prescribed.

CBC, Complete blood count; *ADL,* activities of daily living; *ASA,* acetylsaliclyic acid; *hct,* hematocrit; *hgb, hemoglobin; BUN,* blood urea nitrogen.

Table 34-10 Standard of Care for the Patient Receiving Chemotherapy for Vaginal Cancer—cont'd

Patient Problem and Outcomes	Nursing Interventions and Rationales	Patient Education Instructions
High Risk for Inadequate Nutrition Less the Body Requirements		
Related to: 1. Inadequate intake a. Decreased appetite b. Nausea/vomiting c. Mucositis d. Dysphagia 2. Increased excretion a. Vomiting b. Diarrhea 3. Increased requirements a. Fever b. Infection c. Stress Patient will: • Exhibit minimal signs and symptoms of malnutrition as evidenced by maintaining or increasing pretreatment body weight. • Demonstrate knowledge about how to maintain adequate nutrition.	1. Assess patient for signs of nutritional deficits including: a. Lack of interest in food b. Problems or difficulties with eating: (1) Anorexia (2) Nausea and vomiting (3) Dysphagia (4) Early satiety (5) Alteration in oral membranes 2. Monitor intake and output: a. Obtain diet history, noting patterns in appetite and food preferences, aversions, and food that are well tolerated b. Note best time to eat during the day 3. Measure height and weight on admission and weight weekly. 4. Evaluate dietary patterns. 5. Obtain a dietary consult. 6. Monitor laboratory values: serum albumin, electrolytes, urinalysis, hemoglobin, hematocrit, serum total protein concentration. 7. Observe for signs of dehydration: a. Decreased skin turgor b. Dry mouth and mucous membranes c. Thirst d. Scanty, concentrated urine 8. Perform oral care before meals. 9. Administer antiemetic 30 minutes before meal as ordered. 10. Medicate with topical/systemic analgesics as ordered. 11. Position patient before meals for comfort. 12. Encourage patient to maintain a diet high in calories, protein and vitamins. 13. Provide between meals supplements. 14. Offer small, frequent meals. 15. Determine whether any other symptoms interfere with eating and use strategies to prevent the symptoms: a. Fatigue b. Pain c. Mucositis d. Diarrhea e. Anxiety f. Depression	1. Instruct patient on eating hints and provide the booklet by the National Cancer Institute, "Eating Hints."

Continued

TABLE 34-10 Standard of Care for the Patient Receiving Chemotherapy for Vaginal Cancer—cont'd

Patient Problem and Outcomes	Nursing Interventions and Rationales	Patient Education Instructions
Alteration in Body Image Related to Alopecia		
Patient will: • Verbalize feelings related to hair loss. • Utilize appropriate coping strategies to deal with alopecia.	1. Inform the patient when hair loss is expected to begin and the anticipated degree and duration of the hair loss. 2. Inform patient after temporary hair loss that hair regrowth may differ in color and texture. 3. Assess the importance of hair to patient/significant other. 4. Encourage the patient to verbalize feelings about alopecia. 5. Identify possible measures to take during hair loss: a. Wig b. Scarf, hat or turban c. Use makeup 6. Encourage patient to maintain self-image by: a. Socialization b. Wearing own clothes/pajamas	1. Teach the patient to use the following interventions to minimize hair loss: a. Use mild shampoo followed by a conditioner every 3-5 days b. Avoid excessive shampooing c. Minimize the use of electric hair dryer d. Discontinue the use of electric curlers and curling irons, hair clips, bobby pins, and barrettes e. Hair spray, hair dye, or bleach may increase the fragility of the hair and should be avoided f. Combing with wide-tooth comb is preferred; avoid excessive brushing and combing of the hair g. Use a satin pillowcase
Fatigue		
Patient will: • Be able to identify the factors with the potential to cause fatigue. • Maintain optimal function and comfort.	1. Perform a fatigue assessment including pattern of fatigue, onset, duration, intensity, aggravating and alleviating factors and impact of fatigue on the patient's activity level and assess for contributing factor(s) such as dyspnea, degree of anemia, infection, fever, anorexia, cachexia, and chronic pain. 2. Encourage patient to set priorities and choose activities. 3. Plan intermittent rest periods as needed. 4. Assist the patient with activities as needed. 5. Provide emotional support. 6. Assess for the presence of anemia. 7. Administer packed red blood cells as prescribed. 8. Administer oxygen as prescribed. 9. Provide patient with feedback and encouragement in identifying abilities and limitations.	1. Instruct patient to coordinate realistic daily activities. Teach patient to recognize fatigue and pace herself. 2. Instruct patient to avoid doing too much too soon.
High Risk for Alteration in Renal Function Related to Nephrotoxic or Urotoxic Effects of Chemotherapy		
Patient will: • Maintain fluid intake of 2-3 L unless contraindicated. • Maintain urine output of 100 ml/hr or more.	1. Encourage adequate fluid intake. 2. Monitor intake and output. 3. Administer fluids as prescribed. 4. Assess urine and report changes (e.g., color, sediment). 5. Monitor renal status.	
Potential Alteration in Respiratory Status Secondary to Chemotherapy		
Patient's respiratory status will be within normal limits.	1. Assess respiratory status. 2. Monitor for dyspnea. 3. Monitor pulmonary function test as ordered. 4. Administer O_2 as ordered.	1. Teach patient relaxation and breathing exercises.

CBC, Complete blood count; *ADL,* activities of daily living; *ASA,* acetylsalicylic acid; *hct,* hematocrit; *hgb,* hemoglobin; *BUN,* blood urea nitrogen.

most vulnerable (Chamorro, 1990). Incisions may separate and require debridement and dressings before granulation and healing occur.

Nursing management of the patient undergoing surgery for vaginal cancer is summarized in Table 34-9 . The patient undergoing surgery may need information and education on pain management and sexuality.

Another major postoperative nursing issue is the care of patients with reconstructed vaginas. This procedure may be performed at the time of the initial surgery or several months later. Vaginal packing is placed immediately after the procedure, with stents positioned later. Postoperative care includes bed rest and a constipating diet. At 6 months, if the patient is having intercourse at least twice a week, the stents are no longer used (Hampton, 1986).

Chemotherapy

Patients undergoing chemotherapy receive it as an outpatient. The response rate is disappointing, and, if possible, patients should have the opportunity to participate in a clinical trial. Health care providers must obtain informed consent and explain risks and benefits of participating in a clinical trial. When administering chemotherapy, the patient and significant other(s) must be educated on the side effects and strategies to manage them. The management plan for patients with vaginal cancer receiving chemotherapy is summarized in Table 34-10.

HOME CARE ISSUES

Depending on the treatment approaches used to manage vaginal cancer, the patient and caregivers will be faced with several issues in the home setting. The major teaching issues for patients with reconstructive vagina surgery are listed in Box 34-2.

Sexual Dysfunction

Sexual dysfunction involves not only the patient, but also the patient's sexual partner (Hughes, 1996, Lamb, 1995). The vaginal canal has been identified as one of the main areas of concern related to sexual function after radiation therapy (Lamb, 1990). The effects of radiation on the vaginal epithelium result in a progressive narrowing of the vaginal canal with a significant decrease in elasticity and sensation. Pelvic stenosis and fibrosis cause both decreased blood flow and vaginal secretions, resulting in decreased vaginal sensation and dyspareunia (Cartwright-Alcarese, 1995). Women who are sexually active are encouraged to resume sexual intercourse as soon as the discomfort has resolved. Lamb (1990) noted that women who are not sexually active should be instructed in the use of a vaginal dilator with a water-soluble lubricant. See Table 34-11 for the management of vaginal stenosis.

In addition to being knowledgeable and comfortable in addressing sexual dysfunction in women treated with radiation and/or surgery for vaginal cancer, nurses must assume responsibility for making appropriate referrals to sex counselors, supportive psychotherapy, and support groups forwomen with genital cancer, as well as providing written literature (e.g., *Sexuality and Cancer: For the Woman Who Has Cancer and Her Partner,* a booklet available through the American Cancer Society).

PROGNOSIS

The prognosis for women with squamous cell vaginal carcinoma depends primarily on the extent of the disease at the time of diagnosis. According to Bengtson (1995), women with stage I disease treated with radiation therapy have a 5-year survival rate of 80% to 90%. For women with stage II, 5-year survival rates are 45% to 58%. A decreased 5-year survival rate of 25% to 40% is seen in women diagnosed

Box 34-2
Major Teaching Issues for Patients with Reconstructive Vaginal Surgery

Wound care
Maintain adequate nutrition (high protein, high calorie)
Manage/cope with stents/vaginal molds
Prevent/manage stenosis
- Use of vaginal dilators
- Insertion of estrogen cream
- Resume sexual intercourse

Manage vaginal odors/discharge
- Douche with dilute vinegar

Psychosocial issues
- Discuss change in body image and altered sensation
- Allow patient and her partner to verbalize their feelings
- Experiment using different positions during intercourse to enhance comfort

Provide support for the patient and her partner

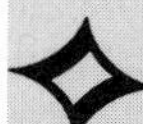

TABLE 34-11 Patient Preparation for the Management of Vaginal Stenosis

Reason for vaginal stenosis: Radiation therapy causes the vaginal canal to narrow. This narrowing results in a decrease in elasticity and a decrease in sensation as well as pain during intercourse.

Instructions for the Patient:

1. Resume sexual activity as soon as your doctor gives you permission to do so.
2. The use of a vaginal dilator may help to prevent vaginal stenosis.
3. Before using the vaginal dilator, warm the dilator by running it under hot water. Coat the dilator with a water-based lubricant (e.g., K-Y jelly) or with an estrogen cream (if your doctor has prescribed the cream). Insert the dilator as far as possible and, using an in-and-out motion, repeat the insertion for 10 to 15 minutes. Clean the dilator with soap and water.

TABLE 34-12 Quality of Care Evaluation for a Patient Receiving External Beam Radiation and/or Interstitial Brachytherapy

Disciplines participating in the quality of care evaluation
☐ Nursing ☐ Radiation Oncology ☐ Social Services

Data from:
☐ Mailed Questionnaire ☐ Patient Interview

CRITERIA	YES	NO
1. Did the doctor or nurse explain to you that you might experience some of the following side effects from your radiation therapy:		
a. Fatigue	☐	☐
b. Diarrhea	☐	☐
c. Cystitis	☐	☐
d. Proctitis	☐	☐
e. Alteration in vaginal mucous membranes	☐	☐
2. Were you taught to manage the side effects?	☐	☐
3. Were you taught to use a vaginal dilator?	☐	☐
4. Were you asked if you want to see a sex counselor?	☐	☐

with stage III disease, and only up to a 10% survival rate can be expected for women diagnosed with stage IV disease. The overall 5-year survival rate is approximately 30% to 35%.

Recurrence carries a poor prognosis, and approximately 50% of squamous cell carcinomas recur within 2 years (DiSaia & Creasman, 1993). Women with recurrent disease in the central pelvic region may be candidates for pelvic exenteration or irradiation.

Similarly, the prognosis for women diagnosed with clear cell adenocarcinoma is related to the extent of the disease at the time of diagnosis. Women with stage I tumors confined to the vaginal wall have a 5-year survival rate of approximately 90% (Bengtson, 1995). For women with stage II disease, 5-year survival rates are 80%, and for stage III disease the rate drops to 37%. The follow-up of many of these cases is still too short for calculating mean 5-year survival rates. However, at the present time, the overall survival rate is 80% and much higher than for squamous cell carcinoma. The better prognosis may be the result of early detection, because it occurs mainly in young women exposed to DES (DiSaia & Creasman, 1993).

EVALUATION OF THE QUALITY OF CARE

Accreditation organizations, such as the Joint Commission for the Accreditation of Health Care Organizations, require that the quality of care provided to patients be evaluated. Because the care provided to patients with vaginal cancer requires input from a multidisciplinary team, an evaluation for the quality of care provided should include aspects of care provided by various members of the team. Tables 34-12 and 34-13 provide examples of quality of care evaluation tools that can be used in the inpatient and outpatient settings.

TABLE 34-13 Quality of Care Evaluation for a Patient Undergoing Radical Hysterectomy, Bilateral Lymphadenectomy, and Reconstructed Vagina

Disciplines participating in the quality of care evaluation
☐ Nursing ☐ Surgery ☐ Sexual Counselor ☐ Social Services

I. Postoperative Management Evaluation

Data from:
☐ Medical Record Review ☐ Patient/Family Interview

CRITERIA	YES	NO
1. Were you provided with preoperative information about:		
a. Diagnostic tests	☐	☐
b. Use of pneumatic calf compression stockings	☐	☐
c. Reconstruction of neovagina	☐	☐
2. Were you provided with postoperative information about:		
a. Wound care	☐	☐
b. Management of stents/vaginal molds	☐	☐
c. Use of vaginal dilators	☐	☐
3. Did the patient experience the following complications:		
a. Pulmonary embolism	☐	☐
b. Wound infection	☐	☐

II. Patient/Family Satisfaction

Data from:
☐ Patient Interview ☐ Family Interview

CRITERIA	YES	NO
1. On a scale of 0 to 10 with 0 being totally dissatisfied and 10 being totally satisfied, how satisfied were you with the pain management you received? ______		
2. Were you told to call the nurse if you experienced pain?	☐	☐
3. Were you instructed to resume sexual intercourse as soon as you were comfortable or to use a vaginal dilator?	☐	☐

RESEARCH ISSUES

Numerous research issues surrounding the diagnosis and management of vaginal cancer require further investigation. Currently there is no effective screening method for early detection of vaginal cancer. Continued research is needed to identify sensitive and specific screening methods so that the potential for cure is enhanced.

Chemotherapy for recurrent vaginal cancer has been disappointing. Randomized clinical trials are needed to identify effective agents and better response rates.

The scarcity of published nursing research on sexual dysfunction following radiation for gynecologic malignancies has been addressed by Cartwright-Alcarese (1995) and signifies the need for future research. Studies are needed to identify the actual incidence of specific sexual dysfunction, strategies to overcome it, and outcomes. In addition, research is warranted to evaluate whether educational programs for nurses (e.g., conferences, workshops, films and books) increase their knowledge and comfort in addressing patients concerns regarding sexuality.

The physiologic and psychological challenges facing the patient with vaginal cancer demand that oncology nurses be knowledgeable, comfortable, and sensitive in providing interventions to this patient population. We must explore the relationship between quality of life and treatment.

REFERENCES

Barber, H. R. K. (1982). Pelvic exenteration. *Cancer Investigation, 5,* 331-338.

Bell, J., Bernd-uwe, S., Averette, H., & Nadji, M. (1984). Vaginal cancer after hysterectomy for benign disease. *Obstetrical Gynecology, 64,* 699-702.

Bengtson, J. M. (1995). The vagina. In K. J. Ryan, R. S. Berkowitz, & R. L. Barbieri (Eds.), *Kistner's gynecology principles and practice.* St. Louis: Mosby Company.

Cartwright-Alcarese, F. (1995). Addressing sexual dysfunction following radiation therapy for a gynecologic malignancy. *Oncology Nursing Forum, 22,* 1227-1232.

Chamorro, T. (1990). Cancer of the vulva and vagina. *Seminars in Oncology Nursing, 6*(3), 198-205.

Deppe, G. & Lawrence, W. D. (1988). Cancer of the vagina including DES-related lesions. In S. B. Ginsberg, H. M. Shingleton, & D. Gunter (Eds.), *Female genital cancer.* New York: Churchill Livingston.

DiSaia, P. J. & Creasman, W. T. (1993). Invasive cancer of the vagina and urethra. In P. J. DiSaia & W. T. Creasman (Eds.), *Clinical gynecologic oncology.* St. Louis: Mosby Company.

Dow, K. H. S. & Hilderley, L. J. (1992). *Nursing care in radiation oncology.* Philadelphia: W. B. Saunders Company.

Hall, K. L., Dewar, M. A., & Perchalski, J. (1992). Screening for gynecologic cancer. *Primary Care Clinics in Office Practice, 19,* 607-619.

Hampton, B. G. (1986). Nursing management of a patient following pelvic exenteration. *Seminars in Oncology Nursing, 2,* 281-286.

Herbst, A. L., Anderson, D., & Hubby, M. M. (1986). Risk factors for the development of diethylstilbestrol-associated clear cell adenocarcinoma: A case-control study. *American Journal of Obstetrical Gynecology, 154,* 814-822.

Herman, J., Homesley, H., & Dignan, M. (1986). Is hysterectomy a risk factor for vaginal cancer? *Journal of American Medical Association, 256,* 601-603.

Hughes, M. K. (1996). Sexuality issues: Keeping your cool. *Oncology Nursing Forum, 23,* 1597-1600.

Lamb, M. A. (1990). Psychosexual issues: The woman with gynecologic cancer. *Seminars in Oncology Nursing, 6,* 237-243.

Lamb, M. A. (1995). Effects of cancer on the sexuality and fertility of women. *Seminars in Oncology Nursing, 11,* 120-127.

Lee, J. Y., Perez, C. A., & Ettinger, N. (1982). The risk of second primaries subsequent to irradiation for cervix cancer. *International Journal Radiation Oncology, 8,* 207-211.

Mahon, S. M. (1996). Educating about early detection of gynecologic cancers using a brochure. *Oncology Nursing Forum, 23,* 529-535.

Martello, J. Y. & Vasconez, H. C. (1995). Vulvar and vaginal reconstruction after surgical treatment for gynecologic cancer. *Clinics in Plastic Surgery, 22,* 129-140.

Martin, L. K. & Braly, P. S. (1991). Gynecologic cancers. In S. B. Baird, R. McCorkle, & M. Grant (Eds.), *A comprehensive textbook.* Philadelphia: W. B. Saunders Company.

Melnick, S., Cole, P., Anderson, D., & Herbst, A. (1987). Rates and risks of diethylstilbestrol-related clear-cell adenocarcinoma of the vagina and cervix. An update. *New England Journal of Medicine, 316,* 514-516.

Merino, M. J. (1991). Vaginal cancer: The role of infectious and environmental factors. *American Journal of Obstetrical Gynecology, 165,* 1255-1262.

Nail, L. M. (1993). Coping with intracavitary radiation treatment for gynecologic cancer. *Cancer Practice, 1,* 218-234.

Perez, C. A., Gersell, D. J., Hoskins, W. J., & McGuire, W. P. (1992). Vagina. In W. J. Hoskins, C. A. Perez, & R. C. Young (Eds.), *Principles and practice of gynecologic oncology.* Philadelphia: J. B. Lippincott Company.

Philips, T. L., Dattatreyuda, N. J., & Peschel, R. E. (1990). Carcinoma of the vagina and vulva. *Interstitial brachytherapy.* New York: Raven Press.

Pride, G. L., Schultz, A. E., & Chuprevich, T. W. (1979). Primary invasive squamous carcinoma of the vagina. *Obstetrical Gynecology, 53,* 218.

Walczak, R. J. & Klemm, P. R. (1993). Gynecologic cancers. In S. L. Groenwald, M. H. Frogge, M. Goodman, & C. H. Yarbro (Eds.), *Cancer nursing principles and practice.* Boston: Jones and Bartlett Publishers.

Zaino, R. J., Robboy, S. J., Bentley, R., & Kurman, R. J. (1994). Diseases of the vagina. In R. J. Kurman (Ed.), *Brainstein's pathology of the female genital tract.* New York: Springer-Verlag.

Vulvar Cancer

Cecilia Gatson Grindel, RN, PhD

INTRODUCTION

Vulvar cancer accounts for 4% to 5% of all gynecologic malignancies and 1% to 2% of all malignancies in women; it is the fourth most common malignancy of the female genital tract (Hacker & Berek, 1995; McLellan & Rosenshein, 1991; Tobias, Smith, Jones, Anderson, Runowicz, & Goldberg, 1995). It is a rare cancer, and the incidence of the disease increases with age (Giles & Kneals, 1995). However, during the last 2 decades, the incidence of vulvar intraepithelial neoplasia (VIN) has increased.

Although the incidence of vulvar cancer is relatively small, it can have profound effects on the patient. Survival is relatively good, but morbidities after surgical treatment can be devastating, especially for the elderly patient.

EPIDEMIOLOGY

To clarify the discussion of vulvar cancer, it is important to understand the types of lesions that can be present in the vulva. The first type is noninvasive. These lesions can be nonneoplastic epithelial disorders or VIN. Nonneoplastic epithelial disorders include such changes as leukoplakia, leukoplakia vulvitis, sclerotic dermatosis, and others. These conditions are not of a cancerous nature and will not be discussed here. VIN is of interest to this discussion because squamous cell carcinoma in situ (stage 0) fits into this classification.

The International Society for the Study of Vulvar Disease (ISSVD) has recommended use of the term *vulvar intraepithelial neoplasia* to end confusion about nomenclature related to vulvar dystrophies. Carcinoma in situ (CIN), or severe dysplasia of the vulva, is designated as squamous VIN 3 (Hacker & Berek, 1995; van der Velden & Hacker, 1994). During the last 2 decades, there has been an increase in the incidence of VIN 3, with younger patients in the 30- and 40-year-old age groups affected (Hacker & Berek, 1995; Giles & Kneals, 1995). CIN is most often seen in younger patients (ages 30 to 60 years), characteristically around 51 years of age (McLellan & Rosenshein, 1991). The occurrence of CIN is strongly related to the sexually transmitted human papilloma virus (HPV) and smoking. Smoking is believed to interact synergistically with HPV infection and *Condylomata acuminata* (genital warts) to produce CIN (Giles & Kneals, 1995; McLellan & Rosenshein, 1991; Sturgeon, Brinton, Devesa, & Kurman, 1992). It is important to note that CIN of the vulva does not automatically progress to invasive cancer (Hacker & Berek, 1995; McLellan & Rosenshein, 1991) and that it is strongly associated with HPV infection (Giles & Kneals, 1995; Hording, Junge, Poulsen, & Lundvall, 1995; Ogunbiyi, Scholefield, Robertson, Smith, Sharp, & Rogers, 1994).

Paget's disease is another vulvar dystrophy that has implications to cancer. This disease is characterized by the development of pathognomonic large, pale Paget's cells that are seen within the epidermis and skin adnexa. Paget's disease is a neoplasm in which the cell types reproduced are of the apocrine glands. This lesion is seldom invasive; however, when it does invade, it is a highly aggressive lesion with massive node involvement early in its clinical course and a poor prognosis (McLellan & Rosenshein, 1991). This disease predominately affects postmenopausal white women. In 20% to 29% of patients, Paget's disease is associated with an underlying adenocarcinoma or invasive cancer in other sites (Hacker & Berek, 1995; Hart & Millman, 1977).

Similar to other gynecologic cancers, no specific etiologic agent has been associated with the development of vulvar cancer. Research supports the hypothesis that two different etiologic types of vulvar cancer exist. The first and most common of the two types is seen frequently in elderly women, with the greatest number of cases occurring in the 75 to 79 age group (McLellan & Rosenshein, 1991). Although many etiologic factors may be associated with the development of vulvar cancer in older women, it is typically not associated with VIN or HPV (Rusk, Sutton, Look, & Roman, 1991). On the other hand, invasive vulvar carcinoma seen in younger women (Apgar & Cox, 1996; Costa, Syrjanen, Vendra, Chang, Guida, & Hippelainen et al., 1995; Giles & Kneals, 1995) is often associated with HPV and VIN, suggesting that two distinct etiologic factors may result in the development of vulvar cancer in these women (Anderson, Franquemont, Williams, Taylor, & Crum, 1991; Bloss, Liao, Wilczynski, Macri, Walker, & Peake et al., 1991; Franquemont, Anderson, Williams, Taylor, & Crum, 1991; Hording, Junge, Poulsen, & Lundvall, 1995; Sherman, Daling, Chu, Weiss, Ashley, & Corey, 1991).

RISK FACTORS

Historically, vulvar cancer has been associated with obesity, hypertension, diabetes mellitus, arteriosclerosis, and menopause at an early age (Franklin & Rutledge, 1972; Green, Ulfelder, & Meigs, 1958). However, recent studies have failed to definitively support all of these risk factors (Brinton, Nasca, Mallin, Baptiste, Wilbanks, & Richart, 1990). Data from the Cancer Surveillance Program in Los Angeles have shown that women of lower socioeconomic status experience rates of vulvar cancer that are three times higher than women with the higher socioeconomic status (McLellan & Rosenshein, 1991). The incidence of vulvar cancer is reported to be three times higher in separated women than in single, married, or divorced women (McLellan & Rosenshein, 1991). Studies have also reported that vulvar cancer is associated with a higher incidence of nulliparity, vulvar leukoplakia, vulvar or vaginal inflammatory disease, and other cancers, especially cervical cancer (Mabuchi, Bross, & Kessler, 1985; McLellan & Rosenshein, 1991). Other risk factors include a history of venereal disease (i.e., granuloma inguinale, lymphogranuloma venereum, or a positive serology for syphilis) and vulvar dystrophies (a group of disorders of uncertain etiology characterized by severe dermal inflammation and scarring with apparent devascularization and either epithelial hyperplasia or thinning) (McLellan & Rosenshein, 1991; Lynch, 1987).

The typical profile of a woman with invasive vulvar cancer suggests that the woman is greater than 60 years of age with hypertension, obesity, diabetes mellitus, and nulliparity and has a history of a positive serology, a malignancy elsewhere in the female genital tract, and/or a vulvar dystrophy (McLellan & Rosenshein, 1991). The development of invasive vulvar carcinoma in younger women would suggest a history of smoking, HPV infection, and VIN (Monk, Burger, Lin, Parham, Vasilev, & Wilczynski, 1995; McLellan & Rosenshein, 1991). The numerous clinical conditions that are associated with vulvar cancer make it difficult to clearly define risk factors. It does, however, highlight the importance of a thorough health history, regular vulvar self-examination, and immediate medical attention for nonresolving pruritus and/or unusual findings on the vulvar self-examination. Further studies are needed to isolate more specific risk factors.

PATHOPHYSIOLOGY

Normal Anatomy and Physiology

The parameters of the area of the vulva include the mons pubis anteriorly, the anus posteriorly, and the inguinal-gluteal folds laterally (Fig. 35-1). The major structures of the vulva are the labia majora and minora, the clitoris with its prepuce

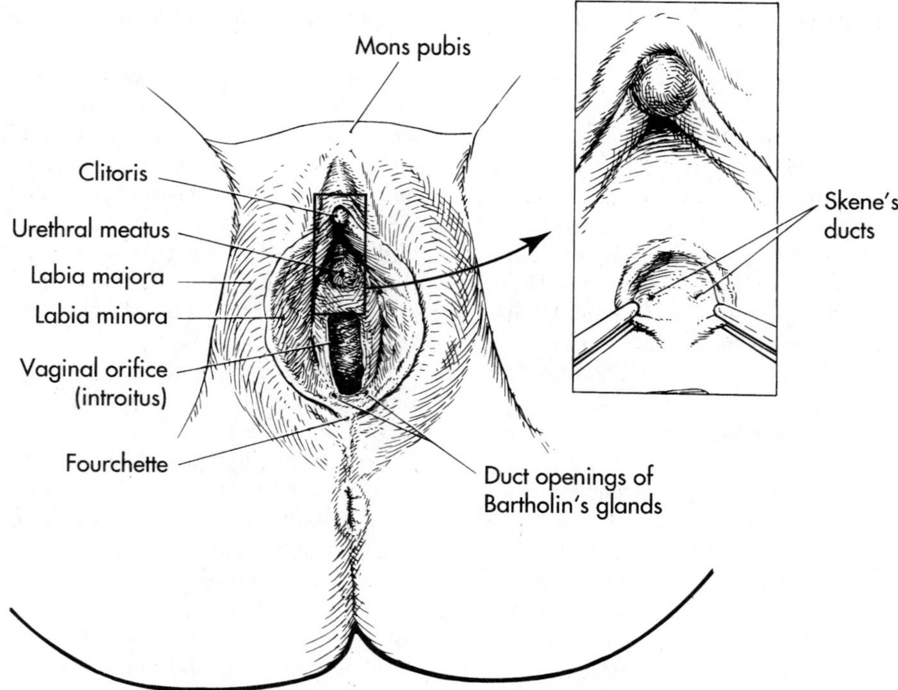

Fig. 35-1 Anatomy of the vulva. (From Kurman, R. J., Norris, H. J., & Wilkinson, E. J. [1992]. *Tumors of the cervix, vagina, and vulva: Atlas of tumor pathology.* Washington, D. C.: Armed Forces Institute of Pathology.)

and frenulum, and the urethral meatus. The vulvar vestibule is that portion of the vulva that extends from the most medial external edge of the hymenal ring laterally to the vestibular line of Hart on the medial aspects of the labia minora. The vestibule extends anteriorly to the frenulum and posteriorly to the perineal body. Within the vestibule are the orifices of the Bartholin's glands, as well as the urethra, the periurethral orifices of Skene glands, and the orifices of the minor vestibular glands (Kurman, Norris, & Wilkinson, 1992).

The femoral and inguinal lymph nodes provide the major lymphatic drainage system for the vulva. Lymphatic channels that drain the anterior labia minor and the clitoris join channels that drain the prepuce and the labia majora. These channels then drain laterally into the inguinal and femoral lymph nodes. The lymphatic drainage system for the vulva is primarily ipsilateral. The 8 to 10 superficial lymph nodes receive most of the drainage from the vulva and are the primary nodes involved in a metastatic tumor from the vulva (Kurman, Norris, & Wilkinson, 1992).

The Process of Carcinogenesis

Keratinized, stratified, squamous epithelium covers the vulva (Kurman, Norris, & Wilkinson, 1992). In cases of CIN, lesions develop on the vulva, which are characterized by disorganization of the epithelial structure. Giant cells with abnormal nuclei, multinucleated cells, formation of corps ronds, and disorders of cytoplasmic and nuclear maturation are all present to varying degrees (Friedrich, 1976). In most cases, these changes extend throughout the full thickness of the epithelium (Hacker & Berek, 1995). The potential for CIN of the vulva to become malignant is unclear. Some reports (Buscema, Woodruff, Parmley, & Genadry, 1980) suggest that only a small percentage of women with CIN will develop invasive carcinoma of the vulva. When it does progress to invasive cancer, the perianal tissue seems to be at particular risk (Hacker & Berek, 1995).

In the initial development of invasive squamous cell carcinoma of the vulva, the invading cells have a capacity to exhibit motility. These cells are characterized by a large amount of pink staining cytoplasm that contains actin and myosin microfibrils. This histologic feature and the presence of inflammation and a disorientation of the basal layer allow for the diagnosis of early-stage invasive carcinoma (McLellan & Rosenshein, 1991). Tumors that develop are usually well-differentiated lesions that are less aggressive and have a lower incidence of lymph node metastasis to the groin (Sedlis, Homesley, Bundy, Marshall, Yordan, & Hacker et al., 1987).

Types of Vulvar Cancer

Two types of vulvar dystrophies are central to a discussion of vulvar cancer. The first type, CIN, is a squamous intraepithelial neoplasia. The second type, Paget's disease, is a nonsquamous intraepithelial neoplasia. Box 35-1 lists the classification system for vulvar diseases.

Box 35-1
Classification of Vulvar Diseases

Nonneoplastic epithelial disorders of skin and mucosa:
- Lichen sclerosus
- Squamous hyperplasia, not otherwise specified
- Other dermatoses

Mixed nonneoplastic and neoplastic epithelial disorders
Intraepithelial neoplasia
- Squamous intraepithelial neoplasia:
  - -VIN 1
  - -VIN 2
  - -VIN 3 (severe dysplasia or carcinoma in situ)

Nonsquamous intraepithelial neoplasia
- Paget's disease
- Tumors of melanocytes, noninvasive

Invasive tumors

From Committee on Terminology, International Society for the Study of Vulvar Disease. (1989). New nomenclature for vulvar disease. *International Journal of Gynecologic Pathology, 8,* 83-84.

Distinctions can be made between the different histologic types of vulvar carcinoma: squamous cell carcinoma, basal cell carcinoma, verrucous carcinoma, malignant melanoma, adenocarcinoma, Bartholin's gland carcinoma, and vulvar sarcoma. Approximately 90% of all invasive vulvar cancers are squamous cell carcinomas, whereas 5% are malignant melanomas (McLellan & Rosenshein, 1991). Malignant melanomas of the vulva can occur in both the nodular and the superficially spreading varieties. Basal cell carcinoma produces the classic rodent ulcer with rolled pearly edges. This lesion rarely involves regional nodes. The verrucous carcinoma is a mature lesion that is often indistinguishable from *C. accuminata* (McLellan and Rosenshein, 1991) Adenosquamous carcinomas of the vulva tend to be highly aggressive tumors, with a higher rate of lymph node metastases (Hacker & Berek, 1995). The Bartholin's gland is composed of columnar epithelium, so adenocarcinomas, squamous cell carcinomas, and transitional cell carcinomas may arise from the gland (Hacker & Berek, 1995). Vulvar sarcomas represent 1% to 2% of vulvar malignancies. The most common histologic type is the leiomyosarcoma, which usually presents in the labia majora or the Bartholin's gland (Hacker & Berek, 1995).

ROUTES OF METASTASES

Cancer of the vulva generally spreads along predictable pathways of the lymphatic system. The incidence of inguinal node metastasis is strongly correlated with tumor thickness, histologic grade, vascular space involvement, clitoral or perineal location, and the presence of clinically suspicious nodes (Sedlis et al., 1987). Because the drainage system in the vulva is primarily unilateral, if the tumor is localized in the labia and the adjacent nodes are negative, then spread of the disease may be localized to one side, (Sedlis et al., 1987). Metastases to the pelvic lymph nodes are uncommon (Hacker & Berek, 1995). Spread of the disease through the blood usually occurs late in vulvar carcinoma and rarely occurs in the absence of lymphatic metastases (Hacker & Berek, 1995).

ASSESSMENT

Overview of the Assessment Process

An evaluation of a patient for vulvar cancer should include a history, physical examination, and appropriate diagnostic tests. A concise approach to the assessment of a patient for vulvar cancer is outlined in Table 35-1. Specific assessment parameters for the various types of vulvar cancer are summarized in the next sections of this chapter.

Definitive diagnosis is obtained following a careful inspection of the vulva and biopsy of abnormal areas. A vulvoscopy or colposcopic examination of the entire vulva is warranted, particularly in patients whose complaints of pruritus are not accompanied by gross abnormalities. These tests also assist in ruling out multicentric lesions (Hacker & Berek, 1995). A thorough health history, with particular attention to a history of sexually transmitted diseases, is essential.

Carcinoma In Situ

There is no characteristic clinical appearance of women presenting with VIN 3 or CIN. These women most often complain of pruritus. In some cases the vulva may appear reddened. When lesions are present, they may appear red, white, pink, gray, or brown (Hacker & Berek, 1995). Gross "warty" tumors have been seen in approximately 30% of cases (Buscema, Woodruff et al., 1980). Confluent or multicentric lesions appear in about two thirds of cases (Friedrich & Wilkinson, 1980), whereas perianal involvement has been reported in 25% of cases (Kaplan, Kaufman, Birken, & Simkin, 1981; Morrow, 1981).

Paget's Disease

Women with Paget's disease seek medical attention with complaints of pruritus and tenderness of the vulva. These conditions may be present for a long time. The affected area of the vulva is usually well demarcated and has the appearance of eczema, with white plaquelike lesions. The disease may be localized, but progressive growth of the lesions results in extension to the greater part of the vulva. These more extensive lesions are usually elevated and have a velvety texture. Persistent weeping is a distressing feature of these extensive lesions (Hacker & Berek, 1995).

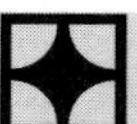

TABLE 35-1 Assessment of the Patient for Vulvar Cancer

	Assessment Parameters	Typical Abnormal Findings
History	A. Personal and social history 1. Age 2. Previous medical history 3. Socioeconomic status B. Evaluation of the female genital tract	A. Personal and social risk factors 1. Disease increases with age. 2. Previous or concurrent medical conditions that increase the risk for vulvar cancer: obesity, hypertension, diabetes mellitus, nulliparity, vulvar leukoplakia, vulvar or vaginal inflammatory disease, or another cancer of the female genital tract. 3. Women of lower socioeconomic status experience higher rates of vulvar cancer. B. Common symptoms include chronic vulvar pruritus and tenderness of the vulva.
Physical Examination	A. Physical examination of the female genital tract 1. Palpation of inguinal lymph nodes	A. The vulva may appear reddened. When lesions are present, they may vary in size, color, shape, and consistency 1. Lymph nodes may be palpable and indicate metastatic disease.
Diagnostic Tests	A. Excisional biopsy B. Wedge biopsy C. Cystoscopy and proctoscopy D. Skeletal radiographs and magnetic resonance imaging or computed tomography scan	A. Done for lesions of 1 cm or less in diameter. B. Biopsy includes the lesion and some surrounding skin and dermis and connective tissue so that the pathologist can adequately evaluate the depth and nature of stromal invasion. C. Tests may be used to evaluate the extent of invasion of the primary tumor. D. Tests may be used as part of a metastatic workup if bone pain is suspected.

Invasive Carcinoma of the Vulva

In the case of invasive vulvar carcinoma, most women present with a vulvar mass or lump. They often report a history of long-standing pruritus. Less common symptoms include vulvar bleeding, discharge, or dysuria. In situations in which the patient has delayed treatment, a large fungating vulvar lesion or lump in the groin may be present. Most lesions appear on the labia majora, with the labia minora the second most common site. Lesions may appear on the clitoris and the perineum (Hacker & Berek, 1995).

A complete health history is the first step in the assessment. Further evaluation includes a thorough inspection of the vulva, with attention to the inguinal lymph nodes. A local excisional biopsy of each of the lesions is done. A Papanicolaou smear with a thorough examination of the cervix, vagina, and pelvis is warranted. A vulvoscopy or colposcopy is often done, as these tests may be useful in defining areas for biopsy. Evaluation of the primary tumor may also include a cystoscopy or proctoscopy, or both, and/or a rectal or bladder biopsy. The metastatic workup should include chest and skeletal radiographs and magnetic resonance imaging (MRI) or computed tomography (CT), particularly if bone pain is suspected (Hacker & Berek, 1995).

STAGING

The clinical staging of vulvar cancer (Table 35-2) is based on the clinical assessment of the primary tumor and regional lymph nodes and a limited search for distant metastases (Hacker & Berek, 1995). A surgical staging system for vulvar cancer (Table 35-3) was adopted by the Federation of Obstetricians and Gynecologists (FIGO) in 1988 (Hacker & Berek, 1995). Clinical assessment for nodes is inherently unreliable. Reports have indicated that approximately 17% of patients with clinically negative nodes had positive nodes and 41% of patients who were thought to have clinically positive nodes were node-negative during surgical staging (Sedlis et al., 1987).

TABLE 35-2 TNM Classification of Carcinoma of the Vulva

T	Primary tumor
TIS	Preinvasive carcinoma (carcinoma in situ)
T_1	Tumor confined to the vulva and/or perineum, 2 cm or less in greatest dimension
T_2	Tumor confined to the vulva and/or perineum, more than 2 cm in greatest diameter
T_3	Tumor of any size with adjacent spread to the urethra and/or vagina and/or to the anus
T_4	Tumor of any size infiltrating the bladder mucosa and/or the rectal mucosa, including the upper part of the urethral mucosa and/or fixed to the bone
N	Regional lymph nodes
N_0	No nodes palpable
N_1	Unilateral regional lymph node metastasis
N_2	Bilateral regional lymph nodes metastasis
M	Distant metastasis
M_0	No clinical metastasis
M_1	Distant metastasis (including pelvic lymph node metastasis)

From McLellan, R. & Rosenshein, N.B. (1991). Vulvar cancer. In A.R. Moossa, S. Schimpff, & M. C. Robson (Eds.), *Comprehensive textbook of oncology* (Vol. 2.). Baltimore: Williams & Wilkins.

MEDICAL MANAGEMENT

Discussion of the medical management for vulvar cancers includes an overview of appropriate surgical, radiation, and chemotherapy interventions followed by a brief discussion of the treatments for the specific cancers. The treatment of premalignant vulvar lesions may include surgical management as described later or other methods such as cautery, laser surgery, cryosurgery, or topical 5-fluorouracil (5-FU). These alternative methods are presented in Table 35-4.

Surgical Management

The overriding theme for therapy for vulvar cancers is that the treatment be conservative and individualized for effective disease control, with minimum disruption and morbidity (Farias-Eisner & Berek, 1993; McLellan & Rosenshein, 1991; DiSaia, 1987). The objective in patients with CIN, microinvasive cancer, and early cancer of the vulva is to achieve optimal results without the morbidity associated with an en bloc dissection of the vulva and inguinal femoral

TABLE 35-3 Surgical Staging for Vulvar Cancer

Stage 0	
TIS	Carcinoma in situ, intraepithelial carcinoma
Stage I	
$T_1N_0M_0$	Tumor confined to the vulva and/or perineum, 2 cm or less in greatest dimension; nodes are not palpable
Stage II	
$T_2N_0M_0$	Tumor confined to the vulva and/or perineum, more than 2 cm in greatest dimension; nodes are not palpable
Stage III	
$T_3N_0M_0$ $T_3N_1M_0$ $T_1N_1M_0$ $T_2N_1M_0$	Tumor of any size with (a) adjacent spread to the lower urethra and/or vagina or the anus, and/or (b) unilateral regional lymph node metastasis
Stage IVA	
$T_1N_2M_0$ $T_2N_2M_0$ $T_3N_2M_0$ T_4 any N M_0	Tumor invades any of the following: upper urethra, bladder mucosa, rectal mucosa, pelvic bone, and/or bilateral regional node metastasis
Stage IVB	
Any T Any N M1	Any distant metastasis including pelvic lymph nodes

From McLellan, R. & Rosenshein, N.B. (1991). Vulvar cancer. In A.R. Moossa, S.C. Schimpff, & M.C. Robson (Eds.), *Comprehensive textbook of oncology* (Vol. 2.). Baltimore: Williams & Wilkins.

TABLE 35-4 Alternative Treatment Methods for Premalignant Vulvar Lesions

Therapy	Advantages	Disadvantages
Destructive cautery	Excellent cosmetic result	Necrotic ulcer may develop
Laser		2-5 treatments required General anesthesia required because of pain Bleeding and infection
Cryosurgery		Pain
Topical 5-fluorouracil		Pain with denudation Lengthy healing period Poor patient compliance Must be applied three times per day for 1 month

Data from DiSaia, P.J. & Creasman, W.T. (1989). *Clinical gynecologic oncology* (3rd ed.). St. Louis: Mosby.

lymph nodes and associated loss of function (McLellan & Rosenshein, 1991). Preservation of sexual function and a satisfactory cosmetic outcome are some of the major goals of surgical management.

One of three surgical approaches is used to manage preinvasive, microinvasive, and invasive carcinomas of the vulva. The first and most radical approach is a total vulvectomy that entails surgical removal of the entire vulva (labia majora, labia minora, clitoris) to the depth of Colle's fascia. This approach is used if there is concern about possible progression to invasive disease. This procedure is associated with a recurrence rate of about 10%, a high rate of postoperative morbidity, and long-term physical and emotional sequelae (McLellan & Rosenshein, 1991). In recent years, a modified vulvectomy (a radical local excision) has been used (van der Velden & Hacker, 1994; Stehman, Bundy, Dvoretsky, & Creasman, 1992). The decision to use the radical or more conservative approach is based primarily on the presence or absence of pathology in the remainder of the vulva (van der Verden & Hacker, 1994). Research indicates that a modification of the standard radical vulvectomy does not result in higher recurrence rates but does result in fewer complications (van der Velden & Hacker, 1994).

The second surgical approach is a skinning vulvectomy in which the excision is more limited in depth and extent. The excision is followed by a skin graft. The advantage of this procedure is that the subcutaneous fat is not removed (McLellan & Rosenshein, 1991). Tissue-flap reconstruction of the vulva has expanded the surgeon's ability to radically resect large cancers with less morbidity and functional impairment (Burke, 1992; Shepherd, Van Dam, Jobling, & Breach, 1990).

The third surgical approach is a wide local excision. This approach is most preferable for the treatment of preinvasive lesions, as it allows for the retention of healthy portions of the vulva without compromising long-term prognosis or quality of life. Recurrences, which are no more frequent than with a total vulvectomy, can be easily detected and treated by repeat excision (McLellan & Rosenshein, 1991).

Surgical management of the inguinal and femoral lymph nodes may be necessary to ensure that the disease is eradicated or arrested. Concurrent with any of the surgeries discussed previously, the physician may elect to perform a bilateral inguinal-femoral lymphadenectomy. Inguinal-femoral lymphadenectomy should be done on all patients if the primary tumor is more than 2 cm in diameter and in patients with T_1 disease in whom the depth of the invasion is greater than 1 mm (Hacker & van der Velden, 1993). The method of choice is the use of two incisions in the groin area for dissection of the nodes (Fig. 35-2). This method is preferred to the traditional en bloc dissection to decrease the incidence of wound breakdown (Hacker & Berek, 1995; Siller, Alvarez, Conner, McCullough, Kilgore, & Partridge et al., 1995). Intraoperative lymphatic mapping is being used to identify the sentinel node (i.e., those nodes most likely to be invaded first by the cancer cells) and to define the extent of superficial inguinal lymphadenectomy (Benjamin & Rubin, 1995; Levenback, Burke, Morris, Malpica, Lucas, & Gershenson, 1995). A pelvic lymphadenectomy is rare and reserved for patients with positive groin nodes (Hacker & Berek, 1995; Morley, 1976).

Radiation Therapy

The use of radiation for the primary treatment of vulvar cancer is rare. However, radiation has been used as adjuvant treatment for some clinical situations. Elective radiation to the inguinofemoral and pelvic nodes has been combined with a radical vulvectomy in patients with stage I or stage II disease (Petereit, Mehta, Buchler, & Kinsella, 1993; Mariani, Lombardi, Atlante, & Atlante, 1993; McLellan & Rosenshein, 1991; Daly & Million, 1974). In patients with locally advanced disease, including disease involving the rectovaginal septum or upper urethra, preoperative radiation may shrink the primary tumor, saving the patient more extensive surgery (Lupi, Raspagliesi, Zucali, Fontanelli, Paladini, & Kenda et al., 1996; Hacker & Berek, 1995; Hacker, Berek, Jullard, & Lagasse, 1984; Boronow, 1982). Postoperative radiation to the groin and pelvis may be appropriate for patients with multiple positive nodes (Hacker & Berek, 1995; van der Velden & Hacker, 1994). In patients with advanced disease, radiation has been used in combination with surgery that would require surgical interventions beyond vulvectomy and inguinofemoral node dissection (McLellan & Rosenshein, 1991; Boronow, 1982). Studies indicate that the use of brachytherapy (i.e., the use of implants of radioactive materials, such as radium, cesium, iridium, or gold at the site) is an effective treatment for patients who decline surgery or for whom surgery is contraindicated (Pohar, Hoffstetter, Peiffert, Luporsi, & Pernot, 1995).

An alteration in skin integrity is a common complication of radiation therapy. In severe cases, radionecrosis occurs. Surgical intervention is required to manage this condition (Roberts, Hoffman, LaPolla, Russ, Fiorica, & Cavanagh, 1991). Skin-sparing radiation techniques are used to prevent

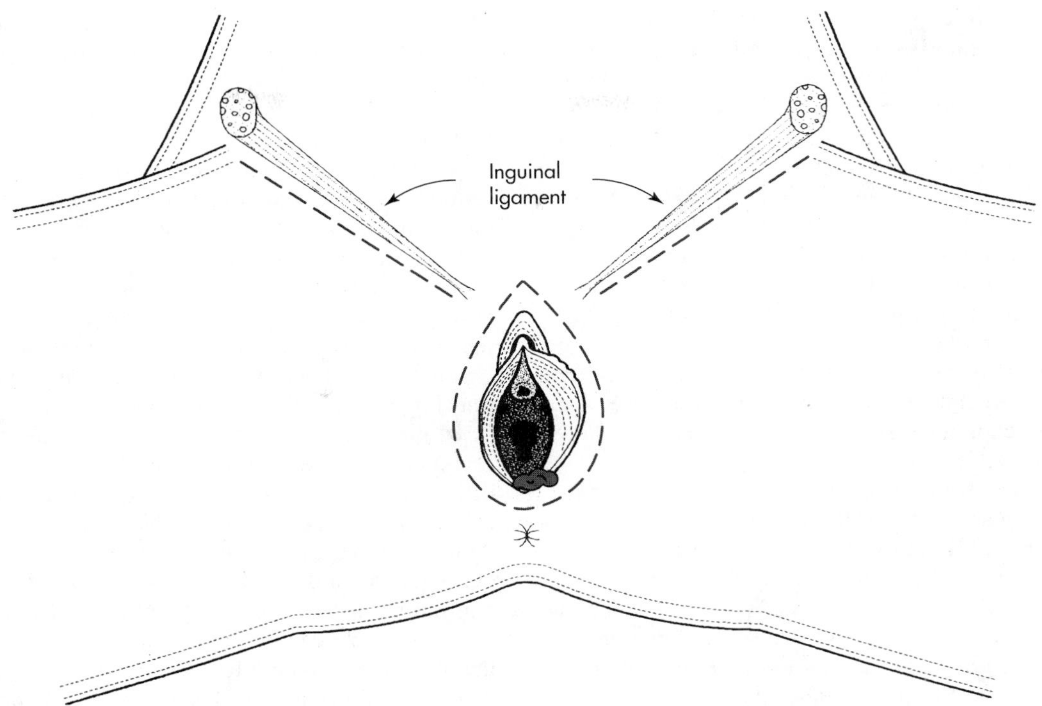

Fig. 35-2 Skin incisions for a bilateral inguinal-femoral lymphadenectomy. (From Hacker, N. F. & Berek, J. S. [1995]. Vulva. In C. M. Haskell & J. S. Berek [Eds.], *Cancer Treatment* [4th ed.]. Philadelphia: W. B. Saunders.)

this complication (Spencer, Pareek, Brezovich, Larson, Kim, & Plott et al., 1991).

Chemotherapy

The use of chemotherapy for the treatment of vulvar cancer has been limited, perhaps in part because many of the patients are elderly women who are in poor health. Effective treatment has been reported with the use of bleomycin in combination with other agents (Deppe, Cohen, & Bruckner, 1979; Trope, Johnsson, Larsson, & Simonsen, 1980; Thigpen, 1991). A recent study reported successful treatment with the combination of bleomycin, methotrexate, and CCNU. However, toxicities (e.g., mucositis, infection, hematologic, and pulmonary) were considerable (Durrant, Mangioni, Lacave, van der Burg, Guthrie, & Rotmenz et al., 1990). Studies have concluded that a combination of chemotherapy and radiation given before radical surgery may be effective for locally advanced squamous cell carcinoma if treatment-related morbidity can be decreased (Lupi et al., 1996; Koh, Wallace, Greer, Cain, Stelzer, & Russell et al., 1993). Further studies are necessary to define the role of chemotherapy in the treatment of vulvar cancer.

Specific Therapies for VIN

Carcinoma In Situ (VIN 3). The mainstay of treatment for carcinoma in situ is local excision of the individual lesions. This approach is effective, as microscopic disease rarely extends beyond the macroscopic lesion. The incidence of recurrence is about 30% (Buscema et al., 1980) When lesions are extensive, a procedure called *skinning vulvectomy* is performed. For this procedure, the skin is removed and replaced by a split-thickness graft (DiSaia & Rich, 1981; Rutledge & Sinclair, 1968). As with the local excision, the recurrence rate is about 30% (Hacker & Berek, 1995). Laser therapy has been used, with particular success with small lesions (Baggish & Dorsey, 1981; Townsend, Levine, Richart, Crum, & Petrelli., 1982). Regardless of the treatment method, routine long-term surveillance of the entire lower genital tract is recommended.

Paget's Disease. A wide local excision is required to decrease the likelihood of recurrence of Paget's disease, as the extent of the disease is wider than is clinically apparent in most cases (McLellan & Rosenshein, 1991). If the disease is extensive, a wide superficial vulvectomy may be required. If the patient's condition does not allow for a vulvectomy, a palliative local excision may be preferred. Recurrence is usually limited and can be treated by minor local excision or laser therapy, if it is detected early. If an underlying invasive cancer is present, treatment is similar to other invasive cancers that may require a radical vulvectomy and bilateral inguinal-femoral lymphadenectomy (Hacker & Berek, 1995; McLellan & Rosenshein, 1991).

Specific Therapies for Invasive Carcinoma of the Vulva

Squamous Cell Carcinoma. Approximately 90% of all invasive vulvar cancers are squamous cell carcinomas. The management of this disease is based on the extent of the disease. In superficially invasive disease (e.g., a lesion ≤ 2 cm in diameter with stromal invasion ≤ 5 mm), the course of treatment is controversial. Some physicians recommend the standard radical vulvectomy with bilateral inguinofemoral lymphadenectomy (Jafari & Cartnick, 1976; Yazigi, Piver, & Tsukada, 1978), whereas others believe that a wide local excision alone is satisfactory (van der Velden & Hacker, 1994). The 5-year survival rate following stages I and II treatment with a radical vulvectomy and bilateral groin dissection is excellent, at 95% and 85%, respectively (Homesley, Bundy, Sedlis, Yordan, Berek, & Jashan et al., 1991). However, morbidity after the standard radical vulvectomy is high. Wound breakdown ranges between 18% and 91%, chronic leg edema occurs in 8% to 70% of patients, lymphocysts develop in 0% to 31%, and mortality rates range from 0% to 12% (Morrow & Townsend, 1987). Further complicating the treatment morbidities is the presence of a high level of psychologic distress as a consequence of radical vulvectomy (Anderson & Hacker, 1983a, b).

Radical local excision has proven to be an adequate treatment for the primary tumor (DiSaia, Creasman, & Rich, 1979; Hacker, Berek, Lagasse, Leuchter, & Moore, 1983), with local recurrence rates approximately the same as with a vulvectomy. The advantages to the patient include a marked improvement in body image and sexual function associated with preserving some vulvar tissue (Hacker, Berek, Lagasse, Nieberg, & Leuchter, 1984). The omission of a groin dissection may be justified if the lesion is a unifocal tumor no more than 2 inches diameter with a depth of invasion less than 1 mm because the risk of metastasis is low in these situations (van der Velden & Hacker, 1994).

Frankly, invasive carcinomas of the vulva are treated with a radical vulvectomy and a bilateral inguinofemoral lymphadenectomy. A pelvic lymphadenectomy is controversial and is usually reserved for patients with positive groin nodes (Hacker & Berek, 1995; Morley, 1976). Adjuvant radiation is often ordered, particularly if the patient has two or more positive groin nodes or one large positive node (Hacker & Berek, 1995). If a CT scan and frozen section of enlarged groin nodes confirm the presence of metastases, adjuvant radiation to the groin and pelvis is given postoperatively (van der Velden & Hacker, 1994).

Although the use of the two-incision lymphadenectomy has reduced the incidence of wound breakdown (Hacker, Leuchter, Berek, Castaldo, & Lagasse, 1981; Rutledge, Smith, & Franklin, 1970), other complications do occur. Seromas occur in 10% to 15% of cases. Other less frequent complications of a radical vulvectomy and bilateral groin resection include cellulitis, anterior thigh anesthesia from femoral nerve injury, thrombophlebitis, and pulmonary embolus (Hacker & Berek, 1995).

Adenosquamous Carcinoma. Unlike its counterpart that appears on the exposed skin, adenocarcinomas of the vulva are highly aggressive tumors that are generally at more advanced stages at the time of diagnosis. They have a high rate of lymph node metastases and are associated with a poor prognosis (Hacker & Berek, 1995). The 5-year survival rate has been reported as low as 5.5% (Underwood, Adcock, & Okagaki, 1978). Treatment includes radical vulvectomy with bilateral inguinofemoral lymphadenectomy.

Verrucous Carcinoma. Verrucous carcinoma is a variant of squamous cell carcinoma. The tumors have a cauliflower-like appearance. Without a histologic examination, it is often difficult to differentiate this carcinoma from *C. acuminata* or squamous papilloma. Although the cause of this carcinoma is unclear, it is similar to *C. acuminata* (genital warts), which have been associated with HPV. A possible viral link is suspected.

Verrucous carcinomas are slow-growing but persistent lesions. They relentlessly grow to invade adjacent tissues, including the bone. Widespread destruction results. Metastases to the lymph nodes are rare (Gallousis, 1972). A wide local excision of the primary tumor is the basic treatment. However, if suspicious groin nodes exist, a bilateral inguinofemoral lymphadenectomy is recommended. Radiation therapy is contraindicated, as it may induce anaplastic transformation in the lesions (Hacker & Berek, 1995).

Malignant Melanoma. Malignant melanoma is found primarily in postmenopausal white women. This rare disease of the vulva accounts for 0.05% to 0.5% of all cancers of the female genital organs (Hacker & Berek, 1995). Although rare, it is the second most common cancer to occur in the vulva. In 80% of cases, the site of origin is the labia minora or the clitoris (McLellan & Rosenshein, 1991). This carcinoma can spread through the lymphatic system or the blood (McLellan & Rosenshein, 1991). Three histologic types of malignant melanoma are (1) superficial spreading melanoma; (2) a flat, frecklelike lesion that can become extensive but remains superficial; and (3) a nodular melanoma, which is a raised tumor that penetrates deeply and carries a poorer prognosis (Hacker & Berek, 1995).

Women presenting with a malignant melanoma are usually asymptomatic, with pigmented lesions that may have changed character. Some patients present with a groin mass. Any pigmented lesion on the vulva requires biopsy and histologic analysis (Hacker & Berek, 1995). Staging differs for this cancer, since the lesions are often smaller than those seen with squamous cell carcinoma of the vulva. Also these lesions tend to metastasize earlier than squamous cell lesions (Hacker & Berek, 1995).

Prognosis is related to the depth of invasion, the size of the lesion, and the extent of local extension. Superficial lesions less than 0.75 mm thick have a low risk of local recurrence or nodal metastasis and can be treated conservatively (McLellan & Rosenshein, 1991). For deeper lesions, a radical vulvectomy and bilateral inguinofemoral lymphadenectomy are recommended (Hacker & Berek, 1995). If the metastatic workup suggests spread of the disease beyond the vulva or groin, surgical interventions are usually limited to palliative wide local excisions of the primary and metastatic groin lesions (Hacker & Berek, 1995). Overall prognosis is poor if positive lymph nodes or signs of other metastatic disease are evident. Adjuvant chemotherapy (Hacker & Berek, 1995) and tamoxifen therapy (Masiel, Buttrick, & Bitran, 1981; Nesbit, Woods, Tattersall, Fox, Forbes, & MacKay et al., 1979) have been tried, but further studies are indicated to determine their effectiveness in treating malignant melanomas of the vulva.

Bartholin's Gland Carcinoma. Because of the nature of the columnar epithelium of Bartholin's gland, adenocarcinomas, squamous cell carcinomas, and, rarely, transitional cell carcinomas can occur in the gland (Hacker & Berek, 1995). Cancer of the Bartholin gland is extremely rare in all women (Visco & Del Priore, 1996). Women as young as 14 years of age have been reported with the disease, but it is most likely to occur during the fourth and fifth decades of life (Leuchter, Hacker, Voet, Berek, Townsend, & Lagasse et al., 1982). Initial treatment for an enlargement of the Bartholin's gland should be drainage and selective biopsy because of the rare occurrence of the disease (Visco & Del Priore, 1996). These cancers may be mistaken for benign cysts or abscesses; when this occurs, treatment is delayed. Because of the deep location of the Bartholin's gland, cases tend to be more advanced at the time of diagnosis; however, the prognosis is no different. The basic treatment is a radical vulvectomy and bilateral inguinofemoral lymphadenectomy. A pelvic lymphadenectomy is reserved for patients with positive groin nodes (Hacker & Berek, 1995). Good results have been reported using more conservative therapy. A hemivulvectomy or radical local excision for the primary tumor, followed by local postoperative radiation, has been reported to be effective (Copeland, Sneig, Gershenson, McGuffee, Abdul-Karim, & Rutledge et al., 1986).

Basal Cell Carcinoma. Basal cell carcinoma of the vulva occurs in about 2% of the vulvar cancers. White, postmenopausal women presenting with this type of vulvar cancer have lesions that appear as rolled-edge "rodent" ulcers. This cancer is locally aggressive, but nonmetastasizing. Usually a wide local excision is adequate treatment, but recurrence occurs in about 20% of cases. Basal cell carcinomas are associated with a high incidence of preceding or concurrent malignancies in other parts of the body, indicating a need for a thorough metastatic workup (Hacker & Berek, 1995).

Vulvar Sarcoma. Vulvar sarcomas are represented by many histologic types, including leiomyosarcomas, fibrosarcomas, neurofibrosarcomas, liposarcomas, rhabdomyosarcomas, angiosarcomas, and epithelioid sarcomas (Friedrich, 1976). The most common histologic type is leiomyosarcomas. Patients present with a painful mass, usually in the area of the labium majus or Bartholin's gland. Treatment is usually a wide local excision. Lymphatic metastases are uncommon. Recurrence is associated with lesion size, tumor contour, and mitotic activity. Lesions that are most likely to recur are greater than 5 cm in diameter, have infiltrating margins, and demonstrate a higher level of mitotic activity.

Rare Vulvar Malignancies. In addition to the common vulvar cancers listed previously, a few rare varieties have been reported: small cell carcinoma (Cliby, Soisson, Berchuck, & Clarke-Pearson, 1991), plasmacytomas (Doss, 1978), and endodermal sinus tumors (Underwood, Adcock, & Okagaki, 1978). The nature of the tumor gives direction to treatment, but generally the treatment plan is individualized to the tumor type and patient condition. A wide local excision followed by adjuvant chemotherapy or radiation is the general direction of the treatment plan (Hacker & Berek, 1995)

ONCOLOGIC EMERGENCIES

Vulvar cancer does not result in any of the major oncologic emergencies. However, elderly patients, who may have a compromised immune status, may be at risk for the development of septic shock when they undergo a surgical procedure. The risk of infection is high because of the presence of catheters/drains in the surgical wound and because the wound is located in the warm, moist environment of the perineum. Monitoring the surgical wound for signs of infection is a priority nursing activity.

Sepsis occurs as a response to a disseminated infection, usually a gram-negative organism. Initial signs and symptoms of sepsis include irritability; restlessness; confusion; fever; chills; warm, dry skin; red, flushed face; tachycardia; decreased blood pressure; and decreased urine output. As the syndrome of septic shock develops, the signs and symptoms that may appear include a decrease in cardiac output with a subsequent decrease in tissue perfusion; dry, cool skin that progresses to cold, clammy skin; peripheral edema; oliguria; tachycardia, and hypotension.

The diagnosis of sepsis and septic shock focuses on identifying the causative organism through cultures of blood, urine, and the surgical wound. Management of sepsis and septic shock focuses on administration of antibiotics, maintenance of the patient's ventilatory status, and maintenance of adequate perfusion to vital organs (e.g., brain, heart, kidney).

NURSING MANAGEMENT

Screening and Early Detection Activities

Nurses play an important role in the prevention and early detection of cancer in women. Nurses have many opportunities to incorporate primary, secondary, and tertiary prevention methods within their practice, regardless of the setting (Mahon, 1995). As the general public is less aware of interventions for the detection and prevention of vulvar cancer, nurses are key to informing women about how to screen for these cancers.

Health promotion education for women has included emphasis on breast self-examination and regular gynecologic checkups. Although cancer of the vulva occurs less frequently, women should be informed of the need to do regular vulvar self-examinations. These examinations can be done at the same time of the month that the woman completes her breast self-examination. The Center for Vulvar Diseases at the University of Michigan Medical Center has developed patient instructions for vulvar self-examinations (Table 35-5). For some women, it might be helpful if these instructions are accompanied by visual aids to point out the specific aspects of the anatomy of the vulva. In addition to monthly vulvar self-examination, women should be told to seek treatment for unresolving pruritus (i.e., itching that lasts more than 2 weeks). Immediate medical attention is warranted with the presence of lesions or lumps, bleeding, or pain in the area of the vulva.

Some women may be uncomfortable with vulvar self-examination. Understanding their attitudes about vulvar self-examination is the first step in preparing women to participate in this examination. Stressing the importance of this health promotion activity in the context of the woman's at-

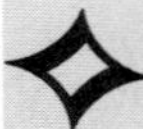

Table 35-5 Patient Preparation for Vulvar Self-Examination

Description of the Procedure: Just as you would examine your breasts or skin for changes that could suggest cancer, you should examine your vulva. Many different diseases of the vulva have similar symptoms. The vulvar self-examination will help you be aware of any changes in the vulvar area that may need further evaluation. This is especially important if you have ever had vulvar disease before. Some changes in the vulva may mean cancer. Tell your physician if you see any changes or have symptoms that do not go away, such as itching, bleeding, or discomfort. If a problem does occur, catching it at an early stage (when treatment is most successful) is in your best interest. Learning how to do a vulvar self-examination can best accomplish this goal.

Procedural Considerations:

1. Wash your hands carefully before you begin. Lie or sit in a comfortable position in good lighting with a hand mirror (a magnifying mirror may work best). It may help to prop up your back with pillows, or you can squat or kneel. The important thing is to find a comfortable position in which you can clearly see the vulvar area, perineum, and anus. At first, just look and learn. Things may appear different from what you expect, and that does not necessarily mean they are abnormal.
2. Gently separate the outer lips of the vulva. Look for any redness, swelling, dark or light spots, blisters, bumps, or other unusual colors.
3. Next, separate the inner lips and look carefully at the area between them for the same changes. Also, look at the entrance of the vagina.
4. Gently pull back the hood of the clitoris and examine the area under the hood at the tip of the clitoris.
5. Be sure to also inspect the area around the urethra, the perineum, the anus, the outside of the labia majora and the mons pubis.

Center for Vulvar Disease, University of Michigan Medical Center, Department of Obstetrics and Gynecology. *Internet communication.* July 15, 1996.

titudes about performing vulvar self-examination is essential for patient adherence. Vulvar self-examination enhances the probability of early detection and treatment if vulvar cancer occurs.

Management of the Common Problems Associated with Treatment of Vulvar Cancer

Treatment for vulvar cancer can be distressing for the patient. The diagnosis of cancer, as well as sensitivity about the location of the disease and the physical aspects of surgery, are emotionally trying for the patient. The goals of nursing care include providing supportive care, as well as the management of medical treatment. The management of a patient undergoing vulvar surgery is summarized in Table 35-6.

Skin Problems. Surgical treatment, whether it is a radical vulvectomy or a radical wide excision, poses many challenges for the patient, her family, and the nursing staff. The risk of infection is high because of the presence of catheters and/or drains, and the warm, moist environment of the perineum. Morbidities can be high, particularly with more extensive surgery. Reports indicate that as high as 85% of groin wounds have to be opened surgically, with healing by secondary intention (Podratz, Symmonds, & Taylor, 1982). This high morbidity rate, added to the fact that many of these patients are elderly women whose immune response may be altered by other medical problems, enhances the need for intense wound care.

Wound care is dictated by the extent of the surgery. Generally, the vulvar area must be kept clean and dry. Skin care may include wound irrigations and/or wound packing. After cleaning the wound, a heat source such as a hair dryer can be used to keep the perineum and the wound dry. Particular attention to signs and symptoms of wound infection is essential.

The patient experiencing a skin graft to the perineum may require bed rest for up to 6 days. Skin care includes careful assessment of the area for suppuration under the graft. Again, the goal is to see that the perineum remains clean and dry. The donor site, which is usually the buttocks, is covered with a Xeroform® gauze or transparent dressing. Patients report pain at the donor site when the graft site is exposed to air.

Short hospital stays enhance the importance of ensuring that the patient can manage skin care at home. Preparation for this activity should begin during hospitalization. Teaching should begin with an assessment of the woman's sensitivities about her "private areas." Gradually the nurse should encourage the patient to take part in her skin care. The surgical procedure causes a major change in the appearance of the vulva. Therefore the first step is to have the patient look at the wound. The first look at the wound site may be distressing for the patient. The patient should gradually be encouraged to participate in wound care. Initially holding supplies for the nurse is a good introduction to patient participation. Later steps include touching the area and gradually doing wound care independently. Patient education on the importance of skin care and the techniques used to do wound care is essential.

Alterations in skin integrity can also result from radiation therapy. Although skin sparing techniques are used, patients may develop skin changes that range from redness to radionecrosis. Treatment for alterations in skin integrity ranges from local therapy for minor to moderate skin conditions to more extreme surgical treatment that may be necessary if radionecrosis occurs (Roberts et al., 1991).

Fatigue. Women receiving surgery, radiation, or chemotherapy for vulvar cancer experience fatigue. Fatigue is characterized by multiple and interacting causes that include disease-, treatment-, biophysical-, functional-, symptom-, psychological-, social-, and occupational-related causes that interact over time (Winningham, 1996). Managing fatigue should be individualized to the patient. However, nurses should speak to patients about their fatigue experience, as-

TABLE 35-6 Standard of Care for the Patient Undergoing Vulvar Surgery

Patient Problem and Outcome	Nursing Interventions and Rationales	Patient Education Instructions
Surgical Wound Patient's wound will heal without an infection.	1. Assess the incision site frequently for signs of bleeding and infection. The risk of wound infection is high because of the presence of catheters/drains and the warm, moist environment of the perineum. 2. Perform wound care as per the surgeon's instructions or institutional protocol: a. Keep the wound clean. b. Keep the wound dry. May use a heat source such as a hair dryer to keep the wound dry. 3. Provide an overhead trapeze to lift and move to prevent shearing of the skin. 4. Maintain bed rest with head of bed elevated 30 to 45 degrees. 5. Provide pressure relief mattress. 6. Instruct patient not to cross her legs. 7. Place pillow between knees while positioned on side. 8. Change dressings immediately if soiled with urine or stool. 9. Avoid chair sitting, if a skin graft has been done, to prevent ischemic pressure areas on the buttocks. 10. Avoid straining at stool; provide stool softeners to prevent the development of anal fissures and bleeding associated with constipation.	1. Discuss with patient the changes that will occur in the anatomy of the vulva before surgery. 2. Have patient gradually participate in wound care: a. Assist by holding supplies. b. Have patient view the wound. c. Have patient perform wound care, if possible. 3. Instruct patient and family members about the signs and symptoms they should report to a health care provider including: a. Unusual odor b. Fresh bleeding c. Perineal pain d. Elevated temperature e. Increased swelling of operative site/groin 4. Instruct patient to elevate legs periodically, avoid prolonged chair sitting, and to not cross legs. 5. Avoid heavy lifting. 6. Discuss patient and caregiver's ability to perform wound care and determine whether a home care referral is needed.
Lymphedema Patient will experience a limited amount of lower extremity swelling and minimal discomfort.	1. Assess lower extremities for swelling and measure the extremity at consistent, anatomic landmarks. 2. Elevate lower extremities when appropriate after incision has healed. 3. Use elastic stockings or compression garments or devices, as prescribed. 4. Obtain a referral to a physical therapist for massage and physical therapy.	1. Discuss with patient the reasons for the swelling in the lower extremities. 2. Teach patient the importance of reporting and signs or symptoms of infection. 3. Emphasize the importance of excellent skin care to prevent infections. 4. Review lower extremity exercises to reduce lymphedema.
Anticipatory grieving related to lifestyle changes, decreased physical abilities, changes in physical appearance and life-threatening prognosis Patient will: • Be able to progress through the stages of grieving. • Demonstrate effective coping strategies.	1. Be sensitive to the changes the patient is experiencing and encourage her to express her feelings. 2. Provide a therapeutic environment that is conducive to open discussion with patient and her partner (if appropriate). 3. Provide information regarding support groups. 4. Collaborate with other professionals (social worker, clergy, psychologist) to provide support and facilitate the grieving process. 5. Support adaptive behaviors that suggest progression and resolution of the grieving process.	1. Explain the normal stages of the grieving process. 2. Teach patient effective coping strategies to help manage the grieving process. 3. Discuss community resources and support groups for the patient and her family.

Modified from Tucker, S.M., Canobbio, M.M., Paquette, E.V., & Wills, M.F. (1996). *Patient care standards: Collaborative practice planning guides* (6th ed.). St. Louis: Mosby.

suring them that it is an expected symptom and working with them to identify strategies to manage their fatigue.

Incontinence. The surgery experience can result in urinary incontinence. A radical vulvectomy itself does not cause incontinence, but when a portion of the urethra is removed, the incidence of urinary incontinence increases (Reid, DeLancey, Hopkins, Roberts, & Morely, 1990). Stress or total incontinence resulting from surgical intervention is more permanent in nature. Urinary incontinence causes additional distress to the patient who is already overwhelmed with the threat of vulvar cancer and its treatment. Supportive nursing care can help the patient cope with incontinence. Patient teaching is also needed to ensure that the patient maintains good skin integrity.

Lymphedema. Women experiencing a lymphadenectomy, particularly a groin lymph node dissection, may experience lymphedema. The incidence of lower extremity lymphedema has decreased since surgical approaches have become more conservative. Studies report the presence of only mild or moderate lymphedema in about 20% of the cases after groin dissection (Karakousis, Heiser, & Moore, 1983).

In addition to a groin lymph node resection (Rogers, 1994; Larson, Weinstein, Goldberg, Silver, Recht, & Cady et al., 1986), radiation therapy after lymphadenectomy also predisposes the patient to lymphedema (Larson et al., 1986). Other risk factors include age (Greenfield, 1994; Gottlieb & Patel, 1991), obesity (Greenfield, 1994), and infections (Kissin, Querici della Rovere, Easton, & Westburg, 1986; Simon & Cody, 1992). Lymphedema causes mild discomfort to severe pain. The swelling can be quite severe, causing the woman to change her clothing style and/or wear a supportive stocking. The edema can be activity related, causing an adjustment to lifestyle, omitting or altering some activities. Temperature shifts in the environment or infections in the extremity can also precipitate swelling (Kalinowski, 1996).

Lymphedema can range from mild to severe. The goals of treatment are to reduce swelling and discomfort and promote lymphatic circulation. Therapeutic approaches to managing mild lymphedema include elevation of the extremity, compression garments or devices, massage and physical therapy (Kalinowski, 1996). Elevation can be achieved via the use of pillows or wedge-shaped cushions. When up in a chair, patients should be instructed to elevate their feet on a stool. Effective compression apparatus include sequential pneumatic compression devices, which are usually limited to hospital use, and elastic stockings (Lerner, 1992; Richmond, O'Donnell, & Zelikowski, 1985). Patients should be instructed to remove the elastic stockings if they are too tight, are causing pain, or are causing decreased circulation to the feet. Size and fit of the elastic stockings should be checked periodically to ensure that they fit properly (Kalinowski, 1996). Manual compression of the extremity may be recommended. A physical therapist trained to manage lymphedema can give nursing staff, the patient, and the family direction in implementing this intervention (Kalinowski, 1996).

Pneumatic compression pumps are the method of choice to control moderate lymphedema to the lower extremity. Severe lymphedema exists when the diameter of the affected extremity is 5 to 6 cm larger than the unaffected extremity. Severe lymphedema is uncomfortable and causes pain and alterations in mobility. Management of severe lymphedema includes all the strategies used for mild edema. More aggressive physical therapy is initiated. Pain management includes the use of nonsteroidal antiinflammatory drugs (NSAIDs), transcutaneous electrical nerve stimulation (TENS) units, and positional measures. Severe lymphedema that has progressed to the stage of hard, fibrotic swelling, accompanied by tough, brawny skin may require surgical intervention to diminish the swelling and promote lymphatic circulation (Kalinowski, 1996).

Psychological Adjustment. The diagnosis of vulvar cancer and its treatment is distressing for each woman experiencing it. Extensive surgical interventions complicate dealing with a potentially life-threatening disease. Physical alterations of the vulva can be overwhelming immediately postoperatively as well as posthospitalization. Preparing the patient for the medical management of vulvar cancer should begin before hospitalization. The primary goal is to support the woman so that she can return to her home, family, and occupation and is able to deal with her altered body appearance and functions. Sensitivity to the woman's feelings about vulvar cancer and its treatment is critical to providing supportive therapy. Nurses are in a position to discuss the treatment and its effects with the patient, listening to her and supporting her and her significant others. Nurses are also key to making referrals to other health care providers who can assist the patient and her family in coping with this cancer experience.

HOME CARE ISSUES

Depending on the treatment approaches used to manage vulvar cancer, the patient's age, and the patient's general state of health, the patient and her family caregivers will be faced with several issues in the home care setting.

Skin Care

Healing in the perineum can occur over an extended period. Patient teaching is essential to ensure that the perineum remains clean and dry. Specific instructions for wound care must accompany the patient home. Before discharge, the patient should demonstrate wound care to the nurse to ensure that she not only understands the procedure, but that she can also perform the wound care. These instructions should be accompanied by specific direction for doing the procedure at home. If supplies and equipment are needed, the patient should receive information regarding resources.

The elderly patient may not be able to care independently for her surgical site. After a thorough assessment of the patient's support systems, a family member or friend can be identified to assist with wound care. The family member or friend can be invited to participate in this care in the hospital or taught the procedure by the home care nurse. In identifying this support person, it is important to be sensitive to the patient's social relationships. For some women, asking their partner or a family member to perform wound care for the perineal area is difficult. The patient may find it embarrassing. Recognizing the patient's feelings about assistance is the first step in supporting her and ensuring proper skin care.

Body Image Disturbance

Alterations with body image are associated with physical changes in the perineum and lymphedema, if present. These physical changes not only affect appearance, but also may alter sexual functioning and elimination patterns. Adjustments to working patterns and responsibilities may also be necessary, depending on the demands of the woman's job. Information that can assist the nurse and the health care team in supporting the patient include data about her support systems, sexual relationships, and coping strategies; her attitudes about herself; her attitudes about her relationship with her spouse/significant other; and her routine activities and work responsibilities (Miller & Pazdur, 1989).

Adjustment to alterations in body image occurs over time. Discharge from the hospital often stimulates thoughts about the realities of treatment and how these realities affect lifestyle. Ongoing support is important if the woman and her family are to effectively cope with this disease and its treatment.

Sexual Dysfunction

A radical vulvectomy is a particularly mutilating surgery that results in a loss of sexually responsive tissue. Even more conservative wide excision procedures affect sexual functioning, particularly if a clitoridectomy is performed. The human sexual response is a total body vasocongestive-neuromuscular response mediated through the autonomic nervous system. The loss of parasympathetic nerves and pelvic vasculature may delay the physiologic response, but gynecologic surgery does not destroy sexual function. (Lamont, DePetrillo, & Sargent, 1978; Glasgow, Halfin, & Althausen, 1987; Miller & Pazdur, 1989). Supportive therapy may be necessary to assist the patient and her partner to adjust to changes in sexual responses. This therapy should begin before surgery (Miller & Pazdur, 1989).

Little attention has been given to the psychosexual responses of women having various surgical treatments for vulvar cancer. Clearly disfiguring surgery can make the woman feel unattractive, affecting the way that she interacts with her partner. The physical, social, and sexual impact of a radical vulvectomy has been described (Springer, 1982). Alterations in body image and sexual function were reported. When distal portions of the vagina were removed, sensory perceptions important to foreplay were lost. The removal of the clitoris resulted in the loss of orgasmic potential and introital stenosis made intercourse painful or difficult for some women (Springer, 1982). In another study, interviews with 18 women who received surgery for vulvar cancer revealed that these women experienced psychologic distress similar to women who had undergone pelvic exenteration. The women with vulvar cancer reported a decrease in sexual activity, lower sexual arousal, sexual anxiety, limited sexual satisfaction, and a disruption of body image (Anderson & Hacker, 1983a, b). The effect of more conservative surgery on sexual functioning has not been reported.

The male partner's response to the extensive surgery must also be examined. The partner may have to confront his own emotions regarding the disease and its treatment. His feelings about the woman may be evaluated. He too will have to adjust to the physical changes and sexual responses of his partner. His willingness to make adjustments to the traditional coital experience to which he was accustomed must be assessed (Miller & Pazdur, 1989). Strong marital relationships are essential to sexual rehabilitation after surgery for vulvar cancer. If there are preexisting problems in the relationship, the surgical treatment may be the focus for all the marital problems (Miller & Pazdur, 1989).

The psychosocial adjustment of the woman and her partner must begin before surgery. Continuity of care should be ensured by a team approach in managing the disease and its treatment. A member of the team should be an expert in dealing with sexual problems that can follow surgery. Expert sexual counseling is essential to psychosexual adjustment. Because of the sensitive nature of sexual intimacy, the patient and her partner may not request assistance in this area. They may be too embarrassed to indicate that sexual functioning may be a concern. However, the astute nurse will recognize the need for such expertise and will make appropriate referrals. It has been suggested that a psychosexual counselor see the woman before and after surgery, every 2 to 4 weeks after discharge for 6 months, and every 3 to 6 months thereafter (Lamont, DePetrillo, & Sargent, 1978).

Many women experiencing vulvar cancer are elderly. Yet age does not preclude that sexual functioning and intimacy are unimportant. Regardless of age or marital status, women treated for vulvar cancer must deal with alterations in sexual functioning. Referrals to experts in sexuality are important in ensuring enhanced quality of life for these women.

Women can be fully rehabilitated sexually after surgery for vulvar cancer if proper education and support are given to the patient and her partner. Nurses are key to initiating appropriate referrals to ensure this rehabilitation. However, nurses may be somewhat reluctant to discuss sexual issues with patients and their partners. This reluctance can result in lack of treatment and a less than satisfactory quality of life for the woman and her partner.

Infertility after treatment for vulvar cancer can be a major concern for younger women experiencing the disease. Discussion of infertility following cancer treatment is beyond the scope of this chapter; other resources can be consulted for an overview of this topic (Howard, 1991; Kaempfer, Wiley, & Hoffman, 1985; Kaempfer & Major, 1986).

PROGNOSIS

The prognosis of vulvar cancer correlates with the stage of the disease, the size of the primary lesion, and the patient's lymph node status. The overall survival for patients with vulvar cancer is 47.3% when including patients treated with vulvar cancer and 47.3% when including patients treated palliatively. When stratified by number of positive nodes, patients with one microscopic node have a 5-year survival rate of 94.6%. In contrast, patients with two and three or more positive nodes have 5-year survival rates of approximately 80% and 15%, respectively. The overall 5-year survival rate of patients with positive lymph nodes is 50.8% (Hacker et al., 1981; Hacker et al., 1984; Hacker et al., 1984; Homesley, Bundy, Sedlis, & Adcock, 1986; Rutledge, Smith, & Franklin, 1970).

EVALUATION OF THE QUALITY OF CARE

Accreditation organizations such as the Joint Commission for the Accreditation of Healthcare Organizations require that the quality of care provided to patients be evaluated. Because the care provided to patients with vulvar cancer requires input from a multidisciplinary team, an evaluation of the quality of care provided to these patients should include aspects of the care provided by the various members of the team. Table 35-7 provides an example of a quality of care evaluation tool that can be used in the inpatient setting.

TABLE 35-7 Quality of Care Evaluation for a Patient Undergoing Vulvar Surgery

Disciplines participating in the quality of care evaluation:
☐ Nursing ☐ Surgery
☐ Physical Therapy ☐ Social Services

Data from:
☐ Medical Record Review ☐ Patient/Family Interview

Criteria	Yes	No
1. Wound care done according to surgeon's prescription or institutional policies.	☐	☐
2. Patient placed on a pressure relief mattress.	☐	☐
3. Patient experienced the following complications:		
a. Wound infection	☐	☐
b. Pressure ulcer	☐	☐

RESEARCH ISSUES

Research issues related to the management of vulvar cancer include topics in self-care and symptom management. Although vulvar cancer is relatively rare, and large sample sizes are not available, research is needed to explore the management of wound care in the home. Elderly patients receiving treatment may have more difficulty in managing wound care than their younger counterparts. Understanding what these women need as far as resources and support systems can lead to implementation of interventions that prevent complications and enhance the patient's quality of life.

Disfigurement of the perineum occurs in all women receiving surgical management of the area. Studies that examine the actual limitations caused by surgery and the methods patients use to cope with these limitations would provide health care workers with a knowledge base to enhance adjustment for future patients with this disease.

Little research is available regarding the psychosexual issues of women receiving treatment for vulvar cancer. A new complement of younger women diagnosed with the disease and new surgical techniques suggest that research to examine alterations in sexual functioning is essential. From such descriptive research, interventions to enhance sexual functioning and quality of life can be developed and tested.

Diagnosis and treatment of vulvar cancer are frightening. Nurses who are sensitive to the realities of this experience can enhance the patient's quality of life by ensuring continuity and quality patient care.

REFERENCES

Anderson, W. A., Franquemont, D. W., Williams, J., Taylor, P. T., & Crum, C. P. (1991). Vulvar squamous cell carcinoma and papillomaviruses: Two separate entities? *American Journal of Obstetrics and Gynecology, 165* (2), 329-335.

Anderson, B. L. & Hacker, N. F. (1983a). Psychosexual adjustment of gynecologic oncology patients: A proposed model for future investigation. *Gynecologic Oncology, 15,* 214-223.

Anderson, B. L. & Hacker, N. F. (1983b). Psychosexual adjustment after vulvar surgery. *Obstetrics and Gynecology, 62,* 457-462.

Apgar, B. S. & Cox, J. T. (1996). Differentiating normal and abnormal findings of the vulva. *American Family Physician, 53*(4), 1171-1180.

Baggish, M. S. & Dorsey, J. H. (1981). CO_2 laser for the treatment of vulvar carcinoma in situ. *Obstetrics and Gynecology, 57*(3), 371-375.

Benjamin, I. & Rubin, S. C. (1995). Advances in surgery for gynecologic malignancies. *Current Opinions in Oncology, 7*(5), 473-477.

Bloss, J. D., Liao, S. Y, Wilczynski, S. P., Macri, C., Walker, J., Peake, M., & Berman, M. L. (1991). Clinical and histologic features of vulvar carcinomas analyzed for human papillomavirus status: Evidence that squamous cell carcinoma of the vulva has more than one etiology. *Human Pathology, 22*(7), 711-718.

Boronow, R. C. (1982). Combined therapy as an alternative to exenteration for locally advanced vulva-vaginal cancer: Rationale and results. *Cancer, 49,* 1085-1091.

Brinton, L. A., Nasca, P. C., Mallin, K., Baptiste, M. S., Wilbanks, G. D., & Richart, R. M. (1990). Case-control study of cancer of the vulva. *Obstetrics and Gynecology, 75,* 859-866.

Burke, T. W. (1992). Changing surgical approaches to vulvar cancer. *Current Opinions in Obstetrics and Gynecology, 4*(1), 86-90.

Buscema, J., Woodruff, J. D., Parmley, T. H., & Genadry, R. (1980). Carcinoma in situ of the vulva. *Obstetrics and Gynecology, 55*(2), 225-230.

Cliby, W., Soisson, A. P., Berchuck, A., & Clarke-Pearson, D. L. (1991). Stage I small cell carcinoma of the vulva treated with vulvectomy, lymphadenectomy and adjuvant chemotherapy. *Cancer, 67*(9), 2415-2417.

Committee on Terminology, International Society for the Study of Vulvar Disease. (1989). New nomenclature for vulvar disease. *International Journal of Gynecologic Pathology, 8,* 83-84.

Copeland, L. J., Sneig, N., Gershenson, D. M., McGuffee, V. B., Abdul-Karim, F., & Rutledge, F. N. (1986). Bartholin gland carcinoma. *Obstetrics and Gynecology, 67*(6), 794-801.

Costa, S., Syrjanen, S., Vendra, C., Chang, F., Guida, G., Hippelainen, M., Terzano, P., Tervahauta, A., Yliskoski, M., & Syrjanen, K. (1995). Human papillomavirus infections in vulvar precancerous lesions and cancer. *Journal of Reproductive Medicine, 40*(4), 291-298.

Daly, J. W. & Million, R. R. (1974). Radical vulvectomy combined with elective node irradiation for TxNo squamous carcinoma of the vulva. *Cancer, 34,* 161-165.

Deppe, G., Cohen, C. J., & Bruckner, H. W. (1979). Chemotherapy of squamous cell carcinoma of the vulva: A review. *Gynecologic Oncology, 7,* 345-348.

DiSaia, P. J. (1987). The case against the surgical concept of en bloc dissection for certain malignancies of the reproductive tract. *Cancer, 60,* 2025-2034.

DiSaia, P. J., Creasman, W. T., & Rich, W. M. (1979). An alternative approach to early cancer of the vulva. *American Journal of Obstetrics and Gynecology, 133*(7), 825-832.

DiSaia, P. J. & Rich, W. M. (1981). Surgical approach to multifocal carcinoma in situ of the vulva. *American Journal of Obstetrics and Gynecology, 140*(2), 136-145.

Doss, L. L. (1978). Simultaneous extramedullary plasmacytomas of the vagina and vulva: A case report and review of the literature. *Cancer, 41*(6), 2468-2474.

Durrant, K. R., Mangioni, C., Lacave, A. J., van der Burg, M. E. L., Guthrie, D., Rotmenz, N., Dalesio, O., & Vermorken, J. B. (1990). Bleomycin, methotrexate, and CCNU in advanced inoperable squamous cell carcinoma of the vulva: A phase II study of the EORTC Gynaecologic Cancer Cooperative Group (GCCG). *Gynecologic Oncology, 37,* 359-362.

Farias-Eisner, R., & Berek, J. S. (1993). Current management of invasive squamous carcinoma of the vulva. *Clinics in Geriatric Medicine, 9*(1), 131-143.

Franklin III, E. W. & Rutledge, F. D. (1972). Epidemiology of epidermoid carcinoma of the vulva. *Obstetrics and Gynecology, 39,* 165-172.

Franquemont, D. W., Anderson, W. A., Williams, J., Taylor, P. T., & Crum, C. P. (1991). Vulvar carcinoma: Two separate etiologies? [Abstract]. *Laboratory Investigation, 64,* 57A.

Friedrich, E. G. & Wilkinson, E.J. (1980). Carcinoma in situ of the vulva: A continuing challenge. *American Journal of Obstetrics and Gynecology, 136* (7), 830-843.

Friedrich, E. G. (1976). *Vulvar disease.* Philadelphia, PA: W. B. Saunders Co.

Gallousis, S. (1972). Verrucous carcinoma: Report of three vulvar cases and a review of the literature. *Obstetrics and Gynecology, 40*(4), 502-507.

Giles, G. G. & Kneals, B. L. (1995). Vulvar cancer: The Cinderella of gynaecological oncology. [See comments]. *Australian and New Zealand Journal of Obstetrics and Gynaecology, 35*(1), 71-75.

Glasgow, M., Halfin, V., & Althausen, A. (1987). Sexual response and cancer. *CA: Cancer Journal for Clinicians, 37,* 322-333.

Gottlieb, L, J. & Patel, P. K. (1991). Lymphedema following axillary surgery: Elephantiasis chirurgica. In J. Harris, S. Hellman, & I. C. Henderson et al. (Eds.), *Breast diseases* (2nd ed.). 820-827). Philadelphia: J. B. Lippincott.

Green, T. H., Ulfelder, H., & Meigs, J. (1958). Epidermoid carcinoma of the vulva: An analysis of 238 cases. Part II. Therapy and end results. *American Journal of Obstetrics and Gynecology, 75,* 834-847.

Greenfield, L, J. (1994). Venous and lymphatic disease. In S. I. Schwartz, T. G. Shires, F. C. Spencer, & W. C. Husser (Eds.), *Principles of surgery* (6th ed.). New York: McGraw-Hill.

Hacker, N. F. & Berek, J. S. (1995). Vulva. In C. M. Haskell, (Ed.), *Cancer treatment* (4th ed). Philadelphia: W. B. Saunders.

Hacker, N. F., Berek, J. S., Jullard, J. F., & Lagasse, L. D. (1984). Preoperative radiation therapy for locally advanced vulvar cancer. *Cancer 54,* 2056-2061.

Hacker, N. F., Berek, J. S., Lagasse, L. D., Nieberg, R. K., & Leuchter, R. S. (1984). Individualization of treatment for stage I squamous cell vulvar carcinoma. *Obstetrics and Gynecology, 63,* 155-162.

Hacker, N. F., Berek, J. S., Lagasse, L. D., Leuchter, R. S., & Moore, J. G. (1983). Management of regional lymph nodes and their prognostic influence in vulvar cancer. *Obstetrics and Gynecology, 39,* 65-68.

Hacker, N. F., Leuchter, R. S., Berek, J. S., Castaldo, T. W., & Lagasse, L. D. (1981). Radical vulvectomy and bilateral inguinal lymphadenectomy through separate groin incisions. *Obstetrics and Gynecology, 58,* 574-579.

Hacker, N. E. & van der Velden, J. (1993). Conservative management of early vulvar cancer. *Cancer, 71*(Suppl. 4), 1673-1677.

Hart, W. R. & Millman, J. B. (1977). Progression of intraepithelial Paget's disease of the vulva to invasive carcinoma. *Cancer, 40*(5), 2333-2337.

Homesley, H. D., Bundy, B. N., Sedlis, A., & Adcock, L. (1986). Radiation therapy versus pelvic node resection for carcinoma of the vulva with positive groin nodes. *Obstetrics and Gynecology, 68,* 733-740.

Homesley, H. D., Bundy, B. N., Sedlis, A., Yordan, E., Berek J. S., Jashan, A., & Mortel, R. (1991). Assessment of current International Federation of Gynecology and Obstetrics staging of vulvar carcinoma relative to prognostic factors for survival (a Gynecologic Oncology Group study). *American Journal of Obstetrics and Gynecology, 164,* 997-1004.

Hording, U., Junge, J., Poulsen, H., & Lundvall, F. (1995). Vulvar intraepithelial neoplasia III: A viral disease of underdetermined progressive potential. *Gynecologic Oncology, 56*(2), 276-279.

Hording, U., Kringsholm, B., Andreasson, B., Visfeldt, J., Daugaard, S., & Bock, J. E. (1993). Human papillomavirus in vulvar squamous cell carcinoma and in normal vulvar tissues: A search for a possible impact of HPV on vulvar cancer prognosis. *International Journal of Cancer, 55*(3), 394-396.

Howard, G. (1991). Fertility following cancer therapy. *Clinical Oncology, 3,* 283-287.

Jafari, K. & Cartnick, E. N. (1976). Microinvasive squamous cell carcinoma of the vulva. *Gynecologic Oncology, 4*(2), 158-166.

Kaempfer, S., Wiley, F., & Hoffman, D. (1985). Fertility considerations and procreative alternatives in cancer care. *Seminars in Oncology Nursing, 1*(1), 25-34.

Kaempfer, S. & Major, D. (1986). Fertility considerations in the gynecologic oncology patients. *Oncology Nursing Forum, 13*(1), 23-27.

Kalinowski, B. H. (1996). Lymphedema. In S. L. Groenwald, M. H. Frogge, M. Goodman, & C. H. Yarbro (Eds.), *Cancer symptom management.* Boston: Jones and Bartlett.

Kaplan, A. L., Kaufman, R.H., Birken, R.A., & Simkin, S. (1981). Intraepithelial carcinoma of the vulva with extension to the anal canal. *Obstetrics & Gynecology, 58*(3), 368-371.

Karakousis, C. P., Heiser, M. A., & Moore, R. H. (1983). Lymphedema after groin dissection. *American Journal of Surgery, 145,* 205-208.

Kissin, M. W., Querici della Rovere, G., Easton, D., & Westburg, G. (1986). Risk of lymphedema following the treatment for breast cancer. *British Journal of Surgery, 73*(7), 580-584.

Koh, W. J., Wallace, H. J. III, Greer, B. E., Cain, J., Stelzer, K. J., Russell, K. J., Tamini, H. K., Figge, D. C., Russell, A. H., & Griffin, T. W. (1993). Combined radiotherapy and chemotherapy in the management of local-regionally advanced vulvar cancer. *International Journal of Radiology: Oncology,-Biology-Physics, 28*(5), 809-816.

Kurman, R. J., Norris, H. J., & Wilkinson, E. J. (1992). *Tumors of the cervix, vagina, and vulva: Atlas of tumor pathology.* Washington, D. C.: Armed Forces Institute of Pathology.

Lamont, J. A., DePetrillo, A. D., & Sargent, E. J. (1978). Psychosexual rehabilitation and exenterative surgery. *Gynecologic Oncology, 6,* 236-242.

Larson, D., Weinstein, M., Goldberg, I., Silver, B., Recht, A., Cady, B., Silen, W, & Harris, J. R. (1986). Edema of the arm as a function of the extent of axillary surgery in patients with stage I-II carcinoma of the breast treated with primary radiotherapy. *International Journal of Radiology: Oncology,-Biology-Physics, 12*(9), 1575-1582.

Lerner, R. (1992). The ideal treatment for lymphedema. *Massage Therapy Journal, Winter,* 37-39.

Leuchter, R. S., Hacker, N. F., Voet, R. L., Berek, J. S., Townsend, D. E., & Lagasse, L. D. (1982). Primary carcinoma of the Bartholin gland: A report of 14 cases and review of the literature. *Obstetrics and Gynecology, 60*(3), 361-368.

Levenback, C., Burke, T. W., Morris, M., Malpica, A., Lucas, K. R., & Gershenson, D. M. (1995). Potential applications of intraoperative lymphatic mapping in vulvar cancer. *Gynecologic Oncology, 59*(2), 216-220.

Lupi, G., Raspagliesi, F., Zucali, R., Fontanelli, R., Paladini, D., Kenda, R., & di Re, F. (1996). Combined preoperative chemoradiotherapy followed by radical surgery in locally advanced vulvar carcinoma: A pilot study. *Cancer, 77*(8), 1472-1478.

Lynch, P.J. (1987). Vulvar dystrophies and intraepithelial neoplasias. *Dermatologic Clinics, 5,* 789.

Mabuchi, K., Bross, D. D., & Kessler, I. I. (1985). Epidemiology of cancer of the vulva: A case-control study. *Cancer, 55,* 1843-1848.

Mahon, J. M. (1995). Prevention and early detection of cancer in women. *Seminars in Oncology Nursing, 11*(2), 88-102.

Mariani, L., Lombardi, A., Atlante, M., & Atlante, G. (1993). Radiotherapy for vulvar carcinoma with positive inguinal nodes: Adjunctive treatment. *Journal of Reproductive Medicine, 38*(6), 429-436.

Masiel, A., Buttrick, P., & Bitran, J. (1981). Tamoxifen in the treatment of malignant melanoma [Letter]. *Cancer Treatment Reports, 65*(5-6), 531-532.

McLellan, R. & Rosenshein, N. B. (1991). Vulvar cancer. In A. R. Moossa, S. C. Schimpff, M. C. Robson, (Eds.), *Comprehensive textbook of oncology* (Vol. 2). Baltimore: Williams & Wilkins.

Miller, N. J. & Pazdur, M. (1989). Gynecologic malignancies. In S. L. Groenwald, (Ed.), *Cancer nursing: Principles and practices.* Boston: Jones & Bartlett.

Monk, B. J., Burger, R. A., Lin, F., Parham, G., Vasilev, S. A., & Wilczynski, S. P. (1995). Prognostic significance of human papillomavirus DNA in vulvar carcinoma. *Obstetrics and Gynecology, 85*(5, Part 1), 709-715.

Morley, G. W. (1976). Infiltrative carcinoma of the vulva: Results of surgical treatment. *American Journal of Obstetrics and Gynecology, 124*(8), 874-888.

Morrow, C. P. (1981). *Synopsis of gynecologic oncology* (2nd ed.). New York: John Wiley & Sons.

Morrow, C. P. & Townsend, E. E. (1987). Malignant tumors of the vulva. In *Synopsis of Gynecologic Oncology.* New York: John Wiley & Sons.

Nesbit, R. A., Woods, R. L., Tattersall, M. H., Fox, R. M., Forbes, J. F., MacKay, I. R., & Goodyear, M. (1979). Tamoxifen in malignant melanoma [Letter]. *New England Journal of Medicine, 301*(22), 124-1242.

Ogunbiyi, O. A., Scholefield, J. H., Robertson, G., Smith, J. H., Sharp, F., & Rogers, K. (1994). Anal human papillomavirus infection and squamous neoplasia in patients with invasive vulvar cancer. *Obstetrics and Gynecology, 83*(2), 212-216.

Petereit, D. G., Mehta, M. P., Buchler, D. A., & Kinsella, T. J. (1993). Inguinofemoral radiation of N0, N1 vulvar cancer may be equivalent to lymphadenectomy if proper radiation technique is used. *International Journal of Radiation: Oncology-Biology-Physics, 24*(4), 963-967.

Podratz, K. C., Symmonds, R. E., & Taylor, W. F. (1982). Carcinoma of the vulva: Analysis of treatment failures. *American Journal of Obstetrics and Gynecology, 143,* 814-817.

Pohar, S., Hoffstetter, S., Peiffert, D., Luporsi, E., & Pernot, M. (1995). Effectiveness of brachytherapy in treating carcinoma of the vulva. *International Journal of Radiology: Oncology-Biology-Physics, 32*(5), 1455-1460.

Reid, G. C., DeLancey, J. O., Hopkins, M. P., Roberts, J. A., & Morley, G. W. (1990). Urinary incontinence following radical vulvectomy. *Obstetrics and Gynecology, 75*(5), 852-858.

Richmond, D. M., O'Donnell, T. F., & Zelikowski, A. (1985). Sequential pneumatic compression for lymphedema. *Archives of Surgery, 120,* 1116-1119.

Roberts, W. S., Hoffman, M. S., LaPolla, J. P., Russ, E., Fiorica, J. V., & Cavanagh, D. (1991). Management of radionecrosis of the vulva and distal vagina. *American Journal of Obstetrics and Gynecology, 164*(5, Pt 1), 1235-1238.

Rogers, R. (1994). Gynecology. In S. I. Schwartz, T. G. Shires, F. C. Spencer, & W. C. Husser (Eds.), *Principles of surgery* (6th ed.). New York: McGraw-Hill.

Rusk, D., Sutton, G. P., Look, K. Y., & Roman, A. (1991). Analysis of invasive squamous cell carcinoma of the vulva and vulvar intraepithelial neoplasia for the presence of human papilloma virus DNA. *Obstetrics and Gynecology, 77,* 918-922.

Rutledge, F., Smith, J. P., & Franklin, E. W. (1970). Carcinoma of the vulva. *American Journal of Obstetrics and Gynecology, 106,* 1117-1130.

Rutledge, F. & Sinclair, M. (1968). Treatment of intraepithelial carcinoma of the vulva by skin excision and graft. *American Journal of Obstetrics and Gynecology, 102*(6), 807-818.

Sedlis, A., Homesley, H., Bundy, B. N., Marshall, R., Yordan, E., Hacker, N., Lee, J. H., & Whitney, R. (1987). Positive groin lymph nodes in superficial squamous cell vulvar cancer: A Gynecologic Oncology Group study. *American Journal of Obstetrics and Gynecology, 156,* 1159-1164.

Shepherd, J. H., Van Dam, P. A., Jobling, T. W., & Breach, N. (1990). The use of rectus abdominus myocutaneous flaps following excision of vulvar cancer. *British Journal of Obstetrics and Gynecology, 97*(11), 1020-1025.

Sherman, K. J., Daling, J. R., Chu, J., Weiss, N. S., Ashley, R. L., & Corey, L. (1991). Genital warts, other sexually transmitted diseases, and vulvar cancer. *Epidemiology, 2*(4), 257-262.

Siller, B. S., Alvarez, R. D., Conner, W. D., McCullough, C. H., Kilgore, L. C., Partridge, E. E., & Austin, J. M. (1995). $T_{2/3}$ vulvar cancer: A case control study of triple incision versus en block radical vulvectomy and inguinal lymphadenectomy. *Gynecologic Oncology, 57*(3), 335-339.

Simon, M. S. & Cody, R. L. (1992). Cellulitis after axillary lymph node dissection for carcinoma of the breast. *American Journal of Medicine, 93*(5), 543-548.

Spencer, S. A., Pareek, P. N., Brezovich, I., Larson, B. J., Kim, R. Y., Plott, W. G., Meredith, R. F., Smith, J. W., Weppelmann, B., & Soong, S. J. (1991). Three-port perineal sparing technique. *Radiology, 180*(2), 563-566.

Springer, M. O. (1982). Radical vulvectomy: Physical, psychological, social and sexual implications. *Oncology Nursing Forum, 9*(2), 19-29.

Stehman, F. B., Bundy, B. N., Dvoretsky, P. M., & Creasman, W. T. (1992). Early stage I carcinoma of the vulva treated with ipsilateral superficial inguinal lymphadenectomy and modified radical hemivulvectomy: A prospective study of the Gynecologic Oncology Group. *Obstetrics and Gynecology, 79*(4), 490-497.

Sturgeon, S. R., Brinton, L. A., Devesa, S. S., & Kurman, R. J. (1992). In situ and invasive vulvar cancer incidence trends (1973-1987). *American Journal of Obstetrics and Gynecology, 166*(5), 1482-1485.

Thigpen, J. T. (1991). Systemic therapy in the management of cancer of the vulva. In *Malignancies of the vulva* (pp. 153-158). New York: George Thieme Verlag Stuttgart.

Tobias, D. H., Smith, H. O., Jones, J. G., Anderson, P., Runowicz, C. D., & Goldberg, G. L. (1995). Cutaneous metastases from squamous cell carcinoma of the vulva: A case report and review of the literature. *European Journal of Gynaecological Oncology, 16*(5), 382-386.

Townsend, D. E., Levine, R. U., Richart, R. M., Crum, C. P., & Petrilli, E. S. (1982). Management of vulvar intraepithelial neoplasia by carbon dioxide laser. *Obstetrics and Gynecology, 60*(1), 49-52.

Trope, C., Johnsson, J. E., Larsson, G., & Simonsen, E. (1980). Bleomycin alone or combined with mitomycin C in treatment of advanced or recurrent squamous cell carcinoma of the vulva. *Cancer Treatment Reports, 64,* 639-642.

Tucker, S. M., Cannobbio, M. M., Paquette, E. V., & Wells, M. F. (1996). *Patient care standards: Collaborative practice planning guides* (6th ed.). St. Louis: Mosby.

Underwood, J. W., Adcock, L. L., & Okagaki, T. (1978). Adenosquamous carcinoma of skin appendages (adenoid squamous cell carcinoma, pseudoglandular squamous cell carcinoma, adenocanthoma of sweat gland of Lever) of the vulva: A clinical and ultrastructural study. *Cancer, 42*(4), 1851-1858.

van der Velden, J. & Hacker, N. F. (1994). Update on vulvar carcinoma. In M. L. Rothenberg (Ed.), *Gynecologic oncology: Controversies and new developments.* Boston: Kluwer Academic.

Visco, A. G. & Del Priore, G. (1996). Postmenopausal Bartholin gland enlargement: A hospital-based cancer risk. *Obstetrics and Gynecology, 87*(2), 286-290.

Winningham, M. L. (1996). Fatigue. In S. L. Groenwald, M. H. Frogge, M. Goodman, & C. H. Yarbro (Eds.), *Cancer symptom management.* Boston: Jones and Bartlett.

Yazigi, R., Piver, M. S., & Tsukada, Y. (1978). Microinvasive carcinoma of the vulva. *Obstetrics and Gynecology, 51*(3), 368-370.

Anal Cancer

Mary Garlick Roll, RN, MSN

INTRODUCTION

Anal cancer is a rare and treatable neoplasm that occurs in both men and women. Its incidence is rising in young men in the United States. Where previously radical surgery was the treatment of choice, innovations in combination therapy using radiation and chemotherapy have dramatically improved survival for patients with early-stage disease. It is imperative that both oncologists and primary care providers have good understanding of this disease to promote early diagnosis, treatment, and long-term survival.

EPIDEMIOLOGY

Cancer of the anal region is rare. In the United States, only 1% to 2% of digestive system cancers arise in this area; however, it accounts for 3.9% of all anorectal cancers. The American Cancer Society estimates that 3300 new cases of anal cancer will be diagnosed in the United States in 1998.

Most anal cancers occur in individuals in their 50s and 60s, with an overall incidence occurring between the ages of 35 and 90. Annual incidence increases steadily after the age of 30, reaching 4.7/100,000 after the age of 85.

Typically, more females than males are diagnosed with anal cancer. Of the 3300 new cases estimated in 1998, 1900 will occur in females, and 1400 in males. Women are more likely to have cancers of the anal canal, whereas men are more likely to develop tumors on the outer portion of the anus. In the United States in the 1980s and 1990s, there has been an increased incidence in men under 45 years of age, particularly homosexual men who engage in anal-receptive intercourse (Strigle, 1994). This trend has reversed the typical gender ratio for individuals in this age group.

Although anal cancer is rare, approximately 500 Americans (300 women, 200 men) will die from the disease in 1998. Treatment for many cases is effective, with 70% of patients receiving radiation therapy or radiation therapy plus chemotherapy surviving for 5 years or longer after diagnosis.

RISK FACTORS

For most patients with anal cancer, no definitive risk factors other than age can be identified. Several studies have suggested that male anal-receptive intercourse may play a role.

A suspected causative agent is the human papilloma virus (HPV) (Strigle, 1994). This virus has been associated with the development of *condylomata acuminata,* which can evolve into squamous cell carcinoma of the anus after many years. HPV is almost universal in homosexual and bisexual men who have tested positive for human immunodeficiency virus (HIV), as well as in approximately 60% of HIV-negative men who engage in anal-receptive intercourse. Women at high risk for the development of anal cancer include those with high-grade cervical disease and vulvar disease. It is speculated that women who engage in anal-receptive intercourse may also be at increased risk (Tabbarah, 1995).

Anal cancer has been associated with anal fistulas and other benign conditions (Shank, Cunningham, & Kelsen, 1997), although the extent of the risk and whether there is more than a temporal relationship are unknown. Prior radiation therapy and immunosuppression may also play a role in the development of anal cancer. Immune-suppressed renal transplant recipients have a 100-fold increase in anogenital tumors compared with the general population (Frisch, Olsen, Bautz, & Melbye, 1994; Penn, 1986; Tucker, 1995).

Smoking has been identified as a major risk factor (Daling, Weiss, Hislop, Maden, Coates, & Sherman, 1987). Anal canal carcinomas have also been associated with prior irradiation, as well as other benign conditions including anal fissures, abscesses, hemorrhoids, and lymphogranuloma venereum. Relative risk has not been determined (Box 36-1) (Tabbarah, 1995).

Prevention

Early detection depends on the patient and primary caregiver's awareness of risk factors. Annual anal examination may be required and yearly anoscopy may be indicated for those at high risk (Tabbarah, 1995).

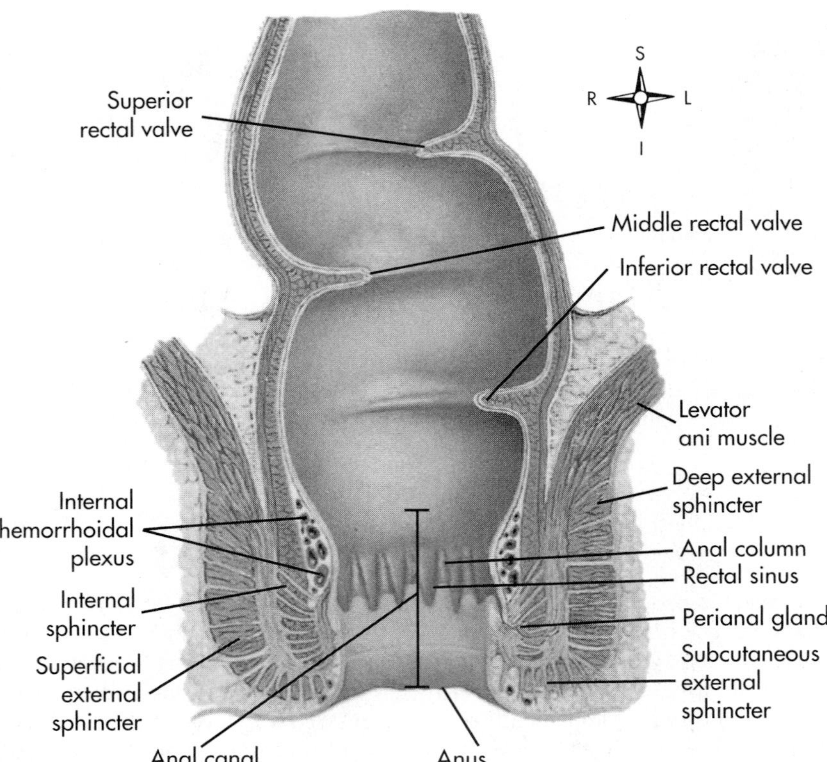

Fig. 36-1 The rectum and anus. (From Thibodeau, G. A. & Patton, K. T. [1996]. *Anthony's textbook of anatomy and physiology* [15th ed.]. St Louis: Mosby.)

Box 36-1
Risk Ractors for Anal Cancer

Prior irradiation
Disease such as anal fissures, chronic local inflammation, hemorrhoids, Crohn's, lymphogranuloma venereum, condylomata acuminata, carcinoma of cervix, carcinoma of the vulva
Infectious agents such as human papillomavirus (HPV), human immunodeficiency virus (HIV), *Chlamydia trachomatis* in women, gonorrhea in men
Immune suppression, kidney transplant recipients
Cigarette smoking
Anal receptive intercourse among men

From Tabbarah, H. J. (1995). Gastrointestinal tract cancers. In D. A. Casciato, and B. B. Lowitz (Eds.), *Manual of clinical oncology* (3rd ed.). Boston: Little, Brown and Company.

TABLE 36-1 World Health Organization Classification of Anal Carcinomas

Anal Canal	
Malignant Epithelial Tumors	**Adenocarcinoma**
Squamous cell carcinoma	Rectal type
Large cell keratinizing	Small cell carcinona
Large cell nonkeratinizing	Undifferentiated
Basaloid	
Anal Margin	
Malignant Epithelial Tumors	
Squamous cell carcinoma	
Giant condyloma	
Basal cell carcinoma	
Bowen's disease	
Paget's disease	
Others	

NORMAL ANATOMY

It is important to understand the anatomy of the anal canal and anal margin, since the cancers that occur there have different natural histories. Fig. 36-1 depicts the anatomic landmarks of the anal region.

The anal canal is shaped like a cylinder and is approximately 4 to 5 cm long, extending from the anal verge to just below the level of the puborectalis muscle (Tarazi & Nelson, 1994). The canal's upper portion is lined by the columnar epithelium of the rectum. At the level of the dentate, it is lined by a mixture of columnar and squamous epithelium. Most anal cancers occur near this dentate line. Tumors below the dentate line are considered *anal margin carcinomas.* The transitional zone is a 6- to 12-mm portion of the canal where the columnar epithelium changes into squamous cells. At the anal orifice, the nonkeratinized squamous epi-

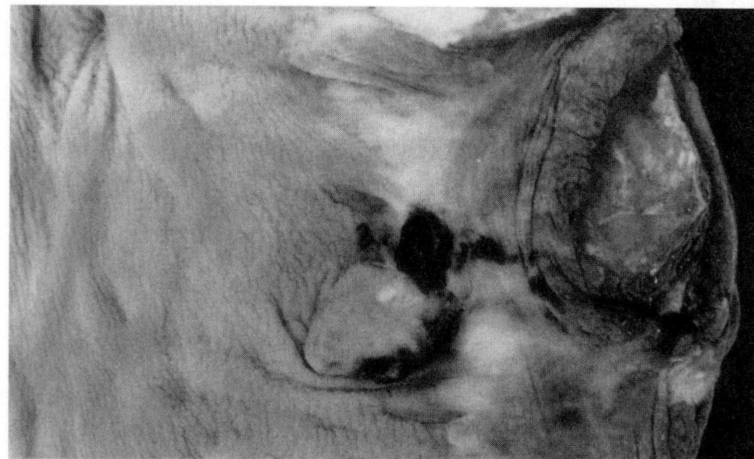

Fig. 36-2 Malignant melanoma of anal canal. This specimen presented with a brief history of episodic rectal bleeding. A hard mass was palpable in the lateral wall of the anal canal, and an adbominoperineal resection was performed. The anal canal has been opened to show a flattened, void nodul (2 cm in diameter) arising at about the level of the dentate line. The edge of the tumor shows obvious melanotic pigmentation, and an irregular streak of pigment extends from the nodule to the anal margin. Anorectal melanoma is rare. (From Skarin S. A. [1996]. *Atlas of diagnostic oncology* [2nd ed.]. St Louis: Mosby-Wolfe.)

thelium changes to epidermis with hair follicles and sweat glands.

The anus meets the rectum at the anorectal ring. This junction lies at approximately the level of the muscular floor of the pelvis, known as the *pelvic diaphragm.* At this point, the anal canal changes into more of a barrel shape as it becomes the rectum (Shank & Enker, 1997).

HISTOLOGY

The World Health Organization classification of anal carcinomas is summarized in Table 36-1. However, some tumors may exhibit mixed features, suggesting that a system implying a single predominant differentiation may be imperfect.

Anal Melanoma

Anal canal carcinoma can be divided into keratinizing and nonkeratinizing squamous cancers. The well-differentiated tumors are keratinizing. Anal margin cancers are most often keratinizing. Among the nonkeratinizing types, squamous, basaloid, or cloacogenic carcinomas are most common (Figs. 36-2 and 36-3).

More rare histologic types include lymphoma and small cell carcinomas (Shank, Cunningham, & Kelsen, 1997). Melanomas may account for 1% to 2% of anal carcinomas. Although extremely rare, anal melanoma is associated with a 5-year survival rate of less than 12%.

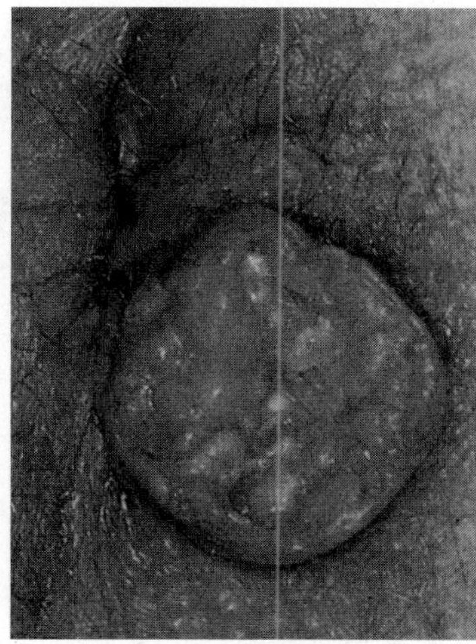

Fig. 36-3 Squamous carcinoma of anal margin. Squamous cancers of the anus are divided into tumors arising in the anal canal (most often above the dentate line) and those arising in the skin at the anal margin. This lesion measures 1 cm across. Neoplasms at this site tend to be slow growing and metastasize to inguinal lymph nodes. Patients have a 5-year survival rate of approximately 70%. (From Skarin S. A. [1996]. *Atlas of diagnostic oncology* [2nd ed.]. St Louis: Mosby-Wolfe.)

ROUTES OF METASTASES

Regional

At the time of diagnosis, many anal carcinomas have already spread, infiltrating the sphincter muscle and adjacent soft tissue (Williams & Talbot, 1994). As many as 10% to 15% of patients may have regional lymph node involvement at the time of diagnosis. Anal margin tumors are most likely to spread to the inguinal lymph nodes, whereas those in the canal tend to involve the hemorrhoidal nodes. Nodal drainage follows from the pararectal and inguinal lymph nodes to the abdominal system.

Anal carcinomas tend to spread to local structures. They may invade the anal sphincter or extend into the ischiorectal space laterally and the vagina anteriorly. Large tumors may invade almost any adjacent structure including the vagina and urinary tract.

Lymphatic Dissemination

Lymphatic dissemination can occur in a variety of ways. Cancer may spread via the superficial inguinal lymph nodes. From the upper anal canal, cancer may spread to the superior hemorrhoidal vessels and the mesorectal lymph nodes. Cancer can also spread to the internal iliacs and laterally to the obturator lymph nodes. It is thought that approximately one third of patients have lymph node involvement at the time of presentation.

Hematogenous Spread

Hematogenous spread is less common, with few patients (5% to 10%) presenting with distant metastatic disease (Keuhn, Eisenberg, & Reed, 1968). Hematogenous spread occurs most often in patients whose tumors arise at or above the dentate line. Hematogenous spread results in metastatic sites in the liver, lung, and skin, as tumor cells travel via the portal system. Distant metastases occur independent of histologic type, although metastasis is rarely seen in patients with anal margin tumors.

Staging

The TNM (tumor, node, metastasis) system of staging for anal cancer is defined in Table 36-2. The staging system for anal cancer has been described by the American Joint Committee on Cancer and the tumor size and invasion into other organs and tissues (Table 36-3). N classification subdivides the regional lymph nodes, recognizing the poor prognosis of inguinal node involvement (American Joint Committee on Cancer, 1988).

ASSESSMENT

Anal Bleeding

Many patients present without symptoms, with abnormal findings noted on physical examination. The most common presenting symptom, bleeding from the anal/rectal area, occurs in more than half of patients. Bleeding rarely includes hemorrhage and is often dismissed by the patient as representing hemorrhoidal irritation (Tabbarah, 1995).

Co-existing Conditions

Other common symptoms include change in bowel habits, discomfort with bowel movements, tenesmus, and pruritus. The patient may also complain of development of a new skin lesion or condyloma, fissure, or fistula. Because benign anal conditions such as hemorrhoids may be coexistent in many patients, diagnosis of cancer may be delayed.

TABLE 36-2 TNM Definitions for Anal Cancer Staging

Primary Tumor (T)	Regional Lymph Nodes (N)	Distant Metastasis (M)
TX: Primary tumor cannot be assessed	NX: Regional lymph nodes cannot be assessed	MX: Presence of distant metastis cannot be assessed
T0: no evidence of primary tumor	N0: No regional lymph node metastasis	M0: No distant metastasis
Tis: Carcinoma in situ	N1: Metastasis in perirectal lymph node(s)	M1: Distant metastasis
T1: Tumor 2.0 cm or less in greatest dimension	N2: Metastasis in unilateral internal iliac and/or inguinal lymph node(s)	
T2: Tumor more than 2.0 cm but not more than 5.0 cm in greatest dimension	N3: Metastasis in perirectal and inguinal lymph nodes and/or bilateral internal iliac and/or inguinal lymph nodes(s)	
T3: Tumor more than 5.0 cm in greatest dimension		
T4: Tumor of any size that invades adjacent organ(s), e.g. vagina, urethra, (bladder involvement of the sphincter muscle(s) alone is not classified as T4)		

TABLE 36-3 Staging of Anal Cancer

Stage 0	Stage I	Stage II	Stage IIIA	Stage IIIB	Stage IV
Carcinoma in situ. (Tis, No, Mo)	T1, N0, M0	T2, N0, M0 T3, N0, M0	T1, N1, M0 T2, N1, M0 T3, N1, M0 T4, N0, M0	T4, N1, M0 Any T, N2, M0 Any T, N3, M0	Any T, any N, M1

From American Joint Committee on Cancer, (1988). Colon and rectum. In O. H. Beahrs, D. E. Hensen, and R. V. Hutter et al. (Eds.), *Manual for staging of cancer.* Philadelphia: J. B. Lippincott; American Joint Committee on Cancer (1992). Anal Canal. In O. H. Beahrs, D. E. Hensen, R. V. Hutter, and P. Kennedy, (Eds.), *Manual for staging of cancer* (4th ed.). Philadelphia: J. B. Lippincott.

Co-existent conditions are common and may include anorectal fistula, anal fissure, or hemorrhoids. Most often, patients report rectal bleeding or a sense of feeling a mass. Pain or spasm may impede rectal examination. A high index of suspicion in the presence of a mass is warranted.

Examination under anesthesia may be needed if the pain or fear impairs the patient's ability to tolerate rectal examination. Patients often also treat themselves with a variety of over-the-counter remedies and delay evaluation because of embarrassment.

If the patient is at increased risk for anal cancer or presents with symptoms, several assessment questions should be posed. Family history of gastrointestinal and gynecologic cancers and familial and hereditary conditions should be investigated. The patient's history of bowel habits, sexual practices, and familial and hereditary conditions should be assessed. Specifically, the patient should be asked about history and nature of constipation or diarrhea, nutritional habits, any pain or discomfort in the anal and perianal area with or without bowel movements, pain or discomfort with intercourse, number and type of sexual partners, and use of safe sex practices (Table 36-4) (Tabbarah, 1995).

Perineal Pain

Perineal pain should be investigated by physical examination. Differential diagnosis includes hemorrhoids, fissures, intertrigo, eczema, condyloma, vaginitis, cystocele, injury or rupture of the urethra, urethral calculus, cystitis, prostatitis, and proctalgia fugax (Patt & Jain, 1990).

Visual Inspection and Digital Rectal Examination

Physical examination should include visual inspection of the anal and perianal area and digital rectal examination (DRE). The most common finding on physical examination is an intraluminal mass. Inspection should be done with and without anal specula. To inspect the perineum, the buttocks should be spread wide apart. The skin should be inspected for signs of local inflammation, ulceration, warts, hyperpigmentation, hypopigmentation (leukoplakia), sinuses, fistulas, and bulges. The mucocutaneous junction may be seen by exerting tension on the skin on each side of the anus.

Lesions such as flat condyloma and low-grade anal intraepithelial neoplasia may be difficult to visualize with the

TABLE 36-4 Assessment of the Patient for Anal Cancer

	Assessment Parameters	Typical Abnormal Findings
History	A. Personal and social history 1. Sexual activity 2. Immunosuppression 3. Family history of gastrointestinal and gynecologic cancers.	A. Personal and social risk factors 1. History of anal receptive intercourse 2. History of human immunosuppressive virus 3. Positive familial history
Physical Examination	A. Evaluation of the anal rectal area	A. Common symptoms 1. Rectal bleeding, 50%. Rectal bleeding is similar to hemorrhoidal irritation and often dismissed by the patient not be serious 2. Pain, 40%. Differential diagnosis should include hemorrhoids, fissures, intertrigo, eczema, condyloma, vaginitis, cystocele, or rupture of the urethra, urethral calculus, cystitis, prostatitis, proctagra fugax 3. Sensations of mass, 25% 4. Pruritis, 15% 5. Asymptomatic, 25% 6. Change in bowel habits, with discomfort with bowel movements, tenesmus, and pruritus 7. Skin lesions, condyloma, fissures or fistulas
Diagnostic Testing	A. Digital anorectal examination and anoscopy. B. Palpation of inguinal lymph nodes. C. Incisional biopsy of inguinal lymph nodes D. Bilateral pelvic examination	A. An anorectal examination can reveal palpable mass. May need to be performed under sedation or general anesthesia in patients with severe pain and anal spasm. B. Palpation of inguinal lymph notes may reveal mass C. An incisional biopsy is necessary and preferable to confirm the diagnosis of anal cancer. If aspiration is negative, surgical biopsy may be performed D. Rule out vaginal fistula

From Tabbarah, H. J. (1995). Gastrointestinal tract cancers. In D. A., Casciato, and B. B. Lowitz (Eds.), *Manual of clinical oncology* (3rd ed.). Boston: Little, Brown and Company.

naked eye. Application of a 3% to 5% acetic acid solution to the perianal skin can highlight areas of atypical epithelium (Strigle, 1994). Atypical lesions should be sampled in a manner similar to a cervical Papanicolaou (Pap) smear. Table 36-5 provides an educational guide to prepare patients for this procedure.

The perineum should be gently palpated. The tip of the gloved examining finger is then lubricated with surgical jelly and inserted into the anus, pointing toward the umbilicus. This should not be painful unless fissures or thrombosed hemorrhoids are present. The patient may be positioned in the left lateral prone (Sims'), which permits inspection of the perianal region and the anal mucosa with or without a speculum. However, it is difficult to perform a DRE in this position, as masses tend to fall away from the examination finger. The lithotomy position is more useful for routine examination. Palpation of the rectum is necessary for feeling the peritoneal contents. It cannot be used with the specula. Although uncomfortable for the patient, the knee-chest position is most useful for specula examination.

DRE is capable of detecting 15% to 20% of anal carcinomas within a 7-cm area from the anal verge. Vaginal examination in women is important when the patient's complaints are consistent with a fistula. Rectal cancer extending to the abdominal side walls can be better evaluated by vaginal examination. Physical examination should include a search for supraclavicular adenopathy, hepatomegaly, abdominal masses or ascites, inguinal adenopathy, and satellite lesions in the intergluteal folds or leading to the inguinal region, as well as a careful assessment of the primary lesion by DRE, anoscopy, and proctoscopy. The primary lesion should be evaluated for size, location, depth of invasion, and presence of inguinal lymphadenopathy. Any suspicious lesion should be biopsied (Shank, Cunningham, & Kelsen, 1997).

Anascopy

The anal canal should be inspected when external signs, palpable masses, sphincter spasm, pain, or bleeding prompt further investigation. An anoscope is about 9 cm long; it is available in a variety of diameters, with or without built-in illumination. Plastic, disposable anoscopes are usually clear, allowing visualization of the anal walls.

The tip of the obturator is lubricated with surgical jelly and gently inserted into the anus, again aiming toward the umbilicus. Once inserted completely (about 2 to 3 inches), the obturator is removed and the anal walls inspected. The anoscope is slowly withdrawn while the anal walls are inspected as they collapse behind the receding tube.

Examination of Stool for Occult Blood

Stool should be tested for occult blood, although a negative result does not preclude the existence of cancer. Routine laboratory studies include a complete blood count and serum chemistries including liver function tests. The carcinoembryonic antigen is not a useful marker for anal cancer and is not included. In patients with suspected colon cancer, flexible sigmoidoscopy and barium enema or colonoscopy should be considered.

Abdominal Assessment

The initial physical examination includes inspection of the abdomen for distention, visible masses, and visible and enlarged veins indicative of portal hypertension and distant disease. The abdomen is auscultated in all four quadrants. The abdomen is palpated and percussed for masses, enlargement, and the occurrence and location of discomfort.

TABLE 36-5 Standard of Care for the Patient with Anal Cancer

Patient Problems and Outcomes	Nursing Interventions and Rationales	Patient Education Instructions
Knowledge Deficit		
Patient will verbalize understanding of the purpose, benefits and risks of multimodality therapy	1. Assess patient's knowledge level regarding radiation therapy and chemotherapy	1. Describe the procedures that can be expected in multimodality therapy a. consultation with medical oncologist b. consultation with radiation oncologist c. informal consent d. treatment procedures
	2. Assess patient's fears and concerns	2. Describe the major side effects associated with this multimodality therapy. a. diarrhea b. skin reaction c. fatigue d. nausea

Proctoscopy and Transrectal Ultrasound

Proctoscopy and transrectal ultrasound may also be used to evaluate anal symptoms and palpable lesions. On endoscopy, tumors may appear as flat or slightly raised lesions, as raised lesions with indurated borders, or as polypoid lesions (Shank, Cunningham, & Kelsen, 1997). Ultrasound may be used to assess infiltration of surrounding structures. Laparoscopic surgery may be used to perform biopsy (partial or total excision) of intraabdominal lesions and partial colon resections (Price & Rubio, 1994).

Staging and metastatic workup include a computed tomography (CT) scan of the abdomen and pelvis. The chest CT scan or a chest x-ray study may be performed to evaluate for metastasis. A bone scan is not indicated, since metastatic spread to the bones is extremely rare.

MEDICAL MANAGEMENT

Therapy options for anal carcinoma include surgery, radiation, and chemotherapy alone or in combination with therapy. As multimodality approaches using chemotherapy and irradiation have improved the primary treatment of patients with anal cancer, radical surgery has become less common (Zuro, Terry, & Saclarides, 1992).

Abdominal-Perineal Resection

Because many anal cancers recur locally, wide excision using abdominal-perineal (A-P) resection was previously the treatment of choice. This extensive surgery resulted in placement of a colostomy and sometimes required use of myocutaneous flaps to close wound defects. Adjacent organs were often resected, including the vagina and bladder. Morbidity associated with A-P resection may be as high as 20%. Microscopic residual disease and lymphatic involvement, however, often led to tumor recurrence and/or persistence despite extensive local resection (Tarazi & Nelson, 1994). Today, A-P resection is reserved for patients who have developed local recurrence after combined modality radiotherapy and chemotherapy. For these patients, A-P resection may offer definitive therapy.

Recurrence after extensive surgery as primary treatment (Shank, Cunningham, & Kelsen, 1997) may be as high as 40%, with median time to recurrence 12 to 15 months. Surgical resection is used for treatment of lesions in the perianal area not involving the anal sphincter. Local excision may be used for small tumors of the perianal skin. When small, superficial lesions are selected for local therapy; excision alone is associated with a 60% to 90% survival rate (Shank & Enker, 1997). In the vast majority of these patients, primary wound closure is possible, without need for skin or muscle grafting. An adequate margin of normal tissue, approximately 1 cm, is excised around the tumor. Local recurrences can be treated with reexcision, with more extensive A-P resection reserved for bulky tumors.

Multimodality Treatment

The majority of tumors with or without regional lymph node involvement require multimodality treatment. These therapies preserve the anal sphincter while incurring minimal toxicity. Surgical intervention in these situations includes only initial biopsy of the primary lesion, with biopsy of suspicious lymph nodes. Tumors that involve the anal sphincter or that are too large for local excision may be treated with radiation therapy with or without chemotherapy, with cure rates reaching 80% to 90% (Tanum, Tevit, Karlsen, & Hauer-Jensen, 1991).

Interstitial radiation therapy using iridium or radium may be used to treat lesions that are localized or that have spread only to regional lymphatics. Recurrence rates, however, are relatively high for lesions greater than 5 cm in diameter (77% local recurrence) (Shank & Enker, 1997). Interstitial therapy is associated with increased risk of local tissue necrosis.

The "gold standard" for multimodality treatment for anal cancer external beam radiation therapy plus chemotherapy, usually 5-fluorouracil (5-FU) and mitomycin, is a protocol designed by Nigro (Nigro, Vaitkeviceus, & Considine, 1974). Typical radiation dose is 45 to 50 Gy, using photons or electron beam with bolus mitomycin-C at 10 to 15 mg/m^2 on day 1 alone or in combination with continuous infusion 5-FU at 1000 mg/m^2 for 2 to 4 days at the beginning and end of radiotherapy.

Nigro Protocol

The Nigro protocol uses the sensitizing effects of chemotherapy to allow delivery of lower radiation doses. Common treatment-related toxicities include diarrhea and thrombocytopenia. Patients with incomplete responses or recurrent disease may then proceed to surgical resection, which may include A-P resection with colostomy (Nigro, Vaitkeviceus, & Considine, 1974).

Treatment for stage III anal cancer may include radiation therapy, chemotherapy, and surgery (Arnell & Stamos, 1996). The patient may be treated initially with a combination chemotherapy and radiation therapy followed by surgical resection for residual disease, or with surgery as the primary treatment followed by combination chemotherapy and radiation therapy. Patients with stage IV anal cancer may be treated with chemotherapy, radiation therapy, or a combination for palliative purposes. Surgery may also be used, particularly if a mass results in obstruction or bleeding. Clinical trials should also be considered for these patients.

ONCOLOGIC EMERGENCIES

The major oncologic emergency associated with anal cancer is sepsis resulting from the immunosuppression of chemotherapy or A-P resection of the anorectum. Sepsis arises from the systemic inflammatory response to infection, which can be the result of invasive microorganisms, extensive tissue damage and necrosis, or various cellular byproducts produced as a result of these conditions (see Chapters 11).

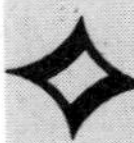

TABLE 36-6 Patient Preparation for Anal Pap Smear

You are being tested for the possibility of anal cancer. This is a preliminary test to let the physician know if you will need further evaluation.

This test is performed in the physician's office and is not a painful procedure. No special preparation is needed before you go to the physician. You may eat or drink what you like. Wear clothing that is easily removed.

You will be asked to remove all clothing below the waist. You will be placed on examination table and your legs spread wide so that the rectum is visible to the physician.

A large cotton swab is gently placed about 1 to 1½ inches into the anus and rotated as it is withdrawn to obtain samples of tissue for anaysis.

Take deep breaths if you become anxious during this procedure. It is performed in minutes.

NURSING MANAGEMENT

Prevention

Anal carcinomas continue to be a health problem in the United States despite improved treatment techniques. The emphasis must be on prevention and early detection. Nurses are uniquely positioned to use available information to encourage prevention and diminish risk. Surveillance of those patients with HPV and/or history of anal-receptive intercourse is indicated. Some authors recommend surveillance of patients with a history of anal fistula and surgical evaluation of anal pain (Tarazi & Nelson, 1994).

Until recently, standard treatment for anal cancer had been A-P resection. However, other therapies are now being used with equitable or improved survival rates. A treatment program involving external beam radiotherapy combined with mitomycin-C and 5-FU infusion (Nigro's protocol) has provided evidence of tumor regression and poses challenges for the oncology nurse caring for this patient (Table 36-6).

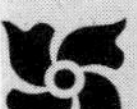

TABLE 36-7 Standard of Care for the Patient Receiving External Examination and/or Nigro's Protocol for Anal Cancer

Patient Problem and Outcome	Nursing Interventions and Rationales	Patient Education Instructions
Enhanced skin reaction	Provide Rx for antidiarrheas to decrease the frequency of stools	Explain to patient and caregivers that moist desquamation is an expected consequence of this therapy
Patient will be able to prevent infection and promote healing	Cleanse area with appropriate antimicrobial skin cleanser. Avoid products containing chlorhexidine (may cause irritation) Sitz bath twice daily After cleansing and/or sitz bath, apply a hydrophilic cream (e.g., Aquaphor) or Aquaphor gauze. Dressings can be held in place with cotton underwear or knit pants.	Explain to patient and caregiver that there is much that they can do to promote healing and prevent infection

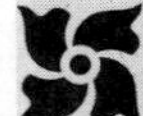

TABLE 36-8 Standard of Care for the Patient Receiving External Beam Radiation and/or Nigro's Protocol (Combined Modality Therapy) for Anal Cancer

Patient Problem and Outcome	Nursing Interventions and Rationales	Patient Education Instructions
Diarrhea	1. Assess elimination patterns a. frequency b. quality c. quantity	1. Explain to patient and caregiver that diarrhea is an expected consequence of this therapy
Patient will maintain fluid balance and weight	1. Obtain consult with dietitian before initiation of treatment 2. Indicate low-residue/lactose-free diet 3. Keep written record of weight Weekly weights to assess for weight loss Provide Rx for antidiarrheal medication 4. Explain usage and provide written instructions a. diphenoxylate hydrochloride b. tincure of opium	1. Assess for understanding of dietary restrictions 2. Assess for understanding of how to administer antidiarrheal medications

Table 36-7 describes the standard of care for enhanced skin reactions occurring as a result of combined modality treatment. Moist desquamation of the perineum and the perirectal area occur approximately 2 weeks after initiation of external beam therapy. Diarrhea will exacerbate moist desquamation, thereby delaying healing and increasing risk for infection (Keane, 1991). Nursing management is focused on promoting comfort and healing, as well as reducing infection risk (Table 36-8).

HOME CARE ISSUES

As the health care delivery system continues to change, the role of the home care nurse becomes increasingly significant. Coordination of care among the outpatient radiation oncology nurse, medical oncology nurse, and home care nurse is pivotal to provide continuity of care. The inpatient nurse will become involved if the patient requires hospitalization.

Regular assessment by the oncology nurse occurs when home care referral is needed. Support for the caregiver is often the primary reason for referral. As the population ages, issues associated with caring for the elderly will predominate. Appropriate and timely referral is a benchmark for care.

The role of the oncology nurse covers the spectrum from prevention through surveillance and treatment. Sensitivity for age, cultural influences, and caregiver needs, as well as patient needs, education, support, and timely referral provide the foundation for care of the person at risk for or who has a diagnosis of anal cancer.

EVALUATION OF THE QUALITY OF CARE

It is important that aspects of patient care be evaluated to monitor quality of care. Table 36-9 provides examples of quality of care evaluation tools that can be used for patients receiving treatment for anal cancer.

PROGNOSIS

Prognosis for patients with anal cancer is correlated with size, site, and differentiation of the primary lesion. Patients with lesions smaller than 2 cm have a significantly better prognosis than those with larger lesions (Shank, Cunningham, & Kelsen, 1997).

Histologic cell type is not as important as tumor size with regard to prognosis. Location of tumor may be of some significance. No difference in survival by gender has been described. Because anal cancer is rare, reports of metastatic disease are uncommon. In such cases, single agent chemotherapy has yielded responses (Shank & Enker, 1997).

FUTURE TRENDS

Many advances have been made in the treatment of anal cancer. Williams and Talbot (1994) recommended further investigation of anal intraepithelial neoplasia in anal cancer etiology. They also identified the effect of HIV on the immune response to HPV-related lesions as an area for further research. The lack of a tumor marker is another area of interest for researchers.

Nursing research in screening for, prevention of, and surveillance of high-risk populations is indicated. Nurses are uniquely positioned to conduct significant research in these areas.

TABLE 36-9 Quality of Care Evaluation for a Patient with Diarrhea as a Result of Radiation

Disciplines participating in the quality of care evaluation:
☐ Nursing ☐ Physician ☐ Dietary

Data from: Medical Record Review ☐
Patient/Family Interview ☐

Criteria	Yes	No
1. Patient provided with information about:		
a. possibility of significant diarrhea	☐	☐
b. signs and symptoms of significant diarrhea	☐	☐
c. measures to reduce diarrhea	☐	☐
d. measures to reduce skin care breakdown as a result of diarrhea	☐	☐
2. The following assessments are made at each visit:		
a. weight	☐	☐
b. dietary intake	☐	☐
c. skin dreakdown in rectal area	☐	☐
d. understanding of dietary and skin care instructions	☐	☐
e. review of medications prescribed to protect skin in anal area	☐	☐
3. Patient experienced the following complications:		
a. topical infections in rectal area	☐	☐
b. weight loss, dehydration	☐	☐
c. loss of function status due to weakness	☐	☐

Patient/Family Satisfaction
Data from: ☐ Patient Interview ☐ Family Interview

Criteria	Yes	No
1. On a scale of 0 to 10, with 0 being totally dissatisfied and 10 being totally satisfied, how satisfied were you with the diarrhea management you received?		
2. Were you told to call the nurse if your diarrhea exceeded 1 L/day?	☐	☐
3. Were you taught to drink at least 2 L (6 large glasses) of fluid every day?	☐	☐
4. Were you given comfort measures to protect the skin in the anal area against infection and pain as a result of your diarrhea?	☐	☐

From Tabbarah, H. J. (1995). Gastrointestinal tract cancers. In D. A. Casciato & B. B. Lowitz (Eds.), *Manual of clinical oncology* (3rd ed.). Boston: Little, Brown and Company.

REFERENCES

American Joint Committee on Cancer. (1988). Colon and rectum. In O. H. Beahrs, D. E. Hensen, R. V. Hutter, & P. Kennedy (Eds.), *Manual for staging of cancer* (4th ed.). Philadelphia: Lippincott.

American Joint Committee on Cancer. (1992). Anal canal. In O. H. Beahrs, D. E. Hensen, R. V. Hutter, & P. Kennedy (Eds.), *Manual for staging of cancer* (4th ed.). Philadelphia: JB Lippincott.

Arnell, T. D. & Stamos, M. J. (1996). Alternatives in therapy for low rectal cancer. *Journal of Wound, Ostomy and Continence Nurses Society, 23,* (3), 150-155.

Daling, J. R., Weiss, N. S., Hislop, G., Maden, C., Coates, R. J., & Sherman, K. J. (1987). Sexual practices, sexual transmitted diseases, and the incidence of anal cancer. *New England Journal of Medicine, 317,* 973.

Frisch, M., Olsen, J. H., Bautz, A., & Melbye, M. (1994). Benign anal lesions and the risk of anal cancer. *New England Journal of Medicine, 331,* 300-302.

Keane, K. S. (1991). Moist desquamation related to combined modality treatment for anal cancer. *Oncology Nursing Forum, 18*(3), 602-603.

Keuhn, P. G., Eisenberg, H., & Reed, J. F. (1968). Epidermoid carcinoma of the perianal skin and anal canal. *Cancer, 22,* 932-938.

Nigro, N. D., Vaitkeviceus, V. K., & Considine, B. (1974). Combined therapy for cancer of the anal canal: A preliminary report. *Diseases of the Colon and Rectum, 17,* 354-356.

Patt, R. & Jain, S. (1990). Long term management of a patient with perineal pain secondary to anal cancer. *Journal of Pain and Symptom Management, 5* (2), 127-128.

Penn, I. (1986). Cancers of the anogenital region in renal transplant patients. *Cancer, 58,* 611-616.

Price, A. L. & Rubio, P. A. (1994). Laparoscopic colo-rectal surgery: A challenge for ET nurses. *Journal of Wound, Ostomy and Continence Nurses Society, 9,* 179-182.

Shank, B. & Enker, W. E. (1997). Neoplasms of the anus. In J. F. Holland, R. C. Bast, D. L. Morton, E. Frei, D. W. Kufe, & R. R. Weichselbaum (Eds.), *Cancer medicine* (4th ed.). Baltimore: Williams & Wilkins.

Shank, B., Cunningham, J. D., & Kelsen, D. P. (1997). Cancer of the anal region. In V. T. DeVita, S. Hellman, & S. A. Rosenberg (Eds.), *Cancer: Principles and practice of oncology* (5th ed.). New York: Lippincott-Raven.

Skarin S. A. (1996). *Atlas of diagnostic oncology* (2nd ed.). St Louis: Mosby-Wolfe.

Strigle, S. M. (1994). Anal neoplasia in homosexual and bisexual men: An overlooked pathology in the spectrum of HIV infection and AIDS. *AIDS Patient Care, 8,* 185-195.

Tabbarah, H. J. (1995). Gastrointestinal tract cancers. In D. A., Casciato, & B. B. Lowitz (Eds.), *Manual of clinical oncology* (3rd ed.). Boston: Little, Brown.

Tanum, G., Tevit, K., Karlsen, K. O., & Hauer-Jensen, M. (1991). Chemoradiotherapy of anal carcinoma: Survival and late morbidity. *Cancer, 67,* 2462-2466.

Tarazi, R. & Nelson, R. L. (1994). Anal adenocarcinoma: A comprehensive review. *Seminars in Surgical Oncology, 10,* 235-240.

Thibodeau, G. A. & Patton, K. T. (1996). *Anthony's textbook of anatomy and physiology* (15th ed.). St Louis: Mosby.

Tucker, M. (1995). Benign anal lesions and anal cancer [Letter to the editor]. *New England Journal of Medicine, 332,* 190.

Williams, G. & Talbot, I. C. (1994). Anal carcinoma: A histological review. *Histopathology, 25,* 507-516.

Zuro, L. M., Terry, C. D., & Saclarides, T. J. (1992). Transanal endoscopic microsurgery. *AORN Journal, 56,*(3), 466-475.

37

Rectal Cancer

Sue M. Schlesselman, RN, MSN, OCN

EPIDEMIOLOGY

Colorectal cancers are a major cause of illness and death in the United States. About one third of colorectal cancers occur exclusively in the rectum (Givel, 1990). The number of new cases of rectal cancer in the United States was estimated at 36,000 in 1997, and 8800 deaths were projected (American Cancer Society [ACS], 1998). Even though mortality from rectal cancer in the United States appears to be declining, the incidence is slowly increasing (Greenwald, 1992; Funkhouser & Cole, 1992).

Rectal cancer occurs predominately at an advanced age, with a majority of individuals diagnosed over the age of 60 years. However, rectal cancer can be diagnosed in younger individuals, especially those with predisposing risk factors such as a familial history of colorectal cancer, polyp or adenoma conditions, or inflammatory bowel disease (Givel, 1990). There is a slight predominance of males vs females, with a ratio of 1.4 to 1.0 (Takahashi, Mori, & Moosa, 1991). Statistics indicate that whites have higher rates of rectal cancer than blacks, but when blacks are diagnosed with rectal cancer, the cancer tends to be late stage with poorer prognosis (Devesa & Chow, 1993; Jessup, Menck, Fremgen, & Winchester, 1997).

RISK FACTORS

The major risk factors associated with the development of rectal cancer are listed in Box 37-1. Risk factors for rectal cancer are presented. A sample patient education tool is presented in Box 37-2. Rectal cancer is distinct in some of its clinical signs and methods of treatment, but it does share several risk factors associated with colon cancer.

Increasing Age

Age is an important risk factor in the development of rectal cancer. Most rectal cancers are diagnosed in individuals over the age of 50 years. According to Corman (1993), the mean age at diagnosis was 63 years for men and 62 years for women. Malignancies occurring in those younger than 30 years old tend to be difficult to control and usually are associated with a poor prognosis (Beart, 1991). Screening guidelines for rectal cancer take into account the age differences associated with the disease.

Geographic Distribution

The incidence of rectal cancer varies greatly in geographic regions around the world. The incidence of colon cancer varies more geographically than that of rectal cancer (Bresalier & Kim, 1993). These differences suggest some differences in etiologies between colon cancer and rectal cancer. In reference to colorectal cancer overall, the highest rates for both sexes are reported from Connecticut, and the lowest rates are from Utah. Worldwide, higher rates of rectal cancer are common in more developed countries of North America, Western Europe, Australia, and New Zealand. Lower rectal cancer rates are noted in Eastern Europe, Asia, Africa, and parts of South America. For cancer of the rectum, incidence rates range from 1.2 per 100,000 in Nigeria to 18.2 per 100,000 in the United States (Winawer, Enker, & Levin, 1992).

Dietary Factors

Dietary factors have been noted to be significant in the development of rectal cancer (Burnstein, 1993). Even though studying the dietary factors related to colorectal cancer is complicated, several epidemiologic studies suggest correlations of fiber, fat, selenium, and alcohol in the development of rectal cancer.

Fiber. Even though several epidemiologic studies strongly or moderately support the protective role of fiber in colorectal cancer, further research is needed (Trock, Lanza, & Greenwald, 1990; Vargas & Albert, 1992). Dietary fiber is a substance derived from a variety of fruit, grain, and legume sources that is resistant to human digestive enzymes (Weiss & Itzkowitz, 1995). It is theorized that dietary fiber exerts positive effects by increasing stool volume, diluting

Box 37-1
Risk Factors for Rectal Cancer

Increasing age
Residence in developed, Western countries
Low-fiber intake
High-fat intake
Low selenium levels
Alcohol (especially beer)
Adenomatous polyps
Prior history of colorectal cancer
Family history/inheritance
- Familial adenomatous polyposis
- Gardner's syndrome
- Sporadic cancer

Inflammatory bowel disease

harmful substances, and speeding colorectal transit time (Mahut & Stearn, 1996).

Even though it is speculated that all sources of fiber are probably protective to the bowel, there is some controversy as to whether soluble fiber or insoluble fiber provides more protection (Mahut & Stearn, 1996). Because Americans on average consume only 10 g of fiber daily, in contrast to the recommended 20 to 30 g, any source of fiber should be encouraged and consumed (Smigel, 1990).

Fat. There is evidence that diets containing high amounts of fat increase the risk of colorectal cancer. In countries where colorectal cancer rates are high, the average fat intake composes 40% to 45% of total caloric intake, whereas in low-risk cohorts, fat intake accounts for only 10% to 15% of dietary calories (Shike, Winawer, Greenwald, Block, Hill, & Swaroop, 1990). Dietary fat has been noted to lead to greater levels of fecal bile acids and free fatty acids, which may potentiate and support malignant processes in the bowel (Burnstein, 1993; Levin & Raijman, 1995). Cholesterol is one component of dietary fat; a positive association has been noted between serum cholesterol level (>275 mg/dl) and the risk of rectal cancer in men; however, this association has not been consistently demonstrated (Tornberg, Holm, Carstensen, & Eklund, 1986; Winawer, Flehinger, Buchelter, Herbert, & Shike, 1990).

Selenium. Inadequate levels of selenium, a micronutrient, have been associated with cancer of the rectum. Selenium is an antioxidant that prevents free radical damage to tissue. Cereal grains and seafood are the main dietary sources of selenium (Burnstein, 1993). Recommended doses of selenium to optimally decrease the risk of rectal cancer have not been established; thus research continues.

Alcohol. The association between beer consumption and the development of rectal cancer has been proposed by some studies (Enstrom, 1977; Pollack, Nomura, Heilbrun, Stemmermann, & Green, 1984). In a prospective study evaluating the development of colorectal cancer in more than 100,000 subjects, a relative risk for rectal cancer of 3.17 was identified compared with a relative risk of 1.71 for colon cancer. These results were based on daily consumption of three or more alcoholic beverages per day. The type of alcohol consumed was not controlled (Klatsky, Armstrong, Friedman, & Hiatt, 1988).

Box 37-2
Facts About Rectal Cancer

Rectal cancer occurs in approximately 37,000 Americans annually. Most rectal cancer is diagnosed after the age of 50, but it can occur in younger individuals. Men are slightly more likely to develop the disease than women. Early detection of rectal cancer allows for more effective treatment.

The Rectum

The lowest portion of the digestive tract is known as the *large intestine*. The last 8 to 10 inches of the large intestine is known as the *rectum*. When solid waste from digested food is moved through the intestines, it will be stored temporarily in the rectum until the body signals that it is time for the waste to be eliminated from the body.

Early Detection of Rectal Cancer

Currently the American Cancer Society recommends the following guidelines to detect rectal cancer early in individuals who have no symptoms:

- After age 40, an annual digital rectal examination by a physician or health care practitioner.
- After age 50, the fecal occult blood test to analyze stool for hidden blood is recommended. The specimen is obtained by the individual and returned to a health care center for testing.
- After age 50, sigmoidoscopy should be performed every 3 to 5 years. This procedure allows visualization of the rectum.

Individuals with an increased risk of rectal cancer should ask their physician about early detection tests and schedules. Anyone with symptoms of rectal cancer should notify his or her physician immediately.

Risk Factors for Rectal Cancer

Increasing age
Low dietary fiber intake
High dietary fat intake
High alcohol intake (especially beer)
Intestinal polyps
Family history of polyps
Inflammatory bowel disease (ulcerative colitis, Crohn's disease)

Signs and Symptoms of Rectal Cancer

Rectal bleeding
Blood in the stool
Change in bowel habits (constipation and/or diarrhea, change in size or quantity of stool)
A sensation that the rectum is still full even after having a bowel movement

Adenomatous Polyps

Most rectal cancers develop in adenomatous polyps. Adenomatous polyps are associated with abnormal cellular proliferation and are made up of dysplastic epithelium (Bresalier,

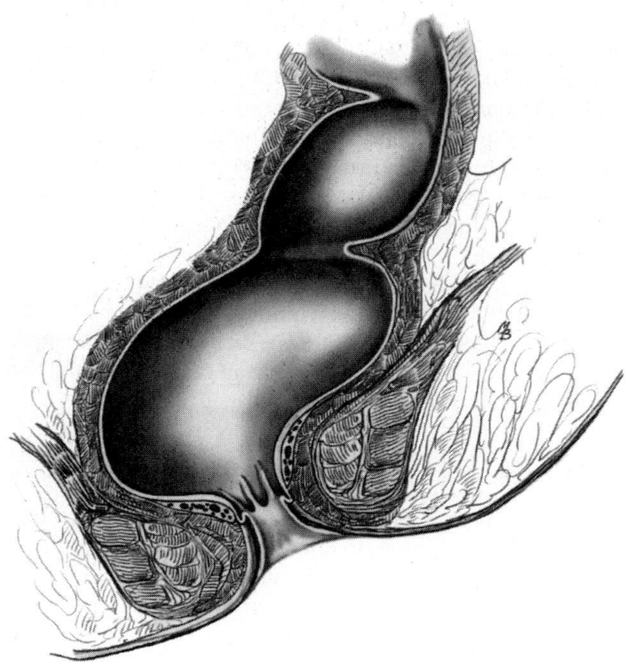

Fig. 37-1 Diagrammatic representation of the rectum.

1996). Biologic evidence of chromosome deletions and *ras*-oncogene mutations support the idea that an adenocarcinoma sequence of progression from normal epithelium to adenoma carcinoma is present in colorectal cancers (Fig. 37-1). Cancer risk increases with larger adenomas (Markowitz & Winawer, 1997).

Prior History of Colorectal Cancer

Individuals who have a history of colorectal cancer are at risk for developing another colorectal neoplasm at a later time. Even though the recurrence of colorectal lesions may be premalignant polyps, it is imperative that colorectal examination and polyp removal be completed to minimize cancer recurrence. A strict follow-up course is needed with individuals with a previous history of colorectal cancer to monitor changes in the bowel (Motwani, Shafir, Merrick, Tepper, & Bruckner, 1997).

Family History

It appears that inheritance functions as a critical factor in the development of adenomatous polyps, the precursors to colorectal cancer. The delineation of the development of colon cancer vs rectal cancer is not always easily understood, but etiologies from predisposing genetic conditions probably play a role. There are three clinical patterns of inheritance: familial adenomatous polyposis, hereditary nonpolyposis colorectal cancer, and the so-called sporadic cancer (Burt, Bishop, Cannon-Albright, Samowitz, Lee, & DiSario et al., 1992).

Familial adenomatous polyposis (FAP) and its variant, Gardner's syndrome, are characterized by the development of hundreds to thousands of adenomatous polyps in the colon and rectum. This is transmitted in an autosomal dominant manner and usually begins manifesting in young adulthood (Mahut & Stern, 1996). Usually within a decade of the appearance of adenomas, cancer development is inevitable. A total colectomy is advocated to properly treat this condition to prevent a recurrence of cancer in the rectum (Bresalier, 1996). In addition to numerous colorectal adenomatous polyps, Gardner's syndrome has other manifestations including fibromas, lipomas, osteomas, and desmoid tumors (Mahut & Stern, 1996).

Hereditary nonpolyposis colorectal cancer (HNPCC) is an inherited disorder in which one or several (but not hundreds) of adenomatous polyps arise in the colon and rectum. HNPCC is characterized by early-onset (before age 50) colorectal cancer involving at least two generations, and the involvement of three or more relatives diagnosed with colorectal cancer. In addition, primary tumors outside the bowel may arise.

Sporadic colorectal cancer is a term that describes malignancies that do not follow FAP or HNPCC patterns; however, sporadic colorectal cancer is hereditary. Population studies have shown a twofold to threefold risk of colorectal cancer in first-degree relatives of individuals diagnosed with colorectal cancer (Bresalier, 1996). A careful family history is imperative to properly follow individuals who have a family history of colorectal cancer.

Inflammatory Bowel Disease

Individuals with a history of inflammatory bowel disease are at an increased risk for colorectal cancer. Even though the mechanisms of pathophysiology are not totally understood, chronic bowel inflammation is suspected (Mahut & Stern, 1996). The risk of cancer correlates most closely with ulcerative colitis. The association with Crohn's disease is not as strongly established, but some colorectal cancer risk is suspected (Bresalier, 1996).

Summary

Although some risk factors associated with the development of rectal cancer (i.e., increasing age and family history) cannot be modified, other risk factors may be reduced through lifestyle changes. For example, reduction of dietary fat, increase in fiber intake, and moderation of alcohol can be attained with the proper teaching and support.

CHEMOPREVENTION

Chemoprevention efforts related to colorectal cancer are fairly new. Studies have been designed to address detoxification of carcinogens, modification of carcinogen formation, and the process of the development of colorectal cancer (Levin, 1992). Chemoprevention studies for colorectal cancer are summarized in Table 37-1. Agents being studied include types and amount of dietary fiber, vitamins, aspirin, sulindac, and calcium (Weiss & Itzkowitz, 1995).

TABLE 37-1 Chemoprevention Studies of Colorectal Neoplasm

Agent Dose/Schedule	Study Population
Wheat bran 25 g/day	Adenoma recurrence
Fat calories < 25% daily Beta-carotene 20 mg/day	Rectal epithelial cell proliferation
Wheat bran 13.5 g/day	Adenoma recurrence Rectal epithelial cell proliferation
Fat calories 20% daily	Adenoma recurrence
Dietary fiber 18 g/1000 kcal/day 5-8 servings fruits and vegetables daily	Rectal epithelial cell proliferation
Calcium 1200 mg/day	Previous colorectal polyps
Beta-carotene 30 mg/day; ascorbic acid 1 g/day; vitamin E 400 mg/day	Previous colorectal adenomas

From Levin, B. & Raijman, I. (1995). Malignant tumors in the colon and rectum. In W. S. Haubrich, F. Schaffner, & J. E. Berk (Eds.), *Gastroenterology* (5th ed.). Philadelphia: WB Saunders; Weiss, N. & Itzkowitz, S. (1995). Clinical aspects of colorectal cancer. In A. K. Rustgi (Ed.), *Gastrointestinal cancers: Biology diagnosis and therapy.* Philadelphia: Lippincott-Raven.

SCREENING

Screening procedures for colorectal cancer can be categorized into two groups: high-risk individuals and average-risk individuals. High-risk individuals have a known risk factor for colorectal cancer such as family history of colorectal cancer or a history of inflammatory bowel disease. Screening methods and schedules should be closely monitored by the individual's physician. Furthermore, as more genetic testing becomes available, physicians will need to explore carefully the psychosocial aspects of screening (Motwani et al., 1997).

Screening for average-risk individuals with no symptoms of colorectal cancer is controversial. There are questions as to the consistency and cost of screening, even though some population studies have indicated earlier detection of colorectal cancers (Winawer, Schottenfeld, & Flehinger, 1991). Despite concerns in evaluating the effectiveness of screening methods, basic screening efforts are still supported. The American Cancer Society recommends that individuals over 40 years of age have an annual digital rectal examination and that individuals over the age of 50 have their stool tested annually for occult blood as well as have a sigmoidoscopy performed every 3 to 5 years (American Cancer Society, 1998).

PATHOPHYSIOLOGY

Normal Anatomy and Physiology of the Rectum

The large intestine is the organ responsible for processing and eliminating waste products produced by nutrient digestion. Anatomically, the rectum begins at the midsacral area and is attached to the sigmoid colon (Fry, Fleshman, & Kodner, 1989). The rectum spans 12 to 15 cm where it attaches distally to the anal canal. In males, the prostate gland is adjacent to the distal part of the rectum (Doughty & Jackson, 1993). Commonly the rectum may be divided into thirds (lower, middle, and upper). Many rectal tumors are located in the lower third (6 cm) of the rectum (Givel, 1990). An illustration of the rectum is presented in Fig. 37-2.

Two main functions of the rectum are to store stool and to assist in the defecation process. When enough stool causes rectal distention, an urge to defecate is signaled. From the rectal distention, the internal sphincter will relax, allowing fecal contents to enter the anal canal. At an appropriate time, the individual will relax the external sphincter, allowing passage of stool (Doughty & Jackson, 1993).

The Process of Carcinogenesis

The development of colorectal cancer is a complex process. As bowel cells rapidly slough and regenerate, genetic and environmental influences moderate the process, with eventual progression to dysplastic changes and malignant cells (Bresalier, 1996). This multistage process has been named the *adenocarcinoma sequence* or the *dysplastic carcinoma sequence* (Lewin, Riddell, & Weinstein, 1992).

It appears that colorectal cancer often arises in a single cell that often is an adenoma. Adenomas are frequently found in association with carcinoma (Milsom, 1993). The development of colorectal cancer involves genetic mutations that can be classified into two general groups of dominant and recessive. Oncogenes are examples of dominant mutations, whereas tumor suppressor genes are examples of recessive mutations. The deleted gene on chromosome 5 in patients with familial adenomatous polyposis is a recessive gene. There is evidence that this is the initial event that inactivates the gene that leads to epithelial cell proliferation and an adenoma (Markowitz & Winawer, 1997). *Ras* oncogenes on chromosome 12 are proto-oncogenes (Milsom, 1993). Other molecular abnormalities in colorectal cancer include oncogene activation as a result of an alteration in the Ki-*ras* gene and mutations of chromosome 18 by removing the DCC (deleted in colorectal cancer) gene, deletion of P53 from chromosome 17, mutations in chromosome 5q21, changes in the MCC (mutated in colorectal cancer) gene, and deletion of the familial adenomatous gene on chromosome 5 (Levin & Raijman, 1995).

Numerous other genetic changes occur during adenoma development and cancer progression. A proposed sequence of events in rectal cancer carcinogenesis is outlined in Fig. 37-2.

ROUTES OF METASTASES

Cancer of the rectum can initially spread by penetrating the rectal wall with the potential to invade adjacent tissues such as the peritoneal cavity, prostate, vagina, bladder, or ureters (Smith, 1992). Metastatic spread can also occur through both lymphatic and hematogenous routes (Lev & Lee, 1995).

Lymphatic spread is the most common route of spread of colorectal cancer. The pararectal group of lymph nodes is a

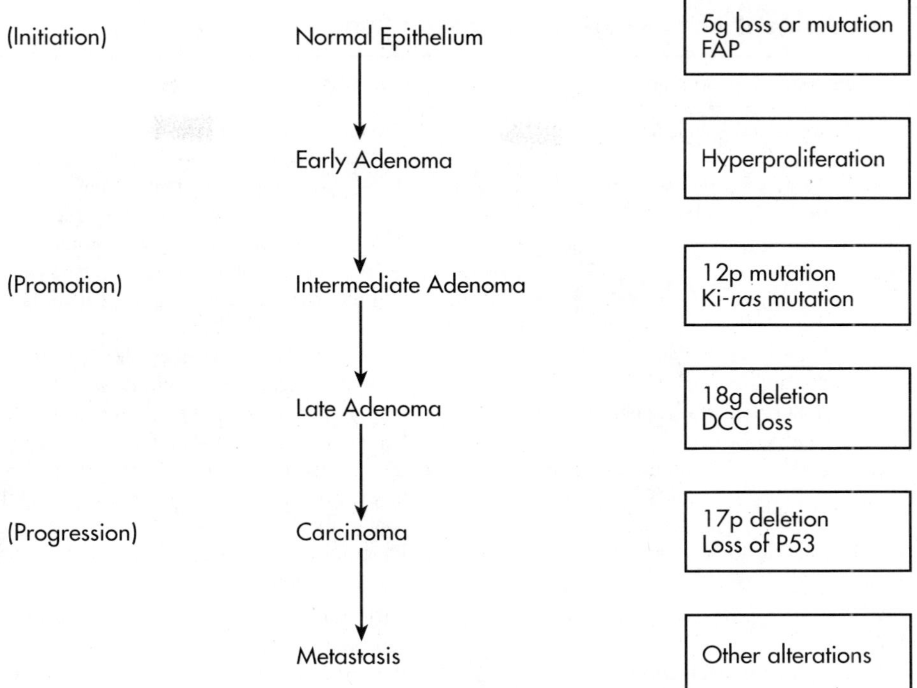

Fig. 37-2 Proposed molecular events involved in the development of rectal cancer.

frequent site of metastasis from rectal cancer. Node metastasis in rectal cancer is approximately 50% at the time of diagnosis (Takahashi, Mori, & Moosa, 1991).

Tumor cells may be carried by the blood to distant organs, with the liver and lung being the most common sites (Smith, 1992). It is postulated that when rectal cancer invades the full thickness of the bowel wall and reaches tributaries of the superior hemorrhoidal veins, transport of disease can occur. Also, invasion of rectal cancer via the venous plexus of the sacrum has been reported (Takahashi, Mori, & Moosa, 1991).

ASSESSMENT

Components of a clinical evaluation of a patient includes a detailed health history, a thorough physical examination, and a variety of diagnostic tests. The signs and symptoms present in the patient often depend on the stage of disease at the time of diagnosis (Table 37-2).

History

The patient should be evaluated for all of the identified risk factors for rectal cancer. Specific attention to the patient's dietary habits, such as fat, fiber, and alcohol intake, is important subjective data to complement the assessment process. Information about involuntary weight loss may indicate metastatic disease. In addition, a careful history of the lower gastrointestinal system should be obtained.

Rectal bleeding is the most common complaint with rectal cancer (Corman, 1993). This symptom can occur from frank hematochezia to subtle spotting in the toilet or on bathroom tissue. It is important to assess for rectal bleeding with the following questions: When did the rectal bleeding start? How much bleeding occurred (i.e., spotting to frank oozing)? Is the bleeding associated with bowel movements? (Weiss & Itzkowitz, 1995).

A change in bowel habits is often associated with rectal cancer. Patients with rectal cancer may experience constipation alternating with diarrhea, increased morning urgency to defecate, a feeling of rectal fullness with or without tenesmus, and fecal incontinence. Questions used to ascertain bowel habits and any changes include the following: What is your usual bowel elimination pattern? Have there been changes in the frequency, size, or consistency of your stools? Do you have voluntary control of your bowels? Do you experience any unusual sensations or pain with your bowel movements? Is there mucus in your stool?

A patient may experience abdominal symptoms with rectal cancer, even though this is a poor prognostic factor. Abdominal symptoms include pain and/or cramping. Assessment questions may include the following: When did the abdominal symptoms begin? What is the pain or cramping like? Is it constant? Do you have other symptoms such as nausea or weakness? Does anything relieve the symptoms?

A history concerning the genitourinary system is necessary to obtain because, in some cases, the rectal cancer may have advanced into the prostate, vagina, or bladder. Assessment questions should address whether the patient is experiencing urinary frequency, hesitancy, urgency, or nocturia. Furthermore, questions regarding impotence, painful inter-

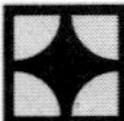

TABLE 37-2 Assessment of the Patient for Rectal Cancer

	Assessment Parameters	Typical Abnormal Findings
History	A. Personal and social history	A. Personal and social risk factors
	1. Age	1. Usually over the age of 60
	2. Gender	2. Slightly more prevalent in men
	3. Place of residence	3. Industrialized, Western countries
	4. Family history	4. Positive family history of colorectal cancer, familial adenamutous polyposis, Gardner's syndrome, hereditary nonpolyposis colorectal cancer, inflammatory bowel disease
	5. Dietary factors	5. High-fat diet, low-fiber diet, high alcohol intake
	6. Involuntary weight loss	6. May indicate metastatic disease
	B. Evaluation of lower gastrointestinal system	B. Common symptoms include rectal bleeding, change in bowel habits, abdominal discomfort.
	C. Evaluation of genitourinary system	C. Symptoms may include urinary frequency, urgency, hesitancy, nocturia, painful intercourse, impotence, vaginal discharge.
	D. Evaluation for pain	D. Patients with metastatic disease may complain of low back, pelvic, or perianal pain.
Physical Examination	A. Digital rectal examination (DRE)	A. DRE may reveal lesions where size, location, and mobility can be assessed.
	B. Lymph node evaluation	B. Presence of inguinal or supraclavicular nodes may indicate metastatic disease.
	C. Abdominal evaluation	C. Presence of ascites or hepatomegaly may indicate metastatic disease.
Diagnostic Tests	A. Rigid sigmoidoscopy	A. Useful in locating rectal cancers. May be more accurate than flexible sigmoidoscopy in determining location of tumor in rectum visualize up to 25 cm in bowel.
	B. Flexible sigmoidoscopy	B. Allows for more visualization in the bowel: up to 60 cm. Increased patient comfort is noted with this procedure.
	C. Colonoscopy	C. Allows for full visualization of bowel. Used to determine disease has spread beyond rectum.
	D. Double contrast	D. Bowel lesions, especially those over 1 cm in diameter, are located.
	E. Endorectal or transrectal ultrasound	E. Distinct layers of the rectum can be visualized; thus depth of rectal wall invasion can be assessed.
	F. Computed tomography	F. Metastatic disease to the pelvis and abdomen may be found
	G. Magnetic resonance imaging	G. Recurrent disease is detected.
	H. Intravenous pyelogram	H. Metastatic disease to ureters and bladder may be found.
	I. Carcinoembryonic antigen assay	I. May be elevated in patients with rectal cancer.
	J. Gastrointestinal cancer antigen (19-9)	J. Primary and metastatic rectal cancer is detected.
	K. Radiolabeled antibody imaging	K. The procedure is sensitive to locating primary and metastatic disease
	L. Fecal occult blood testing	L. In asymptomatic individuals, may indicate blood in the stool. Not needed if individuals already present with rectal bleeding.
	M. Chest x-ray study	M. At the time of diagnosis, 10% of patients have lung metastasis.
	N. Bone scan	N. Bone scan will be positive with disease spread to bone
	O. Liver scan	O. Liver scan will be positive with disease spread to the liver

course, vaginal discharge, or pelvic/flank pain are also important (Mahut & Stern, 1996).

A thorough evaluation for pain is imperative. Patients with rectal cancer that has spread to the sacral area will complain of low back or pelvic pain. Perianal pain is also a poor prognostic indicator. Assessment for pain includes the following questions: Where is the pain? What does the pain feel like? What makes the pain better or worse? Can you rate the pain on a scale of 1 (no pain) to 10 (excruciating pain)?

Physical Examination

Digital rectal examination (DRE) is a crucial component of the physical examination. The examination involves visual inspection of the perianal area including the skin condition and presence of hemorrhoids. Palpation of the rectum occurs when a gloved index finger is inserted into the anal canal and advanced into the rectum. Normal findings of the rectum include regular sphincter function, smooth rectal walls free of lesions or lumps, and soft, nonswollen lymph nodes.

A DRE may reveal abnormalities such as a lesion that may be assessed for approximate location, size, and mobility. Information about whether the lesion occupies the whole or a part of the rectal circumference can be found through DRE (Corman, 1993). Tumor extension into the prostate or vagina can be examined via DRE. Finally, careful palpation may reveal hard or inflamed lymph nodes.

As part of a thorough physical examination for diagnosing rectal cancer, lymph nodes and the abdomen should be specifically assessed. Metastatic rectal cancer may manifest through enlarged lymph nodes in the inguinal and supraclavicular areas (Mahut & Stern, 1996). Also, metastatic disease may be indicated by abdominal ascites and hepatomegaly (Corman, 1993).

Diagnostic Tests

A range of diagnostic tests is available to evaluate the possibility of rectal cancer. It is important to note that practitioners may use the diagnostic tests in combinations they believe best fit the patient situation.

Sigmoidoscopy. Sigmoidoscopy examination is an important diagnostic tool in the evaluation of rectal cancer. A sigmoidoscopy can be conducted using a rigid or flexible instrument. The rigid sigmoidoscope is used only in specific cases to assess the rectum. When the rigid sigmoidoscope is passed to its full length, approximately 25 cm, the examination may reveal inflammatory changes, lesions, polyps, fistulas, fissures, and hemorrhoids (Corman, 1993). This test can be uncomfortable for the patient. Some practitioners believe the rigid sigmoidoscope is better for assessing the rectum (Givel, 1990).

Because of its greater length and flexibility, the flexible sigmoidoscope has been assuming a greater role in the diagnosis of colorectal cancer. The flexible sigmoidoscopy permits visualization of the gastrointestinal tract from the anus to 60 cm. Advantages of flexible sigmoidoscopy include minimal bowel preparation, no sedation required, increased patient comfort, and more visualization of the rectum to sigmoid (Boland, 1995). A guide for preparing the patient for sigmoidoscopy is presented in Table 37-3.

Colonoscopy. The colonoscopy is a diagnostic test that involves the insertion of a flexible fiberoptic tube through the anus into the gastrointestinal tract. This procedure allows the entire colon to be examined. During the test, tissue samples can be taken as well as the removal of small polyps; thus definite diagnosis can be made (Corman, 1993). Bowel preparation is achieved through several means, often oral agents. Intravenous sedation and analgesia are used during the examination.

Double Contrast Barium Enema. Even though use of the double contrast barium enema has been shown to be useful in the diagnosis of colorectal cancer, controversy exists over its use. Some practitioners view this procedure in conjunction with a sigmoidoscopy as an alternative to colonoscopy (Bresalier, 1996). Others believe that the double-contrast barium enema cannot yield as accurate results as can colonoscopy (Corman, 1993). A double contrast barium enema consists of filling the intestine with barium from an enema tube followed by the introduction of air to enlarge the intestines. General patient preparation includes a clear liquid diet and gastrointestinal catheterization (Heaton, 1995).

Endorectal or Transrectal Ultrasound. An endorectal or transrectal ultrasound may be useful in the assessment of patients with rectal cancer. Because each layer of the rectum can be visualized with ultrasound, rectal wall lesions as well as regional lymph nodes can be assessed. Even though this procedure cannot distinguish between benign and malignant lesions, it demonstrates specificity of bowel wall disease. A probe is introduced into the rectum after the patient receives a small-volume enema. This procedure may assist in better diagnosing limited rectal cancer, thus facilitating local treatment (Corman, 1993).

Other Radiologic Studies. Radiologic studies may be used in many combinations for the practitioner to diagnose accurately and make optimal treatment decisions. Computed tomography (CT) of the abdomen and pelvis may be used to evaluate metastatic disease from rectal cancer. Magnetic resonance imaging has not been shown to be advantageous over CT except in diagnosing recurrent disease (Fry, Fleshman, & Kodner, 1989). An intravenous pyelogram may be advised in patients with cancer of the rectum to evaluate spread of the disease to the ureters or bladder (Corman, 1993). Chest x-rays may be used to delineate spread to the lungs. Approximately 10% of patients with rectal cancer will have a pulmonary metastasis (Vignati & Roberts, 1993). Also, scans may be used to evaluate disease spread to the bones or liver.

Tumor Markers. Carcinoembryonic antigen assay (CEA) is a glycoprotein that is present in fetal tissue and colorectal cancer, but it is absent in normal colonic tissue (Fry, Fleshman, & Kodner, 1989). Plasma concentrations of CEA may be elevated in individuals with colorectal cancer, but CEA can also be elevated in conditions such as diverticulitis, pancreatitis, uremia, cirrhosis, and fibrocystic breast disease and in individuals who smoke (Vignati & Roberts, 1993).

CEA levels can be applied relevantly in assessing the prognosis of individuals with colorectal cancer. Preoperative levels of CEA correlate with the degree of differentiation and size of rectal cancers. Studies have indicated that high CEA levels noted preoperatively correlates with poorer survival in patients with rectal cancer. After curative resection, CEA levels should return to normal levels within 4 to 6 weeks, and persistently elevated CEA levels may indicate residual disease (Vignati & Roberts, 1993).

Gastrointestinal cancer antigen is a modified blood group

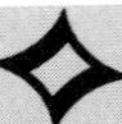

TABLE 37-3 Patient Preparation for a Sigmoidoscopy

Description of the Procedure: A sigmoidoscopy involves the passage of a rigid or flexible scope for direct visualization of mucosa of the sigmoid colon, rectum, and anal canal.

Patient Preparation:

1. Explain the purpose of the procedure.
2. Explain that preparation for the procedure may vary slightly according to the suspected diagnosis or physician preference.
3. Inform the patient that a light meal the evening before the test and clear liquids the morning of the procedure are allowed. Discuss the need if the patient needs to be NPO 8 hours before the procedure.
4. Inform the patient that a bowel preparation of a laxative and enema may be administered the night before the test while one or two small-volume sodium phosphate (Fleets) enemas may be administered 1 to 2 hours before the procedure.

Procedural Considerations:

1. Verify informed consent has been obtained.
2. Reassure the patient that privacy and safety will be ensured.
3. Instruct the patient that a light sedative or analgesic may be administered.
4. The patient needs to disrobe below the waist or wear a hospital gown.
5. Assist the patient to a knee-chest position for rigid sigmoidoscopy or to a left lateral position for flexible sigmoidoscopy.
6. Explain that a digital rectal examination will be completed first followed by the insertion of the lubricated scope into the rectum.
7. Explain that an urge to defecate may be experienced and that deep, slow mouth breathing may minimize this symptom.
8. Explain that air may be injected into the bowel to improve visualization. Also, inform the patient that tissue biopsies and photographs may be taken during the procedure.
9. When the examination is done, the scope is removed and the perineal area cleansed.

Postprocedural Care:

1. The patient may rest in a supine position for about 1 hour before being assisted to sit up.
2. Provide the patient with both written and verbal instructions including the following:
    - Rectal bleeding or blood in the stool may occur up to 48 hours after the test.
    - The patient should avoid vigorous activity on the day of the procedure.
    - The patient may consume a diet as tolerated unless otherwise instructed by the physician.
    - Abdominal pain or distention, fever, sweating, or pallor should be reported to the contact physician or nurse.
    - The name and telephone number of the contact physician or nurse.

Modified from Watson, J. & Jaffe, M. (1995). *Nurse's manual of laboratory and diagnostic tests.* Philadelphia: F.A. Davis.

antigen that can be recognized by a monoclonal antibody labeled 19-9 (Hackford, 1993). To date, there is no evidence to suggest that this tumor marker is more effective than CEA in predicting disease prognosis or recurrence, but this test may hold some promise as a screening tool in the future (Corman, 1993).

Radiolabeled antibody imaging is a process by which a radiolabeled monoclonal antibody is attached to colorectal cells or other antigens to locate tumors within the body (Hackford, 1993). This technique is sensitive for locating primary tumors and metastatic disease (Corman, 1993).

Fecal Occult Blood Testing. In some cases, initial testing of blood in the stool may help to determine further testing for an individual with colorectal cancer who may otherwise be asymptomatic (Corman, 1993). Fecal occult blood testing (FOBT) is not a test for cancer, but a test for blood in the stool, which may be indicative of a malignant disease. The FOBT may result in false-negative or false-positive results for cancer; thus individuals must comply with dietary and medication restrictions for the test. This procedure lends itself more as a screening tool than a diagnostic test. In fact, in patients with a history of rectal bleeding, this test is not needed to confirm the presence of blood (Boyd, 1995).

Diagnosis of Rectal Cancer. The diagnosis of rectal cancer is suggested by an abnormal DRE, elevated CEA level, or abnormal findings from a sigmoidoscopy, double-contrast barium enema, colonoscopy, or transrectal ultrasound. Proper tissue sampling and biopsy are crucial to the appropriate diagnosis of rectal cancer.

STAGING

Two major staging systems, Dukes and TNM System, are used with rectal cancer (Table 37-4). The original Dukes classification system of rectal cancers was proposed in 1932, with subsequent modifications implemented in later years to provide more diagnostic information (Giardiello, 1995). Dukes noted in his classification system the importance of lymph node involvement and the penetration depth of the cancer. Three stages were originally described by Dukes (1932):

1. Involvement of the mucosa with invasion into, but not through the muscularis propria (rectal wall), no lymph node involvement
2. Invasion through the muscularis propria (rectal wall), no lymph nodes involved
3. Regardless of tumor invasion depth into the bowel wall, lymph nodes are noted to contain metastatic disease

Revisions of this classification by Dukes and others have been proposed to provide more accurate prognostic data.

TABLE 37-4 Staging and Grading for Rectal Cancer

Primary Tumor (T)

Tis	Carcinoma in situ: intraepithelial or invasion of the lamina propria
T1	Tumor invades the submucosa
T2	Tumor invades the muscularis propria
T3	Tumor invades through the muscularis propria into the subserosa or into nonperitonealized pericolic or perirectal tissues
T4	Tumor directly invades other organs or structures and/or perforates the visceral peritoneum

Regional Lymph Nodes (N)

N0	No regional lymph node metastasis
N1	Metastasis in one to three pericolic or perirectal lymph nodes
N2	Metastasis in four or more pericolic or perirectal lymph nodes
N3	Metastasis in any lymph node along the course of a named vascular trunk and/or metastasis to apical node(s) (when marked by the surgeon)

Distant Metastasis (M)

M0	No distant metastasis
M1	Distant metastasis

Primary Tumor (T)
Stage Grouping

AJCC/UICC				Dukes
Stage 0	Tis	N0	M0	—
Stage I	T1	N0	M0	A
	T2	N0	M0	
Stage II	T3	N0	M0	B
	T4	N0	M0	
Stage III	Any T	N1	M0	C
	Any T	N2	M0	
	Any T	N3	M0	
Stage IV	Any T	Any N	M1	—

Grading

G_1	Well differentiated
G_2	Moderately well differentiated
G_3	Poorly differentiated
G_4	Very poorly differentiated

From the American Joint Committee on Cancer. (1992). *Manual for staging cancer* (4th ed.). Philadelphia: Lippincott-Raven.
AJCC, American Joint Committee on Cancer; *UICC,* International Union Against Cancer.

The Astler-Coller modification is one modified version of the Dukes system (Astler & Coller, 1954). The Astler-Coller system is staged as follows:

1. Lesion confined to wall of bowel
2. Lesion extends into, but not through, muscularis propria; no lymph nodes involved
   - Lesion extends through the muscularis propria, no lymph nodes involved
3. Lesion extends into, but not through, the muscularis propria; lymph nodes are involved with the tumor
   - Lesion extends through the muscularis propria, lymph nodes are involved with the tumor

TABLE 37-5 General Treatment Recommendations for Rectal Cancer

Stage of Disease	Treatment Regimen
I. (Dukes A)	Surgery
II. (Dukes B)	Surgery
III. (Dukes C)	Chemoradiation (5-FU and radiation)
	Surgery
	Chemoradiation (5-FU and radiation)

5-FU, 5-fluouracil.

In an effort to provide a more uniform manner to classify colorectal cancers, the American Joint Committee on Cancer (AJCC) and the International Union Against Cancer (UICC) proposed the TNM System for staging (Mahut & Stern, 1996). The system classifies the extent of the primary tumor (T), the status of regional lymph nodes (N), and the presence or absence of metastatic disease (M) (American Joint Committee on Cancer, 1992). Stages of disease ranging from 0 to 4 are also correlated with the levels of TNM staging.

In addition to staging, histologic grading is important. Descriptive terms such as *well differentiated, moderately differentiated, poorly differentiated,* and *undifferentiated* may be used to describe the relative appearance of colorectal cancers. Well-differentiated and moderately differentiated cancers are associated with better prognostic factors. Most rectal cancers are well to moderately differentiated (Winawer, Enker, & Levin, 1992).

MEDICAL MANAGEMENT

Several treatment choices are available for a patient with rectal cancer. Factors affecting treatment options include the age, gender, and health status of the patient, as well as the tumor type, tumor location, and disease stage (Mahut & Stern, 1996). The main treatment for rectal cancer is surgical excision, but the use of radiation and chemotherapy is increasing (Freedman & Coia, 1995; Levin & Raijman, 1995). A summary of general treatment options is presented in Table 37-5.

Surgical Management

The goals of surgical management of rectal malignancies include curative resection of the primary tumor and regional lymph nodes and tissue while preserving maximal rectal function (DeCrosse, Tsioulias, & Jacobson, 1994). When the extent of disease precludes a goal for cure, a palliative resection of rectal cancer is performed to manage symptoms such as bleeding, pain, and obstruction (Bleday & Steele, 1995).

Curative treatment for rectal cancer cannot be achieved unless the tumor is completely removed with adequate surgical margins. Because the rectum lies within the confines of the pelvis with closely approximated adjacent organs, acquisition of surgically accepted tissue margins is challenging (Orkin, 1996). Although a margin of 5 cm of involved tissue is recommended as a surgical margin, a 2 cm margin is accepted in rectal cancer surgery (Abcarian, 1992). However, local recurrence after excision of rectal cancer is common. Studies indicate that there is a strong relationship between the extent of tissue margins removed and disease recurrence rates (Guillem, Paty, & Cohen, 1997). In an attempt to control local recurrence, adjuvant radiation and chemotherapy are being used (Orkin, 1996).

The three major surgical curative options for rectal cancer include local excision, sphincter-saving procedures, and abdominoperineal resection (APR). To obtain the best surgical results, it is important to determine the stage of the rectal cancer including depth of tumor invasion into the rectal wall, presence or absence of regional lymph node disease, size and appearance of the cancer, and distance above the anal verge (Billingham, 1992; Givel, 1990).

Local Excision. Local treatment of rectal cancer eliminates major resectional surgery and the subsequent clinical sequelae. An 87%, 5-year disease-free survival rate has been reported using local excision of small rectal cancers (Willett, Compton, Shelito, & Efird, 1994). Rectal lesions suitable for local treatment should meet the following criteria: less than 4 cm in diameter, within 8 cm of the anal verge, well to moderately well-differentiated, mobile, not ulcerated, and not involving more than one third of the rectal circumference (Guillem, Paty, & Cohen, 1997).

A major advantage of local surgical excision vs other local treatments, such as electrocoagulation, is that the cancer specimen can be removed essentially intact, thus allowing for tissue study. Histologic examination is crucial in determining depth of invasion and lymph node involvement (Billingham, 1992). If the pathologic examination reveals that the rectal cancer is confined to the mucosa, with tumor-free margins and negative lymph nodes, local excision alone can be considered acceptable treatment. Tumors involving the submucosa require adjuvant therapy, usually radiation in addition to the local excision (Guillem, Paty, & Cohen, 1997). Rectal lesions that extend beyond the submucosa or do not meet the previously named criteria must be treated with radical surgical excision as determined by the surgeon (Corman, 1993).

The transanal approach is the most common method used for local surgical excision of rectal cancer. The procedure involves a full-thickness excision of the cancer including the rectal wall and perirectal fat. A 1- to 2-cm margin beyond the tumor edge is also sought (Murray & Stahl, 1993). Further resection may be needed if the margins test positive for malignant cells using a frozen tissue section (Bleday & Steele, 1995).

Sphincter-Sparing Procedures. Sphincter-sparing procedures for the resection of midrectal and some distal rectal cancers are increasing. Procedures such as low anterior resection, coloanal anastomosis, and electrocoagulation have demonstrated acceptable outcomes for treating rectal cancer (Mahut & Stern, 1996).

A low anterior resection is appropriate for tumors located in the distal sigmoid and upper rectum (approximately 6 to 11 cm from the anal verge) (Smith, 1992). The involved rectum is excised via the abdomen with reanastomosis of the descending colon to the remaining rectum occurring low in the pelvis (Bleday & Steele, 1995). This sphincter-preserving technique is accomplished by the use of circular stapling devices, which have allowed surgeons to reconnect bowel ends closer to the anal canal (Givel, 1990). Although patients with a low anterior resection may need to have a temporary diverting colostomy, the need for permanent colostomies has been avoided with this procedure. Complications of low anterior resection include fecal incontinence, bowel hyperactivity, anastomotic leakage, bleeding, and obstruction (Orkin, 1996).

In patients in whom the rectal cancer is very low lying with no invasion of the sphincter muscle, a coloanal procedure is used. It is possible for surgeons to perform the anastomosis transanally in patients in whom the rectal cancer and anorectal tissue are within 2 to 3 cm of each other (Smith, 1992). As with low anterior resection, complications of coloanal anastomosis include anastomic leakage, which occurs in 2% to 11% of patients. In addition, anastomic stenosis and fecal incontinence are complications of this procedure (Orkin, 1996).

Electrocoagulation is a sphincter-sparing procedure used to treat rectal cancer involving the distal rectum. The objective of electrocoagulation is to ablate the tumor using electric cautery (Givel, 1990). For this procedure to be used appropriately, the tumor should be small (<4 cm), mobile, noninvasive, and not extending beyond 10 cm of the anal verge (Bleday & Steele, 1995). The procedure is performed with the patient under spinal or general anesthesia. Generally two to four treatments are needed to destroy the cancerous tumor. Potential complications of this procedure include rectovaginal fistulas in women, injury to the prostate in men, fecal incontinence, and rectal bleeding (Murray & Stahl, 1993). One disadvantage of electrocoagulation is that an intact specimen for histologic analysis cannot be obtained because the tumor tissue is eradicated (Mahut & Stern, 1996).

APR. APR is used when rectal cancer is fixed or adjacent to a sphincter mechanism, involves the pelvic floor, or includes tumors that are 8 cm from the anal verge (Corman, 1993). APR is an extensive surgical procedure involving a transabdominal and perineal approach. In the APR procedure, the tumor and rectum are removed via a perineal incision while the remaining sigmoid colon is brought through an abdominal incision. Because the anal orifice is sutured closed, a stoma is created to facilitate fecal evacuation (John, 1993). In some cases in which rectal cancer is locally advanced and bulky in size, the APR will be extended into a total pelvic exenteration, which includes removal of the entire colon, rectum, bladder, ureters, female or male genitalia, lymph node, and perineum (Staniunas & Schoeltz, 1993).

Several postoperative complications can occur from APR: hemorrhage, wound infection, urinary dysfunctions, ostomy problems, thromboembolism, and sexual dysfunction. Specifically, perineal wounds may become a significant problem because some are left open to heal by secondary intention. This process prolongs healing up to 8 months and may require wound irrigation and packing (Orkin, 1996).

Sexual dysfunction after APR is especially common in men (Corman, 1993). A rate of postoperative sexual dysfunction has been reported to be 59% for men and 50% for women (Cunsolo, Bragaglia, Manara, Poggioli, & Gozzetti, 1990. It has been suggested that the occurrence of postoperative sexual dysfunction is related to preoperative libido and sexual function (Corman, 1993). Injury to the nerves in the sacral area may manifest as erectile difficulty, retrograde ejaculation, and total impotence in men, whereas women experience decreased libido and orgasm difficulties (Winawer, Enker, & Levin, 1992).

Radiation Therapy

Radiation therapy for the treatment of rectal cancer is beginning to play a more important role and may be the sole treatment used in some cases. More frequently, however, radiation therapy is used as an adjuvant treatment with surgery. Radiation may be delivered preoperatively, postoperatively, or both; the last approach is referred to as the sandwich technique. Intraoperative radiation is also used. Additionally, radiation therapy may be delivered with chemotherapy, which is called *chemoradiation.*

Preoperative Radiation. Advantages of the use of preoperative radiation for the treatment of rectal cancer include the following:

1. The risk of tumor cells spreading is reduced.
2. Sphincter-sparing surgical procedures can be performed more often.
3. There is less tumor volume, thus potentially improving prognosis.
4. There is improved radiosensitivity of the tumor.
5. There is improved sensitivity of chemotherapy (especially 5-fluorouracil [5-FU]).
6. The risk of local recurrence is less (Cummings, 1993; Kuske, 1996).

Studies conducted using preoperative radiation for rectal cancer have shown varied results. A Swedish study found a statistically significant reduction in local recurrence of rectal cancer with the use of preoperative radiation. Furthermore, the research indicated that in some cases, the preoperative radiation allowed surgeons to perform sphincter-conserving procedures more often (Stockholm Rectal Cancer Study Group, 1990). Even though randomized trials of preoperative radiation have shown statistically significant decreases in the local recurrence rate of rectal cancer, 5-year survival rates have not shown increases (Cummings, 1992). Results from a consensus conference on colorectal cancer indicate that moderate to high doses of preoperative radiotherapy resulted in decreased local recurrence rates (NIH Consensus Conference, 1990).

Recommendations for preoperative radiation note that 40 to 45 cGy delivered over 4 to 6 weeks with subsequent surgical resection of the rectal cancer 6 to 8 weeks after the radiation appeared to be optimal treatment (Corman, 1993).

Postoperative Radiation. Advantages of postoperative radiation include the following:

1. Histologic assessment including prognostic information if available.
2. Patients with noninvasive rectal cancer may be spared from unnecessary treatment.
3. At the time of surgery, clips or mesh can be placed at margin sites to improve radiation treatment planning and implementation.
4. Surgery does not have to be delayed (Cummings, 1993; Kuske, 1996).

Postoperative radiation is generally used in patients whose rectal cancer has penetrated the bowel wall and/or have positive lymph nodes. Studies have indicated that a reduction in local recurrence can be achieved with postoperative radiation, but metastasis continues to be problematic and changes in survival rates cannot be substantiated (Cummings, 1992; Bresalier & Kim, 1993). It is recommended that patients receive 45 to 60 cGy over 5 to 6 weeks. Treatment should begin no sooner than 4 weeks after surgery so as not to impede wound healing (Corman, 1993). More consistent results from more recent studies indicate that postoperative radiation therapy combined with chemotherapy is effective in reducing local recurrence rates and positively affecting survival rates in patients with stage II and stage III rectal cancer (Freedman & Coia, 1995).

Preoperative and Postoperative Radiation Therapy. The use of both adjuvant preoperative and postoperative radiation is referred to as the *sandwich technique.* With this procedure, low-dose radiation is used preoperatively to decrease tumor spread, whereas postoperative radiation is used if the disease stage indicates locally advanced disease (Cummings, 1992). Researchers at Memorial Sloan Kettering noted a 92% 3-year survival rate for rectal cancer patients treated with the sandwich technique compared with 82% of patients with similar stage disease treated only with preoperative radiation (Shank, Enker, Santana, Morrissey, Daly, & Quan et al., 1987). Other studies have not shown benefit from this treatment; thus further research is needed (Cummings, 1992).

Intraoperative Radiation Therapy. For patients who have fixed, unresectable rectal lesions, intraoperative radiation therapy may be beneficial. Intraoperative radiation therapy consists of surgically removing the cancerous tumor with the immediate irradiation of the operative area (Corman, 1993). With this treatment regimen, a patient completes 4 to 6 weeks of 40 to 50 cGy preoperative radiation followed by a 10 to 20 cGy intraoperative dose of radiation. A 12% 5-year failure rate has been reported using this process vs a 29% local failure rate in control groups. Another intraoperative method of radiotherapy is the placement of interstitial iridium-192 implants (Kuske, 1996).

Endocavitary Radiation Therapy. As an alternative to surgery, endocavitary radiation is used to treat small rectal tumors (<5 cm) that are located within 10 cm of the anal verge. A treatment tube through which radiation is transmitted is placed in the rectum next to the tumor (Kuske, 1996). An absorption depth of the radiation is approximately 2 cm. This outpatient procedure usually involves three to five insertions spread over 6 to 7 weeks. Each treatment lasts about 5 minutes, with 20 to 30 cGy delivered (Sischy, 1982). Complications of this procedure include mild proctitis and bleeding.

Chemoradiation. Several studies have supported the use of multimodality treatment for patients with rectal cancer. The initial large randomized study indicating an advantage to using postoperative chemoradiation on patients with Dukes B2 or C rectal cancer was conducted by the Gastrointestinal Tumor Study Group (GITSG). Recurrence rates for patients who received no postoperative treatment compared with those who received chemoradiation were 55% and 33%, respectively (GITSG, 1986). Similarly, a study by the North Central Cancer Treatment Group (NCCTG) demonstrated a significant reduction in both local and distant disease recurrence in patients who received postoperative chemoradiation vs radiation alone (Krook, Moertal, Gunderson, Wieand, Collins, & Beart, 1991). The chemotherapeutic agents used in these studies included 5-FU and semustine. The National Institutes of Health (NIH) Consensus Conference regarding adjuvant therapy for colorectal cancer concluded that sufficient data were available to justify the use of 5-FU and radiation as adjuvant treatment for rectal cancer (NIH Consensus Conference, 1990). However, the use of semustine was not advocated because of its leukemogenic potential. Even though optimal schedules and doses have yet to be defined, use of chemoradiation in stages II and III rectal cancer is considered standard practice (Findley & Cunningham, 1993). Currently, postoperative adjuvant therapy consists of intravenous injection of 5-FU, 500 mg/m^2/day for 5 consecutive days during weeks 1 and 5, followed on week 9 by radiation therapy of 50 to 54 cGy with concurrent 5-FU, 500 mg/m^2/day for 3 consecutive days during weeks 1 and 5 of radiation, followed by two more cycles of 5-FU, 450 mg/m^2/day for 5 days.

To manage advanced colorectal cancer, 5-FU in combination with leucovorin is used. This regimen has provided partial response rates in 35% of patients with metastatic disease (Hamilton & Grem, 1996). In addition, irinotecan, a camptothean analog, has produced partial responses in patients refractory to 5-FU treatments. The major dose-limiting toxicity of irinotecan is diarrhea (Motwani et al., 1997).

ONCOLOGIC EMERGENCIES

A potential oncologic emergency associated with rectal cancer is disseminated intravascular coagulation (DIC). DIC is an inappropriate, accelerated, and systemic activation of the clotting cascade that produces simultaneous clotting and bleeding (Shelton, 1995). DIC always occurs secondary to another condition. Adenocarcinomas of the rectum and rectal tumors producing mucin are two factors that can cause DIC in patients with rectal cancer. Once the clotting cascade is stimulated, fibrin clots are produced and transported to the microcirculation where fibrinolysis breaks the clot down causing bleeding. During the DIC process, platelets and clotting factors are being used; thus if the process is not interrupted, the individual will die of hemorrhage because the body no longer has hemostatic defenses to prevent bleeding (Belcher, 1992).

Signs of bleeding may range from oozing to frank bleeding. Petechiae, ecchymosis, purpura, and hematomas may be noted. Oozing of blood from incisions, puncture sites, and mucous membranes may become evident. Late signs of DIC include organ dysfunction from ischemia, which may manifest as pain, altered mental status, oliguria, and muscle pain (Shelton, 1995). DIC is confirmed by laboratory tests. No single test can diagnose DIC; thus a group of tests are usually done to detect DIC. Generally test results indicate a prolonged prothrombin time/partial thromboplastin time, lowered platelet count, lowered fibrinogen level, and an elevated level of fibrin-split products.

Early recognition of signs and symptoms of DIC is imperative to control it. Prompt diagnosis based on laboratory tests is also crucial. Medical management includes replacement of clotting factors through fresh frozen plasma infusions and platelet infusions. Furthermore, heparin is used in DIC because it inhibits thrombin activity, which will subsequently shut down the inappropriate actions of the clotting cascade (Shelton, 1995).

Another oncologic emergency that can occur with rectal cancer is septic shock. Septic shock is an unstable condition caused by the invasion of the blood by microorganisms, usually gram-negative bacteria. It is characterized by hemodynamic instability, cellular abnormalities, and coagulation alterations. Septic shock mortality rates range from 50% to 75% (Schafer, 1994). Patients with rectal cancer are predisposed to life-threatening infections when the body's defense mechanisms are disrupted by progression of the rectal cancer, surgery, chemotherapy, and radiation.

Fever may be the only early sign of an infection. Initial signs and symptoms of septic shock include chills, confusion, malaise, hyperglycemia, tachycardia, tachypnea, and warm, dry skin (Miaskowski, 1997). As shock progresses, the skin becomes cool and clammy, there is progressive hypotension, peripheral edema occurs, and there is deterioration of neurologic and cardiovascular systems (Shelton, 1995).

Early detection and treatment of septic shock are imperative for patients' recovery. Medical management includes fluid volume replacement, broad-spectrum antibiotics, and hemodynamic and respiratory support (Schafer, 1994).

NURSING MANAGEMENT

Patients with rectal cancer have unique needs that require nursing interventions and patient education. Although a portion of the patient's care will occur in the inpatient setting, the majority of the patient's care occurs in the outpatient and home care setting.

Early in the course of the patient's disease, the focus of nursing care may be on helping the patient understand the different treatment options. As the disease progresses, patients need information about disease interventions and strategies for managing disease or treatment-related side effects. Because surgical and radiation treatments for rectal cancer pose unique patient problems, the major issues associated with these treatments are discussed with standards of care provided in this chapter.

Surgery

Patients undergoing APR are hospitalized for several days. The major focus of inpatient nursing care is to prevent postoperative complications including bleeding, infection, thrombophlebitis, and pulmonary emboli. Follow-up care in the outpatient setting requires that nurses evaluate patients for impotence/sexual dysfunction, ostomy management, and skin and wound care. The nursing management of the patient undergoing surgery for rectal cancer is summarized in Table 37-6.

Radiation Therapy

Postoperative external beam radiation therapy is provided on an outpatient basis. The major problems associated with external beam radiation include fatigue, diarrhea, cystitis, and altered sexual function. Patients require much education to understand the precaution that must be instituted while they are receiving their therapy. The nursing management of the patient with rectal cancer who is receiving external beam radiation is summarized in Table 37-7.

HOME CARE ISSUES

Discharge Information

Discharge planning is a critical component of successful home management of the patient with rectal cancer. Specifics of discharge teaching depend on the patient's individual treatment plan. Patients who have undergone an APR need to be taught that rectal suppositories, thermometers, or enemas should not be used because the rectum has been removed. Patients with an ostomy need verbal and written instructions regarding ostomy management, type of pouching system, ostomy retailers, and follow-up with the enterostomas and home health nurse. Referrals to support groups such as The United Ostomy Association and the American Cancer Society are also useful. Patient teaching about other treatment modalities such as chemotherapy and radiation therapy should be started at discharge.

Skin Care

Management of skin integrity and surgical wounds is paramount to prevent infection and promote healing. Patients who have undergone an APR have an abdominal incision, a perineal incision, and a stoma. In the initial postoperative period, the abdominal wound needs to be assessed for suture integrity, as well as signs and symptoms of infection. Teaching patients and significant others about these issues and when to phone their health care provider about problems is imperative. It is also important to emphasize to patients and caregivers the need for follow-up appointments for suture removal and care. Instruction about a diet that includes foods that can be tolerated and that are of high nutritive value is critical to facilitate wound healing.

The degree of perineal wound care depends on whether the incision has been left open, partially closed with open drainage, or totally closed with closed drainage. This wound may cause more physical and psychological discomfort than the abdominal wound or stoma because the daily care is detailed, the healing may take up to 8 months, and phantom rectal sensations may be experienced. (Heitkemper & Sawchuck, 1996). Patient and caregiver teaching regarding sterile technique, packing/dressing materials, irrigation methods, drain care, and signs and symptoms of infection is important. Also, measures to promote comfort such as sitz baths, antipruritic medications, and analgesics need to be taught. A procedure for perineal wound care is presented in Box 37-3, p. 858.

Ostomy Care

A patient with a new ostomy faces many issues. An overall nursing priority is to provide patient and caregiver teaching and support that facilitates adaptation (Hamptom & Bryant, 1992). Follow-up monitoring with an enterostomal nurse is important. Specifically, home care management includes stoma assessment, pouching system procedures, skin protection, ostomy irrigations, and lifestyle management.

The patient needs to be taught components of assessing the stoma. Stoma color should range from pink to beefy red with a moist appearance. A dusky-blue stoma may indicate ischemia and a pale stoma may indicate a low hemoglobin level (Hampton & Bryant, 1992). In general, stomas should be round, with minimal edema or bleeding.

A cost-effective, secure pouching system that promotes patient self-care is a major goal in choosing a pouching product. Pouching systems must fit snugly to prevent stomal leakage. Reinforcement of patient teaching that occurred in the hospital and consistent support are crucial to the success of patients handling and managing their selected pouching systems (Heitkemper & Sawchuck, 1996).

Skin care of the periostomal area is a high priority. It is important to relay information that periostomal skin is to be intact with no skin alterations such as redness, maceration, rashes, ulcerations, or blisters. Discussion about skin care products such as pastes, powders, gels, foams, sprays, wafers, or wipes help patients use the products optimally (Hampton & Bryant, 1992).

If the patient is to perform colostomy irrigations to regulate bowel function, the patient needs information with regard to this procedure. The patient should not be rushed in performing colostomy irrigations. Ideally, a return demon-

Text continued on p. 858

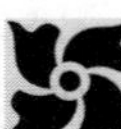

TABLE 37-6 Standard of Care for the Patient Undergoing Abdominoperineal Resection

Patient Problem and Outcomes	Nursing Interventions and Rationales	Patient Education Instructions
Anxiety Patient will: • Verbalize an understanding of the surgical procedure. • Express feelings of decreased anxiety. • Identify strategies to cope with anxiety.	1. Assess patient's level of understanding of the surgical procedure. 2. Give patient the opportunity to ask questions or verbalize concerns. 3. Determine which coping strategies the patient has used effectively in the past to decrease anxiety and reinforce the use of these coping strategies. 4. Administer pharmacologic agents to decrease anxiety, if necessary.	1. Utilize a diagram of the anatomy of the abdomen and rectum to explain the procedure. 2. Provide patient with information about the preoperative routine: a. Diagnostic tests b. Bowel prep c. Anesthesiology consult d. Use of antiembolism stockings e. NPO after midnight f. Stoma marking 3. Teach patient coughing and deep breathing exercises and obtain a return demonstration. 4. Provide patient with information about the postoperative plan of care: a. Pain management b. Management of ostomy c. Use of indwelling catheter d. Surgical incision e. Intravenous hydration f. Use of nasogastric tube
Pain Patient will experience optimal pain relief with minimal side effects.	1. Assess pain intensity using a 0 to 10 verbal rating scale, every 2 to 4 hours for the first 48 hours after surgery, then at least once a shift. 2. Administer opioid analgesics around-the-clock for the first 24 to 48 hours postoperatively. 3. Monitor for analgesic side effects and administer medications to prevent or treat: a. Nausea b. Pruritus c. Constipation	1. Teach patient to inform the nurse if he or she is experiencing pain. 2. Teach patient the importance of taking pain medication on a regular basis to keep pain under control.
High Risk for Hemorrhage Patient will: • Maintain a normal hemoglobin and hematocrit. • Maintain hemodynamic stability.	1. Check hemoglobin, hematocrit, and platelet count. 2. Check surgical incision and dressings for excessive drainage.	1. Teach patient to avoid strenuous exercises for 6 weeks after surgery. 2. Teach patient to report excessive bleeding from wound or ostomy.
High Risk for Pulmonary Embolism Patient will maintain normal arterial blood gases.	1. Apply antiembolic or compression stockings to both legs. 2. Perform active range-of-motion leg exercises to prevent deep vein thrombophlebitis. 3. Assess for leg pain and signs of thrombophlebitis.	1. Teach patient the importance of wearing antiembolic or compression stockings and the rationale for performing range-of-motion leg exercises.

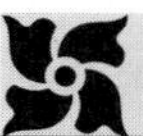

TABLE 37-6 Standard of Care for the Patient Undergoing Abdominoperineal Resection—cont'd

Patient Problem and Outcomes	Nursing Interventions and Rationales	Patient Education Instructions
High Risk for Impotence		
Patient will be able to engage in alternative forms of sexual expression.	1. Obtain a sexual history including: a. Sexual activity b. Impact of previous therapies on sexual functioning c. Onset of the impotency d. Course of the events e. Patient's perception of the problem 2. Encourage alternative methods of sexual expression. 3. Make referrals to appropriate agencies for sexual counseling and rehabilitation for the patient and his partner.	1. Explain to the patient that nerves controlling erection and ejaculation may be damaged by rectal surgery. Explain that erectile dysfunction may be temporary or long term.
Body Image Disturbance		
Patient will express feelings and concerns about living with an ostomy.	1. Assist the patient to express feelings and concerns. 2. Assist the patient to recognize strengths and assets in appearance.	1. Teach the patient methods to express feelings such as anger, frustration, and disappointment. 2. Provide information and guidance on how to access resources for support (United Ostomy Association).
Knowledge Deficit (Related to Ostomy Care)		
Patient will: • Verbalize understanding of stoma appearance and function. • Demonstrate ability to properly care for ostomy on a daily basis. • State signs and symptoms to report to the health care provider.	1. Consult enterostomal therapist. 2. Assess ability to do independent ostomy care (vision, dexterity, strength). 3. Implement ostomy teaching as soon as patient is alert and has physical strength to participate. 4. Provide demonstrations of ostomy products and their use.	1. Teach the patient about normal/ostomy anatomy and function. 2. Teach the patient and significant others about location and characteristics of the stoma. 3. Teach the patient and significant others about stoma/ostomy care including product use, daily routines, dietary recommendations, skin care, and psychosexual implications. 4. Provide information and guidance on how to access resources (United Ostomy Association, American Cancer Society).
High Risk for Skin Integrity Impairment		
Patient will: • Maintain normal skin integrity to peristomal skin. • Identify measures to minimize and prevent impaired skin integrity.	1. Assess patient's skin with special attention to area surrounding the ostomy. 2. Incorporate skin protection measures when caring for patient (gently remove ostomy appliances, cleanse with water, pat dry). 3. Administer pharmacologic agents to treat periostomal skin problems (topical agents, systemic antimicrobials). 4. Assess the patient's knowledge level and ability to care for the stoma and periostomal skin.	1. Teach the patient and significant others about skin assessment (especially periostomal skin). 2. Teach the patient and significant others that periostomal skin damage is evidenced by redness, rash, maceration, ulceration, or blister formation. 3. Teach the patient and significant others that periostomal skin damage can occur from chemical or mechanical damage. 4. Provide reinforcement teaching if the patient is not caring for stoma and skin in an optimal manner. (Review products to prevent stoma leakage, correct site to cut and fit ostomy appliance, when to empty ostomy pouch.)

Continued

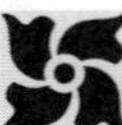

Table 37-6 Standard of Care for the Patient Undergoing Abdominoperineal Resection—cont'd

Patient Problem and Outcomes	Nursing Interventions and Rationales	Patient Education Instructions
High Risk for Altered Patterns of Urinary Elimination		
Patient will: • Void at normal intervals. • Verbalize no complaints of bladder fullness or suprapubic discomfort.	1. If urinary catheter is present, maintain patency of catheter. 2. Determine patient's usual urinary elimination pattern. 3. Assess for signs and symptoms of urinary retention (bladder fullness, dribbling of urine, frequent voiding of less than 50 ml of urine). 4. Assist patient to void using normal position in a relaxed atmosphere (privacy, run water, pour warm water over perineum). 5. Consult with physician to report signs/symptoms or urinary retention and need for intermittent catheterization or insertion of indwelling catheter.	1. Teach patient to inform the nurse of problems voiding. 2. Teach patient to void when the urge is first felt. 3. Teach patient relaxation interventions to promote voiding. 4. Teach patient procedure for self-intermittent urinary catheterization. 5. Teach patient indwelling catheter care.
High Risk for Infection		
Patient will remain infection free as evidenced by: • Absence of fever/chills • Presence of normal breath sounds • Voiding clear, yellow urine without burning, frequency, urgency • Absence of pain, drainage, redness, or swelling in any area • White blood cell and differential count within normal limits	1. Assess and report signs and symptoms of infection. 2. Maintain hydration status (encourage PO intake of at least 2500 ml/day). 3. Maintain a septic technique during invasive procedures (catheterization, injections, IV therapy, wound care). 4. Maintain optimal nutrition status 5. Implement strategies to prevent respiratory complications.	1. Teach the patient signs and symptoms of infection and when to notify health care providers. 2. Teach the patient that adequate hydration helps prevent infection. 3. Teach patient proper hand washing techniques. 4. Teach the patient proper methods to change dressings and provide wound care. 5. Teach the patient about foods and fluids to promote healing. 6. Reinforce preop teaching of coughing, turning, deep breathing.

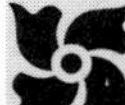

Table 37-7 Standard of Care for the Patient Receiving External Beam Radiation Therapy for Rectal Cancer

Patient Problem and Outcomes	Nursing Interventions and Rationales	Patient Education Instructions
Knowledge Deficit		
Patient will verbalize an understanding of the purpose, benefits, and risks of radiation therapy.	1. Assess patient's level of knowledge about radiation therapy. 2. Assess patient's concerns and fears about radiation therapy.	1. Describe the routine procedures involved in radiation therapy: a. Consultation b. Simulation procedure c. Treatment procedures and routines 2. Describe the major side effects associated with radiation therapy, the importance of notifying the nurse should side effects occur, and self-care measures to manage the side effects of: a. Diarrhea b. Sexual dysfunction c. Fatigue d. Cystitis

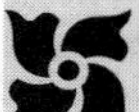

TABLE 37-7 Standard of Care for the Patient Receiving External Beam Radiation Therapy for Rectal Cancer—cont'd

Patient Problem and Outcomes	Nursing Interventions and Rationales	Patient Education Instructions
Fatigue		
Patient will be able to maintain normal activities of daily living and engage in activities to enhance his quality of life	1. Assess patient's level of fatigue using a 0 (not at all tired, full of pep) to 10 (total exhaustion) rating scale. 2. Evaluate patient's sleep and activity pattern to be able to teach patient ways to conserve energy.	1. Inform patient that he is likely to experience fatigue toward the end of treatment and for several weeks following treatment. 2. Teach patient energy conservation strategies including: a. Going to bed at a regular time b. Taking short naps during the day c. Exercising at regular intervals during the day
Diarrhea		
Patient will maintain adequate fluid balance weight, and energy level.	1. Assess elimination patterns including frequency, quality, and quantity. 2. Initiate a low-residue diet at the start of treatment, including: a. Limit foods high in roughage b. Limit fried or highly seasoned food c. Avoid uncooked fruits and vegetables d. Limit rich desserts 3. Obtain a consult with a dietitian. 4. Administer antidiarrheal medication (e.g., diphenoxylate and atropine [Lomotil] 2.5 mg tablets; 1 to 2 tablets after each loose bowel movement; not to exceed 8 tablets per day). 5. Obtain weights weekly. 6. Institute a lactose-free diet if diarrhea becomes severe (i.e., greater than 8 bowel movements per day). 7. Administer tincture of opium (0.5 to 1.0 ml every 4 hours until diarrhea is controlled for severe diarrhea).	1. Inform patient that diarrhea occurs within a few weeks of treatment, usually when a dose of 1500-3000 cGy is reached 2. Teach patient to maintain a low-residue diet until bowel patterns return to normal (usually 2 to 6 weeks after the completion of radiation therapy). 3. Teach patient to evaluate for a pattern to the diarrhea and concentrate the administration of antidiarrheal medication to that time of day.
Cystitis		
Patient will experience relief of urinary symptoms	1. Assess for symptoms of frequency, burning on urination, and urgency. 2. Evaluate for the presence of a urinary tract infection and initiate appropriate antibiotic therapy if an infection is present. 3. Administer urinary antiseptics and antispasmodics: a. Phenazopyridine 200 mg, three times a day, after meals b. Oxybutin 5 mg, 2 to 3 times per day (not to exceed 20 mg/day)	1. Inform patient that urinary symptoms may occur after 3000 cGy have been administered. 2. Teach patient that phenazopyridine (an azo dye with local anesthesia of the urinary mucosa) turns urine an orange-red color. 3. Teach patient that antispasmodics like oxybutynin can cause drowsiness, dry mouth, constipation, and urinary retention.
High Risk for Sexual Dysfunction		
Patient will be able to engage in alternative forms of sexual expression	1. Obtain a sexual history including a. Sexual activity b. Impact of previous therapies on sexual functioning 2. Encourage alternative methods of sexual expression. 3. Make referrals to appropriate agencies for sexual counseling and rehabilitation for the patient and significant other.	1. Explain to the patient that changes in hormone status, fatigue, and area of treatment may all contribute to alterations in sexual functioning. 2. Teach women that lubricants and vaginal dilators may be needed to prevent painful intercourse.

Box 37-3

Perineal Wound Care at Home

Purpose of the Procedure

As part of your rectal surgery, a surgical incision/wound was created in your anal, rectal, and buttock area, otherwise known as the *perineal area*. For proper healing to take place, daily perineal wound care is needed. This procedure will guide you regarding perineal wound care. Many times another person will need to assist with this procedure.

Steps to Follow

1. Gather the required supplies. Depending on your perineal wound, supplies may include an irrigation solution of normal saline or hydrogen peroxide, absorbent dressings such as gauze or thick pads, and tape or mesh undergarments to hold the items in place over the wound.
2. Take your pain medication as prescribed about 30 minutes before the procedure.
3. With gloves on, remove the previous dressing from the perineal area and soak the wound area in a warm, not hot, sitz bath for 10 to 20 minutes.
4. Wash your hands with soap and water.
5. Carefully open and prepare the supplies needed for wound care.
6. Put on latex or other medically approved gloves.
7. Look at the perineal wound for changes in drainage or appearance.
8. Gently irrigate the perineal wound with the prescribed solution, if ordered by your physician.
9. Place the absorbent dressing (gauze, thick absorbent pads) over the perineal wound.
10. Secure the dressing in place with tape or by putting on mesh underpants to hold the dressing in place.

Data from Heitkemper, M. & Sawchuck, L. (1996). Problems of absorption and elimination. In S. Lewis, I. Collier, & M. Heitkemper (Eds.), *Medical surgical nursing: Assessment and management of clinical problems*. St. Louis: Mosby.

stration by the patient is desired to validate understanding of the procedure (Heitkemper & Sawchuck, 1996).

Issues of lifestyle management incorporate the patient's perceptions of the situation, available support systems, and coping mechanisms. Each patient adapts to the ostomy on an individual basis.

Patients with colostomies have few dietary restrictions. However, an understanding of a well-balanced diet, adequate fluid intake, and foods that cause odor or gas is important for the nurse to reinforce (Hampton & Bryant, 1992).

Patients with an ostomy may encounter feelings of low self-concept due to a change in their perceived body image. Nurse interactions that foster a positive, warm regard are important. Interactions that facilitate patients to verbalize positive self-attributes, integrate the ostomy into their lives, and develop problem-solving skills to deal with the ostomy are essential in supporting a patient with body image concerns (Carpenito, 1995).

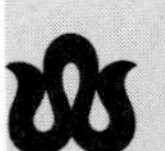

Table 37-8 Quality of Care Evaluation for a Patient Undergoing Abdominoperineal Resection

Disciplines participating in the quality of care evaluation:
☐ Nursing ☐ Surgery
☐ Physical Therapy ☐ Social Services

I. Postoperative Management Evaluation

Data from:
☐ Medical Record Review ☐ Patient/Family Interview

Criteria	Yes	No
1. Patient provided with preoperative information about:		
a. Diagnostic tests	☐	☐
b. Bowel preparation	☐	☐
c. Use of antiembolic stockings	☐	☐
d. Stoma markings	☐	☐
2. Hemoglobin and hematocrit evaluated postoperatively	☐	☐
3. Patient experienced the following complications:		
a. Urinary retention	☐	☐
b. Pulmonary embolism	☐	☐
c. Infection	☐	☐

II. Patient/Family Satisfaction

Data from:
☐ Patient Interview ☐ Family Interview

Criteria	Yes	No
1. On a scale of 0 to 10, with 0 being totally dissatisfied and 10 being totally satisfied, how satisfied were you with the pain management you received? ______		
2. Were you told to call the nurse if you experienced stoma problems?	☐	☐
3. Were you taught to avoid strenuous exercise for 4-6 weeks after surgery?	☐	☐

Sexual Dysfunction

Several treatments for rectal cancer can affect the patient's sexual functioning. Pelvic and rectal resection can cause damage to nerves and blood supply that are involved with sexual arousal and function. Men often experience erectile and ejaculation dysfunction, whereas women infrequently may experience changes in vaginal function. Usually genital pleasure from sexual interaction is not disrupted by pelvic surgery. Additionally, stoma surgery can leave patients concerned about acceptance, sexual activity, cleanliness, and disclosure about the stoma (Hampton & Bryant, 1992).

Systemic effects of chemotherapy can affect sexual functioning with adverse effects such as fatigue, weight changes, nausea and vomiting, diminished libido, mucositis, and myelosuppression. Similarly, external beam radiation also affects sexual functioning. Fatigue, alteration in hormone levels, vaginal changes, cystitis, erectile dysfunctions, skin changes, and diarrhea influence one's body image and perceptions of sexuality (Bruner & Iwamoto, 1996). Finally, medications such as antiemetics and analgesics may affect a patient's sexuality.

To address sexual concerns, nurses must be able to assess a patient's sexual health. Open, trusting communication can assist patients to share information and accept teaching. An initial evaluation that assesses the patient's past and current sexual functioning is important. In addition to taking a sexual health history, interventions that involve patient teaching to facilitate adaptation is imperative. Providing opportunities to express concerns about sexuality is important. Suggestions that affect personal communication, stoma care with sexual activity, alternative methods of sexual/intimate expression, use of a penile prosthesis, sexual counseling, changing medication schedules, and use of support systems can promote sexual integration into the patient's daily life (Hamptom & Bryant, 1992).

TABLE 37-9 Quality of Care Evaluation for a Patient Receiving External Beam Radiation Therapy

Disciplines participating in the quality of care evaluation:
☐ Nursing ☐ Surgery
☐ Physical Therapy ☐ Social Services

Data from:
☐ Mailed Questionnaire ☐ Patient Interview

Criteria	Yes	No
1. Did the doctor or nurse explain to you that you might experience some of the following side effects from your radiation therapy?		
a. Fatigue	☐	☐
b. Diarrhea	☐	☐
c. Cystitis (inflammation of the bladder)	☐	☐
d. Sexual alterations	☐	☐
2. Were you asked if you wanted to see a sex counselor?	☐	☐
3. Were you taught to report any new problems to your doctor or nurse?	☐	☐

PROGNOSIS

The prognosis for patients with rectal cancer varies depending on the stage of disease at the time of diagnosis, the patient's age, and coexistent medical problems. The stage at the time of diagnosis is related to the degree of bowel wall penetration and whether regional lymph nodes or distant metastases are involved. Other factors that may influence a patient's prognosis are serum CEA levels, tumor size, and cell histology (Bresalier, 1996). The 5-year survival rate for localized rectal cancer detected early is 87%. If the malignancy has spread to regional lymph nodes or tissues, the 5-year survival rate is 53%. After the cancer has metastasized to distant organs, the 5-year survival rate is 7% (Boyd, 1995).

EVALUATION OF THE QUALITY OF CARE

It is important that aspects of patients' care be evaluated to monitor quality of care. Tables 37-8 and 37-9 provide examples of evaluation tools that can be used for patients receiving treatment for rectal cancer.

RESEARCH ISSUES

Several issues regarding the prevention, diagnosis, and treatment of rectal cancer require further investigation. The genetic basis of rectal cancer and the risk factors associated with rectal cancer development remain to be further defined. The optimal approach to screening and early detection, including diagnostic techniques and genetics, remains to be identified. Additional research is needed to determine the value of dietary and chemopreventive agents.

Continued research into the appropriateness and effectiveness of multimodality treatment for the various stages of rectal cancer is paramount. Specifically, inquiry into chemoradiation dosages and methods is critical. However, with any rectal cancer research cannot overlook the issues of cost effectiveness, symptom management, and quality of life issues.

REFERENCES

Abcarian, H. (1992). Operative treatment of colorectal cancer. *Cancer, 70,* 1350-1354.

American Cancer Society. (1998). *Cancer facts and figures-1998.* Atlanta: American Cancer Society.

American Joint Committee on Cancer. (1992). *Manual for staging of cancer* (4th ed.). Philadelphia: Lippincott-Raven.

Astler, V. B. & Coller, F. A. (1954). The prognostic significance of direct extension of carcinoma of the colon and rectum. *Annals of Surgery, 139,* 846-851.

Beart, R.W. (1991). Colorectal cancer. In A. I. Holleb, D. J. Fink, & G. P. Murphy (Eds.), *Clinical oncology.* Atlanta: American Cancer Society.

Belcher, A. (1992). *Cancer nursing.* St. Louis: Mosby.

Billingham, R. D. (1992). Conservative treatment of rectal cancer. *Cancer, 70,* 1355-1363.

Bleday, R. & Steele, G. (1995). Colorectal cancer surgery. In A. K. Rustgi (Ed.), *Gastrointestinal cancers: Biology, diagnosis, and therapy.* Philadelphia: Lippincott-Raven.

Boland, C. R. (1995). Malignant tumors of the colon. In T. Yamada (Ed.), *Textbook of gastroenterology.* (2nd ed.). Philadelphia: Lippincott-Raven.

Boyd, M. D. (1995). Colorectal cancer. In C. Varricchio, M. Pierce, C. Walker, & T. Ades (Eds.), *A cancer source book for nurses* (7th ed.). Atlanta: American Cancer Society.

Bresalier, R. S. & Kim, Y. S. (1993). Malignant neoplasms of the large intestine. In M. H. Sleisenger & J. S. Fordtran (Eds.), *Gastrointestinal disease: Pathophysiology, diagnosis, management* (5th ed.). Philadelphia: W.B. Saunders.

Bresalier, R. S. (1996). Diseases of the colon and rectum. In J. H. Grendell, K. R. McQuaid, & S. L. Friedman (Eds.), *Current diagnosis and treatment in gastroenterology.* Stamford: Appleton-Lange.

Bruner, D. W. & Iwamoto, R. R. (1996). Altered sexual health. In S. L. Groenwald, M. H. Frogge, M. Goodman, & C. H. Yarbro (Eds.), *Cancer symptom management.* Boston: Jones and Bartlett.

Burnstein, M. J. (1993). Dietary factors related to colorectal neoplasms. *Surgical Clinics of North America, 73,* 13-29.

Burt, R. W., Bishop, D. T., Cannon-Albright, L., Samowitz, W. S., Lee, R. L., DiSario, J. A., & Skolnick, M. H. (1992). Hereditary aspects of colorectal adenomas. *Cancer, 70,* 1296-1299.

Carpenito, L. J. (1995). *Nursing care plans and documentation: Nursing diagnoses and collaborative problems.* Philadelphia: Lippincott-Raven.

Corman, M. L. (1993). *Colon and rectal surgery.* Philadelphia: Lippincott-Raven.

Cummings, B. J. (1992). Adjuvant radiation therapy for colorectal cancer. *Cancer, 70,* 1372-1383.

Cummings, B. J. (1993). Radiation therapy for colorectal cancer. *Surgical Clinics of North America, 73,* 167-181.

Cunsolo, A., Bragaglia, R. B., Manara, G., Poggioli, G., & Gozzetti, G. Urogenital dysfunction after abdominoperineal resection for carcinoma of the rectum. (1990). *Diseases of the Colon and Rectum, 33,* 918-922.

DeCrosse, J. J., Tsioulias, G. J., & Jacobson, J. S. (1994). Colorectal cancer: Detection, treatment, and rehabilitation. *CA: A Cancer Journal for Clinicians, 44,* 27-42.

Devesa, S. & Chow, W. (1993). Variation in colorectal incidence in the United States by subsite of origin. *Cancer, 71,* 3819-3826.

Doughty, D. B. & Jackson, D. B. (1993). *Gastrointestinal disorders.* St. Louis: Mosby.

Dukes, C. E. (1932). The classification of cancer of the rectum. *Journal of Pathology, 35,* 323-332.

Enstrom, J. E. (1977). Colorectal cancer and beer drinking. *British Journal of Cancer, 35,* 674-683.

Findley, M. & Cunningham, D. (1993). Current advances in the treatment of gastrointestinal malignancy. *Critical Review of Oncology and Hematology, 14,* 127-152.

Freedman, G. M. & Coia, L. R. (1995). Adjuvant and neoadjuvant treatment of rectal cancer. *Seminars in Oncology, 22,* 611-624.

Fry, R. D., Fleshman, J. W., & Kodner, I. J. (1989). Cancer of the colon and rectum. *Clinical Symposia, 41,* 2-32.

Funkhouser, E. & Cole, P. (1992). Declining mortality rates for cancer of the rectum in the United States: 1940-1985. *Cancer, 70,* 2597-2601.

Gastrointestinal Tumor Study Group (1986). Survival after postoperative combination treatment of rectal cancer. *New England Journal of Medicine, 315,* 1294-1295.

Giardiello, F. M. (1995). Gastrointestinal polyposis syndromes and hereditary nonpolyposis colorectal cancer. In A. K. Rustgi (Ed.), *Gastrointestinal cancers: Biology, diagnosis, and therapy.* Philadelphia: Lippincott-Raven.

Givel, J. C. (1990). Rectal tumors. In M. C. Mosti & J. C. Givel (Eds.), *Surgery of anorectal diseases.* New York: Springer-Verlag.

Greenwald, P. (1992). Colon cancer overview. *Cancer, 70,* 1206-1215.

Guillem, J. G., Paty, P. B., & Cohen, A. (1997). Surgical treatment of colorectal cancer. *CA: A Cancer Journal for Clinicians, 47,* (2), 113-127.

Hackford, A.W. (1993). Biochemical markers for colorectal cancer: Diagnostic and therapeutic implications. *Surgical Clinics of North America, 73,* 85-102.

Hamilton, J. M. & Grem J. L. (1996). Lower gastrointestinal cancer. In J. M. Kirkwood, M. T. Lotze, & J. M. Yasko (Eds.), *Current cancer therapeutics.* Philadelphia: Churchill Livingstone.

Hampton, B. G. & Bryant, R. A. (1992). *Ostomies and continent diversions: Nursing management.* St. Louis: Mosby.

Heaton, J. W. (1995). Diagnostic tests in gastroenterology. In S. M. Tilkian, M. B. Conover & A. G. Tilkian (Eds.), *Clinical and nursing implications of laboratory tests.* St. Louis: Mosby.

Heitkemper, M. & Sawchuck, L. (1996). Problems of absorption and elimination. In S. Lewis, I. Collier, & M. Heitkemper (Eds.), *Medical surgical nursing: Assessment and management of clinical problems.* St. Louis: Mosby.

Jessup, J. M., Menck, H. R., Fremgen, A., & Winchester, D. P. (1997). Diagnosing colorectal carcinoma: Clinical and molecular approaches. *CA: A Cancer Journal for Clinicians, 47,* (2), 71-92.

John, M. (1993, November/December). Focus on colon and anorectal cancers. *Cope, 6,* 24-25.

Klatsky, A. L., Armstrong, M. A., Friedman, G. D., & Hiatt, R. A. (1988). The relations of alcoholic beverage use to colon and rectal cancer. *American Journal of Epidemiology, 128,* 1007-1015.

Krook, J. E., Moertel, C. G., Gunderson, L. L., Wieand, H. S., Collins, R. T., Beart, R. W., Kubista, T. P., Poon, M. A., Meyers, W. C., Mailliard, J. A., Twito, D. I., Morton, R. F., Veeder, M. H., Witzig, T. E., Cha, S., & Vidyarthi, S. C. (1991). Effective surgical adjuvant therapy for high-risk rectal carcinoma. *New England Journal of Medicine, 324,* 709-715.

Kuske, R. R. (1996). Acute and late toxicity of radiation therapy in rectal cancer. In T. C. Hicks, D. E. Beck, F. G. Opelka, & A. E. Timmeke (Eds.), *Complications of colon and rectal surgery.* Baltimore: Williams and Wilkins.

Lev, R. & Lee, M. (1995). Colorectal carcinoma pathology. In A. K. Rustgi (Ed.), *Gastrointestinal cancers: Biology, diagnosis, and therapy.* Philadelphia: Lippincott-Raven.

Levin, B. (1992). Inflammatory bowel disease and colon cancer. *Cancer, 70,* 1313-1316.

Levin, B. & Raijman, I. (1995). Malignant tumors of the colon and rectum. In W. S. Haubrich, F. Schaffner, & J. E. Berk (Eds.), *Gastroenterology* (5th ed.). Philadelphia: W. B. Saunders.

Lewin, K. J., Riddell, R. H., & Weinstein, W. M. (1992). *Gastrointestinal pathology and its clinical implications.* New York: Jacku-Shoin.

Mahut, C. & Stern, H. S. (1996). Cancer of the colon, rectum, and anus. In J. C. Harvey & E. J. Beattie (Eds.), *Cancer surgery.* Philadelphia: W. B. Saunders.

Markowitz, A. J. & Winawer, S. J. (1997). Management of colorectal polyps. *CA: A Cancer Journal for Clinicians, 47,* (2), 93-112.

Miaskowski, C. (1997). *Oncology nursing: An essential guide for patient care.* Philadelphia: W. B. Saunders.

Milsom, J. W. (1993). Pathogenesis of colorectal cancer. *Surgical Clinics of North America, 73,* 1-11.

Motwani, B. T., Shafir, M., Merrick, M., Tepper, J., & Bruckner, H. W. (1997). Adenocarcinoma of the colon and rectum. In J. F. Holland, R. C. Bast, D. L. Morton, E. Frei, D. W. Kufe, & R. R. Weichselbaum (Eds.), *Cancer medicine* (4th ed.). Baltimore: Williams & Wilkins.

Murray, J. J. & Stahl, T. J. (1993). Sphincter-saving alternatives for treatment of adenocarcinoma involving distal rectum. *Surgical Clinics of North America, 73,* 131-144.

NIH Consensus Conference. (1990). Adjuvant therapy for patients with colon and rectal cancer. *Journal of the American Medical Association, 264,* 1444-1450.

Orkin, B. A. (1996). Resection for colorectal cancer. In T. C. Hicks, D. E. Beck, F. G. Opelka, & A. E. Timmeke (Eds.), *Complications of colon and rectal surgery.* Baltimore: Williams & Wilkins.

Pollack, E. S., Nomura, A., Heilbrun, L. K., Stemmermann, G. N., & Green, S. B. (1984). Prospective study of alcohol consumption and cancer. *New England Journal of Medicine, 310,* 617-621.

Schafer, S. L. (1994). Oncologic complications. In S. E. Otto (Ed.), *Oncology nursing.* St. Louis: Mosby.

Shank, B., Enker, W., Santana, J., Morrissey, K., Daly, J., Quan, S., & Knapper, W. (1987). Local control with preoperative radiotherapy alone vs "sandwich" radiotherapy for rectal carcinoma. *International Journal of Radiation Oncology, Biology, Physics, 13,* 111-115.

Shelton, B. (1995). Oncologic emergencies. In C. Varricchio, M. Pierce, C. Walker, & T. Ades (Eds.), *A cancer source book for nurses.* Atlanta: American Cancer Society.

Shike, M., Winawer, S. J., Greenwald, P. H., Bloch, A., Hill, J., & Swaroop, W. V. (1990). Primary prevention of colorectal cancer. *Bulletin of the World Health Organization, 68,* 377-385.

Sischy, B. (1982). The place of radiotherapy in the management of rectal adenocarcinoma. *Cancer, 50,* 2631-2637.

Smigel, K. (1990). Experts review national cancer institute's dietary guidelines. *Journal of the National Cancer Institute, 82,* 344-345.

Smith, L. E. (1992). Colorectal cancer: Surgical approach. In J. D. Ahlgren & J. S. Macdonald (Eds.), *Gastrointestinal oncology.* Philadelphia: Lippincott-Raven.

Staniunas, R. J. & Schoelz, D. J. (1993). Extended resection for carcinoma of colon and rectum. *Surgical Clinics of North America, 73,* 117-129.

Stockholm Rectal Cancer Study Group. (1990). Preoperative short-term radiation therapy in operable rectal cancer. *Cancer, 66,* 49-55.

Takahashi, T., Mori, T., & Moosa, A. (1991). Tumors of the colon and rectum: Clinical features and surgical management. In A. R. Moosa, S. C. Schimpff, & M. C. Robson (Eds.), *Comprehensive Textbook of Oncology.* Baltimore: Williams and Wilkins.

Tornberg, S. A., Holm, L. E., Carstensen, J. M., & Eklund, G. A. (1986). Risks of cancer of the colon and rectum in relation to serum cholesterol and beta-lipoprotein. *New England Journal of Medicine, 315,* 1629-1633.

Trock, B., Lanza, E., & Greenwald, P. (1990). Dietary fiber, vegetables, and colon cancer: Critical review and meta-analyses of the epidemiologic evidence. *Journal of the National Cancer Institute, 82,* 650-661

Vargas, P. A. & Albert, D. S. (1992). Primary prevention of colorectal cancer through dietary modification. *Cancer, 70,* 1229-1235.

Vignati, P. V. & Roberts, P. L. (1993). Preoperative evaluation and postoperative surveillance for patients with colorectal carcinoma. *Surgical Clinics of North America, 73,* 67-84

Watson, J. & Jaffe, M. (1995). *Nurse's manual of laboratory and diagnostic tests.* Philadelphia: F. A. Davis.

Weiss, A. A. & Itzkowitz, S. H. (1995). Clinical aspects of colorectal cancer. In A. K. Rustgi (Ed.), *Gastrointestinal cancers: Biology, diagnosis, and therapy.* Philadelphia: Lippincott-Raven.

Willett, C. G., Compton C. C., Shelito, P. C., & Efird, J. T. (1994). Selection factors for local excision or abdominoperineal resection of early stage rectal cancer. *Cancer, 73,* 2716-2720.

Winawer, S. J., Flehinger, B. J., Buchelter, J., Herbert, E., & Shike, M. (1990). Declining serum cholesterol levels prior to diagnosis of colon cancer. *Journal of the American Medical Association, 263,* 2083-2085.

Winawer, S. J., Schottenfeld, D., Flehinger, B. J. (1991). Colorectal cancer screening. *Journal of the National Cancer Institute, 83,* 243-253.

Winawer, S. J., Enker, W. E., & Levin, B. (1992). Colorectal cancer. In S. J. Winawer & R. C. Kurtz (Eds.), *Gastrointestinal cancer.* New York: Gower Medical Publishing.

Colon Cancer

Mary Garlick Roll, RN, MSN

EPIDEMOLOGY

Colon cancer is the third most common cancer in males and females following prostate and lung cancer in males and breast and lung cancer in females. The incidence is greater in densely populated states such as New York, New Jersey, Massachusetts, and the Great Lakes States. For reasons that remain unclear, the incidence is higher in African-American men. When there is an adjustment made for stage at diagnosis, African-American men continue to have an increased mortality rate almost 20% higher than white men (Mayberry, Coates, Hill, Click, Chen, & Austin, 1995). Although cancer of the colon can occur at any age, there is a positive correlation with advancing age, with 93% of new cases occurring in men and women over the age of 50. Two religious groups in the United States have a decreased incidence of colon cancer—Seventh-Day Adventists and Mormons. The reasons for this lower incidence are not certain. It may be due to dietary restrictions, limiting alcohol, coffee, and meat. Overall in the United States in 1996, approximately 94,500 new colon cancer cases were diagnosed, representing 15% of all new cancer cases (Parker, Murray, Bolden & Wingo, 1998).

Colon cancer is the third leading cause of cancer deaths in both males and females, with approximately 46,400 deaths expected in 1998 (Parker et al., 1998). A recent National Cancer Institute (NCI) age-adjusted analysis of Surveillance, Epidemiology, and End Results (SEER) data from the years 1991 to 1995 indicate a first time ever decrease in overall cancer mortality rates (*Overall US Cancer Mortality Rate,* 1996). Because the population in the United States continues to grow proportionally older, and because colon cancer is primarily a disease of older adults, the actual number of colon cancer cases may increase, but the age-adjusted mortality rates are likely to continue to decline. The NCI SEER data analysis indicates the following combined figures for cancers of the colon and rectum:

- In persons over 65 years of age, a decrease in mortality of 4.9%
- Less than 65 years, a decrease of 8.5%
- In all ages combined, a total decrease in mortality of 6.4%.

The overall 5-year survival rate of all cases of colon cancer remains about 54%.

Colon cancer poses a significant public health concern. No definitive etiologic factors for colon cancer have been identified; however, when colon cancer is diagnosed early, the disease is curable by surgical intervention. Therefore efforts to detect this disease early are important. Identification of certain risk factors and of individuals who are at high risk for colon cancer is warranted.

RISK FACTORS

The major risk factors associated with the development of colon cancer are listed in Box 38-1. A strong inherited or genetic influence may account for many colon cancers. Sporadic colon cancer, which occurs in the remainder of cases, are influenced by environment, diet, and lifestyle. Secondary preventive activities, such as monitoring high-risk individuals and groups, and developing better diagnostic tools, have a significant impact on the incidence, morbidity, and mortality of this disease.

Genetic/Hereditary Factors

Family History of Colon Cancer. Individuals who have a first-degree relative (mother, father, sister, or brother) with colon cancer have a threefold to fourfold increase in their individual risk of developing colon cancer compared with the general population. There may also be an increased risk if family members have had breast or female genital cancers.

Familial Adenomatous Polyposis. Familial adenomatous polyposis (FAP), previously known as *familial polyposis coli,* is an autosomal dominant inherited genetic disorder that accounts for about 1% of total colon cancer incidence. During childhood, hundreds to thousands of adenomatous polyps develop on the colon. Approximately 10

Box 38-1
Risk Factors for Colon Cancer

Genetic/Hereditary
- Family history of colon cancer
- Familial adenomatous polyposis
- Hereditary nonpolyposis colorectal cancer

Inflammatory Bowel Disease
- Ulcerative colitis
- Crohn's disease

Personal History
- Age
- Colon cancer
- Noncancer surgery
- Polyps

Diet
- High-fat, low-fiber

to 15 years after this process begins, usually after the age of 20, all individuals will need surgical intervention to prevent the 100% occurrence of cancer. Other concurrent abnormalities may also occur including desmoid tumors, lipomas, sebaceous cysts, and osteomas (Cohen, Minsky, & Schilsky, 1997). Variants of FAP include Gardner's syndrome, Oldfield's syndrome, Tarcot's syndrome, and Zanca's syndrome (Fitzsimmons, 1992). Flat adenoma syndrome may also be a variant.

Hereditary Nonpolyposis Colorectal Cancer. Hereditary nonpolyposis colorectal cancer (HNPCC) is an autosomal dominant inherited genetic disorder characterized by early age of onset, right-sided lesions, and an excess of primary and metachronous lesions, accounting for 10% of the total colorectal cancer burden (Lynch & Lynch, 1995). Two subsets of HPNCC occur, Lynch I, which is site specific, and Lynch II, which is non–site specific (Fitzsimmons, 1992). Patients also have a higher incidence of endometrial, ovarian, ureteral, hepatobiliary, gastric, and small bowel cancers (Rodriquez-Bigas, Lee, O'Malley, Weber, Okhee, & Anderson et al., 1996). HNPCC is the most common form of hereditary colorectal cancer.

Inflammatory Bowel Disease

Ulcerative Colitis. Ulcerative colitis is a chronic inflammatory disease of the mucosa and submucosa of the colon, resulting in severe bouts of bloody diarrhea (Meissner, 1994). The increased risk of colon cancer in patients with ulcerative colitis has been well established, with an estimated incidence of cancer between 0.5% to 1% each year after the first decade of active ulcerative colitis. Patients who are at the highest risk are those who were diagnosed at a young age and have extensive, severe, and long duration of disease. Screening guidelines consist of colonoscopy at 1 to 2 years after the first decade of disease (Bernstein & Rogers, 1996). Data continue to be evaluated to identify a specific method of determining which high-risk patient will actually develop disease, and in whom surgical intervention is recommended.

Crohn's Disease. The risk for developing colon cancer in patients with Crohn's disease continues to be evaluated. There does seem to be a certain subset of this population who are at higher risk and who develop colon cancer at a younger age when compared with the general population. Included in this group are individuals with early-age onset of Crohn's disease; long-term inflammation in the colon; fistulas, strictures, and obstructions in the colon; and right-sided colon disease.

Currently, there is no consensus regarding endoscopic surveillance for Crohn's disease. Screening colonoscopy remains a controversial issue (Bernstein & Rogers, 1996). There appears to be a trend toward screening patients with Crohn's disease using the guidelines previously mentioned for patients with ulcerative colitis (Ribeiro, Greenstein, Sachar, Barth, Balasubramanian, & Harpaz et al., 1996).

Personal History

Age. Age is an important risk factor for the development of colon cancer. Ninety-three percent of colon cancer cases are diagnosed in persons over 50 years of age. Colon cancer is extremely rare in individuals younger than 40. Screening guidelines for colon cancer take into account the age differences associated with the development of the disease. The American Cancer Society's (ACS) recommendation for screening of asymptomatic patients are as follows:

- For individuals over 40, an annual digital rectal examination (DRE)
- For individuals over 50, an annual DRE plus annual stool guaiac test and flexible sigmoidoscopy every 3 to 5 years; after two initial negative sigmoidoscopies 1 year apart.

Colon Cancer. Numerous studies have indicated that the risk for developing another primary colon cancer in patients who have been previously diagnosed and treated for colon cancer are three times greater than in the general population (Cohen, Minsky, & Schilsky, 1997). Careful screening and follow-up for such patients is warranted.

Noncancer Surgery. Patients who have had previous ureterosigmoidostomy for urinary diversion, or a cholecystectomy may have an increased risk of colon cancer. The mechanism for this increased incidence continues to be evaluated. It may be due to the high concentrations of promoting factors in the surgical secretions (Cohen, Minsky, & Schilsky, 1997).

Polyps. Polyps are described as flat, sessile lesions or pedunculated with a stemlike connection to the colon mucosa and a characteristic mushroom shape. Polyps of the colon are divided into two major categories: hyperplastic and adenomatous. Hyperplastic polyps have always been considered harmless. When removed and examined by a pathologist, they consist of normal colon tissue with an increased number of cells, or hyperplasia. The clinical significance of hyperplastic polyps continues to be evalu-

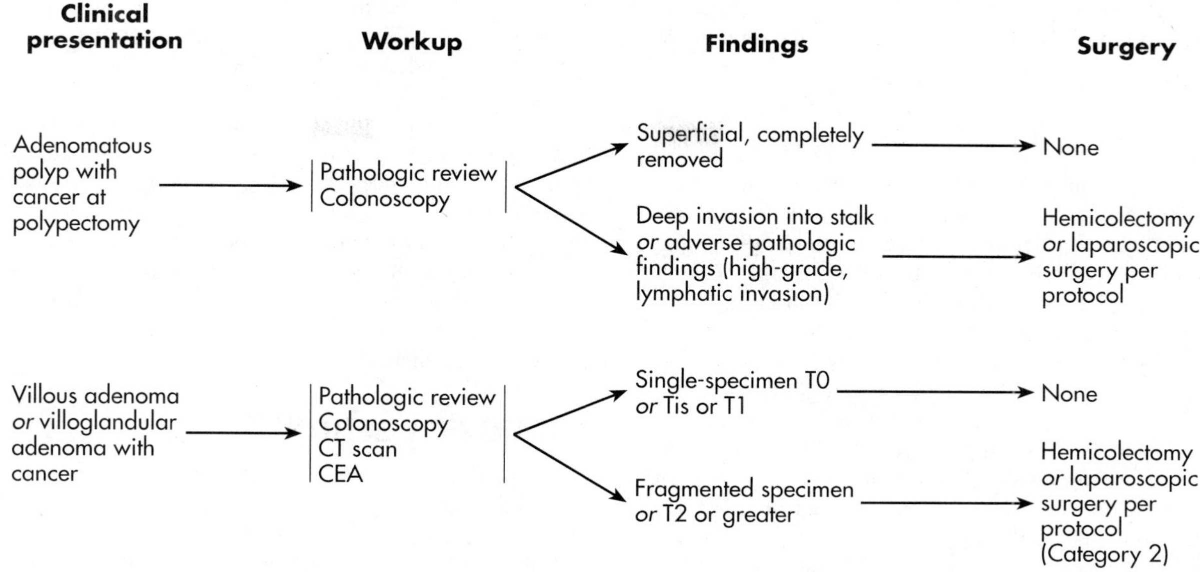

Fig. 38-1 Guidelines for patients with polyps. (From National Comprehensive Cancer Network. [1996]. *Oncology, 10* [Suppl. 11], 147.)

ated. One study concluded that the presence of hyperplastic polyps may be a marker for populations who are at higher risk for colon cancer (Kearney, Giovannucci, Rimm, Stampfer, Colditz, & Ascherio et al., 1995). Adenomatous polyps are precancerous lesions that account for most, if not all, colon cancers that develop in a process known as the *adenoma to carcinoma sequence.* Adenomatous polyps are either tubular, villous, or a combination of both known as *tubulovillous adenoma.* Tubular adenomas are smaller, more common, and more evenly distributed throughout the colon, whereas villous adenomas are larger and are found more commonly in the rectum. In general, the larger the polyps, the more potential there is for malignancy.

Polyps should be removed during an endoscopic procedure, preferably a full colonoscopy, as the presence of one polyp indicates the potential of additional polyps in about 25% of cases (Cohen, Minsky, & Schilsky, 1997). Follow-up strategies continue to be evaluated and are often based on the presence of additional high-risk factors. Current guidelines for care of patients with adenomatous polyps, from the National Comprehensive Cancer Network (NCCN), are presented in Fig. 38-1. In one study, persons with a large polyp (4.5 cm) developed cancer at a rate four times higher than expected (Otchy, Ransohoff, Wolff, Weaver, Illstrup, & Carlson et al., 1996). In such cases, follow-up screening recommendations may differ from those for persons who are at less risk of colon cancers.

Diet

Epidemiologic studies of population groups and their migration patterns to and from countries with high and low incidences of colon cancer have given credence to the protective effect of a high-fiber, low-fat diet. This protective effect is probably due to the decrease in exposure of the colon mucosa to cancer promoters. The incidence is higher in the United States and other Western countries where there is an increased intake of refined carbohydrates and meat and a decrease in fiber. In countries such as Japan and Africa, the incidence of colon cancer is lower.

Dietary fiber, found in plants, is soluble in the digestive process, (i.e., gums, pectins, and some of the hemicelluloses) or insoluble (i.e., cellulose, ligmin, and the remainder of the hemicelluloses). Soluble and insoluble fibers may have different mechanisms of action that contribute to their protective effect. Fiber increases fecal bulk, diluting fecal carcinogens; and accelerates the transit time of feces, limiting the time the colon is exposed to cancer promoters. Fiber is also thought to be protective by reducing food pH; changing bile acid metabolism and bacterial composition, which deactivates carcinogenic metabolites; and changing the rate of cell proliferations in the colon mucosa (Cohen, Minsky, & Schilsky, 1997).

Fat is considered a promoter of colon cancer and not a carcinogen itself. A diet high in fat intake increases the presence of bile acids, which are necessary for fat metabolism, and thereby increases the exposure of the colon mucosa to those bile acids. A low-fat diet continues to be evaluated to determine the mechanisms responsible for the protective effect against colon cancer. Some areas of interest are the total percentage of fat calories; a decreased intake in total calories; the combination of calories from protein, carbohydrates and fat; the different types of fat (such as saturated and unsaturated); energy expenditure; and the correlation between fat intake, age, and history of consumption. Studies are ongoing regarding the type and combination of fat and fiber, which is most protective against colon cancer.

In addition, several other dietary studies are underway to investigate the effect of specific dietary by-products on colon cancers formation. In one such preclinical study,

Bowman-Birk, which is a type of protease inhibitor, has been shown to inhibit colon carcinogenesis (Fitzsimmons & Fales, 1993).

Other

Several investigations continue to evaluate factors that may be protective for the development of colon cancers, such as exercise and physical activity (Thune & Lund, 1996) and history of childbearing in women (Broeders, Lambe, Baron, & Leon, 1996). The potential negative effect of being overweight has been investigated (Shike, 1996). It has been noted that colon cancer patients had a very low cholesterol level. Investigators were involved in trying to determine whether low cholesterol was a potential cause of colon cancer. Results from a current study indicate that these low cholesterol levels are the result of the colon cancer process, not the cause of the cancer (Niendorf, Nagele, Gerding, Meyer-Pannwitt, & Gebhardt, 1995). Ongoing investigation regarding risk factors will not only enable the targeting of individuals for early detection, but may lead to future preventive techniques.

Screening

Currently, guidelines for colon cancer are based on average risk asymptomatic individuals. The ACS recommends the following screening tests for these asymptomatic individuals: for those 40 to 49 years of age, an annual DRE; for those over the age of 50, an annual DRE and annual fecal occult blood test (FOBT) and a sigmoidoscopy every 3 to 5 years after two consecutive annual negative examinations. Recently, an expert panel was convened to promote the publication of new guidelines for colorectal cancer screening (Anonymous, 1996). These guidelines were developed by the American Gastroenterological Association (AGA), American Society for Gastrointestinal Endoscopy, American Society of Colon and Rectal Surgeons, American College of Gastroenterology, and the Society of American Gastrointestinal Endoscopic Surgeons. The AGA has divided the screening guideline into the following categories: average risk (65% to 75% of individuals) and moderate risk (20% to 30% of individuals), and further divided the high-risk individuals into three categories. It is expected that the ACS proposed changes to its current guidelines will be similar to the AGA guidelines. Table 38-1 presents a comparison of the current ACS and new AGA screening guidelines. Despite the publication of these and similar guidelines, a recent study suggests that physicians do not consistently adhere to the guidelines, and that gender of patients and physicians may influence screening (Borum, 1996). Female resident physicians statistically performed more flexible sigmoidoscopies on patients of both sexes when compared with male residents physicians who performed more DRE on male patients only (Borum, 1996). Research is needed to evaluate the role of gender on screening to ensure gender equity in health care.

CHEMOPREVENTION

Chemoprevention is defined as the administration of natural or synthetic chemical agents to prevent the initiation or promotion of events that occur during carcinogenesis (Boone, Kelloff, & Malone, 1990). A number of different investigations have examined the potential preventive influence of several agents: vitamin C, vitamin E, other antioxidants, estrogen, calcium, and low-fat, high-fiber diet not only on the formation of colon cancer but also on the rate of polyp formation and polyp prevention (Kearney, Giovannucci, Rimm, Ascherio, Stampfer, & Colditz et al., 1996)

Polyp Prevention Trial

The National Cancer Institute (NCI) recently completed the Polyp Prevention Trial, a 4-year, multi-institutional, randomized control study involving 2000 men and women who previously had a polyp removed. The diet intervention group was counseled and evaluated regarding a low-fat, high-fiber diet, including five to eight servings of fruits and vegetables each day. Results from this study are being analyzed.

Colorectal Adenoma Trial

The NCI is sponsoring a new colorectal cancer chemoprevention trial, the Colorectal Adenoma Trial, to evaluate whether aspirin can decrease the number of adenomatous polyps and/or prolong disease-free survival in patients who have had a previous corrective surgical resection (*Subjects sought for four cancer chemoprevention trials,* 1996).

TABLE 38-1 Colorectal Cancer Screening Guidelines for Asymptomatic Average Risk Individuals

Age	Current American Cancer Guidelines	New American Gastroenterologists Guidelines
40-49	Annual DRE	None
Over 50	Annual DRE and Annual FOBT	None
	Sigmoidoscopy every 3 to 5 years	Annual FOBT or flexible sigmoidoscopy every 5 years, or both
		Double contrast barium enema every 5 to 10 years
		Colonoscopy every 10 years

DRE, digital rectal examination; *FOBT*, fecal occult blood test; *AGA*, American Gastroenterologists Association.

PATHOPHYSIOLOGY

Normal Anatomy and Physiology of the Colon

The colon is also known as the *large intestine*. The final stages of digestion take place in the colon, where liquid waste and fibers that were not digested by the small intestine are broken down by the large numbers of normal bacteria that reside in the colon. Salt and water are reabsorbed from this semiliquid stool, forming a more solid stool that passes through the entire colon and is excreted. This process can take between 4 and 15 hours.

The colon is approximately 4 to 5 feet long and 1 to 3 inches in diameter. The first portion of the colon is the cecum, a blind pouch that is connected to the ileum, the last segment of the small intestine, via the ileocecal valve. Attached to the cecum is a narrow 3-inch tube known as the *vermiform appendix*. The colon is divided into four segments: the ascending, transverse, descending, and the sigmoid colon.

The ascending colon is smaller in diameter than the cecum. It ascends up the right side of the abdominal cavity, behind the right kidney, to the under surface of the right lobe of the liver. At this point, with the gallbladder lying on the right, the ascending colon makes a sharp turn to the left, known as the *hepatic flexure,* to begin the transverse colon.

The transverse colon is the largest segment of the colon. It transverses right to left across the width of the abdominal cavity until it begins to curve downward at the splenic flexure near the great curvature of the stomach and the lower end of the spleen.

The descending colon descends downward on the left side of the abdominal cavity. Compared with the ascending colon, the descending colon is smaller in diameter and more deeply placed as it descends along the outer border of the left kidney to the level of the crest of the ileum, terminating at the sigmoid flexure.

The sigmoid colon is the narrowest segment of the colon, an S shape that curves forward, downward, and inward, forming a loop that varies in length and position and ending at the rectum (Gray, 1995).

The colon is composed of four layers of tissue types. The inner most layer is the mucosa, which is subdivided into the epithelial layer, which is continually being replaced by rapid cell growth; the lamina propria, which is the connective tissue containing large numbers of blood and lymph vessels; and the muscularis mucosa, which contains muscles that form the mucous membrane into small folds, increasing the surface area of the colon. The second layer is the submucosa, a highly vascular, dense connective tissue. The muscularis propria, the third layer, is made of two layers of smooth muscle, the inner ring of circular fibers, and outer sheet of longitudinal fibers. Contraction of the muscularis propria, known as *peristalsis,* helps with the movement and elimination of waste products from the colon. The fourth and final outer layer of the colon is derived from the peritoneum and is called the *serosa.* The serosa completely covers the cecum, transverse colon, and sigmoid loop. Quite often there is no serosa covering the posterior ascending hepatic flexure, the descending colon, and splenic flexure.

The Process of Carcinogenesis

Just like other cancers, the development of colon cancer is a multistage process of initiation, promotion, and progression. This process has been widely studied in colon cancer owing to the availability of actual tumor tissue from surgical specimens and actual polyps from polypectomies. In addition, concurrent advances in molecular biology have led to further understanding of this process. Several factors must be present for colon cancer to evolve: the activation of oncogenesis and the inactivation of tumor suppressive genes; the mutation in at least four or five of these genes; and although a frequent, similar sequence may occur, it is the long-term accumulation of events that is important (Fearon & Vogelstein, 1990).

Genetic alterations occur during the multistage process of colon carcinogenesis. At an early stage, the tumor suppresser gene APC (adenomatous polyposis coli) is mutated and the activation of the *ras* K oncogene occurs. During later stages, there is inactivation of the tumor suppresser genes DCC (deleted in colorectal carcinoma), and inactivation of P53 (Cooper, 1995).

In colon cancer, molecular analysis of tumor tissue indicates a deletion of chromosome 17p where the P53 gene is located, and deletions of 18q and 5q (Cooper, 1995). Ongoing studies continue to try to determine whether the tumor suppresser gene MCC (mutated in colorectal cancers) is responsible for 5q 21 mutations found in some colon cancers, and the significance of the fact that the gene responsible for HNPCC located in chromosome 2p is not a tumor-suppressive gene. (Cooper, 1995).

ROUTES OF METASTASES

Ninety-five percent of colon cancers are adenocarcinomas, tumors that arise from the glandular epithelial tissue of the mucosa. Colon cancer metastasizes by direct extension, hematogenous and lymphatic spread, and implantation (Fig. 38-2)

Direct Extension

During direct extension, two series of events may occur. Because the initial tumor growth occurs in the mucosa, the tumor takes the path of least resistance and begins to grow into the inside lumen of the bowel, accounting for many of the patient's presenting signs and symptoms (Box 38-2). The tumor also begins to penetrate through the four layers of the bowel walls, inside through the mucosa, submucosa, muscularis propria, and finally through the serosa to adjacent structures. Local invasion of neighboring structures occurs in 10% to 20% of cases. Because there are a large number of contiguous organs near the cecum and rectosigmoid, local invasion occurs more often in these areas. As the tumor begins its penetration through the bowel wall, it gains access to the blood and lymph channels in the sub-

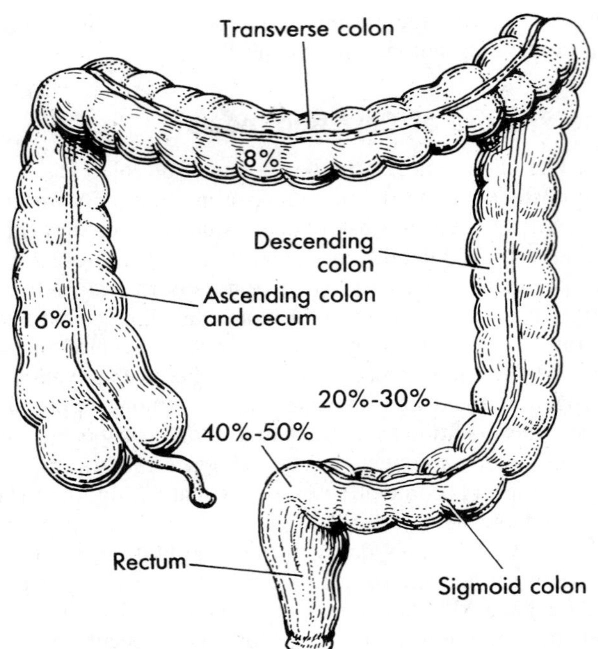

Fig. 38-2 Routes of metastasis for colon cancer.

mucosa, a major reason many patients present with distant metastasis.

Hematogenous

Hemotologic spread primarily occurs via embolization of the tumor cells through the venous system. The incidence of arterial invasion is less than 1% (Cohen, Minsky, & Schilsky, 1997). The liver is the most frequent site of hematologic spread, occurring in approximately 15% to 25% of patients, with an additional 20% to 30% of patients developing liver metastasis after curative surgical resection. The lungs receive their major supply of venous blood by way of the liver; therefore, the lungs are the second most common site of metastasis. Occasionally, the brain, bones, and adrenal glands may be affected once the liver and lung are involved. It is rare that these additional sites would be involved in the absence of liver and lung metastasis (Cohen, Minsky, & Schilsky, 1997).

Lymphatic

Lymphatic spread to the lymph nodes is common, occurring in approximately 50% of patients. Lymph channels follow major arterial routes. The three most common groups of lymph node metastatic spread are the pericolic, intermediate, and central (Cohen, Minsky, & Schilsky, 1997). Perineural invasion occasionally occurs along nerve pathways.

Implantation

Implantation happens when primary tumor cells are released and deposited on other surfaces. During surgery, tumor cells can be deposited on wound surfaces. Serosal penetration followed by tumor shedding may result in peritoneal seeding. Tumor cells that shed from the mucosal surfaces of the primary tumor can cause intraluminal spread to fistulas and abscess in the distal bowel (Cohen, Minsky, & Schilsky, 1997).

Box 38-2
Colon Cancer: Site-Specific Signs and Symptoms

Right Colon
Vague, dull uncharacteristic pain
Dark or mahogany red blood in the stool
Anemia
Mass in right lower quadrant

Left Colon
"Gas" pain, "cramps"
Bright red blood coating surface of stool
Decrease in caliber of stools
Change in bowel habits; increased use of laxatives
Acute large bowel obstruction may occur causing progressive abdominal distention, pain, vomiting, and constipation

ASSESSMENT

Clinical evaluation of the patient involves a detailed family history and a personal history, including the presence of signs and symptoms, a thorough physical examination and a variety of diagnostic tests (Table 38-2).

Personal History

A family history of colon cancer in a first-degree relative, (mother, father, sister, brother) confers a three to four times greater risk to an individual for developing colon cancer. Obtaining this history, as well as a family history of female genital and breast cancers, is an important part of history taking. A personal history of all identified risk factors for colon cancer then follows. Although most patients are asymptomatic during the early stages of colon cancer, with advancing disease, a careful history of presenting signs and symptoms is often a clue to the location of the cancers. Box 38-2 provides the most common site-specific signs and symptoms for the left and right colon. Additional information that should be obtained from the patient involves questions about bowel patterns such as change in bowel habits; laxative use, change in the character of stool, diarrhea, constipation, pencil-shaped stools, blood in the stool; gas pains, bloating, abdominal cramping; and rectal bleeding.

Physical Examination

A thorough examination begins by inspecting the abdomen for distension and obvious masses, and in thin individuals, for evidence of peristaltic waves. Bowel sounds are then evaluated by auscultation, listening for high pitch or tingling bowel sounds, which indicate a partial obstruction.

TABLE 38-2 Assessment of the Patient for Colon Cancer

	Assessment Parameters	Typical Abnormal Findings
History	A. Family History 1. History of colon cancer	A. Family risk factors. 1. First-degree relative (mother, father, brother, sister) increase risk 3 to 4 times.
	B. Personal history of risk factors 1. Age 2. Colon cancer 3. Noncancer surgery 4. Polyps	B. Individuals are categorized as average, moderate or high risk. 1. Usually over age 50 2. Previous colon cancer increases risk for new disease, recurrent disease, or metastatic disease 3. Previous ureterosigmoidostomy and cholelcystectomy may increase risk 4. Polyps should be evaluated yearly and removed
	C. Evaluation of presenting signs and symptoms	C. May be absent in early disease. Signs and symptoms reflect the location of the tumor. Right side include vague, dull, uncharacteristic pain, dark or mahogany red blood mexed in the stool, anemia, mass in right lower quadrant Left side symptoms include: "gas" pain, "cramps," bright red blood coating surface of stool, decrease in caliber of stools, change in bowel habits; increased use of laxatives; acute large bowel obstruction may occur causing progressive abdominal distention, pain, vomiting, and constipation.
Physical Examination	A. Inspect abdomen	A. Distention, obvious masses, in thin individuals, absence or presence of peristaltic waves.
	B. Auscultation of bowel sounds	B. Partial obstruction: high pitch or tingling sound. Total obstruction: absent bowel sounds.
	C. Palpation and percussion	C. Hepatomegaly, splenomegaly, obvious masses along path of colon.
	D. Digital rectal examination (DRE)	D. Presence of masses: a stony hard mass, known as *rectal shelf,* indicating metastatic pelvic disease.
Diagnostic Tests	A. Fecal occult blood test (FOBT)	A. Positive for hidden blood in the stool.
	B. Double contrast barium enema	B. Visualization of polyps and tumors.
	C. Sigmoidoscopy	C. Direct visualization of polyps and tumors in first 60 cm of the bowel.
	D. Colonoscopy	D. Direct visualization of polyps and tumors in the entire large bowel.
	E. Chest radiograph	E. Rule out lung metastasis.
	F. Computed tomography	F. Presence of disease in abdomen, pelvis, liver, or lungs.
	G. Ultrasound of liver	G. Small lesions can be identified and differentiated between solid tumor and cystic lesion.
	H. Carcinoembryonic antigen (CEA)	H. CEA elevated at diagnosis or within 1 week of surgical colectomy is used as a follow-up procedure every 3 months for 2 years, then annually for 5 years.
	I. Complete blood count and chemistries	I. Colon cancers bleed intermittently leading to a decrease in hemoglobin and hematocrit. Disease that has metastasized to the liver may be indicated by elevated liver function tests.

The absence of bowel sounds in all four quadrants while listening for 5 minutes indicates an impending total obstruction. Palpation and percussion of the abdomen follow inspection and auscultation, feeling for the presence or absence of hepatomegaly, splenomegaly, and obvious masses along the path of the colon.

Finally, a DRE allows for palpation of the rectum and lower sigmoid colon. On the interior wall of the rectum, and in the cul-de-sac of women, a stony hard mass known as the rectal shelf may be felt and is an indication that the cancer has metastasized to the pelvic floor (Cohen, Minsky, & Schilsky, 1997).

Diagnostic Tests

Fecal Occult Blood Tests. The standard FOBT measures blood in the stool by indirectly measuring the peroxidase activity of hemoglobin. For a patient to perform the test correctly, a number of medication and dietary restrictions are necessary. False-positive reactions are caused by aspirin, antiinflammatory drugs, iron, fruits (apples, apricots, cantaloupe, pears), and vegetables (broccoli, cabbage, horseradish, potatoes, turnips), which contain high peroxidase, and meat, which contains animal blood. False-negative reactions can be caused by antibiotics. Because cancers bleed intermittently, it is important to test three consecutive bowel movements. If patients have more than one bowel movement in a day, they should test their stool after each movement. Newer FOBT tests are currently being evaluated, including the HemeSelect (SmithKline Diagnostics, Sunnyvale, CA). HemeSelect is an FOBT that selects for human hemoglobin instead of animal hemoglobin, which is found in patients whose diets include meat. An enzyme-linked immunosorbant assay using monoclonal antibodies (MoAbs) derived from feces of colon cancer patients, specifically FE14, has been developed. The MoAb assay has many advantages because of its ability to differentiate between upper and lower gastrointestinal bleeding and the fact that there are no dietary requirements. Results are impressive, especially when combining MoAb with HemeSelect, which then increases the sensitivity of the tests to 100% (Xing, Young, Ho, Sinatra, Hoj, & McKenzie, 1996). Currently, the ACS recommends the yearly use of FOBT in asymptomatic individuals over the age of 50.

Box 38-3

Double Contrast Barium Enema: Patient Information Guide

The barium enema (lower gastrointestinal series) is an x-ray of the large intestine (bowel). To make the bowel easier to see when radiographed, liquid barium and air are put in the bowel through a small enema tube inserted into the rectum. During the procedure, you may feel some discomfort, but there is usually no pain.

Getting Ready

Before the barium enema is done, the bowel must be cleansed. This is important for accurate x-ray results and to prevent having to repeat the procedure. You will be given a prescription for a Prep Kit, which contains the medications needed to cleanse your bowel. Please follow the Prep Kit instruction carefully.

Two Days Before the Examination

- Eat a light breakfast (small amounts of white turkey, chicken, fish, white bread; plain water, black coffee or tea, Popsicles, clear juices [apple, cranberry], clear soups [fat-free], plain Jello, soda pop [ginger ale, 7-Up]).
- Clear liquid lunch (no solid food)
- Clear liquid dinner (no solid food)

Day Before the Examination

- Clear liquid breakfast (no solid food).
- Drink 8 ounces of clear liquid at 9, 10, and 11 AM.
- 12:30 PM (or 30 minutes before lunch)—take 1½ oz. of Fleet PhosphoSoda in one half glass of water, followed by a full glass of water.
- Clear liquid lunch (no solid foods).
- Drink 8 ounces of clear liquid at 2, 3, and 4 PM.
- 6 PM—Clear liquid dinner (no solid foods).
- After dinner, take the four Fleet Bisacodyl tablets with a full glass of water. Do not chew or dissolve tablets.

Day of the Examination

- Do not eat solid food. You may have water or clear juice until 1 hour before the procedure.

One Hour Before the Examination

- Use the Fleet Bisacodyl suppository, as follows:
  -Remove the foil wrap.
  -Lie on your left side.
  -Insert the rounded end of the suppository into your rectum.
  -Use the middle finger of your right hand to gently push the suppository in as far as possible.
  -Wait for 15 minutes before releasing the suppository, even if the urge is strong.

Before the Examination

- Tell your doctor or radiologist if:
  -You might be pregnant.
  -You have abdominal cramping (pain in the stomach)
  -You have ever had rectal surgery.
  -You have ever had a spastic colon (intestinal cramping).
  -You have ever had chronic colitis.

During the Examination

- Remove all of your clothes, put on a hospital gown, and lie on a large x-ray table, which will be moved in different positions during the procedure.
- The liquid barium and air will be given through an enema tube placed in your rectum. This tube will remain in your rectum throughout the procedure. The liquid barium and air will make you feel very full and you may have mild cramps and a strong urge to have a bowel movement. These feelings are natural and happen to everyone who has this exam. Breathing slowly and deeply will help decrease these feelings.
- After the x-rays have been taken and the rectal tube is removed, you will pass the barium in the bathroom. When you have passed the barium, the final x-ray will be taken. The exam takes between 30 minutes and 1 hour.

After the Examination

- Drink plenty of liquids (at least four 8-ounce glasses) during the first 8 hours after the exam.
- Your first bowel movement may be white or pale. This is normal. Laxatives might also be required.
- You may resume your regular diet.
- The radiologist will review the x-ray studies and your physician will discuss the results with you.

Modified from Roswell Park Cancer Institute, Department of Nursing, Buffalo, New York.

Double Contrast Barium Enema. Instilling radiopaque barium into the colon is called a barium enema. Instilling both barium and air is called a double contrast barium enema. The double contrast barium enema allows for better visualization of smaller tumors and polyps when compared with barium enema alone. Patients need to begin to prepare their bowel 2 days before the actual procedure. For an example of a patient information guide, see Box 38-3.

Sigmoidoscopy. A sigmoidoscopy is an examination of the lower portion of the colon with a fiberoptic scope, which allows the health care practitioner to visualize the inside of the bowel and remove polyps or tissue samples for biopsy. Sigmoidoscopies are rigid or flexible. Flexible scopes allow for easier manipulation in the S-shaped sigmoid colon, and also increase patient comfort. For an example of a patient information guide, see Box 38-4.

To *identify* colon cancer, the combination of double contrast barium enema and flexible sigmoidoscopy has been useful. However, the complete evaluation and visualization of the entire colon, via colonoscopy is the recommended procedure for *diagnosis* of colon cancer (Box 38-5). For asymptomatic, average risk patients over the age of 50 years, the ACS recommends sigmoidoscopy in patients every 3 to 5 years after two initial negative examinations.

Colonoscopy. A colonoscopy is an examination of the entire large bowel from rectum to the ileocecal valve, which connects the large and small intestine. A flexible fiberoptic colonoscope is used, allowing the entire colon to be visualized and polyps to be removed and tissue sample obtained for biopsy. A colonoscopy cannot be performed unless the entire colon is completely empty. Therefore, patients are given a Prep Kit, which contains medications and detailed instructions, and a patient information guide. The patient information guide found in Box 38-6 assists patients with recording fluid and medication intake.

Colonoscopy is the definitive procedure for diagnosing colon cancer. Colonoscopy should be used to evaluate abnormal findings after a barium enema or sigmoidoscopy, for patients who present with hematochezia, (red blood in the stool) or melena (black tarry stools), or as a follow-up for

Box 38-4
Sigmoidoscopy: Patient Information Guide

Introduction

Sigmoidoscopy is an examination of the lower part of the large intestine (bowel) with a fiber optic instrument called a *sigmoidoscope.* Because the sigmoidoscope is a long, thin, flexible tube with a light at one end and an eyepiece at the other, it is possible to see inside the bowel. Small tissue samples and/or polyps can be removed during a sigmoidoscopy.

Getting Ready

Day Before the Examination

- Eat and drink normally and take your regular medications, if any.

Day of the Examination

- Eat and drink normally and take your regular medications.
- Before you leave home, give yourself two Fleet enemas, 30 minutes apart, following the directions on the package.

During the Examination

- Remove your clothing, put on a hospital gown and lie on the examining table on your side or stomach.
- Your doctor will examine your rectal area using a gloved finger, and then insert the lubricated tip of the sigmoidoscope into your large bowel.
- The examination is painless, but you may feel some pressure and have the urge to move your bowels.
- The examination takes about 20 minutes.

After the Examination

- Resume your normal diet and activities
- Complications from a sigmoidoscopy are rare. If you should suddenly feel severe stomach pain or have rectal bleeding, report it to your doctor or nurse immediately.
- If you have questions, please ask your doctor or nurse at the time of the examination.

Modified from Roswell Park Cancer Institute, Department of Nursing, Buffalo, New York.

Box 38-5
Colonoscopy: Patient Information Guide

Introduction

Colonoscopy is an examination of the lining of the large intestine through a fiberoptic instrument called a *colonoscope.* This long, thin, flexible tube has a light on one end and an eyepiece on the other. Using the colonoscope, specially-trained doctors can examine the entire length of the large intestine (5 to 7 feet) and take small tissue and cell samples of suspicious areas. This procedure provides valuable information with minimal discomfort.

Getting Ready

Colonoscopy cannot be performed unless the intestine is completely empty. Emptying the intestine requires 2 full days of a clear liquid diet, with laxatives on the second day. This combination causes very loose, watery stools. An enema is taken the morning of the exam.

Do not eat solid foods or opaque liquids. Liquids that you can see through, including black coffee or tea, broth, plain Jello, apple and cranberry juices, ginger ale, soda pop, Popsicles and water are allowed. Three quarts of liquid each day are needed to soften stool and to provide fluid.

Measure the amount of liquid taken in and record it on the chart on the back panel (1 oz = 30 ml). Check off each step as it is completed

The Day of the Examination

- Do not eat or drink anything before the examination. Take a soap suds enema in 2 quarts of tap water. If the return is not clear, repeat the enema with tap water only.

Modified from Roswell Park Cancer Institute, Department of Nursing, Buffalo, New York.

Box 38-6
Surgical Procedures for Colon Cancer

Before the Examination

- The doctor will explain the procedure and its possible complications, answer your questions and ask you to sign a consent form.
- A nurse will check your temperature, pulse, and blood pressure; start an intravenous route to relax you; and give medications during the procedure.
- You will be escorted to the operating room, where you will be assisted onto a special table.
- You will receive medication to make you sleepy, but you will be awake enough to follow instructions.

During the Examination

- A nurse and doctor will stay with you during the examination.
- The operating room lights will be dimmed to help the doctor see better through the eyepiece of the colonoscope. The lighted end is gently inserted into the rectum and then slowly advanced.
- Air is used to straighten out small folds in the intestine and you may feel mild cramping.
- When the exam is completed, the colonoscope is removed.

After the Examination

Following the examination, you will be taken to the recovery room. The entire examination and recovery takes about 2 hours.

When you are fully awake the doctor will explain the results of the examination to you.

Patients usually go home after the examination; however, some are asked to stay overnight for observation. Do not drive for about 12 hours. Plan to have someone available to drive you home. Gradually resume your regular diet.

You may notice some minimal spot bleeding. If you have a large amount of bleeding or sharp pain in the abdomen, report it to your doctor or nurse.

Liquid Intake Chart

First Day

Clear liquid breakfast	____ oz
Clear liquid lunch	____ oz
Clear liquid dinner	____ oz
Clear liquid snacks (anytime all day)	____ oz
TOTAL (at least 96 oz or 2880 ml)	____ oz

Second Day

Clear liquid breakfast	____ oz
Clear liquid lunch	____ oz
9 AM—Drink 8 oz clear liquid	8 oz
10 AM—Drink 8 oz clear liquid	8 oz
11 AM—Drink 8 oz clear liquid	8 oz
NOTE: 30 minutes before lunch, take Fleet Phospho Soda (1.5 oz) in a half glass of water followed by a full glass of water.	
Clear liquid lunch	____ oz
2 PM—Drink 8 oz clear liquid	8 oz
3 PM—Drink 8 oz clear liquid	8 oz
4 PM—Drink 8 oz clear liquid	8 oz
NOTE: Take four biscodyl tablets with a full glass of water.	
Clear liquid snacks (anytime until midnight)	____ oz
TOTAL (at least 96 oz or 2880 ml)	____ oz

previous colon cancer patients or in patients who have had previous removal of a polyp.

Chest Radiographs. The second most common site of distant metastasis is the lungs. A chest radiograph is routinely used to rule out lung metastasis.

Computed Tomography. Computed tomography of the abdomen, pelvis, lungs, or liver, with or with out contrast dye, can be used to establish a presumptive diagnosis of colon cancer (tissue biopsy confirms the diagnosis) or as follow-up surveillance.

Magnetic Resonance Imaging. Magnetic resonance imaging may be useful in certain instances when the evaluation of vascular involvement assists the surgeon in preoperative planning.

Ultrasound of the Liver. Ultrasound of the liver, obtained with state-of-the-art equipment by an experienced nuclear medicine physician, is an effective, noninvasive radiologic test for detecting hepatic metastasis. Quite often lesions as small as 1 cm can be detected. When there is a question of malignancy, an ultrasound-guided liver biopsy can be obtained to differentiate between solid tumor tissue and cystic lesions or hemangiomas. Intraoperative ultrasound is extremely useful in detecting lesions deep within the liver that may be difficult for a surgeon to palpate.

Radioimmunoguided Surgery. Detecting occult, nonvisible colorectal tumor deposits is an important outcome of colon cancer surgery. In a study by Cote, Houchens, Hitchcock, Saad, Nines, & Greenson et al (1996), patients were injected 3 weeks before surgery with a radiolabeled antibody to the TAG-72 antigen (CC49). During surgery, a hand-held γ-detecting probe was used to evaluate locally disseminated disease. Lymph nodes were analyzed for occult metastases and evaluated histologically. None of the radioimmunoguided surgery (RIGS)–negative lymph nodes had occult metastases. RIGS-positive lymph nodes had a significant association with the presence of tumor cells. Evaluation of such new investigative techniques continues.

Carcinoembryonic Antigen. During the early 1960s, colorectal cancer patients were found to have detectable carcinoembryonic antigen (CEA) levels in their blood. At that time it was thought that these CEA levels were predictive of colorectal cancer. It is now known that elevated

Table 38-3 Monitoring and Surveillance Guidelines for the Patient with Colon Cancer

1. Physical examination, including DRE with stool occult blood test every 3 mo for 2 yr, then every 6 mo to 5 yr (category 2)
2. CBC + chemistries every 3 mo for 2 yr, then every 6 mo to 5 yr (category 2)
3. If CEA was elevated at diagnosis or within 1 week of colectomy, repeat CEA every 6 mo for 2 yr, then annually for 5 yr (category 2)
4. Chest radiograph (category 2):
   Every 12 mo for 5 cycles if stage B_2 or C *or*
   Every 6 mo for 10 cycles if resected liver or abdominal metastases *or*
   Every 3 mo for 20 cycles if resected lung metastases
5. Abdominal CT (category 2):
   Every 6 mo for 4 cycles, then annually for 3 yr if resected liver or abdominal metastases *or*
   Every 6 mo for 4 cycles, then annually for 3 yr if resected rectal tumor
6. Chest CT (category 2) every 6 mo for 4 cycles if resected lung metastases
7. Colonoscopy (category 2) in 1 yr; repeat in 1 yr and every 3 yr if:
   Negative for multiple synchronous polyps *or*
   Patient with new polyp on surveillance colonoscopy

From National Comprehensive Cancer Network. (1996). *Oncology, 10*(11 Suppl), 157.

Table 38-4 Colon Cancer: Tumor Node Metastasis (TNM) Staging

Tumor	
TX	Primary tumor cannot be assessed
T0	No evidence of primary tumor
Tis	Carcinoma in situ
T1	Tumor invades submucosa
T2	Tumor invades muscularis propria
T3	Tumor invades through the muscularis propria into the subserosa, or into nonperitonealized pericolic or perirectal tissues
T4	Tumor perforates the visceral peritoneum and/or directly invades other organs or structures
Nodes	
NX	Regional lymph nodes cannot be assessed
N0	No regional lymph node metastasis
N1	Metastasis in 1 to 3 pericolic or perirectal lymph nodes
N2	Metastasis in ≥4 pericolic or perirectal lymph node
N3	Metastasis in any lymph node along the course of a named vascular trunk, and or metastasis to apical node (when marked by surgeon)
Metastasis	
MX	Presence of distant metastasis cannot be assessed
M	No distant metastasis
M1	Distant metastasis

T, tumor size; *N,* lymph node involvement; *M,* degree of metastasis

CEA levels occur in many types of cancers, as well as in chronic smokers. Conversely, in some patients with advanced colon cancer, the CEA may not be elevated.

The major value of CEA levels may be in evaluating patients after surgical resection, as a rising CEA may be the first sign of recurrent disease. Current recommendation regarding the monitoring of CEA levels and the overall surveillance of patients who had previous colon cancer are listed in Table 38-3.

Complete Blood Count and Chemistries. Complete blood count and chemistries are obtained preoperatively. Quite often right-sided colon cancer has been bleeding intermittently for weeks and months, with a resultant decease in hemoglobin and hematocrit. Results of chemistries may indicate elevated liver function tests, necessitating further evaluating of the liver for potential metastases.

STAGING

Duke's Classification and Modifications

The staging of colorectal cancer began with the Duke's classification in 1932, a relatively simple method of A, B, C, with *A* as penetration into, but not through, the bowel wall; *B;* as penetration through the wall; and *C* as any lymph node involvement. Various modifications have been made over the years (Cohen, Minsky, & Schilsky, 1997).

TNM Classification

In 1987 the American Joint Committee on cancer (AJCC) and the Union Internationale Contra le Cancer (UICC) began using the tumor, node, metastasis (TNM) system, with additional modifications incorporated in 1992. The issue of which staging system to use continues to be somewhat controversial. Most literature reports results using the AJCC/UICC TNM staging system. However, for purposes of clarity, quite often TNM is correlated with the Duke's A, B, and C, and with the modified Astler-Coller (MAC). An easy, quick way to remember the staging of colon cancer is to associate stage I with A, stage II with B, stage III with C, and stage IV with D, distant metastasis. Tables 38-4 and 38-5 present a more in-depth look at the TNM staging, correlating stage with both Duke's and MAC systems.

MEDICAL MANAGEMENT

Genetic Counseling

Before treatment decisions are discussed with patients and families, the ramifications of genetic testing for family members often becomes a topic of concern. Genetic testing for many types of cancers is now available outside of clinical trials. This represents a challenge for both patients and their families, as well as for health care professionals. In April 1994, the Workshop on Hereditary Breast, Ovarian,

TABLE 38-5 Tumor Node Metastasis (TNM) Staging Colon Cancer Comparison of TNM and Duke's, Modified Astler-Collier (MAC)

Cancer Involvement	Stage	TNM			Duke's MAC	
Carcinoma in situ	Stage 0	Tis		M0	N0	1
Cancer of the mucosa, submucosa, or muscularis propria	Stage I	T1	N0	M0	A	A
		T2	N0	M0	A	B_1
Cancer invades subserosa or penetrates bowel wall	Stage II	T3	N0	M0	B	B_2
		T4	N0	M0	B	B_3
Cancer involves lymph node or extends into nearby tissue and organs	Stage III	T1-2	N1-2	M0	C	C_1
		T3	N1-3	M0	C	C_2
		T4	N1-3	M0	C	C_3
Cancer spreads to distant sites	Stage IV	Any T	N1-2	M1	D	D

and Colon Cancers was held in Washington, D.C. The following recommendations were made: (1) educate the public in basic genetic concepts, (2) include predisposition testing and counseling as a routine part of health care benefits, (3) train multidisciplinary health care providers, (4) involve consumers, and (5) develop standardized DNA testing (Biesecker & Garber, 1995). In addition, there were discussions regarding the importance of full informed consent, gene- or cancer-specific protocols, realization that genetic testing should not be an isolated point and that other risk factors still need to be considered, the importance of a pre-genetic testing cancer diagnostic examination, and the potential, powerful psychosocial and emotional impact of genetic testing (Biesecker & Garber, 1995). One study demonstrated the complex emotional and psychological impact of genetic testing when first-degree relatives were asked if they would choose to be tested and why or why not (Lerman, Marshall, Audrain, & Gomez-Caminero, 1996). Those who chose to be tested did so to determine whether additional individual screening would be necessary, to determine whether children were at risk, and to be reassured (Lerman et al., 1996). Those who chose not be tested had concerns about insurance, questions regarding accuracy, and worry about the reaction of family members (Lerman et al., 1996). To indicate how complicated this issue becomes, individuals also stated that if they were positive for the gene mutation, they were concerned about dealing with depression, or if they did not have the gene, they were concerned they might feel guilty and still continued to worry (Lerman et al., 1996).

The importance of developing a comprehensive method of dealing with gene testing is obvious. A hereditary cancer clinic is one method to identify families at high risk. Genetic testing would occur, and those who carried the mutated gene would then be offered both standard and innovative screening (Narod, 1995). The Workshop on Hereditary Breast, Ovarian, and Colon Cancers recommended three time points for counseling, pretest education, risk notification, and follow-up (Biesecker & Garber, 1995).

Genetic testing and the implications of commercial availability have far-reaching consequences. Health care professionals need to be educated in this new arena to facilitate thoughtful decision making for patients and their families who need information and support before, during, and after considering genetic testing.

The treatment of colon cancer depends on several factors including clinical presentation, results of workup, surgical options, and pathologic stage. Additionally, the issues of adjuvant therapy, salvage therapy, and follow-up and surveillance continues to be evaluated. The NCCN recently published an excellent article that summarizes practice guidelines and provides more in-depth information regarding the management of colon (and rectal) cancer.

Surgical

Surgical intervention with negative microscopic margins as wide as possible, with or without adjuvant therapy, is the only method of obtaining a cure for colon cancer. Approximately 75% of all patients have some type of surgery.

Polyps that contain cancer and have been completely removed may not require further surgery. Polyps that contain cancer and were removed in fragments or have invaded into the muscularis propria (T2) may require a partial colectomy (see Fig. 38-1).

Presumed or confirmed colon cancers that are deemed resectable require an en bloc resection of the colon, removal of the local and regional draining lymph nodes, and resection of a portion of any contagious organ to which the tumor adheres. The curative goal of colon surgery is to achieve wide microscopic negative margins.

Patients whose colon is resectable, but who have distant metastasis (liver, lung, abdomen) (stage IV, Duke's [IV-D] disease), may still be a candidate for a colon resection. Furthermore, depending on additional factors, they may be candidates for liver resection (1 to 4 nodules), pulmonary resection (1 to 3 nodules), (Wade, Virgo, Li, Callander, Longo, & Johnson, 1996); hepatic cryosurgery may also be an option. Laparoscopic colon cancer surgery continues to be evaluated and may be an option in limited disease.

Patients who are deemed unresectable for cure, those with a nonresectable lesion, or those with extensive distant metastasis, (stage IV-D disease) may be candidates for limited colon resection to alleviate symptoms caused by the colon tumor. Quite often a colostomy is performed as a method of diverting the stool in such cases. Fig. 38-3 de-

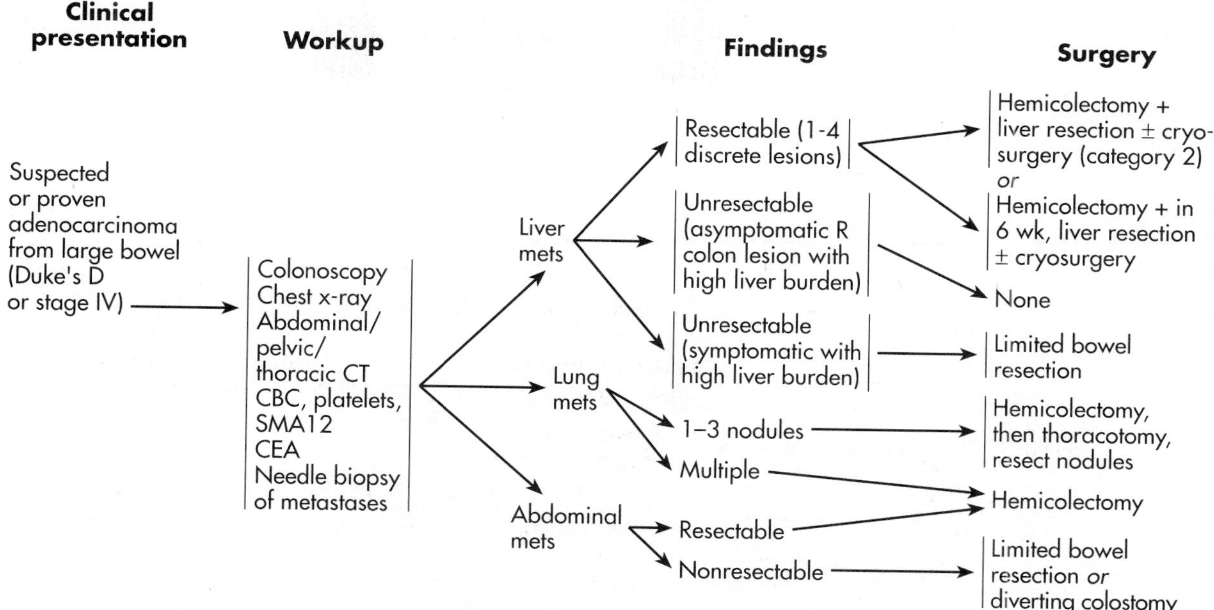

Fig. 38-3 Available options for patients with stage IV, Duke's (IV-D) disease who may or may not be resectable.

picts various options for patients with stage IV-D disease who may or may not be candidates for resection.

Adjuvant Treatment

Adjuvant therapies that are administered before or after curative-intent surgery are chemotherapy, radiation, and immunotherapy (NIH Consensus Conference, 1990). Decisions regarding the utility of adjuvant treatment are based on the evaluation of more than 20 years of data using current methods of meta-analysis. The single most important indicator of the potential effectiveness of adjuvant therapy continues to be the pathologic staging of the disease using the combination of TNM, stage IV-D, and MAC.

Patients with stage 0 and stage I do not require adjuvant therapy, as their overall survival with surgery alone is 90% for stage 0 and 80% for stage I. In stage II (subset B_2), it remains unclear if the benefit of delaying future symptoms resulting from recurrence of tumor outweighs the potential risk in terms of treatment toxicity.

In patients with stage II (subset B_3)and stage III, the standard by which all other treatments are evaluated remains 5-fluorouracil (5-FU) plus levamisole (NIH Consensus Conference, 1990). The substitution of 5-FU plus leucovorin plus radiation continues to be evaluated in patients with T4 lesions that directly invade other organs and/or perforate the visceral peritoneum (stage II B_3 and stage III C_3) (NIH Consensus Conference, 1990).

Finally, adjuvant therapy may be appropriate for certain patients with stage IV-D disease who have undergone resection for distant metastases. The standard treatment in this situation is 5-FU plus leucovorin. Patients with resected liver metastasis continue to be evaluated for the effectiveness of hepatic artery infusion.

To summarize, adjuvant therapy has been effective in certain patients with colon cancer. The dose, timing, and combination of drugs continue to be evaluated and investigated. The "standard" treatment of 5-FU plus levamisole in patients with surgical curative local disease and the "standard" treatment of 5-FU plus leucovorin in surgical-curative distant disease are the best available treatments at this time. Figs. 38-4 and 38-5 summarize adjuvant therapy recommendations based on staging. However, the cure rates and response rates leave room for much improvement. Therefore the NCCN consensus committee has unanimously recommended that placing patients on clinical trials has priority over the current "standard" adjuvant treatments.

Salvage Therapy

Salvage therapy is a term used by health care professionals to describe therapy administered when previous treatments have failed and the disease has recurred, or in certain instances when no previous treatment was initiated because of the nature of metastatic disease.

Salvage surgical resection is a reasonable approach when there is a recurrence in a suture line or in an isolated lesion confined to one organ. When surgical resection is not feasible and patients have not had prior chemotherapy, 5-FU plus leucovorin or continuous infusion 5-FU is appropriate. If patients have had prior chemotherapy and had progression of disease, the drug CPT-11, irinotecan (Camptosar), which has recently been approved by the Food and Drug Administration, is the treatment of choice (*New Drugs Show,* 1996). In all cases of salvage therapy, supportive care or enrollment in a phase I or II clinical trial is appropriate. Fig. 38-6 summarizes the current recommendations of the NCCN regarding salvage therapy.

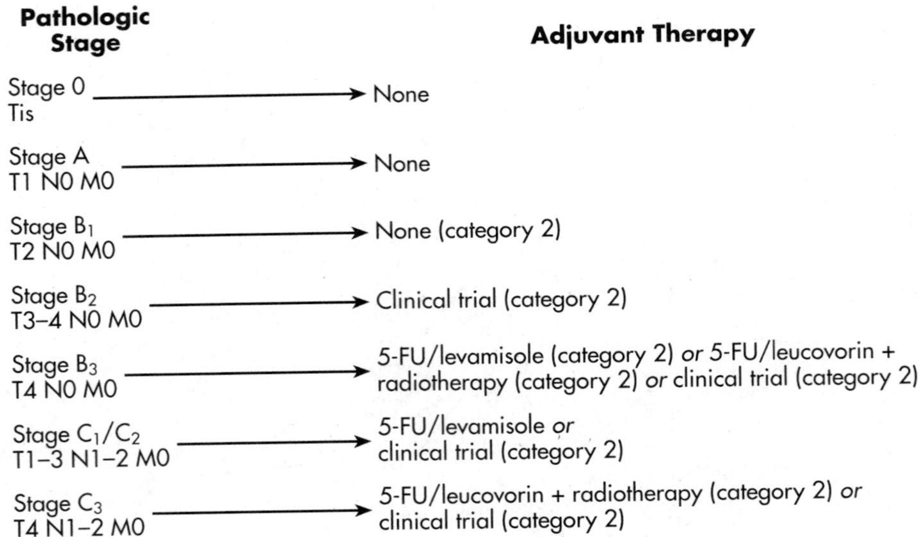

Fig. 38-4 Adjuvant therapy recommendations based on staging.

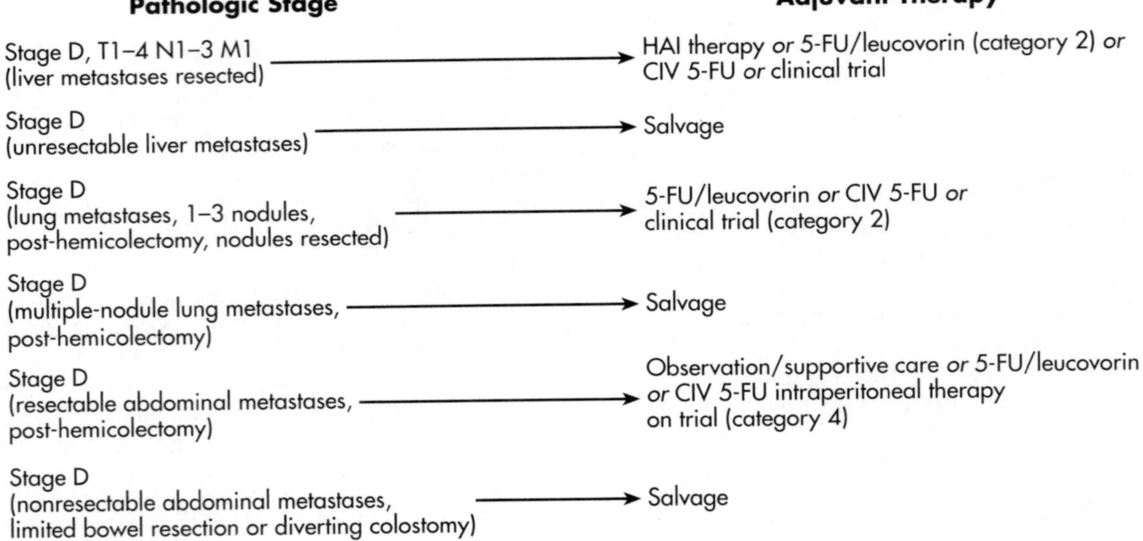

Fig. 38-5 Adjuvant therapy recommendations based on staging.

Monitoring and Surveillance

The medical management of colon cancer extends to the monitoring and surveillance of patients following their curative surgical resection. The recommended guidelines are presented in Table 38-3 (p. 873).

ONCOLOGIC EMERGENCIES

Bowel Obstruction

The major oncologic emergency associated with colon cancer is bowel obstruction. An untreated bowel obstruction can lead to ischemia, perforation, necrosis, shock, and death.

Obstruction is infrequent in right-sided colon cancers where the ascending colon is large in diameter and the stool is liquid and able to pass through the large bulky tumor, which grows into the lumen of the bowel. Tumors in this area typically resemble an apple core lesion. Obstruction in the transverse colon is more frequent compared to the ascending colon, because the transverse colon is smaller in diameter and the stool is becoming more solid and has difficulty passing by the hepatic and splenic flexures. Obstruction is most common in the descending and sigmoid colons where the lumen is smaller and the stool is more solid. Tumors in this legion typically resemble a napkin ring.

When a bowel obstruction occurs, the proximal bowel

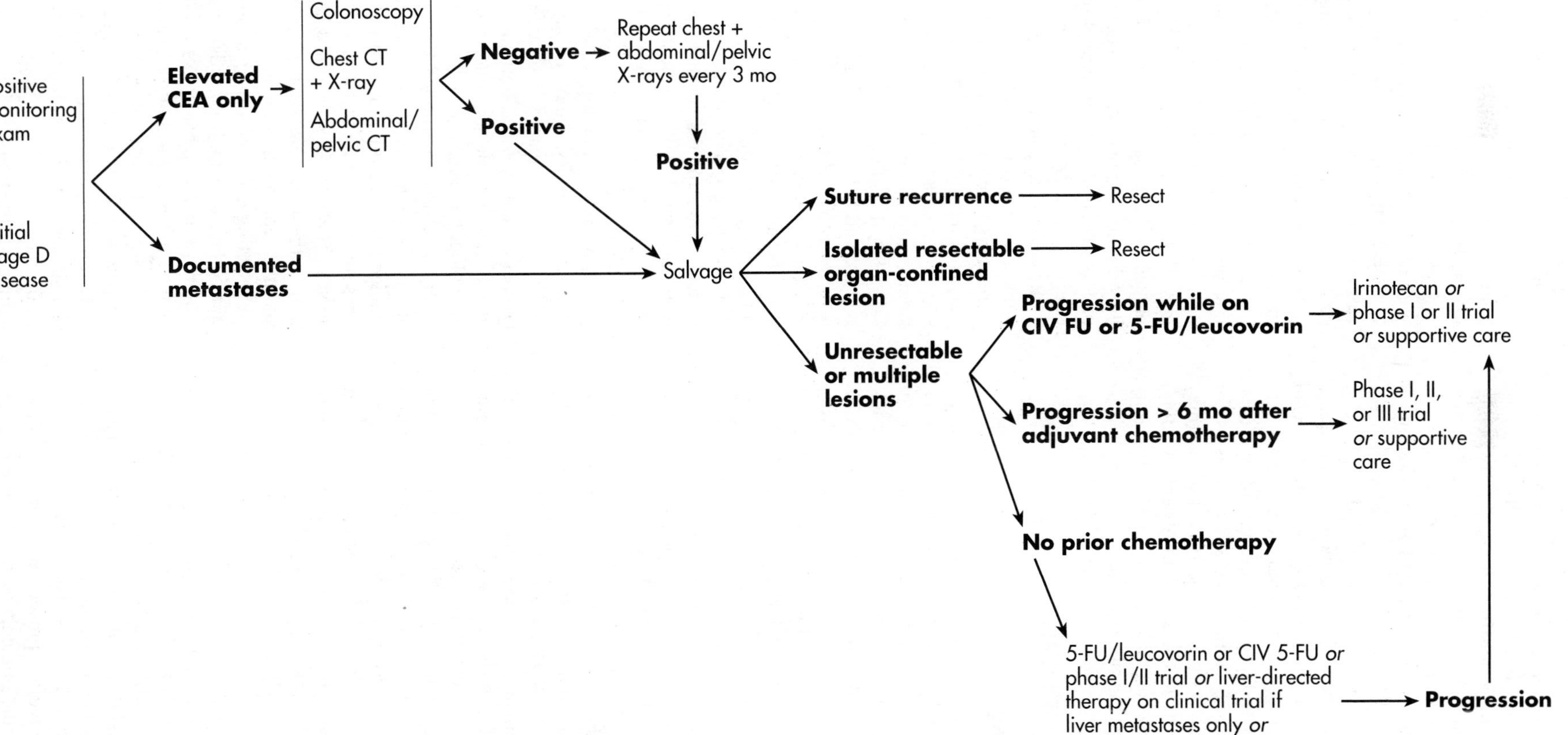

Fig. 38-6 Current recommendations of the NCCN regarding salvaging therapy.

becomes distended with an accumulation of gas and fluid, with a resultant vascular dehydration. Distally the blood flow is impeded causing intestinal ischemia. Ischemia, which lasts 30 to 60 minutes, impairs or destroys the intestinal mucosal barrier, allowing bacteria and toxins to invade the peritoneal cavity and systemic circulation (Cumbie & Clement, 1996; McConnell, 1994)

Patients may present with some or all of the following signs and symptoms: severe abdominal pain and cramping, abdominal distension, nausea, vomiting of brown fecal smelling material, dry mucous membranes, and poor skin turgor. Vital signs may indicate hypotension, tachycardia, and shallow respiration, all compensatory mechanisms for impending hypovolemic or septic shock. Bowel sounds may be high pitched in a partial obstruction or absent in a total obstruction. Emergency surgical intervention is the only treatment for total intestinal obstruction.

NURSING MANAGEMENT

Genetic Counseling

Genetic counseling for patients with colon cancer requires a multidisciplinary team approach, and nurses are often integral team members. A professional nursing organization of registered nurses with an interest and expertise in genetics, the International Society of Nurses in Genetics (ISONG), has emerged to educate nurses in genetic counseling. After acquiring genetics training, oncology nurses can be excellent genetic counselors. Oncology nurses have a rich history of counseling patients and families regarding many life changing decisions. Genetic counseling will become an intricate part of patient care in the near future.

Medical management of colon cancer is extremely complex and variable. A portion of the patient's care occurs in the inpatient setting; but the majority of care occurs in the outpatient and home settings. Early in the course of the disease, the focus of nursing care may be in helping the patient understand various treatment options. As the disease progresses, patients need information about the rationale for different types of intervention and strategies for managing the side effects associated with disease or treatments. Because each major type of treatment for colon cancer (i.e., surgery, adjuvant therapy, salvage therapy) poses unique patient problems, the major issues associated with these treatments are discussed separately, although nursing care issues related to each type of treatment may overlap.

Surgical

Patients undergoing an uncomplicated en bloc colon resection are usually hospitalized for 5 to 7 days. The major focus of inpatient care is on the prevention of postoperative complications, including dehydration, pneumonia, anastomotic leakage, wound infection, hemorrhage, and postresection obstruction (Quinless, 1994; Meissner, 1996).

Discharge planning involves presenting information that helps patients deal with the immediate physical implication of their surgery and their disease (Galloway & Graydon, 1996). Thus, patients need to be told to avoid activities that could damage the anastomosis; heavy lifting should be avoided, driving an automobile is not recommended for 4 to 6 weeks, and straining during defecation should be avoided, with some patients requiring a stool softener (not a laxative). Patients are asked to note the frequency, amount, and character of bowel movements and to report substantial changes. Progressively worsening abdominal pain and distension should be reported. A normal diet can be resumed; gas-producing foods and carbonated beverages should be avoided. Because an extensive bowel resection may interfere with the ability to absorb nutrients, some patients may need to take a multiple vitamin/mineral supplement (Quinless, 1994). Follow-up in the outpatient setting requires that nurses evaluate patients for their usual dietary patterns and bowel patterns postsurgery. The nursing management of the patient under going a colectomy for colon cancer is summarized in Table 38-6.

Resecting the colon may not be feasible in some patients with colon cancer; therefore a diverting colostomy may be necessary. Placement of the colostomy stoma depends on the anatomic location of the tumor. The selection of a stoma site is often made by enterostomal therapy nurses who consider many factors. Stomas need to be placed away from skinfolds, the suture line, scars, bony prominences, the umbilicus, and belt line, and in a location that the patient can readily see (Hoebler, 1997) (Fig. 38-7).

Colostomies can be single barreled, with one opening onto the abdomen, or double barreled, with the proximal functioning opening used for evacuation of stool and the distal opening as a nonfunctioning (in terms of stool) stoma, which allows for the normal ongoing secretion of mucus from the bowel. A loop colostomy is a third type of colostomy in which a loop of bowel is brought out through the abdominal wall.

Postoperative nursing care consists of assessing the stoma for viability. A normal healthy stoma is red to pink and is often edematous and large, although the edema decreases each day, with a normal stoma appearing in approximately 6 weeks. Because the stoma is the fragile mucosa of the colon, there may be a small amount of normal bleeding when the a stoma is rubbed. An indication that the stoma is not receiving adequate blood supply to support viability is a change in color from red to purple, gray, or black. Assessing the skin surrounding the stoma is another responsibility for nurses. The skin should look like the rest of the patient's skin on the abdomen. Redness or excoriated skin is not normal and requires treatment.

Selecting an appropriate appliance to cover the stoma and collect the stool depends on several factors and often requires a period of trial and error. Irrigation of some stomas may be necessary to induce evacuation of some solid stool or to establish a pattern of evacuation that is conducive to the patient's individual schedule.

Discharge planning includes the observation of at least two supervised sessions during which the patient performs all the steps involved in stoma care. During these sessions, written instructions and equipment should be provided.

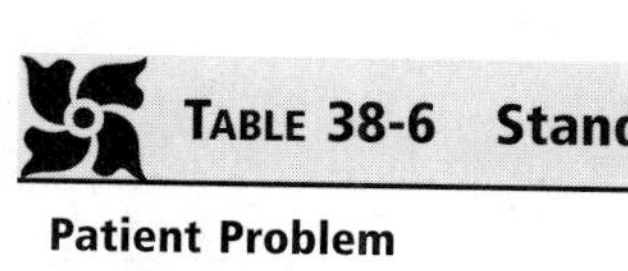

TABLE 38-6 Standard of Care for the Patient Undergoing Colon Resection

Patient Problem and Outcome	Nursing Interventions and Rationales	Patient Education Instruction
Anxiety Patient will: • Verbalize an understanding of the surgical procedure. • Express feeling of decreased anxiety. • Identify strategies to cope with anxiety.	1. Assess patient's level of understanding of the surgical procedure. 2. Give patient the opportunity to ask questions or verbalize concerns. 3. Determine which coping strategies the patient has used in the past to decrease anxiety and reinforce the use of these coping strategies.	1. Use a diagram of the anatomy of the colon to explain the surgical resection procedure. 2. Provide the patient with information about the preoperative routine: a. Diagnostic tests b. Bowel preparalin c. Anesthesiology consult d. Use of antiembolism stocking e. Nothing by mouth after midnight 3. Teach patient coughing and deep breathing exercises and obtain a return demonstration. 4. Provide patient with information about postoperative plan of care: a. Intravenous hydration b. Nasogastric tube c. Surgical incision d. Colostomy care e. Postresection obstruction
Bowel Obstruction Patient will: • Have adequate nasogastric tube drainage • Have bowel sounds on day 2 to 3 • Begin fluid intake day 3 • Begin solid foods day 4	1. Assess patient for nasogastric tube drainage. 2. Remove nasogastric tube on third postoperative day. 3. Assess patient for bowel obstruction: a. Distended abdomen b. Hypoactive or hyperactive bowel sounds c. Intermittent pain relieved by vomiting d. Crampy pain after eating with hypermotility suggests a partial obstruction e. Obtain baseline abdominal girth measurement f. Intake and output measurements	1. Teach patient: a. Avoid kinking of nasogastric tube b. Expected color and amount of drainage c. Call nurse if vomiting occurs d. Call nurse if abdominal pain, distention e. Walking to encourage return of peristalsis
Pain Patient will: • Experience optimal pain relief with minimal side effects	1. Assess origin of pain to rule out impending bowel obstruction. 2. Assess postoperative pain intensity using a 0 to 10 verbal rating scale, every 2 to 4 hours for the first 48 hours after surgery, then at least once a shift. 3. Administer opioid analgesics around-the-clock for the first 24 to 48 postoperative hours. 4. Monitor for analgesic side effects and administer medications to prevent or treat: a. Nausea b. Constipation	1. Teach patient to inform the nurse if experiencing pain. 2. Teach patient the importance of taking pain medication on a regular basis to control pain.
Body Image Disturbance/Ostomy Patient will demonstrate: • Physical ability to apply appliance to stoma. • Verbalize, over time, decreased feelings of anxiety.	1. Assess the patient's ability to apply appliance to stoma: a. Require two return demonstrations before discharge. 2. Assess the patient's level of comfort when caring for stoma: a. Provide a nonjudgmental environment for patient to discuss feelings. b. Determine if referrals for pyschological interventions are appropriate.	1. Provide written, as well as verbal instructions for stoma care. 2. Provide information regarding the variety of available appliances. 3. Encourage participation in support groups.

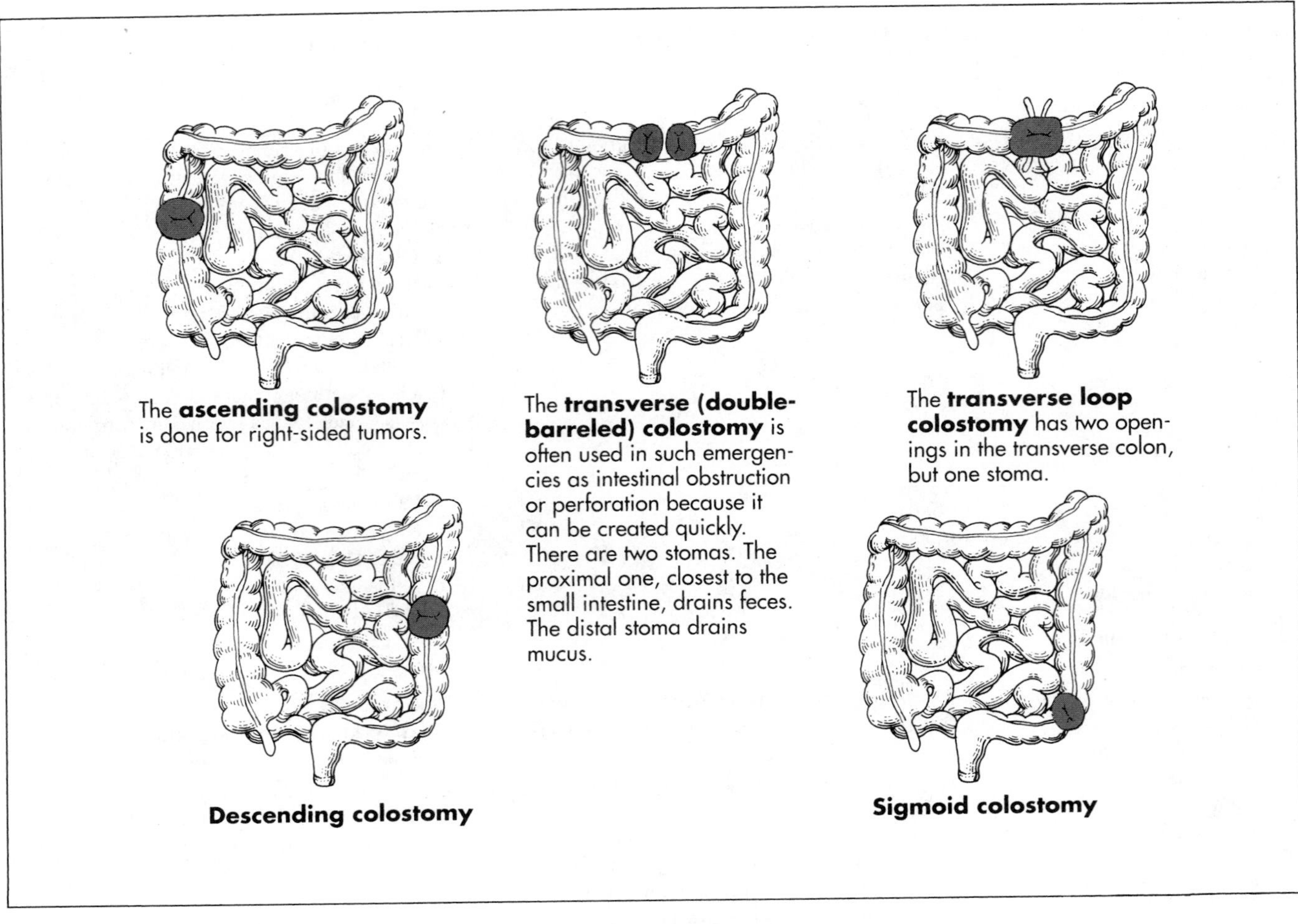

Fig. 38-7 Selection of stoma site.

Home health care visits are often provided until the first preoperative visit. Patients should be made aware of the existence of the United Ostomy Association. Follow-up care in the outpatient setting requires an evaluation of the stoma viability, an evaluation of the patient's ability to handle the appliance and irrigation, and an evaluation of the patient's psychological acceptance of the stoma.

Adjuvant Treatment

Adjuvant therapies administered before or after curative-intent surgery consist of various chemotherapy regimens, plus or minus radiation therapy and perhaps immunotherapy. Most patients receive such treatment in the outpatient setting. Patients need to be taught the rationale for each treatment modality. In addition, strategies must be developed with the patient and the family to manage the side effects associated with the different treatments. Enrollment in clinical trials should be encouraged.

Salvage Therapy

As with adjuvant therapy, patients need to be taught the rationale for each new treatment modality. In three phase II trials, CPT-11 had an overall response rate of 13%, with an additional 50% of patients having stable disease for a median period of 6 months before there was additional progression of disease (*New Drugs Shows,* 1996). As always, enrollment into any available NCI sponsored or endorsed clinical trial is of high priority. Nurses need to be educated regarding the rationale for clinical trials in order for them to share such information with patients or families. The NCI has an excellent patient educational pamphlet that explains the purposes of clinical trials (NCI, 1994).

Supportive care is a reasonable option for patients with colon cancer who have recurrent disease or extensive metastatic disease. Although the term *supportive care* has often been associated with end-of-life care, in a new quarterly publication, *Supportive Cancer Care,* supportive care is described as "the core of cancer practice," encompassing any effort to maximize the physical and emotional reserves of cancer patients and their families (Engelking, 1996). Patients with colon cancer who decide to seek active treatment for their disease can be supported by a multidisciplinary team devoted to meeting a variety of these needs. Patients who decide against active treatment for their disease can still be supported by this same process.

Nurses are often the ones who discuss end-of-life issues

Box 38-7
Glossary of Terms

Caput medusae: A bluish-purple discoloration of the peristomal skin resulting from dilation of cutaneous veins (peristomal varices).
Convexity: The outward curing of a faceplate that begins at the opening of the stoma. The depth of the convexity may be shallow, moderate, or deep.
Faceplate: The component of a pouching system that is in contact with the skin surface. The faceplate may consist of a skin barrier wafer, adhesive surface, or synthetic (e.g., plastic, rubber) ring with varying degrees of rigidity.
Flat peristomal plane: An area around the stoma that is not retracted or rounded.
Flush stoma: A stoma without height or protrusion; a flush stoma lies flat in relation to the peristomal skin plane.
Loop stoma: A stoma constructed when both ends of the bowel are exteriorized without being completely separated during stoma construction. Generally, the distal loop is sutured close to the skin, inferior to the functioning loop. The distal loop may then secrete mucus at skin level and compromise the adhesive seal.
Mucocutaneous junction: The point at which the stoma is sutured to the skin.
Mucocutaneous separation: A disruption of the suture line at the mucocutaneous junction. This may result from suturing techniques, poor wound healing, abscess formation, or trauma.
Peristomal hernia: A bulging of skin near or around the stoma indicating the passage of one or more loops of bowel through a fascial defect around the stoma and into subcutaneous tissues.
Peristomal plane: A surface area located under the faceplate of the pouching system. This surface area of the skin extends out from the base of the stoma; approximately a 4 × 4 inch area around the stoma.
Peristomal plane dynamics: Movement-induced changes in the area around the stoma that may disrupt the interface of the faceplate and skin surface. For example, when a patient moves into a sitting position, a pronounced crease may become apparent.
Retracted stoma: The action of pulling backward or downward so that the stoma moves inward or draws back into the abdomen. A retraction may create a valley or moat around the stoma.
Rounded peristomal plane: Refers to an outward contouring of the area. Whether convexity is needed in this situation is dependent on abdominal muscle tone.
Rounded stoma: Refers to the round shape of a stoma.
Telescoping stoma: A stoma that has become longer and then may retract below the skin surface. The bowel is actually telescoping, as opposed to retracting.
Stoma prolapse: A significant elongation of the stoma that may reduce in size when the patient is lying or when the stoma is mechanically placed back into the abdomen.

From Rolstad, B. S. & Boarini, J. (1996). Principles and techniques of convexity. *Ostomy/Wound Management, 42*(1), 25.

with patients and their families. Nurses should encourage patients to write down a list of questions they need to address with their physician and further clarify these issues and suggest appropriate end-of-life referrals; home health care, hospice care, the use of a living will, or other documentation regarding life support. Forty-six percent of all patients with colon cancer die as a direct result of their disease. Terminal care provided by experienced oncology nurses is extremely useful for patients and families as they face this difficult situation.

Monitoring and Surveillance

An important aspect of nursing care is to educate patients regarding the importance of future follow-up. Patients need to know not only when they require monitoring, but also why this surveillance is important. Additionally, nurses provide valuable emotional support for both patients and families at each follow-up visit. The recommended guidelines for monitoring and surveillance are presented in Table 38-3.

HOME CARE ISSUES

Seamless care between inpatient, outpatient, and home care provides an important foundation for home care. Depending on the treatment approaches used to manage colon cancer, the patient and family care providers may be faced with the following issues in the home care setting.

Reestablishing Normal Patterns

Patients with a resected colon may encounter varying degrees of difficulty reestablishing a normal food intake and bowel movement pattern. Problems range from frequent bowel movements, which may be liquid in nature, to infrequent movements, which may require the use of a stool softener. Patients and families need to begin the process of adding foods to the diet and evaluating their effect on the bowel. It may take 4, 6, or 8 weeks to establish a pattern that allows for adequate absorption of nutrients, which will facilitate a return to normal peristaltic bowel movements. Patients and families can be encouraged to monitor a timed record of food and water intake and correlate this information with bowel movements.

Colostomy Care

A major issue for patients and their significant other is the management of a stoma. The physical dexterity needed to maintain a predictable, secure pouch is one aspect that affects overall quality of life (Rolstad & Boarini 1996). Box 38-7 provides an excellent glossary of terms that will enable the nurse to understand and thereby explain to patients and families the various ostomy appliance techniques that are recommended. Table 38-7 provides a method of evaluating various equipment options. The patient's psychological adjustment with regard to body image and sexuality is another issue that needs to be adequately addressed. The psychoso-

TABLE 38-7 Equipment Options for Achieving Degrees of Convexity and Support

Degree of Convexity	Equipment Options	Degree of Support
None	Addition of skin barrier paste to a flat, all flexible system	None
Shallow	An insert in a two-piece pouching system	Firm
Shallow	A one-piece pouch with a plastic gasket and karaya seal ring attached	Firm
Shallow	Addition of a karaya-, pectin- or silicone-based barrier to a flat pouching system	Soft
Shallow/Moderate	A reusable faceplate with shallow convexity	Firm
Moderate	Additon of a karaya-, pectin- or silicone-based skin barrier to a shallow insert in a two-piece system	Firm
Moderate/Deep	A one-piece pouching system with integrated convexity	Firm
Deep	Additon of a karaya-, pectin- or silicone-based skin barrier to moderate convexity system	Firm
Deep	A reusable faceplate with deep convexity	Firm

From Rolstad, B. S. & Boarini, J. (1996). Principles and techniques of convexity. *Ostomy/Wound Management, 42*(1), 30.

cial sexual adjustment of the patient's significant other is another aspect of stoma adjustment. Patients and families need to be made aware of the support groups such as the United Ostomy Association, and referrals to appropriate professional counseling may be needed as well.

Chemotherapy and Radiation

Patients who are undergoing chemotherapy and/or radiation therapy may require home care for acute bouts of nausea, vomiting, diarrhea, anemia, and fatigue. Such care is often monitored in the outpatient setting.

Fatigue

Fatigue is a multifactorial symptom that has become the number one complaint of cancer patients (Winningham, Nail, Burke, Brophy, Cimprich, & Jones et al., 1994). Patients with colon cancer can experience a minimal amount of fatigue or a fatigue that profoundly affects their overall quality of life. When ever possible, fatigue should be treated by both pharmacologic and nonpharmacologic methods (Table 38-8). Treating all of the components of fatigue appropriately improves a patient's quality of life. No matter how minimal or severe the fatigue may be for an individual, the use of energy conservation methods allows the patient to "save" energy when performing certain activities in order to expend more energy for activities they are obligated to perform or for an activity that brings them peace and joy. Box 38-8 provides and excellent energy conservation resource for patients.

TABLE 38-8 Fatgue Intervention

Potential Causes of Fatigue	Suggested Interventions for Patients
Inadequate food intake	Drink fluids, six small meals
Decreased level of energy	Mild exercise as tolerated Energy conservation
Depression	Express feelings and fears Participate in patient support groups Medication as prescribed
Pain	Take pain medicine around the clock
Inadequate sleep	Re-establish normal sleep-wake patterns Remain awake and dressed during the day except for specific short rest periods. Take sleep medicine
Infection	Take antibiotics as prescribed until completely finished
Anemia	Resue therapy with transfusions Proactive treatment with Procrit (Epoetin alfa) to begin 4 weeks before expected decrease in hemoglobin.

Terminal Care

During terminal stages of colon cancer disease, pain control is a high priority. Maintaining patency of the bowel to foster normal elimination becomes important during terminal stages, and patients and families need information regarding obstruction. Various options regarding treatment for obstruction need to be explained so that patients can make informed decisions about the most appropriate care for them. Some of these options are surgical resections and diverting colostomy, use of a cantor tube to divert the stool around the obstruction, use of laxatives or softeners, and increased water intake to encourage the stool to be more liquid.

Patients with colon cancer are often somewhat active and ambulatory during disease progression until death is imminent. A peaceful death can occur for patients with liver metastasis as the liver slowly becomes unable to function, and a build up of toxins causes patients to "die in their sleep."

Box 38-8

Suggestions for Energy Conservation

Basic Activities of Daily Living

Bathing

- Wash hair in shower, not in sink
- Sit to dry off
- Use a terry robe instead of drying off
- Use shower organizer over the shower head to avoid leaning or reaching
- Use safety strips on the floor of the tub
- Install a grab rail
- Use a shower bench or lawn chair to sit while showering
- Use moderate temperature water, rather than hot
- Use long-handled sponge or brush to reach feet and back

Grooming/Hygiene

- Sit
- Don't lean forward unsupported
- Rest elbows on counter or dressing table
- Use long-handled brushes or combs to avoid holding arms overhead
- Use elevated commode seat

Dressing

- Loose fitting clothes allow you to breathe more easily
- Organize early so you won't have to rush
- Lay out clothes before starting to avoid extra steps
- Bring your foot to your knee to apply shoes and socks so you won't have to lean over
- Wear slip-on shoes
- Use a long-handled shoe horn and sock aid
- Fasten bra in front then turn to back
- Wear button front shirts rather than pullovers
- Use a reacher and/or a dressing stick

Mobility

- Wear low-heeled shoes
- Wear shoes with a shock absorbent sole or insole
- Use a wheelchair for long trips (e.g., the mall)
- Maintain good posture when driving
- Use cruise control if possible
- Install hand rails
- Install ramps
- Place chairs strategically to allow rest stops (along a long hallway)
- Disconnect automatic door closing mechanisms

Advanced activities of daily living

Housekeeping

- Spread tasks out over the week
- Do a little bit each day
- Delegate heavy work
- Hire help
- Use a wheeled car or carpenter's apron to carry supplies
- Do whatever you can sitting
- Use long-handled dust pan

Shopping

- Make a list first
- Organize the grocery list by store aisle
- Use the grocery cart for support
- Use a power scooter if the store has one
- Request store assistance with shopping and getting to the car
- Shop less busy times
- Shop with a friend
- Delegate shopping

Meal Preparation

- Assemble all ingredients before you start
- Use mixes or prepackaged foods
- Use cookware you can serve from
- Use smaller appliances (mixers, toaster oven, microvave)
- Use electric knife and can opener
- Buy ergonomically designed utensils
- Transport items on a rolling cart
- Store frequently used items at chest level to avoid bending and stretching
- Line ovens and burner drip pans with aluminum foil
- Sit while preparing food
- Rest elbows on table or counter
- Let dishes soak rather than scrubbing
- Let dishes air dry
- Use a dishwasher
- Delegate dishwashing
- Use a jar opener
- Use rubber mat or wet towel under mixing bowl to help steady it while stirring or mixing
- Don't lift heavy pans off the stove, ladle the food out at the stove
- Use mitten pot holders to take advantage of the entire hand to lift
- Use lightweight utensils
- Prepare double portions and freeze half for later
- Leave heavy containers where they can be accessed without lifting (e.g., on the countertop)
- Drag garbage bags instead of lifting (or use wheeled can)

Laundry

- Use a laundry cart on wheels
- Use an automatic washer and dryer, if possible
- Sit to transfer clothes to the dryer, if possible
- Use commercial prewash instead of scrubbing
- Wash bras and socks in a lingerie bag to avoid tangling
- Drain hand washables and press the water out instead of wringing
- Sit to iron
- Adjust the ironing board height
- Use an iron with a spray attachment
- Slide the iron onto an asbestos pad between items to avoid lifting
- Use a lightweight iron
- Hang clothes on the doorknob instead of the top of door

Modified from Eileen Donovan. (1997). *Personal communication.* The University of Texas M. D. Anderson Cancer Center.

Continued

Box 38-8
Suggestions for Energy Conservation—cont'd

Child care
- Plan activities around the table or in the living room to allow sitting
- Instead of going to the zoo, go to the beach where you can sit or lie down
- Delegate some of the child care responsibilities, if possible
- Take advantage of programs like Mother's day out
- Teach smaller children to climb up on lap instead of being lifted
- Teach children to make a game of some of the household chores

Workplace
- Plan workload around your best times of the day
- Arrange workspace ergonomically
- Take periodic rest breaks

Leisure
- Wear comfortable clothing
- Use adaptive equipment
- Select less strenuous activities
- Go with a friend
- Use a wheelchair or golf cart

Modified from Eileen Donovan. (1997). *Personal communication.* The University of Texas M. D. Anderson Cancer Center.

Any and all individualized patient information regarding terminal care will help patients and families share in a death with dignity.

PROGNOSIS

Stage at Diagnosis

Fifty-four percent of all patients with colon cancer survive for 5 years or longer. Although many variables are being investigated, it is primarily the stage of disease at diagnosis that is the most accurate predictor of survival and prognosis. The degree of penetration through the bowel wall, lymph node involvement, and presence or absence of distant metastasis (stage of disease)—but not the size of the tumor—affect prognosis. In most studies, age and sex when analyzed by stage adjusted data, does not seem to be an independent predictor of prognosis and survival. The prognosis of patients with synchronous colon cancer, when the highest stage of the synchronous tumor is considered, seems to indicate that the survival is the same for such an individual based on stage alone (Passman, Pommier, & Vetto, 1996).

Degree of differentiation is both an independent variable and a variable in conjunction with stage of disease, which adversely effects prognosis. There are three grades of differentiation of colon cancer tumors: grade 1, well differentiated; grade 2, moderately differentiated; and grade 3, poorly differentiated. Some studies indicate there may be a difference in prognosis for the wartlike exophytic tumors and ulcerating tumors. Others argue that because exophytic tumors are more often limited to the bowel wall and ulcerating tumors have a higher frequency of penetration of the bowel wall, these characteristics are probably not independent predictors of survival and prognosis, but, again, a reflection of the overall stage of disease. Two classic studies have shown that obstruction, irrespective of stage of disease, is an independent predictor that has a negative impact on survival (Steinberg, Barkin, & Kaplan, 1986; Wolmark, Wieand, & Rockette, 1993). An interesting look at patients with colorectal liver metastasis in a London hospital noted that the patients who exhibited high quality of life indicators provided a better estimate of improved survival when compared with tumor size alone (Earlam, Glover, Fordy, Burke, & Allen-Mersh, 1996).

Table 38-9 offers a brief overview of 5-year survival data based solely on stage of disease. Primary prevention and early detection are high priorities in efforts to improve prognosis and survival

Recurrent Disease

Another major factor that affects prognosis for patients with colon cancer is the recurrence of disease. Therefore, another strategy to improve prognosis is to identify patients who are high risk of recurrence and initiate aggressive adjuvant treatment. Several studies are ongoing in an effort to identify such predictors of recurrence (independent of stage). For example, one study has examined a subset of Duke's B patients who are at high risk for recurrence when there has been an allelic loss of chromosome 18q (Bosman, 1995). Another group of investigators looked at node-negative patients who had an increase in angiogenesis, which was an indication of a higher risk for recurrence (Frank, Saclarides, Leurgans, Speziale, Drab, & Rubin, 1995). Information such as this may lead to future treatment of this subgroup with adjuvant chemotherapy.

Currently, such node-negative patients do not routinely receive adjuvant chemotherapy. Nori, Merimsky, Samala, Saw, Cortes, & Chen et al (1995) have concluded that a subset of Duke's B_2 colon cancer patients, in whom aneuploidy was discovered, were at high risk for tumor recurrence and therefore an overall decrease in survival. In another study, patients with right-sided colon cancer whose tumor had Crohn's-like lymphoid reaction, had a more favorable prognosis (Harrison, Dean, el-Zeky, & Vander Zwaag, 1995). Studies continue to explore the role of whole abdominal radiation therapy (plus or minus chemotherapy) on the local recurrence rate of C_2 patients in an effort to identify the subset who would benefit from this approach (Estes, Giri, & Fabian, 1996).

Although the vast majority of colon cancer patients have adenocarcinoma, it has been well established that certain other types of colon cancer have a poorer prognosis. Mucinous cancer, also known as colloid cancer, signet cell, or

Table 38-9 Colon Cancer 5-Year Survival Rates

TNM	Duke's	Survival (%)
Stage 0	—	100
Stage I	A	80 to 90
Stage II	B	60 to 77
Stage III	C	30 to 56
Stage IV	D	10

signet ring carcinoma, carries a poor prognosis (Sun, Carstensen, Stal, Zhang, Boeryd, & Nordenskjold, 1996).

Patients who have untreated liver metastasis have a life expectancy of 3 to 24 months, with a median survival of 8 months. Metastatic disease carries a poor prognosis of 10% 5-year survival.

EVALUATION OF THE QUALITY OF CARE

Accreditation organizations, such as the Joint Commission for the Accreditation of Healthcare Organizations, require evaluation of the quality of care provided to patients. Because the care provided to patients with colon cancer takes place in the inpatient and outpatient setting, Tables 38-10 and 38-11 provide an example of tools used by patients to evaluate enterostomal cancer in both of these settings. Table 38-12 is an example of a Continuous Quality Improvement tool that assesses the quality of educational preparation that nursing staff reserves receive regarding colostomy irrigation.

RESEARCH ISSUES

Numerous research issues regarding the diagnosis and management of colon cancer require further investigation. Research endeavors involve primary prevention of colon cancer through dietary manipulation with various supplements and a low-fat, high-fiber diet. Screening and early detection efforts are ongoing in an effort to establish meaningful guidelines for asymptomatic and high-risk patients. Developing new and more effective screening methods remains a priority. Surgical intervention, the only current effective cure for colon cancer, continues to be evaluated in an effort to develop more sophisticated technology that would allow for the discovery of micrometastasis. Adjuvant therapy remains an important area of investigation. New and more effective chemotherapy agents need to be identified. The appropriate use of radiation, biotherapy, and genetic intervention must be evaluated. Metastatic stage IV Duke's D disease requires additional investigation to improve both survival time and quality of life for patients. During prevention, early detection and screening, surgery, adjuvant treatment, and treatment of metastatic disease, patients should be enrolled, whenever, possible, in well-developed, clinical trials sponsored or endorsed by the NCI. Such research endeavors will ultimately result in a cure for colon cancer.

Table 38-10 Roswell Park Cancer Institute Department of Nursing Continuous Quality Improvement Enterostomal Therapy (ET) Discharge Evaluation

1. Did the preoperative teaching by the ET nurse alleviate some of your anxiety regarding ostomy surgery?
   YES ________ NO ________
2. Was the ET nurse courteous and unhurried in her approach to your ostomy care?
   YES ________ NO ________
3. Did the ET nurse give you sufficient information about the care of your ostomy? (e.g., diet booklet, dealer booklet, *Managing Your Ostomy* booklet)
   YES ________ NO ________
4. Did the ostomy videos reinforce the teaching by the ET nurse?
   YES ________ NO ________ COMMENT: ________
   ____
5. Do you feel the ET nurse made adequate attempts to make your feel confident in assuming self-care of your ostomy?
   YES ________ NO________ COMMENT: ________
   ____
6. Do you feel the ET nurse made adequate attempts to protect your privacy while doing your ostomy care?
   YES ________ NO ________ COMMENT: ________
   ____
7. Did you have any difficulty in caring for your ostomy at home?
   YES ________ NO ________
   If yes, please explain your problem:
   ____
   ____
   ____
   ____

Modified from Roswell Park Cancer Institute, Department of Nursing, Buffalo, New York.

Nursing research is ongoing with regard to effective, quality nursing care delivery for patients with colon cancer. The effect of telemedicine remains to be seen, as nurses begin to care for patients across boundaries (Burdick, Mahmud, & Jenkins, 1996). How patients perceive the nurse and her or his caring behaviors may have a future impact on nursing care, as patients become more proactive and select hospital settings based on their perception of caring behaviors (Andrews, Daniels, & Hall, 1996). Using this type of nursing research enables nurses to help prevent patient dissatisfaction and identify potential difficulties in the nurse-patient relationship (Andrews et al., 1996). Reading the literature and translating current research into practical clinical applications will become more important as health care delivery continues to be refined and each patient encounter needs to be efficient, effective, and meaningful. The new journal, *Clinical Journal of Oncology Care,* available from the Oncology Nursing Society, devotes one section to presenting nursing research and then suggests methods to

TABLE 38-11 Roswell Park Cancer Institute Department of Nursing Patient Clinic Visit Satisfaction Survey for Enterostomal Therapy (ET) Nurse Services

DATE OF VISIT: ____________________
RESON FOR REQUEST: ____________________
CLINIC VISITED: ____________________

1. Did the ET nurse respond to the clinic in a timely manner?
   YES ______ NO ______ COMMENTS: ______
2. Did the ET nurse identify herself?
   YES ______ NO ______ COMMENTS: ______
3. Did the ET nurse address your concern/problem?
   YES ______ NO ______ COMMENTS: ______
4. Did the ET nurse provide and/or explain instruction in regard to your concern/problems?
   YES ______ NO ______ COMMENTS: ______
5. Did the ET nurse offer and provide safe and courteous care with patient confidentially?
   YES ______ NO ______ COMMENTS: ______
6. Do you feel that follow-up care by the ET nurse in a clinic setting would be beneficial?
   YES ______ NO ______ COMMENTS: ______

Modified from Roswell Park Cancer Institute, Department of Nursing, Buffalo, New York.

TABLE 38-12 Roswell Park Cancer Institute Department of Nursing Continuous Quality Improvement for Colostomy Irrigation Utilizing Stoma Care

1. Is irrigating equipment easily obtainable and organized for staff?
   YES ______ NO ______ COMMENTS: ______
2. Is staff experiencing difficulty performing irrigation using stoma cone?
   YES ______ NO ______ COMMENTS: ______
3. Are results of bowel preps adequate using cone technique?
   YES ______ NO ______ COMMENTS: ______
4. Was in-service on colostomy irrigation adequate to prepare staff to perform irrigation using stoma cone?
   YES ______ NO ______ COMMENTS: ______
5. Your comments, concerns, and suggestions on colostomy irrigation using the stoma cone
   COMMENTS: ____________________

Modified from Roswell Park Cancer Institute, Department of Nursing, Buffalo, New York.

apply this new knowledge in the clinical arena. *The Oncology Nursing Scan,* a quarterly journal, presents abstracts of current literature of interest for cancer nurses, who can then read some of the articles that interest them and apply the research to their clinical practice. Applying such research will encourage nurses to eliminate nonproductive behaviors. For example, research has shown that enhancing colon cancer knowledge using video information or a booklet is much more effective than using verbal instructions alone (Meade, McKinney, & Barnas, 1994). Therefore, using this research data will allow nurses to delete the use of verbal instructions only from their routine patient care techniques and justify budgetary requests for patient education materials.

Research of all types must continue for the purpose of providing quality care to patients with colon cancer during their entire spectrum of care.

REFERENCES

Andrews, L., Daniels, P., & Hale, A. (1996). Nurse caring behaviors: Comparing five tools to define perception. *Journal of Extended Patient Care Management, 42,* 29-37.

Anonymous. (1996). Screening for colorectal cancer—United States, 1992-1993, and new guidelines. *Morbidity & Mortality Weekly Report, 45,* 107-110.

Bernstein, D. & Rogers, A. (1996). Malignancy in Crohn's disease. *The American Journal of Gastroneterology, 91,* 434-438.

Biesecker, B. B. & Garber J. E. (1995). Testing and counseling adults for heritable cancer risk. *Journal of the National Cancer Institute Monographs, 17,* 115-117.

Boone, C., Kelloff, G., & Malone, W. (1990). Identification of candidate cancer chemoprevention agents and their evaluation on animal models and human critical trials: A review. *Cancer Research, 50,* 2-9.

Borum, M. L. (1996). Patient and physician gender may influence colorectal cancer screening by resident physicians. *Journal of Women's Health, 5,* 363-367.

Bosman, F. T. (1995). Prognostic value of pathological characteristics of colon cancer tumors. *European Journal of Cancer, 31A* (7-8), 1216-21.

Broeders, M. J., Lambe, M., Baron, J. A., & Leon, D. A. (1996). History of childbearing and colorectal cancer risk in women aged less than 60: An analysis of Swedish routine registry data 1960-1984. *International Journal of Cancer, 66,* 170-175.

Burdick, A. E., Mahmud, K., & Jenkins, D. P. (1996). Telemedicine: Caring for patients across boundaries. *Ostomy/Wound Management, 42,* 26-37.

Cohen, A. M., Minsky, B. C., & Schilsky R. L. (1997) In V. T. DeVita, S. Hellman, & S. A. Rosenberg,. (Eds.). *Cancer: Principles & practice of oncology* (5th ed., pp. 1144-1197). Philadelphia: J. B. Lippincott Company.

Cooper, G. M. (1995). *Oncogenes.* Boston & London: Jones & Bartlett Publishers.

Cote, R. J., Houchens, D. D., Hitchcock C. L., Saad, A. D., Nines, R. G., Greenson, J. K., Schneebaum, S., Arnold, M. W., & Martin E. W. Jr. (1996). Intraoperative detection of occult colon cancer micrometastases using 125 I-radiolabled monoclonal antibody CC49. *Cancer, 77,* 613-620.

Cumbie, B. & Clement, S. (1996). Actionstat. *Nursing96,* 21, 33.

Earlam, S., Glover, C., Fordy, C., Burke, D., & Allen-Mersh, T. G. (1996). Relation between tumor size, quality of life, and survival in patients with colorectal liver metastases. *Journal of Clinical Oncology, 14,* 171-175.

Engelking, C., (1996). Supportive care: The core of cancer practice. *Developments in Supportive Cancer Care, 1* (1) 1-10.

Estes, N. C., Giri, S., & Fabian, C. (1996). Patterns of recurrence for advanced colon cancer modified by whole abdominal radiation and chemotherapy. *American Surgeon, 62,* 546-549.

Fearon, E. R. & Vogelstein, B. (1990). A genetic model for colorectal tumorigenesis. *Cell Press, 61,* 759-767.

Fitzsimmons, M. L. & Fales, L. (1993). Colon cancer prevention update. *Seminars in Oncology Nursing, 9,* 163-168.

Fitzsimmons, M. L. (1992). Hereditary colon cancers. *Seminars in Oncology Nursing, 8,* 252-257.

Frank, R. E., Saclarides, T. J., Leurgans, S., Speziale, N. J., Drab, E. A., & Rubin, D. B. (1995). Tumor angiogenesis as a predictor of recurrence and survival in patients with node-negative colon cancer. *Annals of Surgery, 222,* 695-699.

Galloway, S. C. & Graydon, J. E. (1996). Uncertainty, symptom distress, and information needs after surgery for cancer of the colon. *Cancer Nursing, 19,* 112-117.

Gray, H. (1995). *Gray's anatomy.* New York: Williams and Wilkins.

Harrison, J. C., Dean, P. J., El-Zeky, F., & vander Zwaag, R. (1995). Impact of the Crohn's-like lymphoid reaction on staging of right-sided colon cancer: Results of multivariate analysis. *Human Pathology, 26,* 31-38.

Hoebler, L. (1997). Colon and rectal cancer. In S. L. Groenwald, M. H. Frogge, M. Goodman, & C. H. Yarbro (Eds.), *Cancer nursing principles and practice* (4th ed.). Boston: Jones and Bartlett Publishers.

Kearney, J., Giovannucci, E., Rimm, E. B., Ascherio, A., Stampfer, M.. J., Colditz, G. A., Wing, A., Kampman, E., & Willett, W. C. (1996). Calcium, vitamin D, and dairy foods and the occurrence of colon cancer in men. *American Journal of Epidemiology, 143,* 907-917.

Kearney, J., Giovannucci, E., Rimm, E. B., Stampfer, M. J., Colditz, G. A., Ascherio, A., Bleday, R., & Willett, W. C. (1995). Diet, alcohol, and smoking and the occurrence of hyperplastic polyps of the colon and rectum (United States). *Cancer Causes and Control, 6,* 45-56.

Lerman, C., Marshall, J., Audrain, J., & Gomez-Caminero, A. (1996). Genetic testing for colon cancer susceptibility: Anticipated reactions of patients and challenges to providers. *International Journal of Cancer, 69,* 58-61.

Lynch, H. T. & Lynch, J. F. (1995). Clinical implications of advances in the molecular genetics of colorectal cancer. *Tumori, 81,* (Suppl.) 19-29.

Mayberry, R. M., Coates, R. J., Hill, H. A., Click, L. A., Chen, V. W., Austin, D. F., Redmond, C. K., Fenoglio-Preiser, C. M., Hunter, C. P., Haynes, M. A., (1995). Determinants of black/white differences in colon cancer survival. *Journal of the National Cancer Institute, 87,* 1686-1693.

McConnell, E. A. (1994). Loosing the grip of intestinal obstructions. *Nursing 94,* 34-41.

Meade, C. D., McKinney, W. P., & Barnas, G. P. (1994). Educating patients with limited literacy skills: The effectiveness of printed and videotaped materials about colon cancer. *American Journal of Public Health, 84,* 119-121.

Meissner, J. E. (1994). Caring for patients with ulcerative colitis. *Nursing 94,* 54-55.

Meissner, J. E. (1996). Caring for patients with colorectal cancer. *Nursing 96,* 60-61.

Narod, S. A. (1995). Screening for cancer in high risk families. (Review). *Clinical Biochemistry, 28,* 367-372.

National Cancer Institute. (1994). *What you need to know about cancer of the colon and rectum.* (Publication No. 94-1552). Bethesda, MD: U.S. Department of Health and Human Services.

National Comprehensive Cancer Network. (1996). Oncology practice guidelines. *Oncology, 10,* (Suppl).

National Institutes of Health Consensus Conference Adjuvant Cancer Therapy. (1990). Adjuvant therapy for patients with colon and rectal cancer. *Journal of American Medical Association, 264,* 1444-1450.

New drugs show promise in front-and-second line treatment of colon cancer, (1996). *Oncology News International, 5,* 3.

Niendorf, A., Nagele, H., Gerding, D., Meyer-Pannwitt, U., & Gebhardt, A. (1995). Increased LDL receptor mRNA expression in colon cancer is correlated with a rise in plasma cholesterol levels after curative surgery. *International Journal of Cancer, 61,* 461-464.

Nori, D., Merimsky, O., Samala, E., Saw D., Cortes, E., Chen, E., & Turner, J. W. (1995). Tumor ploidy as a risk factor for disease recurrence and short survival in surgically-treated Dukes' B_2 colon cancer patients. *Journal of Surgical Oncology, 59,* 239-242.

Otchy, D. P., Ransohoff, D. F., Wolff, B. G., Weaver, A., Ilstrup, D., Carlson, H., & Rademacher, D. (1996). Metachronous colon cancer in persons who have had a large adenomatous polyp. *American Journal of Gastroenterology, 91,* 448-454.

Overall US cancer mortality rate falls for the first time. (1996). *Oncology News International, 5,* 1.

Parker, S. L., Murray T, Bolden S., & Wingo, P. A. (1998). Cancer Statistics, 1996. *CA Cancer Journal For Clinicians, 46,* 5-27.

Passman, M. A., Pommier, R. F., & Vetto, J. T. (1996). Synchronous colon primaries have the same prognosis as solitary colon cancers. (Review). *Diseases of the Colon & Rectum, 39,* 329-334.

Quinless, F. W. (1994). When your patient undergoes a bowel resection. *Nursing94,* 32C-D.

Ribeiro, M. B., Greenstein, A. J., Sachar, D. B., Barth J., Balasubramanian, S., Harpaz, N., Heimann, T. M., & Aufses, A. H. Jr. (1996). Colorectal adenocarcinoma in Crohn's disease. *Annals of Surgery, 223,* 186-193.

Rodriquez-Bigas, M. A., Lee, P. H. U., O'Malley, L., Weber, T. K., Okhee, S., Anderson, G.R., & Petrelli, N. J. (1996). Establishment of a hereditary nonpolyposis colorectal cancer registry. *Dis Colon Rectum,* 20, 649-652.

Rolstad, B. S. & Boarini, J. (1996). Principals and techniques in the use of convexity. *The Journal of Extended Patient Care Management, 42,* 24-32.

Shike, M. (1996). Body weight and colon cancer. *American Journal of Clinical Nutrition, 63,* (3 Suppl.), 442S-444S.

Steinberg, S. M., Barkin, J. S., Kaplan, R. S., (1986). Prognostic indicators of colon tumors: The gastrointestinal tumor group experience. *Cancer, 57,* 1866-1870.

Subjects sought for four cancer chemoprevention trials. (1996). *Oncology News International, 5,* 49.

Sun, X. F., Carstensen, J. M., Stal, O., Zhang, H., Boeryd, B., & Nordenskjold, B. (1996). Interrelations of clinicopathologic variables and their prognostic value in colorectal adenocarcinoma. *APMIS, 104,* 35-38.

Thune, I. & Lund, E., (1966). Physical activity and risk of colorectal cancer in men and women. *British Journal of Cancer, 73,* 1134-1140.

Wade, T. P., Virgo, K. S., Li, M. J., Callander, P. W., Longo, W. E., & Johnson, F. E., (1996). Outcomes after detection of metastatic carcinoma of the colon and rectum in a national hospital systems. *Journal of the American College of Surgeons, 182,* 353-361.

Winningham, M. L., Nail, L. M., Burke, M. B., Brophy, L., Cimprich, B., Jones, L. S., Pickard-Holley, S., Rhodes, V., St. Pierre, B., Beck, S., Glass, E. C., Mock, V. L., Mooney, K. H., & Piper, B. (1994). Fatigue and the cancer experience: The state of the knowledge. *Oncology Nursing Forum, 21,* 23-36.

Wolmark, N., Wieand, H. S., Rockette, H. E., (1993). The prognostic significance of tumor and location and bowel obstruction in Dukes B and C colorectal cancer: Findings from the NSABP clinical trials. *Annals of Surgery, 198,* 743-752.

Xing, P.X., Young, G. P., Ho, D., Sinatra, M. A., Hoj, P. B., & McKenzie, I. F. (1996). A new approach to fecal occult blood testing based on the detection of haptoglobin. *Cancer, 78,* 48-56.

Esophageal Cancer

Susan Weiss Behrend RN, MSN

EPIDEMIOLOGY

Esophageal cancer is the seventh most common cancer worldwide. It accounts for 1% of all cancer in the United States, with an incidence of 3.2 per 100,000, and causes 2% of all cancer deaths. Although the statistics appear lower than those for other cancer diagnoses, the significance of esophageal cancer should not be minimized. A comparison of esophageal cancer and rectal cancer demonstrates that the incidence of rectal cancer is four times higher; however, there are more reported deaths annually from esophageal cancer (approximately 11,000) than from rectal cancer (approximately 8000) (American Cancer Society, 1977). The incidence of esophageal cancer depends on age, sex, and race. Esophageal cancer is a disease of mid to late adulthood. Mortality rates increase with age, and the disease is rarely seen in individuals younger than 25 years (Blot, 1994). Esophageal cancer occurs more often among men; in all global reporting regions, rates are typically two to four times higher among males than females. Racial background differences also exist. Esophageal cancers occur more often in blacks than whites. Blacks have a higher incidence of squamous cell carcinomas, and adenocarcinoma is more common amongst whites. Younger black males have a higher rate of esophageal cancer than white males. This diagnosis is one of the most common malignancies among black men under age 55, second only to lung cancer (Blot, 1994) (Box 39-1).

Esophageal cancers are typically adenocarcinomas or squamous cell carcinomas. Historically, about 90% were squamous cell, and 10% adenocarcinomas. A recent shift in the United States has demonstrated approximately 50% of esophageal cancers to be squamous cell in origin. It is estimated that the rate of adenocarcinomas of the esophagus is increasing 10% annually, primarily among white men. This change is puzzling but may be attributed to high incidences of smoking and alcohol consumption in the United States (Blot, 1994). Adenocarcinomas occur commonly in the distal esophagus, although they frequently originate in the stomach. This pathologic shift is of tremendous importance for the development of new research protocols and treatment regimens for clinical disease management.

In addition, rare tumors of the esophagus exist and include undifferentiated small cell carcinoma, adenoid cystic carcinoma, mucoepidermoid carcinoma, leiomyosarcoma, and lymphoma (Klimstra, 1994) (Table 39-1).

RISK FACTORS

Risk factors associated with squamous cell carcinoma include alcohol and tobacco use, ingestion of pickled foods, low-calorie and low-protein diets, and consumption of hot beverages such as tea in Asia and in South Africa a drink known as *mate*. It has been suggested that a diet rich in citrus fruit and leafy green vegetables may decrease the risk factors (Blot, 1994) (Table 39-2).

Greater than half of all esophageal cancer occurs among ethnic populations (Cheng, 1994). In mainland China it is the second most common cancer, and it is endemic in the Linxian of Henan province. Almost half of all cancer deaths in this locality are esophageal. Ethnic Chinese in the United States experience a rate that exceeds that of whites (Cheng, 1994). Research investigations have studied the potential risk factors among this population and have found varied reasons for such endemic figures. These range from diet-related risks such as ingesting pickled vegetables containing N-nitroso compounds to drinking excessively hot beverages. Ingestion of Chinese liquor called "Samsu" amongst Chinese males and smoking Chinese cigarettes by Chinese females have been identified as additional lifestyle risk factors (Cheng, 1994; Frank-Stromborg, 1989).

Additional conditions associated with esophageal cancer include the following: tylosis—a rare genetic disorder characterized by palmar hyperkeratosis (Maesawa, Masuda, Tamura, Satodate, Ishida, & Saito, 1992); achalasia—a dysfunction of the peristalsis of the autonomic musculature of the esophagus; Plummer-Vinson syndrome—a rare type of iron deficiency anemia in Swedish women associated with cancer of the cervical esophagus; and Barrett's esophagus—replacement of smooth squamous epithelium with abnormal

Box 39-1
Epidemiology/Esophageal Cancer

- Seventh most common cancer worldwide
- Second most common of all U.S. cancer deaths
- U.S. incidence: 3.2 per 100,000
- Incidence 4 times greater than rectal cancer
- 11,000 deaths, esophageal cancer; 8,000 deaths, rectal cancer
- M > F; old > young; black > white
- *Endemic:* Lin Xian region—Central China East Coast-Southern Africa

Data from Roth, J. A., Putman, J. B., Rich, T. A., & Forastiere, A. A. (1997). Cancer of the esophagus. In V. T. DeVita, S. Hellman, & S. A. Rosenberg (Eds.), *Cancer: Principles & practice of oncology* (5th ed). Philadelphia: Lippincott-Raven.

columnar epithelium in the distal esophagus. Barrett's esophagus is associated with chronic gastroesophageal reflux predisposing individuals to the development of esophageal adenocarcinoma at a rate of 0.8%. Endoscopic examination of Barrett's esophagus demonstrates smooth pink tissue with an orange hue (Rosen, 1994; Spechler, 1994).

Greater than 90% of esophageal adenocarcinomas occur in the distal one third of the esophagus. These individuals often have a history of duodenal ulcer and hiatal hernia and may also be at risk for developing proximal gastric cancer.

Prevention, detection, and screening of esophageal cancer are limited. Unlike many other cancer diagnoses, limited emphasis has been placed on its diagnosis and control. Prevention and early diagnosis suggestions should include counseling regarding alcohol and tobacco use, reporting difficulty or pain with swallowing, modifying the diet, and seeking prompt multidisciplinary evaluations for any of the aforementioned symptoms. Screening has only occurred in global areas such as Asia, where this disease has been considered endemic, and has included brushing techniques.

Summary

Several esophageal cancer risk factors can be modified through lifestyle changes. Heretofore there are no studies identifying genetic risk factors. The prevalence of endemic rates of esophageal cancer among Chinese people is of particular significance for oncology nurses demonstrating multicultural competence within clinical practice. In addition, the high rates of this diagnosis among African American males (below age 55) (Blot, 1994) requires that the oncology nurse develop methodic care programs that are sensitive to diverse populations. Individuals with this diagnosis present tremendous challenges to the health care team. It is vital that comprehensive care planning occur that includes identification of multicultural risk factors and appropriate interventions to modify behaviors.

TABLE 39-1 Histology

Incidence	Percent
Adenocarcinoma	55
Squamous cell carcinoma	45
Rare histologies	<1
• Squamous cell with sarcomatoid features	
• Adenoid cystic carcinoma	
• Mucoepidermoid carcinoma	
• Small cell carcinoma	
• Sarcomas (leiomyosarcoma)	
• Lymphoma	

Data from Roth, J. A., Putman, J. B., Rich, T. A., & Forastiere, A. A. (1997). Cancer of the esophagus. In V. T. DeVita, S. Hellman, & S. A. Rosenberg (Eds.), *Cancer: Principles & practice of oncology* (5th ed.). Philadelphia: Lippincott-Raven.

TABLE 39-2 Etiology/Risk Factors: Squamous Cell Carcinoma

Increased Risk	Lessened Risk
Alcohol	Citrus fruit
Tobacco	Leafy greens
Pickled foods	Vegetables
Low calorie/low protein	
Hot beverages (Tea in Asia, mate in South America)	

PATHOPHYSIOLOGY

The normal anatomy and physiology of the esophagus are summarized in Fig. 39-1.

The esophagus is a hollow muscular tube that is flat in the resting state. It is composed of striated muscle in the upper part and smooth muscle in the lower. There is a sphincter mechanism at both ends, and there are areas of natural narrowing near the aorta and left mainstem bronchus.

The esophagus is innervated by the tenth and eleventh cranial nerves and also has sympathetic nervous fibers from the cervical and thoracic areas. Although pressure within the esophagus is lower than that within the stomach, stomach contents do not normally regurgitate into the esophagus because of pressure at the cardiac sphincter. The act of swallowing initiates a wave of peristalsis, which moves down the esophagus to the stomach. This contraction is preceded by a wave of relaxation. Food from the esophagus is propelled into the stomach by this peristaltic wave, gravity, and the opening of the cardiac sphincter during the wave of relaxation (Agur & Lee, 1991; Basmajian & Slonecker, 1989; Luckmann & Sorensen, 1993).

The esophagus starts at the cricopharyngeus muscle just below the larynx and extends to the gastroesophageal junction (see Fig. 39-1). It ranges from 22 to 29 cm from pharynx to stomach. It is divided into three principal regions: the cervical and upper thoracic esophagus; the mid-thoracic esophagus; and the lower esophagus. Each region and lesion is measured as a function of distance from the incisors (Coia & Moylan, 1994; Medvec, 1988).

The cervical/upper thoracic esophagus extends from the cricopharyngeus muscle (15 cm from incisors) to the thoracic inlet (18 cm from incisors), and the upper thoracic

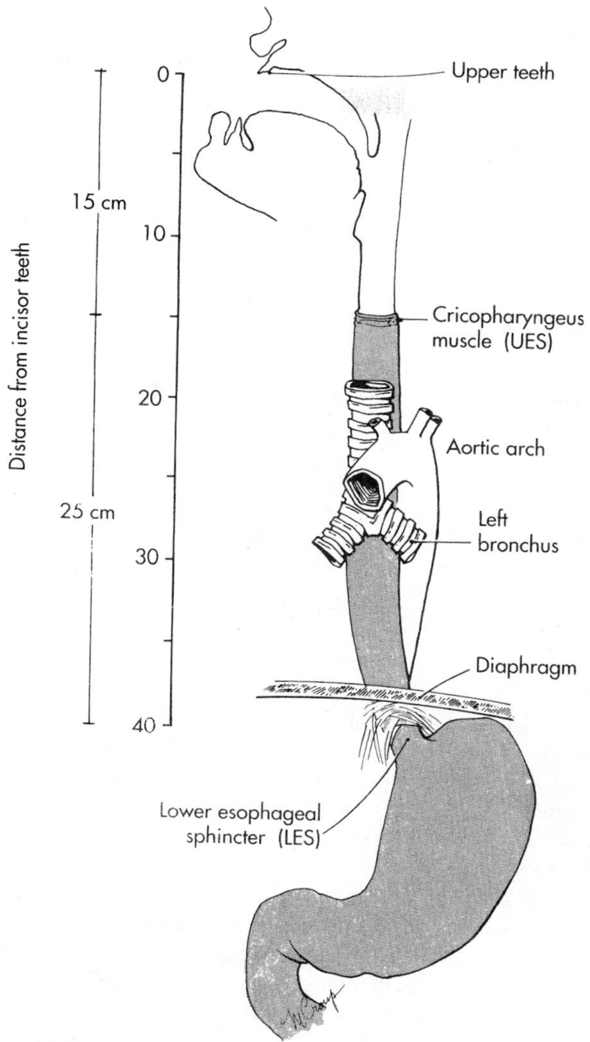

Fig. 39-1 Gross structure and anatomic relationships of the esophagus. (From Price, S. A.: [1997]. *Pathophysiology: Clinical concepts of disease processes* [5th ed]. St. Louis: Mosby.)

esophagus extends from the thoracic inlet to the carina (25 cm from incisors). The mid-thoracic esophagus extends from the thoracic inlet to 10 cm above the esophagogastric junction (or 32 cm from incisors, to the top of the T8 vertebral body). The lower thoracic esophagus extends from 10 cm above the esophagogastric junction to the esophagogastric junction (38 to 40 cm from incisors) (Coia & Moylan, 1994; Perez & Brady, 1992).

Each region of the esophagus accounts for a different percentage of malignancies from varied pathology and routes of local regional metastasis. The cervical/upper esophagus yields approximately 15% of all esophageal cancers, which are mainly squamous cell in origin. The pattern of lymph node spread from this region is as follows: cervical, 10%; supraclavicular, 40%; super mediastinum, 30%; middle mediastinum, 28%; lower mediastinum, 29%; and gastric nodes, 32%. The mid-thoracic esophagus yields approximately 35% of esophageal cancers, which are both squamous and adenocarcinomas. The pattern of lymph node spread from this region is as follows: supraclavicular, 25%; superior mediastinum, 11%; middle mediastinum, 21%; lower mediastinum, 33%; gastric, 33%; and celiac, 4%. The lower thoracic esophagus yields approximately 50% of all esophageal cancers, with 90% of adenocarcinoma pathology. The pattern of lymph node spread from this region is as follows: supraclavicular, 10%; superior mediastinum, 10%; middle mediastinum, 14%; lower mediastinum, 27%; gastric, 61%; and celiac, 21% (Akiyama, Tsurumaru, Kawamura, & Ono, 1981).

Table 39-3 Pattern of Spread vs Length

Length (cm)	Localized	Locally Advanced	DM's
<5	40%	25%	35%
>5	10%	15%	75%

Coia, L.R. (1996). Esophageal cancer: Refresher course. Paper presented at the American Society for Therapeutic Radiology and Oncology, Los Angeles

Pattern of Spread

Cancer of the esophagus can be devastating. This diagnosis is fatal because of both local progression and distant metastases. Unfortunately, fewer than 20% of those diagnosed have disease confined to the esophagus. Approximately 40% have regional lymph node involvement, and distant metastases are present in greater than 50% of patients. Patterns of metastatic spread depend on the length of the tumor, which is determined by barium swallow. If the tumor is less than 5 cm long, 40% are localized, 25% are locally advanced, and 35% have distant metastases. If greater than 5 cm, very few are localized (Coia, 1996) (Table 39-3).

Esophageal cancer typically spreads very rapidly along the axis of the esophagus through the wall and is aided by a rich lymphatic supply. Spread along the esophagus and through the esophageal wall is correlated with distant metastases and regional lymph node spread. Although squamous cell carcinoma was the most common pathology seen, the frequency of adenocarcinoma is rising, and the ratio is now approximately equal. Both of these tissue types are very aggressive, commonly penetrate through the wall of the esophagus, frequently involve nodes, and usually have occult systemic microscopic disease. The specific sites of nodal and distant metastases for adenocarcinoma differ from those of squamous cell carcinoma, with a greater propensity for developing brain metastasis reported in patients with adenocarcinoma. Table 39-4 summarizes distribution of metastases by anatomic site.

The Process of Carcinogenesis

The genetic lesions leading to the development of esophageal cancer have not been extensively identified (Rosen, 1994). It is likely that carcinoma of the esophagus develops from an accumulation of mutations in multiple suppressor

TABLE 39-4 Distribution of Metastases by Anatomic Site

Site	Number of Patients	Percent	Site	Number of Patients	Percent
Lymph nodes	8	73	Thyroid	5	6
Lung	41	52	GI serosa	5	6
Liver	37	47	Aorta	4	5
Adrenals	16	20	Peritoneum	4	5
Diaphragm	15	19	Small bowel	4	5
Bronchus	13	17	Appendix	2	3
Pleura	13	17	Brain	1	1
Stomach	12	15	Skin	1	1
Bone	11	14	Thoracic wall	1	1
Kidneys	10	13	Prostate	1	1
Trachea	10	13	Omentum	1	1
Pericardium	9	11	Large bowel	1	1
Pancreas	9	11	Bladder	1	1
Heart	7	9	Ureter	1	1
Spleen	6	8			

Coia, L. R. (1996). Esophageal cancer: Refresher course. Paper represented at the American Society for Therapeutic Radiology and Oncology, Los Angeles.

genes and proto-oncogenes (Rosen, 1994). The association with smoking among the prevailing risk factors may associate the diagnosis with a variety of mutations (Rosen, 1994). In addition, the increasing incidence of adenocarcinomas of the distal esophagus in a young population within the United States has been associated with Barrett's esophagus and chronic esophagitis. As a result of this shift in pathology, it has been hypothesized that a different sequence of causative molecular lesions exist for squamous cell carcinoma than for adenocarcinoma (Rosen, 1994).

The study of familial cancer traits may help to identify molecular events initiating carcinogenesis. Tylosis and Barrett's esophagus are two clinical presentations with genetic inheritance, suggesting the importance for identifying causal genes in the study of the genetic basis of esophageal cancer (Rosen, 1994). Esophageal cancer has been shown to have multiple chromosomal breaks and deletions. Aneuploidy is another sign that frequent mutations have occurred during tumor development. Aneuploidy reflects the presence of multiple genetic lesions and an increased genomic instability (Rosen, 1994). Significant aneuploidy can be detected in esophageal carcinoma (69% to 87%). This is correlated with prognosis, with diploid tumors having the longest survival. This phenotype may be associated with less of P53 and other suppressor genes (Coia, 1996; Rosen, 1994). P53 mutation can be indicative of an early lesion in the progression of some esophageal carcinomas. It has demonstrated overexpression in carcinoma in situ and in some patients with Barrett's esophagus (Flejou, Potet, & Muzeau, 1993; Ramal, Reid & Sanchez, 1992; Rosen, 1994). It is unknown if P53 overexpression leads to carcinoma. However, the existence of this suppressor gene may be responsible for the accumulation of other cellular mutations, as well as the resistance of esophageal carcinoma to cytotoxic treatment (Rosen, 1994).

Epidermal growth factor receptor (EGFR) and transforming growth factor antigen (TGFA) are biomarkers that are evident in esophageal cancer (Coia, 1996). EGFR and TGFA have been found to be overexpressed in squamous cell carcinoma of the esophagus and correlate with worse prognosis in patients undergoing esophagectomy (Coia, 1996; Rosen, 1994). Decreased expression of EGFR and TGFA following chemoradiation has been associated with longer survival (Coia & Moylan, 1994).

Elevated serum tumor markers have been identified among some individuals with squamous cell carcinoma of the esophagus (i.e., carcinoembryonic antigen CEA [39%], CA-50 [41%], and CA 19-9 [13%]. These studies can be helpful in identifying the correct diagnosis and for monitoring therapeutic response (Coia, 1996).

The process of carcinogenesis, including patterns of genetic alterations of esophageal carcinoma, has not been completely identified. Continuing this area of research is vital to correlate cellular behavior and clinical intervention. It is hoped that future applications of this research will lead to the development of cytotoxic regimens with the ability to inhibit the oncoproteins that sustain the malignant process of esophageal carcinoma (Rosen, 1994).

ASSESSMENT

A complete clinical assessment of the individual suspected to have a diagnosis of esophageal carcinoma begins with a detailed history and physical examination (Table 39-5). Frequently this diagnosis is insidious, and patients may report weight loss and difficulty swallowing that have been longstanding but not reported.

History

The individual should be identified for all of the known risk factors for esophageal cancer. In addition, a detailed history of the alimentary system should be documented. Dysphagia

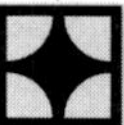

TABLE 39-5 Assessment of the Patient for Esophageal Cancer

	Assessment Parameters	Typical Abnormal Findings
History	A. Personal and social history 1. Age 2. Ethnicity/sex 3. Social and dietary	A. Personal and social risk factors 1. Usually over age 55 2. Blacks > whites males > females 3. History of alcohol consumption and cigarette use, extensive use of antacids, nitrate-laden foods, and hot beverages
	B. Evaluation of alimentary system	B. Common symptoms include: Dysphagia, odynophagia; weight loss; cough induced by swallowing; hoarseness; radiating back pain
	C. Evaluation for distant metastases	C. Patients with metastatic disease frequently complain of radiating back pain (which may indicate extra esophageal spread), dyspnea, bone pain, and abdominal distention.
Physical Examination	A. Thorough head and neck examination	A. 10%-15% of patients with esophageal cancer will develop a secondary primary malignancy within the aerodigestive tract.
	B. Weight	B. Baseline weight loss, which is a predictor of performance status.
	C. Lymph node evaluation	C. Presence of supraclavicular lymph nodes indicates metastatic disease.
	D. Liver palpation lung auscultation	D. Enlarged and painful liver and pulmonary compromise may indicate metastatic disease
Diagnostic Tests	A. Double-contrast esophagogram	A. Rules out fistula formation able to detect ulcerative, cytophytic, and superficial tumors
	B. Panendoscopy (esophagoscopy) with biopsy and brushings	B. Either rigid or flexible Determines pathologic diagnosis Examination of oral cavity, pharynx, larynx, tracheobronchial tree
	C. Computed tomograhy (CT) scan of chest and upper abdomen	C. Useful for preoperative staging and assessment of mediastinal and abdominal lymph nodes and liver metastases; clinical accuracy is as follows: 90% mediastinal involvement 78% abdominal node involvement 98% liver metastases
	D. Magnetic resonance imaging	D. Used as an alternative to CT for staging; provides less detail than CT scan
	E. Endoscopic ultrasound	E. Assesses mucosal and intramural lesions Vital for assessing depth of wall penetration and periesophageal nodes
	F. Bronchoscopy	F. Assess upper and middle thoracic tumors Evaluate tracheoesophageal fistula
	G. Percutaneous biopsy (CT guided)	G. Used to biopsy the neck and abdomen Accurate for diagnosis of squamous cell cancer of the esophagus
	H. Chest x-ray	H. Detects lung metastasis or secondary primary lung tumors
	I. Bone scan	I. Only ordered if patient complains of bone pain or an alkaline phosphatase is elevated
	J. Pulmonary function studies; routine blood studies	J. Pulmonary function test—lung involvement Anemia may indicate bleeding Abnormal chemistry—nutritional depletion

is the most common presenting symptom (it may include odynophagia); however, it does not occur until the circumference of the esophagus is narrowed one half to one third of normal. This symptom, including weight loss (potentially greater than 10%), may have been present up to 5 months before presentation (Coia & Moylan, 1994; Medvec, 1988). Cough induced by swallowing may indicate tracheoesophageal fistula. Hoarseness may be due to recurrent laryngeal nerve involvement. Radiating back pain may be indicative of extraesophageal spread (Coia & Moylan, 1994). The most common sites of distant metastases are lung, bone, or liver. Therefore individuals may report dyspnea, bone pain, and abdominal distention, which may be associated with malignant ascites.

Physical Examination

Although technologically advanced imaging techniques are vital to clinically diagnose esophageal cancer, a thorough physical examination should be the first diagnostic intervention performed. Emphasis should be placed on a detailed head and neck examination, since 10% to 15% of patients with esophageal cancer will develop a second primary malignancy within the upper aerodigestive tract (Coia & Moylan, 1994). In addition, examination includes potential sites of metastasis, such as supraclavicular lymph nodes, the liver, and lungs (Lightdale, 1994). Pulmonary function studies and nutritional and functional assessment should be performed. Laboratory tests can yield information regarding liver or bone metastasis, as well as identify chronic or acute anemia, which may indicate an active bleeding site (Coia & Moylan, 1994; Lightdale, 1994).

Diagnostic Studies

Several diagnostic studies are invoked to clinically evaluate patients with esophageal cancer. A thorough clinical investigation must include a battery of invasive and noninvasive procedures. Superb clinical expertise by the health care team coupled with detailed patient education materials should ensure safe, prompt, and accurate information delivery. A summary of diagnostic procedures for esophageal cancer is summarized in Table 39-6.

Esophagoscopy. Esophagoscopy is the most important study performed to measure and localize the disease. Biopsies and cytologic brushings are obtained, including a search for skip metastasis. Sometimes a secondary tumor is identified within a few centimeters from the primary tumor because of spread through the submucosal lymphatic network. If concern exists about tumor extension through to the aorta and other structures, a rigid technique is used (Coia & Moylan, 1994).

Double-Contrast Esophagogram. This is a barium swallow that is used for measuring and localizing the tumor. The esophagogram assesses patency and degree of circumferential involvement. This information is vital when ruling out fistula formation. In addition, this study may detect a second tumor. The type of macroscopic tumor morphology detected includes ulcerative, exophytic, and superficial. This pertinent diagnostic study is of importance to radiation oncologists for the purposes of treatment planning (Coia & Moylan, 1994).

Computed Tomography Scan of the Chest and Upper Abdomen. The computed tomography (CT) scan of the chest and upper abdomen is important for preoperative staging, as well as for the assessment of mediastinal and abdominal lymph node involvement, including liver metastasis (Thompson & Halvorsen, 1994). Accurate assessment of extraesophageal spread ideally requires a fat plane between the esophagus and surrounding structures. Unfortunately, most of the patients are nutritionally depleted, which may compromise this aspect of the study. Occasionally tumor extension into the trachea or bronchi can be seen on the CT scan, as well as the leakage of the contrast material outside the confines of the esophageal lumen and into the mediastinum (Coia & Moylan, 1994). This study is not as accurate in determining spread through the esophageal wall (longitudinal spread) or penetration of the various layers of the esophagus (radial spread). Clinical accuracy of the CT scan is as follows: mediastinal involvement, 90%; abdominal node involvement, 78%; and liver metastasis, 98%.

Magnetic Resonance Imaging. Magnetic resonance imaging (MRI) has been identified as an alternative to CT for staging purposes; however, it is unable to produce a detailed view of the mediastinum and upper abdomen at the same time. For this reason, CT scans are considered to be of greater use (Thompson & Halvorsen, 1994).

TABLE 39-6 Diagnostic Procedures for Esophageal Cancer

Method	Comments	Recommendation
Computed tomography (CT) scan	Useful in determining distant metastases to liver and lung and in assessing tumor width	Yes
Double-contrast esophagogram	Useful to detect and define primary lesion extent (length) and exclude presence of tracheoesophageal fistula; occasionally demonstrates a second tumor	Yes
Endoscopic ultrasound	More accurate than other studies in determining depth of wall penetration and peri-esophageal nodal involvement; cannot be used in about one fourth of patients because of stenosis	Yes
Bronchoscopy	Useful for upper thoracic and middle thoracic tumors to assess for evidence of tracheoesophageal fistula	In selected cases
Esophagoscopy	Essential in obtaining biopsy and localizing lesion	Yes
Percutaneous biopsies (CT guided)	Invasive but very accurate for squamous cell; rarely used in the chest, but may be used in the neck or abdomen	In selected cases
Chest x-ray	Useful for detecting metastases or second lung primary	Yes
Bone scan	Only useful if clinical signs warrant or unexplained elevation in alkaline phosphatase	In selected cases

Data from Roth, J. A., Putnam, J. B., Rich, T. A., & Forastiere. (1997). Cancer of the esophagus. In V. T. DeVita, S. Hellman, & S. A. Rosenberg (Eds.), *Cancer: Principles & practice of oncology* (5th ed.). Philadelphia: Lippincott-Raven.

In addition, the sensitivity and accuracy for the detection of aortic and pericardial invasion were similar for both CT and MRI scans. The use of CT scans is more cost effective because they are more readily available; thus CT scans remain the diagnostic study of choice (Thompson & Halvorsen, 1994).

Endoscopic Ultrasound. Endoscopic ultrasonography (EUS) has been identified as a new addition to diagnostic gastrointestinal endoscopy. EUS allows the assessment of mucosal and intramural lesions deep to the mucosa and esophageal wall penetration (Lightdale, 1994). EUS is not readily available in all institutions, but it is considered a vital staging study for determination of the depth of wall penetration and peri-esophageal nodal involvement.

EUS uses a water-filled balloon approximately 1.2 cm, which is around the ultrasound transducer, with the forward-oblique optics behind the transducer. The balloon provides acoustic contact and pushes the esophageal wall away from the transducer to bring it into focus (Jaklitsch, Harpole, Healy & Sugarbaker, 1994; Lightdale, 1994). This procedure enables visualization of the five layers of the esophageal wall: the first two layers are the superficial and deep mucosa, the third layer is the submucosa, the fourth is the muscularis propria, and the fifth is the serosa/adventitia (Jaklitsch et al., 1994; Lightdale, 1994). EUS is unique because of its ability to provide a view of the wall of the esophagus more detailed than any other method. This is very important information, as depth of wall penetration is associated with survival in this patient population. The accuracy of the determination of wall penetration is approximately 85% for T stage and approximately 75% for N stage, which indicates peri-esophageal node involvement (Coia, 1996).

Although EUS is considered an integral part of the diagnostic investigation for determining the degree of esophageal involvement, it does have some limitations. EUS is unable to make the distinction between neoplastic tissue and inflammation/fibrosis and hence should be invoked after a pathologic diagnosis is rendered. EUS complements the use of the CT scan and is considered more sensitive for evaluating T and N stages; however, is not appropriate to use for staging of distant metastases and abdominal nodes. In addition, in approximately one fourth of patients the inability to pass the probe (1.2 cm) because of stenotic/obstructing lesions can limit its clinical use (Jaklitsch et al., 1994; Lightdale, 1994).

Additional diagnostic and staging studies may include the following:

- Bronchoscopy is useful in selected cases to assess upper thoracic and middle thoracic tumors and to evaluate tracheoesophageal fistula formation. Bronchoscopy is not used if the patient has an adenocarcinoma of the distal third esophageal region.
- Percutaneous biopsies (CT guided) are used in selected cases. This is an invasive procedure that is rarely used in the chest but may be used in the neck or abdomen. It is accurate for diagnosing squamous cell cancer.
- A chest x-ray is useful for detecting metastases or second primary lung tumors.
- Bone scans are usually ordered only if the patient reports bone pain or if there is an unexplained elevation in alkaline phosphatase. In addition, pulmonary function studies and routine blood studies are obtained.

The numerous procedures used to stage the individual suspected of having esophageal cancer are diverse and require different dimensions of education and preparation. These studies may be done in hospital departments or ambulatory settings. Patients and families must receive detailed information regarding expectations to allay fears and misconceptions. A system for prompt retrieval of results should be provided so that the workup occurs swiftly and interventions are planned without delay. The oncology nurse working with this patient population should be dedicated to developing individualized approaches that appeal to a variety of adaptation skills during a most stressful experience. Patients are often evaluated by a multitude of health care teams, each having different expertise regarding the tests that must be performed. Preparation to consent and proceed with this complicated workup should be planned by the oncology nurse at the initial meeting so that a forum is created for exchange of queries and for the development of trusting professional relationships. Examples of patient education tools are outlined in Box 39-2 and Tables 39-7 and 39-8.

Box 39-2
What is Endoscopy?

What is Endoscopy?

A medical procedure used to explore the inside of an organ or body cavity.

What is an Endoscope?

- It is the instrument used during endoscopy.
- It is a long, flexible tube with an eyepiece at one end and a lens at the other.
- Tiny glass fibers within the tube can transmit light around curves.

Endoscopes Contain Special Instruments

- Forceps (to take tissue samples)
- Brushes (to sample cells)
- Cautery instruments (to stop bleeding)
- The eyepiece of the endoscope may also be fitted with a camera so results of examinations can be recorded on slides or photographs.

Endoscopy is an important tool for diagnosing disease. Endoscopy helps reduce the need for surgery because endoscopes can be passed through a body opening or small incision. Endoscopes are used to detect or study:

Lesions	Internal injuries
Tumors	Abscesses
Growths	Functional disorders
Malformations	Cause of pain or bleeding

Modified from *Manual of gastrointestinal procedures* (1989). (2nd Ed). New York: Society of Gastroenterology Nurses and Associates, Inc.

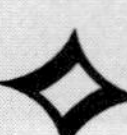

TABLE 39-7 Patient Preparation for Upper Gastrointestinal Endoscopy or Esophagogastroduodenoscopy

Description of the Procedure: EGD visualizes the lining of the esophagus (food tube), stomach, and first part of the small intestine (duodenum). It can help diagnose ulcers, gastritis, tumors, polyps, and lesions. It can also gather specimens for study.

Preparation: You may be instructed not to eat or drink anything for a specified period before the examination.

Before the Examination:

1. The test will be explained and you'll be asked to sign a consent form.
2. Your medical history will be taken. Report allergies and medications you are taking.
3. Remove dentures or partial plates and eyeglasses.
4. Your blood pressure and vital signs will be checked.
5. A needle for intravenous medicines will be placed in your vein before the procedure. Medicine will be given through this needle to help you relax and become sleepy.
6. Your throat may be sprayed or you will gargle with a numbing medicine.

During the Procedure:

1. You will lie on your left side. The doctor will place a small mouthpiece between your teeth. You will be able to breathe normally.
2. The doctor will help you to swallow the flexible endoscope tube, and the upper digestive system will be examined.
3. The study will take between 15 minutes and 1 hour.
4. A biopsy specimen (tiny bit of tissue) may be taken for microscopic examination. You will not feel any sensation or discomfort.

Special Considerations:

1. Many people do not recall any of the procedure because of the effect of the medication.
2. You may feel drowsy and sleep after the procedure.
3. Your tongue and throat may feel sore and swollen, and you may feel bloated, but the discomfort will pass.
4. The doctor will discuss the findings and the gastrointestinal nurse will give you written instructions.
5. If you have any questions, you must ask the health care team.
6. Complications are rare, but report any bleeding, pain, or fever after the procedure immediately.

Modified from *Manual of gastrointestinal procedures* (1989). (2nd Ed.). New York: Society of Gastroenterology Nurses and Associates, Inc.

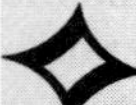

TABLE 39-8 Patient Preparation for Esophageal Dilation

Description of the Procedure: The procedure involves the dilation (stretching) of a narrowed area in your esophagus (food tube).

Preparation: You may be instructed not to eat or drink anything starting the night before the examination.

Before the Procedure:

1. Remove dentures or partial plates and remove eyeglasses.
2. The procedure will be explained and you'll be asked to sign a consent form.
3. Your medical history will be taken. Report allergies and medications you are taking.
4. Your blood pressure and vital signs will be checked.

During the Procedure:

1. You will be sitting in a chair or lying on your left side during the procedure.
2. Your throat will be sprayed or you will gargle with a numbing medicine.
3. The doctor will guide the flexible dilating tube through your mouth and into the narrowed area of your esophagus.
4. The tube will be withdrawn, and two or three slightly larger tubes will be passed and withdrawn the same way.
5. The procedure takes about 10 minutes and is well tolerated.
6. The dilation is repeated over time until the narrowed area is stretched to a bigger size.

Special Considerations:

1. Sometimes esophageal dilation is done following upper endoscopy.
2. Balloon dilators may be used; these are passed through the endoscopes over a guidewire.
3. Your doctor will inform you of the method used.
4. If fluoroscopy (x-ray) is used to assist in passing the dilator, you will lie on a special x-ray table, and the x-ray machine will be turned on during the procedure.
5. The physician and registered nurse will be with you at all times.

Adapted from Manual of gastrointestinal procedures (1989). (2nd Ed.). New York: Society of Gastroenterology Nurses and Associates, Inc.

STAGING

Precise staging of esophageal cancer is necessary to determine approporiate management and prognosis. The most common method of staging is based on the TNM staging system, which defines the anatomic extent of disease. *T* indicates the depth of primary tumor invasion. Squamous cell carcinoma and adenocarcinoma are staged similarly; they both arise in the mucosa and invade the deeper layers of the gastrointestinal tract wall. *N* indicates the spread of cancer to specified regional lymph nodes. In esophageal cancer any regional lymph node metastasis is considered N1. *M* indicates distant metastases to lymph nodes outside specified regional nodes or to distant organs not involved by direct extension from the primary tumor (Lightdale, 1994).

Two staging systems have been identified for esophageal cancer, shown in Tables 39-9 to 39-11. The 1983 American Joint Committee on Cancer (AJCC) (American Joint Committee on Cancer, 1983) staging system and the 1988 AJCC system (American Joint Committee on Cancer, 1988). The 1983 system is clinically useful and is based on axial and circumferential tumor spread. In this system tumor length correlates with local control and survival; however, it does not account for wall penetration or nodal involvement. The

Table 39-9 TNM Staging for Esophageal Cancer: 1983 AJC Staging System

Primary tumor (T)	
T0	No demonstrable tumor
TIS	Carcinoma in situ
T1	Tumor involves 5 cm or less of esophageal length with no obstruction; no circumferential involvement; no extraesophageal spread
T2	Tumor involves more than 5 cm of esophagus and produces obstruction with circumferential involvement of the esophagus but not extra esophageal spread
T3	Tumor with extraesophageal spread
Regional lymph nodes (N)	
Cervical esophagus (cervical and supraclavicular lymph nodes)	
N0	No nodal involvement
N1	Unilateral involvement (movable)
N2	Bilateral involvement (movable)
N3	Fixed nodes
Thoracic esophagus (nodes in the thorax, not those of the cervical, supraclavicular, or abdominal areas)	
NX	Nodes cannot be assessed
M0	No metastases
M1	Distant metastases. Cancer of thoracic esophagus with cervical, supraclavicular, or abdominal lymph node involvement is classified as M1

1988 AJCC staging system is based on wall penetration and nodal involvement; however, this system is based on pathologic findings after surgery; therefore it is not useful for nonsurgical treatment regimens or adjuvant protocols using radiation and/or chemotherapy. A modified 1983 AJCC system has been suggested for staging esophageal cancer. Table 39-12 provides a comparison of T-staging systems for esophageal cancer.

In addition to the AJCC staging system, complementary clinical prognostic factors are vital when evaluating patients. Karnofsky performance status, anatomic location of the tumor, age, gender of the individual (females have better prognoses than males), degree of mechanical dysphagia associated with anorexia and cachexia, and general physical well-being are important indicators for protocol eligibility and ability to withstand the rigors of multidisciplinary treatment.

MEDICAL MANAGEMENT

Treatment and Results

Patients with cancer limited to the esophagus (stage I or II) may be treated with curative intent. Palliation is the only realistic goal in patients with extraesophageal spread (stage III) or distant metastases (stage IV). The median survival for patients treated with surgery alone or radiation alone is less than 1 year. Five-year survival is generally less than 10% (Coia & Moylan, 1994).

Table 39-10 Stage Grouping for Esophageal Cancer

Stage I	Tumor that involves less than 5 cm of esophagus without obstruction; no circumferential, extraesophageal, or nodal involvement and no metastases
Stage II	*Cervical esophagus:* No extraesophageal involvement with movable regional lymph nodes (T1N1, T2N1) but no distant metastases, or a T2 tumor without lymph node involvement (T2N0)
	Thoracic esophagus: Any tumor that is greater than 5 cm in length or produces obstruction or involves the entire circumference of the esophagus without extraesophageal spread (T2NXM0)
Stage III	Any esophageal cancer with extraesophageal spread (T3NX) or, for cervical esophagus, any esophageal cancer with fixed nodes (any N3)
Stage IV	Presence of distant metastases (any T, any N, M1)

Table 39-11 TNM Staging for Esophageal Cancer: 1988 AJC Staging System

Primary tumor (T) classification	
T1	Tumor invades lamina propria or submucosa
T2	Tumor invades muscularis propria
T3	Tumor invades adventitia
T4	Tumor invades adjacent structures
Nodal (N) pathologic classification	
N0	No regional metastases
N1	Regional node metastases (celiac, abdominal nodes, and supraclavicular nodes are considered distant metastasis for tumors of the thoracic esophagus)
Distant metastases (M) classification	
M0	No distant metastases
M1	Distant metastases
Stage grouping	
Stage I	T1, N0, M0
Stage IIA	T2, N0, M0
	T3, N0, M0
Stage IIB	T1, N1, M0
	T2, N1, M0
Stage III	T3, N1, M0
	T4, Any N, M0
Stage IV	Any T, any M, M1

Surgery

Contemporary management of esophageal cancer commonly involves a multimodal approach. Surgical resection is considered the standard of care for operable patients with squamous cell carcinoma of the esophagus. Although esophagectomy offers effective palliation for many patients,

TABLE 39-12 Staging: A Comparison of T-Staging Systems for Esophageal Cancer*

T Stage	1988 AJC	1983 AJC	CT System
T1	Into submucosa	<5 cm, no obstruction, not circumferential	Intraluminal mass
T2	Into muscularis propria	>5 cm, obstruction or circumferential	Mass and wall thickening >5 mm
T3	Into adventitia	Clinical extraesophageal spread	Into adjacent structures
T4	Into adjacent structures	—	Distant metastases

From the American Joint Commerce on Cancer (1988). *Manual for staging of cancer* (3rd Ed.). Philadelphia: J.B. Lippincott.
*Note that these staging systems are significantly **different**. For example, at least 50% of T1 tumors by the 1983 AJC system are T3 tumors by the 1988 AJC system.

local disease control and survival are poor (Coia, 1989). Surgical mortality and morbidity are significant, and only 40% to 60% of patients undergo attempted "curative" resection. This is because the lesions often turn out to be more extensive at surgery than initially staged. Surgical removal of lesions less than 4 cm are more likely to be curative, whereas tumors longer than 9 cm have a worse outcome (Bremmer & DeMeester, 1991; Daniel & Shuey, 1993). Local recurrence following esophagectomy ranges from 16% to 67% and occurs within 2 years (Coia, 1996). In one trial local recurrence was seen in 33% of patients (23/70) undergoing esophagectomy alone, whereas local recurrence as a component of failure was reported at 67% (47/70) (Gignoux, Roussel, Paillot, Gillet, Schlag, Favre, et al., 1987). Many patients have relief from dysphagia after surgery, although swallowing is not normal and may require dietary modification. This complication is often accompanied by gastrointestinal reflux (Coia, 1996; Daniel, 1994).

Several surgical procedures exist for removing the esophagus. Surgeons frequently do not know before surgery whether the goals of cure or tumor debulking will be accomplished. Major surgical decisions that must be made include the following: identifying individuals who are appropriate surgical candidates, the most effective technique to use, and whether neoadjuvant treatment will be prescribed (Whyte & Orringer, 1994).

The esophagus is not easily accessible. It is located near the trachea, recurrent laryngeal nerves, thoracic duct, aorta, and pulmonary vessels. The major surgical procedures are esophagectomy (removal of a part of the cervical or upper two thirds of the thoracic esophagus) (Fig. 39-2) and esophagogastrectomy (removal of the lower third of the thoracic esophagus and the cardia of the stomach). End-to-end anastomosis of the remaining upper-to-lower esophagus and cardia is performed after esophagectomy (gastric pull-up). After esophagogastrectomy, the remaining esophagus is anastomosed to the posterior wall of the stomach. Another surgical option is colon interposition, a two-stage operation in which the esophagus is bypassed by a part of the colon in the first stage and removed in the second stage (Fig. 39-3). In this procedure the colon is used as a substitute for the resected esophagus instead of the stomach. This is an available option, especially for individuals who have had prior gastric surgery. If a colon interposition is chosen, either the right or left colon is used. Transposed segments of colon can elongate and result in obstructive symptoms that may require surgical revision of the cologastric anastomosis (Whyte & Orringer, 1994).

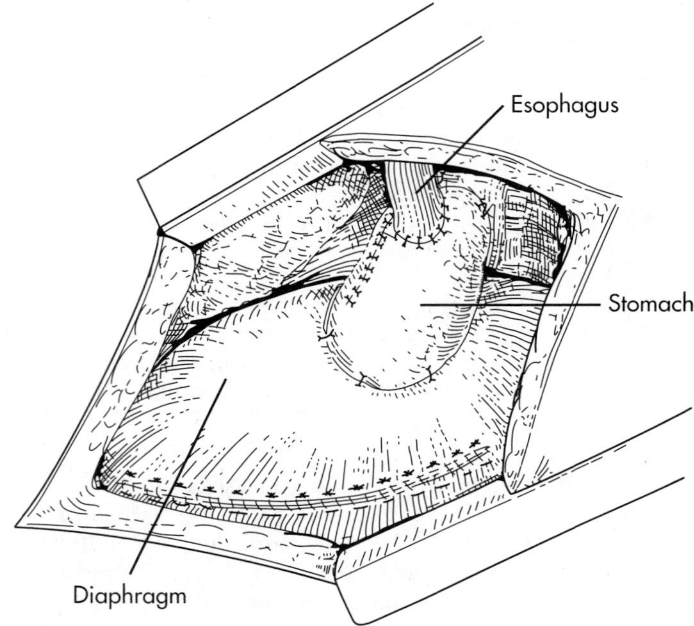

Fig. 39-2 The remaining distal portion of the stomach is mobilized into the chest through the hiatus and suspended to the prevertebral fascia. The esophagogastric anastomosis is constructed away from the line of gastric transsection. The stomach is sutured to the edge of the diaphragmatic hiatus to prevent subsequent herniation of the abdominal viscera into the chest. The diaphragm is reapproximated with heavy nonabsorbable mattress sutures and reinforced with a second, running whipstitch. (From Whyte, R. I. & Orringer, M. B. [1994]. Surgery for carcinoma of the esophagus: The case for transhiatal esophagectomy. *Seminars in Radiation Oncology, 4,* 146-156.)

Surgical approaches may include the Ivor-Lewis, transthoracic, and transhiatal approaches. The Ivor-Lewis procedure is basically a thoracoabdominal approach. Thoracotomy is performed on the right side, along with an abdominal incision.

Sometimes the surgeon may include a cervical incision to facilitate completion of cervical anastomoses. An alternative thoracoabdominal approach uses a left, instead of right, thoracotomy, providing the surgeon with more operative room when the tumor is above the esophagogastric junction (Daniel, 1994).

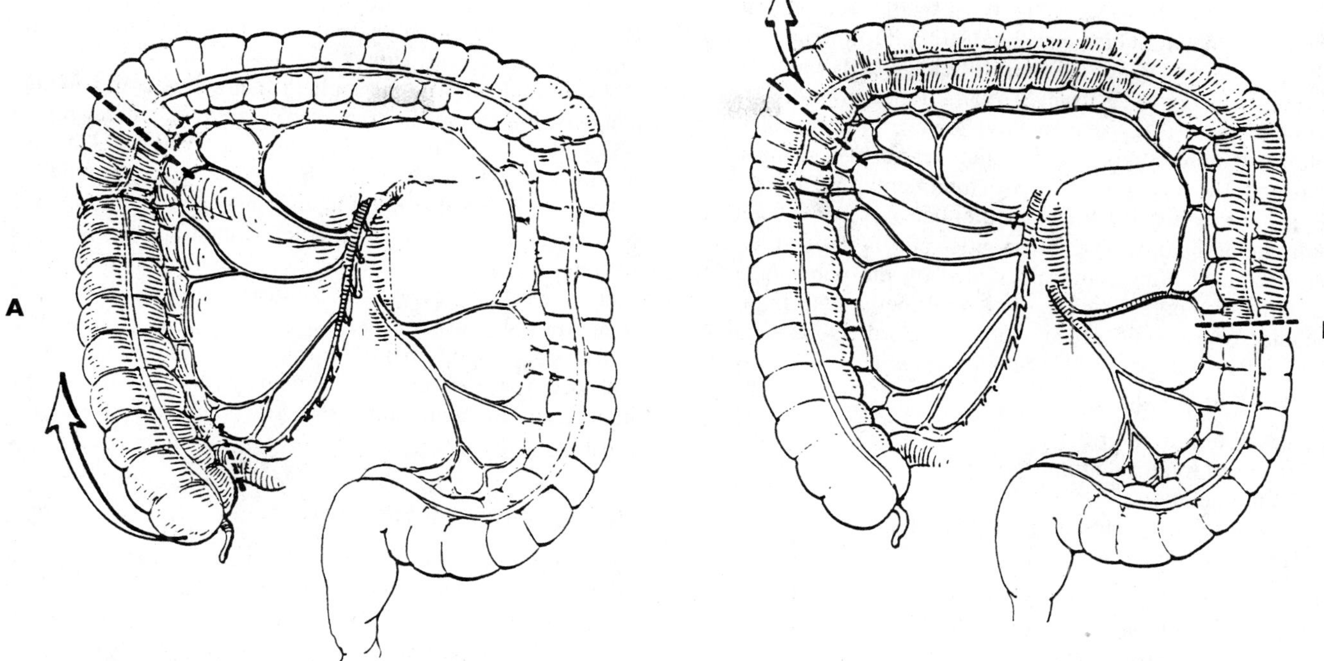

Fig. 39-3 Segments of colon can be used as esophageal substitutes. **A,** The right colon with its vascular supply, which is based on the right branch of the middle colic artery, is rotated as an isoperistaltic segment. **B,** The left colon with its vascular supply, which is based on the ascending branch of the left colic artery, is brought up in an isoperistaltic fashion. (From Whyte, R. I., & Orringer, M. B. [1994]. Surgery for carcinoma of the esophagus: The case for transhiatal esophagectomy. *Seminars in Radiation Oncology, 4,* 146-156.)

The transthoracic approach consists of thoracotomy alone and is generally performed in conjunction with an esophagogastrectomy. Unfortunately, approaches that include thoracotomy are accompanied by increased postoperative pain. The third alternative, especially for tumors located in the cervical or upper thoracic esophagus, is the transhiatal approach, which coincidentally has a lower mortality rate than the other approaches, with an average postsurgical hospital stay of 10 days (Whyte & Orringer, 1994). In this procedure cervical and abdominal incisions are performed to free the esophagus and facilitate tumor removal. Part of the procedure includes a blind dissection. Operating time for the transhiatal approach is significantly less than that for the transthoracic approach and has fewer postoperative complications (Daniel, 1994). The transhiatal approach has gained popularity among surgeons because it avoids thoracotomy and the potential for mediastinitis and sepsis. In addition, operative mortality rates associated with Ivor-Lewis and left thoracotomy are similar to those associated with the transhiatal technique (Whyte & Orringer, 1994). The major advantages associated with the transhiatal approach include low mortality if an anastomotic leak occurs and avoidance of the pulmonary complications of a thoracotomy. This approach is applicable to essentially all lesions of the esophagus and the gastric cardia, whereas thoracotomy approaches expose only one part of the esophagus (Whyte & Orringer, 1994).

Summary

Surgical approaches that treat esophageal cancer provide palliation and tumor control with varied rates of morbidity and mortality. Surgical resection alone does not result in long-term survival; therefore the need for combined modality therapy to control local-regional and micro-metastatic disease has evolved using varied combinations of neoadjuvant and adjuvant chemotherapy and radiation together with surgery or in combination, with omission of surgery, if clinically appropriate.

RADIATION

Although radiotherapy (RT) has been used to manage esophageal cancer since the discovery of radium as a single treatment modality, it is only moderately effective when used to control esophageal cancer. Local control of disease is stage dependent and ranges as follows:

Stage I	50%-75%
Stages II-III	9%-36%

Median survival is:

Stage I	20 months
Stage II-III	8-12 months

The results cannot be compared directly with surgical series because these patients had a lower performance status and tumors that were considered unresectable. RT alone has been shown to be inferior to the use of chemoradiation (Araujo, Souhami, Gil, Carvalho, Garcia, Froimtchuk et al., 1991; Herskovic, Martz, al-Sarraf, Leichman, Brindle, Vaitkevicius et al., 1992; Sischy, Ryan, Haller, Smith, Dayal, Schutt et al., 1990). Occasionally, however, patients are unable to tolerate combined modality treatment and must be managed by RT alone. Precise treatment planning techniques are required if RT is used either alone or combined with chemotherapy. The therapeutic ratio is defined as the percentage of tumor control divided by the percentage of normal tissue complications. Potential methods to improve the therapeutic ratio are as follows (Corn, Coia, Chu & et al., 1991; Gaspar, 1994; Smalley, Gunderson, Reddy & Williamson, 1994):

Increased tumor control:
- Increased total radiation dose
- Chemoradiation
- Accelerated/hyperfractionated radiation
- Brachytherapy

Decreased normal tissue complications:
- Improved radiation planning/delivery
  - Patient positioning
  - Reduction of volume of normal tissues irradiated
  - Three-dimensional treatment planning
- Hyperfractionation
- Brachytherapy

Brachytherapy

Intraluminal brachytherapy provides the benefit of delivering a high dose of radiation directly to the primary esophageal cancer in relation to the adjacent lung and spinal column (Gaspar, 1994). Renewed interest in this modality has recently evolved with the use of small high-activity sources in computerized afterloading machines that provide dose distributions able to conform to the size and shape of the primary lesion. In addition, safety for personnel and refinement of technical planning have been optimized. External beam RT may be supplemented by intracavitary brachytherapy, which is used primarily as a boost following external beam radiation. There have been no randomized trials comparing external beam alone with external beam and brachytherapy (Gaspar, 1994). Traditionally the brachytherapy "boost" volume includes the tumor and 1 to 2 cm of normal esophagus proximally and distally.

Esophageal brachytherapy has been described using low- (LDR), intermediate-, and high-dose rate (HDR) techniques. No evidence exists to determine that one dose rate is superior to another in terms of local control or morbidity (Gaspar, 1994). The dose rate range is as follows: LDR, 0.4 to 2 Gy/hr; IDR, 2 to 12 Gy/hr; HDR, greater than 2 Gy/min. LDR brachytherapy takes 1 to 2 days and is usually done on an inpatient basis in one or two treatments. HDR brachytherapy is completed within minutes but should be given in two to three fractions and requires repeated placement of the esophageal applicator (Coia, 1996; Gaspar, 1994). The choice of applicator diameter is important. A small applicator (less than 0.5 cm diameter) will result in a very high mucosal dose, leading to increased risk of stricture formation and ulceration. Brachytherapy in combination with chemotherapy can lead to severe mucosal toxicity.

Contraindications to esophageal brachytherapy include stenosis that cannot be bypassed, fistula, or patient refusal (Gaspar, 1994). Reports claiming improved local control or survival following brachytherapy may be attributed to selection bias (Nakajima, Fukuda, Hosono, Tsumura, Tada, Nishita et al., 1992). Methodic evaluation of risks and benefits must occur when prescribing brachytherapy regimens for esophageal cancer. Focus on side-effect management and supportive care must be primary and include nutritional support, pain control, and psychosocial issues. Respect for the patients' integrity and desires while maintaining ethical standards for practice and research must prevail.

Preoperative Radiation

Preoperative RT for esophageal cancer has been found to decrease local recurrence. However, randomized trials have failed to show improved resectability or survival. The following table summarizes four preoperative adjuvant RT trials. Patients who are thought to be resectable and are randomized to either preoperative RT or surgery alone have a poor survival, with the medians ranging from 10 to 12 months and 5-year survivals of 10% to 15%.

Postoperative Radiation

Two randomized trials of postoperative RT for carcinoma of the esophagus have been completed. Teniere found a decrease in local failure but no difference in overall survival. Fok found no difference in local recurrence rates between patients treated with curative resection alone and those treated with curative resection and postoperative RT. In addition, there was an increased risk of gastric complications with postoperative RT (37% vs 6%).

There is no indication among the six trials involving preoperative and postoperative radiation that an impact on survival occurred. The possibility of any undetected survival benefit would be small and offset by the morbidity and cost of treatment (Smalley et al., 1994). The routine use of adjuvant RT as a single-modality treatment is not warranted on the basis of these trials. Occasional patients with gross or microscopic disease have been cured with postoperative RT; therefore in this select population this therapy may be warranted (Smalley et al., 1994).

CHEMOTHERAPY

Research and clinical experience have demonstrated that the currently available chemotherapeutic agents for treating esophageal cancer are moderately effective (Ajani, 1994). The need to develop protocols that will deliver optimal doses and ample duration coupled with the development of new agents may provide an enhanced outlook for treating a refractory disease. The most effective therapeutic approach has not been defined; however, a focus on using combination chemotherapy with surgery or RT or both may be an appropriate goal.

Several challenges exist when considering the use of chemotherapy to treat esophageal cancer. The rarity of the disease and the high rates of morbidity and mortality have slowed drug development. A small percentage, approximately 15%, of phase II test agents over the past two decades have been tested against esophageal cancer (Ajani, 1994). The majority of drugs were tested on squamous cell carcinoma and may not apply to adenocarcinoma. The variance of chemosensitivity between adenocarcinoma and squamous cell carcinoma has not been studied adequately. Because of the rising predominance of adenocarcinoma, it will be imperative to address this when chemotherapeutic agents are prescribed (Ajani, 1994). Squamous cell carcinoma of the esophagus is sensitive to various single-agent and combination chemotherapies. Fifteen chemotherapeutic agents have been investigated predominantly in patients with squamous cell carcinoma of the esophagus. Single agents are considered active if they demonstrate a partial or complete response rate of at least 20% in previously untreated patients with carcinoma of the esophagus. Eight active agents identified are as follows: bleomycin, cisplatin, 5-fluorouracil, methotrexate, methyl-GAG, mitomycin-C, paclitaxel, and vindesine (Ajani, 1994).

Limited numbers of studies in patients with adenocarcinoma of the esophagus suggest that it is also chemosensitive (Ajani, 1994). The natural history of squamous cell carcinoma and adenocarcinoma varies and impacts upon the efficacy of treatment. Carcinoma of the cervical esophagus acts similarly to head and neck cancer, causing local morbidity and less metastases when compared with carcinoma of the thoracic esophagus (Ajani, 1994).

Small-cell carcinoma of the esophagus is highly chemosensitive and radiosensitive. It is similar to small cell lung cancer and responds to many chemotherapeutic agents, including etoposide and cisplatin.

Combination chemotherapy demonstrates similar limitations to those of single-agent usage. Some of these issues are a limited number of studies in patients with adenocarcinoma and the lack of controlled randomized studies to demonstrate survival advantage. Results cannot be generalized between the histologic types, and more studies focusing on treating adenocarcinoma are necessary (Ajani, 1994).

Two regimens have been studied extensively in patients with squamous cell carcinoma. These include bleomycin + cisplatin + vindesine and 5-FU + cisplatin. The former regimen has demonstrated a 48% response rate. Because of toxicities, this regimen has been stopped and replaced with the latter. The 5-FU + cisplatin regimen for squamous cell carcinoma of the esophagus demonstrates results within a 50% to 60% response rate. This regimen should be considered the standard for patients with squamous cell carcinoma of the esophagus (Ajani, 1994). In addition, both drugs have radio-enhancing effects and have been studied with the concomitant use of RT compared to RT alone (Herskovic et al., 1992).

No standard regimen for adenocarcinoma of the esophagus exists. An undocumented clinical perception may exist that reflects the refractory profile of adenocarcinoma to chemotherapy; however, no data exist to support or disagree with this thought (Ajani, 1994). The number of studies for adenocarcinoma of the esophagus are few, with limited patients enrolled. Some regimens studied, which are cisplatin-based, demonstrate a response rate between 40% to 50% (Ajani, 1994; Ajani, Roth, Putnam, Ryan, Walsh, Lynch et al., 1992; Ajani, Roth, Ryan, Putnam, Pazdur, Levin et al., 1993). It is of the utmost need to create new regimens using paclitaxel, 5-FU, and cisplatin. New agents, including topoisomerase-I inhibitor and other new agents in pharmaceutical development, may be used to treat adenocarcinoma of the esophagus.

If chemotherapy is given before surgery, the surgical specimen will provide information about the pathologic response. A significant survival advantage is paramount to the effectiveness of the treatment regimen. Continued research to develop new drugs and less toxic regimens are vital to ultimately finding appropriate treatment regimens required to control, palliate, and potentially cure this difficult disease. Additional research questions that require answers include how many chemotherapy cycles are necessary and why has tolerance of preoperative chemotherapy improved, whereas that for postoperative administration has not.

Chemotherapy as a combination regimen has created significant improvements in patient management. The benefit of preoperative chemotherapy alone has not demonstrated any survival benefit; however, results of radiotherapy oncology group (RTOG) trial to answer this query are pending. The rise in adenocarcinoma requires that treatment regimens study the distinct histologies of esophageal cancer (squamous and adenocarcinoma) without assuming similar chemosensitive profiles. New product development should be rapidly developed to promote pathologic response rates and maintain low side-effect profiles. In addition, the effective sequencing of chemotherapeutic regimens with other treatment modalities must be identified and applied clinically.

Preoperative Chemoradiation

Several phase II trials using preoperative chemoradiation have been published. These studies have shown a pathologic complete response rate of approximately 25% to 35%. The median survival of such patients was greater than that for patients with residual cancer, and in some studies only those patients who had pathologically negative specimens were long-term survivors. Postoperative mortality was significant (10% to 30%) (Coia & Moylan, 1994). Cisplatin-containing regimens have been found to be the most effective. Low-dose RT (30 Gy) combined with chemotherapy (infusional 5-FU and mitomycin or cisplatinum) used before surgery produced some promising results, but these results were not substantiated in large group studies. High-dose preoperative radiation and concurrent chemotherapy have also produced some promising results, especially in patients with adenocarcinoma of the esophagus (Coia & Moylan, 1994). Concomitant chemoradiation produces acute toxicities, which must be intensely managed.

Superior results using preoperative chemoradiation were reported from Forastiere (1994). In this study, conventional radiation to 44 Gy was given concurrently with 4 weeks of continuous-infusion 5-FU (300 mg/m2) and continuous-infusion cisplatin (130 mg/m^2) for the first and last 5 days of radiation. Transhiatal esophagectomy was performed 4 weeks later. The pathologic complete remission (CR) rate was 40%, and median survival was 35 months.

Two phase III randomized trials of preoperative chemoradiation vs. surgery (Bosset, 1994; Urba, 1995) have shown no improvement in overall survival. However, the accrual was small and with only brief follow-up times.

In summary, with notable exceptions of the Michigan pilot study (Forastiere, 1994) and the most recent study from Johns Hopkins, most studies in multimodality therapy for esophageal cancer fail to demonstrate significant improvement in survival and results are similar to the poor results achieved with standard therapies. However, they have shown that a high pathologic confirmed complete response rate of 25% to 35% can be obtained with modest doses of radiation and concurrent chemotherapy. The survival in responders was significantly better than that in nonresponders, and in several studies the only long-term survivors were those without evidence of tumor in the resected specimen. These studies raise two important related questions. The first is, "Can we avoid esophagectomy?" The second is, "Can higher doses of radiation result in an even higher rate of complete disappearance of local disease?" Contemporary research investigating the use of chemotherapy and radiation without surgery is a promising field that may provide improved clinical responses (Coia, 1996).

Chemoradiation without Surgery

The use of chemotherapy and RT to treat esophageal cancer without surgery is gaining clinical respect as a result of the refinement of systemic and local-regional treatment techniques. Although surgery has always been the standard of care for resectable esophageal tumors, the associated acute and long-term side effects impair quality of life significantly without affecting long-term survival. No prospective randomized trial exists comparing chemoradiation with surgery; however, distinct advantages and disadvantages are present for both (Coia & Moylan, 1994).

The following advantages of chemoradiation have been identified: wider applicability compared with surgical resection; treatment of both systemic and local-regional disease at the earliest stage; lower treatment-related mortality; potential for improved swallowing in long-term survivors; and possibility of surgical salvage in patients with persistent local disease without distant metastases (Coia & Moylan, 1994).

Potential disadvantages to chemoradiation as primary management of esophageal cancer are as follows: surgical resection may provide rapid relief of dysphagia along with a lower local failure rate than some chemoradiation regimens (Herskovic et al., 1992; Sischy et al., 1990); radiation may diminish the ability to give adjuvant chemotherapy and potentially impede the effectiveness of systemic chemotherapy; acute toxicities can be substantial; and the impact of these side effects has not been compared with the morbidity of surgical resection (Coia & Moylan, 1994). The majority of studies using chemoradiation have been done with patients with squamous cell carcinoma of the esophagus. Limited experience with the use of chemoradiation as primary management of adenocarcinoma of the esophagus exists, even though the incidence of this type of esophageal cancer is rising the United States (Coia & Moylan, 1994).

Chemotherapy and RT are combined according to the following three conceptual models: concurrent, sequential, and alternating. Concurrent use of chemotherapy with RT is the most frequent way these modalities are combined in the treatment of esophageal cancer. Four factors have been described that illustrate concurrent use of chemotherapy and RT to yield improved treatment results:

1. Spatial cooperation of chemotherapy and RT is important because of the propensity of this cancer to progress both locally and distantly.
2. Independent toxicity may occur; although acute esophageal toxicities are worse with chemotherapy and RT, there is no evidence that late toxicities are increased.
3. Enhanced tumor activity may result from the use of drugs such as cisplatin or 5-FU and also with such drugs as mitomycin.
4. Normal tissue protection with protective drugs such as WR-2721 is under investigation (Steel & Peckham, 1979).

Sequential use of early intensive chemotherapy involves the neoadjuvant use of chemotherapy and is based on studies that have demonstrated that resistance to chemotherapy develops over a narrow range of cell growth (Goldie & Coldman, 1983). One disadvantage to this approach is that, during the weeks of chemotherapy, the possibility exists for accelerated repopulation of tumor clonogens before the start of RT. There are relatively few publications on the use of neoadjuvant chemotherapy before RT alone or before chemoradiation, but this approach is under investigation (Coia & Moylan, 1994).

Alternating chemotherapy with RT in an attempt to maximize advantages and minimize side effects has been tested (Looney, Hopkins & Kovaca, 1983). This involves treating with chemotherapy during the days of rest from split-course radiation. Some of the toxicity of concurrent treatment may be minimized. Using this schedule, overall treatment time does not need to be lengthened, and the total RT dosage is not reduced. This schedule has been clinically applied with the treatment of cancer of the head and neck and minimally with treatment of the esophagus (Coia & Moylan, 1994).

Treatment Results: Chemoradiation Without Surgery

Three early studies on the use of concurrent chemoradiation were reported in 1980. The first to report the use of infusional 5-FU and radiation for esophageal cancer (Byfield, Barone, Mendelsohn, Frankel, Quinol, Sharp et al., 1980) found a complete response rate in five of six patients (83%) treated with RT combined with continuous infusion 5-FU. This was a split-course treatment, as it was given every other week for a total of 60 Gy over 11 weeks. This treatment regimen was well tolerated, with the primary toxicity consisting of hematologic suppression. One patient was alive without disease at 22 months. A series of small randomized trials followed that reported examining the use of RT alone vs RT plus bleomycin, RT plus adriamycin, or RT plus bleomycin and adriamycin (Kolaric, Maricic, Roth & Dujmovic, 1980). The response rate to concurrent chemotherapy and RT, regardless of the drugs used, was superior to that of RT alone, with a slight improvement in survival. A larger phase III cooperative group trial failed to corroborate the advantage of concurrent bleomycin and radiation over radiation alone (Earle, Gelber, & Moertel, 1980). The median survival in this study was poor and nearly identical in both treatment arms (i.e., concurrent treatment, 6.2 months, vs RT alone, 6.4 months).

Several investigators began to examine the use of concurrent RT and chemotherapy without surgery. At Fox Chase Cancer Center, a pilot study was begun in 1980 using conventional RT to 60 Gy with two 96-hour infusions of 5-FU (1 g/m^2) on days 2 to 5 and 29 to 32, with bolus mitomycin-C (10 mg/m^2) on day 2. These results for both patients with squamous cell cancer and adenocarcinoma of the esophagus have been previously reported (Coia, 1984; Coia, Engstrom, & Paul, 1987; Coia, Paul, & Engstrom, 1988). In the most recent published series, 90 patients were treated prospectively with this regimen, with a median follow-up time of 45 months (Coia, Engstrom, Paul, Stafford & Hanks, 1991). Fifty-seven patients with stage I/II disease received 60 Gy in 6 to 7 weeks. Thirty-three patients with stage II/IV disease received 50 Gy. All patients were treated with the concurrent chemotherapy regimen described here.

Results of this study are encouraging. Approximately 90% of patients had an improvement in dysphagia. The median time to improvement was less than 2 weeks. Median survival of stage I/II patients was 18 months. The actuarial freedom from local relapse rate was 73% at 1 year and 60% at 3 years. Of the 25 patients with more than 1 year follow-up, 68% were asymptomatic. Only 25% had some dysphagia to solids, and 12% had some dysphagia to soft foods. Median survival for stage III patients was 9 months and for stage IV patients, 7 months. Symptomatically, 77% of these patients were rendered free of dysphagia. Sixty percent were without dysphagia until death with a median time of 5 months. Eleven of 90 patients (12.2%) experienced severe acute toxicities. Three patients required hospitalization for management of treatment-related complications. There were no deaths due to treatment. Failure analysis revealed distant metastases as the predominant site of failure. Isolated local regional failure was rare. Of 29 patients who developed recurrent disease, 14 had local regional failure as a component, and 21 had distant metastases as a component of failure.

Four randomized Eastern Cooperative Oncology Group (ECOG) and Radiation Therapy Oncology Group (RTOG) trials comparing definitive chemoradiation vs RT alone have been completed. Both the trials have shown an improvement in median survival in the chemoradiation arm vs the RT alone arm. The ECOG conducted a randomized trial of concurrent chemotherapy with 5-FU and mitomycin and RT to 60 Gy using a treatment regimen essentially the same as used at Fox Chase vs RT alone to 60 Gy (Sischy et al., 1990). With 127 patients who were able to be evaluated, there was a statistically significant improvement in median survival from 9 months in patients treated with RT alone to 14.9 months in patients treated with concurrent RT and chemotherapy. In the RTOG trial (Herskovic et al., 1992), there was a significant difference in overall survival between the chemoradiation vs RT alone arms (25% vs 0% at 5 years). In addition, chemoradiation provided better local control (50% vs 25% at 2 years) and freedom from distant metastases (75% vs 25% at 2 years). However, there were more toxicities associated with the chemoradiation arm. These were predominantly that of mucositis of the upper aerodigestive tract (33% vs. 18%) and hematologic (8% vs 0%). It should be noted that in the combined arm the radiation dose was decreased to 50 Gy from 64 Gy in the RT alone arm.

In a study from Brazil (Araujo et al., 1991), 59 patients were randomized over a 3-year accrual to receive either RT alone to 50 Gy vs. RT to 50 Gy with concurrent 5-FU, mitomycin, and bleomycin. There was almost a threefold improvement in 5-year survival from 6% to 16%. However, because of the small numbers of patients in treatment arms, the power to detect the difference between these treatment arms, even with this large difference in survival, was less than 50%. To detect a 50% improvement in median survival with an 80% power, approximately 90% patients would need to be accrued to each treatment arm.

A trial conducted by the EROTC (Gill, Denham, Jamieson, Devitt & Olweny, 1992) involving over 200 patients with inoperable squamous cell carcinoma of the esophagus randomized patients to 20 Gy/5 fx/5d given twice with a 15-day rest plus cisplatin (100 mg/m^2) given before each course of RT and every 3 to 4 weeks to a total of six cycles. There was a significant improvement in local control and freedom from progression but not in survival with chemoradiation in these patients with advanced cancer.

A recent intergroup phase III randomized study comparing combined chemotherapy plus RT treatment vs RT only in patients with locally advanced esophageal cancer was just completed (al-Sarraf, Martz, Herskovic, Leichman, Brindle, Vaitkevicius et al., 1997).

Adenocarcinoma. The standard treatment of adenocarcinoma of the esophagus has been surgery. Local recurrence rates for adenocarcinoma are similar to those of squamous cell carcinoma. Distant metastases have been found more frequently in adenocarcinomas. Adenocarcinomas spread to pleura, bone, liver, lung, brain, and peritoneum. Prognosis is poor, with median survival in the range of 15 to 18 months.

There have been attempts at trimodality treatment (chemoradiation before or after surgery). In a nonrandomized design, the Fox Chase Cancer Center has compared the results of chemoradiation alone vs chemoradiation followed by esophagectomy in potentially resectable patients. Conventional RT to 60 Gy was given concurrently with infusional 5-FU and bolus mitomycin-C. There was no difference in median survival (19 months of chemoradiation vs

15 months of chemoradiation and surgery). However, there have been only 35 patients treated with these two regimens (Algan, Coia, Keller, Engstrom, Weiner, Schultheiss et al., 1995). These data suggest that chemoradiation may be as effective as surgery, although there is a higher rate of local failure with chemoradiation alone. In the chemoradiation group all eight evaluated patients had no difficulty swallowing. In the chemoradiation and esophagectomy group, 8 of 11 patients had no difficulty swallowing, whereas 3 patients had dysphagia. Surgical salvage in the event of local regional failure after chemoradiation remains an option (Algan et al., 1995).

An additional phase I/II study began 4 years ago at Fox Chase Cancer Center that involved treating patients with adenocarcinoma of the esophagus (Investigational Review Board [IRB] Protocol 94088, 1993). The study involved administering taxol, cisplatin, and 5-FU along with RT to 60 Gy before esophagectomy. Specifically the doses were as follows: 5-FU at 226 mg/m^2 as a continuous infusion during the course of RT and weekly taxol on a dose-escalated schedule from 10 mg up to 60 mg/m^2 and daily RT to 60 Gy. The patients were then reevaluated, and, if they did not have progressive disease, they proceeded to esophagectomy. The planned accrual of 50 patients was achieved, and the study closed in 1996. This regimen was rigorous and required tremendous supportive care. Patients required nutritional support, including parenteral feedings, as well as hematologic support and pain control. A multidisciplinary approach was required to administer this type of aggressive treatment. It is too soon to predict results; the hope is that taxol will prove to be an important new agent in combination regimens.

A prospective randomized trial comparing multimodal therapy and surgery for esophageal adenocarcinoma was conducted in an attempt to validate that a combination of chemotherapy and RT improves the survival of patients with esophageal adenocarcinoma (Walsh, Noonan, Hollywood, Kelly, Keeling & Hennessy et al., 1996). Patients assigned to multimodal therapy received two courses of chemotherapy in weeks 1 and 6 consisting of 5-fluorouracil, 15 mg/kg daily for 5 days, and cisplatin, 75 mg/m^2 on day 7 and a course of radiotherapy 40 Gy, in 15 fractions over 3 weeks beginning concurrently with the first course of chemotherapy, followed by surgery. Patients assigned to surgery had no preoperative therapy. Thirteen of 52 patients (25%) who underwent surgery after multimodal therapy had complete responses as determined pathologically. At the time of surgery, 42% of patients treated with preoperative multimodal therapy had positive nodes or metastases, as compared with 82% who underwent surgery alone. The median survival of patients assigned to multimodal therapy was 16 months, as compared with 11 months for those assigned to surgery alone. At 1, 2, and 3 years, 52%, 37%, and 32%, respectively, of patients assigned to multimodal therapy were alive, as compared with 44%, 26%, and 6% of those assigned to surgery, with the survival advantage favoring multimodal therapy reaching significance at 3 years. The conclusions of this study validate that multimodal treatment is superior to surgery alone for patients with resectable adenocarcinoma of the esophagus (Walsh et al., 1996).

Chemoradiation is an effective and relatively well-tolerated regimen in the treatment of esophageal cancer. Survival and enhanced local control appear to be greater when a combination of modalities is used than when RT is used alone. No successfully completed randomized trial involving surgery vs definitive RT and concurrent chemotherapy exists. However, the results reported thus far suggest that chemoradiation provides a viable alternative to esophagectomy in the primary management of squamous cell carcinoma of the esophagus. With limited data, chemoradiation also appears to be effective in the treatment of patients with adenocarcinoma of the esophagus, offering significant palliation and the potential for long-term survival (Coia & Moylan, 1994).

PALLIATION

Palliative care for patients with advanced esophageal cancer has been very successful and includes surgery, radiation, chemotherapy, and endoscopic procedures. These interventions are sometimes used alone or in combination and depend on the patients' willingness to receive aggressive treatment, performance status, medical history, and stage of disease.

Surgery

Esophagectomy or bypass surgery results in reasonably good palliation of dysphagia but demonstrates significant morbidity and mortality (Bown, 1991; Coia & Moylan, 1994; Orringer, 1984; Segalin, Little, Ruol, Ferguson, Bardini, Norberto et al., 1989). The rate of palliation is 70% to 80% with severe complication rates of 20% to 50% and mortality rates of 10% to 20%. Thirty-percent of patients will subsequently have recurrence of dysphagia and require further treatment. Therefore surgical bypass is rarely used in patients with advanced disease (Stoller & Brumwell, 1984). In addition, because of many less invasive treatments available, surgery is not routinely recommended in patients whose life expectancy is short. Palliative esophagectomy or bypass is still used when a curative intent demonstrates extensive disease intraoperatively (Ahmad, Goosenberg, Frucht, & Coia, 1994).

Radiation Alone

Radiation alone is an effective modality in palliating advanced esophageal cancer, with symptomatic improvement in 50% to 76% of cases. Duration of palliation is 5 to 10 months. There is better palliation with the use of higher doses (45 to 50 Gy) vs lower doses. However, 30% to 50% of radiated patients will develop benign or malignant strictures requiring dilation. Radiation therapy for advanced esophageal cancer is much less morbid than surgery and has almost equivalent rates of palliation. Radiation alone has been recognized as an effective palliative modality in treating advanced esophageal cancer. Radiation can provide successful palliation of dysphagia (70% to 89%) in patients who are unresectable due to advanced disease or poor health (Ahmad et al., 1994). The duration of symptomatic relief varies (Ahmad et al., 1994).

Chemoradiation

In patients with adequate performance status, chemoradiation is superior to RT alone. Chemoradiation for stage III/IV disease can achieve effective palliation in 60% to 70%. Coia et al. (1991) have used 50 to 60 Gy in conventional fractionation with concurrent 5-FU and mitomycin-C. Seventy-seven percent of patients were palliated with a median duration of 5 months. Morbidity from the combined therapy included esophagitis, nausea and vomiting, and myelosuppression. Severe acute toxicity requiring hospitalization occurred in only 7% of patients (Coia et al., 1991).

Endoscopic and Endocavitary Palliation

Endoscopic procedures provide significant therapeutic palliation for patients with advanced esophageal cancer. These procedures are helpful when obstructive symptoms occur or if a tracheosophageal fistula develops. Referrals for endoscopic therapy are made after patients fail primary treatment, and the clinical presentation includes local failure with recurrent dysphagia or stricture (Ahmad et al., 1994). Primary endoscopic modalities are often suggested for patients with a poor performance status as they are usually unable to tolerate aggressive treatment. Endoscopy has not shown improvement in survival; however, the safety, efficacy in symptom control, and ability to perform these procedures in ambulatory settings designates them as valuable for providing symptomatic palliation of a very difficult disease (Ahmad et al., 1994).

Esophageal Dilation. The primary advantage of endoscopic dilation of esophageal strictures is immediate relief of dysphagia. This outpatient palliative technique can be done with ease and requires inexpensive and readily available equipment. Dilation usually precedes other endoscopic modalities to widen the stenotic area before laser or stent placement. Esophageal dilation only provides transient symptomatic relief and frequently needs to be repeated. Dilators enlarge the esophageal lumen by tearing soft tissue. This can lead to perforation. Bacteremia occurs frequently, and for this reason the American Heart Association recommends antibiotic prophylaxis to reduce the potential risk of endocarditis (Dajani, Bisno, Chung & et al., 1990; Neu, 1989).

The most commonly used dilators are polyvinyl dilators, rubber bougienage catheters, and hydrostatic balloons. Polyvinyl dilators are passed over an endoscopically placed flexible guidewire with the tip being advanced into the stomach with fluoroscopic guidance. Rubber bougienage catheters filled with mercury are passed blindly through the stricture into the stomach. Disadvantages associated with these mercury-filled catheters include limited use on straight strictures with large diameters to avoid perforation and their need to be recycled because of expiration dates (Ahmad et al., 1994).

Hydrostatic balloon dilators are passed using a standard gastroscope; dilation then occurs with the balloon across the stricture. Tortuous or very long strictures are difficult to dilate with balloons and may require fluoroscopy to confirm adequate balloon placement. If a lesion is longer than the length of the balloon, repositioning may be required. The balloon dilators can open strictures to as large as 18 mm (Ahmad et al., 1994).

Esophageal Stenting. Stents are used to maintain patency of esophageal dilations. Stenting is of particular importance for patients who have not received adequate symptomatic relief from dilations. Exophytic tumors, extrinsic strictures, and lesions at least 2 cm from the upper esophageal sphincter are the most amenable to stenting. Lesions must have an adequate tumor shelf to anchor the stent (Ahmad et al., 1994).

Conventional plastic stents are rigid plastic tubes reinforced with metal coils and are the only ones currently approved for clinical use in the United States. These stents are placed across the malignant stricture after dilation with polyvinyl dilators over a guidewire. Fluoroscopic guidance is used to position the stent across the stricture. Endoscopy is done after stent placement to confirm the presence of benign mucosa above and below the stent. Placement confirmation with contrast occurs once the patient has awakened. Cough suppressants are prescribed after the procedure because coughing can cause stent dislodgment. Patients are encouraged to eat slowly and chew thoroughly within a few days after insertion. Fluids should be used to propel food (Ahmad et al., 1994).

The success rate with conventional stents is greater than 90%. The procedure-related complication rate (20%) and mortality rate (8.6%) are significant (Low & Kozarek, 1988).

Stents can successfully treat tracheoesophageal fistulas. Those with an inflatable cuff are used to occlude this type of fistulae, manage arterial bleeding from gastric tumors, and control iatrogenic endoscopic perforations (Sargeant, Thorpe, & Bown, 1992).

New expandable metal stents have been developed but not approved for clinical use. These metal stents are compressed at placement and expand over a 24-hour period after insertion. Because of their expandable property, they do not require predilation and are able to be used in angulated tumors that are inaccessible to conventional stents (Kozarek, Ball, & Patterson, 1992). Metal stents have been coated with silicon or urethane to reduce tumor growth and ease stent removal. It is necessary to monitor these stents for possible migration because of their smooth surface (Fleischer & Bull-Henry, 1992). Ease of placement, improved patient comfort, and lower mortality may indicate that metal stents will replace conventional stents in the future (Ahmad et al., 1994).

Endoscopic Laser Therapy. Endoscopic laser therapy (ELT) used to open malignant esophageal strictures use a Nd:YAG source. The efficacy of establishing a patent lumen (94%) and temporarily eliminating dysphagia (81%) has been prospectively shown (Rutgeerts, Vantrappen, Broeckaert, Muls, Geboes, Coremans et al., 1988). Short straight strictures (less than 6 cm in length) located in the mid or distal esophagus or at the surgical anastomoses are the most amenable to laser treatment. Laser treatment may require a single or multiple applications and depend on the thermal energy delivered to achieve total palliation of the stricture (Overholt, 1992). Contraindications to ELT include tracheoesophageal fistulae, submucosal tumors, and angulated lesions that are prone to perforation. Extensive ventilation is required in endoscopic units where laser therapy is performed because of the possibility that tumor cells and infectious agents may be transmissible in the smoke that is created during the procedure (Ahmad et al., 1994).

The complication rate associated with laser therapy ranges from 2% to 9%. This includes perforation, fistula formation, hemorrhage, and sepsis (Overholt, 1992). Bacteremia and sepsis are more likely associated with dilation prelaser treatment; the procedure-related mortality rate is approximately 1% (Ahmad et al., 1994).

Comparisons of ELT with stenting have found the procedures comparable to providing symptomatic relief. Stenting may provide palliation of longer duration and may not require as many applications (Alderson & Wright, 1990).

Bicap Tumor Probe. Tumor probes provide the direct application of electrical current to circumferential tumors by using short vertical metal strips. This technique is only recommended for use on circumferential tumors to avoid burning the normal mucosa, perforation, or formation of fistulas. Advantages include the ability to treat and shrink both submucosal and mucosal tumors. The probe is passing through the stricture under endoscopic guidance and dilated to the diameter of the probe (up to 15 mm). The probe is withdrawn stepwise while heat is applied to the tumor, treating the entire stricture. If contrast swallow demonstrates adequate luminal patency, without treatment complications patients can eat within 24 hours. Treatments are repeated as needed (Ahmad et al., 1994). The tumor probe has demonstrated a lower complication rate than that of the Nd:YAG laser, with comparable efficacy and wider versatility to treat submucosal, proximal cervical, and long strictures that are not treatable by laser (Jensen, Machicado, Randall, Tung, & English-Zych, 1988).

Photodynamic Therapy. Photodynamic therapy (PDT) involves the intravenous administration of an agent that sensitizes tumors to the light of certain wavelengths. PDT can be used to treat mucosal and superficial lesions. During PDT, laser light is delivered at a nonthermal wavelength through a fiberoptic endoscope. Cell kill occurs through the production of cytotoxic singlet oxygen (Overhold, 1992). Phase II trials are in progress using dihematoporphyrin ether (DHE), whose fluorescent properties are useful in tumor localization (Ahmad et al., 1994). Forty-eight hours after intravenous administration of DHE, endoscopy for laser application is done; it is then repeated in 2 to 3 days to débride the treated area and to treat any residual tumor (Overholt, 1992).

PDT is the only endoscopic technique that has been evaluated as a curative intervention in treating superficial esophageal cancers and for palliation of advanced lesions (Ahmad et al., 1994).

TABLE 39-13 Endoscopic and Endocavitary Modalities

Procedure	Success Rate	Complication Rate	Complications	Most Suitable Tumors
Dilation	90%-100%	5%	Perforation, bleeding	Any stenosis Lesion must allow guidewire to pass through for savary dilation
Stent	≥90%	13.8%	Early: perforation, bleeding, dyspnea from tracheal compression, tube migration, occlusion by tumor Late: tube migration/erosion with bleeding or perforation, tumor overgrowth, chronic aspiration, occlusion by food bolus	Long strictures
Laser therapy	75%-100%	2%-9%	Perforation, fistula, hemorrhage, sepsis	Mucosal tumors; short, straight strictures; mid or distal esophagus
BICAP tumor probe	87%	10.5%	Perforation, fistula, strictures, gastroesophageal reflux	Circumferential tumors; thickened esophageal wall; submucosal or extrinsic lesions; mucosal or submucosal lesions
Photodynamic therapy	80%-90%	NA	Photosensitivity (in all patients: lasts ≥ 1 mo, newer agents do not have this problem), chest pain, fever, transient dysphagia, stricture, perforation	Mucosal and superficial lesions

From Overholt, B. F. (1992). Photodynamic therapy and thermal treatment of esophageal cancer. *Gastrointestinal Endoscopy Clinics of North America. 2,* 433-455.

Photosensitivity is the main limiting complication of PDT using DHE as a sensitizer. Patients must not have direct or reflected sun exposure for at least 1 month after PDT. Systemic side effects include chest pain, fever (caused by periesophageal inflammation), and dysphagia. PDT does not cause the more serious complications associated with other endoscopic modalities such as strictures or perforations. PDT is very costly and requires a second laser unit; therefore the use of this modality will limit availability (Ahmad et al., 1994).

A summary of the endoscopic and endocavitary modalities used to treat esophageal cancer is included in Table 39-13.

ONCOLOGIC EMERGENCIES

Tracheoesophageal Fistulae

The major oncologic emergency associated with esophageal cancer is the development of a tracheoesophageal fistula (TEF). Approximately 5% to 15% of patients with esophageal cancer develop a TEF (Burt, Diehl, Martini, Bains, Ginsberg, McCormack et al., 1991; Gschossman, Bonner, Foote, Shaw, Mortenson, Su et al., 1993). This is a fistula formation between the esophagus and the bronchial tree. This abnormal anatomic communication creates contamination of the bronchial tree with saliva and food. The clinical situation becomes complicated by cough and aspiration pneumonia. If left untreated, median survival is 6 weeks; if treated, median survival is 2 to 5 months (Burt et al., 1991).

Treatment options described include stent placement, esophageal bypass surgery, and RT (with or without chemotherapy). Surgery or RT appears to improve survival. In the past it has been stated that RT was contraindicated in the presence of TEF because of the potential of worsening the TEF by shrinking away the tumor and enlarging the fistula. However, a recent study demonstrates this to be untrue (Burt et al., 1991; Gschossman et al., 1993; Yamada, Takai, Ogawa, Kakuto, & Sakamoto, 1989). Similarly, chemotherapy is not contraindicated to treat TEF. For patients with poor performance status, esophageal stenting only is recommended. If the patient has a good performance status, more aggressive treatment of the TEF is warranted.

The development of a TEF constitutes an oncologic emergency with a poor prognostic outcome. Treatment options exist; however, only radiation therapy and bypass surgery prolong survival. Radiation therapy does not worsen the TEF and may be more easily tolerated by most patients than surgery. If patients are too ill for aggressive management, prompt esophageal stenting is a practical and relatively safe procedure to alleviate symptoms. Nursing assessment of TEF must be keen and swift. The patient must be provided with a prompt multidisciplinary approach to survive this potentially fatal emergency. It is vital that the nurse attempt to allay patient fears, offer acute interventions to alleviate symptoms, and appropriately suggest the correct treatment option that considers the patient's physical performance and personal desires.

NURSING MANAGEMENT

The medical management of esophageal cancer is complex. Treatment options vary and depend on many aspects of a patient's clinical presentation and underlying health history.

Care of these patients and their families is demanding and requires the professional expertise of a cohesive multidisciplinary health care team. Access to research protocols that can provide viable choices is beneficial due to the refractory nature of esophageal cancer to standard treatment. The management of patients with esophageal cancer has been reviewed in the nursing literature (Daniel, 1994; Frank-Stromborg, 1989; Frogge, 1997; Medvec, 1988). It is apparent that patients with esophageal cancer experience a myriad of physical and psychological challenges. These issues are the domain of nursing care and require the expertise of nurses dedicated to managing complicated clinical situations and able to direct the activities of the multidisciplinary team to render complete and appropriate care. Patients with esophageal cancer receive treatment both in acute and ambulatory settings. Coordination of communication between the professionals that staff these environments is an additional integral part of nursing management.

Nursing management for this disease trajectory begins before diagnosis and occurs with the primary prevention of esophageal cancer by taking an active part in smoking and alcohol cessation and identifying high-risk individuals. Prevention and detection strategies can be accomplished both at an individual and group level. Nurses can assist in primary prevention efforts by encouraging government efforts to prevent esophageal cancer, documenting the need for funding to boost research efforts, developing educational programs, treating professionals and lay people involved in educational plans, and assisting with community and regional program planning (Frank-Stromborg, 1989). In addition, nurses can identify individuals with histories of etiologic factors that increase their risk for the development of esophageal cancer.

Once the diagnosis is made, the nurse will be needed to assist the patient and family to choose the appropriate treatment course. Establishing the goals of treatment/cure, control, and palliation is necessary to create a mutually understanding and cooperative environment. Multimodal approaches are commonly used; this requires that patients are provided with both written and oral explanations of different types of interventions and strategies for managing the side effects of the disease or treatments. This educational effort is on a continuum and therefore constantly changes as the clinical situation requires. Treatment options for esophageal cancer vary, and each poses unique patient needs requiring specific symptom management. A review of surgery, RT, and chemotherapy follows, along with standards of care for each modality.

Surgery

Patients undergoing esophagectomy or esophagogastrostomy require an aggressive preoperative evaluation to alleviate postoperative complications. This workup includes pulmonary physiotherapy with incentive spirometry, deep-breathing exercises, and smoking cessation 2 to 4 weeks before surgery. Age is not a factor for eliminating a patient as a surgical candidate; however, underlying chronic illnesses must be stabilized. Preoperative oral hygiene clearance includes a dental evaluation and removal of any dental caries. Enteral or parenteral nutrition may be required to support this patient population, which commonly exhibits moderate to severe weight loss before surgery (Medvec, 1988).

The major focus of acute nursing management is the prevention of postoperative complications such as pain, arrhythmias, emboli, infection, pulmonary complications, diarrhea or dumping syndrome, anastomotic leaks, and nutritional alteration. Surgical complications vary with the type of procedure performed; therefore patients require meticulous follow-up nursing care once discharged to avoid the development of chronic problems. The nursing management of the patient undergoing surgery for esophageal cancer is summarized in Table 39-14.

Radiation Therapy

Side effects associated with external beam RT include esophagitis, pneumonitis, pericarditis, dysphagia, tracheoesophageal fistula, and late esophageal stricture. During treatment the acute side effects that are most distressing are difficulty swallowing caused by esophageal irritation, skin irritation, and fatigue. Radiation treatments are given on an outpatient basis and, depending on the goal of treatment, typically range from 4 to 6 weeks. Supportive care measures are vital and should focus on symptom management, including comprehensive nutritional support, pain management, and allaying potential incapacity caused by fatigue and depression.

Sometimes patients receive intraluminal brachytherapy to provide a boost dose of treatment after external beam RT. These patients require admission to the short-procedure endoscopy unit, where implants are endoscopically placed or high-dose afterloading techniques are used. These patients require astute observation during and after the procedure for potential acute effects such as bleeding, perforation, and cough. In addition, difficulty swallowing may occur from the instrumentation and then subside once the esophageal irritation subsides. Patients receiving RT for esophageal cancer require tremendous educational support coupled with emotional understanding. Providing time to teach, encourage, listen, and advocate should be prioritized as nursing management goals. The nursing management of the patient receiving external beam RT for esophageal cancer is summarized in Table 39-15.

Chemotherapy

Chemotherapy is typically used as part of multimodal therapy either adjuvantly (following surgery) or neoadjuvantly (before surgery) or in combination with RT with or without surgery. The clinical applicability of chemotherapy in these settings allows for enhanced control of micrometastatic disease and the ability to shrink the primary tumor, which enhances surgical resectability. Multiple drugs have been studied both as single agents and in multi-drug regimens. Cisplatin is the most effective single agent and serves as the basis for many combination protocols. Cisplatin, 5-fluorouracil, adriamycin, vindesine, bleomycin, etoposide, mitomycin, methotrexate, and taxol are examples of agents being used and studied. Nurses must know the side-effect profile of these drugs to teach patients how to prevent or minimize side effects, instruct about what symptoms to report, and monitor patients for both acute and long-term related reactions. Toxic effects depend on the agents used and may include anorexia, nausea, vomiting, stomatitis, fatigue, alopecia, myelosuppression, nephrotoxicity, ototoxicity, peripheral neuropathy, and hypersensitivity reactions. Colony-stimulating factors such as G-CSF are being used more often with chemotherapeutic agents associated with neutropenia. Nurses must be prepared to instruct patients in the self-administration of these injectable agents. The management plan for the esophageal cancer patient receiving chemotherapy is summarized in Table 39-16.

Managing the Dysphagic Patient. Dysphagia is a complex manifestation of difficulty swallowing, which is related to possible defects in the head, neck, and esophageal regions (Bloch, 1993). Two types of dysphagia exist: malfunction of the neuromuscular mechanisms involving the mouth, pharynx, and upper esophageal sphincter (oropharyngeal dysphagia); and structural dysfunction of the smooth esophageal muscles and esophageal sphincter (esophageal dysphagia). In oropharyngeal dysphagia, patients have difficulty transferring food from the mouth to the upper esophagus. Esophageal dysphagia causes difficulties transporting ingested food because of diminished peristalsis or obstruction of luminal flow (Bloch, 1993).

Symptoms associated with dysphagia are prevalent in patients with esophageal cancer. Typical complaints that indicate dysphagia include having trouble with food "passing down," food "getting stuck" in the throat or mediastinal region of the chest, heartburn, or abdominal fullness sometimes accompanied by vomiting. Esophageal dysphagia occurs as a result of structural or neuromuscular compromise of esophageal smooth muscle and possible defects in the lower esophageal sphincter. These abnormalities create obstacles for food transport. Strictures, obstructing tumor growth, rings, spasms, and achalasia are some conditions that cause obstruction to the luminal flow and therefore disrupt peristaltic progression of food through the esophagus (Bloch, 1993).

Swallowing involves four phases that allow food to be placed in the mouth; chewed; positioned; and propelled from the lips, through the mouth and throat, and into the esophagus and stomach (Bloch, 1993; Logemann, 1989). The four phases of swallowing are oral preparation, oral, pharyngeal, and esophageal. Each phase of swallowing must be assessed for abnormalities if dysphagia is suspected. Dietary modification and treatment depend on identifying the specific swallowing defect. Each swallowing limitation demands different food choice modifications (Bloch, 1993; Logemann, 1989).

Assessing the Dysphagic Patient. Assessing the patient who is experiencing esophageal dysphagia requires

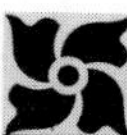

Table 39-14 Standard of Care for the Patient Undergoing Esophagectomy

Patient Problem and Outcomes	Nursing Interventions and Rationales	Patient Education Instructions
Knowledge Deficit Related to Surgical Procedure		
Patient will: • Verbalize knowledge of preoperative and postoperative procedures and expectations. • Express feelings of high and low anxiety. • Identify ways to cope with anxiety and knowledge deficit.	1. Assess barriers to learning. 2. Assess preconceived ideas and experiences. 3. Assess baseline knowledge. 4. Determine which coping strategies the patient has previously used to decrease anxiety and reinforce the use of these. 5. Teach patient to recognize continuum of anxiety level and to match coping strategies to degree of anxiety. 6. Administer antianxiety agents if prescribed by physician and if multidisciplinary team agrees.	Provide patient with verbal explanation and written information on: 1. Preoperative routine: a. Diagnostic tests b. Anesthesiology c. Antiembolic hose d. NPO after midnight 2. Use a diagram of the anatomy of the aerodigestive tract to explain esophagectomy. 3. Postoperative routine: a. Pulmonary toilet b. Diet/enteral feeding c. Pain management d. Range-of-motion exercises (thoracotomy patients only) e. Surgical incision 4. Teach patient complementary relaxation techniques: a. Deep breathing b. Music therapy c. Massage 5. Encourage patients to become self-advocates by promoting self-care and teaching them to feel comfortable asking questions.
Pain Related to Surgical Procedure		
Patient will have a postoperative pain scale rating less than 5/10	1. Assess pain intensity and obtain pain scale rating: a. Use a 0-10 verbal rating scale b. On admission to unit c. Every 2-4 hours if patient controlled anesthesia (PCA) is in use d. Before and within 1 hour after intermittent medication administration 2. Assess response to pain relief measures. 3. Anticipate need for pain medication before ambulation and uncomfortable procedures. 4. Administer opioid analgesics around the clock for the first 24-48 hours before surgery. 5. Monitor for analgesic side effects and administer medications to prevent or treat: a. Nausea b. Pruritus c. Constipation	1. Teach the patient to communicate pain level to the nurse. 2. Teach patient the importance of taking pain medication regularly to keep pain controlled.
Ineffective Airway Clearance Related to Incisional Pain		
Patient will maintain/achieve adequate respiratory function.	1. Document respiratory status every 8 hours and PRN during acute changes. 2. Encourage respiratory exercises every 1-2 hours while awake and every 4 hours if asleep; do not suction unless prescribed in postoperative instructions. 3. Administer O_2 as required. 4. Assess and document amount, color, and consistency of sputum.	1. Teach patient the importance of using oxygen treatment. 2. Teach patient technique of incentive spirometry. 3. Reinforce respiratory therapists' regimen. 4. Explain access system to contact nurse if patient experiences difficulty breathing or coughing.

Continued

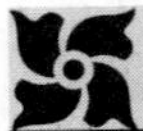

TABLE 39-14 Standard of Care for the Patient Undergoing Esophagectomy—cont'd

Patient Problem and Outcomes	Nursing Interventions and Rationales	Patient Education Instructions
Potential for Infection Related to Surgical Incision, Chest Tube, J-Tube Site		
Patient will have infection-free postoperative course.	1. Assess incision and tube sites BID for signs and symptoms of infection and for healing process. 2. Monitor vital signs 3. Assess incision: Document appearance BID Clean with soap and water BID; if drainage is present, clean more frequently with alcohol or Betadine; if crusting is present, clean with hydrogen peroxide. 4. Assess chest tube site: Remove initial dressing after 48 hours. Document appearance of site. Clean site with alcohol or Betadine with each dressing change. Continue dressing change every 8 hours and PRN until tubes are discontinued. 5. Assess J-tube site: Document appearance BID. Clean around insertion site BID with soap and water; if drainage is present, clean more frequently with alcohol or Betadine; if crusting is present, clean with hydrogen peroxide.	1. Teach patient to report the following symptoms: a. Elevated temperature b. Weakness c. Headache d. Heart palpatations 2. Tell patient to inform the nurse if leakage occurs at invasion site or tube sites. 3. Teach patient self-care measures related to dressing changes and wound care.
Altered Nutrition; Less Than Body Requirements Related to Disease Process and Surgery		
Patient will maintain or increase weight.	1. Monitor daily weight. 2. Record intake and output every shift. 3. Monitor hydration status. 4. Maintain J-tube feedings at prescribed rate and strength. 5. Maintain head of bed at 30 to 45 degrees. 6. Obtain dietary consult. 7. Take calorie counts.	Teach patient to: 1. Obtain weekly weight after discharge from hospital 2. Design adequate nutritional plan to maintain body weight 3. Recognize symptoms of dehydration: a. Fatigue/lethargy b. Shortness of breath c. Excessive thirst

astute observation and prompt intervention. The following pivotal aspects of the clinical presentation should be considered when assessing for dysphagia. Muscular atrophy may occur as a result of fatigue, which causes a weakness and diminished functioning of the pharynx and esophagus. If the pharyngeal sac retains food due to an outpouching of the esophageal wall, symptoms of coughing, neck fullness, throat gurgling, regurgitation, and aspiration are common. Repeated pressure may be required to empty the sacs, with the potential for esophageal obstruction likely (Bloch, 1993) (Box 39-3).

Assessment questions to pose when evaluating a patient for esophageal dysphagia include the following: "What kind of food causes the symptoms, solid or liquid? Is the dysphagia intermittent or progressive? Is heartburn associated with the dysphagia?"

Esophageal motility problems usually present as slowly progressive dysfunction for liquids and solids. Mechanical obstruction usually presents with dysphagia to solids initially and then progresses to more restrictive episodes (Bloch, 1993). Box 39-4 summarizes key assessment queries.

Common characteristics of esophageal dysphagia include difficulty eating solid, bulky, dry foods, accompanied by the inability to swallow saliva. Weight loss, regurgitation, aspiration pneumonia, and odynophagia are additional

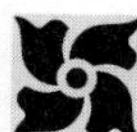

TABLE 39-14 Standard of Care for the Patient Undergoing Esophagectomy—cont'd

Patient Problem and Outcomes	Nursing Interventions and Rationales	Patient Education Instructions
Potential for Feeding Intolerance Patient will: • Recognize early signs and symptoms of feeding intolerance • Adequately tolerate feedings after surgery	1. Assess for: Abdominal discomfort Nausea/vomiting Diarrhea Cramping 2. Assess bowel sounds every shift. 3. Notify surgeon of suspected feeding intolerance. 4. Obtain dietary consult.	1. Patient will be taught to recognize early feeding intolerance with verbal instructions. 2. Patient will be taught the importance of prompt reporting to the health care team should this occur.
Knowledge Deficit Related to Postoperative Home Care Patient and/or caregiver will: • Verbalize knowledge of postoperative home care • Demonstrate and verbalize knowledge of enteral feedings	1. Initiate discharge planning, contact necessary personnel (discharge planning nurse, social worker, home care nurse). 2. Give patient appropriate emergency contact numbers so that health care team can be contacted promptly. 3. Provide patient with assessment of required medical equipment. 4. Establish clear parameters of communication between patient, home care providers, and acute care professionals. 5. Assess patient/caregiver knowledge of J-tube care and tube feeding procedure. 6. Demonstrate to patient/caregiver J-tube care and feeding.	1. Provide written information on all aspects of home care program. 2. Instruct patient about symptoms to report to surgeon/health care team: Tube feeding intolerance Prolonged diarrhea Weight loss >10% of current body weight, or ≥5 lbs Temperature < 101° F Drainage from incisions/J-tube site 3. Instruct patient to weigh weekly at home 4. Assess feeding tube: Care of tube site Irrigation of tube with water before and after feedings or every 8 hours Signs/symptoms of infection/feeding intolerance, aspiration 5. Give enteral feeding instruction: Patency of J-tube Preparation of formula Rate of administration and use of pump (if applicable) Return demonstration of tube feeding administration

symptoms that may accompany this symptom complex. Assessment of the patient's ability to meet his or her nutritional needs is important to design an effective supplementary diet. It is vital to discern exactly what symptoms the patient is experiencing, whether solids or liquids are tolerated, and if supplementation is necessary.

Six grades of functional esophageal dysphagia are described and summarized in Table 39-17. These categories are useful for streamlining assessment and establishing appropriate parameters for interventions before, during, and on completion of treatment. Interventions to ease swallowing need to be tailored to the functional grade of dysphagia. Suggestions for facilitating swallowing are summarized in Box 39-5. Operative procedures may require specific interventions related to nutritional support and treatment of dysphagia. Suggestions for oral intake postesophagogastrectomy are summarized in Box 39-6.

If a patient experiences progressive dysphagia caused by obstructive symptoms from esophageal cancer, his or her diet may regress from normal food intake to intake of moist, soft foods, to thin liquids, to the inability to ingest orally. He or she may require enteral nutrition to meet nutritional demands. Enteral nutrition is a viable option for the support and management of progressive dysphagia. The individual may have a nasoenteric tube or a percutaneous endoscopically placed gastrostomy or jejunostomy tube (PEG or PEJ).

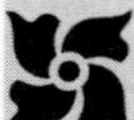

TABLE 39-15 Standard of Care for the Patient Receiving External Beam Radiation Therapy for Esophageal Cancer

Patient Problem and Outcomes	Nursing Interventions and Rationales	Patient Education Instructions
Knowledge Deficit Patient will verbalize an understanding of the purpose, benefits, and risks of radiation therapy.	1. Assess patient's level of knowledge about radiation therapy. 2. Assess patient's concerns and fears about radiation therapy.	1. Describe a "walk-through treatment": a. Initial consultation b. Simulation/Treatment planning c. Treatment routines 2. Describe major side effects associated with radiation therapy, the importance of notifying the nurse should side effects occur, and self-care measures to manage the side effects of: a. Esophagitis/dysphagia b. Skin reaction/changes c. Fatigue d. Nausea/vomiting
Esophagitis/Dysphagia Patient will be able to maintain adequate nutritional intake during treatment and maintain weight, fluid balance and energy level.	1. Assess for choking or regurgitation during or after meals. 2. Obtain daily weights and dietary consultation for calorie count and dietary modification. 3. Offer six to eight small feedings/day of high-calorie, high-protein liquefied foods and supplements. 4. Avoid eating before bedtime. 5. Assess for fatigue, altered mental status, weight loss of 2 lbs or more/day, and decreased serum albumin. 6. Obtain dietary consult for evaulation of alternate routes of nutrition (enteral feedings via nasogastric or gastrostomy tubes or total parenteral nutrition).	1. Instruct patient to sit upright for meals and 30 minutes after meals. If in bed, raise head to at least 45-degree angle. 2. Teach patient to use oral suction if fear of aspiration. 3. Provide oral and written instructions of measures to maintain stable nutritional status and prevent aspiration. 4. Instruct patient/caregiver to administer feedings. 5. Instruct patient/caregiver to provide oral hygiene frequently. 6. Instruct patient/caregive to report any untoward effects promptly.
Skin Reaction Patient will not experience serious radiation skin reaction.	1. Assess skin pretreatment. 2. Offer appropriate topical ointments for treating skin reactions.	1. Teach patient to moisturize erythematous reaction with nonperfumed lotion (Aquaphor). 2. Teach patient to cleanse skin well with nonperfumed soap. 3. Teach patient to use the following agents if moist desquamation occurs: a. Vigilon wound dressing b. Carrington carraderm c. Adaptic gauze d. Silvadene cream® 1%
Fatigue Patient will be able to maintain normal activities of daily living and engage in activities to enhance quality of life.	1. Assess patient's level of fatigue using a 0 (not at all tired, full of pep) to 10 (total exhaustion) rating scale. 2. Evaluate patient's sleep and activity pattern to be able to teach patient ways to conserve energy.	1. Inform patient that he or she is likely to experience fatigue toward the end of treatment and for several weeks following. 2. Teach energy conservation: a. Regular bedtime b. Brief daytime naps c. Regular intervals of daily exercise
Nausea/Vomiting Patient will maintain adequate oral intake throughout course of treatment.	1. Assess patient's gastrointestinal sensitivities before treatment. 2. Recommend small, frequent feedings. 3. Suggest the avoidance of fat-rich foods. 4. Involve the use of antiemetics.	1. Teach appropriate dietary interventions 2. Teach patient to recognize symptoms of dehydration 3. Teach patient appropriate timing and use of antiemetic agents

TABLE 39-16 Standard of Care for the Patient Receiving Chemotherapy for Esophageal Cancer

Patient Problem and Outcomes	Nursing Interventions and Rationales	Patient Education Instructions
Nausea/Vomiting Patient will be able to maintain nutritional input.	1. Obtain pretreatment history of dietary sensitivities. 2. Encourage use of antiemetics.	1. Teach signs and symptoms of dehydration. 2. Explain use of antiemetics. 3. Involve relaxation techniques.
Myelosuppression Patient will receive treatment without delay because of suppressed blood values.	1. Assess laboratory values weekly. 2. Monitor for onset of infectious process. 3. Be prepared to hold treatment if needed. 4. Use colony-stimulating factors.	1. Teach signs and symptoms of a. Fatigue/weakness b. Bleeding c. Shortness of breath d. Elevated temperature 2. Teach self-administration of colony-stimulating factors.
Nephrotoxicity Patient will not experience kidney failure.	1. Assess laboratory values: creatinine, BUN. 2. Monitor intake and output.	1. Teach importance of adequate urinary output. 2. Encourage reporting of symptoms.
Peripheral Neuropathy Patient will be able to cope with potential of this side effect.	1. Assess for tingling, numbness in fingers and toes. 2. Involve use of vasodilators.	1. Teach safety measures: sharp and hot objects. 2. Offer supportive measures.
Alopecia Patient will be able to cope with this side effect.	1. Provide scalp care instructions. 2. Assess patient's coping skills regarding altered body image. 3. Allow for discussion regarding body image changes.	1. Explain reality of hair loss. 2. Provide information with details of wig and beauty suppliers. 3. Offer information on Look Good/Feel Good Makeover programs. 4. Encourage that hair regrowth is temporary. 5. Teach scalp care.

Box 39-3
Common Characteristics of Esophageal Dysphagia

- Difficulty ingesting solid, bulky, dry foods
- Inability to swallow saliva
- Weight loss, regurgitation, aspiration, pneumonia, odynophagia

Bloch, A. S. (1993). Nutritional management of patients with dysphagia. *Oncology* (Suppl.), *7*(11), 127-134.

Liquid feeding preparations may be carefully selected; consider the patients' nutritional needs, as well as underlying health history that may preclude certain nutrients and additives. Frequently this choice is made by a multidisciplinary nutrition support team in conjunction with patient and family input.

Dysphagia is a debilitating symptom laden with serious physical and psychosocial compromise. Therefore it is vital that nursing management prioritize this clinical problem. The development of viable interventions requires mul-

Box 39-4
Assessment of Dysphagia

Fatigue may cause weakness of pharynx and esophagus.
Pharyngeal sac may retain food.
Signs and symptoms:
- Persistent coughing
- Neck fullness
- Throat gurgling
- Regurgitation
- Aspiration
- Slowly progressive for liquids and solids

What kind of food produces the symptoms—liquids or solids?
Is the dysphagia intermittent or progressive?
Is there associated heartburn?
Can the patient meet nutritional needs?
Are solids and liquids easily tolerated?
Is supplementation indicated?
What symptoms is patient experiencing?

Bloch, A. S. (1993). Nutritional management of patients with dysphagia. *Oncology* (Suppl.), *7*(11), 127-137)

TABLE 39-17 Functional Grades of Esophageal Dysphagia

Grade I:	Eating normally
Grade II:	Requires liquids with meals
Grade III:	Able to take only semi-solids
Grade IV:	Able to take only liquids
Grade V:	Unable to take liquids, able to swallow saliva
Grade VI:	Unable to swallow saliva

Bloch, A. S. (1993). Nutritional management of patients with dyphasia. *Oncology* (Suppl.), *7*(11), 127-137.

Box 39-5
Hints to Ease Swallowing

- Moist, soft foods
- Sauces and gravies
- Avoid sticky foods
- Small bites; chew thoroughly
- Sip liquids with meals
- Sit upright during meals
- Food at room temperature

Bloch, A. S. (1993). Nutritional management of patients with dysphagia. *Oncology* (Suppl.), *7*(11), 124-137.

Box 39-6
Hints for Eating Following an Esophagogastrectomy

- Eat small, frequent meals.
- Chew well, eat slowly.
- Limit liquid intake with meals.
- Gradually add milk.
- Gradually add sweets.
- Adhere to a low-fat diet.
- Avoid acidic foods, spicy foods, caffeine.
- Fluids in between meals.

Bloch, A. S. (1993). Nutritional management of patients with dysphagia. *Oncology* (Suppl.) *7*(11), 127-137.

tidisciplinary planning, including patient and family participation.

HOME CARE ISSUES

Depending on the modalities used to treat esophageal cancer, the patient and family caregivers will be challenged with many issues within the home setting. Complex treatment regimens are given on an ambulatory basis, and patients are required to be able to manage their symptoms and recognize reportable situations so that prompt attention is sought by the appropriate health care professionals. Home care issues are numerous and varied because of the differences in therapeutic regimens and individual patient requirements. A few common challenges include transportation to daily RT treatments that can span 4 to 6 weeks in duration), monitoring of venous access devices and portable chemotherapy pump infusions, and management of enteral nutrition programs and postoperative home care.

Transportation

Daily transportation to treatment sessions can be accomplished through the use of ride services provided by local transportation companies, volunteer drivers (e.g., Wheels) and American Cancer Society driver programs. Some hospitals provide temporary housing (furnished apartments) that can be rented for a nominal fee during the course of therapy for patients and family caregivers living too far to travel on a daily basis. The institution social work department is usually involved in providing transportation information. Assessment of transportation needs should be made at the initial patient interview, and proper referrals promptly made.

Venous Access Devices and Portable Chemotherapy Pump Infusions

Chemoradiation protocols may require continuous infusion of chemotherapeutic regimens. Patients and family caregivers must be taught basic psychomotor skills to care for required equipment such as venous access devices and portable pumps and equipment. In addition, patients must be fully aware of specific side-effect profiles of the chemotherapeutic drugs and the requirement for close monitoring procedures.

HOME ENTERAL NUTRITION MANAGEMENT

Patients with esophageal cancer commonly require enteral nutritional supplementation because of dysphagia associated with the obstructive nature of esophageal cancer and treatment side effects. Patients need to receive information regarding feeding tube care and enteral feeding preparation and administration. They must be taught the signs and symptoms of infection, feeding intolerance, and aspiration.

Postoperative Home Care

Patients and their family caregivers will have a knowledge deficit on discharge related to home care during the immediate postoperative period. It is advisable that written and oral information be given at the initiation of the discharge planning phase. Reportable symptoms should include prolonged diarrhea, weight loss greater than 10% of current body weight or greater than or equal to 5 lbs, temperature greater than 101° F, and drainage from incisions/J-tube sites. Refer to Chapter 3.

Home care issues should be considered the domain of the multidisciplinary team caring for the esophageal cancer patient and family caregivers. Professional oncology home care nurses should be the coordinators of this effort by identifying and prioritizing the pertinent issues and providing immediate interventions to enhance symptom management within this environment.

TABLE 39-18 Quality of Care Evaluation for a Patient Receiving Radiation Therapy for Esophageal Cancer

Disciplines participating in the Quality of Care Evaluation:
☐ Nursing ☐ Radiation Oncologists ☐ Social Services

Data from:
☐ Patient Interview ☐ Mailed Form

Criteria	Yes	No
1. Did the nurse or doctor explain to you that you might experience some of the following side effects from your radiation treatments?		
a. Difficulty swallowing	☐	☐
b. Skin irritation	☐	☐
c. Fatigue	☐	☐
2. Were you given instructions for a modified diet?	☐	☐
3. Were you taught how to take care of your skin during treatment?	☐	☐
4. Were you offered suggestions for coping with excessive fatigue?	☐	☐

PROGNOSIS

The prognosis for surviving esophageal cancer is not high. In the United States survival has improved over time; however, the survival statistics are still low. Only 12% of white patients and 8% of black patients survived 5 or more years (Parker, Tong, Bolden & Wingo, 1997). Survival rates remain low for both men and women and white and blacks, although slightly better for women and whites (Blot, 1994). High fatality means that incidence and mortality rates are nearly equal. Unpublished surveillance epidemiology end results (SEER) data from August 1993 shows that similar rates of survival from squamous cell carcinomas and adenocarcinomas exist with 5-year relative survival rates among white males of 9% and 10% respectively (Blot, 1994). Five-year relative survival rates by stage are as follows: localized disease has a 22% rate, regional metastatic disease has an 11% rate, and distant metastatic disease has a 2% rate (American Cancer Society, 1977).

EVALUATION OF THE QUALITY OF CARE

Accreditation organizations require that the quality of care provided to patients be monitored and evaluated. Esophageal cancer patients require multidisciplinary care; therefore an evaluation of the quality of this effort should be multidimensional. Tables 39-18 and 39-19 provide examples of evaluation tools for quality of care that can be implemented both in acute and ambulatory settings.

RESEARCH ISSUES

Numerous research issues surrounding the diagnosis and management of esophageal cancer have been successful in achieving control palliation and cure of this difficult disease. Presently there is evidence that the combination of RT and infusional 5-FU and mitomycin is an effective and well-tolerated regimen in the treatment of esophageal cancer. There appears to be greater survival and better local control with chemoradiation than with the use of RT alone. There has been no successfully completed randomized trial involving surgery vs. definitive radiation and concurrent chemotherapy. However, the results reported thus far suggest that concurrent radiation plus chemotherapy represents a reasonable alternative to esophagectomy in the primary management of squamous cell carcinoma of the esophagus and is an effective regimen in the treatment of patients with adenocarcinoma of the esophagus as well (Coia, 1996).

The following issues must be prioritized and addressed in the future: the challenge of the rise in adenocarcinoma of the esophagus; recognition that chemoradiation is superior to RT alone in squamous cell cancer of the esophagus and offers a chance for long-term palliation and occasional sur-

TABLE 39-19 Quality of Care Evaluation for a Patient Undergoing Esophagectomy

Disciplines participating in quality of care evaluation:
☐ Nursing ☐ Surgery ☐ Radiology ☐ Laboratory
☐ Respiratory Therapy ☐ Physical Therapy ☐ Social Services

I. Postoperative Management Evaluation
Data from:
☐ Medical Record Review ☐ Patient/Family Interview

Criteria	Yes	No
1. Patient given preoperative information about:		
a. Surgical procedure	☐	☐
b. Diagnostic tests	☐	☐
c. Pain management	☐	☐
d. Pulmonary toilet	☐	☐
e. Diet	☐	☐
f. Range-of-motion exercises		
g. Postoperative expectations	☐	☐
2. Nutritional status monitored after surgery	☐	☐
3. Patient experienced the following complications:	☐	☐
a. Infection at surgical incision site	☐	☐
b. Tube feeding intolerance	☐	☐
c. Prolonged diarrhea	☐	☐

II. Patient/Family Satisfaction
Data from:
☐ Patient Interview ☐ Family Interview

1. On a scale of 0 to 10, with 0 being totally dissatisfied and 10 being totally satisfied, how satisfied were you with the care you received after your surgery

vival in patients with adenocarcinoma; the need to evaluate aggressive preoperative chemoradiation in phase III trials, the need to minimize late effects of treatment, and investigations of the clinical effectiveness of new chemotherapy agents and new RT plans. These research issues should consider effectiveness on prolonging quality survival times along with monetary implications, ethical aspects, and the quantification of associated morbidities. In addition, patient and family caregivers' desires and responses should always be prioritized.

REFERENCES

Agur, A. M. R. & Lee, M. J. (1991). *Grant's atlas of anatomy.* Baltimore: Williams & Wilkins.

Ahmad, N. F., Goosenberg, E. B., Frucht, H., Coia, L. R. (1994). Palliative treatment of esophageal cancers. *Seminars in Radiation Oncology, 4*(3), 202-214.

Ajani, J. A. (1994). Contributions of chemotherapy in the treatment of carcinoma of the esophagus: Results and commentary. *Scandinavian Journal of Urology and Nephrology, 21,* 474-482.

Ajani, J. A., Roth, J., Putnam, J., Ryan, B., Walsh, G., Lynch, P. et al. (1992). Feasibility of five courses of preoperative chemotherapy in patients with resectable adenocarcinoma of the esophagus or gastroesophageal junction. *Proceedings of AACR, 33,* 218.

Ajani, J. A., Roth, J., Ryan, M. B., Putnam, J. B., Pazdur, R., Levin, B. et al. (1993). Intensive preoperative chemotherapy with colony-stimulating factor for resectable adenocarcinoma of the esophagus or gastroesophageal junction. *Journal of Clinical Oncology, 8,* 1231-1238.

Akiyama, H., Tsurumaru, M., Kawamura, T., & Ono, Y. (1981). Principles of surgical treatment for carcinoma of the esophagus: Analysis of lymph node involvement. *Annals of Surgery, 194,* 438-446.

al-Sarraf, M., Martz, K., Herskovic, A., Leichman, L., Brindle, J. S., Vaitkevicius, V. K. et al. (1997). Progress report of combined chemoradiotherapy versus radiotherapy alone in patients with esophageal cancer: An intergroup study. *Journal of Clinical Oncology, 15*(1), 277-284.

Alderson, D. & Wright, P. D. (1990). Laser recanalization versus endoscopic intubation in the palliation of malignant dysphagia. *British Journal of Surgery, 77,* 1151-1153.

Algan, O., Coia, L. R., Keller, S. M., Engstrom, P. F., Weiner, L. M., Schultheiss, T. E. et al. (1995). Management of adenocarcinoma of the esophagus with chemoradiation alone or chemoradiation followed by esophagectomy: Results of sequential non-randomized phase II studies. *International Journal of Radiation Oncology, Biology, Physics, 32*(3), 753-761.

American Cancer Society. (1977). *Cancer Facts and Figures.* Atlanta: American Cancer Society.

American Joint Committee on Cancer. (1983). *Manual for staging of cancer.* (2nd ed.). Philadelphia: J.B. Lippincott.

American Joint Committee on Cancer. (1988). *Manual for staging of cancer.* (3rd ed.). Philadelphia: J.B. Lippincott.

Araujo, C. M., Souhami, L., Gil, R. A., Carvalho, R., Garcia, J. A., Froimtchuk, M. J. et al. (1991). A randomized trial comparing radiation therapy versus concomitant radiation therapy and chemotherapy in carcinoma of the thoracic esophagus. *Cancer, 67,* 2258-2261.

Basmajian, J. & Slonecker, C. E. (1989). *Grant's method of anatomy.* Baltimore: Williams and Wilkins.

Bloch, A. S. (1993). Nutritional management of patients with dysphagia. *Oncology (Supplement), 7*(11), 127-137.

Blot, W. J. (1994). Esophageal cancer trends and risk factors. *Seminars in Oncology, 21*(4), 403-410.

Bosset. (1994). Randomized phase III clinical trial comparing surgery alone vs. preoperative combined radiochemotherapy. *ASCO Proceedings, 13,* 197.

Bown, S. G. (1991). Palliation of malignant dysphagia: Surgery, radiotherapy, laser, intubation alone or in combination? *Gut, 32,* 841-844.

Bremner, R. M. & DeMeester, T. R. (1991). Surgical treatment of esophageal carcinoma. *Gastroenterology Clinics of North America, 20,* 743-763.

Burt, M., Diehl, W., Martini, N., Bains, M. S., Ginsberg, R. J., McCormack, P. M. et al. (1991). Malignant esophagorespiratory fistula: Management options and survival. *Annals of Thoracic Surgery, 52,* 1222-1229.

Byfield, J. E., Barone, R., Mendelsohn, J., Frankel, S., Quinol, L., Sharp, T. et al. (1980). Infusional 5-fluorouracil and x-ray therapy for non-resectable esophageal cancer. *Cancer, 45,* 703-708.

Cheng, K. K. (1994). The etiology of esophageal cancer in Chinese. *Seminars in Oncology, 21, 4* (411-415).

Coia, L. R. (1984). A pilot study of combined radiotherapy and chemotherapy for esophageal carcinoma. *American Journal of Clinical Oncology, 7,* 653-659.

Coia, L. R. (1989). Esophageal cancer: Is esophagectomy necessary? *Oncology, 3,* 101-109.

Coia, L. R. (1996). *Esophageal cancer—Refresher course.* Paper presented at the American Society for Therapeutic Radiology and Oncology, Los Angeles.

Coia, L. R. & Moylan, D. J. (1994). *Introduction to clinical radiation oncology.* (2nd ed.). Wisconsin: Medical Physics.

Coia, L. R., Engstrom, P. F., & Paul, A. (1987). Nonsurgical management of esophageal cancer: Reports of a study of combined radiotherapy and chemotherapy. *Journal of Clinical Oncology, 5,* 1783-1790.

Coia, L. R., Paul, A. R., & Engstrom, P. F. (1988). Combined radiation and chemotherapy as primary management of adenocarcinoma of the esophagus and gastroesophageal junction. *Cancer, 61*(4), 643-649.

Coia, L.R., Engstrom, P. F., Paul, A. R., Stafford, P. M., & Hanks, G. E. (1991). Long-term results of infusional 5-FU, mito- mycin-C and radiation as primary management of esophageal carcinoma. *International Journal of Radiation Oncology, Biology, Physics, 20,* 29-36.

Corn, B. J., Coia, L. R., Chu, J. C., Hwang, C. C., Stafford, P. M., & Hanks, G. E. (1991). Significance of prone positioning in planning treatment for esophageal cancer. *International Journal of Radiation Oncology, Biology, Physics, 2,* 1303-1309.

Dajani, A. S., Bisno, A. L., Chung, D. J., Durack, D. T., Free, D. M., Gerber, M. et al. (1990). Prevention of bacterial endocarditis: Recommendations by the American Heart Association. *Journal of the American Medical Association, 264,* 2919-2122.

Daniel, B. T. (1994). Gastrointestinal cancers. In S. E. Otto (Ed.), *Oncology Nursing,* (2nd ed.). St. Louis: Mosby.

Daniel, B. T. & Shuey, K. M. (1993). Role of the nurse in managing the patient with esophageal cancer. *Nursing Interventions in Oncology, 5,* 14-22.

Earle, J., Gelber, R., Moertel, C. (1980). A controlled evaluation of combined radiation and bleomycin therapy for squamous cell carcinoma of the esophagus. *International Journal of Radiation Oncology, Biology, Physics, 6,* 821-826.

Fleischer, D. A. & Bull-Henry, K. (1992). A new coated self-expanding metal stent for malignant esophageal strictures. *Gastrointestinal Endoscopy, 38,* 494-496.

Flejou, J. F., Potet, F., & Muzeau, F. (1993). Overexpression of p53 protein in Barrett's syndrome with malignant transformation. *Journal of Clinical Pathology, 46,* 330-333.

Forastiere, A. A. (1994). A 4-week intensive preoperative chemoradiation program for locoregional cancer of the esophagus. *Proceedings of the American Society of Clinical Oncology, 13,* 195.

Frank-Stromborg, M. (1989). The epidemiology and primary prevention of gastric and esophageal cancer. A worldwide perspective. *Cancer Nursing, 12*(2), 53-64.

Frogge, M. H. (1997). Gastrointestinal cancer: Esophagus, stomach, liver and pancreas. In S.L. Groenwald, M. Goodman, M. H. Frogge, & C. H. Yarbro (Eds.), *Cancer Nursing Principles and Practice,* (4th ed.). Boston: Jones and Bartlett.

Gaspar, L. E. (1994). Radiation therapy for esophageal cancer: Improving the therapeutic ratio. *Seminars in Radiation Oncology, 4,* 192-201.

Gignoux, M., Roussel, A., Paillot, B., Gillet, M., Schlag, P., Favre, J. P. et al. (1987). The value of preoperative radiotherapy in esophageal cancer; Results of a study of the EORTC. *World Journal of Surgery, 11,* 426-432.

Gill, P. G., Denham, J. W., Jamieson, G. G., Devitt, P. G., Yeoh, E. et al. (1992). Patterns of treatment failure and prognostic factors associated with the treatment of esophageal carcinoma with chemotherapy and radiotherapy either as sole treatment of, or followed by surgery. *Journal of Clinical Oncology, 10*(7), 1037-1043.

Goldie, J. H. & Coldman, A. J. (1983). Quantitative model for multiple levels of drug resistance in clinical tumors. *Cancer Treatment Reports, 67,* 923-931.

Gschossman, B. S., Bonner, J. A., Foote, R. L., Shaw, E. G., Martenson, J. A., Su, J. et al. (1993). Malignant tracheoesophageal fistula in patients with esophageal cancer. *Cancer, 72,* 1513-1521.

Herskovic, A., Martz, K., al-Sarraf, M., Leichman, L., Brindle, J., Vaitkevicius, V. et al. (1992). Combined chemotherapy and radiotherapy compared with radiotherapy alone in patients with cancer of the esophagus. *New England Journal of Medicine, 326,* 1593-1598.

IRB 94088. (1993). Phase I/II evaluation of taxol, cisplatinum, and 5-FU given in combination with RT (60 Gy) prior to surgery in patients with resectable esophageal adenocarcinoma.

Jaklitsch, M. T., Harpole, M. T., Healy, E. A., & Sugarbaker, D. J. (1994). Current issues in the staging of esophageal cancer. *Seminars in Radiation Oncology, 4,* 135-145.

Jensen, D. M., Machicado, G., Randall, G., Tung L. A., & English-Zych, S. (1988). Comparison of low-power YAG laser and BICAP tumor probe for palliation of esophageal cancer strictures. *Gastroenterology, 94*(6), 1263-1270.

Klimstra, D. S. (1994). Pathologic prognostic factors in esophageal carcinoma. *Seminars in Oncology, 21*(4), 425-430.

Kolaric, K., Maricic, Z., Roth, A., & Dujmovic, I. (1980). Combination of bleomycin and adriamycin with or without radiation in the treatment of inoperable esophageal cancer. *Cancer, 45,* 2265.

Kozarek, R. A., Ball, T. J., & Patterson, D. J. (1992). Metallic self-expanding stent application in the upper gastrointestinal tract: Caveats and concerns. *Gastrointestinal Endoscopy, 38,* 1-6.

Lightdale, C.J. (1994). Staging of esophageal cancer: Endoscopic ultrasonography. *Seminars in Oncology Nursing, 10,* 438-446.

Logemann, J. A. (1989). Swallowing and communication rehabilitation. *Seminars in Oncology Nursing, 5*(3), 205-212.

Looney, W. P., Hopkins, H. A. & Kovaca, C. J. (1983). Single and combined (radiation-cyclophosphamide) modality therapy in experimental solid tumors. *Advances in Radiation Biology, 10,* 305-311.

Low, D. E. & Kozarek, R. A. (1988). Esophageal endoscopy, dilatation, and intraesophageal prosthetic devices. In L. E. Hill, R. W. McCallum, D. E. Mercer, & R. A. Kozarek (Eds.), *The esophagus: medical and surgical management.* New York: W. B. Saunders.

Luckmann, J. & Sorensen, K. C. (1993). *Medical-surgical nursing: A psychophysiologic approach.* (4th ed.). Omaha: W. B. Saunders.

Maesawa, C., Masuda, T., Tamura, G., Satodate, R., Ishida, K., & Saito, K. (1992). Prognostic assessment of superficial squamous cell carcinoma of the esophagus using karyometric analysis and nucleolar organizer regions. *Journal of Surgical Oncology, 51,* 164-168.

Medvec, B. (1988). Esophageal cancer: Treatment and nursing interventions. *Seminars in Oncology Nursing, 4,* 246-256.

Nakajima, T., Fukuda, H., Hosono, M., Tsumura, M., Tada, T., Nishita, T. et al. (1992). Intralumina irradiation to T2M0 esophageal cancer: Effect of patient selection on prognosis. *Radiation Medicine, 10,* 123-128.

Neu, H. C. (1989). Recommendations for antibiotic prophylaxis before endoscopy. *American Journal of Gastroenterology, a84,* 1488-1489.

Orringer, M. B. (1984). Substernal gastric bypass of the excluded esophagus: Results of an ill-advised operation. *Surgery, 96,* 467-471.

Overholt, B. F. (1992). Photodynamic therapy and thermal treatment of esophageal cancer. *Gastrointestinal Endoscopy Clinics of North America, 2,* 433-455.

Parker, S. L., Tong, T., Bolden, S., & Wingo, P. A. (1997). Cancer statistics, 1997. *CA: A Cancer Journal for Clinicians, 47*(1), 5-27.

Perez, C. A. & Brady, L. W. (1992). *Principles and practice of radiation and oncology.* (2nd ed.). Philadelphia: J. B. Lippincott.

Ramal, S., Reid, B. J., & Sanchez, C. A. (1992). Evaluation of p53 protein expression in Barrett's esophagus by two-parameter flow cytometry. *Gastroenterology, 102,* 1220-1228.

Rosen, N. (1994). The molecular basis for cellular transformation: Implications for esophageal carcinogenesis. *Seminars in Oncology, 21*(4), 416-424.

Rutgeerts, P., Vantrappen, G., Broeckaert, L., Muls, M., Geboles, K., Coremans, G. et al. (1988). Palliative Nd:YAG laser therapy for cancer of the esophagus and gastroesophageal junction: Impact on the quality of remaining life. *Gastrointestinal Endoscopy, 34,* 87-90.

Sargeant, I. R., Thorpe, S., & Bown, S. G. (1992). Cuffed esophageal prosthesis: A useful device in desperate situations in esophageal malignancy. *Gastrointestinal Endoscopy, 38,* 669-675.

Segalin, A., Little, A. G., Ruol, A., Ferguson, M. K., Baordini, R., Norberto, L. et al. (1989). Surgical and endoscopic palliation of esophageal carcinoma. *Annals of Thoracic Surgery, 48,* 267-271.

Sischy, B., Ryan, L., Haller, D., Smith, T., Dayal, Y., Schutt, A. et al. (1990). Interim report of EST phase III protocol for the evaluation of combined modalities in the treatment of patients with carcinoma of the esophagus. *Proceedings of the American Society of Clinical Oncology, 9, A407.*

Smalley, S. R., Gunderson, L. I., Reddy, E. K., & Williamson, S. (1994). Radiotherapy alone in esophageal carcinoma: Current management and future directions of adjuvant, curative, and palliative approaches. *Seminars in Oncology, 21,* 467-473.

Spechler, S. J. (1994). Barrett's esophagus. *Seminars in Oncology, 21*(4), 431-437.

Steel, G. G. & Peckham, M. J. (1979). Exploitable mechanisms in combined radiotherapy-chemotherapy: The concept of additivity. *International Journal of Radiation Oncology, Biology, Physics, 5,* 85-91.

Stoller, J. L. & Brumwell, M. L. (1984). Palliation after operation and after radiotherapy for cancer of the esophagus. *Canadian Journal of Surgery, 27,* 491-495.

Thompson, W. M. & Halvorsen, R. A. (1994). Staging esophageal carcinoma II: CT and MRI. *Seminars in Oncology, 21,* 447-452.

Urba, S. (1995). A randomized trial comparing transhiatal esophagectomy to preoperative concurrent chemoradiation followed by esophagectomy in local-regional esophageal cancer. *Proceedings of the American Society of Clinical Oncology, 14,* 199.

Walsh, T. N. et al. (1996). A comparison of multimodal therapy and surgery for esophageal adenocarcinoma. *New England Journal of Medicine, 335*(7), 462-467.

Whyte, R. I. & Orringer, M. B. (1994). Surgery for carcinoma of the esophagus: The case for transhiatal esophagectomy. *Seminars in Radiation Oncology, 4,* 146-156.

Yamada, S., Takai, Y., Ogawa, Y., Kakuto, Y., & Sakamoto, K. (1989). Radiotherapy for malignant fistula to other tract. *Cancer, 64,* 1026-1028.

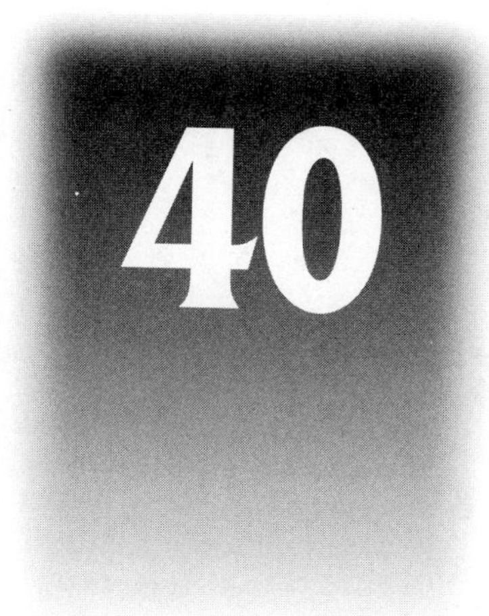

Cancer of the Gallbladder

Christine Miaskowski, RN, PhD, FAAN

EPIDEMIOLOGY

Cancer of the gallbladder is a relatively rare malignancy accounting for approximately 6900 new cases and 3500 deaths per year in the United States (Parker, Tong, Bolden, & Wingo, 1997). The incidence of gallbladder cancer ranges from 0.55% to 1.91% based on a study of 112,713 patients whose gallbladders were examined during surgery or at autopsy (Piehler & Crichlow, 1978).

Gallbladder cancer occurs more frequently in females than in males (ratio ranges from 1.5:1 to 2:1). This cancer usually occurs within the sixth and seventh decades of life (Curley, Levin, & Rich, 1995; Douglas, Kim, & Meropol, 1997). Cancer of the gallbladder is the second most common gastrointestinal malignancy in Native Americans who live in the Southwestern United States. The incidence of gallbladder cancer in this population is six times higher than that in non-Native American populations. The disease has been found in 6% of Native Americans of the Southwest who undergo surgery of the biliary tract (Nelson, Porvaznik, & Benfield, 1971). In addition, cancer of the gallbladder is quite common in Hong Kong (Koo, Wong, Cheng, & Ong, 1981), Bolivia, Mexico, and Chile (Strom, Soloway, Rios-Dalenz, Rodriguez-Martinez, West, & Kinman et al., 1996).

RISK FACTORS

The major risk factor for cancer of the gallbladder appears to be a history of gallstones. Animal studies have shown that more than 50% of animals who were fed a gallstone-inducing diet developed cancer of the gallbladder (Enomoto, Naoe, Harado, Miyata, Saito, & Noguchi, 1974). In humans, a history of gallstones is associated with the development of cancer of the gallbladder. In one study (Nagorney & McPherson, 1988), gallstones were present in 74% to 92% of patients with gallbladder cancer. In addition, the risk of developing cancer of the gallbladder increases directly with increasing gallstone size (Diehl, 1983). Patients with gallstones 2.0 to 2.9 cm in diameter have a 2.4 times higher relative risk of developing cancer of the gallbladder, whereas patients with gallstones greater than 3.0 cm in diameter have a 10.1 times higher risk of developing cancer of the gallbladder (Diehl, 1983).

PATHOPHYSIOLOGY

Normal Anatomy and Physiology

The gallbladder is a pear-shaped sac located below the liver (Fig. 40-1). The function of the gallbladder is to concentrate and store bile. The gallbladder can hold approximately 45 ml of bile. Bile consists of conjugated bilirubin, water, cholesterol, bile salts, electrolytes, and phospholipids. Bile salts are needed for the emulsification and digestion of fat. Bile is released from the gallbladder into the cystic duct and moves down the common bile duct to enter the duodenum at the ampulla of Vater where it aids in the digestion of fat (Elrod, 1996).

The Process of Carcinogenesis

The exact mechanisms underlying the development of cancer of the gallbladder are unknown. However, given the association between gallstones and the development of cancer of the gallbladder, it seems reasonable that gallstones or other factors that cause chronic inflammation of the mucosa of the gallbladder may induce a series of premalignant changes. If a cholecystectomy is not done, these premalignant lesions may progress to invasive cancer of the gallbladder (Curley, Levin, & Rich, 1995). In one study (Albores-Saavedra, Alcantra-Vazquez, Cruz-Ortiz, & Herrara-Goepfert, 1980), epithelial dysplasia, atypical hyperplasia, and carcinoma in situ were found in the gallbladder mucosa of 83%, 13.5%, and 3.5%, respectively, of patients who underwent cholecystectomy for cholelithiasis or cholecystitis. In addition, areas of mucosal dysplasia have been observed in more than 90% of patients with invasive cancer of the gallbladder (Curley et al., 1995).

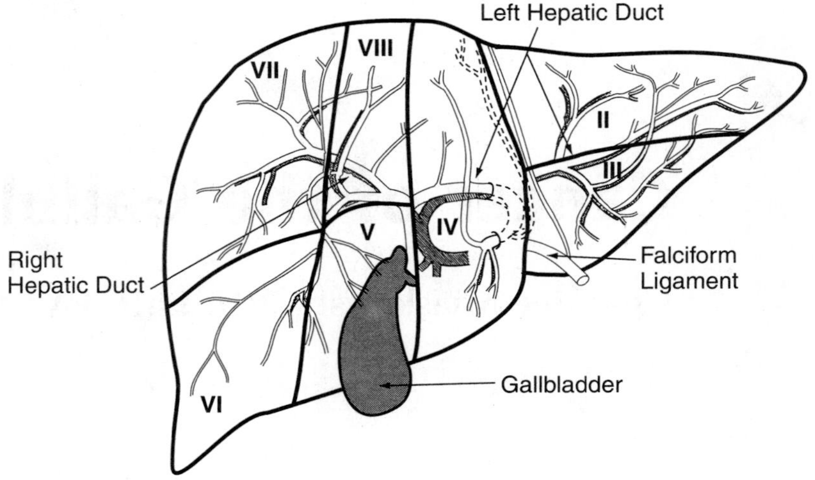

Fig. 40-1 The gallbladder lies at the junction of the right and left lobes of the liver. The relationship of the gallbladder to Couinaud's liver segments is illustrated. A wedge resection of the liver around the gallbladder would result in removal of segment V and the lower portion of segment IV. (The caudate lobe, segment I, is not visualized in this anterior view.) (From Dawes L. G., & Joehl, R. J. [1995]. Gallbladder cancer. In J. L. Cameron (Ed.), *Current surgical therapy* [5th ed.]. St Louis: Mosby.)

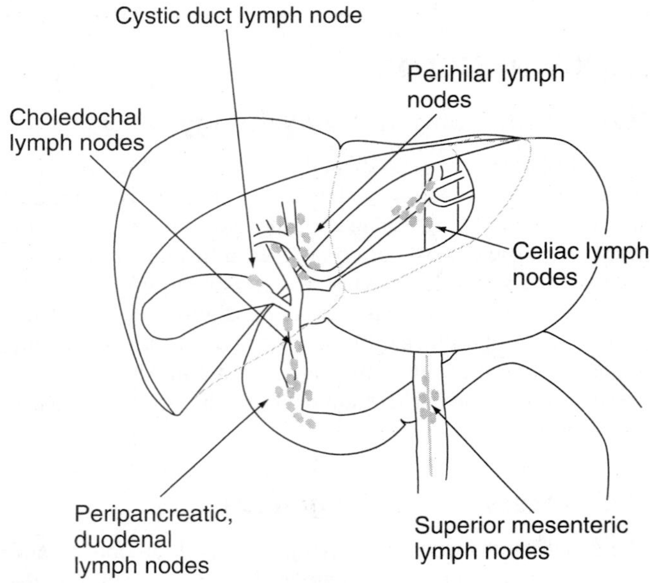

Fig. 40-2 Gallbladder cancer can metastasize to regional lymph nodes. Spread is seen to the cystic duct, choledochal and perihilar lymph nodes (level I nodes), and later to the peripancreatic duodenal lymph nodes and to the celiac and superior mesenteric lymph nodes (level II nodes). (From Dawes L. G., & Joehl, R. J. [1995]. Gallbladder cancer. In J. L. Cameron (Ed.), *Current surgical therapy* [5th ed.]. St Louis: Mosby.)

ROUTES OF METASTASES

Cancer of the gallbladder spreads by local extension. A common mode of spread is by direct extension into the liver. Sixty-five percent to 95% of patients with cancer of the gallbladder have liver metastases. In addition, the tumor can spread through the venous system of the gallbladder. Lymphatic invasion can also occur, with metastasis seen in the cystic duct, choledochal, periportal, or hilar lymph nodes. In addition, the superior and posterior peripancreatic, celiac, superior mesenteric, or periaortic nodes can be involved in cancer of the gallbladder (Fig. 40-2). Intra-abdominal disease can occur as a result of direct extension into the stomach, duodenum, omentum, or colon. Distant metastases can occur in the lung and bone (Dawes & Joehl, 1995).

ASSESSMENT

Clinical evaluation of the patient involves a detailed history, a thorough physical examination, and a variety of diagnostic tests (Table 40-1). The signs and symptoms present in the patient often depend on the stage of the disease at the time of diagnosis.

History

Unfortunately, the most common signs and symptoms reported by patients with cancer of the gallbladder are nonspecific. Signs and symptoms are often vague or may be absent. In many cases, when symptoms are present, they are associated with gallstones. Patients may complain of right upper quadrant abdominal pain that may or may not be exacerbated by eating a fatty meal. Right upper quadrant abdominal pain is the predominant symptom in 75% to 95% of patients (Nagorney & McPherson, 1988; Piehler & Crichlow, 1978). Additional symptoms include nausea, vomiting, anorexia, and weight loss.

Physical Examination

A complete physical examination is warranted, with particular attention to the abdominal examination. Right upper

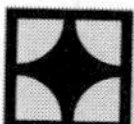

TABLE 40-1 Assessment of the Patient for Cancer of the Gallbladder

	Assessment Parameters	Typical Abnormal Findings
History	A. Personal and social history	
	1. Age	1. Usually occurs in the sixth and seventh decades of life
	2. Gender	2. More common in females
	3. Ethnicity	3. Second most common gastrointestinal malignancy in Native Americans who live in the southwestern United States
	4. History of gallstones	4. Major risk factor for cancer of the gallbladder
	B. Common symptoms	
	1. Right upper quadrant abdominal pain	1. Present in 75%-97% of patients; may be exacerbated by eating a fatty meal
	2. Nausea, vomiting, and anorexia	2. Present in 40%-67% of patients
Physical Examination	A. Skin examination	A. Jaundice is seen in 45% of patients.
	B. Abdominal examination	B. Right upper quadrant abdominal tenderness may be present.
	C. Weight loss	C. Approximately 37%-77% of patients report a weight loss of greater than 10% of their normal body weight.
Diagnostic Tests	A. Serum bilirubin	A. Approximately 70% of patients will have an elevated serum bilirubin at least two times greater than normal.
	B. Serum alkaline phosphatase	B. Elevated in approximately two thirds of patients.
	C. Serum alanine aminotransferase	C. Elevated in one third of patients; may indicate advanced disease with hepatic metastasis.
	D. Serum aspartate aminotransferase	D. Elevated in one third of patients; may indicate advanced disease with hepatic metastasis.
	E. Serum carcinoembryonic antigen (CEA)	E. Serum CEA is elevated in 80% of patients with advanced disease.
	F. Ultrasound of the gallbladder	F. Early tumors as small as 5 cm can be detected as a polypoid mass projecting into the gallbladder lumen or as a focal thickening of the gallbladder. Patients with locally advanced cancer of the gallbladder may exhibit bile duct obstruction, regional lymphadenopathy, direct hepatic extension of tumor, and hepatic metastasis.
	G. Abdominal computed tomography (CT) scan	G. CT scan characteristics include diffuse or focal thickening of the wall of the gallbladder, gallbladder wall contrast enhancement, an intraluminal mass, direct liver invasion by tumor, regional lymph node involvement, or evidence of abdominal metastases.

quadrant abdominal tenderness may be present. Clinically evident jaundice is present in 45% of patients. Weight loss of greater than 10% of normal body weight is found in 37% to 77% of patients (Curley et al., 1995).

Diagnostic Tests

Laboratory tests should include a serum bilirubin, as well as serum alkaline phosphatase, alanine aminotransferase, and aspartate aminotransferase levels. Serum carcinoembryonic antigen levels generally are obtained only in patients diagnosed preoperatively with advanced stage disease (i.e., TNM stage III or IV).

Ultrasonography is the primary imaging study for symptomatic patients to rule out cholelithiasis vs cancer. A high-resolution ultrasound can detect early and locally advanced cancer of the gallbladder (Koga, Yamauchi, Izumi, & Hamanaka, 1985). Preoperative ultrasound can suggest the correct diagnosis in up to 75% of patients with cancer of the gallbladder. Patients with symptoms atypical of cholecystitis may undergo a computed tomography (CT) scan of the abdomen.

CANCER STAGING

Most cancers of the gallbladder (about 90%) are adenocarcinomas; none are squamous or adenosquamous carcinomas. Other less common types of gallbladder cancer include anaplastic (undifferentiated) cancers, carcinoids, or clear cell carcinomas. Adenocarcinoma can be further subdivided into papillary, nodular, papillary infiltrating, or nodular infiltrating tumors. Papillary adenocarcinomas or well-differentiated tumors generally have a better prognosis (Dawes & Joehl, 1995).

Two staging systems are commonly used to clinically stage cancer of the gallbladder, the American Joint Commission on Cancer (AJCC) TNM staging system (Table 40-2) and the Nevin-Moran staging system (Box 40-1). The approximate equivalence of the two staging systems is listed in Table 40-3. However, transposing patients from one sys-

TABLE 40-2 AJCC Staging of Cancer of the Gallbladder

Primary Tumor			
TX	Primary tumor cannot be assessed		
T0	No evidence of primary tumor		
Tis	Carcinoma in situ		
T1a	Tumor invades mucosa		
T1b	Tumor invades muscularis		
T2	Tumor invades perimuscular connective tissue; no extension beyond serosa or into liver		
T3	Tumor penetrates serosa, invades one adjacent organ or extends into liver less than 2 cm, or both		
T4	Tumor extends more than 2 cm into liver, involves two or more adjacent organs (e.g., bile ducts, liver, omentum)		
Lymph Nodes			
NX	Regional nodes cannot be assessed		
N0	No lymph node metastases		
N1	Metastases in cystic duct, pericholedochal, and/or hilar lymph nodes only		
N2	Metastases in peripancreatic (head of pancreas only), periduodenal, periportal, celiac, and/or superior mesenteric lymph nodes		
Metastases			
MX	Distant metastases cannot be assessed		
M0	No distant metastases		
M1	Distant metastases		
Stage 0	Tis	N0	M0
Stage I	T1	N0	M0
Stage II	T2	N0	M0
Stage III	T1-2	N1	M0
	T3	N0-1	M0
Stage IVA	T4	N0-1	M0
Stage IVB	T1-4	N2	M0
	T1-4	N0-2	M1

From American Joint Commission on Cancer. (1993). *Manual for staging of cancer* (4th ed.). Philadelphia: J. B. Lippincott.

tem to another should be considered only an approximation (Douglas et al., 1997).

MEDICAL MANAGEMENT

Treatment of cancer of the gallbladder depends on the stage of the disease at the time of diagnosis. Disease in an early stage is amenable to surgical intervention with or without adjuvant therapy. However, many patients with cancer of the gallbladder are diagnosed with advanced disease that is not amenable to a surgical intervention. In those cases, palliative procedures and aggressive management of symptoms become the mainstay of treatment.

Surgery

Surgical interventions may vary depending on whether the cancer is diagnosed preoperatively, discovered by the surgeon during cholecystectomy, or identified by the pathologist after the surgical procedure. If the diagnosis of cancer of the gallbladder is suspected preoperatively, a CT scan should be performed to evaluate for spread of disease into the liver as well as for distant metastases. Findings of liver involvement and distant metastases may preclude a surgical resection. In these cases, palliative measures should be instituted to minimize symptoms and maximize comfort (Dawes & Joehl, 1995).

TABLE 40-3 Approximate Equivalence of Staging Systems

AJCC Stage	Nevin-Moran Stage
0	I
IA	II
IB	II
II	III
III	IV
IV	V

From Douglas, H. O., Kim, S. Y., & Meropol, N. J. (1997). Neoplasms of the gallbladder. In J. F. Holland, R. C. Bast Jr, D. L. Morton, E. Frei, III, D. W. Keefe, & R. R. Weichselbaum (Eds.), *Cancer medicine* (4th ed.). Baltimore: Williams & Wilkins.

Box 40-1
Nevin-Moran Staging of Gallbladder Cancer

Stage I	Intramucosal cancer
Stage II	Involvement of the mucosa and muscularis
Stage III	Involvement of all three layers
Stage IV	Involvement of all three layers and cystic duct lymph nodes
Stage V	Involvement of liver or metastases to other organs

A large majority of surgeons consider simple cholecystectomy to be an adequate treatment for cancer of the gallbladder confined to the mucosa (T1aN0M0). The 5-year survival rate for patients undergoing simple cholecystectomy for cancer confined to the mucosa ranges from 57% to 100% (Gagner & Rossi, 1991; Gall, Kockerling, Scheele, Schneider, & Hohenberger, 1991; Ogura et al., 1991; Yamaguchi & Tsuneyoshi, 1992). However, some authors recommend that an extended cholecystectomy (see later) be performed to treat patients with these early-stage lesions (Bergdahl, 1980; Ouchi, Owada, Matsuno, & Sato, 1987).

If the cancer extends into the muscularis or serosa (AJCC classification Stage II or III), a radical or extended cholecystectomy is performed. An extended cholecystectomy includes a wedge resection of the liver, with resection of a 2- to 3-cm margin of liver adjacent to the gallbladder (liver segments IV and V, Fig. 40-1), and a lymph node dissection. The lymph node dissection should include the cystic duct, choledochal, periportal, and hilar lymph nodes in addition to the peripancreatic, duodenal, celiac, and superior mesenteric lymph nodes (Fig. 40-2). The 5-year survival rate after extended cholecystectomy for AJCC stages II and III cancer of the gallbladder ranges from 7.5% to 37% (Donohue, Nagorney, Grant, Tsushima, Ilstrup, & Adson, 1990; Gagner & Rossi, 1991; Gall et al., 1991; Ogura et al., 1991; Ouchi et al., 1987). Patients with AJCC stage II or III cancers of the gallbladder who were treated with simple cholecystectomy alone had a 0 to 5% 5-year survival rate compared with a 29% 5-year survival rate for patients treated with extended cholecystectomy (Donohue et al., 1990).

An extremely radical procedure, namely hepatopancreaticoduodenectomy, has been proposed for patients with extensive disease (i.e., AJCC stages III and IV). However, the operative mortality for this radical procedure is at least 15%, with a greater than 90% incidence of major postoperative morbidity. The 5-year survival rate associated with this radical surgery is 14% (Nimura, Hayukawa, Kamiya, Maeda, Kondo, & Yasui et al., 1991; Ogura et al., 1991).

According to Douglas and colleagues (1997), for the patient in whom cancer of the gallbladder is found by the pathologist subsequent to the closure of the abdomen, consideration of a re-exploration should be limited to patients with T3 tumors (i.e., tumor penetrates the serosa, invades one adjacent organ or extends into the liver less than 2 cm, or both). The morbidity and mortality associated with re-exploration must be weighed against the limited efficacy of a second surgical procedure. Most commonly, the lesions found by the pathologist are small tumors and often are confined to the mucosa or submucosa, for which there is still no evidence of benefit from re-exploration.

Laparoscopic cholecystectomy has revolutionized the management of patients with gallstones and chronic cholecystitis (Grace, Quereshi, Coleman, Keane, McEntee, & Broe et al., 1991). Although this procedure reduces postoperative morbidity, it eliminates the surgeon's ability to palpate the gallbladder and adjacent tissues for evidence of tumor or lymph node metastases. A surgeon performing a laproscopic cholecystectomy who suspects a malignancy should not hesitate to close and refer the patient or convert to an open procedure of extended cholecystectomy (Fong, Brennan, Turnbull, Colt, & Blumgart, 1993).

Laparoscopic removal of a previously undiagnosed cancer of the gallbladder can lead to implants in trocar sites (Clair, Lautz, & Brooks, 1993; Fong et al., 1993; Targarona, Pons, Viella, & Trias, 1994) or in the peritoneum (Fong et al., 1993; Pezet, Fondrinier, Rotman, Guy, Lemesle, & Lointier et al., 1992; Wade, Comitalo, Andrus, Goodwin, & Kaminski, 1994). It is estimated that 70,000 laparoscopic cholecystectomies are performed each year in the United States (Grace et al., 1991). On average, cancer of the gallbladder is diagnosed in 2% of patients who undergo cholecystectomy for presumably benign disease (Piehler & Crichlow, 1978). Therefore, approximately 1400 patients who undergo laparoscopic cholecystectomy annually could suffer inadvertent dissemination of cancer of the gallbladder.

Radiation Therapy

Research on the use of radiation therapy as an adjuvant therapy following surgical resection for cancer of the gallbladder is extremely limited. In one study (Bosset, Mantion, Gillet, Pelisser, Boulenger, & Maingon et al., 1989), five of seven patients who received postoperative radiation therapy were alive with no evidence of disease at 5, 9, 11, 31, and 58 months. Treatment consisted of 4600 cGy followed by a 900 Gy external beam boost to the gallbladder tumor bed. The treatment was well tolerated by the patients. According to Douglas and colleagues (1997), although data are limited, conclusions from individual studies suggest the need for adjuvant radiation therapy following complete resection. Although older adjuvant therapy trials used 30 to 45 cGy (Hanna & Rider, 1978; Kopelson, Harisiadis, Tretter, & Chang, 1977), newer trials recommend treatment with 45 to 55 Gy.

Few studies have evaluated the use of palliative radiation therapy for cancer of the gallbladder. In one study of five patients who were treated with primary radiation therapy for cancer of the gallbladder (Kopelson et al., 1977), four patients achieved palliation in terms of pain, pruritus, or mass effect. The dose of radiation ranged from 38 to 50 Gy.

Chemotherapy

The use of chemotherapy has not been explored in a systematic fashion for the management of cancer of the gallbladder. However, a variety of chemotherapeutic agents have been used for the treatment of cancer of the gallbladder. In one early study using mitomycin as a single agent (Crooke & Bradner, 1976), a response rate of 47% was seen in 15 patients with biliary cancers. However, this response rate was not confirmed in later studies (Taal, Audisio, Bleiberg, Blijham, Neijt, & Duez et al., 1991). Additional studies using 5-fluorouracil (5-FU) for the treatment of cancer of the gallbladder demonstrated a response rate of approximately 10% (Falkson, MacIntyre, & Moertel, 1984).

Several combination chemotherapy regimens have been tried in the treatment of cancer of the gallbladder. These combinations include epirubicin, methotrexate, 5-FU, and leucovorin (Kajanti & Pyrhonen, 1994) or 5-FU, doxorubicin, and cisplatin (Moertel, Rubin, O'Connell, Schutt, & Wieand, 1986). The results of these studies were not encouraging in terms of response rates.

Given that the blood supply to the gallbladder derives largely from the hepatic artery, regional intra-arterial therapy has been tried to treat cancer of the gallbladder. Chemotherapy agents that have been used in an intra-arterial infusion include mitomycin C (Kairaluoma, Leinonen, Niemela, Kiviniemi, Siniluoto, & Stahlberg, 1988; Makela & Kairaluoma, 1993), 5-FU and mitomycin C (Smith, Bukowski, Hewlett, & Groppe, 1984), 5-fluorodeoxyuridine (Reed, Vaitkevicius, al-Sarraf, Vaughn, Singhakowinta, & Sexon-Porte et al., 1981; Seeger, Woodcock, Blumenreich, & Richardson, 1989), or doxorubicin (Garnick, Ensmenger, & Israel, 1979). As with systemic administration of chemotherapy, the response rates were extremely poor.

ONCOLOGIC EMERGENCIES

Cancer of the gallbladder can produce biliary obstruction by direct extension of the tumor into the extrahepatic biliary tree or by compression produced by lymph node metastasis.

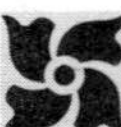

TABLE 40-4 Standard of Care for the Patient with Advanced-Stage Cancer of the Gallbladder

Patient Problems and Outcomes	Nursing Interventions and Rationales	Patient Education Instructions
Pruritus		
• Patient will experience as little pruritus as possible	1. Obtain a history regarding pruritus, including: a. Onset b. Duration c. Intensity d. Sensation e. Pattern f. Location 2. Develop a skin care regimen a. Use mild soaps and rinse well b. Use a bath oil or lubricating emollient cream 3. Use topical ointments (e.g., topical steroids) as prescribed 4. Use moisturizing agents (Aveeno, Aquaphor, Prax, Sarna, Gold Bond). 5. Administer antihistamines, as prescribed.	1. Explain that the exact mechanism underlying itching is not completely understood. 2. Avoid taking very hot baths and to bathe in moderation (not less than 10 minutes and not greater than 20 minutes). 3. Recommend the use of Aveeno Colloidal Oatmeal baths because they tend to be soothing and help the skin to hold moisture. 4. Avoid the use of perfumes, cosmetics, starch-based powders, and deodorants. 5. Encourage the use of loose fitting clothing and the avoidance of harsh fabrics. 6. Maintain a cool environment because increased temperature causes vasodilation and drying of the skin. 7. Avoid scratching to prevent skin injury. a. Keep fingernails short b. Wear cotton mittens on hands 8. Increase fluid intake to at least 3000 ml/day and maintain an adequate nutritional intake. 9. Teach the use of relaxation exercises or guided imagery.
Pain		
• Patient will maintain an optimal level of comfort	1. Perform a pain assessment, including: a. Description b. Location and radiation c. Severity d. Aggravating and relieving factors e. Previous treatment modalities and effectiveness f. Associated symptoms 2. Ascertain the cause of the pain to determine the most appropriate pain management plan. 3. Have patient keep a diary of pain intensity and analgesic use. Review diary and make adjustments in the treatment plan.	1. Explain the cause of the pain and the rationale for each of the pain management interventions. 2. Discuss concerns regarding the meaning of the pain and the differences between tolerance, physical dependence, and addiction. 3. Explain the reason for taking pain medications on a regular schedule. 4. Teach relaxation exercises and guided imagery techniques.
Decreased Nutritional Intake		
• Patient will maintain an adequate nutritional intake	1. Obtain a nutritional history a. Food preferences b. Symptoms that interfere with nutritional intake: nausea, anorexia, taste changes, feelings of fullness, fatigue 2. Weigh patient weekly. 3. Obtain serum albumin level. 4. Evaluate the need for an appetite stimulant (e.g., megestrol acetate). 5. Evaluate the need for a feeding tube if oral intake is compromised.	1. Teach strategies to increase dietary intake: a. Eat small meals, five to six times per day. b. Drink liquids before or after meals to avoid feeling full while eating. c. Plan meals with favorite foods. d. Eat high-protein foods. e. Use food supplements between meals. f. Eat in a pleasant environment. 2. Exercise before meals to stimulate appetite. 3. Teach use of jejunostomy feeding tube (refer to Table 40-5).

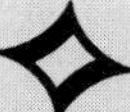

TABLE 40-5 Patient Preparation for Feeding a Patient Using a Jejunostomy Tube

Description: A jejunostomy tube is a hollow tube that is placed through the wall of the abdomen into a part of the intestine (called the jejunum) so that liquid food can be given to the patient.

Procedure:

1. Wash hands.
2. Prepare tube feeding in the administration bag and fill the tubing. If tube feeding is to be administered through a pump, connect bag to pump.
3. Insert large syringe into the feeding tube and pull back gently on the plunger. Check for fluid in the syringe. Do not feed the patient if more than a full syringe of food is removed.
4. Connect the tube feeding bag to the jejunostomy tube and give the tube feeding at the rate that the doctor has recommended. Do not let the feeding bag hang for more than 12 hours.
5. Keep the head of the patient's bed at a 30- to 45-degree angle.
6. Clean the skin around the jejunostomy tube with warm water and put on a gauze dressing.
7. Keep a record of how much food and water the patient takes in through the jejunostomy tube, as well as the patient's urine output.
8. If the patient needs to get his/her medicines through the jejunostomy tube, crush all pills and mix with some water before giving them through the tube. Rinse the tube with water after giving the medicine.

If unresectable disease is found at the time of surgery, a biliary bypass procedure can produce effective palliation of jaundice. A choledochojejunostomy or hepaticojejunostomy can be used to relieve jaundice when extrahepatic obstruction is the cause of the problem. When there is obstruction of the common bile duct near the cystic duct junction, a Roux-en-Y loop of jejunum is anastomosed to the common hepatic duct or to the left hepatic duct (Dawes & Joehl, 1995).

Approximately 30% to 50% of patients with advanced cancer of the gallbladder develop a clinically significant gastroduodenal obstruction (Jones, 1991). The obstruction can be treated with a surgical bypass procedure such as gastrojejunostomy or by the placement of a decompressing gastrostomy tube and a feeding jejunostomy tube.

NURSING MANAGEMENT

Surgical Management

Patients diagnosed with early-stage cancer of the gallbladder undergo a cholecystectomy or extended cholecystectomy. These patients require routine postoperative care that focuses on pain management, early ambulation, implementation of strategies to prevent infection, and wound care. After surgery, the patient may require dietary counseling. The amount of fat in the postoperative diet depends on the patient's tolerance of fat. A low-fat diet may be helpful if the flow of bile is reduced or the patient is overweight. Foods that may need to be avoided include whole milk, cream, butter, whole milk cheese, and ice cream; fried foods; rich pastries and gravies; and nuts.

Palliative Care

Patients diagnosed with advanced stages of cancer of the gallbladder most often receive palliative care. Symptom management becomes a major priority in terms of nursing care (Table 40-4). The major problems that require nursing interventions include pruritus associated with biliary obstruction and jaundice, pain from obstruction or distant metastasis (i.e., to bone), and decreased nutritional intake associated with anorexia and gastroduodenal obstruction.

HOME CARE ISSUES

Home care issues may surface in the management of patients diagnosed with the advanced stages of cancer of the gallbladder. These patients may require the coordinated services provided by hospice. A referral to hospice services is particularly useful because of their expertise in symptom management.

Nutritional management of patients with advanced disease may become a significant issue in the home. If the patient experiences a gastroduodenal obstruction, the patient may undergo a gastrojejunostomy. A gastrojejunostomy involves a partial gastrectomy with removal of the distal two thirds of the stomach and anastomosis of the gastric stump to the jejunum. If surgical treatment is not warranted, the obstruction can be treated with the placement of a decompressing gastrostomy tube and a feeding jejunostomy tube. The patient's family members will need to be taught how to feed the patient using the jejunostomy tube (Table 40-5).

PROGNOSIS

The prognosis for cancer of the gallbladder depends on the stage of the disease at the time of diagnosis. The curative resection rates for cancer of the gallbladder range from 10% to 30% (Barr & Wright, 1984; Hamrick, Liner, Hastings, & Cohn, 1982; Klamer & Max, 1983). Most patients are not candidates for curative resection because of extensive local-regional disease, liver metastasis, or distant metastasis at the time of diagnosis. The overall survival rate for cancer of the gallbladder is about 5%, and the median survival is approxi-

Table 40-6 Quality of Care Evaluation for a Patient with Advanced-Stage Cancer of the Gallbladder

Disciplines participating in the quality of care evaluation:
☐ Nursing ☐ Oncologist ☐ Social Worker ☐ Dietitian

Data from:
☐ Medical record review ☐ Patient/family interview

Criteria	Yes	No
1. Was an assessment done for the following patient problems:		
a. Pruritus	☐	☐
b. Pain	☐	☐
c. Nutritional deficit	☐	☐
2. Did the patient/family members receive instructions on skin care?	☐	☐
3. Was the patient taught to take the pain medication on a regular schedule?	☐	☐
4. Was the patient/family members taught to do relaxation exercises or guided imagery to decrease pruritus or pain?	☐	☐
5. Was a dietary consultation made?	☐	☐
6. Does the patient have a nutritional plan to optimize his dietary intake?	☐	☐

mately 6 months (Burgess, Murphy, & Clauge, 1991; Silk, Douglass, Nava, Driscoll, & Tartarian, 1989).

EVALUATION OF THE QUALITY OF CARE

Accreditation organizations, such as the Joint Commission for the Accreditation of Health Care Organizations, require that the quality of care provided to patients be evaluated. Because the care provided to patients with cancer of the gallbladder requires input from a multidisciplinary team, an evaluation of the quality of care provided should include aspects of care provided by various team members. Table 40-6 provides an example of a quality of care evaluation tool for a patient with cancer of the gallbladder.

RESEARCH ISSUES

Research on the most appropriate treatment options for cancer of the gallbladder is thwarted by the small number of patients diagnosed with this disease. The picture is complicated by the fact that some cancers of the gallbladder appear radiosensitive, whereas others are radioresistant. A similar dimorphism is seen with the administration of chemotherapy. Therefore, studies of the molecular biology of cancers of the gallbladder are necessary to design more promising clinical trials.

REFERENCES

Albores-Saavedra, J., Alcantra-Vazquez, A., Cruz-Ortiz, H., & Herrera-Goepfert, R. (1980). The precursor lesions of invasive gallbladder carcinoma: Hyperplasia, atypical hyperplasia, and carcinoma in situ. *Cancer, 45*(5), 919-927.

American Joint Commission on Cancer. (1993). *Manual for staging of cancer* (4th ed.). Philadelphia: J. B. Lippincott Company.

Barr, L. H. & Wright, F. H. (1984). Carcinoma of the gallbladder. *American Surgeon, 50*(5), 275-276.

Bergdahl, L. (1980). Gallbladder carcinoma first diagnosed at microscopic examination of gallbladders removed from presumed benign disease. *Annals of Surgery, 191*(1), 19-22.

Bosset, J. F., Mantion, G., Gillet, M., Pelissier, E., Boulenger, M., Maingon, P., Corbion, O., & Schraub, S. (1989). Primary carcinoma of the gallbladder: Adjuvant postoperative external irradiation. *Cancer, 64*(9), 1843-1847.

Burgess, P., Murphy, P. D., & Clauge, M. B. (1991). Adenocarcinoma of the gallbladder: A 5-year review of outcome in Newcastle upon Tyne. *Journal of the Royal Society of Medicine, 84*(2), 84-86.

Clair, D. G., Lautz, D. B., & Brooks, D. C. (1993). Rapid development of umbilical metastases after laparoscopic cholecystectomy for unsuspected gallbladder carcinoma. *Surgery, 113*(3), 355-358.

Crooke, S. T. & Bradner, W. T. (1976). Mitomycin C: A review. *Cancer Treatment Reports, 3*(3), 121-139.

Curley, S. A., Levin, B., & Rich, T. A. (1995). Liver and bile ducts. In M. D. Abeloff, J. O. Armitage, A. S. Lichter, & J. E. Neiderhuber (Eds.), *Clinical oncology.* New York: Churchill Livingstone.

Dawes, L. G. & Joehl, R. J. (1995). Gallbladder cancer. In J. L. Cameron (Ed.), *Current surgical therapy* (5th ed.). St. Louis: Mosby.

Diehl, A. K. (1983). Gallstone size and the risk of gallbladder cancer. *Journal of the American Medical Association, 250*(17), 2323-2326.

Donohue, J. H., Nagorney, D. M., Grant, C. S., Tsushima, K., Ilstrup, D. M., & Adson, M. A. (1990). Carcinoma of the gallbladder. *Archives of Surgery, 125*(2), 237-241.

Douglas, H. O., Kim, S. Y., & Meropol, N. J. (1997). Neoplasms of the gallbladder. In J. F. Holland, R. C. Bast, Jr., D. L. Morton, E. Frei, III, D. W. Keefe, & R. R. Weichselbaum (Eds.), *Cancer medicine* (4th ed.). Baltimore, Maryland: Williams & Wilkins.

Elrod, R. (1996). Nursing assessment: Gastrointestinal system. In S. M. Lewis, I. C. Collier, & M. M. Heitkemper (Eds.), *Medical-surgical nursing: Assessment and management of clinical problems* (4th ed.). St. Louis: Mosby.

Enomoto, M., Naoe, S., Harada, M., Miyata, K., Saito, M., & Noguchi, Y. (1974). Carcinogenesis in extrahepatic bile duct and gallbladder: Carcinogenic effect of N-hydroxy-2-acetamidofluorene in mice fed a "gallstone-inducing" diet. *Japanese Journal of Experimental Medicine, 44*(1), 37-54.

Falkson, G., MacIntyre, J. M., & Moertel, C. G. (1984). Eastern Cooperative Oncology Group experience with chemotherapy for inoperable gallbladder and bile duct cancer. *Cancer, 54*(6), 965-969.

Fong, Y., Brennan, M. F., Turnbull, A., Colt, D. G., & Blumgart, L. H. (1993). Gallbladder cancer discovered during laparoscopic surgery: Potential for iatrogenic tumor dissemination. *Archives of Surgery, 128*(9), 1054-1056.

Gagner, M. & Rossi, R. L. (1991). Radical operations for carcinoma of the gallbladder: Present status in North America. *World Journal of Surgery, 15*(3), 344-347.

Gall, F. P., Kockerling, F., Scheele, J., Schneider, C., & Hohenberger, W. (1991). Radical operations for carcinoma of the gallbladder: Present status in Germany. *World Journal of Surgery, 15*(3), 328-336.

Garnick, M. B., Ensmenger, W. D., & Israel, M. (1979). A clinical-pharmacological evaluation of hepatic arterial infusion of Adriamycin. *Cancer Research, 39*(10), 4105-4110.

Grace, P. A., Quereshi, A., Coleman, J., Keane, R., McEntee, G., Broe, P., Osborne, H., & Bouchier-Hayes, D. (1991). Reduced postoperative hospitalization after laparoscopic cholecystectomy. *British Journal of Surgery, 78*(2), 160-162.

Hamrick, R. E., Liner, J., Hastings, P. R., & Cohn, I. (1982). Primary carcinoma of the gallbladder. *Annals of Surgery, 195*(3), 270-273.

Hanna, S. S. & Rider, W. B. (1978). Carcinoma of the gallbladder or extrahepatic bile ducts: The role of radiotherapy. *Canadian Medical Association Journal, 118*(1), 59-61.

Jones, R. S. (1991). Palliative operative procedures for carcinoma of the gallbladder. *World Journal of Surgery, 15*(3), 348-351.

Kairaluoma, M. I., Leinonen, A., Niemela, R., Kiviniemi, H., Siniluoto, T., & Stahlberg, M. (1988). Superselective intra-arterial chemotherapy with mitomycin C in liver and gallbladder cancer. *European Journal of Clinical Oncology, 14*(1), 45-50.

Kajanti, M. & Pyrhonen, S. (1994). Epirubicin-sequential methotrexate-5-fluorouracil-leucovorin treatment in advanced cancer of the extrahepatic biliary system. *American Journal of Clinical Oncology, 17*(3), 223-226.

Klamer, T. W. & Max, M. H. (1983). Carcinoma of the gallbladder. *Surgery, Gynecology, and Obstetrics, 156*(5), 641-645.

Koga, A., Yamauchi, S., Izumi, Y., & Hamanaka, N. (1985). Ultrasonographic detection of early and curable carcinoma of the gallbladder. *British Journal of Surgery, 72*(9), 728-730.

Koo, J., Wong, J., Cheng, F. C. Y., & Ong, G. B. (1981). Carcinoma of the gallbladder. *British Journal of Surgery, 68*(3), 161-165.

Kopelson, G., Harisiadis, L., Tretter, P., & Chang, C. H. (1977). The role of radiation therapy in cancer of the extra-hepatic biliary system: An analysis of 13 patients and a review of the literature on the effectiveness of surgery, chemotherapy, and radiotherapy. *International Journal of Radiation Oncology, Biology, Physics, 2*(9-10), 883-894.

Makela, J. T. & Kairaluoma, M. I. (1993). Superselective intra-arterial chemotherapy with mitomycin for gallbladder cancer. *British Journal of Surgery, 80*(7), 912-915.

Moertel, C. G., Rubin, J., O'Connell, M. J., Schutt, A. J., & Wieand, H. S. (1986). A phase II study of combined 5-fluorouracil, doxorubicin, cisplatin in the treatment of advanced upper gastrointestinal adenocarcinomas. *Journal of Clinical Oncology, 4*(7), 1053-1057.

Nagorney, D. M. & McPherson, G. A. D. (1988). Carcinoma of the gallbladder and extrahepatic bile ducts. *Seminars in Oncology, 15,* 106-109.

Nelson, B. D., Porvaznik, J., & Benfield, J. R. (1971). Gallbladder disease in southwestern American Indians. *Archives of Surgery, 103*(1), 41-43.

Nevin, J. E., Moran, T. J., Kay, S., & King, R. (1976). Carcinoma of the gallbladder. Staging, treatment, and prognosis. *Cancer, 37,* 141-148.

Nimura, Y., Hayakawa, N., Kamiya, J., Maeda, S., Kondo, S., Yasui, A., & Shionoya, S. (1991). Hepatopancreaticoduodenectomy for advanced carcinoma of the biliary tract. *Hepatogastroenterology, 38*(2), 170-175.

Ogura, Y., Mizumoto, R., Isaji, S., Kusuda, T., Matsuda, S., & Tabata, M. (1991). Radical operations for carcinoma of the gallbladder: Present status in Japan. *World Journal of Surgery, 15*(3), 337-343.

Ouchi, K., Owada, Y., Matsuno, S., & Sato, T. (1987). Prognostic factors in the surgical treatment of gallbladder carcinoma. *Surgery, 101*(6), 731-737.

Parker, S. L., Tong, T., Bolden, S., & Wingo, P. A. (1997). Cancer statistics, 1997. *CA: A Cancer Journal for Clinicians, 47,* 5-27.

Pezet, D., Fondrinier, E., Rotman, N., Guy, L., Lemesle, P., Lointier, P., & Chipponi, J. (1992). Parietal seeding of carcinoma of the gallbladder after laparoscopic cholecystectomy. *British Journal of Surgery, 79*(3), 230.

Piehler, J. M. & Crichlow, R. W. (1978). Primary carcinoma of the gallbladder. *Surgery, Gynecology, and Obstetrics, 147*(6), 929-942.

Reed, M. L., Vaitkevicius, V. K., Al-Sarraf, M., Vaughn, C. B., Singhakowinta, A., Sexon-Porte, M., Izbicki, R., Baker, L., & Straatsma, G. W. (1981). The practicality of chronic hepatic artery infusion therapy of primary and metastatic hepatic malignancies: Ten-year results of 124 patients in a prospective protocol. *Cancer, 47*(2), 402-409.

Seeger, J., Woodcock, T. M., Blumenreich, M. S., & Richardson, J. D. (1989). Hepatic perfusion with FUdR utilizing an implantable system in patients with liver primary cancer or metastatic cancer confined to the liver. *Cancer Investigation, 7*(1), 1-6.

Silk, Y. N., Douglass, H. O., Nava, H. R., Driscoll, D. L., & Tartarian, G. (1989). Carcinoma of the gallbladder: The Roswell Park experience. *Annals of Surgery, 210*(6), 751-757.

Smith, G. W., Bukowski, R. M., Hewlett, J. S., & Groppe, C. W. (1984). Hepatic artery infusion with 5-fluorouracil and mitomycin C in cholangiocarcinoma and gallbladder carcinoma. *Cancer, 54*(8), 1513-1516.

Strom, B. L., Soloway, R. D., Rios-Dalenz, J. L., Rodriguez-Martinez, H. A., West, S. L., Kinman, J. L., Crowther, R. S., Taylor, D., Polansky, M., & Berlin, J. A. (1996). Biochemical epidemiology of gallbladder cancer. *Hepatology, 23,* 1402-1411.

Taal, B. G., Audisio, R. A., Bleiberg, H., Blijham, G. H., Neijt, J. P. C. H. N., Duez, N., & Sahmoud, T. (1991). Phase II trial of mitomycin C (MMC) in advanced gallbladder and biliary tree carcinoma. An EORTC gastrointestinal tract cancer cooperative group. *Annals of Oncology, 4*(7), 607-609.

Targarona, E. M., Pons, M. J., Viella, P., & Trias, M. (1994). Unsuspected carcinoma of the gallbladder: A laparoscopic dilemma. *Surgical Endoscopy, 8*(3), 211-213.

Wade, T. P., Comitalo, J. B., Andrus, C. H., Goodwin, M. N., & Kaminski, D. L. (1994). Laparoscopic cancer surgery: Lessons from gallbladder cancer. *Surgical Endoscopy, 8*(6), 698-701.

Yamaguchi, K. & Tsuneyoshi, M. (1992). Subclinical gallbladder carcinoma. *American Journal of Surgery, 163*(4), 382-386.

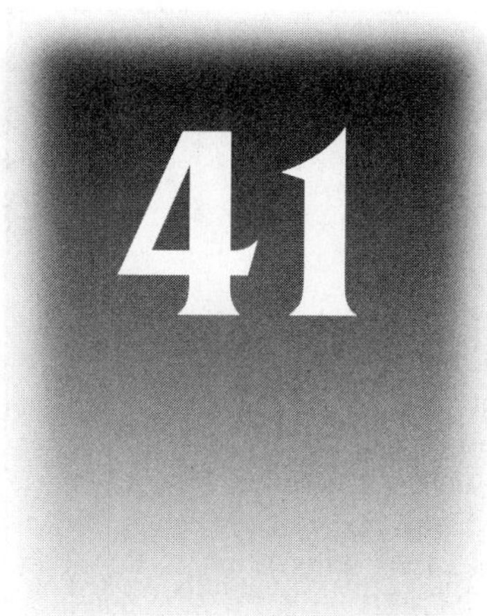

Hepatocellular Cancer

Patricia Collins, RN, MS

EPIDEMIOLOGY

Numerous synonyms for hepatocellular cancer exist, including hepatoma, malignant hepatoma, liver cell carcinoma, primary hepatocellular carcinoma, and primary hepatic carcinoma. The term *hepatoma* does not denote the cell of origin. Therefore, the term *hepatocellular cancer* is preferred when referring to the most common primary epithelial malignancy of the liver (Craig, Peters, & Edmondson, 1989).

Primary liver cancer, specifically, hepatocellular cancer (HCC), is the most frequent cancer worldwide and is responsible for more than 1 million deaths annually (Fong, 1996). There is considerable geographic variation in the incidence of HCC. Although relatively uncommon in the United States, HCC is the most predominant cause of cancer mortality in Southeast Asia and in sub-Saharan Africa (Niederhuber, 1995) (Table 41-1). The incidence rates of HCC are highest in geographic areas where hepatitis is endemic and aflatoxin-contaminated foods are ingested (Groopman & Kensler, 1996).

RISK FACTORS

HCC is almost always associated with chronic underlying liver disease, most frequently with cirrhosis. Therefore, the major risk factors for HCC are those agents that cause prolonged liver damage such as hepatitis B virus (HBV) and hepatitis C virus (HCV) (Venook, 1994).

HBV is a powerful carcinogen, and chronic infection with HBV is the major etiologic agent for human HCC (Beasley, 1988). Moreover, chronic aflatoxin exposure and HBV infection probably work synergistically to promote carcinogenesis (Aguilar, Harris, Sun, Hollstein, & Cerutti, 1994). HCV is also proving to be a potent carcinogen. The unfortunate individuals who have both chronic hepatitis B and C infection are probably at greater risk for developing HCC than are those who have a single infection (Nishiguchi, Kuroki, Nakatani, Morimoto, Takeda, & Nakajima et al., 1995). Other risk factors of varying and perhaps questionable degrees include a positive family history of HCC, tobacco smoking, use of alcohol, exposure to chemicals and toxins, and genetic diseases (Groopman & Kensler, 1996). Box 41-1 lists numerous agents and conditions that can potentially damage liver cells, thus predisposing the organ to the development of tumors.

Chronic Hepatitis/Cirrhosis

Hepatitis B and hepatitis C infections are two of the major risk factors for HCC. Chronic hepatitis B accounts for the majority of HCC cases worldwide. *Chronic hepatitis* is defined as a chronically active necroinflammatory process directed toward the hepatocyte, with or without fibrosis, lasting longer than 6 months. The causes of hepatitis are viral, autoimmune, drug induced, and genetic (Box 41-2). The four major types of chronic hepatitis are chronic persistent hepatitis, chronic lobular hepatitis, chronic active hepatitis, and cirrhosis (Boyer & Reuben, 1993).

Cirrhosis is defined as a chronic liver disease in which diffuse destruction and regeneration of hepatic parenchymal cells have occurred and in which a diffuse increase in connective tissue results in disorganization of the lobular and vascular architecture of the liver. The major causes of cirrhosis are alcohol use, viral hepatitis, use of hepatotoxic drugs, venous outflow obstruction, hemochromatosis, Wilson's disease, and the late stages of parasitic diseases (Conn & Atterbury, 1993). Between 30% and 70% of patients with HCC also have cirrhosis. Overall, the risk of developing HCC is about 40 times greater in a person with cirrhosis than in an individual without cirrhosis (Oberfield, Steele, Gollan, & Sherman, 1989).

Of the five known hepatitis viruses (A, B, C, D, and E), only B, C, and D cause chronic infection and chronic liver damage (Boyer & Reuben, 1993). HCV may be more carcinogenic than HBV (Takano, Yokosuka, Imazeki, Tagawa, & Omata, 1995). Hepatitis D virus (HDV) requires HBV to survive, and HDV may act with HBV to cause more severe liver injury than HBV alone. The role of HDV in the pathogenesis of HCC is unknown (Koff, 1993).

Hepatitis B. HBV is considered a primary carcinogen because it integrates itself into the DNA of the host genome.

TABLE 41-1 Incidence Rates of Hepatocellular Cancer in Males in Various Areas of the World

Area	Estimated Cases Per 100,000/Year
South Africa	
• Mozambique	112
• Zimbabwe	64
• Gambia	33
• Senegal	25
• Cape Bantu	26
Malaysia	
• Singapore (Chinese)	31
• Singapore (Malay)	15
• Singapore (Indian)	14
China	
• Hong Kong	32
• Shanghai	34
Nagasaki, Japan	25
Pacific Polynesian Islands	26
Manila, Philippines	20
Korea	13
Geneva, Switzerland	10
Zaragoza, Spain	7
Hamburg, Germany	4
United States	
• San Francisco (Chinese)	19
• San Francisco (Blacks)	4
• San Francisco (Japanese)	3
• San Francisco (Whites)	3

Modified from Okuda, K., Kojiro, M., & Okuda, H. (1993). Neoplasms of the liver. In L. Schiff & E. Schiff (Eds.), *Diseases of the liver* (Vol 2). Philadelphia: J. B. Lippincott Company.

Box 41-1
Etiologic Factors for Hepatocellular Cancer

Chronic hepatitis B*†
Chronic hepatitis C*†
Mycotoxins
- Aflatoxins*†
- O-demethylsterigmatocystin
- Spertoxin
- Sterigmatocystin
- Luteoskyrin
- Cyclochlorotine

Algal toxin
- Microcystin

Cirrhosis (caused by many of the toxins or conditions listed on this table)
Plant carcinogens
- Pyrrolizidine alkaloids (genus *Senecio*)
- Cycasin (in cycad plants)
- Safrole (in many plant oils)

Synthetic hepatocarcinogens
- AZO dyes
- Aromatic amines
- Chlorinated hydrocarbons (e.g., vinyl chloride)
- Pesticides (e.g., dichlorodiphenyltrichloroethane [DDT], aldrin, dieldrin, heptachlor)
- Hydrazine (rocket fuel)
- Trichoroethylene (dry cleaning solvent)

Oral contraceptives
Anabolic steroids†
Alcohol†
Internal alpha and beta radiation
- Thorotrast†

Tobacco
Alpha-antitrypsin deficiency†
Hemochromatosis†
Budd-Chiari syndrome
Porphyria cutanea tarda†
Types 1 and 3 glycogen storage disease†
Autoimmune chronic active hepatitis†
Primary biliary cirrhosisTyrosinemia†
Family history
Male gender
Malnutrition

*Responsible for the majority of HCC cases worldwide.
†Indicates high to moderate risk for developing HCC

Liver damage occurs when the presence of the virus in the hepatocyte stimulates an immune response that destroys the cell. Some infected hepatocytes may survive, and the ongoing immunologic battle leads to chronic hepatitis (Koff, 1993). People at risk for chronic hepatitis B infection include males, male homosexuals, drug abusers, and the immunologically compromised. The younger the age that one acquires the infection, the higher the risk. If one is generally healthy, the risk of developing chronic hepatitis from an acute infection is approximately 1% (Maddrey, 1993).

In Europe, Latin American, and endemic areas such as Asia and Africa, the major modes of HBV transmission are perinatal, sexual, and close family contact during the first 5 years of life (Boyer & Reuben, 1993). Acquisition of the virus at such a young age invariably leads to the development of chronic hepatitis and thus puts the person at increased risk for HCC (Maddrey, 1993).

In the United States, Japan, and the former Soviet Union, the major mode of HBV transmission is percutaneous, usually from infected blood or blood products. Effective screening and testing of blood have reduced this route of infection. Other important methods of transmission include needle-sharing, occupational exposure, and sexual activity, especially anal sex among male homosexuals (Box 41-3). In the United States, 30% of HBV infections are not associated with an identifiable risk factor (Boyer & Reuben, 1993). The major groups of people at risk for HBV infection are parenteral drug abusers, health care workers, male homosexuals, immunosuppressed individuals, and infants of mothers infected with HBV (Maddrey, 1993).

The major objectives in treating chronic hepatitis infections are to reduce the patient's viral load, to lessen or elimi-

Box 41-2
Some Causes of Chronic Hepatitis

Viral

Hepatitis viruses B, C, and D
Yellow fever
Epstein-Barr
Rubella
Cytomegalovirus

Autoimmune Liver Disease

Classic autoimmune (type 1)
Anti-liver-kidney microsome 1 or type 2 autoimmune hepatitis
Antisoluble liver antigen
Cryptogenic steroid responsive

Drug-Induced Chronic Hepatitis

Oxyphenisatin
Methyldopa
Nitrofurantoin
Dantrolene
Isoniazid

Genetic Disorders

Alpha$_1$-antitrypsin deficiency
Wilson's disease

Modified from Boyer, J. & Reuben, A. (1993). Chronic hepatitis. In L. Schiff & E. Schiff (Eds.), *Diseases of the liver* (Vol. 1). Philadelphia: J. B. Lippincott.

Box 41-3
Transmission of Hepatitis B and C
Blood-to-Blood Inoculation

- Blood/Blood Products Transfusions
- Sexual Transmission
- Maternal-Neonatal
- Transplanted Organs
- Contaminated Needles/Syringes (e.g., illicit drug use, needle/syringe sharing, improper decontamination of medical equipment)
- Occupational Contacts
  - Needle sticks during procedures
  - Scalpel cuts during surgical procedures
  - Blood spillage on mucous membranes or cut skin surfaces
  - Contamination during dental work
  - Smoking/nail biting in blood-contaminated areas
  - Hemodialysis
    - Blood transfusions
    - Infected new patients or staff
    - Intraunit contamination
    - Needle sticks
    - Contamination during refuse collection
  - Contaminated acupuncture needles
  - Contaminated manicurists' equipment
  - Contaminated barbers' razor/clippers
  - Contaminated body-piercing equipment
  - Contaminated tattoo needles/equipment

Modified from Maddrey, W. C. (1993). Chronic hepatitis. *Disease-a-Month, 39*(2), 74, 93; Alter, M. J. (1995). Epidemiology of hepatitis C in the west. *Seminars in Liver Disease, 15*(1), 5-10; Koff, R. S. (1993). Viral hepatitis. In L. Schiff & E. Schiff (Eds.), *Diseases of the liver* (Vol 1). Philadelphia: J. B. Lippincott.

nate symptoms, and to prevent progression to cirrhosis (Fried & Hoofnagle, 1995). Interferons (INF), which have antiviral, antiproliferative, and immunomodulatory properties, can induce a remission in a small portion of patients with chronic HBV. The group of patients who have the best results from treatment with INF, as identified by a loss of serum hepatitis markers, are: females who are HIV negative, individuals who acquire the infection in adulthood versus childhood, and individuals with a high alanine aminotransferase (ALT) level but a low HBV burden (Boyer & Reuben, 1993).

There are numerous ways to prevent HBV transmission. Safer procedures in dialysis units and medical settings can be implemented. People can avoid occupational, sexual, and drug-related routes of transmission. Organ donors, blood, and blood products can be screened for hepatitis viruses. Fortunately, there is a vaccine for HBV. The challenge is to make it accessible and affordable for the world's population.

Hepatitis C. Formerly called *non-A, non-B hepatitis,* this RNA virus is directly cytopathic (Schluger & Bodenheimer, 1995). Chronic HCV causes at least one third of all cases of chronic liver disease in the United States (Boyer & Reuben, 1993). Ninety percent of the present cases of transfusion-related hepatitis are thought to be related to HCV and other yet unidentified viruses. Transplanted organs may be infected with HCV, and this virus is a major cause of hepatitis in dialysis centers. HCV from contaminated blood products has caused many liver cancers in Japan (Groopman & Kensler, 1996). Sexual or household contact spread occurs but is probably less common than that seen with HBV. Perinatal transmission of HCV continues to be the subject of study (Koff, 1993). Chronic HCV infection is often asymptomatic, yet progression of the disease is persistent. Studies report 20% to 70 % of patients develop cirrhosis within 10 years after the onset of an HCV infection (Maddrey, 1993; Fried & Hoofnagle, 1995).

Whereas patients with HBV have high rates of mortality and recurrence after liver transplantation, patients with HCV do much better. Therefore, transplantation is a consideration for those patients with chronic HCV and severe cirrhosis (Boyer & Reuben, 1993).

IFN-alpha induces a temporary remission in chronic HCV, as evidenced by a loss of HCV RNA from serum, normalization of aminotransferase levels, and improvement in liver histology (Fried & Hoofnagle, 1995). In a study by Nishiguchi et al. (1995), IFN-alpha improved liver function in chronic active hepatitis C with cirrhosis and resulted in a decreased incidence of HCC. IFN is the only therapy effective in achieving remission in about 50% of patients. However, half of these patients experience relapse after treatment (Boyer & Reuben, 1993). Questions remain about when patients should begin INF, what dosages should be prescribed, and how long treatment should last.

Prevention of HCV includes developing safer procedures in dialysis units and medical settings, having individuals avoid risky behaviors, screening organ donors, and screening blood and blood products for HCV.

Aflatoxin Exposure

Mycotoxins are among the most potent of all known carcinogens, and chronic aflatoxin exposure is common in parts of the world where HCC rates are the highest. Aflatoxins are molds produced by the fungi *Aspergillus flavus* and *Aspergillus parasiticus*. Aflatoxin B_1 is the most common, toxic, and carcinogenic of the aflatoxin derivatives (Okuda, Kojiro, & Okuda, 1993). This mold grows in hot, humid climates on foods such as corn, peanuts, peanut oil, soy sauce, and fermented soy beans, and is not killed by cooking (Beasley, 1988; Yu, 1995). Aflatoxin B_1 is not only carcinogenic by itself but acts as a synergistic co-carcinogen with the hepatitis virus (Groopman & Kensler, 1996). Epidemiologic studies confirm the relationship between HCC, chronic exposure to aflatoxins, and the presence of hepatitis B and C infection. Studies have shown that aflatoxin exposure causes mutations in the tumor suppressor gene, P53 (Aguilar et al., 1994; Groopman & Kensler, 1996).

Efforts continue to educate the public in high-exposure regions about aflatoxins and to encourage people to switch from corn to rice and to avoid foods commonly contaminated with this mold (Yu, 1995). Researchers have developed molecular biomarkers of aflatoxin exposure, which can be used in screening high-risk populations. (Groopman & Kensler, 1996). In the United States, aflatoxin contamination is uncommon due to climate and food-storage conditions and because the Food & Drug Administration monitors foods for mold contamination (Beasley, 1988).

At least six studies have confirmed that people who drink pond-ditch water (e.g., people in China) experience higher rates of HCC. Recently, the contaminant microcystin (MCYST), a blue-green algal toxin, was identified as a strong promoter of HCC. MCYST causes intrahepatic hemorrhages and liver necrosis, thus leaving the liver cells vulnerable to oncogenesis. Preventive strategies focus on encouraging people to drink deep-well water instead of pond-ditch water (Yu, 1995).

Gender and Age

HCC is more common in males than in females and the ratio between the genders is greater in high-incidence areas than in low-incidence areas. Hormones, genetics, and exposure to carcinogenic environmental stimuli may be other predisposing factors (Okuda, Kojiro, & Okuda, 1993).

The peak age at time of diagnosis varies greatly, according to geographic location. In high-incidence areas, HCC is most common in males between the ages of 25 and 34. In areas where HCC is less prevalent, the disease is seen in people over 50 years of age. This age difference can probably be accounted for by variations in age at time of exposure of hepatitis as it relates to the ultimate development of HCC. Hepatitis infection in children is common in high-incidence areas. In contrast, HCC in childhood and adolescence is rare in the United States. When HCC does occur, the disease is usually the fibrolamellar variation. Worldwide, children under the age of 5 years develop hepatoblastoma versus HCC (Okuda et al., 1993). Although pregnant women occasionally develop HCC, this is a rare occurrence. This finding is probably due to the predominance of HCC in males and to the late age at which HCC usually presents in women. Furthermore, advanced cirrhosis is commonly associated with HCC, and women are less fertile when they have cirrhosis (Lau, Leung, Ho, Lam, Li, & Johnson et al., 1995).

Positive Family History

Family history of HCC has been identified as a risk factor for the development of HCC. However, the pathogenesis of the disease is unknown. In a study of 721 asymptomatic family members of individuals diagnosed with HCC, primary liver cancer was found in 6. This incidence was higher than that observed in the general population. Furthermore, 335 of those studied were hepatitis surface antigen (HBsAg) positive, including those newly diagnosed with HCC. This incidence of HBsAg positivity was also higher than that in the general population. The authors concluded that being a male, having a sibling with HCC, and having cirrhosis are the factors associated with the highest risk for developing HCC. Hepatitis B virus may be the most important factor predisposing an individual to HCC (Hung, Lin, & Chiu, 1995).

Oral Contraceptive Use

The link between oral contraceptives and HCC is controversial. Some authors contend that there is an association, and others believe it is merely coincidental. Researchers have failed to produce HCC in animals who are given contraceptive steroids (Okuda et al., 1993). If there is any risk, it is small and limited to women who have used oral contraceptives for many years (Lau et al., 1995).

Alcohol Use

Alcohol use alone probably does not cause HCC, but it may act as a co-carcinogen. Studies have explored the possible role of concomitant hepatitis B or C virus infections and alcohol-related cirrhosis in the pathogenesis of HCC, but no conclusions have been reached (Mendenhall, 1993). One third of 2319 patients with HCC in Japan surveyed during 1986 and 1987 had a history of an alcohol intake of more than 85 g/day for more than 10 years (Okuda et al., 1993). Alcohol probably acts as a risk factor for HCC when it causes cirrhosis (Simonetti, Camma, Fiorello, Cottone, Rapicetta, & Marino, et al., 1992).

Tobacco Use

Several studies showed an increased incidence of HCC among smokers compared with nonsmokers. However, other studies showed no association. Like the role of alcohol use, the role of tobacco use in HCC is still being debated (Kaklamani, Trichopoulos, Tzonou, Zavitsanos, Koumantaki, & Hatzakis et al., 1991; Tsukuma, Hiyama, Tanaka, Nakao, Yabuuchi, & Kitamura et al., 1993).

Genetic Diseases

Hemochromatosis is an abnormal deposition of iron storage, primarily in liver cells. The causes of hemochromatosis are genetic, secondary to other conditions, or transfusion-related (Tavil, 1993). HCC develops in about 30% of individuals with hemochromatosis (Okuda et al., 1993).

Alpha-1-antitrypsin is a plasma glycoprotein that inhibits proteolytic enzymes and is synthesized primarily by the hepatocyte. A deficiency of this substance predisposes individuals to emphysema, glomerulonephritis, liver disease, and, rarely, HCC. Liver transplantation is recommended for patients with this disease (Schwarzenberg & Sharp, 1993).

Porphyrias are hereditary and acquired disorders in which excessive porphyrins and their precursors accumulate in the liver as a result of abnormalities in the pathway of heme biosynthesis. Patients with porphyria cutanea tarda or the acute porphyrias are at risk for HCC (Bloomer, Straka, & Rank, 1993).

Hereditary tyrosinemia is a metabolic disorder that occurs in acute and chronic forms. Hepatic failure leads to death at an early age. One third of patients with the chronic form of hereditary tyrosinemia develop HCC in their childhood. Liver transplantation is recommended before the age of 2 years (Conn & Atterbury, 1993).

The association of Budd-Chiari syndrome with HCC was first identified in Japanese patients with membranous obstruction or narrowing of the inferior vena cava. HCC may cause this syndrome or be a result of this syndrome. Budd-Chiari syndrome has many possible causes, including thrombosis, tumors, vena caval web, and radiation (Reynolds, 1993). It is thought that obstruction to hepatic venous outflow produces hepatocyte death necessitating liver cell regeneration, which eventually leads to cancer (Okuda et al., 1993).

PREVENTIVE STRATEGIES

The majority of primary liver cancer cases in the world result from chronic viral hepatitis B. Therefore, the major preventive strategy must focus on preventing HBV infection. Preventive measures include meticulous blood-donor screening and blood testing, proper sterilization of medical equipment, practicing safe sex, screening high-risk expectant mothers for HBsAg and if positive treating both mother and child, prompt administration of anti-HBs immune globulin after exposure to the virus, and, ideally, administration of the hepatitis B vaccine worldwide (Koff, 1993). For a large-scale program of mass immunizations to be effective, countries must be committed to the effort in terms of funding and delivery mechanisms. However, while Africa supports immunization, the continent is unable to obtain adequate funding. Conversely, Malaysia, Singapore, Taiwan, China, Thailand, and the Philippines are seeing a reduction in carrier rates due to effective national immunization programs. In Taiwan, the rate of liver cancer in children has already declined (Pajeau & Bennett, 1995). In the United States, hepatitis B vaccine is included in standard childhood immunizations and is strongly recommended for individuals at risk (e.g., health care workers).

EARLY DETECTION AND MASS SCREENING OF HIGH-RISK INDIVIDUALS

Mass screening of high-risk individuals is controversial because current screening tests have significant false-positive and false-negative rates. Even if HCC is identified early, there is little evidence that screening decreases mortality from HCC (Sherman, Peltekian, & Lee, 1995). Despite this grim statement, many individuals have benefited from early detection of an operable HCC lesion (Tang & Yang, 1995). The key to early diagnosis and possibly subsequent cure is to identify individuals at high risk for HCC and to tailor their screenings and diagnostic workups accordingly.

Persons at highest risk for HCC are those with chronic hepatitis or cirrhosis, a family history of HCC, the presence of one of the genetic diseases mentioned earlier, or exposure to aflatoxin or chemical hepatocarcinogens. The recommended frequency of screening for HCC in Western countries is based on the individual's degree of risk. Those individuals in the high-risk category are males over the age of 50 who have any of the following risk factors: cirrhosis, anti-HCV positive status, HbsAg-positive status, acquired HBV in childhood, or hemochromatosis with cirrhosis. Those in the moderate risk group are females over the age of 50 with cirrhosis who are HBsAg positive or who acquired HBV in adulthood. The high-risk group should have their alpha-fetoprotein (AFP) levels checked and a liver ultrasound performed every 6 months. The moderate-risk group should undergo the same tests every 6 to 12 months (Ramsey & Wu, 1995).

The two most common vehicles for screening large populations at risk are ultrasound examination of the liver and testing of AFP levels. Ultrasound has several advantages as an imaging modality. It can detect small lesions, it costs less than other imaging tools, it does not expose patients to radiation, the procedure is noninvasive, and no contrast medium is needed (Liu, Lo, & Fan, 1996).

AFP is a tumor marker for HCC, but it has significant false-positive and false-negative rates. Levels are elevated in only one third of patients with lesions less than 5 cm (Liu et al., 1996). Despite this limitation, AFP is the best serum marker at the present time. AFP-L3, a fractionation of AFP, has been shown to be more specific for HCC. Nevertheless, the presence of AFP-L3 levels is a poor prognostic sign because this marker is significantly elevated when the tumor is moderately or poorly differentiated rather than when it is well differentiated (Yamashita, Tanaka, Satomura, & Tanikawa, 1996). Investigations are underway to evaluate pairing AFP with other serum indicators such as abnormal serum prothrombin (PIVKA-II) to improve tumor detection (Ramsey & Wu, 1995).

PATHOPHYSIOLOGY

Normal Anatomy and Physiology of the Liver

The liver is the largest organ in the body, weighing approximately 15 g and measuring 10 cm × 15 cm × 20 cm. Located in the right upper quadrant of the abdomen, the liver is partially protected by the rib cage and extends from the fifth intercostal space in the mid-clavicular line down to the right costal margin. Glisson's capsule, a tough, fibrous sheath of tissue, covers the liver. The liver is divided into two major lobes, the right and the left, and into two smaller lobes, the caudate and quadrate. The hepatic artery and the portal vein supply the liver with blood, which, after coursing among the liver cells, drains through the hepatic vein into the vena cava. About 1100 ml of portal blood and 350 ml of hepatic artery blood flow through the liver each minute. The portal circulation brings blood from the gastrointestinal system to the liver, where endothelial cells and phagocytic Kupffer cells remove bacteria, worn-out cells, and other foreign matter from the blood. Hepatic arterial blood flow supplies nutrition to the liver (Guyton, 1991; Ishak & Markin, 1996) (Fig. 41-1).

The functional unit of the liver can be described in terms of two models: the lobule and the acinus models. The lobule is a cylindrical structure several millimeters in length and width and consists of hepatocytes, a hepatic arteriole, a portal venule, a bile ductule, lymph vessels, and nerves. Hepatocytes within the lobule are arranged in plates, with sinusoids on each side exposing each hepatocyte to portal blood. Bile canaliculi between the hepatocytes conduct bile to the larger bile ducts. These canaliculi form the right and left hepatic ducts, which, in turn, join to form the common hepatic duct. The cystic duct from the gallbladder connects with the common hepatic duct to become the common bile duct, which together with the duct from the pancreas, empties into the duodenum (Barwick & Rosai, 1996).

The acinus model, first articulated by Rappaport, offers a better description of microanatomy from a hemodynamic viewpoint. According to this model, the hepatic acinus is a mass of parenchyma arranged around an axis consisting of a terminal hepatic arteriole, a portal venule, bile ductules, lymph vessels, and nerves. The acinus resides in parts of several adjacent lobules. The acinus has three circulatory zones (1, 2, and 3), with zone 1 cells receiving the blood with the most oxygen and nutrients and zone 3 cells receiving the blood with the least amount of oxygen and nutrients. In addition, the zones function differently. A complex acinus is composed of at least three simple acini (Rappaport & Wanless, 1993).

The liver performs more than 400 functions for the body. These activities can be divided into vascular, secretory, metabolic, and storage functions (Guyton, 1991). Box 41-4 summarizes the major functions of the liver.

The Process of Carcinogenesis

HCC originates in the parenchymal cells of the liver that have sustained prolonged cellular injury, such as that caused by hepatitis viruses and cirrhosis. Continuous hepatocyte necrosis and compensatory regenerative activities provoke a preneoplastic process that is destined to result in cancer if the person lives long enough. Cellular damage from viruses appears to involve alterations in double-stranded DNA sequences, whereas damage from chemical carcinogens

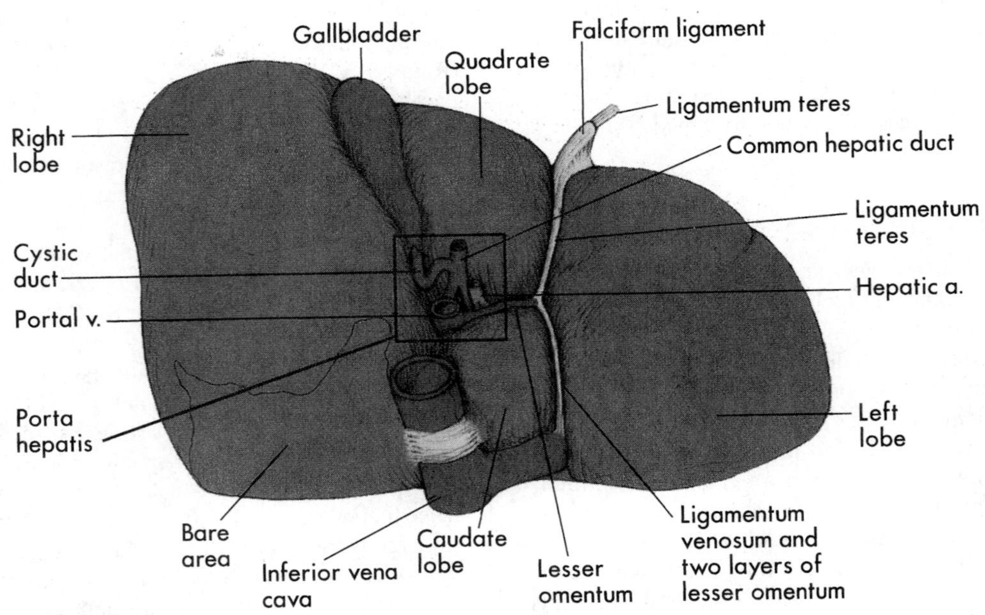

Fig. 41-1 The relationship of the hepatic artery, bile duct, and portal vein exposed by removal of the lesser omentum and the peritoneum on the posterior abdominal wall. (From Williams, P., Dyson, M., Warwick, R., & Bannister, L. [1989]. *Gray's anatomy* [37th ed.]. Edinburgh: Churchill Livingstone.)

evokes single-strand DNA transformations (Okuda et al., 1993).

The development of HCC, as with other cancers, takes place in stages. Although no single oncogene has been identified as always being associated with HCC, the activation of proto-oncogenes is most certainly involved in carcinogenesis. Another important factor in carcinogenesis is mutations of tumor suppressor genes, specifically P53. Mutations vary according to tumor types and within tumors. For example, a high number of individuals with HCC who were exposed to aflatoxins have an AGG to AGT mutation at codon 249 of the P53 tumor suppression gene. In contrast, individuals with HCC who were not exposed to aflatoxin did not have this particular mutation (Aguilar et al., 1994; Groopman & Kensler, 1996).

Box 41-4
Functions of the Liver

Blood Filtration

Removes excess nutrients from the blood
Phagocytizes bacteria and worn-out blood cells

Secretory Functions

Formation of bile
Secretion of bilirubin
Conjugation of bilirubin
Formation of urea

Metabolic Functions

Carbohydrate metabolism
- Storage of glycogen
- Conversion of galactose and fructose to glucose
- Gluconeogenesis

Fat metabolism
- Oxidation of fatty acids and formation of acetoacetic acid
- Formation of lipoproteins
- Formation of cholesterol and phospholipids
- Conversion of carbohydrates and proteins to fat

Protein metabolism
- Deamination of amino acids
- Formation of urea for removal of ammonia from the body
- Formation of plasma proteins
- Synthesize amino acids and other chemical compounds as needed

Other metabolic functions
- Synthesis of coagulation factors (factors II, VI, VII, VIII, IX, X)
- Removal of activated clotting factors
- Detoxification of drugs, hormones and other substances
- Reduction and conjugation of adrenocortical and gonadal steroid hormones
- Synthesis of 25-hydroxycholecalciferol

Storage Functions

Blood
Glucose
Vitamins (A, B_{12}, D, E, K)
Iron and magnesium

Modified from Guyton, A. (1991). *Textbook of medical physiology* (8th ed.). Philadelphia: W. B. Saunders.

ROUTES OF METASTASES

HCC spreads by direct extension within the liver and surrounding tissues. Metastatic spread occurs through both lymphatic and hematogenous routes. Primary liver cancer spreads mainly to the lungs, but can also be found in regional lymph nodes, adrenal glands, bone tissue, kidneys, brain, heart, pancreas, and stomach. Metastatic disease does not usually kill the patient. Death occurs from liver failure (i.e., cachexia, hemorrhage, hepatic coma) resulting from uncontrolled tumor growth in the liver or the underlying cirrhosis (Choi, 1996; Oberfield et al., 1989).

ASSESSMENT

The assessment of a patient for HCC is summarized in Table 41-2. The clinician should take a careful history and perform a thorough examination. With this information, the clinician is better able to determine the appropriate diagnostic tests.

History

Information obtained from a detailed history can help determine the patient's exposure to the risk factors associated with HCC. Sample questions that can be used to evaluate for potential risk factors are listed in Box 41-5. Recent immigrants from high-risk areas, such as Asia and sub-Saharan Africa require more intense questioning about the incidence of hepatitis and history of exposure to aflatoxin-contaminated foods. One should also ask if the patient has received the hepatitis B vaccine.

Physical Examination

Patients with early HCC lesions are typically asymptomatic. Unfortunately, the typical patient presents with advanced disease and appears chronically ill with painful

Box 41-5
Sample Questions to Assess for Risk Factors for HCC

Has anyone in your family ever had liver cancer?
Do you have hepatitis?
Have you ever had jaundice?
Have you ever had problems with your liver?
Have you ever received a blood transfusion or other blood products?
What is your occupation?
Have you ever been exposed to toxic chemicals?
Have you ever shared needles or syringes?
Have you ever used steroids or sex hormones?
What is your alcohol intake?
Do you smoke tobacco?
Do you have any genetic diseases?

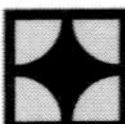

TABLE 41-2 Assessment of the Patient for Hepatocellular Cancer

	Assessment Parameters	Typical Abnormal Findings
History	A. Personal and social history	A. Personal and social risk factors
	1. Age	1. Usually over age 50.
	2. Sex	2. Usually male.
	3. Ethnicity	3. More prevalent in Asia and sub-Saharan Africa.
	4. Family history	4. Positive family history increases the risk.
	5. History of hepatitis B or C	5. Chronic hepatitis is one of the major risk factors for HCC.
	6. History of receiving blood or blood products	6. Hepatitis B and C viruses can be transmitted in blood or blood products.
	7. History of parenteral drug use	7. Needle-sharing is a risk factor for hepatitis.
	8. History of promiscuous sex or male homosexual	8. Hepatitis viruses can be transmitted sexually.
	9. Occupational history	9. Health care workers and people exposed to liver toxic or carcinogenic agents are at risk for hepatitis, cirrhosis, and HCC.
	10. History of alcohol/tobacco use	10. These substances may increase the risk for cirrhosis and HCC.
	11. Presence of genetic diseases	11. Certain genetic diseases increase the risk of developing HCC (hemochromatosis, alpha-1 antitrypsin disease, porphyrias, hereditary tyrosinemia, Budd-Chiari syndrome).
	12. Aflatoxin exposure if recent immigrant from Asia or sub-Saharan Africa	12. Chronic aflatoxin exposure is high-risk factor for HCC.
	B. Evaluation of systems	B. Common signs and symptoms include abdominal pain, weight loss, weakness, fullness, anorexia, abdominal swelling, jaundice, vomiting, hepatomegaly, hepatic bruit, ascites, splenomegaly, jaundice, wasting, and fever.
Physical Examination	A. Palpation of the liver (assess hepatic size, presence of masses, hepatic nodularity, tenderness, and presence of hepatic bruit)	A. Painful hepatomegaly is a common presenting symptom.
	B. Evaluation of abdomen (assess presence of ascites, splenomegaly, dilated abdominal veins)	B. Ascites is a common presenting symptom.
	C. Evaluation of skin and sclera	C. Jaundice may be present.
	D. Evaluation of remaining systems for abnormalities: gastrointestinal (e.g., for esophageal varices), endocrine, respiratory	D. Complications of HCC involve other systems; hence hematemesis, menstrual disorders, testicular atrophy, gynecomastia, wasting, and pleural effusions may occur. Fever may be present.
Diagnostic Tests		
	A. Serum alpha-fetoprotein level	A. May be elevated in patients with HCC.
	B. Ultrasound (US) of the liver	B. Ultrasound can detect small lesions. Intraoperative ultrasound is very useful during liver surgery.
	C. Computed tomography (CT scan) (various types: arterial portography/angiography; Lipiodol-enhanced; spiral CT)	C. Hepatic arteriogram with Lipiodol CT imaging can pick up lesions the US missed and also help determine resectability.
	D. Magnetic resonance imaging (MRI)	D. MRI can help differentiate a hemangioma from HCC and to determine blood flow within the liver.
	E. Chest x-ray and/or CT scan of chest	E. The lungs are a common metastatic site.
	F. Bone scan	F. The bones are a common metastatic site.
	G. Miscellaneous laboratory tests	G. A paraneoplastic syndrome could be present; as a result, erythrocytosis, hypoglycemia, hypercalcemia or other biochemical or hematologic abnormalities may be evident.

hepatomegaly, has a history of weight loss, and shows the presence of ascites. The enlargement of the liver stretches Glisson's capsule, often resulting in organ tenderness. One must use care when palpating a large liver because of the potential for hemorrhage. Obstruction of the portal vein is usually the cause of the ascites and can be readily diagnosed with venous phase angiography or ultrasonography (Lotze, Flickinger, & Carr, 1993; Runyon, 1993). Portal hypertension is caused by obstruction of the portal vein and is a common complication of HCC (Runyon, 1993). In addition to ascites, signs and symptoms of portal hypertension include splenomegaly, dilated abdominal veins, a Cruveilhier-Baumgarten murmur, and a hyperdynamic circulatory state (i.e., bounding pulses; warm, well-perfused extremities; and arterial hypotension). No laboratory tests are used to diagnose portal hypertension. The most common way to measure portal pressure is to indirectly measure the hepatic vein pressure gradient by catheterizing the hepatic vein with a balloon-tipped catheter (Genecin & Groszmann, 1993).

Other signs and symptoms that may help to indicate the degree of liver damage and the presence or absence of metastatic disease include a hepatic bruit, general malaise, anorexia, a feeling of fullness, nausea, vomiting, gastrointestinal bleeding, weight loss, muscle wasting, fever, jaundice, dyspnea, palmar erythema, spider nevi, gynecomastia, testicular atrophy, peripheral edema, hematemesis, bone pain, and pleural effusion (Lotze et al., 1993; Okuda et al., 1993).

Diagnostic Tests

The diagnosis of HCC is made by a carefully taken history and physical examination in association with abnormal AFP levels, a positive lesion seen with imaging tests, and pathologic confirmation through a liver biopsy. It is possible to diagnose HCC without obtaining a biopsy if imaging techniques reveal a space-occupying lesion in a cirrhotic liver and if the patient has elevated serum AFP levels or abnormal serum prothrombin levels (Okuda et al., 1993).

The main objective of the workup is to determine the amount of residual liver function and whether there is extrahepatic disease or portal venous vascular invasion. These factors influence prognosis and affect treatment decisions (Lotze et al., 1993).

Tumor Markers. AFP is a glycoprotein produced by fetal liver cells and is a serum marker for HCC. After birth the serum concentration drops to less than 20 ng/ml. In HCC and chronic hepatitis and cirrhosis, AFP is again expressed. Values above 400 ng/ml are cause for concern. AFP is elevated in only one third of patients with lesions less than 5 cm (Liu et al., 1996). Further, because elevated AFP levels are seen in chronic liver disease, serial levels must be determined. If the AFP levels continue to rise, HCC must be considered. Elevated AFP levels are also seen in gastric, pancreatic, testicular, and lung cancers (Oberfield et al., 1989). A more specific AFP test, the lectin-dependent fractionation of AFP, may help differentiate HCC from cirrhosis (Yamashita et al., 1996). In addition, abnormal levels of serum prothrombin (PIVKA-II), a protein induced by the absence of vitamin K, may aid in diagnosis (Ramsey & Wu, 1995). These latter two tests are not available outside of specific clinical trials.

Other laboratory tests that the clinician may obtain include blood chemistries, coagulation studies, electrolytes, and a complete blood cell count. The following chemistries are elevated in the advanced stage of HCC: aspartate aminotransferase, ALT, lactate dehydrogenase, and alkaline phosphatase. The degree of liver damage and extent of disease outside the liver will determine further laboratory abnormalities (Okuda et al., 1993). Paraneoplastic syndromes may be associated with HCC and include hypoglycemia, erythrocytosis, hypercalcemia, hypercholesterolemia, dysfibrinogenemia, carcinoid syndrome, increased thyroxine-binding globulin, decreased libido, and porphyria cutanea tarda (Lotze et al., 1993; Ramsey & Wu, 1995). Geographic factors appear to influence the type of paraneoplastic syndrome exhibited by the patient. For example, up to 38% of sub-Saharan African patients with HCC exhibit hypercholesterolemia (Ramsey & Wu, 1995).

Imaging Studies. Both ultrasonography and computed tomography (CT) are excellent methods for evaluating liver masses because they illustrate anatomic structures and pathologic defects with a fair degree of accuracy. Ultrasound can detect very small lesions and determine whether the blood vessels within the liver have been invaded. Surgeons routinely use intraoperative ultrasound during hepatic surgery to help define the areas to be resected (Liu et al., 1996).

CT scanning is commonly performed when an abdominal mass is discovered. New variations of CT scanning and angiography can detect a high percentage of liver lesions that might otherwise be missed by conventional scanning methods (Sardi, Akbarov, & Conaway, 1996). For example, CT with arterial portography (CTAP) revealed tumors undetected by magnetic resonance imaging (MRI) and CT (Ramsey & Wu, 1995). However, CTAP may have a false-positive rate as high as 42% owing to perfusion defects (Sardi et al., 1996). Another advancement in CT scanning is the spiral CT, which provides a three-dimensional view of the liver. This tool aids the radiologist in gathering anatomic information about the liver, blood vessels, and ducts (Niederhuber, 1995). Spiral CT is excellent for evaluating small lesions, and, when spiral mode CT is combined with arterial portography, tumor detection appears to be enhanced (Sardi et al., 1996). Others suggest that the combination of hepatic arteriography and Lipiodol CT scanning is the most sensitive diagnostic method presently available (Liu et al., 1996). Lipiodol is an iodized oil emulsion, which, when injected into the hepatic artery, is retained by HCC cells and visualized during a CT scan that occurs 1 week after the injection. MRI can be used to differentiate a hemangioma from HCC and to track blood flow within the liver (Ramsey & Wu, 1995).

Biopsy. Percutaneous liver biopsy is generally safe, simple, and inexpensive to perform. In a small percentage of patients with cirrhosis or tumors, hemoperitoneum can be a fatal complication of a liver biopsy (Schiff & Schiff, 1993). Most clinicians prefer the subcostal approach when per-

TABLE 41-3 Patient Preparation for a Liver Biopsy

Description of the Procedure: Percutaneous biopsy of liver tissue with or without guided imaging. The patient lies on his or her back. The physician inserts the needle by way of the intercostal or subcostal route, and a small amount of tissue is aspirated while the patient holds his/her breath after exhaling. It is important that the patient immobilize the chest wall by holding his/her breath to prevent penetration of the diaphragm and laceration of the liver. The major complication of this procedure is hemorrhage.

Patient Preparation:

1. Obtain the patient's written consent.
2. Results of recent coagulation studies should be available. Coagulopathy is a contraindication to this procedure.
3. Patients usually do not require typing and cross-matching for blood. However, a type and cross should be done in cases in which blood would be readily available, if needed.
4. Explain the procedure and postprocedure care to patient.
5. Have the patient practice inhaling and exhaling deeply several times, then holding his/her breath at the end of an expiration.
6. Obtain vital signs prior to performing the procedure.

Procedural Considerations:

1. Obtain items required for the biopsy (biopsy tray and needle, cleansing solution, a local anesthetic, an adhesive bandage, and formalin).
2. Place the patient prone and expose the right side of the upper abdomen.
3. Assist the physician as needed and provide support to the patient.

Postprocedural Considerations:

1. Immediately after the biopsy, help the patient to turn onto his/her right side. This position helps the liver compress against the chest wall to prevent bleeding. Place a pillow or folded towel against the biopsy site to provide a pressure source. Instruct patient to remain in this position as per institution or physician protocol.
2. Monitor vital signs per institution or physician protocol.
3. Immediately report any changes in vital signs or pain, as these signs may indicate bleeding.
4. Administer analgesics as needed.

Modified from Smeltzer, S. C. & Bare, B. G. (1996). *Brunner and Suddarth's textbook of medical-surgical nursing* (8th ed.). Philadelphia: J. B. Lippincott.

forming a liver biopsy because it reduces the risk of pneumothorax. If the patient's lesion is in the superior portion of the liver, the physician uses an intercostal or prone-angled approach (Nissenbaum, vanSonnenberg, & D'Agostino, 1993). Table 41-3 provides a description of the liver biopsy procedure. Transjugular biopsy can be preformed when severe coagulopathy precludes the percutaneous route, although the complication rate is upward of 20% (Conn & Atterbury, 1993). Some clinicians favor laparoscopic biopsy because up to 90% of liver cancers can be seen with the scope. As a result, one can be assured of more accurate sampling of tissue (Schiff & Schiff, 1993).

When the pathologist receives a liver specimen, he or she must determine whether (1) the tissue is representative of a tumor or another process; (2) the sample is tumor; (3) the sample is benign or malignant; (4) the specimen has the characteristics of cancer; (5) the specimen originated in the liver or in another organ; and (6) whether the tumor is primary liver cancer, what type it is, and to what degree it is malignant. HCC cells resemble normal liver cells, with large, round, hyperchromatic nuclei, prominent nucleoli, and abundant granular eosinophilic cytoplasm (Niederhuber, 1995). The histology of HCC varies with any combination of the following features: the structural pattern (i.e., trabecular, pseudoglandular, solid, sclerosing), variation in the degree of cancer cell differentiation or grading (i.e., well, moderately, poorly, undifferentiated), and cytologic variants (i.e., bile production, clear cells, fatty change, cytoplasmic hyalin, ground-glass inclusion, pleomorphism, sarcomatoid) (Okuda et al., 1993). The most important diagnostic features of HCC are a trabecular pattern, the presence of canaliculi between tumor cells, and the identification of bile in canaliculi or in the cytoplasm of tumor cells (Ishak & Markin, 1996).

The most common primary liver tumor is hepatocellular, categorized as a single mass, a diffuse lesion, or a multiple encapsulated tumor (Niederhuber, 1995). A variant of HCC is the fibrolamellar type that occurs in adolescents or young adults and is not associated with cirrhosis. Another primary liver tumor is cholangiocarcinoma. There are also a number of rare tumors: cholangiocellular carcinoma, combined hepatocellular and cholangiocarcinoma, bile duct cystadenocarcinoma, hepatoblastoma, angiosarcoma, epithelioid lymphoma, hemangioendothelioma, rhabdomyosarcoma, fibrosarcoma, leiomyosarcoma, malignant fibrous histiocytosis, liposarcoma, osteosarcoma, undifferentiated sarcoma, and squamous cell carcinoma (Ishak & Markin, 1996).

STAGING

The principal reason for staging the anatomic extent of the tumor is to assist the clinician in determining the optimal treatment. Moreover, staging provides prognostic information, assists in evaluating treatment outcomes, and provides a uniform method for exchanging important findings about that particular cancer within the oncology community (Beahrs, Henson, Hutter, & Kennedy, 1992).

Histologic Staging

Histologic staging for HCC refers to the degree of malignancy of the tumor cells or the grade. G1 is well differentiated, G2 is moderately differentiated, G3 is poorly differentiated, and G4 is undifferentiated (Niederhuber, 1995).

Clinical Staging

Clinical staging of HCC is similar to that for other solid tumors. The TNM staging system is used to determine the extent of spread within the body (Table 41-4). Clinicians obtain this information from clinical examinations and diagnostic tests such as imaging procedures and tissue biop-

TABLE 41-4 TNM Staging System for Liver Cancer

Primary Tumor (T)

TX	Primary tumor cannot be assessed
TO	No evidence of primary tumor
T1	Solitary tumor 2 cm or less in greatest dimension without vascular invasion
T2	Solitary tumor 2 cm or less in greatest dimension with vascular invasion; or multiple tumors limited to one lobe, none more than 2 cm in greatest dimension without vascular invasion; or a solitary tumor more than 2 cm in greatest dimension without vascular invasion
T3	Solitary tumor more than 2 cm in greatest dimension with vascular invasion; or multiple tumors limited to one lobe, none more than 2 cm in greatest dimension, with vascular invasion; or multiple tumors limited to one lobe, any more than 2 cm in greatest dimension, with or without vascular invasion
T4	Multiple tumors in more than one lobe, or tumor(s) involving a major branch of the portal or hepatic vein(s)

Regional Lymph Nodes (N)

NX	Regional lymph nodes cannot be assessed
NO	No regional lymph node metastasis
N1	Regional lymph node metastasis

Distant Metastasis (M)

MX	Presence of distant metastasis cannot be assessed
MO	No distant metastasis
M1	Distant metastasis

Stage Grouping

Stage I	T1	NO	MO
Stage II	T2	NO	MO
Stage III	T1	N1	MO
	T2	N1	MO
	T3	NO	MO
	T3	N1	MO
Stage IVA	T4	Any N	MO
Stage IVB	Any T	Any N	M1

From Beahrs, O. H., Henson, D. E., Hutter, R. V. P., & Kennedy, B. J. (Eds.) (1992). *American Joint Committee on Cancer manual for staging of cancer* (4th ed.). Philadelphia: J. B. Lippincott.

sies, as well as from findings at the time of surgery. Ideally, the clinician would like to know the clinical stage of the disease before attempting to resect a liver lesion(s) because tumor invasion of hepatic blood vessels usually precludes resection (Niederhuber, 1995).

MEDICAL MANAGEMENT

At first glance, there appear to be many treatment options for HCC. However, only one of these options offers patients any chance for cure—surgical resection (Fong, 1996). Moreover, only 20% to 30% of individuals diagnosed with HCC are candidates for surgery (Farmer & Busuttil, 1994; Liu et al., 1996). In addition, not all patients who undergo surgery leave the operating room having had their cancer resected.

Treatments for HCC are relatively unsuccessful for several reasons. First, patients often present at a late stage in the disease process. HCC tends to be a heterogenous tumor, and there may be an overexpression of the multidrug resistance gene. In addition, subclinical micrometastatic disease is often present at the time of diagnosis (Venook, 1994). Oberfield and colleagues (1989) noted that 70% of resected patients had pulmonary metastasis. Despite improvements in imaging techniques, clinicians are still unable to determine the full extent of the disease in many patients. Most treatments are focused only on the liver, leaving cancer cells outside the treatment area unharmed. Systemic chemotherapy is essentially worthless. Fewer than 20% of patients respond even temporarily to the best drugs, doxorubicin and cisplatin (Choi, 1996; Farmer & Busuttil, 1994).

Deciding which treatment to recommend is difficult owing to the lack of standardization in clinical trail data. Researchers often fail to stratify the variables known to influence treatment outcomes. As a result, it is hard to determine precisely how response rates and survival rates reflect the efficacy of a particular treatment. For instance, patients may participate in the same clinical trial without accounting for the stage of the cancer or concomitant disease. Because of this omission, clinicians are unable to draw conclusions as to at which stage patients would best benefit from a particular treatment. The same concerns are true for other confounding factors such as the use of divergent treatment techniques, the incomplete staging of patients, and unknown variables related to individual patient differences (Sardi et al., 1996).

Similarly, the treatments recommended by experts can be confusing. Venook (1994) writes ". . . cryosurgery and percutaneous ethanol injections (PEI) have not yet been shown to offer any advantage . . ."(p. 1323). Ramsey & Wu (1995) disagree, asserting that ". . . percutaneous ethanol injection has consistently been the most effective (nonsurgical treatment) . . ."(p. 87). The literature is replete with contradictory advice.

Notwithstanding these problems, most experts do agree that if an HCC is resectable, it should be removed. If the tumor is not resectable, the clinician is faced with a dilemma. Treatment at this point may be potentially curable, according to some experts, or palliative, according to others. Should the patient be entered into a clinical trial? Which treatment modality should the clinician recommend? Often, the physician bases the decision not on the often conflicting results of clinical trials, but on local expertise, interest, and experience (Dusheiko, Hobbs, Dick, & Burroughs, 1992). One researcher goes so far as to say that ". . . while there are many treatment options for patients with HCC, none except surgical resection are to be recommended outside of the clinical research setting" (Venook, 1994, p.1330). On the other hand, researchers, who were conducting a study on PEI, wrote "many, even outlying, hospitals can perform PEI without need for referral" (Livraghi, Giorgi, Marin, Salmi, de Sio,

& Bolondi et al., 1995). Clearly a large amount of research on the management of HCC needs to be done.

HCC is a difficult tumor to treat, and no single modality is optimal. Fig. 41-2 illustrates the algorithm used by the University of Miami Center for Liver Diseases to determine treatment (Personal communication, R. Reddy, MD, December, 1996). The best chance for cure is with complete resection. Otherwise therapy is generally palliative except in rare instances. The most promising palliative and occasionally curable nonsurgical treatments are PEI and hepatic arterial chemoembolization. A general overview of PEI and hepatic artery chemoembolization and other treatment modalities for HCC is summarized in Table 41-5.

Surgical Management

Liver Resection. The best candidate for surgery is a patient less than 65 years of age, with a unifocal, well-differentiated, encapsulated tumor measuring less than 5 cm and located in a healthy liver, with no vascular invasion or extrahepatic spread. An AFP level less than 200 g/ml is also helpful, as is having the fibrolamellar variant of HCC (Livraghi et al., 1995; Sardi et al., 1996). Failing these criteria, a patient with one or two small lesions in an otherwise healthy liver and no intrahepatic or extrahepatic spread is the next best candidate (Fong, 1996). Because micrometastatic disease is impossible to find, clinical understaging is common. Despite modern imaging techniques, some patients show evidence of additional tumors at the time of surgery. The following conditions usually rule out surgical resection: lesions located in the middle of the right lobe, numerous lesions, very large lesions, Child's B or C liver disease, intra- or extrahepatic spread, and portal hypertension (Lotze et al., 1993; Bruix, Castells, Bosch, Feu, Fuster, & Garcia-Pagan et al., 1996). The Child-Pugh grading system is used to determine the severity of liver disease (Table 41-6).

Surgical mortality and morbidity have decreased because of several factors including better screening of potential surgical candidates, perioperative parenteral nutrition, and improved intraoperative procedures (e.g., subcostal incision rather than thoracotomy, which eliminates the need for chest tubes, use of an ultrasonic dissector, cell savers, and rapid transfusers) (Liu et al., 1996). Up to 85% of the liver can be resected. Regeneration begins in the immediate postoperative period, and 50% of the liver will have regenerated within 2 to 4 months (Oberfield et al., 1989). The skill of the surgeon is also critical to patient survival. Fortner (1996) makes this appeal: "Finally, it cannot be overemphasized that patients with primary or secondary liver cancer should be treated at medical centers by experienced liver surgeons. The complexity of liver surgery and the good therapeutic results achieved at these centers with low mortality are the bases for this plea. The occasional liver surgeon is a dangerous person who cannot do justice to patients with liver tumors."

Even though there is better preoperative screening for resectable patients, a high proportion of patients experience relapse after surgery for "localized" HCC. Adjuvant or neoadjuvant approaches using regional or systemic chemotherapy continue to be evaluated (Lotze et al., 1993; Takenaka, Yoshida, Nishizaki, Korenaga, Hiroshige, & Ikeda et al., 1995).

Total Hepatectomy with Orthotopic Liver Transplantation. As mentioned previously, only those patients with small lesions and a healthy liver (Child's A liver disease is usually acceptable) are candidates for resection. For other patients, who have multifocal disease and/or decompensating cirrhosis yet show no evidence of extrahepatic disease, orthotopic liver transplantation (OLT) may be an option. An advantage of OLT is that it treats both tumor and cirrhosis. However, early trials demonstrated high recurrence rates and discouraging long-term survival (Olthoff, Rosove, Shackleton, Imagawa, Farmer, & Northcross et al., 1995). Poor outcome is partially due to the presence of undiagnosed micrometastatic disease at the time of surgery. Furthermore, experts speculate that when the cancerous liver is removed, tumor cells may be released and graft onto the donor liver. Sparked by this latter theory, ongoing studies are testing whether pretransplant and/or posttransplant adjuvant chemotherapy and/or immunotherapy will improve prognosis. Using PEI, chemoembolization, or cryotherapy before transplantation is also being tested (Carr, 1995; Farmer & Busuttil, 1994; Mazzaferro, Regalia, Doci, Andreola, Pulvirenti, & Bozzetti et al., 1996; Olthoff et al., 1995).

Added to the biologic problems associated with liver transplantation are the problems of organ availability and the costs associated with the procedure. In parts of the world where HCC rates are the highest, organ donation is the lowest, as a result of cultural taboos (Fong, 1996).

Cryotherapy. Cryotherapy has been suggested as a possible treatment modality when patients cannot undergo resection because of the location of the tumors or because they have poor liver function (Sotomayor & Ravikumar, 1996). Fong (1996) advises that if a patient is in surgery and is deemed inoperable, cryotherapy should be used if it is available. At present, most procedures are performed at laparotomy, although some surgeons are evaluating the laparoscopic approach for small tumors in accessible locations (Sotomayor & Ravikumar, 1996). Further trials are required to compare this approach with PEI and chemoembolization.

Nonsurgical Management

Percutaneous Alcohol Injections. Absolute alcohol injected directly into small liver tumors causes extensive necrosis. The indications for PEI are reduction or elimination of tumors. PEI can be used alone or in conjunction with other surgical or medical procedures. This treatment method has resulted in equivalent survival compared with surgical resection (Nissenbaum et al., 1993, Livraghi et al., 1995). The best results are found in patients with single HCCs that are 3 cm or smaller, because alcohol injection rarely kills all of the tumor cells in larger tumors (Bartolozzi, Lencioni, Caramella, Vignali, Cioni, & Mazzeo et al., 1995). Compared with surgery and chemoembolization, this procedure is generally safer, is potentially as effective, is less expensive, and is easier for the patient to tolerate (Livraghi et al., 1995; Ramsey & Wu, 1995). Livraghi and colleagues

Text continued on p. 945

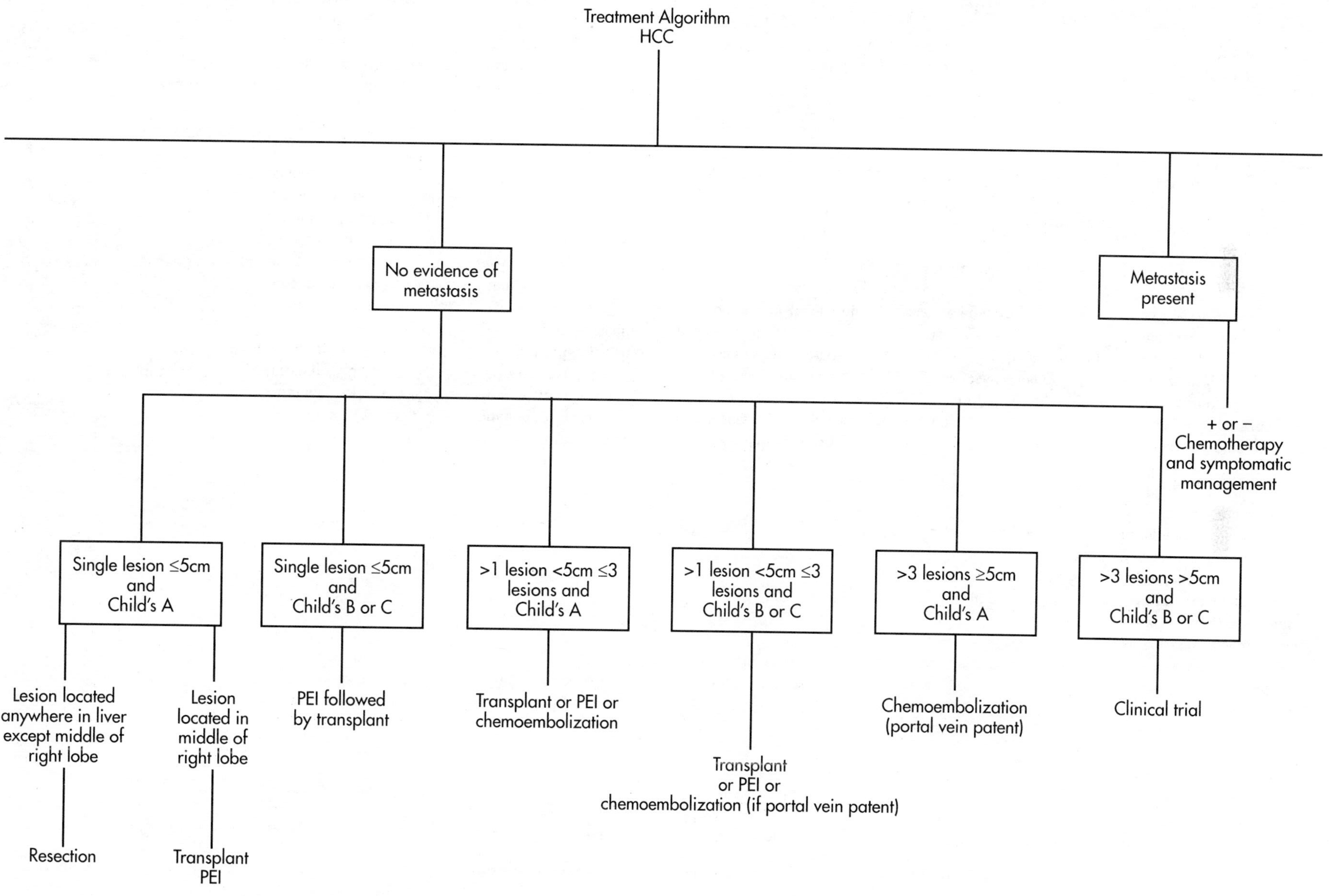

Fig. 41-2 Treatment algorithm. (Algorithm courtesy Rhaender Reddy, MD, University of Miami Center for Liver Diseases, Miami, FL.)

TABLE 41-5 Treatment Modalities for HCC

Modality	Description	Treatment Goals	Tumor Characteristics and Patient Factors	Advantages	Disadvantages
Hepatic resection	Surgical removal of the portion of liver containing the tumor	To remove the tumor To improve survival	Solitary lesions Absence of cirrhosis No evidence of extrahepatic spread	Potentially curable treatment	Mortality (5%-10%) and morbidity from surgery Some patients are not resectable at the time of surgery Recurrence is common
Total hepatectomy with orthotopic liver transplantation	Surgical removal of patient's entire liver and replacement by a donor liver	To remove the tumor To improve survival	Small unresectable lesions in a patient with cirrhosis	Potentially curable Treats both the cancer and the liver disease	Mortality (as high as 20%) and morbidity from surgery Tumor cell dissemination during surgery leading to recurrence in the grafted liver Persistent micrometastasis Immunosuppression Not enough organs available High costs
Percutaneous ethanol injection	Approximately 5 ml of absolute alcohol is percutaneously injected through a 22-gauge needle into the liver lesion using ultrasound guidance. Treatment is repeated once or twice a week for a total of 3 to 8 sessions, depending on the size of the lesion(s).	To reduce or eliminate tumor by causing tumor necrosis and vasoocclusion from alcohol-induced dehydration and intracellular coagulation of tumor	1 or 2 small lesions in a patient with cirrhosis Treatment of choice for patients with small lesions who are not candidates for resection or transplantation	Survival rates about the same as those for surgery Less expensive than many other treatment methods Can be done in outpatient settings and in smaller hospitals. Thus may be more convenient for the patient Can be repeated when new lesions are diagnosed No risk of damage to remaining liver tissue	Recurrence common Cannot be used with large tumors May require numerous treatment sessions Some discomfort associated with procedure Possible side effects and complications: transient increase in liver function tests, liver abscess, cholangitis, bleeding, liver infarction, neoplastic seeding
Systemic chemotherapy	Intravenous chemotherapy (i.e., doxirubicin, cisplatin, or mitomycin-C) Subcutaneous interferon alpha	To reduce tumor recurrence rates in surgical patients To attempt to reduce tumor burden Palliation	Adjuvant or neoadjuvant therapy with surgery Other options are contraindicated	Some reduction of tumor in 20% of patients Cheaper than other therapies for HCC Minimally invasive	Lower response rates Responses are not durable—relapses frequent May adversely affect the patient's quality of life due to the toxicities of therapy

Hepatic artery infusion of chemotherapy	Infusion of chemotherapy through the hepatic artery during angiography or by using an implanted delivery system	Delivers higher doses of drug directly to tumor while reducing systemic toxicity	Unresectable tumors in patient with or without portal vein thrombosis No evidence of extrahepatic spread	Reduction in tumor size in about 40%-50% of patients	Invasive procedure Some discomfort associated with procedure Implanted devices cumbersome and surgery required to place the device Responses are not durable—relapse is common Costly Possible complications: infection, sclerosis, narrowing of bile ducts, hepatic toxicity, ulcer and gastritis (the latter occurs if drug is accidentally diverted to gastric or splenic artery)
Hepatic artery embolization	Injection of an embolizing material (e.g., Gelfoam) into the artery feeding the tumor	To cause tumor cell necrosis by inducing ischemia To relieve pain	Unresectable tumors Small lesions in patients with no portal vein thrombosis or hepatic dysfunction	Reduction in tumor size in about 50% of patients Survival almost comparable to stage II patients who had resections Reduces pain in about 65% of cases	Invasive procedure Some discomfort associated with procedure Implanted devices cumbersome and surgery required to place the device Responses are not durable Costly May result in postembolization syndrome: abdominal pain, nausea, vomiting, fever, elevation in liver enzymes

Continued

TABLE 41-5 Treatment Modalities for HCC—cont'd

Modality	Description	Treatment Goals	Tumor Characteristics and Patient Factors	Advantages	Disadvantages
Hepatic artery chemoembolization with or without Lipiodol	Hepatic artery infusion of chemotherapy followed by injection of an embolizing material (e.g., Gelfoam) With Lipiodol: hepatic artery infusion of a mixture of Lipiodol and chemotherapy (e.g., doxirubicin), followed by an injection of Gelfoam	To deliver higher doses of drug directly to tumor while reducing systemic toxicity To cause tumor cell necrosis by inducing ischemia With Lipiodol, to increase dwell time of chemotherapy in tumor cells	Unresectable tumors Small lesions in patients with no portal vein thrombosis or hepatic dysfunction No evidence of extrahepatic spread	Reduction in tumor size in about 30%-50% of patients	Invasive procedure Some discomfort associated with procedure Responses are not durable Costly Possible side effects/complications: pain, infection, sclerosis, nausea, vomiting, fever, elevation of liver enzymes, liver failure, pancreatitis, pulmonary edema, narrowing of bile ducts, cholecystitis, abscess, tumor rupture, hepatic toxicity, ulcer and gastritis (the latter occurs if drug is accidentally diverted to gastric or splenic artery)
Cryotherapy	Ablation of tumor with liquid nitrogen delivered by an ultrasound guided probe during laparotomy or laparoscopy	To destroy tumor To shrink tumor, thus allowing for subsequent resection To palliate the disease	Unresectable lesions in patients with hepatic dysfunction If patient is found to be unresectable at time of surgery, cryoablation can be done instead	Well-tolerated procedure Spares normal tissue Long-term survival rates of over 20% may be achieved Mortality and complications rare	Requires special equipment, laparotomy, and specially trained physicians Recurrence common Costly Possible complications: hemorrhage due to liver capsule cracking, myoglobinuria, bile leakage, infection, renal failure, hypothermia, coagulopathy, increase in liver enzymes
Conformal radiation therapy with hepatic artery floxuridine (radiation sensitizer)	Three-dimensional radiation treatment planning that minimizes scatter to normal liver, thereby permitting therapeutic dosing to tumor. A continuous intra-arterial infusion of floxuridine is administered during the treatment cycle.	To reduce tumor To palliate the disease	Unresectable tumors	Permits normal liver to be excluded from treatment area; therefore, a higher dose of radiation can be administered May increase survival	Requires expensive equipment Time-consuming for patient Costly Floxuridine can damage the bile ducts

TABLE 41-6 Child-Pugh System for Grading the Severity of Liver Disease

Variable	Points Scored
Encephalopathy	
None	1
1-2	2
3-4	3
Ascites	
Absent	1
Slight	2
Moderate	3
Serum Bilirubin (mg/dl)	
1.0-2.0	1
2.1-3.0	2
>3.1	3
Serum Albumin (g/L)	
>35	1
28-35	2
<28	3
Prolongation of Prothrombin Time (sec)	
1-3	1
4-10	2
>10	3

Scoring: Class A = 5-6 points (good hepatic function); Class B = 7-9 points (intermediate hepatic function); Class C = 10-12 points (poor hepatic function).

Modified from Mazzaferro, V., Regalia, E., Doci, R., Andreola, S., Pulvirenti, A., & Bozzitti, F. et al., (1996). Liver transplantation for the treatment of small hepatocellular carcinomas in patients with cirrhosis. *The New England Journal of Medicine, 334*(11), 694.

(1995) proposed that PEI is the treatment of choice for patients with small lesions who are not surgical candidates.

Systemic Chemotherapy. As mentioned earlier, systemic chemotherapy generally is not effective in the treatment of HCC; however, there may be times when its use is appropriate. For example, the clinician might prescribe a couple of courses of doxorubicin for a motivated patient with a good performance level who is not a candidate for surgery, PEI, intra-arterial treatment, or a clinical trial.

Because HCC cells have hormone receptors, some clinical trials include the administration of tamoxifen in their treatment protocols. Results have been variable (Ramsey & Wu, 1995). Meanwhile, in other studies, INF has been combined with chemohormonal therapy with some beneficial effects (Kountouras, Boura, Karolides, Zaharioudaki, & Tsapas, 1995). Oral 5-fluouracil has resurfaced as a treatment for HCC and is a component of some clinical trials.

Hepatic Artery Infusion of Chemotherapy. HCC derives the bulk of its blood supply from the hepatic artery. Therefore, a major treatment modality for this tumor is injecting chemotherapy directly into the hepatic artery. Doxorubicin, cisplatin, mitomycin-C, floxuridine, leucovorin, and INF-alpha (INF is given subcutaneously) appear to be partially effective. These treatments are administered either through an implantable pump system or intermittently through a percutaneously placed arterial catheter. This treatment method is also used in some preresection and pretransplant protocols (Farmer & Busuttil, 1994).

Hepatic Artery Embolization. Another way to kill cancer cells is to cut off the tumor's blood supply by injecting pieces of Gelfoam into the feeding vessel during hepatic arteriography. This method is most useful when the lesion is small and there is no severe hepatic dysfunction or portal vein thrombosis. Hepatic artery embolization is the most widely used treatment modality in Asia, and survival rates are nearly as good as surgery for stage II patients (Okuda et al., 1993). In the palliative setting, embolization is effective in reducing pain in 65% of cases (Johnson, 1996). Gelfoam is the most common material used in hepatic artery embolization. Other materials that have also been tried include starch, polyvinyl alcohol, autologous blood clots, and collagen (Venook, 1994).

Hepatic Artery Chemoembolization with or Without Lipiodol. Researchers have hoped that by combining chemotherapy and embolization, they could destroy more tumor cells than with either method alone. They developed numerous techniques, among them injecting chemotherapy first, followed by Gelfoam, and injecting Gelfoam that had been soaked in a chemotherapeutic drug.

One method of hepatic artery chemoembolization involves injection of Lipiodol, an oil-based contrast medium used for visualizing the lymphatic system during lymphangiograms. Coincidentally, this contrast medium is retained by HCC cells. As a result of this property, Lipiodol can be used not only for diagnosing HCC, but also for its treatment. In transcatheter oily chemoembolism, a mixture of chemotherapy (doxorubicin, mitomycin, or cisplatin) and Lipiodol is administered intra-arterially. The theory behind this approach is that the chemotherapy, when mixed with the Lipiodol, will remain in the tumor longer. In fact, doxorubicin has been found in resected tumors 1 and 2 months after treatment (Niederhuber, 1995). During the procedure, Gelfoam may be injected after the mixture is instilled. However, Lipiodol itself may act as an embolizer by reducing blood flow at the capillary level (Johnson, 1996; Ramsey & Wu, 1995).

Chemoembolization is contraindicated in patients with portal vein obstruction and advanced liver disease because of the high risk that the procedure will worsen liver function (Chung, Park, Han, Choi, & Han, 1995). Although some studies of chemoembolization have shown improved tumor responses and increased survival rates, other studies have not demonstrated positive effects. More studies are needed to determine the role of chemoembolization in the treatment of HCC (Choi, 1996; Johnson, 1996; Sardi et al., 1996).

Radiation Therapy. Historically, radiation therapy to the liver has been limited owing to the radiosensitivity of normal hepatocytes. The maximum tolerance of hepatocytes is 35 cGy. When this dose is exceeded, radiation hepatitis is likely to develop. Conformal high-dose radiation is a new approach for treating liver tumors. This technique consists of three-dimensional radiation treatment planning, which has two advantages. It provides for the radiation beam to enter from several angles, and it specifically targets the tumor. Because the normal liver is excluded from the treatment ports, higher doses of radiation can be administered. For example, Lawrence, Kessler, and Robertson (1993) have given patients at least 70 cGy without producing significant radiation hepatitis. Their protocol includes the arterial administration of floxuridine, a radiation sensitizer.

Other Investigational Therapies. Numerous trials are exploring potential therapies for HCC. These treatments include: microwave coagulation (Seki, Wakabayashi, Nakagawa, Itho, Shiro, & Sato et al., 1994; Sato, Watanabe, Ueda, Iseki, Abe, & Sato et al., 1996), gene therapy (Wills, Huang, Harris, Machemer, Maneval, & Gregory 1995), liposomes, radioimmunotherapy (Venook, 1994), radioimmunoguided surgery (Sardi et al., 1996), Yttrium microspheres (Johnson, 1996), and hepatic arterial perfusion with hepatic venous isolation and extracorporeal chemofiltration (Choi, 1996).

ONCOLOGIC EMERGENCIES

The major oncologic emergency associated with HCC is hemorrhage from ruptured esophageal or gastric varices. Tumor obstruction of the portal vein causes portal hypertension because the mass blocks venous blood flow from the intestinal tract and spleen. The liver forms new passages (i.e., collateral channels) to redirect blood flow, ultimately to the right atrium. Unfortunately, these channels send blood to low-pressure veins in the submucosal layer of the lower esophagus and upper part of the stomach, and the resulting strain causes these vessels to become tortuous and fragile. Hematemesis and melena are clinical signs of ruptured varices. Blood loss can be massive and lead to shock. Emergency endoscopy is usually performed to determine the source of bleeding, which is treated with sclerotherapy. Other ways to manage the hemorrhaging include treating it pharmacologically with vasopressin, somatostatin, or propranolol; using a balloon tamponade; performing repeated endoscopic sclerotherapy; and performing transjugular intrahepatic portosystemic shunting. Despite the high mortality rate, surgeons may have to intervene for patients who fail to respond to nonsurgical approaches. Portosystemic shunting and esophageal transection with or without devascularization are two surgical procedures used to treat bleeding varices (Genecin & Groszmann, 1993, Siegel & Veerappan, 1993).

NURSING MANAGEMENT

Nursing management of the patient with HCC depends on how far the disease has progressed and related symptomology, as well as what treatment the patient is receiving, the patient's learning needs, psychosocial factors, and where the patient receives nursing care.

During the diagnostic workup, the patient may require information about the tests and general information about the disease. Treatment issues then emerge as test results indicate whether the patient is a candidate for surgery or other treatment options. Nursing care will then focus on assisting the patient through the treatment. The focus of nursing care is palliative, with the emphasis on helping patients achieve their goals at a time when they may be suffering from increasing symptoms. Unfortunately, many patients with HCC ultimately die from the disease, some of them fairly quickly.

Surgery

Liver Resection. The principal focus of inpatient nursing care is to prevent or recognize postoperative complications as soon as possible. Patients undergoing liver resection usually stay for several days in the critical care unit, where they can receive intensive nursing care and be monitored for complications. Some patients are on a ventilator, and most patients will have an arterial line, a nasogastric tube, an indwelling urinary catheter, one or two bile drains, and a central venous catheter. Surgery may have been lengthy; hence, the patient may be acidotic from lactic acid buildup. Hypoglycemia often occurs in the immediate postoperative period due to liver ischemia resulting from the isolation procedures used in surgery. Fluid overload may be a problem if the patient required a lot of blood replacement during surgery. Postoperative recovery is greatly dependent on residual liver function. A patient with cirrhosis (recall that many HCC patients have this disease) is at great risk for liver failure. The nurse must be alert for signs of acidosis, coagulopathies, jaundice, ascites, sepsis, and renal failure (Frogge, 1993).

Patient/family education begins preoperatively and continues throughout the course of recovery. Among the topics that need to be covered are what to expect in the intensive care unit, patient self-care, which signs and symptoms to report to the medical team, and what follow-up measures to take at home. The nursing management of the patient undergoing a liver resection is summarized in Table 41-7.

Cryotherapy. Most patients go to the critical care unit after undergoing cryotherapy. Because myoglobinemia may occur after this procedure, the urine is alkalized with intravenous sodium bicarbonate. Low-dose dopamine and mannitol may be prescribed to ensure adequate renal perfusion (Weaver, Atkinson, & Zemel, 1995). Along with serum electrolytes, urine myoglobin levels may be requested. The nurse monitors intake and output, assesses the surgical site, observes for bleeding, monitors vital signs, and evaluates laboratory results.

Nonsurgical Therapies

Percutaneous Alcohol Injections. The primary foci of nursing care for the patient receiving PEI therapy are patient education, assisting with the procedure, and postpro-

Text continued on p. 951.

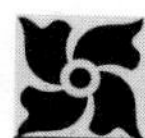

TABLE 41-7 Standard of Care for the Patient Undergoing Liver Resection

Patient Problem and Outcomes	Nursing Interventions and Rationales	Patient Education Instructions
Preoperatively		
Anxiety Patient will: • Verbalize an understanding of the surgical procedure. • Express feelings of decreased anxiety. • Identify strategies to cope with anxiety.	1. Assess patient's level of understanding of the surgical procedure. 2. Give patient the opportunity to ask questions or verbalize concerns. 3. Determine which coping strategies the patient has used effectively in the past to decrease anxiety and reinforce the use of these strategies. 4. Provide any of the following if appropriate: a. Relaxation tapes b. Quiet environment for meditation c. Spiritual intervention d. Music e. Family/significant other visit f. Pharmacologic agents	1. Reinforce surgeon's explanation of surgical procedure if needed. 2. Provide patient with information about the preoperative routine: a. Diagnostic tests b. Bowel prep c. Anesthesiology consult d. Incentive spirometer/importance of deep breathing, coughing, and activity postoperatively e. Antiembolic stockings 3. If patient desires, teach him or her about various relaxation techniques.
Knowledge Deficit Regarding Postoperative Pain Management, Alterations of Body Integrity, Possible Complications, Length of Hospital Stay, and Home Care Needs		
Patient will: • Verbalize an understanding of how his or her pain will be managed. • Verbalize an understanding of the type of incision and tubes/drains to expect postoperatively as well as the monitoring equipment that will be in place. • Verbalize an understanding of the possible complications related to hepatic resection and signs and symptoms to report.	1. Assess patient's knowledge, attitudes, beliefs and desires about his postoperative pain management. 2. Assess patient's knowledge and expectations about the incision, drains and monitoring postoperatively. 3. Assess patient's level of understanding about possible postoperative complications and the signs and symptoms to report.	1. Provide written information about postoperative pain management if available and teach patient the following: a. Inform nurse when pain is present b. Inform nurse if pain is not relieved to his satisfaction c. Take pain medication at regular intervals when the pain is severe, especially during the first few days postoperatively. d. Use a variety of pain-reducing interventions, if desired. e. Report any side effects related to analgesics or other pain-reducing interventions. 2. Provide patient with information about what to expect postoperatively. Use preprinted information or drawings as needed for teaching a. Type of incision b. Tubes and drains c. Monitoring equipment 3. Reinforce surgeon's instructions about possible surgical complications and signs and symptoms to report.

Modified from Gillespie, P. (1995). Hepatocellular cancer. In C. Miaskowski (Ed.), *Oncology nursing*. Albany, NY: Delmar; Smeltzer, S. & Bare, B. (1996). Assessment and management of patients with hepatic and biliary disorders. In S. Smeltzer & B. Bare (Eds.), *Brunner and Suddarth's textbook of medical-surgical nursing* (8th ed.). Philadelphia: J. B. Lippincott.

Continued

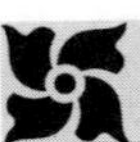

TABLE 41-7 Standard of Care for the Patient Undergoing Liver Resection—cont'd

Patient Problem and Outcomes	Nursing Interventions and Rationales	Patient Education Instructions
Postoperatively		
Bleeding If bleeding occurs, patient will have this complication promptly recognized by the nurse.	1. Monitor vital signs q1h until stable, then q4h. 2. Monitor hemodynamic parameters. 3. Examine skin and extremities for perfusion. 4. Inspect dressings and examine patient for signs of bleeding q2h and as observation requires. 5. Avoid invasive procedures, if possible. Apply pressure to puncture sites. 6. Measure abdominal girth q shift. 7. Monitor laboratory studies (blood cell count, coagulation studies). 8. Notify surgeon immediately if abnormal bleeding is present.	1. Tell patient to inform nurse if he or she feels any of the following: faint, heart beating fast, fullness in abdomen. 2. Instruct patient to report overt bleeding immediately. 3. Explain to patient reasons for various nursing interventions. 4. Teach patient that for a couple weeks, he or she may bleed easily as a result of the surgery' effect on the liver's ability to produce clotting factors. Instruct him or her on measures to reduce bleeding and instances when he or she should notify the physician.
Fluid and Electrolyte Imbalance Patient will maintain adequate fluid and electrolyte balance.	1. Monitor hemodynamic parameters. 2. Monitor blood chemistries. 3. Maintain accurate intake and output. 4. Monitor for signs and symptoms of displaced or occluded biliary drains: excess or decrease of drainage, pain, and fever. 5. Monitor patient's mental status. 6. Promptly report abnormalities to surgeon.	1. Instruct patient to inform the nurse if he or she notices a lot of drainage or lack of drainage at incision/drain site or if he or she is experiencing pain or increased pressure at surgical site. 2. Explain to patient the purpose for the drains.
Potential for Liver Failure Patient will have normal liver function. If liver failure occurs, the patient will have it promptly recognized by the nurse.	See Table 41-8	See Table 41-8
Portal Hypertension If portal hypertension occurs, the patient will have it promptly recognized by the nurse.	1. Monitor hemodynamic parameters. 2. Watch patient closely for overt and subclinical signs of bleeding. 3. Report any abnormalities promptly to surgeon.	1. Instruct patient to report any bleeding, especially from the surgical site and gastrointestinal system.

Modified from Gillespie, P. (1995). Hepatocellular cancer. In C. Miaskowski (Ed.), *Oncology nursing.* Albany, NY: Delmar; Smeltzer, S. & Bare, B. (1996). Assessment and management of patients with hepatic and biliary disorders. In S. Smeltzer & B. Bare (Eds.), *Brunner and Suddarth's textbook of medical-surgical nursing* (8th ed.). Philadelphia: J. B. Lippincott.

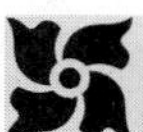

TABLE 41-7 Standard of Care for the Patient Undergoing Liver Resection—cont'd

Patient Problem and Outcomes	Nursing Interventions and Rationales	Patient Education Instructions
Pain		
Patient will experience optimal pain relief with minimal side effects.	1. Assess pain every 2-4 hours while patient is awake using the following parameters: location, quality, severity (0-10 scale) and aggravating/relieving factors. Examine the painful area when pain is reported. Distinguish postoperative pain from pain caused from a complication. 2. Administer analgesics routinely for first 24-48 hours postoperatively. 3. Assist patient with other pain-reducing interventions as appropriate (e.g., positioning, relaxation techniques, music). 4. Monitor for analgesic side effects and toxic effects and treat as required (e.g., respiratory depression, nausea, vomiting, sedation, constipation). 5. Obtain a change in analgesic, dose or frequency, if pain persists.	1. Reinforce preoperative teaching: that the patient should: a. Inform nurse when pain is present b. Inform nurse if pain is not relieved to his or her satisfaction c. Take pain medication at regular intervals when the pain is severe, especially during the first few days postoperatively. d. Use a variety of pain-reducing interventions. e. Report any side effects related to analgesics or other pain-reducing Interventions.
Pulmonary Complications (i.e., pneumonia, atelectasis)		
Patient will have absence of pulmonary complications.	1. Ensure that patient complies with procedures to maintain adequate gas exchange and lung expansion (e.g., incentive spirometry, deep breathing, coughing, ambulation by providing assistance, and encouragement. Medicate before ambulation if necessary. 2. Assess lung sounds q2h during the first 24-72 hours then q shift. Monitor pulse oximetry, if applicable. 3. Report any abnormalities promptly to surgeon.	1. Reinforce the importance of incentive spirometry, deep breathing, coughing and activity for maintaining good respiratory function.
Infection		
If an infection occurs, the patient will have it promptly recognized by the nurse.	1. Monitor for signs and symptoms of infection (e.g., fever; abnormal amount and appearance of drainage; redness of incision site, increase in pain, elevation of white blood cell count). 2. Report any abnormalities to surgeon promptly.	1. Teach patient signs and symptoms to report to health care professional (e.g., abnormal amount and appearance of drainage; redness of incision site, increased pain, malaise).
Potential Abscess Formation		
If an abscess forms, the patient will have this situation promptly recognized by the nurse.	1. Monitor for signs and symptoms of an abscess (e.g., abnormal amount and character of bile drainage, low-grade fever, sharp pain). 2. Promptly report any abnormalities to surgeon.	1. Instruct patient that fever, increase in pain or any sudden change in the amount or appearance of the drainage should be immediately reported to the surgeon.

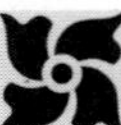

TABLE 41-8 Standard of Care for the Patient Experiencing Hepatic Failure

Patient Problem and Outcomes	Nursing Interventions and Rationales	Patient Education Instructions
Knowledge Deficit Related to Impaired Skin Integrity: Jaundice, Pruritus		
Patient will experience relief from symptoms.	1. Provide frequent skin care, bed baths without soap, and applications of emollient lotion or oil. 2. Administer antipruritic medications and monitor for effectiveness. Some medications commonly prescribed may not be effective and, in fact, may cause added problems.	1. Instruct patient on ways to reduce skin irritation: a. Avoid soaps, hot baths, harsh detergents and irritating clothing. b. Put a little vinegar in the rinse cycle of the washing machine. c. Use emollient lotion and oil. d. Humidify environment if dry. e. Use distraction techniques. f. Use medications if effective (i.e., antihistamines, cholestyramine, corticosteroids).
Knowledge Deficit Related to Fluid Volume Deficit: Ascites		
Patient will experience some relief from ascites.	1. Administer diuretics and monitor for effectiveness: weigh patient, measure abdominal girth, assist with paracentesis, provide safe environment. Aldactone is the preferred diuretic because it is potassium-sparing. 2. Monitor laboratory studies.	1. Instruct patient to restrict sodium intake.
Knowledge Deficit Related to High Risk for Bleeding: Altered Clotting Factors		
Patient will maintain hemodynamic stability.	1. Avoid or minimize trauma to skin and mucous membranes. 2. Monitor laboratory studies. 3. Observe and report any signs or symptoms of spontaneous or excessive bleeding. 4. Administer vitamin K as prescribed to promote clotting.	1. Teach patient the significance of being at risk for bleeding. 2. Instruct patient on ways to prevent bleeding. 3. Instruct patient to report bleeding. 4. Explain purpose of vitamin K.
Knowledge Deficit Related to Altered Thought Processes: Increased Serum Ammonia		
Patient will demonstrate improved mental status.	1. Restrict dietary protein to reduce source of ammonia. 2. Administer lactulose until diarrhea occurs; then adjust dose and frequency based on assessment. Lactulose acidifies colonic contents; hence ammonia moves from the blood into the colon. 3. Provide protective perianal care before diarrhea begins. 4. Clean, dry, and apply ointment to perianal area after each bowel movement. Consider use of a rectal pouch. 5. Provide safe environment.	1. Explain purpose of dietary restrictions. 2. Explain purpose and dosing of lactulose. 3. Instruct patient on perianal care.

Modified from Bord, M., McCray, N., & Shaffer, S. (1991). Alteration in comfort: pruritus. In J. McNally, E. Somerville, C. Miaskowski, & M. Rostad (Eds.), *Guidelines for oncology nursing practice.* Philadelphia: W. B. Saunders; Gillespie, P. (1995). Hepatocellular cancer. In C. Miaskowski (Ed.), *Oncology nursing.* Albany, NY: Delmar; Smeltzer, S. & Bare, B. (1996). Assessment and management of patients with hepatic and biliary disorders. In S. Smeltzer & B. Bare (Eds.), *Brunner and Suddarth's textbook of medical-surgical nursing* (8th ed.). Philadelphia: J. B. Lippincott.

cedure monitoring. Patients treated with this modality require education about the procedure and its potential complications. Patients often undergo this procedure on an outpatient basis. Therefore, it is important that they understand what signs and symptoms to report because complications or side effects may arise after they leave the hospital or clinic.

Intra-Arterially Administered Therapies. Chemotherapy, embolizing materials, or a combination of the two are given through a catheter that has been inserted into the hepatic artery either surgically or percutaneously during angiography. Nursing care of patients undergoing these treatments includes patient education, assisting with the procedure, and postprocedural monitoring. The nurse must be cognizant of potential side effects and complications. By being able to recognize the symptoms of a postembolization syndrome, the nurse can provide prompt symptom management with analgesics, antipyretics, and/or antiemetics. Knowing what drug(s) the patient received enables the nurse to structure nursing care and the patient teaching plan accordingly. Other common nursing measures entail assessing pedal pulses postangiography, observing the patient for bleeding, monitoring vital signs, and evaluating laboratory results. Patients require education about the procedure and its potential complications and side effects (Rospond & Mills, 1995). Patients also need to understand their postprocedural responsibilities, especially if they have an implantable pump.

Radiation Therapy. High-dose conformal radiation therapy with intra-arterial floxuridine is a rigorous therapy that usually requires the patient to go to the radiation therapy department twice a day, 5 days a week, for several weeks. Furthermore, the patient receives concurrent intra-arterial floxuridine through an implanted or external catheter/pump system. Nursing care includes patient education about the basics of the procedure, its possible side effects and complications, self-care instructions, and how to manage the pump, if applicable. The radiation therapy nurse will assess the patient's skin, check pump operation, evaluate laboratory results, elicit patient feedback, and observe for bleeding and infection.

For many patients, enduring the procedures outlined previously is their final effort at trying to control or palliate this disease. Consequently, the patient, family, and loved ones may require a great deal of emotional support and information about available resources.

Nursing Care Related to Impaired Hepatic Function

Impaired liver function results from increasing tumor growth or from worsening of the underlying liver disease. Liver failure is a frequent cause of death in patients with HCC (Groupe d'Etude et de Traitement du Carcinome Hepatocellulaire, 1995). Symptoms of liver failure can be particularly distressing. Patients can have yellow-tinged skin and sclerae from the excess bilirubin in the extracellular fluids because liver cells can no longer clear it from the blood. The accumulated bile salts subsequently irritate cutaneous nerve endings, resulting in intense itching (Bord, McCray, & Shaffer, 1991; Gillespie, 1995).

Another distressing symptom is ascites, which is caused when blood cannot leave the liver due to a blockage. The high pressure in the liver sinusoids causes plasma to weep from the surface of the liver into the peritoneal cavity. The high colloidal osmotic pressure in the fluid pulls even more fluid into the abdomen (Guyton, 1991). Serum albumin is decreased. Patients experience dyspnea when the excess fluid pushes up against the diaphragm.

Bleeding occurs when the liver is no longer able to form coagulation factors or to store vitamin K. Many patients also have anemia and thrombocytopenia, further compounding the problem (Nettina, 1996; Tucker, Cannobbio, Paquette, & Wells, 1996).

The patient's mental state changes when the liver cannot convert the ammonia into urea. The ammonia is toxic to the cerebral metabolism and results in hepatic coma if unchecked (Smeltzer & Bare, 1996). Table 41-8 summarizes the nursing management of these problems.

HOME CARE ISSUES

Home care issues are determined by treatment requirements, side effect and symptom management, disease effects on quality of life, financial issues, and the presence or absence of support from family/significant others. The patient may require home nursing care during treatment cycles, as mentioned previously. The patient and family will be especially challenged if symptoms related to liver failure occur. Hospice care may be indicated when it is clear that further efforts aimed at controlling tumor growth are futile.

PROGNOSIS

Prognosis is determined largely by the stage of the disease at the time of diagnosis. Presumably, the earlier the stage, the better the prognosis. However, unless the tumor has been totally removed or destroyed, or a miraculous spontaneous remission occurs, history tells us that HCC marches forward relentlessly. The original tumor expands and new lesions develop or, as happens most frequently, hepatic failure occurs as an end result of cirrhosis. In fact, according to Johnson (1996), the single greatest determinant of survival is the functional reserve of the nonmalignant liver. The median survival after the onset of symptoms related to liver failure (i.e., painful hepatomegaly, ascites, jaundice) is 3 to 6 months (Sardi et al., 1996).

Researchers have conducted numerous studies to identify factors that could potentially predict prognosis. These factors include age, sex, hormonal receptor status, AFP level, degree of cirrhosis, bilirubin levels, presence of portal vein thrombosis, tumor size, macroscopic appearance, histologic features, resection margin, and lymph node metastasis (Choi, 1996, Liu et al., 1996). Prognosis may also be influenced by the expertise of the treating physicians and their access to the latest diagnostic and therapeutic modalities. Similarly, because some therapies impart significant morbidity, knowing when not to use this technology is important.

Table 41-9 Quality of Care Evaluation for a Patient Undergoing Liver Resection

Disciplines participating in the quality of care evaluation:
☐ Nursing ☐ Surgery
☐ Respiratory Therapy ☐ Social Services

I. Postoperative Management Evaluation

Data from:
☐ Medical Record Review ☐ Patient/Family Interview

Criteria	Yes	No
1. Was the patient provided with preoperative information about:		
a. Diagnostic tests	☐	☐
b. Bowel prep	☐	☐
c. Use of incentive spirometer/ importance of deep breathing, coughing, activity	☐	☐
d. Use of antiembolic stockings	☐	☐
e. Pain management	☐	☐
2. Were liver function studies, blood counts, and coagulation studies evaluated:		
a. Preoperatively	☐	☐
b. Postoperatively	☐	☐
3. Did patient experience the following complications:		
a. Bleeding	☐	☐
b. Liver failure	☐	☐
c. Portal hypertension	☐	☐
d. Pulmonary complications	☐	☐
e. Infection	☐	☐

II. Patient/Family Satisfaction

Data from:
☐ Patient Interview ☐ Family Interview

Criteria	Yes	No
1. On a scale of 0 to 10, with 0 being totally dissatisfied and 10 being totally satisfied, how satisfied were you with the pain management you received?	______	
2. Were you told to call the nurse if you experienced bleeding from anywhere or leakage of fluid at your incision?	☐	☐
3. Regarding home care instructions, were you instructed on:		
a. How to manage your drains, if present?	☐	☐
b. Signs and symptoms to report to doctor (e.g., bleeding, pain, swelling of abdomen, yellowing of skin, or anything else unusual)	☐	☐

Box 41-6 Research Questions Related to Hepatocellular Cancer

- What is the most efficient and cost-effective method of vaccinating people against hepatitis B (and eventually hepatitis C when the vaccine is developed)?
- What is the effect of interferon on viral replication? When should patients begin interferon therapy? What dosages should be prescribed? How long should the treatment last?
- Are there other cost-effective screening tools that are more sensitive and specific to hepatocellular cancer than current tools?
- Is there a way to detect subclinical micrometastasis?
- What are the characteristics of the people who respond well to therapy? Can we categorize these people into groups?
- Should patients who have had liver resections and transplants be given adjuvant or neoadjuvant therapy?
- What is the best therapy for patients who are not surgical candidates?
- What are the effects of various therapies on the patient's quality of life?

EVALUATION OF THE QUALITY OF CARE

Accreditation organizations, such as the Joint Commission for the Accreditation of Health Care Organizations, require that the quality of care proved to patients be evaluated. Because the care provided to patients with HCC requires input from a multidisciplinary team, an evaluation of the quality of care provided to these patients should include aspects of care provided by various members of the team. Table 41-9 provides an example of a quality of care evaluation tool.

RESEARCH ISSUES

Literally thousands of clinical trials are underway worldwide to investigate prevention, screening, detection, and treatment of HCC. Well-designed clinical trials are the only way that clinicians will one day be able to answer treatment questions with confidence. Some questions that urgently need to be answered are listed in Box 41-6.

REFERENCES

Aguilar, F., Harris, C., Sun, T., Hollstein, M., & Cerutti, P. (1994). Geographic variation of p53 mutational profile in nonmalignant human liver. *Science, 264,* 1317-1318.

Bartolozzi, C., Lencioni, R., Caramella, D., Vignali, C., Cioni, R., Mazzeo, S., Carrai, M., Maltinti, G., & Conte, P.F. (1995). Treatment of Large HCC: Transcatheter arterial chemoembolization combined with percutaneous ethanol injection versus repeated transcatheter arterial chemoembolization. *Radiology, 197* (3), 812-818.

Barwick, K. & Rosai. (1996). Liver. In J. Rosai (Ed.), *Ackerman's surgical pathology* (8th ed.). St. Louis: Mosby.

Beahrs, O., Henson, D., Hutter, R., & Kennedy, B.J. (1992). Liver (Including intrahepatic bile ducts). *Manual for staging of cancer* (4th ed.). Philadelphia: J. B. Lippincott Company.

Beasley, R. P. (1988). Hepatitis B virus: The major etiology of hepatocellular carcinoma. *Cancer, 61*(10), 1942-1956.

Bloomer, J., Straka, J., & Rank, J. (1993). The porphyrias. In L. Schiff,. & E. Schiff (Eds.), *Diseases of the liver* (Vol. 2). Philadelphia: J. B. Lippincott Company.

Bord, M., McCray, N., & Shaffer, S. (1991). Alteration in comfort: pruritus. In J. McNally, E. Somerville, C. Miaskowski, & M. Rostad (Eds.), *Guidelines for oncology nursing practice.* Philadelphia: W. B. Saunders Company.

Boyer, J. & Reuben, A. (1993). Chronic hepatitis. In L. Schiff & E. Schiff (Eds.), *Diseases of the liver* (Vol. 1). Philadelphia: J. B. Lippincott Company.

Bruix, J., Castells, A., Bosch, J., Feu, F., Fuster, J., Garcia-Pagan, J., Bru, C., & Rodes, J. (1996). Surgical resection of hepatocellular carcinoma in cirrhotic patients: Prognostic value of preoperative portal pressure. *Gastroenterology, 111,* 1018-1022.

Carr, B. (1995). Chemo plus transplant promising for advanced hepatocellular ca. *Oncology News International, 4*(9), 2, 21.

Choi, J. (1996). Regional transcatheter therapy of hepatic neoplasms. *Cancer Control, 3* (5), 407-413.

Chung, J., Park J. H., Han, J. K., Choi, B. I., & Han, M. C. (1995). Hepatocellular carcinoma and portal vein invasion: Results of treatment with transcatheter oily chemoembolization. *American Journal of Roentgenology, 165*(2), 315-321.

Conn, H. O. & Atterbury, C. E. (1993). Cirrhosis. In L. Schiff, & E. Schiff (Eds.), *Diseases of the liver* (Vol. 2). Philadelphia: J. B. Lippincott Company.

Craig, J. R, Peters, R. L., & Edmondson, H. (1989). *Tumors of the liver and intrahepatic bile ducts.* Washington, D.C.: Armed Forces Institute of Pathology.

Dusheiko, G., Hobbs, K., Dick, R., & Burroughs, A. (1992). Treatment of small hepatocellular carcinomas. *Lancet, 340,* 285-288.

Farmer, D. & Busuttil, R. (1994). The role of multimodal therapy in the treatment of hepatocellular carcinoma. *Cancer, 73*(11), 2669-2670.

Fong, Y. (1996). Surgical management of hepatocellular carcinoma. *Proceedings of the American Society of Clinical Oncologists.* Philadelphia: American Society of Clinical Oncologists.

Fortner, J. (1996). The Sardi/Akbarov/Conaway article reviewed. *Oncology, 10*(6), 929-930.

Fried, M. & Hoofnagle, J. (1995). Therapy of hepatitis C. *Seminars in Liver Disease, 15*(1), 82-91.

Frogge, M. H. (1993). Gastrointestinal cancers: Esophagus, stomach, liver, and pancreas. In S. Groenwald, M. Frogge, M. Goodman, & C. Yarbro (Eds.), *Cancer nursing: Principles and practice.* Boston: Jones and Bartlett Publishers.

Genecin, P. & Groszmann, R. (1993). Portal hypertension. In L. Schiff, & E. Schiff (Eds.), *Diseases of the liver* (Vol. 2). Philadelphia: J. B. Lippincott Company.

Gillespie, P. (1995). Hepatocellular cancer. In C. Miaskowski & K. Gettrust (Eds.), *Oncology nursing.* Albany, NY: Delmar Publishers.

Groopman, J. & Kensler, T. (1996). Hepatoma: Linkage of chemical-viral etiology and opportunities for prevention. *Proceedings of the American Society of Clinical Oncologists.* Philadelphia: American Society of Clinical Oncologists.

Groupe d'Etude et Traitement du Carcinome Hepatocellulaire. (1995). A comparison of Lipiodol chemoembolization and conservative treatment for unresectable hepatocellular carcinoma. *The New England Journal of Medicine, 332*(19), 1256-1261.

Guyton, A. (1991). The liver as an organ. *Textbook of medical physiology* (8th ed.). Philadelphia: W. B. Saunders Company.

Hung, Y., Lin, D., & Chiu, C. (1995). Risk factors of hepatocellular carcinoma with familial tendency. *Chang Gung Medical Journal, 18*(1), 8-13.

Ishak, K. & Markin, R. (1996). Liver. In I. Damjanov & J. Linder (Eds.), *Anderson's pathology* (10th ed.). St. Louis: Mosby.

Johnson, P. (1996). Management of inoperable hepatocellular carcinoma. *Proceedings of the American Society of Clinical Oncologists.* Philadelphia: American Society of Clinical Oncologists.

Kaklamani, E., Trichopoulos, D., Tzonou, A., Zavitsanos, X., Koumantaki, Y., Hatzakis, A., Hsieh, C. C., & Hatziyannis, S. (1991). Hepatitis B and C viruses and their interaction in the origin of hepatocellular carcinoma. *Journal of the American Medical Association, 265*(15), 1974-1976.

Koff, R. Viral hepatitis. (1993). In L. Schiff, & E. Schiff (Eds.), *Diseases of the liver* (Vol. 1). Philadelphia: J. B. Lippincott Company.

Kountouras, J., Boura, P., Karolides, A., Zaharioudaki, E., & Tsapas, G. (1995). Recombinant α2 interferon (α-INF) with chemo-hormonal therapy in patients with hepatocellular carcinoma (HCC). *Hepato-Gastroenterology, 42* (1), 31-36.

Lau, W. Y., Leung, W. T., Ho, S., Lam, S. K., Li, C. Y., Johnson, P. J., Williams, R., & Li, A. K. C. (1995). Hepatocellular carcinoma during pregnancy and its comparison with other pregnancy-associated malignancies. *Cancer, 75*(11), 2669-2675.

Lawrence, T., Kessler, M., & Robertson, J. (1993). Conformal high-dose radiation plus intraarterial floxuridine for hepatic cancer. *Oncology, 7*(10), 51-63.

Liu, C., Lo, C., & Fan, S. (1996). Surgical resection of hepatocellular carcinoma. *Cancer Control, 3*(5), 399-406.

Livraghi, T., Giorgio, A., Marin, G., Salmi, A., de Sio, I., Bolondi, L., Pompili, M., Brunello, F., Lazzaroni, S., Torzillo, G., & Zucchi, A. (1995). Hepatocellular carcinoma and cirrhosis in 746 patients: Long-term results of percutaneous ethanol injection. *Radiology, 197,* 101-108.

Lotze, M., Flickinger, J., & Carr, B. (1993). Hepatobiliary neoplasms. In V. DeVita, S. Hellman, & S. Rosenberg, *Cancer: Principles and practice of oncology* (4th ed.). Philadelphia: J. B. Lippincott Company.

Maddrey, W. (1993). Chronic hepatitis. *Disease-a-Month, 39*(2), 53-126.

Mazzaferro, V., Regalia, E., Doci, R., Andreola, S., Pulvirenti, A., Bozzetti, F., Montalto, F., Ammatuna, M., Morabito, A., & Gennari, L. (1996). Liver transplantation for the treatment of small hepatocellular carcinomas in patients with cirrhosis. *The New England Journal of Medicine, 334*(11), 693-699.

Mendenhall, C. (1993). Alcoholic hepatitis. In L. Schiff & E. Schiff (Eds.), *Diseases of the liver* (Vol. 2). Philadelphia: J. B. Lippincott Company.

Nettina, S. (1996). Hepatic, biliary, and pancreatic disorders. In S. Nettina (Ed.), *The Lippincott manual of nursing practice* (6th ed.). Philadelphia: J. B. Lippincott Company.

Niederhuber, J. (1995). Tumors of the liver. In G. Murphy, W. Lawrence, & R. Lenhard (Eds.), *American Cancer Society textbook of clinical oncology.* Atlanta: The American Cancer Society.

Nishiguchi, S., Kuroki, T., Nakatani, S., Morimoto, H., Takeda, T., Nakajima, S., Shiomi, S., Seki, S., Kobayashi, K., & Otani, S. (1995). Randomized trial of effects of interferon on incidence of hepatocellular carcinoma in chronic active hepatitis C with cirrhosis. *Lancet, 346,* 1051-1055.

Nissenbaum, M., vanSonnenberg, E., & D'Agostino, H. (1993). Interventional radiology in the liver, biliary tract, and gallbladder. In L. Schiff & E. Schiff (Eds.), *Diseases of the liver* (Vol 1). Philadelphia: J. B. Lippincott Company.

Oberfield, R. A., Steele, G., Gollan, J., & Sherman, D. (1989). Liver cancer. *Ca-A Cancer Journal for Clinicians 39*(4), 206-218.

Okuda, K., Kojiro, M., & Okuda, H. (1993). Neoplasms of the liver. In L. Schiff & E. Schiff (Eds.), *Diseases of the liver* (Vol. 2). Philadelphia: J. B. Lippincott Company.

Olthoff, K., Rosove, M., Shackleton, C., Imagawa, D., Farmer, D., Northcross, P., Pakrasi, A., Martin, P., Goldstein, L., Shaked, A., & Busuttil, R. (1995). Adjuvant chemotherapy improves survival after liver transplantation for hepatocellular carcinoma. *Annals of Surgery, 221*(6), 734-741.

Pajeau, T. & Bennett, C. (1995) Preventing hepatitis B, hepatocellular cancer: Made in Taiwan. *Oncology News International, 4*(9), 21.

Ramsey, W., & Wu, G. (1995). Hepatocellular carcinoma: Update on diagnosis and treatment. *Digestive Diseases, 12*(2), 81-91.

Rappaport, A., & Wanless, I (1993). Physioanatomic considerations. In L. Schiff & E. Schiff (Eds.), *Diseases of the liver* (Vol. 1). Philadelphia: J. B. Lippincott Company.

Reddy, R., Dr., University of Miami Center for Liver Diseases, Miami, FL. Personal Communication, December 18, 1996.

Reynolds, T. (1993). Budd-Chiari syndrome. In L. Schiff & E. Schiff (Eds.), *Diseases of the liver* (Vol. 2). Philadelphia: J. B. Lippincott Company.

Rospond, R. M., & Mills, S. (1995). Hepatic artery chemoembolization therapy for hepatic tumors. *Association of Operating Room Nurses Journal, 61*(3), 573-576.

Runyon, B. (1993). Ascites. In L. Schiff, & E. Schiff (Eds.), *Diseases of the liver* (Vol 2). Philadelphia: J. B .Lippincott Company.

Sardi, A., Akbarov, A., & Conaway, G. (1996). Management of primary and metastatic tumors to the liver. *Oncology, 10*(6),911-925.

Sato, M., Watanabe, Y., Ueda, S., Iseki, S., Abe, Y., Sato, N., Kimura, S., Okubo, K., & Onji, M. (1996). Microwave coagulation therapy for hepatocellular carcinoma. *Gastroenterology, 110,* 1507-1514.

Schiff, G. (1993). Hepatitis caused by viruses other than hepatitis A, hepatitis B, and non-A, non-B hepatitis viruses. In L. Schiff, & E. Schiff (Eds.), *Diseases of the liver* (Vol. 1). Philadelphia: J. B. Lippincott Company.

Schiff, E. & Schiff, L. (1993). Needle biopsy of the liver. In L. Schiff & E. Schiff (Eds.), *Diseases of the liver* (Vol. 1). Philadelphia: J. B. Lippincott Company.

Schluger, L. & Bodenheimer, H., Jr. (1995). Tackling liver cancer with interferon. *Lancet, 346,* 1049-1050.

Seki, T., Wakabayashi, M., Nakagawa, T., Itho, T., Shiro, T., Sato, M., Uchiyama, S., & Inoue, K. (1994). Ultrasonically guided percutaneous microwave coagulation therapy for small hepatocellular carcinoma. *Cancer, 74*(3), 817-825.

Schwarzenberg, S. & Sharp, H. (1993). α_1-Antitrypsin deficiency. In L. Schiff & E. Schiff (Eds.), *Diseases of the liver* (Vol. 1). Philadelphia: J. B. Lippincott Company.

Sherman, M., Peltekian, K., & Lee, C. (1995). Screening for hepatocellular carcinoma in chronic carriers of hepatitis B virus: Incidence and prevalence of hepatocellular carcinoma in a North American urban population. *Hepatology, 22*(2), 432-438.

Siegel, J., & Veerappan, A. (1993). Gastrointestinal endoscopy in the diagnosis and management of hepatobiliary disease. In L. Schiff, L. & E. Schiff (Eds.), *Diseases of the liver* (Vol. 1). Philadelphia: J. B. Lippincott Company.

Simonetti, R., Camma, C., Fiorello, F., Cottone, M., Rapicetta, M., Marino, L., Fiorentino, G., Craxi, A., Ciccaglione, A., Giuseppetti, R., Stroffolini, T., & Pagliaro, L. (1992). Hepatitis C virus infection as a risk factor for hepatocellular carcinoma in patients with cirrhosis. *Annals of Internal Medicine, 116*(2) 97-101.

Smeltzer, S., & Bare, B. (1996). Assessment and management of patients with hepatic and biliary disorders. In S. Smeltzer & B. Bare (Eds.), *Brunner and Suddarth's textbook of medical-surgical nursing* (8th ed.). Philadelphia: J. B. Lippincott Company.

Sotomayor, R. & Ravikumar, T. (1996). Cryosurgery in the treatment of hepatic tumors. *Cancer Control, 3*(5), 414-420.

Takano, S., Yokosuka, O., Imazeki, F., Tagawa, M., & Omata, M. (1995). Incidence of hepatocellular carcinoma in chronic hepatitis B and C: A prospective study of 251 patients. *Hepatology, 21*(3), 650-655.

Takenaka, K., Yoshida, K., Nishizaki, T., Korenaga, D., Hiroshige, K., Ikeda, T., & Sugimachi, K. (1995). Postoperative prophylactic Lipiodolization reduces the intrahepatic recurrence of hepatocellular carcinoma. *American Journal of Surgery, 169,* 400-404.

Tang, Z. & Yang, B. (1995). Secondary prevention of hepatocellular carcinoma. *Journal of Gastroenterology and Hepatology, 10*(6), 683-690.

Tavil, A. (1993). Hemochromatosis. In L. Schiff, & E. Schiff (Eds.), *Diseases of the liver* (Vol 1). Philadelphia: J. B. Lippincott Company.

Tsukuma, H., Hiyama, T., Tanaka, S., Nakao, M., Yabuuchi, T., Kitamura, T., Nakanishi, K., Fujimoto, I., Inoue, A., Yamazaki, H., & Kawashima, T. (1993). Risk factors for hepatocellular carcinoma among patients with chronic liver disease. *The New England Journal of Medicine, 328*(25), 1797-1801.

Tucker, S., Canobbio, M, Paquette, E., & Wells, M. (1996). *Patient care standards* (6th ed.). St. Louis: Mosby.

Venook, A. (1994). Treatment of hepatocellular carcinoma: Too many options? *Journal of Clinical Oncology, 12*(6),1323-1334.

Weaver, M. L, Atkinson, D., & Zemel, R. (1995). Hepatic cryosurgery in treating colorectal metastases. *Cancer, 76*(2), 210-214.

Williams, P., Dyson, M., Warwick, R., & Bannister, L. (1989). *Gray's anatomy* (37th ed.). Edinburgh: Churchill Livingstone.

Wills, K., Huang, W., Harris, M., Machemer, T., Maneval, D., & Gregory, R. (1995). Gene therapy for hepatocellular carcinoma: Chemosensitivity conferred by adenovirus-mediated transfer of the HSV-1 thymidine kinase gene. *Cancer Gene Therapy, 2*(3), 191-197.

Yamashita, F., Tanaka, M., Satomura, S., & Tanikawa, K. (1996). Prognostic significance of *lens culinaris* agglutinin A-reactive α-fetoprotein in small hepatocellular carcinomas. *Gastroenterology, 111,* 996-1001.

Yu, S, (1995). Primary prevention of hepatocellular carcinoma. *Journal of Gastroenterology & Hepatology 10*(6), 674-82.

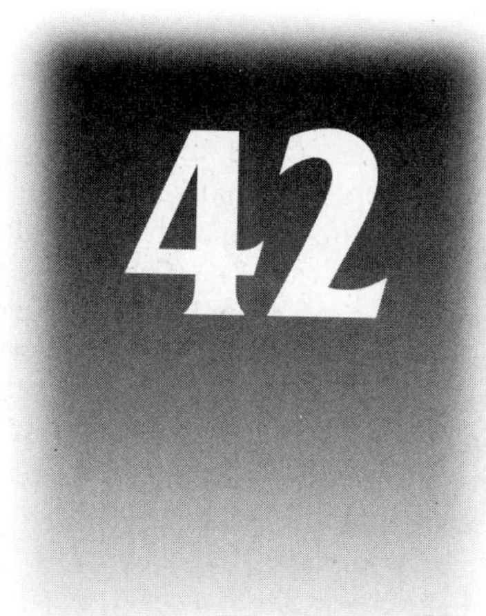

Pancreatic Cancer

Barbara Hawkins, RN, MS, OCN

EPIDEMIOLOGY

Pancreatic cancer ranks ninth among all cancers, accounting for approximately 2% of all cancers in the United States and resulting in 5% of all cancer deaths (after lung, colorectal, breast, and prostate cancers). The number of new cases of cancer of the pancreas are estimated at 29,000, and approximately 28,900 die annually of this disease (Landis, Murray, Bolden & Wingo, 1998).

The incidence of pancreatic cancer has increased steadily for unknown reasons over the last 60 years worldwide. In the United States the incidence doubled from the 1930s to the 1980s. The rate has now steadied at nine per 100,000 and is starting to decline, although the reduction has been entirely among males. Incidence among white females, black men, and black females has not fallen (Murr, Sarr, Oishi, & van Heerden, 1994). These changes have been small, however, and the prognosis remains grim, with a median survival of 4.1 months.

In 1985, the last year for which comprehensive figures are currently available, there were approximately 185,000 new cases of pancreatic cancer worldwide, with a death rate of approximately 0.99:100,000 (Ahlgren, 1996). It is a disease that is treatable if diagnosed early, but is rarely curable. Because of difficulties in diagnosis, the aggressiveness of pancreatic cancer, and the lack of effective systemic therapies, only 1% to 4% of patients with adenocarcinoma of the pancreas will be alive 5 years after the diagnosis. Unfortunately, incidence rates and mortality rates are virtually identical (Evans, Abbruzzese, & Rich, 1997).

RISK FACTORS

The major risk factors associated with the development of pancreatic cancer are listed in Box 42-1. Evidence supporting these risk factors and the nursing implications for prevention and early detection are discussed.

Increasing Age

Age is an important risk factor in the development of pancreatic cancer. The peak incidence occurs in the seventh and eighth decades of life. It is a rarity before the age of 40. Although this is primarily a disease of adults, rare childhood cases have been reported (Ahlgren, 1996). In addition, pancreatic cancer is more common in men than in women by 30% (McLaughlin, 1994).

Ethnic Differences

The incidence of pancreatic cancer is 1.5 to 2.0 times higher in the black population in the United States than for any other ethnic group. As a consequence, the American black male has one of the highest risks of pancreatic cancer in the world; however, the incidence of pancreatic cancer in the native African population is generally quite low. Japanese immigrants to the United States also have a higher incidence than native whites. The Korean population in Los Angeles also has a high incidence (16.4 : 100,000), whereas the lowest rate in the world is in India (0.7 : 100,000) (Murr et al., 1994). Epidemiological studies have shown some clustering in parts of Louisiana, a higher incidence in urban areas, and a higher incidence in American counties with a significant portion of residents of Scandinavian or Russian descent (Coleman, 1997).

Tobacco Use

Smoking is the only factor that has consistently been reported to increase the risk for the development of pancreatic cancer. Current estimates suggest that approximately 30% of pancreatic cancer cases are due to smoking. Recent studies have shown that the risk of pancreatic cancer increases as the amount and duration of smoking increase, and that long-term smoking cessation (more than 10 years) reduces risk by approximately 30% compared with the risk for current smokers (Evans, Abbruzzese, & Rich, 1997). The mechanism for this has not been clearly determined, but several theories have been offered: carcinogens (nitrosureas) excreted in the bile and refluxing into the pancreas, carcinogens arriving via the blood stream to the pancreas, or an indirect effect of smoking causing hyperlipidemia that could promote the development of a pancreatic tumor (Garcia & Egner, 1995).

Research currently being done for lung cancer will hopefully provide a greater specificity in linking tobacco exposure with the development of pancreatic cancer, and may facilitate the study of chemoprevention strategies (Evans, Abbruzzese, & Rich, 1997).

Dietary Carcinogens

There is a possible relationship between the consumption of dietary fat and protein from meat intake and the development of pancreatic cancer. Although the mechanisms of this relationship remain unclear, it has been suggested that this type of diet can stimulate the release of cholecystokinin and other hormones that act to increase pancreatic cell turnover and thereby increase the susceptibility of the pancreas to the effects of carcinogens. A protective effect from citrus fruits, vegetables, fiber, and vitamin C has been reported (Ahlgren, 1996; McLaughlin, 1994). The association of diets high in citrus with a reduced risk of pancreatic cancer is particularly interesting given the recent observation that limonene, a natural product found in citrus fruits, is a potent inhibitor of the K-*ras* oncoprotein (Evans, Abbruzzese, & Rich, 1997).

Alcohol and Coffee Consumption

The association between the development of pancreatic cancer and the consumption of either alcohol or coffee has been shown to be tenuous. Cigarette smoking is common among heavy alcohol users and is a known etiologic factor in cancer of the pancreas. Unless there is adequate control for cigarette smoking, studies of the relationship between alcohol and pancreatic cancer cannot be considered reliable. The current available evidence does not show a relationship in the development of pancreatic cancer and the consumption of caffeinated or decaffeinated coffee or tea (Ahlgren, 1996).

Box 42-1
Risk Factors for Pancreatic Cancer

1. Increasing age
2. Gender
3. Ethnicity
4. Tobacco use
5. Dietary carcinogens (high dietary fat and meat protein)
6. Alcohol and coffee consumption (association)
7. Occupational exposure (association)
8. Positive family history
9. Diabetes
10. Radiation
11. Chronic pancreatitis
12. Other medical factors

Data from Evans, D., Abbruzzese, J., Rich, T. (1997) Cancer of the pancreas. In V. DeVita, S. Hellman, & S. A. Rosenberg (Eds.). *Cancer: Principles and practice of oncology.* Philadelphia: Lippincott-Raven.

Occupational Exposure

Several occupations have been implicated as possibly increasing the risk for pancreatic cancer. These include chemical and coke plant workers, chemists, and dry cleaning workers, as well as those who are exposed to solvents, gasoline, petroleum compounds, 2-naphthylamine, benzidine, and dichlorodiphenyltrichlorethane (DDT) (Garcia & Egner, 1995; Gold, 1995). Currently, most newly diagnosed patients with pancreatic cancer do not have evidence of a specific chemical exposure or relevant occupational history. Other factors such as smoking and diet will probably play a much greater overall role in determining individual risk of pancreatic cancer (Evans, Abbruzzese, & Rich, 1997).

Inherited Predisposition

Although a genetic predisposition to pancreatic cancer appears to exist, it is unusual. There has been reported familial clustering of pancreatic cancer (Murr et al., 1994). Patients with this type of cancer are 5 to 13 times more likely to report a family history of pancreatic cancer than is the control group. It is currently estimated that familial traits account for approximately 4% of pancreatic cancer patients (Douglass, Kim, & Meropol, 1997). Gene mutations and other chromosomal abnormalities are being delineated with increasing frequency. Abnormalities in the expression of the tumor suppression gene P53 and the oncogenes, K-*ras* and *c-erB-2* are occurring with a frequency of greater than 50% (Ahlgren, 1996; Garcia & Egner, 1995).

Diabetes

An apparent association of diabetes and pancreatic cancer has been reported by many investigators, but this has not been a consistent finding. One difficulty in studying this link is related to problems with establishing cause and effect. It has been suggested that diabetes is more likely to result as a consequence of the pancreatic tumor, rather than the reverse. This reflects that pancreatic endocrine insufficiency is secondary to the cancer. A recent study comparing 760 patients who have pancreatic cancer with 720 patients in a control group gives a good perspective. Of the patients, 164 (22.8%) had diabetes compared with 60 control-group patients (8.3%). The relationship between pancreatic cancer and diabetes becomes insignificant for all patients (male and female) who have had diabetes for more than 3 years. The odds ratio did continue to decrease for an increasing duration of diabetes, so there does not appear to be a causative relationship (Ahlgren, 1996).

Screening costs for pancreatic cancer would depend on the volume of the appropriate population and the screening tests that would be used. For instance, if screening ultrasounds were used with new-onset diabetics, a large number of negative screening tests would result. If other clinical features were used to select new-onset diabetics suspected of harboring pancreatic malignancies, the size of the screening cohort and the cost of the screening program would be decreased. For example, if diabetes associated with pancreatic cancer is typically characterized by a negative family history for diabetes, then screening only those with nondiabetic parents would eliminate approximately 96% of new-onset diabetics over the age of 45. Physicians should be alerted by newly diabetic patients without obesity or family history and/or those who require unusually aggressive insulin-dependent management. These diabetics should be screened for pancreatic cancer (Noy & Bilezikian, 1993).

Radiation

Radiation may modestly increase the risk of pancreatic cancer, although the evidence is not conclusive. In a study of survivors of the atomic bombings of Hiroshima and Nagasaki, there was a small increased risk, but the relative risk is much lower than for other malignancies such as leukemia and bone cancers. There appears to be minimal increased risk of developing cancer of the pancreas among patients receiving radiation therapy for ankylosing spondylitis or for cancer of the cervix (Ahlgren, 1996; Gold, 1995).

Chronic Pancreatitis

The relationship of chronic pancreatitis to pancreatic cancer has been of considerable interest. Pancreatic calcifications associated with chronic pancreatitis have been described in 3% of patients with pancreatic cancer. In patients with chronic pancreatitis, the diagnosis of pancreatic cancer may be difficult because of the similarity of presenting symptoms (Lowenfels, Maisonneuve, & Cavalline, 1993). It is also of note that patients who die of pancreatic cancer may have evidence of pancreatitis, but this may be a result of the obstructive changes caused by the cancer itself (Ahlgren, 1996; Gold, 1995).

Other Medical Factors

Tonsillectomy and various allergic disorders, such as asthma or hay fever, have been suggested as offering a possible protective effect for pancreatic cancer. This may suggest an immunologic mechanism because the tonsils can be a source of antigenic stimulus. More study is required to establish a clearer connection (Ahlgren, 1996; Gold, 1995).

Summary

Although several risk factors associated with the development of pancreatic cancer (i.e., increasing age, ethnicity, and gender) cannot be modified, other risk factors may be reduced through making modifications in life-style. For example, cigarette smoking is a clear risk factor. Oncology nurses need to be active in smoking-cessation programs or programs for teenagers that target the benefits of not smoking at all.

PATHOPHYSIOLOGY

Normal Anatomy and Physiology of the Pancreas

The pancreas is a racemose gland located in the retroperitoneum. It is approximately 15 cm in length and 2 to 3 cm in thickness, and it weighs about 90 g. It is shaped like a slender pear lying on its side. The pancreas is divided into a head, body, and tail. The head is positioned over the vena cava and is tucked into the first three portions of the duodenum on the right side. The body crosses in front of the spine, and the thin tail lies in front of the left kidney but behind the stomach and almost touches the spleen (Fig. 42-1).

The pancreas is a single organ that performs both endocrine and exocrine functions. The endocrine portion consists of a specialized group of cells (islets of Langerhans) that secrete the hormones insulin and glucagon directly into the bloodstream. Cancer of the endocrine pancreas is very rare and is not discussed in this text.

The exocrine portion, which releases secretions outside the organ via a duct, makes up about 99% of the pancreas. The secretory cells, called *acini,* line the multiple small al-

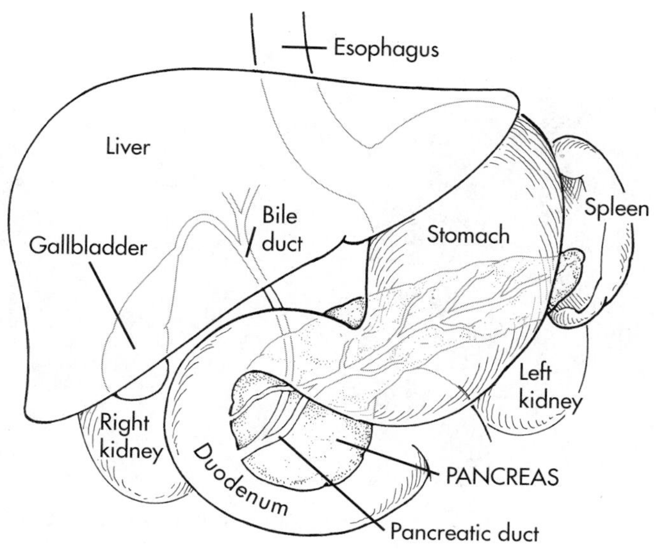

Fig. 42-1 Diagrammatic representation of the location of the pancreas within the abdominal cavity.

veoli that together form the lobules of the exocrine pancreas. These lobules contain small ducts receiving secretions from the alveoli. These small ducts empty pancreatic secretions into the Wirsung's canal, which runs from the tail to the head and empties into the duodenum. This main duct joins the common bile duct, which carries bile from the liver and gallbladder to the duodenum.

Each day, 300 to 800 ml of pancreatic juice are secreted directly in the duodenum. The major exocrine components are electrolytes and the digestive enzymes trypsin, amylase, and lipase. These enzymes are responsible for the hydrolysis of protein, starch, glycogen, and fats (Coleman, 1997; Schellenberg & Garnett, 1994).

The Process of Carcinogenesis

Just as with other cancers, the development of cancer of the pancreas appears to occur as a multistage process (Fig. 42-2). Most (95%) malignant neoplasms of pancreatic origin arise from the exocrine portion of the gland and are consistent with adenocarcinomas. Much more infrequent are tumors arising from the endocrine cells of the pancreas (islets of Langerhans). The predominant morphologic type is adenocarcinoma of ductal cell origin. Box 42-2 lists the histologic classifications of common tumors of the pancreas.

Attempts to identify premalignant ductal lesions of the pancreas in humans have been limited to autopsy studies, which have produced inconclusive results indicating a possible stepwise progression of ductal dysplasia to malignancy. Many histopathologic changes in the proliferating ductal epithelium can be identified. These changes may range from nonpapillary ductal hyperplasia to papillary hyperplasia, atypical papillary hyperplasia, and carcinoma in situ (Evans, Abbruzzese, & Rich, 1997).

The majority of patients with pancreatic cancer have been identified as having mutated K-*ras* deoxyribonucleic acid (DNA). This may be a possible tool by which these hyperproliferative states can be assessed for their malignant potential based on the frequency of the K-*ras* mutations. Patients who are found to have this mutation can be studied to determine if they will develop invasive pancreatic cancer. These data are suggesting that it may be possible to capitalize on the evolving understanding of the early molecular events that characterize exocrine pancreatic carcinogenesis to develop an effective means of detecting the disease at an early, potentially curable point. For example, the detection of mutated K-*ras* in bile or pancreatic ductal secretions could suggest the presence of an underlying pancreatic lesion. With the application of appropriate screening strategies, small, minimally invasive carcinomas could be identified, and would increase the number of patients who could have curative surgical or other interventions (Evans, Abbruzzese, & Rich, 1997).

The P53 gene is the most commonly mutated gene in human cancer. Seventy percent of pancreatic adenocarcinomas contain mutations in P53. These mutations are more com-

Box 42-2
Histologic Classification of Epithelial Tumors of the Exocrine Pancreas

Malignant

Ductal adenocarcinoma
Mucinous cystadenocarcinoma
Acinar cell carcinoma
Small cell carcinoma
Pancreatoblastoma

Uncertain Malignant Potential

Duct-ectatic mucin-hypersecreting tumor
Mucinous cystadenoma
Papillary cystic neoplasm

Benign

Serous cystadenoma

From Evans, D., Abbruzzese, J., Rich, T. (1997). Cancer of the pancreas. In V. DeVita, S. Hellman, & S. A. Rosenberg (Eds.). *Cancer: Principles and practice of oncology.* Philadelphia: Lippincott-Raven.

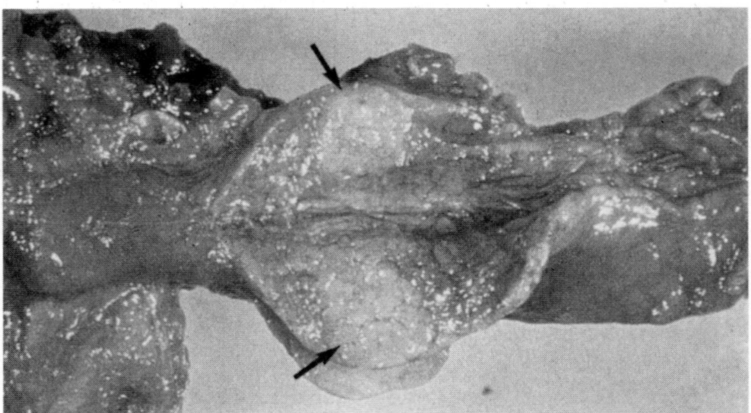

Fig. 42-2 Pancreatic carcinoma. (Skarin, A. T. [1996]. *Atlas of diagnostic oncology* [2nd ed.]. St. Louis: Mosby-Wolfe.)

monly seen in poorly differentiated pancreatic tumors. Based on the frequency with which mutations in K-*ras,* P53, and the oncogene, P16 are found, a model of pancreatic carcinogenesis has been suggested. It is proposed that the malignant clone evolves from cells driven by a dominant oncogene (K-*ras*) with subsequent deregulation of cell growth precipitated by abnormal cell-cycle control resulting from mutations in P53 or P16 or both.

A recently discovered tumor suppressor gene is *DCPA.* The exact functional role of this gene remains unclear, but it may be related to the signaling pathway that is necessary for normal cellular growth (Evans, Abbruzzese, & Rich 1997). It is still not clear how the molecular alterations in pancreatic cancer interact during pancreatic carcinogenesis. The hope is that studies designed to correct these alterations may lead to more effective treatment options.

ROUTES OF METASTASES

In pancreatic cancer, it is usually the metastatic symptoms that lead to the awareness of the presence of the cancer. Pancreatic cancer spreads early to regional and paraduodenal lymph nodes and later develops in mesocolic, peripancreatic, paraaortic, mesenteric and posterior mediastinal nodes. Supraclavicular nodes may be involved with carcinoma of the body and tail more often than with tumors of the head of the pancreas. Box 42-3 discusses nodal spread of pancreatic cancer. Peritoneal seeding by metastatic deposits can occur. Subclinical liver metastases are present in the majority of patients at the time of diagnosis, even when findings from imagining studies are normal.

Adenocarcinomas commonly invade the entire pancreas, obliterate the lobulated tissue and obstruct the common bile duct and Wirsung's canal. Invasion of the retroperitoneal lymphatics is the most common route of cancer dissemination. At the time of detection, large tumor masses may be fixed to the retropancreatic tissues or the vertebral column. The tumor may directly invade the spleen, kidney, or diaphragm. Metastasis to the lung, pleura, abdominal viscera, adrenal glands, and bones are common (Coleman, 1997). Most patients with this type of tumor invasion have neural invasion of the celiac nerve plexus, which may be the cause of the pain associated with carcinomas of the body and tail of the pancreas. Carcinoma eventually may infiltrate the duodenal musculature, stomach, transverse colon, portal vein, and the superior mesenteric vein. At the time of diagnosis, pancreatic cancer has invaded locally or metastasized in most patients. Patients with metastatic disease have a short survival (3 to 6 months), the length of which depends on the extent of the disease and performance status at the time of diagnosis (Douglass, Kim, Meropol, 1997).

Box 42-3
Sites of Regional Lymph Node Metastases in Pancreatic Cancer Patients

Lymph Nodes of Head of Pancreas

Lymph nodes superior to pancreatic head
Lymph nodes inferior to pancreatic head
Anterior pancreaticoduodenal lymph nodes
Pyloric, infrapyloric, and subpyloric lymph nodes
Posterior pancreaticoduodenal lymph nodes
Pericholedochal lymph nodes
Proximal mesenteric lymph nodes
Lymph nodes along hepatic artery
Celiac lymph nodes

Regional Lymph Nodes of All Portions of the Pancreas

Superior mesenteric lymph nodes
Lymph nodes adjacent to and surrounding uncinate process
Lymph nodes along splenic artery and superior border of pancreas
Lateral aortic lymph nodes
Retroperitoneal lymph nodes

Lymph Nodes of Body and Tail of Pancreas

Pancreatolineal lymph nodes
Splenic hilar lymph nodes

Lymph Nodes Superior and Posterior to Tail of the Pancreas

From Douglass, H., Kim, S., & Meropol, N. (1997). Neoplasms of the exocrine pancreas. In J. Holland, R. Bast, D. Morton, E. Frei, D. Kufe, & R. Weichselbaum (Eds.), *Cancer medicine* (4th ed.). Baltimore: Williams & Wilkins.

ASSESSMENT

Clinical evaluation of the patient involves a detailed history, a thorough physical examination, and a variety of diagnostic tests (Fig. 42-3 and Table 42-1). Cancer of the pancreas has an insidious onset. The early signs and symptoms are often referred to other organs or systems.

History

The clinician needs to conduct an extensive inquiry into the character, onset, duration, and modulators of presenting signs and symptoms. Manifestations of the disease differ according to the location of the tumors in the pancreas. A classic triad of symptoms is apparent with cancer of the head of the pancreas: pain, profound weight loss, and progressive jaundice and usually indicate advanced disease. Pain is often an early symptom in most patients. This pain is initially in the epigastric region, is dull and intermittent in nature, and is often ignored or self-treated as indigestion or gaseous distention. The pain becomes much more distinctive as the disease progresses, possibly as a result of tumor invasion of the celiac plexus. At this point, the pain is often continuous and radiates to the right upper quadrant of the abdomen or to the dorsolumbar area. The pain is described as being colicky, dull, or vague. It is affected by activity, eating, and posture. It often becomes worse in the supine position and is relieved by sitting forward (Lillemoe, 1994). This is usually the symptom that prompts the patient to seek medical attention.

Approximately 75% to 90% of patients with carcinoma of the head of the pancreas have jaundice as a presenting

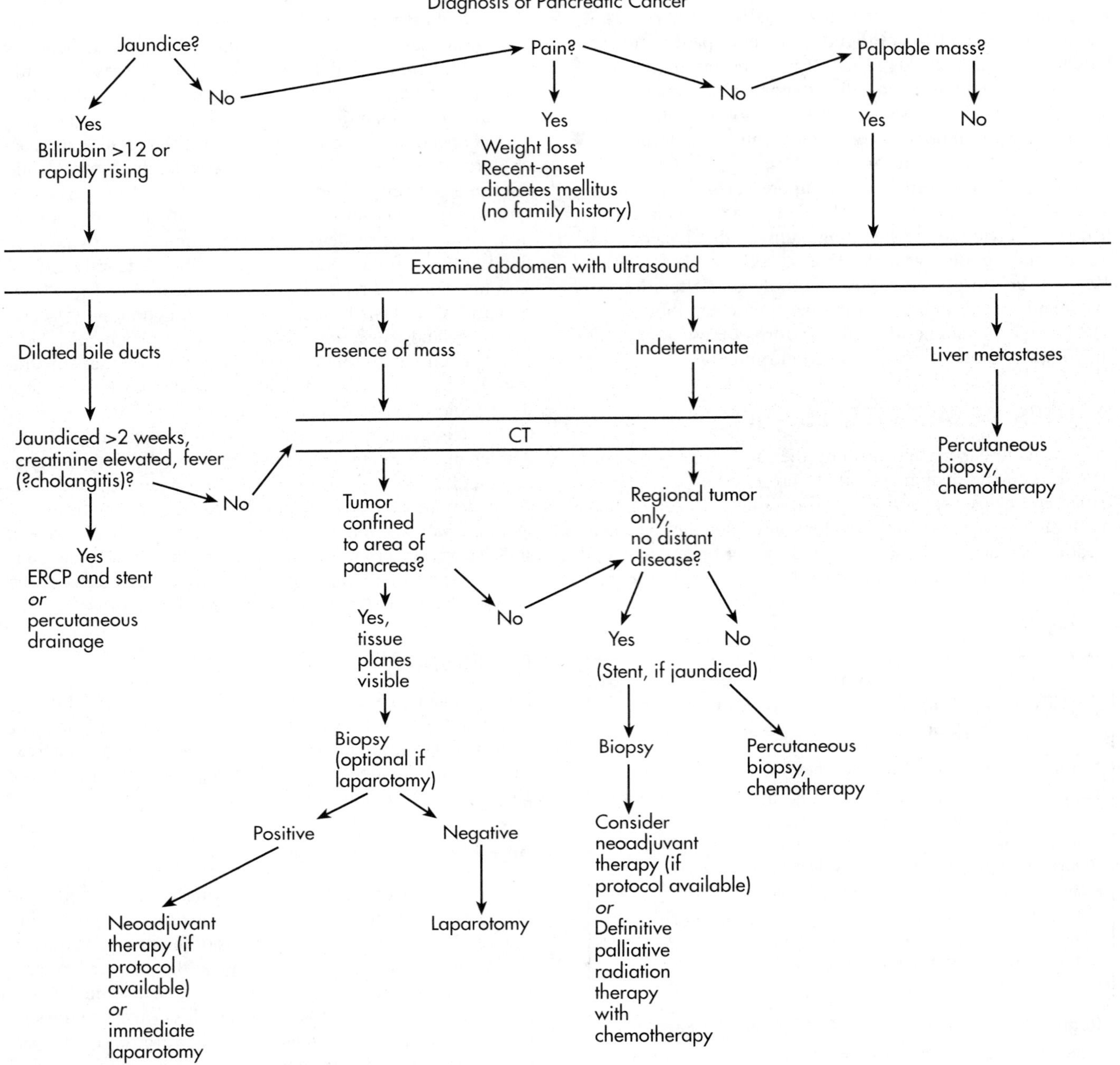

Fig. 42-3 Algorithm of initial treatment of pancreatic cancer by stage. (From Douglass, H., Kim, S., & Meropol, N. [1997]. Neoplasms of the exocrine pancreas. In J. Holland et al. [Eds.], *Cancer medicine* [4th ed.]. Baltimore: Williams & Wilkins.)

symptom. The jaundice is a result of the obstruction of the common bile duct. "Painless jaundice" has been a classical symptom attributed to pancreatic cancer; however, the vast majority of patients do indeed have pain with jaundice (Moossa & Gamagami, 1995). The evolution of jaundice with pancreatic cancer is distinctive. It appears first on the mucous membranes, then on the palms of the hands, and then gradually becomes generalized. The face, genitals, and linea alba are more discolored than other areas. The jaundice is progressive and persistent and leads to severe pruritus, dark urine, and clay-colored stools (Coleman, 1997). Jaundice potentially could be a early symptom of cancer of the head of the pancreas, and surgical resection may be a possibility.

Weight loss is the third classic symptom of cancer of the head of the pancreas. The weight loss is often dramatic (e.g., more than 10% of ideal body weight over the period of several months) and may be explained in part by anorexia, mal-

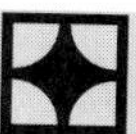

TABLE 42-1 Assessment of the Patient for Pancreatic Cancer

	Assessment Parameters	Typical Abnormal Findings
History	A. Personal and social history 1. Age 2. Ethnicity 3. Tobacco use B. Evaluation for pain	A. Personal and social risk factors 1. Usually occurs after age 70 2. More prevalent in blacks than whites 3. Smokers have increased risk B. Patients with pancreatic cancer often describe significant abdominal pain.
Physical Examination	C. Weight B. Jaundice C. Abdominal palpation D. Lymph node evaluation	A. Weight loss is common and may be dramatic. B. Jaundice may be an early symptom of cancer of the head of the pancreas. C. An enlarged gallbladder or a hard well-defined mass may be palpated. D. Presence of supraclavicular, periumbilical, rectovaginal, or rectovesical nodes may indicate advanced disease.
Diagnostic Tests	A. Abdominal ultrasound B. Abdominal computed tomography (CT scan) C. Endoscopic retrograde cholangiopancreatography (ERCP) D. Tumor marker-CA 19-9	A. Localized enlargement of the pancreas may be an initial finding. B. CT scan is useful in the diagnosis and staging of pancreatic cancer. C. Invasive examination is the most sensitive test for the diagnosis of pancreatic cancer. D. Blood levels of CA 19-9 are most commonly elevated in patients with pancreatic cancer greater than 3 cm.

digestion due to exocrine insufficiency, and/or the presence of impaired glucose tolerance (McLaughlin, 1994). Tumor involvement of the pancreas or common bile duct prevents secretion of digestive enzymes and often diminishes insulin production. Malabsorption can lead to diarrhea, constipation, steatorrhea, and muscle weakness. Metabolic disturbances such as hyperglycemia, glycosuria, and hypoalbuminemia may occur (Coleman, 1997).

Tumors in the body of the pancreas produce signs and symptoms late in the disease process. By the time these are brought to the attention of the physician, the tumor may be large enough to be palpated. Severe epigastric pain is the first and predominant symptom. This pain generally occurs 3 to 4 hours after eating. It is excruciating and often accompanied by vomiting. The painful episodes are short in duration and more frequent at night.

Carcinoma in the tail of the pancreas often mimics other diseases. Metastases to the liver, lungs, bone, peritoneum, and other organs may be the first symptoms. These patients complain of generalized weakness, gripping upper abdominal pain, vague indigestion, anorexia, and unexplained weight loss. Pain is not as common in cancer of the tail of the pancreas as it is in cancer of the head and body of the pancreas. Upper gastrointestinal bleeding, splenomegaly, and signs of portal hypertension or ascites may result from thrombosis of the portal system of extensive liver damage (Coleman, 1997).

Jaundice as a symptom of cancer of the body and tail of the pancreas occurs in only about 6% of the patients and usually reflects inoperability due to hepatic metastases and/or lymph node involvement at the porta hepatis (Moossa & Gamagami, 1995).

Physical Examination

Physical examination of the pancreas itself is difficult because it is situated deep in the retroperitoneal space. In many patients with cancer of the head of the pancreas, however, the clinician may be able to palpate an enlarged gallbladder and a smooth liver. With tumors of the body and tail of the pancreas, a hard and well-defined mass may be palpated in the subumbilical or left hypochondrial region. An abdominal bruit may be heard on auscultation of the left hypochondrium if the tumor has compressed or involved the splenic artery (Coleman, 1997). Evidence of distant metastasis may be seen in Trousseaux's sign, which is a migrating thrombophlebitis. This is never an early sign, and it can occur in patients with advanced cancer at any site. Palpable supraclavicular lymphadenopathy or Virchow's node, a periumbilical mass (Sister Mary Joseph's nodule) or palpable rectovaginal or rectovesical nodularity due to pelvic cul-de-sac seeding (Blumer's shelf) can be late presentations of pancreatic cancer (Moossa & Gamagami, 1995).

No clear-cut clinical features on physical examination reliably establish a diagnosis of pancreatic cancer. The clinician should perform further diagnostic tests for the patient population at high risk. This includes patients (1) over the age of 40; (2) who have a history of heavy cigarette smoking; (3) who present with obstructive jaundice; (4) who have unexplained weight loss of greater than 10% of body weight; (5) who have unexplained upper abdominal or lumbar back pain; (6) who have new-onset dyspepsia; and/or (7) who have sudden onset of diabetes mellitus or glucose intolerance (Moossa & Gamagami, 1995).

Diagnostic Tests

Ultrasonography of the Abdomen. Ultrasonography of the abdomen is an excellent imaging technique for the initial evaluation of upper abdominal pain or obstructive jaundice, especially for lesions located in the head of the pancreas. A localized enlargement in the pancreas is the most common finding. Ultrasounds can detect lesions as small as 1 to 1.5 cm. This examination does not entail exposure to ionizing radiation and is less costly and time consuming than computed tomography (CT) scans; however, as many as 25% of the studies will be nondiagnostic. This may be a result of bowel gas interference, obesity, previous operations, or the skill of the operator. The visualization of the body, tail, and uncinate process of the pancreas is often marginal (Moossa & Gamagami, 1995; Garcia & Egner, 1995).

Computed Tomography. Improved CT technology over the last decade has resulted in this being the study of choice to determine the extent of disease and resectability status in patients with pancreatic cancer. Image resolution has improved considerably. The development of helical or spiral scanning has increased the speed and accuracy of the diagnostic images (Evans, Abbruzzese, & Rich, 1997).

Optimal results can be achieved only if the radiologist is aware of the underlying clinical problem and undertakes the appropriate measures for establishing pancreatic scans at the appropriate increments using both intravenous (IV) bolus enhancement and oral contrast. The sensitivity of the CT scan is diminished for lesions less than 1 cm in size. It can define the level of obstruction; demonstrate the presence of a pancreatic mass, peripancreatic nodal involvement, and varices from portal hypertension; and detect liver metastasis greater than 1 cm. CT scans have some ability to detect local invasion of cancer into arteries and veins (Fig. 42-4). At present, CT scanning has proven itself in the determination of tumor unresectability with an accuracy of approximately 95%. About one third of tumors considered resectable by CT scan were found to be unresectable at the time of surgery (Lillemoe, 1994; Moossa & Gamagami, 1995; Thoeni & Blakenberg, 1993).

Magnetic Resonance Imaging. Magnetic resonance imaging (MRI) is being evaluated as a diagnostic tool in pancreatic cancer, but at this time offers no advantage over the CT scan and is not commonly used. This modality may be useful for follow-up in selected postsurgical patients in whom multiple clip artifacts need to be eliminated (Moossa & Gamagami, 1995).

Endoscopic Retrograde Cholangiopancreatography. Endoscopic retrograde cholangiopancreatography (ERCP) is the most sensitive diagnostic test for pancreatic cancer. This invasive procedure requires a skilled clinician with proper radiologic equipment and patient preparation. Even in the best of circumstances it carries a morbidity of 2% to 3%, most commonly from pancreatitis and cholangitis. If an abnormality has been detected by a noninvasive diagnostic examination, the ERCP serves three useful functions: (1) direct visualization of the duodenum and ampulla; (2) delineation of pancreatic and biliary ductal anatomy and findings such as stenosis and/or obstruction can be demonstrated radiologically; and (3) brush and/or aspiration cytology can be obtained (Table 42-2).

Endoscopic Ultrasonography. The modality of endoscopic ultrasonography (EUS) has emerged as another diagnostic test for pancreatic cancer. It may more accurately confirm the presence of a tumor, especially when still 1 to 2 cm in size and is located in the head of the pancreas. EUS will need to be more widely available before its true impact on the diagnosis and treatment of pancreatic cancer can be fully assessed (Douglass, Kim, & Meropol, 1997; Palazzo, Roseau, & Gayet, 1993).

Tumor Markers. Tumor markers are molecules that can be detected in body fluids and are biochemical indicators of neoplastic cells. No tumor marker is specific because they are all present normally at low levels and can be increased in various tumors. CA 19-9 is a glycoprotein that can be increased in several gastrointestinal tumors. Blood

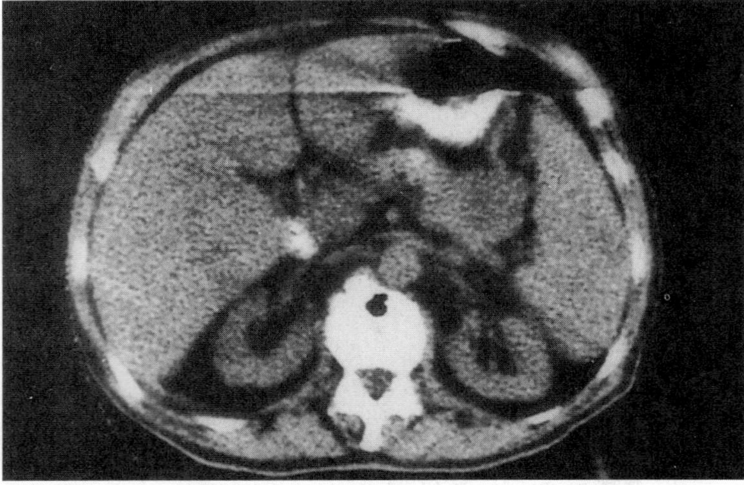

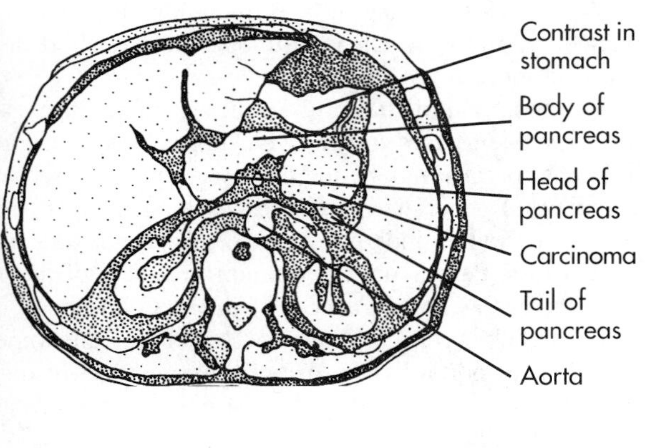

Fig. 42-4 Abdominal computerized tomography. (From Skarin, A. T. [1996] *Atlas of diagnostic oncology* [2nd ed.]. St. Louis: Mosby-Wolfe.)

levels of CA 19-9 are commonly elevated primarily in patients in whom the pancreatic cancer measures 3 cm or greater. Thus, its utility is limited in the detection of a potentially resectable tumor. CA-19-9 is of value in estimating the prognosis of a patient after pancreatic resection. In one study of patients in whom an elevated preoperative CA-19-9 level returned to normal after pancreatectomy, seven of eight remained alive longer than 18 months. In contrast all six patients whose serum CA 19-9 levels remained elevated following resection died in less than 12 months (Douglass, Kim, & Meropol, 1997).

As a potential for screening for pancreatic cancer, CA 19-9 has been a disappointment. Many patients with potentially curable stages I and II cancers have normal CA 19-9 values. Some patients will also have negative CA 19-9 values even in the presence of metastatic disease, whereas elevation of CA 19-9 is found in patients with pancreatitis (Douglass, Kim, & Meropol, 1997).

The glycoprotein antigen CA 494 has shown early promise as a marker for pancreatic cancer, and at this point compares favorably with CA 19-9. Because of its higher specificity, CA 494 may better differentiate chronic pancreatitis from pancreatic cancer. It is also not elevated in patients with type I or II diabetes without malignant pancreatic lesions. The preliminary results of this tumor marker have been encouraging but have yet to stand the test of time (Moosa & Gamagami, 1995).

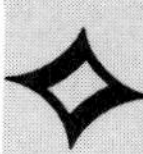

TABLE 42-2 Patient Preparation of Endoscopic Retrograde Cholangiopancreatography

Description of the Procedure: ERCP studies the ducts of the gallbladder, pancreas, and liver through an endoscope into which contrast material is injected and radiographs are taken.

Patient Preparation: Instruct the patient to fast for at least 6 hours before the procedure and make arrangements for someone to drive him or her home after the examination.

Procedural Considerations:

1. Obtain informed consent.
2. Discuss any allergy to iodine-containing drugs/foods.
3. Assist patient to disrobe and wear a gown.
4. Application of local anesthetic to throat (optional).
5. Administer intravenous (IV) sedation and/or antibiotics.
6. Assist patient onto x-ray table. Position patient on their left side.
    - Assist physician and support patient as the endoscope is passed through the mouth, esophagus, and stomach into the duodenum.
    - Air is introduced through the endoscope.
    - Contrast dye is infected via the endoscope.
    - Radiographs are taken.

Women of childbearing age must inform their physician if they may be pregnant.

Modified from Understanding ERCP (Endoscopic Retrograde Cholangiopancreatography) (1995). American Society for Gastrointestinal Endoscopy. Manchester, MA: Eli Lilly.

Diagnosis of Pancreatic Cancer. The diagnosis of pancreatic cancer is suggested by elevated CA 19-9 and an abnormal ERCP or CT scan. A histologic confirmation is required to make an actual diagnosis. Fine-needle aspiration when guided with CT scan or ultrasound has been a safe reliable method to confirm the histologic presence of pancreatic cancer. Laparoscopy is also used to diagnose this type of cancer. This technique is also able to detect small peritoneal involvement that would have been undetected by other means. Also, patients who undergo laparoscopy and are found to have unresectable disease are spared major surgery (Garcia & Egner, 1995).

STAGING

The current staging system for pancreatic cancer is the tumor, node, metastases (TNM) system used by the Cancer of the Pancreas Task Force of the American Joint Committee on Cancer Staging and End-Results (Table 42-3). This classifies pancreatic cancer according to tumor size, extent of local invasion, presence or absence of regional lymph node

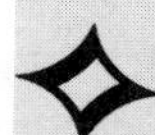

TABLE 42-3 TNM Classification System for Cancer of the Pancreas

Primary Tumor (T)

TX	Primary tumor cannot be assessed
T0	No evidence of primary tumor
T1	Tumor limited to the pancreas
	T1a Tumor 2 cm or less in greatest dimension
	T1b Tumor more than 2 cm in greatest dimension
T2	Tumor extends directly to any of the following: duodenum, bile duct, or peripancreatic tissues
T3	Tumor extends directly to any of the following: duodenum, stomach, spleen, colon, or adjacent large vessels

Lymph Node (N)

NX	Regional lymph nodes cannot be assessed
N0	No regional lymph node metastasis
N1	Regional lymph node metastasis

Distant Metastasis (M)

MX	Presence of distant metastasis cannot be assessed
M0	No distant metastasis
M1	Distant metastasis

Stage Grouping

I	T1	N0	M0
	T2	N0	M0
II	T3	N0	M0
III	Any T	N1	M0
IV	Any T	Any N	M1

From Beahrs, O. H., Henson, D. E., Hutter, K., & Meyers, M. (1993). *Handbook for staging cancer.* Philadelphia: J. B. Lippincott.

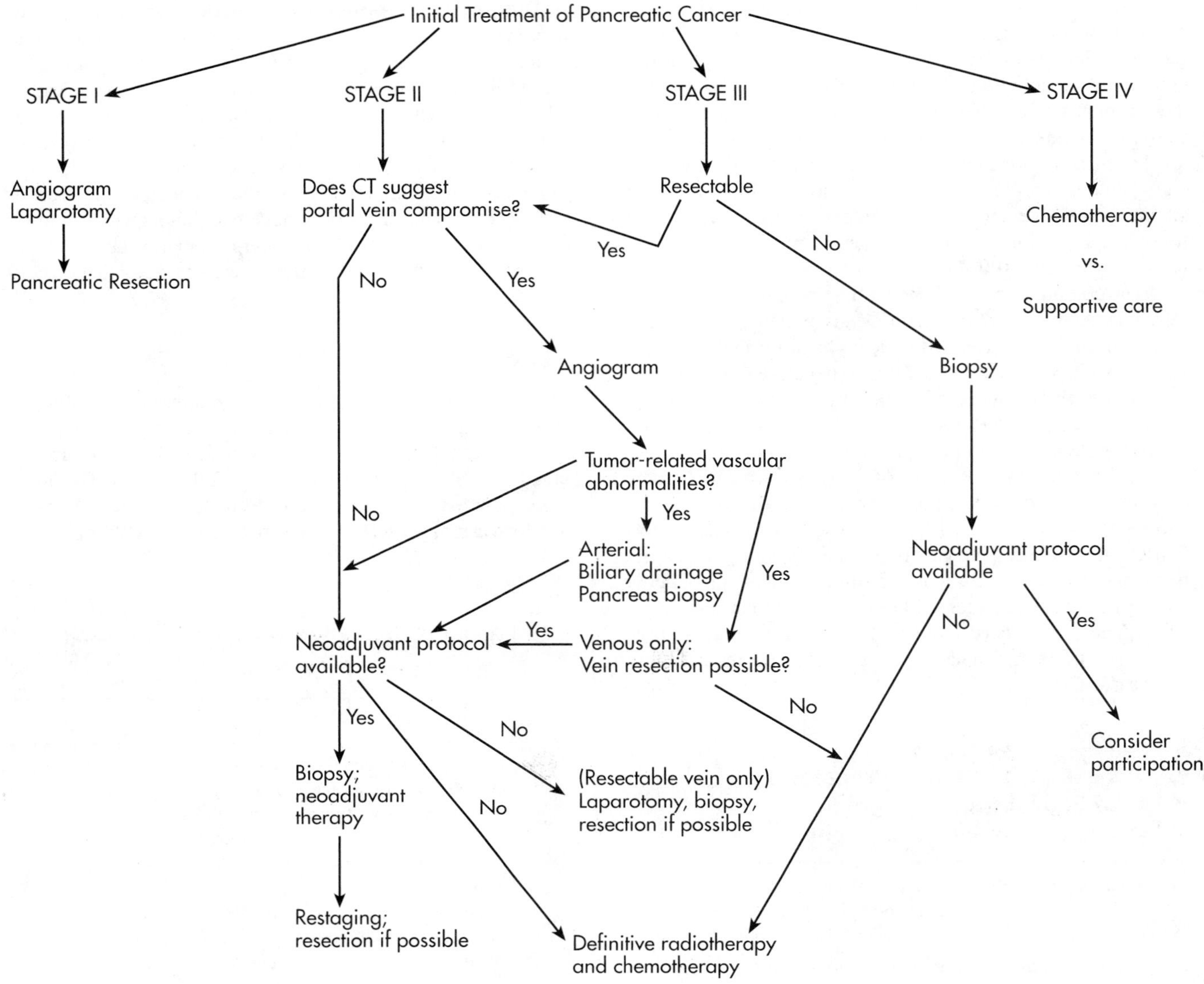

Fig. 42-5 Algorithm of initial treatment of pancreatic cancer by stage. (From Douglass, H., Kim, S., & Meropol, N. [1997]. Neoplasms of the exocrine pancreas. In J. Holland, R. Blast, D. Morton, E. Frei, D. Kufe, & R. Weichselbaum. [Eds.], *Cancer medicine* [4th ed.]. Baltimore: Williams & Wilkins.)

metastases and the presence or absence of distant nonnodal metastatic disease. These parameters are the most important factors that influence the resectability and prognosis of the disease (Fig. 42-5) (Beahrs, Henson, Hunter, & Meyers, 1993). Preoperative staging is essential because patients without evidence of unresectability who are good operative candidates should be offered possible curative resection. Conversely, the patient who is a poor operative candidate should be considered for nonoperative palliation when the preoperative staging shows local tumor invasion or distant metastases (Murr et al., 1994).

MEDICAL MANAGEMENT

The treatment of pancreatic cancer depends on several factors including the patient's age, nutritional status, hematologic status, liver function, and concomitant disease. Tumor volume, extent, classification, and staging are also carefully evaluated before initiation of treatment. If the disease is believed to be potentially curable, the therapy will be radical and may include surgery, radiation therapy, and chemotherapy. Palliation for pancreatic cancer can also be achieved with these modalities.

Only a small portion of patients with pancreatic cancer have early-stage disease suitable for curative resection. At the time of diagnosis, the tumor is confined to the pancreas in fewer than 10% of patients, 40% have locally advanced disease, and more than 50% have distant spread. More than 95% of patients eventually die of their disease. Even after resection for cure, the median length of survival is only 18 to 20 months. Unfortunately these statistics have changed little in the last 25 years.

Some improvements in early diagnosis have been made with the diagnosis being made up to 6 months earlier than it was a decade ago, probably due to improved diagnostic tests such as CT scan and ERCP (Reber, Ashley, & McFadden, 1995).

When definitive surgery is not possible, surgical biliary bypass procedures such as choledochojejunostomy or cholecystojejunostomy prove to be effective palliation of obstructive symptoms in many patients (Ellis & Cunningham, 1994). Gudjonsson (1995) has compared results from 340 papers that deal with survival rates. The best overall survival rate in surgical studies reported in detail is only 3.6%, and for a nonsurgical study it was 1.7%. The average excess cost for each resection was at least $150,000. With only one in 30 patients who underwent resection living for 5 years, the cumulative cost per "successful" resection was therefore approximately $4.5 million. The patient facing radical surgery must be physically and psychologically capable of withstanding the therapy.

Surgical Management

Cure is the objective of therapy if the tumor is localized and not fixed to other structures and if there is no evidence of regional or distant metastases (T1-T3, N0, M0). Radical surgical resection will be performed and may be supplemented with neoadjuvant or adjuvant radiation or chemotherapy. Despite sophisticated preoperative staging methods, most patients (60% to 70%) with adenocarcinoma of the pancreatic head that appears to be resectable preoperatively are found to have metastatic or locally invasive disease at laparotomy, which precludes resection (Murr et al., 1994).

Whipple Procedure. During the first 30 years after the original description of the procedure by Whipple and coworkers in 1935, the pancreaticoduodenectomy evolved from a resection of a limited portion of the duodenum and adjacent head of the pancreas to a more extensive resection that includes the distal stomach; the entire duodenum; the distal common bile duct and gallbladder; and the head, neck, and uncinate process of the pancreas. This surgery should also include the lymph nodes superior to the head of the pancreas and the pyloric and anterior pancreaticoduodenal lymph nodes. With minor extension of the operation, lymph nodes from the mesentery are also removed (Douglass, Kim, & Meropol, 1997; McGrath, Sloan, & Kenady, 1996). This procedure should be considered only in patients with a good performance status (Karnofsky performance score of 70% or higher) and as part of a multimodality treatment program that includes either preoperative or postoperative chemoradiation. Published perioperative mortality rates support the referral of patients with potentially resectable disease to centers that are experienced with the operative management of pancreatic cancer and that perform at least nine major pancreatic resections a year (Lieberman, Kilburn, Lindsey, & Brennan, 1995).

Total pancreatectomy allows removal of the splenic hilar lymph nodes and of the lymph nodes adjacent to the pancreatic tail. The retropancreatic lymph nodes, which are located behind the uncinate process contiguous with the common hepatic lymph nodes, can be a first site of metastatic disease, yet are often not removed. It has been suggested that patients undergoing radical pancreatectomy with more extensive lymph node dissection have improved survival stage-for-stage than patients undergoing a more conventional operation. Although the use of radical pancreatectomy is controversial and has not generally found acceptance in the Western hemisphere, one possible explanation for the improved survival would be the more extensive removal of locoregional disease (Abrams & Grochow, 1995).

In this surgery, the entire abdominal cavity is carefully explored to detect the presence of tumors outside the limits of the Whipple procedure. The peritoneal surfaces are inspected and palpated for peritoneal seeding. In addition, bimanual palpation of the liver is performed to detect metastatic disease. After a thorough exploration has excluded the presence of clinically evident distant metastases, the resectability of the primary tumor needs to be determined. If the tumor involves the inferior vena cava, the aorta, the superior mesenteric artery or vein, or the portal vein, complete surgical resection would not be performed (McGrath, Sloan, & Kenady, 1996).

Reconstruction after the Whipple procedure requires anastomoses between the pancreatic remnant and the jejunum and between the common hepatic duct and the jejunum, as well as re-establishment of gastrointestinal continuity through a gastrojejunostomy. Total pancreatectomy reduces on anastomoses that needs to be constructed (Fig. 42-6) (Douglass, Kim, & Meropol, 1997).

There has been a precipitous drop in hospital mortality after pancreaticoduodenectomy from before 1980 to after the 1980 era. Critical care anesthesia is clearly better and all tertiary care medical centers now have intensive care units. Better nutritional support is available preoperatively, and postoperatively if complications develop. This procedure has in part become regionalized, so tertiary care centers are now gaining more experience with the surgery, and fewer are being done in community hospitals. This has led to a small group of surgeons performing virtually nothing but liver, bilary, and pancreatic surgery. They have become more experienced in the techniques of the procedure, understand the anatomy more thoroughly, and perhaps better anticipate postoperative complications. Today the Whipple procedure can be performed with the expectation of a hospital mortality of less than 5% (Cameron, 1995).

The major complications of pancreatic resection surgery include pancreatic fistula, delayed gastric emptying, intra-abdominal abscess, infection, pancreatitis, or anastomotic leak (Pitt, 1995). In the immediate postoperative period, hemorrhage, hypovolemia, and hypotension pose the greatest threats (Table 42-4).

Hemorrhage may occur from leakage at the surgical anastomosis or from generalized coagulopathy. Abdominal distention, shock hematemesis, bloody stool, bloody drainage, or bleeding from the incision site are immediate nursing care issues. Retroperitoneal bleeding will be seen as a bluish-brown discoloration on either or both flanks.

Hypovolemia can develop from the loss of fluids during surgery or from "third spacing" (the shift of fluid from the

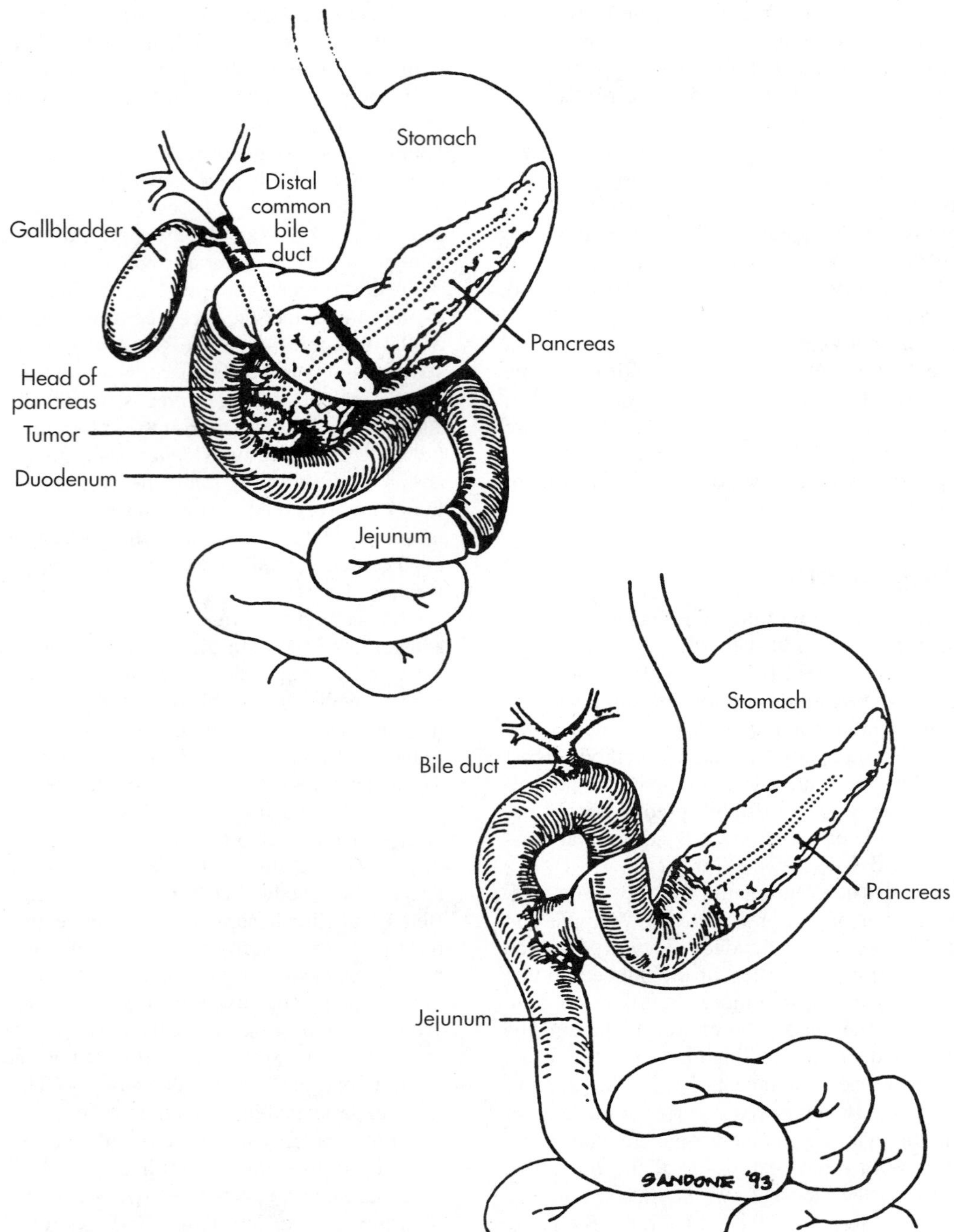

Fig. 42-6 Pylorus-preserving pancreatoduodenectomy anatomy of resected area and reconnected digestive tract with end-to-end pancreatojejunostomy. (From Pitt, H. [1995]. Curative treatment for pancreatic neoplasms. *Surgical Clinics of North America 75*[5]:891-904.)

vascular space to the interstitial space). Low levels of circulating plasma proteins usually account for third spacing. The first phase of fluid shifting begins immediately after surgery and can last for 48 to 72 hours. The nurse will need to be aware of decreased blood pressure, increased pulse rate, low central venous pressure, decreased urine output, increased specific gravity, low levels of serum albumin, and hemoconcentration. When the plasma protein is replaced and levels return to normal, the fluid will be reabsorbed. Urine output will suddenly and dramatically increase, and will greatly exceed input; therefore the patient will need to be monitored closely for signs of circulatory overload.

The severance of the sympathetic nerve fibers of the mesenteric complex is thought to be the cause for hypotension. Vital signs and urine output should be frequently monitored.

It is common for pancreatic resection patients to experience pulmonary complications, possibly due to immobility and inadequate lung expansion secondary to pain and splinting. Vigorous pulmonary toilette and ambulation are extremely important (Coleman, 1997).

TABLE 42-4 Complications After Pancreatioduodenectomy

Common	Uncommon
Delayed gastric emptying	Fistulas
Pancreatic fistula	Biliary
Intra-abdominal abscesses	Duodenal
Hemorrhage	Gastric
Wound infection	Organ failure
Metabolic	Cardiac
Diabetes	Hepatic
Pancreatic exocrine insufficiency	Pulmonary
	Renal
	Pancreatitis
	Marginal ulceration

Common complications are typically seen in more than 10% of patients, whereas "uncommon" complications occur in less than 10% of patients. The list of uncommon complications is not complete.

All patients develop complete pancreatic endocrine and exocrine insufficiency, and often, these patients have insulin resistance, and control of blood sugars may be difficult. This may be a temporary or permanent condition.

Radiation Therapy

External Radiation. Radiation therapy can be standard treatment of unresectable pancreatic cancer, in the palliation of symptoms, and the prolongation of life. 5-fluorouracil (5-FU) is often used in combination with external beam radiation therapy as a radiosensitizer. A high incidence of local-regional failure is found to be the cause of relapse in pancreatic cancer in spite of complete surgical resection. This may be a result of the difficulty in obtaining wide margins because of the presence of major blood vessels that could not be sacrificed and the high potential for residual cancer in unresected lymph nodes.

The Gastrointestinal Tumor Study Group conducted a classic prospective randomized study assessing the value of postoperative adjuvant combined chemotherapy and radiation therapy after complete resection (Box 42-4). Randomization was between no treatment vs 40 cGy of radiation delivered as a split course of 20 cGy in 10 fractions over 2 weeks with a 2-week break between courses. The 5-FU was added as a radiosensitizer during day 1 through day 3 of each course of radiation at a dose of 500 mg/m^2 per day. In addition, 5-FU was given weekly for 2 years. There was evidence that the adjuvant therapy arm demonstrated an increase in survival from 10 months to 20 months and an improved 2-year survival rate from 18% without adjuvant treatment to 43% with postoperative chemotherapy and radiation therapy (Douglass, Kim, & Meropol, 1997; Garcia & Egner, 1995). The limited radiation tolerance of the kidneys, liver, stomach, small bowel, and spinal cord limit the dosage that can be routinely administered (Abrams, 1995).

Preoperative Radiation Therapy. Preoperative radiotherapy appears to hold some possibilities for treatment.

BOX 42-4
Radiation Therapy for Locally Unresectable Pancreatic Cancer

1. Radiation 20 Gy × 3 over 10 weeks
2. Radiation 20 Gy + 5-FU at 500 mg/m^2/day for 1-3 days over 10 weeks, then 5-FU at 500 mg/m^2/week beginning week 14 until recurrence
3. Radiation 20 Gy + 5-FU at 500 mg/m^2/day for 1-3 days over 2 to 6 weeks, then 5-FU (500 mg/m^2/wk) beginning week 10

Adapted from Evans, D., Abbruzzese, J., & Rich, T. (1997). Pancreatic cancer. In V. DeVita, S. Hellman, & S. Rosenberg (Eds.). *Cancer: Principles and practice of oncology.* Philadelphia: Lippincott-Raven.

Fox Chase Cancer Center conducted an aggressive program of preoperative irradiation and concurrent chemotherapy of 5-FU and mitomycin C on 27 pancreatic cancer patients. Twenty-five patients completed therapy, of which 13 underwent complete resections. Of the resected patients, 60% survived 1 year, and 43% survived for 2 years. These encouraging results have led the Eastern Cooperative Oncology Group (ECOG) to undertake a multi-institution phase II study (Thomas, 1996).

Interstitial Irradiation. High doses of radiation can be delivered to the pancreas using seed implantation at the time of laparotomy. Theoretically, this method of treatment should have advantages since the lesion is directly visualized and normal tissues can avoid irradiation. The most commonly used isotope is ^{125}I, and external radiation and chemotherapy are given as well. The experience with this modality have not been impressive. Infusion brachytherapy using ^{32}P has begun to be evaluated with doses between 230 and 500 cGy (Thomas, 1996).

Intraoperative Radiation Therapy. Additional boost irradiation can be given to an unresectable pancreatic cancer during surgery with external beam intraoperative radiation therapy (IORT). The use of IORT with or without external beam radiation has been extensively studied. In combination, the survival rate appears to improve compared with surgery or IORT alone. Studies show that IORT is well tolerated, and survival times and local control were minimally improved.

Overall, the results of radiation therapy in all forms in the treatment of pancreatic cancer either alone or in combination therapy have been disappointing. It is clear that patients who receive radiation do somewhat better than those who do not. The future will depend on the development of successful chemotherapy and other modalities that can be combined with radiation therapy (Thomas, 1996; Evans, Abbruzzese, & Rich, 1997).

Chemotherapy

For the last 20 years many chemotherapeutic agents have been evaluated in phase II trials in the treatment of locally advanced pancreatic tumors. 5-FU has been the most widely used agent in gastrointestinal cancers. Treatment of pancreatic cancer with 5-FU has shown only limited response. Leukovorin and interferon have been studied in combination with 5-FU, and again limited response was noted. Most combination chemotherapy regimens contain 5-FU. Two of the most widely used regimens have been 5-FU, doxorubicin, and mitomycin (FAM) and streptozotocin, mitomycin, and 5-FU (SMF). These, too, have shown only limited success.

The most exciting new agent being studied in pancreatic cancer is gemcitabine. Several trials have been undertaken with this drug. In a study comparing gemcitabine to 5-FU, clinical benefit was reported in 23.8% of the patients treated with gemcitabine vs 4.8% of those treated with 5-FU. Median survival was 5.65 months vs 4.4 months respectively. Gemcitabine is arousing interest not only because it produces partial antitumor responses, but also because it appears to improve quality of life by reducing the amount of pain medication needed, improving performance status, and weight gain (Schnall & MacDonald, 1996). Gemcitabine is indicated as a first-line treatment for patients with locally advanced, unresectable stage II or stage III, or metastatic (stage IV) adenocarcinoma of the pancreas. Structurally, it is very similar to cytarabine (Ara-C). However, gemcitabine appears to have greater efficacy against solid tumors, whereas cytarabine is more effective against hematologic cancers. Gemictabine exhibits cell-cycle specificity, primarily killing cells in the S-phase. In pancreatic cancer clinical trials, doses were started at 800 to 1000 ml/m^2 weekly for up to 7 weeks or until toxicity necessitated holding a dose, followed by a week of rest. Subsequent cycles consisted of weekly IV injections for 3 consecutive weeks out of every 4 weeks.

Myelosuppression is the principle dose-limiting toxicity. Dosage reduction for hematologic toxicities is necessary. Nausea and vomiting were reported in 70% of patients and were usually mild to moderate. Mild diarrhea was reported in 20% of patients, and mild stomatitis was reported in 11%. One of the most common adverse effects is a flu-like syndrome consisting of low-grade fever, chills, headache, malaise, fatigue, myalgias and arthralgias. Onset of symptoms is about 4 to 24 hours after drug administration and lasts from 12 hours to 3 days. These symptoms are often responsive to acetaminophen. Rash occurs in about 30% patients and mild alopecia in about 15% of patients. Edema may occur in up to 20% of patients. Gemcitabine is not a vesicant, and there have been no reports of injection site necrosis in the patients in whom the drug extravasated (Rothenberg, Moore, Cripps, Andersen, Portenoy, Burns et al., 1995). It is hoped that this new agent will have a greater impact on pancreatic cancer than other agents that have been used in the past.

NURSING MANAGEMENT

As has been illustrated, the medical management of pancreatic cancer is extremely complex and variable depending on the patient's age, clinical condition, and stage of the cancer at the time of diagnosis. Patients with cancer of the pancreas have numerous problems that require nursing interventions and patient education. Patients who have abdominal surgery will be hospitalized, but most of the patient's care will occur in the outpatient and home care settings.

Early in the course of the patient's disease, the focus of nursing care may be on helping the patient and family understand the diagnosis and possible treatment options available. As the disease progresses, patients need information about nutritional support and pain management interventions. Since each type of major treatment of pancreatic cancer (i.e., surgery, radiation therapy, and chemotherapy) poses unique patient problems, the major issues associated with these treatments are discussed and three standards of care are provided in this chapter.

Surgery

Patients undergoing pancreatic resection may be hospitalized for 14 days or more, with the goal of the patient returning to a normal diet at the time of discharge (Lillemoe & Barnes, 1995). The major areas of inpatient surgery nursing care include the prevention and/or treatment of postoperative complications. These complications include infection, delayed gastric emptying, pulmonary emboli, and bleeding. Other inpatient admissions for pancreatic cancer are for terminal care and pain control. The nursing management of the patient undergoing pancreatic resection is summarized in Table 42-5.

Radiation Therapy

Patient problems will vary depending on whether the patient is receiving external beam radiation therapy or brachytherapy. External beam radiation is done in the outpatient setting. The major problems associated with external beam radiation are small bowel toxicities, diarrhea and nausea. Interstitial brachytherapy of intraoperative radiation will occur in the inpatient setting (Table 42-6).

Chemotherapy

The administration of chemotherapy is primarily accomplished in the out patient setting. The side effects the patient will experience depend of the specific chemotherapeutic agent(s) the patient receives. The nursing management of the patient with cancer of the pancreas who is receiving chemotherapy is summarized in Table 42-7.

Management of Pancreatic Cancer Pain

Much attention is paid to the effective and timely relief of the pain often associated with pancreatic cancer. Table 42-8 illustrates a pain assessment plan for patients with pancreatic cancer. The prevalence of pain in patients with advanced disease is as high as 85%. The appropriate use of oral analgesic agents can be successful in most patients. Patients with significant constant pain should receive their medications on an around-the-clock basis as opposed to an as-needed basis. The use of long-acting morphine derivative compounds appears to be the analgesic mainstay. Since pancreatic secretion is modulated by prostaglandins, prosta-

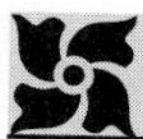

TABLE 42-5 Standard of Care for the Patient Undergoing Pancreatic Resection

Patient Problem and Outcomes	Nursing Interventions and Rationales	Patient Education Instructions
High Risk for Pancreatic Fistula		
Patient will have decreasing amount of drainage.	1. Assess drainage volume (pancreatic fistula is commonly recognized between postoperative day 3 to day 7 when persistent drainage is 50 m/day), appearance (drainage due to pancreatic fistula is milky in appearance). 2. Assess for intra-abdominal sepsis or hemorrhage. 3. Check all drainage tubes, incision, and dressing for excessive drainage. 4. Administer medications as needed.	1. Teach patient that oral intake will be prohibited, and total parenteral nutrition may be initiated. 2. Teach patient that placement and care of the tube(s) is essential. 3. Teach patient that some patients will require surgical intervention if complications fistula healing occur.
High Risk for Delayed Gastric Emptying		
Patient will require nasogastric decompression for less than 10 days.	1. Assess for postoperative emesis that requires reinsertion of nasogastric tube. 2. Assess patient's comfort level. 3. Administer medications as needed.	1. Teach patient that nasogastric tube placement will occur postoperatively. 2. Teach patient that emesis after nasogastric tube removal may require tube replacement.
High Risk for Hemorrhage		
Patient will: • Maintain a normal hemoglobin and hematocrit. • Maintain hemodynamic stability.	1. Assess tube(s) for drainage, including color and presence of clots. 2. Check hemoglobin, hematocrit, and platelet counts. 3. Check surgical incision and dressings for excessive drainage.	1. Teach patients that bleeding should steadily decrease. 2. Teach patient to inform health care team if he or she notices any increased bleeding.
Pain		
Patient will experience optimal pain relief with minimal side effects.	1. Assess pain intensity using a 0 to 10 verbal rating scale, every 2 to 4 hours and as needed. 2. Administer opioid and/or adjuvant analgesics around the clock. 3. Monitor for analgesic side effects and administer medications to prevent or treat: a. Nausea b. Pruritus c. Constipation	1. Teach the patient to inform the nurse if he or she is experiencing pain. 2. Teach patient that pain relief is a high priority of the health care team. 3. Teach patient the importance of taking pain medication on a regular basis to keep pain under control.

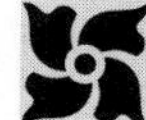

TABLE 42-6 Standard of Care for the Patient Undergoing Radiation Therapy for Pancreatic Cancer

Patient Problem and Outcomes	Nursing Interventions and Rationales	Patient Education Instructions
Diarrhea		
Patient will maintain adequate fluid balance and weight.	1. Assess elimination patterns including frequency, quality, and quantity. 2. Obtain a consult with a dietitian. 3. Initiate low-residue diet at start of treatment, if appropriate. 4. Administer antidiarrheal medication (e.g., difenoxylic hydrochloride 2.5 mg tablets, one to two tablets after each loose stool, not to exceed 8 tablets per day)	1. Inform patient that diarrhea may occur within a few weeks of treatment. 2. Teach patient to maintain diet recommended by dietitian. 3. Teach patient to evaluate pattern of diarrhea and concentrate the administration of antidiarrheal medication to that time of day.

TABLE 42-7 Standard of Care for the Patient Receiving Gemcitabine for Pancreatic Cancer

Patient Problem and Outcomes	Nursing Interventions and Rationales	Patient Education Instructions
Pruritus		
Patient will not experience symptoms of pruritus.	1. Assess for generalized rash that presents as an erythematous, pruritic, maculopapular rash involving the neck and extremities. 2. Administer topical steroids as ordered. 3. Notify physical of rash since dose of gemcitabine may be reduced.	1. Teach patients that a generalized rash may occur within 48 to 72 hours of receiving gemcitabine. 2. Teach patient that the skin rash is reversible and can be treated.

TABLE 42-8 Pain Assessment

Initial Pain Assessment

Assessment of Pain Intensity and Character

1. Onset and temporal pattern: When did your pain start? How often does it occur? Has the intensity changed?
2. Location: Where is your pain? Is it in more than one site?
3. Description: What does your pain feel like? What words would you use to describe your pain?
4. Intensity: On a scale of 0 to 10, with 0 being no pain and 10 being the worst pain you can imagine, how much does it hurt right now? How much does it hurt at its worst? How much does it hurt at its best?
5. Aggravating and relieving factors: What makes your pain better? What makes your pain worse?
6. Previous treatment: What types of treatment have you tried to relieve your pain? Were and are they effective?
7. Effect: How does the pain affect physical and social function?

Psychological Assessment (Should Include the Following):

1. Effect and understanding of the cancer diagnosis and treatment on the patient and caregiver.
2. The meaning of the pain to the patient and the family.
3. Significant past instances of pain and their effect on the patient.
4. The patient's typical coping response to pain or stress.
5. The patient's knowledge of, curiosity about, preferences for, and expectations about pain management methods.
6. The patient's concerns about using controlled substances such as opioids, anxiolytics, or stimulants.
7. The economic effect of the pain and its treatment.
8. Changes in mood that have occurred as a result of the pain (e.g., depression, anxiety).

Physical and Neurologic Examination

1. Examine site of pain and evaluate common referral patterns.
2. Perform pertinent neurologic evaluation:
   - Head and neck pain: cranial nerve and fundoscopic evaluation
   - Back and neck pain: motor and sensory function in limbs, rectal and urinary sphincter function

Diagnostic Evaluation

1. Evaluate recurrence or progression of disease or tissue injury related to cancer treatment:
   - Tumor markers and other blood tests
   - Radiologic studies
   - Neurophysiologic (e.g., electromyography) testing
2. Perform appropriate radiologic studies and correlate normal and abnormal findings with physical and neurologic examination.
3. Recognize limitations of diagnostic studies:
   - Bone scan: false negatives in myeloma, lymphoma, previous radiotherapy sites
   - Computed tomography (CT): good definition of bone and soft tissue, but difficult to imagine entire spine.
   - Magnetic resonance imaging: bone definition not as good as CT, but better images of spine and brain.

Ongoing Pain Assessment

Pain Should Be Assessed and Documented.

1. At regular intervals after starting the treatment plan.
2. With each new report of pain.
3. At a suitable interval after each pharmacologic or nonpharmacologic intervention, such as 25 to 30 minutes after parenteral drug therapy and 1 hour after oral administration.

Modified from Agency for Health Care Policy Research (1994). *Management of cancer pain.* (Clinical Practice Guideline No. 9). U.S. Department of Health and Human Services, Public Health Services.

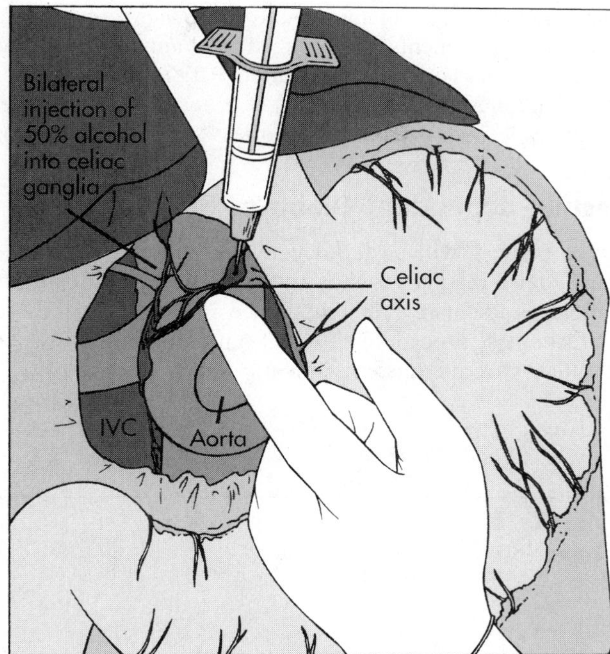

Fig. 42-7 Alcohol block for pancreatic cancer pain. (From Lillemoe, K., Cameron, J., Kaufman, H. S., Yeo, C. J., Pitt, H. A., & Sauter, P. K. [1993]. Chemical splanchnicectomy in patients with unresectable pancreatic cancer: A prospective randomized trial. *Annals of Surgery 217,* 447-457.)

Table 42-9 Suggested Opioid Analgesic Agents for Use in Moderate to Severe Pain

Drug	Route	Starting Dose
Morphine	PO	30 mg every 3 to 4 hr
	IM	10 mg every 3 to 4 hr
Morphine, sustained release	Sustained	90 to 120 mg every 8 to 12 hr
	PO	7.5 mg every 3 to 4 hr
	IM	1.5 mg every 3 to 4 hr
Methadone	PO	20 mg every 6 to 8 hr
	IM	10 mg every 6 to 8 hr
Levorphanol	PO	4 mg every 6 to 8 hr
	IM	2 mg every 6 to 8 hr
Fentanyl	Transdermal	75 mcg every 3 days
Codeine (Tylenol No. 3) 30 mg/tab	PO	180-200 mg every 3 to 4 hr
	IM	130 mg every 3 to 4 hr
Oxycodone 5 mg/tab	PO	30 mg every 3 to 4 hr
	IM	

Modified from Alter, C. (1996). Palliative and supportive care of patients with pancreatic cancer. *Seminars in Oncology, 23* (2), 229-240.

Box 42-5
Agents Used in the Management of Pancreatic Cancer Pain

Chemotherapy
Surgical procedures (e.g., gastrojejunostomy for obstruction)
Opioid and nonopioid analgesics
Celiac plexus blocks
External beam radiation therapy
Splenic nerve blocks

glandin inhibitors such as aspirin or other nonsteroidal anti-inflammatory drugs (NSAIDs) may occasionally relieve pain when opiates do not.

The pain experienced by patients with pancreatic cancer tends to be multifactorial and dynamic, which indicates treatment will often include a combination of pharmacologic, surgical, anesthetic, and other supportive measures (Box 42-5). The pain management plan needs to remain flexible and responsive to the patients changing needs (Alter, 1996).

Many patients will also benefit from nonpharmacologic methods of pain management. These may include celiac blocks and neuroablative procedures. Celiac blocks may be performed at the time of surgery or at a later date using a radioscopically controlled percutaneous technique (Fig. 42-7). In a randomized study, splenic injection of 50 ml of alcohol provided significant benefit over placebo. Pain scores in the treated group were lower than the controls at 2-, 4-, and 6-month follow-up. Almost half of these patients were able to reduce or avoid the use of opioids. Unfortunately, two thirds of patients with significant preoperative pain experienced a recurrence of pain before they died.

A recent development is the injection of analgesics and local anesthetics into the right pleural cavity. This procedure has relieved pain in a number of cases. Chronic infection is possible through an interpleural catheter attached to a port or pump (Douglass, Kim, & Meropol, 1997; Garcia & Egner, 1995; McGrath, Sloan, & Kenady, 1996). Endoscopic pancreatic stenting may be considered an effective alternative for palliation in selected patients with "obstructive" pain that does not respond to analgesics (Lichenstein & Carr-Locke, 1995). External beam radiation and/or chemotherapy may also be used in the palliative setting for pain relief. The most common approach used in the management of pancreatic cancer is summarized in Table 42-9.

It is necessary to be aggressive and timely in the use of pharmacologic and nonpharmacologic methods of pain control. This is one of the most important aspects of care in many patients with pancreatic cancer.

HOME CARE ISSUES

Depending on the treatment approaches used to manage pancreatic cancer, the patient and caregivers are faced with several issues in the home care setting. Patients recovering from pancreatic surgical resections may have many postoperative needs.

Nutritional Support

A primary concern for patients with pancreatic cancer is their nutritional status, because nutrition plays a significant role in postsurgical healing and recovery. Many patients will present with a significant and unintentional weight loss of over 10% of body weight. Total parental nutrition is often initiated within 48 hours of surgery to alleviate the catabolic stress response to surgery and prevent the starvation state from occurring. Early tolerance to oral feeding may be limited because of anorexia, early satiety, delayed gastric emptying, and diarrhea. Nutritional supplementation may be necessary via gastric or jejunal tube. Dumping syndrome may occur in patients who have undergone the Whipple procedure. Additionally, patients need to take pancreatic digestive enzyme replacements, including lipase, amylase, and protease, as soon as oral intake is started. Patients need to understand that these replacements must be taken each time they eat or drink foods that contain calories (McLaughlin, 1994).

Insulin-dependent Diabetes Mellitus

Some patients will be faced with fluctuating blood sugars that require regular monitoring and insulin injections. The patient and/or caregivers should be instructed on how to perform these procedures. Box 42-6 provides a step-by-step technique for administering insulin injections.

Box 42-6

Giving an Insulin Injection

Preparing the Insulin

1. Gather all of your equipment:
   - Syringe
   - Alcohol swab
   - Insulin
2. Wash your hands.
3. Roll the bottle of insulin gently between the palms of your hands. This will mix the insulin well. Do not shake. Shaking leaves air bubbles that can get into the syringe.
4. Take the needle cap off the syringe. Hold syringe with needle pointing toward the ceiling. Keep syringe at eye level, so you can easily see the markings on the barrel.
5. Put air into the insulin bottle before you get the insulin out of the bottle. First, pull the syringe plunger down until the top of the black tip crosses the mark of the dose to be taken. This draws air into the syringe.
6. Turn the syringe tip down. Put the needle through the rubber stopper of the insulin bottle. Push down all the way on the plunger, and hold the plunger in. This puts air into the bottle.
7. Turn the bottle and syringe upside down, so the bottle is on the top and the syringe is on the bottom. Leave the needle in the bottle with the plunger pushed all the way in.
8. Place the tip of the needle in the insulin. Pull down slowly on the plunger. This brings insulin into the syringe. Pull it down until the black tip is 2 or 3 units past your dose.
9. Push all of the insulin back into the bottle.
10. Pull down slowly on the plunger to the exact line of your insulin dose. The right amount of insulin should now be in your syringe.
11. Look in the syringe for air bubbles. If you see air bubbles, push the insulin back into the bottle. Then pull the plunger back to the exact line of your insulin dose. If bubbles are still in the syringe, repeat the process until they are gone.
12. When all the bubbles are out and you have the right dose, pull the bottle straight up and off the needle. Put the needle cap back on the syringe over the needle. Put the syringe down. Check to be sure that you have the right dose. You will know that it is right if the top of the plunger crosses the right mark on the syringe and there are no air bubbles.
13. Now you are ready to give yourself your shot. Take a deep breath and let it out slowly to help you relax.

Giving the Injection

1. You will inject yourself in your abdomen. Insulin is absorbed most evenly from this site. Your abdomen also has fewer nerves than other places, and a pad of fat underneath. Pick a spot from the chart, and then find this spot on yourself. Pick a spot at least 1 inch from the place you gave your last shot.
2. Clean the spot with alcohol. Let dry.
3. Remove the top from the needle. Hold the syringe in one hand as you would hold a pencil.
4. With your other hand, pinch up a couple of inches of skin.
5. Stick the needle straight into the pinched skin. Put the needle all the way in through the skin with one smooth motion.
6. Relax the pinch, and slowly push the plunger all the way down. Be sure the insulin is in, remove the needle.
7. Lightly press down on the site. Don't rub the spot. Don't worry if a drop of blood appears where the needle was.
8. When you are ready to discard your used needles and syringes, put them into a hard plastic or metal container with a screw-on lid. Label and discard according to local regulations.
9. Record the insulin dose you just gave yourself in your diabetes diary.

Depression

Alter (1996) has stated that it is believed that patients with pancreatic cancer have an increased rate of depressive disorders thought to predate the diagnosis of the tumor. The presence of pain did not in any way predict the presence of depression in the study group. Numerous theories have been put forth that correlate possible enzyme, hormonal, neurotransmitter, and acid-base imbalances present in pancreatic cancer with the presence of depression and anxiety. There appears to be evidence that if the pancreatic tumor is excised, many of these symptoms may abate.

Patients may also develop symptoms of depression secondary to pain, terminal illness, other aspects of treatment, and other life stressors. The presence of depression, agitation, hopelessness, and guilt or other emotional complaints must be evaluated and taken seriously (Alter, 1996).

Hospice care is intended for both the home and inpatient settings and is provided to patients whose disease is deemed to have a prognosis of 6 months or less as determined by a physician. These patients are thought to be beyond curative intervention and have needs for physical or emotional symptom management. Many studies show that patients with pancreatic cancer do not receive timely referrals for hospice. Kinzbrunner (1994) suggests that rather than seeing hospice care as separate from treatment for cancer, it should be thought of as a therapeutic option in and of itself. He has developed a five-point category scale based on disease characteristics and specific diagnoses. For instance, *category 1* is defined as malignancies that are treatable with a high or moderate expectation of cure. Included are such entities as testicular cancer or Hodgkin's disease, which would have a low likelihood for referral to hospice. *Category 5* includes malignancies that are virtually untreatable, as well as malignant melanoma and pancreatic cancer. It has been suggested that these patients be offered hospice as an option at the time of diagnosis. Rather than focusing on what hospice does not do, one should be thinking of hospice as a routine and usual part of treatment that may include surgery, chemotherapy, or radiation therapy. An introduction of the hospice concept early in the discussions about care and disease progression between patients and health care providers makes it a more viable and realistic option for the patient, family, and physician. Hospice may be the most effective means of offering relief of pain and other symptoms, hence ensuring hope for quality of life and being viewed as a positive aspect of care (Alter, 1996).

PROGNOSIS

The prognosis for patients with pancreatic cancer varies depending on the stage of the disease at the time of diagnosis, the patient's age, and coexisting medical conditions. Other factors that influence a patient's prognosis are the involvement of local or distant lymph nodes, or metastatic disease. In general, pancreatic cancer is not usually curable. Patients diagnosed with stage I disease have a 3-year survival of 15%, whereas stages II and III have a 3-year survival rate of 2%. Stage IV offers a 3-year survival rate of less than 1%. The median survival time for patients with pancreatic cancer without treatment is measured in a matter of months (Coleman, 1997).

EVALUATION OF THE QUALITY OF CARE

Accreditation organizations such as the Joint Commission for the Accreditation of Health Care Organizations require that the quality of care provided to patients is evaluated. Since the care provided to patients with pancreatic cancer requires input from a multidisciplinary team, the evaluation of the quality of care should include aspects of care provided by various team members. Tables 42-10 and

TABLE 42-10 Quality of Care Evaluation for a Patient Undergoing Pancreatic Cancer Surgical Resection

Disciplines participating in the quality of care evaluation:
☐ Nursing ☐ Surgery ☐ Social Services ☐ Dietary

Postoperative Management Evaluation

Data from:
☐ Medical Record Review ☐ Patient/Family Interview

Criteria	Yes	No
1. Patient provided with preoperative information about:		
a. Bowel preparation	☐	☐
b. Pain management (patient-controlled analgesic [PCA])	☐	☐
c. Dietary consult	☐	☐
2. Hemoglobin and hematocrit evaluated postoperatively	☐	☐
3. Patient experienced the following complications:		
a. Pulmonary embolism	☐	☐
b. Pancreatic fistula	☐	☐
c. Hemorrhage	☐	☐
d. Sepsis	☐	☐

Patient/Family Satisfaction

Data from: ☐ Patient Interview ☐ Family Interview

Criteria	Yes	No
1. On a scale of 0 to 10, with 0 being totally dissatisfied and 10 being totally satisfied, how satisfied were you with the pain management you received in the hospital?	______	
2. On a scale of 0 to 10, with 0 being totally dissatisfied and 10 being totally satisfied, how satisfied were you with the pain management teaching you received at discharge?	______	
3. Were you adequately taught to manage your dietary needs at discharge?	☐	☐

TABLE 42-11 Quality of Care Evaluation for a Patient Receiving Gemcitabine for Pancreatic Cancer

Disciplines participating in the quality of care evaluation:
☐ Nursing ☐ Medical Oncology ☐ Dietary ☐ Social Services

Data from: ☐ Mailed Questionnaire ☐ Patient Interview

Criteria	Yes	No
1. Did the doctor or nurse explain to you that you might experience some of the following side effects from your chemotherapy?		
a. Reduced blood counts	☐	☐
b. Nausea/vomiting	☐	☐
c. Rash or itching	☐	☐
d. "Flue-like" symptoms	☐	☐
2. Were you taught to report any new pain problems to your doctor or nurse?	☐	☐
3. Were you taught how to care for yourself if your blood counts became low?	☐	☐

42-11 provide examples of quality of care evaluation tools that can be used in the inpatient and outpatient settings, respectively.

RESEARCH ISSUES

Numerous research issues surrounding the diagnosis and management of cancer of the pancreas require further investigation. Areas of continuing research include genetics and risk factors associated with the development of pancreatic cancer. Unfortunately, early detection of this type of cancer remains abysmal. Screening techniques for high-risk patients need to be refined and used. The link between smoking and pancreatic cancer will be strengthened by lung cancer research.

Numerous randomized clinical trials are desperately needed to determine the most effective treatments for pancreatic cancer, especially systemic therapy for metastatic disease. All studies need to consider the effectiveness of the treatment in improving patients' survival, as well as quality of life. The costs of the treatments, as well as their associated side effects, also need to be included in these studies.

REFERENCES

Abrams, R. & Grochow, L. (1995). Adjuvant therapy with chemotherapy and radiation therapy in the management of carcinoma of the pancreatic head. *Surgical Clinics of North America, 75*(5), 925-938.

Agency for Health Care Policy Research (1994). *Management of cancer pain* (Clinical Practice Guideline No. 9). U.S. Department of Health and Human Services, Public Health Services.

Ahlgren, J. (1996). Epidemiology and risk factors in pancreatic cancer. *Seminars in Oncology, 23*(2), 241-250.

Alter, C. (1996). Palliative and supportive care of patients with pancreatic cancer. *Seminars in Oncology, 23*(2), 229-240.

Boring, C., Squires, T., Tong, T., & Montgomery, S. (1994). Cancer statistics. *CA: A Cancer Journal for Clinicians, 44,* 7-26.

Beahrs, O., Henson, D., Hunter K., & Myers, M. (1993) Exocrine pancreas. In *Handbook for staging cancer.* Philadelphia: J. B. Lippincott.

Cameron, J. (1995). Long-term survival following pancreaticoduodenectomy for adenocarcinoma of the head of the pancreas. *Surgical Clinics of North America, 75*(5), 939-951.

Coia, L., Hoffman, J., Scher, R., Weese, J., Solin, L., Weiner, L., Eisenberg, B., Paul, A., & Hanks, G. (1994). Preoperative chemoradiation for adenocarcinoma of the pancreas and duodenum. *International Journal of Radiation Oncology Biologic Physics, 30,* 161.

Coleman, J. (1997). Esophageal, stomach, liver, gallbladder, and pancreatic cancers. In S. L. Groenwald, M. H. Frogge, M. Goodman, & C. H. Yarbro (Eds.), *Cancer nursing: Principles and practice.* Sudbury, MA: Jones and Bartlett.

Douglass, H., Kim, S., & Meropol, N. (1997). Neoplasms of the exocrine pancreas. In J. Holland, R. Bast, D. Morton, E. Frei, D. Kufe, & R. Weichselbaum (Eds.), *Cancer medicine* (4th ed.). Baltimore: Williams & Wilkins.

Ellis, P. & Cunningham, D. (1994). Management of carcinomas of the upper gastrointestinal tract. *British Medical Journal, 308,* 834-838.

Evans, D., Abbruzzese, J., & Rich, T. (1997). Cancer of the pancreas. In V. DeVita, S. Hellman, & S. A. Rosenberg (Eds.), *Cancer, principles and practice of oncology* (4th ed.). Philadelphia: Lippincott-Raven.

Garcia, A. & Egner, J. (1995). Pancreatic cancer and primary care providers, *Cancer Practice, 3*(1), 37-41.

Gold, E. (1995). Epidemiology of and risk factors for pancreatic cancer. *Surgical Clinics of North America, 75*(5), 819-843.

Green, M. (1996). Gemcitabine: We've reached the end of the beginning. *Seminars in Oncology, 23*(5), 99-100.

Gray, J., Coldman, A., & MacDonald, W. (1992). Cigarette and alcohol use in patients with adenocarcinoma of the gastric cardia or lower esophagus. *Cancer, 69,* 2227-2231.

Gudjonsson, B. (1995). Carcinoma of the pancreas: Critical analysis of costs, results of resections, and the need for standardized reporting. *Journal of the American College of Surgeons, 181*(6) 483-503.

Jacox, A., Carr, D., & Payne, R. (1994). New clinical-practice guidelines for the management of pain in patients with cancer. *New England Journal of Medicine,* 330. 651-655.

Kinzbrunner, B. (1994). What to do when anticancer therapy is no longer appropriate, effective, or desired. *Seminars in Oncology, 21,* 792-798.

Landis, S. H., Murray, T., Bolden, S., & Wingo, P. A. (1998) Cancer statistics, 1998. *CA: A Cancer Journal for Clinicians, 6,* 29.

Lee, M., Mueller, R., & vanSonnenberg, E. (1993). CT-guided celiac ganglion block with alcohol. *American Journal of Roentgenology, 161,* 633-636.

Lichtenstein, D. & Carr-Locke, D. (1995). Endoscopic palliation for unresectable pancreatic cancer. *Surgical Clinics of North America, 75*(5), 969-988.

Lieberman, M., Kilburn, H. Lindsey, M., & Brennan, M. (1995). Relationship of perioperative deaths to hospital volume among patients undergoing pancreatic resection for malignancy. *American Surgery,* 222-238.

Lillemoe, K., Cameron, J., Kaufman, H. et al. (1993). Chemical splanchnicectomy in patients with unresectable pancreatic cancer: A prospective randomized trial. *Annals of Surgery 217,* 447-457.

Lillemoe, K. (1994). Current management of pancreatic cancer. *Annals of Surgery, 221*(2), 133-148.

Lillemoe, K. & Barnes, S. (1995). Surgical palliation of unresectable pancreatic carcinoma. *Surgical Clinics of North America, 75*(5), 953-968.

Lowenfels, A., Maisonneuve, P., & Cavalline, G. (1993). Pancreatitis and the risk of pancreatic cancer: International Pancreatitis Study Group. *New England Journal of Medicine, 328,* 1433-1437.

McGrath, P., Sloan, D., Kenady, D. (1996). Surgical management of pancreatic cancer. *Seminars in Oncology, 23*(2), 200-212.

McLaughlin, S. (1994). Pancreatic cancer and diabetes. *The Diabetes Educator, 20*(1), 20-26.

Moossa, A. & Gamagami, R. (1995). Diagnosis and staging of pancreatic neoplasms. *Surgical Clinics of North America 75*(5), 871-890.

Murr, M., Sarr, M., Oishi, A., & van Heerden, J. (1994). Pancreatic cancer. *CA: A Cancer Journal for Clinicians, 44*(5), 304-317.

Noy, A. & Bilezikian, J., (1993). Diabetes and pancreatic cancer: Clues to early diagnosis of pancreatic malignancy. *Journal of Clinical Endocrinology and Metabolism, 79*(5),1223-1231.

Palazzo, L., Roseau, G., & Gayet, B. (1993). Endoscopic ultrasonography in the diagnosis and staging of pancreatic carcinoma. *Endoscopy, 25,* 143-150.

Pitt, H. (1995). Curative treatment for pancreatic neoplasms. *Surgical Clinics of North America, 75*(5), 891-904.

Rothenberg, M. L., Moore, M. J., Cripps, M. C., Andersen, J. S., Portenoy, R. K., Burris, H. A. III, Green, M. R., Tarassoff, P. G., Brown, T. D., Casper, E. S., Storniolo, A. M., & Von Hoff, D. D. (1996). A phase II trial of gemcitabine in patients with 5-FU-refractory pancreas cancer. *Annals of Oncology 7*(4): 347-353.

Reber, H., Ashley, S., & McFadden, D. (1995). Curative treatment for pancreatic neoplasms. *Surgical Clinics of North America,* 75 (5), 905-911.

Scarpa, A., Capelli, P., & Mukai, K. (1993). Pancreatic adenocarcinoma frequently shows p53 gene mutations. *American Journal of Pathology, 142,* 1534-1543.

Schellenberg, D. & Garnett, L. (1994). Pancreatic cancer: Hunting a killer. *Harvard Health Letter, 7,* 4-6.

Schnall, S. & MacDonald, J. (1996). Chemotherapy of adenocarcinoma of the pancreas. *Seminars in Oncology, 23*(2), 220-238.

Shumate, C. & Baron, T. (1996). Palliative procedures for pancreatic cancer: when and which one? *Southern Medical Journal, 89*(1), 27-32.

Skarin, A. T. (1996). *Atlas of diagnostic oncology* (2nd ed.). St. Louis: Mosby–Wolfe.

Thomas, P. (1996). Radiotherapy for carcinoma of the pancreas. *Seminars in Oncology, 23*(2), 213-219.

Thoeni, R. & Blakenberg, F. (1993). Pancreatic imaging, computed tomography and magnetic resonance imaging. *Radiologic Clinics of North America, 31,* 1085-1113.

Yeo, C. (1995). Management of complications following pancreaticoduodenectomy. *Surgical Clinics of North America, 75*(5), 913-924.

Zatonski, W., Boyle, P., & Przewozniak, K. (1993). Cigarette smoking, alcohol, tea, and coffee consumption and pancreas cancer risk: A case-control study from Opole, Poland. *International Journal of Cancer, 53,* 601.

Adenocarcinoma of the Small Intestine

Marnie McHale, RN, MS, AOCN
Sharon A. Aronovitch, PhD, RN, CETN

EPIDEMIOLOGY

Malignant and benign tumors of the small intestine are considered remarkably rare and make up fewer than 10% of all gastrointestinal (GI) tumors, depending on whether autopsy data is included (Ellis, 1987). Approximately two thirds of all small intestine tumors are malignant, accounting for less than 0.3% of all malignancies in general. Although the small intestine makes up more than 75% of the total length of the GI tract and more than 90% of its mucosal surface, it accounts for less than 2% of primary GI malignancies. In 1997, the number of new cases of small intestine cancer in the United States was 4900, and approximately 1140 people died of the disease. Of these new cases, there was a slight predominance of males (53%) over females (47%) (Landis, Murray, Bolden, & Wingo, 1998).

Four major histologic types of cancer occur in the small intestine: adenocarcinoma, malignant carcinoid tumor, lymphoma, and sarcoma. Of these four types, adenocarcinoma is the most common primary malignancy in the small intestine, accounting for slightly less than 50% of all primary small intestine malignancies. The duodenum is the most commonly affected portion of the small intestine, with approximately 15% of small intestine adenocarcinomas occurring in the first portion of the duodenum, 40% in the second portion, and 45% in the distal duodenum, a distribution that parallels the relative length of each portion of the duodenum (Ouriel & Adams, 1984). The jejunum and ileum together account for the remainder of small intestine adenocarcinomas, with one series reporting that 33% of these tumors were located in the early portion of the jejunum in close proximity to the ligament of Trietz (Herbsman, Wetstein, Rosen, Orecs, Alfonsoe, & Iyer et al., 1980). Interestingly, the distribution of adenocarcinomas in the proximal small intestine suggests the possibility that the small intestine may be susceptible to carcinognens. This distribution pattern correlates with the length of contact of the small intestine mucosa with pancreaticobiliary secretions, implicating bile as a possible carcinogen (Ross, Hartnett, Bernstein, & Henderson, 1991).

Tumors of the small intestine have been primarily investigated in the United States using hospital-based reviews. Information from these types of studies has the potential for compromise because of the selection bias that occurs when reporting on rare cancers. A recent epidemiologic investigation using population-based data collected between 1973 and 1990 from the Surveillance, Epidemiology, and End-Results (SEER) Program (1993) confirmed that cancers of the small intestine are rare. The investigation also noted that during the last two decades, a slow increase in the incidence of adenocarcinomas, malignant carcinoids, and lymphomas in white men, black men, and black women has occurred, along with increases in malignant carcinoids and lymphomas in white women (Chow, Chen, Ahsan, & Neugut, 1996). In addition, the study reported that small intestine adenocarcinomas in black women composed nearly 50% of all cases, but less than 40% in black men, white men, or white women. Interestingly, the incidence of adenocarcinoma of the small intestine has remained stable in white women, along with the incidence of sarcomas in all groups except black women, for which it has declined. In men, the increase in incidence of duodenal adenocarcinomas may be related to the similar rise of adenocarcinomas of the colon during this same period. The precise reasons for these findings is somewhat unclear, although they may represent variations in lifestyle and sociocultural factors.

Small intestine cancers are extremely rare in the first three decades of life. At presentation, the average age of patients with either benign or malignant small intestine tumors is within the fifth and sixth decades (Hart & Levin, 1993). The 1973-1990 SEER data revealed that more than 90% of the cases occurred in people over the age of 40. The peak incidence for adenocarcinoma of the small intestine is within the sixth and seventh decades of life (Herbsman et al., 1980; DiSario, Burt, Vargas, & McWhorter, 1994).

The rarity of small intestine malignancies has been considered quite interesting by the medical community and has been the basis for scientific speculation since 1973, when Lowenfels first offered his hypotheses regarding the rarity. Normally, it might be expected that the incidence of cancer of the small intestine would be considerably higher due to the highly proliferative nature of the small intestine cells, the carcinogenic potential of the human diet, and the location of the small intestine between such high cancer sites as the stomach and colon.

Several hypotheses have been formulated to possibly explain this observation (Lowenfels, 1973; Gabos, Berkel, Band, Robson, & Whittaker, 1993). First, faster transit time through the small intestine compared with the colon may reduce the exposure of the small intestine mucosa to potential ingested carcinogens. Second, the presence of large volumes of liquid chyme in the small intestine may dilute carcinogenic substances, thereby creating a less mechanically irritating liquid against the small intestine mucosa compared with solid stool against the colonic mucosa. Third, the small, metabolically inactive bacterial population present in the small intestine may not be capable of transforming procarcinogens into their active components. Fourth, acid neutralization by pancreatic and small intestine secretions may protect against the carcinogenic effects of nitrosamines, which normally require the presence of acids for activity. Fifth, the presence of high concentrations of enzymes such as benzopyrene hydroxylase and diamine oxidase may play an active role in detoxifying carcinogens. Finally, the presence of abundant lymphoid tissue and high concentrations of secretory immunoglobulins (IgA) in the distal ileum may create a local immunosurveillance system that prevents the development of malignancies (Ashley & Wells, 1988; Coit, 1993).

RISK FACTORS

The major risk factors associated with the development of adenocarcinoma of the small intestine are listed in Box 43-1. Although the majority of patients with malignant small intestine cancers have no apparent risk factors, several diseases, including Crohn's disease, celiac disease, inherited familial GI syndromes, and immunodeficiency states, have been implicated as factors predisposing to the development of small intestine cancer in general, and in some cases adenocarcinoma specifically. In addition, both increasing age and a history of colorectal cancer or adenocarcinomas have shown some relationship to the occurrence of small intestine cancer (Donohue & Kelly, 1991; Hart & Levin, 1993).

Box 43-1
Risk Factors for Adenocarcinoma of the Small Intestine

Crohn's disease
Celiac disease
Inherited familial gastrointestinal (GI) syndromes
Peutz-Jeghers syndrome
Familial adenomatous polyposis
Gardner's syndrome
Hereditary nonpolyposis colon cancer
Increasing age
History of colorectal cancer or adenocarcinoma

From Donohue, J. H., & Kelly, K. A. (1991). Cancer of the small intestine. In A. R. Moosa, S. C. Schimpff, & M. C. Robson (Eds.), *Comprehensive textbook of oncology* (2nd ed.). Baltimore: Williams & Wilkins; Hart, R. & Levin, B. (1993). Neoplasms of the small intestine. In P. Calabresi, & P. Schein (Eds.), *Medical oncology: Basic principles and clinical management of cancer* (2nd ed.). New York: McGraw-Hill.

Crohn's Disease

The chronic inflammation of the small intestine seen in Crohn's disease has been implicated as predisposing to malignant transformation. Crohn's disease, which is also known as *regional enteritis,* is a transmural, predominantly submucosal inflammation that may affect any part of the GI tract, but occurs most commonly in the terminal ileum. Although the exact cause of Crohn's disease remains unknown, the associated inflammation of the intestine spreads slowly and progressively, with periods of remission often alternating with exacerbation. More than half of all patients with Crohn's disease eventually need surgery because the disease progression has caused permanent structural damage to the intestine. Surgery may be required to correct an intestine perforation, fistula formation, hemorrhage, or an acute intestinal obstruction (Society of Gastrointestinal Nurses & Associates, 1993).

In 1982 a report of 62 cases of small intestine adenocarcinomas occurring in patients with Crohn's disease was published (Fresko, Lazarus, Dotan, & Reingold, 1982). Unlike small intestine tumors in the general population, the tumors in patients with Crohn's disease developed at a younger age (mean: 47 years) and predominantly in the ileum (76%). Patients who had segments of intestine surgically bypassed for the treatment of Crohn's disease were at particular risk for developing adenocarcinomas. The causal relationship between Crohn's disease and cancer is strengthened by the pattern of intestine involvement seen in regional enteritis and cancer, and the dysplasia and carcinoma in situ found in these patients. The risk of small intestine cancer in a patient with Crohn's disease is estimated at 100 times that of the normal population. It has been stressed that special attention be given to the pathologic examination of resected intestine in Crohn's disease because small intestine adenocarcinomas can often be clinically occult and found only on microscopic examination of the specimen.

Celiac Disease

Celiac sprue is characterized by poor food absorption and intolerance of gluten, a protein found in wheat and wheat products. The exact cause of celiac sprue is unknown, but is believed to result from a combination of environmental factors and genetic predisposition. The primary treatment is lifelong elimination of gluten from the patient's diet, combined with appropriate supportive therapy, such as supplemental iron, vitamin B_{12}, folic acid, and/or electrolyte and fluid replacement as needed. In 1983, a multi-institutional review reported on 235 patients with celiac disease who had 259 malignancies (Swinson, Slavin, Coles, & Booth, 1983). Over half of those cancers were lymphomas, the majority of them originating in the small intestine; 19 of the 62 known GI carcinomas were small intestine adenocarcinomas. In general, the majority of cancer patients with a diagnosis of celiac disease have been diagnosed with their celiac disease years before the cancer has developed. Unfortunately, a positive response to a gluten-free diet does not appear to prevent the development of malignancy (Cooper, Holmes, Ferguson, & Cooke, 1980).

Inherited Familial Gastrointestinal Syndromes

Peutz-Jeghers syndrome has been described as the familial association of mucocutaneous melanin pigmentation, primarily of the face, lips, and buccal mucosa, in conjunction with polyps, which are most common in the jejunum and ileum (Jeghers, McKusick, & Katz, 1949). This syndrome is inherited as a single, dominant, pleiotrophic gene with a high degree of penetrance. Although the small intestine tumors of Peutz-Jeghers syndrome were originally thought to be malignant, they are now generally agreed to be hamartomas, with the possible presence of an adenomatous component. Although small intestine carcinomas have been reported in association with this syndrome, most cancers have occurred away from any identifiable polyp (Dozois, Judd, Dahlin, & Bartholomew, 1969) and are believed to be the result of malignant evolution of the adenomatous component of the hamartoma (Spigelman, Murday, & Phillips, 1990). No current evidence exists for increased risk for small intestine cancer in patients with Peutz-Jeghers syndrome (Perzin & Bridge, 1982). Treatment of the hamartomas of Peutz-Jeghers syndrome is primarily a conservative approach directed at relieving the complications of bleeding and obstruction that occur as a result of intussusception of the small intestine.

Adenomatous polyps of the small and large intestine with a marked malignant potential occur frequently in patients with either familial adenomatous polyposis syndrome (FAP) or Gardner's syndrome. Both syndromes are inherited as an autosomal dominant trait, with 90% penetrance in FAP. Gardner's syndrome occurs with half the frequency of familial adenomatous polyposis syndrome and includes other clinical features such as desmoid tumors of the mesentery and abdominal wall, multiple epidermoid cysts and connective tissue tumors of the skin, osteomas of the skeletal system, and dental abnormalities. Adenomatous polyps occurring in the duodenum of patients with either FAP or Gardner's syndrome tend to be small and difficult to detect without endoscopy (Yao, Ida, Ohsato, Watanabe, & Omae, 1977). In addition, when duodenal tumors occur in patients with either of these syndromes, the tumors tend to be ampullary adenocarcinomas and not true small intestine cancers (Schnur, David, Brown, Beahrs, Remine, & Harrison, 1973).

The most common form of hereditary colorectal cancer is hereditary nonpolyposis colorectal cancer (HNPCC), sometimes referred to as *Lynch syndrome I* and *II*. This subclassification of HNPCC is based on the absence or presence of extracolonic malignancies, respectively. Lynch syndrome I is characterized by an autosomal dominant inherited susceptibility to colorectal cancer with early age of onset, proclivity of colorectal cancer in the proximal colon, and a marked excess of synchronous and metachronous colonic cancers. Families with the same Lynch syndrome I features, but who also show an integral association with carcinomas of the endometrium and other organs, have been referred to as having Lynch syndrome II. Adenocarcinomas of the small intestine have been reported in Lynch syndrome II (Lynch, Smyrk, Lynch, Lanspa, & Boman et al., 1989). Extracolonic cancers observed in some Lynch II families have also included transitional cell carcinoma of the ureter and renal pelvis; adenocarcinomas of the stomach, ovary, pancreas, and biliary tract; and hematologic malignancies (Watson & Lynch, 1993).

Immunodeficiency

Immunosuppressed patients have an increased risk of small intestine cancer, in particular lymphomas. The immunosuppression can result from inherited immunodeficiency syndromes such as Wiskott-Aldrich, immunosuppressive regimens after transplantation, or acquired immune deficiency syndrome. Although the occurrence of extranodal lymphoma involving the small intestine is generally recognized in this patient population, the incidence and pattern of intestine involvement in these immunodeficient states vary considerably. Alexander and Altemeier (1968) reported that 83 of 112 patients with a primary tumor of the small intestine had another independent neoplasm at the time of death. Speculation is that there is some connection between the second primary tumor and the suspected defect in the immunosurveillance system of the small intestine. At this time, adenocarcinoma of the small intestine does not appear to be related to immunodeficiency.

Increasing Age

In general, increasing age is considered an important risk factor in the development of cancer. It has been suggested that the marked increase in cancer with advancing age is the result of some aspect of the aging process that increases the susceptibility of cancer through the impairment of the body's immune function. In addition, the importance of duration of exposure of carcinogens and long induction periods helps explain the increase in cancer with increasing age. With the peak incidence of adenocarcinoma of the small intestine occurring during the sixth and seventh decades of life, it appears that with the aging process, there is some failure of the normal small intestine physiologic factors that have been hypothesized to protect the small intestine from the development of cancer. Because of the low incidence of tumors of the small intestine, it is difficult to determine the precise impact of increasing age on the occurrence of small intestine cancer.

History of Colorectal Cancer or Adenocarcinomas

There is an increased risk for adenocarcinomas of the small intestine in individuals with a history of colorectal cancer and vice versa (Neugut & Santos, 1993), as well as persons with a previous history of adenocarcinomas (Chen, Neugut, & Rotterdam, 1994). In addition, the trend for the rising incidence of duodenal adenocarcinomas is similar to the incidence trends of colon adenocarcinomas, which suggests that there are similar risk factors for cancers in these regions (Chow et al., 1996).

CHEMOPREVENTION

Chemoprevention is the use of defined noncytotoxic nutrients and/or pharmacologic agents to inhibit or reverse the process of carcinogenesis (Loescher, 1997). It is one of the most tested and promising approaches to altering the body's internal environment to prevent the initiation or progression of cancer. Chemopreventive agents can affect carcinogenesis in many ways through the use of dietary constituents (e.g., beta-carotene), vitamins (e.g., vitamins A, C,and E), or micronutrients (e.g., selenium), as well as synthetic retinoids (e.g., isotretinoin), antiestrogens (e.g., tamoxifen), or nonsteroidal anti-inflammatory drugs. Although at present numerous chemoprevention trials are being conducted by the National Cancer Institute that include other portions of the GI tract, such as the colon and the esophagus, there are no chemoprevention trials specifically directed at the small intestine. The rarity of small intestine tumors combined with the remarkable disparity in incidence between small and large intestine carcinomas suggests that the small intestine would not be a high priority for chemoprevention trials at this time.

PATHOPHYSIOLOGY

Normal Anatomy and Physiology of the Small Intestine

The small intestine is a tubular structure with two concentric layers of smooth muscle that extends from the pyloric sphincter to the cecum. The small intestine measures about 6.7 to 7.0 m (22 to 23 feet) in length, and about 1.9 to 3.8 cm (0.75 to 1.5 in) in diameter. The wall of the small intestine consists of four layers: the outer serous layer (serosa) composed of peritoneum and connective tissue; the muscular layer (muscularis externa), which contains outer longitudinal and inner circular muscles, separated by a nerve network called the *myenteric plexus;* the submucosal layer, which consists of connective tissue containing blood vessels, lymphatics, and a submucosal nerve plexus; and the inner mucosal layer, which contains columnar epithelium, a layer of connective tissue known as lamina propria, and a thin layer of smooth muscle (muscularis mucosae), which separates the mucosa from the submucosa (Fig. 43-1). All three embryonic germ layers give rise to the structures within the small intestine, including the endoderm, which gives rise to the columnar epithelium of the mucosa; the mesoderm, which gives rise to the connective, vascular, lymphatic, and muscular tissues; and the ectoderm, which gives rise to the enterochromaffin cells and nerve cells of the small intestine (Society of Gastrointestinal Nurses & Associates, 1993).

The mucosa of the small intestine is highly folded, with the surface of the folds creating fingerlike projections known as *villi* (Fig. 43-2). The surface of each villus is covered with a single layer of epithelial cells whose surface membranes form small projections known as *microvilli.* The total surface area of the small intestine available for absorption is increased 600-fold through the combination of the mucosal folds, villi, and microvilli. The crypts of Lieberkuhn, small, tubular glands that lie between each villi, contain extremely mitotic cells responsible for replacement of the surface epithelium every 32 hours, as well as Paneth's cells that may play a role in regulating intestinal flora.

GI-associated lymphoid tissue makes up approximately 25% of the intestinal mucosa and includes three distinct populations. Peyer's patches, aggregated lymph nodes that lie in the mucosa and submucosa of the ileum, participate in the body's immune response through antibody synthesis. Lymphocytes and plasma cells located in the lamina propria produce immunoglobulin A (IgA), which is the primary immunoglobulin located in intestinal secretions. This secretory IgA plays an important role in the resistance of the mucous membranes to pathologic microorganisms and dietary antigens. The intraepithelial lymphocytes that lie between the intestinal epithelial cells are primarily T lymphocytes, which play a role in cell-mediated immunity (Society of Gastrointestinal Nurses & Associates, 1993).

The small intestine is divided into three segments: the duodenum, the jejunum, and the ileum. The duodenum, the shortest and widest segment of the small intestine, consists of the first 30 cm (12 inches) of the small intestine, beginning at the pyloric sphincter and ending at the ligament of Treitz. Most of its length is fixed and in the retroperitoneum while making a C-shaped curve around the head of the pancreas. The duodenum is usually divided into four segments, with the pancreatic and biliary ducts draining into the ampulla of Vater located in the second, descending portion of the duodenum (Donohue & Kelly, 1991).

After the duodenum, the next 40% of the small intestine is considered the jejunum, and the remaining 60% is the ileum. The division between the jejunum and the ileum is arbitrary. The small intestine is supported by a fold of the peritoneum, the mesentery. Whereas the duodenum has no mesentery and is only partially covered by peritoneum, the jejunum and ileum are attached to the retroperitoneum by the mesentery. The jejunum usually occupies the periumbilical region, and the ileum resides in the hypogastrium and pelvis. Beginning with the jejunum and continuing until the ileocecal valve, there are progressive decreases in both small intestine diameter and thickness along with increases in the amount of lymphatic tissue (Society of Gastrointestinal Nurses & Associates, 1993).

The duodenum receives arterial blood from the hepatic artery, and the rest of the small intestine derives its blood supply from the superior mesenteric artery. Blood from the entire small intestine drains through the mesenteric vein (Society of Gastrointestinal Nurses & Associates, 1993).

The small intestine has three important functions: absorption, secretion, and motility. The primary function is the absorption of nutrients from the chyme, a solution of

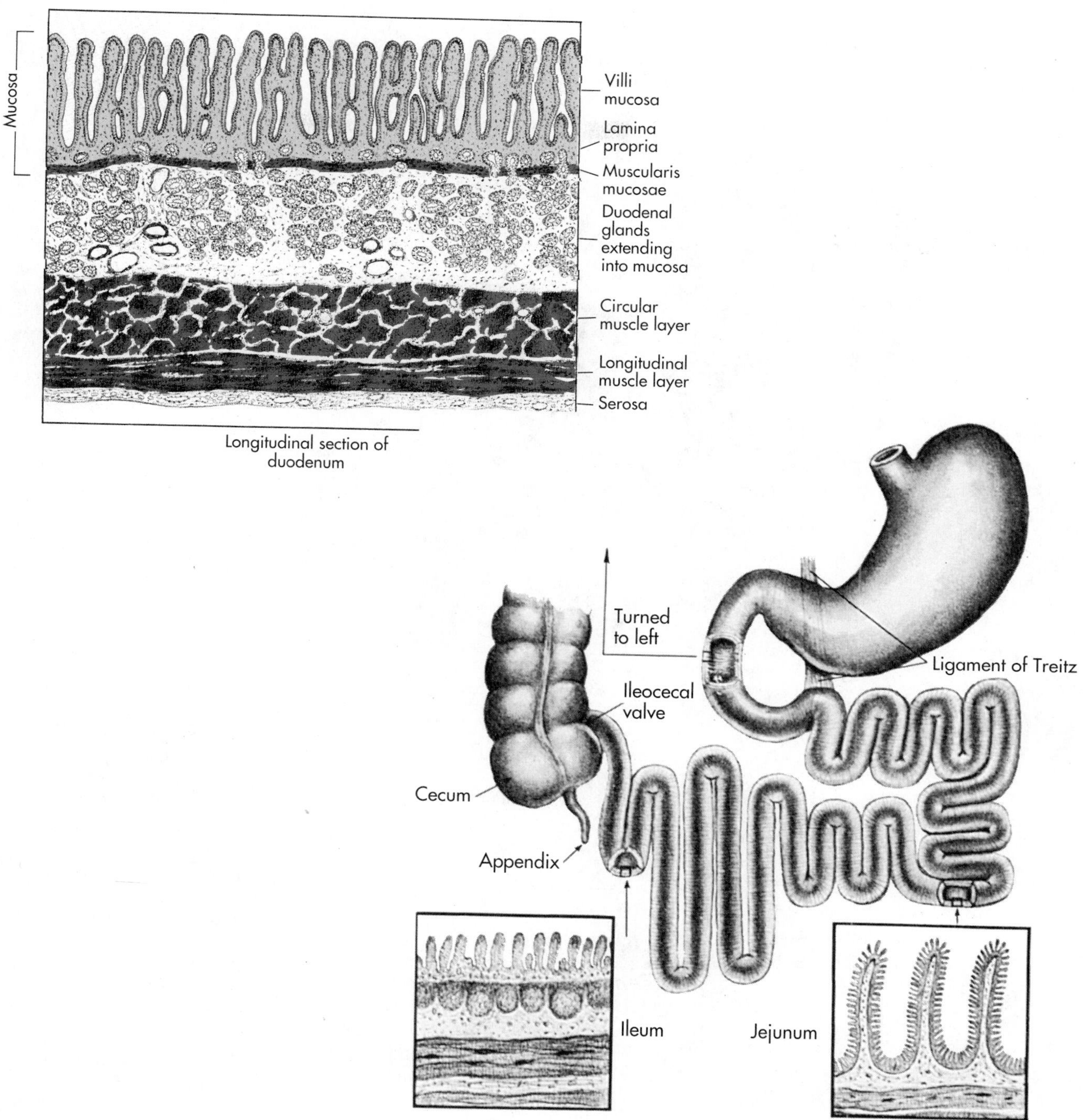

Fig. 43-1 The small intestine. (From McCance, K. L. [1998]. *Pathophysiology: The biologic basis for disease in adults and children* (3rd ed.). St Louis: Mosby.)

partially digested food created in the lumen of the stomach before being propelled into the intestines. Although the small intestine receives up to 8 L of fluid per day, it passes only 500 to 1000 ml on to the large intestine, with the rest of the fluid being absorbed by the columnar cells of the villous epithelium. Throughout the small intestine, the absorption of nutrients takes place in different locations. The duodenum is the primary site of iron and calcium absorption; the jejunum is the site of fat, protein, and carbohydrate absorption; and the ileum absorbs vitamin B_{12} and bile acids. The process of absorption through the wall of the small intestine occurs through a variety of mechanisms including hydrolysis, nonionic movement, passive diffusion, facilitated diffusion, active transport, or combinations thereof (Society of Gastrointestinal Nurses & Associates, 1993).

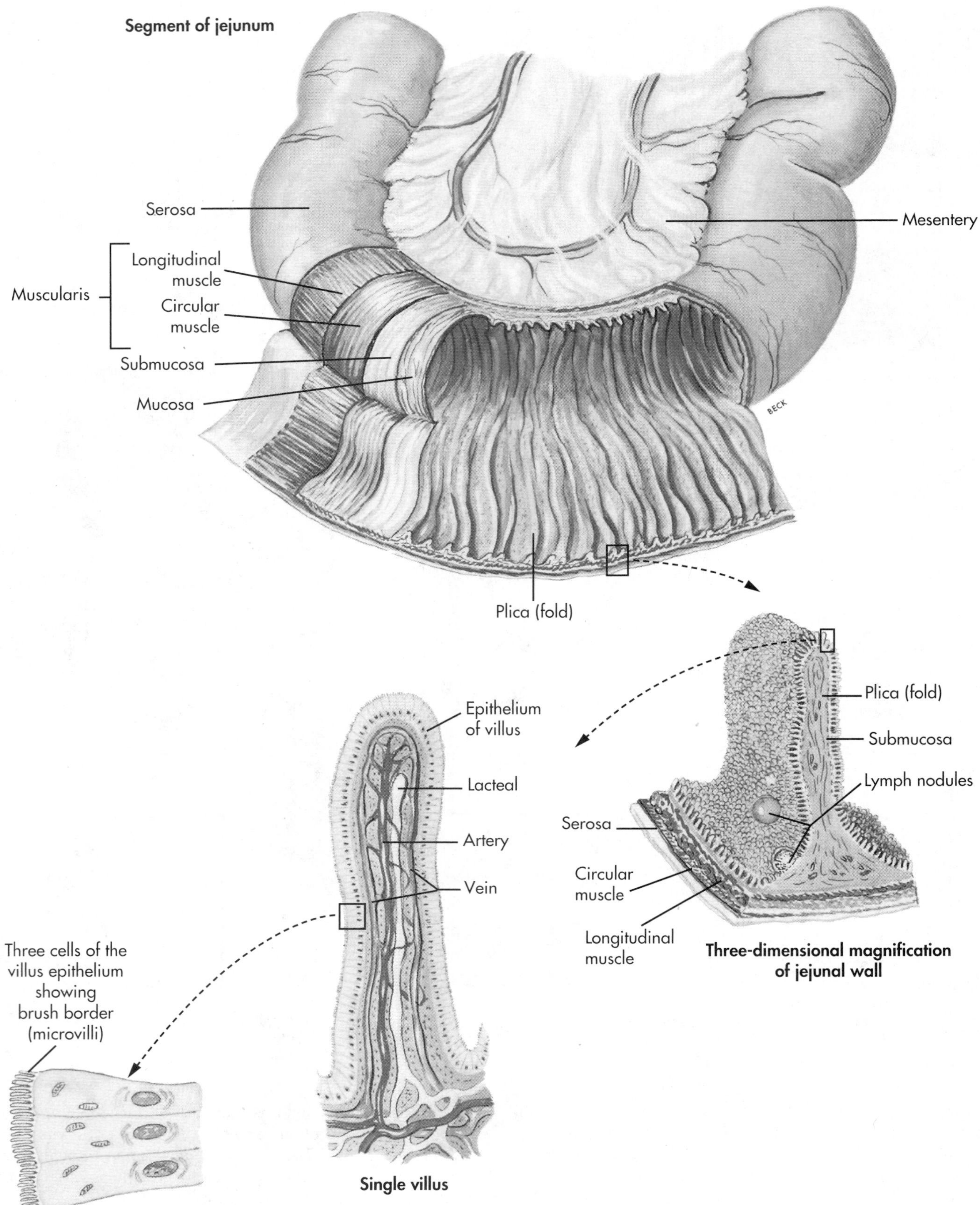

Fig. 43-2 Wall of the small intestine. Folds of mucosa are covered with villi and each villus is covered with epithelium, which increases the surface area for absorption of food. (From Thibodeau, G. A. & Patton, K. T. (1996). *Anatomy & physiology* (3rd ed.). St. Louis: Mosby.

The cells of the small intestine are responsible for the secretion of digestive juices, mucus, and a variety of hormones and peptides; they also receive secretions from the liver and the pancreas. Brunner's glands, located in the proximal duodenum, secrete a clear, viscous, alkaline fluid that protects the duodenal mucosa from gastric acid secretions. Goblet cells located on or between the mucosal villi provide additional protection to the mucosal surface through the secretion of a protective mucus. The crypts of Lieberkuhn, responsible for the production of numerous peptides and hormones, secrete a watery fluid that supplies a carrier substance for the absorption of nutrients when the villi come in contact with the chyme. The microvilli secrete enzymes that aid in the digestion of proteins and carbohydrates (Society of Gastrointestinal Nurses & Associates, 1993).

Various movements of the small intestine wall contribute to the mixing of the chyme. These movements include concentric, segmenting contractions of the jejunum, which help mix the chyme particles with the secretions of the small intestine; peristaltic contractions of the first portion of the duodenum and the jejunum, which slowly push the chyme in the direction of the colon; and ongoing shortening and lengthening of the villi, which stirs the intestinal contents (Society of Gastrointestinal Nurses & Associates, 1993)

The Process of Carcinogenesis

Thorough understanding of the biology and method of spread of small intestine cancer is considered incomplete because of the rarity of small intestine malignancies. Because different regions of the small intestine seem to react to carcinogenesis differently, the etiology of small intestine tumors remains unknown (Chow et al., 1996). Adenocarcinomas of the small intestine typically arise from the crypts of the mucosa and are generally well to moderately differentiated with recognizable glandular structures and mucin production (Hart & Levin, 1993). They are usually histologically similar to colonic adenocarcinomas. Given the differences in length between the different segments of the small intestine, the mucosa of the duodenum shows a substantially higher propensity toward malignant transformation compared with the jejunum and ileum. Adenocarcinomas are either polypoid intraluminal masses or, more frequently, infiltrative annular constricting lesions (Hart & Levin, 1993). The polyp-cancer sequence for tubular polyps has not been established for small intestine adenocarcinomas.

ROUTES OF METASTASES

Small intestine lesions can metastasize to anywhere in the body, but are especially likely to affect the lymph nodes, liver, and lung. By the time of diagnosis, the majority of adenocarcinomas have already metastasized to regional lymph nodes, liver, or the peritoneal surface. Duodenal adenocarcinomas frequently infiltrate the pancreas because of their close proximity. Because the small intestine is very mobile from the ligament of Trietz down to the cecum, tumors in this portion of the small intestine do not as readily invade other areas of the GI tract.

TABLE 43-1 Malignant Tumors and Their Original Sites

Site Involved	Origin of Tumor
Duodenum	Colon Stomach Pancreas Kidney Retroperitoneum
Jejunum	Colon Stomach Pancreas Kidney
Ileum	Colon Pelvis Retroperitoneum

Modified from Coit, D. G. (1997). Cancer of the small intestine. In V. T. DeVita, S. Hellman, & S. A. Rosenberg (Eds.), *Cancer: Principles and practice of oncology* (4th ed.). Philadelphia: J. B. Lippincott, Co.

In addition to primary malignancies, the small intestine may be involved by malignant tumors that originate in adjacent organs as described in Table 43-1 (Hart & Levin, 1993). The small intestine may be the site for metastatic disease arising from primary neoplasms of other organs, most frequently the uterus, cervix, lung, breast, kidney, urinary bladder, ovary, and skin (Viamonte & Viamonte, 1992; Haskell, Lavey, & Ramming, 1995).

ASSESSMENT

Patient History

Complete evaluation of the patient involves obtaining a detailed personal and family medical history for the presence of high-risk GI diseases, completing a thorough physical examination and review of the patient's GI system, and performing a variety of diagnostic tests (Table 43-2). For patients with a preexisting history of Crohn's disease, celiac disease, colorectal cancer, or adenocarcinoma of another organ who are already under the care of a physician at the time of noticing changes in their GI functioning, the primary focus of care should be directed toward obtaining the necessary diagnostic tests to fully evaluate their GI symptoms.

Signs and Symptoms

Clinical detection of both benign and malignant small intestine tumors can be difficult and requires special attention to various signs and symptoms. Although fewer than half the patients with benign small intestine tumors develop symptoms, more than 90% of patients with malignant tumors of the small intestine are symptomatic before diagnosis (Coit, 1993). Most benign tumors of the small intestine are undiagnosed in the lifetime of the patient and are usually discov-

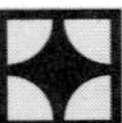

TABLE 43-2 Assessment of the Patient for Adenocarcinoma of the Small Bowel

	Assessment Parameters	Typical Abnormal Findings
History	A. Personal and social history 1. Age 2. Ethnicity 3. Family history 4. Prior history	A. Personal and social risk factors 1. Sixty to 70 years of age. 2. Countries with high fat intake (e.g., Norway, Denmark, Sweden). 3. Familial gastrointestinal (GI) syndromes. 4. Chrohn's disease, celiac disease and immunodeficiency states may be predisposing factors.
	B. Evaluation of GI tract	B. Symptoms depend on location and tumor size. Common symptoms include intermittent abdominal pain, vague and indistinct cramping, which may be due to partial small intestine obstruction due to tumor infiltration and adhesions, intermittent nausea and vomiting, and change in intestine habits; unexplained weight loss due to anorexia and tumor growth; pallor, dyspnea, shortness of breath due to anemia from chronic blood loss due to mucosal ulceration. C. Weakness, malaise, and fatigue.
Physical Examination	A. Palpation of abdominal area	A. Rarely reveals mass.
	B. Weight	B. Weight loss may indicate of tumor growth in the presence of other symptoms.
	C. Pallor, dyspnea, shortness of breath	C. May indicate anemia secondary to chronic bleeding.
Diagnostic Tests	A. Upper GI series	A. May reveal suspicion of duodenum adenocarcinoma.
	B. Upper GI endoscopy with total duodenoscopy	B. May allow for histologic confirmation of tumor.
	C. Radiographic films	C. May show mass and localize tumor.
	D. Complete blood count	D. Microcytic, hypochromic anemia associated with chronic blood loss of small bowel malignancy.
	E. Liver function tests	E. May be elevated due to biliary obstruction or hepatic metastasis.

From Ashley, S. W. & Wells, S. A. (1988). Tumors of the small intestine. *Seminars in Oncology, 15*(2), 116-128; DiSario, J. A., Burt, R. W., Vargas, H., & McWhorter, W. P. (1994). Small bowel cancer: Epidemiological and clinical characteristics from a population-based registry. *The American Journal of Gastroenterology, 89*(5), 699-701.

ered as incidental findings at the time of autopsy (Haskell, Lavey, & Ramming, 1995). The symptoms of malignant small intestine lesions can be insidious and nonspecific, often resulting in a significant delay in diagnosis. In a review of 77 patients with small intestine malignancy, the average delay between onset of symptoms and presentation to the physician was 1 month, but the average interval from seeing the physician to final diagnosis was 7.8 months (Maglinte, O'Connor, Bessette, Chernish, & Kelvin, 1991). On average, patients frequently report symptoms for 6 to 12 months before the diagnosis is made (Ashley & Wells, 1988).

The presenting symptoms associated with small intestine malignancies depend on the location and size of the tumor and its growth pattern. The most common symptom is intermittent abdominal pain, generally vague and indistinct but occasionally cramping in nature, which may stem from a partial small intestine obstruction due to tumor infiltration and adhesions (Ashley & Wells, 1988). Compared with cancers in other regions of the gut, small intestine cancers may cause symptoms of obstruction earlier due to the small luminal diameter (DiSario et al., 1994). The incidence of small intestine obstruction varies considerably due to malignant tumors (15% to 35%) compared with benign small intestine tumors (40% to 70%). It is important to note that benign small intestine tumors are the most common cause of intestine intussusception in adults. The infiltrative pattern of growth seen with adenocarcinomas are more likely to produce apple core lesions similar to those observed in the colon, as opposed to the extrinsic intestine compression and dysmotility due to nerve invasion seen in lymphomas (Peacock, Keller, & Asbury, 1993). Complete intestine obstructions are more common in adenocarcinomas of the small intestine (Donohue & Kelly, 1991). Because intestine obstructions due to malignant small intestine tumors can often be intermittent and partial, patients may also report abdominal pain in the absence of intestine obstruction, along with intermittent nausea and vomiting, and changes in intestine habits.

The second most common symptom associated with small intestine malignancy is unexplained weight loss due to anorexia and tumor growth. Although weight loss is more commonly associated with the malabsorption syndromes seen in lymphoma patients, it can occur in up to 50% of all patients with small intestine malignancy. Chronic blood loss and anemia, although common in all forms of small intestine malignancy, primarily result from mucosal ulceration when seen with adenocarcinomas (Donohue & Kelly, 1991). Frank upper GI hemorrhage is unusual. Patients may also report additional constitutional symptoms such as weakness, malaise, and fatigue.

Obstruction of the common bile duct due to duodenal adenocarcinoma is the most frequent cause of jaundice, although jaundice can also be a sign of advanced hepatic metastasis from a either a primary small intestine malignancy or another primary tumor. A movable, palpable mass in the abdomen is present in about 10% to 20% of patients, although this is usually the result of dilated proximal small intestine rather than the tumor itself (Ashley & Wells, 1988). Intestine perforation, usually localized, occurs in 10% or fewer of patients and is more commonly seen with lymphomas or sarcomas.

At present, routine screening examinations do not exist for small intestine malignancy. Because of the nonspecific nature of the presenting signs and symptoms, the diagnosis of small intestine malignancy is often difficult to make preoperatively. If a small intestine malignancy is suspected based on the patient's medical history, physical examination, and reported GI symptoms, appropriate diagnostic tests should be ordered.

Radiography

Radiographic abnormalities are present at diagnosis in about 75% of small intestine cancers. Although plain films of the abdomen may reveal a mass effect from a large sarcoma or lymphoma, obstruction, or free air from a perforation, small intestine barium follow-through studies are considered the best method for localizing the tumor within the intestine (Donohue & Kelly, 1991; Martin, 1994). The probability of tumor detection on a small intestine series increases with a more proximal location. Unfortunately, redundancy of the small intestine frequently obscures the ability to detect small intestine lesions during an upper GI examination with small intestine follow-through study (Peacock, Keller, & Asbury, 1993). Hypotonic duodenography using glucagon enhances the diagnostic accuracy of the conventional upper GI series by retarding duodenal motion, allowing subtle mucosal abnormalities to be better visualized (Hart & Levin, 1993). Because the distal ileum is not always well-visualized on conventional small intestine studies, a reflux barium enema can be used if reflux through the ileocecal valve can be obtained.

Endoscopy

With more sophisticated forward- and side-viewing fiberoptic instruments, endoscopy is more frequently used in the investigation of small intestine disease. Upper GI endoscopy with total duodenoscopy is the mainstay for detection, diagnosis, and occasionally treatment of proximal neoplasms (Bowden, 1989). When evaluating a duodenal lesion, histologic confirmation of a small intestine malignancy can often be obtained by endoscopy, whereas proximal and distal lesions of the jejunum or ileum often require a laparotomy to histologically confirm diagnosis

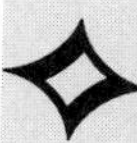

TABLE 43-3 Patient Preparation for the Patient Undergoing Diagnostic Gastrointestinal Procedures

Description of the Procedure: Suspected small intestine tumors may be evaluated using both invasive and noninvasive gastrointestinal diagnostic procedures, which may include radiography, endoscopy, computed tomography (CT), or ultrasonography.

Patient Preparation: Patient is usually instructed to refrain from fluid and food for a predetermined period before the procedure, as well as preparation of the intestine for better visualization during the procedure.

Procedural Considerations:

1. Review patient medical and surgical history along with current mediations for any potential contraindications to performing the diagnostic procedure.
2. Review laboratory results for any abnormalities that would preclude performing the diagnostic procedure.
3. Thoroughly explain diagnostic procedure to patient, including:
   - The purpose and approximate length of the test.
   - The type of positioning and special techniques to be used.
   - Anticipated effect of any medications or anesthetics that will be used.
   - Any sensations the patient may experience during and after the procedure
   - Potential risks and complications that may be encountered during or after the procedure.
4. Obtain informed consent.
5. Confirm length of NPO status and adherence to preprocedural dietary restrictions.
6. Verify completion of specified bowel preparation if indicated.
7. Obtain baseline vital signs and establish patient intravenous (IV) line if indicated.

(Ross, Hartnett, Bernstein, & Henderson, 1991; Coit, 1993). The diagnosis of lymphoma in the terminal ileum can be enhanced by the use of colonoscopy with retrograde ileoscopy as performed by a physician experienced in endoscopy (Coit, 1993). Table 43-3 provides a patient teaching tool for diagnostic testing for adenocarcinoma of the small intestine.

Laboratory Tests

Routine blood tests rarely show any abnormality, with the exception of microcytic, hypochromic anemia associated with the chronic blood loss of small intestine malignancy. Hyperbilirubinemia may occur with periampullary duodenal tumors. Mild or moderate elevations of liver function tests may occur with biliary obstruction or hepatic metastasis. No specific serologic tests exist for small intestine cancers. Carcinoembryonic antigen and other tumor-associated antigens lack the specificity and sensitivity needed for the diagnosis of small intestine adenocarcinomas (Donohue & Kelly, 1991).

Enteroscopy

Although small intestine enteroscopy is still in the developmental stage, it can be performed on withdrawal of a special endoscope that is passed orally and allowed to migrate with peristalsis. Approximately 50% of the mucosal surface can be reliably evaluated, but biopsies of lesions cannot be done. Currently, this procedure is tedious and time consuming, but it will likely become more widely available in the future as technical improvements continue (Hart & Levin, 1993).

Computed Tomography

Although computed tomography (CT) is more accurate in detecting small intestine tumors, it is not particularly helpful unless the lesion is large, as with lymphomas. In addition, it does not conclusively determine that a malignancy exists. Small intestine adenocarcinomas have been described on CT findings as a partially obstructing concentric narrowing in the proximal small intestine. CT is best suited for detecting tumors larger than 3 cm in diameter (Laurent, Raynaud, Biset, Boisserie-Lacroix, Grelet, & Drouillard, 1991).

Angiography is rarely helpful in the diagnosis of nonvascular small intestine tumors, except in the case of active GI bleeding (Coit, 1993). Magnetic resonance imaging is of no value because of intestine motion (Peacock, Keller, & Asbury, 1993).

STAGING

Because primary cancers of the small intestine are rare, a staging system was not published until 1992 by the American Joint Committee on Cancer (Table 43-4). Before then, the classification of small intestine tumors used the Dukes classification system for colorectal cancers with correlation to their histopathologic tumor type. Currently, primary small intestine carcinomas are staged according to their depth of penetration and involvement of adjacent structures or distant sites. Lateral spread from the duodenum into the jejunum or jejunum into the ileum is not considered in the classification, only the depth of tumor penetration. Of note, GI lymphomas have been traditionally staged using a modification of the Ann Arbor system.

Differences between the small intestine staging system and that of the colon should be noted. Unlike the large intestine, there is no subdivision of the N category. Also, in the colon, T applies to intraepithelial (in situ) lesions as well as intramucosal spread. In the small intestine, intramucosal spread is listed as T1. The T1 definition for the small intestine is the same as the T1 category as defined for the stomach. Invasion through the wall is staged the same as the colon. Discontinuous metastasis or seeding is coded as M1.

Histologic staging is used to determine the grade or biologic aggressiveness of the tumor. The following classification applies to all carcinomas arising in the small intestine: GX, grade not assessed; G1, well differentiated; G2, moderately differentiated; G3, poorly differentiated; and G4, undifferentiated. Lymphomas, carcinoid tumors, and sarcomas are not included in this classification system (Beahrs, Henson, Hutton, & Kennedy, 1992).

TABLE 43-4 American Joint Committee on Cancer TNM Staging System Primary

TX	Primary cancer cannot be assessed		
T0	No evidence of primary tumor		
Tis	Carcinoma in situ		
T1	Tumor invades lamina propria or submucosa		
T2	Tumor invades muscularis propria		
T3	Tumor invades through the muscularis propria into the subserosa or in to the nonperiotionealized perimuscular tissue (mesentery or retroperitoneum) with extension 2 cm or less		
T4	Tumor perforates the visceral peritoneum or directly invades other organs or structures (includes other loops of the small intestine, mesentery, or retroperitoneum more than 2 cm, and the abdominal wall by way of the serosa; for the duodenum only, includes invasion of the pancreas).		
Regional Lymph Nodes (N)			
NX	Regional lymph nodes cannot be assessed		
N0	No regional lymph node metastasis		
N1	Regional lymph node metastasis		
Distant Metastasis (M)			
MX	Presence of distant metastasis cannot be assessed		
M0	No distant metastasis		
M1	Distant metastasis		
Stage Grouping			
Stage 0	Tis	N0	M0
Stage I	T1	N0	M0
	T2	N0	M0
Stage II	T3	N0	M0
	T4	N0	M0
Stage III	Any T	N1	M0
Stage IV	Any T	Any N	M1

NOTE: The nonperitonealized perimuscular tissue is, for the jejunum and ileum, part of the mesentery and, for the duodenum in areas where serosa is lacking, part of the retroperitoneum.
From Beahrs, O. H., Henson, D. E., Hutton, R., & Kennedy, B. J. (1992). *Handbook of staging of cancer: From the manual for staging of cancer* (4th ed.). American Joint Committee on Cancer. Philadelphia: J. B. Lippincott.

MEDICAL MANAGEMENT

Surgery

Because of the low prevalence and diverse nature of small intestine cancers, the majority of recommendations for treating these tumors have come from small hospital-based reviews gathered over the last two decades. Although surgical resection is considered the standard treatment for adenocarcinomas of the small intestine, the infrequency of small intestine tumors has made comparative surgical analysis difficult. In adenocarcinoma of the small intestine, thorough intraoperative examination of the entire abdomen must be performed to determine whether there is any tumor spread, particularly to the liver and lymph nodes, or peritoneal seeding (Martin, 1994). Outcome in these patients is determined by resectability, lymph node involvement, and histologic grade (Lai, Doty, Irving, & Tompkins, 1988).

As a rule, extended segmental resection is the treatment of choice for malignant lesions (Haskell, Lavey, & Ramming, 1995). The principles of surgical resection include attainment of negative surgical margins and wide resection of the corresponding mesentery of the involved segment of intestine (Coit, 1993). When the lesion is large and extends beyond the wall of the intestine, efforts are made to avoid removal of any more intestine than is necessary. Any mesentery that contains lymph nodes draining the area in which the lesion is located should be removed, recognizing that the removal of too much mesentery can jeopardize the maintenance of the blood supply to the small intestine. An end-to-end anastomosis of the remaining intestine is usually possible, except in certain cases of ileocolic anastomosis, which may require end-to-side anastomosis. Repeated anastomoses in the small intestine using stapling devices can interrupt peristalsis, leading to devastating, prolonged ileus (Haskell, Lavey, & Ramming, 1995).

Patients with adenocarcinomas in the first and second portion of the duodenum often require a more extensive surgical procedure known as *pancreaticoduodenectomy (Whipple procedure);* those with tumors of the third and fourth portions of the duodenum may be resected with segmental duodenectomy and primary anastomosis (Coit, 1993). Adequate local excision of the primary tumor with wide resection of the adjacent mesentery to include regional lymph nodes is the preferred operation for jejunal or ileal adenocarcinomas (Hart & Levin, 1993). When malignant tumors of the terminal ileum are part of the operative procedure, a right colectomy is usually included because the removal of lymph nodes that drain the ileum can interfere with the blood supply to the ascending colon. Unfortunately, tumor extension into the mesentery may involve blood vessels that cannot be resected without sacrificing large segments of the small intestine (Hart & Levin, 1993).

Pancreaticoduodenectomy, more commonly known as the *Whipple procedure,* was first performed in 1935 and has since become the most commonly performed operation for carcinoma of the pancreas. Classic pancreaticoduodenectomy involves removal of the head, neck, and unicate process of the pancreas, the duodenum, the gastric antrum and pylorus, the gallbladder, the common bile duct, and lymph nodes in the pancreaticoduodenal groove (Coleman, 1997).

One important complication in the treatment of small intestine tumors is perforation. This is more likely in adenocarcinomas or lymphomas. Perforations are considered emergency situations; segmental resection is preferred, although intestine sidetracking and drainage may be all that is possible.

Box 43-2

Potential Acute Complications After Surgery for Small Bowel Cancer and Their Signs and Symptoms

General

Cardiopulmonary

Atelectasis: dyspnea, anxiety, cyanosis, diaphoresis, tachycardia

Pneumonia: cough, sputum production, pleuritic chest pain, chills, fever

Pulmonary embolus: dyspnea, bloody sputum, chest pain tachycardia, fever

Congestive heart failure: dyspnea, orthopnea, hypoxia, cough, high blood pressure, palpitations, wheezes, crackles

Wound infection: redness, swelling, tenderness, purulent discharge, chills, fever, foul-smelling drainage

Septicemia: *early signs:* fever, chills, nausea, vomiting, diarrhea, oliguria; *late signs:* restlessness, irritability, apprehension, tachycardia, tachypnea, hypotension, thirsted, altered consciousness, anuria, hypothermia

Small Bowel

Intraperitoneal hemorrhage: decreased hematocrit, increased abdominal distention, peritoneal irritation, hypovolemic signs

Anastomotic leaks: peritonitis, abscess, fistula formation, abdominal pain

Peritonitis: sudden, severe abdominal pain, weakness, pallor, diaphoresis, decreased intestinal motility, low blood pressure, tachycardia, rebound tenderness, fever

Intra-abdominal abscess: recurring or persistent fever more than 72 hours postoperatively, leukocytes with high bands count; no abdominal pain or tenderness

Hypoxic bowel: guaiac-positive diarrhea, general signs and symptoms of infection

Small bowel obstruction: abdominal pain, nausea, vomiting, distention, tenderness, audible bowel sounds with rushes

Modified from Hoebler, L. & Irwin, M. M. (1992). Gastrointestinal tract cancer: Current knowledge, medical treatment, and nursing management. *Oncology Nursing Forum, 19*(9), 1403-1415.

In nonresectable lesions, palliative bypass should be performed to relieve the symptoms of obstruction, perforation, or GI bleeding. Primary resection for metastatic lesions is justified to prevent or relieve the complications of obstruction or bleeding. Box 43-2 describes potential acute complications after surgery for small intestine cancer.

Radiation Therapy

Radiation therapy is difficult in these patients because of the mobile nature of the small intestine mesentery and the inability to localize the target field. Adjuvant radiotherapy may be of benefit in patients with minimal residual disease following surgical resection, but the tolerance of normal tissues to radiation limits the dose that can be administered. Intraoperative radiotherapy (IORT) may be more useful because normal tissue can be protected from the beam, but there is still no conclusive evidence that IORT is beneficial in the management of these tumors. Mucin-producing adenocarcinomas of the small intestine are usually radioresistant.

Chemotherapy

The use of adjuvant chemotherapy such as 5-flurouracil and nitrosureas after curative surgical resection has not been recommended because they have been found to be of little benefit (Hart & Levin, 1993). At present, no effective single-agent or combination chemotherapy has been found for advanced or metastatic small intestine carcinomas. Further evaluation of these modalities will require multi-institutional trials.

ONCOLOGIC EMERGENCIES

Oncologic emergencies are primarily due to the interruption of the GI system as a result of intestine obstruction, intestine perforation, or GI hemorrhage. Medical management of these emergent situations usually requires surgical intervention aimed at relieving the obstruction, repairing the perforation, and/or controlling GI bleeding. Nursing interventions aimed at managing these oncologic emergencies are based on the nature of the treatment. Additional psychosocial support for the patient and family may be required because of the emergent nature of the situation and the stage of the disease at the onset of the oncologic emergency.

NURSING MANAGEMENT

Nursing interventions aimed at managing patients diagnosed with adenocarcinoma of the small intestine are guided primarily by the stage of the disease at the time of diagnosis, the type of treatment chosen, the existing prognostic factors, and the presence of preexisting, underlying medical conditions that might have placed the patient at higher risk for the development of small intestine cancer. The psychosocial responses of the patient and family or significant others along with the presence or absence of adequate support systems also determine appropriate nursing interventions. Nursing care for the patient with small intestine cancer can be delivered in the inpatient, outpatient, or home care setting depending on the nature of the treatment and the physical and emotional condition of the patient. Table 43-5 describes the standard of care for patients with small intestine adenocarcinoma.

Early Detection

As with all cancers, early detection is the key to obtaining an accurate diagnosis in order to begin appropriate medical treatment. Because of the difficulty detecting small intestine cancer owing to its vague and nonspecific GI symptoms, careful nursing assessment in the primary care outpatient setting can play an important role in preventing any delay in diagnosis. Nurses should monitor all patients for early signs of unexplained weight loss, change in intestine habits, and/or persistent abdominal complaints. Additionally, patients with medical histories that place them at high risk of developing GI malignancies should be systematically identified as high-risk patients in their outpatient charts to routinely initiate prevention and early detection efforts by members of their health care team.

Diagnosis

The diagnostic period can be physically and mentally stressful for the patient with a suspected GI malignancy while undergoing an extensive invasive and noninvasive diagnostic workup. Diagnostic procedures that are now routinely done in the outpatient setting, such as the upper GI series with small intestine follow-through, can be lengthy and physically challenging for many patients. Nursing interventions for all patients, especially the medically compromised or elderly patient, should include thorough preprocedure instruction, comfort and safety measures during the procedure itself, and planning for sufficient postprocedure instruction and support. Psychosocial support should also be provided to help the patient and family cope with the anxiety, fear, and worry commonly experienced during the diagnostic period.

Preoperative Care

Small intestine endoscopic examination and biopsy are currently limited to duodenal and some ileal lesions because of the available fiberoptic equipment and techniques. Because the definitive diagnosis of small intestine adenocarcinoma cannot be made until a tissue sample from the tumor has been obtained, some patients with a suspected small intestine malignancy may be scheduled for abdominal surgery without definitive diagnosis or extent of malignancy. Nursing care during the preoperative period should be directed at assessing the patient's physical and emotional status, explaining the surgical procedure to the patient and family, and preparing the patient and family for the anticipated short- and long-term postoperative sequelae.

Patient assessment should included general physical condition, presence of concomitant disease, nutritional status, cardiopulmonary status, and psychosocial responses to actual or potential diagnosis. The patient and family should have the surgical procedure verbally and visually explained, and the anticipated length of hospital stay should be discussed. The patient should be prepared for postoperative care, which includes respiratory and circulatory exercises, pain control, wound and drain care, catheter care, intravenous lines, and nutritional support. Unfortunately, the patient requiring surgical intervention for the diagnosis and treatment of adenocarcinoma of the small intestine may present in a significantly malnourished state secondary to weight loss associated with the disease process itself, delay in diagnosis, and/or the presence of advanced disease at the time of diagnosis.

Postoperative Care

Nursing care in the acute postoperative period primarily focuses on the prevention and early detection of potential surgical complications. The nursing management of patients

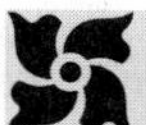

TABLE 43-5 Standard of Care for the Patient with Short Bowel Syndrome

Patient Problem and Outcome	Nursing Interventions and Rationale	Patient Education Instructions
Malabsorption of Nutrients Patient will: • Verbalize an understanding of the normal function of the GI tract. • Identify signs and symptoms of electrolyte imbalance. • Identify signs and symptoms of dehydration.	1. Assess patient's level of understanding of the normal GI tract. 2. Provide patient the opportunity to ask questions. 3. Determine patient's ability to identify complications of chronic diarrhea and the relationship to short bowel syndrome.	1. Use a diagram of the GI system to explain the normal function. 2. Provide patient with information on short bowel syndrome. 3. Instruct patient on normal absorption of nutrient and fluid 4. Instruct patient on usual output from intestinal tract (consistency, volume) 5. Instruct patient on signs and symptoms of electrolyte imbalance 6. Instruct patient on signs and symptoms of dehydration
Weight loss Patient will: • Verbalize an understanding of the reason for potential weight loss. • Maintain acceptable weight for height, age and, sex.	1. Access patient's level of understanding of malabsorption and diarrhea in relation to weight loss. 2. Weigh weekly. 3. Maintain accurate input and output. 4. Collaborate with dietitian to obtain appropriate calories and nutrients during a 24-hour period.	1. Provide patient with information on caloric intake related to malabsorption and chronic diarrhea. 2. Instruct patient to weigh self daily and record. 3. Instruct patient on maintaining an accurate record of intake (nutrients and fluids) and output (urine and stool).
Infection Patient will: • Verbalize the signs and symptoms of infection. • Demonstrate aseptic care of central or IV line. • Demonstrate clean technique in hanging intravenous fluids and/or hyperalimentation.	1. Assess central and/or venous catheter as per institution's policy. 2. Change dressing of central and/or venous catheter per hospital policy. 3. Obtain and assess vital signs and appropriate laboratory values.	1. Provide patient with written instructions on care of central line and/or intravenous line. 2. Provide patient with the opportunity to change central and/or intravenous line dressing and solutions under nursing supervision.
Diarrhea Patient will verbalize an understanding of the relationship between diarrhea and the removal of more than 30% of the small intestine.	1. Determine patient's level of understanding related to diarrhea and small bowel syndrome. 2. Provide patient with the opportunity to ask questions.	1. Provide patient with information on small bowel syndrome.
Alteration in Skin Integrity Patient will: • Demonstrate appropriate perianal skin care following each episode of diarrhea. • Identify the resource person to call for assistance in managing skin irritation.	1. Provide patient with the needed equipment for performing perianal hygiene (i.e., a no-rinse perianal cleanser, moisture barrier). 2. Provide patient with the name and telephone number of the wound/skin care nurse. 3. Assess perianal skin every shift and as needed.	1. Instruct patient on proper care of perianal skin using demonstration. 2. Arrange a meeting with the wound/skin care nurse for patient to become familiar with this resource person.

undergoing cancer surgery has been summarized in several publications (Hoebler & Irwin, 1992; Polomano, Weintraub, & Wurster, 1994; Frogge & Kalinowski, 1997). Because the exact location of the tumor within the small intestine and the involvement of surrounding tissue or organs determine the extent of the surgery, the oncology nurse needs to know exactly what surgical procedure was performed so that he or she can know what to assess from various drains and tubes placed during surgery. Box 43-2 outlines the general and specific acute complications of small intestine surgery, along with their associated signs and symptoms (Hoebler & Irwin, 1992).

Nutritional repletion in the immediate postoperative period is most crucial for surgical oncology patients undergoing radical procedures resulting in extensive tissue trauma, alterations in the GI tract, and lengthy hospitalizations (Polomano et al., 1994). Unfortunately, preoperative malnutrition is associated with poor surgical outcomes such as sepsis, wound complications, ileus, and more lengthy hospital stays (Chen, Souba, & Copeland, 1991).

Nutrition

Nutritional care of the cancer patient should always be considered supportive, regardless of whether the goal is cure or palliation. The purpose of nutritional care is to support the patient's nutritional status, body composition, functional status, and quality of life. Although a host of factors may play a role in the occurrence of nutritional depletion in the patient with adenocarcinoma of the small intestine, the primary factors involve abnormalities of small intestine digestion and absorption along the small intestine along with tumor involvement by accessory organs such as the liver and pancreas. Because of the delay in diagnosis of small intestine cancers, nutritional compromise often already exists at the time of confirmed diagnosis.

Inadequate caloric and protein intake is the primary basis for clinically evident nutritional depletion in malignancy, with anorexia being the most common symptom contributing to poor nutrient intake (Ottery, 1995). Nutrition impact symptoms that impede oral intake include common GI complaints such as nausea/vomiting, stomatitis/mucositis, dysphagia, and diarrhea/constipation; sensory changes such as taste and olfaction; and problems with pain and anorexia. Ottery recommends standardized, cost-efficient nutritional assessment and aggressive symptom management to identify nutritional risk or deficit early enough to prevent progressive nutritional deterioration.

Nutritional impact symptoms in the patient with suspected or confirmed adenocarcinoma of the small intestine include the potential nausea, vomiting, and abdominal pain associated with a partial or complete intestine obstruction. Prompt relief of the intestine obstruction via intestine decompression or surgical intervention can restore the capacity for adequate intake of proper nutrients. In addition, the diarrhea and malabsorption associated with the underlying disruption of the absorptive function of the small intestine secondary to the tumor or the impact of surgical resection of the small intestine can have significant nutritional consequences. Adequate monitoring and appropriate replacement of fluids, electrolytes, vitamins, and minerals are critical to successful management of the impact of diarrhea and malabsorption in this patient population. Table 43-6 describes the nutritional and dietary considerations to decrease the occurrence and impact of diarrhea.

TABLE 43-6 Nutritional and Dietary Considerations for the Management of Diarrhea

Eat low-residue foods that are high in protein and calories.
Attempt small, frequent snacks rather than three large meals.
Avoid foods that irritate or stimulate the gastrointestinal tract.
Avoid extreme temperatures in foods or beverages.
Eliminate foods that are highly spiced or greasy.
Ensure adequate intake of uncarbonated beverages (2 to 3 quarts/day).
Eliminate lactose-containing foods and beverages to prevent lactose intolerance.
Utilize nutritional supplements to increase calorie and protein intake.
Consider a liquid diet or enteral nutritional support if diarrhea becomes severe.

From Doughty, D. B. & Jackson, D. B. (1993). *Gastrointestinal disorders.* St. Louis: Mosby.

TABLE 43-7 Management of Short Bowel Syndrome

Stage	Medical Management
Stage 1 (Postoperative phase)	NPO status NG suction during initial postoperative period IV fluids and TPN to supply nutrients, vitamins, minerals, fluids and electrolytes Careful monitoring of hemodynamic status
Stage 2 (2 months to 1-2 years postoperatively)	Gradual advancement of oral intake of nutrients and fluids Decrease in volume of TPN based on tolerance Begin with simple electroyte and carbohydrate solutions Advance to solutions of chemically defined diets with short-chain peptides and simple amino acids Progress to high-carbohydrate, high-protein, moderate-fat, low-lactose diet (Note: solids should be given separately from lipids) Supplement with short-chain and medium-chain triglycerides Monitor nutritional status closely
Stage 3 (Long-term management)	Oral intake as tolerated Oral intake sufficient to compensate for malabsorbed nutrients Enteral and/or parenteral supplementation for patients unable to maintain weight with oral feedings

Data from Doughty, D. B. & Jackson, D. B. (1993). *Gastrointestinal disorders.* St. Louis: Mosby.
NPO, nothing by mouth; *NG,* nasogastric; *IV,* intravenous; *TPN,* total parenteral nutrition.

Short Intestine Syndrome

Short intestine syndrome is a condition of malabsorption and malnutrition that follows major small intestine resection. This syndrome results when the length of functional small intestine is insufficient to provide adequate absorption of nutrients, vitamins, minerals, fluids, and electrolytes (Doughty & Jackson, 1993). Although much controversy exists over the precise length of intact intestine that is required for adequate absorptive capacity, it is now recognized that the minimal amount of small intestine required to maintain life without long-term parenteral nutrition support varies among patients. Factors that increase the risk of short intestine syndrome include resection of 75% or more of the small intestine (with residual length of less than 100 cm) and resection of the terminal ileum and ileocecal valve. If the duodenum, distal ileum, and ileocecal valve remain intact, most patients can tolerate the loss of 40% or more of the small intestine (Doughty & Jackson, 1993). Although short intestine syndrome occurs most commonly as a result of massive small intestine resection for management of medical conditions such as mesenteric vascular disease, volvulus, strangulated hernias, or massive abdominal trauma, the patient requiring surgical resection for small intestine adenocarcinoma should be monitored for signs and symptoms of short intestine syndrome during the immediate postoperative period, as well as 1 to 2 years after small intestine surgery.

Short intestine syndrome is characterized by steatorrhea, weight loss, malabsorption, malnutrition, and fluid-electrolyte abnormalities. In terms of clinical presentation, short intestine syndrome is commonly divided into three stages. Stage 1, characterized by massive diarrhea, begins immediately after resection of the small intestine and continues for about 2 months. The major challenge during this stage is to maintain fluid and electrolyte stability. Stage 2 typically begins about 2 months after the small intestine resection and lasts for 12 months or longer. This stage begins when the fecal output has stabilized at 2 L or less a day and signals the beginning of intestine adaptation. Stage 3 is considered the stabilization and long-term management phase and begins about 1 to 2 years after the intestine resection. Medical management throughout the various stages of short intestine syndrome is described in Table 43-7.

Although the specific manifestations of short intestine syndrome depend on the length and specific segment of small intestine that has been resected, one of the most debilitating effects of short intestine syndrome is intractable diarrhea. Diarrhea associated with this syndrome can be due to the loss of absorptive surface from the small intestine, the increase in fluid load to the colon, the increase in solute load due to undigested nutrients, hypermotility due to resection of the ileocecal valve, and the depletion of bile salts from the terminal ileum causing impaired fat absorption and steatorrhea. Massive small intestine resection resulting in fat intolerance can also lead to malabsorption of the fat-soluble vitamins A, D, E, and K. Water-soluble vitamins, although absorbed much more readily than fat-soluble vitamins, can also become deficient, as described in Table 43-8 (Doughty & Jackson, 1993). In addition, patients undergoing partial or total duodenectomy can develop mineral deficiencies of iron, calcium, and folic acid.

In addition to the malabsorption of micronutrients, other complications of short intestine syndrome include fluid and electrolyte imbalance, gastric hypersecretion, transient changes in liver function, cholelithiasis, and calcium oxalate renal stones. Patients with short intestine syndrome may initially lose as much as 5 L of fluid daily through the stool, resulting in hypovolemia, hypokalemia, hyponatremia, and metabolic acidosis. Proximal small intestine resections generally produce less long-term imbalance than distal small intestine resections (Doughty & Jackson, 1993). Gastric hypersecretion, a common secondary effect of short intestine syndrome, can result in complicating peptic ulcer disease, diffuse mucosal damage, and/or impaired intraluminal lipid digestion (Society of Gastroenterology Nurses and Associates, 1993). Although the exact etiology is not known, hy-

TABLE 43-8 Symptoms of Water-Soluble Vitamin Deficiencies

Vitamin	Function	Signs of Deficiency
B_1 (thiamine)	Supports carbohydrate and amino acid metabolism; required for growth	Muscle weakness, paralysis, neuritis
B_2 (riboflavin)	Involved in citric acid cycle	Fissures at corners of mouth, eye disorders
Pantothenic acid (component of B_2 complex)	Promotes gluconeogenesis and synthesis of steroid hormones; constituent of coenzyme A	Fatigue, neuromuscular dysfunction
B_3 (niacin)	Supports metabolic processes (glycolysis and citric acid cycle)	Diarrhea, dermatitis, mental confusion
B_6 (pyridoxine)	Amino acid metabolism	Dermatitis, growth retardation, nausea
Folic acid	Hematopoiesis and nucleic acid synthesis	Macrocytic anemia
B_{12} (cobalamin)	Erythrocyte production; nucleic acid and amino acid metabolism	Pernicious anemia, nervous system disorders (e.g., peripheral neuropathy)
C (ascorbic acid)	Collagen synthesis; protein metabolism	Delayed wound healing, capillary fragility, defective bone formation
H (biotin)	Fatty acid and purine synthesis; citric acid cycle	Fatigue, nausea, mental and muscle dysfunction

From Doughty, D. B. & Jackson, D. B. (1993). *Gastrointestinal disorders.* St. Louis: Mosby.

perbilirubinemia and jaundice are common developments during the initial period following small intestine resection. In addition, resection of the terminal ileum leads to the loss of bile salt reabsorption, which increases the potential for gallstone production. The incidence of calcium oxalate renal stones is also increased in the presence of steatorrhea secondary to the inability of dietary oxalate to bind with calcium in the intestine lumen, resulting in increased reabsorption of oxalate (Doughty & Jackson, 1993).

HOME CARE ISSUES

Significant changes in long-term oncology patient care, including the shift from the inpatient settings, to the outpatient and home care settings, play a significant role in the long-term management of the patient diagnosed with small intestine adenocarcinoma. Home care needs of the patient diagnosed with small intestine malignancy depend on the stage of the patient's disease. Because of the primary role that surgery plays in the treatment of small intestine adenocarcinomas, care of the postoperative patient in the home is typically the most significant home care issue in the early period after diagnosis (see Chapter 3).

PROGNOSIS

Prognosis for small intestine adenocarcinomas is grim; 5-year survival rate ranges from 5% to 32%. Disease stage and regional lymph node involvement are the most critical prognostic factors (Donohue & Kelly, 1991). Ouriel and Adams (1984) reported some of the more positive results, with 65% considered amenable to curative resection and an overall 5-year survival rate of 30%. When nodes were negative, 70% were alive at 5 years, whereas only 13% with positive nodes lived as long. When analyzed stage for stage, survival was similar to that for patients with colonic carcinoma, suggesting that the poorer prognosis is related for the most part to the greater delay in diagnosis of small intestine lesions.

EVALUATION OF THE QUALITY OF CARE

External accreditation organizations such as the Joint Commission for the Accreditation of Health Care Organizations, along with internal hospital-based Quality Monitoring departments, require that quality of care provided to patients be evaluated. Because of the integral role that surgery and home care play in the management of the patient with adenocarcinoma of the small intestine, the evaluation of quality of care provided to these patients should incorporate input from a multidisciplinary team, including the surgical oncologist, oncology nurse, anesthesiologist, dietitian, pain service, physical therapist, discharge planner, and home care nurse. Table 43-9 provides examples of tools that can be used in the treatment setting.

TABLE 43-9 Quality of Care for the Patient with Short Bowel Syndrome

Prospective chart review for documentation. Compliance demonstrated by score of 80%.
Disciplines participating in the quality of care evaluation:
☐ Nursing ☐ Surgery ☐ Dietary

Criteria	YES	NO
1. Was there an assessment of perianal skin every 8 hours?	☐	☐
2. Was there an application of skin protectant after each bowel movement and as needed?	☐	☐
3. Was there an accurate input and output for last 24 hours?	☐	☐
4. Was there an assessment of serum electrolytes?	☐	☐
5. Did the patient have a consultation with a nutritionist?	☐	☐
6. Was the patient educated with relation to changes in bowel patterns?	☐	☐
7. Was there intravenous line care?	☐	☐
8. Was there an assessment of hydration status every 8 hours?	☐	☐
9. Was there an initiation of discharge planning?	☐	☐
10. Was there an assessment of surgical site and drains?	☐	☐

RESEARCH ISSUES

Because small intestine malignancies are so rare, major research questions directed at diagnosis and treatment are somewhat limited. Increased understanding of the risk factors associated with small intestine malignancy, including the relationship with diet, environment, and underlying genetic-related medical history, may increase the knowledge regarding other GI malignancies. In addition, *Helicobacter pylori* has been linked closely to gastric cancer, yet appears to be unrelated to colorectal cancer. Because its relationship to small intestine malignancies is unknown, further research may be warranted (Chow et al., 1996).

REFERENCES

Alexander, J. W. & Altemeier, W. A. (1968). Association of primary neoplasms of the small intestine with other neoplastic growths. *Annals of Surgery, 167*, 958-964.

Ashley, S. W. & Wells, S. A. (1988). Tumors of the small intestine. *Seminars in Oncology, 15*(2), 116-28.

Bagg, A. (1988). Whipple's procedure: Nursing guidelines. *Critical Care Nurse, 8*(5), 34-45.

Beahrs, O. H., Henson, D. E., Hutton, R., & Kennedy, B. J. (1992). *Handbook for staging of cancer: From the manual for staging of cancer.* American Joint Committee on Cancer. (4th ed.). Philadelphia: J. B. Lippincott.

Bowden, T. A. (1989). Endoscopy of the small intestine. *Surgical Clinics of North America, 69*(6), 1237-1247.

Chen, C. C., Neugut, A. I., Rotterdam, H. (1994). Risk factors for adenocarcinomas and malignant carcinoids of the small intestine: Preliminary findings. *Cancer Epidemiology, Biomarkers, and Prevention, 3*(3), 205-207.

Chen, M. K., Souba, W. W., & Copeland, E. M. (1991). Nutritional support of the surgical oncology patient. *Hematology-Oncology Clinics of North America, 5*(1), 125-145.

Chow, J. S., Chen, C. C., Ahsan, H., & Neugut, A. I. (1996). A population-based study of the incidence of malignant small intestine: SEER, 1973-1990. *International Journal of Epidemiology, 25*(4), 722-728.

Coit, D. G. (1993). Cancer of the small intestine. In V. T. DeVita, S. Hellman, & S. A. Rosenberg (Eds.), *Cancer: Principles and practice of oncology* (4th ed.). Philadelphia, J.B. Lippincott.

Coleman, J. (1997). Esophageal, stomach, liver, gallbladder, and pancreatic cancer. In S. Groenwald, M. Frogge, M. Goodman, & C. Yarbro C. (Eds.), *Cancer nursing: Principles and practice* (4th ed.). Boston: Jones & Bartlett.

Cooper, B. T., Holmes, G. K. T., Ferguson, R., & Cooke, W. T. (1980). Celiac disease and malignancy. *Medicine, 59*(4), 249-261.

DiSario, J. A., Burt, R. W., Vargas, H., & McWhorter, W. P. (1994). Small bowel cancer: Epidemiological and clinical characteristics from a population-based registry. *American Journal of Gastroenterology, 89*(5), 699-701.

Donohue, J. H. & Kelly, K. A. (1991). Cancer of the small intestine. In A. R. Moossa, S. C. Schimpff, & M. C. Robson (Eds.), *Comprehensive textbook of oncology* (2nd ed.). Baltimore: Williams & Wilkins.

Doughty, D. B. & Jackson, D. B. (1993). *Gastrointestinal disorders.* St. Louis: Mosby.

Dozois, R. R., Judd, E. S., Dahlin, D. C., & Bartholomew, L. G. (1969). The Peutz-Jeghers syndrome. Is there a predisposition to the development of intestinal malignancy. *Archives of Surgery, 98*(4), 509-517.

Ellis, H. (1987). Tumors of the small intestine. *Seminars in Surgical Oncology, 3*(1), 12-21.

Fresko, D., Lazarus, S. S., Dotan, J., & Reingold, M. (1982). Early presentation of carcinoma of the small bowel in Crohn's disease ("Crohn's carcinoma"): Case reports and review of literature. *Gastroenterology, 82*(4), 783-789.

Frogge, M. & Kalinowski, B. (1997). Surgical therapy. In S. Groenwald, M. Frogge, M. Goodman, & C. Yarbro (Eds.), *Cancer nursing: Principles and practice* (4th ed.). Boston: Jones & Bartlett.

Gabos, S., Berkel, J., Band, P., Robson, D., & Whittaker, H. (1993). Small bowel cancer in western Canada. *International Journal of Epidemiology, 22*(2), 198-206.

Hart, R. & Levin, B. (1993). Neoplasms of the small intestine. In P. Calabresi & P. Schein, (Eds.), *Medical oncology: Basic principles and clinical management of cancer* (2nd ed.). New York: McGraw-Hill.

Haskell, C. M., Lavey, R. S., & Ramming, K. P. (1995). Small intestine. In C. M. Haskell (Ed.), *Cancer treatment* (4th ed.). Philadelphia: W.B. Saunders.

Herbsman, H., Wetstein, L., Rosen, Y., Orecs, H., Alfonsoe, A. E., Iyer, S. K., & Gardner, B. (1980). Tumors of the small intestine. *Current Problems in Surgery, 17*(3), 121-182.

Hoebler, L. & Irwin, M. M. (1992). Gastrointestinal tract cancer: Current knowledge, medical treatment, and nursing management. *Oncology Nursing Forum, 19*(9), 1403-1415.

Jeghers, H., McKusick, V. A., & Katz, K. H. (1949). Generalized intestinal polyposis and spots of oral mucosa, legs, and digits: Syndrome of diagnostic significance. *New England Journal of Medicine, 291,* 993-996.

Lai, E. C., Doty, J. E., Irving, C., & Tompkins, R. K. (1988). Primary adenocarcinoma of the duodenum: Analysis of survival. *World Journal of Surgery, 12*(5), 695-699.

Landis, S. H., Murray, T., Bolden, S., & Wingo, P. A. (1998). Cancer statistics, 1998. *CA: A Cancer Journal for Clinicians, 48,* 6-10.

Laurent, F., Raynaud, M., Biset, J. M., Boisserie-Lacroix, M., Grelet, P., & Drouillard, J. (1991). Diagnosis and categorization of small bowel neoplasms: Role of computed tomography. *Gastrointestinal Radiology, 16*(2), 115-119.

Loescher, L. (1997). Dynamics of cancer prevention. In S. Groenwald, M. Frogge, M. Goodman, & C. Yarbro (Eds.), *Cancer nursing: Principles and practice* (4th ed.). Boston: Jones & Bartlett.

Lowenfels, A. B. (1973). Why are small-bowel tumours so rare? *Lancet, 1*(7793), 24-26.

Lynch, H. T., Smyrk, T. C., Lynch, P. M., Lanspa, S. J., Boman, B. M., Ens, J., Lynch, J. F., Strayhorn, P., Carmody, T., & Cristofaro, G. (1989). Adenocarcinoma of the small intestine in Lynch syndrome II. *Cancer, 64*(10), 2178-2183.

Lynch, J. (1997). The genetics and natural history of hereditary colon cancer. *Seminars in Oncology Nursing, 13*(2), 91-98.

Maglinte, D. D., O'Connor, K., Bessette, J., Chernish, S. M., & Kelvin, F. M. (1991). The role of the physician in the late diagnosis of primary malignant tumors of the small intestine. *American Journal of Gastroenterology, 86*(3), 304-308.

Martin, R. G. (1994). Malignant tumors of the small bowel. In R. J. McKenna & G. P Murphy (Eds.), *Cancer surgery.* Philadelphia: J. B. Lippincott.

Neugut, A. I. & Santos, J. (1993). The association between cancers of the small and large bowel. *Cancer Epidemiology, Biomarkers, & Prevention, 2*(6), 551-553.

Ottery, F. D. (1995). Supportive nutrition to prevent cachexia and improve quality of life. *Seminars in Oncology, 22*(Suppl. 3), 98-111.

Ouriel, K. & Adams, J.T. (1984). Adenocarcinoma of the small intestine. *American Journal of Surgery,* 147(1), 66-71.

Peacock, J.L., Keller, J.W., & Asbury, R.F. (1993). Alimentary cancer. In P. Rubin (Ed.), *Clinical oncology: A multidisciplinary approach for physicians and students* (7th ed.). Philadelphia: W. B. Saunders.

Perzin, K. H. & Bridge, M. F. (1982). Adenomatous and carcinomatous changes in hamartomatous polyps of the small intestine (Peutz-Jeghers syndrome): A report of a case and review of the literature. *Cancer, 49*(5), 971-983.

Polomano, R., Weintraub, F.N., & Wurster, A. (1994). Surgical critical care for cancer patients. *Seminars in Oncology Nursing, 10*(3), 165-176.

Ross, R. K., Hartnett, N. M., Bernstein, L., & Henderson, B. E. (1991). Epidemiology of adenocarcinomas of the small intestine: Is bile a small bowel carcinogen? *British Journal of Cancer, 63*(1), 143-145.

Schnur, P. L., David, E., Brown, P. W., Beahrs, O. H., Remine, W. H., & Harrison, E. G. (1973). Adenocarcinoma of the duodenum and the Gardner syndrome. *Journal of the American Medical Association, 223*(11), 1229-1232.

Sellner, F. (1990). Investigations on the significance of the adenoma-carcinoma sequence in the small intestine. *Cancer, 66*(4), 702-705.

Society of Gastroenterology Nurses & Associates (1993). *Gastroenterology nursing: A core curriculum.* St Louis: Mosby.

Spigelman, A. D., Murday, V., & Phillips, R. K. (1990). Cancer and the Peutz-Jeghers syndrome. *Gut, 30*(11), 1588-1590.

Surveillance, Epidemiology, & End Results (SEER) Program. (1993). Special public use tape (1973-1990). Bethesda, MD: National Cancer Institute, DCPC, Surveillance Program, Cancer Statistics Grant, November 1993.

Swinson, C. M., Slavin, G., Coles, E. C., & Booth, C. C. (1983). Coeliac disease and malignancy. *Lancet, 1*(8316), 111-115.

Viamonte, M. & Viamonte, M. (1992) Primary squamous-cell carcinoma of the small bowel: Report of a case. *Diseases of the Colon & Rectum, 35*(8), 806-809.

Watson, P. & Lynch, H. T. (1993). Extracolonic cancer in hereditary nonpolyposis colorectal cancer. *Cancer, 71*(3), 677-685.

Yao, T., Ida, M., Ohsato, K., Watanabe, H., Omae, T. (1977). Duodenal lesions in familial polyposis of the colon. *Gastroenterology, 73*(5), 1086-1092.

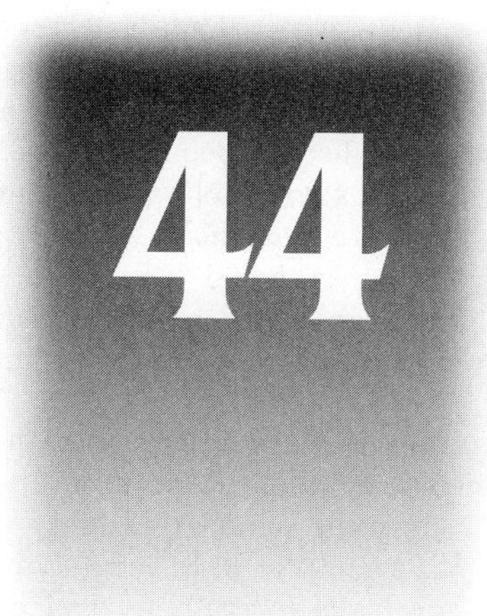

44 Lymphoma of the Small Intestine

Sharon A. Aronovitch, PhD, RN, CETN

EPIDEMIOLOGY

Chow and associates reported in the Surveillance, Epidemiology, and End-Results (SEER) study (Chow, Chen, Ahsan, & Neugut, 1996) that, although the occurrence of small intestine tumors is very low, the annual rate of incidence is 9.9 per 1 million people, an increase from the reported rate of 1.6 cases per million people in 1987 (Donohue & Kelly, 1991). The annual incidence rate of lymphoma was 1.1 per million people. The rarity of small intestine cancer is attributed to its inherent protective mechanism related to its rapid transit time of food stuffs, relatively low level of microorganisms, and alkalinity of intestinal fluid, which decrease the intensity of mucosal exposure to carcinogenics (Donohue & Kelly, 1991; Ashley & Wells, 1988; Lowenfels, 1973).

Lymphoma of the small intestine can be either a primary tumor, although it is rarely a solitary lesion, or a manifestation of an extensively disseminated systemic disease such as non-Hodgkin's type lymphoma. As a primary lesion, lymphomas measure more than 5 cm and typically extend beneath the mucosa to a great extent (Ashley & Wells, 1988; Herbsman, Wetstein, Rosen, Orecs, Alfonsoe, & Iyer et al., 1980). Microscopic examination of the small intestine reveals diffuse infiltration of the intestinal wall.

A primary lymphoma of the small intestine constitutes less than 4% of gastrointestinal (GI) malignancies and accounts for 17% of all small intestine malignancies (Coit, 1997). It is estimated that the number of new cases of small intestine malignancies diagnosed in 1996 was 4600, which resulted in 1140 deaths (Daniel, 1997).

The average age for small intestine cancer is 57 years, but the range has been documented from 1 to 84 years old (Daniel, 1997). Survival at 5 years is 20% and drops to 5% with a late diagnosis (Hawks, 1997), although a study completed using the Utah Cancer Registry reported 5-year survival rates of 54% (DiSario, Burt, Vargas, & McWhorter, 1994).

The incidence of primary small intestine lymphoma increases as the tumor is more distal from the stomach; the primary site is the ileum (Coit, 1997). This is an obvious site given the amount of lymphatic tissue located at this area. Between 1985 and 1990, the incidence of small intestine lymphoma nearly doubled (Coit, 1997). It is speculated that this has occurred because of an increase in the immunocompromised patient population (i.e., acquired immune deficiency syndrome [AIDS], transplantations) and the immigration of individuals from developing countries. Lymphoma of the small intestine can be divided into five distinct subtypes: adult Western type, pediatric type (Burkitt's lymphoma), immunoproliferative small intestinal disease (IPSID), enteropathy associated T-cell lymphoma, and Hodgkin's lymphoma.

The most common type, the Western type, occurs predominately in men between the ages of 54 and 61 years (Coit, 1997). Two thirds of this type are of B-cell origin and the rest are of T-cell origin (Sarna & Kagan, 1995). T-cell lymphoma is reported to have a poorer prognosis than the B-cell type (Sarna & Kagan, 1995). Tumors found in the distal small intestine are of B-cell origin and are high grade (Sarna & Kagan, 1995). Patients typically present with complaints of abdominal pain related to a partial intestine obstruction, and the most common finding is a mass. Ten percent of these patients also have a perforation and 90% have anemia (Coit, 1997).

Childhood lymphoma is the second major type of lymphoma of the small intestine (Coit, 1997). It generally occurs in children under the age of 15 years. On histologic examination, nearly half of these lymphomas resemble Burkitt's lymphoma. Prognosis for this form of lymphoma is improving with the use of combination therapies such as surgery and chemotherapy.

Immunoproliferative, or Mediterranean, lymphoma ranks third and is the most common lymphoma in the Middle East and African countries. Its occurrence is equal between the sexes and is most often found in young adults; the median age is 30 years. Mediterranean lymphoma generally involves the entire small intestine. Patients present with a mass (Coit, 1997). It is theorized that the tumor may evolve from IPSID, which is manifested by diarrhea, malabsorption, clubbing, and plasma cell infiltration of the small intestine (Sarna & Kagan, 1995). This form of lymphoma is occasionally associated with monoclonal alpha chains in the blood. It is presumed that the etiology is related to parasites or other infections, as well as a racial and genetic predisposition (Sarna & Kagan, 1995).

Enteropathy-associated T-cell lymphoma is rare and most often seen in the Middle East (Coit, 1997). It is typically associated with a history of malabsorption and celiac disease. It is theorized that unrestricted proliferation of the T-cell clones from the reactive T-cell population in the enteropathic intestine is the precursor to malignancy (Coit, 1997).

Primary Hodgkin's lymphoma of the small intestine is very rare and accounts for less than 3% of all small intestine lymphomas (Coit, 1997). It usually is not a primary tumor, but represents impingement of mesenteric lymphadenopathy (Coit, 1997).

RISK FACTORS

Disease and environmental factors predisposing to small intestine lymphoma are specific to the intestinal tract (Box 44-1). Crohn's disease and celiac sprue are two of the most often identified intestinal diseases. Nontropical sprue has also been indicated as a possible intestinal risk factor. Alteration of the immune system secondary to drug therapies required after transplantation surgeries or human immunodeficiency virus infection are considered to be risk factors. Environmental factors have focused on developing nations and Mediterranean countries (Chen, Neugut, & Rotterdam, 1994).

Crohn's disease is a nonsegmental ulceration of the alimentary tract that can occur from mouth to anus. It is known as a *transmural disease* because it affects all layers of the intestine. Forty percent of patients will have involvement of the ileocecal area of the small intestine, with the vast majority having involvement of the ileum and in particular the terminal ileum (Farmer, 1989). There is an increased risk of 3% to 5% for the development of cancer from irritable intestine disease that has involved the entire colon for 10 years (Blackstone, 1989).

Celiac disease is an intestinal disorder characterized by intolerance of gluten, a protein found in wheat and wheat products (see Chapter 43). Patients with a long history of celiac disease have a 7% to 10% lifetime risk of developing cancer (Anonymous, 1996). Because lymphoma develops in only a small percentage of these patients, its course is rapid and malignant. Although the progression of celiac disease to lymphoma is not known, it is theorized that this disease may be a low-grade lymphoma of intraepithelial lymphocytes (Anonymous, 1996) or a premalignant disorder (Cooper, Holmes, Ferguson, & Cooke, 1980; Swinson, Slavin, Coles, & Booth, 1983).

Immunosuppression related to AIDS or organ transplantation, as well as immunoproliferative small intestine disease or enteropathy T-cell lymphoma, are risk factors for malignancy. Although the occurrence of extranodal lymphoma involving the small intestine is generally recognized in this patient population, the incidence and pattern of intestine involvement in these immunodeficient states vary considerably. Alexander and Altemeier (1968) reported that 83 of 112 patients with a primary tumor of the small intestine had another independent neoplasm at the time of death. It is speculated that there is some connection between the second primary tumor and the suspected defect in the immunosurveillance system of the small intestine.

Box 44-1
Risk Factors for Lymphoma of the Small Bowel

Crohn's disease
Celiac disease
Nontropical sprue
Immunocompromised patient
- Human immunodeficiency virus
- Posttransplant
- Immunoproliferative disorder of small intestine

Environmental factors
- Developing nations
- Mediterranean countries

From Coit, D. G. (1997). Cancer of the small intestine. In V. T. DeVita, S. Hellman, & S. Rosenberg (Eds.), *Cancer: Principles and practice of oncology* (5th ed.). Philadelphia: J. B. Lippincott.

CHEMOPREVENTION

Chemoprevention has been defined as the use of noncytotoxic nutrients and/or pharmacologic agents to inhibit or reverse the process of carcinogenesis (Loescher, 1997). The majority of research in this area has focused on cancers related to the bladder, breast, cervix, colon, head and neck, lung, prostate, and skin. It is not known when research will be conducted on chemoprevention related to the small intestine. Given the fact that small intestine cancer is rare compared with breast, colon, or lung cancer, the search for prevention is not a priority at this time.

PATHOPHYSIOLOGY

Normal Anatomy and Physiology of the Small Intestine

The small bowel is a tubular structure that extends from the pyloric sphincter to the ileal cecal valve, measuring about 6.7 to 7.0 m (22 to 23 feet) in length and about 1.9 to 3.8 cm (0.75 to 1.5 in) in diameter. The wall of the small bowel consists of four layers: the outer serous layer (serosa), the muscular layer (muscularis externa), the submucosal layer, and a thin layer of smooth muscle (muscularis mucosae), which separates the mucosa from the submucosa (see Fig. 43-1)

The small intestine is divided into three segments: the duodenum, jejunum, and ileum. The duodenum, the shortest and widest segment of the small intestine, consists of the first 30 cm (12 in) of the small intestine, beginning at the pyloric sphincter and ending at the ligament of Treitz. The jejunum is the next 40% of small intestine and the remaining 60% is the ileum. The division between the jejunum and the ileum is arbitrary.

The primary function of the small intestine is the absorption of nutrients from the chyme. Although the small intestine receives up to 8 L of fluid per day, it passes only 500 to 1000 ml on to the large intestine, with the rest of the fluid absorbed by the columnar cells of the villous epithelium. The process of absorption through the wall of the small intestine occurs through a variety of mechanisms including hydrolysis, nonionic movement, passive diffusion, facilitated diffusion, active transport, or combinations thereof (Society of Gastrointestinal Nurses & Associates, 1993).

The cells of the small intestine are not only responsible for the secretion of digestive juices, mucus, and a variety of hormones and peptides, but they also receive secretions from the liver and the pancreas. Movements of the small intestine wall contribute to the mixing of the chyme. The concentric, segmenting contractions of the jejunum help mix the chyme particles with the secretions of the small intestine. The peristaltic contractions of the first portion of the duodenum and the jejunum slowly push the chyme in the direction of the colon. The ongoing shortening and lengthening of the villi stirs the intestinal contents.

The Process of Carcinogenesis

Given the differences in length between the different segments of the small intestine, the mucosa of the duodenum shows a substantially higher propensity toward malignant transformation compared with the jejunum and ileum. The pathophysiology of small intestine lymphoma has been classified using the Rappaport system, which classifies it into three types: non-Hodgkin's lymphomas (60%), lymphocytic tumors (25%), and mixed type (15%). Forty percent of non–Hodgkin's lymphoma of the small intestine can be diffuse large cell, and 20% are immunoblastic.

The Kiel system classifies lymphomas by morphology and cell surface markers (Coit, 1997). Lymphomas are typically graded as intermediate or high grade. Although histologic grading of this type of tumor is still evolving, grading of lymphoma is still predictive of long-term outcome.

ROUTES OF METASTASES

Small intestine lymphoma is most likely to metastasize to the lymph nodes. Distant metastasis is most often found near the diaphragm and spleen. Patients with a primary neoplasm of the small intestine are more prone to development of a primary neoplasm in another site of the body (Alexander & Altemeier, 1968). The small intestine is the site for metastatic disease arising from primary neoplasms of other organs, primarily the uterus, cervix, lung, breast, kidney, urinary bladder, ovary, and skin (Haskell, Lavey, & Ramming, 1995).

ASSESSMENT

Patients typically present with surgical emergencies owing to the difficulty in diagnosing small intestine lymphoma. Symptoms of intestine obstruction, perforation, and massive hemorrhage bring the patient to the hospital for immediate treatment. Definitive diagnosis is made at the time of laparotomy. The most frequently reported symptoms not requiring emergent surgery are weight loss, weakness, lower abdominal pain, and bleeding (Hoebler & Irwin, 1992). Radiologic tests are inconclusive because this disease is easily confused with other segmental diseases of the small intestine such as Crohn's disease. Also, many times an incorrect test or reading of the x-ray film has resulted in misdiagnosis (Maglinte, O'Connor, Bessette, Chernish, & Kelvin, 1991). A computerized tomography (CT) scan provides a better means of differentiating between segmental intestine diseases.

Patient History

The assessment of a patient suspected of having an lymphoma of the small intestine includes obtaining a detailed personal and family medical history for the presence of high-risk GI diseases, completing a thorough physical examination and review of the patient's GI system, and performing a variety of diagnostic tests. For patients with a preexisting history of Crohn's disease, celiac disease, or immunosuppression who present with symptoms of possible GI changes while under the care of their primary physician, the primary focus of care should be directed toward obtaining the necessary diagnostic tests to fully evaluate their GI symptoms. Table 44-1 illustrates a guideline for patients with suspected lymphoma of the small intestine.

Signs and Symptoms

Clinical detection of both benign and malignant small intestine tumors can be difficult and requires special attention to various signs and symptoms. Unlike with other types of small intestine carcinomas, patients usually present when symptoms have lasted less than 6 months (Donahue & Kelly, 1991). The majority of patients present with generalized symptoms of fatigue, malaise, anorexia, and weight loss. Complaints of interrupted intestine function include cramping, nausea, vomiting, constipation, diarrhea, and malabsorption. Occult blood in the stool and hemorrhage are the more common presentations (Donahue & Kelly, 1991). A palpable abdominal mass can be felt in 20% to 60% of patients (Donahue & Kelly, 1991). Patients with a known diagnosis of celiac disease who present with generalized symptoms and worsening of malabsorption should be evaluated for small intestine lymphoma (Donahue & Kelly, 1991).

Diagnostic Tests

Radiography. An upper GI series with small intestine follow-through can detect abnormalities caused by lymphoma in 90% of cases (Hoebler & Irwin, 1992; Donahue & Kelly, 1991). The presenting picture is of an aneurysmal dilation of an involved loop (Donahue & Kelly, 1991). A CT scan accurately locates the small intestine lymphoma and

TABLE 44-1 Assessment of the Patient for Lymphoma of the Small Bowel

	Assessment Parameters	Typical Abnormal Findings
History	A. Personal and social history 1. Age 2. Ethnicity 3. Family history 4. Prior history	A. Personal and social risk factors 1. 60-70 years of age 2. Mediterranean countries 3. Familial gastrointestinal syndromes 4. Crohn's disease, celiac disease and immunodeficiency states may be predisposing factors.
	B. Evaluation of gastrointestinal tract	B. Symptoms depend on location and tumor size. Common symptoms include intermittent abdominal pain; vague and indistinct cramping, which may be due to partial small bowel obstruction due to tumor infiltration and adhesions; intermittent nausea and vomiting; change in bowel habits; unexplained weight loss due to anorexia and tumor growth; and pallor, dyspnea, shortness of breath due to anemia from chronic blood loss due to mucosal ulceration. Weakness, malaise, and fatigue
Physical Examination	A. Palpation of abdominal area B. Weight	A. Rarely reveals mass B. Weight loss may indicate tumor growth in the presence of other symptoms
	C. Pallor, dyspnea, shortness of breath.	C. May indicate anemia secondary to chronic bleeding
Diagnostic Tests	A. Upper gastrointestinal series B. Upper gastrointestinal endoscopy with total duodenoscopy	A. May reveal suspicion of duodenum adenocarcinoma B. May allow for histologic confirmation of tumor
	C. Radiographic films D. Complete blood count	C. May show mass and localized tumor D. Microcytic, hypochromic anemia associated with chronic blood loss of small bowel malignancy
	E. Liver function tests	E. May be elevated due to biliary obstruction or hepatic metastasis

From Ashley, S. W. & Wells, S. A. (1988). Tumors of the small intestine. *Seminars in Oncology, 15* (2), 116-128; DiSario, J. A., Burt, R. W., Vargas, H., & McWhorter, W. P. (1994). Small bowel cancer: Epidemiological and clinical characteristics from a population-based registry. *American Journal of Gastroenterology, 89*(5), 699-701.

may be helpful in the staging process. Table 44-2 presents a teaching guide for patients undergoing upper GI radiographic tests.

Endoscopy. An endoscopy is not typically used for diagnosis of lymphoma given the usual location of the terminal ileum and ileocecal valve. However, it is useful in diagnosis for patients with celiac disease or Mediterranean lymphoma.

Laboratory Tests

Routine blood tests rarely show any abnormality, with the exception of microcytic, hypochromic anemia associated with the chronic blood loss of small intestine malignancy. No specific serologic tests exist for small intestine cancers, except for the possibility of high levels of serum immunoglobulin A, which would clue the clinician into further investigating the patient's presenting symptoms.

STAGING

Staging of lymphomas of the small intestine can be accomplished using one of two staging systems: Ann Arbor or Blackledge. The Ann Arbor system (Table 44-3) has been traditionally used to stage lymphomas, but the tool was modified for this purpose and not specifically designed for staging small intestine lymphoma. In light of this problem, the Blackledge staging system was developed to capture the prognostic significance or intestine perforation (Table 44-4).

A modification of the Ann Arbor classification was developed to identify the extent of a GI lymphoma in relation to the patient's probable prognosis (Table 44-5). The Dukes system of staging has been used most often; however, it does not accurately describe the characteristics found in small intestine lymphoma.

MEDICAL MANAGEMENT

Optimal therapy for management of small intestine lymphoma has not been established. Most clinicians agree that surgery is the preferred management; however, some institutions are beginning to give patients adjunctive therapies.

Surgery

The principles of surgical resection include attainment of negative surgical margins and wide resection of the corresponding mesentery of the involved segment of intestine

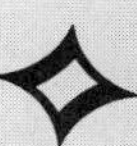

TABLE 44-2 Patient Preparation for Undergoing Diagnostic Gastrointestinal Procedures

Description of the Procedure: Suspected small bowel tumors may be evaluated using both invasive and noninvasive gastrointestinal diagnostic procedures, which may include radiography, endoscopy, computerized tomography (CT), or ultrasonography.

Patient Preparation: The patient is usually instructed to refrain from fluid and food for a predetermined period before the procedure and is instructed on preparation of the bowel for better visualization during the procedure.

Procedural Considerations:

1. Review past medical and surgical history along with current medications for any potential contraindications to performing the diagnostic procedure.
2. Review laboratory results for any abnormalities that would preclude performing the diagnostic procedure.
3. Thoroughly explain the diagnostic procedure to patient, including:
   - the purpose and approximate length of the test.
   - the type of positioning and special techniques to be used.
   - anticipated effect of any medications or anesthetics that will be used.
   - any sensations the patient may experience during and after the procedure, and
   - potential risks and complications that might be encountered during or after the procedure.
4. Obtain informed consent.
5. Confirm length of NPO status and adherence to preprocedural dietary restrictions.
6. Verify completion of specified bowel preparation if indicated.
7. Obtain baseline vital signs and establish patent IV line if indicated.

(Coit, 1997). Mesentery containing lymph nodes draining the area in which the lesion is located are removed; note that removal of large amounts of mesentery jeopardizes the blood supply to the small intestine. An end-to-end anastomosis of the remaining intestine is usually possible, except in some cases of ileocolic anastomosis, which may require end-to-side anastomosis.

When malignant tumors of the terminal ileum are part of the operative procedure, a right colectomy is usually included because the removal of lymph nodes that drain the ileum can interfere with the blood supply to the ascending colon (Hampton & Bryant, 1992). Tumor extending into the mesentery may involve blood vessels that cannot be resected without sacrificing large segments of the small intestine.

In nonresectable lesions, palliative bypass should be performed to relieve the symptoms of obstruction, perforation, or GI bleeding. Primary resection for metastatic lesions is justified to prevent or relieve the complications of obstruction or bleeding (Sarna & Kagan, 1995).

TABLE 44-3 Ann Arbor Staging System

Stage	Description
I	Single nodal group or single nodal site (IE)
II	More than one nodal group on the same side of diaphragm or single extranodal site with one or more nodal groups on the same side of diagram (IIE)
III	Nodes on both sides of diaphragm, with or without extranodal sites (IIIE), spleen (IIIS), or both (IIIES)
IV	Diffuse involvement of viscera or bone marrow

Modified from Coit, D. G. (1997). Cancer of the small intestine. In V. T. DeVita, S. Hellman, & S. A. Rosenberg (Eds.), *Cancer: Principles and practice of oncology* (5th ed.). Philadelphia: J. B. Lippincott.

TABLE 44-4 Blackledge Staging System

Stage	Description
I	Confined to gastrointestinal (GI) tract
II	Local mesenteric nodal involvement
III	Perforation at tumor site
IV	Distant nodal involvement (para-aortic and beyond)
V	Visceral or bone marrow involvement

Modified from Coit, D. G. (1997). Cancer of the small intestine. In V. T. DeVita, S. Hellman, & S. A. Rosenberg (Eds.), *Cancer: Principles and practice of oncology* (5th ed.). Philadelphia: J. B. Lippincott.

TABLE 44-5 Classification of Gastrointestinal Lymphoma

Stage	Extent of Disease
I_E	Confined to bowel
II_{1E}	Adjacent lymph node involvement
II_{2E}	Regional, nonadjacent lymph node involvement
III	Lymph node involvement on both sides of diaphragm, localized extralymphatic nodes, and/or spleen involvement
IV	Diffuse or disseminated disease

Modified from Donohue, J.H. & Kelly, K.A. (1991). Cancer of the small intestine. In A. R. Moossa, S. C. Schimpff, & M. C. Robson (Eds.). *Comprehensive textbook of oncology* (2nd ed.). Baltimore: Williams & Wilkins.

Radiation Therapy

Typically, lymphoma of the small intestine is resistant to radiation therapy. Lower levels of external radiation are being administered to provide palliation of symptoms such as pain or obstruction when alternative therapies are limited (Hoebler & Irwin, 1992). Studies are now

TABLE 44-6 Standard of Care for the Patient with Potential Alteration in Skin Integrity

Patient Problem and Outcome	Nursing Interventions and Rationale	Patient Education Instructions
Potential Risk for Pressure Ulcer		
Patient will maintain intact skin integrity.	1. Complete a skin risk assessment tool on admission and with any untoward change in patient's condition. 2. Provide supportive devices per institution's policy.	1. Instruction on what pressure ulcers are and how a pressure ulcer can be prevented.
Malnutrition		
Patient will: • Verbalize an understanding of the effect of poor nutrition on intact skin. • Maintain acceptable weight for height, age and, gender.	1. Assess patient's level of understanding of malnutrition and relation to potential loss of intact skin integrity. 2. Weigh weekly. 3. Maintain accurate intake and output. 4. Collaborate with dietician to obtain appropriate calories and nutrients during a 24-hour period. 5. Provide patient with the opportunity to ask questions.	1. Provide patient with information on nutrition related to skin integrity and healing. 2. Instruct patient to weigh self daily and record. 3. Instruct patient on maintaining an accurate record of intake (nutrients and fluids) and output (urine and stool).
Decreased Serum Albumin (Less than 2.8 gm/dl)		
Patient will: • Verbalize an understanding of the relationship between low serum albumin and high risk of skin breakdown. • Identify foods high in protein.	1. Monitor serum albumin weekly. 2. Collaborate with dietitian to provide patient with favorite foods that are high in protein.	1. Provide patient with information on foods high in protein.
Hydration		
Patient will: • Maintain adequate hydration of tissues. • Describe the effect of dehydration on the skin.	1. Monitor intake and output. 2. Encourage oral fluid intake of at least six to eight 8-oz glasses per day. 3. Assess mucous membranes every 8 hours. 4. Observe for signs of lethargy, increased fatigue. 5. Monitor serum Hct and Hgb for any increase.	1. Instruction on the importance of adequate fluid intake.

demonstrating that intraoperative radiation therapy is more beneficial in long-term survival rates (Hoebler & Irwin, 1992).

Adjuvant radiotherapy may be of benefit in patients with nonbulky stages I_E and II_{1E} tumors (Donahue & Kelly, 1991). For patients with stage IV tumors, radiation is considered palliative. Total abdominal radiation for Mediterranean lymphoma can achieve a complete response and disease-free survival beyond 1 year (Sarna & Kagan, 1995).

Chemotherapy

Systemic chemotherapy is given to patients with GI tumor classifications of stages II_{2E}, III, and IV. Multiple chemotherapy regimens, similar to those provided for nodal lymphomas, are now being given to patients to increase their survival rates. Nearly 90% of patients with complicating celiac disease are diagnosed at surgery with stage IV lesions. For these patients, chemotherapy is the primary choice of therapy, with surgical treatment being limited to diagnosis and palliation of disease (i.e., debulking) (Donahue & Kelly, 1991).

In patients with alpha chain disease (Mediterranean lymphoma or immunoproliferative small instestinal disease [IPSID] in early stage, with no evidence of tumor nodules or distant metastasis, treatment consists of a broad-spectrum antibiotic, antiparasitic drugs, and corticosteroids. A low dose of cyclophosphamide is added if there is no response in 6 months or minimal response after 1 year of treatment (Donahue & Kelly, 1991).

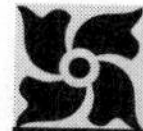

TABLE 44-6 Standard of Care for the Patient with Potential Alteration in Skin Integrity—cont'd

Patient Problem and Outcome	Nursing Interventions and Rationale	Patient Education Instructions
Decreased mobility Patient will: • Ambulate or perform body shifts in bed/chair at least every 4 hours. • Maintain muscle strength and joint range of motion. • Maintain intact skin integrity.	1. Encourage and/or assist patient to ambulate or perform body shifts in bed/chair. 2. Perform range of motion exercises every 4 hours while awake if patient is not ambulatory. 3. Lift patient's body when moving to avoid shear force. 4. Use preventive/support surfaces (i.e., foam mattress, alternating air pressure mattress) as indicated for patient's care.	1. Provide patient with information on the effects of immobility on intact skin. 2. Instruction on the proper way to accomplish body shifts in bed/chair without causing shear injury.
Skin Care Patient will: • Identify the reason for cleansing skin when soiled. • Identify at least two reasons to moisturize the skin.	1. Cleanse skin using a mild soap. 2. Collaborate with patient on frequency and time of bathing (if incontinence is not an issue). 3. Instruct patient on the differences in moisturizers (lotion, cream, ointment). 4. Encourage patient to apply moisturizer to skin at least 4 times per day. 5. Assist patient in application of moisturizer if unable to perform self care. 6. Assess skin at least every 8 hours for possible changes in skin integrity.	1. Provide a list of appropriate cream moisturizers (i.e., Lubriderm, Alpha Keri cream). 2. Instruction on the effectiveness of moisturizers to maintain skin pliability and decrease tissue injury.
Knowledge Deficit Patient will verbalize an understanding of risk factors related to pressure ulcers.	1. Assess patient's level of understanding of pressure ulcers, etiology, and risk factors. 2. Provide patient the opportunity to ask questions.	1. Provide patient with information on pressure ulcers: • Etiology • Prevention • Skin care • Nutrition • Skin inspection • Avoidance of rubber rings • Reporting skin changes to healthcare provider

ONCOLOGIC EMERGENCIES

Oncologic emergencies are due primarily to the interruption of the GI system as a result of intestine obstruction, intestine perforation, or GI hemorrhage. Surgical intervention is the primary modality used to relieve the obstruction, repair the perforation, and/or control GI bleeding. Nursing interventions are directed at managing these oncologic emergencies by preparing both the patient and family for an unplanned surgical intervention. After the emergent surgery, the patient's care is similar to any patient recovering from surgery, although it depends on the hemodynamic condition during and immediately after surgery. Additional psychosocial support for the patient and family is necessary because of the emergent nature of the situation and the stage of the disease at the onset of the oncologic emergency.

NURSING MANAGEMENT

Nursing interventions aimed at managing patients diagnosed with lymphoma of the small intestine are guided primarily by the stage of the disease at the time of diagnosis, the type of treatment chosen, the existing prognostic factors, and the presence of preexisting or underlying medical conditions that might have placed the patient at higher risk for the development of small intestine cancer (Table 44-6). The psychosocial responses of the patient and family or significant others along with the presence or absence of adequate support systems also determine appropriate nursing inter-

TABLE 44-7 Potential Acute Complications Following Surgery for Small Bowel Cancer and Their Signs and Symptoms

A. General
  1. Cardiopulmonary
     - Atelectasis: dyspnea, anxiety, cyanosis, diaphoresis, tachycardia
     - Pneumonia: cough, sputum production, pleuritic chest pain, chills, fever
     - Pulmonary embolus: dyspnea, bloody sputum, chest pain tachycardia, fever
  2. Congestive heart failure: dyspnea, orthopnea, hypoxia, cough, high blood pressure, palpitations, wheezes, crackles
  3. Wound infection: redness, swelling, tenderness, purulent discharge, chills, fever, foul-smelling drainage
  4. Septicemia: early signs: fever, chills, nausea, vomiting, diarrhea, oliguria; late signs: restlessness, irritability, apprehension, tachycardia, tachypnea, hypotension, thirsted, altered consciousness, anuria, hypothermia

B. Small Bowel
  1. Intraperitoneal hemorrhage: decreased hematocrit, increased abdominal distention, peritoneal irritation, hypovolemic signs
  2. Anastomotic leaks: peritonitis, abscess, fistula formation, abdominal pain
  3. Peritonitis: sudden, severe abdominal pain, weakness, pallor, diaphoresis, decreased intestinal motility, low blood pressure, tachycardia, rebound tenderness, fever
  4. Intra-abdominal abscess: recurring or persistent fever more than 72 hours postoperatively, leukocytes with high bands count; no abdominal pain or tenderness
  5. Hypoxic bowel: guaiac-positive diarrhea, general signs and symptoms of infection
  6. Small bowel obstruction: abdominal pain, nausea, vomiting, distention, tenderness, audible bowel sounds with rushes

Modified from Hoebler, L. & Irwin, M. M. (1992). Gastrointestinal tract cancer: Current knowledge, medical treatment, and nursing management. *Oncology Nursing Forum, 19*(9), 1403-1415.

ventions. Nursing care for the patient with small intestine lymphoma can be delivered in the inpatient, outpatient, or home care setting depending on the nature of the treatment and the physical and emotional condition of the patient. Typically these patients present to the hospital in a medical emergency and require immediate surgical intervention for both diagnosis and treatment.

Preoperative Care

Nursing care during the preoperative period should be directed at assessing the patient's physical and emotional status, explaining the surgical procedure to the patient and family, and preparing the patient and family for the anticipated short- and long-term postoperative sequelae.

Patient assessment should include general physical condition, presence of concomitant disease, nutritional status, cardiopulmonary status, and psychosocial responses to actual or potential diagnosis. The patient and family should have the surgical procedure verbally and visually explained, and the anticipated length of hospital stay should be discussed. The patient should be prepared for postoperative care that includes respiratory and circulatory exercises, pain control, wound and drain care, catheter care, intravenous lines, and nutritional support. Unfortunately, the patient requiring surgical intervention for the diagnosis and treatment of lymphoma of the small intestine may present in a significantly malnourished state secondary to weight loss associated with the disease process itself, delay in diagnosis, and/or the presence of advanced disease at the time of diagnosis (Polomano, Weintraub, & Wurster, 1994).

Postoperative Care

Nursing care in the acute postoperative period focuses primarily on the prevention and early detection of potential surgical complications. The nursing management of patients undergoing cancer surgery has been summarized in both general surgical nursing texts and publications. Because the exact location of the tumor within the small intestine and the involvement of surrounding tissue or organs determines the extent of the surgery, it is important for the oncology nurse to know exactly what surgical procedure was performed so that he or she can assess the patient based on various drains and tubes placed during surgery. Table 44-7 outlines the general and specific acute complications of small intestine surgery, along with their associated signs and symptoms.

Nutritional repletion in the immediate postoperative period is important for surgical patients undergoing radical procedures resulting in extensive tissue trauma, alterations in the GI tract, and lengthy hospitalizations. Unfortunately, preoperative malnutrition is associated with poor surgical outcomes such as sepsis, wound complications, ileus, and more lengthy hospital stays (Chen, Souba, & Copeland, 1991; Bryant, 1992).

Nutrition

Nutritional care of the cancer patient should always be considered supportive, regardless of whether the goal is cure or palliation. The purpose of nutritional care is to support the patient's nutritional status, body composition, functional status, and quality of life. Because of the delay in diagnosis of small intestine cancers, nutritional compromise already exists in this patient population at the time of confirmed diagnosis.

PROGNOSIS

Prognosis for the patient with small intestine lymphoma depends entirely on the stage of the disease. The presence of a large tumor that involved other organs at the time of surgery adversely affects the patient's long-term outcome. Tumor-related complications such as perforation and severe malnutrition also worsen the prognosis. Patients who undergo resection at the earliest stages of disease have a more favorable outcome, with 5-year survival rates reaching 80% (Donahue & Kelly, 1991), although a 40% to 50% survival rate is more typical (Sarna & Kagan, 1995). Stages III and IV tumors are fatal, and patients are provided with palliative care.

EVALUATION OF THE QUALITY OF CARE

Hospitals and other agencies require monitoring of the quality of care provided to patients. The type of monitoring involved depends on the data to be collected and the patient circumstances. The evaluation of quality care provided to these patients should incorporate input from a multidisciplinary team, including the surgical oncologist, oncology nurse, anesthesiologist, dietitian, pain service, physical therapist, discharge planner, and home care nurse (Table 44-8).

TABLE 44-8 Quality of Care: Immediate Postoperative Care (First 72 Hours)

Prospective chart review for documentation. Compliance demonstrated by score of 80%.
Disciplines participating in the quality of care evaluation:
☐ Nursing ☐ Surgery ☐ Dietary

Criteria	Yes	No
1. Was there assessment of perianal skin every 8 hours?	☐	☐
2. Was there assessment of serum hemoglobin and hematocrit?	☐	☐
3. Was there an accurate input and output for last 24 hours?	☐	☐
4. Was there an assessment of serum electrolytes?	☐	☐
5. Was there consultation with nutritionist?	☐	☐
6. Was a discharge teaching plan initiated?	☐	☐
7. Was there intravenous line care?	☐	☐
8. Was there an assessment of hydration status every 8 hours?	☐	☐
9. Was a Skin Risk Assessment Tool completed?	☐	☐
10. Was there an assessment of surgical drains?	☐	☐

RESEARCH ISSUES

Research directed at small intestine lymphoma is currently directed at fact finding, such as case studies and reporting on incidence. Questions that focus on the relationship between Crohn's disease and small intestine lymphoma need to be asked, particularly because the etiology of Crohn's disease is unknown. An understanding of the risk factors associated with small intestine lymphoma and the variation in types of GI lymphomas may increase knowledge about other GI malignancies.

REFERENCES

Alexander, J. W. & Altemeier, W. A. (1968). Association of primary neoplasms of the small intestine with other neoplastic growths. *Annals of Surgery, 167,* 958-964.

Anonymous. (1996). Weekly clinicopathological exercises: Case 15-1996: A 79-year-old woman with anorexia, weight loss, and diarrhea after treatment of celiac disease. *New England Journal of Medicine, 334,* 20.

Ashley, S. W. & Wells, S. A. (1988). Tumors of the small intestine. *Seminars in Oncology, 15*(2), 116-128.

Blackstone, M. O. (1989). Endoscopy. In Bayless, T. M. (Ed.), *Current management of inflammatory bowel disease.* Philadelphia: B.C. Decker.

Bryant, R. (Ed.). (1992). *Acute and chronic wounds: Nursing management.* St. Louis: Mosby.

Chen, C. C., Neugut, A. I., & Rotterdam, H. (1994). Risk factors for adenocarcinomas and malignant carcinoids of the small intestine: Preliminary findings. *Cancer Epidemiology, Biomarkers, and Prevention, 3*(3), 205-207.

Chow, J. S., Chen, C. C., Ahsan, H., & Neugut, A. I. (1996). A population-based study of the incidence of malignant small bowel: SEER, 1973-1990. *International Journal of Epidemiology, 25*(4), 722-728.

Coit, D. G. (1997). Cancer of the small intestine. In V. T. DeVita, S. Hellman, & S. A. Rosenberg (Eds.), *Cancer: Principles and practice of oncology* (5th ed.). Philadelphia, J.B. Lippincott, Co.

Cooper, B. T., Holmes, G. K. T., Ferguson, R., & Cooke, W. T. (1980). Celiac disease and malignancy. *Medicine, 59*(4), 249-261.

Daniel, B. T. (1997). Gastrointestinal cancers. In Otto, S. (Ed.), *Oncology nursing* (3rd ed.). St. Louis: Mosby.

DiSario, J. A., Burt, R. W., Vargas, H., & McWhorter, W. P. (1994). Small bowel cancer: Epidemiological and clinical characteristics from a population-based registry. *American Journal of Gastroenterology, 89*(5), 699-701.

Donohue, J. H. & Kelly, K. A. (1991). Cancer of the small intestine. In A. R. Moossa, S. C. Schimpff, & M. C. Robson (Eds.), *Comprehensive textbook of oncology* (2nd ed.). Baltimore: Williams & Wilkins.

Farmer, R. G. (1989). Small bowel disease: Medical therapy. In T. M. Bayless (Ed.), *Current management of inflammatory bowel disease.* Philadelphia: B.C. Decker.

Hampton, B. & Bryant, R. (1992). *Ostomies and continent diversions: Nursing management.* St. Louis: Mosby.

Haskell, C. M., Lavey, R. S., & Ramming, K. P. (1995). Small intestine, In C. M. Haskell (Ed.), *Cancer treatment* (4th ed.). Philadelphia, W.B. Saunders.

Hawks, J. H. (1997). Nursing care of clients with intestinal disorders. In J. M. Black, & E. Matassarin-Jacobs (Eds.), *Medical-surgical nursing clinical management for continuity of care* (5th ed.). Philadelphia: W.B. Saunders.

Herbsman, H., Wetstein, L., Rosen, Y., Orecs, H., Alfonsoe, A. E., Iyer, S. K., & Gardner, B. (1980). Tumors of the small intestine. *Current Problems in Surgery, 17*(3), 121-182.

Hoebler, L. & Irwin, M. M. (1992). Gastrointestinal tract cancer: Current knowledge, medical treatment, and nursing management. *Oncology Nursing Forum, 19*(9), 1403-1415.

Loescher, L. (1997). Dynamics of cancer prevention. In S. Groenwald, M. Frogge, M. Goodman, & C. Yarbro (Eds.), *Cancer nursing: Principles and practice* (4th ed.). Boston: Jones & Bartlett Publishers.

Lowenfels, A. B. (1973). Why are small-bowel tumours so rare? *Lancet, 1*(7793), 24-26.

Maklebust, J. & Sieggreen, M. Y. (1996). *Pressure ulcers: Guidelines for prevention and nursing management* (2nd ed.). Springhouse: Springhouse Corp.

Maglinte, D. D., O'Connor, K., Bessette, J., Chernish, S. M., & Kelvin, F. M. (1991). The role of the physician in the late diagnosis of primary malignant tumors of the small intestine. *American Journal of Gastroenterology, 86*(3), 304-308.

Polomano, R., Weintraub, F. N., & Wurster, A. (1994). Surgical critical care for cancer patients. *Seminars in Oncology Nursing, 10*(3), 165-176.

Sarna, G. P. & Kagan, A. R. (1995). Extranodal lymphomas. In C. M. Haskell (Ed.), *Cancer treatment* (4th ed.). Philadelphia, W.B. Saunders.

Society of Gastroenterology Nurses & Associates. (1993). *Gastroenterology nursing: A core curriculum.* St. Louis: Mosby.

Swinson, C. M., Slavin, G., Coles, E. C., & Booth, C. C. (1983). Coeliac disease and malignancy. *Lancet, 1*(8316), 111-115.

Sarcoma of the Small Intestine

Linda A. House, RN, BSN

INTRODUCTION

Sarcoma of the small intestine is a smooth muscle tumor that is often underdiagnosed and undertreated, and subsequently has a poor survival rate. Diagnostic tools currently available to the medical community render the overall diagnostic, treatment, and prognostic situation an oncologic challenge. The purpose of this chapter is multidimensional and will describe the epidemiology, risk factors, clinical signs and symptoms, and diagnoses of this obscure cancer. This chapter also defines current prognostic factors and nursing considerations.

ANATOMY

The small intestine is the major digestive organ (Marieb, 1992). It is the part of the gastrointestinal (GI) tract that facilitates the transport of nutrients, GI secretions, and waste products from the pyloric sphincter outlet of the stomach, through the ileocecal valve, and into the large intestine (Marieb, 1992). This section of intestine is composed of the largest portion of smooth muscle in the body (Horowitz, Spellman, Driscoll, Velez, & Karakousis, 1995) mucous membrane, mucosal glands, lymph nodules, and a rich blood supply. The primary function of the small intestine is to remove essential elements (e.g., fluid, electrolytes) from the ingested content and pass the waste to the large intestine (Fig. 45-1).

Remarkably, the small intestine accounts for between 75% and 90% of the total length of the GI tract (Chami, Ratner, Henneberry, Smith, Hill, & Katz, 1994; Gabos, Berkel, Band, Robson, & Whittaker, 1993; Marcilla, Bueno, Aguilar, & Paricio, 1994; Chow, Chen, Ahsan, & Neugut, 1996; O'Riordan, Vilor, & Herrera, 1996; Rivkind, Admon, Yarom & Schreiber, 1994). Furthermore, the small intestine comprises between 90% to 98% of the total mucosal surface which, according to Marieb (1992) is "equal to the floor space of an average two-story home."

With respect to the size and function of the small intestine, it is amazing to realize that the small intestine is nine times the size of the colon, but the incidence of colorectal carcinoma is 40 times more common than that of the small intestine (Basson, 1993).

TYPES OF SARCOMA OF THE SMALL INTESTINE

Sarcoma of the small intestine is a rare situation that accounts for approximately 14% of all cancers of the small intestine (Scott, 1997). To put this statistic into perspective, Chow and colleagues (1996) report the age-adjusted incidence rate of colon cancer to be 303 : 1,000,000, whereas the incidence rate of cancer of the stomach is 7 : 1,000,000. The average annual age-adjusted incidence rate for all small intestine malignancies was 9.9 per million with sarcomas accounting for 1.3 per million (Chow et al., 1996). Within the definition of small intestine sarcoma, there are several subcategories, which are identified in this section. However, these subtypes are extremely rare and are included in the broad sarcoma category for the purpose of this review.

Leiomyosarcoma

Leiomyosarcoma is the most common type of small intestine sarcoma and the fourth most common type of small intestine malignancy (O'Riordan, Vilor, & Herrera, 1996). Leiomyosarcoma accounts for approximately 150 new cases annually in the United States. This subtype is responsible for between 22% and 27% of the small intestine sarcomas (Matsuo, Eto, Tsunoda, Kanematsu, & Shinozake, 1994; Ng, Pollock, Munsell, Atkinson, & Romsdahl, 1992; Serour, Dona, Birkenfeld, Balassiano, & Krispin, 1992). Leiomyosarcoma is a malignant tumor that develops from any smooth muscle (Scott, 1997). It is important to note that a leiomyosarcoma can develop in any area of the body, but with the amount of smooth muscle contained in the small intestine, it is understandable how this histologic type is the most common type of small intestine sarcoma.

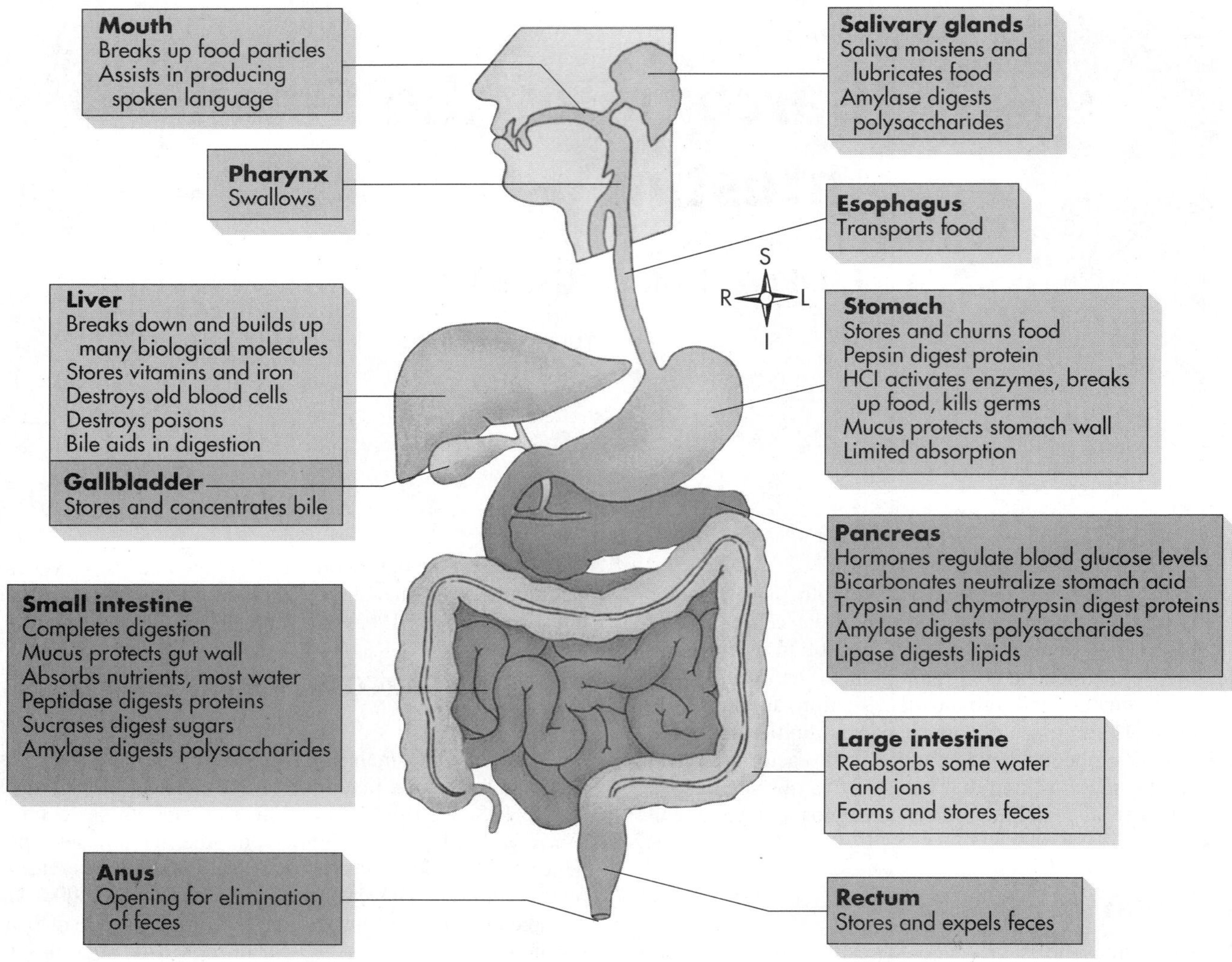

Fig. 45-1 Functions of the small intestine. (From Thibodeau, G. A. & Patton, K. T. [1996]. *Anatomy and Physiology* [3rd ed.]. St. Louis: Mosby.)

Angiosarcoma

Angiosarcoma is another rare subtype of small bowel sarcoma. Scott (1997) defines this tumor as arising either from blood vessels (hemangiosarcoma) or lymph vessels (lymphangiosarcoma). A reference to the anatomy of the small intestine would explain this origination. A review of the literature reveals that studies performed over several years found only a few patients to have a primary angiosarcoma of the small intestine. Researchers at Roswell Park Memorial Institute reported 19 patients with sarcomas over a 44-year period and no angiosarcoma patients were identified (Chami et al., 1994). Similarly, studies from Vanderbilt University Hospital in Nashville, Tenn., reported only one patient with an angiosarcoma in a span of 28 years (Chami et al., 1994).

Another subtype of small intestine sarcoma is granulocytic sarcoma, which is the result of the rich lymphatic system in the small intestine. This is actually a situation where the primary tissue is invaded by acute nonlymphocytic leukemia cells (Rottenberg & Thomas, 1994). Rottenberg (1994) reports that any organ could experience this type of invasion, but the most common areas are the GI tract and the lymph nodes.

Other Sarcomas of the Small Intestine

Liposarcoma of the small intestine is a malignant lesion originating from adipose tissue (Scott, 1997). It is extremely rare. The symptoms are often mistaken for appendicitis (Rivkind et al., 1994). Thomas and colleagues discuss the subtype plexosarcoma (or GI autonomic nerve tumor) as a rare tumor whose characteristics suggest "origin from neurons of the enteric plexus" (Thomas, Mrak, & Libuit, 1994). This subtype is so rare that from the first description of it by Herrera et al in 1984 until the 1994 article of Thomas and colleagues, fewer than 12 cases have been identified (Thomas, Mrak, & Libuit, 1994). Fibrosarcoma is a tumor that is composed of cell and fibers derived from fibrocytes (Scott, 1997). Although extremely rare, this type of sarcoma has been identified as a primary malignancy of the small intestine.

Finally there are malignant tumors of the neural sheath defined as *malignant schwannoma, malignant neurilemomas, neurogenic sarcomas,* and *neurofibrosarcomas.* (Scott, 1997).

EPIDEMIOLOGY

The incidence of malignancy of the small intestine accounts for between 1% and 5% of all GI malignancies. Sarcoma of the small intestine accounts for only 11% to 14% of the 1% to 5% (Basson, 1993; Chami et al., 1994; Rivkind et al., 1994; Scott, 1997). When placed into numerical perspective, there will be an estimated 4500 new cases of small intestine cancer and 1200 deaths as a result of small intestine cancer in 1997. Based on the 11% cited by Scott, this translates into 539 new cases and 125 small intestine sarcoma–related deaths in 1997.

It is interesting to note that the overall estimated new cases and deaths concerning small intestine sarcoma have increased in number from 1990 to 2800 new cases and 900 deaths (Ciresi & Scholten, 1995), but the rates of sarcoma of the small intestine have remained consistent (Chow et al., 1996).

A number of studies have reported a gender differentiation for cancers of the small intestine. In 1998 the incidence of projected new cases for males and females are 2600 and 2300, respectively, and the projected deaths are 540 and 600, respectively (Landis, Murray, Bolden, & Wingo, 1998). It is interesting to note that most studies cite gender incidence rates specifically for sarcoma of the small intestine to be similar to the above. There is a slightly higher incidence of sarcoma of the small intestine in males vs females, with the ratio being 1.6:1 (Horowitz et al., 1995).

A review of the literature reveals consistent reporting of the age incidence of small intestine sarcoma. This disease affects most patients between the fifth and seventh decades of life (O'Riordan et al., 1996; Serour et al.,1992; Horowitz et al., 1995), but cases have been reported as early as the fourth decade of life (Maglinte, O'Connor, Bessett, Chernish, & Kelvin, 1991). In addition to the gender and age statistics, all studies consistently cite an increased incidence in whites over blacks.

RISK FACTORS

The exact risk factors of sarcoma of the small intestine are not differentiated from the other forms of cancer of the small intestine. The elements contained in bile salts are suggested as having a potential carcinogen risk (Gabos et al., 1993). Bile salts are a required element for proper fat digestion in the small intestine. After completing their objective in coordination with the bacteria in the small intestine, the bile salts are reabsorbed in the ileum. It is during this "activation" phase that the bile salts are changed to substances that are identified as carcinogens (Gabos et al., 1993).

In addition to the carcinogenic nature of bile salts in GI secretions, Gabos and colleagues (1993) cite the continuous entry of GI secretions, particularly bile and pancreatic secretions, as a possible irritant causing cellular damage. Their study further refers to the constant factors required for tissue healing as a potential risk for tumor development.

Situations that result in a less-than-desirable small intestinal emptying, are also implicated as potential causes (Gabos et al., 1993). GI secretions are believed to play in the development of tumors of the small intestine. Conditions causing such concerns include diverticulosis, Crohn's disease, scleroderma, intestinal obstruction, and cirrhosis of the liver, to name a few.

In 1993, hereditary syndromes were identified as potential risk factors. In particular, von Recklinghausen's neurofibromatosis has been associated with the development of malignant schwannoma (Scott, 1997). Coit (1993) identifies this syndrome as an autosomal dominant situation that has an incidence rate of 1 per 3000 births. Approximately 10% to 15% of patients with von Recklinghausen's neurofibromatosis will experience the development of a malignant schwannoma (Coit, 1993).

Physical conditions or medications that result in immunosuppression have also been listed as potential risk factors for the development of cancer of the small intestine (Serour et al., 1992). There are other risk factors for cancers of the small intestine such as familial polyposis, but these conditions are listed primarily as precursors for adenocarcinoma of the small intestine.

PROTECTIVE FACTORS

Considering the length and surface area of the small intestine, coupled with the risk factors associated with cancer of the small intestine, it is truly amazing that incidence rates are low. A number of inherent protective factors within the small intestine are hypothesized to create an environment hostile to the development of cancer. A number of these situations will be discussed here.

The first hypothesized protective mechanism of the small intestine is the time the GI contents are actually present in the small intestine. The time it takes for the contents to travel from the opening of the small intestine to large intestine is relatively short. This quick travel time decreases the length of exposure of intestinal mucosa to potential carcinogenic material found in the GI material (Chow et al., 1996; Gabos et al., 1993; O'Riordan et al., 1996).

The actual content of the GI secretions at the level of the small intestine is the basis of several other protective theories. The contents of the digestive matter at this level are very fluid-rich. It is felt that the liquid is less irritating to the intestinal mucosa than the more solid waste found in the large intestine (Chow et al., 1996; O'Riordan et al., 1996). A second thought about the secretion issue is that the large volume of contents and liquid actually serve to dilute the potential carcinogens to make the contents less toxic to the small intestine (Chow et al., 1996). Another detoxification theory of the gut involves the presence of benzopyrene hydroxylase and diamine oxidase. It is felt that the abundance of these enzymes play a role in the inhibition of carcinogenesis (Chow et al., 1996; Gabos et al., 1993; O'Riordan et al., 1996). Finally, the contents of the small intestine are alkaline by nature. This alkalinity is believed to play a role in protecting the small intestine from a cancerous predisposition (Gabos et al., 1993; O'Riordan et al., 1996).

The small intestine has an abundance of lymph nodes. The rich supply of immunoglobulin A (IgA) secreted by these lymph nodes is felt to produce a local immune environment hostile to a the development of malignancies (Chow et al., 1996; Gabos et al., 1993; O'Riordan et al., 1996).

The "normal" small intestine is found to have fewer and different bacteria than what is found in the large intestine. Since it is the function of bacteria to break down the contents of the GI tract into potentially carcinogenic substances, the decreased amount of bacteria translates into less of the carcinogen-producing metabolic activity (Chow et al., 1996; Gabos et al., 1993; O'Riordan et al., 1996).

SIGNS AND SYMPTOMS

The signs and symptoms of cancer of the small intestine are variable, vague, and present in only 40% to 70% of the patients (Ciresi & Scholten, 1995). Marcilla et al. (1994) report that a patient will experience symptoms for an average of 3 to 6 months before diagnosis. O'Riordan et al (1996) report this window to be closer to 6 to 8 months. One of the most commonly cited symptoms is abdominal pain. The experience of pain has been reported as vague to severe when associated with intestinal obstruction or perforation (Serour et al., 1992). The occurrence rates reported range from 30% to 85% (O'Riordan et al., 1996).

The second most commonly cited sign is GI hemorrhage. As with pain the degree of severity varies with the extension of the disease. Hemorrhage is more common in a patient with leiomyosarcoma than in a patient with another type of small intestine cancer (O'Riordan et al., 1996).

An intestinal perforation in patients with leiomyosarcoma is commonly seen in patients who have a lesion that is termed *exometric,* or outside of the inner intestinal cannula. This emergency situation is often the presenting sign for a number of sarcoma patients. It is during the emergency intervention that a patient is found to have a cancer of the small intestine (O'Riordan et al., 1996).

A second emergency surgical situation in which patients are often found to have cancer of the small intestine is that of intestinal obstruction. Coit (1993) notes that obstructions are more common with endoenteric lesions (lesions inside the GI tract), which can be partial or complete and can recur. Approximately 15% to 35% occur as a complete obstruction, although it can be partial rather than complete (O'Riordan et al., 1996). Perhaps the presentation and absolution of symptoms could be a reason for the often misleading symptoms of this disease.

Patients report a number of common and vague symptoms that are associated with any number of conditions (Box 45-1). The vague symptoms coupled with less than ideal diagnostic tools are felt to be responsible for the delay in diagnosis and subsequent poor survival rates.

Box 45-1
Common Signs and Symptoms of Sarcoma of the Small Intestine

Signs

Anemia
Bloating
Gastrointestinal hemorrhage
Intestinal obstruction
Intestinal perforation
Jaundice
Palpable abdominal mass
Weight loss

Symptoms

Abdominal pain
Constipation
Diarrhea
Reported nausea and vomiting

DIAGNOSIS

The diagnosis of sarcoma of the small intestine remains a concern in the medical community (Table 45-1). Maglinte et al. (1991) report that medical practitioners may error in not making the correct diagnosis for 6 months after patient presentation of symptoms. Maglinte et al (1991) demonstrated that the lag time between symptom appearance and diagnosis was delayed by the patient one seventh of the total time and the clinician six sevenths of the time. The delay was attributed primarily to either physicians' not ordering appropriate diagnostics coupled with misinterpreting examination results. The results of the study led to recommendation to consider small intestine studies when any feature of a patient's GI symptoms remain undiagnosed, are atypical, or are unresponsive to a brief empiric treatment trial.

Enteroclysis

A number of diagnostic tools are helpful to identify small intestine lesions. Enteroclysis is accepted as the most sensitive diagnositic method. The patient undergoes a pretest preparation, followed by the passing of a flexible tube through the nose, past the stomach, and into the small intestine. A contrast substance is injected through the tube so that examination can be performed by fluoroscopy. Accuracy rates are noted to be 90%.

Upper Gastrointestinal Series

A second diagnostic tool is the upper GI series with small intestine follow through. During this procedure, the patient ingests a contrast substance, and a series of radiographs are taken at various points of upper GI clearance. This test allows visualization of the stomach and small intestine. Success rate for this procedure are reported to be 53% to 83% for identification of an abnormality and 30% to 44% for identification of a small intestine tumor.

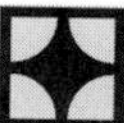

TABLE 45-1 Assessment of the Patient for Sarcoma of the Small Intestine

	Assessment Parameters	Typical Abnormal Findings
History	1. Age 2. Gender 3. Race 4. Patient history	1. Usually effects persons in fifth to seventh decade 2. Male:Female 1.6:1 3. More prevalent in whites than in African Americans 4. Family history of gastrointestinal (GI) disease Family History of von Recklinghausen's syndrome • Neurofibromatosis Patient history of GI disease (obstruction, Chron's, etc.) • Immunosuppression
Physical Examination	Evaluate patient for signs and symptoms 1. Interview 2. Weight 3. Assess laboratory values 4. Determine bowel patterns 5. Abdominal assessment 6. Monitor vital signs	• Abdominal pain • Anemia • Fatigue • Bloating • Constipation • Diarrhea • GI hemorrhage • Intestinal obstruction • Intestinal perforation • Jaundice • Nausea and vomiting • Palpable abdominal mass • Weight loss
Diagnostic Tests	1. Enteroclysis 2. Upper GI barium study 3. Computed tomography (CT) scan 4. Angiography 5. Duodenography 6. Transabdominal ultrasound 7. Upper endoscopy 8. Surgery	1. 90% accurate 2. 30% to 44% accurate for tumors 3. 80% accurate 4. Useful to determine blood-rich tumors 8. Up to 90% of tumors are found at the time of surgery

Computed Tomography

A computed tomography (CT) scan is given an accuracy rating of 80% for diagnostic purposes (Basson, 1993). It may be helpful to use CT scans in conjunction with one of the above contrast studies to provide an accurate picture of both the internal lumen and external mucosal wall of the small intestine (Scott, 1997).

Angiography

Angiography is specific to the diagnosis of leiomyosarcoma of the small intestine. This tool is useful in identifying this particular tumor type due to it's excessive vascular supply (Serour et al., 1992). Box 45-2 includes alternative endoscopic procedures.

Surgery

Ninety percent of patients with small intestine cancer are diagnosed with their disease at the time of surgery (Gawdat & Corey, 1993; Ng et al., 1992) compared with a preoperative diagnosis of 21% to 53% (Ciresi & Scholten, 1995; Matsuo et al., 1994). In a review of 61 patients treated for surgical emergencies, 32 where found to have sarcoma of the small intestine (Gawdat & Corey, 1993; Ng et al., 1992). This reinforces the surgical emergency identification, but also points out the discovery of intestinal tumors at the time of elective surgery.

Box 45-2
Diagnostics for Sarcoma of the Small Intestine

Enteroclysis
Upper GI barium study
CT scan
Angiography
Surgery
Duodenography
Transabdominal ultrasound
Upper endoscopy

ROUTES OF METASTASES

The tumor location and metastatic growth patterns of sarcoma of the small intestine are not complex. Sarcomas are found evenly distributed throughout the small intestine (Matsuo et al., 1994). When comparing the sites of the duodenum, jejunum, and ileum, studies done by both Maglinte et al. (1991) and Horowitz et al. (1995) demonstrate the ileum as the common site of sarcomas of the small intestine. With current diagnostic imitations and delay in treatment, it is not surprising that some studies identify as high as a 50% metastatic rate at the time of diagnosis (Serour et al., 1992). Metastatic growth is usually accomplished by direct tumor invasion or by spread throughout the bloodstream, with the most common sites of metastatic development being the liver, lung, and bone (O'Riordan et al., 1996). Both Horowitz et al. (1995) and O'Riordan et al. (1996) state that lymph node metastasis occurs in less than 15% of the sarcoma population, but Serour et al. (1992) report finding several patients with mesenteric or retroperitoneal lymph node metastasis during their study.

STAGING AND TREATMENT

The system traditionally used for mapping cancer disease stages is not typically utilized for sarcoma of the small intestine. The TNM staging method (*T,* tumor size; *N,* lymph node involvement; *M,* distant metastasis) is used to determine adenocarcinoma of the small intestine, but the remainder of small intestinal cancers, such as sarcomas, are referenced by histologic type and size rather that stage. The treatment for sarcoma of the small intestine is largely dependent on the extent of the disease. The National Cancer Institute (NCI) (1996) cites treatment options according to resectable primary disease, unresectable primary disease, or unresectable metastatic disease.

The literature repeatedly stresses that a complete resection is the only treatment option for potential cure of sarcoma of the small intestine (O'Riordan et al., 1996; Maglinte et al., 1991). For the most effective result, the surgery must be radical and in the early stages of tumor development (Serour et al., 1992). If a complete resection is not a possibility, a number of surgical options are available, though less effective. One such option is incomplete resection in which as much of the tumor as possible is removed. This treatment is offered with or without the addition of radiation or chemotherapy. A second surgical intervention is bypass surgery where the tumor is circumvented to allow the passage of intestinal contents through the small intestine. This intervention is primarily palliative in nature and can be accompanied by radiation therapy (National Cancer Institute, 1997).

Chemotherapy

Chemotherapy for the treatment of sarcoma of the small intestine is an option, however Coit (1993), Horowitz et al. (1995), and Ng et al (1992) report that there has not been a benefit to adding adjuvant chemotherapy as a treatment option. The use of chemotherapy for palliative treatment in symptomatic metastatic disease is noted by Coit (1993); this method uses doxorubicin-based combinations with or without high-dose ifosfamide. The response rates of these regimens are listed to be as high as 40% (Scott, 1997). It is also important to note that at the time of this writing, there are currently three clinical trials that list criteria for small bowel tumors, but on questioning one lead investigator, it was discovered that sarcomas were not currently being enrolled due to the lack of response (National Cancer Institute, 1997).

Radiation

The option of radiation therapy as a treatment of sarcoma of the small intestine is similar to that of chemotherapy. It is reserved primarily for palliative care and demonstrates little effectiveness as an adjuvant therapy.

In review, the treatment of choice for sarcoma of the small intestine is currently wide, radical resection. Adjuvant chemotherapy and radiation therapy have been added with little effect on recurrence rates. The NCI lists surgical bypass with radiation therapy as the treatment for unresectable primary disease, palliative surgery, radiation therapy, and/or chemotherapy for unresectable metastatic disease, and clinical trial options with chemotherapy or biotherapy for unresectable primary, metastatic, or recurrent disease (NCI, 1997).

PROGNOSIS

The prognosis for patients with sarcoma of the small intestine is as varied as the other aspects of this disease. The literature reveals many different opinions, but there is agreement that the prognosis is dependent on more than the disease name itself. A review of the literature demonstrates the highest overall 5-year survival rate to be 45% to 50% (DiSario, Burt, Vargas, & McWhorter, 1994; O'Riordan et al., 1996), with the majority of references noting a 5-year survival rate of between 18% and 28% (Ng et al., 1992; Serour et al., 1992; Scott, 1997).

Although the prognosis for patients with sarcoma of the small intestine has remained the same for the past 40 years (Basson, 1993), there is information about some factors that can identify which patients will have a better prognostic outlook. Ng et al. (1992) identified four issues that demonstrate a more positive prognostic outlook for a patient with sarcoma of the small intestine, specifically leiomyosarcoma: (1) resectability of the tumor with or without rupture, (2) size of the tumor, (3) grade of the tumor (Dahllof & Ringden, 1997), and (4) localization of the lesion. According to this group, there is a significant prognostic benefit to the patient if the tumor can be completely resected (no evidence of gross disease postoperatively) and the tumor is not ruptured. The median survival time for the patient with complete resection without tumor rupture was 46 months, compared with the patient with complete resection and tumor rupture, who has a median survival of 17 months. Even those patients with disease extension who underwent complete resection without tumor rupture experienced an improved median survival of 36 months from the patients with tumor rupture. Ng et al. (1992) furthered their work to develop a

TABLE 45-2 Overall and Disease-Free Survival Based on M. D. Anderson Cancer Center Staging Classification for Gastrointestinal Leiomyosarcoma

Stage	TGM	N(%)	5 years	8 years	10 years	2 years	4 years
I	T1/G1/M0	10	89%	28%	75%	56%	28%
II	T2/G1/M0	12(9)	52%	28%	28%	57%	34%
III	T1-2G2/M0 T3 any G/M0	47(34)	28%	14%	14%	47%	18%
IVA	M1 or residual disease after surgery	46(33)	12%	4%	0	—	—
IVB	T4	24(17)	7%	—	—	19%	19%

T, tumor size and extra-organ involvement: T1 = localized, <5 cm; T2 = localized, ≥5 cm; T3 = contiguous organ invasion or peritoneal implants, any size; T4 = tumor ruptured, any size.
G, tumor grade: G1 = low grade; G2 = high.
M, distant metastases: M0 = no metastasis; M1 = metastasis present.
From Ng, E. (1992). Prognostic factors influencing survival in gastrointestinal leiomyosarcomas: Implications for surgical management and staging. *Annals of Surgery, 215*(1), 68-77.

staging system to determine a patient's survival potential. They based their system on a T (tumor), G (grade), M (metastasis) method (Table 45-2), which then could be used to predict survival based on several different factors.

The size of the tumor played an important role in the study done by Ng et al. (1992). Patients with tumors smaller than 5 cm had median survival times of 68 months as opposed to tumor sizes of 5 to 10 cm and larger than 10 cm, where the median survival times were 32 and 27 months respectively. With regard to localization of the tumor and tumor grade as they effect survival, Ng et al. (1992) and Horowitz et al. (1995) cite these issues as prognostic indicators. Ng et al. (1992) report an improved prognosis in the patient whose tumor was localized as opposed to those who had peritoneal seeding or metastasis. They list median survival rates as 46 months, 23 months, and 19 months respectively. Finally, both Ng and Horowitz agree that the lower the tumor grade, the better the prognosis. Horowitz et al. (1995) cite a 44% 5-year survival for low-grade tumors vs 0% 5-year survival for high-grade tumors.

When comparing prognosis of patients with sarcoma of the small intestine to those with adenocarcinoma or malignant lymphoma of the small intestine, Matsuo et al. (1994) discovered the prognosis to be a more positive 17.2 months as compared with 8.7 months for adenocarcinoma and 9 months for lymphoma.

EVALUATION OF THE QUALITY OF CARE

Accreditation organizations, like the Joint Commission for the Accreditation of Health Care Organizations, require that the quality of care provided to patients be evaluated. Since the care provided to patients with prostate cancer requires input from a multidisciplinary team, an evaluation of the quality of care provided to these patients should include aspects of care provided by various members of the team. Table 45-3 lists evaluation tools that can be used in the inpatient and outpatient settings.

TABLE 45-3 Quality of Care Evaluation for a Patient Experiencing Fatigue

Disciplines participating in the quality of care evaluation:
☐ Nursing ☐ Social Services
☐ Physician ☐ Patient/Support Person

Criteria	Yes	No
1. Was the patient/support person given information about fatigue?		
a. Risk factors	☐	☐
b. Early indicators	☐	☐
2. Was the patient given a thorough fatigue assessment?		
a. Interview/rating	☐	☐
b. Laboratory assessment	☐	☐
3. Was the patient informed about early intervention?		
a. Diet	☐	☐
b. Fluid intake	☐	☐
c. Activity	☐	☐
d. Journal maintenance	☐	☐
4. Does the patient record indicate fatigue intervention education?	☐	☐
5. Does the patient indicate satisfaction with fatigue management?		
a. Assessment	☐	☐
b. Intervention	☐	☐
c. Education	☐	☐
(Please rate satisfaction on a scale of 0 [very dissatisfied] to 10 [very satisfied])		
6. How would you rate your fatigue on this particular day? (Please rate your fatigue on a scale of 0 [no fatigue] to 10 [worst possible fatigue])	☐	☐

ONCOLOGIC EMERGENCIES

The major oncologic emergency associated with sarcoma of the small intestine is bowel obstruction. Surgical intervention is usually the treatment of choice, but it is associated with subsequent wound infection, dehiscence, sepsis, enterocutaneous fistulae, peritoneal abscess, anastomsis dehiscence, and GI bleeding. Deep venous thrombus with or without pulmonary embolism may occur (Ripamoni, 1998). Chapter 3 offers a complete discussion on the medical treatment and nursing care of patients presenting with this problem.

NURSING MANAGEMENT

A review of the nursing literature specific for the care of the patient with sarcoma of the small intestine is sparse to nonexistent. For the purpose of this review, basic concepts surrounding the nursing care of patients with sarcoma of the small intestine with the primary focus on disease-related issues are explored. Nursing care of a patient begins at the time the patient presents with subtle and confounding symptoms in a physician's office or in a life-threatening situation such as emergency department. Table 45-4 illustrates patient education guidelines. With the identified time from symptom appearance to diagnosis, the patient's fear and anxiety issues need to be addressed. Once diagnosis occurs, the patient and family members require education and emotional support about the illness, treatment options, prognosis, and future planning. Table 45-5 offers a standard of care. Attentive nursing focused on the level of need can combat some of the issues of confusion and depression that are common during this time.

The oncology nurse can provide assistance to the patient and family member on the rationale and process of diagnostic tools, as well as treatment options accompanied by statistical outcomes. A large portion of education focuses on nutrition topics because of the nature of the disease. Patients should be encouraged to monitor their intake, measure their weight, and call their practitioner for problems or concerns. Depending on the individual situation, a diet high in protein and calories should be attempted. It may be more comfortable for the patient to take daily requirements in small, frequent meals rather than larger, less frequent meals. All vitamin and mineral supplements should be reviewed with the health care practitioner before starting use.

Symptom management is a large focus of nursing considerations. Pain management, in the event of surgery, bowel obstruction, or nerve innervation by tumor, is a critical nursing responsibility. See Chapter 15 for a complete discussion of symptom management in the cancer patient. Nursing assessment includes patient rating of the pain, as well as a detailed description that includes location, duration, intensity, and causative and relief factors.

Fatigue is a complaint that is often overlooked in this patient population. A number of patient self-assessment scales are available and range in structure from 0 to 10 rating scales to more sophisticated self-assessment linear analogue scales (Table 45-6). Treatment is directed toward addressing the underlying cause if applicable or by working with the patient to maximize nutrition, activity, rest, and alternative options (i.e., massage therapy, humor therapy).

Nausea and vomiting are symptoms that can accompany the disease itself or be the result of therapy. A number of medications are now available but often it is the nurse who interacts with the patient to identify the most effective and affordable medication. A number of studies address the effects of symptom distress on a patient's quality of life, and it should be the responsibility of the practitioner to work with the patient to minimize symptom distress and maximize functional capacity and quality of life.

Quality Assurance

Diagnosis and treatment of sarcoma of the small intestine remains an oncologic challenge. This review has raised the awareness of the practitioner to the vague symptomatology and challenges that occur with the diagnosis of this disease. It identifies the current treatment options and resulting prognostic situations that will allow the practitioner to identify and focus on issues that are affecting a patient's holistic situation.

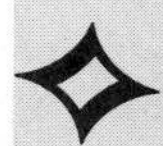

TABLE 45-4 Patient Preparation for the Diagnosis of Sarcoma of the Small Intestine

Your doctor has discovered that you have a sarcoma of the small intestine. This is a cancerous tumor that is found in the part of your bowel that is located between the stomach and the large bowel or colon. You have a number of choices regarding your treatment, and it is important that you speak with your doctor and nurse about these options. It is important that you take good care of yourself during this time. This worksheet is a guide to help you understand some of the choices you will be asked to make and some of the things you can do to take care of yourself. Talk to your health care professional to learn all that you can about your disease.

Your treatment options are:

1. **Surgery**—An operation is performed to remove the diseased area. All or a part of the tumor is removed. If you are having a problem with a blockage of the intestine, the surgeon can operate to reopen the blockage.
2. **Chemotherapy**—Medication (chemotherapy) is given (usually through a vein in your arm) to destroy the cancer cells. Chemotherapy can be given in addition to surgery or by itself.
3. **Radiation therapy**—A radiation beam is used to destroy cancer cells. Unlike chemotherapy, it is not given through your veins, but is given by a machine in the radiation oncology department.
4. **Biotherapy**—Medication to stimulate your body's own defenses to fight the cancer. Many of these treatments are experimental, so talk to your doctor about any specific requirements you might have.

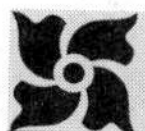

TABLE 45-5 Standard of Care for the Patient with Sarcoma Having a Bowel Resection

Patient Problem and Outcomes	Nursing Interventions	Patient Education
Pain Patient will state that pain is relieved by medication and other pain relief measures.	1. Assess effectiveness of pain relief obtained by medications. 2. Consult with appropriate clinicians about changes in pain medication, if inadequate pain relief is not obtained. 3. Promote nonpharmacologic techniques to reduce pain.	1. Teach patient preoperatively that bowel resection is a painful procedure, that he or she may be uncomfortable. 2. Assure patient that asking for increases in pain medication is appropriate and acceptable. 3. Change patient positions, use distraction techniques, guided imagery, back rubs, touch, massage.
Respiratory Status Lungs will be clear to auscultation.	1. Reinforce preoperative teaching concerning the importance of deep breathing, coughing, and turning. 2. Promote and assist patient to turn, cough, deep breath every hour. 3. Assist patient in changing positions every hour. 4. Splint the patient's incision to help him or her cough effectively. 5. Assist patient with use of incentive spirometer. 6. Auscultate lungs every 4 hours. 7. Monitor intake and output, color of urine.	1. Teach patient that the effects of anesthesia and pain related to surgery can decrease mobility and increase risk of respiratory problems.
Infection Patient will be discharged from hospital infection free.	1. Explain and demonstrate care of abdominal incision. 2. Wash margins of wound carefully with prescribed soap. 3. Use sterile technique. 4. Avoid bending and lifting until told otherwise by surgeon. 5. Describe nutritional diet. 6. Teach symptoms to be reported to health care provider: a. Wound separation, redness, swelling, warmth, or discharge b. Fever, chills c. Increasing cough d. Urinary frequency, burning e. Pain, swelling in legs	1. Teach patient and family caregiver the rationale of wound care. 2. Teach patient and family signs and symptoms of postoperative complications: wound dehiscence, pneumonia, urinary tract infection and deep vein thrombus.
Patient will have to assess cancer support system after discharge from hospital.	1. Give patient phone numbers and e-mail address of support group for psychological support: a. Cancer Information Center 1-800-4-CANCER b. Cancer Fax® 1-301-402-5874 c. CancerNet http://nci.nih.gov	Teach patient and family the advantages of support groups with patients having had bowel resections for sarcoma.
Fatigue Patient will have an understanding of the impact and management of fatigue.	1. Raise patient's awareness that fatigue is a result of disease, anesthesia, and recovery: a. Prioritize activities; do only important tasks first b. Keep mobile, walk as soon and as far possible c. Ask for help when needed d. Discuss fatigue with health care provider 2. Monitor patient complete blood counts.	Explain to patient that fatigue is an expected outcome of surgery and cancer treatment.

Modified from Sands, J. (1995). Management of persons with problems of the intestine. In, W. J. Phipps, V. Cassmeyer, J. K. Sands, & M. K. Lehman (Eds.), *Medical-surgical nursing: Concepts and clinical practice.* St. Louis: Mosby.

TABLE 45-6 Patient Self-Assessment Scale for Fatigue

The patient moves the arrow to indicate the level of fatigue currently experienced.

No Fatigue	
1	
2	
3	
4	⇦
5	
6	
7	
8	
9	
10	

Courtesy Orthobiotech, Raritan, NY, 1996.

REFERENCES

Basson, M. D. (1993). Small bowel tumors. *Current Opinion in General Surgery,* 219-224.

Chami, T. N., Ratner, L. E., Henneberry, J., Smith, D. P., Hill, G., & Katz, P. O. (1994). Angiosarcoma of the small intestine: A case report and literature review. *American Journal of Gastroenterology, 89*(5), 797-800.

Chow, J. S., Chen, C. C., Ahsan, H., & Neugut, A. (1996). A population-based study of the incidence of malignant small bowel tumors: SEER, 1973-1990. *International Journal of Epidemiology, 25,* 722-728.

Ciresi, D. L. & Scholten, D. J. (1995). The continuing clinical dilemma of primary tumors of the small intestine. *American Surgeon, 61,* 698-703.

Coit, D. G. (1993). Cancer of the small bowel. In V. T. DeVita, S. Hellman, & S. A. Rosenberg (Eds.), *Cancer: Principles and practice of Oncology* (3rd ed., pp. 915-928). Philadelphia: J. B. Lippincott Company.

DiSario, J. A., Burt, R. W., Vargas, H., & McWhorter, W. P. (1994). Small bowel cancer: Epidemiological and clinical characteristics from a population-based registry. *American Journal of Gastroenterology, 89*(5), 699-701.

Gabos, S., Berkel, J., Band, P., Robson, D., & Whittaker, H. (1993). Small bowel cancer in western Canada. *International Journal of Epidemiology, 22*(2), 198-206.

Gawdat, K. & Corey, C. J. (1993). Small bowel sarcomas presenting as a diverticular abscess [Letter to the editor]. *Journal of Clinical Gastroenterology, 16*(3), 272-274.

Herrera, A., Sålad-Celigny, P., Brousse, N., Renoux, M., Dehrmy, D., Theodore, C. Breil, P., Bernard, J. F., Paolaggi, J. A. (1984). Primary lymphomas of the digestive tract: Therapeutic results of 35 cases. *Gastroenterology of Clinical Biology, 8,* 407-413.

Horowitz, J., Spellman, J. E., Driscoll, D. L., Velez, A. F., & Karakousis, C. P. (1995). An institutional review of sarcomas of the large and small intestine. *Journal of the American College of Surgeons, 180,* 465-471.

Landis, S. H., Murray, T., Bolden, S., & Wingo P. A. (1998). Cancer statistics, 1998. *CA: A Cancer Journal For Clinicians, 48*(1), 6-30.

Maglinte, D. T., O'Connor, K., Bessett, J., Chernish, S. M., & Kelvin, F. M. (1991). The role of the physician in the late diagnosis of primary malignant tumors of the small intestine. *American Journal of Gastroenterology, 86*(3), 304-308.

Marcilla, J. A., Bueno, F. S., Aguilar, J., & Paricio, P. P. (1994). Primary small bowel malignant tumors. *European Journal of Surgical Oncology, 20,* 630-634.

Marieb, E. N. (1992). *Human anatomy and physiology* (2nd ed.). Redwood City, CA: Benjamin/Cummings.

Matsuo, S., Eto, T., Tsunoda, T., Kanematsu, T., & Shinozake, T. (1994). Small bowel tumors: An analysis of tumor-like lesions, benign and malignant neoplasms. *European Journal of Surgical Oncology, 20,* 47-51.

National Cancer Institute. (1997). PDQ cancer treatment summary for health professionals: Small intestine cancer (208/01175). Bethesda, MD: National Cancer Institute.

National Cancer Institute. (1996). PDQ cancer treatment summary for patients: Small intestine cancer (208/01175). Bethesda, MD: National Cancer Institute.

Ng, E. (1992). Prognostic factors influencing survival in gastrointestinal leiomyosarcomas: Implications for surgical management and staging. *Annals of Surgery, 215*(1), 68-77.

Ng, E., Pollock, R. E., Munsell, M. F., Atkinson, E. N., & Romsdahl, M. M. (1992). Prognostic factors influencing survival in gastrointestinal leiomyosarcomas: Implications for surgical management and staging. *Annals of Surgery, 215*(1), 68-77.

O'Riordan, B. G., Vilor, M., & Herrera, L. (1996). Small bowel tumors: An overview. *Digestive Diseases, 14,* 245-257.

Ripamoni, C. (1998). Bowel obstruction. In A. Berger, R. K. Portnoy, & Weissman (Eds.). *Principles and practice of supportive oncology.* Philadelphia: Lippincott-Raven.

Rivkind, A. I., Admon, D., Yarom, R., & Schreiber, L. (1994). Myxoid liposarcoma of the small intestine mimicking acute appendicitis: Case report. *European Journal of Surgery, 160,* 251-252.

Rottenberg, G. T. & Thomas, B. M. (1994). Case report: Granulocytic sarcoma of the small bowel—A rare presentation of leukemia. *Clinical Radiology, 49.*

Scott, D. G. (1997). Cancer of the small intestine. In V. T. DeVita, S. Hellman, & S. A. Rosenberg (Eds.), *Cancer: Principles and practice of oncology* (5th ed.). Philadelphia: Lippincott-Raven.

Serour, F., Dona, G., Birkenfeld, S., Balassiano, M., & Krispin, M. (1992). Primary neoplasms of the small bowel. *Journal of Surgical Oncology, 49,* 29-34.

Thomas, J. R., Mrak, R. E., & Libuit, N. (1994). Gastrointestinal autonomic nerve tumor presenting as high-grade sarcoma: Case report and review of the literature. *Digestive Diseases and Sciences, 39*(9), 2051-2055.

Ueyama, T., Guo, K. J., Hashimoto, H., Daimaru, Y., & Enjoji, M. (1992). A clinicopathologic and immunohistochemical study of gastrointestinal stromal tumors. *Cancer, 69,* 947-955.

Stomach Cancer

Barbara Hawkins, RN, MS, OCN

EPIDEMIOLOGY

Gastric cancer ranks as the seventh most common cancer and accounts for only about 2% of all cancers in the United States; yet, in 1930, gastric cancer was the country's most common cancer. Over the last 50 years, there has been a steady decline of the disease, with a plateau in 1985. This same pattern also occurred in Canada, Australia, and New Zealand (Bruckner, Kondo, & Kondo, 1997). In 1995 the number of new cases of gastric cancer in the United States was 22,800, with over 14,700 deaths predicted (Alexander, Kelsen, & Tepper, 1997). African Americans, Hispanic Americans, and Native Americans are 1.5 to 2.5 times more likely than Caucasians to develop gastric cancer (Fuchs & Mayer, 1995).

Gastric cancer remains the second most common cancer globally. Until 1988 it was the leading cause of cancer death worldwide, and in the 1980s an estimated 670,000 new cases developed annually. It is a leading cause of cancer deaths in Central and South America, parts of eastern Europe, Iceland, the Chinese population in Singapore, and the Maoris of New Zealand. It is the most prevalent cancer in Korea, southern China, and Japan. With the exception of Costa Ricans, the Japanese have the highest incidence of gastric cancer in the world. The incidence rate in Japan is 100 per 100,000, vs 10 per 100,000 in the United States and western Europe (Bruckner, Kondo, & Kondo, 1997; Alexander, Kelsen, & Tepper, 1997). In Japan, aggressive early screening for gastric cancer is routine and gastric resection can be curative. In the United States, only about 20% of patients who have gastric cancer could undergo potentially curative resections (Parsonnet, 1993). Early symptoms of gastric cancer are vague and often ignored. Most patients are diagnosed with stage III or stage IV disease when long-term survival is uncommon.

The incidence of gastric cancer in first- and second-generation Japanese who move to the United States is much lower than those who live in Japan. This points to a possible environmental cause. A new area for investigators has opened with the promising study of the role of *Helicobacter pylori* infection in gastric cancer (Sawyers, 1995). Gastric cancer is a disease of poverty that affects developing nations and areas in the industrial world with low socioeconomic conditions. In Peru, Mexico, and Columbia, the rate of gastric cancer is almost epidemic. Virtually all adults in these areas are infected with the *H. pylori* bacteria. In high-risk areas, the infection is acquired in early childhood and causes stomach inflammation and ulcers, which may play a role in the development of gastric cancer (Parsonnet, 1993).

RISK FACTORS

In 1965, Lauren described two distinct histologic types of stomach adenocarcinomas: *intestinal* and *diffuse*. This provides a model for a better understanding of the etiology and epidemiology of this disease. The intestinal type arises from precancerous conditions such as gastric atrophy or intestinal metaplasia in the stomach. This occurs more commonly in men than in women and more frequently in an older population, and it is representative of the dominant histologic type in geographic areas where stomach cancer is epidemic. This suggests a primarily environmental etiology. The diffuse form does not actually arise from precancerous conditions and represents the major histologic type in the geographic areas where gastric cancer is endemic. It is slightly more common in women and in younger patients. There is an increased association of this form of gastric cancer with familial occurrence (blood type A); therefore it appears to have a genetic link. The major risk factors associated with the development of gastric cancer are listed in Box 46-1 (Maehara, Yasunori, Tomisaki, Oshiro, Kakeji, & Ichiyoshi et al., 1996).

Increasing Age

Starting at the fourth decade, the incidence of stomach cancer increases with advancing age. It has a peak incidence in the seventh decade in men and a slightly later peak incidence in women (Alexander, Kelsen, & Tepper, 1997; Sano, Sasako, Kinoshita, & Maruyama, 1993).

Box 46-1
Risk Factors for Gastric Cancer

Genetic and Environmental Factors

- Family history of gastric cancer
- Blood type A and achlorhydria (lack of stomach acid)
- Low socioeconomic status
- Low consumption of fruits and vegetables
- Consumption of salted, smoked, or poorly preserved foods
- Cigarette smoking
- Increased age
- Ethnic differences
- Gender

Precursor Conditions

- Chronic atrophic gastritis and intestinal metaplasia
- Pernicious anemia
- Partial gastrectomy for benign disease
- *Helicobacter pylori* infection
- Ménétrier's disease
- Gastric adenomatuous polyps
- Barrett's esophagus

From Fuchs, C., & Mayer, R. (1995). Gastric carcinoma. *The New England Journal of Medicine, 333,* 32-41.

Ethnic Differences

Stomach cancer occurs more frequently in African-American men in the United States than in Caucasian men (1.5:1). The incidence is also higher among Hispanic Americans and Native Americans (1:2.5) (Alexander, Kelsen, & Tepper, 1997).

Gender Differences

Men have a higher incidence of gastric cancer than women by a ratio of 2:1.

Chronic Atrophic Gastritis and Intestinal Metaplasia

Studies of specimens obtained at surgery or autopsy have suggested that gastric cancers often develop in the context of other conditions. Chronic atrophic gastritis and its associated abnormality, intestinal metaplasia, are more closely linked to an increased risk of gastric cancer. Atrophic gastritis usually begins as a multifocal process in the stomach. As foci coalesce, reduced gastric acid production results. This condition may progress to metaplasia, dysplasia, and ultimately carcinoma. The incidence of atrophic gastritis and gastric metaplasia is highest in regions of the world that have the highest rates of gastric cancer (Fuchs & Mayer, 1995).

Pernicious Anemia

Studies have shown that patients with pernicious anemia are two to three times more likely to develop stomach cancer (Fuchs & Mayer, 1995).

Partial Gastrectomy for Benign Disease

Controversy exists regarding the association between gastric ulcer and gastric cancer. There is an increased risk of stomach cancer in patients who have had a partial gastrectomy for benign disease. This risk remains low until 15 to 20 years after the resection, but steadily increases after that to the range of 1.5:3. This delay may be due to the time it would take for the gradual progression of normal mucosa to metaplasia to dysplasia to cancer that is a result of acholrhydria and enterogastric reflux. Some investigators advocate endoscopic screening for these patients, but given the small relative risk associated with partial gastrectomy, as well as scant evidence that would offer support, this routine screening does not appear to be justified (Fuchs & Mayer, 1995; Miwa, Hattori, & Miyazaki, 1995).

Helicobacter Pylori Infection

Studies show a consistent association between *H. pylori* infection and the risk of gastric cancer. People with *H. pylori* infection are three to six times more likely to develop stomach cancer than those without this infection. It appears there is a strong association between *H. pylori* infection and stomach cancer in women and African Americans. The role of *H. pylori* in gastric carcinogenesis is unclear, although it is associated with the development of chronic atrophic gastritis. Gastric carcinoma develops only in a small portion of infected persons, so genetic or environmental cofactors are also required (Parsonnet, 1993; Correa, 1995).

Ménétrier's Disease

Numerous cases link gastric cancer with Ménétrier's disease, or hypertrophied gastropathy. Ménétrier's disease is quite rare, and it has been difficult to determine the strength of this relationship (Fuchs & Mayer, 1995).

Gastric Adenomatous Polyps

Considerable evidence also indicates an increased risk of gastric cancer among patients with adenomatous polyps of the stomach. The size of the polyp and the degree of dysplasia appear to be related to the malignant potential of the adenomas (Sawyers, 1995; Lee, Nascimento, Farnell, Carney, Harmsen, & Ilstrup, 1995).

Barrett's Esophagus

An increased incidence of adenocarcinoma of the gastric cardia and distal esophagus has been noted in patients with Barrett's esophagus. The incidence of cancer with this condition is approximately 0.8% a year. Further research is required to identify the patients who are at risk (Fuchs & Mayer, 1995).

Family History of Gastric Cancer

Considerable evidence supports the role of genetics in the development of gastric cancer. There are historic reports of family clustering. Among the most notable is the Bonaparte family, with Napoleon, his father, and grandfather dying of this disease. Studies indicate that first-degree relatives of patients with gastric cancer are two to three times more likely to develop this cancer (Hoebler, 1997).

Blood Type A

Studies also support a slight increased risk of gastric cancer among people with blood type A.

Low Socioeconomic Status

Worldwide, the risk of gastric cancer is inversely associated with socioeconomic status. It probably reflects the contributing aspects of overcrowding, poor sanitation, methods of food preservation, and poor nutrition. A startling contrast is evident with the increasing incidence of adenocarcinoma in the distal esophagus and the gastric cardia among higher socioeconomic classes. This remains largely unexplained (Fuchs & Mayer, 1995).

Low Consumption of Fruits and Vegetables

Data regarding diet and gastric cancer have been difficult to interpret because most of the studies are retrospective and rely on the patient's recollection of early eating habits. However, studies show that diets rich in raw (not cooked) fruits, vegetables, citrus fruits, and dietary fiber result in the lowest risk of gastric cancer. Diets rich in vitamins A and C are also associated with a lower risk (Alexander, Kelsen, & Tepper, 1997).

Consumption of Salted, Smoked, or Poorly Preserved Foods

Diets rich in salted, smoked, or poorly preserved foods are associated with a higher risk of developing the disease. The consumption of highly salted or pickled foods over a long period may lead to atrophic gastritis, which makes the gastric mucosa more susceptible to the development of cancer. Nitrates and nitrites were previously used to preserve meat, fish, and vegetables; however, during this century the use of these compounds has declined by 75%. Long-term use of refrigeration and improved methods of food preservation are associated with the decline of gastric cancer in industrial countries (Fuchs & Mayer, 1995; Fay, Fennerty, Emerson, & Larez, 1994).

Cigarette Smoking

The role of smoking in the development of gastric cancer remains equivocal. Some studies show that smokers are one and a half to three times more likely to develop gastric cancer. Studies about the relationship of alcohol consumption with gastric cancer are largely inconclusive (Fuchs & Mayer, 1995, Fay et al., 1994).

CHEMOPREVENTION

Few primary strategies, with the exception of quitting cigarette smoking, are recommended for the prevention of gastric cancer for Caucasian natives of the United States. Dietary avoidance of heavily processed or cured foods containing nitrates is recommended, and a diet with adequate amounts of fresh vegetables and fruits is advised. Patients at high risk, such as Japanese newly located in this country who have eaten traditional Japanese foods, may be advised to have fluoroscopic and endoscopic screening for gastric cancer. Patients older than 40 years of age with undiagnosed weight loss or a history of documented gastric ulcers may also be candidates for screening (Tabbarah, 1995).

PATHOPHYSIOLOGY

Normal Anatomy and Physiology of the Stomach

The stomach is a hollow, pouchlike reservoir that extends from the esophageal (cardiac) sphincter to the duodenal (pyloric) sphincter. It is divided into three major areas: the fundus, corpus or body, and antrum (Fig. 46-1).

The stomach wall is composed of four layers: the serosa, muscle, submucosa, and mucosa. Close to, or in contact with, the stomach are the liver, diaphragm, left suprarenal gland, kidney, pancreas, duodenum, and transverse colon. The stomach is rich with a lymphatic system running through the mucosal, submucosal, muscular, and serosal layers. These lymphatic networks communicate freely with each other, as well as with the esophagus and duodenum, and thereby serve as a route for metastatic spread. Blood vessels approximate the same course as the lymphatic vessels shown in Fig. 46-2. Approximately 95% of gastric cancers are adenocarcinomas; the other 5% are leiomyosarcomas, lymphomas, squamous cell cancers, or other rare types (Tabbarah, 1995).

The pathophysiology of gastric cancer in the United States tends to differ from gastric cancer in Japan, where it is endemic. Japan has a vigorous screening program, which results in higher rates of stomach cancer that are detected earlier, leading to higher survival rates.

In the United States, gastric cancer is more aggressive and invasive. It tends to infiltrate into the submucosa of the stomach, where detection by endoscopy is more difficult and the risk of metastatic spread is high. In the United States, 37% of gastric tumors originate in the upper third of the stomach, 20% in the middle third, and 30% in the lower third, and 12% involve the entire stomach. The 5-year survival rate after resection is 20% to 25% for tumors in the distal portion of the stomach, 10% for proximal tumors, and less than 5% if the entire stomach is involved. The diminished survival rate for tumors in the proximal stomach may due to the aggressiveness of tumors in that site, or it may be explained by the surgical difficulty of resection of that area, as well as the difficulty of obtaining sufficiently wide surgical margins (Fuchs & Mayer, 1995).

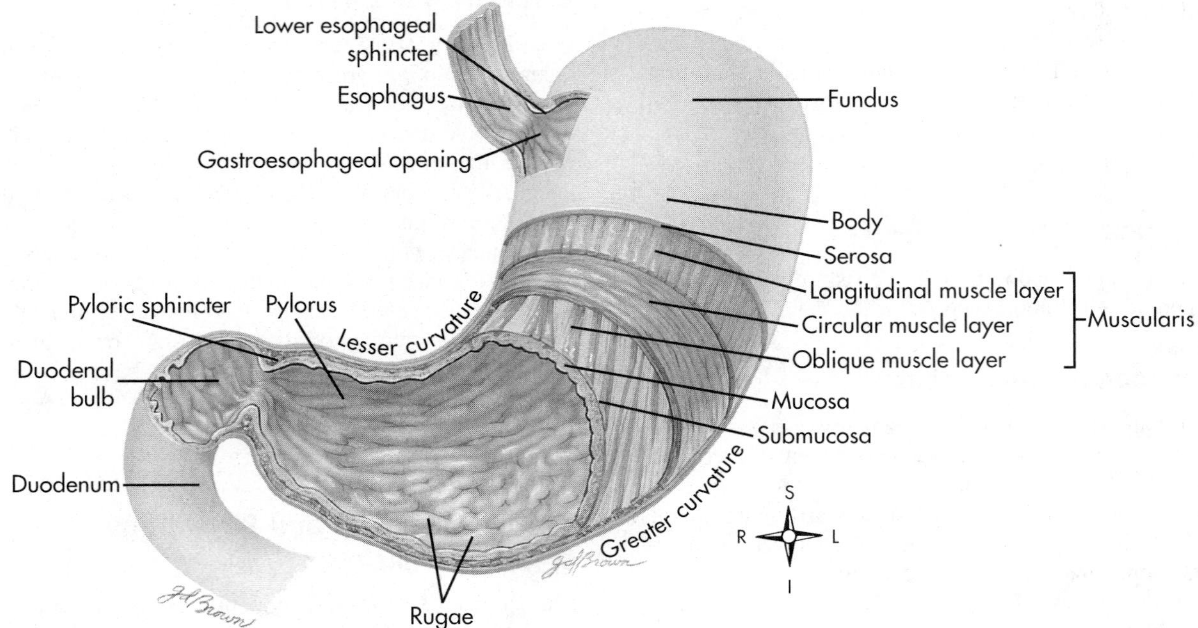

Fig. 46-1 Stomach: A portion of the anterior wall has been cut away to reveal the muscle layers of the stomach wall. (From Thibodeau, G. A. & Patton, K. T. [1996]. *Anatomy and Physiology* [3rd ed.]. St. Louis: Mosby.)

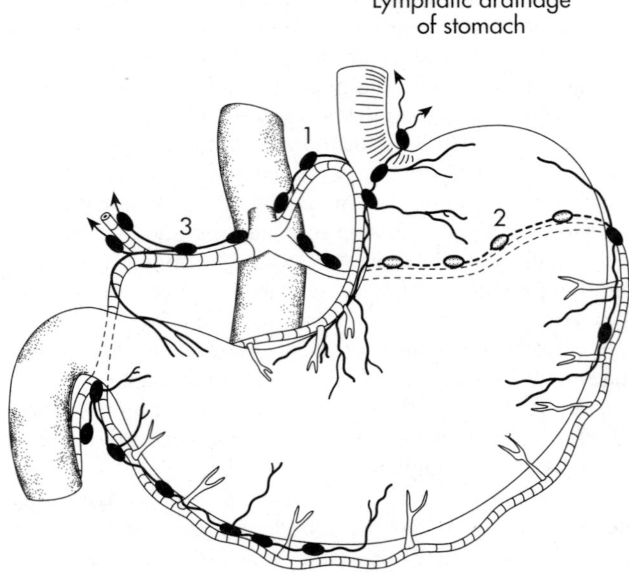

Fig. 46-2 Lymphatic drainage of the stomach showing (1) collecting trunks of the gastric artery, (2) splenic artery, and (3) hepatic artery. (Adapted from Lawrence, W. & Zfass, A. [1995]. Gastric Neoplasms. In G. P. Murphy, W. Lawrence & R. E. Lenhard [Eds.]. *American Cancer Society Textbook of Clinical Oncology*. Atlanta: The American Cancer Society.)

The Process of Carcinogenesis

Recent epidemiologic evidence indicates that *H. pylori* infection increases the risk for gastric cancer. There are several potential mechanisms of gastric carcinogenesis by *H. pylori:* (1) Metabolic products of the organisms directly transform the mucosa; (2) analogous to carcinogenesis by viral pathogens, *H. pylori* deoxyribonucleic acid (DNA) is incorporated into the host cells, causing transformation; or (3) *H. pylori* induces an inflammatory response that is genotoxic. Chronic inflammation has been causally linked with diverse malignancies, such as colon cancer following ulcerative colitis and squamous cell carcinoma following chronic osteomyelitis. These chronic inflammatory processes are thought to induce cancer by causing cell proliferation and increasing free-radical formation. Proliferation puts cellular DNA at risk for spontaneous replication error. In experiments in vitro and in vivo, *H. pylori* causes increased cell proliferation. Most DNA damage is corrected by the body's normal protective mechanisms, but the capacity to survey and repair is less than perfect. The longer the duration of the infection, the higher the likelihood of inadequate repair and subsequent malignant transformation. *H. pylori* infection increases the rate of proliferation of the gastric epithelial cells and decreases the gastric secretion of ascorbic acid. This process may modulate the process of carcinogenesis. People infected with *H. pylori* at a young age who generate a marked inflammatory response may be at risk for gastric cancer. If these people consume diets high in potential carcinogens and low in antioxidants, their risk is higher. Although infection or diet alone could explain gastric cancer in some individuals, a combination of these cofactors could have a synergistic effect (Parsonnet, 1993; Veldhuyzen & Sherman, 1994; Correa, 1995). This process is outlined in Fig. 46-3.

The role of the tumor-suppressor protein, P53, in the carcinogenesis of gastric cancer has received considerable attention. Higher rates of the P53 abnormality correlate directly with the stage of the disease. The clinical significance of P53 accumulation may be helpful preoperatively to identify patients at high risk of metastatic spread to regional

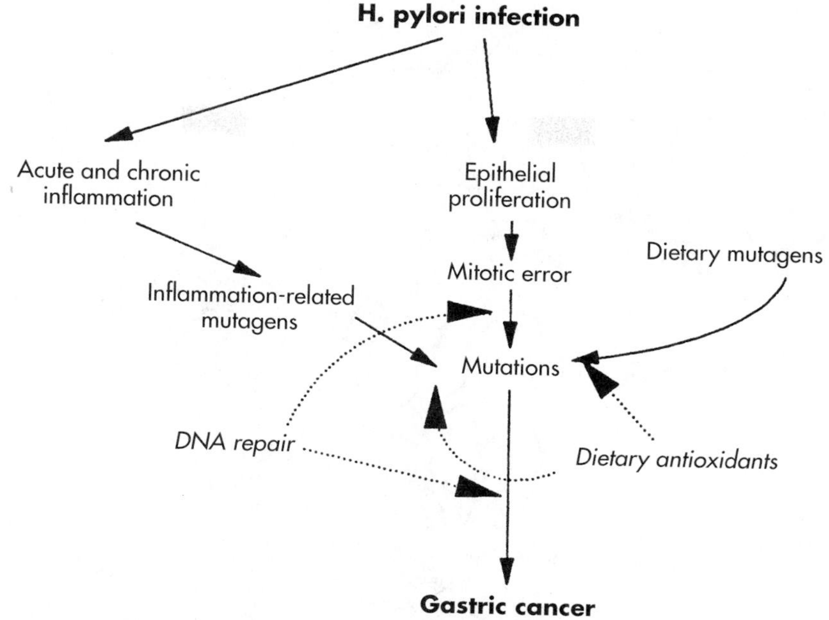

Fig. 46-3 A model for gastric carcinogenesis incorporating *H. pylori* infection. The *solid arrows* indicate detrimental factors, and the *dotted arrows* indicate protective factors. *H. pylori,* by causing both proliferation and inflammation, would increase the risk for mutation and eventual malignant transformation. (From Parsonnet, J. [1993]. *Helicobactor pylori* and gastric cancer. *Gastroenterology Clinics of North America, 22,* 89-104.)

lymph nodes and to identify those with an equally poor prognosis. This marker may allow for the appropriate planning of better treatment strategies (Starzynska, Markiewski, Domagala, Marlicz, Mietkieski, & Roberts et al., 1996; Thompson, van Heerden, & Sarr, 1993).

In a recent report, epidermal growth factor (EGF) was found in about 26% of patients with gastric cancer. The presence of EGF in these patients correlated with the degree of gastric wall invasion and lymph node metastasis. The 5-year survival for patients with EGF-positive tumors is worse than for those with EGF-negative tumors. This represents a higher malignant potential for gastric cancer when EGF is present. About 12% of the gastric cancers in this study were also positive for c-*erb*B-2. This type of tumor has frequent metastasis and a poorer prognosis than tumors negative for the c-*erb*B-2 one α gene (Tokunaga, Onda, Okuda, Teramoto, Fujita, & Mizutani et al., 1995).

Although surgery remains the treatment of choice for gastric cancer, most patients suffer a relapse after the procedure. TNM staging is currently used to determine patient selection for surgery; however, the status of lymph nodes is very difficult to establish before surgery. A better understanding of the carcinogenesis of gastric cancer leads to more effective methods of treatment.

ROUTES OF METASTASES

Gastric tumors are aggressive and metastasize early by lymph spread or by direct extension. Spread through the lymphatic vessels may be quite extensive, reaching as far as 10 to 15 cm from the primary gastric lesion.

There are several characteristic routes by which gastric cancer progresses and metastasizes: (1) by extension and infiltration along the mucosal surface and stomach wall or lymphatics; (2) through lymphatic or vascular embolism, probably to regional lymph nodes, occurring in approximately two thirds of patients: (3) by direct extension into adjacent structures such as the pancreas, esophagus, spleen, colon, gallbladder, adjacent mesenteries, or most commonly to the liver; or (4) through the bloodstream (Fuchs & Mayer, 1995).

As with other cancers, the metastatic spread of gastric cancer is correlated with the size and location of the tumor. Tumors of the distal stomach usually metastasize to infrapyloric, inferior gastric, and celiac nodes. Lesions in the proximal stomach often metastasize to the pancreatic, pericardial, and gastric lymph nodes. In advanced gastric cancer, there may be involvement of the left supraclavicular nodes. This is a classic sign of inoperability (Virchow's node). Fig. 46-4 shows the nodal spread of gastric cancer. The lungs, adrenal glands, liver, pancreas, bones, and peritoneal cavity are the usual sites of distant metastasis. A Krukenberg tumor is gastric cancer that has spread to the ovary. Direct extension into the colon may be associated with foul-smelling emesis or passage of recently ingested material in the stool. A tumor that has spread along the peritoneal surfaces and results in a periumbilical node is known as *Sister Mary Joseph's node* (Lawrence, 1991). Fig. 46-5 diagrams the routes of gastric cancer spread.

ASSESSMENT

Table 46-1 summarizes the assessment of a patient for gastric cancer. The clinical evaluation needs to include a de-

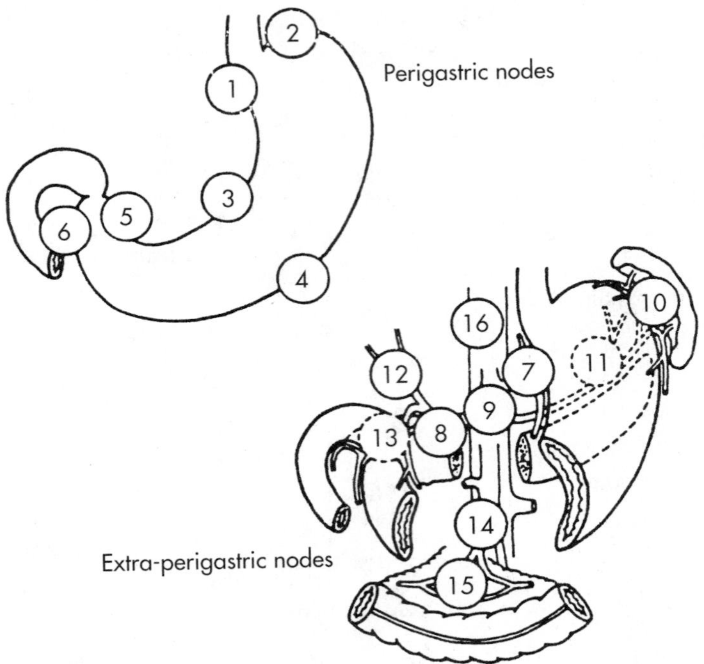

Fig. 46-4 Nodal spread of gastric cancer. Top: perigastric lymph nodes 1-6; bottom: extragastric lymph nodes; left gastric artery; 8, 11, splenic artery; 12, hepatoduodenal ligament; 13, retropancreatic; 14, root of mesentery; 15, middle colic artery; 16, para-aortic. (From Thompson, G., van Heerden, J., & Sarr, M. [1993]. Adenocarcinoma of the stomach: Are we making progress?" *The Lancet, 342,* 713-718.)

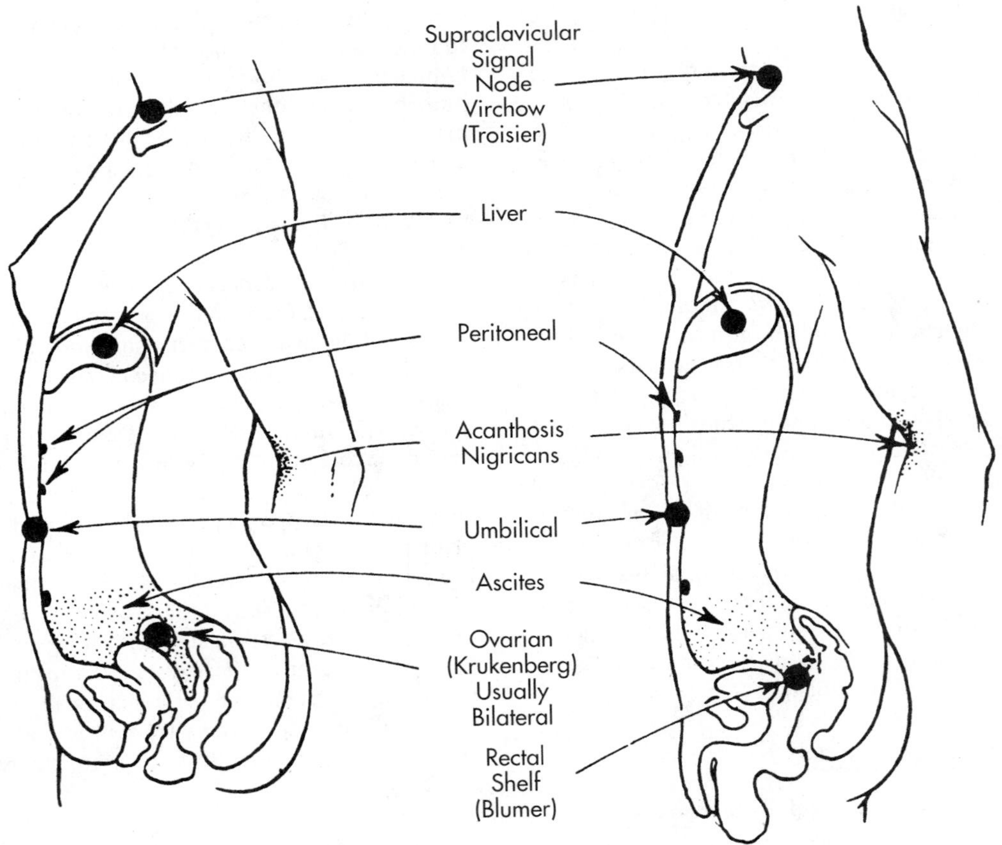

Fig. 46-5 Gastric cancer routes of spread. (From Lawrence, W. [1995]. Gastric neoplasms. In G. P. Murphy, W. Lawrence, & R. E. Lenhard [Eds.]. *American Cancer Society Textbook of Clinical Oncology,* Atlanta: The American Cancer Society, 279-292.)

TABLE 46-1 Assessment of the Patient for Gastric Cancer

	Assessment Parameters	Typical Abnormal Findings
History	A. Personal and social history 1. Age 2. Ethnicity 3. Family history 4. Gender 5. Evaluation of nutritional status	A. Personal and social risk factors 1. Usually over age 40 years 2. More prevalent in African Americans and Asians than Causasians in the United States 3. Positive family history increases the risk 4. More common in males 5. Common symptoms include sense of fullness, feeling of heaviness, distention after meals, nausea, vomiting, change in appetite, dysphagia, hematemesis, melena, and change in bowel habits.
Physical Examination	A. Abdominal palpation	A. Palpable abdominal mass and/or hepatomegaly may indicate advanced disease. Peristalsis moving in left-to-right direction could indicate pyloric obstruction.
	B. Lymph node evaluation	B. The presence of abdominal nodes and palpation of supraclavicular or axillary nodes could indicate sites of metastatic disease.
	C. Weight	C. Weight loss may be a sign of advanced disease.
	D. Rectal examination	D. Palpation of the tumor on rectal shelf may indicate metastatic deposits.
Diagnostic Tests	A. Upper gastrointestinal series	A. Filling defects and stomach wall rigidity suggest malignant involvement.
	B. Flexible endoscopic gastroscopy	B. Presence of gastric lesion may be visualized.
	C. Computed tomographic scanning (CT scan)	C. Delineation of the extent of the primary gastric tumor and any lymph node involvement or distant metastasis can be detected.

tailed patient and family history, a thorough physical examination, and a battery of diagnostic tests. Because the initial symptoms are vague, the diagnosis and treatment are often delayed. Although the incidence of gastric cancer is decreasing, it is necessary to provide aggressive preventative health care to high-risk individuals.

History

The patient needs to be assessed for all the known risk factors for gastric cancer. To establish a clinical picture, a complete assessment of the patient's nutritional status should be done. This in-depth nutritional assessment and history assists in identifying the subtle changes in dietary habits or contributory signs such as pain or bowel changes that may be indicative of gastric cancer. About two thirds of patients usually have epigastric pain after eating. Unlike the epigastric pain of peptic ulcers, this pain is vague, with a feeling of fullness or discomfort after eating (Sawyers, 1995).

Individuals usually delay several months between the onset of symptoms and the initial medical consultation. Pain in the epigastric, back, or retrosternal area is often an early symptom that is ignored or responds temporarily to symptomatic treatment. The individual may complain of a vague, uneasy sense of fullness, a feeling of heaviness, and moderate distention after eating. Antacids and other home remedies are successful for awhile and are used until the symptoms become more definitive. As the disease advances, progressive weight loss may occur as a result of decreased appetite, nausea, and vomiting. Weakness, fatigue, and anemia are also common findings. Tumors in the proximal portion of the stomach often cause dysphagia. Patients sometimes report hematemesis, melena, or a change in bowel habits. Unfortunately, the definitive clinical signs occur with advanced disease (Fuchs & Mayer, 1995; Sawyers, 1995; Hoebler, 1997). Table 46-2 shows common symptoms of gastric cancer at the time of diagnosis.

TABLE 46-2 Common Signs and Symptoms at the Time of Initial Diagnosis of Gastric Cancer

Symptom	Frequency (%)
Weight loss	61.6
Abdominal pain	51.6
Palpable abdominal mass	37
Nausea	34.3
Anorexia	32.0
Dysphagia	26.1
Melena	20.2
Early satiety	17.5
Ulcer type of pain	17.1
Anemia	10.0
Lower-extremity edema	5.9

Physical Examination

The physical examination is normal in most patients until the gastric cancer is advanced enough to show metastatic spread. Unfortunately, these findings are frequently those of disease so advanced that cure is not possible (Sawyers, 1995). The physical examination includes palpation of the abdomen and lymph nodes, particularly the supraclavicular and axillary lymph nodes because they can be sites of metastatic disease. An abdominal mass and/or hepatomegaly may be palpated. A rectal examination may reveal a shelf of metastatic deposits. Peristaltic activity moving in a left-to-right direction may be detected if there is an obstruction in the pyloric area. Anemia and jaundice are usual signs of advanced gastric cancer (Hoebler, 1997).

Diagnostic Tests

Any signs or symptoms of an upper gastrointestinal nature that are suggestive of gastric cancer, particularly in the over 40 age group, need to be investigated by diagnostic procedures to identify the source of the symptoms. About 5% to 10% of gastric cancer patients may have complaints similar to those of patients with peptic ulcer disease. Another 10% have nonspecific symptoms of chronic disease, such as weight loss, anemia, and weakness. A small number of patients first present with an acute intraabdominal problem, such as massive upper gastrointestinal bleeding, acute obstruction of the esophagus or pylorus, or gastric perforation, often requiring emergency surgery. The only observation that may lead to an early diagnosis of gastric cancer is a positive stool occult blood test (Alexander, Kelsen, & Tepper, 1997).

Upper Gastrointestinal Examination

The first test performed to investigate the signs and symptoms of gastric cancer is a double-contrast upper gastrointestinal series. This reveals the mucosal pattern, character of mobility, distensibility, and flexibility of the stomach walls. Patients with dyspepsia or other upper gastrointestinal symptoms who fail to respond to an emperic trial of medical therapy need to undergo a diagnostic workup. Table 46-3 reviews the patient preparation for this procedure (Levine, 1995).

Flexible Endoscopic Gastroscopy

An endoscopic examination should be considered if the upper gastrointestinal examination indicates the possibility of a tumor or if a previously noted lesion has not healed completely in 6 weeks. A fiberoptic endoscopy and biopsy have a reported accuracy rate of 95%. The accuracy of the diagnosis increases with the number of biopsy samples obtained. During this procedure the clinician is able to view the lesion directly and obtain multiple biopsies and brushings for cytology (Levine, 1995; Nicholson & Shorvon, 1993).

Computed Tomography

A computed tomograpy (CT) scan of the abdomen delineates the extent of the primary gastric tumor and also any node involvement or distant metastasis. When preoperative CT scans are compared with findings from gastric resections, the scans underestimate the extent of the disease, primarily due to radiographically undetectable lymph nodes and metastasis in the liver and omentum. Investigators use a high-frequency ultrasound probe to determine the depth of tumor penetration and lymph node metastasis, but this pro-

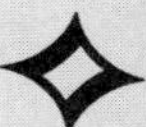

TABLE 46-3 Patient Preparation for Upper Gastrointestinal Endoscopy

Description of the Procedure: An upper endoscopy (also known as an *upper GI endoscopy, esophagogastroduodenscopy [EGD],* or *panendoscopy*) is a procedure that enables the physician to examine the lining of the upper part of the gastrointestinal tract (i.e., the esophagus, stomach, and duodenum [first portion of the small intestine]) using a thin, flexible tube with its own lens and light source. It is usually performed to evaluate symptoms of persistent upper abdominal pain, nausea, vomiting, or difficulty swallowing. It is also used to find the cause of bleeding from the upper gastrointestinal tract.

Patient Preparation: The patient must have a completely empty stomach and will need to fast for approximately 6 hours before the examination. The patient needs to alert the physician if antibiotics are required for dental procedures because antibiotics may be needed prior to an upper endoscopy as well. Topical anesthetics, analgesics, or sedatives are administered to facilitate endoscopic instrumentation and to make the patient comfortable. After the procedure, the patient receives nothing to eat or drink until the gag reflex returns. Hoarseness from throat irritation can be relieved by lozenges or warm saline gargling after the effects of anesthesia dissipate.

Procedural Considerations:

1. Obtain informed consent.
2. Place the patient in a gown.
3. Ask the patient to remove dentures or partial plates.
4. Spray the patient's throat with a local anesthetic, and administer intravenous (IV) medication to assist in relaxation before the test begins, if appropriate.
5. Assist the patient into a comfortable position on his or her side.
6. Pass the endoscope through the mouth, and then through the esophagus, stomach, and duodenum. Most patients consider the test to be only slightly uncomfortable, and many patients fall asleep during the procedure.
7. Monitor the patient after the test until most of the effects of the medication have worn off. The patient's throat may feel sore, and he or she may feel bloated immediately after the procedure due to the air introduced in the stomach during the test.
8. Arrangements for someone to accompany the patient home may be necessary.
9. Most patients will be able to resume their regular diet after the procedure.

Modified from American Society for Gastrointenstinal Endoscopy. (1995). *Understanding upper GI endoscopy.* Manchester, MA: American Society for Gastrointestinal Endoscopy.

cedure does not examine the entire abdomen and is unable to identify distant metastasis, as can a CT scan.

Tumor Markers

Tumor markers are not useful in the diagnosis of early gastric cancer. Carcinoembryonic antigen (CEA) levels are less frequently elevated than in colon cancer, although elevated levels (<5% per dl) have been reported in 40% to 50% of patients with metastatic gastric cancer. Similar elevations are noted in 10% to 20% of patients with surgically resectable disease. CEA levels are not used in the diagnostic phase of gastric cancer, but they may be of some value in postoperative follow-up.

The α-fetoprotein level (found in germ-cell and hepatocellular tumors) and CA 19-9 (found in pancreatic cancer) are elevated in 30% of patients with incurable gastric cancer. These markers are not useful in the early detection phase of gastric cancer. Investigators are examining gastric juices for the presence of tumor markers that may be helpful in the diagnosis of stomach cancer.

Magnetic Resonance Imaging

Magnetic resonance imaging (MRI) has been disappointing in the diagnostic workup for gastric cancer. This procedure may be used to evaluate the presence of hepatic metastasis.

STAGING

Clinical staging of gastric cancer is based on the extent of the disease, as shown by physical examination, as well as radiologic and endoscopic studies. However, the more accurate staging classification is contingent on the extent of the disease found at the time of the surgical exploration of the abdomen and the histologic study of the excised surgical specimens.

The positive findings of a cervical lymph node, liver, and/or peritoneal metastasis establish a stage IV disease, for which palliative treatment only is indicated. Such findings are not usually apparent until the time of gastric surgery.

Analyses from multiple clinical trials confirm the importance of the depth of tumor penetration into the gastric wall and the presence of metastasis to regional or distant sites in the prediction of survival rates (Fuchs & Mayer, 1995) (Fig. 46-6). The size or location of the primary gastric tumor ("T" in the staging classification) is of less significance in the prediction of a prognosis. Nodal involvement is, however, a significant prognostic factor in the staging process. The degree of nodal involvement ranges from no lymphatic metastasis (N0), to lymphatic spread to immediately adjacent nodes (N1), to the presence of positive nodes in the perigastric area on the lesser and greater gastric curvatures (N2), to more distant positive nodes (N3). Distant metastasis to the peritoneal surfaces, liver, or other sites detected at surgery is categorized as M1 and is a very poor prognostic indicator. (Table 46-4 contains the TNM classification for gastric cancer.)

The American Joint Commission on Cancer gastric cancer staging system is accepted in the United States and is recommended by the Joint Commission on Hospitals. The Japanese use the UICC (Union Internationale Caotre le Cancer) staging system. It is important to note the differences in these systems and that they are not to be considered equal.

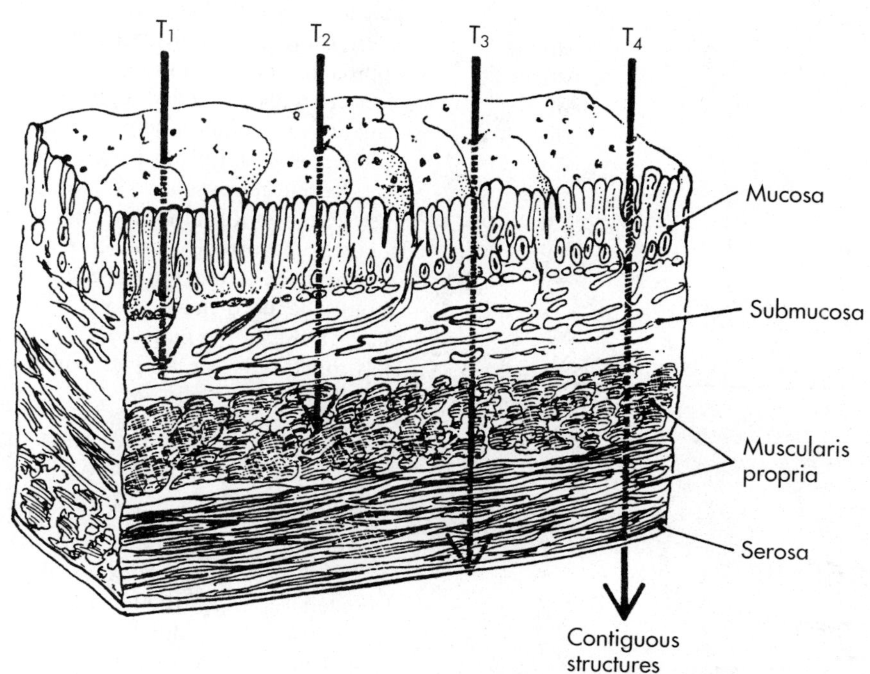

Fig. 46-6 Definition of "T" stage based on depth of penetration of the gastric wall. (From Alexander, H., Kelsen, D., & Tepper, J. [1997]. Cancer of the stomach. In V. T. Devita, S. Hellman, & S. A. Rosenberg [Eds.]. *Cancer: Principles and practice of oncology,* Philadelphia: Lippincott-Raven.)

TABLE 46-4 Staging for Gastric Cancer

Definitions			
Primary Tumor (T)			
TX	Primary tumor cannot be assessed		
T0	No evidence of primary tumor		
Tis	Carcinoma in situ: intraepithelial tumor without invasion of lamina propria		
T1	Tumor invades lamina propria or submucosa		
T2	Tumor invades the muscularis propria or the subserosa		
T3	Tumor penetrates the serosa (visceral peritoneum) without invasion of adjacent structures		
T4	Tumor invades adjacent structures		
Node (N)			
NX	Regional lymph node(s) cannot be assessed		
N0	No regional lymph node metastasis		
N1	Metastasis in perigastric lymph node(s) within 3 cm of the edge of the primary tumor		
N2	Metastasis in perigastric lymph node(s) more than 3 cm from the edge of the primary tumor, or in lymph nodes along the left gastric, common hepatic, splenic, or celiac arteries		
Metastasis (M)			
MX	Presence of distant metastasis cannot be assessed		
M0	No distant metastasis		
M1	Distant metastasis		
Stage System			
Stage 0	Tis	N0	M0
Stage 1A	T1	N0	M0
Stage 1B	T1	N1	M0
	T2	N0	M0
Stage II	T1	N2	M0
	T2	N1	M0
	T3	N0	M0
Stage IIIA	T2	N2	M0
	T3	N1	M0
	T4	N0	M0
Stage IIIB	T3	N2	M0
	T4	N1	M0
Stage IV	T4	N2	M0
	Any T	Any N	M1

Adapted from Alexander, H. R., Kelsen, D. G., & Tepper, J. C. [1997]. Cancer of the Stomach. In V. T. DeVita, S. Hellman, & S. A. Rosenberg [Eds.]. *Cancer: Principles and practice of oncology.* Philadelphia: Lippincott-Raven.

MEDICAL MANAGEMENT

Surgical Management

Surgery remains the most effective method of treatment of early and advanced gastric cancer. For localized lesions, surgery alone or in combination with chemotherapy or radiotherapy may provide cure. Effective palliation for advanced gastric cancer may be obtained by surgery combined with chemotherapy. The treatment of this cancer depends on the stage of the disease, the general condition of the patient, and the current available techniques in surgery, radiotherapy, and chemotherapy. Table 46-5 reviews the treatment of gastric cancer based on the stage of the disease.

Before any treatment option is initiated, the patient and family need to receive a complete explanation of the anticipated course of therapy and the expected outcomes. Ongoing investigation continues in regard to the differences in the extent of surgical approaches for gastric cancer. Controversy remains among those who favor a more radical surgical approach and those who support a more conservative resection. In many cases, resectability for cure or for palliation can only be definitively assessed at the time of abdominal surgery. Many of the patients with gastric cancer may be offered exploratory surgery. This is not a usual option for patients with documented liver metastasis or other proven distant metastases (i.e., cervical lymph nodes). Generally, the choice of surgical procedures is based on the location and extent of the disease (Alexander, Kelsen, & Tepper, 1997).

Total Gastrectomy

The major surgical options for gastric cancer are distal radical subtotal gastric resection, proximal subtotal esophagogastrectomy, or total gastrectomy. If the lesion is resectable and located in the body of the stomach, a total gastrectomy is usually performed. The entire stomach is removed "en bloc," along with supporting mesentery and lymph nodes (Fig. 46-7). The esophagus is anastomosed to the jejunum. A thoracic approach is often necessary to perform the esophagojejunostomy. Overall mortality rates are 10% to 15% for total gastrectomy surgery. Pneumonia, infection, anastomotic leak, hemorrhage, and reflux aspiration are frequent surgical complications. An even more radical surgical approach is common in Japan. A more extended lymph node dissection and extended regional resection that includes the pancreas is commonly performed. Surgery that includes splenectomy and distal pancreatectomy remains controversial. Recent retrospective studies lead to the conclusion that the resection of adjacent organs for contiguous spread seems to be of value only in patients with otherwise early gastric disease undergoing potentially curative surgery and should be used selectively (Thompson, van Heerden, & Sarr, 1993). In the palliative setting, total gastrectomies are performed only for patients with gastric bleeding or proximal gastric obstructions.

Subtotal Gastrectomy

Biillroth I. A radical subtotal gastrectomy, a Billroth I or Billroth II procedure, is performed for lesions located in the middle and distal portions of the stomach. The Billroth I procedure, or gastroduodenostomy, involves resecting the first portion of the duodenum, distal stomach, pylorus, and supporting circulatory and lymph vessels. The remaining stomach is anastomosed to the duodenum (Hoebler, 1997). Fig. 46-8 illustrates this procedure. Because it is not as extensive as the Billroth II, the Billroth I surgery is usually

TABLE 46-5 Treatment of Gastic Cancer Based on Stage of the Disease

Stage	Involvement	Therapeutic Option
Stage 0		
Tis, N0, M0	In situ tumor has not spread beyond, limiting membrane of the stomach (the mucosa)	Gastrectomy
Stage 1		
T1, N0, M0 (Stage 1A) T1, N1, M0 T2, N0, M0 (Stage 1B)	Cancer confined to wall of the stomach and no lymph nodes are involved	Radical subtotal gastrectomy Total gastrectomy plus, at minimum, removal of omentum and lymph nodes Chemotherapy Radiation therapy
Stage II		
T1, N2, M0 T2, N1, M0 T3, N0, M0	Cancer confined to wall of stomach, does not involve adjacent tissues; lymph nodes may be involved	Radical subtotal gastrectomy Total gastrectomy plus, at minimum, removal of omentum and lymph nodes Chemotherapy Radiation therapy
Stage III		
T2, N2, M0 T3, N1, M0 T4, N0, M0 T3, N2, M0 T4, N1, M0	Cancer involves tissues adjacent to stomach and/or lymph nodes close to or in stomach	Subtotal radical gastrectomy Total gastrectomy Chemotherapy Radiation therapy
Stage IV		
T4, N2, M0 Any T, any N, M1	Cancer has spread to adjacent tissues and lymph nodes or has spread to distant sites	Palliative surgery Chemotherapy Radiation therapy

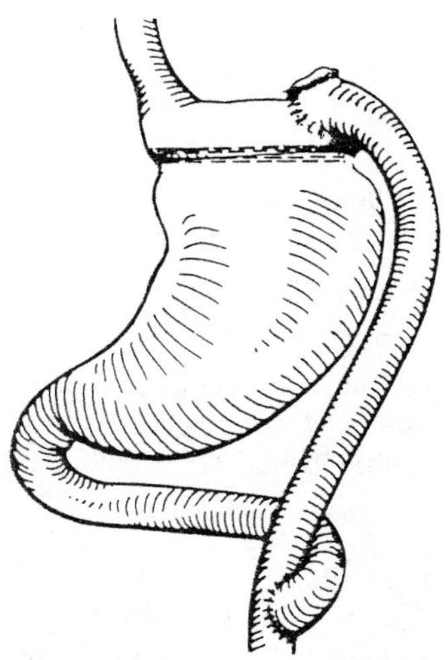

Fig. 46-7 Total gastrectomy reconstruction with a "Roux-En-Y" procedure to prevent bile from entering the esophagus. (Adapted from Rosenbaum, E. H. & Dollinger, M. [1994]. Stomach cancer. In M. Dollinger, E. H. Rosenbaum, & G. Cable. *Everyone's Guide to Cancer Therapy,* Kansas City: Andrews and McNeel, 591-601.)

performed on elderly or debilitated patients when the intraoperative time needs to be more closely controlled.

Billroth II. The Billroth II is the procedure performed for those who can tolerate and require a more radical surgery. About 75% of the stomach is resected, thus reducing the possibility of nodal or metastatic recurrence. The antrum, pylorus, first portion of the duodenum, supporting circulatory structures, and all visible and palpable lymph nodes are removed. The remaining stomach is anastomosed end-to-end to the jejunum. The duodenal stump is closed with sutures (Fig. 46-9).

The Billroth I and Billroth II procedures affect gastric emptying. All postgastrectomy syndromes result in the same potential complications and sequela: stoeatorrhea, dumping syndrome, nausea, vomiting, diarrhea, vitamin deficiency, and anastomotic leak.

Subtotal Esophagogastrectomy

Resectable tumors in the proximal stomach or cardia have a characteristic behavioral pattern, which usually requires a subtotal esophagogastrectomy. In some cases a total gastrectomy and distal esophagectomy are selected for more extensive resection. This procedure entails an "en bloc" removal of the lower portion of the esophagus and supporting circulatory and lymphatic structures, removal of most of the greater and lesser omental, and sometimes a total gastrectomy. The esophagus is sutured to the duodenum or jejunum, often requiring a thoracoabdominal approach. Potential complications include pneumonia, anastomotic leak, infection, reflux aspiration, and esophagitis.

Before any gastric surgery, the patient needs to have fluid and electrolyte imbalances, as well as anemia from chronic

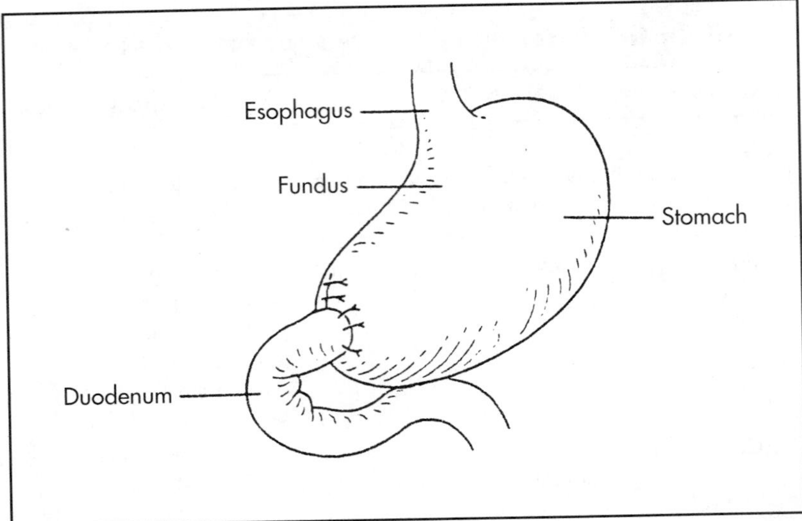

Fig. 46-8 A Billroth I, or gastroduodenostomy, involves resection of the proximal duodenum, distal stomach, pylorus, and supporting structures. (From Coleman, J. [1997]. Esophageal, stomach, liver, gallbladder, and pancreas cancers. In *Cancer nursing principles and practice* [4th ed]. Sudbury: Jones and Barlett.

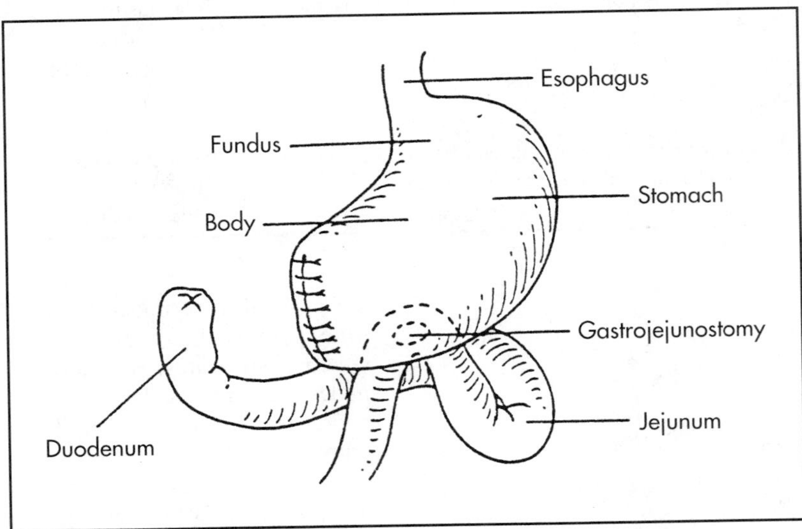

Fig. 46-9 A Billroth II, or gastrojejunostomy, is a wider resection of the Billroth I. Up to 75% of the stomach can be resected. The remaining stomach is then anastomosed end-to-end to the jejunum. (From Coleman, J. [1997]. Esophageal, stomach, liver, gallbladder, and pancreas cancers. In *Cancer nursing principles and practice* [4th ed]. Sudbury: Jones and Bartlett.

blood loss, corrected. The patient also needs to have vigilant attention paid to nutritional status. Weight loss, emaciation, and malnutrition require aggressive intervention.

Radiation Therapy

Despite the radiosensitivity of gastric adenocarcinoma, radiation therapy does not play a primary role in the treatment of the disease. The tumors are usually deep in the abdomen and often widely disseminated. The stomach, liver, kidneys, and spinal cord are radiation dose–limited organs. Radiation therapy to the upper abdomen is technically very difficult and is poorly tolerated by patients. This treatment achieves better local control and survival when it is combined with chemotherapy than when it is used alone. Postoperative radiation therapy alone adds little to the 5-year survival of gastric tumor patients. Many tumors decrease in size with 4000 cGy administered in fractionated doses over a 4- to 5-week period, but the overall survival of the patient is not increased. Radiation therapy may be used to alleviate the pain that is caused by bone metastases from the gastric cancer (Hoebler, 1997; Bruckner, Kondo, & Kondo, 1997).

Special techniques using intraoperative radiotherapy (IORT) are being used most extensively in Japan. Residual lesions after this procedure are irradiated using high-energy electrons. This technique is feasible and considered safe, but it is still investigational for patients with locally advanced gastric tumors. Hemorrhage and the development of fistulas

TABLE 46-6 Adjuvant Therapy for Resected Gastric Cancer Clinical Study

ARM I	ARM II
Observation	Chemotherapy 5-FU + leucovorin (One course only) Chemotherapy/radiation therapy Radiation therapy + 5-FU Concomitant chemotherapy 5-FU + Leucovorin (Repeated ×2 at 28-day intervals)

are the most common potential complications. IORT is available at only a few institutions in the United States because of the special equipment, operating room, and extensive professional collaboration that are required (Bruckner, Kondo, & Kondo, 1997).

Chemotherapy

There is a continued interest in the role of chemotherapy in the treatment of gastric cancer. No specific chemotherapeutic regimen alone has been shown to have a clear effect on patient survival. Single agents (5-fluorouracil [5-FU], doxorubicin, cisplatin, etoposide, and mitomycin-C) have been studied, but it appears that combination therapy is superior. Response rates of 30% to 50% have been observed with combination chemotherapy, compared with a 20% response rate with single agents (Hoebler, 1997). Median survival associated with multidrug chemotherapy has generally ranged from 6 to 10 months (Fuchs & Mayer, 1995). Toxicities depend on the drug used and the dosages given. In a trial conducted by the Gastrointestinal Tumor Study Group, the combination of IV 5-FU and radiation therapy offered improved survival. In this setting, simultaneous chemotherapy and radiation therapy may decrease the burden of residual microscopic disease after gastric resection, which contributes to the prevention of local and regional recurrences and distant metastases (Fuchs & Mayer, 1995).

The National Cancer Institute through the Southwest Oncology Group currently has a randomized study of the "Trial of Adjuvant Chemotherapy After Gastric Resection for Adenocarcinoma" that compares surgery alone with postoperative radiation therapy in combination with 5-FU–based chemotherapy (Table 46-6). Several controlled trials are in progress or have been recently completed using combination chemotherapy in the treatment of gastric cancer. Preliminary data show no difference in the survival of patients after 3 years of follow-up. There is an urgent need for further research in more progressive methods of the treatment of gastric cancer.

ONCOLOGIC EMERGENCIES

The most serious and persistent problem occurring in patients with gastric cancer relates to nutrition. Most patients die from bronchopneumonia or from lung abscesses due to malnutrition and/or immobility. Occasionally, deep-vein thrombosis, pulmonary emboli, anastomotic rupture, or even a secondary primary tumor may also cause death in these patients. (See Chapter 11 for a complete discussion of oncologic emergencies.)

NURSING MANAGEMENT

The nursing management of patients with gastric cancer is complicated by the fact that most of these patients have advanced disease at diagnosis. Whereas gastric surgery usually occurs in the inpatient setting, radiation therapy and chemotherapy are commonly performed in the outpatient setting. Most of the patient's care occurs in the outpatient and home care areas. Patient and family education needs to take place at the time of diagnosis to understand the treatment options that are open to the patient based on the stage of the cancer and the patient's co-morbidities.

Surgery

Because surgery is the mainstay treatment for gastric cancer, most of the nursing care is concentrated in this phase. Patients undergoing gastric resection are usually admitted to the hospital the morning of the surgery. They undergo at-home bowel preparation, usually with Go-Lytely (Braintree Laboratories, Inc., Braintree, Mass.), the night before the operation. Intravenous antibiotics are initiated in the surgery's holding room and continued for the next 1 to 3 days (Sawyers, 1995). Uncomplicated gastric surgeries usually require about 1 week in the hospital. Nursing care is focused on the prevention of postoperative complications, including pneumonia, infection, anastomotic leak, hemorrhage, or reflux aspiration. Table 46-7 reviews the standard of therapy for patients undergoing gastric surgery.

RADIATION THERAPY

Radiation therapy is usually administered as an adjuvant therapy in conjunction with chemotherapy or surgery for patients with locally advanced or recurrent disease. The major problems associated with radiation for gastric cancer include abdominal cramps, diarrhea, anorexia, nausea, or vomiting. The nutritional management of these patients is the most challenging nursing priority. Table 46-8 outlines a standard of care for patients receiving external beam radiation therapy for gastric cancer.

Chemotherapy is most commonly used in combination with gastric resection and/or radiation therapy. The overall response rate of gastric cancer to chemotherapy has been low, and this treatment is not a standard clinical option but is used in the clinical trial setting. Table 46-9 reviews a standard of care for the patient receiving chemotherapy for gastric cancer.

HOME CARE ISSUES

Many patients with gastric cancer undergo surgery. The issues facing the patients and their family caregivers are similar to those for patients recovering from other abdominal

TABLE 46-7 Standard of Care for the Patient Undergoing Gastric Surgery

Patient Problems and Outcomes	Nursing Interventions and Rationales	Patient Education Instructions
Nausea due to dumping syndrome	1. Assess the patient's level of understanding about dumping syndrome. 2. Consult with a registered dietician about the diet.	1. Explain that after gastric surgery, patients may lose the functioning of the pyloric valve. This allows food and fluid to pass too rapidly into the small bowel. It most commonly occurs 1 to 3 weeks after surgery. 2. Provide patient nutritional information: a. Eat six small meals a day. b. Drink no liquids 30 to 40 minutes before or after meals. c. Eat a diet low in carbohydrates and salt, moderate in fat, and high in protein. d. Include foods containing pectin, citrus fruits, yellow vegetables, bananas, apricots, apples, cherries, and beans. e. Eat food slowly; chew well. f. Lie down after meals for approximately 30 minutes.

TABLE 46-8 Standard of Care for the Patient Receiving External Beam Radiation for Gastric Cancer

Patient Problems and Outcomes	Nursing Interventions and Rationales	Patient Education Instructions
Nausea and Vomiting Patient will have minimal weight loss and maintain adequate hydration	1. Assess the patient for nausea and vomiting patterns. 2. Initiate preventive therapies, including the following: a. Change positions slowly. (Rapid movement stimulates the afferent vestibulocerebellar pathway with resultant stimulation of the chemoreceptor trigger zone.) b. Provide good oral hygiene after each emesis and before meals. c. Avoid serving foods with an overpowering aroma. d. Eat small, frequent meals. e. Avoid foods/liquids that irritate the gastric mucosa. 3. Consult with a registered dietician to teach the patient dietary parameters and guidelines. 4. Institute methods to control nausea/vomiting: a. Take slow, deep breaths. b. Sip carbonated beverages. c. Eat dry foods (toast, crackers), and avoid drinking fluids with meals. 5. Administer antiemetic medication (i.e., prochlorerazine 10 mg, one tablet every 6 hours as needed; or ondansectran 8 mg, one tablet before treatment and one to three times a day as needed). 6. Monitor weight. 7. Monitor dietary intake amounts and choices. 8. Add nutritional supplements.	1. Inform the patient that nausea and vomiting occurs within 1 to 3 hours after treatment. 2. Teach the patient methods to prevent nausea and vomiting. 3. Teach the patient to evaluate for a pattern of nausea/vomiting and concentrate the use of medication to prevent occurrences.

surgeries. (See Chapter 3 for a complete discussion of the care of the surgical oncology patient.)

Nutrition

Many, but not all, patients who have had subtotal gastrectomies or total gastrectomies have "dumping syndrome," characterized by sweating and weakness after eating. Small, frequent feedings of low-carbohydrate, high-fat, high-protein foods are recommended. It is important to restrict liquids for 30 to 40 minutes before and after a meal to avoid the effects of dumping syndrome. Vitamin B_{12} deficiency will occur; therefore monthly parenteral replacement therapy is necessary.

Because most patients diagnosed with gastric cancer in the United States are diagnosed at an advanced stage, a rapid physical deterioration may occur. Nursing considerations focus on nutrition and maintaining optimal functions

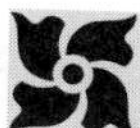

TABLE 46-9 Standard of Care for the Patient Receiving Chemotherapy for Gastric Cancer

Patient Problems and Outcomes	Nursing Interventions and Rationales	Patient Education Instructions
Mucositis		
Patient will have clean mucosa or have mucosal lesions healing progressively	1. Assess the patient's oral cavity with a tongue blade and light moisture for the presence of lesions. 2. Initiate a prophylactic oral hygiene regimen. 3. Assess the pain level and ability to swallow. Assess for antifungal or antibacterial agents.	1. Explain that mucositis generally occurs 5 to 7 days after chemotherapy and lasts up to 10 days. 2. Instruct the patient to do the following: a. Brush teeth with soft bristle toothbrush. b. Use only alcohol-free mouthwashes. c. Apply lip lubricant every 2 hours while awake.

for as long as possible for the patient. The lack of gastric secretions leads to enzymatic and nutrient deficiencies. Malnutrition that is a result of the disease decreases the patient's ability to fight infections, withstand any cancer treatment options, or even perform the activities of daily living.

Emotional Support

Because the insidious symptoms that mark the development of gastric cancer are often ignored and are temporarily relieved with over-the-counter medications, patients and their family members may feel a sense of guilt or negligence that medical attention has been delayed until the disease has advanced. The nurse can dispel any misconceptions and assist the patient and family to realize their goals and achieve a realistic sense of hope. Many end-stage patients are eligible to enroll in a hospice program if it is available. This provides the services for the patient and family members that will enable them to receive the care needed during the terminal phases of life. The acceptance of a diagnosis of a life-limiting disease and the emotional transition that takes place are facilitated by a skilled hospice staff as well as assistance with the physical care issues presented by the patient.

PROGNOSIS

In a 1993 report from the American College of Surgeons, the survival rates of over 18000 patients with gastric cancer were compared in the United States and Japan. The 5-year survival rates in the United States were similar to the rates in other Western countries that were studied. Stage I patients had a survival rate of 50%, compared with a 29% survival rate for stage II patients. Stages III and IV patients had 5-year survival rates of 13% and 3%, respectively. Overall, the 5-year survival rate for gastric cancer is 19%. The Japanese series had improved survival rates for each stage, with an overall survival rate of 56% (Fuchs & Mayer, 1995; Sawyers, 1995).

EVALUATION OF THE QUALITY OF CARE

The quality of care that is provided to patients requires evaluation. The "Continuous Quality Improvement" aspects of patient care are multidisciplinary, and each member of the team needs to be accountable and able to evaluate the outcomes of his or her care. Table 46-10 provides an example of a quality of care evaluation tool that can be used.

TABLE 46-10 Quality of Care Evaluation for a Patient Undergoing Gastric Resection

Disciplines participating in the quality of care evaluation
☐ Nursing ☐ Surgery ☐ Dietary ☐ Social Services

I. Postoperative Management Evaluation

Data from ☐ Medical Record Review
☐ Patient/Family Interview

Criteria	YES	NO
1. Patient provided with preoperative information about the following:		
a. Diagnostic tests	☐	☐
b. Bowel preparation	☐	☐
c. Pain management	☐	☐
2. Hemoglobin and hematocrit evaluated postoperatively	☐	☐
3. Patient experienced the following complications:		
a. Pulmonary embolism	☐	☐
b. Anastomotic leak	☐	☐

II. Patient/Family Satisfaction

Data from ☐ Patient interview
☐ Family interview

Criteria	YES	NO
1. On a scale of 0 to 10, with 0 being totally dissatisfied and 10 being totally satisfied, how satisfied were you with the pain management you received?	☐	☐
2. Did you receive a consultation from a registered dietitian about "dumping syndrome"?	☐	☐
Did you receive clear instructions about nutrition at home after surgery?	☐	☐

RESEARCH ISSUES

There is a continuing urgent need for the development of novel diagnostic and treatment options for gastric cancer. The emerging role of ultrasonic endoscopy assists in the accurate staging of primary tumors without the need for abdominal surgery. Progress has been made in the area of perioperative chemotherapy as well as in the area of intraoperative radiation therapy. Advances in chemotherapy, as well as in biologic agents and their possible combinations before and/or after surgery, may contribute to the reduction of recurrences after surgical intervention. Research trials continue to study the efficacy of combined chemotherapy regimens and the role of radiation therapy. The identification of high-risk patients for the development of gastric cancer may allow for appropriate specific investigational therapies that can be targeted for this population (Ellis & Cunningham, 1994).

REFERENCES

Alexander, H., Kelsen, D., & Tepper, J. (1997). Cancer of the stomach. In V. T. DeVita, S. Hellman, & S. A. Rosenberg (Eds.), *Cancer: Principles and practice of oncology.* Philadelphia, New York: Lippincott-Raven.

Bruckner, H., Kondo, T., & Kondo, K. (1997). Neoplasms of the stomach. In J. E. Holland, R. C. Bast, D. L. Morton, & E. Frei (Eds.), *Cancer medicine.* Baltimore: Williams and Wilkins.

Correa, P. (1995). *Helicobactor pylori* and gastric carcinogenesis. *American Journal of Surgical Pathology, 19,* S37-43.

Ellis, P. & Cunningham, D. (1994). Management of carcinomas of the upper gastrointestinal tract. *British Medical Journal, 308,* 834-838.

Fay, M., Fennerty, M., Emerson, J., & Larez, M. (1994). Dietary habits and the risk of stomach cancer: A comparison study of patients with and without intestinal metaplasial. *Gastroenterology Nursing, 16,* 158-162.

Fuchs, C. & Mayer, R. (1995). Gastric carcinoma. *The New England Journal of Medicine, 333,* 32-41.

Hoebler, L. (1997). Colon rectal cancer. In S.L. Groenwald, M.H. Frogge, M. Goodman, & C. H. Yarbro (Eds.), *Cancer nursing.* Sudbury, MA: Jones and Bartlett.

Lawrence, W. & Zfass, A. (1995). Gastric neoplasms. In G. P. Murphy, W. Lawrence & R. E. Lenhard (Eds.) *American Cancer Society textbook of clinical oncology.* Atlanta: The American Cancer Society.

Lee, J., Nascimento, A., Farnell, M., Carney, J., Harmsen, W., & Ilstrup, M. (1995). Epithelioid gastric stromal tumors: A study of fifty-five cases. *Surgery, 118,* 660-661.

Levine, M. (1995). Role of double-contrast upper gastrointestinal series in the 1990's. *Gastroenterology Clinics of North America, 24,* 289-308.

Maehara, Y., Yasunori, E., Tomisaki, S., Oshiro, T., Kakeji, Y., Ichiyoshi, Y., & Sugimachi, K. (1996). Age-related characteristics of gastric carcinoma in young and elderly patients, *Cancer, 77,* 1774-1780.

Miwa, K., Hattori, T., & Miyazaki, I. (1995). Duodenogastric reflux and foregut carcinogenesis. *Cancer 75,* 1426-1432.

Nicholson, D. & Shorvon, P. (1993). Review article: endoscopic ultrasound of the stomach. *British Journal of Radiology, 66,* 487-492.

Parsonnet, J. (1993). *Helicobactor pylori* and gastric cancer. *Gastroenterology Clinics of North America, 22,* 89-104.

Rosenbaum, E., & Dollinger, M. (1994). *Stomach cancer: Everyone's guide to cancer therapy.* Kansas City: Somerville House Books.

Sano, T., Sasako, M., Kinoshita, T., & Maruyama, K. (1993). Recurrence of early gastric cancer: Follow-up of 1475 patients and review of the Japanese literature. *Cancer 72,* 3174-3178.

Sawyers, J. (1995). Gastric cancer. *Current Problems in Surgery, 32,* 106-178.

Solcia, E., Fiocca, R., Villani, L., Luinetti, O., & Capella, C. (1995). Hyperplastic, dysplastic, and neoplastic enterochromaffin-like-cell proliferations of the gastric mucosa. *American Journal of Surgical Pathology,* 19 Suppl. 1: S1-7.

Starzynska, Y., Markiewski, M., Domagala, W., Marlicz, K., Mietkieski, J., Roberts, S., & Stern, P. (1996). The clinical significance of p53 accumulation in gastric cancer. *Cancer 77,* 2005-2012.

Tabbarah, H.J. (1995). Gastrointestinal tract cancers. In D. A. Casciato & B. B. Lowitz (Eds.), *Manual of clinical oncology* (3rd ed.). Boston: Little, Brown.

Thompson, G., van Heerden, J., & Sarr, M. (1993). Adenocarcinoma of the stomach: Are we making progress? *The Lancet, 342,* 713-718.

Tokunaga, A., Onda, M., Okuda, T., Teramoto, T., Fujita, I., Mizutani, T., Kiyama, T., Yoshiyuki, T., Nishi, K., & Matsukura, N. (1995). Clinical significance of epidermal growth factor (EGF) ECG receptor, and c-*erb*B-2 in human gastric cancer. *Cancer 75,* 1418-1428.

Veldhuyzen, S., & Sherman, P. (1994). Helicobacter pylori infection as a cause of gastric duodenal ulcer, gastric cancer, and nonulcer dyspepsia: A systematic overview. *Canadian Medical Association Journal, 150,* 177-185.

Superficial Bladder Cancer

Stacey Young-McCaughan, RN, PhD, OCN, Lt. Col.*

EPIDEMIOLOGY

In 1998, an estimated 54,400 new cases of bladder cancer were diagnosed, and 12,500 people died from this disease (Landis, Murray, Bolden, & Wingo, 1998). Bladder cancer accounts for only 5% of all new cases of cancer among men and 3% of all new cases of cancer among women, yet it is the fourth most prevalent cancer in men (after prostate, lung, and colon cancers) and the sixth most prevalent cancer in women (after breast, lung, and colon cancer; the gynecologic malignancies; and lymphoma) (Landis et al., 1998). Men are three times more likely than women to develop bladder cancer (American Cancer Society, 1996; Fleshner, Herr, Stewart, Murphy, Mettlin, & Menck, 1996; Hartge, Harvey, Linehan, Silverman, Sullivan, & Hoover, et al., 1990; Melicow, 1974). In addition, whites are more likely to develop bladder cancer than blacks, Asians, Hispanics, and American Indians (American Cancer Society, 1996; Fleshner et al., 1996; Harris, Chen-Backlund, & Wynder, 1990; Silverman, Hartge, Morrison, & Devesa, 1992). Approximately two thirds of patients diagnosed with bladder cancer are 60 years of age or older (Fleshner et al., 1996; Melicow, 1974; Silverman et al., 1992), except for patients with chronic urinary schistosomiasis, who are commonly diagnosed with bladder cancer between the ages of 40 and 50 (Makhyoun, 1974).

Over the past 20 years, the incidence of bladder cancer has increased 11%, although with improved treatments, the mortality from this disease has decreased 19.4% (Devesa, Blot, Stone, Miller, Tarone, & Fraumeni, 1995). With the long latency between carcinogen exposure and the development of bladder cancer (Cohen & Johansson, 1992), one possible explanation for the increasing incidence of bladder cancer is that the effects of past carcinogen exposure, primarily cigarette smoking, are just now becoming evident. Women, who began smoking in large numbers later than men, may now be at particularly high risk for bladder cancers as well as other tobacco-related diseases.

RISK FACTORS

Known and suspected risk factors for bladder cancer are listed in Box 47-1.

Occupational Exposure to Chemical Carcinogens

In 1895, Rehn observed an increase in the incidence of bladder cancer among German textile workers exposed to aniline dyes. Over the next 40 years, an increased incidence of bladder cancer was also seen in the dye and textile workers of Switzerland, Great Britain, and the United States. In 1938, Hueper demonstrated that the arylamines used in making the dyes caused bladder tumors in dogs (Cohen & Johansson, 1992; Lower, 1982). Arylamines are metabolized in the liver and excreted in the urine. Compounds related to the arylamines that are also known or strongly suspected to be bladder carcinogens are listed in Box 47-1.

In addition to dye and textile workers, other workers believed to be at increased risk for bladder cancer are listed in Box 47-2. Like those employed in the dye and textile industry, these workers can be exposed to arylamines at the work site. Arylamines were once used in the rubber and tire industries as a hardening antioxidant (Lower, 1982; Wallace, 1988). Although these compounds are no longer commonly used in making tires, some workers may still risk exposure from working with recycled tires or from working with other antioxidants contaminated with small amounts of the carcinogenic arylamines (Wallace, 1988). Other occupations, such as leather workers, bootblacks, painters, and hairdressers, are at risk because of the dyes they may use in their work. Arylamines have also been found in environmental pollution, especially tobacco smoke and diesel exhaust (Cohen & Johansson, 1992; Wallace, 1988). Although governmental agencies have attempted to reduce exposure to these compounds, one study estimated that between 21%

*The views of the author are her own and do not purport to reflect the position of the Army Medical Department, Department of the Army, or Department of Defense.

Box 47-1
Known and Suspected Risk Factors for Bladder Cancer

Known Risk Factors

Occupational exposure to chemical carcinogens listed below:
- 2-naphthylamine
- 4-aminobiphenyl
- Benzidine
- Chlornaphazine
- 4-chloro-o-toluidine
- O-toluidine
- 4,4'-methylene bis (2-chloroaniline)
- Methylene dianiline
- Benzidine-derived azo dyes

(Occupations known to use these chemicals are listed in Box 47-2.)

Cigarette smoking

Chronic infection with *Schistosoma haematobium*

Family history

Suspected Risk Factors

Dietary factors:
- Coffee drinking
- Consumption of artificial sweeteners (saccharin & cyclamate)
- Alcohol drinking
- High cholesterol intake
- High meat consumption (particularly pork and beef)

Urologic conditions:
- Frequent urinary tract infections
- Urinary stasis

Infection with the human papillomaviruses (HPVs) 16 & 18

Drug use:
- Use of phenacetin-containing analgesics
- Prolonged use of cyclophosphamide

Radiation exposure

Drinking water:
- Water contaminated with pesticides
- Highly chlorinated drinking water

Modified from Cohen, S. M. & Johansson, S. L. (1992). Epidemiology and etiology of bladder cancer. *Urologic Clinics of North America, 19*(3), 421-428; Scher, H. I. (1994). Editorial comment. *Journal of Urology, 152*(2), 569; Silverman, D. T., Hartge, P., Morrison, A. S., & Devesa, S. S. (1992). Epidemiology of bladder cancer. *Hematology Oncology Clinics of North America, 6*(1), 1-30; Song-ting, Y., Ming-ming, W., & Li-ming, L. (1993). Prevalence of human papilloma viruses 16 and 18 in transitional cell carcinoma of bladder. *Chinese Medical Journal, 106*(7), 494-496.

and 25% of bladder cancer diagnosed among white men in the United States could be attributed to occupational exposure (Silverman, Levine, Hoover, & Hartge, 1989).

Cigarette Smoking

Large epidemiologic studies have identified consistently that smokers have 2 to 10 times the risk of developing bladder cancer compared with nonsmokers (Burch, Rohan, Howe, Risch, Hill, & Steele et al., 1989; Clavel, Cordier, Boccon-Gibod, & Hemon, 1989; González, López-Abente, Errezola, Escolar, Riboli, & Izarzugaza et al., 1989; Harris et al., 1990; Hartge, Silverman, Hoover, Schairer, Altman, & Austin, et al., 1987; Howe, Burch, Miller, Cook, Esteve, & Morrison et al., 1980; Kantor, Hartge, Hoover, & Fraumeni, 1985, 1988; Mills, Beeson, Phillips, & Fraser, 1991; Morrison, Buring, Verhoek, Aoki, Leck, & Ohno et al., 1984; Piper, Matanoski, & Tonascia, 1986; Wynder & Goldsmith, 1977). Although the mechanisms by which cigarette smoking might induce bladder cancer are not known, aromatic amines that are present in dyes and known to cause bladder cancer in dye and textile workers are also present in tobacco smoke (Patrianakos & Hoffmann, 1979).

Box 47- 2
Occupations Associated with an Increased Risk of Bladder Cancer

Textile workers
Dye workers
Tire & rubber workers
Leather workers
Bootblacks
Painters
Truck drivers
Drill press operators
Chemical workers
Petroleum workers
Hairdressers

Modified from Cohen, S. M., & Johansson, S. L. (1992). Epidemiology and etiology of bladder cancer. *Urologic Clinics of North America, 19*(3), 421-428.

The risk of developing bladder cancer appears to increase with the number of cigarettes smoked (Auerbach & Garfinkel, 1989; Burch et al., 1989; Clavel et al., 1989; Howe et al., 1980; Kantor et al., 1985, 1988; Mills et al., 1991; Morrison et al., 1984), as well as for smokers who inhale deeply (Burch et al., 1989; Clavel et al., 1989; Morrison et al., 1984). The use of unfiltered cigarettes, compared with the use of filtered cigarettes, increased the risk of bladder cancer in one study but did not affect the risk of developing bladder cancer in two other studies. The use of other tobacco products, such as pipes, cigars, chewing tobacco, or snuff, has not been associated with an increased risk of bladder cancer. Neither has passive smoking been associated with an increased risk (Burch et al., 1989; Hartge et al., 1987; Morrison et al., 1984).

It is estimated that one third to half of bladder cancers are attributable to cigarette smoking (Burch et al., 1989; Hartge et al., 1987; Wynder & Goldsmith, 1977). The importance of encouraging patients to stop smoking cannot be emphasized enough. In addition to being associated with bladder cancers, smoking has also been implicated as a possible cause of cancers of the lung, mouth, pharynx, larynx, esophagus, pancreas, cervix, and kidney (American Cancer Society, 1996).

Smokers cite a health care provider's advice to stop smoking as a potent motivation for quitting, yet only approximately half of current smokers report ever having been asked by their primary care provider if they smoked (Fiore, Bailey, Cohen, Dorfman, Goldstein, & Gritz et al., 1996). Even fewer smokers have received guidance on how to quit. Nurses can advise all their patients who smoke to stop, and can provide information on nicotine replacement therapy as well as support groups and programs available for smokers interested in quitting (Fiore, Jorenby, Baker, & Kenford, 1992; Kottke, Battista, DeFriese, & Brekke, 1988; Ockene, 1987; Risser, 1996). Great strides have been made in banning smoking in public places such as hospitals, schools, government agencies, stores, and restaurants. Nurses can support this trend and continue to support tobacco control measures at the local, state, and federal levels (Gallagher & Holm, 1996). Nurses can also support individuals who do not allow smoking in their homes; the more difficult it is to find a comfortable place to smoke, the more likely it is that smokers are going to abandon the habit.

Chronic Bladder Infection with *Schistosoma Haematobium* (Bilharziasis)

A relatively rare form of bladder cancer, squamous cell carcinoma, has been associated with chronic bladder infections with the blood fluke *S. haematobium* (Makhyoun, 1974; Tanagho, 1995b). The fluke lives in a fresh-water snail and infects humans working or recreating in infested water (Tanagho, 1995b). Once inside its host, the fluke migrates in the blood and lymph systems to the bladder, where it deposits its ova in the bladder wall. These ova eventually hatch and are excreted in the urine back into the water supply. The ova are an irritation to the bladder, resulting in a chronic urothelial inflammation. This irritation and inflammation are believed to predispose the host to squamous cell carcinoma of the bladder (Tanagho, 1995b). Although *S. haematobium* is not a common infection in the United States, these infections are endemic along the northern coast of Africa, Saudi Arabia, Israel, Jordan, Lebanon, and Syria. Because of emigration, schistosomiasis is seen with increasing frequency in Europe and the United States (Tanagho, 1995b), and the incidence of this particular type of bladder cancer may increase in the future.

Family History

Epidemiologic studies have shown that a family history of bladder cancer increases the risk of bladder cancer, even when the risk from both smoking and occupational exposure are statistically controlled (Kantor et al., 1985; Kiemeney & Schoenberg, 1996; Lynch, Kimberling, Lynch, & Brennan, 1987). For people with a positive family history and who also smoke, the risk of bladder cancer increased dramatically in one study (Kantor et al., 1985).

People who have a history of bladder cancer in their family need to be advised that they may be at increased risk for the disease. They should be strongly encouraged not to smoke and to monitor their work site for possible exposure to bladder carcinogens.

Suspected Risk Factors

Also listed in Box 47-1 are a host of possible risk factors for bladder cancer that have been noted in the literature. Dietary factors that have been associated with an increased risk of bladder cancer include coffee drinking; consumption of artificial sweeteners, particularly saccharin and cyclamate; alcohol drinking; a high cholesterol intake; and a diet high in meat (Silverman et al., 1992). The findings from studies reporting these dietary risk factors for bladder cancer are highly variable, contradicting each other in some instances. The following factors lead to the conclusion that if there are dietary risk factors for bladder cancer, the risk is relatively small: lack of consistent results, failure to control for confounding variables such as cigarette smoking, and the risk of identifying statistically significant risks only because of the large number of people studied (Silverman et al., 1992).

Urologic conditions such as frequent urinary tract infections and urinary stasis have also been suggested as risk factors for bladder cancer (Kantor, Hartge, Hoover, Narayana, Sullivan, & Fraumeni et al., 1984; Kantor et al., 1988). Presumably, if carcinogens are present in the urine, frequent and prolonged exposure of the urothelium to these carcinogens increases the likelihood of neoplastic changes in the bladder. However, as with studies of dietary factors, the results of these studies are also inconsistent and definitive conclusions are impossible.

There is a great deal of clinical and epidemiologic evidence that infection with human papillomavirus (HPV) types 16 and 18 is associated with an increased risk of cervical cancer. There has also been some speculation that HPV 16 and 18 are associated with an increased risk of some bladder cancers (Furihata, Inoue, Ohtsuki, Hashimoto, Terao, & Fujita, 1994; Song-ting, Ming-ming, & Li-ming, 1993). Possibly, the HPV inactivates the p53 suppressor gene, allowing neoplastic changes of the urothelium to go unchecked (Scher, 1994). However, much more work needs to be done before HPV infections can definitively be considered a risk factor for bladder cancer.

Drugs that have been associated with an increased risk of bladder cancer include phenacetin-containing analgesics (Piper, Matanoski, & Tonascia, 1986) and the antineoplastic chemotherapeutic drug cyclophosphamide (Fairchild, Spence, Solomon, & Gangai, 1979; Fernandes, Manivel, Reddy, & Ercole, 1996; Levine & Richie, 1989; Pedersen-Bjergaard, Ersbøll, Hansen, Sørensen, Christoffersen, & Hou-Jensen et al., 1988). Western countries no longer allow phenacetin to be sold, obviating its role as a possible bladder carcinogen. In contrast, cyclophosphamide is currently used to treat many different cancers as well as various nonmalignant diseases (e.g., autoimmune disorders such as rheumatoid arthritis, systemic lupus erythematosus, and thrombocytopenic purpura). Cyclophosphamide is metabolized by the liver into acrolein that is excreted in the urine. Acrolein has long been identified as a bladder irritant, and prolonged exposure to acrolein can lead to cystitis. Aggressive hydration to promote frequent urination is a routine part of care for patients being treated with cyclophosphamide. Acrolein may also be carcinogenic, especially if the urothelium is exposed to high concentrations of this metabolite over a prolonged time.

Individual cases of bladder cancer in women who received pelvic radiation for dysfunctional uterine bleeding or gynecologic cancers have been reported in the literature (Boice, Engholm, Kleinerman, Blettner, Stovall, & Lisco et al., 1988; Inskip, Monson, Wagoner, Stovalla, Davis, &

Kleinerman et al., 1990; Quilty & Kerr, 1987). Also, an increased incidence of bladder cancer has been seen in patients treated with radioactive iodine-131 for thyroid cancer (Edmonds & Smith, 1986; Piper, Matanoski, & Tonascia, 1986). It is very likely that during treatment the bladder was inadvertently exposed to small doses of radiation, predisposing the urothelium to neoplastic changes.

Some epidemiologic studies have identified people who live in rural areas and drink water contaminated with pesticides (Mills et al., 1991) and people who drink highly chlorinated water (Crump & Guess, 1982) as being at an increased risk of developing bladder cancer. However, these findings are not consistent between studies. If either drinking water in rural areas or drinking highly chlorinated water is a risk factor for bladder cancer, the risk is relatively small.

Studies of known and suspected risk factors for bladder cancer have been extensively reviewed by Silverman and colleagues (1992), and the interested reader is referred to this article as well as the others cited in Box 47-1 for more detailed information.

CHEMOPREVENTION

Chemoprevention refers to the use of various drugs to either prevent malignant changes in cells or to prolong the time it takes malignant changes to occur in cells (Kelloff, Boone, Malone, Steele, & Doody, 1992). Bladder cancers offer a unique opportunity to test various chemopreventive agents because even after complete resection of the tumor, half to three quarters of patients suffer a recurrence of their disease (Heney, Nocks, Daly, Prout, Newall, & Griffin et al., 1982; Lamm, Blumenstein, Crawford, Montie, Scardino, & Grossman et al., 1991). In animal studies, many drugs have shown promise in reducing bladder cancer recurrence, including alpha-difluoromethylornithine (DFMO), oltipraz (which contains the same active ingredient as cruciferous vegetables), and various nonsteroidal anti-inflammatory drugs (NSAIDs) such as ibuprofen, indocin, and piroxicam (Kelloff et al., 1992). Yet, the few human clinical trials that have been done using DFMO (Loprinzi & Messing, 1992), 13-cis-retinoic acid (Prout & Barton, 1992), and N-(4-hydroxyphenyl) retinamide (4-HPR) (Decensi, Bruno, Giaretti, Torrisi, Curotto, & Gatteschi, et al., 1992) showed only a modest reduction in tumor recurrence, if any at all. The Chemoprevention Branch of the National Cancer Institute (NCI) is continuing to test new compounds in the hope that one will effectively prevent malignant changes in the urothelium, thereby preventing primary bladder cancer as well as reducing the recurrence of bladder cancer in patients already diagnosed with the disease.

PATHOPHYSIOLOGY

Normal Anatomy and Physiology of the Bladder

The bladder is a hollow, muscular organ that expands to hold approximately 300 ml of urine at low pressures (Bates, 1991; Harrison & Abrams, 1994; Tanagho, 1992). The bladder is located on the floor of the pelvic cavity behind the peritoneum. In men, the bladder is located ventral to the rectum, and in women ventral to the vagina and uterus, as indicated in Fig. 47-1 (see also Figs. 48-1 and 48-2). The upper portion of the bladder is named the *fundus*. Two ureters, one from each kidney, enter the bladder posteriorly, as also depicted in Fig. 47-1. The trigone is a triangular area on the posterior bladder wall, bounded superiorly by the two ureters and inferiorly by the urethra. The trigone closes the ureteral openings during micturition, thereby preventing urine from being forced back into the ureters and renal pelvis. The urethra exits the bladder at the bladder neck.

The urethra is a muscular tube that carries urine from the bladder out of the body. It functions as a sphincter, contracting to hold urine in the bladder and relaxing to allow urine to flow out of the bladder. In men, the urethra is 20 cm long, traversing the prostate gland and the length of the penis before exiting the body; whereas in women, the urethra is only 4 cm long.

Specialized transitional cells line the renal pelvis, both ureters, the bladder, and the urethra, preventing various metabolites and toxins excreted in the urine from being reabsorbed into the circulation. Three to six layers of transitional cells, called the *urothelium,* line the urinary tract, allowing for expansion and contraction of the bladder while maintaining the integrity of the system.

As more than 300 ml of urine accumulates in the bladder, the smooth muscle of the bladder (the detrusor muscle) is stretched, pressure in the bladder rises, and the urge to void becomes conscious. In cognitively intact adults, the brain can inhibit the detrusor muscle from contracting until the maximum bladder capacity of 400 to 500 ml is reached (Bates, 1991).

As both men and women age, bladder capacity decreases, causing urinary frequency. Emptying of the bladder is more difficult due to weakened bladder muscles, resulting in urinary retention (Whitbourne, 1985).

The Process of Carcinogenesis

As with the development of many different cancers, evidence suggests that the evolution of bladder cancer depends on a series of genetic events. Papillary bladder cancers have a very different natural history compared with carcinoma in situ (CIS). Although the majority of both papillary tumors and CIS are considered early-stage superficial bladder tumors, papillary tumors rarely recur or progress, whereas CIS very often recurs and progresses to a higher-stage invasive tumor. Molecular genetic differences between papillary tumors and CIS may explain the reason the natural history of these two tumors is so different. Papillary bladder carcinomas are more likely to have mutations in the tumor suppressor gene p16 on chromosome 9q, whereas CIS is more likely to have mutations of the tumor suppressor gene p53 on chromosome 17p. These differences in natural history and molecular biology support a two-pathway model for the pathogenesis and progression of bladder cancer, as shown in Fig. 47-2 (Israel, Natale, & Skinner, 1995; Spruck, Ohneseit, Gonzalez-Zulueta, Esrig, Miyao, & Tsai, et al., 1994). Although the majority of papillary tumors rarely recur or progress, the few that do transform into a more aggressive

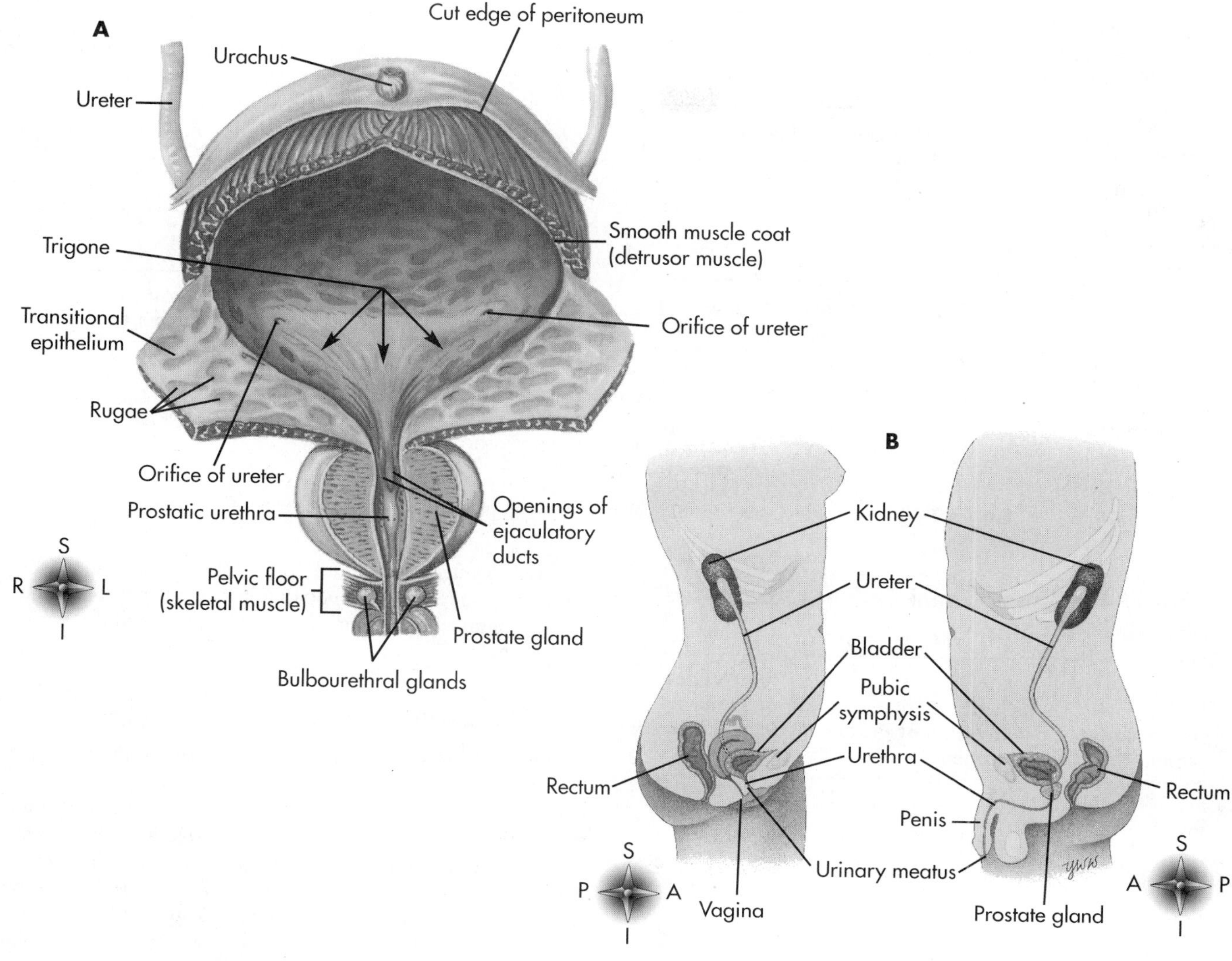

Fig. 47-1 **A** and **B,** Male anatomy and relations of the bladder, prostate, seminal vesicles, penis, urethra, and scrotal contents. **B,** Female anatomy and relations of the bladder, urethra, uterus, ovary, vagina, and rectum. (From Tanagho, E. A. [1995a]. Anatomy of the genitourinary tract. In E. A. Tanagho & J. W. McAninch [Eds.], *Smith's general urology* [14th ed.]. Norwalk, CT: Appleton & Lange.)

tumor acquire mutations of gene P53. Other chromosomal changes have been associated with bladder tumors and are listed in Table 47-1, but p16 and P53 mutations have been the most widely studied.

Both p16 and P53 mutations involve inactivation of a tumor suppressor gene. Without these tumor suppressor mechanisms, malignant cells in the urothelium go unchecked. Only one proto-oncogene, H-*ras*, located on the short arm of chromosome 11 has been studied as a possible initiator of bladder malignancies.

ASSESSMENT

The assessment of a patient for bladder cancer is summarized in Table 47-2. Clinical evaluation of the patient involves a detailed history, a physical examination, and a variety of diagnostic tests. Definitions of commonly experienced bladder symptoms are provided in Table 47-3. These symptoms can occur as evidence of bladder cancer, as side effects of therapy for bladder cancer (particularly intravesical therapy), or with a bladder infection. Usually, further urinary testing is needed to determine the etiology of these symptoms and to treat the cause as well as the symptoms appropriately.

History

Approximately 75% of patients with bladder cancer seek medical care, complaining of hematuria (Fair, Fuks, & Scher, 1993; Wallace & Harris, 1965). Hematuria in bladder cancer is often intermittent, deceiving practitioners into believing that the cause is benign (Lamm & Torti, 1996). Between 20% and 30% of patients have irritative bladder symptoms (IBSs) such as dysuria, frequency, or urgency (Cummings, Barone, & Ward, 1992; Fair, Fuks, Scher, 1993). In women, these symptoms can be mistaken for in-

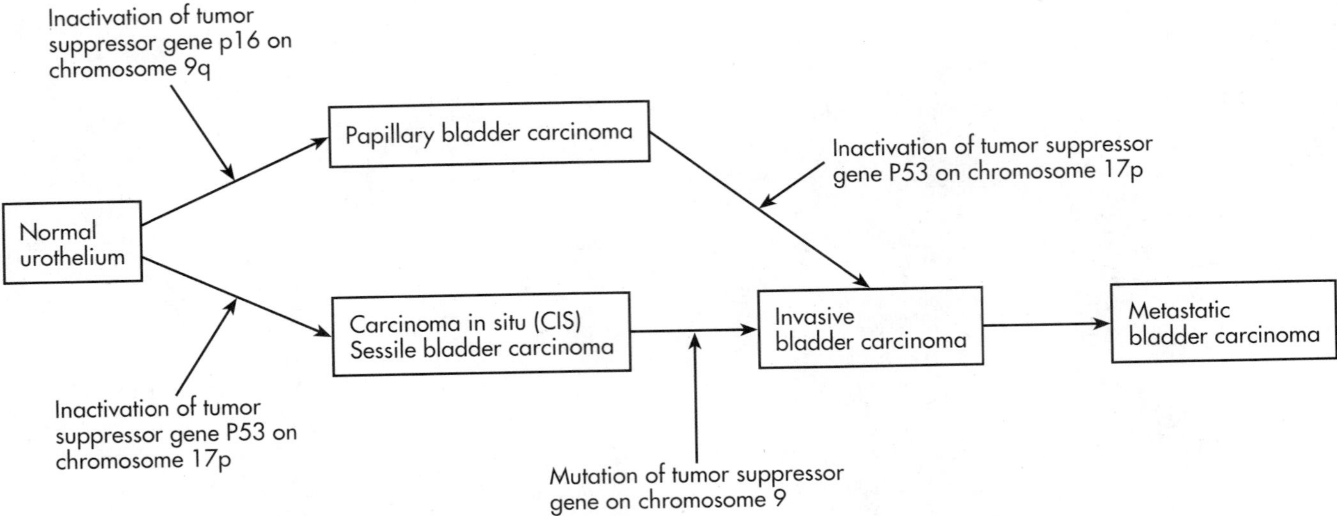

Fig. 47-2 Two-pathway model for the pathogenesis and progression of bladder cancer.

TABLE 47-1 Chromosomal Changes Associated with Bladder Cancer

Chromosomal Region	Activation of Proto-Oncogene	Inactivation of Tumor Suppressor Gene
1q		
3p		
5p		
6		
7		
8p		
9p & 9q		p16
10q		
11p	H-*ras*	
13q		Rb
17p &17q		P53
18q		
Y		

p, Short arm of chromosome; *q,* long arm of chromosome; *Rb,* retinoblastoma suppressor gene.
Information for this table was taken from the following reviews of the molecular biology of bladder cancer: Borland, R. N., Brendler, C. B., & Isaacs, W. B. (1992). Molecular biology of bladder cancer. *Hematology Oncology Clinics of North America, 6*(1), 31-39; Perucca, D., Szepetowski, P., Simon, M. P., & Gaudray, P. (1990). Molecular genetics of human bladder carcinomas. *Cancer Genetics and Cytogenetics, 49*(2), 143-156; Sandberg, A. A. (1992). Chromosome changes in early bladder neoplasms. *Journal of Cellular Biochemistry, Suppl. 16 I,* 76-79; Sidransky, D. & Messing, E. (1992). Molecular genetics and biochemical mechanisms in bladder cancer: Oncogenes, tumor suppressor genes, and growth factors. *Urologic Clinics of North America, 19*(4), 629-639.

terstitial cystitis. Lamm and Torti (1996) warn against dismissing these relatively innocuous symptoms without an adequate diagnostic workup in an attempt to reduce health care costs.

Physical Examination

A bimanual examination is done to determine the presence of a pelvic mass, bladder wall thickening, and whether the bladder is freely mobile or fixed to the pelvic sidewall (Fair et al., 1993). This examination is best done with the patient anesthetized for patient comfort and so that the pelvic muscles are relaxed (Israel, Natale, & Skinner, 1995; Lamm & Torti, 1996). Part of the staging workup for bladder cancer is a transurethral resection of the bladder (TURB), which is done with the patient anesthetized. The bimanual physical examination is generally done at this time.

Diagnostic Tests

All patients suspected of having bladder cancer should be assessed with urine cytology, an intravenous urogram (IVU), and cystoscopy (Israel, Natale, & Skinner, 1995).

Urine Cytology. The transitional cells that line the renal pelvis, ureters, bladder, and urethra are constantly being exfoliated and excreted in the urine. Urine cytology examines these cells to identify malignant changes. One technique uses a Papanicolaou stain to examine the cells under a microscope. Another technique uses flow cytometry, which treats the cells with a dye that binds to nucleic deoxyribonucleic acid (DNA), then passes the cells through a sensor that is able to quantify the amount of DNA in the cells. Malignant cells have an abnormally high amount of DNA because more of these cells are in the process of dividing (Walther, 1992). In addition to flow cytometry, another molecular method that is being investigated to detect malignant changes in exfoliated transitional cells uses polymerase chain reaction (PCR) technology to amplify specific

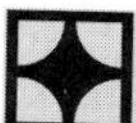

TABLE 47-2 Assessment of the Patient for Bladder Cancer

	Assessment Parameters	Typical Abnormal Findings
History	A. Personal and social history: 1. Gender 2. Ethnicity 3. Age 4. Occupation 5. Cigarette smoking 6. Family history B. Evaluation of genitourinary system	A. Personal and social risk factors: 1. More prevalent in men than women 2. More prevalent in whites than blacks, Asians, Hispanics, and American Indians 3. Usually over age 60 4. High-risk occupations listed in Box 47-2 5. Increased risk from smoking cigarettes 6. Increased risk from positive family history B. Common symptoms include hematuria, dysuria, frequency, and urgency.
Physical Examination	A. Bimanual examination under anesthesia	A. Bladder wall thickening and abnormal masses are indicative of possible extension of disease or metastasis.
Diagnostic Tests	A. Urine cytology B. Intravenous urogram C. Cystoscopy D. Transurethral resection of the bladder	A. Malignant cells are present. B. Filling defects may be detected, indicating a space-occupying lesion. C. Tumors may be flat, papillary, or sessile. CIS can appear as a velvety, mossy, erythematous lesion. During cystoscopy, the location, size, appearance, and condition of the surrounding mucosa should be evaluated for each lesion. D. Malignant cells are present in tissue that has undergone biopsy.

regions of DNA known to mutate in bladder cancer, thereby making DNA alterations easier to identify. One study (Mao, Schoenberg, Scicchitano, Erozan, Merlo, & Schwab et al., 1996) reported that this type of microsatellite analysis identified specific DNA alterations in 95% of a small sample of patients with bladder cancer, whereas routine urine cytology detected cancer cells in only 50% of the samples.

Urine cytology cannot determine the size or location of malignant tumors, only the presence of malignant cells in the urinary tract. However, it is possible to screen for malignant cells being shed by lesions in the ureters or renal pelvis, parts of the urinary tract not visualized with cystoscopy. The best urine specimen for cytologic examination is a freshly voided sample. Prolonged exposure of exfoliated cells to urine can complicate the pathologic interpretation. Because of this, urine specimens should not be sent from the first morning void or from catheter bags (Itoku & Stein, 1992; Murphy, 1990).

Currently, some form of urine cytology is a routine part of the diagnostic workup of patients suspected of having bladder cancer, and it is also used in the follow-up of patients previously treated for bladder cancer to assess for recurrence. In the future, urine cytology using molecular techniques could be part of a screening examination for people at high risk for bladder cancer based on their smoking habits, occupation, and family history.

Intravenous Urogram. An IVU, also known as an *intravenous pyelogram (IVP),* is done routinely in the diagnosis and staging of bladder cancer to evaluate the architecture and filling pattern of the urinary system. Although only 60% of bladder tumors are visualized with urography (Israel, Natale, & Skinner, 1995), these dye studies can iden-

TABLE 47-3 Bladder Symptoms

Symptom	Description
Dysuria	Painful and/or burning sensations during urination
Frequency	Voiding more often than every 2 hours; daytime frequency sometimes described as *diurnal* frequency; *nocturia* used to describe nighttime voiding more than once if under 65 years of age and more than twice if over 65 years of age
Urgency	Compelling feeling of the need to urinate as soon as possible
Irritative bladder symptoms	A symptom index generally including dysuria, urgency, and frequency
Cystitis	Inflammation of the bladder urothelium
Hematuria	Blood in the urine; can be microscopic or visible to eye alone as pink-tinged or red urine, with or without clots
Hemorrhagic cystitis	An often sudden onset of hematuria combined with bladder pain and irritative bladder symptoms

From Berry, D. L. (1996). Bladder disturbances. In S. L. Groenwald, M. H. Frogge, M. Goodman, & C. H. Yarbro (Eds.), *Cancer symptom management.* Sudbury, MA: Jones and Bartlett.

tify suspicious lesions that might otherwise be missed. Space-occupying lesions within the urinary tract or external to the system that are obstructing the flow of urine can be identified with this test. Bladder wall expansion can also be evaluated. Asymmetric expansion may be indicative of a deeply invasive bladder tumor (Israel, Natale, & Skinner, 1995). Preparation of the patient undergoing an IVU is outlined in Table 47-4.

Cystoscopy. Central to the diagnosis, staging, treatment, and follow-up of patients with bladder cancer is cystoscopy. A flexible cystoscope is routinely used, making it possible to perform the procedure in an outpatient setting with the patient under local anesthesia. During the procedure, the entire bladder and urethra are visualized. Every lesion should be described in detail, noting the location, size, appearance, and condition of the surrounding mucosa (Itoku & Stein, 1992). Approximately 70% of tumors are located on the lateral and posterior walls, 20% on the trigone, and 10% in the bladder dome (Fleshner et al., 1996; Melicow, 1974). During cystoscopy, bladder washings can also be obtained and sent for cytology (Table 47-5).

If suspicious lesions are identified during the initial cystoscopy, a TURB with the patient under spinal or general anesthesia is planned. (Transurethral resection of the bladder is discussed in more detail in the Medical Management and Nursing Management sections.)

Need for Additional Imaging Studies. For superficial tumors extending no further than the lamina propria, additional imaging studies (e.g., cystography, computed axial tomography, magnetic resonance imaging, ultrasonog-

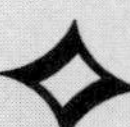

Table 47-4 Patient Preparation for Intravenous Urogram (IVU)

Description of the Procedure: The architecture and filling pattern of the kidneys, renal pelvis, ureters, and bladder are visualized on a timed series of plain radiograph films with the help of radiopaque iodine contrast that concentrates in the urine after being injected intravenously.

Patient Preparation: Patients are usually instructed to take a laxative the evening before the examination and an enema the next morning to clear the bowel of stool and gas, which can obscure the radiographs. Patients are also instructed to abstain from food and fluids 12 hours before the examination so that the contrast will concentrate in the urinary tract.

Procedural Considerations:

1. Explain the procedure to the patient. Query the patient about allergies to contrast media.
2. Obtain informed consent.
3. Take a radiograph with the patient in a supine position to ensure that the bowel is empty and the location of the kidneys can be visualized.
4. Inject radiopaque iodine contrast intravenously.
5. Over the next 20 to 30 minutes, take a series of at least three radiographs.
6. After the patient voids, take a final radiograph.

Special Considerations:

1. Contraindications to an IVU include the following:
   a. Hypersensitivity or allergy to iodine preparations
   b. Renal and hepatic disease
   c. Oliguria
   d. Renal failure with a creatinine greater than 1.5 mg per dl and/or a blood urea nitrogen greater than 40 mg per dl
   e. Patients receiving drug therapy for chronic bronchitis, emphysema, or asthma
2. The patient may experience warmth, flushing, a salty taste, and/or nausea shortly after the contrast media is injected. Usually these feelings quickly resolve and no treatment is needed.
3. Resuscitation supplies and equipment should be readily available in case the patient has an anaphylactic reaction to the contrast media.

Modified from Fischbach, F. T. (1996). *A manual of laboratory and diagnostic tests* (5th ed.). Philadelphia: J. B. Lippincott.

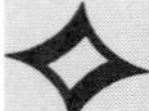

Table 47-5 Patient Preparation for Diagnostic Cystoscopy

Description of the Procedure: A thin, lighted scope is passed through the urethra into the bladder to visualize the urethra, interior of the bladder, and ureteral orifices. The cystoscope is usually a flexible, fiberoptic instrument, although rigid cystoscopes of various diameters are also available.

Patient Preparation: For cystoscopies done under local anesthesia, liquids should be encouraged until the time of the procedure to promote urine formation. If other forms of anesthesia are planned, the patient may need to be NPO.

Procedural Considerations:

1. Explain the procedure to the patient.
2. Obtain informed consent.
3. Instruct the patient to disrobe below the waist, and then help the patient into a lithotomy position with his or her legs in stirrups.
4. Clean the external genitalia with an antiseptic solution, such as povidone-iodine (Betadine) or chlorhexidine (Hibiclens).
5. Instill anesthetic jelly, such as lidocaine, into the urethra.
6. Connect the scope to an irrigation system, and flush with an isotonic, clear solution such as normal saline or glycine.
7. Pass the scope through the urethra and into the bladder.
8. The patient may experience a strong urge to void during the procedure because of the presence of the scope as well as fluids that are used to irrigate the scope and bladder.
9. After the procedure, the patient may experience urethral burning, dysuria, frequency, and/or some hematuria that should resolve within a couple of days.

Modified from Fischbach, F. T. (1996). *A manual of laboratory and diagnostic tests* (5th ed.). Philadelphia: J. B. Lippincott.

raphy, and bone or liver scans) are neither necessary nor cost effective (Lamm & Torti, 1996).

STAGING

Bladder cancer is considered a heterogeneous disease of the urothelium, indicating that multiple tumors can develop simultaneously in different areas of the bladder. Approximately 30% of patients have multiple tumors at the time of diagnosis (Fair, Fuks, & Scher, 1993; Heney et al., 1982; Itoku & Stein, 1992). Each lesion needs to be characterized as to its (1) pathology or cell type, (2) morphology or appearance, (3) invasiveness into the bladder wall and surrounding tissue, and (4) grade or degree of cytologic abnormality.

Pathology

The pathology of bladder cancers is outlined in Table 47-6 and described below.

Transitional Cell Carcinoma (TCC). More than 90% of tumors of the bladder arise from the urothelium, a specialized transitional epithelium lining the bladder and urinary tract (Fleshner et al., 1996; Lynch & Cohen, 1995; Melicow, 1974; Silverman et al., 1992). The urothelium is believed to be susceptible to malignant changes because of the constant exposure to urinary waste products. These tumors are amenable to a variety of treatments.

Squamous Cell Carcinoma. Squamous cell carcinoma accounts for less than 5% of bladder carcinomas in the United States (Lynch & Cohen, 1995; Melicow, 1974). In countries where *S. haematobium* is endemic, the percentage of bladder cancers that are squamous cell in origin is much higher (Ghoneim, 1995). Unfortunately, this type of bladder cancer is usually not diagnosed until it is at an advanced stage. More than 90% of squamous cell bladder tumors are invasive at the time of diagnosis (Faysal, 1981; Newman, Brown, Jay, & Pontius, 1968). Surgery is the primary treatment modality because squamous cell tumors are generally unresponsive to radiation therapy or chemotherapy (Brodsky, 1992; Lamm & Torti, 1996).

Adenocarcinoma and Others. Other, even less common carcinomas of the bladder include adenocarcinomas, spindle cell carcinomas, small cell carcinomas, carcinoid tumors, pheochromocytomas, choriocarcinomas, and germ cell neoplasms (Brodsky, 1992). Like squamous cell carcinomas, surgery is the primary treatment modality for these tumors because they are generally unresponsive to radiation therapy or chemotherapy (Bane, Rao, & Hemstreet, 1996; Brodsky, 1992; Lamm & Torti, 1996).

TABLE 47-6 Pathology of Bladder Cancers

Pathology	Percent of Tumors
Transitional cell:	90%-95%
• Papillary	
• Carcinoma in situ	
• Sessile	
Squamous cell	2%-5%
Adenocarcinoma	1%-2%
Rare bladder carcinomas, including small cell carcinoma, neuroendocrine spindle cell carcinoma, carcinoid carcinoma, pheochromocytomas, choriocarcinomas, germ cell neoplasms, villous adenomas	<1%

Modified from Brodsky, G. L. (1992). Pathology of bladder carcinoma. *Hematology Oncology Clinics of North America, 6*(1), 59-80; Fleshner, N. E., Herr, H. W., Stewart, A. K., Murphy, G. P., Mettlin, C., & Menck, H. R. (1996). The national cancer data base report on bladder carcinoma. *Cancer, 78*(7), 1505-1513; Lynch, C. F. & Cohen, M. G. (1995). Urinary system. *Cancer, 75(Suppl. 1)*, 316-329; Melicow, M. M. (1974). Tumors of the bladder: A multifaceted problem. *Journal of Urology, 112*(4), 467-478; Silverman, D. T., Hartge, P., Morrison, A. S., & Devesa, S. S. (1992). Epidemiology of bladder cancer. *Hematology Oncology Clinics of North America, 6*(1), 1-30.

Morphology

The morphology, or appearance, of bladder tumors can be flat, papillary, or sessile. These descriptions, confirmed with pathologic examination, help to characterize the primary tumor for staging.

Carcinoma in Situ. Nonpapillary CIS is a flat tumor that has been described as a velvety, mossy, erythematous lesion (Itoku & Stein, 1992; Lamm, 1992a). These changes in the bladder mucosa can be very subtle; many times the urothelium appears completely normal, and it is only with pathologic evaluation of bladder washings and random bladder wall biopsies that CIS is diagnosed. Patients are likely to complain of IBS, which brings them to seek medical care and an evaluation. Carcinoma in situ is staged Tis, as indicated in Table 47-7.

The prevalence of CIS is difficult to determine because it can occur as a primary focal lesion, as diffuse urothelial disease, or adjacent to either a papillary or sessile lesion (Fair et al., 1993). Often, Tis and small papillary Ta tumors are reported together as Stage 0 disease. One prospective study of 2454 patients with bladder cancer reported that only 10% of the patients had an initial diagnosis of CIS (Utz & Farrow, 1984). This form of bladder cancer is considered a highly variable and unpredictable malignancy with the potential for rapid progression and invasion that demands aggressive treatment and close follow-up (Itoku & Stein, 1992; Lamm, 1992a).

Papillary Tumors. As the name suggests, papillary tumors grow on stalks. Depending on their size and location, papillary tumors can intermittently obstruct the ureters or urethra as they bend with the flow of urine. Papillary tumors account for 70% to 80% of bladder carcinomas (Fleshner et al., 1996; Melicow, 1974). They are usually staged Ta, as indicated in Table 47-7. The base of a papillary tumor generally does not invade the lamina propria or detrusor muscle, although this is possible. If the base of the stalk extends beyond the epithelium, the tumor is upstaged according to the degree of bladder wall invasion, as outlined in Table 47-7.

TABLE 47-7 Tumor Staging Systems for Bladder Cancer

Jewett-Strong-Marshall Classification	TNM Classification	
	Primary Tumor (T)	
	TX	Primary tumor cannot be assessed
	T0	No evidence of primary tumor
0	Tis	Tumor in situ (flat tumor) or carcinoma in situ
	Ta	Noninvasive papillary carcinoma limited to epithelial layer
A	T1	Tumor invades subepithelial connective tissue extending to the lamina propria
B1	T2	Tumor invades superficial muscle extending less than halfway through the detrusor muscle
B2	T3a	Tumor invades deep muscle extending more than halfway through the detrusor muscle
C	T3b	Tumor invades perivesical fat
	T4a	Tumor invades prostate, uterus, vagina
D1	T4b	Tumor invades the pelvic or abdominal wall
	Lymph Nodes (N)	
	NX	Lymph nodes cannot be assessed
	N0	No regional lymph node metastasis
	N1	Metastasis in a single lymph node <2 cm in greatest dimension
	N2	Metastasis in a single lymph node >2 cm but not >5 cm in greatest dimension or multiple lymph nodes
	N3	Metastasis in lymph node >5 cm in greatest dimension
	Distant Metastasis (M)	
	MX	Presence of distant metastasis cannot be assessed
	M0	No distant metastasis
D2	M1	Distant metastasis

Modified from American Joint Committee on Cancer. (1992). Urinary bladder. In O. H. Beahrs, D. E. Henson, R. V. P. Hutter, & B. J. Kennedy (Eds.), *Manual for staging of cancer* (4th ed.). Philadelphia: J. B. Lippincott; Marshall, V. F. (1952). The relation of the preoperative estimate to the pathologic demonstration of the extent of vesical neoplasms. *Journal of Urology, 68*(4), 714-723.

Sessile Tumors. The remaining 20% to 30% of bladder tumors have a broad base and commonly invade the subepithelial connective tissue (Melicow, 1974). These tumors are called *sessile* and are staged according to the extent of tumor invasion, as indicated on Fig. 47-2 and in Table 47-7. A sessile morphology is a poor prognostic feature, indicating that the cancer may already be invasive.

TNM Staging

The earliest classification of bladder cancers was the Jewett-Strong Classification developed in 1946 (Jewett & Strong, 1946), modified by Jewett in 1952 (Jewett, 1952), and again by Marshall in the same year (Marshall, 1952). The Jewett-Strong-Marshall Classification describes Stages 0, A, B, C, and D according to the depth of tumor invasion into the bladder wall and metastasis to adjacent structures. More recently, most health care providers have adopted the American Joint Committee on Cancer (AJCC) Classification System to uniformly communicate cancer statistics internationally. The AJCC Classification System describes the stage of cancer according to the size of the primary tumor (T), the presence or absence of disease in regional lymph nodes (N), and the presence or absence of distant metastasis (M) (American Joint Committee on Cancer, 1992). Table 47-7 compares the two staging systems, and Table 47-8 shows how the stage of disease is determined according to the TNM system for bladder cancer.

Both staging systems depend on a bladder wall biopsy to determine whether the tumor has invaded the muscle. Clinical staging with cystoscopy alone is notoriously inaccurate in determining the degree of tumor invasion into the bladder wall. In a combined series of four studies with a total of 465 patients with bladder cancer, clinical staging agreed with pathologic staging for less than 50% of the patients (Fair, Fuks, & Scher, 1993). More than one third of the patients would have been understaged without the benefit of a bladder wall muscle biopsy, resulting in insufficient treatment.

TABLE 47-8 Stage Grouping for Bladder Cancer

Stage	Tumor (T)	Lymph Node (N)	Metastasis (M)
0is	Tis	N0	M0
0a	Ta	N0	M0
I	T1	N0	M0
II	T2	N0	M0
	T3a	N0	M0
III	T3b	N0	M0
	T4a	N0	M0
IV	T4b	N0	M0
	Any T	N1	M0
	Any T	N2	M0
	Any T	N3	M0
	Any T	Any N	M1

Modified from American Joint Committee on Cancer. (1992). Urinary bladder. In O. H. Beahrs, D. E. Henson, R. V. P. Hutter, & B. J. Kennedy (Eds.), *Manual for staging of cancer* (4th ed.). Philadelphia: J. B. Lippincott.

TABLE 47-9 Histologic Staging of Bladder Carcinoma

Grade	Defining Characteristics*
I	Mildly dysplastic, as evidenced by an increase in the number of urothelial cell layers (greater than seven), slight cytologic dysplasia, and rare mitoses
II	Moderately dysplastic, as evidenced by moderate cytologic dysplasia and greater mitotic activity
III	Severely dysplastic, as evidenced by focal high-grade nuclear dysplasia and frequent mitoses

*Based on the following features: number of cell layers, polarity, denudation, cytoplasmic clearing, nuclear size, nuclear crowding, nuclear notching, chromatin pattern, nucleoli, and mitoses.

Modified from Bane, B. L., Rao, J. Y., & Hemstreet, G. P. (1996). Pathology and staging of bladder cancer. *Seminars in Oncology, 23*(5), 546-570; Murphy, W. M., & Soloway, M. S. (1982). Developing carcinoma (dysplasia) of the urinary bladder. *Pathology Annual, 17*(1), 197-217.

Histologic Staging

The fourth major consideration in describing a bladder cancer is the grade, or the degree of cellular dysplasia of the tumor (Bane, Rao, & Hemstreet, 1996; Brodsky, 1992). Pathologists determine a histologic grade of I, II, or III based on 10 pathologic features listed in Table 47-9. Some classification systems assign a grade between I and IV, but because the biologic behavior of grade III and grade IV tumors are so similar, the World Health Organization has combined them into a single grade (Fair, Fuks, & Scher, 1993).

The higher the grade, the more dysplastic and less differentiated the tumor appears. The higher the grade, the worse the prognosis for the patient. The TNM staging of bladder cancer (0, I, II, III, IV) does *not* describe the grade of the tumor (I, II, III). Both features of the cancer are important to characterize and help the urologist and patient plan appropriate therapy. It is important to note that, whereas papillary and sessile tumors can histologically be grade I, II, or III, CIS is always considered a grade III lesion (Bane, Rao, & Hemstreet, 1996; Lamm, 1992a).

MEDICAL MANAGEMENT

As shown in Table 47-10, approximately two thirds of patients with bladder cancer have superficial, stage 0 or stage I, disease involving only the bladder mucosa or submucosa (Fleshner et al., 1996). The vast majority of these tumors are TCC. They can appear flat or papillary. Superficial bladder cancers can be grade I, II, or III. These cancers have long been recognized as unpredictable. Some tumors are eradicated by surgery alone, whereas others have a propensity for recurrence and progression. The urologist must carefully consider each patient's disease characteristics before offering a specific treatment plan. Table 47-11 outlines possible treatment approaches according to the stage of disease and tumor characteristics. Patients must understand that even with successful treatment of the primary tumor, the risk of disease recurrence can be very high, and lifelong medical surveillance is imperative to detect and treat any recurrence as soon as possible.

TABLE 47-10 Percentage of Cases by Stage at Diagnosis in 1993

Stage	Cases by Stage at Diagnosis in 1993
0	32.5%
I	28.9%
II	12.5%
III	6.6%
IV	6.1%
Unknown	13.4%

Modified from Fleshner, N. E., Herr, H. W., Stewart, A. K., Murphy, G. P., Mettlin, C., & Menck, H. R. (1996). The national cancer data base report on bladder carcinoma. *Cancer, 78*(7), 1505-1513.

Surgery

Transurethral Resection of the Bladder. If a bladder tumor is detected during cystoscopy, a TURB is scheduled. Although most patients can tolerate a flexible cystoscopy with only local anesthesia, spinal or general anesthesia is required for a TURB. Not only is the patient more comfortable, the anesthesia relaxes the pelvic floor, abdominal wall, and bladder, allowing the urologist to do a

Table 47-11 Treatment Options According to Stage of Disease and Tumor Characteristics

Stage	Tumor Characteristics	Possible Treatment Approaches
0	Tis (CIS)	TURB and intravesical BCG
	• Persistent disease after BCG	• Cystectomy with bladder reconstruction
	• First recurrence	• Re-treatment with intravesical BCG
	• Multiple recurrences	• Intravesical chemotherapy, photodynamic therapy, alternative immunotherapies, cystectomy with bladder reconstruction
0	Ta	TURB
	• Incomplete resections, size greater than 3 cm, grade II or III, multiple tumors, and/or abnormal cells in random biopsies	• Intravesical BCG
	• Multiple recurrences	• Laser surgery, PDT, or cystectomy with bladder reconstruction
I	T1	TURB
	• Incomplete resections, size greater than 3 cm, grade II or III, multiple tumors, and/or abnormal cells in random biopsies	• Intravesical BCG
	• Multiple recurrences	• Laser surgery, PDT, or cystectomy with bladder reconstruction

CIS, Carcinoma in situ; *BCG,* Bacillus Calmette-Guérin; *TURB,* transurethral resection of the bladder; *PDT,* photodynamic therapy.
Modified from Fair, W. R., Fuks, Z. Y., & Scher, H. I. (1993). Cancer of the bladder. In V. T. DeVita, Jr., S. Hellman, & S. A. Rosenberg (Eds.), *Cancer: Principles and practice of oncology* (4th ed.). Philadelphia: J. B. Lippincott; Israel, V. K., Natale, R. B., & Skinner, D. G. (1995). Bladder. In M. D. Abeloff, J. O. Armitage, A. S. Lichter, & J. E. Niederhuber (Eds.), *Clinical oncology.* New York: Churchill Livingstone; Itoku, K. A., & Stein, B. S. (1992). Superficial bladder cancer. *Hematology Oncology Clinics of North America, 6*(1), 99-116; Lamm, D. L. (1992a). Carcinoma in situ. *Urologic Clinics of North America, 19*(3), 499-508.

complete bimanual physical examination and biopsy of the bladder wall without the risk of stimulating the obturator reflex and perforating the bladder (Soloway & Patel, 1992).

After the patient is anesthetized adequately, a bimanual physical examination is done to determine the presence of a pelvic mass or bladder wall thickening and whether the bladder is freely mobile or fixed to the pelvic sidewall (Fair, Fuks, & Scher, 1993). The cystoscope is then inserted through the urethra and into the bladder. This cystoscope has various components and attachments, including a light source, at least two viewing lenses (30° and 70°), electric wire cutting loops, and bladder irrigating and draining capabilities (Soloway & Patel, 1992). Care must be taken to perform an adequate biopsy of the bladder wall muscle, yet not perforate the bladder.

Additional biopsies of the tissue surrounding the tumor, as well as random bladder wall biopsies, are usually also taken. Biopsies from normal-appearing mucosa can be pathologically abnormal in 14% to 33% of patients (Heney, Daly, Prout, Nieh, Heaney, & Trebeck, 1978; Murphy, Nagy, Rao, Soloway, Parija, & Cox et al., 1979; Soloway, Murphy, Rao, & Cox, 1978; Wallace, Hindmarsh, Webb, Busuttil, Hargreave, & Newsam, et al., 1979). "Cold-cup" biopsies are recommended to minimize cautery distortion of small pieces of tissue (Fair, Fuks, & Scher, 1993; Israel, Natale, & Skinner, 1995; Lamm & Torti, 1996). In men, a biopsy of the prostatic urethra should also be done to guide treatment decision making (Lamm & Torti, 1996). One study (Wood, Montie, Pontes, Medendorp, & Levin, 1989) found that 43% of 84 men undergoing radical prostatectomies for bladder cancer had involvement of the prostatic urethra. Women should also have a biopsy performed on the urethra.

After a TURB, an indwelling catheter is placed to drain urine and monitor for bleeding. The patient may be hospitalized overnight, but more commonly the patient will be discharged home from the Post Anesthesia Care Unit (PACU). (The nursing care of these patients will be discussed in the Nursing Management section.)

Laser Therapy. For patients who have had repeated recurrences of superficial bladder cancer without a change in stage or grade, another treatment option is laser therapy ablation (Benson, 1995; Itoku & Stein, 1992). Laser surgery has several advantages compared with repeated TURB for recurrent superficial disease. Laser procedures can be done as part of a flexible cystoscopy under local anesthesia in an outpatient setting, the risk of perforating the bladder wall is very small, and an indwelling catheter is rarely necessary postoperatively because bleeding does not occur. The major disadvantage of laser surgery is that the tumor is completely obliterated; therefore no tissue is obtained from the procedure for pathologic evaluation (Itoku & Stein, 1992).

Argon, potassium-titanyl-phosphate (KTP), and neodymium:yttrium-aluminum-garnet (Nd:YAG) lasers have all been used to treat superficial bladder tumors (Benson, 1995; Itoku & Stein, 1992). The argon laser has a penetration depth of only 1 mm, whereas the KTP laser has a penetration depth of 2 to 3 mm and the Nd:YAG laser a penetration of 4 to 5 mm.

Intravesical Therapy

Intravesical therapy, instilling drugs directly into the bladder, is part of the primary treatment of CIS and an adjuvant therapy for high risk Ta and T1 superficial bladder cancers. Both chemotherapeutic and immunologic agents have been successfully used intravesically. The advantage of intravesical therapy is the ability to provide intimate contact of the drug with the tumor without the toxicities of systemic therapy. In the past, radical cystectomy was the recommended treatment for superficial CIS bladder cancers. Today, however, intravesical therapy has replaced cystectomy as the primary treatment of CIS, thereby preserving the bladder for the majority of patients with this disease. Box 47-3 outlines the indications for intravesical therapy in the management of superficial bladder cancer.

Chemotherapy. Intravesical chemotherapy was first introduced in the 1960s (Jones & Swinney, 1961; Veenema, Dean, Roberts, Fingerhut, Chowhury, & Tarassoly, 1962). The chemotherapy is believed to be directly cytotoxic to tumor cells (Lamm & Torti, 1996). Various clinical trials have found thiotepa, doxorubicin (Adriamycin), and mitomycin (Mutamycin) to be effective in prolonging disease-free survival (Kurth, 1995; Reijke & Kurth, 1995; Soloway, 1995), but these drugs have not altered long-term disease progression rates (Lamm, 1992c; Nseyo & Lamm, 1996).

Intravesical chemotherapy can begin 1 to 4 weeks after TURB. Treatment schedules vary, but most induction regimens include weekly drug installations for 4 to 8 weeks, which may be followed by a maintenance regimen (Herr, 1992). Table 47-12 provides typical doses of the various drugs used. The actual administration of intravesical therapy is discussed under the Nursing Management section.

The side effects of intravesical chemotherapy depend on the drug instilled, dosage, and frequency of treatment. Irritative bladder symptoms are the most commonly reported side effects, occurring in between 10% and 50% of patients (Thrasher & Crawford, 1992). Urinary function usually returns to normal after treatment is completed. Systemic effects of intravesical chemotherapy are possible if the drug is absorbed through the bladder wall and into the blood circulation. Patients with large areas of denuded bladder epithelium or who are treated within 1 week of TURB are at higher risk for systemic toxicities. The lower the molecular weight of the drug, the more likely it is to be absorbed systemically. Intravesical thiotepa, a drug that has a very low molecular weight, has been reported to cause leukopenia (white blood cell count less than 4000 per cubic mm) in 8% to 54% of patients and thrombocytopenia (platelet count less than 100,000 per cubic mm) in 3% to 31% of patients (Thrasher & Crawford, 1992). Myelosuppression is rare in patients receiving doxorubicin or mitomycin because of the higher molecular weight of these drugs. Contact dermatitis can occur if the drug spills or splashes on the perineum or hands during or after treatment (Nissenkorn, Herrod, & Soloway, 1981). This adverse effect can be avoided by careful administration and immediately washing the hands and perineum after treatment and after each urination. Thrasher and Crawford (1992) recently reviewed the complications of intravesical therapy, and the interested reader is referred to this reference for more detailed information on the side effects of intravesical thiotepa, doxorubicin, and mitomycin, as well as epirubicin, ethoglucid (Epodyl), and mitoxantrone (Novantrone).

Box 47-3
Indications for Intravesical Therapy in the Management of Superficial Bladder Cancer

Therapeutically, to treat existing disease such as the following:
- Diffuse CIS
- Large tumors that cannot be completely resected with TURB
- Numerous tumors that cannot be completely resected with TURB
- Patients with persistently positive urine cytology after TURB

Prophylactically, to prevent disease recurrence and progression in patients with completely resected tumors but when the tumor had any of the following pathologic characteristics:
- CIS
- Multifocality
- High grade
- T1 in size, of any grade

CIS, Carcinoma in situ; *TURB,* transurethral resection of the bladder.

Modified from Badalament, R. A., Ortolano, V., & Burgers, J. K. (1992). Recurrent or aggressive bladder cancer: Indications for adjuvant intravesical therapy. *Urologic Clinics of North America, 19*(3), 485-498; Herr, H. W. (1992). Intravesical therapy. *Hematology Oncology Clinics of North America, 6*(1), 117-127; Lamm, D. L. (1992a). Carcinoma in situ. *Urologic Clinics of North America, 19*(3), 499-508; Nseyo, U. O. & Lamm, D. L. (1996). Therapy of superficial bladder cancer. *Seminars in Oncology, 23*(5), 598-604.

Table 47-12 Intravesical Drug Doses

Drug	Dose (Diluted in Sterile Saline to a Concentration of 1 mg/ml)
Thiotepa	30-60 mg
Adriamycin (Doxorubicin)	20-80 mg
Mitomycin (Mutamycin)	20-60 mg
Bacillus Calmette Guérin (BCG)*	
Pasteur	75-150 mg
Tice	50 mg
Connaught	120 mg
Armand Frappier	120 mg

*10^7-10^9 viable colony-forming units (CFUs).

Modified from Fair, W. R., Fuks, Z. Y., & Scher, H. I. (1993). Cancer of the bladder. In V. T. DeVita, Jr., S. Hellman, & S. A. Rosenberg (Eds.), *Cancer: Principles and practice of oncology* (4th ed.). Philadelphia: J. B. Lippincott; Herr, H. W. (1992). Intravesical therapy. *Hematology Oncology Clinics of North America, 6*(1), 117-127; Israel, V. K., Natale, R. B., & Skinner, D. G. (1995). Bladder. In M. D. Abeloff, J. O. Armitage, A. S. Lichter, & J. E. Niederhuber (Eds.), *Clinical oncology.* New York: Churchill Livingstone.

Immunotherapy. Bacillus Calmette-Guérin (BCG) was identified as a useful agent in the treatment of superficial bladder cancer in 1976 (Morales, Eidinger, & Bruce,

1976) and has since replaced chemotherapy as the primary treatment for CIS, as well as tumors at high risk for recurrence. Although no one clinical trial has compared the efficacy of BCG with that of thiotepa, adriamycin, or mitomycin, the benefit of BCG therapy compared with the other chemotherapies can be appreciated from Table 47-13, which summarizes data from many studies evaluating these drugs.

BCG is a vaccine containing attenuated, live tuberculosis bacilli. The exact mechanism of action of BCG in the treatment of bladder cancer is unknown, but the patient's immunologic response against the bacillus is believed to destroy the cancer cells as well (Brosman, 1992). Because effective therapy depends on the patient having a competent immune system, BCG intravesical therapy is not an option for patients who are severely immunocompromised, such as those with human immunodeficiency virus (HIV) or those on chronic steroid therapy. Also, patients taking antibiotics or fibrin clot inhibitors (including warfarin, indomethacin, ibuprofen, salicylates, and dipyridamole) should not be treated with BCG because these drugs render the BCG inactive (Brosman, 1992; Hudson, Yuan, Catalona, & Ratliff, 1990).

Intravesical immunotherapy can begin 1 to 4 weeks after TURB. Doses between 50 and 120 mg (10^7 and 10^9 viable colony-forming units), depending on the substrain of BCG, are instilled weekly for 6 weeks (Brosman & Lamm, 1990; Herr, 1992). (Table 47-12 provides common dosages of several different strains.) Because BCG is a biologic product and the response to this therapy depends on the patient's immune response, treatment should be tailored to the individual patient.

The goal is to induce an inflammatory immunologic response within the bladder, which may happen with fewer than six treatments or may require more than six treatments. There is no benefit to an exaggerated inflammatory response to the BCG (Brosman, 1992). Induction therapy may be followed by a maintenance regimen of BCG installations. Some urologists give three to six additional weekly installations, some give monthly installations for 1 to 2 years, some give one to three installations every 3 to 6 months for 1 to 2 years, and still others give no additional therapy (Brosman, 1992). At least one prospective, randomized trial failed to demonstrate any benefit of maintenance BCG therapy given monthly for 2 years after induction therapy as compared with close follow-up of the patient after induction therapy (Badalament, Ortolano, & Burgers, 1987). Other studies are needed to test different maintenance schedules to determine whether a different regimen might prolong disease-free survival.

Compared with the side effects of intravesical chemotherapy, the side effects associated with intravesical BCG immunotherapy occur more frequently and are more severe. Almost all patients experience IBS, half have hematuria, one quarter have a fever up to 102° F, and one quarter report malaise (Lamm, Stogdill, Stogdill, & Crispen, 1986; Lamm, van der Meijden, Morales, Brosman, Catalona, & Herr et al., 1992). Symptoms usually begin after two or three installations and persist for about 2 days. After a patient experiences IBS, he or she is more likely to have symptoms with the next and subsequent treatments (Berry, Blumenstein, Magyary, Lamm, & Crawford, 1996; Böhle, Balck, von Wietersheim, & Jocham, 1996). Medications that can be taken for relief of IBS include urinary analgesics such as phenazopyridine (Pyridium), antispasmodics such as oxybutynin (Ditropan) or flavoxate (Urispas), or anticholinergics such as propantheline (ProBanthine) (Lamm et al., 1992). Patients should increase their fluid intake if they experience hematuria and can take acetaminophen or diphenhydramine (Benadryl) for flu-like symptoms (Lamm, 1992b).

Patients should be advised not to take analgesics that are also fibrin clot inhibitors (e.g., salicylates, ibuprofen, and indomethacin) because these drugs may interfere with the anti-tumor effects of BCG (Hudson, Yuan, & Catalona et al., 1990). If any of these symptoms are unusually severe or if they do not resolve in 48 hours, isoniazid (300 mg) can be given daily until the symptoms improve. The BCG treatment should be held until all side effects from previous installations have resolved (Lamm, 1992c).

TABLE 47-13 Effects of Intravesical Therapy on Recurrence and Progression

Agent	Number of Patients	Controls	Treated	Net Benefit
Effect on Recurrence (tumor free more than 1 year)				
Thiotepa	757	48	56	8%
Doxorubicin (Adriamycin)	860	59	69	1%
Mitomycin (Mutamycin)	880	46	58	12%
Bacillus Calmette-Guérin (BCG)	318	30	72	42%
Effect on Progression Rate (tumor free more than 1 year)				
Thiotepa	513	6	4.5	NS
Doxorubicin (Adriamycin)	455	11.2	12.9	NS
Mitomycin (Mutamycin)	455	5	2.4	NS
Bacillus Calmette-Guérin (BCG)	329	28	14	14%

From Fair, W. R., Fuks, Z. Y., & Scher, H. I. (1993). Cancer of the bladder. In V. T. DeVita, Jr., S. Hellman, & S. A. Rosenberg (Eds.), *Cancer: Principles and practice of oncology* (4th ed.). Philadelphia: J. B. Lippincott.

Less than 5% of patients treated with BCG intravesical therapy experience serious complications such as fever greater than 102° F (38.8° C), sepsis, hepatitis, or permanent bladder contracture (Lamm et al., 1986; Lamm et al., 1992). BCG installations should be avoided after a traumatic catheterization because of a higher reported incidence of serious side effects (Lamm et al., 1992). Treatment recommendations for selected BCG-related complications can be found in Table 47-14.

Other immunologic agents that have been instilled intravesically in an attempt to control superficial bladder cancer include interferon, keyhole limpet hemocyanin (KLH), and oral bropirimine (Lamm & Sosnowski, 1995). The role of these agents in the treatment of this disease remains to be established (Nseyo & Lamm, 1996).

Photodynamic Therapy (PDT). Another type of intravesical therapy involves the intravenous administration of a photosensitizer followed by activation using whole-bladder laser therapy with visible light (Benson, 1995; Dachowski & DeLaney, 1992; Nseyo, 1992; Nseyo & Lamm, 1996). The photosensitizer is preferentially taken up by low-density lipoprotein receptors in tumor cells. Light activates the photosensitizing agent, generating singlet oxygen and free radicals that are cytotoxic (Nseyo, 1992; Nseyo & Lamm, 1996).

Photodynamic therapy has been used for the treatment of recurrent or refractory superficial bladder cancer, as well as for prophylaxis of recurrent superficial disease. Long-term data on the prevention, recurrence, and progression of bladder cancer after PDT therapy are not yet available (Nseyo & Lamm, 1996). Local side effects of PDT include urinary frequency, urgency, nocturia, and bladder spasm. Permanent bladder contracture is also possible and was reported in 10% of 101 patients who were treated under various treatment protocols (Nseyo, 1996). Patients are also at risk for cutaneous photosensitivity and should be advised to avoid sunlight for 4 to 6 weeks after therapy to avoid severe sunburn.

Follow-Up

Because of the propensity for recurrence and the risk of disease progression, the management of superficial bladder cancer should include lifelong surveillance. One recommended protocol includes cystoscopy and urine cytology studies every 3 months for 2 years, then every 6 months for 2 years, and yearly thereafter (Brosman, 1992; Itoku & Stein, 1992). Urinalysis, looking for microscopic hematuria, and urine cytology should be performed at the time of each cystoscopy. Any positive findings warrant a complete diagnostic workup and appropriate treatment.

TABLE 47-14 Treatment Recommendations for Selected BCG-Related Complications

Complication	Recommended Treatment
IBS (e.g., dysuria, frequency, urgency)	Urinary analgesic such as phenazopyridine (Pyridium) Antispasmodic such as oxybutynin (Ditropan) or flavoxate (Urispas) Anticholinergic such as propantheline (ProBanthine) If symptoms are severe or have not resolved within 48 hours, consider isoniazid 300 mg every day. Hold BCG until symptoms have resolved.
Hematuria	Increase fluid intake. If symptoms are severe or have not resolved within 48 hours, consider isoniazid 300 mg every day. Hold BCG until symptoms have resolved.
Flu-like symptoms (e.g., fever <102° F (38.8° C), aching in muscles and joints, malaise, or fatigue)	Acetaminophen or diphenhydramine (Benadryl) as needed for patient comfort If symptoms are severe or have not resolved within 48 hours, consider isoniazid 300 mg every day. Hold BCG until symptoms have resolved.
Fever >102° F (38.8° C)	Isoniazid 300 mg every day for 3 months May resume BCG when patient is asymptomatic
Acute, severe illness	Isoniazid 300 mg, rifampin 600 mg, and ethambutol 1200 mg, all by mouth every day for 3 months Discontinue BCG.
Sepsis	Isoniazid 300 mg, rifampin 600 mg, ethambutol 1200 mg, and cycloserine 500 mg, all by mouth twice a day Consider prednisolone 40 mg intravenously. Discontinue BCG.

IBS, Irritative bladder symptom; *BCG,* Bacillus Calmette-Guérin.
Modified from Lamm, D. L. (1992b). Complications of bacillus Calmette-Guérin immunotherapy. *Urologic Clinics of North America, 19*(3), 565-572; Lamm, D. L., van der Meijden, P. M., Morales, A., Brosman, S. A., Catalona, W. J., Herr, H. W., et al. (1992). Incidence and treatment of complications of bacillus Calmette-Guérin intravesical therapy in superficial bladder cancer. *Journal of Urology, 147*(3), 596-600.

Table 47-15 Standard of Care for the Patient Undergoing a Transurethral Resection of the Bladder (TURB)

Patient Problem and Outcomes	Nursing Interventions and Rationales	Patient Education Instructions
Knowledge Deficit		
Patient will verbalize an understanding of the surgical procedure.	1. Determine who the patient's support person is, and have this person present when teaching is done. 2. Assess the patient's level of understanding of the surgical procedure. 3. Give the patient the opportunity to ask questions or verbalize concerns.	1. Use a gender-specific diagram of the anatomy of the pelvis to explain the procedure. 2. Provide the patient with information about the preoperative routine: a. Diagnostic tests b. Anesthesiology consult 3. Provide the patient with information about the postoperative plan of care: a. Anticipated discharge, either immediately after surgery or the following day b. Home care of indwelling catheter (see Box 47-5) c. Possibility of hematuria d. Management of bladder spasms e. Management of pain
Hematuria		
Patient will experience a minimum of hematuria.	1. Assess degree of hematuria every 2-4 hours while the patient is hospitalized. 2. Maintain patency of urinary catheter.	1. Advise the patient to drink 3-4 L of fluid per day.
Bladder Spasms		
Patient will experience a minimum of bladder spasms.	1. Assess for bladder spasms every 2-4 hours while the patient is hospitalized. 2. Administer antispasmodics as the patient requires to minimize bladder spasms.	1. While the patient is hospitalized, teach the patient to inform the nurse if he or she is experiencing bladder spasms. 2. Teach the patient to take the prescribed antispasmodic medication to control and minimize bladder spasms.
Pain		
Patient will experience optimal pain relief with minimal side effects.	1. Assess pain intensity using a 0-10 verbal rating scale every 2-4 hours while the patient is hospitalized. 2. Administer opioid analgesics as the patient requires to keep the pain intensity below 2 or 3 on the 0-10 scale. 3. Monitor for analgesic side effects, and administer medications to prevent or treat: a. Constipation b. Pruritus c. Nausea	1. While the patient is hospitalized, teach the patient to inform the nurse if he or she is experiencing pain. 2. Teach the patient to take the prescribed pain medication often enough to control the pain. 3. Teach the patient that there may be side effects from the pain medication and how to manage side effects if they occur.
Anxiety		
Patient will: • Express feelings of decreased anxiety. • Identify strategies to cope with anxiety.	1. Complete patient teaching of the procedure so that the patient is not anxious due to a knowledge deficit. 2. Determine which coping strategies the patient has used effectively in the past to decrease anxiety, and reinforce the use of these coping strategies. 3. Administer pharmacologic agents to decrease anxiety, if necessary.	

NURSING MANAGEMENT

Although the prognosis for patients with superficial bladder cancer is very good, the patient must be actively involved in the management of the disease and diligent in keeping follow-up appointments. Nurses play an important role in educating the patient and family about the disease, assisting with various diagnostic and therapeutic procedures, and helping the patient manage side effects of therapy (Hossan & Striegel, 1993; Kelly & Miaskowski, 1996; Leek, Sebastian, Kawachi, & Sullivan, 1996; Lind, Kravitz, & Greig, 1993; Moore, Newton, Grant, & Keetch, 1993; Tootla & Easterling, 1992).

Surgery

A standard of care for the patient undergoing a TURB is outlined in Table 47-15. The major concerns are knowledge deficit, hematuria, bladder spasms, pain, and anxiety. Patients may be hospitalized after this procedure with an indwelling catheter to monitor for bleeding, but more commonly patients will be discharged home from the PACU with an indwelling catheter and expected to care for themselves. Usually, several different nurses in various settings accomplish the preoperative, postoperative, and follow-up nursing care of these patients. These nurses can work in the urology clinic, in the preadmission unit, in the PACU, in the surgical in-patient ward, and with home care agencies. Communication between these nurses is crucial to provide consistent care. An interdisciplinary clinical pathway might be one way to organize the treatment of these patients across the trajectory of care.

Intravesical Therapy

Patients with stage 0 CIS, as well as patients with stage I papillary tumors at high risk for recurrence, are treated with intravesical therapy after TURB. The nurse is integrally involved in teaching the patient about the therapy and in ensuring safe handling and administration of the prescribed intravesical agent. The majority of patients receive intravesical immunotherapy with BCG. Box 47-4 outlines the procedure for preparing and administering intravesical BCG, and Table 47-16 outlines the standard of care for the patient undergoing this therapy. The major concerns are knowledge deficit, IBS, hematuria, and flu-like symptoms. During subsequent weekly treatments, a physician may not examine the patient, so it is important that the nurse obtain a precise history of any adverse reactions the patient experienced after the previous treatment.

If BCG is contraindicated for a particular patient or if BCG therapy has not been effective, intravesical chemotherapy may be prescribed. The nursing care of these patients is similar to that of patients receiving BCG. Because chemotherapy does not use a live agent, the equipment used to administer the drug does not need to be soaked in bacteriocidal detergent before being disposed of as hazardous waste, and the patient does not need to use bleach in the toilet after urinating. Patient teaching should be specific to the drug administered.

HOME CARE ISSUES

Medical care of the patient with superficial bladder cancer is accomplished primarily in out-patient clinics. Although nurses may see patients frequently, time with the patient and family may be limited. Before the TURB, the nurse must schedule time to discuss with the patient and family what to expect before, during, and after the procedure. Likewise, before initiating intravesical therapy, the nurse should again schedule time to discuss with the patient and family what to expect.

Urination

Following TURB. Following TURB, the majority of patients have an indwelling catheter to decompress the bladder of urine and monitor for bleeding. The patient will very likely be discharged home with the catheter and will need to know how to care for it. Box 47-5 provides a sample patient teaching guide for the patient going home with an indwelling catheter. Several days after surgery the catheter is removed. If the amount of residual urine following the next void is less than 50 ml, the catheter does not need to be replaced. If the volume of residual urine is greater than 50 ml, the urologist should be consulted to consider replacing the catheter for 1 to 2 more days before again attempting to remove the catheter and letting the patient void spontaneously.

Following Intravesical Therapy. Following intravesical therapy, fluids and frequent urination should be encouraged to flush out the bladder. The patient should wash his or her hands and perineum thoroughly after urinating to minimize skin irritation. For the next 6 (Giglione, 1991) to 24 hours (Brosman, 1992), patients should use a single toilet facility in their home. The patient should sit down while urinating to minimize splashing. A bottle of household bleach should be kept close by the toilet, and after urinating the patient should pour 1 or 2 cups of bleach into the toilet and let it stand for 15 to 20 minutes before flushing (Brosman, 1992; Giglione, 1991; LeBouton, 1990). These measures are also aimed at protecting household members from BCG exposure, although there have not been any reported incidents of patients inoculating household members with BCG (Brosman, 1992). Sexual activity may be resumed 48 hours after treatment (Brosman, 1992). Sexual transmission of BCG has not been reported. However, some clinicians recommend using a condom for 1 week to protect the patient's partner against possible exposure (Lamm et al., 1992).

Following intravesical chemotherapy (i.e., with thiotepa, doxorubicin, mitomycin, or another antineoplastic agent), the patient does not need to pour bleach in the toilet. Otherwise, the patient home care instructions are the same as for the patient receiving BCG therapy and for the same purposes of minimizing side effects, reducing the chance of skin irritation, and protecting household members from drug exposure.

Box 47-4
Preparing and Administering Intravesical Bacillus Calmette-Guérin (BCG) to a Patient With Superficial Bladder Cancer

Patient Preparation

1. The patient should restrict fluids 6 to 8 hours before the BCG instillation to ensure that the BCG remains concentrated and the patient can retain the BCG solution for 2 hours.
2. If the patient regularly takes diuretics, he or she may want to consider waiting to take the diuretic until after the BCG instillation is completed.
3. If the patient has difficulty retaining the BCG instillation for 2 hours, an anticholinergic drug such as oxybutynin (Ditropan) can be taken 1 hour before treatment.

Patient Assessment

1. Have the patient submit a urine specimen for urinalysis.
2. Review the urinalysis. Pyuria and/or micro-hematuria, due to the BCG-induced inflammatory response, are normal and can be expected; however, BCG instillation should be withheld for bacturia, and a physician should examine the patient.
3. Interview the patient about symptoms experienced after the last BCG instillation. BCG instillation should be withheld for any current reports of gross hematuria or bladder irritability, and a physician should examine the patient.
4. Take and record the patient's vital signs. BCG instillation should be withheld for a temperature greater than 101° F, and a physician should examine the patient.

Preparation and Handling

1. Don a protective gown, gloves, and a mask.
2. Reconstitute the BCG with 1 ml of sterile, preservative-free normal saline under a Class II biologic safety cabinet (BSC) with vertical laminar airflow.
3. Dilute the contents with sterile, preservative-free normal saline to a volume of 50 ml.
4. Place the BCG in a glass bottle. (When plastic containers have been used, there have been reports of a cloudy precipitation possibly due to residues from the plastic reacting with the BCG.)
5. If clumping and/or marked opacity occur, discard the solution and prepare a new vial.
6. Instill the solution immediately after reconstitution. Therefore the patient should be available and ready for instillation before the BCG is reconstituted.
7. After the BCG solution is prepared, wipe down the laminar flow hood with 70% alcohol, glutaraldehyde (Cidex), bleach, or a similar disinfectant to prevent the possibility of contaminating solutions that will subsequently be prepared in the same area.

Administration of BCG

1. Have the patient urinate to empty his or her bladder.
2. Assemble all required equipment. Have a cytotoxic drug spill kit and appropriate disinfectant available to immediately clean up any spills.
3. Don a protective gown, gloves, and a mask.
4. Flush the IV tubing with sterile, preservative-free normal saline, and then spike the BCG glass bottle.
5. Assist the patient onto the examination table in a supine position.
6. Prep the patient's genitals with povidone-iodine (Betadine) or chlorhexidine (Hibiclens).
7. Drape the patient.
8. Pass a well-lubricated 14 French catheter into the bladder. Lidocaine jelly can be used for local anesthesia during catheter insertion if the patient prefers. Note the amount of residual urine drained.
9. If the catheterization is traumatic, withhold the BCG instillation.
10. Insert the IV tubing into the catheter. An adaptor may be necessary to obtain a tight seal.
11. Allow the BCG solution to flow into the bladder via gravity. Do not force the solution into the bladder.
12. When the BCG has been instilled into the bladder, flush the IV tubing of all BCG into the bladder with sterile, preservative-free normal saline.
13. Remove the catheter.
14. Immediately place the catheter, IV tubing, and IV bottle in 70% alcohol, glutaraldehyde (Cidex), bleach, or a similar disinfectant. The next day, discard the catheter, IV tubing, and IV bottle into a hazardous waste container.
15. Clean the patient's genitals with soap and water to wash away any BCG solution that might have spilled when the catheter was removed.
16. Have the patient change positions every 15 minutes for 2 hours from prone to supine and from side to side to ensure that the BCG is equally distributed throughout the bladder.
17. After 2 hours, have the patient urinate completely. If during the initial catheterization the volume of residual urine was greater than 100 ml, recatheterize the patient at the end of the 2-hour dwell time to ensure that no BCG is retained longer than 2 hours.

Modified from Brosman, S. A. (1992). Bacillus Calmette-Guérin immunotherapy: Techniques and results. *Urologic Clinics of North America, 19*(3), 557-564; Brosman, S. A. & Lamm, D. L. (1990). The preparation, handling and use of intravesical bacillus Calmette-Guérin for the management of stage Ta, T1, carcinoma in situ and transitional cell cancer. *Journal of Urology, 144*(2), 313-315; LeBouton, J. (1990). Nursing aspects of bacillus Calmette-Guérin immunotherapy for superficial bladder cancer. *Urologic Nursing, 10*(4), 9-14; Powel, L. L. (Ed.). (1996). *Cancer chemotherapy guidelines and recommendations for practice.* Philadelphia: Oncology Nursing Press; Giglione, L. (1991). Home bacillus Calmette-Guérin therapy for the treatment of superficial bladder cancer. *Home Health Care Nurse, 9*(5), 50-52.

Table 47-16 Standard of Care for the Patient Undergoing Intravesical Therapy with Bacillus Calmette-Guérin (BCG)

Patient Problem and Outcomes	Nursing Interventions and Rationales	Patient Education Instructions
Knowledge Deficit		
Patient will verbalize an understanding of the procedure.	1. Determine who the patient's support person is, and have this person present when teaching is done. 2. Assess the patient's level of understanding of the procedure. 3. Give the patient the opportunity to ask questions and verbalize concerns.	1. Use a gender-specific diagram of the anatomy of the bladder to explain the procedure. 2. Provide the patient information about the procedure: a. Preprocedure urinalysis b. Catheter insertion c. BCG installation 3. Provide the patient with information about the postprocedure plan of care: a. Encourage patient to drink 3-4 L of fluid per day b. Toileting precautions c. Sexual activity
Irritative Bladder Symptoms (IBS)		
Patient will experience relief of urinary symptoms.	1. Assess the patient for dysuria, frequency, and urgency. 2. Administer urinary analgesics, antispasmodics, and/or anticholinergics as prescribed.	1. Inform the patient that these symptoms are expected and occur as a result of irritation to the bladder from the BCG. 2. Advise the patient to avoid foods and other substances that can also irritate the bladder, such as coffee, tea, alcoholic beverages, and tobacco. 3. Tell the patient to telephone the nurse or physician in the Urology Clinic if symptoms worsen or do not resolve within 72 hours.
Hematuria		
Patient will be able to manage hematuria.	1. Assess the degree of hematuria.	1. Inform the patient that these symptoms are expected and occur as a result of irritation to the bladder from the BCG. 2. Encourage the patient to drink 3-4 L of fluid per day. 3. Tell the patient to telephone the nurse or physician in the Urology Clinic if symptoms worsen or do not resolve within 72 hours.
Flu-like Symptoms		
Patient will be able to manage flu-like symptoms.	1. Assess the patient for achiness, low-grade fever, and fatigue. 2. Administer acetaminophen as the patient requires to be comfortable.	1. Inform the patient that these symptoms occur as a result of the body's inflammatory response to the BCG. 2. Tell the patient to telephone the nurse or physician in the Urology Clinic if symptoms worsen or do not resolve within 48 hours.

Modified from Brosman, S. A. (1992). Bacillus Calmette-Guérin immunotherapy: Techniques and results. *Urologic Clinics of North America, 19*(3), 557-564; Brosman, S. A. & Lamm, D. L. (1990). The preparation, handling and use of intravesical bacillus Calmette-Guérin for the management of stage Ta, T1, carcinoma in situ and transitional cell cancer. *Journal of Urology, 144*(2), 313-315; LeBouton, J. (1990). Nursing aspects of bacillus Calmette-Guérin immunotherapy for superficial bladder cancer. *Urologic Nursing, 10*(4), 9-14; Giglione, L. (1991). Home bacillus Calmette-Guérin therapy for the treatment of superficial bladder cancer. *Home Health Care Nurse, 9*(5), 50-52; Miaskowski, C. (1995). Bladder cancer. In C. Miaskowski (Ed.), *Oncology nursing*. Albany, NY: Delmar.

Urinary Symptoms

Following intravesical therapy with either BCG or chemotherapy, IBS and mild hematuria are commonly experienced. Flu-like symptoms, including a low-grade fever, aching in the muscles and joints, malaise, and fatigue, are also possible. As previously discussed, the incidence of these symptoms is much greater with intravesical BCG immunotherapy compared with intravesical chemotherapy. These symptoms can be very uncomfortable and generally occur after the patient has left the clinic and is at home.

The patient should be aware that these symptoms can oc-

Box 47-5
Indwelling Urinary Catheter Care

Patient Name: ____________________

Symptom and Description
An indwelling urinary catheter is a tube that continuously drains urine from your bladder into a collection bag. Some people need a catheter after certain surgeries. Others may have a catheter placed because using the bathroom is too difficult or impossible, or because urine leakage cannot be controlled.

Learning Needs
You can help the catheter work safely by preventing blockage and infection of the catheter.

Management
Equipment
- Wash your hands with soap and water before and after handling the catheter, tubing, or bag.
- Use a leg bag during the day and the larger bedside bag at night or if you will be resting in bed more than 2 hours. Any drainage bag must be kept below the level of the bladder. Hang the larger bag on the bed, or place it on a low stool. Do not lay the bag on the floor. Check the tubing for kinks that might stop the flow of urine.
- Empty the leg bag at least every 2 hours and the bedside bag at least every morning. After emptying, clean the end of the drainage tube with a cotton ball and povidone-iodine (Povidone-iodine [Betadine]®) or 70% alcohol.
- When you change from one type of drainage bag to the other, follow these directions to clean the bag that is not being used. If you are not using both a leg bag and a bedside bag, clean the drainage bag about once a week. (1) Rinse the bag with cold water; wash with warm, soapy water; and rinse very well with cold, clear water. (2) Then fill the bag with a solution of one part vinegar to four parts water, and soak for 30 minutes. (3) Empty the bag and let it air dry.
- Store any green or blue protection caps in a container of 70% alcohol.

Drinking fluids
- Keep your bladder flushed with plenty of fluids. Drink at least 1½ quarts of water (48 ounces or 6 cups, or about 1½ L) each day.
- Ask your physician or nurse about drinking more or taking drinks that will make you urinate more acid. If you are not at risk for irritative bladder symptoms, you may be able to avoid problems with bladder infections by drinking certain juices.

Hygiene and self-washing
- You may take a shower or any kind of bath with the catheter in place. Also, wash the pubic area with a soapy washcloth and dry well twice a day.
- *Women* should wipe the length of the catheter with the washcloth, starting where the catheter enters the body. Then wipe the pubic area from front to back, starting where the catheter enters the body, cleaning the folds around the vagina as well.
- *Men* should wipe the length of the catheter with the washcloth, starting where the catheter enters the body. Uncircumcised men should pull back the foreskin and wash the end of the penis. Then wash the penis, scrotum, and groin areas.

Follow-Up
Talk to your physician or nurse about bacteria and infections related to the catheter. People with an indwelling catheter often have some bacteria in their urine. A urinary tract infection occurs when enough bacteria grow to cause symptoms, such as fever or blood in the urine. Call your physician or nurse right away if you notice any of the following symptoms:
- Low back pain or stomach pain
- Cloudy, bad-smelling urine
- Material (sediment) in the urine
- Blood in the urine
- Fever or chills

Phone Numbers
Nurse: ____________________ Phone: ____________
Physician: ____________________ Phone: ____________
Other: ____________________ Phone: ____________

Comments
Patient's Signature: ____________________ Phone: ____________
Nurse's Signature: ____________________ Phone: ____________

Modified from Berry, D. L. (1996). Bladder disturbances. In S. L. Groenwald, M. H. Frogge, M. Goodman, & C. H. Yarbro (Eds.), *Cancer symptom management.* Sudbury, MA: Jones and Bartlett.

cur, but that they are usually self-limiting, resolving within 48 hours. Hematuria should signal the patient to increase his or her fluid intake. As previously described in the Medical Management section, various medications may be prescribed to help manage the IBS and flu-like symptoms. The patient typically arrives home with multiple medications and needs to have a clear understanding and written instructions of when to take a particular medication. The patient also needs to know to call the clinic to speak with a physician or nurse for gross hematuria, for a temperature greater than 101° F (38.3° C), or if symptoms are unusually severe or do not resolve within 48 hours.

PROGNOSIS

As indicated in Table 47-17, the prognosis for patients with superficial stage 0 and I bladder cancer is very good, with more than 85% of patients surviving more than 5 years (Fleshner et al., 1996). The greatest concern for patients with superficial bladder cancer is disease recurrence and/or progression.

For patients with Tis (CIS), more than 80% initially have a complete response to one or two courses of induction intravesical therapy with BCG (Lamm, 1992a). For the 20% of patients with persistent CIS even after intravesical therapy, a cystectomy is recommended. For the patients who achieve a complete response with intravesical therapy, careful follow-up is warranted because 55% of these patients have recurrent disease within the succeeding 5 years (Lamm et al., 1991). Treatment options for patients with recurrent CIS include re-treatment with BCG or cystectomy with bladder reconstruction. Patients can be re-treated safely with intravesical therapy one or two times, although the patient must be informed that there is a 25% chance of subsequent tumor recurrences being muscle-invasive or metastatic (Catalona, Hudson, Gillen, Andriole, & Ratliff, 1987).

For patients with Ta or T1 disease, 70% of patients treated with TURB have disease recurrence within 5 years of diagnosis (Heney et al., 1982). Treatment options for patients with recurrent Ta or T1 disease include repeat TURB or laser surgery, possibly with adjuvant intravesical therapy. Specific tumor characteristics associated with a higher risk of recurrence and poorer prognosis include tumor size greater than 3 cm, tumor grades II or III, tumor stage T1, the presence of multiple tumors, and the presence of abnormal cells found in random biopsies (Heney et al., 1982; Herr, 1992; Itoku & Stein, 1992; Nseyo & Lamm, 1996). Once diagnosed with superficial bladder cancer, patients must be willing to undergo regular medical examinations and testing to detect and immediately treat any recurrences of the disease. Diligent follow-up is essential to the long-term survival of these patients.

TABLE 47-17 Five-Year Cumulative Survival Rates for Bladder Cancer According to Stage of Disease at Diagnosis

Stage of Disease at Diagnosis	5-Year Survival Rates
0	90.2%
I	86.6%
II	65.1%
III	47.9%
IV	23.2%

Modified from Fleshner, N. E., Herr, H. W., Stewart, A. K., Murphy, G. P., Mettlin, C., & Menck, H. R. (1996). The national cancer data base report on bladder carcinoma. *Cancer, 78*(7), 1505-1513.

EVALUATION OF THE QUALITY OF CARE

Accreditation organizations, like the Joint Commission for the Accreditation of Health Care Organizations, require that the quality of care provided to patients be evaluated. Because the care provided to patients with bladder cancer requires input from an interdisciplinary team, an evaluation of the quality of this care should include aspects of care provided by various members of the team. Tables 47-18 and 47-19 provide examples of quality of care evaluation tools that can be used after TURB and for a patient undergoing intravesical therapy with BCG.

RESEARCH ISSUES

Many medical and nursing issues remain to be resolved in the diagnosis, treatment, and continuing care of the patient with superficial bladder cancer. The cellular mechanisms that regulate activation of proto-oncogenes and inactivation of tumor suppressor genes in bladder cancer remain largely unknown. Basic research is investigating the cascade of events associated with the development of this heterogeneous disease. Hopefully, affordable molecular screening tools will be available in the next few years to identify patients who may be developing malignant changes in their urothelium. These same molecular tools may also provide information about which patients are at highest risk for disease recurrence and warrant aggressive treatment.

Almost all patients undergoing intravesical immunotherapy with BCG experience side effects from treatment. Although various medications can be prescribed to help manage side effects, the efficacy of these drugs has not been described. Neither have nonpharmaceutical interventions to control treatment side effects been explored. Only recently has an instrument been developed to measure IBS (Berry, Moinpour, Blumenstein, Thrasher, & Ellis, 1997), which will allow reliable and valid assessments of IBS and meaningful comparisons of treatment effectiveness.

The risk of bladder cancer recurrence remains very high. Adjuvant therapies improve the chances of disease-free sur-

TABLE 47-18 Quality of Care Evaluation for a Patient Following Transurethral Resection of the Bladder (TURB)

Disciplines participating in the quality of care evaluation:
☐ Nursing (Urology Clinic)
☐ Nursing (Preadmission Unit)
☐ Nursing (Postanesthesia Care Unit)
☐ Nursing (In-Patient Unit)
☐ Urology

I. Postprocedure Management Evaluation

Data from:
☐ Medical Record Review
☐ Patient/Family Interview

Criteria	Yes	No
1. Patient provided with preprocedure information about:		
a. Anticipated discharge date	☐	☐
b. Type of anesthesia	☐	☐
2. Patient experienced the following complications:		
a. Fever >101° F	☐	☐
b. Need for postoperative blood transfusion	☐	☐
c. Rehospitalization	☐	☐

II. Patient/Family Satisfaction

Data from:
☐ Patient Interview
☐ Family Interview

Criteria	Yes	No
1. On a scale of 0 to 10, with 0 being totally dissatisfied and 10 being totally satisfied, how satisfied are you with the care you received? ______________		
2. Were you prepared to care for your urinary catheter while you were at home?	☐	☐

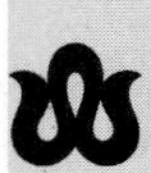

TABLE 47-19 Quality of Care Evaluation for a Patient Undergoing Intravesical Therapy With Bacillus Calmette-Guérin (BCG)

Disciplines participating in the quality of care evaluation:
☐ Nursing (Urology Clinic)
☐ Urology

I. Postprocedure Management Evaluation

Data from:
☐ Medical Record Review
☐ Patient/Family Interview

Criteria	Yes	No
1. Patient provided with preprocedure information about:		
a. Catheter insertion	☐	☐
b. BCG dwell time	☐	☐
2. Preprocedure urine sample checked for bacteriuria	☐	☐
3. Patient experienced the following complications:		
a. Traumatic catheter insertion	☐	☐
b. Fever >101° F (38.3° C)	☐	☐
c. Gross hematuria	☐	☐

II. Patient/Family Satisfaction

Data from:
☐ Patient Interview
☐ Family Interview

Criteria	Yes	No
1. On a scale of 0 to 10, with 0 being totally dissatisfied and 10 being totally satisfied, how satisfied are you with the care you received? ______________		
2. Following a BCG instillation, which of the following precautions were you instructed to take when urinating:		
Use only one toilet facility?	☐	☐
Sit down while urinating?	☐	☐
Pour bleach in the toilet after each void?	☐	☐
Wash your hands and perineum after urinating?	☐	☐
3. Were you taught how to manage the irritative bladder symptoms (dysuria, frequency, urgency) you might experience after BCG intravesical therapy?	☐	☐

vival for some patients, but research to develop even more effective adjuvant treatments is ongoing. Early results from PDT show that recurrence rates are reduced with this therapy (Nseyo, 1992). The methods to deliver PDT are still being refined, aided by technologic advances in biomedical engineering.

Following treatment for superficial bladder cancer, many patients return to work. Patients will very likely face social and physical barriers (Berry & Catanzaro, 1992). Patients' experiences rejoining the work force have only recently been described (Berry, 1993) and warrant further investigation.

Although the mortality from bladder cancer is decreasing, the incidence of the disease is increasing. Important work remains to be done in the diagnosis, treatment, and follow-up of these patients, focusing on the quality of care that can be provided in a managed care environment.

REFERENCES

American Cancer Society. (1996). *1996 cancer facts & figures.* New York: ACS.

American Joint Committee on Cancer. (1992). Urinary bladder. In O. H. Beahrs, D. E. Henson, R. V. P. Hutter, & B. J. Kennedy (Eds.), *Manual for staging of cancer* (4th ed.). Philadelphia: J. B. Lippincott.

Auerbach, O. & Garfinkel, L. (1989). Histologic changes in the urinary bladder in relation to cigarette smoking and use of artificial sweeteners. *Cancer, 64*(5), 983-987.

Badalament, R. A., Herr, H. W., Wong, G. Y., Gnecco, C., Pinsky, C. M., Whitmore, W. F., Fair, W. R., & Oettgen, H. F. (1987). A prospective randomized trial of maintenance versus nonmaintenance intravesical bacillus Calmette-Guérin therapy of superficial bladder cancer. *Journal of Clinical Oncology, 5*(3), 441-449.

Badalament, R. A., Ortolano, V., & Burgers, J. K. (1992). Recurrent or aggressive bladder cancer: Indications for adjuvant intravesical therapy. *Urologic Clinics of North America, 19*(3), 485-498.

Bane, B. L., Rao, J. Y., & Hemstreet, G. P. (1996). Pathology and staging of bladder cancer. *Seminars in Oncology, 23*(5), 546-570.

Bates, B. (1991). *A guide to physical examination* (5th ed.). New York: J. B. Lippincott.

Benson, R. C. (1995). Laser therapy. In J. M. Fitzpatrick & R. J. Krane (Eds.), *The bladder.* Edinburgh: Churchill Livingstone.

Berry, D. L. (1993). Return-to-work experiences of people with cancer. *Oncology Nursing Forum, 20*(6), 905-911.

Berry, D. L. (1996). Bladder disturbances. In S. L. Groenwald, M. H. Frogge, M. Goodman, & C. H. Yarbro (Eds.), *Cancer symptom management.* Sudbury, MA: Jones and Bartlett.

Berry, D. L., Blumenstein, B. A., Magyary, D. L., Lamm, D. L., & Crawford, E. D. (1996). Local toxicity patterns associated with intravesical bacillus Calmette-Guérin: A Southwest Oncology Group study. *International Journal of Urology, 3*(2), 98-100.

Berry, D. L. & Catanzaro, M. (1992). Persons with cancer and their return to the workplace. *Cancer Nursing, 15*(1), 40-46.

Berry, D. L., Moinpour, C., Blumenstein, B. A., Thrasher, B., & Ellis, W. J. (1997). Measurement of irritative bladder symptoms [Abstract]. *Oncology Nursing Forum, 24*(2), 319.

Böhle, A., Balck, F., von Wietersheim, J., & Jocham, D. (1996). The quality of life during intravesical bacillus Calmette-Guérin therapy. *Journal of Urology, 155*(4), 1221-1226.

Boice, J. D., Engholm, G., Kleinerman, B. R., Blettner, M., Stovall, M., Lisco, H., Moloney, W. C., Austin, D. F., Bosch, A., Cookfair, D. L., Krementz, E. T., LaTourette, H. B., Merrill, J. A., Peters, L. J., Schulz, M. D., Storm, H. H., Björkholm, E., Pettersson, F., Bell, C. M. J., Coleman, M. P., Fraser, P., Neal, F. E., Prior, P., Choi, N. W., Hislop, T. G., Koch, M., Kreiger, N., Robb, D., Robson, D., Thomson, D. H., Lochmüller, H., von Fournier, D., Frischkorn, R., Kjørstad, K. E., Rimpela, A., Pejovic, M. H., Kirn, V. P., Stankusova, H., Berrino, F., Sigurdsson, K., Hutchison, G. B., & MacMahon, B. (1988). Radiation dose and second cancer risk in patients treated for cancer of the cervix. *Radiation Research, 116*(1), 3-55.

Borland, R. N., Brendler, C. B., & Isaacs, W. B. (1992). Molecular biology of bladder cancer. *Hematology Oncology Clinics of North America, 6*(1), 31-39.

Brodsky, G. L. (1992). Pathology of bladder carcinoma. *Hematology Oncology Clinics of North America, 6*(1), 59-80.

Brosman, S. A. (1992). Bacillus Calmette-Guérin immunotherapy: Techniques and results. *Urologic Clinics of North America, 19*(3), 557-564.

Brosman, S. A., & Lamm, D. L. (1990). The preparation, handling and use of intravesical bacillus Calmette-Guérin for the management of stage Ta, T1, carcinoma in situ and transitional cell cancer. *Journal of Urology, 144*(2), 313-315.

Burch, J. D., Rohan, T. E., Howe, G. R., Risch, H. A., Hill, G. B., Steele, R., & Miller, A. B. (1989). Risk of bladder cancer by source and type of tobacco exposure: A case-control study. *International Journal of Cancer, 44*(4), 622-628.

Catalona, W. J., Hudson, M. A., Gillen, D. P., Andriole, G. L., & Ratliff, T. L. (1987). Risks and benefits of repeated courses of intravesical bacillus Calmette-Guérin therapy for superficial bladder cancer. *Journal of Urology, 137*(2), 220-224.

Clavel, J., Cordier, S., Boccon-Gibod, L., & Hemon, D. (1989). Tobacco and bladder cancer in males: Increased risk for inhalers and smokers of black tobacco. *International Journal of Cancer, 44*(4), 605-610.

Cohen, S. M. & Johansson, S. L. (1992). Epidemiology and etiology of bladder cancer. *Urologic Clinics of North America, 19*(3), 421-428.

Crump, K. S. & Guess, H. A. (1982). Drinking water and cancer: Review of recent epidemiological findings and assessment of risks. *Annual Review of Public Health, 3,* 39-57.

Cummings, K. B., Barone, J. G., & Ward, W. S. (1992). Diagnosis and staging of bladder cancer. *Urologic Clinics of North America, 19*(3), 455-465.

Dachowski, L. J. & DeLaney, T. F. (1992). Photodynamic therapy: The NCI experience and its nursing implications. *Oncology Nursing Forum, 19*(1), 63-67.

Decensi, A., Bruno, S., Giaretti, W., Torrisi, R., Curotto, A., Gatteschi, B., Geldo, E., Polizzi, A., Costantini, M., Bruzzi, P., Nicolò, G., Costa, A., Boccardo, F., Giuliani, L., & Santi, L. (1992). Activity of 4-HPR in superficial bladder cancer using DNA flow cytometry as an intermediate endpoint. *Journal of Cellular Biochemistry, Suppl. 16 I,* 139-147.

de Reijke, T. M., & Kurth, K. (1995). Intravesical agents for superficial bladder cancer: Anthracyclines. In J. M. Fitzpatrick & R. J. Krane (Eds.), *The bladder.* Edinburgh: Churchill Livingstone.

Devesa, S. S., Blot, W. J., Stone, B. J., Miller, B. A., Tarone, R. E., & Fraumeni, J. F., Jr. (1995). Recent cancer trends in the United States. *Journal of the National Cancer Institute, 87*(3), 175-182.

Edmonds, C. J. & Smith, T. (1986). The long-term hazards of the treatment of thyroid cancer with radioiodine. *British Journal of Radiology, 59*(697), 45-51.

Fair, W. R., Fuks, Z. Y., & Scher, H. I. (1993). Cancer of the bladder. In V. T. DeVita, Jr., S. Hellman, & S. A. Rosenberg (Eds.), *Cancer: Principles and practice of oncology* (4th ed.). Philadelphia: J. B. Lippincott.

Fairchild, W. B., Spence, C. R., Solomon, H. D., & Gangai, M. P. (1979). The incidence of bladder cancer after cyclophosphamide therapy. *Journal of Urology, 122*(2), 163-164.

Faysal, M. H. (1981). Squamous cell carcinoma of the bladder. *Journal of Urology, 126*(5), 598-599.

Fernandes, E. T., Manivel, J. C., Reddy, P. K., & Ercole, C. J. (1996). Cyclophosphamide associated bladder cancer—a highly aggressive disease: Analysis of 12 cases. *Journal of Urology, 156*(6), 1931-1933.

Fiore, M. C., Bailey, W. C., Cohen, S. J., Dorfman, S. F., Goldstein, M. G., Gritz, E. R., Heyman, R. B., Holbrook, J., Jaen, C. R., Kottke, T. E., Lando, H. A., Mecklenburg, R., Mullen, P. D., Nett, L. M., Robinson, L., Stitzer, M. L., Tommasello, A. C., Villejo, L., & Wewers, M. E. (1996). *Smoking cessation.* Clinical Practice Guideline No 18. Agency for Health Care Policy and Research (AHCPR) Publication No. 96-0692. Rockville, MD: U. S. Department of Health and Human Services, Public Health Service.

Fiore, M. C., Jorenby, D. E., Baker, T. B., & Kenford, S. L. (1992). Tobacco dependence and the nicotine patch: Clinical guidelines for effective use. *Journal of the American Medical Association, 268*(19), 2687-2694.

Fischbach, F. T. (1996). *A manual of laboratory and diagnostic tests* (5th ed.). Philadelphia, J. B. Lippincott.

Fleshner, N. E., Herr, H. W., Stewart, A. K., Murphy, G. P., Mettlin, C., & Menck, H. R. (1996). The national cancer data base report on bladder carcinoma. *Cancer, 78*(7), 1505-1513.

Furihata, M., Inoue, K., Ohtsuki, Y., Hashimoto, H., Terao, N., & Fujita, Y. (1994). High-risk human papilloma virus infections and over expression of p53 protein as prognostic indicators in transitional cell carcinoma of the urinary bladder. *Journal of Urology, 152*(2), 568-569.

Gallagher, J. & Holm, L. (1996). Power of one: Nurses and tobacco control. *Seminars in Oncology Nursing, 12*(4), 270-275.

Ghoneim, M. A. (1995). The urinary bladder in bilharziasis. In J. M. Fitzpatrick & R. J. Krane (Eds.), *The bladder.* Edinburgh: Churchill Livingstone.

Giglione, L. (1991). Home bacillus Calmette-Guérin therapy for the treatment of superficial bladder cancer. *Home Health Care Nurse, 9*(5), 50-52.

González, C. A., López-Abente, G., Errezola, M., Escolar, A., Riboli, E., Izarzugaza, I., & Nebot, M. (1989). Occupation and bladder cancer in Spain: A multi-center case-control study. *International Journal of Epidemiology, 18*(3), 569-577.

Harris, R. E., Chen-Backlund, J. Y., & Wynder, E. L. (1990). Cancer of the urinary bladder in blacks and whites: A case-control study. *Cancer, 66*(12), 2673-2680.

Harrison, S. C. W. & Abrams, P. (1994). Bladder function. In G. R. Sant (Ed.), *Pathophysiologic principles of urology.* Boston: Blackwell Scientific.

Hartge, P., Harvey, E. B., Linehan, W. M., Silverman, D. T., Sullivan, J. W., Hoover, R. N., & Fraumeni, J. F. Jr. (1990). Unexplained excess risk of bladder cancer in men. *Journal of the National Cancer Institute, 82*(20), 1636-1640.

Hartge, P., Silverman, D., Hoover, R., Schairer, C., Altman, R., Austin, D., Cantor, K., Child, M., Key, C., Marrett, L. D., Mason, T. J., Meigs, J. W., Myers, M. H., Narayana, A., Sullivan, J. W., Swanson, M. G. M., Thomas, D., & West, D. (1987). Changing cigarette habits and bladder cancer risk: A case-control study. *Journal of the National Cancer Institute, 78*(6), 1119-1125.

Heney, N. M., Daly, J., Prout, G. R., Nieh, P. T., Heaney, J. A., & Trebeck, N. E. (1978). Biopsy of apparently normal urothelium in patients with bladder carcinoma. *Journal of Urology, 120*(5), 559-560.

Heney, N. M., Nocks, B. N., Daly, J. J., Prout Jr., G. R., Newall, J. B., Griffin, P. P., Perrone, T. L., & Szyfelbein, W. A. (1982). Ta and T1 bladder cancer: Location, recurrence and progression. *British Journal of Urology, 54*(2), 152-157.

Herr, H. W. (1992). Intravesical therapy. *Hematology Oncology Clinics of North America, 6*(1), 117-127.

Hossan, E. & Striegel, A. (1993). Carcinoma of the bladder. *Seminars in Oncology Nursing, 9*(4), 252-266.

Howe, G. R., Burch, J. D., Miller, A. B., Cook, G. M., Esteve, J., Morrison, B., Gordon, P., Chambers, L. W., Fodor, G., & Winsor, G. M. (1980). Tobacco use, occupation, coffee, various nutrients, and bladder cancer. *Journal of the National Cancer Institute, 64*(4), 701-713.

Hudson, M. A., Yuan, J. J., Catalona, W. J., & Ratliff, T. L. (1990). Adverse impact of fibrin clot inhibitors on intravesical bacillus Calmette-Guérin therapy for superficial bladder tumors. *Journal of Urology, 144*(6), 1362-1364.

Inskip, P. D., Monson, R. R., Wagoner, J. K., Stovall, M., Davis, F. G., Kleinerman, R. A., & Boice, J. D. (1990). Cancer mortality following radium treatment for uterine bleeding. *Radiation Research, 123*(3), 331-344.

Israel, V. K., Natale, R. B., & Skinner, D. G. (1995). Bladder. In M. D. Abeloff, J. O. Armitage, A. S. Lichter, & J. E. Niederhuber (Eds.), *Clinical oncology.* New York: Churchill Livingstone.

Itoku, K. A. & Stein, B. S. (1992). Superficial bladder cancer. *Hematology Oncology Clinics of North America, 6*(1), 99-116.

Jewett, H. J. (1952). Carcinoma of the bladder: Influence of depth of infiltration on the 5-year results following complete extirpation of the primary growth. *Journal of Urology, 67*(5), 672-676.

Jewett, H. J., & Strong, G. H. (1946). Infiltrating carcinoma of the bladder: Relation of depth of penetration of the bladder wall to incidence of local extension and metastases. *Journal of Urology, 55*(4), 366-372.

Jones, H. C., & Swinney, J. (1961). Thiotepa in the treatment of tumours of the bladder. *Lancet, II*(7203), 615-618.

Kantor, A. F., Hartge, P., Hoover, R. N., & Fraumeni, J. F., Jr. (1985). Familial and environmental interactions in bladder cancer risk. *International Journal of Cancer, 35*(6), 703-706.

Kantor, A. F., Hartge, P., Hoover, R. N., & Fraumeni, J. F., Jr. (1988). Epidemiological characteristics of squamous cell carcinoma and adenocarcinoma of the bladder. *Cancer Research, 48*(13), 3853-3855.

Kantor, A. F., Hartge, P., Hoover, R. N., Narayana, A. S., Sullivan, J. W., & Fraumeni, J. F., Jr. (1984). Urinary tract infection and risk of bladder cancer. *American Journal of Epidemiology, 119*(4), 510-515.

Kelloff, G. J., Boone, C. W., Malone, W. F., Steele, V. E., & Doody, L. A. (1992). Development of chemopreventive agents for bladder cancer. *Journal of Cellular Biochemistry, Suppl. 16 I,* 1-12.

Kelly, L. P., & Miaskowski, C. (1996). An overview of bladder cancer: Treatment and nursing implications. *Oncology Nursing Forum, 23*(3), 459-468.

Kiemeney, L. A., & Schoenberg, M. (1996). Familial transitional cell carcinoma. *Journal of Urology, 156*(3), 867-872.

Kottke, T. E., Battista, R. N., DeFriese, G. H., & Brekke, M. L. (1988). Attributes of successful smoking cessation interventions in medical practice: A meta-analysis of 39 controlled trials. *Journal of the American Medical Association, 259*(19), 2882-2889.

Kurth, K. (1995). Intravesical agents for superficial bladder cancer: Thiotepa. In J. M. Fitzpatrick & R. J. Krane (Eds.), *The bladder.* Edinburgh: Churchill Livingstone.

Lamm, D. L. (1992a). Carcinoma in situ. *Urologic Clinics of North America, 19*(3), 499-508.

Lamm, D. L. (1992b). Complications of bacillus Calmette-Guérin immunotherapy. *Urologic Clinics of North America, 19*(3), 565-572.

Lamm, D. L. (1992c). Long-term results of intravesical therapy for superficial bladder cancer. *Urologic Clinics of North America, 19*(3), 573-580.

Lamm, D. L., Blumenstein, B. A., Crawford, E. D., Montie, J. E., Scardino, P., Grossman, H. B., Stanisic, T. H., Smith, J. A., Sullivan, J., Sarosdy, M. F., Crissman, J. D., & Coltman, C. A. (1991). A randomized trial of intravesical doxorubicin and immunotherapy with bacille Calmette-Guérin for transitional-cell carcinoma of the bladder. *New England Journal of Medicine, 325*(17), 1205-1209.

Lamm, D. L., van der Meijden, P. M., Morales, A., Brosman, S. A., Catalona, W. J., Herr, H. W., Soloway, M. S., Steg, A., & Debruyne, F. M. J. (1992). Incidence and treatment of complications of bacillus Calmette-Guérin intravesical therapy in superficial bladder cancer. *Journal of Urology, 147*(3), 596-600.

Lamm, D. L. & Sosnowski, J. T. (1995). Intravesical agents for superficial bladder cancer: Bacillus Calmette-Guérin Immunotherapy, keyhole limpet hemocyanin, and interferon. In J. M. Fitzpatrick & R. J. Krane (Eds.), *The bladder.* Edinburgh: Churchill Livingstone.

Lamm, D. L., Stogdill, V. D., Stogdill, B. J., & Crispen, R. G. (1986). Complications of bacillus Calmette Guérin immunotherapy in 1,278 patients with bladder cancer. *Journal of Urology, 135*(2), 272-274.

Lamm, D. L. & Torti, F. M. (1996). Bladder cancer, 1996. *CA-A Cancer Journal for Clinicians, 46*(2), 93-112.

Landis, S.H., Murray, T., Bolden, S. & Wingo, P.A. (1998). Cancer Statistics, 1998. *CA: A Cancer Journal for Clinicians, 48(1):*6-32.

LeBouton, J. (1990). Nursing aspects of bacillus Calmette-Guérin immunotherapy for superficial bladder cancer. *Urologic Nursing, 10*(4), 9-14.

Leek, C. L., Sebastian, W., Kawachi, M. H., & Sullivan, L. (1996). Genitourinary cancers. In R. McCorkle, M. Grant, M. Frank-Stromborg, & S. B. Baird (Eds.), *Cancer nursing: A comprehensive textbook* (2nd ed.). Philadelphia: W. B. Saunders.

Levine, L. A. & Richie, J. P. (1989). Urological complications of cyclophosphamide. *Journal of Urology, 141*(5), 1063-1069.

Lind, J., Kravitz, K., & Greig, B. (1993). Urologic and male genital malignancies. In S. L. Groenwald, M. H. Frogge, M. Goodman, & C. H. Yarbro (Eds.), *Cancer nursing: Principles and practice* (3rd ed.). Boston: Jones & Bartlett.

Loprinzi, C. L. & Messing, E. M. (1992). A prospective clinical trial of difluoromethylornithine (DFMO) in patients with resected superficial bladder cancer. *Journal of Cellular Biochemistry, Suppl. 16 I,* 153-155.

Lower, G. M. (1982). Concepts in causality: Chemically induced human urinary bladder cancer. *Cancer, 49*(5), 1056-1066.

Lynch, C. F. & Cohen, M. G. (1995). Urinary system. *Cancer, 75(Suppl. 1),* 316-329.

Lynch, H. T., Kimberling, W. J., Lynch, J. F., & Brennan, K. (1987). Familial bladder cancer in an oncology clinic. *Cancer Genetics and Cytogenetics, 27*(1), 161-165.

Makhyoun, N. A. (1974). Smoking and bladder cancer in Egypt. *British Journal of Cancer, 30*(6), 577-581.

Mao, L., Schoenberg, M. P., Scicchitano, M., Erozan, Y. S., Merlo, A., Schwab, D., & Sidransky, D. (1996). Molecular detection of primary bladder cancer by microsatellite analysis. *Science, 271*(5249), 659-662.

Marshall, V. F. (1952). The relation of the preoperative estimate to the pathologic demonstration of the extent of vesical neoplasms. *Journal of Urology, 68*(4), 714-723.

Melicow, M. M. (1974). Tumors of the bladder: A multifaceted problem. *Journal of Urology, 112*(4), 467-478.

Miaskowski, C. (1995). Bladder cancer. In C. Miaskowski (Ed.), *Oncology nursing*. Albany, NY: Delmar.

Mills, P. K., Beeson, L., Phillips, R. L., & Fraser, G. E. (1991). Bladder cancer in a low risk population: Results from the Adventist health study. *American Journal of Epidemiology, 133*(3), 230-239.

Moore, S., Newton, M., Grant, E. G., & Keetch, D. W. (1993). Treating bladder cancer: New methods, mew management. *American Journal of Nursing, 93*(5), 32-39.

Morales, A., Eidinger, D., & Bruce, A. W. (1976). Intracavitary bacillus Calmette-Guérin in the treatment of superficial bladder tumors. *Journal of Urology, 116*(2), 180-183.

Morrison, A. S., Buring, J. E., Verhoek, W. G., Aoki, K., Leck, I., Ohno, Y., & Obata, K. (1984). An international study of smoking and bladder cancer. *Journal of Urology, 131*(4), 650-654.

Murphy, W. M. (1990). Current status of urinary cytology in the evaluation of bladder neoplasms. *Human Pathology, 21*(9), 886-896.

Murphy, W. M. Nagy, G. K., Rao, M. K., Soloway, M. S., Parija, G. C., Cox, C. E., & Friedell, G. H. (1979). "Normal" urothelium in patients with bladder cancer: A preliminary report from the National Bladder Cancer Collaborative Group A. *Cancer, 44*(3), 1050-1058.

Murphy, W. M., & Soloway, M. S. (1982). Developing carcinoma (dysplasia) of the urinary bladder. *Pathology Annual, 17*(1), 197-217.

Newman, D. M., Brown, J. R., Jay, A. C., & Pontius, E. E. (1968). Squamous cell carcinoma of the bladder. *Journal of Urology, 100*(4), 470-473.

Nissenkorn, I., Herrod, H., & Soloway, M. S. (1981). Side effects associated with intravesical mitomycin C. *Journal of Urology, 126*(5), 596-597.

Norton, J. M. (1995). Urologic disorders. In A. D. Linton, M. A. Matteson, & N. K. Maebius (Eds.), *Introductory nursing care of adults*. Philadelphia: W. B. Saunders.

Nseyo, U. O. (1992). Photodynamic therapy. *Urologic Clinics of North America, 19*(3), 591-599.

Nseyo, U. O. & Lamm, D. L. (1996). Therapy of superficial bladder cancer. *Seminars in Oncology, 23*(5), 598-604.

Ockene, J. K. (1987). Physician-delivered interventions for smoking cessation: Strategies for increasing effectiveness. *Preventive Medicine, 16*(5), 723-737.

Patrianakos, C. & Hoffmann, D. (1979). Chemical studies on tobacco smoke LXIV. On the analysis of aromatic amines in cigarette smoke. *Journal of Analytical Toxicology, 3*(4), 150-154.

Pedersen-Bjergaard, J., Ersbøll, J., Hansen, V. L., Sørensen, B. L., Christoffersen, K., Hou-Jensen, K., Nissen, N. I., Knudsen, J. B., & Hansen, M. M. (1988). Carcinoma of the urinary bladder after treatment with cyclophosphamide for non-Hodgkin's lymphoma. *New England Journal of Medicine, 318*(16), 1028-1032.

Perucca, D., Szepetowski, P., Simon, M. P., & Gaudray, P. (1990). Molecular genetics of human bladder carcinomas. *Cancer Genetics and Cytogenetics, 49*(2), 143-156.

Piper, J. M., Matanoski, G. M., & Tonascia, J. (1986). Bladder cancer in young women. *American Journal of Epidemiology, 123*(6), 1033-1042.

Powel, L. L. (Ed.). (1996). *Cancer chemotherapy guidelines and recommendations for practice.* Philadelphia: Oncology Nursing Press.

Prout, G. R., Jr., & Barton, B. A. (1992). 13-*cis*-Retinoic acid in chemoprevention of superficial bladder cancer. *Journal of Cellular Biochemistry, Suppl. 16 I,* 148-152.

Quilty, P. M., & Kerr, G. R. (1987). Bladder cancer following low or high dose pelvic irradiation. *Clinical Radiology, 38*(6), 583-585.

Risser, N. L. (1996). Prevention of lung cancer: The key is to stop smoking. *Seminars in Oncology Nursing, 12*(4), 260-269.

Sandberg, A. A. (1992). Chromosome changes in early bladder neoplasms. *Journal of Cellular Biochemistry, Suppl. 16 I,* 76-79.

Scher, H. I. (1994). Editorial comment. *Journal of Urology, 152*(2), 569.

Sidransky, D. & Messing, E. (1992). Molecular genetics and biochemical mechanisms in bladder cancer: Oncogenes, tumor suppressor genes, and growth factors. *Urologic Clinics of North America, 19*(4), 629-639.

Silverman, D. T., Hartge, P., Morrison, A. S., & Devesa, S. S. (1992). Epidemiology of bladder cancer. *Hematology Oncology Clinics of North America, 6*(1), 1-30.

Silverman, D. T., Levine, L. I., Hoover, R. N., & Hartge, P. (1989). Occupational risks of bladder cancer in the United States: I. white men. *Journal of the National Cancer Institute, 81*(19), 1472-1480.

Soloway, M. S. (1995). Intravesical agents for superficial bladder cancer: Mitomycin. In J. M. Fitzpatrick & R. J. Krane (Eds.), *The bladder.* Edinburgh: Churchill Livingstone.

Soloway, M. S., Murphy, W., Rao, M. K., & Cox, C. (1978). Serial multiple-site biopsies in patients with bladder cancer. *Journal of Urology, 120*(1), 57-59.

Soloway, M. S., & Patel, J. (1992). Surgical techniques for endoscopic resection of bladder cancer. *Urologic Clinics of North America, 19*(3), 467-471.

Song-ting, Y., Ming-ming, W., & Li-ming, L. (1993). Prevalence of human papillomaviruses 16 and 18 in transitional cell carcinoma of bladder. *Chinese Medical Journal, 106*(7), 494-496.

Spruck, C. H., Ohneseit, P. G., Gonzalez-Zulueta, M., Esrig, D., Miyao, N., Tsai, Y. C., Lerner, S. P., Schmütte, C., Yang, A. S., Cote, R., Dubeau, L., Nichols, P. W., Hermann, G. G., Steven, K., Horn, T., Skinner, D. G., & Jones, P. A. (1994). Two molecular pathways to transitional cell carcinoma of the bladder. *Cancer Research, 54*(3), 784-788.

Tanagho, E. A. (1992). Anatomy of the lower urinary tract. In P. C. Walsh, A. B. Retik, T. A. Stamey, & E. D. Vaughan, Jr. (Eds.), *Campbell's urology* (6th ed.). Philadelphia: W. B. Saunders.

Tanagho, E. A. (1995a). Anatomy of the genitourinary tract. In E. A. Tanagho & J. W. McAninch (Eds.), *Smith's general urology* (14th ed.). Norwalk, Conn.: Appleton & Lange.

Tanagho, E. A. (1995b). Specific infections of the genitourinary tract. In E. A. Tanagho & J. W. McAninch (Eds.), *Smith's general urology* (14th ed.). Norwalk Conn.: Appleton & Lange.

Thrasher, J. B. & Crawford, E. D. (1992). Complications of intravesical chemotherapy. *Urologic Clinics of North America, 19*(3), 529-539.

Tootla, J., & Easterling, A. (1992). Current options in bladder cancer management. *RN, 55*(4), 42-48.

Utz, D. C. & Farrow, M. D. (1984). Carcinoma in situ of the urinary tract. *Urologic Clinics of North America, 11*(4), 735-740.

Veenema, R. J., Dean, Jr., A. L., Roberts, M., Fingerhut, B., Chowhury, B. K., & Tarassoly, H. (1962). Bladder carcinoma treated by direct instillation of thio-tepa. *Journal of Urology, 88*(1), 60-63.

Wallace, D. M. A. (1988). Occupational urothelial cancer. *British Journal of Urology, 61*(3), 175-182.

Wallace, D. M. A. & Harris, D. L. (1965). Delay in treating bladder tumours. *Lancet, II*(7407), 332-334.

Wallace, D. M. A., Hindmarsh, J. R., Webb, J. N., Busuttil, A., Hargreave, T. B., Newsam, J. E., & Chisholm, G. D. (1979). The role of multiple mucosal biopsies in the management of patients with bladder cancer. *British Journal of Urology, 51*(6), 535-540.

Walther, P. J. (1992). The role of flow cytometry in the management of bladder cancer. *Hematology Oncology Clinics of North America, 6*(1), 81-98.

Whitbourne, S. K. (1985). *The aging body: physiological changes and psychological consequences.* New York: Springer-Verlag.

Wood, D. P., Montie, J. E., Pontes, J. E., Medendorp, S. V., & Levin, H. S. (1989). Transitional cell carcinoma of the prostate in cystoprostatectomy specimens removed for bladder cancer. *Journal of Urology, 141*(2), 346-349.

Wynder, E. L. & Goldsmith, R. (1977). The epidemiology of bladder cancer: A second look. *Cancer, 40*(3), 1246-1268.

Invasive Bladder Cancer

Stacey Young-McCaughan, RN, PhD, OCN, Lt. Col.*

EPIDEMIOLOGY

In 1998 an estimated 54,400 new cases of bladder cancer were diagnosed, and 12,500 people died from this disease (Landis, Murray, Bolden, & Wingo, 1997). Bladder cancer accounts for only 5% of all new cases of cancer among men and 3% of all new cases of cancer among women, yet it is the fourth most prevalent cancer in men (after prostate, lung, and colon cancers) and the sixth most prevalent cancer in women (after breast, lung, and colon cancer, the gynecologic malignancies, and lymphoma) (Landis et al., 1997). Men are three times more likely than women to develop bladder cancer (American Cancer Society, 1996; Fleshner, Herr, Stewart, Murphy, Mettlin, & Menck, 1996; Hartge, Harvey, Linehan, Silverman, Sullivan, & Hoover et al., 1990; Melicow, 1974). In addition, whites are more likely to develop bladder cancer compared with blacks, Asians, Hispanics, and American Indians (American Cancer Society, 1996; Fleshner et al., 1996; Harris, Chen-Backlund, & Wynder, 1990; Silverman, Hartge, Morrison, & Devesa, 1992).

Approximately two thirds of patients diagnosed with bladder cancer are 60 years of age or older (Fleshner et al., 1996; Melicow, 1974; Silverman et al., 1992), except for patients with chronic urinary schistosomiasis, who are commonly diagnosed with bladder cancer between the ages of 40 and 50 (Makhyoun, 1974).

Over the past 20 years, the incidence of bladder cancer has increased 11%, although with improved treatments, the mortality from this disease has decreased 19.4% (Devesa, Blot, Stone, Miller, Tarone, & Fraumeni, 1995). With the long latency between carcinogen exposure and the development of bladder cancer (Cohen & Johansson, 1992), one possible explanation for the increasing incidence of bladder cancer is that the effects of past carcinogen exposure, primarily cigarette smoking, are just now becoming evident. Women, who began smoking in large numbers later than men, may be a group now at particularly high risk for bladder cancers, as well as other tobacco-related diseases.

RISK FACTORS

Known and suspected risk factors for bladder cancer are listed in Box 47-1.

Occupational Exposure to Chemical Carcinogens

In 1895, Rehn observed an increase in the incidence of bladder cancer among German textile workers exposed to aniline dyes. Over the next 40 years, an increased incidence of bladder cancer was also seen in the dye and textile workers of Switzerland, Great Britain, and the United States. In 1938, Hueper demonstrated that the arylamines used in making the dyes caused bladder tumors in dogs (Cohen & Johansson, 1992; Lower, 1982). Arylamines are metabolized in the liver and excreted in the urine. Compounds related to the arylamines that are known or strongly suspected to also be bladder carcinogens are also listed in Box 47-1.

In addition to dye and textile workers, other workers believed to be at increased risk for bladder cancer are listed in Box 47-2. Like those employed in the dye and textile industry, these workers can be exposed to arylamines at the work site. Arylamines were once used in the rubber and tire industries as a hardening antioxidant (Lower, 1982; Wallace, 1988). Although these compounds are no longer commonly used in making tires, some workers may still risk exposure from working with recycled tires or from working with other antioxidants contaminated with small amounts of the carcinogenic arylamines (Wallace, 1988). Others, such as leather workers, bootblacks, painters, and hairdressers, are at risk because of the dyes they may use in their work. Arylamines have also been found in environmental pollution, especially tobacco smoke and diesel exhaust (Cohen & Johansson, 1992; Wallace, 1988). Although governmental agencies have attempted to reduce exposure to these com-

*The views of the author are her own and do not purport to reflect the position of the Army Medical Department, Department of the Army, or the Department of Defense.

pounds, one study estimated that between 21% and 25% of bladder cancer diagnosed among white men in the United States could be attributed to occupational exposure (Silverman, Levine, Hoover, & Hartge, 1989).

Cigarette Smoking

Large epidemiologic studies have identified consistently that smokers have 2 to 10 times the risk of developing bladder cancer compared with nonsmokers (Burch, Rohan, Howe, Risch, Hill, & Steele et al., 1989; Clavel, Cordier, Boccon-Gibod, & Hemon, 1989; González, López-Abente, Errezola, Escolar, Riboli, & Izarzugaza et al., 1989; Harris, Chen-Backlund, & Wynder, 1990; Hartge, Silverman, Hoover, Schairer, Altman, & Austin et al., 1987; Howe, Burch, Miller, Cook, Esteve, & Morrison et al., 1980; Kantor, Hartge, Hoover, & Fraumeni, 1985, 1988; Mills, Beeson, Phillips, & Fraser, 1991; Morrison, Buring, Verhoek, Aoki, Leck, & Ohno et al., 1984; Piper, Matanoski, & Tonascia, 1986; Wynder & Goldsmith, 1977). Although the mechanisms by which cigarette smoking might induce bladder cancer are not known, aromatic amines present in dyes and known to cause bladder cancer in dye and textile workers are also present in tobacco smoke (Patrianakos & Hoffmann, 1979).

The risk of developing bladder cancer appears to increase with the number of cigarettes smoked (Auerbach & Garfinkel, 1989; Burch et al., 1989; Clavel et al., 1989; Howe et al., 1980; Kantor et al., 1985, 1988; Mills et al., 1991; Morrison et al., 1984) as well as for smokers who inhale deeply (Burch et al., 1989; Clavel et al., 1989; Morrison et al., 1984). The use of unfiltered cigarettes, compared with the use of filtered cigarettes, increased the risk of bladder cancer in one study (Hartge et al., 1987) but did not affect the risk of developing bladder cancer in two other studies (Burch et al., 1989; Morrison et al., 1984). The use of other tobacco products such as pipes, cigars, chewing tobacco, or snuff has not been associated with an increased risk of bladder cancer (Burch et al., 1989; Morrison et al., 1984). Neither has passive smoking been associated with an increased risk (Burch et al., 1989).

Approximately one third to half of bladder cancers are attributable to cigarette smoking (Burch et al., 1989; Hartge et al., 1987; Wynder & Goldsmith, 1977). The importance of encouraging patients to stop smoking cannot be emphasized enough. In addition to being associated with bladder cancers, smoking has also been implicated as a possible cause of cancers of the lung, mouth, pharynx, larynx, esophagus, pancreas, cervix, and kidney (American Cancer Society, 1996). Smokers cite a health care provider's advice to stop smoking as a potent motivator for quitting, yet only approximately half of current smokers report ever having been asked by their primary care provider if they smoked (Fiore, Bailey, Cohen, Dorfman, Goldstein, & Gritz et al., 1996). Even fewer smokers have received guidance on how to quit. Nurses can advise all their patients who smoke to stop and can provide information on nicotine replacement therapy as well as support groups and programs available for smokers interested in quitting (Fiore, Jorenby, Baker, & Kenford, 1992; Kottke, Battista, DeFriese, & Brekke, 1988; Ockene, 1987; Risser, 1996). Great strides have been made in banning smoking in public gathering places such as hospitals, schools, government agencies, stores, and restaurants. Nurses can support this trend and continue to support tobacco-control measures at the local, state, and federal levels (Gallagher & Holm, 1996). Nurses can also support individuals who do not allow smoking in their homes. The more difficult it is to find a comfortable place to smoke, the more likely smokers are going to abandon the habit.

Chronic Bladder Infection with *Schistosoma Haematobium* (Bilharziasis)

A relatively rare form of bladder cancer, squamous cell carcinoma, has been associated with chronic bladder infections with the blood fluke *Schistosoma haematobium* (Makhyoun, 1974; Tanagho, 1995b). The fluke lives in a fresh-water snail and infects humans working or recreating in infested water (Tanagho, 1995b). Once inside its host, the fluke migrates in the blood and lymph systems to the bladder, where it deposits its ova in the bladder wall. These ova eventually hatch and are excreted in the urine back into the water supply. The ova are an irritation to the bladder, resulting in a chronic urothelial inflammation. This irritation and inflammation are believed to predispose the host to squamous cell carcinoma of the bladder (Tanagho, 1995b). Although *Schistosoma haematobium* is not a common infection in the United States, these infections are endemic along the northern coast of Africa, Saudi Arabia, Israel, Jordan, Lebanon, and Syria. Because of emigration, schistosomiasis is being seen with increasing frequency in Europe and the United States (Tanagho, 1995b), and the incidence of this particular type of bladder cancer may increase in the future.

Family History

Epidemiologic studies have shown that a family history of bladder cancer increases the risk of bladder cancer, even when the risk from both smoking and occupational exposure are statistically controlled (Kantor et al., 1985; Kiemeney & Schoenberg, 1996; Lynch, Kimberling, Lynch, & Brennan, 1987). For people with a positive family history and who also smoke, the risk of bladder cancer increased dramatically in one study (Kantor et al., 1985).

People who have a history of bladder cancer in their family need to be advised that they may be at increased risk for the disease. These people should be strongly encouraged not to smoke and to monitor their work site for possible exposure to bladder carcinogens.

Suspected Risk Factors

Also listed in Box 47-1 are a host of possible risk factors for bladder cancer that have been noted in the literature. Dietary factors that have been associated with an increased risk of bladder cancer include coffee drinking, consumption of artificial sweeteners (particularly saccharin and cyclamate), alcohol drinking, a high cholesterol intake, and a diet high in meat (Silverman et al., 1992). The findings from studies reporting these dietary risk factors for bladder cancer are highly variable, contradicting each other in some instances. Lack of consistent results, failure to control for confounding variables such as cigarette smoking, and the risk of identifying statistically significant risks only because of the large number of people studied, lead to the conclusion that if there are dietary risk factors for bladder cancer, the risk is relatively small (Silverman et al., 1992).

Urologic conditions such as frequent urinary tract infections and urinary stasis have also been suggested as risk factors for bladder cancer (Kantor, Hartge, Hoover, Narayana, Sullivan, & Fraumeni, 1984; Kantor et al., 1988). Presumably, if carcinogens are present in the urine, frequent and prolonged exposure of the urothelium to these carcinogens increases the likelihood of neoplastic changes in the bladder. However, as with studies of dietary factors, the results of these studies are also inconsistent and definitive conclusions are impossible.

There is a great deal of clinical and epidemiologic evidence that infection with human papillomavirus (HPV) types 16 and 18 is associated with an increased risk of cervical cancer. There has also been some speculation that HPV 16 and 18 are associated with an increased risk of some bladder cancers (Furihata, Inoue, Ohtsuki, Hashimoto, Terao, & Fujita, 1994; Song-ting, Ming-ming, & Li-ming, 1993). Possibly, the HPV inactivates the p53 suppressor gene, allowing neoplastic changes of the urothelium to go unchecked (Scher, 1994). However, much more work needs to be done before HPV infections can definitively be considered a risk factor for bladder cancer.

Drugs that have been associated with an increased risk of bladder cancer include phenacetin-containing analgesics (Piper, Matanoski, & Tonascia, 1986) and the antineoplastic chemotherapeutic drug, cyclophosphamide (Fairchild, Spence, Solomon, & Gangai, 1979; Fernandes, Manivel, Reddy, & Ercole, 1996; Levine & Richie, 1989; Pedersen-Bjergaard, Ersbøll, Hansen, Sørensen, Christoffersen, & Hou-Jensen et al., 1988). Western countries no longer allow phenacetin to be sold, obviating its role as a possible bladder carcinogen. In contrast, cyclophosphamide is currently used to treat many different cancers as well as various nonmalignant diseases (e.g., autoimmune disorders such as rheumatoid arthritis, systemic lupus erythematosus, and thrombocytopenic purpura). Cyclophosphamide is metabolized by the liver into acrolein that is excreted in the urine. Acrolein has long been identified as a bladder irritant, and prolonged exposure to acrolein can lead to cystitis. Aggressive hydration to promote frequent urination is a routine part of care for patients being treated with cyclophosphamide. Acrolein may also be carcinogenic, especially if the urothelium is exposed to high concentrations of this metabolite over a prolonged period.

Individual cases of bladder cancer in women who received pelvic radiation for dysfunctional uterine bleeding or gynecologic cancers have been reported in the literature (Boice, Engholm, Kleinerman, Blettner, Stovall, & Lisco et al., 1988; Inskip, Monson, Wagoner, Stovall, Davis, & Kleinerman et al., 1990; Quilty & Kerr, 1987). Also, an increased incidence of bladder cancer has been seen in patients treated with radioactive iodine-131 for thyroid cancer (Edmonds & Smith, 1986; Piper, Matanoski, & Tonascia, 1986). It is very likely that, during treatment, the bladder was inadvertently exposed to small doses of radiation, predisposing the urothelium to neoplastic changes.

Some epidemiologic studies have identified people who live in rural areas drinking water contaminated with pesticides (Mills et al., 1991) and people who drink highly chlorinated water (Crump & Guess, 1982) as being at an increased risk of developing bladder cancer. However, these findings are not consistent between studies. If either drinking water in rural areas or drinking highly chlorinated water is a risk factor for bladder cancer, the risk is relatively small.

Studies of known and suspected risk factors for bladder cancer have been extensively reviewed by Silverman and colleagues (1992), and the interested reader is referred to this article as well as the others cited in Box 47-1 for more detailed information.

CHEMOPREVENTION

Chemoprevention refers to the use of various drugs to prevent malignant changes in cells or to prolong the time required for malignant changes to occur in cells (Kelloff, Boone, Malone, Steele, & Doody, 1992). Bladder cancers offer a unique opportunity to test various chemopreventive agents because even after complete resection of the tumor, half to three quarters of patients suffer a recurrence of their disease (Heney, Nocks, Daly, Prout, Newall, & Griffin et al., 1982; Lamm, Blumenstein, Crawford, Montie, Scardino, & Grossman et al., 1991). In animal studies, many drugs have shown promise in reducing bladder cancer recurrence, including alpha-difluoromethylornithine (DFMO), oltipraz (which contains the same active ingredient as cruciferous vegetables), and various nonsteroidal anti-inflammatory drugs (NSAIDs), such as ibuprofen, indocin, and piroxicam (Kelloff et al., 1992). Yet, the few human clinical trials that have been done using DFMO (Loprinzi & Messing, 1992), 13-*cis*-retinoic acid (Prout & Barton, 1992), and N-(4-hydroxyphenyl)retinamide (4-HPR) (Decensi, Bruno, Giaretti, Torrisi, Curotto, & Gatteschi et al., 1992) showed only a modest reduction in tumor recurrence, if any at all. The Chemoprevention Branch of the National Cancer Institute (NCI) is continuing to test new compounds in the hope that one will effectively prevent malignant changes in the urothelium, thereby preventing primary bladder cancer as well as reducing the recurrence of bladder cancer in patients already diagnosed with the disease.

PATHOPHYSIOLOGY

Normal Anatomy and Physiology of the Bladder

The bladder is a hollow, muscular organ that expands to hold approximately 300 ml of urine at low pressures (Bates, 1991; Harrison & Abrams, 1994; Tanagho, 1992). The bladder is located on the floor of the pelvic cavity behind the peritoneum. In men the bladder is located ventral to the rectum and in women ventral to the vagina and uterus. The upper portion of the bladder is named the *fundus*. Two ureters, one from each kidney, enter the bladder posteriorly, as depicted in Fig. 47-1. The trigone is a triangular area on the posterior bladder wall, bounded superiorly by the two ureters and inferiorly by the urethra. The trigone closes the ureteral openings during micturition, thereby preventing urine from being forced back into the ureters and renal pelvis. The urethra exits the bladder at the bladder neck.

The urethra is a muscular tube that carries urine from the bladder out of the body. It functions as a sphincter, contracting to hold urine in the bladder and relaxing to allow urine to flow out of the bladder. In men the urethra is 20 cm long, traversing the prostate gland and the length of the penis before exiting the body; whereas in women the urethra is only 4 cm long.

Specialized transitional cells line the renal pelvis, both ureters, bladder, and urethra, preventing various metabolites and toxins excreted in the urine from being reabsorbed into the circulation. Three to six layers of transitional cells (called the *urothelium*) line the urinary tract, allowing for expansion and contraction of the bladder, while maintaining the integrity of the system.

As more than 300 ml of urine accumulates in the bladder, the smooth muscle of the bladder (the detrusor muscle) is stretched, pressure in the bladder rises, and the urge to void becomes conscious. In cognitively intact adults the brain can inhibit the detrusor muscle from contracting until the maximum bladder capacity of 400 to 500 ml is reached (Bates, 1991).

As both men and women age, bladder capacity decreases, causing urinary frequency. Emptying of the bladder is more difficult due to weakened bladder muscles, resulting in urine retention (Whitbourne, 1985).

The Process of Carcinogenesis

As with the development of many different cancers, evidence suggests that the evolution of bladder cancer depends on a series of genetic events. Papillary bladder cancers have a very different natural history compared with carcinomas in situ (CIS). Although the majority of both papillary tumors and CIS are considered early-stage superficial bladder tumors, papillary tumors rarely recur or progress, whereas CIS very often recurs and progresses to a higher stage invasive tumor. Molecular genetic differences between papillary tumors and CIS may explain how the natural history of these two tumors is so different. Papillary bladder carcinomas are more likely to have mutations in the tumor suppressor gene p16 on chromosome 9q, whereas CIS is more likely to have mutations of the tumor suppressor gene P53 on chromosome 17p. These differences in natural history and molecular biology support a two-pathway model for the pathogenesis and progression of bladder cancer, as shown in Fig. 47-2 (Israel, Natale, & Skinner, 1995; Spruck, Ohneseit, Gonzalez-Zulueta, Esrig, Miyao, & Tsai et al., 1994). Although the majority of papillary tumors rarely recur or progress, the few that do transform into a more aggressive tumor acquire mutations of gene P53. Other chromosomal changes have been associated with bladder tumors and are listed in Table 47-1, but p16 and P53 mutations have been the most widely studied.

Both p16 and P53 mutations involve inactivation of a tumor suppressor gene. Without these tumor suppressor mechanisms, malignant cells in the urothelium go unchecked. Only one proto-oncogene, H-*ras*, located on the short arm of chromosome 11 has been studied as a possible initiator of bladder malignancies.

ROUTES OF METASTASES

After it invades the muscle wall, a bladder tumor can extend locally to the pelvic organs and/or use the lymphatic and hematologic systems to metastasize to other areas of the body.

Local Extension to Pelvic Organs

Primary bladder tumors can extend through the bladder wall and into adjacent pelvic organs such as the prostate and seminal vesicle in men; the uterus, ovary, cervix, and vagina in women; and the perivesical tissue, rectum, colon, ileum, and psoas in both genders (Melicow, 1974). In addition to invading these adjacent organs, tumors can compress various organs, disrupting normal functioning. Constipation, hydronephrosis, lower extremity edema, and pain have been reported when bladder tumors invade or compress adjacent organs.

Distant Metastasis

The most common sites of distant metastasis in patients with invasive bladder cancer are the lungs, followed by the liver, bone, and brain (Bane, Rao, & Hemstreet, 1996). On autopsy, metastatic bladder cancer has also been found in the adrenal glands, heart, kidneys, colon, and pancreas (Babaian, Johnson, Llamas, & Ayala, 1980; Melicow, 1974).

ASSESSMENT

Table 47-2 summarizes the assessment of a patient with bladder cancer. Clinical evaluation of the patient involves a detailed history, a physical examination, and a variety of diagnostic tests. Definitions of commonly experienced bladder symptoms are provided in Table 47-3. These symptoms can occur as evidence of bladder cancer, as side effects of therapy for bladder cancer, or with a bladder infection. Usually, further urinary testing is needed to determine the etiology of these symptoms and to appropriately treat the cause as well as the symptoms.

History

Approximately 75% of patients with bladder cancer seek medical care complaining of hematuria (Fair, Fuks, & Scher, 1993; Wallace & Harris, 1965). Hematuria in bladder cancer is often intermittent, deceiving practitioners into believing that the cause is benign (Lamm & Torti, 1996). Between 20% and 30% of patients present with irritative bladder symptoms (IBSs) such as dysuria, frequency, or urgency

(Cummings, Barone, & Ward, 1992; Fair, Fuks, & Scher, 1993). In women, these symptoms can be mistaken for interstitial cystitis. Lamm and Torti (1996) warn against dismissing these relatively innocuous symptoms in an attempt to reduce health care costs without an adequate diagnostic workup.

Patients with advanced bladder cancer can present with pelvic, rectal, flank, or bone pain. Hydronephrosis and flank pain can occur if the tumor is obstructing a ureter. Difficulty voiding can occur with a bladder outlet obstruction. Constipation can occur if the tumor compresses the rectum. Occasionally with advanced disease, obstruction of lymphatic and venous drainage can cause lower extremity and genital edema (Fair, Fuks, & Scher, 1993; Israel, Natale, & Skinner, 1995).

Physical Examination

A bimanual examination is done to determine the presence of a pelvic mass and bladder wall thickening, as well as whether the bladder is freely mobile or fixed to the pelvic sidewall (Fair, Fuks, & Scher, 1993). This examination is best done with the patient anesthetized for comfort and so that the pelvic muscles are relaxed (Israel, Natale, & Skinner, 1995; Lamm & Torti, 1996). Part of the staging workup for bladder cancer is a transurethral resection of the bladder (TURB), which is done with the patient anesthetized. The bimanual physical examination is generally done at this time.

Diagnostic Tests

All patients suspected of having bladder cancer should be assessed with urine cytology, an intravenous urogram (IVU), and cystoscopy (Israel, Natale, & Skinner, 1995). Additional radiologic imaging and a bone scan are tests indicated for patients suspected of having invasive bladder cancer.

Urine Cytology. The transitional cells that line the renal pelvis, ureters, bladder and urethra are constantly being exfoliated and excreted in the urine. Urine cytology examines these cells to identify malignant changes. One technique uses a Papanicolaou stain to examine the cells under a microscope. Another technique uses flow cytometry, which treats the cells with a dye that binds to nucleic deoxyribonucleic acid (DNA), then passes the cells through a sensor that is able to quantify the amount of DNA in the cells. Malignant cells have an abnormally high amount of DNA because more of these cells are in the process of dividing (Walther, 1992). In addition to flow cytometry, another molecular method that is being investigated to detect malignant changes in exfoliated transitional cells uses polymerase chain reaction (PCR) technology to amplify specific regions of DNA known to mutate in bladder cancer, thereby making identification of DNA alterations easier. One study (Mao, Schoenberg, Scicchitano, Erozan, Merlo, & Schwab et al., 1996) reported that this type of microsatellite analysis identified specific DNA alterations in 95% of a small sample of patients with bladder cancer, whereas routine urine cytology detected cancer cells in only 50% of the samples.

Urine cytology cannot determine the size or location of malignant tumors, only the presence of malignant cells in the urinary tract. However, it is possible to screen for malignant cells being shed by lesions in the ureters or renal pelvis, parts of the urinary tract not visualized with cystoscopy. The best urine specimen for cytologic examination is a freshly voided sample. Prolonged exposure of exfoliated cells to urine can complicate the pathologic interpretation. Because of this, urine specimens should not be sent from the first morning void or from catheter bags (Itoku & Stein, 1992; Murphy, 1990).

Currently, some form of urine cytology is a routine part of the diagnostic workup of patients suspected of having bladder cancer, and it is also used in the follow-up of patients previously treated for bladder cancer to assess for recurrence. In the future, urine cytology using molecular techniques could be part of a screening examination for people at high risk for bladder cancer based on their smoking habits, occupation, and family history.

Intravenous Urogram. An IVU, also known as an *intravenous pyelogram (IVP)*, is routinely done in the diagnosis and staging of bladder cancer to evaluate the architecture and filling pattern of the urinary system. Although only 60% of bladder tumors are visualized with urography, these dye studies can identify suspicious lesions that might otherwise be missed. Space-occupying lesions within the urinary tract or external to the system obstructing the flow of urine can be identified with this test. Bladder wall expansion can also be evaluated. Asymmetric expansion may be indicative of a deeply invasive bladder tumor (Israel, Natale, & Skinner, 1995). Preparation of the patient undergoing an IVU is outlined in Table 47-4.

Cystoscopy. Central to the diagnosis, staging, treatment, and follow-up of patients with bladder cancer is cystoscopy. A flexible cystoscope is routinely used, making it possible to perform the procedure in an outpatient setting with the patient under local anesthesia. During the procedure the entire bladder and urethra are visualized. Every lesion should be described in detail, with the location, size, appearance, and condition of the surrounding mucosa being noted (Itoku & Stein, 1992). Approximately 70% of tumors are located on the lateral and posterior walls, 20% on the trigone, and 10% in the bladder dome (Fleshner et al., 1996; Melicow, 1974). During cystoscopy, bladder washings can also be obtained and sent for cytology. Preparation of the patient undergoing a diagnostic cystoscopy is outlined in Table 47-5.

If suspicious lesions are identified during the initial cystoscopy, a TURB with the patient under spinal or general anesthesia is planned. (TURB is discussed in more detail in the Medical Management section.)

Radiologic Imaging. Patients with invasive bladder cancer should have a chest radiograph looking for possible metastasis to the lungs. Ultrasound (US), computed tomography (CT) scans, and magnetic resonance imaging (MRI) have been used to scan the abdomen for enlarged lymph nodes, as well as for discrete lesions in distant organs such as the liver, colon, adrenal glands, and kidneys (Bane, Rao, & Hemstreet, 1996; Fair, Fuks, & Scher, 1993; Israel, Natale, & Skinner, 1995). MRI provides the best differentiation between the tumor and the bladder (Barentsz, Jager, Witjes, & Ruijs, 1996). However, when Bane, Rao, and Hemstreet (1996) reviewed radiologic imaging techniques, they concluded that for the majority of patients, MRI's small improvement in sensitivity and specificity compared with CT scanning did not warrant the additional cost of MRI. They recommended CT scans to screen for distant disease in the majority of patients with invasive bladder cancer. CT scans of the chest or brain are indicated only for patients with localizing pulmonary or neurologic findings (Bane, Rao, & Hemstreet, 1996).

Bone Scan. A bone scan to screen for metastatic disease is warranted for patients with an elevated serum alkaline phosphatase (Bane, Rao, & Hemstreet, 1996; Fair, Fuks, & Scher, 1993; Israel, Natale, & Skinner, 1995). However, for patients with a normal serum alkaline phosphatase, the likelihood of bone metastasis is very low; therefore many practitioners forego the expense of a bone scan.

STAGING

Bladder cancer is considered a heterogeneous disease of the urothelium, indicating that multiple tumors can develop simultaneously in different areas of the bladder. Approximately 30% of patients present with multiple tumors at the time of diagnosis (Fair, Fuks, & Scher, 1993; Heney et al., 1982; Itoku & Stein, 1992). Each lesion needs to be characterized as to its (1) pathology or cell type, (2) morphology or appearance, (3) invasiveness into the bladder wall and surrounding tissue, and (4) grade or degree of cytologic abnormality.

Pathology

The pathology of bladder cancers is outlined in Table 47-6 and described in the following sections.

Transitional Cell Carcinoma (TCC). More than 90% of tumors of the bladder arise from the urothelium, a specialized transitional epithelium lining the bladder and urinary tract (Fleshner et al., 1996; Lynch & Cohen, 1995; Melicow, 1974; Silverman et al., 1992). The urothelium is believed to be susceptible to malignant changes because of the constant exposure to urinary waste products. These tumors are amenable to a variety of treatments.

Squamous Cell Carcinoma. Squamous cell carcinoma accounts for less than 5% of bladder carcinomas in the United States (Lynch & Cohen, 1995; Melicow, 1974). In countries where *Schistosoma haematobium* is endemic, the percentage of bladder cancers that are squamous cell in origin is much higher (Ghoneim, 1995). Unfortunately, this type of bladder cancer is usually not diagnosed until it is at an advanced stage. More than 90% of squamous cell bladder tumors are invasive at the time of diagnosis (Faysal, 1981; Newman, Brown, Jay, & Pontius, 1968). Surgery is the primary treatment modality because squamous cell tumors are generally unresponsive to radiation therapy or chemotherapy (Brodsky, 1992; Lamm & Torti, 1996).

Adenocarcinoma and Others. Other, even less common carcinomas of the bladder include adenocarcinoma, spindle cell carcinoma, small cell carcinoma, carcinoid tumors, pheochromocytomas, choriocarcinoma, and germ cell neoplasms (Brodsky, 1992). Like squamous cell carcinomas, surgery is the primary treatment modality for these tumors because they are generally unresponsive to radiation therapy or chemotherapy (Bane, Rao, & Hemstreet, 1996; Brodsky, 1992; Lamm & Torti, 1996).

Morphology

The morphology, or appearance, of bladder tumors can be flat, papillary, or sessile. These descriptions, confirmed with pathologic examination, help to characterize the primary tumor for staging.

Carcinoma in Situ. Nonpapillary CIS is a flat tumor that has been described as a velvety, mossy, erythematous lesion (Itoku & Stein, 1992; Lamm, 1992). These changes in the bladder mucosa can be very subtle; often the urothelium appears completely normal, and it is only with pathologic evaluation of bladder washings and random bladder wall biopsies that CIS is diagnosed. Patients are likely to complain of IBS, which brings them to seek medical care and an evaluation. CIS is staged Tis, as indicated in Table 47-7.

The prevalence of CIS is difficult to determine because it can occur as a primary focal lesion, as diffuse urothelial disease, or adjacent to a papillary or sessile lesion (Fair, Fuks, & Scher, 1993). Often, Tis and small papillary Ta tumors are reported together as stage 0 disease. One prospective study of 2454 patients with bladder cancer reported that only 10% of the patients had an initial diagnosis of CIS (Utz & Farrow, 1984). This form of bladder cancer is considered a highly variable and unpredictable malignancy with the potential for rapid progression and invasion that demands aggressive treatment and close follow-up (Itoku & Stein, 1992; Lamm, 1992).

Papillary. As the name suggests, papillary tumors grow on stalks. Depending on their size and location, papillary tumors can intermittently obstruct the ureters or urethra as they bend with the flow of urine. Papillary tumors account for 70% to 80% of bladder carcinomas (Fleshner et al., 1996; Melicow, 1974). They are usually staged Ta, as indicated in Table 47-7. The base of a papillary tumor generally does not invade the lamina propria or detrusor muscle, although this is possible. If the base of the stalk extends beyond the epithelium, the tumor is upstaged according to the degree of bladder wall invasion, as outlined in Table 47-7.

Sessile. The remaining 20% to 30% of bladder tumors present with a broad base that commonly invade the subepithelial connective tissue (Melicow, 1974). These tumors are called *sessile* and are staged according to the extent of tumor invasion, as indicated in Table 47-7. A sessile morphology is a poor prognostic feature, indicating that the cancer may already be invasive.

TNM Staging

The earliest classification of bladder cancers was the Jewett-Strong Classification developed in 1946 (Jewett & Strong, 1946) and modified by Jewett in 1952 (Jewett, 1952), and again by Marshall in the same year (Marshall, 1952). The Jewett-Strong-Marshall classification describes Stages 0, A, B, C, and D according to the depth of tumor invasion into the bladder wall and metastasis to adjacent structures. More recently, most health care providers have adopted the American Joint Committee on Cancer (AJCC) Classification System to uniformly communicate cancer statistics internationally. The AJCC Classification System describes the stage of cancer according to the size of the primary tumor (T), the presence or absence of disease in regional lymph nodes (N), and the presence or absence of distant metastasis (M) (American Joint Committee on Cancer, 1992). Table 47-7 compares the two staging systems, and Table 47-8 shows how the stage of disease is determined according to the TNM system for bladder cancer.

Both staging systems depend on a bladder wall biopsy to determine whether the tumor has invaded the muscle. Clinical staging with cystoscopy alone is notoriously inaccurate in determining the degree of tumor invasion into the bladder wall. In a combined series of four studies with a total of 465 patients with bladder cancer, clinical staging agreed with pathologic staging for less than 50% of the patients (Fair, Fuks, & Scher, 1993). More than one third of the patients would have been understaged without the benefit of a bladder wall muscle biopsy, resulting in insufficient treatment.

Histologic Staging

The fourth major consideration in describing a bladder cancer is the grade, or the degree, of cellular dysplasia of the tumor (Bane, Rao, & Hemstreet, 1996; Brodsky, 1992). Pathologists determine histologic grade of I, II, or III based on 10 pathologic features listed in Table 47-9. Some classification systems assign a grade between I and IV, but because the biologic behavior of grade III and grade IV tumors is so similar, the World Health Organization has combined them into a single grade (Fair, Fuks, & Scher, 1993).

The higher the grade, the more dysplastic and less differentiated the tumor appears. The higher the grade, the worse the prognosis for the patient. The TNM staging of bladder cancer (0, I, II, III, IV) does *not* describe the grade of the tumor (I, II, III). Both features of the cancer are important to characterize and help the urologist and patient plan appropriate therapy. Whereas papillary and sessile tumors can histologically be grade I, II, or III, CIS is always considered a grade I lesion (Bane, Rao, & Hemstreet, 1996; Lamm, 1992).

MEDICAL MANAGEMENT

As shown in Table 47-10, approximately one third of patients with bladder cancer present with invasive stage II, III, or IV disease involving the detrusor muscle (Fleshner et al., 1996). A variety of surgical and radiologic approaches, outlined in Table 48-1, have been employed in the primary treatment of invasive bladder cancer. Each approach can claim some measure of success, but 5-year survival rates show that no one approach stands out as the definitive treatment for invasive bladder cancer. Table 48-2 outlines possible treatment approaches according to the stage of disease and tumor characteristics. Before the urologist and patient decide on a treatment approach that offers the best length and quality of survival, the following must be assessed: the physical status of the patient, the patient's ability and willingness to undergo multiple procedures, the patient's desire to maintain his or her own bladder versus undergoing a bladder reconstruction, and the patient's willingness to risk postoperative sexual dysfunction.

TABLE 48-1 Five-Year Survival Rates in Patients with Invasive Bladder Cancers According to Treatment

	Size of Primary Tumor		
Primary Treatment	T2	T3a	T3b
Repeat TURB	57%-70%	14%-57%	2%-7%
Partial cystectomy	43%-60%	14%-45%	<1%
Radical cystectomy	50%-88%	26%-60%	6%-40%
Radiation therapy	19%-57%	0%-36%	0%-6%

TURB, Transurethral resection of the bladder.
Modified from Whitmore, W. F. (1990). Selection of treatment for muscle infiltrating transitional cell bladder cancer. *Archivos Espanoles de Urologia, 43*(Suppl. 2), 219-222.

Surgery

Transurethral Resection of the Bladder. If a bladder tumor is detected during cystoscopy, a TURB is scheduled. Although most patients can tolerate a flexible cystoscopy with only local anesthesia, spinal or general anesthesia is required for a TURB. Not only is the patient more comfortable, but the anesthesia relaxes the pelvic floor, abdominal wall, and bladder, allowing the urologist to do a complete bimanual physical examination and biopsy of the bladder wall without the risk of stimulating the obturator reflex and perforating the bladder (Soloway & Patel, 1992).

After the patient is anesthetized adequately, a bimanual physical examination is done to determine the presence of a pelvic mass and bladder wall thickening, as well as whether the bladder is freely mobile or fixed to the pelvic sidewall (Fair, Fuks, & Scher, 1993). The cystoscope is then inserted through the urethra and into the bladder. This cystoscope has various components and attachments, including a light source, at least two viewing lenses (30° and 70°), electric wire-cutting loops, and bladder irrigating and draining capabilities (Soloway & Patel, 1992). Care must be taken to perform an adequate biopsy of the bladder wall muscle, yet not perforate the bladder.

Additional biopsies of the tissue surrounding the tumor as well as random bladder wall biopsies are usually also taken. Biopsies from normal-appearing mucosa can be pathologically abnormal in 14% to 33% of cases (Heney, Daly, Prout, Nieh, Heaney, & Trebeck, 1978; Murphy, Nagy, Rao, Soloway, Parija, & Cox et al., 1979; Soloway, Murphy, Rao, & Cox, 1978; Wallace, Hindmarsh, Webb, Busuttil, Hargreave, & Newsam et al., 1979). "Cold-cup" biopsies are recommended to minimize cautery distortion of small pieces of tissue (Fair, Fuks, & Scher, 1993; Israel, Natale, & Skinner, 1996). In men, a biopsy of the prostatic urethra should also be done to guide treatment decision making (Lamm & Torti, 1996). One study (Wood, Montie, Pontes, Medendorp, & Levin, 1989) found that 43% of 84 men undergoing radical prostatectomies for bladder cancer had involvement of the prostatic urethra. Women should also have a biopsy performed on the urethra.

After a TURB, an indwelling catheter is placed to drain urine and monitor for bleeding. The patient may be hospitalized overnight, but more commonly the patient is discharged home from the Post Anesthesia Care Unit (PACU).

TURB is most often used to establish a diagnosis of bladder cancer and to stage the disease. As shown in Table 48-1, however, TURB may itself cure some patients with invasive bladder cancer. For patients with lesions that were originally less than 5 cm, a restaging TURB can be performed 3 to 4 weeks after the diagnostic TURB (Herr, 1992). During this second TURB the urologist again resects the site of the primary tumor to identify any residual tumor. Patients without residual tumor do not need further therapy and can be safely followed with urine cytology and cystoscopy every 3 months.

Herr (1987) reported on 217 patients with invasive bladder cancer who underwent a second TURB. About 21% (45) of the 217 patients did not have residual disease and were managed conservatively with close observation. At median of 5 years after the second TURB, 82% (37) of the 45 patients were tumor free and 67% (30) of the 45 patients were able to maintain their own bladder. However, this is not an option for the majority of patients with invasive bladder cancer. Almost 80% of Herr's 217 patients who underwent a second TURB suffered from residual disease and subsequently had a partial or radical cystectomy. Yet, repeat TURB may be curative surgery for a subset of patients with invasive bladder cancer.

Partial Cystectomy. Partial cystectomy, also known as *segmental resection of the bladder*, removes a portion of the bladder and pelvic lymph nodes through an abdominal incision. A partial cystectomy is indicated for patients with invasive or high-grade bladder cancer who have a solitary tumor in a region of the bladder where complete resection with adequate margins can be accomplished (Bales, Kim, & Steinberg, 1996; Fair, Fuks, & Scher, 1993; Israel, Natale, & Skinner, 1995; Sweeney, Kursh, & Resnick, 1992). Most patients are not candidates for a partial cystectomy because they have multiple tumors, CIS, disease in the prostatic urethra, a lesion invading the trigone, or a lesion located near one of the ureteral openings, necessitating ureteral reimplantation to completely resect the tumor. In a review of

TABLE 48-2 Treatment Options According to Stage of Disease and Tumor Characteristics

Stage	Tumor Characteristics	Possible Treatment Approaches
II	T2 or T3a	Repeat TURB Partial cystectomy Cystectomy with continent urinary diversion Primary radiation therapy Neoadjuvant chemotherapy and bladder preservation as part of a clinical trial
III	T3b or T4a	Repeat TURB Partial cystectomy Cystectomy with continent urinary diversion Primary radiation therapy Neoadjuvant chemotherapy and bladder preservation as part of a clinical trial Adjuvant chemotherapy as part of a clinical trial
IV	T4 Lymph node negative	Repeat TURB Partial cystectomy Cystectomy with continent urinary diversion Primary radiation therapy Neoadjuvant chemotherapy and bladder preservation as part of a clinical trial Adjuvant chemotherapy as part of a clinical trial
IV	T4 Lymph node positive	Repeat TURB Partial cystectomy Cystectomy with continent urinary diversion for pelvic control of disease Primary radiation therapy Chemotherapy

TURB, Transurethral resection of the bladder.
Modified from Sternberg, C. N. (1996). Neoadjuvant and adjuvant chemotherapy in locally advanced bladder cancer. *Seminars in Oncology, 23*(5), 621-632.

seven studies, only between 6% and 19% of patients met these criteria for treatment with partial cystectomy (Sweeney, Kursh, & Resnick, 1992).

In the past, partial cystectomy was a means to preserve normal bladder function in patients with limited disease

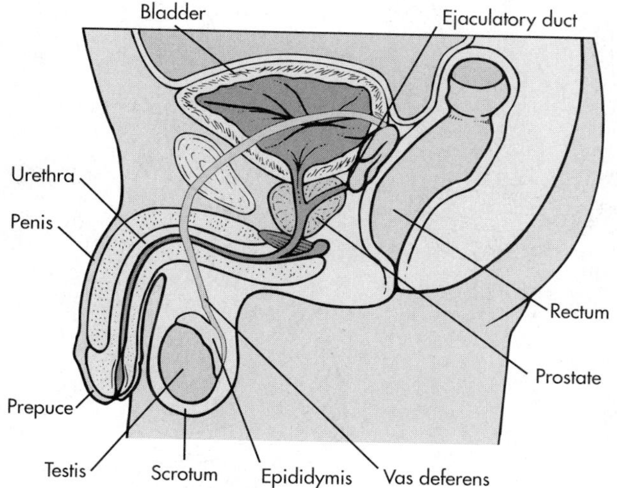

Fig. 48-1 Male anatomy and relations of the bladder, prostate, seminal vesicles, penis, urethra, and scrotal contents. (From Tanagho, E. A. [1995a]. Anatomy of the genitourinary tract. In E. A. Tanagho & J. W. McAninch [Eds.], *Smith's general urology* [14th ed.]. Norwalk, CT: Appleton & Lange.)

who objected to cystectomy and urinary diversion with an ileal conduit. However, between 38% and 78% of patients who underwent a partial cystectomy suffered disease recurrence (Sweeney, Kursh, & Resnick, 1992). Today, with the option of bladder reconstruction, partial cystectomy does not have any advantages over more radical surgery and therefore plays a very limited role in the surgical treatment of patients with invasive bladder cancer.

Radical Cystectomy. Radical cystectomy has historically been the primary treatment for invasive bladder cancer. This procedure involves removing the bladder with contiguous organs and tissues en bloc. In men the prostate, seminal vesicles, vas deferens, and 1 to 2 cm of the urethra are removed with the bladder. In women the uterus, fallopian tubes, ovaries, anterior vaginal wall, and entire urethra are removed with the bladder (Fair, Fuks, & Scher, 1993; Israel, Natale, & Skinner, 1995; Richie, 1992). Surgical margins for men and women are outlined in Figs. 48-1 and 48-2. A regional, bilateral lymph node dissection is part of the radical cystectomy to examine pelvic nodal tissue (Richie, 1992). The presence of nodal metastasis increases the patient's risk of disease recurrence; therefore these patients may want to consider further therapy. The incidence of nodal metastasis increases as the size of the primary tumor increases. As indicated in Table 48-3, in a review of 591 consecutive patients who underwent cystectomy and lymph node dissection for bladder cancer, 20% of patients with T2 tumors had positive lymph nodes, whereas 45% of patients with a T4 tumor had lymph node involvement

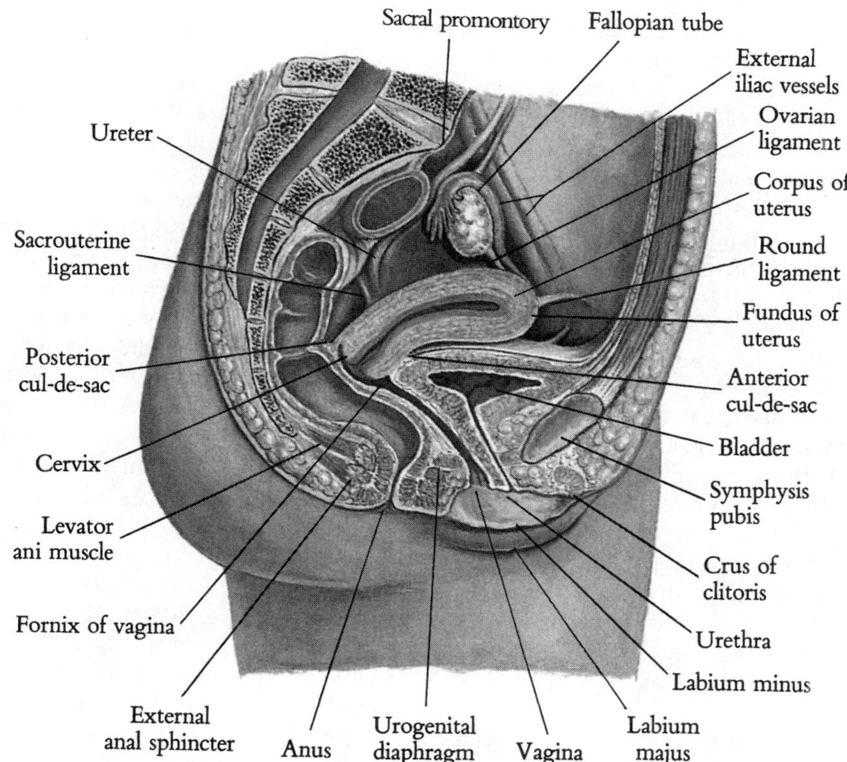

Fig. 48-2 Female anatomy and relations of the bladder, urethra, uterus, ovary, vagina, and rectum. (From Tanagho, E. A. [1995a]. Anatomy of the genitourinary tract. In E. A. Tanagho & J. W. McAninch [Eds.], *Smith's general urology* [14th ed.]. Norwalk, CT: Appleton & Lange.)

Table 48-3 Incidence of Nodal Metastases According to Pathologic Bladder Tumor State in 592 Patients Who Underwent Radical Cystectomy

Pathologic Tumor Stage	Patients Undergoing Radical Cystectomy with En Bloc Lymph Node Dissection Who Had Positive Lymph Nodes (%)
T0	0
Tis	0.75
T1	13
T2	20
T3a	24
T3b	42
T4	45

Data from Lerner, S. P., Skinner, D. G., Lieskovsky, G., Boyd, S. D., Groshen, S. L., Ziogas, A., Skinner, E., Nichols, P., & Hopwood, B. (1993). The rationale for en bloc pelvic lymph node dissection for bladder cancer patients with nodal metastases: Long-term results. *Journal of Urology, 149*(4), 758-765.

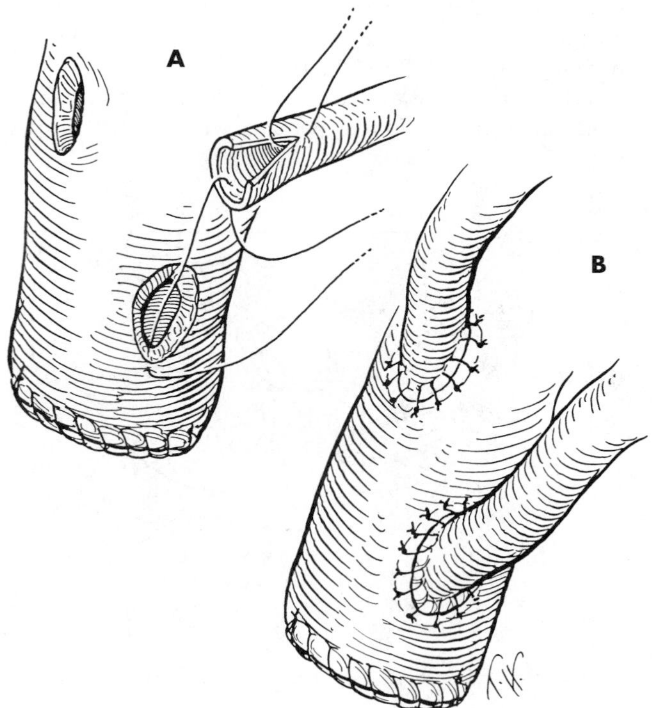

Fig. 48-3 Bricker procedure for ureteroileal anastomosis. **A,** One-centimeter–staggered elliptoid incisions are made in the ileum. Following spatulation of the ureter, 4-0 absorbable apical sutures are placed at the 6 and 12 o'clock positions. **B,** Additional sutures are placed in an interrupted fashion. (From Gillenwater, J. T. [1996]. *Adult and pediatric urology* [3rd ed.]. St. Louis: Mosby.)

(Lerner, Skinner, Lieskovsky, Boyd, Groshen, & Ziogas et al., 1993).

Between 1950 and 1980, an ileal conduit to an abdominal stoma was the standard for urinary diversion following cystectomy (Bricker, 1950, 1978). Although many patients were successfully treated for their bladder cancer with this procedure, patients' quality of life was adversely affected by having to manage a stoma and wear an external urine collection bag (Boyd, Feinberg, Skinner, Lieskovsky, Baron, & Richardson, 1987; Månsson, Johnson, & Månsson, 1988; Smith & Babaian, 1989). Furthermore, virtually all men were impotent after cystectomy. Over the intervening 20 years, advances in surgical procedures have taken place that allow patients today to have many more choices for urinary diversion. In addition, nerve-sparing surgical techniques preserve potency in the majority of men undergoing cystectomy.

Although an ileal conduit is not the urinary diversion of choice for the majority of patients, some conduits are still indicated for patients with renal insufficiency, gastrointestinal disease, or liver disease, and for patients unable or unwilling to care for a reconstructed bladder (Benson & Olsson, 1992; Richie, 1992). The surgical procedure to construct a Bricker ileal conduit begins with isolating a 15- to 20-cm segment of distal ileum, preserving the blood supply to this bowel segment. The ureters are anastomosed to the isolated segment of ileum that will form the conduit. One end of the conduit is closed, and the open end is brought out through the abdomen and fashioned into a stoma (Benson & Olsson, 1992; Bricker, 1978; Carroll & Barbour, 1995) (Fig. 48-3).

Immediate postoperative surgical complications are relatively uncommon, but can include infection, urinary extravasation, intestinal obstruction, and stomal ischemia (Bales, Kim, & Steinberg, 1996; Carroll & Barbour, 1995). Late complications of an ileal conduit can include pyelonephritis and upper urinary tract deterioration from urine refluxing up the ureters and into the renal pelvis. Stomal complications such as stenosis, hernia formation, skin irritation, and infections are also possible (Carroll & Barbour, 1995). One descriptive study of 144 patients who underwent an ileal conduit urinary diversion reported that 33% of the patients experienced early complications, whereas 28% of the patients experienced late complications. Almost 20% of the patients required another surgical procedure to revise the urinary diversion (Nurmi, Puntala, & Alanen, 1988).

In 1982, Kock described a procedure to construct a continent urine reservoir in patients undergoing cystectomy (Kock, Nilson, Nilsson, Norlén, & Philipson, 1982; Skinner, Boyd, & Lieskovsky, 1984; Skinner, Lieskovsky, & Boyd, 1984, 1987, 1989). The procedure Kock described is similar to that for constructing a continent ileostomy. As depicted in Fig. 48-4, a 60- to 70-cm segment of bowel is isolated with its blood supply intact. The middle portion of the isolated bowel is cut lengthwise and reconfigured into a U-shaped pouch. By reshaping the bowel, the pouch can hold a greater volume of urine as compared with the intact, cylindrical bowel. Also, with the bowel detubularized, the reconstructed reservoir cannot generate an organized peristaltic contraction and leak urine from the pouch.

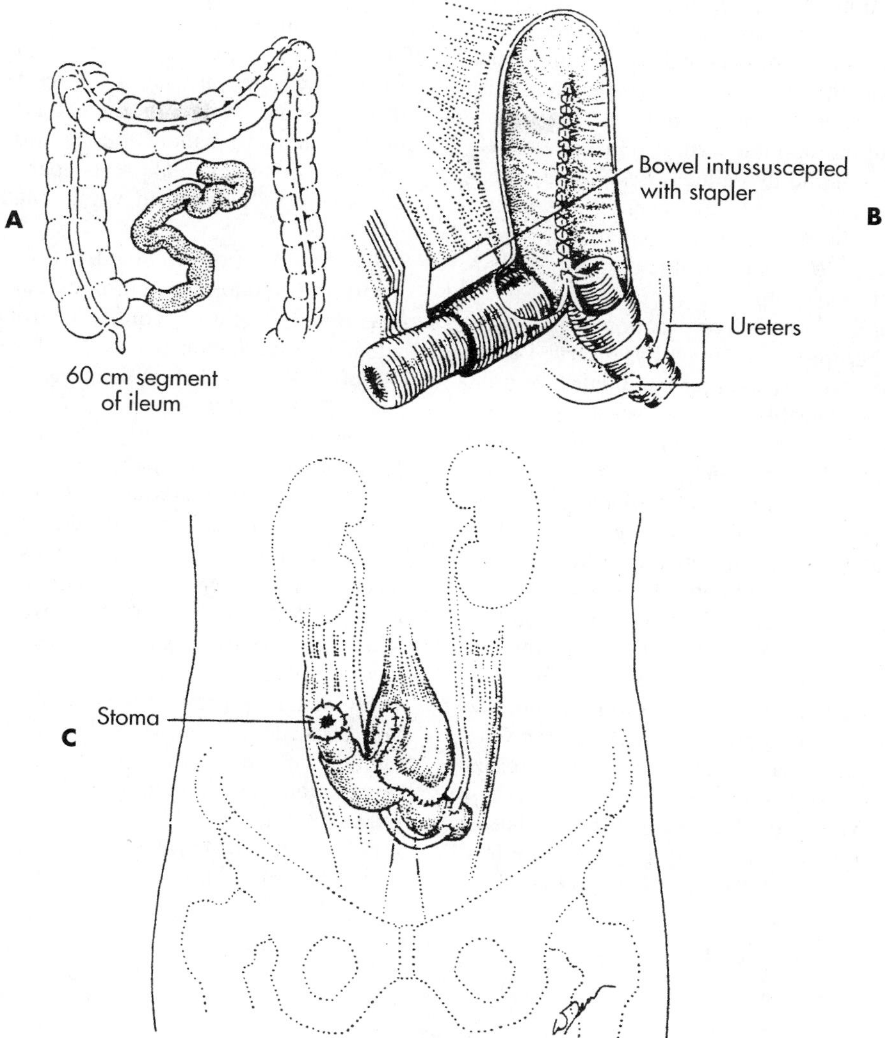

Fig. 48-4 Surgical construction of the Kock pouch urinary reservoir. **A,** A 60- to 70-cm section of small intestine is selected and dissected. **B,** The middle portion of the isolated bowel is cut lengthwise and reconfigured into a U-shaped reservoir. One end of the bowel is intussuscepted and fashioned into a nonrefluxing, afferent valve. The ureters are implanted distal to the afferent valve. The other end of the bowel is also intussuscepted and fashioned into a nonrefluxing, efferent valve that exits the reservoir as an abdominal stoma. **C,** The completed reservoir. (From Carroll, P. R., & Barbour, S. [1995]. Urinary diversion and bladder substitution. In E. A. Tanagho & J. W. McAninch [Eds.], *Smith's general urology* [14th ed.]. Norwalk, CT: Appleton & Lange.)

One end of the bowel segment is intussuscepted and fashioned into a nonrefluxing afferent valve. The ureters are anastomosed to the reservoir through this valve. This valve prevents urine from being forced back up the ureters and into the renal pelvis. The other end of the bowel segment is also intussuscepted and fashioned into a nonrefluxing efferent valve. The efferent valve exits through an abdominal stoma. This valve holds urine in the reservoir until the patient catheterizes the stoma through the efferent valve and drains the reservoir. The pouch holds approximately 500 ml of urine. The patient does not need to wear an external bag. However, many patients wear a small stoma covering to protect clothing from mucus and any accidental urine leakage.

The Mainz (Thüroff, Alken, Riedmiller, Engelmann, Jacobi, & Hohenfellner, 1985, 1986; Thüroff, Alken, Riedmiller, Jacobi, & Hohenfellner, 1988), Indiana (Ahlering, Weinberg, & Razor, 1989, 1991; Rowland, Mitchell, Bihrle, Kahnoski, & Piser, 1987), and Penn (Benson & Olsson, 1992) reservoirs are similar to the Kock reservoir in that they exit through an abdominal stoma that must be periodically catheterized. These reservoirs use different sections of bowel to make the reservoir and valves in an attempt to make the reservoir compliant to larger volumes of urine, improve continence, and reduce the need for surgical revisions of the reservoir. The major disadvantage of these reservoirs remains infection from repeated catheterizations.

To reduce the infection rate in these continent reservoirs and to even more closely approximate normal bladder function, Camey (1985) described a procedure to anastomose an ileal reservoir to the patient's own urethra. The patient voids by relaxing the pelvic floor muscles, and a Valsalva's maneuver forces urine out through the urethra. This type of reconstructed bladder is commonly called a *neobladder* (i.e., new bladder) or an *orthotopic bladder* (i.e., tissue transplanted to function as a bladder in its normal anatomic position). Fig. 48-5 shows a W-shaped ileal neobladder with a planned anastomosis to the urethra.

Originally, orthotopic bladder reconstructions were done only for men where the urethra is routinely preserved with cystectomy. Today, however, women are candidates for urethral sparing and orthotopic bladder reconstruction (Cancrini, de Carli, Fattahi, Pompeo, Cantiani, & von Heland, 1995; Stenzl, Colleselli, Poisel, Feichtinger, Pontasch, & Bartsch, 1995). The Kock, Mainz, and Indiana reservoirs can be anastomosed to the patient's own urethra. Other types of reservoirs that can be constructed to form an orthotopic bladder include the Hautmann orthotopic bladder (Hautmann, Egghart, Frohneberg, & Miller, 1988; Wenderoth, Bachor, Egghart, Frohneberg, Miller, & Hautmann, 1990), the Studer orthotopic bladder (Benson & Olsson, 1992), the sigmoid pouch (Reddy, 1987; Reddy, Lange, & Fraley, 1991), and the gastric pouch (Hauri, 1996). The characteristics and unique features of each of these reservoirs are outlined in Table 48-4.

Depending on the type of bladder reconstruction that is done, construction of a continent urinary reservoir requires 1½ to 3 additional hours of operative time beyond that of an ileal conduit (Razor, 1993). In addition to being able to tolerate the longer surgery, patients must have adequate renal function, as indicated by a serum creatinine less than 2.5 mg per dl. The mucosal wall of the reservoir will reabsorb fluids and urinary waste products, and the patient's kidneys must be able to handle the additional load. A complete gastrointestinal evaluation is part of the preoperative assessment of patients in whom bladder reconstruction is considered.

Contraindications to bladder reconstruction include malabsorptive syndromes, chronic diarrhea, irritative bowel syndrome, ulcerative colitis, neuropathic bowel disease, extensive diverticular disease, or bowel cancer (Benson & Olsson, 1992; Israel, Natale, & Skinner, 1995; Razor, 1993; Richie, 1992). Patients must have adequate motor coordination to perform intermittent self-catheterization. This requirement is true even for patients who have an orthotopic bladder anastomosed to their urethra. This is because catheterization is needed frequently as the patient learns to interpret the sensations of the reconstructed bladder (Israel, Natale, & Skinner, 1995; Razor, 1993; Richie, 1992) and check for residual volumes of urine while learning to urinate with the new bladder (Benson & Olsson, 1992).

Immediate postoperative complications of bladder reservoir constructions occur in 16% to 28% of patients and can include excessive bleeding, urinary extravasation, intestinal obstruction, and infection (Ahlering, Weinberg, & Razor, 1989; Skinner, Lieskovsky, & Boyd, 1989). The patient must be actively involved in his or her postoperative care and in learning how to drain the reconstructed bladder

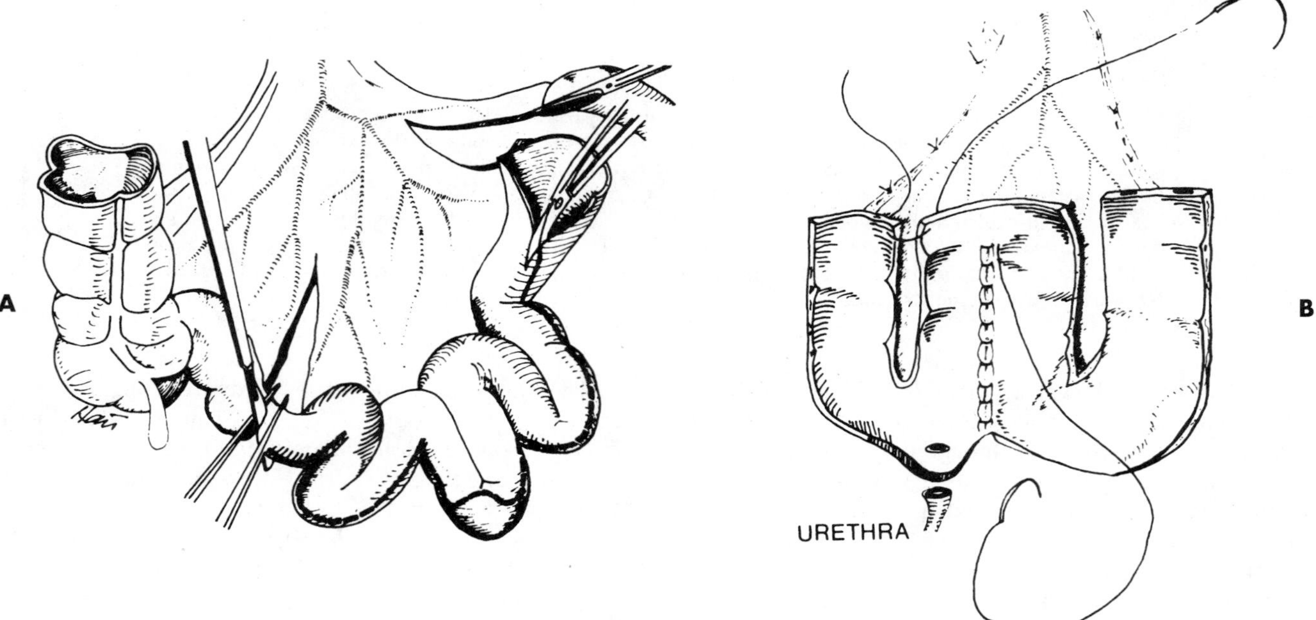

Fig. 48-5 Surgical construction of an ileal, orthotopic neobladder. **A,** A 60- to 70-cm section of small intestine is selected and dissected. **B,** The bowel has been rearranged in a W-shape. A U-shaped flap is identified for anastomosis to the urethra. (From Gillenwater, J. T. [1996]. *Adult and pediatric urology* [3rd ed.]. St. Louis: Mosby.)

TABLE 48-4 Urinary Diversions

Type of Urinary Diversion	Characteristics	Unique Features
Bricker Ileal Conduit (Bricker, 1950, 1978)	*Conduit:* ileum (15 to 20 cm) *Ureters:* anastomosed to ileum *Outlet:* abdominal stoma	The ileal conduit is considered the gold standard of urinary diversion. This is a relatively simple surgical procedure with few immediate postoperative complications. However, over time there is a risk of urine refluxing up the ureters, causing upper tract deterioration. Also, patients' quality of life is adversely affected managing a stoma and wearing an external urinary collection device.
Kock Continent Reservoir (Benson & Olsson, 1992; Kock, Nilson, Nilsson, Norlén, & Philipson, 1982; Skinner, Boyd, & Lieskovsky, 1984; Skinner, Lieskovsky, & Boyd, 1984, 1987, 1989)	*Reservoir:* U-shaped segment of ileum (60 to 70 cm) *Ureters:* anastomosed to an intussuscepted ileal segment to form a nonrefluxing nipple valve *Outlet:* intussuscepted ileum used to construct a catheterizable abdominal stoma or urethra	The Kock pouch is a continent reservoir that is emptied at a time convenient to the patient. The patient still has an abdominal stoma that must be catheterized four to six times a day. There is a risk of nipple valve failure necessitating surgical revision of the reservoir in between 15% and 20% of patients. Also, there is a risk of metabolic and nutritional deficiencies. More recently, the Kock pouch has been used to construct an orthotopic bladder that empties through the urethra.
Mainz Continent Reservoir or Orthotopic Bladder Reservoir (Benson & Olsson, 1992; Thüroff, Alken, Riedmiller, Engelmann, Jacobi, & Hohenfellner, 1985, 1986; Thüroff, Alken, Riedmiller, Jacobi, & Hohenfellner, 1988)	*Reservoir:* spherical segment of ileum (20 to 30 cm) and cecum/ascending colon (10 to 15 cm) *Ureters:* tunneled to form in a nonrefluxing anastomosis *Outlet:* ileocecal valve used to construct a catheterizable abdominal stoma or anastomosed to the urethra	The Mainz pouch has an increased reservoir capacity because of its spherical shape. When the reservoir is drained through an abdominal stoma, the ileocecal valve is used to construct the stoma, eliminating one of the nipple valves and reducing the need for subsequent surgeries to revise malfunctioning valves.
Indiana Continent Reservoir (Ahlering, Weinberg, & Razor, 1989, 1991; Benson & Olsson, 1992; Rowland, Mitchell, Bihrle, Kahnoski, & Piser, 1987)	*Reservoir:* U-shaped segment of ileum (8-18 cm) and cecum/ascending colon (20-30 cm) *Ureters:* tunneled into tenia of the colon to form a nonrefluxing anastomosis *Outlet:* tapered ileocecal valve used to make continent catheterizable abdominal stoma or anastomosed to the urethra	Like the Mainz pouch, the Indiana pouch uses the ileocecal valve to construct the abdominal stoma or to anastomose the reservoir to the urethra. In constructing the Indiana reservoir, the ileocecal valve is tapered to improve continence.
Penn Continent Reservoir (Benson & Olsson, 1992; Duckett & Snyder, 1986)	*Reservoir:* ileum and cecum/ascending colon or entire ascending colon *Ureters:* tunneled to form a nonrefluxing anastomosis *Outlet:* appendix used to construct a catheterizable abdominal stoma	The Penn pouch uses the appendix to construct the abdominal stoma. The appendix is naturally tapered, which improves the continence of the reservoir without the need for surgical tapering.
Camey II Orthotopic Bladder Reservoir (Benson & Olsson, 1992; Camey, 1985)	*Reservoir:* U-shaped segment of ileum (65 cm) *Ureters:* tunneled to form a nonrefluxing anastomosis *Outlet:* urethra	The Camey pouch was the first reservoir that drained through the patient's own urethra. The incidence of reservoir infection was reduced by eliminating the need to catheterize the reservoir.
Ileal Neobladder, or the Hautmann Orthotopic Bladder Reservoir (Benson & Olsson, 1992; Hautmann, Egghart, Frohneberg, & Miller, 1988; Wenderoth, Bachor, Egghart, Frohneberg, Miller, & Hautmann, 1990)	Reservoir: M- or W-shaped segment of ileum (60 to 70 cm) *Ureters:* tunneled to form a nonrefluxing anastomosis *Outlet:* urethra	The surgery to construct an ileal neobladder is a shorter procedure because the reconfigured ileum is simply sutured without an attempt to create water-tight suture lines. Patients have ureteral stints in place at least 3 weeks to divert urine while the reservoir is healing.

Continued

TABLE 48-4 Urinary Diversions—cont'd

Type of Urinary Diversion	Characteristics	Unique Features
Studer Orthotopic Bladder Reservoir (Benson & Olsson, 1992)	*Reservoir:* intact segment of ileum (60 cm) is folded up onto itself *Ureters:* simple anastomosis to ileum *Outlet:* urethra	The intact rostral end of the Studer reservoir continues to have peristaltic muscle contractions that prevent ureteral urine reflux, but that are not so strong as to cause increased incontinence.
Sigmoid Pouch (Benson & Olsson, 1992; Reddy, 1987; Reddy, Lange, & Fraley, 1991)	*Reservoir:* U-shaped segment of sigmoid colon (30 to 35 cm) detubularized *Ureters:* tunnelled to form a nonrefluxing anastomosis *Outlet:* urethra	Creating a reservoir from this section of colon is an easier surgery to perform because of the location of the sigmoid colon relative to the ureters and urethra. Patients usually do not experience any change in their bowel habits after this surgery and are not at risk for nutritional deficiencies as a result of this surgery. Patients may be at a higher risk for colon cancer of the reservoir.
Gastric Pouch (Hauri, 1996)	*Reservoir:* trapezoidal segment of stomach (10-15 cm along the greater curvature), the serosa is incised crosswise to increase capacity *Ureters:* tunneled to form a nonrefluxing anastomosis *Outlet:* urethra	Because the parietal cells of the stomach secrete hydrochloric acid, the urine stored in the reservoir is kept at a lower pH and patients have fewer urinary infections.

through a stoma or the urethra. Immediate postoperative incontinence is common, but over time, approximately 90% of patients achieve day continence and 85% of patients achieve night continence (Bales, Kim, & Steinberg, 1996). The long-term complication rate of urinary reservoir construction is between 15% and 22% (Bales, Kim, & Steinberg, 1996; Skinner, Lieskovsky, & Boyd, 1989; Wenderoth et al., 1990) and can include metabolic disorders, stomal stenosis, pyelonephritis, renal calculi, and renal deterioration (Carroll & Barbour, 1995), necessitating medical treatment and often additional surgery.

Radiation Therapy

Primary Radiation Therapy. Because of the survival advantage definitive surgery offers patients with invasive bladder cancer, radiation therapy is often not considered a primary treatment of this disease. However, as shown in Table 48-1, primary radiation therapy can offer some patients long-term survival and is the treatment of choice for patients who refuse surgery, cannot tolerate surgery because of other medical conditions, or have widespread pelvic disease that cannot be surgically resected (Gospodarowicz & Warde, 1992; Israel, Natale, & Skinner, 1995; Wesson, 1992). In countries other than the United States, particularly Great Britain and Canada, radiation therapy is considered the primary treatment for invasive bladder tumors, and cystectomy is reserved for patients who fail to respond to radiation therapy (Lamm & Torti, 1996; Sternberg, 1996; Wesson, 1992).

Doses of external beam radiation used to treat bladder tumors are between 6000 and 7000 cGy in daily fractions of 180 to 200 cGy over 7 to 8 weeks (Fair, Fuks, & Scher, 1993; Gospodarowicz & Warde, 1992; Wesson, 1992). Four field-treatment techniques (anterior, posterior, right lateral, and left lateral) permit higher doses of radiation to be delivered to the bladder while minimizing the dose to the rectum, small bowel, and local tissues (Gospodarowicz & Warde, 1992). The patient should be instructed to empty his or her bladder just before treatment to ensure that the radiation dose is consistently delivered to the intended treatment field.

Between 50% and 70% of patients treated with external beam radiation experience acute, self-limiting side effects specific to the urinary tract and lower gastrointestinal tract, including IBS, diarrhea, and rectal irritation (Fair, Fuks, & Scher, 1993; Gospodarowicz, Hawkins, Rawlings, Connolly, Jewett, & Thomas et al., 1989; Sell, Jakobsen, Nerstrøm, Sørensen, Steven, & Barlebo, 1991). In addition, skin reactions in the radiation treatment ports are possible, and most patients report fatigue. IBS can be treated with a urinary analgesic such as phenazopyridine (Pyridium). Care must be taken to rule out a urinary tract infection before prescribing a medication to treat the symptoms. Diarrhea can be treated with kaolin and pectin (Kaopectate), loperamide (Imodium), or diphenoxylate hydrochloride with atropine sulfate (Lomotil).

Late toxic effects of external beam radiation occurring 3 months to 3 years after treatment can affect bladder and bowel function. Patients can experience a reduction in bladder capacity accompanied by severe urinary frequency, hematuria, persistent diarrhea, bowel obstruction, bowel necrosis, and/or bowel perforation (Duncan & Quilty, 1986; Gospodarowicz & Warde, 1992). Late radiation-related bladder and bowel complications requiring treatment can occur in 3% to 20% of patients (Duncan & Quilty, 1986; Gospodarowicz et al., 1989; Sell et al., 1991).

For patients who do not respond to primary radiation therapy or whose cancer recurs some time after radiation therapy, a salvage cystectomy with bladder reconstruction is recommended (Gospodarowicz & Warde, 1992). There has been some concern that construction of a urinary reservoir might not be possible in these patients. However, prior radiation therapy does not appear to increase the incidence of complications in patients undergoing cystectomy and bladder reconstruction (Ahlering, Kanellos, Boyd, Lieskovsky, Skinner, & Bernstein, 1988; Gospodarowicz & Warde, 1992; Gschwend, May, Paiss, Gottfried, & Hautmann, 1996).

Other radiation techniques that have been used to treat patients with invasive bladder cancer include intraoperative external beam therapy, hyperfractionization of doses, and brachytherapy (Gospodarowicz & Warde, 1992; Israel, Natale, & Skinner, 1995; Wesson, 1992). To date, however, these techniques have neither improved the long-term survival nor reduced the toxicity of standard external beam therapy.

Preoperative Radiation Therapy. Over the previous 2 decades, numerous retrospective reviews have suggested that preoperative radiation therapy reduced intraoperative tumor seeding and thereby improved long-term survival of patients with invasive bladder cancer. However, various prospective randomized studies have failed to demonstrate any benefit of preoperative radiation therapy (Crawford, Das, & Smith, 1987; Gospodarowicz & Warde, 1992). Currently, preoperative radiation therapy for invasive bladder cancer is not recommended routinely (Crawford, Das, & Smith, 1987; Fair, Fuks, & Scher, 1993; Israel, Natale, & Skinner, 1995).

Systemic Chemotherapy

Bladder carcinoma is considered a chemotherapy-sensitive tumor, and yet the role of chemotherapy in the treatment of this disease is not clearly defined. Chemotherapy is not a primary treatment of invasive bladder cancer, but rather is an adjunct to definitive surgery and/or radiation therapy. Whether chemotherapy is best used before primary therapy, after definitive therapy, or only in patients with widespread metastatic disease is not known. Various clinical trials are currently underway to address these issues.

Table 48-5 outlines the typical chemotherapy treatment protocols used to treat a patient with invasive bladder cancer. Combinations of the drugs methotrexate, vinblastine, doxorubicin (Adriamycin), and cisplatin (MVAC) or cisplatin, methotrexate, and vinblastine (CMV) are considered the most effective regimens in the treatment of transitional cell carcinoma (Sternberg, 1995). Between 40% and 70% of patients with measurable disease respond to combination chemotherapy regimens (Roth, 1996; Sternberg, 1995). Whether chemotherapy lengthens a patient's disease-free or long-term survival is currently under investigation.

Patients receiving chemotherapy can experience significant toxicities, including myelosuppression (from doxorubicin, methotrexate, and vinblastine), renal toxicity (from cisplatin), mucositis (from methotrexate), nausea and vomiting (from cisplatin and doxorubicin), alopecia (from doxorubicin), taste alterations (from cisplatin), fatigue (from cisplatin, doxorubicin, methotrexate, and vinblastine), and ototoxicity (from cisplatin). Patients must be able to tolerate aggressive hydration to reduce the risk of renal toxicity from cisplatin. Adriamycin is a cardiotoxic agent, and cardiac function should be monitored with left ventricular ejection fraction (LVEF), especially in patients with a history of cardiac dysfunction. Substituting carboplatin for cisplatin and mitoxantrone for adriamycin reduces a patient's risk for renal toxicity and cardiotoxicity, but whether the long-term survival for patients receiving regimens with these drugs is equivalent to that of patients receiving regimens containing cisplatin and adriamycin is not known (Small, Fippin, Ernest, & Carroll, 1996). Use of the hematopoietic growth factors has reduced the number of days patients are neutropenic and the incidence of mucositis, thereby allowing more patients to receive full doses of therapy (Gabrilove, Jakubowski, Scher, Sternberg, Wong, & Grous et al., 1988). However, this approach has not improved overall response rates to these drugs. Neither has escalating the dose of drugs while supporting patients with hematopoietic growth factors improved overall response rates (Loehrer, Elson, Dreicer, Hahn, Nichols, & Williams et al., 1994; Seidman, Scher, Gabrilove, Bajorin, Motzer, & O'Dell et al., 1993).

The use of chemotherapy to treat invasive bladder cancer has been reviewed extensively by Roth (1996), and the interested reader is referred to this source for more detailed information about specific agents that have been used singly or in combination.

Neoadjuvant Chemotherapy. Neoadjuvant chemotherapy is administered before definitive surgery to downstage the tumor and treat micrometastatic disease that may be present at the time of diagnosis (Fair, Fuks, & Scher, 1993; Smith & Kantoff, 1995; Sternberg, 1996). The use of chemotherapy before surgery enables better delivery of drugs to the tumor than is possible after surgery that may damage the vascular bed (Scher, 1990). Patients can better tolerate chemotherapy before major pelvic surgery, allowing the full dose of the drug to be administered on schedule (Smith & Kantoff, 1995; Sternberg, 1996). Generally three cycles of MVAC or CMV are administered. However, the primary tumor serves as a marker of response to therapy guiding the optimal duration of chemotherapy before attempting surgery. One disadvantage of neoadjuvant chemotherapy is that patients who have a complete response to neoadjuvant chemotherapy may refuse definitive surgery (Fair, Fuks, & Scher, 1993). Also, for patients who do not respond to neoadjuvant chemotherapy, 2 or 3 months may be wasted before definitive surgery can be performed (Sternberg, 1996).

Sternberg (1996) has reviewed 11 neoadjuvant chemotherapy trials. These trials report overall response rates of between 60% and 70% with complete response rates of 30%. However, this treatment approach has not yet been

TABLE 48-5 Adjuvant Chemotherapy Treatment Regimens for Invasive Bladder Cancer

Regimen	Dose of Drug and Day in Cycle of Treatment	Cycle Interval
MVAC		
*M*ethotrexate	30 mg/m^2 on days 1, 15, and 22	28 days
*V*inblastine (Velban)	3 mg/m^2 on days 2, 15, and 22	
Doxorubicin (*A*driamycin)	300 mg/m^2 on day 2	
*C*isplatin (Platinol, CDDP)	70 mg/m^2 on day 2	
CMV		
*C*isplatin (Platinol, CDDP)	70-100 mg/m^2 on day 2	21 days
*M*ethotrexate	30 mg/m^2 on days 1 and 8	
*V*inblastine (Velban)	3-4 mg/m^2 on days 1 and 8	
MVNC		
*M*ethotrexate	50 mg/m^2 on days 1 and 15	28 days
*V*inblastine (Velban)	3 mg/m^2 on day 1	
Mitoxantrone (*N*ovantrone)	10 mg/m^2 on day 1	
*C*arboplatin (Paraplatin)	200 mg/m^2 on day 1	

MVAC information modified from Herr, H. W. & Scher, H. I. (1994). Neoadjuvant chemotherapy and partial cystectomy for invasive bladder cancer. *Journal of Clinical Oncology, 12*(5), 975-980; Logothetis, C. J., Dexeus, F. H., Finn, L., Sella, A., Amato, R. J., Ayala, A. G. et al. (1990). A prospective randomized trial comparing MVAC and CISCA chemotherapy for patients with metastatic urothelial tumors. *Journal of Clinical Oncology, 8*(6), 1050-1055; Roth, B. J. (1996). Chemotherapy for advanced bladder cancer. *Seminars in Oncology, 23*(5), 633-644; Sternberg, C. N., Arena, M. G., Calabresi, F., Carli, P. D., Platania, A., & Zeuli, M. et al. (1993). Neoadjuvant M-VAC (methotrexate, vinblastine, doxorubicin, and cisplatin) for infiltrating transitional cell carcinoma of the bladder. *Cancer, 72*(6), 1975-1982; Sternberg, C. N., Yagoda, A., Scher, H. I., Watson, R. C., Herr, H. W., & Morse, M. J., et al. (1988). M-VAC (methotrexate, vinblastine, doxorubicin, and cisplatin) for advanced transitional cell carcinoma of the urothelium. *Journal of Urology, 139*(3), 461-469; Sternberg, C. N., Yagoda, A., Scher, H. I., Watson, R. C., Geller, N., & Herr, H. W., (1989). Methotrexate, vinblastine, doxorubicin, and cisplatin for advanced transitional cell carcinoma of the urothelium: Efficacy and patterns of response and relapse. *Cancer, 64*(12), 2448-2458.
CMV information modified from Freiha, F., Reese, J., & Torti, F. M. (1996). A randomized trial of radical cystectomy versus radical cystectomy plus cisplatin, vinblastine and methotrexate chemotherapy for muscle invasive bladder cancer. *Journal of Urology, 155*(2), 495-500; Harker, W. G., Meyers, F. J., Freiha, F. S., Palmer, J. M., Shortliffe, L. D., & Hannigan J.F. et al. (1985). Cisplatin, methotrexate, and vinblastine (CMV): An effective chemotherapy regimen for metastatic transitional cell carcinoma of the urinary tract: A Northern California Oncology Group study. *Journal of Clinical Oncology, 3*(11), 1463-1470.
MVNC information modified from Roth, B. J. (1996). Chemotherapy for advanced bladder cancer. *Seminars in Oncology, 23*(5), 633-644; Small, E. J., Fippin, L. J., Ernest, M. L., & Carroll, P. R. (1996). A carboplatin-based regimen for the treatment of patients with advanced transitional cell carcinoma of the urothelium. *Cancer, 78*(8), 1775-1780.

shown to improve overall survival (Smith & Kantoff, 1995; Sternberg, 1996).

Adjuvant Chemotherapy. In contrast to neoadjuvant chemotherapy, which is administered before definitive surgery, adjuvant chemotherapy is administered after removal of the primary tumor, when no residual disease can be identified but when the patient is at a high risk for disease recurrence (Fair, Fuks, & Scher, 1993; Smith & Kantoff, 1995; Sternberg, 1996). Up to 50% of patients with bladder cancer develop metastasis after cystectomy (Prout, Griffin, & Shipley, 1979; Sternberg, 1995). Two thirds of these relapsing patients develop distant metastases, indicating that micrometastasis had already occurred at the time of the initial surgery (Sternberg, 1995). This group of patients seems to be a population that would benefit from adjuvant chemotherapy. However, although disease-free survival has been lengthened in a subset of high-risk patients, an overall survival benefit has not been shown in patients who received adjuvant chemotherapy. It has been difficult to recruit enough patients for adjuvant chemotherapy clinical trials to make meaningful comparisons between treatment arms while controlling for confounding factors such as the physical condition of the patient, disease stage, and tumor grade (Smith & Kantoff, 1995; Sternberg, 1996). It is very difficult for patients who have recently undergone major pelvic surgery to tolerate full-dose chemotherapy on schedule. Two studies designed to test the benefits of adjuvant chemotherapy reported that less than half of the patients randomized to receive chemotherapy completed the planned four cycles of therapy (Skinner, Daniels, Russell, Lieskovsky, Boyd, & Nichols et al., 1991; Stöckle, Meyenburg, Wellek, Voges, Rossmann, & Gertenbach et al., 1995).

Sternberg (1996) has reviewed six trials of adjuvant chemotherapy. These trials suggest that patients with T2 or T3a disease do not benefit from adjuvant therapy, but patients with stage T3b or T4 disease or those who have nodal disease may benefit from adjuvant chemotherapy (Smith & Kantoff, 1995; Sternberg, 1996).

Chemotherapy for Recurrent or Metastatic Disease

Only approximately 5% of patients present with clinically evident metastases at the time they are diagnosed with bladder cancer (Fleshner et al., 1996). However, up to 50% of patients who present with muscle-invasive bladder tumors

TABLE 48-6 Average Costs of Bladder Cancer Treatment in Europe, Japan, and the United States

Treatment	Holland	Japan	United States
Three cycles of MVAC chemotherapy	$ 4,285	$4,960	$ 5,240
Radical radiotherapy(6000 cGy)	$ 2,335	$1,500	$ 1,670
Radical cystectomy with bladder reconstruction	$10,800	$8,400	$11,850

From Sternberg, C. N., Raghavan, D., Ohi, Y., Bajorin, D., Herr, H., & Kato, T. et al (1995). Neo-adjuvant and adjuvant chemotherapy in locally advanced disease: what are the effects on survival and prognosis. *International Journal of Urology, 2*(Suppl. 2), 76-88.

develop metastatic disease, usually within 2 years of diagnosis (Prout, Griffin, & Shipley, 1979; Sternberg, 1995). Combination chemotherapy, with either MVAC or CMV, is the primary treatment for patients with metastatic disease. Between one third and two thirds of patients have a complete response or a partial response to chemotherapy with a median survival of 8 to 12 months (Harker et al., 1985; Loehrer, Einhorn, Elson, Crawford, Kuebler, & Tannock et al., 1992; Loehrer et al., 1994; Logothetis et al., 1990; Sternberg, Yagoda, Scher, Watson, Geller, & Herr et al., 1989).

As discussed previously, patients can experience severe toxicities from these drugs. Although chemotherapy can prolong a patient's life for several months, the patient's quality of life can be adversely affected by the side effects of therapy, such as infection, nausea, mucositis, alopecia, taste alterations, and fatigue. For patients debilitated by their disease or with other medical conditions, symptomatic management of their metastatic bladder cancer may be a better option than an aggressive combination chemotherapy regimen. Patient characteristics associated with higher response rates to chemotherapy and longer survival are high performance status (Karnofsky Performance Status greater than 90), normal alkaline phosphatase, stable weight, and absence of lung, liver, and bone metastasis (Geller, Sternberg, Penenberg, Scher, & Yagoda, 1991; Loehrer et al., 1992, 1994).

Combined Modality Treatment for Bladder Preservation

Three bladder-preserving strategies in the treatment of invasive bladder cancer have already been discussed: repeat TURB, partial cystectomy, and primary radiation therapy. A fourth approach to treatment of invasive tumors that preserves bladder function combines chemotherapy and radiation therapy after TURB (Douglas, Kaufman, Zietman, Althausen, Heney, & Shipley, 1996; Bales, Kim, & Steinberg, 1996). Chemotherapy not only reduces the risk of recurrence by treating micrometastatic disease at the time of diagnosis, but chemotherapy also serves as a radiosensitizer, increasing the likelihood that radiation therapy will eradicate the tumor in the bladder.

Typically, patients are given two 28-day cycles of CMV (cisplatin, methotrexate, and vinblastine). This is followed by 4000 cGy of radiotherapy to the bladder and pelvic lymphatic system with cisplatin (70 mg/m^2) administered concurrently as a radiosensitizer on day 0 and on day 22 of radiation therapy (Kachnic, Kaufman, Heney, Althausen, Griffin, & Zietman et al., 1997; Kaufman, Shipley, Griffin, Heney, Althausen, & Efird, 1993; Tester, Caplan, Heaney, Venner, Whittington, & Byhardt et al., 1996). Patients then undergo another cystoscopy, and those with complete responses receive an additional 3000 cGy of radiotherapy again with cisplatin (70 mg/m^2). Patients who do not respond to induction therapy are referred for cystectomy. In four clinical trials involving almost 450 patients (Dunst, Sauer, Schrott, Kühn, Wittekind, & Altendorf-Hofmann, 1994; Housset, Maulard, Chretien, Dufour, Delanian, & Huart et al., 1993; Kachnic et al., 1997; Kaufman et al., 1993; Tester, Porter, Asbell, Coughlin, Heaney, & Krall et al., 1993; Tester et al., 1996), between 53% and 80% of patients responded to induction therapy and were able to preserve their own bladders. Of these patients, between 62% and 89% were alive 4 years after diagnosis with a functioning, tumor-free bladder. Bladder-preserving surgery and adjuvant therapy may be an option for selected patients, offering long-term survival and an excellent quality of life (Bales, Kim, & Steinberg, 1996; Douglas et al., 1996).

Cost Comparisons

A comparison of the costs of the various treatments is shown in Table 48-6. Radical radiotherapy is by far the least expensive of the treatment options, although the costs quickly escalate if the patient fails primary radiation therapy and requires a salvage cystectomy with bladder reconstruction. This type of analysis plays an increasingly important role in the future for individuals facing their own treatment decisions as well as for managed care institutions making policy decisions for their beneficiaries (Sternberg, 1996).

ONCOLOGIC EMERGENCIES

The major oncologic emergency associated with invasive bladder cancer is urinary obstruction. Obstruction of the ureters usually occurs when the primary lesion has extended beyond the bladder wall and externally compresses the ureter. Patients may experience a dull backache, but more commonly they do not report any symptoms. An IVU shows poor drainage from the renal pelvis and a dilated ureter above the obstruction. A CT scan shows the compressed ureter as well as the dimensions of the mass causing the obstruction. Ureteral stints can be placed radiologically to drain the kidney until definitive treatment can be initiated.

An acute obstruction of the urethra is rare. Usually, patients experience hesitancy, decreased force of their urine stream, and frequency, which brings them to medical attention before the urethra is completely occluded. If the urethra is obstructed by a tumor in the bladder or by a tumor externally compressing the urethra, an indwelling or suprapubic catheter can be placed to drain urine until definitive treatment can be instituted.

NURSING MANAGEMENT

The patient with invasive bladder cancer has many physical and psychological concerns that require nursing interventions. Nurses are integrally involved in educating, treating, and supporting the patient and family during various surgical, radiation, and chemotherapy procedures and treatments (Broadwell & Jackson, 1982; Hossan & Striegel, 1993; Kelly & Miaskowski, 1996; Leek, Sebastian, Kawachi, & Sullivan, 1996; Lind, Kravitz, & Greig, 1993; McGinn, 1985; Miaskowski, 1995; Moore, Newton, Grant, & Keetch, 1993; Razor, 1993; Smith & Johnson, 1986; Tootla & Easterling, 1992; Watt, 1986).

Surgery

The major concerns are knowledge deficit, altered urinary elimination, altered bowel function, pain, potential for fluid and electrolyte imbalance, potential for respiratory complications, and potential for anxiety (Table 48-7).

Preoperatively, the nurse should review the surgical procedure with the patient and family and what to expect postoperatively. If an ileal conduit or reservoir that empties through an abdominal stoma is planned, preoperative assessment for stoma site selection is essential. The urologist often consults with a specially trained enterostomal therapy nurse to determine with the patient where the stoma should be placed. Usually, a site in the lower right abdominal quadrant on an imaginary line extending between the umbilicus and the anterior superior iliac spine is chosen. The site should be as far lateral as possible, while still allowing the stoma to be brought through the abdominal rectus muscle for support (Benson & Olsson, 1992; Carroll & Barbour, 1995).

As shown in Fig. 48-6, postoperatively patients have a nasogastric tube to decompress the stomach, a longitudinal abdominal incision, a surgical drain (e.g., Penrose, Jackson Pratt) to drain fluid from the surgical field, and some type of urinary drainage. Patients with a reconstructed bladder emptying through an abdominal stoma have a drainage tube (e.g., Malecot, Medena, Robinson) through the stoma to drain urine. Patients with a reconstructed bladder anastomosed to the urethra have a Foley catheter sutured in place to drain urine. Most surgeons also place ureteral stints that divert urine from the reservoir and maintain the patency of the ureters while the surgical incisions heal. These stints may be externalized through a separate abdominal stab wound, or they may drain directly into the reconstructed

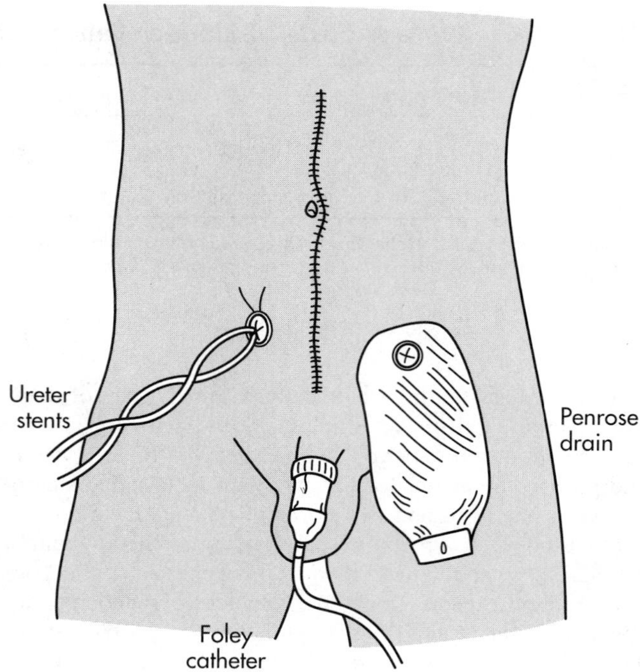

Fig. 48-6 Postoperative abdomen. Reservoir to urethra with stents exteriorized to skin surface and sutured in place. Penrose pouched. Parachute cord stabilizing Foley catheter. (From Razor, B. R. [1993]. Continent urinary reservoirs. *Seminars in Oncology Nursing, 9*[4], 277.)

bladder and not be visible. These stints can become obstructed with blood and sediment and, if accessible, need to be irrigated with 3 to 5 ml of sterile normal saline every 4 to 6 hours, or as prescribed by the surgeon (Razor, 1993). A reconstructed bladder initially produces large amounts of mucus. Immediately postoperatively, the tube draining the reservoir (i.e., Malecot, Medena, Robinson, Foley catheter) needs to be flushed with 30 to 120 ml of saline every 4 to 8 hours and as needed to keep the tube patent and free of mucus (Benson & Olsson, 1992; Razor, 1993). A new reservoir's capacity is usually between 150 and 250 ml, and this volume should not be exceeded when performing repeated irrigations.

The patient is also at risk for fluid and electrolyte imbalance because fluid and urinary wastes can be reabsorbed thorough the reconstructed bladder. The patient's risk for metabolic imbalances depends in part on the section of bowel that was used for the bladder reconstruction. Table 48-8 outlines immediate and long-term metabolic imbalances specific to the bowel used in the reconstruction. The patient's serum electrolytes and creatinine should be monitored and the patient assessed for signs and symptoms of imbalance.

Patients are usually hospitalized for 7 days or until bowel function returns. Approximately 1 week after surgery, radiologic contrast studies are done to evaluate the ureteral anastomoses and the reservoir sutures. If there is no extravasation of the contrast dye, the ureteral stints and the surgical drain are removed (Benson & Olsson, 1992). If there is any

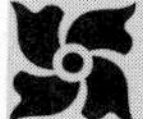

Table 48-7 Standard of Care for the Patient Undergoing a Cystectomy with Bladder Reconstruction

Patient Problem and Outcomes	Nursing Interventions and Rationales	Patient Education Instructions
Knowledge Deficit		
Patient will verbalize an understanding of the surgical procedure and how the orthotopic bladder will function.	1. Determine who the patient's support person is, and have this person present when teaching is done. 2. Assess the patient's level of understanding of the surgical procedure. 3. Give the patient the opportunity to ask questions or verbalize concerns.	1. Use a gender-specific diagram of the anatomy of the pelvis to explain the procedure. 2. Provide the patient with information about the preoperative routine: a. Gastrointestinal workup b. Anesthesiology consult c. Mechanical and antibiotic bowel preparation (clear liquid diet 1 to 3 days before surgery and purging enemas the day before surgery) d. For the patient who will have reservoir to stoma: stoma site marking e. For the patient who will have reservoir to urethra: Kegal exercises 3. Provide patient with information about the postoperative plan of care: a. Management of pain b. Home care of surgical drains and catheters c. Anticipated discharge d. Follow-up with Urology Service
Altered Urinary Elimination		
Patient will demonstrate an understanding of the urinary diversion as evidenced by the ability to care for the orthotopic bladder and identify signs and symptoms of complications.	1. Using sterile technique, flush the ureteral stints as prescribed (e.g., every 4 to 6 hours with 3 to 5 ml of sterile saline) and as needed to keep the stints patent and free of blood and sediment. 2. Using clean technique, flush the reservoir catheter as prescribed (e.g., every 4 to 8 hours with 30 to 120 ml of saline) and as needed to keep the catheter patent and free of mucus. 3. Assess for stoma viability. 4. Assess for urine extravasation through surgical drain.	1. Teach the patient how to care for ureteral stints, stoma catheter (e.g., Malecot, Medena, or Robinson), and/or urethral catheter (e.g., Foley catheter). 2. Encourage the patient to continue Kegal exercises. 3. About 7 to 12 days after surgery, the stints and catheters will be removed and the patient taught by the urologist or urology nurse how to void by relaxing the pelvic muscles and performing a Valsalva maneuver.
Altered Bowel Function		
Patient will have normal bowel function as evidenced by bowel sounds, bowel movements, and the ability to eat without nausea or vomiting.	1. Maintain patency of nasogastric tube. 2. Ambulate patient three times a day, increasing the frequency as the patient can tolerate.	1. After bowel function has returned and the nasogastric tube has been removed, teach the patient to take actions to facilitate gastrointestinal mobility: a. Ambulate three times a day. b. Drink between 1500 and 2000 ml of fluid each day. c. Eat foods high in fiber such as whole grains, fruits, and vegetables.

Continued

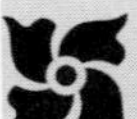

TABLE 48-7 Standard of Care for the Patient Undergoing a Cystectomy With Bladder Reconstruction—cont'd

Patient Problem and Outcomes	Nursing Interventions and Rationales	Patient Education Instructions
Pain		
Patient will experience optimal pain relief with minimal side effects	1. Assess pain intensity using a 0-10 verbal rating scale every 2 to 4 hours while the patient is hospitalized. 2. Administer opioid analgesics as the patient requires to keep pain intensity below 2 or 3 on the 0-10 scale. 3. Monitor for analgesic side effects, and administer medications to prevent or treat the following: a. Constipation b. Pruritus c. Nausea	1. While the patient is hospitalized, teach him or her to inform the nurse if experiencing pain. 2. Teach the patient to take the prescribed pain medication often enough to control the pain. 3. Teach the patient that there may be side effects from the pain medication and how to manage side effects if they occur.
Potential for Altered Fluid and Electrolyte Imbalance (depending on the section of bowel used for the reconstruction)		
Patient will have a stable weight, fluid intake approximately equal to urine output, and serum electrolyte measures within normal limits	1. Daily weights 2. Monitor intake and output. 3. Monitor serum electrolytes and creatinine. 4. Assess the patient for nausea, vomiting, anorexia, and muscle weakness.	1. Depending on the section of the bowel used for reconstruction, teach the patient to monitor for signs and symptoms of fluid and electrolyte imbalance as outlined in Table 48-8.
Potential for Respiratory Complications		
Patient will not experience atelectasis, pneumonia, or pulmonary embolus	1. Apply intermittent compression stockings to both legs. 2. Encourage the patient to turn, cough, breathe deeply, and use incentive spirometry every 2 hours while awake. 3. Perform active range-of-motion leg exercises to prevent deep vein thrombophlebitis. 4. Ambulate the patient twice a day, increasing the frequency as the patient can tolerate. 5. Prohibit smoking.	1. Encourage the patient to continue pulmonary toilet, range-of-motion leg exercises, and ambulation. 2. Encourage the patient not to smoke, and provide information on available local smoking cessation programs.
Potential for Anxiety		
Patient will: • Express feelings of decreased anxiety • Identify strategies to cope with anxiety	1. Complete patient teaching of the procedure so that the patient's anxiety is not due to a knowledge deficit. 2. Determine which coping strategies the patient has used effectively in the past to decrease anxiety, and reinforce the use of these coping strategies. 3. Administer pharmacologic agents to decrease anxiety, if necessary.	

question of extravasation, the stints are left in place an additional 5 days. Patients are discharged with a drainage tube (i.e., Malecot, Medena, Robinson, Foley catheter) to keep the new urinary reservoir decompressed while it continues to heal. This drainage tube needs to be flushed with normal saline at least two to three times a day to keep the tube patent and free of mucus. The patient and family need to be instructed on how to care for these tubes and allowed time to practice while the patient is still hospitalized.

Approximately 3 weeks after surgery, 2 weeks after discharge, the patient returns to the urologist to have another radiologic contrast study of the reservoir. If there is no extravasation of the contrast dye, the urinary drainage tube is removed and the patient taught stomal catheterization or how to void through their urethra by relaxing the pelvic muscles and performing a Valsalva maneuver.

Patients who have a reservoir that empties through an abdominal stoma are instructed to catheterize the reservoir ev-

TABLE 48-8 Potential Metabolic and Nutritional Imbalances in Patients with a Urinary Diversion

Bowel Segment Used to Construct the Urinary Diversion	Possible Fluid and Electrolyte Imbalance	Signs and Symptoms	Treatment
Stomach	1. Hypergastremia 2. Decreased production of intrinsic factor 3. Decreased hydrochloric acid secretion	1. Peptic ulcer disease 2. Vitamin B_{12} deficiency 3. Maldigestion of protein and incomplete release and solubilization of iron and calcium from foods: a. Iron deficiency anemia b. Hypocalcemia	1. H_2 antagonists 2. Vitamin B_{12} replacement 3. Iron replacement 4. Calcium replacement
Ileum	1. Decreased absorption of bile salts resulting in malabsorption of fat and fat-soluble vitamins (i.e., A & D) 2. Increased oxalate absorption because fatty acids bind to calcium 3. Vitamin B_{12} deficiency 4. Hyperchloremia and hypernatremia	1. Secretory diarrhea and/or steatorrhea 2. Urolithiasis 3. Megaloblastic anemia, neurologic injury, glossitis, and anorexia	1. Cholestyramine to bind free bile salts, low-fat diet (<40 g/day), loperamide, codeine, or diphenoxylate to decrease gastrointestinal motility 2. Adequate hydration, alkalinize urine, avoid foods high in oxalate, oral calcium citrate supplements 3. B_{12} replacement
Large intestine	1. Dehydration	1. Diarrhea	1. Antidiarrheal medications

Modified from Carroll, P. R. & Barbour, S. (1995). Urinary diversion and bladder substitution. In E. A. Tanagho & J. W. McAninch (Eds.), *Smith's general urology* (14th ed.). Norwalk, CT: Appleton & Lange; Steiner, M. S. & Morton, R. A. (1991). Nutritional and gastrointestinal complications of the use of bowel segments in the lower urinary tract. *Urologic Clinics of North America, 18*(4), 743-754.

ery 2 hours day and night the first week. The patient then decreases the frequency of catheterization by 1 hour each week until the patient is catheterizing the reservoir every 6 hours by the fifth week (Razor, 1993). Initially, patients should continue to irrigate the reservoir with saline once a day to keep the reservoir free of mucus. By the fifth week, patients should need to irrigate the reservoir only 3 to 7 times a week.

Patients who have a reservoir anastomosed to their own urethra must practice a new voiding technique. Invariably, patients are incontinent at times and need suggestions for how to protect their clothing, bedding, and pride. Over time, approximately 90% of patients achieve day continence, and 85% of patients achieve night continence (Bales, Kim, & Steinberg, 1996). The reader interested in more detailed patient teaching guidelines for all types of bladder reconstructions is referred to Lind, Kravitz, and Greig (1993) and Razor (1993).

A home health care consult to assess how the patient and family are managing at home and to reinforce teaching provided in the hospital is appropriate. The inpatient primary care nurse should closely coordinate care with the enterostomal therapy nurse, urology nurse, and home health care nurse to ensure consistent and coordinated follow-up with the patient and family.

Radiation Therapy

A standard of care for the patient undergoing radiation therapy as primary treatment of invasive bladder cancer is outlined in Table 48-9. The major concerns are knowledge deficit, IBS, diarrhea, fatigue, skin reactions, and potential for anxiety. If radiation is part of a combined treatment approach, the patient may experience more severe side effects, especially if a radiosensitizer such as cisplatin is administered concurrently with the radiation. The nurse can play an important role in communicating care between urology, medical oncology, radiation oncology, and nursing services to ensure consistent and coordinated care.

Systemic Chemotherapy

A standard of care for the patient undergoing chemotherapy as primary treatment of invasive bladder cancer is outlined in Table 48-10. The major concerns are knowledge deficit and potential for anxiety. Chemotherapy regimens can be very difficult for patients to tolerate, especially for those who have recently undergone pelvic surgery. As previously discussed, fewer than half of the patients randomized to receive chemotherapy in adjuvant chemotherapy trials completed the planned therapy (Skinner et al., 1991; Stöckle et al., 1995).

One particular side effect of the drug methotrexate peculiar to patients with a reconstructed urinary tract is mucositis of the bowel segment used in the reconstruction. Although the bladder is not normally considered part of the gastrointestinal tract, patients receiving methotrexate who have had an ileal conduit or urinary reservoir constructed from bowel are susceptible to mucositis of their recon-

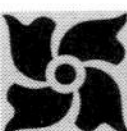

TABLE 48-9 Standard of Care for the Patient Undergoing Radiation Therapy

Patient Problem and Outcomes	Nursing Interventions and Rationales	Patient Education Instructions
Knowledge Deficit		
Patient will verbalize an understanding of the purpose, benefits, and risks of radiation therapy.	1. Determine who the patient's support person is, and have this person present when teaching is done. 2. Assess the patient's level of understanding of the radiation therapy. 3. Give the patient the opportunity to ask questions or verbalize concerns.	1. Use a gender-specific diagram of the anatomy of the pelvis to explain the procedure. 2. Describe the routine procedures involved in radiation therapy: a. Consultation b. Simulation procedure c. Treatment procedures and routines 3. Provide the patient with information about possible side effects of therapy, when to expect these side effects, the importance of notifying the nurse if side effects occur, and self-care measures to manage the side effects of the following: a. IBS b. Diarrhea c. Fatigue d. Skin reactions
Irritative Bladder Symptoms (IBS)		
Patient will experience relief of urinary symptoms.	1. Assess the patient for dysuria, frequency, and urgency. 2. Evaluate for the presence of a urinary tract infection, and refer the patient to the urologist for appropriate antibiotic therapy if an infection is present. 3. Administer urinary analgesics, antispasmodics, and/or anticholinergics as prescribed.	1. Inform the patient that urinary symptoms may occur after 3000 cGy have been administered. 2. Teach the patient to take prescribed medications for IBS.
Diarrhea		
Patient will maintain adequate fluid balance, weight, and energy level.	1. Assess elimination patterns, including frequency, quality, and quantity. 2. Obtain weekly weights. 3. Obtain a consult with a dietician. 4. Administer anti-diarrheal medication (e.g., Imodium as directed on the box, or Lomotil as prescribed by the physician).	1. Inform the patient that diarrhea occurs within a few weeks of treatment, usually when a dose of 1500 to 3000 cGy is reached. 2. Teach the patient to eat a low-residue diet until bowel patterns return to normal, usually 2 to 6 weeks after therapy is complete: a. Avoid foods high in fiber. b. Avoid fatty foods and rich deserts. c. Avoid foods that increase bowel activity, such as spicy foods, caffeinated beverages, and alcohol.

structed urinary tract. Blood in the urine or a reddened, excoriated stoma may be the only signs of mucositis in these patients. The urologist should evaluate any suspicion of mucositis in a reconstructed bladder.

In addition to chemotherapy, colony-stimulating factors (CSFs) such as granulocyte colony-stimulating factor (G-CSF) may also be used to minimize neutropenia and reduce the patient's risk of infection. If prescribed, the nurse will also have to teach the patient and family how to administer the CSFs subcutaneously and monitor for possible side effects.

HOME CARE ISSUES

Urination

Following Transurethral Resection of the Bladder. The majority of patients have an indwelling catheter after TURB to decompress the bladder of urine and monitor for bleeding. It is very likely that the patient will be discharged home with the catheter and will need to know how to care for it. Several days after surgery the catheter is removed. If the amount of residual urine after the next void is less than 50 ml, the catheter does not need to be replaced. If the vol-

TABLE 48-9 Standard of Care for the Patient Undergoing Radiation Therapy—cont'd

Patient Problem and Outcomes	Nursing Interventions and Rationales	Patient Education Instructions
		3. Increase fluid intake to 1500 to 2000 ml each day. 4. Teach the patient to evaluate for a pattern to the diarrhea, and concentrate the administration of anti-diarrheal medication to that time of day. 5. Instruct the patient to wash after each bowel movement and keep the skin clean and dry.
Fatigue Patient will be able to maintain normal activities of daily living and engage in activities to enhance his or her quality of life	1. Assess the patient's level of fatigue using a 0 (not at all tired, full of pep) to 10 (total exhaustion) rating scale. 2. Evaluate the patient's sleep and activity pattern to be able to teach the patient ways to conserve energy.	1. Inform the patient that he or she is likely to experience fatigue toward the end of treatment and for several weeks after treatment. 2. Teach the patient energy conservation strategies, including the following: a. Going to bed at a regular time b. Taking short naps during the day c. Exercising at regular intervals during the day
Skin Reactions Patient will not experience moist desquamation	1. Assess all radiation skin ports (i.e., anterior, posterior, and both lateral ports).	1. Teach the patient to do the following: a. Keep skin clean and dry, avoiding any lotions or powders b. Wear loose-fitting cotton clothing that does not abrade treated skin
Potential for Anxiety Patient will: • Express feelings of decreased anxiety • Identify strategies to cope with anxiety	1. Complete patient teaching of the procedure so that the patient's anxiety is not due to a knowledge deficit. 2. Determine which coping strategies the patient has used effectively in the past to decrease anxiety and reinforce the use of these coping strategies. 3. Administer pharmacologic agents to decrease anxiety, if necessary.	

ume of residual urine is greater than 50 ml, the urologist should be consulted to consider replacing the catheter for 1 to 2 more days before again attempting to remove the catheter and letting the patient void spontaneously.

Ileal Conduit. Patients with an ileal conduit wear an external collection device draining into a leg bag during the day and a Foley bag at night. Ideally, an enterostomal therapy nurse is consulted preoperatively to meet the patient and plan placement of the stoma. Normally, this nurse continues to follow the patient postoperatively and decide on the optimal stoma wafer and urine collection device, making adjustments in supplies as needed.

Typically, the urine collection bag is changed twice a day, usually when switching between the day leg bag and the night Foley bag. When not in use, the urine collection bag should be washed with soap and water and allowed to air dry. With properly selected and fitting supplies, the wafer around the stoma should need to be changed no more frequently than every 3 days (Lind, Kravitz, & Greig, 1993). Stomal complications can include skin irritation and infection (Carroll & Barbour, 1995). A poorly placed stoma, one that recedes or is herniated, can be difficult to fit with a wafer and urine collection device, predisposing the patient to stomal complications. An

TABLE 48-10 Standard of Care for the Patient Undergoing Chemotherapy with MVAC (Methotrexate, Vinblastine, Adriamycin, and Cisplatin)

Patient Problem and Outcomes	Nursing Interventions and Rationales	Patient Education Instructions
Knowledge Deficit Patient will verbalize an understanding of the chemotherapy treatments, possible side effects, and how to manage side effects if they occur.	1. Determine who the patient's support person is, and have this person present when teaching is done. 2. Assess the patient's level of understanding about chemotherapy. 3. Give the patient the opportunity to ask questions or verbalize concerns.	1. Provide the patient with information about the specific chemotherapy agents, possible side effects, and how to manage side effects: a. Myelosuppression from doxorubicin, methotrexate, and vinblastine b. Renal toxicity from cisplatin c. Mucositis from methotrexate d. Nausea and vomiting from cisplatin, and doxorubicin e. Alopecia from doxorubicin f. Taste alterations from cisplatin g. Fatigue from doxorubicin, methotrexate, and vinblastine h. Ototoxicity from cisplatin
Anxiety Patient will: • Express feelings of decreased anxiety. • Identify strategies to cope with anxiety.	1. Complete patient teaching of the procedure so that the patient's anxiety is not due to a knowledge deficit. 2. Determine which coping strategies the patient has used effectively in the past to decrease anxiety, and reinforce the use of these coping strategies. 3. Administer pharmacologic agents to decrease anxiety, if necessary.	

enterostomal therapy nurse should be consulted to determine a plan of care.

The patient should be encouraged to drink up to 2 L of fluid each day to help keep the reservoir cleared of mucus. Some patients notice a strong odor to the urine. Adequate hydration helps dilute the urine and minimize this odor. The majority of conduits are colonized with gastrointestinal pathogens (e.g., *Escherichia coli*) and are susceptible to periodic urinary tract infections. Taking 500 to 2000 mg of vitamin C each day and drinking at least a quart of acidic fruit juice such as orange, grapefruit, or cranberry juice may lower bacterial counts in the urinary diversion (Lind, Kravitz, & Greig, 1993). Patients should monitor for signs and symptoms of infection (e.g., cloudy or tea-colored urine, foul-smelling urine, abdominal or flank pain, fever, or chills) and immediately call the urologist or urology nurse for evaluation and treatment.

Reservoir to Stoma. Patients with continent urinary diversions have an internal reservoir for urine collection that is periodically drained through an abdominal stoma, which needs to be catheterized to drain the reservoir. Patients should wash their hands, clean the stoma with povidone-iodine (Betadine) solution, and then insert a clean, straight catheter. Urine can be drained directly into the toilet. When the reservoir is empty, the catheter is removed and the stoma is covered with a small dressing to protect clothing from mucus and accidental incontinence. The used catheter is washed with soap and water and allowed to air dry. Patients should drain their reservoir between four and six times a day and at least once during the night to prevent overfill incontinence. Irrigating the reservoir with 60 to 100 ml of normal saline 3 to 7 days per week helps keep the reservoir free of mucus. Just as for patients with an ileal conduit, patients should be encouraged to drink up to 2 L of fluids each day to help keep the reservoir free of mucus. Daily doses of vitamin C (500 to 2000 mg) and drinking acidic fruit juices (e.g., orange, grapefruit, or cranberry juice) may lower bacterial counts in the urinary diversion and help prevent infection (Lind, Kravitz, & Greig, 1993). Patients should be taught to monitor for signs and symptoms of infection (e.g., cloudy or tea-colored urine, foul-smelling urine, abdominal or flank pain, fever, or chills) and immediately call the urologist or the urology nurse for evaluation and treatment.

Reservoir to Urethra. Patients with orthotopic bladder substitutions such as the Mainz or Hautmann pouch have an internal reservoir for urine collection that is drained through the patient's own urethra when the patient relaxes the pelvic muscles and performs a Valsalva maneuver. Patients experience fewer infections with an orthotopic bladder substitution compared with reservoirs that drain through a stoma because catheterization is not necessary. Patients must still drain their reservoir between four and six times a day and at least once during the night to prevent overfill incontinence. Again, just as for patients with an ileal conduit or a reconstructed reservoir that drains through an abdominal stoma, patients with a reservoir reanastomosed to their own urethra should be encouraged to drink up to 2 L of fluids each day to help keep the reservoir free of mucus. Daily doses of vitamin C (500 to 2000 mg) and drinking acidic fruit juices (e.g., orange, grapefruit, or cranberry juice) may lower bacterial counts in the urinary diversion and help prevent infection (Lind, Kravitz, & Greig, 1993). Patients should be taught to monitor for signs and symptoms of infection (e.g., cloudy or tea-colored urine, foul-smelling urine, abdominal or flank pain, fever, or chills) and immediately call the urologist or urology nurse for evaluation and treatment.

Sexual Dysfunction

Patients who have undergone surgery, radiation therapy, and/or chemotherapy for treatment of invasive bladder cancer are at risk for sexual dysfunction (Lind, Kravitz, & Greig, 1993; Ofman, 1993; Schover, 1987; Smith & Babaian, 1989). Before 1980, virtually all men who underwent a radical cystectomy were impotent postoperatively (Richie, 1992). In the intervening years, new surgical approaches have been developed that spare the neurovascular bundles supplying the corpora cavernosum (Walsh & Donker, 1982), thus preserving potency without increasing the risk of tumor recurrence (Brendler, Steinberg, Marshall, Mostwin, & Walsh, 1990). Men experience a "dry ejaculation" without the emission of semen because the prostate and seminal vesicles are removed as part of the cystectomy. In one study of 76 men who underwent nerve-sparing radical cystoprostatectomies, two thirds of men who were potent preoperatively recovered potency within a year of surgery (Brendler et al., 1990; Marshall, Mostwin, Radebaugh, Walsh, & Brendler, 1991). Still, approximately one third of men who are potent preoperatively do not regain sexual function following surgery. Whether this dysfunction is due to inadvertent damage to the neurovascular bundles supplying the corpora cavernosum, psychological inhibition, or some other factor is unknown.

Sexual dysfunction in women after cystectomy has not been researched extensively or written about. The clitoris may be inadvertently injured during surgery because of its proximity to the urethral meatus (Swanson, 1981). If the woman can achieve an orgasm postoperatively, the quality of the orgasm may be changed. As part of the cystectomy, the anterior vaginal wall is removed. To close the vagina, either the edges of the posterior wall are approximated, significantly narrowing the vaginal vault, or the upper half of the posterior wall is folded down to rebuild a vagina of normal diameter but reduced length (Schover, 1986). With either of these reconstructions, women may experience pain with intercourse. Premenopausal women receiving chemotherapy as part of their treatment are at risk for ovarian failure and premature menopause accompanied with vasomotor instability (i.e., hot flashes), vaginal dryness, and dyspareunia (i.e., painful intercourse) (Feldman, 1989; Sherins, 1993).

Treatment options for men with erectile dysfunction include the insertion of a penile prosthesis (Lind, Kravitz, & Greig, 1993). Both semi-rigid and inflatable protheses can successfully restore a man's ability to have vaginal coitus. Treatment options for women depend on the nature of the problem. Women with a narrowed or shortened vagina may be able to gradually expand the vaginal vault over several weeks and months using vaginal dilators. For women experiencing the menopausal symptoms of vaginal dryness and dyspareunia, various over-the-counter products are now available. Replens (Warner Wellcome, Morris Plains, NJ), Gyne-Moistrin (Health Care Products, Memphis, TN), Lubrin (Kenwood Laboratories, Fairfield, NJ), and KY vaginal moisturizer (Johnson & Johnson, Skillman, NJ) are designed to be used regularly to maintain vaginal moisture. Astroglide (Bio Film, Vista, CA), AquaLube (Mayer Laboratories, Oakland, CA), and KY liquid (Johnson & Johnson, Skillman, NJ) are water-based, glycerine lubricants designed to be used during intercourse. Prescribed estrogen replacement therapy may also be an option for these women (Schover, 1986).

Patients with an abdominal stoma as part of an ileal conduit or continent reservoir will likely have concerns about how to manage the stoma, and possibly an external collection bag, during sexual intimacy and intercourse. Box 48-1 provides some practical suggestions that can be discussed with couples.

Men and women and their partners should be encouraged to discuss sexual functioning concerns preoperatively and after they have recovered from surgery. Referral to a sexual therapist or counselor can help patients deal with their feelings about their body and sexual self after radical treatment (Schover, Evans, & von Eschenbach, 1986; Schover & von Eschenbach, 1985).

PROGNOSIS

As indicated in Table 47-17, only 65% of patients with stage II disease, 48% of patients with stage III disease, and 23% of patients with stage IV disease will be alive 5 years after diagnosis. Although these tumors are radiosensitive and chemotherapy sensitive, the majority of patients with invasive bladder cancer die of their disease. Advances in surgical techniques and supportive therapies have improved the quality of life for these patients. Hopefully the results of ongoing clinical trials of combined therapy will provide some insight into how to offer these patients longer quality survival.

TABLE 48-11 Quality of Care Evaluation for a Patient Following Cystectomy with Bladder Reconstruction

Disciplines participating in the quality of care evaluation:
☐ Nursing (Urology Service) ☐ Nursing (Inpatient Unit)
☐ Nursing (Enterostomal Therapy)
☐ Nursing (Home Health) ☐ Urology

Data from:
☐ Medical Record Review ☐ Patient/Family Interview

I. Postprocedure Management Evaluation

Criteria	YES	NO
1. Patient provided with preprocedure information about the following:		
a. Postoperative care (i.e., surgical drains and catheters, pain management, intermittent compression stockings, incentive spirometry, ambulation)	☐	☐
b. Home care of surgical drains and catheters	☐	☐
c. Plan for urination rehabilitation	☐	☐
2. Patient experienced the following complications:		
a. Fever >101° F (38° C)	☐	☐
b. Pulmonary embolus	☐	☐
c. Stomal stenosis, hernia, skin irritation, or fungal infections	☐	☐
d. Rehospitalization	☐	☐
e. Need for additional surgery	☐	☐

II. Patient/Family Satisfaction

Data from:
☐ Patient Interview ☐ Family Interview

Criteria	YES	NO
1. On a scale of 0 to 10, with 0 being totally dissatisfied and 10 being totally satisfied, how satisfied are you with the care you received? ________	☐	☐
2. Were you prepared to care for your surgical drains and catheters when you went home?	☐	☐
3. Do you feel you received adequate information about how to urinate with your reconstructed bladder?	☐	☐
4. What percentage of the time are you continent during the day? ________ What percentage of the time are you continent at night? ________		

Box 48-1 Pragmatic Advice for Patients with Ostomy Appliances and Their Partners to Ease Resumption of Sexual Activity

1. The ostomy pouch should be emptied before sexual activity. A well-fitting seal prevents any odor. Abstinence from foods causing smelly urine, such as asparagus, as well as use of deodorants and perfumes may further add to the patient's confidence.
2. Usually, the smallest pouch available suffices for the duration of sexual interaction. Cloth ostomy covers can be sewn from any material following patterns that are available from most enterostomal therapists.
3. Taping the pouch sideways to the body keeps the appliance out of the way and prevents distracting flapping.
4. Crotchless panties for women and boxer shorts for men completely cover the pouch.
5. Use positions for intercourse that minimize friction on the ostomy appliance. A small cushion placed over the ostomy appliance when using the missionary position also helps deflect friction.
6. Having a rubber undersheet or an absorbing towel in the bed may add to the couple's level of comfort and reduce concerns about what to do when leakage occurs.
7. Planning of a mutual response if a pouch leak occurs may help ease tension for both partners.

Modified from Ofman, U. S. (1993). Psychosocial and sexual implications of genitourinary cancers. *Seminars in Oncology Nursing, 9*(4), 286-292.

EVALUATION OF THE QUALITY OF CARE

Accreditation organizations, like the Joint Commission for the Accreditation of Health Care Organizations, require that the quality of care provided to patients be evaluated. Because the care provided to patients with bladder cancer requires input from an interdisciplinary team, an evaluation of the quality of care provided to these patients should include aspects of care provided by various members of the team. Tables 47-18 and 48-11 provide examples of quality of care evaluation tools that can be used following TURB and for a patient after cystectomy with bladder reconstruction.

RESEARCH ISSUES

Many medical and nursing issues remain to be resolved in the diagnosis, treatment, and continuing care of the patient with invasive bladder cancer. The cellular mechanisms that regulate activation of proto-oncogenes and inactivation of tumor suppressor genes in bladder cancer remain largely unknown. Basic research is investigating the cascade of events associated with the development of this heterogeneous disease (Sternberg, 1996). Hopefully, affordable molecular screening tools will be available in the next years to identify patients who may be developing malignant changes in their urothelium. These same molecular tools may also provide information about which patients are at highest risk for disease recurrence and warrant aggressive treatment.

For patients currently diagnosed with invasive bladder cancer, the most urgent research issue remains how to reduce the rate of metastatic disease recurrence. The results of neoadjuvant and adjuvant chemotherapy clinical trials will help better define the role of chemotherapy in the treatment of bladder cancer and determine the direction of future clinical trials.

Health care agencies will be carefully following this research. Costs for bladder cancer treatment vary greatly depending on the treatment approach. Health policy research will be needed to ensure that the efficacy of treatment and the quality of life afforded the patients by a particular treatment as well as the cost of the treatment are all considered before policy decisions are made. Important work remains to be done in the diagnosis, treatment, and follow-up of patients with bladder cancer, focusing on the quality of care that can be provided in a managed care environment.

REFERENCES

Ahlering, T. E., Kanellos, A., Boyd, S. D., Lieskovsky, G., Skinner, D. G., & Bernstein, L. (1988). A comparative study of perioperative complications with Kock pouch urinary diversion in highly irradiated versus nonirradiated patients. *Journal of Urology, 139*(6), 1202-1204.

Ahlering, T. E., Weinberg, A. C., & Razor, B. (1989). A comparative study of the ileal conduit, Kock pouch and modified Indiana pouch. *Journal of Urology, 142*(5), 1193-1196.

Ahlering, T. E., Weinberg, A. C., & Razor, B. (1991). Modified Indiana pouch. *Journal of Urology, 145*(6), 1156-1158.

American Cancer Society. (1996). *1996 cancer facts & figures*. New York: ACS.

American Joint Committee on Cancer. (1992). Urinary bladder. In O. H. Beahrs, D. E. Henson, R. V. P. Hutter, & B. J. Kennedy (Eds.), *Manual for staging of cancer* (4th ed.). Philadelphia: J. B. Lippincott.

Auerbach, O. & Garfinkel, L. (1989). Histologic changes in the urinary bladder in relation to cigarette smoking and use of artificial sweeteners. *Cancer, 64*(5), 983-987.

Babaian, R. J., Johnson, D. E., Llamas, L., & Ayala, A. G. (1980). Metastases from transitional cell carcinoma of urinary bladder. *Urology, 16*(2), 142-144.

Bales, G. T., Kim, H., & Steinberg, G. D. (1996). Surgical therapy for locally advanced bladder cancer. *Seminars in Oncology, 23*(5), 605-613.

Bane, B. L., Rao, J. Y., & Hemstreet, G. P. (1996). Pathology and staging of bladder cancer. *Seminars in Oncology, 23*(5), 546-570.

Barentsz, J. O., Jager, G. J., Witjes, J. A., & Ruijs, J. H. J. (1996). Primary staging of urinary bladder carcinoma: The role of MRI and a comparison with CT. *European Radiology, 6*(2), 129-133.

Bates, B. (1991). *A guide to physical examination* (5th ed.). New York: J. B. Lippincott.

Benson, M. C. & Olsson, C. A. (1992). Urinary diversion. *Urologic Clinics of North America, 19*(4), 779-795.

Berry, D. L. (1996). Bladder disturbances. In S. L. Groenwald, M. H. Frogge, M. Goodman, & C. H. Yarbro (Eds.), *Cancer symptom management*. Sudbury, MA: Jones and Bartlett.

Boice, J. D., Engholm, G., Kleinerman, B. R., Blettner, M., Stovall, M., Lisco, H., Moloney, W. C., Austin, D. F., Bosch, A., Cookfair, D. L., Krementz, E. T., LaTourette, H. B., Merrill, J. A., Peters, L. J., Schulz, M. D., Storm, H. H., Björkholm, E., Pettersson, F., Bell, C. M. J., Coleman, M. P., Fraser, P., Neal, F. E., Prior, P., Choi, N. W., Hislop, T. G., Koch, M., Kreiger, N., Robb, D., Robson, D., Thomson, D. H., Lochmüller, H., von Fournier, D., Frischkorn, R., Kjørstad, K. E., Rimpela, A., Pejovic, M. H., Kirn, V. P., Stankusova, H., Berrino, F., Sigurdsson, K., Hutchison, G. B., & MacMahon, B. (1988). Radiation dose and second cancer risk in patients treated for cancer of the cervix. *Radiation Research, 116*(1), 3-55.

Borland, R. N., Brendler, C. B., & Isaacs, W. B. (1992). Molecular biology of bladder cancer. *Hematology Oncology Clinics of North America, 6*(1), 31-39.

Boyd, S. D., Feinberg, S. M., Skinner, D. G., Lieskovsky, G., Baron, D., & Richardson, J. (1987). Quality of life survey of urinary diversion patients: Comparison of ileal conduits versus continent Kock ileal reservoirs. *Journal of Urology, 138*(6), 1386-1389.

Brendler, C. B., Steinberg, G. D., Marshall, F. F., Mostwin, J. L., & Walsh, P. C. (1990). Local recurrence and survival following nerve-sparing radical cystoprostatectomy. *Journal of Urology, 144*(5), 1137-1141.

Bricker, E. M. (1950). Bladder substitution after pelvic evisceration. *Surgical Clinics of North America, 30*, 1511-1521.

Bricker, E. M. (1978). The evolution of the ileal segment bladder substitution operation. *American Journal of Surgery, 135*(6), 834-841.

Broadwell, D. C., & Jackson, B. S. (1982). *Principles of ostomy care*. St. Louis: Mosby.

Brodsky, G. L. (1992). Pathology of bladder carcinoma. *Hematology Oncology Clinics of North America, 6*(1), 59-80.

Burch, J. D., Rohan, T. E., Howe, G. R., Risch, H. A., Hill, G. B., Steele, R., & Miller, A. B. (1989). Risk of bladder cancer by source and type of tobacco exposure: A case-control study. *International Journal of Cancer, 44*(4), 622-628.

Camey, M. (1985). Bladder replacement by ileocystoplasty following radical cystectomy. *World Journal of Urology, 3*(3), 161-166.

Cancrini, A., de Carli, P., Fattahi, H., Pompeo, V., Cantiani, R., & von Heland, M. (1995). Orthotopic ileal neobladder in female patients after radical cystectomy: 2-year experience. *Journal of Urology, 153*(3), 956-958.

Carroll, P. R. & Barbour, S. (1995). Urinary diversion and bladder substitution. In E. A. Tanagho & J. W. McAninch (Eds.), *Smith's general urology* (14th ed.). Norwalk, CT: Appleton & Lange.

Clavel, J., Cordier, S., Boccon-Gibod, L., & Hemon, D. (1989). Tobacco and bladder cancer in males: Increased risk for inhalers and smokers of black tobacco. *International Journal of Cancer, 44*(4), 605-610.

Cohen, S. M. & Johansson, S. L. (1992). Epidemiology and etiology of bladder cancer. *Urologic Clinics of North America, 19*(3), 421-428.

Crawford, E. D., Das, S., & Smith, J. A. (1987). Preoperative radiation therapy in the treatment of bladder cancer. *Urologic Clinics of North America, 14*(4), 781-787.

Crump, K. S., & Guess, H. A. (1982). Drinking water and cancer: Review of recent epidemiological findings and assessment of risks. *Annual Review of Public Health, 3*, 39-57.

Cummings, K. B., Barone, J. G., & Ward, W. S. (1992). Diagnosis and staging of bladder cancer. *Urologic Clinics of North America, 19*(3), 455-465.

Decensi, A., Bruno, S., Giaretti, W., Torrisi, R., Curotto, A., Gatteschi, B., Geldo, E., Polizzi, A., Costantini, M., Bruzzi, P., Nicolò, G., Costa, A., Boccardo, F., Giuliani, L., & Santi, L. (1992). Activity of 4-HPR in superficial bladder cancer using DNA flow cytometry as an intermediate endpoint. *Journal of Cellular Biochemistry, Suppl. 16 I*, 139-147.

Devesa, S. S., Blot, W. J., Stone, B. J., Miller, B. A., Tarone, R. E., & Fraumeni, J. F., Jr. (1995). Recent cancer trends in the United States. *Journal of the National Cancer Institute, 87*(3), 175-182.

Douglas, R. M., Kaufman, D. S., Zietman, A. L., Althausen, A. F., Heney, N. M., & Shipley, W. U. (1996). Conservative surgery, patient selection, and chemoradiation as organ-preserving treatment for muscle-invading bladder cancer. *Seminars in Oncology, 23*(5), 614-620.

Duckett, J. W. & Snyder, H. M. III. (1986). Continent urinary diversion: Variations on the Mitrofanoff principle. *Journal of Urology, 136*(1), 58-62.

Duncan, W. & Quilty, P. M. (1986). The results of a series of 963 patients with transitional cell carcinoma of the urinary bladder primarily treated by radical megavoltage x-ray therapy. *Radiotherapy and Oncology, 7*(4), 299-310.

Dunst, J., Sauer, R., Schrott, K. M., Kühn, R., Wittekind, C., & Altendorf-Hofmann, A. (1994). Organ-sparing treatment of advanced bladder cancer: A 10-year experience. *International Journal of Radiation Oncology Biology Physics, 30*(2), 261-266.

Edmonds, C. J. & Smith, T. (1986). The long-term hazards of the treatment of thyroid cancer with radioiodine. *British Journal of Radiology, 59*(697), 45-51.

Fair, W. R., Fuks, Z. Y., & Scher, H. I. (1993). Cancer of the bladder. In V. T. DeVita, Jr., S. Hellman, & S. A. Rosenberg (Eds.), *Cancer: Principles and practice of oncology* (4th ed.). Philadelphia: J. B. Lippincott.

Fairchild, W. B., Spence, C. R., Solomon, H. D., & Gangai, M. P. (1979). The incidence of bladder cancer after cyclophosphamide therapy. *Journal of Urology, 122*(2), 163-164.

Faysal, M. H. (1981). Squamous cell carcinoma of the bladder. *Journal of Urology, 126*(5), 598-599.

Feldman, J. E. (1989). Ovarian failure and cancer treatment: Incidence and interventions for the premenopausal woman. *Oncology Nursing Forum, 16*(5), 651-657.

Fernandes, E. T., Manivel, J. C., Reddy, P. K., & Ercole, C. J. (1996). Cyclophosphamide associated bladder cancer — a highly aggressive disease: Analysis of 12 cases. *Journal of Urology, 156*(6), 1931-1933.

Fiore, M. C., Bailey, W. C., Cohen, S. J., Dorfman, S. F., Goldstein, M. G., Gritz, E. R., Heyman, R. B., Holbrook, J., Jaen, C. R., Kottke, T. E., Lando, H. A., Mecklenburg, R., Mullen, P. D., Nett, L. M., Robinson, L., Stitzer, M. L., Tommasello, A. C., Villejo, L., & Wewers, M. E. (1996). *Smoking cessation.* Clinical Practice Guideline No 18. Agency for Health Care Policy and Research (AHCPR) Publication No. 96-0692. Rockville, MD: U. S. Department of Health and Human Services, Public Health Service.

Fiore, M. C., Jorenby, D. E., Baker, T. B., & Kenford, S. L. (1992). Tobacco dependence and the nicotine patch: Clinical guidelines for effective use. *Journal of the American Medical Association, 268*(19), 2687-2694.

Fleshner, N. E., Herr, H. W., Stewart, A. K., Murphy, G. P., Mettlin, C., & Menck, H. R. (1996). The national cancer data base report on bladder carcinoma. *Cancer, 78*(7), 1505-1513.

Freiha, F., Reese, J., & Torti, F. M. (1996). A randomized trial of radical cystectomy versus radical cystectomy plus cisplatin, vinblastine and methotrexate chemotherapy for muscle invasive bladder cancer. *Journal of Urology, 155*(2), 495-500.

Furihata, M., Inoue, K., Ohtsuki, Y., Hashimoto, H., Terao, N., & Fujita, Y. (1994). High-risk human papilloma virus infections and over expression of p53 protein as prognostic indicators in transitional cell carcinoma of the urinary bladder. *Journal of Urology, 152*(2), 568-569.

Gabrilove, J. L., Jakubowski, A., Scher, H., Sternberg, C., Wong, G., Grous, J., Yagoda, A., Fain, K., Moore, M. A. S., Clarkson, B., Oettgen, H. F., Alton, K., Welte, K., & Souza, L. (1988). Effect of granulocyte colony-stimulating factor ion neutropenia and associated morbidity due to chemotherapy for transitional-cell carcinoma of the urothelium. *New England Journal of Medicine, 318*(22), 1414-1422.

Gallagher, J., & Holm, L. (1996). Power of one: Nurses and tobacco control. *Seminars in Oncology Nursing, 12*(4), 270-275.

Geller, N. L., Sternberg, C. N., Penenberg, D., Scher, H., & Yagoda, A. (1991). Prognostic factors for survival of patients with advanced urothelial tumors treated with methotrexate, vinblastine, doxorubicin, and cisplatin chemotherapy. *Cancer, 67*(6), 1525-1531.

Ghoneim, M. A. (1995). The urinary bladder in bilharziasis. In J. M. Fitzpatrick & R. J. Krane (Eds.), *The bladder.* Edinburgh: Churchill Livingstone.

González, C. A., López-Abente, G., Errezola, M., Escolar, A., Riboli, E., Izarzugaza, I., & Nebot, M. (1989). Occupation and bladder cancer in Spain: A multi-center case-control study. *International Journal of Epidemiology, 18*(3), 569-577.

Gospodarowicz, M. K., Hawkins, N. V., Rawlings, G. A., Connolly, J. G., Jewett, M. A. S., Thomas, G. M., Herman, J. G., Garrett, P. G., Chua, T., Duncan, W., Buckspan, M., Sugar, L., & Rider, W. D. (1989). Radical radiotherapy for muscle invasive transitional cell carcinoma of the bladder: Failure analysis. *Journal of Urology, 142*(6), 1448-1454.

Gospodarowicz, M. K. & Warde, P. (1992). The role of radiation therapy in the management of transitional cell carcinoma of the bladder. *Hematology Oncology Clinics of North America, 6*(1), 147-168.

Gschwend, J. E., May, F., Paiss, T., Gottfried, H. W., & Hautmann, R. E. (1996). High-dose pelvic irradiation followed by ileal neobladder urinary diversion: Complications and long-term results. *British Journal of Urology, 77*(5), 680-683.

Harker, W. G., Meyers, F. J., Freiha, F. S., Palmer, J. M., Shortliffe, L. D., Hannigan, J. F., McWhirter, K. M., & Torti, F. M. (1985). Cisplatin, methotrexate, and vinblastine (CMV): An effective chemotherapy regimen for metastatic transitional cell carcinoma of the urinary tract: A Northern California Oncology Group study. *Journal of Clinical Oncology, 3*(11), 1463-1470.

Harris, R. E., Chen-Backlund, J. Y., & Wynder, E. L. (1990). Cancer of the urinary bladder in blacks and whites: A case-control study. *Cancer, 66*(12), 2673-2680.

Harrison, S. C. W. & Abrams, P. (1994). Bladder function. In G. R. Sant (Ed). *Pathophysiologic Principles of Urology*. Boston: Blackwell Scientific.

Hartge, P., Harvey, E. B., Linehan, W. M., Silverman, D. T., Sullivan, J. W., Hoover, R. N., & Fraumeni, J. F., Jr. (1990). Unexplained excess risk of bladder cancer in men. *Journal of the National Cancer Institute, 82*(20), 1636-1640.

Hartge, P., Silverman, D., Hoover, R., Schairer, C., Altman, R., Austin, D., Cantor, K., Child, M., Key, C., Marrett, L. D., Mason, T. J., Meigs, J. W., Myers, M. H., Narayana, A., Sullivan, J. W., Swanson, M. G. M., Thomas, D., & West, D. (1987). Changing cigarette habits and bladder cancer risk: A case-control study. *Journal of the National Cancer Institute, 78*(6), 1119-1125.

Hauri, D. (1996). Can gastric pouch as orthotopic bladder replacement be used in adults? *Journal of Urology, 156*(3), 931-935.

Hautmann, R. E., Egghart, G., Frohneberg, D., & Miller, K. (1988). The ileal neobladder. *Journal of Urology, 139*(1), 39-42.

Heney, N. M., Daly, J., Prout, G. R., Nieh, P. T., Heaney, J. A., & Trebeck, N. E. (1978). Biopsy of apparently normal urothelium in patients with bladder carcinoma. *Journal of Urology, 120*(5), 559-560.

Heney, N. M., Nocks, B. N., Daly, J. J., Prout, Jr., G. R., Newall, J. B., Griffin, P. P., Perrone, T. L., & Szyfelbein, W. A. (1982). Ta and T1 bladder cancer: Location, recurrence and progression. *British Journal of Urology, 54*(2), 152-157.

Herr, H. W. (1987). Conservative management of muscle-infiltrating bladder cancer: Prospective experience. *Journal of Urology, 138*(5), 1162-1163.

Herr, H. W. (1992). Transurethral resection in regionally advanced bladder cancer. *Urologic Clinics of North America, 19*(4), 695-700.

Herr, H. W., & Scher, H. I. (1994). Neoadjuvant chemotherapy and partial cystectomy for invasive bladder cancer. *Journal of Clinical Oncology, 12*(5), 975-980.

Hossan, E., & Striegel, A. (1993). Carcinoma of the bladder. *Seminars in Oncology Nursing, 9*(4), 252-266.

Housset, M., Maulard, C., Chretien, Y., Dufour, B., Delanian, S., Huart, J., Colardelle, F., Brunel, P., & Baillet, F. (1993). Combined radiation and chemotherapy for invasive transitional-cell carcinoma of the bladder: A prospective study. *Journal of Clinical Oncology, 11*(11), 2150-2157.

Howe, G. R., Burch, J. D., Miller, A. B., Cook, G. M., Esteve, J., Morrison, B., Gordon, P., Chambers, L. W., Fodor, G., & Winsor, G. M. (1980). Tobacco use, occupation, coffee, various nutrients, and bladder cancer. *Journal of the National Cancer Institute, 64*(4), 701-713.

Inskip, P. D., Monson, R. R., Wagoner, J. K., Stovall, M., Davis, F. G., Kleinerman, R. A., & Boice, J. D. (1990). Cancer mortality following radium treatment for uterine bleeding. *Radiation Research, 123*(3), 331-344.

Israel, V. K., Natale, R. B., & Skinner, D. G. (1995). Bladder. In M. D. Abeloff, J. O. Armitage, A. S. Lichter, & J. E. Niederhuber (Eds.), *Clinical oncology*. New York: Churchill Livingstone.

Itoku, K. A. & Stein, B. S. (1992). Superficial bladder cancer. *Hematology Oncology Clinics of North America, 6*(1), 99-116.

Jewett, H. J. (1952). Carcinoma of the bladder: Influence of depth of infiltration on the 5-year results following complete extirpation of the primary growth. *Journal of Urology, 67*(5), 672-676.

Jewett, H. J., & Strong, G. H. (1946). Infiltrating carcinoma of the bladder: Relation of depth of penetration of the bladder wall to incidence of local extension and metastases. *Journal of Urology, 55*(4), 366-372.

Kachnic, L. A., Kaufman, D. S., Heney, N. M., Althausen, A. F., Griffin, P. P., Zietman, A. L., & Shipley, W. U. (1997). Bladder preservation by combined modality therapy for invasive bladder cancer. *Journal of Clinical Oncology, 15*(3), 1022-1029.

Kantor, A. F., Hartge, P., Hoover, R. N., & Fraumeni, J. F., Jr. (1985). Familial and environmental interactions in bladder cancer risk. *International Journal of Cancer, 35*(6), 703-706.

Kantor, A. F., Hartge, P., Hoover, R. N., & Fraumeni, J. F., Jr. (1988). Epidemiological characteristics of squamous cell carcinoma and adenocarcinoma of the bladder. *Cancer Research, 48*(13), 3853-3855.

Kantor, A. F., Hartge, P., Hoover, R. N., Narayana, A. S., Sullivan, J. W., & Fraumeni, J. F., Jr. (1984). Urinary tract infection and risk of bladder cancer. *American Journal of Epidemiology, 119*(4), 510-515.

Kaufman, D. S., Shipley, W. U., Griffin, P. P., Heney, N. M., Althausen, A. F., & Efird, J. T. (1993). Selective bladder preservation by combination treatment of invasive bladder cancer. *New England Journal of Medicine, 329*(19), 1377-1382.

Kelloff, G. J., Boone, C. W., Malone, W. F., Steele, V. E., & Doody, L. A. (1992). Development of chemopreventive agents for bladder cancer. *Journal of Cellular Biochemistry, Suppl. 16 I*, 1-12.

Kelly, L. P. & Miaskowski, C. (1996). An overview of bladder cancer: Treatment and nursing implications. *Oncology Nursing Forum, 23*(3), 459-468.

Kiemeney, L. A. & Schoenberg, M. (1996). Familial transitional cell carcinoma. *Journal of Urology, 156*(3), 867-872.

Kock, N. G., Nilson, A. E., Nilsson, L. O., Norlén, L., J., & Philipson, B. M. (1982). Urinary diversion via a continent ileal reservoir: Clinical results in 12 patients. *Journal of Urology, 128*(3), 469-475.

Kottke, T. E., Battista, R. N., DeFriese, G. H., & Brekke, M. L. (1988). Attributes of successful smoking cessation interventions in medical practice: A meta-analysis of 39 controlled trials. *Journal of the American Medical Association, 259*(19), 2882-2889.

Lamm, D. L. (1992). Carcinoma in situ. *Urologic Clinics of North America, 19*(3), 499-508.

Lamm, D. L., Blumenstein, B. A., Crawford, E. D., Montie, J. E., Scardino, P., Grossman, H. B., Stanisic, T. H., Smith, J. A., Sullivan, J., Sarosdy, M. F., Crissman, J. D., & Coltman, C. A. (1991). A randomized trial of intravesical doxorubicin and immunotherapy with bacille Calmette-Guérin for transitional-cell carcinoma of the bladder. *New England Journal of Medicine, 325*(17), 1205-1209.

Lamm, D. L., & Torti, F. M. (1996). Bladder cancer, 1996. *CA-A Cancer Journal for Clinicians, 46*(2), 93-112.

Landis, S.H., Murray, T., Bolden, S., & Wingo P.A. (1998). Cancer statistics, 1998. *CA: A Cancer Journal for Clinicians,* 48:6-29.

Leek, C. L., Sebastian, W., Kawachi, M. H., & Sullivan, L. (1996). Genitourinary cancers. In R. McCorkle, M. Grant, M. Frank-Stromborg, & S. B. Baird (Eds.), *Cancer nursing: A comprehensive textbook* (2nd ed.). Philadelphia: W. B. Saunders.

Lerner, S. P., Skinner, D. G., Lieskovsky, G., Boyd, S. D., Groshen, S. L., Ziogas, A., Skinner, E., Nichols, P., & Hopwood, B. (1993). The rationale for en bloc pelvic lymph node dissection for bladder cancer patients with nodal metastases: Long-term results. *Journal of Urology, 149*(4), 758-765.

Levine, L. A. & Richie, J. P. (1989). Urological complications of cyclophosphamide. *Journal of Urology, 141*(5), 1063-1069.

Lind, J., Kravitz, K., & Greig, B. (1993). Urologic and male genital malignancies. In S. L. Groenwald, M. H. Frogge, M. Goodman, & C. H. Yarbro (Eds.), *Cancer nursing: Principles and practice* (3rd ed.). Boston: Jones & Bartlett.

Loehrer, P. J., Sr., Einhorn, L. H., Elson, P. J., Crawford, E. D., Kuebler, P., Tannock, I., Raghavan, D., Stuart-Harris, R., Sarosdy, M. F., Lowe, B. A., Blumenstein, B., & Trump, D. (1992). A randomized comparison of cisplatin alone or in combination with methotrexate, vinblastine, and doxorubicin in patients with metastatic urothelial carcinoma: a Cooperative Group study. *Journal of Clinical Oncology, 10*(7), 1066-1073.

Loehrer, P. J., Sr., Elson, P., Dreicer, R., Hahn, R., Nichols, C. R., Williams, R., & Einhorn, L. (1994). Escalated dosages of methotrexate, vinblastine, doxorubicin, and cisplatin plus recombinant human granulocyte colony-stimulating factor in advanced urothelial carcinoma: An Eastern Cooperative Oncology Group trial. *Journal of Clinical Oncology, 12*(3), 483-488.

Logothetis, C. J., Dexeus, F. H., Finn, L., Sella, A., Amato, R. J., Ayala, A. G., & Kilbourn, R. G. (1990). A prospective randomized trial comparing MVAC and CISCA chemotherapy for patients with metastatic urothelial tumors. *Journal of Clinical Oncology, 8*(6), 1050-1055.

Loprinzi, C. L. & Messing, E. M. (1992). A prospective clinical trial of difluoromethylornithine (DFMO) in patients with resected superficial bladder cancer. *Journal of Cellular Biochemistry, Suppl. 16 I*, 153-155.

Lower, G. M. (1982). Concepts in causality: Chemically induced human urinary bladder cancer. *Cancer, 49*(5), 1056-1066.

Lynch, C. F., & Cohen, M. G. (1995). Urinary system. *Cancer, 75*(Suppl. 1), 316-329.

Lynch, H. T., Kimberling, W. J., Lynch, J. F., & Brennan, K. (1987). Familial bladder cancer in an oncology clinic. *Cancer Genetics and Cytogenetics, 27*(1), 161-165.

Makhyoun, N. A. (1974). Smoking and bladder cancer in Egypt. *British Journal of Cancer, 30*(6), 577-581.

Månsson, A., Johnson, G., & Månsson, W. (1988). Quality of life after cystectomy: Comparison between patients with conduit and those with continent caecal reservoir urinary diversion. *British Journal of Urology, 63*(3), 240-245.

Mao, L., Schoenberg, M. P., Scicchitano, M., Erozan, Y. S., Merlo, A., Schwab, D., & Sidransky, D. (1996). Molecular detection of primary bladder cancer by microsatellite analysis. *Science, 271*(5249), 659-662.

Marshall, V. F. (1952). The relation of the preoperative estimate to the pathologic demonstration of the extent of vesical neoplasms. *Journal of Urology, 68*(4), 714-723.

Marshall, F. F., Mostwin, J. L., Radebaugh, L. C., Walsh, P. C., & Brendler, C. B. (1991). Ileocolic neobladder post-cystectomy: continence and potency. *Journal of Urology, 145*(3), 502-504.

McGinn, K. A. (1985). *The ostomy book for nurses*. Palo Alto, CA: Bull.

Melicow, M. M. (1974). Tumors of the bladder: A multifaceted problem. *Journal of Urology, 112*(4), 467-478.

Miaskowski, C. (1995). Bladder cancer. In C. Miaskowski (Ed.), *Oncology nursing*. Albany, NY: Delmar.

Mills, P. K., Beeson, L., Phillips, R. L., & Fraser, G. E., (1991). Bladder cancer in a low risk populations: Results from the Adventist health study. *American Journal of Epidemiology, 133*(3), 230-239.

Moore, S., Newton, M., Grant, E. G., & Keetch, D. W. (1993). Treating bladder cancer: New methods, mew management. *American Journal of Nursing, 93*(5), 32-39.

Morrison, A. S., Buring, J. E., Verhoek, W. G., Aoki, K., Leck, I., Ohno, Y., & Obata, K. (1984). An international study of smoking and bladder cancer. *Journal of Urology, 131*(4), 650-654.

Murphy, W. M. (1990). Current status of urinary cytology in the evaluation of bladder neoplasms. *Human Pathology, 21*(9), 886-896.

Murphy, W. M., Nagy, G. K., Rao, M. K., Soloway, M. S., Parija, G. C., Cox, C. E., & Friedell, G. H. (1979). "Normal" urothelium in patients with bladder cancer: A preliminary report from the National Bladder Cancer Collaborative Group A. *Cancer, 44*(3), 1050-1058.

Murphy, W. M. & Soloway, M. S. (1982). Developing carcinoma (dysplasia) of the urinary bladder. *Pathology Annual, 17*(1), 197-217.

Newman, D. M., Brown, J. R., Jay, A. C., & Pontius, E. E. (1968). Squamous cell carcinoma of the bladder. *Journal of Urology, 100*(4), 470-473.

Norton, J. M. (1995). Urologic disorders. In A. D. Linton, M. A. Matteson, & N. K. Maebius (Eds.), *Introductory nursing care of adults*. Philadelphia: W. B. Saunders.

Nurmi, M., Puntala, P., & Alanen, A. (1988). Evaluation of 144 cases of ileal conduits in adults. *European Urology, 15*(1-2), 89-93.

Ockene, J. K. (1987). Physician-delivered interventions for smoking cessation: Strategies for increasing effectiveness. *Preventive Medicine, 16*(5), 723-737.

Ofman, U. S. (1993). Psychosocial and sexual implications of genitourinary cancers. *Seminars in Oncology Nursing, 9*(4), 286-292.

Patrianakos, C. & Hoffmann, D. (1979). Chemical studies on tobacco smoke LXIV. On the analysis of aromatic amines in cigarette smoke. *Journal of Analytical Toxicology, 3*(4), 150-154.

Pedersen-Bjergaard, J., Ersbøll, J., Hansen, V. L., Sørensen, B. L., Christoffersen, K., Hou-Jensen, K., Nissen, N. I., Knudsen, J. B., & Hansen, M. M. (1988). Carcinoma of the urinary bladder after treatment with cyclophosphamide for non-Hodgkin's lymphoma. *New England Journal of Medicine, 318*(16), 1028-1032.

Perucca, D., Szepetowski, P., Simon, M. P., & Gaudray, P. (1990). Molecular genetics of human bladder carcinomas. *Cancer Genetics and Cytogenetics, 49*(2), 143-156.

Piper, J. M., Matanoski, G. M., & Tonascia, J. (1986). Bladder cancer in young women. *American Journal of Epidemiology, 123*(6), 1033-1042.

Prout, G. R., Jr. & Barton, B. A. (1992). 13-*cis*-Retinoic acid in chemoprevention of superficial bladder cancer. *Journal of Cellular Biochemistry, Suppl. 16 I*, 148-152.

Prout, G. R., Jr., Griffin, P. P., & Shipley, W. U. (1979). Bladder carcinoma as a systemic disease. *Cancer, 43*(6), 2532-2539.

Quilty, P. M. & Kerr, G. R. (1987). Bladder cancer following low or high dose pelvic irradiation. *Clinical Radiology, 38*(6), 583-585.

Razor, B. R. (1993). Continent urinary reservoirs. *Seminars in Oncology Nursing, 9*(4), 272-285.

Reddy, P. K. (1987). Detubularized sigmoid reservoir for bladder replacement after cystoprostatectomy: Preliminary report of new configuration. *Urology, 29*(6), 625-628.

Reddy, P. K., Lange, P. H., & Fraley, E. E. (1991). Total bladder replacement using detubularized sigmoid colon: Technique and results. *Journal of Urology, 145*(1), 51-55.

Richie, J. P. (1992). Surgery for invasive bladder cancer. *Hematology Oncology Clinics of North America, 6*(1), 129-145.

Risser, N. L. (1996). Prevention of lung cancer: The key is to stop smoking. *Seminars in Oncology Nursing, 12*(4), 260-269.

Roth, B. J. (1996). Chemotherapy for advanced bladder cancer. *Seminars in Oncology, 23*(5), 633-644.

Rowland, R. G., Mitchell, M. E., Bihrle, R., Kahnoski, R. J., & Piser, J. E. (1987). Indiana continent urinary reservoir. *Journal of Urology, 137*(6), 1136-1139.

Sandberg, A. A. (1992). Chromosome changes in early bladder neoplasms. *Journal of Cellular Biochemistry, Suppl. 16 I*, 76-79.

Scher, H. I. (1990). Chemotherapy for invasive bladder cancer: Neoadjuvant versus adjuvant. *Seminars in Oncology, 17*(5), 555-565.

Scher, H. I. (1994). Editorial comment. *Journal of Urology, 152*(2), 569.

Schover, L. R. (1986). Sexual rehabilitation of the ostomy patient. In D. B. Smith & D. E. Johnson (Eds.), *Ostomy care and the cancer patient: Surgical and clinical considerations*. Orlando, FL: Grune & Stratton.

Schover, L. R. (1987). Sexuality and fertility in urologic cancer patients. *Cancer, 60*(3), 553-558.

Schover, L. R., & von Eschenbach, A. C. (1985). Sexual function and female radical cystectomy: A case series. *Journal of Urology, 134*(3), 465-468.

Schover, L. R., Evans, R., & von Eschenbach, A. C. (1986). Sexual rehabilitation and male radical cystectomy. *Journal of Urology, 136*(5), 1015-1017.

Seidman, A. D., Scher, H. I., Gabrilove, J. L., Bajorin, D. F., Motzer, R. J., O'Dell, M., Curley, T., Dershaw, D. D., Quinlivan, S., Tao, Y., Fair, W. R., Begg, C., & Bosl, G. J. (1993). Dose-intensification of MVAC with recombinant granulocyte colony-stimulating factor as initial therapy in advanced urothelial cancer. *Journal of Clinical Oncology, 11*(3), 408-414.

Sell, A., Jakobsen, A., Nerstrøm, B., Sørensen, B. L., Steven, K., & Barlebo, H. (1991). Treatment of advanced bladder cancer category T2 T3 and T4a. *Scandinavian Journal of Urology and Nephrology, Suppl. 138*, 193-201.

Sherins, R. J. (1993). Gonadal dysfunction. In V. T. DeVita, Jr., S. Hellman, & S. A. Rosenberg (Eds.), *Cancer: Principles and practice of oncology* (4th ed.). Philadelphia: J. B. Lippincott.

Sidransky, D., & Messing, E. (1992). Molecular genetics and biochemical mechanisms in bladder cancer: Oncogenes, tumor suppressor genes, and growth factors. *Urologic Clinics of North America, 19*(4), 629-639.

Silverman, D. T., Hartge, P., Morrison, A. S., & Devesa, S. S. (1992). Epidemiology of bladder cancer. *Hematology Oncology Clinics of North America, 6*(1), 1-30.

Silverman, D. T., Levin, L. I., Hoover, R. N., & Hartge, P. (1989). Occupational risks of bladder cancer in the United States: I. white men. *Journal of the National Cancer Institute, 81*(19), 1472-1480.

Skinner, D. G., Boyd, S. D., & Lieskovsky, G. (1984). Clinical experience with the Kock continent ileal reservoir for urinary diversion. *Journal of Urology, 132*(6), 1101-1107.

Skinner, D. G., Daniels, J. R., Russell, C. A., Lieskovsky, G., Boyd, S. D., Nichols, P., Kern, W., Sakamoto, J., Krailo, M., & Groshen, S. (1991). The role of adjuvant chemotherapy following cystectomy for invasive bladder cancer: A prospective comparative trial. *Journal of Urology, 145*(3), 459-467.

Skinner, D. G., Lieskovsky, G., & Boyd, S. (1984). Technique of creation of a continent internal ileal reservoir (Kock pouch) for urinary diversion. *Urologic Clinics of North America, 11*(4), 741-749.

Skinner, D. G., Lieskovsky, G., & Boyd, S. (1987). Continuing experience with the continent ileal reservoir (Kock pouch) as an alternative to cutaneous urinary diversion: An update after 250 cases. *Journal of Urology, 137*(6), 1140-1145.

Skinner, D. G., Lieskovsky, G., & Boyd, S. (1989). Continent urinary diversion. *Journal of Urology, 141*(6), 1323-1327.

Small, E. J., Fippin, L. J., Ernest, M. L., & Carroll, P. R. (1996). A carboplatin-based regimen for the treatment of patients with advanced transitional cell carcinoma of the urothelium. *Cancer, 78*(8), 1775-1780.

Smith, D. B. & Babaian, R. J. (1989). Patient adjustment to an ileal conduit after radical cystectomy. *Journal of Enterostomal Therapy, 16*(6), 244-246.

Smith, D. B. & Johnson, D. E. (1986). *Ostomy care and the cancer patient: Surgical and clinical considerations*. Orlando, FL: Grune & Stratton.

Smith, M. R. & Kantoff, P. W. (1995). Neoadjuvant and adjuvant chemotherapy for invasive bladder cancer. *Seminars in Oncology, 22*(6), 625-632.

Soloway, M. S., Murphy, W., Rao, M. K., & Cox, C. (1978). Serial multiple-site biopsies in patients with bladder cancer. *Journal of Urology, 120*(1), 57-59.

Soloway, M. S. & Patel, J. (1992). Surgical techniques for endoscopic resection of bladder cancer. *Urologic Clinics of North America, 19*(3), 467-471.

Song-ting, Y., Ming-ming, W., & Li-ming, L. (1993). Prevalence of human papillomaviruses 16 and 18 in transitional cell carcinoma of bladder. *Chinese Medical Journal, 106*(7), 494-496.

Spruck, C. H., Ohneseit, P. G., Gonzalez-Zulueta, M., Esrig, D., Miyao, N., Tsai, Y. C., Lerner, S. P., Schmütte, C., Yang, A. S., Cote, R., Dubeau, L., Nichols, P. W., Hermann, G. G., Steven, K., Horn, T., Skinner, D. G., & Jones, P. A. (1994). Two molecular pathways to transitional cell carcinoma of the bladder. *Cancer Research, 54*(3), 784-788.

Steiner, M. S. & Morton, R. A. (1991). Nutritional and gastrointestinal complications of the use of bowel segments in the lower urinary tract. *Urologic Clinics of North America, 18*(4), 743-754.

Stenzl, A., Colleselli, K., Poisel, S., Feichtinger, H., Pontasch, H., & Bartsch, G. (1995). Rationale and technique of nerve sparing radical cystectomy before an orthotopic neobladder procedure in women. *Journal of Urology, 154*(6), 2044-2049.

Sternberg, C. N. (1995). The treatment of advanced bladder cancer. *Annals of Oncology, 6*(2), 113-126.

Sternberg, C. N. (1996). Neoadjuvant and adjuvant chemotherapy in locally advanced bladder cancer. *Seminars in Oncology, 23*(5), 621-632.

Sternberg, C. N., Arena, M. G., Calabresi, F., Carli, P. D., Platania, A., Zeuli, M., Giannarelli, D., Cancrini, A., & Pansadoro, V. (1993). Neoadjuvant M-VAC (methotrexate, vinblastine, doxorubicin, and cisplatin) for infiltrating transitional cell carcinoma of the bladder. *Cancer, 72*(6), 1975-1982.

Sternberg, C. N., Raghavan, D., Ohi, Y., Bajorin, D., Herr, H., Kato, T., Kuroda, M., Logothetis, C. H., Scher, H., Splinter, T. A, & van Oosterom, A. T. (1995). Neo-adjuvant and adjuvant chemotherapy in locally advanced disease—what are the effects on survival and prognosis. *International Journal of Urology, 2*(Suppl. 2), 76-88.

Sternberg, C. N., Yagoda, A., Scher, H. I., Watson, R. C., Herr, H. W., Morse, M. J., Sogani, P. C., Vaughan, E. D., Jr., Bander, N., Weiselberg, L. R., Geller, N., Hollander, P. S., Lipperman, R., Fair, W. R., & Whitmore, W. F., Jr. (1988). M-VAC (methotrexate, vinblastine, doxorubicin, and cisplatin) for advanced transitional cell carcinoma of the urothelium. *Journal of Urology, 139*(3), 461-469.

Sternberg, C. N., Yagoda, A., Scher, H. I., Watson, R. C., Geller, N., Herr, H. W., Morse, M. J., Sogani, P. C., Vaughan, E. D., Bander, N., Weiselberg, L., Rosado, K., Smart, T., Lin, S., Penenberg, D., Fair, W. R., & Whitmore, W. F., Jr. (1989). Methotrexate, vinblastine, doxorubicin, and cisplatin for advanced transitional cell carcinoma of the urothelium: Efficacy and patterns of response and relapse. *Cancer, 64*(12), 2448-2458.

Stöckle, M., Meyenburg, W., Wellek, S., Voges, G. E., Rossmann, M., Gertenbach, U., Thüroff, J. W., Huber, C., & Hohenfellner, R. (1995). Adjuvant polychemotherapy of nonorgan-confined bladder cancer after radical cystectomy revisited: Long-term results of a controlled prospective study and further clinical experience. *Journal of Urology, 153*(1), 47-52.

Swanson, D. A. (1981). Cancer of the bladder and prostate: The impact of therapy on sexual function. In A. C. von Eschenbach & D. B. Rodriguez (Eds.), *Sexual rehabilitation of the urologic cancer patient*. Boston: G. K. Hall.

Sweeney, P., Kursh, E. D., & Resnick, M. I. (1992). Partial cystectomy. *Urologic Clinics of North America, 19*(4), 701-711.

Tanagho, E. A. (1992). Anatomy of the lower urinary tract. In P. C. Walsh, A. B. Retik, T. A. Stamey, & E. D. Vaughan, Jr. (Eds.), *Campbell's urology* (6th ed.). Philadelphia: W. B. Saunders.

Tanagho, E. A. (1995a). Anatomy of the genitourinary tract. In E. A. Tanagho & J. W. McAninch (Eds.), *Smith's general urology* (14th ed.). Norwalk, CT: Appleton & Lange.

Tanagho, E. A. (1995b). Specific infections of the genitourinary tract. In E. A. Tanagho & J. W. McAninch (Eds.), *Smith's general urology* (14th ed.). Norwalk, CT: Appleton & Lange.

Tester, W., Caplan, R., Heaney, J., Venner, P., Whittington, R., Byhardt, R., True, L., & Shipley, W. (1996). Neoadjuvant combined modality program with selective organ preservation for invasive bladder cancer: Results of Radiation Therapy Oncology Group phase II trial 8802. *Journal of Clinical Oncology, 14*(1), 119-126.

Tester, W., Porter, A., Asbell, S., Coughlin, C., Heaney, J., Krall, J., Martz, D., Venner, P., & Hammond, E. (1993). Combined modality program with possible organ preservation for invasive bladder carcinoma: Results of RTOG protocol 85-12. *International Journal of Radiation Oncology Biology Physics, 25*(5), 783-790.

Thüroff, J. W., Alken, P., Riedmiller, H., Engelmann, U., Jacobi, G. H., & Hohenfellner, R. (1985). The Mainz-pouch (mixed augmentation ileum 'n zecum) for bladder augmentation and continent diversion. *World Journal of Urology, 3*(3), 179-184.

Thüroff, J. W., Alken, P., Riedmiller, H., Engelmann, U., Jacobi, G. H., & Hohenfellner, R. (1986). The Mainz-pouch (mixed augmentation ileum and cecum) for bladder augmentation and continent diversion. *Journal of Urology, 136*(1), 17-26.

Thüroff, J. W., Alken, P., Riedmiller, H., Jacobi, G. H., & Hohenfellner, R. (1988). 100 cases of Mainz pouch: Continuing experience and evolution. *Journal of Urology, 140*(2), 283-288.

Tootla, J. & Easterling, A. (1992). Current options in bladder cancer management. *RN, 55*(4), 42-48.

Utz, D. C. & Farrow, M. D. (1984). Carcinoma in situ of the urinary tract. *Urologic Clinics of North America, 11*(4), 735-740.

Wallace, D. M. A. (1988). Occupational urothelial cancer. *British Journal of Urology, 61*(3), 175-182.

Wallace, D. M. & Harris, D. L. (1965). Delay in treating bladder tumours. *Lancet, II*(7407), 332-334.

Wallace, D. M. A., Hindmarsh, J. R., Webb, J. N., Busuttil, A., Hargreave, T. B., Newsam, J. E., & Chisholm, G. D. (1979). The role of multiple mucosal biopsies in the management of patients with bladder cancer. *British Journal of Urology, 51*(6), 535-540.

Walsh, P. C. & Donker, P. J. (1982). Impotence following radical prostatectomy: Insight into etiology and prevention. *Journal of Urology, 128*(3), 492-497.

Walther, P. J. (1992). The role of flow cytometry in the management of bladder cancer. *Hematology Oncology Clinics of North America, 6*(1), 81-98.

Watt, R. C. (1986). Nursing management of a patient with a urinary diversion. *Seminars in Oncology Nursing, 2*(4), 265-269.

Wenderoth, U. K., Bachor, R., Egghart, G., Frohneberg, D., Miller, K., & Hautmann, R. E. (1990). The ileal neobladder: Experience and results of more than 100 consecutive cases. *Journal of Urology, 143*(3), 492-497.

Wesson, M. F. (1992). Radiation therapy in regionally advanced bladder cancer. *Urologic Clinics of North America, 19*(4), 725-734.

Whitbourne, S. K. (1985). *The aging body: physiological changes and psychological consequences*. New York: Springer-Verlag.

Whitmore, W. F. (1990). Selection of treatment for muscle infiltrating transitional cell bladder cancer. *Archivos Espanoles de Urologia, 43*(Suppl. 2), 219-222.

Wood, D. P., Montie, J. E., Pontes, J. E., Medendorp, S. V., & Levin, H. S. (1989). Transitional cell carcinoma of the prostate in cystoprostatectomy specimens removed for bladder cancer. *Journal of Urology, 141*(2), 346-349.

Wynder, E. L. & Goldsmith, R. (1977). The epidemiology of bladder cancer: A second look. *Cancer, 40*(3), 1246-1268.

49 Renal Cell Cancer

Mary Monaghan, RN, APN, AOCN

EPIDEMIOLOGY

Renal cell cancer, a relatively rare malignancy, is the tenth most common cancer and represents 2% to 3% of all adult neoplasms. In 1997 the number of new cases of renal cell cancer in the United States was approximately 28,800, with 11,300 deaths from the disease (Parker, Tong, Bolden, & Wingo, 1997). Renal cell cancer's peak incidence is between 60 and 70 years of age, with progressive increases after the age of 40 (Glick & de Vere White, 1997; McDougal & Garnick, 1996). It occurs twice as frequently in men than in women for both black and white races (Pack, 1993). Age-adjusted incidence rates are highest in Iceland, Denmark, and Sweden, and the lowest incidence rates are reported in Japan. The United States, Canada, and most countries of western Europe have intermediate risk levels. Although native Scandinavians have high incidence rates, migrants to the western United States have incidence rates similar to other white populations of this region (Paganini-Hill, Ross, & Henderson, 1988).

Renal cell cancer is more common among urban than rural residents (Madajewicz, 1995). Its incidence has steadily increased at about 2% per year in the past few decades, which is believed to be due in part to advances in diagnostic imaging techniques that have improved the detection of early-stage disease (LaFollette, 1992; Linehan, Shipley, & Parkenson, 1993; Couillard & de Vere White, 1993).

Some controversy exists regarding the effect of socioeconomic status as a risk factor for renal cell cancer. Paganini-Hill, Ross, and Henderson (1988) reported an increased risk in men in higher socioeconomic classes, but not in women. Mellemgaard and colleagues (1994), however, reported an increased risk in men and women in lower socioeconomic groups.

Renal cell cancer occurs in sporadic and familial forms. Familial renal cell cancer is a rare autosomal-dominant inherited disorder. There is an increased incidence of renal cell cancer with von Hippel-Lindau (VHL) syndrome and polycystic kidney disease. These familial cancer syndromes tend to occur at an earlier age and are often bilateral (Martz, 1992; Linehan, Shipley, & Parkenson, 1993), with an increased risk seen in both men and women (Mellemgaard et al., 1994).

Renal cell cancer, also known as *kidney cancer, renal adenocarcinoma, hypernephroma,* or *Grawitz tumor,* accounts for approximately 85% of all adult kidney cancers and is found in the renal parenchyma (Pack, 1993). Kidney cancer is one of the least studied major cancers in the United States (Paganini-Hill, Ross, & Henderson, 1988).

RISK FACTORS

The major risk factors associated with the development of renal cell cancer are listed in Box 49-1. Environmental, hormonal, cellular, and hereditary factors have been studied as possible risk factors in the development of renal cell cancer. The evidence supporting each risk factor is not always conclusive, but rather suggestive in many cases. Most etiologic studies of renal cell cancer have been conducted in Western countries, with obesity and cigarette smoking the most consistently reported risk factors (McLaughlin, Gao, Gao, Zheng, Ji, & Blot et al., 1992).

Increasing Age

Age is the most important demographic risk factor for renal cell cancer. In persons under the age of 35, its incidence is rare. After age 35, and into old age, there is a steady increase in risk (Paganini-Hill, Ross, & Henderson, 1988).

Smoking

Cigarette smoking is the only risk factor consistently linked to renal cell cancer in epidemiologic studies. According to some studies, the relative risk has been small and a dose-response relationship has not always been observed (Paganini-Hill, Ross, & Henderson, 1988; McLaughlin et al., 1992; Hiatt, Tolan, & Quesenberry, 1994). Although the particulate matter from cigarette smoke is known to contain numerous carcinogens, the exact mechanism by which cigarettes induce kidney cancer is unclear. The higher risk of re-

Box 49-1
Risk Factors for Renal Cell Cancer

- Increasing age
- Tobacco use
- Obesity (association)
- Positive family history
- Cadmium exposure (? association)
- Use of prescription diuretics (? association)
- Non-narcotic analgesic use

nal cell cancer in men compared with that in women is believed to be due to the increased use of tobacco earlier in this century (Paganini-Hill, Ross, & Henderson, 1988).

Non-Narcotic Analgesic Use

There may be an association between heavy use of non-narcotic analgesics and cancer of the kidney. Phenacetin, a pain-relieving drug, was most often indicated in these studies, but the exact analgesic ingredient responsible for this increased risk was not always clearly established (Paganini-Hill, Ross, & Henderson, 1988; McLaughlin et al., 1992).

Occupation

Occupational and environmental exposure to chemicals has been associated with the development of renal cell cancer. Cadmium, a chemical used in batteries and rust-proof electroplating, is the chemical most frequently mentioned (Paganini-Hill, Ross, & Henderson, 1988; Mandel, McLaughlin, Schlehofer, Mellemgaard, Helmert, Lindblad et al., 1995). Because the kidney concentrates cadmium more heavily than any other organ and inhibits growth-regulating enzymes, a potential mechanism for carcinogenesis may exist (Paganini-Hill, Ross, & Henderson, 1988).

Other occupational studies have indicated a possible link in increased kidney cancer in lead smelter workers (Steenland, Selevan, & Landrigan, 1992; Mandel et al., 1995), coke oven workers, iron and steel industry workers, asbestos insulation workers, and those exposed to petroleum products and dry cleaning solvents (Mandel et al., 1995). However, current evidence suggests that very few cases of renal cell cancer are caused by occupational exposure (Paganini-Hill, Ross, & Henderson, 1988).

Obesity

Early studies have shown a strong association between obesity and renal cell cancer, especially in women, but this finding needs further confirmation (Paganini-Hill, Ross, & Henderson, 1988; Muscat, Hoffman, & Wynder, 1995; Chow, McLaughlin, Mandel, Blot, Niwa, & Fraumeni, 1995; Mellemgaard et al., 1994). An alternative mechanism for the association between obesity and renal cell cancer may be renal damage from obesity-related artherosclerosis or increased use of diuretics (Paganini-Hill, Ross, & Henderson, 1988; Finkle, McLaughlin, Rosgon, Yeoh, & Low, 1993).

Other researchers (Finkle et al., 1993; Hiatt, Tolan, & Quesenberry, 1994) have reported an association between diuretic use and renal cell cancer, especially in women.

Family History

There is an increased risk of renal cell cancer in certain hereditary disorders. These disorders include adult polycystic disease, horseshoe kidney, acquired renal cystic disease, and VHL disease, in which 30% to 35% of patients may develop renal cell cancer (McDougal & Garnick, 1996).

VHL disease is a rare autosomal-dominant hereditary disorder in which affected individuals are genetically predisposed to develop tumors or tumorlike cysts. Most of these tumors are nonmalignant but may undergo a malignant transformation. Renal cell cancer is one of the most common manifestations of VHL and is frequently bilateral, occurring at a younger age (Linehan, Shipley, & Parkenson, 1993). Martz (1992) suggests that oncology nurses should maintain a high index of suspicion for hereditary disorders when they see patients who have unusual disease manifestations with early age of onset. This may allow potential hereditary cancer syndromes to be identified sooner, making earlier surveillance and intervention possible.

PATHOPHYSIOLOGY

Normal Anatomy and Physiology of the Kidneys

The kidneys are paired reddish-brown, bean-shaped organs located on the posterior wall of the abdominal cavity on either side (Fig. 49-1) of the vertebra column between T_{12} and L_3 (Fig. 49-2). They are under the dome of the diaphragm and protected by the lowest two ribs. An adult kidney weighs about 150 gm (5 ounces) and is approximately 12.5 cm (5.0 inches) long, 7 cm (3.0 inches) wide, and 2.5 cm (1.0 inch) thick. The right kidney is slightly lower than the left because of the space occupied by the liver. The lateral surface of the kidney is convex; the medial surface is concave with a vertical cleft called the *hilus*. The ureters, renal artery and vein, lymphatics, and nerves enter or exit the kidney at the hilus. The adrenal glands are situated over the upper pole of each kidney and are distinctly separate functionally (Marieb, 1991).

Three layers of supportive tissue surround each kidney. The renal capsule, the layer closest to the kidney, is smooth, transparent, and fibrous. It acts as a barrier that prevents infections in surrounding regions from spreading to the kidneys and plays a minor role in protecting the kidneys from physical trauma. The middle layer is a fatty mass called the *adipose capsule,* which helps hold the kidney in place against the posterior trunk muscles and protect it from trauma. The outermost layer, the renal fascia (fascia of Gerota), is dense fibrous connective tissue. It surrounds the kidney and adrenals, and it anchors them to surrounding structures (Marieb, 1991).

The kidney is divided into three regions: the renal cortex,

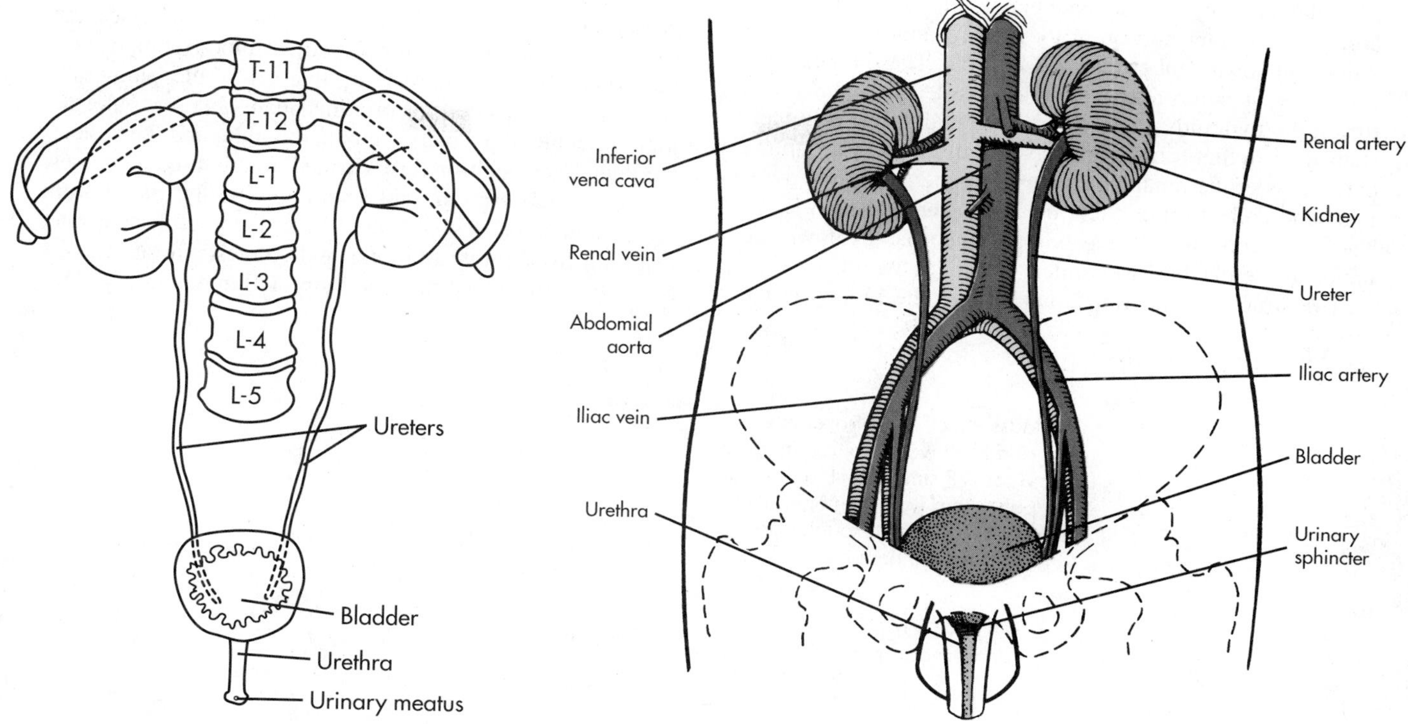

Fig. 49-1 The kidneys, anatomic relations.

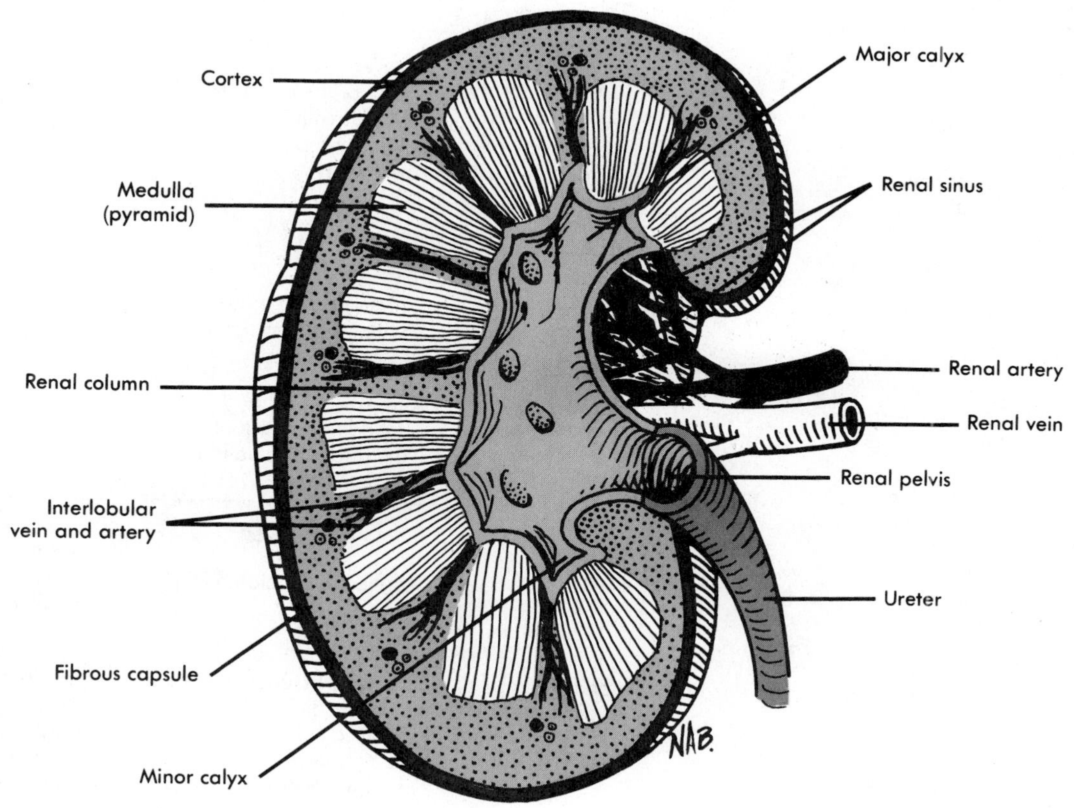

Fig. 49-2 Gross structure of the kidney, longitudinal section.

the renal medulla, and the renal pelvis (Fig. 49-3). The renal cortex is the outer portion of the kidney, and the renal medulla contains the tubes that collect urine. These tubes form a number of cone-shaped structures called *pyramids.* The tips of the pyramids point toward the renal pelvis, a funnel-shaped basin that forms the upper end of the ureter. Cuplike extensions of the renal pelvis surround the tips of the pyramids and collect urine; these extensions are called *calyces.* The urine collects in the pelvis and then passes down the ureter to the bladder (Memmler, Cohen, & Wood, 1996).

The structural and functional unit of the kidney is the nephron. Each kidney contains over 1 million blood-processing nephrons, which carry out the processes that form urine and simultaneously adjust blood composition. Each nephron is composed of five parts: the glomerular (Bowman's) capsule, the proximal convoluted tubule, the loop of Henle, the distal convoluted tubule, and the collecting duct. Each nephron forms urine through three processes: filtration, reabsorption, and secretion. Briefly, blood from glomerular arterioles is filtered in the glomerular capsule, resulting in a filtrate of water and solutes. Filtrate travels through the proximal tubules, loop of Henle, and distal tu-

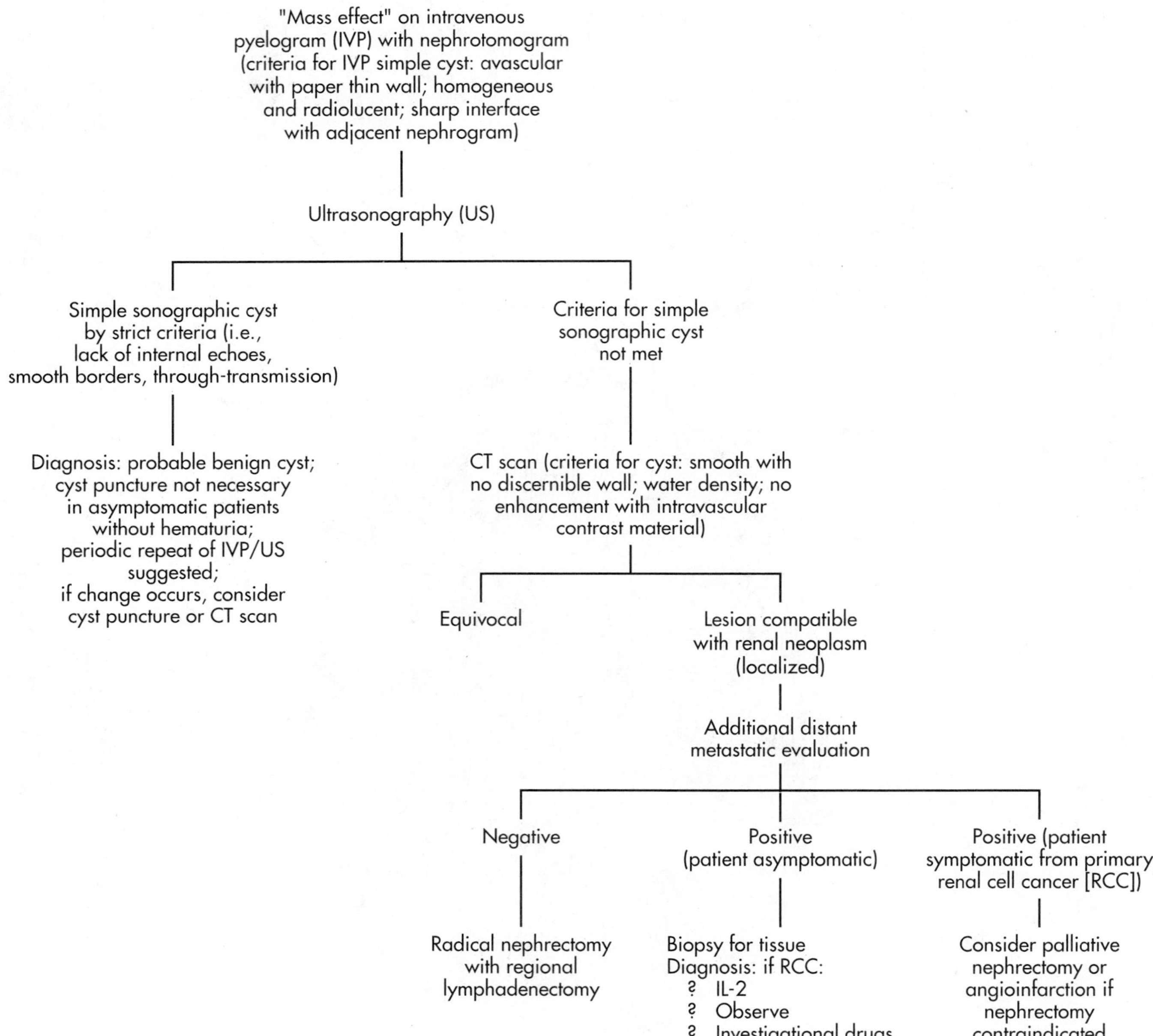

Fig. 49-3 Flow chart for the diagnosis evaluation and therapeutic approach to patients with mass lesions of the kidney. (From Garnick, M., & Richie, J. [1996]. Renal neoplasia. In B. Brenner [Ed.], *The kidney* [5th ed.]. Philadelphia: W. B. Saunders.)

bule, where the majority of the reabsorption of water and solutes takes place. In the collection duct the unwanted water, solutes, and waste products are excreted as urine. The kidneys process about 180 L (45 gallons) of blood-derived fluid daily. Of this amount, only about 1% (1.5 L) leaves the body as urine; the rest is returned to circulation.

The primary functions of the kidney include the following:

1. Excretion of unwanted substances such as waste products from cell metabolism, excess salts, and toxins
2. Maintenance of water balance
3. Regulation of acid base balance of body fluids
4. Production of renin, an enzyme that is important in the regulation of blood pressure
5. Production of the hormone erythropoietin, which stimulates the production of red blood cells in the bone marrow. This hormone is produced when the kidneys do not get enough oxygen (Memmler, Cohen, & Wood, 1996).

The Process of Carcinogenesis

The initiation, promotion, and progression of cancer is determined by balance between the activation and inactivation mechanism, the efficiency of the deoxyribonucleic acid (DNA) repair process, and the ability of the immune system to eliminate abnormal cells (Madajewicz, 1995).

In renal cell cancer, there is indirect evidence of the role of the immune system in this disease. Spontaneous regression occurs more often in renal cell cancer than in any other solid tumor. Oliver, Nethersell, and Bottomley (1989) reported on a series of 73 patients with metastatic renal cell cancer who were followed without therapy. Results showed that, without treatment, 4% of patients had a complete response (CR), 3% a partial response (PR), and 5% had a prolonged period (>12 months) of stable disease. Some of the responses in the absence of treatment may be evidence of the immune system at work. Other indirect evidence is in the many cases where metastasis develops 10, 20, or more years after resection of a localized cancer. It is presumed that the cancer had metastasized before the nephrectomy, but that the metastatic foci had remained in check by the immune system. The occasional dramatic regression of disease seen with patients treated with IL-2 immunotherapy is further evidence of the role of the immune system in the natural history of renal cell cancer (Bander, 1996).

Growth Factors

For many patients with renal cell cancer, there is evidence of tumor-produced factors that have systemic effects. Fever, cachexia, abnormal liver function, anemia, hypercalcemia, neuromyopathy, and amyloidosis have been reported with renal cell cancer. Hypercalcemia is thought to be caused by transforming growth factor (TGF) α and β, which may be related to the development of renal cell cancer (Madajewicz, 1995). The interaction between TGF-α and the epithelial growth factor receptor plays a role in promoting transformation and/or proliferation of renal cell cancer, possibly by an autocrine mechanism (Belldegrun, Abi-ad, Figlin, & de Kernion, 1991).

Madajewicz (1995) reports that studies of renal cell cancer tissues have demonstrated abnormally high expression of proto-oncogenes, including c-*myc,* c-*fos,* c-Ha-*ros,* c-Ki-*ros,* c-*fms,* and c-*erb* B-1. Expression of interleuken 6 (IL-6) was confirmed in kidney tumor cells. Patients with enhanced expression of the IL-6 gene showed increased incidence of lymph node metastasis.

Molecular Genetics

Studies indicate that deletions and translocations involving the short arm of chromosome 3 are important in the oncogenesis of sporadic and familial renal cell cancer and VHL disease. This information may suggest that a tumor suppressor gene helps play a role in sporadic and familial renal cell cancer (Walther, Jennings, Guarra, Zbar, & Linehan, 1996).

ROUTES OF METASTASES

Renal cell cancer is thought to originate in the proximal convoluted tubule in the parenchyma of the kidney and spread inward toward the renal medulla and cortex, directly invading normal kidney structures. It can further spread from its primary lesion in the kidney by direct extension into the renal vein, up the inferior vena cava, and occasionally into the right atrium of the heart. This tumor thrombus in the renal vein occurs in 15% to 20% of patients; inferior vena cava thrombi occur in 8% to 15% of patients (Couillard & de Vere White, 1993; McDougal & Garnick, 1996). Metastatic spread also occurs through lymphatic and hematogenous routes. Lymphatic spread begins in the nodal region in the renal hilum. Lymph node drainage of the kidney is variable, with metastatic disease reported in iliac, hilar, intraaortocaval, supraclavicular, and subdiaphragmatic areas. This makes a regional lymph node dissection less likely curative (McDougal & Garnick, 1996).

The sites of metastases with their approximate frequency

TABLE 49-1 Sites and Frequency of Metastasis in Renal Cell Cancer

Site	Percent
Lung	50-60
Lymph nodes	30-40
Liver	30-40
Bone	30-40
Adrenal	20
Opposite kidney	10
Brain	5

From McDougal, W. & Garnick, M. (1996). Clinical signs and symptoms of renal cell carcinoma. In M. Vogelzang, P. Sardini, W. Shipley, & D. Coffey (Eds.), *Comprehensive Textbook of Genitourinary Oncology.* Baltimore: Williams and Wilkins.

are listed in Table 49-1. Approximately 25% to 33% of patients have metastasis at the time of diagnosis (McDougal & Garnick, 1996).

ASSESSMENT

Routine and specific diagnostic tests are performed based on assessment findings and patient symptoms (Table 49-2). Early-stage cancer, specifically early stage renal cell cancer, may be asymptomatic. Approximately one third of renal cell cancers are discovered as incidental findings on imaging studies of the abdomen for nonurologic complaints (Glick & de Vere White, 1997).

History

For all patients, symptomatic and asymptomatic, a thorough history and review of systems is obtained. A detailed family medical history, including a family history of cancer, is an important component of this database. Health habits, which include a smoking history as well as the occupational or environmental exposure to carcinogens or toxins, should be obtained. This information not only helps assess cancer risk, but will add to existing epidemiologic data.

A general review of systems is obtained, with specific attention directed toward the following:

- Weight–present, usual, recent gain/loss
- Performance status–present and previous level of activity; note any weakness, fatigue, malaise, fevers
- Endocrine system–sweating, tachycardia, palpitations, flushing
- Musculoskeletal system–"lumps or bumps," flank mass; pain or tenderness in area
- Gastrointestinal system–appetite; note recent decrease
- Urinary tract and bladder–hematuria

In addition, asymptomatic individuals should be specifically queried about cancer's seven warning signals. This information adds to the assessment data and reinforces cancer-specific screening guidelines for patients and their families.

After a comprehensive database is obtained, the patient's symptoms are assessed. The classic triad of pain, hematuria,

TABLE 49-2 Assessment of the Patient for Renal Cell Cancer

	Assessment Parameters	Typical Abnormal Findings
History	A. Personal and social history: 1. Age 2. Family history 3. Patient's health history B. Evaluation of genitourinary system symptoms or presence of paraneoplastic symptoms	A. Personal and social risk factors: 1. Peak incidence 60-70 years of age 2. Renal disease or VHL Symptoms may include hematuria, intermittent fever, hypertension, weight loss, or hypercalcemia.
Physical Examination	Palpation of flank or abdominal mass	It is most readily palpated in thin adults and tumors of the lower pole of the kidney. The mass is generally firm, nontender, and hemogenous and moves with respiration. Occasionally, palpation of the mass may cause severe pain.
	Variocele	Acute onset of scrotal variocele that fails to empty in the recumbent position; usually on the left side
Diagnostic Tests	A. CBC	A. Anemia is present in many patients. Erythrocytosis is rare.
	B. Chemistry Liver/renal profile	Hypercalcemia due to bone metastasis or paraneoplastic syndrome Elevation of serum alkaline phosphatase, prothrombin time, and bilirubin values may indicate paraneoplastic syndrome.
	C. Plain abdominal film, KUB	May show mass effect that changes renal profile or generalized unilateral enlargement of kidney.
	Intravenous urography	The most significant diagnostic finding is distortion of the collection system.
	Ultrasound	This modality has improved the ability to differentiate between a simple benign cyst and a solid tumor. Needle aspiration of a cyst for cytology may be performed with ultrasound guidance.
	CT of abdomen	CT may demonstrate normal renal parenchyma and associated mass lesions. It may determine regional node involvement.
	MRI	MRI may be useful in the evaluation of renal masses, but especially useful in the evaluation of renal vein or inferior vena cava involvement with the tumor.

VHL, von Hippel-Lindau; *CBC,* complete blood count; *KUB,* kidneys, ureters, and bladder; *IVP,* intravenous urography; *CT,* computed tomography; *MRI,* magnetic resonance imaging.

and flank mass is found in less than 10% of patients at diagnosis and usually only in patients with advanced disease (McDougal & Garnick, 1996; Garnick & Richie, 1996). Painless hematuria is the most common presenting symptom, with gross hematuria occurring in 40% to 50% of patients (McDougal & Garnick, 1996). Hemorrhage into the tumor results in significant pain, with clot colic secondary to ureteral obstruction common (Glick & de Vere White, 1996). Flank pain is present in 35% to 40% of patients, and less than one third have a palpable abdominal or flank mass (Leder & Walther, 1996). Paraneoplastic syndromes occur in approximately 10% to 40% of presentations and are occasionally the initial finding that leads to a diagnosis (Table 49-3). These symptoms are due to humoral and local effects of renal cell cancer. Anemia may be present and is out of proportion to blood loss secondary to hematuria. It is normocytic and normochromic, but associated with decreased serum iron and iron-biding capacity and thought to be related to a decrease in erythropoietin production by the kidney (Chisholm & Roy, 1971). A small percentage of patients have erythrocytosis because of an erythropoietin-secreting tumor (Glick & de Vere White, 1996). Hypertion is common and may be renin mediated or secondary to arteriovenous fistula (Garnick & Richie, 1996). Fever may be secondary to the production of endogenous pyrogen by the tumor. It is usually intermittent without a constant pattern. Hypercalcemia may be due to bone metastasis, elevation of prostaglandins, or the production of a parathyroid-like hormone by the tumor (Glick & de Vere White, 1997). The cause of hepatic dysfunction (Stauffer's syndrome) manifested by abnormal liver functions tests is unknown and is occasionally associated with hepatosplenomegaly. Its presence does not imply metastatic disease to the liver, and liver function tests often return to normal after nephrectomy (McDougal & Garnick, 1996; Glick & de Vere White, 1997).

The acute appearance of a variocele, usually on the left side, is a presenting sign in 2% to 11% of patients. This is caused by obstruction of the left gonadal vein by the tumor.

TABLE 49-3 Paraneoplastic Syndromes Associated with Renal Cell Cancer

Syndrome	Incidence (%)
Anemia	20-40
Cachexia, fatigue, weight loss	33
Fever	30
Hypertension	24
Hypercalcemia	10-15
Hepatic dysfunction (Stauffer's Syndrome)	3-6
Amyloidisis	3-5
Erychrocytosis	3-4
Enteropathy	3
Neuromyopathy	3

From McDougal, W., & Garnick, M. (1996). Clinical signs and symptoms of renal cell carcinoma. In M. Vogelzang, P. Sardini, W. Shipley, & D. Coffey (Eds.), *Comprehensive Textbook of Genitourinary Oncology.* Baltimore: Williams and Wilkins.

The presence of a right-sided variocele occurs less frequently (Glick & de Vere White, 1997). Other rare systemic or endocrine effects may include a polyneuromyopathy manifested by neurologic complaints, secondary amyloidosis, and enteropathy.

Signs of vena cava obstruction occur in 7% to 36% of patients and include edema, abdominal distention with ascites, liver dysfunction, nephrotic syndrome, venous collaterals on the abdominal wall, variocele, malabsorption, pulmonary embolus, and jugular venous distention.

Physical Examination

Following inspection, palpation and ascultation as appropriate, renal cell cancer–specific assessment includes: Presence of costal-vertebral angle (CVA) tenderness, palpation of spine, genitourinary (GU) examination, palpation of flank and abdomen.

A physical examination may reveal a palpable mass in the upper quadrant, a variocele that does not subside on assuming a supine position, adenopathy, or bone pain suggestive of metastatic disease.

Diagnostic Tests

In addition to a complete blood count (CBC), blood chemistry, renal and liver profile, and urinalysis, the following diagnostic tests are performed:

- A *KUB (kidney, ureter, bladder) radiograph* may be the first diagnostic test performed to evaluate urologic symptoms. It may suggest unilateral enlargement or a mass effect that alters the renal profile.
- An *intravenous pyelogram (IVP)* is also frequently the first study used to detect renal cell cancer in patients who have flank pain or hematuria. The IVP is used to evaluate function, anatomy, and possible kidney or ureter obstruction. A mass effect as evidenced by distortion of the calices, lack of visualization of part of the collecting system, or distortion of the renal outline should be evaluated by a diagnostic workup (Glick & de Vere White, 1997). The IVP is neither specific nor sensitive for small to medium renal tumors that may be present despite a normal IVP. Fig. 49-4 presents a flow chart for the evaluation of renal masses.
- *Renal ultrasound* may be the first diagnostic test for patients with a contrast dye allergy or renal failure. Ultrasound is highly accurate in differentiating cystic from solid renal masses. Criteria for a simple cystic mass include a smooth wall with lack of separation, absence of internal echoes, good sound transmission, a round or oval shape, and acoustic shadowing at the edges of the cyst. When these criteria are met, there is a 98% chance that it is a benign cyst (McDougal & Garnick, 1996). For doubtful lesions, cyst aspirations may be performed, with fluid sent for cytology.
- The *computed tomography (CT) scan* also differentiates between a cyst and a tumor. In addition, it is the most common means of staging the primary tumor and assess-

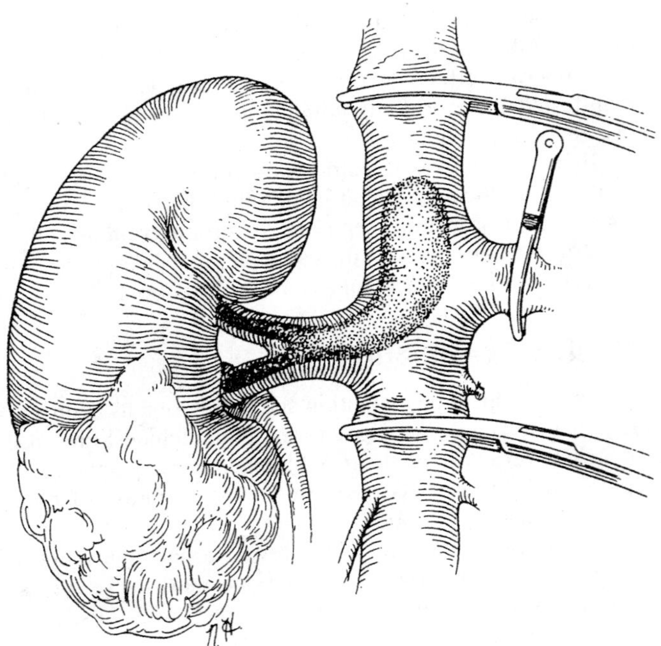

Fig. 49-4 Surgical removal of a kidney tumor that has extended through the renal vein into the inferior vena cava. (Modified from Linehan, W., Shipley, W., & Parkenson, D. [1993]. Cancer of the kidney and ureter. In V. DeVita, S. Hellman, & S. Rosenberg [Eds.], *Cancer principles and practice of oncology.* Philadelphia: J. B. Lippincott.)

Table 49-4 Comparison of Modified Robson and TNM Staging Systems of Renal Adenocarcinoma

Modified Robson Stage		T	N	M
I	Confined to renal capsule	T1 < 2.5 cm T2 > 2.5 cm	N0	M0
II	Through renal capsule, confined to Gerota's fascia	T3a	N0	M0
IIIA	Renal vein involvement	T3b	N0	M0
IIIB	Lymphatic involvement	T1-3b	N1-4	M0
IIIC	Vein and node involvement	T3b	N1-4	M0
IVA	Continguous organ involvment	T1-3b	N0-4	M0
IVB	Metastatic spread	T1-3b	N0-4	M1

From McDougal, W., & Garnick, M. (1996). Clinical signs and symptoms of renal cell carcinoma. In M. Vogelzang, P. Sardini, W. Shipley, & D. Coffey (Eds.), *Comprehensive Textbook of Genitourinary Oncology.* Baltimore: Williams and Wilkins.

ing nodal involvement, as well as renal vein and vena cava involvement with tumor thrombus.

- *Magnetic resonance imaging (MRI)* is being used more frequently in the evaluation of solid renal masses. MRI has the advantage over CT of being able to move in multiple planes, as well as having more accuracy in determining the presence and level of tumor invasion into vascular structures. (Glick & de Vere White, 1997).
- A *chest x-ray film* is routinely taken preoperatively or as part of a metastatic workup.
- A *bone scan* is performed only in the presence of bone pain or elevated serum alkaline phosphatase.

Diagnosis of Renal Cell Cancer.. Renal cell cancer, known as the *internist's tumor* because of its often broad and nonspecific presenting signs and symptoms, is often a diagnostic challenge. Subtle presenting symptoms such as hypertension, fever, and weakness are part of a parneoplastic syndrome and often represent advanced disease. The early detection of renal cell cancer when it is still localized and potentially curable is most often a fortuitous event found by imaging techniques evaluating a nonurologic complaint. After renal cell cancer is suspected, various radiographic techniques allow further characterization of suspicious pathology, as well as staging of known neoplastic disease prior to consideration of treatment options.

STAGING

As with any malignancy, the total volume of a tumor or the extent of disease influences survival. The staging of renal cell cancer is based on clinical and pathologic evidence of disease extent. Staging is necessary to determine appropriate treatment, as well as to provide prognostic information. Two systems have been used to stage renal cell carcinoma: the TNM classification and the Robson classification (Table 49-4). Historically in the United States, the staging system most commonly used was Robson's modification of the Flocks and Kadesky system (Robson, Churchill, & Anderson, 1969). A brief summary of this system is as follows: A stage I tumor is confined to the renal capsule; a stage II tumor extends through the renal capsule but is confined to Gerota's fascia; a stage III tumor involves the renal vein, inferior vena cava, or the local hilar lymph nodes; and a stage IV tumor involves spread to local, adjacent organs or to distant sites. A disadvantage of this staging system is that it fails to give consistent prognostic information in Stage III, combining tumors of renal vein involvement with those of regional lymph node involvement (Glick & de Vere White, 1997).

The TNM staging system was developed to classify the extent of a tumor more accurately. This method is used by the American Joint Committee on Cancer Staging and End Results Reporting Classification (Table 49-5). It has an advantage over the modified Robson classification in that it allows for separation of nodal involvement from vascular invasion and more clearly defines the anatomic extent of disease (Beahrs, Henson, Hutter, & Kennedy, 1992).

Pathologic staging includes the histologic examination of the resected tumor and confirmation of the extent of disease. Resection of the primary tumor, kidney, Gerota's fascia, perinephric fat, renal vein, and lymph nodes is required. Renal cell cancers have been histologically typed as clear cell, granular, sarcomatoid, and papillary types. The histologic types are commonly mixed, except for the papillary type (McDougal & Garnick, 1996).

TABLE 49-5 TNM Staging for Renal Cell Cancer

Primary Tumor (T)			
TX	Primary tumor cannot be assessed		
T0	No evidence of primary tumor		
T1	Tumor 2.5 cm or less in greatest dimension limited to the kidney		
T2	Tumor more than 2.5 cm in greatest dimension limited to the kidney		
T3	Tumor extends into major veins or invades adrenal gland or perinephric tissues, but not beyond Gerota's fascia		
T3a	Tumor invades adrenal gland or perinephric tissues, but not beyond Gerota's fascia		
T3b	Tumor grossly extends into renal vein(s) or vena cava below diaphragm		
T3c	Tumor grossly extends into vena cava above diaphragm		
T4	Tumor invades beyond Gerota's fascia		
Lymph Node (N)			
NX	Regional lymph nodes cannot be assessed		
N0	No regional lymph node metastasis		
N1	Metastasis in a single lymph node, 2 cm or less in greatest dimension		
N2	Metastasis in a single lymph node, more than 2 cm but not more than 5 cm in greatest dimension, or multiple lymph nodes, none more than 5 cm in greatest dimension		
N3	Metastasis in a lymph node more than 5 cm in greatest dimension		
Distant Metastasis (M)			
MX	Presence of distant metastasis cannot be assessed		
M0	No distant metastasis		
M1	Distant metastasis		
Stage Grouping			
I	T1	N0	M0
II	T2	N0	M0
III	T1	N1	M0
	T2	N1	M0
	T3a	N0	M0
	T3a	N1	M0
	T3b	N0	M0
	T3b	N1	M0
	T3c	N0	M0
	T3c	N1	M0
IV	T4	Any N	M0
	Any T	N2	M0
	Any T	N3	M0
	Any T	Any N	M1

MEDICAL MANAGEMENT

Complete surgical resection is the only potentially curative therapy for localized renal cell cancer. Patients with tumors confined to the kidney have the most hopeful prognosis. The site and volume of metastatic disease (solitary versus multiple metastatic sites), as well as the age and general physical health of the patient, are prognostic variables that affect further treatment decisions. Immunotherapy and radiotherapy are possible options in the treatment of metastatic renal cell cancer.

Localized Renal Cell Cancer

Radical nephrectomy is the most common surgical technique used in the treatment of renal cell cancer and is the procedure of choice for localized disease. It routinely involves the ligation of the renal artery and vein, as well as the removal of the kidney, ipsilateral adrenal gland, perinephric fat, Gerota's fascia, and at most institutions, regional lymph nodes (Glick & deVere White, 1997; Sokoloff, de Kernion, Figlin, & Belldegrum, 1996; Kassabian & Graham, 1995). In the past a simple nephrectomy had been reported as adequate treatment. This procedure included removal of the kidney from the perinephric fat, the adrenal gland, and regional lymph nodes. There are no randomized studies comparing simple versus radical nephrectomy, but because renal tumors often invade the perinephric fat, there is no benefit to leaving Gerota's fascia (Sokoloff et al., 1996; Glick & deVere White, 1997; Couillard & deVere White, 1993).

The risk of ipsilateral adrenal gland involvement with renal cell cancer is relatively rare and is related to the size, location, and malignant potential of the kidney primary. The need for routine ipsilateral adrenalectomy is currently being debated. At this time in the absence of long-term data suggesting otherwise, the adrenal gland is usually removed as part of the radical nephrectomy (Sokoloff et al., 1996; Glick & deVere White, 1997).

The necessity of regional lymphadenectomy also remains controversial. Although its role in improving staging accuracy is important, its effectiveness in prolonging survival has not been clearly demonstrated and the survival rate for patients with positive nodes is poor (Glick & de Vere White, 1997; Linehan, Shipley, & Parkenson, 1993).

The most common surgical approaches for a radical nephrectomy are the anterior transperitoneal approach, the flank approach, and the throcoabdominal approach. The choice is based on the surgeon's preference, the location and size of the tumor, and the body habitus of the patient. A flank incision, with or without removal of part of the tenth or eleventh rib, may be used for small tumors without venous involvement. A transabdominal approach with a midline or bilateral subcoastal incision is used for bilateral renal surgery, parenchyma-sparing surgery, and left-sided carcinoma with a thrombus in the renal vein or proximal vena cava. A right intrapleural thorocabdominal approach can be used for right-sided lesions with extensive involvement of the inferior vena cava.

Renal cell cancer has a tendency to form a thrombus, which may involve the renal vein (Fig. 49-5) or the inferior vena cava and may extend into the right atrium. Extension into the renal vein occurs in 15% to 20% of patients (Couillard & deVere White, 1993) and thrombi involving the vena cava in 8% to 15% of patients (Glick & deVere White, 1997). Signs of vena cava obstruction occur in 7% to 36% of patients and include edema, abdominal distention with ascites, liver dysfunction, nephrotic syndrome, venous col-

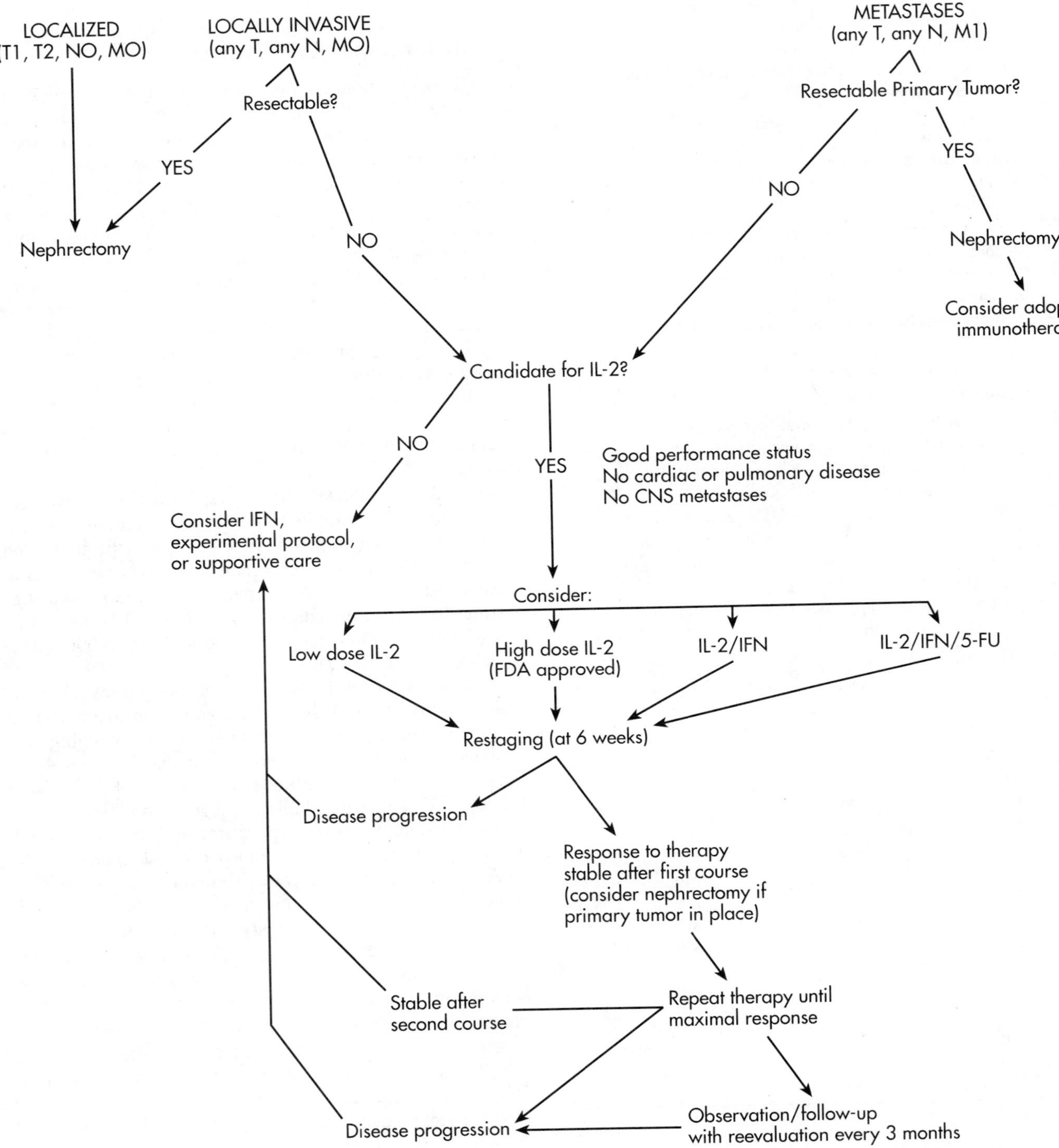

Fig. 49-5 Management algorithm used at UCLA when treating a patient with advanced renal cell carcinoma. (From Sokoloff, M., Figlin, R., & Belldegrum, A. [1996]. Treatment of metastatic renal cell carcinoma. In E. Crawford & S. Das [Eds.], *Current genitourinary cancer surgery.* Baltimore: Williams and Wilkins.)

laterals on the abdominal wall, variocele, malabsorption, pulmonary embolus, and jugular venous distention (McDougal & Garnick, 1996).

The outcome of the surgical procedure in these patients is determined by the size of the primary tumor. Vena cava involvement without evidence of nodal or distant metastasis of itself is not necessarily a poor prognostic sign and justifies an aggressive surgical approach (Couillard & deVere White, 1993). Preoperative assessment of the precise extent of the tumor thrombus is necessary before determining the feasibility of the surgery, as well as the surgical approach, which may require a cardiopulmonary bypass. Although vena cava involvement can be suspected based on clinical signs, symptoms, and CT findings, MRI is the diagnostic test of choice for assessing the extent of the thrombus (Glick & deVere White, 1993; McDougal & Garnick, 1996).

Nelson and Marshall (1996) summarized complications from a large series of patients who underwent surgical resection of renal cell cancer extending into the superior vena cava. Operative mortality rates from 1.4 to 13 were reported, with deaths occurring intraoperatively. The postoperative complications range from 30% to 60%, with sepsis, retroperitoneal hemorrhage, and hepatic dysfunction the most commonly reported complications.

Partial Nephrectomy

The nephron-sparing surgical procedure, or partial nephrectomy, was developed for patients who had tumors in solitary kidneys. The goal of the procedure was to totally excise the tumor, leaving enough renal parenchyma to function and obviate the need for renal dialysis. This procedure produced some encouraging results and is gradually becoming an accepted method of therapy for selected patients with renal cell cancers less than 3 cm and normal contralateral kidneys (Sokoloff et al., 1996; Klein & Novick, 1996; Steinback, Stockle, & Hohenfellner, 1995).

In a review of the results of 259 nephron-sparing operations, the most common postoperative complications were urinary fistula formation and acute renal failure. The majority of fistulas resolved spontaneously or with placement or removal of a uretheral stint. Renal failure resolved spontaneously in a majority of patients. The risk of developing significant complications was considered low for small tumors in the periphery of the kidney (Klein & Novick, 1996).

Renal Artery Embolization

Embolic occlusion of the renal circulation has been used before nephrectomy to shrink large hypervascular tumors. It has also been used in patients who are not surgical candidates and have life-threatening A-V fistulas, bleeding, and other severe symptoms (Nelson & Marshall, 1996; Linehan, Shipley, & Parkenson, 1993).

Although a variety of techniques have been used to occlude the renal artery, generally an angiographic catheter is advanced to the renal artery through a transfemoral approach. Agents such as Gelfoam, stainless steel pellets, barium, silicone, or rubber are injected for transcatheter embolization. The procedure is done under fluoroscopic control (Nelson & Marshall, 1996).

A postinfarction syndrome may occur almost immediately after the procedure; this syndrome consists of pain, fever, gastrointestinal complaints, and malaise (Garnick & Richie 1996). The major risk associated with embolization is potential emboli (Garnick & Richie, 1996; Nelson & Marshall, 1996). Other reported complications include renal failure, renal abscess, aneurysm formation, prolonged hypertension, paraplegia, and colonic infarction (Nelson & Marshall, 1996).

Bilateral Renal Cell Cancer

The incidence of bilateral renal cell cancer is approximately 2%. Surgical options for bilateral synchronous tumors include the following: unilateral partial nephrectomy followed by contralateral nephrectomy, bilateral partial nephrectomy, or bilateral radical nephrectomy followed by renal dialysis (Glick & deVere White, 1997; Couillard & deVere White, 1993). The goal is to preserve as much functioning kidney as possible while removing all of the cancer. Although treatment decisions are difficult, the long-term risks of hemodialysis are considerable.

Metastatic Renal Cell Cancer

About one third of patients with renal cell cancer have metastatic disease at the time of diagnosis, with approximately 3% of these patients presenting with a solitary metastasis. Surgical resection may be appropriate in selected patients; nephrectomy and resection result in few cures, but frequently produce some long-term survivors (Linehan, Shipley, & Parkenson, 1993; Sokoloff, Figlin, & Belldegrum, 1996).

Radiation Therapy

The role of radiation therapy in the local management of renal cell cancer is usually palliative. For some, renal cell cancer is considered to be a radioresistant tumor (Garnick & Richie, 1996). To date, no study has shown a survival advantage with the adjuvant postoperative radiotherapy or for primary radiotherapy for locally extensive disease (Sokoloff, deKernion, Figlin, & Belldegrum, 1996). For patients with symptomatic metastasis, external beam irradiation has reported objective or subjective response in half to two thirds of patients (Linehan, Shipley, & Parkenson, 1993).

Chemotherapy

The success rate for single agent or combination chemotherapy in the treatment of renal cell cancer has been poor. This has led to researchers describing renal cell cancer as a *chemotherapy-resistant tumor* (Gorsch & Ernstoff, 1996; Linehan, Shipley, & Parkenson, 1993; Yogoda, Petrylak, & Thompson, 1993). In a review of 72 agents used singly or in a limited number of two-drug combinations in over 3500 patients treated between 1983 and 1992, an objective response (complete and partial remissions) rate of 5.6% was noted. This response was usually of short duration (Yogoda, Petrylak, & Thompson, 1993; Sokoloff, deKernion, Figlin, & Belldegrum, 1996). The reason for this lack of response to chemotherapy may be related to evidence suggesting that a transmembrane glycoprotein is actively involved in pumping drugs out of cells. Research overcoming multidrug resistance may lead to more effective chemotherapy-based treatment for renal cell cancer (Linehan, Shipley, & Parkenson, 1993; Glick & de Vere White, 1997).

Hormonal Therapy

There are no studies showing that treating renal cell cancer with progestational agents or tamoxifen has been more than anecdotally useful (Gorsch & Ernstoff, 1996; Glick & de Vere White, 1997; Linehan, Shipley, & Parkenson, 1993).

Immunotherapy

Unique immunologic factors associated with renal cell cancer include occasional spontaneous regression, circulating hormonal and cellular elements, temporary regression of metastatic lesions after nephrectomy, and widely variable doubling times. The acknowledgment of these factors, manipulation of the immune system, and potential benefit of biologic response modifier therapy continue to be investigated in the management of metastatic disease.

Recombinant DNA technology, with the ability to produce large quantities of cytokines, has resulted in the widespread use of cytokines as they become an approved treatment modality for metastatic disease. At present, most studies investigating cytokines in the treatment of metastatic renal cell cancer have used Interferon α (IFNα), IL-2, combinations of these, or adoptive immunotherapy with tumor-infiltrating lymphocytes (TILs) or lymphokine-activated killer cells (LAKS) (Sokoloff, deKernion, Figlin, & Belldegrum, 1996).

IL-2 was the first cytokine to demonstrate antitumor effects on the host immune system. Rosenberg and colleagues (1994) summarized their experiences with high-dose IL-2, showing an overall response rate of 20%. Better response rates were seen in patients with good performance status and small volume disease. The significant side effects of this therapy, which were dose related, included hypotension, pulmonary edema, renal failure, fluid retention, myocardial infarction, gastrointestinal bleeding and perforation, and death. Other side effects included fever, chills, anorexia, mental status changes, and tachycardia (Sokoloff, deKernion, Figlin, & Belldegrum, 1996).

IL-2 has gained approval by the U.S. Food and Drug Administration for the treatment of metastatic renal cell cancer in patients with good performance status. Since the approval of IL-2, studies have been published with response rates of 10% to 35% in patients with excellent performance status, previous nephrectomy, and minimal pulmonary or lymph node disease (Garnick & Richie, 1996).

Combining IL-2 with IFNα was investigated as a means of reducing the toxicity of treatment with IL-2 alone. Results of studies at UCLA using a low-dose outpatient regimen showed an average response rate of 25% with a median response duration of 23 months and median survival duration of 34 months or more (Figlin et al., 1992). The side effects of therapy included fever, chills, nausea, anorexia, and hypotension, which were less severe than those of high-dose IL-2 therapy (Sokoloff, deKernion, Figlin, & Belldegrum, 1996). The combination of IL-2, IFNα, and 5-fluorouracil has shown response rates of over 45% and continues as an area of ongoing research (Sella, Zakewski, & Robinson, 1994).

Sokoloff, deKernion, Figlin, & Belldegrum, (1996) at UCLA reported progressive increases in responses to immunotherapy for renal cell cancer over the past 2 decades as therapy has evolved from systemic IFNα (16%), combination IFNα/IL-2 (25%) to current treatment regimens using bulk TILs (33%) and CD8+/TILs (40%). Although further investigation of immunotherapy treatment for renal cell cancer is still needed, current treatment protocols have produced significant and lasting remissions in selected patients.

ONCOLOGIC EMERGENCIES

The major oncologic emergency associated with renal cell cancer is hypercalcemia. The presence of hypercalcemia may be due to osseous metastasis or a paraneoplastic syndrome resulting from the secretion of a variety of hormonal agents. Patients who are symptomatic or those with serum calcium levels of 13 mg/dl require emergency treatment. Symptoms of hypercalcemia are progressive, with early symptoms including anorexia, nausea, vomiting, abdominal pain, constipation, lethargy, and polyuria. Later symptoms include dehydration, confusion, stupor, convulsions, bradycardia, tachycardia, and orthostatic hypotension. Intensive medical management includes vigorous saline hydration and may include furosemide, mithranycin, or calcitonin. When hypercalcemia is due to a paraneoplastic syndrome, removal of the primary tumor may eliminate the syndrome.

Skeletal metastases are seen in approximately 50% of patients with renal cell cancer (Kozlowski, 1996), with 5% of these lytic metastatic lesions responsible for spinal cord compression (Nielsen, Munro, & Tannock, 1991). The vertebral bodies of the lumbar thoracic spine are most often involved in this process (Cybulski, 1989). Back pain is the most common presenting symptom. Emergency treatment includes radiation therapy with or without a surgical decompression. Because spinal cord compression is one of the most common oncologic emergencies for all patients with cancer, prompt recognition, evaluation, and treatment of this complaint is necessary to preserve neurologic function, which greatly affects the quality of life.

NURSING MANAGEMENT

The medical management of renal cell cancer depends on the patient's stage of disease at diagnosis and performance status. The nursing management of patients with renal cell cancer has been summarized in several publications (LaFollette, 1992; Davis, 1993, 1994; Lind, Kravitz, & Greig, 1993; Gale & Charette, 1995). As with all oncology nursing care, nurses caring for patients with renal cell cancer must be familiar with the disease process and medical management. Nursing assessment, patient teaching, and patient advocacy are geared toward the individual patient and the treatment setting. Providing a copy of the National Cancer Institute publication *Kidney Cancer* may assist in providing baseline information to patients and families. The major treatment modalities for renal cell cancer are surgery and immunotherapy. The major issues associated with immunotherapy are discussed elsewhere in this text. Unique patient problems associated with radical nephrectomy for renal cell cancer are discussed as follows, with four standards of care provided.

Surgery

Surgical excision, or radical nephrectomy, is the only potentially curative therapy for patients with renal cell cancer. Patients undergoing this procedure are hospitalized for 5 to 7 days. The perioperative goal of nursing care is to provide and assess patient education regarding the preoperative evaluation, the surgical procedure, and pertinent surgical findings, as well as the specific expectations and procedures that are part of the postoperative period. Nursing interventions (Table 49-6) for patients undergoing a radical nephrectomy focus on assessment, management, and prevention of postoperative complications, which may include pain, pneumothorax, pneumonia, atelectasis, hemorrhage, ileus, renal insufficiency, and third-space fluid shifts.

Postoperative complications and care after radical nephrectomy include possible management of pleural injuries that escaped notice during the surgical procedure, resulting in a pneumothorax that may require chest tube placement. Nasogastric suction continues until peristalsis returns. Parenteral fluid replacement should consider the large volume of protein-rich transudate loss from the renal fossa and retroperitoneum. Replacement with plasma or albumin may be necessary. Vigorous pulmonary toilet and early ambulation are necessary to prevent respiratory compromise (Das, 1997). Other postoperative complications may include secondary hemorrhage, wound dehiscence, and intercostal neuralgia. Less common complications include CVA, precipitation of congestive heart failure (CHF), myocardial infarction, pulmonary embolus, atelectasis, and pneumonia (Heppe & Crawford, 1997).

Oncology nurses should allow patients to express their feelings about their diagnosis and the planned treatment. Patients undergoing nephrectomy should be assessed for anxiety regarding the loss of a kidney and reassured that a normal life is possible with one functioning kidney.

Radiation Therapy

At present the role for radiotherapy in renal cell cancer is primarily associated with symptom management and palliation in metastatic disease. Objective or subjective response rates are reported in half to two thirds of patients receiving palliative radiation therapy for pain or bleeding. The nursing care and assessment for patients receiving this treatment modality depend on the individual's symptoms and the specific area being treated. Nursing interventions are not specific to renal cell cancer and are discussed elsewhere in this text.

Immunotherapy

Nurses play a critical role in the care of patients receiving immunotherapy for renal cell cancer. For these patients with known advanced disease, this treatment is physically and emotionally challenging, and patients may consider discontinuing therapy prior to completion of the planned course. Careful patient and family education provided in an empathetic manner, combined with prompt intervention in side effect management, can help patients continue therapy and improve their potential for a positive clinical outcome (Reiger, 1995).

Various immunologic agents currently used include Interferons, Interleukin 2 (IL-2), or TILs. Side effects of treatment may include fever, chills, nausea, anorexia, hypotension, mental status changes, and hematologic changes. Specific nursing interventions and rationale are discussed in Chapter 7.

HOME CARE ISSUES

An assessment of the patient's and family's perception of the diagnosis and understanding is needed to ensure continuity of care for medical follow-up. Patients having undergone radical nephrectomy for potentially curative renal cell cancer need reassurance of the possibility of a normal life with one functioning kidney. Postoperative discharge instructions include the importance of fluid intake to 2500 ml/day to ensure renal perforation, pain management for incision, not lifting for 4 weeks to avoid wound adhesion, a low-fat diet, and wound pain management if a dressing remains in place. A list of potentially renal toxic drugs for the patient to avoid can be obtained from the pharmacist with instructions to avoid their use. Routine blood pressure assessment to monitor the function of the remaining kidney is important in signaling hypertensive and impending renal dysfunction. Symptoms such as uncontrolled pain, changes in respiratory status, increased wound drainage and fever, decreased urinary output, fluid retention, and hypertension require immediate medical assessment. Patients require guidance in reporting these problems to appropriate medical personnel (i.e., home care nurses or physicians).

Evaluation following a radical nephrectomy includes laboratory studies, chest x-ray, and physical examination every 6 months for 2 years, then annually (Montie, 1994) and abdominal CT scans every 12 months for 2 years, then every 2 years are necessary to monitor for disease recurrence. After a partial nephrectomy, laboratory studies and a physical examination are recommended every 3 months, with an abdominal CT scan obtained at 1, 6, 12, 18, and 24 months, then annually (Sokoloff et al., 1996). The American Cancer Society, programs such as "I Can Cope," and the National Kidney Cancer Association can offer patients and families supportive services to remind them of the need for follow-up.

For patients receiving biologic response modifiers therapy, extensive patient/family assessment and education

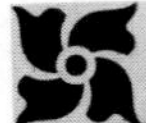

TABLE 49-6 Standard of Care for the Patient Undergoing Radical Nephrectomy

Patient Problem and Outcome	Nursing Interventions and Rationale	Patient Education/Instruction
Patient is at high risk for the following: • Pneumothorax • Atelectasis • Pneumonia Patient will maintain optimal respiratory status.	1. Assess for evidence of pneumothorax. Monitor for the following: • Restlessness • Anxiety • Increased diaphoresis • Shock • Sudden, sharp chest pain 2. Assess for evidence of atelectasis/pneumonia: • Shortness of breath • Fever • Cough • Blueness of lips/fingertips 3. If there is a chest tube in place, assess the drainage. 4. Assist patient to turn, cough, and deep breathe every 2 hours. (Administer analgesia 30 minutes prior. Splint incision with pillows.) 5. Monitor the rate, rhythm, depth, and effort of respirations. 6. Auscultate breath sounds, and note the type and location of adventicious sounds. 7. Incentive spirometer. 8. Ambulation.	1. Teach the patient about the risk of pneumothorax due to the close location of the kidney to the diaphragm, with the possibility of fluid/air in the pleural space. 2. Teach the patient to report the following: • Change in respiratory pattern or effort • Increased pulmonary secretions • Increased pain
Alteration in Comfort: Pain The patient will experience optimal pain relief with minimal side effects.	1. Assess/document the pain intensity using a 0-10 verbal rating scale every 2 hours for 48 hours postoperatively. 2. Administer opiod analgesia for first 48 hours postoperatively (consider PCA). 3. Assess/document the level of pain relief with each intervention. 4. Monitor analgesia side effects: prevent or treat. 5. Use massage/pillows to support the back when lying on the side.	1. Teach the patient that incisional pain as well as aches and discomfort from positioning during surgery may be relieved. 2. Review the explanation of the pain intensity scale: "0" = no pain; "10" = worst pain imaginable. 3. Teach the patient to inform the nurse of the presence of breakthrough pain.
High Risk for Hemorrhage Patient will maintain hemoglobin and hematocrit at an acceptable level.	1. Monitor for signs and symptoms of hemorrhage/shock: • Increasing respiratory rate • Increasing pulse with decreasing blood pressure • Palor; sweating; cool, clammy, or cyanotic skin • Restlessness, agitation, change in mentation • Dizziness, fainting • Urine output less than 30 cc/hr 2. Monitor the fluid status: • Intake (parenteral/oral) • Output—urine, vomitus, chest tube drainage 3. Assess the surgical site for distention and bleeding dehiscense. 4. Monitor the hemoglobin and hematocrit.	1. Teach the patient that monitoring for possible postoperative complications allows early intervention. 2. Teach the patient to inform the nurse if he/she experiences the following: • Weakness • Heart palpations • Chest pain 3. Explain the rationale for blood transfusions (i.e., low hematocrit). 4. Discuss possible signs and symptoms of transfusion reaction that should be reported immediately.
High Risk for Paralytic Ileus Patient will be assessed/treated to minimize complications.	1. Monitor for signs of paralytic ileus: • Absent or decreased bowel sounds • Abdominal discomfort • Abdominal distention 2. Keep the patient NPO until bowel sounds are present. 3. Monitor for vomiting, and note the type and amount of emesis.	1. Teach the patient that paralytic ileus is a possible complication of manipulation of the bowel during surgery, anesthesia, or narcotic analgesia. 2. Inform the nurse of the following: • Increasing abdominal discomfort • Nausea/vomiting

PCA, patient controlled analgesia; *NPO,* nothing by mouth.

is completed prior to discharge. Specific verbal and written instructions on side effects of treatment, management strategies, and mechanisms for reporting adverse events should be reviewed.

PROGNOSIS

The most important prognostic variable identified for patients with renal cell cancer is the stage of disease at the time of diagnosis. Patients with disease confined to the kidney and thus able to be completely resected have significantly better survival than those with nodal or metastatic spread. Demographic variables such as the patient's age, race, gender, performance status, and presenting symptoms appear to have less effect on the patient's ultimate survival. Unique tumor features such as nuclear grade, histologic pattern, tumor size, cell type, DNA content, and nuclear morphometry have been reported to affect survival to a variable extent. Controversy exists about the prognostic importance of renal vein, inferior vena cava, and renal pelvis involvement (Thrasher & Paulson, 1993). The actuarial 10-year survival of all patients diagnosed with renal cell cancer is 50% (McDougal & Garnick, 1996).

The reported 5-year survival rates for patients with organ-confined disease (stages I, II, IIIA) who undergo nephrectomy range from 56% to 90% (Thrasher & Paulson, 1993; Sokoloff et al., 1996; McDougal & Garnick, 1996). The stage IIIB 5-year survival rate reportedly ranges from 30% to 45% and stage IIIC from 16% to 20% (Couillard & de Vere White, 1993).

Patients with metastatic disease (Stage IV) have a 5-year survival of approximately 3% to 10% (Thrasher & Paulson, 1993; Glick & de Vere White, 1997; McDougal & Garnick, 1996).

Other variables such as the site of metastatic disease, the number of metastatic lesions, the time interval from the diagnosis to the appearance of metastatic disease, the grade of the primary tumor, and the presence of weight loss have been reported to affect survival (Thrasher & Paulson, 1993).

Patients who have disease spread by direct extension into the perinephric fat have a survival advantage over those with lymph node involvement but do worse than those with organ-confined disease (Thrasher & Paulson, 1993). Approximately 1.5% to 3.5% of patients with renal cell cancer have a solitary metastasis that is amenable to surgical resection. For these patients who have a nephrectomy and removal of their solitary metastatic lesion, the 5-year survival rate reportedly ranges from 34% to 59% (McDougal & Garnick, 1996). Renal cell cancer's growth rate is unpredictable, and it may remain localized for many years. There are reports of rare instances where the tumors or metastases have spontaneously shrunk or disappeared.

EVALUATION OF THE QUALITY OF CARE

Patients undergoing a radical nephrectomy for renal cell cancer require the expert care of a multidisciplinary team. All significant aspects of quality care should be documented in the interdisciplinary medical record. Further evaluation of this care can be gathered by patient survey. Table 49-7

TABLE 49-7 Quality of Care Evaluation for a Patient Undergoing Radical Nephrectomy

Part I: Data Documented in Medical Record

Disciplines participating in the quality of care evaluation:

☐ Nursing ☐ Urologic Surgeon
☐ Radiology ☐ Respiratory Therapy

Criteria	Yes	No
1. Patient provided with information about the following:		
a. Preoperative diagnostic tests	☐	☐
b. Significance of findings; rationale for surgery	☐	☐
c. Operative procedure; postoperative care/expectations	☐	☐
d. Pain management policy	☐	☐
2. Patient experienced the following complications:		
a. Postoperative pneumothorax requiring chest tube placement	☐	
b. Hemorrhage	☐	☐
c. Pneumonia	☐	☐
3. Patient experienced uncontrolled post-operative pain, as evidence by pain rating an average of 6 during a 24-hour interval.	☐	☐

Part II: Patient/Family Satisfaction

Data from the following:

☐ Patient interview prior to discharge ☐ Patient mailed survey

Criteria	Yes	No
1. Were you informed preoperatively about the hospital's pain management policy and the 0-10 pain assessment scale?	☐	☐
2. Were your questions about your diagnosis answered satisfactorily by the following:		
a. Doctor	☐	☐
b. Nurse	☐	☐
3. Were your questions about your care answered satisfactorily by the following:		
a. Nurse	☐	☐
b. Doctor	☐	☐
c. Respiratory therapist	☐	☐
4. Did you receive satisfactory pain control after your surgery?	☐	☐
5. Were you informed of the importance of the postoperative follow-up and schedule?	☐	☐

TABLE 49-8 Quality of Care Evaluation for Patients Receiving BRM Therapy

Disciplines participating in the quality of care evaluation:
☐ Nursing ☐ Medical Oncology ☐ Social Service
☐ Pharmacy

Data from: ☐ Mailed questionnaire ☐ Patient interview

Criteria	Yes	No
1. Did your doctor or nurse discuss the following possible side effects of your therapy with you or your family?		
a. Fever	☐	☐
b. Nausea	☐	☐
c. Fatigue	☐	☐
d. Loss of appetite	☐	☐
e. Mental status changes	☐	☐
f. Flu-like symptoms		
• Fever	☐	☐
• Muscle aches	☐	☐
Were you given written information on these side effects?	☐	☐
2. Were you instructed to take acetaminophen prior to each dose of interferon?	☐	☐
3. Were you instructed on ways to help manage the following side effects?		
a. Fatigue	☐	☐
b. Nausea	☐	☐
c. Decreased appetite	☐	☐
4. Were you given emergency instructions and a phone number?	☐	☐
5. Were you given information on individual or family support groups (i.e., "I Can Cope")?	☐	☐

(Parts I and II) provides an evaluation tool that can be used after radical nephrectomy. Patients with metastatic renal cell cancer may be candidates for therapy with biologic response modifier therapy, and Table 49-8 provides an evaluation tool that may be used for patients receiving this treatment modality.

RESEARCH ISSUES

Renal cell cancer is one of the least studied of all the major cancers in the United States. Studies are needed to define the environmental, occupational, immunologic, and genetic risk factors of renal cell cancer more specifically, as well as to demonstrate possible early intervention or prevention strategies.

Data continue to be evaluated regarding the role of various surgical techniques used in the treatment of localized renal cell cancer. This includes radical versus simple nephrectomy, versus nephron-sparing procedures, as well as limited versus extensive lymphectomy.

There is strong indirect evidence that the host immune system is involved in the natural history of renal cell cancer (Bander, 1996). Research continues into the role of the immune system and immunotherapy, as well as the use of monoclonal antibodies in the diagnosis and possible treatment of renal cell cancer.

Studies suggest that quality of life (QOL) and quality of care (QOC) are independent concepts and that a patient's QOL assessment is not necessarily predictive of the perception of QOC, or vice versa (Rieker, Clark, & Fogeberg, 1992). Further study is needed on QOL/QOC concepts as they relate to patients receiving at times aggressive biologic and surgical therapies for metastatic renal cell cancer.

REFERENCES

Bander, N. H. (1996). Immunology of renal cell carcinoma. In N. Vogelzang, P. Sardino, W. Shipley, & D. Coffey, (Eds.), *Comprehensive textbook of genitourinary oncology.* Baltimore: Williams and Wilkins.

Beahrs, O., Henson, D., Hutter, R., & Kennedy, B. (1992). *Manual for staging of cancer* (4th ed.). Philadelphia: J. B. Lippincott.

Belldegrun, A., Abi-ad, A., Figlin, R., & de Kernion, J. (1991). Renal cell carcinoma: Basic biology and current approaches to therapy. *Seminars in Oncology, 18*(5), 96-101.

Chisholm, G. & Roy, R. (1971). The systemic effects of malignant renal tumors. *British Journal of Urology, 43,* 687.

Chow, W., McLaughlin, J., Mandel, J., Blot, W., Niwa, S., & Fraumeni, J. (1995). Reproductive factors and the risk of renal cell cancer among women. *International Journal of Cancer, 60*(3), 321-324.

Couillard, D. & de Vere White, R. (1993). Surgery of renal cell carcinoma. *Urologic Clinics of North America, 20*(2), 263-272.

Cybulski, C. (1989). Methods of surgical stabilization for metastatic disease of the spine. *Neurosurgery, 25,* 240-252.

Das, S. (1997). Radical nephrectomy; thoracoabdominal extrapleural approach. In E. Crawford & S. Das (Eds.), *Current genitourinary cancer surgery.* Baltimore: Williams and Wilkins.

Davis, M. (1993). Renal cell carcinoma. *Seminars in Oncology Nursing, 9*(4), 267-271.

Davis, M. (1994). Genitourinary cancers. In S. Otto (Ed.), *Oncology nursing.* St. Louis: Mosby.

Finkle, W., McLaughlin, J., Rasgon, S., Yeoh, H., & Low, J. (1993). Increased risk of renal cell cancer among women using diuretics in the United States. *Cancer Causes and Control 4*(6), 555-558.

Gale, D. & Charette, J. (1995). *Genitourinary cancer: Oncology nursing care plans.* El Paso: Skidmore-Roth.

Garnick, M. & Richie, J. (1996). Renal neoplasia. In B. Brenner (Ed.), *The kidney* (5th ed.). Philadelphia: W. B. Saunders.

Glick, S. & de Vere White, R. (1997). Primary renal cell cancer. In E. D. Crawford & S. Das (Eds.), *Current genitourinary cancer surgery.* Baltimore: Williams and Wilkins.

Gorsch, S. & Ernstoff, M. (1996). Chemotherapy, hormonal therapy, and interferons. In N. Vogelzang, P. Scardino, W. Shipley, & D. Coffey (Eds.), *Comprehensive textbook of genitourinary oncology.* Baltimore: Williams and Wilkins.

Heppe, R. & Crawford, E. (1997). Radical nephrectomy, throabdominal approach. In E. Crawford & S. Das (Eds.), *Current genitourinary cancer surgery* (2nd ed.). Baltimore: Williams and Wilkins.

Hiatt, R., Tolan, K., & Quesenberry, C. (1994). Renal cell carcinoma and thiazide use: A historical, case control study. *Cancer Causes and Control, 5*(4), 319-325.

Kassabian, V.S. & Graham, S. D. (1995). Urologic and male genital cancers. In G. Murphy, W. Lawrence, & R. Lenhard (Eds.), *American cancer society textbook of clinical oncology.* Atlanta: American Cancer Society.

Klein, E. & Novick, A. (1996). Surgical management of localized disease. In M. Vogelzang, P. Sardini, W. Shipley, & D. Coffey (Eds.), *Comprehensive textbook of genitourinary oncology.* Baltimore: Williams and Wilkins.

Kozlowski, J. (1996). Surgical resection of metastatic disease. In N. Vogelzang, P. Scardino, W. Shipley, & D. Coffey (Eds.), *Comprehensive textbook of genitourinary oncology.* Baltimore: Williams and Wilkins.

LaFollette, S. (1992). Kidney cancer, an overview of the disease, treatment. *AORN Journal 56*(1), 31-48.

Leder, A. & Walther, P. (1996). Radiologic imaging of renal cell carcinoma: Its role in diagnosis, staging and management. In M. Vogelzang, P. Sardini, W. Shipley, & D. Coffey (Eds.), *Comprehensive textbook of genitourinary oncology.* Baltimore: Williams and Wilkins.

Lind, J., Kravitz, K., & Greig, B. (1993). Urologic and male genital malignancies. In S. Groenwald, M. Goodman, M. Frogge, & C. Yarboro (Eds.), *Cancer nursing principles and practice* (3rd ed.). Boston: Jones and Bartlett.

Linehan, W., Shipley, W., & Parkenson, D. (1993). Cancer of the kidney and ureter. In V. DeVita, S. Hellman, & S. Rosenberg (Eds.), *Cancer: Principles and practice of oncology.* Philadelphia: J. B. Lippincott.

Madajewicz, S. (1995). Genitourinary cancer. In P. Greenwald, B. Kramer, & D. Weed (Eds.), *Cancer: Prevention and control.* New York: Marcel Dekker.

Mandel, J., McLaughlin, J., Schlehofer, B., Mellemgaard, A., Helmert, A., Lindblad, P., McCredie, M. (1995). International renal-cell cancer study IV, Occupation. *International Journal of Cancer, 61*(5), 601-605.

Marieb, E. (1991). *The kidney: Essentials of human anatomy and physiology* (3rd ed.). Menlo Park, CA: Benjamin/Cummings.

Martz, C. (1992). Von Hippel-Lindau disease: A genetically transmitted multisystem neoplastic disorder. *Seminars in Oncology Nursing, 8*(4), 281-287.

McDougal, W. & Garnick, M. (1996). Clinical signs and symptoms of renal cell cancer. In M. Vogelzang, P. Sardini, W. Shipley, & D. Coffey (Eds.), *Comprehensive textbook of genitourinary oncology.* Baltimore: Williams and Wilkins.

McLaughlin, J., Gao, Y., Gao, R., Zheng, W., Ji, B., Blot, W., & Fraumeni, J. (1992). Risk factors for renal cell cancer in Shanghai, China. *International Journal of Cancer, 52,* 562-565.

Mellemgaard, A., Engholm, G., McLaughlin, J., & Olsen, J. (1994). Risk factors for renal-cell carcinoma in Denmark: Role of weight, physical activity and reproductive factors. *International Journal of Cancer, 56*(1), 66-71.

Memmler, R., Cohen, B., & Wood, D. (1996). *The urinary system and body fluids. Structure and function of the human body* (6th ed.). Philadelphia: J. B. Lippincott.

Montie, J. (1994). Follow up after partial or total nephrectomy of renal cell carcinoma. *Urologic Clinics of North America, 2,* 589-592.

Muscat, J., Hoffman, D., & Wynder, E. (1995). The epidemiology of renal cell carcinoma: A second look. *Cancer, 75*(10), 2552-2557.

Nelson, J. & Marshall, F. (1996). Surgical treatment of locally advanced renal cell carcinoma. In M. Vogelzang, P. Sardini, W. Shipley, & D. Coffey (Eds.), *Comprehensive textbook of genitourinary oncology.* Baltimore: Williams and Wilkins.

Nielsen, O., Munro, A., & Tannock, I. (1991). Bone metastasis: Pathophysiology and management policy. *Journal Clinical Oncology, 9,* 509-524.

Oliver, R., Nethersell, A., & Bottomley, J. (1989). Unexplained spontaneous regression and alpha-interferon as a treatment for metastatic renal carcinoma. *British Journal of Urology, 63,* 128-131.

Pack, R. (1993). Descriptive epidemiology of genitourinary cancers. *Seminars in Oncology Nursing,. 9*(4), 218-223.

Paganini-Hill, A., Ross, R., & Henderson, B. (1988). Epidemiology of renal cancer. In D. Skinner & G. Lieskovsky (Eds.), *Diagnosis and management of genitourinary cancer.* Philadelphia: W. B. Saunders.

Parker, S. L., Tong, T., Bolden, S., & Wingo, P.A. (1997). Cancer statistics 1997. *CA-A. Cancer Journal for Clinicians, 47*(1), 5-27.

Rieger, P. (1995). *Interleukin-2: A paradigm for developing nursing strategies for patient management.* USA: Pro Ed Communications.

Rieker, P., Clark, E., & Fogeberg, P. (1992). Perceptions of quality of life and quality of care for patients with cancer receiving biological therapy. *Oncology Nursing Forum, 19*(3), 433-440.

Robson, C. J., Churchill, B. M., & Anderson, W. (1969). Results of radical nephrectomy for renal cell carcinoma. *Journal of Urology, 101,* 297.

Sella, A., Zukiwski, A., Robinson, E. et al. (1994). Interleukin 2 (IL-2) with interferon α and 5-fluoruracil (5-FU) in patients with metastatic renal cell cancer. *Proceedings of the American Society of Clinical Oncologists,* (13), 237.

Sokoloff, M., de Kernion, J., Figlin, R., & Belldegrum, A. (1996). Current management of renal cell carcinoma. *CA: A Cancer Journal for Clinicians, 46*(5), 284-303.

Sokoloff, M., Figlin, R., & Belldegrum, A. (1996). Treatment of metastatic renal cell carcinoma. In E. Crawford & S. Das (Eds.), *Current genitourinary cancer surgery.* Baltimore: Williams and Wilkins.

Steenland, K., Selevan, S., & Landrigan, P. (1992). The mortality of lead smelter workers: An update. *American Journal of Public Health, 82*(12), 1641-1644.

Steinbach, F., Stockle, M., & Hohenfellner, R. (1995). Clinical experience with nephron-sparing surgery in the presence of a normal contralateral kidney. *Seminars in Urologic Oncology, 13*(4), 288-291.

Thrasher, J. B. & Paulson, D. (1993). Prognostic factors in renal cell cancer. *Urologic Clinics of North America, 20*(2), 247-261.

Walther, M., Jennings, S., Guarra, J., Zbar, B., & Linehan, W. (1996). Molecular genetics of renal cell carcinoma. In M. Vogelzang, P. Sardini, W. Shipley, & D. Coffey (Eds.), *Comprehensive textbook of genitourinary oncology.* Baltimore: Williams and Wilkins.

Yogoda, A., Petrylak, D., & Thompson, S. (1993). Cytotoxic chemotherapy for advanced renal cell carcinoma. *Urologic Clinics of North America, 20*(2), 303-321.

Ureteral Cancer

Jamie S. Myers, RN, MN, AOCN

EPIDEMIOLOGY

Cancer of the ureter is rare. It is often categorized with cancer of the renal pelvis and accounts for only 1% of all upper genitourinary tract malignancies (Linehan, Shipley, & Parkinson, 1997). Because of the limited incidence of ureteral cancer, it is not considered separately from kidney and other urinary cancers for prediction of new cases or related deaths. Estimates for new cases of all renal and urinary tract cancers in 1998 are 300 for males and 700 for females. Estimated cancer deaths from urinary tract cancers in 1998 are 300 and 300, respectively. Ureteral cancer predominately occurs in the sixth, seventh, and eighth decades of life. It occurs twice as often in males. About 70% occur in the lower third of the ureter, and less than 1% are bilateral (American Cancer Society, 1998; Linehan et al., 1997).

The renal pelvis and ureters are lined with transitional cells. Transitional cell carcinomas make up over 90% of ureteral cancers. About 20% of these have squamous cell differentiation and are often associated with chronic calculus disease and infection. Approximately 8% are pure squamous cell, and 1% are adenocarcinomas (Table 50-1). The incidence of ureteral cancer appears to be increasing, but this may be due to increased detection through improved diagnostic techniques.

RISK FACTORS

The cause of ureteral cancer is unknown. It is assumed that the risk factors are the same as for other urothelial cancers (Box 50-1). Relationships are suspected with cigarette smoking, coffee drinking, leather working, vesical schistosomiasis (a parasitic infestation), Balkan nephropathy (chronic tubular interstitial nephropathy geographically restricted to areas of Bulgaria, Romania, and Yugoslavia), and exposure to phenacetin and aniline dyes (Linehan et al., 1997; Lang, 1991). There is an association between primary ureteral cancers and prior bladder cancers in up to 50% of patients (Kassabian & Graham, 1995).

About 60% to 90% of patients have gross, painless hematuria. Approximately 35% experience flank pain from the passage of blood clots or the rapid onset of ureteral obstruction, and 50% experience lower tract irritative symptoms of urinary frequency or dysuria (Linehan et al., 1997; Jennings & Linehan, 1996; Paulson, 1991).

PATHOPHYSIOLOGY

Normal Anatomy and Physiology of the Ureter

The primary function of the ureters is to transport urine from the kidneys to the bladder. Like the kidneys, the ureters are paired structures. These 25- to 30-cm long tubes extend in a tortuous course from the renal pelvis to the bladder. The ureters are composed of three layers: the inner mucosal layer, the muscular layer, and the outer adventitial layer. The inner layer is lined with transitional cell epithelium and is called the *urothelium.* Four natural sites of intraluminal narrowing occur: (1) the ureteropelvic junction, (2) the area where the ureter crosses anteriorly to the iliac vessels, (3) the ureterovesical junction, and (4) the ureteral meatus (Clayman & Bagley, 1996). The ureters descend medially from the kidneys and lie on the psoas muscle. They are supplied with blood from a number of segmental arteries that arise from the aorta. Lymphatic drainage along the ureteral tract occurs in the lateral aortic, lumbar, and iliac nodes (Weiss & Coolsaet, 1996). Peristalsis in the ureters conducts the urine distally through the ureterovesical junction, which prevents retrograde flow of urine (Redman, 1996).

Process of Carcinogenesis

It is now generally accepted that cancer occurs as a multistage process involving both initiating and promoting events or agents. It is also known that malignant cells are not restricted from growth and division by the phenomenon of contact inhibition. Cancer cells are not controlled by the normal feedback mechanisms that inhibit cell growth and multiplication. Oncogenes are genetic segments that are ca-

TABLE 50-1 Classification of Malignant Ureteral Tumors

Type of Tumor	Percentage
Epithelial	
Transitional cell carcinoma	71%
Transitional cell carcinoma with differentiation	20%
• Squamous differentiation	
• Glandular differentiation	
• Mixed	
Squamous cell carcinoma (pure)	
Adenocarcinoma	8%
Undifferentiated carcinoma	1%
	1%
Mesodermal	
Leiomyosarcoma	

Modified from Linehan, W.M., Shipley, W.U., & Parkinson, D.R. (1997). Cancer of the Kidney. In V.T. Devita, S. Hollman, & S.A. Rosenberg (Eds.). (1997). *Cancer: Principles and practice of oncology* (5th ed.). Philadelphia: J. B. Lippincott.

Box 50-1
Risk Factors for Ureteral Cancer

- Prior history of bladder cancer
- Cigarette smoking
- Coffee
- Leather working
- Vesical schistosomiasis
- Balkan nephropathy
- Phenacetin exposure
- Aniline dye exposure
- Chronic calculus disease
- Chronic urothelial infection

pable of transforming normal cells into cancer cells. Antioncogenes, or tumor suppressor genes, normally function to suppress the progression of normal cells to malignant cells. Initiating and promoting events may function to stimulate oncogenes and/or inhibit tumor suppressor genes, thus promoting the dedifferentiation and formation of malignant cells (DeWolf, 1996).

Recent research has indicated that a decrease or loss of E-cadherin (ECD) might contribute to the malignant character of renal, ureteral, and bladder tumor cells and lead to tumor progression (Wakatsuki, Watanabe, Saito, Katagiri, & Sato, 1996). Recent findings also suggest that infection with the human papillomavirus or mutation of the P53 protein may be related to tumor-cell growth and progression of urothelial cancers (Furihata, Yamasaki, Ohtsuki, Sonobe, Morioka, & Yamamoto, 1995).

ROUTES OF METASTASES

Ureteral cancer metastasizes through direct extension as well as hematologic and lymphatic invasion. As tumors in the ureter grow, the ureteral wall is penetrated and surrounding fat and adjacent organs are invaded. Blood vessel and lymphatic involvement leads the disease to spread primarily to the lungs, but also to bones and liver.

ASSESSMENT

Patient History

It is important to elicit the patient's work history to determine whether there has been exposure to leather working products or aniline dyes (Table 50-2). A history of vesical schistosomiasis or primary bladder cancer is related to an increased incidence of ureteral cancer. The practitioner should elicit information concerning the presence of any gross, painless hematuria or flank pain. Other symptoms to investigate include urinary frequency or dysuria.

Physical Examination

Ureteral tumors are rarely palpable, but the clinician may be able to palpate the resultant hydronephrosis from ureteral obstruction (Bushman & Wyker, 1996).

Diagnostic Tests

A diagnosis of ureteral cancer primarily depends on radiographic studies. A urinalysis can show microscopic hematuria. There are no known tumor markers or paraneoplastic syndromes. The intravenous urogram is the primary screening study. It can be used to visualize the entire ureteral course bilaterally (Kellum, Fisher, & Tegtmeyer, 1996). The results in ureteral cancer are as follows: intraluminal filling defect (19%), hydronephrosis (34%), and nonvisualization of the kidney (46%). These results can also be caused by blood clots, calculi, varices, and extrinsic masses (Linehan et al., 1997). The retrograde ureterogram is used to delineate accurately the precise location of the ureteral lesion. Results can show an intraluminal mass that is displaced by contrast, giving a wine goblet image or a more diffuse area of stricture. Cystoscopy is used to diagnose synchronous bladder tumors or ureteral tumors that are exiting the ureteral orifice. Angiography has been of little benefit. Computed tomography (CT) and magnetic resonance imaging (MRI) are used more for staging than for initial diagnosis. After a diagnosis has been confirmed, a chest radiograph, CT of the abdomen, and bone scan are required to rule out distant metastasis (Lang, 1991).

The newest technique for diagnosis, and in limited situations for treatment, is ureteronephroscopy. Advances in the development and use of rigid and flexible endoscopes have made it possible to inspect and manipulate the entire urinary tract. Rigid endoscopes are best used to inspect the distal ureter. Flexible deflatable endoscopes vary in size from 8.5 to 10.8 French with a range of tip deflection from 160 to 280 degrees. These can be used to inspect the proximal ureter

Table 50-2 Assessment of the Patient for Ureteral Cancer

	Assessment Parameters	Typical Abnormal Findings
History	A. Personal and social history 1. Age 2. Gender 3. Infection 4. Cancer B. Evaluation of urinary system	A. Personal and social risk factors: 1. Usually over age 60. 2. Twice as common in males. 3. Vesical shistomiasis. 4. Bladder cancer. B. Common symptoms include painless hematuria, flank pain, urinary frequency, and dysuria.
Physical Examination	A. Palpation	A. May be able to palpate hydronephrosis from ureteral obstruction.
Diagnostic Tests	A. Urinalysis B. Intravenous urogram C. Retrograde ureterogram D. Cystoscopy E. Computed tomography, magnetic resonance imaging F. Bone scan	A. Hematuria: B. Typical results: 1. Intraluminal filling defect (19%). 2. Hydronephrosis (34%). 3. Nonvisualization of the kidney (46%). C. Results: 1. Wine goblet sign or diffuse stricture. 2. Urine cytology is performed during the procedure. D. Synchronous bladder tumors or those at ureteral orifice. E. Useful in staging for direct extension of tumor, lymphadenopathy, or metastases to the lung or liver. F. Useful for staging hematogenous spread to the bone.

and kidney. The scopes can be used for brushings and biopsy. Some low-grade, low-stage transitional cell cancers of the distal ureter may be treated by excision during endoscopy (Clayman & Bagley, 1996; Grossman, Schwartz, & Konnak, 1992). A urine culture is performed to rule out bacteriurias prior to endoscopic procedures. A urine cytology is performed before the procedure as well. If grade 3 or 4 transitional cell carcinoma is detected, it is more prudent to proceed to open surgical intervention. (Patient instructions for nephroureteroscopy can be found in Table 50-3.)

STAGING

As with other transitional cell cancers, ureteral cancer is histologically graded as 1 (low grade) through 4 (high grade), indicating the degree of differentiation of the malignant cells (Table 50-4). Two clinical staging systems are currently in use for ureteral cancer. Since 1993 the TNM staging system, developed by the American Joint Committee on Cancer (AJCC) (1992) and the International Union Against Cancer (UICC), has been required for any hospital seeking accreditation by the AJCC. Another staging system still commonly used by physicians was cited by Batata, Whitmore, Hilaris, Tokita, & Grabstald (1975). (The two staging systems are outlined in the table.)

MEDICAL MANAGEMENT

Treatment for ureteral cancer is similar to that for renal urothelial cancer. The standard treatment for ureteral cancer is nephroureterectomy, or segmental ureterectomy. Ureteral cancer in the proximal two thirds of the ureter is considered to be multifocal disease. These tumors are typically high grade and/or high stage, and there is significant incidence of distal ureteral recurrence. However, the contralateral kidney and ureter have only a 1% to 3% incidence of recurrence (Crawford, 1991). Nephroureterectomy is recommended as the primary treatment. Lymphadenectomy has been of more value for prognostic evaluation than for enhanced survival. For low-grade/low-stage tumors of the distal one third of the ureter, segmental ureterectomy with reimplantation of the distal ureter can be considered. It is important to accurately determine the grade and stage preoperatively. The advantages of more conservative surgery are the preservation of the kidney and bilateral renal function. The risk for potential recurrence in the remaining portion of the ureter is estimated between 12% and 40%. Segmental ureteroscopy is also considered for patients who have only one kidney or who have decreased renal function. Ureteral carcinoma in situ can be effectively treated by endoscopic resection and/or fulguration. Care must be taken during the diagnostic workup to verify the degree of invasion and anaplasia before proceeding (Linehan et al., 1997).

Radical nephroureterectomy (Figs. 50-1 and 50-2) includes removal of the kidney, the entire contents of Gerota's fascia, the ureter, the bladder cuff (including the ureteral orifice), and the intramural ureter. As discussed above, regional lymph nodes may be resected for prognostic purposes.

There are no current standards for treating extensive regional disease. Some studies have shown radiation therapy to decrease the incidence of local recurrence and increase

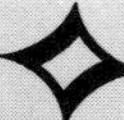

TABLE 50-3 Patient Preparation for Nephroureteroscopy

Description of the Procedure: A cystoscope is inserted through the urethra and into the bladder. A guidewire is passed through the cystoscope and into the ureter. The ureter is dilated, and a rigid or flexible endoscope is inserted to the desired location to inspect and/or perform a biopsy on the lesion.

Patient Preparation: A urine culture is done to ensure that the urine is sterile. The patient also receives one preoperative dose of antibiotics to ensure sterile urine. The patient is instructed not to eat or drink after midnight prior to the day of the procedure. Elderly patients may require intravenous hydration during this time. The patient is informed that the procedure will not be completed if the ureter goes into a spasm. In this situation a ureteral stent is placed and the procedure is delayed for 3 to 7 days. The patient is informed of the risks and potential complications of the procedure.

Risks and Potential Complications: About 1% to 3% of patients undergoing nephroureteroscopy develop a ureteral stricture within 6 months. This can be treated with balloon dilatation. If dilatation is unsuccessful, open surgical correction may be required. There is a risk of loss of renal function or the need for a nephrectomy if surgical correction fails. About 10% to 15% of patients experience a perforation of the ureter. A ureteral stent can be placed. Most perforations seal within 48 to 72 hours. There is a chance for instrument breakage during the procedure. This must be corrected endoscopically or surgical correction is required. Most patients experience hematuria for 1 to 3 days after the procedure due to mucosal abrasion. About 3% experience fever, but only 1.3% develop a bacteriuremia.

Procedural Considerations:

1. Obtain informed consent.
2. General anesthesia is preferred for proximal ureteral lesions. It relaxes the pelvic musculature and prevents unexpected movement or cough during the procedure. Regional anesthesia is usually acceptable for distal ureteral lesions.
3. Place the patient in the dorsal lithotomy position with the leg opposite the involved ureter in a slightly abducted position.

Postprocedural Considerations:

1. A ureteral catheter is commonly placed, as is an indwelling Foley catheter to which the ureteral catheter is attached. These are left in place for 24 to 48 hours, until hematuria clears. A ureteral stent may be placed instead. This may be removed cystoscopically in the office after 3 days. Dysuria, frequency with urgency, and flank pain during urination due to urine reflux are more common with ureteral stents.
2. Aching in the lower quadrant or flank on the affected side is common. Severe pain is not usual and may indicate obstruction by a blood clot or ureteral stricture.
3. About 3 to 6 weeks after the procedure, the ureters should be radiographically evaluated to rule out silent ureteral stricture.

Special Consideration: Nephroureteroscopy is *never* performed when there is bacteriuria. A sterile urine culture must be obtained before the procedure.

Modified from Clayman, R.V. & Bagley, D.H. (1996). Ureteronephroscopy. In J.Y. Gillenwater & J.T. Grayhack (Eds.), *Adult and pediatric urology* (3rd ed.). St. Louis: Mosby.

the 5-year survival for patients with poor-risk (high-stage or high-grade) transitional cell cancer of the renal pelvis and ureter. These patients may be eligible for clinical trial consideration. Other treatment modalities undergoing evaluation include intraluminal instillation of cytoxic agents (thiotepa, mitomycin, doxorubicin) or immunologic/inflammatory agents (bacille Calmette-Guéron [BCG], interferon) because these have proven useful in superficial tumors of the bladder (*Transitional cell cancer of the renal pelvis and ureter,* 1996). Patients with metastatic ureteral cancer may respond to systemic chemotherapy with M-VAC (methotrexate, vinblastine, adriamycin, and cisplatin). This regimen has demonstrated some success for patients with metastatic transitional cell cancer of the bladder.

ONCOLOGIC EMERGENCIES

Because ureteral cancer metastasizes to the bone, the patient may be at risk for developing hypercalcemia as calcium is released into the serum when bone is destroyed. Any patient who has bony metastasis may also be at risk for developing cord compression from vertebral involvement. See Chapter 11 for a discussion on oncologic emergencies.

NURSING MANAGEMENT

Patients diagnosed with cancer have many fears and concerns related to the potential of dying from their disease. The nurse's role includes helping the patient and family understand the stage of the disease, the treatment plan, and the anticipated outcome. Many patients with ureteral cancer must prepare for the surgical removal of the involved ureter, the kidney, and a portion of the bladder. Significant fears are associated with the loss of a kidney. The nurse is in an excellent position to reassure and teach the patient about the ability of the remaining kidney to handle the body's excretion (Lind, Kravitz, & Greig, 1993).

Preoperative Care

Instructing patients to stop smoking at least 2 weeks before surgery is essential, as are deep-breathing and coughing

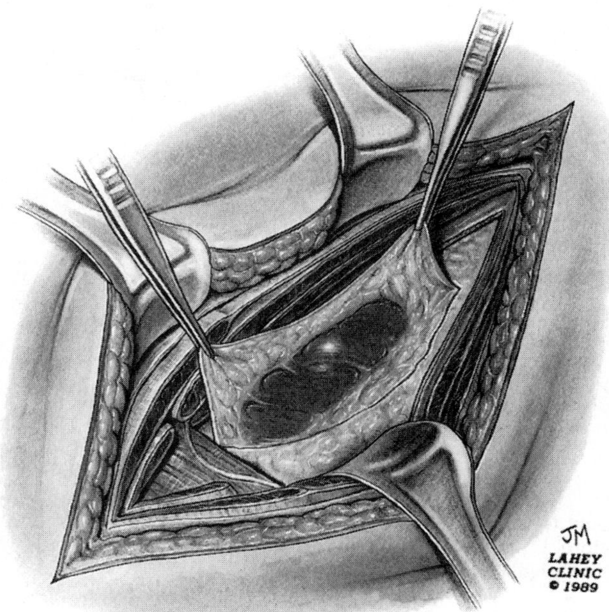

Fig. 50-1 Longitudinal incision through Gerota's fascia exposing perirenal fat and kidney. (From Libertino, J. A. [1998]. *Reconstructive urologic surgery* [3rd ed.]. St. Louis: Mosby.)

techniques. The flank incision for nephroureterectomy is very near the diaphragm and makes postoperative pulmonary toilet and turning more painful than an abdominal incision. A complete blood count, electrolyte panel, creatinine, creatinine clearance, urinalysis, and culture are recommended for all patients being prepared for renal surgery (Crawford, 1991; Smeltzer & Bare, 1996).

Perioperative Care

Nephroureterectomy may be performed with three types of incisions (Fig. 50-3). The patient may be positioned on his or her side in a hyperextended position. This elevates the flank with the twelfth rib centered over a kidney rest and the break in the table (Fig. 50-4). The kidney rest is raised until the flank muscles become tensed. The upper leg is straight and positioned over a pillow, and the lower leg is slightly flexed (Cass, 1990). An alternative patient position is a modified flank position so that the body forms a 45-degree angle with the flexed table (Fig. 50-5) (Lang, 1991). Perioperative positioning contributes to the patient's pain postoperatively. Muscle aches and pains are experienced in addition to incisional pain (Smeltzer & Bare, 1996).

Postoperative Care

Postoperative care is similar for patients undergoing a laparotomy. The primary nursing concerns are hemorrhage, pain, atelectasis, fluid balance, bowel function, and incisional care (Table 50-5) (Smeltzer & Bare, 1996).

TABLE 50-4 Staging Systems for Carcinoma of the Renal Pelvis and Ureter

TNM Staging System			
Primary Tumor (T)			
TX	Primary tumor cannot be assessed		
T0	No evidence of primary tumor		
Tis	Carcinoma in situ		
Ta	Papillary noninvasive carcinoma		
T1	Tumor invades subepithelial connective tissue		
T2	Tumor invades muscularis		
T3	Tumor invades beyond muscularis into periureteric or peripelvic fat or renal parenchyma		
T4	Tumor invades adjacent organs or through the kidney into perinephritic fat		
Regional Lymph Nodes (N)			
NX	Regional lymph node(s) cannot be assessed		
N0	No regional lymph node metastasis		
N1	Metastasis in a single lymph node, 2 cm or less in greatest dimension		
N2	Metastasis in a single lymph node, more than 2 cm but not more than 5 cm in greatest dimension, or multiple lymph nodes, none more than 5 cm in greatest dimension		
N3	Metastasis in a lymph node more than 5 cm in greatest dimension		
Distant Metastasis (M)			
MX	Presence of distant metastasis cannot be assessed		
M0	No distant metastasis		
M1	Distant metastasis		
AJCC Stage Groupings			
Stage 0	Tis	N0	M0
	Ta	N0	M0
Stage I	T1	N0	M0
Stage II	T2	N0	M0
Stage III	T3	N0	M0
	T4	N0	M0
Stage IV	Any	N1-N3	M0
	T	Any N	M1
	Any T		
Histopathologic Grade			
GX	Grade cannot be assessed		
G1	Well differentiated		
G2	Moderately differentiated		
G3-4	Poorly differentiated or undifferentiated		
Batata Staging System			
Stage 0	Limited to mucosa		
Stage 1	Lamina propria invasion		
Stage 2	Confined to muscularis		
Stage 3	Invasion through muscularis with involvement of adjacent structures		
Stage 4	Metastatic		

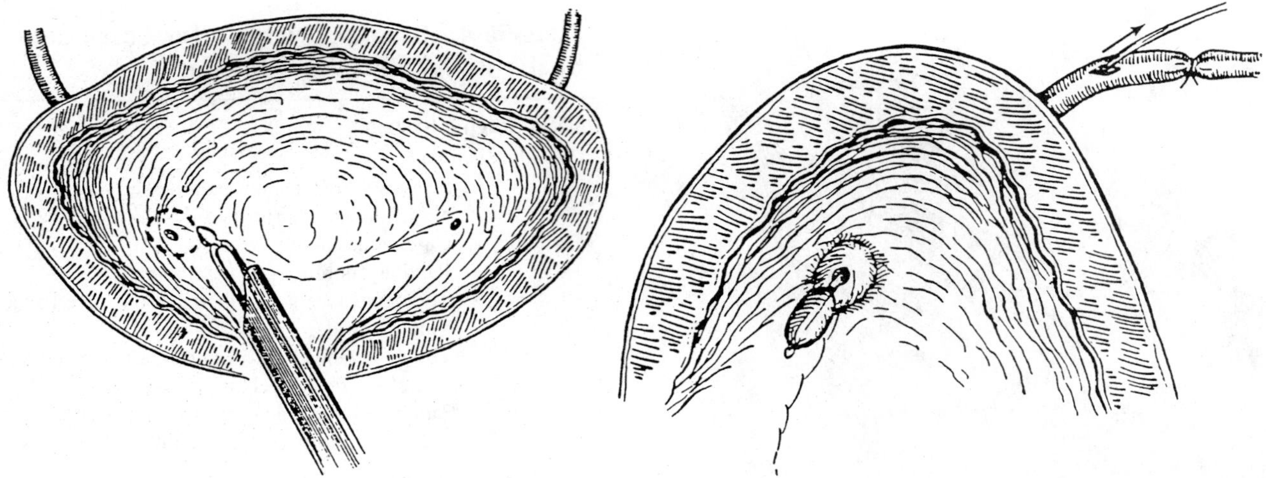

Fig. 50-2 Renal dissection. The kidney, surrounding fat and fascia, lymph nodes, and adrenal gland are lifted out of the wound, attached by the ureter. (From Crawford, E.D. [1991]. Nephrectomy and nephroureterectomy. In J. F. Glenn [Ed.], *Urologic surgery* [4th ed.]. Philadelphia: J. B. Lippincott.)

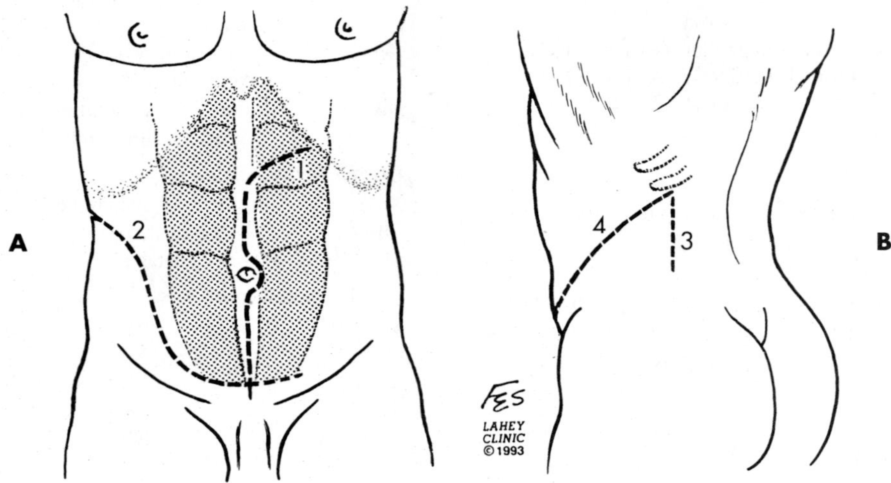

Fig. 50-3 **A,** *1,* Transperitoneal incision with an oblique left lateral extension offers the most versatile approach for access to the ureter. *2,* The oblique anterior extraperitoneal incision with extension into the flank for exposure of the lumbar and pelvic ureter. **B,** *3,* Posterior incision of Simon is used for limited exposure of the upper ureter and renal pelvis. *4,* Classic extraperitoneal subcostal flank incision is used for unilateral exposure of the renal pelvis and upper two thirds of the ureter. (From Libertino, J. A. [1998]. *Reconstructive urologic surgery* [3rd ed.]. St. Louis: Mosby.)

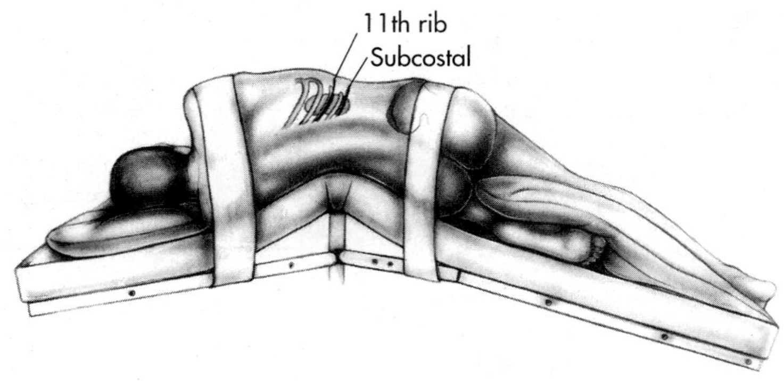

Fig. 50-4 Patient positioning for a modified flank incision. (From Libertino, J. A. [1998]. *Reconstructive urologic surgery* [3rd ed.]. St. Louis: Mosby.)

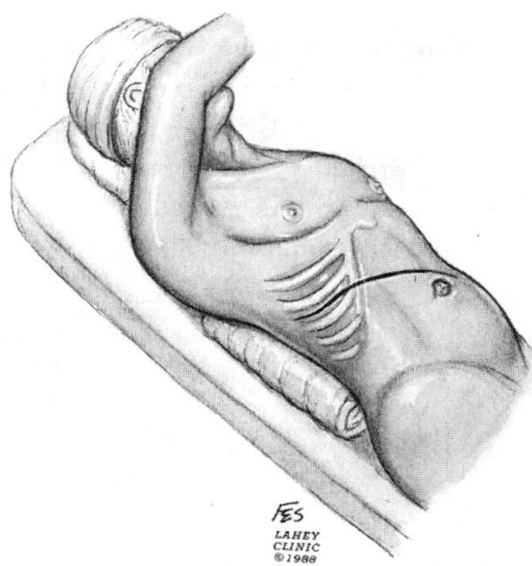

Fig. 50-5 Position for thoracoabdominal approach. (From Libertino, J. A. [1998]. *Reconstructive urologic surgery* [3rd ed.]. St. Louis: Mosby.)

Chemotherapy

Patients with high-grade/stage or metastatic disease may be offered adjuvant or palliative therapy with chemotherapy. Cisplatin has been the most efficacious single agent for transitional cell cancers of the urothelium. However, the most effective multiagent treatment regimen is currently M-VAC (Box 50-2). It has been shown to have increased response and median survival rates for transitional cell bladder cancer as compared with cisplatin alone (Loehrer, Einhorn, Elson, Crawford, Kuebler, & Tannock, 1992; Sternberg, Yagoda, Scher, Watson, Geller, & Herr, 1989). Nursing care issues for patients receiving this regimen include cardiac assessment, prevention/control of nausea and vomiting, management of mucositis, prevention/management of infection, and patient teaching around the issues of immunosuppression, hair loss, fatigue, and loss of appetite. Some of these issues are addressed in Table 50-6. Patients may also experience knowledge deficit as a result of chemotherapy (Somerville, 1991). Research is currently being conducted by the Eastern Cooperative Oncology Group (ECOG) as a phase II study comparing the addition of paclitaxel (Taxol) to cisplatin (Cheson, 1996).

Radiation Therapy

Radiation may be indicated for treating extensive regional disease. Side effects depend on the treatment volume and location. Radiation therapy to the abdomen and pelvis can cause nausea and vomiting, diarrhea, and skin reactions. Knowledge deficit can also be a side effect of radiation therapy, particularly if full-body radiation is administered (Shell, 1991). Table 50-7 outlines the nursing care for common side effects.

Palliative Care

Patients with advanced disease may develop symptom management problems from pain due to bony metastases or respiratory distress from lung involvement. Regularly scheduled analgesia should be used to control the patient's pain. Oxygen therapy, antianxiolytics, and narcotics can decrease discomfort from air hunger. Patients and families dealing with end-stage disease may benefit from supportive care provided by local hospice agencies.

Box 50-2
M-VAC Regimen

Methotrexate 30 mg/m^2 on day 1
Vinblastine 3 mg/m^2 on day 2
Cisplatin 70 mg/m^2 on day 2 (after hydration)
Repeat vinblastine and methotrexate on days 15 and 22 (if white blood cell and platelet counts sufficient).
Repeat cycle every 28 days.

Box 50-3
Home Care Instructions for Patients Who Have Had a Nephroureterectomy

1. Observe your urine and report any signs of blood to your physician.
2. Drink 2-3 quarts of fluid each day.
3. Observe the incision, and report any signs of infection, such as redness, swelling, drainage, or an elevated temperature.
4. Avoid strenuous exercise for 2-3 weeks after surgery. Discuss when to resume exercise with your physician.
5. Urinate frequently (every 2-4 hours). It will take several months for your bladder to expand after surgery.
6. Avoid fad diets that are high in proteins. Talk with your physician before starting any new diet.
7. Call your physician if you have any trouble breathing, cough up blood, or have bone pain.
8. Have regular check-ups frequently. Have a computed tomographic (CT) scan of the abdomen and pelvis periodically as a part of your follow-up.

HOME CARE ISSUES

After nephroureterectomy, bladder capacity is decreased to 60 ml. Bladder elasticity allows the bladder to gradually expand to 200 to 400 ml in several months. Patients should be taught to empty their bladder frequently to prevent undue tension on the operative area. Patients must learn to protect their remaining kidney by drinking 2500 to 3000 ml of fluid each day and avoiding fad diets that may result in excess protein catabolism. Patients with a prior history of hypertension should have frequent blood pressure checks because the nephrotic pressure gradient may change with only one kidney. Postoperative follow-up includes periodic CT scans of the chest and abdomen. Patients should report any signs of potential disease progression, such as respiratory distress, hemoptysis, pain, or fracture. (A tool for home care instructions is described in Box 50-3.)

Patients being treated for regional or metastatic disease experience the side effects of adjuvant treatment, as well as the emotional aspects of a less positive prognosis. It is im-

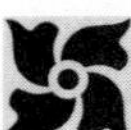

TABLE 50-5 Standard of Care for the Patient Undergoing Nephroureterectomy

Patient Problems and Outcomes	Nursing Interventions and Rationales	Patient Education Instructions
Pain Patient will experience pain relief with minimal side effects (Table 50-3).	1. Ongoing assessment of pain control. Use a scale of 0-10. Assess 30 minutes after administration of pain medication and q 2-4 hours for first 48 hours postoperatively. 2. Administer regularly scheduled pain medication for 48 hours postoperatively. Gradually decrease analgesia based on patient's needs and response. 3. Assess patient/family concerns about opioids.	Instruct patient: 1. To rate pain on 0-10 scale. 2. On the importance of preventing severe pain, which can lead to respiratory complications. 3. That there is no risk of addiction.
High Risk for Atelectasis Patient will maintain clear lung sounds bilaterally.	1. Regularly assess lung sounds. 2. Assist the patient with turn, cough, deep-breathing regimen q 2-4 hours. 3. Monitor for temperature elevation. 4. Assess for shortness of breath and signs of decreased tissue oxygenation (blue lips, low pulse oximetry). 5. Encourage and assist with early ambulation.	Instruct patient: 1. On the importance of deep breathing and coughing to promote drainage of secretions. 2. To splint incision(s) with hands or small pillow when deep breathing and coughing.
High Risk for Hemorrhage Patient will maintain stable VS, Hgb, and Hct.	1. Regularly turn patient and assess dressing for bloody drainage. 2. Monitor for elevation in pulse and decrease in blood pressure. 3. Monitor patients for other signs of shock (dizziness, cold/clammy skin, fainting).	Instruct patient to: 1. Report wet dressings 2. Report blood in urine after discharge.
High Risk for Alteration in Renal Function (Cass, 1990) Patient will maintain urinary output > 30 ml/hr.	1. Accurate I&O. Output should be greater than 30 ml/hr. 2. Observe for signs of renal insufficiency (hiccoughs, decrease in locus of control). 3. Monitor for increased BUN and serum Cr. 4. Once nasal gastric tube discontinued, force fluids to 2500-3000 ml/day. 5. Weigh daily. 6. Regularly assess heart and lung sounds.	Instruct patient to: 1. Drink 2500-3000 ml fluid/day.
High Risk for Ileus Patient will regain normal bowel function within 48-72 hours.	1. Maintain nasal gastric tube suction. 2. Regularly assess for bowel sounds. 3. Assess patient for tolerance of nasal gastric tube clamping when ordered by physician. 4. Assist patient with turning and ambulation to promote relief of flatus. Apply heat for comfort. 5. Use topical anesthetic spray to soothe throat pain from nasogastric tube.	Instruct patient in the importance/need for gastric suction until effects off anesthesia diminish.
Risk for Infection Patient will remain afebrile and free from infection.	1. Keep incisional dressing dry and intact. 2. Observe and document condition of incision. 3. Maintain closed urinary drainage system. 4. Assist patient in turning and ambulating to prevent dislodgement of ureteral stent or catheter.	Instruct patient: 1. To observe for redness, swelling, and drainage on discharge. 2. On care of urinary drainage system if not discontinued prior to discharge.

VS, vital signs; *Hgb,* hemoglobin; *Hct,* hematocrit; *I & O,* input and output; *Cr,* creatinine.

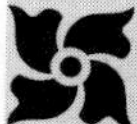

TABLE 50-6 Standard of Care for the Patient Receiving M-VAC Chemotherapy for Ureteral Cancer

Patient Problems and Outcomes	Nursing Interventions and Rationales	Patient Education Instructions
Alopecia (Chernecky, 1993) Patient will: • Describe the cause, expected degree, and duration of alopecia. • Cope effectively with the effect of alopecia.	1. Assess the patient for anticipated effect of alopecia. 2. Allow the patient time and opportunity to verbalize feelings about alopecia.	Instruct patient that: 1. Hair loss occurs in days to weeks after chemotherapy. 2. Regrowth occurs 6-8 weeks after last chemotherapy. 3. Color and texture may change with regrowth. To slow the occurrence of hair loss, instruct the patient to: 1. Avoid excessive shampooing. 2. Avoid electric hair dryers, or use at coolest setting. 3. Avoid excessive hair manipulation through brushing, electric rollers, curling irons, hair dyes, and permanent solutions. To minimize the effect of hair loss: 1. Encourage the patient to prepare for hair loss prior to occurrence. 2. Inform the patient about resources for obtaining wigs, hats, and scarves/turbans to cover the scalp. (The local American Cancer Society may be a source for wigs and turbans. The American Cancer Society may also have a "Look Good, Feel Better" program to assist women with wig styling and makeup application during chemotherapy.) 3. Inform the patient that insurance may reimburse for wigs if they are prescribed by a physician. 4. Instruct the patient to protect the scalp from sun exposure.
Nausea and Vomiting (Hogan, 1993) Patient will maintain adequate fluid intake.	1. Administer prophylactic antiemetic 30 minutes prior to chemotherapy. 2. Obtain a prescription for antiemetics for the patient to take at home for 24-72 hours after chemotherapy. Cisplatin causes delayed nausea and vomiting. Some effective agents include oral ondansetron, dexamethosone, and metaclopramide.	Instruct patient to: 1. Continue regular antiemetic administration for 24-72 hours after chemotherapy. 2. Report prolonged vomiting and intake < 2000 ml of fluid/day. 3. Eat cold or room temperature foods to decrease nausea induced by aromas.

Continued

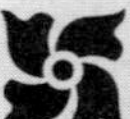

TABLE 50-6 Standard of Care for the Patient Receiving M-VAC Chemotherapy for Ureteral Cancer—cont'd

Patient Problems and Outcomes	Nursing Interventions and Rationales	Patient Education Instructions
Neutropenia		
Patient will • Promptly report signs and symptoms of infection to the health care team. • Describe strategies to prevent exposure to infection.	1. Monitor the absolute neutrophil count (ANC). 2. Implement neutropenic precautions when ANC <500, including the following: a private room, good handwashing, no dietary raw fruits or vegetables, and no cut flowers/ plants or other sources of stagnant water in the room. 3. Monitor vital signs every 4 hours. If febrile, obtain peripheral and central (venous access device) blood cultures and initiate intravenous antibiotics ASAP as ordered. Urine and sputum cultures may also be ordered. 4. Assess skin and mucous membranes daily. 5. Assess respiratory status every 4 hours. 6. Monitor for urinary symptoms of frequency, dysuria, urgency, or cloudiness.	Instruct patient to: 1. Monitor temperature at home, and notify physician if it is 101° F (38° C) or above. 2. Avoid crowds and potential exposure to colds or flu. 3. Maintain fluid intake of 2-3 L/day. 4. When ANC <500, avoid sexual intercourse, use of tampons, constipation, and contact with animal excretia.
Potential for Cardiomyopathy		
Patient will report weight gain, lower extremity swelling, and shortness of breath.	1. Monitor electrocardiogram for changes in S-T wave or other abnormalities, and notify physician. 2. Assess heart and lung sounds. 3. Weigh patient daily. 4. Maintain accurate I&O. 5. Monitor vital signs for increased blood pressure and pulse. 6. Perform ongoing tabulation of cumulative doxorubicin dose (not to exceed 550 mg/m^2).	Instruct patient to: 1. Report weight gain, edema, and shortness of breath.
Mucositis (Miller, 1993)		
Patient will: • Describe strategies to minimize mucositis. • Report signs and symptoms of infection to the health care team.	1. Assess the status of oral mucosa daily (7-10 days after chemotherapy). 2. Assess the level of pain, and ask the patient to rate on a scale of 0-10. 3. Assess the nutritional intake and hydration status. 4. For mild mucositis, obtain mouth rinse with topical anesthetic, topical coating agent, and anti-inflammatory agent (viscous xylocaine, substrate of antacid, and Benadryl elixer). 5. For moderate to severe mucositis, oral care should be done every 2 hours. Use a sponge-tipped swab instead of a toothbrush. Obtain topical and systemic antifungal and antiviral agents as prescribed. Administer analgesics on a regular schedule to control pain.	Instruct patient to have any necessary dental work done prior to the initiation of chemotherapy (14 days) if possible. 1. Use a soft-bristle toothbrush. 2. Perform oral care 30 minutes after meals and at night. 3. Avoid lemon/glycerine and commercial mouthwash preparations (alcohol content dries oral mucosa). Better mouth rinses include salt water (1 tsp in 500 ml), baking soda and water (½ tsp in 500 ml), or a combination of both. 4. Drink 2-3 L/day. 5. Minimize mucous membrane trauma by avoiding alcohol, tobacco, and foods that are hot (temperature) or irritating (spicy, acidic, hard, or sharp edged).

TABLE 50-7 Standard of Care for the Patient Receiving Radiation Therapy for Ureteral Cancer

Patient Problem and Outcomes	Nursing Interventions and Rationales	Patient Education Instructions
Diarrhea (Culhane, 1993) Patient will: • Maintain adequate hydration. • Maintain optimal nutritional status.	1. Monitor intake and output. 2. Monitor serum potassium level. 3. Administer antidiarrheal agents every 6 hours until diarrhea subsides for 12 hours. 4. Administer intravenous hydration as ordered.	Instruct patient to: 1. Eat foods that are low in residue and high in protein and calories. 2. Avoid foods that may stimulate/irritate the gastrointestinal tract. 3. Report >3 liquid stools a day. 4. Drink 2-3 L fluid/day.
Skin Reaction (Daeffler & Landrum, 1990) Patient will: • Verbalize expected changes in the treatment field. • Describe strategies to minimize skin problems.	1. Assess skin integrity daily.	Teach patient/family about expected skin reactions: 1. Confined to treatment field. 2. Greater occurrence in sensitive and moist areas like skin folds. 3. Mild erythema may occur 1-3 weeks after starting treatment. Teach patient/family to: 1. Limit washing of affected area, use tepid water, and pat dry. 2. Use water-based ointment or lubricant. 3. Avoid metal-based products. 4. Avoid irritation of skin. Wear soft, loose clothing. Avoid shaving of skin in treatment field. Avoid extreme temperatures and sun exposure to treatment field. Avoid creams or deodorants not approved by the health care team.
Fatigue (Mädeya & Britton, 1993) Patient will learn to plan priority activities around rest periods.	1. Assess the pattern of fatigue (time it is greatest, length of time it persists, intensity, aggravating or alleviating factors). 2. Assess the effect of fatigue on lifestyle patterns.	Instruct patient to: 1. Prioritize activities (plan rest periods around activities the patient finds most important or enjoyable). 2. Avoid caffeine-containing foods/beverages after 6 P.M. and strenuous exercise before bedtime. 3. Rest when fatigued but also try to maintain usual patterns of rest and sleep.

portant to inform patients and families about local resources. American Cancer Society divisions may provide supplies, wigs and turbans, and transportation to and from radiation and chemotherapy treatments. Local hotels may provide free guest rooms for people who live a great distance from the treatment facility. Local support groups may be available for patients and families and can assist people in learning coping strategies (Lind, Kravitz, & Greig, 1993).

Box 50-4
Ureteral Cancer
Five-Year Survival by Stage

Stage 0 or A: 90% to 100%
Stage B: 45% to 85%
Stage C: 25% to 30%
Stage D: 0 to 5%

PROGNOSIS

Primary ureteral cancer has a 30% chance of recurrence in the retained portion of the ureter and a 50% chance of recurrence in the bladder. Superficial ureteral tumors that are confined to the ureter have a 90% cure rate. Deeply invasive tumors penetrating the urothelial wall or with distant metastasis are not curable with currently available treatment (DeVita, 1993). The chance of 5-year survival depends on the grade and stage of the disease. Variables of gender and age are insignificant. The 5-year survival rate based on the stage of disease is summarized in Box 50-4.

TABLE 50-8 Quality of Care Evaluation for a Patient Undergoing Nephroureterectomy

Disciplines participating in the quality of care evaluation:
☐ Nursing ☐ Surgery ☐ Physical Therapy ☐ Social Services

I. Postoperative Management Evaluation

Data from:
☐ Medical Record Review ☐ Patient/Family Interview

Criteria	YES	NO
1. Patient provided with information about:		
a. Turn, cough, deep breath, and incentive spirometry procedure	☐	☐
b. Nasogastric suction	☐	☐
2. Patient's Hgb and Hct were evaluated postoperatively.	☐	☐
3. Patient's pain was assessed q 2-4 hrs × 48 hours postoperatively.	☐	☐

II. Patient/Family Satisfaction

Data from: ☐ Patient Interview ☐ Family Interview

Criteria	YES	NO
1. On a scale of 0-10, how satisfied were you with the pain management you received in the hospital? ____________		
2. Were you instructed to observe your urine and notify your physician of any blood in your urine after returning home?	☐	☐
3. Were you taught to avoid strenuous exercise for 2-3 weeks after surgery?	☐	☐

EVALUATION OF THE QUALITY OF CARE

Pain control and postoperative instructions are two important facets of care for the patient treated for ureteral cancer. Facilities accredited by the Joint Commission for the Accreditation of Health Care Organizations are required to define and monitor objective quality indicators for the care provided. See Table 50-8 for an evaluation tool for patients who undergo nephroureterectomy.

RESEARCH ISSUES

There is an ongoing need for clinical trials to evaluate treatment options for patients with locally advanced and metastatic disease. Outcomes for radiation therapy, chemotherapy, and immunotherapy are needed to define best practice.

REFERENCES

American Cancer Society. (1998). *Facts and figures.* Atlanta: American Cancer Society.

American Joint Committee on Cancer. (1992). Renal pelvis and ureter. *Manual for staging of cancer* (4th ed.). Philadelphia: J.B. Lippincott.

Batata, M.A., Whitmore, W.F., Hilaris, B.S., Tokita, N., & Grabstald, H. (1975). Primary carcinoma of ureter: A prognostic study. *Cancer, 35,* 1626-1632.

Bushman, W., & Wyker, A., Jr. (1996). Standard diagnostic considerations. In J.Y. Gillenwater & J.T. Grayhack (Eds.), *Adult and pediatric urology* (3rd ed.). St. Louis: Mosby.

Cass, A.S. (1990). Nephrectomy: A review of the surgical approaches. *Today's O.R. Nurse, 12,* 6, 16-21.

Chernecky, C.C. (1993). Alopecia. In J.M. Yasko (Ed.), *Nursing management of symptoms associated with chemotherapy* (3rd ed.). Philadelphia: Meniscus Health Care Communications.

Cheson, B.D. (1996). Newly approved clinical trials. *Oncology News, 5,* 8, 21.

Clayman, R.V. & Bagley, D.H. (1996). Ureteronephroscopy. In J.Y. Gillenwater & J.T. Grayhack (Eds.), *Adult and pediatric urology* (3rd ed.). St. Louis: Mosby.

Crawford, E.D. (1991). Nephrectomy and nephroureterectomy. In J.G. Glenn (Ed.), *Urologic surgery* (4th ed.). Philadelphia: J.B. Lippincott.

Culhane, B. (1993). Diarrhea. In J.M. Yasko (Ed.), *Nursing management of symptoms associated with chemotherapy* (3rd ed.). Philadelphia: Meniscus Health Care.

Daeffler, R.J., & Landrum B. (1990). Impaired skin and/or tissue integrity. In R.J. Daeffler & B.M. Petrosino (Eds.), *Manual of oncology nursing practice: Nursing diagnoses and care.* Rockville, MD: Aspen Publishers.

DeWolf, W.C. (1996). Malignancy: Underlying concepts of etiology, natural history, and treatment. In J.Y. Gillenwater & J.T. Grayhack (Eds.), *Adult and pediatric urology* (3rd ed.). St. Louis: Mosby.

Furihata, M., Yamasaki, I., Ohtsuki, Y., Sonobe, H., Morioka, M., & Yamamoto, A. (1995). p53 and human papillomavirus DNA in renal pelvic and ureteral carcinoma including dysplastic lesions. *International Journal of Cancer, 64,* 5, 298-303.

Grossman, H.G., Schwartz, S.L., & Konnak, J.W. (1992). Ureteroscopic treatment of urothelial carcinoma of the ureter and renal pelvis. *The Journal of Urology, 148,* 275-277.

Hogan, C.M. (1993). Nausea and vomiting. In J.M. Yasko (Ed.), *Nursing management of symptoms associated with chemotherapy* (3rd ed.). Philadelphia: Meniscus Health Care.

Jennings, S.B. & Linehan, W.M. (1996). Renal, perirenal, and ureteral neoplasms. In J.Y. Gillenwater & J.T. Grayhack (Eds.), *Adult and pediatric urology* (3rd ed.). St. Louis: Mosby.

Kassabian, V.S. & Graham, S.D. (1995). Urologic and male genital cancers. In G.P. Murphy, W. Lawrence, & R.E. Lenhard (Eds.), *American Cancer Society textbook of clinical oncology* (2nd ed.). Atlanta: The American Cancer Society.

Kellum, C.D., Fisher, L.M., & Tegtmeyer, C.J. (1996). Excretory urography. In J.Y. Gillenwater & J.T. Grayhack (Eds.), *Adult and pediatric urology* (3rd ed.). St. Louis: Mosby.

Lang, P.H. (1991). Carcinoma of the renal pelvis and ureter. In J.F. Glenn, *Urologic surgery* (4th ed.). Philadelphia: J.B. Lippincott.

Lind, J., Kravitz, K., & Greig, B. (1993). Urologic and male genital malignancies. In S.L. Groenwald, M. Frogge, M. Goodman, & C.H. Yarbro. (Eds.), *Cancer nursing principles and practice* (3rd ed.). Boston: Jones and Bartlett.

Linehan, W.M., Shipley, W.U., & Parkinson, D.R. (1997). Cancer of the kidney and ureter. In V.T. DeVita, S. Hellman, & S.A. Rosenberg (Eds.), *Cancer: Principles & practice of oncology* (5th ed.). Philadelphia: J.B. Lippincott.

Loehrer, P.J., Sr., Einhorn, L.H., Elson, P.J., Crawford, E.D., Kuebler, P., & Tannock, I. (1992). A randomized comparison of cisplatin alone or in combination with methotrexate, vinblastine, and doxorubicin in patients with metastatic urothelial carcinoma: A cooperative group study. *Journal of Clinical Oncology, 10,* 7, 1066-1073.

Madeya, M.L. & Britton, D. (1993). Fatigue. In J.M. Yasko (Ed.), *Nursing management of symptoms associated with chemotherapy* (3rd ed.). Philadelphia: Meniscus Health Care.

Miller, S.E. (1993). Stomatitis and esophagitis. In J.M. Yasko (Ed.), *Nursing management of symptoms associated with chemotherapy* (3rd ed.). Philadelphia: Meniscus Health Care.

Paulson, D.F. (1991). The urinary system. In D.C. Sabiston (Ed.), *Textbook of surgery* (14th ed.). Philadelphia: W.B. Saunders.

Redman, J.F. (1996). Anatomy of the genitourinary system. In J.Y. Gillenwater & J.T. Grayhack (Eds.), *Adult and pediatric urology* (3rd ed.). St. Louis: Mosby.

Shell, J.A. (1991). Knowledge deficit related to radiation therapy. In J.C. McNally, E.T. Somerville, C.C. Miaskowski, & M.M. Rostad. (Eds.), *Guidelines for oncology nursing practice* (2nd ed.). Philadelphia: W.B. Saunders.

Smeltzer, S.C. & Bare, B.G. (Eds.). (1996). *Brunner & Suddarth's textbook of medical-surgical nursing* (8th ed.). Philadelphia: J.B. Lippincott.

Somerville, E.T. (1991). Knowledge deficit related to chemotherapy. In J.C. McNally, E.T. Somerville, C.C. Miaskowski, & M.M. Rostad. (Eds.), *Guidelines for oncology nursing practice* (2nd ed.). Philadelphia: W.B. Saunders.

Sternberg, C.N., Yagoda, A., Scher, H.I., Watson, R.C., Geller, N., & Herr, H.W. (1989). Methotrexate, vinblastine, doxorubicin, and cisplatin for advanced transitional cell carcinoma of the urothelium: Efficacy and patterns of response and relapse. *Cancer, 64,* 2448-2458.

Transitional cell cancer of the renal pelvis and ureter. CancerNet from the National Cancer Institute, PDQ Information for Professionals, July 3, 1996.

Wakatsuki, S., Watanabe, R., Saito, K., Katagiri, A., & Sato, S. (1996). Loss of human E-cadherin (ECD) correlated with invasiveness of transitional cell cancer in the renal pelvis, ureter and urinary bladder. *Cancer Letter, 103,* 1, 11-17.

Weiss, R.M. & Coolsaet, B.L.R.A. (1996). The ureter. In J.Y. Gillenwater & J.T. Grayhack (Eds.), *Adult and pediatric urology* (3rd ed.). St. Louis: Mosby.

51 Laryngeal Cancer*

Dianna Wellen, RN, MS, OCN

EPIDEMIOLOGY

Laryngeal cancer is the most common head and neck cancer (skin excluded) and is second only to the oral cavity as the most frequent site of cancer of the head and neck. In the United States the number of new cases of laryngeal cancer in 1998 is estimated at 11,100 with approximately 4,300 deaths. Of all estimated cancer deaths in 1998, cancer of the larynx accounts for 0.7% and represents nearly 1% of all estimated new cancer cases (Landis, Murray, Bolden & Wingo, 1998). The glottic larynx is the most common site. Although laryngeal cancer constitutes a small percentage of all cancers, it poses a visible and significant physical and psychological threat to the lifestyle and quality of life of the patient (Norris & Cady, 1991). Men develop laryngeal cancer more frequently than women. In 1986/1987 the male-to-female ratio was 4:1. However, this ratio is decreasing. The decrease can be attributed to the overall rising incidence of tobacco and alcohol consumption in women. In 1992 the male-to-female ratio was 3.7:1.

The geographic distribution for laryngeal cancer closely resembles the high-risk areas for lung cancer. In the United States the distribution shows excess occurrences in the northeast, particularly in northern New Jersey, New York City, and along the Hudson River. The rates are also high along the southeastern Atlantic coast and the Gulf coast (Million, Cassisi, & Mancuso, 1994).

RISK FACTORS

Over 95% of laryngeal cancers are squamous cell carcinomas (SCCs). Other cell types include verrucous carcinoma, carcinosarcoma, adenocarcinoma, lymphoma, small cell carcinoma, and sarcoma. SCCs have a strong association with alcohol and tobacco use and rarely develop in the absence of tobacco use. Consequently, this disease is often considered a result of "self-determined exposures" (Mashberg & Samit, 1995; Vines, 1988).

Because of the self-determined attributes of the disease, laryngeal cancer is an excellent one to target for prevention and detection. To prevent tobacco use, as recently described by Bal, Lloyd, & Manley (1995), the health care professional is urged to "denormalize" smoking by lowering its acceptability in various social circumstances. Within the context of denormalization, smoking cessation is viewed as an outcome as opposed to an intervention. For health care professionals, strategies and responsibilities toward smoking cessation are outlined in the free National Cancer Institute (NCI) publication referenced at the end of this chapter (NCI, 1994).

Tobacco and Alcohol

Over the past 20 years numerous studies have supported the relationship between cigarette tobacco, alcohol, and cancer of the upper aerodigestive tract (i.e., oral cavity, pharynx, larynx, and esophagus). Nondrinking smokers have two to four times the risk of developing SCC as abstainers of alcohol and tobacco. Heavy-drinking smokers have a risk six to fifteen times greater than that for abstainers (Hoffman & Karnell, 1996; Mashberg & Samit, 1995).

The effect of multiple carcinogenic factors can be synergistic. However, the elimination of even a single factor can greatly influence the overall risk to the patient (Norris & Cady, 1991). Table 51-1 highlights the estimated proportion of cancer mortality attributable solely to cigarette smoking by site, including the larynx and oral cavity.

Synchronous Primaries. Mashberg and Samit (1995) summarized the risk of developing synchronous or metachronous multiple primary cancers encountered by men and women who consume 40 or more cigarettes and three or more whiskey equivalents per day (Box 51-1). Patients who consume the above amounts for 30 years or more have a relative risk 3.9 times greater than that of patients exposed to fewer than 20 cigarettes and less than three whiskey equivalents per day of developing multiple primary cancers. The association with tobacco most probably explains the 10% to 20% frequency with which patients who have a pri-

*The author acknowledges IMPAC Medical Systems, Inc. for their generosity and support in the writing of this chapter.

TABLE 51-1 Estimated Percentage of Cancer Mortality Attributed to Cigarette Smoking, by Site

Site	Percent (%)
Lung	85
Larynx and oral cavity	50-70
Esophagus	50
Bladder and Kidney	30-40
Pancreas	30
Cervix	?
All cancer deaths	30

Modified from Ernster, V. L. & Cummings, S. R. (1991). Smoking and cancer. In A. Holleb, D. Fink & G. Murphy (Eds.), *American Cancer Society textbook of clinical oncology.* Atlanta: American Cancer Society.

BOX 51-1
Alcohol Consumption

Alcohol consumption is defined in terms of Whiskey Equivalents (WEs).

1 Whiskey Equivalent = 1 oz. 86-proof whiskey
OR
4 oz. dry wine (11% to 12% alcohol)
OR
12 oz. beer.

A moderate to heavy drinker will consume 6 or more Whiskey Equivalents per day.

Data from Mashberg, A. & Samit, A. (1995). Early diagnosis of asymptomatic oral and oropharyngeal squamous cancers. *CA: A Cancer Journal for Clinicians, 45,* 328-351.

mary carcinoma of the larynx develop another cancer at some other time in their lives (Johnson, 1994).

The presence of a first cancer in the upper aerodigestive tract signifies an increased risk of developing or having a second cancer in the same region. Heavy smoking and drinking promote significant dysplastic changes throughout the aerodigestive epithelial field. The initially detected lesion signals a susceptibility to other SCCs. Consequently, a successfully treated patient monitored for an initial carcinoma can be challenged with synchronous or metachronous multiple primaries. Even after successful primary therapy for early-stage or locally advanced tumors, 30% to 50% of patients have local or regional recurrence. Of these patients, 20% to 30% have distant metastasis, and 10% to 40% develop a second primary tumor.

Primary carcinoma of the larynx is associated with additional synchronous cancers of the lung, pharynx, and esophagus. When patients with stage I or II carcinomas succumb to cancer, the lesion(s) directly responsible for their death are almost always synchronous primary tumors of the hypopharynx, lung, or esophagus (Gluckman, Crissman, & Donegan, 1980; Mashberg & Samit, 1995).

Age, Ethnicity, Gender, and Income

Age is an important risk factor, with 90.5% of all reported cases in 1992 occurring in patients at and over 50 years of age. Most patients reported in 1992 were non-Hispanic whites (83.1%), and 35.8% of all patients were between the ages of 60 and 69. Persons with low and middle incomes have the highest incidence (86%) of laryngeal carcinoma. The percentage of advanced-stage SCC of the larynx was higher among ethnic minorities and patients in the lowest income bracket (Table 51-2). The risk of the disease being more advanced at the time of diagnosis was greater for women and middle-aged patients (Hoffman & Karnell, 1996).

Other risk factors have been listed as strong possibilities; however, definitive scientific studies have yet to validate their likelihood. Box 51-2 lists the known risk factors for laryngeal cancer, as well as those that are highly suspected as being associated with the development of this disease.

CHEMOPREVENTION

A clear association between smoking, excessive alcohol consumption, and the development of laryngeal carcinoma has been established. It is also known that if a patient with a single cancer does continue to smoke and drink, not only does the likelihood for a cure diminish, but the risk of a second tumor is increased (Spitz, 1994). Approximately 25% of head and neck cancer patients with a controlled primary lesion will go on to develop a second primary tumor, usually of the aerodigestive tract (Hong, Lippman, & Itri, 1990). Over 70% of these second primary tumors occur in the tobacco-exposed field.

13-*Cis*–Retinoic Acid

The retinoids are a class of over 3000 naturally and synthetically derived analogs of vitamin A. They have a potent effect on premalignant and malignant cell growth, thought to be due to the modulation of gene expression. The connection between retinoids and chemoprevention was solidified by the discovery of the presence of nuclear retinoid receptors. It appears that these nuclear receptors are the primary mediators of the effects of the retinoid on carcinogenesis.

In the late 1950s, early chemoprevention trials for premalignant oral lesions were done using systemic or topical vitamin A. In 1986 Hong, Endicott, Itri, Doos, Batsakis, & Bell et al. reported the effects of 13-*cis*–retinoic acid on oral leukoplakia in a randomized trial with 44 patients. Thirteen of the 24 patients on 13-*cis*–retinoic acid had reversal of their dysplasia on biopsy, whereas only 2 of the 20 patients who received a placebo had the same results.

Based mostly on positive oral leukoplakia data, Hong, Lippman, & Itri (1990) designed an adjuvant chemoprevention study in head and neck cancer patients to determine the effectiveness of 13-*cis*–retinoic acid in the prevention of second primary tumors. The tolerable dose of 13-*cis*–retinoic acid was shown to be 50 mg/m^2 per day, with skin dryness, cheilitis, hypertriglyceridemia, and conjunctivitis being the dose-limiting toxicities. At a median follow-up of

TABLE 51-2 Percentage of 1992 Laryngeal Squamous Cell Cancer Cases by Age, Gender, Ethnicity, and Income

	Stage Group					
	0	**I**	**II**	**III**	**IV**	**Total %**
Age						
0-39	10.4	34.8	14.8	16.5	23.5	100
40-49	4.5	33.2	17.3	14.8	30.2	100
50-59	3.4	33.7	17.5	19.1	26.3	100
60-69	4.7	36.7	19.0	17.7	21.9	100
70-79	6.3	41.2	17.2	16.4	18.9	100
80+	5.0	45.5	21.5	13.8	14.2	100
TOTAL	**4.9**	**37.5**	**18.2**	**17.2**	**22.2**	100
Gender						
Male	5.0	39.6	18.0	16.5	20.9	100
Female	4.4	29.8	19.0	19.6	27.2	100
Ethnicity						
Non-Hispanic White	5.0	39.0	18.4	17.0	20.6	100
Hispanic	5.3	38.6	11.1	15.0	30.0	100
African American	3.3	26.7	18.0	20.0	32.0	100
Native American	0.0	16.7	33.3	16.7	33.3	100
Asian	2.4	35.7	16.7	19.0	26.2	100
Unknown	7.8	33.7	21.7	13.3	23.5	100
Income						
Low	3.1	30.3	17.9	21.3	27.4	100
Middle	5.2	39.0	17.9	16.5	21.4	100
High	5.7	42.7	18.8	15.4	17.4	100
Unknown	4.7	33.4	20.9	16.2	24.8	100

Modified from Hoffman, H. & Karnell, L. (1996). Laryngeal cancer. In G. D. Steele, J. D. Jessup, D. P. Winchester, H. R. Menck & G. P. Murphy (Eds.), *National Cancer Data Base: Annual review of patient care 1995*. Atlanta: American Cancer Society.

55 months only 7 of the 51 patients receiving 13-*cis*–retinoic acid developed second primary tumors, whereas 16 of the 49 patients receiving placebo developed second primary tumors (14% vs 31%, $p = 0.04$). However, recurrence of the primary disease (local, regional, or distant) was not significantly different between the two arms. Studies thus far proclaim that retinoid treatment has achieved a 54% reduction in the annual rate of second primary tumor development of the head and neck (Lippman, Clayman, Huber, Benner, & Hong, 1995).

The threat of a second primary malignancy remains troublesome in the laryngeal cancer patient population, and chemoprevention is a promising new strategy to manage the emergence of a second primary tumor. The role of the nurse in monitoring 13-*cis*–retinoic acid toxicities, in patient education, and in encouraging patients to adhere to the therapeutic regimen cannot be underestimated.

Box 51-2
Risk Factors for Developing Squamous Cell Carcinoma of the Larynx

Cigarette smoking combined with alcohol consumption*
Cigarette smoking*
Presence of leukoplakia, erythroplakia, or keratosis*
Age greater than 40*
- Passive smoking (sd)
- Chronic laryngeal irritation (sd)
  - -Gastroesophageal reflux (sd)
  - -Inhalation of toxic fumes (sd)
- Viral infection (sd)
  - -Herpes viruses (sd)
  - -Human papilloma virus (sd)
- Marijuana smoking (dd)

Modified from Shah, J. & Lydiatt, W. (1995). Treatment of cancer of the head and neck. *CA: A Cancer Journal for Clinicians, 45*(6), 352-368; and Hoffman, H. & Karnell, L. (1996). Laryngeal cancer. In G. D. Steele, J. D. Jessup, D. P. Winchester, H. R. Menck, & G. P. Murphy (Eds.), *National Cancer Data Base: Annual review of patient care 1995*. Atlanta: American Cancer Society.

*Known; *sd,* strongly indicated; *dd,* confounded by simultaneous use of cigarettes.

PATHOPHYSIOLOGY

Anatomy and Physiology of the Larynx

The larynx begins at the superior tip of the epiglottis and extends to the inferior margin of the cricoid cartilage. It is divided into three regions: supraglottic, glottic, and subglottic. Anatomically the supraglottic larynx consists of the epiglottis, the false vocal cords, the ventricle of Morgagni, the aryepiglottic folds, and the arytenoids. The glottis includes the true vocal cords and the anterior commissure. The subglottic area is located below the vocal cords and contains the cricoid cartilage and subglottic space (Fig. 51-1).

There exists an embryologic basis for the separation of these anatomic regions of the larynx. In fact, due to the separate embryologic origin of its two sides, the right and left sides of the larynx do not communicate through the submucosal space (Weber & Callender, 1992).

Of clinical significance is the fact that these three regions have different vascular, lymphatic, and structural topographies that affect the pattern of tumor growth within the larynx. The rates and regions of expected metastases, symptom occurrence, and prognosis are also affected by these differ-

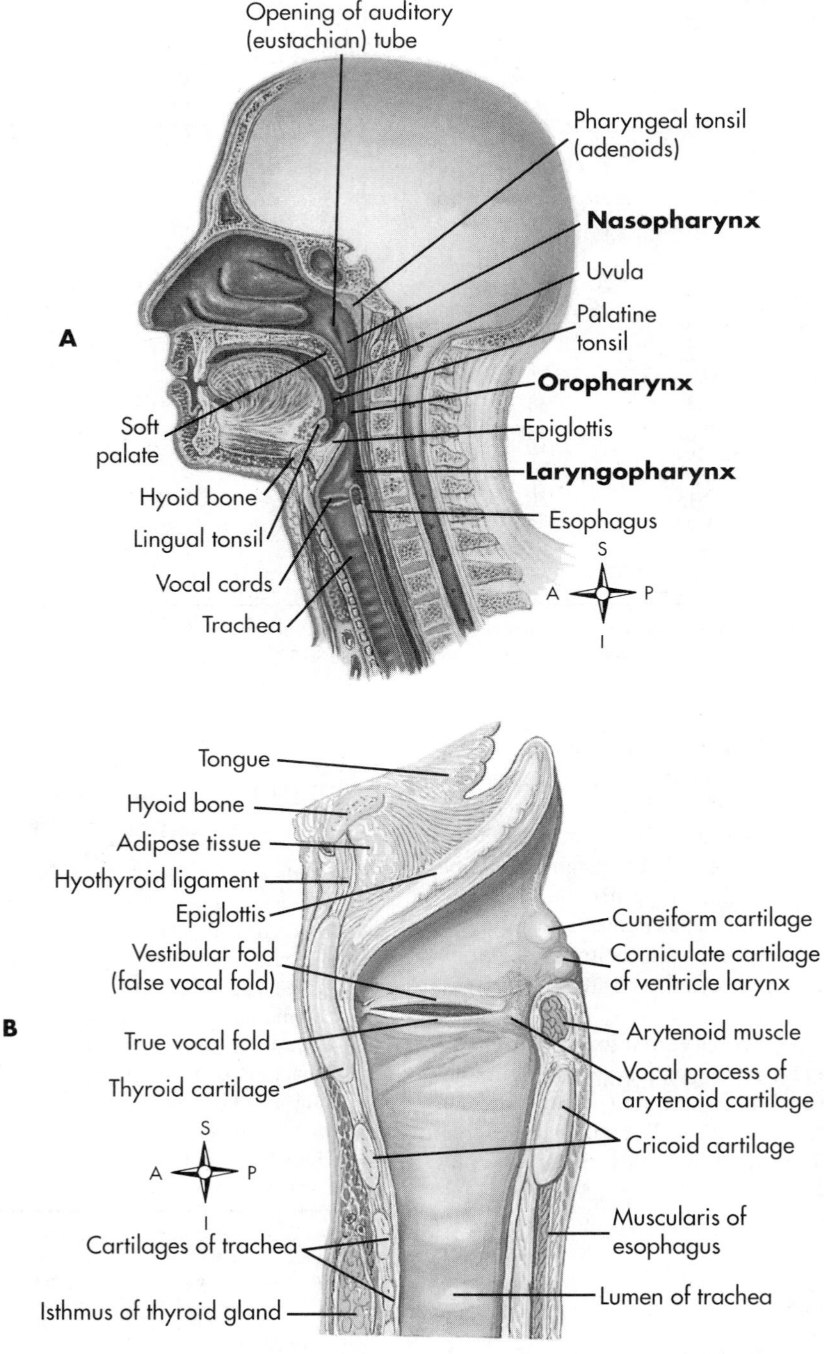

Fig. 51-1 **A,** Pharynx. This midsagittal section shows the three divisions of the pharynx (nasopharynx, oropharynx, and laryngopharynx) and nearby structures. **B,** Larynx (sagittal section). (From Thibodeau, G. A. & Patton, K. T. [1998]. *Anatomy and physiology.* St. Louis: Mosby.)

ing anatomies (Table 51-3). In the United States the supraglottic, glottic, and subglottic regions of the larynx have an approximate tumor occurrence ratio of 40:58:2, respectively (Olson & Wolf, 1995).

The vocal cords act as the line of demarcation between the supraglottic larynx and the glottis. The division between the glottis and subglottis is ill defined but considered to begin 5 mm below the free margin of the vocal cords. The vocal cords are approximately 2.2 cm in length in men and 1.8 cm in women. At their thickest point they are 3 to 5 mm in width. The cricothyroid muscle, an exterior muscle responsible for tensing the vocal cords, is innervated by a branch of the superior laryngeal nerve. Damage to the superior laryngeal nerve will cause a "bending" of the true vocal cord, leading to hoarseness. The internal muscles of the larynx are innervated by the recurrent laryngeal nerve (Million, Cassisi, & Mancuso, 1994).

Lymphatic Drainage and Routes Of Metastases. The structures in the supraglottic region have a rich capillary lymphatic drainage system (Fig. 51-2). The lymphatic collecting trunks terminate in the subdigastric node and the posterior supraclavicular chain. Consequently, the risk of cervical metastatic disease in patients with supraglottic carcinoma is high and depends on the stage of the primary tumor. There are more abundant lymphatics in the posterior larynx than in the anterior region. Consequently, metastasis through lymphatic spread is more likely when tumors occur within this region. In fact, the risk of cervical node metastasis in patients with T1, T2, T3, or T4 tumors is 20%, 40%, 60%, and 80%, respectively (Johnson, 1994). Between 52% and 72% of all patients with supraglottic carcinoma of the larynx present with positive cervical lymph nodes. Furthermore, 38% of patients who present with clinically negative nodes have positive nodes when they undergo biopsy (Zagars, Norante, Smith, & McDonald, 1993).

The true vocal cords have no capillary lymphatics. Consequently, lymphatic spread from cancer in the glottic region occurs only after the tumor extends to either the supraglottic or subglottic regions. This observation correlates with an extremely low rate of cervical lymph node metastases for early true vocal cord lesions. Less than 8% of patients with T1 and T2 glottic carcinoma will develop cervical metastases. The distribution of positive neck nodes in 150 patients with supraglottic and glottic carcinoma undergoing elective neck dissection is illustrated in Fig. 51-3 (Johnson, 1994; Million, Cassisi, & Mancuso, 1994; Olson & Wolf, 1995).

The subglottic region has abundant lymphatics that freely transport across the midline of the trachea. Lymphatic drainage migrates to the middle and lower jugular nodes and the paratracheal and pretracheal nodes. Accordingly, there is a higher rate of cervical lymph node metastasis and an increased tendency for bilateral cervical node metastasis. However, primary tumors in the subglottis account for less than 5% of all laryngeal cancers. (Johnson, 1994).

The Process of Carcinogenesis

Carcinogens and Promoters in Tobacco Products. Genotoxic carcinogens are deoxyribonucleic acid (DNA) reactive and act directly to alter the structure of DNA and support mutations. Tobacco smoke contains a number of powerful carcinogens and mutagens such as benzo(a)pyrene or dibenzo(a,h)anthracene. Unburned chewing and snuff tobacco and tobacco smoke also contain several potent nitrosamines such as nitrosonornicotine and carcinogenic heterocyclic amines. These chemicals are all genotoxic carcinogens and mutagens, keys in the initiation and development of specific types of cancer (Templeton & Weinberg, 1991).

The nature of the conversion from normal cells to a malignancy is believed to be a multistep progression (Templeton & Weinberg, 1991). In the case of carcinoma of the larynx, the combined use of the toxins alcohol and tobacco serve to promote the development of keratosis and subsequent epithelial dysplasia.

Precancerous lesions (keratosis) have a predicted conversion rate to malignant disease of approximately 4% of cases.

TABLE 51-3 Three Subdivisions of the Larynx as They Relate to Function, Symptom Occurrence, and Prognosis

Laryngeal Region	Function	Symptom Occurrence	Prognosis
Supraglottic	Air passage, shield and protect airway	Sore throat and dysphagia present at late and more advanced stage of disease; unilateral otalgia	Poor; late appearance of symptoms, two thirds of patients are diagnosed at later stages of disease
Glottic	Phonation, airway protection during swallowing/cough	Early, usually hoarseness, dysphonia, and cough; sore throat, otalgia	Good; sparse lymphatics, rare nodal metastasis
Subglottic	Air conduit	Respiratory stridor; usually represents extension from glottis	Poor; rich lymphatic network draining into multiple lymph nodes

Modified from Johnson, J. (1994). Larynx. In J. Gluckman, P. Gullane, & J. Johnson (Eds.), *Practical approach to head and neck tumors.* New York: Raven Press; and Norris, C. M. & Cady, B. (1991). Head, neck, and thyroid cancer. In A. Holleb, D. Fink & G. Murphy (Eds.), *American Cancer Society textbook of clinical oncology.* Atlanta: American Cancer Society.

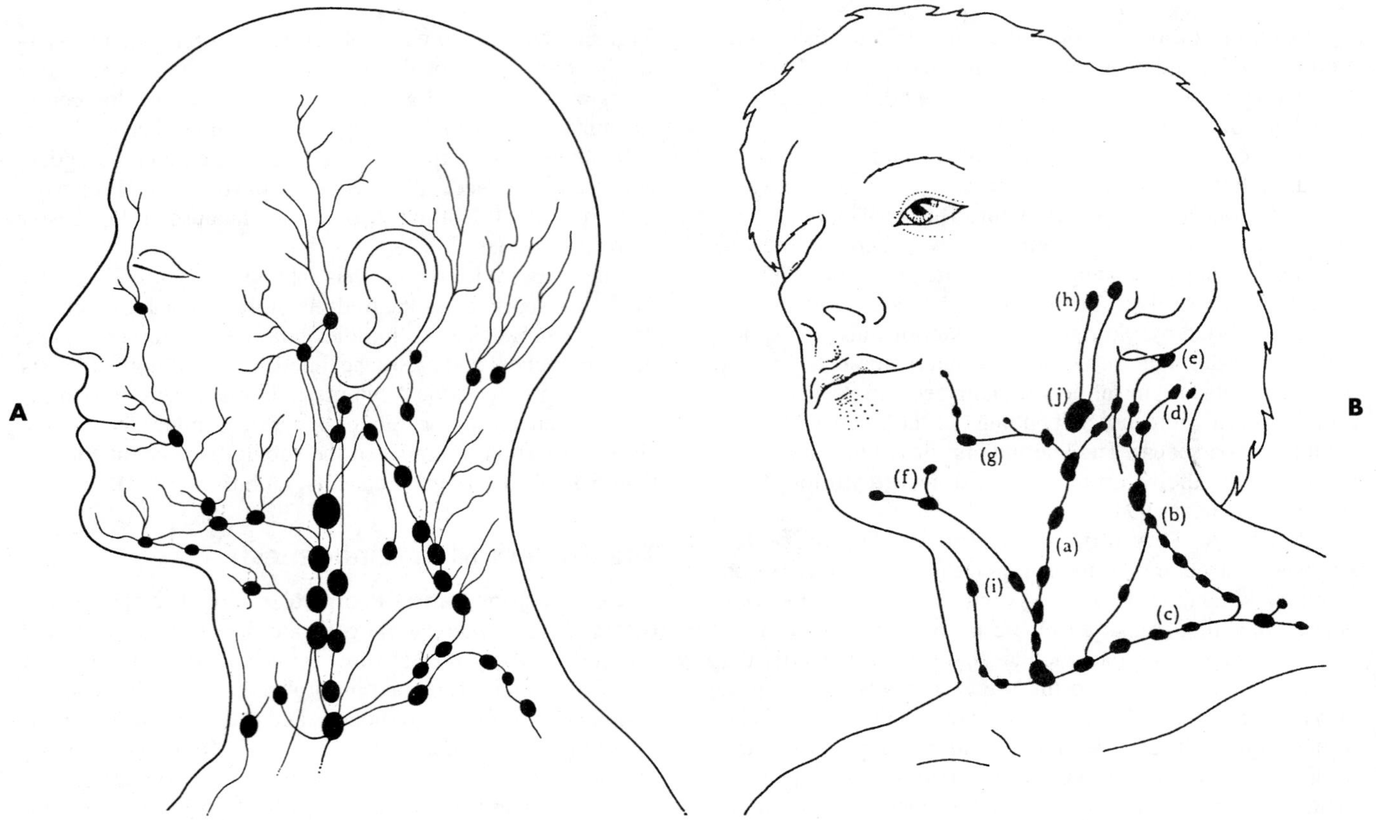

Fig. 51-2 Lymphatic drainage of the head and neck. **A,** Neck. **B,** Head and neck. (a) Lateral cervical midjugular; (b) midposterior cervical; (c) supraclavicular; (d) occipital; (e) posterior auricular; (f), submental; (g) submandibular; (h) preauricular; (i) anterior cervical; (j) subdigastric. (From Goodman, M. [1990]. Head and neck cancer. In S. L. Groenwald, M. H. Frogge, M. Goodman, & C. H. Yarbro [Eds.], *Cancer nursing: Principles and practice* [2nd ed.]. Boston: Jones and Bartlett.)

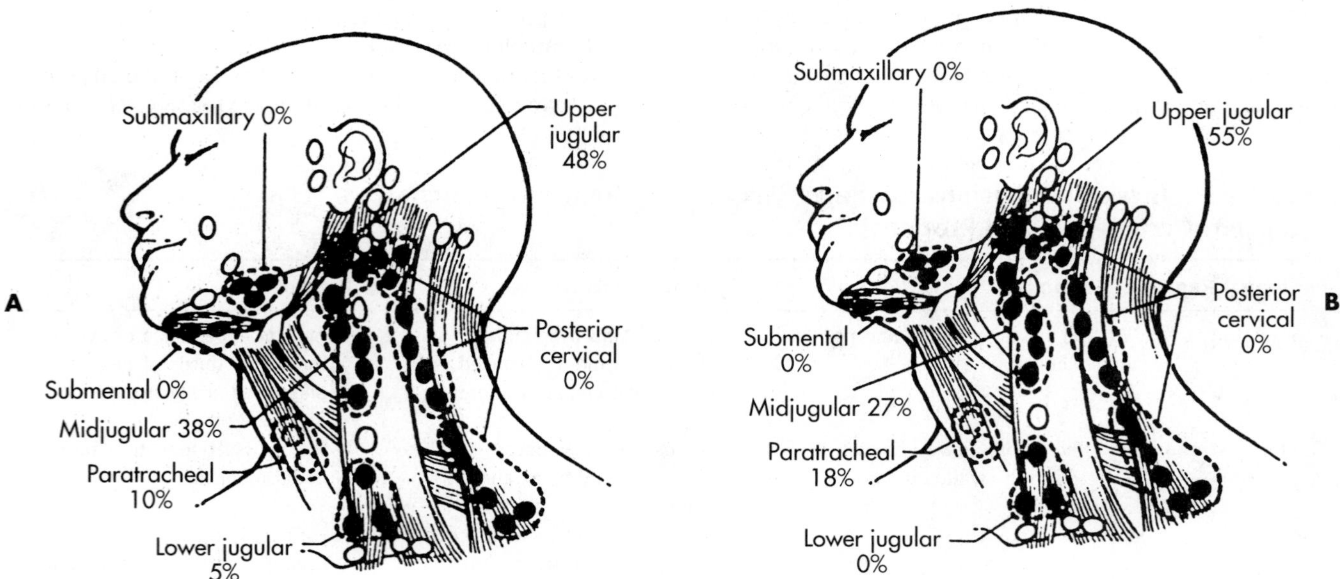

Fig. 51-3 The distribution of positive neck nodes in elective neck dissections of a total of 150 patients with carcinoma of the supraglottic and glottic larynx. **A,** Ninety-three patients underwent supraglottic larynx dissection, and **B,** 57 underwent glottic dissection. (From Million, R., Cassisi, N., & Mancuso, A. [1994]. Larynx. In R. Million & N. Cassisi [Eds.], *Management of head and neck cancer: A multidisciplinary approach.* Philadelphia: J. B. Lippincott.)

When keratotic, leukoplakic, or erythroplakic lesions demonstrate epithelial dysplasia, the risk for subsequent malignancy increases 30% to 50%, especially in patients who continue to smoke (Olson & Wolf, 1995). Once transformed, malignant cells have eight basic qualities that serve to enhance their survival. These properties are listed in Box 51-3.

ROUTES OF METASTASES

When lymphatic spread goes beyond the local region, the three most common distant metastatic sites include the lung, liver, and bone, respectively. The lung is by far the most common site of distant metastasis, accounting for 52% of the first recognized metastatic sites for SCC of the head and neck (Million, 1994).

ASSESSMENT

History and Physical Examination

A behavioral history includes questions about alcohol and tobacco use and occupational exposure to specific known carcinogens. A complete physical examination includes an evaluation of the scalp, facial and neck skin, regional lymph nodes, thyroid gland, salivary glands, and cranial nerves. The oral cavity and oropharynx are carefully examined, and a mirror examination of the nasal cavity is performed. Table 51-4 provides a summary of the assessment of the patient for laryngeal cancer.

Box 51-3
Basic Properties of Malignant Cells

1. Malignant cells have an altered cell structure.
2. Malignant cells display altered interactions with neighboring cells.
3. Malignant cells have a reduced requirement for growth.
4. Malignant cells are "immortal."
5. Malignant cells must escape immune surveillance.
6. Malignant cells exhibit some features of cell differentiation.
7. Malignant cells have an altered metabolism.
8. Malignant cells are capable of invasion and metastasis.

Data from Templeton, D. J. & Weinberg, R. A. (1991). Principles of cancer biology. In A. Holleb, D. Fink, & G. Murphy (Eds.), *American Cancer Society textbook of clinical oncology.* Atlanta: American Cancer Society.

TABLE 51-4 Assessment of the Patient for Laryngeal Cancer

	Assessment Parameters	Typical Abnormal Findings
History	A. Personal and social history	A. Personal and social risk factors
	1. Gender	1. Men develop laryngeal cancer more frequently than women (M:F ratio = 3.7:1).
	2. Tobacco and alcohol use	2. Nondrinking smokers have 2 to 4 times the risk of developing laryngeal cancer compared to abstainers of alcohol and tobacco; heavy-drinking smokers have a risk 6 to 15 times greater than abstainers
	3. Age	3. Over 90% of the cases of laryngeal cancer occur in persons at or over 50 years of age.
	4. Ethnicity	4. Most cases (83.1%) are reported in non-Hispanic whites
	5. Socioeconomic status	5. Persons with low and middle incomes have the highest incidence of laryngeal cancer
	B. Evaluation of the head and neck region	B. Common symptoms include deep-seated ear pain, dysphagia, hoarseness, neck mass, slow-healing sore, unilateral pain
Physical Examination	A. Head and neck examination 1. Examination of the scalp 2. Examination of skin of the face and neck 3. Palpation of regional lymph nodes, thyroid gland, and salivary glands 4. Evaluation of cranial nerve functioning	A. With metastatic disease, regional lymph nodes may be palpable
Diagnostic Tests	A. Indirect laryngoscopy and fiberoptic laryngoscopy	A. Primary tumor can often be visualized by indirect laryngoscopy
	B. Computerized tomography	B. Use of intravenous contrast allows for pronunciation of the primary tumor margins
	C. Direct laryngoscopy	C. Done to determine tumor extension and to obtain a biopsy of a suspected lesion
	D. Chest x-ray examination	D. Done to rule out metastatic lung disease

Diagnostic Tests

Indirect Laryngoscopy And Fiberoptic Laryngoscopy. In most patients with cancer of the larynx, the primary tumor can be visualized by a careful and thorough head and neck examination. Indirect laryngoscopy through the use of a mirror and photography is the most important method for the detection and diagnosis of laryngeal cancer. For patients unable to tolerate indirect mirror laryngoscopy, flexible fiberoptic laryngoscopy has become a valuable addition as a diagnostic tool (Johnson, 1994; Zagars et al., 1993).

Additional Diagnostic And Staging Procedures. In previous years laryngeal imaging was done by plain film tomography and contrast laryngography. Recently these imaging techniques have been replaced by contrast-enhanced computed tomography (CT) and supplemental magnetic resonance imaging scans that should be done before biopsy. The intravenous contrast-enhanced CT scan allows for the pronunciation of the primary tumor at the margins of otherwise healthy tissue. The entire course of the vagus and recurrent laryngeal nerve can also be visualized.

Direct laryngoscopy under general anesthesia is needed to determine tumor extension and obtain a biopsy of the suspected lesion. Additional tumor "debulking" of the lesion with a CO_2 laser or forceps is not recommended unless the airway is compromised by the mass. Vocal cords are also assessed for mobility and lesion location (Zagars et al., 1993).

Patients need a chest x-ray film to rule out metastatic lesions in the lung and/or synchronous primary tumors. Pulmonary function studies are done for patients suspected of having jeopardized pulmonary function resulting from tobacco use. Hematologic studies include a complete blood count to assess for anemia, as well as renal and liver function studies as a prequel to surgery and/or chemotherapy administration. (Million, Cassisi, & Mancuso, 1994; Zagars et al., 1993).

TABLE 51-5 Staging of Larynx Cancer

Primary Tumor	
TX	Primary tumor cannot be assessed
T0	No evidence of primary tumor
Tis	Carcinoma in situ
Supraglottis	
T1	Tumor limited to one subsite of supraglottis with normal vocal cord mobility
T2	Tumor invades more than one subsite of supraglottis or the glottis, with normal vocal cord mobility
T3	Tumor limited to larynx with vocal cord fixation and/or invades postcricoid area, medial wall of pyriform sinus, or pre-piglottic tissue
T4	Tumor invades through thyroid cartilage and/or extends to other tissues beyond the larynx (e.g., to soft tissues of the neck)
Glottis	
T1	Tumor limited to vocal cord(s) (may involve anterior or posterior commissures) with normal mobility
T1a	Tumor limited to one vocal cord
T1b	Tumor involves both vocal cords
T2	Tumor extends to supraglottis and/or subglottis and/or with impaired vocal cord mobility
T3	Tumor limited to the larynx with vocal cord fixation
T4	Tumor invades through thyroid cartilage and/or extends to other tissues beyond the larynx (e.g., soft tissues of the neck)
Subglottis	
T1	Tumor limited to the subglottis
T2	Tumor extends to vocal cord(s) with normal or impaired mobility
T3	Tumor limited to larynx with vocal cord fixation
T4	Tumor invades through cricoid or thyroid cartilage and/or extends to other tissues beyond the larynx (e.g., soft tissues of the neck)

From Hoffman, H. & Karnell, L. (1996). Laryngeal cancer. In G. D. Steele, J. D. Jessup, D. P. Winchester, H. R. Menck, & G. P. Murphy (Eds.), *National Cancer Data Base: Annual review of patient care 1995*. Atlanta: American Cancer Society.

STAGING

More than any other factor, the staging of laryngeal cancer determines the course of treatment. Consequently, accurate pretreatment clinical staging is crucial. Numerous classical clinical studies have demonstrated that classification by anatomic site is important in predicting the probable spread of laryngeal cancer (Weber & Callender, 1992). An underestimate of local disease extension may result in inappropriate consent and treatment (e.g., a patient is prepared for partial laryngectomy, and intraoperative findings necessitate a more extensive surgical procedure). In a group of patients with a supraglottic primary, 38% of those who were clinically staged as node negative actually had pathologically node-positive disease (Zagars et al., 1993). This finding coincides with the fact that most patients who present with symptoms of supraglottic carcinoma do so at a relatively advanced stage of the disease. In contrast, clinical overstaging rarely occurs (Norris & Cady, 1991).

In general, tumors of the larynx are staged by the extent of their local extension to adjacent sites and regions (Table 51-5). In contrast, tumors of the oral cavity are staged by their surface dimension. The diagnosis and staging of SCCs of the larynx has improved over the past decade. Yet in 1992 two thirds of the reported cases were diagnosed as stage III or IV disease (Dimery & Hong, 1993).

Any firm and enlarged cervical lymph node (greater than 1 cm) in an adult is thought to be malignant until proven otherwise. Careful palpation, measurement, and mapping of cervical lymph nodes is a necessary part of the diagnostic workup, and the number of palpable nodes is an important prognostic factor. The risk of distant metastasis correlates with nodal stage: less than 10% with N0 or N1 disease and 30% or greater with N2 or N3 disease (Tables 51-6 and 51-7). In patients with T4 lesions or extensive cervical lymphadenopathy, the presence of distant metastases in the lungs, liver, or bone should be ruled out before aggressive

Table 51-6 Staging of Cervical Node Metastases

	Regional Lymph Nodes (N)
NX	Regional lymph nodes cannot be assessed
N0	No regional lymph node metastases
N1	Metastasis in a single ipsilateral lymph node ≤3 cm in greatest dimension
N2	
• N2a	Metastasis in a single ipsilateral lymph node >3 cm but <6 cm in greatest dimension
• N2b	Metastasis in multiple ipsilateral lymph nodes, none >6 cm in greatest dimension
• N2c	Metastasis in bilateral or contralateral lymph nodes, none >6 cm in greatest dimension
N3	Metastasis in a lymph node >6 cm in greatest dimension

From Hoffman, H. & Karnell, L. (1996). Laryngeal cancer. In G. D. Steele, J. D. Jessup, D. P. Winchester, H. R. Menck, & G. P. Murphy (Eds.), *National Cancer Data Base: Annual review of patient care 1995*. Atlanta: American Cancer Society.

Table 51-7 Clinical Tumor Stage and Groupings for Head and Neck Cancer

Stage 0	Tis	N0	M0
Stage 1	T1	N0	M0
Stage 2	T2	N0	M0
Stage 3	T3	N0	M0
	T1-3	N1	M0
Stage 4	T4	Any N	M0
	Any T	N2,3	M0
	Any T	Any N	M1

From Hoffman, H. & Karnell, L. (1996). Laryngeal cancer. In G. D. Steele, J. D. Jessup, D. P. Winchester, H. R. Menck, & G. P. Murphy (Eds.), *National Cancer Data Base: Annual review of patient care 1995*. Atlanta: American Cancer Society.

local or regional therapy is instituted (Vokes, Weichselbaum, Lippman, & Hong, 1993; Zagars et al., 1993).

MEDICAL MANAGEMENT

The goal of treatment in laryngeal cancer is cure with the best functional result and the least risk of a serious complication. Eradication of the cancer, maintenance of adequate function, and achievement of a socially acceptable cosmetic result are major concerns for patients with this disease. Surgery and radiation therapy are the major curative modalities, and recently chemotherapy has been shown to be an effective adjuvant to standard treatment (Million, Cassisi, & Mancuso, 1994; Zagars et al., 1993).

The management of head and neck cancer increasingly and appropriately involves the participation and judgment of multiple disciplines, including radiation oncology, head and neck surgery, medical oncology, oncology nursing, dentistry, maxillofacial prosthodontics, nutrition, smoking cessation, speech therapy, social work, and hospice care. The main factors that need to be considered in the selection of treatment(s) for laryngeal carcinomas include regional location, stage and extent of the primary tumor, presence of nodal and distant metastases, anticipated functional and cosmetic results of treatment, overall health, performance status, and preferences of the patient and family. Arguably, the most important treatment goal is that of cure. However, quality of life issues need to assume a major role in the treatment decision-making process (Million & Cassisi, 1994; Norris & Cady, 1991).

The patients with laryngeal cancer tend to be elderly, undernourished users of excessive amounts of tobacco and alcohol. Medical problems such as diabetes, pulmonary disease, and cardiovascular disease are often present. The need for an expert treatment team is evident from the point of assessment onward. The optimal course of medical treatment can vary greatly on the basis of a single factor, such as the presence of positive cervical lymph nodes. It is incumbent on the physician and nurse to educate the patient and family about the subtitles of treatment planning and assure them that, once all of the necessary data have been collected, a total treatment strategy will be presented to them for discussion and consent. Critical factors that need to be evaluated when making judgments about medical treatment outcomes include voice quality, deglutition, disfigurement, and the potential for complications associated with treatment such as aspiration, dysphagia, and radiation necrosis (Weber & Callender, 1992).

Surgery or radiation therapy alone are the only curative treatments for SCC of the larynx. Chemotherapy, when used alone, is not curative and only plays an adjunctive role to surgery and/or radiation therapy. Assuming that the cure rates are comparable, Million & Cassisi (1994) compare and contrast the advantages of surgery and radiation therapy in the management of this disease (Table 51-8).

Practice Variability

In both early- and advanced-stage laryngeal cancers, there are a variety of options for the clinician and patient to consider, all of which contribute to practice variation. In a study done by O'Sullivan, Mackillop, Gilbert, Gaze, Lundgren, Atkinson et al. (1994), otolaryngologists and radiation oncologists from six geographic locations were surveyed concerning their management of specific scenarios for T1-T4 SCC of the larynx. Treatment options included radiation (single modality), conservation laryngectomy, and total laryngectomy. As expected, treatment approaches varied as a function of tumor stage. However, treatment selection within each specific tumor stage varied significantly, depending on the physician's specialty and geographic location.

From the perspective of the patient, total laryngectomy is one of the most feared operations, and rehabilitation using esophageal speech, an electrolarynx, and tracheoesophageal puncture is often seen as less desirable than the initial surgical procedure. Consequently, in the hopes of avoiding the

TABLE 51-8 Comparative Advantages of Surgery and Radiation

Advantages of Surgery	Advantages of Radiation Therapy
Advantages *may* include the following: 1. A limited amount of tissue is exposed to treatment. 2. Treatment time is shortened. 3. The risks of the sequelae of radiation therapy are avoided. 4. Irradiation can be reserved for subsequent head and neck primary tumors that may not be suitable for surgical intervention. 5. Pathologic tissue examination permits identification of patients with more extensive disease than originally determined and immediate postoperative irradiation can be added. 6. There is a small risk of radiation-induced malignancy in young patients. If radiation is given after the age of 30, the risk is small. This risk must be balanced against the immediate mortality risk of anesthesia, surgery, blood transfusions, etc.	Advantages *may* include the following: 1. The threat of a major operation is avoided. 2. No tissues are removed. Surgical resection of a small lesion may produce a functional or cosmetic defect. This problem must be weighed against the risk of radiation necrosis. 3. Elective irradiation of the lymph nodes can be included with little added morbidity, whereas the surgeon must "wait and see" or perform an elective neck dissection. 4. The surgical salvage of irradiation treatment failures is more likely to succeed than the salvage of a surgical failure. 5. The total cost of radiotherapy is often less than surgery. Some patients are able to work. 6. Multiple simultaneous primary lesions can be more easily encompassed. An odd distribution of node metastases often clues to a second primary.

Data from Million, R., & Cassisi, N. (1994). General principles for treatment of cancers of the head and neck: The primary site. In R. Million & N. Cassisi, (Eds.), *Management of head and neck cancer: A multidisciplinary approach.* Philadelphia: J. B. Lippincott.

surgery, alternative therapies are often considered, even if they are clinically less effective (Weeks & Pfister, 1996). Table 51-9 highlights the fact that, regardless of the choice of treatment, the potential for physical impairment exists.

Surgical Management

Small laryngeal lesions with no fixation or lymph node involvement can be successfully treated with surgery alone, including laser excision surgery. For patients with T1 and T2 disease the likelihood of undisclosed nodal disease is minimal (<10%). Consequently, limited surgery may be preferable, provided that the soundness of the larynx can be maintained. Examples of conservative procedures include partial laryngectomy, hemilaryngectomy, and laryngofissure. Fig. 51-4 outlines the intricate steps taken for a patient undergoing a hemilaryngectomy. However, current treatment philosophy leans toward initial radiation therapy to preserve the voice, leaving surgery for salvage treatment when there is recurrence of the disease. Regardless of the surgical procedure chosen, the involvement of a multidisciplinary team in the assessment and management of each individual patient cannot be underestimated.

A variety of curative surgical procedures may be considered, and some are capable of being successful while preserving the natural lung-powered voice. For example, a supraglottic laryngectomy may be considered for a patient with a supraglottic carcinoma that does not involve the true vocal cords. The absence of cervical metastases and the overall pulmonary function of the patient must also be considered. The appropriate surgical procedure must take into account the anatomic extent of the disease, the expertise of the surgeon, and the performance status of the patient.

Recent endoscopic excisions of small lesions of the mobile vocal cord with CO_2 lasers have shown good results. Carcinoma in situ arising on the true vocal cord can be treated endoscopically by stripping the involved segment of

TABLE 51-9 Categories of Potential Physical Impairment Due to Treatment of Laryngeal Carcinoma

Alteration in:	Area(s) of Impairment*
Speech	
Phonation	Larynx
Articulation	Tongue, teeth, palate, lips
Chewing	Jaw, teeth, salivary lubrication, relevant musculature
Swallowing	
Deglutition	Tongue, palate, pharynx, esophagus, salivary lubrication, larynx, esophagus;
Airway protection	coordinated reflexes and sensation
Breathing	Larynx, esophagus; coordinated reflexes and sensation
Senses	Taste, smell, sight, hearing

*Secondary effects on nutrition, chronic pulmonary health, and physical appearance must also be considered when measuring treatment against proven outcome(s).
Modified from Norris, C. M. & Cady, B. (1991). Head, neck, and thyroid cancer. In A. Holleb, D. Fink, & G. Murphy (Eds.), *American Cancer Society textbook of clinical oncology.* Atlanta: American Cancer Society.

the vocal cord. If the carcinoma in situ persists, further microlaryngoscopy at 5- to 6-week intervals can be performed until evidence of the tumor is gone. However, careful observation, expertise with the technique, and close patient observation are essential in the management of patients using this approach (Johnson, 1994; Shah & Lydiatt, 1995; Vokes et al., 1993).

Table 51-10 lists the current standard surgical treatment options for patients with carcinoma of the supraglottic, glottic, and subglottic regions. When a combined modality ap-

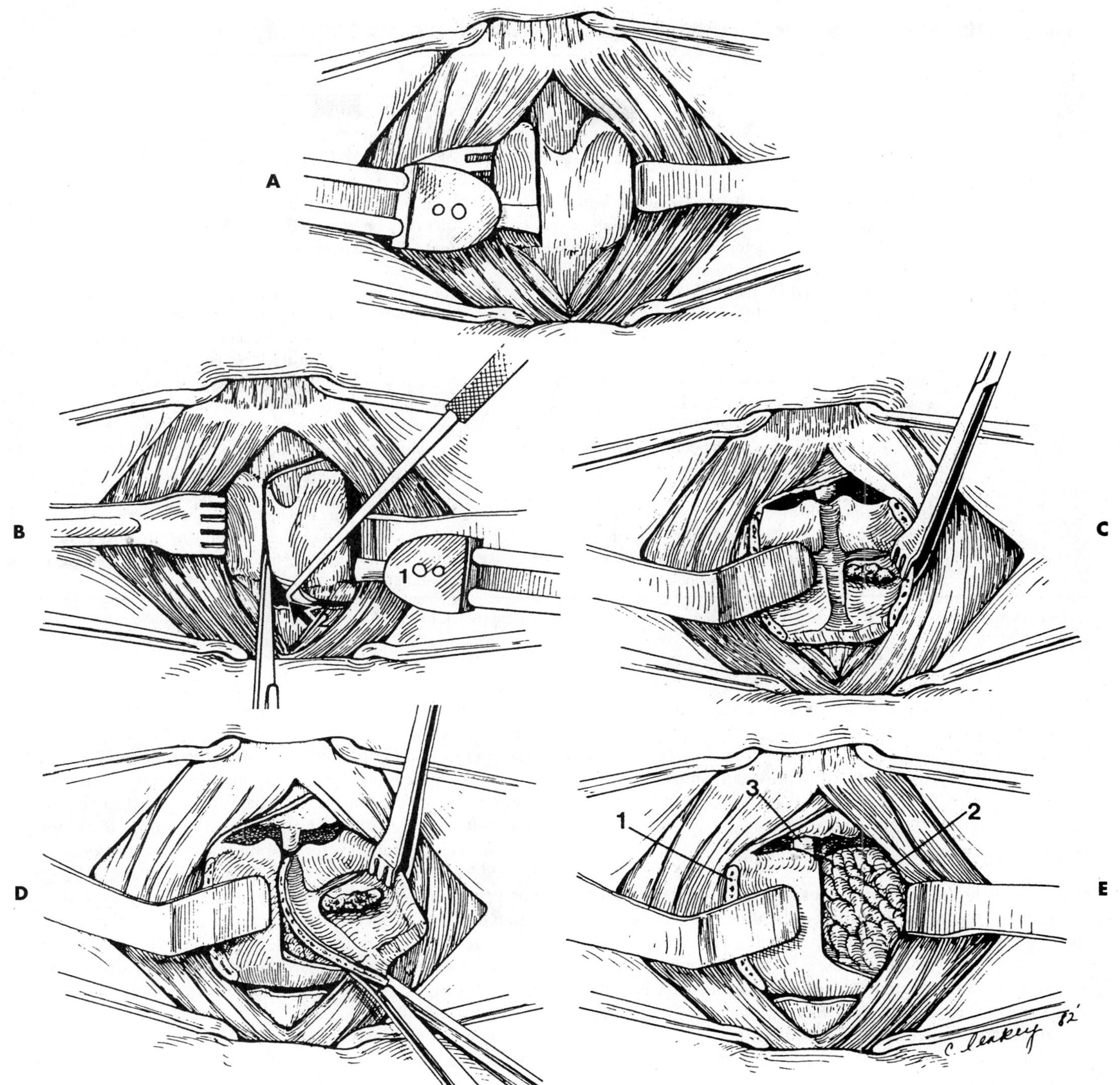

Fig. 51-4 Hemilaryngectomy for carcinoma of the left vocal cord with extension to the anterior commissure. **A,** Strap muscles are retracted, exposing the thyroid cartilage. Perichondrium on the left is preserved. A saw cut is made just to the right of the midline. **B,** A saw cut is made through the posterior edge of the thyroid cartilage, leaving 2 to 3 mm of cartilage posteriorly *(1)*. The larynx is then entered anteriorly through the cricothyroid membrane *(2)*. The lesion can then be viewed through a 1-cm exposure. A knife cut through the mucosa to the right of the midline is made under direct vision, and the incision is joined superiorly and inferiorly to the posterior cut. **C,** The thyroid laminae are retracted, and the lesion is exposed. The posterior extent is now clearly visible. **D,** The posterior mucosal cut is made along the line of the posterior cartilage cut. The final cut may include the arytenoid, if it is involved. **E,** Surgical defect after the specimen has been removed. Closure is completed by suturing the perichondrium from the left side to the perichondrium and thyroid cartilage on the right side *(1)*. *(2),* Mucosa of the pharyngeal wall; *(3),* nasogastric tube. (From Million, R., Cassisi, N., & Mancuso, A. [1994]. Larynx. In R. Million & N. Cassisi [Eds.], *Management of head and neck cancer: A multidisciplinary approach.* Philadelphia: J. B. Lippincott.)

TABLE 51-10 Standard Surgical Treatment Options Based on Disease Stage and Anatomic Region

Region	Stage I	Stage II
Supraglottic	Supraglottic laryngectomy; total laryngectomy reserved for patients unable to tolerate potential respiratory complications of surgery or the supraglottic laryngectomy	Supraglottic laryngectomy or total laryngectomy; depends on location of the lesion, clinical status of the patient, and expertise of the treatment team
Glottic	Cordectomy for carefully selected patients with limited and superficial T1 lesions; partial or hemilaryngectomy or total laryngectomy; depends on anatomic considerations; laser excision	Partial or hemilaryngectomy, total laryngectomy; depends on anatomic considerations; laser microsurgery may be appropriate
Subglottic	Surgery is reserved for radiotherapy failures or for patients in whom follow-up is likely to be difficult	Laryngectomy plus isolated thyroidectomy and node dissection followed by postoperative radiation therapy; for nonsurgical candidates salvage can be planned for local or neck recurrences
	Surgery with or without postoperative radiotherapy; surgery for salvage of radiation failures	Total laryngectomy with postoperative radiotherapy; may consider induction chemotherapy for organ preservation
	Surgery with or without postoperative radiotherapy; surgery for salvage of radiation failures	Total laryngectomy with postoperative radiotherapy; May consider induction chemotherapy for organ preservation
	Laryngectomy plus isolated thyroidectomy and node dissection usually followed by postoperative radiation therapy; surgical salvage planned for nonsurgical candidates with local or neck recurrences	Laryngectomy plus isolated thyroidectomy and bilateral node dissection usually followed by postoperative radiation therapy; some patients are not surgical candidates

Modified from Johnson, J. (1994). Larynx. In J. Gluckman, P. Gullane, & J. Johnson (Eds.), *Practical approach to head and neck tumors.* New York: Raven Press.

proach is planned (i.e., postoperative irradiation), the surgeon should not rely on irradiation to eradicate gross residual disease. If treatment is to have curative potential, all bulky, visible disease must be removed (Johnson, 1994; Zagars et al., 1993).

Radiation Therapy

When considering radiation therapy, the preservation of function and the cosmetic effects of treatment depend on the specific effects of irradiation on muscle, nerve, bone, and major blood and lymphatic vessels. One of the overall advantages of radiation therapy is its ability to successfully treat carcinomas without undue complications. One of the overall disadvantages, according to patients, is the seemingly long (i.e., 4 to 6 weeks; Monday through Friday) treatment schedule.

Although the risk of a second primary cancer is high among the head and neck cancer patient population (for some the relative risk is 3.9 times higher than that for the general population), adult patients with SCC treated by high-dose radiation therapy alone have no greater chance of a second head and neck cancer than the same patients treated with surgery or combined modalities. There is essentially no difference in the risk of a second cancer at the initial site, in a marginal site, or in a remote head and neck site (Mashberg & Samit, 1995; Million & Cassisi, 1994; Parker & Enstrom, 1988).

Radiation therapy of at least 6000 cGy is effective for recurrent disease or second primary lesions. When irradiation is unsuccessful in treating a primary lesion, the cancer almost always recurs in the core of the original lesion. A rescue operation may then be done, but with greater risk for a serious complication. The rescue operation may even entail a more severe functional or cosmetic loss than if the operation had been performed initially. For example, if an epiglottic lesion suitable for supraglottic laryngectomy is treated by radiation therapy and the treatment fails, the rescue procedure is often a total laryngectomy. Prior high-dose irradiation to the head and neck area is usually a contraindication to recurrent radiation therapy. Curative reirradiation is rarely successful, and risk of major tissue necrosis is high. Salvage surgery should be the treatment of choice (Million & Cassisi, 1994).

Radiation therapy should include irradiation of the bilateral regions of the neck at risk for metastases. Patients with a preradiation hemoglobin level >13 g/dl experience better local control of the disease and higher survival rates when compared to patients who are anemic (Fein, Lee, & Hanlon, 1995). Tobacco and alcohol users who continue these habits during treatment have a slightly higher risk of developing radiation necrosis or edema. The practicing alcoholic is likely to refuse a major operation but is also rather intolerant of the acute effects of irradiation once treatment is started. About 50% of the patients who smoke are able to stop immediately when advised to do so, about 25% decrease their tobacco use, and the remaining 25% do not alter their habit (Million & Cassisi, 1994).

Treatment of Early, Localized Disease. Radiotherapy is used in various regimens for early, localized (T1 and T2) laryngeal carcinomas. Patients who have compromised pulmonary function or who present a high surgical risk because of concurrent medical problems should be treated with radiation therapy as opposed to surgery. Consequently, for surgically unsafe T1 and T2 patients with no known nodal involvement (N0), radiation therapy is the primary treatment of choice.

Radiation therapy is also used with curative intent for T1 and T2 glottic and subglottic cancers. Radiation for vocal cord (glottic) cancer is delivered by small portals that cover only the primary lesion (Fig. 51-5). Generally, portal sizes larger than 6 × 6 cm increase the risk of edema without increasing the rate of cure. Since the incidence of lymph node involvement is so rare, elective irradiation of lymph nodes is not the standard procedure. It should be noted that subglottic cancers are rare and their diagnosis at an early stage is even more infrequent. For curative purposes it is common to prescribe between 5500 and 7000 cGy over a 6- to 7-week period (Million et al., 1994; Norris & Cady, 1991; Olson & Wolf, 1995).

Treatment of Moderately Advanced Disease. Fixed-cord lesions (T3) are further subdivided for voice preservation into early, favorable lesions and unfavorable lesions. Unfavorable lesions are extensive and bilateral, may include invasion of cartilage, and may be compromising the patient's airway. Radiation therapy is usually less successful if cartilage has been invaded by the tumor. Surgical intervention is the primary method of treatment for patients with unfavorable lesions. The major difficulty with the use of irradiation for the more advanced glottic lesions is the ability of the clinician to distinguish between radiation edema and local recurrence during follow-up examinations (Million et al., 1994).

Favorable T3 lesions have a tumor confined to one side of the larynx with minimal-to-no airway compromise. Patients with favorable T3 disease can be offered a full course of radiation therapy with the option of salvage surgery and immediate total laryngectomy for radiation failure. Using radiation therapy, the local control rate with voice preservation is reported to be between 50% and 70%. Fifty to 70% of the radiation failures are then cured with surgical salvage and total laryngectomy.

Patients are advised that there may be a reduction in their 5-year survival rate compared with those who have had an immediate total laryngectomy (5% to 10%). Should salvage laryngectomy be required, the risk of complications following radiation therapy is greater as a result of the impeded healing response in previously irradiated tissue (Johnson, 1994; Million, Cassisi, & Mancuso, 1994).

Continuous Irradiation, Fractionation, and Hyperfractionation. *Continuous irradiation* is defined as treatment that is not interrupted over a prescribed period of time. A common prescription may be 6000 cGy delivered over a 6-week period (Monday through Friday) at 200 cGy per day (30 fractions × 200 cGy = a total dose of 6000 cGy). Studies have shown that continuous irradiation yields more favorable results when compared with interrupted course schedules of radiation therapy.

Hyperfractionation, on the other hand, refers to *continuous* treatment fractions delivered on a twice daily basis. The rationale behind hyperfractionation is that it allows healthy tissue to recover enough over a 6-hour period to tolerate an additional radiation treatment on the same day. In addition, an attempt is made to overcome resistance to radiation by administering the radiation in a more intensive schedule. In fact, increased overall dosage may be achieved by slightly increasing the total daily dose fractions. If the prescription described in the previous paragraph were delivered at a tolerable 110 cGy twice daily for 30 fractions, the total dose would then equal 6600 cGy. Preliminary results are showing improved 3-year survival rates (i.e., from 43% to 59%) with the use of hyperfractionation in some head and neck studies (Zagars et al., 1993).

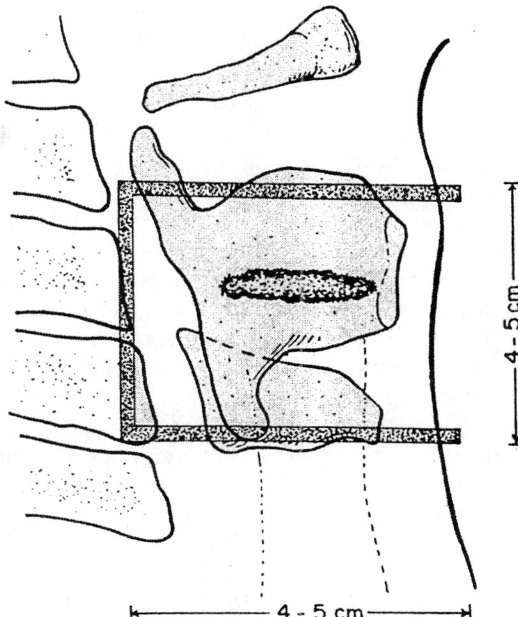

Fig. 51-5 Radiation for vocal cord (glottic) cancer delivered by small portals that cover only the primary lesion. (From Million, R., Cassisi, N., & Mancuso, A. [1994]. Larynx. In R. Million & N. Cassisi [Eds.], *Management of head and neck cancer: A multidisciplinary approach.* Philadelphia: J. B. Lippincott.)

Chemotherapy

The role of chemotherapy in the treatment of laryngeal cancer continues to evolve. For locally recurrent disease, for which surgical treatment and radiation therapy are no longer possible, chemotherapy is the standard treatment, and palliation of symptoms is the goal. The use of systemic antineoplastic agents is believed to prolong local disease control and eradicate micrometastases. However, Zagars et al. (1993) point out the difficulty in proving absolute effectiveness due to the advanced clinical stage of the disease and the poor nutritional status of most patients with locally recurrent tumors of the head and neck (Vokes et al., 1993; Zagars et al., 1993).

Neoadjuvant Therapy. *Neoadjuvant (induction) therapy* is the term used to describe chemotherapy that is administered as a first-line modality before planned irradiation or surgery in patients with advanced (stage III or IV) head and neck cancers. Neoadjuvant therapy is given to preserve the affected organ, possibly avoid surgical intervention, or treat inoperable tumors. The most common neoadjuvant regimen for head and neck tumors is cisplatin (100 mg/m^2 on day 1) and 5-fluorouracil (5-FU; 1000 mg/m^2/day by continuous infusion for 5 days) (Dimery & Hong, 1993; Jacobs & Pinto, 1995; Rooney, Kish, Jacobs, Kinzie, Weaver, Cressman et al., 1985; Zagars et al., 1993).

Although neoadjuvant chemotherapy before definitive surgery produces high induction response rates of 60% to 90%, it has not translated into improved survival rates for patients with head and neck cancer. The majority of patients do have tumor shrinkage from the induction chemotherapy. However, the prognostic significance of this response is still under investigation. A significant reduction in the rate of metastatic disease also occurs. However, improved survival is again hampered by the lack of impact of the therapy on local control of the disease and the 10% to 40% rate of second primaries in this patient population (Dimery & Hong, 1993; Jacobs & Pinto, 1995; Zagars et al., 1993).

Adjuvant and Concomitant Therapies. Chemotherapy in early stage disease (I or II) is used as an adjuvant treatment with standard surgery and/or irradiation. The goal of chemotherapy is the eradication of micrometastatic disease that remains after effective local-regional control with standard treatment. The use of chemotherapy in the adjuvant setting does offer improved survival (Zagars et al., 1993).

Concomitant therapy generally involves the use of single-agent chemotherapy (cisplatin or fluorouracil) at a low or moderate dose *during* radiation therapy treatment. The goals of treatment are to eliminate microscopic disease while simultaneously enhancing the cytotoxic effects of irradiation against gross disease in the head and neck (i.e., chemosensitization). Systemic toxicity does increase with concomitant therapy. However, some studies also report a small increase in disease-free survival. The most frequently reported dose-limiting toxicity of concomitant therapy is mucositis (Vokes et al., 1993; Zagars et al., 1993).

Research is currently being conducted on the use of combination chemotherapy with concomitant radiation therapy. It is being compared to induction chemotherapy (with the same antineoplastic agents) followed by standard radiation therapy. Preliminary results indicate a better disease-free or overall survival for the group that receives combination chemotherapy with concomitant radiation therapy (Vokes et al., 1993a; Pinto & Jacobs, 1995).

Commonly Used Single Agents. Methotrexate, cisplatin, vinblastine, doxorubicin, cyclophosphamide, and bleomycin are all active single agents for advanced laryngeal carcinoma (Table 51-11). Methotrexate (MTX) is the most widely used agent and is considered a standard for judging the efficacy of new regimens. With the use of this antimetabolite, response rates of 40% to 50% are seen with advanced lesions. However, the use of high-dose MTX with leucovorin rescue has not been shown to be more effective and adds cost and increased risks of toxicities in patients who do not adhere to the leucovorin regimen (Zagars et al., 1993).

Treatment with single-agent chemotherapy can be considered acceptable palliative therapy, assuming, of course, that the patient's corresponding quality of life is not diminished as a result of the toxic effects of the prescribed antineoplastic treatment. Although single agents are active in laryngeal cancer, the response lasts only an average of 3 months when used on advanced disease. This statistic is an important fact for the multidisciplinary team to realize as they support the "newly hopeful and responding" patient, all the while knowing that this reprieve will be transient (Vokes et al., 1993; Zagars et al., 1993).

TABLE 51-11 Active Single Antineoplastic Agents and Associated Response Rates in Patients with Advanced Laryngeal Carcinoma

Chemotherapeutic Agent	Percentage Response Rate*
Methotrexate	40-50
Cisplatin	30-40
Bleomycin	20-40
Cyclophosphamide	20-40
Vinblastine	20-40
Doxorubicin	20-40

Modified from Zagars, G., Norante, J., Smith, J. L., & McDonald, S. (1993). Tumors of the head and neck. In P. Rubin (Ed.), *Clinical oncology for medical students and physicians: A multidisciplinary approach* (7th ed.). Philadelphia: W. B. Saunders.
*>50% reduction in tumor volume.

Combination Agents Leading to Organ Preservation. Over the past 10 years the most dramatic change in the approach to the delivery of chemotherapy involves the use of combination regimens with cisplatinum and 5-FU. Cisplatinum combinations produce the highest responses, and overall response rates of 60% to 90% have been reported. However, despite these impressive response rates, there is no evidence that the duration of response or survival is improved (Vokes et al., 1993; Zagars et al., 1993).

Although neoadjuvant chemotherapy has not improved overall survival in advanced head and neck cancer, it has a clear role in the management of patients with SCC of the larynx. The Department of Veterans Affairs Laryngeal Cancer Study Group (1991) described a randomized trial that included 332 patients treated with either surgery/radiation or induction chemotherapy followed by irradiation. The induction chemotherapy regimen included the combination of cisplatin and 5-FU every 21 days for a total of three cycles. The two study arms had the same 68% survival rate at 2 years. The 3-year survival rates for the two groups are comparable at 53% to 56%. However, the chemotherapy group had significantly fewer distant metastases and more local recurrences. Although no survival benefit was realized, the results of the trial were important because 64% of the patients treated with chemotherapy were able to preserve their larynx, thus eliminating the need for a risky and disfiguring surgical procedure. The impact on the quality of life of those individuals cannot be underestimated. On analysis, the pretreatment clinical factors that were predictive of unsuccessful larynx preservation include more advanced tumor stage and prior tracheostomy (Department of Veterans Affairs Laryngeal Cancer Study Group, 1991; Wolf, Hong, & Fisher, 1993).

Because of the promising results of the Department of Veterans Affairs study, Eisbruch, Thornton, Urba, Esclamado, Carroll, & Bradford (1996) treated advanced laryngeal cancer patients with accelerated fractionated radiation therapy after two to three cycles of cisplatin and fluorouracil. The purpose of accelerated treatment (i.e., 7040 cGy delivered over 5.5 weeks) was to minimize the repopulation of clonogenic tumor cells during prolonged total treatment time. Compared with standard chemotherapy and radiation therapy, accelerated radiation therapy after chemotherapy increased both acute and long-term morbidity rates. In addition, local/regional tumor control and survival were not improved. Consequently, neoadjuvant chemotherapy with continuous standard-dose radiation therapy remains the option for laryngeal preservation.

Combined Modality Treatment

Every patient with laryngeal cancer does not require treatment with surgery, irradiation, and chemotherapy. Small primary lesions (T1 and T2) with a clinically negative neck are best managed with a single modality; and combination therapy under these conditions may result in overtreatment, inviting the unnecessary risk of complications.

Large primary lesions (T3 and T4) or cervical lymphatic involvement may require a planned approach that combines multiple treatment modalities. Currently the most frequent multimodal treatment regimen is high-dose preoperative or postoperative irradiation and radical surgery. Standard surgical techniques may need some modification when radiation is administered because of changes in tissue strength and healing capacity.

ONCOLOGIC EMERGENCIES

Airway Obstruction

Newly diagnosed patients with laryngeal cancer rarely possess the threat of immediate airway obstruction unless they present with a stage IV tumor and multiple, large cervical neck metastases. In this situation an emergency tracheostomy is performed. After a patent airway has been established, patients are staged to evaluate the extent of their disease. Palliative therapy can generally be offered in the form of irradiation or chemotherapy.

Other patients with laryngeal cancer are at risk for airway obstruction as a result of a number of potential clinical scenarios. Box 51-4 summarizes several situations that can lead to this oncologic emergency. Regardless of the source, the treatment remains the same. The health care team must be able to establish a patent airway, or death is imminent. Consequently, a patient who learns to care for his or her own tracheostomy must be able to demonstrate ways to maintain a patent airway in situations in which high anxiety and panic may be present because of vomiting and aspiration that may lead to an obstructed airway.

Box 51-4

Clinical Scenarios for the Patient with Laryngeal Cancer That May Lead to the Oncologic Emergency: Airway Obstruction

Supraclavicular lymph node and tissue edema as a result of:
- Surgery
- Radiation therapy
- Infection

Inability to clear mucus and aspiration as a result of:
- Surgical denervation
- Loss of hypoglossal reflex

Trismus (locking of the jaw muscle) due to radiotherapy
Esophageal stricture

Aspiration Pneumonia

In an otherwise healthy population, aspiration pneumonia is considered an acute-nonemergent event. However, patients who have had a laryngectomy have a host of characteristics that cause aspiration pneumonia to be considered an oncologic emergency.

The most significant complication following supraglottic laryngectomy is life-threatening aspiration. When supraglottic laryngectomy must extend to include a part of the base of the tongue, the risk for aspiration increases. If a patient with marginal baseline pulmonary function elects to have surgery, minimal amounts of aspiration can lead to life-threatening pneumonia. Aspiration pneumonia is treated with aggressive nursing care aimed at promoting ambulation, as well as deep breathing and pulmonary toilet. Initially the tracheotomy cuff should remain inflated, and the patient should be fed through a nasogastric or gastrostomy feeding tube. Appropriate antibiotics are administered as scheduled. If the patient aspirates on a chronic basis, the pulmonary and digestive systems may need to be separated permanently by having the patient undergo a total laryngectomy (Goodman, 1990; Johnson, 1994).

NURSING MANAGEMENT

The nursing care of the patient with cancer of the larynx occurs in distinct phases, depending on the stage of the disease and the treatment methods chosen to manage the disease. Throughout a course of treatment, the patient with laryngeal cancer might require the expertise of a surgical oncology nurse, a radiation oncology nurse, an oncology nurse skilled in the administration of multiple chemotherapeutic agents, and a hospice nurse.

Often the role of the oncology nurse is to shepherd the patient through the health care system, ensuring the completion of assigned procedures and tests throughout the course of treatment. The oncology nurse will have the patient's entire treatment plan in mind as he or she introduces the patient to the various phases of their care and the staff members associated with it. The overall plan of care can be quite complex and may last well over 6 months. Consequently, it is incumbent on the oncology nurse to monitor the patient throughout the experience and ensure that proper referrals are in place as the need arises.

Surgical Management

The location of the laryngeal tumor and the extent of the patient's disease guide the surgical treatment options available to the patient (see Table 51-10). Consequently, the surgical oncology nurse may be caring for a patient with laryngeal cancer who is undergoing a procedure as minimally invasive as laser microsurgery to remove a small, mobile vocal cord lesion or an extremely invasive procedure such as a total laryngectomy with a thyroidectomy and extensive node dissection.

Regardless of the specific surgical procedure required, there are several areas of overlap when considering the nursing management of the head and neck patient who undergoes surgery. Box 51-5 lists the potential complications that can occur following head and neck surgery.

Supraglottic Laryngectomy, Hemilaryngectomy, Total Laryngectomy. Patients who have a supraglottic laryngectomy undergo resection of the part of the larynx that is responsible for sphincteric action. This procedure automatically predisposes the patient to aspiration. The recurrent laryngeal nerve becomes responsible for the total innervation of the larynx since the internal branches of the superior laryngeal nerves are paralyzed. Unfortunately, some patients may never be able to swallow secretions and nutrition without the risk of chronic aspiration. If this syndrome develops, the patient will have to undergo a second surgery for a total laryngectomy. Consequently, supraglottic laryngectomy is contraindicated in patients who have substandard pulmonary function and in whom pneumonia would become a life-threatening complication. Therefore a preoperative pulmonary evaluation provides essential information to help determine the most appropriate surgical procedure (Goodman, 1990; Johnson, 1994). During the immediate postoperative period, the patient has a laryngectomy tube in place for at least 3 to 4 days. This tube allows for a complete stoma and minimizes trauma caused by suctioning. If the laryngeal sphincter does not function as a result of surgery, the patient is unable to elevate intrabronchial pressure to a level necessary for effective coughing and clearing of the airway. As a result, the force of the cough is much less effective. The patient will have problems managing thickened secretions caused by postanesthesia effects, local edema, pain, and fear. He or she will need to be able to suction the oral cavity and thus should demonstrate proficiency with suctioning as a part of the preoperative preparation. Postoperative nasal secretions are also a problem because of the continued secretion of mucus by the nose in tandem with the inadequacy of normal mucus drainage channels. Consequently, mucus drains out of the nose. Nasal hygiene includes the gentle removal of crusting with a gauze that is soaked in saline. The nares are swabbed daily with a mixture of eucalyptol in a mineral base (Goodman, 1990; Johnson, 1994). A standard of care for a patient undergoing supraglottic laryngectomy is summarized in Table 51-12.

Box 51-5
Potential Complications Following Surgery for the Laryngeal Cancer Patient

Immediate Postoperative Complications*

1. Wound infection
2. Fistula formation
3. Sloughing of skin flap
4. Exposure and rupture of the carotid artery
5. Tenacious nonclearing secretions
6. Aspiration pneumonia
7. Pulmonary embolism
8. Alcohol withdrawal (sd)

Chronic, Long-Term Complications

1. Superficial infection due to loss of mucous membrane moisture
2. Chronic neck pain
3. Shoulder disability

*Local complications occur more frequently in the previously irradiated patient.

sd, Patient may have been unable to report the average daily amount of alcohol consumed. Lack of management can lead to withdrawal symptoms within 48 hours after surgery.

The development of fistulas in the postoperative period will delay the patient's discharge and increase the risk for aspiration, infection, and pneumonia. For example, a small fistula in a patient with laryngectomy usually heals without extraordinary measures. However, if the site has been irradiated previously, the fistula may progress, requiring a second surgical procedure for reconstruction. Fistulas contribute to additional scarring and may lead to esophageal stricture and dysphagia. Drying of the mucous membranes and infection can lead to chronic bronchitis. The use of aerosolized saline and room humidifiers together with adequate fluid intake can help to maintain the moistness of the mucous membranes.

Following total laryngectomy, serious postoperative wound complications can occur in approximately 5% of the cases. Proper and patent wound drainage facilitates wound healing, and the administration of antibiotics helps to prevent the development of systemic sepsis (Johnson, 1994).

Postoperative Nutrition. Postoperative nutrition is delivered through a nasogastric (NG) or a percutaneous gastric tube (G-tube). The type of feeding device that will be used is chosen before surgery and is based on the clinical scenario facing the treatment team. A thorough preoperative nutritional assessment provides the dietitian with the necessary information to calculate the precise number of calories required to promote recovery and tissue healing. The dietitian and speech/swallowing therapist are integral members of the multidisciplinary team.

The NG tube remains in place for 7 to 10 days. Antiemetics may be needed to prevent episodes of emesis since the muscular strain of vomiting can lead to trauma, dislodgment of the NG tube, and possible puncture of suture lines. Previously irradiated patients have prolonged healing times and are at greater risk for fistula formation. Consequently,

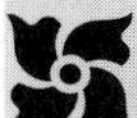

TABLE 51-12 Standard of Care for the Patient with Laryngeal Cancer Undergoing Supraglottal Laryngectomy

Patient Problem and Outcomes	Nursing Interventions and Rationales	Patient Education Instructions
Anxiety Related to Surgery		
Patient will: • Be able to discuss the rationale for surgery. • Discuss current habits (alcohol and tobacco) that will impact on recovery. • Obtain list of smoking and alcohol cessation experts from the health care team. • List behaviors viewed as realistic and necessary to support postoperative recovery	1. Evaluate patient's level of understanding. 2. Allow patient time to honestly discuss their use of alcohol and tobacco. 3. Aside from tobacco and alcohol, work with patient to construct a list of familiar, trusted coping strategies. 4. Provide patient with a list of smoking and alcohol cessation professionals. 5. If applicable, discuss the ways that alcohol withdrawal will be managed during the recovery period.	1. Use simple, clearly labeled pictures to show patient basic steps and planned results of surgery. 2. Allow patient to tour the intensive care unit if he or she expresses a desire to do so. 3. Meet with patient/family and discuss: a. Preoperative examinations: dental, anesthesia, pulmonary, nutrition b. Nasogastric (NG) or G-tube placement c. Temporary tracheostomy and temporary loss of speech d. Rehabilitation and follow-up care
Dysphagia, Impaired Swallowing		
Patient will: • Receive preoperative teaching instructions. • State expectations and probable results of surgical procedure, including temporary tracheostomy. • Demonstrate effective oral suctioning before supraglottic laryngectomy. • Be able to discuss pain management strategies used by health care team for their comfort and recovery. • Be able to explain the rationale for frequent respiratory therapy. treatments and deep suctioning during the postoperative recovery period.	1. Consistently place oral self-suctioning device within easy reach of patient. 2. Encourage patient to self-suction, if able. 3. Administer narcotics and other prescribed medications to minimize pain caused by surgery and postoperative edema. 4. Administer antianxiety agents, if needed. 5. Rinse and swab oral cavity and nares on an hourly basis with a nondrying saline solution. 6. Maintain patient elevated at $\geq$45 degrees. 7. Provide tracheostomy care per unit policy and procedure. 8. Offer communication board.	1. Provide patient with information about the following: a. Self-oral suctioning technique. Patient is not able or advised to swallow for the first 48 hours after surgery without supervision and coaching. b. Pain control plan, including patient-controlled analgesia. c. Importance of deep breathing and mild coughing (violent coughing can disrupt surgical incision). d. Nutritional needs met via NG or G-tube. Report all sensations of nausea to avoid vomiting and aspiration. e. Use of communication board for communication with unit staff.
Partial Airway Obstruction and Pulmonary Infection		
Patient will: • Alert staff to changes is respiratory status. • Safely and correctly perform self-suction with handheld oral suction device. • Maintain head of bed elevated. • Request pain and antianxiety medications when needed. • Alert staff to initial sensation of nausea that may lead to vomiting, aspiration, and pneumonia.	1. Monitor oxygen saturation, lung sounds, vital signs, and other indicators of a decline in respiratory status. 2. Perform tracheostomy suctioning per unit protocol. 3. Assess patient for potential nausea and vomiting due to: a. Anesthesia effects b. Pain medications c. Tube-feeding reflux d. Withdrawal symptoms 4. Instruct patient to request antiemetics at the first sign of nausea. 5. Evaluate patient for signs of aspiration pneumonia such as fever, elevated white blood cell count, sweating and pallor, and chest x-ray film results.	1. Provide patient with information about the following: a. Self-oral suctioning technique b. Importance of deep breathing and mild coughing (violent coughing can disrupt surgical incision) c. Reporting of all sensations of nausea to obtain medications to prevent vomiting and aspiration pneumonia d. Possibility of frequent chest x-ray films

the additional irritation caused by an NG tube is generally avoided, and a G-tube is placed during the surgical procedure. During the rehabilitation phase, if the NG tube is discontinued and the patient is unable to coordinate swallowing without aspiration, the NG tube will need to be reinserted. This process is often psychologically defeating for the patient, who interprets the reinsertion of the tube to mean that the treatment has failed (Johnson, 1994).

Hyposmia (i.e., loss of the olfactory sense) is usually permanent and is believed to be due to motor denervation of the larynx or to vascular changes in the mucous membranes. A less mature, secondary olfactory sense will eventually develop and allow for the detection of strong, pronounced odors. The ability to taste is also modified because of the relationship between the olfactory cells and taste discrimination. Hyposmia is even more pronounced in patients who have had previous irradiation to the pharynx and larynx (Goodman, 1990; Johnson, 1994).

Laryngeal rehabilitation. The rehabilitation processes around vocalization and swallowing begin with the decannulation of the tracheostomy. After 5 to 7 days the cuff of the tracheostomy tube is deflated, and, when the patient tolerates the deflation overnight, the tracheotomy is downsized and plugged. Patients who can sleep comfortably overnight with a plugged tracheotomy tube can then be decannulated.

Oral feeding should not begin until the tracheotomy stoma has completely healed. The sealed stoma greatly enhances the patient's ability to cope with the inevitable episodes of aspiration. Oral intake is carefully monitored by the nursing staff and the swallowing therapist. Initial oral intake should be made up of foods that have the consistency of applesauce or pudding. These foods are easier to control than liquids, and their texture allows for ease of movement down the esophagus (Johnson, 1994).

Vocal rehabilitation is a critical part of the management plan for patients with laryngeal cancer. Speech therapists should be involved early in the course of the patient's treatment. They should evaluate and educate the patient before surgery. Voice rehabilitation options for patients who require total laryngectomy include esophageal speech, electric artificial laryngeal devices, and the creation of tracheoesophageal shunts.

Up to 75% of patients with laryngectomy are able to develop understandable esophageal speech. Spasms and the inability to control the upper esophageal sphincter as a result of scarring create problems for the other 25%. Esophageal speech requires the swallowing of air and then the abdominal thrusting of this air through the nasal and oral cavities. The process of swallowing air can lead to gastric distress and distention, but patients eventually learn how to control their abdominal muscles to minimize distention. Even if esophageal speech is excellent, some patients also use a hand-held electrolarynx for ease in conversation and more rapid speech (Goodman, 1990; Iwamoto, 1992; Johnson, 1994).

Some patients receive a tracheoesophageal puncture at the time of their laryngectomy. A 14F rubber catheter is temporarily placed to create a stoma that is suited for later surgical insertion of a speech prosthesis. The prosthesis is placed 2 to 3 weeks after surgery, and, in the interim, patients are instructed in the use of an electrolarynx for communication (Johnson, 1994).

Radiation Therapy

The role of the radiation oncology nurse in the management of patients with laryngeal cancer cannot be underestimated. Patient education, constant and consistent assessments, symptom management, dental hygiene referrals, psychological support during treatment, and counseling about smoking cessation are just a few of the areas in which expert oncology nurses intervene in the management of these patients.

A standardized tool to document the assessment and care of the patient undergoing radiation therapy to the head and neck was created by the Radiation Oncology Special Interest Group of the Oncology Nursing Society. The Radiation Therapy Patient Care Record allows for consistent assessment and documentation of repeated problem areas such as alterations in comfort, mucous membranes, nutrition, sensory, skin, bleeding, and infection. The computerized version of this tool allows for the recording of assessment data that can be filtered and queried and the documentation of treatment information that can be used for instant and comprehensive outcome reports. Data collected in this fashion also allow for immediate, real-time monitoring of the quality of care that the patient receives.

Continued and Excessive Use of Alcohol. The continued use of alcohol impairs wound healing, destroys the oral mucosa, has negative effects on liver function, and provides no nutritional value. Patients who continue to use excessive amounts of alcohol may be in a social situation where there is little or no support for a healthy lifestyle transition. Consequently, the patient is at risk for self-care deficits after the initial diagnosis, as well as during the entire course of treatment. This situation will become more apparent to the staff in the radiation oncology center who see the patient on a daily basis. The staff need to document their awareness of the patient's alcohol use, as well as the steps taken to support the patient. The patient's support system and significant others need to be assessed to assist the patient through the entire course of treatment. An objective plan of care should be developed by the staff in consultation with experts in the field of substance abuse.

Symptom Management. Patients undergoing radiation therapy to the head and neck region are at great risk of developing a myriad of symptoms, including mucositis, trismus, dysphagia, and osteoradionecrosis. A thorough discussion of these symptoms and nursing standards of care can be found in Chapter 53, Oral Cavity Cancer.

Xerostomia. Saliva is necessary for the lubrication of food during chewing and swallowing. Saliva is also important for taste, digestion, teeth cleaning, maintenance of denture stability and retention, and speech. Without saliva, dental caries can be severe. Xerostomia (dryness of the mouth) occurs when the salivary glands are affected by irradiation. When it is present, there is an increased risk for dental caries, periodontal diseases, stomatitis, disturbed oral sensations, dysphagia, and altered taste. It is ubiquitous in patients receiving greater than 5000 cGy to any field involving the major salivary glands. Patients can average an 83% reduction in saliva flow after 6 weeks of irradiation at 1000 cGy/week. Xerostomia has been reported by patients after 1 week or 1000 cGy of radiation therapy.

The quality of the saliva changes to an acidic, thick, ropy substance. Prolonged therapy leads to complete atrophy and fibrosis of the salivary glands. The xerostomia can last for months, but symptoms peak at the end of the course of radiation and begin to become less bothersome after 1 to 2 years. Anaerobic microbes populate the mouth in the presence of xerostomia, and an increase in candidiasis is also reported. Prevention of infection by a meticulous oral hygiene regimen cannot be overemphasized because, once the salivary glands are infected, their function is generally lost forever (Iwamoto, 1992; Manne, 1996).

Patients with xerostomia should be taught to follow a few basic self-care measures that will greatly increase their comfort level. Encourage the patient to increase fluid intake of water and diluted, low-acid fruit juices. Avoid thick, dry food such as crackers, peanut butter, and popcorn and caffeine-based liquids such as coffee, tea, and cola. Salivary production is stimulated by chewing sugarless gum or sucking on citrus-flavored sugarless candy. Because of their drying effect, alcohol-containing commercial mouthwashes and lemon-glycerine swabs should not be used.

Saliva substitute can be used. However, it is important to teach the patient that the effect is temporary, lasting only a few minutes. Fluoride may be added to the cellulose lubrication to assist in the prevention of dental caries. Saliva substitute is useful before meals to assist with lubrication while chewing, and it can facilitate swallowing. Patients can use sauces and gravies to assist with the lubrication of food and to add calories to their diet. In addition, patients should be taught to drink fluids with all meals (Iwamoto, 1992).

As opposed to surface lubrication, salivary production is stimulated by pilocarpine hydrochloride. Pilocarpine hydrochloride (Salagen tablets, 5 mg tid) is a cholinergic alkaloid that is useful in relieving the symptoms of xerostomia with fewer side effects than its stronger cousin, pyridostigmine. Some patients experience symptomatic relief within a few weeks. However, it may take 1 to 3 months for others to realize significant improvement. The most common side effect of pilocarpine hydrochloride is sweating. If the patient sweats excessively, without the ability to replace fluids, dehydration may develop. Pilocarpine hydrochloride is contraindicated in patients with uncontrolled asthma and glaucoma. It may also cause visual disturbances at night that can impair driving ability (Johnson, Ferretti, & Nethery, 1993).

Chemotherapy

The patient with laryngeal cancer who undergoes chemotherapy generally fits into one of four clinical situations. Individuals are receiving neoadjuvant therapy for organ preservation, adjuvant therapy for the management of micrometastasis, concomitant low-dose chemotherapy to augment radiation, or palliative chemotherapy for end-stage disease.

Patients with laryngeal cancer who undergo concomitant chemotherapy present with unique nursing care needs that are summarized in the next section of this chapter.

Management of the Patient Who Undergoes Concomitant Therapy. Special attention must be paid to patients undergoing combined therapies. The risk for toxicities increases, along with the chances for disease-free survival. 5-FU–based regimens are known to cause painful mucositis, and patients with xerostomia resulting from irradiation are at greater risk of developing intolerable toxicities from the treatment. The patient may be unable to cope with the compounded toxicities of mucositis, xerostomia, infection, pain, and weight loss caused by dysphagia. Consequently, the patient is at risk for stopping treatment altogether. The nurse must thoroughly assess the patient during each visit, teach the patient symptom management strategies, and alert the physician at the first sign that the patient is having difficulty coping. Patients should be instructed to alert the staff should they notice any changes in their oral status.

Patients undergoing concomitant therapy often receive nutritional support through a percutaneous G-tube. Enteral feedings provide the patient with adequate nutrition during the months of guaranteed dysphagia. Unfortunately, the patient may grow to expect mild diarrhea as a side effect of the enteral feedings and neglect to report it as a symptom of 5-FU toxicity. Patient education and relentless nursing assessments are the keys to the prevention of dehydration and the sloughing of gastrointestinal tissue. Aggressive nutritional support is necessary because median weight loss in one combined chemotherapy/radiation therapy study was reported to be 11% during the concomitant phase of the treatment (Eisbruch et al., 1996).

If the patient has a history of years of alcohol and tobacco use, baseline liver and renal function tests must be evaluated carefully. If a platinum-based regimen is prescribed and the patient has compromised renal function, the nurse should expect a corresponding reduction in the dose of chemotherapy.

Posttreatment Follow-Up. Regardless of the specific treatment plan, the chance for recurrence within the first 2 years after treatment or the development of a second primary lesion remains high for patients with laryngeal cancer (Pinto & Jacobs, 1995b). Therefore close monitoring of patients after treatment is an essential component of their care. When recurrences are detected early, the chance for successful salvage treatment improves. A standard follow-up schedule would be: *once* a month for *1* year; every *2* months during the *second* year; every *3* months during the *third* year; and every *4* to *6* months during the *fourth, fifth,* and *sixth* years.

This follow-up schedule is easy to remember due to the consistency of the months and years. Patients and family members can be provided with follow-up cards containing this plan to reinforce the importance of keeping their scheduled clinic appointments.

A follow-up examination includes a search for recurrences at the primary site. Any change in voice or vocal cord mobility or new onset of pain should prompt an evaluation with CT studies and endoscopic biopsy. In patients with persistent edema of the larynx after radiation therapy, tumor is found 40% to 50% of the time. Early biopsy to detect the tumor allows for a higher chance of successful salvage (Olson & Wolf, 1995).

HOME CARE ISSUES

Active Treatment

As a result of impressive treatment advances coupled with shortened hospital stays, the patient with laryngeal cancer usually undergoes outpatient treatment with chemotherapy and irradiation. If the patient lives a great distance from the health care facility and is undergoing standard chemotherapy (cisplatin, 100 mg/m^2 day 1, and 5-FU, 1000 mg/m^2/day by continuous infusion for 5 days), the oncologist may use the support services of a home care agency nurse. Clinical areas that require the expertise of an oncology nurse in the home care setting are outlined in Box 51-6.

Patients who receive the standard chemotherapy regimen listed in the previous paragraph in the clinic setting will receive platinum along with hydration and an aggressive antiemetic regimen. Delayed nausea and vomiting are common and can occur for 48 hours after therapy. The goals of the home care nurse are to maintain the patient's hydration status and minimize the amount of nausea and vomiting associated with the chemotherapy regimen. The nurse should emphasize the importance of adhering to an around-the-clock antiemetic regimen and assess the patient for dehydration. A patient diary to record the intensity of symptoms and responses to treatment serves as a useful tool to facilitate communication between the patient and clinicians about nonwitnessed yet profoundly distressing problems for the patient.

Box 51-6
Home Care Nursing Issues for the Patient with Laryngeal Cancer Who Is Undergoing a Continuous Infusion of 5-FU and Platinum

1. Safely manage the continuous infusion of an antineoplastic agent by being able to:
   a. Competently manage a wide variety of vascular access devices
      (1) Able to draw blood from vascular access device for laboratory testing
      (2) Able to troubleshoot potentially occluded, pinched, leaking, infected, or slow infusing catheters
   b. Use safety precautions when handling chemotherapeutic agents and their containers
      (1) Instruct in safe handling of emesis, oral secretions, chemotherapy (containers and tubing), and linens if there is a cytotoxic spill
2. Expertly assess and monitor the patient for signs and symptoms of chemotherapy toxicity, including but not limited to:
   a. Delayed nausea and vomiting (increased potential 48 hours after platinum)
   b. Infection and fever (know when the chemotherapeutic nadir will occur)
   c. Mucositis, diarrhea, and dehydration
3. Instruct the patient on self-care measures, including adherence to postplatinum antiemetic regimen, oral hygiene, pain management, increased fluid intake, high protein/calorie intake, pulmonary health, and signs and symptoms of potential infection.
4. Monitor the patient's planned treatment schedule and visit during the 5-FU infusion period and at the time of discontinuance. Telephone follow-up should be planned for symptom assessment during the time of patient nadir.

5-FU, 5-fluorouracil

Palliative Care and Hospice

It is possible to manage patients with stage IV laryngeal cancer at home with the support of a competent caregiver and an expert home hospice staff. SCC of the head and neck does respond to single-agent chemotherapy for a few months (see Table 51-11). Even though a hospice patient has end-stage disease, use of chemotherapy can be an effective palliative therapy. It is the role of the hospice nurse to constantly evaluate the patient's response to therapy from *the patient's* quality of life standpoint. Patients who tolerate single-agent therapy with minimal side effects experience a much more positive outcome than patients who experience severe, debilitating mucositis while receiving "palliative" treatment. On the other hand, if the fear, pain, and suffering that stem from a slowly closing airway can be minimized by chemotherapy and the side effects kept to a minimum, the patient outcome is much more favorable.

In the home, untreated aspiration pneumonia is a common cause of death. Management strategies to maintain comfort in the patient with pneumonia includes antipyretics, as well as medications to minimize oral and bronchial secretions, pain, and tachypnea.

If patients are suffering from locally metastatic disease of the larynx, they are at risk for airway obstruction and carotid erosion and bleeding. The nursing care of the hospice patient who has the potential for an external carotid bleed presents a unique set of challenges. The caregiver(s) must be told of the potential for a bleed and be given simple, clear, and concise instructions. Given the inherent stress of this situation, the instructions provided in Table 51-13 were designed with ease of readability and understanding in mind. The computed Flesch-Kincaid grade level for the instructions in Table 51-13 is grade school level 3 (Cooley, Moriarty, Berger, Selm-Orr, Coyle, & Short, 1995). The teaching document may be used by the hospice team with the family caregivers to help guide their actions in the event that this traumatic experience occurs before the patient's death.

When managing the patient with a potential for a carotid bleed, one of the goals of the hospice nurse is to clearly communicate the possibility of the bleed without causing overdue alarm. The nurse can review items on the list provided in Table 51-13 while reminding the caregivers that they cannot harm the patient in any way. The nurse needs to reassure the caregiver that, although the immediate care is visually and emotionally frightening, the patient becomes

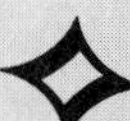

Table 51-13 Patient Preparation for a Hospice Patient with a Carotid Bleed

Procedural Considerations:

1. Call the 24-hour hospice number: ________ if you begin to notice blood oozing or leaking from the neck and wound area. If there is a bandage on the neck, do not take it away.
2. Get a stack (four to six) of dark hand towels and keep them within reach of the bed or chair where the patient spends most of his or her time. If you use these towels, you will throw them away.
3. If the bleeding begins, gently place the towels on the neck, two at a time. Call the 24-hour hospice number: ________ if you have not already done so. The nurse will be there as soon as possible.
4. If you wish, call a friend who can come over to be with you. Make sure you have asked that person ahead of time and that they know what might be happening. That person is ________ Phone # ________.
5. The patient will become unconscious very quickly. If you can, raise the head and shoulders up on a few pillows. The patient does not know what you are doing, and he or she is not suffering.
6. Talk to the nurse about other things that might happen and what you will do about them. You may want to make a few notes on the other side of this page.
7. DO NOT CALL 911. Make sure you can find the Do Not Resuscitate papers at your home if someone does call 911 by mistake.

NOTE: Flesch-Kincaid Index: Grade School Level 3. The index computes readability based on the average number of syllables per word and the average number of words per sentence. From Cooley, M. E., Moriarty, H., Berger, M. S., Selm-Orr, D., Colye, B., & Short, T. (1995). Patient literacy and the readability of written cancer education materials. *Oncology Nursing Forum, 22*(9), 1345-1351

unconscious very rapidly and is not suffering. Because of the trauma and insult witnessed by the caregiver at the end of the patient's life, the caregiver may be at risk for bereavement complications, and the hospice team should support the caregiver accordingly.

A frequent sign of an impending external bleed is the oozing and trickling of blood at a previously dry area within the carotid region. Consequently, the caregiver is instructed to call the hospice nurse when he or she notices this problem. If dressings are used in the carotid area, they should be moist-to-moist saline dressings or moist gauze and sterile petroleum gel dressings. These types of dressings will prevent the unwanted removal of tissue. A stack of four to six dark towels can be used to soak up the blood. The contrasting sight of bright red blood against a white towel is quite distressing and can create unwanted anxiety and panic. The hospice nurse should rehearse with the caregivers the steps listed on the instruction sheet and fill in all of the appropriate names and phone numbers. The "No Code" order should be documented per hospice protocol, and the necessary legal paperwork should be available in the patient's home.

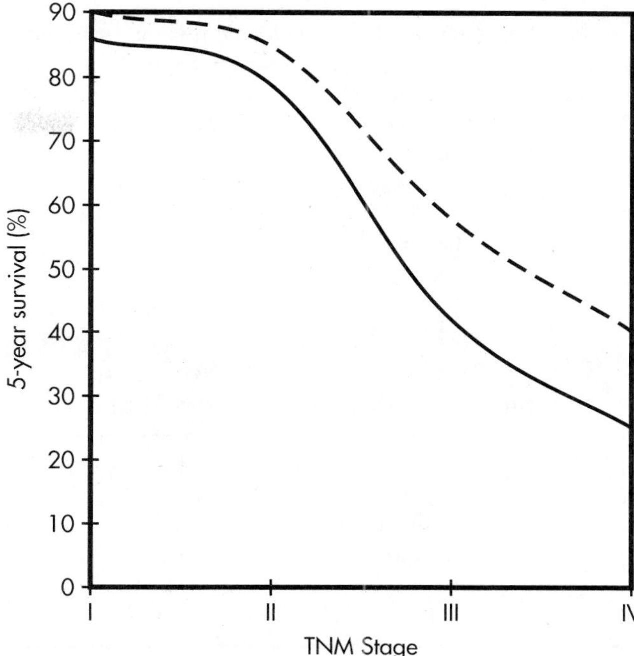

Fig. 51-6 Graphic representation of the similarity in 5-year survival for surgery *(top)* and radiation therapy *(bottom)* in squamous cell carcinomas of the head and neck and the diminishing efficacy of both treatments in advanced stage disease. (From Shah, J. & Lydiatt, W. [1995]. Treatment of cancer of the head and neck. *CA: A Cancer Journal for Clinicians, 45*[6], 352-368.)

Remind the caregiver not to activate the EMS system (do not call 911).

An expert home hospice team is skilled in the area of symptom management and becomes an invaluable asset in the care of the patient. The nurse caring for a patient with laryngeal cancer may deal with some or all of the following symptoms: pain, respiratory distress, aspiration pneumonia, mucositis, excessive mucus secretion, poor mucus drainage, severe facial edema, local wound infection, anxiety, and extreme distress.

PROGNOSIS

Patient prognosis is directly linked to the TNM stage at the time of diagnosis and to timely intervention (Fig. 51-6). Other major factors that influence prognosis include the development of a synchronous primary and the continued use of alcohol and tobacco. Recall that the relative risk for developing multiple primary cancers is 3.9 times greater in patients with laryngeal cancer who consume 40 or more cigarettes and 3 or more whiskey equivalents per day (Mashberg & Samit, 1995).

Prognosis cannot be discussed with the patient in an isolated manner. His or her current and future lifestyle habits must be taken into consideration. This discussion provides an excellent opportunity for the nurse to educate the patient on the damaging effects of continued tobacco use. Smoking cessation then becomes a cancer "treatment" that the patient can self-administer.

EVALUATION OF THE QUALITY OF CARE

A thorough discussion of the systematic review, evaluation, and measurement of clinical practice is beyond the scope of this chapter. In general, patient care standards and guidelines are the framework used to develop a quality assurance monitoring tool. The nurse chooses a high-frequency event requiring observation or a high incidence problem that demands evaluation and attention. With the focus on patient outcomes, the process involves using a monitoring tool to systematically collect data on specific aspects of the patient's care. The nurse is then able to analyze the data, draw conclusions, make recommendations, and develop an action plan. Ideally, any changes made in clinical practice will result in improved care (Miaskowski & Donovan, 1992).

An example of quality-of-care evaluation tools for the monitoring of patient education and symptom management activities for patients with laryngeal cancer can be found in Tables 51-14 and 51-15, respectively.

TABLE 51-14 Quality of Care Evaluation for a Patient with Laryngeal Cancer Who Is Undergoing Radiation Therapy

Disciplines participating in the quality of care evaluation:
☐ Nursing ☐ Radiation Therapy ☐ Radiation Oncology
☐ Nutritional Therapy ☐ Social Services

I. Pretreatment Symptom Prevention and Management
Data from:
☐ Medical Record Review ☐ Patient/Family Interview

Criteria	Yes	No
1. Patient/family provided with verbal and written information about:		
a. Dental hygiene	☐	☐
b. Mucositis prevention and management	☐	☐
c. Xerostomia management	☐	☐
d. Weight loss management	☐	☐
e. Smoking cessation N/A ____	☐	☐
2. Patient scheduled for pretreatment dental evaluation	☐	☐
3. Patient scheduled for pretreatment nutritional evaluation	☐	☐
4. Patient scheduled for pretreatment social services evaluation	☐	☐

II. Patient/Family Satisfaction
Data from:
☐ Patient Interview ☐ Family Interview

Criteria	Yes	No
1. On a scale of 0 to 10, with 0 being totally dissatisfied and 10 being totally satisfied, how satisfied were you with the *verbal* education you received about symptoms you may have? ____	☐	☐
2. On a scale of 0 to 10, with 0 being totally dissatisfied and 10 being totally satisfied, how satisfied were you with the *written* education you received about symptoms you may have? ____	☐	☐
3. If you were interested in knowing, were you told about the smoking cessation programs available to you and your family? N/A ____	☐	☐

RESEARCH ISSUES

With the exception of the Department of Veterans Affairs study (1991), little recent research exists that directly impacts the current course of treatment for patients with laryngeal cancer. Surgery, radiation therapy, and chemotherapy remain the three main treatments. Fig. 51-6 illustrates that the survival rates for patients treated with surgery versus radiation therapy remain in close enough proximity to ask the following question: "What is the patient's perceived quality of life while undergoing surgery as compared to radiation therapy?" The asking and answering of questions such as this perhaps will guide the treatment team in their preferences and recommendations.

TABLE 51-15 Quality Of Care Evaluation for the Patient with Laryngeal Cancer and Mucositis and/or Xerostomia

Disciplines participating in the quality of care evaluation:
☐ Nursing ☐ Radiation Therapy
☐ Radiation Oncology ☐ Nutritional Therapy

I. Symptom Management
Data from: ☐ Medical Record Review
☐ Patient/Family Interview

Criteria	Yes	No
1. Patient/family states they were provided with verbal and written information about ways to prevent and manage mucositis.	☐	☐
2. Patient/family states they were provided with verbal and written information about ways to manage xerostomia.	☐	☐
3. Documentation of the following exists:		
a. Oral assessment three times per week	☐	☐
b. Oral pain assessment three times per week	☐	☐
c. Patient Instructed on oral care regimen	☐	☐
d. Patient able to provide a return demonstration on oral care	☐	☐
e. Patient provided with necessary prescriptions and/or supplies	☐	☐

REFERENCES

American Cancer Society. (1996). *Cancer facts and figures—1996.* Atlanta: The Society.

Bal, D. G., Lloyd, J. C., & Manley, M. W. (1995). The role of the primary care physician in tobacco use prevention and cessation. *CA: A Cancer Journal for Clinicians, 45*(6), 369-374.

Cooley, M. E., Moriarty, H., Berger, M. S., Selm-Orr, D., Coyle, B., & Short, T. (1995). Patient literacy and the readability of written cancer education materials. *Oncology Nursing Forum, 22*(9), 1345-1351.

Department of Veterans Affairs Laryngeal Cancer Study Group. (1991). Induction chemotherapy plus radiation compared with surgery plus radiation in patients with advanced laryngeal cancer. *The New England Journal of Medicine, 324*(24), 1685-1690.

Dimery, I. W. & Hong, W. K. (1993). Overview of combined modality therapies for head and neck cancer. *Journal of the National Cancer Institute, 85*(2), 95-106.

Eisbruch, A., Thornton, A. F., Urba, S., Esclamado, R. M. , Carroll, W. R., & Bradford, C. R. (1996). Chemotherapy followed by accelerated fractionated radiation for larynx preservation in patients with advanced laryngeal cancer. *Journal of Clinical Oncology, 14,* 2322-2330.

Ernster, V. L. & Cummings, S. R. (1991). Smoking and cancer. In A. Holleb, D. Fink, & G. Murphy (Eds.), *American Cancer Society textbook of clinical oncology.* Atlanta: American Cancer Society, Inc.

Fein, D. A., Lee, W. R., & Hanlon, A. L. (1995). Pretreatment hemoglobin level influences local control and survival of T1-T2 squamous cell carcinomas of the glottic larynx. *Journal of Clinical Oncology, 13*(8), 2077-2083.

Gluckman, J. L., Crissman, J. D., & Donegan, J. O. (1980). Multicentric squamous cell carcinoma of the upper aerodigestive tract. *Head and Neck Surgery, 3,* 90-96.

Goodman, M. (1990). Head and neck cancer. In S. L. Groenwald, M. H. Frogge, M. Goodman, & C. H. Yarbro (Eds.), *Cancer nursing: Principles and practice* (2nd ed.). Boston: Jones and Bartlett.

Hoffman, H. & Karnell, L. (1996). Laryngeal cancer. In G. D. Steele, J. D. Jessup, D. P. Winchester, H. R. Menck, & G. P. Murphy (Eds.), *National cancer data base: Annual review of patient care 1995.* Atlanta: American Cancer Society.

Hong, W. K., Endicott, J., Itri, L. M., Doos, W., Batsakis, J. G., Bell, R., Fofonoff, S., Byers, R., Atkinson, E. N., & Vaughn, C. (1986). 13-*cis*-Retinoic acid in the treatment of oral leukoplakia. *New England Journal of Medicine, 315,* 1501-1505.

Hong, W. K., Lippman, S. M., & Itri, L. M. (1990). Prevention of second primary tumors with isotretinoin in squamous-cell carcinoma of the head and neck. *New England Journal of Medicine, 323,* 795-801.

Iwamoto, R. (1992). Altered nutrition. In D. Dow & L. J. Hilderley (Eds.), *Nursing care in radiation oncology.* Philadelphia: W. B. Saunders.

Jacobs, C. & Pinto, H. (1995). Adjuvant and neoadjuvant treatment of head and neck cancer: The next chapter. *Seminars in Oncology, 22*(6), 540-552.

Johnson, J. (1994). Larynx. In J. Gluckman, P. Gullane, & J. Johnson (Eds.), *Practical approach to head and neck tumors.* New York: Raven Press.

Johnson, J. T., Ferretti, G. A., & Nethery, W.J. (1993). Oral pilocarpine for post-irradiation xerostomia in patients with head and neck cancer. *New England Journal of Medicine, 329,* 390-395.

Landis, S. H., Murray, T., Bolden, S., & Wingo, P.A. (1998). Cancer statistics, 1998. *CA: A Cancer Journal for Clinicians, 48,* 6-29.

Lippman, S. M., Clayman, G. L., Huber, M. H., Benner, S. E., & Hong, W. K. (1995). Biology and reversal of aerodigestive tract carcinogenesis. In W. K. Hong & R. S. Weber (Eds.), *Head and neck cancer: Basic and clinical aspects.* Boston: Kluwer Academic Publishers.

Manne, D. (1996). Down in the mouth: Oral complications experienced by patients with head and neck cancer. *Oncology Nursing Society Special Interest Group Newsletter: Radiation,7*(3), 3.

Mashberg, A. & Samit, A. (1995). Early diagnosis of asymptomatic oral and oropharyngeal squamous cancers. *CA: A Cancer Journal for Clinicians, 45,* 328-351.

Miaskowski, C. & Donovan, M. (1992). Implementation of the American Pain Society Quality Assurance Standards for Relief of Acute Pain and Cancer Pain in Oncology Nursing Practice. *Oncology Nursing Forum, 19*(3), 411-415.

Million, R. (1994). Natural history of squamous cell carcinoma. In R. Million & N. Cassisi (Eds.), *Management of head and neck cancer: A multidisciplinary approach.* Philadelphia: J. B. Lippincott.

Million, R. & Cassisi, N. (1994). General principles for treatment of cancers of the head and neck: The primary site. In R. Million & N. Cassisi (Eds.), *Management of head and neck cancer: A multidisciplinary approach.* Philadelphia: J. B. Lippincott.

Million, R., Cassisi, N., & Mancuso, A. (1994). Larynx. In R. Million & N. Cassisi (Eds.), *Management of head and neck cancer: A multidisciplinary approach.* Philadelphia: J. B. Lippincott.

National Cancer Institute (1994). The health professional's responsibility in smoking cessation: Strategies for office and community. In J. W. Richards, T. P. Houston, & A. Blum (Eds.), *Smoking and tobacco control: tobacco and the clinician: interventions for medical and dental practice 5.* NCI-NIH Publication No. 94-3693. Bethesda, Md.

Norris, C. M. & Cady, B. (1991). Head, neck, and thyroid cancer. In A. Holleb, D. Fink, & G. Murphy (Eds.), *American Cancer Society textbook of clinical oncology.* Atlanta: American Cancer Society, Inc.

Olson, T. & Wolf, G. T. (1995). Cancer of the larynx. In M. C. Brain & P. P. Carbone (Eds.), *Current therapy in hematology/oncology* (5th ed.). St. Louis: Mosby.

O'Sullivan, B., Mackillop, W., Gilbert, R., Gaze, M., Lundgren, J., Atkinson, C., Wynne, C., & Fu, H. (1994). Controversies in the management of laryngeal cancer: Results of an international survey of patterns of care. *Radiotherapy and Oncology, 31*(1), 23-32.

Parker, R. G. & Enstrom, J. E. (1998). Second primary cancers of the head and neck following treatment of initial primary head and neck cancers. *International Journal of Radiation Oncology, Biology, Physics, 14,* 561-564.

Pinto, H. A. & Jacobs, C. (1995a). Combined modality therapy and chemotherapy. In M. C. Brain & P. P. Carbone (Eds.), *Current therapy in hematology/oncology* (5th ed.). St. Louis: Mosby.

Pinto, H. A. & Jacobs, C. (1995b). Head and neck cancer, basic and clinical aspects. In W. K. Hong & R. S. Weber (Eds.), *Head and neck cancer: Basic and clinical aspects.* Boston: Kluwer Academic Publishers.

Rooney, M., Kish, J., Jacobs, J., Kinzie, J., Weaver, A., Cressman, J., & Al-Sarraf, M. (1985). Improved complete response rate and survival in advanced head and neck cancer after three-course neoadjuvant chemotherapy with 120-hour 5-FU infusion and cisplatin. *Cancer, 55,* 1123-1128.

Shah, J. & Lydiatt, W. (1995). Treatment of cancer of the head and neck. *CA: A Cancer Journal for Clinicians, 45*(6), 352-368.

Spitz, M. R. (1994). Epidemiology and risk factors for head and neck cancer. *Seminars in Oncology, 21,* 281-288.

Templeton, D. J. & Weinberg, R. A., (1991). Principles of cancer biology. In A. Holleb, D. Fink, & G. Murphy (Eds.), *American Cancer Society textbook of clinical oncology.* Atlanta: American Cancer Society, Inc.

Vines, G. (1988). Interaction of alcohol and tobacco in laryngeal cancer. *American Journal of Epidemiology, 115,* 380-388.

Vokes, E. E., Weichselbaum, R. R., Lippman, S. M., & Hong, W. K. (1993). Head and neck cancer. *New England Journal of Medicine, 328,* 184-193.

Weber, R. S., & Callender, D. L. (1992). Laryngeal conservation surgery. *Seminars in Radiation Oncology, 2,* 149-157.

Weeks, J. & Pfister, D. G. (1996). Outcomes research studies. *Oncology, 10*(Suppl. 11), 29-34.

Wolf, G., Hong, W., & Fisher, S. (1993). Larynx preservation with induction chemotherapy and radiation (XRT) in advanced laryngeal cancer: Final results of the VA laryngeal cancer study group cooperative trial. *Proceedings of the American Society of Clinical Oncology, 12,* 277-281.

Zagars, G., Norante, J., Smith, J. L., & McDonald, S. (1993). Tumors of the head and neck. In P. Rubin (Ed.), *Clinical oncology for medical students and physicians: A multidisciplinary approach, 7.* Philadelphia: W. B. Saunders.

Nasopharyngeal Cancer

Gayle H. Shiba, RN, PhD, OCN

EPIDEMIOLOGY

Head and neck cancers represent about 5% of all cancers in the United States. Cancer of the nasopharynx is one of many cancers that occur in the head and neck region. The distribution of head and neck cancer is shown in Table 52-1. Nasopharyngeal cancer occurs less often in the United States; however, there is a high incidence of nasopharyngeal carcinoma among people living in parts of southern China and immigrants to the United States from these regions. Because of the anatomy of the nasopharynx, tumors arising in this area are frequently large and have spread beyond the nasopharynx before symptoms from the tumor occur. Therefore patients at the time of diagnosis frequently have advanced disease. The management of nasopharyngeal carcinoma provides significant challenges to health care professionals because of the location of the nasopharyngeal tumor and the significant treatment morbidity that affects the patient's physical and emotional well-being.

In the United States, nasopharyngeal cancer accounts for approximately 2% of all squamous cell carcinomas occurring in the head and neck region, or approximately 0.5 to 2 cases per 100,000 people (Clayman, Lippman, Laramore, & Hong, 1997). Nasopharyngeal carcinoma is uncommon in North America and Europe. However, the incidence of nasopharyngeal carcinoma in southern China has been reported to be between 12 to 15/100,000 per year (Lo, Mok, Huang, Liu, Choi, & Lee et al., 1992) and 25 to 50/100,000 per year (Fandi, Altun, Azli, Armand & Cvitkovic, 1994). This difference may be partially explained by genetic, environmental, and viral factors that may contribute to the development of nasopharyngeal carcinoma. The age-adjusted incidence for nasopharyngeal carcinoma by race or ethnicity in the United States indicates elevated rates in the Chinese population, intermediate rates among Filipinos, and low rates among African Americans, Hispanics, and Japanese (Muir, Waterhouse, & Mack, 1987).

A high risk of nasopharyngeal carcinoma is maintained among first-generation Chinese immigrants to countries, including the United States, and an elevated risk is reported in subsequent generations compared with the general population (Collins, Dougherty, Stupp, Weichselbaum, & Vokes, 1995). The risk for nasopharyngeal carcinoma among Chinese-American males is six times higher than that for other ethnic groups (Levine, McKay, & Connelly, 1987).

The incidence of nasopharyngeal carcinoma in the United States has remained relatively unchanged over the years. Nasopharyngeal carcinoma has a tendency toward early regional and distant spread (Clayman et al., 1997). Therefore most cases of nasopharyngeal carcinoma are advanced at the time of diagnosis and have spread beyond the region of the nasopharynx. In spite of advanced disease at the time of diagnosis, improved treatment techniques and the use of combined treatment modalities have been quite successful in treating nasopharyngeal carcinoma.

RISK FACTORS

A number of factors may be associated with increased risk for nasopharyngeal carcinoma (Box 52-1). Awareness of these factors is important when evaluating patients who are suspected of having nasopharyngeal cancer because symptoms suggestive of nasopharyngeal carcinoma are often vague and easily attributed to other problems.

Age

Carcinomas of the nasopharynx occur in a younger age group than other head and neck cancers, with up to 20% of patients being under the age of 30 (Cassisi, 1987; Fandi & Cvitkovic, 1995). Peak incidence occurs between ages 40 and 50, with a bimodal age distribution occurring at 10 to 24 and 40 to 60 years of age. This incidence by age varies between Chinese and non-Chinese people, with the incidence in non-Chinese populations being highest at 40 to 50 years of age, and in Chinese populations being highest at 20 to 30 years of age. However, nasopharyngeal carcinoma can occur at almost any age (Ayan & Altun, 1996; Fandi & Cvitkovic, 1995). In children, nasopharyngeal carcinoma accounts for less than 1% of all childhood malignancies.

TABLE 52-1 Distribution of Head and Neck Cancers

Site	Percentage (%)
Larynx	25
Tongue	13
Lips	11
Oropharynx	10
Floor of mouth	7
Salivary	7
Hypopharynx	5
Nasopharynx	4
Nose and sinus	4
Buccal	4
Gingiva	4
Other	3-5

Modified from McQuarrie, D. G. (1992). Head and neck cancer: An overview for the perioperative nurse. *AORN, 56,* 79-97. 1992.

Gender

As with other head and neck cancers, nasopharyngeal carcinoma occurs more frequently in men than women. Nasopharyngeal carcinoma occurs two to three and a half times more frequently in men than in women in all populations (Collins et al., 1995; Fandi & Cvitkovic, 1995). The male-to-female ratio in the Chinese population is 3:1, whereas in non-Chinese populations the ratio is 2:1.

Ethnicity

Nasopharyngeal carcinoma is rare in the United States and Europe. However, the incidence of nasopharyngeal carcinoma is high in southern China (between 12 to 50/100,000), and the incidence remains high for descendants of immigrants from that region (Fandi & Cvitkovic, 1995; Lo et al., 1992). In the United States, Chinese-American males have a six-fold increased risk of developing nasopharyngeal carcinoma compared with other ethnic groups. There is a higher incidence of nasopharyngeal carcinoma, World Health Organization (WHO) classification type 2 or 3, among Chinese Americans as opposed to a higher incidence of WHO type 1 nasopharyngeal carcinoma among non–Chinese Americans.

Genetic Predisposition

There may be a genetic predisposition for the development of nasopharyngeal carcinoma. The increased risk of nasopharyngeal carcinoma in genetically distinct subgroups of Chinese origin lends support to this belief and suggests that genetic susceptibility is necessary for the development of nasopharyngeal carcinoma. In addition, there is an increased incidence of nasopharyngeal carcinoma in people who have a family member with a history of nasopharyngeal carcinoma. A correlation between certain human lymphocyte antigens (HLAs), which are genetically determined, and the occurrence of nasopharyngeal carcinoma also supports this view. HLA-A2 and HLA-BSin2 have been associated with an increased incidence of nasopharyngeal carcinoma. The HLA types AW19, BW46, and B17 are associated with increased risk. A2-BW46 antigens are associated with a two-fold increased risk for nasopharyngeal carcinoma in southern China, whereas the BW46 antigen is uncommon in Caucasian Americans or Europeans (Collins et al., 1995). However, the high-risk HLA pattern is not present in all patients with nasopharyngeal carcinoma and has been found in some individuals without nasopharyngeal carcinoma.

Box 52-1
Risk Factors for Nasopharyngeal Cancer

Age
Gender
Ethnicity/geographic
Genetic predisposition
Epstein-Barr virus
Dietary habits
Tobacco and alcohol

Epstein-Barr Virus

There is evidence that the Epstein-Barr virus (EBV) is an etiologic agent for nasopharyngeal carcinoma. A relationship between the EBV and nasopharyngeal carcinoma has been shown. However, this relationship appears to occur almost exclusively with the less differentiated and undifferentiated form of nasopharyngeal carcinoma (i.e., WHO, types 2 and 3) and to a lesser degree with the squamous cell carcinoma form of nasopharyngeal carcinoma (i.e., WHO, type 1). A greater than 90% correlation in endemic areas and proof of incorporation of EBV antigens into nasopharyngeal carcinoma tumors provided the evidence to support the strong association between the EBV and the undifferentiated form of nasopharyngeal carcinoma (Collins et al., 1995).

Epstein-Barr virus infections are common in China, with almost all children under the age of 5 years having been infected by the virus. Antibody titers to EBV antigens are elevated in patients with nasopharyngeal carcinoma, regardless of geographic or ethnic origin. The association of the EBV with nasopharyngeal carcinoma has been studied, and high IgA antibody levels to EBV viral capsid antigen (VCA) and early antigen (diffuse) have provided a screening tool for the detection of nasopharyngeal carcinoma in high-risk populations (Fee, 1993).

Diet

Dietary habits may be linked to the development of nasopharyngeal carcinoma. People living in regions where nasopharyngeal carcinoma is prevalent have diets characterized by the cooking and eating of salt-cured and dried foods, especially fish and meats. The cooking of such foods releases nitrosamines. Nitrosamines are suspected of having a role in the development of nasopharyngeal carcinoma when they are inhaled and distributed over the nasopharyngeal mucosa (Schantz, Harrison, & Hong, 1993). Zheng and associates (1994), studying people from southern China, reported that consumption of salted fish and herbal tea, and the early exposure to wood fires, were significantly related to the undifferentiated form of nasopharyngeal carcinoma. Lee, Gourley, Duffy, Esteve, Lee, & Day (1994) also reported an increased risk of nasopharyngeal carcinoma in Chinese adults whose diet consisted of frequent amounts of salted foods. However, in a study of patients with nasopharyngeal carcinoma in the Philippines, no correlation was found between the intake of salted foods (primarily fish) and the development of nasopharyngeal carcinoma (West, Hildesheim, & Dosemeci, 1993). The authors stated that these results may indicate an interaction between environmental and other factors in the development of nasopharyngeal carcinoma.

Tobacco and Alcohol

The more differentiated squamous cell form of nasopharyngeal carcinoma (i.e., WHO type 1) has been associated with the patient's use of tobacco and alcohol products (Fandi & Cvitkovic, 1995; Nam, McLaughlin, & Blot, 1992). Chow, McLaughlin, Hrubec, Nam, & Blot (1993) found a positive correlation between cigarette smoking and the development of nasopharyngeal carcinoma when they studied United States veterans. However, the development of nasopharyngeal carcinoma in high-risk populations (i.e., WHO type 2 or 3) does not appear to be associated with the patient's use of tobacco or alcohol products.

Summary

Most of the risk factors associated with the development of nasopharyngeal cancer (i.e., age, gender, ethnicity, genetic predisposition, EBV exposure) cannot be modified, and the modification of other factors may have varied effects on nasopharyngeal carcinoma development in high-risk populations. In the United States, there is no routine screening test for nasopharyngeal carcinoma. Eliminating smoking tobacco and drinking alcoholic beverages may reduce the risk of nasopharyngeal carcinoma for certain groups of people, and the reduction of salted and cured foods, especially among Chinese, may also decrease the risk. As modifiable risk factors are identified, oncology nurses will need to develop programs to address these factors. In addition, if people fall into the high-risk categories, they should be educated about the possible signs and symptoms associated with nasopharyngeal carcinoma. Because the symptoms of nasopharyngeal carcinoma tend to be vague and are not necessarily concerning, people may not seek medical attention in a timely fashion even if they know they are at greater risk for developing nasopharyngeal carcinoma.

PATHOPHYSIOLOGY

Normal Anatomy and Physiology of the Nasopharynx

The nasopharynx is an area of the pharynx that is cuboidal, lies behind the nasal cavity, and is posterior and superior to the soft palate (see Fig. 51-1). The dimensions of the nasopharynx are approximately 2.5 to 3.5 cm (anteroposterior diameter), 4.0 to 5.5 cm (at its widest transverse diameter), and 4 cm in height. The soft palate forms the inferior border of the nasopharynx, whereas the anterior border is located at the junction of the soft and hard palates. The lateral walls include the eustachian tube openings. Its roof is bordered by the base of the skull, extends continuously to the posterior pharyngeal wall, and continues inferiorly to the lower border of the second cervical vertebrae at the level of the uvula. The nasopharynx is continuous with the oropharynx, nasal cavity, and middle ear through the eustachian tubes. Ciliated columnar epithelium containing mucous and seromucous glands line the nasopharynx. The primary blood supply to the nasopharynx is from the ascending pharyngeal branch of the external carotid artery, the artery of the pterygoid canal, and the sphenopalatine artery.

The nasopharynx has a rich lymphatic supply. The lymphatic system drains into ipsilateral and contralateral nodes. The lymphatics from the nasopharynx follow three major pathways. One pathway is through the lateral pharyngeal wall, to the lateral pharyngeal nodes, and then to the retropharyngeal space and nodes. This nodal group is close in proximity to cranial nerves IX, X, XI, and XII. The next pathway is to the deep posterior cervical nodes and spinal accessory and jugular lymph node chains. The third pathway includes the jugulodigastric node. Because of the presence of this lymphatic plexus, a high incidence of neck metastases at the time of diagnosis is not uncommon.

The Process of Carcinogenesis

Epidemiologic studies have suggested a multifactoral etiology to the development of nasopharyngeal carcinoma involving infection by the EBV, environmental risk factors, and a genetic susceptibility (de The, 1987; Liebowitz, 1994; Pearson, 1993; Simons, Wee, Goh, Shanmugaratnam, Day, & de The, 1976). The genetic susceptibility involves the HLA-associated risk and potential suppressor genes located on chromosome 3, whereas the environmental risk factors include those discussed previously, such as dietary habits and chemical exposure.

Regardless of the level of endemic incidence, the association between EBV and nasopharyngeal carcinoma is specific and constant, indicating a causal relationship, even in low-incidence areas (de The, 1987). This association between the EBV and nasopharyngeal carcinoma is based on the high incidence of elevated EBV titers in patients with nasopharyngeal cancers. Pearson (1993) reported that patients with nasopharyngeal carcinoma were infected with EBV and had antibody titers to various EBV antigens that were higher than in control populations. These findings were seen regardless of the patient's geographic origin.

An HLA-associated risk for nasopharyngeal carcinoma has been shown for the southern Chinese (Simons et al., 1976). The joint occurrence of HLA-A2 and HLA-BSin2 resulted in relative risk of 2.35 for nasopharyngeal carcinoma compared with matched controls (Liebowitz, 1994), but the risk for nasopharyngeal carcinoma is only increased if both of the antigens are inherited on the same chromosome (Simons et al., 1976). The HLA-BSin2 antigen is rare in Caucasians but prevalent among Chinese. Increased risk for nasopharyngeal carcinoma is also associated with HLA types AW19, BW46, and B17, whereas HLA-A11 is associated with a decreased risk of developing nasopharyngeal carcinoma (Collins et al., 1995; Lu, Day, Degos, Lepage, Wang & Chan et al., 1990).

The evidence of the role of EBV in the development of nasopharyngeal carcinoma, and the EBV's possible relationship with the environmental and genetic factors associated with nasopharyngeal carcinoma, have provided a model for hypothesizing the development of nasopharyngeal carcinoma through a multistep process. However, little is known about the molecular events surrounding the development of nasopharyngeal carcinoma, and research continues to be focused in this area.

The EBV is a human herpesvirus that infects and establishes a persistent infection in individuals. During the acute infection, the EBV infects the epithelium of the oropharynx and the nasopharynx. The virus replicates in the epithelium and infects the B lymphocytes by a yet unknown process. Studies of EBV gene expression in infected B lymphocytes have identified six nuclear proteins (EBV nuclear antigens [EBNA-1 through -6]) and three membrane proteins (latent membrane proteins [LMP1-2-3]) that likely facilitate the EBV effects on cellular proliferation (Liebowitz, 1994). LMP1 has significant growth-stimulating effects when studied in vitro and is thought to have a similar effect on the epithelium of the nasopharynx. As these cells are stimulated to divide, the presence of EBNA-1 allows for the replication of the viral genome and its distribution to the new cells. To reach full malignant potential, the dividing nasopharyngeal cells may acquire the cellular genetic changes of the tumor suppressor genes on chromosome 3. It is believed that the risk for developing alterations in these genes may be increased by viral exposure as well as by exposure to environmental carcinogens (de The, 1987).

This model of carcinogenesis for nasopharyngeal carcinoma helps in the understanding of the possible interactions of the genetic, environmental, and viral factors involved in oncogenic cellular transformation in nasopharyngeal carcinoma. Future research will help to further elucidate the specific mechanisms involved in this process.

ROUTES OF METASTASES

Because of the location of the nasopharynx, nasopharyngeal carcinoma when diagnosed is often locally advanced or has already spread to the lymph nodes. Tumors confined to the nasopharynx and with no clinically involved lymph nodes account for less than 15% of all cases of nasopharyngeal carcinoma (Collins et al., 1995; Schantz, Harrison, & Hong, 1993).

Nasopharyngeal cancers usually arise from the superior wall or in the lateral posterior wall of the nasopharynx. The tumor may involve the mucosa or occur submucosally. The spread of nasopharyngeal carcinoma generally occurs early by invading adjacent tissues and structures and spreading along the lateral walls of the pharynx and pharyngeal muscles down to the oropharynx and tonsillar pillars or into the nasal cavity. Extension into the nasal cavity is common. Invasion of the retropharyngeal space has been shown by computed tomography (CT) scanning to occur in more than 80% of patients (Sham & Choy, 1991).

Nasopharyngeal cancers may spread laterally and superiorly and directly invade the base of the skull. Intracranial invasion may also occur (Sham & Choy, 1991; Teo, Leung, Yu, Lee, & Shiu, 1991). Tumors invading the base of skull can extend directly into the middle cranial fossa with involvement of cranial nerves III, IV, V, and VI. Based on radiographic studies, approximately 25% of the cases have spread into or through the base of the skull at the time of diagnosis (Neel, 1985).

Because lymph drainage for the nasopharyngeal region occurs primarily through the high upper cervical, jugulodigastric, and retropharyngeal lymph nodes, the initial spread of nasopharyngeal cancer occurs generally along these routes, spreading then to the internal jugular and spinal accessory or posterior cervical chain lymph nodes (Fig. 52-1). Inferior spinal accessory, lower cervical, and supraclavicular nodes are the next group of nodes in the drainage pattern that can become involved. Because lymphatic channels cross the midline, there may be contralateral or bilateral lymph node involvement. Patients with nasopharyngeal cancers rarely have clinically involved lymph nodes in the submaxillary, submandibular, or parotid regions, although parotid involvement may occur due to the lymphatic drainage patterns of the eustachian tube. About 70% to 90% of patients develop metastatic nodes during the course of their disease, and approximately 30% to 50% have bilateral nodal involvement (Collins et al., 1995; Clayman et al., 1997; Schantz, Harrison, & Hong, 1993).

Cranial nerves IX (glossopharyngeal), X (vagus), XI (spinal accessory), and XII (hypoglossal) are in close proximity to the superior retropharyngeal lymph nodes. Therefore any involvement of these nodes may affect these cranial nerves. If the nasopharyngeal tumor extends superiorly to the lateral wall of the cavernous sinus, cranial nerves III (oculomotor), IV (trochlear), and VI (abducens), as well as portions of the V (trigeminal), may be affected. Cranial nerve involvement of the lateral wall of the cavernous sinus or the base of the skull indicates more advanced disease (Perez, 1992; Clayman et al., 1997).

Distant spread of the nasopharyngeal carcinoma occurs more frequently than with other head and neck cancers, with metastases occurring most often to the bone, followed by the lung and liver. Although the presence of distant metastases at the time of diagnosis has been reported to occur in about 35% of all nasopharyngeal cancers, less than 3% of

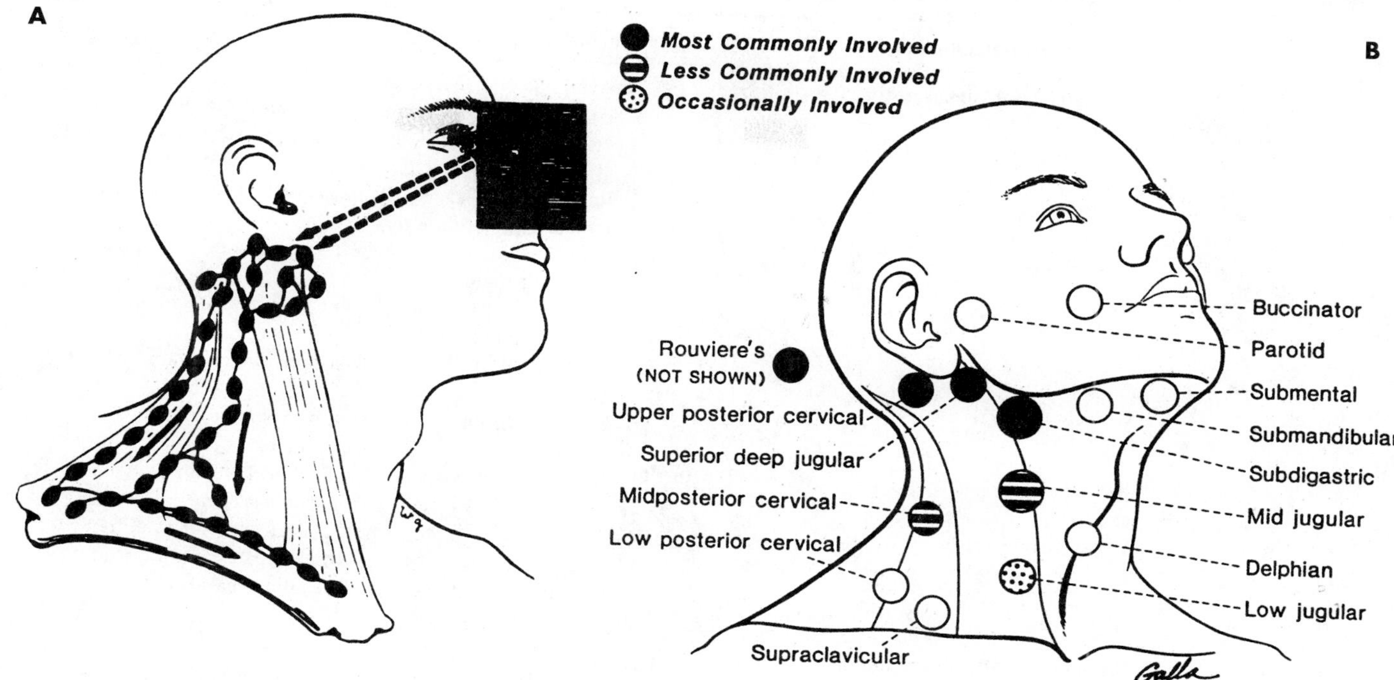

Fig. 52-1 **A,** Pathways for the lymphatic spread of carcinoma of the nasopharynx. (From Batsakis, J. G. [1979]. *Tumors of the head and neck* [2nd ed.]. Baltimore: Williams and Wilkins.) **B,** Important group of lymph nodes involved by nasopharyngeal cancer. (From Wang, C.C. [1997]. *Radiation therapy for head and neck neoplasms* [3rd ed.]. New York: Wiley-Liss.)

North American patients have clinical evidence of distant metastases at the time of diagnosis (Neel, 1985). The incidence of distant metastases is not related to the stage of the primary tumor but is highly correlated with the extent of cervical lymph node involvement. Distant metastases in 25% to 50% of patients with advanced cervical lymph node involvement have been reported (Bedwinek, Perez, & Keys, 1980; Hoppe, Goffinet, & Bagshaw, 1976; Perez, Devineni, Marcial-Vega, Marks, Simpson, & Kucik, 1992).

SCREENING

There are no routine screening indications or methods recommended for nasopharyngeal carcinoma. However, the anti-EBV serologic profile (high IgA antibody levels to EBV viral capsid antigen [VCA] and early antigen [diffuse]) has been used to screen and detect nasopharyngeal carcinoma in high-incidence/high-risk populations (Fandi & Cvitkovic, 1995; Fee, 1993). Although a highly positive anti-EBV serologic profile is not specific for nasopharyngeal carcinoma, it is indicative that the patient has been exposed to and has produced an antibody response to EBV, and this result is highly correlated with the development of nasopharyngeal carcinoma. Because the development of nasopharyngeal carcinoma is related to a number of factors discussed previously, the presence of a positive anti-EBV serologic profile alone does not mean that an individual has or will develop nasopharyngeal carcinoma. However, individuals with a positive anti-EBV serologic profile and who possess positive genetic and environmental factors related to the development of nasopharyngeal carcinoma would be considered at high risk for developing the disease and may be candidates for screening. In addition to the serologic studies, screening for this high-risk group should include a clinical head and neck examination and visualization of the nasopharynx (i.e., mirror examination, fiberoptic nasopharyngoscope) at prescribed intervals.

ASSESSMENT

The assessment of the patient for nasopharyngeal cancer is summarized in Table 52-2. Clinical evaluation of any patient with a possible nasopharyngeal cancer requires a detailed history, physical examination (especially of the head and neck region), visualization of the nasopharynx, and a number of diagnostic tests and studies.

History

The patient should be evaluated for the identified risk factors for nasopharyngeal carcinoma. A careful history of any head and neck symptoms should be obtained.

The presenting symptoms are often varied, vague, and nonspecific (Table 52-3). In more than 50% to 90% of cases, nasopharyngeal carcinoma presents as a painless mass or swelling in the neck (Cassisi, 1987; Schantz, Harrison, & Hong, 1993). Other presenting symptoms include nasal discharge, nasal stuffiness, obstruction with bloody drainage, or alterations in hearing associated with serous otitis media (Schantz, Harrison, & Hong, 1993; Fandi & Cvitkovic,

Table 52-2 Assessment of the Patient for Nasopharyngeal Cancer

	Assessment Parameters	Typical Abnormal Findings
History	A. Personal and social history:	A. Personal and social risk factors:
	1. Age	1. Peak incidence occurs between ages 40 to 50 years of age, with a bimodal age distribution at 10 to 24 years and 40 to 60 years of age.
	2. Gender	2. Ratios are 3:1 male to female in Chinese and 2:1 male to female in non-Chinese.
	3. Ethnicity	3. Higher incidence in southern Chinese and descendants from that region.
	4. Diet	4. Higher risk for those people consuming salted and salt-cured fish and meats.
	5. Family history	5. Positive family history of nasopharyngeal carcinoma increases risk.
	6. Epstein-Barr virus (EBV)	6. EBV infections associated with nasopharyngeal carcinoma.
	7. Tobacco and alcohol	7. Increased risk associated with World Health Organization (WHO) type 1 category of nasopharyngeal carcinoma.
	B. Evaluation for head and neck signs/ symptoms.	B. Common signs/symptoms noted: neck mass or swelling; blockage or feeling of fullness in the ear, ear pain, hearing loss (usually unilateral); nasal bleeding; nasal obstruction; nasal speech.
Physical Examination	A. Palpation of primary tumor	A. May feel fullness or bulging of soft palate. If tumor extends to tonsillar pillar or oropharynx, may feel mass or fullness.
	B. Evaluation of lymph nodes.	B. The most likely groups to be involved are the upper jugular, subdigastric, posterior cervical, and retropharyngeal lymph nodes. Nodes may have firm to hard consistency, have limited mobility, or be fixed; they may feel spherical, matted, or ill defined. Generally, nodes are not painful. Presence of nodes indicates metastatic disease.
	C. Inspection of nasopharynx, oral cavity, and oropharynx using mirror and fiberoptic nasopharyngoscope.	C. May visualize tumor as a mass in the nasopharynx; or if the tumor occurs in the submucosa, it may appear as a fullness. Tumor mass may extend to tonsillar pillar and to oropharynx.
	D. Testing of cranial nerves, especially III through VI and IX through XII.	D. Cranial nerves V (trigeminal) and VI (abducens) most frequently involved. Findings vary depending on cranial nerves involved (e.g., diplopia, eye muscle abnormalities, eye or orbital pain, difficulty swallowing, asymmetric tongue protrusion, hoarseness, paralysis of sternocleidomastoid and trapezius muscles).
	E. Inspection of tympanic membranes.	E. Bulging or retraction of tympanic membrane (unilateral). Serous otitis media (unilateral).
Diagnostic Studies	A. Computed tomography (CT) scan.	A. Often better for evaluating extent of neck disease.
	B. Magnetic resonance imaging (MRI) scan.	B. Used if a primary nasopharyngeal carcinoma is suspected but the tumor cannot be visualized by nasopharyngoscopy. In staging nasopharyngeal carcinoma, MRI is better for evaluating muscle, nerve, and intracranial extension. It is also preferred for diagnosis of locoregional recurrences.
	C. Chest x-ray.	C. Positive chest x-ray indicative of distant spread.
	D. Bone scan is done in patients with advanced locoregional disease or if laboratory studies or clinical findings (i.e., bone pain) suggest bone involvement.	D. At time of diagnosis, 3% of patients have distant metastases.
	E. Liver scan is done only if laboratory studies (liver function studies) or clinical findings (i.e., enlarged liver) suggest liver involvement.	E. Liver scan would be abnormal in patients with metastatic disease.
	F. Epstein-Barr virus (EBV)–specific serology: IgA and IgG antibody titers to viral capsule antigen (VCA) and diffused early antigen (EA[D]).	F. Elevated in greater than 75% to 80% of patients with WHO type 2 and 3 nasopharyngeal carcinoma histology.
	G. Liver function studies.	G. Elevated in patients with liver metastases.

TABLE 52-3 Most Frequently Occurring Signs and Symptoms of Nasopharyngeal Carcinoma

Sign/Symptom	Percentage (%)
Mass in the neck	60-80
Unilateral hearing loss or otitis media	40
Nasal obstruction, epistaxis, difficulty breathing, or nasal speech	30
Cranial nerve(s) involvement	15-30

1995). Patients may report problems with hearing or difficulty in equalizing pressure in the inner ear, which, if present, is usually unilateral and occurs as a result of obstruction of the eustachian tube. Nasal congestion or stuffiness, nasal drainage, and epistaxis may be present and result from local effects of the tumor. A report of a sore throat may be indicative of tumor extension into the oropharynx. Trismus and proptosis may also occur from muscle and cranial nerve invasion. The signs and symptoms the patient conveys at the time of diagnosis may vary considerably depending on the location of the tumor in the nasopharynx and the extent of the disease beyond the nasopharynx and into surrounding tissues and structures.

The presence of pain, its characteristics and severity, should be determined. Pain may be present as a result of compression of nerves or as a result of bone invasion. Facial pain and headaches (occipital and temporal) are the most common pain complaints. Pain associated with lifting the head and extending the neck may be present if tumor invasion of the prevertebral muscle has occurred.

Patients can present with metastatic disease in the neck but have no visible primary lesion in the nasopharynx. The presence of only a high jugular node mass or a posterior cervical node mass, with no overt signs of any other head and neck tumor, suggests an occult primary tumor in the nasopharynx (Rao & Levitt, 1986).

Physical Examination

The oral cavity should be examined thoroughly using visual inspection and palpation. The tongue and floor of the mouth should be palpated with a gloved finger, feeling for any abnormalities, swelling, or masses. Extension of a nasopharyngeal carcinoma to the tonsillar pillars or oropharynx may be seen directly and may be felt on palpation.

The use of a fiberoptic nasopharyngoscope allows for indirect examination of the nasopharynx. Tumors of the nasopharynx are often submucosal (appearing as fullness in the nasopharynx), are less frequently lobulated, and are rarely ulcerated (de The, 1987). Early lesions usually occur on the lateral wall or roof of the nasopharynx. The extent of the tumor outside the nasopharynx involving the tonsillar pillars and oropharynx, or the nasal cavity, may also be seen. Vocal cord mobility can also be assessed during this examination.

The cranial nerves (CNs) should be evaluated, especially those at greatest risk for involvement (i.e., III through VI and IX through XII). Assessment of extraocular movements evaluates the functioning of CN III through CN VI and may indicate disease involving the base of the skull. Cranial nerves V and VI are most commonly involved. An evaluation of CN IX and branches of CN X is done by examining the elevation of the palate, and CN XII can be checked by having the patient stick out his or her tongue and observing for any abnormalities or deviations. To check cranial components of the vagus nerve (X), vocal cord mobility must be evaluated. This evaluation can be done by using a laryngeal mirror or fiberoptic nasopharyngoscope to visualize the vocal cords.

Examination of the ears should be done with all patients, especially those reporting problems with hearing (often unilateral), obstructions, or pain in the ears. Abnormal findings may include bulging or retraction of the tympanic membrane or serous otitis media, both of which may be unilateral.

A thorough examination of the neck for the presence of neck masses or nodes should be conducted. All of the neck nodes, especially nodal groups at high risk for involvement, should be palpated. The presence of a mass or masses most likely indicates metastatic disease.

Diagnosis of Nasopharyngeal Cancer

A definitive diagnosis of nasopharyngeal carcinoma is established by a biopsy of the tumor in the nasopharynx. The use of a fiberoptic nasopharyngoscope for examination and biopsy is done usually under local anesthesia in the outpatient setting. The procedure is easy to perform and is well tolerated by the patient. However, biopsy of a submucosal mass or the necessity for multiple random biopsies of the nasopharynx may require that the patient be examined under general anesthesia.

Diagnostic/Pretreatment Studies

When a cancer of the nasopharynx is suspected but is not found on the outpatient examination, a CT scan or magnetic resonance imaging (MRI) scan should be performed to locate a mass before an examination under anesthesia and biopsy. If a mass is not found, but a neck node is present, tissue from the neck node can be obtained by fine-needle aspiration and subjected to a laboratory examination (polymerase chain reaction) to detect the presence of the viral genome of EBV associated with nasopharyngeal carcinoma (Feinmesser, Miyazaki, Cheung, Freeman, Noyek, & Dosch, 1992). Testing for EBV-specific serology may be a useful diagnostic tool in patients at high risk for nasopharyngeal carcinoma or those with symptomatology consistent with nasopharyngeal carcinoma but without an apparent nasopharyngeal mass. An elevated EBV-specific IgA antibody titer suggests a diagnosis of nasopharyngeal carcinoma, which can help guide the diagnostic workup.

Imaging Studies. Accurate staging of nasopharyngeal cancers requires imaging studies of the nasopharynx, nasal cavity, paranasal sinuses, base of the skull, and neck nodes. These studies are also necessary for treatment planning for nasopharyngeal cancers. CT and MRI are essential

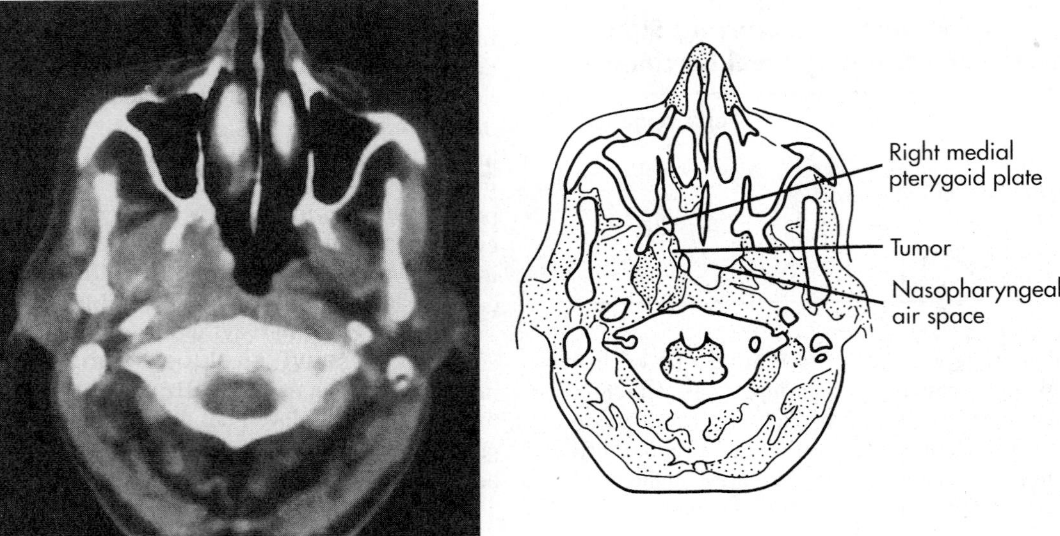

Fig. 52-2 Squamous cell carcinoma of nasopharynx. A 64-year-old woman presented with a resistant serous effusion of the right middle ear. An axial CT scan demonstrates a soft tissue mass in the right lateral aspect of the nasopharynx in the region of the fossa of Rosenmuller. The tumor infiltrates deeply and involves the eustachian tube. Note that the fascial planes have been destroyed by the advancing neoplasm (compare with normal left side). (From Skarin, A. T. [1996]. *Atlas of diagnostic oncology.* St. Louis: Mosby.)

in diagnosing and determining the extent of tumor involvement. Tumor extension to the parapharyngeal and retropharyngeal spaces, the oropharynx, and the orbits can be detected early using these techniques (Mendenhall, Million, Mancuso, & Stringer, 1994; van den Brekel, Castelijns, & Snow, 1994).

MRI has greater sensitivity than CT in detecting small lesions. It is superior to a CT scan in differentiating a tumor from inflammatory tissue, and in detecting muscle, nerve, or intracranial extension (Fandi & Cvitkovic, 1995). In addition, MRI is better than CT for diagnosing locoregional recurrences and evaluating lymphoid tissue. However, CT is often the imaging study of choice for evaluating the neck nodes when one is attempting to stage the extent of disease in the neck. Fig. 52-2 depicts a CT scan of a squamous cell cancer of the nasopharynx (van den Brekel, Castelijns, & Snow, 1994).

Chest X-Ray. Because nasopharyngeal cancer has a likelihood to metastasize early to distant sites, especially the lungs, a chest x-ray film is taken to determine whether there is spread to the lungs. A chest CT scan would be indicated with positive x-ray findings to determine the extent of involvement. Distant spread would be an indication for the use of chemotherapy as part of the treatment regimen.

Epstein-Barr Virus–Specific Serology. Immunoglobulin (Ig)A and IgG antibody titers to VCA and diffused early antigen (EA[D]) should be obtained in patients suspected of nasopharyngeal carcinoma and in patients already diagnosed with the disease. For patients with nasopharyngeal carcinoma, this test may be used as a marker for determining the response to treatment and recurrence of the disease (de Vathaire, Sancho-Garnier, de The, Pieddeloup, Schaab, & Ho et al., 1988).

Liver Function Studies and Liver Scan. Elevated liver function studies are indicative of possible liver metastases. Patients with elevated liver function tests should have a liver scan to determine whether there is tumor spread to the liver.

Bone Scan. A bone scan is recommended for patients with advanced locoregional disease or if there are any laboratory studies or clinical findings (i.e., bone pain) that suggest bone metastases. As stated previously, any distant metastases would be an indication for using chemotherapy as part of the treatment regimen.

Dental Examination. All patients who will be receiving radiation therapy as part of their treatment should have a pretreatment dental evaluation and begin dental prophylaxis. All necessary dental work (e.g., extractions, fillings) should be completed, if possible, prior to the initiation of radiation therapy treatments due to the increased risk for osteoradionecrosis after treatment.

STAGING

The staging of nasopharyngeal cancer involves the use of a histopathologic staging system (i.e., WHO typing system) as well as a clinical staging system. In the United States, Canada, and Europe, the clinical staging system used is the one developed by the American Joint Committee on Cancer (1992). In other parts of the world, particularly China, other staging systems have been developed and are used to stage nasopharyngeal carcinoma.

BOX 52-2
World Health Organization (WHO) Classification System for Nasopharyngeal Carcinoma

WHO type 1, keratinizing squamous cell carcinoma
WHO type 2, a nonkeratinizing carcinoma that includes transitional carcinoma
WHO type 3, undifferentiated carcinoma or lymphoepitheliomas

Histopathologic Staging

Histologic staging is determined by a pathologist examining a biopsy specimen(s) from the nasopharynx. The purpose of this type of staging is to determine the biologic characteristics of the tumor. The majority of malignant tumors of the nasopharynx arise from the epithelium, can be considered variants of squamous cell carcinoma, and include a variety of histologic cell types (Rao & Levitt, 1986). These range from well-differentiated keratinizing and nonkeratinizing squamous cell carcinomas to undifferentiated carcinomas, including lymphoepitheliomas. As shown in Box 52-2, the WHO introduced a three-item classification of nasopharyngeal carcinomas based on the degree of differentiation of the tumor (World Health Organization, 1978).

Mixed histologic patterns are commonly found. About 75% of nasopharyngeal carcinomas are type 1 or 2, or a combination of these two types. WHO type 1 accounts for one third to one half of all nasopharyngeal carcinomas in low-risk populations but accounts for less than 5% of nasopharyngeal carcinomas in high-risk populations (Fandi & Cvitkovic, 1995). The presence of keratin (WHO type 1) is associated with a poorer prognosis. The undifferentiated form of nasopharyngeal carcinoma is found more commonly among high-risk populations and younger patients (i.e., those less than 20 years old at the time of diagnosis).

The metastatic potential of nasopharyngeal carcinoma is governed by this classification system. WHO type 1 is more likely to spread locally than to distant sites, in contrast to WHO types 2 and 3. For WHO types 2 and 3, metastatic spread is reported in 80% to 90% of patients, compared with only 60% in patients with WHO type 1 tumors (Baker, 1980; Neel, 1985). WHO type 3 has a higher rate of advanced locoregional disease and the presence of distant metastasis at the time of diagnosis than the other WHO types (Ayan & Altun, 1996; Ingersoll, Wood, Donaldson, Giesler, Maor, & Goffinet et al., 1990; Pao, Hustu, Douglass, Beckford, & Kun, 1989).

Other cancers found in the nasopharynx are lymphomas (10%), salivary gland tumors, plasmacytomas, and adenocarcinomas. In children, rhabdomyosarcomas may occur in this region (Collins et al., 1995).

Clinical Staging. The clinical staging system used for nasopharyngeal cancer is the TNM system developed by the American Joint Committee on Cancer (1992). This system is used to determine the extent of disease and is shown in Table 52-4. Clinical staging is generally used in nasopharyn-

TABLE 52-4 TNM Staging System for Nasopharyngeal Cancer

Primary Tumor (T)			
TX	Primary tumor cannot be assessed		
T0	No evidence of primary tumor		
T1	Tumor limited to one subsite of nasopharynx		
T2	Tumor invades more than one subsite of nasopharynx		
T3	Tumor invades nasal cavity and/or oropharynx		
T4	Tumor invades skull and/or cranial nerve(s) (Subsites of nasopharynx are the superior wall, posterior wall, lateral wall, and anterior wall.)		
Lymph Node (N)			
NX	Regional lymph nodes cannot be assessed		
N0	No regional lymph node metastasis		
N1	Metastasis in a single ipsilateral lymph node, 3 cm or less in greatest diameter		
N2	Metastasis in a single ipsilateral lymph node, more than 3 cm but not more than 6 cm in greatest dimension; or in multiple ipsilateral lymph nodes, none more than 6 cm in greatest dimension; or in bilateral or contralateral lymph nodes, none more than 6 cm in greatest dimension		
N2a	Metastasis in a single ipsilateral lymph node, more than 3 cm but not more than 6 cm in greatest dimension		
N2b	Metastasis in multiple ipsilateral lymph nodes, none more than 6 cm in greatest dimension		
N2c	Metastasis in bilateral or contralateral lymph nodes, none more than 6 cm in greatest dimension		
N3	Metastasis in a lymph node, more than 6 cm in greatest dimension		
Distant Metastasis (M)			
MX	Presence of distant metastasis cannot be assessed		
M0	No distant metastasis		
M1	Distant metastasis		
Stage Grouping			
0	Tis	N0	M0
I	T1	N0	M0
II	T2	N0	M0
III	T3	N0	M0
	T1	N1	M0
	T2	N1	M0
	T3	N1	M0
IV	T4	N0	M0
	T4	N1	M0
	Any T	N2	M0
	Any T	N3	M0
	Any T	Any N	M1

From American Joint Committee on Cancer. (1992). *Pharynx (including base of tongue, soft palate, and uvula). Manual for staging of cancer* (4th ed.). Philadelphia: J. B. Lippincott.

geal cancers because this tumor is generally treated by nonsurgical means. Assessment is based primarily on inspection, examination, palpation, and imaging studies. Neurologic evaluation of cranial nerves is required.

MEDICAL MANAGEMENT

Medical management of nasopharyngeal carcinoma is primarily determined by the stage of the disease at the time of diagnosis (Fig. 52-3). Staging is based on AJCC criteria.

Surgery

In general, cancers of the head and neck region (especially squamous cell carcinomas) are aggressive, and treatment failures are usually due to locoregional recurrence. Treatment modalities that target locoregional disease, such as surgery or radiation therapy, or both, have been considered standard therapy. However, surgery is used infrequently to treat definitively nasopharyngeal carcinoma due to the location of the nasopharynx and the extent of disease at the time of diagnosis. The anatomic borders of the nasopharynx usually do not allow for adequate surgical resection with the adequate margins required for curative treatment. There is also considerable treatment morbidity associated with nasopharyngeal surgery. Therefore the treatment modality of choice for nasopharyngeal carcinoma is radiation therapy, using external beam radiation therapy alone or in combination with intracavitary brachytherapy. For the more advanced stages of disease, chemotherapy in addition to radiation therapy is recommended.

A radical or modified radical neck dissection may be used as part of the treatment plan for residual nodal disease. This procedure is recommended if the primary tumor is controlled (Wang, 1997).

External Beam Radiation Therapy

Because of the anatomic location and tendency for early bilateral lymph node metastases, radiation therapy is the pri-

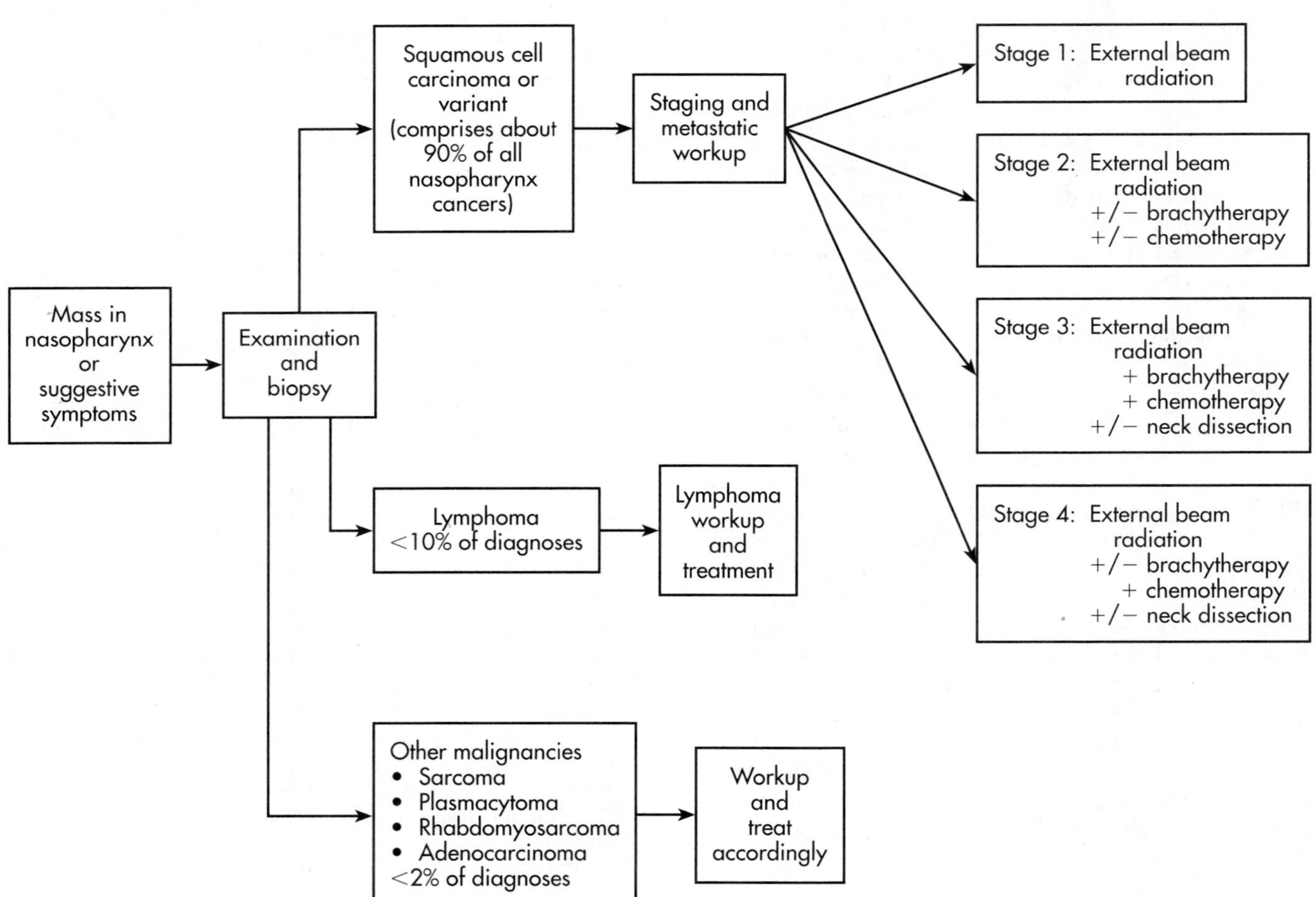

Fig. 52-3 Medical management for a patient with nasopharyngeal cancer. (Modified from Rao, Y. & Levitt, S. [1986]. Nasopharyngeal carcinoma. In D. G. McQuarrie, G. L. Adams, A. R. Shons, & G. A. Browne [Eds.], *Head and neck cancer: Clinical decisions and management principles.* Chicago: Mosby.)

mary treatment modality for nasopharyngeal carcinoma. In general, nasopharyngeal carcinoma is very radioresponsive and radiocurable, even with metastatic disease to the lymph nodes. Optimal field size, dose, and fractionation regimens can vary (Kaasa, Kragh-Jensen, Bjordal, Lund, Evensen, & Vermund et al., 1993; Yamashita, Kondo, Inuyama, & Hashimoto, 1986). A combination of external beam radiation therapy followed by an intracavitary implant is recommended for most patients with nasopharyngeal cancer.

The treatment volume for external beam radiation therapy should encompass the tumor, including a disease-free margin, as well as regional lymph nodes, especially the cervical lymph nodes where metastases occur frequently. Nodal irradiation is recommended even in clinically node-negative patients (Perez et al., 1992; Collins et al., 1995; Wang, 1997). Treatment fields include the nasopharynx and the upper and lower portions of the neck, including the retropharyngeal, bilateral cervical, posterior jugular, spinal accessory, and supraclavicular lymph nodes.

Radiation therapy treatments are given 5 days a week at doses of 180 to 200 cGy for 6 to 7 weeks. The primary tumor and clinically involved lymph node regions are treated to a total dose of 6500 to 7500 cGy. For clinically uninvolved lymph nodes, but those at high risk for metastatic disease, a total radiation dose of 4500 to 5000 cGy is delivered. T3 and T4 lesions (tumors extending beyond the nasopharynx) and keratinizing squamous cell carcinomas are usually irradiated to a higher dose than T1 or T2 lesions (i.e., tumors confined to the nasopharynx) and the nonkeratinizing undifferentiated carcinomas or lymphoepitheliomas (Table 52-5) (Fu, 1987; Mendenhall et al., 1994). Because almost all nasopharyngeal carcinomas in children are lymphoepitheliomas, the total dose of external beam radiation recommended for the primary tumor in children is 6000 cGy for T1 and T2 lesions and 6500 cGy for T3 and T4 lesions (Mendenhall et al., 1994).

The most common side effects reported by patients undergoing radiation therapy include sore throat, xerostomia, taste changes, mucositis, mucositis-related pain, dysphagia, and fatigue (Hilderley, 1993; Mendenhall et al., 1994; Strohl, 1989). The problems of taste changes, mucositis, and mucositis pain (especially when swallowing) contribute to the patient's inability to eat and drink adequate amounts of food and fluid, which can result in significant weight loss. Because the eustachian tube is in the radiation field, patients may experience obstruction of the tube, resulting in hearing loss or otitis media. Symptoms related to treatment usually occur starting at the end of the second or beginning of the third week of treatment and resolve several weeks after treatment (Strohl, 1989; Wang 1997). Newer treatment techniques such as the use of three dimensional (3-D) conformal treatment planning may enhance local control, while minimizing the effects to normal tissues (Clayman et al., 1997).

Table 52-5 Doses of Radiation Used to Treat Patients with Nasopharyngeal Carcinoma

Area	Dose (cGy)
Nasopharynx	6500-7500
Brachytherapy	600-700
Neck Nodes	
Not palpable	5000-6000
5 cm or less	6000+
Greater than 5 cm	6000-7000

Data from Mendenhall, W. M., Million, R. R., Mancuso, A.A., & Stringer, S.P. (1994). Nasopharynx. In R.R. Million & N.J. Cassisi (Eds.), *Management of head and neck cancer: A multidisciplinary approach* (2nd ed.). Philadelphia: J.B. Lippincott; Perez, C. A. (1992). Nasopharynx. In C. A. Perez & L. W. Brady (Eds.), *Principles and practice of radiation oncology* (2nd ed.). Philadelphia: J.B. Lippincott; Wang, C. C. (1997). *Radiation therapy for head and neck neoplasms* (3rd ed.). New York: Wiley-Liss.

Late complications of radiation therapy are relatively rare. Most patients experience permanent xerostomia that can be severe. Patients are prone to developing dental caries as a consequence of decreased saliva production and alteration in salivary consistency. Trismus resulting from fibrosis and contracture of the pterygoid muscles occurs with varying degrees and has been reported in about 10% of patients (Mesic, Fletcher, & Goepfert, 1981). Hypothyroidism occasionally occurs due to the effects of radiation on the thyroid gland or through an indirect effect on the pituitary gland. Radiation myelitis of the cervical spinal cord or brain and brain necrosis are the most severe complications resulting from treatment and occur in less than 1% to 2% of the cases (Mendenhall et al., 1994).

The overall effects of treatment are very demanding on the patient, and it may take several months before patients begin to regain their optimal sense of well-being. At the completion of the radiation therapy treatments, patients receiving concurrent radiation and chemotherapy treatment may still be scheduled to receive additional courses of chemotherapy and their recovery period will be prolonged. For patients receiving chemotherapy treatments concurrently with radiation therapy, the side effects of treatment may be more severe. The acute side effects caused by the treatments are difficult management issues for the health professional and patient.

Brachytherapy

The use of intracavitary implants with cesium-137 (low dose rate) or high dose rate (HDR) iridium is indicated for most patients with nasopharyngeal cancer. However, implants are not recommended for patients with nasopharyngeal cancers that invade the base of the skull or extend into the cranial cavity (Mendenhall et al., 1994; Wang, 1997).

The purpose of the intracavitary implants is to deliver a high dose of radiation or "boost" the dose of radiation to the primary tumor while minimizing the side effects to surrounding normal tissues. The intracavitary implants, which are temporary, are done within a few weeks after the completion of external beam radiation therapy. Low dose rate (LDR) intracavitary implants using cesium-137 or iridium-192 require the patient to be hospitalized for several days while the radioactive sources are in place. The HDR iridium delivers high doses of radiation in a short time. The procedure is done on an outpatient basis in the radiation therapy department. The patient receives one to two fractions of HDR iridium, lasting only minutes, and each session is separated by 6 hours (Wang, 1997).

HDR iridium has advantages over LDR brachytherapy because it improves radiation safety, decreases treatment time, allows for outpatient scheduling, is cost effective, and is an effective treatment (Hilderley & Dow, 1996). In addition, the procedure is more comfortable and less tedious for the patient because of the reduced treatment time. It is also less disruptive to the patients' routine because they are not hospitalized for several days.

Patients who undergo intracavitary implants receive an external beam radiation therapy dose of up to 70 Gy and an additional 6 to 7 Gy by implant. Patients who do not receive an intracavitary implant receive external beam radiation therapy to a dose of 72 to 75 Gy (Wang, 1997).

The potential acute side effects associated with intracavitary brachytherapy include discomfort related to the placement of the catheters that hold the radioactive sources; irritation of the nasal passage and oropharynx; and nasal drainage.

Chemotherapy

Although radiation therapy is effective in achieving long-term survival for patients in the early stages of nasopharyngeal carcinoma, long-term survival rates for patients with advanced stages of the disease at the time of diagnosis are considerably worse because these patients tend to develop distant metastatic disease. Studies on the use of chemotherapy for patients with nasopharyngeal carcinoma have resulted in findings that have been less than definitive. Therefore the indications for the use of chemotherapy for adjuvant treatment of nasopharyngeal carcinoma remain controversial. Several studies of patients with nasopharyngeal cancer investigated different drug regimens in an adjuvant setting prior to radiation therapy or after completion of radiation therapy. These studies did not show any significant improvement in overall survival. In addition, patients reported significant treatment-associated morbidities (Dimery, Legha, Peters, Goepfert, & Oswald, 1987; International Nasopharynx Cancer Study Group, 1996; Tannock, Payne, Cummings, Hewitt, Panzarella, & Beale et al., 1987).

Recently, the preliminary results of a Radiation Therapy Oncology Group study (RTOG 88-17) of 191 patients with stage III or stage IV nasopharyngeal carcinoma showed that the administration of chemotherapy concurrently with radiation results in significantly improved progression-free survival (Fu, Cooper, Marcial, Laramore, Pajak, & Jacobs et al., 1996). This study evaluated complete response rate, time to treatment failure, overall survival, and acute and late toxicities between radiation therapy alone and radiation therapy plus chemotherapy. The chemotherapy regimen consisted of cisplatin (100 mg/m^2) every 3 weeks during radiation therapy, followed by three cycles of adjuvant chemotherapy with cisplatin and 5-fluorouracil (5-FU; 1000mg/m^2/day). The 5-FU was given as a continuous infusion over 96 hours. Although the acute treatment-related morbidity was more severe for the patients receiving combined treatment, the acute side effects resolved and the overall benefits to the patient appeared to outweigh the treatment toxicities. While progression-free survival was significantly improved, differences in overall survival have yet to be determined. As a result of the findings of this study and indications that concurrent chemotherapy is beneficial in treating late-stage nasopharyngeal carcinoma, chemotherapy is often included as part of the treatment regimen for patients with stage III or IV nasopharyngeal carcinoma where metastases outside the locoregional area are more likely to occur.

The use of chemotherapy to treat earlier stages of nasopharyngeal carcinoma is still debatable. Without definitive evidence that the combination treatment is better than radiation therapy alone in improving progression-free survival or overall survival, recommending such treatment to patients may be more difficult in view of the increased morbidity associated with combination treatment. Further study of the use of chemotherapy for early-stage nasopharyngeal carcinoma needs to done. The need for an effective systemic therapy is evidenced by the high recurrence rates for nasopharyngeal carcinoma despite the high initial response rates associated with primary therapy (Clayman et al., 1997).

Treatment of Recurrent Nasopharyngeal Cancer

Local or Regional Recurrence. Permanent iodine-125 (^{125}I) implants are often used for discrete local recurrence of nasopharyngeal carcinoma. Permanent implants provide the advantage of limiting the radiation dose to normal tissues in the surrounding areas while delivering high doses of radiation to the area of recurrence.

Because patients who develop local recurrence do not usually have a discrete, localized lesion, a second course of radiation therapy combining external beam radiation therapy and brachytherapy sources may be recommended (Mendenhall et al., 1994). Significant palliation and the potential for long-term survival may be achieved. It is necessary to deliver a high dose of radiation (5000 to 6000 cGy) to obtain good results (Wang, 1997).

The use of surgery for locally recurrent nasopharyngeal carcinoma is limited to a small local recurrence that is amenable to surgery. Otherwise, other treatment modalities should be considered. For regional recurrence (i.e., lymph node recurrence), surgery is recommended if the tumor can be resected. This goal may require a neck dissection (Mendenhall et al., 1994; Moss, 1994). Chemotherapy may also be recommended for treatment of locoregional recurrence because distant spread of disease is likely.

Locoregional Recurrence with Distant Metastases or Distant Metastases Only. For recurrences of nasopharyngeal carcinoma at the primary site or in the neck with distant metastases or distant metastases alone, systemic

Box 52-3
Chemotherapy Drugs Used to Treat Nasopharyngeal Carcinoma

Cisplatin
Adriamycin
Bleomycin
5-Fluorouracil
Epirubicin
Methotrexate
Vincristine

chemotherapy is indicated (Schantz, Harrison, & Hong, 1993). Box 52-3 lists chemotherapy drugs that have been effective in the treatment of recurrent nasopharyngeal carcinoma. These drugs have been used as single agents or in combination with each other, with varying treatment schedules. The highest response rates recorded occur with platinum-based chemotherapy regimens; therefore such a drug regimen should be used to treat patients with recurrent nasopharyngeal carcinoma (Schantz, Harrison, & Hong, 1993; Clayman et al., 1997).

The time from initial treatment to recurrence is prognostically significant. In a study of patients with nasopharyngeal cancer (Wang, 1997), those who developed recurrence more than 2 years after initial treatment had 5-year survival rates of 66%, whereas only 13% of the patients who experienced recurrence within 2 years of initial treatment were 5-year survivors.

Treatment of Children with Nasopharyngeal Carcinoma

Standard treatment for children with nasopharyngeal carcinomas generally follows the same guidelines established for adults. The treatment regimen consists of external beam radiation therapy to the nasopharynx and involved cervical lymph nodes, with a lesser radiation dose to noninvolved lymph nodes. Higher doses of radiation therapy in children are associated with significant morbidity in long-term survivors. These effects include endocrine dysfunction manifested by stunted growth and thyroid dysfunction, soft tissue fibrosis, bone and dental problems, and second malignancies (Ayan & Altun, 1996).

ONCOLOGIC EMERGENCIES

Airway Obstruction

Newly diagnosed patients with nasopharyngeal cancer rarely experience an airway obstruction. However, patients may experience an airway obstruction from edema in supraclavicular nodes or tissues as a result of radiation therapy or infection, trismus due to radiation therapy, or an esophageal stricture. Regardless of the etiology of the airway obstruction, the treatment remains the same. The health care team must be able to establish a patent airway; otherwise, death is imminent.

NURSING MANAGEMENT

Nursing care of the patient with nasopharyngeal carcinoma is generally grouped with the care of the patient who has head and neck cancer. Although patients with other types of head and neck cancers are treated similarly or with the same treatment modalities as patients with nasopharyngeal carcinoma, the problems or needs specific to the patient with nasopharyngeal carcinoma are not always the same. As illustrated in Fig. 52-3, the medical management of nasopharyngeal carcinoma varies, primarily based on the patient's stage of disease at the time of diagnosis. The management of these patients provides the oncology nurse with many challenges (Bildstein, 1993; Reese, 1996). Patients and their families experience numerous problems that require patient education and nursing interventions. Because treatment for patients with nasopharyngeal carcinoma occurs predominantly in an outpatient setting, the role of the oncology nurse is instrumental in assisting patients and caregivers to deal with and manage successfully the problems and issues they may encounter.

Diagnostic Workup

During the diagnostic process, patients should be assessed for their understanding of what will occur and the needs they have surrounding this process. The oncology nurse provides appropriate information about the different tests and procedures the patient will undergo. Patients and caregivers should be properly instructed and prepared for these tests and procedures because this eases the fear and anxiety that patients and caregivers may experience.

After a diagnosis is made, patients and caregivers need to consider the treatment options. Patients need information about the treatment. The treatment for the majority of patients with nasopharyngeal carcinoma consists of radiation therapy (external beam with or without brachytherapy) alone or radiation therapy and chemotherapy. Patients need to be aware of and understand the different treatments that they will receive and the possible side effects they may encounter. They need to be instructed in self-care strategies for managing possible side effects and problems from their treatment or disease when they are at home.

External Beam Radiation Therapy

External beam radiation therapy is the major treatment modality for this disease and can result in numerous side effects and problems for the patient. The major problems resulting from external beam radiation therapy include mucositis, mucositis-related pain, xerostomia, taste changes, dysphagia, loss of appetite, skin erythema and desquamation, and fatigue. Patients frequently lose significant amounts of weight during treatment due to a combination of treatment-related side effects that makes it difficult for patients to maintain an adequate caloric intake. (A standard of care form for a patient undergoing external beam radiation therapy for nasopharyngeal cancer is provided in Table 52-6.)

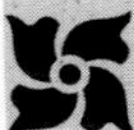

TABLE 52-6 Standard of Care for the Patient Undergoing External Beam Radiation Therapy for Nasopharyngeal Cancer

Patient Problem and Outcomes	Nursing Interventions and Rationales	Patient Education Instructions
Knowledge Deficit Patient will verbalize an understanding of the purpose, benefits, and risks of radiation therapy.	1. Assess patient's level of knowledge about radiation therapy treatments that will be administered. 2. Assess patient's concerns and fears about radiation therapy.	1. Describe the procedures involved in radiation therapy: a. Consultation. b. Simulation. c. Treatment procedures and routines. 2. Describe the common side effects associated with radiation therapy treatments and self-care measures to manage the side effects of the following: a. Painful mucositis. b. Decreased nutritional intake. c. Fatigue. d. Skin reactions. e. Xerostomia. f. Taste changes.
Painful Mucositis Patient will: • Experience optimal pain. • Maintain adequate nutritional intake.	1. Monitor for oral changes. 2. Assess for other factors that may contribute to the development of mucositis and mucositis pain (i.e., chemotherapy). 3. Examine the oral cavity for the development of mucositis. 4. Assess oral cavity for signs and symptoms of oral infection (i.e., candida, herpes). 5. Assess pain intensity using a 0 to 10 verbal rating scale. 6. Initiate appropriate topical and systemic analgesics for mucositis. 7. Monitor effectiveness of topical and systemic analgesics. 8. Modify diet as needed to minimize irritation to painful mucosa.	1. Inform patient that mucositis usually occurs during the later part of the second or beginning of the third week of radiation therapy. 2. Instruct patient to do oral care and mouthrinses with non-alcoholic mouthrinse three to four times a day. 3. Instruct patient in the use of mouthrinses or topical anesthetics to minimize mucositis pain, especially prior to eating. 4. Teach patient the importance of taking pain medication regularly to keep pain under control. 5. Instruct patient to inform the nurse if pain persists and is not relieved with interventions. 6. Instruct patient about dietary modifications (e.g., softer diet, dietary supplements) that minimize irritation to the oral mucosa.
Inadequate Nutritional Intake Patient will maintain adequate nutritional intake and weight.	1. Obtain baseline weight prior to the start of therapy. 2. Assess patient's nutritional/caloric intake. 3. Assess patient's ability for oral intake. 4. Assess for factors contributing to decreased oral intake (e.g., taste changes, decreased appetite, pain with eating and swallowing, mucositis, xerostomia). 5. Obtain weekly weights.	1. Teach patient the importance of maintaining adequate nutritional intake during treatment. 2. Discuss with patient ways to increase proteins and calories in diet. 3. Inform patient that intake of 2000 calories or more a day is necessary. 4. Instruct patient to eat numerous small feedings throughout the day instead of three large meals per day.

TABLE 52-6 Standard of Care for the Patient Undergoing External Beam Radiation Therapy for Nasopharyngeal Cancer—cont'd

Patient Problem and Outcomes	Nursing Interventions and Rationales	Patient Education Instructions
Inadequate Nutritional Intake—cont'd		
	6. Treat problems identified in No. 3 that contribute to patient's inability to maintain adequate nutrition and lead to weight loss. 7. Obtain nutritional consultation. 8. Have a nasogastric tube or percutaneous endogastric tube placed if patient is unable to maintain an adequate nutritional intake.	5. If nasogastric tube or percutaneous endogastric tube is necessary, teach patient and caregivers how to use and care for such tubes.
Fatigue		
Patient will maintain normal activities of living and optimal quality of life.	1. Assess for fatigue prior to the start of therapy and throughout therapy using a 0 to 10 rating scale. 2. Monitor for and treat other factors that contribute to fatigue (e.g., inadequate nutritional intake, sleep problems, pain, xerostomia, stress of illness and treatment).	1. Teach patient that fatigue is one of the most common side effects of radiation treatment. 2. Inform patient that fatigue is self-limiting and resolves within months after treatment is completed. 3. Encourage patient to maintain normal level of activity as tolerable. 4. Encourage patient to make lifestyle changes as necessary to maximize energy levels. Such changes can include taking naps during the day or spacing out activities during the day or over a few days.
Skin Reactions		
Patient will maintain normal skin integrity.	1. Assess for and monitor skin reactions. 2. Apply a skin care product to affected intact skin three to four times a day (e.g., Sween cream, Lubriderm, aloe vera). 3. Institute skin care regimen for moist desquamation as determined by institution (e.g., Domboros soaks, A & D ointment, aloe vera).	1. Instruct patient about skin care guidelines that may help to minimize the reaction: a. Avoid wearing constrictive clothing over the area. b. Do not shave the treated area. c. Do not use any skin care products on the treated skin without checking with the nurse. d. Avoid exposing the area to the sun. e. Gently care for the treated skin. f. Avoid exposing skin to extreme hot or cold temperatures. g. Do not scratch skin if it becomes dry or itchy. 2. Inform patient that skin reactions usually occur starting during the second or third week of treatment with moist desquamation, if it occurs, happening during the fifth or sixth week of treatment. Skin reactions resolve after the completion of treatment. 3. Teach patient how to manage the various skin reactions.

Continued

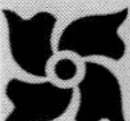

TABLE 52-6 Standard of Care for the Patient Undergoing External Beam Radiation Therapy for Nasopharyngeal Cancer—cont'd

Patient Problem and Outcomes	Nursing Interventions and Rationales	Patient Education Instructions
Xerostomia		
Patient will maintain adequate mouth moisture and optimal quality of life.	1. Assess for xerostomia using a 0 to 10 scale. 2. Initiate measures to increase salivary flow: a. Chewing sugar-free gum and eating sugarless hard candies. b. Medications (e.g., pilocarpine as directed). 3. Initiate measures to provide moisture to the oral mucosa: a. Rinse oral cavity with water every 2-3 hours. b. Use saliva substitutes or mouth moisturizers (e.g., Oralbalance, Salivart, Moistir). c. Drink more fluids. d. Use a humidifier. e. Dietary modifications (e.g., softer, moister foods; foods with gravies or sauces; drinking more fluids with meals). 4. Monitor the effectiveness of the above measures. 5. Assess for factors that may contribute to mouth dryness: a. Medications (e.g., antihistamines, diuretics, antihypertensives, antidepressants). b. Chemotherapy. c. Alcohol. d. Smoking.	1. Inform patient that mild xerostomia may be experienced during the first week of treatment and generally worsens over the course of treatment. 2. Teach the importance of a good oral hygiene program consisting of brushing, flossing, regular dental care, and daily fluoride treatments for life because patients are more prone to caries. 3. Teach measures to increase salivary flow and provide moisture to oral cavity. 4. Inform patient that xerostomia may be permanent.
Taste Alterations		
Patient will maintain taste acuity and maintain an adequate oral intake.	1. Monitor for taste alterations. 2. Assess for other factors that may contribute to taste alterations: a. Chemotherapy. b. Medications. c. Alcohol. d. Smoking 3. Obtain a dietary consultation. 4. Institute and experiment with dietary changes that may enhance taste acuity.	1. Inform patients that taste alterations may occur beginning the first week of treatment and will not resolve completely for several months after the treatments are completed. 2. Teach patients strategies to deal with taste alterations: a. Seasoning foods. b. Experimenting with different seasoning and flavors. c. Trying different types of foods. d. Experimenting with different food temperatures. e. Eating small, frequent meals. 3. Inform patients of the importance of eating even if they cannot taste or have an altered taste.

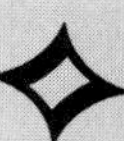

TABLE 52-7 Patient Preparation for Intracavitary Nasopharyngeal Brachytherapy

Description of the Procedure: Afterloading intracavitary brachytherapy uses cesium-137 or high dose rate (HDR) iridium-192 sources to deliver high doses of radiation to the primary tumor site. The use of these afterloading sources allows a high dose of radiation to be delivered to the primary site while minimizing the radiation dose to the surrounding normal tissues.

Patient Preparation: Patient should be NPO for 6 to 8 hours prior to procedure.

Procedural Considerations:

1. Obtain informed consent.
2. Patient should wear a gown.
3. A peripheral intravenous line may be started (at the discretion of the physician).
4. Patient may be premedicated.
5. Patient should be positioned in a Fowler's or semi-Fowler's position.
6. The oropharyngeal mucosa is anesthetized with a topical anesthetic
7. 5% cocaine is topically applied to nasal and nasopharyngeal mucosa to shrink the mucous membranes and anesthetize the area.
8. Endotracheal tubes are inserted into the nasopharynx through the nares.
9. After the endotracheal tube is correctly positioned, the balloon is inflated.
10. Insert dummy sources for treatment planning and adjustment of sources.
11. After tube placements are verified, sources are loaded into catheters for prescribed treatment time.
12. At the completion of treatment, the tubes are removed gently.

It is essential for the oncology nurse to assess and monitor these patients closely. The ineffective management of side effects may result in the worsening of side effects that cause delays or changes in treatment that could compromise the effectiveness of the overall treatment plan.

Brachytherapy

Patients undergoing LDR or HDR intracavitary brachytherapy require special instructions about precautions that will be used while they are receiving this treatment. Patients receiving LDR brachytherapy are hospitalized for up to several days during the time the radioactive sources are in place. Patients treated with HDR brachytherapy are treated as outpatients in the radiation therapy department where the HDR radioactive sources are inserted into the catheters. The patients receiving HDR receive one or two (separated by 6 hours) treatments lasting a few minutes (Wang, 1997). Table 52-7 contains a guideline for preparing patients for the intracavitary nasopharyngeal brachytherapy procedure.

BOX 52-4
General Guidelines for Patients with a Sealed Radioactive Implant

- Assign the patient to a private room with a private bath.
- Place a "Caution: Radioactive Material" sign on the door of the patient's room.
- Wear a dosimeter film badge at all times while caring for patients with implants.
- Pregnant nurses should not care for these patients; do not allow children under 18 years or pregnant women to visit.
- Limit each visitor to ½ hour per day. Be sure that visitors are at least 6 feet from the radioactive source.
- Never touch the radioactive source with bare hands. In the rare instance that it is dislodged, use long-handled forceps to retrieve it. Deposit the radioactive source in the lead container that is kept in the patient's room.
- Save all dressings and bed linens until after the radioactive source is removed. Then dispose of dressings and linens in the usual manner. Other equipment can be removed from the room at any time.

From Hassey, K. (1985). Demystifying care of patients with radioactive implants. *American Journal of Nursing, 85,* 792.

The procedure for inserting the catheters (endotracheal tubes) that hold the radioactive sources is essentially the same whether the radiation treatment requires the patient to be hospitalized for several days or treated with the HDR technique in the outpatient setting. The insertion of the applicators is generally done in the radiation therapy department with the patient awake. The patient may be given premedication prior to the start of the insertion process. Patients receiving LDR brachytherapy are placed in a shielded room. (General guidelines for patients with a sealed radioactive implant are listed in Box 52-4.)

Patients who undergo the HDR procedure and receive two treatments generally wait between treatments in the radiation therapy department. These patients have their catheters in place between treatments but are not radioactive because the sources are only inserted when they are in the treatment room. The patient should be provided with privacy and comfort measures. Patients should be monitored for any discomfort they may experience and be medicated as needed. Patients need to breathe through their mouths while the catheters are in place, which may cause some discomfort. Suction should be available because patients may have difficulty clearing oral secretions.

After the treatment is completed, patients should be informed of potential side effects (i.e., swelling or irritation of the nasal passage and nasopharynx, nasal drainage, and pain or soreness in the nasopharynx and oropharynx) and be taught self-care measures to manage these side effects.

Chemotherapy

Patients who receive concurrent chemotherapy with external beam radiation therapy not only have to deal with the side effects accompanying their radiation treatments, but also with side effects that occur from their chemotherapy treatments. Patients may experience acute side effects earlier in the treatment course, and these side effects may be more severe with combined treatment (Hirschfield-Bartek, 1992). Patients receiving combination therapy often report a poorer general sense of well-being and worse side effects from their treatment than patients receiving radiation therapy alone. Anecdotally, patients appear to feel worse immediately following and up to 1 week after their chemotherapy treatment and begin to improve until the next course of chemotherapy.

Currently, patients with nasopharyngeal carcinoma can receive their chemotherapy treatments every 3 weeks, starting at the initiation of radiation therapy. Depending on which chemotherapy drugs patients receive, the side effects they experience may vary. The oncology nurse must have knowledge of the chemotherapy drugs the patient is receiving and the potential side effects of those drugs in order to anticipate potential problems that may be compounded by combined treatment. In addition, the oncology nurse assists the patient and caregiver to assess for and deal with any treatment-related problems that may occur. For instance, the combination of radiation therapy and cisplatin can increase the patient's risk of developing hearing problems because each treatment alone has the potential for causing this problem. In such a case, patients should have a baseline hearing test done before the initiation of treatment and be instructed to report any hearing changes during their therapy.

At the completion of their course of radiation therapy, patients who continue to receive additional courses of chemotherapy may experience more severe side effects because of the radiation therapy. Patients with nasopharyngeal cancer who are treated with subsequent cycles of chemotherapy (especially with 5-FU) frequently experience an enhanced mucositis or skin reaction in the area treated with radiation therapy, even though they may have completed their radiation therapy treatments weeks to months earlier. This phenomenon is a result of the sensitization of the tissues by the radiation therapy treatments. Patients need to be instructed about this potential problem.

Patients receiving chemotherapy for recurrent nasopharyngeal cancer experience side effects specifically related to the drugs they receive. Patients may receive a single agent or a combination of drugs. See Table 52-5 for a list of drugs that are active against nasopharyngeal carcinoma. A platinum-containing regimen is usually recommended (Schantz, Harrison, & Hong, 1993). Patients need to be prepared and instructed about the chemotherapy, possible side effects, and self-care measures to deal with such effects.

Surgery

Because surgery is not a standard part of the treatment for nasopharyngeal carcinoma, the patient needs to be informed about any surgical procedure that may be proposed. For patients with bulky or residual nodal disease, some form of neck dissection may be recommended. Patient problems vary depending on the extent of the surgery, location of the tumor, and amount of disease present. Therefore the nursing care for these patients varies accordingly. Patients who require some form of neck dissection are generally hospitalized for several days and require routine postoperative nursing care, in addition to care specific to the surgical procedure performed.

HOME CARE ISSUES

Depending on the treatment modalities used in the management of nasopharyngeal cancer, patients and their caregivers are required to deal with multiple issues during the course of treatment and for a period of time after the treatment. Because the major portion of the treatment for patients with nasopharyngeal carcinoma is delivered in an outpatient setting, most of the problems and issues faced by patients and their caregivers are those discussed in the nursing management section of this chapter. Although the oncology nurse manages and deals with disease and treatment problems that patients with nasopharyngeal carcinoma encounter when they are in the hospital or outpatient setting, a majority of the success in managing patient problems relies on the patients and their caregivers to perform self-care measures successfully at home. Educating and instructing patients and caregivers about specific care issues, accurately monitoring their ability to successfully provide the care, and modifying the care as appropriate are crucial to the success of patients managing problems at home.

Eardley (1986), in a study of 30 patients with head and neck cancer who were 7 weeks post–external beam radiation therapy, reported patients still had significant symptoms related to their treatment (Table 52-8). These findings are important because these are the problems that patients and their caregivers will be facing at home.

TABLE 52-8 Problems Reported by Head and Neck Radiation Therapy Patients 7 Weeks After the Completion of Treatment

Complaint or Problem	Percent Reporting
Unable to eat normally	83%
Unable to resume normal activity	70%
Impaired taste/altered taste	60%
Unable to eat certain foods/takes longer to eat	60%
Tired/weak	50%
Additional expenses due to side effects	50%
Depressed	47%
Soreness in mouth	30%
Not prepared for the severity of side effects	23%
Only able to eat soft foods	17%

From Eardley, A. (1986). Patients and radiotherapy: Part 3. Patients' experiences after discharge. *Radiography, 52,* 17-19.

Nutritional Considerations

All patients receive radiation therapy, and the majority of these patients develop a series of side effects, including mucositis, mucositis-related pain, dysphagia, xerostomia, and taste changes or taste loss. These side effects contribute to patients having difficulty eating and drinking adequate amounts of food and fluids to maintain their weight. Patients and caregivers must monitor these side effects and their effect on the patient's nutritional intake. Instructions about dietary modifications, such as a softer diet and the use of dietary supplements to increase caloric intake, need to be discussed with patients and their caregivers. If significant weight loss occurs, the placement of a nasogastric (NG) or percutaneous endogastric tube (PEG) may be necessary to provide supplemental feedings to the patient. The patient and caregiver need to learn to care for the tube and how to use the tube for feedings. Patients may not feel hungry as long as they continue regular tube feedings. However, as treatment-related side effects resolve, patients need to be encouraged to gradually resume a normal diet.

Continued nutritional supplementation may be necessary for weeks and up to several months after radiation therapy has been completed for patients to maintain an adequate caloric intake. Patients should be encouraged to introduce regular foods into their diet gradually as soon as symptoms begin to resolve. Patients and caregivers may need assistance with dietary instructions and modifications, and a combination of dietary supplements and regular foods may be necessary until a normal diet can be resumed.

Treatment-Related Side Effects

Patients and caregivers must be taught that the side effects from treatment, especially those from radiation therapy, may continue or worsen for several weeks after the treatments are completed. Patients frequently think that once the treatments are completed, the side effects should start to improve immediately. Although that can occur, it is more likely that patients will experience no significant changes in side effects or a worsening of side effects for a period of time. Reporting on patients with head and neck cancer 7 weeks post–radiation therapy, Eardley (1986) stated that some patients experienced worsened side effects after completing radiation (53%), most had side effects still noticeable (70%), and less than a third (30%) had resumed normal activities.

Patients may experience a worsening of their mucositis for several weeks after the completion of treatment, as well as continued pain with swallowing. It may take at least 4 to 6 weeks for patients to feel that treatment-related side effects are improving, and it may take months for the side effects to resolve completely. Loss of taste or taste changes and fatigue may take 4 to 6 months or longer in some patients to resolve completely.

Patients may continue to experience significant pain related to radiation-induced mucositis. This pain may last for weeks after the completion of therapy. Patients must continue to take their systemic pain medications regularly while they are experiencing pain. In addition, they should be instructed to continue taking prescribed topical or oral care treatments until the pain resolves.

As stated previously, for patients receiving chemotherapy concurrently with radiation therapy, the side effects from treatment (e.g., mucositis, taste changes, skin reactions, fatigue, xerostomia) may be more severe. They may experience other side effects such as nausea and vomiting and lowered blood counts that, in combination with the enhanced side effects of combined treatment, may negatively affect their overall well-being and quality of life. Patients must be instructed to take their medications for side effects as directed and use self-care measures that may minimize these effects.

Patients who require a surgical procedure need assistance directly related to the surgical intervention performed. Patient and caregiver education and nursing interventions should address the expected postoperative course at home, as well as possible problems or issues that may require attention, such as infections, problems with healing, or increased pain or swelling.

The patient may be faced with rehabilitation therapies or permanent lifestyle modifications that need to be continued in the home care setting. Neck exercises and mouth exercise (for trismus) are activities that the patient needs to do continually to maintain maximum mobility and function of these areas. Daily fluoride treatments, as well as regular dental visits, are necessary for these patients for the remainder of their life because they are more prone to dental problems and osteoradionecrosis.

PROGNOSIS

Although nasopharyngeal cancers are extremely radiosensitive and respond well to chemotherapy, the prognosis for patients with this disease varies depending on a number of factors. These factors include the histology of the tumor, the stage of the disease at the time of diagnosis, the extent of lymph node involvement at the time of diagnosis, serologic and biologic factors, and the techniques used in the treatment plan (Vokes, Weischselbaum, Lippman, & Hong, 1993).

Early-stage nasopharyngeal cancers are generally curable. However, most nasopharyngeal cancers when diagnosed are usually advanced or have metastasized to areas outside the nasopharynx. Local control is achieved in greater than 80% of patients with T1 and T2 lesions (Fu, 1987).

Overall disease-free survival for patients with nasopharyngeal carcinoma is about 50% at 5 years (Lee, Law, Ng, Chan, Poon, & Foo et al., 1992; Mesic, Fletcher, & Goepfert, 1981), with 5-year survival rates post recurrence ranging between 21% and 41%. Approximately 20% of the patients develop distant metastatic disease. Cervical lymph node size is a prognostic factor for the development of distant metastases, with a reported incidence of 25% in patients with nodes 3 to 6 cm, 50% for nodes larger than 6 cm, and only 10% for nonpalpable or small (less than 3 cm) nodes (Sweeney, Haraf, Vokes, Dougherty, & Weichselbaum, 1994).

Histologically, patients with a differentiated squamous

cell carcinoma (WHO type 1) do worse in terms of local control as well as overall survival than patients with a more undifferentiated carcinoma (WHO, types 2 and 3) when treated with radiation therapy alone or with radiation therapy and neoadjuvant chemotherapy (Gallo, Bianchi, Giannini, Gallina, Libonati, & Fini-Storchi, 1991; Johansen, Mestre, & Overgaard, 1992).

In general, younger patients have a better outcome even if a greater proportion of advanced stages of disease are seen in childhood (Perez et al., 1992). However, patients younger than 20 years seem to have worse outcomes from their disease (Martin & Shah, 1994). Female patients with nasopharyngeal carcinoma appear to have better outcomes than males (Johansen, Mestre, & Overgaard, 1992).

In conclusion, patients diagnosed with advanced disease fare worse than patients with early-stage disease. In addition, although nasopharyngeal carcinoma is very responsive to treatment, by the time patients are diagnosed with nasopharyngeal carcinoma the disease is usually advanced, with the cancer spread outside the nasopharynx as well as to distant sites. The ability to diagnose nasopharyngeal carcinoma sooner and at an early stage would have a significant effect on the overall survival of these patients.

EVALUATION OF THE QUALITY OF CARE

Organizations such as the Joint Commission for the Accreditation of Health Care Organizations require that the quality of care that patients receive be evaluated in order for health care facilities to receive accreditation. Because of this requirement, all departments or disciplines of accredited health care institutions should have a formal mechanism in place to evaluate the care provided within their area. Patients with nasopharyngeal cancer receive similar treatments and care, experience similar problems, and should be evaluated accordingly.

Because nasopharyngeal carcinoma is a head and neck cancer, documentation and quality of care evaluations are designated under the head and neck category. Figs. 52-4 and 52-5 are examples of documentation tools (developed by the Oncology Nursing Society's Radiation Oncology Special Interest Group) for patients with head and neck cancer who are undergoing radiation therapy. The first includes the teaching and instructions for patients with head and neck cancer, and the second is the patient care record that can be used to monitor patients throughout the course of their treatment. (An example of a quality of care evaluation tool to assess for alterations in nutrition for the patients undergoing head and neck radiation therapy is provided in Table 52-9.)

TABLE 52-9 Quality of Care Evaluation for a Patient Undergoing Head and Neck Radiation Therepy: Alteration in Nutrition

Disciplines participating in the quality of care evaluation:
☐ Nursing ☐ Radiation Oncologist
☐ Dietary ☐ Social Services

I. Treatment Management Evaluation

Data from:
☐ Medical Record Review ☐ Patient/Caregiver Interview

Criteria	YES	NO
1. Baseline information obtained prior to start of treatment:		
a. Baseline weight	☐	☐
b. Weight loss over past 3 months	☐	☐
c. Any problems or difficulty with eating	☐	☐
2. Patient weighed weekly.	☐	☐
3. Dietary consult obtained if weight loss >10% of body weight.	☐	☐
4. Dietary teaching documented.	☐	☐
5. Side effects related to treatment affecting nutritional intake evaluated:		
a. Anorexia	☐	☐
b. Mucositis	☐	☐
c. Taste changes/loss	☐	☐
d. Xerostomia	☐	☐
e. Fatigue	☐	☐
6. Patient required:		
a. Oral dietary supplements	☐	☐
b. Nasogastric or percutaneous endogastric tube	☐	☐

RESEARCH ISSUES

There are several areas of research currently being considered or pursued in addressing issues surrounding the diagnosis and management of nasopharyngeal cancers. The controversy surrounding the use of chemotherapy for nasopharyngeal carcinoma in general continues to be discussed. Although significant improvement has been seen in progression-free and disease-free survival, overall survival has not always been affected. Continued study in this area is required to determine more definitely the benefits of this treatment. Another question asked is about the treatment of patients with stage II tumors (tumors confined to the nasopharynx but invading more than one subsite of the nasopharynx). The question is whether these patients would benefit from receiving chemotherapy added to their initial treatment because the 5-year local control rates are 65%, with patients experience local recurrence or distant metastatic disease (Clayman et al., 1997; Lee et al., 1992).

Another area of research being pursued involves methods for early detection of a nasopharyngeal carcinoma. Within the last decade, the research on the etiologic factors for nasopharyngeal carcinoma (as well as the focus on and interaction among the genetic, environmental, and viral factors) has helped to identify patients at high risk for developing the disease. Additional research in this area to identify markers for nasopharyngeal carcinoma and the development of early screening methods, especially for high-risk patients, is being conducted and would be beneficial if cost effective. The potential for increases in long-term survival and even cure for patients with nasopharyngeal carcinoma would be greatly increased with early diagnosis and treatment.

RADIATION THERAPY PATIENT CARE RECORD — HEAD & NECK

Dx: ____________________

SITE: ____________________

NAME: **MR #/RT#:**

ASSESSMENTS (Date/rad or Gy)											
Comfort Alteration Fatigue											
Pain Rating											
Pain Treatment											
Pain Relief											
Mucous Membrane Alteration Esophagitis/Pharyngitis											
Laryngitis											
Mucositis											
Taste Changes											
Xerostomia											
Nutrition Alteration Anorexia											
Nausea											
Vomiting											
Weight											
Sensory Alteration Hearing Changes											
Skin Alteration Skin Reaction											
Injury, Potential Bleeding/Infection CBC DATE											
WBC											
Hemoglobin/Hematocrit	/	/	/	/	/	/	/	/	/	/	/
Platelets											
Other											
INITIALS											

Pre-existing Conditions/Medical Information

Date: Ht = BP = P = R = Concurrent Chemotherapy: Yes No

( ) ( ) ( )

Signature **Initials** **Signature** **Initials** **Signature** **Initials**

Fig. 52-4 Example of a patient care record form for head and neck radiation therapy patients. (From Oncology Nursing Society Radiation Therapy Special Interest Group, Pittsburgh, Penn.)

NAME: ____ MR #/RT#: __________

TEACHING AND INSTRUCTIONS — HEAD & NECK

	DATE/ INITIALS	METH	EVAL	PLAN	DATE/ INITIALS	METH	EVAL	PLAN	EDUCATIONAL MATERIALS
GENERAL Simulation									
Initial Treatment									
Self Care Information									
Nutrition									
Social Service									
Discharge Instructions									
SITE-SPECIFIC Side Effects									
Dental Hygiene									
Esophagitis Management									
Fatigue Management									
Hearing Loss Management									
Laryngitis Management									
Mucositis Management									
Pain Management									
Skin/Scalp Care									
Taste Management									
Xerostomia Management									
Weight Loss Management									
OTHER/PREVENTION BSE/TSE									
Smoking Cessation									

Method Codes:
A. Person: Person Session
B. Family Conference
C. Booklet (specify)
D. Demonstration
E. Audio/Visual

Evaluation Codes:
UE: Unable to evaluate (explain)
V: Verbalizes concept accurately
D: Demonstrates skill accurately
R: Needs review
NR: Not receptive to learning at this time (explain)

Plan Codes:
RC: Reinforce Concept
RD: Return Demonstration
LOM: Learning objective met
RF: Referral to other health care givers (specify)
O: Other (specify)

DATE	COMMENTS

Signature	( ) Initials	Signature	( ) Initials	Signature	( ) Initials

Fig. 52-5 Example of a teaching instruction record for head and neck radiation therapy patients. (From Oncology Nursing Society Radiation Therapy Special Interest Group, Pittsburgh, Penn.)

Finally, an area of research in which oncology nurses could have a vital role is that aimed at effective symptom management of treatment-related side effects. The areas of pain management and nutritional management are just two of a number of problems that patients with nasopharyngeal carcinoma experience and need to be investigated. Finding effective strategies to deal with these two major problems could enhance the patients' physical well-being and overall quality of life. The ineffective management of symptoms in general can be costly and result in the need for treatment delays or changes that can compromise the effectiveness of the treatment plan.

REFERENCES

American Joint Committee on Cancer (1992). Pharynx (including base of tongue, soft palate, and uvula). *Manual for staging of cancer* (4th ed.). Philadelphia: J. B. Lippincott.

Ayan, I. & Altun, M. (1996). Nasopharyngeal carcinoma in children: Retrospective review of 50 patients. *International Journal of Radiation Oncology, Biology, Physics, 35,* 485-492.

Baker, S. R. (1980). Nasopharyngeal carcinoma: Clinical course and results of therapy. *Head and Neck Surgery, 3,* 8-14.

Bedwinek, J. M., Perez, C. A., & Keys, D. J. (1980). Analysis of failure after definitive irradiation for epidermoid carcinoma of the nasopharynx. *Cancer, 45,* 2725-2729.

Bildstein, C. Y. (1993). Head and neck malignancies. In S. L. Groenwald, M. H. Frogge, M. Goodman, & C. H. Yarbro (Eds.), *Cancer nursing: Principles and practice* (3rd ed.). Boston: Jones and Bartlett.

Cassisi, N. J. (1987). Clinical evaluation of pharyngeal tumors. In S. E. Thawley & W. R. Panje (Eds.), *Comprehensive management of head and neck tumors* (Vol. 1). Philadelphia: W. B. Saunders.

Chow, W. H., McLaughlin, J. K., Hrubec, Z., Nam, J. M., & Blot, W. J. (1993). Tobacco use and nasopharyngeal carcinoma in a cohort of U.S. veterans. *International Journal of Cancer, 55,* 539-540.

Clayman, G. L., Lippman, S. M., Laramore, G., & Hong, W. K. (1997). Head and neck cancer. In J. F. Holland, R. C. Bast, Jr., D. Morton, E. Frei, III, D. W. Kufe, & R. R. Weichselbaum (Eds.), *Cancer medicine* (4th ed.). Baltimore: Williams & Wilkins.

Collins, S. L., Dougherty, M., Stupp, R., Weichselbaum, R. R., & Vokes, E. E. (1995). Head and neck cancer. In M. D. Abeloff, J. O. Armitage, A. S. Lichter, & J. E. Niederhuber (Eds.), *Clinical oncology*. New York: Churchill Livingstone.

de The, G. (1987). Cancer of the nasopharynx. In S. Ariyan (Ed.), *Cancer of the head and heck.* St. Louis: Mosby.

de Vathaire, F., Sancho-Garnier, H., de The, H., Pieddeloup, C., Schaab, G., Ho, J. H., Elloz, R., Micheau, E., Cammoun, M., & Cachin, Y. (1988). Prognostic value of EBV markers in the clinical management of nasopharyngeal carcinoma (nasopharyngeal carcinoma): A multicenter follow-up study. *International Journal of Cancer, 42,* 176-181.

Dimery, I. W., Legha, S. S., Peters, L. J., Goepfert, H., & Oswald, M. J. (1987). Adjuvant chemotherapy for advanced nasopharyngeal carcinoma. *Cancer, 60,* 943-949.

Eardley, A. (1986). Patients and radiotherapy: Part 3. Patients' experiences after discharge. *Radiography, 52,* 17-19.

Fandi, A., Altun, M., Azli, N., Armand, J. P., & Cvitkovic, E. (1994). Nasopharyngeal cancer: Epidemiology, staging, and treatment. *Seminars in Oncology, 21,* 382-397.

Fandi, A. & Cvitkovic, E. (1995). Biology and treatment of nasopharyngeal cancer. *Current Opinion in Oncology, 7,* 355-363.

Fee, W. E. (1993). Nasopharyngeal carcinoma. In J. T. Johnson & M. S. Didolkar (Eds.), *Head and neck cancer* (Vol. III). London: Elsevier Science.

Feinmesser, R., Miyazaki, I., Cheung, R., Freeman, J.L., Noyek, A. M., & Dosch, H. M. (1992). Diagnosis of nasopharyngeal carcinoma by DNA amplification of tissue obtained by fine-needle aspiration. *New England Journal of Medicine, 326,* 17-21.

Fu, K. K. (1987). Treatment of tumors of the nasopharynx: Radiation therapy. In S. E. Thawley & W. R. Panje (Eds.), *Comprehensive management of head and neck tumors* (Vol. 1). Philadelphia: W. B. Saunders.

Fu, K. K., Cooper, J. S., Marcial, V. A., Laramore, G. E., Pajak, T. F., Jacobs, J., Al-Sarraf, M., Forastiere, A. A., & Cox, J. D. (1996). Evolution of the Radiation Therapy Oncology Group clinical trials for head and neck cancer. *International Journal of Radiation Oncology, Biology, Physics, 35,* 425-438.

Gallo, O., Bianchi, S., Giannini, A., Gallina, A., Libonati, G.A., & Fini-Storchi, O. (1991). Correlations between histopathological and biological findings in nasopharyngeal carcinoma and its prognostic significance. *Laryngoscope, 101,* 487-493.

Hilderley, L. J. (1993). Radiotherapy. In S. L. Groenwald, M. H. Frogge, M. Goodman, & C. H. Yarbro (Eds.), *Cancer nursing: Principles and practice* (3rd ed.). Boston: Jones and Bartlett.

Hilderley, L. J., & Dow, K. H. (1996). Radiation oncology. In R. McCorkle, M. Grant, M. Frank-Stromborg, & S. B. Baird (Eds.), *Cancer nursing: A comprehensive textbook* (2nd ed.). Philadelphia: W. B. Saunders.

Hirschfield-Bartek, J. (1992). Combined modality therapy. In K. H. Dow & L. J. Hilderley (Eds.), *Nursing care in radiation oncology.* Philadelphia: W. B. Saunders.

Hoppe, R. T., Goffinet, D. R., & Bagshaw, M. A. (1976). Carcinoma of the nasopharynx: Eighteen years experience with megavoltage radiation therapy. *Cancer, 37,* 2605-2612.

Ingersoll, L., Wood, S. Y., Donaldson, S., Giesler, J., Maor, M. H., Goffinet, D., Cangir, A., Goepfert, H., Oswald, M. J., & Peters, L. J. (1990). Nasopharyngeal carcinoma in the young: A combined M. D. Anderson and Stanford experience. *International Journal of Radiation Oncology, Biology, Physics, 19,* 881-887.

International Nasopharynx Cancer Study Group: VUMCA I Trial. (1996). Preliminary results of a randomized trial comparing neoadjuvant chemotherapy (cisplatin, epirubicin, bleomycin) plus radiotherapy vs. radiotherapy alone in stage IV (≥N2, M0) undifferentiated nasopharyngeal carcinoma: A positive effect on progression-free survival. *International Journal of Radiation Oncology, Biology, Physics, 35,* 463-469.

Johansen, L. V., Mestre, M., & Overgaard, J. (1992). Carcinoma of the nasopharynx: Analysis of treatment results in 167 consecutively admitted patients. *Head and Neck, 14,* 200-207.

Kaasa, S., Kragh-Jensen, E., Bjordal, K., Lund, E., Evensen, J. F., Vermund, H., Monge, O., & Boehler, P. (1993). Prognostic factors in patients with nasopharyngeal carcinoma. *Acta Oncologica, 32,* 531-536.

Lee, A. W., Law, S. C. K., Ng, S. H., Chan, D. K. K., Poon, Y. F., Foo, W., Tung, S. Y., Cheung, F. K., & Ho., J. H. (1992). Retrospective analysis of nasopharyngeal carcinoma treated during 1976-1985: Late complications following megavoltage irradiation. *British Journal of Radiology, 65,* 918-928.

Lee, H. P., Gourley, L., Duffy, S. W., Esteve, J., Lee, J., & Day, N. E. (1994). Preserved foods and nasopharyngeal carcinoma: A case-control study among Singapore Chinese. *International Journal of Cancer, 59,* 585-590.

Levine, P. H., McKay, F. W., & Connelly, R. R. (1987). Patterns of nasopharyngeal cancer mortality in the United States. *International Journal of Cancer, 39,* 133-137.

Liebowitz, D. (1994). Nasopharyngeal carcinoma: The Epstein-Barr virus association. *Seminars in Oncology, 21,* 376-381.

Lo, K., Mok, C., Huang, D. P., Liu, Y., Choi, P. H. K., Lee, J. C. K., & Tsao, S. (1992). p53 Mutation in human nasopharyngeal carcinomas. *Anticancer Research, 12,* 1957-1964.

Lu, S., Day, N. E., Degos, L., Lepage, V., Wang, P. C., Chan, S. H., Simons, M., McKnight, B., Easton, D., Seng, Y., & de The, G. (1990). Linkage of a nasopharyngeal carcinoma susceptibility locus to the HLA region. *Nature, 346,* 470-471.

Martin, W.M. & Shah, K.J. (1994). Carcinoma of the nasopharynx in young patients. *International Journal of Radiation Oncology, Biology, Physics, 28,* 991-999.

Mendenhall, W. M., Million, R. R., Mancuso, A. A., & Stringer, S. P. (1994). Nasopharynx. In R. R. Million & N. J. Cassisi (Eds.), *Management of head and neck cancer: A multidisciplinary approach* (2nd ed.). Philadelphia: J. B. Lippincott.

Mesic, J. B., Fletcher, G. H., & Goepfert, H. (1981). Megavoltage irradiation of epithelial tumors of the nasopharynx. *International Journal of Radiation Oncology, Biology, Physics, 7,* 447-453.

Moss, W. T. (1994). The nasopharynx. In J D. Cox (Ed.), *Moss' radiation oncology: Rationale, technique, results* (7th ed.). St. Louis: Mosby.

Muir, C., Waterhouse, J., & Mack T. (1987). *Cancer incidence in five continents, Volume V: IARC Scientific Publication No. 88.* Lyon, France: World Health Organization.

Nam, J., McLaughlin, J. K., & Blot, W.J. (1992). Cigarette smoking, alcohol, and nasopharyngeal carcinoma: A case-control study among U.S. whites. *Journal of the National Cancer Institute, 84,* 619-622.

Neel, H. B. (1985). Nasopharyngeal carcinoma: Clinical presentation, diagnosis, treatment and prognosis. *Otolaryngology Clinics of North America, 18,* 479-490.

Pao, W. J., Hustu, H. O., Douglass, E. C., Beckford, N. S., & Kun, L. E. (1989). Pediatric nasopharyngeal carcinoma: Long-term follow-up of 29 patients. *International Journal of Radiation Oncology, Biology, Physics, 17,* 299-305.

Pearson, G. R. (1993). Epstein-Barr virus and nasopharyngeal carcinoma. *Journal of Cellular Biochemistry, Supplement, 17F,* 150-154.

Perez, C. A. (1992). Nasopharynx. In C. A. Perez & L. W. Brady (Eds.), *Principles and practice of radiation oncology* (2nd ed.). Philadelphia: J. B. Lippincott.

Perez, C. A., Devineni, V. R., Marcial-Vega, V., Marks, J.E., Simpson, J. R., & Kucik, N. (1992). Carcinoma of nasopharynx: Factors affecting prognosis. *International Journal of Radiation Oncology, Biology, Physics, 23,* 271-280.

Rao, Y. & Levitt, S. (1986). Nasopharyngeal carcinoma. In D. G. McQuarrie, G. L. Adams, A. R. Shons, & G. A. Browne (Eds.), *Head and neck cancer: Clinical decisions and management principles.* Chicago: World Book.

Reese, J. L. (1996). Head and neck cancers. In R. McCorkle, M. Grant, M. Frank-Stromborg, & S. B. Baird (Eds.), *Cancer nursing: A comprehensive textbook* (2nd ed.). Philadelphia: W.B. Saunders.

Schantz, S. P., Harrison, L. B., & Hong, W. K. (1993). Cancer of the head and neck. In V. T. DeVita, Jr., S. Hellman, & S. A. Rosenberg (Eds), *Cancer: Principles and practice of oncology* (4th ed.). Philadelphia: J. B. Lippincott.

Sham, J. S. T. & Choy, D. (1991). Prognostic value of paranasopharyngeal extension of nasopharyngeal carcinoma on local control and short-term survival. *Head and Neck, 13,* 298-310.

Simons, M. J., Wee, G. B., Goh, E. H., Shanmugaratnam, K., Day, N. E., & de The, G. (1976). Immunogenetic aspects of nasopharyngeal carcinoma: IV. Increased risk in Chinese of nasophayrngeal carcinoma associated with a Chinese-related HLA profile (A2, Singapore). *Journal of the National Cancer Institute, 57,* 977-980.

Strohl, R.A. (1989). Radiation therapy for head and neck cancers. *Seminars in Oncology Nursing, 5,* 166-173.

Sweeney, P. J., Haraf, D. J., Vokes, E. E., Dougherty, M., & Weichselbaum, R. R. (1994). Radiation therapy in head and neck cancer: Indications and limitations. *Seminars in Oncology, 21,* 296-303.

Tannock, I., Payne, D., Cummings, B., Hewitt, K., Panzarella, T., Beale, F., Clark, R., Fitzpatrick, P., Garret, P., Harwood, A., Keane, T., & Rider, W. (1987). Sequential chemotherapy and radiation for nasopharyngeal cancer: Absence of long-term benefit despite a high rate of tumor response to chemotherapy. *Journal of Clinical Oncology, 5,* 629-634.

Teo, P., Leung, S. F., Yu, P., Lee, W. Y., & Shiu, W. (1991). A retrospective comparison between different stage classifications for nasopharyngeal carcinoma. *British Journal of Radiology, 64,* 901-908.

van den Brekel, M. W. M., Castelijns, J. A., & Snow, G. B. (1994). The role of modern imaging studies in staging and therapy of head and neck neoplasms. *Seminars in Oncology, 21,* 340-348.

Vokes, E. E., Weichselbaum, R. R., Lippman, S. M., & Hong, W. K. (1993). Head and neck cancer. *New England Journal of Medicine, 328*(3), 184-194.

Wang, C. C. (1997). *Radiation therapy for head and neck neoplasms* (3rd ed.). New York: Wiley-Liss.

West, S., Hildesheim, A., & Dosemeci, M. (1993). Non-viral risk factors for nasopharyngeal carcinoma in the Philippines: Results from a case-control study. *International Journal of Cancer, 55,* 722-727.

World Health Organization. (1978). *World Health Organization: International histological classification of tumors: No. 19. Histological typing of upper respiratory tract tumors.* Geneva: World Health Organization.

Yamashita, S., Kondo, M., Inuyama, Y., & Hashimoto, S. (1986). Improved survival of patients with nasopharyngeal squamous cell carcinoma. *International Journal of Radiation Oncology, Biology, Physics, 16,* 307-312.

Zheng, Y. M, Tuppin, P., Hubert, A., Jeannel, D., Pan, Y. J., Xeng, Y., & de The, G. (1994). Environmental and dietary risk factors for nasopharyngeal carcinoma: A case-control study in Zangwu County, Guangxi, China. *British Journal of Cancer, 69,* 508-514.

Ocular Cancers

Kathleen McNamara, RN, BS, OCN

EPIDEMIOLOGY

Cancers of the eye and orbit are rare, relative to the total number of estimated new cancer cases in the United States for 1998. Of the total number of estimated new cancers, only 2,100 of the nearly 1,220,000 cases will involve the eye and orbit. Male numbers will be slightly greater, accounting for 1,100 of the total cases. The estimated death rate is projected to be approximately 300 this year, with twice as many males dying as females (Landis, Murray, Bolden, & Wingo, 1998; Stephans & Shields, 1992).

Cancers that result from metastatic seeding from distant primaries are far more common and representative of the all-encompassing term *ocular malignancy* (Ferry & Font, 1974). This chapter focuses on the most common of all adult intraocular primary tumors, melanoma of the uveal tract.

RISK FACTORS

Uveal tract melanoma is the most common primary intraocular cancer in the Caucasian adult population. The incidence of intraocular melanoma in this population in the United States and Europe is about 5 to 7.5 persons per million per year. In people over 50 years of age the incidence soars to 21 persons per million. The risk for uveal melanoma has been 8 to 15 times greater in Caucasian adults than African Americans. Caucasians have a three-fold increase of intraocular melanoma over their Asian counterparts. (Other risk factors for the development of ocular melanoma are listed in Box 53-1.)

PATHOPHYSIOLOGY

Normal Anatomy of the Uveal Tract

Melanoma is defined as any group of cancers arising from melanocytes, which are cells able to make melanin. Melanomas of the uveal tract arise from the melanocytes that give pigmentation to the structures of the tract, iris, ciliary body, and choroid. The melanocytes originate in the same embryonic layer, the ectothelium, as that of the skin and conjunctiva (Loescher & Booth, 1992).

The uveal tract is divided into two portions. The anterior portion contains the iris. The ciliary body and choroid make up the posterior uveal tract.

The iris is a thin, round contractile diaphragm that lies behind the cornea and is suspended in the aqueous humor. The iris forms the circular frame for the pupil. The anterior surface of the iris is composed of flattened endothelial cells on a hyaline membrane. This pigmented portion gives characteristic color to an individual's eyes. The posterior surface of the iris is more deeply pigmented because it is lined with two layers of columnar epithelium. The iris is contiguous with the ciliary body around its circumference.

The ciliary body extends from the edges of the iris to the margin of the retina. It connects the iris with the choroid. The ciliary body contains the thickened vascular portion of the uveal tract and the ciliary muscle. This muscle holds the suspensory ligament of the lens in place.

The choroid is a thin, darkly pigmented and highly vascular membrane covering the vast majority of the posterior uveal tract. The choroid's outer surface adheres to the sclera and is attached to pigmented retinal cells on its interior surface.

Histology and Prognostic Factors of Uveal Melanomas

Major cell types composing uveal melanomas were first recognized by Callender (1931). His work on cell histology led to a system of cellular classification that had a degree of prognostic significance for patients post enucleation. Three categories of cell types characterized by Callender were identified. He described Spindle A cells as uniform, cohesive cells with nuclei that are small, slender, and spindle-shaped. Mitotic figures are rare, and no distinct nucleoli are present. He described Spindle B cells as plumper, cohesive, spindle-shaped cells with larger, oval nuclei that contain a chromatin network and a nucleolus. Often, mitotic figures

Box 53-1
Risk Factors for Ocular Melanoma

- Increasing age
- Ethnicity
- Family history
- Exposure to ambient solar ultraviolet radiation
- Hormonal influence, such as estrogen exposure (i.e., pregnancy and/or estrogen replacement)
- Ocular nevi
- Metal exposure (nickel, platinum, radium)

Data from Sahel, J. A., Earle, J. D., & Albert, D. M. (1997). Intraocular melanoma. In V. T. DeVita, S. Hellman, & S. A. Rosenberg, (Eds.), *Cancer: Principles and practice of oncology.* (5th ed.) Philadelphia: J. B. Lippincott.

Table 53-1 Uveal Melanoma Cell Type Morphology and Prognosis

Spindle A cells	• Cohesive • Small nuclei • Indistinct nucleoli • Rare mitotic figures	• Slow growing • Low malignant potential
Spindle B cells	• Cohesive yet plump • Oval nuclei • ± Chromatin network • Nucleolus present • Mitotic figures seen	• Slow growing • Greater malignant potential due to increased mitotic activity
Epithelioid cells	• Poorly cohesive • Larger • Round nuclei with single or multiple nucleoli • Abundant mitotic figures	• Greatest malignant potential due to increasingly aneuploid morphology

Data from Sahel, J. A., Earle, J. D., & Albert, D. M. (1993). Intraocular melanoma. In V. T. DeVita, S. Hellman, & S. A. Rosenberg (Eds.), *Cancer: Principles and practice of oncology.* (4th ed.) Philadelphia: J. B. Lippincott.

are seen. Epithelioid cells are poorly cohesive, are larger in size, and are increasingly pleomorphic. They contain eosinophilic cytoplasm. The cells are polygonal and have round nuclei with single or multiple nucleoli. Mitotic figures are found in abundance (Table 53-1).

Three categories of tumor types were derived through Callender's work. They are Spindle cell melanomas types A and B, or A/B; mixed cell melanomas containing spindle and epithelioid cells; and epithelioid cell melanoma.

Callender's (1931) work relating cell type and prognosis was further supported by Gamel and McLean (1984). Using computed cytomorphology of the uveal melanoma, the nucleolar area was measured and evaluated statistically. Later work incorporated the mean measurement of the ten largest nucleoli seen in the specimen. This is thought to be an objective and reliable determinant of a tumor's malignant potential. This finding reinforced Callender's thought that a tumor with greater epithelioid content signaled a poorer prognosis (Coleman, Baak, van Diest, & Mullaney, 1996). Lesions that extended into the sclera, involved the ciliary body, or exceeded 10 mm at its largest dimension also related to poor prognostic features (Sahel, Earle, & Albert, 1993).

MELANOMA OF THE ANTERIOR UVEAL TRACT

Melanoma of the Iris

Melanoma of the iris is the most common primary malignancy of the iris. It is also the most rare uveal tract melanoma, followed by that of the ciliary body and choroid (Geisse & Robertson, 1985; Bomanji, Hungerford, Granowska, & Britton, 1987).

Melanomas of the iris are usually small at the time of diagnosis. Frequently, a patient or family member notices a change in the shape, color, or pigmented irregularity of the affected iris, often prompting a physician's evaluation. Lesions of the iris are thought to be relatively benign for the following reasons. First, these lesions are often discovered while very small. Small lesion size is suggestive of a slower rate of growth (Kersten, Tse, & Anderson, 1985). Second, these lesions are comprised predominately of Spindle A cell type (Shields, 1983), which have low malignancy potential, as discussed previously in this chapter. Metastasis of anterior uveal tract melanoma is rare due to decreased vascularity of the area, absence of lymphatic channels, and cell type.

ROUTES OF METASTASES

Melanoma of the uveal tract can metastasize in two ways. Disease can travel by the hematogenous route, with the liver being the major organ of spread, followed by the lungs. Disease may also travel by direct extension into surrounding tissue. Melanoma of the iris spreads by direct extension in its early stages. If detected very late, it may gain access to the bloodstream or lymphatic channels. However, iris melanoma is thought to be relatively benign because of its favorable cell histology and frequency of early detection.

Posterior uveal tract melanomas have a greater propensity to metastasize than those of the iris. The choroid and ciliary body are contiguous with major intraocular structures such as the sclera and retina, allowing for direct extension of the tumor into these areas. The posterior uveal tract is highly vascular, with evidence of hematogenous spread most frequently found in the liver (Zimmerman, 1986). Approximately 2% of patients with posterior uveal tract melanoma have metastatic disease at the time of diagnosis (Gragoudas, Egan, Seddon, Glynn, Walsh, & Finn, 1991; Pach & Robertson, 1986).

ASSESSMENT OF MELANOMA OF THE IRIS

Melanomas of the anterior uveal tract can most often be successfully managed with a conservative approach. Evaluation of the lesion includes careful examination and ophthal-

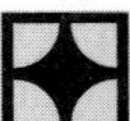

TABLE 53-2 Assessment of the Patient for Intraocular Melanoma

	Assessment Parameters	Typical Abnormal Findings
History	A. Personal and social history	A. Personal and social risk factors 1. Older age 2. Caucasian 3. Positive family history 4. Estrogen exposure (pregnancy or estrogen replacement) 5. Exposure to nickel, platinum, radium
	B. Evaluation of the eye	B. Patient may notice change in the shape, color, or pigment irregularity of iris.
Physical examination	A. Ophthalmologic examination through a dilated pupil	A. Astute clinical evaluation is optimal for early diagnoses. Lesion may be visible on examination.
Diagnostic tests	A. Fluorescein angiography	A. Orange lesion over tumor margin and bright pigment changes. Notes irregular vascular pattern of lesion.
	B. Slit lamp and gonioscopy inspection with slit lamp photography	B. Documents baseline tumor size and location.
	C. Ultrasound	C. Confirms diagnosis and differentiates between hemangiomas and metastatic melanomas.
	D. Fine-needle biopsy	D. Not reliable and rarely done
	E. Immunologic testings	E. Not reliable and rarely done

Data from Sahel, J. A., Earle, J. D., & Albert, D. M. (1997). Intraocular melanoma. In V. T. DeVita, S. Hellman, & S. A. Rosenberg (Eds.), *Cancer: Principles and practice of oncology.* (5th ed.) Philadelphia: J. B. Lippincott.

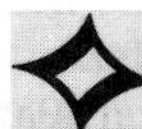

TABLE 53-3 Patient Preparation for a Fluorescein Angiography

Purpose of Procedure: A fluorescein angiography is a specialized procedure used in the diagnosis, monitoring, and treatment of the eye. The test is safe and takes approximately 1 hour to complete.

Patient Preparation:

1. Explain the procedure to the patient.
2. Query the patient about allergies to contrast media.
3. Obtain informed consent.

Procedural Considerations:

1. The pupil is dilated with special eyedrops so that the fundus of the eye is more visible for examination.
2. Fluorescein contrast is injected intravenously and travels the arteries in the eyes to visualize possible abnormalities.
3. Photographs are taken with a specially designed camera called a *fundus camera.*
4. The patient is placed in a chair with a chin rest, with the forehead placed against a bar, while a rapid series of photographs are taken to see the movement of dye in the eyes. Patients are asked to keep their head still and move their eyes only when instructed by the ophthalmic photographer.

Special Considerations:

1. The patient may experience the following:
   a. Temporary deceased visual acuity after the photographs because of the dazzled effect from the flashing lights.
   b. Light sensitivity for several hours after the test due to the dilation. Instruct the patient to avoid bright light and wear sunglasses until normal vision returns, usually in a few hours.
   c. Jaundiced skin and urine 24 hours after the test from the contrast media. Instruct the patient to drink at least eight glasses of water 12 hours after the test.

Data from Allen, M. (1995). Assessment of the visual system. In W. J. Phipps, V. L. Cassmeyer, J. K. Sands, & M. K. Lehman (Eds.), *Medical-surgical nursing: Concepts and clinical practice.* (5th ed.) St. Louis: Mosby.

mologic studies (Table 53-2). Baseline assessment includes size, location, and vascular properties of the lesion. Fluorescein angiography evaluates vascular patterns of the lesion. Slit lamp and gonioscopy inspection with serial slit lamp photography document the baseline tumor size and location. These parameters govern treatment at the time of diagnosis. Changes in these baseline measurements may warrant more aggressive approaches than frequent, careful observation. (Table 53-3 illustrates a teaching tool for patients having a fluorescein angiography.) However, observation of this tumor is quite acceptable when certain criteria are met. Sahel, Earle, and Albert (1993) have listed the following favorable observation criteria:

- No evidence of growth in size of lesion
- No evidence of increased vascularization of cornea
- Vision not compromised by lesion
- No evidence of complication, such as hemorrhage into anterior chamber, glaucoma due to pressure, or obvious involvement of other structures such as lymph node
- Vision only in affected eye
- Location of the lesion near the pupil

Medical Treatment

For patients in whom tumor growth has been documented, excisional surgery is indicated. Iridectomy is performed to remove the portion of the iris containing the tumor. Surgical expertise is critical to prevent tumor cell dissemination into the eye or incision. If the trabeculae become involved, clearly the tumor is growing. The trabecula is the area of the eye in the angle of the iris and cornea (Sahel et al., 1997). Secondary glaucoma may develop as a result. This condition necessitates iridotrabeculectomy because blindness may occur as a consequence of glaucoma (Territo, Shields, Shields, Augsburger, & Schroeder, 1988).

If the ciliary body is involved at the time of diagnosis, an iridocyclectomy is performed. Tumors that invade the cornea or fill the anterior chamber angle in addition to the ciliary body should be more aggressively excised. Sahel, Earle, and Albert (1993) cite enucleation as the prudent course of treatment for melanoma of the iris under the following conditions:

1. More than half the iris is involved, and the anterior chamber angle is also affected.
2. The tumor is too bulky to be handled by excision. (The affected eye is blind.)
3. Cell histology shows increased malignant potential, thereby signaling increased risk of recurrence.
4. The tumor has recurred despite previous surgical removal.

MELANOMA OF THE POSTERIOR UVEAL TRACT

Melanoma of the Ciliary Body and Choroid

Melanomas of the posterior uveal tract present a greater challenge to the patient, physician, and nurse than those of the iris. These lesions are less likely to be diagnosed early and may contain a larger percentage of mixed cells or epithelioid cells, which have greater malignant potential (Gamel, McCurdy, & McLean, 1992). Ciliary body and choroid tumors are most often diagnosed on clinical examination after pupil dilatation. Photographing the fundus is useful in detecting and evaluating nevi and small malignant melanomas with the fluorescein dye. Angiography may be helpful in differentiating tumors from other nonmalignant conditions such as choroid hemorrhage or in identifying a metastatic carcinoma from a distant primary. Ultrasonography can be useful in distinguishing characteristic melanoma patterns from other space-occupying lesions. Computed tomography may detect a tumor that has extended into extraocular tissue or the optic nerve.

Small Melanomas of the Posterior Uveal Tract

The tumor size at the time of diagnosis plays an important part in determining treatment and can be prognostic, as mentioned previously. Lesions are carefully measured at the initial diagnosis for elevation and basal size. Small tumors measure 2 to 2.5 mm elevated and $<$16 mm at the base. Medium tumors measure $\geq$2.5 to $\leq$10 mm elevated and $<$16 mm at the base, whereas large tumors are $>$10 mm elevated and $>$16 mm at the base (Sahel, Earle, & Albert, 1993).

For small tumors of the ciliary body or choroid, observation may be the treatment of choice. Observation every 3 months is prudent for tumors that appear to be quiescent, are asymptomatic to the patient, or occur in the patient's only useful eye. More aggressive treatment is warranted when a small tumor increases in size beyond 3 mm in elevation and 10 mm at the base or if the tumor is rapidly growing.

Visual impairment, which has not been noted previously, may also signal the need for increasingly aggressive therapy to preserve the patient's sight. When observation is no longer an option, radiation therapy offers an additional treatment modality. Excellent short-term survival has been achieved using radioactive applicators of Cobalt-60 or Iodine-125 sources. However, no long-term survival data is available at this time (Packer, Stoller, Lesser, Mandel, & Finger, 1992). Comparable encouraging results have been reported using β particles from Rubidium-106 and Ruthenium applicators (Lommatzsch, 1983).

Enucleation of a patient's eye is recommended if the lesion is rapidly growing or is nearing the optic nerve. The eye should be enucleated if extraocular spread is suspected. The decision of enucleation must take into account the patient's visual prospects after the procedure and the patient's decision after informed consent. Box 53-2 lists factors influencing prognostic indicators and affecting enucleation (Shammas & Blodi, 1977).

Medium Melanomas of the Posterior Uveal Tract

Medium melanomas have posed a dilemma among clinicians regarding the optimal treatment approach. Although observation is acceptable in small lesions and large lesions have a clear treatment mandate, these lesions do not.

Because no treatment plan is universally embraced as most favored, medium choroidal melanoma is the subject of clinical trials. The Collaborative Ocular Melanoma Study (COMS) is currently comparing enucleation to Iodine-125 plaque irradiation for treatment of these lesions. Irradiation

Box 53-2
Significant Factors Influencing Prognosis of Posterior Uveal Tract Melanoma after Enucleation

- Age of patient at enucleation
- Location of tumor
- Location of anterior border of tumor
- Largest diameter of tumor in contact with sclera
- Height and basal measurement of tumor
- Integrity of Bruch's membrane
- Cell type composition of tumor
- Scleral infiltration by tumor

From Shammas, H. F., & Blodi, F. C. (1977). Prognostic factors in choroidal and ciliary body melanoma. *Archives of Ophthalmology, 95*(1), 63-69.

may be a viable alternative to progressive disease in patients who refuse enucleation or have vision only in the affected eye (Fine, 1996).

Large Melanomas of the Posterior Uveal Tract

Enucleation remains the standard method of treatment for large choroidal melanomas. However, owing to advances in radiation therapy techniques, the COMS has sought to compare enucleation with enucleation preceded by external beam irradiation. COMS has enrolled more than 1,000 patients since 1994. It is hoped that long-term survival data may be enhanced by the addition of irradiation to the area preoperatively. This may furnish clinicians with definitive information needed for optimal patient outcomes (Fine, 1996).

NURSING MANAGEMENT

Nursing care of the patient with a uveal tract melanoma clearly depends on the treatment of choice (Table 53-4).

Observation of clinically stable tumors requires scrupulous baseline documentation by the nurse of the size and location of the anterior uveal tract. The nurse should report any increase in size or number of lesions to the patient's physician. Stable tumors are evaluated approximately every 3 months, as described previously. Patients and/or caregivers should be educated to report their observations of changes as soon as they observe them. Changes in visual acuity or feelings of pain or pressure experienced by the patient should be reported immediately. These may be indicative of tumor growth or the development of secondary glaucoma.

Patients who require surgical resection of the lesions and affected tissue require nursing care similar to all surgical patients (see Chapter 3). Information about the disease process, the need for surgical intervention, and an explanation of the procedure should all be included in the patient's and caregivers' surgical experience.

Patients receiving radiation therapy as treatment for their disease should be cared for in accordance with established nursing practice for the specific type of radiation the patient will receive (Chapter 4).

EVALUATION OF THE QUALITY OF CARE

Accreditation organizations, such as the Joint Commission for the Accreditation of Health Care Organizations, require that the quality of care provided to patients be evaluated. Because the care provided to patients with ocular cancer requires input from a multidisciplinary team, an evaluation of the quality of care provided to these patients should include aspects of care provided by various members of the team. (Table 53-5 provides evaluation tools that can be used in the inpatient and outpatient setting.)

PROGNOSTIC FACTORS

A number of key factors influence prognosis and treatment for patients with uveal melanoma. The size of the tumor is most crucial when planning treatment despite the location of the lesion. Size may determine whether a tumor can be carefully observed at specific intervals, surgically excised, or treated with enucleation. Tumor location is another important consideration when planning treatment. A certain location of a lesion may allow for surgical excision or deem enucleation necessary to preserve the patient's sight. Cell type, discussed earlier, is critical to planning treatment because of its influence on malignant potential and the patient's prognosis. The presence or absence of extraocular disease also dictates treatment decisions and prognosis (see Box 53-2) (Gragoudas, Seddon, Egan, Glynn, Goitein, & Munzenrider, 1988).

RESEARCH ISSUES IN OCULAR MELANOMA

In addition to the COMS trials, other areas of concern are being investigated. Diagnosis of ocular melanoma is being further fine-tuned for accuracy using technetium-99m (^{99m}TC) tagged cutaneous melanoma antibody fragment (Bomanji et al., 1987). The authors of the study sought to differentiate ocular melanoma from similar lesions by using monoclonal antibodies and immunoscintigraphy. The results show this imaging method may have a part to play in differentiating uveal melanomas from other similar tumors.

Prevention of metastasis and subsequent treatment of liver metastases are being investigated. Marble (1997) describes the research being done according to which uveal melanoma metastasis is being inhibited. Using gene-transfer techniques, plasminogen activator inhibitor type 1 is injected directly into intraocular spaces of clinically relevant models. Metastasis is prevented by disrupting plasminogen activator function, which promotes invasion of tissue barriers. This research could have a great effect on the prevention of liver metastases, most deadly to the patient with uveal tract melanoma.

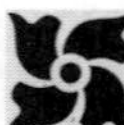

TABLE 53-4 Standard of Care for the Patient Undergoing Enucleation

Patient Problems and Outcomes	Nursing Interventions and Rationales	Patient Education Instructions
Anxiety Patient will: • Verbalize an understanding of the surgical procedure. • Express feelings of decreased anxiety. • Identify strategies to cope with anxiety.	1. Assess the patient's level of understanding of the surgical procedure. 2. Give the patient the opportunity to ask questions or verbalize concerns. 3. Determine which coping strategies the patient has used effectively in the past to decrease anxiety, and reinforce the use of these coping mechanisms. 4. Administer relaxation techniques, visual imagery, and pharmacologic agents, if necessary.	1. Use a diagram of the anatomy of the eye to explain enucleation. 2. Orient the patient to the components of the postoperative room and locating personal belongings after surgery. 3. Prepare the patient for diminished eyesight. 4. Provide the patient with information about the preoperative routine: a. Facial scrubs b. Anesthesiology consultation c. NPO after midnight 5. Teach the patient deep-breathing exercises, and obtain a return demonstration. 6. Provide the patient with information about the postoperative plan of care: a. Pain management b. Intravenous fluids
Pain Patient will: • Experience optimal pain relief with minimal side effects.	1. Assess the pain intensity using a 0 to 10 verbal rating scale, every 2-4 hours for the first 48 hours after surgery, then at least once a shift. 2. Administer opioid analgesics around-the-clock for the first 24-48 hours postoperatively. 3. Monitor for analgesic side effects, and administer medications to prevent or treat the following: a. Nausea. b. Pruritus. c. Constipation.	1. Teach the patient to inform the nurse if he or she is experiencing pain. 2. Teach the patient the importance of taking pain medication regularly to keep pain under control.
High Risk for Infection	1. Change dressings with aseptic technique. Administer antibiotics as directed. 2. Take vital signs q4h.	1. Teach the patient to report shaking chills.
High Risk for Meningitis Due to Thrombosis of Blood Vessels	1. Assess the patient for pain on the operative side of the head.	1. Teach the patient to report pain on the operative side of the head immediately.
High Risk for Hemorrhage	1. Apply pressure dressing for 1 or 2 days to help control possible hemorrhage.	1. Teach the patient to report loosening of the dressing, so that the dressings can be reinforced.
High Risk for Depression Due to Visual Impairment	1. Arrange for social support and education classes for the visually impaired. Arrange for prostatic eyes, if the patient desires. 2. Prepare the patient to adjust to monovision in activities of daily living.	1. Teach the patient the necessity of social and emotional support. 2. Teach the patient about supportive organizations such as the Lions Eye Bank and referrals to occupational therapists.

Data from Allen, M. (1995.) Assessment of the visual system. In W. J. Phipps, V. L. Cassmeyer, J. K. Sands, & M. K. Lehman (Eds.), *Medical-surgical nursing: Concepts and clinical practice* (5th ed.). St. Louis: Mosby.

TABLE 53-5 Quality of Care Evaluation for a Patient Having a Placement of a Prosthetic Eye

Disciplines participating in the quality of care evaluation:
☐ Nursing ☐ Physician ☐ Occupational Therapists

Data from:
☐ Medical Record Review ☐ Patient/Family Interview

Criteria	YES	NO
1. Patient provided with information about the following:		
a. Removing and cleaning a prosthetic eye	☐	☐
b. Guidelines for care of the prosthetic eye	☐	☐
c. Wearing of a protective patch or goggle when swimming, diving, or water skiing	☐	☐
d. Signs and symptoms of infection	☐	☐
e. Measures to adjust to loss of eye	☐	☐
f. Names, addresses, and phone numbers of support groups in your area	☐	☐

Patient/Family Satisfaction

Data from: ☐ Patient Interview ☐ Family Interview

Criteria	YES	NO
1. On a scale of 0 to 10, with 0 being totally dissatisfied and 10 being totally satisfied, how satisfied were you with the care you received during your surgery? ________		
2. Were you told to call the nurse if you experienced pain on the operative side of your head?	☐	☐
3. Were you given information on support groups in your area to help you adjust to your partial loss of vision?	☐	☐
4. Were you given clear instructions to orient yourself to your hospital room so that you could find your belongings and the bathroom after your surgery?	☐	☐
5. Did you feel you were given adequate instructions about the care of your prosthesis?	☐	☐

REFERENCES

Allen, M. Assessment of the visual system. In W. J. Phipps, V. L. Cassmeyer, J. K. Sands, & M. K. Lehman (Eds.), *Medical-surgical nursing: Concepts and clinical practice.* (5th ed.). St. Louis: Mosby.

Beras, O. H. & Myer, M. H. (1983). *Manual for staging cancer* (2nd ed.). Philadelphia: J. B. Lippincott.

Bomanji, J., Hungerford, J. L., Granowska, M., & Britton, K. E. (1987). Radioimmunoscintigraphy of ocular melanoma with 99ntC labeled cutaneous melanoma antibody fragments. *British Journal of Ophthalmology, 71*(9), 651-658.

Callender, G. R. (1931). Malignant melanotic tumors of the eye: A study of histologic types in 111 cases. *Transactions—American Academy of Ophthalmology and Otolaryngology, 3,* 131-142.

Coleman, K., Baak, J. P., van Diest, P. J., & Mullaney, J. (1996). Prognostic value of morphometric features and the Callender classification in uveal melanoma. *Ophthalmology, 103*(10), 1634-1641.

Ferry, A. P. & Font, R. L. (1974). Carcinoma metastatic to the eye and orbit: A clinicopathologic study of 227 cases. *Archives of Ophthalmology, 92,* 276-286.

Fine, S. L. (1996). No one knows the preferred management for choroidal melanoma. [Editorial]. *American Journal of Ophthalmology, 122* (July), 106.

Gamel, J. W. & McLean, I. W. (1984). Modern developments in histopathologic assessment of uveal melanomas. *Ophthalmology, 91*(6), 679-684.

Gamel, J. W., McCurdy, J. B., & McLean, I. W. (1992). A comparison of prognostic covariants for uveal melanoma. *Investigative Ophthalmology and Visual Science, 33*(6), 1919-1922.

Geisse, L. J. & Robertson, D. M. (1985). Iris melanomas. *American Journal of Ophthalmology, 99*(6), 638-648.

Gragoudas, E. S., Egan, K. M., Seddon, J. M., Glynn, R. J., Walsh, S. M., & Finn, S. M. (1991). Survival of patients with metastases from uveal melanoma. *Ophthalmology, 98*(3), 383-390.

Gragoudas, E. S., Seddon, J. M., Egan, K. M., Glynn, R. J., Goitein, M., & Munzenrider, J. (1988). Metastasis from uveal melanoma after proton beam irradiation. *Ophthalmology, 95*(7), 992-999.

Kersten, R. C., Tse, D., & Andersen, D. R. (1985). Iris melanoma: Nevus or malignancy? *Survey of Ophthalmology, 29,* 423-433.

Landis, S. H., Murray, T., Bolden, S., & Wingo, P. A. (1998). Cancer statistics 1998. *Ca-A Journal for Clinicians, 48,* No. 1, 6-10.

Loescher, J. J. & Booth, A. (1992). Skin cancer. In S. L. Groenwald, M. Goodman, M. Frogge, & C. Yarbro (Eds.), *Cancer nursing principles and practice.* Boston: Jones and Bartlett.

Lommotzsch, P. K. (1983). Beta irradiation of choroidal melanoma with 106 Ru/106 Rh applicators: 16 years experience. *Archives of Ophthalmology, 101*(5), 713-717.

Marble, M. (1997). Intraocular melanomas offer excellent target for gene therapy. *Cancer Weekly Plus,* Oct. 27, 2-7.

Pach, J. M. & Robertson, D. M. (1986). Metastases from untreated uveal melanoma. *Archives of Ophthalmology, 104,* 1624-1625.

Packer, S., Stoller, S., Lesser, M. L., Mandel, F. S., & Finger, P. T. (1992). Long-term results of iodine 125 irradiation of uveal melanoma. *Ophthalmology, 99*(5), 767-774.

Sahel, J. A., Earle, J. D., & Albert, D. M. (1993). Intraocular melanoma. In V. T. DeVita, S. Hellman, & S. A. Rosenberg (Eds.), *Cancer, principles and practice of oncology.* Philadelphia: J. B. Lippincott.

Shammas, H. F. & Blodi, F. C. (1977). Prognostic factors in choroidal and ciliary body melanoma. *Archives of Ophthalmology, 95*(1), 63-69.

Shields, J. A. (1983). Melanocytic tumors of the iris. In *Diagnosis and management of intraocular tumors.* St. Louis: Mosby.

Stephens, R. F. & Shields, C. L. (1992). *Intraocular tumors: A text and atlas.* Philadelphia: W. B. Saunders.

Stephens, R. F. & Shields, J. A. (1979). Diagnosis and management of cancers metastatic to the uvea: A study of 70 cases. *Ophthalmology, 86,* 1336-1349.

Territo, C., Shields, C. L., Shields, J. A., Augsburger, J. J., & Schroeder, R. P. (1988). Natural course of melanocytic tumors of the iris. *Ophthalmology, 95,* 1251.

Thibodeau, G. A. & Patton, K. T. (1996). *Anatomy & physiology* (3rd ed.). St. Louis: Mosby.

Zimmerman, L. E. (1986). Malignant melanomas of the uveal tract. In W. H. Spencer (Ed.), *Ophthalmologic pathology.* Philadelphia: W. B. Saunders.

Oral Cavity Cancer

Mikaela Olsen, RN, MS

EPIDEMIOLOGY

Oral cancers, which include oral and oropharyngeal carcinomas, account for approximately 6% of all cancers diagnosed each year in the United States (Alvi, Myers, & Johnson, 1996). An estimated 30,300 new cases of oral cancer were diagnosed in 1998 (Landis, Murray, Bolden, & Wingo, 1998). Approximately 8,000 deaths occurred in 1998 as a result of oral cancer (Landis, Murray, Bolden, & Wingo, 1998). Oral cancer is primarily a disease of the elderly, occurring in the sixth and seventh decades of life in many instances (Goodman, Yellowitz, & Horowitz, 1995). The incidence of oral cancer is expected to rise as our aging population increases (Wong & Feussner, 1994).

Oral cancer occurs more often in men than women by 2:1. Because of the increased use of tobacco in women since the 1950s, there has been an increased incidence in oral cancer in this population (Fig. 54-1). Overall relative 5-year survival rates for oral cancer have increased slightly over the past 30 years from 45% to 55% in Caucasians. The overall relative 5-year survival rate for African Americans is 33% (American Cancer Society, 1996). This difference may be related to limited access to health care or socioeconomic status. Higher mortality rates from oral cancer occur in people with little or no access to health care (Smart, 1993). In general, the populations included are those with low financial income, low education, age greater than 65 years, minority status, and those who lack private health insurance (Bloom, Gift, & Jack, 1992). Furthermore, Medicare and Medicaid do not cover oral health care or screening. People with poor access to health care are often involved in high-risk behaviors, putting them at greater risk for oral cancer.

In other countries the incidence of oral cancer is much higher than that in the United States. In countries of the Far East (Singapore, Hong Kong) and Europe (France, Hungary), age-adjusted death rates from oral cancer are triple those in the United States (Dibb, Urba, & Wolf, 1995). Approximately 50% of all cancers in India are of the oral cavity. In France, oral cancer is the third most common cause of cancer in the male population and the second most common cause of cancer death (Jensen, Esteve, Moller, & Renard, 1990). The widespread habit of betel quid chewing has led to the increased incidence of oral cancer in India and other parts of southeast Asia. Betel quid contains tobacco and a component called *slaked lime.* In addition to tobacco being a known etiologic factor in the development of oral cancer, slaked lime has also been implicated.

The initial diagnosis of oral cancer usually occurs in the more advanced stages, limiting the efficacy of current treatment options. In the early stages, oral cancer responds well to surgery or radiation therapy and is highly curable. Unfortunately, oral cancers are not diagnosed in most cases until they have advanced. Trends over the past 10 years have shown little alteration in incidence, survival, or mortality (Silverman, 1994).

It has been estimated that the costs for treatment and rehabilitation of patients with oral cancer are greater than half a billion dollars annually. Oral cancer is a preventable disease in most cases. Approximately 75% to 80% of all squamous cell carcinomas of the oral cavity are a result of tobacco and alcohol use (Blot, McLaughlin, Winn, Austin, Greenburg, & Preston-Martin et al., 1988; Thomas, 1995). As is the case with lung cancer, mortality could be drastically reduced with the cessation of tobacco use and the use of alcohol only moderately.

RISK FACTORS

The major known risk factors for oral cancer as well as potential risk factors are listed in Table 54-1. Increasing age, tobacco, and alcohol are major risk factors for the development of oral cavity cancer (Binnie, Rankin, & MacKenzie, 1983; Blot et al., 1988; Boffetta, Mashberg, Winklemann, & Garfinkel, 1992; Miller, 1983).

Increasing Age

Greater than 95% of all oral cancers occur in people over 40 years of age. The average age at the time of diagnosis is 63 years (Alvi, Myers, & Johnson, 1996). Compounding this is the fact that the number of people age 65 years or greater is

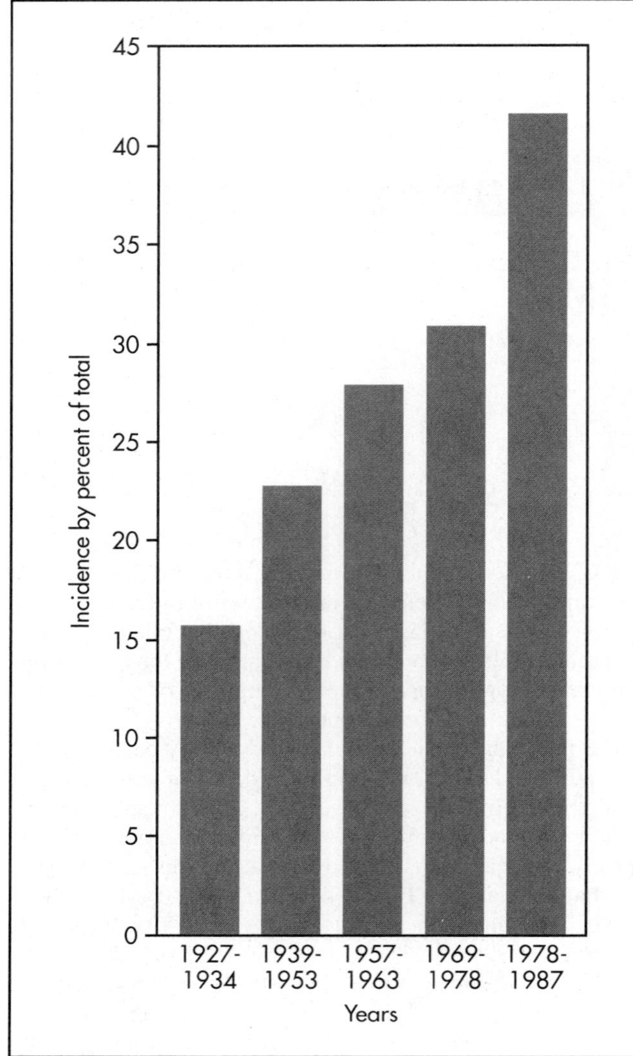

Fig. 54-1 Increasing incidence of squamous cell carcinoma of the oral cavity in females. (From Shah, J. P. & Lydiatt, W. [1995]. Treatment of head and neck cancer. *CA: Cancer Journal for Clinicians, 45*[6], 354; data from Franceschi, D., Gupta, R., Spiro, R. H., & Shah, J.P. [1993]. Improved survival in the treatment of squamous carcinoma of the oral tongue. *American Journal of Surgery, 166,* 36-365.)

around 30 million in the United States today and rising (Silverman, 1994). This population must be carefully evaluated for factors that could further affect the risk for oral cancer.

Tobacco Use

Tobacco as an etiologic factor in the development of oral cancer is demonstrated well throughout the literature (Boffetta et al., 1992). Worldwide, there are over 1 billion smokers and 600 million tobacco chewers (Centers for Disease Control, 1993). The use of tobacco in any form, including pipe smoking, tobacco chewing, and cigarette smoking, increases the risk of oral cancer. Cancer risks are 5 to 25 times higher for heavy smokers compared with nonsmokers. The use of nonfiltered cigarettes increases the risk of oral cancer (Rothman, Cann, Flanders, & Fried, 1980).

Table 54-1 Risk Factors of Oral Cancer

Known	Potential
Increasing age	Lower socioeconomic status
Alcohol use (past and present)	Poor oral hygiene
Exposure to sun (lip)	Spicy foods
Tobacco—cigarettes, cigars, pipes, chewing tobacco, snuff	Alcohol-based mouthwashes
	HSV1
Occupation—plumbers, workers in steel, textiles, coal, and metal	HPV

HPV, Human papilloma virus; HSV1, herpes simplex virus type 1.
Modified from Spitz, M. (1995). Risk factors and genetic susceptibility. In W. K. Hong & R. S. Weber (Eds.), *Head and neck cancers.* Boston: Kluwer Academic.

Synergistic effects of tobacco and alcohol are well demonstrated (Mashberg, Garfinkel, & Harris, (1981). In 1988, the International Agency for Research on Cancer concluded from research studies that tobacco was carcinogenic to humans. People who quit smoking show a steady decline in the risk of oral cancer. The risk can equal that of nonsmokers after 15 years of cessation.

Throughout the world, tobacco is used in many different variations. As previously mentioned, tobacco in betel quid is responsible for a large number of oral cancers in Asia. The most frequent sites of occurrence in these populations are the buccal mucosa, anterior tongue, and oropharynx. In betel quid users who also smoke tobacco, the risk of developing oral cancer is 23 to 35 times higher (Moore, 1971; Reichart, 1995).

In the past 20 years, smokeless tobacco use has nearly tripled. This form of tobacco is not only highly addictive, it contains major carcinogens (Department of Health and Human Services, 1992). The amount of nicotine in smokeless tobacco is 2 to 15 times greater than that of cigarettes. Smokeless tobacco can not only cause oral cancer, but can also lead to nicotine addiction. The public education regarding the use of smokeless tobacco should stress the importance of not substituting this form of tobacco for cigarettes. The use of smokeless tobacco is most common in people ages 18 to 24 and is associated with low socioeconomic status (Spangler & Salisbury, 1995). It has been estimated that 24% of white male high school students use smokeless tobacco. Risk factors for use of smokeless tobacco include white or native American; male; use by family members, peers or role models; or participation in baseball leagues (Spangler & Salisbury, 1995). In young native Americans, the use of smokeless tobacco is a cultural factor and begins as early as kindergarten. Clearly, the use of smokeless tobacco among people of any age is a health hazard.

The risk of buccal mucosa and gingival cancer in smokeless tobacco users is 50 times that of nonusers (Spitz, 1995). Cancer of the floor of the mouth is seen much more frequently in people who use snuff compared with nonusers. The development of oral leukoplakia in smokeless tobacco users should be scrutinized carefully as a premalignant lesion. Oral leukoplakias are discussed in more detail under the assessment of patients section.

The role of marijuana as a carcinogenic agent is unknown. It has been difficult to study as a single agent due to the fact that many marijuana users also use tobacco and alcohol. However, it has been postulated to have carcinogenic effects similar to those of tobacco.

Alcohol Use

Alcohol is thought to impair the ability of cells to repair deoxyribonucleic (DNA) damage. In combination with smoking, alcohol may potentiate the carcinogenic effects of tobacco. Alcohol is associated with a higher risk of oral cancer, particularly in people who also use tobacco (Choi & Kahyo, 1991). In a large study the risk of oral cancer was multiplied with an increased number of drinks per week in men and women (Blot et al., 1988).

An increased risk of oral cancer in regular and heavy users of alcohol has been established. The International Agency for Research on Cancer published a review of pertinent studies in 1988. Of the 10 studies reviewed, all demonstrated the correlation between alcohol and oral cancers. Heavy alcohol use is a common finding in patients diagnosed with oropharyngeal cancers (Civantos & Goodwin, 1996).

The correlation between oral cancer and excessive alcohol consumption was first noticed when assessing its incidence in individuals who worked in the alcohol trading industry (Blot et al., 1988). Alcohol has been implicated in the development of oral cancer in nonsmokers. It was suggested that alcohol may be contaminated with carcinogens. Hard liquor, wine, and beer consumption have all been linked to oral cancer. As the use of alcohol and tobacco increase, the risk of squamous cell carcinoma of the oral cavity rises significantly (Fig. 54-2). Heavy alcohol and tobacco users have a six-fold to fifteen-fold risk of oral cavity cancer (Mashberg & Samit, 1995). Alcohol consumed in large quantities is commonly associated with improper nutritional intake, thereby decreasing the protective effects of antioxidant nutrients. Liver damage due to excessive alcohol use may impair the liver's ability to detoxify the potential carcinogenic components of alcohol. When liver function is diminished and nutritional status is altered as a result of heavy alcohol use, this situation may promote immune suppression, further placing the patient at risk (Thomas, 1995).

Of interest, Mashberg & Samit (1995) also found that if a smoker doubles the amount of alcohol consumed, the risk of oral cancer is significantly greater than if the smoker doubles the number of cigarettes.

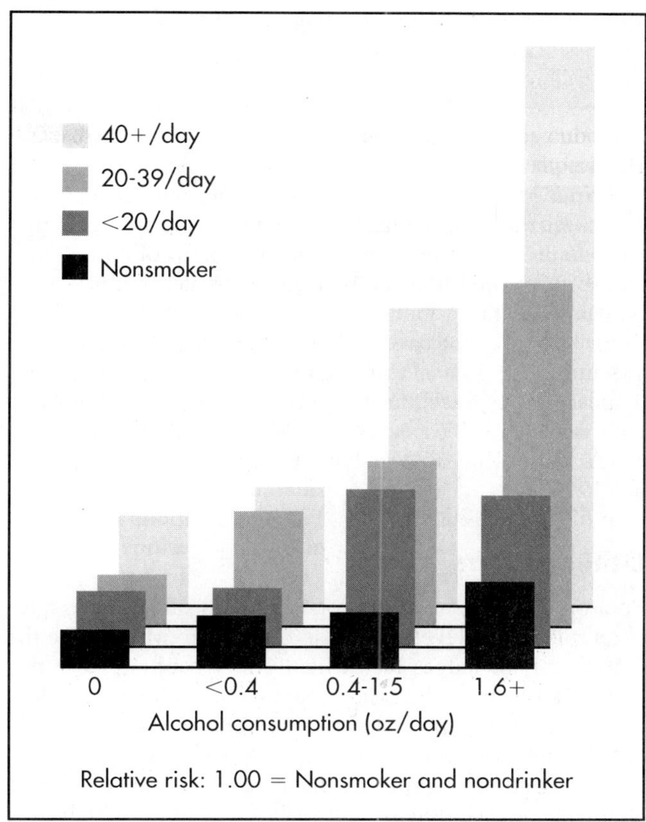

Fig. 54-2 Relative risk of cancer as it relates to tobacco and alcohol usage. (From Shah, J. P. & Lydiatt, W. [1995]. Treatment of head and neck cancer. *CA: Cancer Journal for Clinicians, 45*[6], 355; data from Rothman, K. & Keller, A. [1972]. The effect of joint exposure to alcohol and tobacco on risk of cancer of the mouth and pharynx. *Journal of Chronic Diseases, 25,* 711-716.)

Occupational Exposure

An increased rate of oral carcinomas has been observed in a number of occupations, including plumbers and steel, coal, metal, and textile workers. More studies are needed to establish a correlation between oral cancer and these occupations while carefully controlling for alcohol and tobacco use (Mahboudi & Sayed, 1982).

Diet

A number of epidemiologic studies have implicated dietary and nutritional deficiencies in the development of oral cancer. Many of these studies are case-control studies in which groups of individuals with oral cavity cancer are compared with individuals without oral cancer. Retrospective information is obtained regarding diet, alcohol and tobacco use, and other risks. A consistent finding among these case-controlled studies was the protective effect of fruit intake. Individuals with a high intake of fruit had a 20% to 80% reduction in the risk of oral cancer (Franco, Kowalski, Oliveira, Curado, Pereira, & Silva et al., 1989; Gridley, McLaughlin, Block, Winn, Greenberg, & Schoenberg et al.,

1990; Lavecchia, Negri, D'Avanzo, Boyle, & Franceschi, 1991; McLaughlin, Gridley, Block, Winn, Preston-Martin, & Schoenberg et al., 1988). A decreased intake of vitamin A in diets has been linked to a two-fold increase in the incidence of oral cancers (Winn, Ziegler, Pickle, Gridley, Blot, & Hoover, 1984).

Fruits contain vitamin C, β-carotene, and other carotenoids that are antioxidants. Antioxidants are nutrients that work to protect the body, when in the process of normal metabolism, oxygen-induced damage to tissues occurs. Antioxidants are thus believed to have some protective abilities in the formation of cancer (Lavecchia et al., 1991; Tanaka, 1995; Willitt, 1994). Current recommendations to protect against oral cancer include eating at least five servings of fruit and vegetables each day (Marshall & Boyle, 1996; MacFarlane, Zheng, Marshall, Bofetta, Niu, & Brasire et al., 1995).

Other Factors

Poor oral hygiene and dentition have been suggested as having a role in the development of oral cancer. Most of the literature acknowledges the difficulty in separating these potential causes from the concurrent use of alcohol or tobacco. It is believed that poor oral hygiene in association with alcohol and/or tobacco use increases a person's risk for oral cancer. Controlled studies in this area are needed to show a significant association. Mouthwashes containing a high content of alcohol (>25%) have been implicated in oral cancer (Winn, Blot, McLaughlin, Austin, Greenburg, & Preston-Martin et al., 1991; Weaver, Fleming, & Smith, 1979). In a study of 200 people with head and neck cancer, 11 of which did not use tobacco or alcohol, 10 patients had used mouthwashes with a high alcohol content at least two times a day for over 20 years (Weaver, Fleming, & Smith, 1979). Additional research is needed to provide more conclusive evidence as to the role of mouthwashes and oral cancer.

It has been estimated that three fourths of patients with oral cancer have the human papillomavirus (HPV). However, a clear-cut association between oral cancer and HPV has not been established. Some research suggests that HPV may be involved in the growth of benign and malignant lesions in the oral cavity (Balaram, Nalinakumari, Abraham, Balan, Harcendran, & Bernard et al., 1995) Herpes simplex virus is also being studied in relationship to the development of oral cancer. This relationship needs further investigation.

Sun exposure has been strongly associated with cancer of the lip. An increased incidence of lip cancer is noted in people with outdoor occupations. This risk is decreased among ethnic groups with dark skin as a result of the protective effects of melanin. The use of lipstick or lip balm with sun-screening agents can protect outdoor workers from lip cancer (Alvi, Myers, & Johnson, 1996).

CHEMOPREVENTION

In the 1980s the National Cancer Institute began to study chemoprevention to identify and evaluate anticarcinogenic agents. Cancer chemoprevention is the use of natural or chemical agents prior to cancer invasion to slow or actually halt the carcinogenic process (Frank-Stromberg & Cohen, 1993; Tanaka, 1995). Chemoprevention trials in premalignant oral cavity changes have been in existence for over 40 years (Silverman, Renstrip, & Pindburg, 1963). Among these trials, retinoids are the compounds that are studied most frequently.

Retinoids

Retinoids are structural analogues of vitamin A that affect the growth, maturation, and differentiation of various cell types (Tanaka, 1995). Within the oral cavity specifically, epithelial cells require vitamin A for normal cellular differentiation (Amos & Lotan, 1991). The exact mechanism by which retinoids modulate carcinogenesis is not understood completely. Prior randomized trials using retinoids show statistically significant evidence that retinoids are effective in treating oral leukoplakias or erythroplakias. *Oral leukoplakia* is defined by the World Health Organization (WHO) as "a white patch or plaque that cannot be rubbed off." Many leukoplakias will not progress to an oral malignancy. This condition cannot be considered malignant until a histologic diagnosis has been made. Conditions that more commonly transform to oral cancer are erythroplakia, speckled leukoplakia, and severe dysplasia. These conditions occur less frequently than the common leukoplakias. With the initiation of a chemopreventive agent to reverse all oral leukoplakias and erythroplakia, including the large proportion that will remain benign and not be problematic, the amount of toxicity should be negligible.

Studies are being conducted to determine the effectiveness of the chronic use of retinoids after initial therapy. This approach is due to the fact that after primary therapy for oral leukoplakias or erythroplasias, many patients have relapses. Whether the reversal of these premalignant lesions will result in decreased risks of oral cancer is being investigated (Chiesa, Tradati, & Marazza, 1992).

The retinoid 13-*cis*-retinoic acid reverses oral leukoplakias. However, in high doses it has been associated with significant side effects to the patient. Presently, the use of high-dose 13-*cis*-retinoic acid to reverse premalignant oral lesions followed by a low-dose 13-*cis*-retinoic acid to maintain response is being studied (Lippman, Clayman, Huber, Benner, & Hong, 1995). Dose-limiting toxicities of high-dose 13-*cis*-retinoic acid include cheilitis (dry lips), skin dryness and peeling, pruritus, conjunctivitis, and arthralgias (Dorr & VonHoff, 1994).

Vitamin C, E, and β-Carotene

Less toxic agents currently being investigated are vitamin C, vitamin E, and β-carotene. These antioxidant nutrients are nontoxic, less costly, and easy to administer. A more recent indication for these agents may be for the prevention of second malignancies, which occur in many patients with head and neck cancer. (DePalo & Formelli, 1995; Lippman, Heyman, Korie, Benner, & Hong, 1995). These second malignancies are thought to be the result of diffuse abnormal mucosa due to exposure to alcohol or tobacco, which is termed *field cancerization* (Slaughter, Southwick, & Smejkal, 1953). In other words, the entire area exposed to carcinogenic agents, which can include many different anatomic locations, can generate malignant cells. Antioxidants used in the prevention of second malignancies may aid in the reversal of the extensive mucosal damage that occurs in field cancerization.

Randomized placebo-controlled trials are underway to establish the activities of these chemopreventive agents. Chemoprevention of oral cancer is not accepted as a current standard of practice. However, results of studies done to date are encouraging. More studies are underway to delineate the efficacy of less toxic retinoids as chemoprevention in oral cancer.

PATHOPHYSIOLOGY

Normal Anatomy and Physiology of the Oral Cavity

The oral cavity is the port of entry into the digestive system and extends from the junction of skin and vermilion of the anterior lips to the junction of the hard and soft palate. The oral cavity specifically includes the lips, anterior two thirds of the tongue, floor of the mouth, gingiva hard palate, retromolar trigone, and buccal mucosa. Tumors in these anatomic regions have similar biologic characteristics and prognostic factors (Fig. 54-3).

The lips contain a rich supply of lymphatics draining into the submandibular, submental, preauricular, and periparotic nodes. Tumors located near the midline of the lip are frequently associated with bilateral metastasis (Alvi, Myers, & Johnson, 1996). The lips function primarily in speech and articulation. The tongue is the largest structure in the oral cavity. Tongue cancer accounts for 20% to 50% of all oral cavity cancers. The anterior two thirds is the movable portion of the tongue, extending to the floor of the mouth. Lymphatic drainage in this region is extensive, including submental, submandibular, and upper and deep jugular nodes. As a result of anastomosis, drainage often enters contralateral lymph nodes. The floor of the mouth involves a superficial and deep lymphatic drainage system, including ipsilateral submandibular, upper jugular, jugulodigastric, and jugulocerotid nodes (Alvi, Myers, & Johnson, 1996). The buccal mucosa is the inner surface of the cheeks and lips. Lymphatics from this area drain into the periparotid, submental, and submandibular nodes. The lymphatic drainage of the retromolar trigone is primarily circulated to the deep jugular nodes. The hard palate is a nonmovable structure forming the anterior portion of the roof of the mouth. Lymphatics in this area are scant. However, they do involve the jugular and retropharyngeal nodes.

The oropharynx begins where the oral cavity ends posteriorly. Anatomic structures in the oropharyngeal region are the soft palate, base of the tongue, tonsils, and posterior pharyngeal wall (Alvi, Myers, & Johnson, 1996). Carcinomas in this region tend to spread from level II of cervical lymph nodes to levels III and IV, respectively.

As illustrated in Fig. 54-4, the oral cavity has an extensive lymphatic drainage system. Lymphatic drainage from the oral cavity is relatively consistent. This observation led to the discovery that most oral cavity cancers metastasize in an orderly fashion. (The levels of cervical lymph nodes are shown in Fig. 54-4.)

Carcinogenesis

The oral cavity mucosa constantly undergoes repair and restructuring due to everyday wear and tear, as well as damage from toxic exposure. Most oral cancers begin on the surface epithelium. The epithelium undergoes premalignant changes or dysplasia that can begin to occur many years before a malignancy develops. Dysplasia is disorganized cell growth; cells vary in size, shape, and appearance. The degree of dysplasia is relative to the risk of a lesion being malignant. Over 90% of oral cancers are squamous cell carcinomas. Prior to the occurrence of the malignancy, the surface epithelium initiation, promotion, and progression must occur. Alterations in the thickness of the lining of the oral epithelium result in atrophy. Sites of the oral cavity more susceptible to damage from carcinogens are those that have a thin epithelium and lack keratin, submucosa, and fat (Mashberg & Samit, 1995).

Currently, a specific tumor marker to identify or predict malignant transformation in patients at risk for oral cancer does not exist (Wright, 1994). Health care providers rely on visual and microscopic examination to diagnose these carcinomas. Two common variations in the oral cavity tissue that occur are leukoplakia (LK) and erythroplasia, as mentioned previously. Only about 3% to 6% of all oral LKs will eventually transform into a malignancy. These data illustrate the fact that most oral LKs are benign histologic conditions, making oral carcinomas even more difficult to diagnose (Gupta, Mehta, Daftary, Pindburg, Bhonsle, & Jalnawalla et al., 1980; Roed-Peterson, 1971). Conditions or appearance of the oral cavity that should heighten a clinician's suspicion include red, raised, erosive areas. Oral LK can be confused with candida albicans. The link between oral carcinoma and oral candida has not been established in the literature. Areas with oral LK most commonly associated with carcinomas are the lower lip from the lateral and ventral surface of the tongue (Wright, 1994). Management of oral LK varies widely. Risk factors, appearance, location, and size of the oral LK can be used to determine the most appropriate management.

Erythroplakia is defined as a "red mucosal lesion which cannot be clinically or pathologically diagnosed as a specific disease or condition" (Wright, 1994). Roed-Peterson (1971) reported higher rates of malignant transformation in erythroplakia than in LK. Erythroplakia can be difficult to distinguish from inflammatory conditions caused by infection, physical or chemical insult, or immune reactions. Erythematous lesions or mixed leukoplakia/erythroplastic lesions should be viewed as highly suspicious and analyzed through a biopsy.

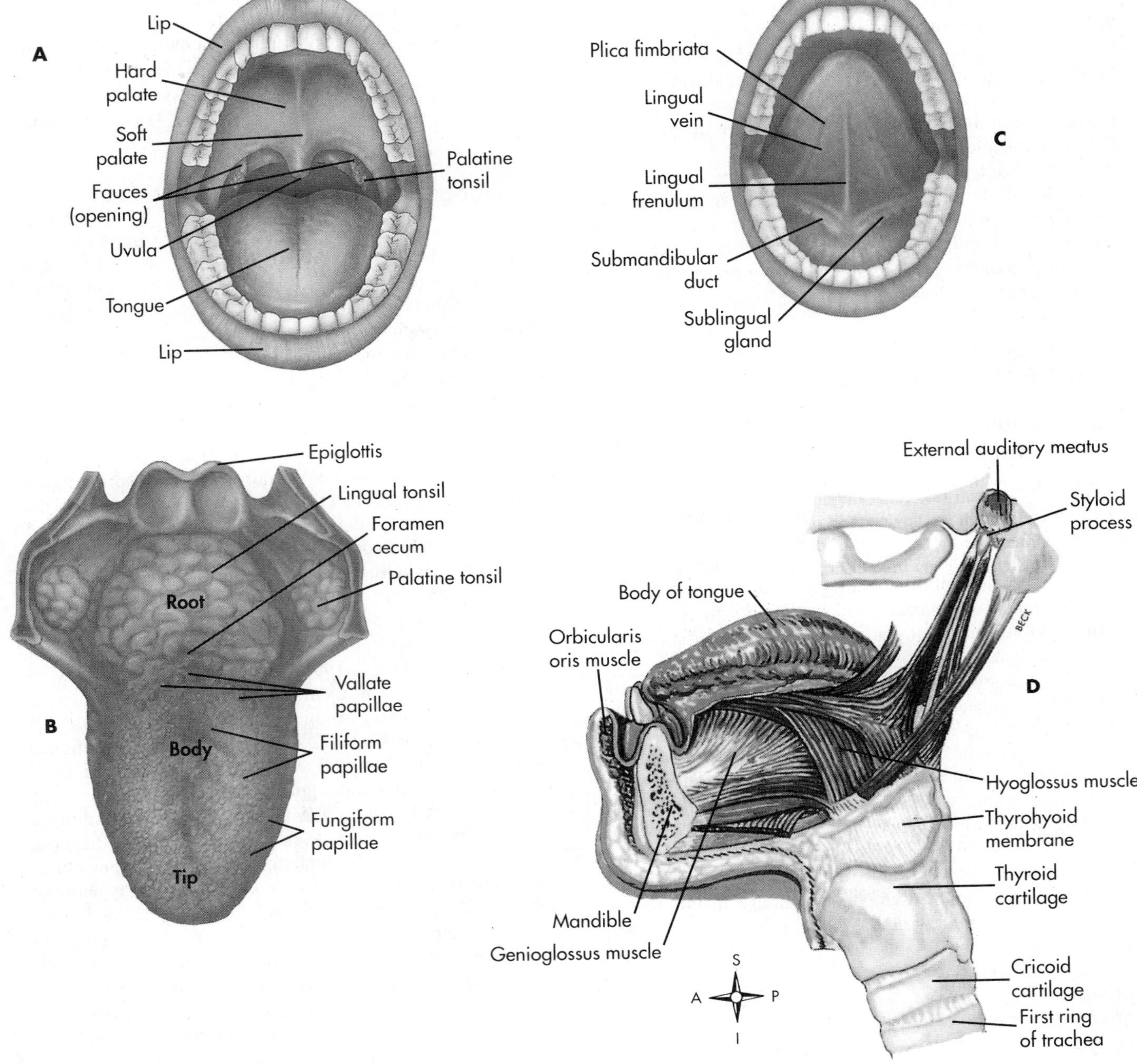

Fig. 54-3 Oral cavity and oropharynx anatomy. **A,** Open mouth view. **B,** Tongue elevated showing the floor of the mouth. **C,** Tongue elevated showing the floor of the mouth. **D,** Extrinsic muscles of the tongue. (From Thibodeau, G. A. & Patton, K. T. [1995]. *Anatomy and physiology* [4th ed.]. St. Louis: Mosby.)

Genetic Alterations

Abnormal mutations and deletions in DNA are associated with uncontrolled tumor growth. An accepted genetic marker for oral cavity cancer has not yet been identified (Alvi, Myers, & Johnson, 1996). Tumor suppresser gene p53 alterations have been demonstrated in premalignant and malignant oral cavity lesions. This gene in squamous cell carcinoma of the oral cavity has been correlated with alcohol and tobacco use (Brennan, Sessions, Spitznagel, & Harvey, 1991). Oncogenes that have been identified in head and neck carcinomas include *int-2,* c-*myc,* H-*ras,* and *bcl-1* (Alvi, Myers, & Johnson, 1996; Shin, & Tainsky, 1995). These oncogenes are currently being studied to determine their value in the diagnosis and prognosis of oral cancer.

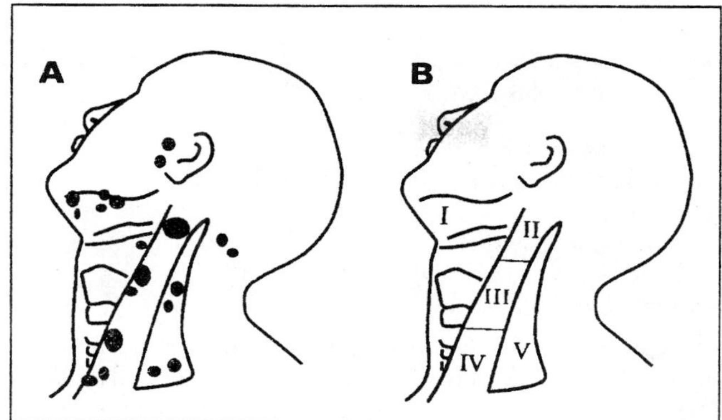

Fig. 54-4 **A,** Regional lymphatic pattern in the head and neck. **B,** Neck levels of the head and neck. (From Shah, J. P. & Lydiatt, W. [1995]. Treatment of head and neck cancer. *CA: A Cancer Journal for Clinicians, 45*[6], 357.)

ROUTES OF METASTASES

Regional Metastases

The most important prognostic factor in patients with oral cancer is the extent of cervical lymph node involvement. The presence of cervical lymph node involvement lowers cure rates by as much as 50% (Johnson, Barnes, Meyers, Schramm, Borochovitz, & Sigler, 1981). For a review of the levels of cervical lymph nodes I through IV, see Fig. 54-4.

Most commonly in oral cancer, lymph node involvement occurs in levels I, II, and III. In patients with oral cancer, cervical lymph node metastasis is present in approximately 30% of patients at the time of presentation (Alvi, Myers, & Johnson, 1996). An exception to this is the lip and hard palate areas that have less lymphatics involved and thus a decreased likelihood of lymphatic spread. However, if lip and tongue cancers with lymph node metastasis are located near the midline, they commonly have bilateral lymph node involvement. The tongue, floor of the mouth, and retromolar trigone are commonly associated with cervical lymphatic metastasis and are the most common sites of oral cancer in drinkers and smokers (Boffetta et al., 1992). Oral malignancies in these areas should be carefully staged and treated for any neck involvement. Cervical lymph node metastasis is an important factor in the failure of treatment of oral cancer. The risk of lymphatic spread may be influenced by the site of the primary oral cancer. A thorough understanding of the patterns of lymphatic spread from various cancerous sites in the oral cavity can assist in developing the most effective treatment.

Distant Metastases

Distant metastases in patients with oral carcinoma are relatively rare. Approximately 15% to 20% of patients with oral cancer eventually develop distant metastasis (Alvi, Myers, & Johnson, 1996; Brennan & Sessions, 1991). Squamous cell carcinoma of the oral cavity usually remains localized at the primary site and lymph nodes for some time. In a number of studies by Crile in 1906, distant metastasis was discovered in very few patients. In fact, in patients with early-stage oral cancer, the risk of dying from a second primary cancer is greater than the risk of death from distant metastasis or the original primary cancer (Lippman & Hong, 1989). The most common sites of distant metastasis in patients with oral cancer are the lung, liver, and bone. Metastasis can also occur in the adrenals, kidney, spleen, bowel, and heart. A thorough metastatic workup for distant metastasis in these patients is not recommended unless they are symptomatic or it is highly suspected. More important is the practice of a careful evaluation to ensure that second primaries are not present.

ASSESSMENT

History

The assessment of the patient for oral cancer is summarized in Table 54-2. Currently, a definitive screening examination or test for the early detection of oral cancer is not recommended due to the relatively low incidence of oral carcinomas. To date, screening tests have not been able to establish a cost benefit. However, a simple oral examination incorporated in a cancer-related checkup can be a valuable tool in the diagnosis of localized oral cancer in high-risk individuals. Cancers of the oral cavity are frequently not diagnosed in the early stages when they are most amenable to treatment (Box 54-1). Health care providers and patients often overlook oral carcinomas. Furthermore, recommendations for oral cancer screening are inconsistent (Spangler, 1995). (Refer to Table 54-3 for an overview of current recommendations.) The existence of nonstandardized oral cancer screening guidelines does not assist in promoting the use of routine oral examinations. Family practitioners, as well as dentists, play a pivotal role in the early detection of oral cancer in high-risk individuals. Increased awareness among physicians and nurses of patients at risk for developing oral cancer is necessary to increase early detection (Yellowitz, Goodman, Horowitz, & Al-Tannir, 1995; Maguire & Roberts, 1994). In addition, the public lacks knowledge regarding the risk factors as well as signs and symptoms of oral cancer (Goodman, Yellowitz, & Horowitz, 1995).

On routine examination of patients, primary care providers and dentists have a responsibility to assess individual risk factors for patients to better educate and inform them. In addition to promoting or suggesting cessation of alcohol or tobacco use, primary care providers need to inform patients of signs and symptoms specific to oral cancer that should be reported. As previously stated, many high-risk groups also lack access to health care, further inhibiting the likelihood of early diagnosis. In a screening program of 672,000 veterans, oral examinations were performed, resulting in the diagnosis of 814 oral squamous cell cancers. The results demonstrated that, in high-risk patients who use large amounts of tobacco and alcohol and are greater than 40 years of age, rates of detection can be as high as 1 in 200 to 250 patients (Mashberg & Barsa, 1984).

The identification of high-risk groups when obtaining a patient history followed by patient education regarding

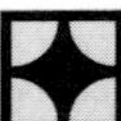

TABLE 54-2 Assesment of the Patient for Oral Cancer

	Assessment Parameters	Typical Abnormal Findings
History	A. Personal and social history	A. Personal and social risk factors:
	1. High-risk behaviors	1. Use of any form of tobacco or excessive alcohol intake; excessive exposure to sun without sunscreen.
	2. Age	2. Average age at diagnosis is 60 years.
	3. Ethnicity	3. African Americans have a greater risk than Caucasians.
	4. Gender	4. Male-to-female ratio is 2:1.
Physical Examination	A. Evaluation of the oral cavity	A. Common signs and symptoms: soreness, bleeding, burning, dysphagia, numbness, swelling, difficulty chewing, weight loss, trismus.
	B. Bimanual palpation and visual assessment	B. Unusual lesions, lumps or thickening in buccal mucosa, white or red patches located on the gums, tongue, or lining of the mouth.
	C. Lymph node evaluation	C. Submental, submandibular, superior deep jugular, and superior cervical nodes are the most common lymph nodes involved in oral cancer; upper deep jugular nodes can be involved in oropharyngeal carcinomas.
	D. Evaluation of patient for trismus (lockjaw) or nerve palsies	D. Pain with palpation—if present, could indicate deep tumor involvement.
Diagnostic Tests	A. Computed tomography (CT) scan	A. Can detect extent of tumor invasion, bone and lymph node involvement.
	B. Magnetic resonance imaging (MRI)	B. Can detect soft tissue and perineural involvement of tumor.
	C. Tissue biopsy	C. Mandatory prior to treatment; more than 90% of oral cavity cancers are squamous cell cancers.
	D. Toluidine blue (TCI)	D. Stains neoplastic tissues, inexpensive; high false-positive rate due to the fact that inflamed and noncancerous lesions will also stain blue.
	E. Chest x-ray	E. To rule out metastasis or a concurrent primary lung cancer in patients who use tobacco; to evaluate invasion of mandible.
	F. Liver function tests	F. Hepatic disease can be a common problem in patients with oral cavity cancer secondary to intake alcohol.
	G. Laryngoscopy, bronchoscopy, or esophagoscopy	G. Can be used to determine extent of tumor involvement or to rule out concurrent primary cancer in the larynx, lung, or esophagus.

TABLE 54-3 Recommendations for Oral Cancer Screening

Institution	Recommendations
American Academy of Family Physicians U.S. Preventive Services Task Force	Complete oral cavity examination only on adults at increased risk for oral cancer due to tobacco and/or alcohol exposure.
National Cancer Institute and National Institute of Dental Research	Complete oral examination with periodic health physicals of all adults starting at age 50.
American Cancer Society	Individuals 20-39 years old should have a complete oral examination included in a cancer checkup every 3 years; >40 years of age should have oral examination annually.

Modified from Goodman, H.S., Yellowitz, J.A., & Horowitz, A.M. (1995). Oral cancer prevention: The role of family practitioners. *Archives of Family Medicine, 4,* 628-632.

Box 54-1
Reasons Early Diagnosis of Oral Cancer Has Been Limited

1. Individuals at high risk are not targeted by health care providers.
2. High-risk sites of the oral cavity are not monitored closely.
3. Lack of knowledge concerning erythroplasia and its tendency to be malignant versus an overemphasis on leukoplakia that is usually benign.
4. Inconsistent recommendations for screening among health care providers for high-risk individuals.

Modified from Goodman, H. S., Yellowitz, J. A., & Horowitz, A. M. (1995). Oral cancer prevention: The role of family practitioners. *Archives of Family Medicine, 4,* 628-632.

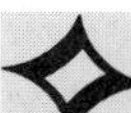

TABLE 54-4 Patient Preparation/Education on the Cessation of Smokeless Tobacco Use

Tips on How to Stop Using Smokeless Tobacco

Why Is It Hard to Quit Using Smokeless Tobacco?

Compared with cigarettes, smokeless tobacco (snuff or chewing tobacco) puts more nicotine into your bloodstream. For this and other reasons, people who chew tobacco regularly often say that quitting smokeless tobacco is even harder than quitting cigarette smoking. But many smokeless tobacco users have quit successfully—and so can you. Your family physician can help you quit.

Why Is It Important for Me to Stop Using Smokeless Tobacco?

The use of *any* tobacco product has both immediate and long-term effects on your health and overall well-being. Smokeless tobacco stains and wears down your teeth, causes your gums to recede, and produces mouth sores. Bad breath is a common problem. Over time, the use of smokeless tobacco can cause mouth cancer. Nicotine from smokeless tobacco also raises blood pressure and cholesterol levels and can make it more likely that you will have a heart attack.

It is important for you to have your own reasons for wanting to stop using smokeless tobacco. In addition to health effects, you may be concerned about saving money, giving up an addictive habit, or setting a good example for family members and friends. Write down your reasons for wanting to quit using smokeless tobacco—and keep your list in places where you can see it often during your efforts to stop.

What Can I Do to Get Ready to Quit Using Smokeless Tobacco?

Set a date to quite—and stick to it. Choose a date 1 to 2 weeks from today.

Quitting can be hard, so develop a plan that works for you. Anticipate times when you will want to chew or dip, and plan what you will do instead. Prepare yourself for quitting by recognizing the times when you will want smokeless tobacco the most. Plan to avoid those situations or to have tobacco substitutes with you (such as sunflower seeds or chewing gum). Get rid of all your chewing tobacco or snuff before your quit date. Start cutting down now on the amount you chew or dip to prepare for stopping.

Get support from your family, friends, and physician. Even better, have a friend or family member stop chewing or dipping with you. Studies have shown that quitting is more successful with the support of family or friends.

What Can I Use To Replace Smokeless Tobacco?

You might think about using nicotine gum or the nicotine patch. Nicotine addiction can be tough to overcome. Talk to your physician about whether the nicotine patch or gum is right for you. Generally, people who use three or more tins, or pouches, a week, people who use smokeless tobacco within 30 minutes after they wake up, and people who usually swallow tobacco juice benefit most from the nicotine gum or patch.

Find an oral substitute for smokeless tobacco that you enjoy. This may be non-tobacco mint-leaf snuff, sugarless gum or hard candy, beef jerky, or sunflower seeds. Don't substitute cigarette smoking for smokeless tobacco. Stop using *all* tobacco products.

Find activities to do when you want to chew. Many people chew or dip when they are bored. Instead, take a walk or a quick jog, lift weights, take a hot shower to relax—or do any activity you enjoy that will keep your mind off smokeless tobacco.

What If I Slip Up and Start Using Smokeless Tobacco Again?

You may slip up and start using smokeless tobacco again. This is normal. Learn from your slip! Think about what you can do to avoid that situation next time. Plan how you can handle things without going back to using smokeless tobacco.

Once you have quit, congratulate yourself. Celebrate beating the habit. You've worked hard! Use the money you would have spent on smokeless tobacco to buy yourself a present that you enjoy.

This information provides a general overview on quitting smokeless tobacco and may not apply to everyone. Talk to your family physician to find out if this information applies to you and to get more information on this subject.

Courtesy American Academy of Family Physicians (1995).

avoidance of potential carcinogens are the most tangible approaches to decreasing mortality from oral cancers. (For an example of a patient information sheet to assist with the cessation of smokeless tobacco, refer to Table 54-4. Signs and symptoms of oral cancer are outlined in Box 54-2.) A lack of knowledge in the general population concerning the signs and symptoms of oral cancer promotes delays in diagnosis. Most patients delay seeking professional advice for more than 3 months after becoming aware of an oral sign or symptom (Silverman & Dillon, 1990).

Box 54-2
A Patient Guide to Signs and Symptoms of Oral Cancer

If you notice any of the following signs and symptoms in your mouth, cheeks, gums, or lips, notify your physician immediately:

- A sore or irritation that does not heal or bleeds
- White or red lesions that cannot be rubbed off and do not go away
- A lump, thickening, or crusty lesion
- Pain, tenderness, or numbness
- Difficulty chewing, swallowing, speaking, or moving the jaw
- Sore throat

Modified from Goodman, H. S., Yellowitz, J. A., & Horowitz, A. M. (1995). Oral cancer prevention: The role of family practitioners. *Archives of Family Medicine, 4,* 628-632.

Physical Examination

An accurate physical examination of the oral cavity requires careful visualization. Adequate lighting with the use of dental lights or fiberoptic light systems provides the ideal environment for detection of early lesions. According to Mashberg and Samit (1995), lamps and penlights do not provide the effective lighting required to detect subtle mucosa alterations. A tongue blade and a 2 × 2-inch gauze sponge can be useful to properly examine all areas of the oral cavity. In early oral carcinomas that are usually nonpalpable, proper visual examination is imperative. After visual examination and bimanual palpation of any visible tumors to determine size and depth, the neck must be thoroughly palpated to detect cervical adenopathy. The presence of trismus and nerve palsies can indicate deep tumor invasion. Patients with lip cancer often have a sore on the lower lip that fails to heal and forms a dry seal that bleeds when removed. Buccal mucosa carcinomas are frequently in or near leukoplakia. Tumors in these areas often become large before the patient is symptomatic. Cancers in the floor of the mouth are also frequently in or near leukoplakia and erythroplakia and can be asymptomatic in the early stages. Tumors of the tongue most commonly occur in the middle third and lateral aspects. Noticeable pain and decreased mobility of the tongue are symptoms that usually do not develop in cancers of the tongue and floor of the mouth until late stages of the disease. Advanced tongue cancers can also radiate to the ear, causing pain.

Oropharyngeal tumors most commonly cause throat soreness or discomfort. Lesions of the tonsils and tongue base are often difficult to assess. These tumors often go undetected until advanced. Because oropharyngeal carcinoma invades muscle in the late stages of the disease, patients may complain of dysphagia, pain radiating to the ear, trismus, bleeding, aspiration, or airway obstruction. As previously mentioned, cervical lymph node involvement occurs through levels II, III, and IV, respectively. Cervical lymph node metastasis is not uncommon in oropharyngeal cancer (Table 54-5).

Diagnostic Tests

The World Health Organization (1982) outlines a systematic technique for examining the oral cavity. Diagnostic tests in oral cancer are used to evaluate the histologic type of tumor as well as to define the extent of tumor involvement.

Computed Tomography Scan. Computed tomography (CT) can be useful in determining the extent of tumor, as well as any bone and cervical lymph node involvement. Most commonly, CT is used to determine bone involvement. CT can also be used to evaluate the liver or lungs if the chest x-ray film or liver function tests are abnormal and further staging is indicated.

Magnetic Resonance Imaging. Magnetic resonance imaging (MRI) is used to evaluate stages II through IV tumors. The MRI can define soft tissue planes, perineural involvement, and anatomic abnormalities that may exist. The CT and the MRI have equal specificity when used to detect mandibular involvement. The MRI can be particularly useful in evaluating thickness of oral cancers of the tongue.

Tissue Biopsy. The diagnosis of oral carcinoma must always be confirmed histologically. This confirmation is usually obtained by performing an incisional biopsy. Incisional biopsies allow for a sample of normal as well as abnormal tissue. These biopsies should be deep enough to determine the extent of the carcinoma. An intraoral biopsy can be obtained easily with the patient under local anesthesia. An excisional biopsy usually is not done in oral cancers unless the tumor is extremely small, making complete removal curative. Most oral malignancies are not detected early enough for this procedure to be beneficial (Mashberg & Samit, 1995). Suspicious lesions that are analyzed through a biopsy and have normal results should be further investigated, and a repeat biopsy may be required.

Toluidine Blue. A 1% aqueous solution of toluidine blue can be painted on suspicious areas in the oral cavity (Fig. 54-5). Toluidine blue stains malignant tissues without involving normal tissue. However, areas with inflammation or irritation may also stain, which can lead to false-positive

Table 54-5 Incidence of Cervical Adenopathy at the Time of Presentation: Primary Site

Site	Percentage
Soft palate	44%
Tonsillar fossa	76%
Anterior pillar/retromolar trigones	45%
Tongue base	78%
Oropharyngeal walls	59%

Adapted from data in Department of Veteran Affairs Laryngeal Cancer Study Group (VALCS). (1991). *New England Journal of Medicine, 324,* 1685-1690.

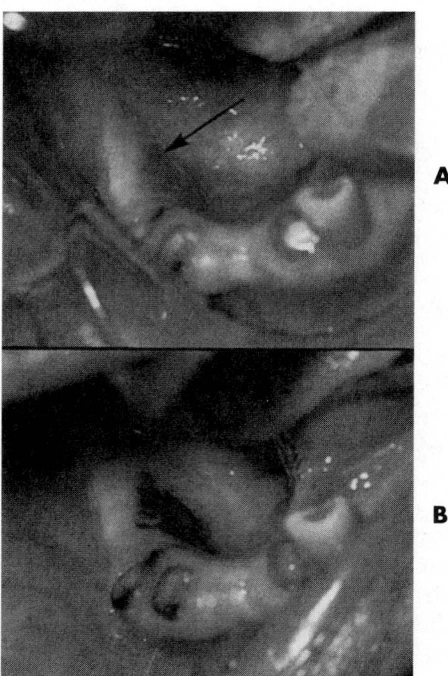

Fig. 54-5 **A,** Granular erythroplastic area at junction of alveolus and floor of the mouth. **B,** Site stained by toluidine blue application; biopsy revealed carcinoma. (From Mashberg, A. & Samit, G. [1995]. Early diagnosis of asymptomatic oral and oropharyngeal squamous cancers. *CA: A Cancer Journal Clinicians, 45*[6], 346.)

results. The sensitivity and specificity using toluidine blue has been estimated at 93% to 98% and 73% to 93%, respectively (Rosenberg & Cretin, 1989). Restaining suspicious or previously stained positive areas after a waiting period is one way to determine whether the lesion may be malignant (Mashberg & Samit, 1995). After an area is stained positive and irritation or inflammation has been ruled out, a biopsy is needed to confirm any carcinoma. Toluidine blue may be helpful in the screening of high-risk individuals if used properly. Toluidine blue could also be used to guide the physician to perform a biopsy on a suspicious lesion.

Other Diagnostic Tests. A chest x-ray and liver function tests (LFTs) are taken commonly in patients who present for a workup of a potential oral carcinoma. If the patient is a heavy drinker, the use of LFTs to determine co-existing liver damage is an important factor. A chest x-ray film is used to determine the presence of a second primary malignancy or metastasis (Alvi, Myers, & Johnson, 1996). A secondary primary tumor can be further investigated with the use of a laryngoscopy, bronchoscopy, or esophagoscopy.

Oral cancer is difficult to diagnose unless the patient has specific complaints of irritation or discomfort. Unfortunately, by the time many lesions are symptomatic, they are stage II and many already have cervical node metastasis (Mashberg & Samit, 1995). Early detection and treatment of oral cancer gives patients the best chance of cure, increased survival, and decreased dysfunction. Unfortunately, early diagnosis does not occur in many patients.

STAGING

Accurate staging of all tumors is pertinent to the selection of appropriate treatment in oral malignancy and factual reporting of results.

Histologic Staging

Histologic staging refers to the examination of tissue obtained during biopsy. For tumors that are visible and accessible, a tissue biopsy provides the most definitive histologic diagnosis. A fine-needle biopsy can be performed if the tumor is not apparent and the patient has known cervical lymph adenopathy (Davidson, Spiro, Patel, Patel, & Shah, 1994). A histologic diagnosis can be obtained with a fine-needle aspiration, an excisional biopsy, or an incisional biopsy.

Approximately 90% of oral cancers are squamous cell carcinomas (Silverman, 1994). Other types that are less common include melanoma, salivary gland origin, lymphoma, and bone cancers. (This chapter does not discuss the diagnosis and treatment of these less common oral malignancies.) Premalignant lesions may precede squamous cell carcinomas. Lesions are then divided into noninvasive (carcinoma in situ) and invasive carcinomas. Invasive carcinomas are then graded according to their resemblance to normal cells. Tumor grading using Broder's classifications include well-differentiated (G1), moderately well-differentiated (G2), poorly differentiated (G3), and undifferentiated (G4) (Broder, 1920). The value of histologic grading in determining prognosis of oral cancers is limited. Attempts are being made to redefine the histologic grading of oral cancer to make it more useful. Squamous cell carcinomas are usually regarded as exophytic or ulcerative. Ulcerative squamous cell carcinoma invades deeply and has a higher histologic grade than exophytic types of squamous cell carcinomas. Basaloid squamous cell carcinoma is an aggressive subtype of squamous cell carcinoma. It presents as an ulcerative lesion. This subtype of squamous cell carcinoma of the oral cavity is associated with a less favorable prognosis.

Verrucous carcinoma, also a subtype of squamous cell carcinoma, is rare, accounting for only 5% of all oral cancers (Elliott, MacDougall, & Elliott, 1973). Verrucous carcinomas occur most commonly in the buccal mucosa and are usually low grade and associated with a better prognosis than other squamous cell carcinomas.

Clinical Staging

The TNM Staging System is used consistently in patients with head and neck cancer to develop treatment options, assess prognosis, and compare results of treatment between institutions. *T* refers to the size of the tumor, *N* is the cervical node involvement, and *M* is the absence or presence of distant metastasis as a result of a primary oral cancer (American Joint Committee on Cancer, 1993). The T in the TNM Staging System differs among various head and neck cancers. Each T is specifically designed to denote not only the tumor size, but also the presence of deep muscle or bone invasion. See Tables 54-6 and 54-7 for the TNM staging classification for oral and oropharyngeal carcinomas.

MEDICAL MANAGEMENT

Overview

In treating oral cancers, the primary goal is cure. Secondary goals that greatly affect the patient are preservation of function and form, maintenance of quality of life, and prevention of secondary primaries. Surgery and radiation therapy alone or in combination have been used in the treatment of oral cavity cancer. Surgery and radiation are the treatments of choice for small T1 and T2 lesions, resulting in 5-year survival rates of 50% to 70% (Liggett & Forastiere, 1995). Chemotherapy continues to be under investigation and is used in combination with surgery and radiation therapy. Gene therapy and immunotherapy are also being studied.

The location of the tumor, depth of invasion, presence or absence of nodal involvement, distant metastasis, and histologic grade are all important factors in defining appropriate treatment options. The patient's age, physical performance status, and support system must be evaluated prior to treatment to ensure a successful outcome (Box 54-3). The treatment of oral cavity cancers by stage and site vary. Treatment options are summarized in Tables 54-8 and 54-9. In early-stage oral cancer, surgery and radiation therapy are equally efficacious (Fig. 54-6). Early-stage T1 and T2 oral tumors have responded well to single-modality treatment with surgery or radiation therapy. Unfortunately the diagnosis of T1 and T2 oral tumors occurs in only one third of patients. The

Table 54-6 Oral Cavity TNM Classification

Primary Tumor (T)	
TX	Primary tumor cannot be assessed
T0	No evidence of primary tumor
Tis	Carcinoma in situ
T1	Tumor 2 cm or less in greatest dimension
T2	Tumor more than 2 cm but not more than 4 cm in greatest dimension
T3	Tumor more than 4 cm in greatest dimension
T4	(lip) Tumor invades adjacent structures (e.g., through cortical bone, tongue, skin of neck)
T4	(oral cavity) Tumor invades adjacent structures (e.g., through cortical bone, into deep [extrinsic] muscle of tongue, maxillary sinus, skin)
Regional Lymph Nodes (N)	
NX	Regional lymph nodes cannot be assessed
N0	No regional lymph node metastasis
N1	Metastasis in a single ipsilateral lymph node, 3 cm or less in greatest dimension
N2	Metastasis in a single ipsilateral lymph node, more than 3 cm but not more than 6 cm in greatest dimension; or in multiple ipsilateral lymph nodes, none more than 6 cm in greatest dimension; or in bilateral or contralateral lymph nodes, none more than 6 cm in greatest dimension
N2a	Metastasis in single ipsilateral lymph node more than 3 cm but not more than 6 cm in greatest dimension
N2b	Metastasis in multiple ipsilateral lymph nodes, none more than 6 cm in greatest dimension
N2c	Metastasis in bilateral or contralateral lymph nodes, none more than 6 cm in greatest dimension
N3	Metastasis in a lymph node more than 6 cm in greatest dimension
Distant Metastasis (M)	
MX	Presence of distant metastasis cannot be assessed
M0	No distant metastasis
M1	Distant metastasis

From American Joint Committee on Cancer (1993). Handbook for staging of cancer. In *The manual for staging of cancer* (4th ed.). Philadelphia: J. B. Lippincott.

Box 54-3
Factors That Impact the Type of Treatment Used in Oral Cancers

- Age
- Concurrent medical conditions
- Physical performance status
- Patient acceptance
- Support system

Modified from Mashberg, A. & Samit, G. (1995). Early diagnosis of asymptomatic oral and oropharyngeal squamous cancers. *CA: A Cancer Journal for Clinicians, 45*(6), 328-351.

Table 54-7 Oropharynx TNM Classification

Primary Tumor (T)	
TX	Primary tumor cannot be assessed
T0	No evidence of primary tumor
Tis	Carcinoma in situ
Oropharynx	
T1	Tumor 2 cm or less in greatest dimension
T2	Tumor more than 2 cm but not more than 4 cm in greatest dimension
T3	Tumor more than 4 cm in greatest dimension
T4	Tumor invades adjacent structures (e.g., through cortical bone, soft tissues of neck, deep [extrinsic] muscle of tongue)
Nasopharynx	
T1	Tumor limited to one subsite of nasopharynx
T2	Tumor invades more than one subsite of nasopharynx
T3	Tumor invades nasal cavity and/or oropharynx
T4	Tumor invades skull and/or cranial nerve(s)
Hypopharynx	
T1	Tumor limited to one subsite of hypopharynx
T2	Tumor invades more than one subsite of hypopharynx or an adjacent site, without fixation of hemilarynx
T3	Tumor invades more than one subsite of hypopharynx or an adjacent site, with fixation of hemilarynx
T4	Tumor invades adjacent structures (e.g., cartilage or soft tissues of neck)
Regional Lymph Nodes (N)	
NX	Regional lymph nodes cannot be assessed
N0	No regional lymph node metastasis
N1	Metastasis in a single ipsilateral lymph node, 3 cm or less in greatest dimension
N2	Metastasis in a single ipsilateral lymph node, more than 3 cm but not more than 6 cm in greatest dimension; or in multiple ipsilateral lymph nodes, none more than 6 cm in greatest dimension; or in bilateral or contralateral lymph nodes, none more than 6 cm in greatest dimension
N2a	Metastasis in a single ipsilateral lymph node more than 3 cm but not more than 6 cm in greatest dimension
N2b	Metastasis in multiple ipsilateral lymph nodes, none more than 6 cm in greatest dimension
N2c	Metastasis in bilateral or contralateral lymph nodes, none more than 6 cm in greatest dimension
N3	Metastasis in a lymph node more than 6 cm in greatest dimension
Distant Metastasis (M)	
MX	Presence of distant metastasis cannot be assessed
M0	No distant metastasis
M1	Distant metastasis

From American Joint Committee on Cancer (1993). Handbook for staging of cancer. In *The manual for staging of cancer* (4th ed.). Philadelphia: J. B. Lippincott.

TABLE 54-8 Medical Management of Oral Cancer Based on Stage of Disease

Stage	Treatment
Stage I	
Lip	Surgery and radiation have equal cure rates
Anterior tongue	Wide local excision transorally for small lesions
	Surgery or radiation therapy for larger lesions
	Radiation may be external beam or radiation implant
Buccal mucosa	<1 cm, surgery alone if only one side of the oral cavity is involved
	If tumor invades opposite side of oral cavity, radiation therapy including implantable radiation is considered
	Larger T1 lesions are treated with surgical excision and skin grafting or radiation therapy
Floor of mouth	Surgery and radiation have similar cure rates for T1 lesions
	Small lesions (<0.5 cm) may be treated with excision alone
	If lesion involves tongue, radiation therapy is used
Retromolar trigone	For lesions without bone involvement, resection of the mandible is done
	Radiation may be substituted if resection is extensive
Upper gingiva & hard palate	Surgical resection.
	+/− Postoperative radiation
Stage II	
Lip	T2 or < = surgery
	If reconstructive surgery is required due to extensive surgical removal of tumor, radiation may be substituted (external beam or implanted radiation)
Anterior tongue	T2 lesions are treated with radiation therapy
	Surgery is used if radiation is not successful
	+/− neck resection
	If T2 lesions are invasive, treatment can be surgery, radiation, or a combination of these
Buccal mucosa	Small T2 (<3 cm) lesions = radiation
	Large T2 (>3 cm) lesions = surgery, radiation, or a combination
Floor of the mouth	Small T2 lesions = surgery or radiation
	Large T2 lesions = surgery or radiation; if surgery is used on large T2 lesions, external beam or implanted radiation is considered in addition
Gingiva & hard palate	Small lesions = surgical resection
	+/− Postoperative radiation therapy
Retromolar trigone	Lesions without bone invasion = partial resection of mandible
	If greater surgical resection is necessary, radiation can be used
Stages III and IV	
Lip +/− bone, nerve, nodal involvement	Combination surgery and radiation (external beam or implanted radiation)
	Clinical trials using chemotherapy preoperatively/postoperatively or before radiation are done
	Superfractionated radiotherapy
Anterior tongue	External beam radiation +/− implanted radiation
	Lesions with greater infiltration are treated with surgery and postoperative radiation
	For advanced and extensive lesions, palliative radiation therapy may be indicated
Buccal mucosa	Radical surgical resection
	Radiation therapy
	Radical surgical resection and radiation postoperatively
	Chemotherapy preoperatively/postoperatively or in addition to radiation is under investigation
	Chemotherapy with radiation therapy is being studied.
	Surgery includes rim resection, partial mandibulectomy with nodal dissection
	Radiation includes external beam alone or combined with a local radiation implant
	Surgery and radiation combined
Gingiva/retromolar trigone	Radical surgical resection and preoperative/postoperative radiation

Modified from Alvi, A., Myers, E. N., & Johnson, J. T. (1996). Cancer of the oral cavity. In E. N. Meyers & J. Y. Suen (Eds.), *Cancer of the head and neck* (3rd ed.). Philadelphia: W. B. Saunders; The National Cancer Institute, Physician Data Query, Nov. 1996.

TABLE 54-9 Medical Management of Oropharyngeal Cancer Based on Stage of Disease

Stage	Treatment
Stage I	Surgery or radiation therapy Radiation may be chosen over surgery to avoid associated morbidity
Stage II	Surgery or radiation
Stage III	Surgery with postoperative radiation External beam radiation +/− interstitial radiation. Neck dissection +/− Neoadjuvant chemotherapy is under investigation
Stage IV	Surgery with postoperative radiation Neck dissection +/− Neoadjuvant chemotherapy is under investigation Unresectable tumors may be treated with radiation +/− chemotherapy

Modified from Alvi, A., Myers, E. N., & Johnson, J. T. (1996). Cancer of the oral cavity. In E. N. Meyers & J. Y. Suen (Eds.), *Cancer of the head and neck* (3rd ed.). Philadelphia: W. B. Saunders; The National Cancer Institute, Physician Data Query, Nov. 1996.

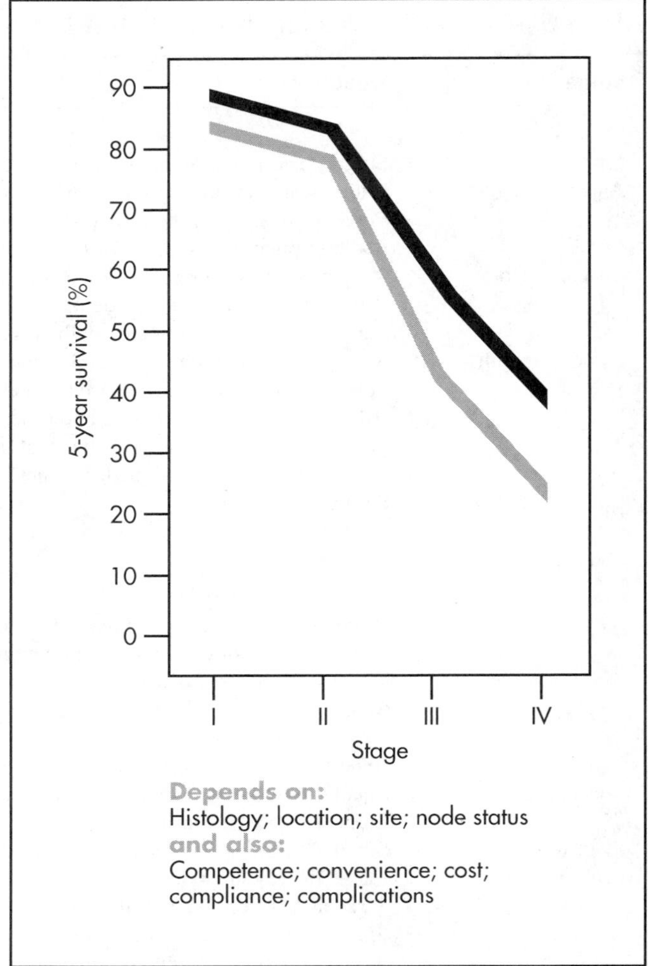

Fig. 54-6 Graphic representation of the similarity in 5-year survival for surgery *(black)* and radiotherapy *(gray)* and the reduction in effectiveness of both treatments in advanced disease. (From Shah, J. P., & Lydiatt, W. [1995]. Treatment of head and neck cancer. *CA: A Cancer Journal for Clinicians, 45*[6], 360.)

majority of patients have cervical node involvement, making combination treatment the only option.

In T1, NO lesions of the oral cavity, laser surgery can be successful and is associated with less dysfunction. In most advanced oral cancers, combined treatment with surgery and radiation are indicated. T3 and T4 tumors are generally less responsive to radiation and require surgical resection with or without adjuvant implanted radiation. Patients with advanced oral lesions frequently have nodal metastasis and require nodal radiation or neck dissection. Despite treatment, many oral cancers can recur. Salvage treatment for recurrences has not been successful in most patients. Chemotherapy, immunotherapy, and radiosensitizers are currently under investigation in patients with advanced oral cancer. Treatment for oral cavity cancer today is associated with less morbidity than in the past; however, survival rates have remained relatively unchanged.

Surgical Management

Factors that affect the type of surgery used in oral cancers include the size and location of the tumor, presence of bone invasion, and neck metastasis. Surgical procedures used in oral cavity cancers are outlined in Table 54-10.

Surgical Approaches. Small oral tumors less than 2 cm and located toward the opening of the mouth can be excised periorally. Tumors not accessible by this approach may require transcervical or transmandibular surgery.

Postoperative psychological and functional difficulties in patients who undergo radical resections of advanced oral carcinomas are common. Problems with deglutition, dysphagia, aspiration, and articulation can severely affect these patients. If resection of the mandible is required, the effect on physical appearance can be remarkable. Schuller and colleagues (1983) reported that after undergoing a radical or modified radical neck dissection, as many as 41% of patients were dissatisfied by their appearance, 30% to 70% experienced difficulty lifting their arm, and up to 40% reported neck numbness. Surgery for advanced oral cancer must be carefully contemplated. The patient needs to fully understand the outcomes of various treatment modalities, as well as their effect on quality of life and overall survival.

Improvements in surgery for the treatment of advanced oral cancer have not had a great effect on cure rates. However, the decreases in surgical mortality and morbidity rates have been significant. Surgical techniques used for oral cancers include intraoral, lower cheek flap, visor flap, mandibulotomy, and upper cheek flap (Fig. 54-7).

Resection of any part of the mandible is called a *mandibulotomy.* This surgical technique is used to treat oral cav-

TABLE 54-10 Surgical Treatment of Oral Cancer

Procedure	Description	Rationale
Laser excision—For transorally accessible oral cavity tumors	Powerful laser light is used in place of a scalpel to cut through tissue	Decreased pain, bleeding, swelling and scarring associated with other surgical techniques
Transoral resection	Removal of the tumor through the mouth	Can remove small tumors that are located anteriorly and are well defined; used to remove some oropharyngeal tumors that are not deeply infiltrating
Upper/lower cheek flap	Turning back a portion of the cheek	To expose large tumors; for excision, can aid in excision of anterior and lateral tumors
Visor flap	Dissection into the neck to access the oral cavity	
Mandibulectomy—Marginal segmental	Resection of a part of the mandible; can be used to gain access to oropharyngeal tumors	For primary tumors of the mandible, base of the tongue, and tonsils, or metastasis to the mandible
Mandibulotomy	Mandible is split in the midline and retracted	To access moderate to large proximally located tumors without bone invasions; mandible is then returned to normal position
Glossectomy—Total Glossectomy—Partial	Total removal of the tongue Partial removal of the tongue	For tumors involving the entire tongue or the tongue and floor of the mouth; partial for tumors involving a portion of the tongue
Alveolectomy	Removal of a portion of the gingiva	
Palatectomy	Removal of a portion or all of the hard palate with prosthetic device application	Prosthesis allows for tongue to make contact, improving speech and swallowing functions
Transhyoid pharyngotomy Lateral pharyngotomy	Alternative surgical approaches to access the oropharyngeal area	Can be used to remove base of tongue tumors
Radical neck dissection	Resection of all nodal groups I-V	For treatment of advanced tumors with neck metastasis; N2 and N3
Supraomohyoid neck dissection	Removal of nodal groups I-III	For treatment of early neck metastasis, or prophylactic for N0; less morbidity than N0; not indicated for advanced disease; predictable pattern of nodal spread in oral cavity cancers; has allowed less radical approaches to be viable in some patients

Modified from Alvi, A., Myers, E. N., & Johnson, J. T. (1996). Cancer of the oral cavity. In E. N. Meyers & J. Y. Suen (Eds.), *Cancer of the head and neck* (3rd ed.). Philadelphia: W. B. Saunders.

ity tumors with mandible invasion (Fig. 54-8). Mandibular reconstruction is performed after resection to decrease morbidity associated with surgery. The anterior mandible is necessary to support the tongue. Defects of the anterior mandible produce significant speech and swallowing problems. The integrity of the mandible also affects facial appearance. Mandibular defects can result in emotionally and physically devastating sequelae. Conversely, the lateral mandible defects result in less dysfunction and may not require reconstruction (Larsen & Sanger, 1995). Mandibulectomy can be performed to gain access to tumors not obtainable through an intraoral approach. This procedure is called a *mandibular swing*. Reconstruction of the mandible is currently performed with microvascular composite free grafts. The fibula and iliac crest are commonly used (Shah & Lydiatt, 1995). Because of the significant amount of swelling postoperatively, many patients undergoing reconstruction of the mandible require a temporary tracheostomy. After reconstruction the mandible must be immobilized 4 to 6 weeks to ensure stability.

Advances in reconstruction of the mandible have greatly affected the management of oral cancers involving the mandible. Other reconstructive techniques used in oral cavity cancer include the radical forearm microvascular free flap, split-thickness skin graft, primary closure, or regional myocutaneous flaps (Shah & Lydiatt, 1995). A review of common surgical techniques and reconstructive methods are summarized in Table 54-11.

A transoral laser partial glossectomy can be performed to treat early cancer of the tongue in patients with local control rates of about 79%. Tongue cancers that have advanced often require treatment with surgery and radiation. Surgical treatment may include a partial or complete glossectomy, marginal or segmental mandibulectomy, and neck dissection. Severe dysfunction in swallowing and speech can occur with treatment for advanced tongue carcinomas. A prosthesis is needed to aid in swallowing, as well as for speech in patients who receive a total glossectomy. Chemotherapy used in combination with radiation is being studied to preserve function and decrease morbidity.

Neck Dissection. Nodal metastasis is an extremely important prognostic indicator in patients with oral cancer. Crile first described the radical neck dissection in 1906. This procedure has been the treatment of choice for patients with head and neck cancer with cervical node metastasis for many years. Functional and cosmetic morbidity associated with the radical neck dissection has prompted increased investigation into the spread of nodal metastasis with head and neck cancers. Important discoveries concluded that cervical lymph node metastasis occurred through fairly predictable routes. It became apparent that not all patients required such a drastic procedure. Radical neck dissection involves the removal of cervical lymph nodes I to V (see Fig. 54-4). Most metastases to cervical lymph nodes that are a result of oral cancer occur in levels I to III. Oropharyngeal lymph node metastasis follows a slightly different pattern. The use of limited neck dissections in patients with minimal lymph node involvement is performed and compared with radical dissections in relationship to morbidity, mortality, local recurrence, and overall survival.

Oral cancers of the floor of the mouth that cross the midline may require bilateral neck dissection due to the common occurrence of ipsilateral spread. In general, T3 and T4 tumors, as well as some T2 tumors, require some form of neck dissection.

Generally, radical neck dissections are not performed when there are positive distant metastases or if the primary oral cancer is unresectable. However, radical neck dissection remains an important treatment option in patients with advanced oral cancer without distant metastasis (Box 54-4).

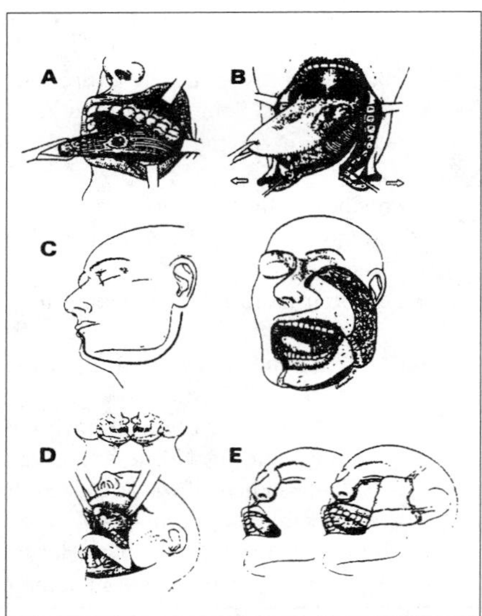

Fig. 54-7 Surgical approaches to the oral cavity. **A,** Per oral; **B,** median mandibulotomy; **C,** lower cheek flap; **D,** visor flap; **E,** upper cheek.

Radiation Therapy

Radiation therapy is used when morbidity rates are improved and survival rates exceed or are equal to those of surgery. Radiation therapy is generally associated with less functional disability than surgery. With T3 or T4 tumors, due to the degree of invasiveness, radiation therapy alone is less effective. If small T1 and T2 tumors are not easily accessible, radiation is usually indicated. Doses of external beam radiation are usually 2 Gy/day for 5 to 7 weeks (Alvi, Myers, & Johnson, 1996). For tumors of the gingiva, hard palate, and retromolar trigone, a tendency toward bone involvement early in the course of the disease can preclude radiation from being a single-treatment option. These patients require surgical resection in most cases.

Local radiation therapy in the treatment of oral cancer can be delivered by external beam or interstitial beam radiation. Interstitial beam radiation, also called *brachytherapy,* includes the placement of radioactive materials directly into or near the tumor. This type of radiation is often used in combination with surgery or external beam radiation for the treatment of tumors of the floor of the mouth and the tongue. The timing of radiation therapy has been controversial. Pre-

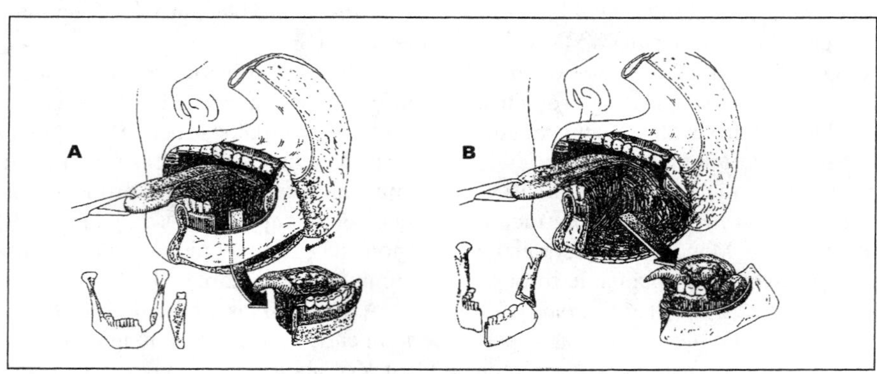

Fig. 54-8 Manibular resection. **A,** Marginal mandibulectomy. **B,** Segmental mandibulectomy. (From Shah, J. P. & Lydiatt, W. [1995]. Treatment of head and neck cancer. *CA: A Cancer Journal for Clinicians, 45*[6], 361.)

operatively, radiation treatment has been more effective because tumor cells unmanipulated by surgery are better oxygenated. The downside to preoperative radiation has been the increased risk of problems, such as impaired wound healing and infection. Tumor margins are also less visible during surgery when preoperative radiation has been used (Alvi, Myers, & Johnson, 1996).

Postoperative radiation has been used to remove residual tumor cells. For maximum effect, postoperative radiation is usually administered within the first 6 weeks after surgery. Radiation after surgery for oral cavity cancer is a more common practice. A disadvantage of postoperative radiation is the decreased oxygenation of the tumor cells manipulated by surgery. Higher doses of radiation are generally used postoperatively due to radioresistance (Alvi, Myers, & Johnson, 1996).

Other important considerations in choosing radiation as a treatment for oral cancer include the health of the patient's mouth. Osteoradionecrosis occurs when bone is destroyed as a result of radiation. This complication of radiation treatment can be even more problematic for patients with poor dental health. Radiation damages osteoclasts and osteoblasts, resulting in loss of bone cells. This process causes a decrease in the thickness and the strength of bone. If many bone cells are damaged, bone necrosis can occur. The mandible is the most common bony structure in the oral cavity that is involved. Factors that increase the risk of osteoradionecrosis are the dosage used, tumor invasion of the bone, and infection.

Nutritional deficits also need to be identified prior to treatment for oral cancer. These defects may be coexistent secondary to alcohol use and/or the actual oral tumor impeding the normal chewing or swallowing functions. To decrease complications associated with surgery and radiation therapy, these patients should have concurrent dietary supplements and be evaluated by a dietitian.

In older patients with coexisting pulmonary and/or cardiovascular problems, surgery may be contraindicated, making radiation the only available treatment option. Conversely, if patients have xeroderma pigmentosa, vitiligo, or other sun disorders, external beam radiation may need to be avoided (Beyers, 1995).

In early cancer of the tongue, T1 and T2, without nodal metastasis, radiation can be curative. External beam radiation or interstitial radiation (brachytherapy) can be used singly or in combination. Brachytherapy in tongue cancer can cause a large amount of edema to the tongue, making a tracheostomy necessary during treatment. In a study by Piedbois and colleagues (1991), stages I and II cancers of the tongue were treated with brachytherapy and neck dissection if indicated. The local control rate was 87% for patients at approximately 3 years. Long-term sequelae of radiation treatment can be difficult and permanent. Xerostomia, mucositis, hypoguesesthesia, and osteoradionecrosis can greatly affect these patients' quality of life. Approximately 12 to 14 days after the initiation of radiation, mucositis begins to occur with the beginnings of erythema and fibrinous exudate. Skin reactions occur at about 3 weeks after radiation has been started due to the slow turnover of cells in the

Box 54-4

Possible Complications of Radical Neck Dissection

Short-Term Surgical Complications

- Hemorrhage
- Pain
- Airway obstruction
- Infection
- Thoracic duct leakage
- Nerve injury

Chronic Problems

- Neck contractore
- Loss of neck contours
- Shoulder droop
- Subluxation
- Chronic shoulder pain

TABLE 54-11 Surgical Reconstructive Techniques after Surgery for Oral Cancer

Procedure	Description	Rationale
Microvascular composite-free grafts	Grafts from the iliac crest, fibula, or radial forearm	For mandibular repair after mandibulectomy; necessary in anterior defects because of resulting speech and swallowing disabilities
Primary closure	Wound closed primarily	For small tumors located anteriorly; minimal functional loss
Split-thickness skin graft	Sewing tissue in to cover the surgical defect	Used to repair large defects in oral cavity cancer
Prosthesis	Used after resection of the hard palate and/or alveous; plates are used after resection of the mandible	Can aid in decreasing eating, chewing, swallowing, and talking dysfunction
Regional myocutaceous flaps	Skin and muscle used to replace large defects in the oral cavity	

Modified from Alvi, A., Myers, E. N., & Johnson, J. T. (1996). Cancer of the oral cavity. In E. N. Meyers & J. Y. Suen (Eds.), *Cancer of the head and neck* (3rd ed.). Philadelphia: W. B. Saunders.

skin compared with those of the mucosa. Erythema is followed by dry desquamation and in some cases ulceration. The rapidly growing cells of the integumentary system are very radiosensitive, making them vulnerable to the adverse effects of radiation. Because of the advancements in the quality of external beam radiation, severe skin reactions are less common than in the past.

Xerostomia is a result of radiation damage to the salivary and mucous glands. Saliva becomes decreased, thick, and sticky. A decrease in saliva begins to occur 2 to 3 days after receiving radiation. A decrease in saliva can cause problems with swallowing, chewing, and speaking, as well as dental caries. Hypoguesesthesia, or loss of taste sensations, occurs with most patients receiving external radiation to the oral cavity. This problem may be due not only to the radiation damage, but also to the decreased production of saliva, which can hinder the ability to taste foods.

Chemotherapy

Chemotherapy continues to be studied for use in oral cancer. Adjuvant, neoadjuvant, and concurrent use of chemotherapy are all under investigation with surgery and radiation. Although surgery and radiation have been beneficial for patients, these types of treatment are locally administered and have limited use in oral cancers that reoccur or have metastasis. Researchers have been hopeful that chemotherapy might have some benefit for this group of patients. In the past, chemotherapy has been used for patients with recurrent or metastatic oral cavity cancer. The use of chemotherapy for local control of oral cancer has not demonstrated an increase in overall survival (Alvi, Myers, & Johnson, 1996; Liggett & Forastiere, 1995). Although the use of chemotherapy in oral cancer remains unclear, there is hope that this treatment modality may be helpful in providing palliation for patients with recurrent disease or patients at high risk for relapse. Further large, randomized studies are needed to substantiate the role of chemotherapy in patients with oral cancer. The chemotherapeutic agents that have shown activity in head and neck cancers are carboplatin, cisplatin, bleomycin, methotrexate, and 5-fluorouracil. Many more are being studied.

The concurrent use of chemotherapy with radiation may result in radiosensitization of tumor cells, thereby increasing the efficacy of radiation. Clinical trials are being conducted comparing radiation alone to chemotherapy and radiation in the treatment of patients with locally advanced nonresectable head and neck cancer. Currently, chemotherapy may play a role in the management of patients with oral cancer and distant metastasis. In a National Cancer Institute study, patients with oral cancer and with limited nodal status treated with adjuvant chemotherapy had significant improvement in 3-year disease-free survival from 67% vs 49% in the group without chemotherapy (Jacobs & Makuch, 1990). Findings from these and other studies suggest that there may be a role for chemotherapy in select patients with oral cancer. However, an increased overall survival has not been demonstrated. Clinical trials are underway to further investigate chemotherapy as a treatment option in oral cavity cancer and to identify patients who would benefit from this treatment modality.

Gene Therapy

The role of gene therapy in oral cancer is the subject of much interest. Scientists have theorized that the risk for oral cancer in the presence of alcohol and/or tobacco use may be influenced by the person's ability to repair damaged DNA. Clearly, not all people who use tobacco and/or alcohol get oral cancer. Further investigation into what affects individual susceptibility to oral cancer could allow for the use of gene therapy (Shillitoe, Lapeyre, & Adler-Storthz, 1994).

ONCOLOGIC EMERGENCIES

In oral cancer the most serious oncologic emergency is airway obstruction. Several factors could place a patient at risk for an airway obstruction, including tumor obstruction, blood clots, mucus plugs, or edema as a result of surgery or radiation treatment. A tracheostomy may be placed during surgery or interstitial radiation treatment when large amounts of tissue swelling and difficulty clearing secretions are anticipated. Nursing assessment of the patient's oral cavity and respiratory status should be done routinely to recognize any signs of occlusion. The patient and family should be instructed on this potentially life-threatening complication (Table 54-12). Patients with any symptoms of ineffective airway clearance should be treated immediately.

NURSING MANAGEMENT

The nursing management of the patient with oral cancer requires a thorough knowledge of the treatment options and side effects. Nursing care and patient education are essential in these patients not only to ensure a successful outcome, but also to empower patients and family members to provide the high levels of self-care that are required. The patient with oral cancer will likely receive radiation, surgery, or a combination of these treatments. The nursing care of the patient undergoing surgery and/or radiation involves many challenging problems. The care of a patient with oral cancer receiving radiation or surgery is reviewed, and standards of care are provided to guide nursing management.

Patients receiving radiation treatment have varying side effects, depending on whether the radiation is external beam or interstitial irradiation (brachytherapy). Interstitial irradiation is most commonly used in combination with radiation or surgery for small cancers of the floor of the mouth or tongue and has also been used in lip and buccal mucosa carcinomas. The major problems that occur in patients receiving external beam radiation for oral cavity cancer include xerostomia, hypoguesesthesia, stomatitis, and skin problems. Nursing management of patients receiving external beam radiation is summarized in Table 54-12.

Xerostomia, or dryness of the mouth as a result of decreased saliva production, can be a very disturbing side effect of radiation therapy, affecting eating, swallowing, and

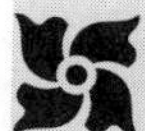

TABLE 54-12 Standard of Care for the Patient With Oral Cancer Receiving External Beam Radiation Therapy

Patient Problem and Outcomes	Nursing Interventions and Rationales	Patient Education Instructions
Knowledge Deficit Patient will: • Understand external beam radiation therapy as well as side effects and self-care measures.	1. Assess the patient's understanding of external beam radiation, side effects, and self-care measures. 2. Reinforce teaching. 3. Encourage self-care. 4. Assess the patient's resources and ability to comply with the treatment plan and self-care measures.	1. Describe the process of radiation treatment: a. Consultation with radiation oncologist. b. Simulation to localize the tumor and determine volume to be treated. c. Treatment—explain time involved in proposed treatment. 2. Review side effects of external beam radiation specific to the oral cavity: a. Xerostomia b. Hypoguesesthesia c. Stomatitis d. Skin desquamation e. Osteoradionecrosis f. Fatigue g. Trismus 3. Encourage self-care measures to minimize side effects.
Xerostomia Patient will: • Maintain adequate fluid balance and experience a decrease in severity of xerostomia.	1. Assess for xerostomia and associated complaints of dysphagia, taste alterations, and difficulty chewing. 2. Assess amount and characteristics of saliva—thick, sticky, scant. 3. Assess patient comfort and anxiety regarding effects of xerostomia. 4. Assess patient for complications of xerostomia; saliva contains immunoglobulins and bacteriostatic enzyme properties; without the protective ability of saliva, plaque buildup occurs, increasing the risk of dental carries & other infections.	1. Describe how xerostomia occurs, the onset, and symptoms. 2. Teach the patient self-care measures to alleviate or minimize xerostomia: a. Frequent oral intake of fluids b. Use of hard sugar-free candies or gum c. Moisten foods with liquids, sauces, gravies, or soups before eating d. Frequent mouth care e. Use of artificial saliva f. Prophylactic oral antibacterial rinses g. Avoidance of alcohol, tobacco, and temperature extremes h. Apply K-Y jelly or lanolin to the lips
Hypoguesesthesia (A Decrease in Taste Sensations) Patient will: • Verbalize ways to decrease the severity of hypoguesesthesia.	1. Assess the oral cavity for dryness or any concomitant infections that can also affect taste buds. 2. Obtain a dietary consultation to assess daily intake and assist with food choices. 3. Encourage frequent mouth care. 4. Obtain weekly weights & monitor. 5. Assess laboratory values that may affect hypoguesesthesia: a. Zinc b. Nickel c. Copper d. Niacin e. Vitamin A	1. Explain to the patient that destruction of the taste buds occurs with doses of 1000 cGy and is temporary, usually lasting about 2-3 months. 2. Teach the patient that sweet is the first taste to recover, followed by bitter, sour, & salty, respectively. 3. Review self-care measures to decrease the severity of hypoguesesthesia: a. Use spices and flavoring to increase the sensitivity of taste buds. b. Avoid bland foods and temperature extremes. c. Foods that may have a metallic taste include meats; these may need to be avoided. d. Fish, poultry, soybeans, eggs, legumes, and cheeses can be high-protein additions to the diet. e. Drink liquids with meals to keep the mouth moist. f. Encourage frequent mouth care.

Modified from Bloch, A. S. (1990). *Nutrition management of the cancer patient.* Rockville, MA: Aspen; Bucholtz, J. D. (1992). Implications of radiation therapy for nursing. In J. C. Clark & R. R. McGee (Eds.), *Core curriculum for oncology nursing.* Philadelphia: W. B. Saunders; Goodman, M., Ladd, L. A., & Purl, S. (1993). Integumentary and mucous membrane alterations. In S. Groenwald, M. H. Frogge, M. Goodman, & L. H. Yarbro (Eds.), *Cancer nursing principles and practice.* Boston: Jones and Bartlett.

Continued

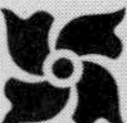

TABLE 54-12 Standard of Care for the Patient with Oral Cancer Receiving External Beam Radiation Therapy—cont'd

Patient Problem and Outcomes	Nursing Interventions and Rationales	Patient Education Instructions
Stomatitis (Inflammation of the Oral Cavity Mucous Membrane)		
Patient will: • Experience a decrease in the severity of mucositis. • Not develop oral infections.	1. Assess for redness, edema, tenderness, or infection of the oral cavity, and report any suspected infections. 2. Encourage frequent mouth care. 3. Obtain a dietary consultation. 4. Assess patient comfort and administer topical analgesics to decrease pain and allow for mouth care to be performed: a. 1% diclone 5 cc swish & spit prior to mouth care or eating b. Benadryl, Mylanta, viscous lidocaine	1. Explain the rationale for the occurrence of stomatitis with radiation treatment; onset 2 weeks. 2. Review side effects associated with oral cavity radiation treatment. 3. Teach the patient how to assess the oral cavity and to inform the nurse of any burning, pain, redness, odor, white patches, sores, or lesions. 4. Teach the patient ways to manage & minimize stomatitis induced by radiation therapy & avoid infection: a. Frequent mouth care four to five times a day can include a baking soda, salt water rinse, soft toothbrush. b. Soft, bland, nonirritating foods, if area is tender; high calorie and protein foods are preferable. c. Avoid temperature extremes. d. Avoid alcohol-based mouthwashes, tobacco, and caffeine. e. Avoid lemon-glycerin swabs that can further dry the mouth.
Skin Desquamation Due to External Beam Radiation Therapy		
Patient will: • Experience a decrease in discomfort related to skin changes caused by radiation. • Provide proper self-care of the skin to prevent worsening of skin problems.	1. Assess skin daily for erythema, edema, ulcerations, pruritus, infection, drainage, dryness, moisture, or other changes. 2. Assess patient comfort. 3. Encourage fluid intake. 4. Assess the need for topical therapies, such as water-soluble lubricants or topical steroids.	1. Describe the effects of radiation therapy to the oral cavity on the skin: a. Erythema b. Dry desquamation c. Pruritus d. Hyperpigmentation e. Moist desquamation 2. Teach the patient how to care for the skin involved in the radiation treatment area: a. Keep the skin clean and dry. b. Report redness, pain, blistering, drainage, and wet areas of itching. c. Avoid temperature extremes and sun exposure. d. Avoid the use of lotions, powders, deodorants, or other skin-care products unless checking with a nurse or physician. e. Wear loose-fitting, cotton clothing. f. Avoid washing off radiation markings.

Modified from Bloch, A. S. (1990). *Nutrition management of the cancer patient.* Rockville, MA: Aspen; Bucholtz, J. D. (1992). Implications of radiation therapy for nursing. In J. C. Clark & R. R. McGee (Eds.), *Core curriculum for oncology nursing.* Philadelphia: W. B. Saunders; Goodman, M., Ladd, L. A., & Purl, S. (1993). Integumentary and mucous membrane alterations. In S. Groenwald, M. H. Frogge, M. Goodman, & L. H. Yarbro (Eds.), *Cancer nursing principles and practice.* Boston: Jones and Bartlett.

talking. Hypoguesesthesia, or a loss of taste sensations, is caused by the destruction of the taste buds by radiation. Waste products that occur as a result of cellular destruction from radiation and/or chemotherapy alter taste sensations. Compounding this problem, the lack of saliva makes it difficult to taste foods. Stomatitis, or an inflammation of the oral cavity membrane, can occur after radiation therapy to the oral cavity or chemotherapy for oral cancer. Xerostomia promotes the growth of bacteria and the buildup of debris in the oral cavity. Without the antibacterial properties and the

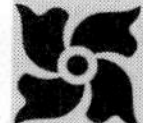

TABLE 54-12 Standard of Care for the Patient with Oral Cancer Receiving External Beam Radiation Therapy—cont'd

Patient Problem and Outcomes	Nursing Interventions and Rationales	Patient Education Instructions
Osteoradionecrosis (Bone Damage as a Result of Radiation)		
Patient will: • Have normal swallowing and chewing capabilities.	1. Assess patient chewing and swallowing abilities. 2. Evaluate for the presence of infections; initiate antibiotics if infection present. 3. Encourage frequent mouth care with an antibacterial mouth rinse.	1. Explain to the patient the effects of osteoradionecrosis: a. Impaired ability to chew or swallow b. Weight loss c. Infection 2. Review ways to decrease the severity of osteoradionecrosis and to promote healing: a. Frequent mouth care four to five times a day b. Use of antibiotics 3. Educate patient on reportable signs and symptoms: a. Difficulty chewing b. Difficulty swallowing c. Pain
Trismus (Inability or Difficulty in Moving the Jaw)		
Patient will: • Maintain adequate nutritional intake.	1. Assess the mobility of the patient's jaw and ability to safely ingest foods. 2. Administer tube feeding to prevent weight loss and malnutrition. 3. Assess tolerance to tube feedings.	1. Teach the patient that trismus can result from radiation fibrosis of the oral cavity. 2. Explain to the patient the rationale for tube feedings. 3. Instruct the patient on adverse reactions to tube feedings that should be reported to the nurse. 4. Instruct the patient on range-of-motion exercises for the jaw to be done twice daily during radiation and as long as stiffness occurs.
Airway Obstruction		
Patient will: • Recognize and seek prompt treatment for signs of ineffective airway clearance.	1. Assess the oral cavity and ability to swallow every day or with each visit. 2. Assess the patient for respiratory disease. 3. Assist the patient with oral irrigation and suctioning as needed.	1. Teach the patient the signs & symptoms of ineffective airway clearance or obstruction: a. Difficulty breathing b. Inability to clear secretions c. Ineffective cough 2. Instruct the patient on measures to maintain a patent airway: a. Elevate the head of the bed 45° to 90°. b. Encourage coughing & deep breathing. c. Humidify air to loosen secretions.

cleansing abilities of saliva, the oral cavity can become a problematic area leading to pain, tenderness, and infections.

The degree of skin changes that occur as a result of radiation therapy depends on many factors. The dosage of radiation used, site, type of equipment, age, and nutritional status of the patient are just a few important considerations. Skin changes caused by radiation therapy to the oral cavity can involve dry and moist desquamation, pruritus, erythema, and hyperpigmentation. The nurse plays a pivotal role in providing upfront and ongoing patient education. The patient's ability to manage these problems can be inhibited greatly by a lack of self-care education about strategies.

Interstitial irradiation, or brachytherapy, is a technique where a radioactive source is placed into the tumor. The patient is prepared under general anesthesia, and catheters are placed to harbor the radioactive source. Damage to normal tissue is minimized with interstitial irradiation. Due to swelling in the oral cavity, this type of radiation may require a temporary tracheostomy.

As reviewed in the medical management section, the surgical treatment of the patient with oral cancer can be diverse. Depending on the location, size, extension, and presence of nodal metastasis, surgical procedures can vary. The use of laser surgery (light amplification of stimulated emission of radiation) for intraoral resection of small oral lesions has resulted in significantly less blood loss, pain, wound drainage, and functional disability (Alvi, Myers, & Johnson, 1996). Nursing management of the patient undergoing surgery for oral cancer not only involves preoperative and postoperative management, but also complex nutritional assessment.

Rehabilitation Issues

Intensive rehabilitation of speech and swallowing is often necessary in patients with oral cancer. For rehabilitation to be successful, interdisciplinary members of the health care team, such as speech therapists, dietitians, and occupational therapists, must be involved in the pretreatment period. Patient education should start prior to radiation, surgery, or chemotherapy. A thorough assessment of the patient's swallowing, speech, and dentition is performed prior to treatment, after treatment, and routinely throughout rehabilitation. Rehabilitation includes ways to improve swallowing and speech.

Unfortunately, xerostomia as a result of radiation therapy in these patients is often a permanent sequela. Xerostomia can make swallowing and speech difficult. Speech and swallowing therapists play an extremely valuable role in assessing and teaching patients effective ways to minimize these problems.

The nature of the surgical procedure performed determines the type and amount of rehabilitation needed. As previously discussed, many surgeries of the oral cavity result in speech, chewing, and swallowing dysfunction. When reconstruction of the oral cavity includes tissue transplantation from a different part of the body, swallowing can be affected because these new tissues do not have sensory capabilities. Patients may not be able to feel the food in these areas, making it difficult to swallow. A maxillofacial prosthodontist is often involved in assessing the need for a prosthesis to improve oral cavity function. Patients with oropharyngeal cancer experience similar problems as a result of surgery. However, the risk of aspiration is greater in this group of patients postoperatively because of the location of treatment. A comprehensive swallowing evaluation with subsequent rehabilitation is essential.

Psychosocial support is fundamental in the treatment and rehabilitation of patients with oral or oropharyngeal cancer. Patients are frequently not prepared for the functional disability and expect to return to normal after treatment. Nursing education of these patients preoperatively and postoperatively can help enable them to deal with side effects and long-term sequelae of treatment.

TABLE 54-13 Quality of Care Evaluation for a Patient Undergoing External Beam Radiation Therapy

Interdisciplinary members of the quality of care evaluation:
☐ Nursing ☐ Radiation Therapy
☐ Dietary ☐ Social Services

I. Postradiation management evaluation
Data from: ☐ Medical record ☐ Patient/family

Criteria	Yes	No
1. Patient provided with information before radiation concerning side effects:		
a. Xerostomia	☐	☐
b. Skin changes	☐	☐
c. Stomatitis	☐	☐
d. Hypoguesesthesia	☐	☐
e. Osteoradionecrosis	☐	☐
f. Trismus	☐	☐
g. Fatigue	☐	☐
2. Patient provided with information on how to minimize and manage side effects of radiation therapy.	☐	☐
3. Patient received a dietary consultation prior to radiation therapy.	☐	☐

II. Patient/Family Satisfaction
Data from: ☐ Patient ☐ Family

Criteria	Yes	No
1. On a scale of 0-10, with 0 being not satisfied at all and 10 being completely satisfied, how satisfied were you with the education on how to manage problems related to your radiation therapy? ________		
2. Were you told about decreased salivation and how to manage this problem?	☐	☐
3. Were you instructed on choosing foods that are high in protein and calories?	☐	☐

HOME CARE ISSUES

The challenges that patients and families encounter in the home to a large degree depend on the extent of the disease, the necessary treatment, and their functional status. Patients diagnosed with early-stage oral cancer who receive radiation or surgery for curative purposes are less likely to experience significant problems at home. Patients undergoing daily radiation treatments need to identify and mobilize appropriate resources to ensure appointments are met. Social workers and case managers can be extremely valuable members of the interdisciplinary team involved in the care of the patient with oral cancer. Instructions on self-care measures to minimize and manage the side effects of radiation therapy, xerostomia, hypoguesesthesia, and stomatitis need to be given to all patients. Education of the patient prior to radiation and continued reinforcement at each home visit are essential. Invasive surgical procedures reviewed previously can drastically affect these patients' quality of life. These patients may require reconstructive surgery followed by intensive rehabilitation to resume speech, swallowing, and eating. Occupational, speech, and physical therapy rehabilitation may be required in the home care setting for a period of time. If chemotherapy is used, the patient may experience problems with nausea, vomiting, stomatitis, diarrhea, and neutropenia. Ways to minimize the risk of infection if neutropenia occurs must be taught to patients who are in the home setting.

Although some of the care for these patients may occur in the inpatient setting, a large part of their care occurs in the outpatient or home environment. It is important for the nurse to assess the patient's needs, provide instruction and guidance, and promote self-care in the home setting.

Patient Resources

Patients may obtain information on oral cancer from the Cancer Information Service (CIS), 1-800-4-CANCER; American Cancer Society (ACS), 1-800-ACS-2345; National Institute of Dental Research; and American Dental Association (1994). Tobacco educational resources are also available to assist health care workers in teaching patients about the hazards of tobacco. These materials are available through the National Cancer Institute as well as the American Dental Association (1995).

PROGNOSIS

The prognosis for patients with oral cancer depends on many factors. Early diagnosis of oral cancer can result in significant improvements in survival rates and morbidity associated with treatment. However, despite the use of surgery, radiation and chemotherapy overall survival rates for Caucasians and African Americans are 55% and 34%, respectively (Mashberg & Samit, 1995) (see Fig. 54-6).

EVALUATION OF QUALITY OF CARE

Monitoring the quality of patient care is essential to continue to improve and provide safe and effective care to patients. Table 54-13 is an example of a quality of care evaluation tool that can be used when caring for the patient undergoing external beam radiation therapy for oral cavity cancer.

RESEARCH ISSUES

Research continues to be needed in many areas for this patient population. Studies examining early diagnosis, initiation of successful tobacco and alcohol cessation programs, treatment options, and quality of life are extremely important to improve the outcome for patients with oral cancer. Improvements in screening techniques and standardized approaches to early detection of oral cancer are essential. Randomized clinical trials are also needed to determine the effect of chemopreventive agents used with premalignant lesions, as well as for the prevention of second malignancies. Head and neck cancers are thought to have decreased oxygenation, making them resistant to chemotherapy and radiotherapy. The use of agents to make tumor cells more sensitive to current treatments is a topic of interest that is currently under investigation.

REFERENCES

Alvi, A., Myers, E. N., & Johnson, J. T. (1996). Cancer of the oral cavity. In E.N. Meyers & J. Y. Suen (Eds.), *Cancer of the head and neck* (3rd ed.). Philadelphia: W. B. Saunders.

American Dental Association. (1995). *Smoking can do a real number on your mouth.* Location: The Association.

American Dental Association. (1994). *What you should know about oral cancer.* Chicago: The Association.

American Joint Committee on Cancer. (1993). Handbook for staging of cancer. In *The manual for staging of cancer* (4th ed.). Philadelphia: J. B. Lippincott.

Amos, B. & Lotan, R. (1991). Retinoid-sensitive cells and cell lines. *Methods in Enzymology, 190,* 217-225.

Balaram, P., Nalinakumari, K. R., Abraham, E., Balan, A., Harcendran, N. K., Bernard, H. U., & Chan, S. Y. (1995). Human papilloma virus in 91 oral cancers from Indian betal quid chewers—high prevelence and multiplicity of infections. *International Journal of Cancer, 61,* 450-454.

Beyers, R. M. (1995). Factors affecting the choice of initial therapy in oral cancer. *Seminars in Surgical Oncology, 11,* 183-189.

Binnie, W. H., Rankin, K. V., & Mackenzie, I. C. (1983). Risk factors in head and neck cancer. *New England Journal of Medicine, 306,* 1151-1155.

Bloch, A. S. (1990). *Nutrition management of the cancer patient.* Rockville, MA: Aspen.

Bloom, B., Gift, H. C., & Jack, S. S. (1992). Dental services and oral health: United States, 1989. *Vital Health Statistics, 10*(183), 1-95.

Blot, W. J., McLaughlin, J. K., Winn, D. M., Austin, D. F., Greenburg, R. S., Preston-Martin, S., Bernstein, L., Schoenberg, J. B., Sternhagen, A., & Fraumeri, J.F., Jr. (1988). Smoking and drinking in relation to oral and pharyngeal cancer. *Cancer Research, 48,* 3282-3287.

Boffetta, P., Mashberg, A., Winklemann, R., & Garfinkel, L. (1992). Carcinogenic effect of tobacco smoking and alcohol drinking on anatomic sites of the oral cavity and oropharynx. *International Journal of Cancer, 52,* 530-533.

Brennan, C. T., Sessions, D. G., Spitznagel, E. L., & Harvey, J. E. (1991). Surgical pathology of cancer of the oral cavity and oropharynx. *Laryngoscope, 101,* 1175-1197.

Broder, A. C. (1920). Squamous cell epithelioma of the lip. *Journal of the American Medical Association, 74,* 656-664.

Buchholtz, J. D. (1992). Implications of radiation therapy for nursing. In J. C. Clark & R. F. McGee (Eds.), *Core curriculum for oncology nursing*. Philadelphia: W. B. Saunders.

Centers for Disease Control. (1993). Cigarette smoking among adults, United States, 1991. *Morbidity and Mortality Weekly Reports, 42,* 230-233.

Chiesa, F., Tradati, N., & Marazza, M. (1992). Prevention of local relapses and new localizations of oral leukoplakias with synthetic retinoid fenertinide (4-HPR): Preliminary results. *Oral Oncology European Journal of Cancer, 28B,* 97-102.

Choi, S. Y. & Kahyo, H. (1991). Effect of cigarette smoking and alcohol consumption in the aetiology of cancer of the oral cavity, pharynx, and larynx. *International Journal of Epidemiology, 20*(4), 878-885.

Civantos, F. J. & Goodwin, J. W. (1996). Cancer of the oropharynx. In E. N. Meyers & J. Y. Suen (Eds.), *Cancer of the head and neck* (3rd ed.). Philadelphia: W.B. Saunders.

Crile, G. (1906). Excision of cancer of the head and neck with special reference to the plan of dissection based on one hundred and thirty-two operations. *Journal of American Medical Association, 47,* 1780-1786.

Davidson, B. J., Spiro, R. M., Patel, S., Patel, K., & Shah, J. P. (1994). Cervical metastasis of occult origin: The impact of combined modality therapy. *American Journal of Surgery, 168,* 395-399.

DePalo, G. & Formelli, F. (1995). Risks and benefits of retinoids in the chemoprevention of cancer. *Drug Safety, 13*(4), 245-256.

Department of Health and Human Services, Office of the Inspector General. (1992). *Spit tobacco and youth* (DHHS Publication No. OEI 06-92-00500). Washington, DC: Author.

Department of Veteran Affairs Laryngeal Cancer Study Group (VALCS). (1991). *New England Journal of Medicine, 324,* 1685-1690.

Dibb, C.R., Urba, S., & Wolf, G.T. (1995). Organ preservation in advanced head and neck cancer. In W.K. Hong & R.S. Weber (Eds.), *Head and neck cancer: Basic and clinical aspects.* Boston: Kluwer Academic.

Dorr, R. T. & VonHoff, D. D. (1994). *Cancer chemotherapy handbook* (2nd ed.). Norwalk, CT: Appleton & Lange.

Elliott, G. V., MacDougall, J. A., & Elliott, J. D. (1973). Problems of verrucous squamous carcinoma. *Annals of Surgery, 177,* 21-29.

Franceschi, D., Gupta, R., Spiro, R. H., & Shah, J. P. (1993). Improved survival in the treatment of squamous carcinoma of the oral tongue. *American Journal of Surgery, 166,* 360-365.

Franco, E. L., Kowalski, L. P., Oliveira, B. V., Curado, M. P., Pereira, R. N., Silva, M.E., & Fava, A. S. (1989). Risk factors for oral cancer in Brazil: A case control study. *International Journal of Cancer, 43,* 992-1000.

Frank-Stromberg, M. & Cohen, R. F. (1993). Assessment and interventions for cancer prevention and detection. In S. L. Groenwald, M. Froggs, M. Goodman, & C. Yarbro Henke (Eds.), *Cancer nursing principles and practice* (3rd ed.). Boston: Jones and Bartlett.

Goodman, H. S., Yellowitz, J. A., & Horowitz, A. M. (1995). Oral cancer prevention: The role of family practitioners. *Archives of Family Medicine, 4,* 628-632.

Goodman, M., Ladd, L. A., & Purl, S. (1993). Integumentary and mucous membrane alterations. In S. Groenwald, M. H. Frogge, M. Goodman, & L. H. Yarbro (Eds.), *Cancer nursing principles and practice.* Boston: Jones and Bartlett.

Gridley, G., McLaughlin, J. K., Block, G., Winn, D. M., Greenberg, R. S., Schoenberg, J. B., Preston-Martin, S., Austin, D. F., & Fraumeni, J. F. (1990). Diet and oral and pharyngeal cancer among blacks. *Nutrition Cancer, 14,* 219-225.

Gupta, P. C., Mehta, F. S., Daftary, D. K., Pindburg, J. J., Bhonsle, R. B., Jalnawalla, P.N., Sinor, P.N., Pitkar, V.K., Murti, P.R., & Irani, R.R. (1980). Incidence rates of oral cancer and natural history of oral precancerous lesions in a 10-year follow-up study of Indian villagers. *Community Dental and Oral Epidemiology, 8,* 283-333.

International Agency for Research on Cancer. (1988). *Monographs on the evaluation of carcinogenic risks to humans,* Vol. 44. Lyons, France.

Jacobs, C. & Makuch, R. (1990). Efficacy of adjuvant chemotherapy for patients with resectable head and neck cancer: A subject analysis of the Head and Neck Contracts Program. *Journal of Clinical Oncology, 8,* 838-847.

Jensen, O.M., Esteve, J., Moller, H., & Renard, M. (1990). Cancer in the European community and its member states. *European Journal of Cancer, 26,* 1167-1256.

Johnson, J.T., Barnes, L., Meyers, E.N., Schramm, V.L. Borochovitz, D., & Sigler, B.A. (1981). The extracapsular spread of tumors in cervical node metastasis. *Archives of Otolaryngology, 107,* 725-729.

Larsen, D.L. & Sanger, J.R. (1995). Management of the mandible in oral cancer. *Seminars in Surgical Oncology, 11,* 190-199.

Lavecchia, C., Negri, E., D'Avanzo, B., Boyle, P., & Franceschi, S. (1991). Dietary indicators of oral and pharyngeal cancer. *International Journal of Epidemiology, 20,* 1, 39-44.

Liggett, W., Jr. & Forastiere, A.A. (1995). Chemotherapy advances in head and neck oncology. *Seminars in Oncology, 11,* 265-271.

Lippman, S.M., Clayman, G.L., Huber, M.H., Benner, S.E., & Hong, W.K. (1995). Biology and reversal of aerodigestive tract carcinogenesis. In W.K. Hong & R.S. Weber (Eds.), *Head and neck cancer.* Boston: Kluwer Academic.

Lippman, S.M., Heyman, R.A., Korie, J.M., Benner, S.E., & Hong, W.K. (1995). Retinoids and chemoprevention: Clinical and basic studies. *Journal of Cellular Biochemistry, Suppl. 22,* 1-10.

Lippman, S.M. & Hong, W.K. (1989). Second malignant tumors in head and neck squamous cell carcinoma: The overshadowing threat for patients with early stage disease. *International Journal of Radiation Oncology and Biophysics, 17,* 691-694.

MacFarlane, G.J., Zheng, T., Marshall, J.R., Bofetta, P., Niu, S., Brasire, J., Merletti, F., & Boyle, P. (1995). Alcohol, tabacco, diet and the risk of oral cancer: A pooled analysis of three case control studies. *European Journal of Cancer, Part B. Oral Oncology, 31B,* 181-187.

Maguire, B.P. & Roberts. (1994). Dentists' examination of the oral mucosa to detect oral cancer. *Journal of Public Health Dentation, 53,* 115.

Mahboudi, E. & Sayed, G.M. (1982). Oral cavity and pharynx. In D. Scotterfeld & J.F. Fraumeri, Jr. (Eds.), *Cancer epidemiology and prevention.* Philadelphia: W. B. Saunders.

Marshall, J.R. & Boyle, P. (1996). Guidelines on diet, nutrition, and cancer prevention: Reducing the risk of cancer with healthy food choices and physical activity. *CA: ACancer Journal for Clinicians, 46*(6), 325-341.

Mashberg, A. & Barsa, P. (1984). Screening for oral and oropharyngeal squamous carcinomas. *CA: A Cancer Journal for Clinicians, 34*(5), 262-268.

Mashberg, A., Garfinkel, L., & Harris, S. (1981). Alcohol as a primary risk factor in oral squamous carcinoma. *CA: A Cancer Journal for Clinicians, 31,* 146-155.

Mashberg, A. & Samit, G. (1995). Early diagnosis of asymptomatic oral and oropharyngeal squamous cancers. *CA: A Cancer Journal for Clinicians, 45*(6), 328-351.

McLaughlin, J.K., Gridley, G., Block, G., Winn, D.M., Preston-Martin, S., Schoenberg, J.B., Greenberg, R.S., Stemhagen, A., Austin, D.F., & Erslow, A.G. (1988). Dietary factors in oral and pharyngeal cancer. *Journal of the National Cancer Institute, 80,* 1237-1243.

Miller, A.B. (1983). Trends in cancer mortality and epidemiology. *Cancer, 51,* 2413-2418.

Moore, C. (1971). Cigarette smoking and cancer of the mouth, pharynx, and larynx. *American Journal of Surgery, 114,* 510.

Piedbois, P., Majeron, J.J., & Haddad, E. (1991). Stage I-II squamous cell carcinoma of the oral cavity treated by Iridium-192: Is elective neck dissection indicated? *Radiotherapy Oncology, 21,* 100-106.

Reichart, P.A. (1995). Oral cancer and precancer related to betel and miang chewing in Thailand: A review. *Journal of Oral Pathology Medicine, 24,* 241-243.

Roed-Peterson, B. (1971). Cancer development in oral leukoplakia: Follow-up of 331 patients. *Journal of Dental Research, 50,* 711.

Rosenberg, D. & Cretin, S. (1989). Use of meta-analysis to evaluate tolonium chloride in oral cancer. *Cancer Causes Control, 4,* 63-66.

Rothman, K.J., Cann, C.I., Flanders, D., & Fried, M.P. (1980). Epidemiology of laryngeal cancer. *Epidemiology Review, 2,* 195-209.

Schuller, D.E., Reiches, N.A., Hamaker, R.C., Lingeman, R.E., Weisberger, E.C., Suen, J.Y., Conley, J.J., Kelly, D.R., & Miglets, A.W. (1983). Analysis of disability resulting from treatment including radical neck dissection or modified neck dissection. *Head Neck Surgery, 6,* 551.

Shah J.P. & Lydiatt, W. (1995). Treatment of head and neck cancer. *CA: A Cancer Journal for Clinicians, 45*(6), 352-368.

Shillitoe, E.J., Lapeyre, N., & Adler-Storthz, K. (1994). Gene therapy—Its potential in the management of oral cancer. *Oral Oncology, European Journal of Cancer, 30B,* 143-154.

Shin, D.M., Tainsky, M.A. (1995). Molecular phenotyping of head and neck cancer. In W.K. Hong & R.S. Weber (Eds.), *Head and neck cancer.* Boston: Kluwer Academic Publishers.

Silverman, S. (1994). Oral cancer. *Seminars in Dermatology, 13*(2), 132-137.

Silverman, S., Jr., & Dillon, W.P. (1990). Diagnosis. In S. Silverman, Jr. (Ed.), *Oral cancer* (3rd ed.). Atlanta: American Cancer Society.

Silverman, S., Renstrip, G., & Pindburg, J.J. (1963). Studies in oral leukoplakia. *Acta Odontologica Scandinavica, 21,* 271-292.

Slaughter, D.P., Southwick, H.W., & Smejkal, W. (1953). "Field cancerization" in oral stratified squamous-cell epithelium: Clinical implications of muticentric origin. *Cancer, 5,* 963-68.

Smart, C.R. (1993). Screening for cancer of the aerodigestive tract. *Cancer, 72*(Suppl.), 1061-1065.

Spangler, J.G. (1995). Open your mouth and say "Ahhhh . . .": Oral cancer screening and family physicians. *Archives of Family Medicine, 4,* 585-586.

Spangler, J.G. & Salisbury, P.L. (1995). Smokeless tobacco: Epidemiology, health effects and cessation strategies. *American Family Physician, 152,* 1421-1429.

Spitz, M. (1995). Risk factors and genetic susceptibility. In W.K. Hong & R.S. Weber (Eds.), *Head and neck cancers.* Boston: Kluwer Academic Publishers.

Tanaka, T. (1995). Chemoprevention of oral carcinogenesis. *Oral Oncology, European Journal of Cancer, 31B,* 3-15.

Thomas, D.B. (1995). Alcohol as a cause of cancer. *Environmental Health Perspectives, 103*(Suppl. 8), 153-159.

Weaver, A., Fleming, S.M., & Smith, D.B. (1979). Mouthwash and oral cancer: Carcinogen or coincidence? *Journal of Oral Surgery, 37,* 250-253.

Willet, W.C. (1994). Micronutrients and cancer risk. *American Journal of Clinical Nutrition, 59*(Suppl. 5), 1162S-1165S.

Winn, D.M., Blot, W.J., McLaughlin, J.K., Austin, D.F., Greenburg, R.S., Preston-Martin, S., Schoenberg, J.B., & Fraumeni, J.F. (1991). Mouthwash use and oral conditions in the risk of oral and pharyngeal cancer. *Cancer Research, 51,* 3044-3047.

Winn, D.M., Ziegler, R.G., Pickle, L.W., Gridley, G., Blot, W.J., & Hoover, R.N. (1984). Diet in the etiology of oral and pharyngeal cancer among women in the southern U.S. *Cancer Research, 44,* 1216-1222.

Wong, J.G.,& Feussner, J.R. (1994). Screening for oral cancer: It takes more than just a look. *North Carolina Medical Journal, 55,* 65-67.

World Health Organization. (1982). *Oral mucosa manual.* Geneva: Author.

Wright, J.W. (1994). Oral precancerous lesions and conditions. *Seminars in Dermatology, 13*(2), 125-131.

Yellowitz, J.A., Goodman, H.S., Horowitz, A.M., & Al-Tannir, M.A. (1995). Assessment of alcohol and tobacco use in dental schools' health and history forms. *Journal of Dental Education, 59,* 1091-1096.

55 Thyroid and Parathyroid Cancer

Julie Painter, RN, MSN, OCN

THYROID CANCER

EPIDEMIOLOGY

Thyroid cancer is the most common cancer of the endocrine system, accounting for 90% of all endocrine neoplasms. Cancer of the thyroid may affect any age group but is much more serious in the elderly. Thyroid cancer can occur in the very young but is relatively rare (Schlumberger, Challeton, De Vathaire, & Parmentier, 1995). Even though thyroid cancer can occur in the young and the elderly, it remains most common between the fourth and fifth decades of life. Although the incidence has risen slightly over the last 4 decades, the malignancy remains rare (Norton, Levin, & Jensen, 1993). It accounts for approximately 1% of the total cancer incidence and approximately 0.2% of the cancer deaths (Silverberg & Luber, 1989).

Thyroid cancer affects women twice as often as men, with the majority of the occurrences between ages 25 and 65. In 1998, thyroid cancer was estimated to occur in approximately 17,200 persons in the United States. Deaths from this cancer were estimated to be 1,200 in 1998. Thyroid cancer is classified as one of the following cellular origins: papillary, follicular, medullary, and anaplastic cancer, with various subgroups under each cellular type. These classifications are listed in Box 55-1.

RISK FACTORS

The risk factors for thyroid cancer are difficult to establish. This is most likely due to the low incidence of the disease and the lack of understanding of the etiology (Franceschi, Boyle, La Vecchia, Burt, Kerr, & MacFarlane, 1993). Thyroid cancer occurrences are correlated with the risk factors of radiation exposure, family history of thyroid disease, goiter (hyperthyroidism), iodine consumption, and oncogenes. Risk factors are listed in Box 55-2.

Radiation Exposure

Radiation exposure is considered to be the most common risk factor for thyroid cancer. Over the decades, radiation has been used for the treatment of thymic enlargement, enlarged tonsils and adenoids, mastoiditis, sinusitis, hemangiomas, lymphadenopathy, tinea capitis, keloid, pertussis, and acne (Sloan, Schwartz, McGrath, & Kenady, 1995). Many persons have received radiation treatment for these diagnoses. In 1950, Duffy (1950) collected research data regarding children who had received radiation therapy for thymic enlargement. In the report of 28 children, nine were diagnosed with thyroid cancer. Age is an important risk modifier; it has been noted that when persons under the age of 5 are exposed to radiation, they have a greater likelihood of developing thyroid cancer (Ron, Modan, Preston, Alfandry, Stovall, & Boice, 1989). In a group of 2634 patients treated with radiation before the age of 16 years, 1043 had thyroid nodules (309 of which were malignant). The conclusion is that radiation exposure in early life, especially before age 5 years, significantly increases a person's risk of developing thyroid cancer (Schneider, Shore-Freedman, Beckerman, Favus, & Pinsky, 1985).

No other event validates the risk of radiation exposure as does the Chernobyl nuclear disaster in 1986. More than 100 cases of thyroid cancer in children were diagnosed in the 3 years after disaster. The previous rate in children had been one to two cases per year (Gagel, Goepfert, & Callender, 1996).

Iodine

Papillary carcinoma of the thyroid has been theorized to be more common in countries that use iodized salt (United States) or products high in iodine (Sweden). The incidence of follicular carcinoma of the thyroid has been higher in countries that characteristically are iodine deficient, such as Switzerland. A feasible correlation would be the prolonged stimulation of thyroid-stimulating hormone (TSH) (Harach,

Escalant, Onatavia, Lederer-Outes, Saravia-Day, & Williams, 1985). Research data have correlated iodine deficiency and thyroid carcinomas, specifically in Switzerland and Austria (Langsteger, Koltringer, Wolf, Dominik, Buchinger, & Binter, 1993). In Iceland and Hawaii, where high iodine–containing diets are common, an increased incidence of thyroid cancer exists. These data could show that iodine deficiency and excess may enhance the risk of thyroid cancer. However, in countries deficient in iodine, the introduction of iodized salt caused a decline in the thyroid cancer mortality rate (Franceschi et al., 1993).

Goiters

Laboratory studies in animals have demonstrated an increase in cancers of the thyroid with the use of antithyroid agents. These agents increase the secretion of TSH, causing a prolonged exposure of the thyroid to the TSH. Other studies have indicated a higher proportion of anaplastic and follicular carcinomas of the thyroid gland in areas with endemic goiter (Meisner, 1984; Rallison, Dobyns, Keating, Rall, & Tyler, 1975; Rojeski & Ghanb, 1985; Liechty, Stoffel, Zimmerman, & Silverberg, 1977; DeGroot, Reilly, Pinnameneni, & Refetoff, 1983). Several studies have suggested that the development of anaplastic thyroid cancer is more likely in a person with a history of nodular goiter (LiVolsi, Brooks, & Arendash-Durand, 1987).

Enlargement of the thyroid gland is one of the most common clinical presentations of health care visits. Among adults, more than 6% of women and 2% of men have palpable thyroid nodules, and up to 35% of women have nodules on ultrasonography (Vander, Gaston, & Dawber, 1968; Bruneton, Balu-Maestro, Marcy, Melia, & Mourou, 1994). This clinical presentation is believed to be the result of an autoimmune disorder and/or certain neoplastic thyroid disorders, as well as endemic goiter due to iodine deficiency. The practitioner needs to determine between benign disease and malignant disease.

Box 55-1
Classifications of Thyroid Cancer

Well-Differentiated Thyroid Cancer

Papillary or Mixed Papillary-Follicular

1. Variants of papillary with good prognosis
   - Micropapillary
   - Encapsulated
   - Solid
   - Follicular
2. Variants of papillary with poor prognosis
   - Tall cell
   - Columnar
   - Diffuse sclerosing
   - Insular

Follicular

1. Good prognosis without invasive growth.
   - Hurthle cell

Medullary (Cancer of the Parafollicular C-Cells)
Anaplastic (Undifferentiated)
Other Cancers Metastasized to Thyroid

Modified from Horsely J. S. & Fratkin, M. J. (1995). Cancer of the thyroid and parathyroid glands. In G. P. Murphy, W. Lawrence, and R. R. Lenhard (Eds.). *American cancer society textbook of clinical oncology* (2nd ed.). Washington D.C.: Pan American Health Organization Publications; Norton, J. A., Levin, B., & Jensen, R. T. (1997). Cancer of the endocrine system. In V. T. DeVita, S. Hellman, & S. A. Rosenberg (Eds.), *Cancer: Principles and practice.* (5th ed.) Philadelphia: J. B. Lippincott.

Familial Risk Factors

Recent research has shown that the development of thyroid cancer may be related to a genetic abnormality. Medullary thyroid carcinoma is the most genetically influenced cancer of the thyroid (Nelkin, deBustros, Mabry, & Baylin, 1989; Jackson, Norum, O'Neal, Nikolai, & DeLaney, 1988). Research has linked the centromere of chromosome 10. Medullary thyroid cancer is genetically transmitted through a variant of the multiple endocrine neoplasia (MEN) type 2 gene. About 25% to 35% of persons diagnosed with medullary thyroid cancer have a variant of the MEN type 2 gene syndrome. These syndromes are classified as MEN 2A (medullary thyroid cancer, pheochromocytoma, hyperparathyroidism) and MEN 2B (medullary thyroid cancer, pheochromocytoma, mucosal neuromas, and marfanoid-like features) (Sipple, 1984; Steiner, Goodman, & Powers, 1968). Medullary thyroid cancer is inherited through an autosomal dominant gene, and approximately 90% of persons who have the MEN type 2 gene develop medullary thyroid cancer within their lifetime.

The correlation between Gardner's syndrome (familial colonic polyposis) and Cowden disease (familial goiter) provide well-defined examples of disease processes related to differentiated thyroid cancers (Camiel, Mule, Alexander, & Beninghoff, 1968; Plail, Bussey, Glazer, & Thomson, 1987). An increased occurrence of papillary thyroid cancer is noted in patients with family histories of breast, ovarian, renal, or central nervous system malignancies (Lote, Anderson, Nordal, & Brennhovd, 1980; McTiernan, Weiss, & Daling, 1987). This may suggest that the causative genes of these disorders are somehow linked to the cellular changes that occur in the development of thyroid cancer. Also, a relationship between Hashimoto's thyroiditis and the devel-

Box 55-2
Risk Factors for Thyroid Cancer

1. Radiation exposure, especially at an early age
2. Iodine
3. Familial history of thyroid cancers
4. Goiter
5. Multiple endocrine neoplasia (MEN) type 2 gene
   - MEN 2A (medullary thyroid cancer, pheochromocytoma, hyperparathyroid)
   - MEN 2B (medullary thyroid cancer, pheochromocytoma, mucosal neuromas, marfanoid-like features)
6. Oncogenes

opment of medullary thyroid cancer may exist (Weiss & Weinberg, 1983).

Oncogenes

The role of the RET proto-oncogene is being clinically explored to determine the relationship with molecular and cellular changes that may result in neoplastic alterations in the thyroid gland, resulting in cancer (Cote, Wohlik, Evans, Geopfert, & Gagel, 1995). Models in research for tumorigenesis imply that there is, in fact, a series of alterations that occur genetically during the progression from normal cell to neoplastic cells (Eng, Smith, Mulligan, Healey, Zvelebil, & Stonehouse, 1995).

Mutations have been noted in three of the RAS oncogenes (K-RAS, H-RAS, and N-RAS) occurring in thyroid cancers, as well as other malignancies. Several studies have been completed while others remain in progress related to the genetic mutations that occur in the development of thyroid cancer (Namba, Gutman, Matsuo, Alvarez, & Fagin, 1988; Namba, Rubin, & Fagis, 1990; Karga, Lee, Vickery, Thor, & Jameson, 1991; Wright, Williams, Lemoine, & Wynford-Thomas, 1991; Bongarzone et al., 1989). Aside from radiation exposure, there have been no epidemiologic validations of any other risk factor (Franceschi & La Vecchia, 1994). Research must continue to determine other causes of this disease.

CHEMOPREVENTION

Chemoprevention is defined as the administration of natural or synthetic chemical agents to prevent the initiation or promotion of events that occur during carcinogenesis. Currently, no chemoprevention trials exist for thyroid cancer.

PATHOPHYSIOLOGY

Normal Anatomy of the Thyroid Gland

The thyroid gland is a bilobular gland (Fig. 55-1) located in the interior midline of the neck and below the larynx. The two lateral lobes are connected by the isthmus, which is positioned over the trachea. The four parathyroid glands are located on the posterior surface of the gland. The gland is covered by skin and platysma muscle and lies posterior to the sternohyoid and sternothyroid muscles. The sternocleidomastoid muscles provide boundaries on either side of the gland. The thyroid is a rich vascular network. The superior thyroid artery, which arises from the external carotid artery and the inferior thyroid artery, from the thyrocervical trunk enters the midsection of the gland providing the main arterial blood supply. Deep thyroid veins (superior, middle, and inferior) drain into the internal jugular vein.

There is an extensive lymphatic drainage network from the thyroid gland (Fig. 55-2). The lymph glands extend vertically, from the upper neck and down to the mediastinum, and horizontally, from the lateral neck and into the retropharyngeal area of the contralateral side of the neck (Horsely & Fratkin, 1995; Shelton, Shivnan, & Kozlowski, 1993).

The thyroid is composed of thyroid follicles, which are separated by the parafollicular cells. The synthesis of the primary thyroid hormones, triiodothyronine (T3) and thyroxine (T4), occurs in the center of each follicle. The hormones influence growth and metabolic function of the body. Thyroid

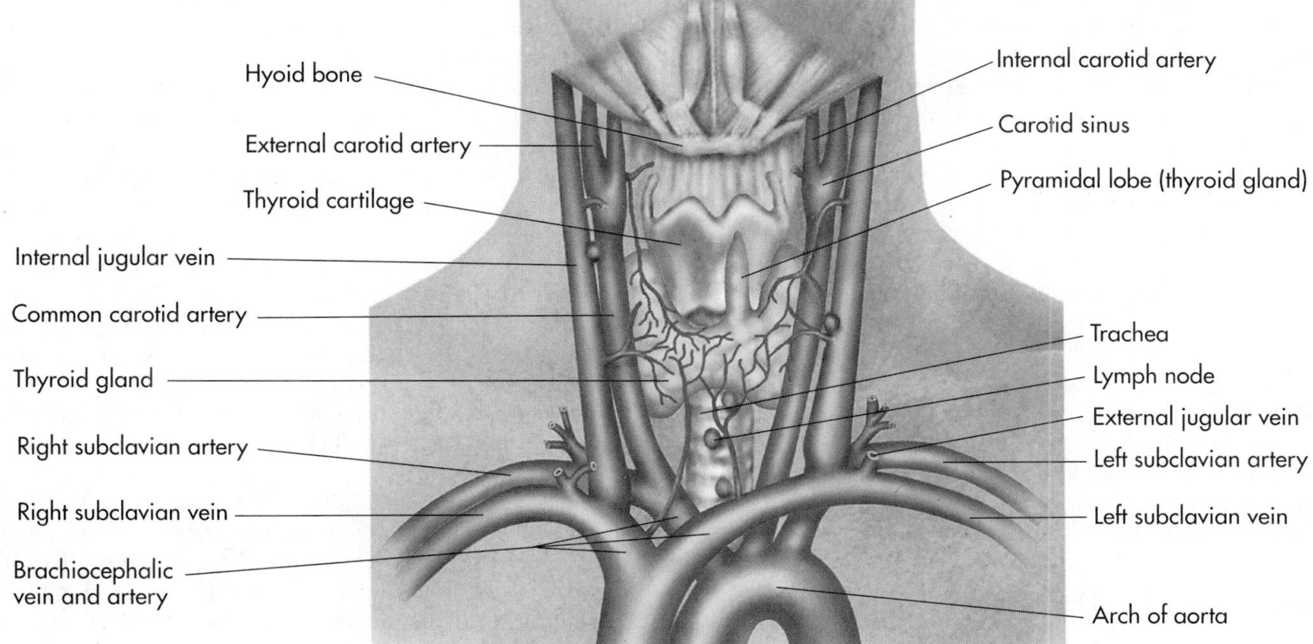

Fig. 55-1 Underlying structures of the neck. (From Seidel, H. M., Ball, J. W., Dains, J. E., & Benedict, G. W. [1998]. *Mosby's guide to physical examination* [3rd ed.]. St. Louis: Mosby.)

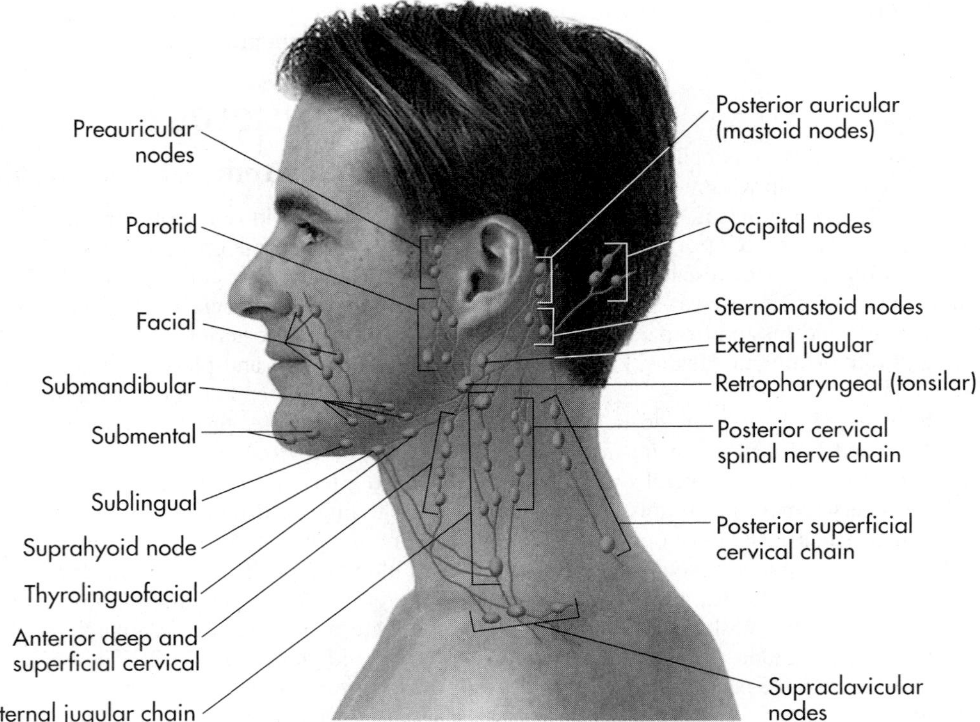

Fig. 55-2 Lymphatic drainage system of the head and neck. If the group of nodes is often referred to by another name, the second name appears in parentheses. (From Seidel, H. M., Ball, J. W., Dains, J. E., & Benedict, G. W. [1998]. *Mosby's guide to physical examination* [3rd ed.]. St. Louis: Mosby.)

hormone levels are controlled by the hypothalamus, the pituitary gland, iodine transport capabilities, and calcium levels (Shelton, Shivnan, & Kozlowski, 1993). The levels of these hormones are maintained by a feedback loop system.

Thyroxine (T3) is released and regulates the function of the thyroid by three mechanisms. Mechanism one, the high level of thyroxine, inhibits the release of the thyrotopin-releasing hormone (TRH) from the hypothalamus. This then cues the anterior pituitary to stop the release of thyroid stimulating hormone (TSH). The second mechanism is the way that thyroxine inhibits the release of TSH. This is done by sending messages to the anterior pituitary gland. Then the stimulated pituitary gland signals the hypothalamus that there is enough thyroxine in the system. T3 and T4 are separated from thyroglobulin (TRG) and become activated after the stimulation of the thyroid by TSH (Shelton, Shivnan, & Kozlowski, 1993).

Iodine levels are influential on the function of thyroid hormones. A decline in the amount of iodine in the diet results in an inability of the thyroid hormone to bind to thyroid binding globulin (TBG) in the follicular cells. Without this mechanism the hormones cannot respond to the TSH levels appropriately, resulting in alterations of metabolic functions.

THE PROCESS OF CARCINOGENESIS

Similar to the causation of other cancers, genetics is thought to play a major role in the transformation of thyroid cells to cancerous cells. Cell growth and differentiation regulatory factors may influence cellular mutations.

RET proto-oncogene is the most recognized for transformational signals causing mutational changes. Researchers have noted two mutations that may occur due to the role of RET proto-oncogene, resulting in the transformation of follicular cells and parafollicular (C) cells into papillary thyroid cancer and medullary thyroid cancer (Gagel, Goepfert, & Callender, 1996).

It is believed that the RET proto-oncogene encodes a receptor for tyrosine kinase, a gene that is usually not released from the follicular cells of the thyroid. This results in rearrangements of the genes. The tyrosine kinase portion of the RET proto-oncogene is then put under control of a promoter for one of three genes expressed in the follicular cell. This results in a chromosome 10 rearrangement, known as the *papillary thyroid carcinoma oncogene* (Simpson, Kidd, Goodfellow, McDermid, Myers, & Kidd, 1987). Each of the rearrangements affects the normal regulatory events, causing an alteration in the order of encoding of the extracellular components, resulting in an increased release of tyrosine kinase from the affected follicular cell (Gagel, Goepfert, & Callender, 1996).

It has been noted that in 95% of persons diagnosed with medullary thyroid cancer, there are germline point mutations in the RET proto-oncogene. These mutations then affect one of the five cysteines (codons 609, 611, 618, 620, or 634) located in the cysteine-rich region of the RET tyrosine kinase receptor and activate it, causing transformation (Mulligan, Kwok, Healey, Elsdon, Eng, & Gardner, 1993).

Mutation of codon 634 is the most commonly observed mutation and is found in about 80% of persons with hereditary medullary thyroid cancer (Gagel & Cote, 1994; Gagel, Cote, Martins-Bugalho, Boyd, Cummings, & Goepfert, 1995; Mulligan, Eng, Healey, Clayton, Kwok, & Gardner, 1994). Familial medullary thyroid cancer has been correlated with the codon 768 and 804 point mutations (Eng et al., 1995). Another area identified as a mutation-causing cancerous transformation is codon 918. Codon 918 (somatic mutation only) is noted in 95% of persons with MEN 2B and in about 25% to 30% of persons with sporadic medullary thyroid cancer (Hofstra, Landsvater, Ceccherini, Stulp, Stelwagen, & Luo, 1994).

Immunohistochemical and biochemical studies have established that thyroid tissue, both normally and in the cancerous process, contains estrogen receptors. Noting that thyroid cancer occurs twice as often in women as in men, the studies are ongoing to determine the role of estrogen and thyroid cancer, if any (Inoue, Oshimo, Miki, Kawano, & Monden, 1993; Metaye, Millet, Kraimps, Aubouin, Barbier, & Begon, 1993). At this time the data have not statistically validated the role of estrogen in thyroid cancer development.

ROUTES OF METASTASES

The regional lymph nodes are the most common site of metastasis for thyroid cancer. Metastatic spread outside the region of the neck occurs in approximately 10% to 15% of patients with differentiated thyroid cancer; almost half of these are present at the time of the initial diagnosis (Schlumberger et al., 1995). Distant metastases to the lung and bone occur in approximately 4% of patients with papillary thyroid carcinoma and 16% with follicular thyroid carcinoma (Box 55-3) (Horsely & Fratkin, 1995).

Metastases to the brain, liver, or skin often occur in persons who have had previous metastatic disease to the lung and bone. It is key to note that the elderly person with thyroid cancer has a higher frequency of distant metastasis (Sugino, Yoshio, Iwasaki, Mimura, Matsumato, & Ito, 1995). In a study attempting to determine variables that influence the risk of distant metastases, it was found that among factors such as age, gender, tumor size, and number of involved lymph nodes, the only statistically significant variable was age.

Because of the vascular supply of the thyroid gland, it becomes a common site for secondary or metastatic tumors from other primary locations. Common sources of cancer that spread to the thyroid include malignant melanoma and cancer of the lung, breast, and esophagus. The thyroid may be the site of a lymphoproliferative disease, thyroid lymphoma. Thyroid lymphoma accounts for approximately 5% of all thyroid cancers (Wortofsky, 1994).

Studies have demonstrated the crucial need to differentiate between primary thyroid cancer and metastatic disease at the time of diagnosis. The histologic make-up of various other types of cancers can masquerade the appropriate diagnosis by mimicking the symptoms of primary thyroid carcinoma. Metastases to the thyroid gland most likely occur more often than known. Therefore a thorough evaluation and fine-needle aspirate sampling assist in the definitive diagnosis (Michelow & Leiman, 1995).

Box 55-3
Common Sites of Metastasis in Thyroid Cancer

- Regional lymph nodes
- Bone
- Lung
- Brain
- Liver
- Skin

ASSESSMENT

History

The objective of obtaining a history on patients with symptoms of possible thyroid cancer is to assess the patient to discriminate between malignant and benign thyroid disorders. A definitive diagnosis cannot be made with the history and physical examination alone, but these provide a firm basis of data related to risk factors, appropriate laboratory tests, and necessary diagnostic tests.

The gathering of a history should prompt information that assesses the patient's symptoms, complaints, onset, change in lifestyle, and quality of life (Younger, 1995). Information related to possible risk factors such as childhood irradiation, radiation exposure, autoimmune conditions, history of Hashimoto's thyroiditis, and familial history of thyroid cancer should be gathered in the initial assessment. Age and gender are crucial; patients younger than 40 years and males have a greater risk of a malignant finding. The patient may complain of symptoms such as hoarseness, dysphagia, or obstruction. Inquire whether there is a lump or nodule that is new or one that is rapidly changing in the anterior aspect of the throat.

Physical Assessment

The neck and area of the thyroid are first observed for any enlargement. The neck is noted as the patient swallows because the thyroid raises and lowers with swallowing. The thyroid is then gently palpated to allow the fingers to glide across the gland. The thyroid is assessed for size, shape, configuration, consistency, tenderness, and the presence of nodules. To palpate the isthmus, the body of the gland, and the lateral lobes, the examiner should stand in front of or behind the patient. The lobes of the thyroid gland should be small, smooth, and free of nodules. The gland should rise freely with swallowing. This assessment may be facilitated if the patient sips water through a straw slowly (Clinical Guidelines, 1995).

The thyroid at its broadest dimension is approximately 4 cm, and the right lobe may be approximately 25% larger than the left. Thyroid tissue should be firm, yet pliable. The patient should be positioned comfortably in a sitting position, relaxing the sternocleidomastoid, with the neck flexed slightly forward and laterally toward the side being examined. Using the pads of the first two fingers, the examiner should palpate the left lobe with the right hand and then the right lobe with the left hand. Any nodules should be classi-

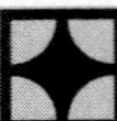

TABLE 55-1 Assessment of the Patient for Thyroid Cancer

	Assessment Parameters	Typical Abnormal Findings
History	A. Personal history 1. Age/gender 2. Exposure to radiation 3. Age of exposure 4. Length of exposure 5. Familial history of thyroid disease 6. Hyperthyroidism 7. Hashimoto thyroiditis	A. Risk factors 1. The greatest risk is between the ages of 25 and 65. It affects women 2 times more often than men, although men with nodules are at greatest risk to have a malignant nodule. 2. Past exposure to radiation increases the risk of developing thyroid cancer. 3. Early age of exposure and/or dose increases risks. 4. The length of radioactive exposure and/or dose increases risks. 5. Genetics is a major risk factor. Medullary cancer is more genetically linked.
	B. Evaluation of personal symptoms	B. Common symptoms include a solitary nodule that is new or rapidly growing, hoarseness, dysphagia, obstruction, neck pain, and stridor.
Physical Examination	A. Inspection of neck	A. Inspect the patient's neck for fullness and symmetry, as well as the patient's ability for range of motion of the neck.
	B. Palpation 1. Thyroid glands and isthmus 2. Lymph node evaluation	B. Thyroid cancer most commonly presents as a fixed or rapidly enlarging neck mass. Also palpate the cervical lymph nodes and areas embedded with sternocleidomastoid. Note any difficulty in swallowing.
Diagnostic Tests	A. Cytopathology—fine-needle aspiration (FNA)	A. FNA—allows for determination of benign or malignant cells. It is the most valuable tool; it serves as a histology report that will guide further treatment.
	B. Laboratory tests	B. Laboratory tests are used only to document the presence or absences of underlying thyroid disease. A serum T3 is indicated only if hyperthyroidism is suspected. A serum T4 is drawn to diagnose hyperthyroidism or hypothyroidism. T4 secretions occur in response to TSH. Serum calcitonin is evaluated in medullary thyroid cancer and may also be used as a tumor marked after the diagnosis.
	C. Ultrasound	C. Ultrasound determines whether the cancer is fluid filled or a solid nodule. Also, ultrasound can detet the number of nodules and their size.
	D. Thyroid scan	D. A radioactive isotope detects nodules.
	E. Radioactive iodine uptake scan	E. A tumor marker monitors the response; it is given orally.
	F. Thyroid suppression test	F. Oral thyroxine is used to suppress TSH secretion and reduce the size of the thyroid. No response may indicate malignant growth. For other possible tests, see Fig. 55-3.

fied as to number, size, location, smooth or irregular surface, and soft or hard feeling. If enlargement is noted, the neck should be auscultated for vascular sounds because a hyperthyroid state may result in increased blood supply and a bruit, or soft, rushing sound may be observed. Increased vascularity and blood flow may occur in a hypermetabolic state (Seidel et al., 1995). Standards for patient assessment are outlined in Table 55-1 and patient education in Table 55-2 (Ashcraft & Van Herle, 1981a).

Diagnostic Testing.

Fine-Needle Aspiration. Differentiation between benign and malignant thyroid nodules is virtually impossible on clinical evidence alone. The use of cytopathology examination serves as the hallmark of diagnostics for the thyroid nodule. Fine needle aspiration (FNA) biopsy is a valuable tool for the evaluation of patients with thyroid nodules and is surpassing radionuclide scanning as the preferred initial evaluation of single thyroid nodules. Not only is FNA the best initial test, but it is cost effective as well. FNA allows histologic diagnosis, yet has the prerequisite of a cytopathologist experienced in thyroid needle aspirations. The use of FNA as an initial diagnostic test allows for the specification of cancerous versus noncancerous nodules and therefore reduces the need for exploratory surgery (Hershman, Ladenson, & Paulshock, 1992; Silverman, West, Larkin, Park, Finley, & Swanson et al., 1986; Van Herle, Rich, Ljung, Ashcraft, Solomon, & Keeler, 1982; Willems & Lowhagen, 1981). An excisional biopsy would be a reasonable approach for a thyroid nodule that yielded suspicious cytology and would avoid more costs related to fur-

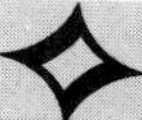

TABLE 55-2 Patient Preparation for a Thyroid Biopsy

Thyroid Biopsy: This test permits microscopic examination of a thyroid tissue specimen. The physician uses this procedure for people with thyroid enlargement or nodules, breathing and swallowing difficulties, vocal cord paralysis, weight loss, and a sensation of fullness in the neck. It is commonly performed when noninvasive tests (tests that do not enter the body), such as thyroid ultrasound and scans, are abnormal or inconclusive.

Thyroid tissue may be obtained from the neck with a hollow needle while the patient is under local anesthesia or during an open (surgical) biopsy while the patient is under general anesthesia. An open biopsy provides more information than a needle biopsy. It also permits a direct examination and immediate excision of suspicious tissue.

Why Is This Test Done?

A thyroid biopsy may be performed for the following reasons:

- To help the doctor differentiate between benign and malignant thyroid disease.
- To help diagnose Hashimoto's thyroiditis, subacute granulomatous thyroiditis, hyperthyroidism, and nontoxic nodular goiter.

What Should the Patient Know Before the Test?

- The patient will not need to change his or her diet before the test (unless a general anesthetic will be given).
- The test takes 15 to 30 minutes, and results should be available in 1 day.
- The nurse will ask the patient to sign a consent form and will check the patient's history for hypersensitivity to anesthetics or pain relievers.
- The patient will receive a local anesthetic to minimize pain during the procedure, but some pressure may be experienced when the specimen is withdrawn.
- The patient may have a sore throat the day after the test.
- The patient will be given a sedative 15 minutes before the biopsy.

What Happens During the Test?

- For a needle biopsy, the patient lies on his or her back, with a pillow under the shoulder blades and the head back.
- As the examiner prepares to inject the local anesthetic, the patient is warned not to swallow.
- The examiner withdraws a specimen with a needle and sends it to the laboratory.

What Happens After the Test?

- The nurse will apply pressure to the biopsy site to stop bleeding, and then apply a bandage.
- The patient will be told to avoid straining the biopsy site by putting both hands behind the neck when sitting up.

What Are the Normal Results?

A microscopic examination of normal tissue shows fibrous networks dividing the gland.

What Do Abnormal Results Mean?

Malignant tumors appear as well-encapsulated, solitary nodules of uniform, but abnormal, structure. The test may also show benign tumors and patterns that indicate diseases such as thyroiditis and hyperthyroidism. Because thyroid cancers are frequently small and scattered, a negative report does not rule out cancer.

Modified from Springhouse Corporation. (1996). *Everything you need to know about medical tests: A consumer reference.* Springhouse, PA: Springhouse Corporation.

ther FNA and scanning (Mandreker, Nadkarni, Pinto, & Menezes, 1995).

Laboratory Tests. Thyroid function studies, with measurement of serum TSH, triiodothyronine (T3), thyroxine (T4), and free T4 are usually the first laboratory tests done. Most persons with a malignant thyroid nodule have normal serum levels of these hormones. If the patient has elevated serum levels of T3 and T4 with low levels of TSH, a thyroid scan is indicated to determine whether the nodule is hot (hyperfunctional). Hot nodules should be removed surgically, yet are rarely malignant.

Serum levels of thyroglobulin can be of use in persons with well-differentiated thyroid cancer and nodular disease of the thyroid that is the result of previous neck irradiation. Thyroglobulin levels are elevated in persons with differentiated thyroid tumors that arise from follicular epithelium and are normal or low in persons with anaplastic or medullary tumors. The thyroglobulin levels cannot predict benign or malignant nodules (Collachi, Lo Gerfo, & Feind, 1980).

Serum calcitonin levels are used as a tumor marker for the diagnosis and evaluation of the treatment response for patients with medullary thyroid cancer. It is also used as a screening test for familial forms of medullary thyroid cancer.

Thyroid Gland Suppression. Thyroid gland suppression is performed through the administration of exogenous thyroid hormone (thyroxine) for several months. Thyroxine then suppresses the secretion of TSH. The belief is that benign nodules shrink in size, whereas malignant nodules will not. Suppression therapy is most likely to be used on small nodules that have a benign appearance upon cellular aspiration. If malignancy is suspected upon aspiration, surgical intervention is appropriate (Norton, Levin, & Jensen, 1993).

Radionuclide Imaging. Radionuclide imaging can be used to determine whether a nodule is cold, warm, or hot. The majority of cancerous thyroid nodules are cold. If a nodule appears warm, an oblique view scan, a T3 suppression test, or a biopsy may be necessary. Hot nodules are rarely cancerous, and a biopsy is not needed for a warm or hot nodule. Although these nodules are rarely cancerous, further evaluation and follow-up are needed to evaluate the function of the gland and the need for appropriate therapy (Hershman, Ladenson, & Paulshock, 1992).

Radionuclide imaging is most commonly performed with three isotopes for thyroid scanning: iodine-123, iodine-131, and sodium pertechnetate Tc 99m. The isotopes image the thyroid nodules and tissues because they have an ability to trap iodine (Parker, Mettler, Christie, & Williams, 1984). Thyroid scanning cannot differentiate between a benign and malignant nodule. Scanning provides a probability of malignancy based on the function of the nodule and is not used as part of the initial workup. Thyroid scanning may only be recommended initially if the patient has elevated serum thyroid hormone levels, which may indicate possible hyperthyroidism (Ashcraft & Van Herle, 1981b).

Ultrasonography. Ultrasonography allows the thyroid gland to be examined for measurement of the size of the nodule, determination of whether the nodule is solid or fluid filled, and detecting of the actual number of nodules. Ultrasonography, like radionuclide imaging, cannot determine the difference between a benign and malignant lesion. The test is noninvasive and sensitive but is not specific. It is best in measuring the size of the lesion in the patient on thyroid suppression and can be used to guide the FNA or biopsy of some lesions. This test has a role in the evaluation and follow-up of thyroid carcinomas (Norton, Levin, & Jensen, 1993). See Table 55-3 for a list of tests.

STAGING

Primary carcinomas of the thyroid are classified as differentiated thyroid cancers (papillary and follicular), medullary thyroid carcinomas, and undifferentiated or anaplastic car-

TABLE 55-3 Diagnostic Studies and Nursing Interventions

Test	Significance	Nursing Intervention
Fine-needle aspiration (FNA)	Provides sample for histologic studies; fine-gauge needle is used to aspirate cells; false positives are rare.	Patient education: describe process and possible feelings of pressure; observe site afterward for bleeding, swelling, and redness.
Cutting-needle aspiration	Large-bore needle used to aspirate cells from large lesions (greater than 3 cm); when FNA is nondiagnostic or for rapidly growing tumors; causes more trauma than FNA.	May require local anesthesia; observe for indication of tissue trauma.
Ultrasound	Identifies presence of nodules, differentiates solid tumors from fluid-filled cysts, and provides accurate assessment of nodule size.	Patient education: review noninvasive nature of procedure to minimize patient anxiety.
Thyroid scan	Injection of radioactive isotope (usually technetium) to detect nodules.	Assure patient that he or she will not be radioactive: keep patient NPO if ordered.
Serum triiodothyronine (T3)	Very specific radioimmunoassay; T3 secretion occurs in response to thyroid-stimulation hormone (TSH) secretion by the pituitary gland; used to diagnose hyperthyroidism or hypothyroidism.	None.
Serum thyroxine (T4)	T4 secretion occurs in response to TSH secretion by pituitary gland; used to diagnose hyperthyroidism or hypothyroidism.	None.
Thyroid suppression test	Administration of oral T4 to suppress TSH secretion and reduce size of thyroid.	Reinforce to patient the importance of taking medication.
Radioactive iodine uptake	Tumor marker used to monitor treatment response; tracer dose given orally; after 24 hours, scintillation-counter measures radioactive emissions.	Reassure patient that radioactive dose is small and harmless; test is contraindicated in pregnant women; obtain 24-hour urine collection.
Barium swallow	Outlines displacement or fixation of trachea.	Describe procedure; maintain NPO status if ordered.
Soft tissue films	Reveal psammoma bodies associated with follicular carcinoma, stenosis, and calcifications lateral to trachea.	None.
Direct laryngoscopy	Assesses vocal cord function and possible tumor invasion.	May require general anesthesia with appropriate preparation and monitoring.
Magnetic resonance imaging (MRI) and computed tomography (CT)	Provide details of size, shape, and characteristics of thyroid mass; identify cartilage invasion; localize vascular structures; provide image of structures in several different planes; can provide information for preoperative diagnoses or postoperative evaluation.	Maintain NPO status from midnight before; assess for allergies to contrast medium and for history of claustrophobia.

Modified from Baker, K. H. & Feldman, J. E. (1993). Thyroid cancer: A review, *Oncology Nursing Forum, 20,* 95-104.

cinomas. Less frequent classifications are Hurthle cell carcinomas, squamous cell carcinomas, lymphomas, other hematopoietic lesions, and other unusual carcinomas and soft tissue sarcomas (Gagel, Goepfert, & Callender, 1996).

The development of various classification and staging systems has facilitated the identification of key prognostic factors that can guide therapy. Some of the more widely used systems include the following:

- AMES (age, metastases, extracapsular extent, size)
- DAMES (D=DNA ploidy and AMES)
- pTNM (postsurgical tumor, node, metastases)
- AGES/MACIS—AGES based the formula on age at the time of diagnosis, histologic tumor grade, extent of the disease at the time of presentation, and tumor size. The MACIS scoring model from the Mayo Clinic defines a mechanism for scoring the prognostic scoring and the prediction of mortality from papillary thyroid cancer.
- MACIS (presence of metastases, age of patient, completeness of resection, invasion, size)—With MACIS, the higher the score, the poorer the survival prognosis (Hay, Bergstrahl, Goellner, Ebersold, & Grant, 1993). The MACIS system was developed because the AMES system was difficult to apply to various patient populations because of the infrequent use of tumor grading across all facilities (Table 55-4) (Sloan et al., 1995; Gagel, Goepfert, & Callender, 1996).

TABLE 55-4 Staging Classification of Thyroid Carcinomas

Primary Tumor (T)	
TX	Primary tumor cannot be assessed
T0	No evidence of primary tumor
T1	Tumor 1 cm or less in greatest dimension limited to the thyroid
T2	Tumor more than 1 cm but not more than 4 cm in greatest dimension limited to the thyroid
T3	Tumor more than 4 cm in greatest dimension limited to the thyroid
T4	Tumor of any size extending beyond the thyroid capsule
Regional Lymph Nodes (N)	
Regional lymph nodes are the cervical and upper mediastinal lymph nodes.	
NX	Regional lymph nodes cannot be assessed
N0	No regional lymph node metastasis
N1	Regional lymph node metastasis
	N1a Metastasis in ipsilateral cervical lymph node(s)
	N1b Metastasis in bilateral, midline, or contralateral cervical or mediastinal lymph node(s)
Distant Metastasis (M)	
MX	Presence of distant metastasis cannot be assessed
M0	No distant metastasis
M1	Distant metastasis

From Beahrs, O. H., Henson, D. E., Hutter, R. V. P., & Kennedy, A. O. (1993). *Manual for staging of cancer* (3rd ed.). Philadelphia: J. B. Lippincott.

The system proposed by the American Joint Commission of Cancer for staging thyroid cancer is vastly used because of its inclusion of the prognostic factors of age and histologic type (Beahrs, Henson, Hutter, & Kennedy, 1993).

One system may not be applicable to all patient populations (Hannequin, Liehn, & Delisle, 1986). Younger age at diagnosis, smaller size of the primary tumor, absence of extrathyroidal extension, complete gross resection at the time of initial surgery, and lack of nodal or distant metastasis are key factors to determine prognostic outcomes.

MEDICAL MANGEMENT

The treatment of thyroid cancer depends on various factors. These factors include histologic diagnosis, stage, size of the original lesion, presence of metastasis, age, and gender of the patient. Following is a brief review of each classification of thyroid cancer and modalities of treatment used.

Papillary Thyroid Cancer

Papillary thyroid cancer is the most common of the thyroid cancers (60%) and presents as slow growing, usually nonencapsulated, and may spread to structures in the neck, especially the regional lymph nodes. In most cases the cancer remains localized for a long time before spread to the cervical and/or upper mediastinal lymph nodes. Recommendations for treatment of papillary carcinoma are as follows:

- Lesions less than 2 cm in diameter usually can be treated by lobectomy and isthmectomy, with exploration of the ipsilateral lymph nodes.
- For larger lesions and those with extension through the thyroid capsule into the periglandular tissues, a total lobectomy can be performed on the involved side and a subtotal or nearly total thyroidectomy on the contralateral side.
- These patients are usually considered for Iodine 131 treatment, as well as resection of normal tissue.
- All patients should have exploration of the lymph nodes, with resection of any involved nodes.

Follicular Thyroid Cancer

Follicular cancer is the second most common cancer of the thyroid (20%). This type of cancer commonly includes follicles, is encapsulated, and differs from benign follicular adenoma by the presence of capsulation and/or vascular invasion. The histologic grading of follicular cell carcinoma is reliant on the amount of follicular differentiation and the presence of Hürthle cell transformation in the cytoplasm. Hürthle cell carcinoma is a variant of follicular carcinoma and tends to invade locally and have an increased incidence of recurrence after surgery. Follicular cell cancer is more likely to have hematogenous spread, perhaps presenting with metastatic disease. Locations of spread can include the lung, bone, and/or central nervous system. Like papillary thyroid cancer, the larger the lesion the worse the prognosis.

Treatment for follicular cell cancer needs to be aggressive. Treatment should include a total or near total thyroidectomy, followed with radioiodine ablation. There have been noted improvements in survival of patients receiving a total resection compared with those receiving only partial resection. Thyroxine replacement therapy is required for patients after total thyroidectomy (Wortofsky, 1994; Sloan et al., 1995).

Medullary Thyroid Cancer

Medullary cancer of the thyroid comprises approximately 2% to 5% of thyroid malignancies. Medullary thyroid cancer tends to be bilobular, yet may only affect one lobule. Patients with medullary thyroid cancer are likely to have elevated serum calcitonin levels. The elevation of serum calcitonin correlates to the degree of thyroid involvement.

Medullary carcinomas are treated by total thyroidectomy and removal of soft tissue and nodes in the central portion of the neck and upper mediastinum. A partial thyroidectomy is recommended only if the tumor is not completely resectable. A modified radical neck dissection may be indicated for persons with cervical lymph node involvement. Patients require thyroid hormone replacement following thyroid resection. Surgery is the only treatment option for medullary carcinoma, with external radiation and chemotherapy reserved for patients with residual disease or recurrence. Medullary thyroid cancer has the potential for metastasis to the cervical lymph nodes, liver, bones, and adrenal glands (Wortofsky, 1994; Sloan et al., 1995).

Anaplastic Thyroid Cancer

Anaplastic thyroid cancer is the least common thyroid cancer, yet the most highly malignant. Anaplastic cancers are rapid growing and may coexist with papillary and follicular cell carcinomas.

Persons with anaplastic cancer usually have extensive lesions that are not capable of being treated with surgery alone. Metastatic spread may occur to lymph nodes, lungs, bone, and liver. Despite radical surgery, the prognosis is poor. Surgical interventions are for palliative purposes only. Chemotherapy may be used for palliation after surgery, but external radiation offers little improvement because the disease is rapid growing, invasive, and resistant to the radiation (Wortofsky, 1994; Gupta, 1995; Sloan et al., 1995).

The oncologist usually treats patients who have other types of cancers that have metastasized to the thyroid. Treatment is based on the primary cancer site. Most commonly these patients are given chemotherapy and/or radiation therapy.

ONCOLOGIC EMERGENCIES

Although oncologic emergencies rarely occur with thyroid cancer, it is still important to be aware of situations that could occur. Oncologic emergencies with the patient with thyroid cancer include airway obstruction due to an enlargement of the gland and/or nodules related to the malignant process. Hypercalcemia may occur in patients with medullary thyroid cancer related to the elevated levels of the serum calcitonin, and the patient with a hyperthyroid state is at risk for thyroid storm. Each of these situations can be life threatening, and immediate treatment is necessary.

Nursing Management

The medical management for thyroid cancer depends on various factors, such as age, classification, stage, and the patient's overall health status at the time of diagnosis. Nursing management varies based on the modality of treatment selected. Nursing care has been documented specifically to thyroid cancer in various publications (Baker & Feldman, 1993; Groenwald, Frogge, Goodman, & Yarbro, 1995). The nursing care is planned according to the medical events as they occur: admission for appropriate surgical intervention, radioactive iodine, and chemotherapy. Radiation therapy (external) occurs on a daily outpatient basis. Outpatient care focuses on maintenance of self-care abilities, monitoring of surgical sites, and symptom and side effect management for radiation and/or chemotherapy treatments.

In the initial phase of diagnosis the focus of nursing care should be on assisting patients to gain a better understanding of their disease and the required modalities of treatment. It is critical to assess the current knowledge base related to the disease and the specific concerns of patients. Addressing the patient's and family's concerns initially provides them with information, allowing a sense of security and comfort. Educational interventions should be individualized to meet their needs. Educational needs vary based on educational level; past health history and experiences; psychosocial, physical, cultural, spiritual, religious, and financial status; perceived threat of the illness; and access to resources.

In the initial phase, education should focus on specific information related to the disease process and the proposed modality of treatment. Educational efforts can be complemented with brochures and handouts, but the determination of reading abilities is crucial. Effective education should include a variety of educational mediums and never be composed of verbal instruction alone. Discussion follows, related to the recommended therapies for thyroid cancer. Standards of care are contained as well.

Surgery

Total and subtotal thyroidectomy are the hallmark treatments for thyroid cancer. Surgery is indicated if the fine-needle aspirate is cancerous; airway obstruction, dysphagia, or hoarseness is present; the diagnosis occurred in a patient who was exposed to low-dose radiation of the neck; or the thyroid enlarges regardless of TSH suppression (Baker & Feldman, 1993). The extent of surgery depends on the histologic findings and extent of the disease. A total or subtotal thyroidectomy is the initial treatment for all differentiated thyroid cancers, whereas lobectomy is recommended in undifferentiated cancer (anaplastic) (Groenwald et al., 1995).

Complications postoperatively may include hemorrhage, damage to parathyroid glands resulting in hypercalcemia, laryngeal nerve damage resulting in vocal cord paralysis, airway obstruction, and/or hypothyroidism. A standard of care for the patient receiving surgical intervention for thy-

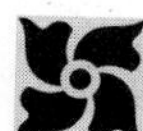

TABLE 55-5 Standard of Care for the Patient Undergoing Thyroidectomy

Patient Problem and Outcomes	Nursing Interventions and Rationales	Patient Education Instructions
Anxiety Patient will: • Verbalize an understanding of the surgical procedure. • Express feelings. • Identify strategies to cope with anxiety.	1. Assess the patient's level of understanding of the surgical procedure. 2. Give the patient the opportunity to ask questions or verbalize concerns. 3. Determine which coping strategies the patient has used effectively in the past to decrease anxiety and reinforce the use of these coping strategies. 4. Administer pharmacologic agents to decrease anxiety as ordered.	1. Use a diagram of the anatomy of the thyroid gland to explain the thyroidectomy procedure. 2. Provide the patient with information about the preoperative routine: a. Diagnostic tests b. Bowel preparation c. Anesthesiology consultation d. Use of antiembolism stockings e. NPO after midnight 3. Teach the patient coughing and deep-breathing exercises, and obtain a return demonstration. 4. Provide the patient with information about the postoperative plan of care: a. Pain management b. Management of bleeding c. Surgical incision d. Intravenous hydration
Pain Patient will: • Experience optimal pain relief with minimal side effects.	1. Assess the pain intensity using a 0 to 10 verbal rating scale, every 2-4 hours for the first 48 hours after surgery, then at least once a shift. 2. Administer opioid analgesics around-the-clock for the first 24-48 hours postoperatively as ordered. 3. Monitor for analgesic side effects, and administer medications to prevent or treat the following: a. Nausea b. Pruritus c. Constipation	1. Teach the patient to inform the nurse if he or she is experiencing pain. 2. Teach the patient the importance of taking pain medication regularly to keep pain under control. Review with the patient the availability of medications and the rationale for use. 3. Teach the patient possible side effects and what to report.
High Risk for Hemorrhage Patient will: • Maintain normal hemoglobin and hematocrit levels. • Maintain hemodynamic stability.	1. Check the hemoglobin, hematocrit, and platelet count. 2. Check the surgical incision and dressings for excessive drainage.	1. Teach the patient that slight hematuria may occur for up to 2 weeks. 2. Teach the patient to avoid strenuous exercises for 2-3 weeks after surgery.
Airway Obstruction Patient will: • Experience optimal airway function.	1. Assess the patient's level of respiratory function, including cough, sputum, respiratory rate, depth, lung sounds, color of skin and membranes, and capillary refills.	1. Teach the patient pertinent signs and symptoms to report to the health care team: a. Increased shortness of breath on exertion or at rest b. Change in sputum color c. Persistent, nonproductive cough d. Feeling of tightness in neck and throat e. Changes in swallowing

TABLE 55-6 Standard of Care for the Patient Receiving Radioiodine Treatment for Thyroid Cancer

Patient Problems and Outcomes	Nursing Interventions and Rationales	Patient Education Instructions
Knowledge Deficit Patient will: • Verbalize an understanding of the rationale for the use of radioiodine and the plan of treatment.	1. Assess the patient's knowledge and understanding of Iodine 131 treatment.	1. Explain the procedures and the following to the patient: a. Ingestion of Iodine 131 b. Radioactives precautions c. Review how therapy works d. Provide brochures
• Verbalize an understanding of the care after discharge.	2. Assess the patient's level of understanding and provide him or her with written guidelines, phone numbers of the healthcare team, and signs and symptoms about which to call the team.	2. Review guidelines with the patient. For 3 days after, the patient should do the following: a. Remain off work for at least a few days after discharge. b. Use separate toilet for 3 days. c. Rinse tub after use for 3 days. d. Do not share linen for 3 days. e. Sleep separately for 3 days. f. Do not share eating utensils and wash separately for 3 days. g. Wash bed and bath linen separately. h. Avoid prolonged contact with others, especially children for 3 days. i. Drink plenty of fluids. j. Avoid pregnancy for 6 months to 1 year, until thyroid levels are stable.
Potential for Injury Patient will: • Maintain a safe environment according to NCR guidelines while patient in radiation precautions	1. Review nuclear medicine orders, and ensure that all are fulfilled.	1. Prepare the patient's room and explain to the patient the following: a. Admit to private room. b. Postradioactive material sign on door and on front of patient chart. c. Do not allow pregnant staff members or visitors into the room. d. Cover mattress and pillows with protective materials (rubber or plastic). e. Alert Environmental Services department about precautions. f. Alert Dietary Services for patient use of all disposable items. g. Put plastic liners in linen and waste basket.

roid cancer is contained in Table 55-5 (Groenwald et al., 1995; Clark & McGee, 1992).

Radiation Therapy

Internal radiation is given through the ingestion of an oral radioisotope, Iodine 131. The treatment is used as a primary treatment or as an alternative to thyroidectomy in patients who have metastatic thyroid carcinoma. This occurs approximately 6 months after surgery. Patients who are receiving thyroid hormone replacement therapy have the medications discontinued before the iodine ingestion. The iodine is in the form of a drink for the patient to ingest. Discharge normally occurs within 72 hours, when the radioactive emission readings are adequately low. Complications can include nausea, vomiting, fatigue, headache, inflammation of the salivary glands, bone marrow suppression, and, in rare instances, pulmonary radiation fibrosis and leukemia (Table 55-6).

External radiation may be used as a single or combination therapy, for residual disease after iodine therapy, and/or for palliation and treatment of metastatic disease. Effects of radiation therapy most commonly include erythema of the skin, mucositis, xerostomia, dysphagia, anorexia, and fatigue. Nursing management of the patient receiving radia-

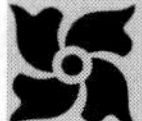

Table 55-6 Standard of Care for the Patient Receiving Radioiodine Treatment for Thyroid Cancer—cont'd

Patient Problems and Outcomes	Nursing Interventions and Rationales	Patient Education Instructions
Potential for Injury—cont'd		2. Complete the following guidelines and inform the patient: a. Survey the room for exposure rates. b. Mark the "safe distance" line by placing tape on the floor. The nursing staff members should remain outside this line at all times, unless an absolute emergency occurs. Emergency care takes precedence over radiation safety guidelines. c. In an emergency, notify the radiation safety office immediately. d. The patient should: • Be given daily changes of pajamas, disposable footwear, and linens. • Remain in the room and in bed, especially when visitors or staff members are in the room. • Not share any food with anyone. • Not be permitted to smoke. e. The nurse should: • Wear a film badge or dosimeter when in the room. • Stay outside the floor-marker (usually 1 to 2 meters away from the patient) and remain in the room no longer than 30 minutes at any one time. • Monitor visitors (no children or pregnant women). • Use only disposable items in the patient's room. • Ensure that items taken into the room remain there. • Wear rubber or plastic gloves when handling items touched by the patient or when handling waste products and body fluids. Specimens such as blood or urine may be collected, labeled "RADIOACTIVE," and sent to Nuclear Medicine at that department's request. • Notify Radiation Safety of any spills. Spills need immediate attention to prevent contamination that might cause the room to become unavailable for a period. • Coordinate discharge plans for Radiation Safety, Nuclear Medicine, and other departments involved in the care of the patient. 3. Review discharge instructions: a. Do not remove any items from the room. b. Place clothes and linen in laundry bags; place disposable items in designated trash containers. c. Leave nondisposable items in the room so they can be checked by Radiation Safety personnel.

tion therapy is in Table 55-7 (Baker & Feldman, 1993; Donehower, 1990).

Chemotherapy

The use of chemotherapy for the treatment of thyroid cancer is minimal. The agent most likely to be used is doxorubicin (Adriamycin). Doxorubicin is considered a vesicant agent with the potential to cause alopecia, nausea, vomiting, bone marrow suppression, stomatitis, and cardiotoxicity (Barton-Burke, Wilkes, Berg, Bean, & Ingwersen, 1991).

Potential radiation recall may occur in an area of the body previously irradiated. The nursing care should include education related to the treatment, side effects, follow-up appointment, and information regarding side effects and symptoms to report to the physician.

HOME CARE ISSUES

The home care needs for patients with thyroid cancer should be individualized. Needs should be determined by the age, comorbid conditions, disease extent, modality of therapy,

TABLE 55-7 Standard of Care for the Patient Receiving External Beam Radiation Therapy for Thyroid Cancer

Patient Problem and Outcomes	Nursing Interventions and Rationales	Patient Education Instructions
Knowledge Deficit Patient will: • Verbalize an understanding of when and what side effects to report to healthcare team	1. Assess the patient's level of knowledge about radiation therapy.	1. Describe the routine procedures involved in radiation therapy: a. Consultation b. Simulation procedure c. Treatment procedures and routines d. Laboratory tests, x-ray films, etc.
	2. Assess the patient's concerns and fears about radiation therapy.	2. Describe the major side effects associated with radiation therapy, the importance of notifying the nurse if side effects occur, and self-care measures to manage the side effects of the following: a. Erythema of skin b. Stomatitis c. Esophagitis d. Fatigue e. Taste alteration f. Dysphagia g. Hoarseness
	3. Assess the patient's willingness and capability to learn.	3. Describe the treatment plan: a. Number of total treatments b. Daily/time c. Allow to view room and machine d. Evaluation of disease response—how/when
	4. Assess the patient's level of understanding related to side effects and management of side effects.	4. Explain reasons to call the physician: a. Bleeding b. Shortness of breath c. Unresolved nausea/vomiting d. Difficulty swallowing; tightness in throat e. Sudden onset of pain
		5. Describe effective ways to care for side effects: a. Skin care b. Oral care c. Good nutrition d. Fluid intake e. Promote rest to decrease fatigue

and resources for care. It is critical to assess every patient for the possibility of home care service. Much of the therapy and care of the patient with thyroid cancer is done within the confines of the health care facility, yet with the decline in acute care length of stay, thorough assessment is critical.

The goal of all endeavors should be to promote the self-care abilities and function of patients within their home setting. Assessment data can be gathered through the physician's office, case manager, social services, and family. The assessment is helpful in planning for interventions to occur in a time-efficient manner without delays in care or injury to the patient.

PROGNOSIS

The prognosis for patients with thyroid cancer depends on many factors. These include age, classification, stage of cancer, extent of disease, and response to treatment. Younger age at diagnosis, smaller size of the primary tumor, absence of extrathyroidal extension, complete gross resection during initial surgery, and lack of nodal or distant metastasis are common factors correlated with low risk for tumor recurrence or disease mortality (Gagel, Goepfert, & Callender, 1996; Gupta, 1995). Others have noted a poor prognosis with patients who have the following: (1) tumor >5 cm in diameter; (2) distant metastasis at the time of initial diagnosis and treatment; (3) >40 years of age; and (4) extracapsular tumor extension (Rodriguez-Cuevas, Labastida Almendaro, Reyes Cardoso, & Rodriguez Maya, 1993).

EVALUATION OF THE QUALITY OF CARE

All accredited health care organizations are required by specific accrediting organizations to collect data related to vari-

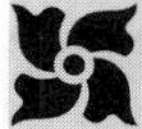

TABLE 55-7 Standard of Care for the Patient Receiving External Beam Radiation Therapy for Thyroid Cancer—cont'd

Patient Problem and Outcomes	Nursing Interventions and Rationales	Patient Education Instructions
Dysphagia Patient will: • Exhibit stable nutritional status. • Identify measures to obtain adequate nutrition. • Identify signs and symptoms to report to the health care team.	1. Assess weight at least once per week 2. Give the patient the opportunity to meet with a dietician (nutritional consultant). 3. Assess swallowing ability: a. Check gag reflex b. Check cough reflex 4. Assess oral mucosa for alteration.	1. Teach basic nutritional needs and the importance of a balanced daily diet. 2. Offer options of nutritional supplements to enhance calorie/protein intake. 3. Discuss signs and symptoms to report: a. Choking when swallowing liquids b. Pain in swallowing c. Tenderness and pain with lesions in oral cavity d. Food sticking in esophagus e. Fear of choking
Skin Desquamation Patient will: • Demonstrate knowledge related to potential impairment of skin integrity. • Maintain skin integrity.	1. Assess the patient's knowledge and level of understanding related to impairment of skin integrity.	1. Teach the patient the indications of skin impairment and what to report to the health care team: a. Erythema b. Scaling c. Tenderness d. Weeping e. Break in skin
	2. Assess the patient's knowledge of ways and ability to prevent impairment of skin integrity.	2. Provide the patient with information to prevent skin irritation/breakdown: a. Avoid constricting clothing over irradiated skin. b. Avoid irritating substances on irradiated skin (perfume, soap, deodorant, powder, etc.). c. Wear soft, cotton clothing over area that is irradiated. d. Avoid heat or cold application to area. e. Avoid oil-based creams, ointments, and lotions. f. Avoid sun exposure. g. Keep area dry and exposed to air when possible.
	3. Determine whether the patient is appropriately following skin care guidelines.	3. Teach the patient methods to prevent skin impairment.

ous outcomes and indicators. These measurements of outcomes evaluate the patient care quality, documentation, satisfaction, specific interventions, time efficiency, and other outcomes as determined by the organization. Currently, many health care institutions are using care maps (pathways, critical paths) to guide care. These documents provide information related to interventions of care that must occur in a timely, cost-effective manner to move the patient along the care continuum. Measurement of key outcomes assists in the evaluation of care and identifies possible areas of improvement. The development of care maps extends across the continuum, providing care management for preadmission, admission, and discharge; findings on follow-up care; and frequent reviews to make necessary changes in care to enhance quality, safety, and patient satisfaction.

Patient/family satisfaction tools are valuable and can be easily developed in cooperation with the marketing component of the institution.

Regardless of the mechanism of gathering data, the data must be useful. Data may be collected prospectively or retrospectively through a variety of methodologies.

Table 55-8 is an example of a retrospective evaluation tool. In the future it will be critical to develop methods of gathering data that provide immediate access to data and span across the care continuum.

RESEARCH ISSUES

Alhough thyroid cancer comprises a minimal portion of all cancers, research surrounding various issues must continue. Research endeavors need to continue to determine the relationship between genetics and other risk factors to the development of thyroid cancer. Data collection occurring over

TABLE 55-8 Quality of Care Evaluation for a Patient Undergoing Radioactive Treatment

Health care providers participating in the quality of care evaluation

☐ Nursing ☐ Medical ☐ Social Services/Case Management
☐ Nuclear Medicine ☐ Other ____________

I. Postradioiodine Treatment Evaluation

Date from:
☐ Patient Medical Record ☐ Patient/Family Interview

Criteria	Yes	No
1. Patient/family provided with educational information before radioiodine treatment about the following:		
a. Purpose of treatment	☐	☐
b. Precautions needed	☐	☐
c. Possible side effects	☐	☐
d. Education documented	☐	☐
2. Radioactive precautions maintained throughout length of stay:		
a. Documentation to validate	☐	☐
b. Room cleaned upon patient discharge after clearance from nuclear medicine	☐	☐
3. Complications/side effects and management documented:		
a. Patient assessed at least once per shift for nausea/vomiting or other side effects	☐	☐
b. Documented management of each	☐	☐
4. Patient received information upon discharge related to guidelines for care and following appointment:		
a. Documented on appropriate discharge form	☐	☐
II. Patient/Family Satisfaction		
Data obtained from:		
☐ Patient interview (phone)		
☐ Family interview (phone)		
☐ Written patient satisfaction tool		
1. Did you receive adequate information about your admission and treatment?	☐	☐
2. Were members of the health care team attentive to your needs/concerns?	☐	☐
3. Were you satisfied with your level of comfort?	☐	☐
4. Were you given information to help you upon discharge?	☐	☐

the life span of persons is necessary to monitor environmental factors and patients predisposed genetically to thyroid cancer.

Studies focused on the genetic influence in the development of thyroid cancer are warranted to study the RAS proto-oncogene, MEN 2 gene, and other possible genetic mutations. Results of such studies would clearly assist the expansion of genetic counseling and early detection of high-risk populations for thyroid cancer.

Currently, there are no screening tests for thyroid cancer, and the low occurrence of the disease would not validate the costs of mass screenings. However, future genetic research may assist in determining who is in the high-risk population(s) and allow early detection with better prognostic implications.

PARATHYROID CANCER

EPIDEMIOLOGY

The occurrence of parathyroid cancer is rare and comprises only approximately 1% to 4% of all cases of hyperparathyroidism. The distribution of occurrence between genders is nearly equal, and the majority of patients are between the ages of 30 and 60 years (Wang & Gaz, 1985; Cady & Rossi, 1991; Obara & Fujimoto, 1991).

RISK FACTORS

The actual causative factors of parathyroid cancer are unknown, yet there is some evidence related to previous radiation exposure to the head and neck. Parathyroid cancer may also occur as a component of the MEN syndromes (Donehower, 1990).

PATHOPHYSIOLOGY

Normal Anatomy

The parathyroid glands are closely associated with the thyroid gland. The majority of persons have four glands (80%), and others may have three to five glands. The superior parathyroid glands are superior and lateral to the recurrent laryngeal nerve and the inferior thyroid artery. The inferior thyroid glands are inferior and medial to the recurrent laryngeal nerve and the inferior thyroid artery (Norton, Levin, & Jensen, 1993).

Clinical Presentation

Cancer of the parathyroid is most likely to be detected by a serum calcium. The majority of persons have hyperparathyroidism, noted by the elevated calcium and parathormone (PTH) levels (Horsely & Fratkin, 1995). Only about 30% of patients have a palpable mass, although rare pain can occur as well. Approximately 50% of patients have bone disease, which may be apparent on x-ray film. The bone disease is correlated to the bone resorption that occurs, releasing calcium into the serum. Because of the hypercalcemia, patients may have renal compromise due to calcium deposits in the renal calculi.

Metastases may occur in the form of deposits in the lung. These may be surgically removed, yet may reoccur. The major effect with this disease is the continuous elevation of calcium related to bone resorption, causing bone disease with pain and possibility of fractures.

DIAGNOSIS

The diagnosis of parathyroid cancer is difficult due to identical symptomatology clinically and chemically as the benign parathyroid diseases (Chan & Tsang, 1995). Parathyroid adenomas usually have a significantly lower level of calcium than the malignancy. Distinguishing histologic findings for cancer include a trabecular pattern, mitotic figures, thick fibrous bands, and capsular and blood vessel invasion (Wang & Gaz, 1985; Levin, 1987). Mortality with parathyroid cancer is most likely due to hypercalcemia.

MEDICAL MANAGEMENT

Preoperatively the goal of medical management is to decrease the patient's serum calcium level. The use of agents such as gallium nitrate and etidronate may be useful in decreasing the calcium level. Hydration and the use of furosemide have also offered temporary effects. Hypercalcemia is a chronic problem and requires ongoing assessment and treatment (Horsely & Fratkin, 1995; Gucalp, Ritch, Wiernik, Sarma, Keller, & Richman, 1992).

Surgical resection is the treatment of choice. Surgical intervention is to be an en bloc resection of abnormal parathyroid tissue (usually thyroid lobectomy) and excision of tracheoesophageal tissue, lymph nodes, and the adjoining thymus.

Radiation and chemotherapy have not been effective in the treatment regimen of parathyroid cancer. Recurrence is likely in approximately 30% to 65% of patients, even after the surgical resection. Complications postoperatively can include hemorrhage, hypoparathyroidism, and laryngeal nerve damage (Donehower, 1990). There is a 5-year survival rate of 25% to 50% (Cady & Rossi, 1991). Most deaths are related to the metabolic complications caused by the disease.

Currently, it is important that health care professionals identify patient populations at risk and strive for early detection and early appropriate surgical intervention. Research endeavors will be minimal related to the rarity of this type of cancer.

REFERENCES

Ashcraft, M. W. & Van Herle, A. J. (1981a). Management of thyroid nodules I: History, physical examination, blood tests, x-rays, and ultrasonograph. *Head & Neck Surgery, 3,* 216.

Ashcraft, M. W. & Van Herle, A. J. (1981b). Management of thyroid nodules II: scanning techniques, thyroid suppression therapy, and fine needle aspiration. *Head & Neck Surgery, 3,* 297.

Baker, K. H. & Feldman, J. E. (1993). Thyroid cancer. *Oncology Nursing Forum, 20,* 95-104.

Barton-Burke, M., Wilkes, G. M., Berg, D., Bean, C. K., & Ingwersen, K. (1991). *Cancer chemotherapy: A nursing process approach.* Boston: Jones & Barlett.

Beahrs, O. H., Henson, D. E., Hutter, R. V. P., & Kennedy, A. O. (Eds.). (1993). *Manual for staging of cancer* (3rd ed.). Philadelphia: J. B. Lippincott.

Bongarzone, I., Pierotti, M. A., Monzini, N., Mondellini, P., Manenti, G., Donghi, R., Pilotti, S., Grieco, M., Santoro, M., & Fusco, A. (1989). High frequency of activation of tyrosine kinase oncogenes in human papillary thyroid carcinoma. *Oncogene,* 4(12), 1457-1462.

Bruneton, J. N., Balu-Maestro, C., Marcy, P. Y., Melia, P., & Mourou, M. Y. (1994). Very high frequency (13 mhz) ultrasonographic examination of the normal neck: detection of normal lymph nodes and thyroid nodules. *Journal of Ultrasound in Medicine, 13,* 87-90.

Cady, B. & Rossi, R. L. (1991). *Surgery of thyroid and parathyroid glands* (3rd ed.). Philadelphia: W. B. Saunders.

Camiel, M. R., Mule, J. E., Alexander, L. L., & Beninghoff, D. L. (1968). Association of thyroid carcinoma with Gardener's syndrome in siblings. *New England Journal of Medicine, 278,* 1056-1058.

Chan, J. K. C. & Tsang, W. Y. W. (1995). Endocrine malignancies that may mimic benign lesions. *Seminars in Diagnostic Pathology, 12,* 45-63.

Clark, J. C. & McGee, R. F. (1992). *Core curriculum for oncology nursing* (2nd ed.). Philadelphia: W. B. Saunders.

Clinical Guidelines. (1995). Adult screening for cancer detection: Thyroid examination and function. *Nurse Practitioner, 20,* 64-67.

Collachi, T. A., Lo Gerfo, P., & Feind, C. R. (1980). Fine needle cytologic diagnosis of thyroid nodules: Review and report of 300 cases. *American Journal of Surgery, 140,* 568-571.

Cote, G. J., Wohlik, N., Evans, D., Goepfert, H., & Gagel, R. F. (1995). RET proto-oncogene mutations in multiple endocrine neoplasia type 2 and medullary thyroid carcinoma. *Bailleres Clinical Endocrinology and Metabolism, 9,* 609-630.

DeGroot, L. J., Reilly, M., Pinnameneni, K., & Refetoff, S. (1983). Retrospective and prospective study of radiation-induced thyroid disease. *American Journal of Medicine, 74,* 852.

Donehower, M. G. (1990). Endocrine cancer. In S. L. Groenwald, M. H. Frogge, M. Goodman, & C. H. Yarbro (Eds.), *Cancer nursing principles & practice* (2nd ed.). Boston: Jones & Barlett.

Duffy, B. J., Jr. & Fitzgerald, P. J. (1950). Cancer of the thyroid in children: a report of 28 cases. *Journal of Clinical Endocrinology and Metabolism,* 10:1296.

Eng, C., Smith, D. P., Mulligan, L. M., Healey, C. S., Zvelebil, M. J., & Stonehouse, T. J. (1995). A novel point mutation in the tyrosine kinase domain of the RET proto-oncogene in sporadic medullary thyroid carcinoma and in a family with FMTC. *Oncogene, 10,* 509-513.

Franceschi, S., Boyle, P., La Vecchia, C., Burt, A. D., Kerr, D. J., & Macfarlane, G. J. (1993). The epidemiology of thyroid cancer. *Critical Review in Oncogenesis, 4,* 25-52.

Franceschi, S. & La Vecchia, C. (1994). Thyroid cancer. *Cancer Surveys, 19/20,* 393-422.

Gagel, R. F. & Cote, G. C. (1994). Decision making in multiple endocrine neoplasia type 2A. In E. L. Massaferi (Ed.), *Advances in endocrinology and metabolism.* St. Louis: Mosby.

Gagel, R. F., Cote, G. J., Martins-Bugalho, M. J., Boyd, A. E., III, Cummings, T., & Goepfert, H. (1995). Clinical use of molecular information in the management of multiple endocrine neoplasia type 2A. *Journal of Internal Medicine, 238,* 333-341.

Gagel, R. F., Goepfert, H., & Callender, D. L. (1996). Changing concepts in the pathogenesis and management of thyroid carcinoma. *CA Cancer Journal for Clinicians, 46,* 261-283.

Groenwald, S. L., Frogge, M. H., Goodman, M., & Yarbro, C. H. (Eds.). (1995). *Comprehensive cancer nursing review* (2nd ed.). Boston: Jones & Bartlett.

Gucalp, R., Ritch, P., Wiernik, P. H., Sarma, P. R., Keller, A., & Richman, S. P. (1992). Comparative study of pamidronate disodium and etidronate disodium in the treatment of cancer related hypercalcemia. *Journal of Clinical Oncology, 10*(1), 134-142.

Hannequin, P., Liehn, J. C., & Delisle, M. J. (1986). Multifactorial analysis of survival in thyroid cancer: Pitfalls of applying the results of published studies to another population. *Cancer, 58,* 1749-1755.

Harach, H. R., Escalant, D. A., Onatavia, A., Lederer-Outes, J., Saravia-Day, E., & Williams, E. D. (1985). Thyroid carcinoma and thyroiditis in an endemic goiter region before and after iodine prophylaxis. *Acta Endocrinologica, 108,* 55-60.

Hay, I. D., Bergstrahl, E. J., Goellner, J. R., Ebersold, J. R., & Grant, C. S. (1993). Predicting outcome in PTC: development of a reliable prognostic scoring system in a cohort of 1779 patients surgically treated at one institution during 1940-1989. *Surgery, 114,* 1050-1058.

Hershman, J. M., Ladenson, P. W., & Paulshock, R. Z. (1992). A savvy approach to thyroid testing. *Patient Care,* 134-151.

Hofstra, R. M., Landsvater, R. M., Ceccherini, I., Stulp, R. P., Stelwagen, T., & Luo, Y. (1994). A mutation in the RET proto-oncogene associated with multiple endocrine neoplasic type 2B and sporadic medullary thyroid carcinoma. *Nature, 367,* 319-320.

Horsely, J. S. & Fratkin, M. J. (1995). Cancer of the thyroid and parathyroid glands. In G. P. Murphy, W. Lawrence, & R. R. Lenhard (Eds.), *American Cancer Society textbook of clinical oncology* (2nd ed.). Washington D.C.: Pan American Health Organization.

Inoue, H., Oshimo, K., Miki, H., Kawano, M., & Monden, Y. (1993). Immunohistochemical study of estrogen receptors and the responsiveness to estrogen in papillary thyroid carcinoma. *Cancer, 72,* 1364-1368.

Jackson, C. E., Norum, R. A., O'Neal, L. W., Nikolai, T. F., & DeLaney, J. P. (1988). Linkage between MEN 2B and chromosome 10 markers linked to MEN 2A. *American Journal of Human Genetics, 43,* 147.

Karga, H., Lee, J. K., Vickery, A. L., Jr., Thor, A. G., & Jameson, J. L. (1991). Ras oncogene mutations in benign and malignant thyroid neoplasms. *Journal of Clinical Endocrinology and Metabolism, 73,* 8832.

Langsteger, W., Koltringer, P., & Wolf, G., Dominik, K., Buchinger, W., & Binter, G. (1993). The impact of geographical, clinical, dietary and radiation-induced features in epidemiology of thyroid cancer. *European Journal of Cancer, 29A,* 1547-1553.

Levin, K. E., Galante, M., & Clark, O. H. (1987). Parathyroid carcinoma versus parathyroid adenoma in patients with profound hypercalcemia. *Surgery. 101,* 649-660.

Liechty, R. D., Stoffel, R. T., Zimmerman, D. E., & Silverberg, S. G. (1977). Solitary thyroid nodules. *Archives of Surgery, 112,* 59.

LiVolsi, V. A., Brooks, J. J., & Arendash-Durand, B. (1987). Anaplastic thyroid tumors immunohistology. *American Journal of Clinical Pathology, 87,* 434.

Lote, K., Anderson, K., Nordal, E., & Brennhovd, I. O. (1980). Familial occurrence of papillary thyroid carcinoma. *Cancer, 46,* 1291-1297.

Mandreker, S. R. S., Nadkarni, N. S., Pinto, R. G. W., & Menezes, S. (1995). Role of fine needle aspiration cytology as the initial modality in the investigation of thyroid lesions. *The Journal of Clinical Cytology and Cytopathology, 39,* 898-904.

McTiernan, A., Weiss, N. S., & Daling, J. R. (1987). Incidence of thyroid cancer in women in relation to known or suspected risk factors for breast cancer. *Cancer Research, 47,* 292-295.

Meisner, W. A. (1984). Tumors of the thyroid gland. *Atlas of tumor pathology.* Washington, D.C.: Armed Forces Institute of Pathology.

Metaye, T., Millet, C., Kraimps, J. L., Aubouin, B., Barbier, J., & Begon, F. (1993). Estrogen receptors and cathepsin D in human thyroid tissue. *Cancer, 72,* 1991-1996.

Michelow, P. M. & Leiman, G. (1995). Metastases to the thyroid gland: diagnosis by aspiration cytology. *Diagnostic Cytology, 13,* 209-213.

Mulligan, L. M., Eng, C., Healey, D. S., Clayton, D., Kwok, J. B., & Gardner, E. (1994). Specific mutations of the RET proto-oncogene are related to the disease phenotype MEN type 2A and FMTC. *National Genetics, 6,* 70-74.

Mulligan, L. M., Kwok, J. B., Healey, C. S, Elsdon, M. J., Eng, C., & Gardner, E. (1993). Germ-line mutations of the RET proto-oncogene in multiple endocrine neoplasia type 2A. *Nature, 363,* 458-460.

Namba, H., Gutman, R. A., Matsuo, K., Alvarez, A., & Fagin, J. A. (1988). H-ras proto-oncogene mutations in human thyroid neoplasms. *Journal of Clinical Endocrinology and Metabolism, 48,* 4459.

Namba, H., Rubin, S. A., & Fagis, J. A. (1990). Point mutations of ras oncogenes are an early event in thyroid tumorigenesis. *Molecular Endocrinology, 4,* 1474.

Nelkin, B. D., deBustros, A. C., Mabry, M., & Baylin, S. B. (1989). The molecular biology of medullary thyroid carcinoma. *Journal of the American Medical Association, 261,* 3130.

Norton, J. A., Levin, B., & Jensen, R. T. (1993). Cancer of the endocrine system. In V. T. DeVita (Ed.), *Cancer principles & practice.* Philadelphia: J. B. Lippincott.

Obara, T., & Fujimoto, Y. (1991). Diagnosis and treatment of patients with parathyroid carcinoma: An update and review. *World Journal of Surgery, 15,* 738-744.

Parker, T. W., Meltler, F. A., Jr., Christie, J. H., & Williams, A. G. (1984). Radionuclide thyroid studies: A survey of practice in the United States in 1981. Special Report. *Radiology. 150*(2), 547-550.

Plail, R. O., Bussey, H. J., Glazer, F., & Thomson, J. P. (1987). Adenomatous polyposis: An association with carcinoma of the thyroid. *British Journal of Surgery, 74,* 377-380.

Rallison, M. L., Dobyns, B. M., Keating, F. R., Rall, J. E., & Tyler, F. H. (1975). Thyroid nodularity in children. *Journal of the American Medical Association, 233,* 1069-1072.

Rodriguez-Cuevas, S., Labastida Almendaro, S., Reyes Cardoso, J., & Rodriguez Maya, E. (1993). Papillary thyroid cancer in Mexico: Review of 409 cases. *Head & Neck, 15,* 537-545.

Rojeski, M. T. & Ghanb, H. (1985). Nodular thyroid disease. *New England Journal of Medicine, 313,* 428.

Ron, E., Modan, B., Preston, D., Alfandry, E., Stovall, M., & Boice, J. D. (1989). Thyroid neoplasia following low-dose radiation in childhood. *Radiation Research, 120,* 516-531.

Schlumberger, M., Challeton, C., De Vathaire, F., & Parmentier, C. (1995). Treatment of distant metastases of differentiated thyroid carcinoma. *Journal of Endocrinological Investigation, 18,* 170-172.

Schneider, A. B., Shore-Freedman, R. Y. O., Beckerman, C., Favus, M., & Pinsky, S. (1985). Radiation-induced tumors of the head and neck following childhood irradiation: Prospective studies. *Medicine, 64,* 1-15.

Seidel, H. M., Ball, J. W., Dains, J. E., & Benedict, G. W. (1995). *Mosby's guide to physical examination* (2nd ed.). St. Louis: Mosby.

Shelton, B. K., Shivnan, J., & Kozlowski, L. (1993). The endocrine system. In J. E. Wright & B. K. Shelton (Eds.), *Critical care nursing.* Boston: Jones & Barlett.

Silverberg, E. & Luber, J. (1989). Cancer statistics. *Cancer, 39,* 3-20.

Silverman, J. F., West, R. L., Larkin, E. W., Park, H. K., Finley, J. L., Swanson, M. S., & Fore, W. W. (1986). The role of fine needle aspiration biopsy in the rapid diagnosis and management of thyroid neoplasm. *Cancer, 57,* 1164-1170.

Simpson, N. E., Kidd, K. K., Goodfellow, P. J., McDermid, H., Myers, S., & Kidd, J. R. (1987). Assignment of multiple endocrine neoplasia type 2A to chromosome 10 by linkage. *Nature, 328,* 528-530.

Sipple, J. H. (1984). Multiple endocrine neoplasia type 2 syndromes: Historical perspectives. *Henry Ford Medical Journal, 32,* 219-221.

Sloan, D. A., Schwartz, R. W., McGrath, P. C., & Kenady, D. E. (1995). Diagnosis and management of thyroid and parathyroid hyperplasia and neoplasia. *Current Opinion in Oncology, 7,* 47-55.

Steiner, A. L., Goodman, A. D., & Powers, S. R. (1968). Study of a kindred with pheochromocytoma, medullary thyroid carcinoma, hyperparathyroidism, and Cushing's disease: Multiple endocrine neoplasia, type 2. *Medicine, 47,* 371-409.

Sugino, K., Yoshio, K., Iwasaki, H., Mimura, T., Matsumato, A., & Ito, K. (1995). Metastases to the regional lymph nodes, lymph node recurrence, and distant metastases in nonadvanced papillary thyroid carcinoma. *Surgery Today, 25,* 324-328.

Van Herle, A. J., Rich, P., Ljung, B. M., Ashcraft, W., Solomon, D. H., & Keeler, E. B. (1982). The thyroid nodule. *Annals of Internal Medicine, 96,* 221-232.

Vander, J. B., Gaston, E. A., & Dawber, T. R. (1968). The significance of nontoxic thyroid nodules: A final report of a 15 year study of the incidence of thyroid malignancy. *Annals of Internal Medicine, 69,* 537-540.

Wang, C. A. & Gaz, R. D. (1985). Natural history of parathyroid carcinoma: Diagnosis, treatment, and results. *American Journal of Surgery, 149,* 522-527.

Weiss, L. M. & Weinberg, D. S. (1983). Medullary carcinoma arising in a thyroid with Hashimoto's disease. *American Journal of Clinical Pathology, 80,* 534-538.

Willems, J. S. & Lowhagen, T. (1981). The role of fine needle aspiration in the management of thyroid disease. *Clinical Endocrinology & Metabolism, 10,* 267-273.

Wortofsky, L. (1994). Diseases of the thyroid. In K. J. Isselbacher, E. Braunwald, J. D. Wilson, J. B. Martin, A. S. Fauci, & D. L. Kasper (Eds.), *Harrison's principles of internal medicine* (13th ed.). New York: McGraw Hill.

Wright, P. A., Williams, E. D., Lemoine, N. R., & Wynford-Thomas, D. (1991). Radiation associated and spontaneous human thyroid carcinomas show a different pattern of ras oncogene mutation. *Oncogene, 6,* 471.

Younger, J. (1995). Endocrinologic problems. In A. H. Goroll, L. A. May, & A. G. Mulley (Eds.), *Primary care medicine: Office evaluation and management of the adult patient* (3rd ed.). Philadelphia: J. B. Lippincott.

Acute Leukemia

Kathleen Dietz, RN, MA, MS, AOCN

EPIDEMIOLOGY

Leukemias represent 2% of all adult cancers, and the occurrence of leukemia is higher in men than women. It was estimated that there would be 28,700 new cases of leukemia diagnosed in 1998; of these patients, 12,500 would be diagnosed with acute leukemia. Although often thought of as a disease of children, 24,800 of those diagnosed with acute or chronic leukemia will be adults (Landis, Murray, Bolden, & Wingo, 1998).

RISK FACTORS

The exact etiology of leukemia remains unknown. There are, however, certain predisposing factors that place a person in a high-risk group (Box 56-1).

Exposure to Ionizing Radiation

Unfortunately, there was a fifty-fold increase in the development of acute myelogenous leukemia (AML) as a result of the atomic bombs that were dropped on Hiroshima and Nagasaki during World War II (1945). The peak incidence was seen at 5 to 7 years but continued for up to 14 years (Mitus & Rosenthal, 1995). More recently, after the nuclear accident at Chernobyl in 1986, there had been speculation that there would be an increase in the incidence of leukemia in the area where fallout occurred. This has not yet been documented, but studies are ongoing. Before precautionary measures were instituted, there was an increased incidence of leukemia among U.S. radiologists and radium workers. An increased risk of leukemia has also been seen in patients who have received radiation therapy for ankylosing spondylitis, thymic enlargement, menorrhagia, polycythemia vera, and malignancy (Heath, 1991; Keating, Esyet, & Kantarjian, 1993). Secondary leukemia resulting from chemotherapy and irradiation has been noted in Hodgkin's disease, lymphoma, myeloma, and ovarian and breast cancer, with the peak incidence occurring 4 to 5 years after the diagnosis of the initial malignancy. When radiation therapy is given in combined modality with alkylating agents, the risk of leukemia also increases (Keating, Esyet, & Kantarjian, 1993; Scheinberg, Maslak, & Weiss, 1997). About 85% of secondary AML cases occur within 10 years after therapy (Scheinberg, Maslak, & Weiss, 1997).

Exposure to Chemicals

Benzene is a known chemical leukomogen that is used in paint shops and petroleum products and is present in lead-free gasoline. There is speculation that exposure to radon may also be associated with an increased risk of leukemia (Mitus & Rosenthal, 1995; Keating, Esyet, & Kantarjian, 1993). Cigarette smoke contains many carcinogens, and it is speculated that 20% of the AML cases may be attributed to cigarette smoke, particularly in patients over the age of 60 years (Scheinberg, Maslak, & Weiss, 1997).

Chemotherapy

The alkylating agents (especially melphalan, cyclophosphamide, and mechlorethamine) and the nitrosureas (such as carmustine) have been implicated as leukemogenic. Cytogenetic abnormalities and preceding myelodysplasia are often seen with secondary leukemia associated with these chemotherapeutic agents. Recently, children treated for acute lymphocytic leukemia (ALL) with VP 16 (etoposide) and VM 26 (tenopiside) have also had an increased risk for developing AML 1 to 4 years after receiving these agents (Mitus & Rosenthal, 1995; O'Donnell, 1996; Scheinberg, Maslak, & Weiss, 1997).

Genetics (Congenital Disorders)

Persons with Down syndrome have a twenty-fold increase in the incidence of leukemia, and higher rates have also been noted in children with Fanconi's anemia, Bloom's syndrome, and Siskott-Aldrich syndrome (Mitus & Rosenthal, 1995; O'Donnell, 1996; Keating, Esyet, & Kantarjian, 1993; Cortes & Kantarjian, 1995). Also, there is an increased chance of developing leukemia if one twin has the

Box 56-1
Risk Factors for Acute Leukemia

Ionizing Radiation

Atomic bomb radiation
Therapeutic radiation

Chemicals

Benzene
Cigarette smoke

Chemotherapy

Alkylating agents
Nitrosureas
Etoposide, teniposide

Genetic Syndromes

Down syndrome
Fanconi's anemia
Bloom's syndrome
Ataxia telangiectasia
Family clustering, twins

Viruses

Human T-cell leukemia virus-1 (HTLV-1)

From Mitus, A. J. & Rosenthal, D. S. (1995). The adult leukemias. In G. P. Murphy, W. Lawrence, R. E. Lenhard (Eds.), *American Cancer Society textbook of clinical oncology* (2nd ed.). Atlanta: The American Cancer Society.

disease. Clusters in families have been noted, although the leukemogenic mechanism is unknown (O'Donnell, 1996; Cortes & Kantarjian, 1995).

Viruses

The feline leukemia virus has long been identified, but until recently there was not a proven virus in humans. In the early 1980s, the human T-cell leukemia virus (HTLV-1) was isolated in some adult cases of T-cell leukemias and lymphomas. Also, the HTLV-2 virus is sometimes seen in hairy cell leukemia (Keating, Esyet, & Kantarjian, 1993). The finding of these retroviruses has strengthened speculation of a viral cause of the disease. There may also be an association between specific human leukocyte antigen (HLA) types and cytogenetically defined subgroups of AML (Scheinberg, Maslak, & Weiss, 1997).

PATHOPHYSIOLOGY

Normal hematopoeisis in children takes place in the bone marrow throughout the body. In adults, bone marrow activity is limited to the base of the skull, the ribs and sternum, the vertebrae, and the iliac crests. The most primitive blood-forming cells are pluripotent stem cells, which in the bone marrow commit to differentiate along the myeloid or lymphoid pathway in the presence of the colony-forming unit granulocyte-erythrocyte-macrophage-megakaryocyte (CFU-GEMM), or the colony-forming unit, lymphoid (CFU-L). Hematopoeitic growth factors and cytokines promote further differentiation of these cells into the myeloid series (erythrocytes, platelets, monocyte-macrophages, neutrophils, eosinophils, basophils) or the lymphoid series (T lymphocytes, B lymphocytes, and plasma cells) (Rothstein, 1993).

Normal Anatomy and Physiology

Leukemia is a clone of abnormal hematopoetic cells in the bone marrow. Leukemias are classified according to morphology (cell type) and the stage at which maturation arrest occurs. When a bone marrow aspiration is done, the cells are examined microscopically and special cytochemical tests are done. In acute leukemia the cells are very immature and they proliferate (divide) quickly. These young cells are called *blast cells.* A leukemia is acute when there are 30% or more blast forms in the marrow or peripheral blood (Ghaddar & Estey, 1995). Chronic leukemias initially have fewer blast cells and more mature, normal cells in the bone marrow. Therefore they generally have a longer clinical course before becoming an aggressive leukemia (Fig. 56-1).

In acute leukemia, cell differentiation is blocked at an early state and there is an accumulation of blast cells (Fig. 56-2). In chronic leukemia, there is unregulated proliferation of differentiated cells, and some blast cells as well. These leukemic cells (Fig. 56-3) have the ability to expand at the expense of normal lymphoid and myeloic cell lines. The exact mechanism by which this happens is unknown, but it is hypothesized that it is either a "crowding out" effect or that the abnormal clone secretes a growth-suppressing factor affecting the normal population of cells.

Acute Myelogenous Leukemia

AML is also referred to as *acute non-lymphocytic leukemia (ANLL).* This disease was first described in 1897 by Virchow as *weisses blood* (white blood) (Mitus & Rosenthal, 1995). In AML the clonal abnormality stems from the myeloid committed stem cell, and usually one cell type predominates. In 1976, French, American, and British (FAB) physicians established criteria for the diagnosis and classification of AML. The FAB system uses morphology and cytochemical staining to classify the eight types of AML (Table 56-1). More recently, cytogenetic banding techniques allow the detection of chromosomal abnormalities, which aid in the diagnosis and prognostication of AML. Cells may express surface markers, and immunophenotyping with monoclonal antibodies (MABs) offers another diagnostic tool to define lineage (Mitus & Rosenthal, 1995; O'Donnell, 1996; Keating, Esyet, & Kantarjian, 1993).

The incidence of AML is 2.3 per 100,000 persons, and there is an exponential rise in the disease after the age of 40 years (O'Donnell, 1996). However, complete remission of the disease may be achieved in 60% to 80% of patients (O'Donnell, 1996; Ghaddar & Estey, 1995). Prognostic factors for resistance to chemotherapy include karyotype, prior myelodysplastic syndrome (MDS), history of treatment with chemotherapy or radiation, abnormal blood counts

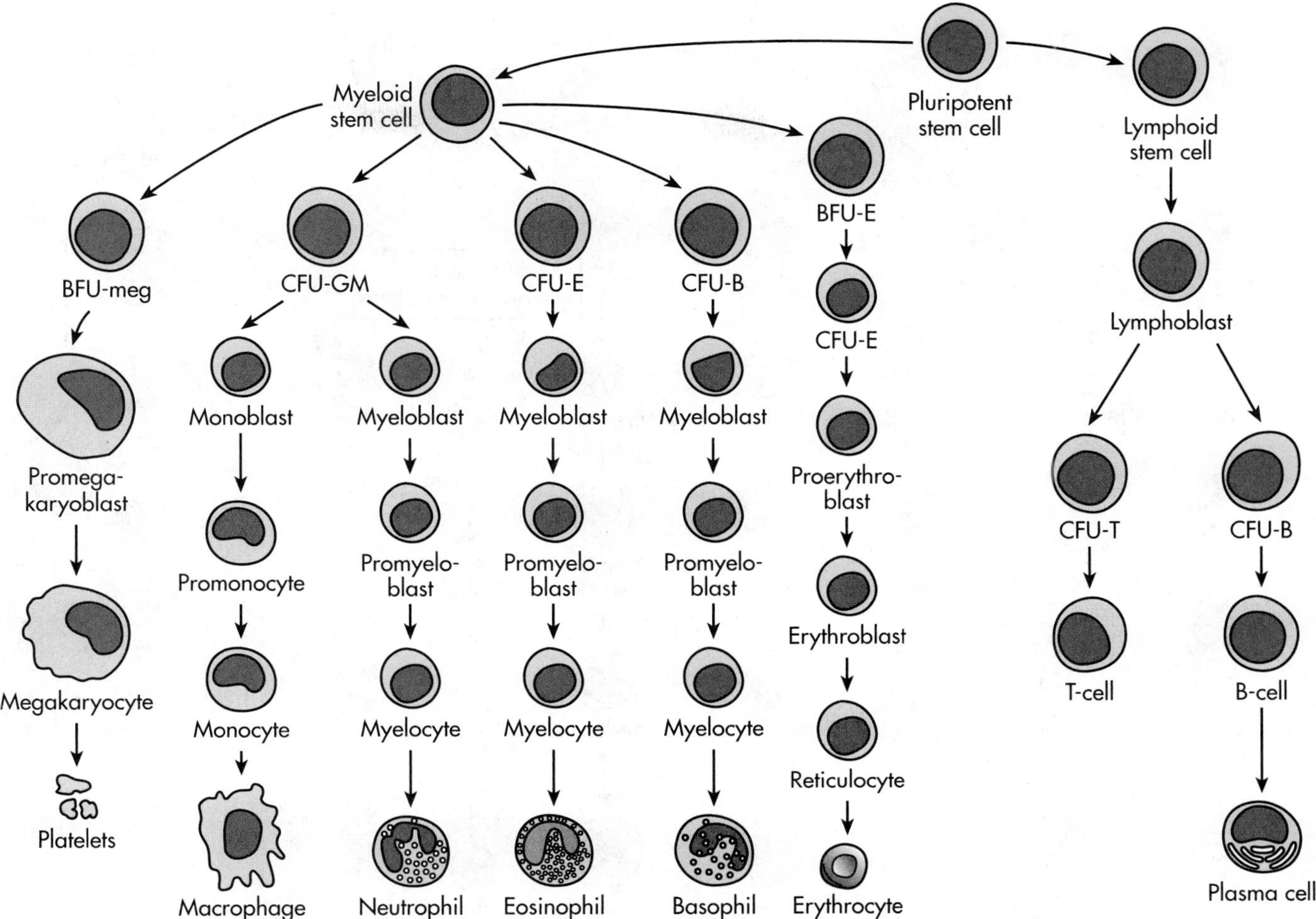

Fig. 56-1 Hematopoietic growth chart. (Courtesy OrthoBiotech, Raritan, NJ.)

TABLE 56-1 French American British Classification of Acute Myeloid Leukemia

Subtype	>30% Blasts (Bone Marrow Morphology)
M0	Acute undifferentiated leukemia
M1	Acute myelogenous leukemia
M2	Acute myelogenous leukemia (with >10% maturing granulocytes)
M3	Acute promyelocytic leukemia
M4	Acute myelomonocytic leukemia
M5	Acute monoblastic leukemia
M6	Acute erythroblastic leukemia
M7	Acute megakaryocytic leukemia

From Scheinberg, D., Mazslak, P., & Weiss, M. (1997). Acute leukemias. In V. T. DeVita, S. Hellman, & S. A. Rosenberg (Eds), *Cancer: Principles and practice of oncology* (5th ed.). Philadelphia: Lippoincott-Raven.

more than 1 month before AML diagnosis related to a hematologic disorder, age, and performance status. Poor performance status, age over 60 years, and abnormal organ function are also predictors of early death during chemotherapy (Ghaddar & Estey, 1995).

Acute promyelocytic leukemia (APL or M3) is a subset of AML characterized by the halt of differentiation at the promyelo cyte stage and translocation of chromosomes 15 and 17. Disseminated intravascular coagulopathy (DIC) is common before or as chemotherapy is initiated. Patients who are successfully supported through the induction phase tend to have improved remission and survival rates (Degos, Dombret, Chomienne, Daniel, Miclea, & Chastang, 1995; Warrell, Maslak, Eardley, Heller, Miller, & Frankel, 1994). Recently, promising results have been reported with an agent that stimulates cell differential of APL blasts into neutrophils rather than causing cytoreduction as with conventional chemotherapy (Degos et al., 1995; Warrell et al., 1994).

Although central nervous system (CNS) involvement is rare in patients with AML, those diagnosed with acute monoblastic leukemia (AMOL, or M5) or with inverted chromosome 16 tend to be at risk for this and for skin infiltration with monoblasts (Mitus & Rosenthal, 1995). Acute erythroleukemia (M6) often follows MDS, and acute megaloblastic leukemia (M7) is associated with myelofibrosis (Keating, Esyet, & Kantarjian, 1993).

In acute biphenotypic leukemia, the leukemic clone arises in the pluripotent stem cell because cells have morphologic and cytochemical features of two populations, myeloid and lymphoid (Keating, Esyet, & Kantarjian, 1993).

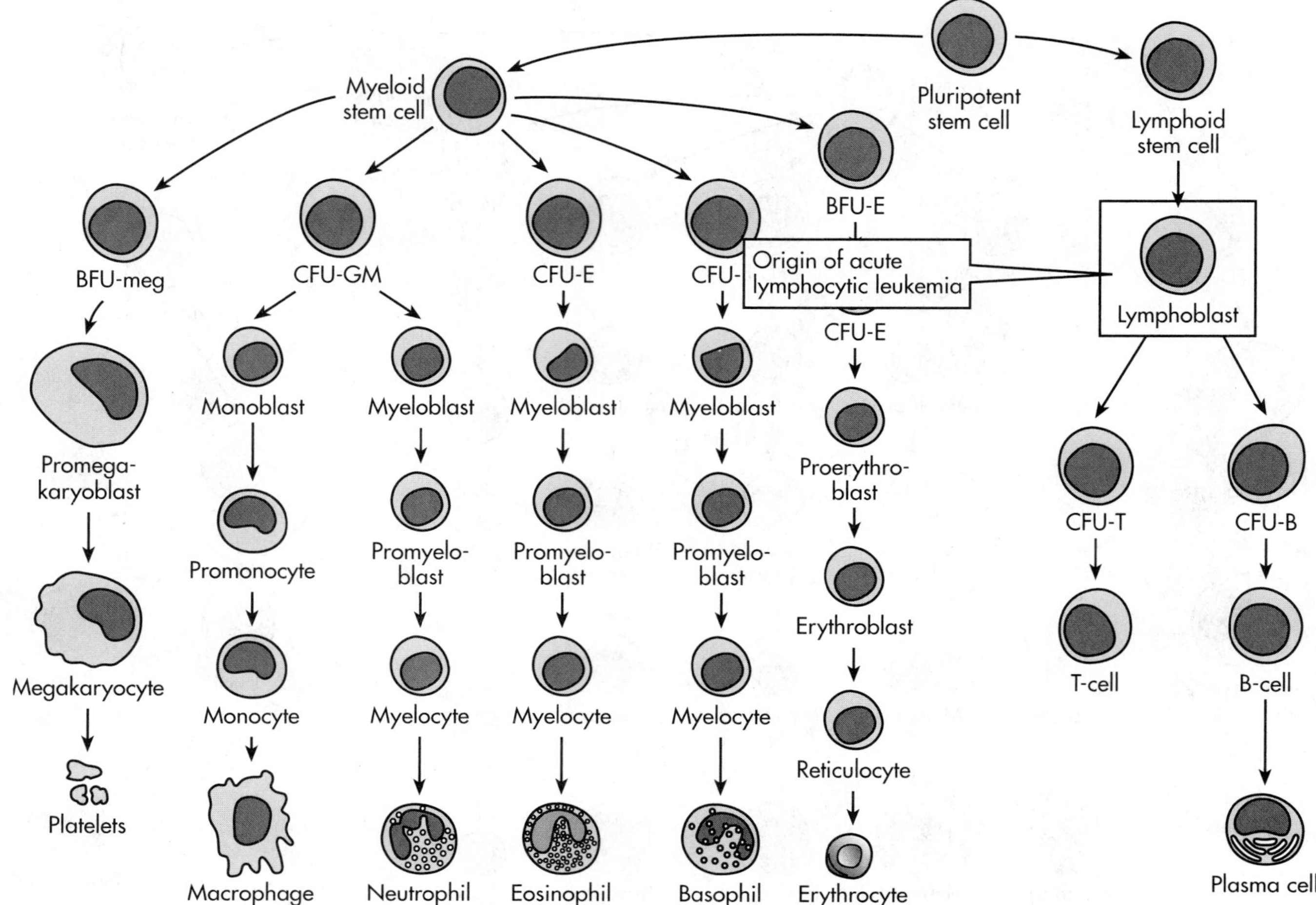

Fig. 56-2 Growth chart highlighting the origin of acute lymphocytic leukemia. (Courtesy OrthoBiotech, Raritan, NJ.)

This type of leukemia is also called *acute mixed lineageleukemia,* or *Ph' + ALL.* Leukemias in this category are very undifferentiated and carry a poor prognosis.

Acute Lymphoblastic Leukemia

ALL is the childhood form of leukemia that occurs in 80% of children with leukemia and only 20% of adults. ALL is the most common childhood cancer and accounts for one fourth of all childhood malignancies. ALL is more common in males and has a bimodal peak at 3 to 5 years of age and again over the age of 50 years. When one identical twin under the age of 1 year is diagnosed with ALL, there is a 100% chance that the other sibling will develop the disease within 1 year. This percentage declines as age increases over 4 years when the overall risk for all siblings is 20% (Cortes & Kantarjian, 1995).

In ALL, there is a clonal proliferation of immature lymphoid precursors and concurrent maturation arrest. These cells can arise from either B-cell or T-cell lineage and marrow involvement with more than 25% lymphoblasts differentiating ALL from lymphoblastic lymphoma. In adults with ALL, 75% have B-cell disease, whereas T-cell ALL accounts for 25% of all cases (O'Donnell, 1996). The leukemic clone expands at the expense of normal hematopoeisis, and there is infiltration of nonhematopoietic tissues. The FAB classification for ALL identifies the following three subgroups (Table 56-2):

- LI, which is seen in 85% of children and 30% of adults with ALL
- L2, which is seen in 60% of adults and less than 30% of children with ALL
- L3 (Burkitt's lymphoma), which is seen in less than 5% of all cases (Cortes & Kantarjian, 1995)

CNS involvement is seen in 5% of children and less than 10% of adults with ALL. However, before the standard practice of CNS prophylaxis, there was a 40% risk of patients with ALL having CNS infiltration with leukemic cells. The testes are a *sanctuary site* for lymphoblastic leukemia in children treated with systemic therapy. Persistent leukemia or site of relapse has been reported in up to 15% of children, but testicular involvement is rare in adults (Cortes & Kantarjian, 1995).

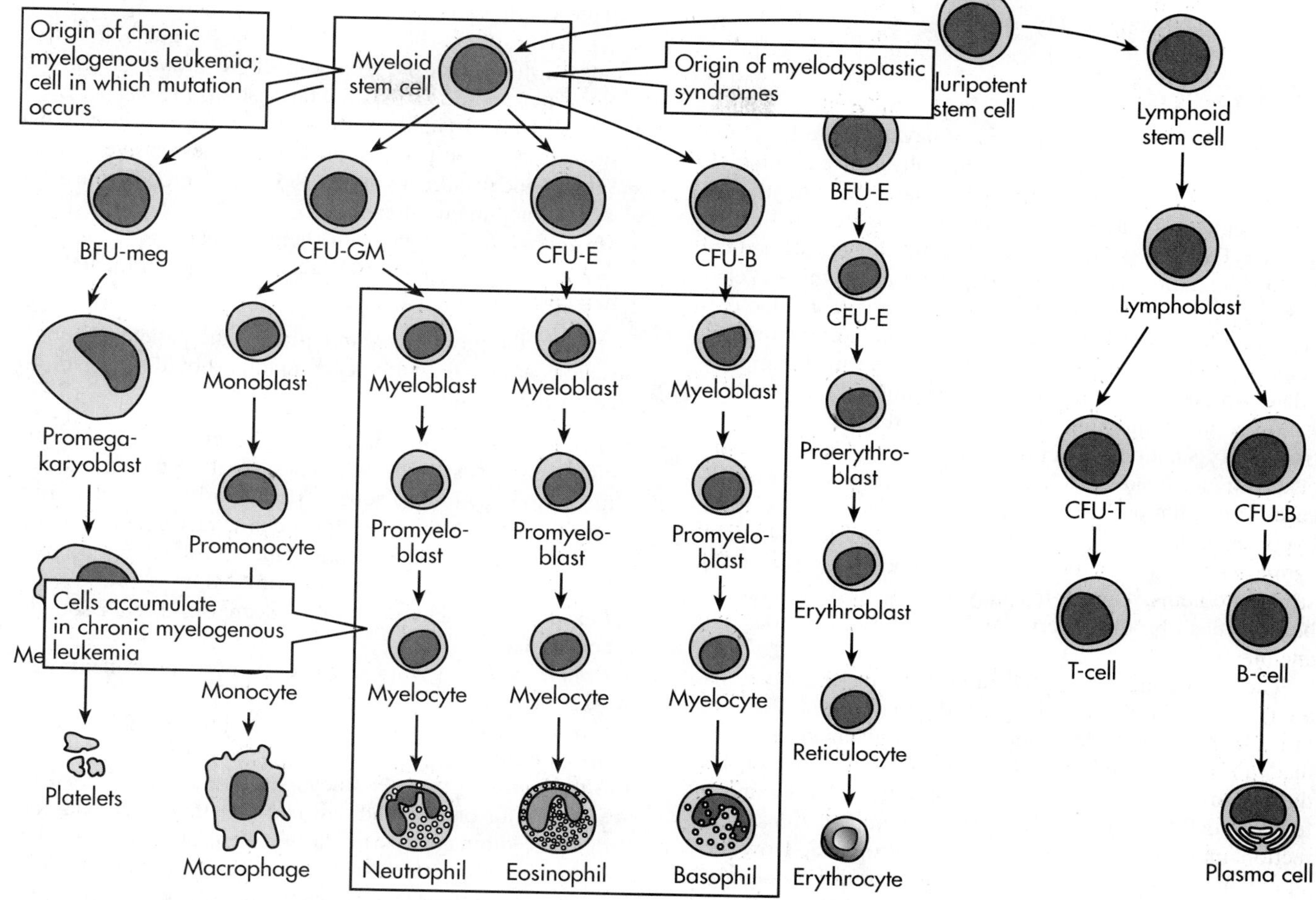

Fig. 56-3 The origin of chronic myelogenous leukemia. (Courtesy OrthoBiotech, Raritan, NJ.)

TABLE 56-2 French American British Classification of Acute Lymphoblastic Leukemia

Subtype	Bone Marrow Morphology
L1	Small cells with minimal cytoplasm Rare nucleoli 30% of adult acute lymphocytic leukemia
L2	Larger cell with moderate amounts of cytoplasm and vacuoles B-cell or Burkitt's leukemia, 5% of acute lymphocytic leukemia

Modified from Cortes, J. E. & Kantarjian, H. (1995). Acute lymphocytic leukemia. In R. Pazdur (Ed.), *Medical oncology: A comprehensive review.* New York: PRR.

Box 56-2
Acute Lymphoblastic Leukemia Poor Prognostic Factors

White blood cell count greater than 20,000/ml at presentation
Age less than 1 year or over 9 years; age over 60 years
Time to achieve complete remission (CR) (more than 4 weeks)
Male gender
Chromosome abnormality

Modified from Cortes, J. E. & Kantarjian, H. (1995). Acute lymphocytic leukemia. In R. Pazdur (Ed.), *Medical oncology: A comprehensive review.* New York: PRR.

Hyperdiploidy (>50 chromosomes) is a good prognostic sign in children with ALL, but this is rarely seen in adults. The cytogenetic abnormalities t(4;11) and t(9;22) carry a poor prognosis in adults with ALL. Although the long-term outcome is good for children with ALL and better than AML in adults, certain indicators are predictive of early relapse of the disease (Box 56-2). These include the following:

- White blood cell (WBC) count greater than or equal to 20,000 at diagnosis
- Age less than 1 year or greater than 9 years; greater than 60 years at diagnosis
- Time to achieve complete remission (CR): greater than 4 weeks

- Male gender
- Chromosome abnormality

ASSESSMENT

Assessment of patients suspected of having acute leukemia begins with a thorough history and physical examination (Table 56-3). The majority of newly diagnosed patients with acute leukemia have had symptoms for fewer than 3 months. Patients should be asked about their past medical history, including malignancy, exposure to chemicals, chemotherapy, radiation therapy, family history of genetic disease, and a current list of medications, including over-the-counter medications. Signs and symptoms are commonly related to anemia, infection, and bleeding.

Signs and symptoms of anemia are related to impaired tissue oxygenation. Chief complaints may include malaise, fatigue, headache, lightheadedness, dizziness, tachycardia, palpitations, dyspnea at rest or with exertion, hypersensitivity to cold, exercise intolerance, abdominal symptoms (nausea, constipation), impotence, and menstrual problems. Symptoms may be nonspecific and will be influenced by the severity and acuteness of the onset of anemia.

The most commonly affected systems in leukopenic patients are the oropharynx, lungs, and perianal area. Bacterial infections and oral ulcerations are the only manifestations that can be attributed to neutropenia. The incidence of life-threatening infections correlates with a neutrophil count of fewer than 0.5×10^9/L cells. Common clinical signs of infection may be absent because of neutropenia. However, chief complaints often include fever greater than or equal to 100.4° F (38° C), chills, sweats, malaise, and fatigue. In the review of systems, patients should be questioned about the following:

- *HEENT:* Sore throat, oral sensitivity or ulcerations, esophageal burning, dysphagia, sinus tenderness
- *Respiratory:* Productive or nonproductive cough, shortness of breath, dyspnea on exertion
- *Gastrointestinal:* Urinary frequency, dysuria, flank pain, vaginal or penile discharge
- *Musculoskeletal:* Myalgias, arthralgias
- *Skin:* Erythema, edema, heat, tenderness, drainage where skin integrity has been altered
- *Central nervous system:* Headache, change in vision, photophobia, nuchal rigidity

The severity and frequency of bleeding associated with thrombocytopenia correlates to the platelet count. Spontaneous hemorrhage is most likely to occur when platelet counts are fewer than 50,000/μl, whereas uncontrollable hemorrhage is most likely with counts of 10,000/μl or less (Cortes & Kantarjian, 1995). Patients may also have bleeding related to DIC, particularly when the diagnosis is APL. Symptoms that may be indicative of bleeding include the following:

- *HEENT:* Change in or loss of vision, spots in front of eyes, epistaxis, gingival bleeding spontaneously or with brushing
- *Respiratory:* Blood-flecked sputum or frank hemoptysis, acute shortness of breath, inspiratory pain
- *Gastrointestinal:* Blood flecks in emesis, guaiac-positive emesis, hematemesis, guaiac-positive stool, bright red blood per rectum (BRBPR), tarry stool, melena
- *Genitourinary:* Guaiac-positive urine, hematuria, vaginal spotting between periods, prolonged or excessive menses
- *Skin:* Petechiae, ecchymoses, oozing of blood from sites where integument altered
- *Musculoskeletal:* Joint pain (hemarthrosis)
- *Central nervous system:* Headache, change in mental status, parasthesia

During the physical examination of the patient, the various signs associated with pancytopenia should be noted, including the following:

- *HEENT:* Pallor of conjunctivas and circumoral mucosa, sinus tenderness with palpitation, oral erythema, edema, ulcerations, white plaques (particularly oral pharynx), tongue, periorbital petechiae, conjunctival hemorrhage, retinal hemorrhage, epistaxis, gingival bleeding; gingival hypertrophy prominent feature of AMOL
- *Respiratory:* Tachypnea, rales, decreased breath sounds, consolidation
- *Lymph nodes:* Lymphadenpathy, more prominent with ALL or AMOL
- *Cardiovascular:* Tachycardia, accentuated S_1, systolic flow murmur
- *Abdomen:* Hepatosplenomegaly, more common in ALL
- *Skin:* Pallor of face and nail beds, erythema, edema, tenderness, drainage (particularly where skin integrity has been altered), petechiae, ecchymoses, oozing of blood from injection sites (especially in APL); patients with AMOL have skin inspected and palpated for infiltrates
- *Rectal:* Circumanal erythema, ulceration, tenderness with palpation
- *Musculoskeletal:* Edema, erythema, decreased range of motion if related to bleeding
- *Central nervous system:* Neurologic deficits related to leukemic infiltration or bleeding more common in ALL, AMOL, or APL, respectively

Complete Blood Count with Differential

An elevated or a low WBC count with circulating blasts accompanied by anemia and thrombocytopenia should alert the practitioner to the possibility of acute leukemia.

Bone Marrow Aspiration and Biopsy

Bone marrow aspiration with smears is performed in patients suspected of having leukemia. Table 56-4 illustrates a procedure for preparing a patient for this test. This test is done to identify the morphologic composition of the marrow, whereas bone marrow biopsy is best for evaluating cellularity. In AML and ALL the marrow is usually hypercellular with more than 50% blast cells. Immunophenotyping of the leukemic cells determines the presence of myeloid and/or lymphoid surface markers. Marrow aspirate is also studied using flow cytometry to determine the percent-

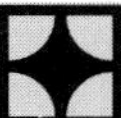

TABLE 56-3 Assessment of the Patient for Acute Leukemia

Acute Leukemia Assessment	Assessment Parameter	Typical Abnormal Findings
History	A. Personal history	A. Personal history risk factors
	1. Past medical history	1. History of malignancy (e.g., Hodgkin's disease, myelodysplasia, myeloma, breast cancer, ovarian cancer. Treatment with radiation. Treatment with chemotherapy: alkylating agents, etoposide, tenopiside, nitrosureas.
	2. Exposure to carcinogens	2. Benzene, radon, cigarette smoke, radiation.
	3. Family history	3. Family history of leukemia.
	4. Genetics	4. History of Down, Bloom's, or Wiskott-Aldrich syndromes, or Fanconi's anemia.
	5. Virus	5. Human T-cell leukemia virus-1.
	B. Evaluation of bone marrow function	
	1. Anemia; signs and symptoms are related to impaired tissue oxygenation.	1. Chief complaints may include malaise, fatigue, headache, lightheadedness, dizzyness, tachycardia, palpatations, dyspnea at rest or with exertion, hypersensitivity to cold, exercise intolerance, nausea, constipation, impotence, and menstrual problems.
	2. Neutropenia; most commonly affected systems include oropharynx, lungs, and perianal area.	2. Incidence of life-threatening infection correlates with a neutrophil count $<0.5 \times 10^9$ cells (500). Chief complaints include fever $\geq$100.4° F (38° C), chills, fatigue, sore throat, esophageal burning, dysphagia, sinus tenderness, cough, SOB, DOE, abdominal pain, nausea, vomiting, diarrhea, rectal tenderness, urinary frequency, dysuria, flank pain, vaginal or penile discharge, myalgias, tenderness and edema where skin integrity has been altered, headache, photophobia, and nuchal rigidity.
	3. Thrombocytopenia 2° to acute leukemia or DIC.	3. Spontaneous hemorrhage when platelet count <50,000 μL; uncontrolled hemorrhage with platelet count <10,000 μL. Chief complaints include change in or loss of vision, spots in front of eyes, epistaxis, gingival bleeding, blood flecks in sputum or hemoptysis, guaiac-positive emesis, stool, urine, petechiae, oozing of blood from sites where integument has been altered, vaginal spotting between periods, prolonged or excessive menses, headache, change in mental status, and paresthesia.
Physical Examination	A. HEENT	A. Signs of marrow dysfunction include pallor of conjuntiva and oral mucosa, oral edema, ulceration, white plaques of candida, and gingival bleeding. Sinus tenderness with palpation can be indicative of fungal infection. Periorbital petechiae and retinal or conjunctival hemorrhage can be signs of risk of CNS bleeding. Gingival hypertrophy is a sign of AMOL.
	B. Lymph nodes	B. Lymphadenopathy occurs more likely in ALL or monocytoid leukemia.
	C. Respiratory	C. Tachypnea, rales, decreased breath sounds, or consolidation may develop with pulmonary infection.
	D. Cardiovascular	D. Tachycardia and systolic flow murmur are associated with anemia.
	E. Abdomen	E. Hepatosplenomegaly is more common in ALL.

ALL, Acute lymphocytic leukemia; *AMOL;* acute monoplastic leukemia (mo); *CNS,* central nervous system; *DIC,* disseminated intravascular coagulation; *DOE,* dyspnea on exertion; *HEENT,* head, eyes, ears, nose, throat; *SOB,* shortness of breath.

Continued

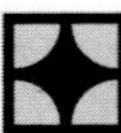

TABLE 56-3 Assessment of the Patient for Acute Leukemia—cont'd

Acute Leukemia Assessment	Assessment Parameter	Typical Abnormal Findings
	F. Skin	F. Petechiae, ecchymoses, oozing of blood from injection or marrow aspiration sites is common in APL 2° to DIC. Patients with AMOL may have skin infiltrates. Erythema, tenderness and edema may indicate infection. Pus is not seen 2° to neutropenia, abnormal functioning of WBC count
	G. Rectal	G. Circumanal erythema, ulceration, or tenderness with palpation indicates anal fissure or infection.
	H. Assessment parameter	H. Typical abnormal findings
	I. Musculoskeletal	I. Myalgias and muscle tenderness are symptoms of diffuse fungal infection. Joint edema, erythema, and decreased range of motion may be symptoms of bleeding into joint.
	J. Central nervous system	J. Nerve palsy or paresthesia 2° to leukemia infiltrate is more common in ALL and AMOL. Cerebral bleeding may occur in APL 2° to DIC.
Diagnostic Tests	A. Bone marrow aspiration and biopsy	A. Hypercellular marrow with ≥30% blasts and decreased number of pronormoblasts and megakaryocytes.
	B. Complete blood count with differential	B. Elevated or low WBC count with blast forms. Decreased RBC, hemoglobin, hematocrit, platelet counts.
	C. Lactate dehydrogenase	C. Elevated in most patients with acute leukemia. Prognostic factor in ALL reflecting high tumor burden and risk of CNS involvement.
	D. Blood urea nitrogen and creatinine	D. If common causes of elevation are ruled out (e.g., dehydration), may be caused by leukemic infiltration of kidneys. Renal ultrasound may be indicated.
	E. Albumin	E. About 30%-40% of patients with leukemia will have hypoalbuminemia at diagnosis.
	F. Calcium	F. Hypercalcemia is seen in T-cell ALL.
	G. Uric acid, potassium, phosphorus, calcium	G. Baseline parameter to rule out TLS. Elevated uric acid, potassium, and phosphorous with decreased calcium is indicative of TLS. More commonly seen in ALL or AMOL.
	H. Prothrombin and partial thromboplastin level	H. Baseline parameter to rule out DIC. If abnormal, draw full coagulation profile. Increased PT, PTT, thrombin time, and fibrin split products with low fibrinogen are indicative of DIC. Occurs in 85% of patients with APL, especially when WBC count is >10,000. DIC should also be anticipated in patients with AMOL or ALL.
	I. Lumbar puncture	I. Diagnostic spinal tap for patients with ALL with instillation of intrathecal Ara-C or methotrexate. Diagnostic tap for AML when CNS symptoms are present. Blast cells or red cells in spinal fluid are indicative of leukemia or bleeding, respectively. When patients are thrombocytopenic, lumbar puncture must be done under platelet coverage.
	J. Chest x-ray	J. Mediastinal mass is common in T-cell ALL.
	K. Cytomegalovirus serology	K. Baseline; to determine positive or negative for transfusion therapy.
	L. HLA typing	L. Patient and family; to determine eligibility for allogeneic BMT or for matched platelets in refractory patients.

APL, Acute promyelacytic leukemia; *Ara-C,* cytosine arabinoside; *BMT,* bone marrow transplantation; *HLA,* human leukocyte antigen; *RBC,* red blood cell; *PT,* prothrombin time; *PTT,* partial prothrombin time; *TLS,* tumor lysis syndrome; *WBC,* white blood cell.

age of cycling cells and the labeling index (proportion in S phase). Cytogenetic studies using Giemsa or quinacrine banding techniques determine whether there is an abnormal karotype in the leukemic cells. Histochemical staining may also help differentiate between myeloid and lymphoid cells. If more than 3% of the blast cells stain myeloperoxidase positive, a diagnosis of AML is likely. If terminal deoxynucleotidyl transferase (tdt) is positive, ALL is suspected. At times, however, the leukemic population may be comprised of mixed lineage cells (biphenotypic or PH' +

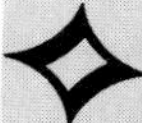

TABLE 56-4 Patient Preparation for a Bone Marrow Aspirate

Description of Procedure: A needle is inserted into the bone marrow space, usually in the hip bone or occasionally the sternum or breastbone.

Patient Preparation: Instruct the patient to bring soothing music, a family member, or friend to offer support.

1. Obtain informed consent.
2. Request the patient to loosen clothes from the waist down.
3. Request the patient to lie flat on the stomach.
4. Examine the iliac crest for the exact area to aspirate.
5. Cleanse the skin with povidine or iodine solution, wait for it to air-dry, clean it again with alcohol, and air dry.
6. Prepare heparin and lidocaine solutions to anesthetize the patient.
7. Inject the local skin area with lidocaine.
8. After the skin is numb, inject anesthesia into the bone.
9. When the patient is comfortable, insert the trocar needle into the marrow space.
10. Ask the patient to take a deep breath; aspiration of marrow begins.
11. After the specimen is obtained, the needle is removed and pressure applied to the area to prevent bleeding.
12. Apply an appropriate bandage.

ALL) or undifferentiated cells (AUL) (Keating, Esyet, & Kantarjian, 1993).

Blood Chemistries

Lactate dehydrogenase (LHD) is elevated in most patients with acute leukemia and is a prognostic factor in ALL, reflecting high tumor burden and increased risk of CNS involvement. Elevated blood urea nitrogen (BUN) and serum creatinine at the time of presentation may be indicative of renal impairment or infiltration with leukemic cells. About 30% to 40% of patients have hypoalbuminemia at the time of presentation. Hypercalcemia is suggestive of T-cell ALL. Baseline parameters for tumor lysis syndrome are performed, as well as prothrombin (PT), partial thromboplastin (PTT), and possibly full coagulation screen to rule out DIC.

MEDICAL MANAGEMENT

Acute Myelogenous Leukemia

Treatment of AML consists of the administration of a combination of various drugs. Induction chemotherapy is given to decrease the number of blast cells to fewer than 5% and normalize the peripheral blood environment, the criteria for complete remission (CR) (Schiffer, 1997). The mainstay treatment for AML since the 1960s has been cytosine arabinoside (Ara-C) (Box 56-3). In the early 1970s, anthracycline development ensued, and Ara-C in intermediate or high dose was combined with Ara-C with promising results (Berman, Heller, Santorsa, McKenzie, Gee, & Kempin, 1991). When CR is achieved with one or two induction

Box 56-3
Acute Myelogenous Leukemia

Treatment
Daunorubicin
Idarubicin
Ara-C (standard or high dose)
Etoposide
Mitoxantrone
Allogeneic or autologous BMT

Ara-C, cytosine arabinoside; *BMT,* bone marrow transplantation.

courses, consolidation therapy is usually given at 5-week intervals to promote durable remissions. The same combination of these aforementioned chemotherapeutic agents may be used, or combinations of etoposide, mitoxantrone, and Ara-C. Maintenance therapy is not effective in AML. In some protocols a late intensification course of therapy is given. Because the rate of relapse remains high in patients treated with chemotherapy alone, allogeneic or autologous bone marrow transplantation (BMT) is recommended for persons under 50 years of age in first CR. Potential transplant candidates and their families should be HLA typed soon after the diagnosis to determine the patient's eligibility for BMT (Schiffer, 1997; Scheinberg, Maslak, & Weiss, 1997). Anti-CD 33 monoclonal antibody is also being tested to treat patients with minimal residual disease, those in relapse, or as a purging method for autologous BMT (Jurcic & Scheinberg, 1995).

Acute Promyelocytic Leukemia

All-trans-retinoic acid (ATRA), a differentiating agent, is more effective than chemotherapy in inducing complete remission in patients with APL. However, treatment with ATRA 45 mg/m^2 daily does not sustain CR, and consolidation therapy with several courses of Ara-C and an anthracycline is recommended (Warrell et al., 1994). A complete discussion of this agent that works on the gastrointestinal system, reproduction, epithelial cell differentiation, and immune function is found in Chapter 5. Disease-free survival using this regimen is greater than 4 years (Degos et al., 1995).

Treatment with ATRA is associated with retinoic acid syndrome in up to 40% of patients. The early mortality rate is 10% to 15% in this group. This potentially fatal syndrome consists of fever, respiratory distress, weight gain, lower extremity edema, pleural or pericardial effusions, hypotension, and sometimes renal failure. The syndrome is most commonly seen when there is leukocytosis; however, these symptoms have been demonstrated in patients when the WBC count is less than 10,000/μL. Retinoic acid syndrome may be treated by intravenous dexamethasone 10 mg every 12 hours for 3 or more days, or by giving chemotherapy concurrently with ATRA in patients having or developing high WBC counts (Warrell et al., 1994; Degos et al., 1995; Fine, Fielding, Machin, Goldstone, Solomon, & Gann, 1994). Serious complications are preventable when steroids are administered at the first sign of this problem (Warrell, 1996).

Other symptoms associated with ATRA include headache and focal bone pain several hours after ingesting the drug that may require narcotic analgesia or steroids. However, patients develop tolerance to these symptoms, and ATRA therapy can be continued through them. Nausea, vomiting, dry skin, and inflammation of the lips are also common. A small number of patients may develop pseudotumor cerebri, manifested by papilledema, severe headache, and increased cerebrospinal fluid pressure. This has been successfully managed with corticosteroids and lumbar punctures to relieve symptoms (Frankel, Eardley, Heller, Berman, Miller, & Dimitrovsky, 1994).

Acute Lymphoblastic Leukemia

The first successful treatment regimens for the treatment of ALL included vincristine (VCR) and prednisone (Box 56-4). With the addition of anthracyclines using either doxorubicin or daunorubicin, in combination with cyclophosphomide and asparaginase, CR rates continued to improve. Most induction regimens include these drugs and are followed by consolidation courses with Ara-C and methotrexate. Other chemotherapy known to be effective in ALL includes mitoxantrone, etoposide, tenipodide, and amsacrine, and these agents are combined in many induction and consolidation protocols (Weiss, Maslak, Feldman, Berman, Bertino, & Gee, 1996). Maintenance therapy administered for an average of 2 years with methotrexate (MTX) mercaptopurine, vincristine, and prednisone is necessary to sustain CR. Ongoing CNS prophylaxis with intrathecal (IT) MTX or IT Ara-C either alone or in combination with whole brain radiation therapy (WBRT) shortly after diagnosis has decreased the incidence of CNS relapse (Cortes & Kantarjian, 1995; Larson, Dodge, Burns, Lee, Stone, & Schulman, 1995). Frequently, an Ommaya reservoir is placed into the ventricle of the brain to aid in administering intrathecal therapy. This is done during induction therapy if the platelet count and coagulation parameters allow.

Box 56-4
Acute Lymphoblastic Leukemia Treatment

Vincristine
Prednisone
Cytoxan
Adriamycin
L-asparaginase
Methotrexate
Mitoxantrone
Etoposide
Idarubicin
Daunorubicin
Amsacrine
Ara-c (standard or high dose)
Teniposide

CNS Prophylaxis (IT Methotrexate or Ara-c; Whole Brain Radiation Therapy)

Allogeneic bone marrow transplant; high-risk patients, first remission standard-risk patients, second remission

Ara-c, cytosine arabinoside; *CNS,* central nervous system; *IT,* intrathecal.

Allogeneic BMT may be an effective therapy for patients with ALL. There is controversy, however, as to when this aggressive therapy is indicated because the morbidity and mortality rates are significant (Cortes & Kantarjian, 1995; Zhang, Hoelzer, Horowitz, Gale, Messerer, & Klein, 1995). Patients at high risk of relapse because of poor prognostic factors may benefit from BMT in first CR, whereas those with a standard risk are maintained with chemotherapy. If relapse occurs, this group may be reinduced with chemotherapy before allogeneic BMT. Autologous BMT does not seem to be advantageous over chemotherapy (Borgmann, Schmid, Hartman, Baumgarten, Hermann, & Klingebeil, 1995).

Supportive measures to decrease infectious complications during neutropenic periods resulting from chemotherapy in ALL include prophylactic trimethoprim-sulfamethoxazole when long-term prednisone is tapered and granulocyte colony-stimulating factors during induction (Weiss et al., 1996; Ottman, Hoelzer, Gracien, Ganser, Kelley, & Reutzel, 1995).

ONCOLOGIC EMERGENCIES

DIC is predominately seen in patients with APL but should also be considered when the WBC count is high in patients with monocytoid leukemia (M4 or M5) or ALL, when chemotherapy is initiated (Keating, Esyet, & Kantarjian, 1993; Sarris, Kempin, Berman, Michaeli, Little, & Andreeff, 1992; Sarris, Kantarjian, Cortes, Pierce, Stass, & Andreef, 1993; Rhodes & Manzullo, 1995). This complication is discussed in detail in Chapter 11.

In APL the release of plasminogen activators from the granules of promyelocyte cells initiates the clotting cascade and is exacerbated when cells are lysed. One report has correlated the incidence of DIC to a WBC count greater than 10,000 (Rhodes & Manzullo, 1995). Interestingly, the incidence of DIC has not decreased with the use of ATRA (Warrell et al., 1994).

Tumor lysis syndrome (TLS) may be seen in both AML and ALL, although it is more common in patients with ALL. It is associated with a rapid proliferation index and large tumor burden, as evidenced by a high WBC count and an elevated lactic dehydrogenase (LDH), and is more severe when the renal function is impaired. In AML, TLS is more common in patients with monocytoid leukemia (Keating, Esyet, & Kantarjian, 1993; Rhodes & Manzullo, 1995).

Hypercalcemia occurs rarely in acute leukemia but is associated with T-cell ALL (Keating, Esyet, & Kantarjian, 1993; O'Donnell, 1996). HTLV-1 should be looked for in T-cell ALL patients who have hypercalcemia and lytic bone lesions (O'Donnell, 1996).

Sepsis syndrome and septic shock may occur in patients with acute leukemia, owing to profound, prolonged neutropenia, use of indwelling catheters, and in the older patient comorbid conditions (e.g., diabetes mellitus, chronic obstructive pulmonary disease).

NURSING MANAGEMENT

The nursing management of patients with acute leukemia is related to the prevention and treatment of symptoms related to pancytopenia. Standards of care for potential and actual problems caused by leukopenia, anemia, and thrombocytopenia in patients with leukemia were first introduced in the nursing literature in the early 1970s and have been applied to a gamut of patients receiving chemotherapy for hematologic and solid malignancies, as well as bone marrow and peripheral stem cell transplantation. These standards have been well documented in the nursing literature (Yeager & Miaskowski, 1994; Whedon, 1996; Wujcik, 1996).

Care of the patient with acute leukemia requires a tremendous emotional commitment and dedicated effort with meticulous attention to detail. Early on, the patient is taught self-care measures to reduce the risk of infection and bleeding. However, the profound pancytopenia quickly leads to debilitation, requiring intensive nursing care and daily infusion of multiple antibiotics, repletion of minerals, and blood product support. The symptomatology leading to the diagnosis of acute leukemia develops rapidly, and treatment is initiated immediately, so the patient is often overwhelmed with facing the ramifications of this potentially fatal illness. Intensive psychological support is necessary to help patients and families adjust to the diagnosis of acute leukemia, the intensity of the treatment, and the potential for relapse in the adult population.

An induction course of chemotherapy typically requires hospitalization of the patient for 4 to 8 weeks. After a brief respite for physical recuperation, a 5- to 7-day consolidation chemotherapy course is given for treatment of infection, followed by a nadir, which may require hospital admission for antibiotic therapy. Although treatment regimens vary, generally two or three consolidation courses are administered. As noted previously, maintenance therapy is not given in AML, but in ALL outpatient therapy may continue for 2 to 3 years. Nurses can help patients plan for their outpatient treatment so that the effect on daily routines and work schedules is minimal. Likewise, leisure and vacation time should be planned to occur when blood counts are normal and side effects few.

Patients who are eligible for allogeneic or autologous BMT (Chapters 9 and 10) need counseling to aid them in making the decision to choose this modality because there is significant morbidity and mortality associated with this treatment. Some specific standards of nursing care for patients with acute leukemia receiving treatments are outlined in Table 56-5.

HOME CARE ISSUES

The use of indwelling long-term catheters is controversial because they are often removed when an infection fails to clear with antibiotic therapy or when there is recrudescence with the same organism. When these access devices are used, patients are taught to manage them with aseptic dressing change and intermittent intravenous saline or heparin flushes.

Numerous patients are given recombinant colony-stimulating factors to reduce periods of neutropenia after chemotherapy. In spite of early fears, hematopoietic growth factors have not increased the incidence of drug-resistant

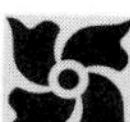

TABLE 56-5 Standard of Care for the Patient with Acute Leukemia

Patient Problem and Outcomes	Nursing Interventions and Rationale	Patient Education Instructions
Impaired Gas Exchange Related to Retinoic Acid Syndrome		
Patient will • Report shortness of breath and lower extremity edema as early symptoms if retinoic acid syndrome develops. • Have normal gas exchange and normal breath sounds.	1. Monitor for shortness of breath. 2. Monitor for fever, hypotension, and techypnea q4 hours and report promptly. 3. Weigh daily to assess for pulmonary overload. 4. Monitor for fluid retention. Check for the following: a. Sacral or lower extremity edema b. Distended neck veins c. Decreased breath sounds 2° to pleural effusion; rales d. Pericardial rub 2° pericardial effusion 5. Monitor intake and output q shift or more frequently prn. 6. Encourage assisted ambulation, deep breathing and coughing, turning side to side. 7. Administer decadron 10 mg IV q12 hours for 3 days, as ordered, and monitor effects.	1. Inform the patient about the potential for retinoic acid syndrome and the importance of reporting early signs, which include fever, shortness of breath, and sudden weight gain. 2. Teach the patient to report fever, shortness of breath, weight gain, or ankle edema promptly. 3. Inform the patient that although this syndrome is life threatening, early intervention with steroids is very effective treatment.

Continued

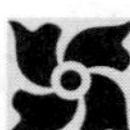

TABLE 56-5 Standard of Care for the Patient with Acute Leukemia—cont'd

Patient Problem and Outcomes	Nursing Interventions and Rationale	Patient Education Instructions
High Risk for Bleeding Related to DIC and Thrombocytopenia		
Patient will: • Report early signs and symptoms of bleeding. • Decrease potential for injury. • Maintain hemodynamic stability.	1. Monitor vital sign q4 hours and prn. 2. Report early signs of bleeding. 3. Alleviate symptoms that increase intracranial pressure (e.g., cough, retching, straining). 4. Monitor output for guaiac. 5. Assisted ambulation after receiving medication that may cause orthostatic hypotension or when dizzy or lightheaded. 6. Inspection for prolonged bleeding or applying pressure to where integument has been altered (e.g., bone marrow or IV punctures sites). 7. Institute bleeding precautions. 8. Monitor platelet count, coagulation profile (fibrinogen, fibrin split products). 9. Administer blood products (platelets, fresh frozen plasma, red blood cells) as ordered. 10. Administer continuous heparin infusion when ordered for DIC. Heparin infusion should be discontinued immediately if headache or signs of frank bleeding develops (e.g., hemoptysis, hematemesis).	1. Teach the patient importance of the following: a. Reporting early signs of bleeding b. Alleviating symptoms that increase intracranial pressure (e.g., cough, retching, straining while having a bowel movement) c. Monitoring stools for blood d. Assisted ambulation after receiving medication that may cause orthostatic hypotension or when dizzy or lightheaded e. Inspecting for prolonged bleeding or applying pressure to where integument has been altered (e.g., bone marrow or IV punctures sites)
Anxiety		
Patient will: • Verbalize an understanding of acute leukemia, induction chemotherapy, and side effects of treatment. • Verbalize feelings of decreased anxiety. • Identify strategies to cope with anxiety.	1. Assess the patient's level of understanding about acute leukemia and induction chemotherapy. 2. Give the patient the opportunity to ask questions or verbalize concerns. 3. Determine which coping strategies the patient has used effectively in the past to decrease anxiety, and reinforce the use of these coping strategies. 4. Encourage the patient to attend an existing support group for patients with leukemia. 5. Ask a patient who has completed treatment for acute leukemia to talk with this newly diagnosed patient. The LSA has begun the First Connection program to aid newly diagnosed patients and families by connecting them with a peer who has undergone a similar experience. 6. Administer pharmacologic agents to decrease anxiety, if necessary.	1. Use printed patient education material about acute leukemia. The Leukemia Society of America (LSA) publishes the following booklets: a. Acute Myelogenous Leukemia b. Acute Lymphocytic Leukemia Topics covered in this booklet include the incidence of AML or ALL, a description of the illness and symptoms, procedures to diagnose and treat leukemia, possible causes and risk factors, and coping with the illness. 2. Provide the patient with information about the following: a. Bone marrow aspiration and biopsy b. Long-term central venous catheter care c. Ommaya reservoir (ALL patients) d. HLA typing (AML and high-risk ALL) e. Neutropenic and bleeding precautions f. Head prosthesis consultants g. LSA patient financial aid program

LSA, Leukemia Society of America.

leukemia when given to patients with acute leukemia (Schiffer, 1996). When these medications are covered by medical insurance, injections may be self-administered in the home with nursing follow-up.

Because induction chemotherapy causes significant morbidity requiring prolonged hospitalization, many patients become physically incapacitated and can benefit from follow-up with a physical therapist. Patients who have received multiple doses of vincristine and long-term prednisone may have significant peripheral neuropathy and large muscle wasting and require additional intervention. Likewise, patients treated with high-dose Ara-C may develop cerebellar toxicity, making ambulation difficult or temporarily impossible, and referral to a physical therapist and an occupational therapist may be helpful.

Patients must be knowledgeable about signs and symptoms of infection and bleeding. They must also be reliable to call the physician or nurse when discharged from the hospital after consolidation therapy because their blood will again nadir. When a patient's physical condition is stable, nadir fever without documented bacteremia after consolidation courses may be treated with home intravenous antibiotic therapy (Freifeld & Pizzo, 1996; Malik, Khan, Karim, Aziz, & Khan, 1995).

The Leukemia Society of America (LSA) is a national voluntary health agency that provides public and professional educational material about leukemia and current therapies. A patient aid program reimburses blood component therapy support, drugs, transportation, and parking up to $750 annually for leukemia patients treated as outpatients. The LSA funds research grants and lobbies the federal government to increase funding for leukemia research. This organization works closely with the National Marrow Donor Program and local support groups.

PROGNOSIS

Complete remission data for patients with AML treated with one or two induction courses of chemotherapy ranges from 60% to 80% (Ghaddar & Estey, 1995; Scheinberg, Maslak, & Weiss, 1997; Berman, 1995). Patients with the cytogenetic translocations of 15, 17 (APL), 8, 21, or inversion 16 seem to have a higher CR rate and longer median remission duration, whereas patients with monosomy 5 or 7, or trisomy 8, have a lower CR rate and shorter remission duration. The rate and duration for patients with normal karyotype or other cytogenetic abnormalities lie somewhere in between (O'Donnell, 1996; Scheinberg, Maslak, & Weiss, 1997). Fewer than 50% of patients with therapy-related AML achieve CR, and the median duration is only 5 months (O'Donnell, 1996).

Approximately 25% of patients with AML relapse within 2 years from the time of the diagnosis. For patients under the age of 50 years, allogeneic or autologous BMT has increased the chance of long-term survival to 50% to 60% (Keating, Esyet, & Kantarjian, 1993; Scheinberg, Maslak, & Weiss, 1997).

Patients with APL historically had a poor prognosis because of DIC, which is exacerbated by chemotherapy. More recent reports cite improved long-term survival when the

TABLE 56-6 Quality of Care Evaluation for a Patient with Acute Promyelocytic Leukemia Receiving ALL-Trans Retinoic Acid

Disciplines participating in the quality of care evaluation:
☐ Nursing ☐ Medical Oncology ☐ Social Services

I. Induction Therapy Evaluation

Data from:
☐ Medical Record Review ☐ Patient/Family Interview

Criteria	Yes	No
1. Patient provided with information about the following:		
a. Retinoic acid syndrome and its symptoms	☐	☐
b. Need to report early symptoms promptly	☐	☐
c. Effective treatment with steroids	☐	☐
2. Vital signs every 4 hours	☐	☐
3. Monitored for fluid retention:		
a. Daily weight	☐	☐
b. Intake and output every shift or more frequently, prn	☐	☐
c. Sacral or lower extremity edema	☐	☐
d. Distended neck veins	☐	☐
e. Decreased breath sounds or rales	☐	☐
f. Pericardial rub	☐	☐
4. Patient experienced complications of retinoic acid syndrome:		
a. Fever	☐	☐
b. Shortness of breath	☐	☐
c. Weight gain	☐	☐
d. Pleural effusion	☐	☐
e. Pericardial effusion	☐	☐
f. Renal failure	☐	☐

II. Patient/Family Satisfaction

Data from:
☐ Patient Interview ☐ Family Interview

Criteria	Yes	No
1. On a scale of 0 to 10, with 0 being totally dissatisfied and 10 being totally satisfied, how satisfied were you with the care you received during your induction therapy with ALL-transretinoic acid for acute promyelocytic leukemia?	☐	☐
2. Were you told that you could experience retinoic acid syndrome?	☐	☐
3. Were you taught to report fever, shortness of breath, weight gain, or ankle edema promptly?	☐	☐

patient is successfully supported through coagulapathy and infectious complications. Patients treated with high-dose daunomycin (DNR) have a 61% survival rate at 9 years with no relapses after 3 years, although there were a high number of early deaths (Head, Kopecky, Weick, Files, Ryan, & Foucar, 1995). Treatment with ATRA followed by anthracycline containing chemotherapy has a CR rate of 75% to 90%, and it appears that patients who die early because of bleeding or infection, or those who are misdiagnosed, are the only treatment failures (Warrell, 1996). Because the majority of patients with APL have prolonged remissions, BMT is not recommended in this group (Degos et al., 1995).

More than 90% of children with ALL achieve CR, and 60% to 80% of them enjoy long-term remission or cure. About 60% to 85% of adults achieve CR with standard therapy; however, disease-free survival is reported from 25% to 50% when stratified for patient age, WBC count, cytogenetics, and other prognostic signs (Cortes & Kantarjian, 1995; Weiss et al., 1996; Larson et al., 1995). Long-term (9 years) follow-up of adults with ALL treated in first CR with chemotherapy or HLA-identical sibling BMT showed a relapse rate of 66% with chemotherapy versus 30% for transplantation. Mortality associated with BMT was much higher than with chemotherapy; however, leukemia-free survival data for both groups was 32% to 34% (Zhang et al., 1995). Although the timing of BMT remains controversial in patients with ALL, many treatment centers perform BMT on patients at high risk for relapse in first CR (Cortes & Kantarjian, 1995). For these high-risk patients, disease-free survival may be as high as 60% (O'Donnell, 1996).

EVALUATION OF THE QUALITY OF CARE

Accreditation organizations, such as the Joint Commission for the Accreditation of Healthcare Organizations (JCAHO), require that the quality of care provided to patients be evaluated. Because the care provided to patients with acute leukemia requires a multidisciplinary approach, an evaluation of the quality of care should include aspects of care provided by various team members. Table 56-6 provides an example of a quality of care evaluation tool for a patient taking ALL-transretinoic acid.

RESEARCH ISSUES

Disease-free survival curves in adults with acute leukemia treated with chemotherapy have not changed in the past 20 years, despite various combinations of chemotherapy. BMT has improved survival in some subsets of patients but not without significant treatment-related mortality. Other retinoids and vitamin D analogs may also be inducers of myeloid differentiation and should be clinically tested (Warrell, 1996). Likewise, monoclonal antibodies may prove to be adjuncts to chemotherapy and BMT by selectively targeting and destroying malignant cells (Jurcic & Scheinberg, 1995).

REFERENCES

Berman, E. (1995). Chemotherapy in acute myelogenous leukemia: High dose, higher expectation? *Journal of Clinical Oncology, 13*(1), 1-4.

Berman, E., Heller, G., Santorsa, J., McKenzie, S., Gee, T., & Kempin, S. (1991). Results of a randomized trial comparing idarubicin and cytosine arabinoside with daunorubicin and cytosine arabinoside in adult patients with newly diagnosed acute myelogenous leukemia. *Blood, 77,* 1666-1674.

Borgmann, A., Schmid, H., Hartman, R., Baumgarten, E., Hermann, K., & Klingebeil, T. (1995). Autologous bone-marrow transplants compared with chemotherapy for children with acute lymphoblastic leukemia in a second remission: A matched-pair analysis. *The Lancet, 346,* 873-876.

Cortes, J. E. & Kantarjian, H. (1995). Acute lymphocytic leukemia. In R. Pazdur (Ed.), *Medical oncology: A comprehensive review.* New York: PRR.

Degos, L., Dombret, H., Chomienne, C., Daniel, M. T., Miclea, J. M., & Chastang, C. (1995). All-trans-retinoic acid as a differentiating agent in the treatment of acute promyelocytic leukemia. *Blood, 85*(10), 2643-2653.

Fine, L. J., Fielding, A., Machin, S. J., Goldstone, A. H., Solomon, E., & Gann, A. (1994). Acute promyelocytic leukemia. *The Lancet, 344,* 1615-1618.

Frankel, S. R., Eardley, A., Heller, G., Berman, E., Miller, W. H., & Dimitrovsky, E. (1994). All-trans-retinoic acid for acute promyelocytic leukemia: Results of the New York study. *Annals of Internal Medicine, 120*(4), 278-286.

Freifeld, A. G. & Pizzo, P. A. (1996). The outpatient management of febrile neutropenia in cancer patients. *Oncology, 10*(4), 599-616.

Ghaddar, H. M. & Estey, E. H. (1995). Acute myelogenous leukemia. In R. Pazdur (Ed.), *Medical oncology: A comprehensive review.* New York: PRR.

Head, D., Kopecky, K. J., Weick, J., Files, J. C., Ryan, D., & Foucar, K. (1995). Effect of aggressive daunomycin therapy on survival in acute promyelocytic leukemia. *Blood, 86*(5), 1717-1728.

Heath, C. (1991). Epidemiology and hereditary aspects of acute leukemia. In P. Wiernik, G. Canellos, R. Kyle, & C. Schiffer (Eds.), *Neoplastic diseases of the blood.* New York: Churchill Livingstone.

Jurcic, J. G. & Scheinberg, D. A. (1995). Monoclonal antibody therapy of myeloid leukemias. *PPO Updates, 9*(2), 1-12.

Keating, M. J., Esyet, E., & Kantarjian, H. (1993). Acute leukemia. In V. T. Devita, S. Hellman, & S. A. Rosenberg (Eds.), *Cancer: Principles and practice of oncology* (4th ed.). Philadelphia: J. B. Lippincott.

Landis, S. H., Murray, T., Bolden, S., & Wingo, P. A. (1998). Cancer Statistics, 1998. *CA: A Cancer Journal for Clinicians, 48:*6-9.

Larson, R. A., Dodge, R. K., Burns, C. P., Lee, E. J., Stone, R. M., & Schulman, P. (1995). A five-drug remission induction regimen with intensive consolidation for adults with acute lymphoblastic leukemia Group B study 8811. *Blood, 85*(8), 2025-2037.

Malik, I. A., Khan, W. A., Karim, M., Aziz, Z., & Khan, M. A. (1995). Feasibility of outpatient management of fever in cancer patients with low risk neutropenia: Results of a randomized trial. *American Journal of Medicine, 98*(3), 224-231.

Mitus, A. J. & Rosenthal, D. S. (1995). The adult leukemias. In G. P. Murphy, W. Lawrence, & R. E. Lenhard (Eds.), *American Cancer Society textbook of clinical oncology* (2nd ed.). Atlanta: The American Cancer Society.

O'Donnell, M. R. (1996). Acute leukemia. In R. Pazdur, L. R. Coia, W. J. Hoskins, & L. D. Wagman (Eds.), *Cancer management: A multidisciplinary approach.* New York: PRR.

Ottman, O. G., Hoelzer, D., Gracien, E., Ganser, A., Kelley, K., & Reutzel, R. (1995). Concomitant granulocyte colony-stimulating factor and induction chemoradiotherapy in adult acute lymphoblastic leukemia: A randomized phase III trial. *Blood, 86*(2), 444-450.

Rhodes, V. & Manzullo, E. (1995). In R. Pazdur (Ed.), *Medical oncology: A comprehensive review.* New York: PRR.

Rothstein, G. (1993). Origin and development of the blood and blood-forming tissues. In G. R. Lee, T. C. Bithell, & J. Foerster (Eds.), *Wintrobe's clinical hematology* (9th ed.). Philadelphia: Lea & Febiger.

Sarris, A. H., Kantarjian, H. M., Cortes, J. E., Pierce, S., Stass, S., & Andreef, M. (1993). Successful treatment of the DIC of adult ALL with fresh-frozen plasma, cryoprecipitate, and platelets. *Blood, 82*(suppl. 1), 253a.

Sarris, A. H., Kempin, S., Berman, E., Michaeli, J., Little, C., & Andreeff, M. (1992). High incidence of disseminated intravascular coagulation during remission induction of adult patients with acute lymphoblastic leukemia. *Blood 79,* 1305-1310.

Scheinberg, D. A., Maslak, P., & Weiss, M. (1997). Acute leukemias. In D. T. Devita, S. Hellman, & S. A. Rosenberg (Eds.), *Cancer: Principles and practice of oncology* (5th ed.). Philadelphia: Lippincott-Raven.

Schiffer, C. A. (1996). Hematopoietic growth factors as adjuncts to the treatment of acute myeloid leukemia. *Blood, 88*(10), 3675-3685.

Schiffer, C. A. (1997). Acute myeloid leukemia in adults. In J. F. Holland, E. Frei, & R. C. Blast (Eds.), *Cancer medicine* (4th ed.). Baltimore: Williams and Wilkens.

Warrell, R. (1996). Use of retinoic acid in acute promyelocytic leukemia patients triples overall survival rates. *Oncology News International, 5*(12), 2, 23.

Warrell, R. P., Maslak, P., Eardley, A., Heller, G., Miller, W. H., & Frankel, S. R. (1994). Treatment of acute promyelocytic leukemia with all-trans retinoic acid: An update of the New York experience. *Leukemia, 8*(6), 929-933.

Weiss, M., Maslak, P., Feldman, E., Berman, E., Bertino, J., & Gee, T. (1996). Cytarbine with high dose mitoxantrone induces rapid complete remission in adult acute lymphoblastic leukemia without the use of vincristine or prednisone. *Journal of Clinical Oncology, 14*(9), 2480-2485.

Whedon, M. B. (1996). Nursing role in management, hematologic problems. In S. M. Lewis, I. C. Collier, & M. M. Heitkemper (Eds.), *Medical surgical nursing assessment and management of clinical problems* (4th ed.). St. Louis: Mosby.

Wujcik, D. (1996). Update on the diagnosis and therapy for acute promyelocytic leukemia and chronic myelogenous leukemia. *Oncology Nursing Forum, 23*(3), 478-487.

Yeager, K. A. & Miaskowski, C. (1994). Advances in understanding the mechanisms and management of acute leukemia. *Oncology Nursing Forum, 21*(3), 541-548.

Zhang, M., Hoelzer, D., Horowitz, M. M., Gale, R. P., Messerer, D., & Klein, J. P. (1995). Long-term follow-up of adults with acute lymphoblastic leukemia in first remission treated with chemotherapy or bone marrow transplantation. *Annals of Internal Medicine, 123*(6), 428-431.

57 Chronic Myelogenous Leukemia

Deborah Chielens, RN, OCN

EPIDEMIOLOGY

The median age for chronic myelogenous leukemia (CML) incidence is 50 to 53 years. However, it can occur at any age. There is a slight male prevalence; the male-to-female ratio is estimated to be 1.4-2.2:1. CML is responsible for about 7% to 15% of all leukemias The incidence of CML has remained constant for the last 50 years (Cortes, Talpaz, & Kantarjian, 1996).

RISK FACTORS

The cause of CML remains a mystery. Children of CML patients do not have an increased risk of developing the disease (Cortes, Talpaz, Kantarjian, 1996). The survivors of Hiroshima and Nagasaki have a higher incidence of CML, as do patients who have had radiation treatment for other malignancies. However, Rundles (1982) showed that only 1 in 15 or 20 patients developing CML actually has had any unusual exposure to any form of radiation. There also have been cases documented of patients who have had occupational exposure to benzene. However, in most cases the cause is unclear. Risk factors for CML are as follows:

- Age: Peaks in fourth or fifth decade of life
- Males
- Possible radiation exposure

NORMAL ANATOMY AND PHYSIOLOGY

To fully understand the pathophysiology of CML, normal hematopoiesis must be examined. Normal production of blood cell lines can be traced through a study of hematopoiesis (see Fig. 56-1, p. 1225). In normal bone marrow, there are regulatory mechanisms that ensure hematopoietic cell proliferation, differentiation, and maturation. Chapter 9 offers a complete discussion of hematopoiesis. Hematopoietic cells are initiated by the pluripotent stem cell, the smallest and most immature cell responsible for differentiating into the myeloid or lymphoid cell lines. The myeloid and lymphoid cell lines further differentiate and mature. The myeloid line produces erythrocytes, granulocytes, monocytes, or megakaryocytes. The lymphoid line produces B or T lymphocytes. As cells mature, they migrate into the bloodstream at a rate matching the death of old cells. With the exception of T lymphocytes, hematopoietic cells are not released from the bone marrow until they are fully matured. T lymphocytes leave the bone marrow at a relatively immature state and then mature in the thymus gland before entering the peripheral circulation.

PATHOPHYSIOLOGY

CML, also called *chronic granulocytic leukemia,* is classified as a hematologic malignancy. The common characteristic of all leukemias is an unregulated proliferation in the bone marrow of the cell of hematologic origin (Rapaport, 1987). The malignant clones take over normal marrow function. Therefore all cell lines are affected. Leukemias are classified according to the cell of origin. Most leukemias arise from the white cell line, and in CML, the myeloid stem is a dysfunctional stem. Approximately 90% of all CML patients have a diagnostic marker of the Philadelphia chromosome. Fig. 56-3, p. 1227, illustrates the cell of origin for CML.

CML, discovered in 1960 by Peter Nowell and David Hungerford, is the first disease to have a consistent chromosomal abnormality in human cancer (Mitelman, 1994). The Philadelphia chromosome is described as the G group chromosome; number 22 is missing a portion of the long arm (q), which has been translocated to the long arm of 9. When the proto-oncogene c-abl is translocated from 9 to 22, a new oncogene, bcr-abl, is formed. This new gene produces a protein that is associated with starting growth factor receptors. Fig. 57-1 illustrates the translocation of genes in patients with CML. Fig. 57-2 demonstrates a peripheral bone marrow transplant aspiration slide suggesting a diagnosis of CML. These are events that lead up to the uncontrolled proliferation of white cells (Foon & Casciato, 1995).

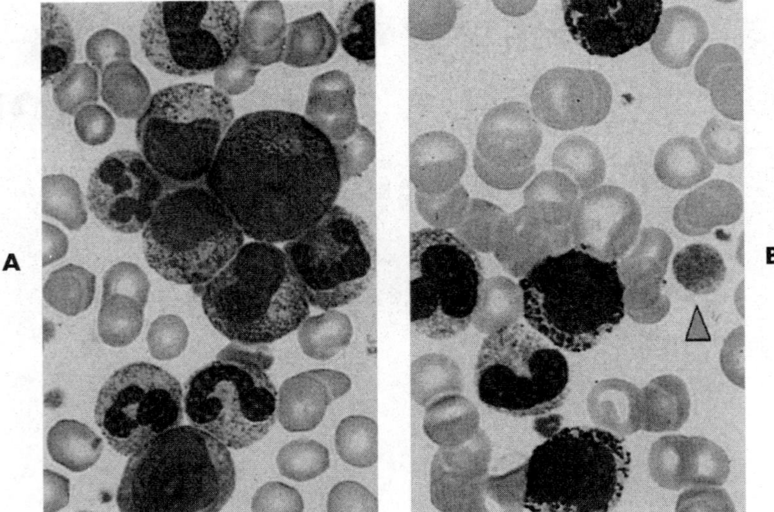

Fig. 57-1 Chronic myelogenous leukemia. Peripheral blood films show **A,** a myeloblast, promyelocytes, myelocytes, metamyelocytes, and band and segmented neutrophils, as well as **B,** basophils and a giant platelet *(arrow)*. (From Skarin, A. T. [1996]. *Atlas of diagnostic oncology* [2nd ed.]. St. Louis: Mosby.)

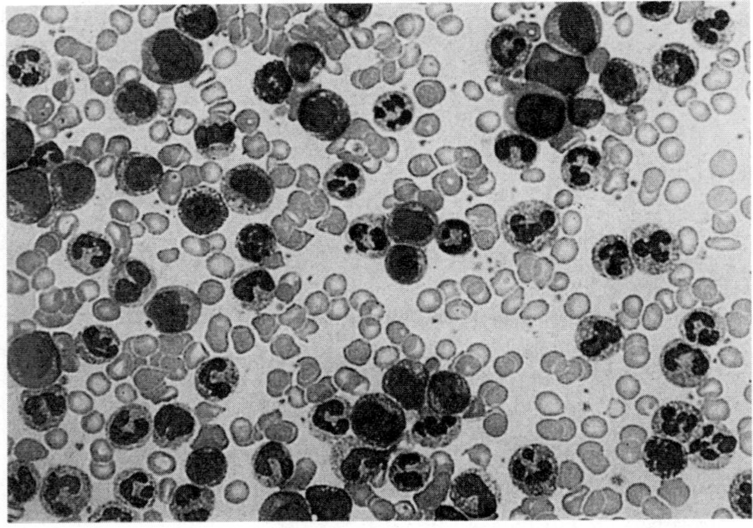

Fig. 57-2 Chronic myelogenous leukemia. Peripheral blood film shows cells at all stages of granulopoietic development. (From Skarin, A. T. [1996]. *Atlas of diagnostic oncology* [2nd ed.]. St. Louis: Mosby.)

ROUTES OF METASTASES

Because CML is a hematologic malignancy, its primary sites are the bone marrow and the peripheral blood. However, in blast crisis, extramedullary infiltrates can occur in the central nervous system, lymph nodes, bone, and skin (Wujcik, 1997).

ASSESSMENT

In about 20% of patients, CML is diagnosed while patients are asymptomatic and undergoing routine physical examination for a variety of reasons. There is no single tool that can diagnose CML; the diagnosis is determined by the presence of a constellation of symptoms and the results of clinical tests. A careful patient history is important because the vagueness of symptoms such as fatigue, malaise, abdominal fullness, anorexia, or early satiety present a confounding picture. An essential part of the physical examination is palpation of the spleen and liver to assess for classic lymphadenopathy and splenomegaly associated with CML. Lymphadenopathy results from the collection of B and T lymphocytes within the lymph drainage system. Splenomegaly is seen in 50% of patients as a result of massive production and destruction of hematologic cells (Fig. 57-3). Hepatomegaly is seen in 20% of patients. One of the most important diagnostic keys to CML is to obtain a complete blood count (CBC) with a full differential to assess for shifts in white cells that may exceed 30,000/μL, indicating

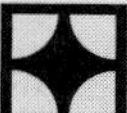

TABLE 57-1 Assessment of the Patient for Chronic Myelogenous Leukemia

	Assessment Parameters	Typical Abnormal Findings
History	A. Personal and social history 1. Age 2. Occupation 3. Evaluation of constitutional symptoms	A. Personal and social factors 1. Older patients. 2. Radiation exposure has been implicated but it is not definitive. 3. Patient may report flulike sumptoms: malaise, fatigue, bone or joint pain, left upper quadrant pain, early satiety, anorexia and abdominal fullness, night sweats, fever, and weight loss.
Physical Examination	1. Spleen 2. Appetite 3. Lymph system 4. Neurologic examination	1. Enlarged spleen secondary to sequestering of hematopoietic cells. 2. Poor appetite and weight loss due to enlarged spleen impinging on gastrointestinal tract. 3. Lymphadenopathy from accumulation of white cells. 4. Priapism, tinnitus, stupor, visual changes (rare).
Diagnostic Tests	A. Complete blood count B. Bone aspiration and biopsy	A. Leukocytosis. B. Hypercellular marrow with Philadelphia positive chromosome.

Modified from Deisseroth, A. B., Kantarjian, H., Andreeff, M., Talpaz, M., Keating, M. J., & Khouri, I. (1997). Chronic leukemias. In V. T. DeVita, S. Hellman, & S. A. Rosenberg (Eds.), *Cancer: Principles and procedures of oncology* (5th ed.), Philadelphia: Lippincott-Raven.

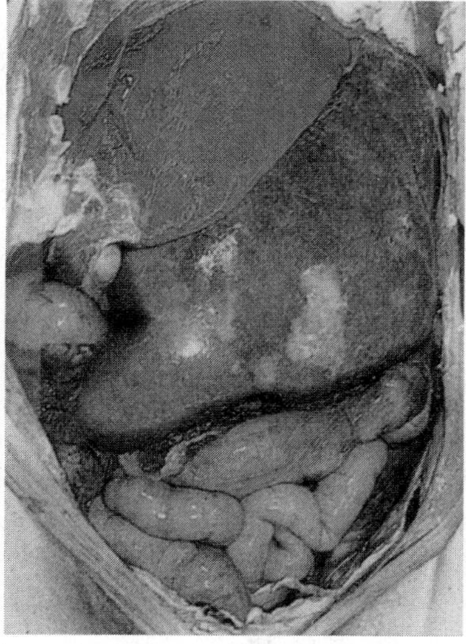

Fig. 57-3 Splenic involvement of chronic myelogenous leukemia. (From Skarin, A. T. [1996]. *Atlas of diagnostic oncology* [2nd ed.]. St. Louis: Mosby.)

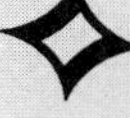

TABLE 57-2 Patient Preparation for a Bone Marrow Aspirate

Description of Procedure: A needle is inserted into the bone marrow space, usually in the hip bone, or occasionally the sternum or breastbone is used.

Patient Preparation: The patient can bring soothing music, a family member, or friend to hold a hand. A gentle message or ice can be used for distraction.

1. Obtain informed consent
2. Request that the patient loosen clothes from the waist down.
3. Request the patient to lie flat on the stomach.
4. Examine the iliac crest to determine the area to aspirate.
5. Cleanse the skin with povidone or iodine solution twice.
6. Draw up and inject heparin and lidocaine solutions.
7. Insert the trocar needle into the marrow space.
8. Aspirate marrow and determine whether the sample is adequate.
9. Once marrow is obtained, remove the needle, apply pressure to the area to stop bleeding, and apply an appropriate bandage.

an overcrowded and underfunctioning marrow. Platelets may exceed 1,000,000 μL, further raising the suspicion of a chronic leukemia. A bone marrow aspiration with cytogenetic analysis, seeking the possible presence of the Philadelphia chromosome, is essential to make a differential diagnosis. Table 57-1 outlines steps in patient assessment for CML. Table 57-2 illustrates a teaching tool for patients having bone marrow aspiration for a diagnosis of CML.

STAGING

CML is known to have three phases: chronic, acute, and blast crises. Table 57-3 describes these phases with their clinical manifestations (Mitus & Rosenthal, 1955). The chronic phase is usually the initial phase, which eventually leads to a blastic phase, which is similar to an acute leukemia. The *chronic phase* is defined as 30% blasts in the bone marrow or the peripheral blood. Often, patients have extramedullary infiltration occurring in the central nervous system, lymph nodes, bones, skin, and infrequently in the bone marrow and peripheral blood blasts. Patients in blast crisis, without treatment, usually die in approximately 3 to 6 months. There are two other staging systems used in CML: the synthesis staging system for CML (Table 57-4) and the Sokal prognostic risk system, which is not as clinically useful as phases staging or the synthesis staging system, secondary to its complexity.

TABLE 57-3 Phases and Clinical Manifestations of Chronic Myelogenous Leukemia

Characteristic	Chronic Phase (Ph+)	Chronic Phase (Ph−)	Blastic Phase
Median age of onset	50	60	–
Signs/symptoms	Fatigue, malaise, headache, weight loss, early satiety, and left upper quadrant fullness	Same as chronic phase (Ph+)	Fatigue, weakness, fever, night sweats, weight loss, easy bruising, and splenic and bone pain
Bone marrow status	<20% immature myeloid cells; hypercellular	Increased myeoblasts and myelofibrosis	>20% circulating or bone marrow myeloblasts; >30% circulating white blood cells; or >50% of bone marrow blasts and progranulocytes
Mean WBC count	225,000	50,000-75,000	>50,000
Mean platelet count	>450,000 in 50% of patients; >1,000,000 in 25% of patients; normal or slightly elevated in 25% of patients	170,000	<100,000
Other laboratory values	Increased LDH, uric acid, and vitamin B_{12} levels; increased vitamin B_{12} binding capacity; decreased LAP	Normal or slightly increased LAP	Normal or increased LAP
Organomegaly	Splenomegaly common; hepatomegaly rare	Splenomegaly less common	Splenomegaly and hepatomegaly common
Median survival (untreated)	40-45 months	10-19 months	2-4 months

LAP, Leucocyte adhesion protein; *LDH,* lactate dehydrogenase; *PH,* Philadelphia chromosome.
Modified from Wujcik, D. (1996). Update on the diagnosis of and therapy for acute promyelocytic leukemia and chronic myelogenous leukemia. *Oncology Nursing Forum, 23*(3), 477-485.

TABLE 57-4 Synthesis Staging System for Chronic Myelogenous Leukemia

	Stage	Definition
Chronic Phase		
Age >60 years	1	0 or 1
Characteristics:		
Spleen >10 cm below costal margin		
Blasts >3% in blood or 5% in marrow	2	2 Characteristics
Basophils >7% in blood or >3% in marrow		
Platelets >700 × 10 9/L	3	> 3 Characteristics
Accelerated Phase	4	>1 Characteristic defines accelerated phase
Cytogenic clonal evolution		
Blasts >15% in blood		
Blasts + promyelocytes >30% in blood phase; basophils >20% in blood		
Platelets <100 × 109/L		

Modified from Deisseroth, A. B., Kantarjian, H., Andreeff, M., Talpaz, M., Keating, M. J., Khouri, I. et al. (1997). Chronic leukemias. In V. T. DeVita, S. Hellman, & S. A. Rosenberg (Eds.), *Cancer: Principles and procedures of oncology* (5th ed.). Philadelphia: Lippincott-Raven.

MEDICAL MANAGEMENT

Chemotherapy

For many years, the standard treatment for patients with CML was busulfan or hydroxyurea. Busulfan provides long periods of hematologic control of the white count and is an affordable treatment option. However, adverse effects include lung, marrow, heart fibrosis, and an Addison-like disease. Busulfan is given orally, either daily (4 to 8 mg per day) or in 2-week courses. Busulfan is associated with unpredictable prolonged myelosuppression, pulmonary fibrosis, and Addison-like disease. A dose of 0.1 mg per kg per day is often used initially. The dose is halved as the white blood cell (WBC) count drops by half and is discontinued when the WBC count drops below 20,000.

Hydroxyurea provides good hematologic control of the disease but has had only a transient response in patients with the Philadelphia+ chromosome. Patients treated with hydroxyurea usually have prolonged chronic phases. Hydroxyurea is given daily by mouth (1 to 3 g/day as a single dose on an empty stomach). Hydroxyurea is superior to busulfan in the chronic phase of CML, with significantly longer median survival and significantly fewer severe adverse effects. A dose of 40 mg/kg per day is often used initially and often results in a rapid reduction of the WBC count. When the WBC count drops below 20,000 per cubic mm, the hydroxyurea is often reduced and titrated to maintain a WBC count between 5,000 and 20,000 μL. However, in a randomized trial in which the hydroxyurea dose was adjusted to normalize the WBC count, no difference in survival was seen between a group treated with hydroxyurea and a group treated with interferon-alpha. This suggests that a more aggressive application of hydroxyurea may lead to additional benefits (Hehlmann, Heimpel, Hasford, Kolb, Pralle, Hossfeld et al., 1994). More research is needed in this area. Because of its lower toxicity, hydroxyurea is the drug of choice for patients who are candidates for bone marrow transplantation.

Other Chemotherapy

Other chemotherapeutic agents administered are melphalan 6 mercaptopurine alone or used in combination with busulfan. Thiotepa has been studied in clinical trials but was found to cause severe thrombocytopenia. Continuous infusion of low-dose cytarabine was studied and found to have controlled hematologic symptoms such as infection and bleeding, and some patients had some level of cytogenetic response. However, out of five patients, only one had a complete response (CR) and the others had a partial response (Hehlmann, et al., 1994).

Interferon-Alpha

Interferon-alpha (IFN-α), a biologic response modifier (discussed thoroughly in Chapter 7), has been used to treat patients with CML since 1985 and has shown significant improvements in these patients. In two trials comparing interferon alpha with conventional chemotherapy (hydroxyurea or busulfan), patients in the chronic phase who received IFN-α had more karyotypic responses, more delay of disease progression, and prolonged overall survival. Another randomized study confirmed the advantage of alpha interferon (median survival 5.5 years) over busulfan (median survival 3.8 years), but it did not detect a significant difference between interferon and hydroxyurea (median survival 4.7 years). About 20% of the chronic-phase patients treated with IFN-α have significant cytogenetic remissions with temporary disappearance of Philadelphia + cells in the marrow, and in about 10% of the patients, these cytogenetic responses are quite long lasting. However, using molecular methods of analysis, small numbers of Ph+ cells can still be detected in the majority of patients having long-term cytogenetic remissions, and longer follow-up is required to ascertain whether the disease will reoccur. Patients older than 60 years with chronic phase CML have a hematologic and cytogenetic response rate and duration of cytogenetic response similar to that in younger patients; however, the incidence of complications is greater in elderly patients (Kantarjian, Smith, O'Brien, Beran, Pierce, & Talpaz, 1995; Kantarjian, Deisseroth, Zurzrock, Estrov, & Talpaz, 1993).

IFN-α has significant toxic effects that can result in dosage modification or discontinuation therapy in many cases. Common side effects include influenza-like syndrome, nausea, anorexia, and weight loss. Immune-mediated complications, such as hyperthyroidism, hemolysis, and connective tissue diseases, may occur rarely after long-term treatment. Table 57-5 lists a patient teaching guide for patients receiving IFN-α and Table 57-6 illustrates a nursing care plan for patients receiving this therapy. IFN-α is costly, and daily subcutaneous injections can be troublesome, but pharmaceutical companies are often committed to reimbursement support through assisting patients with billing issues, determination of insurance carrier policies, assistance with preapproval of claims, and assistance in the appeals of claims that have been denied.

Splenectomy

Splenectomy, performed during the chronic phase of CML, may be beneficial to control hypertension caused by the infiltrative character of lympocyte disorders, but it neither delays the onset of blastic transformation nor prolongs survival. Splenectomy during the accelerated phase in not indicated (Palackdharry, 1995) and has been used as a surgical method to control disease. However, it has not been curative.

Bone Marrow or Stem Cell Transplantation

There is no cure for CML, and the treatment of choice for selected patients with CML is allogeneic or syngeneic bone marrow transplantation (BMT). The outcome of BMT for matched sibling transplants depends on the stage of the disease at the time of the transplant. The best results are in patients who are in the chronic phase, with moderate results for those receiving a transplant in the accelerated phase. The least favorable results are transplants done in the blast crisis. In Seattle, since 1985, 400 patients receiving transplants for CML in the chronic phase had a 5-year survival rate of 75%. Of those 400 receiving transplants in the accelerated phase, the 5-year survival rate was 50%, and the rate was 10% for those receiving transplants in blast crisis. Prior exposure to busulfan has been documented as an adverse risk for BMT (Applebaum, 1996) (Fig. 57-4). The major conclusion of this experience is to give CML patients transplants as early as possible in the chronic phase so that disease acceleration does not occur. Even further, the experience shows that transplantation within 6 months of the diagnosis has superior results (Appelbaum, 1996).

Unrelated Bone Marrow Transplantation

Results of the use of unrelated donor transplants for patients with CML have been studied. Initially, data were disappointing, and morbidity associated with graft versus host disease and treatment-related complications were discouraging. However, more recent results demonstrate a disease-free survival of 65% of patients receiving transplants.

Autologous Marrow or Stem Cell Transplantation

The possibility of eradicating the leukemic cell population during the chronic phase by intensive treatment followed by rescue with autologous marrow or peripheral blood

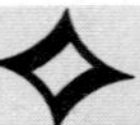

TABLE 57-5 Patient Preparation for Symptoms Associated with IFN-α Administration

Symptom Management for Patients: This is a list of common side effects or symptoms seen with interferon. Some of these symptoms can be associated with leukemia and/or could be a result of hypothyroidism. Some of these symptoms can occur, and there is not much that can be done to alleviate them.

Symptoms	What to Do
Fatigue	Take naps during the day. If fatigue occurs at a certain time of the day, plan that part of the day to be more restful, if possible.
Aches of Muscle and Joints	Take Tylenol or ibuprofen. Report to the physician if symptoms become severe.
Low-Grade Fevers	Take Tylenol and report to the physician persistent fevers after 1 week of starting interferon.
Flulike Symptoms	Take Tylenol before treatment and every 4 hours as needed. Drink fluids to prevent dehydration.
Gastrointestinal Symptoms, Lack of Appetite, Weight Loss	Weight will be monitored by your primary physician.
Diarrhea	Take Lomotil or Imodium.
Constipation	Start with increasing fiber in your diet (i.e., fruits, vegetables, grains) and also increasing fluid intake. Stool softeners or Metamucil could be taken.
Dry Mouth	Drink liquids and rinse frequently. Take artificial saliva preparations or sugarless hard candies.
Dry Cough, Postnasal Drip	Take Sudafed. If these symptoms become severe, call the primary physician.
Blood Counts Dropping	Your primary care physician will draw your CBC (complete blood cell count) once a week. Your interferon dose can be adjusted accordingly. Bone marrow aspirations are done every 3 months.
Bleeding or Infections	Report to your physician.
Central Nervous System Symptoms	Report these symptoms to your physician if they become worse.
Transient Tingling and Numbness	Antidepressants can be prescribed (e.g., Paxil, Zoloft, or Prozac).
Depression	
Insomnia	Try warm baths, warm milk, or herbal teas before bed.
Memory Defects, Reduced Attention Span	Report to your physician. Your blood pressure should be checked.
Dizziness	
Sex (Lack of Libido Desire)	Impotence (lack of ability to have sex) should be reported to your physician.
Hair Loss, Thinning of Hair	This occurs in about 25% of the patient population. Avoid hot hair dryers or towel dry before dryer use; use mild shampoos and conditioners.

GENERAL SUGGESTION: If symptoms occur after interferon injection, time the injection right before sleep so symptoms can occur during the night.

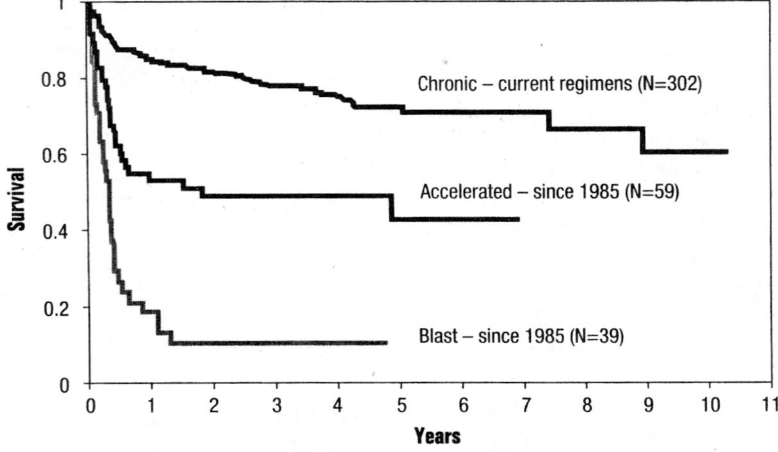

Fig. 57-4 Survival of 400 patients receiving transplants in Seattle from matched siblings for treatment of chronic myelogenous leukemia. Current regimens include cyclophosphamide plus 12 Gy total body irradiation or cyclophosphamide plus busulfan. As for most other hematologic malignancies, survival after transplantation is highest among patients receiving transplants earlier in the disease course. (From Appelbaum, F. R., Clift, R., Radich, J., Anasetti, C., & Buckner, C. D. [1995]. Bone marrow transplantation for chronic myelogenous leukemia. *Seminars in Oncology, 22*(4):405-411.)

TABLE 57-6 Nursing Care Plan for Patients with Chronic Myelogenous Leukemia Receiving Interferon Alfa-2a

Nursing Diagnosis	Desired Patient Outcome	Nursing Interventions
Knowledge deficit regarding subcutaneous or intramuscular injection	Patient will correctly self-administer IFNα-2a	1. Teach the patient dose preparation. 2. Teach the patient/family about medication handling and storage (no shaking or freezing; refrigeration). 3. Teach the patient/family proper administration techniques using appropriate teaching tools (videotapes, flip charts, models). 4. Plan for a return demonstration to ensure proper administration. 5. Teach the patient/family about proper disposal of syringes and needles, such as placement in a puncture-proof container and returning them to the health care setting.
Risk for flulike syndrome (fever, chills, myalgias) related to side effects of IFNα-2a	Patient's symptoms of flulike syndrome will be controlled or minimized.	1. Manipulate the dose, schedule, and route to determine the best effect with minimal discomfort. 2. Premedicate as indicated: a. Fever/myalgia: Prostaglandin inhibitor and nonsteroidal antiinflammatory drugs b. Chills/rigors: Meperidine c. Headache: Antihistamines and prostaglandin inhibitor 3. Use other comfort measures as needed, such as extremity wraps, hydration, relaxation, distraction, education, and reassurance.
Risk for bone marrow suppression related to side effects of IFNα-2a	Patient will remain infection free.	1. Arrange for regular blood drawing; monitor white blood cell counts. 2. Perform regular physical assessment. 3. Teach the patient/family the signs and symptoms of infection to report.
Risk for fatigue related to side effects of IFNα-2a	Patient will participate in activities of daily living as desired and as is consistent with disease status.	1. Perform baseline and ongoing assessment to evaluate the activity status. 2. Manipulate the dose, schedule, and route to maximize the effect and minimize fatigue. 3. Educate the patient to be aware of activities that increase or decrease fatigue; assist with priority and goal setting that is realistic and consistent with the patient's desires. 4. Teach and support activities that decrease fatigue, such as proper nutrition and rest, scheduling of activities, and energy conservation measures. 5. Encourage the patient to exercise within individual limitations.

Modified from Wujcik, D. (1996). Update on the diagnosis of and therapy for acute promyelocytic leukemia and chronic myelogenous leukemia. *Oncology Nursing Forum, 23*(3), 477-485.

stem cells has also been considered. Various methods have been instituted to eliminate or reduce residual leukemic cells in the autografts, including ex vivo treatment with cytotoxic drugs and various immunologic or biologic purging methods. Although some of the early reports appear promising, they are based on relatively small numbers of selected patients, and the follow-up period is too short to be sure late relapses will not occur. Autologous BMT is increasingly being studied, but little or no data exist to suggest that, with current approaches, this technique can lead to long-term cures for patients with CML (Viele, 1996).

ONCOLOGIC EMERGENCIES

Several potential oncologic emergencies can exist for patients with CML. Chapter 11 gives a complete review of these conditions. The most common oncologic emergencies for CML are discussed here.

Septic Shock

Patients with CML have compromised immune systems from their disease and treatments for their disease placing them at life-threatening risk for infection. Septic shock is manifested by hemodynamic instability and alternations in cellular metabolism. The typical signs and symptoms of infection may be absent due to pancytopenia, but early signs and symptoms include anxiety, restlessness, confusion, and a decreased level of consciousness progressing to chills, fever, tachycardia, widening pulse pressure, warm flushed skin, rales, chronic cough, and wheezes. Late signs and symptoms include disorientation and lethargy, dyspnea, cyanosis, and increased pulmonary congestion. Management includes administration of intravenous fluids such as normal saline solution or lactated Ringers solution and colloids to restore the patient's hemodynamic stability. Dopamine may be required to increase cardiac contractility, peripheral vascular resistance, and renal blood flow. Administration of antibiotics sensitive to the specific organism cultured from the blood is imperative. Oxygen support may be required (Clark & McGee, 1992).

Patient and caregiver information about the risks for infection and possible septic shock is imperative. Education includes a list of symptoms to report immediately, in particular shaking chills without a fever, and methods to access emergency care. Strategies to minimize the risk of infection, such as aseptic central venous catheter management, scrupulous personal hygiene, practicing safe sex, avoiding infectious persons, and adherence to medication schedules, are critical to the safety of these immunosuppressed patients.

Tumor Lysis Syndrome

Tumor lysis syndrome (TLS) is a metabolic imbalance that occurs with the rapid release of intracellular potassium, phosphorus, and nucleic acid into the blood stream as a result of tumor kill. This syndrome includes hyperkalemia, hyperphosphatemia, hyperuricemia, hypocalcemia leading to seizures, renal failure, and cardiac arrest. CML recipients receiving high doses of chemotherapy or those who are recipients of bone marrow transplants are at a high risk for TLS immediately after the transplant as a result of high-dose conditioning regimens. Preventive measures when high tumor burden is suspected are taken to increase the patient's oral and intravenous fluid intake. Allopurinol given before chemotherapy can maintain the pH of the urine at greater than 7, helping to prevent renal failure. Nursing assessment of early renal failure symptoms such as decreased urine output, increased weight, changes in mental status, anorexia, nausea, vomiting, and diarrhea is critical to the life of the patient. Symptoms of cardiac arrthymias include decreased blood pressure, increased pulse rate, irregular pulse, chest pain, or shortness of breath (Maquire-Eisen & Edmonds, 1992).

Disseminated Intravascular Coagulation

Disseminated intravascular coagulation (DIC) can occur in response to infection or the malignancy in patients with CML. DIC is described as the inappropriate accelerated and systemic activation of the coagulation cascade, resulting in simultaneous hemorrhage and thrombosis (Finley, 1992). Treatment for the underlying cause of DIC, such as antibiotics to treat the infection, chemotherapy to treat the malignancy, and replacement of coagulation factors and platelets, is essential. Treating DIC requires the infusion of platelets, cryoprecipitate, which provides fibrinogen and factor VIII, and red blood cells (Finley, 1992).

NURSING MANAGEMENT

The nursing management of patients with CML has been described by Wujcik, Viele, Maquire-Eisen, and Edmonds (Maquire-Eisen & Edmonds, 1992; Viele, 1996; Wujcik, 1997). Nursing care of the patient with CML begins at the time of assessment and diagnosis. Nursing management includes an assessment of possible risk factors, a physical examination, preparation and evaluation of laboratory testing, treatment options including entry into clinical trials, and emotional support for the patient and family caregiver. The patient and family can be further assisted in learning about the disease and treatment through cancer organizations such as the National Cancer Institute, the Leukemia Society of America (LSA), and bone marrow transplantation support groups. A growing number of cancer centers have educational programs with patient access to the World Wide Web.

After treatment begins, care is centered around supporting the patient through the adverse effects of treatment, such as infection, bleeding, fatigue, nausea and vomiting, and diarrhea. Self-care measures to decrease the incidence and severity of symptoms are particularly important because a large portion of care is administered in the outpatient or home care setting (Table 57-7).

As treatment for CML patients with BMT increases, comprehensive preparation is needed for candidates of this procedure. BMT is discussed in depth in Chapter 8 of this text. Table 57-7 illustrates the components of a preparation program for a patient with BMT.

HOME CARE ISSUES

Nursing concerns in the home care environment depend on specific treatment the patient has undergone. Patients require knowledge about all medications and their side effects, assistance with venous catheter devices, knowledge of reportable symptoms associated with their therapy or relapse, access to care, and disposal of hazardous wastes. BMT recipients may be required to remain near the transplant center in temporary housing for weeks after treatment and require administration of blood component therapy, IV antimicrobials, and daily assessments by specially trained nursing staff members. Patients receiving IFN-α therapy can have fevers as a normal side effect; this is not a cause for concern. Emotional support can be provided by most medical centers, such as the LSA, Cancer Lifeline, and American Cancer Society.

Fatigue for the patient and family can be overwhelming, especially if the patient is not forewarned of the debilitating symptoms. Patients receiving IFN-α, an agent known to cause significant fatigue, may need daily encouragement to

TABLE 57-7 Standard of Care for the Patient Undergoing a Bone Marrow Transplantation for Chronic Mylogenous Leukemia

Patient Problems and Outcomes	Nursing Interventions	Patient Education Instructions
Anxiety Patient will: • Verbalize an understanding of the transplant procedure. • Express feelings of decreased anxiety. • Identify strategies to cope with anxiety.	1. Assess the patient's level of understanding for the transplant process. 2. Give the patient the opportunity to ask questions or verbalize concerns. 3. Determine which coping strategies the patient has used effectively in the past to decrease anxiety, and reinforce the use of these skills. 4. Administer pharmacologic agents to decrease anxiety, if necessary.	1. Use a diagram of the human body to define where the bone marrow exists and how the hematologic system functions in the body. 2. Provide the patient with a description of the pretransplant care: a. Describe how the hematophoetic system functions. b. Describe how chemotherapy and radiation prepare the body for the new cell growth.
Potential for Infection Patient will: • Understand infection and methods to prevent infection.	1. Assess vital signs q4 hours reporting fevers >100.4° F (38°C) or decreasing blood pressure. 2. Administer prophylactic antibiotic and antiviral medications as ordered: a. Nystatin by mouth to prevent fungal overgrowth b. Administer TMX for prevention of *Pneumocystis carinii* pneumonia. c. Administer acyclovir for prevention of herpetic reactivation. d. Administer ganciclovir for prevention of cytomegalovirus (CMV). e. Administer growth factors GMCSF or GCSF to prevent infection. 3. Perform routine surveillance cultures for bacteria, fungi, and viruses. 4. Transfuse CMV-negative blood products to patients who have negative CMV titers.	1. Teach the patient the role of white blood cells in the human body. 2. Teach the patient how to do mouth care using saline rinses and toothettes. 3. Teach the patient and family to avoid contact with small children and people who are ill.
Altered Mucous Membranes Patient will: • Verbalize an understanding of the reason mucositis occurs.	1. Assess oral mucosal membranes for erythema and integrity twice a day. 2. Assess the patient with normal saline rinses. 3. Assess the patient's level of discomfort. 4. Administer analgesics as necessary for pain.	1. Teach the patient the rationale for cells breaking down quickly in the mouth. 2. Teach the patient how to do normal saline rinses and use toothettes. 3. Avoid food or fluids that are irritating to the mucous membranes.
Potential Bleeding Patient will: • Understand the potential for bleeding in the posttransplant setting and the need for platelet and/or red blood cell transfusions.	1. Assess the complete blood cell and platelet counts daily. 2. Assess the patient daily for bleeding. 3. Administer platelets and red blood cells as necessary.	1. Teach the patient to avoid any potential risk of injury (i.e., avoid razors when platelet count is low and use toothettes not a hard tooth brush).

ATG, Antithymocyte globulin; *CMV,* cytomegalovirus; *GCSF,* granulocytic colony-stimulating factor; *GMCSF,* granulocyte-macrophage colony-stimulating factor; *GVHD,* graft vs host disease; *MTX,* methotrexate; *TMX,* trimethoprim.

Continued

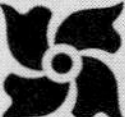

Table 57-7 Standard of Care for the Patient Undergoing a Bone Marrow Transplantation for Chronic Mylogenous Leukemia—cont'd

Patient Problems and Outcomes	Nursing Interventions	Patient Education Instructions
Graft vs Host Disease Patient and family will: • Have knowledge of what GVHD means in the posttransplant setting.	1. Administer prophylactic medications for GVHD (i.e., cyclosporin, MTX, ATG, FK506). 2. Assess the skin daily for the presence of erythema, maculopapular rashes, dryness, and pruritus. 3. Follow liver function tests for rising bilirubin and transaminases. 4. Assess for gastrointestinal symptoms such as nausea and vomiting, cramping, and green spinach type of diarrhea, which is guiac positive. 5. Prepare the patient for any interventions to a diagnosis of gastrointestinal GVHD, such as endoscopy. 6. Administer treatment medication for GVHD per the physician's order.	1. Teach the patient and caregivers to report symptoms that might be important in the diagnosis of GVHD (i.e., pruritus, cramping, and nausea).
Nausea and Vomiting Patient will: • Understand the need to report symptoms of nausea and vomiting.	1. Assess the patient for nausea. 2. Administer antiemetics such as ondansetron or granisetron q4 hour prn in immediate postchemotherapy time. 3. Ensure accurate intake and output. 4. Take postural blood pressure checks.	1. Teach the patient that nausea and vomiting is a normal side effect from the chemotherapy and radiation.
Altered Body Image as a Result of Chemotherapy and Radiation Patient will: • Gain an understanding of the changes his or her body will go through during the transplant process.	1. When alopecia starts to occur, help the patient to be more comfortable by offering to shave the head or cut long hair. 2. Ensure frequent bedding changes. 3. Offer scarves, hats, or head coverings of some sort. 4. Keep the patient's skin clean, dry, and moisturized.	1. Teach the patient that hair will be lost in 7-14 days. 2. Hair loss can include all body hair. 3. Hair will grow back, although the color and texture may be different.

ATG, Antithymocyte globulin; *CMV,* cytomegalovirus; *GCSF,* granulocytic colony-stimulating factor; *GMCSF,* granulocyte-macrophage colony-stimulating factor; *GVHD,* graft vs host disease; *MTX,* methotrexate; *TMX,* trimethoprim.

continue administration of this drug. Nurses can teach the patient to minimize unnecessary rest, balance energy expenditures with engineer conservation, ensure periods of uninterrupted rest and quiet, minimize emotional drains, and maximize priorities (Winningham, 1997).

PROGNOSIS

In the past, survival for patients diagnosed with CML was approximately 3 years, and fewer than 20% were expected to be alive at 5 years after the diagnosis. CML is not curable with conventional chemotherapy, but the use of allogeneic BMT and IFN-α have changed the natural course of this disease. Survival after the development of an accelerated phase is usually less than 1 year and only a few months after blastic transformation, although patients with lymphoblastic transformation may live longer with appropriate treatment (Deisseroth et al., 1997). Today, secondary to early diagnosis, improved treatment options and better supportive care result in an increase in survival.

EVALUATION OF THE QUALITY OF CARE

Accreditation organizations, such as the Joint Commission on Accreditation of Healthcare Organizations, require that the quality of care provided to patients be evaluated. Because the care provided to patients with CML requires input from a multidisciplinary team, an evaluation of the quality of care should include aspects of care provided by various members of the team. Table 57-8 illustrates quality of care tools for patients being treated with IFN-α.

RESEARCH ISSUES

BMT is considered the cure for CML when an appropriate donor is available. However, relapse occurs in 10% to 30% of those patients. Treatment failure forces a discussion of alternative treatments. Several options are available, but the risk vs benefit ratio requires careful consideration. A second BMT is an option. However, this therapy is not recommended within the first year after initial BMT because the mortality rate exceeds 50% as a result of toxicities of conditioning regimens. Donor lymphocyte infusion (DLI), or buffy coat infusion, appears promising. However, a 10% to 20% mortality rate is associated with this treatment. DLI produces a complete remission only when a GVHD response occurs, which can often require long-term immunosuppression. There is also a possibility that DLI can cause aplasia, thus requiring a second transplant (Ranjeny & Lipsky, 1996).

IFN-α is also being studied in this group that relapses after BMT. The response rate is good, particularly in groups that have minimal residual disease. For example, for patients who have a full clinical relapse, the complete response rate is 33%. For patients who have only a cytogenetic relapse, the response rate is much improved at 80% (Higano, Chielens, Raskind, Bryant, Flowers, & Radich et al., 1997).

Currently, an investigation looking at a predictor of relapse and thus a treatment to prevent that relapse is being conducted. Radich documented that if the bcr-abl transcript detected by the polymerase chain reaction (PCR) is positive at 6 to 12 months after BMT, a 40% to 60% chance of relapse exists. Treating this population with interferon for 1 year to determine the relapse rate decrease is the subject of ongoing clinical trials. More studies are needed to evaluate the treatment and prevention of relapse in CML. Nursing research aimed at identifying meaningful quality of life issues during all stages of the patient's treatment and subsequent outcomes is essential to the care of the patient and family.

TABLE 57-8 Quality of Care Management for Chronic Myelogenous Leukemic Patients Receiving IFN-α

Disciplines participating in the quality of care evaluation:
☐ Nursing ☐ Medical ☐ Dietary

Criteria	Yes	No
1. Were you taught the adverse effects of interferon-alpha?		
a. Flulike symptoms (fever, chills, or headache)	☐	☐
b. Fatigue	☐	☐
c. Gastrointestinal effects	☐	☐
2. Were you taught that fever may be a sign of infection or from interferon-alpha?	☐	☐
3. Were you given tips to manage flulike symptoms, such as bedtime administration so that you could sleep during the time of most symptoms?	☐	☐
4. Were you told that acetaminophen may prevent or partially alleviate fever and headache?	☐	☐
5. Were you told that fatigue is a major problem after interferon-alpha administration?	☐	☐
6. Were you given strategies to manage fatigue, such as energy conservation tips?	☐	☐
7. Did a nurse of physician explain that interferon alpha may cause diarrhea, anorexia, nausea, abdominal pain, or vomiting?	☐	☐
8. Did a nurse or dietitian tell you that drinking fluids, drinking high-calorie or high-protein drinks, eating soft foods, or eating small, frequent meals or snacks may help minimize the gastrointestinal side effects?	☐	☐
9. Did a health care person talk to you about alternative ways to manage the gastrointestinal side effects, such as relaxation techniques or music therapy?	☐	☐
10. Sometimes interferon-alpha causes depression, impaired concentration or forgetfulness. Did your nurse or physician make you aware of this problem?	☐	☐

REFERENCES

Appelbaum, F. R., Clift, R., Radich, J., Anasetti, C., & Buckner, C. D. (1995). Bone marrow transplantation for chronic myelogenous leukemia. *Seminars in Oncology, 22,* 405-411.

Appelbaum, F. R. (1996). The use of bone marrow and peripheral blood stem cell transplantation in the treatment of cancer. *CA: A Cancer Journal for Clinicians, 46*(3), 142-164.

Clark, J. C. & McGee, R. F. (1992) (Eds.), *Core curriculum for oncology nursing* (2nd ed.). Philadelphia: W. B. Saunders.

Cortes, G. E., Talpaz, M., & Kantarjian, H. (1996). Chronic myelogenous leukemia: A review: *The American Journal of Medicine, 100,* 555-568.

Deisseroth, A. B., Kantarjian, H., Andreeff, M., Talpaz, M., Keating, M. J., Khouri, I., & Champlin, R. B. (1997). Chronic leukemias. In V. T. DeVita, S. Hellman, & S. A. Rosenberg (Eds.), *Cancer: Principles and procedures of oncology* (5th ed.). Philadelphia: Lippincott-Raven.

Foon, K. A. & Casciato, D. A. (1995). Chronic leukemias. In D. A. Casciato & B. Lowitz (Eds.), *Manual of clinical oncology* (3rd ed.). Boston: Little, Brown.

Giralt, S., Kantarjian, H., & Talpaz, M., (1995). Treatment of chronic myelogenous leukemia. *Seminars in Oncology, 22,* 396-404.

Hehlmann, R., Heimpel, H., Hasford, J., Kolb, H. J., Pralle, H., Hossfeld, D. K., Queisser, W., Loffler, H., Hoehhaus, A., & Heinze, B. (1994). Randomized comparison of interferon-alpha with busulfan and hydroxurea in chronic myelogenous leukemia. The German CML Study Group. *Blood, 84*(12):4064-4077.

Higano, C. S., Chielens, D., Raskind, W., Bryant, E., Flowers, E. D., Radich, J., Clift, R., & Appelbaum, F. (1997). Use of alfa-2a-interferon to treat cytogenetic relapse of chronic myelogenous leukemia after marrow transplantation. *Blood. 90*(7):2549-2554.

Kantarjian, H. M., Smith, T. L., O'Brien, S., Beran, M., Pierce, S., & Talpaz, M. (1995). Prolonged survival in chronic myelogenous leukemia after cytogenetic response to IFN-α therapy. *Annals of Internal Medicine, 122*(4): 254-261.

Kantarjian, H. P., Deisseroth, A., Kurzrock, R., Estrov, Z., & Talpaz, M. (1993). Chronic myelogenous leukemia: A concise update. *Blood 82,* 691-703.

Maquire-Eisen, M. & Edmonds, K. (1992). Leukemias. In J. C. Clark & R. F. McGee (Eds.), *Core curriculum for oncology nursing* (2nd ed.). Philadelphia: W. B. Saunders.

Mitelman, F. (1994). Chromosomes, genes and cancer. *CA-A Cancer Journal for Clinicians, 44,* 133-135.

Mitus, A. J. & Rosenthal, D. S. (1955). The adult leukemias. In G. P. Murphy, W. Lawrence, & R. E. Lenhard (Eds.), *American Cancer Society textbook of clinical oncology* (2nd ed.). Atlanta: American Cancer Society.

Palackdharry, C. S. (1995). Chronic leukemias. In R. T. Skee & N. A. Lachart (Eds.), *Handbook of cancer chemotherapy* (4th ed.). Boston: Little, Brown.

Ranjeny, T. & Lipsky, P. (1996). Dendritic cells: Origin and differentiation. *Stem Cells, 14,* 196-206.

Rapaport, S. I. (1987). *Introduction to hematology.* Philadelphia: J. B. Lippincott.

Rundles, R. W. (1982). *Hematology.* New York: McGraw-Hill.

Sullivan, K. M., Appelbaum, F. R, & Thomas, E. D. (1995). Polymerase chain reaction detection of the BCR-ABL fusion transcript after allogeneic marrow transplantation for chronic myelogenous leukemia: Results and implications in 346 patients. *Blood, 85,* 2632-2638.

Viele, C. (1996). Chronic myelogenous leukemia and acute promyelocytic leukemia: new bone marrow transplantation options. *Oncology Nursing Forum, 23*(3), 488-492.

Winningham, M. L. (1997). New concepts in the nursing care of fatigue. In T. R. Rieger (Ed.), *Fighting fatigue.* Beechwood, Ohio: Pro ED Communications.

Wujcik, D. (1997). Leukemia. In S. W. Gronewald, M. H. Frogge, M. Goodman, & C. H. Yarbro (Eds.), *Cancer nursing: Principles and practice* (4th ed.). Boston: Jones and Bartlett.

Chronic Lymphocytic Leukemia

Carolyn K. Pittinger, RN, MS, AOCN

INTRODUCTION

Chronic lymphocytic leukemia (CLL) is a malignant hematologic disorder characterized by an accumulation of relatively normal-appearing lymphocytes that are immunologically incompetent. The majority of cases (95%) are neoplasms of B lymphocytes, whereas the remaining 5% are T-lymphocyte lymphoproliferative disorders (Rossman & Montserrat, 1995). CLLs include numerous types of mature clonal proliferations, including B-lymphocyte CLL, T-lymphocyte CLL, hairy cell leukemia, prolymphocytic leukemia, small cleaved cell leukemia, Sezary syndrome, and large granular lymphocytic leukemia (Foon & Casciato, 1995).

The course of the disease varies; some patients have a normal life expectancy, but others may die within 5 years of diagnosis. Patients with CLL have a two-fold incidence of visceral cancers and eight-fold increase of skin carcinoma compared with the normal population. Until recently, there has been little enthusiasm for finding a cure for this often indolent disease. Important advances are being made now to understand the biology, natural history, and treatment of CLL (Foon & Cascatio, 1995). The purpose of this chapter is to discuss CLL B-lymphocyte leukemia because this type of CLL is the most common chronic leukemia malignancy, accounting for 30% of adult leukemias (Palackdharry, 1995). Other chronic leukemias are discussed in Part II of this text.

EPIDEMIOLOGY

CLL is the most common adult chronic leukemia documented in western Europe and North America and now represents 25% of all leukemias. With an annual incidence of 2.9 persons in 100,000 diagnosed per year, CLL constitutes about 0.9% of all cancers (Mitus & Rosenthall, 1995) The apparent increasing incidence of CLL over the past 50 years is probably related to improved diagnostic criteria such as surface marker and cytogenic analyses (Deisseroth et al., 1997).

RISK FACTORS

The etiologic factors of CLL remains unknown. However, there are certain causative factors being considered. (Foon & Casciato, 1995).

Age and Gender

Age plays an important role as a risk factor associated with CLL and is seen more commonly in men, with a ratio of 2.5:1. The median age at time of diagnosis is 64 years, after which the incidence continues to increase. Only 10% of patients are diagnosed before the age of 50. Since the majority of patients diagnosed are elderly, 30% die of the disease. Survival is closely correlated with the state of disease at time of diagnosis (Foon & Casciato, 1995).

Ethnic Differences

The incidence of CLL varies widely in different regions of the world, ranging from 2.5% of all leukemias in Japan and other eastern countries and Africa, to 38% in Denmark (Faguet, 1994).

Family History. Familial clusters of CLL have been noted. The incidence in first-degree relatives of leukemic patients is two- to three-fold greater than the normal population (Foon & Casciato, 1995).

Occupational Hazards. There is a suggested risk of CLL reported in populations with agricultural, asbestos, and other occupational exposures (Faguet, 1994). However, populations exposed to radiation do not have an increased exposure to the incidences of CL (Foon & Casciato, 1995), nor is there evidence for a retroviral cause of the disease (Deisseroth et al., 1997).

Heredity

There are data to support a genetic basis, but no causative genes have been yet identified (Flynn & Grever, 1996). Cytogenetic and gene rearrangement studies have demon-

Box 58-1
Risk Factors for Chronic Lymphocytic Leukemia

- Increasing age (most common >50 yrs)
- Ethnicity (Caucasian >Asians)
- Positive family history for leukemias (1st degree relatives)
- Occupational exposures to asbestos (?association)
- Inherited, acquired immunodeficient syndromes and lymphoproliferative neoplasms

From Deisseroth, A. B., Kantarjian, H., Andreeff, M., Talpaz, M., Keating, M. J., Khouri, I., & Champlin, R. B. (1997). Chronic leukemias. In V. T. DeVita, S. Hellman, and S. A. Rosenberg (Eds.), *Cancer: Principles and procedures of oncology* (5th ed.). Philadelphia: Lippincott-Raven.

strated abnormalities in patients with CLL. Trisomy 12 is the most frequent cytogenetic abnormality, followed by abnormalities of chromosomes 13 and 14 (Juliusson, Oscier, Fitchett, Ross, Stockdill, Mackie, & Parker et al., 1990). Immunologic factors associated with CLL include hereditary diseases, acquired immunodeficiency syndrome (AIDS), and other lymphoproliferative neoplasms. A strong correlation has been noted between CLL and autoimmune diseases such as systemic lupus erythematosus and Sjogren's syndrome. Since CLL is an acquired disease and there are no established risk factors, one must be aware of the familial history, genetic disposition, and occupation exposure of patients presenting with symptoms of CLL. See Box 58-1 for risk factors for CLL.

ANATOMY AND PHYSIOLOGY

To fully understand the pathophysiology of CLL, normal hematopoiesis should be examined. Normal production of blood cell lines can be traced through a study of hematopoiesis (see Fig. 56-1, p. 1225). In normal bone marrow, there are regulatory mechanisms that ensure hematopoietic cell proliferation, differentiation, and maturation. Chapter 9 offers a complete discussion of hematopoiesis. Hematopoietic cells are initiated by the pluripotent stem cell, the smallest and most immature cell responsible for differentiating into the myeloid or lymphoid cell lines. The myeloid and lymphoid cell lines further differentiate and mature. The myeloid line produces either erythrocytes, granulocytes, monocytes, or megakaryocytes. The lymphoid line produces B or T lymphocytes. As cells mature, they migrate into the bloodstream at a rate matching the death of old cells. With the exception of T lymphocytes, hematopoietic cells are not released from the bone marrow until they are fully matured. T lymphocytes leave bone marrow at a relatively immature stage and mature in the thymus gland before entering the peripheral circulation.

PATHOPHYSIOLOGY

CLL is a clonal disorder. The cells of disease origin are small, mature-appearing lymphocytes that have reached the final stage of development but are nonfunctional. Fig. 58-1 depicts a hematologic growth chart highlighting the origin of CLL. Disease progress in CLL is less rapid than in the acute leukemias because the affected cells are more mature than lymphoblasts. Consequently, their proliferation and accumulation in the bone marrow, blood, lymph nodes, and spleen occur more slowly. Abnormal or excessive reproduction of any cell type disrupts the delicate balance. The nurse must be aware of the familial history, genetic disposition, and occupational exposure (Foon & Casciato, 1995)

In patients with CLL, normal hematopoietic regulatory mechanisms are absent or abnormal, resulting in (1) arrest of cells in early phases of maturation that cause an accumulation of immature cells; (2) abnormal proliferation of these immature cells; (3) crowding of other marrow elements, which results in inhibited growth or function; and eventually (4) replacing bone marrow with leukemic cells (Foon & Casciato, 1995; Wheeler, 1997).

ROUTES OF METASTASES

As the disease progresses, abnormal lymphocytes accumulate in the bone marrow, lymph nodes, and other organs such as the liver and spleen. In 95% of cases seen, there is clonal expansion of neoplastic B lymphocytes (Rai & Han, 1990). The degree of symptoms a patient exhibits on diagnosis is representative of the spread of the disease and the prognosis. The progression of disease begins with symptomatic lymphadenopathy, splenomegaly, and hepatomegaly (Fig. 58-2). The white blood cell count increases and anemia and thrombocytopenia become apparent as the bone marrow becomes infiltrated (Rossman & Montserrat, 1995). Progressive disease is accompanied by deterioration of both humoral and cell-mediated immunity. As the disease progresses, patients develop progressive pancytopenia, persistent fevers, and infection. Herpes zoster is the cause of 10% of infection in CLL patients, whereas bacterial pathogens associated with hypogammaglobulinemia represent the majority of infections. *Pneumocystis carinii* may be the causative infectious agent in patients with pulmonary infiltrates. During the latter stages of disease, cytotoxic chemotherapy is generally effective, so dosages are restricted because of pancytopenia. Death is usually caused by infection, bleeding, or other complications of the disease (Foon & Casciato, 1995).

ASSESSMENT

Twenty-five percent of patients with early stage CLL are usually asymptomatic and may be serendipitously diagnosed on routine physician examinations and blood tests. Others present with complaints of flu-like symptoms that include fatigue, night sweats, weight loss, frequent bacterial and viral infections, and bleeding tendencies. Lymphadenopathy is found in almost 80% of patients and frequently prompts the diagnostic investigation (Faguet, 1994). Patients with more advanced stages of the disease may experience weight loss, frequent infections as a result of neutropenia, bleeding episodes resulting from thrombocytopenia, and shortness of breath from anemia. Symp-

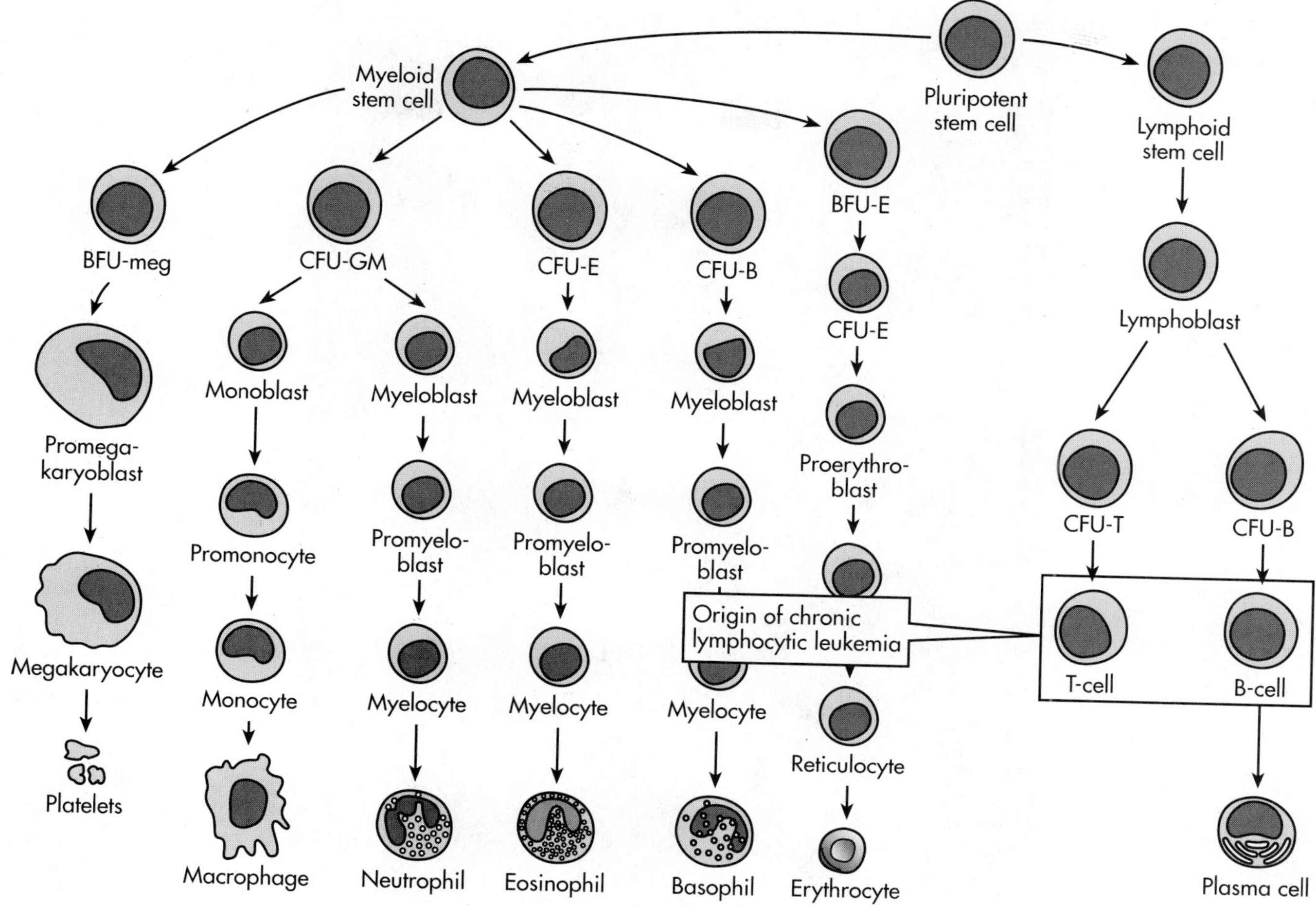

Fig. 58-1 Growth chart highlighting origin of chronic lymphocytic leukemia. (Courtesy Orthobiotech, Raritan, New Jersey.)

toms of malaise, fatigue, and anorexia are noted due to the bone marrow infiltration. Splenomegaly, accompanied by symptoms of abdominal discomfort and early satiety are caused by the spleen's infringement on the gastrointestinal tract. Edema or thrombophlebitis may result from obstruction of lymphatic or venous channels by enlarged lymph nodes (Foon & Casciato, 1995). The cervical, axillary, inguinal, and femoral nodes are palpable and described as mobile, nontender, and discrete. (Rai & Han, 1990). Table 58-1 lists assessment guidelines for patients who may have CLL.

Diagnostic tests include a complete blood count (CBC) with differential, liver function tests (LFTs), Coombs' (antiglobulin) tests, serum proteins assessment, bone marrow aspiration, and biopsy. The demonstration of B lymphocyte monoclonality with an absolute lymphocyte count of more than 5000/mm^3 sustained for at least a month may be sufficient for a diagnosis of early-stage CLL. Hemoglobin levels and platelet counts are below normal (Palackdharry, 1995). Immunological assays can determine whether the leukemic cells are derived from B or T lymphocytes. Flow cytometry analysis of peripheral blood demonstrates clonal B lymphocytes that differ from normal B lymphocytes in their characteristic expression of the T-lymphocyte antigen CD5. Furthermore, these analyses can distinguish CLL from other B-lymphocyte leukemias such as hairy cell leukemia. Finally, immunologic testing can determine whether patients are at an increased risk for infections. The diagnosis of CLL also includes staging the disease, which is important to determine the appropriate treatment and prognosis. Bone marrow aspirates reflect patchy or focal infiltrates of lymphocytes. Progressive disease is marked by the appearance of a "packed marrow" with few normal hematopoietic cells and the presence of more than 30% lymphocytes in the marrow. A lymphocyte count greater than 10,000/mm^3 indicates CLL (Fig. 58-3).

The clinical course and prognosis of B-lymphocyte CLL is variable and depends on the disease stage at diagnosis. Patients with early-stage CLL are known to live 10 or more years without treatment, whereas those with more aggressive, advanced disease usually succumb within 2 years (Foon & Casciato, 1995).

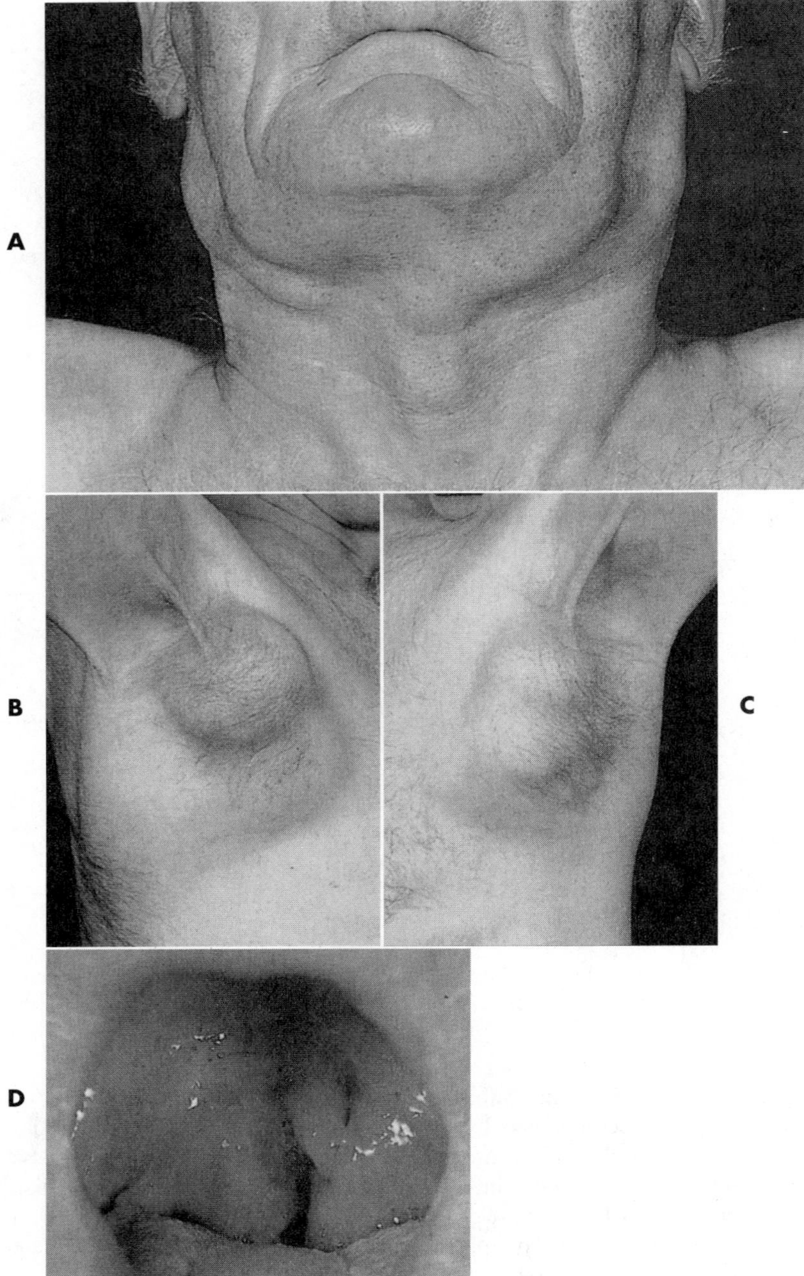

Fig. 58-2 Lymphadenopathy. This 65-year-old man with CLL presented with bilateral **A,** cervical; **B** and **C,** axillary lymphadenopathy; and **D,** massive enlargement of the pharyngeal tonsils.

STAGING

The staging of CLL involves the use of one of the two most widely used staging systems—the Binet and modified Rai approaches. The link between tumor burden and survival lead to these disease staging systems that form the basis for therapy (Faguet, 1994). The modified Rai staging system places patients into low-, intermediate-, and high-risk categories based on their clinical presentation. These categories, which correspond to Rai's initial stage 0, I plus II, and III plus IV, respectively, represent 30%, 60%, and 10% of newly diagnosed patients. Associated with these percentages are 10-, 6-, and 2-year survival rates (Rai, & Han, 1990) (Table 58-2).

The Binet staging system is based on areas of lymph node involvement and the presence of thrombocytopenia and/or anemia. Patients with three or more of the five areas of potential infiltration (e.g., cervical, axillary, or inguinal nodes; spleen; or liver) are classified as stage A or B, respectively. Those patients with thrombocytopenia or anemia are stage C. Binet's stages A, B, and C account for 60%,

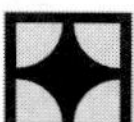

TABLE 58-1 Assessment of the Patient with Chronic Lymphocytic Leukemia

	Assessment Parameters	Typical Abnormal Findings
History	A. Personal and social history 1. Age 2. Ethnicity 3. Family history	A. Personal and social history 1. Usually over age 50 2. More prevalent in Caucasians than Asians 3. Frequently seen when first-degree relatives have history of leukemias or autoimmune diseases
	B. Evaluation of infections	B. Common symptoms include: Flu-like syndrome, frequent bacterial or viral infections, fevers, fatigue
	C. Evaluation of bleeding	C. Extended period of bleeding, oozing, and frequent ecchymoses
Physical Examination	A. Weight	A. Continued weight loss
	B. Lymph node evaluation	B. Enlarged lymph nodes, described as palpable, discrete, mobile, and nontender
	C. Palpation of abdomen/pelvis	C. Splenomegaly and hepatomegaly seen in advanced disease
Diagnostic Tests	A. Complete blood count with differential	A. Increased white blood cell count (>100,000 mm^3); anemia associated with low hematocrit, decreased platelet count, and an abnormal differential
	B. Bone marrow aspirate and biopsy	B. Packed marrow with few normal mature cells

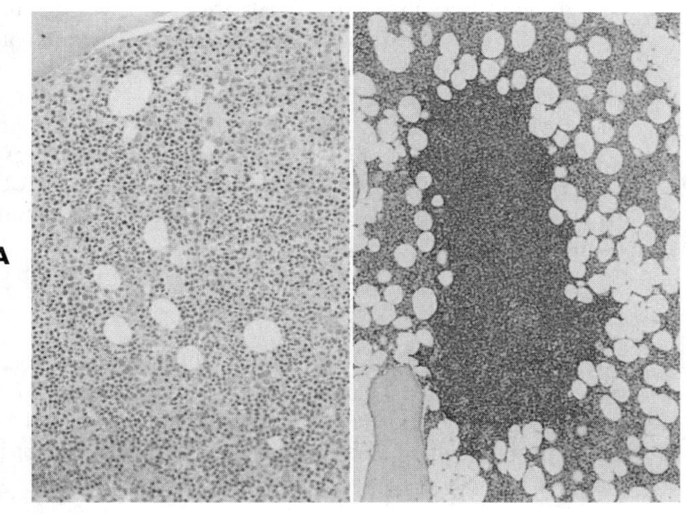

Fig. 58-3 Bone marrow. Biopsy specimens of CLL in **A,** early and **B,** late stages (hematoxylin and eosin, × 75). **A,** Interstitial infiltration by lymphocytes, sparing other hematopoietic precursors and fat cells. **B,** Diffuse replacement of all marrow components by the neoplastic lymphocytes.

TABLE 58-2 The Modified RAI Staging System for CLL

RAI Stage	Three-stage System	Clinical Features	Medial Survival (Years)
0	Low-risk	Lymphocytosis only in blood and marrow	>10
I	Intermediate-risk	Lymphocytosis + lymphadenopathy +	
II		splenomegaly ± hepatomegaly	7
III	High-risk	Lymphocytosis + anemia	1.5
IV		+ thrombocytopenia	

From Foon, K. & Casciato, D. A. (1995). Chronic leukemias. In D. A. Casciato & B. B. Lowitz (Eds.), *Manual of clinical oncology.* Boston: Little, Brown.

TABLE 58-3 The Binet Staging System

Stage	Clinical Features	Medial Survival (Years)
A	Fewer than three areas of clinical lymphadenopathy; no anemia or thrombocytopenia	>10
B	Three or more involved node areas; no anemia or thrombocytopenia	7
C	Hemoglobin ≤10 g/dl and/or platelets <100,000/μl	2

From Foon, K. & Casciato, D. A. (1995). Chronic leukemias. In D. A. Casciato & B. B. Lowitz (Eds.), *Manual of clinical oncology*. Boston: Little, Brown.

30%, and 10 % of newly diagnosed cases but show comparable median survival rates of 9, 5, and 2 years, respectively (Faguet, 1994) (Table 58-3).

MEDICAL MANAGMENT

Although disease staging can indicate tumor bulk, the dynamics and clinical course of CLL varies among individual patients. Observation or watchful waiting is recommended for asymptomatic patients. Clinical trials have shown "early-stage" treatment to be of little to no benefit in relation to survival and deemed harmful (Shustik, Mick, Silver, Sawitsky, Rai, & Shapiro, 1988). Treatment usually begins once patients demonstrate progressive cytopenias and organomegaly. The standard treatment for patients with CLL has been chlorambucil (CHL), which is available in tablet form and is rapidly and almost completely absorbed from the gastrointestinal tract, with peak plasma concentration occurring within 1 hour.

The alkylating agent cyclophosphamide (CYA) is often administered as first-line therapy for patients with CLL. However, it has had minimal evaluation as a single agent and is often combined with vincristine and prednisone in the cyclophosphamide/vincristine/prednisone (CVP) regimen if CHL fails. CHL is administered in mg per kg or 3 mg/m^2 orally daily and CYA administered at a dose of 2 to 3 mg/kg orally daily. Corticosteroids such as prednisone added to these agents appear to be effective in reducing symptoms related to lymphadenopathy and splenomegaly (Faguet, 1994). Most patients respond to therapy, including at least one half of patients with high-risk disease. Combination chemotherapy regimens such as CHOP (CYA, doxorubicin, vincristine, and prednisone), CAP (cyclophosphamide, doxorubicin, and prednisone), DHAP (dexamethasone, high-dose cytarabine, and asparaginase) and the M2 protocol (melphalan, CYA, carmustine, and prednisone) are used for higher-stage patients (Faguet, 1994; Rossman & Montserrat, 1995). None of these regimens showed improved survival statistics compared with CHL alone (Faguet, 1994).

Newer agents that include the purine analogues, fludarabine (Flurdara), cladribine (2-chlorodeosyadenosine [2-CDA), and 2'Deoxycoformycin (Pentostatin), are beginning to show significant activity in refractory and untreated patients with CLL. Fludarabine can produce response rates of 50% to 60% in patients who are treated for relapse or refractory disease (O'Brien, Kantarjian, Feldman, Beran, Robertson, Koller et al., 1995). Preliminary data suggests 2-CDA may halt disease progression for those patients who have failed on fludarabine therapy (Caguioa, Tansan, & McCaffery, 1994).

2-CDA is usually administered at 4 mg/m^2/day for 7 days as a continuous infusion (Rossman &, Monserrat, 1995). Pentostatin is administered intravenous push (IVP) and dosages vary according to clinical trial protocols (Burke, Wilkes, Berg, Bean, & Ingwersen, 1991). Virtually all CLL patients become resistant to the above therapies.

Biotherapy

The use of biotherapy is offering new treatment approaches for patients with CLL, but much research is needed in this area. Interleukin-2 appears ineffective, and responses to IFN-α remain disappointing. The response rates are usually partial and thus this area needs further investigation. (Deisseroth et al., 1997). There are a number of monoclonal antibodies (MoAbs) directed against CLL-associated antigens, including CD5, cCLLA, CD19, CD20, lym-1, lym-2 and CAMPATH binding protein. Encouraging results are now evident, but additional data from conjugated MoAb trials are needed to support the utility of these agents in CLL. Patients receiving these agents should be entered into clinical trials.

Radiation

The role of radiation for treatment of CLL is limited. Local radiation therapy for patients with CLL is recommended to reduce lymph node masses that threaten vital organs and respond poorly to chemotherapeutic agents. This treatment is palliative and short-lived (Foon & Casciato, 1995)

Surgery

Splenectomy is performed for patients with immune hemolytic anemia or thrombocytopenias who are or have become resistant to chronic corticosteroid therapy or immunosuppressive and cytotoxic therapies. Splenectomy may also be helpful in patients with problematic hypersplenism (Foon & Casciato, 1995)

Bone Marrow and Stem Cell Transplantation

More than 300 BMTs for patients with CLL have been performed to date (*Blood and Marrow Transplant Newsletter,* 1997). Michallet and colleagues (1996) reported the results of a retrospective study of human leukocyte antigen (HLA)–matched allogeneic recipients transplanted in 30

European and North American centers. Approximately one half of the patients achieved complete remission after BMT. The investigators concluded that BMT from HLA-identical siblings can result in hematologic remission and survival in persons with CLL but were uncertain how these results compare with those of conventional therapy. Several studies are under way to test the graft versus leukemic effect in patients who have failed conventional therapy for CLL and who are consequently transplanted in relapse. If the studies prove to be successful, it may be reasonable to treat early stage CLL patients with BMT with less toxic conditioning regimens, thereby circumventing the significant adverse of this therapy. Chapter 8 offers a complete description of the graft versus luekemic effect in BMT recipients. Few BMTs have been performed for autologous patients because of the major concern that CLL cells may be collected from the patient and reinfused during the transplant. Many centers are investigating ways to eliminate the malignant cells by purging techniques.

Hypogammaglobulinemia associated with this disease is the factor most responsible for infections (Faguet, 1994). Bacterial infections associated with hypogammaglobulinemia include *Streptococcus pneumoniae, Staphylococcus aureus,* and *Haemophilus influenzae.* Herpes zoster is the cause of 20% of infections, and *P. carinii* may be the causative infectious agent in patients with pulmonary infiltrates. Prevention and treatment of septic episodes is key in preventing significant morbidity and mortality in neutropenic patients. Prophetic antibiotics, recombinant colony-stimulating factors and intravenous immunoglobulin (IVIG) have been administered to this patient population to decrease risk of serious bacterial infections, The use of IVIG, however, remains controversial. Vaccinations against pneumonococcus, *H. influenzae,* and meningococcus are advised. Live vaccines are to be avoided because they can cause severe localized necrotizing vasculitis or a potentially fatal system illness (Mitus & Rosenthal, 1995).

ONCOLOGIC EMERGENCIES

The two most common life-threatening complications in patients with CLL are septic shock and hemorrhage. Each problem results from progressive pancytopenia. Chapter 11 contains a complete discussion of the dynamics of each of these complications. Typically, when patients reach this point in their disease progress, chemotherapy is ineffective and doses are restricted because of persistent pancytopenia. Death is usually imminent.

NURSING MANAGEMENT

Patients with CLL have multiple problems that require comprehensive nursing assessment and intervention skills, as well as patient and family caregiver education (Tables 58-4 and 58-5). The majority of care for these patients is delivered in outpatient settings beginning at time of diagnosis and often this trend continues throughout treatment. As discussed earlier, patients with CLL present with "flu-like" symptoms, and patients are usually not prepared for the possible fatal diagnosis of a malignant disease. Explanations of the natural history of the disease, treatment options, possible entry into clinical trials, and requisite lifestyle adjustments need to be assimilated by the patient and the caregiver. Patients with early-stage indolent disease who may not require immediate treatment often require considerable psychological support during the "watch and wait" period.

Once treatment begins the nursing care of patients receiving chemotherapy, radiation, and surgical procedures for their disease is aimed at initial patient assessments, pharmacologic knowledge of chemotherapies and their adverse reactions, and prevention and management of adverse effects of their disease and treatments. Patients are taught the signs and symptoms of infection and given specific instructions relative to their institution for management in the home environment. Patients taking corticosteroids are at particular risk for sudden onset of septic shock and often do not manifest the classic symptoms such as shaking chills that herald imminent sepsis. Knowledge of the hallmarks of bleeding episodes such as oozing from the nose or gums and low platelet counts are also imperative.

Nelson & Hogan (1995) have described in detail the nursing care for patients receiving cladribine. Management of this agent's adverse effects such as myelosuppression, particularly neutropenia, and fever is a principle nursing responsibility. Nadirs are usually manifested approximately 14 days after therapy is initiated, and white counts return to normal values within 1 to 2 months after therapy. Fever associated with neutropenia is often reported approximately 7 days after therapy. Infection as a cause of fever must be ruled out, especially in those patients who are neutropenic. Fever develops but is usually transient and easily treated with acetaminophen. Phlebitis, skin rashes, nausea, and fatigue have also been reported with this therapy. Anemia and thrombocytopenia are also experienced by patients receiving this therapy, and monitoring of hemoglobin, platelet levels, and body temperature are imperative (Wujcik, 1996).

Radiation therapy is used to treat lymphadenopathy and/or painful organomegaly. Problems associated with radiation therapy include skin irritation or breakdown and abdominal discomfort. Nursing management is targeted at methods to provide prevention and treatment techniques to assure and maintain skin integument (Frogge & Kalinowski, 1997).

Splenectomy is performed in CLL patients when the disease is refractory to systemic therapy. Nursing care is aimed at observation for signs and symptoms of postoperative bleeding and infection. Patient care includes frequent skilled physical assessments, and close monitoring of CBCs to monitor for pending infection or bleeding problems (Frogge & Kalinowski, 1997).

HOME CARE ISSUES

Today's health care environment often dictates that a large portion of patient care be given in outpatient and home care settings. Early recognition of symptoms can determine patient mortality throughout the disease process and its treatment. Assisting caregivers in creative ways to encourage op-

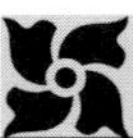

TABLE 58-4 Standard of Care for the Patient with CLL Receiving Chemotherapy

Patient Problems and Outcomes	Nursing Interventions and Rationales	Patient Education Instructions
Nausea/Vomiting Patient will: • Verbalize understanding of each drug given and it's potential for ematogenicity. • Have three or less episodes of nausea/vomiting during treatment. • Identify strategies to help decrease the potential for nausea/vomiting.	1. Assess the patient's level of understanding about chemotherapy. 2. Identify the patient's fears and preconceived ideas about chemotherapy. 3. Administer antiemetic drugs before and after treatment as needed to ensure maximal coverage. 4. Use relaxation therapy as necessary to prevent anxiety. 5. Continually reassess patient after therapy to maintain nausea-free status.	1. Use booklets and pamphlets (various learning and culturally oriented tools are available) for explaining chemotherapy 2. Provide specific drug information and side effects. 3. Alleviate fears and anxieties regarding chemotherapy. 4. Teach relaxation therapy, and provide other available resources (e.g., massage therapy, acupuncture).
Fatigue Patient will: • Verbalize an understanding that energy is decreased. • Identify strategies to cope with this symptom. • Maintain energy levels by having frequent rest periods and conserving energy.	1. Prioritize activities to allow for rest periods. 2. Pace activities in relationship to energy levels. 3. Monitor physical and mental status. 4. Teach use of assistive measures to conserve energy (i.e., take showers rather than baths). 5. Request assistance from family members or support persons.	1. Teach patients to delegate nonessential activities. 2. Provide ways to reduce environmental stimuli. 3. Encourage documentation (e.g., journal records) of patterns of fatigue to aid in planning professional and personal responsibilities.
Body Image Disturbance Patient will: • Verbalize expected body changes, alopecia, and weight gain. • Be allowed to ventilate grief/anger toward changes. • Use resources for feeling of helplessness or hopelessness.	1. Assess level of understanding toward body image changes. 2. Give permission to grieve. 3. Monitor for ineffective coping. 4. Initiate referrals as necessary.	1. Provide information of what body image changes are expected and how long they can last. 2. Provide a resource list to obtain support as needed. 3. Teach strategies to detect and manage self-destructive behavior.

timal environments and to decrease infection provides optimal nutritional intake and combats adverse effects of the disease. Treatment either maintains or improves the quality of life of these patients. Encouraging periods of rest and discussions about fatigue help decrease stress on family members. Depending on the treatment approach used for a CLL patient, the care needed at home will vary.

Patients who receive central lumen catheters require instructions in aseptic catheter management techniques, obtaining supplies, manipulating needles and syringes, and disposing of hazardous materials (Table 58-6). Education includes learning to take frequent temperatures and recognizing signs and symptoms of infection (Wujcik, 1996). Postoperative care after a splenectomy consists of monitoring the operative site for possible infection or bleeding (Frogge & Kalinowski, 1997). Fatigue, particularly among those patients requiring radiation therapy is a common and often unexpected complication for patients. Patients may not be able to work or perform their customary roles because of treatment schedules or discomfort associated with organomegaly. Role reversal may occur within the family structure. Alopecia and skin changes from chemotherapy can occur and these symptoms, although not permanent, can present body image concerns (University of California-San Francisco School of Nursing, 1996; Winningham, 1996).

Referrals to support groups to assist patients and families with medical transportation, cosmetic consultations, and psychological support groups within the local community can be helpful. Many composites of resources are now

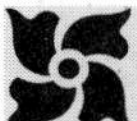

TABLE 58-5 Standard of Care for the Patient Undergoing Splenectomy

Patient Problem and Outcomes	Nursing Interventions and Rationales	Patient Education Instructions
Anxiety Patient will: • Verbalize an understanding of planned surgical procedure. • Demonstrate knowledge of preoperative routine. • Express feelings of decreased anxiety. • Identify strategies to cope with anxiety.	1. Assess level of understanding of splenectomy. 2. Provide time to discuss concerns/questions. 3. Discuss coping strategies and what has been helpful in the past. 4. Administer medications to decrease anxiety as necessary.	1. Discuss preoperative routine to include the following: a. Diagnostic tests b. Anesthesia consult c. NPO status 2. Explain surgical procedure with teaching diagram. 3. Teach postoperative breathing exercises; obtain return demonstration. 4. Provide patient with written information regarding the following: a. Postoperative pain b. Surgical incision c. Intravenous medication/hydration
Infection Patient will: • Remain infection free for postoperative period. • Verbalize signs and symptoms of infection.	1. Monitor vital signs for symptoms of infection (e.g., fever, chills). 2. Use aseptic technique for patient care and treatments. 3. Administer antibiotics prophylactically as ordered. 4. Institute measures to minimize exposure to exogenous/endogenous organisms.	1. Teach handwashing and personal hygiene to decrease potential of infection. 2. Demonstrate ability to use and read a thermometer accurately. 3. Teach sign and symptoms of infection and to report immediately. 4. Discuss relationship between cellular immunity, chronic disease, and infection. 5. Provide educational brochures to enhance teaching.

NPO, nothing by mouth.

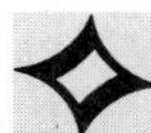

TABLE 58-6 Patient Preparation for Home Care of Central Venous Catheters

Purpose: To maintain functional catheter and prevent catheter contamination and infection from occurring while the catheter is in place.

Patient Preparation

1. Be aware of the catheter type (Groshong, peripherally inserted central catheter (PICC), Hickman, or Port-a-cath).
2. Gather equipment needed to do a dressing change.
   a. Betadine swabs
   b. Op-site/transparent dressing
   c. Alcohol swabs
   d. Gloves (nonsterile)
   e. 5 ml syringes for flushing as necessary
   f. Heparin flush 10 units/ml.
3. Clean area in examination room where dressing is to be changed.
4. Wash hands. Remove old dressing. Observe site for redness, swelling, or drainage.*
5. Cleanse site from center where the catheter is inserted to the outside area of skin with betadine in a circular pattern. Cleanse three times, using a new swab each time, and do not go back over the area you have cleansed with the same swab. Let Betadine dry.
6. Wipe Betadine area clean with the alcohol now, using the same instructions as above.
7. Apply transparent dressing, and secure tube with tape as necessary.

Procedural Considerations: Flush each catheter lumen with 5 ml of heparin, once a week if the catheter is not being used (Groshong catheters do not need heparin flushes.)

*If you suspect that there is something wrong with the catheter or if the area around the catheter is draining bloody or yellow fluid, report this to your doctor immediately. If your catheter does not flush, report this to your nurse immediately.

TABLE 58-7 Quality of Care Evaluation for Patient with Chronic Lymphocytic Leukemia Undergoing a Splenectomy

Disciplines participating in quality of care evaluation:
☐ Nursing ☐ Surgery

I. Postoperative Management Evaluation

Data from:
☐ Medical record ☐ Patient/family interview

Criteria	Yes	No
1. Patient provided with preoperative information about:		
a. Possible transfusion of blood products	☐	☐
b. NPO status	☐	☐
c. Postoperative site care needed for home	☐	☐
2. Patient instructed about follow-up physician visits and laboratory draws.	☐	☐
3. Patient experienced the following complications:		
a. Bleeding	☐	☐
b. Infection	☐	☐

NPO, Nothing by mouth.

TABLE 58-8 Quality of Care Evaluation for a Patient Receiving Chemotherapy

Disciplines participating in quality of care evaluation:
☐ Nursing ☐ Oncologist ☐ Pharmacist ☐ Social worker

Data from:
☐ Mailed questionaire ☐ Patient interview

Criteria	Yes	No
1. Information given/explained regarding chemotherapy		
A. Specific drug information	☐	☐
B. Side effects of each drug		
a. Alopecia	☐	☐
b. Fatigue	☐	☐
c. Nausea/vomiting	☐	☐
d. Neutropenia/infection	☐	☐
2. Resources available to you were discussed with social worker	☐	☐
3. Teaching done in regard to monitoring for infections postchemotherapy.	☐	☐

available through organizations such as the Leukemia Society of America and American Cancer Society (ACS), as well as through internet links (Leukemia Society of America, 1994a; 1994b). The ACS publishes materials related to specific cancer types and can provide educational avenues to assist in further learning for patients and their families. Bereavement groups for family members and friends are available in the event of the patient's death.

PROGNOSIS

The prognosis for patients with CLL is grim. There is no "cure," but improved survival due to early treatment and interventions for symptomatic patients is increasing (Flynn & Grever, 1996). New therapies and high remission rates from aggressive treatment warrant further studies. New cytotoxic agents, MoAb conjugates, IL-2 toxin fusion proteins, IFNs, and judicious use of BMT are bringing optimism to achieving longer periods of survival (Caguioa, Tansan, & McCaffrey, 1994).

EVALUATION OF THE QUALITY OF CARE

Much attention is focused on the quality of health care to assure that the patient achieves optimal care. Accreditation organizations such as the Joint Commission of American Hospital Organizations, as well as most universities and hospitals, require that the quality of care provided be evaluated. Tables 58-7 and 58-8 offer examples of quality of care evaluation tools that can be used for patients with CLL across care settings.

RESEARCH ISSUES

Numerous research studies are underway for patients with CLL. Randomized trials for patients with stages II, III, and IV disease are currently ongoing, using biologic modifiers and hematologic marrow and stem cell transplantation. For example, a National Cancer Institute-sponsored phase IB/II trial of humanized anti-Tac MoAb for CLL and other leukemias and lymphoma are being studied to assess the safety and tolerability of a multidose regimen of humanized anti-Tac (HAT) MoAb. The study objectives are to describe the pharmacokinetics and pharmacodynamics in a multidose schedule, evaluate the immunogenicity of HAT, and identify immunologic parameters that correlate with efficacy. Considerable research is needed in this area before wide application can be assured.

Considerable interest exists in stem cell transplantation for patients with CLL. Full acceptance of this treatment awaits further evaluation through documentation of long-term engraftment and improved outcomes compared with traditional chemotherpay and radiation.

REFERENCES

Burke, M. B., Wilkes, G. M., Berg, D., Bean, C., & Ingwersen, K. (Eds.). (1991). *Cancer chemotherapy: A nursing process approach.* Sudbury, MA: Jones and Bartlett.

Deisseroth, A. B., Kantarjian, H., Andreeff, M., Talpaz, M., Keating, M. J., Khouri, I., & Champlin, R. B. (1997). Chronic leukemias. In V. T. DeVita, S. Hellman, & S. A. Rosenberg (Eds.), *Cancer: Principles and procedures of oncology.* (pp. 2321-2343.) Philadelphia: Lippincott-Raven.

Faguet, G. (1994). Chronic lymphocytic leukemia: An updated review. *Journal of Clinical Oncology, 12*(9), 1974-1990.

Flynn, I. & Grever, M. (1996). Chronic lymphocytic leukemia. *Cancer Treatment Reviews, 22,* 1-13.

Foon, K. & Casciato, D. A. (1995). Chronic leukemias. In D. A. Casciato & B. B. Lowitz (Eds.), *Manual of clinical oncology.* (pp. 402-417) Boston: Little, Brown.

Frogge, M. H. & Kalinowski, B. H. (1997). Surgery therapy. In S. L. Groenwald, M. H. Frogge, M. Goodman, & C. H. Yarbro (Eds.), *Cancer nursing: Practices and principles.* (4th ed.). Sudbury, MA: Jones and Bartlett.

Juliusson, G., Oscier, D.G., Fitchett M., Ross, F. M., Stockdill, G., Mackie, M. J. Parker A. C., Castoldi, G. L. Guneo, A., & Knuutila, S. (1990). Prognosis subgroups in B-cell by specific chromosomal abnormalities. *New England Journal of Medicine, 323* (11), 720-740.

Leukemia Society of America. (1994a). *Chronic lymphocytic leukemia.* New York: Leukemia Society of America.

Leukemia Society of America. (1994b). *What everyone should know about leukemia.* New York: Leukemia Society of America.

Michallet, M., Archimbaud, E., Bandini. G., Rowlings, P. A., Deeg, H. J., Gahrton, G., Montserrat, E., Rozman C., Gratwohl, A., & Gale, P. R. (1996). HLA-identical transplantation in younger patients with chronic lymphocytic leukemia. European Group for Blood and Marrow Transplantation and the International Bone Marrow Transplant Registry. *Annals of Internal Medicine, 124,* 311-315.

Mitus, A. J. & Rosenthal, D. S. (1995), The adult leukemias. In G. P. Murphy, W. Lawrence, & R. E. Lenhard (Eds.), *American Cancer Society textbook of clinical oncology.* Atlanta: American Cancer Society.

National Cancer Institute (1997). Cancerlit.R Biblographic Database Search Results.

Nelson, M. & Hogan, D. (1995). The role of Cludarabine in the treatment of lymphoids. *Oncology Nursing Forum, 22*(9), 1395-1400.

O'Brien, S., Kantarjian H., Feldman E., Beran, M., Robertson, L. E., Koller, C., Lerner, S., & Keating, M. J. (1995). Interferon maintenance therapy for patients with chronic lymphocytic leukemia in remission after Fludarabine therapy. *Blood 86*(4), 1298-1300.

Palackdharry, C. S. (1995). Chronic leukemias. R. T. Skee & N. A. Lachart (Eds.), *Handbook of cancer chemotherapy* (4th ed.). Boston: Little, Brown.

Rai, K. R. & Han, T. (1990). Prognostic factors and clinical staging in chronic lymphocytic leukemia. *Hematology Oncology Clinics of North America, 4,* 447-456.

Rossman C, Montserrat, E. (1995). Chronic lymphocytic leukemia. *New England Journal of Medicine, 333,* 1052-1057.

Shustik, C., Mick, R., Silver, R., Sawitsky, A., Rai, K., & Shapiro, L. (1988). Treatment of early chronic lymphocytic leukemia: intermittent chlorambucil versus observation. *Hematology Oncology,* 6, 7-12.

(1997). Treating CLL with BMT. *Blood and Marrow Transplant Newsletter, 8*(2):1-5.

University of California-San Francisco School of Nursing (1996). *Managing the side effects of chemotherapy and radiation therapy.* San Francisco: University of California-San Francisco Press.

Wheeler, V. S. (1997). Biotherapy. In S. L. Groenwald, M. H. Frogge, M. Goodman, & C. H. Yarbro, (Eds.), *Cancer nursing: Practices and principles.* (4th ed.). Boston: Jones and Bartlett.

Winningham, M. L. (1996). Fatigue. In (Eds.) S. L. Groenwald, M. H. Frogge, M. Goodman, & C. H. Yarbro (Eds.), *Cancer symptom management.* Sudbury, MA: Jones and Bartlett.

Wujcik, D. S. (1996). Infection. S. L. Groenwald, M. H. Frogge, M. Goodman, & C. H. Yarbro (Eds), *Cancer symptom management.* Sudbury, MA: Jones and Bartlett.

Hairy Cell Leukemia

Denise K. Reinke, RN, BSN, OCN
Eva Gallagher, RN, MS, AOCN

EPIDEMIOLOGY

Hairy cell leukemia (HCL), also known as *leukemic reticuloendotheliosis* (Bouroncle, Wiseman, & Doan, 1958), is a chronic malignant lymphoproliferative disorder primarily of the B lymphocyte (Gollard, Lee, Piro, & Saven, 1995). When viewed under the microscope, the affected lymphocytes have unusual cytoplasmic projections, coined "hairy cells" by Shreck and Donnelly in 1966 (American Cancer Society [ACS], 1994). It is a rare disorder with approximately 500 to 600 new cases identified in the United States annually, accounting for 2% of all adult leukemias (ACS, 1994). No evidence of increasing incidence of HCL has been noted at this time; the number of new cases annually has remained stable (Staines & Cartwright, 1993).

HCL occurs four times more often in males than females, and the median age of onset is between the ages of 50 and 55 years (Mitus & Rosenthal, 1995). Although cases have been reported in patients 20 to 80 years of age (ACS, 1997), HCL has not been reported in children or teenagers (Kipps & Robbins, 1995).

Data were compiled from 208 cases of HCL diagnosed in Los Angeles County between 1972 and 1987 (Bernstein, Newton, & Ross, 1990). These data supported previous study results regarding incidence and male/female distribution of HCL. These conclusions regarding race, religion, and occupation have not been replicated.

Staines and Cartwright (1993) conducted a case-controlled study of 50 cases of HCL and 95 controls in the Yorkshire and Trent Regional Health Authority. Overall, Staines and colleagues (1993) concluded that, "Previous results on the ætiology of hairy cell leukæmia were not supported by this study, with the exception of an association between hairy cell leukaemia and exposure to organic solvents, petrochemicals and related products" (p. 714).

Epidemiologic data generally include a discussion of mortality rate, which is the number of deaths that occur in the population at risk in a specific period (Cartnel & Reid, 1997). Although no discussion of death rates was noted in the literature reviewed, Hess (1993) notes, that on the basis of the therapeutic success achieved to date with pentostatin, and the preliminary results with 2-chlorodeoxyadenosine, the prognosis for patients with HCL could approach that of age-matched controls.

RISK FACTORS

The etiologic factors of HCL remain unknown (Kipps & Robbins, 1995). Patients diagnosed with HCL have been retrospectively studied in an attempt to determine possible risk factors (Oleske, Golumb, Farber, & Levy, 1985). Although several potential factors have been identified, a high relative risk has not been determined (Box 59-1).

According to Hess (1993), familial predisposition is suggested by reports of the disorder in a father and son, a mother and daughter, a mother and son, two brothers, and three siblings, all with the same haplotype, A1, B7. Although the development of HCL is not associated with any single human leukocyte antigen (HLA) haplotype, affected family members generally share the same HLA haplotype (Kipps & Robbins, 1995).

Although HCL is primarily a disease of B lymphocytes, a small number of cases have been reported in which the T lymphocyte was the cell of origin. In these cases, the human T-cell leukemia/lymphoma (HTLV-2) virus has been isolated, implicating a potential viral link (Yarbro, 1997).

The possibility of a relationship between HCL and radiation exposure remains controversial (Hess, 1993). Although one study suggested an association of radiation exposure and HCL, a subsequent larger survey did not verify these findings (Kipps & Robbins, 1995). Oleske and colleagues (1985) reported that epidemiologic studies suggest a correlation between HCL with a history of infectious mononucleosis, chronic anemia, woodworking, farming, routine use of aspirin or tranquilizers, and prior exposure to chemicals.

As noted, the study by Staines and Cartwright (1993) did not support previous studies on the possible etiologic factors of HCL except for an association between HCL and exposure to organic solvents, petrochemicals, and related products. To increase their understanding of pesticide use and its

Box 59-1
Potential Risk Factors for Hairy Cell Leukemia*

- Familial predisposition
- Exposure to organic solvents, petrochemical and related products (linked with farming or woodworking)
- Viral link
- Radiation exposure
- Routine use of aspirin or tranquilizers
- Infectious mononucleosis
- Chronic anemia

*No high relative risk has been determined for hairy cell leukemia.

From Foon K. A. & Casciato D. A. (1995). Chronic leukemias. In Casciato D. A. and Lowitz, B. B. (Eds.), *Manual of clinical oncology* (3rd ed.). Boston: Little Brown.

potential health effects, Garry and colleagues (1994) conducted a survey of 1,000 randomly selected pesticide workers in Minnesota. Two cases of HCL were identified in this study group (annual incidence of HCL in Minnesota is 0.67 : 100,000). These data raised questions as to whether chronic immunostimulation leading to B lymphocyte proliferation and exposure to genotoxic pesticides can be a setting for development of tumors of the immune system (Garry, Kelly, Sprafka, Edwards, & Griffith 1994). The hypothesis of a connection between HCL and agricultural work is further supported by data from an ongoing case control study of agricultural workers in Sweden (Garry et al., 1994).

Clearly, epidemiologic studies to date have not revealed specific correlates on which actions can be taken to reduce the risk of developing HCL. It is the goal of cancer epidemiology to attempt to determine causative factors. This information is useful in developing nursing interventions specific to prevention and detection activities (Cartmel & Reid, 1997). This is an area that warrants further monitoring and ongoing surveillance of those diagnosed with HCL.

CHEMOPREVENTION

Chemoprevention, a relatively new field, targets a particular disease before it progresses and becomes invasive. It is defined as the attempt to intervene using natural and synthetic compounds early in the precancerous stages of carcinogenesis (Greenwald, 1996). To date, there is no published research on chemoprevention efforts related to HCL.

PATHOPHYSIOLOGY

Anatomy and Physiology of the Bone Marrow, Immune System, and Spleen in Hairy Cell Leukemia

To better understand the pathophysiology of HCL, it is helpful to know the anatomy and physiology of the key organs and systems affected by HCL.

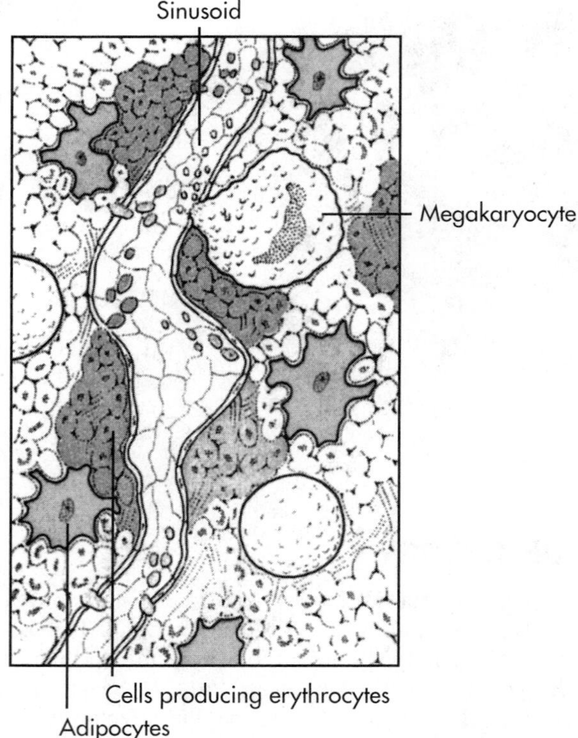

Fig. 59-1 The structure of bone marrow.

Bone Marrow

The red bone marrow, which is located in the medullary cavity of selected adult bones, is the site of hematopoiesis (Jacob, 1992). Structurally, the red marrow consists of an irregular network of hematopoietic cells and vascular-like spaces called *sinusoids* (Jacob, 1992). Between the network of connective tissue fibers are spaces filled with colonies of cells that are dividing and maturing (Jacob, 1992) (Fig. 59-1). In HCL, the hairy cells multiply within the network of the bone marrow. The bone marrow in HCL is laced with a fine fibrosis in which fibers are closely linked to the individual hairy cells (Burthem & Cawley, 1994). Burthem et al. (1994) stated that hairy cells synthesize and assemble matrix in a manner analogous to fibroblasts (fiber-forming cells), and that a substance called *fibronectin* (present in large amounts in hairy cells) contributes to the distinctive pattern of fibrosis that is classic of HCL.

This fibrotic pattern makes it difficult to obtain cell material from the bone marrow (Gollard, Lee, Piro, & Saven, 1995; Hess, 1993). Fibrosis, coupled with the rarity of HCL and the usually low number of circulating cells, has lead to limited investigation of chromosomal abnormalities (Haglund, Julliusson, Stellan, & Gahrton, 1994). Haglund et al. (1994) analyzed the cytogenics of bone marrow specimens from 36 patients, concluding that clonal abnormalities were common and structural abnormalities were largely caused by inversions and deletions and only rarely translocations.

The pattern of bone marrow infiltration is also distinct from other chronic lymphoproliferative disorders (Hess,

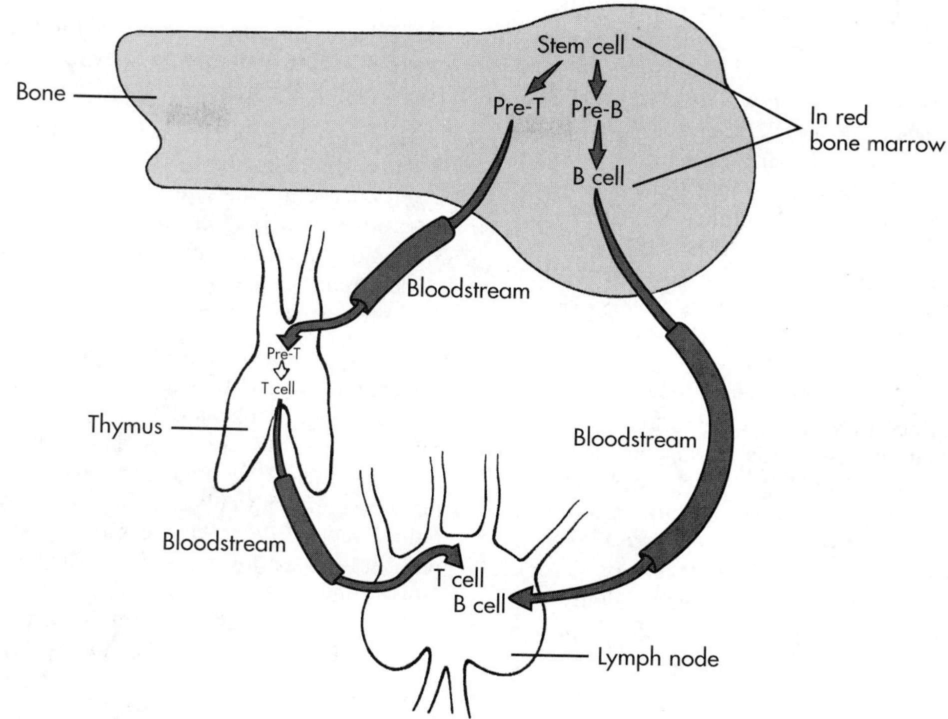

Fig. 59-2 Origin and processing of B lymphocytes and T lymphocytes. Both B lymphocytes and T lymphocytes originate in red bone marrow. B lymphocytes are processed in the red marrow, whereas T lymphocytes are processed in the thymus. Both cell types circulate to other lymphatic tissues.

1993). It tends to be diffuse and has a honeycomb appearance with each hairy cell nucleus surrounded by a halo of pale cytoplasm (Hess, 1993). Generally, the marrow cellularity in HCL is increased; however, some patients may have a hypocellular marrow (Kipps & Robbins, 1995).

All blood cells are derived through the process of hematopoiesis from the pluripotent stem cells in the red bone marrow (Seeley, Stephens, & Tate, 1991). Hematopoiesis can be impaired by hairy cells within the bone marrow. Both marrow infiltration and fibrosis contribute to the cytopenias associated with HCL (Hess, 1993). Kipps & Robbins (1995) note that pancytopenia can be caused by cytokines produced by the hairy cells. Marrow cells of patients with HCL often demonstrate reduced numbers of erythroid colony-forming units (CFU-E). High levels of tumor necrosis factor-α (TNF-α), presumably produced by the leukemic hairy cells in vitro, are found in these cell cultures (Kipps & Robbins, 1995).

In HCL, the cell of origin had been uncertain for many years (Migone, Guilbellino, Casorati, Tassinari, Lauria, & Foa, 1987). The advent of monoclonal antibodies (MoAbs) and molecular technologies at the DNA level has definitively clarified this debated issue (Migone, Guilbellino, Casorati, Tassinari, Lauria, & Foa, 1987). Immunoglobulin (Ig) gene analysis has verified the presence of monoclonal membrane immunoglobulins, which confirms the B lymphocyte origin of hairy cells, although the specific clone of the B lymphocyte that transforms into HCL has not been identified (Visser, Shaw, Slupsky, Vos, & Poppema, 1989).

Immune System

The immune system functions to protect the body from invading microorganisms that may damage the body (Male, 1986). The leukocytes and accessory cells, which are located throughout the organs of the body, coordinate the immune response to eliminate pathogens or minimize the damage it may cause (Male, 1986).

The function of B lymphocytes in the immune response is antibody production (Seeley, Stephens, & Tate, 1991). B lymphocytes are derived from stem cells in the red bone marrow. Mature B lymphocytes are released from the bone marrow and move through the circulation to secondary lymphoid tissues, where they respond to antigens by dividing and differentiating into plasma cells (Male, 1986) (Fig. 59-2). There is evidence to suggest that small groups of identical B lymphocytes or T lymphocytes, called *clones,* are formed during embryonic development and each clone can respond only to a particular antigen (Seeley, Stevens, & Tate, 1991). When a macrophage is exposed to a new antigen, a lymphocyte is stimulated to synthesize antibodies specific to the antigen, then begin production of clonal cells (Rogers, 1992). HCL is a monoclonal (single clone) proliferation of B lymphocytes (Burthem, Baker, Hunt, & Cawley, 1994).

When a specific clone B lymphocyte binds with an antigen, the B lymphocyte begins the process of differentiating into a plasma cell stimulating the production of antibodies (Sherwood, 1993). Antibodies eventually are secreted into the blood or the lymph where they are known as *immuno-*

globulins or *gamma globulins* (Sherwood, 1993). Antibody proteins are structurally composed of polypeptide chains—two long, heavy chains and two short, light chains that are arranged in the shape of a Y (Sherwood, 1993). DiCelle, Reato, Raspadori, Carbone, Rondelli, Lauria, & Foa, (1994) noted that there is monoclonal rearrangement of Ig chain genes on the hairy cell, both heavy and light chain, and these can be useful in monitoring the clinical course of HCL at the deoxyribonucleic acid (DNA) level.

Lymphocytes are also identified by surface markers that are designated human lymphocyte surface proteins recognized by antibodies (Male, 1986). To distinguish classes of lymphocytes, a uniform system of nomenclature has been developed (Abbas, Lichtman, & Pober, 1994). According to this system a surface marker is assumed to a particular lineage or differentiation stage. This marker has a defined structure and is recognized by a group of Mo Abs called *cluster of differentiation* (CD) (Abbas, Lichtman, & Pober, 1994). Distinct patterns of surface markers are expressed in HCL, and hairy cells express high levels of CD11c, CD22, CD25, and CD103 surface antigens along with pan-B-cell antigens CD19, CD20, or CD22 (Kipps & Robbins, 1995).

Spleen

The spleen is a lymphatic organ located in the left upper quadrant of the abdomen (Seeley, Stephens & Tate, 1991). The primary functions of the spleen are as follows:

1. Exchange lymphocytes with blood (removes, stores, produces and adds them)
2. Produce antibodies and sensitized T lymphocytes (by resident lymphocytes)
3. Remove microbes and other particulate debris (by resident macrophages)
4. Store a small percentage of red blood cells

Two specialized types of lymph tissue located within the spleen, the white pulp and the red pulp, perform these functions (Seeley, Stephens & Tate, 1991). The white pulp surrounds the splenic arteries and contains lymph nodules that in turn contain B lymphocytes (Jacob, 1992). Blood is filtered and any particulate matter is phagocytosed in the red pulp (Jacob, 1992). All the blood passes through the red pulp before leaving the spleen (Seeley, Stephens & Tate, 1991) (Fig. 59-3).

Like HCL infiltration within the bone marrow, the pattern of hairy cell involvement in the spleen is unique (Hess,

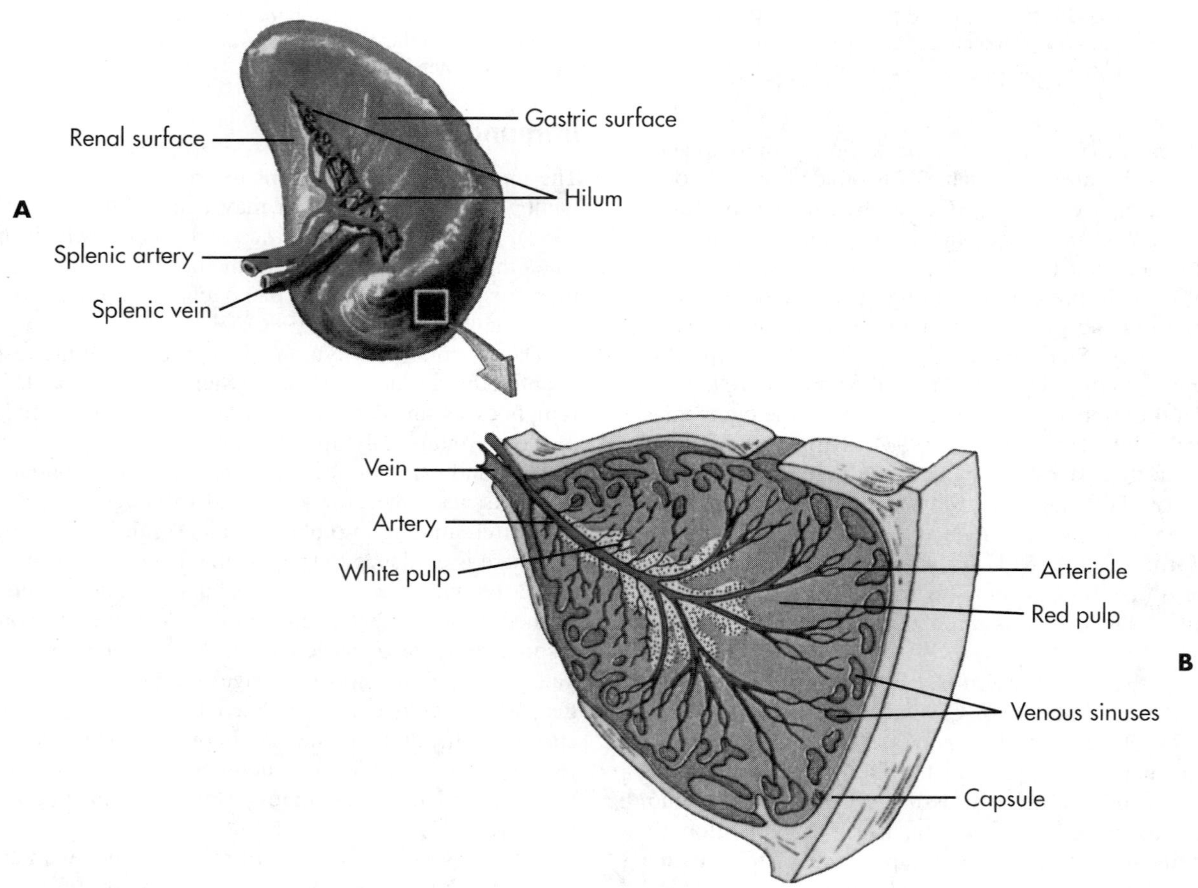

Fig. 59-3 The spleen. **A,** Inferior view of the spleen. **B,** Section showing the arrangement of arteries, veins, white pulp, and red pulp.

1993). The infiltrates are confined to the red pulp, and the white pulp is usually atrophic (Hess, 1993). In an enlarged spleen, hairy cells infiltrate the red pulp cords and sinuses (Kipps & Robbins, 1995).

Peripheral cytopenias identified in patients with HCL are multifactoral, and can be a manifestation of pooling of blood within the red pulp of the spleen (Hess, 1993). In those with HCL, apparently because of the formation of blood-filled pseudosinuses by the hairy cells, a greater proportion of the peripheral red cell volume (as much as 48%) may be pooled in a massively enlarged spleen. Hess (1993) explains that the normal cells (platelets, red cells, and granulocytes) are not destroyed within the spleen at an increased rate but are released into the blood stream at a slower rate.

The Process of Carcinogenesis

The development of some cancers can be delineated through the multistage process of carcinogenesis, but a careful review of the literature does not address this process for HCL. The literature is rich with information regarding the features of the hairy cell (Gollard, Lee, Piro, & Saven, 1995; Haikman, Tallman, Kiley, & Peterson, 1993; Hess, 1993; Kipps & Robbins, 1995; Saven & Piro, 1992), and it is noted that this syndrome is a clinically and morphologically well-defined entity. However, researchers note that no normal equivalent has been identified for the hairy cell (Hess, 1993; Visser et al., 1989).

The initial stage of carcinogenesis (initiation) is characterized by damage to DNA (Yarbo, 1997). Without a specifically identified normal cell, it is not possible to examine the process of change that leads not only to the initiation of HCL, but further analysis of the promotion and progression of this disease. Haglund and colleagues (1994) note that there have been few investigations into the chromosome abnormalities associated with HCL. This is related to, in part, the rarity of the disease and difficulty in obtaining cell material because of the low number of circulating cells and bone marrow fibrosis (Haglund, Juliusson, Stellan, & Gahrton, 1994).

ROUTES OF METASTASES

HCL spreads through both the lymphatic and hematogenous route. The hairy cell closely resembles a mature B cell just before terminal differentiation into a plasma cell (Hess, 1993). Hairy cells are released into circulation just as normal B lymphocytes. Given the level of maturity of the cells, hairy cells move through the lymphatic system and through the hematogenous route in the same fashion as normal B lymphocytes.

Hairy cells have a distinctive pattern of tissue infiltration (Burthem, Baker, Hunt, & Cawley, 1994). Burthem et al. (1994) note that hairy cells have a predilection for bone marrow, splenic red pulp, and hepatic sinusoids. Additionally, these cells act as adhesive cells with a particular affinity for basement membranes and reticular fibers of the bone marrow and spleen. Their research revealed that there are specific adhesive-protein/integrin-receptor interactions that lead to this pattern of mobility and infiltration that is distinctive to HCL (Burthem, Baker, Hunt & Cawley, 1994).

ASSESSMENT

The assessment of the patient for HCL is summarized in Table 59-1. Clinical evaluation of the patient involves performing a detailed history, a thorough physical examination, and diagnostic testing. Both splenomegaly and cytopenias are the primary causes of clinical manifestations of HCL (Hess, 1993). A patient may have any of the presenting symptoms described in the following paragraph or may be asymptomatic. HCL may be diagnosed during a routine examination.

History

The patient should be evaluated for the common symptoms that occur with HCL. These symptoms include fatigue, weakness, lethargy, abdominal fullness or pain, weight loss, bruising, or recurrent infections (Hess, 1993; Jaiyesimi, Kantarjian, & Estey, 1993; Kipps & Robbins, 1995). The leading cause of death for patients with HCL is recurrent infections. Frassoldati and colleagues (1994) note that approximately 25% of patients with HCL will present with some type of infection. Nearly all (80%) patients present with a complaint of fatigue or weakness (Nelson, 1993). Splenomegaly to varying degrees occurs in approximately 85% of patients (Frassoldati, Lamparelli, Federico, Annino, Capnist, & Pagnucco et al., 1994), and about one fourth of patients with HCL complain of resultant left upper quadrant pain or abdominal fullness (Hess, 1993). Hess noted that abdominal fullness may lead to anorexia, causing weight loss in 20% to 35% of patients (Hess, 1993).

Physical Examination

Physical examination of the patient with HCL classically reveals splenomegaly without peripheral lymphadenopathy (Hess, 1993). In only a small percentage of normal adults is the spleen palpable below the left costal margin (Bates, 1991). However, with HCL, splenomegaly occurs in nearly all (85%) patients, and 25% of the time the spleen is massive and extends 8 cm or more below the left costal margin (Kipps & Robbins, 1995). In contrast, the liver is enlarged only 30% of the time (Hess, 1993). Assessment of the abdomen requires techniques to distinguish an enlarged spleen compared with an enlarged liver. Palpation of the spleen may note the following (Bates, 1991):

1. A notch on the medial border
2. Extension beyond midline
3. Dullness to percussion
4. The ability to get the fingers deep into its medial and lower borders but not between the mass and the costal margin

Definitive differentiation, however, cannot be made on this clinical criteria alone.

Following the examination of the abdomen, a lymph node evaluation is performed. The absence of lymph node swelling is an important negative finding due to the fact that peripheral lymphadenopathy is rare in patients with HCL. When found, lymphadenopathy is minimal and localized (Kipps & Robbins, 1995). Extensive retroperitoneal, abdominal, and mediastinal lymphadenopathy may be found (Hess, 1993).

During the physical examination, evaluation of the skin is important because cutaneous lesions are common in patients with HCL. These lesions include petechiae and ecchymosis due to thrombocytopenia, skin infections, and vasculitis, but that lesions caused by infiltration of hairy cells into the skin are uncommon. If present, they are usually disseminated, and diagnosis can be confirmed with skin biopsy (Hess, 1993).

Diagnostic Tests

Complete Blood Count. Patients with HCL often present with altered blood counts manifested by one or more of the following: a decreased white blood count, red blood count, hemoglobin, and platelets. These cytopenias (decreased cell counts) are multifactorial and include the following (Hess, 1993):

1. Hairy cell infiltration of the bone marrow
2. Reticulin fibrosis
3. Pooling of normal peripheral blood cells
4. Plasma volume expansion

Two thirds of patients with HCL demonstrate moderate to severe pancytopenia. The patient's hematocrit is usually between 20% to 35%. Thrombocytopenia, either mild or moderate, is common; however, platelet counts below 20,000/μl are rare. A white blood cell count of less than 4,000/μl is usually typical and in rare cases, patients may have profound leukocytosis (abnormal increase in the number of circulating white blood cells) of greater than 200,000/μl. The percent of hairy cells in the blood may vary, however, in patients with low white cell counts, hairy cells usually account for less than 20% of the lymphocytes. In patients with high white cell counts (those exceeding 10,000/μl), they represent the predominant leukocyte population (Kipps & Robbins, 1995).

TABLE 59-1 Assessment of the Patient for Hairy Cell Leukemia

	Assessment Parameters	Typical Abnormal Findings
History	A. Personal and social history 1. Age 2. Gender	A. Personal and social risk factors 1. Typically occurs in middle age; median age is 50 years 2. 4:1 male predominance
	B. Evaluation of symptoms	B. Common symptoms include fatigue, lethargy, weakness, abdominal fullness or pain, weight loss, anorexia, ecchymosis, petechiae, and a history of recurrent infections.
Physical Examination	A. Palpation of spleen	A. Approximately 80% of patients have splenomegaly at the time of diagnosis. Patients may also have abdominal fullness or discomfort caused by splenomegaly.
	B. Palpation of the liver	B. Approximately 30% of patients have hepatomegaly.
	C. Lymph node evaluation	C. Retroperitoneal and mediastinal adenopathy is occasionally reported.
	D. Weight	D. Weight loss occurs in 20% to 35% of patients with HCL.
	E. Skin involvement	E. Cutaneous lesions due to thrombocytopenia, infection, or vasculitus are common; lesions caused by infiltration of the skin by hairy cells are uncommon (5% of HCL patients).
	F. Lytic bone lesions	F. Lesions are uncommon (3% of HCL patients).
Diagnostic Tests	A. Complete blood count	A. Patients often present with anemia (Hgb between 7 and 10 g/dl) and thrombocytopenia (platelet count below $8.0 \times 10^9/L^6$).
	B. Peripheral blood morphology	B. Presence of hairy cells—when treated with tartrate acid, hairy cells characteristically retain acid phosphatase. Therefore they are identified as tartrate-resistant, acid phosphatase (TRAP)–positive because their cytoplasm stains strongly for TRAP.
	C. Bone marrow biopsy	C. Bone marrow biopsy is the most reliable diagnostic tool to confirm HCL. The bone marrow is usually hypercellular, and the myeloid-to-erythroid ratio is usually <1. Hairy cells are round, oval, or spindle-shaped nuclei and are separated by abundant amounts of pale cytoplasm, which separates individual cells, a pattern of infiltration referred to as *fried egg*.

Hgb, Hemoglobin.

Peripheral Blood Morphology. Patients with HCL typically (90%) demonstrate hairy cells on a peripheral blood smear. The most important diagnostic finding is the appearance of hairy cells on a Wright's stained peripheral blood smear (Hess, 1993). When treated with tartrate acid, hairy cells retain acid phosphatase and are identified as tartrate resistant acid phosphatase (TRAP)–positive (Nelson, 1993). The nuclear membrane and the Golgi area is where the tartrate concentrates, and 95% of patients with HCL stain positive for tartrate (Hess, 1993).

Hairy cells typically are mononuclear with an unusually large amount of pale blue-gray agranualar cytoplasm. They have elongated (hairy) projections, and the diameter ranges from 10 to 25 μm. The nucleus is usually round, oval, or dumbell-shaped (Hess, 1993). When hairy cells are compared with normal mature lymphocytes or the lymphocytes seen in classic chronic lymphocytic leukemia (CLL) and prolymphocytic leukemia (PLL), the nuclear chromoplasm pattern of the hairy cell is homogeneous, less clumped, and lighter staining (Hess, 1993; Kipps & Robbins, 1995).

Immunophenotyping. Unfortunately, there is no individual antibody that identifies an antigen found only on the hairy cell. There are patterns of surface marker expression, however, that can be used to distinguish these leukemic hairy cells from those of other B-lymphocyte lymphoproliferative disorders. Most distinctively, hairy cells express high levels of the CD11c, CD22, and CD103 surface antigens (Kipps & Robbins, 1995). In nearly all patients with HCL, strong expression of these antigens is present on the leukemic B cells. In other B-lymphocyte leukemias and lymphomas, CD11c and CD25 may also be expressed, but hairy cells are distinctive due to the intensity and uniformity with which they express these antigens (Kipps & Robbins, 1995).

Bone Marrow Biopsy. The diffuse pattern of bone marrow involvement in HCL patients is unique to this disease (Hess, 1993). At time of diagnosis, the bone marrow is often hypercellular. However, in a few cases the bone marrow is excessively hypocellular, and it may be similar to that of a patient with aplastic anemia, or the marrow may show isolated hairy cells invading between the marrow fat cells (Kipps & Robbins, 1995).

When comparing HCL with other chronic lymphoproliferative disorders, the pattern of infiltration is unique (Hess, 1993). The individual hairy cells have been described as resembling a "fried egg" or a honeycomb with the nucleus of each hairy cell surrounded by a halo of cytoplasm (Hess, 1993). Special staining for reticulin, a substance found in the connective fibers of reticular tissue, reveals diffuse reticulin fibrosis without a collagen fibrosis (Hess, 1993). This fibrosis is the reason why clinicians may fail to obtain an adequate aspirate or they may get a "dry tap" (Hess, 1993). Additionally, infiltration of red cells into areas of hairy cell invasion is common (Kipps & Robbins, 1995).

Diagnosis of Hairy Cell Leukemia. Diagnosis of HCL is not usually difficult and is suspicious when splenomegaly is associated with pancytopenia and an absence of peripheral lymphadenopathy (Hess, 1993). In most cases, hairy cells are found in the peripheral blood of a routine blood smear (Nelson, 1993). Hairy cells will be tartrate resistant, acid phosphatase positive. A tartrate-resistant acid phosphatase stain involving at least 2 cells with greater than 40 granules or with many granules obscuring the nucleus is most often diagnostic of HCL (Gollard, Lee, Piro, & Saven, 1995). Biopsy of the bone marrow will reveal a diffuse, focal, or interstitial pattern of infiltration of hairy cells. Antibodies analysis is necessary when examination of bone marrow is atypical or when the cells stain TRAP -negative (Hess, 1993).

STAGING

In general, the literature does not refer to the staging of HCL. Leukemias are usually classified as acute versus chronic, and myeloid versus lymphocytic. This classification, along with the presence of specific clinical features, guides the treatment of leukemia (Pui, 1995). In HCL, treatment decisions are based on the presence of specific clinical features; if a patient does not have any of these clinical features, no therapy may be necessary (Kipps & Robbins, 1995).

In 1982, Jansen and Hermans proposed a three-stage system for HCL based on hemoglobin levels and spleen sizes. They analyzed data from 391 patients with HCL with the purpose of defining a clinical staging system to assist in identifying patients who would most benefit from splenectomy (Jansen & Hermans, 1982) (Table 59-2).

Chemotherapy for HCL in 1982 had not been studied thoroughly and splenectomy was essentially the only form of treatment that resulted in an improvement in symptoms and survival (Hess, 1993; Jansen & Hermans, 1982). The favorable results obtained with the purine analogs such as fludarabine and 2-chlorodeoxgadenosine (2 CdA) has led to the use of systemic therapy over splenectomy as first-line therapy (Golumb, 1994). Current literature, which primarily focuses on systemic therapy, does not classify HCL by the Jansen staging system.

TABLE 59-2 Jansen Clinical Staging for Hairy Cell Leukemia

Stage	Findings at the Time of Diagnosis
I	Hb > 12.0 g/dl + spleen ≤ 10 cm UCM
	OR
	Hb > 8.5 g/dl + spleen < 4 cm UCM
II	Hb > 12.0 g/dl + spleen > 10 cm UCM
	OR
	Hb 8.5 − 12.0 g/dl + spleen 4 − 10 cm UCM
	OR
	Hb < 8.5 g/dl + spleen < 4 cm UCM
III	Hg 8.5 − 12.0 g/dl + spleen > 10 cm UCM
	OR
	Hg < 8.5 g/dl + spleen ≥ 4 cm UCM

UCM, Under costal margin
Jansen, J. & Hermans, J. (1982). Clinical staging system for hairy-cell leukemia. *Blood, 60* (3), 571-577.

MEDICAL MANAGEMENT

In approximately 10% of patients, the medical management of HCL entails only regular follow-up evaluation to monitor for development of cytopenias or disease progression (Nelson, 1993) (Fig. 59-4). These patients do not have any of the key clinical features (HCL) such as lymphadonapathy and no immediate therapy is necessary (Kipps & Robbins, 1995). Patients who do not require treatment often include older adults with small spleens and with few circulating hairy cells (Saven & Piro, 1992).

Indications for systemic therapy include the following:

- Symptomatic splenomegaly (i.e., decreased satiety, abdominal fullness)
- *Anemia* defined as a hemoglobin less than 10 g/dl
- *Thrombocytopenia* defined as a platelet count less than 100,000/μl
- Granulocytopenia with recurrent opportunistic infections
- Leukemic phase of HCL with a white blood cell count greater than 20,000/μl
- Associated autoimmune complications
- Tissue infiltration with hairy cells (Kipps & Robbins, 1995).

The exact values of the above noted hematologic parameters vary by institution (Saven & Piro, 1992; 1993; 1994).

HCL was resistant to most drugs available before the mid-1980s (Nelson, 1993). Rarely did a patient respond to chemotherapeutic agents that were successful treatment in other lymphoproliferative disorders (Hess, 1993). Splenectomy was the treatment of choice, and this procedure did result in an improvement in symptoms and survival in most patients (Nelson, 1993). With the advent in the mid-1980s of new drugs to which hairy cells responded, the prognosis of patients with HCL has improved dramatically, and HCL is now considered a potentially curable disease (Kipps & Robbins, 1995).

Splenectomy. Splenectomy has been standard therapy for most patients with HCL before the development of purine analogues as discussed above (Kipps & Robbins, 1995). In 1958, the first successful splenectomy was reported (Saven & Piro, 1992). An enlarged spleen is problematic because it causes peripheral cytopenias due to increased seclusion or pooling of blood cells within the spleen, reentry of cellular elements into circulation at a slower rate, and dilution of cellular components of the peripheral blood (Hess, 1992). Splenectomy causes a decrease in the blood plasma volume, and it eliminates the reservoir effect of the enlarged spleen (Hess, 1993). Additionally, the spleen has the potential to alleviate patient sweating, weight loss due to early satiety and hypermetabolism, and abdominal discomfort (Hess, 1993).

Following splenectomy, rapid changes in the blood counts are noted. Kipps and Robbins (1995) documented that in more than 90% of patients postsplenectomy, improvement of blood counts occured, and in 40% to 77% of these patients, normalization of all blood counts also occurred. The duration of response after splenectomy is variable. Some poor prognostic indicators include increased postoperative bone marrow cellularity (greater than 85%) and low platelet counts (less than 60,000/μl) (Hess, 1993).

Many patients who undergo this procedure will be asymptomatic for years (Nelson, 1993). However, it does not decrease the number of leukemia cells in the marrow, and more importantly, it is not curative (Kipps & Robbins, 1995). Approximately one third of HCL patients postsplenectomy have only a minimal response or relapse a few months after the splenectomy (Hess, 1993).

With improved systematic therapy, the indications for splenectomy in patients with HCL have become much more limited. Splenectomy is a major operative procedure with significant mortality and morbidity (Hess, 1993). Currently, splenectomy is only considered in patients who have a massive, painful, or ruptured spleen; those with pancytopenia and an active infection due to an opportunistic pathogen; or individuals who have failed systemic therapy (Kipps & Robbins, 1995).

Interferon-α. HCL was one of the first malignancies to show significant response to therapy with IFN-α. Before IFN-α, results of treatment with other chemotherapeutic agents in HCL were generally unsuccessful (Kipps & Robbins, 1995). In 1984 a small but significant report rated a response to IFN-α in seven out of seven patients. Three patients achieved a complete remission, and the other four achieved a partial remission (Jaiyesimi, Kantarjian & Estey, 1993). IFN-α has been proven effective in both splenectomized and nonsplenectomized patients with a median duration of response of 25 months (Hess, 1993).

Despite the proven activity of IFN-α in HCL, this agent is not curative (Jaiyesimi, Kantarjian & Estey, 1993), and nearly half of all patients successfully treated have a clinical relapse in less than 2 years following discontinuation of therapy (Kipps & Robbins, 1995). If a patient with HCL does relapse or have disease progression, restarting IFN-α is effective in promoting a partial response in 50% of patients (Kipps & Robbins, 1995). One potential danger in the use of IFN-α is the development of anti-IFN antibodies. The significance of this finding is controversial (Hess, 1993).

In studies evaluating the effectiveness of various agents

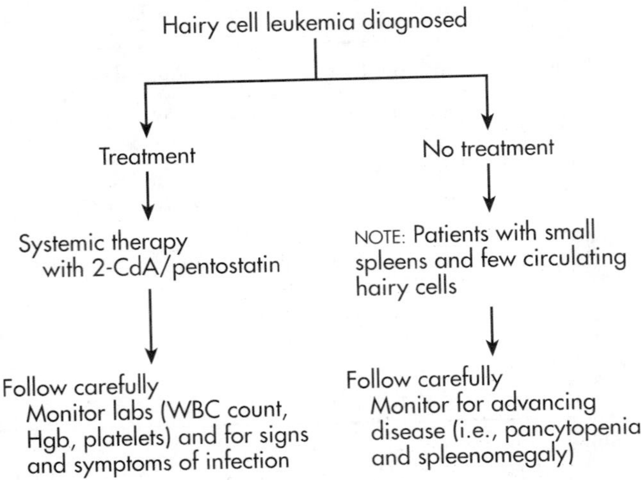

Fig. 59-4 Algorithm for hairy cell leukemia management.

in patients with HCL, *partial response* is defined as significant improvement in the pancytopenia, a reduction in the size of the spleen, and improvement in immunologic function (Hess, 1993). Although the response rate is 80% to 90% in HCL patients, only 5% to 10% of these patients have a complete response (Hess, 1993). IFN-α causes the percentage of hairy cells in the bone marrow to decrease, but rarely do all of the hairy cells disappear and often, evidence of reticulin fibrosis persists (Hess, 1993). The recommended dose is 3×10^6 units per day (Kipps & Robbins, 1995). This dose can be self-administered subcutaneously three to seven times a week for 12 months (Hess, 1993).

Most patients will experience some toxicity, which may limit patient compliance (Gollard, Lee, Piro & Saven, 1995). Severity of side effects with IFN-α use are both age- and dose-related, with virtually all patients experiencing some toxicity (Kipps & Robbins, 1995). Side effects in order of most prevalent to least prevalent include flu-like symptoms, leukopenia, nausea, vomiting, central nervous system symptoms, diarrhea, cardiovascular symptoms, skin involvement, anemia, and thrombocytopenia (Hess, 1993). Chronic fatigue syndrome is also prevalent and is increasingly severe when treatment lasts for more than 1 year (Hess, 1993).

It has recently been reported that there is an unusually high incidence of second neoplasms found in patients following treatment with IFN-α. The neoplasms reported include both those of hematopoietic and lymphatic origin. The increased frequency of these malignancies may be due to the longer length of survival of these patients who are immunocompromised due to the HCL adenocarcinomas (Gollard et al. 1995). In view of the superior effectiveness of the purine analogs (discussed below), the future use of IFN-α in the treatment of HCL may be for patients who initially are too ill with infections to tolerate these agents (Kipps & Robbins, 1995).

Purine Analogs. 2-chlorodeoxyadenosine (cladribine, 2-CdA) is a purine nucleoside analog (Fig. 59-5) that has emerged as the optimal treatment for HCL due to the high incidence of durable and complete remissions that follow infusion of this drug (Gollard et al., 1995). The mechanism of action revolves around nucleosides, which are important precursors in DNA synthesis. For DNA synthesis to occur, the nucleoside deoxyadenosine must be phosphoralated three times, forming deoxyadenosine-monophosphate (dAMP), deoxyadenosine-diphosphate (dADP), and deoxyadenosine-triphosphate (dATP) (Fig. 59-6). Nucleosides, such as deoxyadenosine, are essential for the cell proliferation.

2-CdA is resistant to adenosine deaminase (ADA), and it accumulates as 2-chlorodeoxyadenosine triphosphate (2-CdATP) in cells (Jaiyesimi, Kantarjian & Estey, 1993). (Fig. 59-7). 2-CdATP is the substance that is actually toxic to the cells causing: (1) generation of strand breaks in the DNA of the lymphocyte; (2) depletion of intracellular nucleoside adenine phosphate (NAD) and adenosine triphosphate (ATP), which leads to cytotoxicity (damage to tissue cells); and (3) a decrease in the synthesis of ribonucleic acid (RNA) (Jaiyesimi, Kantarjion & Estey, 1993). In contrast to most other chemotherapeutic agents, which are toxic only to dividing cells, 2-CdATP is toxic to both dividing and resting cells, making it ideal for HCL, a chronic leukemia. However, 2-CdA does target only certain types of cells, namely lymphocytes and monocytes. Therefore side effects characteristic of most chemotherapeutic agents (i.e., nausea and vomiting or hair loss) are not found.

2-CdA was first administered in 1986 to two splenectomized HCL patients who both achieved a complete remission (Saven & Piro, 1993). Then in 1990, 12 HCL patients with evidence of active disease were treated with 2-CdA, and 11 of the 12 achieved complete remissions (Saven & Piro, 1993). Since that time, research has shown that nearly all patients with HCL respond to a single 7-day course of 2-CdA administered via continuous IV infusion 4 mg/m^2

Fig. 59-5 Cladribine, 2-chlorodeoxyadenosine.

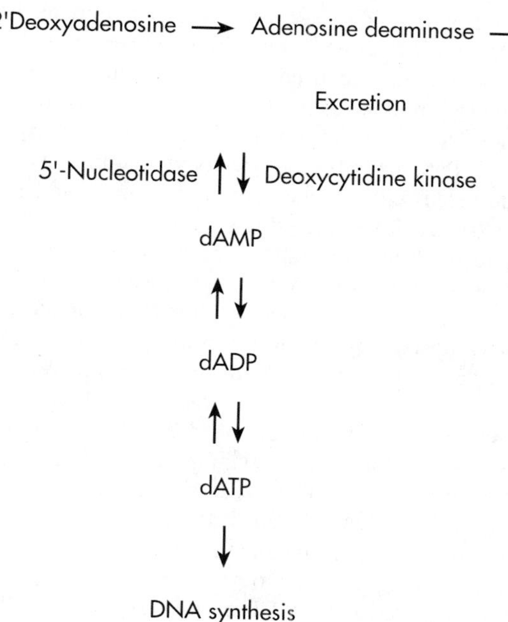

Fig. 59-6 Pathway of deoxyadenosine metabolism.

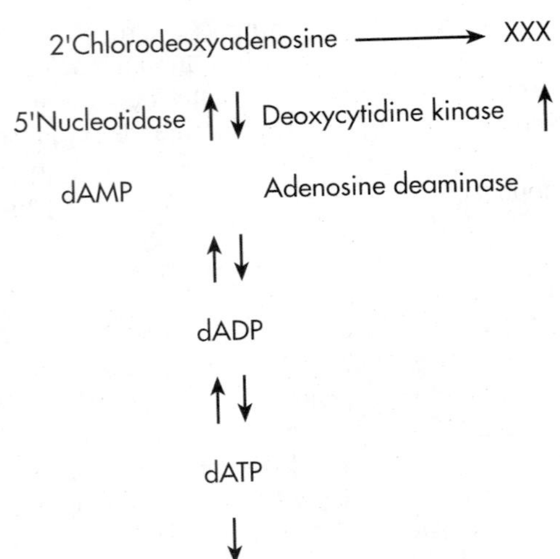

Fig. 59-7 Pathway of 2-CdA metabolism.

daily (Foon & Casciato, 1995). In more than 75% of patients treated with 2-CdA, a complete and durable remission was observed. In some studies, the complete response rate exceeded 90%. Response to therapy is not affected by prior splenectomy, and patients who are refractory to other agents such as pentostatin and IFN-α can achieve complete remission following a 1 week course of 2-CdA (Kipps & Robbins, 1995).

Side effects of 2-CdA are minimal. The primary hematologic side effect is myelosuppression and associated fever. Investigators have also noted increased incidence of opportunistic infections in patients immediately following therapy with 2-CdA (Kipps & Robbins, 1995). With further follow-up, these patients are found to have profound CD4 and CD8 lymphopenia that can last for years after treatment (Foon & Casciato, 1995). Since this drug targets lymphocytes, 2-CdA should not be used in patients who already have weakened immune systems (such as patients with acquired immunodeficiency syndrome [AIDS] or organ transplant recipients). Patients whose lymphocyte count has already been depleted with another purine analog should also not receive 2-CdA. Rare side effects include peripheral neuropathy, late bone marrow failure, and isolated incidences of severe proximal myopathy (Foon & Casciato, 1995).

2′-Deoxycoformycin (pentostatin, DCF), a purine analog, is synthesized by streptomyces antibioticus, a substance that is structurally related to adenosine (Kipps & Robbins, 1995). This drug is a tight binding inhibitor of adenosine deaminase, an enzyme important in lymphocyte purine metabolism that is found in all lymphoid cells (Nelson, 1993; Saven & Piro, 1993). The exact mechanism of this drug, however, is unknown (Saven & Piro, 1993).

The typical dose for patients treated with pentostatin for HCL is 2 to 4 mg/m^2 every other week by intravenous (IV) bolus after hydration with 1 L of 5% dextrose with 0.5 normal saline. Following administration of the drug, 500 ml of the same solution is given (Foon & Casciato, 1995; Kipps & Robbins, 1995). Patients are often hospitalized the first time the drug is administered to evaluate patient tolerance.

Nearly half of the patients have a complete response, and nearly all have a partial response within 4 months of therapy. These numbers include those patients who have failed to respond to IFN-α and/or those who had undergone splenectomy (Kipps & Robbins, 1995).

Within 2 months of treatment with pentostatin, patients achieve normal blood cell counts, and they often have a 50% to 95% decrease in the number of hairy cells found in their marrow (Kipps & Robbins, 1995). In addition to ridding the bone marrow of hairy cells, patients who receive pentostatin have resolution of neutropenia. Although a patient can relapse in the marrow after this therapy, additional therapy may not be required for more than 1 year (Kipps & Robbins, 1995).

Myelosuppression, nausea and vomiting, fevers, neurologic toxicity, skin rash, reversible renal dysfunction, conjunctivitis, and mild hepatic toxicity can be seen within the first two to three cycles (Kipps & Robbins, 1995). T-cell depletion has been reported, particularly of the CD4+ helper T-lymphocyte group (Kipps & Robbins, 1995).

ONCOLOGIC EMERGENCIES

Oncologic emergencies are a rare occurrence with HCL and its treatment. The most common presenting symptoms are splenomegaly and pancytopenia (Kipps & Robbins, 1995), neither of which usually lead to an oncologic emergency. Treatment for HCL with INF-α does not typically cause an oncologic emergency either.

Occasionally, a patient with HCL will present with a very high proportion of hairy cells, and treatment will be immediately initiated because of the risk of the oncologic emergency of leukostasis (Gollard, Lee, Piro, & Saven, 1995). Leukostasis develops in patients with blast crisis when peripheral blast counts exceed 50,000 to 100,000/μl. If counts are greater than 60,000/μl, there is an increased likelihood of pulmonary hypoxemia and intracerebral hemorrhage.

There are currently two options in the treatment of leukostasis. To decrease leukostasis when it involves the brain and the lungs, chemotherapy must be started immediately in an effort to decrease the cell count. Leukapheresis is also useful to decrease the cell count but does not prevent the growth of leukemic 1 (Deisseroth, Keating, Andreeff, Kantarjian, Champlin, & Khouri et al., 1997).

NURSING MANAGEMENT

The medical management of HCL is variable depending on a patient's clinical condition at the time of diagnosis. Patients with HCL manifest complications that require comprehensive nursing interventions and patient education. HCL is primarily treated in the outpatient setting; therefore the patient must be equipped with adequate knowledge for self-care in the home setting.

Early in the course of the patient's disease, the focus of nursing care is helping the patient understand the disease process and it's treatment (Table 59-3). With the initiation

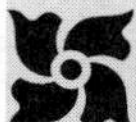

TABLE 59-3 Standard of Care for the Patient Receiving Systemic Chemotherapy with a Purine Analog-Knowledge Deficit

Patient Problem and Outcomes	Nursing Interventions and Rationales	Patient Education Instructions
Knowledge Deficit Patient will verbalize an understanding of HCL and potential therapeutic effects and potential side effects of treatment with purine analog.	1. Assess educational level, ability, and desire to learn. 2. Assess significant other's educational level, ability, and desire to learn. 3. Determine understanding of anatomy/physiology related to hairy cell leukemia and effect of purine analogs and provide information. 4. Assess attitudes/expectations related to the outcome of treatment.	1. Develop a teaching plan at an appropriate level of understanding. 2. Using diagram of bone marrow, lymph system, and spleen, explain the anatomy/physiology of HCL: a. It is a disease of B lymphocyte b. Cells have "hairy" like projections when viewed under the microscope c. Malignant cells move through the lymph system d. Hairy cells effect normal hematopoeisis 3. Provide oral and written information regarding purine analogs, route of administration, frequency, and duration of administration. 4. Explain mode of action of purine analog: a. Acts on rapidly dividing cells b. Affects normal lymphocyte cells, as well as hairy cells 5. Explain potential side effects: a. Decreased white blood cell count b. Potential for infection

TABLE 59-4 Standard of Care for the Patient Receiving Systemic Chemotherapy with a Purine Analog-Neutropenia

Patient Problem and Outcomes	Nursing Intervention and Rationales	Patient Education Instructions
Neutropenia/Infection Patient will: • Remain infection-free. • Verbalize understanding of strategies to prevent infection.	1. Encourage proper handwashing. 2. Assess for signs and symptoms of infection. 3. Monitor lab values.	1. Teach patient to monitor temperature and signs of inflammation and/or infection, and report immediately: a. Fever (per institution) b. Sore throat c. Inflammation d. Shaking chills e. Painful urination f. Cough, shortness of breath (SOB), or rapid breathing 2. Describe role of white blood cells in fighting infection and implication of neutropenia. 3. Instruct to avoid crowds and people with known infection. 4. Inform of need to avoid fresh unpeeled fruits, raw vegetables, flowers, and houseplants.

of therapy, patients need information about managing side effects, as well as complications caused by the disease itself. The major side effect in the patient with HCL being treated with a purine analog is neutropenia (Table 59-4). Other nursing concerns in an HCL patient related to the disease itself are abdominal fullness, fatigue, and weakness. These issues are discussed in the Standards of Care Tables 59-5 and 59-6 (Nelson, 1993).

HOME CARE ISSUES

Home care issues in the patient with HCL are dependent on the treatment approach taken. Patients with HCL and their caregivers need to be educated about the disease and potential side effects of the treatment.

The first cells to regenerate following treatment for HCL are the platelets, followed by the leukocytes, and lastly the red cells (Saven & Piro, 1993). In patients who are treated

TABLE 59-5 Standard of Care for the Patient with Hairy Cell Leukemia

Patient Problem and Outcomes	Nursing Interventions and Rationales	Patient Education Instructions
Abdominal Fullness/Anorexia		
Patient will verbalize: • Understanding of the etiologic factors of abdominal fullness and resulting anorexia. • Strategies to manage discomfort and anorexia. Patient will: • Maintain weight • Achieve personally satisfactory control of pain/discomfort	1. Assess splenomegaly. 2. Monitor weight. 3. Assess pain/ discomfort. 4. Consult dietician as necessary.	1. Teach patient correlation between splenomegaly and abdominal fullness/anorexia. 2. Encourage strategies to decrease abdominal fullness associated with dietary intake: a. Eat small amounts 6 to 8 times per day b. Drink beverages between meals instead of with meals c. Avoid strenuous exercise immediately following meals to allow for adequate digestion d. Avoid gas-producing foods e. Avoid fried/greasy foods 3. Discuss elements of nutritious diet. 4. Instruct patient regarding pain: a. Can be controlled b. Highly individual and variable c. Record pattern, duration, intensity, and relieving factors d. As spleen decreases in size, associated pain will diminish/resolve

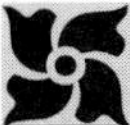

TABLE 59-6 Standard of Care for the Patient with Hairy Cell Leukemia

Patient Problems and Outcomes	Nursing Interventions and Rationales	Patient Education Instructions
Fatigue/Weakness		
Patient will verbalize strategies to reduce and cope with fatigue and weakness.	1. Obtain patient history/review for potential physiologic basis of fatigue (anemia, electrolyte imbalance, medication); intervene to correct as appropriate. 2. Assess pattern, duration, intensity, relieving factors, and impact of fatigue.	1. Instruct patient that fatigue and weakness can be a presenting symptom of hairy cell leukemia and can persist through the period of pancytopenia. 2. Instruct patient to monitor pattern of fatigue and report symptoms to healthcare providers. 3. Discuss strategies to reduce and cope with fatigue: a. Energy conservation b. Effective energy utilization c. Energy restoration

TABLE 59-7 Home Care Issues for the Patient with Low Blood Counts

Issue	Definitions	Action
Neutropenia	Low white blood cell count	• Good handwashing • Keep skin intact • Take temperature every day at the same time
Thrombocytopenia	Low platelet count	• Avoid injury to the skin • Use a soft bristle toothbrush and avoid dental floss • Be sure dentures fit properly to avoid irritation • Keep bowels soft and regular
Anemia	Low red cell count	• Tell your doctor if you have any of the following symptoms: -Fatigue -Shortness of breath -Difficulty staying warm -Chest pain • Pace your activities limiting the amount of work you do in a day

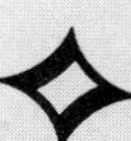

TABLE 59-8 Patient Preparation for Symptoms Associated With Cladribine (2-Chlordeoxyadenosine)

Rationale: Cladribine (2-Chlordeoxyadenosine) is a common agent used in the treatment of hairy cell leukemia and other chronic leukemias. Knowledge of the possible adverse effects of this therapy helps you and your family be aware of possible problems and to report them to your health care team as soon as you notice them.

Common Adverse Reactions	Signs and Symptoms
1. Infection	Sore throat, cough, stuffy nose; shaking chills, diarrhea, temperature over 100.5°F (38°C), burning eyes,
2. Bleeding	Bruises; bleeding gums, nosebleeds, blood in vomit or stool, vision changes, increased menstrual flow
3. Anemia	Excess fatigue, dizziness and light-headedness; chilling, insomnia, nervousness
4. Fever	Temperature over 100.5°F (38°C)
5. Breathing problems	Shortness of breath, dry cough when walking fast
6. Injection site symptoms	Swelling, redness, warmth, and pain over skin

Report any of the above symptoms to your nurse or physician.

Modified from: School of Nursing, University of California at San Francisco (1996). *Managing the side effects of chemotherapy and radiation therapy.* University of California, San Francisco: University of California San Francisco Press.

TABLE 59-9 Quality of Care Evaluation for a Patient Undergoing Therapy With 2-CdA

Disciplines participating in the quality of care evaluation:
☐ Nursing ☐ Hematology ☐ Social Services

I. Post-therapy Management Evaluation

Data from:
☐ Medical Record Review ☐ Patient/Family Interview

Criteria	Yes	No
1. Patient experienced to following pre-therapy information		
a. Side effect information	☐	☐
b. Explanation of laboratory values	☐	☐
2. Patient experienced the following complications:		
a. Fever	☐	☐
b. Infection	☐	☐
3. Blood counts during nadir		
a. White blood cell count	☐	☐
b. Platelets	☐	☐
c. Red blood cell count	☐	☐

II. Patient/Family Satisfaction

Data from:
☐ Patient Interview ☐ Family Interview

Criteria	Yes	No
1. On a scale of 1 to 10, with 0 being totally dissatisfied and 10 being totally satisfied, how satisfied were you with the symptom management you received?________		
2. Were you told to call the nurse if your temperature rose above 100°F	☐	☐
3. Were you told to call your nurse if you experienced chills, new cough or production of sputum, a sore throat, more than three loose stools a day, or burning on urination?	☐	☐

with splenectomy, only 40% to 60% have normalization of their blood counts (Gollard, Lee, Piro, & Saven, 1995). Depending on the therapy used, an explanation of the purpose and potential problems related to the white cells, the red cells, and the platelets should be reviewed (Table 59-7).

The family caregivers of a patient with HCL should be included in patient teaching. They need to thoroughly understand the disease, treatment options, and their adverse reactions, as well as their roles in the patients care management. The caregiver can help process information that can be overwhelming (Table 59-8). Many community resources are available to cancer patients and those who support them. Persistence is needed to find the organization that fits with ones individual needs.

PROGNOSIS

Before the availability of systemic therapy, HCL was a chronic, progressive, fatal disorder with a median survival of 53 months; today HCL has become a treatment model for indolent lymphoid malignancies (Gollard et al., 1995). In a 1994 editorial in Annals of Internal Medicine, Dr. Harvey Golomb noted the following:

> If HCL can not be cured with IFN, Pentostatin, or 2-CdA alone, then is some combination of these three likely to cure it? This question will probably not be able to be answered as the disease is so well controlled with any of these agents in sequence for such a long period of time that a randomized study to answer the question asked can not probably be completed.

Frassoldati et al. (1994) reviewed data on 725 patients with HCL diagnosed over 25 years; once documented the overall 5- and 10- year survivals at 66.3% and 54.8% respectively. Data were grouped into five periods: A (1965-

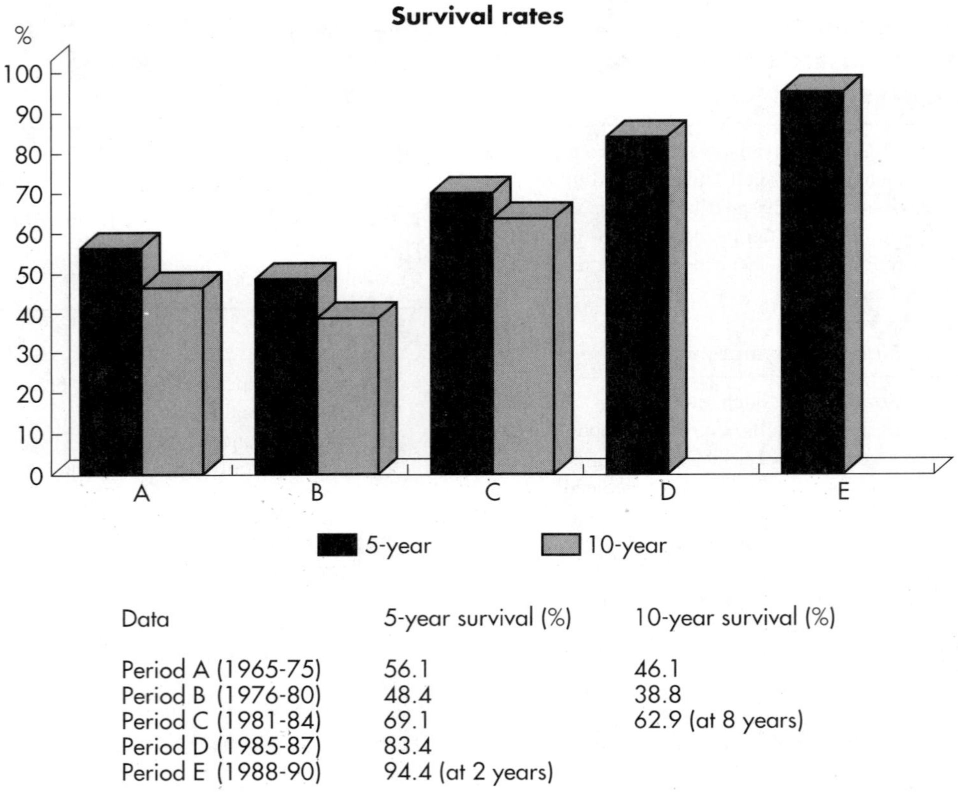

Data	5-year survival (%)	10-year survival (%)
Period A (1965-75)	56.1	46.1
Period B (1976-80)	48.4	38.8
Period C (1981-84)	69.1	62.9 (at 8 years)
Period D (1985-87)	83.4	
Period E (1988-90)	94.4 (at 2 years)	

Fig. 59-8 Summary of survival rates: hairy cell leukemia. (Modified from Frassoldati, A., Lamparelli, T., Federico, M., Annino, L., Capnist, G., Pagnucco, G. et al. [1994]. Hairy cell leukemia: A clinical review based on 725 cases of the Italian Cooperative Group [ICGH CL]. *Leukemia and lymphoma, 13,* 307-316.)

75), B (1976-80), C (1981-84), D (1985-87), and E (1988-90). These groupings were divided according to the time of diagnosis and correlate with the evolution of treatment for HCL:

> Thus, period A (when, in the absence of strict diagnostic criteria the disease was often confused with other clinico-pathologic entities), period B (characterized by better diagnostic criteria and by a wide spectrum of therapeutic approaches), period C (almost all patients treated with splenectomy), period D (characterized by IFN availability, but uncertainty about its use at the onset of the disease), and period E (when IFN was considered the standard initial therapy for HCL) (Frassoldati et al.)

Analysis of the data reveals an overall improvement in survival associated with improved therapy (Fig. 59-8).

EVALUATION OF THE QUALITY OF CARE

The Joint Commission for the Accreditation of Health Care Organizations (JCAHO) is an accreditation organization that requires the quality of care provided to patients be evaluated. An evaluation of the quality of care provided to patients with HCL needs to include all of the team members: nursing, medicine, and social services. Table 59-9 is an example of a tool that can be used in the outpatient setting.

RESEARCH ISSUES

Various issues surrounding treatment of HCL require further investigation. Although treatment with purine analogs has yielded high complete remission (CR) in many patients, further study and monitoring is needed to determine whether these therapies will translate into a cure. Research into the methods for detection of minimal residual disease would further clarify if a CR has been achieved or whether methodology to date does not detect the presence of minimal disease. Given the immunosuppression associated with purine analogs, optimal subsequent therapy for relapse in patients who present with cytopenia also needs to be determined. The best approach to managing patients diagnosed with HCL is enrollment into ongoing clinical trials to determine optimal therapy to confirm the possible curative role of the purine analogs.

As with any cancer survivor, nurses should monitor HCL survivors for related physical or psychosocial survivorship issues. Because of the relative rarity of this disease, issues specific to this population require collaboration among various cancer centers to correlate data specific to HCL survivors and subsequent problems.

REFERENCES

Abbas, A., Lichtman, A., & Pober, J. (1994). *Cellular and molecular immunology* (2nd ed.). Philadelphia: W. B. Saunders.

American Cancer Society, Document 004280, *Leukemia-hairy cell,* 1994.

Bates, B. (1991). *A guide to physical examination and history taking.* 356). Philadelphia: J. B. Lippincott.

Bernstein, L., Newton, P., & Ross, R. (1990). Epidemiology of hairy cell leukemia in Los Angeles county. *Cancer Research, 50,* 3605-3609.

Bouroncle, B. A., Wiseman, B. K., & Doan, C. A. (1958). Leukemic reticuloendotheliosis. *Blood, 13,* 609-630.

Burthem, J., Baker, J., Hunt, J. & Cawley, J. (1994). Hairy cell interactions with extracellular matrix: Expression of specific integrin receptors and their role in the cell's response to specific adhesive proteins. *Blood, 84(3),* 873-882.

Burthem, J., Baker, P., Hunt, J. & Cawley, J. (1994). The function of c-fms in hairy-cell leukemia: Macrophage colony-stimulating factor stimulates hairy-cell movement. *Blood, 83(5),* 1381-1389.

Burthem, J. & Cawley, J. (1994). The bone marrow fibrosis of hairy-cell leukemia is caused by the synthesis and assembly of a fibronectin matrix by the hairy cells. *Blood, 83(2),* 497-504.

Deisseroth, A., Keating, M., Andreeff, M., Kantarjian, H., Champlin, R., Khouri, I. & Talpaz, M. (1997). In V. T. DeVita, S. Hellman, & S. A. Rosenberg (Eds.), *Cancer: Principles and practice of oncology* (4th ed.). Philadelphia: J. B. Lippincott.

DiCelle, P., Reato, G., Raspadori, D., Carbone, A., Rondelli, D., Lauria, F., & Foa, R. (1994). Molecular evaluation of clonal remission in hairy cell leukemia patients treated with 2-CdA. *Leukemia and Lymphoma, 14* (1), 139-142.

Frassoldati, A., Lamparelli, T., Federico, M., Annino, L., Capnist, G., Pagnucco, G., Dini, E., Resegotti, L., Damasio, E. & Silingardi, V. (1994). Hairy cell leukemia: a clinical review based on 725 cases of the Italian Cooperative Group (ICGHCL). *Leukemia and Lymphoma, 13,* 307-316.

Foon, K. A. & Casciato, D. A. (1995). Chronic leukemias. In D. A. Casciato & B. B. Lowitz (Eds.), *Manual of clinical oncology* (3rd ed.). Boston: Little, Brown.

Garry, V., Kelly, J., Sprafke, J., Edwards, S. & Griffith, J. (1994). Survey of health and use characterization of pesticide appliers in Minnesota. *Archives of Environmental Health, 49* (5), 337-44.

Gollard, R., Lee, T., Piro, L., & Saven, A. (1995). The optimal management of hairy cell leukemia. *Drugs, 49 (6),* 921-29.

Golumb, H. (1994). Do we know the treatment of choice for hairy cell leukemia? *Annals of Internal Medicine, 5,* 676-77.

Greenwald, P. (1996). Chemoprevention of cancer. *Scientific American,* September, 1996.

Haglund, U., Juliusson, G., Stellan, B., & Gahrton, G. (1994). Hairy cell leukemia is characterized by clonal chromosome abnormalities clustered to specific regions. *Blood, 83*(3), 2637-2645.

Hakimian, D., Tallman, M., Kiley, C., & Peterson, L. (1993). Detection of minimal residual disease by immunostaining of bone marrow biopsies after 2-chlorodeoxyadenosine for hairy cell leukemia. *Blood, 82*(6), 1798-1802.

Hess, C. (1993). Hairy cell leukemia, malignant histiocytosis, and related disorders. In G. R. Lee, T. C. Bithell, J. Foerster, J. W. Athens, & J. N. Lukens (Eds.), *Wintrobe's clinical hematology.* Philadelphia: Lea and Febiger.

Jacob, S. (1992). The spleen, bone marrow and thymus. In A. Rogers (Eds.), *Textbook of anatomy.* New York: Churchill Livingstone.

Jaiyesimi, I., Kantarjian, H., & Estey, E. (1993). Advances in therapy for hairy cell leukemia. *Cancer, 72,* 1, 5-13.

Jansen, J. & Hermans, J. (1982). Clinical staging system for hairy-cell leukemia. *Blood, 60*(3), 571-77.

Kipps, T. J. & Robbins, B. A. (1995). Hairy-cell leukemia. In E. Beutler, M. A. Lichtman, B. S. Coller, & T. J. Kipps (Eds.), *William's hematology* (5th ed.). New York: McGraw-Hill.

Lenhard, R., Lawrence, W. & McKenna, R. (1995). General approach to the patient. In G. Murphy, W. Lawrence, & R. Lenhard (Eds.). *American Cancer Society textbook of clinical oncology* (2nd ed.). Atlanta: American Cancer Society.

Male, D. (1986). *Immunology: an illustrated outline.* Toronto: Mosby.

Migone, N., Guibellino, M., Casorati, G., Tassinari, A., Lauria. F. & Foa, R. (1987). Configuration of the immunoglobulin and T cell receptor gene regions in hairy cell leukemia and B-chronic lymphocytic leukemia. *Leukemia, 1,* 393-94.

Mitus, A. & Rosenthal, D. (1995). The adult leukemias. In G. Murphy, W. Lawrence, & R. Lenhard (Eds.), *American Cancer Society textbook of clinical oncology.* Atlanta: American Cancer Society.

Nelson, M. (1993). New therapies for the anemia of chemotherapy and hairy cell leukemia (Monograph). Beachwood, Ohio: Pro Ed Communications.

Oleske, D., Golumb, H., Farber, M., & Levy, P. (1985). A case control study into the etiology of hairy cell leukemia. *American Journal of Epidemiology, 121,* 675-83.

Pui, C. (1995). Childhood leukemias. In G. Murphy, W. Lawrence, & R. Lenhard (Eds). *American Cancer Society textbook of clinical oncology.* Atlanta: American Cancer Society.

Rogers, A. (1992). *Textbook of anatomy.* New York: Churchill Livingstone.

Saven, A. & Piro, L. (1993). 2-chlorodeoxyadenosine in the treatment of hairy cell leukemia. *Cancer Investigation, 11,* 5, 559-564.

Saven, A. & Piro, L. (1994). Newer purine analogues for the treatment of hairy-cell leukemia. *New England Journal of Medicine, 330,* 10, 691-696.

Saven, A. & Piro, L. (1992). Treatment of hairy cell leukemia. *Blood, 79,* 5, 111-1120.

Seeley, R., Stephens, T., & Tate, P. (1991). *Essentials of anatomy and physiology* St. Louis: Mosby.

Sherwood, L. (1993). *Human physiology: From cells to systems* (2nd ed.). St. Paul: West.

Staines, A. & Cartwright, R. (1993). Hairy cell leukemia: a descriptive epidemiology and a case-control study. *British Journal of Haematology, 85,* 714-17.

Visser, L., Shaw, A., Slupsky, J., Vos, H., & Poppema, S. (1989). Monoclonal antibodies reactive with hairy cell leukemia. *Blood, 74,* 1, 320-5.

Wujcik, D. (1997). Leukemia. In S. W. Groenwald, M. H. Frogge, M. Goodman, & C. H. Yarbro (Eds), *Cancer nursing* (4th ed.). Boston: Jones and Bartlett.

Yarbro, J. (1997). Carcinogenesis. In S. L. Groenwald, M. H. Frogge, N. Goodman, & C. H. Yarbro (Eds). *Cancer nursing* (4th ed.). Boston: Jones and Bartlett.

Myelodysplastic Syndromes

Ellen W. Leum, ARNP, MSN, OCN
Susan Rudder Randolph, RN, MSN, CS

EPIDEMIOLOGY

Myelodysplasia, or myelodysplastic syndrome (MDS), encompasses a group of rare hematologic disorders. Characteristic features of MDS include hyperproliferative and ineffective hematopoiesis, resulting in peripheral blood cytopenias of one or more cell lineages and an increased risk of transformation into acute myeloblastic leukemia (AML).

Over 80% of patients diagnosed with MDS are over 60 years of age (Utley, 1996). The overall incidence of MDS is 2 to 4 per 100,000 each year, with a steep rise in the elderly population. The incidence rate for persons over 70 years is 20 to 30 per 100,000 each year, demonstrating that MDS is a common hematologic finding in this age group (Aul, Gattermann, & Schneider, 1995). Median survival rates are listed in Table 60-1.

MDS is rare in children, and true incidence is unknown but believed to be approximately 3% of all pediatric hematologic malignancies (Locatelli, Zecca, Pession, Maserati, DeStefano, & Severi, 1995). Approximately 17% of all pediatric AML cases are believed to have had a previous myelodysplastic phase (Locatelli et al., 1995). Significant differences exist in the classification, progression, and cytogenetic findings of pediatric MDS compared with adult MDS. The median age for presentation in children is 6 years, with a 16% probability of survival 3 years after the diagnosis (Hasle, 1994).

MDS primarily occurs de novo but may develop as a secondary or treatment-related condition from prior chemotherapy or radiation treatment. It predominately affects male adults and female children (Cole, Sateren, & Delzell, 1995; Hasle, 1994).

The incidence of secondary MDS is increasing, and several factors contribute to this trend (Kantarjian, Estey, & Keating, 1993). First, there are increased survival rates for cancer patients treated with both conventional chemotherapy and radiation therapy, as well bone marrow transplantation. There are expanding indications for the use of autologous transplantation, increasing the numbers of persons exposed to marrow ablative chemotherapy preparative regimens (Kelley, 1996). Rates of treatment-related or secondary MDS are estimated between 2% and 10% and depend on the dose, duration, and type of chemotherapeutic agent (Ballen & Antin, 1993). In addition, close follow-up of oncology patients allows for early detection of MDS before AML transformation.

The exact reason the incidence of primary MDS is increasing remains unclear. However, the increasing age of the general population, clinical awareness, and exposure to environmental or occupational carcinogens may explain part of the increased incidence.

RISK FACTORS

The exact cause of MDS is unknown. The major risk factors associated with the development of MDS are listed in Box 60-1. The evidence supporting each of these risk factors is reviewed, and the nursing implications for prevention and early detection activities are discussed.

Increasing Age

As previously stated, MDS is seen with increased frequency in the elderly. Exact age-dependent changes in the hematopoietic system are unknown. However, it is theorized that with increased aging, there is a reduction in the size of the stem cell pool, compromising the marrow reserve and increasing proliferative activity. The remaining cells may be vulnerable to mutagenic insults. In addition, immunologic attacks on stem cells, mitochondrial deoxyribonucleic acid (DNA) mutations, and other regulatory influences on the microenvironment may contribute to early stages of MDS (Aul, Gattermann, & Schneider, 1995).

Occupational Exposure

Epidemiologic studies have attempted to determine environmental and occupational risk factors in the development of leukemia. Historically, exposure to the chemical benzene has been strongly linked with the development of hematologic abnormalities and malignancies (Ballen & Antin,

Table 60-1 Myelodysplastic Syndrome—Median Survival and Incidence of Leukemic Progression

MDS Subtype	Subtype Abbreviation	Median Survival (Months)	Survival Range (Months)	Percentage Developing Leukemic Progression
Refractory anemia	RA	50	18-64	12
Refractory anemia with ringed sideroblasts	RA-S RARS	51	14-76+	8
Refractory anemia with excess blasts	RAEB	11	7-16	44
Refractory anemia with excess blasts in transformation	RAEB-T	5	2.5-11	60
Chronic myelomonocytic leukemia	CMML	11	9-60+	14

Modified from Utley, S. (1996). Myelodysplastic syndromes. *Seminars in Oncology Nursing 12*(1), 52.

Box 60-1
Risk Factors for Development of Myelodysplasia

Increased Age
>60 years

Occupational Exposure
Radiation
Halogenated organic agents

Previous Treatment
Chemotherapeutic agents
Radiation therapy

Human Immunodeficiency Virus
HIV virus
Drug toxicity
Opportunistic infections

1993). West, Stafford, Farrow, & Jacobs (1995) did a case-control study of occupational and environmental exposures and myelodysplasia. Their findings added to the call for minimizing exposures to radiation and halogenated organics (West et al., 1995).

Previous Chemotherapy or Radiation Therapy

Secondary or treatment-related MDS commonly occurs 4 to 5 years after chemotherapy for bone marrow transplantation (BMT), Hodgkin's disease, and other cancers (Applebaum, 1994). Alkylating agents, high-dose chemotherapy (HDC), and prolonged treatment with chemotherapeutic agents and radiation therapy are factors that increase the risk of developing secondary MDS (Kantarjian, Estey, & Keating, 1993; Kelley, 1996; Utley, 1996). Close follow-up of these patients has assisted in the identification of these risk factors.

Human Immunodeficiency Virus Variant

Persons with human immunodeficiency virus (HIV) infection can exhibit a hematopoietic disorder characterized by dysmaturation and peripheral cytopenias, but without the propensity for leukemic transformation (Kouides & Bennett, 1992). This presentation is similar to primary MDS, and there are multiple risk factors contributing to the development of this condition, including the underlying HIV infection, drug toxicity, and opportunistic infection (Goasguen & Bennett, 1992; Utley, 1996).

Signs and Symptoms

Some patients are diagnosed with MDS without any obvious findings during the physical examination. However, 75% to 100% of the patients are symptomatic at the time of diagnosis and have signs and symptoms classically associated with the underlying cytopenias (Ballen & Antin, 1993).

Anemia. *Anemia,* defined as a hemoglobin less than 10 g/dl, is seen in 80% to 85% of patients (Ganser & Hoelzer, 1992). The anemia is normocytic or macrocytic, with a low reticulocyte count, and the erythrocytes may be disfigured and hypochromic (Greenberg, 1995). In addition, an elevated mean corpuscular volume (MCV) serves as a warning sign that damage to the stem cell has occurred and a person may be at risk for developing MDS (Ballen & Antin, 1993). Patients may exhibit clinical manifestations that include fatigue, malaise, weakness, shortness of breath, pallor, chest pain, rapid heart rate, dizziness, and fainting.

Thrombocytopenia. Thrombocytopenia, or a platelet count less than 100,000 mm^3, occurs in approximately 60% of patients (Greenberg, 1995). Patients with thrombocytopenia may experience increased bruising, petechiae, nose bleeds, bleeding gums, bloody stool, or hemorrhage from trauma.

Neutropenia. The absolute neutrophil count (ANC) is less than 1000 in 60% of newly diagnosed MDS patients, placing them at an increased risk of infection (Greenberg, 1995). Even in patients with normal white blood cell (WBC) counts, there is an increased infection rate believed to be caused by the functional abnormalities found in the neutrophils of MDS patients (Ganser & Hoelzer, 1992). Fever is the predominant clinical presentation, and bacterial infections due to normal host flora are common (Utley, 1996).

Other Clinical Manifestations. Fewer than 20% of patients exhibit splenomegaly or hepatomegaly at the time of the diagnosis, and approximately 10% of patients with MDS exhibit a rheumatic phenomenon (Applebaum, 1994; Castro, Conn, & Su, 1991). These clinical findings include cutaneous vasculitis, lupus-like syndrome, and other neuropathies (Utley, 1996).

CHEMOPREVENTION ACTIVITIES

There are currently no chemoprevention activities for this particular disease. However, close monitoring of patients previously treated for oncologic diseases has led to early detection of secondary MDS.

PATHOPHYSIOLOGY

Normal Anatomy and Physiology of the Hematopoietic System

The human hematopoietic system is made up of various precursor and mature, functional components, including the erythrocytes, leukocytes, and thrombocytes. These mature cells are responsible for carrying out the functions of the human blood–producing and immune systems. These activities include carrying oxygen throughout the body to all cells, forming clots, and fighting off infection and invasion from foreign antigens.

One of the unique and amazing features of the hematopoietic system is that all of these cell lines are derived from the same basic cell, known as the *stem cell.* The stem cell is pluripotent, able to self-replicate, and responsible for replication and differentiation of all the cell lines. There are two theories on how the pluripotent stem cell differentiates. Some researchers believe external influences (e.g., hormones) dictate stem cell development, whereas others believe it is a random process (Golde, 1991). In either case, the stem cell initially divides into the myeloid and lymphoid cell lines.

The myeloid cell line further differentiates into the erythrocytes, thrombocytes, and phagocytic leukocytes (neutrophils, basophils, eosinophils, monocytes, and macrophages). The lymphoid cell line differentiates into B lymphocytes and T lymphocytes, which are responsible for the humoral and cell-mediated components of the immune system. Each of the mature cells produced from the parent stem cell pool plays an integral role, and disruption or alterations of any individual or all these cell lines can result in life-threatening illness.

The Process of MDS

MDS is believed to be caused by a malignant transformation at or close to the point of stem cell differentiation, resulting in myeloid and lymphoid cell lines arising from an altered clone (Tefferi, Thibodeau, & Solbert, 1990). There is some debate about this theory because some studies evaluating the expression of chromosomal abnormalities (e.g., karyotyping and fluorescent in situ hybridization) have not found abnormal karyotype in the lymphoid cells (Weimar, Bourhis, De Gast, & Gerritsen, 1994). However, experiments with X-linked restriction fragment length polymorphism (RFLP) have demonstrated clonal deletions in all cell lineages, indicating that MDS is a stem cell disorder, and these results have been duplicated through molecular biologic techniques such as polymerase chain reaction (PCR) (Weimar et al., 1994). The lesions responsible for the initial alteration in the disease process are unknown, and further cytogenetic and molecular biologic studies will assist in providing the answer to the exact fundamental pathogenesis of MDS.

The pathophysiology of MDS is therefore characterized by the expansion of an abnormal clone, which leads to dysmaturation of cell lines and pancytopenia. The following abnormalities may be detected on microscopic evaluation of the marrow: dyserythropoiesis with ringed sideroblasts, dysgranulopoiesis with hypogranulation, dysmegakaryocytopoiesis with micromegakaryocytes, and Auer rods (Applebaum, 1994). MDS has the propensity to progress into AML in approximately 20% to 30% of cases (Locatelli et al., 1995).

Diagnosis

The diagnosis of MDS is based on laboratory studies, morphologic features, cytogenetic studies, and molecular biologic techniques. A complete blood count (including differential, platelet, and reticulocyte counts), peripheral blood smear, bone marrow aspirate, and biopsy are necessary tests and procedures to determine the diagnosis, and cytogenetic and molecular studies can assist in determining the prognosis (Utley, 1996).

Differentiation Between MDS and Myeloproliferative Disorders

It is important to differentiate between myelodysplastic and myeloproliferative disorders. Myeloproliferative disorders include polycythemia vera, essential thrombocytosis, agnogenic myeloid metaplasia with myelofibrosis, and juvenile chronic myeloid leukemia, and are characterized by a progressive increase of a single-lineage hematopoietic cell, increasing peripheral blood counts. This slow expansion increases the affected myeloid cell line and can develop into a myeloid blast crisis (Applebaum, 1994). MDS, on the other hand, is multilineage, is clonal, and results in cytopenias.

Chromosomal Abnormalities Associated with MDS

There are cytogenetic abnormalities reported in approximately 55% to 60% of all patients who have MDS (Hoagland, 1995). The feature primarily seen is loss of genetic material as a result of deletion or chromosomal monosomy. The most common deletions are reported in chromosomes 5, 7, and 20. Deletions have been reported less frequently in chromosomes 11, 12, and 13 (Boultwood & Fidler, 1995).

ROUTES OF METASTASES

One of the classic features of MDS is its propensity to develop into AML. The risk of AML transformation depends on the MDS subtype and may take weeks to months to occur. Table 60-1 lists each MDS subtype and the percentage that transforms into AML.

ASSESSMENT OF THE PATIENT

The assessment of the patient with MDS is summarized in Table 60-2. Clinical evaluation of patients with MDS includes a comprehensive description of their current illness or chief complaint for seeking care, a detailed review of present and past health status, a review of systems, and a physical examination. It is also important to obtain a list of the current medications the patient is taking for the treatment of other diseases. A thorough description of the chief complaint elicits the onset of signs and symptoms, their quality and quantity, aggravating or alleviating factors, interference with the ability to carry on activities of daily living, and the patient's interventions to alleviate symptoms. The type and severity of cytopenias and their subsequent clinical manifestations depend on the French-American-British (FAB) classification of MDS at the time of presentation. Prompted by subjective findings such as fatigue or malaise, as well as objective signs such as pallor, tachycardia, or petetchiae, nursing assessment and physical examination are directed at uncovering abnormalities of the hematopoietic system. A complete blood count with differential, blood smears, and bone marrow aspiration establish abnormalities in cellular morphology. Subsequent cytogenetic studies of the bone marrow reveal abnormal cellular karotypes that confirm the diagnosis.

History

A thorough review of systems includes data collection about the patient's physical systems, functional status, and social systems (i.e., occupational history and recreational activities or hobbies). Social systems data can provide additional information about identified risk factors for MDS that may not be obtained during a routine review of systems intake. Age is a primary risk factor that should not be overlooked. The incidence of MDS increases significantly with age. The overall incidence of MDS is about 2 to 4 people per 100,000 each year. However, after the age of 70 years, incidence rates increase to approximately 20 to 30 people per 100,000 each year (Aul, Gattermann, & Schneider, 1995).

A variety of medications alter platelet production or function and therefore can exacerbate platelet dysfunction in patients with MDS. They include classes of antimicrobial medications, such as penicillin and cephalosporins, antiinflammatory agents, and over-the-counter products containing aspirin (Lin & Beddar, 1996). The patient's current medication profile, along with his or her past medication history, is an important part of the health history. Adequate nutritional intake is essential for the functioning hematopoietic system.

A detailed review of the hematopoietic system investigates the incidence of bleeding tendencies, bruising, history of infection, and exposure to radiation and other occupational or environmental hazards. Dyshemopoiesis of platelet, red blood cell, and granulocyte cell lines is a prevalent characteristic of all subtypes of MDS. Nurses must be aware of the implications; the signs and symptoms related to anemia, granulocytopenia, or thromboctyopenia; and other factors that affect the function, replication, and maturation of hematopoietic stem cells.

Fatigue, weakness, bleeding, bruising, or recurrent infections are common symptoms of MDS (Ballen & Antin, 1993). Nonspecific complaints of malaise suggest a problem with erythropoiesis, as well as the potential for refractory anemia (RA) or refractory anemia with ringed sideroblasts (RARS). Patient reports of recurrent infection and bleeding imply potential problems associated with severe neutropenia and thrombocytopenia. Data collection regarding alterations in the gastrointestinal, genitourinary, and pulmonary systems can lead to positive findings that support dyshematopoiesis. Clinical manifestations such as abdominal pain, diarrhea, dysuria, and shortness of breath can be signs of underlying infection. Patients with clinical findings of severe pancytopenia often have more aggressive forms of MDS, such as refractory anemia with excess blasts (RAEB), refractory anemia with excess blasts in transformation (RAEB-t), or chronic myelomonocytic leukemia (CMML).

Physical Examination

Physical examination of the patient with MDS is organized from a head-to-toe body direction to determine clinical findings associated with ineffective multipotent stem cell hematopoiesis. It is not focused in one organ or organ system. Instead, the examination follows a multisystem approach, using a combination of examination techniques (i.e., inspection, palpation, auscultation, and percussion). Symptomatic patients should be assessed relative to life-threatening versus non–life-threatening cytopenias and age. Key assessment parameters center on the patient's risk for infection, bleeding, and anemia, as well as the manifestation of their respective signs and symptoms, throughout the all-body system. The appearance of signs and symptoms apparent at the time of the physical examination depends on the type of MDS and the degree of disease progression.

General inspection begins with observing the patient while the clinician explains what interactions will be occurring during the patient visit (Barkauskas, Bauman, Stolenberg-Allen, & Fisher-Darling, 1994). The examiner notes an overall impression presented by the patient's appearance relative to chronologic age, nutritional status, posture and gait, affect, and general state of health. The examiner can quickly assess whether the patient is in acute distress or chronically ill.

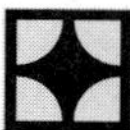

TABLE 60-2 Assessment of the Patient with Myelodysplastic Syndrome

	Assessment Parameters	Typical Abnormal Findings
History	A. Personal and social history	A. Personal and social risk factors
	1. Age	1. Usually greater than 70 years old.
	2. Past health history	2. History of cancer, cancer treatment with alkylating chemotherapeutic agents, topoisomerase inhibitors, HIV infection.
	3. Occupational or environmental exposure	3. Exposure to radiation, benzene compounds at work or exposure during leisure activity.
	B. Evaluation of hematopoietic system	B. Common symptoms include malaise, fatigue, dizziness, lightheadedness, fever, bleeding tendencies, bruising.
Physical Examination	A. Inspection	A. Clinical manifestations of anemia, thrombocytopenia, and infection depend on the MDS subtype, the affected stem cell line, and the disease progression.
	1. Skin	1. Pallor, cyanotic nail beds, bruising of extremities, petechiae, localized erythema, lesions, inflammation, exudate.
	2. Oral cavity	2. Pale mucous membranes and hard palate, erythema inflammation or exudate of buccal mucosa, tonsillar arches, bleeding gums.
	3. Eyes	3. Pale conjunctiva, scleral hemorrhage, exudate.
	4. Lungs	4. Increased respiratory rate, shortness of breath, asymmetric respiratory movements.
	B. Palpation	
	1. Skin	1. Cool, clammy, localized warmth or tenderness.
	2. Radial pulses	2. Hyperkinetic: bounding, or hypokinetic, thready and weak, irregular.
	3. Frontal & maxillary sinuses	3. Pain, tenderness.
	4. Liver	4. Palpable below the right anterior costal margin.
	5. Spleen	5. Palpable below the left anterior costal margin.
	6. Lungs	6. Increased tactile fremitus with pneumonia, decreased tactile fremitus with pneumothorax.
	C. Auscultation	
	1. Lungs	1. Adventitious, increased, decreased, or absent breath sounds.
	2. Heart (apical impulse)	2. Presence of extra heart sounds, dysrhythmias, murmurs.
	D. Vital signs	D. Increase in temperature, pulse, or respiration, and an increased or decreased blood pressure with infection, anemia, or bleeding.
Diagnostic Tests	A. Complete blood count (CBC), differential, reticulocyte count	A. Peripheral cytopenias in one or more cell lines are a classic feature of MDS. Anemia, along with thrombocytopenia or neutropenia, may be evident at diagnosis.
	1. Hemoglobin (Hgb)	1. A Hgb level <10 g/dl is a common finding. • Normal Hgb values: Adult males: 14-18 g/dl Adult females: 12-16 g/dl Children (1-10 years): 11-16 g/dl
	2. Red blood cell (RBC) indices	2. RBC mean cell volume (MCV) can be increased >100. • Normal MCV range 76-99.
	3. Reticulocyte count	3. A decreased reticulocyte count (<0.5%) is common with MDS. Normal reticulocyte values: • Adults: 0.5%-1.5% • Children 2.0%-6.0%
	4. White blood cell (WBC) count & differential	4. WBCs may be normal or decreased (less than 4500/mm^3) except in the CMML subtype.
	5. Neutrophils	5. An absolute neutrophil count of <1000 is common.
	6. Monocytes	6. A monocyte count of greater than 1000 μ/l is a feature associated with chronic myelomonocytic leukemia. • Normal monocyte range: 200-1000 μ/l.
	7. Platelets	7. Platelet count can be normal (150,000-400,000/mm^3) or decreased (less than 100,000/mm^3).

Continued

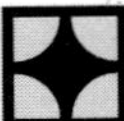

TABLE 60-2 Assessment of the Patient with Myelodysplastic Syndrome—cont'd

	Assessment Parameters	Typical Abnormal Findings
Diagnostic Tests—cont'd	B. Vitamin or nutritional deficiencies	
	1. Folate	1. Adequate levels of folate (3-14 ng/nl) are essential for the production of RBCs. Inadequate folate can result in decreased RBC production and anemia.
	2. Vitamin B12	2. Adequate levels of vitamin B12 (200-800 pg/ml) are necessary for the production of RBCs. A vitamin B12 deficiency can contribute to anemia.
	C. Bone marrow aspiration	
	1. Cellularity	1. Bone marrow cellularity is usually increased; occasionally, it is decreased.
	2. Morphology	2. Dysplastic changes in hematopoeitic precursors are characteristic of MDS.
	• Refractory anemia (RA)	• Bone marrow contains less than 5% leukemic blasts.
	• Refractory anemia with ringed sideroblasts (RARS)	• Bone marrow is composed of 15% or more of ringed sideroblasts.
	• Refractory anemia with excess blasts (RAEB)	• Bone marrow consists of 5%-20% leukemia blasts.
	• Refractory anemia with excess blasts in transformation (RAEB-t)	• Bone marrow consists of greater than 20% but not more than 30% leukemic blasts and contains Auer rods.
	• Chronic myelomonocytic leukemia (CMMOL)	• Bone marrow contains less than 20% leukemic blasts.
	D. Cytogenetics	D. The incidence of chromosomal aberrations differs with primary and secondary MDS. The translocation of genetic material usually involves chromosomes 8, 17, 11, 12, and 21, whereas chromosomes 5 and 7 are deleted (Utley, 1996).

Focused examination begins with obtaining a baseline set of vital signs. Vital signs are indicators of normal body function (Barkauskas et al., 1994). They represent internal homeostasis and reveal the patient's overall general well-being. Alterations in vital signs can reveal problems associated with infection, hypovolemia, and bleeding. All skin surfaces and mucous membranes should be inspected for color, lesions, petechiae, bruising, eccyhmosis, erythema, and exudate. The skin assessment includes palpation for temperature, turgor, pain, and tenderness. Pale, cool, or clammy skin may indicate complications associated with anemia or infection. It is important to keep in mind that patients with severe neutropenia may not exhibit the classic signs and symptoms of infection (i.e., erythema, swelling, pain, and purulence). Examine the lips, total buccal mucosa, gums, tongue, sublingual area, hard and soft palate, and tonsillar area for color, characteristics, and condition. Note any lesions, exudate, erythema, inflammation, and tenderness. Inspect the outer chamber of the eye for inflammation, drainage, and signs of bleeding. Sclera are typically white. Conjunctiva may appear pale, rather than pink or red, due to anemia.

Nail beds should be observed for cyanosis and tested for capillary refill. The presence of sluggish capillary refill can be associated with an abnormally low red blood cell (RBC) volume. Alterations in cardiopulmonary status are apparent due to the body's inability to compensate for decreased RBC production or function. Initially, tachycardia, exertional dyspnea, and palpitation may be evident. As the level of hemoglobin decreases, clinical manifestations of chronic oxygen deficiency are obvious in multiple body systems. Signs and symptoms of severe anemia (hemoglobin less than or equal to 7 g/dl) are outlined in Table 60-3.

Clinicians should palpate the radial pulse and auscultate the apical pulse. The pulse rate rhythm and amplitude should be documented. The heart rate is increased during fever, anemia, hypoxia, and low-volume states (shock). Dysrhythmias, cardiac murmurs, or a third heart sound (S_3) may be present. An S_3 heart sound can occur with high cardiac output conditions such as anemia (Barkauskas et al., 1994).

Pulmonary inspection should note the rate, quality, and symmetry of respiration. Pulmonary assessment includes auscultation of the lungs for adventitious breath sounds. The presence of rales, rhonchi, or decreased breath sounds suggests the potential for infection. Hepatomegaly and splenomegaly occur in less than 20% to 25% of patients with MDS (Applebaum, 1994; Ganser & Hoelzer, 1992). However, the abdomen should be palpated to determine the presence or absence of hepatosplenomegaly. Lymphadenopathy is not usually present.

TABLE 60-3 Signs and Symptoms of Severe Anemia

Body System	Signs/Symptoms
Cardiovascular	Systolic ejection murmur Palpitations at rest Exercise intolerance Respiratory Dyspnea at rest
Skin/mucous membranes	Hypersensitivity to cold Pallor
Central nervous system	Dizziness Headaches Irritability Difficulty sleeping or concentrating
Gastrointestinal system	Anorexia Indigestion
Genitourinary system	Menstrual problems Male impotence

Modified from *Clinical Advances in Anemia (Epoetin alfa).* (1995). Raritan, NJ: Ortho Biotech.

Diagnostic Tests

Complete Blood Count with Differential. A complete blood count (CBC) with differential enumerates and identifies hematopoeitic cells circulating in the peripheral blood produced by the bone marrow. The presence of MDS can dramatically alter the number and function of circulating peripheral blood cells. The severity of the effect on peripheral cytopenias and the hematopoietic cell line depends on the MDS subtype and level of disease progression.

Hemoglobin. Hemoglobin levels are measured to determine the oxygen-carrying capacity of blood and to assess for anemia. Anemia is diagnosed when a decreased hemoglobin, hematocrit, or erythrocyte count is detected. Decreased hemoglobin levels can be the result of marrow failure, hemolysis, hemorrhage, and vitamin or nutritional deficiencies. Patients should be screened for vitamin B12 and folate deficiencies to rule out these anomalies as an underlying etiology for anemia.

Anemia is a universal symptom associated with all MDS subtypes. A hemoglobin level less than 10 g/dl is noted in greater than 80% of patients with MDS (Ganser & Hoelzer, 1992). Through microscopic inspection, RBCs may appear hypochromic and dysmorphic. The anemia of MDS may be classified as *normocytic* or *macrocytic* (Greenberg, 1995). Macrocytic anemia is characterized by an MCV of greater than 100, whereas patients with normocytic features reflect a normal MCV of 76 to 99 (Bakerman, 1994).

Reticulocyte count. The reticulocyte count is an index for erythropoiesis. A decreased reticulocyte count can result from a variety of conditions. The decreased production of reticulocytes is apparent with marrow dysplasia, replacement of erythroid precursors with leukemic blasts, toxins, infection, renal disease, and disorders of erythroid maturation (Bakerman, 1994). A decreased reticulocyte response is a common laboratory finding associated with MDS (Applebaum, 1994; Greenberg, 1995).

TABLE 60-4 Normal Number of Leukocytes and Percentage of Types of Leukocytes

Total Number of Leukocytes	4.5-11.0/mm³
Polymorphonuclear neutrophils	62.0%
Polymorphonuclear eosinophils	2.3%
Polymorphonuclear basophils	0.4%
Monocytes	5.3%
Lymphocytes	30.0%

From Bakerman, S. (1994). *ABC's of Interpretive Laboratory Data* (3rd ed.). Myrtle Beach, SC: Interpretive Laboratory Data; Chapman and Hall. (1996).

White Blood Cell/Leukocyte Count. The analysis of the total number of circulating WBCs (leukocytes) is useful in the evaluation myleodysplastic disorders, as well as in the diagnosis and management of infection and hematopoeitic malignancies. Adequate levels of leukocytes and a sufficient number of different types of WBCs are required to protect the body from invading antigens. There are six classifications of WBCs that are normally present in the blood. Table 60-4 outlines the normal percentages of the different types of WBCs.

The concentration of each type of WBC in the blood remains constant with homeostasis. With myelodysplastic syndrome the total number of WBCs can be altered, as can the functional properties of WBCs. The total number of circulating WBCs may be normal or diminished (less than 4500/mm^3) in all MDS subtypes, with the exception of the CMML subtype. With CMML the WBC is usually elevated (Utley, 1996).

Neutrophils. The total number of neutrophils (ANC) reflects the body's ability to fight infection. Neutrophils are derived from the myeloid lineage. Their major defensive property is the phagocytosis of bacteria, viruses, and other foreign antigens. A decrease in the number of blood neutrophils places patients at an increased risk of infection. An absolute neutrophil count of less than 1000 is common in approximately 60% of patients with MDS (Utley, 1996).

Monocytes. Monocytes comprise a small percentage of the myeloid leukocytes whose major function includes the mediation of the inflammatory response and phagocytosis. A monocyte count of greater than 1000 μ/l is a common feature associated with chronic myelomonocytic anemia.

Platelets. An essential requirement for normal hemostasis is the production of an adequate number of functional platelets. The primary function of platelets is the formation of a platelet plug at the site of injury to prevent bleeding. Thrombocytopenia (platelet count of less than 100,000) is a platelet anomaly that is the result of an aberrant production

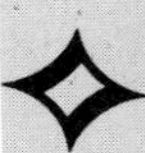

TABLE 60-5 Patient Preparation for the MDS Patient Receiving a Bone Marrow Aspiration/Biopsy

Description of the Procedure: Bone marrow aspiration and biopsy provide access to the hematopoietic cells in the marrow space where cellular proliferation, differentiation, and maturation occur. The posterior iliac crests are the most common sites for obtaining marrow samples. Marrow aspirate is examined for the number of hematopoietic cells present, their maturity level, and cytogenetic abnormalities.

Patient Preparation: In adults, usually no special instructions or interventions are required before a bone marrow aspiration/biopsy. However, pediatric patients are instructed to not take anything to eat or drink for several hours before the procedure if they will be receiving sedation or a short-acting general anesthesia. All patients should be instructed about the nature of the procedure and the potential discomfort they can experience during and after bone marrow aspiration and/or biopsy. It is important to teach patients how to care for the aspiration site, along with the reportable signs and symptoms of infection at the aspiration site.

Procedural Considerations:

1. Obtain informed consent.
2. Ascertain whether the patient has any allergies to medications or anesthetics.
3. The patient needs to disrobe below the waist or wear a gown.
4. The patient is assisted into a supine position.
5. The aspiration site (posterior iliac crest) is cleaned using betadine and alcohol swabs applied in concentric motions, working from the aspiration site outward.
6. A local anesthetic is injected into subcutaneous tissue and bone to alleviate pain and discomfort during the procedure.
7. After the site is numb, a large-gauge hollow needle is inserted into the subcutaneous tissue and twisted through the bone into the marrow cavity.
8. A syringe is attached to the hollow needle, and marrow is aspirated back and plated on glass slides.

Modified from Alkire, K. (1993). Physiology of bone marrow. In D. Wujcik (Ed.), *Nursing issues in adult acute leukemia.* Huntington, NY: PRR.

of platelets, or the deviation in the functional ability or quality of platelets (Lin & Beddar, 1996). In MDS, defective platelet maturation results in abnormal-sized megakaryocytes and thrombocytopenia. The platelet count is usually normal or diminished (less than 100,000/mm^3) in approximately 60% of patients with MDS (Greenberg, 1995).

Bone Marrow Aspiration and Biopsy. Bone marrow aspiration and biopsy is used to evaluate the cellularity and morphologic features of hematopoeitic components. The preparation of a patient for a bone marrow aspiration and biopsy is outlined in Table 60-5. Variations in the quantity of cellular elements and the form or structure of hematopoeitic cells signal bone marrow pathology that results in an array of clinical diseases. Bone marrow cellularity is usually increased in MDS due to clonal proliferation and neoplastic transformation of the multipotent stem cell and multilineage progenitor cells. Sometimes the bone marrow appears hypocellular (Applebaum, 1994). The MDS subtypes RA, RARS, RAEB, and RAEB-t display common characteristics. Morphologic alterations in the quality and quantity of erythropoeitic, granulocytic, and platelet precursors result in ringed sideroblasts, hypogranualtion, and micromegakaryocytes, respectively (Applebaum, 1994).

Cytogenetic analysis of somatic chromosomes in the bone marrow aspirate reveals multiple aberrations in patients with MDS and aids in characterizing a patient's prognosis. The translocation (transfer of a broken portion of a chromosome to a different part of the same or a different chromosome) of chromosomes 8, 17, 11, 12, and 21 and deletion (a loss of a chromosome in an otherwise paired diploid cell) of chromosomes 5, 7, and 20 are common cytogenetic features associated with MDS (Kelley, 1996; Boultwood & Fidler, 1995).

STAGING

The most widely recognized classification or staging system for MDS was developed in 1982 by the FAB Cooperative Group. It is based primarily on the presence and percentage of marrow blasts. This classification system is listed in Table 60-6. There are numerous criticisms of this system, including its lack of prognostic indicators, limited ability to

TABLE 60-6 Classification of Myelodysplastic Syndrome by The French-American-British (FAB) Cooperative Group (1982)

Classification (with Abbreviation)	Bone Marrow Blasts	Peripheral Blood Blasts	Ringed Sideroblasts >15% of Bone Marrow	Monocytes >1000 μl
Refractory anemia (RA)	<5%	<1%	Absent	Absent
Refractory anemia with ringed sideroblasts (RARS)	<5%	<1%	Present	Absent
Refractory anemia with excess blasts (RAEB)	5%-20%	<5%	Present or absent	Absent
Refractory anemia with excess blasts in transformation (RAEB-T)	20%-30% (or RAEB + Auer rods)	<5% (may have Auer rods)	Present or absent	Present or absent
Chronic myelomonocytic leukemia (CMML)	≤20%	mt5%	Present or absent	Present

categorize all patients (especially pediatric patients), and inclusion of CMML, which some researchers believe should be classified under chronic myeloproliferative disorders (Taylor, Rodwell, Taylor, & Seeley, 1994; Applebaum, 1994; Kouides & Bennett, 1992). Despite these criticisms, this classification system remains the most universally accepted staging mechanism for MDS.

MEDICAL MANAGEMENT

Factors that must be considered when choosing a treatment option are disease subtype, patient age, and whether symptoms are life threatening. No single or combination treatment, aside from supportive care, has emerged as the standard of care for the MDS patient. Although other therapies such as chemotherapy, hematopoietic growth factor (HGF), and interferons have been used with varying degrees of success, supportive care has been and continues to be the hallmark of medical management.

Supportive Care

Antimicrobial therapy, hemotherapy, patient monitoring, education, and anticipatory guidance are primary supportive care interventions. These interventions are primarily aimed at alleviating or managing complications arising from peripheral cytopenias.

Symptomatic thrombocytopenia and anemia are managed with platelet and packed red blood cell (PRBC) transfusions. Parameters for transfusions vary among centers. However, indications for PRBC transfusions may include symptomatic anemia alone or with a hemoglobin less than 8 g/dl. Platelets are indicated for active bleeding, prophylactically if less than 10,000 mm^3, or prior to an invasive procedure if less than 50,000 mm^3 (Utley, 1996). Supportive care requirements for patients requiring hemotherapy include close monitoring of complete blood counts with differential, platelet, and reticulocyte counts; liver function tests; viral titers; serum iron levels; and other organ functions studies (e.g., echocardiogram).

Patients may require irradiated, cytomegalovirus (CMV)-negative, or leukocyte-depleted blood products. Irradiation prevents transfusion-related graft-versus-host disease in an immunocompromised patient, and CMV screening prevents transmission of CMV to a CMV-negative patient. Leukodepletion is important, especially in patients with high transfusion requirements or candidates for bone marrow transplantation (BMT), to decrease exposure to foreign antigens and prevent antibody development (Utley, 1996).

Patients requiring long-term use of PRBCs may develop iron overload in numerous organ systems, including the heart, liver, spleen, and pancreas. Administration of an iron-chelating agent (e.g., defersoamine) may be required to prevent significant organ dysfunction.

Leukocyte transfusions are not part of hemotherapy for neutropenic MDS patients. Patients and family members are taught signs and symptoms of infections, and the appropriate antimicrobial therapy is administered when infections arise. There is no consensus on the use of prophylactic antimicrobial therapies.

Hematopoietic Growth Factors

One of the newer treatment modalities for MDS is HGF. Erythropoietin (EPO), granulocyte-macrophage colony stimulating factor (GM-CSF), granulocyte colony-stimulating factor (G-CSF), and interleukin-3 (IL-3) have been used individually or in combination with varying response rates.

EPO has been most effective in treating the RA or RARS subtypes, with 20% to 30% of patients treated exhibiting decreased transfusion requirements or becoming red cell independent (Stein, 1994). EPO administration involves subcutaneous injections daily or three times a week with minimal toxicity (Mittelman & Lessin, 1994).

GM-CSF has been the most extensively studied agent, demonstrating an increase in granulocyte counts in up to 80% of patients treated (Greenberg, 1995). Up to 15% of patients also have an increase in platelet and reticulocyte counts with a decrease in RBC transfusion requirements (Applebaum, 1994). Unfortunately, these hematopoietic effects are limited in duration to approximately 6 months and are associated with adverse effects, including skin rash, bone pain, and general malaise (Utley, 1996).

G-CSF studies suggest similar results in increasing neutrophil function. However, there have been minimal to no responses in the other cell lines. Bone pain and headaches are the most commonly reported side effects, and treatment is generally well tolerated. A few IL-3 studies have shown increased granulocytes, but unlike the other HGF, considerable side effects have affected patient compliance (Ganser, Seipelt, & Lindemann, 1990).

Several issues are important to consider with the use of HGF for the treatment of MDS. The first is the high cost associated with the pharmaceutical agents related to the variable response rates. Second are the questions concerning the possible acceleration of AML progression with HGF use. Patients treated with greater than 15% blasts in their bone marrow have exhibited an increase in marrow blasts (Applebaum, 1994). This trend usually reverses when treatment is discontinued. Despite these issues, HGF remains an area for medical research, and newer agents or combination therapy may provide a more adequate, long-term treatment.

Differentiation-Inducing Agents

Agents such as 13-Cis retinoic acid (13-CRA), all-trans-retinoic acid (ATRA), and vitamin D analogues have been used in MDS treatment clinical trials. These agents are believed to promote hematopoietic cell maturation. Minimal responses of short duration were noted in 20% of patients treated in studies with 13-CRA (Koeffler, Heitjan, & Mertelsmann, 1988). Similar results were reported in studies using ARTA (Aul, Runde, & Gattermann, 1993). One study evaluated the use of alfacalcidol, a vitamin D analogue. The results indicated no improvement in blood counts, and hypercalcemia was a significant side effect (Yoshida, Oguma, & Uchino, 1993). The future use of differentiating agents is unknown, and current clinical trials are evaluating the effectiveness as part of combination therapy (Utley, 1996).

Interferons

Interferons (alpha and gamma) have been used in clinical trials to treat MDS. The treatment schedule is usually a subcutaneous injection three times a week, with fever, chills, and general malaise as primary side effects. Similar to HGF, there have been transient elevations in blood counts in 30% to 50% of patients, and further research is warranted (Utley, 1996).

Hormone Therapy

Hormone therapy has been used in the MDS population with limited success. Corticosteroid treatment has yielded minimal response with an increased rate of infection and is currently not indicated for use in MDS (Cheson, 1990). Androgen therapy, most notably danazole (a synthetic androgen), has been found to improve platelet counts in a small percentage of MDS patients who are moderately thrombocytopenic and have less than 20% bone marrow blasts (Cines, Cassileth, & Kiss, 1985). The exact action of danazole is unknown, and the future role of hormone therapy for this disease process is uncertain.

Chemotherapy

Numerous protocols have been tried using chemotherapeutic agents to treat MDS. These treatments range from single low-dose therapy to aggressive antileukemic therapy using multiple agents.

Cytosine arabinoside (ara-C) has been extensively studied as a continuous infusion or as a subcutaneous low-dose treatment. Overall, a summary of this treatment demonstrates a 16% complete response (CR) and 20% partial response (PR), with a 10% mortality rate related to therapy. One randomized trial compared low-dose ara-C with supportive care, and no difference in survival was noted in the treatment group (Cheson, Jasperse, Simon, & Friedman, 1986).

Other single agents studied recently include homoharringtonne and 5-azacytidine. The results of the homoharringtonne trial yielded high toxicities and concluded that the treatment doses in this study were not recommended (Feldman, Seiter, Ahmed, Baskind, & Arlin, 1996). 5-Azacytidine was administered subcutaneously daily for 7 days and repeated every 28 days. Early results in this study demonstrate a trilineage response of 31% and 38% in high-risk patients (RAEB and RAEB-t) surviving at 2 years (Silverman, Holland, Demakos, Mandeli, Castro-Malaspina, & Gattani et al., 1995). Currently, phase III trials are testing these observations.

Aggressive combination AML induction chemotherapeutic protocols have had CR rates between 13% and 52%, with the duration of response averaging 12 months (Applebaum, 1994). The best responders to therapy are younger patients with primary MDS.

There are numerous issues associated with the use of chemotherapy, most notably the average age of the patients at the time of diagnosis. MDS primarily affects the geriatric population and often has an indolent course. These factors often preclude the use of aggressive treatment because there is usually low tolerance, poor marrow recovery, and a short response to therapy (Greenberg, 1995).

Bone Marrow/Stem Cell Transplantation

Allogeneic bone marrow transplantation is the only known curative treatment for MDS with an event-free survival ranging from 40% to 67% (Applebaum, 1994). There are currently a few prospective studies evaluating the use of autologous bone marrow or peripheral blood stem cell transplantation after a patient has achieved a remission (DeWitte, 1994). Unfortunately, with a predominately elderly population, age and functional status do not permit extensive use of this therapy.

For younger MDS patients, selection criteria, timing of the transplant, conditioning regimens, and complications are significant concerns. Patients who are physiologically and psychologically fit and are under the age of 55 to 60 years are candidates for BMT, especially if they have high-risk disease. This includes patients with a predicted survival of less than 1 year, greater than 10% bone marrow blasts, less than 40,000 mm^3 platelets, or less than 1,000 granulocytes (Applebaum, 1994). Research has demonstrated that patients with the best outcome are those who have a shorter time between the diagnosis and the transplant, and those receiving transplants in remission or early-disease stages (DeWitte, 1994; Applebaum, 1994; Utley, 1996). Donor availability is an issue, and human leukocyte antigen (HLA)-matched sibling donors are the ideal source of donor stem cells (Uberti, 1994). There have also been successes using HLA-matched unrelated donors, as well as one-antigen mismatched-related donors (Fung, Shepherd, Nantel, Spinelli, Sutherland, & Klingemann et al., 1995). Conditioning regimens vary, but there is a consensus that marrow ablative therapy is necessary to achieve disease control (DeWitte, 1994). Cyclophosphamide (CY) and total body irradiation (TBI) have been the most extensively used protocols. However, due to a high rate of disease recurrence with RAEB and RAEB-t subtypes and increasing numbers of treatment-related or secondary MDS, several nonradiotherapy regimens or triple-agent regimens have been trialed. Bulsulfan/cyclophosphamide (BU/CY) and bulsulfan, cytosine arabinoside, and cyclophosphamide (BAC) have both been successful as pretransplant conditioning, especially for patients who have previously received dose-limiting radiation therapy (Uberti, 1994; O'Donnell, Long, Parker, Niland, Nademanee, & Amylon et al., 1995). In addition, cytosine arabinoside, bulsulfan, and etoposide have been added to CY/TBI regimens to decrease disease recurrence.

Despite the type of conditioning regimen used for transplantation, there is significant treatment toxicity. There is a 25% to 45% incidence of treatment-related death from interstitial pneumonia, graft-versus-host disease, or disease recurrence (Applebaum, 1994). Veno-occlusive disease (VOD) is another significant side effect, especially for patients treated for secondary MDS (O'Donnell et al., 1995). The use of transplantation, therefore, must be measured against supportive care, prognosis, and its place in the continuum of MDS treatment measured on an individual patient basis.

ONCOLOGIC EMERGENCIES

Life-threatening emergencies associated with MDS are infection and hemorrhage (Utley, 1996). These complications are directly related to the pancytopenia seen in MDS. Fever is the hallmark symptom of infection, and uncontrolled bleeding, usually from trauma or an invasive procedure, is the classic sign of hemorrhage. Unfortunately, these symptoms may precede the diagnosis, and appropriate medical interventions may be delayed.

If MDS transforms to AML, the patient is then at risk for the development of oncologic emergencies related to that diagnosis (e.g., tumor lysis syndrome). Refer to Chapter 11 for further discussion of these complications.

NURSING MANAGEMENT

The medical management of myelodysplastic disorders is extremely complex and variable. Treatment interventions are based on the MDS subtype, the patient's age, the degree of clinical disease progression, and the propensity for transformation to acute leukemia. Curative treatments are limited for patients with MDS. Low-dose cytarabine may be helpful in deterring disease progression, whereas intensive antileukemia chemotherapy may result in short-term disease remission (Greenberg, 1995; Juneja, Jodhani, Gardner, Trevarthen, & Schottstedt, 1994). Only allogeneic bone marrow transplantation offers the hope of a potential cure. The treatment options available for patients diagnosed with MDS include (1) supportive care, (2) allogeneic bone transplantation, and (3) clinical trials with cytotoxic agents, biologic therapy, or differentiation-inducing agents.

Supportive care interventions are the mainstay of treatment for patients with MDS due to the older patient's inability to tolerate toxicities associated with intensive chemotherapy or bone marrow transplantation. Most patients with MDS receive supportive care treatment in an ambulatory care setting, an outpatient department, or the physician's office or home. Patients are usually hospitalized for aggressive treatments such as bone marrow transplantation, intensive chemotherapy, or as the result of complications related to progressive cytopenias (i.e., infection or an acute bleeding episode). Nursing management of the patient with MDS integrates an understanding of the disease process, degree and type of marrow dysplasia associated with the MDS subtype, and treatment choices. Nursing care interventions depend on the type of medical management, disease progression, and health setting.

Patients with myelodysplastic syndrome have numerous problems that require nursing interventions and patient education. Upon initial diagnosis, nursing interventions assist patients and their significant others in understanding the clinical implications of MDS, the disease's trajectory, and available treatment options. Considerable time should be allotted to patients and families so they can assimilate the information and verbalize the potential effect on activities of daily living and their quality of life. As cytopenias progress or leukemia progression ensues, patients require knowledge about alternate treatment strategies and new medications, their potential risks and benefits, and efforts to minimize and manage complications.

There are a diverse number of treatment options available to patients with MDS. Each modality (i.e., supportive care, cytotoxic chemotherapy, allogeneic bone marrow transplantation, and clinical trials with new agents) imposes a particular perplexity for the patient. The outstanding problems are discussed in the following sections. Standards of care (Tables 60-7, 60-8, and 60-9) detail the nursing management of supportive care interventions, the use of hematopoietic growth factors, and blood component therapy.

Supportive Care

Hemotherapy, antimicrobial therapy, and the administration of growth factors are the cornerstones of supportive care interventions. The goals of supportive care focus on managing peripheral cytopenias and their complications (Utley, 1996). Patient problems vary, depending on the hematopoeitic cell lines that are affected and the subsequent development of anemia, thrombocytopenia, or neutropenia. Nursing management requires astute evaluation for infection, bleeding, and acute or chronic blood loss. Fever is a medical emergency. Patients require a thorough review of systems, blood, urine, and other cultures, and possibly a chest x-ray examination before antimicrobial therapy is initiated. Patients need to be closely monitiored for a response to antimicrobial therapy.

Interventions are aimed at early recognition of signs and symptoms of cytopenias and a prompt, appropriate course of action. Most supportive care measures are administered in an ambulatory care setting unless an acute event such as hemorrhage or infection precipitates hospitalization.

Hemotherapy. The potential complications of allogeneic blood component therapy pose significant immediate and delayed adverse effects. The immediate onset of platelet and red blood cell transfusion reactions such as fever and urticaria are manageable and usually void of negative sequelae. However, immediate reactions to red blood cell transfusion, such as respiratory distress, fluid volume overload, hemolytic transfusion reaction, and anaphylaxis, support significant life-threatening patient outcomes. The delayed complications of allogeneic blood component therapy are usually more insidious than immediate transfusion reactions. Late complications of hemotherapy include infection, alloimmunization, possible immunosuppression, graft versus host disease, and hemosiderosis (iron overload) with chronic RBC replacement. Although the literature describes a variety of numerical parameters for the automatic administration of packed red blood cells (PRBCs) and platelets in patients with MDS, the decision to transfuse patients with red blood cells or platelets should be carefully considered. General therapeuticprinciples for packed red blood cell transfusion, established by the American College of Physicians (1992), recommend the elimination of an automatic transfusion trigger (i.e., transfusion threshold). The decision to transfuse should

TABLE 60-7 Standard of Care for the Patient with Myelodysplastic Syndrome

Patient Problem and Outcomes	Nursing Interventions and Rationales	Patient Education and Instruction
Knowledge Deficit Patient will: • Verbalize an understanding of MDS and the hematologic complications associated with the MDS subtype. • Identify strategies to manage complications associated with peripheral cytopenias. • Understand the available treatment options, the related potential benefits, and complications.	1. Instruct the patient about the role of bone marrow in hematopoiesis, as well as the function of red blood cells, white blood cells, and platelets. 2. Identify common clinical manifestations associated with the patient's MDS classification. 3. Discuss therapeutic and self-care strategies to minimize or prevent complications related to anemia, neutropenia, and thrombocytopenia. 4. Clarify the patient's understanding of his or her diagnosis and disease process.	1. Use a diagram of the hematopoietic cascade to explain normal hematopoiesis and dyshematopoiesis that results with MDS. 2. Provide the patient with information about the following: a. Normal CBC laboratory values b. Signs and symptoms of anemia, infection, and bleeding (Table 60-1) c. Signs and symptoms that require immediate reporting 3. Review self-care activities: a. Bleeding precautions b. Neutropenic precautions c. Fatigue management 4. Teach the patient about appropriate treatment strategies, rationale, and potential complications: a. Blood component therapy b. Growth factors c. Chemotherapy d. Bone transplantation e. Participation in clinical trials 5. Encourage the patient to ask questions and verbalize an understanding of the diagnosis.

be based on a thorough assessment of the patient's clinical condition, symptomology, and hemoglobin, instead of solely on a predetermined hemoglobin/hematocrit level. For patients with MDS, the transfusion history coupled with the patient's response to red blood cells (RBCs) and platelets should be evaluated too. The judicious use of blood products can delay the onset of hemosideriosis and alloimmunization and minimize the risk of transfusion-related infection.

Other significant issues related to hemotherapy are the need for specialized blood products (i.e., irradiated blood products, leukocyte-depleted RBCs, frozen washed RBCs, HLA platelets) in heavily transfused patients or patients awaiting bone marrow transplantation. Cost and availability are key considerations in light of a limited blood supply and the current economic-health environment.

Patient education focuses on the complications related to anemia, infection, and bleeding, as well as the way patients can minimize or avoid serious complications with self-care activities. Patients must understand the signs and symptoms of hematologic complications (anemia, thrombocytopenia, and neutropenia) that warrant immediate reporting to the health care and expedient intervention.

Growth factors. Most patients receiving growth factors (i.e., G-CSF, GM-CSF, and epoetin alfa) exhibit advanced cytopenias of one or more hematopoietic cell lines. Patients with RA may only receive epoetin alfa because of erythroid dysplasia, whereas patients with RAEB may receive other growth factors such as G-CSF or GM-CSF because of significant myeloid dysplasia. Patients with neutropenia should be instructed about the risk of infection as it relates to the degree of neutropenia and absolute neutrophil count, potential sources of infection, and measures to prevent infection. The administration of hematopoeitic growth factors mandates the reinforcement of neutropenic and/or bleeding precautions, along with fatigue-management strategies for anemia.

Growth factors are usually administered in an outpatient setting or at home. Patient education requires instruction regarding the rationale of therapy, the action of different growth factors, and their associated side effects. Interventions to alleviate adverse effects of growth factors such as bone pain, skin irritation at the injection site, fever, and malaise should be discussed as well.

Cytotoxic Chemotherapy

The treatment regimen administered and its associated complications dictate the nursing care of the patient receiving cytotoxic therapy for MDS. Nurses must recognize the hallmark side effects for each chemotherapy and provide care to alleviate potential or actual clinical manifestations of toxicities. Patients should understand the goal of treatment (i.e., palliation or preparation for bone marrow transplantation) and be instructed about the potential side effects and inter-

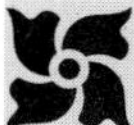

Table 60-8 Standard of Care for the Myelodysplastic Patient Receiving Blood Component Therapy

Patient Problem and Outcomes	Nursing Interventions and Rationales	Patient Education Instructions
Anemia Patient will: • Maintain homeostasis. • Maintain an appropriate hemoglobin/hematocrit level. • Verbalize signs and symptoms of anemia, as well as interventions and strategies to alleviate. • Understand the benefits and risks of transfusion. • Verbalize concerns and apprehension regarding RBC transfusion. • Understand interventions to prevent and minimize complications related to RBC transfusion.	1. Assess the etiology of anemia: a. Patient history b. Physical examination c. Laboratory data • Hemoglobin/ hematocrit • RBC • RBC indices (MCV, MCH, MCHC) • Peripheral smear • Iron, folate, B12, ferritin, TIBC 2. Transfuse packed red blood cells as ordered: • Obtain informed consent. 3. Discuss blood screening and administration procedures with the patient to allay anxiety.	1. Provide the patient with information about anemia and how it is a common manifestation of MDS. 2. Instruct the patient regarding the objective and subjective findings associated with a low red blood cell count: a. Objective signs and symptoms • Tachycardia, dyspnea with or without exertion, pallor, headache, exercise intolerance, palpitations b. Subjective signs and symptoms • Fatigue, malaise, sensitivity to cold, irritability, difficulty concentrating or sleeping, anorexia 3. Teach the patient fatigue-management strategies: a. Eat a balanced diet with adequate fluids. b. Balance periods of activity with rest. c. Plan activities of daily living. d. Identify important life events, and plan energy expenditure. e. Use stress-management techniques. 4. Instruct the patient about the acute and delayed transfusion reactions and strategies to prevent or treat complications: a. Acute reactions • Hemolytic—chills, fever, low back pain, flushing, tachycardia, tachypnea, hypotension, vascular collapse, renal failure, cardiac arrest, death • Nonhemolytic—chills, fever, headache, flushing, muscle pain • Allergic—flushing, itching, urticaria • Anaphylactic—anxiety, urticaria, wheezing, cyanosis, shock, possible cardiac arrest • Circulatory overload—cough, dyspnea, rales, headache, hypertension, tachycardia • Sepsis—sudden onset of chills, fever, vomiting, diarrhea, hypotension, shock b. Delayed reactions • Hemolytic—fever, jaundice usually 7-14 days after transfusion • Hepatitis B—increased SGPT & SGOT, anorexia, malaise, nausea, vomiting, fever, dark urine, jaundice • Hepatitis C—similar to hepatitis B, but symptoms are usually less severe • HIV infection—flu-like symptoms 2 to 4 weeks after transfusion • Iron overload—congestive heart failure, arrhythmias, impaired thyroid and gonadal function, diabetes, cirrhosis • Graft versus host disease—fever, rash, diarrhea, hepatitis 5. Inform the patient about blood screening: a. ABO and Rh compatibility b. Antibody screen c. Blood screen for HIV, hepatitis d. Preparation and administration procedures to prevent infectious contamination 6. Instruct the patient about interventions to prevent complications: a. Use of blood filters, leukocyte depletion b. Administration of premedications such as diphenhydramine hydrochloride, acetaminphen, etc. c. Use of chelation therapy with defersoamine to prevent iron overload

Continued

TABLE 60-8 Standard of Care for the Myelodysplastic Patient Receiving Blood Component Therapy—cont'd

Patient Problem and Outcomes	Nursing Interventions and Rationales	Patient Education Instructions
Bleeding Patient will: • Understand the risks of bleeding associated with thrombocytopenia. • Verbalize the signs and symptoms of bleeding and manifestations that warrant immediate reporting. • Verbalize interventions to prevent or minimize bleeding. • Maintain an appropriate platelet count.	1. Monitor the platelet count and assess the patient's risk for bleeding. 2. Monitor the patient for clinical manifestations of bleeding. 3. Examine the oral cavity, bodily excretions, sclerae, and skin for signs and symptoms of bleeding. 4. Assess the neurologic status and level of consciousness. 5. Identify factors that interfere with platelet function (i.e., medications, fever, sepsis). 6. Instruct the patient to avoid or prevent injury by altering self-care activities. 7. Transfuse platelets as ordered. 8. Monitor the patient for adverse reaction and response to platelet transfusion. 9. Minimize invasive procedures. 10. Assess the patient's home for environmental hazards that place the patient at risk for injury.	1. Provide the patient with information about the risk for bleeding: a. Potential for bleeding if the platelet count is <100,000 mm^3 b. Increased risk if platelet count is <50,000 mm^3 c. Serious risk if the platelet count is <20,000 mm^3 2. Instruct the patient about the signs and symptoms of bleeding: a. Ecchymosis b. Petechiae c. Vaginal or rectal bleeding d. Hematuria e. Bleeding gums f. Epistaxis g. Scleral hemorrhage h. Headache i. Visual changes j. Behavioral changes 3. Teach the patient measures to avoid injury and prevent bleeding: a. Use an electric razor for shaving. b. Avoid straining with bowel movements, use stool softeners, and increase fluid, fiber, and roughage in diet. c. Avoid blowing nose with force. d. Avoid contact sports and strenuous physical activity. e. Apply pressure to puncture sites. f. Avoid use of rectal suppositories and enemas. 4. Discuss home safety strategies with the patient: a. The availability of basic needs, water, phone access, electricity, etc. b. Physical layout of the home environment c. Safety devices such as fire detectors, fire extinguishers, electrical hazards d. Area for medication storage e. Infection-control measures • Personal hygiene measures • Interaction with pets f. Support systems

ventions to allay complications. Regardless of the cytotoxic regimen administered (low-dose chemotherapy versus aggressive treatment), nurses should anticipate the emergence of anemia, thrombocytopenia, and neutropenia. Myelosuppresssion may be prolonged in this patient population due to the inherent defects in bone marrow function.

Bone Marrow Transplantation

Allogenic bone marrow transplantation is a viable treatment option for a limited subset of patients with MDS. The use of BMT is usually restricted due to a patient's increased age and the availability of a suitable donor. BMT for MDS is performed in the inpatient setting, although the pretransplant evaluation and testing, along with posttransplant care, take place in the outpatient setting. Historically, allogeneic bone marrow transplant recipients remained in close proximity to the transplant center to receive follow-up care for 100 days after transplantation. Currently, transplant recipients are being discharged to referring physicians for follow-up care approximately 50 to 70 days after transplantation (Kelleher, 1994). At this time, patients continue to re-

TABLE 60-9 Standard of Care for the Patient Receiving Hematopoietic Growth Factors for Myelodysplastic Syndromes

Patient Problems and Outcomes	Nursing Intervention and Rationales	Patient Education Instructions
Knowledge of Deficit Related to the Administration of Hematopoietic Growth Factors (HGFs)		
Patient will: • Verbalize the mechanism of action and therapeutic effects of the prescribed HGF. • Maintain increased levels of neutrophils and decreased incidence of infection with the administration of granulocyte factors. • Maintain an adequate hemoglobin level to diminish signs and symptoms of anemia and maintain quality of life.	1. Provide the patient with information about the off-label use of hematopoietic growth factors as supportive care interventions for neutropenia and anemia. 2. Instruct the patient about the use of HGFs that stimulate G-CSF, GM-CSF, or Epoetin alfa as appropriate. 3. Provide information about the preparation, administration, and side effects of the prescribed HGF therapy. 4. Monitor targeted hemoglobin and neutrophil counts relative to the HGF. 5. Monitor the patient for side effects of the appropriate HGF. 6. Provide interventions to minimize or eliminate side effects: a. Administer acetaminophen for pain. b. Monitor injection sites. c. Reinforce fatigue-management strategies.	1. Inform the patient about the role of HGFs in normal hematopoiesis and their clinical application in MDS. 2. Review the development and function of granulocytes, red blood cells, and platelets. 3. Reinforce the signs and symptoms of anemia, infection, and bleeding. 4. Explain that HGFs have been successful in increasing levels of hemoglobin and neutrophils in subsets of patients with MDS. 5. Teach the patient the following: a. rHu G-CSF regulates the development of neutrophils. b. rHu GM-CSF regulates the development of neutrophils and macrophages. c. rHu Epo regulates the development of red blood cells. 6. Instruct the patient regarding the following: a. Reconstitution of medication b. Storage and disposal of medication c. Self-injection d. Medication's side effects e. Monitoring of therapy f. Rotation of injection sites 7. Instruct the patient about the dose and side effects related to HGF therapy (N.B. G-CSF, GM-CSF, and Epoetin alfa are used off label for patients with MDS; dosage and administration schedules may vary from package insert). Check the institution protocol. a. rHu Gm-CSF • Usual dose range 250 μm^2-500 μ/m^2, IV or S Q • Side effects—flulike symptoms, headache, myalgia, arthralgia • Monitor CBC × 2 weekly, titrate to targeted ANC b. rHu G-CSF • Usual dose range 5 μ/kg-10 μ/kg I V or S Q • Side effects—mild to moderate bone pain, skin reaction, or breakdown at the injection site c. Monitor CBC with differential × 2 weekly, titrate dose to targeted ANC d. rHu EPO • Usual dose range 150 μ/kg-300 μ/kg S Q × 3 weekly, titrate to targeted hemoglobin level • Side effects—possible hypertension with a rapid rise in hemoglobin e. Monitor blood pressure, hemoglobin, hematocrit, and reticulocyte count at weeks 2 and 4 weeks after the start of treatment, then monthly. If the hemoglobin rise is $<$1.0 g/dl, consider increasing the HGF up to a maximum dose of 300 μ/kg.

quire close monitoring for the acute and chronic complications associated with BMT.

Care of the patient receiving a BMT depends on the phase of the patient's transplantation that the nurse encounters. In the pretransplant phase, nursing care is directed at preparing the patient for the procedure, orchestrating diagnostic tests, and administering supportive treatments preceding transplantation. Patients should be instructed regarding the transplant process, the rationale for the pretransplant evaluation, conditioning regimens, marrow reinfusion, engraftment, and recovery. During the transplant phase, which includes conditioning regimens, marrow infusion, and engraftment, care of the patient is focused on the assessment, monitoring, and management of acute complications associated with the conditioning regimen, organ system(s) toxicities, and graft versus host disease. In the recovery phase, nursing management continues relative to the clinical manifestations of the affected organ system. A number of patients require continued treatment with intravenous antibiotics and immunoglobulins, blood component therapy, and the management of multisystem graft versus host disease (Buchsel, Leum, & Randolph, 1996). An extensive review of the bone marrow transplant process, associated morbidity and mortality, and the nursing management of complications is contained in the literature (Buchsel & Whedon, 1995; Buschsel, Leum, & Randolph, 1996; Franco & Gould, 1994; Wujcik, Ballard, & Camp-Sorrell, 1994.)

HOME CARE ISSUES

Patient Education

The patient, family, and caregivers are faced with numerous issues in the home care setting. The first challenge is patient education. Patients are increasingly being managed on an outpatient basis, requiring monitoring for compliance and comprehension of the disease process, as well as actual care issues, being performed in the home (Council on Scientific Affairs, 1990). Patients must understand the disease process and hematologic guidelines associated with their stage of MDS. In addition, they will live with the uncertainty of whether their disease will progress to AML. There is currently no cure for MDS, except BMT, and therefore education on high-tech supportive care such as home hemotherapy, intravenous antimicrobial therapy administration, and central venous catheter care may become necessary.

Caregiver Issues

The caregiver must be taught parameters for supportive care and self-care that the patient is taught. In addition, he or she must be guided on the way to respond to an emergency situation and where to seek the appropriate medical care. In addition, there may not be a caregiver because the primary population is elderly, a partner may be deceased, and the family may live a distance away.

Home Care Provider

The home care provider should have experience with caring for geriatric and immunocompromised patients. The patient, support systems, and environment should be assessed on the first visit (Table 60-10). All home care providers (skilled nurses, nurses aids, etc.) should be aware of all the hematologic and supportive care guidelines set forth by the managing medical team. Any issues identified in the home should be communicated to the medical team immediately.

Financial Issues

Patients with MDS are predominately elderly and on fixed incomes. The amount of medical coverage for hospitalization, pharmaceutical support, and home care vary depending on whether Medicare is primary or secondary coverage.

Costs for home care range significantly depending on the stage of disease and the supportive care or treatment chosen. If the patient is young and undergoes a BMT, average costs (autologous and allogeneic combined), including evaluation, procurement, hospital stay, follow-up, and home care, are approximately $217,000 (Hauboldt, 1996). Patients should be aware of their home care benefits, as well as coverage for physician, inpatient, outpatient, pharmaceutical, and durable medical equipment because the use of home care is rapidly increasing (Lonergan, McBride, Kelley, & Randolph, 1996).

PROGNOSIS

Survival is variable in patients with MDS; some patients live for several years, and others die in months. Transformation to AML or complications related to pancytopenia, most notably infection and hemorrhage, are the leading causes of death in patients with MDS. Poor prognostic factors include greater than 10% blasts, platelets less than 40,000, or granulocytes less than 1000/μl, and these patients usually have survival rates of less than 1 year (Applebaum, 1994). Patients exhibiting complex chromosomal abnormalities at the time of diagnosis and patients with secondary or treatment-related MDS are subgroups with a high risk of short survival, leukemic transformation, and overall poorer prognosis (Musilova, Michalova, Zemanova, Neuwirthova, & Dohnalova, 1995; Utley, 1996). Diagnosis at a younger age is associated with an increased probability of leukemic progression, but also with a longer survival (Musilova et al., 1995). Table 60-1 lists the median survival and survival ranges, in months, for each of the MDS subtypes.

EVALUATION OF THE QUALITY OF CARE

Accreditation organizations, like the Joint Commission for the Accreditation of Health Care Organizations, require that the quality of care provided to the patient be evaluated. Tables 60-11 through 60-13 provide examples of quality of

TABLE 60-10 Coram Healthcare Environmental Assessment Form

Patient:
Referral Source:
Date:
Nurse:

Assessment Category	Observed/Discussed	Verbalized Understanding	Action Required	Comments
Home environment basic needs: 1. Electricity 2. Heat 3. Water 4. Gas 5. Phone access 6. Emergency service access (e.g., 911) 7. Outside access 8. Other				
Home environment physical layout: 1. Bedroom 2. Bathroom 3. Stairs 4. Doorways/halls 5. Other				
Home safety: 1. Fire detector 2. Fire hazards 3. Electric hazards 4. Furnace type/care 5. Area for medication storage 6. Tobacco products 7. Other				
Home infection control: 1. General condition of home 2. Area for medical supply preparations 3. Presence of pets or plants 4. Evidence of rodents/insects 5. Visitor restrictions 6. Cleaning requirements: • Shower • Toilet • Sink • Vacuuming • Dusting • Carpets • Floors • Bed linens • Pillows 7. Person(s) available for cleaning				

Courtesy Coram Healthcare, Chicago, Illinois.

TABLE 60-10 Coram Healthcare Environmental Assessment Form—cont'd

Patient:
Referral Source:
Date:
Nurse:

Assessment Category	Observed/Discussed	Verbalized Understanding	Action Required	Comments
Personal hygiene: 1. General appearance 2. Hair/skin/clothing 3. Use of own towels/soap 4. Use of own thermometer 5. Personal habits: • Alcohol • Drugs • Tobacco • Caffeine • Other *Support systems:* 1. Primary caregiver • Available • Capable • Limitations 2. Family/family roles 3. Friends 4. Community 5. Medical personnel 6. Religion related 7. Other				
Ancillary needs: 1. Transportation 2. Grocery services 3. Pharmacy services *Education:* 4. Transplant center guidelines pre and post transplant				

Signature Date

Courtesy Coram Healthcare, Chicago, Illinois.

care evaluation tools that can be used in the inpatient and outpatient settings, respectively.

RESEARCH ISSUES

Numerous research issues regarding the pathogenesis, diagnosis, and treatment of MDS require further investigation. Research shows myelodysplastic syndrome is a malignant abnormality of the pluripotent stem cell that results in progressive cytopenias in one or more cell lines. However, the mechanism that initiates and promotes disease progression is unclear (Taylor et al., 1994). A study by Silverman and others (1995) revealed that stromal cells, the microenvironment of the bone marrow, is significantly impaired in MDS. Additional studies are required to address abnormalities affecting the microenvironment in MDS.

Supportive care intervention with growth factors such as G-CSF, GM-CSF, and Epoetin alfa have palliated the effects of neutropenia and anemia for a limited duration. These positive effects are well documented. Subsequent clinical trials are warranted to evaluate the effect of growth factors on total survival time and the patient's quality of life. The clinical application of other growth factors needs continued

TABLE 60-11 Quality of Care Evaluation for a Patient Receiving Blood Component Therapy

Disciplines participating in the quality of care evaluation:
☐ Nursing ☐ Hematology Service
☐ Social Services ☐ Home Care

Data from:
☐ Medical Record Review ☐ Patient Interview

Criteria	Yes	No
1. The patient has been provided with information regarding red blood cell and platelet transfusion:		
a. Benefits and potential immediate and delayed complications explained	☐	☐
b. Informed consent for transfusion obtained	☐	☐
c. Interventions and strategies to prevent or minimize risks of complications discussed	☐	☐
2. Hemoglobin and hematocrit levels were evaluated at prescribed intervals and maintained at targeted levels.	☐	☐
3. The platelet count was evaluated at prescribed intervals and maintained at targeted levels.	☐	☐
4. The patient experienced the following complications:		
a. Chills, fever, heartache, tachycardia, tachypnea, hypotension	☐	☐
b. Sepsis, sudden onset of chills, high fever, hypotension	☐	☐
c. Facial/body flushing, itching, urticaria	☐	☐
d. Wheezing, cyanosis, shock	☐	☐
e. Signs and symptoms of hepatitis, CMV disease, HIV	☐	☐
f. Graft versus host disease	☐	☐
g. Iron overload	☐	☐

TABLE 60-12 Quality of Care Evaluation for a Patient Receiving Hematopoietic Growth Factors

Disciplines participating in the quality of care evaluation:
☐ Nursing ☐ Hematology Service
☐ Social Services ☐ Home Care

Data from:
☐ Mailed Questionnaire ☐ Patient Interview

Criteria	Yes	No
1. Did the physician or nurse explain to you that you might experience some of the following side effects?		
a. Flu-like symptoms, headache, aches in your muscles and bones, and a possible skin reaction at the injection site with the medication G-CSF	☐	☐
b. Mild to moderate pain in your bones or skin reaction at the injection site with the medication GM-CSF	☐	☐
c. Hypertension with the administration of Epoetin alfa	☐	☐
2. Were you instructed to report medication side effects to the nurse or physician?	☐	☐
3. Did the physician or nurse discuss how to prevent or alleviate the side effects of the medication you are taking?	☐	☐
4. Were you instructed about the follow-up care and blood count monitoring that was required while you were taking hematopoietic growth factor?	☐	☐

exploration. There are limited clinical trials that test the efficacy of interleukin-2, interleukin-3, and interleukin-6, alone or in combination with other agents in the treatment of MDS.

Buttafarano and others (1995) showed that the high level of tumor necrosis factor (TNF) alpha was associated with a significant number of hematopoietic cell and marrow stem cell deaths. Treatment with cyclosporine or pentoxifyline showed a reduction in the TNF levels and a spectrum of clinical response in patients. It is essential that clinical trials continue to explore and define the efficacy of other treatments such as differentiating agents, the application of aggressive chemotherapy and postremission transplantation, and immune modulators.

A variety of treatment options are available for patients with MDS, but only bone marrow transplantation offers a potential cure. Current research recommendations regarding the timing of allogeneic transplantation, patient age, and disease status at the time of transplantation are unclear. Findings from one study recommend allogenic transplantation from a related or unrelated donor early in the course of the disease in patients less than 40 years of age (Anderson, Applebaum, & Storb, 1995). Another study revealed that the interval from the diagnosis to BMT, prior intensive chemotherapy, age, and conditioning regimen did not predict event-free survival (Fung et al., 1995). It is clear that further research is indicated to identify when patients can benefit most from BMT.

TABLE 60-13 Quality of Care Evaluation for a Patient Receiving Supportive Care Interventions

Disciplines participating in the quality of care evaluation:
☐ Nursing ☐ Hematology Service
☐ Social Services ☐ Home Care

I. Patient Education Instruction Evaluation

Data from:
☐ Medical Record Review ☐ Patient/Family Interview

Criteria	Yes	No
1. The patient is provided with information about the following:		
a. Myelodysplastic syndrome and MDS subtype, as well as the abnormal production and function of hematopoietic cells	☐	☐
b. Function of red blood cells, white blood cells, and platelets	☐	☐
c. Treatment options	☐	☐
2. The patient verbalizes the signs and symptoms of infection, anemia, and thrombocytopenia.	☐	☐
3. The patient describes therapeutic and self-care strategies to minimize complications related to anemia, neutropenia, and thrombocytopenia.	☐	☐

II. Patient/Family Satisfaction

Data from:
☐ Patient Interview ☐ Family Interview

Criteria	Yes	No
1. Did the physician or nurse explain to you the hematologic complications associated with MDS and your MDS subtype?	☐	☐
a. Do you and your family feel the explanation was adequate?	☐	☐
b. Will you be able to manage your treatment, follow-up care, and activities of daily living?	☐	☐
2. Were you told to speak with your physician or nurse if you had any additional questions or concerns about your diagnosis and treatment?	☐	☐

REFERENCES

Alkire, K. (1993). Physiology of bone marrow. In D. Wujcik (Ed.), *Nursing issues in adult acute leukemia.* Huntington, NY: PRR.

American College of Physicians. (1992). Practice strategies for elective red blood cell transfusion. *Annuals of Internal Medicine, 116,* 403-406.

Anderson, J. B., Applebaum, F. R., & Storb, R. (1995). An update on allogeneic marrow transplantation for myelodysplastic syndrome. *Leukemia and Lymphoma. 17*(1-2), 95-99.

Applebaum, F. R. (1994). Allogeneic bone marrow transplantation for myelodysplastic and myeloproliferative disorders. In G. Forman, K. G. Blume, & E. D. Thomas (Eds.), *Bone marrow transplantation.* Boston: Blackwell Scientific.

Aul, C., Gattermann, N., & Schneider, W. (1995). Epidemiological and etiological aspects of myelodysplastic syndromes. *Leukemia & Lymphoma, 16*(13-14), 247-262.

Aul, C., Runde, V., & Gattermann, N. (1993). All-trans retinoic acid in patients with myelodysplastic syndromes: Results of a pilot study. *Blood, 82,* 2967-2974.

Bakerman, S. (1994). *ABC's of Interpretive Laboratory Data* (3rd ed.). Myrtle Beach, SC: Interpretive Laboratory Data.

Ballen, K. K., & Antin, J. H. (1993). Treatment of therapy related acute myelogenous leukemia and myelodysplastic syndrome. *Hematology/Oncology Clinics of North America, 7,* 447-493.

Barkauskas, V. H., Bauman, L. C., Stolenberg-Allen, K., & Fisher-Darling, C. (1994). *Health and physical assessment.* St. Louis: Mosby.

Boultwood, J. & Fidler, C. (1995). Chromosomal deletions in myelodysplasia. *Leukemia & Lymphoma, 17*(1-2), 71-78.

Buchsel, P. C., Leum, E. W., & Randolph, S. R. (1996). Delayed complications of bone marrow transplantation: An update. *Oncology Nursing Forum 23*(8), 1267-1291.

Buchsel, P. C. & Whedon, M. B. (1995). *Bone marrow transplantation: Administrative and clinical strategies.* Boston: Jones and Bartlett.

Buttafarano, R. J., Kim, S. K., Dahlberg, P. S., Farbee, M. S., Ratz, C. A., Johnston, J. W., & Dunn, D. L. (1995). Lymphocyte derived cytokines augment macrophage tumor necrosis factor-alpha and interleukin-6 secretion during experimental gram-negative bacterial sepsis. *Journal of Surgical Research, 58*(6) 739-745.

Castro, M., Conn, D., & Su, W. (1991). Rheumatic manifestations in myelodysplastic syndrome. *Journal of Rheumatology, 18,* 721-727.

Cheson, B. (1990). The myelodysplastic syndrome: current approaches to therapy. *Annals of Internal Medicine 112,* 932-941.

Cheson, B., Jasperse, D., Simon, R., & Friedman, M. (1986). A critical appraisal of low-dose cytosine arabinoside in patients with acute nonlymphocytic leukemia and myelodysplastic syndromes. *Journal of Clinical Oncology, 4,* 1857-1864.

Cines, D., Cassileth, P., & Kiss, J. (1985). Danazole therapy in myelodysplasia. *Annals of Internal Medicine 103,* 58-60.

Cole, P., Sateren, W., & Delzell, E. (1995). Epidemiologic perspectives on myelodysplastic syndromes and leukemia. *Leukemia Research, 19*(6), 361-365.

Council on Scientific Affairs. (1990). Home care in the 1990's. *Journal of the American Medical Association, 263,* 1241-1244.

DeWitte, T. (1994). New treatment approaches for myelodysplastic syndrome and secondary leukemias. *Annals of Oncology, 5*(5), 401-408

Feldman, E., Seiter, K., Ahmed, T., Baskind, P., & Arlin, Z. (1996). Homoharringtonine in patients with myelodysplastic syndrome (MDS) and MDS evolving to acute myeloid leukemia. *Leukemia, 10*(1), 40-42.

Franco, F. & Gould, A. (1994). Allogeneic bone marrow transplantation. *Seminars in Oncology Nursing 10*(1), 3-11.

Fung, H., Shepherd, J., Nantel, S., Spinelli, J., Sutherland, H., Klingemann, H., Reece, D., Phillips, G., & Barnett, M. (1995). Allogeneic bone marrow transplantation (BMT) for adults with myelodysplastic syndrome (MDS) (meeting abstract). *Proceedings of the Annual Meeting of the American Society of Clinical Oncologists, 14,* A7.

Ganser, A. & Hoelzer, D. (1992). Clinical course of myelodysplastic syndromes. *Hematology/Oncology Clinics of North America, 6,* 107-115.

Ganser, A., Seipelt, G., & Lindemann, A. (1990). Effects of recombinant human interleukin-3 in patients with myelodysplastic syndromes. *Blood, 76,* 455-462.

Goasguen, J. & Bennett J. (1992). Classification and morphologic features of the myelodysplastic syndromes. *Seminars in Oncology, 19,* 4-13.

Golde, D. (1991). The stem cell. *Scientific American, 265*(6), 86-93.

Greenberg, P. (1995). Myelodysplastic syndrome. In R. Hoffman, E. J. Benz, S. J. Shattile, B. Furie, H. J. Cohen, & L. E. Siberstein (Eds.), *Hematology: Basic principles and practice* (2nd ed.). New York: Churchill Livingstone.

Hasle, H. (1994). Myelodysplastic syndromes in childhood: classification, epidemiology, and treatment. *Leukemia & Lymphoma, 13*(1-2), 11-26.

Hauboldt, R. (1996). *Research report: Cost implications of human organ and tissue transplantation, an update.* New York: Milliman & Robertson.

Hoagland, H. (1995). Myelodysplastic (preleukemia) syndromes: the bone marrow factory failure problem. *Mayo Clinic Proceedings, 70*(7), 673-676.

Juneja, H. S., Jodhani, M., Gardner, F. H., Trevarthen, D., & Schottstedt, M. (1994). Low-dose ARA-C consistently induces hematologic responses in the clinical 5q-syndrome. *American Journal of Hematology 46*(4), 338-342.

Kantarjian, H., Estey, E., & Keating, M. (1993). Treatment of therapy-related leukemia and myelodysplastic syndrome. *Hematology/Oncology Clinics of North America, 7,* 81-105.

Kelleher, J. (1994). Issues for designing marrow transplant programs. *Seminars in Oncology Nursing, 10*(1), 64-71.

Kelley, C. (1996). Commentary: Therapy-related myelodysplastic syndrome. *Oncology Nursing Forum, 23,* 1529-1530.

Koeffler, H., Heitjan, D., & Mertelsmann, R. (1988). Randomized study of 13 cis retinoic acid v placebo in the myelodysplastic disorders. *Blood, 71,* 703-708.

Kouides, P., & Bennett, J. (1992). Morphology and classification of myelodysplastic syndromes. *Hematology/Oncology Clinics of North America, 6,* 485-499.

Lin, E. M. & Beddar, S. M. (1996). Abnormalities in homeostasis and hemorrhage. In R. McCorkle, M. Grant, M. Frank-Stromberg, & S. B. Baird (Eds.), *Cancer nursing: A comprehensive textbook.* Philadelphia: W. B. Saunders.

Locatelli, F., Zecca, M., Pession, A., Maserati, E., DeStefano, P., & Severi, F. (1995). Myelodysplastic syndromes: The pediatric point of view. *Haematologica, 80,* 268-279.

Lonergan, J., McBride, L., Kelley, C., & Randolph, S. (1996). *Homecare management of the bone marrow transplant patient* (2nd ed.). Sudbury, MA: Jones and Bartlett.

Miller, K., Kim, K., & Morrison, F., et al. (1988). Evaluation of low dose ara-C versus supportive care in the treatment of myelodysplastic syndromes: An intergroup study by the Eastern Cooperative Oncology Group and the Southwest Oncology Group. *Blood, 72,* 215-222

Mittelman, M. & Lessin, L. (1994). Clinical application of recombinant erythropoietin in myelodysplasia. *Hematology Oncology Clinics of North America 8*(5), 993-1009.

Musilova, J., Michalova, K., Zemanova, Z., Neuwirthova, R., & Dohnalova, A. (1995). Karyotype at diagnosis, subsequent leukemic transformation and survival in myelodysplastic syndrome. *Leukemia Research, 19*(5), 303-308.

O'Donnell, M. R., Long, G. D., Parker, P., Niland, J., Nademanee, A., Amylon, M., Chao, N., Negrin, R. S., Schmidt, G. M., & Slovak M. L. (1995). Busulfan/cyclophosphamide as conditioning regimen for allogeneic bone marrow transplantation for myelodysplasia. *Journal of Clinical Oncology, 13*(12), 2973-2979.

Silverman, L., Holland, J., Demakos, E., Mandeli, J., Castro-Malaspina, H., Gattani, A., & Cuttner, J. (1995). Subcutaneous 5-azacytidine in myelodysplastic syndromes (MDS): The experience at Mount Sinai Hospital, New York (meeting abstract). *Proceedings of the Annual Meeting of the American Society of Clinical Oncologists, 14,* A1021.

Stein, R. (1994). Clinical use of growth factors in the myelodysplastic syndromes. *American Journal of Medical Science, 307,* 360-367.

Taylor, K., Rodwell R., Taylor, D., & Seeley, G. (1994). Myelodysplasia. *Current Opinion in Oncology, 6*(1), 32-40.

Tefferi, A., Thibodeau, S., & Solbert, L. (1990). Clonal studies in a myelodysplastic syndrome using X-linked restriction fragment length polymorphisms. *Blood, 75,* 1770-1773.

Uberti, J. (1994). Allogeneic bone marrow transplantation in patients with myelodysplastic syndromes. *Leukemia & Lymphoma, 14*(5-6), 379-385.

Utley, S. (1996). Myelodysplastic syndromes. *Seminars in Oncology Nursing, 12*(1), 51-58.

Weimar, I., Bourhis, J., De Gast, G., & Gerritsen, W. (1994). Clonality in myelodysplastic syndromes. *Leukemia & Lymphoma, 13*(3-4), 215-221.

West, R., Stafford, D., Farrow, A., & Jacobs, A. (1995). Occupational and environmental exposures and myelodysplasia: A case-control study. *Leukemia Research, 19*(2), 127-139.

Wujcik, D., Ballard, B., & Camp-Sorrell, D. (1994). Selected complications of allogeneic bone marrow transplantation. *Seminars in Oncology Nursing 10*(1), 28-41.

Yoshida, Y., Oguma, S., & Uchino, H. (1993). A randomized study of alfacalcidol in the refractory myelodysplastic anaemias: A Japanese cooperative study. *International Journal of Clinical Pharmacology Resources 13,* 21-27.

Small Cell Lung Cancer

Tamie R. Bressler, RN, MN, OCN

INTRODUCTION

Lung cancer is the second most common cancer and has the highest mortality rate for men (1 in 13) and women (1 in 24). It is the leading cause of death for people over the age of 35 years. Small cell lung cancer represents 25% of the lung cancers. Only 12% to 15% of patients with lung cancer are being cured with today's treatments (Garfinkel & Silverberg, 1991). In the United States, 178,100 new cases of lung cancer and 160,400 deaths from lung cancer are estimated for 1998. The survival rate is 46% for cases detected in a localized stage, but only 15% of lung cancers are discovered that early (American Cancer Society, 1998).

Small Cell Lung Cancer

Small cell lung cancer (SCLC) is a unique form of lung cancer characterized by rapid growth, dissemination at the time of diagnosis, and poor responsiveness to radiotherapy and chemotherapy due to rapid cell division. It has the most aggressive clinical course of any type of pulmonary tumor, accounts for about one quarter of all primary lung cancers, and left untreated, results in the shortest survival of any pulmonary neoplasm, with a median survival of 2 to 4 months (Hinson & Perry, 1993). SCLC is aggressive, not generally resectable, and not considered a target for early detection or screening.

SCLC is also called *oat cell carcinoma* because the cells are shaped like grains of oats. The tumors are usually located in central regions of the lung, often at the hilum. Tumors typically grow submucosally with early intralymphatic invasion. Because of their central location and early lymphatic metastases, small cell tumors often occur as hilar or perihilar masses. These rapidly growing central tumors can cause bronchial obstruction and pneumonia.

Small cell cancers have a poor prognosis because of their high growth rate and tendency to metastasize early and widely. Lymphatic and distant metastases are usually present at the time of diagnosis. Short-term relapses are common, even though these tumors are the most sensitive of the histologic types to radiation and chemotherapy (Ihde, Pass, & Glatstein, 1997).

EPIDEMIOLOGY

Epidemiologic studies related to lung cancer indicate alarming trends. The incidence of lung cancer has risen dramatically since the turn of the century. The peak incidence in males is 50 to 60 years of age, although it is not uncommon to diagnose lung cancer in individuals under or near 40 years of age. The incidence increases rapidly after age 50 and is found most frequently (75%) in individuals 50 to 75 years of age (Glover & Miaskowski, 1994). SCLC has historically been much more prevalent in males, but smoking among women has led to a predictable increase in women with SCLC. Lung cancer in women began to increase in the late 1960s, and the mortality rate among women in the United States has increased over 400% since the mid 1950s. The projected peak for mortality rates in women will not occur until 2010 (Brown & Kessler, 1988). Lung cancer mortality rates are higher for African Americans than for Caucasians. Mahaney (1992) suggests that the mortality rate for African Americans is not expected to fall until after the year 2000. Incidence rates for lung cancer have been declining for African-American males since the mid 1980s, leveling off in African-American women in younger age groups (Boring, Squires, & Heath, 1992).

Lung cancer is highly virulent and rapidly fatal. There is a close relationship between incidence and death rates, indicating that most individuals (90%) die of the disease. The length of time from a person's initial exposure to a carcinogen to the onset of lung cancer can take 10 to 30 years to develop. Each individual who succumbs loses an average of 15 years of life (Horm & Sondik, 1989).

ETIOLOGIC FACTORS

Lung cancers most commonly occur after repeated exposure to substances that cause tissue irritation and inflammation.

Lung tissues are exposed to these substances primarily as they are inhaled with ambient air. Lung cancer develops when the genetic material (deoxyribonucleic acid) of normal cells has been damaged repeatedly. Most lung cancers develop in the epithelium of the lungs and tracheobronchial tree, which is directly exposed to inhaled air and is a target for airborne carcinogens.

RISK FACTORS

The major risk factors/populations at risk associated with the development of lung cancer are listed in Box 61-1 (Fink, 1992; Elpern, 1993; Frank-Stromborg & Cohen, 1993). In addition, several proposed steps to reduce the development of smoking behavior are detailed in Box 61-2.

Tobacco Smoke

Numerous epidemiologic studies have shown an irrefutable causal relationship between cigarette smoking and lung cancer. Factors linked to this conclusion are benzopyrene and other carcinogens in combusted tobacco, histologic changes in the bronchial epithelium of heavy smokers, increased incidence of other smoking-related diseases and cancer, and experimental production of tumors in animals after the internal and cutaneous application of tobacco condensates.

The incidence of lung cancer has been greatly affected by the mass production and marketing of cigarettes, as well as the practice of repetitive inhalation of cigarette smoke. The relationship of smoking to lung cancer has a dose-response nature. The relative risk of lung cancer increases with the number of cigarettes smoked per day and the number of years of smoking history. Lung cancer increases proportionately to the history of packs smoked per year, and the risk decreases in those who stop smoking (Mulley, 1995). Two-pack-a-day smokers who have smoked over 40 years have 20 times the risk compared with nonsmokers (Wolpaw, 1996). After 5 years of smoking cessation, the risk of SCLC steadily declines and continues to decrease as the period of abstinence increases (Public Health Service, 1990). The rate of decline of the risk after cessation of smoking is determined by the cumulative smoking exposure before cessation, the age when smoking began, and the degree of inhalation (Rogot, 1974). About 15 years of nonsmoking may elapse before lungs return to normal (Wynder & Stellman, 1979).

To determine an individual's risk for lung cancer, several factors need to be considered (Box 61-3) (Elpern, 1993). The number of pack years is calculated by multiplying the packs of cigarettes consumed per day by the number of years of smoking. Individuals who start smoking before age 15 years have a greater risk of lung cancer than those who start after age 25 years. The size of the puff, depth of inhalation, time of breath holding, amount and type of cigarette smoked, tar and nicotine content, and filtered or nonfiltered cigarettes must be taken into consideration. The people at highest risk began smoking in their teens, inhale deeply, and smoke at least half a pack a day.

Cigarette smoke contains more than 3600 chemicals, and many are carcinogens (43) or mutagens. The potential interactive effects of inhalation of these chemicals with environmental or genetic factors increase the risk. The mechanism by which tobacco smoke causes cancer is unclear, even though the incidence of lung cancer clearly correlates to smoking habits. SCLC occurs almost exclusively in smok-

Box 61-1

Risk Factors/Populations at Risk for Small Cell Lung Cancer

Tobacco Smoke

Passive Smoking

Air Pollution

- The sulfur-oxide/particulate complex arising from the combustion of sulfur-containing fuels
- Photochemical oxidants related to motor vehicle emissions
- Miscellaneous pollutants from localized sources such as refineries and manufacturing plants

Occupational Factors

- Radon
- Uranium
- Asbestos
- Cadmium
- Chromium
- Sulfur dioxide
- Silica
- Formaldehyde
- Copper
- Alkylating compounds
- Halo ethers

Constitutional Factors

- Family history
- Pre-existing lung disease and prior lung cancer
- Age

Box 61-2

Proposed Steps to Reduce the Development of Smoking Behavior

- Reduce the easy availability of cigarettes to young people.
- Encourage parents and important role models to set the example of not smoking.
- Reduce the intensity of emotionally charged proscriptions of smoking, which serve to stimulate contrary action.
- Stress the costs associated with smoking without denying the benefits. Encourage the achievement of these benefits in less damaging ways.
- Avoid stereotyping smoking and smokers in ways that turn youth away from antismoking "do-gooders."
- Help young people develop insight into their perception of smoking as attractive. Encourage them to seek alternative means of satisfying this need.

ers and is usually dose related. The risk of SCLC increases in direct proportion to the total amount of exposure to cigarette smoke. Total exposure encompasses the age smoking started, number of cigarettes smoked, products smoked, and inhaling pattern (Samet, 1993). There are no safe levels of smoking.

Pipe and Cigar Smoking

Those who smoke pipes and cigars have a twofold increased risk over nonsmokers of developing lung cancer, but much less so than cigarette smokers. Pipe or cigar smoking, or even smokeless tobacco, is not an acceptable alternative to cigarette smoking.

Passive Smoking

Passive smoking refers to the involuntary exposure of nonsmokers to tobacco combustion products (Ingle, 1997). The 1986 Report of the Surgeon General indicated that sidestream smoke is qualitatively similar to mainstream smoke inhaled by the smoker. Although the smoke breathed in by involuntary smokers is not as concentrated as that inhaled directly by smokers, it contains the same carcinogens. Second-hand smoke accounts for an estimated 3000 lung cancer deaths annually in nonsmoking adults (American Cancer Society, 1998). Approximately 17% of lung cancers among nonsmokers can be attributed to high levels of exposure to cigarette smoke during childhood and adolescence (Janerich, Thompson, & Varela, 1990). Second-hand smoke poses health hazards for unborn and young children. It is classified as a class A cancer-causing agent by the Environmental Protection Agency (EPA). Nonsmoking wives have a 35% higher risk of lung cancer if their husbands smoke. An increased incidence of lung cancer in nonsmokers who have lived with smokers and an increased frequency of respiratory infections and symptoms in children whose parents smoke highlight this health risk. In 1988, a federal bill was passed banning smoking on commercial airline flights of 120 minutes or less. To be accredited by the Joint Commission of Healthcare Organizations, hospitals must be smoke free. Antismoking policies are also appearing in corporations and other work-related environments. Hopefully, the growing intolerance of the public for smoking and continuing public policy initiatives will help drastically reduce the number of smokers in the United States. Examples of smoking-cessation strategies are listed in Box 61-4.

Box 61-3
Risk Factors Related to Tobacco Smoke

Number of Pack Years
Age at Onset of Smoking
Smoking Practices

- Size of puff
- Depth of inhalation
- Time of breath holding
- Amount of cigarette smoked

Type of Cigarette
Tar Content
Filtered
Nonfiltered

Air Pollution

Air pollution is a complex mixture that varies from place to place and over time. The three major sources and types of air pollution are listed in Box 61-1 (Elpern, 1993). Carcinogens have been identified in atmospheric pollution. In addition, there is evidence that the incidence of lung cancer increases in polluted urban areas. It is unclear whether air pollution functions as a promoter or as a carcinogen in the development of lung cancer.

Occupational Factors

Chemicals associated with lung cancer and the occupations that result in exposure are listed in Box 61-1 (Crowley, 1992; Fink, 1992; Elpern, 1993). SCLC is the most common type of lung cancer in uranium miners (Archer, Saccomanno, & Jones, 1974). Death from bronchogenic lung cancer among asbestos workers is seven times more frequent than in the general population, resulting from a combination of smoking and asbestos fibers. Occupational exposure to these chemicals and a long latency period can lead to tumor induction. Environmental factors such as temperature, humidity, and ventilation may also affect the amount or type of exposure. The interactive and synergistic effects of smoking and occupational exposure are seen with lung cancer causation, stressing the enhanced carcinogenic potential of these agents. It has been estimated that occupational exposures may cause 15% of male and 5% of female lung cancers (Doll & Peto, 1981).

Radon

Radon is a naturally occurring, colorless, odorless, and tasteless radioactive gas produced by uranium decay in soil and rocks. Radon and its radioactive decay products can be inhaled directly or attached to air particles and transported

Box 61-4
Smoking-Cessation Strategies and Interventions

Example setting:

- Limiting smoking in the workplace; direct, face-to-face advice and suggestions on smoking cessation
- Identification of high-risk individuals; smoking-cessation self-help materials that are culturally and educationally relevant to the person

Referral to community smoking-cessation programs
Referral of smokers motivated to quit
Drug therapy when appropriate (nicotine gum, nicotine patch)
Scheduled reinforcement with the smoker

into the lungs, causing cell damage that may lead to cancer. Uranium and fluorspar miners, especially those who smoke, are at an increased risk of lung cancer.

Radon moves through small spaces in soil and rock, seeping into buildings through dirt floors, cracks in concrete, and floor drains. It can migrate up through porous soils and enter homes through basement or foundation cracks, sumps, drains, or deep private wells. Tight insulation and poor ventilation can increase household radon levels. Radon levels vary by the geographic location, climate, season, and type of heating and ventilation system. As with several of the lung cancer risk factors, a synergistic effect exists between radon exposure and cigarette smoking, as well as between other agents such as uranium and fluorspar. The longer the period of radon exposure, the greater the risk; yet cancer risk decreases with time after cessation of exposure. Radon exposure may be the most significant risk factor for the nonsmoker that can be readily reduced (Harley & Harley, 1990), because indoor radon is estimated to be responsible for 9,000 to 13,000 lung cancer cases per year (Samet, 1989). Detection devices are now available for home monitoring.

Asbestos

Asbestos is a group of minerals that occur naturally as fibers. Asbestos is considered the second most important etiologic, or causal, agent associated with lung cancer after tobacco. These fibers tend to break easily into particles that float in the air and stick to clothes when the particles are inhaled. They can lodge in the lungs, damaging cells and increasing the risk for lung cancer. Exposure has been observed in industries such as shipbuilding, asbestos mining and manufacturing, insulation work, sheet metal work, and brake repair (Ingle, 1997).

Constitutional Factors

Evidence is emerging that certain individuals may be genetically predisposed to lung cancer, especially in the presence of an environmental stimulus such as smoking or an occupational carcinogen (Sellers, Potter, & Bailey-Wilson, 1992). Multiple cases of lung cancer in the same family have been used as supportive data, yet sufficient evidence to confirm this hypothesis is lacking (Birrer & Minna, 1988). Primary lung cancer patients are at risk (3%) of developing a second primary lung cancer.

Preexisting lung disease may also increase the risk of developing lung cancer. Chronic obstructive pulmonary disease may be a risk factor independent of the smoking history (Skillrud, Offord, & Miller, 1986). The exact mechanisms underlying this risk are not known, but impaired mucociliary transport with enhanced deposition of carcinogens, chronic inflammation and scarring, and genetic predisposition to mucosal injury are thought to be involved. Individuals who smoke and have bullous emphysema and other preexisting lung diseases may also be at risk for lung cancer. This may be attributed to poor clearance of carcinogens from areas of destroyed lung. In addition, studies by Baumm and Medsger (1985) suggest an association between progressive systemic sclerosis (PSS) and lung cancer. Also, a scarred area of the lung caused by a prior inflammatory process increases the risk of a "scar" cancer, usually an adenocarcinoma.

Social Class/Education

For Caucasian and African-American males, and African-American females, age-adjusted lung cancer incidence rates are significantly associated with socioeconomic status and education. The highest rates are among those with the lowest socioeconomic status and least education. However, with Caucasian females, higher lung cancer rates are found in the lower and upper income and education groups (Pierce, Fiore, & Novotny, 1989).

Geographic Location

Caucasian males living in large industrial cities, particularly those with paper, chemical, and petroleum manufacturing, as well as shipbuilding industries, are at an increased risk for lung cancer. This finding reflects the environmental and occupational factors implicated in lung disease. Such cities are located primarily along the Atlantic coast and Gulf of Mexico. Among non-Caucasian males, the highest rates tend to be in the urban areas of the southern states. There appears to be minor geographic variation among females.

Other Factors

In addition, other risk factors for lung cancer have been noted, such as radiation in patients treated for ankylosing spondylitis, body mass index (leanness), alcohol consumption, pet birds in the home, and endocrine factors among women (Kabat, 1993).

PREVENTION

Throughout the lifespan, the probability for developing lung cancer changes as environmental risk factors interact with an individual's biologic characteristics. Carcinogenesis may arise as a result of chemical, physical, biologic, and/or genetic insults to cells (Greenwald, Kelloff, Burch-Whitman, & Kramer, 1995). This multistep process occurs over a wide area in the lung and includes an initiation step followed by a number of promotion and progression steps that lead to malignancy. The promotion stage is usually long and is generally reversible, whereas progression from premalignancy to malignancy involves genetic mechanisms that are irreversible (Lippman, Benner, & Hong, 1994).

Cancer prevention is divided as follows: (1) complete avoidance of carcinogens, (2) reduction of known environmental and lifestyle risks, and (3) efforts to prevent progression from premalignancy to cancer or to prevent recurrence (Loescher, 1993).

Prevention of Smoking

According to Pierce, Fiore, and Novotny (1989), education appears to be one of the strongest predictors of smoking status. For Caucasian and African-American males, and African-American females, age-adjusted lung cancer incidence rates are significantly associated with education. The highest rates are among those with the lowest socioeconomic status and least education. With Caucasian females, higher lung cancer rates are found in the lower and upper income and education groups.

Stopping smoking, recognizing high-risk individuals, and incorporating an aggressive approach to diagnosis and treatment could prevent a significant proportion of lung cancer.

Multiple factors appear to influence the initiation and maintenance of smoking. The reasons an individual starts to smoke are entirely different from those that lead him or her to continue smoking. Activities aimed at reducing the development of smoking behaviors are different from those designed to assist smokers to quit. Initiation of smoking is largely socially determined. Horn (1977) states that smoking behaviors are usually initiated at a fairly young age and in response to opportunity, curiosity, and a need for self-expression. Adolescents begin to smoke for multiple reasons. These include parental smoking, low self-esteem, underestimation of the power of addiction, expressing independence from adults, advertising, curiosity, truancy, alcohol, relative unimportance of school grades, peer pressure, parents in a lower income and education group, a single-parent household, lack of acceptance of health risks, type A and extroversion personality trait, anger, risk-taking orientation, and parental acceptance of smoking experimentation (Risser, 1987). Suggested smoking cessation behaviors are listed in Box 61-4 (Horn, 1977). To reverse the trend of smoking, preventive efforts need to begin before youth experimentation occurs and focus on the broader social arena. Strategies could include enforcement of prohibition of sales to minors, restriction of advertisement and promotion, and increased tobacco taxation (Horowitz, 1993; Institute of Medicine, 1994).

The regular use of cigarettes leads to behavioral and pharmacologic dependence. Smoking becomes a habitual, conditioned response. A chemical dependence on nicotine occurs. Nicotine is a drug with powerful physiologic and psychoactive effects that lead to its compulsive use. Even though more individuals are aware of the serious health hazard that cigarette smoking represents, about one person out of four continues to smoke. The majority of these people indicate a desire to quit smoking, yet only one out of three smokers remains abstinent 1 year after attempting to quit smoking because of the addicting qualities of nicotine (Novello, Davis, & Giovino, 1991).

Approximately 95% of those who quit smoking do so without the aid of an organized program (U.S. Department of Health and Human Services, 1982). Some of the self-help program formats available include self-help manuals, cassettes, books, broadcast media programs, hypnosis, relaxation training, group programs, therapists, and antismoking specialists. Nicotine-replacement products are available to control symptoms of nicotine withdrawal during smoking cessation. The nicotine patch is available to assist smokers in quitting. The nicotine is directly released through the skin or through a membrane system in contact with the skin. Side effects are minimal and include mild-to-moderate sleep disturbances; skin reactions, including transient itching, burning, and erythema; poorly defined body aches; and increased coughing.

Programs designed to reduce tobacco use among children and adults are important aspects of the National Cancer Institute's overall cancer prevention and control efforts. Since the early 1980s, the Smoking and Tobacco Control Program (STCP) of the NCI has awarded over $300 million in an effort to study and document the efficacy of interventions involving schools, the media, and the health care system. Interventions targeted specific populations such as minorities, children, women, smokeless tobacco users, and heavy smokers. Between 1982 and 1990, more than 100 individual research projects were funded by the program (Box 61-5).

Social Policy

Intolerance to smoking is a growing trend in the public sector. Antismoking activist groups exist at the community, state, and national levels and are becoming increasingly vocal and effective at influencing public policy. Government at all levels is also deeply involved in smoking issues. Local and state governments have passed laws that place limitations on public smoking. Government initiatives that control tobacco use are listed in Box 61-5 (*State Tobacco and Prevention Control Activities,* 1991).

Occupation-Related Risk Prevention

Although the number of cases of lung cancer caused by occupational exposure is relatively small, job-related cancer is potentially preventable. To prevent occupational lung dis-

Box 61-5
Government Initiatives to Control Tobacco Use

Regulatory Activities

- Laws restricting smoking in public places
- Policies restricting smoking in government buildings
- Prohibitions on access to tobacco products
- Restrictions on tobacco advertising
- Warning label requirements

Continuing Education/Information

- Public information campaigns
- Smoking-cessation programs

Economic Incentives/Deterrents

- Differential benefits package for nonsmokers
- Tobacco excise taxes

ease, elimination or reduction to lung exposure to toxic substances is necessary. Workers who smoke cigarettes significantly increase the risk of lung cancer from occupational exposure.

The Occupational Safety and Health Act, Federal Mine Safety and Health Act, and Toxic Substances Control Act are steps taken by the federal government to ensure safer working conditions. Landrigan and Selikoff (1986) feel that the prevention of occupational lung cancer may be achieved by a combination of techniques, including premarket toxicologic testing of new compounds, application of industrial hygiene techniques, legal and regulatory approaches, and epidemiologic surveillance.

Nutrition and Lung Cancer

Strong evidence exists that diets high in fruit and vegetables are protective against cancer, particularly lung cancer (Willett, 1990). Individuals who report high intake of all vegetables and fruit, especially all yellow, green, and green leafy vegetables, are at a significantly reduced risk of lung cancer (Block, Patterson, & Subar, 1992).

Chemoprevention

Chemoprevention is the use of natural or synthetic agents, such as defined chemicals or micronutrients that inhibit or reverse the process of carcinogenesis, to reduce the risk of cancer (Loescher & Meyskens, 1991). The term is used to describe attempts at prevention of disease by drugs, chemicals, vitamins, and/or minerals. Chemicals may be useful in disabling the initiated cells from progressing to a malignant form when exposed to a promoter, or preventing the promoter from acting on the initiated cells. The NCI's Chemoprevention Program is designed to study whether some micronutrients and synthetic compounds could reduce cancer incidence. The retinoids (chemical cousins of vitamin A) are one of three classes of preventive agents that have shown promise in clinical trials and are considered priority substances for study as chemopreventive agents.

Vitamin A plays a role in the regulation of cell differentiation. Studies conducted over the last 20 years suggested an inverse relationship between lung cancer and dietary intake of vitamin A (Willett, 1990). Vitamin A deficiency has been associated in particular with small cell carcinoma (Fontham, 1990). Patients with lung cancer appear to consume smaller quantities of foods rich in vitamin A or have lower blood levels of retinol and/or beta-carotene. Retinol (preformed vitamin A) is found in animal foods such as milk, butter, egg yolks, and liver. Carotenoids, such as beta carotene, are converted by the body into vitamin A. It has been thought that these nutrients had the potential to prevent carcinogenesis by absorbing free oxygen radicals produced by tobacco smoke, solvents, and pollutants. Hennekens and colleagues (1996) determined no benefit to the administration of betacarotene supplementation in a 12-year study in healthy men.

Lung cancer chemoprevention remains an experimental approach, yet it is our best hope for reducing the rates of developing lung cancer in those who have been exposed to tobacco smoke. Because survival after a diagnosis of lung cancer is generally poor and early detection is usually not achievable, interventions must be aimed at prevention. Not smoking, avoiding risky occupational exposures, and eating diets high in fruits and vegetables can help prevent lung cancer.

EARLY DETECTION

The earlier disease is detected, the more probable it is that the cancer is localized and the better the chance for cure. Unfortunately, the natural history of lung cancer usually includes years of tumor growth before clinical presentation, and occult or localized lung cancers are diagnosed infrequently. Early detection of lung cancer is very difficult.

Sputum cytologies and chest radiographs, generally used in combination, are screening tests currently available for the diagnosis of asymptomatic lung cancers. Cancerous lesions may be radiographically undetectable because of their small size or because their presence is obscured by other chest structures or abnormalities. The smallest detectable tumor on a chest roentgenogram is 1 cm. In this situation, sputum cytologies are necessary for the detection of these lesions, as well as detecting lung tumors located in the central airways. Multiple specimens must be evaluated for sputum cytologies to be sensitive detectors of lung cancer. Chest radiographs are more effective in detecting peripheral lung tumors. Both of these tests are costly and require special facilities and personnel. Mass screening for lung cancer is considered to be unwarranted, and the cost of performing these screening measures on the general adult population is considered excessive. However, some screening programs do exist. They have achieved earlier diagnoses and longer survival but have demonstrated no reduction in lung cancer mortality. Earlier detection appears to lengthen the interval between the diagnosis and death without increasing the total life span. Asymptomatic chest x-ray examination and sputum cytology have not been effective in increasing the cure rate or reducing the death rate from lung cancer. Neither chest x-ray examination nor sputum cytology can be recommended as an effective or practical method to detect lung cancer in individuals without symptoms. Routine screening for lung cancer in asymptomatic persons is not recommended. Several substances that could be used as tumor markers are being studied.

The NCI is conducting a large-scale screening trial called the *Prostate, Lung, Colorectal and Ovarian Cancer Screening Trial* to determine whether certain tests can detect these cancers early enough to reduce the number of deaths they cause in asymptomatic individuals. The efficacy of annual chest x-ray examinations versus routine medical care for early lung cancer detection is being evaluated. The trial began in 1993 and continues for 16 years (Cleary, Gorenstein, & Omenn, 1996). Approximately 37,000 men will be screened for 4 years for prostate cancer, and 37,000 women will be screened for the same period of time for ovarian cancer. Both groups will be screened for colorectal and lung cancer. A comparison, or control, group of men and women of equal size (74,000) will receive the usual care.

HISTOGENESIS

Over 90% of all primary lung tumors arise from the bronchial epithelium (Groenwald, Frogge, Goodman, & Yarbro, 1995). Normal bronchial epithelial cells serve a lining and protective function. Abnormalities occur in the bronchial epithelium because it is chronically exposed to irritating substances inhaled with ambient air. Inhaled cigarette smoke is the chief irritant.

The bronchial epithelium serves as a protective layer between the body and outer environment. The bronchial epithelium is continually damaged, shed, and replaced. Inhaled irritant substances are deposited in the airways at points of major bronchial bifurcation. Short-term exposure to cigarette smoke may change the ciliary structure or reduce ciliary beating but is principally associated with mucous cell hyperplasia and hypersecretion of mucus. With continued years of smoking, ciliated cells are repeatedly damaged and shed from the basement membrane. More rapid loss of these cells stimulates an increase in the cell turnover rate in the basal cell layer (basal cell hyperplasia). With repeated insult, the rapidly proliferating basal cells have less energy available for differentiation and squamous cell metaplasia occurs (Ingle, 1997).

These dysplastic cells replace the protective ciliated and mucus-producing cells, allowing easier access of irritants and carcinogens. Epithelial injury is not irreversible if the cause is removed, even at the point of squamous metaplasia. With the continuation of heavy smoking, atypia of the epithelial cells progresses to nuclear enlargement, nuclear variability, hyperchromatism, and abnormal mitotic activity. Several sites of fully developed intraepithelial carcinomas that do not invade the basement membrane (carcinoma in situ) can develop in the bronchi of both lungs (Ingle, 1997).

The transformation of the bronchial epithelium occurs over extended periods of time, usually several decades. The developmental period depends on the duration and degree of exposure to lung irritants and/or carcinogens.

HISTOLOGY

Lung tumors are usually referred to as *SCLC* or *non–small cell lung cancer* (NSCLC). Histologic classification depends on the identification of the distinct morphology of tumor cells. Many lung tumors contain more than one cellular element, or the cell type identified at the time of the diagnosis may evolve to a different type with treatment. The presence of multiple cell types in a single tumor mass, as well as the possibility of conversion to other cell types, suggests a common progenitor cell for all lung carcinomas. Also, tumors probably arise from proliferating simple pleuropotential reserve cells and differ only in their degree of differentiation. Yesner and Carter (1982) suggest a spectrum of lung cancer ranging from poorly differentiated small cell cancer that evolves into more differentiated adenocarcinomas and squamous cell tumors, with large cell undifferentiated tumors as intermediate.

ANATOMY AND PHYSIOLOGY OF THE LUNG

Healthy Lung

Air inhaled passes through the trachea and the branching passageways of the lung (bronchi), filling tiny air sacs (the alveoli) at the ends of the bronchi. The average lung has more than 300 million of these air sacs, providing a combined surface area of more than 750 square feet for oxygen to be absorbed into the bloodstream and carbon dioxide to be expelled (Fig. 61-1).

To some extent the lung can clean itself. Mucus produced by some cells in the bronchi traps unfamiliar material, and the movement of the cilia (tiny hairlike structures on other cells) sweeps the mucus toward the throat, where it can be coughed out. The blood and lymph systems carry away other impurities (American Cancer Society, 1987).

Smoke-Damaged Lung

Long-term exposure to cigarette smoke or irritants such as coal dust damage the ciliated cells and mucus-producing cells, resulting in replacement by dysplastic cells. The constant assault of cigarette smoking on the cells lining the bronchi can cause mucus-secreting cells to enlarge and increase the production of mucus. The cilia lining the air passages become worn away and are then unable to sweep foreign particles out of the throat. This causes what is known as *smoker's cough.*

If the smoker quits at the time of these early changes, the inner surface of the bronchi can return to normal. If the irritation continues, the atypia of the epithelial cells progresses to nuclear enlargement, nuclear variability, hyperchromatism, and abnormal mitotic activity. If the smoker continues smoking, many of the air sacs can be destroyed. Smoking beyond this stage can cause the lung cells to form abnormal growth patterns that may eventually become lung cancer.

Cancerous Lung

Cigarette smoke and other carcinogens that enter the lungs damage the respiratory epithelium. Irritants cause transformations in the epithelial cells that result in a progressive change from a benign to a malignant phenotype. When abnormal cells grow through the full thickness of the epithelium, the growth is termed a *carcinoma in situ.* This precedes the development of invasive cancer and is followed by infiltration of cancerous cells into deeper tissue (Mackey, Lukeman, & Ordonez, 1991).

The Pathology Committee of the International Association of the Study for Lung Cancer has divided SCLC into three subtypes: small cell carcinoma (about 90% of the total), mixed small cell/large cell carcinoma, and combined small cell carcinoma (typical SCLC elements mixed with

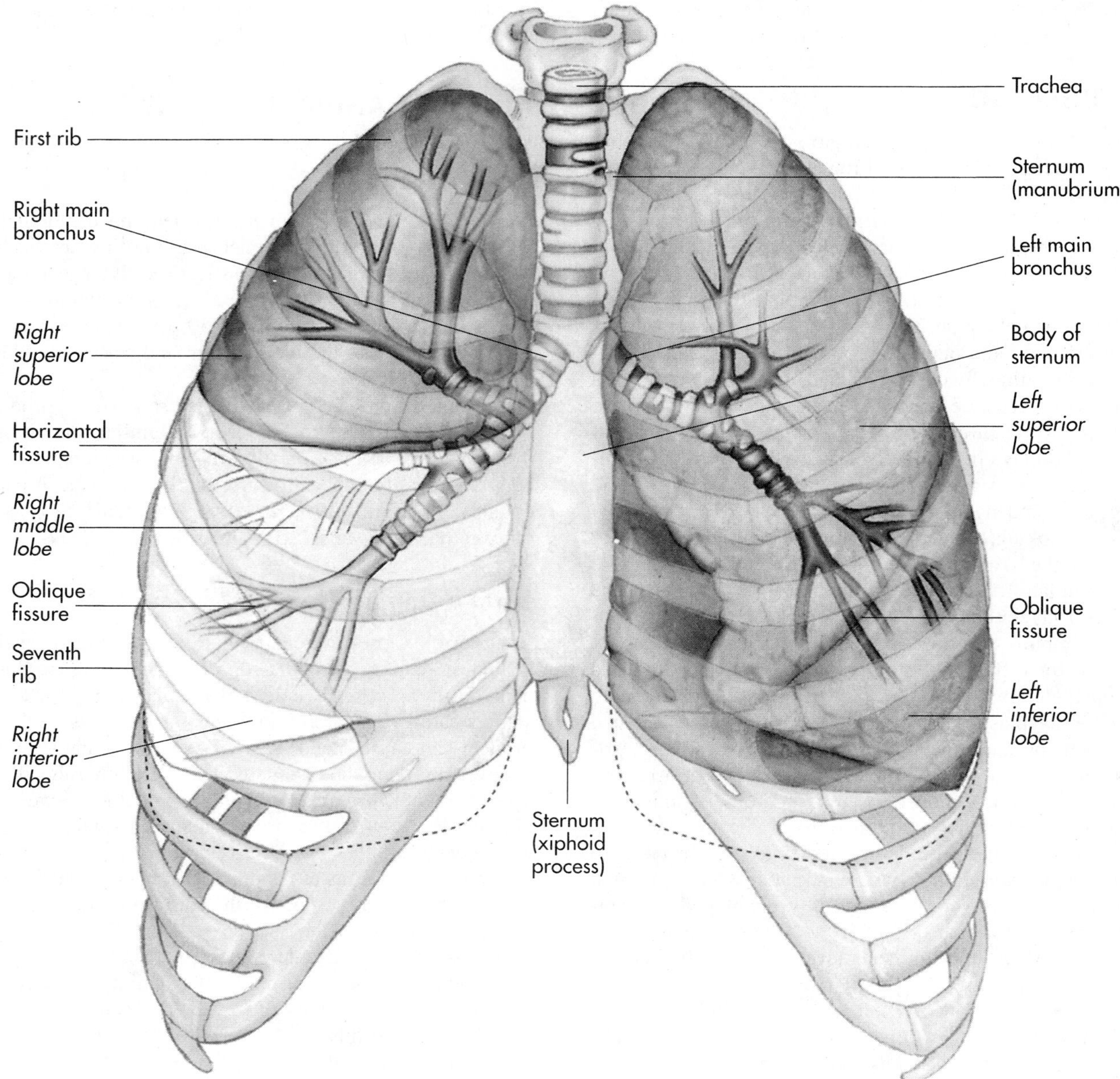

Fig. 61-1 Lungs. The trachea is an airway that branches to form a treelike formation of bronchi and bronchioles. Note that the right lung has three lobes and that the left lung has two lobes. (From Thibodeau, G. A., & Patton, K. T. [1997]. *Structure and function of the body,* [10th ed.]. St. Louis: Mosby.)

areas of differentiated squamous cell carcinoma or adenocarcinoma) (Hirsch, Matthews, Aisner, Campobasso, Elema, & Gazdar, 1988). SCLC has the poorest prognosis in this group.

SCLC develops most often in the bronchial submucosa, which is a layer of tissue beneath the epithelium. SCLC is believed to arise in neuroendocrine cells in the lung. These cells can produce hormones that stimulate their own growth and the growth of neighboring cells. When neuroendocrine cells become cancerous because of damage to their genetic material, the hormones may stimulate the growth of a tumor.

PATHOGENESIS

Carcinogenesis is thought to be a multistep process, involving the development of hyperplasia, metaplasia, dysplasia, carcinoma in situ, invasive carcinoma, and metastatic carcinoma in sequence. These steps are characterized by multiple genetic changes, including activation or overt expression of oncogenes and loss or mutation of tumor suppresser genes. Amplification of one of the myc family oncogenes is common in SCLC. Changes that commonly lead to a loss of tumor suppresser gene function in SCLC include loss, inactivation, or mutation of genes on chromosome 3p (unknown gene or genes), 13q (retinoblastoma gene), and 17p (p53 gene) (Davila & Williams, 1993; Hinson & Perry, 1993).

Lung cancer arises after certain changes have occurred in a cell's chromosomes. These changes may occur in parts of chromosomes called *genes,* or they may affect an entire chromosome. One gene, known as *p53,* appears to be defective in virtually every SCLC. This gene normally functions as a tumor suppresser gene, one of the body's natural defenses against the cancer process. In its defective form, however, p53 allows lung cancer to develop, primarily when environmental factors have damaged the lungs. People who have inherited a strong ability to metabolize the chemical debrisoquine, which is found in cigarette smoke, have a much higher risk of developing lung cancer than people who do not metabolize it readily.

SMALL CELL LUNG CANCER METASTASES

The rich supply of blood vessels and lymphatics in the lungs allows the disease to metastasize rapidly. Lung cancers spread by direct extension, lymphatic invasion, and bloodborne metastases. Tumors spread by direct invasion in the bronchus of origin. Growth can occur such that the lumen is partially or completely filled and occluded. Tumors also extend in a flattened, plaquelike fashion along the inside of the lumen. Others may invade the bronchial wall and encircle and obstruct the airway. Intrapulmonary spread may lead to compression of lung structures other than airways, such as blood or lymph vessels, alveoli, and nerves. Direct extension through the pleura can result in spread over the surface of the lung, chest wall, or diaphragm. Most centrally located tumors spread to the hilar lymph structures, either by direct extension or lymphatic spread. When the tumor invades lymphatic structures, the pattern of subsequent spread depends on the tumor cell type and the anatomic location of the tumor. The central hilar, mediastinal, and paratracheal glands are most commonly affected by lung tumors. Supraclavicular, cervical, and abdominal channels may be invaded. Tumors originating in the lower lobes tend to spread through the lymph channels.

Lung cancer generally has a widespread pattern of hematogenous metastases. This is due to the invasion of the pulmonary vascular system. After tumor cells enter the pulmonary venous system, they can be carried through the heart and disseminated systemically. Tumor emboli can become lodged in areas of organ systems where vessels become too narrow for their passage and/or where blood flow is reduced. Invasion of branches of the pulmonary arteries occurs less commonly. Metastatic lesions outside the thorax frequently involve the liver, adrenals, bone, and brain. Recent studies have shown the following percentages of metastatic sites: Metastases usually involve the bone (35%), bone marrow (17% to 23%), liver (25%), central nervous system (0% to 14%), lymph nodes (3% to 11%), subcutaneous tissue (3% to 11%), or pleura (10%) (Mackey, Lukeman, & Ordonez, 1991; Ihde, Pass, & Glatstein, 1997).

Weakness and weight loss are characteristic of hepatic metastases. Intrahepatic metastases are small and not palpable. Liver involvement may be evidenced by an elevated alkaline phosphatase level. Ribs and vertebrae are the most common bone sites of lung cancer metastases. Patients complain of severe, dull pain aggravated by respiration. Hemiplegia, personality changes, epileptic seizures, confusion, and headaches are manifestations of brain metastases.

Disease Progression

At the time of diagnosis, most tumors have probably progressed through the majority of their life span. By the time a diagnosis is made, about 85% of lung cancer patients have disease that is no longer confined to the lung. SCLC usually occurs endobronchially in a segmental bronchus; however, because of its aggressiveness, hilar and mediastinal nodes are involved in 80% of cases at the time of presentation.

CLINICAL MANIFESTATIONS/ CHARACTERISTICS

Lung cancer rarely gives an early warning of its presence. The earliest symptoms are likely to be so ordinary (coughing or wheezing) that they are often dismissed as minor irritants.

The most typical presenting symptoms of lung cancer in general are a persistent, new, or changing cough; wheezing; stridor; shortness of breath; chest wall pain; dyspnea; and hemoptysis. These symptoms are also seen with cigarette smoking and chronic obstructive pulmonary disease. Other common symptoms of secondary tumor growth include changes in breathing habits, anemia, fever, dysphagia, and weakness. Anorexia, weight loss, and unexplained fatigue are systemic symptoms associated with lung cancer (Grippi, 1990). Recurring attacks of pneumonia are present in nearly 30% of cases (Martin & Comis, 1996). Late, but clinically significant, signs may include hemoptysis, clubbing of the fingers, weight loss, and pleural effusion. Ectopic hormone syndromes and paraneoplastic syndromes are also sometimes seen.

Signs and symptoms of SCLC depend on the size and location of the tumor and the presence and extent of metastases. Patients may have local, regional, or metastatic disease (Hinson & Perry, 1993). The period of time from the first symptoms to the diagnosis is usually 3 to 4 months. Because SCLC tumors most commonly arise in the central endobronchial location, patients who are almost exclusively chronic smokers typically have a persistent new or changing cough, dyspnea, stridor, wheezing, hemoptysis, chest pain, and postobstructive (bronchial) pneumonitis. SCLC chest x-ray films more commonly show a hilar mass, hilar and mediastinal adenopathy, atelectasis, and pneumonitis than do NSCLC films. The less common peripheral tumors, seen more often in NSCLC patients, produce cough and dyspnea, and they may cause pain from pleural or chest wall involvement or pleural effusion. Also, because SCLC is usually located in the submucosa, hemoptysis is observed less often than in NSCLC. Cavitation is rarely seen (Ihde et al., 1981; Green, Kurohara, & George et al., 1972).

SCLC tumor spread intrathoracically to the mediastinum and beyond invariably occurs. This often produces superior vena cava syndrome (SVCS) with head and neck swelling, recurrent laryngeal nerve paralysis/entrapment with resultant hoarseness, dysphagia, phrenic nerve paralysis with diaphragmatic elevation and dyspnea, Horner's syndrome (unilateral ptosis, miosis, loss of facial sweat), Pancoast's syndrome (shoulder pain radiating down an arm along ulnar nerve distribution), obstruction of the trachea or esophagus (tracheo-esophageal or broncho-esophageal fistula), pericardial involvement with effusion and/or tamponade, pleural effusions, spontaneous pneumothorax, and lymphangitic metastases/carcinomatosis (hypoxia and dyspnea) (Grippi, 1990; Hinson & Perry, 1993).

By the time SCLC is diagnosed, widespread dissemination has almost always occurred. An estimated 70% of newly diagnosed patients have metastatic cancer. Symptoms of this spread include localized bone pain or pathologic fracture from skeletal involvement; a rapidly enlarging liver, abdominal discomfort, weight loss, jaundice, anorexia, elevated liver function tests, and nausea and vomiting from liver involvement; bowel symptoms from intestinal involvement; pancytopenia from bone marrow involvement; headache, seizures, and/or neurologic changes from central nervous system metastasis; subcutaneous or oral masses; and metastatic deposits on the fingertips (Mackey, Lukeman, & Ordonez, 1991). Systemic symptoms in more advanced illness also include anorexia, cachexia, and severe fatigue. Nearly 50% of SCLC patients with disseminated cancer develop a pleural effusion during the course of their illness, with associated cough and dyspnea.

Systemic symptoms commonly seen, especially with advanced disease, are anorexia, cachexia, fatigue, and weight loss. Ectopic hormone syndromes and paraneoplastic syndromes may also occur but are infrequent.

Paraneoplastic Syndromes

Paraneoplastic syndromes are caused by hormones or other substances produced by the cancer cells. Paraneoplastic syndromes occur more often in people with SCLC than NSCLC and may be the first sign of lung cancer (Grippi, 1990; Holleb, Fink, & Murphy, 1991; Hinson & Perry, 1993; Thompson, McFarland, Hirsch, & Tucker, 1993; Glover & Miaskowski, 1994). The wide range of paraneoplastic syndromes that occur in lung cancer patients includes disorders of hormone production, the nervous system, the blood, the kidneys, and the skin. Treatment of the SCLC with chemotherapy provides the most significant improvement of the syndromes because the underlying cause of the secretion of all hormones is the carcinoma itself.

Syndrome of Inappropriate Antidiuretic Hormone

The most frequently seen of the paraneoplastic syndromes is the syndrome of inappropriate antidiuretic hormone (SIADH). The incidence of SIADH in SCLC is 11%, which accounts for about ¾ of cancer-related SIADH. Some lung cancer cells produce arginine vasopressin, which causes the body to lose sodium and the kidneys to retain water. The level of sodium in the body becomes very low, causing hyponatremia, abnormal water retention, severe confusion, and coma. Other characteristic findings include concentrated urine, inability to excrete a water load, irritability, lethargy, headache, hyporeflexia, nausea, vomiting, anorexia, diarrhea, and weight gain without edema, weakness, and confusion. Otherwise, the patient may be asymptomatic. The diagnosis is confirmed by a serum sodium level of less than 130 mEq/L, serum osmolarity of less than 280 mOsm/kg H_2O, and a urine sodium level of 20 mEq/L. The most common treatment for SIADH is water restriction, but chemotherapy, antibiotics, hypertonic saline, diuretics, and demeclocycline may also be prescribed. Nursing interventions include accurate intake and output recording, fluid restriction, monitoring laboratory results, and providing safety measures for weak and confused patients.

Cushing's Syndrome

Another paraneoplastic syndrome is caused by adrenocorticotropic hormone (ACTH), the hormone normally produced by the pituitary gland to act on the adrenal glands. Unrestrained ACTH production by lung cancer cells can cause an elevated blood sugar level, diabetes, decreased concentration of potassium in the blood, and an increase in body fat and hair growth. Physiologic manifestations are different from classical Cushing's syndrome. Common signs and symptoms are muscle weakness, glucose intolerance, edema, hypokalemia, hyperpigmentation, and mild hypertension. Cushing's syndrome is associated with a poor response to chemotherapy, a shortened survival time, and an increase in therapy-related complications.

Hypercalcemia

Hypercalcemia, caused by production of a hormonelike substance called *parathormone-related protein,* occurs in about 5% of SCLC cancer patients. Symptoms produced include loss of appetite, nausea, drowsiness, constipation, and mental confusion.

Pancoast's Syndrome and Horner's Syndrome. Pancoast's syndrome causes pain in the posterior shoulder, axilla, and arm. Nerve compression can result in acroparesthesia. Horner's syndrome may result from invasion of the cervical sympathetic plexus and cause unilateral miosis, ptosis, and absence of sweating of the affected side of the neck and face (Fig. 61-2). Patients are treated with a combined surgical-radiation approach (Grippi, 1990; Cleary, Gorenstein, & Omenn, 1996).

ASSESSMENT

Any individual who has a persistent and productive cough, chest pain, weight loss, dyspnea, fever, fatigue, and/or transient hemoptysis has a history of smoking or exposure to carcinogenic agents. If that person complains of pneumonitis that persists longer than 2 weeks despite antibiotic

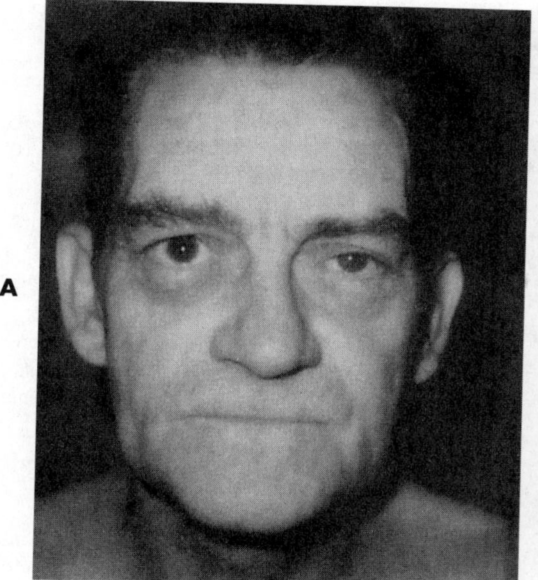

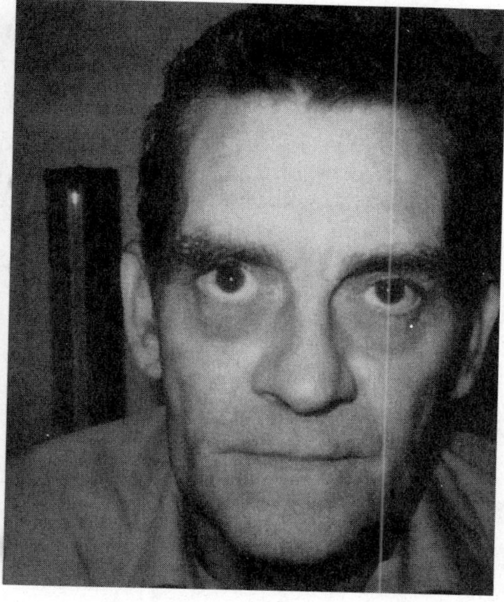

Fig. 61-2 Pancoast tumor. **A,** This 58-year-old man presented with chronic left arm and shoulder pain, along with progressive weakness of his lower arm and hand. Physical examination showed clinical findings of superior sulcus (Pancoast) tumor: ptosis of the left eyelid; miosis of the pupil; decreased sweating of the left face, arm, and upper chest (Horner's syndrome); and a tumor mass in the lung apex that involved the brachial plexus and adjacent rib. **B,** After radiotherapy, the manifestations of Horner's syndrome have resolved. There was also improvement in his pain and neurologic symptoms. Survival is poor with Pancoast tumors (less than 30% at 5 years) due to progressive regional disease, but also distant metastases. (From Skarin, A. T. [1996]. *Atlas of diagnostic oncology* [2nd ed.]. London: Mosby-Wolfe.)

therapy, suspicion of lung cancer is warranted. Some individuals may be asymptomatic when first seen, but a lesion on a routine chest radiograph suggestive of a lung malignancy, or more rarely, a positive sputum cytology, may have been detected. These individuals should receive a complete clinical evaluation, including a history, physical examination, laboratory tests, special diagnostic procedures related to lung cancer diagnosis, and, if lung cancer is confirmed, appropriate tests to determine the stage of the disease, as well as the treatment to be implemented (Table 61-1).

History Assessment

Because smoking and exposure to known carcinogens in the home, the general environment, and the workplace greatly increase the risk for the development of lung cancer, patients should be queried regarding smoking habits, occupational history, and the general respiratory environment in the workplace and home when a history is taken. According to Fielding and Phenow (1988) and Humble, Samet, and Pathak (1987), a detailed history should be taken of the number of smokers in the home and the length of time the individual has been exposed to the smoke environment because of the risks of passive smoking.

Obtaining a lifetime occupational history is recommended for individuals who have worked in shipyards or who have been exposed to asbestos. The exposure is significant even if it was brief or long ago. For individuals exposed to other known carcinogenic respiratory agents (such as clothing, textile, and laundry workers; meat wrappers and cutters; hairdressers; agricultural and chemical workers; electrical machinery manufacturers; and health care workers), a lifetime occupational history should be obtained (Stellman & Stellman, 1983).

Persons over 50 years of age may have been exposed to toxic chemicals or carcinogens that are no longer manufactured or permitted in unsupervised occupational settings. It should be determined whether these individuals had prior employment in settings unregulated by the National Institute of Occupational Safety and Health, the Occupational Safety and Health Act of 1970, or the Toxic Substances Control Act of 1976.

An occupational history includes dates of employment, a list of current and longest-held jobs, average hours worked per week, exposure to potential hazards in the workplace, common illnesses in coworkers, and personal protective equipment worn on the job.

Physical Examination

There are almost no physical signs or symptoms in the early stage of lung cancer. The only early physical finding that strongly suggests lung cancer is wheezing localized to a single lobe of the lung in an elderly person with a long history of smoking. The majority of physical signs the practitioner discovers during physical assessment are the result of late and far-advanced carcinoma of the lung. Pulmonary manifestations seen may include cough, hemoptysis, dyspnea, and pneumonia. Local manifestations seen, related to

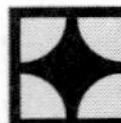

TABLE 61-1 Assessment of the Patient for Small Cell Lung Cancer

	Assessment Parameters	Typical Abnormal Findings
History	A. Personal and social history	A. Personal and social risk factors.
	1. Smoking history	1. Tobacco use: cigarettes, cigars, and pipes.
	2. Lifelong occupational history	2. Exposure to asbestos, radon, passive smoke.
	3. Family history of smoking	3. Exposure to passive household smoke.
	4. Family history of lung cancer	4. Possible genetic risk to lung cancer.
	5. Activities of daily living	5. Inability to climb stairs or walk at reasonable pace.
Physical Examination	A. History and physical	
	1. Patient report of symptoms	1. Typical patient complaints are cough; hemoptysis; chest, shoulder, and arm pain; headaches; seizures; dyspnea; pneumonia; weight loss; hoarseness; and swelling of the face and neck.
	2. Fingers	2. Finger clubbing.
	3. Cushing's syndrome	3. May indicate small cell lung cancer.
	4. Thorax	4. Tenderness may indicate tumor invasion.
	5. Liver	5. Palpation of enlarged liver may indicate metastasis.
	6. Ectopic hormone syndromes	6. Vena cava syndrome, paraneoplastic syndromes, jaundice herald advanced disease, Cushing's syndrome, syndrome of inappropriate antidiuretic hormone, carcinoid syndrome.
	7. Tibia	7. Tenderness of tibia may indicate hypertropic osteoarthropathy.
Diagnostic Tests	A. Chest x-ray examination	A. May demonstrate lung lesion. Comparative chest x-ray films are helpful to determine lung opacity, growth rate, and mediastinal involvement.
	B. Computed tomography	B. Clearly demonstrates presence, size, and shape of mass. Evidence of invasion to adjacent structures is noted.
	C. Magnetic resonance imaging	C. May prove to be superior to computed tomograph to determine invasion of brachial plexus and assessment of the mediastinum without contrast, sparing allergic reactions.
	D. Cytology	D. Can diagnose malignant disease in patients in whom a lung mass is visible on a chest x-ray film.
	E. Fiberoptic examination (bronchoscopy with biopsy, brushing, needle aspiration)	E. Fluoroscopy offers definitive diagnoses in 85% of patients.
	F. Video-assisted thoracoscopic surgery	F. Provides excellent view of chest wall, diaphragm, lung parenchyma, and mediastinal structures, enabling biopsy of viable lesions.
	G. Histology	G. Shows anaplastic undifferentiated (includes oat cell).

Modified from Humphrey, E. W., Ward, H. B., & Perri, R. T. (1995). Lung cancer. In G. P. Murphy, W. Lawrence, & R. E. Lenhard, Jr. (Eds.), *American Cancer Society textbook of clinical oncology* (2nd ed.). United States of America: American Cancer Society.

the growth of the tumor and compression of adjacent structures, may include shoulder pain, arm pain, and SVCS (distention of arm and neck veins; facial, neck, and arm edema; suffusion of mucous membranes).

Laboratory Data

Metabolic complications include an elevated antidiuretic hormone (ADH) level because of ADH-mimic produced by the tumor and an elevated adrenocorticotropic hormone (ACTH) level because of ACTH-mimic produced by the tumor. Blood gas values and pulmonary function test (PFT) results should be evaluated.

RADIOGRAPHIC PROCEDURES

Chest X-Ray Films

A chest x-ray film is obtained for visualization and location of any pathology of the lung, including a suspected mass. The chest x-ray film (anterior/posterior and lateral) is valuable in locating suspected tumors and revealing information about the size and shape of the tumor. It is the primary tool for the diagnosis of lung cancer. Lung cancer usually appears on the x-ray film as a centrally located tumor. An x-ray film can aid in determining whether there is invasion of the chest wall or mediastinum, the widened mediastinum, or a hilar adenopathy.

Tomograms

Tomograms are x-ray films that show one thin layer of the lung at a time. They may reveal a small cancer not visible on a standard x-ray film and can determine the size and location of the primary tumor. A computed tomogram of the chest can aid in determining the precise delineation of the tumor, its density, and the presence of calcium, as well as invasion or compression of vascular structures. Existence of abnormal mediastinal lymph nodes of the upper abdomen can reveal whether metastatic disease exists.

Computed Tomography Scan

Computed tomography (CT) scans can show the relationship of a lung tumor to other structures in the chest, reveal the size and location of the primary tumor, and indicate the extent of the tumor and whether it involves other organs. CT delineates solitary or multiple nodules in the parenchyma and shows any extension to the mediastinum, peribronchial lymph nodes, or distant sites. CT with intravenous contrast has become the standard examination for the evaluation of hilar and mediastinal masses and to demonstrate abnormal masses for investigation at distal sites.

Physical Examination

Examination of the Thorax. Palpation of the thorax includes testing for vocal fremitus and respiratory excursion and compression.

Vocal Fremitus

Decreased or absent vocal fremitus indicates local bronchial obstruction from bronchial carcinomas, adenomas, or foreign bodies. Sound transmission through the bronchus is interrupted. This causes the change in fremitus. Absent vocal fremitus may indicate pleural effusions. Lung tumors immediately adjacent to the visceral pleura often cause early, insidious formation of pleural effusion that is responsible for the initial complaint of dyspnea (Rohwedder, 1977).

Barrel Chest

A barrel chest is characterized by the prominence of the sternum and a barrel-shaped configuration of the chest that appears to be held in a state of full inspiration (Bouchier & Morris, 1976). The barrel chest is seen in individuals with emphysema who have smoked for a lifetime. Pursed lips during breathing, retraction of the intercostal spaces during inspiration, use of accessory muscles during quiet respirations, and audible wheezes are typical findings of emphysema.

Abnormal Breathing

Expiration is prolonged, and inspiration is gasping. This may require the use of the accessory muscles of respiration in the neck and about the shoulder girdle due to obstructive types of pulmonary disease (Buckingham, 1979). These patients may experience breathlessness.

Thoracic Wall

Palpation of the thoracic wall reveals masses. A bulge on the chest may be observed with the use of indirect lighting. A neoplasm of the ribs may protrude and is visible on inspection.

Deviated and Fixed Trachea

Normally, the trachea is located in the midline and is freely movable. Localized disease may produce a tracheal shift, or the trachea may be fixed by disease in the surrounding structures. Carcinoma of the lung rarely causes displacement, except by producing atelectasis (DeGowin & DeGowin, 1987).

Superior Vena Cava Obstruction

This is a common complication of lung cancer. Buckingham (1979) describes the clinical picture as follows: Edema of both eyelids, arms, and hands develops and will "pit" on pressure; the face is a dusky blue color; the lips are deeply cyanotic; and the swollen, blue head sits on a thick "bull neck" that is distended by many large, tense collateral veins. The shoulders, chest, and upper abdomen are covered with a lacy collateral venous pattern. Patients with superior vena cava syndrome are treated with combination chemotherapy with or without radiation therapy.

Dullness

Dullness on percussion usually indicates pleural effusion or a consolidated lung. The normal sound percussed over the lung is resonance. Lung cancer is the most common cause of hemorrhagic pleural effusion in middle-aged and elderly male smokers. The early production of pleural fluid by most tumors produces the classic signs of pleural effusion. These are flatness, absence of fremitus, and breath sounds (DeGowin & DeGowin, 1987).

Whispered Pectoriloquy, Bronchophony, and Egophony

When a lung is consolidated or compressed by a pleural effusion, the transmission of sounds is louder, clearer than usual, and sometimes changed in quality. Changes seen that are common in lung cancer include the following:

1. Whispered Pectoriloquy: The patient whispers numerals (one, two, and three). Normally these sounds are muffled; in consolidation they are clearly transmitted (Bates, 1983).
2. Bronchophony: When the patient says a number (99) the sound normally is muffled. When the sound transmitted is a clear sound of the vocalized numerals, it is created by mucus- or fluid-filled alveoli or by a cellular mass replacing alveolar tissue (Burns & Johnson, 1980).
3. Egophony: The patient says "e," which normally results in a muffled, indistinct sound. In pleural effusion, the "e" sound is heard as a nasal-sounding "a."

Unilateral Wheezing and the Bagpipe Sign

Tumors in the main bronchus may cause a localized expiratory and/or inspiratory wheeze, or "honk," which is sometimes reproduced only when the individual lies on the affected side. When a continuous wheeze is heard at the end of expiration as air continues to whistle out past a partial obstruction, this is known as the *bagpipe sign* (Rohwedder, 1977).

Finger Clubbing

About 5% to 12% of the patients with lung cancer have clubbing of the fingers that may be an early or a late sign of thoracic disease. It may be absent even in the presence of advanced disease. An examination of nail beds may reveal sponginess or a thickened and boggy nail bed in the presence of clubbing. Clubbing usually occurs first in the thumb and index finger and then spreads to the other fingers. Changes associated with clubbing usually occur gradually over many weeks, months, and years. Clubbing is best assessed by viewing the finger from the side. A normal finger viewed from this direction has an angle of about 160 degrees between the base of the nail and the skin next to the cuticle. In clubbing, this base angle is obliterated and becomes 180 degrees or more (Grimes & Burns, 1987).

DIAGNOSTIC STUDIES SPECIFIC TO SMALL CELL LUNG CANCER

Further diagnosis for SCLC is obtained through sputum cytology and pathologic diagnosis by biopsy through a fiberoptic bronchoscopy. A complete blood count; blood chemistries; immunochemical markers; CT scans of the chest, abdomen, and brain; a bone scan; and bilateral bone marrow aspiration and biopsy complete the extensive workup procedure (Martin & Comis, 1996). These latter tests determine the extent of the disease spread.

Radiologic studies are essential in the diagnosis and staging of SCLC. It is usually seen in the hilar or mediastinal regions. CT with intravenous contrast has become the standard examination for the evaluation of hilar and mediastinal masses and to demonstrate abnormal masses for investigation at distal sites, including the head, liver, lymph nodes, and adrenal glands (Harper, Houang, Spiro, Geddes, Hodson, & Souhami, 1981). Radionuclide scans are used for the detection of bony lesions.

Mediastinoscopy/Mediastinotomy

Mediastinoscopy is used to determine whether the cancer has spread to the lymph nodes in the mediastinum. Mediastinoscopy can be performed for the diagnosis of lesions not accessible to flexible fiberoptic bronchoscopy and for the staging of certain mediastinal lesions (Ashbaugh, 1970). The left anterior mediastinotomy (Chamberlain procedure) is a modification that allows access to the aortic window and lower left hilar lesions. Scalene node biopsy and hilar tomography also aid in determining lymph node involvement.

Thoracentesis

Thoracentesis is used to diagnose malignant pleural effusions with a diagnostic accuracy of about 70% (Light, 1983). Ultrasound guidance is used to help detect and localize small effusions.

STAGING

Although NSCLC uses the usual TNM system for staging, the anatomic extent of SCLC is most often described as limited or extensive, using the two-stage system proposed by the Veteran's Administration Lung Cancer Study Group (VALG). This exception is so because all SCLC is treated with chemotherapy. Patients determined to have limited SCLC also usually receive radiotherapy. Therefore sophisticated staging for purposes of therapeutic planning is not required. Limited disease can be treated in a single radiotherapy portal and is generally defined as tumor confined to one hemithorax and regional lymph nodes without pleural effusion.

Limited disease is defined as primary tumor involvement confined to one lung, the mediastinum, ipsilateral hilar lymph nodes, ipsilateral and/or contralateral supraclavicular lymph nodes, ipsilateral and contralateral mediastinal lymph nodes, and pleural effusion. Another criterion is that limited disease can be treated in a single radiotherapy portal. *Extensive disease* refers to spread beyond the criteria for limited disease. Namely, metastases in the contralateral lung and distant metastases (brain, bone, liver, bone marrow, adrenals, and lymph nodes) are considered extensive disease (Mann & Karwande, 1988). This two-stage system provides significant prognostic information. Long-term survival (2 years) in SCLC occurs almost exclusively in the limited disease category. Approximately one third of patients with SCLC have limited disease at the time of diagnosis, and two thirds have extensive disease (Hirsch et al., 1988; Cancer Net, 1996). *Recurrent disease* means that the cancer has come back after it has been treated. It may come back in the lungs or in another part of the body.

Diagnosis

A diagnosis of lung cancer usually is confirmed by tissue that has been studied through biopsy but may be done by cytologic examination. The method of choice for obtaining tissue depends on the location of the suspected tumor. The following procedures are used to obtain tissue for biopsy.

Thoracotomy is performed as an exploratory procedure if other diagnostic methods fail and there is reason to believe cancer is present. The procedure is usually performed only when the surgeon is reasonably sure that if cancer is diagnosed, the tumor can be completely removed.

Staging Procedures

At the time of diagnosis, almost all SCLC patients have regional lymph node involvement. For the most part, individuals with mediastinal node metastases have unresectable disease.

A medical history and physical examination, in conjunction with routine blood chemistries, can be useful techniques in evaluating metastatic spread. Organ scanning is of limited value in detecting unsuspected disease in the absence of signs or symptoms of specific organ involvement. Metastatic disease not detectable by physical examination or biochemical screening is rarely encountered. Organ scans and biopsies may be used to confirm the presence of metastatic disease and for assessment of stage (Ingle, 1997). Procedures include the following: A metastatic workup for staging purposes includes a CT scan of the chest, adrenal glands, liver, and brain, as well as cytologic evaluation of bone marrow aspirate, lymph node biopsy, bilateral biopsies, barium esophogram, and fluoroscopy. Other procedures include evaluation of serum chemistries to determine electrolyte abnormalities, especially hyponatremia secondary to the SIADH, evaluation of renal and hepatic function, evaluation of hematologic profiles, and an electrocardiogram analysis. Radionuclide scans are also used.

Sputum Cytology

Sputum cytology can reveal lung cancers in patients with normal x-ray results, can reveal the type of lung cancer, and can confirm the pathologic diagnosis. Centrally located endobronchial tumors usually yield positive sputum cytologies. In addition, sputum cytology can be done on an outpatient basis. The recommended procedure for outpatient collection of pooled sputum specimens for cytologic examination can be found in Box 61-6 (Elpern, 1993). However, because it cannot pinpoint the tumor's location, a positive sputum cytology test is usually followed up with further diagnostic procedures.

Box 61-6
Recommended Procedure for Outpatient Collection of Pooled Sputum Specimens for Cytologic Examination

1. The individual is given three to five containers, each containing 2 oz of fixative. Each container is labeled to indicate consecutive days of collection. The probability of detecting malignant cells is approximately 75% with three daily specimens and 90% with five consecutive daily specimens.
2. The person is instructed to cough and expectorate into one of the containers, according to the following procedure:
   a. The person should obtain specimens on arising in the morning. This produces the best specimen of secretions from deep in the lungs.
   b. The person should not perform any mouth care, eating, or drinking of fluids other than water before obtaining the specimen.
   c. The person should breathe deeply and cough to raise sputum. Saliva specimens have no benefit in cancer detection. Heated hypertonic aerosol, ultrasonic mist, and postural drainage may be used to assist in sputum induction.
   d. The person should expectorate directly into the specimen container.
3. Additional sputum raised by the individual should be added to the same container during the day.
4. A separate container is used for each day's sputum.

Bronchoscopy

Centrally located tumors are accessible for bronchoscopic visualization, washing, brushing, and biopsy. Samples of cells are obtained, the precise location of the tumor is discovered, and a judgment is made whether the tumor can be completely removed. Bronchoscopy facilitates the acquisition of cytologic material by brush and collection of liquid washings and by biopsy of small specimens from endobronchial and transbronchial lesions. It can confirm the pathologic diagnosis and stage, determine the size and location of the primary tumor, and provide a better specimen for histologic evaluation. Bronchoscopy can also be done as an outpatient procedure.

Needle Biopsy (Aspiration)

Peripherally located tumors may be accessed by percutaneous needle biopsy of the lung. The procedure is guided by a fluoroscope, which is an x-ray machine that projects the image on a fluorescent screen. This procedure is useful for patients who are not likely candidates for surgery because the presence of malignant cells in pleural fluid is considered a contraindication of surgical resection. Pleural fluid is examined, and the pleura is studied through biopsy to confirm the diagnosis of lung cancer. Pleural effusions result from tumor extension to the pleural surface.

Radionuclide scans (nuclear medicine scans) reveal whether cancer has spread to other areas of the body. A small amount of radioactive material is injected where it can be absorbed only by cancer cells. Any cancerous tumors are projected on a small screen. Brain, bone, liver, and spleen scans can identify distant metastases.

Other tests being studied to ascertain their usefulness in determining if and where lung cancer has spread are as follows:

- Complete blood counts and blood chemistries, which provide information on the general level of the individual's health and signs of paraneoplastic syndromes
- Magnetic resonance imaging (MRI), which can determine invasion or compression of vascular structures by the tumor
- Pulmonary angiography
- Monoclonal antibodies
- Immunocytochemical markers (neuron-specific enolase, chromogranin A), which provide information on the histologic diagnosis and maybe the prognosis

MEDICAL MANAGEMENT

The treatment of lung cancer remains a therapeutic challenge. The potential toxicities and risks of aggressive therapy must be carefully weighed and presented when determining the potential benefits. The goal of cancer treatment is based on the potential for cure and a careful assessment of the adverse effects. Fewer than 10% of SCLC patients are cured with standard therapy. At times, less intensive treatment, palliative care, or supportive care (consisting of pain control dyspnea and psychological support) may be the wisest therapeutic choice. Supportive care may not affect the ultimate outcome, but it can allow the patient extended periods of a functional, pain-free life.

Ironically, SCLC is the most responsive of all lung tumors to chemotherapy and radiotherapy. SCLC is considered a systemic disease, and therefore treatment is combination chemotherapy, with or without radiotherapy. Usually, only patients determined to have localized SCLC are given radiotherapy. Surgical resection is not usually used as an adjunctive treatment because about 40% of lung cancers have already spread to other parts of the body at the time of diagnosis (American Cancer Society, 1995). Quite infrequently, surgical resection combined with preoperative and/or postoperative chemotherapy may be considered for the patient with a small peripheral tumor without apparent nodal involvement.

Box 61-7

Principles That Guide Current Therapy for Small Cell Lung Cancer

1. Multiple simultaneously administered chemotherapeutic agents are preferable to single agents in both limited and extensive disease. A regimen is continued if a complete response occurs. A second-line regimen is tried if a lesser response is obtained. Etoposide (VP-16) has demonstrated high activity against small cell lung cancer and therefore is included in most new drug regimens. Ifosfamide is under evaluation in clinical trials.
2. Maximum results require high-dose therapy sufficient to produce serious toxicity. More intensive regimens appear to produce higher response rates. There is a limit to this dose response, above which increased toxicity occurs without improved survival.
3. Tumor regression in response to chemotherapy often occurs quickly. Most individuals who respond relapse in a short time, frequently at the initial intrathoracic site.
4. The development of drug resistance is a common problem. Alternating chemotherapy regimens to prevent the development of drug resistance is a proposed, but not confirmed, strategy.
5. Median survival times are about 14 months for limited disease and 7 to 9 months for extensive disease. Less than 20% of the patients achieve long-term (2 years) survival after initiation of treatment. Typically, there are patients with limited disease who achieve a complete response to therapy. Relapses in long-term survivors are often related to the appearance of nonsmall cell lung cancer.

Chemotherapy

Chemotherapy is the most common treatment for all stages of SCLC. There have been few advances in chemotherapy since the 1970s, although combination chemotherapeutic regimens have had a positive influence on survival. Several clinical trials have been conducted, and the results have demonstrated several principles that guide current therapy. These principles can be found in Box 61-7 (Elpern, 1993). Combination chemotherapy has helped increase the survival time somewhat for about 70% of patients with early-stage lung cancer.

Many active single agents and combination chemotherapeutic protocols are used in the treatment of SCLC. Response rates of greater than 80% to combination chemotherapy have been seen in limited-stage SCLC. About 10% to 25% of patients with limited disease are alive and disease free in 2 years. Response rates of greater than 50% are common in extensive disease. Patients with extensive disease may respond to combination chemotherapy, but they usually relapse. With combination chemotherapy, overall response rates of 70% to 85% for extensive disease have been seen with complete response rates, a necessary requirement for cure, averaging about 50% for limited disease and 20% to 30% for extensive disease (Hinson & Perry, 1993; Cancer Net, 1996).

Etoposide/cisplatin (VP/DDP) is the first-line choice in SCLC, with a median survival from 6 to 10 months and an overall response rate of 40% to 80% (only 10% to 20% of extensive disease patients achieve a complete remission) (Faylona, Loehrer, Ansari, Sandler, Gonin, & Einhorn, 1995). Ifosfamide is an active single agent in extensive SCLC, with 48% to 76% response rates (Nichols, 1995).

Limited (Disease)–Stage Small Cell Lung Cancer. Patients with limited-stage SCLC are treated most effectively with a combination of two or more drugs. Radiation therapy plus combination chemotherapy is more effective than chemotherapy alone in controlling the primary tumor in the lung. Overall objective response rates of 65% to 90%, complete response rates of 45% to 75%, and a median survival time of 12 to 20 months have been seen. SCLC patients with limited disease have a 2-year disease-free survival rate of approximately 15% to 40%. Of all the chemotherapeutic agents, cisplatin and etoposide have produced high response rates and better survival and have become the first-line therapy for SCLC (Einhorn, 1986; Faylona et al., 1995; Cleary, Gorenstein, & Omenn, 1996; Ihde, Pass, & Glatstein, 1997). Carboplatin, etoposide, and paclitaxel (Taxol) are also used. No improvement in survival has been seen when the duration of drug administration exceeds 4 to 6 months. No evidence exists that maintenance chemotherapy is of benefit.

Extensive Stage Small Cell Lung Cancer. Combination chemotherapy is the cornerstone treatment for extensive disease. Combination chemotherapy plus chest radiation does not appear to increase survival over chemotherapy alone. Cytoxan, vincristine, and doxorubicin have been effective. Overall response rates of 60% to 80%, complete response rates of 15% to 20%, and a median survival time of 7 to 11 months have been seen. Disease-free survival for 2 years in extensive disease is uncommon. No improvement in survival has been seen when the duration of drug administration exceeds 6 months. No evidence exists that maintenance chemotherapy is of benefit.

Nonresponsive (Recurrent-Stage) Small Cell Lung Cancer. The prognosis for SCLC that has progressed despite chemotherapy is exceedingly poor, regardless of the stage. The expected median survival time is 2 to 3 months. Patients who are primarily resistant to chemotherapy and those who have received multiple chemotherapeutic regimens rarely respond to additional treatment. Patients who have relapsed more than 6 months after the initial treatment are more likely to respond to additional chemotherapy (Greco, 1993).

Combination chemotherapy has produced a plateau in extensive disease. Simple therapy should be considered for patients with a poor prognosis, without negatively affecting their quality of life. Single-agent treatment is an acceptable therapy for patients with poor performance status or those with other medical risk factors that would increase the risk of treatment toxicites.

To date, there is no single regimen that has proven to be superior. Etoposide-containing regimens appear to be superior to CAV (cyclophosphamide, Adriamycin, vincristine). There is also no clear evidence that alternating chemotherapeutic regimens is more effective than VP/DDP (Giaccone, Dalesio, McVie, Kirkpatrick, Postmus, & Burghouts, 1993).

Radiotherapy

Radiation therapy has an important role in the treatment of lung cancer. It may be given with curative, adjuvant, or palliative intent. SCLC has excellent initial response rates to external beam radiation, but reoccurrence is typical and sensitivity decreases over time. The radiation dose is based on the size and location of the tumor. External beam radiation is given to a wide area that includes the primary tumor and surrounding tissue. After the initial treatments, progressively smaller areas are treated. In the final treatment, or "boost," the treated area may be quite small. Radiation therapy is local treatment because it affects only the cells in the area being treated.

Radiation can be used to kill cancer cells in the lungs or in other parts of the body where the cancer has spread. It may also be used to shrink tumors. Radiation can be used to treat bronchial or tracheal obstructions, hemoptysis, painful bone lesions, central nervous system involvement, and superior vena cava obstructions. Side effects experienced during or after radiation therapy vary depending on the organ systems or normal tissue in the radiation field, the amount and duration of radiation, and the type of concurrent or recent chemotherapy. It is also used as palliation to control symptoms associated with lung cancer, such as severe cough and obstructive pneumonitis, or to prolong the functional life of the individual.

Internal radiation therapy, or brachytherapy, is also used. Brachytherapy is the placement of radioactive sources directly into or adjacent to a tumor. The two principle techniques in use today are (1) interstitial brachytherapy using radioactive seeds or wires implanted directly into the tumor and (2) intracavitary brachytherapy, in which the radioactive source is placed through a catheter or other hollow applicator into a body cavity or lumen. Brachytherapy is a viable option for the treatment of lung cancer. High-dose-rate brachytherapy is used most often as palliative therapy for obstructive symptoms. Endobronchial obstruction by lung cancer is a potentially fatal complication occurring in 20% to 30% of newly diagnosed patients (Mehta, Speiser, & Macha, 1994).

Acute side effects include dyspnea, cough, anorexia, fatigue, esophagitis, dysphagia, and skin changes. Early reactions of external beam radiotherapy include skin irritation; dysphasia (2 to 3 weeks after treatment ends); a dry, sore throat; esophagitis (during treatment); strictures; loss of appetite; nausea; vomiting; weight loss; hair loss in the treated area; a decreased blood count (myelosuppression); fatigue; a nonproductive cough (which may persist throughout the person's life); pneumonitis (occurs 1 to 6 months after treatment has been completed); increased tenacity of bronchial secretions; and inflammation of the pleura and pericardium. Late reactions of radiotherapy include pericardial constriction, damage to the heart muscle, pneumonitis, lung fibrosis, fracture of the ribs, and spinal cord damage. Problems associated with whole-brain irradiation include mild erythema, alopecia, otitis, and neurologic complications (Abner, 1993).

Combined Therapy

Thoracic recurrence is the most significant treatment failure. The majority of SCLCs relapse, with over 60% of recurrences occurring in the chest (Mira, Livingston, Moore, Chen, Bailey, & Bogardus, 1982). Therefore chest irradiation has been combined with chemotherapy to reduce the frequency of intrathoracic relapse after chemotherapy alone. Patients with limited disease usually are treated with combined therapy. A reduced frequency of tumor recurrence in the chest and an increased 2-year survival time have been reported from combined modality therapy for these patients. Radiation therapy in conjunction with chemotherapy is now routinely administered to patients with limited disease (Pignon, Arriagada, Ihde, Johnson, Perry, & Souhami, 1992). The radiation field includes the tumor, mediastinal nodes, and supraclavicular lymph nodes. Combination therapy has its downfalls, with increased toxicity to the skin, esophagus, and lung parenchyma. Patients with extensive disease have not been shown to benefit from the addition of radiation therapy.

Recurrent-Stage Small Cell Lung Cancer. Patients with intrinsic endobronchial obstructing lesions or extrinsic compression due to the tumor have achieved successful palliation with endobronchial laser therapy and/or brachytherapy (Miller & Phillips, 1990). Patients with a progressive intrathoracic tumor after failing initial chemotherapy can achieve significant tumor responses, palliation of symptoms, and short-term control with external-beam radiotherapy. Only the rare patient experiences long-term survival after "salvage" radiotherapy (Ochs, Tester, Cohen, Lichter, & Ihde, 1983).

Metastatic Small Cell Lung Cancer

Central nervous system (CNS) metastases are an important cause of morbidity and mortality in patients with SCLC (Lucas, Robinson, Hoskin, Yarnold, Smith, & Ford, 1986). Brain metastases are found in 10% of the patients at the initial diagnosis (Hirsch, Paulson, Hansen, & Larsen, 1983; Ihde, Pass, & Glatstein, 1997), and the longer the patient with SCLC survives, the greater the likelihood of the development of brain involvement. Prophylactic cranial irradiation has been recommended for patients who have achieved or demonstrated a complete response to chemotherapy. This is done to eliminate the CNS as a site of early relapse. Patients with CNS recurrences can often obtain palliation of symptoms with radiotherapy and/or additional chemotherapy. The majority of patients treated with radiotherapy obtain objective responses and improvement after radiotherapy (Carmichael, Crane, Bunn, Glatstein, & Ihde, 1988). Radiation may reduce the incidence of brain metastases but does not clearly increase survival.

Irradiation remains the cornerstone therapy for CNS metastases and for the therapy of relapsed patients with SVCS or spinal cord compression (SCC). The survival advantage is not necessarily significant and neurotoxicity occurs. PCI side effects include involuntary trembling, loss of muscular coordination, and impairment of memory and thought processes.

Radiation therapy can play an important role in relieving symptoms caused by the primary tumor and by metastatic tumors, especially in the brain and bone. Radiotherapy can also relieve pain and other symptoms. Refined patient selection criteria, biologic improvements with combined therapy, technical improvements in equipment, and radiation delivery systems all offer hope of therapeutic gain in lung cancer treatment (Hilderley, 1996).

Phototherapy (Photodynamic Therapy)

Photodynamic therapy (PDT) is used for palliation of advanced lung cancer. This is a technique that uses an interaction between light and a substance that makes cells more sensitive to light to destroy tumor tissue. The photosensitizing agent is injected into the body and absorbed by all cells. The substance rapidly leaves most cells, but it remains in or around cancer cells for a longer time. It usually takes 48 to 72 hours for the drug to clear healthy tissues and concentrate in malignant cells. Light from a laser is then delivered through a bronchoscope and is absorbed by the photosensitizing agent in the cancer cells, causing a chemical reaction that destroys the cells. The procedure is painless because no tissue is burned or cut. PDT promising features are as follows: (1) Cancer cells can be selectively destroyed while most normal cells are spared; (2) the damaging effect of the photosensitizing agent occurs only when it is exposed to light; and (3) there appear to be few side effects. The photosensitizer causes profound photosensitivity, so patients must avoid sunlight for up to 6 weeks after treatment.

For individuals with far advanced obstructing airway tumors, phototherapy using a neodymium:yttrium-aluminum-garent (YAG) laser has been applied for palliation. The YAG laser is applied through a bronchoscope. It produces thermal necrosis and tumor shrinkage, allowing tumors to be removed through biopsy forceps. As with all invasive procedures, hemorrhage is a complication, but heating helps reduce the blood supply and control bleeding.

PCI had been thought to be safe and effective, but that has been questioned, especially when administered in conjunction with chemotherapy. Cranial irradiation might damage the blood-brain barrier and increase the CNS toxic effects of systemic chemotherapy (Fleck, Einhorn, Lauer, Schultz, & Miller, 1990). In addition, radiation to the brain has significant side effects. According to Livingston, Stephens, Bonnet, Grozea, and Lehene (1984) and Schmidt and Shell (1994), delayed neurologic complications have been reported after PCI. The reported complications include dementia, memory loss, psychomotor retardation, organic brain syndrome, optic atrophy, hemiparesis, confusion, ataxia, occasional falling episodes, speech impairment, inability to concentrate, problems in judgment, parkinsonian symptoms, weakness, depression, dizziness, abnormal gait, and intention tremors. Although PCI may reduce the incidence of brain metastases, it does not appear to increase survival. Few patients live long enough to experience these delayed reactions.

Current Standards of Treatment for Small Cell Lung Cancer

Limited-Stage. For patients with limited disease, the current standard of care is combination chemotherapy plus thoracic radiation therapy (Haraf, Devine, Ihde, & Vokes, 1992). The use of both modalities dictates against the selection of chemotherapeutic drugs whose side effects are enhanced by radiation therapy. Etoposide-cisplatin combinations can be combined with radiation therapy more safely. Response rates are high, yet acute and chronic toxicities are also enhanced. Treatment options include (1) chemotherapy and radiation therapy to the chest with or without radiation therapy to the brain or (2) chemotherapy with or without PCI (National Cancer Institute, 1997). The most important therapeutic advances have occurred in the treatment of limited disease in which etoposide/cisplatin have been combined with concurrent radiation therapy. New agents show promise (paclitaxel, docetaxel, topotecan, CPT-11, gemcitabine, and vinorelbine).

Extensive-Stage Small Cell Lung Cancer. Patients with extensive disease usually receive combination chemotherapy, at least initially. Radiation therapy is usually not used for patients with extensive disease. Treatment options for extensive stage SCLC include the following: (1) combination chemotherapy with or without PCI; (2) combination chemotherapy and chest radiation with or without PCI; (3) radiation therapy to the brain, bone, spine, and other sites of metastasis; and (4) treatment with new drugs under evaluation in clinical trials (National Cancer Institute, 1997).

ONCOLOGIC EMERGENCIES

Recurrent Stage

Treatment options for recurrent patients include the following: (1) palliative radiation therapy to reduce discomfort, (2) a clinical trial testing new drugs in phase I or phase II, (3) salvage chemotherapy, or (4) endobronchial laser therapy and/or brachytherapy (National Cancer Institute, 1997).

Spinal Cord Compression

Spinal cord compression (SCC) from extradural metastases of lung cancer is often treated with radiation therapy. Signs and symptoms of SCC may be gradual and subtle. Epidural cord compression usually results from direct extension of vertebral metastases, which MRI readily shows. Back pain is often the first sign. Progressive back pain may occur up to 6 months before the diagnosis. The pain may be constant and aggravated by movement, lying down, Valsalva maneuver, sneezing, motion, or coughing. Patients develop weakness, sensory loss, and a Babinski's reflex. Bed rest is recommended, and pain may be relieved by sitting upright.

Radiation therapy is usually the treatment of choice for epidural metastases from lung cancer. Neurosurgical consultation and intervention may be indicated if the area of compression has been previously irradiated to maximum tolerance. Surgical decompression may also be indicated if neurologic deterioration occurs during the initiation of radiation therapy (Glick & Glover, 1995). The treatment field extends two vertebral bodies above and below the level of blockage. Corticosteroids are prescribed to reduce swelling and inflammation around the cord.

The prognosis appears to be related to the patient's ability to walk at the time of the diagnosis. Severe or prolonged cord compression can lead to extremity paralysis and loss of sphincter control.

Superior Vena Cava Syndrome

Compression of the superior vena cava by extrinsic compression, intraluminal thrombus, or tumor invasion, resulting in impaired venous drainage of the head, neck, and upper extremities, can lead to the complex of symptoms known as *SVCS* (Fig. 61-3). The more common signs and symptoms include edema of the face, neck, upper thorax, and upper extremities, with neck and thoracic vein distention; dilation of veins in the neck, trunk, or upper extremities; cough; dyspnea; plethora of the face and neck; orthopnea; cyanosis; and tachypnea. Less common complaints include hoarseness, stridor, respiratory distress, nausea, dysphagia, headache, visual disturbances, dizziness, and chest pain. Position changes (bending forward, stooping, or lying down) aggravate symptoms. CNS effects include headache, visual changes, syncope, seizures, and altered states of consciousness. Onset can be gradual, and therefore difficult to recognize, or rapid. The presenting symptom in approximately 4% of all lung cancer patients is SVCS (Komaki & Cox, 1994).

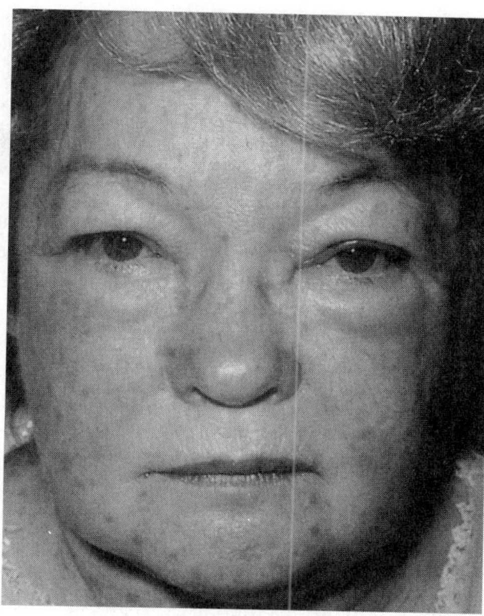

Fig. 61-3 Squamous cell carcinoma (SVC syndrome). A 56-year-old woman with diagnosed lung cancer presented with marked facial edema characteristic of SVC syndrome. (From Skarin, A. T. [1996]. *Atlas of diagnostic oncology* [2nd ed.]. London: Mosby-Wolfe.)

Major considerations in the nursing care of patients with SVCS include recognition of high-risk patients; facilitation and coordination of diagnostic procedures; assessment of respiratory, cardiac, and neurologic systems; administration of therapy; provision of emotional, supportive, and psychosocial support; and patient education (Stewart, 1996). Patient complaints include cyanosis, dyspnea, cough, severe headaches, pain, dysphagia, syncope, and edema of the face, neck (Stokes' collar), arms, and upper thorax. Venous pulsations in the neck are absent.

SVCS is treated as an emergency when there is upper airway edema, brain edema, or decreased cardiac output. CT, MRI, contrast venography, and mediastinoscopy/mediastinotomy confirm the diagnosis.

Combination chemotherapy is the most common and effective means of palliating the symptoms of SVCS caused by SCLC. The patient must be kept in the Fowler's position. Treatment may also include steroids, diuretics, thrombolytics, anticoagulation therapy, stint placement, and surgery.

Chemotherapy

Aggressive, multiagent chemotherapy regimens are used in the treatment of lung cancer. When these regimens are combined with chest irradiation, serious toxicities occur. Preleukemia and postleukemia therapy have been seen. This is indicative of long-term bone marrow toxicity. Individuals most at risk for this occurrence are those treated aggressively with cytotoxic agents, especially alkylating agents.

According to Cooper, White, and Matthay (1986), the risk of pulmonary toxicities from cytotoxic drugs increases with cumulative drug dose, age, use of chest radiotherapy, and concurrent oxygen therapy. Many pharmacologic agents are associated with pulmonary parenchymal damage (Elpern, 1993).

Radiotherapy

One of the most common late effects of chest irradiation is pulmonary fibrosis, which may not occur for months to years after radiation to the thorax. The total dose of radiation and the size of the treatment portal determines the severity of this condition. When chemotherapy and radiation are combined in treatment, there can be a synergistic effect of injury to lung tissue. The changes in pulmonary function are usually a progressive decline in lung volumes and a decrease in lung compliance and diffusing capacity. Dry cough, dyspnea, weakness, hypoxemia, and cor pulmonale are clinical manifestations commonly seen. If curative-dose radiotherapy to the heart or spinal cord was implemented, pericarditis and myelitis may ensue. As doses increase, the frequency of complications increases. However, most of the time, patients die of their cancer before these complications develop.

When cranial irradiation is used, especially in conjunction with chemotherapy, a CNS syndrome of neurologic abnormalities appears. Some of the symptoms are memory loss, tremor, slurred speech, and somnolence.

NURSING MANAGEMENT

Symptom Management

Virtually all individuals with lung cancer encounter distressing physical symptoms. These are associated with the tumor and/or its treatment. The degree of symptomatic distress influences the physical performance, subjective well-being, and quality of life. Cough, pain, dyspnea, hemoptysis, and wheezing are symptoms most commonly experienced by individuals with lung cancer.

Cough

A chronic cough may result from hypersecretion of mucus or stimulation of irritant receptors in the bronchial mucosa through tumor infiltration. Persistent coughing can deprive an individual of sleep, as well as increase musculoskeletal chest pain and hemoptysis. It is not appropriate to suppress a productive cough. However, a dry, persistent, and debilitating cough, usually with narcotic medications such as codeine preparations, is of concern. Inspired air should be warmed and humidified. Cigarette smoking once again should be discouraged. Deep breathing and effective coughing techniques should be taught and reinforced. If an individual's cough is ineffective in removing secretions, tracheal suctioning may be used. Inhaled bronchodilators may be implemented in a patient who has underlying chronic obstructive lung disease and a chronic, nonproductive cough. Nursing measures to minimize the symptoms of cough include increasing oral fluids and using humidifiers or vaporizers.

Pain

Chest pain due to a bronchogenic tumor is dull, poorly localized, and described as an ache. If there is tumor involvement of the bony thorax or parietal pleura, a more sharp and severe type of chest pain is experienced. Pain may increase in intensity and duration with advancing metastatic disease and cancer treatment.

Individuals in pain generally have significant disease and a short life expectancy. Pain is best controlled with the input of several disciplines. If standard cancer therapies fail to relieve or control pain, pharmacologic agents such as dilaudid or morphine are usually added to the regimen. There is no reason to withhold morphine sulfate from people with lung cancer, based on the fear that it depresses respirations. Opioids do not depress respiration in patients with pain because pain stimulates respiration. There is no single maximum dosage of morphine sulfate for hospice patients who require cancer pain management. The right dosage is the one that relieves the pain with minimal side effects. The fear of addiction should not play a role in the dosage ordered and subsequently administered. These individuals should be made as comfortable as possible.

Dyspnea

Dyspnea can be seen as a presenting symptom in some individuals with lung cancer. Others may not develop dyspnea until after the diagnosis. Multiple factors may influence the presence and severity of dyspnea. These factors include airway obstruction, fibrosis, edema, tumor infiltration, pleural effusion, inspiratory muscle fatigue, anxiety, and depression. Foote, Sexton, and Pawlik (1986) have found that in lung cancer patients, the presence of dyspnea is associated with fatigue and decreased energy. Emotional stress may contribute to the production of dyspnea, as well as result from the experience of dyspnea. Thoracentesis, irradiation, chemotherapy, diuretics, steroids, or supplemental oxygen may improve dyspnea, depending on the cause. Measures to control persistent dyspnea include adjustment of lifestyle and environmental factors, activity limitation, energy conservation planning, bronchial hygiene measures, oxygen support, diaphragmatic breathing, a bedside fan, a humidifier, a vaporizer, positioning, systematic relaxation training, meditation, imagery, therapeutic touch, and emotional support.

Hemoptysis

Hemoptysis is caused by tumor erosion into pulmonary blood vessels. These are usually bronchial arteries or their branches. Bleeding appears as streaks, dots, or gross blood loss. The time course and volume of bleeding determine the therapeutic approach to lung cancer patients with hemoptysis.

Mild hemoptysis is considered less than 50 ml in 24 hours. Individuals with mild hemoptysis are usually treated as outpatients using conservative measures. Activities that tend to aggravate bleeding should be avoided. If the hemoptysis is associated with significant coughing, cough suppressants may be recommended. Antibiotics may also be prescribed because blood is a medium for bacterial growth. The frequency and amount of bleeding are monitored on an ongoing basis. Most bleeding stops within several days.

Hospitalization and careful monitoring for increasing blood loss, changes in blood pressure, and pulse and respiratory distress are required for patients with significant bleeding or respiratory compromise. Major bleeding is considered 200 ml in 24 hours. Asphyxiation and shock can occur if immediate steps are not taken. The lung containing the bleeding site should be in a dependent position. The individual is positioned in this manner to prevent spillover of blood into the nonbleeding lung. Angiographic embolization of the bronchial artery source of the bleed or emergency surgery may be needed to control massive bleeding.

Wheezing

If a tumor is partially obstructing a bronchus, unilateral persistent wheezing may occur. Tumor shrinkage through irradiation may relieve this symptom. The individual should be assessed to determine whether wheezing is more severe when the individual lies on one side as opposed to the other. If this is the case, the patient must be positioned to protect bronchial patency. Inhaled bronchodilators, corticosteroids, and mucolytics may provide relief for diffuse wheezing.

Prevention

Nurses are in a strategic position to prevent smoking initiation and influence successful smoking cessation through education, information on the multiple modalities to assist behavioral change, and ongoing reinforcement (Risser, 1996). All nurses can take positive action toward tobacco control. Some of these actions include the following:

1. Target young people and nonsmokers for educational programs to decrease the initiation of tobacco use.
2. Increase tobacco-use cessation through educational and support programs targeted toward smokers.
3. Support public action and legislative changes that restrict the advertising, distribution, and use of tobacco products (Gallagher & Holm, 1996).
4. Propose and support local community initiatives to restrict tobacco use in the workplace and public settings.
5. Act as a role model for patients and the public.

Lung cancer prevention and early detection teaching priorities are as follows:

1. Avoid the use of tobacco.
2. Know environmental carcinogens that increase risk.
3. Realize that personal and family histories are important risk factors.

Nursing care should focus on promoting comfort, as well as preventing and managing disease and treatment complications (Table 61-2).

Rehabilitation

The effective management of short- and long-term side effects from lung cancer treatment is essential for patient rehabilitation. Increasing nursing knowledge relative to the psychosocial effect of lung cancer assists nurses in planning appropriate intervention programs and promoting the optimal use of resources. If patients and their families can overcome treatment barriers, they will be more motivated toward achieving increased and sustained independence.

Some of the modifications of activities of daily living for the patient/family experiencing lung cancer are as follows:

1. Do not treat the patient as an invalid just because his or her activity tolerance has decreased.
2. Encourage significant others to include the patient in family decision making.
3. Help the patient establish a new daily routine with realistic goals.
4. Provide some small activity for the patient to look forward to.
5. Encourage larger-scale activities in moderation.

HOME CARE ISSUES

After the patient has been discharged from the hospital, the family is responsible for provision of the hour-to-hour patient care (Box 61-8 and Table 61-3). The nurse must anticipate problems and work with the patient and family to develop plans for dealing with them. The patient and family should be in a position to manage current problems and prepare for future events while maintaining a sense of control and confidence. Compassionate nursing can assist families to know what to expect and how to deal with these events. Lung cancer patients are often not referred for home care until they are dying. The majority of lung cancer patients experience progressive disease with increasing symptoms, and consequently, increased dependency on others for self-care needs.

Some of the more common symptoms experienced by lung cancer patients being cared for in the home are pain, difficulty eating, respiratory problems (dyspnea, cough, and hemoptysis), nausea and vomiting, constipation, confusion, fatigue/weakness, and family turmoil. The less common symptoms experienced by lung cancer patients are insomnia, anxiety/depression, personality changes, hiccoughs, skin breakdown, incontinence, and diarrhea.

Home care of the patient with advanced disease is common. Treatments once performed only in medical centers are now routine parts of home care. Families are providing sophisticated bedside care under the guidance of the home care clinician. The home care nurse functions as a teacher and coordinator and assists the patient and family to live each day to the fullest (White, 1987).

TABLE 61-2 Small Cell Lung Cancer

Patient Problems and Outcomes	Nursing Interventions and Rationales	Patient Education Instructions
Ineffective Airway Clearance Patient will: • Demonstrate normal respiratory status as evidenced by breath sounds that are clear throughout all lung fields, respirations that are moderate in depth and between 12 and 20 minutes, and decreased dyspnea.	1. Auscultate breath sounds every shift and when needed. 2. Assess the respiratory rate, depth, and rhythm every shift and when needed. 3. Assess the length of the expiratory phase of breathing and pursed-lip breathing. 4. Assess the paradoxical abdominal motion and asynchronous chest and abdominal motions. 5. Ask the patient to rate dyspnea on a scale of 0 to 10 (0 = no dyspnea, 10 = worst dyspnea) and record every 4 hours. 6. Assess the vital capacity through an incentive spizometer. 7. Assess and record the use of dyspnea-reducing strategies found helpful by the patient. 8. Collect sputum for culture as ordered.	Teach patient the following: 1. Teach the patient the use of pursed-lip breathing and slow abdominal-diaphragmatic breathing during periods of dyspnea. 2. Assist and teach patient to turn, cough, and deep breathe every 2 hours; note the type, color, and character of the sputum. 3. Discuss avoidance of smoke and dust with the patient and family or significant other. 4. Encourage the intake of 2 to 3 L of fluid every 24 hours unless fluids are restricted. 5. Monitor the hematocrit and hemoglobin levels daily.
Impaired Gas Exchange Patient will: • Demonstrate optimal gas exchange for condition as evidenced by blood gases within acceptable levels, usual skin color, and usual mental status.	1. Monitor arterial blood gases every shift. 2. Monitor the color of the skin, nailbeds, and mucous membranes of the mouth. 3. Assess the mental status. 4. Assess for complications of oxygen therapy, such as nasal dryness or congestion, epistaxis, and skin breakdown every shift.	Teach patient the following: 1. Maintain bed rest in a quiet environment during exacerbation. 2. Elevate the head of bed 45 to 90 degrees. 3. Administer humidified oxygen per nasal catheter or cannula at prescribed flow.
Pain and Dyspnea Patient will: • Experience relief/control of pain as evidenced by verbalization of pain at a 0, 1, or 2 on scale of 1-10. • Identify strategies to control pain as evidenced by verbalization/use of nonpharmacologic measures for pain relief. • Demonstrate decreased dyspnea as evidenced by relief/control of dyspnea at a 0, 1, or 2 on a scale of 0-10.	1. Assess/record the character, location, duration, frequency of pain, and any other precipitating factors every 4 hours and when needed. 2. Ask the patient to rate the intensity of pain on a scale of 0-10 (0 = absence of pain and 10 = worst pain experienced) and record every 4 hours. 3. Ask the patient to rate dyspnea on a scale of 0-10 (0 = no dyspnea and 10 = worst dyspnea) and record every 4 hours.	Teach patient the following: 1. Administer analgesic/anxiolytic as prescribed, and assess/record the effectiveness. 2. Reduce or eliminate common side-effects of narcotics: a. Constipation: Administer a stool softener as prescribed. b. Nausea and vomiting: Administer an antiemetic as prescribed. c. Dry mouth: Provide good oral hygiene, encourage the patient to rinse the mouth often, and offer sugarless candy for the patient to suck on. 3. Use nonpharmacologic measures for pain relief (e.g., relaxation, imagery, distraction, biofeedback, self-hypnosis). 4. Use energy/conservation techniques.
Altered Nutrition Less Than Body Requirements Patient will: • Maintain an adequate nutritional status as evidenced by weight moving toward normal range for the patient's height, age, and build.	1. Obtain a dietary consultation to assess nutritional requirements and the quality of usual intake. 2. Monitor the percent of meals eaten. 3. Weigh the patient daily. 4. Monitor skin turgor and mucous membranes.	Teach patient the following: 1. Eat favorite foods that are high in carbohydrates and protein as prescribed. 2. Eat small, frequent meals consisting of soft, easily swallowed foods to supplementary feedings. 3. Encourage rest period prior to meals to reduce fatigue.

Modified from: Glover, J., & Miaskowski, C. (1994). Small lung cell cancer: pathophysiologic mechanisms and nursing implications. *Oncology Nursing Forum, 21,* 87-95.

TABLE 61-2 Small Cell Lung Cancer—cont'd

Patient Problems and Outcome	Nursing Interventions and Rationales	Patient Education Instructions
Altered Nutrition Less Than Body Requirements—cont'd		
	5. Monitor bowel function. 6. Monitor for stomatitis. 7. Monitor for results of laboratory studies (serum albumin, total protein concentration, glucose, acetone, 24-hour urinary creatine, nitrogen, and electrolytes). 8. Record the intake and output every shift.	4. Take megesterol acetate as prescribed to increase appetite; monitor for side effects; edema, diffuse rash, menstrual irregularities, impotence in males. 5. Perform oral care 30 minutes before meals and frequently between meals. 6. Take prescribed antiemetic to reduce nausea. 7. Increased fluid intake. 8. Teach the patient and family the following: a. Importance of maintaining adequate calorie intake b. Eating patterns to promote weight gain and positive nitrogen balance
Activity Intolerance Patient will: • Demonstrate an increased activity tolerance as evidenced by the ability to resume activities of daily living (ADL) free from extremes of fatigue or dyspnea.	1. Monitor vital signs before and after periods of increased activity. 2. Monitor the heart and lung sounds with activity. 3. Monitor oxygen saturation with activity, and provide oxygen therapy as prescribed. 4. Monitor for signs of extreme fatigue, chest pain, or diaphoresis.	Teach the patient methods to do the following: 1. Provide optimal rest and limit activity in accordance with the degree of pulmonary dysfunction. 2. Perform active and passive range of motion movement to all extremities one to four times a day. 3. Rest in a chair, rather than a bed. 4. Use pursed-lip breathing and diaphragmatic breathing.
Ineffective Individual/Family Coping Patient/family will: • Demonstrate effective coping as evidenced by expression of feelings and concerns and use of adaptive coping behaviors.	1. Assess the level of anxiety and depression every shift. 2. Assess the presence of biologic factors related to small cell lung cancer that could be causing depression (e.g., parahormone, vasopressin, ACTH, enkephalins, beta-endorphins).	1. Establish a therapeutic relationship to encourage communication with nursing staff every shift. a. Provide an environment conducive to discussing private issues and feelings. b. Provide for continuity of care. 2. Allow the patient/family to react in their own ways without judgment. 3. Encourage the verbalization of fears/concerns. 4. Assist in identifying new coping strategies: a. Active listening: Validate information by reflecting what has been said for clarification and verification. b. Use open-ended questions to elicit emotional expression. c. Assist the patient/family with identifying strengths and coping skills. 5. Assist the patient/family with identifying the nature and strengths of situational supports; collect data from current and potential sources of support. 6. Explain procedures, confirm the patient's understanding, and answer questions or refer to appropriate sources. 7. Involve the patient in the decision-making process regarding care. 8. Administer anxiolytic and antidepressant medications as ordered, and teach the patient relaxation techniques.

Box 61-8
Interventions to Incorporate Patient/Family in Care

1. Help the family to allow the patient to maintain roles and activities most important to him or her:
   a. Place emphasis on short-term goals in daily care and the priority setting.
   b. Refer to the local American Cancer Society or American Lung Association for a respiratory program, if available.
2. Teach supportive care skills:
   a. Instruct the patient and family in the use of oxygen equipment, postural drainage, and a self-pacing program.
   b. Teach the patient general strengthening exercises.
   c. Instruct the patient in relaxation techniques.
   d. Assist the patient to maintain realistic hope, yet prepare for changes in lifestyle if the prognosis is poor.
   e. Assist the patient to resume previous roles and responsibilities if prognostic factors are favorable (small, solitary, isolated lesion).

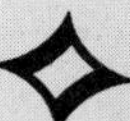

TABLE 61-3 Patient Preparation for Home Care Planning

1. Discourage smoking by the patient and family or significant others.
2. Explain how to cough productively and to perform breathing exercises and other respiratory therapy as prescribed to maintain pulmonary function.
3. Help the patient ambulate, and instruct the patient in the use of assistive devices such as canes and walkers to maintain mobility.
4. Explain how to self-administer medication for pain to maintain comfort.
5. Inform the patient of the need for adequate nutrition (high-calorie, high-protein diet) to maintain energy.
6. Inform the patient of the signs and symptoms of complications or adverse reactions to chemotherapy, radiation therapy, or both so that they can be treated immediately.
7. Help the patient identify resources and support systems to help in rehabilitation and maintenance of the quality of life.
8. Alert the patient to the signs and symptoms of recurrence or metastatic disease, such as shoulder or arm pain, superior vena cava syndrome, liver disease, and central nervous system changes, so that they can be treated as soon as possible.

Hospice is a concept of care for the dying patient that emphasizes the comfort and dignity of the patient and family. This concept accepts death as a natural phenomenon and enables all involved to experience the patient's death in a manner that minimizes emotional trauma while promoting personal growth and closeness with one another (White, 1987).

PSYCHOSOCIAL ISSUES

Limited Survival

Most patients with lung cancer typically have a limited prognosis. Nonetheless, individuals with cancer need to be dealt with honestly and hopefully. Patients not only hope for a cure or an extension of life, but also hope to preserve the quality of their life. Needs of patients vary in importance according to changing phases of illness.

Patients need help in anticipating and planning how to spend their remaining days. Disease progression and impending death cannot be ignored, but constant reminders to patients that their days are limited are also of no value to patients.

Planning for end-of-life care is a process, not an event. Substantial time and discussion are necessary. Accurate information regarding the use of life-sustaining technologies must be presented to patients so that they may formulate their desires regarding the use of these treatments. Anticipatory discussions should occur with patients and family members about the realities, outcomes, and alternatives to critical care before a medical crisis occurs and urgent decisions must be made. The decision to use or not use life-sustaining technologies does not mean a person is choosing treatment versus no treatment. That person is merely deciding on a form of treatment.

Patients should always make the decisions regarding treatment and life-supportive care, if they are able. Actual preferences for treatment and life-supportive care often differ from what family members and caregivers infer them to be. When decisions about care are made without patient participation, treatment may be more or less aggressive than the patient would have desired.

Family Disruptions. Individuals with lung cancer usually experience a rapid disease progression. Major shifts in family roles and dynamics may occur in a short time. This could possibly strain family resources and aggravate conflicts predating the cancer diagnosis. Now that lung cancer management is occurring primarily in the outpatient setting, family coping may become more compromised and stressed by the need to manage tumor- and treatment-related problems at home.

CANCER SUPPORT

Cancer patients may worry about holding jobs, caring for their families, or keeping up with daily activities. Worries about tests, treatments, hospital stays, and medical bills are also common. Patients can meet with social workers, counselors, or members of the clergy to talk about their feelings or discuss their concerns about the future or personal relationships. Physicians, nurses, and other members of the health care team can answer questions and help calm fears about treatment, working, or other activities. Many patients find it helpful to discuss their concerns with others who are facing similar problems. Cancer support groups are available, where patients get together and share what they have learned about coping with cancer and the effects of treatment. Each patient is different. Treatments and ways of dealing with cancer that work for one person may not be right for another.

RESEARCH

Researchers are evaluating combinations of standard and new drugs and variations of doses for drug combinations already in use. Investigators are looking at the possible benefits of combining chemotherapy with surgery to remove the tumor or radiation therapy to destroy it. New radiation therapy schedules are being evaluated for the primary cancer and for metastatic tumors in the brain. Scientists are also studying hormones produced by SCLC cells that act as growth factors for the cancer. Cells obtained by biopsy of a patient's tumor can be grown in test tube cultures and exposed to various anticancer drugs to determine which ones kill the cancer cells. Scientists are investigating the usefulness of this technique.

Some lung cancer patients do not respond well to chemotherapy because their tumor cells are resistant to the drugs that are usually effective against cancer. Researchers are trying to increase the effectiveness of chemotherapy by administering an anticancer agent together with one or more chemosensitizers. Chemosensitizers are drugs that increase the sensitivity of tumor cells to anticancer drugs.

Researchers are also evaluating the usefulness of tumor markers in monitoring the effectiveness of treatment. Elevated levels of these substances are present in the blood of lung cancer patients. They may be useful for detecting a recurrence of lung cancer after treatment. Markers of particular interest include neuron-specific enolase and carcinoembryonic antigen. The current prognosis for patients with SCLC is unsatisfactory, even though considerable improvements in diagnosis and therapy have been made over the past 10 to 15 years. Therefore all patients with SCLC may be considered for inclusion in clinical trials at the time of diagnosis.

QUALITY OF CARE

Quality of care measurements are currently being mandated by a number of government agencies and third-party payers. Unless health care providers can measure positive outcomes relative to the care they provide, these agencies will no longer be chosen as reimbursable entities. Table 61-4 provides examples for patients and caregivers to access small cell lung cancer support systems in their community.

PROGNOSIS

In general, the prognosis for SCLC is poor, and cures are rare. The prognosis and selection of appropriate treatment protocols are based primarily on the anatomic extent or stage of the cancer at the time of diagnosis. The stage of the disease is the most important prognostic indicator. Other indicators include gender, performance status, extent of the disease, number of metastatic sites, amount of weight loss, age, tumor volume, and immune status. The presence of anemia, a low platelet count, hyponatremia, an elevated leu-

TABLE 61-4 Quality of Care Assessment for the Patient with Lung Cancer

Disciplines participating in the quality of care evaluation:
☐Medical ☐Social Workers ☐Nursing

Data from:
Mailed Questionnaire Patient Interview
Collected by: ____________ Position: ____________

Criteria	Yes	No
1. Was the patient given formal education about the risks of smoking and the benefits of quitting?	☐	☐
2. Was the patient given the name of at least two smoking-cessation resources in the respective community?	☐	☐
3. Was the patient given both medication and nonpharmaceutical interventions for pain management, if appropriate?	☐	☐
4. If postural drainage was indicated for the patient, were the patient and caregiver given technique instructions?	☐	☐
5. If the patient was prescribed oxygen therapy, were the patient and caregivers given written and verbal instructions in using the equipment?	☐	☐
6. Was the patient given information regarding the external and internal factors that increase the risk of upper respiratory infection, exposure to crowds, inadequate rest, nutrition, or hydration?	☐	☐
7. Could the patient verbalize the signs and symptoms of upper respiratory infection: fever, cough, and expectoration (yellow or green)?	☐	☐
8. If the patient had radiation therapy, was he or she given written and verbal instructions about the possible complications?	☐	☐
9. Could the patient verbalize methods to treat radiation skin reactions?	☐	☐
10. Could the patient identify foods appropriate for dysphagia and/or esophagitis?	☐	☐
11. Could the patient and caregiver verbalize indicators of hope (constitutional, psychological, and prognostic)?	☐	☐
12. Was the patient given a list of the signs and symptoms of metastatic disease?	☐	☐

kocyte count, raised lactate dehydrogenase, elevated alkaline phosphatase, and raised gamma glutamyl transpeptidase are indicative of low survival rates and reduced survival duration (Rawson & Peto, 1990; Ihde, Pass, & Glatsterin, 1997).

Multiple factors are known to influence the prognosis in SCLC, according to Abrams, Dole, and Aisner (1988). Patients with limited disease usually have a better initial performance status than those with extensive disease. The performance status at the time of diagnosis has been an important independent determinant of the treatment regimen, treatment response, and survival. Patients who stop smoking at the time of diagnosis also improve the prognosis. The prognosis declines with the extent of patient debilitation. Weight loss has had prognostic significance. Poor response to chemotherapy (poor initial response or relapse after treatment) is an adverse prognostic sign. Patients with SCLC have an immune deficit that may contribute to the rapid growth of this cancer.

Extensive disease is the worst prognostic factor. Other adverse prognostic factors include male gender and a poor performance score (2) on the Zubrod Scale (Spiegelman, Maurer, Ware, Perry, Chahinian, & Comis, 1989). Age greater than 70 years is also associated with an adverse likelihood of survival, especially in extensive disease (Maurer & Pajak, 1987; Siu, Shepherd, Murray, Feld, Pater, & Zee, 1996). An interaction between age and disease extent that affected the probability of obtaining a complete response to therapy and long-term survival has been noted (Poplin, Thompson, Whitacre, & Aisner, 1987). Elevated serum lactic dehydrogenase levels, low serum sodium, and elevated alkaline phosphatase levels are thought to be an indication of poor prognosis. Prior chemotherapy is also associated with a low likelihood of response to therapy. Patients with mixed small cell/large cell carcinomas or combined small cell carcinomas do not do as well as those with pure small cell carcinoma. Weight loss greater than 5% of the baseline weight or weight loss of 10 pounds in 6 months is also considered a negative prognostic factor (Greco & Hainsworth, 1994).

Long-term disease-free survival is unusual. Patients who achieve complete response to treatment have the best overall survival (Perry, Eaton, Propert, Ware, Zimmer, & Chahinian, 1987). The cure rate for SCLC ranges from 3% in one study (Ktaslersky, 1995) to 5% to 10% in other studies (Cleary, Gorenstein, & Omenn, 1996). The average cure rate is about 5%.

Most SCLC patients die of their disease. Even though this cancer is one of the most responsive of all tumors to radiotherapy and chemotherapy, it almost always recurs, typically within 2 years of treatment. As would be expected, patients with limited-stage SCLC have the best survival rates. This is especially true for those treated with both radiotherapy and chemotherapy, although they remain at a relatively high risk of a lung recurrence or development of other primary cancers (Lin & Ihde, 1992; Sagman, Lishner, Maki, Shepherd, Haddad, & Evans, 1992).

The 5-year survival rate in limited disease is 7% with a median survival time of 10 to 16 months with current forms of treatment, and in extensive disease it is 1% with a median survival of 6 to 12 months with current forms of treatment (Ihde, Pass, & Glatstein, 1994). The length of survival for extensive disease can be measured in weeks with supportive care alone. The goals of therapy should be palliation and prolongation of useful survival.

Long-Term Evaluation

The primary care physician determines follow-up intervals and testing. Chest x-ray examinations may be done to detect recurrence or new primary lesions. The patient should promptly report any new symptoms. If the patient has not already ceased smoking, he or she should be strongly encouraged to do so. Interventions to monitor disease progression include scheduling follow-up care; discussing the purpose of brain, bone, and liver scans or other surveillance procedures for metastatic disease; and teaching patients and the family signs and symptoms of metastatic disease (changes in affect or personality, bone pain, changes in respiratory status, and jaundice) (Lind, 1992).

Lung cancer research is ongoing and extensive. Researchers are trying to learn more about what causes lung disease and how to prevent it, detect it, and treat it. They are continuing to identify factors that may increase the risk for lung cancer, studying ways to help people lower their risk of lung cancer.

Lung cancer is difficult to diagnose at an early stage, yet scientists are investigating ways of checking for lung cancer in people who have no symptoms of the disease. More effective treatments are being explored. In addition, ways to reduce the side effects of treatment and improve the quality of patients' lives are being investigated.

Clinical trials are under way to study new treatments for patients with all stages of lung cancer. Some trials involve treatments to shrink or destroy the primary tumor. Other tests are exploring ways to prevent lung cancer from coming back in the chest or spreading to other parts of the body after the primary tumor has been treated. Additional trials involve treatments to slow or stop the spread of lung cancer.

Researchers are studying the timing of treatments and new ways to combine various types of treatment. They are also trying new anticancer drugs and drug combinations, new forms of radiation therapy, and drugs that make cancer cells more sensitive to radiation. Photodynamic therapy is being studied with other lasers as a way to open the airways in patients whose tumors block the bronchi. Biologic therapy is being explored further (National Cancer Institute, 1993).

FUTURE DIRECTIONS

Prevention is vital to future change in patient survival rates. A lifestyle free of smoking or cessation of smoking is the best defense against lung cancer. Studies are being undertaken to determine how to help high-risk populations, especially in understanding the addiction process and why smoking is so difficult for some people to quit. Research is concentrating on chemoprevention and immunotherapy.

Promising new chemotherapeutic agents include paclitaxel (Taxol), taxotere, gemcitabine, CPT-11, topotecan, and 9-AC. The use of hematopoietic growth factors with autologous bone marrow or peripheral-blood stem-cell support may permit higher doses of chemotherapy and/or their safer administration, resulting in higher response rates. Accelerated hyperfraction radiation therapy may increase local control with decreased toxicity. Chemoprevention trials offer the potential of decreasing the incidence of second malignancies. Promising new treatment methods based on tumor biology include gene therapies, antibodies against growth factors, and agents that prevent angiogenesis and tissue invasion (Works & Gallucci, 1996). Biologic therapy (biotherapy/immunotherapy) may be used to boost the ability of a cancer patient's immune system to fight the growth of cancer cells, to eliminate or suppress body responses that permit cancer growth, and to increase the ability of the body to produce infection-fighting blood cells to recover from the damaging effects of anticancer drugs.

Areas of active clinical evaluation in SCLC for limited disease include new drug regimens composed of standard and new agents, variation of drug doses in current regimens, and the study of possible benefits of adding surgical resection of the primary tumor or radiotherapy to the chest and other sites to combination chemotherapy. New radiotherapy schedules and the timing of thoracic radiation may allow improved tumor control with less toxicity (Turrisi, 1993).

Areas of active clinical evaluation in SCLC for extensive disease include new drug regimens composed of standard and new agents, variation of drug doses in current regimens, and the study of possible benefits of adding radiotherapy to the chest and other sites to combination chemotherapy.

REFERENCES

Abner, A. (1993). Prophylactic cranial irradiation in the treatment of small-cell carcinoma of the lung. *Chest, 103,* 445-448.

Abrams, J., Dole, L. A., & Aisner, J. (1988). Staging, prognostic factors and special considerations in small-cell lung cancer. *Seminars in Oncology, 15,* 261-277.

American Cancer Society. (1987). *Facts on lung cancer.* Atlanta: American Cancer Society.

American Cancer Society. (1995). *Answering your questions about cancer.* Atlanta: American Cancer Society.

American Cancer Society. (1998). Cancer statistics, 1997. *CA Cancer Journal for Clinicians, 47,* 5-27.

Archer, V. E., Saccomanno, G., & Jones, J. H. (1974). Frequency of different histologic types of bronchogenic carcinoma as related to radiation exposure. *Cancer, 34,* 206-260.

Ashbaugh, D. (1970). Mediastinoscopy. *Archives of Surgery, 100,* 568-573.

Bates, B. (1983). *A guide to physical examination* (3rd ed.). Philadelphia: J. B. Lippincott.

Baumm, A. D. & Medsger, T. A. (1985). Cancer and systemic sclerosis: An epidemiologic study. *Arthritis and Rheumatism, 28,* 1336-1340.

Birrer, M. J. & Minna, J. D. (1988). Molecular genetics of lung cancer. *Seminars in Oncology, 15,* 226-235.

Block, G., Patterson, B., & Subar, A. (1992). Fruit, vegetables and cancer prevention: A review of the epidemiologic evidence. *Nutrition & Cancer, 18,* 1-29.

Boring, C. C., Squires, T. S., & Heath, C. W. (1992). Cancer statistics for African Americans. *Cancer, 42,* 7-17.

Bouchier, I. & Morris, J. (1976). *Clinical skills: A system of clinical examination.* London: W.B. Saunders.

Brown, C. C. & Kessler, L. G. (1988). Projections of lung cancer mortality in the U.S. *Journal of the National Cancer Institute, 80,* 43-51.

Buckingham, W. (1979). *A primer of clinical diagnosis* (2nd ed.). New York: Harper & Row.

Burns, K. & Johnson, P. (1980). *Health assessment in clinical practice* (2nd ed.). Englewood Cliffs, NJ: Prentice-Hall.

Cancer Net: National Cancer Institute. (1996). *PDQ information for health care professionals: Small-cell lung cancer.* gopher://gopher.nih.gov:70/00/clin/cancernet.

Carmichael, J., Crane, J. M., Bunn, P. A., Glatstein, E., & Ihde, D. C. (1988). Results of therapeutic cranial irradiation in small-cell lung cancer. *International Journal of Radiation Oncology, Biology, & Physics, 14*(3), 455-459.

Cleary, J., Gorenstein, L. A., & Omenn, G. S. (1996). Lung cancer: Prevention is the best cure. *Patient Care, 9,* 35-67.

Cooper, J. A., White, D. A., & Matthay, R. A. (1986). Drug induced pulmonary disease: Cytotoxic drugs. *American Review of Respiratory Diseases, 133,* 321-340.

Crowley, M. (1992). Primary prevention in oncology nursing practice. In J.C. Clark & R. F. McGee (Eds.), *Core curriculum for oncology nursing.* Philadelphia: W. B. Saunders.

Davila, D. G. & Williams, D. E. (1993). The etiology of lung cancer. *Mayo Clinic Proceedings, 68,* 170-182.

DeGowin, E. & DeGowin, R. (1987). *Bedside diagnostic examination* (5th ed.). New York: Macmillan.

Doll, R. & Peto, R. (1981). The causes of cancer. Quantitative estimates of avoidable risks of cancer in the United States today. *Journal of the National Cancer Institute, 66,* 1193-1308.

Einhorn, L. H. (1986). Cisplatin and vp-16 in small-cell lung cancer. *Seminars in Oncology, 13,* 3-4.

Elpern, E. H. (1993). Lung cancer. In S. L. Groenwald, M. H. Frogge, M. Goodman, & C. H. Yarbro (Eds.), *Cancer nursing principles and practice* (3rd ed.). Boston: Jones and Bartlett.

Faylona, E. A., Loehrer, P. J., Ansari, R., Sandler, A., Gonin, R., & Einhorn, L. (1995). Phase II study of daily oral etoposide plus ifosfamide plus cisplatin for previously treated recurrent small-cell lung cancer: A hoosier oncology group trial. *Journal of Clinical Oncology, 13,* 1209-1214.

Fielding, J. (1985). Smoking: Health effects and control. *New England Journal of Medicine, 313,* 491-498.

Fielding, J. & Phenow, J. (1988). Health effects of involuntary smoking. *New England Journal of Medicine, 319,* 1452-1460.

Fink, D. (1992). Guidelines for the cancer-related check-up: Recommendations and rationale. *American Cancer Society. CA, 42,* 44-45.

Fleck, J. F., Einhorn, L. H., Lauer, R. C., Schultz, S. M., & Miller, M. E. (1990). Is prophylactic cranial irradiation indicated in small-cell lung cancer? *Journal of Clinical Oncology, 8*(2), 209-214.

Fontham, E. T. (1990). Protective dietary factors and lung cancer. *International Journal of Epidemiology, 19*(Suppl. 1), 532-542.

Foote, M., Sexton, D., & Pawlik, L. (1986). Dyspnea: A distressing sensation in lung cancer. *Oncology Nursing Forum, 13,* 25-31.

Frank-Stromborg, M. & Cohen, R. F. (1993). Assessment and interventions for cancer prevention and detection. In S. L. Groenwald, M. H. Frogge, M. Goodman, & C. H. Yarbro (Eds.), *Cancer nursing principles and practice* (3rd ed.). Boston: Jones and Bartlett.

Gallagher, J. & Holm, L. (1996). Power of one: Nurses and tobacco control. *Seminars in Oncology Nursing, 12*(4), 270-275.

Garewal, H. S. & Meyskens, F. L. (1991). Chemoprevention of cancer. *Hematology/Oncology Clinics of North America, 5*(1), 69-77.

Garfinkel, L. & Silverberg, E. (1991). Lung cancer and smoking trends in the United States over the past 25 years. *Cancer, 41,* 137-145.

Giaccone, G., Dalesio, O., McVie, G. J., Kirkpatrick, A., Postmus, P. E., & Burghouts, J. T. (1993). Maintenance chemotherapy in small-cell lung cancer: Long-term results of a randomized trial. *Journal of Clinical Oncology, 11*(7), 1230-1240.

Glick, J. H. & Glover, D. (1995). Oncologic emergencies. In G. P. Murphy, W. Lawrence, & R. E. Lenhard (Eds.), *Clinical oncology* (2nd ed.). Atlanta: American Cancer Society.

Glover, J. & Miaskowski, C. (1994). Small-cell lung cancer: Pathophysiologic mechanisms and nursing implications. *Oncology Nursing Forum, 21,* 87-95.

Greco, F. A. (1993). Treatment options for patients with relapsed small-cell lung cancer. *Lung Cancer, 9*(Suppl. 1), 85-89.

Greco, F. A. & Hainsworth, J. D. (1994). Practical approaches to the treatment of patients with extensive stage small-cell lung cancer. *Seminars in Oncology, 4*(Suppl. 7), 3-6.

Greenwald, P., Kelloff, G., Burch-Whitman, C., & Kramer, B. S. (1995). Chemoprevention. *Ca-A Cancer Journal for Clinicians, 45,* 31-49.

Grimes, J. & Burns, E. (Eds.). (1987). *Health assessment in nursing practice* (2nd ed.). Boston: Jones and Bartlett.

Grippi, M. (1990). Clinical aspects of lung cancer. *Seminars in Roentgenology, 25,* 12-24.

Groenwald, S. L., Frogge, M. H., Goodman, M., & Yarbro, C. H. (1995). *A clinical guide to cancer nursing.* London: Jones and Bartlett.

Haraf, D. J., Devine, S., Ihde, D. C., & Vokes, E. E. (1992). The evolving role of systemic therapy in carcinoma of the lung. *Seminars in Oncology, 19*(Suppl. 11), 72-87.

Harley, N. H. & Harley, J. H. (1990). Potential lung cancer risk from indoor radon exposure. *Cancer, 40,* 265-275.

Harper, P. G., Houang, F. M., Spiro, S. G., Geddes, D., Hodson, M., & Souhami, L. (1981). Computerized axial tomography in the pretreatment assessment of small-cell carcinoma of the bronchus. *Cancer, 47,* 1775-1780.

Hennekens, C. H., Buring, J. E., Manson, J. E., & Stampfer. (1996). Lack of effect of long-term supplementation with beta carotene on the incidence of malignant neoplasms and cardiovascular disease. *New England Journal of Medicine, 334:*1145-1149.

Hermanson, B., Omenn, G., & Kronmal, R. (1988). Participants in the coronary artery surgery study: Beneficial six-year outcome of smoking cessation in older men and women with coronary artery disease. *New England Journal of Medicine, 319,* 1365-1369.

Hilderley, L. (1996). Radiation therapy for lung cancer. *Seminars in Oncology Nursing, 12*(4), 304-311.

Hinson, J. A. & Perry, M. C. (1993). Small-cell lung cancer. *Ca-A Cancer Journal for Clinicians, 43,* 216-225.

Hirsch, F. R., Matthews, M. J., Aisner, S., Campobasso, O., Elema, J. D., & Gazdar, A. F. (1988). Histopathologic classification of small-cell lung cancer: Changing concepts and terminology. *Cancer, 62,* 973-977.

Hirsch, F. R., Paulson, O. B., Hansen, H. H., & Larsen, O. (1983). Intracranial metastases in small-cell carcinoma of the lung: Prognostic aspects. *Cancer, 51,* 529-533.

Holleb, A. I., Fink, D. J., & Murphy, G. P. (1991). *American Cancer Society textbook of clinical oncology.* Atlanta: American Cancer Society.

Horm, J. W. & Sondik, E. J. (1989). Person-years of life lost due to cancer in the United States, 1970 and 1984. *American Journal of Public Health, 79,* 1490-1493.

Horn, D. (1977). Social and psychologic aspects of starting smoking. In H. E. Nieburgs (Ed.), *Prevention and detection of cancer.* New York: Dekker.

Horowitz, J. C. (1993). Toward a social policy for health. *New England Journal of Medicine, 329,* 130-133.

Humble, C., Samet, J., & Pathak, D. (1987). Marriage to a smoker and lung cancer risk. *American Journal of Public Health, 77,* 598-560.

Huuskonen, M. S. (1992). Screening for occupational cancer. *Scandinavian Journal of Work Environmental Health, 18*(Suppl. 1), 110-114.

Ihde, D. C. & Hansen, H. (1981). Staging procedures and prognostic factors in small-cell carcinoma of the lung. In F. A. Greco, R. K. Oldham, & P. A. Bunn (Eds.), *Small-cell lung cancer.* New York: Grune & Stratton.

Ihde, D. C., Pass, H. I., & Glatstein, E. J. (1997). Small-cell lung cancer. In V. T. DeVita, S. Hellman, & S. Rosenberg (Eds.), *Cancer principles and practice of oncology* (5th ed.). Philadelphia: J. B. Lippincott.

Ingle, R. J. (1997). Lung cancers. In S. L. Groenwald, M. H. Frogge, M. Goodman, & C. H. Yarbro (Eds.), *Cancer: Nursing principles and practice* (4th ed.). Boston: Jones and Bartlett.

Institute of Medicine. (1994). *Growing up tobacco free: Preventing nicotine addiction in children and adults.* Washington, DC: National Academy Press.

Janerich, D., Thompson, W. D., & Varela, L. R. (1990). Lung cancer and exposure to tobacco smoke in the household. *New England Journal of Medicine, 323,* 632-636.

Kabat, G. C. (1993). Recent developments in the epidemiology of lung cancer. *Seminars in Surgical Oncology, 9,* 73-79.

Komaki, R. & Cox, J. D. (1994). The lung and thymus. In J. D. Cox (Ed.), *Moss radiation oncology* (7th ed.). St. Louis: Mosby.

Ktaslersky, J. (1995). Small-cell lung cancer: Can treatment results be improved further? *Seminars in Oncology, 21*(Suppl. 2), 1-2.

Landrigan, P. J. & Selikoff, I. J. (1986). Primary prevention against occupational carcinogens. In P. Bannasch (Ed.), *Cancer risks.* New York: Springer-Verlag.

Light, R. W. (1983). *Pleural diseases.* Philadelphia: Lea & Febiger.

Lin, A. Y. & Ihde, D. C. (1992). Recent developments in the treatment of lung cancer. *Journal of the American Medical Association, 267,* 1661-1664.

Lind, J. (1992). Lung Cancer. In J. C. Clark & R. F. McGee (Eds.), *Core curriculum for oncology nursing* (2nd ed.). Philadelphia: W.B. Saunders.

Lippman, S. M., Benner, S. E., & Hong, W. K. (1994). Cancer chemoprevention. *Journal of Clinical Oncology, 12,* 851-873.

Livingston, R. B., Stephens, R. L., Bonnet, J. D., Grozea, P. N., & Lehene, D. E. (1984). Long-term survival and toxicity in small-cell lung cancer. Southwest Oncology Group Study. *American Journal of Medicine, 77,* 415-417.

Loescher, L. L. (1993). Commentary: Expanding our horizons with an alternative approach to cancer prevention and detection. *Seminars in Oncology Nursing, 9,* 147-149.

Loescher, L. J. & Meyskens, F. L. (1991). Chemoprevention of human skin cancer. *Seminars in Oncology Nursing, 1,* 45-52.

Lucas, C. F., Robinson, B., Hoskin, P. J., Yarnold, J. R., Smith, I. E., & Ford, H. T. (1986). Morbidity of cranial relapse in small-cell lung cancer and the impact of radiation therapy. *Cancer Treatment Reports, 70,* 565-570.

Mackey, B., Lukeman, J., & Ordonez, N. (1991). *Tumors of the lung.* Philadelphia: W. B. Saunders.

Mahaney, F. X. (1992). Lung cancer rates in white males leveling off. *Journal of the National Cancer Institute, 84,* 83-84.

Mann, H. & Karwande, S. V. (1988). The new proposed international staging system for lung cancer. *Seminars in Ultrasound, CT, and MR, 9*(1), 34-39.

Martin, V. R. & Comis, R. L. (1996). Small-cell carcinoma of the lung: An updated overview. *Seminars in Oncology Nursing, 12*(4), 295-303.

Maurer, L. H. & Pajak, T. F. (1987). Prognostic factors in small-cell carcinoma of the lung: A cancer and leukemia group b study. *Cancer Treatment Reports, 65,* 767-774.

Mehta, M. P., Speiser, B. H., & Macha, H. N. (1994). High dose rate brachytherapy for lung cancer. In S. Nag (Ed.), *High dose rate brachytherapy.* New York: Futura.

Miller, J. I. & Phillips, T. W. (1990). Neodymium: YAG laser and brachytherapy in the management of inoperable bronchogenic carcinoma. *Annals of Thoracic Surgery, 50*(2), 190-196.

Mira, J. G., Livingston, R. B., Moore, T. N., Chen, T., Bailey, F., & Bogardus, C. (1982). Influence of chest radiotherapy in frequency and patterns of chest relapse in disseminated small-cell lung carcinoma. Southwest Oncology Group Study. *Cancer, 50,* 1266-1272.

Mulley, A. G. (1995). Screening for lung cancer. In A. H. Goroll, L. A. May, & A. G. Mulley (Eds.), *Primary care medicine.* Philadelphia: J. B. Lippincott.

National Cancer Institute. (1993). *What you need to know about lung cancer.* NIH publication No. 93-1553.

National Cancer Institute. (1997). *PDQ: Small-cell lung cancer: Treatment summaries of patients.* CN-708590.

Nichols, C. R. (1995). The role of ifosfamide in germ cell tumors and small-cell lung cancer. *Seminars in Oncology, 22,* 13-17.

Novello, A. C., Davis, R. M., & Giovino, G. A. (1991). The slowing of the lung cancer epidemic and the need for continued vigilance. *Cancer, 41,* 133-136.

Ochs, J. J., Tester, W. J., Cohen, M. H., Lichter, A. S., & Ihde, D. C. (1983). "Salvage" radiation therapy for intrathoracic small-cell carcinoma of the lung progressing on combination chemotherapy. *Cancer Treatment Reports, 67*(12), 1123-1126.

Perry, M. C., Eaton, W. L., Propert, K. J., Ware, J. H., Zimmer, B., & Chahinian, A. P. (1987). Chemotherapy with or without radiation therapy in limited small-cell carcinoma of the lung. *New England Journal of Medicine, 316*(15), 912-918.

Pierce, J. P., Fiore, M. C., & Novotny, T. E. (1989). Trends in cigarette smoking in the United States: Educational differences are increasing. *Journal of the American Medical Association, 261,* 56-60.

Pignon, J. P., Arriagada, R., Ihde, D. C., Johnson, D. H., Perry, M. C., & Souhami, R. L. (1992). A meta-analysis of thoracic radiotherapy for small-cell lung cancer. *New England Journal of Medicine, 327,* 1618-1624.

Poplin, E., Thompson, B., Whitacre, M., & Aisner, J. (1987). Small-cell carcinoma of the lung: Influence of age on treatment outcome. *Cancer Treatment Reports, 71,* 291-296.

Public Health Service. (1990). *The health benefits of smoking cessation.* Washington, DC: Government Printing Office.

Rawson, N. B. & Peto, J. (1990). An overview of prognostic factors in small-cell lung cancer: A report from the subcommittee for the management of lung cancer of the United Kingdom coordinating committee on cancer research. *British Journal of Cancer, 61,* 597-604.

Risser, N. L. (1987). The key to prevention of lung cancer. *Seminars in Oncology Nursing, 3,* 228-236.

Risser, N. L. (1996). Prevention of lung cancer: The key is to stop smoking. *Seminars in Oncology Nursing, 12*(4), 260-269.

Rogot, E. (1974). Smoking and mortality among U.S. veterans. *Journal of Chronic Diseases, 27,* 189-203.

Rohwedder, J. (1977). Neoplastic disease. In C. Guenter & M. Welch (Eds.), *Pulmonary medicine.* Philadelphia: J. B. Lippincott.

Sagman, U., Lishner, M., Maki, E., Shepherd, F. A., Haddad, R., Evans, W. K., DeBoer, G., Payne, D., Pringle, J. F., & Yeoh, J. L. (1992). Second primary malignancies following diagnosis of small-cell lung cancer. *Journal of Clinical Oncology, 10,* 1525-1533.

Samet, J. M. (1989). Radon and lung cancer. *Journal of the National Cancer Institute, 81,* 745-757.

Samet, J. M. (1993). The epidemiology of lung cancer. *Chest, 103*(Suppl.), 20-29.

Schmidt, S. P. & Shell, J. A. (1994). Lung cancer. In S. E. Otto, *Oncology nursing* (2nd ed.). St. Louis: Mosby.

Sellers, T. A., Potter, J. D., & Bailey-Wilson, J. E. (1992). Lung cancer detection and prevention: Evidence for an interaction between smoking and genetic predisposition. *Cancer Research, 52*(Suppl.), 2694-2697.

Siu, L. L., Shepherd, F. A., Murray, N., Feld, R., Pater, J., & Zee, B. (1996). Influence of age on the treatment of limited stage small-cell lung cancer. *Journal of Clinical Oncology, 14,* 821-828.

Skillrud, D. M., Offord, K. P., & Miller, R. D. (1986). Higher risk of lung cancer in chronic obstructive pulmonary disease. *Annals of Internal Medicine, 105,* 503-507.

Spiegelman, D., Maurer, L. H., Ware, J. H., Perry, M. C., Chahinian, P., & Comis, R. (1989). Prognostic factors in small-cell carcinoma of the lung: An analysis of 1,521 patients. *Journal of Clinical Oncology, 7,* 344-354.

Stellman, J. & Stellman, S. (1983). Occupational lung disease and cancer risk in women. *Occupational Health Nursing, 31,* 40-46.

Stewart, I. E. (1996). Superior vena cava syndrome: An oncologic complication. *Seminars in Oncology Nursing, 12*(4), 312-317.

Thompson, J. M., McFarland, G. K., Hirsch, J. E., & Tucker, S. M. (1993). *Mosby's clinical nursing* (3rd ed.). St. Louis: Mosby.

Turrisi, A. T. (1993). Incorporation of radiotherapy fractionation in the combined-modality treatment of limited small-cell lung cancer. *Chest, 103*(Suppl. 4), 418-422.

U. S. Department of Health and Human Services, Office on Smoking and Health. A Report of the Surgeon General. (1982). *The health consequences of smoking: Cancer (DHHS [PHS] 82-S0179).* Washington, DC: U. S. Government Printing Office.

White, E. J. (1987). Home care of the patient with advanced lung cancer. *Seminars in Oncology Nursing, 3*(3), 216-221.

Willett, W. C. (1990). Vitamin A and lung cancer. *Nutrition Reviews, 48,* 201-211.

Wolpaw, D. R. (1996). Early detection in lung cancer: Case finding and screening. *Medical Clinics of North America, 80*(1), 63-82.

Works, C. R. & Gallucci, B. B. (1996). Biology of lung cancer. *Seminars in Oncology Nursing, 12*(4), 276-284.

Wynder, E. L. & Stellman, S. D. (1979). Impact of long term filter cigarette usage on lung and laryngeal cancer risk. *Journal of the National Cancer Institute, 62,* 471-477.

Yesner, R. & Carter, D. (1982). Pathology of carcinoma of the lung. *Clinics in Chest Medicine, 3,* 257-289.

Non–Small Cell Lung Cancer

Lorie Precht Lindsey, RNC, FNP, OCN
Diva Thielvoldt, RN, MSN, CNS, NP

INTRODUCTION

Lung cancer has become a leading cause of cancer-related death throughout the world. Worldwide, the mortality rate of lung cancer is 88%, exceeded only by cancers of the pancreas, liver, and esophagus (Gazdar & Carbone, 1994). Nationwide, more individuals die from lung cancer than from breast, colon, and prostate cancers combined. In the United States, lung cancer has been the leading cause of cancer-related death in men since about 1960 and in women since about 1987 (Schottenfeld, 1997).

Lung cancer has been described as a disease of the twentieth century. As early as 1912, researchers described lung cancer as a rare disease. However, over the last 70 years, there has been a dramatic progressive increase in primary lung cancer, which is thought to be directly related to cigarette abuse (Burns, Garfinkel, & Samet, 1997).

Recent data on teenage smoking have revealed that between 1995 and 1996, smoking increased among eighth through tenth graders but remained stable and sometimes high among twelfth graders (*Fact Sheet,* 1996; National Institute on Drug Abuse, 1996) (Fig. 62-1). In August 1996, President Bill Clinton launched a major initiative to prevent smoking by minors.

The obligation of health care professionals is to assist in the prevention of lung cancer through increased awareness of smoking-related diseases and to provide better education through smoking-cessation programs.

This chapter provides a review of non–small cell lung cancer (NSCLC), which comprises approximately 80% of all lung cancer cases (Ihde, 1995).

INCIDENCE EPIDEMIOLOGY

It was expected that in 1998, there would be 171,500 new lung cancer cases and an estimated 160,100 lung cancer–related deaths. Respectively, those figures account for 14% of cancer diagnoses and 28% of all cancer deaths. The estimated new lung cancer cases and deaths by gender for all sites in the United States are illustrated in Table 62-1 (American Cancer Society, 1998). Lung cancer incidence has decreased in men, from 87:100,000 in 1984 to 77:100,000 in 1993. Since 1987 the incidence in women has also begun a slight decline, although more women have died annually of lung cancer than breast cancer (Mason, 1994; Yang & Fossella, 1996) (Fig. 62-2).

Lung cancer is divided into two groups, NSCLC and small cell lung cancer (SCLC). The incidence of NSCLC accounts for approximately 80% of total lung cancer cases.

Incidence per cell type was once equally divided. More recently, the number of adenocarcinoma cell types diagnosed has increased. Several theories explaining the histologic changes are discussed later in this chapter. Fig. 62-3 illustrates the incidence of the cell types of lung cancer. The incidence of squamous cell and the unspecified cell types, including large cell, is approaching the incidence of the adenocarcinomas. The SCLC type and related cell types account for approximately one fifth of the total group (Ihde, 1995; Travis, Linder, & Mackay, 1997).

SCREENING AND CHEMOPREVENTION

Lung cancer is generally diagnosed in the later stages of the disease. Many patients present with advanced disease, and treatment up to now has not added to survival in most cases. The poor outcomes for this patient group have led to the investigation of early detection and prevention strategies.

Screening

Numerous screening programs have been conducted in individuals at high risk for lung malignancy with the purpose to improve early diagnosis. These programs have not yielded improvement in long-term survival for these patients. Currently, no randomized trials have demonstrated a reduction in mortality as a result of screening for lung cancer (Ginsberg, Kris, & Armstrong, 1997). Screening procedures using sputum cytology and serial chest radiography have been proposed in high-risk patients, although data have not supported the use in community practice (Cortese, Edell, & Harubumi, 1997; White, 1997).

Primary Prevention

Tobacco is the etiologic carcinogen in 80% to 90% of all lung cancer cases (Burns, Garfinkel, & Samet, 1997). Elimination of this major causative factor, or primary prevention, would decrease the lung cancer incidence dramatically. Unless changes in smoking behavior occur, the incidence of lung cancer will remain a significant health problem well into the twenty-first century, as a result of the latency from exposure to actual development of lung cancer.

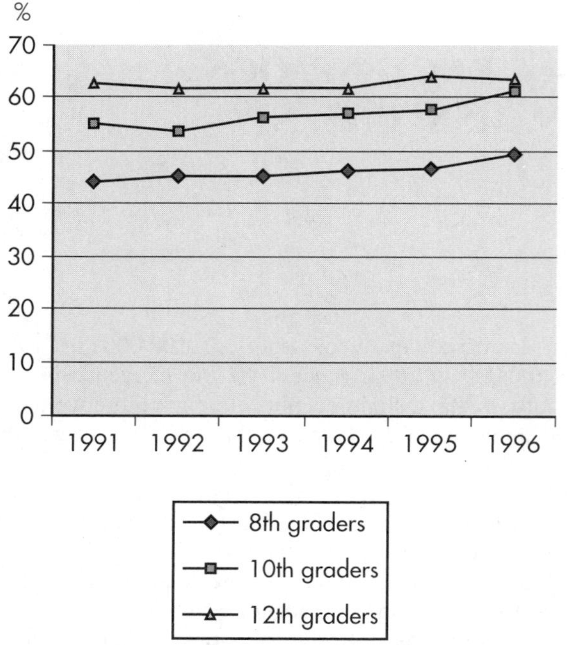

Fig. 62-1 Trends in prevalence of lifetime cigarette usage in eighth, tenth, and twelfth graders. (Modified from the National Institute on Drug Abuse [1996]. *Monitoring the future study.* Bethesda: The Institute.)

Numerous surveys have shown that the majority of current smokers demonstrate desire to stop smoking. An American Cancer Society survey in 1994 revealed that an estimated 69% of current smokers wanted to quit. Intervention through smoking-cessation programs varies in content and efficacy. Many major smoking-cessation guidelines have been evaluated and consequently, in April 1996, the Agency for Health Care Policy on Research (AHCPR) made recommendations to assist health care providers in providing smokers with consistent and effective smoking-cessation guidelines (AHCPR, 1996). Specific guidelines with treatment strategies were recommended by the AHCPR and theses are briefly described in Box 62-1.

Chemoprevention

Chemoprevention, the administration of drugs before the diagnosis of invasive cancer to block or reverse carcinogenesis, has been studied and continues to offer a viable option for decreasing lung cancer incidence and mortality. The efficacy of chemoprevention has not been established and trials are ongoing to determine which agents provide benefit. Among the numerous substances studied for potential chemopreventive actions, retinol (vitamin A) and its synthetic derivative, retinoid, are the most heavily investigated agents (Goodman, 1995; Karp, 1997; Pastorino, 1995).

Beta-carotene, a precursor of vitamin A, is of the carotenoid class. Beta-carotene is converted to vitamin A by the body and is found in fruits and vegetables that are deep yellow, orange, or dark green in color.

TABLE 62-1 Current Morbidity and Mortality Rates for Patients with Non–Small Cell Lung Cancer

Estimated New Cases Both Sexes	Estimated New Cases Male	Estimated New Cases Female	Estimated Deaths Both Sexes	Estimated Deaths Males	Estimated Deaths Female
178,100	98,300	79,800	160,400	94,400	66,000

Modified from American Cancer Society. (1998). *Cancer facts and figures 1998.* Atlanta: The Society.

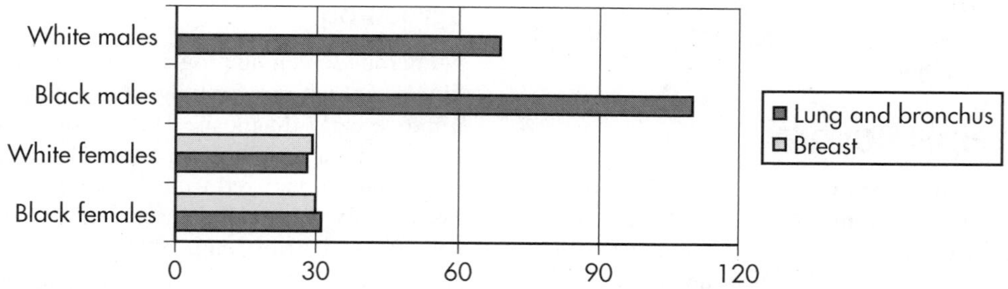

Fig. 62-2 Age-adjusted lung and breast cancer death rates, 1987-1991. (From Shopland, D. R. [1996]. Cigarette smoking as a cause of cancer. In A. H. Harris, B. K. Edwards, W. J. Blot, & L. A. Gloeckler Ries [Eds.], *Cancer rates and risks* [4th ed.]. (NIH Publication No. 96-691.). Washington, D. C.: U. S. Department of Health and Human Services.)

Evidence accumulated from observational studies has proven that individuals who eat more fruits and vegetables that are rich in beta-carotene and retinol have lower incidence of lung cancer. The role of carotenoids and retinoids in the pathogenesis and prevention of lung cancer has not been established.

The Beta-Carotene and Retinol Efficacy Trial (CARET), a large chemoprevention trial, was conducted to find out whether a combination of beta-carotene and vitamin A supplements would prevent lung and other cancers in individuals at high risk. The research participants included 18,314 smokers and former smokers, as well as men with a history of asbestos exposure. Interestingly enough, the CARET study was terminated in January 1996, 21 months early because of clear evidence of no benefit and substantial evidence of possible harm. CARET participants receiving the combination of beta-carotene and vitamin A had no chemopreventive benefit *and* had excess lung cancer incidence and mortality (National Cancer Instutite, 1997).

CAUSAL AGENTS FOR LUNG CANCER

As our country has become more urbanized and industrialized, the incidence of lung cancer has risen. Various agents have been recognized as causal factors, although none as notable as cigarette smoking (Box 62-2).

Our lungs are exposed to airborne environmental particles with every breath. Inhalation of smaller particles (0.5 to 3.0 microns) poses the greatest danger because as smaller causal particles are inhaled, the more likely they are to gain access to the terminal bronchi and bronchioles, causing po-

Box 62-1
Smoking Cessation: A Guide for Primary Care Clinicians

- Ask about smoking.
- Advise tobacco users to quit.
- Assist the patient with a quit plan.
- Offer intensive smoking-cessation programs.
- Provide follow-up to patients.
- Prevent relapse through positive reinforcement.
- Three key treatment strategies were identified in the guidelines:
  1. Nicotine replacement therapy
  2. Clinician-provided social support
  3. Skills training/problem-solving techniques

From Tellervo, K., Su, S., Korhonen, H. J., Utela, A. & Puska, P. (1997). Evaluation of a national quit and win contest: Determinants for successful quitting. *Preventative Medicine, 26,* 556-564.

Box 62-2
Risk Factors/Populations at Risk for Small Cell Lung Cancer

Tobacco smoke
Passive smoking
Air pollution
- The sulfur-oxide/particulate complex arising from the combustion of sulfur-containing fuels
- Photochemical oxidants related to motor vehicle emissions
- Miscellaneous pollutants from localized sources such as refineries and manufacturing plants

Occupational exposure
- Alkylating compounds
- Arsenic
- Asbestos
- Cadmium
- Chromium
- Copper
- Formaldehyde
- Halo ethers
- Radon
- Silica
- Sulfur dioxide
- Tuberculosis
- Uranium

Constitutional factors
- Family history
- Preexisting lung disease and prior lung cancer
- Age

Geographic location
Social class
High-fat diet

From American Cancer Society. (1998). *Cancer facts and figures 1998.* Atlanta: The Society.

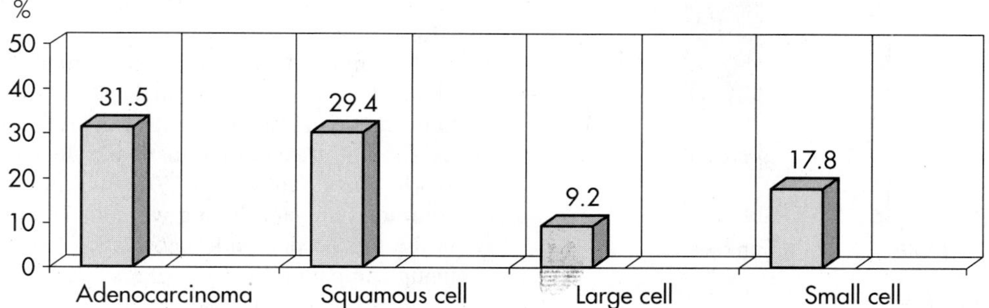

Fig. 62-3 Incidence of lung cancer cell types. Note: Age-adjusted incidence rates per 100,000 person-years for all races and both genders from 1983-1987. (From Shopland, D. R. [1996]. Cigarette smoking as a cause of cancer. In A. H. Harris, B. K. Edwards, W. J. Blot, & L. A. Gloeckler Ries [Eds.]. *Cancer rates and risks* [4th ed.]. (NIH Publication No. 96-691.). Washington, D. C.: U. S. Department of Health and Human Services.)

tential injury. Although lung cancer occurs through a multistep carcinogenic process, inhalation of these causal agents through the tracheobronchial tree causes the initial injury to the bronchial surface epithelium (Groeger, Esposito, Mueller, Caputi, Kaiser, & Giordano, 1997, Shields & Harris, 1993).

Research has led investigators to believe that bronchogenic carcinomas emerge from a pluripotent stem cell of epithelial origin. It is believed that exposure to inhaled carcinogens (i.e., causal agents) often result in premalignant changes throughout the respiratory epithelium, which antecede malignancy (Carbone, 1997).

The probability of bronchogenic cancer developing is also linked to the ability of the individual's bronchopulmonary defense mechanisms and the genetic integrity, as well as exposure amount and duration to the causal agent (Spivak, Fasco, Walker, & Kaminsky, 1997; Groeger et al., 1997).

Tobacco Smoking

An estimated 30% of total cancer deaths and 85% of all lung cancer deaths in the United States are related to tobacco smoking (Gazdar & Carbone, 1994). Compared with nonsmokers, smokers present a dose-dependent risk of mortality increase from other malignancies such as pancreatic, renal, and bladder cancers, as well as leukemia and myelomas (Skaar, Tsoh, Cinciripini, Wetter, Prokhorov, & Gritz, 1996). The percent of lung cancer deaths attributed to cigarette smoking is outlined in Fig. 62-4.

Tobacco, particularly cigarette smoking, has been known as the major cause of lung cancer for 40 years. In 1957, U.S. Surgeon General Leroy E. Burney issued a policy statement that acknowledged and recognized the greater incidence of lung cancer in smokers than nonsmokers (Ginsberg, Kris, & Armstrong, 1997). At that time, the incidence of smoking in the United States was at an all-time high. The National Health Interview Survey has shown that since then, trends in smoking among adults (ages 18 and over) have declined between 1965 and 1990, although between 1990 and 1994 smoking prevalence remained unchanged (American Cancer Society, 1998).

The risk of developing lung cancer is directly related to the number of years an individual has smoked and the number of packs per day. The relative risk factor is measured in terms of pack years (number of years smoked × number of packs per day), and risk is increased after 10 pack years. Former smokers can decrease their risk after 5 years of abstaining from smoking, although it takes 10 to 15 years to equal nonsmokers' risk (Elpern, 1993; White, 1997).

Decreases in cigarette "tar" and nicotine emissions have occurred over the last 40 years. Tar and nicotine emission of cigarettes has decreased from 38 mg and 2.7 mg, respectively, to 12 mg and 0.9 mg. These decreases were presumed to be a result of the addition of filter tips and changes in tobacco blend. The use of filter tips rose from 0.56% in 1950, to 97% in more recent times.

Some hypothesize that the decrease in "tar" and nicotine has caused smokers to change their smoking patterns. Research has revealed that smokers adjust their intake to satisfy addictive needs for nicotine by inhaling deeper and more intensely. Seemingly, the excess volume inhaled delivers increased amounts of carcinogens and toxins to the peripheral lungs (Hoffmann, Djordjevic, & Hoffmann, 1997). The modifications to an individual's smoking patterns are suspect regarding the epidemiologic changes in the major histiologic types of lung cancers. An example of these changes is the increasing incidence of adenocarcinoma cell type in smokers.

The adenocarcinoma lung cancer cell type typically arises in the lung periphery. Researchers suspect the changes in smoking patterns, and subsequent greater exposure of tobacco smoke to the peripheral lung explains the higher incidence (Hoffmann, Djordjevic, & Hoffmann, 1997; Stellman, Muscat, Hoffmann, & Wynder, 1997).

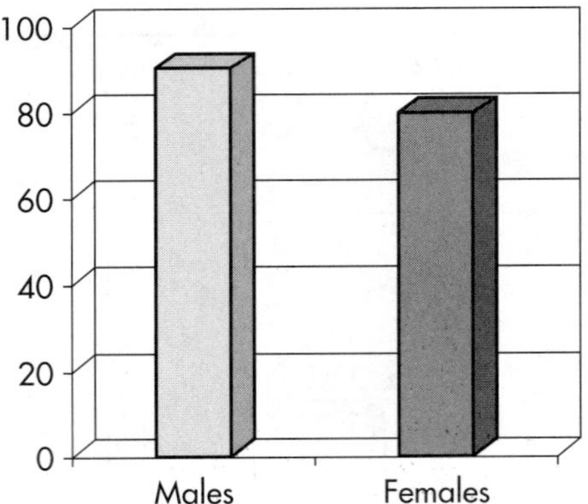

Fig. 62-4 Percentage of lung cancer deaths attributed to cigarette smoking in the United States in 1994. (Modified from Shopland, D. R. [1996]. Cigarette smoking as a cause of cancer. In A. H. Harris, B. K. Edwards, W. J. Blot, & L. A. Gloeckler Ries [Eds.]. *Cancer rates and risks* [4th ed.] (NIH Publication No. 96-691.). Washington, D. C.: U. S. Department of Health and Human Services.)

History of Tobacco

The use of tobacco by Americans predates the arrival of Columbus to the New World. Tobacco use by native Americans was largely ceremonial and religious in contrast to the regular and continuos abuse that typifies cigarette smoking today (Burns, 1994).

The first successful national marketing of a modern blended cigarette, the Camel brand, occurred in 1913. At that time, cigarette smoking was predominantly a male behavior that increased dramatically during and subsequent to World War I. Until the 1930s, smoking was a relatively uncommon behavior among women. The increase in smoking in the female population corresponded with a major advertising campaign, Lucky Strike's "Reach for a Lucky Instead of a Sweet." That advertisement, which presented an inferred message of potential weight loss, encouraged women's interest in cigarette smoking (Burns, Garfinkel, & Samet, 1997). Recent evaluation has confirmed that fear of weight gain in female smokers is a major impediment to smoking cessation (Marcus, King, Albrecht, Parisi, & Abrams, 1997).

Recently, the U.S. government has intervened with a proposal for a tobacco settlement between the 50 states' Attorneys General and the tobacco industry. This settlement ultimately holds the tobacco companies liable for tobacco's potential health hazard. As of this writing, terms for this proposal have not yet been agreed upon.

Carcinogens in Tobacco

Tobacco smoke is comprised of more than 4000 components of which an approximate 50 are carcinogens. In tobacco smoke, the major causal agents of lung cancer are the polynuclear aromatic hydrocarbons (PAHs) and tobacco-specific N-nitrosamines. Tobacco smoking also results in increased exposure to ethylene oxide, aromatic amines, and other agents that cause damage to deoxyribonucleic acid (DNA) (Shields & Harris, 1993; Hoffmann, Djordjevic, & Hoffmann, 1997).

Cigar and Pipe Smoking

Most studies suggest that smokers of strictly pipes and cigars experience some increase in risk of lung cancer compared with nonsmokers. It seems the risk has varied in different studies, depending largely on the amount smoked and depth of inhalation (Wu-Williams & Samet, 1994).

Passive Smoking/Secondhand Smoke

In 1994 an estimated 48 million adults were smokers, and many nonsmokers subsequently were endangered by breathing the cigarette smoke. Each year about 3000 nonsmoking adults die of lung cancer caused from secondhand smoke (American Cancer Society, 1998).

This exposure increases the risks for the children of smokers and becomes an occupational hazard in individuals working in bars and restaurants.

In 1981 the first reports on increased lung cancer risks in nonsmokers married to smokers were published. In 1992 the U.S. Environmental Protection Agency declared secondhand smoke (ETS) to be a human carcinogen.

Secondhand tobacco smoke contains four known human carcinogens (benzene, 2-naphthylamine, 4-aminobiphenyl, and polonium-210); as well as 10 others are classified as probable carcinogens (American Cancer Society, 1998). Many components of ETS are also classified as respiratory irritants (Groeger et al., 1997).

Exposure to ETS is primarily an indoor problem, and level of exposure depends on room size, ventilation, and number of individuals smoking. Short-term concentrations of ETS are extremely high in smoke-filled environments such as bars and nightclubs. It has been estimated that nonsmokers inhale a dose equivalent of 0.1 to 1 cigarette when exposed to high levels of ETS. More than 25 epidemiological studies have been published on the effects of ETS. Combined, these studies suggest a 20% to 30% increased risk of lung cancer in nonsmokers married to smokers. These studies have confirmed that there are no known safe levels of secondhand smoke (Pershagen, 1994).

Public policies to protect others from secondhand smoke have been enacted at many local, state, and federal levels. These polices vary from disallowing smoking in areas not appropriately ventilated to preventing sale of tobacco products to individuals under 18 years of age.

Occupational/Environmental Hazards

Exposure to chemicals in the occupational environment has been proven to increase an individuals risk of lung cancer (see Box 62-1). This risk is relatively small compared with smoking. These occupational agents interact synergistically with tobacco smoking; therefore a smoking individual exposed to these agents has a combined relative risk factor that far exceeds nonsmokers. For example, data have revealed that smokers exposed to asbestos have a risk increase 50 times higher than an unexposed nonsmoker (Warnock & Isenberg, 1986) (see Box 62-2).

Air Pollution

Air pollutants have been suspected as potential causal agents of lung cancers in urbanized and industrialized nations.

Indoor Radon Exposure

Occupational exposure to radon in uranium miners has been associated with a 10-fold or greater risk factor for lung cancer (Gazdar & Carbone, 1994). Indoor exposure from natural ground sources in private residences has become a concern. Radon, a product of radium 226, is produced from the decomposition of rocks and soil. House foundations with cracks have represented a risk for potential exposure. Damage to lung DNA can occur with exposure to radon and consequently risk of lung cancer is increased although presumed small (Darby & Samet, 1994) (see Box 62-2).

Nutrition

Numerous epidemiological studies have suggested a connection between increased consumption of fresh vegetables and fruits and lowered lung cancer risk. Using that premise, various chemoprevention studies were conducted between 1975 and 1993.

A positive association between many malignancies and dietary fat has been identified, and there is some suggestion of increased incidence of lung cancer in patients with high dietary fat intake (Schottenfeld, 1997) (see Box 62-2).

Genetic Predisposition

A smoking relative of an individual with lung cancer assumes an increased risk of developing lung cancer. It has been postulated that the defect in the body's ability to defend against the carcinogens in tobacco smoke may be inherited (Gazdar & Carbone, 1994).

DIAGNOSTIC EVALUATION

Diagnostic evaluation includes obtaining a detailed history and complete physical assessment in addition to other baseline tests (Table 62-2). A thorough history and physical examination may disclose evidence of external signs of malignancy. Visual examination of the patient may reveal evidence of cutaneous signs of malignancy or complications related to tumor development, such as superior vena caval obstruction. Palpation may reveal lymphadenopathy, subcutaneous nodules, or organomegaly secondary to metastasis. Auscultation may reveal wheezing suggestive of endobronchial obstruction and absent or decreased breath sounds, which when paired with percussive dullness, may indicate pleural effusion (Bullock, 1984).

A variety of diagnostic tools are used in determining lung cancer patient's stage and prognosis (American Society of Clinical Oncology [ASCO], 1997). The type and extent of evaluation depends on a variety of factors including physi-

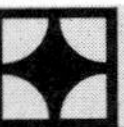

TABLE 62-2 Assessment of the Patient with Non–Small Cell Lung Cancer

	Assessment Parameters	Typical Abnormal Findings
History	A. Personal and social history 1. Smoking history 2. Marijuana use 3. Occupational history	A. Personal and social risk factors 1. Smoking, cigarettes, cigars, pipes—household members who smoke place patient at increased risk for lung cancer. 2. Smoking marijuana places patient at increased risk. 3. Obtain lifelong history of occupations with attention to shipyard work, chalking textile workers, meat packers and cutters, hairdressers, agricultural workers, chemical workers, and electrical machinery manufacturers. B. Common early symptoms include cough, chest pain, weight loss, dyspnea, fever, fatigue, and transient nausea. Common late symptoms include productive cough with hemoptysis or chest pain, wheezes, hoarseness, and nerve disorders due to local tumor invasion.
Physical Examination	A. Pulmonary and lymphatic system	A. Dyspnea; rapid, shallow breathing; intercostal retractions on inspiration indicating obstruction; and bulging innerspaces on expiration indicate outflow obstruction. B. Finger clubbing; skin changes; weight loss; Harner's, Pancoast's, and superior vena cava syndromes; joint swelling consistent with hypertrophic pulmonary osteoarthropathy. C. Palpation for decreased tactile fremitus may indicate pleural effusion or pleural cavity tumor, increased tactile fremitus, and lung mass. D. Auscultation of lungs may indicate decreased or absent breath sounds. E. Pleural rub may indicate inflammatory response to invading tumor.
Diagnostic Tests	A. Sputum cytology	A. Once routine, it has been largely replaced by fiberoptic bronchoscope; may show malignant cells.
	B. Chest x-ray	B. Mass may be shown with persistent infiltrates, particularly in the anterior segments of the upper lobes.
	C. Fiberoptic examination, bronchoscopy or mediastinoscopy with biopsy	C. Determine location and extent of tumor.
	D. Complete blood count	D. Low hematocrit or hemoglobin indicative of anemia
	E. Blood chemistries	E. Elevated LDH
	F. Immunocytochemical markers	F. Presence of neuronspecific markers (enolase, chromogranin) indicate exact histologic diagnosis and possible prognosis.
	G. CT scan of liver and brain	G. Determine liver and brain metastases.
	H. Bone scan with x-rays of abnormal areas	H. Determine bone metastases.
	I. Bilateral bone marrow aspirations	I. Aspirate for metastases disease.
	J. Positive emission tomography	J. Identify occult metastatic disease.

From Harwood, H. V. (1996). Non-small lung cancer: An overview and diagnosis, staging and treatment. *Seminars in Oncology Nursing, 4,* 285-294; White, E. J. (1997). Lung cancer. In C. Varricchio, M. Pierce, C. L. Walker, & T. B. Ades, (Eds.), *A cancer source book for nurses* (7th ed.). Atlanta: American Cancer Society. J. & Fossella, F. V. (1996). Non-small cell lung cancer. *Physician Assistant, 11,* 36-67.
LDH: lactic dehydrogenase.

cian practice style and patient's suspected stage of disease. Initial staging is vital because the decision on the most appropriate therapy is dependent on surgical-pathological staging.

Chest x-ray and sputum cytology may detect asymptomatic lung cancer. Most lung tumors are not visible on chest x-ray until they are approximately 1 cm in diameter. Chest x-rays best locate peripherally located tumors, whereas sputum cytology serves as a better evaluation for centrally located tumors (Shaw, 1995).

Computed tomography (CT) of the chest is used in the evaluation of suspected lung cancer and has proved superior to chest x-ray in detecting multiple intrapulmonary lesions and mediastinal lymphadenopathy. The physician request for extension of the CT view to include the liver and adrenals for evaluation of metastatic disease is usually a standard assessment in most medical centers.

Magnetic resonance imaging (MRI) is similar in its accuracy to CT, although due to its cost and longer examination times, it is not routinely used in evaluating patients with lung cancer (Broderick, Tarver, & Conces, Jr., 1997).

Recently positron emission tomography (PET) with F-18-fluorodeoxyglucose (^{18}FDG) has been used for the imaging of thoracic malignancies. ^{18}FDG is a glucose analog labeled with a positron-emitting fluorine-18 molecule. It is known that tumor cells have increased glucose uptake due to increased metabolic activity. ^{18}FDG is a useful imaging agent because it is taken up and accumulates in the tumor cells to allow visualization of abnormal areas.

Early studies comparing PET-FDG imaging and CT reveals that PET-FDG is more accurate than CT in determining malignant nodal involvement. The use of PET-FDG technology seems promising in the future evaluation of patients with thoracic malignancies (Broderick, Tarver, & Conces, Jr., 1997).

In addition to the tests discussed above, bronchoscopy, mediastinoscopy, and pulmonary tests are also valuable in the staging evaluation. Table 62-2 lists steps in a diagostic evaluation for patients with possible lung cancer.

Flexible fiberoptic bronchoscopy offers visibility of the tracheobronchial tree, usually to the third and fourth bronchi, and bronchoscopic biopsy confirms histological diagnosis in most lung cancer cases (Reed, DeCamp, & Sugarbaker, 1995) (Table 62-3).

A pulmonary or thoracic surgeon usually performs mediastinoscopy, a surgical procedure used in surgical staging similar to bronchoscopy. Patients with earlier stage disease are more likely to undergo mediastinoscopy. Certain absolute and relative indications are recommended before staging patients with mediastinoscopy, and these are listed in Box 62-3 (Webb, 1995; Reed & Sugarbaker, 1997; Ginsberg, Kris, & Armstrong, 1997).

The mediastinoscopy procedure requires a 3- to 4-cm transverse skin incision to be made 1 to 2 cm above the suprasternal notch. It provides view of the regional nodes and allows biopsy of the mediastinal nodes. General anesthesia is usually necessary, although local anesthesia may be used in selected patients. Thoracotomy with surgical resection of tumor often follows mediastinoscopy in a potentially surgically resectable patient (Reed & Sugarbaker, 1997).

Mediastinoscopy is commonly used to document the presence of N2 or N3 disease and allows for identification of patients with early stage disease. Identification of patients with stage IIIA disease has become increasingly important. Clinical trials in this patient group have confirmed the ben-

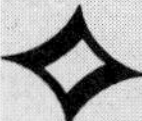

TABLE 62-3 Patient Preparation for a Bronchoscopy

Description of the Procedure: A bronchoscopy test permits visualization of the trachea, bronchi, and select bronchioles with a flexible or rigid bronchoscope. It is performed to diagnose tumors, coin lesions, or granulomatous lesions or to obtain a biopsy or obtain cytologic examinations under local anesthesia. A bronchoscopy is usually performed under conscious sedation.

Patient Preparation:

1. The patient must be NPO for at least 6 hours before the procedure to reduce the risk of aspiration. Gag, cough, and swallowing reflexes are blocked during, and for a few hours after, surgery.
2. Wigs, nail polish, makeup, dentures, jewelry, and contact lenses must be removed before the examination.

Procedural Considerations:

1. A local anesthetic is sprayed and swabbed onto the back of the nose, tongue, pharynx, and epiglottis. If the patient has a history of bronchospasms, steroids and aminophylline are often administered before the procedure.
2. The bronchoscope is inserted through the mouth or nose into the pharynx and trachea.
3. The patient is administered diazepam, midazolam, or meperidine.
4. Arterial blood gases during and after bronchoscopy may be ordered. Sputum specimens or cytologic examination or culture and sensitivity testing may be ordered.

Postoperative Considerations:

1. Assess for swallow, gag, and cough reflexes before allowing patient food or water.
2. Provide gargles to relieve mild pharyngitis.
3. Monitor ECG, blood pressure, temperature, pulse, pulse oximeter readings, skin and nailbed color, lung sounds, and respiratory rate and patterns.
4. Oxygen per mask or nasal cannula may be ordered. Humidified oxygen at specific concentrations up to 100% by mask may be necessary.
5. Provide written discharge instructions.

Special Considerations: Morphine sulfate is contraindicated in patients who have problems with bronchospasm or asthma because it can cause bronchospasm. Analgesics, barbiturates, tranquilizers, sedatives, and atropine may be ordered and administered one half to 1 hour before bronchoscopy. The patient should be as relaxed as possible before and during the procedure but also needs to know that anxiety is normal. Therefore the patient may need additional IV sedatives administered during the procedure.

Modified from Krebs, L. U. & Williams, P. (1997). Lung cancer. In R. Gates & R. M. Fink (Eds.), *Oncology nursing secrets.* Philadelphia: Hanley & Belfus.
NPO, Nothing by mouth; *ECG,* electrocardiogram.

efits of preresectional or neoadjuvant chemotherapy, which has improved resectability and resulted in lower-stage disease (Reed & Sugarbaker, 1997). Table 62-4 illustrates a patient teaching tool for a mediastinascopy.

Recently the ASCO released guidelines for the diagnostic evaluation, treatment, and follow-up care of patients with unresectable NSCLC. These ASCO guidelines confirmed the use of chest x-ray, chest CT scan, and biopsy of enlarged mediastinal lymph nodes (greater than 1 cm in shortest transverse axis) to stage clinically resectable locoregional disease. Recommendations for patients with advanced disease includes evaluation using bone scan for patients with symptoms or elevated serum calcium or serum alkaline phosphatase levels, CT or MRI brain scans for patients with symptoms of central nervous system (CNS) disease, and biopsy of patients with suspicious adrenal or liver masses (ASCO, 1997).

Box 62-3

Indications for Mediastinoscopy

Absolute Indications

- Mediastinal lymph nodes >1.5 cm on computed tomography (CT) scan of the chest

Relative Indications

- T2 tumor or T3 primary lesion that is resectable
- Tumor location within inner one third of lung section
- Preoperative biopsy reveals tumor cell type of adenocarcinoma or undifferentiated large cell
- Multiple primary lesions suspected or synchronous lung tumors
- Primary tumor located in left upper lobe causing vocal cord paralysis

Plan to use adjuvant chemotherapy.

Modified from Reed, M. F. & Sugarbaker, D. J. (1997). Mediastinal staging of lung cancer. In H. I. Pass, J. B. Mitchell, D. H. Johnson, & A. T. Turrisi (Eds.), *Lung cancer principles and practice*. Philadelphia: Lippincott-Raven.

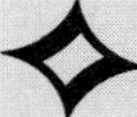

Table 62-4 Patient Preparation for a Mediastinoscopy

Description of the Procedure: A mediastinoscopy is performed under general anesthesia to examine and take a biopsy of mediastinal lymph nodes. Because these nodes receive lymphatic drainage from the lungs, mediastinal biopsies may be diagnosed in staging of lung cancer.

Patient Preparation:

1. Obtain informed consent.
2. The patient must be NPO for 8 or more hours before the test.

Procedural Considerations:

1. Previous mediastinoscopy contraindicates repeat examination because adhesions make satisfactory dissection of nodes extremely difficult or sometimes impossible.
2. Complications can result from the risks associated with general anesthesia or from preexisting conditions.

Postoperative Considerations:

1. Evaluate breathing and lung sounds; check wound for bleeding and hematoma.
2. Instruct patient to call physician if problems occur.

Modified from Carpentino, L. J. (1994). Nursing care plans and documentation—CD-Rom. Philadelphia: Lippincott-Raven.
NPO, Nothing by mouth.

STAGING

Staging of lung cancer is used to assist the practitioner in estimating the patient's prognosis and assigning treatment. After diagnostic evaluation and, subsequently, a precise pathologic diagnosis has been made, complete clinical and or surgical staging can begin. NSCLC is staged through the international TNM staging system, which was revised in 1986 (Ginsberg, Kris, & Armstrong, 1997) (Table 62-5). The international TNM staging system classifies the tumor anatomically and provides information for reproducible clinical outcome. It is based on the T (primary tumor), N (regional lymph node), and M (evidence of distant metastasis) system. (Beahrs, Henson, Hutter, & Kennedy, 1992) Staging conveys information about the site and size of the primary tumor, its cell type, and the anatomic extent of the disease. Proper staging of NSCLC is critical in determining therapy. NSCLC is only curable by surgery; therefore the question of whether the patient's disease is operable or inoperable must be answered before proceeding with therapy. The TNM staging system provides the basis for selecting patients for resection. Generally, patients with stages I and II and occasionally stage IIIA diseases are considered candidates for surgical resection, whereas patients with stages IIIB and IV are not (Ginsberg, Kris, & Armstrong, 1997).

Table 62-5 Lung Cancer Stage Grouping

Occult	TX	N0	M0
Stage 0	Tis	N0	M0
Stage I	T1	N0	M0
	T2	N0	M0
Stage II	T1	N1	M0
	T2	N1	M0
Stage IIIA	T1	N2	M0
	T2	N2	M0
	T3	N0	M0
	T3	N1	M0
	T3	N2	M0
Stage IIIB	Any T	N3	M0
	T4	Any N	M0
Stage IV	Any T	Any N	M1

Ihde, D. D. (1995). Non-small cell lung cancer. In J. S. MacDonald, D. G. Haller, & R. J. Mayer (Eds.), *Manual of oncologic therapeutics* (3rd ed.). Philadelphia: J. B. Lippincott.

Primary Tumor

The general size of the primary tumor is reflected by the T specification. The actual tumor size, location, and whether there is pulmonary or extrapulmonary spread directly affects stage and thus patient's survival.

The TX designator identifies primary tumors that cannot be evaluated or tumors that have been established by the presence of malignant cells in sputum or bronchial washing. The tumor cannot be visualized on radiography or bronchoscopy. This can also be referred to as an *occult tumor.*

T0 represents no evidence of primary tumor. Tis—carcinoma in situ—is specified as stage 0. The T1 listing includes tumors that are 3 cm or less and have no central extension beyond a lobar bronchus. T2 includes tumors 3 cm or smaller that invade visceral pleura. T4 designates further growth of tumor into the major structures (mediastinum, great vessels, trachea, or heart) or if a pleural effusion is present.

Nodes

The classification of regional lymph nodes reflects the progression of the tumor via metastasis or direct extension to particular groups of nodes. N0 designates no evidence of nodal metastasis. N1 designates spread of tumor to hilar and peribronchial nodes, and N2 reflects the continued progression of tumor to the peritracheal, aortic, subcarinal, esophageal, and pulmonary ligament nodes (ipsilateral mediastinal lymph nodes). N3 reflects the involvement of the contralateral hilar, mediastinal, and scalene ipsilateral or contralateral nodes. Extension of tumor to the supraclavicular nodes is also classified as N3 disease.

Distant Metastases

Involvement of distant organ sites (i.e., brain, bone, liver, adrenal, etc.) is associated with the poorest prognosis. M0 reflects no evidence of metastasis, and M1 indicates evidence of distant metastasis (Beahrs et al., 1992).

Stage Grouping

Once the TNM is defined, a stage group of either I, II, III (A/B), or IV is assigned (Table 62-6). This grouping allows an organized method of separating stages, thus offering appropriate management of lung cancer patients.

Stage I. Patients with stage I disease include those patients with smaller primary T1 or T2 tumors. Patients with stage I disease have no nodal or distant spread; therefore tumor resection is the most viable option in these patients. Obviously the earlier stage and thus less structurally involved the tumors is, the greater is the likelihood it can be surgically resected with good survival results. When surgically resected, the smaller tumor, T1 vs T2, is associated with improved patient outcome.

Stage II. Patients with stage II disease have T1 or T2 tumors and metastasis to the ipsilateral peribronchial and/or hilar regional nodes. Approximately 10% to 15% of all patients with NSCLC present with stage II disease.

TABLE 62-6 International TNM Staging System

Primary Tumor (T)	
TX	Primary tumor cannot be assessed; tumor proven by the presence of malignant cells in sputum or bronchial washings but not visualized by imaging or bronchoscopy; occult tumor
T0	No evidence of primary tumor
Tis	Carcinoma in situ
T1	Tumor 3 cm or less in greatest dimension, surrounded by lung or visceral pleura, without bronchoscopic evidence of invasion more proximal than the lobar bronchus (i.e., not in the main bronchus)*
T2	Tumor with any of the following features of size or extent More than 3 cm in greatest dimension Involving main bronchus, 2 cm or more distal to the carina Invading the visceral pleura Associated with atelectasis or obstructive pneumonitis that extends to the hilar region but does not involve the entire lung
T3	Tumor of any size that directly invades any of the following: chest wall (including superior sulcus tumors), diaphragm, mediastinal pleura, or parietal pericardium Tumor in the main bronchus less than 2 cm distal to the carina but without involvement of the carina Associated atelectasis or obstructive pneumonitis of the entire lung
T4	Tumor of any size that invades any of the following: mediastinum, heart, great vessels, trachea, esophagus, vertebral body, carina Tumor with a malignant pleural effusion†
Regional Lymph Nodes (N)	
N0	No regional lymph node metastasis
N1	Metastasis in ipsilateral peribronchial and/or ipsilateral hilar lymph nodes, including direct extension
N2	Metastasis in ipsilateral mediastinal and/or subcarinal lymph node(s)
N3	Metastasis in contralateral mediastinal, contralateral hilar, ipsilateral or contralateral scalene, or supraclavicular lymph node(s)
Distant Metastasis (M)	
M0	No distant metastasis
M1	Distant metastasis

Ihde, D. D. (1995). Non-small cell lung cancer. In J. S. MacDonald, D. G. Haller, & R. J. Mayer (Eds.), *Manual of oncologic therapeutics* (3rd ed.). Philadelphia: J. B. Lippincott.

*The uncommon superficial tumor of any size with its invasive component limited to the bronchial wall, which may extend proximal to the main bronchus, is also classified at T1.

†Most pleural effusions associated with lung cancer are due to tumor. However, there are a few patients in whom multiple cytopathologic examinations of pleural fluid are negative for tumor. In these cases, fluid is non-bloody and is not an exudate. When these elements and clinical judgment dictate that the effusion is not related to the tumor, the effusion should be excluded as a staging element and the patient should be staged as T1, T2, or T3.

Stages IIIA and IIIB. Patients with stage IIIA disease have either T3 tumors with or without metastasis to the ipsilateral peribronchial and/or hilar regional nodes. This group also includes patients that have T1 to T3 tumors with metastasis to the ipsilateral mediastinal or subcarinal lymph nodes.

Patients with stage IIIB disease have either T4 tumors, with or without nodal involvement, or they have any size tumor with metastasis to contralateral mediastinal, hilar, scalene, or supraclavicular nodes (Moore & Lee, 1997; Mountain, 1993). Approximately 20% to 25% of patients present with stages IIIA or IIIB (Surveillance, Epidemiology, and End Results [SEER] Data, 1997).

Stage IV. Patients with stage IV disease can have any T or N classification, although if they have evidence of distant metastasis they are assigned the M1 classification and therefore the stage IV group.

Common distant metastatic sites include the brain, bone, liver, and adrenal glands. Metastatic involvement of the brain, liver, and bone is associated with unfavorable outcomes, with bone metastasis being the most unfavorable site prognostically (Moore & Lee, 1997). Approximately 40% to 45% of all patients present with advanced metastatic disease.

PATHOPHYSIOLOGY

Anatomy and Physiology

Familiarity with the anatomy of the pulmonary structures is important in the nursing assessment and continued management of lung cancer patients. By understanding the anatomy of the pulmonary structures, nursing assessment of factors such as disease stage, progression, and patient symptoms can be facilitated. Below is a brief review of the pulmonary structures.

Thoracic Cavity

The thoracic cavity is divided into two distinct right and left pleural cavities, which are separated by the mediastinum.

Mediastinum

The mediastinum is the partition that originates at the superior portion of the thoracic outlet and extends inferiorly to the diaphragm. Contained within the mediastinum is the heart and its pericardium, the bases of the great vessels, the trachea and bronchi, esophagus, thymus, lymph nodes, thoracic duct, and the phrenic and vagus nerves.

The right and left lungs are located outside the mediastinum (Bullock, 1984).

Hilum

The hilum is the depression bordering the mediastinal portion of the lung where the bronchus blood vessels and nerves enter. On radiologic examination fullness in the hilar region, termed *hilar fullness,* could be indicative of advanced locoregional disease or possibly tumor progression.

Right Lung/Left Lung

The right lung is composed of three lobes: superior, middle, and inferior lobes. The left lung is composed of two lobes: superior and inferior lobes. Each lobe is subdivided into two to five bronchopulmonary segments.

Bronchi

The right main bronchus is shorter, wider, and more vertical when compared with the left main bronchus. The bronchial structures further divide into smaller bronchioles (Bullock, 1984) (Fig. 62-5).

Bronchioles

The foremost bronchioles are about 1 mm in diameter, and branching out, they become progressively smaller. The respiratory bronchioles open directly into thin ducts, with passage into the alveolar ducts and then alveolar sacs. Each bronchiole opens into an alveolar duct from which multiple alveoli radiate (Bullock, 1984; Lee & Hong, 1993).

Alveoli

The alveolar sacs are totally lined with alveoli. The group function of the alveoli is respiratory gas exchange. In the normal adult, alveoli are small (approximately 200 μm across) and have a volume of about 2500 ml (Kelly, 1997). Lungs in the adult contain approximately 300 million alveoli (Malasanos, Barkauskas, Moss, & Stoltenberg-Allen, 1986) (Fig. 62-6).

Great Vessels of the Lungs

The great vessels of the lungs include the aorta, pulmonary artery, superior and inferior caval veins, and certain segments of the right and left pulmonary veins.

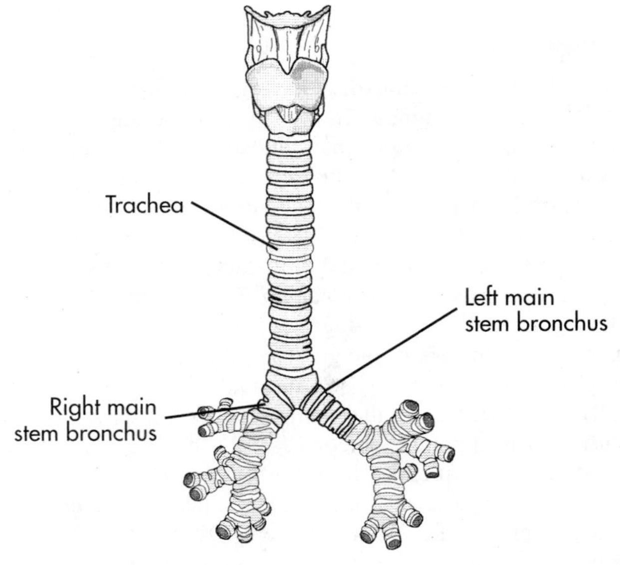

Fig. 62-5 Diagram of trachea and bronchi.

Trachea

The trachea of an adult is approximately 10 cm in length. The esophagus separates the trachea from the vertebral column (see Fig. 62-5).

Carina

The carina is the area in the trachea located anteroposteriorly between the right and left mainstem bronchus. The carina is one of the anatomic markers used in identifying tumor location during staging.

Pleura

The pleural membrane is the thin (less than 20 μm wide), serous membrane that surrounds and lines the thoracic cavity. The visceral pleura is the inner lining that overlies the lung parenchyma, and the parietal pleura is the outer lining. The space within these two layers is termed the *pleural space.* The amount of fluid within the pleural space is normally enough to facilitate the movement of the lungs during ventilation (Bullock, 1984; Malasanos et al., 1986). Tumor invasion can potentially cause abnormal fluid accumulation within this space and is termed *pleural effusion.* Clinical manifestations of a pleural effusion depend on the rate and amount of accumulation in the pleural space.

HISTOLOGY

Accurate pathologic information is extremely vital to the clinician in the management of lung cancer cases. The exact cell type must be known before therapy can be outlined. There are several methods, including light microscopy, electron microscopy, and immunohistochemistry used to evaluate specific cell types of lung cancer (McDuffie, Klaassen, & Dosman, 1990).

There are four histological types of lung cancer: small cell carcinoma, squamous cell carcinoma, adenocarcinoma, and large cell carcinoma. For practical therapeutic reasons, lung cancers are divided into two distinct groups: non–small cell and small cell types. The two different classes of lung cancer have different natural histories, follow different courses, and consequently are managed differently. Non–small cell lung cancer subtypes include squamous cell carcinoma, adenocarcinoma, and large cell carcinoma. This chapter reviews the information specific to NSCLC.

Table 62-7 lists the classification of the various malignant cell types associated with lung cancers. The World Health Organization (WHO) divides lung cancers into four major categories, which include the rare or minor cell types. In this section, discussion is limited to the three primary cell types of NCSLC: squamous, adenocarcinoma, and large cell.

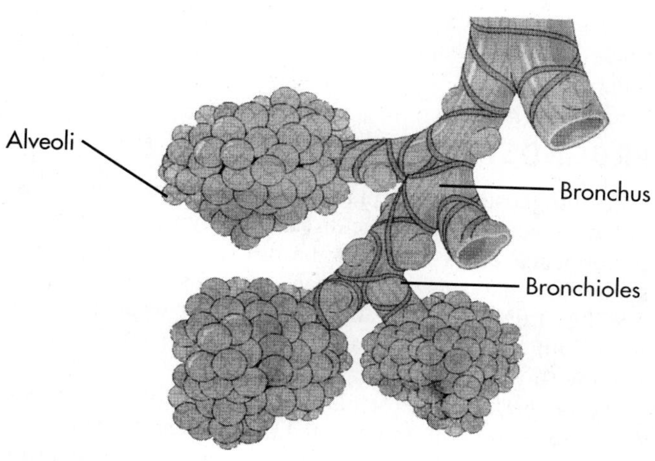

Fig. 62-6 Pulmonary bronchus, bronchioles, and alveoli.

Squamous

Once the most common cell types seen worldwide, the occurrence of squamous cell type has markedly declined within the last 2 decades. Epidemiologically the squamous cell type is most commonly seen in smokers, with predominance in males. Incidence of squamous cell carcinoma is approximately 29.4% of the total incidence. Pathologic evaluation of pulmonary squamous cell carcinomas typically reveals an intermediate to poorly differentiated cell

TABLE 62-7 World Health Organization Classification of Lung Cancer

Squamous Cell Carcinoma
Variant
1. Spindle cell carcinoma

Adenocarcinoma
1. Acinar adenocarcinoma
2. Papillary adenocarcinoma
3. Bronchiolo-alveolar carcinoma
4. Solid carcinoma with mucus formation

Large Cell Carcinoma
1. Solid carcinoma without mucin
2. Giant cell carcinoma
3. Clear cell carcinoma

Small Cell Carcinoma
1. Oatcell carcinoma
2. Intermediate cell type
3. Combined small call carcinoma

Carcinoids
Mesothelioma
1. Epithelial
2. Fibrous (spindle cell)
3. Biphasic

Ihde, D. D. (1995). Non-small cell lung cancer. In J. S. MacDonald, D. G. Haller, & R. J. Mayer (Eds.), *Manual of oncologic therapeutics* (3rd ed.). Philadelphia: J. B. Lippincott.

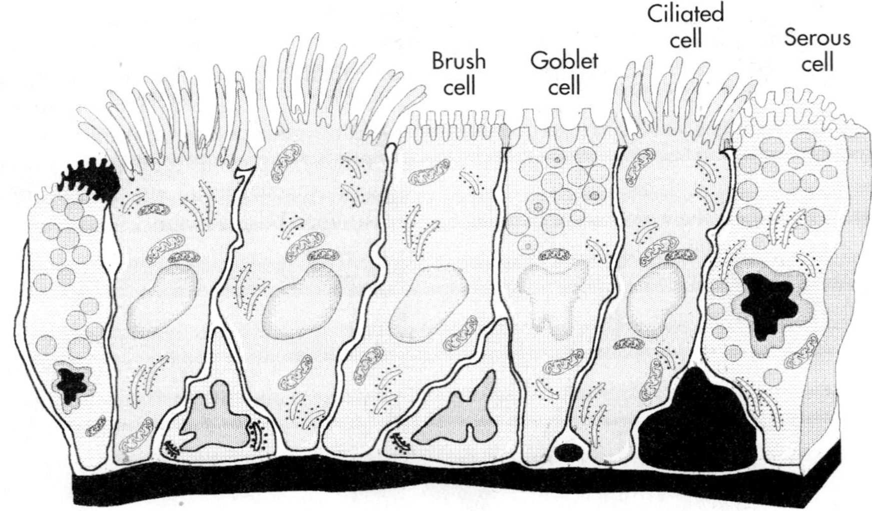

Fig. 62-7 Surface epithelium.

compared with the well-differentiated cell of the squamous cell malignancies involving the head and neck (Carbone, 1997; Linnoila & Aisner, 1995).

There are no squamous epithelial cells in the normal tracheobronchial tree (respiratory epithelium) (Fig. 62-7), although squamous cell carcinomas can arise from metaplastic foci. Over several years of smoking, as the damage to the squamous epithelium occurs in response to multiple factors including injury, infections, and toxins, mucosal changes progress from squamous metaplasia, dysplasia, and carcinoma in situ to invasive carcinoma (Gazdar & Carbone, 1994).

Squamous cell carcinomas usually arise centrally, and although they may grow rapidly, they often remain located within the thoracic cavity. For this reason, curative treatment of the small squamous cell tumor is more likely when compared with other NSCLC types (Linnoila & Aisner, 1995).

Adenocarcinoma

The adenocarcinoma cell type has become the most common form of lung cancer in the United States. Adenocarcinomas in general account for approximately 31.5% of all lung cancers (Carbone, 1997; Travis, Linder, & Mackay, 1997). It is the most common cell type of NSCLC found in women, nonsmokers (even though most adenocarcinoma patients do smoke), and young people.

Adenocarcinoma is composed of four major subtypes: acinar, papillary, bronchoalveolar adenocarcinomas, and solid carcinomas with mucus formation. Of these subtypes, bronchoalveolar carcinoma (BAC) represents 10% to 25% of all adenocarcinomas (Lee & Hong, 1993).

The adenocarcinoma cell as reviewed by light microscopy reveals formation of glands and papillary structures, and the production of substantial amounts of mucin (Linnoila & Aisner, 1995). The majority of adenocarcinomas develop in the peripheral airway or bronchoalveolar region. Since the development of adenocarcinomas usually occurs peripherally, patients have fewer pulmonary symptoms compared with the central obstructive lesions (i.e., squamous cell type) (Gazdar, & Carbone, 1994).

Despite size or cell source, adenocarcinomas often penetrate the pleural lymphatics and subsequently metastasize to distant sites, including brain, bone, and liver.

Large Cell Carcinoma

The histologic diagnosis of large cell lung carcinoma is one often made of exclusion; hence, the large cell group has been labeled the "wastebasket" of all lung cancer cell types. The term *large cell carcinoma* was established in the 1950s to label the lung cancer cell type that exhibited lack of squamous or glandular differentiation. The cells are relatively large, with prominent nucleoli, and have morphologic differentiation. They typically present in peripheral locations and access the lymphatics, which increases their likelihood of distant spread. The majority of the large cell lung cancers are comparable to lung adenocarcinomas when one compares disease characteristics and natural history. Their incidence varies approximately 10% to 20% of lung tumors, depending on the diagnostic criteria used (Carbone, 1998; Linnoila & Aisner, 1995).

PROGNOSTIC FACTORS

Three prognostic factors play a major role in the prognosis of lung cancer: extent of the disease, cell type, and patients' performance status. Stage of the disease and performance status are the most significant prognostic factors for NSCLC. Limited-stage patients have better responses than those with extensive disease even when given the same therapy (Ingle, 1997).

Initial performance status is critical in predicting patients' response both in untreated patients and those undergoing chemotherapy. Patients who are ambulatory tend to do better than those spending more than 50% of their time in bed. Other factors associated with poor prognosis include weight loss of more than 10 pounds in 6 months and generalized weakness (Ginsberg, Kris, & Armstrong, 1997).

Clinical Presentation

The signs and symptoms of lung cancer are usually related to the location of the disease and to the extent of systemic involvement. Approximately 90% of patients present with symptoms at the time of diagnosis (Ingle, 1997). The most common symptoms that cause a patient to seek medical attention include cough, dyspnea, wheezes, and hemoptysis. Cough is present in 75% of patients and, in the absence of other symptoms, can easily be misdiagnosed as the result of a cold (Ingle, 1997). Swelling of the face, neck, and arms with neck and thoracic vein distension are typical symptoms of compression of the superior vena cava by tumor (superior vena cava [SVC] syndrome). SVC syndrome is usually a sign of advanced disease and is a result of either right-side tumors or mediastinal nodal involvement compressing the SVC. If left untreated, SVC syndrome results in cerebral edema and possible death. Increased intracranial pressure, headaches, dizziness, visual disturbances, and alteration in mental status are signs of progressive compression (Stewart, 1996). Radiation of the mediastinum is the treatment of choice for palliation of SVC syndrome (Hilderly, 1996).

Cardiac metastasis occurs in about 25% of the patients. This can result in pericardial temponade, arrhythmias, and congestive heart failure (Pazdur, 1996). Patients presenting with centrally located lesions usually have cough, hemoptysis, wheezing, stridor, dyspnea, and postobstructive pneumonia (Epps, 1992). Peripheral lesions usually cause pain secondary to pleural or chest wall invasion. Patients may also have the presenting symptoms of cough or restrictive dyspnea (Pazdur, 1996). Radiologic destruction of the first and second ribs is also a common finding. Lesions involving the intrathoracic nerves may present with shoulder pain radiating to the arm (Pancoast's syndrome). This is caused by tumor involvement of the eighth cervical and first thoracic nerves in the superior sulcus. Extension of the tumor into the paravertebral sympathetic nerves results in Horner's syndrome, which consists of enophthalmos, ptosis, and miosis. Patients presenting with hoarseness need to be evaluated for recurrent laryngeal nerve involvement. Patients may also present with paralysis, elevation of the hemidiaphragm, and dyspnea secondary to phrenic nerve involvement. Compression of the esophagus often leads to dysphagia.

MEDICAL MANAGEMENT

Since the majority of patients with non–small cell lung cancer present with metastatic disease, symptoms related to systemic involvement are numerous and dependent on the site involved. General signs include anorexia, weight loss, and overall weakness. Bone pain resulting from bone metastasis is common as are symptoms of hepatomegaly and jaundice related to liver involvement. Brain metastasis may present as seizures, nausea, headaches, or focal neurologic signs (Harwood, 1996).

Paraneoplastic Syndromes

Paraneoplastic syndromes are a result of communication between tumor cells and normal cells. This communication is not much different than normal cellular communication with intensification of actions a result of the tumor cells' inability to differentiate (Hall, 1997). The syndromes are usually associated with a histologic type of lung cancer, and clinical signs tend to decrease with successful response of the tumor (Ginsberg, Kris, & Armstrong,1994).

It has been estimated that paraneoplastic syndromes are present at the time of diagnosis in about 10% of patients with malignancy. When patients present with metabolic or generalized paraneoplastic manifestations such as fever, cachexia, and anorexia, these patients most often present with paraneoplastic syndrome. The presenting symptoms associated with these syndromes may include toxic side effects that significantly decrease quality of life in lung patients. Prompt diagnosis of these symptoms and appropriate treatment may improve quality of life and decrease the possibility of life-threatening events.

The endocrine paraneoplastic syndromes are caused by secretion of a hormonelike substance by the tumor. In normal physiology a hormone or hormonelike substance is released into the blood to act on distant tissues. In certain malignancies these substances are released in large quantities, causing an inflated response. Hypercalcemia caused by bone metastasis or early production of parathyroid hormone is a relatively common finding. Other syndromes associated with NSCLC include nephrotic syndrome and hypertropic pulmonary osteoarthropathy (Harwood, 1996).

Surgery resection represents the best chance for cure in stages I and II non–small cell lung cancer. Pulmonary lobectomy with mediastinal lymph node dissection is the most common surgical procedure performed for primary lung cancer, and it offers the potential for cure for those patients presenting with early disease. The overall 5-year survival rate for T1 has been reported to be around 80% and around 68% for T2N0 disease (Feins, 1997). Current data do not support adjuvant chemotherapy for stage I disease. Stage II disease includes a small group of patients presenting with T2N2 involvement. Decreased survival has been reported for patients presenting with general symptoms such as cachexia and weight loss. The Lung Cancer Study Group conducted a postoperative therapy trial of cyclophosmide, doxorubicin, and cisplatin (CAP) vs no treatment in this group of patients and found no difference in survival for patients who received adjuvant chemotherapy (Sheperd, 1994).

Thoracic surgery involves high risk of morbidity; therefore it is important that extensive measures be taken to appropriately stage patients presenting with clinically early disease. The majority of patients with NSCLC already present with metastasis at time of diagnosis and are no longer curable; therefore surgery with this group of patient should only be used in a palliative setting (Fry, Meneck, & Winchester, 1996). Diagnostic tests such as CT scans are not always good predictors of accurate staging. Feins (1997) described that 38% of the time, chest CT scans were incorrect in staging T status, and they were able to predict lymph node status in only 62% of the cases. He also stated that evaluation of distant metastasis, as well as full lymph node dissection at the time of surgery, gives the most accurate staging.

Although surgery remains the best option of treatment for early NSCLG, radiotherapy is indicated for patients who cannot undergo surgery. Studies have reported survival rates as high as 20% when radiotherapy is used in medically inoperable patients (Ruckdeschel, 1997).

STAGES III AND IV

Almost 45% of all cases of NSCLC present with clinically detectable metastasis at diagnosis. These patients are not curable.

The treatment of stage III lung cancer is based on the extent of the disease. Stage IIIA patients with N2 disease were shown to have a 5-year survival of 30%. The majority of the surviving patients were found to have N2 disease at surgery but were clinically N0 or N1. Patients presenting with clinical N2 disease had a dismal survival of only 9%.

Patients with stage IIIA disease include those with peripheral tumors with direct extension into the chest wall and pericardium, as well as patients with ipsilateral mediastinal lymph node metastases. Patients with superior sulcus tumors are also considered to have stage IIIA disease. Patients with stage IIIB disease have direct mediastinal invasion or contralateral intrathoracic nodal involvement. Those patients with distant metastatic disease are classified as stage IV. These patients are not considered to be surgical candidates (Feins, 1997).

Radiation Therapy

For patients with locally advanced, inoperable NSCLC, radiation therapy has been the mainstay of treatment in the United States. Radiation therapy can be given either with palliation or therapeutic intent. However, the result of this modality of therapy as a therapeutic approach has been poor because of either local-regional failure or metastatic failures. The median length survival for patients treated with radiation alone is 10 months. Recent studies of combination suggest that radiation therapy may improve survival of selected patients with NSCLC.

Combination Radiation Therapy

Multimodality treatment of stage III patients combining radiation therapy is an area that has shown promising results. Postoperative radiation is often used for selected groups of stage IIIA patients undergoing surgery, and it has been described as prolonging disease-free survival (Ball & Burmeinster, 1997). The role of combination modalities using radiation has focused on the use of pre- and postoperative addition of radiation therapy. Several studies have compared radiation therapy alone with chemoradiation. In a trial conducted by the Cancer Leukemia Group B (CALGB), 155 patients with inoperable stage III NSCLC were randomly assigned to receive thoracic radiation at 60 Gy over 6 weeks or radiation or radiation preceded by cisplatin at 100 mg/m^2 and vinblastine. After more than 24 months follow-up the median survival was 13.8 months for the combined modality arm and 9.7 months for the radiotherapy group. Survival was 7% for the radiation only group compared with 19% for patients assigned to chemoradiation (Wagner, 1997). Some studies have documented responses of up to 50% for preoperative radiation (Ruckdeschel, 1997). A randomized trial by the lung cancer group suggested that postoperative chemoradiation for stages IIIA and IIIB leads to improved disease-free survival and increased survival.

Chemotherapy for Advanced Non–Small Cell Lung Cancer

The use of chemotherapy in patients with NSCLC is moving from an approach of palliation to that of an effective therapeutic approach when given as multimodality therapy (Treat & Kiser, 1997). The most active agents in the treatment of NSCLC include cisplatin, etoposide, Navelbine, ifosfomide, and vinblastine (Brogden & Nevidjon, 1995). Navelbine, given in combination with cisplatin, has been shown to double the response rate of Navelbine alone (Bunn, 1997).

Recently, randomized trials have shown some benefit using cisplatin-based chemotherapy. Review of the literature shows a 21% response rate for single-agent cisplatin. The NSCLC group of collaborators recently performed a meta-analysis study to answer the question of whether cisplatin-based therapy actually improved survival. More than 9000 patients participating in clinical trials between 1965 and 1992 were included. The group looked at primary therapy alone vs the same treatment with the addition of a cytotoxic agent. For patients using cisplatin-based chemotherapy, there was a 27% reduction in the death rate, corresponding to an improvement in median survival from 6 to 8 months (Harwood, 1996). These results were confirmed by a retrospective analysis by the Southwest Oncology Group. Performance status and gender were found to be prognostic factors in determining survival. Preoperative induction chemotherapy with or without radiotherapy offers survival advantage over surgery or radiotherapy alone (Fossella, Rivera, & Roth, 1996).

Recurrent Non–Small Cell Lung Cancer

The treatment of patients with advanced NSCLC who have failed cisplatin-based chemotherapy remains questionable. Docetaxel (Taxotere) has been used as a frontline for patients with advanced NSCLC, with responses rates ranging from 21% to 38%. The median survival ranges from 25.2 weeks to 47 weeks. These data are consistent with other studies (Ramanathan & Belani, 1997).

Two studies were conducted at M.D. Anderson Cancer Center in Houston, Tex. and the University of Texas in San Antonio to evaluate the efficacy of docetaxel as second-line therapy. Eighty-eight patients were evaluated. Of the patients, 17% achieved a partial response (PR). Median time to PR was 6 weeks, and the median duration of response was 29 weeks (Fossella, Lee, & Hong, 1997). The investigators have concluded that although the results were modest, there was a statistically significant benefit of docetaxel in this setting.

ONOCOLOGIC EMERGENCIES

SVC syndrome is usually a sign of advanced disease and is a result of either right-side tumors or mediastinal nodal involvement compressing the SVC. If left untreated, SVC syndrome results in cerebral edema and possible death. Increased intracranial pressure, headaches, dizziness, visual disturbances, and alteration in mental status are signs of progressive compression (Stewart, 1996). Radiation of the mediastinum is the treatment of choice for palliation of SVC syndrome (Hilderly, 1996). Cardiac metastasis occurs in about 25% of the patients, resulting in pericardial tamponade, arrhythmias, and congestive heart failure (Pazdur, 1996). Chapter 11 offers a complete discussion of SVC and cardiac tamponade.

NURSING MANAGEMENT

Nursing care of the lung patient will depend on the stage of disease and treatment plan. The importance of patient teaching increases as the focus of care shifts from the inpatient to outpatient setting. Patients need to be familiar with the side effects of their disease and treatment, as well as the management techniques, as they may now find themselves more often in the position of triaging when to call for medical help. For early-stage NSCLC, nursing management is related to surgical nursing care. Nursing care for patients undergoing thoracotomy for wedge resection, lobectomy, or pneumonectomy is quite complex. Surgical nursing care begins during the diagnostic phase. Compromised health care places these patients at risk of postoperative complications. It is important to develop aggressive pre- and postoperative nursing care plans to minimize postoperative complications and promote comfort.

Preoperative plans include diagnosis related to knowledge deficits and operative procedure, as well as how to minimize possible complications. This can be achieved by addressing issues such as knowledge deficit, alteration in comfort, potential for impaired gas exchange, potential for infection, alteration in bowel habits, and anxiety. Postoperative plan involves reinforcement of early teachings. Table 62-8 offers a standard of care for patients undergoing a lobectomy for NSCLC. Patients presenting with local-regional advanced or systemic disease are treated with radiation therapy, chemotherapy, or a combination of both.

Patients undergoing radiotherapy require teaching regarding side effects experienced during or after radiation therapy. Information on general side effect management, such as adequate nutritional intake, as well as bone marrow suppression, is important before treatment. Patients also need information on site-specific side effects. Included in the nursing plan should be measures to manage nausea and vomiting, pneumonitis, esophagitis, and cough. Skin erythema with wet desquamation is also often encountered as a complication of radiation treatment for lung cancers. Patients need to know up front that fatigue is a major side effect of radiation and is experienced by 98% of patients undergoing radiation. Patients should be encouraged to set realistic goals to accommodate scheduled rest periods. Fatigue may persist for months after treatment. It is important that patients be prepared appropriately to minimize anxiety associated with thoughts of disease progression (see Chapter 4). Finally, it is important that nurses caring for patients undergoing radiation work closely with members of the multidisciplinary health team to provide patients and their families the emotional support they might need. Educate patient and family members about anxieties and grief associated with response to the illness and treatment.

The addition of chemotherapy increases radiation therapy side effects in patients receiving combined radiotherapy and chemotherapy. The severity of these problems depends on the type of the drug and its dose and timing of administration. It is important that nurses have knowledge of side effects associated with different classes of chemotherapeutic agents to help predict toxicity, which is enhanced by the combination.

Patients with advanced NSCLC are exposed to a variety of single agents or combination chemotherapy with potential lethal side effects. Some of these include myelosuppression, renal problems, nausea and vomiting, anorexia, cardiac problems, pneumonitis, and fibrosis. There are many goals of chemotherapy teaching. Patients need to know what drugs they are taking and what these drugs are supposed to be doing for them. They need to understand the side effects associated with their treatment, as well as the significance of the toxicities. They need to be taught to recognize these signs before they become life threatening (see Chapter 3).

Psychological Issues in Non–Small Cell Lung Cancer

The word *cancer* often strikes fear among patients and their families. Anxiety related to diagnosis of cancer combined with the poor prognosis of advanced NSCLC accounts for a high degree of distress among patients and family members. Emotional responses include a feeling of lack of hope, anxiety, fear, anger, and denial. Fear of pain associated with progression of the disease, as well of death, are common. The goal of nursing in meeting the needs of patient and family members is to identify resources that could help patients meet their psychosocial needs and ways to enhance coping skills. Patient education about the disease process and appropriate referral helps patients and their families become active participants, arming them with tools for setting realistic expectations and goals.

Symptom distress that has been associated with decreased quality of life has included suffering, fear of the disease, and lack of knowledge regarding the disease process, leading to a sense of loss of control. Research is necessary to define stressors contributing to anxiety and suffer-

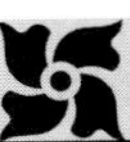

TABLE 62-8 Standard of Care for the Patient with Large Cell Lung Cancer

Patient Problem and Outcomes	Nursing Interventions and Rationales	Patient Education Instructions
Ineffective Airway Clearance		
Patient will demonstrate normal respiratory status as evidenced by breath sounds that are clear throughout all lung fields, respirations that are moderate in depth and between 12 to 20 minutes, and decreased dyspnea.	1. Auscultate breath sounds every shift and when needed. 2. Assess respiratory rate, depth, and rhythm every shift and when needed. 3. Assess length of expiratory phase of breathing, pursed-lip breathing. 4. Assess paradoxical abdominal motion and asynchronous chest and abdominal motions. 5. Ask patient to rate dyspnea on a scale of 0-10 (0—no dyspnea, 10—worst dyspnea) and record every 4 hours. 6. Assess vital capacity via incentive spirometer. 7. Assess and record use of dyspnea-reducting strategies found helpful by the patient. 8. Collect sputum for culture as ordered.	Teach patient to: 1. Teach patient the use of pursed-lip breathing and slow abdominal-diaphragmatic breathing during periods of dyspnea. 2. Assist and teach patient to turn, cough, and deep breathe every 2 hours; note type, color, and character of sputum. 3. Discuss avoidance of smoke and dust with patient and family or significant other. 4. Encourage intake of 2 to 3 L of fluid every 24 hours unless fluids are restricted. 5. Monitor hematocrit and hemoglobin levels daily.
Impaired Gas Exchange		
Patient will demonstrate optimal gas exchange for condition as evidenced by blood gases within acceptable levels, usual skin color, and usual mental status.	1. Monitor arterial blood gases every shift. 2. Monitor color of skin, nailbeds, and mucous membranes of the mouth. 3. Assess mental status. 4. Assess for complications of oxygen therapy, such as nasal dryness or congestion, epistaxis, and skin breakdown every shift.	Teach patient to: 1. Maintain bed rest in quiet environment during exacerbation. 2. Elevate head of bed 45° to 90°. 3. Administer humidified oxygen per nasal catheter or cannula at prescribed flow.
Pain and Dyspnea		
Patient will experience relief/control of pain as evidenced by verbalization of pain at a 0, 1, or 2 on scale of 1 to 10; will identify strategies to control pain as evidenced by verbalization/use of nonpharmacologic measures for pain relief; demonstrate decreased dyspnea, as evidenced by relief/control of dyspnea at a 0, 1, or 2 on a scale of 0-10.	1. Assess/record character, location, duration, frequency of pain, and any other precipitating factors every 4 hours and when needed. 2. Ask patient to rate intensity of pain on a scale of 0 to 10 (0—absence of pain and 10—worst pain experienced) and record every 4 hours. 3. Ask patient to rate dyspnea on a scale of 0 to 10 (0—no dyspnea and 10—worst dyspnea) and record every 4 hours.	Teach patient to: 1. Administer analgesic/anxiolytics as prescribed and assess/record effectiveness. 2. Reduce or eliminate common side-effects of narcotics: a. Constipation: administer a stool softener as prescribed b. Nausea and vomiting: administer an antiemetic as prescribed c. Dry mouth: provide good oral hygiene, encourage patient to rinse mouth often, offer sugarless candy for patient to suck on. 3. Use nonpharmacologic measures for pain relief (e.g., relaxation, imagery, distraction, biofeedback, self-hypnosis). 4. Use energy conservation techniques.

Modified from: Glover, J. & Miaskowski, C. (1994). Small cell lung cancer: Pathophysiologic mechanisms and nursing implications. *Oncology Nursing Forum, 21,* 87-95.
ACTH: adrenocorticotropic hormone.

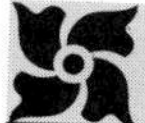

TABLE 62-8 Standard of Care for the Patient with Large Cell Lung Cancer—cont'd

Patient Problem and Outcomes	Nursing Interventions and Rationales	Patient Education Instructions
Altered Nutrition Less Than Body Requirements		
Patient will maintain an adequate nutritional status as evidenced by weight moving toward normal range for patient's height, age, and build.	1. Obtain a dietary consult to assess nutritional requirements and quality of usual intake. 2. Monitor percent of meals eaten. 3. Weight patient daily. 4. Monitor skin turgor and mucous membranes. 5. Monitor bowel function. 6. Monitor for stomatitis. 7. Monitor results of laboratory studies (serum albumin, total protein, glucose, acetone, 24-hour urinary creatine, nitrogen, and electrolytes). 8. Record intake and output every shift.	Teach patient to: 1. Eat favorite foods that are high in carbohydrates and protein as prescribed. 2. Eat small frequent meals consisting of soft, easily swallowed foods to supplement feedings. 3. Encourage rest periods before meals to reduce fatigue. 4. Take megesterol acetate as prescribed to increase appetite; monitor for side effects; edema, diffuse rash, menstrual irregularities, impotence in males. 5. Perform oral care 30 minutes before meals and often between meals. 6. Take prescribed antiemetic to reduce nausea. 7. Increased fluid intake. 8. Teach patient and family: a. Importance of maintaining adequate calorie intake b. Eating patterns to promote weight gain and nitrogen balance.
Activity Intolerance		
Patient will demonstrate an increased activity tolerance as evidenced by the ability to resume activities of daily living (ADL) free from extremes of fatigue or dyspnea.	1. Monitor vital signs before and after periods of increased activity. 2. Monitor heart and lung sounds with activity. 3. Monitor oxygen saturation with activity and provide oxygen therapy as prescribed. 4. Monitor for signs of extreme fatigue, chest pain, or diaphoresis.	Teach patient methods to: 1. Provide optimal rest; limit activity in accordance with degree of pulmonary dysfunction. 2. Perform active and passive range of motion to all extremities one to four times a day. 3. Rest in a chair, rather than bed. 4. Use pursed-lip breathing and diaphragmatic breathing.
Ineffective Individual/Family Coping		
Patient will demonstrate effective coping as evidenced by expression of feelings and concerns and use of adaptive coping behaviors.	1. Assess levels of anxiety and depression every shift. 2. Assess presence of biological factors related to small cell lung cancer that could be causing depression (e.g., parahormone, vasopressin, ACTH, enkephalins, beta-endorphins).	1. Establish therapeutic relationship to encourage communication with nursing staff every shift. a. Provide environment conducive to discussing private issues and feelings. b. Provide for continuity of care. 2. Allow patient/family to react in own ways without judgment. 3. Encourage verbalization of fears/concerns.

Continued

TABLE 62-8 Standard of Care for the Patient with Large Cell Lung Cancer—cont'd

Patient Problem and Outcomes	Nursing Interventions and Rationales	Patient Education Instructions
Ineffective Individual/Family Coping—cont'd		
		4. Assist in identifying new coping strategies. a. Active listening: validate information by reflecting what has been said for clarification and verification. b. Use open-ended questions to elicit emotional expression. c. Assist patient/family with identifying strengths and coping skills. 5. Assist patient/family with identifying nature and strengths of situational supports; collect data about current and potential sources of support. 6. Explain procedures; confirm patient's understanding; answer questions or refer to appropriate sources. 7. Involve patient in decision-making process regarding care. 8. Administer anxiolytic and antidepressant medications as ordered and teach patient relaxation techniques.

Modified from: Glover, J. & Miaskowski, C. (1994). Small cell lung cancer: Pathophysiology mechanisms and nursing implications. *Oncology Nursing Forum, 21,* 87-95.

ing among patients with lung cancer. Symptoms like fatigue and depression are common among these patients. The literature on cancer-related fatigue has focused primarily on breast cancer. With improved survival in patients with advanced lung cancer it becomes important to define lung cancer–related fatigue and activities that will improve fatigue and quality of life. The depression associated with lung cancer is multifactorial. It is important to differentiate depression that is secondary to side effects of fatigue, insomnia, and overall weakness from primary depression. A good history that includes personal and family history of psychiatric illness and inadequate social support can aid the health professional in making an appropriate diagnosis (Ryan, 1996). Nurses can help patients communicate more effectively about their psychological status by teaching them how to keep a diary and reflect accurate information on timing and characteristics of the symptoms. Patients can also be encouraged to quantify their distress with tools such as analog scales for measuring pain.

Home Health Care

With the shift from inpatient therapy to outpatient therapy, a large percentage of lung cancer patients receive their care at home. Home health nursing includes care continuing from diagnosis to the terminal phase of the disease. Nurses caring for this group of patients are often responsible for administration of chemotherapy, as well as managing side effects associated with the treatment and/or advanced disease. Included in home care of these patients is the need to help families care for their loved ones. By close identification, assessment, and management of side effects nurses can help reduce suffering and improve the care of patients at home. Home health nurses are also in the position to facilitate communication between the health care team, patient, and family. It is important that a multidisciplinary approach involving discharge planning be initiated early during the diagnosis, allowing for the most appropriate home referral to be made. The literature supports findings that early referral to oncology home care was associated with a 6-week symptom delay (McCorkle, Benoliel, Donaldson, Georgiadou, Moinpour, & Goodell, 1989). A large percentage of patients with NSCLC-1 eventually experience progressive disease; therefore the preferred home health care allows patients to convert to hospice as their disease progresses and the primary goal of therapy changes to palliation.

EVALUATION OF THE QUALITY OF CARE

The Standards of Oncology Education states that it is the nursing profession's responsibility to ensure that accurate and current information about cancer, cancer-related treatments, and possible complications be available (Oncology

Nursing Society, 1989). Groups that provide accreditation for health care organizations require that quality of care provided to patients be evaluated. Quality of care has become the standard by which care provided to oncology patient is judged. It has become the core of cancer service. Patient education and its effect on quality of life should be incorporated in the evaluation of quality of care. The collection of data using a measurement tool is one way to measure quality of care (Dorsett, 1997). One way to apply this evaluation to the clinical practice is by documenting patient outcome.

The care of patients with lung cancer is largely dependent on the stage of the disease. Evaluation of the quality of care should reflect the patients needs and care provided at different points on the continuum of lung cancer. Table 62-9 provides an example of quality-of-care evaluation tools that can be used at different stages of the disease.

TABLE 62-9 Quality of Care Evaluation of Patients Receiving Radiation Therapy for Non Small Cell Lung Cancer

Disciplines participating in the quality of care evaluation:
☐ Medical ☐ Nursing

Criteria	Yes	No
1. Was the patient assessed for knowledge of radiation therapy treatment and possible side effects?	☐	☐
2. Was the patient informed of treatment schedule, duration, purpose?	☐	☐
3. Did you explain possible side effects, dysphasia, skin reaction, pneumonitis, pulmonary fibrosis?	☐	☐
4. Was the patient instructed on measures how to handle side effects from radiation to the chest?	☐	☐
5. Was the patient provided written information on radiation to the chest and its possible side effects?	☐	☐
Patient/Response		
1. Did the patient verbalize understanding of treatment schedule?	☐	☐
2. Did the patient read information provided?	☐	☐
3. Did family members verbalize an understanding of side effects?	☐	☐

PROGNOSIS

The prognosis of any patient with lung cancer is grim (Krebs & Williams, 1997). Localized lung cancer has the best prognosis. However, up to 90% of all patients with large cell lung cancer eventually relapse and die of disease. Patients with distant metastasis are not curable, and fewer than 5% of patients with stage III mediastinal lymph node involvement are cured. Up to 45% of all patients are at risk for second primary lung tumors.

RESEARCH ISSUES

The goal of therapy for most patients with advanced NSCLC is effective palliation. Several new agents are currently been investigated in phase II trials with optimistic results. Camptothecins, taxanes, gemcitabine, vinorelbine, and edatraxate have been among the new additions to show come clinical activity against NSCLC.

Camptothecins are a new family of plant alkaloids that exert their antitumor activity through inhibition of DNA topoisomerase-I. CPT-11 has been evaluated as either a single agent or in combination with cisplatin for advanced NSCLC. Ardizzoni (1995) reported response rates of up to 41% for CPT-11 given as a single agent and as high as 54% for cisplatin combinations. Dose-limiting toxicities of CPT-11 include diarrhea, myelosuppression, and nausea/vomiting.

The taxanes, paclitaxel and docetaxel, which interfere with normal activity by blocking mitotic division and by blocking cells in the M phase of the cell cycle, have also demonstrated activity against NSCLC. These new agents are derivatives of the yew tree. The main toxicities are neutropenia, alopecia, and hypersensitivity reactions. Paclitaxel requires administration with corticosteroids to minimize allergic reactions. Paclitaxel has been tested in phase II studies with response rates approaching 25%. Hoffman and colleagues (1996) performed a phase II study using ifosfomide and paclitaxel. Thirty-one patients with advanced disease were treated. The dose-limiting toxicity was granulocytopenia. Partial response was seen in 23% of the patients. The authors concluded that this combination was active in advanced NSCLC and compared favorably with cisplatin-based regimens with fewer side effects.

Vinorelbine (Navelbine), a semisynthetic vinka alkaloid, acts by dissolving mitotic spindle. This new drug, which initially was tested in Europe, has been used alone and in combinations in several phase I and phase II trials. The principle toxicity of this drug is neutropenia. Response rates of around 30 % have been observed in previously untreated patients (Brogden & Nevidjon, 1995).

Edatrexate, a methotrexate analog, blocks DNA by inhibiting the synthesis of nucleotides necessary for DNA replication. In phase II trials response rates ranged from 10% to 32% at a dose of 80 mg/m^2 (Sheperd, 1994). Mucositosis has been the dose-limiting side effect.

The antimetabolite gemcitabine has been used in several phase II clinical trials in advanced NSCLC with response rates ranging from 21% to 24% (Bunn, 1997). Gemcitabine has a low-toxicity profile, making it a good choice for treatment in elderly patients. Flu-like symptoms and a rash are some of the most commonly observed side effects.

REFERENCES

Agency for Health Care Policy on Research. (1996). *Smoking cessation: A guide for primary care clinician* (AHCPR Publication No. 96-0693). Bethesda, MD: Public Health Service.

American Cancer Society. (1998). *Cancer facts and figures 1998.* Atlanta: The Society.

American Society of Clinical Oncology (1997). Clinical practice guidelines for the treatment of unresectable non-small cell lung cancer. *Journal of Clinical Oncology, 15*(8), 2996-3018.

Ardizzoni, A. (1995). Camptothecin analogues in the treatment of non-small cell lung cancer. *Lung Cancer, 12*(Suppl 1): 177-185.

Ball, D. L. & Burmeinster, B. H. (1997). Recent advances in managing non-small cell lung cancer. *Medical Journal of Australia, 166,* 11-12.

Beahrs, O. H., Henson, D. E., Hutter, R. V. P., & Kennedy, B. T. (Eds.). (1992). *Manual for staging of cancer.* Philadelphia: J. B. Lippincott.

Broderick, L. S., Tarver, R. D., & Conces, D. J. Jr. (1997). Imaging of lung cancer: Old and new. *Seminars in Oncology 24*(4), 411-418.

Brogden J. M. & Nevidjon, B. (1995). Vinorelbine tartrate (Navelbine): Drug profile and nursing implications of a new vinca alkaloid. *Oncology Nursing Forum, 22*(4), 635-46.

Bullock, B. L. (1984). Normal respiratory function. In B. L. Bullock & P. Philbrook Rosendahl (Eds.), *Pathophysiology adaptations and alterations in function.* Boston: Little, Brown.

Bunn, P. A. (1997). The emerging role of gemcitabine in lung: Part I. *Seminars in Oncology Nursing 24,* S7-1.

Burns, D. M. (1994). Tobacco smoking. In J. M. Samet (Ed.), *Epidemiology of lung cancer.* New York: Marcel Dekker.

Burns, D. M., Garfinkel, L., & Samet, J. M. (1997). Changes in cigarette-related disease risks and their implication for prevention and control. *Monograph 8: Smoking and tobacco control,* (NIH Publication No. 97-4213). Bethesda, MD: Public Health Service.

Carbone, D. P. (1997). The biology of lung cancer. *Seminars in Oncology 24*(4), 388-401.

Carpentino, L. J. (1994). *Nursing care plans and documentation—CD-Rom.* Philadelphia: Lippincott-Raven.

Cortese, D. A., Edell, E. S., & Harubumi, K. (1997). Early detection and treatment of lung cancer: Photodynamic therapy. In H. I. Pass, J. B. Mitchell, D. H. Johnson, & A. T. Turrisi (Eds.), *Lung cancer principals and practice.* Philadelphia: Lippincott-Raven.

Darby, S. C. & Samet, J. M. (1994). Radon. In J. M. Samet (Ed.), *Epidemiology of lung cancer.* New York: Marcel Dekker

Dorsett, D. S. (1997). *Cancer nursing principles and practice* (4th ed.). Sudbury, MA: Jones and Bartlett.

Elpern, E. H. (1993). Lung cancer. In S. L Groenwald, M. H. Frogge, M. Goodman, & C. H. Yarbro (Eds.), *Cancer nursing principals and practice.* Boston: Jones and Bartlett.

Epps, M. E. (1992). Diagnostic testing for patients with lung cancer. *Nursing Clinic of North America, (27),* 615-629.

Feins, R. H. (1997). Surgery for early stage non-small cell lung cancer. *Seminars in Oncology, 24*(4), 419-422.

Fossella, F. V., Lee, J. S., & Hong, W. K. (1997). Management strategies for recurrent non-small cell lung cancer. *Seminars in Oncology, 4,* 455-462.

Fossella, F. V., Rivera, E., & Roth, J. A. (1996). Preoperative chemotherapy for stage IIIA non-small cell lung cancer. *Current Opinion in Oncology, 2,* 106-111.

Fry, W. A., Meneck, H. R., & Winchester, D. P. (1996). The National Data Base Report on lung cancer. *Cancer, 77*(9), 1947-55.

Gazdar, A. F. & Carbone, D. P. (Eds.). (1994). *The biology and molecular genetics of lung cancer.* Austin, TX: R. G. Landes.

Ginsberg, R. J., Kris, M. G., & Armstrong, J. G. (1997). Cancer of the lung. In V. T. Devita, S. Hellman, & S. A. Rosenberg (Eds.), *Cancer: Principles and practice of oncology* (5th ed.). Philadelphia: Lippincott-Raven.

Glover, J. & Miaskowski, C. (1994). Small cell lung cancer: Pathophysiologic mechanisms and nursing implications. *Oncology Nursing Forum, 21,* 87-95.

Goodman, G. E. (1995). The prevention of primary lung cancer. In B. E. Johnson, & D. H. Johnson (Eds.), *Lung cancer.* New York: Wiley-Liss.

Groeger, A. M., Esposito, V., Mueller,.M. R., Caputi, M., Kaiser, H. E., & Giordano, A. (1997). Advances in the understanding of lung cancer. *Anticancer Research, 17,* 2519-2522.

Hall, T. (1997). Paraneoplastic syndromes: Mechanism. *Seminars in Oncology Nursing, 3,* 269-276.

Harwood, H. V. (1996). Non-small lung cancer: An overview and diagnosis, staging and treatment. *Seminars in Oncology Nursing, 4,* 285-294.

Held, J. L. (1995). Caring for a patient with lung cancer. *Nursing, 95*(10), 34-43.

Hilderly, L. J. (1996). Radiation therapy for lung cancer. *Seminars in Oncology Nursing, 12*(4), 304-11.

Hoffmann, D., Djordjevic, M. V., & Hoffmann, I. (1997). The changing cigarette. *Preventative Medicine, 26,* 427-434.

Hoffman, P. C., Masters, G. A., & Drinkard, L. C. (1996). Ifosfomide plus paclitaxel in advanced non-small-cell lung cancer: a phase II study. *Annals of Oncology, 7*(3), 314-5.

Ihde, D. D. (1995). Non-small cell lung cancer. In J. S. MacDonald, D. G. Haller, & R. J. Mayer (Eds.), *Manual of oncologic therapeutics* (3rd ed.). Philadelphia: J. B. Lippincott.

Ingle, R. J. (1997). Lung cancers. In S. L. Groenwald, M. H. Frogge, M. Goodman, & C. H. Yarbo (Eds.), *Cancer nursing: Principles and practice* (4th ed.). Sudbury, MA: Jones and Bartlett.

Karp, D. D. (1997). Lung cancer chemoprevention and management of carcinoma *in situ. Seminars in Oncology 24,*(4), 402-410.

Kelly, K. (1997). Overview of the randomized phase III trials in non-small cell lung cancer in north america. *Seminars in Oncology, 24*(8), S8-3-S8-5.

Krebs, L. U. & Williams, P. (1997). Lung cancer. In R. A. Gates & R. M. Fink (Eds.), *Oncology nursing secrets.* Philadelphia: Hanley & Belfus.

Lee, J. S. & Hong, W. K. (1993). Biology of preneoplastic lesions. In J. A. Roth, J. D. Cox, & W. K Hong (Eds.), *Lung cancer.* Boston: Blackwell Scientific.

Linnoila, R. I. & Aisner, S. C. (1995). Pathology of lung cancer: An exercise in classification. In B. E. Johnson & D. H. Johnson (Eds.), *Lung cancer.* New York: Wiley-Liss.

Malasanos, L., Barkauskas, V., Moss, M., & Stoltenberg-Allen, K. (Eds.). (1986). *Health assessment.* St. Louis: Mosby.

Marcus, B. H., King, T. K., Albrecht, A. E., Parisi, A. F., & Abrams, D. B. (1997). Rationale, design, and baseline data for commit to quit: An exercise efficacy trial for smoking cessation among women. *Preventative Medicine, 26,* 586-597.

Mason, T. J. (1994). The descriptive epidemiology of lung cancer. In J. M. Samet (Ed.), *Epidemiology of lung cancer.* New York: Marcel Dekker.

McCorkle, R., Benoliel, J. Q., Donaldson, G., Georgiadou, F., Moinpour, C, & Goodell, B. (1989). A randomized clinical trial of home nursing care for lung patients. *Cancer, 64*(6), 1375-1382.

McDuffie, H. H., Klaassen, D. J., & Dosman, J. A.. (1990). Determinants of cell type in patients with cancer of the lung. *Chest, 98* (5), 1187-1193.

Moore, D. F. & Lee, J. S. (1997). Staging and prognostic factors: Non-small cell lung cancer. In H. I. Pass, J.B. Mitchell, D.H. Johnson, & A. T. Turrisi (Eds.), *Lung cancer principals and practice.* Philadelphia: Lippincott–Raven.

Mountain, C. F. (1993). Staging of lung cancer. In J. A. Roth, J. D. Cox, & W. K. Hong (Eds.), *Lung cancer.* Boston: Blackwell Scientific.

National Cancer Institute (1996). Beta carotene and vitamin A halted in lung cancer prevention trial. *CancerNet.* Available at http://www.NIH.GOV/ib./su.edu/gov/fidgoo.html

National Institute on Drug Abuse, Monitoring the Future Study. (1996). *Marijuana and tobacco use still rising among eighth and tenth graders.* Available at http://www.NIH.GOV/ib./su.edu/gov/fidgoo.html

Oncology Nursing Society. (1989). *Standards of oncology education: Patient/family and public.* Pittsburgh: Oncology Nursing Press.

Pastorino, U. (1995). In H. H. Hansen (Ed.), *Lung cancer advances in basic and clinical research.* Boston: Kluwer Academic.

Pazdur, R. (1996). *Medical oncology: A comprehensive review.* (2nd ed.). New York: Huntington House.

Pershagen, G. (1994). Passive smoking and lung cancer. In J. M. Samet (Ed.), *Epidemiology of lung cancer.* New York: Marcel Dekker.

Ramanathan, R. K. & Belani, C. P. (1997). Chemotherapy for advanced non-small cell lung cancer: past, present and future. *Seminars in Oncology 24*(4), 440-454.

Reed, M. F. & Sugarbaker, D. J. (1997). Mediastinal staging of lung cancer. In H. I. Pass, J. B. Mitchell, D. H. Johnson, & A. T. Turrisi (Eds.), *Lung cancer principles and practice.* Philadelphia: Lippincott–Raven.

Reed, M. F., DeCamp, M. M., & Sugarbaker, D. J. (1995). Diagnostic procedures related to the thorax. In J. S. MacDonald, D. G. Haller, & R. J. Mayer (Eds.), *Manual of oncologic therapeutics* (3rd ed.). Philadelphia: J. B. Lippincott.

Ruckdeschel, J. (1997). Combined modality therapy in non-small cell lung cancer. *Seminars in Oncology, 24*(4), 429-439.

Ryan, L. S. (1996). Psychosocial issues and lung cancer: A behavior approach. *Seminars in Oncology Nursing 12*(4), 318-323.

Schottenfeld, D. (1997). Epidemiology of lung cancer. In H. I. Pass, J.B. Mitchell, D.H. Johnson, & A. T. Turrisi (Eds.), *Lung cancer principals and practice.* Philadelphia: Lippincott–Raven.

Shaw, G. L. (1995). Screening for lung cancer. In B. E. Johnson & D. H. Johnson (Eds.), *Lung cancer.* New York: Wiley-Liss.

Sheperd, F. A. (1994). Future directions in the treatment of non-small cell lung cancer. *Seminars in Oncology 21*(4), 48-62.

Shields, P. G. & Harris, C. C. (1993). Genetic predisposition to lung cancer. In J. A. Roth, J. D. Cox, & W. K. Hong (Eds.), *Lung cancer.* Boston: Blackwell Scientific.

Shopland, D. R. (1996). Cigarette smoking as a cause of cancer. In A. H. Harris, B. K. Edwards, W. J. Blot, & L. A. Gloeckler Ries (Eds.), *Cancer rates and risks* (4th ed.). (NIH Publication No. 96-691.). Washington, D. C.: U. S. Department of Health and Human Services.

Skaar, K., Tsoh, J., Cinciripini, P., Wetter, D., Prokhorov, A., & Gritz, E. (1996). Current approaches in smoking cessation. *Current Opinion in Oncology, 8,* 434-440.

Spivak, S. D., Fasco, M. J., Walker, V. E., & Kaminsky, L. S. (1997). The molecular epidemiology of lung cancer. *Critical Reviews in Toxicology, 27*(4), 319-365.

Stellman, S. D., Muscat, J. E., Hoffmann, D., & Wynder, E. L. (1997). Impact of filter cigarette smoking of lung cancer histology. *Preventative Medicine, 26,* 451-456.

Stewart, I. E. (1996). Superior vena cava syndrome: An oncology complication. *Seminars in Oncology Nursing, 4,* 312-7.

Tellervo, K., Su, S., Korhonen, H. J., Utela, A. & Puska, P. (1997). Evaluation of a national quit and win contest: Determinants for successful quitting. *Preventative Medicine, 26,* 556-564.

Thun, M. J. & Heath, C. W. (1997). Changes in mortality from smoking in two American cancer society prospective studies since 1959. *Preventative Medicine, 26,* 422-426.

Travis, W. D., Linder, J., & Mackay, B. (1997). Classification, histology, cytology, and electron microscopy. In H. I. Pass, J. B. Mitchell, D. H. Johnson, & A. T. Turrisi (Eds.), *Lung cancer principals and practice.* Philadelphia: Lippincott–Raven.

Treat, J. & Kaiser, L. R. (1997). The role of chemotherapy in the treatment of non-small cell carcinoma of the lung. *Seminars in Thoracic and Cardiovascular Surgery, 1,* 90-100.

Wagner, H. (1997). Radiation therapy in the management of patients with unressectable stage IIIA and IIIB non-small cell lung cancer. *Seminars in Oncology, 24*(4), 23-428.

Warnock, M. L. & Isenberg, B. S. (1986). Asbestos burden and the pathology of lung cancer. *Chest, 89,*(1), 20-26.

Webb, W. R. (1995). Lung cancer staging: The role of imaging. In B. E. Johnson & D. H. Johnson (Eds.), *Lung cancer.* New York: Wiley-Liss.

White, E. J. (1997). Lung cancer. In C. Varricchio, M. Pierce, C. L. Walker, & T. B. Ades, (Eds.), *A cancer source book for nurses* (7th ed.). Atlanta: American Cancer Society.

Wu-Williams, A. H. & Samet, J. M. (1994). Lung cancer and cigarette smoking. In J. M. Samet (Ed.), *Epidemiology of lung cancer.* New York: Marcel Dekker

Yang, Z. J. & Fossella, F. V. (1996). Non-small cell lung cancer. *Physician Assistant, 11,* 36–67.

Burkitt's Lymphoma

Nancy Oksenholt, RN, MSN, CCRN
Florence Seelig, RN, OCN

EPIDEMIOLOGY

Burkitt's lymphoma was first described by Dennis Burkitt in equatorial Africa. These lymphomas were then recognized throughout the world. The endemic form is common and almost always associated with the Epstein-Barr virus (EBV). The nonendemic, or sporadic form, is rare (Weinstein & Tarbell, 1997). Burkitt's lymphoma is classified under non–Hodgkin's lymphoma (NHL), a heterogeneous group of diseases with differing clinical presentation, behavior, pathologies, treatments, and prognoses. (Burkitt's lymphoma NHL is further subdivided into nonendemic [non-African] and endemic [African] cases.)

There are several nomenclatures of Burkitt's lymphoma depending on current classification systems. These include the undifferentiated lymphomas, which are classified using the Modified Rappaport Classification staging system; small noncleaved follicular center lymphomas, which use the Revised European American Classification (REAL) staging system; and small noncleaved cell lymphomas, which uses the Working Formulation staging system (The staging classification systems are detailed under Staging, p. 1358). The incidence of Burkitt's lymphoma is higher in children than adults. In children, Burkitt's lymphoma represents 30% of pediatric lymphomas but only 1% to 2% of NHLs in adults.

RISK FACTORS

The major risk factors associated with the development of NHL are listed in Box 63-1. EBV is thought to be the cause of more than 90% of endemic cases of Burkitt's lymphoma. The evidence supporting each risk factor is reviewed. Table 63-1 shows the comparison of Burkitt's lymphoma in Africa and the United States.

Patients with acquired immunodeficiency syndrome (AIDS) have shown an increasing incidence over the years. The use of antiretroviral therapy as a treatment for opportunistic infections is one reason why the life expectancy of a person with AIDS has increased. New programs encouraging patients with AIDS to seek medical attention about persistent, common signs may lead to early diagnosis of Burkitt's lymphoma. However, diagnosis may be difficult due to the similarities to complications from AIDS.

Patients who have undergone organ and tissue transplantation are predisposed to various cancers, the majority being NHL. The reason for this increase is thought to be the immunosuppressive and chemotherapy agents used and/or the immunostimulation.

Autoimmune Disorders

Patients with autoimmune disorders such as sicca syndrome (Sjogren's syndrome), systemic lupus erythematosis (SLE), Hashimoto's thyroiditis, and rheumatoid arthritis have a higher incidence of NHL. The disease severity among sicca syndrome patients is directly related to the level of lymphoma risk (Hoover, 1992).

Immunodeficiency Syndromes

The immunodeficiency syndromes with the greatest risk of lymphoma are agamma-globulinemia, ataxia-telangiectasia, Wiscott-Aldrich syndrome, and X-linked recessive syndrome. The X-linked recessive syndrome is associated with a variety of sequelae, including fatal infection with infectious mononucleosis of lymphoid malignancy, particularly Burkitt's lymphoma.

Virus. Viruses are implicated in the development of human cancers (Chow 1993). Human immunodeficiency virus (HIV) and the human T-cell leukemia/lymphoma virus-1 (HTLV-1) are associated with increased risk of Burkitt's lymphoma due to the impairment of the immune function. EBV is a B-lymphotropic polyclonal cellular activator that stimulates cell division and transforms lymphocytes into propagating lymphoblastoid cells indefinitely. EBV is a member of the *Herpes viridae* family that is mainly responsible for endemic Burkitt's lymphoma.

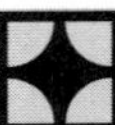

TABLE 63-1 Assessment of the Patient for Burkitt's Lymphoma

	Assessment Parameters	Typical Abnormal Findings
History	A. Personal and social history	A. Personal and social risk factors
	1. Age	1. Most common in children; rare in adults
	2. Gender	2. Female 3:1; males 2
	3. Ethnicity	3. Africans (endemic) American (sporadic)
	4. Immunosuppression	4. May be linked to HIV disease
	5. Pain	5. *Endemic:* jaw and orbital pain *Sporadic:* abdominal pain
	6. Viral	6. Epstein-Barr virus in patients with African Burkitt's; rare in American Burkitt's
Physical Examination	A. Differential diagnosis must be established among non–Hodgkin's lymphoma	A. Lymph node enlargement rare in African but may be seen in American
		B. American Burkitt's lymphoma patients may present with bowel obstruction or perforation due to abdominal involvement of disease
Diagnostic Tests	A. Bone marrow aspiration and biopsy	A. Bone marrow cells show extremely high rate of proliferation and "starry sky" appearance (Fig. 63-1)
	B. Lumbar puncture	B. Patients with Burkitt's lymphoma tend to have positive central nervous system disease
	C. Computed tomography of chest, abdomen, and pelvis	C. Will reveal enlarged nodes or masses if present; these are useful in staging disease
	D. Gallium scan	D. If large masses are detected, they are easily followed for response to therapy via gallium
	E. Lymph node evaluation	E. Lymph node enlargement could be present in any of the following lymph node areas: cervical, supraclavicular, axillary, epitrochlear, retroperitoneal, mesenteric, iliac, inguinal, femoral, and oropharyngeal; malignant lymph nodes are characteristically nontender, firm and rubbery

Box 63-1
Risk Factors for Non–Hodgkin's Lymphoma

Children
Tropical African children
Males 2:3.1
Altered immunologic states
- AIDS
- Organ transplantation
- Autoimmune disorders

Immunodeficiency syndrome viruses
- HTLV-3
- HIV
- Epstein-Barr virus

Chemical exposure
- Agriculture chemicals
- Hair-darkening dyes

Autoimmune disorders
- Treated Hodgkin's disease
- Radiation exposure

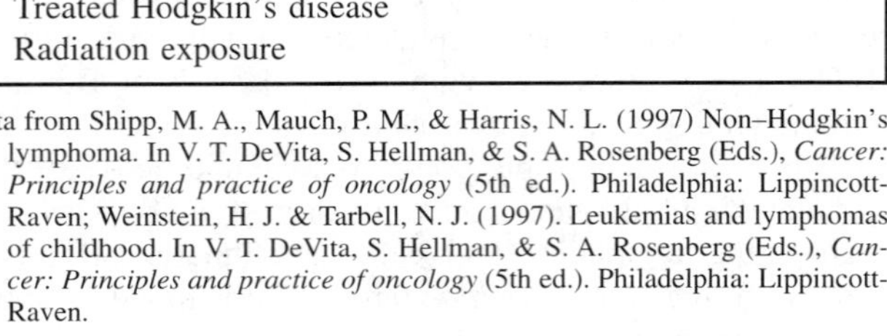

Data from Shipp, M. A., Mauch, P. M., & Harris, N. L. (1997) Non–Hodgkin's lymphoma. In V. T. DeVita, S. Hellman, & S. A. Rosenberg (Eds.), *Cancer: Principles and practice of oncology* (5th ed.). Philadelphia: Lippincott-Raven; Weinstein, H. J. & Tarbell, N. J. (1997). Leukemias and lymphomas of childhood. In V. T. DeVita, S. Hellman, & S. A. Rosenberg (Eds.), *Cancer: Principles and practice of oncology* (5th ed.). Philadelphia: Lippincott-Raven.

AIDS, Acquired immunodeficiency syndrome; *HIV,* human immunodeficiency virus; *HTLV,* human T-lymphocyte virus-3

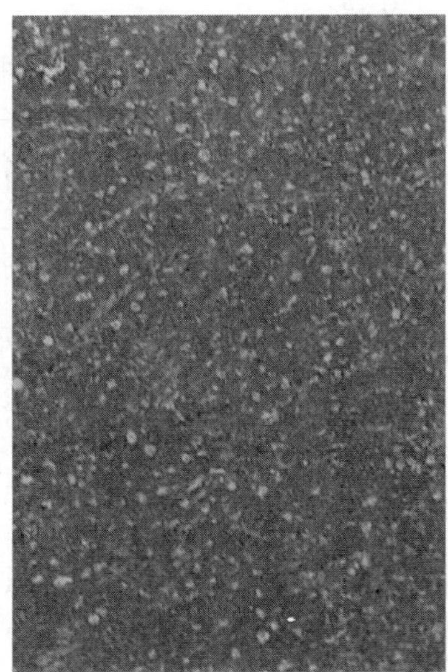

Fig. 63-1 Small, uncleaved cell, Burkitt's type. Low-powered photomicrograph reveals a "starry night" appearance resulting from the presence of benign macrophages, which are active in the phagocytosis of necrotic cells and debris. (Skarin, A. T. [1996]. Atlas of diagnostic oncology [2nd ed.]. St. Louis: Mosby-Wolfe.)

Radiation Exposure

Survivors of the atomic bombing in Hiroshima have also had an increased incidence of NHL. Oncology nurses taking histories should note patients' birthplaces and monitor for side effects.

In addition, akylating therapy for Hodgkin's disease can also be a cause of NHL. Oncology nurses need to be aware of long-term complications following organ transplants, treatment for Hodgkin's disease, and radiation exposure with education for follow-up care. Patients can be informed about the signs and symptoms of Burkitt's lymphomas so that they can report these problems to their physicians.

PATHOPHYSIOLOGY

Normal Anatomy and Physiology of the Lymph System

The lymphatic system consists of a network of vessels that branch throughout the body, with hundreds of small, bean-shaped organs called *lymph nodes.* The colorless, watery fluid that contains lymphocytes is carried by these vessels. The major lymphatic structures include the following: groups and chains of lymph nodes, spleen, thymus, Waldeyer's ring, appendix, bone marrow, tonsils, adenoids and Peyer's patches (Fig. 63-2). The lymph system sets up a complex network that defends the body against infection. The main concern of the lymphocytic cells is immune function; they are the primary cellular component of malignant lymphomas (McFadden 1993).

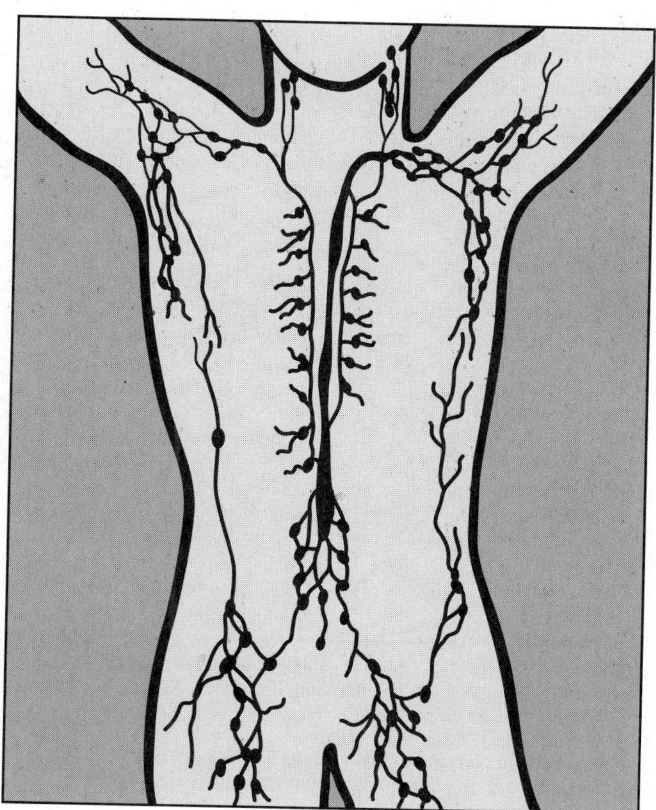

Fig. 63-2 Anatomy of lymphatic systems.

The lymphatic organs are concerned with the growth, development, and deployment of T and B lymphocytes. Lymphatic precursors arise from pluripotent stem cells in the marrow and are carried through the blood to the lymph nodes and spleen. They proliferate and differentiate on contact with antigens. T lymphocytes are memory cells that regulate both antibody production by B lymphocytes and the cell-mediated effector responses of other T lymphocytes. B lymphocytes are memory and plasma cells, which are factories for the production of antibodies.

THE PROCESS OF CARCINOGENESIS

As stated above, NHLs are a diverse group of diseases because of their wide range of cellular origins. NHL is a malignancy of the lymphatic system that causes an uncontrolled proliferation of lymphocytes. The lymphatic system plays a major role in the body's defense against infection and antibody production. Burkitt's lymphoma is classified under NHL as a high-grade lymphoma and is thought to be the fastest growing human malignancy. Burkitt's lymphoma and most of the high-grade lymphomas usually affect B lymphocytes. The B-lymphocyte NHLs represent more than 80% of all lymphomas. Burkitt's lymphoma causes monoclonal B-lymphocyte tumors. In Burkitt's lymphoma the growth pattern of cells is primarily diffuse. Cells are very uniform, with an intermediate size, round/oval nuclei with two to five prominent nucleoli, coarsely reticulated chromatin, and two to five prominent peripheral nucleoli (Prizzere 1995).

When lymph node imprints or bone marrow smears are examined, cytoplasm is noted to contain small vacuoles of neutral lipids. Cell proliferation is consistently associated with a high number of mitoses and a prominent "starry sky" pattern, produced by a scattering throughout of macrophages containing nuclear debris. There is a diffuse pattern of growth. Diffuse, occasional lymphomatous follicles may be evident, implying a possible relationship to germinal centers. Approximately 20% of cases are follicular structures (Prizzere 1995). Burkitt's lymphoma cells are of B lineage, expressing monoclonal immunoglobulin M (IgM), a surface immunoglobulin. Also reported are surface immunoglobulins G (IgG), A (IgA), and D (IgD) (Sarna & Kagan 1995) Tumors of B-lymphocyte origin may cause abnormal antibody secretion. There are five different classes of immunoglobulins. IgM antibodies are the first antibodies to appear after initial exposure to antigens.

Consistent series of cytogenetic translocations and explosive growth are characteristic of Burkitt's lymphoma. Burkitt's lymphoma translocations are between chromosome 8 and chromosome 14, which results in the c-*myc* oncogene being placed in the normal location of the immunoglobulin heavy-chain locus (Lister & Armitage 1995; Melnyk & Rodriguez 1995).

All Burkitt's lymphoma of both the endemic and sporadic variants manifest one of the three translocations t(8;14) (q24;q32), t(8;22) (q24;q11), and t(2;8) (p11-p13; q24) with rare exceptions (Melynk & Rodriguez, 1995; Prizzere, 1995). In more than 90% of the endemic Burkitt's lymphoma tumors, translocation t(8:14) occurs.

EBV is a B-lymphotropic polyclonal cellular activator that stimulates cell division and transforms lymphocytes into indefinitely propagating lymphoblastoid cells. Endemic Burkitt's lymphoma is found in areas such as Africa and Papua New Guinea, which have a high incidence of malaria. Malaria causes a defect in the immune system, which results in an inability to resolve EBV infections that remain persistent in the body. These findings suggest that this subtype of Burkitt's lymphoma can be environmentally determined (Magrath, Jain, & Bhatia 1996). EBV can be detected in more than 90% of endemic Burkitt's lymphoma and 25% to 40% of sporadic and AIDS-associated B lymphomas (Medeiros & Jaffee 1996).

Endemic Burkitt's lymphoma cases have much higher EBV antibody titers. After EBV infection, lymphoma develops when a chromosome translocation brings the c-*myc* oncogene on chromosome 8 into the proximity of an immunoglobulin gene on either side of chromosome 2, 14, or 22 and its regulatory sequence. There is a morphologic variation known as *Burkitt's-like lymphoma,* which shows greater nuclear variability but is not discussed in detail here.

ROUTES OF METASTASES

Metastasis is the production of secondary tumors at distant sites. Dissemination occurs via the lymphatic system; entrapment may occur in the first lymph node encountered, or cells may bypass the first node and reach more distant sites.

The prognosis of NHL depends on the capacity of malignant cells to disseminate, take hold, and grow in distant sites of the body. The main determinant of metastatic spread is the adhesiveness of the tumor cells, and this reflects an important degree of display of CD44, a cell surface glycoprotein that governs the normal pattern of lymphocytes from blood to lymphatic tissues and is the key to metastatic dissemination of lymphoma cells. There is in vitro evidence that EBV may down-regulate adhesion molecules that increase the interaction between virally transferred cells and T lymphocytes. This down-regulation may allow the virally transformed B cells of the Burkitt's lymphoma to evade host immune defenses.

ASSESSMENT

Burkitt's lymphoma is perhaps the most rapidly growing human malignancy. There is an actual doubling time of 66 hours and a mean doubling time of 25.6 hours (Sarna & Kagan, 1995). The implications of a rapid doubling time implies phenomenal cell growth with little resting cell population. This accelerated cell growth may generate signs of bulky disease such as massive lymphadenopathy, viscous perforation, or painful bone involvement and affects the treatment course by having a predilection for tumor lysis syndrome (Yandle, 1996). Clinical workup of the Burkitt's lymphoma patient should be done expeditiously to allow for timely treatment of the disease. Patients in the United States present with advanced disease more than 60% of the time (Levine, Connelly, Berard, O'Connor, Dorfman, & Eastman et al., 1975; Sarna & Kagan, 1995). Evaluation of this patient population encompasses a complete and thorough physical examination, an assessment for any risk factors, a history of the patient that includes recent signs and symptoms, and a review of the number of staging studies that are required. Though the median age of the Burkitt's lymphoma patient has shown this to be a pediatric disease, roughly one third of patients are over age 15 and the disease can be seen in patients into their 70s (Cohen, Bennett, Berard, Ziegler, Vogel, & Sheagren et al., 1969; Levine et al., 1975; Levine, Kamaraju, Connelly, Berard, Dorfman, & Magrath et al., 1982).

Table 63-2 identifies key features of Burkitt's lymphoma. African Burkitt's lymphoma is also known as *equatorial* or *endemic,* and United States and American Burkitt's lymphoma is also referred to as *nonendemic* or *sporadic* Burkitt's lymphoma (Bierman, Vose, & Armitage, 1995; Levine et al., 1975, 1982).

TABLE 63-2 Comparison of Burkitt's Lymphoma in Africa and the United States

Africa (Equatorial and Endemic)	United States (Sporadic and Nonendemic)
Common (100 per 1 million children)	Rare (1 to 2 per 1 million children)
Distribution relates to climate and geography	Distribution apparently unrelated to climate and geography
Male occurrence predominant	Male occurrence predominant
Median age 7, rare to see >15 years of age	Median age 11, 25% >15 years of age
Nearly always associated Nonendemic with Epstein-Barr virus (EBV)	Uncommonly associated with EBV
t(8:14) common	t(8:14) common
Jaw tumors common, marrow involvement rare	Jaw tumors rare, marrow involvement common as is abdominal, gastrointestinal tract
50% prolonged survival with combination therapy	50% prolonged survival with combination therapy
Isolated central nervous system (CNS) relapse common with cyclophosphamide therapy	Isolated CNS relapse uncommon with combination therapy
Multiple relapses not incompatible with eventual prolonged disease-free survival	Survival uncommon after relapse
30% to 50% in advanced stage at presentation	60% in advanced stage presentation

Data from Shipp, M. A., Mauch, P. M., & Harris, N. L. (1997) Non–Hodgkin's lymphoma. In V. T. DeVita, S. Hellman, & S. A. Rosenberg (Eds.), *Cancer: Principles and practice of oncology* (5th ed.). Philadelphia: Lippincott-Raven; Weinstein, H. J. & Tarbell, N. J. (1997). Leukemias and lymphomas of childhood. In V. T. DeVita, S. Hellman, & S. A. Rosenberg (Eds.), *Cancer: Principles and practice of oncology* (5th ed.). Philadelphia: Lippincott-Raven.

HISTORY

An assessment of the patient includes a complete family history, history of past medical or surgical treatments, any significant illnesses (including viral), environmental exposures, and a detailed discussion of presenting symptoms including any "B" symptoms. See Box 63-2 for B symptoms (Shipp, Mauch, & Harris, 1997). American Burkitt's lymphoma patients may present with symptoms of bowel obstruction or perforation due to the abdominal involvement of the disease.

The patient should undergo a complete physical examination with particular emphasis on the evaluation for adenopathy, musculoskeletal lesions, symptoms of abdominal perforation or sanctuary site lesions (e.g., testicular, ocular orbit, or central nervous system [CNS] lesions) (Yandle, 1996). Prompt institution of staging studies should be undertaken and a histological diagnosis should be confirmed. See Table 63-3 for staging procedures (Bierman, Vose, & Armitage, 1995; Long, DeVita, Jaffe, Mauch, & Urba, 1993). Appropriate staging allows the clinician to provide an accurate evaluation of the current stage of the patient's lymphoma and then to prescribe a suitable treatment regimen (Long et al., 1993; Poplack, Kun, Pizzo, & Magrath, 1993; Prizzere, 1995).

Establishment of the diagnosis should be confirmed by the pathologic evaluation of a lymph node, bone marrow sample, or other tissue. A fine-needle aspiration (FNA) may be taken to obtain a tissue sample, or the patient may require surgical excision of an abnormal lymph node. Assessment for clonality, gene rearrangement or chromosomal/cytogenetic translocations or deletions is helpful in establishing the diagnosis in Burkitt's lymphoma. The affected gene is c-*myc* (8q 24) and chromosomal translocations of t(8;14), t(8;22) and t(2;8) are reported. (Melnyk & Rodriguez 1995; Prizzere, 1995).

Box 63-2
"B" Symptoms

Fever (±Pel-Edstein relapsing pattern)
Drenching night sweats
>10% weight loss
Pruritus (not always considered B symptom)

From Hubbard, S. (1996). Current issues and controversies in the management of non–Hodgkin's lymphoma. *Educational Monolith,* 2, 1-39. New York: Tricilinca Communications.

TABLE 63-3 Staging Procedures for Burkitt's Lymphoma

Required	Recommended/ Dependent on Clinical Condition
• Chest x-ray (PA and LAT) • Bone marrow aspirate and biopsy • CBC with platelet count and differential • Lumbar puncture with cytogenetics • Chemistry panel to include liver and renal tests (Alk $P0_4$, SGOT, SGPT, BUN, creatine), electrolytes, LDH, and uric acid levels.	• CT scan of chest and abdomen/pelvis • Bone scan/skeletal survey • Ultrasound of affected areas • Endoscopy/barium studies of GI tract • Myelogram • Lymphangiogram • Gallium scan • IVP • Laparotomy

Data from Shipp, M. A., Mauch, P. M., & Harris, N. L. (1997) Non–Hodgkin's lymphoma. In V. T. DeVita, S. Hellman, & S. A. Rosenberg (Eds.), *Cancer: Principles and practice of oncology* (5th ed.). Philadelphia: Lippincott-Raven; Weinstein, H. J. & Tarbell, N. J. (1997). Leukemias and lymphomas of childhood. In V. T. DeVita, S. Hellman, & S. A. Rosenberg (Eds.), *Cancer: Principles and practice of oncology* (5th ed.). Philadelphia: Lippincott-Raven.
$ALKP0_4$, Alkaline phosphatase; *BUN,* blood urea nitrogen; *CBC,* complete blood count; *CT,* computed tomography; *GI,* gastrointestinal; *IVP,* intravenous pyelogram; *LDH,* lactic dehydrogenase; *SGOT,* serum glutamic-oxaloacetic transaminate; *SGPT,* serum glutamic-pyruvic transaminase.

STAGING PROCEDURES

Bone Marrow Aspirate and Biopsy

Bone marrow constitutes the most extensive tissue in the body. In Burkitt's lymphoma the marrow is often involved. Detection of marrow involvement and subsequent pathologic diagnosis requires more aggressive intervention to obtain tissue for diagnosis. Bone marrow biopsies and aspirates are usually performed on the sternum or posterior iliac crest since those are the most accessible areas of the body for obtaining a marrow sample.

The patient is administered a local anesthetic to the skin and periosteum and an aspirating needle with stylet is introduced under sterile conditions. The needle is advanced into the marrow space, the stylet is removed, and a syringe is attached to the needle. Approximately 2 to 6 ml of liquid marrow are aspirated. The aspirating needle is removed and the procedure is repeated using a biopsy needle and obtaining a marrow core sample. The patient should not require a significant recovery period. Premedication with a mild analgesic or sedative may lessen the patient's anxiety and discomfort.

Complete Blood Count

A CBC that includes a differential is a basic test to assess the patient for the presence of cytopenia. A blood count may be useful in assessing marrow involvement, especially if circulating malignant cells (blast cells) are present.

Blood Chemistries

Blood chemistries, including blood urea nitrogen (BUN), creatinine (CR), serum glutamic oxaloacetic transaminase (SGOT), total bilirubin, alkaline phosphatase, and lactic acid dehydrogenase (LDH), may reveal urerthal obstruction and, less commonly, direct renal involvement. Uric acid is

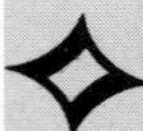

TABLE 63-4 Patient Preparation for a Gallium Scan

Description of the Procedure: Gallium scans involve IV administration of gallium-67–citrate, followed by camera imaging.

Patient Preparation: A gallium scan usually requires two visits to the nuclear medicine department. No special preparation is required by the patient before the study. Assure the patient that gallium is safe and will not harm him or her or family members. On the first day an injection of gallium is administered intravenously. The patients return 2 to 5 days later for imaging.

Procedural Considerations:

1. Explain the procedure to the patient. Determine if patients are allergic to contrast medium.
2. Obtain informed consent.
3. Patient should lie on an imaging table with camera positioned above or below the patient.
4. Multiple images are taken, or the camera may move slowly, scanning the entire length of the body.
5. A tomographic study may be done at this time. This involves having patient lie on a narrow imaging table while camera rotates 360 degrees around the patient.

Special Consideration:

1. Gallium normally is excreted through the bowel and may obstruct images of the abdomen and pelvis on the first day of imaging. The patient may be asked to return for additional imaging.

an end product of metabolism and is elevated during times of rapid cell division and death. An elevated LDH is associated with high tumor burden and rapid cell proliferation rate. (Bierman, Vose, & Armitage, 1995).

Other Tests

Lumbar puncture or spinal taps to assess for CNS disease is imperative to rule out occult lymphomatous involvement of the meninges. Computed tomography (CT) scans are used to assess extent of disease and the presence or degree of adenopathy. A Tc99 bone scan is used to determine bony lesions or areas of widespread involvement. Gallium scans can be useful in reassessing patients after therapy (if scanned pretreatment measures are available for comparison); they often aid in evaluating persistent tumor vs residual fibrotic masses (Table 63-4). Persistent positive uptake of the gallium into areas of disease may indicate ongoing tumor activity. Intravenous pyelogram or urogram may be done to identify urologic structures affected by bulky tumor sites.

Magnetic Resonance Imaging

Magnetic resonance imaging (MRI) may show bone marrow or CNS involvement. Chest x-ray is performed to assess for mediastinal involvement or gross co-morbid disease such as cardiomyopathy, congestive heart failure, or pulmonary disease. Laparotomy for exploratory surgery with resection of bulky intra-abdominal disease or repair of gastrointestinal perforation may be necessary.

STAGING

Staging of Burkitt's lymphoma encompasses several systems. Four of the staging systems are descriptive of all lymphomas (i.e., Ann Arbor staging system, REAL, Working Formulation, and Modified Rappaport Classification) The alternative clinical staging systems for Burkitt's lymphoma are used more often for childhood lymphomas such as Burkitt's lymphoma. The Ziegler staging system is used often and is referred to as the *National Cancer Institute (NCI) staging system* (Casciato & Lowitz, 1988; Murphy, 1980). Because Burkitt's lymphoma is a well-defined entity within the NHLs, the Working Formulation or the REAL staging systems can be used most effectively. New classifications systems that link to the ICD-0 (World Health Organization's International Classification of Disease) are being discussed that would give the same ICD-0 code number to equivalent terms used in different classifications. This would facilitate literature searches and clarify co-joined names in the different classifications.

Due to the rapid pace of Burkitt's lymphoma, staging studies and complete classification may ultimately be completed after initiation of therapy. See Tables 63-3, 63-5, and 63-6 for staging classifications.

MEDICAL MANAGEMENT

Even in patients who do not have marrow or CNS involvement at diagnosis, rapid progression can occur and alter the patient's prognosis. Prompt institution of therapy is necessary to initiate control of the lymphoma. Without treatment, survival is measured in weeks to a few months (Burkitt, 1958).

Surgery

For patients with bulky abdominal disease, the role of debulking surgery before chemotherapy has been debated. In Ziegler's (NCI) classification system, there is a category for patients who have had more than 90% of their abdominal tumor mass resected (Ziegler & Magrath, 1974). Debulking surgery, or excision of the abdominal mass (usually resection of bowel, kidney or ovary), may reduce tumor burden, thus decreasing the risk of tumor lysis syndrome, decreasing the amount of tumor the chemotherapy needs to kill, and diminishing the possibilities of obstruction or intussusception (Kemeny, Magrath, Brennan, 1982; Yandle, 1996; Ziegler, 1981). Tumor reduction may also change the patient's stage to a more favorable one (e.g., stage C to A) (Sarna & Kagan 1995).

Surgery may be required if the patient has resistant or recurrent disease that necessitates the alleviation of an obstruction or diminishes the size of the tumor mass. Finally, surgery may be necessary for the placement of a cen-

TABLE 63-5 Comparison of Non–Hodgkin's Lymphoma Staging Systems

Ann Arbor Staging System		Revised European American Lymphoma	
Stage	**Explanation**	**Classification**	**Working Formulation**
I	Involvement of a single lymph node region (I) or a single extralymphatic organ or site (I_E)	Precursor B-lymphoblastic lymphoma/leukemia	Lymphoblastic
II	Involvement of two or more lymph node regions (II) or localized involvement of an extralymphatic organ or site (II_E), on the same side of the diaphragm.	B-cell chronic lymphocytic leukemia/prolymphocytic leukemia/small lymphotyctic lymphoma	Small lymphocytic, consistent with CLL Small lymphocytic, plasmacytoid
		Lymphoplasmacytoid lymphoma	Small lymphocytic, plasmacytoid Diffuse, mixed small and large cell
III	Involvement of lymph node regions (III) or localized involvement of an extralymphatic organ or site (III_E) on both sides of the diaphragm or spleen (IIIx) or both (III_{SE}).	Mantle cell lymphoma	Small lymphocytic Diffuse, small cleaved cell Follicular, small cleaved cell Diffuse, mixed small and large cell Diffuse, large cleaved cell
IV	Diffuse or disseminated involvement of one or more cell extralymphatic organs, with or without associated lymph node involvement.	Follicular center lymphoma, follicular • Grade I	Follicular, predominantly small cleaved cell
		• Grade II	Follicular mixed, small and large cell
		• Grade III	Follicular, predominantely large cell
		Follicular center lymphoma, diffuse, small cell (provisional)	Diffuse, small cleaved cell Diffuse, mixed small and large cell
		Extranodal marginal zone B-cell lymphoma (low-grade B-cell lymphoma of MALT type)	Small lymphocytic Diffuse, small cleaved cell Diffuse, mixed small and large cell
		Nodal marginal zone B-cell lymphoma (provisional)	Small lymphocytic Diffuse, small cleaved cell Diffuse, mixed small and large cell Unclassified

NOTE: Each stage is divided into an A or B category: A, asymptomatic; B, fever, sweats, weight loss > 10% of body weight.

Rappaport Classification		
• Diffuse well-differentiated lymphocytic	Splenic marginal zone B-cell lymphoma (provisional)	Small lymphocytic Diffuse, small cleaved cell
• Nodular poorly differentiated lymphocytic	Hairy cell leukemia	
• Nodular mixed lymphocytic-histiocytic	Plasmacytoma/myeloma	Extramedullary plasmacytoma
• Nodular histiocytic • Diffuse poorly differentiated lymphocytic	Diffuse large B-cell lymphoma	Diffuse, large cell Large cell immunoblastic Diffuse, mixed small and large cell
• Diffuse mixed lymphocytic-histiocytic	Primary mediastinal large B-cell lymphoma	Diffuse, large cell Large cell immunoblastic
• Diffuse histiocytic	Burkitt's lymphoma	Small, noncleaved cell Burkitt's
• Diffuse histiocytic • Diffuse lymphoblastic • Diffuse undifferentiated	High-grade B-cell lymphoma, Burkitt's-like (provisional)	Small, noncleaved cell, non-Burkitt's Diffuse, large cell Large cell immunoblastic
	Precursor T-lymphoblastic lymphoma/leukemia	Lymphoblastic
	T-cell chronic lymphocytic leukemia/prolymphocytic leukemia	Small lymphocytic Diffuse, small cleaved cell

From Shipp, M. A., Mauch, P. M., & Harris, N. L. (1997). Non–Hodgkin's lymphoma. In V. T. DeVita, S. Hellman, & S. A. Rosenberg (Eds.), *Cancer: Principles and practice of oncology* (5th ed.). Philadelphia: Lippincott-Raven; Weinstein, H. J. & Tarbell, N. J. (1997). Leukemias and lymphomas of childhood. In V. T. DeVita, S. Hellman, & S. A. Rosenberg (Eds.), *Cancer: Principles and practice of oncology* (5th ed.). Philadelphia: Lippincott-Raven.
CLL, Chronic lymphocytic leukemia; *E,* extranodal spread; *NK,* natural killer; *S,* involvement of both localized and extranodal regions.

Continued

TABLE 63-5 Comparison of Non–Hodgkin's Lymphoma Staging Systems—cont'd

		Rappaport Classification—cont'd
	Large granular lymphocytic leukemia • T-cell type • NK-cell type	Small lymphocytic Diffuse, small cleaved cell
	Mycosis fungoides/Sézary syndrome	Mycosis fungoides
	Peripheral T-cell lymphomas, unspecified) (including provisional subtype: subcutaneous panniculitic T-cell lymphoma)	Diffuse, small cleaved cell Diffuse, mixed small and large cell Diffuse, large cell Large cell immunoblastic
	Hepatosplenic γ-δ T-cell lymphoma (provisional)	
	Angioimmunoblastic T-cell lymphoma	Diffuse, mixed small and large cell Diffuse, large cell Large cell immunoblastic

From Shipp, M. A., Mauch, P. M., & Harris, N. L. (1997) Non–Hodgkin's lymphoma. In V. T. DeVita, S. Hellman, & S. A. Rosenberg (Eds.), *Cancer: Principles and practice of oncology* (5th ed.). Philadelphia: Lippincott-Raven; Weinstein, H. J. & Tarbell, N. J. (1997). Leukemias and lymphomas of childhood. In V. T. DeVita, S. Hellman, & S. A. Rosenberg (Eds.), *Cancer: Principles and practice of oncology* (5th ed.). Philadelphia: Lippincott-Raven.
CLL, Chronic lymphocytic leukemia; *E,* extranodal spread; *NK,* natural killer; *S,* involvement of both localized and extranodal regions.

TABLE 63-6 Clinical Staging Systems for Childhood Lymphomas

	Memorial Sloan-Kettering	St. Jude Children's Research Hospital (Murphy, 1990)		National Cancer Institute (Zeigler & Magrath, 1974)
Stage			**Stage**	
I	One single site	• A single tumor (extranodal) or single anatomic area (nodal), with the exclusion of mediastinum or abdomen	A	Single solitary extraabdominal site
II	Two or more sites on the same side of the diaphragm	• A single tumor (extranodal) with regional node involvement • Two or more nodal areas on the same side of the diaphragm • A primary gastrointestinal tract tumor, usually in the ileocecal area, with or without involvement of associated mesenteric nodes only	B	Multiple extraabdominal sites
III	Disseminated disease without marrow or central nervous system (CNS) involvement	• Two single tumors (extranodal) on opposite sides of the diaphragm • All the primary intrathoracic tumors (mediastinal, pleural, thymic) • All extensive primary intraabdominal disease • All paraspinal or epidural tumors regardless of other tumor site(s)	C	Intraabdominal tumor
IV	Any of the above with bone marrow and/or CNS involvement	• Any of the above with initial CNS or bone marrow involvement	D	Intraabdominal tumor with ≥ extra abdominal site
			AR	Intraabdominal tumor >90% tumor surgically resected

From Shipp, M. A., Mauch, P. M., & Harris, N. L. (1997) Non–Hodgkin's lymphoma. In V. T. DeVita, S. Hellman, & S. A. Rosenberg (Eds.), *Cancer: Principles and practice of oncology* (5th ed.). Philadelphia: Lippincott-Raven; Weinstein, H. J. & Tarbell, N. J. (1997). Leukemias and lymphomas of childhood. In V. T. DeVita, S. Hellman, & S. A. Rosenberg (Eds.), *Cancer: Principles and practice of oncology* (5th ed.). Philadelphia: Lippincott-Raven.

tral venous catheter for the administration of chemotherapy, transfusions, or nutrients or to maintain temporary hemodialysis in the advent of renal failure secondary to tumor lysis or obstruction (Kaufman Burgert, & Banks, 1987; Kemeny Magrath, & Brennan, 1982; Shamberger & Weinstein 1992).

Several disadvantages need to be considered for the addition of surgery to the treatment plan. Patients undergoing exploratory laparotomy and resection may require a period of convalescence when the unresected tumor can grow and flourish. If appropriate convalescence does not take

Box 63-3
Poor Prognostic Indicators (High Risk Factors) at Presentation

- Central nervous system involvement
- Bone marrow involvement
- Lactic dehydrogenase ≥ 500 IU/L
- Tumor bulk ≥ 10

Data from Shipp, M. A., Mauch, P. M., & Harris, N. L. (1997) Non–Hodgkin's lymphoma. In V. T. DeVita, S. Hellman, & S. A. Rosenberg (Eds.), *Cancer: Principles and practice of oncology* (5th ed.). Philadelphia: Lippincott-Raven; Weinstein, H. J. & Tarbell, N. J. (1997). Leukemias and lymphomas of childhood. In V. T. DeVita, S. Hellman, & S. A. Rosenberg (Eds.), *Cancer: Principles and practice of oncology* (5th ed.). Philadelphia: Lippincott-Raven.

place, poor wound healing and infections may occur, such as thrombophlebitis, abdominal abscesses, and postoperative wound infection (Sarna & Kagan, 1995). Kemeny and colleagues (1982) reported that gastrointestinal hemorrhage can be a complication occurring from therapy or primary disease. Because of surgical morbidity Frappaz and associates (1995) argue that surgery should be restricted to only three occasions, one being to obtain tissue for initial diagnosis when no other means of diagnosis is possible. The second occasion is to intervene in acute abdominal complications on presentation or secondary to treatment. The final occasion is to ensure complete excision of localized disease. Surgical removal of any residual masses after medical treatment may be considered if bulky disease is left after chemotherapy has ended. Necrotic tissue is found in two thirds of those patients with bulky disease, and when the necrotic mass is totally removed, they have a similar prognosis to those who are in complete remission after completion of therapy (Frappaz, Boufett, Blay, Philip, & Brunat-Mentigny 1995).

Chemotherapy

Chemotherapy is the gold standard of treatment for Burkitt's lymphoma. Patients who have nonendemic (i.e., American, or sporadic) Burkitt's lymphoma can achieve a complete remission (more than 50% to 75%) the majority of time (Sarna & Kagan, 1995; Yandle, 1996). Because of the rapid growth rate of this lymphoma, patients who maintain a complete remission (CR) status for more than 1 year may be considered cured, since relapses are rarely beyond 1 year (Ziegler, 1981; Sarna & Kagan, 1995). In contrast, patients with endemic Burkitt's lymphoma, however, may undergo later relapse. Patients with poor risk disease as defined by LDH > 500 IU/L, bone marrow involvement, meningeal involvement, or leukemic presentation have only a 20% to 40% chance of long-term survival. Box 63-3 lists poor prognostic indicators at presentation (Bierman, Vose, & Armitage 1995). Table 63-7 lists common chemotherapy regimens used in treating adult and childhood Burkitt's lymphoma (Frappaz et al., 1995; Long et. al, 1993; Poplack et al., 1993).

Burkitt's lymphoma is highly responsive to chemotherapy. Clinical remissions often occur early in the course of therapy secondary to the exquisite sensitivity of the tumor cells to chemotherapy. Oncologic complications such as tumor lysis syndrome (which will be reviewed later) may occur strictly because of the rapidity of the tumor response to therapy.

TABLE 63-7 Childhood Chemotherapy Regimens for Lymphomas

COP	Vincristine, cyclophosphamide, prednisone, methotrexate (intrathecal)
COPADEM	Vincristine, cyclophosphamide, prednisone, doxorubicin, methotrexate (systemic and intrathecal), folinic acid
CYM	Cytarabine (systemic and intrathecal), methotrexate (systemic and intrathecal), folinic acid, vincristine, cyclophosphamide, prednisone
APO	Doxorubicin, prednisone, vincristine
Adult Chemotherapy Regimens for Lymphomas	
C-MOPP	Cyclophosphamide, vincristine, procarbazine, prednisone
CHOP	Cyclophosphamide, doxorubicin, vincristine, prednisone
CHOMP	Cyclophosphamide, doxorubicin, vincristine, prednisone, methotrexate (intrathecal)
COMLA	Cyclophosphamide, vincristine, methotrexate, folinic acid, cytarabine
M-BACOD	Methotrexate, folinic acid, bleomycin, doxorubicin, cyclophosphamide, vincristine, dexamethasone
ProMACE-MOPP	Prednisone, methotrexate, folinic acid, doxorubicin, cyclophosphamide, etoposide, mechlorethamine, vincristine, procarbazine, prednisone
COP-BLAM	Cyclophosphamide, vincristine, prednisone, bleomycin, doxorubicin, procarbazine
CAP-BOP	Cyclophosphamide, doxorubicin, procarbazine, bleomycin, vincristine, prednisone
MACOP-B	Methotrexate, folinic acid, doxorubicin, cyclophosphamide, vincristine, prednisone, bleomycin
COP-BLAM	Cyclophosphamide, vincristine, prednisone, bleomycin, doxorubicin, procarbazine
ProMACE-CytaBOM	Prednisone, methotrexate, folinic acid, doxorubicin, cyclophosphamide, etoposide, cytarabine, bleomycin, vincristine
LNA-84	Doxorubicin, cyclophosphamide, prednisone, bleomycin, methotrexate (systemic and intrathecal), vindesine, ifosfamide, etoposide, l-asparaginase, cytarabine

Data from Frappaz, D., Bouffet, E., Blay, J., Philip, T., & Brunat-Mentigny D. (1995) Childhood lymphoma. In M. Abelhoff, J. Armitage, A. Lichter, & J. Niderhuber (Eds.), *Clinical oncology.* New York: Churchill Livingstone; Long., D., DeVita, V. T., Jaffe, E., Mauch, P., & Urba, W. (1993). Lymphocytic lymphomas. In V. T. DeVita, S. Hellman, & S. A. Rosenberg (Eds.), *Cancer: Principles and practice of oncology* (4th ed.). Philadelphia: Lippincott-Raven; Poplack, D., Kun, L., Pizzo, P., & Magrath, I. (1993) Leukemias and lymphomas of Childhood. In V. T. DeVita, S., Hellman, & S. A. Rosenberg (Eds.), *Cancer; Principles and practice of oncology* (4th ed.). Philadelphia: Lippincott-Raven.

CENTRAL NERVOUS SYSTEM PROPHYLAXIS

CNS relapse is a documented problem for patients with Burkitt's lymphoma (Raz, Siegal, & Polliack, 1984). Thus prophylaxis would appear prudent. Intrathecal chemotherapy and cranial irradiation are the current standards of care. Intrathecal chemotherapy can cross or overcome the blood-brain barrier, and the most common agents used for this purpose are methotrexate, cytarabine, thiotepa, or dexamethasone (Koeller & Fields, 1994; Yandle, 1996). Intrathecal chemotherapy should be delivered on a repetitive basis by means of lumbar punctures or via an Ommaya reservoir. (An Ommaya reservoir is a semipermanent subcutaneous access pump that delivers chemotherapy through the cerebral spinal fluid system by means of an intraventricular catheter connected to the reservoir (Yandle, 1996). Ommaya reservoirs may be utilized if lumbar punctures are unsuccessful due to scarring or blockage and provide better delivery of drug throughout cerebrospinal fluid (CSF). The reservoir requires surgical placement and infection is a risk. Long-term or high doses of intrathecal methotrexate are not without complications. According to Yandle, in children, seizures, somnolence, paraperesis, leukoencephalopathy, and even death have been associated with intrathecal methotrexate. In adults, both acute and chronic neurotoxicity has been documented.

Though CNS prophylaxis regimens differ, treatment should be given twice weekly until the CSF is cleared of lymphoma cells in three separate cytologic evaluations on the first visit, weekly for 4 weeks, and finally monthly through the duration of treatment.

Radiation to the craniospinal axis according to Sarna and Kagan (1995), has not been successful as a single modality in preventing meningeal spread by Burkitt's lymphoma cells. In combination with intrathecal or intraventricular (through the Ommaya reservoir) therapy, it may be a useful treatment tool.

Radiation Therapy

Radiation therapy as a single treatment therapy is not effective in Burkitt's lymphoma. The speed at which Burkitt's lymphoma cells grow and divide often produces disseminated disease, which makes it difficult to encompass specific radiation port sites. The rapid growth of the lymphoma may also allow the tumor to "escape" from daily radiation treatments according to Haskell. Attempts at using smaller doses of radiation more often (2 to 3 times per day) to achieve improved local control has not been widely accepted as a successful treatment modality nor has more-extended but lower-dose radiation doses to the abdomen proved effective (Sarna & Kagan, 1995).

Management of Burkitt's Lymphoma Relapse or Treatment Failures

Patients who have a slow response to primary therapy or who have other poor prognostic indicators may be evaluated early on in their course of treatment for marrow or blood stem cell transplant using bone marrow or peripheral blood stem cells (either autologous or allogeneic). Bone marrow and stem cell transplantation has been covered in previous chapters and will be discussed only briefly here.

Salvage therapy, or second-line therapy, should be initiated promptly for relapsed disease. A sample of salvage regimens often used are DHAP (dexamethasone, Ara-C, Platinol) ICE (ifosfamide, carboplatin, etoposide), or CE (cyclophosphamide, etoposide). Immediate initiation of request for insurance or primary financial support of transplant should be done as the duration of response may be short.

Autologous Blood or Bone Marrow Transplant

Autologous blood or marrow transplant for poor-risk or relapsed high-grade lymphomas is a treatment option that offers a potential cure to patients who would otherwise die of their aggressive disease. Patients with refractory Burkitt's lymphoma in relapse who do not respond to salvage chemotherapy appear not to benefit from high-dose therapy and succumb to their disease. Many transplant centers have demonstrated an actuarial survival rate of 10% to 50% disease-free survival for those patients with relapsed or poor-risk, high-grade lymphomas such as Burkitt's lymphoma (Appelbaum, Deisseroth, Graw, Herzig, Levine, & Magrath et al., 1978, Appelbaum, Sullivan, Buckner, Clift, Deeg, & Fefer et al., 1987; Blay & Phillip, 1992; Lister & Armitage 1995; Vose et al., 1993). Myeloablation followed by reinfusion of previously collected adequate numbers of marrow or blood stem cells allows hematopoietic engraftment and neutrophil recovery. Toxicities of transplant, such as infection, hemorrhage, veno-occlusive disease (VOD), or organ failure, are still issues to be overcome. Later complications such as secondary malignancies remain a problem (Darrington, Vose, Anderson, Bierman, Bishop, & Chan et al., 1994; Stone, Neuberg, Soiffer, Takvorian, Whelan, & Rabinowe et al., 1994).

Allogeneic Blood or Bone Marrow Transplant

Marrow grafting is pursued in patients for whom autologous transplant is not the most attractive or feasible option. Myelodysplasia, lymphomatous marrow involvement, or pelvic irradiation may exclude a patient from autologous harvest and transplant (Phillips, Herzig, Lazarus, Fay, Griffith, & Herzig, 1986). A graft versus lymphoma effect may also be sought, leading the practitioner to select allogeneic transplant as the preferred treatment option (Jones, Ambinder, Pitantadosi, & Santos, 1991). Long-term disease from survival rates are similar to those of the autologous population (Antin & Smith 1995; Appelbaum et al., 1987; Blay & Phillip, 1992).

NEW ADVANCES

Bone Marrow Purging

In autologous transplants, malignant clonogenic cells may be reinfused. Given the propensity for Burkitt's lymphoma to involve the bone marrow, many centers are investigating ways to "purge" or rid the blood or marrow stem cells of tumor. Monoclonal antibodies (MoAbs), cytotoxic agents, and cell separation techniques have been used by a variety of centers. No one method has been shown to be superior, and relapse after transplantation most often occurs in sites of previous disease (Blay & Phillip 1992). The role of purging remains controversial (Negrin, Keim, Schmidt-Wolf, Blume, & Cleary, 1991). In allogeneic bone marrow transplantation, T lymphocytes may be purged from the marrow graft by use of MoAbs. Although the incidence of graft versus host disease is decreased, the relapse rate is higher.

Radiolabeled Antibodies

Radiolabeled MoAbs may allow delivery of higher radiation doses to tumor sites. This would attempt to selectively target tumor cells, but the biodistribution of the radiolabeled antibodies may create an uneven pattern and the appropriate dose has not been determined. (Grossbard, Press, Appelbaum, Berstein & Nadler, 1992). Phase I/II trials are under way to evaluate the use of radiolabeled antibodies in autologous transplantation.

Biologic Response Modifiers (Immunotherapy)

Interleukin-2 (IL-2) has been shown to be effective in producing complete or partial responses in some relapsed lymphomas. A phase III trial by the Southwest Oncology Group (SWOG) is under way to assess if treatment with IL-2 post-autologous transplant will eliminate residual tumor cells. These cells may have survived the conditioning regimen or may have been reinfused with the marrow or stem cells.

The goal of the therapy would be to decrease the risk of relapse or eliminate minimal disease after transplant by stimulating an immunomodulating response and graft versus lymphoma effect. (IL-2 augments the function of T lymphocytes and natural killer cells and promotes the production of tumor necrosis factor [TNF] and interferon-γ.)

ONCOLOGIC EMERGENCIES

Tumor lysis syndrome is the most common complication associated with Burkitt's lymphoma. Other most commonly occurring emergent complications are superior vena cava (SVC) syndrome, and spinal cord compression (SCC). Tumor lysis syndrome occurs when rapidly proliferating cells are killed and their intracellular contents are released into the bloodstream. The spill of the intracellular debris into the circulation results in hyperuricemia, hyperkalemia, hyperphosphatemia and hypocalcemia (Moore, 1992; Groenwald, Frogge, Goodman, & Yarbro, 1995). These metabolic abnormalities are worsened in the face of pretherapy azotemia, which may be caused by renal involvement of Burkitt's cells, dehydration, or renal obstruction. If tumor lysis syndrome is not anticipated, observed for, and treated aggressively, renal failure and death can be the sequelae (Sarna & Kagan, 1995).

Pretreatment of tumor lysis syndrome includes the use of allopurinol (Zyloprim), a xanthine oxidase inhibitor that blocks uric acid metabolically, and the use of vigorous intravenous (IV) hydration, or hyperhydration. Alkalization of the urine by adding sodium bicarbonate ($NaHCo_3$) to IV hydration is often recommended; however, according to Sarna & Kagan (1995), this practice may contribute to calcium phosphate precipitation in the renal tubules and may be contraindicated. Close monitoring (every 6 to 8 hours) of metabolic parameters (electrolytes, BUN, CR, phosphatase, LDH, uric acid levels) is critical during treatment to allow for early intervention to correct abnormalities. Early symptoms of tumor lysis syndrome include weakness, muscle cramps, nausea, vomiting, diarrhea, lethargy, and paresthesia. Late symptoms include paralysis, bradycardia, hypotension, oliguria, edema, carpopidal spasm, laryngospasm, flank pain, hematuria, crystalluria, tetany, or convulsions (Moore, 1992).

Spinal Cord Compression

SCC occurs when tumor impinges on the spinal cord. SCC can be classified as to the level of cord involvement (i.e., cauda equina, sacral, lumbar, thoracic, or cervical region) and by the location (i.e., extradural or intradural, extravertebral, or intramedullary) of the compression. Permanent neurologic damage including paralysis can occur without prompt evaluation and emergent care. Presenting symptoms include pain that may be aggravated by coughing, sneezing or the Valsalva maneuver. Paresthesias, bowel or bladder incontinence, and motor weakness are also symptoms of SCC. Evaluation of the patient may include spine film or MRIs and must include a complete neurologic examination. Treatment is initiated quickly and may be multifocal. Steroids, analgesics, radiation therapy, chemotherapy, and/or surgical intervention may be used. Rehabilitation and recovery are improved when therapy initiated before extensive neurologic insult has occurred. Lymphomas account for approximately 12% of SCC cases (Couillard-Getreuer, 1992; Groenwald, Frogge, & Goodman, 1995).

Superior Vena Cava Syndrome

SVC syndrome is caused by obstruction of the great vessels of the chest by tumor, lymphadenopathy, or thrombosis. It results in a decrease in the venous drainage of the upper thorax. The sequela of this decrease is venous drainage, can be life-threatening, and if untreated, it can result in cerebral edema, pulmonary complications or death.

Clinical signs include face, neck, chest and upper extremity edema, as well as development of collateral blood vessels in chest or dilatation of collateral torso vessels. Plethora of the face, neck, chest, and breasts is common. Conjunctiva swelling and redness can occur. Cerebral edema results in headache, visual changes, vertigo, and altered mentation. Cerebral edema signs and symptoms are often late signs of obstruction. Airway obstruction, stridor, cough, hoarseness and respiratory distress are all possible results (Kreamer, 1992).

The treatment should be initiated promptly and may include chemotherapy, radiotherapy, steroids or a combined modality approach. A histologic diagnosis should be made,

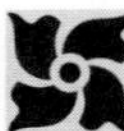

TABLE 63-8 Standard of Care for the Patient Receiving Chemotherapy

Patient Problem and Outcomes	Nursing Interventions and Rationales	Patient Instructions
Knowledge Deficit		
Patient will verbalize an understanding of the purpose, benefits, and risks of diagnostic evaluation, and chemotherapy.	1. Assess patient's level of knowledge about diagnostic tests. 2. Assess patient's level of knowledge about chemotherapy. a. Assess patient's concern and fears about chemotherapy.	1. Describe the procedures involved. a. Computed tomography b. Bone marrow biopsy and aspirate c. Lumbar puncture d. Blood work 2. Describe the following: a. Major side effects associated with chemotherapy. b. Importance of notifying the nurse should side effects occur. c. Self-care measures to manage the side effects of the following: (1) Nausea and vomiting (2) Mucositis (3) Diarrhea (4) Fatigue (5) Fever (6) Bleeding
Nausea and Vomiting		
Patient will be able to maintain adequate nutritional intake to maintain metabolic equilibrium and stable weight.	1. Assess patient's level of understanding regarding immediate or delayed causes of N/V. 2. Assess patient's level of knowledge about chemotherapy. a. Assess patients concern and fears about chemotherapy.	1. Discuss interventions to minimize occurrence, severity, or complications of N/V: a. Modify environment. b. Limit exposure to noxious sights and smells. c. Modify diet; provide bland, cool foods; increase calorie-containing fluids. d. Antiemetics before meals or around the clock per physician direction for periods of increased risk of N/V. e. Instruct patient to observe for signs of dehydration (dry mouth, lightheaded, dizzy, reduction in urine output). f. Report any signs of blood in emesis. g. Teach relaxation techniques (cool cloth to forehead, mental imagery, visualization and breathing exercises). h. Notify health care personnel if above measures ineffective.

N/V, nausea and vomiting.

but emergent therapy can be instituted if syndrome is life-threatening. Resolution of symptoms is dramatic in SVC syndrome due to tumor involvement. If a patient with SVC syndrome is unresponsive, there should be further investigation to discover the exact source of obstruction.

Nursing Management

The nursing management of patients with an NHL of Burkitt's lymphoma has been discussed in detail throughout this decade (Hubbard, 1996; Rahr & Tucker, 1990; Reed & Franco, 1992.). Anxiety, fear, and depression at diagnosis, as well as the rapidity at which diagnosis staging and initiation of therapy occurs can be overwhelming for a patient with Burkitt's lymphoma. Patients do not have time to "adjust" to their disease before plunging headlong into their treatment regimen, they and may appear bewildered or unable to comprehend the multitude of tasks before them. The patient may initially be hospitalized for surgery (if necessary) and for his or her first cycle of chemotherapy. Hospitalization is often desired for initiation of chemotherapy to ensure adequate monitoring for tumor lysis syndrome. The majority of additional therapy will then be undertaken in the outpatient setting (unless transplantation is pursued).

Early on, the focus of nursing care is designed to support patients through their staging workup with descriptions of the tests involved and the preparations required for each examination. A patient's fears may be allayed by explanations of abbreviations for tests and his or her role in the staging process. Patients must learn a new vocabulary that entails

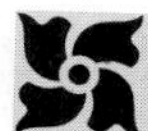

TABLE 63-8 Standard of Care for the Patient Receiving Chemotherapy—cont'd

Patient Problem and Outcomes	Nursing Interventions and Rationales	Patient Instructions
Mucositis		
Patient will maintain adequate oral intake, verbalize comfort, and be without signs of active infection.	1. Assess oral intake including frequency, quality and quantity. 2. Assess patient's level of comfort using a scale of 0 (no pain) to 10 (maximum pain). 3. Assess patient's mucosa for erythema, breakdown, or lesions. 4. Obtain dietary consult, if mucositis is severe.	1. Teach patient to maintain fluid intake diary and monitor for nutritional foods and fluid entered. a. Monitor for signs of dehydration as discussed above. 2. Teach patient to use the following analgesic measures: a. Administer topical analgesia. b. Administer systemic analgesia. c. Administer frequent oral care. d. Modify diet to avoid spicy, acidic, or rough foods. e. Provide alternative means of communication if patient unable to speak. f. Meticulous perianal hygiene (e.g., sitz baths). 3. Teach patient to conduct the following: a. Assess oral mucosa for lesions and assess perianal area for lesions, breakdown, redness or areas of discomfort. b. Report any signs of infection.
Diarrhea		
Patient will maintain adequate fluid intake, weight, and performance status.	1. Assess elimination patterns including amount, frequency, and descriptive characteristics. 2. Adapt diet to avoid foods that are high in fiber or fat, and avoid dairy products, if lactose intolerant. 3. Administer antidiarrheal medication (e.g., Kaopectate, Imodium, or Lomotil) 4. Obtain dietary consult. 5. Assess for sequelae of prolonged periods of diarrhea: a. Electrolyte imbalance b. Weakness c. Dehydration d. Infectious causes	1. Teach patient to modify diet if diarrhea occurs. 2. Teach patient to administer antidiarrheal medications if stool is liquid and estimated volume is greater than 300 ml/24 hours. 3. Teach patient to keep food diary to assess for foods that exacerbate diarrhea. 4. Instruct patient in perianal skin care: a. Sitz baths b. Skin medications (topical) c. External hemorrhoid medications 5. Teach patient to report: a. Persistent diarrhea for greater than 2 days b. Fever greater than 100.4° F (38° C) c. Abdominal discomfort, cramps d. Any open peri-rectal areas

Continued

complicated testing terms, chemotherapy names, and consequences of therapy, which include neutropenia, thrombocytopenia, and anemia. Further education is provided at each juncture in the treatment algorithm, since high-dose chemotherapy (blood or marrow stem cell transplantation) may be considered if patients present with high-risk factors or respond slowly to therapy (Bierman, Vose, & Armitage, 1995; Prizzere 1995). Symptom management is critical to maintain optimal quality of life as the patient moves through therapy. Nausea, vomiting, mucositis, fatigue, pain control, and anxiety are all key components of the patient's experience.

As patients initiate therapy, the most critical standards of care encompass the administration of chemotherapy and its sequelae and the monitoring for and treatment of tumor lysis syndrome. The nursing management is summarized below, and the standards of care can be noted in Tables 63-8 and 63-9.

When patients with Burkitt's lymphoma undergo a surgical procedure (e.g., resection), the nursing care of this patient population is similar to the needs of patients with abdominal tumors. Therefore this discussion will not be covered here.

Chemotherapy Administration

Since antineoplastic therapy is the cornerstone of treatment, nursing interventions must have a multifaceted focus. Knowledge deficits related to diagnosis, staging, and chemotherapy administration, potentials for alterations in pro-

Table 63-8 Standard of Care for the Patient Receiving Chemotherapy—cont'd

Patient Problem and Outcomes	Nursing Interventions and Rationales	Patient Instructions
Fatigue		
Patient will be able to maintain modest activities of daily living.	1. Assess patient's level of fatigue, using a 0 (full of energy) to 10 (total exhaustion) rating scale. 2. Evaluate patient's current sleep pattern and teach energy conservation activities.	1. Inform patient that fatigue is multifactoral and may persist throughout treatment. 2. Teach patient energy conservation strategies: a. Prioritize activity. b. Pace energy expenditures. c. Use frequent rest periods. d. Maximize nutrition. e. Delegate nonessential activities. f. Short periods of exercise daily. g. Correct physiological causes of fatigue (anemia). h. Adjust medications (steroids) to reduce insomnia and side effects and to promote adequate rest. i. Avoid caffeine.
Alteration in Protective Mechanisms		
Patient will verbalize an understanding of the definition of, sequelae, and treatment for anemia, neutropenia, thrombocytopenia.	1. Assess patient's level of knowledge about implications of blood work and different components of CBC, including WBC, RBC, and platelet counts. 2. Assess patient's CBC.	1. Describe the function of each component of the CBC in simple terms: a. RBC b. WBC c. Platelet 2. Describe the major side effects, as well as the medical and nursing management associated with the following: a. Anemia b. Thrombocytopenia c. Neutropenia
Anemia		
Patient will maintain ADLs and be without signs of active bleeding.	1. Assess and evaluate for level of fatigue (see previous patient problem). 2. Monitor patient's blood counts with particular emphasis on hemoglobin and hematocrit. 3. Provide red blood cell support with the following: a. Transfusions b. Nutritional support: vitamins, iron c. Epoetin-alpha NOTE: Administer above on direction of physicians.	1. Educate patient to review medications with each clinic visit. 2. Teach patient to report signs and symptoms of anemia: a. Pale skin b. Shortness of breath c. Sensation of rapid heart rate d. Lightheadedness, dizziness e. Headache, changes in thinking processes f. Any bleeding such as nose bleeding, vaginal bleeding 3. Teach patient safety precautions: a. Avoid sudden change in position. b. Request assistance with ADL and ambulation. c. Avoid driving or operation of machinery if lightheaded or faint.
Thrombocytopenia		
Patient will be without signs of active bleeding.	1. Monitor patient's blood count with particular attention to platelet count. 2. Recognize level of severity and implications of different levels of thrombocytopenia (severe or moderately severe) to educate patient in safety measures.	1. Teach patient to manage thrombocytopenia: a. Explain relationship between platelets and bleeding. b. Explain relationship between a moderately low platelet count and the risk of bleeding. c. Instruct client/family to assess daily for signs and symptoms of bleeding.

ADL, Activity of daily living; *CBC*, complete blood count; *RBC*, red blood cell; *WBC*, white blood cell.

TABLE 63-8 Standard of Care for the Patient Receiving Chemotherapy—cont'd

Patient Problem and Outcomes	Nursing Interventions and Rationales	Patient Instructions
Thrombocytopenia—cont'd		
	3. Provide supportive medical therapy with platelet transfusion. 4. Avoidance of drugs that inhibit platelet function. 5. Monitor patient's blood count with particular attention to platelet count. 6. Recognize level of severity and implications of different levels of thrombocytopenia severe (<20,000 mm^3) or moderately severe (<50,000 mm^3) to educate patient in safety measures. 7. Provide supportive medical therapy with platelet transfusion. 8. Avoid drugs that inhibit platelet function.	2. Discuss measures to prevent bleeding: a. Avoid forceful nose blowing. b. Prevent constipation. c. Use electric razors for shaving; do not use razor blades. d. Avoid tight and restrictive clothing. e. For female patients, use sanitary napkins instead of tampons. f. Use water-based lubricant before sexual intercourse. g. Avoid taking aspirin, non-steroidal anti-inflammatory drugs (e.g., Advil, Motrin, Indocin) and blood thinners (Coumadin) or anything that contains aspirin (e.g., cold and influenza remedies) 3. Describe signs and symptoms that should be reported: a. Bruising, petechiae, hematomas on skin b. Bleeding gums c. Black or red color in stools d. Blood in urine e. Blood in emesis or coffee ground color f. Dizziness or light-headedness especially when standing from a sitting, lying, or stooping position g. Change in mental status—sign of intracranial bleeding h. Scleral bleeding, nose bleeding i. Increased pad count or prolonged menstrual flow j. Signs/symptoms of bleeding after a fall
Neutropenia		
Patient will be without signs of active infection.	1. Monitor patient's blood counts, with particular emphasis on WBCs and differential, to be able to instruct patient as to the risk of infection related to WBCs and, in particular, his or her neutrophil count. 2. Evaluate and assess patient with each visit for any signs or symptoms of infection as reviewed in patient instructions. The nurse should recognize that subtle changes may indicate onset of sepsis, localized symptoms may be absent, and steroid therapy can mask signs of infection.	1. Explain relationship of WBC levels (neutrophils) to the infectious process. 2. Instruct patient/family to assess daily and as needed for signs and symptoms of infection and report to health care professional: a. Temperature more than 100.4° F (38° C) b. Chills c. Cough lasting longer than 2 days d. Pain when urinating or having bowel movement e. Vaginal discharge f. Central catheter erythema, tenderness, or pain g. Rash h. Open skin areas or lesions i. Change in behavior or mentation
Patient will have active signs of infection	1. Monitor patient's blood counts, with particular emphasis on WBCs and differential, to be able to instruct patient as to the risk of infection related to WBCs and, in particular, his or her neutrophil count. 2. Evaluate and assess patient with each visit for any signs or symptoms of infection as reviewed in patient instructions. The nurse should recognize that subtle changes may indicate onset of sepsis; localized symptoms may be absent; and steroid therapy can mask signs of infection.	1. Discuss measures to reduce risk of infection: a. Frequent and appropriate handwashing b. No contact with people who have transmissible diseases c. Avoidance of crowds d. Frequent temperature checks (at least twice a day) e. Avoid use of acetaminophen (may mask fever) f. Scrupulous personal hygiene g. Frequent oral care h. Avoid trauma to rectum (no suppositories or enemas) i. Low-bacteria diet 2. Prompt medical/nursing intervention if any signs of infection

TABLE 63-9 Standard of Care for the Patient at Risk for Tumor Lysis Syndrome

Patient Problem and Outcomes	Nursing Interventions and Rationales	Patient Instructions
Fluid and Electrolyte Imbalance		
Patient will have normal serum electrolytes and close observation of metabolic parameters that enables identification of tumor lysis syndrome.	1. Assess baseline renal function and serum electrolytes to be able to assess deviation from baseline and note duration. 2. Evaluate and assess patient for symptoms of tumor lysis by frequent blood draws and educating patient to rationale for same. 3. Intervene to control tumor lysis syndrome by use of the following: a. Pharmacologic agents (allopurinol, $NaHCO_3$) b. Mechanical means (dialysis, hyperhydration with forced diuresis) c. Correction with metabolic abnormalities	1. Describe to the patient the process of cell breakdown and release of by-products into blood and implication of the same. 2. Provide patient with information as to frequency of laboratory draws, need for vigorous hydration, and close monitoring of intake and output and daily weights. 3. Provide patient with copies of laboratory values to illustrate and explain cellular destruction. 4. Teach patient importance of maintaining adequate oral intake and recognizing significance of the following: a. Low urine output b. Muscle cramps c. Flank pain d. Weakness e. Change in mental status f. Paresthesias g. Seizures

From Miaskowski, C. (1997). Oncologic emergencies. In R. McCorkle, M. Grant, M. Frank-Stromborg, & S. Baird (Eds.), *Cancer nursing: A comprehensive textbook.* (2nd ed.). Philadelphia: W. B. Saunders; Yarbro, C. H. & McFadden, M. E. (1997). Malignant lymphomas. In S. L. Groenwald, M. H. Frogge, M. Goodman, & C. H. Yarbro (Eds.), *Cancer nursing: Principles and practice.* (4th ed.). Boston: Jones and Bartlett.

tective mechanisms, and changes in performance status and quality of life lead the list of experiences with which the patient must be educated and equipped to deal. Complicating factors such as tumor lysis syndrome must be scrupulously monitored for and treated aggressively to prevent renal failure or death of the patient.

HOME CARE ISSUES

The patient receiving chemotherapy for Burkitt's lymphoma requires ongoing assessment in several arenas. Since the chemotherapy treatment intent is to keep the patient on schedule and at maximum doses to achieve optimal benefit, the patient may not have adequate time to recover to full physical, social, and psychological function before initiating the next cycle of therapy.

Patients and caregivers are taught central catheter dressing changes, flushing of central catheters, and even how to draw blood from their catheters and other tasks. Nurses educate patients to observe for signs and symptoms of infection and bleeding and to report them to health care professionals. Patients receive "layered" levels of instructions based on where they are in their chemotherapy cycle and what their degree of risk is for infection or bleeding. Lower levels of platelets or white blood cells indicate different levels of risk, and patients are instructed accordingly for the home setting. See Boxes 63-4 and 63-5 for home care instructions for patients at risk for bleeding and neutropenic episodes.

Nutrition maintenance is an issue for this patient population. Chemotherapy can alter taste sensations, and nausea, vomiting, diarrhea, and mucositis are all common side effects of therapy. Maximizing nutrition is a challenge and may require ongoing dietary manipulations, encouraging personal preferences and dietary consults.

Body image issues rise to the forefront as patients continue in their treatment course. The chemotherapy agents most efficacious in eradicating the disease also cause significant hair loss. The period of hair loss is an emotionally distressing time and usually occurs several weeks after the patient has experienced chemotherapy. Hair loss may also encompass other hair-producing body areas such as the genitalia, chest, nares, and extremities, and it is an ongoing reminder to the patient of his or her illness.

Because of the rapidity of onset of the disease, patients with Burkitt's lymphoma often do not have time to address future fertility issues. Sperm banking and ovum storage are often time-consuming tasks, and it may not be possible to delay treatment to provide adequate assessment for banking and storage time. As the patient completes therapy, this may be an issue that resurfaces (Rahr & Tucker, 1990; Tucker & Rahr, 1990).

Education of the patient and caregiver is an ongoing flow of information throughout the patient's treatment life in the home setting. Initial education focuses on staging studies and the impact of diagnosis. It then moves on to chemotherapy agents to be given and transitions to education as to

Box 63-4
Bleeding Precautions

Platelets help blood clot. A low platelet count means you are at risk for bleeding. *Thrombocytopenia* is another term for having a low platelet count. Thrombocytopenia precautions are rules to follow to lower your risk of bleeding until your platelet counts return to normal.

1. Some drugs like aspirin or ibuprofen lower your clotting ability. Do not take aspirin or other drugs that would increase your bleeding risk without talking with your doctor.
2. Do not take rectal temperatures or insert rectal suppositories or enemas or vaginal douches. If you believe you need to do so, check first with your doctor.
3. It is important that you not get constipated because hard stools can cause you to bleed rectally. You may need to take a stool softener or laxative.
4. Use sanitary napkins instead of tampons for monthly periods
5. Do not use blade razors to shave. Electric razors are appropriate to use.
6. Do not bend over so that your head is lower than your shoulders. Bend with your knees and keep your head up.
7. If you need to blow your nose, do so carefully.
8. Don't wear tight clothes such as underwear with tight elastic or tight jeans.
9. Call a family member to help you in and out of bed if you are at all unsteady. Do not do anything that puts you at risk for a fall or a bump. Walk more slowly than usual so that you do not knock against furniture or equipment. Use a cane or walker if necessary. Report any signs of bleeding to your doctor.
10. Report any of the following right away:
    - Bleeding of the gums that does not stop right away
    - Nosebleeds
    - Black or bloody stools
    - Vomit that looks like it contains coffee grounds
    - Cloudy or reddish urine
    - Petechiae (small bright red spots on your skin)
    - Greater than normal vaginal bleeding
    - Changes in neurologic signs (e.g., drowsiness or vision problems)

If you have any questions, please ask your nurse or doctor.

Box 63-5
Low White Blood Cell Precautions

When your white blood cell (WBC) count gets too low, you are at great risk for infection. To protect you, we suggest the following guidelines that help protect you from infections:

1. Avoid crowds and people with infections.
2. Do not allow people with colds, influenza, diarrhea, or infections to visit you at home. Children are a particular risk to you since they may be exposed to illness at school or play. Talk with your nurse and doctor about your own needs for having visitors.
3. Wash your hands often and practice rigorous hygiene. Family members and visitors should do the same.
4. Do not use suppositories, tampons, or douches.
5. Avoid raw fruits and vegetables unless they can be washed and peeled or cooked.
6. Place plants in a separate room until your white blood cell count improves.
7. Drink regular tap water. Change your glass, water, and straw at least every 4 to 8 hours. Use clean utensils or glasses. Do not share drinks or food, or eat or drink from other people's glasses or plates.
8. Pets can carry diseases that you may catch. If you touch them, wash your hands well afterward. Have someone else take care of pet waste (e.g., kitty litter).
9. Call your doctor right away if you have any of the following:
    - Fever, aching, or chills
    - Tenderness or redness of the central venous catheter site
    - Excessive fatigue
    - Blisters on the lips, mouth sores or sore throat
    - Burning or painful urination
    - Skin sores or rash
    - Cough with sputum production and/or sinus tenderness
    - Earache
    - Drainage from the eyes
    - Unusual or foul smelling vaginal discharge
    - Diarrhea

the sequelae of therapy. It persists with discussions of late effects of therapy in biomedical, psychosocial, economic, and legal aspects. All require ongoing adjustment for the patient and family (Leigh 1992).

EVALUATION OF THE QUALITY OF CARE

The quality of care provided to oncology patients must have an ongoing evaluation by accreditation organizations. These evaluations would focus on the standard of care provided by the Joint Commission for the Accreditation of Healthcare Organizations and the Oncology Nursing Society.

In a patient receiving chemotherapy for Burkitt's lymphoma, side effects from chemotherapy are a big issue and can be addressed by the multidisciplinary team. Oncology nurses represent the key component in the care of cancer patients and have access to the teaching and evaluation of the teaching methods used.

Table 63-10 provides examples of quality-of-care evaluation tools that can be used for patients receiving chemotherapy in inpatient or outpatient settings. If side effects from chemotherapy are not controlled with traditional pharmacologic methods, alternative methods may be employed, such as visual imagery and relaxation techniques. Ways to make the patient comfortable are available, and help from the multidisciplinary team may be initiated.

PROGNOSIS

The prognosis for the patient with Burkitt's lymphoma is reliant on the chemosensitivity of the disease and the number or presence of adverse risk factors. Patients with respon-

TABLE 63-10 Quality of Care Evaluation for a Patient Undergoing Chemotherapy

Disciplines participating in the quality of care evaluation:
☐ Nursing ☐ Pharmacy ☐ Social Services

I. Patient education

Data from: ☐ Medical Record Review
☐ Patient/Family Interview
☐ Pharmacist

Criteria	Yes	No
1. Patient provided with information about chemotherapy:		
a. Antiemetics	☐	☐
b. Oral care	☐	☐
c. Drop in blood counts	☐	☐
2. Complete blood counts evaluated daily	☐	☐
3. Patient experienced the following:		
a. Nausea/vomiting	☐	☐
b. Mucositis	☐	☐
c. Neutropenia	☐	☐

II. Patient/family satisfaction

Data from: ☐ Patient Interview
☐ Family Interview

Criteria	Yes	No
1. On a scale of 0 to 10, with 0 being totally dissatisfied and 10 being totally satisfied, how satisfied were you with the explanation of the side effects of chemotherapy you received. 0 ______________________10		
2. Did the health care provider explain to you that you might experience some of the following side effects from your chemotherapy?		
a. Nausea/vomiting	☐	☐
b. Sore mouth	☐	☐
c. Drop in blood counts	☐	☐
3. Were you told to call the health care provider if you had a fever?	☐	☐
4. Were you taught measures to relieve nausea/vomiting?	☐	☐
5. Were you taught measures to relieve pain with mucositis?	☐	☐

sive disease and without poor prognostic indicators can enjoy long-term, disease-free survival rates of up to 75% (Yandle, 1996; Lister & Armitage, 1995). However, the patients with poor prognostic indicators can expect only approximately 20% chance of long-term, disease-free survival (Lister and Armitage, 1995). The rapid pace of Burkitt's lymphoma may allow for early prognosticating as the patients who do not respond to chemotherapy succumb quickly to their disease.

RESEARCH ISSUES

Research issues abound in the Burkitt's lymphoma area. The role of viruses such as EBV, herpes virus, and HIV is being studied (Aranjo, Foss, Bittencourt, Hummel, Demel, & Mendonca et al., 1996; Kingma,Weiss, Jaffe, Kumar, Frekko, & Raffield, 1996; Nador, Cesarman, Chadburn, Dawson, Ansari, & Said et al., 1996). Detecting minimal residual disease after treatment remains a challenge, even though Burkitt's lymphoma recurs rapidly, if persistent, after primary therapy (Erickson, Dessev, Lisher, Phillips, Robinson, & Drabkin, 1996). Lymphoma vaccines are being investigated and remain a high-priority research area by the NCI, as do other study pathways that attempt to "turn on" the body's immune system (Kwak, Campbell, Czerwinski, Hart, Miller, & Levy, 1992; Staff, 1993). The multidrug resistance gene (mdr 1) and the genomic and cytogenetic abnormalities associated with Burkitt's lymphoma continue to be evaluated with the eventual goal being control of the disease on a molecular level (Yuen & Sikic, 1994).

REFERENCES

Anonymous. (1993). Moving forward with a "second" generation lymphoma vaccine. *Journal of the National Cancer Institute, 85*(2), 91-92.

Antin, J. & Smith, B. (1995). Bone marrow transplantation. In R. Handin, S. Lux, & T. Stossel (Eds.), *Blood principles and practice of hematology.* Philadelphia: J. B. Lippincott.

Appelbaum, F., Deisseroth, A., Graw, R., Herzig, G., Levine, A., Magrath, I., Pizzo, P., Poplack, D., & Ziegler, J. (1978). Prolonged complete remission following high-dose chemotherapy of Burkitt's lymphoma in relapse. *Cancer, 41,* 1059-1063.

Appelbaum, F., Sullivan, K., Buckner, D., Clift, R., Deeg, J., Fefer, A., Hill, R., Mortimer, J., Neiman, P., Sanders, J., Singer, J., Stewart, P., Storb, R., & Thomas, E. D. (1987). Treatment of malignant lymphoma in 100 patients with chemotherapy, total body irradiation, and marrow transplantation. *Journal of Clinical Oncology, 5*(9), 1340-1347.

Aranjo, I., Foss, H., Bittencourt, A., Hummel, M., Demel, G., Mendonca, N., Herbst, H., & Stein, H. (1996). Expression of Epstein-Barr virus gene products in Burkitt's lymphoma in northeast Brazil. *Blood, 87*(12), 5279-5286.

Bierman, P., Vose, J., & Armitage, J. (1995). Clinical manifestations and staging of and therapy for non–Hodgkin's lymphoma. In R. Hoffman, E. Benz, S. Shattil, B. Furie, H. Cohen, & L. Silberstein (Eds.), *Hematology: Basic principles and practice* (2nd ed.). New York: Churchill Livingstone.

Blay, J. & Philip, T. (1992). High-dose therapy in Burkitt's lymphoma. In J. Armitage & K. Antman (Eds.), *High-dose cancer therapy.* Baltimore: Williams and Wilkins.

Burkitt, D. (1958). A sarcoma involving the jaws in African children. *British Journal of Surgery, 46,* 218-223.

Casciato, D. & Lowitz, B. (1988). Non–Hodgkin's lymphoma. In D. Casciato & B. Lowitz (Eds.), *Manual of clinical oncology* (2nd ed.). Boston: Little, Brown.

Chow, V. T. (1993). Cancer and viruses. *Annals of the Academy of Medicine, 22*(2), 163-169.

Cohen, M., Bennett, J., Berard, C., Ziegler, J., Vogel, C., Sheagren, J., & Carbone, P. (1969). Burkitt's tumor in the United States. *Cancer, 23,* 1259-1272.

Couillard-Getreuer, D. (1992). Spinal cord compression. In B. Johnson & J. Gross (Eds.), *Handbook of oncology nursing.* Boston: Jones and Bartlett.

Darrington, D., Vose, J., Anderson, J., Bierman, P., Bishop, M., Chan, W., Morris, M., Reed, E., Sanger, W., Tarantolo, S., Weisenburger, D., Kessinger, A., & Armitage, J. (1994). Incidence and characterization of secondary myelodysplastic syndrome and acute myelogenous leukemia following high-dose chemoradiotherapy and autologous stem cell transplant for lymphoid malignancies. *Journal of Clinical Oncology, 2*(12), 2527-2534.

Erickson, P., Dessev, G., Lisher, R., Phillips, G., Robinson, M., & Drabkin, H. (1996). ETO and AML1 phosphoproteins are expressed in CD34+ hematopoietic progenitors: Implications for t(8;21) leukomogenesis and monitoring residual disease. *Blood, 88*(5), 1813-1823.

Frappaz, D., Bouffet, E., Blay, J., Philip, T., & Brunat-Mentigny D. (1995) Childhood lymphoma. In M. Abelhoff, J. Armitage, A. Lichter, & J. Niderhuber (Eds.), *Clinical oncology.* New York: Churchill Livingstone.

Groenwald, S., Frogge, M.H., Goodman, M., & Yarbro, C. (1995). Manifestation of cancer and its treatment. In S. Groenwold, M. H. Frogge, M. Goodman, & C. Yarbro (Eds.), *A clinical guide to cancer nursing.* Boston: Jones and Bartlett.

Grossbard, M., Press, O, Appelbaum, F., Bernstein, I., & Nadler, L. (1992). Monoclonal antibody–based therapies of leukemias and lymphomas. *Blood, 80*(4), 863-878.

Hoover, R. (1992). Lymphoma risks in population with altered immunity: A search for mechanism. *Cancer Research (Suppl) 52,* 5477s-5478s.

Hubbard, S. (1996). Current issues and controversies in the management of non–Hodgkin's lymphoma. *Educational Monolith, 2,* 1-39. New York: Tricilinca Communications.

Jagannath, S., Velasquez, W., Tucker, S., Fuller, L., McLaughlin, P., Manning, J., North, L., & Cabanillas, F. (1986). Tumor burden assessment and its implication for a prognostic model in advance diffuse large-cell lymphoma. *Journal of Clinical Oncology 4(6),* 859-865.

Jones, R., Ambinder, R., Piantadosi, S., & Santos, G. (1991). Evidence of a graft-versus-lymphoma effect associated with allogeneic bone marrow transplantation. *Blood 77*(3), 649-653.

Kaufman, B., Burgert, E., & Banks, P. (1987). Abdominal Burkitt's lymphoma: Role of early aggressive surgery. *Journal of Pediatric Surgery, 22*(7), 671-674.

Kemeny, M., Magrath, I., & Brennan, M. (1982). The role of surgery in the management of American Burkitt's lymphoma and its treatment. *Annals of Surgery, 196,* 82-86.

Kingma, D., Weiss, W., Jaffee, E., Kumar, S., Frekko, K., & Raffield, M. (1996). Epstein-Barr virus latent membrane protein-1 oncogene deletions: Correlations with malignancy in Epstein-Barr virus–associated lymphoproliferative disorders and malignant lymphomas. *Blood, 88*(1), 242-251.

Koeller, J. & Fields, S. (1994). Alternative routes of chemotherapy administration. In R. Dorr & D. VonHoff (Eds.), *Cancer chemotherapy handbook* (2nd ed.). Norwalk, CT: Appleton and Lange.

Kreamer, K., (1992). Superior vena cava syndrome. In B. Johnson & J. Gross (Eds.), *Handbook of oncology nursing.* Boston: Jones and Bartlett.

Kwak, L., Campbell, M., Czerwinski, D. Hart, S., Miller, R., & Levy, R. (1992). Induction of immune-responses in patients with B-cell lymphoma against the surface-immunoglobulin idiotype expressed by their tumors. *New England Journal of Medicine, 327*(17), 1209-1215.

Leigh, S. (1992). Myths, monsters and magic: Personal perspectives and professional challenges of survival. *Oncology Nursing Forum, 19*(10), 1475-1480.

Levine, P.H., Connelly, A., Berard, C., O'Connor, G., Dorfman, R., Easton, J., & DeVita, V. T. (1975). The American Burkitt's lymphoma registry: A progress report. *Annals of Internal Medicine 83,* 31-36.

Levine, P., Kamaraju, L., Connelly, R., Berard, C., Dorfman, R., Magrath, I., & Easton, J. (1982). The American Burkitt's lymphoma registry: Eight years' experience. *Cancer, 4,* 1016-1022.

Lister, T. & Armitage, J. (1995). Non–Hodgkin's lymphomas. In M. Abeloff, J. Armitage, A. Lichter, & J. Niederhuber (Eds.), *Clinical oncology.* New York: Churchill Livingstone.

Long., D., DeVita, V. T., Jaffe, E., Mauch, P., & Urba, W. (1993). Lymphocytic lymphomas. In V. T. DeVita, S. Hellman, & S. A. Rosenberg (Eds.), *Cancer: Principles and practice of oncology* (4th ed.). Philadelphia: Lippincott-Raven.

Magrath I., Jain, V., & Bhatia, K. (1996). Epstein-Barr virus and Burkitt's lymphoma. *Seminars in Cancer Biology, 3*(5), 285-295.

McFadden, M. (1993). Malignant lymphomas. In L. Groenwald, M. Frogge, M. Goodman, & C. Yarbro (Eds.), *Cancer nursing: Principles and practice* (3rd ed.). Boston: Jones and Bartlett.

Medeiros, L. J. & Jaffe, E. S. (1996). Pathology of non–Hodgkin's lymphomas and Hodgkin's disease. In P. Wiernih, G. Canellos, J. P. Dutcher, & R. Kyke (Eds.), *Neoplastic diseases of the blood* (3rd ed.). Churchill Livingstone.

Melnyk, A. & Rodriguez, A. (1995). Intermediate and high-grade non–Hodgkin's lymphoma. In R. Pazdur (Ed.), *Medical oncology: A comprehensive review* (2nd ed.). Huntington, NY: PRR.

Miaskowski, C. (1997). Oncologic emergencies. In R. McCorkle, M. Grant, M. Frank-Stromborg, & S. Baird (Eds.), *Cancer nursing: A comprehensive textbook.* (2nd ed.). Philadelphia: W. B. Saunders.

Moore, J. (1992) Tumor lysis syndrome. In B. Johnson & J. Gross (Eds.), *Handbook of oncology nursing.* Boston: Jones and Bartlett.

Murphy, S. (1980) Classification, staging and end results of treatment of childhood non–Hodgkin's lymphomas: Dissimilarities from lymphomas in adults. *Seminars in Oncology 7*(3), 2332-2339.

Nador, R., Cesarman, E., Chadburn, A., Dawson, D., Ansari, M., Said, J., & Knowles, D. (1996). Primary-effusion lymphoma: A distinct clinicopathologic entity associated with the Kaposi's sarcoma–associated herpes virus. *Blood 88*(2), 645-656.

Negrin, R., Kiem, H.P, Schmidt-Wolf, I., Blume, K., & Cleary, M., (1991). Use of polymerase chain reaction to monitor the effectiveness of ex-vivo tumor cell purging. *Blood 77*(3), 654-660.

Phillips, G., Herzig, R., Lazarus, H., Fay, J., Griffith, R., & Herzig, G. (1986). High-dose chemotherapy, fractionated total-body irradiation and allogeneic marrow transplantation for malignant lymphoma. *Journal of Clinical Oncology,* 4(4), 480-488.

Poplack, D., Kun, L., Pizzo, P., & Magrath, I. (1993) Leukemias and lymphomas of childhood. In V. T. DeVita, S., Hellman, & S. A. Rosenberg (Eds.), *Cancer; Principles and practice of oncology* (4th ed.). Philadelphia: Lippincott-Raven.

Prizzere, T. (1995). Non–Hodgkin's lymphomas: pathologic features and clinical correlation. In R. Hoffman, E. Benz, S. Shattil, B. Furie, H. Cohen, & L. Silberstein (Eds.), *Hematology basic principles and practice.* (2nd ed.). New York: Churchill Livingstone.

Rahr, V. & Tucker, R., (1990). Non–Hodgkin's lymphoma: Understanding the disease. *Cancer Nursing, 13*(1), 56-61.

Raz, I., Siegal, T., Siegal, T., & Polliack, A., (1984). CNS involvement by non–Hodgkin's lymphoma. *Archives of Neurology, 4,* 1167-1171.

Reed, E. & Franco, T. (1992). Nursing for patients receiving high-dose chemotherapy with hematopoietic rescue. In J. Armitage & K. Antman (Eds.), *High-dose cancer therapy.* Baltimore: Williams and Wilkins.

Sarna, G. & Kagan, A. R., (1995) Small noncleaved cell lymphoma (Burkitt's and non-Burkitt's types). In C. Haskell (Eds.), *Cancer treatment medicine.* Philadelphia: W. B. Saunders.

Shamberger, R. & Weinstein, H., (1992). The role of surgery in abdominal Burkitt's lymphoma. *Journal of Pediatric Surgery, 27*(2), 236-240.

Shipp, M. A., Mauch, P. M., & Harris, N. L. (1997) Non–Hodgkin's lymphoma. In V. T. DeVita, S. Hellman, & S. A. Rosenberg (Eds.), *Cancer: Principles and practice of oncology* (5th ed.). Philadelphia: Lippincott-Raven.

Stone, R., Neuberg, D., Soiffer, T. Takvorian, T., Whelan, M., Rabinowe, S., Aster, J., Lavitt, P., Mauch, P., Freedman, A., & Nadler, L. (1994). Myelodysplastic syndrome as a late complication following autologous bone marrow transplantation for non-Hodgkin's lymphoma. *Journal of Clinical Oncology 12*(12), 2535-2542.

Tucker, R. & Rahr, V. (1990). Nursing care of the patient with non-Hodgkin's lymphoma. A case study. *Cancer Nursing, 13*(4), 229-234.

Weinstein, H. J. & Tarbell, N. J. (1997). Leukemias and lymphomas of childhood. In V. T. DeVita, S. Hellman, & S. A. Rosenberg (Eds.), *Cancer: Principles and practice of oncology* (5th ed.). Philadelphia: Lippincott-Raven.

Vose, J., Anderson, J., Kessigner, A., Bierman. P., Coccia, P., Reed, E., Gordon, B., Armitage, J. (1993). High-dose chemotherapy and autologous hematopoietic stem-cell transplantation for aggressive non–Hodgkin's lymphoma. *Journal of Clinical Oncology 11*(10), 1846-1851.

Yandle, J. (1996). Non–Hodgkin's lymphomas. In Yandle, J. (Ed.), *Textbook of hematology* (2nd ed.). Boston: Little, Brown.

Yarbro, C. H. & McFadden, M. E. (1997). Malignant lymphomas. In S. L. Groenwald, M. H. Frogge, M. Goodman, & C. H. Yarbro (Eds.), *Cancer nursing: Principles and practice* (4th ed.). Boston: Jones and Bartlett.

Yuen, A. & Sikic, B. (1994). Multidrug resistance in lymphoma. *Journal of Clinical Oncology, 12*(11), 2453-2459.

Ziegler, J. & Magrath, I. (1974). Burkitt's lymphoma. *Pathobiology Annual 4,* 129-142.

Ziegler, J. (1981). Burkitt's lymphoma. *New England Journal of Medicine, 305*(13), 735-745.

Ziegler, J. (1972). Chemotherapy of Burkitt's lymphoma. *Cancer, 30,* 1534-1540.

64 Cutaneous T-Cell Lymphoma

Kathy Lilleby, RN

EPIDEMIOLOGY

Cutaneous T-cell lymphoma (CTCL) is a rare malignancy with 800 to 1000 new cases each year (Horm & Weinstock, 1988). It may, however, be underreported due to difficulty in diagnosing the disease (Wilson, Kacinski, Edelson, & Heald, 1997). There are approximately 40,000 to 50,000 people affected with CTCL in the United States (Worobec-Victor, 1989). International statistics for CTCL are unavailable because it is classified with other lymphoproliferative disorders (McFadden, 1991). The majority of patients diagnosed with CTCL are between 40 and 60 years of age, and CTCL is more common in males than in females and in African Americans than in Caucasians (Wilson et al., 1997).

RISK FACTORS

Risk factors such as occupation, viral infection, smoking, and chemical or pesticide exposure have been investigated, and no epidemiologic links have been found (Tuyp, Burgoyne, Aitchison, & MacKie, 1987) (Box 64-1).

PATHOPHYSIOLOGY

Normal Anatomy and Physiology

The two major organ systems involved in CTCL are the lymphatic system (T cells) and the skin. See Chapter 8 for a complete discussion of the function of the hematopoietic system. Fig. 64-1 illustrates the rise of T cells from the pluripotent stem cell, and Fig. 64-2 depicts a microscopic diagram of the skin.

The skin is a thin, flat organ classified as a membrane that is composed of a cutaneous membrane, which has an outer, thinner layer (epidermis) and an inner thicker layer (dermis). The cellular epidermis is an epithelial layer derived from the ectodermal germ layer of the embryo. By the sixteenth week of gestation, the epidermis of the fetus has developed the essential characteristics of an adult (Thibodeau & Patton, 1996.

PATHOBIOLOGY

CTCL is a neoplasm of T lymphoytes that settle in the skin and other T-cell lymphoid tissues. It is a lymphoproliferative disorder of the epidermis with varied clinical symptoms (Wilson et al., 1997). It is the malignant proliferation of helper T cells that invade the skin (Harris & Macey, 1994).

Molecular phenotyping and the ability to define antigens has made it possible to classify some diseases that were previously considered distinct disorders as part of the different clinical presentations of CTCL. These diseases are mycosis fungoides (MF), Sézary syndrome (SzS), reticulum cell sarcoma of the skin, lymphoma cutis, histiocytic lymphoma, and adult T-cell lymphoma (Wilson et al., 1997), the most common being MF and SzS. Pautrier's microabscesses in the epidermis are seen on biopsy (Gilyon & Kuzel, 1991). In 1975, these diseases were labeled *cutaneous T-cell lymphoma* (Stoupa, 1990).

CTCL is a clonal neoplasm of mature CD4+ helper/inducer T cells. Two markers are expressed on most circulating CTCL cells. They are CD45RO, characteristic of memory T cells, and cutaneous lymphoid antigen (CLA), a glycoprotein, which is expressed on the surface of a small number of normal cells in cutaneous infiltrates (Picker, Michie, Rott, & Butcher, 1990). CLA is expressed on the surface of endothelial cells of cutaneous venules during chronic inflammation. CLA on the surface of CTCL cells allow them to adhere to the walls of cutaneous venules, leave the circulation and enter the skin (Wilson et al., 1997).

As CTCL progresses, the cells lose their adhesion capability, so tumor nodules begin to develop, extending deep into the dermis and spreading into visceral organs. At this stage, CTCL may become difficult to distinguish from an aggressive, high-grade B-cell lymphoma (Wilson et al., 1997)

ETIOLOGIC FACTORS

MF was named as such because the first patient diagnosed with it had tumors that looked like mushrooms. The disease,

Box 64-1
Risk Factors for Patients with Cutaneous T-Cell Lymphoma

Occupation in Manufacturing
- Petroleum
- Rubber
- Printing
- Textiles
- Metal
- Machinery

Exposure to Hazardous Chemicals
- Industrial solvents
- Heavy metals

Exposure to Viruses Including Human Immunodeficiency Virus
Lived in Specific Locations
- Southeastern United States
- West Indies
- West Africa
- Southern Japan

however, is not caused by a fungus; rather, its cause is unknown (Stocker, Liegey, & Cooley, 1990).

The malignant cells responsible for this disease seem to be stimulated by chronic exposure to antigens. Prolonged exposure to hazardous chemicals, industrial solvents, heavy metals and drugs, including nicotine, are possible risk factors. Employment in a manufacturing occupation, especially petrochemical, textile, rubber, printing, metal, or machinery, has been associated with high risk. Mortality rates from CTCL are high in counties in the United States with these industries (Greene, Dalager, Lamberg, Argyropoulous, & Fraumeni, 1979; McFadden, 1991).

CTCL presents primarily in areas normally shielded from the sun, such as under a bathing suit, so exposure to the sun does not seem to be a link (Wilson et al., 1997). A history of contact allergies, photosensitivity, and viral or fungal skin infections may be correlated with the development of CTCL (McFadden, (1991). Studies do not confirm a familial basis for the development of CTCL (Wilson et al., 1997); however, four families with a documented association have been identified (Cameron, 1993; Sandbank & Katzenellenbogen, 1968).

Patients infected with human T-cell leukemia virus (HTLV-1) are being investigated, since these patients develop T-cell leukemias with skin involvement, which are difficult to distinguish from CTCL. Geographic HTLV-1 viral clustering has been found in the southeastern United States, the West Indies, parts of west Africa, and southern Japan. This is important when considering that HTLV has been implicated in the development of a particularly aggressive, rapidly fatal, atypical form of CTCL. The relationship between HTLV- and non-HTLV–associated CTCL is not clear, but the symptoms of extensive skin lesions, high leukemic cell counts, and nodal or visceral involvement are the same, suggesting a link (Levi, 1986).

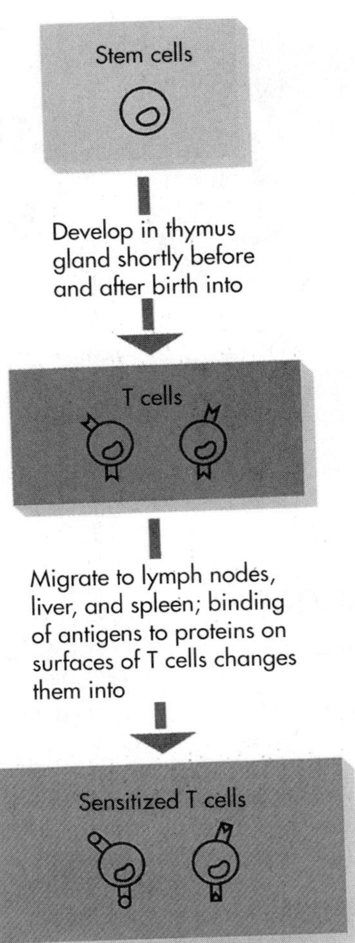

Fig. 64-1 T-cell development. (From Thibodeau, G. A. & Patton, K. T. [1996]. *Anatomy and physiology* [10th ed.]. St. Louis: Mosby.)

ROUTES OF METASTASES

When T cells lose their affinity for the skin, they migrate to the peripheral blood, lymph nodes, or visceral organs (Harris & Macey, 1994). Commonly involved organs are the liver, spleen, and lungs; however, any organ may be affected. Approximately 45% of patients with advanced disease have palpable lymph nodes draining the major sites of skin involvement. Evidence of extracutaneous CTCL is found in the majority of patients at the time of death (Broder & Bunn, 1980).

Secondary malignancies, including second skin cancers, Hodgkin's disease, non–Hodgkin's lymphoma, myeloid leukemia, and lung and colon cancer, are observed in patients with CTCL (Wilson et al., 1997).

ASSESSMENT

The presentation of CTCL may be confused with several related but benign conditions of the skin, including lympho-

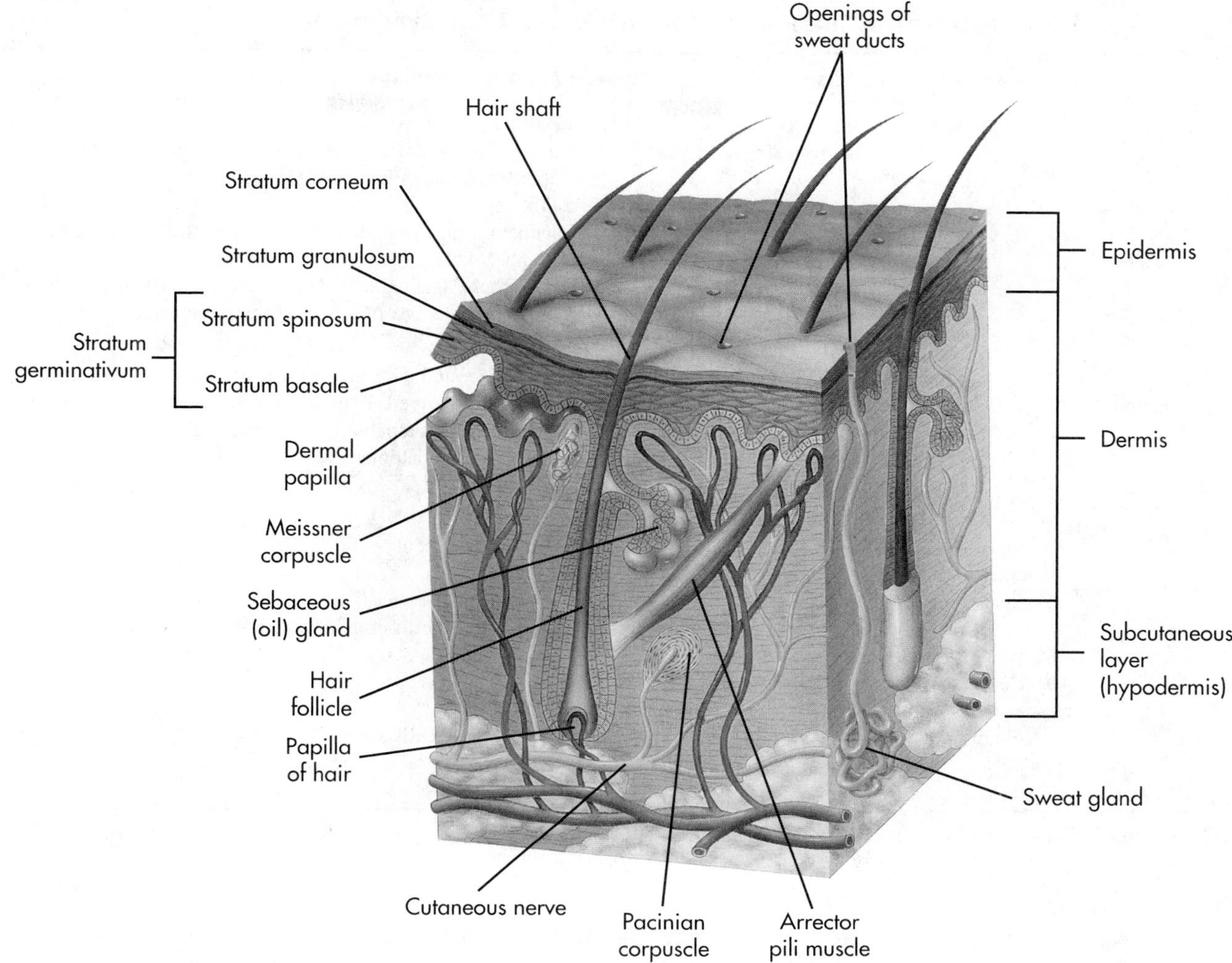

Fig. 64-2 Microscopic diagram of the skin. (From Thibodeau, G. A. & Patton, K. T. [1996]. *Anatomy and physiology* [10th ed.]. St. Louis: Mosby.)

matoid papulosis, alopecia mucinosa/follicular mucinosis, and pagetoid reticulosis. It can also be confused with two other malignant disorders, adult T-cell leukemia/lymphoma (ATLL) and CD30+ anaplastic large cell lymphoma (Wilson et al., 1997).

The classic presentation of CTCL is an erythroderma that may begin suddenly or according to the four phases described in Box 64-2. Tumor nodules are almost never seen without patches or plaque developing first (Wilson et al., 1997). Table 64-1 illustrates an assessment for the presence of CTCL.

The most important factors in staging the disease are the percent of total skin surface involved, lymph node involvement, visceral organs involved, and the number of CTCL cells in the peripheral circulation.

Box 64-2

Four Phases of Mycosis Fungoides Presentation of Cutaneous T-Cell Lymphoma

1. Premycotic phase—Asymptomatic, scaling erythematous macular eruption in sunshielded areas lasting for months to years without histologic confirmation of CTCL
2. Patch phase—Thin, barely palpable, erythematous and eczematous lesions with histologic features consistent with CTCL
3. Plaque phase—Easily palpable erythematous lesions
4. Tumor phase—neoplastic infiltrate extends below the upper dermis

Wilson, L. D., Kacinski, B. M., Edelson, R. L., & Heald, P. W. (1997). Cutaneous T-cell lymphomas. In V. T. DeVita, S. Hellman, S. A. Rosenberg, (Eds.), *Cancer: Principles and practice of oncology* (5th ed). Philadelphia: Lippincott-Raven.

Patient History

A careful history regarding skin lesions is important to document their onset and length and how they have pro-

Table 64-1 Assessment of the Patient for Cutaneous T-Cell Lymphoma

	Assessment Parameters	Typical Abnormal Findings
History	A. Personal and social history 1. Environmental surroundings 2. Occupational history 3. Use of illegal drugs or tobacco 4. Viral exposure	A. Personal and social risk factors 1. Exposure to hazardous chemicals, industrial solvents, heavy metal; living in southeastern United States, west Africa, southern Japan 2. Occupation in manufacturing such as petroleum, rubber, printing, textile, metal, or machinery 3. Use of these agents place patients at risk for cancer 4. Immunosuppression of acquired immunodeficiency syndrome (AIDS) or hepatitis
Physical Examination	A. A complete physical examination with attention to skin, lymph nodes, and abdomen	Note number, size, and distribution of lesions and plaques and percent of skin involved. Lymph node involvement may be suspicious as noted by palpable lymph glands. Palpation of abdomen reveals hepatomegalia.
Diagnostic Tests	A. Skin biopsies B. Complete blood count with differential and smear C. Liver function tests D. Posterior and lateral chest x-rays E. Computed tomography or magnetic resonance imaging F. Lymph node biopsy	A. Routine histology may reveal hematoxylin and eosin histopathology. B. Detects circulating cutaneous T cells C. Detects possible metastasis and identifies sites capable of being biopsied to make a differential diagnosis D. Allow disease to be staged E. Same F. Shows atypical T cells with irregular cerebriform nuclei infiltrating the epidermis and a zone beneath it, forming characteristic Pautrier's microabscesses

Data from Wilson, L. D., Kacinski, B. M., Edelson, R. L., & Heald, P. W. (1997). Cutaneous T-cell lymphomas. In V. T. DeVita, S. Hellman, S. A. Rosenberg, (Eds.), *Cancer: Principles and practice of oncology* (5th ed.). Philadelphia: Lippincott-Raven.

gressed. The patient should be questioned about skin integrity, pruritus, the use of moisturizers and the skin's reaction to extreme temperatures.

Skin Lesion Assessment and Biopsies. The number, size, sites, type (i.e., patchy, plaque, tumor, erythema), and extent of skin involved by CTCL lesions should be evaluated. Biopsies of each patch or plaque are necessary, since the morphology may vary from lesion to lesion. The depth into the dermis of the lesion should be measured. Immunophenotyping has been found to show some correlation between cells and staging. Immunogenotyping by polymerase chain receptor (PCR) of the biopsies can define whether there is a clonal T-cell population in 90% of the samples (Wilson et al., 1997).

Lymph Node Examination and Biopsy. The number, size, and location of lymph nodes should be documented. Biopsies of lymph nodes should be obtained by excision, immunophenotype, and immunogenotype for a clearer diagnosis. Palpation of the abdomen should be done to detect hepatosplenomegaly. Imaging studies with a computed tomography (CT) scan or a magnetic resonance imaging (MRI) scan of the chest, abdomen, and pelvis, as well as chest x-ray, are recommended at diagnosis or for patients with advanced disease (Wilson et al., 1997).

Peripheral Blood. A complete blood count (CBC) with differential and smear is needed at diagnosis, along with liver and renal function tests. The number of circulating CTCL cells, or Sézary cells, is an important evaluation since it correlates with their prognosis (Wilson et al., 1997).

STAGING

Patch Stage

The patch stage is characterized by the insidious onset of irregularly shaped, hyperpigmented patches, with or without scales. The patches may involve the body surface; however, the most commonly affected areas are the bathing suit area, buttocks, thighs, abdomen, and breasts of females. The lesions are raised due to hyperplasia and the intracellular edema within the epidermis (McFadden, 1991) (Fig. 64-3).

Diagnosis is difficult, since the lesions resemble benign dermatoses such as eczema, seborrhea, psoriasis, or contact dermatitis. Patients may experience transient regression and exacerbation, so repeat biopsies are common (Worobec-Victor, 1989).

The predominant symptom is severe pruritus, which is at times out of proportion to the extent of the lesions. This stage lasts 2 to 5 years but may persist as long as 15 to 30 years (Klein & Schwartz, 1982).

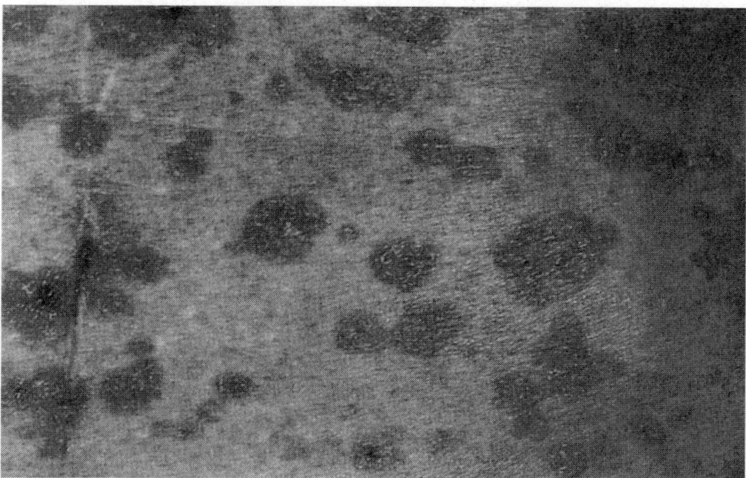

Fig. 64-3 Patch stage of mycosis fungoides with pink, scaly patches, which may exhibit various shapes and sizes. (From Skarin, A. T. [1996]. *Atlas of diagnostic oncology* [2nd ed.]. London: Mosby-Wolfe.)

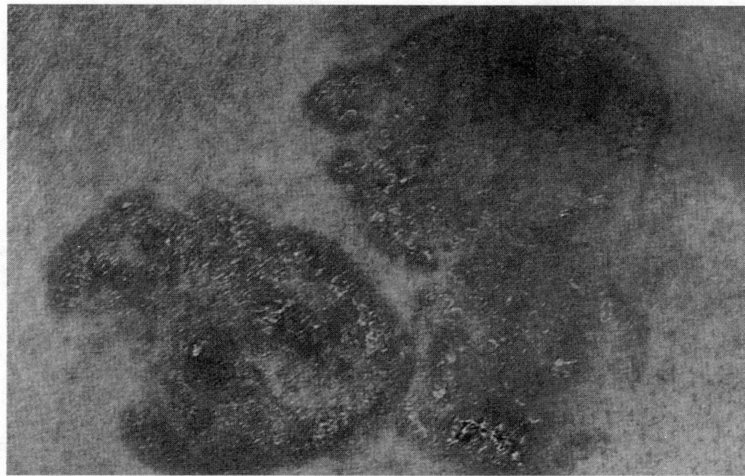

Fig. 64-4 Plaque stage of mycosis fungoides, sometimes called *parapsoriasis en plaque*. (From Skarin, A. T. [1996]. *Atlas of diagnostic oncology* [2nd ed.]. St. Louis: Mosby-Wolfe.)

Plaque Stage

The disease then progresses to indurated plaques that arise from the thickening patches or in areas where there have been no patches. Facial plaques may produce a leonine facies similar to leprosy, and scalp involvement can cause alopecia (Fig. 64-4). Nails show dystrophic changes, and palmoplantar fissures are common (Klein & Schwartz, 1982). The irregular shapes may merge together and appear as doughnut-shaped, rounded, or kidney-shaped rings; curled ribbons; and of various colors such as bluish, yellow, or vivid shades of red (Arnold, Odom, & James, 1990).

During this phase, the disease accelerates and the skin lesions become more widespread (Bunn & Fuks, 1989). The median survival for initial plaque stage diagnosis can be more than 8 years (Sausville, Eddy, Makuch, Fischmann, Schechter, & Matthews et al., 1988).

Erythroderma (Sézary Syndrome)

Sézary & Bouvrain (1938) described the erythroderma as hypotrophy of the epidermis of feet and palms, hyper- or hypopigmentation of the skin, intense pruritus, shedding of the epidermis, and circulating lymphocytes in the blood, which later were called *Sézary cells*. Erythroderma (SzS) may present after the plaque stage, or de novo. It causes a loss of hair and the inability to maintain body temperature. It has been called *red man's disease* (Besnier & Hallopeau, 1982). The nails become dystrophic, and pruritus and a burning sensation of the skin are distressing to the patient (Stoupa, 1990).

Tumor Stage

Tumors are nodules that form within the plaques, as well as on normal skin surfaces anywhere on the body. Tumors are,

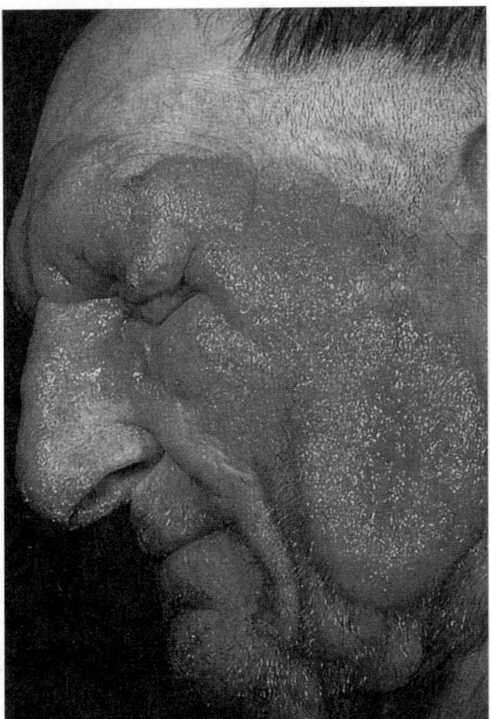

Fig. 64-5 Mycosis fungoides. Late stage. (From Skarin, A. S. [1996]. *Atlas of diagnostic oncology* [2nd ed.]. St. Louis: Mosby-Wolfe.)

however, particularly common on the face, scalp, and body folds and can measure up to 10 cm in diameter, thus causing significant disfigurement (Fig. 64-5). Pruritus and pain are usually absent at this stage. Nodules may erode, ulcerate, and cause severe pain and may be a source of secondary infection. Patients diagnosed at this stage have a median survival of 40 months (Sausville et al., 1988).

Table 64-2 TMN Classification of Cutaneous T-Cell Lymphoma

TNM Definitions	
Skin	
T0	Clinically and/or histopathologically suspicious lesions
T1	Limited plaques, papules, or eczematous patches covering <10% of the skin surface
T2	Generalized plaques, papules or erythematous patches covering >10% of the skin surface
T3	Tumors
T4	Generalized erythroderma
Lymph Nodes	
N0	No clinically abnormal peripheral lymph nodes, negative for CTCL
N1	Clinically abnormal peripheral lymph nodes, pathology negative for CTCL
N2	No clinically abnormal peripheral lymph nodes, pathology positive for CTCL.
N3	Clinically abnormal peripheral lymph nodes, pathology positive for CTCL
Visceral Organs	
M0	No visceral organ involvement
M1	Visceral organ involvement (must have pathology confirmation and organ involvement should be specified)
Staging Grouping	
Stage IA	T1, N0, M0
Stage IB	T2, N0, M0
Stage IIA	T1-2, N1, M0
Stage IIB	T3, N0-1, M0
Stage III	T4, N0-1, M0
Stage IVA	T1-4, N2-3, M0
Stage IVB	T1-4, N0-3, M1

Wilson, L. D., Kacinski, B. M., Edelson, R. L., & Heald, P. W. (1997). Cutaneous T-cell lymphomas. In V. T. DeVita, S. Hellman, S. A., Rosenberg, (Eds.), *Cancer: Principles and practice of oncology.* (5th ed.) (Vol. 2). Philadelphia: Lippincott-Raven Publishers, 2220-2232.

MEDICAL MANAGEMENT

CTCL is a distinct disorder and cannot be treated as a localized B-cell lymphoma. Early-stage disease responds well to local therapy; however, disease that has spread to the lymph nodes or visceral organs can rarely be cured (Wilson et al., 1997). Staging of CTCL is listed in Table 64-2, and treatment according to state is found in Table 64-3.

Dissemination of CTCL to organs occurs earlier than previously thought, so the shorter time between its clinical onset and diagnosis is vital to improve survival rates. There is some debate about how aggressive initial therapy should be so that the disease is eradicated in the early stages, since treatment of recurrent disease is often poorly tolerated by the patient. In the end stages, palliation of the pain may be the better measurement of successful treatment (McFadden, 1991).

Cutaneous Treatment

Local treatment of CTCL is accomplished by destroying the malignant cells by triggering T-cell apoptosis and interference with the production of cytokines necessary for T-cell proliferation and survival (Wilson et al., 1997).

Topical Chemotherapy

The most common topical chemotherapy is mechlorethamine hydrochloride (nitrogen mustard [NM]) because it is effective not only in its treatment of the CTCL cells but also in its decrease in the patient with intense pruritus. The advantages of topical NM are its reasonable cost, availability, minimal toxicity, and ability to be delivered as an outpatient procedure. The disadvantages are the need for daily applications for 6 to 12 months (McFadden,1991), development of hyperpigmentation, and delayed hypersensitivity reaction (Vonderheid, Van Scott, Wallner, & Johnson, 1979).

Topical NM is applied to the whole body except the eyelids, lips, and genitals with a solution of 10 mg in 50 ml tap water. Patients, nurses, or family members should wear latex gloves while applying NM with a cloth or brush. If a delayed hypersensitivity reaction occurs, as it does in 40% of the patients, the treatment may be discontinued temporarily. The patient may be desensitized with one tenth of the dose followed by a gradual return to full strength (Gilyon & Kuzel, 1991). An ointment-based NM (10 mg NM mixed with Aquaphor) is also available, which causes fewer reactions and is stable at room temperature. A neutralizing solution of 5% sodium thiosulfate can be used by nurses or family members if an accidental contact with NM occurs (Gilyon & Kuzel, 1991).

Other side effects of topical NM therapy include a secondary cutaneous malignancy such as squamous cell carcinoma, hyperpigmentation, or hypopigmentation. In patients with T1 and T2 CTCL, 64% to 90% achieve a complete response to topical NM treatment. Maintenance treatment with NM can be used to prevent or delay relapse of CTCL in patients who have achieved a complete remission through total-skin electron beam therapy or to treat minimal patch or plaque recurrences after therapy (Wilson et al., 1997).

Carmustine (i.e., 1,3-bis[2-chlorethyl]-1-nitrosurea, or BCNU) is another topical chemotherapy used to treat CTCL in patients who develop an allergy to NM. It can be given in a 10- to 49-mg/dl ointment or in a solution of 25 to 50 mg/dl of diluted alcohol. The ointment is stable at room temperature indefinitely, and the alcohol solution is stable for at least 3 months when refrigerated.

Hypersensitivity reactions to BCNU are rare; however, erythema in the treated areas occurs in one in three patients treated. Bone marrow suppression is rare but can occur in patients who receive more than 600 mg of BCNU. Monitoring of CBC is recommended (Wilson et al., 1997). Patient teaching guidelines for application of topical chemotherapy are outlined in Table 64-3.

Photochemotherapy

Methoxsalen is activated in the presence of ultraviolet (UV) light, binding with deoxyribonucleic acid (DNA) to cause cell death by inhibiting DNA synthesis and cell division (McFadden, 1991). Psoralens are naturally occurring photoactive substances found in the *Ammi majus* plant. When psoralen is activated by light, it binds to the DNA of the white blood cells (*Physicians Desk Reference,* 1997). Psoralens activated by UV light not only kills T cells but also elicits anti-CTCL cell immune responses. The UV light penetrates only the dermis and epidermis (Gilchrest, Parrish, Tannenebaum, Haynes, & Fitzpatrick, 1976). Photochemotherapy, or PUVA therapy, approved by the Food and Drug Administration (FDA) for the treatment of CTCL, is effective in patients with CTCL at the patch or thin plaque stage (Wilson et al., 1997).

Patients are given 0.6 mg/kg of thoxypsoralen or 8-methoxypsoralen (8-MOP) by mouth 1 to 2 hours before treatment with the UV light at 320 to 400 nm. Therapy is given 3 times per week until most of the lesions respond, then it is decreased to twice a week for 4 to 6 months. If there is no complete remission, other therapy should be added (Wilson et al., 1997). Once maintenance therapy is

TABLE 64-3 Management of Patient with CTCL According to Stage

Stage IA

Limited Patch/Plaque

1. Topical NM
2. If unable to tolerate topical NM: PUVA or topical BCNU
3. If disease progresses or if disease is refractory: TSEB irradiation or PUVA with IFN-α

Stage IB

Generalized Patch/Plaque

Stage IIA

Patch/Plaque without Histologic Node Involvement

A. Chronic disease: topical NM or PUVA
B. Rapidly progressive disease with thick plaques:
   1. TSEB irradiation with follow-up therapy with topical NM, PUVA, or ECP
   2. If refractory to these treatments, add a systemic drug such as IFN-α, a retinoid, or MTX

Stage IIB

Tumors

1. TSEB irradiation with optional follow-up with topical therapy or ECP
2. If refractory tumors, use sequential topical therapies (see Stage Ia)
3. If disease progresses: ECP; if no response, systemic therapy

Stage III

Generalized Erythroderma without Histologic Node Involvement

Sézary Syndrome

Erythroderma, Lymphadenopathy and Circulating Atypical Cells

1. ECP
2. If disease progresses or if unresponsive: add MTX
3. If disease progresses: palliative PUVA or NM, IFN-α, systemic chemotherapy, retinoids, experimental protocols such as fludarabine, monoclonal antibodies, or bone marrow transplant

Stage IVA

Histologic Lymph Node Involvement

1. Palliative treatment
2. Local radiation to local symptomatic disease
3. ECP (response does not correlate with lymph node involvement)
4. Retinoids, experimental protocols as mentioned above

Stage IVB

Visceral Involvement

1. Individualized palliative treatment with chemotherapy
2. Palliative treatment with IFN-α, retinoids or experimental protocols as mentioned above

From Holloway K., Flowers, F., & Ramos-Caro, F. (1992). Therapeutic alternatives in cutaneous T-cell lymphoma. *Journal of American Academy of Dermatology, 27,* 367-378.
BCNU, Carmustine; *ECP,* extracorporeal photopheresis; *IFN-α,* interferon-alpha; *NM,* nitrogen mustard; *PUVA,* photochemotherapy; *TSEB,* total-skin electron beam.

discontinued, there tends to be a prompt relapse (Bunn & Fuks, 1989).

Side effects are minimal and may include mild nausea, generalized pruritus, sunburn-like skin changes, and cataract formation due to binding of psoralens to the lens of the eye. The patient must wear UV-protective goggles for 24 hours after taking the drug. If the patient is seropositive for the herpes simplex virus, the virus may be activated and cause an infection (Vonderheid & Micailey, 1985). Nausea from psoralens may be prevented by taking the drug on a full stomach or with milk. The patient may need antiemetics (Gilyon & Kuzel, 1991). PUVA is expensive and may cause

TABLE 64-4 Standard of Care for the Patient Undergoing PUVA Therapy or Photopheresis

Patient Problem and Outcomes	Nursing Interventions and Rationales	Patient Education Instructions
Anxiety Patient will: • Verbalize an understanding of the procedure. • Express feelings of decreased anxiety.	1. Assess patient's level of understanding of the procedure. 2. Give the patient an opportunity to ask questions or verbalize concerns. 3. Determine which coping strategies the patient has used in the past and reinforce the use of the successful strategies.	1. Explain to the patient what PUVA or ECP is and what it does. 2. Show the patient the PUVA bed or the leukapheresis machine and the radiation equipment. 3. Introduce the staff who will administer the treatment.
Nausea Patient will experience minimal nausea.	1. Psoralens can cause gastric irritation. 2. Offer dry crackers, hard candies, or carbonated beverage. 3. Encourage deep breathing.	1. Instruct the patient to take psoralens on a full stomach or with milk. 2. Instruct the patient to take psoralens 2 hours before the treatment begins.
Photosensitization Patient will have decreased exposure to the sun on the day psoralens is taken.	1. Photosensitization is related to the ingestion of psoralens. 2. Exposure of eyes to sun after taking psoralens can cause cataract formation. 3. Other photosensitive medications should be avoided such as tetracycline, sulfonamides, phenothiazines, coal tar, and furosemide.	1. Instruct patient to wear protective UVA glasses immediately after taking psoralens and continue for 24 hours after the dose. 2. Encourage wearing a wide-brimmed hat to cover ears, nose, and lips. 3. Encourage patient to wear sunscreen with SPF >15. 4. Teach patient to wear trousers and long sleeved shirts of tightly woven fabrics. 5. Instruct patient that sunlight penetrates windows and clouds. 6. Instruct patient to avoid other photosensitive medications.
Pruritus Patient will experience minimal pruritus.	1. PUVA therapy can cause dry skin. 2. PUVA therapy is a long-term treatment that may cause erythema.	1. Teach the patient to use only non–alcohol-containing lotions twice a day. 2. Instruct the patient to call the doctor for medication for severe itching.
Altered Fluid Balance Patients receiving ECP will maintain their fluid balance.	1. Fluid volume may shift during the leukapheresis procedure 2. Patients need to be monitored for hypotension when a large volume of blood is out of their body.	1. Assess for signs and symptoms of fluid volume deficit such as hypotension, tachycardia, restlessness, confusion, or cool, moist skin. 2. Monitor vital signs every 20 minutes during the procedure. 3. Administer IV fluids as needed.

Modified from Macey, W. H. & Harris, J. S. (1995). Photopheresis and the role of the nurse, *Dermatology Nursing* 7(1), 1995.
ECP, Extracorporeal photopheresis; *PUVA,* photochemotherapy; *UVA,* ultraviolet A.

a second nonmelanoma cutaneous malignancy (McFadden, 1991). Patients should be apprised of both situations before therapy. A standard of care for patients undergoing PUVA therapy or photopheresis is illustrated in Table 64-4.

Local External Beam Irradiation

Cutaneous CTCL lesions are very responsive to radiotherapy and a dose-response relationship has been seen. Local x-ray or electron beam therapy is able to clear lesions that failed to respond to PUVA or lesions that recurred after a complete remission to PUVA or total-skin electron beam (TSEB) irradiation. Local treatment of isolated plaques or tumors has a response rate of greater than 90% (Wilson et al., 1997).

Total-Skin Electron Beam Irradiation. Electrons have a limited depth penetration to the epidermis and dermis; therefore in treating with electrons ranging between 4 and 7 MeV, structures below the deep dermis are spared. Treatments are given in six fields over a 2-day cycle with local boosts to the scalp, perineum, and soles of feet, as well as any other areas not exposed by the beam. Corneas are protected by external and internal eye shields to prevent the formation of cataracts. Helmets shield the face and the hands, and feet are shielded 50% of the time. Therapy continues 4 days a week for 9 weeks for a total of 3000 to 4000 cGy (Vonderheid & Micailey, 1992).

Patients must be able to stand in a supportive frame alone in the room where they receive radiation for 45 minutes to 1 hour. The patient may rest in between the six fields that are irradiated to help avoid the risk of becoming dizzy, tired, or faint (Vonderheid & Micailey, 1992).

TSEB irradiation is well tolerated in most patients. Common side effects during or within 6 months after treatment may include red and dry skin, pruritus, erythema, desquamation, alopecia, nail loss, lower extremity edema, bullae of the feet, and impaired function of sweat glands (Vonderheid & Micailey, 1992).

TSEB irradiation is the treatment of choice for patients with diffuse involvement with thick plaques, cutaneous tumors, and symptomatic erythroderma, as well as patients with extensive patches or thin plaques refractory to PUVA or other skin-directed therapies (Wilson et al., 1997)

TSEB irradiation can be used in patients with stages T1 and T2 disease or in combination with systemic chemotherapy. Therapy may also be repeated in patients who relapse.

Secondary malignancies such as squamous and basal cell carcinomas, as well as malignant melanoma, have been seen in patients treated with TSEB irradiation. However the addition of x-ray or electron beam irradiation after TSEB irradiation does not increase the risk of second cutaneous malignancies (Wilson et al., 1997). It is expensive and its availability is limited (McFadden, 1991). Table 64-5 illustrates a standard of care for patients undergoing total electron beam therapy.

Extracutaneous Treatment

Systemic Chemotherapy. Systemic chemotherapy can be used as palliation in patients with CTCL. Common single agents used are methotrexate, mechlorethamine, doxorubicin, vincristine, and etoposide. Preliminary results of the use of high-dose systemic chemotherapy with marrow rescue for visceral disease are not encouraging (Wilson et al., 1997). Overall responses have been less than 12 months, so palliation of symptoms is the most beneficial effect (Levi, 1986).

Combination chemotherapy is another treatment option with standard protocols similar to those of non–Hodgkin's lymphoma, such as MOPP (mechlorethamine hydrochloride, vincristine sulfate, procarbazine hydrochloride, and prednisone), CHOP (cyclophosphamide, vincristine sulfate, and prednisone), CVP (cyclophosphamide, vincristine sulfate, and prednisone) and CVP with bleomycin or methotrexate (Wilson et al., 1997).

Extracorporeal Photopheresis. Extracorporeal photopheresis (ECP) is the use of psoralens followed by leukapheresis. The white blood cells are separated from about 500 ml of blood circulated through the apheresis machine and exposed to UV light for about 1.5 hours, which kills the lymphocytes (Perez, Edelson, La Roche, & Berger, 1989). It is also believed that there is a possible active immunization process that occurs when these photoactivated T cells are returned to the patient.

ECP, FDA-approved in 1987 for the treatment of patients with CTCL, is given once a month until maximum response is seen; then an additional 6 months may be given as consolidation therapy. The interval between ECP treatments is prolonged by 1 week per cycle every three cycles when the disease is stable. When the interval reaches 8 weeks for three cycles, therapy can be discontinued (Wilson et al., 1997)

Transient responses are seen 1 to 2 days after ECP treatment, but sustained responses occur as early as the second month of therapy. A *sustained response* is defined as a decrease in erythema, scaling, and pruritus, or in subtle changes such as the return of body hair, loss of rigors, and return of the ability to sweat (Wilson et al., 1997)

The side effects of ECP are infrequent and minimal, and long-term follow-up has shown no immunosuppression of the patient. Erythema and edema, as well as nausea from psoralens, have been seen. There is a possibility of venous access problems. Some patients experience fever as a result of cell death in the first few treatments. Patients should be monitored for cardiac overload or hypotension due to fluid shifts while their blood is being irradiated and they are receiving IV fluids (Wilson et al., 1997)

ECP is most effective when combined with other therapies such as IFN, methotrexate, etoposide, etretinate, or TSEB irradiation (Harris & Macey, 1994). It is contraindicated in patients with hepatitis or human immunodeficiency virus (HIV) (Dean, 1990).

Biotherapy

Interferon-alpha. Interferon-alpha (IFN-α) has been shown to have active anti-tumor effects in patients with CTCL. The best response rates are seen in previously untreated patients, but IFN-α may also benefit patients with chemorefractory disease (Bunn & Fuks, 1989). IFN-α in 3

TABLE 64-5 Standard of Care for the Patient Undergoing Total Electron Beam Therapy

Patient Problem and Outcomes	Nursing Interventions and Rationales	Patient Education Instructions
Knowledge Deficit Patient will verbalize an understanding of the purpose, benefits and risks of TSEB therapy.	1. Assess patient's level of knowledge regarding TSEB irradiation. 2. Assess patient's concerns and fears about TSEB irradiation. 3. Ensure privacy during the procedure since little or no clothing is worn.	1. Describe the procedure. 2. Instruct the patient about major side effects.
Safety Patient will not be dizzy, tired or weak during procedure.	1. Assess the patient for his or her ability to stand motionless and alone for 45 minutes to 1 hour. 2. Allow for rest periods between fields.	1. Encourage the use of music tapes for distraction during the procedure.
Eyes • Will be protected from radiation. • Will not become dry.	1. TSEB irradiation can increase the risk of cataract formation. 2. Use of eye shields and helmet may prevent cataract formation.	1. Wear eye shields during treatment. 2. Rinse eyes with normal saline after each treatment. 3. Use artificial tears to prevent dry eyes twice a day.
Edema Patient will not have signs of edema.	1. Damage to lymphatic system will lead to edema. 2. Standing for long periods may lead to peripheral edema.	1. Instruct patient to elevate hands and feet after each treatment.
Impaired Skin Integrity Patient will: • Have skin that is intact. • Not experience pruritus.	1. Radiation can cause dryness, which leads to breakdown in the integrity of the skin. 2. Encrusted lesions need to be removed before treatment to allow maximum penetration of the radiation.	1. Apply aloe vera and lanolin lotion before and after therapy. 2. Use lubricating lotion for dry desquamation. 3. Soak in oatmeal bath for pruritus.

to 6 megaunits has also been used to clear lesions that have not responded to PUVA alone.

The side effects of IFN are flu-like symptoms such as fever, myalgia, fatigue, and listlessness, especially during the first week. Persistent mild fatigue is the patient's main complaint. Proteinuria, thrombocytopenia, and anemia have also been seen as complications. Long-term side effects may be neuropathy, dementia, and myelopathy (Wilson et al., 1997).

Interleukin-2. Interleukin-2 (IL-2) is a glycoprotein that mediates its antitumor effects through complex interactions with the immune system. One Japanese study reported a complete remission lasting 13 months with a good response to chemotherapy after a recurrence (McFadden, 1991). Side effects from IL-2 range from flu-like symptoms to capillary leak syndrome.

Monoclonal Antibodies. Monoclonal antibodies (MoAbs) such as anti-CD5, anti-CD4, and anti-TAC have been studied for the treatment of CTCL with varied responses (Wilson et al., 1997). They may be used alone, conjugated to radioisotopes, or chemotherapeutic agents. Transient clinical responses have been seen in the treatment of CTCL (DiJulio, 1988). The side effects of MoAbs are flu-like symptoms.

Combined Modality Therapy

The combination of radiation plus chemotherapy (topical or systemic) has shown some improvement in survival, as has topical NM plus systemic chemotherapy (Wilson et al., 1997)

Retinoids

Retinoids (vitamin A) or etretinate (Tegison) is commonly used to treat CTCL because of its immunomodulatory and antiinflammatory effects. It may be used alone in the early stages (Claudy, Rouchouse, Boucheron, & LePetit, 1983) or in later stages with IFN-α (Dreno, Claudy, Meynadier, Verret, Souteyrand, & Ortonne et al., 1991), with EBT (Jones, McLean, Rosenthal, Roberts, & Sauder, 1992), or with photopheresis.

The side effects include increased liver function test, hepatitis, abnormal vision, myalgias, alopecia, cardiovascular thrombosis and edema. Vitamin A is teratogenic so pregnant women should not take it at high doses.

ONCOLOGIC EMERGENCIES

The major oncologic emergency in patients with advanced CTCL who have open lesions is septic shock resulting from a gram-negative organism that invades the circulation. The patient may present with fever; chills; tachypnea and tachycardia; flushed, warm, dry skin; hypotension; widened pulse pressure; anxiety; restlessness; decreased level of consciousness and later, dyspnea; cool, clammy skin; decreased urine output; and lethargy. Blood cultures, chest x-ray, arterial blood gases, prothrombin time, partial thromboplastin time, and renal function tests should be conducted, and antibiotics should be started immediately (Eriksson, 1994).

NURSING MANAGEMENT

Patient Education

Accurate information about cancer, treatment options, consequences of therapy, potential problems, and resources is necessary for patients and their families from diagnosis through the course of the disease process (McFadden, 1991). One method of treatment may work temporarily, it may fail, and another may be started. In particular, patients and family members should be assured that CTCL is not contagious and that touching the plaques or tumors is safe (Gilyon & Kuzel, 1991).

Skin Assessment

The nurse should assess the skin for change in color, fissures, hair growth, sweating, erythema, dry or moist desquamation, and infection. The site and type of lesions and their progression should be noted. If the patient has encrusted areas of skin, the lesions should be soaked in water or saline to loosen them manually and then they should be debrided before each treatment with TSEB irradiation. This allows the radiation to penetrate the skin (Strohl, 1994). Recommendations for skin care are listed in Box 64-3.

Box 64-3
Skin Care Recommendations

1. Daily whirlpool bath.
2. Use a chair if a whirlpool is not available.
3. Apply non–alcohol-containing lotion such as Eucerin, Lubriderm, aloe vera, and lanolin twice daily.
4. Use hypoallergenic make-up.
5. Use nonadhesive material to cover sheets on bed.
6. Air-fluidized bed system to reduce pressure on skin.
7. Apply silver nitrate to open sores.
8. Debride encrusted lesions before TSEB irradiation.

Pain Control

The major cause of pain is the stimulation of cutaneous skin receptors in the infiltrative lesions (McFadden, 1991). When lesions involve the whole body, painful cracks or fissures in the hands and feet can cause pain that will prevent the patient from moving. Oral opioids should be given at doses that allow patients comfort without sedation so that activities of daily living can be performed. (Stocker, Liegey, & Cooley, 1990). Other methods of pain controls can include relaxation techniques and diversional activities (McFadden, 1991).

Infection Control

The loss of the normal protection of the skin accounts for 50% of all deaths due to bacteremia, septicemia, and pneumonia. The most common pathogens are *Staphylococcus aureus* and *Pseudomonas aeruginosa*, which can be treated with appropriate antibiotic therapy. Empirical treatment with antibiotics should be started at the first sign of a fever. Even in the earliest stages of the disease, the importance of caring for the skin is important because of the sloughing of skin (McFadden, 1991). Herpes simplex can also complicate an already compromised skin lesion (Stocker, Liegey, & Cooley, 1990).

Draining lesions are both uncomfortable and have the potential for causing septicemia. A skin care routine is vital to the patient. The most soothing and cleansing program is a daily whirlpool bath. However, if a patient has open herpes lesions, the patient may sit on a chair under the shower. A cream such as Eucerin or Aquaphor can then be applied to areas of skin that are still intact, and silver nitrate can be applied to open sores. For patients with herpetic lesions, acyclovir (Zovirax) should be applied. A nonadhesive dressing is then applied, or lesions can be exposed to air. It may be more comfortable for the patient to lay on a sheet of nonadhesive material (Stocker, Liegey, & Cooley, 1990). An air-fluidized bed system reduces pressure on the skin and enhances blood flow (McFadden, 1991). Another important impairment to consider is the loss of the skin's normal thermal-regulatory mechanism (McFadden, 1991). Environmental temperature and amount of clothing will need to be regulated. Recommendations for skin care for the patient with pruritus are listed in Box 64-4.

Venous Access

IV fluids and antibiotics are routine for patients with draining lesions. A central catheter is the most convenient venous access for both the patient and the nurse caring for him or her; however, if there are widespread skin lesions, the risk of infection may prevent the use of a central catheter. If ve-

Box 64-4
Nursing Care for the Patient with Pruritus

Dry desquamation
- Cornstarch
- Baby powder
- Eucerin
- Aquaphor
- Lubriderm
- Aloe vera and lanolin
- Oatmeal bath
- Open wet dressings
- Sauna suit
- Atarax

Moist desquamation
- Gentle cleansing with water, saline, and hydrogen peroxide

nipuncture is needed, the patient's arms can be wrapped in warm compresses to dilate the veins to gain venous access. The IV needle should be changed every 3 days to prevent infection (Stocker, Leigey, & Cooley, 1990).

Nutrition and Hydration

A careful nutritional assessment is required for patients with draining lesions or with exfoliation and vasodilation. They may need additional protein, iron, electrolytes and calories, as well as fluids. A dietitian can plan a diet with the patient's favorite foods to meet his or her needs (Stocker, Liegey, & Cooley, 1990). Protein is also essential for skin repair (Dean, 1990).

Emotional Needs

Patients with CTCL are often frustrated at the difficulty and time it takes to find a diagnosis. Then pain, distress, and anger with their physical appearance, as well as depression at their prognosis, should be addressed. Taking time listen to the patient to discover how to meet his or her needs is important. Finding ways to keep the patient's interest in normal activities will help. Letting the patient have some control over his or her daily routine will take away some of the helpless feelings (Stocker, Liegey, & Cooley, 1990).

Issues relating to sexuality and intimacy need to be discussed with patients and their family/caregivers because self-image is greatly affected due to lesions in the advanced stages (McFadden, 1991). Kirchner (1984) defines *self-image* as people's perception of themselves, as well as the image they believe others have of them. This leads to fears of rejection, isolation and unacceptability, which may cause more anxiety than the fear of the disease, pain, or death (Sutherland, 1960).

EVALUATION OF THE QUALITY OF CARE

The quality of a patient's care should be monitored. Specific aspects of care can be evaluated through the use of the tools in Tables 64-6 and 64-7.

Table 64-6 Quality of Care Evaluation of a Patient with CTCL

Disciplines participating in the quality of care evaluation:
☐ Nursing ☐ Physician
☐ Physical Therapy ☐ Social Services

Data from:
☐ Medical Record Review ☐ Patient/Family Interview

Criteria	Yes	No
1. Patient provided with information about:		
a. Photosensitive medication to avoid when receiving PUVA or ECP.	☐	☐
b. Signs and symptoms of radiation burns.	☐	☐
c. Types of lotion or baths to prevent or treat pruritus.	☐	☐
d. How to apply topical chemotherapy.	☐	☐
2. The following assessments are made at each visit:		
a. Extent of erythema, patches, plaques, or tumors	☐	☐
b. Functional status	☐	☐
c. Fluid balance	☐	☐
d. Patients' understanding of instructions	☐	☐
3. Patient experienced the following complications:		
a. Nausea	☐	☐
b. Hypotension during ECP	☐	☐
c. Edema after TSEB irradiation	☐	☐
d. Desquamation of skin	☐	☐

Patient/Family Satisfaction

Data from:
☐ Patient Interview ☐ Family Interview

Criteria	Yes	No
1. On a scale of 0 to 10, with 0 being totally dissatisfied and 10 being totally satisfied, how satisfied were you with the management of pruritus you received? ____________		
2. Were you told to wear protective eye goggles for 24 hours after taking psoralens?	☐	☐
3. Were you taught how to apply topical chemotherapy and how to dispose of the materials used to apply it?	☐	☐

PROGNOSIS

The extent of disease at diagnosis is the principal prognostic factor. This includes the degree of skin and lymph node involvement and evidence of invasion into the peripheral blood or visceral organs (Lamberg, Green, Byar, Block, Clendenning, & Epstein et al., 1979). Patients may live for

10 or more years if there is no lymph node involvement or metastasis to visceral organs. After metastasis, the average survival is 2.5 years (Stocker, Liegey, & Cooley, 1990). For patients with lymph node disease, the median survival rate is less than 2 years. If visceral metastasis is present, the survival rate is less than 1 year (Green, Byar, & Lamberg, 1981; Vonderheid, & Micailey, 1992). Patients presenting with systemic symptoms such as fever, chills, burning sensation, and malaise have an extremely poor prognosis (Strohl, 1994).

Advanced age, black race, prior malignancy, and the presence of Sézary cells at the time of diagnosis are each independently associated with a poor prognosis (Weinstock & Horm, 1988).

The prognosis for patients with less than 10% of the body surface are more likely to be cured than a patient with more than 10% of the body surface involved. Patients with cutaneous tumors or erythroderma have a still poorer prognosis (Wilson et al., 1997).

RESEARCH ISSUES

Since the prognosis of CTCL is so poor, the symptom management is extremely vital to patient comfort and the emotional impact of disfiguring lesions is so great. Therefore the need for effective treatment is much needed. Ways to support patients during advanced stages need to be explored. Approaches to combination treatment modalities to improve overall survival rates are necessary (McFadden, 1991)

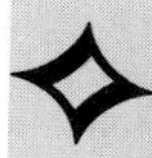

TABLE 64-7 Patient Preparation for Adminstering Topical Mechlorethamine Hydrochloride

Description of the Procedure: Topical treatment for patients in the early stages (plaque) of cutaneous T-cell lymphoma.

Patient Preparation: Patient is instructed about the toxic effects of the treatment on the skin and care of the skin after treatment.

Procedural Considerations

1. Obtain informed consent.
2. Patient needs to disrobe and wear a gown and latex gloves.
3. Topical solution is applied to the whole body except the eye lids, lips, and genitals.
4. Mechlorethamine hydrochloride solution is applied with a brush or cloth.
5. The patient is desensitized with a one-tenth solution of nitrogen mustard until achieving the desired dose.
6. If hypersensitivity occurs, the treatment is temporarily discontinued.
7. A neutralizing solution of 5% sodium thiosulfate is used for nurse or family who have an accidental contact with patient.
8. Gloves and clothes are disposed of in a chemotherapy receptacle.
9. Report any hypersensitivity reactions or erythema to your doctor.

REFERENCES

Arnold, H. L., Odom, R. B., & James, W. D. (1990). Mycosis fungoides, other malignant lymphomas and allied diseases. (8th ed.). *Andrews' diseases of the skin: Clinical dermatology.* Philadelphia: W. B. Saunders.

Besnier, E. & Hallopeau, H. (1982). On the erythroderma of mycosis fungoides. *Journal of Cutaneous Genitourinary Disease, 10,* 453.

Broder, S. & Bunn, P. A. (1980). Cutaneous T-cell lymphomas. *Seminars in Oncology, 7,* 310-327.

Bunn, P. A. & Fuks, Z., (1989). Cutaneous lymphomas. In V. T. DeVita, S. Hellman, & S. A. Rosenberg (Eds.), *Cancer: Principles and practice of oncology* (3rd ed.). Philadelphia: Lippincott-Raven.

Bunn, P. A. & Lamberg, S. I. (1979). Report of the committee on staging and classification of cutaneous T-cell lymphomas. *Cancer Treat Rep, 63,* 725.

Cameron, O. J. (1993). Mycosis fungoides in mother and daughter. *Archives of Dermatology Syph, 27,* 232-236.

Claudy, A., Rouchouse, B., Boucheron, S., & LePetit, J. (1983). Treatment of cutaneous lymphoma with etretinate. *British Journal of Dermatology, 109,* 49-56.

Dean, F. A. (1990). Caring for CTCL patients undergoing photopheresis. *Dermatology Nursing, 2*(1), 26-28.

DiJulio, J. E. (1988). Treatment of B-cell and T-cell lymphomas with monoclonal antibodies. *Seminars in Oncology Nursing, 4,* 102-106.

Dreno, B., Claudy, A., Meynadier, J., Verret, J., Souteyrand, J., Ortonne, J., Kalis, B., Godefroy, W., Beerblock, K., & Thill, L. (1991). The treatment of 45 patients with cutaneous T-cell lymphoma with low doses of interferon-alpha 2a and etretinate. *British Journal of Dermatology, 125,* 456-459.

Dewey, W. C., Ling, C. C., & Meyn, R. E. (1995). Radiation-induced apoptosis: Relevance to radiotherapy. *International Journal of Radiation Oncology, Biology, and Physics, 33,* 781.

Edelson, R. L. (1975). Membrane properties of the abnormal cells of cutaneous lymphoma. *Annals of Internal Medicine, 83,* 536.

Edelson, R. L. (1988). Light-activated drugs. *Scientific American, 8,* 68-75.

Eriksson, J. H. (1994). *Oncologic nursing.* Springhouse, PA: Springhouse.

Gilchrest, B. A., Parrish, J. A., Tannenbaum, L. R., Haynes, H. A., & Fitzpatrick, T. B. (1976). Oral methoxsalen photochemotherapy of *mycosis fungoides. Cancer 38*(4), 683-698.

Gilyon, K. & Kuzel, T. M., (1991). Cutaneous T-cell lymphoma. *Oncology Nursing Forum, 18*(5), 901-908.

Greene, M. H., Dalager, N. A., Lamberg, S. L., Argyropoulous, C. E., & Fraumeni, J. F. (1979). *Mycosis fungoides:* Epidemiologic observations. *Cancer Treat Rep, 63*(4), 597-606.

Green, S., Byar, D., & Lamberg, S. (1981). Prognostic variables in mycosis fungoides. *Cancer, 47*(11), 2671-2677.

Harris, J. S. & Macey, W. H. (1994). Cutaneous T-cell lymphoma: a case study, treatment and nursing implications. *Dermatology Nursing, 6,* 41-49.

Holloway, K., Flowers, F., & Ramos-Caro, F. (1992). Therapeutic alternatives in cutaneous T-cell lymphoma. *Journal of American Academy of Dermatology, 27,* 367-378.

Horm, J. W. & Weinstock, M. A. (1988). *Mycosis fungoides* in the United States: Increasing incidence and descriptive epidemiology. *Journal of the American Medical Association, 260*(1), 42-46.

Jones, G., McLean, J., Rosenthal, D., Roberts, J., & Sauder, D. (1992). Combined treatment with oral etretinate and electron beam therapy in patients with cutaneous T-cell lymphoma (*mycosis fungoides* and Sézary syndrome). *Journal of the American Academy of Dermatology, 26,* 960-967.

Kirchner, W. C. (1984). Sexuality and selected cancer therapies. In N. F. Woods (Ed.), *Human sexuality in health and illness.* St. Louis: Mosby.

Klein, E. & Schwartz, R. A. (1982). Cancer and the skin. In J. F. Holland & E. Frei (Eds.), *Cancer medicine* (2nd ed.). Philadelphia: Lea and Febriger.

Lamberg, S. I., Green, S. B., Byar, D. P., Block, J. B., Clendenning, W. E., Epstein, Jr., E. H., Fuks, Z. Y. Golitz, L. E., Lorincz, A. L., Michel, B., Roenigk, H. H., Jr., Van Scott, E. J., Vonderheid, E. C., & Thomas R.J. (1979). Status report of 376 mycosis fungoides patients at 4 years. *Mycosis Fungoides* Cooperative Group. *Cancer Treatment Reports, 63,* 701-707.

Levi, J. A. (1986). Cutaneous T-cell lymphomas. In A. R. Moosa, M. C. Robson, & S. C. Schimpff, (Eds.), *Comprehensive textbook of oncology.* Baltimore: Williams and Wilkins.

Lutzer, M., Edelson, R., & Schein, P. (1968). Cutaneous T-cell lymphomas: The Sézary syndrome, *mycosis fungoides,* and related disorders. *Annals of Internal Medicine, 83,* 534-552.

Macy, W. H. & Harris, J. S. (1995). Photopheresis and the role of the nurse. *Dermatology Nursing, 7*(1), 13-22.

McFadden, M. (1991). Cutaneous T-cell lymphoma. *Seminars in Oncology Nursing, 1,* 36-44.

Perez, M., Edelson, R., La Roche, L., & Berger, C. (1989). Inhibition of anti-skin allograft immunity by infusions with syngeneic photoinactivated effector lymphocytes. *The Society for Investigative Dermatology, 92*(5), 669-678.

Physicians desk reference (1997). Oradell, N. J.: Medical Economics.

Picker, I. J., Michie, S. A., Rott, L. S., & Butcher, E. C. (1990). A unique phenotype of skin-associated lymphocytes in humans: Preferential expression of the HECA-452 epitope by benign and malignant T cells at cutaneous sites. *American Journal of Pathology, 136,* 1053.

Rosenbaum, M. M., Roenigk, J. J., & Caro, W. (1985). Photochemotherapy in cutaneous T-cell lymphoma and parapsoriasis in plaques. Long-term follow-up in forty-three patients. Journal of *American Academy of Dermatology, 13*(4), 613-622.

Sandbank, M. & Katzenellenbogen, I. (1968). *Mycosis fungoides* of prolonged duration in siblings. *Arch Dermatology 98*(12), 620-627.

Sausville, E. A., Eddy, J. L., Makuch, R. W., Fischmann, A. B., Schechter, G. P., Matthews, H., Glatstein, E., Ihde, D. C., Kaye, F., & Veach, S. R. (1988). Histopathologic staging at initial diagnosis of mycosis fungoides and the Sézary syndrome. *Annals of Internal Medicine, 109,* 372-382.

Sézary, A. & Bouvrain, Y. (1938). Erythroderme avec presence des cellules monstrueuses dans derme et dans sang circulant. *Bulletin for the Society of French Dermatology Symposium, 45,* 254.

Skarin, A. T. (1996). *Atlas of diagnostic oncology* (2nd ed.). St. Louis: Mosby-Wolfe.

Stocker, J., Liegey, C., & Cooley, D. (1990). When little more could be done, we did a lot . . . *mycosis fungoides. RN, 53*(8). 25-27.

Stoupa, R. (1990). Understanding cutaneous T-cell lymphoma. *Dermatology Nursing, 2,* 19-25.

Strohl, R. A. (1994). The role of total skin electron beam radiation therapy in the management of *mycosis fungoides. Dermatology Nursing, 6*(3), 191-194, 196, 220.

Sutherland, A. M. (1960). *The psychological impact of cancer.* New York: American Cancer Society.

Thibodeau, G. A. & Patton, K. T. (1996). *Anatomy and physiology* (10th ed.). St. Louis: Mosby.

Tuyp, E., Burgoyne, A., Aitchison, T., & MacKie, R. (1987). A case-controlled study of possible causative factors in mycosis fungoides. *Archives of Dermatology, 123,* 196-200.

Vonderheid, E. C., Van Scott, E. J., Wallner, P. E., & Johnson, W. C. (1979). A ten-year experience with topical mechlorethamine for mycosis fungoides. *Cancer Treatment Report 63*(4), 691-700.

Vonderheid, E. & Micailey, B. (1985). Treatment of cutaneous T-cell lymphoma. *Dermatology Clinics, 3,* 673-687.

Vonderheid, E. & Micailey, B. (1992). Cutaneous T-cell lymphoma. In Perez, C. (Ed.), *Principles and practice of radiation oncology* (2nd ed.). Philadelphia: J. B. Lippincott.

Weinstock, M. A. & Horm, J. W. (1988). Population-based estimate of survival and determinants of prognosis in patients with *mycosis fungoides. Cancer, 62,* 1658-1661.

Whittmore, A. S., Holly, E., Lee, I. M., Abel, E. A., Adams, R. M., Nickoloff, B. J., Bley, L., Peters, J. M., & Gibney, C. (1989). *Mycosis fungoides* in relation to environmental exposures and immune response: A case-control study. *Journal of the National Cancer Institute, 81,* 1560.

Wilson, L. D., Kacinski, B. M., Edelson, R. L., & Heald, P. W. (1997). Cutaneous T-cell lymphomas. In V. T. DeVita, S. Hellman, & S. A., Rosenberg (Eds.), *Cancer: Principles and practice of oncology* (5th ed.). Philadelphia: Lippincott-Raven.

Worobec-Victor, S. M. (1989). Cutaneous T-cell lymphoma. *New England Journal of Medicine, 86,* 395-400.

Hodgkin's Disease

Nellee M. H. Fine, RN, MA, AOCN
Lynn E. Scallion, RN, MSN, AOCN

Hodgkin's disease (HD) is an uncommon lymphoid malignancy that accounts for 15% of all lymphomas and less than 1% of all cancers (Ries, Miller, & Hankey, 1994). Over the past 40 years of research, a systematic approach to HD has produced one of the best cure rates in oncology and continues to serve as a model for modern cancer therapy. Careful staging and treatment strategies have resulted in a cure rate for all patients with HD as high as 75% (Urba & Longo, 1992) and a cure rate for childhood HD of 90% (Vecchi, Pileri, Burnelli, Bontempi, Comelli, & Testi, 1992). Despite the relatively low overall incidence of HD, it is one of the most common cancers in adolescents and young adults (Jarrett, Armstrong, & Alexander, 1996). Even with a high rate of treatment success, HD remains the fifth leading cause of cancer death in 15- to 34-year-old males (Landis, Murray, Bolden, & Wingo, 1998). Table 65-1 defines differences between HD and non–Hodgkin's disease (NHD).

Despite long-term survival for many patients with HD, curative therapy may result in serious long-term consequences. Second malignancies (skeletal, immune, endocrine, cardiovascular, pulmonary, digestive, and gonadal disorders) are a potential sequelae of treatment (Henry-Amar & Joly, 1996). The goal of current clinical trials is a reduction in treatment-associated toxicity without loss of disease control (Oberlin, 1996). Early identification of patients at high risk for treatment failure is essential to avoid overtreatment and subsequent long-term complications in the majority of patients who do not fall in the high-risk category. In addition, continued assessment of the quality of life of the survivors of HD is critical to a comprehensive plan of care. Designing appropriate and effective interventions enhances long-term well-being and improves the functional status of HD survivors.

HISTORY

In 1832 an English physician, Thomas Hodgkin, published a historic paper, "On Some Morbid Appearances of the Absorbent Glands and Spleen." In this paper he provided a detailed description of postmortem findings for seven patients who had progressive and eventually fatal disorders characterized by enlargement of the lymph nodes, liver, and spleen. From observations of gross anatomy and without the aid of microscopy, he recognized that this disease represented a primary disorder of these lymphoid structures, rather than an infectious process (Zantinga & Coppes, 1996). For over 30 years, his astute observations went unnoticed by colleagues, until Sir Samuel Wilks became aware of Dr. Hodgkin's original paper. In 1865, Wilks published a paper on "Enlargement of the Lymphatic Glands and Spleen (or, Hodgkin's Disease)." At the turn of the century, pathologists Carl Sternberg (1898) and Dorothy Reed (1902) distinguished HD from tuberculosis and other infectious processes. They also identified the characteristic multinucleated giant cell of HD now known as *Reed-Sternberg (RS) cell.*

INCIDENCE

The annual age-adjusted incidence of HD is 2.8 and 2.4 per 100,000 in the United States and United Kingdom, respectively (Ries, Miller, & Hankey, 1994). Internationally, however, incidence rates are 3 to 4 times greater, with the exception of Asian countries (Jarrett, Armstrong, & Alexander, 1996). Worldwide, there are three patterns of incidence for HD. In economically developed countries, HD has a bimodal age distribution with two peaks; the first peak occurs in the age group 15 to 34 years, and the second peak occurs in patients over 55 years (Medeiros & Greiner, 1997). In underdeveloped countries the overall incidence of HD is lower than in developed countries. In these areas a higher incidence rate occurs in children survivors before age 15 years, with only a modest increase throughout adolescence and young adulthood (Jarrett, Armstrong, & Alexander, 1996). In Asia, where the incidence rates are generally low, the first peak is absent (Macfarlane, Evistifeeva, Boyle, & Grufferman, 1995). In the United States, HD is rarely diagnosed in children younger than 5 years; the median age at the time of diagnosis is 32 years.

TABLE 65-1 Differentiating Hodgkin's Disease and NHL

Hodgkin's Disease	Non-Hodgkin's Lymphoma
Age:	
Younger population	Older population
Symptoms:	
B symptoms common: Pel-Ebstein fever Night sweats Weight loss >10%	B symptoms rare More indolent disease
Patients less debilitated at Dx	More debilitated at Dx
Stage:	
Localized disease in 50% to 60% of patients Stage I/II common	Advanced-stage disease in 80% Stage III/IV common
Histopathology:	
Reed-Sternberg cell identified; diagnostic for HD Cell origin: not determined	No Reed-Sternberg cells Cell origin: 90% B cell; 10% T cell
Sites of disease:	
Origin: nodal	Origin: extranodal
Uncommon bone marrow involvement	Common bone marrow involvement
Spleen frequently only organ involved below diaphragm	Diffuse disease
Mesentery rarely involved	Mesentery often involved
Centripetal: axial nodal distribution of disease with neck, mediastinum, and periaortics common	Centrifugal: extensive disease vs axial distribution, mediastinum involvement rare
Uncommon abdominal node involvement	Common abdominal node involvement
Alterations in immune system:	
Defect in cellular immunity (T cell)	Defect in humoral immunity (B cell)
Metastasis:	
Route of metastasis: contiguous lymph node spread	Route of metastasis: follows lymph circulation/distribution throughout body; noncontiguous
Prognosis:	
High cure rate in early-stage disease	Cure varies based on Dx of indolent vs aggressive disease; a therapeutic challenge

Note: The prognosis for HD and NHL varies with the following factors: stage of disease at diagnosis, amount of bulky disease, number of extranodal sites, bone marrow involvement, systemic symptoms, age of patient, performance status, comorbid conditions, sensitivity to standard and salvage chemotherapy, the development of multidrug resistance, patient-family goals, and decisions about initiating or continuing therapy.

The incidence of HD varies with respect to gender, race, age, social class, and histologic subtype. The Surveillance, Epidemiology and End Results (SEER) program of the National Cancer Institute collected 9493 cases of HD between 1973 and 1987 (Medeiros & Greiner, 1995). The overall incidence was slightly higher in males than females. Between 1983 and 1987, the peak in males and females was similar in young adults. In the elderly, males had a higher age-specific incidence rate. Since 1973, the SEER study has demonstrated that the incidence of HD in the United States has markedly increased in the younger age group, particularly in nodular sclerosis subtype; here the incidence rate rose from 1.1 to 1.6 per 100,000 from 1973 to 1987, primarily in young adult women. In the elderly the incidence has decreased in recent years. This is likely due to the improved ability to diagnose and differentiate HD and non–Hodgkin's lymphoma (NHL). Historically, HD has been more common in Caucasians than in African-Americans. Differences in the age distribution between the races were also noted in the SEER data. For Caucasians the age distribution was bimodal. However, the curve was more uniform for African Americans with smaller peaks (Medeiros & Greiner, 1995).

Incidence patterns vary with histologic type. Nodular sclerosis HD (NSHD) exhibits a unimodal incidence curve and accounts for the young adult peak seen in developed countries. In contrast, the other histologic subtypes demonstrate a gradual increased incidence with increasing age. Lymphocyte-predominant and mixed cellularity disease are most common in patients over age 40 years. Mixed cellularity is the most common subtype of HD in the 50-year age group. The lymphocyte-predominant subtype affects all ages; the incidence rate for this histology also correlates with increasing age. The lymphocytic-depletion subtype is rare in patients younger than age 40 years; however, this type increases progressively thereafter (Jarrett, Armstrong, & Alexander, 1996).

EPIDEMIOLOGY

Epidemiologic evidence suggests that HD is at least two different diseases. One disease type occurs in young persons age 15 to 34 years, whereas the second disease affects people over 55 years (Medeiros & Greiner, 1995). The first incidence peak, which is seen in more well-developed countries like the United States, may be the result of delayed exposure to a common infectious agent that is most likely viral in origin. Epidemiologic factors such as social class, small family size, single-family housing, high maternal education, and decreased number of siblings suggest a high standard of living and are associated with an increased risk of HD in young adults (Gutensohn & Cole, 1981; Gutensohn, 1982). These risk factors, however, seem to be restricted to nodular sclerosing HD (Jarrett, Armstrong, & Alexander, 1996). Cozen, Katz, and Mack (1992) found that there was the suggestion of a reverse correlation in children and older adult age groups; increasing socioeconomic status reduced the incidence of HD.

Epstein-Barr Virus

The Epstein-Barr virus (EBV) has been implicated in the pathogenesis of HD. EBV, the causative agent of infectious mononucleosis, is also associated with Burkitt's lymphoma, seen chiefly in central Africa. EBV, a herpesvirus, is known to transform resting human B cells into proliferative lymphoblastoid cell lines (Niedobitek, 1996). Since 1987, a variety of techniques have demonstrated the EBV genome. EBV has been detected in the Reed-Sternberg cells of HD patients; however, the EBV genome is only associated with approximately 40% of all HD cases (Jarrett, Armstrong, & Alexander, 1996; Weiss, Movahad, Warnke, & Sklar, 1989). The absence of EBV in the remaining 60% and the prevalence of EBV infection in the general population suggest that EBV infection may be one of several factors in the pathogenesis of HD. The histologic subtype most suggestive to be the result of an EBV infection is the nodular sclerosis subtype. Yet, the highest proportion of EBV-positive cases are of the mixed cellularity subtype (Herbst, Steinbrecher, Neidobitek, Young, Brooks, & Muller-Lantzsch, 1992; Horning, 1995). In addition, children and older adults are more closely linked with EBV exposure than young adults, which implies the possibility of a different etiology for different age groups (Diehl & Engert, 1996). This observation suggests that another, as yet undiscovered, viral agent may be involved in the natural history of HD (Jarrett, Armstrong, & Alexander, 1996; Pelstring, Zellmer, Sulak, Banks, & Clare, 1991).

Human Immunodeficiency Virus

Patients infected with the human immunodeficiency virus (HIV) are known to be at risk for developing non–Hodgkin's lymphoma. The relationship of HIV to the development of HD is less clear. Interestingly, the EBV is known to be common in HD patients with HIV infection (Audoin, Diebold, & Pallesen, 1992). To determine the relationship between HIV infection and the risk of developing HD, the SEER data from San Francisco County was analyzed separately from other data. The San Francisco data demonstrated an age-adjusted incidence rate increase for all cases of HD from 2.6 to 3.0 per 100,000 between 1978 and 1987. The increase occurred predominantly in males between the ages of 30 and 49 years with mixed cellularity and miscellaneous historic subtypes; this was significantly different from the previously described incidence rate (Medeiros & Grenier, 1997). Additional studies are needed to investigate and confirm this association.

RISK FACTORS

Genetics

Genetic evidence to support an increased susceptibility to HD includes a ninefold increased risk for same-gender siblings and a fivefold increase in opposite-gender siblings. Several investigators found that there was an increased risk among parent-child pairs, but not among spouses (Grufferman, Cole, Smith, & Lukes, 1977; Robertson, Lowman, Grufferman, Kostyu, van der Horst, & Matthews, 1987; Gutterman, Barton, & Eby, 1987).

Infectious Agents

In the past, reports of clusters of HD cases gave rise to suspicions that HD was a contagious disorder (Vianna, Greenwald, & Davies, 1971; Vianna & Polan, 1973). However, data revealed that the clusters were determined to have occurred by chance (Gutterman, Cole, & Levitan, 1979). Other studies have indicated that patients with a prior history of infectious mononucleosis have approximately a threefold increased risk for developing HD (Miller & Beebe, 1973; Rosdahl, Larsen, & Clemmensen, 1974; Munoz, Davidson, Witthoff, Ericsson, & De Th'e, 1978). Recently, reports have suggested that HIV-positive persons, already at an increased risk of developing non–Hodgkins lymphoma, are at a slightly greater risk for developing HD as well (Medeiros & Grener, 1995).

Other Factors

A variety of diverse factors, including woodworking, benzene exposure, and elevated rates after tonsillectomy and appendectomy, have been associated with an increased risk for developing HD (Box 65-1) (Millham & Hesser, 1967; Vianna, Greenwald, & Davies, 1971; Bierman, 1968; Aksoy, Erdern, Dincol, Hepuyksel, & Dincol, 1974). HD has rarely been documented as a second malignancy and has not been associated with immunosuppressive therapy (Mauch & Bonadonna, 1997).

PATHOLOGY

Origin of the Reed-Sternberg Cell

Hodgkin's disease is primarily a disease of the lymph nodes, characterized by the presence of giant, abnormal cells that are binucleate or multinucleated. These cells have prominent eosinophilic nucleoli, which are known as *RS cells,* and were named after the pathologists Reed and Sternberg, who first described the malignant cells. Establishing the presence of RS cells is essential in confirming the diagnosis of HD; however, in contrast to the cellular makeup of other malignancies, neoplastic RS cells comprise only 1% to 2% of the total lymphoid tissue specimen. In addition to the paucity of RS cells, RS cells are not pathognomonic for HD. RS cells have also been reported in benign conditions such as hyperplasia, inflammatory nodes, mononucleosis, other viral infections, and phenytoin (Dilantin) therapy (Strum, Dark, & Rappaport, 1970). The affected lymph node contains mostly normal reactive and inflammatory cells and scar tissue, with rare RS cells interspersed amidst the cellular composition, as shown in Fig. 65-1 (Rosenthal & Eyre, 1995).

Biologic Features of the Reed-Sternberg Cell

Although the cellular origin of the RS cells has been a controversial subject, current research findings indicate that the majority of RS cells are of lymphocyte origin. Immunophenotype fingerprinting has revealed that surface antigen markers expressed by RS cells are a monoclonal population of B cell origin (Diehl & Engert, 1996). RS cells express antigens found on resting or activated lymphocytes, including B cell (CD19, CD20, CD22) and T cell (CD2, CD3, CD4) surface antigens; occasionally RS cells express neither phenotype (Mauch & Bonadonna, 1997). Most RS cells have CD15 and CD30 surface antigens; however, the subtype lymphocyte predominant HD is CD15 negative and CD45 positive (leukocyte common antigen [LCA]) (Haluska, Brufsky, & Canellos, 1994). A summary of HD immunophenotype by histologic subtype is provided in Table 65-2.

Cytogenic Studies

Cytogenic abnormalities are common in RS cells; however, no consistent pattern has been described (Mauch & Bonadonna, 1997). At first presentation, HD is thought to represent both monoclonal and polyclonal cells, which gradually

Box 65-1
Risk Factors for Hodgkin's Disease

- Inherited susceptibility
- Viral exposure (EBV, HIV)
- Occupational exposure (woodworking, benzene)
- History of tonsillectomy or appendectomy (?)

From Millham, S., & Hesser, J. (1967). Hodgkin's disease in woodworkers. *Lancet, 2,* 136; Vianna, N. J., Greenwald, P., & Davies, J. N. P. (1971); Extended epidemic of Hodgkin's disease in high school students. *Lancet, 1,* 1209; Bierman, H. R. (1968). Human appendix and neoplasia. *Cancer, 121,* 109; Aksoy, M., Erden, S., Dincol, K., Hepuyksel, T., & Dincol, G. (1974). Chronic exposure to benzene as a possible contributory etiological factor in Hodgkin's disease, *Blut, 28,* 298; Mauch P. M. & Bonadonna, G. (1997). Hodgkin's disease. In J. F. Holland, R. C. Bast, D. L. Morton, E. Frei, D. W. Kufe, & R. R. Weichselbaum (Eds.), *Cancer medicine.* Philadelphia: Williams & Wilkins.

TABLE 65-2 Hodgkin's Disease Immunophenotype by Histologic Subtype

Antigen	Histologic Subtype			
	LP	NS	MC	LD
CD45 (LCA)	+	−	−	−
CD30 (Ki-1)	−(+)	+	+	+
CD15 (LeuM1)	−	+	+	+
CD20 (L26)	+	−(+)	−(+)	−(+)

Modified from Haluska, F. G., Brufsky, A. M., & Canellos, G. P. (1994). The cellular biology of the Reed-Sternberg cell. *Blood, 84,* 1005.
LP, Lymphocyte predominance, nodular subtype only; *NS,* nodular sclerosis; *MC,* mixed cellularity; *LD,* lymphocyte depletion; +, positive; −, negative; *(+),* some cases positive.

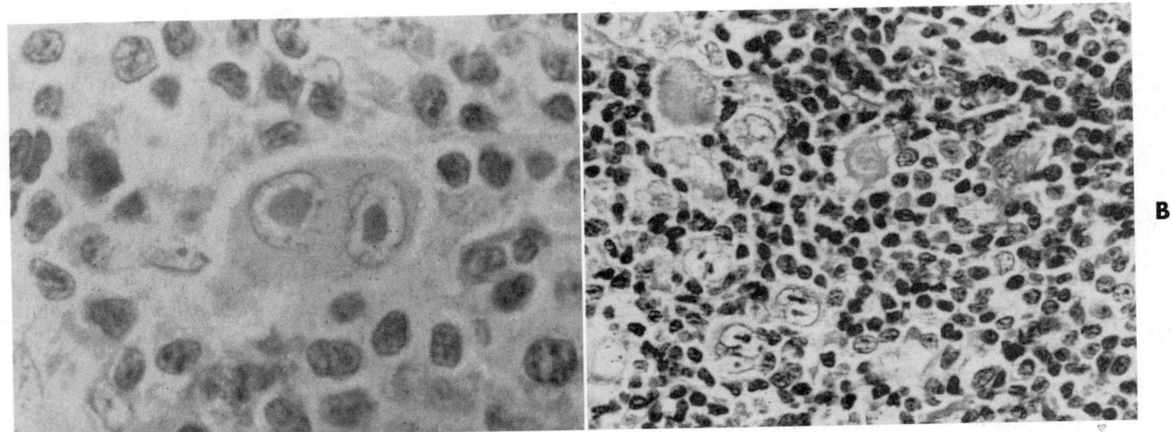

Fig. 65-1 **A,** Diagnostic Reed-Sternberg cell, seen in classic types of Hodgkin's disease (mixed cellularity, nodular sclerosis, lymphocyte depletion). **B,** Variants of Reed-Sternberg cells seen in nodular lymphocyte predominance Hodgkin's disease—popcorn cells, or L and H cells (lymphocytic or histiocytic predominance). Reed-Sternberg cells of the classic type generally are not seen in nodular lymphocyte predominance Hodgkin's disease. (From DeVita, V. T., Hauch, P. M., & Harris, N. L. [1997]. Hodgkin's disease. In V. T. DeVita, S. Hellman, & S. A. Rosenberg [Eds], *Cancer: Principles and practice of oncology* [5th ed.]. Philadelphia: J. B. Lippincott.)

develop into a true monoclonal population (Diehl & Engert, 1996). Establishing HD cell lines for cytogenic studies has been difficult due in part to the task of isolating the rare RS cell from the vast majority of reactive cells in an HD lymph node. In addition, the exceedingly low mitotic yield of these cells inhibits cell culture growth. RS cells also may secrete cytokines that inhibit cell proliferation. The aneuploidy seen in HD may represent replication of deoxyribonucleic acid (DNA) without accompanying nuclear division. This "dead end cell"–like behavior may explain why the monoclonal proliferation, so characteristic of other lymphomas, is diminished in HD cell lines.

RS cells have been reported to express *bcl*-2 oncogene products. The *bcl*-2 oncogene is known to prevent apoptosis, the "programmed death" of a cell; this, in turn, promotes the growth and "immortality" of cells, even though the DNA has been damaged. The translocation t (14;18) found in nodular NHL activates *bcl*-2, but this defect is rare in HD. EBV infection also activates *bcl*-2 and may contribute to the pathogenesis of some forms of HD (Weiss et al., 1989). Recent studies analyzing the distribution of EBV in HD have revealed that in most EBV-positive HD cases, the viral genomes are monoclonal (Niedobetik, 1996). The EBV genome has been identified more often in the RS cells of patients with mixed cellularity (MC) histology than with nodular sclerosis (NS), and are rare in patients with lymphocyte predominance Hodgkin's disease (LPHD) (Staal, Ambinder, Beschorner, Hayward, & Mann, 1989).

Cytokine Secretion

RS cells secrete a variety of cytokines listed in Table 65-3. These substances may contribute to the diverse histologic patterns of HD, as well as the assemblage of nonmalignant cells, marked inflammatory component, and fibrosis in the lymph node specimen (Hsu, Waldron, Hsu, & Hough, 1993). The proliferation of nonneoplastic cells in the lymph node and bone marrow tissue, as well as aberrations of immune response, are linked to cytokine secretion. In turn, these reactive nonmalignant cells produce cytokines that influence RS cells, contributing to the pathogenesis of this disease (Horning, 1995). Cytokine secretion may also be responsible for the classic triad of symptoms of fever, weight loss, and night sweats, experienced by patients with HD. Patients with active HD have increased cytokine production. The cytokine interleukin-2 (IL-2) has been detected in patients' sera and correlates with poor prognosis in children with HD (Pui, Ip, Thompson, Wilimas, Brown, & Dodge, 1989).

TABLE 65-3 Cytokines Produced by Hodgkin's Disease

Cytokine	Relatable Biologic Features
IL-1	Lymphoproliferation, fever, night sweats, immunodeficiency
IL-2	Similar to IL-1, promotes growth of RS cells in culture
IL-4	Unknown
IL-5	Eosinophilic infiltration
IL-6	Promotes growth of RS cells in culture
IL-9	Lymphoproliferation
TNF-alpha	Weight loss
TNF-beta	Weight loss
IFN	Unknown
GM-CSF	Leukocyte or eosinophil infiltration
G-CSF	Myeloproliferation
M-CSF	Unknown
TGF-beta	Fibrosis, potent immunosuppressant

Modified from Diehl, V., von Kalle, C., Fonatash, C., Tesch, H., Juecker, M., & Schaadt. (1990). The cell of origin in Hodgkin's disease. *Seminars in Oncology, 17,* 660.
IL, Interleukin; *TNF,* tumor necrosis factor; *IFN,* interferon; *CSF,* colony stimulating factor; *G,* granulocyte; *M,* macrophage; *TGF,* transforming growth factor.

Abnormalities in Immune Function

As a malignancy of the immune system, Hodgkin's disease involves defects primarily in cellular immunity. Because the total lymphocyte count is depressed, patients are continuously at risk for infectious processes. In 1928, Ewing observed that "tuberculosis follows Hodgkin's disease like a shadow." He noted that 20% of his patients with Hodgkin's disease were infected with tuberculosis. Later, Jackson and Parker (1944) found that despite the presence of active tuberculosis, a positive tuberculin test in HD patients was rare. Table 65-4 shows the functional deficits in cellular immunity and T cell-mediated response that are known to exist in HD patients. Although HD and NHL are malignancies of the immune system, the severity of decreased cellular immune response is greater in HD patients than in patients with NHL. Delayed hypersensitivity response improves in long-term survivors of HD. Yet, other permuta-

TABLE 65-4 Immunologic Dysfunction in Hodgkin's Disease

Disease-Related Immune Dysfunction

Cellular Immunity (T cell)
- Delayed-type hypersensitivity
- Diminished IL-2 production
- Decreased mitogenic response
- Increased monocyte suppressor activity
- Decreased lymphocyte numbers
- Reduced natural killer cell cytotoxicity

Treatment-Related Immune Dysfunction

Humoral Immunity (B cell)
- Decreased antibody production (t-dependent)
- Diminished mitogenic responses
- Impaired vaccine response
- Increased antilymphocyte antibodies
- Increased circulating immune complexes

From DeVita, V. T., Mauch, P. M., & Harris, N. L. (1997). Hodgkin's disease. In V. T. DeVita, S. Hellman, & S. A. Rosenberg (Eds.), *Cancer: Principle and practice of oncology* (5th Ed.), Philadelphia: J. B. Lippincott.

tions of cellular immunity endure, despite successful treatment and disease-free status. NHL patients who have received comparable chemotherapy do not demonstrate the persistence of these abnormalities (Slivnick, Ellis, Nawrocki, & Fischer, 1990).

Deficits in cellular immunity include impairment of delayed hypersensitivity, depressed proliferative responses to T cell mitogen stimulation, decreased natural killer (NK) cell cytotoxicity, and enhanced immunoglobulin production (Slivnick et al., 1990). These abnormalities worsen with advancing disease, suggesting that the immunosuppression demonstrated in untreated HD patients is secondary to chronic overstimulation by cytokines that are secreted primarily by the RS cells (Mauch & Bonadonna, 1997). As yet, it is not known why these immune deficits persist in patients cured of HD. In contrast to cellular immune defects, humoral immunity functions relatively normal in all but the most advanced cases of HD. Defects in humoral response are primarily due to treatment of the neoplasm; depressed humoral immunity is typically transient. Splenectomy (performed as part of staging laparotomy), chemotherapy, and radiation therapy all contribute to impaired humoral immunity (antibody formation) (Aisenberg, 1991). Although splenectomy alone has not been demonstrated to alter B cell function, the combination and intensity of therapies has a negative effect on B cell function (Devita, Mauch, & Harris, 1997).

Vaccines against encapsulated organisms (i.e., pneumococci, *Haemophilus influenzae,* and meningococci) may decrease the risk of developing life-threatening sepsis. Vaccination is recommended for all patients with HD, especially those who will receive intensive or combination chemotherapy and radiotherapy. Because there is a diminished response to vaccines after treatment for HD has begun, vaccines should be administered at least 14 days before initiation of therapy for patients to receive maximal benefit. Also, response to booster vaccinations are ineffective in the first year of treatment for HD. Minor, Shiffman, & McIntosh (1979) demonstrated that patients immunized 3 years after completing therapy responded with a greater than twofold increase in antibody level postimmunization compared with patients who had completed therapy in the past 3 years. Postimmunization antibody production was postulated to return to normal approximately 8 years after completion of curative HD therapy. Unfortunately, neither antibiotic prophylaxis nor vaccination can guarantee the prevention of life-threatening sepsis; therefore all febrile illnesses need to be evaluated promptly in patients with HD. Risk of microbial infection from fungal, protozoal, and other organisms is high due to disease and/or treatment-induced immunodeficiency. "Infection patrol" and "infection control" are priorities of care.

HISTOLOGY

Histopathologic reviews distinguish HD from the less favorable non–Hodgkin's lymphomas and other lymphoproliferative disorders. Histologic classification has correlated well with the natural history and patterns of spread associated with different HD subtypes. Prior to radiotherapy and chemotherapy proficiency, histologic subtyping was an essential guide to determining the therapeutic approach. Over the past 5 decades, three major classification systems of HD have been used: the Lukes-Butler system, the Jackson-Parker system, and the Rye Conference system. A comparison of the histologic subtyping of these systems is shown in Fig. 65-2 (Lukes, Butler, & Hicks, 1966; Lukes, Craver, Hall, Rappaport, & Ruben, 1966; Jackson & Parker, 1944; Carbone, Kaplan, Muschoff, Smithers, & Tubiana, 1971).

Treatment decisions require expedient differentiation of HD from other non–Hodgkin's lymphomas. This need has promoted continued refinement in the histologic classification systems for HD. In 1994 a revised classification of HD

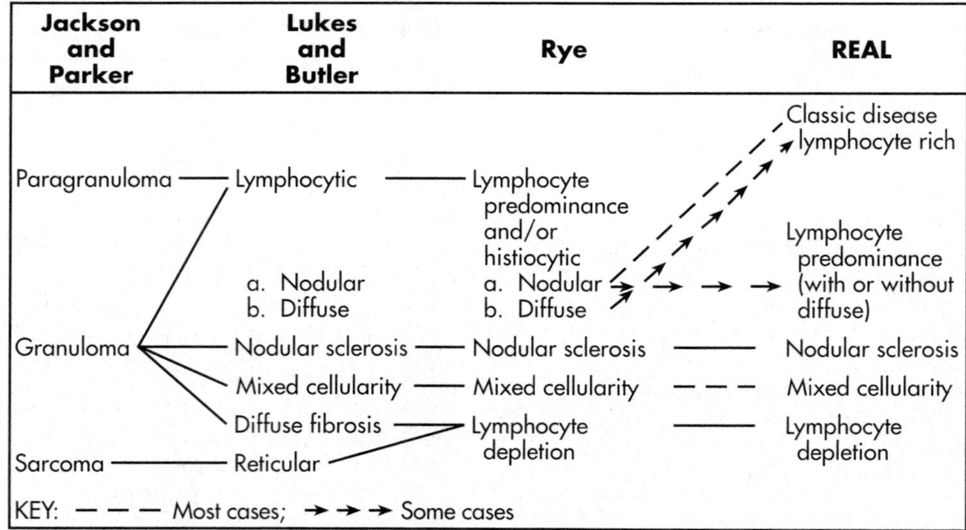

Fig. 65-2 Comparison of histologic classification systems of Hodgkin's disease. (From DeVita, V. T., Hauch, P. M., & Harris, N. L. [1997]. Hodgkin's disease. In V. T. DeVita, S. Hellman, & S. A. Rosenberg [Eds.], *Cancer: Principles and practice of oncology* [5th ed.]. Philadelphia: J. B. Lippincott.)

was introduced that incorporates new immunologic and molecular data (Harris, Jaffe, Stein, Banks, Chan, & Cleary, 1994). The Revised European American Lymphoma (REAL) classification system is expected to provide a basis for further discernment of the HD subtypes. The REAL system uses immunologic and epidemiologic evidence that at least two relatively distinct disease entities exist. REAL classification delineates a classic form of HD, which consists predominantly of NS, MC, and nodular lymphocyte predominant (NPDL) HD. In addition, the REAL classification further distinguishes NPDL by immunophenotype, resulting in a revised category referred to as *lymphocyte-rich classic disease* (DeVita Mauch, & Harris, 1997). Fig. 65-2 shows a comparison of the REAL and Rye classification systems. Advocates of the REAL classification recommend that the unclassifiable HD cases previously contained in the mixed cellularity subtype be renamed *Hodgkin's disease unclassifiable.* Recent evidence suggests that NLPD is a distinct disease entity separate from classic HD and may be more appropriately classified as a non–Hodgkin's lymphoma (Mason, Banks, Chan, Cleary, Delsol, & de Wolf-Peeters, 1994). Although pathologists are using the REAL system for its ability to discriminate more accurately the subtypes of HD, the Rye histopathologic classification system of HD is still the system used predominantly in current clinical practice.

The Rye classification system is composed of four major histologic subtypes of HD: lymphocyte predominant, nodular sclerosing, mixed cellularity, and lymphocyte depleted. Each category varies as to natural history, pattern of spread, and epidemiologic factors. SEER data regarding relative frequency and overall survival rates are shown in Table 65-5.

Nodular Sclerosis

NS involves extensive scarring and is the most common type of HD. This subtype occurs primarily in adolescents and young adults, and it is rare in patients over 50 years of age. In developed countries, NS comprises 40% to 70% of all HD cases and is less common in underdeveloped countries (Mauch & Bonadonna, 1997). The SEER study reports that from 1973 to 1987, the relative frequency of nodular sclerosis rose from 40.3% to 57.7%. The increase was significant in Caucasians (58.7%), but not in African Americans (46.7%). The 1973 to 1987 Seer data indicate that there were more female cases (66.1%) compared with male cases (51.3%) (Medeiros & Greiner, 1997). Nodular sclerosis commonly involves the head and neck lymph nodes and the lymph nodes of the intrathoracic region, including the mediastinum and thymus (Mauch, Kalisch, Kadin, Coleman, Osteen, & Hellman, 1993). At the time of diagnosis, approximately 70% of all patients with NSHD have limited disease and a favorable prognosis (Horning, 1995).

TABLE 65-5 Relative Frequency and Survival Rates of Hodgkin's Disease

Histology	Relative Frequency (%) 1983-1987	Overall 5-Year Survival Rate (%) 1983-1987
Nodular sclerosing	57.7	84.0
Mixed cellularity	23.4	70.0
Lymphocyte predominant	6.0	81.4
Lymphocyte depleted	3.8	34.4

Modified from Medeiros, L. J. & Greiner, T. C. (1997). Hodgkin's disease. *Cancer, 75* (Suppl. 1), 357-369.

Lymphocyte Predominance

Lymphocyte predominance (LPHD) with a diffuse replacement by lymphocytes occurs in approximately 5% to 10% of all HD patients. There are variants in this HD subtype that are characterized by a nodular or diffuse cellular pattern. The LPHD subtype is thought to be closely related to B-cell lymphoma. LPHD is most frequent in males under 15 and over 40 years of age. About 70% of LPHD patients have stage I disease (Horning, 1997). The pattern of spread often is localized to a single peripheral nodal region, with rare involvement of the mediastinal or abdominal lymph node regions (Mauch et al., 1993). LPHD has a unique indolent course with the longest time to recurrence of all HD subtypes. Relapse-free periods, however, do not affect survival. The 10-year survival rate of the lymphocyte predominance subtype is 90%. Some pathologists and clinicians believe that LPHD should be reported separately or reclassified as a non–Hodgkin's lymphoma because it differs in morphology, immunophenotype, and clinical course from classic HD (Horning & Hardy, 1994; Mason et al., 1994).

Mixed Cellularity

As implied in its designation, mixed cellularity HD (MCHD) contains a combination of lymphocytes, epithelial histiocytes, eosinophils, neutrophils, and plasma cells in the cellular material. Mixed cellularity HD is seen in all age groups, with a peak incidence in males 30 to 40 years old. In the United States, this subtype comprises 30% to 50% of all HD cases. It is seen more frequently in underdeveloped countries than in developed countries. More than 50% of patients with MCHD have an advanced stage of disease at the time of diagnosis. Patients commonly experience constitutional B symptoms (fever, sweats, and weight loss). In the past, MCHD was associated with a poorer prognosis than at present. With the advent of newer therapy, these patients now have an overall survival rate of approximately 70% (Medeiros & Grenier, 1997).

Lymphocyte Depleted

Lymphocyte depleted HD (LPHD) has a predominant pattern of large malignant cells, is the least common type of HD, and accounts for less than 5% of all HD cases worldwide.

LPHD is less common in economically developed countries (Mauch & Bonadonna, 1997). The U.S. SEER study

(1983 to 1987) revealed a relative frequency of LPHD of 3.8% (Medeiros & Grenier, 1997). LPHD is more common in the elderly and represents 15% to 20% of all cases of HD in patients after the age of 65 years (Medeiros & Greiner, 1997). LPHD has a uniquely aggressive natural history and often occurs in an advanced stage of disease (Canellos, 1995a). At the time of diagnosis, patients with LDHD may have abdominal adenopathy, spleen, liver, and bone marrow involvement; mediastinal and peripheral adenopathy, however, are rare (DeVita, Mauch, & Harris, 1997). LDHD is the most common type of HD found in HIV-positive patients (Pelstring et al., 1991). LDHD has an overall 5-year survival rate of less than 50% (Rosenthal & Eyre, 1995). The recent advent of immunophenotyping has distinguished LDHD from large cell lymphomas. As a result, the reported incidence rate of LDHD has decreased (Medeiros & Greiner, 1997).

CLINICAL PRESENTATION

Typically, patients with HD have painless cervical or supraclavicular lymphadenopathy. The characteristic lymph nodes are 1 cm or larger, firm, and freely movable, and they may be unilateral or bilateral. If growth has been rapid, the lymph nodes may be tender to palpation. Unlike other lymphoproliferative malignancies, HD is thought to evolve from a single lymph node group, spreading contiguously from one lymph node region to another in a predictable pattern. At presentation, the most common site of lymph node involvement, occurring in 80% of all cases, is above the diaphragm. Lymphadenopathy limited only to the subdiaphragmatic region is infrequent and occurs in less than 10% to 20% of patients. The generalized adenopathy, characteristic of other malignant lymphomas, is rarely seen in HD patients.

Mediastinal adenopathy is found in more than half of all HD patients. It is most common in young women with nodular sclerosis. Mediastinal adenopathy is often difficult to distinguish from normal thymus development in children. To minimize the risk of airway obstruction, careful evaluation of this region is critical before any procedure requiring anesthesia. Mediastinal masses may become large and bulky before the patient reports symptoms of coughing, difficulty swallowing, feeling short of breath, and/or experiencing occasional chest pain. In patients with a large mediastinal mass, cough and orthopnea (shortness of breath that intensifies when lying down and is relieved after sitting up) are common complaints. The involved nodes tend to be rubbery and distensible, which may explain that, despite the size and bulk of these mediastinal masses, superior vena cava syndrome is rare in HD (Canellos, 1995a).

Subdiaphragmatic presentation is uncommon in young patients and is reported at 10%. However, this location represents the only site of disease in 25% of elderly HD cases (Rosenthal & Eyre, 1995). The most common site of abdominal involvement is the spleen. Because the spleen has no afferent lymphatics, splenic involvement results from hematogenous spread of HD. Other organ involvement is uncommon because the RS cell depends on the lymphoid cellular environment. In addition, most organs are relatively lymphocyte poor; the growth of the RS cell at these sites is inhibited (Rosenthal & Eyre, 1995). Involvement of the liver, central nervous system, and retroperitoneal and mesenteric lymph nodes is indicative of advanced HD disease.

Although many HD patients are asymptomatic, constitutional symptoms may accompany the diagnosis of HD in 25% to 40% of all cases. The classic triad of B symptoms (drenching night sweats, fever greater than 100.4°F (38°C), and unexplained weight loss of 10% of the baseline in the preceding 6 months of diagnosis) is of prognostic significance. Approximately one third of all patients experience an irregular, low-grade fever. In rare cases, the classic Pel-Ebstein fever (high fever for 1 to 2 weeks alternating with similar afebrile periods) is seen and is virtually diagnostic of Hodgkin's disease. Patients may also experience fatigue, malaise, weakness, pruritus, erythematous rash, and pain in affected lymph nodes after alcohol consumption. These symptoms have not been of prognostic significance, but like the B symptoms, they may be a result of cytokine secretion by affected lymphocytes.

DIAGNOSTIC EVALUATION

The patient with HD requires a complete history and careful physical examination of all node-bearing areas, including Waldeyer's ring. An excisional biopsy of one or more of the

TABLE 65-6 Staging Evaluation for Hodgkin's Disease

Excisional Lymph Node Biopsy

History and physical examination:
- Presence and duration of B symptoms and pruritus
- Thorough lymph node evaluation

Imaging Studies
- Plain chest radiograph
- CT scan of thorax
- CT scan of abdomen and pelvis
- Bipedal lymphangiogram
- Gallium scan

Laboratory Tests
- CBC
- ESR
- RFT
- LFT
- LDH, albumin, calcium

Optional Procedures
- MRI
- Liver biopsy
- Bone scan
- Staging laparotomy
- Oophoropexy

From Rosen, P. J. (1995). Hodgkin's disease and malignant lymphoma. In D. A. Casciato & B. B. Lauritz (Eds.), *Manual of clinical oncology*. Boston: Little, Brown & Company.

CT, Computed tomography; *CBC,* complete blood count; *ESR,* erythrocyte sedimentation rate; *RFT,* renal function tests; *LFT,* liver function tests; *LDH,* lactate dehydrogenase; *MRI,* magnetic resonance imaging.

largest lymph nodes is performed to provide the pathologist with an adequate specimen. Frequently, multiple biopsies may be necessary because the diseased lymph nodes can exhibit reactive changes that are not diagnostic of HD. Needle biopsy, although simpler, is not recommended because the amount of tissue obtained by this method is inadequate for immunologic and cytogenic examination. After the diagnosis of HD is confirmed, accurate determination of the extent and of disease is essential for planning successful treatment. The recommended procedures and diagnosing staging of patients for HD are outlined in Tables 65-6 and 65-7.

Laboratory Tests

There are no clinical laboratory tests diagnostic for HD. A complete blood count may show nonspecific changes such as granulocytosis, eosinophilia (particularly in patients with pruritus), and thrombocytosis. Because an elevated erythrocyte sedimentation rate (ESR) has been correlated with advanced disease and constitutional symptoms, serial ESR studies may be used to monitor the disease process. Anemia of chronic disease and other cytopenias may result from bone marrow involvement, autoimmune disorders, or hypersplenism. An elevated serum alkaline phosphatase, although often nonspecific, may be associated with lactate dehydrogenase (LDH) and has been associated with a poor prognosis in some studies (Portlock & Yahalom, 1996).

Imaging Studies

A standard anteroposterior and lateral chest radiograph should be performed because greater than 60% of all patients have thoracic involvement on presentation. In addition, chest radiography is a simple, ideal surveillance tool for monitoring patients after therapy. Computed tomographic (CT) scans of the chest should be obtained in patients with abnormal chest x-ray films. Massive mediastinal adenopathy occurs in approximately 20% of the patients with limited clinical stage I or II disease, and these patients are at greater risk of relapse after treatment with radiation therapy alone (Leopold, Canellos, Rosenthal, Shulman, Weinstein, & Mauch, 1989). A gallium scan is useful in pretreatment staging and in monitoring tumor response to therapy. An important role of gallium scanning is to predict early treatment failure by discerning the presence of active, residual tumor in patients who have thoracic radiographic abnormalities after therapy (Hagemeister, Purugganan, Podohoff, Hess, Rodriguez, & McLaughlin, 1994; Hagemeister, Fesus, Lamki, & Haynie, 1990). Ultrasonography has limited usefulness in staging, with the exception of evaluating the presence of pericardial fluid.

Accurate documentation of the tumor below the diaphragm is critical to determining a successful treatment plan. However, CT scanning, lymphangiography, magnetic resonance imaging (MRI), and gallium scanning all have limitations in evaluating abdominal lymph nodes. Bipedal

TABLE 65-7 Assessment of the Patient for Hodgkin's Disease

	Assessment Parameters	Typical Abnormal Findings
History	A. Personal and social history	A. Personal and social factors 1. Age: First occurrence is usually in early 20s. Higher social class, advanced education, small family.
	B. Pain	B. Painless lymphadenopathy involving superficial lymph nodes
	C. Common symptoms reported	C. Night sweats, weight loss, marked fatigue, and general weakness, cough, and shortness of breath.
Physical Examination	A. Examine lymph nodes for size, number, consistency, and tenderness (submental, supraclavicular, infraclavicular, epitrochlear, iliac, femoral popliteal nodes).	A. Waldeyer's ring involvement indicates an endoscopy.
Diagnostic Tests	A. Peripheral node biopsy	A. Histopathologic findings for Hodgkin's disease.
	B. Anteroposterior and lateral chest radiograph	B. Immunophenotyping reveals presence of Hodgkin's disease. About 60% of patients have thoracic involvement. Also provides surveillance after therapy.
	C. Complete blood count	C. Usually nonspecific, but may reveal granulocytoses, eosinophilia, and thrombocytosis. Elevated sedimentation rate may indicate advanced disease. Anemia of chronic disease may indicate bone marrow involvement, autoimmune disorders, or hyperspenic disease.
	D. Serum alkaline phosphatase	D. Elevated levels, although nonspecific, may be associated with liver, bone, or bone marrow involvement.
	E. Serum lactate dehydrogenase	E. Elevated levels may indicate advanced disease.

Modified from DeVita, V. T., Mauch, P. M., & Harris, N. L. (1997). Hodgkin's disease. In V. T. DeVita, S. Hellman, & S. A. Rosenberg (Eds.), *Cancer: Principles and practice of oncology* (5th ed.). Philadelphia: J. B. Lippincott.

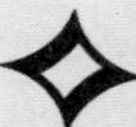

TABLE 65-8 Patient Preparation for Bipedal Lymphangiography

Description of Procedure: Bipedal lymphangiography is a direct method for investigating the lymphatic system using a blue radiopaque iodine contrast oil. The radiopaque dye is injected into the lymphatic channels located near the interdigital webs of the first three toes of each foot. This study is used for staging, and follow-up studies can be performed to monitor results of treatment because the dye can remain in the body for as long as a year.

Patient Preparation: The patient will be asked to lie still for approximately 2 to 3 hours during the dye infusion. Local anesthesia is administered to the feet and a small incision 1 to 2 inches is made on the top of each foot. Slight discomfort is expected at the start of the procedure. A plain x-ray film will be taken after the dye is infused and repeated in 12 to 24 hours.

Procedural Considerations

1. Informed consent is required.
2. Blue dye may discolor the skin, urine, and stool for approximately 48 hours.
3. It is contraindicated in patients with known iodine hypersensitivity, cardiac disease, advanced hepatic or renal disease, orthopnea, and/or restricted lung capacity.
4. Contrast dye fever occurs in approximately 40% of patients within 24 hours of injection.
5. Assess for signs of oil embolism every 4 hours for 24 hours. Instruct the patient to report shortness of breath and chest discomfort immediately.
6. Elevate the legs to prevent swelling for 24 hours, if ordered.
7. Keep the incision lines clean and dry until the sutures are removed.
8. Instruct the patient to report any signs or symptoms of redness or swelling and to wear loose-fitting shoes until the incisions are healed.

lymphangiography is valuable in assessing the architecture of small lymph nodes positive for HD, particularly in the femoral or inguinal region (Table 65-8). However, CT scanning is superior at imaging the celiac axis, splenic hillus, porta hepatis, and mesenteric nodes. The CT scan can discern normal lymph nodes from enlarged, tumor-involved lymph nodes in this region. These imaging studies are complementary diagnostic tools. The quality of the data from gallium scanning used to assess occult abdominal disease is limited by low test sensitivity (false-negative findings in a person with abdominal HD). MRI has test limitations as well, and it is an expensive diagnostic test that is not superior to CT scanning.

STAGING

Following the diagnosis of HD, the patient must undergo a thorough workup detailing the precise location and extent of tumor involvement. This process is known as *staging* and is of particular importance given the ability of HD to spread in a predictable, nonrandom way through contiguous chains of lymph nodes. Accurate documentation of the location of HD is essential in determining the plan of treatment. The purpose of staging HD is to differentiate patients who can benefit from radiation therapy alone from those who require systemic treatment (DeVita, Mauch, & Harris, 1997). The staging system used in HD describes the extent of disease in relation to the diaphragm. These classification systems are based on current understanding of the disease process and mechanisms of metastases. Modifications are based on research findings.

Staging Systems

The first useful staging classification system for HD was developed by Peters, Hasselbach, & Brown in 1968. The involvement of a single lymph node region or lymphoid structure (e.g., thymus, spleen) is designated as stage I. Involvement of two or more lymph node regions on the same side of the diaphragm is classified as stage II. Stage III HD includes the involvement of lymph node regions on both sides of the diaphragm. Additional refinement of the staging system occurred at a meeting in Rye, New York, where stage IV was added to the original system to describe situations where HD had disseminated beyond the lymph node system and involved one or more extranodal organs. The Rye staging system was again modified in 1970, at a conference in Ann Arbor, Michigan (Carbone et al., 1971). At this conference systemic symptoms classified as "B" present or "A" absent were added to the criteria. The constitutional symptoms deemed prognostically important were added to the criteria. The constitutional symptoms deemed prognostically important were as follows: fever above 100.4°F (38°C) for 3 consecutive days, night sweats, or unexplained loss of body weight in the previous 6 months. Other symptoms such as pruritus and pain after ingestion of alcohol contributed less prognostic information and are not included in this classification system. In addition, patients whose disease had spread contiguously, from lymph node chain to adjacent organ, were not considered to have "diffuse dissemination" of disease; the subscript "E" denotes direct extension. Splenic involvement is indicative of hematogenous spread of tumor and is recognized by the subscript "S."

The Ann Arbor Staging system remained the paradigm of classification until 1989, when an international classification system was proposed at a conference held in Cotswold, England. This historic assembly used the knowledge gleaned from the previous decades of research and established the Cotswold Staging classification for HD. This classification system is currently in use today and is described in Table 65-9. The following are some of the recommended modifications of the Ann Arbor system: The subscript "X" denotes the presence of bulky disease (greater than 10 cm diameter); clinical involvement of the liver and/or spleen can be confirmed if two or more imaging techniques demonstrate focal defects; and abnormalities of liver function tests are irrelevant to the staging process (Lister, Crowther, Sutcliffe, Glatstein, Cannellos, & Young, 1989).

The Cotswold classification system acknowledges clinical and pathologic criteria. *Clinical staging (CS)* refers to

TABLE 65-9 Cotswold Staging Classification for Hodgkin's Disease

Stage I	• Involvement of a single lymph node region • Involvement of a single lymphoid structure (e.g., spleen, thymus, Waldeyer's ring [stage I_E])
Stage II	• Involvement of two or more lymph node regions on the same side of the diaphragm (The number of anatomic sites are indicated by a subscript, such as II_2.) • May include extralymphatic involvement on the same side of the diaphragm (stage II_E)
Stage III	• Involvement of lymph node regions or structures on both sides of the diaphragm: III_1: With or without involvement of splenic, hilar, celiac, or portal nodes III_2: With involvement of paraaortic, iliac, or mesenteric nodes
Stage IV	• Diffuse extralymphatic disease (e.g., liver, lung, bone marrow, skin)
Subscripts Applicable to Any Disease Stage:	
A:	No symptoms
B:	Fever, night sweats, weight loss
X:	Bulky disease >⅓ the width of the mediastinum >10 cm maximal dimension of the nodal mass
E:	Involvement of a single extranodal site; contiguous or proximal to a known nodal site
CS:	Clinical stage
PS:	Pathologic stage
Indicators for Extranodal Sites:	
H:	Liver
L:	Lung
M:	Bone marrow
O:	Bone
P:	Pleura
D:	Skin

Modified from Rosen, P. J. (1995). Hodgkin's disease and malignant lymphoma. In D. A. Cascito & B. B. Lowitz (Eds.), *Manual of clinical oncology* (3rd ed.). Boston. Brown, Little, Brown; DeVita, V. T., Mauch, P. M., & Harris, N. L. (1997). Hodgkin's disease. In V. T. DeVita, S. Hellman, & S. A. Rosenberg (Eds.), *Cancer: Principles and practice of oncology* (5th ed.). Philadelphia: J. B. Lippincott.

information derived form the history, physical examination, laboratory tests, imaging studies, and initial diagnostic biopsy. *Pathologic staging (PS)* is based on histopathologic evidence confirmed through biopsy of suspected tumor sites. Although newer and improved imaging techniques are available for evaluating intraabdominal involvement, pathologic staging continues to be the most accurate method for documenting tumor presence.

Staging Laparotomy

The use of a staging laparotomy in Hodgkin's disease is the most precise method for determining occult intraabdominal tumor. In the early 1960s, laparotomies were performed to define the extent of disease, particularly involvement of the liver and spleen. The procedure for a staging laparotomy requires extensive biopsy and dissection of abdominal lymph nodes, wedge and needle biopsies of the liver, and splenectomy. The complications of a staging laparotomy include the risks of general anesthesia and abdominal surgery. Morbidity from infection, wound dehiscence, subphrenic abcess, atelectasis, and small bowel obstruction occurs in approximately 3% to 7% of patients (Leibenhaut, Hoppe, Efron, Halpern, Nelsen, & Rosenberg, 1989). Surgical mortality is rare (less than 1%) when performed by a surgeon skilled in the technique. The most significant long-term complication of laparotomy is postsplenectomy sepsis syndrome. This can be ameliorated if pneumococcal vaccine is administered before surgery (Kaplan, Dorfman, Nelson, & Rosenberg, 1973).

Laparotomy is not a routine staging procedure and is only relevant for early-stage patients who are potential candidates for radiation therapy alone. Even with modern imaging methods (e.g., CT scan, MRI), laparotomy alters the stage of 30% to 35% of patients (25% are upstaged, and 10% to 15% are downstaged) (Mauch, Larson, Osteen, Silver, Yeap, & Canellos, 1990). Still, 20% to 30% of laparotomy-staged patients treated with radiation relapse, despite the more accurate pathologic staging (Murrell, Perry, Muscato, Dorr, Wilkes, & Doll, 1995). Controversy regarding staging laparotomy persists as surgical morbidity from the procedure continues, and the overall survival from HD improves with modern treatment strategies (Murrell et al., 1995; Jockovich, Mendenhall, Somback, Talbert, & Copeland, 1994).

MEDICAL MANAGEMENT

Overview

Significant scientific advances made in the past 30 years of treatment for HD have set the precedent for treating many other malignancies. The goal of HD therapy is optimal efficacy and cure of the disease with minimal toxicity and the least possible secondary complications of treatment. A curative intent is the standard approach to treatment for all patients with HD. The stage of the disease, however, is the most important determining factor in arriving at treatment decisions (Box 65-2). Even though the characteristics of the various subtypes of HD are different, treatment is generally the same and is typically determined by stage rather than subtype. This may not hold true for the lymphocyte-predominant subtype, however, because limited treatment may suffice for this relatively favorable diagnosis (Rosenberg & Canellos, 1998). An overall cure rate of 75% has been achieved with current treatment methods for HD (Horning, 1997). A cure is possible even for patients with advanced-stage disease and for those who relapse when the initial therapy fails (Table 65-10).

Unfavorable prognostic indicators in HD (Table 65-11) include age at diagnosis greater than 50 years, involvement of multiple extranodal sites, B symptoms, stage III or IV disease, and high tumor burden with bulky mediastinal adenopathy (Rosenberg & Canellos, 1998; DeVita, Mauch, &

Box 65-2
Medical Management of Hodgkin's Disease

Treatment Options
Radiation therapy (RT)
Chemotherapy (CT)
Combined modality therapy (CMT):
  Radiation therapy plus chemotherapy
Salvage therapy
  CT if patient had prior RT
  RT if patient had prior CT
  Transplantation: High-dose CT ± RT
    Bone marrow transplant
    Peripheral stem cell transplant
Palliative care
  Symptom management

TABLE 65-10 Treatment for Hodgkin's Disease by Stage

Stage of Disease	Treatment
IA, IIA	
Supradiaphragmatic	RT: Extended mantle and upper abdominal field
Bulky disease	CMT: CT then RT
Infradiaphragmatic	RT
	CMT if spleen involved
IB, IIB	
Supradiaphragmatic	RT: subtotal nodal
Infradiaphragmatic	RT: total nodal
IIIA	
Nonbulky, limited upper abdominal distension	RT: total nodal
	CT
	CMT
Extensive spleen/lymph nodes	CT
	CMT
IIIB	CT
Bulky/incomplete regression	CT + RT
IV	CT
	CT + total nodal RT
	BMT/PSCT

RT, Radiation therapy; *CT,* combination chemotherapy; *CMT,* combined modality therapy: RT plus CT; *BMT,* bone marrow transplantation; *PSCT,* peripheral stem cell transplantation.

Harris, 1997). Refined and increasingly more accurate diagnostic and staging techniques and the use of CT scans have made a significant difference in the success achieved with treatment. These dramatic improvements have led to better overall response and survival rates.

Developments in modern therapeutic regimens, including combined modality therapy with chemotherapeutic agents used in new combinations, along with radiation therapy with more precise blocking of other organs, have led to greater success with fewer complications of treatment. Complications that do arise secondary to therapy are discussed extensively in the next section of this chapter.

TABLE 65-11 Unfavorable Prognostic Indicators in Patients with Hodgkin's Disease

Age greater than 50 years
Male gender
B symptoms
Multiple extranodal sites
Bulky mediastinal mass
Stage III or IV disease
Decreased lymphocyte count
Decreased hemoglobin
Low serum albumen
Increased erythrocyte sedimentation rate
Inguinal node involvement

Modified from DeVita, V. T., Mauch, P. M., & Harris, N. L. (1997). Hodgkin's disease. In V. T. DeVita, S. Hellman, & S. A. Rosenberg (Eds.), *Cancer: Principles and practice of oncology* (5th ed.). Philadelphia: J. B. Lippincott.

Unlike the presentation of the more widely disseminated NHL, the presentation of HD is frequently one of localized disease that spreads predictably to contiguous lymph nodes. Accurate clinical staging provides the basis for the therapeutic plan. The extent and type of the disease determines treatment and prognosis. Early-stage treatment is aimed at the identified nodal area of disease, as well as extended fields (i.e., the site or sites of next predicted involvement). Cure of localized disease (stages I, II, and some IIIA), with radiation therapy (RT) can be accomplished in this manner by including clinically negative sites. The most appropriate method of treating stage IIIA disease remains controversial because equally good results are obtained with either RT or combination chemotherapy.

When HD has progressed to advanced stages (stages IIIB and IV), combination chemotherapy or chemotherapy combined with radiation therapy (combined modality treatment) is necessary to control diffuse lymphadenopathy and extension to extranodal sites. Disseminated stage IV disease may involve multiple extralymphatic organs such as the lungs, liver, and bone marrow. Chemotherapy is also indicated in patients who have been identified as high risk for relapse. Accurate prediction of those patients in this high-risk group is essential for achieving prolonged disease-free survival.

Chemotherapy and/or radiotherapy have historically been the mainstays of HD treatment. Modern treatment also includes the use of bone marrow transplantation (BMT) or peripheral stem cell transplantation (PSCT). Although surgical interventions are not used for HD treatment, surgery does have a significant role in the diagnostic and staging phases. An excisional biopsy of the largest involved lymph nodes is indicated to diagnose HD. Surgery is also performed when a laparotomy, laparoscopy, splenectomy, or oophoropexy is indicated.

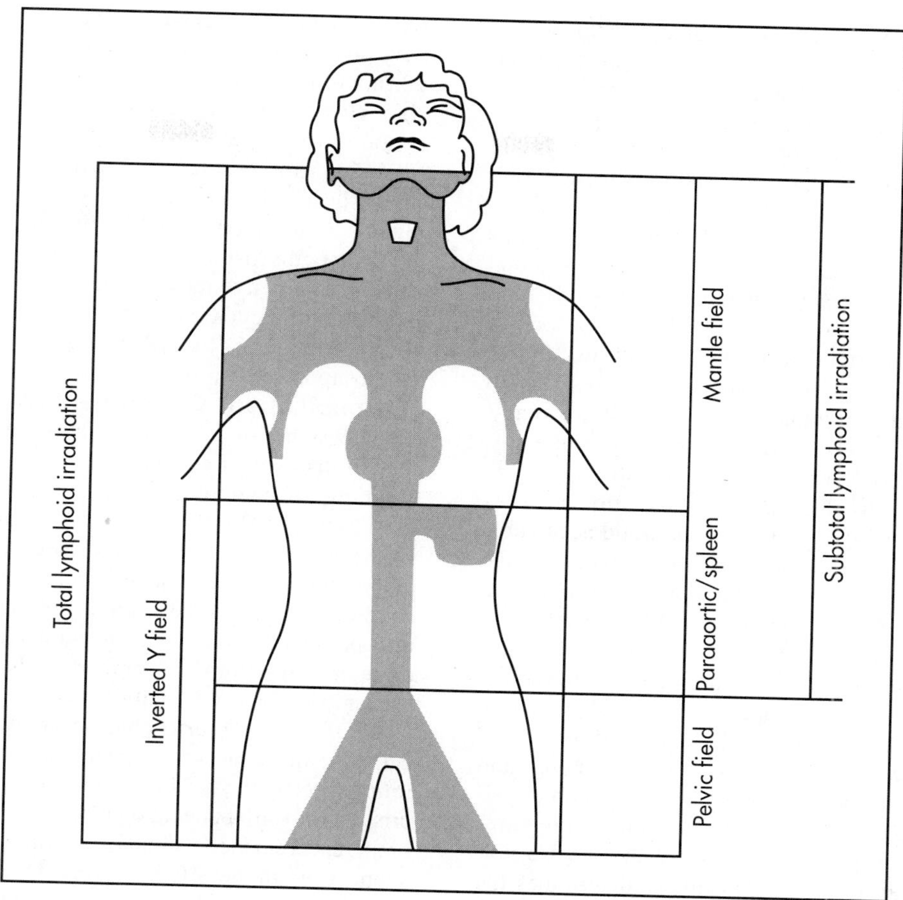

Fig. 65-3 Standard fields of radiation for Hodgkin's disease. (From Portlock, C. & Yahalom, J. [1996]. Hodgkin's disease. In J. Bennett & F. Plum [Eds.], *Cecil textbook of medicine.* Philadelphia: W. B. Saunders.)

Methods of Treatment

Radiation Therapy. Radiotherapy is curative in most patients with early-stage, limited, and localized disease (Rosenthal & Eyre, 1995; Portlock & Yahalom, 1996; Marcus, Buck, & Mauch, 1998). RT was the first effective treatment identified for HD, used as early as the year 1901. It continues to be the primary mode of treatment for early stage HD; however, the role of RT is evolving (DeVita, Mauch, & Harris, 1997).

Fortunately, HD is very sensitive to radiation. Initial success with radiation was enhanced by the recognition that adjacent nodal areas needed to be prophylactically radiated along with the identified site(s) of HD involvement. Supervoltage external beam radiation is administered in approximately 20 daily fractions of the total dose and is delivered through a linear accelerator over 4 or more weeks (Portlock & Yahalom, 1996), typically on an outpatient basis.

The three major fields of treatment include the mantle, paraaortic, and pelvic, or inverted Y, fields. These fields of radiation for HD are illustrated in Fig. 65-3. The mantle field involves the areas above the diaphragm, including the neck, chest, and axilla to treat the submandibular, cervical, supraclavicular, infraclavicular, axillary, mediastinal, and hilar nodes. Side effects of mantle field radiation include pharyngitis or esophagitis, causing problems with swallowing. However, these side effects are usually transient, are relatively easily managed, and resolve gradually after treatment is completed. Salivary changes in patients under age 40 years recover within 6 months of RT. However, in patients over age 40 years, xerostomia may last for a year or more. To prevent dental caries in this time period, daily fluoride treatments during the year and more frequent dental examinations and dental hygienist care three to four times a year are indicated (Marcus, Buck, & Mauch, 1998).

The paraaortic field includes the celiac and paraaortic lymph nodes, from the diaphragm to the aortic bifurcation, as well as the entire spleen if it has not been surgically removed. If a splenectomy has been performed, surgical clips are placed at the time of surgery so that the splenic pedicle is readily identifiable. Radiation is then accurately delivered to the splenic pedicle as well. Nausea and vomiting can be anticipated with paraaortic field RT and treated prophylactically with antiemetics.

The pelvic field includes the iliac, inguinal, and femoral nodes. Transient diarrhea and urinary frequency may develop in some patients treated with pelvic field RT, even though blocks are used to shield the bladder and bowel. Blocks are also placed on the iliac crest to spare the bone marrow during pelvic field radiation. Scatter of radiation to the testes in men and to the ovaries in women, a possibility even with prophylactic oophoropexy, results in infertility in the majority of patients treated with pelvic field radiation (Marcus, Buck, & Mauch, 1998). The paraaortic and pelvic fields together comprise the inverted Y field; however, this field has been used less frequently in recent years. Subtotal lymphoid irradiation therapy includes the mantle and paraaortic fields in treatment (Horning, 1997; Portlock & Yahalom, 1996) and is standard extended field therapy for stages I and IIA disease. Total nodal radiation includes all three fields. Regional consolidative low-dose radiotherapy, indicated for bulky or advanced disease after chemotherapy, may also be used before or after transplantation.

New techniques allow high doses of radiation with reduced scatter to other organs, skin sparing, and acceptable tolerance by normal tissue. Normal tissue is spared by the use of divergent lead blocks that shield and limit radiation exposure to vital organs (e.g., the heart and lungs) and other areas such as the spinal column, larynx, kidneys, and gonads. Of particular importance is the protection of the spinal cord from overdose with overlapping mantle and paraaortic fields of treatment (Marcus, Buck, & Mauch, 1998).

Modern technology includes extensive planning and mapping by radiation oncologists, dosimetrists, and physicists to limit toxicity to nearby organs. Simulation films, taken in the treatment position, document the precise volume of disease to be irradiated. Dosimetry determines the amount, rate, and distribution of radiation based on body size and tumor mass that will provide the most effective cell kill with minimal damage to areas adjacent to the treatment site. Tumoricidal doses are delivered to the sites of identified disease, as well as contiguous lymph nodes, where the disease would next progress if left unchecked (Horning, 1997). Conformal treatment shapes or conforms the field of radiation directly to the patient's anatomy and to the configuration of the tumor. Repeated portal films, viewed periodically by the radiation team, continually reverify treatment field accuracy.

Possible side effects of radiation therapy include fatigue, myelosuppression, hypothyroidism, pericarditis, and pneumonitis. Side effects depend on the total volume, dose, and technique of radiation. The extent and type of chemotherapy, if used, and the age and physiologic stability of the patient are other factors that influence the side effect response. Careful RT planning, delivery, and follow-up are essential elements of radiotherapy. Long-term sequelae from radiation have been reported as late as 15 to 25 years after treatment (Horning, 1997). Consequently, other methods of treatment that result in fewer long-term complications, such as the use of limited radiotherapy in combination with chemotherapy, are currently being investigated.

Chemotherapy. Chemotherapy for advanced-stage HD is aggressive and lengthy, although long-term, disease-free response is possible in a high percentage of patients. Chemotherapy is also effective in patients with early-stage disease who relapse after radiation therapy. Treatment typically involves chemotherapeutic agents that do not have overlapping toxicity used in combination over 6 to 12 months. The optimal duration of chemotherapy is variable. However, it is generally recommended that treatment continue for at least two additional cycles after complete remission to ensure eradication of residual disease. Single-agent chemotherapy is usually not effective in inducing a sustained complete or partial remission beyond a few months from treatment. Yet, single agents may be used as a palliative measure in older people who are unable to withstand the toxic effects of combination chemotherapy or in previously treated patients who remain severely myelosuppressed.

Combination Chemotherapy. Combination chemotherapy has an additive antitumor effect that is more effective than single agents used alone. Many different combinations of chemotherapeutic agents (Table 65-12) have been tried in HD treatment in the attempt to decrease toxicity while maintaining efficacy. Regimens may vary if cardiopulmonary status is severely compromised. For example, combination chemotherapeutic options without bleomycin may be substituted for patients with a history of emphysema or pulmonary fibrosis from previous radiation therapy to prevent pulmonary toxicity.

MOPP, ABVD, and Hybrid Combinations. Historically, the most successful treatment has been with regimens referred to by the acronyms MOPP (mechlorethamine, vincristine, procarbazine, and prednisone) and ABVD (doxorubicin, dacarbazine, cyclophosphamide, and bleomycin). The agents used in the MOPP regimen, the first successful combination chemotherapy in use since the mid 1960s, include nitrogen mustard (Mustargen), which has been used since 1943, vincristine (Oncovin), procarbazine, and prednisone. The multidrug MOPP program provided a 50% long-term cure rate for patients with stages IIIB and IV disease (Canellos, 1995a) but had problems with acute and chronic toxicity. This problem was alleviated somewhat by removing nitrogen mustard and substituting chlorambucil in the regimen ChlVPP (chlorambucil, vinblastine, procarbazine, and prednisone). Vincristine was also substituted for vinblastine for the combination LOPP (chlorambucil, vincristine, procarbazine, and prednisone). Other combinations have included EVAP (etoposide, vinblastine, doxorubicin, and prednisone) and LOPP-EVAP or LOPP-EVA hybrids. EVA has demonstrated effectiveness in patients resistant to MOPP (Mauch & Bonadonna, 1997).

Treatment has slowly moved away from using MOPP toward replacing it with other agents or varying the way in which it is used. In the mid 1970s, a program of MOPP combined with ABVD was developed. The agents used in the ABVD regimen include doxorubicin (Adriamycin), bleomycin, vinblastine (Velban), and dacarbazine (DTIC). Cardiopulmonary toxicity from doxorubicin and bleomycin is problematic with these agents. ABVD and ABVD hybrids, used since the mid 1980s, use ABVD in combination and alternating with MOPP (MOPP-ABVD) or MOPP with ABV without DTIC (MOPP-ABV). These agents have been as or more effective in achieving complete response than MOPP used alone and have the advantage of causing

TABLE 65-12 Combination Chemotherapeutic Regimens Used in Treating Hodgkin's Disease

MOPP Nitrogen mustard (Mustargen) Vincristine (Oncovin) Procarbazine Prednisone	**MVPP** Nitrogen mustard Vinblastine Procarbazine Prednisone	**EPOCH** Etoposide Vincristine Doxorubicin Cyclophosphamide Prednisone
ABVD Doxorubicin (Adriamycin) Bleomycin Vinblastine Dacarbazine (DTIC)	**EVAP** Etoposide Vinblastine Doxorubicin Prednisone	**BEAM** BCNU (Carmustine) Etoposide ARA-C Melphalan
MOPP Plus ABVD Alternating cycles: MOPP: all agents ABVD: all agents	**EVA** Etoposide Vinblastine Doxorubicin	**ABDIC** Doxorubicin Bleomycin Dacarbazine Lomustine (CCNU) Prednisone
MOPP Plus ABV Hybrid Nitrogen mustard Vincristine Procarbazine Prednisone Doxorubicin Bleomycin Vinblastine **Stanford V** Doxorubicin Vinblastine Nitrogen mustard Etoposide Vincristine Bleomycin Prednisone **ChlVPP** Chlorambucil Vinblastine Procarbazine Prednisone	**LOPP** Chlorambucil Vincristine Procarbazine Prednisone **LOPP Plus EVA Hybrid** Vinblastine Chlorambucil Procarbazine Prednisolone Vincristine Doxorubicin Etoposide **BCVPP** BCNU Cyclophos- phamide Vinblastine Procarbazine Prednisone	**VAPEC-B:** Salvage therapy Vincristine Doxorubicin Prednisolone Etoposide Cyclophosphamide Bleomycin Prophylactic: Co-trimoxazole Ketoconazole

Modified from DeVita, V. T. Mauch, P. M., & Harris, N. L. (1997). Hodgkin's disease. In V. T. DeVita, S. Hellman, & S. A. Rosenberg (Eds.), *Cancer: Principles and practice of oncology* (5th ed.). Philadelphia: J. B. Lippincott.

less toxicity to other body organs (Canellos, 1995b). This drug combination remains in use today (Viviani, Bonadonna, Santoro, Bonfante, Zanini, & Devizzi, 1996). In particular, the risks of sterility and secondary nonlymphocytic leukemia are less with ABVD. For young adults who want to preserve fertility, ABVD is preferable to MOPP. ABVD, which is not cross-resistant to MOPP, has the additional benefit of being able to salvage patients who failed to achieve a lengthy remission with MOPP in previous treatment.

Side effects of chemotherapeutic agents include fatigue, myelosuppression, nausea, vomiting, alopecia, sterility, neuropathy, cardiomyopathy, and secondary malignancies, especially acute nonlymphocytic leukemia (ANLL). Dose-limiting factors of chemotherapy include bone marrow toxicity and cardiotoxicity. Myelodysplasia, a precursor to acute leukemia, and sterility are additional problems of MOPP regimens. Long-term side effects of combination chemotherapy are numerous and are discussed later in this chapter.

Combined Modality Treatment with Chemotherapy and Radiation Therapy. Whereas the role of RT as a single therapy in HD is changing, its role as an adjuvant to chemotherapy is increasing. Combination treatment regimens that use radiation therapy and chemotherapy are effective for patients with bulky disease. The definition of *bulk,* however, is vague unless specific measurements or accurate estimates are provided. Mediastinal masses are labeled bulky if they measure greater than one third of the chest wall (ratio of mass to chest wall >1 : 3) on a standard PA (posteroanterior) chest film (Rosenberg & Canellos, 1998). Large masses in other sites, such as the neck, abdomen, or pelvis, are also termed *bulky disease* and are more likely to benefit from combined modality than from RT alone.

For some patients, complete response is more readily achievable with combination therapy than with either treatment modality used alone. Horning (1997) reported that combined modality chemotherapy and radiation therapy resulted in a 70% to 80% cure rate in patients with extensive mediastinal HD, including lung, pericardium, pleura, and chest wall involvement, versus a 40% to 55% cure rate with radiation therapy alone. Chemotherapy may be used in combination with low-dose radiation to treat childhood HD. This avoids the bone growth abnormalities that are evident in children treated with extensive radiation before achieving full skeletal development. Chemotherapy added to low-dose RT for children with HD supplements the effectiveness of the radiation (Rosenberg & Canellos, 1998).

Side effects of combination treatment include the potential for a radiation recall reaction. This results in delayed radiation-induced pneumonitis in some patients who received mantle field radiation before receiving doxorubicin. Additional problems of combination therapy include myelosuppression and an increased incidence of second malignancies, especially ANLL and NHL. The use of hematopoietic growth factors has lessened some of the side effects of treatment, especially susceptibility to infection, and has allowed greater dose intensity with combined-modality therapy.

Stanford V Regimen. A recent abbreviated combination chemotherapeutic regimen, referred to as the *Stanford V* (adriamycin, vinblastine, nitrogen mustard, vincristine, bleomycin, etoposide, and prednisone) has demonstrated effectiveness with HD (Horning, Rosenberg, & Hoppe, 1996). Agents are administered weekly over a shorter time than other combinations. This well-tolerated regimen involves brief 12-week chemotherapy, alternating myelosuppressive and nonmyelosuppressive agents, along with adjuvant consolidative low-dose RT to bulky or advanced disease sites. In addition, a modified mantle field approach to radiation, which excludes the axillae, is used with the Stanford V to reduce the risk of secondary malignancies such as breast cancer. The hematopoietic growth factor G-CSF (colony stimulating factor) is added to the regimen as well. Because the cumulative doses of bleomycin, adriamycin, and nitrogen mustard are lower in the Stanford V regimen than in regimens using MOPP or ABVD and because procarbazine is omitted from the Stanford V, a more favorable toxicity profile is projected (Horning, Rosenberg, & Hoppe, 1996).

The shorter duration of therapy may increase patient satisfaction with treatment; however, further data are needed to establish the efficacy of this therapeutic approach. Although long-term follow-up will be needed to evaluate the effectiveness, it is anticipated that this method of intense 12-week treatment will afford better preservation of fertility and less risk of treatment-related secondary malignancies and other long-term cardiopulmonary complications than standard longer duration combination chemotherapy with or without RT.

Salvage Therapy. Salvage therapy is used for patients who relapse after their primary treatment for HD. About 75% of relapses after radiotherapy occur in the first 3 years of RT (Portlock & Yahalom, 1996). These patients are then treated with combination chemotherapy such as ABVD or with extended-field radiation if the relapse occurs outside of the initial radiation field. Portlock and Yahalom (1996) report a 50% to 60% 10-year relapse-free survival rate for this group of patients. For patients who relapse after chemotherapy, regimens using different chemotherapeutic agents, with or without transplantation, may be used.

The duration of the initial remission and extent of disease at relapse are important prognostic indicators for patients who relapse after chemotherapy. If relapse occurs less than 12 months after the initial remission, the duration of disease-free survival is limited and prognosis is poor. For patients who relapse more than 12 months after remission, longer disease-free survival is possible with retreatment. However, even these remissions are usually not durable. The ability of these patients to respond to subsequent chemotherapy and to maintain response over a period of time from second line chemotherapy results in a survival rate of 45% at 5 years from the additional second course of chemotherapy (Horning, 1997). Data indicate that patients who relapse respond better to salvage therapy if their recurrence is nodal than if it is visceral (Stein, 1995). Patients with a poor performance status and refractory disease are unlikely to benefit from second- or third-line treatment. Increasingly, a standard approach to salvage therapy is autologous bone marrow or peripheral stem cell transplantation. Further studies will be needed, however, to determine the optimal time to initiate this mode of therapy.

Bone Marrow and Peripheral Stem Cell Transplantation. Dose-intensive myeloablative chemotherapy and autologous bone marrow transplantation (ABMT) or PSCT have been effective with documented survival benefits for relapsed HD. Usefulness has been demonstrated in HD that had previously been refractory to treatment, in relapsed disease, and in patients determined to be at high risk for relapse of disease (Vose & Armitage, 1998). Although this combination of high-dose chemotherapy with ABMT or PSCT has been used successfully in other malignancies for a while, including use in NHL, it is a relatively novel method of treating HD. Controversies still surround this method of treating HD, however. The ideal transplant regimen, optimal timing of transplantation, role of RT, and optimal source of the hematopoietic stem cells (bone marrow, peripheral cells, or umbilical cord blood) are some of the unclear and unresolved management issues. According to Mauch and Bonadonna (1997), the best time for high-dose therapy with transplantation is after the initial relapse.

Initial response rates have been promising, but long-term follow-up studies will be needed to predict overall survival and successfulness of this treatment method. It is anticipated that more durable disease-free remission can be maintained with transplantation. CBV with cyclophosphamide, carmustine (BCNU), and etoposide (VP 16) is one combination of drugs used in high-dose regimens with transplantation (Portlock & Yahalom, 1996; Stein, 1995). BEAM (BCNU, VP 16, cytosine arabinoside, and melphalan) and VP-CY-TBI (etoposide, cyclophosphamide, and total-body irradiation) are also used as high-dose treatments (Stein, 1995; Vose & Armitage, 1998).

Optimal timing of transplantation is controversial. For some patients who fail to achieve an initial complete response with conventional therapy or who relapse within 12 months of standard therapy, an improved long-term disease-free survival is achievable with transplantation (Vose & Armitage, 1998). This treatment modality will be an exciting area to follow in the next several years in patients with recurrent or refractory disease and those at high risk for relapse. If high-risk patients are accurately and promptly identified and high-dose chemotherapy with transplantation is initiated early in the treatment plan, progression-free survival may be improved.

Complications of therapy include those related to toxicities of high-dose chemotherapeutic agents used, toxicities of total-body irradiation (TBI) if used in preparative regimens, and those related to BMT or PSCT. Veno-occlusive disease of the liver, failure to engraft, prolonged pancytopenia, increased susceptibility to infectious processes, hemorrhagic cystitis, and refractory secondary myelodysplasia are possible complications of treatment. Other long-term sequelae include sterility, chronic fatigue, chronic graft versus host disease (GHVD), cataracts from TBI, chronic restrictive pulmonary disease, cardiac insufficiency and/or cardiac failure, and secondary malignancies, especially solid tumors or ANLL refractory to treatment.

PSCT has gained recent popularity as a method of treating relapsed HD and has some definite advantages over BMT. Multiple factors have contributed to this therapeutic preference, including an easier process of stem cell collection, shortened hematopoietic recovery due to quicker engraftment, good response to treatment, less transplant-associated mortality, shortened hospitalization time, and overall cost-effectiveness. Outpatient management of PSCT is now available in community oncology practice settings. PSCT will likely continue to be an area of importance in quality of life enhancement for HD survivors in the near future.

Challenging Clinical Problems in HD Treatment

Special circumstances such as the diagnosis of HD in children, pregnancy at the time of diagnosis, and HD in patients previously diagnosed with human immunodeficiency virus/acquired immunodeficiency syndrome (HIV/AIDS) may alter treatment decisions (Rosenberg & Canellos, 1998; DeVita, Mauch, & Harris, 1997; Portlock & Yahalom, 1996). Therapeutic decisions for these groups of patients need to involve medical and nursing clinical specialists as an integral part of the treatment-planning team.

Hodgkin's Disease in Children

The diagnosis of HD in children under age 16 years is relatively uncommon and warrants management by pediatric oncologists. To prevent acute and chronic complications associated with asplenia, a splenectomy may be avoided in children with HD. Chemotherapy and radiation therapy may be significantly modified to protect fertility. Because radiation has a growth inhibitory effect on muscle and bone, attention to these areas is also a primary consideration in children. Combination chemotherapy may be selected over RT as the primary treatment to avoid skeletal and bone impairment. If RT is used, low-dose radiation to the entire bone may prevent serious segmental skeletal damage. Children with HD have an excellent prognosis; therefore effectively minimizing acute and chronic side effects of treatment is a goal in therapeutic selection.

Hodgkin's Disease During Pregnancy

The management of HD during pregnancy requires an individualized plan. Factors that influence treatment decisions include the age and size of the fetus, the volume and site of bulky disease, the extent and involvement of extranodal sites, the aggressiveness of the disease, associated symptoms, and the estimated date of delivery. If the course of disease is indolent and the patient is asymptomatic, treatment may be delayed until delivery. However, if treatment cannot be deferred safely, limited-field radiation, using lead shields to block the uterus, may be used. Single-agent or combination chemotherapy may also be safely administered without adverse effects on the fetus. A therapeutic first-trimester abortion may be advisable if prompt aggressive therapy that would cause serious fetal damage is indicated. Pregnant patients and their family members need to have adequate prognostic, therapeutic, and teratogenic information to arrive at this difficult decision. In contrast, third-trimester pregnancies pose fewer treatment-related problems. Full-term delivery may be possible after partial-dose or full-dose chemotherapy or RT without causing damage to the developing fetus.

Hodgkin's Disease in Patients with HIV/AIDS

Although NHL is diagnosed more frequently than HD in patients with HIV, HIV-associated HD has a more aggressive clinical course than in non-HIV patients. Extranodal involvement is also more prominent in HIV-associated HD. HIV-positive patients are approached with a curative intent, even in the presence of advanced stage Hodgkin's disease. *Pneumocystis carinii* pneumonia prophylaxis is needed for each patient, whereas alterations in combination chemotherapy to avoid pulmonary toxicity may be needed for some. If HIV-positive patients are not immunosuppressed and do not have concomitant opportunistic infections, treatment will be similar to therapy with HIV-negative patients. However, this group of patients may have poor tolerance to marrow-suppressive drugs and will need close monitoring for infections and other associated problems. The administration of zidovudine and other antiviral treatment for HIV is not recommended during chemotherapy (Portlock & Yahalom, 1996). Palliative therapy may be indicated if opportunistic infections, cachexia, or significant T4-lymphocyte depression exist. Because HIV-positive patients often have unusual patterns of tumor involvement and advanced HD, management of the disease and side effects of treatment are challenging. Response to treatment and overall survival may be limited secondary to HIV/AIDS-related complications and refractory Hodgkin's disease.

Treatment Follow-Up

Extensive, regular, periodic follow-up is needed for every patient living with HD to detect disease recurrence early. Typically, patients are seen for follow-up visits every 2 months during the first year, every 3 months during the second year after treatment, and every 4 months in the third year. During the fourth and fifth years, visits every 6 months are recommended. About 5 years after treatment, visits are scheduled biannually or annually thereafter (Torrey, Poen, & Hoppe, 1997). A complete history of any present or recent symptoms, a thorough review of systems, a complete physical examination, laboratory studies including a CBC (complete blood count) and erythrocyte sedimentation rate (ESR, the rate at which red blood cells settle out in a test tube in a specified time), radiologic studies including chest x-ray examinations, and abdominopelvic CT or gallium scans are indicated to detect relapse (Marcus, Buck, & Mauch, 1998). Radionuclide gallium scans, useful in identifying areas of residual disease, are effective in predicting the chance of relapse. Most relapses occur within 5 years from treatment (Torrey Poen, & Hoppe, 1997). A high ESR after treatment is a poor prognostic factor (Rosenberg & Canellos, 1998; DeVita, Mauch, & Harris, 1997). Although the ESR is a nonspecific test that is abnormally elevated in numerous conditions, including infection, inflammation, and age over 60 years, it is useful as an indicator of metastatic disease and as such is a measurement of response to treatment and disease relapse.

Sites of prior bulky disease warrant close observation over time. In addition, biannual thyroid function studies are indicated if the thyroid gland was in the radiation field. Continual careful medical surveillance is needed to monitor for relapse and/or possible long-term sequelae of treatment, including hypothyroidism, heart disease, and secondary malignancies. Follow-up evaluation is expensive and is therefore a concern of case managers who monitor cost-containment issues. Comprehensive follow-up is warranted, however, if early detection of relapse results in improved duration and quality of survival.

Summary of Treatment

When treatment methods have been exhausted without disease remission or cure of HD, palliative therapy is provided for maximal comfort and quality living with the disease. The future of HD treatment may eventually include an identified group of "watchful waiting" patients who seem to tolerate disease that is resistant to treatment for extended periods of time without aggressive therapeutic intervention. The prognosis for those living with HD has continued to improve over the past 30 years due to changes and modifications in treatment plans. Although biologic agents have been tested in NHL, few clinical trials to date have used these agents with HD. Biologic agents may prove to offer utility with HD in the future. The recent advances in PSCT and the use of umbilical cord blood as an excellent source of stem cells have helped move HD treatment forward. The future may look even brighter as additional data on newer methodologies is accumulated and better alternatives identified.

As the management of HD continues to evolve, treatment recommendations will be modified as well to ensure that the incidence and severity of acute and chronic side effects of treatment are as limited as possible. A balanced approach needs to be taken when considering treatment options, especially if additional severe treatment-related sequelae are anticipated. The increasing number of longer-surviving patients has heightened awareness of the need to prevent long-term consequences of HD treatment. For this reason, the aggressiveness of therapy for HD is continually being reevaluated.

ONCOLOGIC EMERGENCIES

Nursing interventions for two significant oncologic emergencies related to HD, sepsis, and epidural spinal cord compression are discussed in Table 65-13. A more detailed discussion of various complications with HD is found in other sections of this chapter.

Sepsis

Sepsis potential, a life-threatening risk for severely immunocompromised patients, is related to significant alterations in host-defense mechanisms. Neutropenic patients, those with an absolute neutrophil count (ANC) of <500 mm^3, are at severe risk for developing infectious complications. Patients with an ANC of <100 are at an even greater sepsis risk. The degree, duration, and rapidity of decline in the neutrophil count predispose the immunocompromised patient to infection from a variety of pathogens. It is important to note that a "normal" range neutrophil count may represent dysfunctional and/or immature, and subsequently ineffective, neutrophils. Infections progress quickly in patients with impaired protective skin and mucous membrane barriers and in those with alterations in the normal microbial flora of the gastrointestinal tract.

Common pathogens that account for the majority of infections in neutropenic oncology patients include gram-positive bacteria *(Staphylococcus, Streptococcus, Enterococcus,* and *Corynebacterium)* and gram-negative bacteria *(Pseudomonas, Escherichia coli,* and *Klebsiella)* (Hughes Armstrong, Bodey, Brown, Edwards, & Feld, 1997). Frequent fungal organisms that cause infections secondary to treatment with broad spectrum antibiotics or cause primary infections include *Aspergillus, Candida,* and *Cryptococcus neoformans.* Herpes simplex, varicella-zoster, and cytomegalovirus are frequently occurring viral infections. Because there is a high morbidity associated with bacterial infections in neutropenic patients, empiric broad-spectrum intravenous antibiotics are initiated promptly in patients with neutrophil counts of <500 and in patients with neutrophil counts in the 500 to 1000 range who are expected to have a further decrease in white count (Hughes et al., 1997).

Overwhelming infection may quickly result in sepsis syndrome (hypotensive septic shock, rapid-onset multisystem organ failure, and death). Activation of coagulation pathways, cell injury and cell death from tissue oxygenation deficits, metabolic alterations, cardiovascular dysfunction, and microvascular perfusion deficits contribute to the septic process. In HD, cellular immunity is altered as a consequence of the disease process and treatment-induced immunosuppression. Ineffective immune responses lead to septicemia, due in part to decreased numbers of functional phagocytic neutrophils. Asplenic and hyposlenic patients, patients with one or more severely debilitating chronic illness(es), and older people are also at an increased risk for sepsis. Early detection and prompt initiation of aggressive polydrug therapy and enhanced tissue perfusion to vital organs is necessary to prevent permanent end-organ damage to the heart, liver, kidneys, and brain.

A complicated cascade of microthrombi formation, fibrinolysis, clot dissolution, consumption of the clotting factors and platelets, and hemorrhage result. Increased capillary permeability due to capillary pressure changes results in fluid shifts to extravascular spaces with progression to pulmonary edema and/or acute respiratory distress syndrome (ARDS). Metabolic acidosis, hyperventilation, respiratory alkalosis, reduced cardiac output, and circulatory collapse ensue. Astute recognition by health care providers of signs and symptoms of late shock (cold shock) is needed to avert progressive decline and morbidity. Physical findings may include irritability; restlessness; confusion; cool, clammy skin; tachycardia; weak pulse; rapid, shallow respirations; increasing respiratory distress; abdominal distension and discomfort/pain; oliguria; and hypoglycemia. A change in the patient's mental status may herald the onset of septicemia before other indicators. Sepsis in the neutropenic patient is a medical emergency, and treatment is aggressive.

Table 65-13 Oncologic Emergencies

Problem	Nursing Interventions
Sepsis	• *Assess* for signs and Sx of infectious processes: fever, shaking chills, malaise, hypotension, altered mentation, headache, pain, SOB, diarrhea, and vomiting. • *Assess* for Sx of late/cold shock: irritability; restlessness; confusion; clammy skin; rapid, shallow respirations; respiratory distress; tachycardia; thready pulse; oliguria; hypoglycemia; and metabolic acidosis. • *Obtain* cultures from all sites: blood, sputum, urine, intravascular and urinary catheters, wounds, and throat. • *Obtain* stat chest x-ray film, CBC with differential, and electrolytes. *Monitor* laboratory values frequently. • *Initiate* stat antibiotics **after** cultures are obtained. *Add* antifungal therapy as indicated. *Intervene* early to prevent circulatory collapse and organ failure. • *Restore* hemodynamic status: *Stabilize* the blood pressure and *monitor* frequently. • *Regulate* intravenous hydration and *monitor* the urine output. • *Monitor* for coagulation, fibrinolysis, and impending disseminated intravascular coagulation (DIC). *Observe* for signs of hemorrhage and clot formation: hematomas, ecchymoses, petechiae, and oozing from mucous membranes. *Observe* for signs of widespread clotting: dyspnea, oliguria, and abdominal pain. *Obtain* platelet, fibrinogen, fibrin degradation products, prothrombin time, and clotting factor levels. *Treat* DIC with platelets, fresh frozen plasma, and cryoprecipitate. *Evaluate* the need for intravenous heparin therapy. • *Initiate* oxygen therapy. *Monitor* oxygenation with a pulse oximeter and arterial blood gases (ABGs). • *Reevaluate* the response to selected antibiotics, including broad-spectrum coverage. *Manage* secondary problems. • *Continue* intensive surveillance and consider transfer of patient to an intensive care unit if the condition rapidly deteriorates (impending circulatory collapse or respiratory failure). • *Provide* information, emotional support, and time for the patient/family to discuss fears of death. *Provide* hopefulness balanced with realism. • *Monitor* the response to treatment.
Spinal cord compression	• *Recognize* early Sx of epidural cord compression. Back pain may be the first indication. Radicular back pain: from compression of sensory nerve roots; retroperitoneal pain, aggravated by lying supine; vertebral pain, increases with standing and movement. • *Recognize* uncommon presentations of cord compression: motor weakness of extremities, sensory deficits, and bowel and bladder dysfunction. • *Complete* a focused neuromuscular physical examination, and document the findings. *Facilitate* Rx promptly, usually radiation therapy, to prevent serious and permanent neurologic dysfunction. • *Provide* education, support, and counsel to the patient/family. • *Monitor* the response to treatment.

Sx, signs and symptoms; *SOB*, shortness of breath; *Rx*, treatment.

Spinal Cord Compression

Although it is more commonly seen in NHL than HD, compression of the spinal cord may result from progressive, late-stage HD (Rosenberg & Canellos, 1998). Symptoms of epidural spinal cord compression (SCC) may be subtle and are related to edema and ischemia of the cord. The health care provider needs to be alert for the presence of back pain, lower extremity weakness and sensory deficits, and hyperreflexia. Back pain may be the first indication of epidural cord compression, and its presence warrants a complete evaluation. Definitive diagnosis of SCC is accomplished by noninvasive MRI and/or CT scanning. The risk of permanent neurologic impairment and paralysis exists if treatment, most often with radiotherapy and high-dose corticosteroids, is not initiated promptly. Steroid intervention decreases the degree of spinal cord edema; this in turn reduces compression-related pain. The degree of neurologic deficit, including permanent paralysis, is significantly increased if early symptoms are missed and treatment is delayed. However, prompt diagnosis and radiotherapy intervention can stop progressive neurologic dysfunction.

NURSING MANAGEMENT

Nursing interventions for patients with HD are discussed in Table 65-14. Complex acute and chronic care needs require a thorough understanding of pathophysiology and pharmacology, as well as proficiency in physical assessment skills, patient education strategies, and documentation of relevant findings and interventions. Because much of the therapy is delivered on an outpatient basis, thorough patient-family education regarding self-care strategies is essential for effective management of treatment-related side effects. Future studies, including the integration of pharmacologic and nonpharmacologic strategies, may determine more adequate control measures of troublesome cancer-related side effects.

Considerable progress has been made in identifying and implementing effective side effect management strategies to improve health-related quality of life. Despite these improvements, however, many patients still experience treatment-related or disease-related nausea, vomiting, chronic fatigue, and pain. The World Health Organization (WHO) three-step analgesic ladder (AHCPR, 1994) has

TABLE 65-14 Standard of Care for the Patient Receiving Chemotherapy for Hodgkin's Disease

Patient Problems and Outcomes	Nursing Interventions and Rationales	Patient Education and Interventions
Anxiety Patient will: • Verbalize an understanding of the effect of disease on self and family. • Express feelings of decreased anxiety. • Identify strategies to cope with anxiety.	1. Assess the patient's understanding of the disease process and accompanying signs and symptoms. 2. Give the patient the opportunity to ask questions or verbalize concerns. 3. Determine which coping strategies the patient has used effectively in the past to decrease anxiety, and reinforce the use of these coping mechanisms. 4. Prepare the patient for possible chemotherapy side effects.	1. Use a diagram of the lymphatic system to explain the disease process and symptoms. The most common signs and symptoms are lymphadenopathy, fever, night sweats, weight loss, pruritus, and alcohol-induced pain. 2. Offer patient support groups to patients and families (i.e., Alliance for Lymphoma Survivors, American Cancer Society). Web sites with Oncolink, Lymphoma Research Foundation of America, and National Cancer Institute.
Infection Patient will acknowledge the high risk for infection.	1. Teach the patient strategies to avoid or decrease the effects of immunosuppression relative to myelosuppression.	1. Teach the patient an overview of the hematologic system, with an emphasis on composition and function of the hematopoietic system. 2. Stress the importance of personal hygiene, especially correct handwashing techniques. 3. Inform the patient of the risk of infection and situations to avoid: crowds, friends/family with colds, and gastrointestinal or upper respiratory flu-like illnesses. 4. Teach the patient to identify signs and symptoms of infection: fever, productive cough, and erythematous and/or warm areas of skin. 5. Teach the patient to inspect mucous membranes frequently throughout therapy. 6. Instruct the patient on effective skin care management, especially sites of central catheter sites. 7. Instruct the patient in subcutaneous injection techniques if colony stimulating factors for the white cell line are prescribed. 8. Provide the patient and caregiver with clear instructions for emergency access to their health care provider.

helped care providers make significant strides in effective pain management. WHO guidelines recommend a standard hierarchy of treatment options that includes starting pain management with nonopioids such as a nonsteroidal antiinflammatory drug (NSAID) with or without an adjuvant, such as an antidepressant, for mild to moderate level 1 pain and an opioid plus a nonopioid with or without an adjuvant for persistent or increased intensity level 2 pain. Use of an opioid with increasing doses with or without a nonopioid and/or an adjuvant is recommended for severe level 3 pain.

As patients develop tolerance and resistance to the analgesic effects of pharmacologic treatment, increasing doses will be needed and should be used to manage pain effectively. However, with elderly patients, especially those with reduced renal clearance, it is necessary to increase dosage slowly, using a "start low, go slow" approach to avoid adverse events. Analgesic adjuncts such as antidepressants, anxiolytics, psychostimulants, and corticosteroids are effective in all phases of a comprehensive pain management plan. Adjuvants enhance analgesic efficacy and treat associated symptoms related to the pain experience.

The acronym PQRST enables the careprovider to fully assess multiple characteristics of cancer-related pain (factors that provoke/palliate pain, the quality of the pain using patient descriptors, radiation of pain to other sites, severity on a 0 to 10 scale, and temporal factors). OLDCART is another useful acronym to make a differential diagnosis of pain (onset, location, duration, characteristics, associated symptoms, and timing). Chronic severe pain is best treated by around-the-clock treatment with long-acting agents combined with

TABLE 65-14 Standard of Care for the Patient Receiving Chemotherapy for Hodgkin's Disease—cont'd

Patient Problems and Outcomes	Nursing Interventions and Rationales	Patient Education and Interventions
Patient will experience no nausea and vomiting or be controlled with antiemetic medication.	1. Determine the emetogenic potential of chemotherapeutic agents used. Identify the most emetogenic agent in combination therapy, and assess the relative potential of other agents. Emetogenicity levels of chemotherapy range from Level 1 (nonemetogenic: <10%) to Level 5 (extremely emetogenic: >90%). 2. Administer antiemetics (e.g., serotonin or dopamine antagonist) 30 minutes before chemotherapy administration. Selective serotonin 5-hydroxytryptamine receptor antagonists (e.g., granisetron and ondansetron). Benzodiazepines (e.g., diazepam or lorazepam) provide an antianxiety and amnesic effect to lessen anticipatory nausea. The addition of corticosteroids contributes to significant reduction in nausea and vomiting. 3. Select and tailor optimal antiemetics. 4. Assess for nausea, vomiting, and ability to eat and drink.	1. Inform the patient of the emetic potential of chemotherapy, and provide assurance of pharmacologic and nonpharmacologic interventions to alleviate symptoms. 2. Teach the patient to report nausea and vomiting. 3. Teach the patient the need to eat and drink small quantities of food. Inform the patient of the emetic potential of chemotherapy, and provide assurance of pharmacologic intervention to alleviate symptoms. 4. Teach the patient progressive muscle relaxation, deep-breathing exercises, visualization, imagery, or cognitive distraction techniques as the patient adjusts to antiemetics. Counseling and hypnosis may be helpful.
Anemia		
Patient will maintain a normal hemoglobin and hematocrit.	1. Monitor complete blood count to ensure that the patient is not anemic as a result of immunosuppression. 2. Monitor for the effect of fatigue on functional capacity 3. Administer red blood cell transfusions, if indicated. 4. Administer the colony stimulating factor, epoetin alpha (Epogen), if indicated	1. Teach the patient the signs and symptoms of anemia: dyspnea on exertion, pallor, and fatigue. 2. Encourage the patient to report fatigue in quantitative amounts. Empower the patient to acknowledge the effects of fatigue in terms of functional capacity, such as not being able to perform activities of daily living. 3. Teach the patient and family caregiver administration techniques, as well as storage and disposal of needles and syringes used for Epogen alfa.

shorter-acting agents for breakthrough pain. Although unrelieved pain is still one of the most common and most feared symptoms associated with cancer, pain can be managed effectively in 90% of patients with cancer-related pain (AHCPR, 1994). Effective pain control throughout the cancer experience prevents unnecessary, unresolved suffering and, in turn, significantly enhances the patient's quality of life.

The fear of nausea and vomiting also ranks high in patient-related concerns throughout HD treatment. Determining the emetogenic potential (high, moderate, or mild) of single chemotherapeutic agents and then using an algorithm to determine the emetogenicity of combination chemotherapy enables the care provider to develop effective antiemetic regimens. Level 5 drugs, such as high-dose cyclophosphamide, have the greatest emetogenic potential; level 1 drugs, such as bleomycin, vincristine, and vinblastine, have the least emetogenic potential. Because each agent used in combination chemotherapy may have an additive emetogenic effect, use of an emetogenic algorithm is helpful to determine the most efficacious antiemetic regimen. During the active chemotherapy treatment phase, prophylactic antiemetic therapy and regularly scheduled antiemetic dosing provide better control of symptoms than does prn dosing. Frequently used drugs in acute antiemetic therapy include the combination of a serotonin antagonist (ondansetron, granisetron, or dolasetron) or a dopamine antagonist (metoclopramide) with a corticosteroid (dexamethasone) plus a benzodiazepine (lorazepam). Effective relief from acute episodes of chemotherapy-induced emesis may prevent the syndrome of anticipatory nausea and vomiting.

HOME CARE ISSUES

Nursing interventions for home care management are addressed in Table 65-15. Referrals to physical, occupational, respiratory, and nutritional therapy, as well as social services, are often needed to adequately meet extensive care needs. Especially for the neutropenic or posttransplant patient, cleanliness and other environmental safety issues, such as adequate heat, ventilation, water, and sanitation, need to be addressed and resolved before sending the patient home from an in-hospital stay. The more knowledge patients and their family members have about minimizing exposure to infection and monitoring for signs of infection, the more effective home management will be.

Information regarding treatments, medication regimens, side effect management, smoking cessation, and follow-up plans need to be reinforced through repetition when patients return for periodic clinic visits. Smoking-cessation information often needs frequent repetition. A brief guide for health care providers to use in assisting patients with smoking cessation is provided in Box 65-3. Data suggest that a depressed mood is strongly related to smoking relapse. Therefore it is important for members of the health care team to complete a thorough assessment of depression and take advantage of every "window of opportunity" to encourage and educate patients in effective "stay quit" measures. Patients who report negative or depressed moods associated with previous quit attempts may benefit from bupropion (Zyban) as an adjunct to nicotine replacement therapy during cessation attempts. It is useful for nurses to be well versed in change theory to better assist smokers in altering their smoking behaviors (Prochaska, DiClemente, & Norcross, 1992).

Some method of organization is needed to help patients locate and use information provided to them regarding their health status. A loose-leaf notebook with pocket folders is a useful tool for helping patients keep track of their questions, information booklets or other handouts, laboratory results, and discharge instructions. Patients can also be encouraged to keep a diary of how they are feeling to monitor their progress. Opportunities need to be provided for patients and family members to ask clarification questions and discuss their concerns or fears during each clinic visit. In addition, because patients and their family members are often curious about the latest herbal "remedy," it is helpful for the nurse to be well-versed in this topic as well.

If the patient is physically or emotionally unable to be independent and self-reliant in personal health care, it will be important to assess the home care provider's knowledge of the patient's strengths, physical limitations, and care requirements. In addition, the desire and abilities of the home care provider to meet care needs in terms of other roles and responsibilities need to be evaluated. The emotional ability and stability of patients and home care providers and their degree of interest in assuming responsibility for care needs are significant determinants in successful home management. If warranted, home visits by nursing staff members can be arranged to evaluate the patient's and family's self-care abilities. Home visitation also provides the opportunity to determine how successfully the patient is able to manage in the home setting and helps determine the need for other community services.

TABLE 65-15 Home Care Issues

Concern	Nursing Interventions
Home care management	• *Discuss* home environment, support systems available, patient-family education to manage daily, and problem situations. • *Provide* the patient and family with clear verbal and written instructions for all home-going medications and treatments. • *Relay* the importance of continuous monitoring for signs of infection (i.e., "infection patrol and infection control"). *Stress* need to report and initiate stat emergency treatment for any infectious processes. • *Provide* information on the need to maintain a clean home environment. *Discourage* visitors with any acute upper respiratory or gastrointestinal illness, visitors with fever, or visitors who recently received live attenuated vaccines (oral poliovirus vaccine [OPV], measles, mumps, rubella [MMR], varicella-zoster vaccines) because the virus may be shed in stool for 4 to 6 weeks after administration, increasing susceptibility in immunocompromised patients. • *Encourage* vaccination with pneumococcal and influenza vaccines for high-risk patients (chronic cardiopulmonary diseases, chronic metabolic disorders, age >65 yrs, alcoholics, other co-morbid chronic illnesses, immunosuppression, splenic dysfunction, or asplenia). • *Provide* home visits periodically to evaluate care in the home, to assess the patient's self-care abilities, to provide counsel and education, and to determine the need for additional community services. • *Monitor* compliance with medications and instructions. • *Facilitate* self-care strategies. • *Stress* the need for continued frequent medical surveillance. • *Encourage* participation in psychoeducational and/or therapeutic groups for cancer survivors to discuss with other survivors the lived experience of transplantation. • *Provide* ongoing education and support.

Box 65-3

Smoking Cessation: A Guide for Health Care Providers with Recommendations for Counseling and Education

Overview

Smoking is the most modifiable cause of premature death in the United States. Most smokers have significant difficulty quitting, and many are reluctant to consider a quit attempt, even in view of the recent news regarding the various hazards of smoking and related risks of inhaling second-hand smoke. Because multiple health risks can be reduced by smoking cessation, it is recommended that health care providers address the issue of smoking during each office visit. First-time success with smoking cessation is, unfortunately, the exception rather than the rule. Repeated quit attempts are usually necessary for behavior modification to occur. (Note: Prochaska, DiClemente, and Norcross' Stages of Change [1992] are used in this guide to explore acceptance of and resistance to behavior change.)

Step 1

Determine the *precontemplation* stage, defined as being unaware of a need to change a behavior, being unwilling to stop smoking, or being discouraged about the ability to make a behavior change.

Action

Assess the desire, readiness, interest, and commitment in making a behavior change to stop smoking.

- The present stage of change will predict the likelihood of success.
- After readiness for change has been determined, interventions can be tailored to the patient's level of interest.
- Internal motivation is a stronger predictor of success than external motivation from loved ones, employment managers, or friends.

Action

- Provide brief information about health consequences of smoking.
- Repeat a brief message at every visit "window of opportunity."
- Provide a flag chart with a red sticker "Smoker" as a reminder to raise the question at each visit.
- Keep information limited if the patient is not interested or ready to process information.
- Provide simple encouragement.

Step 2

Determine the *contemplation* stage, defined as personal consideration of making a change without full readiness for change. Options are being considered and evaluated in terms of risks and benefits.

Action

Provide brief, simple encouragement and advice on possible smoking-cessation methods available:

- Nicotine replacement with patch or gum
- Oral bupropion (Zyban) to relieve withdrawal symptoms and depressed mood
- American Cancer Society (ACS) Fresh Start Smoking Cessation Program of education and peer-to-peer support

Step 3

Determine the *preparation* stage, defined as readiness for change with a definite "just do it" commitment to stop smoking.

Action

- Assist the patient with preparing for the process of change.
- Continue to offer advice, encouragement, and support.
- Provide self-help materials such as handouts and/or booklets with useful "quit tips": suggest that patient avoid contact with smokers, change and vary activities.
- Provide the patient with an ACS phone number to register for Fresh Start, usually offered twice per month in a series of 4 to 5 classes.

Step 4

Determine the *action* stage, defined as actual modifications in behavior.

Action

- Encourage the patient to identify a specific "quit date."
- Provide skills, tools, tricks, and tips to manage nicotine withdrawal.
- Provide brief written handouts on ways to prevent relapse; help identify obstacles such as having another smoker in the home or friends who smoke.
- Assist in developing assertiveness behaviors.
- Provide resources for stress management and conflict-resolution skills.

Step 5

Support the *maintenance* stage, defined as the period of sustaining change.

Action

- Discuss the "one day at a time" concept to stay "quit."
- Remind the patient not to have even one cigarette because one easily leads to one more.
- Provide community resources or support groups for ex-smokers
- Teach several relaxation therapy methods: progressive muscle relaxation, controlled breathing, mindful meditation, yoga, music therapy, graduated exercise program of walking.
- Remind the patient that active efforts will be needed for the next 6 months to 3 years.
- Continue to offer encouragement during each visit.
- If relapse occurs, encourage the patient to start the process again.
- Following relapse, discuss feelings of failure, guilt, and demoralization that may accompany relapsed smoking behaviors.
- Provide information that most people require at least three to four quit attempts for complete and lasting success.
- Recycle through the stages of change as many times as necessary with modifications in the approach to quitting until an effective method is secured.
- Continue to provide a supportive approach with a reminder to "never quit quitting."

Summary

It is essential to identify a patient's stage of change behavior because receptivity to information, commitment, and success is determined by each individual's self-recognition of a problem behavior, increased awareness of adverse effects of continuing the behavior, and internal motivation to get ready for change. The Prochaska, DiClemente, & Norcross model of change behavior is useful in helping health care providers know where to put their time and efforts in helping patients recycle through these stages several times in search of success.

PROGNOSIS

The cure rate for HD is excellent. Therapeutic successes with combination chemotherapy and multimodality treatment for HD became a paradigm for the development of combination chemotherapy/radiotherapy regimens for cancers other than HD. Prognostic variables for HD are listed in Table 65-16. Prognosis varies with the stage of disease at the time of diagnosis, extensiveness of the disease and number of extranodal sites involved, age of the patient, number and significance of co-morbid acute and chronic diseases, and resistance to drug therapy.

EVALUATION OF THE QUALITY OF CARE

Patients may be questioned about their perceptions of care received at any point along the treatment continuum. Al-

TABLE 65-16 Long-Term Complications of Hodgkin's Disease Treatment

Complication	Causes and Risk Factors	Management and Prevention
Immunologic dysfunction	Underlying disease, therapy	Appropriate vaccinations
Herpes zoster or varicella-zoster	Underlying disease, therapy	Systemic antiviral therapy, zoster immunoglobulin
Pneumococcal sepsis	Splenectomy, functional asplenia after RT	Pretherapy pneumococcal vaccine, selected antibiotic prophylaxis, avoid unnecessary staging splenectomy
Nonlymphocytic leukemia	Therapy, older than 40 years	Avoid combined-modality therapy for Hodgkin's disease; supportive care, low-dose chemotherapy, aggressive therapy with or without bone marrow transplantation
Myelodysplastic syndromes	Therapy, older than 40 years	Avoid combined-modality therapy for Hodgkin's disease; supportive care, low-dose chemotherapy, aggressive therapy with or without bone marrow transplantation
Non–Hodgkin's lymphoma	Therapy	Aggressive combination chemotherapy
Solid tumors	Direct or indirect RT exposure	Conventional management
Thymic hyperplasia	Underlying disease, therapy	Resection
Hypothyroidism	Direct or indirect RT exposure	Hormone replacement, thyroid suppression during therapy (?)
Thyroid cancer	Direct or indirect RT exposure, chronic thyroid stimulation	Thyroid suppression
Male infertility	Therapy, underlying disease	Attempt sperm storage, testicular shielding during RT, suppression of spermatogenesis during CT (?), alternative chemotherapeutic regimens
Male impotence	Therapy, underlying disease	Counseling, trial of testosterone
Female infertility	Therapy	Oophoropexy, ovarian suppression during therapy (?), cyclic estrogen replacement
Female dyspareunia	Therapy, underlying disease	Counseling, cyclic estrogen replacement
Pericarditis, acute	Mediastinal RT, recall with CT after RT	Appropriate RT shielding and technique, avoid doxorubicin after RT, antiinflammatory medication, pericardiocentesis
Pericarditis, chronic	Mediastinal RT	Appropriate RT shielding and technique, pericardiectomy
Cardiomyopathy	Mediastinal RT, doxorubicin, recall with CT after RT	Appropriate RT shielding and technique, avoid doxorubicin after RT, monitor for early signs of toxicity, limit cumulative doxorubicin dose, supportive medical management
Pneumonitis, acute	Direct or indirect RT, bleomycin, nitrosoureas, recall with CT after RT	Appropriate RT shielding and technique, monitor for early signs of toxicity, avoid known toxic drugs, avoid excessive Po_2
Pneumonitis, chronic	Same as above	Supportive management
Avascular necrosis	Steroid therapy, underlying disease (?)	Antiinflammatory medications, joint surgery
Growth retardation	Pediatric RT	Minimize RT, use symmetric RT fields
Dental caries	Salivary change after RT	Maintain good oral hygiene, daily fluoride treatments

Modified from DeVita, V. T., Mauch, P., & Harris, N. (1997). Hodgkin's disease. In V. T. DeVita, S. Hellman, & S. Rosenberg (Eds.), *Cancer: Principles and practice of oncology.* Philadelphia: Lippincott-Raven.
RT, Radiation therapy; *CT,* chemotherapy.

though response to mailed questionnaires is often limited in terms of low yield, this type of evaluation, more than direct interpersonal questioning, offers confidentiality of results. Collecting data at various points along the recovery phase, both immediately after treatment and at a designated period of time-out-from-treatment, enhances objectivity. Information obtained from patient evaluations may be incorporated in changes for future care delivery. Selection of a few open-ended questions may provide enough qualitative data for adequate quality assurance feedback. An example of an eleven-item tool is included in Table 65-17. Most of the questions in this tool require a "Yes/No" answer, but room is provided for discussion if the patient chooses to make additional comments.

RESEARCH ISSUES

Clinical trials are ongoing for HD treatment (NCI/PDQ, 1998). The Physician's Data Query (PDQ) computerized database of the National Cancer Institute includes active cancer treatment protocols. Unfortunately, many of the experimental protocols may not be more efficacious than standard treatment methods. Because many of the protocols in the various phases of study in clinical trials are potentially toxic, U.S. Federal regulations protect human subjects by requiring approval of all clinical trials by local institutional review boards (IRBs). It is important to note that laws that protect the rights of humans differ outside the United States.

Information contained in the *Current Clinical Trials* (NCI/PDQ; 1998) represents state-of-the-art data distributed by the International Cancer Information Center, a division of the National Cancer Institute (NCI). It is a bimonthly directory of all currently active cancer clinical trials in the United States and is intended for use by clinical hematology-oncology physicians to refer patients to a contact physician at sites participating in ongoing research studies.

A sampling of current clinical trials for Hodgkin's disease listed in the NCI/PDQ database (1998) includes, among others, the following studies:

- Quality of life and health status evaluation in patients with stage I/IIA HD
- The use of positron emission tomography (PET) to stage and predict treatment outcomes for HD and NHL
- Short-term Stanford V combination chemotherapy followed by modified involved-field RT in favorable limited stage and unfavorable HD
- RT ± ABVD versus ABVD alone in stage IA/IIA HD
- VAPEC-B (vincristine, doxorubicin, prednisolone, etoposide, cyclophosphamide, bleomycin) chemotherapy + involved-field RT versus mantle RT in early-stage HD
- Adjuvant involved-field RT versus no adjuvant therapy following remission induction with MOPP/ABV hybrid in stage III/IV HD
- Coactivated T-cell (COACT) therapy with refractory HD: patients who failed first-line standard therapy, second-line salvage therapy, or experimental treatments
- Aminocamptothecin in refractory or relapsed HD and NHL
- EVA intensification therapy for slowly responding stage III/IV HD with subsequent autologous BMT/PBSC for partial responders without a suitable transplantation donor
- Cytotoxic T-cell infusion with PBSC transplantation for HD and NHL
- Oral versus intravenous empirical antibacterial therapy for granulocytopenic patients with HD and NHL

TABLE 65-17 Quality of Care Evaluation of a Patient with Hodgkin's Disease

Disciplines participating in the quality of care evaluation:
Medical ☐ Nursing ☐ Dietary ☐ Pharmacy ☐

Data from:
☐ Medical Record Review ☐ Patient Family Interview

Criteria	Yes	No
1. Were you able to ask questions about Hodgkin's disease?	☐	☐
2. Were you given sufficient information to make an informed choice about your treatment options?	☐	☐
3. Did your family feel included in your treatment process?	☐	☐
4. Were you given sufficient information about the chemotherapy you received for your disease?	☐	☐
5. Were you told about the possible immediate symptoms, such as immunosuppression and possible nausea and vomiting?	☐	☐
6. Were you given instruction on neutropenia precautions?	☐	☐
7. Did the nurse provide you with education materials?	☐	☐
8. Were education materials helpful to you?	☐	☐
9. Did you receive information about after hours care, the phone number to call, and what symptoms to report?	☐	☐
10. Were you given dietary information?	☐	☐
11. Did pharmacists fill your prescriptions promptly and give your medication instructions?	☐	☐
12. Were told about any of the possible long-term complications of your treatment?	☐	☐
13. What, if anything, would you like to see changed?	☐	☐
14. Were there things about the care you received that you did not like?	☐	☐

- Interleukin 11 (IL-11) for HD/NHL chemotherapy-induced thrombocytopenia
- The use of intravenous allopurinol to prevent/control HD and NHL chemotherapy-induced hyperuricemia in patients unable to tolerate oral allopurinol
- Brief physician-initiated quit-smoking strategies for patients with HD and other cancers

Many other current research trials for HD are listed in the NCI/PDQ database. Exact treatment parameters of each protocol are omitted from the publication so that therapy cannot be initiated based solely on the limited information contained in the overview. Up-to-date data is included regarding screening and prevention, investigational drug treatment, and supportive care. In addition to this comprehensive database for health care providers, PDQ maintains patient information, updated monthly and written in lay terminology, with explanations of specific oncologic diseases, staging, and treatment options. Many patients and family members are expanding their cancer knowledge base from comprehensive overviews that are readily accessed on the Internet. OncoLink, a website maintained by the University of Pennsylvania (http://www.oncolink.upenn.edu), contains links to educational information on Hodgkin's disease for health care providers and patients. OncoLink includes a link to the PDQ database.

LONG-TERM SEQUELAE OF HODGKIN'S DISEASE TREATMENT

Overview

Successful cure rates for HD have provided long-term survivorship to many patients. Overall cure rates have been reported as high as 75% in some forms of the disease (Rosenberg & Canellos, 1998). As a result, increasing numbers of patients are disease free. Some, however, are faced with multiple chronic illnesses and secondary complications that emerge years after the initial treatment. Over time, it will be important to monitor quality of life data to evaluate how the occurrence of secondary medical problems and second cancers affect long-term survival of patients who have been cured of HD. It is anticipated that many late complications will be lessened as treatment plans are continually refined. Treatment modifications include dose reduction, shortened cycle timing, and chemotherapeutic agents with fewer long-term toxicities. However, the development of one or several secondary problems, including the major concern of developing a second malignancy, remains a significant problem of treatment success. While this serious possibility and the potential for cardiopulmonary complications resulting from treatment are often some of the most physically challenging long-term side effects, infertility is frequently one of the most emotionally challenging sequelae, particularly for young adult patients. A challenge for care providers is to provide adequate information to patients and family members so that the uncertainties of the near and distant future can be fully explored early and throughout the course of HD, symptom management, and/or secondary disease. A multidisciplinary team approach with life-long medical surveillance is needed for comprehensive support of the patient-family unit.

Potential complications are listed in Table 65-16 (DeVita, Mauch, & Harris, 1997). Although the list of possible concerns is lengthy, many long-term survivors do not develop serious problems. It is fortunate that HD has changed from a disease that was almost always fatal to a disease that is curable in most patients. However, the risk of developing long-range treatment-induced side effects increases significantly when the combined modalities of intensive chemotherapy and extensive RT are used. Risk of treatment complications is also greater in older patients. Determining an individualized optimal dose of each treatment method, without sacrificing long-term survival, is essential in comprehensive care planning.

Second Malignancies

Patients cured of HD are at an increased risk over the general population of developing a second malignancy such as ANLL, NHL, and various solid tumors including lung, breast, thyroid, stomach, colon, mouth, and pharynx cancer, as well as melanoma (Mauch & Bonadonna, 1997; van Leeuwen, 1997). The increased risk of aggressive melanoma is attributed to immunosuppression that accompanies HD and HD treatment (van Leeuwen, 1997). Dysplastic nevi may occur as precursors to melanoma lesions. Continual screening for skin lesions and biopsies of suspicious lesions are particularly relevant for patients with a history of HD.

All occurrences of second malignancies may not be treatment induced. Some second cancers can be attributed to chance alone, especially in older adults, or to an increased susceptibility from other immunodeficiencies. Unfortunately, all studies do not consistently collect data on second malignancies after HD treatment or do not collect data beyond 5 years out from treatment. Radiation therapy is a known risk factor in the development of solid tumors, including an increased risk of gastrointestinal cancers after paraaortic and pelvic irradiation (van Leeuwen, 1997).

Acute Nonlymphocytic Leukemia. Most secondary leukemias that develop from HD treatment with radiotherapy or chemotherapy are refractory to treatment. Although radiation is known to cause ANLL in some patients, it more commonly develops from alkylating chemotherapeutic agents. There is a seventyfold increased risk of ANLL in patients treated for HD over the general population (van Leeuwen, 1997). Onset of ANLL after chemotherapy typically occurs from 2 to 9 years after the initial chemotherapy, with a peak occurrence of 5 to 7 years after treatment. However, it may be diagnosed up to 15 years after treatment. Risk of acute leukemia, from multiple and repeated insults to the bone marrow, rises with increasing doses of alkylating agents and with increasing age of the patient. DeVita, Mauch, and Harris (1997) reported that age greater than 40 years and prolonged exposure to alkylating agents make the relative risk of secondary leukemia very high, with a cumulative risk ranging from 10% to 40% at 10 years out from treatment. Acute bone marrow toxicity and chronic bone marrow dysfunction contribute to an increased risk of ANLL. In particular, severely thrombocytopenic patients demonstrate an increased risk. Although a specific causal relationship with thrombocytopenia has not been determined, continual bioavailability of chemotherapeutic agents that results in thrombocytopenia is postulated as a prime contributor to ANLL development (van Leeuwen, 1997).

Although the leukemogenicity of chemotherapeutic agents varies, MOPP regimens, especially repeated MOPP cycles, cause a definite increase in the risk of ANLL. Van Leeuwen (1997) reported a three to five times greater risk in patients who received 10 to 12 MOPP cycles than in patients who received 6 cycles of MOPP. ABVD, in use since the 1980s, has a relatively low reported risk of ANLL compared with MOPP used alone (Portlock & Yahalom, 1996). This lower risk also applies to regimens that combine MOPP with ABVD (van Leeuwen, 1997). However, because multiple chemotherapeutic agents are typically used in HD management, it is difficult to attribute the risk of ANLL to a single agent alone. It is hypothesized that splenectomy, as well as hyposplenism that results from radiation, contribute to an increased risk of ANLL due to alterations in immunologic functions (van Leeuwen, 1997). Cumulative data do not indicate that combined modality treatment with chemotherapy plus radiotherapy results in higher risk of ANLL than chemotherapy alone. However, further studies are needed to reevaluate this potential because data from several studies are conflicting regarding the late effects of combination therapy.

Most patients with ANLL secondary to HD are diagnosed within 10 years from the onset of HD treatment (Rosenberg & Canellos, 1998). Typically, the acute leukemia is preceded by a prolonged period of myelodysplasia, especially a slowly developing anemia and thrombocytopenia. The late complication of ANLL has a very poor prognosis for patients with HD because it is resistant even to intensive therapy. Confirmation of this diagnosis is devastating news for patients and their families who need counseling and support to cope with a second major malignancy.

Non–Hodgkin's Lymphoma. A late occurring complication of HD is the development of diffuse, aggressive non–Hodgkin's lymphoma. The incidence of NHL increases over time following treatment and continues even beyond 10 years after therapy. It may occur in patients who have been cured of their HD. According to Rosenberg and Canellos (1998), the risk of NHL secondary to HD is approximately 5% at 25 years, long after the onset of HD and successful treatment or cure of HD. This risk does not decrease over time, nor does it reach a plateau at a particular time period. Patients treated for HD have a nineteenfold increased risk of NHL over the general population, especially in the first 5 years after treatment (van Leeuwen, 1997). Most NHLs secondary to HD are intermediate grade or high grade and often involve abdominal organs. Aggressive treatment with chemotherapy is required. Although the specific cause of NHL has not been identified, it is most likely a consequence of overall immunosuppression resulting both from the HD and HD treatment (van Leeuwen, 1997).

Although rare, HD has occurred subsequent to a previous diagnosis of NHL. Dunphy, Craver, & Emerson (1997) reported a 5- to 7-year median interval time between the two diseases. Although the cause of HD after NHL is unknown, it is hypothesized that this type of HD may have a B-cell origin. It is also thought that two separate unrelated lymph node malignancies exist. Treatment for HD subsequent to NHL includes combination chemotherapy and RT. Because of the small number of cases of HD occurring after NHL in the same individual, prognostic implications have yet to be determined. In a few patients, residual NHL has been detected at the time of an HD diagnosis (Dunphy Craver, & Emerson, 1997).

Solid Tumors. Most solid tumors secondary to treatment are not evident until 10 years after therapy; the risk of developing a solid tumor increases during the second decade of survival after HD (Skeel & Ganz, 1995). The extensiveness of the radiation field is thought to be a significant factor in solid tumor development. The propensity of second neoplasms to develop in the previously irradiated field warrants close observation of this site during follow-up care. Life-long surveillance and cancer screening is necessary to detect disease in its earliest stages.

Lung Cancer. The risk of lung cancer after radiation therapy is four times greater for patients with HD than the general population and is significantly increased in patients who smoke. After HD treatment, the risk of lung cancer continually increases over time out from treatment and may not be apparent until 10 to 15 years from the initial treatment (van Leeuwen, 1997). Smoking, an identified risk factor for lung cancer, appears to have an additive effect with radiation therapy in promoting lung cancer. It is thought that radiation potentiates cellular changes already initiated by smoking. Assessment of smoking status and progress toward smoking cessation needs to be completed with each visit to the health care provider. Smoking cessation before the initiation of treatment is strongly recommended; cessation attempts need continual reinforcement from healthier providers. Repeated efforts to quit using combination treatment with nicotine patches and/or nicotine nasal spray (Nicotrol), hypnosis, behavior modification, or other innovative pharmacologic and nonpharmacologic strategies are often needed for complete success. Nicotine gum has not proved to be as effective when used alone or in combination with other methods as it was initially thought to be. Current smoking-cessation measures include the use of oral bupropion (Zyban), particularly in patients who have a moderate to high level of anxiety associated with addiction and cessation (Box 65-3).

The American Cancer Society's Fresh Start series of four to five educational support group meetings, held within a 2- to 3-week period, explores behaviors associated with smoking and effective ways to quit. The Fresh Start series includes practical information on ways to master cravings and withdrawal symptoms, stress management, conflict resolution, coping skills, relaxation strategies, ways to prevent weight gain, and relapse prevention. Referrals to programs such as Fresh Start, along with continual guidance and support during each repeat quit attempt, are useful patient education measures.

A definite association between radiation and lung cancer exists. Increasing doses of radiation and smoking are also attributed to a higher risk of lung cancer. Data regarding the risk of lung cancer with chemotherapy alone or chemotherapy in combination with radiation therapy are conflicting. Long-term follow-up of treated patients 10 to 20 years from treatment are needed to determine the significance of this relationship.

Breast Cancer. The risk of breast cancer, evidenced approximately 15 years after irradiation, is significantly increased in young girls and young women who have received mantle radiation (van Leeuwen, 1997; Rosenberg & Canellos, 1998). Data from several studies indicate that the site of the majority of breast cancers originated at or in the margin of the anterior mantle radiation field. Because girls younger than 15 years who were treated with radiation for HD are in the highest risk group for breast cancer, early and continual lifetime breast cancer screening is needed. Data indicate that women treated for HD before age 30 years have an increased risk of breast cancer (Horning, 1997). Although women over age 30 years treated for HD are at no increased risk over the general population for developing breast cancer, monthly self breast examination, yearly physical examination by palpation, and mammograms are important clinical tools to assist with early detection. It is essential to initiate screening examinations at an earlier age than is recommended for the general population by standardized American Cancer Society (ACS) and NCI criteria. Prompt detection of early-stage breast cancer improves survival.

Other Sites. Thyroid cancer after neck irradiation for HD has a sixteenfold increased risk over the general population. Children, however, demonstrated a 67 times greater risk of developing thyroid cancer, especially with increased doses and mantle-field radiation (van Leeuwen, 1997). If the thyroid stimulation hormone level rises, thyroid replacement therapy is given to decrease the risk of thyroid cancer (Skeel & Ganz, 1995). The stomach, soft tissue, bones, and skin are other less common sites of radiation-induced second cancers. Alkylating agents, defects in cell-mediated immunity, and surveillance defects are additional contributing factors to the development of secondary tumors. Advances in radiation technology and narrowed fields of irradiation may eventually decrease the incidence of solid tumors after HD treatment.

Cardiopulmonary Complications

Cardiac. Although modern blocking techniques limit the amount of radiation exposure, serious myocardial damage may result from RT and/or anthracycline (DeVita, Mauch, & Harris, 1997; Steinherz & Yahalom, 1997). However, late vascular effects of therapy may be difficult to differentiate from common changes related to an aging circulatory system. Acute or chronic pericarditis may result from mediastinal irradiation, especially if the heart has not been adequately shielded during treatment. Doxorubicin therapy after mediastinal radiation potentiates this problem, especially because it has increasing cardiotoxicity with cumulative drug exposure. Coronary artery disease, cardiomyopathy, valvular disease, ischemia, endothelial damage, and accelerated atherogenesis may result from radiation as well. Doxorubicin combined with mediastinal radiation may produce cardiotoxicity at lower chemotherapeutic doses than with chemotherapy alone. According to Horning (1997), there is an increased risk of death from coronary artery disease and acute myocardial infarction after mediastinal radiotherapy in children and adults. However, current radiotherapy techniques, with better dose-fractionation schedules and reduction of the heart volume radiated, should result in a decreased incidence of pericardial, coronary, and myocardial disease.

Anthracycline-related cardiomyopathy may occur with acute, subacute, or late symptomatology (Steinherz & Yahalom, 1997). The acute phase includes pericardial effusion and friction rub, pleuritic pain, transient dysrhythmias, and myocardial dysfunction that may proceed to transient cardiac failure or death. Pericardiocentesis, antiinflammatory agents, and/or diuretics may be indicated. A pericardiectomy may be necessary if acute changes become chronic and restrictive pericarditis develops. However, the risk of restrictive pericarditis from radiation therapy has decreased significantly with modern radiation techniques (Marcus, Buck, & Mauch, 1998). Symptoms of the more insidious subacute phase may include increasing tachycardia, tachypnea, dyspnea, pulmonary edema, fatigue, low cardiac output, and congestive failure. The onset of congestive heart failure during pregnancy or upon initiation of vigorous exercise in previously treated patients is evidence that cardiac reserve is marginal. The late phase, which may occur 5 years or more after chemotherapy, indicates continued cardiac decompensation from hypertrophy and fibrosis of the myocytes, resulting eventually in cardiac failure.

Thorough cardiac evaluation is necessary before initiating anthracycline therapy, and frequent long-term follow-up is needed to continually evaluate the cardiac status after treatment. Serial echocardiography is a useful noninvasive technique to monitor early and late functional changes and cardiotoxicity. This is particularly useful in children because echo images are more clearly identified through thin chest walls. Radionuclide studies are also useful to detect subtle changes and monitor cardiac status. Nuclear cineangiography is used to periodically monitor effects on the cardiac ejection fraction of the ventricles.

Early diagnosis and therapeutic interventions may successfully limit late cardiac effects of treatment. Patient education to decrease cardiac risk factors includes information on lifestyle modifications such as smoking cessation; dietary alterations to decrease high-fat, high-calorie, high-cholesterol foods; effective hypertension management; stress reduction; and graduated exercise programs. Regular, moderate exercise is a relatively safe and effective method to control high blood pressure. A 30-minute period of exercise, which can be broken down to several smaller units, such as three 10-minute periods, is recommended daily. Exercise also has a positive effect on the management of cancer-related fatigue. Other treatment measures for cardiac problems may include afterload reduction with angiotensin-converting enzyme (ACE) inhibitors that may effectively stabilize cardiac failure secondary to anthracycline chemotherapy (Steinherz & Yahalom, 1997). Marcus, Buck, &

Mauch (1998) recommended routine blood pressure and cholesterol screening to decrease cardiac risk factors in patients treated for HD.

Pulmonary. Bleomycin pulmonary toxicity associated with ABVD may result in fibrotic changes, restrictive lung disease, and a significant decrease in lung diffusion capacity (Portlock & Yahalom, 1996; Mauch & Bonadonna, 1997). These alterations, with functional lung tissue gradually replaced by fibrotic scar tissue, are dose dependent. Respiratory changes are monitored by serial pulmonary function studies. These findings are compared with baseline studies completed before initiating treatment with bleomycin. Symptoms of respiratory deficiencies may be diminished somewhat with early initiation of steroid therapy. Lung fibrosis may also result from radiation therapy alone.

The onset of radiation pneumonitis ranges from 1 to 6 months after the completion of mantle radiation and has an incidence of less than 5% of treated patients (Mauch & Bonadonna, 1997; Marcus, Buck, & Mauch, 1998). This risk increases to 10% to 15% in patients with bulky mediastinal disease and in patients treated with combined chemotherapy and RT (Mauch & Bonadonna, 1997). Typically, the pneumonitis is confined to the areas of lung tissue in the irradiated field. Symptoms include a mild, nonproductive cough, dyspnea on exertion, pleuritic pain, malaise, and low-grade fever. Patients who receive radiation therapy alone have less incidence of radiation-induced pneumonitis than patients who receive combination chemotherapy with MOPP as well as RT. Although data on the degree of pneumonitis associated with regimens of ABVD and RT is still being accumulated, discontinuance of bleomycin is necessary when symptoms of dysfunctional lung disease occur.

Chronic restrictive lung disease, resulting in decreased lung distensibility, may increase the risk of pulmonary infectious processes from viral, bacterial, or fungal organisms, which require aggressive therapy. Pulmonary symptoms that do not respond to steroids may be indicative of *Pneumocystis carinii* or other opportunistic infections (Mauch & Bonadonna, 1997; Marcus, Buck, & Mauch, 1998). Fibrotic lung tissue changes are chronic and result in decreased lung tissue compliance with diminished diffusion capacity, hypoxemia, and hypercapnea. Restrictive lung disease also causes a decrease in total lung capacity. The chronic loss of functional lung parenchyma eventually causes hypoventilation. This, in turn, results in an increased workload necessary for air exchange to meet the body's oxygen demand. Respiratory insufficiency is especially prominent on exertion during exercise and is exacerbated by the aging process. Dyspnea at rest indicates severe pulmonary dysfunction. These energy-depleting respiratory alterations often contribute to or exacerbate generalized fatigue.

Alterations in Sexuality: Infertility, Sterility, Loss of Libido

Chen, Zheng, Chou, Boyle, and Holford (1997) noted an increased incidence of HD in young adults ages 20 to 44 years, particularly in females, since 1970. In view of this trend and the overall prolonged survival in young patients treated for HD, issues surrounding changes in sexuality and fertility secondary to treatment are becoming increasingly more important considerations. Reproductive dysfunction and other changes in sexuality that result from treatment of HD are traumatic for young adult patients who are in their peak reproductive years. This is especially true if patients were not well prepared by health care providers for long-term consequences of gonadal failure resulting in infertility. Decreased libido may be a persistent problem related to fatigue and/or hormonal changes. Additional sexual concerns may center on the question of inheritability of cancer or susceptibility of future children to mutagenic changes if fertility resumes after prolonged azoospermia or amenorrhea. However, no evidence to support either of these concerns exists to date (Henry-Amar & Joly, 1996).

To provide the most accurate information to patients, a sexual and reproductive history, including menstrual cycling, pretreatment fertility, obstetric history, contraceptive use, libido, and past sexually transmitted diseases that may affect reproduction, needs to be completed before predicting future reproductive success. Some health care providers admit to feelings of discomfort when first initiating a discussion on sexual concerns with patients; some also fear offending patients with intimate questioning. Differences in age and culture between patient and care provider may make discussing sexual concerns problematic as well. It is helpful if caregivers are sensitive but direct in their statements to increase the patient/provider comfort level. This facilitates information gathering and patient education, and it legitimizes sexuality as an appropriate topic of discussion. Setting the stage for sexual history taking can be initiated by seeking acceptance from the patient and or spouse to ask potentially sensitive questions. The universality of sexuality and/or fertility concerns and the relationship of these concerns to an overall sense of well-being can be addressed to ease the transition from medical issues to those surrounding sexuality.

Depending on the dose and type of chemotherapeutic agent used, sterility may not be avoidable. This iatrogenic toxicity of treatment has a significant effect on the quality of life of HD survivors and their partners. For male patients, cryopreservation of sperm is an effective option if it is initiated before beginning chemotherapy. Sperm banking requires serial collection of at least three semen samples over the course of 1 to 2 weeks. Several days between specimen collection with a 48-hour period of abstinence between samples are needed to enhance the quality of sperm collected (Koeppel, 1995; Meistrich, Vassilopoulou-Sellin, & Lipshultz, 1997). Although this could necessitate a delay in starting chemotherapy treatment, banking may be accomplished in the intervening days of the diagnostic evaluation phase when preliminary tests and procedures are being completed. Although sperm counts may only be moderately reduced during the first 2 months of cytotoxic chemotherapy, it is advisable to collect sperm for banking before the initiation of chemotherapy. However, it may prove difficult for the patient and his or her partner to focus on future family planning when urgent treatment decisions are also required of them. In addition, the cost of sperm banking, including collection, analysis, and storage fees, is expensive and not presently likely to be covered under the majority of health care plans. Success with cryopreservation of ova has not been achieved to date, and it remains to be seen whether this will be accomplished in future treatment of infertile women who were treated for HD.

The survival of the spermatogenic stem cells and their ability to proliferate, differentiate, and produce spermatozoa directly influence the eventual recovery of adequate sperm production, motility, and viability (Meistrich, Vassilopoulou-Sellin, & Lipshultz, 1997). Survival of spermatogenic stem cells depends on the duration and degree of cytotoxicity. Procarbazine in MOPP regimens and doxorubicin (Adriamycin) in ABVD regimens have the greatest effect on sperm production. Azoospermia is common with mechlorethamine (Nitrogen mustard). Bleomycin and vinblastine cause a temporary reduction in sperm count with negligible stem cell inactivation (Meistrich, Vassilopoulou-Sellin, & Lipshultz, 1997). Prednisone does not seem to have a negative effect on sperm production. Normospermic levels can return within 1 to 3 years after chemotherapy at low doses of agents cytotoxic to sperm stem cells. However, a long duration of azoospermia due to severe stem cell inactivation after treatment diminishes the probability that spermatogenesis will recover adequately for successful conception. Interestingly, many male patients with HD have low sperm counts even before HD treatment has been used. The cause of this problem has not been clearly identified, but because it is found in males with other malignancies as well, it is attributed to the neoplastic process.

Permanent infertility in the majority of male patients treated with MOPP and in a significant number of females has been documented. Azoospermia results after just a few cycles of MOPP in 90% to 100% of male patients (Mauch & Bonadonna, 1997). Although ABVD causes transient azoospermia, it does not usually result in permanent infertility in males. Sperm counts typically increase within the first 2 years after treatment with ABVD. In young women, ABVD may only temporarily disrupt menstrual function without evidence of ovarian failure (Portlock & Yahalom, 1996). However, in older women, ABVD treatment may result in infertility or permanent premature menopause and associated estrogen deficiency. Procarbazine-containing regimens cause permanent ovarian failure.

Irradiation of the ovaries also induces ovarian failure and is age dependent. Translocation of the ovaries (oophoropexy) out of the pelvic radiation port and shielding of the ovaries may provide at least partial fertility preservation in younger women. Without translocation, pelvic and total nodal irradiation results in loss of ovarian function. With modern technology, oophoropexy may be done laparoscopically, as well as by laparotomy, which had been the standard procedure before the advent of and skillfulness with laparoscopy. However, oophoropexy is useful only if the radiation therapist concurs that shielding will protect the ovaries from radiation scatter (Stein, 1995). During the staging workup, one minimally invasive laparoscopic procedure can accomplish paraaortic lymph node dissection, liver biopsy, splenectomy, and oophoropexy (Ramshaw, 1997). Without oophoropexy, radiation therapy has the potential to more significantly damage prepubescent ovaries than does cytotoxic chemotherapy.

Unless contraindicated, estrogen replacement therapy is needed to preserve bone density and cardiac function in menopausal women. Patient education ensures acceptance and compliance with prompt initiation and maintenance of hormone replacement therapy (HRT). If HRT is delayed, estrogen deficiency leads to an increased risk of premature osteoporotic changes and cardiovascular disease. Premature menopause is a strong predictor of developing osteoporosis. This risk is compounded by immobilization, physical inactivity, lack of weight-bearing activity, excessive alcohol intake, smoking, and deficiencies in calcium and vitamin D.

Patients benefit from nutritional education on excellent dietary sources of high-calcium foods. These include cheese, yogurt, sardines, milk, and salmon (Davis & Sherer, 1994). Other useful sources less high in calcium include turnip greens, spinach, oysters, broccoli, and shrimp. Vitamin D is also necessary for calcium absorption. Diets deficient in calcium are a frequent occurrence in an aging population. It is important to halt the progression of osteoporosis before irreversible structural changes to bone occur. Progressive osteoporosis and decreasing bone density increase susceptibility to fractures and vertebral collapse. A graduated program of weight-bearing exercise, such as a walking regimen, has a positive effect on calcium deposits in bone and needs to be encouraged.

Ovarian failure is irreversible when maturing follicles are destroyed by cytotoxic therapy. Amenorrhea is common with mechlorethamine. The combination of RT and MOPP has an additive effect on ovarian failure. Older women are more sensitive to permanent ovarian failure and associated amenorrhea because the total number of follicles decreases as the age of the patient increases. Signs and symptoms of ovarian failure and menopause include hot flashes (also referred to as *hot flushes*), night sweats, insomnia, frequent nighttime waking, occasional sensations of dyspnea, fatigue, headache, palpitations, decreased bone mass, increased bone fragility, decreased libido, skin and vaginal dryness, dyspareunia, stress incontinence, and recurrent bladder infections. Vaginal atrophy, dryness, and thinning of the vaginal walls, which may be accompanied by vaginal itching and burning, can make sexual intercourse a painful event. Over-the-counter water-soluble lubricants may decrease some of this discomfort. During the lengthy course of typical perimenopause and menopause, an 8- to 10-year process, changes are gradual and less noticeable than the sudden abrupt onset of menopause resulting from cancer therapy. Symptoms of menopause can be aggravated by stress and concomitant cancer-related or other medical problems. Psychological concerns associated with menopause may include anxiety, nervousness, changes in mood, irritability, overemotionality, depression, memory loss, and feelings of worthlessness or hopelessness. These feelings may also surface throughout the course of the disease and/or during HD treatment and recovery phases.

Testicular shielding during RT may decrease the incidence of male infertility (DeVita, Mauch, & Harris, 1997).

Cumulative high doses of RT and total-body irradiation before bone marrow transplantation likely result in permanent azoospermia. Multiple structural abnormalities in spermatozoa are seen immediately after radiotherapy. Because RT and combination chemotherapy can cause toxic effects on male and female gonads from additive effects of multiple agents, patients of both genders need adequate counseling and education to increase their awareness of possible fertility options. In vitro fertilization and other assisted reproductive technologies (ARTs) may be the most viable option for women to consider after curative treatment. However, these procedures are expensive and success is limited at present.

Due to a possible mutational risk from cytotoxic therapy, Meistrich, Vassilopoulou-Sellin, & Lipshultz (1997) recommend a 3-month waiting period before conception following cytotoxic therapy for women and a wait of 6 months following therapy for men. Before considering conception, Rosenberg and Canellos (1998) recommend a 2-year period of close observation for disease recurrence because this is a high-risk time for relapse. Contraception methods should be used during this time to avoid pregnancy. For male patients the 6-month period allows a full spermatogenic cycle (from stem cell to sperm) without exposure to cytotoxic agents. The risk of mutagenic alterations may be higher if pregnancy occurs earlier than 6 months out from the male partner's final chemotherapy administration (Meistrich, Vassilopoulou-Sellin, & Lipshultz, 1997). Further research is needed to fully determine the risk of mutagenic alterations caused by combination chemotherapy.

The optimization of fertility after HD treatment, enhanced by modern technology and ART procedures, is an important area of concern for adult patients in child-bearing years. However, success rates, limited to date, need to improve for this to become a realistic goal.

Hypothyroidism

Hypothyroidism, a deficiency of thyroid hormone and/or the loss or destruction of thyroid gland tissue, results from direct cellular injury in approximately 30% of patients who received mantle-field radiation for HD (Horning, 1997; Portlock & Yahalom, 1996). Hypothyroidism may be detected by a rising thyroid-stimulating hormone (TSH) level. The amount of hormone deficiency determines the degree of thyroid dysfunction. This condition is usually effectively managed with thyroid hormone replacement therapy (thyroxine) for patients with elevated TSH levels and is monitored by periodic TSH assays. Because the thyroid hormones thyroxine (T_4) and triiodothyronine (T_3) significantly influence every body system, signs and symptoms of hypothyroidism are varied (Stern, 1996). An overall decreased metabolic rate results from thyroid deficiency. Symptoms such as slowed physical and cognitive processes also may be present and need to be differentiated from similar symptoms of depression.

Patients may have subclinical or clinical symptoms of hypothyroidism. Fatigue, lethargy, and malaise are among the earliest signs of this endocrine problem. Other symptoms include a marked sensitivity or intolerance to cold temperatures, a decreased appetite with a paradoxical mild weight gain, physical-mental-emotional lethargy, dulled thought processes, decreased attention span, alterations in memory, and other cognitive deficits. Additional symptoms include decreased exercise tolerance related to the effects on the cardiovascular system, neuromuscular weakness, and gastrointestinal sluggishness or constipation. Sexuality changes secondary to hypothyroidism include a decrease in both libido and fertility, as well as disorders of menstruation. Skin may appear dry, rough, or edematous, especially in the face, hands, and feet. Susceptibility to infections and a delayed response in wound healing are evident. Increased peripheral vascular resistance results in decreased tissue perfusion. In addition, renal perfusion and glomerular filtration are altered. Overall, there is a decrease in available energy, which then contributes to generalized fatigue and ennui.

OTHER CLINICAL MANAGEMENT PROBLEMS

Postsplenectomy Sepsis Syndrome

Although the development of bacterial postsplenectomy sepsis is seen in a small percentage of patients with HD, it is a serious medical concern. Encapsulated organisms such as pneumococci or *Haemophilus influenzae* are the primary organisms of concern in asplenic patients. Sepsis also occurs rarely as a result of hyposplenism after radiation to the spleen. Sepsis is a medical emergency that develops more frequently in children than in adult patients; it is aggravated by the underlying HD immune defects and immunosuppressive therapy. Ineffective control mechanisms allow the microbial invasion of fungal and protozoal organisms that are frequently found in patients with HD. Particularly in adults, pneumonococcal organisms are the more commonly identified agents. *Pneumocystis carinii,* although uncommon, may also occur. Bacteremia, pneumonia, skin infections, or meningitis may progress quickly. Prompt treatment with multiple intravenous antibiotics and antifungals is needed because the onset of sepsis is rapid and mortality rates are significant. A typical septic clinical presentation includes high fever, shaking chills, headache, malaise, and hypotension. DIC and/or ARDS may progress rapidly (Rosenberg & Canellos, 1998). The cascading interconnected problems of DIC and ARDS often lead to a poor prognostic outcome, even when intervention has been prompt. Attempts to stabilize patients with fulminant sepsis are aggressive and may require intensive care settings to meet acute, complex, multisystem needs.

Patient-family education about signs and symptoms of impending sepsis may facilitate early detection and treatment success. Antibiotic prophylaxis may be successful in preventing infection. It is recommended that polyvalent pneumococcal vaccine be administered before splenectomy or initial treatment for HD to reduce an overwhelming sepsis potential (Rosenberg and Canellos, 1998; Mauch & Bonadonna, 1997; Henry-Amar & Joly, 1996). New vaccines against *Haemophilus influenzae* and *Neisseria* microorganisms have also recently been developed and are useful preventives. Persistent cytopenias after treatment and immunologic impairment due to a decreased number of functionally immunocompetent cells make the possibility of infection and sepsis a long-term threat. If the current trend of performing fewer diagnostic splenectomies continues, a decline in the incidence of sepsis and associated mortality in patients with HD may result.

Herpes Zoster

Herpes zoster (varicella-zoster) is a common complication of a suppressed immune system that occurs in one third of patients with HD (Rosenberg & Canellos, 1998). The presentation is similar to other herpes zoster infections that occur in the general population. Chills, fever, malaise, and pruritus may exist 3 to 4 days before the eruption of vesicular lesions. These lesions typically have an erythematous base and occur in a contiguous dermatomal pattern. However, in aging iinmunocompromised patients with HD, localized infection may result in prolonged episodes of postherpetic neuralgia or severe disseminated disease. Although relatively rare, lung, central nervous system, or other organ involvement with herpes zoster may contribute to mortality. Early pharmaceutical intervention with systemic antiviral acyclovir therapy (Zovirax) is indicated to decrease the morbidity and potential mortality of disseminated herpes. Zoster immunoglobulin may also be used in the management plan.

Lhermitte's Syndrome

Lhermitte's syndrome is a transient, self-limited, mild form of radiation myelitis experienced by approximately 10% to 15% of patients treated with mantle-field radiation (Marcus, Buck, & Mauch, 1998; DeVita, Mauch, & Harris, 1997). This perplexing dysesthesia/paresthesia syndrome is described as a sudden, brief, electrical shocklike painful sensation or numbness that radiates down the backs of both legs, arms, and/or the back when the head is flexed forward.

Lhermitte's syndrome is bothersome to patients, especially if they have not been informed of the possibility of its occurrence. The "pins and needles" and other sensations occur 6 weeks to 3 months after radiation and resolve within months up to 1 to 2 years. Symptoms usually disappear spontaneously without treatment, and the syndrome does not result in permanent damage to the cord. Although no specific cause has been identified, this syndrome may reflect transient demyelination of the cervical spinal cord secondary to radiation-induced damage to the oligodendroglia responsible for myelin formation (Portlock & Yahalom, 1996; Posner, 1996).

Physiologic Changes Related to Aging

The risk of developing HD decreases after the second bimodal incidence peak in the 50- to 55-year age range. However, HD often has a more aggressive clinical course in this age group. In view of a large population of long-term HD survivors, it is imperative that oncologic care providers are attuned to the changing needs of older adult patients. Recognizing the need to periodically complete comprehensive geriatric physical assessments in this age group is an important step in the care of elderly oncology patients. Thorough assessment data enable the care provider to note early changes in physiologic functioning that typically occur in older age and to differentiate these changes from advanced or secondary disease. Because one or several chronic illnesses may confound the clinical picture, arriving at a differential diagnosis through diagnostic reasoning and problem solving is a clinical challenge in caring for elders.

Because there is a reduction in the functional status, size, and weight of the kidneys with aging, dose adjustment of renally excreted drugs requires careful consideration. Older patients may have increased vulnerability to adverse effects of chemotherapy as a result of these changes and the age-related changes in bone marrow reserves. However, these alterations should not rule out chemotherapeutic intervention for this age group. Selection of regimens with moderate levels of toxicity may be preferable to high-dose chemotherapeutic protocols. The aging adult is less able to distribute, metabolize, and excrete medications than younger adults (McDaniel, 1996). Decreased organ efficiency, including diminished circulation of blood to the liver and decreased kidney function, results in varying pharmacokinetic responses to medications in general. Because some agents have a cumulative effect, toxicities to a wide range of drugs may develop. Many older patients are concurrently taking multiple medications for one or more chronic conditions.

Other typical aging changes include osteoporotic vertebral compression with thinning of the intervertebral disks and kyphotic development, decreased bone density, lean muscle mass decline with body fat increase, and alterations in the functional status and perfusion of the heart, liver, lungs, and kidneys. Reduced alveolar ventilation, especially at lung bases, is a typical age-related change. These structural and functional changes put the elderly patient at further risk for the development of respiratory infections.

Older patients may also demonstrate evidence of mental status changes such as progressive dementia or cognitive impairment, which make assessment and patient education challenging. Acute confusion may result from medication administration if degradation of the blood-brain barrier has occurred related to changes of aging. Effective management of the numerous psychobiologic conditions of aging, both related and unrelated to cancer, as well as the ramifications of one or more chronic illnesses, is essential in comprehensive care of the elderly. Because older patients frequently have a higher incidence of adverse reactions to drugs in general than younger patients, dose reduction may be needed to safely manage HD, a second malignancy, or other medical or psychiatric conditions. Yet, many older patients are able to tolerate the side effects of chemotherapy and radiation therapy if the management of their disease is individualized to specific body system changes.

Depression. Depression may accompany usual changes of aging and/or is aggravated by the cancer experience, particularly if re-treatment of either HD or another malignancy is necessary. Older adults are especially vulnerable to depression because they often experience multiple concurrent losses. Diminishing physical functioning, loss of spouse and/or friends to death, reduced income, and changes in the living environment are some of the frequent losses associated with aging. Depression and an accompanying decreased quality of life are frequent problems among the elderly. Depression is characterized by multiple symptoms, including a despondent mood, loss of interest in usual desirable activities, weight loss or weight gain, difficulty sleeping (such as problems falling or staying asleep and/or early waking), a low level of energy, feelings of worthlessness and/or hopelessness, and a diminished ability to concentrate or think clearly.

The Beck Depression Inventory (BDI) and the Zung Self-Rating Depression Scale (ZSRDS) are several commonly used self-report instruments to assess depression. The BDI is an easily administered, brief assessment tool that includes items on sleep disturbance and fatigue. In addition, the use of a focused history on symptoms of depression during the clinical interview often provides more useful information on depression and related problems than the assessment tools used alone. Moore and Blumenthal (1998) recommend combining a structured interview with self-report measures to more accurately detect depression than either the BDI or the ZSRDS used independently. Persistent feelings of extreme sadness and profound loss of interest in both environment and usual enjoyable activities warrants careful evaluation. Psychiatric referral is particularly useful in patients who have had recurrent or severe depressive episodes in the past. Collaboration with social services may be warranted for patients with inadequate funds or insufficient interpersonal sources of support.

Oral antidepressant pharmacotherapy with selective serotonin reuptake inhibitors (SSRIs), such as sertraline (Zoloft) or paroxetine (Paxil), are more useful in treating depression in older adults than the tricyclic antidepressants. SSRIs have fewer untoward cardiac and central nervous system (CNS) side effects than do the tricyclics. Zoloft and Paxil inhibit neuronal uptake of serotonin in the CNS and therefore potentiate the serotonin activity of mood elevation. These agents need to be used cautiously in patients with severe hepatic or renal impairment. CNS psychostimulants such as methylphenidate (Ritalin) have also been used effectively in some patients to manage associated symptoms of depression. Treatment with methylphenidate may also diminish the sensation of cancer-related fatigue and secondary problems of attentional deficits. Improvement in mental alertness and diminished fatigue are anecdotally reported effects of this drug in the elderly. Ritalin is contraindicated in patients with severe cardiovascular disease and should be taken before 6 PM to avoid insomnia and other disruptions in nighttime rest.

Exercise is a cost-effective strategy useful in the management of depression to improve mental and physical well-being. Increased physical activity is also associated with fewer side effects, especially in older adults, than pharmacotherapy. Although few studies to date have examined the effects of exercise specifically in the elderly, anecdotal and study reports from older patients indicate an increased sensation of energy and overall life satisfaction related to exercise. After an extensive review of the literature, Moore and Blumenthal (1998) concluded that exercise is associated with decreased symptomatology of depression and increased psychological functioning. Improved physical fitness that accompanies an exercise program also has a positive effect on patients' sense of mastery and control over life situations related to the cancer experience. Exercise has the added benefit of providing distraction from negative thoughts and emotions that may intrude on living successfully with cancer.

Several examples of patient education materials on managing depression and secondary fatigue through the use of exercise and other behavioral strategies are included in Boxes 65-4 through 65-7. It is important that an exercise program begins with a gradual increase in activity, particularly in patients who have been sedentary for prolonged pe-

Box 65-4

Characteristics Common to Depression, Fatigue, Grief/Loss

Symptoms

- Difficulty concentrating:
  - Cognitive deficits
  - Attentional deficits
  - Problems learning new material
  - Confusion, mental fogginess
- Variability in mood:
  - Irritability, agitation
  - Sadness, anger
  - Flattened affect
- Diminished self-esteem and confidence:
  - Accompanied by feelings of the following:
    - Worthlessness
    - Helplessness
    - Hopelessness
    - Emptiness
    - Guilt, pessimism
- Frequent crying, tearfulness
- Loss of interest or pleasure in the following:
  - Work, leisure activities
  - Family, friends
  - Sexual relationships
  - Appearance
- Vague sensation of discomfort, distress, anxiety
- Lack of energy:
  - Diminished psychomotor activity
  - Unable to contemplate, initiate, or complete tasks
  - Overwhelming sensation of tiredness
- Sleep disturbances:
  - Insomnia
  - Problems falling asleep
  - Difficulty staying asleep
  - Early morning awakening
  - Sleeping too much
- Change in eating habits:
  - Anorexia
  - Diminished appetite
  - Overeating
  - Weight loss or weight gain

Box 65-5
Managing Depression by Mastering Fatigue: A Patient Education Handout

Fatigue, an overwhelming feeling of a lack of energy, is a frequent concern during and after treatment for cancer. Although it is often ignored or undertreated, fatigue has a profound effect on the sense of well-being. Being well-informed is being well-armed in the fight against fatigue. Knowing some of the causes and effects is the first step toward better fatigue management.

Characteristics of Fatigue	Factors That Contribute to Fatigue
Overwhelming lack of energy	Anemia, infections, stress, boredom
Increased need for rest	Side effects of treatment or medications
Inability to regain energy with rest	Inadequate rest, too much activity
Inability to concentrate or do work	Inadequate nutrition or fluid intake
Feelings of guilt if unable to participate	Lack of physical activity or exercise
Inability to join in social activities	Limited social supports, depression

Simple Tips to Fight Fatigue

Exercise: Gradually add physical activity and exercise after discussing this with your care provider. Slowly, work your way up to 30 minutes a day. This can be achieved by accumulating time over the course of each day. Give yourself time to develop your strength and endurance. Stay as active as you can. Make the move to improve physical fitness.

Relaxation: Try out different ways to relax until you find a strategy useful for you. Soothing music, meditation, distraction techniques, car rides, deep breathing, progressive muscle relaxation, visualization, and imagery may help. Give yourself time to practice these new behaviors.

Stress Reduction: Try to avoid things and people that cause you stress. Develop positive thoughts; avoid negative thoughts and negative people. A support group may be useful if members demonstrate caring and concern.

Nutrition: Eat frequent, small, well-balanced meals. Delegate the grocery shopping and meal preparation to others if possible. Stay well-hydrated by drinking plenty of fluids. Eight glasses of water a day is suggested unless not recommended by your care provider.

Rest: Balance activity and rest during the day. Plan brief naps no later than 4 or 5 PM so that nighttime sleep will not be interrupted. During the day, find a room that is dim and quiet, and set an alarm so that you will not sleep too long. Naps for 30 minutes can be refreshing. Reduce any distracting noises; put yourself in brief periods of "time-out" for some quiet time alone.

Conserve Energy: Do things that are most important to you when your energy level is the greatest. Say "yes" to offers of help, and delegate errands and chores whenever you can. Provide suggestions to family and friends on ways they can help. Slowly increase your activity level, and plan some light, enjoyable activity into each day.

Courtesy Lynn Scallion, RN, MSN, AOCN.

riods of time. Individual "Exercise Prescriptions" need to be developed based on patients' needs and abilities. Stationary or regular biking, swimming, the use of a treadmill, or a walking program are effective and appropriate beginning and maintenance strategies for the elderly. Exercise has the potential to alleviate or diminish fatigue, depression, or other psychological distress.

Many patients note lingering cognitive changes and attentional deficits after chemotherapy. Bothersome "fuzzy-headedness" or "mental cloudiness" present problems in accomplishing work and leisure activities. This "mental fog" is especially problematic in attempting completion of detailed tasks and complex cognitive challenges. Some side effects of medications, such as those attributed to procarbazine, include depression, confusion, and alterations in the level of consciousness. Comprehensive assessment is warranted and includes a mental status examination, such as the Mini Mental State Exam (MMSE) (Folstein, Folstein, & McHugh, 1975). The MMSE is a widely used brief method to assess and evaluate cognitive function. It is a graded standardized clinical tool that can detect cognitive impairment, follow cognitive changes, and monitor response to treatment. The MMSE assesses orientation, attention, immediate and short-term recall, language, and the ability to follow simple verbal and written commands. It also includes normative data for different age groups and education levels in its grading scale, making it a useful clinical assessment tool. An evaluation of depression along with a complete assessment of the cognitive, affective, functional, social, environmental, and nutritional status of each patient is needed as well. Incorporating data from the physical examination, history, and review of systems enables the aging patient and care provider to make accurate treatment and symptom management decisions.

SUMMARY

Hodgkin's disease is an acute and a chronic illness. Once uniformly fatal, it is now regularly cured, even in advanced stages. Long-term sequelae, however, may make "living with" HD a continuous psychobiologic challenge. Physical limitations such as pulmonary fibrosis, congestive heart failure, hypothyroidism, and infertility imposed by treatment may be overshadowed by an unrelenting fear of recurrence. Many patients report periods of insomnia, anxiety, and dread with approaching annual physical examination. Each appointment with a health care provider serves as a reminder of continued vulnerability to a possible recurrence or new secondary problems. A strong relationship with a consistent care provider assists patients and their family

Box 65-6

Managing Insomnia: A Patient Education Handout: Promoting Better Sleep

Poor sleep habits can interfere with your daily life and leave you feeling worn out, irritable, short-tempered, and ineffective in achieving your personal and/or professional goals. If you are bothered by sleep problems, have trouble concentrating, or are feeling sluggish and energy depleted, take time to try out new sleep strategies.

Establish a regular sleep schedule: Try to go to bed at about the same time each night and get up at approximately the same time each day, even during the weekend. Be consistent in establishing your sleep-wake cycle. Sleep just long enough to awaken feeling refreshed. Balance time up out of bed and awake with time down resting or sleeping. Create relaxing presleep rituals like taking a warm bath.

Take naps early in the day and limit the duration of napping: Several short naps 30 to 45 minutes long may be more effective than 1- to 2-hour naps. Set your alarm clock so that brief "catnaps" will refresh you without interfering with nighttime rest. Avoid napping after 4 or 5 PM.

Create a restful, relaxing, comfortable bedroom environment: Reserve your bed for sleep or sexual activity. Wear loose-fitting, comfortable night clothes. Replace an old, sagging mattress. Try a new pillow. Regulate your bedroom to a temperature comfortable for you, neither too hot nor too cold. Sleep in a dark, well-ventilated room. Limit clutter and distractions in the room. Keep work-related assignments in a room other than the bedroom.

Limit distracting noise and interruptions: Keep the bedroom quiet. Turn the telephone down or off. Mask noises with soft, soothing music, "white noise," or the hum of a fan. Heavy drapes may help soundproof and darken the room. Avoid stimulating or distressing mental or physical activities close to bedtime.

Incorporate relaxation strategies and stress reduction measures into each day: Spend time winding down before bedtime. Progressive muscle relaxation, slow deep-breathing exercises, meditation, visualization, and imagery are pleasant sleep inducers. Try recalling all the details and sensations of pleasant memories such as past vacations or enjoyable trips to the beach or mountains. Music, prayer, massage, a warm bath, or light reading material may also be helpful.

Refocus negative thinking: Focus your thoughts on positive ideas and affirmative statements to ease your mind. Set aside a brief, specific time during the day to worry. Use this "worry opportunity" for creative problem solving, but do not let worries linger. Distance yourself from worries and concerns by writing them down, along with possible solutions, and depositing them in a "worry jar" before bedtime. Place the jar in a room other than the bedroom.

Develop a program of increased activity and regular exercise: Morning or early afternoon exercise positively influences the quality of nighttime sleep. Walking outside or on a treadmill is a beneficial activity that can be gradually increased in time and speed, based on how you are feeling. Try enlisting a friend or partner in your walking program to make exercise fun. For added energy, you may want to try a short walk instead of napping in the daytime. Avoid strenuous exercise at least 1 hour before bedtime. Try to get some form of exercise each day.

Restrict intake of caffeine, alcohol, or nicotine: Avoid alcohol and stimulants such as coffee, tea, cola products, and chocolate after lunchtime or within 8 hours of bedtime. These products often cause fragmented sleep.

Treat treatable medical problems: Ineffective symptom management may interfere with sleep. Depression, pain, nausea, dehydration, treatment-related side effects, sleep apnea, restless leg syndrome, or medications for one or more chronic illnesses may disrupt sleep. Make an appointment to discuss these concerns with your health care provider.

Use sleeping pills sparingly and only with approval from your care provider: Try other measures first. Avoid repeated and/or prolonged use of sedatives.

Know when to quit struggling with sleep problems: If you are still awake 20 to 30 minutes after trying to fall asleep or return to sleep, get up and do something else. Try getting out of bed and out of the bedroom when sleep is ineffective. Reading, having a light snack, or briefly changing the sleep setting may enable you to return to bed for a restful night. If sleep problems persist, it may be useful to enlist the assistance of a sleep specialist. Be persistent in attempts to get a good night's sleep.

Courtesy Lynn Scallion, RN, MSN, AOCN.

members to recognize symptoms of importance and differentiate these from symptoms of minor illness. The uncertainties of the future may also interfere with establishing and maintaining intimate and other personal relationships. Intimacy may be further hampered by chronic sexual dysfunction. Individual therapy, group therapy, and/or educational support groups may decrease feelings of vulnerability and a sense of aloneness. Shared concerns discussed by support group members often bring about shared insight and creative problem solving to meet the multiple and varied long-term consequences of disease and treatment.

The National Coalition for Cancer Survivorship, the NCI's Cancer Information Service (CIS), and the ACS are useful resources for patients, family members, and professional care providers. Having available several reliable sources of information for questions regarding employment issues, job protection, insurance coverage, economic considerations related to expenses of illness, financial security, rehabilitation, and other survivorship concerns decreases cancer-related anxiety and uncertainty. The combined talents of multidisciplinary team members, with active involvement of nurses, nurse practitioners, other advanced practice nurses, social workers, pharmacists, physicians, physician specialists, physician assistants, psychologists, chaplains, nutritionists, physical and occupational therapists, personal exercise trainers, massage thera-

Box 65-7

Guidelines for Exercise: A Patient Education Handout to Manage Fatigue and Depression

Fatigue remains one of the most common problems experienced by patients with cancer. Light exercise with increasing physical activity is one strategy for successful management of fatigue.

Benefits of Exercise

Increases sense of well-being
Increases feeling of control and independence
Utilizes the "gift of nature"
Enhances restful nighttime sleep
Promotes efficient use of energy
Strengthens muscles
Increases strength and endurance
Enhances coordination
Lifts depression and self-esteem
Enhances weight control

An "Exercise-Lite" Prescription

General guidelines:

Discuss your exercise plans with your care provider first. Collaboratively develop an exercise prescription right for you.

Carefully monitor your response to increased activity, and adjust your program as needed. Be self-paced.

Individualize your exercise program to your level of fitness, health status, and ability.

Start slowly and gradually add more time and intensity.

Realize that developing a habit of exercise will be established slowly. It will take time for you to develop an exercise identity.

Exercise in a safe area; wear comfortable and supportive athletic shoes. Get together with others to socialize during your exercise routine. "Get up, get moving, get out, get started, get together." Exercise with a partner if possible.

Start with a short period to warm up, and end with a cool-down period.

Prevent dehydration by replacing fluids that may be lost during exercise. Avoid exercising outdoors in very warm or very cold weather. Consider walking in an air-conditioned mall or shopping center, but keep walking and save window shopping for later.

Carry identification and emergency phone money with you.

Simple Steps to Fitness with "Exercise-Lite"

Almost any form of physical activity provides health benefits. Walking is an excellent form of exercise and can be done anywhere. Finding an activity you enjoy helps you stay with it.

Exercise time is recommended for 30 minutes each day. Gradually build up to this over the course of several weeks or longer. The 30 minutes of exercise can be accomplished in any amount of time increments: 5 minutes six times a day, or 10 minutes three times a day, for example. Even frequent 2-minute times are useful, and there is no need to accomplish it all at once. It may actually be easier to stick with your exercise program over the long haul if you gradually add activity over the course of your day.

Try to keep a record of the amount of exercise time you are able to accumulate each day. Establish a routine that you are comfortable with so that you will stay with it.

Be aware of contraindications to exercise: Chest pain, shortness of breath, or any other abnormal response to exercise on days of intravenous chemotherapy; metastatic bone involvement; abnormally low platelet, white cell, or red cell blood values; fever; dizziness; or confusion.

Courtesy Lynn Scallion, RN, MSN, AOCN.

pists, music therapists, and/or recreation therapists, are useful resources to meet ever changing needs and concerns.

Optimization of therapeutic effects to induce HD cure without sacrificing overall quality of life is a realistic goal for the entire team. Effective symptom management, continual patient-family education, and emotional/psychosocial support and counsel have a significant effect on promoting positivity, encouragement, and the spirit of hopefulness. The primary goal of these interventions is to enhance the quality of survival for patients living with HD and treatment sequelae. Restorative and supportive interventions help patients and their families regain and maintain the highest possible level of functioning. Maintaining efficacy of treatment while simultaneously reducing the late effects of treatment ensures quality living for HD survivors.

REFERENCES

Agency for Health Care Policy and Research (AHCPR). (1994). U.S. Department of Health and Human Services. *Management of cancer pain.* Publication No. 9.

Aksoy, M., Erden, S., Dincol, K., Hepuyksel, T., & Dincol, G. (1974). Chronic exposure to benzene as a possible contributory etiological factor in Hodgkin's disease. *Blut, 28,* 298.

Audoin, J., Diebold, J., & Palleson, G. (1992). Frequent expression of Epstein-Barr virus latent membrane protein-1 in tumor cells of Hodgkin's disease in HIV-positive patients. *Journal of Pathology, 167,* 381-384.

Bierman, H. R. (1968). Human appendix and neoplasia. *Cancer, 121,* 109.

Canellos, G. P. (1995a). Hodgkin's disease. In J. S. MacDonald, D. G. Haller, & R. J. Mayer (Eds.), *Manual of oncologic therapeutics.* Philadelphia: J. B. Lippincott.

Canellos, G. (1995b). Is ABVD the standard regimen for Hodgkin's disease based on randomized CALGB comparison of MOPP, ABVD, and MOPP alternating with ABVD? *Leukemia 10* (Suppl. 2), 68.

Carbone, P. P., Kaplan, H. S., Muschoff, K., Smithers, D. W., & Tubiana, M. (1971). Report of the committee on Hodgkin's disease staging classification. *Cancer Research, 31,* 1860-1861.

Chen, Y., Zheng, T., Chou, M., Boyle, P., & Holford, T. (1997). The increase of Hodgkin's disease incidence among young adults. *Cancer, 79,* 2209-2218.

Cozen, W., Katz, J., & Mack, T. M. (1992). Risk patterns of Hodgkin's disease in Los Angeles vary by cell type. *Cancer Epidemiology, Biomarkers, and Prevention, 1,* 261-268.

Davis, J. & Sherer, K. (1994). *Applied nutrition and diet therapy for nurses.* Philadelphia: W. B. Saunders.

DeVita, V. T., Mauch, P. M., & Harris, N. L. (1997). Hodgkin's disease. In V. T. DeVita, S. Hellman, & S. A. Rosenberg (Eds.), *Cancer: Principles and practice of oncology* (5th ed.). Philadelphia: J. B. Lippincott.

Diehl, V. & Engert, A. (1996). An overview of the Third International Symposium on Hodgkin's Lymphoma. *Annals of Oncology, 7* (Suppl. 4), S1-S4.

Diehl, V., von Kalle, C., Fonatash, C., Tesch, H. Juecker, M., & Schaadt. (1990). The cell of origin in Hodgkin's disease. *Seminars in Oncology, 17,* 660.

Dunphy, C., Craver, J., & Emerson, W. (1997). Demonstration of composite nodal B-cell lymphoma and subsequent Hodgkin's disease by flow cytometry and immunohistochemistry. *Arch Pathol Lab Med, 121,* 637-640.

Folstein, M., Folstein, S., & McHugh, P. (1975). "Mini-mental state." A practical method for grading the cognitive state of patients for the clinician. *Journal of Psychiatric Research, 12,* 189-198.

Grufferman, S., Cole, P., Smith, P., & Lukes, R. (1977). Hodgkin's disease in siblings. *New England Journal of Medicine, 296,* 248-250.

Gutensohn, N. (1982). Social class and age at diagnosis of Hodgkin's disease: New epidemiologic evidence for the "two disease hypothesis." *Cancer Treatment Report, 66,* 689-695.

Gutensohn, N. & Cole, P. (1981). Childhood social environment and Hodgkin's disease. *New England Journal of Medicine, 304,* 135-140.

Gutterman, S., Barton, J. I., & Eby, N. (1987). Increased sex concordance of sibling pairs with Becket's disease, Hodgkin's disease, multiple sclerosis, and sarcoidosis. *American Journal of Epidemiology, 126,* 365-369.

Gutterman, S., Cole, P., & Levitan, T. R. (1979). Evidence against transmission of Hodgkin's disease. *New England Journal of Medicine, 289,* 499.

Hagemeister, F. B., Fesus, S. M., Lamki, L. M., & Haynie, T. P. (1990). The role of the gallium scan in Hodgkin's disease. *Cancer, 65,* 1090-1096.

Hagemeister, F. B., Purugganan, R., Podohoff, D. A., Hess, M., Rodriguez, M. A., & McLaughlin, P. (1994). The gallium scan predicts relapse in patients with Hodgkins disease treated with combined modality therapy. *Annals of Oncology, 5,* S59-S63.

Haluska, F. G., Brufsky, A. M., & Canellos, G. P. (1994). The cellular biology of the Reed-Sternberg cell. *Blood, 84,* 1005.

Harris, N. L., Jaffe, E. S., Stein, H., Banks, P. M., Chan, J. K., & Cleary, M. L. (1994). A revised European-American classification of lymphoid neoplasms: A proposal from the International Lymphoma Study Group. *Blood, 84,* 1361-1392.

Henry-Amar, M. & Joly, F. (1996). Late complications after Hodgkin's disease. *Annals of Oncology, 7,* (Suppl. 4), S73-S78.

Herbst, H., Steinbrecher, E., Neidobitek, G., Young, L. S., Brooks, L., & Muller-Lantzsch, N. (1992). Distribution and phenotype of Epstein-Barr virus-harboring cells in Hodgkin's disease. *Blood, 80,* 484-491.

Hodgkin, T. (1832). On some morbid appearances of the absorbent glands and spleen. *Medical Chir. Trans., 17,* 68-114.

Horning, S. J. (1995). Hodgkin's disease. In E. B. Beutler, M. A. Lichtman, B. S. Coller, & T. J. Kipps (Eds.). *Williams hematology.* New York: McGraw Hill.

Horning, S. J. (1997). Hodgkin's disease. In W. Kelley (Ed.), *Textbook of internal medicine.* Philadelphia: Lippincott-Raven.

Horning, S. J. & Hardy, R. (1994). Lymphoma: Hodgkin's disease. In M. Dolinger, E. H. Rosenbaum, & G. Cable (Eds.), *Cancer therapy.* Kansas City: Andrews and McMeel.

Horning, S., Rosenberg, S., & Hoppe, R. (1996). Brief chemotherapy (Stanford V) and adjuvant radiotherapy for bulky advanced Hodgkin's disease: An update. *Annals of Oncology 7,* (Suppl. 4), 105-108.

Hsu, S. M., Waldron, J. W. Jr., Hsu, P. L., & Hough, A. J. (1993). Cytokines in malignant lymphomas: Review and prospective evaluation. *Human Pathology, 24,* 1040-1057.

Hughes, W., Armstrong, D., Bodey, G., Brown, A., Edwards, J., & Feld, R. (1997). Guidelines from the Infectious Diseases Society of America. *Clinical infectious diseases, 25,* 551-573.

Jackson, H. J. & Parker, F. J. (1944). Hodgkin's disease pathology. *New England Journal of Medicine, 231,* 35-44.

Jarrett, A. F., Armstrong, A. A., & Alexander, E. (1996). Epidemiology of EBV and Hodgkin's lymphoma. *Annals of Oncology, 7,* (Suppl. 4), S5-S10.

Jockovich, M., Mendenhall, N. P., Somback, M. D., Talbert, J. L., & Copeland, E. M., III. (1994). Long-term complications of laparotomy in Hodgkin's disease. *Annals of Surgery, 219,* 615-624.

Kaplan, H. S., Dorfman, R. F., Nelson, T. S., & Rosenberg, S. A. (1973). Staging laparotomy and splenectomy in Hodgkin's disease: Analysis and patterns of involvement in 285 consecutive, unselected patients. *NCI Monograph, 36,* 291-301.

Koeppel, K. (1995). Sperm banking and patients with cancer. Issues concerning patients and health care professionals. *Cancer Nursing, 18,* 306-312.

Landis, S. H., Murray, T. S., Bolden, P. S., & Wingo, P. A. (1998). Cancer statistics, 1998. *CA: A Cancer Journal for Clinicians, 48,* 6-29.

Leibenhaut, M. H., Hoppe, R. T., Efron, B., Halpern, J., Nelsen, T., & Rosenberg, S. A. (1989). Prognostic indicators of laparotomy findings in clinical stage I-II supradiaphragmatic Hodgkin's disease. *Journal of Clinical Oncology, 7,* 81-91.

Leopold, K. A., Canellos, G. P., Rosenthal, D., Shulman, L. N., Weinstein, H., & Mauch, P. (1989). Stage IA-IIB Hodgkin's disease: Staging and treatment with large mediastinal adenopathy. *Journal of Clinical Oncology, 7,* 1059-1065.

Lister, T. A., Crowther, D., Sutcliffe, S. B., Glatstein, E., Cannellos, G. P., & Young, R. C. (1989). Report of a committee convened to discuss the evaluation and staging of patients with Hodgkin's disease: The Cotswolds meeting. *Journal of Clinical Oncology, 7,* 1630-1636.

Lukes, R., Butler, J., & Hicks, E. (1966). Natural history of Hodgkin's disease as related to its pathological picture. *Cancer, 26,* 317.

Lukes, R., Craver, L., Hall, T., Rappaport, H., & Ruben, P. (1966). Report of the nomenclature committee. *Cancer Research, 26,* 1311.

Macfarlane, G. J., Evistifeeva, T., Boyle, & Grufferman, S. (1995). International patterns in the occurrence of Hodgkin's disease in children and young adult males. *International Journal of Cancer, 61,* 165-169.

Marcus, K., Buck, B., & Mauch, P. (1998). Principles of radiation therapy for lymphomas. In G. Canellos, T. Lister, & J. Sklar (Eds.). *The lymphomas.* Philadelphia: W. B. Saunders.

Mason, D., Banks, P., Chan, J., Cleary, M. L., Delsol, G., & de Wolf-Peeters, C. (1994). Nodular lymphocytic predominance Hodgkin's disease: A distinct clinicopathological entity. *American Journal of Surgical Pathology, 18,* 526-530.

Mauch, P. M. & Bonadonna, G. (1997). Hodgkin's disease. In J. F. Holland, R. C. Bast, D. L. Morton, E. Frei, D. W., Kufe, & R. R. Weichselbaum. In *Cancer medicine.* Philadelphia: Williams & Wilkins.

Mauch, P., Kalisch, L., Kadin, M., Coleman, C., Osteen, R., & Hellman, S. (1993). Patterns of presentation of Hodgkin's disease. *Cancer, 71,* 2062-2071.

Mauch, P., Larson, D., Osteen, R., Silver, B., Yeap, B., & Canellos, G. (1990). Prognostic factors for positive surgical staging in patients with Hodgkin's disease. *Journal of Clinical Oncology, 8,* 257-265.

McDaniel, G. (1996). Biophysical changes of the older adult. In B. Bullock (Ed.), *Pathophysiology: Adaptations and alterations in function.* Philadelphia: Lippincott-Raven.

Medeiros, L. J. & Greiner, T. C. (1997). Hodgkin's disease. *Cancer, 75* (Suppl. 1), 357-369.

Meistrich, M, Vassilopoulou-Sellin, R., & Lipshultz, L. (1997). Gonadal dysfunction. In V. DeVita, S. Hellman, & S. Rosenberg (Eds.), *Cancer: Principles and practice of oncology.* Philadelphia: Lippincott-Raven.

Miller, R. W. & Beebe, G. W. (1973). Infectious mononucleosis and the empirical risk of cancer. *Journal of the National Cancer Institute, 50,* 315.

Millham, S., Jr. & Hesser, J. (1967). Hodgkin's disease in woodworkers. *Lancet, 2,* 136.

Minor, D. R., Shiffman, G., & McIntosh, S. (1979). Response of patients with Hodgkin's disease to pneumococcal vaccines. *Annals of Internal Medicine, 90,* 887-892.

Moore, K. & Blumenthal, J. (1998). Exercise training as an alternative treatment for depression among older adults. *Alternative Therapies, 4,* 48-56.

Munoz, N. D., Davidson, R. J., Witthoff, B., Ericsson, J. E., & De Th'e, G. (1978). Infectious mononucleosis and Hodgkin's disease. *International Journal of Cancer, 22,* 10-13.

Murrell, H. J., Perry, M. C., Muscato, J. J., Dorr, V. J., Wilkes, J. D., & Doll, D. C. (1995). Hodgkin's disease: Is staging laparotomy still necessary? *Seminars in Oncology, 22,* xv-xxiv, xxiv-xxv.

National Cancer Institute/PDQ. (1998). Current clinical trials. *Oncology, 5* (1), 3-4.

Niedobitek, G. (1996). The role of Epstein-Barr virus in the pathogenesis of Hodgkin's disease. *Annals of Oncology, 7* (Suppl. 4), S11-S17.

Oberlin, O. (1996). Present and future strategies of treatment in childhood Hodgkin's lymphoma. *Annals of Oncology, 7* (Suppl. 4), S73-S78.

Pelstring, R., Zellmer, R., Sulak, L., Banks, P. M., & Clare, N. (1991). Hodgkin's disease in association with human immunodeficiency virus infection. *Cancer, 67,* 1865-1873.

Peters, M. V., Hasselbach, R., & Brown, T. C. (1968). The natural history of the lymphomas related to clinical classification. In C. J. D. Zarafonetis (Ed.), *Proceedings of the International Conference on Leukemia-Lymphoma.* Philadelphia: Lea & Febinger.

Portlock, C. S. & Yahalom, J. (1996). Hodgkin's disease. In J. Bennett, F. Plum, et al. (Eds.), *Cecil textbook of medicine.* Philadelphia: W. B. Saunders.

Posner, J. (1996). Nonmetastatic effects of cancer on the nervous system. In J. Bennett & F. Plum, et al. (Eds.), *Cecil textbook of medicine.* Philadelphia: W. B. Saunders.

Prochaska, J., DiClemente, C., & Norcross, J. (1992). In search of how people change. *American Psychologist,* September, 1102-1114.

Pui, C. H., Ip, S., Thompson, E., Wilimas, J., Brown, M., & Dodge, R. K. (1989). High serum interleukin-2 receptor levels correlate with a poor prognosis in children with Hodgkin's disease. *Leukemia, 3,* 481-484.

Ramshaw, B. (1997). Laparoscopic surgery for cancer patients. *Cancer-A Cancer Journal for Clinicians, 47,* 327-350.

Reed, D. M. (1902). On the pathological changes in Hodgkin's disease, with special reference to its relation to tuberculosis. *John Hopkin's Hospital Report, 10,* 133-196.

Ries, L. A. G., Miller, B. A., & Hankey, B. F. (1994). *SEER Cancer Statistics Review, 1973-1991: Tables and Graphs.* N.I.H. Publication No. 94-2789. Bethesda, MD: National Cancer Institute.

Robertson, S., Lowman, J., Grufferman, S., Kostyu, D., van der Horst, C. M., & Matthews, T. J. (1987). Familial Hodgkin's disease: A clinical and laboratory investigation. *Cancer, 59,* 1314-1319.

Rosdahl, N., Larsen, S. O., & Clemmensen, J. (1974). Hodgkin's disease in patients with previous mononucleosis: 30 years experience. *British Medical Journal, 2,* 253.

Rosen, P. J. (1995). Hodgkin's disease and malignant lymphoma. In D. A. Cascito & B. B. Lowitz (Eds.), *Manual of clinical oncology* (3rd ed.). Boston: Little, Brown.

Rosenberg, S. & Canellos, G. (1998). Hodgkin's disease. In G. Canellos, T. Lister, & J. Sklar (Eds.), *The lymphomas.* Philadelphia: W. B. Saunders.

Rosenthal, D. S. & Eyre, H. J. (1995). Hodgkin's disease and non-Hodgkin's lymphoma. In G. P. Murphy, W. Lawrence, & R. E. Lenhard (Eds.), *American Cancer Society text book of clinical oncology.* Atlanta: ACS.

Skeel, R. & Ganz, P. (1995). Systematic assessment of the patient with cancer and long-term medical complications of treatment. In R. Skeel & N. Lachant (Eds.), *Handbook of cancer chemotherapy.* Boston: Little, Brown.

Slivnick, D. J., Ellis, T. M., Nawrocki, J. F., & Fisher, R. I. (1990). The impact of Hodgkin's disease on the immune system. *Seminars in Oncology, 17,* 673-682.

Staal, S. P., Ambinder, R., Beschorner, W. E., Hayward, G. S., & Mann, R. (1989). A survey of Epstein Barr virus DNA in lymphoid tissue. Frequent detection in Hodgkin's disease. *American Journal of Pathology, 91,* 1-5.

Stein, R. (1995). Hodgkin's disease and malignant lymphomas. In R. Skeel & N. Lachant (Eds.), *Handbook of cancer chemotherapy.* Boston: Little, Brown.

Steinherz, L. & Yahalom, J. (1997). Toxicity. In V. T. DeVita, S. Hellman, & S. Rosenberg (Eds.), *Cancer: Principles and practice of oncology.* Philadelphia: Lippincott-Raven.

Stern, C. (1996). Thyroid and parathyroid functions and alterations. In B. Bullock (Ed.), *Pathophysiology: Adaptations and alterations in function.* Philadelphia: Lippincott-Raven.

Sternberg, C. (1898). Uber eine Eigneatige unter dem Bilde Der Pseudoleukamie verlaufende Tuberculose des lymphatischen Aappartes. *Z. Heilk, 19,* 21-90.

Strum, S. B., Dark, J. K., & Rappaport, H. (1970). Observations of cells resembling Sternberg Reed cells in conditions other than Hodgkin's disease. *Cancer, 26,* 176-190.

Torrey, M., Poen, J., & Hoppe, R. (1997). Detection of relapse in early-stage Hodgkin's disease: Role of routine follow-up studies. *Journal of Clinical Oncology, 15,* 1123-1130.

Urba, W. J. & Longo, D. L. (1992). Hodgkin's disease. *New England Journal of Medicine, 362,* 678-687.

van Leeuwen, F. (1997). Second cancers. In V. T. DeVita, S. Hellman, & S. Rosenberg (Eds.), *Cancer: Principles and practice of oncology.* Philadelphia: Lippincott-Raven.

Vecchi, V., Pileri, S., Burnelli, R., Bontempi, N., Comelli, A., & Testi, A. M. (1992). Treatment of pediatric Hodgkin's disease tailored to stage, mediastinal mass and age. *Cancer, 72,* 2049-2057.

Vianna, N. J., Greenwald, P., & Davies, J. N. P. (1971). Extended epidemic of Hodgkin's disease in high school students. *Lancet, 1,* 1209.

Vianna, J. H. & Polan, A. K. (1973). Epidemiological evidence for transmission of Hodgkin's disease. *New England Journal of Medicine, 289,* 499.

Viviani, S., Bonadonna, G., Santoro, A., Bonfante, V., Zanini, M., & Devizzi, L. (1996). Alternating versus hybrid MOPP and ABVD combinations in advanced Hodgkin's disease: Ten-year results. *Journal of Clinical Oncology, 14,* 1421-1430.

Vose, J. & Armitage, J. (1998). Bone marrow transplantation for malignant lymphoma. In G. Canellos, T. Lister, & J. Sklar (Eds.), *The lymphomas.* Philadelphia: W. B. Saunders.

Weiss, L., Movahed, L., Warnke, R., & Sklar, J. (1989). Detection of Epstein Barr viral genomes in Reed-Sternberg cells of Hodgkin's disease. *New England Journal of Medicine, 320,* 502-506.

Wilks, S. (1865). Enlargement of the lymphatic glands and spleen (or, Hodgkin's disease). *Guy's Hospital Report, 1838,* 1156.

Zantinga, A. R. & Coppes, M. J. (1996). Thomas Hodgkin (1798-1866): Pathologist, social scientist, and philanthropist. *Medical and Pediatric Oncology, 27,* 122-27.

Multiple Myeloma

Sandra Malamed, RN, MS, OCN

EPIDEMIOLOGY

Multiple myeloma (MM), or myeloma, is a relatively rare systemic malignancy arising from plasma cells. It is a clonal B-cell disorder and is classified as a non–Hodgkin's lymphoma.

Predictions are that there will be 13,800 new cases of MM in the United States in 1998 and a corresponding 11,030 deaths. MM is a disease of older adults, with the majority of cases occurring in the seventh decade and only rare instances noted in those younger than 40. The median age at diagnosis is between 62 and 68 years. In Caucasians, MM represents approximately 1% of all cancers and 13% of hematologic malignancies; in African Americans, it accounts for 2% of all cancers and 33% of hematologic malignancies (American Cancer Society, 1998; Landis, Murray, Bolden, & Wingo, 1998). As with occurrence rates, the mortality rates in African Americans is twice that of Caucasians (Bubley & Schnipper, 1995). Annual rates of MM have been increasing, and the speculation is that this rise may be the result of earlier detection of the disease and the expansion of the aging population. MM is slightly more common in men than in women.

RISK FACTORS

Although the exact cause of MM remains unknown, several risk factors have been identified. The major risk factors associated with MM are listed in Box 66-1. Age is a predominating factor. The immune system changes with age. One such change may occur in plasma cells, increasing the likelihood of the rise of a malignant clone.

Genetics may play a role in the development of MM. There appears to be an increased risk in the first-degree relatives of patients with MM, and several cases of familial myeloma have been reported. Animal models have demonstrated that alterations in the genes that encode immunoglobulin (Ig) and the *myc* or *ras* genes are associated with plasma cell disorders. Alterations in these same genes have been demonstrated in another B-cell disease, Burkitt's lymphoma, but not with MM (Bubley & Schnipper, 1995; Salmon & Cassady, 1993). There is no definitive evidence at this time that an oncogene is involved in MM (Longo, 1994). This is in contrast to other human B-cell tumors, which have been shown to exhibit certain chromosomal alterations consistently (Hussein, 1994; Longo, 1994).

The increased risk of MM in African Americans in part may be due to genetic predisposition. African Americans have higher average levels of immunoglobulin than do Caucasians. Therefore African Americans probably have more B lymphocytes and thus greater opportunity for a malignant clone to develop (Bubley & Schnipper, 1995). Although these epidemiologic differences between African Americans and Caucasians are clearly demonstrated, it is unclear whether they are the result of genetic makeup or environmental influences (Salmon & Cassady, 1993).

Occupational exposure to petroleum products, rubber, asbestos, and farming and other chemicals may be implicated (Bubley & Schnipper, 1995; Miaskowski, 1997; Salmon & Cassady, 1993). Chronic low-dose exposure to radiation may also pose a risk. Higher than average rates of MM have been reported in radiologists and workers at nuclear power plants. There is a clear connection between exposure to high doses of ionizing radiation and the development of MM. This association has been demonstrated in Japanese survivors of the atomic bomb. People exposed to 100 cGy of radiation demonstrated rates of MM nearly five times normal, occurring after a latency period of 20 years (Bubley & Schnipper, 1995; Salmon & Cassady, 1993).

An animal model has also indicated that a viral cause may be involved. Viral causes have been linked to plasmacytomas and B-cell malignancies in mice (Bubley & Schnipper, 1995; Salmon & Cassady, 1993). Such studies have led to the suspicion of a viral cause in humans, but no direct correlation has been made yet.

A connection may exist between the development of plasma cell neoplasms and chronic antigenic stimulation. Conditions such as chronic or recurrent infections, reactions to allergen hyposensitization injections, and chronic exposure to environmental pollution are possible sources. Although studies on this subject are intriguing, they have

Box 66-1
Risk Factors for Multiple Myeloma

Increasing age
Ethnicity (greater risk for African Americans than Caucasians)
Positive family history
Exposure to high-dose ionizing radiation
Chronic exposure to low-dose ionizing radiation (? association)
Occupational exposure to petroleum products, rubber, farming-related chemicals

been inconclusive thus far (Bubley & Schnipper, 1995; Hussein, 1994; Salmon & Cassady, 1993).

CHEMOPREVENTION

Currently no chemoprevention activities are available for MM. In fact, when a patient is found to have early MM, the approach is to watch and wait. Researchers hypothesize that one benign disease process that often develops into MM, monoclonal gammopathy of unknown significance (MGUS), may actually be a malignancy in a dormant phase (Bergsagel, Smith, Szczepek, Mant, Belch, & Pilarski, 1995). If this is true, it raises the possibility that some forms of MGUS are plausible targets for preventive therapy in the future.

PATHOPHYSIOLOGY

Normal B-Cell Development

Humoral immunity is mediated by B cells, which produce and secrete immunoglobulins (antibodies) in response to antigenic stimulation. Antibody-secreting B cells vary in their appearance, life span, and sites of antibody production (MacLennan, Hardie, Ball, & Drew, 1995). Fig. 66-1 shows the development of normal and myeloma B cells.

Millions of B-cell clones are produced in the bone marrow through a series of developmental steps. These cells migrate to the spleen and other lymphoid tissues, where they await antigenic stimulation. Exposure to an antigen triggers the continuing differentiation of immature B cells and the production of antibodies. The developing B cell digests the antigen and displays a specific receptor to that antigen on its cell surface as part of a major histocompatibility complex. This complex can be recognized by helper T lymphocytes, which in turn produce the factor that promotes the final stages of B-cell development. The end result is the plasma cell, a terminally differentiated B cell that is capable of secreting antibodies (Bubley & Schnipper, 1995). Antibody production continues as long as the antigenic stimulus continues.

Antibody Synthesis and Activity

The genetic coding for immunoglobulin production comes from a series of genetic recombinations that occur during different phases of B-cell development. There is potential for an infinite number of recombinations, and the result is antibody diversity and specificity.

Each antibody contains two identical light chains and two identical heavy chains. Within the immunoglobulin molecule are variable, or V, regions and constant regions that are located in the heavy and light protein chains. The V regions of the heavy and light chains together determine the idiotype (antigen specificity) of the immunoglobulin. There are two types of light chains, defined by their constant regions, k and l. The constant region of the heavy chains defines the five classes of antibodies, IgA, IgG, IgM, IgE, and IgD, and determines their biologic characteristics (Hussein, 1994; Joshua, 1995). The constant region is not involved in antigen recognition (Joshua, 1995). The remainder of the immunoglobulin molecule is identical to that of all other immunoglobulins of the same class. Although immunoglobulins may be very similar in their structure, each class has a different function and is found in different fluids.

Changes that occur as a part of heavy and light chain development ensure that a B cell is capable of producing immunoglobulins that recognize only one specific antigen. Therefore a B cell may produce more than one class of immunoglobulin, but all will be specific to that one antigen.

The first immunoglobulin produced by developing B cells is IgM. Coincidentally it is also the first antibody produced by infants. IgM is produced during the primary immune response. It is also the monoclonal immunoglobulin that is overproduced in Waldenström's macroglobulinemia (Bubley & Schnipper, 1995). As normal B cells mature, genetic changes occur and the cell progresses from producing IgM to making IgG or IgA.

IgA is the first line of local defense; it is present in saliva, tears, and respiratory and gastrointestinal (GI) secretions. IgD is a trace protein in plasma and plays a role in B-cell proliferation and maturation. IgE is another trace protein and plays a part in an allergic response.

IgG is the major immunoglobulin found in serum. It is normally produced during the secondary immune response. IgG is the only immunoglobulin that can cross the placental barrier and thus is the one that provides passive immunity to newborns. Different subclasses of IgG may be produced by a single clone of B cells that are different yet specific to the same antigen. IgG has four such subgroups, each with slightly different properties.

Plasma Cell Dyscrasias

Plasma cell dyscrasias (PCDs) are a group of clonal neoplastic disorders characterized by the overproduction of a specific monoclonal antibody (M protein). M proteins can be complete immunoglobulins or parts of them (e.g., light chains) that may be found in the serum or urine of patients with PCD, including MM. However, even if the M protein is a complete immunoglobulin molecule, it is nonfunctional.

Monoclonal proteins are produced by clones of a B cell. These clones are a population of cells that were all derived from a single parent cell and have identical characteristics. M proteins can vary from one patient to another, even among those who have the same PCD.

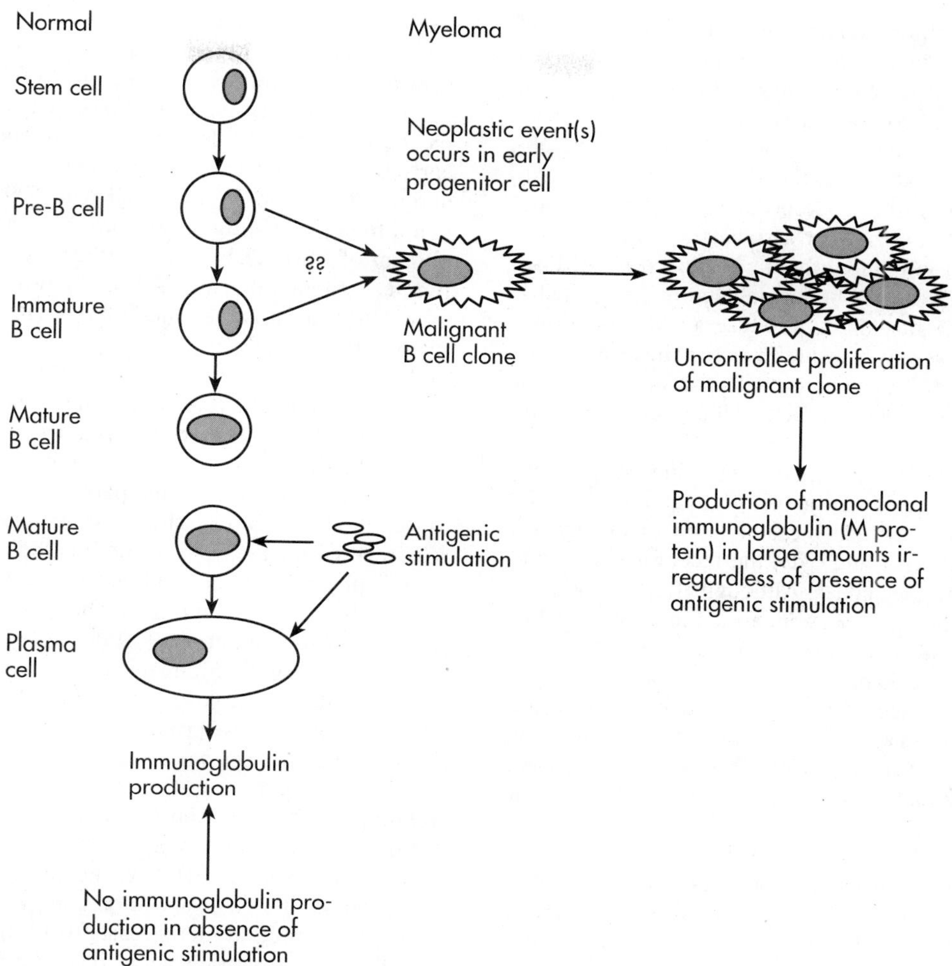

Fig. 66-1 Development of normal and myeloma B cells.

However, in any given patient all molecules of the M protein are identical.

Occasionally the production of monoclonal immunoglobulin may occur in a healthy individual with no specific disease characteristics or defining symptom complex. This condition is known as *monoclonal gammopathy of undetermined significance* (MGUS), or smoldering myeloma. It sometimes progresses slowly to become a specific disease entity; examples include MM, Waldenström's macroglobulinemia, amyloidosis, and non–Hodgkin's lymphoma (Bubley & Schnipper, 1995; Hussein, 1994; Salmon & Cassady, 1993).

M-protein levels are used to monitor the activity of the disease. These levels may remain stable for long periods in patients with MGUS. In the malignant plasma cell diseases, M-protein levels continue to rise and other evidence of disease develops. It is recommended that patients with monoclonal gammopathies receive follow-up care that includes measurement of the M-protein component on a yearly basis to monitor for such a trend (Bubley & Schnipper, 1995; Hussein, 1994). Approximately 11% of patients with MGUS will develop MM, and still others will develop one of the other diseases mentioned earlier (Kyle, 1992; Longo, 1994; Salmon & Cassady, 1993). This type of disease progression was seen in the long-term follow-up of a group of patients with MGUS (Kyle, 1992). The time from the first identification of a benign monoclonal gammopathy to disease progression ranged from 2 years to more than 20 years.

One theory holds that MGUS may not be a benign condition. Pilarski, Masellis-Smith, Szczepek, Mant, & Belch, (1996) propose that some forms of MGUS may be rigorously controlled malignancies. They believe that certain B cells found in patients with MGUS may be malignant cells in a dormant stage of growth. The dormancy of these cells is maintained by immunoregulatory and microenvironmental factors. Frank MM occurs when the regulatory mechanisms fail and the previously dormant malignancy is free to grow and spread. Clonotypal precursors of myeloma B cells have already been discovered in blood. If these cells are proven to be malignant, the popular view of MGUS as a benign condition would need to be reevaluated.

Carcinogenesis

The most common malignant PCD is MM. MM results in the overproduction of monoclonal immunoglobulins and/or light chains. The proliferation and maturation of B cells and immunoglobulin production in PCD occurs in the same sequence as do normal developmental patterns. However, in PCD the B-cell clones continue to proliferate uncontrollably and produce their monoclonal immunoglobulin in the absence of an antigenic stimulus. So much M protein is produced that it results in the underproduction of normal immunoglobulins and causes other associated problems.

The monoclonal immunoglobulins produced in MM are often complete IgG or IgA molecules and/or light chains. Approximately 99% of patients produce an M protein that can be detected in serum or urine or both (Hussein, 1994). Approximately 20% of patients will exhibit only light chains, which are excreted as Bence Jones protein in the urine (Longo, 1994).

The cause of MM is not known. A growing body of evidence, however, suggests that a specific factor may be the key. Possible factors include the activation of oncogenes, deregulation of cytokine and cytokine receptor genes, and loss of tumor suppresser genes. Although specific and consistent genetic events have been identified in several malignant lymphomas and leukemias, none have been found in MM (Tesch, Diehl, & Kibe, 1995).

Many authors agree that several genetic steps are involved in the process of MM development (MacLennan et al., 1995; Salmon & Cassady, 1993; Tesch, Diehl, & Kibe, 1995). However, exactly what the steps are is an issue for debate.

It is suspected that the neoplastic event may occur in early B-cell progenitors, perhaps early multipotential progenitor cells (Bubley & Schnipper, 1995; Longo, 1994). A single malignant B-cell clone may begin the process by escaping normal control mechanisms early in the differentiation process. The fact that it is very rare to find more than one malignant clone in a patient with MM supports the theory of a single cell of origin (MacLennan et al., 1995).

A "two-hit" hypothesis underlies a theory based on the characteristics of MM development and epidemiology. However, researchers disagree about the chronicity of the events. There is evidence that the "first hit" happens when a mutation occurs in the gene that encodes the V region of immunoglobulin in an immature B cell (MacLennan et al., 1995). The final neoplastic event, or a "second hit," occurs later in the cell's development (MacLennan et al., 1995). These alterations in the genes of the cell trigger the production of monoclonal cells that have retained the ability to proliferate and/or have prolonged survival (Tesch, Diehl, & Kibe, 1995).

Some authors suggest that chronic exposure to a particular antigenic stimulus may be the final neoplastic event. The stimulus promotes the terminal differentiation of the B-cell monoclones, enabling them to produce monoclonal immunoglobulins in large amounts (Bataille, 1996; Bubley & Schnipper, 1995).

Another theory suggests that the first hit is exposure to a chronic antigenic stimulus in a susceptible person, giving rise to a benign B-cell monoclone. The increased population of monoclonal B cells is then subjected to the second hit, a mutagenic or transforming event that results in the progression to myeloma (Salmon & Cassady, 1993). This theory implies that antigenic stimulation can promote the malignant transformation of an immature B cell.

Some argue that this is not possible because they think it has been established that the transformation occurs in very early B cells, ones that are too immature to be stimulated by antigens (Herriton, Weiss, & Olshan, 1995). However, that is not to say that antigen exposure has no role in the development of MM. These same authors do agree that chronic immune stimulation can result in the progression of the disease. One reason is that interleukin-6 (IL-6) is produced by many different cells in response to various stimuli and antigens (Herriton, Weiss, & Olshan, 1995).

IL-6 is a potent stimulator of myeloma growth (Bataille, 1996; Herriton, Weiss, & Olshan, 1995; Sporeno, Savino, Ciapponi, Paonessa, Gabibbo, & Lahm et al., 1996). It is believed to play a role in the pathogenesis of MM, chronic autoimmune diseases, and postmenopausal osteoporosis (Sporeno et al., 1996). IL-6 inhibits the chemotaxis of malignant plasma cell lines and may explain the localization of MM cells in the bone marrow, where large amounts of IL-6 are found (Sporeno et al., 1996).

The effect of IL-6 on myeloma cells has been demonstrated by the in vitro use of antisense IL-6 messenger RNA (mRNA). When these proteins are successfully inserted into human myeloma cell nuclei, the result is a significant suppression of myeloma cell proliferation in vitro (Bubley & Schnipper, 1995; Salmon & Cassady, 1993; Sopreno et al., 1996). Antisense technology involves the engineering of a deoxyribonucleic acid (DNA) molecule that fouls the normal process of DNA translation and prevents the synthesis of a selected protein (in this case, IL-6). In vivo studies have also demonstrated the role of IL-6. Anti–IL-6 monoclonal antibody can temporarily suppress myeloma cell proliferation and reduce tumor mass in patients with advanced MM (Bataille & Klein, 1995; Klein, Wijdenes, Zhang, Jourdan, Boiron, & Brochier et al., 1991).

Studies suggest that a myeloma cell can produce and display an IL-6 receptor and synthesize IL-6, indicating an autocrine mechanism (Bubley & Schnipper, 1995; Tesch, Diehl, & Kibe, 1995). Others support a theory of a paracrine mechanism in which IL-6 is produced by the bone marrow, where MM cells are found, and not by the myeloma cells themselves (Klein, 1995). It is possible that both mechanisms are at play (Salmon & Cassady, 1993).

Further studies are directed at investigating the usefulness of IL-6 receptor evaluation as a prognostic indicator for MM (Sporeno et al., 1996). High levels of serum IL-6 are found predominantly in patients with advanced disease (Tesch, Diehl, & Kibe, 1995).

In the future, IL-6 inhibitors may have a role in the treatment of MM. The potential efficacy of inhibitors to IL-6 production, IL-6 activity, and IL-6 receptors are all areas of interest (Bataille & Klein, 1995).

IL-1 inhibitors and receptor antagonists are also being studied. The IL-1 preparations have been shown to suppress osteoclast activity and may have an effect on myeloma cells (Torcea, Lucibello, Vannier, Fabiani, Miliani, & Guidi et al., 1996).

Variants

Immunoglobulin D Myeloma. IgD myeloma is often diagnosed in the late phases of its course. This may be one of the reasons why its median survival is less than that of IgG and IgA myelomas. The incidence of plasma cell leukemia, amyloidosis, and extramedullary plasmacytomas is more common in this patient group (Kyle, 1995).

Nonsecretory Myeloma. Nonsecretory myeloma is a rare (1%) variant of MM in which no M protein is identified in the serum or urine (Bartyl, Frisch, & Wilmans, 1995). These may be light-chain myelomas in which the M protein, a light chain, is catabolized by the kidney and therefore undetectable in the urine (Longo, 1994). Survival is similar to that of MM or longer (Kyle, 1995).

Plasma Cell Leukemia. Plasma cell leukemia is defined as >20% plasma cells in the peripheral blood. There are two classifications, primary and secondary. Primary plasma cell leukemia is one that is diagnosed in the leukemic phase. The primary form is more common than the secondary. It tends to occur in younger patients. Hepatosplenomegaly and lymphadenopathy are common. In contrast with MM, there are fewer bone lesions and a smaller M component. Primary plasma cell leukemia responds well to treatment with chemotherapy regimens similar to those used to treat MM. Survival is longer than in the secondary form, yet the survival is still short (Kyle, 1995).

Rarely (2%) during the late phases of the disease, secondary plasma cell leukemia may develop (Bartl, Frisch, & Wilmans, 1995). Affected patients have most likely received multiple courses of chemotherapy in the past. They rarely respond to current chemotherapy because they have previously developed resistance to it (Kyle, 1995).

Osteosclerotic Myeloma. Osteosclerotic myeloma is a rare variant of MM occurring in only 1.4% of patients (Hussein, 1994). It is characterized by a syndrome of polyneuropathy, organomegaly, endocrinopathy, M protein, and skin changes (POEMS) (Kyle, 1995).

Other Plasma Cell Neoplasms

Waldenström's Macroglobulinemia. Waldenström's macroglobulinemia is a malignant PCD characterized by the production of an M protein (IgM), hyperviscosity, and hepatosplenomegaly. It is much less common than MM. Waldenström's macroglobulinemia has a pathogenic mechanism similar to that of MM; however, there is a stronger familial susceptibility. Although MM and Waldenström's macroglobulonemia both involve the bone marrow, there are several differences in the two. Waldenström's macroglobulinemia does not cause lytic bone lesions and hypercalcemia, renal failure is uncommon, hyperviscosity syndrome accompanied by bleeding is very common, and few patients (20%) excrete light chains. Treatment is similar to that of MM and chronic lymphocytic leukemia, with oral alkylating agents used alone or in combination with prednisone (Salmon & Cassady, 1993). Plasmapheresis is used to control hyperviscosity.

Solitary Plasmacytoma of Bone. Solitary plasmacytoma of bone differs from MM in a number of ways. It tends to occur in younger people, and a smaller number of patients (30% vs 97%) are found to have M protein in their serum or urine (Salmon & Cassady, 1993). Treatment includes high-dose local radiation or surgery. Patients with solitary plasmacytomas of bone have a survival that is significantly longer than that of patients with MM. Unfortunately, most patients will eventually develop systemic disease.

Extramedullary Plasmacytoma. This rare (3%) plasma cell neoplasm usually occurs in the nasopharynx, tonsils, or paranasal sinuses. Like solitary bone plasmacytomas, extramedullary plasmacytoma tends to occur at a younger age than MM, and fewer patients produce an M protein. Treatment is most often radiation therapy to the lesion and the surrounding lymph nodes. A majority of patients have a long disease-free survival.

Amyloidosis. Approximately 15% of patients with MM develop systemic amyloidosis (Hussein, 1994). Amyloidosis is characterized by the deposition of fibrous amyloid protein in various parts of the body, production of an M protein, and plasmacytosis. Because of their similarities, amyloidosis and MM are considered to be parts of the same disease process (Hussein, 1994).

Symptoms of amyloidosis include weakness, weight loss, ankle edema, dyspnea, paresthesia, light-headedness, syncope, and carpal tunnel syndrome. Physical examination may reveal an enlarged liver and tongue, skin nodules or plaques, evidence of congestive heart failure, and purpura. Diagnosis is made by either rectal biopsy or aspiration of abdominal fat. Myeloma therapy generally has no effect on shrinking amyloid deposits; however, it may slow their progression (Hussein, 1994).

Clinical Manifestations

The characteristic clinical manifestations of MM are caused by the direct expansion of the tumor mass and the production of M protein and cytokines as part of the disease process. The major characteristics of MM are outlined in this section and summarized in Table 66-1.

Skeletal Changes. Bone pain is the most common symptom of MM and affects 70% of patients. It is thought to be due to microfractures in bones weakened by osteolytic activity and tumor cell proliferation. The pain, usually centered around the back and the ribs, is precipitated by movement.

Myeloma cells produce osteoclast activating factors, which cause unusual bone destruction and inhibit new bone formation (Bataille, 1996; Bubley & Schnipper, 1995; Longo, 1994). The imbalance of bone breakdown and inadequate bone formation results in the development of lytic lesions. Myeloma cells also stimulate the recruitment, differentiation, and resorptive activity of osteoclasts, which become large in number and aggressive by nature (Bataille, 1996). Because osteoclasts produce organic acids that demineralize bone, hypercalcemia, both acute and chronic, is a problem in patients with MM.

IL-1β, tumor necrosis factor-β, and IL-6 are major bone-resorbing factors produced in excess in MM, and they di-

TABLE 66-1 Clinical Manifestations of Multiple Myeloma

	Clinical Features		Disease Process	
Body System	**Assessment Findings/Patient Complaints**	**Laboratory/ Radiographic Findings**	**Underlying Cause**	**Pathologic Mechanism**
Skeletal	1. Bone pain, decreased range of motion, decreased mobility, inability to bear weight 2. Swelling, mass over vertebrae, ribs, sternum	1. Multiple "punched out" lesions on plain film x-rays, CT scan, or MRI	1, 2. Tumor expansion in bone	1, 2. Secretion of osteoclast activating factor by tumor cells, increased bone breakdown in absence of bone repair
Hematologic	1. Fatigue, pallor, weakness	1. Normocytic, normochromic anemia; altered iron profile; rouleau bodies	1, 2, 3. Myelophthisis 1. Anemia of chronic disease	1, 2, 3. Replacement of hematopoietic cells in bone marrow by plasma cells 1. Decreased production and increased destruction
	2. Infection	2. Leukopenia, immunoelectrophoresis (M spike)	2. Immunosuppression	2. Hypogammaglobulinemia, decreased neutrophil migration
	3. Bleeding, petechiae, ecchymosis	3. Normal to low platelet count	3. Platelet dysfunction	3. Immunoglobulin coating of platelets (PTS), interference with clotting factors
Renal	1. Ranges from asymptomatic uremia to nausea and vomiting, fatigue, confusion	1. Elevated BUN, creatinine, Ca^{++}, uric acid, urine light-chain electrophoresis > 1 g/24 hr	1. Renal insufficiency, renal failure	1. Excretion of nephron-damaging tumor products; amyloid deposits (rare), renal infiltration of plasma cells
Nervous	1. Severe localized back pain, motor weakness, autonomic dysfunction	1. Evidence of spinal nerve compression on radiographic study	1. Extradural tumor or compression fracture	1. Spinal cord compression

rectly inhibit bone formation (Barlogie & Beck, 1993; Bataille, 1996). It is possible that other bone-damaging factors are also produced by myeloma cells, but they are yet to be discovered.

Bone destruction in MM can have two clinical presentations. Approximately 20% of patients initially have generalized osteoporosis without distinct lesions (Hussein, 1994). In the remainder of patients there is excessive resorption of bone only in the vicinity of myeloma cells, giving rise to the characteristic "punched out" appearance that MM lesions exhibit on x-ray film. These x-ray findings are typically different from those of the lytic lesions found in other malignancies, which may have some evidence of an attempt at bone repair at the borders of the lesion and may be less well defined.

Some patients initially demonstrate a normal skeletal survey because considerable demineralization must occur before it becomes radiographically detectable. However, this does not mean that no bone pathologic evidence is present. Histologic examination of the bone tissue still shows destructive changes because >30% of bone calcium must be lost before the pathologic evidence can be seen on x-ray film (Bataille, 1996; Hussein, 1994).

A small number of patients (15%) develop firm, localized plasma cell tumors that can be palpated (Hussein, 1994). Expansile lesions are most commonly found on the skull, clavicles, and sternum, where the involved bone is close to the skin.

The axial skeleton is a primary site of damage because the distribution of the disease correlates with normal sites of red marrow (Dahnert, 1995). Vertebrae may become weak and collapse. These compression fractures cause significant pain, and the patient may lose several inches in height. At times these fractures may result in spinal cord compression, with the potential for permanent neurologic damage.

Radiographic evaluation is an important part of the diagnosis, staging, and evaluation of the response to therapy in MM. Plain film skeletal survey is typically used to detect lytic bone lesions. However, computed tomography (CT) and magnetic resonance imaging (MRI) are more sensitive in detecting bone destruction, and they are more useful in identifying soft tissue disease once an area of suspicion is localized (Dahnert, 1995; Hussein, 1994). Studies involving the use of radiopharmaceuticals (e.g., bone scans) are not effective in detecting bone lesions in MM because the lytic lesions of MM are hypovascular and do not have increased metabolic activity, as do the blastic lesions of other metastatic cancers (Bubley & Schnipper, 1995; Dahnert, 1995).

The management of skeletal manifestations of MM includes the use of appropriate analgesics, assistive devices that promote mobility, and measures to control hypercalcemia. Severe localized bone pain can be treated with radiotherapy (x-ray therapy), with approximately 2500 cGy given over 7 to 10 days (Hussein, 1994). Newly diagnosed patients with severe bone pain are often given chemotherapy first; if the response is unsatisfactory, x-ray therapy is performed (Hussein, 1994). X-ray therapy may also be used to prevent pathologic fractures in areas where a great deal of bone destruction has occurred (Hussein, 1994). At times it may be necessary to treat a pathologic fracture surgically, particularly if it occurs in a weight-bearing bone such as the femur.

The use of pamidronate, a diphosphonate, in MM has been studied. It is an effective treatment for hypercalcemia and has added benefits in the treatment of MM. Berenson, Lichtenstein, Porter, Dimopoulous, Bordini, George, and colleagues (1996) studied its use as an adjunct to chemotherapy. Pamidronate was given on a monthly basis along with chemotherapy, whether or not the patient had hypercalcemia. The study showed that 90 mg of pamidronate given as a 4-hour intravenous infusion significantly reduced the number of skeletal events (e.g., pathologic fractures, irradiation or surgery on a bone, spinal cord compression, hypercalcemia, and bone pain). Additionally, patients had a more stable performance status and a better quality of life. Based on these results and others, some researchers have advocated the use of pamidronate in all patients with MM, whether or not they exhibit measurable osteolytic disease (Bataille, 1996).

Anemia. Anemia is the prevailing hematologic manifestation of MM and is a presenting symptom in more than 75% of patients (Garton, Gertz, Witzig, Greipp, Lust, & Schroeder et al., 1995; Longo, 1994). It is most often a normochromic-normocytic anemia indicative of a hypoproliferative state (Bubley & Schnipper, 1995; Salmon & Cassady, 1993). A combination of factors contribute to the development of anemia in myeloma, including myelophthisis, renal failure, myelosuppressive chemotherapy, and anemia of chronic diseases (ACD) (Barlogie & Beck, 1993; Bunn, 1994).

ACD is a cytokine-induced anemia and may be the major active factor in MM (Barlogie & Beck, 1993). It occurs in the presence of chronic systemic inflammatory disorders, including malignancy, and can be corrected only if the primary condition is reversible. The severity of the anemia is proportional to the duration and severity of the inflammatory process (Bunn, 1994).

Because ACD is a hypoproliferative disorder, the corrected reticulocyte count is low (Bunn, 1994). Calculating the corrected reticulocyte count makes the reticulocyte value relative to the degree of anemia and therefore more meaningful. This measure can be determined by multiplying the reticulocyte count (%) by the patient's hemoglobin count divided by the expected normal hemoglobin. In most cases a corrected reticulocyte count <2 to 3 is indicative of hypoproliferation, a relative marrow failure in which there is an inadequate response to the presence of anemia (Roodman & Spivak, 1991).

Characteristics of ACD include the decreased availability of iron for heme synthesis despite an abundance of stored iron. Laboratory values will indicate normal ferritin levels and decreased iron-binding capacity. This block of iron use is most likely mediated by IL-1, a cytokine released as part of the inflammatory process (Bunn, 1994). A second feature of ACD is the moderately short erythrocyte life span, probably caused by increased phagocytosis by monocytes (Bunn, 1994). Finally, there is inadequate production of erythropoietin (EPO), the hormone that stimulates red cell production and maturation (Barlogie & Beck, 1993; Bunn, 1994). Fig. 66-2 shows an EPO feedback loop.

Other factors in MM can affect the EPO response. Approximately 90% of EPO is synthesized in the kidney, and the acute or chronic renal failure that is common in MM can cause a decrease in or absence of EPO production. Likewise, renal failure causes the accumulation of toxins that affect bone marrow function (Brenner & Lazarus, 1994).

IL-6 may play a role in the anemia associated with MM. It appears to suppress erythropoiesis while stimulating platelet production. Studies have shown that the administration of anti–IL-6 monoclonal antibodies to patients with MM reversed anemia while worsening thrombocytopenia (Klein, 1995). Barlogie and Beck (1993) suggest that the abundant supply of IL-6 found in the bone marrow of patients with MM may explain why thrombocytopenia is not more of a problem in MM.

Increased plasma viscosity can contribute to the anemia in two ways. It results in the inhibition of EPO production and causes hemolysis. It can also expand the plasma volume, causing hemodilution, and can give the false impression of anemia (Salmon & Cassady, 1993).

In the past the treatment of anemia in patients with cancer relied on the use of packed red blood cell (RBC) transfusion. Concerns about the hazards of blood product transfusion and the need to preserve the blood supply have inspired strategies to reduce RBC use. Guidelines of the American College of Physicians recommend treating anemia based on symptoms, not in relation to an absolute hemoglobin value (American College of Physicians, 1992). These guidelines call for using RBC transfusion in acute anemia if the volume depletion cannot be corrected with the use of crystalloids. For chronic anemia the guidelines recommend the use of epoetin alfa and hematinics first and RBC transfusion as a rescue therapy. A summary of recommendations for the use of RBC preparations given by the American Red Cross, the Council of Community Blood Centers, and the American Association of Blood Banks (1994) is presented in Table 66-2.

Epoetin alfa has been shown to be effective in treatment of anemia in patients with MM and other cancers (Barlogie & Beck, 1993; Garton et al., 1995; Osterborg, Boogaerts, Cimino, Essers, Holowiecki, & Juliusson et al., 1996). Dos-

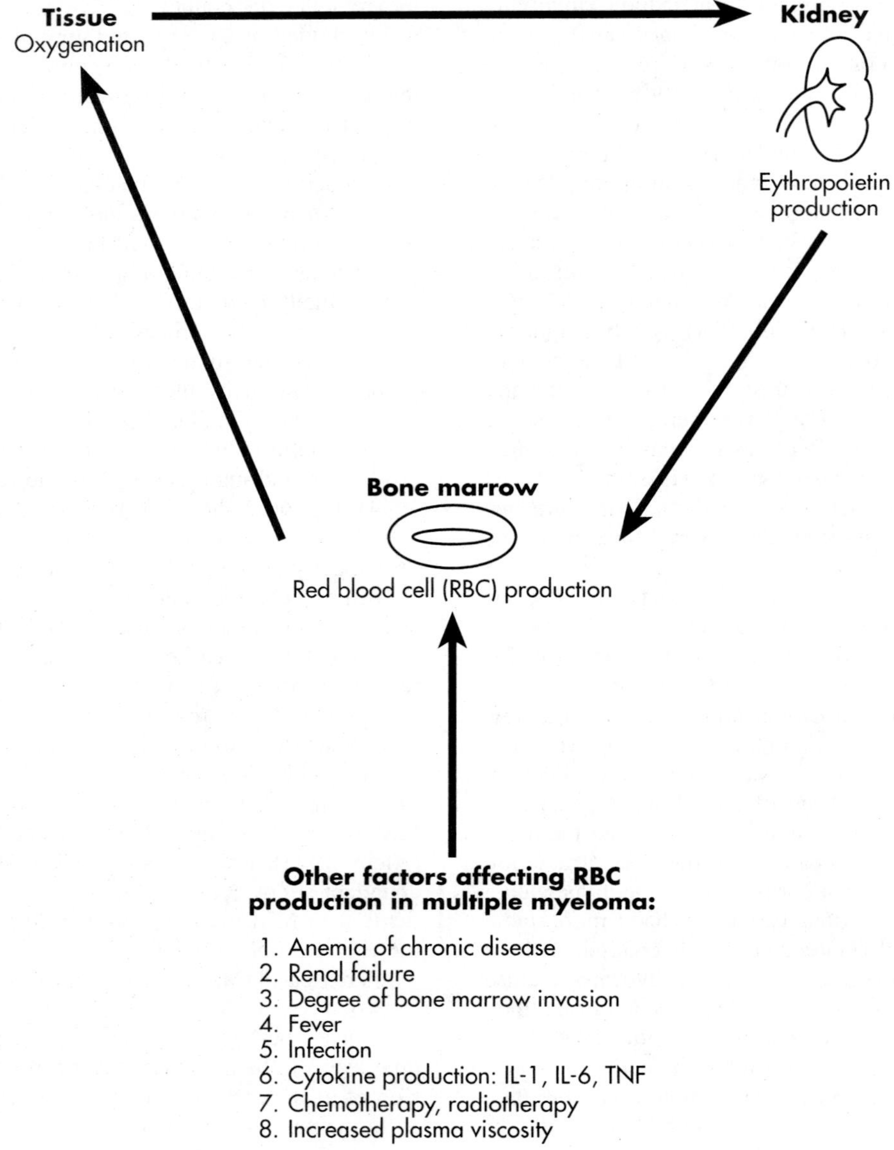

Fig. 66-2 Multiple myeloma.

ing recommendations made in the various studies vary. For patients with cancer, the drug package insert (Ortho Biotech, 1993) currently recommends a starting dose of 150 μ/kg given subcutaneously three times a week. The dose can be titrated up to a maximum of 300 μ/kg three times a week if a satisfactory rise in hemoglobin is not seen after 8 weeks of therapy. Patients with lower endogenous EPO levels (<200 mU/ml) respond more vigorously to therapy. Patients need adequate iron stores or supplementation to achieve the best response. Barlogie and Beck (1993) recommend that epoetin alfa should be considered for all newly diagnosed patients who are severely anemic and undergoing chemotherapy, regardless of the predicted response to antineoplastic therapy.

Blood transfusion therapy is reserved for patients who require immediate correction of their anemia. Patients with cardiopulmonary disease are less tolerant of anemia; however, they may also be at risk for fluid volume complications stemming from blood transfusion. Hussein (1994) suggests that patients at risk for pulmonary edema may require simultaneous plasmapheresis when blood transfusion is necessary. Blood transfusion is generally not used in patients with immunohemolytic anemia because transfused RBCs will be quickly hemolyzed (Roodman & Spivak, 1991).

Other Hematologic Complications. Fewer than 5% of patients with MM develop a hyperviscosity syndrome (HVS) (Salmon & Cassady, 1993). This occurs most commonly in patients who produce IgM, IgG1, IgG3, and IgA paraproteins in very large amounts (Bubley & Schnipper, 1995). Signs and symptoms include lassitude, confusion, retinal hemorrhage, and unusual bleeding (Hussein, 1994). The presentation of HVS can be an oncologic emergency.

Table 66-2 Recommended Use of Red Blood Cell Preparations

Component	Major Indications	Not Indicated for	Hazards
Red blood cells	Symptomatic anemia	Pharmacologically treatable anemia, coagulation deficiencies	Infectious diseases; septic/toxic, allergic, febrile reactions; graft versus host disease
Red blood cells, leukocytes removed	Symptomatic anemia, febrile reactions from leukocyte antibodies	Same as above	Infectious diseases; septic/toxic, allergic, reactions (unless plasma also removed)
Red blood cells, adenine-saline	Symptomatic anemia with volume deficit	Same as above	Infectious diseases; septic/toxic, allergic, febrile reactions; circulatory overload; graft versus host disease

Modified from American Red Cross, Council of Community Blood Centers, & American Association of Blood Banks. (1994). *Circular of information for the use of human blood and blood components.* Atlanta: American Cancer Society.

Refer to the oncologic emergencies section of this chapter and Chapter 11 for more information about its management.

Normal plasma is twice as viscous as water. Symptoms of hyperviscosity occur when plasma viscosity increases to roughly three to four times that of water, with plasma concentrations of immunoglobulin between 4 and 7 g/dl, depending on the immunoglobulin subtype (Longo, 1994). Blood sludging and rouleau formation are two problems associated with increased viscosity (Bubley & Schnipper, 1995). Rouleau formation occurs when erythrocytes become coated with M protein, causing them to stack up like a roll of coins, clogging the microvasculature and resulting in hemolysis (Malpas, 1995).

Chemotherapy administration is generally effective in reducing immunoglobulin levels and reducing the risk of HVS. However, if chemotherapy is ineffective in inducing remission, regular plasmapheresis may become necessary to maintain an acceptable plasma viscosity (Hussein, 1994). Myeloma-induced thrombocytopenia and leukopenia are less common than anemia. They most often occur when the disease is fairly advanced or by the administration of antineoplastic therapy (Longo, 1994; Sheridan, 1996). Clotting can be impaired despite a normal platelet count because antibody-coated platelets are unable to aggregate normally. In addition, M protein can interfere with the function of a number of clotting factors (Longo, 1994). Mild granulocytopenia is common and is exacerbated by the administration of chemotherapy (Hussein, 1994).

Circulatory problems and Raynaud's phenomenon may be observed if the M protein forms cryoglobulins (Longo, 1994). Cryoglobulins are proteins, usually immunoglobulins or M proteins that precipitate when cooled or in the presence of hyperviscosity (Bolognia & Braverman, 1994). This can lead to hemorrhagic infarcts of the fingers and toes. Raynaud's phenomenon is characterized by spasm of peripheral arterioles with blanching, cyanosis, and pain and numbness of the affected area, most commonly the fingers and toes (Creager & Dzau, 1994).

Immunosuppression. The presenting complaint of some patients may be a history of recurrent infections, commonly of the sinuses or lungs (Seiden & Anderson, 1995). Humoral immunodeficiency results in the susceptibility to significant infections and bacterial sepsis. The risk is compounded by the initiation of myelosuppressive chemotherapy. Infection is both a serious and common accompaniment to MM. More than 75% of patients experience a serious infection at some time in their disease course, and 50% of MM-related deaths can be attributed to infection (Bubley & Schnipper, 1995; Longo, 1994).

The crowding of the bone marrow by malignant cells suppresses other hematopoietic cells. This reduces the number of monocytes and neutrophils and increases the risk of bacterial infection. Although there is diffuse hypergammaglobulinemia of the M component, normal antibodies are underproduced. At the same time catabolism of normal antibodies is increased. The result is a poor antibody response to polysaccharide antigens, such as those present on bacterial cell walls (Longo, 1994). In addition, there may be suppression of certain CD4+ T cells, slowed granulocyte migration, inhibition of B cells by a plasma cell factor, and abnormalities of complement function, all of which contribute to the immune deficiency (Bubley & Schnipper, 1995).

A biphasic pattern of infection appears to occur in MM (Savage, Lindenbaum, & Garrett, 1982; Oken, Pomeroy, Weisdorf, & Bennett, 1996). The first phase occurs in the early part of the disease, either in untreated patients or nonneutropenic patients. The predominating pathogens are *Streptococcus pneumoniae* and *Haemophilus influenzae* (Salmon & Cassady, 1993). Twice as many infections occur during the first 2 months of chemotherapy than during the remainder of the disease; one third of these serious infections are fatal (Oken et al., 1996). The second phase occurs later in the disease, when patients are either refractory to treatment or neutropenic. During this time *Staphylococcus aureus* and gram-negative bacteria are more common (Salmon & Cassady, 1993; Savage, Lindenbaum, & Garrett, 1982).

Because of the serious nature of infection in MM, prompt diagnosis and initiation of appropriate antibiotic therapy is crucial. When infections are detected early, outpatient management with broad-spectrum oral antibiotics is appropriate. Severe infections require hospitalization and initiation of intravenous multidrug therapy. If such a regimen includes an aminoglycoside, particular attention must be paid to renal function and dosing should be based on peak and trough serum levels (Salmon & Cassady, 1993). Patients with repeated infection may benefit from having an oral antibiotic prescribed for them that they can self-initiate at the onset of symptoms. Oken and colleagues (1996) advocate the prophylactic use of trimethoprim-sulfamethoxazole (TMP-SMX) during the early months of therapy. They found that TMP-SMX significantly reduced the rates of serious infection, was inexpensive, and was generally well tolerated by study participants.

The prophylactic use of intravenous gamma globulin in MM is controversial. Some argue that although the therapy raises hope, it is expensive and has not been proven to be efficacious and therefore is not recommended (Longo, 1994; Salmon & Cassady, 1993; Seiden & Anderson, 1995). In contrast, Chapel, Lee, Hargreaves, Pamphilon, and Prentice (1994) conducted a randomized trial and found it to be effective in significantly reducing the risk of recurrent infections in a subset of patients.

Because *S. pneumoniae* is the most common infectious pathogen in patients with MM, pneumococcal vaccination has also been tried. However, humoral immunosuppression usually prevents patients with MM from making adequate antibodies to provide immunity (Salmon & Cassady, 1993; Seiden & Anderson, 1995).

Renal Failure. Renal failure occurs in approximately 20% of patients with MM, and an additional 50% exhibit some degree of renal pathologic condition during the course of disease (Salmon & Cassady, 1993; Longo, 1994). Renal failure at the time of diagnosis is considered an indicator of poor prognosis and has a negative impact on survival, regardless of when it occurs. It is second to infection as a leading cause of death (Kyle, 1995). Renal failure in MM often develops in a subtle manner but progresses rapidly. For those patients with normal renal function or limited dysfunction, the prevention of further renal damage is a high priority.

The most common causes of renal failure are hypercalcemia and Bence-Jones (light chain) proteinuria. Hypercalcemia is the result of the demineralization of bone. It causes tubulointerstitial damage and progressive renal insufficiency. The death of tubular cells leads to obstruction of nephrons and the stasis of intrarenal urine. This promotes the precipitation of calcium salts and infection, which can further damage the kidney (Hostetter & Brenner, 1994).

Both acute and chronic severe hypercalcemia cause a decrease in the glomerular filtration rate and renal blood flow. Hypercalciuria often accompanies hypercalcemia and can lead to the development of renal calculi. Calcium deposits can occur in the interstitium, glomeruli, and renal arterioles. Renal dysfunction that results from acute hypercalcemia can often be completely reversed; however, the progressive renal insufficiency that accompanies chronic hypercalcemia may not be reversed (Hostetter & Brenner, 1994).

Bence Jones proteinuria, myeloma cast nephropathy, and myeloma kidney are all synonyms describing the damage caused by the excretion of light chains (Bubley & Schnipper, 1995; Salmon & Cassady, 1993). Under normal conditions light chains are filtered, reabsorbed in the tubules, and catabolized; however, large amounts of light chains can overwhelm the kidney. Hard casts form inside the tubules and result in cell death and tubular rupture. This in turn leads to interstitial inflammation, fibrosis, and, ultimately, renal failure (Bubley & Schnipper, 1995). Dehydration can compound the problem by causing the precipitation of light chains and calcium in the tubules. Patients are advised to drink at least 2 L of water a day to help flush out light chains and to avoid bed rest, if possible, to reduce the risk of hypercalcemia.

Other causes of renal damage include infection, hyperuricemia following the initiation of antineoplastic therapy, and amyloidosis. Renal amyloid deposits occur in 30% of patients and are found in the tubules, renal vessels, interstitium, and glomeruli (Bubley & Schnipper, 1995). These deposits can lead to proteinuria and nephrosis.

Management and prevention techniques include maintaining adequate hydration and using allopurinol to control hyperuricemia, glucocorticoids for hypercalcemia, and chemotherapy to control myeloma and reduce M-protein excretion (Hussein, 1994). Acute renal failure that results from Bence Jones nephropathy can often be partially reversed by restoration of renal perfusion and the cautious use of loop diuretics (Bubley & Schnipper, 1995). Plasmapheresis can reduce the volume of light chains and reduce the demand on the kidney. Dialysis may be necessary at times when renal failure is severe.

Secondary Malignancies. There is a significantly increased risk of developing acute nonlymphocytic leukemia and myelodysplasia in patients with MM. Although a few patients may develop leukemia in the absence of therapy, treatment with alkylating agents (melphalan in particular) appears to be the primary risk factor (Salmon & Cassady, 1993; Seiden & Anderson, 1995). Leukemia is difficult to treat under these conditions because the patients are older, have compromised bone marrow reserve, are immunosuppressed, and have some degree of renal insufficiency (Salmon & Anderson, 1993).

ROUTES OF METASTASES

Although plasma cells are widely distributed in the body, MM is primarily contained in the bone and bone marrow (Longo, 1994). Invasive cells are capable of entering and exiting the blood and lymph system without restriction. Only the blood system passes through the bone marrow; therefore the spread of MM is by hematogenous dissemination throughout the skeletal system (Bergsagel et al., 1995). It is reasonable to expect, then, that myeloma cells or their precursors could be found in the blood (Pilarski et al., 1996). However, bone marrow plasma cells show an affinity toward being anchored in the bone marrow and lack the receptors required for malignant spread (Bergsagel et al., 1995). There are very few myeloma cells in the bone marrow that divide, which suggests that little contribution to generation of new malignant cells comes from this site (Pilarski et al., 1996). This raises questions about which cells are responsible for the generation of new and distant tumor sites. Bone marrow plasma cells do not appear to have the capabilities of a self-renewing stem cell, which can migrate between bone sites; thus there must be another source (Pilarski et al., 1996). It makes sense, then, that there is no correlation between decreases in the number of plasma cells or the amount of M protein and survival (Pilarski et al., 1996).

In their research Bergsagel and colleagues (1995) found that between 50% and 88% of circulating B cells are clonal relatives of the malignant bone marrow plasma cells in MM. The myeloma-related B cells found in blood are resistant to chemotherapy, persist throughout the course of the disease, and are active migratory cells with the behavior and receptors required for hematogenous dissemination. Although these cells have not been proven to be malignant, they possess characteristics that suggest they may be the cells that mediate the spread of myeloma throughout the skeleton (Pilarski et al., 1996).

Common skeletal sites of myeloma lesions include the skull, proximal humeri and femurs, vertebrae, and thoracic cage. Rarely MM spreads to the brain or kidney or causes splenomegaly and lymphadenopathy (Hussein, 1994; Longo, 1994).

ASSESSMENT

Diagnosis of Multiple Myeloma

A number of diagnostic tests and observations are necessary to reach a diagnosis of MM. These include tissue pathologic studies obtained through bone marrow aspiration, urine immunoelectrophoresis (IEP), and serum evaluations (complete blood cell count [CBC], IEP, erythrocyte sedimentation rate [ESR], electrolyte panel, coagulation studies) and radiographic studies (plain film, CT scan, or MRI) of the skeletal system. Table 66-3 outlines the instructions for preparation of the patient for serum and urine protein electrophoresis testing. Tests used to determine tumor burden are outlined in the prognosis section of this chapter.

Identification of a monoclonal protein in the serum or urine is a first step in the process of making a definitive diagnosis. This is accomplished by electrophoretic testing. The M protein appears as a sharp spike on the electrophoresis tracing (Fig. 66-3). However, a number of nonmyelomatous diseases result in the production of M proteins (Hussein, 1994). In fact, monoclonal gammopathies are common in older adults and individuals with autoimmune disorders (Bubley & Schnipper, 1995). Occasionally, no M protein is identified in the serum or urine, indicating nonsecretory MM, a rare variant (Bartyl, Frisch, & Wilmans, 1995). Once an M spike has been confirmed, further studies must be completed to determine if the patient has MGUS, indolent or active myeloma, or one of a number of diseases associated with an M protein (Hussein, 1994).

Serum electrophoresis is the basic screening test for M protein in blood. It is followed by immunoelectrophoresis (IEP), the most commonly used technique to confirm a monoclonal band or an M spike (Joshua, 1995). IEP is also used to detect M protein in urine. With this technique a 24-hour urine collection is used to determine the amount of M protein excreted. The amount of M protein found in the serum or urine in patients with MM has a positive correlation with tumor cell burden (Longo, 1994). Immunofixation is a newer and more sensitive technique that is useful in the investigation of abnormal protein bands, making interpretation easier, although it is not widely available at this time (Joshua, 1995).

Because MM can present in a variety of ways, the system used for diagnosis is based on both major and minor criteria (Table 66-4). A definitive diagnosis of MM requires either (1) a minimum of one major and one minor criteria or (2) three minor criteria, which must include bone marrow plasmacytosis and M spike (Hussein, 1994; Salmon & Cassady, 1993). The morphologic diagnosis of MM is commonly made based on the percentage of plasma cells in bone marrow aspirates (Bartyl, Frisch, & Wilmans, 1995). The criteria for the percentage of cells diagnostic of MM may vary from one institution or cooperative group to another. Table

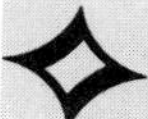

TABLE 66-3 Patient Preparation for Protein Electrophoresis

Description of the Procedure: An electrophoretic test to identify a monoclonal protein in the serum or urine. It is a first step in a definitive diagnosis for multiple myeloma. The M protein appears as a sharp spike on the electrophoresis tracing. Once an M spike has been confirmed, further studies are done to determine if the patient has MGUS, indolent or active myeloma, or one of a number of diseases associated with an M protein. This test is followed by IEP to detect of M proteins in urine. In this technique a 24-hour urine collection is used to determine the amount of M protein excreted. The amount of M protein found in the serum or urine in patients with multiple myeloma has a correlation with tumor cell burden.

Patient Preparation: There are no specific instructions to the patient for the electrophoresis serum test. Instruct patient to obtain 24-hour urine collection kit for urine electrophoresis test.

Procedural Considerations

1. The serum electrophoresis test is preliminary and must be followed by the electrophoresis urine test.
2. Instruct the client to void and discard the specimen at the beginning of the collection.
3. The 24-hour collection begins with the first discarded voiding.
4. Toilet paper should not be dropped into the container used to catch the urine.
5. The collection container should be refrigerated or kept on ice throughout the 24-hour collection time.
6. This retards bacterial growth and stabilizes the analysis.
7. The collection is taken to the laboratory as soon as possible.

From Longo, D. L. (1994). Plasma cell disorders. In K. J. Isselbacher, E. Braunwald, J. D. Wilson, J. B. Martin, A. Fauci, & D. L. Kaspter (Eds.), *Harrison's principles of internal medicine* (13th ed.). New York: McGraw Hill.

IEP, Immunoelectrophoresis; *MGUS,* monoclonal gammopathy of unknown significance.

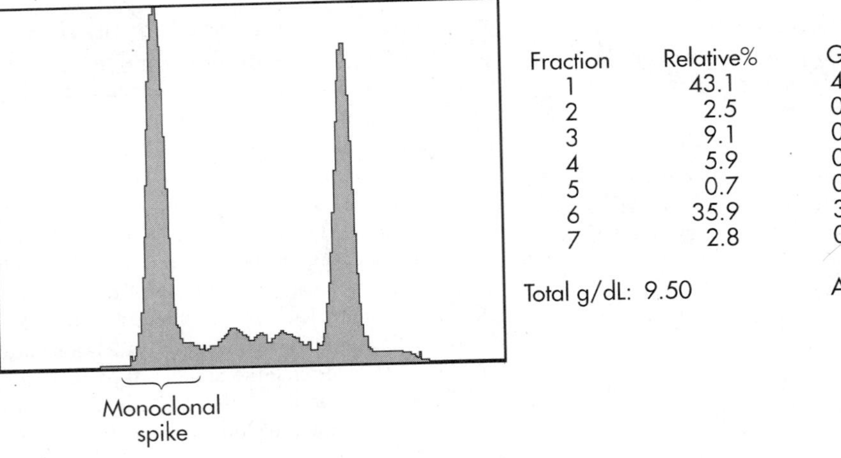

Fraction	Relative%	G/dL
1	43.1	4.09
2	2.5	0.24
3	9.1	0.86
4	5.9	0.56
5	0.7	0.07
6	35.9	3.41
7	2.8	0.27

Total g/dL: 9.50 A/G: 0.76

Fig. 66-3 Serum protein electrophoresis of a patient with multiple myeloma. Sharp spike to left indicates the presence of an M protein, either a complete or partial immunoglobulin (i.e., light chain).

TABLE 66-4 Diagnostic Criteria for Multiple Myeloma*

Major criteria	Minor criteria
1. Plasmacytoma confirmed by tissue biopsy	1. 10%-30% plasma cells in bone marrow
2. >30% plasma cells in bone marrow	2. M spike present but to a lesser degree than above
3. M spike on serum protein electrophoresis: IgG >3.5 g/dl, IgA >2 g/dl	3. Lytic bone lesions
4. κ or λ light chains >1 g/24 hr on urine electrophoresis	4. Hypogammaglobulinemia (normal immunoglobulin)

Modified from Bubley, G. J. & Schnipper, L. E. (1995). Multiple myeloma. In G. P. Murphy, W. Lawrence, & R. E. Lenhards (Eds.), *American Cancer Society textbook of clinical oncology.* Atlanta: American Cancer Society; Salmon, S. E. & Cassady, J. R. (1993). Plasma cell neoplasms. In V. T. DeVita, S. Hellman, & S. A. Rosenberg (Eds.), *Cancer: Principles and practice of oncology.* Philadelphia: J. B. Lippincott.

*Further criteria differentiate multiple myeloma from indolent and smoldering myeloma.

66-5 presents a summary of assessment parameters and typical abnormal findings for the patient with MM.

Nursing Assessment

Patients with MM may experience repeated episodes of acute and chronic disease and a number of related complications. The goals of treatment will change during the acute, chronic, and terminal phases of the disease. The early recognition of disease complications and treatment toxicities is one goal of nursing care that remains constant throughout the disease course. Effective patient and family education can aid the nurse in meeting this objective.

Skilled nursing assessments and interventions are essential in the care of the patient with MM. The early recognition of hypercalcemia can minimize renal damage. Identifying the impact of anemia on a patient's functional status can avoid unnecessary immobility. Finding an early infection before it creates sepsis can save a life. Providing a systematic approach to pain management prevents unnecessary suffering. Knowing when a patient or family member needs help to cope with the physical or emotional demands of an incurable illness can nurture inner strength and hope. It is not difficult to see what an impact nurses can have in minimizing morbidity and maximizing quality of life in this patient population.

The skeletal disease that is a hallmark of MM is a prime example of how nursing assessment can make a difference. A majority of patients experience bone pain. Pain can be an indicator of response to treatment or disease progression; therefore it is important to conduct and document pain assessments regularly. For example, steadily increasing back pain can precede spinal cord compression. Likewise, persistent localized pain suggests pathologic fracture.

High-dose steroids are often used in the treatment of patients with MM. Nurses need to observe for signs and symptoms of steroid toxicity. These might include fluid retention and weight gain. Monitoring the patient's intake/output and weight aids in identifying the problem earlier than observing for edema or abnormal lung sounds. Preventing severe fluid retention can be particularly important in patients who are prone to congestive heart failure. Steroids can also cause GI toxicities such as gastritis. Home management strategies include taking steroids on a full stomach and antacids and H_2-blockers as prescribed by the oncologist. Care must be taken in administering magnesium-based antacids to patients with renal failure. Patients should be instructed to report GI symptoms that progress to the point of nausea and vomiting or intense abdominal pain. Steroids can induce the formation of gastric ulcers and significant bleeding when their administration is not closely monitored.

Other common chemotherapy toxicities that need to be monitored include bone marrow suppression, which can complicate disease-induced anemia and immunosuppres-

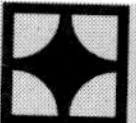

TABLE 66-5 Assessment of the Patient for Multiple Myeloma

	Assessment Parameters	Typical Abnormal Findings
History	A. Personal and social history 1. Age 2. Ethnicity 3. Occupational/environmental exposure 4. Family history	A. Personal and social risk factors 1. Usually >age 60 2. More prevalent in African Americans 3. Increased risk with chronic exposure to ionizing radiation, farming-related chemicals, petroleum products, etc. 4. Increased risk in first-degree relatives
	B. Evaluation for pain	B. The majority of patients present with complaints of pain, usually centered around the back and ribs. The pain is precipitated by movement.
	C. Infection	C. Complaint of recurrent infection (especially sinorespiratory) is common at presentation.
Physical Examination	A. Assess for pallor of conjunctiva, nailbeds, and/or palms	A. Most patients present with some degree of anemia.
	B. Palpate back and rib cage	B. Occasionally patients will develop palpable mass lesions in areas where bones are close to the skin.
Diagnostic Tests	A. Electrophoresis of serum and/or urine	A. Monoclonal spike, 99% of patients will produce an M protein, which can be detected in serum or urine.
	B. Complete blood count	B. Most patients will be anemic. There may also be mild leukopenia and thrombocytopenia in some patients.
	C. BUN/creatinine	C. Renal insufficiency and failure are common; blood uric sodium and creatinine can be elevated.
	D. Skeletal survey, CT scan, or MRI	D. Multiple "punched out" (lytic) bone lesions
	E. Bone marrow aspiration	E. Plasmacytosis with >5% plasma cells

sion. Patients who have had repeated or prolonged chemotherapy or extensive radiotherapy experience more severe myelosuppression. Neurotoxicity should be evaluated in patients receiving vincristine. Interferon (IFN) can cause neurotoxicity in addition to the classic flu-like syndrome, fatigue, and thrombocytopenia. Since many patients with MM may be unable to tolerate IFN, careful assessment is warranted.

In addition to assessment of the patient's physical signs and symptoms, it is important to evaluate the psychosocial aspects of the patient's and the family's well-being. Although the patient with MM may respond to treatment, relapse usually occurs. Patients suffer from considerable disability, and caregiver burden can be an issue. For this reason it is important to monitor the patient's functional capacity and make appropriate referrals when necessary. Assessment of the available support systems and early intervention with supportive services can be a lifeline for patients and families. When coping issues are identified, referral to local support groups or a counseling service is appropriate.

STAGING

The staging of MM is based on laboratory findings, not the anatomic staging system of solid tumors. The Durie-Salmon staging system, which has been widely accepted, distinguishes three stages of MM based on tumor burden, hemoglobin and calcium levels, bone lesions, renal function, and rate of immunoglobulin production (Durie & Salmon, 1975) (Table 66-6). Another staging method uses the evaluation of serum β_2-microglobulin (β_2-M). Serum β_2-M levels <0.4 mg/ml represent stage 1, and levels >0.4 mg/ml indicate stage 2. Although the initial patient presentation may occur at any disease stage, a majority of patients are first diagnosed during a phase of indolent tumor growth.

MEDICAL MANAGEMENT

Although a great deal is known about the biologic aspects of MM, researchers disagree on a number of important issues regarding its treatment. This section presents a summary of the current thinking regarding MM therapy and attempts to find some middle ground or at least a majority opinion.

General Principles of Myeloma Therapy

Systemic chemotherapy, particularly the use of alkylating agents, is the mainstay of myeloma therapy. A great deal has been learned from the study of numerous therapies, including those supported by stem cell transplantation. Yet MM remains an incurable disease with a relatively poor prognosis. As a result, the best available strategy may be to achieve frequent remissions that can be maintained for several years and then to control relapses repeatedly with a series of effective treatments (Alexanian & Weber, 1996).

The question of when to begin therapy is not always an easy one to answer. Many authors agree that treating asymp-

TABLE 66-6 Myeloma Staging System

Stage	Criteria	Estimated Tumor Burden ($\times 10^{12}$ cells/m^2)	Median Survival
I	All the following: 1. Hemoglobin >10 g/dl 2. Serum calcium <12 mg/dl 3. Normal bone structure (scale 0) on x-ray or solitary lesion 4. Low M-component production a. IgG level <5 g/dl b. IgA level <3 g/dl c. Urine light chain electrophoresis <4 g/24 hr	<0.6 (low)	IA: 61 months; 5 yr survival: 25%-40%
II	Fitting neither stage I or stage III	0.6-1.2 (intermediate)	IIA,B: 55 months; 5 yr survival: 15%-30%
III	Any one or more of the following: 1. Hemoglobin <8.5 g/dL 2. Serum calcium >12 mg/dL 3. Advanced lytic bone lesions (more than three) 4. High M component production a. IgG level >7 g/dl b. IgA level >5 g/dl c. Urine light chain electrophoresis >12 g/24 hr	>1.2 (high) (1×10^{12} equals 1 kg of tumor)	IIIA: 30 months; IIIB: 15 months; <5 yr survival: <10%-25%
Subclassification Based on Renal Function			
A = Relatively normal (serum creatinine <2 mg/dl)			
B = Abnormal (serum creatinine >2 mg/dl)			

Durie, B. G., & Salmon, S. E. (1975). A clinical staging system for multiple myeloma. *Cancer, 36,* 842-954; Longo, D. L. (1994). Plasma cell disorders. In K. J. Isselbacher, E. Braunwald, J. D. Wilson, J. B. Martin, A. Fauci, & D. L. Kaspter (Eds.), *Harrison's principles of internal medicine* (13th ed.). New York: McGraw-Hill.

tomatic early MM is not warranted (Kyle, 1995; Longo, 1994; Salmon & Cassady, 1993; Seiden & Anderson, 1995). Treatment begins when the patient develops physical symptoms or when there is other evidence of disease progression, such as a rising M component. If it is unclear whether or not therapy is indicated, treatment is withheld and the patient is re-evaluated in 2 to 3 months. At times it may be necessary to delay the initiation of primary therapy. If the patient initially has an emergent complication such as significant infection, long bone fractures requiring stabilization, or spinal cord compression, these need to be dealt with before therapy can be started (Salmon & Cassady, 1993).

Myeloma is radiosensitive and chemosensitive. X-ray therapy is used primarily to treat painful bone lesions that were not palliated by chemotherapy and spinal cord compression (Salmon & Cassady, 1993; Seiden & Anderson, 1995). However, it is the primary treatment for patients with solitary plasmacytomas.

A plateau effect is often seen in patients with MM who respond to induction chemotherapy. A drug-sensitive phase is followed by a plateau period of stable tumor burden and M-protein levels. The plateau appears to be unaffected by chemotherapy (Bubley & Schnipper, 1995). It can continue for a period of several months and is followed by a relapse phase, when cells have an increased growth fraction and have become drug resistant (Bubley & Schnipper, 1995; Malpas, 1995; Salmon & Cassady, 1993). At presentation, between 15% and 20% of patients have disease that is resistant to chemotherapy; however, most are drug sensitive for 2 to 3 years before resistance develops (Salmon & Cassady, 1993). Common chemotherapeutic regimens for MM are outlined in Table 66-7.

Evaluation of the Response to Treatment

As with diagnosis, no single test is adequate to evaluate the response to treatment. In addition to a thorough history and physical examination, the evaluation typically includes bone marrow biopsy, several laboratory tests, and a skeletal survey. Laboratory tests include a CBC with differential, serum and/or urine M-component evaluations, and serum calcium, creatinine, or blood urea nitrogen levels (Salmon & Cassady, 1993).

A complete response is defined as <5% plasma cells in the bone marrow and the absence of M protein on IEP (Seiden & Anderson, 1995). Complete responses are seldom seen with conventional-dose chemotherapy (Seiden & Anderson, 1995). The definition of *partial response* varies among cooperative groups, but it falls in the range of 50% to 75% reduction in M protein.

TABLE 66-7 Common Chemotherapy Regimens Used in Multiple Myeloma

Melphalan and Prednisone			
Melphalan	8-10 mg/m²	PO	Days 1-4
Prednisone	60 mg/m²	PO	Days 1-4
(Because of varying bioavailability of oral melphalan, the dose must be increased to induce hematologic toxicity, absolute granulocyte counts <2000/μL, or significant under dosing may occur.)			
Repeat every 21-28 days.			
Multiple dosing and time schedules for the MP regimen are employed, a common alternative uses the same doses of melphalan and prednisone on days 1-7, repeated every 6 weeks			
VAD			
Vincristine	0.4 mg/m²	24 hr infusion	Days 1-4
Doxorubicin	9 mg/m²	24 hr infusion	Days 1-4
Dexamethasone	40 mg	PO	Days 1-4, 9-12, 17-20
To reduce the risk of hypercorticism, the frequency of administration of dexamethasone should be decreased once a clinical response is reached.			
Repeat every 28 days.			
VBMCP or M2			
Vincristine	1.2 mg/m² (up to 2 mg)	IV	Day 1
Melphalan	8 mg/m²	PO	Days 1-7
Cyclophosphamide	400 mg/m²	IV	Day 1
BCNU	20 mg/m²	IV	Day 1
Prednisone	40 mg/m²	PO	Days 1-7 all cycles
	20 mg/m²	PO	Days 8-14 cycles 1-3 only
Repeat every 5 weeks.			
Changes in doses of the M2 protocol are used.			
Glucocorticoids			
Dexamethasone	20 mg/m²	PO	Days 1-4, 9-12, 17-20
Methylprednisolone	2 g	IV	3 times/wk
Continued at least 4 weeks, if response is seen, dose is reduced to once or twice weekly.			

Data from Kyle, R. A. (1995). Multiple myeloma and other plasma cell disorders. In R. Hoffman & L. E. Silberstein (Eds.), *Hematology.* New York: Churchill Livingstone; Oken, M. M. (1995). Multiple myeloma and other plasma cell dyscrasias. In R. R. Skeel & N. A. Lachant (Eds.), *Handbook of cancer chemotherapy.* Boston: Little Brown; Seiden, M. V. & Anderson, K. C. (1995). Plasma cell dyscrasias. In J. S. MacDonald, D. G. Haller, & R. J. Mayer (Eds.), *Manual of oncology therapeutics.* Philadelphia: J. B. Lippincott.

Induction Chemotherapy

Conventional chemotherapy is effective in palliating the complications of MM. Therapy is given until a best response, the plateau phase, is reached. This requires up to 12 months of therapy in most cases. Although response rates are high, complete responses are rare and most patients undergo relapse (Seiden & Anderson, 1995).

Standard treatment usually involves administration of a combination of an alkylating agent (melphalan, cyclophosphamide, or chlorambucil) and prednisone. Steroids increase response rates to melphalan substantially but do not have a significant impact on survival (Bubley & Schnipper, 1995; Salmon & Cassady, 1993). The alkylating agents appear to have similar degrees of activity, but resistance to one often means resistance to all. Dose adjustments are frequently necessary for the alkylating agents, and they are based on bone marrow toxicity. There are fewer factors that have an impact on the steroid dose, and it appears that higher doses are more effective (Longo, 1994).

Melphalan plus prednisone (MP) has been the standard of care for more than 30 years. It is a safe and effective regimen that yields response rates between 40% and 60% and a median survival of 2 to 3 years (Attal, Harousseau, Stoppa, Sotto, Fuzibet, & Rossi et al., 1996; Seiden & Anderson, 1995). Many different schedules for MP have been developed, with no one of them demonstrating superiority (Seiden & Anderson, 1995). It is important to note that the absorption of oral melphalan can be erratic and renal failure increases its toxicity. For these reasons doses should be individually titrated. Melphalan should be taken on an empty stomach to enhance absorption.

The melphalan dose is escalated until myelosuppression occurs to ensure that the bioavailability of the dose is adequate to induce a response. Myelosuppressive toxicity is cumulative with repeated courses of melphalan and may require a switch to another alkylating agent. Some clinicians (Bergsagel et al., 1995; Longo, 1994) favor the use of cyclophosphamide over melphalan because they think that it is less marrow toxic and less likely to cause myelodysplastic syndrome.

Oral melphalan is given every 4 to 6 weeks. Sheridan (1996) makes a number of suggestions for improving patient compliance during the MP regimen. These include assessing the patient's ability to administer the medications safely at home and providing a 6-week calendar outlining drug administration times and follow-up appointment schedules.

Extensive studies done to compare the efficacy of MP and conventional-dose combination chemotherapy have conflicting results. Earlier analysis of such studies determined that although some combination regimens induce a more rapid response and may prolong remission, they have failed to improve survival rates and have more associated toxicities (Gregory, Richards, & Malpas, 1992). However, the VBMCP (vincristine, BCNU, melphalan, cyclophosphamide, and prednisone), or M2 regimen, is reported to have a higher response rate (72% vs 51%) and a better 5-year survival rate (26% vs 19%) than MP (Oken, 1995). The M2 regimen is employed both as a primary and a salvage therapy. Other recent studies claim better response and survival with high-dose therapy (HDT) and bone marrow or peripheral blood stem cell (PBSC) support.

Patients who have very high tumor burdens or life-threatening hypercalcemia may benefit from a combination regimen because this approach induces a more rapid response and clinical improvement (Seiden & Anderson, 1995). An example of one such regimen is VAD (vincristine, doxorubicin, dexamethasone). This popular regimen is most commonly used to treat resistant myeloma. As with many of the combination therapies, this regimen yields higher response rates than does MP, but it offers no significant improvement in overall survival (Alexanian & Dimopoulos, 1995). An advantage to VAD is that it is less marrow toxic than some of the other regimens. A disadvantage is that it is more complicated to administer because the vesicants vincristine and doxorubicin are given by continuous infusion for 4 consecutive days. This requires central venous access and necessitates hospitalization in most cases.

The addition of interferon- (INF-) to the MP and combination regimens does not improve survival, but it may modestly prolong the plateau phase (Kyle, 1995; Nordic Myeloma Study Group, 1996; Seiden & Anderson, 1995). Studies evaluating the value of INF- as a part of myeloma therapy are ongoing.

It is recommended that the therapy chosen for the initial treatment of MM be continued until a best response or plateau is achieved. This may take more than 12 months, and it is recommended that induction chemotherapy continue for at least 1 year (Oken, 1995).

The disappointing results of conventional-dose chemotherapy raised interest in HDT and bone marrow transplantation. HDT with bone marrow transplantation offers hope for some, but many patients are excluded from participation. Most of these protocols require that patients be <65 years old, have a functional status <3 (Eastern Cooperative Onlcology Group [ECOG] scale), and have acceptable cardiac, pulmonary, and liver function. Currently, <20% of patients with MM are potential candidates for treatment intensification with HDT and autotransplant based on these acceptance criteria (Blade, San Miguel, Fontanillas, Alcala, Moldanado, & Conde et al., 1996). Even fewer patients (5% to 10%) are eligible for allogeneic transplant (Kyle, 1995).

The pretransplant therapy usually consists of high-dose alkylating agents and total body irradiation. Patients who appeared to be resistant to standard doses of melphalan will often respond to escalated doses, and therefore it is often used (Bubley & Schnipper, 1995). Melphalan doses used in HDT (with or without BMT or PBSC support) range from 80 to 140 mg/m^2 intravenously; this is noted in comparison to conventional doses of 8 to 10 mg/m^2 (Salmon & Cassady, 1995).

One of the questions still to be answered is whether or not HDT offers significant improvement over conventional therapies. Opinions are strong on this matter, and no consensus can be reached at this time. It is not difficult to find one protransplant study for each antitransplant study.

Blade and colleagues (1996) evaluated the outcome of patients treated with conventional therapy who were eligible for HDT with autotransplant. They found that the survival of their conventionally treated patients was very similar to the reported survival rates of patients treated with HDT and autologous or PBSC transplant. Their conclusion mirrors popular opinion. Although the use of HDT raises hope for some patients, the impact that it can have on survival has not been established and more time is needed to evaluate this treatment approach. One of the criticisms of studies of HDT in MM is the significant selection bias for the HDT group.

However, complete response rates of 20% to 30% compels researchers to attempt to perfect the use of HDT (Bubley & Schnipper, 1995). Attal and colleagues (1996) conducted a randomized prospective trial to evaluate the use of autotransplant in patients with newly diagnosed disease. Twenty-six percent of patients who were randomized to the HDT group had to be excluded because they did not tolerate the pretransplant therapy. Despite this fact, the results of this study support the use of HDT in newly diagnosed patients. Based on their results, the authors concluded that HDT plus autotransplant improves response rates, event-free survival, and overall survival of patients with MM when compared to conventional chemotherapy. They also reported that the duration of bone marrow aplasia may be shorter in patients who receive PBSC support than in those who have autologous marrow transplant. Another study comparing HDT followed by autologous bone marrow and PBSC also reported faster bone marrow recovery in patients who received peripheral stem cells (Bensinger, Rowley, Demirer, Lilleby, Schiffman, & Clift, et al., 1996).

Autologous bone marrow transplant may be most useful in patients who do not have drug-resistant disease (Bubley & Schnipper, 1995; Kyle, 1995). Several factors related to drug resistance have an impact on success rates. Those associated with a negative outcome include more than two regimens of prior therapy, having more than eight cycles of prior treatment, time to transplant longer than 3 years from diagnosis, and having had prior radiation (Bensinger et al., 1996). These adverse prognostic indicators suggest that HDT may produce better results when it is used as an early intervention.

Advantages of autologous and PBSC over allogeneic transplant include the ability to perform transplantation in patients of older age and the avoidance of graft versus host disease (GVHD). A disadvantage in autologous transplant is that the graft may be contaminated with myeloma cells. Methods used to purge autologous marrow and PBSC of plasma cells may improve the patient's duration of remission (Bubley & Schnipper, 1995).

Allogeneic transplant has also been used in the treatment of MM. Despite the advantage of having a graft that is free of tumor cells, patients still relapse. In addition, transplant-related mortality is high. Enrollment in allogeneic transplant protocols is limited by the availability of a compatible donor and the patient's age. Despite these problems, allogeneic transplant is associated with high complete response rates (40%), and some patients enjoy prolonged disease-free survival (Bubley & Schnipper, 1995). Oken (1995) suggests that allogeneic transplant should be discussed with every patient younger than 55 who has a matched donor.

Among the many questions raised about intensification therapy with transplant is: When is the optimal time to administer such therapy? HDT has been used both in early disease and following relapse. The suggestions for future study made by researchers to improve the outcome with HDT and bone marrow or PBSC transplant include earlier intervention, improved posttransplant therapies (including maintenance therapy), and the use of sequential HDT (double transplant) (Attal et al., 1996; Bensinger et al., 1996; Blade et al., 1996).

Maintenance Therapy

Another unanswered question in the treatment of MM is: How long should chemotherapy be continued? Many authors agree that although the ideal duration of chemotherapy is unknown, induction chemotherapy should continue until a plateau is reached (Bubley & Schnipper, 1995; Kyle, 1995; Seiden & Anderson, 1995). When chemotherapy is stopped, relapse usually follows (Kyle, 1995). Oken (1995) suggests continuing the induction regimen for 2 years or to a maximal response but recommends decreasing the frequency of administration to every 6 to 8 weeks during the second year. Long-term therapy with alkylating agents is thought to increase the risk of developing myelodysplastic syndrome or leukemia and results in no further improvement.

There has been a great deal of interest in the use of INF-, which has shown some activity in the treatment of MM. Many studies have evaluated the value of INF- in maintaining remission. Several investigators report that INF- was able to prolong remission in patients who had responded to induction chemotherapy but that overall survival was not improved (Alexanian & Weber, 1996; Kyle, 1995; Seiden & Anderson, 1995). Further study may uncover the most appropriate role for INF- in myeloma therapy. The search continues to find a more effective therapy.

In the meantime more questions remain about the cost/benefit ratio. INF- therapy is expensive and has a significant side effect profile. The Nordic Myeloma Study Group (1996) evaluated a combination therapy of MP with INF-. There was significant toxicity in the INF- group, with 30% of patients unable to tolerate the therapy.

Systemic radiation therapy has also been tried as a remission consolidation treatment. Whole-body or hemibody x-ray therapy results in myelotoxicity that is much more severe than maintenance chemotherapy. The survival outcome is inferior to that of chemotherapy, and therefore the practice has been abandoned (Salmon & Anderson, 1993).

Treatment of Refractory or Relapsed Multiple Myeloma

Chemotherapy frequently eradicates myeloma cells, but cure occurs rarely, if ever, and the disease recurs. There does not appear to be a correlation between (1) the number of myeloma cells in the bone marrow, (2) how much treatment decreases the number of myeloma cells or M protein, and (3) survival (Bergsagel et al., 1995). Destroying myeloma cells in the bone marrow relieves the patient's symptoms. However, the relapse rate for myeloma suggests that the generative population of myeloma cells may not be in the bone marrow and is not being eliminated. The clonotypal B cells found in the blood by Bergsagel et al. (1995) persist in the blood even when the patient has minimal disease. These authors theorize that it is these cells that are the key to regeneration of myeloma cells and that eradicating them may offer longer survival. If future research is able to identify a malignant subset of these B cells, this information may be a valuable tool for evaluating the efficacy of new therapies.

Refractory myeloma can be categorized into two groups. Primary refractory myeloma never achieves a response and continues to progress during induction chemotherapy. Approximately 30% of patients fail to respond to induction chemotherapy. Patients with secondary refractory myeloma are those who did respond to induction therapy but have relapsed and are currently refractory to a previously effective chemotherapy regimen. In patients with secondary refractory disease, the myeloma growth rate increases with each subsequent relapse and remissions become increasingly shorter. Only a few of those with primary refractory disease will respond to further chemotherapy. These patients have a poorer prognosis, with a median survival of <1 year.

Both of these groups of patients require alternate therapy. Refractory disease is usually treated with the same agents used in the initial treatment. Alternative doses, scheduling, and combinations of these drugs may be attempted. Up to 80% of patients will achieve a second response after relapse (Longo, 1994).

The most effective therapy for patients who are resistant to alkylating agents may be the VAD regimen (Kyle, 1995; Seiden & Anderson, 1995). It boasts a response rate of 75% in resistant myeloma (Hussein, 1994). Unfortunately, the response is often of short duration. Although most of the activity in this regimen comes from dexamethasone, the dose must often be reduced to use in only days 1 through 4 because of toxicity (Kyle, 1995). Another option is the M2 regimen, considered to be a conservative therapy that provides a 20% response rate in patients in their first relapse or those who have failed initial MP therapy (Oken, 1995).

High-dose pulsed glucocorticoids are also used for treatment of MM. Glucocorticoids may be particularly useful in patients with little bone marrow reserve because they are not myelotoxic. Steroids typically employed include prednisone, methylprednisolone, and dexamethasone. Methylprednisolone has fewer side effects than dexamethasone. Forty percent of patients will respond to therapy with glucocorticoids (Kyle, 1995; Salmon & Anderson, 1993).

The use of HDT therapy with bone marrow or PBSC support has also been tried in patients with MM relapse and has had mixed results. Its use in relapse may be limited because it appears to be most effective in patients whose disease is still sensitive to chemotherapy (Bubley & Schnipper, 1995). Studies intended to define the role of HDT in refractory MM are continuing.

The use of IFN- has produced disappointing results in patients refractory to alkylating agents (Kyle, 1995). Only 10% of patients can expect to achieve an objective response with INF-2 (Oken, 1995).

Future and Developing Therapies

A number of research questions about HDT, with or without bone marrow or PBSC support, are currently being investigated. Such therapies offer promise to patients with MM, but they need to be perfected so that the comparison of efficacy with standard therapy and the risk/benefit ratio are more clearly understood. Aggressive research into the use of HDT is ongoing.

A number of agents have demonstrated activity in MM in phase II trials. These include pentostatin, epirubicin, peptichemio, and teniposide (Salmon & Anderson, 1993). These agents are capable of inducing remission in 10% of patients with relapsed MM. Studies continue to define their activity more clearly. A recent study of Z-Dex (oral idarubicin and dexamethasone) concluded that this regimen is an oral equivalent of VAD (Cook, Sharp, & Tansey, 1996). If these results can be replicated, this new regimen may provide an alternative to VAD that is easier to administer.

In vitro studies of IL-6 receptor superantagonists show promise that there may be a way of blocking this myeloma cell growth factor (Sopreno et al., 1996). Antisense mRNA and anti–IL-6 monoclonal antibodies have already shown the ability to suppress myeloma cell proliferation in vivo (Bataille & Klein, 1995; Bubley & Schnipper, 1995; Klein et al., 1991). Research on the relationship between IL-6 and myeloma cells has greatly increased our knowledge of the biologic aspects of MM. In the future these techniques may be perfected and developed as primary therapy for MM. In the meantime access to these protocols is available in a only few research sites.

ONCOLOGIC EMERGENCIES

Oncologic emergencies that occur in patients with MM include spinal cord compression, hypercalcemia, sepsis, and hyperviscosity. The following discussion is specific to MM. For more detailed information about the pathophysiology and management of oncologic emergencies, see Chapter 11.

Spinal Cord Compression

Spinal cord compression (SCC) in MM occurs as a result of extradural plasma cell tumors or compression fracture. Because of the frequency and severity of bone destruction that often affects the spinal column, an assessment for signs and symptoms of SCC should be made at each encounter with patients with MM. It is also advisable to educate the patient and family members about such symptoms and instruct them to report symptoms immediately. Failure to diagnose SCC promptly and accurately can result in permanent neurologic damage. When SCC occurs, immediate intervention with radiation therapy and high-dose steroids is indicated (Bubley & Schnipper, 1995; Longo, 1994; Salmon & Anderson, 1993).

Hypercalcemia

Hypercalcemia is a common complication of MM. Lytic bone disease and immobility are two major causes. Prevention of serious morbidity relies on good assessment and early intervention. Because hypercalcemia can be expected to occur, regular laboratory assessment should be done and nurses should be alert to early manifestations. It is important to recognize that the clinical manifestations of hypercalcemia can vary depending on serum levels and the speed at which the condition has developed.

Standard therapy includes vigorous hydration and diuresis. The addition of corticosteroids is useful because they have a direct effect on myeloma cells and block osteoclast activity (Salmon & Anderson, 1993). For patients whose myeloma is not actively being treated, the initiation of chemotherapy can bring hypercalcemia under control. Patients with severe hypercalcemia (serum levels τ13.5 mg/dl) or patients who fail to respond to standard therapy can be treated with plicamycin, gallium nitrate, calcitonin, or diphosphonates. As mentioned earlier, pamidronate may be the preferred treatment choice in patients with MM. Chronic hypercalcemia can be managed with oral phosphates, provided the patient has adequate renal function and normal serum phosphate levels (Salmon & Anderson, 1993).

Sepsis

Recurrent bacterial infection is the cause of death for 20% to 50% of patients with MM (Hussein, 1994; Seiden & Anderson, 1995). Patients exhibiting symptoms of bacterial infection, such as a productive cough or a fever, should have cultures and a chest x-ray film taken immediately. It must be kept in mind that steroids can mask the signs of infection. If infection is suspected, empiric antibiotic therapy should be started without delay to avoid serious complications.

Hyperviscosity

Hyperviscosity is caused by large amounts of M protein in the serum. It can result in serious neurologic and cardiac complications and significant bleeding. Emergent therapy is usually plasmapheresis, and the long-term control of plasma viscosity relies on the efficacy of chemotherapy (Salmon &

Cassady, 1993). Chronic hyperviscosity can occur in patients who do not respond to chemotherapy. These patients can sometimes be adequately managed with regular plasmapheresis (Hussein, 1994; Salmon & Cassady, 1993).

NURSING MANAGEMENT

Nursing diagnoses for the patient with MM are centered on the biophysical manifestations of the disease and the psychological sequelae of terminal illness. Most of the care for the patient with MM is provided in the outpatient center. Inpatient care usually focuses on management of acute complications. At times it may be necessary to admit patients for extended infusions of vesicant chemotherapeutic agents. Major issues associated with care of the patient with MM are discussed in the following section. Three standards of care are provided in this chapter. (See Tables 66-6 through 66-9.)

As with all cancers, nursing care must be dynamic and responsive to the changing needs of the patient. For the most part MM is a predictable disease. This aids in the anticipation of the physical needs that must be addressed. Psychosocial care must be individually tailored to the patient's personal characteristics and resourcefulness and the support system available.

Educating the Patient

Nursing management during the early stages of the disease focuses on the presenting symptoms, patient education, and interventions to promote effective coping. Patient education about the disease process, diagnostic procedures, and treatment options is an early nursing goal. It is crucial that the patient and family have a clear understanding of home management techniques to control and assess the various manifestations of MM, such as hypercalcemia, lytic bone disease, anemia, infection, and renal failure. These complications are likely to occur and can cause serious morbidity if they are not recognized early.

The patient needs to be taught not only what symptoms to expect, but their significance and relevance to therapy. Making consistent systematic assessments at regular intervals can help to identify trends that signal a developing problem. Nursing research has demonstrated that patient self-report is an effective means of information gathering. The results of a chemotherapy toxicity self-report assessment developed by Brinkman, Hay, and Laubinger (1994) demonstrated that self-reported information is accurate and more complete than that gained through patient interview. Asking a patient to keep a symptom diary may be helpful in obtaining information that the patient might otherwise fail to report.

Patients can receive overwhelming amounts of verbal and written information. Ideally patient education is tailored to an individual's educational needs, priorities of care, and level of sophistication. Unfortunately, the written materials available to oncology nurses are limited and require the gathering of multiple brochures and pamphlets to cover each area of importance adequately (Griffiths & Leek, 1995). Additional problems facing nurses is that the reading level of most written materials may not be appropriate for their patient population (Cooley, Moriarity, Berger, Orr, Coyle, & Short, 1995). These factors combined with the increasing demands on nurses' time make providing quality patient education a challenge.

Oncology nurses face a difficult task in helping patients manage the overwhelming amount of information available to them from a variety of sources, including the Internet. A brief exploration of the Internet reveals hundreds of thousands of documents related to cancer. There are many that are specific to MM, some of which are written specifically for patients. Other documents are of a highly technical nature and are intended for health care professionals; these include a listing of open myeloma protocols from the National Cancer Institute. Patients who access such information may require a great deal of assistance to interpret and sort out what is applicable to their situation. Patients may demand enrollment in protocols about which they have read. They may inquire about why they were not enrolled in protocols for which they felt they would have been eligible in the past, wondering if that approach would have been more effective than the one chosen. In addition, patients can participate in a number of on-line self-help groups. If such chat groups and information services are prepared by an unqualified persons, patients may be exposed to misinformation or poor advice from well-meaning individuals.

The International Myeloma Foundation (IMF) maintains a site on the Internet. The IMF is self-described as a nonprofit organization dedicated to improving the QOL for multiple myeloma patients and ultimately to prevent and cure myeloma. Patients are invited to call or write with questions or concerns. Information from the IMF is available in both English and Spanish. The organization publishes a journal entitled *Myeloma Today*. Articles from this journal are summarized on the Internet. The information is current and very informative; however, it is also presented at a level of significant sophistication.

Pain Management

Pain management in MM includes pharmacologic and nonpharmacologic measures. Bone pain that was present at the time of diagnosis often subsides soon after the initiation of chemotherapy. At other times it may be necessary to use x-ray therapy to manage bone pain in MM (Table 66-10). Opiates are most effective in controlling pain. It is important to note that nonsteroidal antiinflammatory agents are associated with a higher incidence of renal failure in MM (Salmon & Cassady, 1993). Pamidronate, used to treat hypercalcemia, has also been shown to provide significant decreases in bone pain in MM by inhibiting bone destruction (Berenson et al., 1996).

Promoting Mobility and Independence

The pathologic aspects of bone and bone pain can have a significant impact on the patient's mobility and comfort level. Several nursing care issues for the patient with MM

TABLE 66-8 Standard of Care for the Patient with Extensive Lytic Bone Disease

Patient Problem and Outcomes	Nursing Interventions and Rationales	Patient Education Instructions
Pain Patient will: • State relief of pain with medications and comfort measures • Understand and report pain that is indicative of disease complications	1. Assess pain using a standardized tool (e.g., 1-10 visual analog scale) at each visit. Monitor for trends and/or evidence of disease progressing. 2. Assess effectiveness of pain medications, titrate to comfort. 3. Consult with physical/occupational therapist about the use of a back brace if appropriate. 4. Evaluate patient's understanding of teaching and reinforce as needed.	1. Instruct patient on proper use of pain medications and side effects, including what to do if medications become ineffective. 2. Educate patient on the cautious use of nonsteroidal medications, which is associated with increased occurrence of renal failure in MM. 3. Teach patient to report steadily increasing back pain, which can precede spinal cord compression, and persistent localized pain, suggesting pathologic fracture.
Hypercalcemia Patient will have serum calcium within normal limits	1. Monitor serum calcium, evaluate trends, notify physician if serum calcium exceeds normal limits (>11.5 mg/dl after correction for serum albumin). 2. Administer therapy to control hypercalcemia as ordered. 3. Encourage patient to ambulate as tolerated to promote bone strength and slow demineralization. 4. Evaluate patient's understanding of teaching and reinforce as needed	1. Instruct patient to drink at least 2 L of fluid per day to facilitate excretion of calcium. 2. Instruct patient to report early signs and symptoms of hypercalcemia: nausea and vomiting, anorexia, constipation, lethargy, drowsiness, restlessness, mood changes, muscle weakness, fatigue, bradycardia, polyuria, polydipsia.
Impaired Physical Mobility Patient will maintain an optimal level of functioning and independence	1. Monitor functional status and rate on a standardized scale (e.g., Karnofsky score or Eastern Cooperative Group score) at each visit. 2. Consult with physical therapist to institute a program to minimize deconditioning throughout the disease process. 3. Consult with physical therapist to provide assistive devices if necessary. 4. Provide prompt treatment for symptoms that inhibit mobility (e.g., pain, anemia, pathologic fracture). 5. Evaluate patient's understanding of teaching and reinforce as needed.	1. Instruct patient about the importance of maintaining physical activity early in the disease. 2. Instruct patient to report changes in activity level, symptoms that impair mobility. 3. If patient is not ambulatory, encourage range-of-motion exercises, and strategies to promote independendence. 4. If patient is bedridden, teach family member how to safely pivot patient in and out of bed.
High Risk for the Development of Pathologic Fractures Patient will maintain safety precautions to help reduce the risk of pathologic fractures	1. Assess for new complaints of pain at each visit; report complaints of persistent localized pain or steadily increasing back pain to physician. 2. Consult with physical therapist to institute a program of strengthening and reconditioning. 3. Evaluate the need for assistive devices. 4. Evaluate patient's understanding of teaching and reinforce as needed.	1. Explain to patient that he or she is at risk for the development of pathologic fractures because of bone lesions. 2. Teach measures to reduce the potential for fractures, including: a. Avoid trauma to sites of known bone lesions. b. Avoid moving/lifting heavy objects. c. Avoid performing the Valsalva maneuver. d. Change position gradually. e. Use good body mechanics. 3. Teach patient methods to safety-proof the home (e.g., remove scatter rugs) to avoid falls.

TABLE 66-9 Standard of Care for the Management of the Hematologic Complications of Multiple Myeloma

Patient Problem and Outcomes	Nursing Interventions and Rationales	Patient Education Instructions
Anemia		
Patient will maintain a hemoglobin level sufficient to prevent activity intolerance	1. Monitor hemoglobin level. If it falls below 10 g/dl or if patient is symptomatic, notify physician. 2. Assess patient for symptoms of anemia: fatigue, tachycardia, tachypnea, pallor, cold intolerance, or changes in activity level. Determine the impact of these symptoms on mobility and quality of life. 3. Administer therapy for anemia as ordered. 4. Evaluate patient's level of fatigue at each visit using a standardized scale (e.g., 1-10 visual analog scale). 5. Evaluate patient's understanding of teaching and reinforce as needed.	1. Teach patient that anemia is very common in patients with multiple myeloma. 2. Educate patient about the treatment of anemia with epoetin alfa or blood transfusion. 3. Teach self-administration of epoetin alfa injections if ordered. 4. Teach fatigue management strategies: a. Energy conservation, use of shower chair, organizing daily activities, use of assistive devices b. Prioritizing activities, including leisure activities c. Ensure adequate uninterrupted rest. d. Accept offers of help from others.
Immunosuppression		
Patient will receive prompt treatment of infection to avoid serious complications	1. Assess for signs and symptoms of infection at each visit. 2. Monitor laboratory values and report white blood cell count <2000 to physician. 3. Administer antiinfective therapy as ordered. 4. Evaluate patient's understanding of teaching and reinforce as needed.	1. Teach patient to identify and promptly report signs of infection (e.g., cough, fever, dysuria). 2. Teach patient strategies to minimize the risk of infection (e.g., avoid crowds, maintain adequate nutrition). 3. If patient is to self-initiate antibiotic therapy, teach appropriate and prudent use, and instruct patient to notify physician. 4. Teach patient to administer granulocyte colony stimulating factor (G-CSF) injection if ordered.
Bleeding		
Patient will maintain safety precautions to help reduce the risk of bleeding	1. Assess the patient for signs of unusual bleeding (e.g., petechiae, bruising). 2. Monitor coagulation studies and platelet counts. 3. Evaluate patient's understanding of teaching and reinforce as needed.	1. Teach the patient about the increased risk for bleeding related to the M protein and/or chemotherapy. 2. Teach measures to reduce the potential for bleeding, including: a. Use an electric razor. b. Use a soft tooth brush. c. Avoid trauma from bumping into things or from aggressive sports or activities. d. Avoid performing the Valsalva maneuver. 3. Teach patient methods to safety-proof the home (e.g., remove scatter rugs) to avoid falls.

center on mobility. Promoting and preserving the patient's mobility is of extreme importance.

Physical rehabilitation and the use of assistive devices can be helpful in maintaining normal activity and promoting self-care. Medical management of bone disease, including x-ray therapy and stabilization of pathologic fractures, may be necessary, and these methods are warranted to achieve this goal (Salmon & Cassady, 1993).

Oncology rehabilitation, once considered a novelty, is slowly gaining acceptance by the health care community. An example of such endorsement was made by the Oncology Nursing Society when it issued its position statement on the rehabilitation of people with cancer (Mayer & Kelleher, 1993). This organization emphasizes the need to promote optimal functioning and wellness to address the needs of cancer survivors. However, the terminal cancer patient can also benefit from rehabilitation. Maintaining a patient's mobility, even in the terminal phase of disease, can prevent unnecessary morbidity and maximize independence (Gerber, Levinson, Hicks, Gabelli, Whitehurst, & Scheib et al., 1993).

Promoting activity, specifically ambulation, has other benefits for the patient with MM, and bed rest should be

TABLE 66-10 Standard of Care for the Patient Receiving High-Dose Steroids

Patient Problem and Outcomes	Nursing Interventions and Rationales	Patient Education Instructions
Fluid and Electrolyte Imbalance: Iatrogenic Hypercorticism		
Patient will demonstrate knowledge of the appropriate use of measures to control fluid retention and when to notify physician of symptoms	1. Monitor intake and output, daily weights. 2. Assess for signs and symptoms of infection (NOTE: steroids may mask signs of infection). 3. Monitor serum sodium, potassium, calcium. 4. Assess for fluid retention: auscultate lung sounds, assess for peripheral edema, closely monitor patients at risk for congestive heart failure. 5. Closely monitor diabetic patients for hyperglycemia. 6. Evaluate patient's understanding of teaching and reinforce as needed.	1. Teach patient to record intake and output and daily weight. 2. If ordered, instruct patient on proper use of diuretics and/or restricted sodium diet. 3. Instruct patient to report weight gain of 2 to 3 pounds over a few days and/or peripheral edema.
Infection		
Patient will receive prompt treatment of infection to avoid serious complications	1. Monitor for signs and symptoms of infection. 2. Administer antiinfective therapy as ordered. 3. Evaluate patient's understanding of teaching and reinforce as needed.	1. Teach patient to identify and promptly report signs of infection (e.g., cough, fever, dysuria). 2. Teach patient strategies to minimize the risk of infection (e.g., avoid crowds, maintain adequate nutrition).
Gastritis		
Patient will demonstrate knowledge of the management of steroid-induced gastrointestinal symptoms and when to notify physician	1. Evaluate the patient's understanding of teaching and reinforce as needed. 2. Obtain guaiac stools, emesis.	1. Instruct patient on the proper administration of steroids and side effects. 2. Instruct patient to take steroids on a full stomach. 3. Teach patient how to properly use prescribed antacids of H_2 antagonist. 4. Teach patient to promptly report nausea and vomiting, hematemesis, severe or persistent stomach pain, or tarry stools.

avoided as much as possible. Even 1 or 2 days of bed rest can cause fluid and electrolyte imbalances, precipitate hypercalcemia, and lead to the rapid deterioration of the patient's general condition (Bubley & Schnipper, 1995; Nail & Winningham, 1995; Salmon & Cassady, 1993). On the other hand, ambulation enhances skeletal strength and greatly benefits the patient with MM (Salmon & Cassady, 1993). One week of bed rest can lead to enough muscle atrophy to prevent a patient from walking even short distances. Each week that a patient is immobile can require up to 1 month of rehabilitation to restore the functional mobility that was lost (Gerber et al., 1993).

Maintenance of mobility and promotion of ambulation, therefore, are two logical goals of nursing care. Fatigue is a complicated and bothersome symptom experienced by cancer patients and can have a profound impact on mobility. Fatigue is currently recognized as the most commonly reported symptom of cancer and its treatment (Winningham, Nail, Burke, Brophy, Cimprich, & Jones et al., 1994). Ferrell, Grant, Dean, Funk, and Ly (1996) conducted a study to evaluate specifically the impact of fatigue on quality of life. They concluded that fatigue is not an isolated physical symptom but a force that has an impact on all dimensions of quality of life: physical, psychological, social, and spiritual. Bone pathologic factors, pain, immobility, anemia, repeated infection, and prolonged treatment with chemotherapy can contribute to the fatigue problem in patients with MM. For a complete discussion of the management of fatigue, refer to Chapter 13.

Clinically prescribed and monitored exercise programs have been shown to ameliorate fatigue, increase energy levels, decrease weakness, and improve overall quality of life in cancer patients (Gerber et al., 1993; Smith, 1996; Winningham, 1991). It is generally advisable to screen patients adequately and seek appropriate referrals before recommending an exercise prescription (Smith, 1996). Rehabilitation programs typically require patients to meet certain criteria to be eligible for participation. Included in these criteria are restrictions based on the patient's blood counts. Exercise restrictions are warranted in both thrombocytopenic and anemic patients. Gerber and colleagues (1993) recommend that patients with cancer refrain from resistive exercise (functional strengthening) when their platelet count falls below 50,000/ml and avoid exercise completely when platelets number <20,000/ml. Anemic patients with a hemoglobin level <10 g/dl should be restricted or excluded from endurance exercise (e.g., stationary bicycle, cross-country skiing, treadmill). Anemia is a common and persistent problem in patients with MM. Since anemia can have a negative impact on the patient's activity tolerance, energy levels, and quality of life, early intervention is warranted. Treatment with epoetin alfa may have an advantage over blood transfusion in meeting this objective if the agent can be titrated to maintain a steady hemoglobin level.

Psychosocial Issues

Patients with MM experience the many emotional challenges faced by individuals diagnosed with cancer. The special emotional needs that these patients may face include issues related to an incurable illness, such as a relatively short life expectancy and periods of "watch and wait." Despite new aggressive treatment regimens, the number of patients with MM who experience long-term disease-free survival is relatively small. Chapter 16 specifically addresses the psychosocial needs of cancer patients, including those of the terminally ill.

For those patients with stable disease, the period of watch and wait that occurs before treatment is initiated can be a very difficult time. The thoughts of some patients may be dominated by worries that their myeloma will return at any moment, whereas others may feel insecure when they are not actively fighting their disease. Nursing intervention, including education and ongoing support and encouragement, can help to manage these feelings of helplessness and loss of control. To be most effective, the nurse caring for patients with MM needs to be aware of the disease and its treatment course and the related psychosocial implications for patient care. Although one-to-one interaction with a primary caregiver is very important, patients may find great comfort in a support group for those with leukemia and lymphoma, where issues specific to their disease can be addressed.

HOME CARE ISSUES

The complexity of care combined with cost and reimbursement issues have changed the face of cancer treatment and made home care part of the cancer experience for many patients. Home care issues in the patient with MM focus on mobility and self-care, pain management, administration of drugs and other treatments, and hospice care. With the introduction of more sophisticated technologies into the home, the demands on the home care nurse are also increasing. Home care nurses need both a broad base of knowledge and specific oncology-focused training and experience to care for this complex patient group competently (McEnroe, 1996).

Pain Management

Pain management services have been available through home care agencies for many years. Patients with MM can experience both acute and chronic pain and may benefit from referral to a home care agency for pain management. Qualities of a good home pain management service include competent staff, 24-hour access, and collaboration with the primary site of care (Magrum, Bentzen, & Landmark, 1996).

Promoting Mobility and Independence

Patients with MM benefit from interventions directed toward maintaining and promoting mobility and functional capacity. Home care nurses have the distinct advantage of being able to assess the patient in his or her own environment, and they have the opportunity for key insights into how the patient is managing. Home care nurses are responsible for assessing and promoting the patient's level of functioning. It is necessary to include cancer rehabilitation concepts in the initial home care assessment. When deficits are identified, nursing interventions are instituted based on the patient's level of disability, disfigurement, and life expectancy (Blesch, 1996). Referral to appropriate rehabilitation services may be warranted. If the home care nurse or home physical therapist has not had a great deal of experience with cancer patients, it may be necessary to enlist the assistance of an experienced oncology nurse. Guidance and education about the specific complications and manifestations of MM and their relevance to the rehabilitation program can be helpful to family members and professional and ancillary workers involved in the home care.

In a study of hospice services, McMillan (1996) found that patients were least satisfied with the physical/functional aspects of quality of life. McMillan identifies an opportunity and need for nurses to develop and use interventions directed at these aspects of care.

Home Infusion Services

Infusion services that may be used in the home care of the patient with MM include parenteral pain management therapies, gamma globulin infusions, chemotherapy, and blood product administration. Although the role of gamma globulin therapy in the prophylaxis of infection in MM remains unclear, it continues to be used. At times it may be necessary to administer this agent in the home setting. Gamma globulin can take several hours to infuse, and a number of precautions for its use are recommended by the manufacturer (Armour Pharmaceutical, 1990). These include detailed instructions for reconstitution, which can take up to 20 minutes, and the need for an anaphylaxis protocol. Therefore home therapy with gamma globulin places a number of demands on home care staff and the patient and family.

The transfusion of blood products in the home should be restricted to those patients who are truly homebound, alert, oriented, and cooperative and who have a responsible adult available in the home during and after the procedure (Gorski & Grothman, 1996). Blood transfusions pose a number of complications to the home care staff. Gorski and Grothman (1996) summarize home transfusion therapy as labor-intensive, requiring a great deal of planning, coordination, and attention to detail, and not being without risk.

Hospice Care

MM is a terminal illness, and many affected patients may choose to enter hospice care in the final phase of their illness. Hospice and home care are distinct entities with differences in focus, types of nursing care provided, length and availability of service, use of volunteers, and several other factors (McNally, Bohnet, & Lindquist, 1996). Promoting and preserving quality of life is a focal point of hospice care. As outlined earlier, patients with MM have a number of physical and emotional issues that can impair their quality of life.

Some nursing researchers have identified hospice needs beyond physical comfort that could greatly enhance the quality of life of patients and their families. In addition to providing attention to the physical, emotional, and comfort needs of the patient, hospice nurses should assess and attend to several issues related to caregivers. Support that includes attention to the physical, emotional, social, and financial concerns of caregivers improves the caregivers' quality of life (McMillan & Mahon, 1994; Steele & Fitch, 1996). Caregivers need encouragement and guidance to help them maintain a positive attitude about providing care and a sense of hope so that they can continue caregiving (Steele & Fitch, 1996). This can be particularly true if the anticipated period of caregiving responsibility is a long one, as with a debilitating illness such as MM. The quality of life of the caregiver and that of the patient are interrelated. Thus efforts by the hospice nurse to improve the caregiver's quality of life will also have a positive effect on the patient (McMillan & Mahon, 1994). In addition, McMillan (1996) found that nursing interventions designed to enhance the caregiver's ability to assess the patient's status are important to support the outcomes of hospice care.

PROGNOSIS

Despite discoveries in the biologic aspects of MM, the diagnosis remains synonymous with poor prognosis. Survival can range from a few months to more than 10 years, with a median survival of 2.5 to 3 years (Hussein, 1994; Kyle, 1995). Several prognostic indicators have been employed in MM. They are based on tumor burden and intrinsic features of the disease. Of the available indicators, only two, plasma cell labeling index and β_2-microglobulin, have independent prognostic significance (Kyle, 1995).

Plasma Cell Labeling Index

The in vivo labeling index (LI) estimates the number of myeloma cells in S phase (growth fraction) and is one of the most powerful independent prognostic indicators in MM (Hussein, 1994; Klein, 1995). An LI $<0.8\%$ indicates a good prognosis, and one $>2\%$ correlates with a poor prognosis (Bergsagel et al., 1995). At presentation, most patients have an LI between 1% and 5% (Bubley & Schnipper, 1995). Although patients with a low LI take longer to respond to treatment, both the duration of response and the survival are longer (Bubley & Schnipper, 1995). Myeloma is characteristically a low-growth-fraction tumor, and a low LI at diagnosis is predictive of a long survival, regardless of the patient's response to treatment (McIntyre, 1995).

β_2-Microglobulin

β_2-M is a component of the class I histocompatibility antigens that are present in the cell membranes of all nucleated cells (Boccadoro & Pileri, 1995). It is released from dying cells and excreted in urine (Bergsagel, 1994). Myeloma cells produce β_2-M, and serum levels are elevated in patients with active disease (Hussein, 1994). β_2-M levels are highly accurate in predicting survival; the higher the level, the poorer the prognosis (Kyle, 1995; McIntyre, 1995). Patients with serum β_2-M levels <0.4 mg/ml have a median survival of 43 months, and those with levels >0.4 mg/ml survive a median of only 12 months (Longo, 1994).

C-Reactive Proteins and Interleukin-6

The production of C-reactive proteins by the liver is controlled by IL-6 (Hussein, 1994). Because of this relationship, serum C-reactive protein levels are a direct indicator of IL-6 production (Hussein, 1994; McIntyre, 1995). This surrogate test for IL-6 concentration is correlated with both disease activity and prognosis (McIntyre, 1995). Assay tests specifically for IL-6 are preferable, but they are not widely available at this time. Concentrations of the receptors for IL-6 can also be measured, and high levels indicate a poor prognosis (Klein, 1995).

Thymidine Kinase

The serum thymidine kinase (TK) level is another test to determine the number of myeloma cells in S phase. The TK level correlates with the hemoglobin level, tumor cell mass, and survival, and a high value is a negative prognostic indicator (McIntyre, 1995).

Renal Function

Renal failure at the time of diagnosis is a prognostic indicator of short survival. Likewise, the development of renal failure at any point during the course of disease is indicative of a less favorable outcome. Serum creatinine levels can be used as a measure of renal function, and an elevation in this value is an adverse prognostic factor (Kyle, 1995).

Lactate Dehydrogenase

A high serum lactate dehydrogenase (LDH) level has been established as an adverse prognostic sign (Oken, 1995). Elevations in LDH are associated with aggressive disease, high tumor mass, and poor response to chemotherapy (Kyle, 1995).

Karyotype

Although no specific and consistent gene mutation has been identified in MM, when mutations are present, they are most often observed in chromosomes 1, 11, and 14 (Hussein, 1994; Tesch, Diehl, & Kibe, 1995). Patients with abnormal karyotypes have a shorter mean survival (Hussein, 1994).

EVALUATION OF THE QUALITY OF CARE

The care of the patient with MM requires a multidisciplinary approach to be effective. Likewise, it is important that the evaluation of the quality of care include measures to assess the effectiveness of all team members. Table 66-11 presents an example of a quality of care evaluation tool that can be implemented in the inpatient or outpatient setting. The use of evaluation tools is helpful in meeting the requirements of accreditation organizations such as the Joint Commission on Accreditation of Healthcare Organizations.

RESEARCH ISSUES

Randomized clinical trials are needed to determine the most effective treatments for the various stages of MM. Included in these studies should be a determination of the benefit of and best therapy for remission maintenance. Additional studies are warranted to determine the appropriate and most efficacious use of HDT, with or without bone marrow or PBSC transplant, and INF. These studies should include information about the phase of the disease at which these therapies should be implemented.

Because MM remains a terminal illness with a relatively short survival, studies focused on quality of life issues are relevant. Nursing research might focus on comfort measures and methods to preserve function, such as oncology rehabilitation programs.

TABLE 66-11 Quality of Care Evaluation for Patient with Extensive Lytic Bone Disease

Disciplines participating in the quality of care evaluation:
☐ Nursing ☐ Physician
☐ Physical therapy ☐ Social services

Data from:
☐ Medical record review ☐ Patient/family interview

Criteria	Yes	No
1. Patient provided with information about:		
a. Proper use of pain medications and comfort measures	☐	☐
b. Signs and symptoms of hypercalcemia	☐	☐
c. Measures to promote optimal level of functioning	☐	☐
d. Measures to reduce the risk of pathologic fractures	☐	☐
2. The following assessments are made at each visit:		
a. Pain	☐	☐
b. Serum calcium and/or ionized calcium	☐	☐
c. Functional status	☐	☐
d. Patient's understanding of instructions	☐	☐
3. Patient experienced the following complications:		
a. Accidental overdose of narcotic	☐	☐
b. Dehydration	☐	☐
c. Unrecognized pathologic fracture	☐	☐
d. Fall with injury	☐	☐
e. Other	☐	☐

Patient/family satisfaction

Data from:
☐ Patient interview ☐ Family interview

Criteria	Yes	No
1. On a scale of 0 to 10, with 0 being totally dissatisfied and 10 being totally satisfied, how satisfied were you with the pain management you received? ________		
2. Were you told to call the nurse if your pain was not controlled by the measures taught to you?	☐	☐
3. Were you taught to drink at least 2 L (6 large glasses) of fluid every day?	☐	☐

REFERENCES

Alexanian, R. & Dimopoulos, M. A. (1995). Management of multiple myeloma. *Seminars in Hematology, 32,* 20-30.

Alexanian, R. & Weber, D. (1996). Whither interferon for myeloma and other hematologic malignancies? *Annals of Internal Medicine, 124*(2), 264-265.

American Cancer Society. (1998). *Cancer facts and figures 1998.* Atlanta: Author.

American College of Physicians. (1992). Practice strategies for elective red blood cell transfusion. *Annals of Internal Medicine, 116,* 403-406.

American Red Cross, Council of Community Blood Centers, & American Association of Blood Banks. (1994). *Circular of information for the use of human blood and blood components.* Bethesda, MD: American Association of Blood Banks.

Armour Pharmaceutical. (1990). *Gammar: Immune globulin (human)* [package insert]. Kankakee, IL: Author.

Attal, M., Harousseau, J. L., Stoppa, A. M., Sotto, J. J., Fuzibet, J. G., Rossi, J. F., Casassus, P., Maisonneuve, H., Facon, T., Ifrah, N., Payen, C., & Bataille, R. (1996). A prospective, randomized trial of autologous bone marrow transplantation and chemotherapy in multiple myeloma. *New England Journal of Medicine, 335*(2), 91-97.

Barlogie, B. & Beck, T. (1993). Recombinant human erythropoietin and the anemia of multiple myeloma. *Stem Cells, 11*(2), 88-94.

Bartyl, R., Frisch, B., & Wilmans, W. (1995). Morphology of multiple myeloma. In J. S. Malpas, D. E. Bergsagel, & R. A. Kyle (Eds.), *Myeloma: Biology and management.* New York: Oxford University Press.

Bataille, R. (1996). Management of myeloma with biophosphonates. *New England Journal of Medicine, 334*(8), 529-530.

Bataille, R. & Klein, B. (1995). Cytokine therapy in myeloma. In J. S. Malpas, D. E. Bergsagel, & R. A. Kyle (Eds.), *Myeloma: Biology and management.* New York: Oxford University Press.

Bensinger, W. I., Rowley, S. D., Demirer, T., Lilleby, K., Schiffman, K., Clift, R. A., Applebaum, F. R., Fefer, A., Barnett, T., Storb, R., Chauncy, T., Maziarz, R. T., Klarnet, J., McSweeney, P., Holmberg, L., Maloney, D. G., Weaver, C. H., & Buckner, C. D. (1996). High-dose therapy followed by autologous hematopoietic stem-cell infusion for patients with multiple myeloma. *Journal of Clinical Oncology,14*(5), 1447-1456.

Berenson, J. R., Lichtenstein, A., Porter, L., Dimopoulos, M. A., Bordoni, R., George, S., Lipton, A., Keller, A., Ballester, O., Kovacs, M. J., Blacklock, H. A., Bell, R., Simeone, J., Reitsman, D. J., Heffernan, M., Seaman, J., & Knight, R. D. (1996). Efficacy of pamidronate in reducing skeletal events in patients with advanced multiple myeloma. *New England Journal of Medicine, 334*(8), 488-493.

Bergsagel, P. L., Smith, A. M., Szczepek, A., Mant, M. J., Belch, A. R., & Pilarski, L. M. (1995). In multiple myeloma, clonotypic B lymphocytes are detectable among CD19+ peripheral blood cells expressing CD38, CD56, and monotypic immunoglobulin light chains. *Blood, 85,* 436-447.

Blad'e, J., San Miguel, J. F., Fontanillas, M., Alcala, A., Moldanado, J., Conde, J. G., Conde, E., Brito, G. C., Moro, M. J., Escuerdo, M. L., Trujillo, J., Pascual, A., Rozman, C., Estape, J., & Montserrat, E., (1996). Survival of multiple myeloma patients who are potential candidates for early high-dose therapy intensification/autotransplantation and who were conventionally treated. *Journal of Clinical Oncology, 14*(7), 2167-2173.

Blesch, K. S. (1996). Rehabilitation of the cancer patient at home. *Seminars in Oncology Nursing, 12*(3), 219-225.

Boccadoro, M. & Pileri, A. (1995). Prognostic factors in multiple myeloma. In J. S. Malpas, D. E. Bergsagel, & R. A. Kyle (Eds.), *Myeloma: Biology and management.* New York: Oxford University Press.

Bolognia, J. & Braverman, I. M. (1994). Skin manifestations of internal disease. In K. J. Isselbacher, E. Braunwald, J. D. Wilson, J. B. Martin, A. Fauci, & D. L. Kaspter (Eds.), *Harrison's principles of internal medicine* (13th ed.). New York: McGraw-Hill.

Brenner, B. M. & Lazarus, J. M. (1994). Chronic renal failure. In K. J. Isselbacher, E. Braunwald, J. D. Wilson, J. B. Martin, A. Fauci, & D. L. Kaspter (Eds.), *Harrison's principles of internal medicine* (13th ed.). New York: McGraw-Hill.

Brinkman, P., Hay, D., & Laubinger, P. (1994). Chemotherapy toxicity assessment using a self-report tool. *Oncology Nursing Forum, 21*(10), 1731-1736.

Bubley, G. J. & Schnipper, L. E. (1995). Multiple myeloma. In G. P. Murphy, W. Lawrence, & R. E. Lenhard (Eds.), *American Cancer Society textbook of clinical oncology.* Atlanta: American Cancer Society.

Bunn, H. F. (1994). Anemia associated with chronic disorders. In K. J. Isselbacher, E. Braunwald, J. D. Wilson, J. B. Martin, A. Fauci, & D. L. Kaspter (Eds.), *Harrison's principles of internal medicine* (13th ed.). New York: McGraw-Hill.

Chapel, H. M., Lee, M., Hargreaves, R., Pamphilon, D. H., & Prentice, A. G. (1994). Randomized trial of intravenous immunoglobulins as prophylaxis against infection in plateau-phase multiple myeloma. *Lancet, 343,* 1059-1063.

Cooley, M. E., Moriarity, H., Berger, M. S., Orr, D. S., Coyle, B., & Short, T. (1995). Patient literacy and the readability of written cancer education materials. *Oncology Nursing Forum, 22*(9), 1345-1351.

Cook, G., Sharp, R. A., Tansey, P., & Franklin, I. M. (1996). A phase I/II trial of z-Dex (oral idarubicin and dexamethasone), an oral equivalent of VAD, as initial therapy at diagnosis or progression in multiple myeloma. *British Journal of Haematology, 93*(4), 931-934.

Creager, M. A. & Dzau, V. J. (1994). Vascular diseases of the extremities. In K. J. Isselbacher, E. Braunwald, J. D. Wilson, J. B. Martin, A. Fauci, & D. L. Kaspter (Eds.), *Harrison's principles of internal medicine* (13th ed.). New York: McGraw-Hill.

Dahnert, W. (1995). *Radiology review manual.* Baltimore: Williams & Wilkins.

Durie, B. G. & Salmon, S. E. (1975). A clinical staging system for multiple myeloma. *Cancer, 36,* 842-954.

Ferrell, B. R., Grant, M., Dean, G. E., Funk, B., & Ly, J. (1996). "Bone tired": The experience of fatigue and its impact on quality of life. *Oncology Nursing Forum, 23*(10), 1539-1547.

Garton, J. P., Gertz, M. A., Witzig, T. E., Greipp, P. R., Lust, J. A., Schroeder, G., & Kyle, R. A. (1995). Epoetin alfa for the treatment of the anemia of multiple myeloma. *Archives of Internal Medicine, 155,* 2069-2074.

Gerber, L. H., Levinson, S., Hicks, J. E., Gallelli, P., Whitehurst, J., Scheib, D., & Sonies, B. C. (1993). Evaluation and management of disability: Rehabilitation aspects of cancer. In V. T. DeVita, S. Hellman, & S. A. Rosenberg (Eds.), *Cancer: Principles and practice of oncology.* Philadelphia: J. B. Lippincott.

Gorski, L. A. & Grothman, L. (1996). Home infusion therapy. *Seminars in Oncology Nursing, 12*(3), 193-202.

Gregory, W. M., Richards, M. A., & Malpas, J. S. (1992). Combination chemotherapy versus melphalan and prednisone in the treatment of multiple myeloma: An overview of published trials. *Journal of Clinical Oncology,10,* 334-342.

Griffiths, M. & Leek, C. (1995). Patient education needs: Opinions of oncology nurses and patients. *Oncology Nursing Forum, 22*(1), 139-144.

Herriton, L. J., Weiss, N. S., & Olshan, A. F. (1995). Epidemiology of multiple myeloma. In J. S. Malpas, D. E. Bergsagel, & R. A. Kyle (Eds.), *Myeloma: Biology and management.* New York: Oxford University Press.

Hostetter, T. H. & Brenner, B. M. (1994). Tubulointerstitial diseases of the kidney. In K. J. Isselbacher, E. Braunwald, J. D. Wilson, J. B. Martin, A. Fauci, & D. L. Kaspter (Eds.), *Harrison's principles of internal medicine* (13th ed.). New York: McGraw-Hill.

Hussein, M. (1994). Multiple myeloma: An overview of diagnosis and management. *Cleveland Clinic Journal of Medicine, 61*(4), 285-298.

Joshua, D. E. (1995). Immunoglobulins. In J. S. Malpas, D. E. Bergsagel, & R. A. Kyle (Eds.), *Myeloma: Biology and management.* New York: Oxford University Press.

Klein, B. (1995). Cytokine and cytokine receptors in human multiple myeloma. In J. S. Malpas, D. E. Bergsagel, & R. A. Kyle (Eds.), *Myeloma: Biology and management.* New York: Oxford University Press.

Klein, B., Wijdenes, J., Zhang, H. G., Jourdan, M., Boiron, J. M., Brochier, J. M., Liautard, J., Merlin, M., Clement, C., Morel-Fournier, B., Lu, Z. Y., Mannoni, P., Sany, J., & Bataille, R. (1991). Murine anti–interleukin-6 monoclonal antibody therapy for a patient with plasma cell leukemia. *Blood, 78,* 1198-1204.

Kyle, R. A. (1992). Diagnostic criteria of multiple myeloma. *Hematology Oncology Clinics of North America, 6,* 347-358.

Kyle, R. A. (1995). Multiple myeloma and other plasma cell disorders. In R. Hoffman & L. E. Silberstein (Eds.), *Hematology.* New York: Churchill Livingstone.

Landis, S. H., Murray, T., Bolden, S., & Wingo, P. A. (1998). Cancer statistics, 1998. *CA: A Cancer Journal for Clinicians, 48*(1), 6-29.

Longo, D. L. (1994). Plasma cell disorders. In K. J. Isselbacher, E. Braunwald, J. D. Wilson, J. B. Martin, A. Fauci, & D. L. Kaspter (Eds.), *Harrison's principles of internal medicine* (13th ed.). New York: McGraw-Hill.

MacLennan, I. C., Hardie, D. L., Ball, J., & Drew, M. (1995). Antibody-secreting cells and their origin. In J. S. Malpas, D. E. Bergsagel, & R. A. Kyle (Eds.), *Myeloma: Biology and management.* New York: Oxford University Press.

Magrum, L. C., Bentzen, C., & Landmark, S. (1996). Pain management in home care. *Seminars in Oncology Nursing, 12*(3), 202-219.

Malpas, J. S. (1995). Clinical presentation and diagnosis. In J. S. Malpas, D. E. Bergsagel, & R. A. Kyle (Eds.), *Myeloma: Biology and management.* New York: Oxford University Press.

Mayer, D. K. & Kelleher, L. O. (1993). *Rehabilitation of people with cancer: An ONS position statement.* Pittsburgh: Oncology Nursing Society.

McEnroe, L. E. (1996). Role of the oncology nurse in home care: Family-centered practice. *Seminars in Oncology Nursing, 12*(3), 188-193.

McIntyre, O. R. (1995). Laboratory investigation of myeloma. In J. S. Malpas, D. E. Bergsagel, & R. A. Kyle (Eds.), *Myeloma: Biology and management.* New York: Oxford University Press.

McMillan, S. C. (1996). The quality of life of patients with cancer receiving hospice care. *Oncology Nursing Forum, 23*(8), 1221-1228.

McMillan, S. C. & Mahon, M. (1994). The impact of hospice services on the quality of life of primary caregivers. *Oncology Nursing Forum, 21*(7), 1189-1195.

McNally, J. C., Bohnet, N. L., & Lindquist, M. E. (1996). Hospice nursing. *Seminars in Oncology Nursing, 12*(3), 238-243.

Miaskowski, C. (1997). *Oncology nursing: An essential guide for patient care.* Philadelphia: W. B. Saunders.

Nail, L. M. & Winningham, M. L. (1995). Fatigue and weakness in cancer patients: The symptom experience. *Seminars in Oncology Nursing, 11*(4), 272-278.

Nordic Myeloma Study Group. (1996). Interferon-alpha-2b added to melphalan-prednisone for initial and maintenance therapy in multiple myeloma. *Annals of Internal Medicine, 124*(2), 212-222.

Oken, M. M. (1995). Multiple myeloma and other plasma cell dyscrasias. In R. R. Skeel & N. A. Lachant (Eds.), *Handbook of cancer chemotherapy.* Boston: Little, Brown.

Oken, M. M., Pomeroy, C., Weisdorf, D., & Bennett, J. M. (1996). Prophylactic antibiotics for the prevention of early infection in multiple myeloma. *American Journal of Medicine, 110*(6), 624-628.

Ortho Biotech. (1993). *Procrit: Epoetin alfa for injection* [package insert]. Raritan, NJ: Author.

Osterborg, A., Boogaerts, M. A., Cimino, R., Essers, U., Holowiecki, J., Juliusson, G., Jager, G., Najman, A., & Peest, D. (1996). Recombinant human erythropoietin in transfusion-dependent anemic patients with multiple myeloma and non–Hodgkin's lymphoma: A randomized multicenter study. *Blood, 87*(7), 2675-2682.

Pilarski, L. M., Masellis-Smith, A., Szczepeck, A., Mant, M. J., & Belch, A. R. (1996). Circulating clonotypic B cells in the biology of multiple myeloma: Speculations on the origin of myeloma. *Leukemia and Lymphoma, 22*(5-6), 375-383.

Roodman, G. D. & Spivak, J. L. (1991). *Handbook of anemia.* New York: CoMedica.

Salmon, S. E. & Cassady, J. R. (1993). Plasma cell neoplasms. In V. T. DeVita, S. Hellman, & S. A. Rosenberg (Eds.), *Cancer: Principles and practice of oncology.* Philadelphia: J. B. Lippincott.

Savage, D. G., Lindenbaum, J., & Garrett, T. J. (1982). Biphasic pattern of bacterial infection in multiple myeloma. *Annals of Internal Medicine, 96,* 47-50.

Seiden, M. V. & Anderson, K. C. (1995). Plasma cell dyscrasias. In J. S. Macdonald, D. G. Haller, & R. J. Mayer (Eds.), *Manual of oncology therapeutics.* Philadelphia: J. B. Lippincott.

Sheridan, C. A. (1996). Multiple myeloma. *Seminars in Oncology Nursing, 12*(1), 59-70.

Smith, S. L. (1996). Physical exercise as an oncology nurse intervention to enhance quality of life. *Oncology Nursing Forum, 23*(5), 771-786.

Sporeno, E., Savino, R., Ciapponi, L., Paonessa, G., Gabibbo, A., Lahm, A., Pulkki, S. R., Sun, R. X., Toniatti, C., Klein, B., & Ciliberto, G. (1996). Human interleukin-6 receptor superantagonists with high potency and wide spectrum on multiple myeloma cells. *Blood, 87*(11), 4510-4519.

Steele, R. G. & Fitch, M. I. (1996). Coping strategies of family caregivers of home hospice patients with cancer. *Oncology Nursing Forum, 23*(6), 955-960.

Tesch, H., Diehl, V., & Kibe, D. (1995). Molecular biology of myeloma. In J. S. Malpas, D. E. Bergsagel, & R. A. Kyle (Eds.), *Myeloma: Biology and management.* New York: Oxford University Press.

Torcea, M., Lucibello, M., Vannier, E., Fabiani, S., Miliani, A., Guidi, G., Spada, O., Dower, S. K., Sims, J. E., Shaw, A. R., Dinarello, C. A., Garaci, E., & Cozzolino, F. (1996). Modulation of osteoclast activating factor activity of multiple myeloma bone marrow cells by different interleukin-1 inhibitors. *Experimental Hematology, 24*(8), 868-874.

Winningham, M. L. (1991). Walking program for people with cancer: Getting started. *Cancer Nursing,14,* 270-276.

Winningham, M. L., Nail, L. M., Burke, M. B., Brophy, L., Cimprich, B., Jones, L. S., Holley, S. P., Rhodes, V., St. Pierre, B., Beck, S., Glass, E. C., Mock, V. L., Mooney, K. H., & Piper, B. (1994). Fatigue and the cancer experience: The state of the knowledge. *Oncology Nursing Forum, 21*(1), 23-36.

Non–Hodgkin's Lymphoma

Denise K. Hogan, RN, MS, OCN

The diagnosis of non–Hodgkin's lymphoma (NHL) includes a diverse group of neoplasms arising from the lymphoreticular system. Each of these diseases is identified by the clonal expansion of a developmental compartment of one of the lymphoid lineages (Aisenberg, 1995). Representing a broad spectrum of disease, these lymphomas range from rapidly progressive and often fatal malignancies to some of the most indolent of human tumors.

During the late nineteenth and early twentieth centuries, no distinction was made between Hodgkin's lymphoma (HD) and NHL. Various terms, such as *lymphosarcoma* and *reticulum cell sarcoma,* were some of the first introduced to distinguish lymphoproliferative diseases from others (Kundrat, 1893; Roulet, 1930). However, by the 1950s, NHL was recognized as a disease entity, identified by the absence of the characteristic HD Reed-Sternberg cell, in addition to other pathologic features (Greer, Macon, List, & McCurley, 1993; Rosenberg, 1993; Armitage, 1995). Merely differentiating between HD and NHL does not completely identify this complicated disease. Examining histopathologic features, reviewing clinical characteristics, and classifying accordingly have become the greatest challenges in successfully managing patients with this disease.

EPIDEMIOLOGY

The malignant lymphomas are the sixth most common cause of death from cancer in the United States (American Cancer Society, 1997). Incidence rates for HD have declined since the early 1970s (American Cancer Society, 1997). However, the incidence rates for NHL have increased approximately 75% over the same period. This has been observed to be the most rapid of all increases in cancer incidence (Hartge, Devesa, & Fraumeni, 1994). The increases have been seen in both males and females, but in different proportions (Aisenberg, 1995; American Cancer Society, 1997; Weisenburger, 1994). The largest increase in cancer incidence has been among elderly, white males. From 1947 through 1950 and from 1984 through 1988, incidence rates in white males age 75 years and older increased nearly 400% (Rabkin, Devesa, Zahm, & Gail, 1993). These disproportionate increases may be due to the fact that the diagnosis of NHL may have been missed more frequently in the older population because of less rigorous diagnostic evaluations.

In the past four decades a steady rise in age-adjusted mortality rates has been consistent with increased occurrence (Hartge, Devesa, & Fraumeni, 1994). In 1998 there were an estimated 55,400 new cases diagnosed and approximately 24,900 deaths from this disease (American Cancer Society, 1998). The changing mortality rates represent an increase of approximately 2% per year (Miller, Ries, Hankey, Kosary, & Edwards, 1992). These statistics, plus the young average age—42 years—of the lymphoma population ranks this disease fourth in terms of economic effects among cancers in the United States (Longo, DeVita, Jaffe, Mauch, & Urba, 1993).

Cases of NHL involving peripheral lymph nodes are more common in adults than in children and are usually of B cell origin (Greer, et al., 1993). Children often present with gastrointestinal involvement (small non-cleaved cell, B cell) or mediastinal widening (lymphoblastic lymphoma, T cell). Also, adults with NHL often have a more variable histologic appearance. They frequently present with low-grade, nodular patterns consisting of primarily small, dormant lymphocytes. In contrast, children usually have high-grade diffuse patterns in which the cells have a "blastic," or transformed, appearance and a high mitotic rate.

Whites have higher survival rates than African-Americans and women higher rates than men (Rabkin et al., 1993). In addition, the median age at diagnosis is younger in the African-American population than in the white population. Continued research is needed in this area to explain the rationale for these differences.

RISK FACTORS

The risk factors for NHL are largely unknown, but a variety of risk factors play a role in the etiologic factors of NHL, some with a more definitive association than others. These include viruses, immunosuppressive states (both genetic and acquired), family history, and occupational exposure to

Box 67-1
Risk Factors for Non–Hodgkin's Lymphoma

Inherited immunodeficiency disease
Acquired immunodeficiency states
Viral exposure (HIV, HTLV I, EBV)
Occupational exposure (pesticides, insecticides, solvents)
Hair dyes (? association)

Modified from American Cancer Society (1997). *Cancer facts and figures.* Atlanta: The Society; Hartge, P., Devesa, S. S., & Fraumeni, J. F. (1994). Hodgkin's and non–Hodgkin's lymphomas. *Cancer Surveys, 19-20,* 423-453; Rabkin, C. S., Devesa, S. S., Zahm, S. H., & Gail, M. H. (1993). Increasing incidence of non-Hodgkin's lymphoma. *Seminars in Hematology, 30*(4), 286-296.

HIV, Human immunodeficiency virus; *HTLV I,* human t-cell lymphotrophic virus, type 1; *EBV,* Epstein-Barr virus.

herbicides and pesticides (Box 67-1) (American Cancer Society, 1997; Hartge, Devesa, & Fraumeni, 1994; Rabkin et al., 1993; Weisenburger, 1994).

Immunosuppression

Immunosuppression has the strongest link to the increase in NHL (Rabkin et al., 1993). Genetic disorders characterized by a depressed immune system, such as Wiskott-Aldrich syndrome, ataxia telangiectasia, acute combined immunodeficiency, x-linked lymphoproliferative syndrome, and common variable immunodeficiency, have a significant predisposition to NHL (Filipovich, Mather, Kamat, & Shapiro, 1992). In addition, immunosuppressive states that result from therapy for an underlying disease (transplant recipients, autoimmune disorders such as rheumatoid arthritis, and Sjögren's and Hodgkin's disease) increase the risk of NHL (Levine & Hoover, 1992; Weisenburger, 1992).

Viruses

Several viruses have been identified as likely etiologic factors in the occurrence of NHL. Human immunodeficiency virus (HIV) infection, the cause of AIDS, has probably had a significant effect on the number of cases of NHL (primarily immunoblastic and small non-cleaved cell) since the early 1980s and will continue to in the future (Hartge, Devesa, & Fraumeni, 1994; Rabkin, et al., 1993). Human T lymphotrophic virus type I (HTLV I), a virus that has been relatively stable with low infectivity in the United States, is implicated in a small number of lymphoma cases, specifically adult T cell leukemia-lymphoma (ATL) (Hartge, Devesa, & Fraumeni, 1994). Japan and the Caribbean are considered high-risk areas of the world for this virus. Epstein-Barr virus (EBV), the probable cause of Burkitt's lymphoma, is frequently associated with lymphomas, which complicate immunodeficiency disorders.

Occupational Exposure

A variety of occupations with exposure to toxins, pesticides, solvents, hair dyes, and chemicals associated with woodworking are thought to increase the risk of NHL (Hartge, Devesa, & Fraumeni, 1994; Rabkin, et al., 1993). Contact with phenoxyacetic acid herbicides, specifically 2, 4 dichlorophenoxyacetic acid, may be responsible for this association (Zahm & Blair, 1992). Blair et al. reported excesses of NHL cases in groups working with industrial machinery production and in the dry-cleaning business (Blair, Linos, Stewart, Burmeister, Gibson & Everett et al., 1992). There also has been an increased incidence noted in persons who use hair coloring products (Zahm, Weisenberger, Babbitt, Saal, Vaught & Blair, 1992). In a study done by Zahm et al., there were significant risks observed for overall use of hair coloring products, with even higher risk noted for permanent, dark hair colors. The mechanisms causing these increased incidences are as yet unconfirmed and need further investigation.

PATHOPHYSIOLOGY

Normal Anatomy and Physiology of the Immune System

The body's immune system is a sophisticated mechanism of defense against invading microorganisms, with the potential to destroy malignant cells. The key components of the immune system are the T and B lymphocytes. These cells originate from a pluripotent stem cell in the bone marrow and undergo a process of differentiation where they mature into either the myeloid or lymphoid cell lines. Once determined to be of lymphoid nature, these cells are processed through the primary organs of the lymph system, namely the thymus and the bone marrow (Fig. 67-1). T and B lymphocytes also migrate to and populate the secondary lymphoid organs, which include the lymph nodes, spleen, oropharyngeal lymphoid tissues, and lymphoid aggregates in the fibrous connective tissue and submucosa of the respiratory and gastrointestinal tracts. The organs in the gastrointestinal tract are referred to as *Peyer's patches.* With the exception of the central nervous system (CNS), practically all tissues contain lymphocytes as part of the interstitial elements (Longo et al., 1993).

The immune function of lymphocytes is twofold. T lymphocytes are responsible for the cell-mediated immune responses. Recognition of foreign antigens, such as tumor cells or virally infected cells, and the ability to directly lyse or destroy them is the function of cytotoxic T cells. A different sublineage of T cells, termed *helper T cells,* have regulatory functions and act as helpers or suppressors for other lymphoreticular cells, such as B cells, macrophages, and other T cells.

The humoral immune system is the other arm of the immune system and is regulated by the B lymphocytes. As B lymphocytes differentiate and mature into plasma cells, they develop the ability to produce immunoglobulins or antibodies specific to various antigens. On encountering a foreign antigen, these B lymphocytes then produce antibodies against the antigen.

Lymph, the clear, watery fluid found in lymphatic vessels, is carried into and out of the nodes and organs via the afferent and efferent vessels (Fig. 67-2). Size and structure of lymph

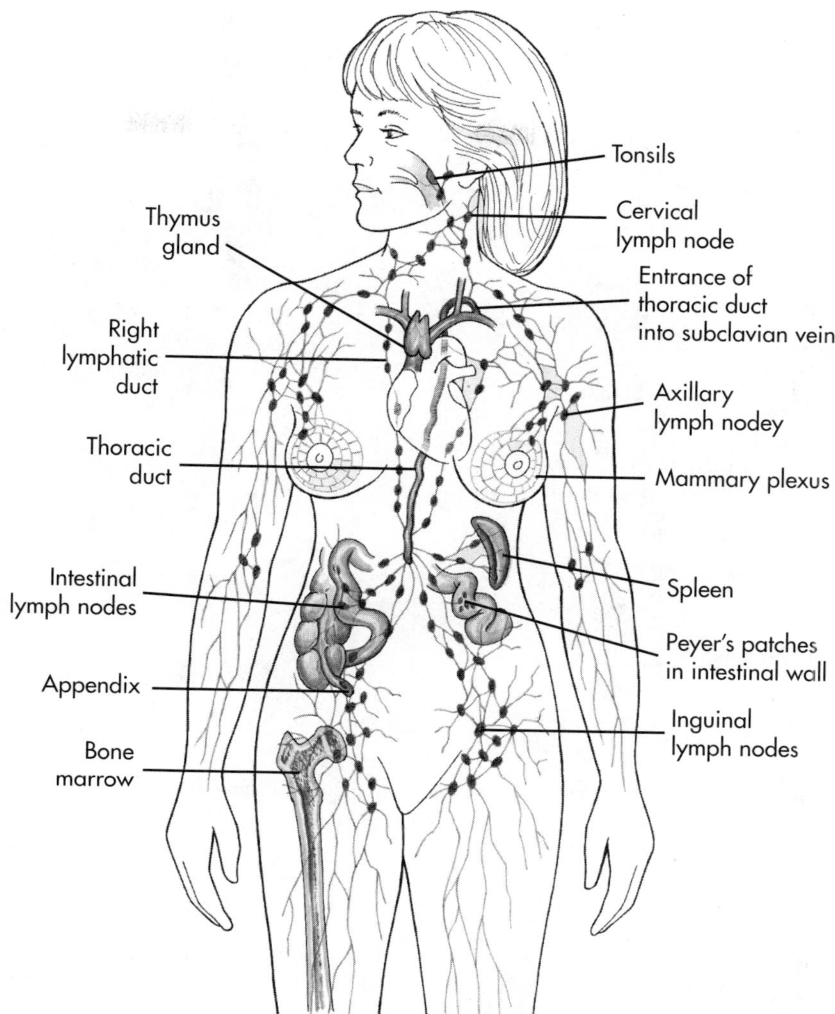

Fig. 67-1 Principal organs of the lymphatic system. (From Thibodeau, G. A., Patton, K. T. [Eds.]. [1996]. *Anatomy and physiology* [3rd ed.]. St. Louis: Mosby.)

nodes vary from 2 to 20 mm, depending upon the location and person's age. Lymph nodes in the abdomen, neck, and inguinal areas experience frequent antigenic stimulation and have proportionally larger and more numerous germinal centers (Miller, 1995). In contrast, mesenteric nodes have fewer germinal centers and wider medullary sinuses.

The distribution of T and B cells within the lymph node compartments is distinct. Peripheral node T cells are normally found in the paracortical and interfollicular areas (Miller, 1995). Concentration of B cells is usually in the lymphoid follicles and medullary zones. Specific cell marker staining is part of the identification process when determining cell type. Examining the architecture of lymph nodes is helpful in differentiating between a malignant process and a reactive one.

Process of Carcinogenesis

Evidence shows that neoplastic transformation is a multistep process that reflects the contribution of many factors. Several have been specifically implicated in the pathogenesis of NHL. They include cytogenetic abnormalities, molecular genetic events, viruses, immune suppression, oncogenes, and regulators of gene transcription and the cell cycle (Aisenberg, 1995).

Mutations in the chromosomal structure, such as translocations, deletions, or base-pair substitutions, are suspected as specific causes of NHL. This occurs through the transformation or loss of critical genes responsible for growth and differentiation (oncogenes and antioncogenes) (Greer et al., 1993). Several NHL subtypes are associated with specific chromosomal abnormalities. Examples include t(8;14)(q24;q32) in small non-cleaved B cell lymphomas, t(14;18) in follicular B cell lymphomas, and t(11;14)(q13;q32) in intermediate forms (Longo et al., 1993).

Activation of oncogenes can occur through chromosomal translocation, application, and point mutation (Gaidano, Pastore, Volpe, 1995). Chromosomal translocation is the most common mechanism in hematopoietic tumors. Oncogenes activated by chromosomal translocation include the

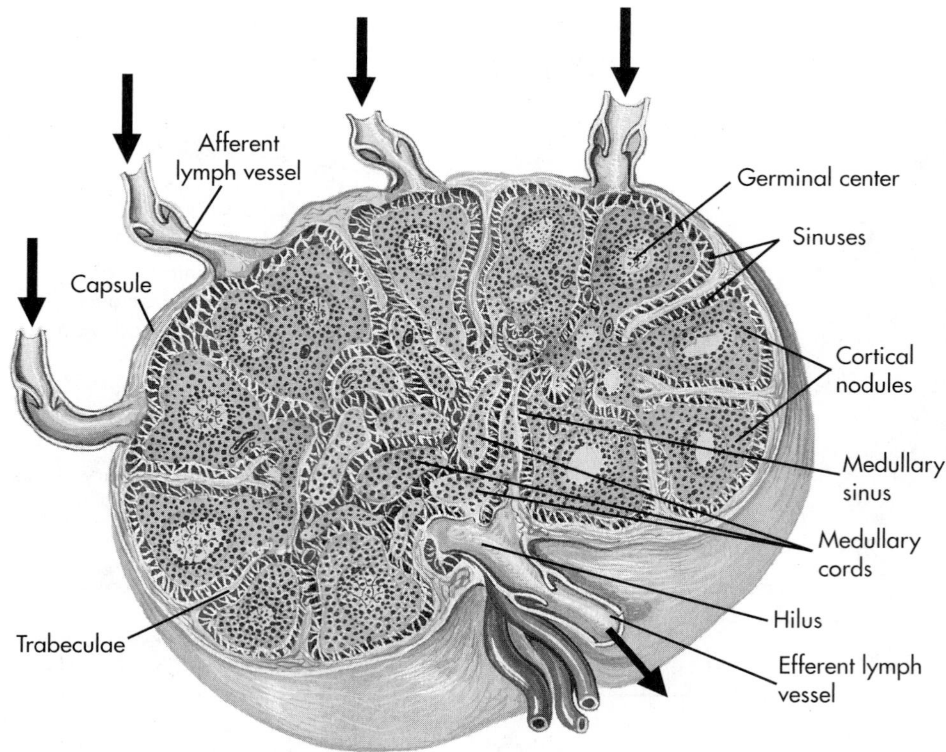

Fig. 67-2 Sites of lymphocyte transformation in the lymph node. (From Groenwald, S.L., Frogge, M.H., Goodman, M., Yarbro, C.H. [Eds.]. [1993]. *Cancer nursing: Principles and practice* [3rd ed.]. Boston: Jones and Barlett.)

c-*myc* oncogene associated with t(8;14) translocations, the B-cell leukemia lymphoma-2 gene (bcl 2) oncogene associated with t(14;18) translocation, and the bcl1 oncogene involved with the t(11;14) translocation (Longo et al., 1993). bcl2 and bcl1 are activated in certain subsets of low-grade NHL and the c-*myc* in a proportion of intermediate and high-grade lymphomas (Gaidano & Dalla-Favera, 1993). It is because of the deregulation of these genes that cell growth is promoted and programmed cell death is prevented.

ROUTES OF METASTASES

In contrast to HD, the predictable spread of disease in NHL is different. HD spreads contiguously from lymph node to lymph node. NHL's pattern of spread mimics that of the normal lymphocyte circulation and distribution throughout the entire body. As with solid tumors, which spread by direct invasion, local symptoms can occur as a result of compression from a diseased node or organ or the presence of extranodal disease.

ASSESSMENT

To properly manage the patient with NHL, a careful and complete diagnostic assessment needs to be performed. Table 67-1 outlines the requirements. The signs and symptoms reported are more closely related to the specific type of NHL than to the stage of the disease.

History

Obtaining a thorough social history on the patient helps identify any of the risk factors already mentioned. It is imperative to evaluate the patient for the occurrence of night sweats, fevers, nausea and vomiting, abdominal pain, and metabolic wasting leading to greater than 10% loss in body weight within the past 6 months. These characteristics are called "B" symptoms and confer a worse prognosis (Foon & Fisher, 1995). Other symptoms associated with NHL are listed in Box 67-2.

Physical Examination

Physical examination of all lymph node areas, including the cervical, supraclavicular, axillary, epitrochlear, retroperitoneal, mesenteric, iliac, inguinal, femoral, popliteal, and oropharyngeal (Waldeyer's ring), should be done to detect lymph node enlargement (Longo et al., 1993; Rosenberg, 1993). Lymph nodes positive for malignant cells are usually non-tender, firm, and rubbery (Foon & Fisher, 1995). Extranodal sites (skin, CNS) may be involved in intermediate- and high-grade lymphomas and therefore should be evaluated as appropriate.

TABLE 67-1 Assessment of the Patient for Non–Hodgkin's Lymphoma

	Assessment Parameters	Typical Abnormal Findings
History	A. Personal and social history 1. Age 2. Gender 3. Ethnicity 4. Immunosuppression	A. Personal and social risk factors 1. Over age 75 2. Males greater than females 4. Whites have greatest prevalence 4. Genetically caused immunosuppressed states such as Wiskott-Aldrich syndrome, ataxia telangiectasia, acute combined immunodeficiency, x-linked lymphoproliferative syndrome and common variable immunodeficiency or acquired immunosuppressed states that result from therapy for an underlying disease such as organ transplants, autoimmune diseases, and Hodgkin's disease.
	5. Environmental exposure to viruses	5. HIV, HTLV I, and EBV have all been implicated as potential etiologic factors.
	6. Occupational exposure to viruses	6. Exposure to toxins, pesticides, and solvents is thought to increase risk of NHL.
	B. Evaluation of occurrence of "B" symptoms	B. B symptoms include night sweats, fevers, metabolic wasting leading to greater than 10% loss in body weight in 6 months, and significant fatigue.
Physical Examination	A. Lymph node evaluation	A. Lymph node enlargement could be present in any of the following lymph node areas: cervical, supraclavicular, axillary, epitrochlear, retroperitoneal, mesenteric, iliac, inguinal, femoral, and oropharyngeal. B. Malignant lymph nodes are characteristically not tender, firm and rubbery.
Diagnostic Tests	A. Routine chemistry and hematology studies	A. Anemia, thrombocytopenia, or reticulocytosis could be present as a result of an autoimmune process or marrow replacement. 1. Elevated LDH levels are not uncommon in intermediate- and high-grade lymphomas.
	B. Lymph node biopsy	B. Excisional biopsy of largest lymph node or mass lesion is essential to confirm a diagnosis.
	C. Bone marrow biopsy	C. Bone marrow involvement may be characteristic of the NHL subtype or it may be an indicator of a more advanced stage.
	D. Lumbar puncture	D. Intermediate- and high-grade lymphomas with positive marrow involvement tend to have positive CNS disease.
	E. Chest x-ray	E. Will be abnormal if lymphadenopathy present in chest.
	F. CT of chest, abdomen, and pelvis	F. Will reveal enlarged nodes or masses if present; these are useful in staging disease.
	G. Gallium scan	G. If large masses are detected, they are easily followed for response to therapy via gallium.
	H. Upper gastrointestinal series with small bowel follow-through and barium enema	H. Patients with gastrointestinal symptoms or Waldeyer's ring involvement often have gastrointestinal lymphoma.
	I. Leukocyte common oncogene test	I. Distinguishes between lymphoid and nonlymphoid malignancies using monoclonal antibodies.
	J. Ki-67 test	J. Measures cellular proliferation with monoclonal antibodies.

From Hubbard, S. M. (1996). Current issues and controversies in the management of non–Hodgkin's lymphoma. In *Management for the oncology nurse* (2nd ed.). New York: Triclinica.

HIV, Human immunodeficiency virus; *HTLV* I, human t-cell leukemia/lymphoma virus; *EBV,* Epstein-Barr virus; *LDH,* lactic dehydrogenase; *CT,* computed tomography; *CNS,* central nervous system

Laboratory

Routine chemistry and hematology studies are indicated. If anemia or reticulocytosis is detected, a Coomb's test should be performed to rule out the presence of autoimmune hemolytic anemia. Thrombocytopenia could also be present as a result of an autoimmune process, or it could be caused by marrow replacement or hypersplenism. Autoimmune problems in addition to marrow involvement are more common in low-grade lymphomas (Foon & Fisher, 1995). An elevated serum lactic dehydrogenase level, which is a poor prognostic factor, is more common in intermediate- and high-grade lymphomas and may indicate to the physician rapid cell turnover or a large tumor burden and a need to hydrate before treatment (Longo et al., 1993; Foon & Fisher, 1995).

Lymph Node Biopsy

An excisional biopsy of the largest lymph node or mass lesion is usually essential to establish an accurate diagnosis. Extranodal disease may require a surgical biopsy of the area involved to provide the pertinent information. Needle biopsy and aspiration are not recommended for an initial diagnosis because the sample may not reveal the nodal architecture, which has important implications, and because these samples are small and could possibly miss disease. In addition, small sample sizes limit the number of ancillary studies that can be performed. This could alter data interpretation and, in turn, result in a less-effective treatment choice. Examples of routine and ancillary studies to be performed that may be critical for an accurate diagnosis include histologic, immunologic, molecular, immunoglobulin and T-cell receptor gene rearrangement, oncogene rearrangement, cytogenetics, and flow cytometry (Foon & Fisher, 1995). Patient preparations for a lymph node biopsy are included in Table 67-2.

Bone Marrow Biopsy

Bone marrow involvement in NHL may vary, depending upon the disease subtype and stage. Focal or spotty involvement of the marrow is not uncommon, especially early in the disease course. Therefore, bilateral bone marrow biopsies are generally required for staging. Indolent lymphomas have a higher incidence (20% to 95%) of bone marrow involvement than the more aggressive lymphomas (10%) (Foon & Fisher, 1995). Patients with intermediate- and high-grade lymphomas and marrow involvement have a greater likelihood of CNS disease and should undergo a lumbar puncture (Rosenberg, 1993; Foon & Fisher, 1995).

Radiographic Studies

All patients with NHL should have chest roentgenograms (CXR). About one fourth of the cases will have abnormalities, the most frequent being mediastinal adenopathy (18%), followed by pleural effusions (8%), and parenchymal involvement (4%) (Longo et al., 1993). If a CXR proves to be questionable, a chest computed tomographic (CT) scan should be performed for greater detail and to identify any other involved areas. A lymphangiogram was once used for this purpose but has been eliminated from the diagnostic regimen (Longo et al., 1993; Foon & Fisher, 1995). CT of the abdomen and pelvis is recommended in all patients to evaluate for enlarged nodes or masses. Abdominal CT scans are especially useful in patients with mesenteric nodal disease or kidney, bone, spleen, or liver involvement.

Gallium scans may also be useful in detecting large masses or disseminated disease. In addition, gallium scanning has shown to be beneficial in evaluating tumor response, especially when a residual mass is noted. Ultrasonography and magnetic resonance imagery may complement or clarify other test results or be more appropriate for evaluating certain body systems, such as the renal collecting system (Rosenberg, 1993).

Gastrointestinal lymphoma is not an unusual occurrence and is frequently associated with those patients with Waldeyer's ring involvement. As a result, anyone with gastrointestinal symptoms, mesenteric lymphadenopathy, or Waldeyer's ring lymphoma should have an upper gastro-

Box 67-2

Common Presenting Symptoms of Patients with Non–Hodgkin's Lymphoma

1. Flu-like symptoms, fatigue, "B" symptoms, night sweats, fever, and weight loss
2. Enlarged, "rubbery," painless lymph nodes in the neck, axilla, or groin that are unresponsive to antimicrobial therapy
3. Decreased appetite, weight loss, abdominal fullness, indigestion, abdominal pain, or bloating
4. Pressure or pain in lower back, extending down the legs; headache and diplopia
5. Pruritus
6. Cough, congestion in the face, neck, and upper chest

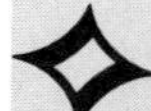

TABLE 67-2 Patient Preparation for an Excisional Lymph Node Biopsy

Description of the Procedure: Excisional lymph node biopsy is the total removal of a lymph node to test for malignant disease.

Patient Preparation: If your doctor plans on giving you medication through your veins to help you relax, you may be asked not to eat or drink anything for 8 hours before the test.

Procedural Considerations

1. You will be asked to sign an informed consent.
2. The procedure may be done in an outpatient surgical area or in the doctor's office.
3. The doctor injects medication into the area of the lymph node so that you feel nothing when the incision (cut) is made.
4. An incision is made, and the entire lymph node and possibly some tissue around it is removed.
5. The incision is then closed with surgical thread.
6. A sterile dressing is placed over the site for 24 hours.
7. Your doctor will ask you to watch for any bleeding, unusual swelling, or foul-smelling drainage.
8. You will be given a phone number to contact your physician on a 24-hour basis if you are having problems.
9. You will be asked to return in approximately 1 week to have your stitches removed.

intestinal series with a small bowel follow-through and barium enema. Staging laparotomies are rarely indicated.

STAGING

Ann Arbor Classification

The Ann Arbor staging classification (Table 67-3), which is used for Hodgkin's disease, is the standard staging system used for NHL (Carbone, Kaplan, Musshof, Smithers, & Tubiana, 1971). The number of involved sites and their relation to the diaphragm, the presence of B symptoms, and the existence of extranodal disease are all part of this staging classification. No adequate alternative staging systems have been developed for NHL despite the fact that there are noted deficiencies in the Ann Arbor model (Longo et al., 1993; Rosenberg, 1993; Foon & Fisher, 1995). This system is useful in defining patient composition but inadequate in conveying prognostic information needed to determine therapeutic decisions (Longo et al., 1993; Rosenberg, 1993). Size or bulk of the lymphoma mass at presentation, bone marrow involvement, performance status, and serum LDH levels are important prognostic factors not included in the Ann Arbor system (Greer et al., 1993; Longo et al.,1993; Rosenberg, 1993). These features may be indicative of tumor load, chemotherapy tolerance potential, aggressiveness of disease, and the ability to achieve and maintain a remission.

Histopathologic Classification

The histopathologic classification of NHL is one of the most important areas of study and at the same time one of the most complicated. NHL is subdivided in such a way as to predict prognosis and guide treatment. Characteristics identified as key in classifying various forms of NHL include the absence or presence of follicular structure, cell size, and details of nuclear and cytoplasmic structure (Aisenberg, 1995; Rosenberg, 1993). Over the past 150 years, six different pathologic classification systems have been developed and used throughout the world (Aisenberg, 1995; Longo et al., 1993; Rosenberg, 1993). This has made analysis and comparison of clinical trial data difficult and less meaningful.

TABLE 67-3 Ann Arbor Staging System

Stage I	Restricted to one lymph node–bearing area
Stage II	Two or more areas of nodal involvement on one side of the diaphragm
Stage III	Lymphatic involvement on both sides of the diaphragm
Stage IV	Liver, marrow, or other extensive, extranodal disease
Symptom status A	Absence of fevers, sweats, or weight loss
Symptom status B	Unexplained fevers higher than 38° C, drenching night sweats, weight loss of more than 10% of body weight in the preceding 6 months
Clinical stage	The assigned stage based only on history, physical findings, and laboratory and radiologic studies
Pathologic stage	The assigned stage based only on areas of biopsy-proven involvement
Substage E	Localized, extranodal disease

Modified from Carbone, P. P., Kaplan, H. S., Musshof, K., Smithers, D. W., & Tubiana, M. (1971). Report of the committee on Hodgkin's staging classification. *Cancer Research, 31,* 1860.

Rappaport Classification

The Rappaport classification, developed approximately 50 years ago, has been the most popular classification in the United States (Longo et al., 1993; Rosenberg, 1993). It proved useful for about 20 years until advances in cellular immunology took place, resulting in a greater understanding of the immune system and consequently a recognition of the inaccuracies of the Rappaport scheme. Between the 1970s and the 1980s several other classification schemes were introduced, none of which were unanimously accepted. In the early 1980s an international study undertaken by the National Cancer Institute resulted in the development of the Working Formulation, a classification scheme that attempts to provide morphologic classification with prognostic relevance, utilizing common language that allows translation from one classification scheme to another (Box 67-3). Although useful, the Working Formulation also has limitations, such as excluding new disease entities and inaccurate groupings of histologically related subtypes (Greer et al., 1993; Longo et al., 1993). The current major subtypes of NHL are classified in Table 67-4. As a result, no scheme is universally agreed upon, making the classification of NHL still a clinical challenge.

Box 67-3
Working Formulation of Tumor Grading

Low Grade

Small lymphocytic consistent with CLL
Plasmacytoid
Follicular, predominantly small cleaved cell
Follicular, mixed small cleaved and large cell

Intermediate Grade

Follicular, large cell
Diffuse, small cleaved cell
Diffuse, large cell

High Grade

Large cell immunoblastic
Lymphoblastic
Small noncleaved cell
- Burkitt's
- Non-Burkitt's

TABLE 67-4 Major Subtypes and Frequency of Non–Hodgkin's Lymphoma

Subtype	Frequency (%)
Diffuse large B cell	31
Follicular	22
Marginal zone < mucosa-associated lymphoid tissue	8
Peripheral T cell	7
Small lymphocytic (B cell)	7
Mantle cell	6
Primary mediastinal large B cell	2
Anaplastic large T/NK-cell	2
High-grade, B cell Burkitt's-like	2
Marginal zone, nodal	2
Lymphoblastic, T cell	2
Burkitt's	<1

Modified from Armitage, J. O. (1995.) The changing classification of non–Hodgkin's lymphomas. Non–Hodgkin's lymphoma. *CA: A cancer Journal for Clinicians. 47(6)*: 323-325.

MEDICAL MANAGEMENT

To determine the most effective treatment approach, the tumor histology, stage of the disease, and age and physiologic status of the patient should be considered. The histologic diagnosis is probably the best single prognostic indicator (Longo et al., 1993). Even though most NHL subtypes are responsive to chemotherapy and/or radiation therapy, an accurate histologic diagnosis can distinguish between indolent and aggressive disease and subsequently guide the physician in the selection of the most effective treatment choice. The Working Formulation classifies NHL subtypes according to their natural histories and responsiveness to treatment. In this way the likelihood of a patient responding to a certain treatment regimen can be anticipated, based on responses of comparable patients.

The second determinant reviewed when deciding appropriate treatment is disease extent. For cases of indolent lymphomas, accurate identification of stage I and stage II disease could mean a cure with radiation therapy only. The importance of distinguishing between stages III and IV in the indolent lymphomas is less crucial because there are many acceptable treatment options, all with a low likelihood of cure. For those with intermediate-grade lymphoma, staging also affects therapeutic options. In cases of high-grade lymphoma, most patients have disseminated disease at diagnosis, and all of these cases receive high-dose combination chemotherapy (Longo et al., 1993).

The third and final component of the treatment approach to be evaluated is the patient's physiologic status. Many patients with lymphoma are older than 65 years of age at diagnosis. However, advanced age is not an indication to withhold a potentially effective combination chemotherapy program (Longo et al., 1993). The lymphomas seen in older people are often the types curable with aggressive chemotherapy. Underlying medical problems, such as pulmonary, cardiac, renal, or hepatic disease may complicate the choice of therapy for older adults with lymphoma. If this is the case, choosing an alternative therapy such as one with less toxicity or reduced doses is the recommendation. Myelotoxicity tends to be increased in the older patient population. Therefore dose reductions may be appropriate.

Treatment of NHL is determined primarily by histologic stage and grade. The various treatment options are presented in this manner.

Low-Grade Lymphomas

The management of low-grade lymphomas is an area of great controversy. The disease is characterized by a long median survival, but a survival that slowly and continuously declines (Greer et al., 1993). Treatment of early-stage (I and II) disease does not present questions. Whether any treatment can induce long-term, disease-free survival in those with advanced-stage (III and IV) disease is the issue of debate.

Low-grade lymphomas are relatively rare in younger individuals, as evidenced by the median age being between 50 and 70 years old (Weisenburger, 1991). More than 80% of the low-grade cases will present as a clinical stage III or IV. Marrow involvement is dependent upon the histologic subtype. The greatest incidence of marrow involvement (70% to 80%) is seen in those patients with small lymphocytic (SL), and the lowest incidence (25% to 35%) in those with follicular mixed (FML) and large cleaved cell lymphoma (Weisenburger, 1991).

Radiation Therapy. Early-stage, low-grade NHL accounts for approximately 10% to 20% of the indolent lymphomas (Paryani, Hoppe, Cox, Colby, Rosenberg, & Kaplan, 1983; Stein, Greer, Cousar, Hendey, Wehner, & Flexner et al., 1989). Radiation therapy (>3000 cGy), which is considered standard treatment, is a potentially curable therapy in this population of patients, producing complete remissions (CR) of significant length (Longo et al., 1993). The extent of irradiation and the efficacy of combination chemotherapy are controversial. Complete staging and an accurate diagnosis are of great importance to avoid overtreating occult stage IV disease.

Most clinical trials involving early-stage, low-grade NHL involve patients with follicular small cleaved (FSCL) and FML. In a study of patients from Stanford with stage I or II follicular lymphoma, survival at 5, 10, and 15 years was 84%, 68% and 42%, respectively (Paryani et al., 1983). In 80% of those who were 40 years old or younger, involved-field, extended-field, or total nodal irradiation (TNI) appeared to cure them. Because some patients treated with less than TNI tend to relapse outside of the field limits, controversy regarding the size of the radiation field has arisen (Longo et al., 1993). The role of adjuvant chemotherapy and its effects on long-term survival in patients with early-stage, low-grade lymphoma has not yet been established.

As stated earlier, the majority of patients with low-grade lymphomas present with advanced stage III or IV disease, which responds to single-agent chemotherapy, multiple-agent chemotherapy, radiation therapy, and combined modality therapy. Although many of the treatment options produce 60% to 75% CR rates, these are of short duration and have not been shown to improve patient survival (Longo et al., 1993; Fisher & Oken, 1995). Relapse rates of approximately 10% to 15% per year are found regardless of therapy (Longo et al., 1993).

Chemotherapy. Standard chemotherapy for low-grade lymphoma utilizes the alkylating agents, alone or in combination. As single agents, chlorambucil and cyclophosphamide are the drugs of choice. Used separately, complete clinical responses can be achieved, though very slowly. The advantage to this approach is the low incidence of acute toxicities. But because these drugs are often administered daily for prolonged periods of time, these patients are at an increased risk of acute myelogenous leukemia and other diseases (Fisher & Oken, 1995). Combination chemotherapy for advance-stage, low-grade lymphoma has been shown to induce remissions more quickly than single-agent chemotherapy but has resulted in no difference in relapse-free or overall survival (Longo et al., 1993).

Radiation therapy in the forms of total lymphoid irradiation (TLI) and total body irradiation (TBI) are other options for treatment of stage III and stage IV low-grade lymphoma. They can be used alone or in combination with chemotherapy. When used alone, neither has resulted in durable complete remissions (Longo et al., 1993).

Watch and Wait. Lack of treatment-related improvements in disease-free and overall survival prompted a study led by Rosenberg and colleagues to evaluate a "watch and wait" approach in comparison to other treatment regimens (Portlock & Rosenburg, 1979). Survival in the "watch and wait" patient group was approximately the same as for patients receiving other therapies. For those patients who do not undergo initial therapy upon diagnosis, frequent medical evaluations are recommended so as not to neglect progressive disease symptoms (Fisher & Oken, 1995). Median time before therapy is required is 3 years, and approximately 20% of patients will not require any therapy for up to 10 years.

There appear to be advantages and disadvantages to instituting the "watch and wait" approach (Longo et al., 1993). One advantage is avoidance of therapy side effects such as myelosuppression and possible second tumors. In a patient who experiences a spontaneous regression, it would mean avoidance of unnecessary therapy or, in the case of a patient whose disease transforms to a higher-grade lymphoma, it would mean avoidance of potentially ineffective treatment. Disadvantages include persistent discomfort from bulky disease, problems associated with chronic administration of alkylating agents once therapy is begun, and data suggesting that two groups (FM and any stage III) may experience long-term, disease-free survival after appropriate therapy.

The transformation of a low-grade lymphoma to a high-grade lymphoma is often termed *Richter's syndrome.* Diffuse large cell or immunoblastic are the most frequently occurring types. Approximately 25% of patients with SL will show evidence of this progression at autopsy (Garvin, Simon, & Osborne, 1983). A rapid enlargement of one or more involved nodal sites and the development of new symptoms characterize this phenomenon.

Other therapies being investigated for use in the treatment of low-grade lymphomas include bone marrow and stem cell transplantation (allogeneic and autologous), monoclonal antibodies, interferon, and several new chemotherapeutic agents. Each is briefly explained below.

Bone Marrow or Peripheral Stem Cell Transplantation. The use and timing of allogeneic or autologous peripheral stem cell or bone marrow transplants in patients with low-grade lymphomas are still under debate. At present, bone marrow and stem cell transplants are being considered in those cases in which other systemic treatment regimens have failed. There is no evidence that indolent lymphoma is curable by a bone marrow transplant, but long, disease-free remission has resulted (Fisher & Oken, 1995). The question of final outcome has yet to be determined (see Chapters 8 and 9).

Monoclonal Antibodies. Monoclonal antibodies (MoAbs) have been used to treat low-grade, B-cell lymphoma patients with limited success. As stated by Grossbard and Nadler (1993), the majority of patients receiving MoAb therapy have undergone extensive prior therapy and have disease that is refractory to conventional therapies. It was noted that these treatments could be safely administered to patients, and that there were some transient responses, with occasional complete responses and partial responses. It remains to be seen if MoAb-bases therapies can produce significant, lasting clinical responses.

Biologic Therapy. Interferon $\propto$ (IFN$\propto$) alone, and in combination with chemotherapy, has shown activity in low-grade lymphoma. There has been a prolongation of time to treatment failure seen in patients treated with combined IFN-chemotherapy but no strong survival benefit noted (Parkinson, Sznol, & Cheson, 1993). As observed by Parkinson, Sznol and Cheson, a more appropriate application of IFN $\propto$ in the treatment of hematologic malignancies may be following induction of complete remission by chemotherapy.

Purine Analogues. Although low-grade lymphoma usually responds to chemotherapy, most patients will eventually relapse and die of either their disease or a complication of their disease (Fisher & Oken, 1995). As a result, new drugs and drug combinations are being investigated for use in the treatment of low-grade NHL. Several promising agents in the category of purine analogues have demonstrated activity in relapsed and refractory low-grade NHL. They are fludarabine, deoxycoformycin (DCF), and 2-chlorodeoxyadenosine (2CdA) (Longo et al., 1993; Fisher & Oken, 1995; Cheson, 1993). Fludarabine and 2CdA have shown significant activity in chronic lymphocytic leukemia (CLL) and relapsed low-grade lymphoma, but further research in less heavily treated or untreated patients is needed to accurately evaluate the benefits of these new drugs (Cheson, 1993).

Intermediate-Grade Lymphomas

The three diseases classified as intermediate-grade lymphomas according to the Working Formulation include follicu-

TABLE 67-5 Adverse Prognostic Factors

Age > 60	B symptoms
Stage III or IV disease	Masses ≥ 10 cm
Two or more extranodal sites	
Poor performance status	
Abnormal serum lactate dehydrogenase	
Intermediate- or high-grade histology	

Modified from Foon, K. & Fisher, R. (1995). Lymphomas. In E. Beutler, M. A Lichtman, B. S. Coller, & T. J. Kipps, (Eds.), *William's hematology* (5th ed.). New York: McGraw-Hill.

lar predominantly large cell, diffuse small cleaved-cell, and diffuse large cell lymphoma. However, immunoblastic lymphoma, although classified as high-grade, is treated similarly to intermediate-grade lymphomas based upon response to treatment and prognosis. The most common of these is the diffuse large cell type, a rather invasive form that could compress blood vessels and airways (Fisher & Oken, 1995). Many patients with intermediate-grade lymphomas who achieve a CR with therapy may be cured. Choice of therapy should be based upon clinical stage rather than histologic subtype (Foon & Fisher, 1995). Prognosis for those patients with early-stage disease, specifically stages I and II (good prognostic factors) is better than for those with advanced-

TABLE 67-6 Chemotherapy Regimens for Non–Hodgkin's Lymphoma

Agent(s)	Dose	Route	Day(s) of Treatment
CVP			
Cyclophosphamide	400 mg/m^2	PO	1-5
Vincristine	1.4 mg/m^2 (maximum 2 mg)	IV	1
Prednisone	100 mg/m^2	PO	1-5
CHOP			
Cyclophosphamide	750 mg/m^2	IV	1
Doxorubicin	50 mg/m^2	IV	1
Vincristine	1.4 mg/m^2 (maximum 2 mg)	IV	1
Prednisone	100 mg	PO	1-5
ProMACE/CYTABOM			
Cyclophosphamide	650 mg/m^2	IV	1
Doxorubicin	25 mg/m^2	IV	1
Etoposide	120 mg/m^2	IV	1
Cytarabine	300 mg/m^2	IV	8
Bleomycin	5 mg/m^2	IV	8
Vincristine	1.4 mg/m^2	IV	8
Methotrexate	120 mg/m^2	IV	8
Leucovorin	25 mg/m^2	PO	9(q6h × 4)
Prednisone	60 mg/m^2	PO	1-14
Cotrimoxazole	2 PO bid		
MACOP-B			
Methotrexate	400 mg/m^2	IV	8, 36, 64
Leucovorin	15 mg/m^2	PO (q6h × 6)	9, 37, 65
Doxorubicin	50 mg/m^2	IV	1, 15, 29, 43, 57, 71
Vincristine	1.4 mg/m^2	IV	8, 22, 36, 50, 64, 78
Bleomycin	10 mg/m^2	IV	22, 50, 78
Prednisone	75 mg	PO	1-84 (tapered over days 70-84)
Cotrimoxazole	2 PO bid		
m-BACOD			
Methotrexate	200 mg/m^2	IV	8, 15
Leucovorin	10 mg/m^2	PO (q6h × 6)	9, 16
Bleomycin	4 mg/m^2	IV	1
Doxorubicin	45 mg/m^2	IV	1
Cyclophosphamide	600 mg/m^2	IV	1
Vincristine	1 mg/m^2	IV	1
Dexamethasone	6 mg/m^2	PO	1-5

Modified from Foon, K. & Fisher, R. (1995). Lymphomas. In E. Beutler, M. A Lichtman, B. S. Coller, & T. J. Kipps, (Eds.), *William's hematology* (5th ed.). New York: McGraw-Hill.

stage disease, specifically stages II (one or more poor prognostic factors), III, and IV. Adverse prognostic factors are listed in Table 67-5.

Initially, patients with localized intermediate-grade lymphoma were treated with involved-field or extended-field radiation. Those who relapsed were doing so at distant sites. Therefore investigators chose to incorporate chemotherapy, usually CHOP (cyclophosphamide, doxorubicin, vincristine, prednisone)–based regimens, into the treatment plan and response rates improved (Table 67-6). Chemotherapy alone proved to be sufficient. Ongoing studies are now investigating the optimal number of cycles of CHOP chemotherapy for these patients (Foon & Fisher, 1995).

Chemotherapy. For those patients with advanced-stage intermediate lymphoma, chemotherapy can be curative. Much research has been conducted over the years comparing various chemotherapy regimens for efficacy and long-term survival. The first generation of chemotherapy regimens, developed in the mid 1960s and 1970s, included four or five chemotherapeutic agents and produced CR rates in approximately half of the patients. Assuming that a more intensive regimen with a greater number of chemotherapy agents would improve CR rates, several new, complex treatment plans were developed. These included ProMACE-CytoBOM (prednisone, methotrexate; doxorubicin, cyclophosphamide, and etoposide followed by cytarabine,

TABLE 67-6 Chemotherapy Regimens for Non–Hodgkin's Lymphoma—cont'd

Agent(s)	Dose	Route	Day(s) of Treatment
ESHAP (for relapsed lymphoma)			
Etoposide	60 mg/m^2	IV/2 h	1-4
Methylprednisolone	500 mg/m^2	IV	1-4
Cytarabine	2 g/m^2	IV/3 h	5
Cisplatin	25 mg/m^2	CIV	1-4
DHAP (for relapsed lymphoma)			
Dexamethasone	40 mg	PO or IV	1-4
Cisplatin	100 mg/m^2	CIV	1
Cytarabine	2 g/m^2	IV/q12h × 2	2
MIME (for relapsed lymphoma)			
Methyl-GAG	500 mg/m^2	IV	1, 14
Ifosfamide	1 g/m^2	IV	1-5
Methotrexate	30 mg/m^2	IV or IM	3
Etoposide	100 mg/m^2	IV	1-3
MINE (for relapsed lymphoma)			
Mesna	1.33 g/m^2 mixed with ifosfamide	IV	1-3
	500 mg	PO	1-3, 4 h after ifosfamide
Ifosfamide	1.33 g/m^2		
Mitoxantrone	8 mg/m^2	IV/1h	1-3, over 1 h
Etoposide	65 mg/m^2	IV/15 min.	1
		IV/1h	1-3
DICE (for relapsed lymphoma)			
Dexamethasone	10 mg	IV bolus q6h	1-4
Ifosfamide	1 g/m^2 (maximum, 1.75 g)	IV	1-4
Mesna	200 mg/m^2	IV	1 h before each ifosfamide infusion, days 1-4, immediately followed by a continuous infusion of 900 mg/m^2/d, and continued for 12 h after last dose of ifosfamide
Cisplatin	25 mg/m^2	IV	1-4
Etoposide	100 mg/m^2	IV	1-4
ICE (for relapsed lymphoma)			
Ifosfamide (with mesna uroprotection)	2 g/m^2	IV	Divided doses, days 1 and 2
Carboplatin	400 mg/m^2	IV	Divided doses, days 1 and 2
Etoposide	600 mg/m^2	CI	Divided doses, days 1 and 2

bleomycin, vincristine, and methotrexate with leucovorin rescue) and ProMACE-MOPP (prednisone, methotrexate, doxorubicin, cyclophosphamide, and etoposide alternating with nitrogen mustard, vincristine, procarbazine, and prednisone). MACOP-B (methotrexate with leucovorin rescue, doxorubicin, cyclophosphamide, vincristine, prednisone, and bleomycin), and m-BACOD (methotrexate with leucovorin rescue, bleomycin, doxorubicin, cyclophosphamide, vincristine, and dexamethasone). For various combination chemotherapy regimens, see Table 67-6. Phase II trials utilizing these new regimens resulted in very encouraging results. However, single-institution trials may have been biased by patient selection issues such as age and limited stage. It became evident that some form of phase III trial was needed to compare first-, second-, and third-generation treatment regimens.

In 1984 the Eastern Cooperative Oncology Group started a randomized controlled clinical trial of patients with advanced diffuse NHL to determine differences in CR rates, survival, and toxicity of those patients treated with CHOP versus m-BACOD. Results reported by Gordon et al. indicated no difference between the two regimens in complete response rates, overall survival, time to treatment failure, or disease or disease-free survival (Gordon, Harrington, Andersen, Colgan, Glick, & Neiman et al., 1992). However, significant differences were noted in severe and life-threatening toxicities: the m-BACOD group experienced more grades 3 and 4 pulmonary toxicity, infection, leukopenia, stomatitis, and thrombocytopenia. In 1986, the Southwest Oncology Group and Eastern Cooperative Oncology Group conducted a study comparing CHOP and three other combinations—m-BACOD, ProMACE-CYTABOM, and MACOP-B—in patients with intermediate- and high-grade NHL (Fisher, Gaynor, Dalberg, Oken, Grogan, & Mize, et al., 1993). The results yielded similar failure-free and overall survival rates, but CHOP was less costly and less severely toxic. Therefore CHOP prevailed as the best available treatment option for patients with advanced-stage, intermediate-grade NHL.

Bone Marrow or Peripheral Stem Cell Transplantation. Refractory and relapsed patients may need alternative therapy such as bone marrow or peripheral stem cell transplantation. Complete responses and cures using these approaches are more likely to occur if a patient does not have bone marrow involvement, has no or minimal residual disease, is not of advanced age or in poor medical condition, and has responded well to initial and salvage chemotherapy regimens. For those not suitable to be transplanted, salvage chemotherapy is the typical course. However, if a patient is eligible, bone marrow transplantation has shown to increase event-free and overall survival (Philip, Guglielmi, Hagenbeek, Somers, Van Der Lelie, & Bron et al., 1995).

High-Grade Lymphomas

Referring to the Working Formulation, the three diseases included in the high-grade lymphoma category include large cell immunoblastic, lymphoblastic, and small non-cleaved cell (SNC) lymphomas. As stated earlier in the text, immunoblastic lymphoma is commonly treated as an intermediate-stage disease.

Lymphoblastic lymphoma, basically all of a T-cell variety, is characteristically very similar to T-cell acute lymphocytic leukemia. It often presents with a mediastinal mass and widespread dissemination, including bone marrow and CNS disease. In contrast, SNC lymphomas are primarily B-cell disorders and can be separated into Burkitt's and non-Burkitt's types. Burkitt's tends to be more prominent in children in the United States.

Because of poor median survival rates, the treatment of lymphoblastic lymphoma has evolved from the more common lymphoma treatment choices of cyclophosphamide, vincristine, and prednisone (CVP) and CHOP to much more aggressive protocols similar to those used in treating acute lymphoblastic leukemia. These regimens include induction, consolidation, and maintenance phases, in addition to CNS prophylaxis with intrathecal methotrexate and cranial radiation. This approach has improved survival in patients with lymphoblastic lymphoma. The questions that remain to be answered are the type of CNS prophylaxis, the role of radiation therapy to the mediastinum, and the necessity, length, and type of maintenance therapy (Peter, Willemze, & Colly, 1987).

Chemotherapy. Encouraging results have been reported from studies evaluating various chemotherapy regimens for the treatment of SNC lymphoma. Complete remission rates range from 45% to 84%, with results varying due to age differences, stage, number of HIV-positive patients, and intensity of therapy (Greer et al., 1993). A variety of drugs are utilized, and most studies include intrathecal therapy as CNS prophylaxis, not radiation therapy. McMaster and colleagues developed a high-intensity, brief-duration combination chemotherapy regimen that includes cyclophosphamide, doxorubicin, etoposide, vincristine, bleomycin, methotrexate, and prednisone (McMaster, Greer, Greco, Johnson, Wolff, & Hainsworth, 1991). The complete response rate was 85%, with 65% of the patients disease-free at 29 months.

Bone Marrow or Peripheral Stem Cell Transplantation. The role of stem cell or bone marrow transplantation in this setting is still uncertain. For those patients who were unable to achieve a CR after receiving conventional therapy or for those with poor prognostic factors at high risk for relapse, bone marrow or stem cell transplantation may improve results. Table 67-7 illustrates the standard of care for those undergoing marrow harvest for marrow or stem cell transplantation.

Salvage Chemotherapy

Patients who have relapsed after a complete remission are receiving a variety of salvage chemotherapy regimens. Some are conventional-dose drug combinations such as DHAP (dexamethasone, cytarabine, cisplatin), MIME (methyl-GAG, ifosfamide, methotrexate, etoposide), MINE (mesna, ifosfamide, Novantrone [mitoxantrone], etoposide) followed by consolidation with ESHAP (etoposide, methylprednisolone [Solu-Medrol], cytarabine [ara-C], cisplatin

TABLE 67-7 Standard of Care for the Patient Undergoing Storage of Bone Marrow for Possible Transplantation

Patient Problems and Outcomes	Nursing Interventions and Rationales	Patient Education and Interventions
Anxiety Patient will: • Verbalize an understanding of the bone marrow harvest procedure • Express feelings of decreased anxiety • Identify strategies to cope with anxiety	1. Assess patient's understanding of marrow harvest. 2. Give the patient the opportunity to ask questions or verbalize concerns. 3. Determine which coping strategies the patient has used effectively in the past to decrease anxiety and reinforce use of these coping mechanisms.	1. Use a skeletal iliac crest to explain the method of marrow harvest. Reassure the patient that although numerous aspirations are done, only 5-6 entries through the skin are made. Reassure patient that scarring is minimal and the procedure is safe. 2. Reassure patient that the shelf-life of stored marrow is indefinite. 3. Reassure patient information about the preoperative routine: a. Electrocardiogram and chest rays to determine patient's ability to undergo general anesthesia. b. Skin prep with providone iodine (Betadine) scrub to reduce skin bacteria, thereby decreasing infection risk. c. Nothing by mouth after midnight. d. Clear instructions of time and place of procedure. e. Caregiver or responsible person to accompany patient home at time of discharge.
Infection Patient will be infection free	1. Assess surgical sites for possible infection of surgical sites. 2. Take routine vital signs. 3. Administer antibiotics, if indicated.	1. Teach patient to change dressing and swab operative sites with Betadine or other antibacterial agent.
Patient will experience no nausea and vomiting or be controlled with antiemetic medication	1. Assess for nausea, vomiting, and ability to eat and drink. 2. Administer opioid analgesics around the clock for the first 24-48 hours postoperatively. 3. Monitor for analgesic side effects and administer medications to prevent or treat: a. Nausea b. Pruritus c. Constipation	1. Teach patient to report nausea and vomiting. 2. Teach patient need to eat and drink small quantities of nutrition and gradually increase diet.
Anemia Patient will maintain a normal hemoglobin and hematocrit	1. Monitor complete blood counts to ensure that patient is not anemic from surgical blood loss. Administer red blood cells, if indicated.	1. Teach patients the signs and symptoms of anemia: dyspnea on exertion, pallor, and fatigue. 2. Teach patient to report symptoms to primary health care provider. 3. Teach patient the need to take iron supplements for 2-3 months after marrow harvest.
Pain Patient will experience optimal pain relief with minimal side effects	1. Assess patient for pain, especially at surgical sites.	1. Teach patient to inform the nurse if he or she is experiencing pain. 2. Teach patient the importance of taking pain medication on a regular basis for pain control.

From Buchsel, P. C. (1998). Marrow and peripheral stem cell transplantation. B. L. Johnson & J. Gross (Eds.), *Handbook of oncology nursing* (3rd ed). Sudbury, MA: Jones and Bartlett.

[Platinol]), DICE (dexamethasone, ifosfamide with mesna, cisplatin, and etoposide); and ICE (ifosfamide with mesna, carboplatin, and etopside). Other strategies under evaluation are utilizing high-dose therapy followed by either bone marrow or stem cell transplants.

Mantle Zone Lymphoma

Mantle zone lymphoma is an intermediate-grade lymphoma with distinct immunologic and cytogenetic features. Some behave as indolent lymphomas, some more aggressively. It constitutes between 2% and 8% of all lymphomas and occurs predominantly in males (Foon & Fisher, 1995). Other characteristics of this disease include generalized lymphedema, splenomegaly, hepatomegaly, and gastrointestinal and bone marrow involvement.

Malignant Histiocytosis

Malignant histiocytosis is a form of NHL made up of cells that morphologically look like histiocytes (macrophages). It is very rare and is usually treated as an aggressive large cell lymphoma (Foon & Fisher, 1995). It tends to be in advanced stages, involving extranodal sites such as lungs, CNS, skin, and soft tissue (Greer et al., 1993).

Extranodal Disease

Extranodal presentations of NHL occur in approximately 30% to 40% of patients (Fisher & Oken, 1995). Most of these forms of NHL are of the B lineage. Primary lesions have been described in the testes, thyroid, lung, bone, CNS, and female reproductive system. In the CNS, the most common manifestation is an extranodal tumor mass compressing the spinal cord. Primary CNS lymphomas are usually associated with AIDS. Any involvement of the CNS is a poor prognostic factor.

ONCOLOGIC EMERGENCIES

There are a variety of oncologic emergencies that may complicate the disease course of NHL. Some of these—such as spinal cord compression (SCC), superior vena cava syndrome (SVC), and pericardial effusions—occur as a result of the disease process itself. Two other oncologic emergencies seen in NHL patients that can result from treatment modalities are tumor lysis syndrome and septic shock. Regardless of the cause, all of these situations are life threatening and must be treated emergently to reduce permanent impairments and prevent death.

An enlarged lymph node or extranodal disease pressing on the spinal column between the vertebral bodies is the cause of SCC in NHL patients. Any section of the spinal cord can be involved. Pain is the most common initial symptom in the majority of patients. The nature of the pain may differ, depending upon where the tumor is and how extensive the involvement (i.e., local or nerve root involvement). If the SCC is not diagnosed with the complaints of pain, the symptoms can progress to motor deficits, paralysis, and bowel and bladder dysfunction. Emergent radiation therapy combined with steroids is usually the treatment approach used for most patients. Whatever the treatment, palliation of symptoms and preservation of function and quality of life are the main goals.

SVC is the obstruction of venous flow through the superior vena cava, which in turn results in impaired venous drainage from the head, neck, and upper extremities. Occlusion secondary to extrinsic pressure is probably the mechanism causing SVC in NHL patients. Signs and symptoms include edema of the head and upper extremities, prominent chest wall veins, headaches, shortness of breath on exertion, chest pain, dysphagia, and cyanosis of the upper body due to venous stasis. Radiation and chemotherapy are the primary treatment modalities utilized in most SVC cases. Regardless of the treatment, maintaining airway patency and ensuring adequate oxygenation are the most critical needs in a patient with SCC that need to be addressed.

NHL can metastasize to the pericardium and therefore has the potential to cause pericardial effusions. An accumulation of fluid in the pericardial sac can lead to increased intrapericardial compression and subsequent decreased cardiac output. Tachycardia, pulsus paradoxus, jugular venous distention, and hypotension are the main clinical findings leading to the diagnosis of pericardial effusions. Treatment options vary, depending upon the severity of the effusion, aggressiveness of the primary disease, prior treatment, and physical condition of the patient. Removing the fluid and restoring normal hemodynamic functioning are the desirable outcomes.

Tumor lysis syndrome (TLS) is a metabolic cascade of events and usually occurs as a consequence of high cell turnover during chemotherapy. Intracellular contents are released into the blood, resulting in hyperuricemia, hyperphosphatemia, hyperkalemia, and hypocalcemia. If left untreated, TLS could result in renal failure or death. TLS is preventable with adequate hydration, alkalinization, and allopurinol. If it does occur, establishing normal electrolyte levels and preventing or reversing acute renal failure are the immediate goals.

As a result of the neutropenic periods a patient with NHL may experience from their treatment regimens, they are susceptible to septicemia and potentially to septic shock. Septic shock is a consequence of either gram-positive bacteria or gram-positive bacteria in the bloodstream. The effects of these can cause hemodynamic, cellular, metabolic, and humoral changes that can lead to circulatory collapse and respiratory failure. Early recognition of the various signs and symptoms of septic shock and prompt treatment can prevent the life-threatening scenario associated with this complication.

NURSING MANAGEMENT

Similar to the medical management of NHL, nursing management of the patient can be quite complex and can vary greatly from patient to patient. An excellent and complete nursing perspective for patients with NHL is given by Hubbard (1996). The complications or clinical issues that face this patient population are dictated by the histologic subtype, the areas of disease involvement, the treatment regimen chosen, and the physiologic status of the patient. Because health care trends are moving away from the necessity to be treated as an inpatient, management of NHL patients will more often occur in outpatient and home-care environments.

As is the situation with the new diagnosis of any disease state, education of the patient and family is a key component of the nurse's role. Because of the many factors that contribute to a confirmed diagnosis and treatment plan, patients and families are anxious and have many questions about rationale for diagnostic tests, interpretation of results (Jacobs, 1993), toxicities of the chosen treatment, and expected outcomes. This need for information continues throughout the course of their disease. The main treatment modalities for NHL, chemotherapy and radiation therapy, are briefly discussed below.

Chemotherapy

Chemotherapy is the mainstay in treatment for NHL. Many agents, alone and in combination, are extremely active against this disease. As a result of the numerous chemotherapy agents used for treating NHL, and because chemotherapy is administered with different goals in mind (cure, control, palliation), the toxicity profiles from this treatment will greatly vary. Nursing management of these patients will focus on preventing, minimizing, and controlling chemotherapy's many side effects. Possible toxicities include nausea, vomiting, diarrhea, stomatitis, myelosuppression, fatigue, anorexia, weight loss or gain, organ system toxicities (central nervous system, cardiac, renal, hepatic, pulmonary, reproductive, integumentary), and the potential for the development of secondary malignancies. Specific problems and interventions are outlined in Chapter 5.

Radiation Therapy

As in the case of patients receiving chemotherapy for NHL, those undergoing radiation therapy may be doing so with the hopes of cure, control, or merely palliation of their disease. The goal may in part dictate the dose of radiation therapy. The dose, area being irradiated, and patient's performance status will collectively determine the side effects experienced. External beam radiation therapy is used. Major problems that may be encountered include skin irritation, anorexia, fatigue, and symptoms specific to the area being irradiated (i.e., esophagitis, pneumonitis, gastritis, nausea, vomiting, diarrhea, cystitis). Interventions are outlined in Chapter 4.

The psychosocial dilemma of a diagnosis of NHL is a constant issue of concern in the lives of patients and families. Adapting to the lifestyle changes that occur as a result of NHL diagnosis is difficult. Providing patients with accurate information regarding the treatment and disease, encouraging them to verbalize their fears and concerns, and assuring the adequacy of their support systems are all necessary interventions. Referrals to support groups and/or utilization of other professionals such as social workers or psychologists for emotional support, financial aid, or other needs is often of great benefit.

HOME CARE ISSUES

Because of the movement toward outpatient and home care, fewer and fewer NHL cases are being treated in a controlled hospital setting unless there is risk of a life-threatening complication. Therefore the majority of disease and treatment-related problems will be dealt with at home by the patient and family caregiver.

Side Effect Management

Managing the side effects of the various treatment modalities can be accomplished by the patient and family alone or in coordination with a home healthcare agency. Specific instructions on type, amount, and frequency of medications to be taken at home; nutritional tips; guidelines for energy conservation; oral care; and skin care, in addition to what side effects to report to the nurse or physician, will help prevent unnecessary trips to the physician's office or the hospital. Educating the patient and family is a necessity but often has the added benefit of decreasing anxiety.

At times, care of the patient at home may be beyond the family's abilities. The need for antiemetics, pain medications, growth factors, antibiotics, and any type of intravenous fluid may require a referral to a home healthcare or intravenous therapy agency.

Infection. One of the most serious problems that NHL patients face in the home is that of infection. Because both the disease and treatments are immunosuppressive, patients must be educated on prevention strategies and the signs and symptoms to report to their physician. Providing them with written guidelines to use as a reference at home is of great importance (Box 67-4). Instructing them on what period of time they will be most susceptible to infection, good handwashing techniques, avoidance of others with infections, minimizing the intake of uncooked or unpeeled fruits and vegetables during their most vulnerable time period, and signs and symptoms of a potential infection to report (such as a cough or elevated temperature), are critical nursing responsibilities.

The patient may encounter a variety of other problems. For those receiving radiation therapy for their NHL, daily transportation to and from treatments may be difficult. Elderly patients who live alone or merely need assistance with normal activities of daily living could benefit from local meal delivery services or visits from a home health aide. Referrals to agencies such as the American Cancer Society, Department of Social Services, and the United Way may be appropriate to obtain information regarding local programs for these patients.

PROGNOSIS

Clinical research has led to greater knowledge about genetics and immunology and thus improvements in the manage-

Box 67-4
Home Care Instructions to Reduce Infection Risks

Mark your calendar for those days when your blood counts are expected to be at their lowest.

Diet

Avoid eating any uncooked fruits or vegetables (if you are able to peel it, such as a banana or orange, it is permitted).

People Contact

Avoid close contact with any person who has a cold, cough, or known infection.

Avoid contact with any person who has recently received a vaccination against disease. EXAMPLES: polio, rubella, measles, mumps.

Do not change diapers (or wear gloves if you must change diapers) of a child who has received the live oral polio vaccine. This virus is found in bowel movements (stools) for 2 to 4 weeks after vaccination.

Handwashing/Personal Cleanliness

Always wash your hands well after using the bathroom and before meals.

Fever/Infection

Report a fever of >101°F to your nurse or doctor.

Report chills or shakes.

Report any problems that may mean an infection is starting. Examples: cough, sore throat, runny nose, pain or burning after you urinate, any redness, rash or drainage from your skin.

TABLE 67-8 Treatment Options for Non–Hodgkin's Lymphoma

Category	Option
Low Grade	
Stage I or II	Radiation
Stage III or IV	Watch and wait or combination chemotherapy or local radiation or ? BMT
Intermediate Grade	
Stage I or II	CHOP ± radiation
Stage II, bulky, III, IV	CHOP
High Grade	
Lymphoblastic	Combination chemotherapy + CNS prophylaxis ± radiation or BMT for high-risk
Small noncleaved cell (Burkitt's)	Combination chemotherapy

BMT, Bone marrow transplantation; *CHOP,* cyclophospamide, hydroxydaunomycin, Oncovin (vincristine), and prednisone; *CNS,* central nervous system.

TABLE 67-9 Quality of Care Evaluation for a Patient Receiving Radiation Therapy for Non-Hodgkin's Lymphoma

Disciplines participating in the quality of care evaluation:
☐ Nursing ☐ Radiation Oncology ☐ Social Services

I. Post treatment Management Evaluation

Data from:
☐ Medical Record Review ☐ Patient/Family Interview

Criteria	Yes	No
1. Patient was provided with pretreatment information about the following:		
a. Radiation therapy markings	☐	☐
b. Treatment schedule	☐	☐
c. Expected side effects	☐	☐
2. A complete blood count was performed weekly	☐	☐
3. Patient experienced the following problems:		
a. Lack of transportation to and from radiation treatments	☐	☐
b. Skin burn	☐	☐

II. Patient/Family Satisfaction

Data from:
☐ Patient Interview ☐ Family Interview

Criteria	Yes	No
1. On a scale of 0-10, with 0 being totally dissatisfied and 10 being totally satisfied, how satisfied were you with management strategies used for your esophagitis? ________		
2. Were you given nutritional information appropriate for patients with esophagitis?	☐	☐
3. Were you informed of side effects of fatigue?	☐	☐

ment of patients with NHL. Because of the many variables that play a part in the treatment decisions, such as the wide spectrum of histologic subtypes, stage, and age, it is difficult to make generalizations about success. Most patients with NHL are very responsive to therapy, namely chemotherapy and radiation therapy. A significant number are actually curable, and those that are not can receive very good palliative benefit and have an acceptable quality of life. General treatment options are presented in Table 67-8.

Intermediate- and high-grade lymphomas are potentially curable diseases (Fisher & Oken, 1995; Portlock, 1992). Initiation of therapy should be prompt after an accurate diagnosis is made. Without an accurate diagnosis, optimal treatment is unlikely. In the low-grade lymphomas, a curative outcome is less certain. Although patients with low-grade lymphoma are responsive to therapy, intensive treatment remains controversial. No adequate documentation of cure exists in advanced stages of low-grade lymphomas.

EVALUATION OF THE QUALITY OF CARE

Evaluating the quality of patient care is a basic requirement of accreditation organizations such as the Joint Commission for the Accreditation of Healthcare Organizations and the American College of Surgeons. As with any cancer patient, care provided to those with NHL involves a multidisciplinary team approach. Therefore an evaluation of the quality of care given to these patients should include input from the various disciplines. Table 67-9 is an example of a quality of care evaluation tool that can be used with the NHL patient population.

RESEARCH ISSUES

The future will be a challenging but exciting one in the area of NHL (Box 67-5). Various studies investigating the use of different antibodies to cell surface markers and the use of interleukin 2 and lymphokine-activated killer cells have yielded positive results (Aisenberg, 1995). Polymerase chain reaction (PCR) sensitivity is proving very helpful in detecting minimal disease, one of the most important pieces of data needed for selecting appropriately intense treatments. PCR probes that are specific for identified NHL oncogenes such as *bcl*-1, *bcl*-2, and c-*myc* may aid in determining prognosis and eventually could provide the basis for a new lymphoma classification system (Aisenberg, 1995). These advances in biotechnology, in addition the ongoing clinical trials of new agents and modifications of existing regimens, will hopefully result in new treatment regimens for NHL to extend survival and improve the patient's quality of life.

Box 67-5
Treatment Options Under Research for Non–Hodgkin's Lymphoma

1. Marrow and stem cell transplantation.
2. Chemosensitizers such as calcium-channel blockers (verapamil, azidopine, tiapamil), calmodulin antagonists (trifluoperazine, chlorpromazine), lysosomotropic agents (chloroquine), noncytotoxic drug analogs (vindoline)
3. Less toxic and more potent modulators (e.g., cyclosporine analog PS833)
4. Recombinant cytokines such as interferon and interleukin-2
5. B-cell lymphoma vaccines
6. New chemotherapy options (e.g., fludarabine, pentostati, and 2-chlorodeoxyadenosine)
7. Synthetic peptides to deliver toxins or isotopes to tumor cells

From Hubbard, S. M. (1996). Current issues and controversies in the management of non–Hodgkin's lymphoma. In *Management for the oncology nurse* (2nd ed.). New York: Triclinica.

REFERENCES

Aisenberg, A. J. (1995). Coherent view of non–Hodgkin's lymphoma. *Journal of Clinical Oncology, 13*(10), 2656-2675.

American Cancer Society (1998). *Cancer facts and figures.* Atlanta: The Society.

Armitage, J. O. (1995.) The changing classification of non–Hodgkin's lymphomas. Non–Hodgkin's lymphoma. *CA: A Cancer Journal for Clinicians. 47*(6): 323-325.

Blair, A. Linos, A., Stewart, P. A., Burmeister, L. F., Gibson, R., Everett, G., Schuman, L., & Cantor, K. P. (1992). Comments on occupational and environmental factors in the origin of non–Hodgkin's lymphoma. *Cancer Research, 52,* 5501s-5502s.

Buchsel, P. C. (1998). Marrow and peripheral stem cell transplantation. B. L. Johnson & J. Gross (Eds.), *Handbook of oncology nursing* (3rd ed). Sudbury, MA: Jones and Bartlett.

Carbone, P. P., Kaplan, H. S., Musshof, K., Smithers, D. W., & Tubiana, M. (1971). Report of the committee on Hodgkin's staging classification. *Cancer Research, 31,* 1860.

Cheson, B. D. (1993). New chemotherapeutic agents for the treatment of low-grade non–Hodgkin's lymphomas. *Seminars in Oncology, 20* (Suppl. 5), 96-110.

Filipovich, A. H., Mather, A., Kamat, D., & Shapiro, R. S. (1992). Primary immunodeficiencies: Genetic risk factors for lymphoma. *Cancer Research, 52*(Suppl.), 5465s-5467s.

Fisher, R. I., Gaynor, E. R., Dalberg, S., Oken, M. M., Grogan, T. M., Mize, E. M., Glick, J. H., Coltman, C. A., & Miller, T. P. (1993). Comparison of standard regimen (CHOP) with three intensive chemotherapy regimens for advanced non–Hodgkin's lymphoma. *New England Journal of Medicine, 328,* 1002-1006.

Fisher, R. I. & Oken, M. M. (1995). Clinical practice guidelines: Non–Hodgkin's lymphomas. *Cleveland Clinic Journal of Medicine, 62*(Suppl. 1), 1-48.

Foon, K. & Fisher, R. (1995). Lymphomas. In E. Beutler, M. A Lichtman, B. S. Coller, & T. J. Kipps, (Eds.), *William's hematology* (5th ed.). New York: McGraw-Hill.

Gaidano, G. & Dalla-Favera, R. (1993). Biologic and molecular characterization of non–Hodgkin's lymphoma. *Current Opinions in Oncology, 5,* 776-784.

Gaidano, G., Pastore, C., & Volpe, G. (1995). Molecular pathogenesis of non–Hodgkin's lymphoma: A clinical perspective. *Haematologica, 80,* 454-472.

Gordon, L. I., Harrington, D., Andersen, J., Colgan, J., Glick, J., Neiman, R., Mann, R., Resnick, G. D., Barcos, M., Gottlieb, A., & O'Connell, M. (1992). Comparison of a second generation combination chemotherapeutic regimen (mBACOD) with a standard regimen (CHOP) for advanced diffuse non–Hodgkin's lymphoma. *New England Journal of Medicine, 327*(19), 1342-1349.

Greer, J. P., Macon, W. R., List, A. F., & McCurley, T. L. (1993). Non–Hodgkin's Lymphomas. In G. R. Lee, T. C. Bithell, J. Foerster, J. W. Athens & J. N. Lukens (Eds.), *Wintrobe's clinical hematology*. Philadelphia: Lea and Febiger.

Grossbard, M. L. & Nadler, L. M. (1993). Monoclonal antibody therapy for indolent lymphomas. *Seminars in Oncology, 20*(Suppl. 5), 118-135.

Hartge, P., Devesa, S. S., & Fraumeni, J. F. (1994). Hodgkin's and non–Hodgkin's lymphomas. *Cancer Surveys, 19-20,* 423-453.

Hubbard, S. M. (1996). Current issues and controversies in the management of non–Hodgkin's lymphoma. In *Management for the oncology nurse* (2nd ed.). New York: Triclinica.

Jacobs, P. (1993). Hodgkin's disease and the malignant lymphomas. *Disease of the Month, 39*(4), 213-297.

Kundrat, H. (1893). Uber lympho-sarkomatosis. *Wein Klin Wochenschr, 6,* 211.

Levine, P. H. & Hoover, R. N. (1992). The emerging epidemic of non–Hodgkin's lymphoma: Current knowledge regarding etiologic factors. *Cancer Research, 52*(Suppl.), 5425s-5474s.

Longo, D. L., DeVita, V. T., Jaffe, E. S., Mauch, P., & Urba, W. J. (1993). Lymphocytic lymphomas. In V. T. DeVita, S. Hellman, & S. A. Rosenberg (Eds.), *Cancer: Principles and practice of oncology* (4th ed.). Philadelphia: J. B. Lippincott.

McMaster, M. L., Greer, J. P., Greco, F. A., Johnson, D. H., Wolff, S. N., & Hainsworth, J. D. (1991). Effective treatment of small-non-cleaved-cell lymphoma with high intensity, brief duration chemotherapy. *Journal of Clinical Oncology, 9,* 941-946.

Miller, K.B. (1995). Reactive lymphocyte disorders and lymphadenopathy. In R. I. Handin, T. P. Stossel, S. E., Lux, S. E. (Eds). *Blood: Principles and practice of hematology*. Philadelphia: J. B. Lippincott.

Miller, B. A., Ries, L. A. G., Hankey, B. F., Kosary, C. L., & Edwards, B. K. (1992). Cancer statistics review: 1973-1989 (NIH Pub. No. 92-2789). Bethesda, MD: National Cancer Institute.

Non–Hodgkin's Lymphoma Pathologic Classification Project. (1982). National Cancer Institute Sponsored Study of Classifications of Non-Hodgkin's Lymphomas. *Cancer, 99(*10), 2112-2135.

Parkinson, D. R., Sznol, M., & Cheson, B. D. (1993). Biologic therapies for low-grade non-Hodgkin's lymphomas. *Seminars in Oncology, 20*(Suppl. 5), 111-117.

Paryani, S. B., Hoppe, R. T., Cox, R. S., Colby, T. V., Rosenberg, S. A., & Kaplan, H. S. (1983). Analysis of non–Hodgkin's lymphomas with nodular and favorable histologies, Stages I and II. *Cancer, 52,* 2300-2307.

Peter, N. G., Willemze, R., & Colly, L. P. (1987). Intermediate and high-dose cytosine arabinoside-containing regimens for induction and consolidation therapy for patients with acute lymphoblastic leukemia and lymphoblastic non–Hodgkin's lymphoma: The Leyden experience and review of the literature. *Seminars in Oncology, 14,* 86-91.

Philip, T., Guglielmi, C., Hagenbeek, A., Somers, R., Van Der Lelie, H., Bron, D., Sonneveld, P., Gisselbrecht, C., Cahn, J. Y., Harousseau, J. L., Coiffier, B., Biron, P., Mandelli, F., & Chauvin, F. (1995). Autologous bone marrow transplantation as compared with salvage chemotherapy in relapses of chemotherpy-sensitive non–Hodgkin's lymphoma. *New England Journal of Medicine, 333* (23), 1540-1545.

Portlock, C. S. (1992). Management of non–Hodgkin's lymphoma. *International Journal of Clinical and Laboratory Research, 22,* 81-83.

Portlock, C. S. & Rosenburg, S. A. (1979). No initial therapy for Stage III and IV non-Hodgkin's lymphoma of favorable histologic types. *Annals of Internal Medicine, 90,* 10-13.

Rabkin, C. S., Devesa, S. S., Zahm, S. H., & Gail, M. H. (1993). Increasing incidence of non-Hodgkin's lymphoma. *Seminars in Hematology, 30*(4), 286-296.

Rosenberg, S. A. (1993). Non-Hodgkin's lymphoma. In P. Calabrese & P. S. Schein (Eds.), *Medical oncology: Basic principles and clinical management of cancer* (2nd ed.). New York: McGraw-Hill.

Roulet, F. (1930). Das primare retothelsarkom der lymphknoten. *Virchows Arch [A], 277,* 15.

Stein, R. S., Greer, J. P., Cousar, J. B., Hendey, G. W., Wehner, J. H., Flexner, J. M., & Collins, R. D. (1989). Malignant lymphomas of follicular center cell origin. VII. Prognostic features in small cleaved cell lymphoma. *Hematological Oncology, 7,* 381-391.

Thibodeau, G. A., Patton, K. T. (Eds.). (1996). *Anatomy and physiology* (3rd ed.). St. Louis: Mosby.

Weisenburger, D. D. (1994). Epidemiology of non–Hodgkins' lymphoma: Recent findings regarding an emerging epidemic. *Annals of Oncology, 5*(Suppl. 1), 19-24.

Weisenburger, D. D. (1992). Pathological classification of non-Hodgkin's lymphoma for epidemiological studies. *Cancer Research, 52* (Suppl.), 5456s-5464s.

Weisenburger, D. D. (1991). Non–Hodgkin's lymphomas of mantle zone origin. In P. P. Rosen & R. E. Fechner, (Eds.), *Pathology annual, 26.* Norwalk, CT: Appleton & Lange.

Zahm, S. H. & Blair, A., (1992). Pesticides and non-Hodgkin's lymphoma. *Cancer Research, 52*(Suppl.), 5485s-5488s.

Zahm, S. H., Weisenberger, D. D., Babbitt, P. A., Saal, R. C., Vaught, J. B, & Blair, A. (1992). Use of hair coloring products and the risk of lymphoma, multiple myeloma, chronic lymphocytic leukemia. *American Journal of Public Health, 82,* 990-997.

Prostate Cancer

Christine Miaskowski, RN, PhD, FAAN

EPIDEMIOLOGY

Prostate cancer is the most common cancer and the second-leading cause of cancer deaths in men. In 1996 the number of new cases of prostate cancer in the United States was 317,100, and approximately 41,000 men died of the disease (Parker, Tong, Bolden, & Wingo, 1996). The diagnosis and management of prostate cancer is extremely controversial. Controversy exists, in part, because prostate cancer tends to be diagnosed at a median age of 66 years, and if the cancer is confined to the gland, the disease may not adversely affect the patient's survival until 10 to 15 years after the initial diagnosis. In fact, in autopsy studies, 30% of men between the ages of 50 and 70 years, with no overt evidence of prostate cancer before death, had pathologic evidence of prostate cancer. Perhaps due to the natural history of this disease, many men will die from diseases other than prostate cancer. This fact has led some clinicians to suggest that a "less interventional approach" or "a watchful waiting approach" be taken toward the management of prostate cancer (Adolfsson, Cartensen, & Lowhagen, 1992).

Needless to say, prostate cancer represents a significant public health problem. Twelve years ago, prostate cancer was the tenth most frequent cancer in the world. Today it is the most common cancer in the world and the most common cancer in men in the United States. In the United States men have a one in five lifetime probability of receiving a diagnosis of prostate cancer (Parker et al., 1996). The exact reason for the increase in the incidence of prostate cancer remains unclear. Because the disease is largely diagnosed in older men, the aging population may explain part of the increased incidence. Additional factors that may contribute to the increased incidence of prostate cancer include improvements in the clinical diagnosis of the disease and increased awareness of the disease (Maxwell, 1993; Mettlin, Murphy, Ho, & Menck, 1996).

RISK FACTORS

The major risk factors associated with the development of prostate cancer are listed in Box 68-1. The evidence supporting each of these risk factors is reviewed, and the nursing implications for prevention and early detection activities are discussed. A sample patient education tool that summarizes the risk factors, prevention activities, and signs and symptoms of prostate cancer is found in Box 68-2.

Increasing Age

Age is an important risk factor in the development of prostate cancer. Eighty percent of the cases of prostate cancer are diagnosed in men over 65 years of age. The median age at the time of diagnosis is 70 years. Recent estimates suggest that prostate cancer is present in 80% of men over 80 years of age (Maxwell, 1993; Moon, 1992). Prostate cancer is extremely rare in men younger than age 40. Screening guidelines for prostate cancer take into account the age differences associated with the development of the disease.

Ethnic Differences

African-American men have the highest prostate cancer rate in the world. In contrast, Japanese and Chinese men native to those countries have the lowest incidence of prostate cancer. There is a 30- to 50-fold difference in the risk of developing prostate cancer between African-American men and Asian men. As illustrated in Fig. 68-1, among racial and ethnic groups living in Los Angeles, California, African Americans had the highest prostate cancer rate, whereas white men, either Latino or non-Latino, had roughly half that rate, and Japanese-American and Chinese-American men had half or less the rate for whites (Ross, Coetzee, Reichardt, Skinner, & Henderson, 1995).

Research findings suggest that variations in the secretion and metabolism of androgens and/or the regulation of androgen activity may explain some of the ethnic differences in the incidence of prostate cancer. In one study, the mean testosterone level of African-American men was found to be 15% higher than in whites. Differences of this magnitude, if sustained for a long period of time, may explain the 50% to 70% increase in prostate cancer in African-American men

Box 68-1
Risk Factors for Prostate Cancer

Increasing age
Ethnicity (African Americans > Whites > Asian men)
Positive family history
Vasectomy (? association)
Cadmium exposure (? association)
Tobacco use (? association)
High dietary fat intake

(Ross, Bernstein, Judd, Hanisch, Pike, & Henderson, 1986). This hypothesis is supported by research findings that show that testosterone induces the development of prostate cancer in experimental animal models (Noble, 1977).

Another factor that may explain the increased incidence of prostate cancer in African-American men is the fact that African-American women are known to have markedly elevated levels of testosterone during early pregnancy (i.e., 50% higher than white women). Again, the higher levels of testosterone during intrauterine development may contribute to the development of prostate cancer (Henderson, Bernstein, Ross, Depue, & Judd, 1988).

The most recent data suggest that ethnic differences in prostate cancer incidence may be explained by differences in the expression of genes for an enzyme called *5-alpha reductase*. This enzyme is involved in the metabolism of testosterone. Further research in this area is currently in progress (Ross et al., 1995).

Although nothing can be done to change an individual's ethnic group, cancer-screening programs can be targeted to high-risk groups. One approach for successfully recruiting African-American men to a prostate screening program has been described recently (Powell, Gelfand, Parzuchowski, Heilbrun, & Franklin, 1995).

Positive Family History

Several studies have found that men with prostate cancer are more likely to have one or more relatives who had prostate cancer. Men with a father or brother who had prostate cancer are two to three times more likely to develop the disease than men without a positive family history. In addition, among men younger than 65 years who had a brother with prostate cancer before age 65, the relative risk for prostate cancer was 6.0. In addition, the risk for prostate cancer increases as the affected number of first-degree relatives increases. The risk is doubled for men with one first-degree relative, it increases five times for those with two first-degree relatives, and increases eleven times for those with three affected relatives (Giovannucci, 1995). The strong positive family history suggests a genetic predisposition for the development of prostate cancer. In fact, recent evidence suggests that in families at high risk for prostate cancer there is evidence of a genetic linkage to the long arm of chromosome 1 (i.e., 1q24-25) (Smith, Freije, Carpten, Grönberg, Xu, & Isaacs et al., 1996).

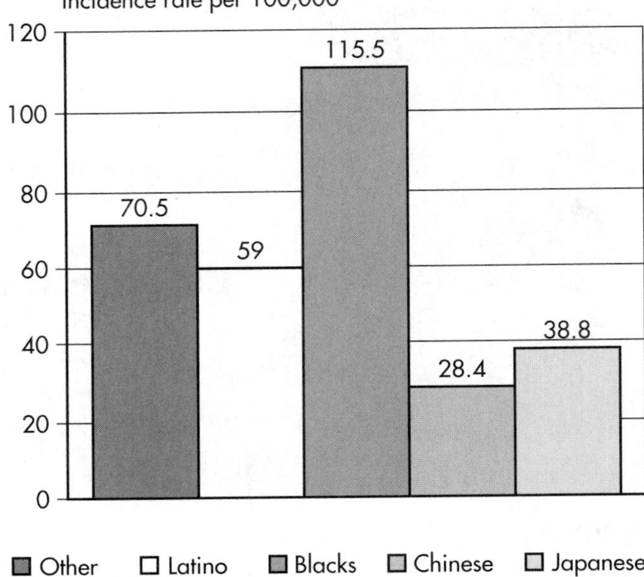

Fig. 68-1 Average annual age adjusted incidence rates for prostate cancer by race-ethnicity in Los Angeles County (1972-1987). (From Ross, R. K., Coetzee, G. A., Reichardt, J., Skinner, E., & Henderson, B. E. [1995]. Does the racial ethnic variation in prostate cancer risk have a hormonal basis? *Cancer, 75,* 1778-1782.)

Vasectomy

Some epidemiologic studies (Wolf, 1960; Mettlin, Natarajan, & Huben, 1990; Rosenberg, Palmer, Zauber, Warshauer, Stolley, & Shapiro, 1990; Spitz, Fueger, Babaian, & Newell, 1991; Hayes, Pottern, Greenberg, Schoenberg, Swanson, & Liff et al., 1993; Giovannucci, Tosteson, Speizer, Ascherio, Vessey, & Colditz, 1993; Giovannucci, Ascherio, Rimm, Colditz, Stampfer, & Willett, 1993) have suggested a positive relationship between vasectomy and the development of prostate cancer. However, in other studies (Ross, Paganini-Hill, & Henderson, 1983; Nienhaus, Goldacre, Seagroatt, Gill, & Vessey, 1992; Sidney, Queensberry, Sadler, Guess, Lydick, & Cattolica, 1991), an increased risk was not observed. Because more than 15% of men in the United States over age 40 have had a vasectomy, knowledge of an association between vasectomy and increased risk of prostate cancer would be important from a cancer prevention and early detection perspective.

According to Giovannucci (1995), the association between vasectomy and prostate cancer found in epidemiologic studies is unlikely to be due to chance, but whether vasectomy actually causes an individual to develop prostate cancer remains controversial. Part of the difficulty in establishing a more definitive relationship between vasectomy and prostate cancer is that a biologic mechanism that would explain such a relationship remains unclear. One proposal suggests that vasectomy may result in prolonged exposure of the prostate gland to carcinogenic substances in prostatic fluid that are no longer secreted. An alternative mechanism

Box 68-2

Public Information Brochure About the Early Detection of Prostate Cancer

Information to Help You Defend Yourself Against Cancer

Prostate cancer occurs in about one out of every ten men, so every man should consider himself at risk. Most often prostate cancer is diagnosed after age 50, but it can occur in younger men. It is important to remember that when prostate cancer is diagnosed early, treatment is usually most effective and men can expect to continue to live productive lives.

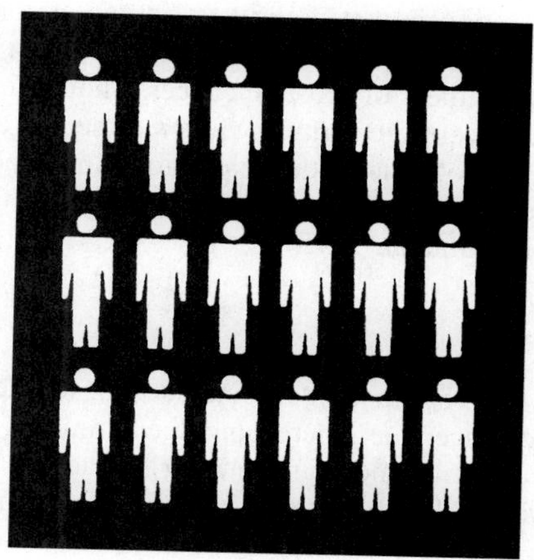

What Is The Prostate?

The prostate is a walnut-size sex gland which is located just below the bladder. The prostate surrounds part of the urethra which is the tube that drains urine from the bladder. The primary function of the prostate is to provide fluid and nutrients for the sperm. The normal function of the prostate depends on the male hormone testosterone which is made by the testicles.

Prostate function is not necessary after a man has finished having children. As a man grows older, it is not uncommon for him to experience some enlargement of the prostate. This is called benign prostatic hypertrophy.

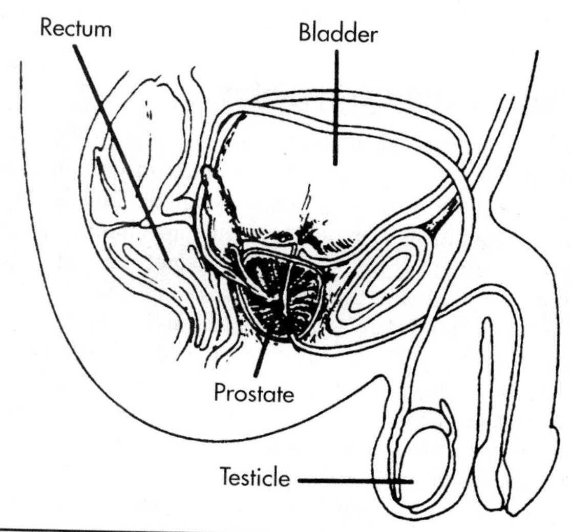

What Should You Do To Detect Prostate Cancer Early?

Currently the American Cancer Society recommends two tests to detect prostate cancer in its earliest stages when treatment is most effective. These tests are designed for men who are not having any signs or symptoms of prostate cancer. Remember prostate cancer is most easily treated in its early stages and in the early stages often the man will not have any symptoms of prostate cancer.

All men should have a digital rectal examination every year beginning at age 40. Beginning at age 50 all men should have a digital rectal examination *and* a Prostate Specific Antigen (PSA) blood test every year.

This digital rectal examination will not only help detect prostate cancer early, but may also find an early rectal cancer. To examine the prostate the examiner places a gloved, lubricated finger into the patient's rectum to feel the size and shape of the prostate. The examination takes less than one minute and causes only minimal discomfort.

The PSA is a blood test which measures the body's level of Prostate Specific Antigen. The PSA level may be high in prostate cancer. The PSA level may also be high in benign prostatic hypertrophy or in prostate infections or irritations.

If either of these tests are abnormal or suspicious your doctor will order other tests to help distinguish between benign and cancerous conditions of the prostate.

Signs and Symptoms of Prostate Cancer

In the earliest stages of prostate cancer you may not notice any of the symptoms of prostate cancer. It is also important to remember that these symptoms may be the same as those seen with benign enlargement of the prostate. That is why you need to be sure you get a check-up for prostate cancer. If you notice any of these symptoms be sure to talk to your doctor right away.

- A need to urinate more frequently especially at night.
- Difficulty starting urination.
- A weak or interrupted flow of urine.
- Blood or pus in the urine.
- Continuing pain in the lower back, hips or upper thighs.

Who Is At Risk For Prostate Cancer?

All men are at risk for developing prostate cancer. However some men have a higher risk. Having a risk factor does not mean you will develop prostate cancer but it does mean you should be sure to have regular check-ups.

- Age is a major determinant. Most prostate cancers occur after age 50 and the average age of diagnosis is about age 70.
- A man with a family history of prostate cancer is at higher risk.
- Black Americans have the highest incidence among all men.
- A high fat diet may increase risk.
- Occupational exposure to cadmium (through welding, electroplating or battery production) or rubber increases risk.

Screening recommendations may be modified for individuals with several risk factors or a strong family history of prostate cancer.

From Mahon, S. M. (1995). Using brochures to educate the public about early detection of prostate and colorectal cancer. *Oncology Nursing Forum, 22*(9), 1413.

that has been proposed is that sperm antigens formed following vasectomy may enhance tumor growth by blocking antibodies or tumor suppressor cells (Giovannucci et al., 1993). Additional epidemiologic research is needed to evaluate the relationship between vasectomy and prostate cancer risk because vasectomy is an otherwise safe procedure and an important contraceptive option.

Occupational Exposure

Occupational studies have not yielded consistent associations between specific exposures and prostate cancer risk. The three areas that have been studied the most are occupational exposure to cadmium, farming, and rubber manufacturing.

Cadmium is a trace element that may antagonize the action of zinc in the prostate gland. Zinc, which is highly concentrated in the prostate gland, appears to be required in several enzymatic reactions that are involved in the replication and repair of DNA and RNA. If cadmium levels are increased, the action of zinc would be antagonized, and DNA and RNA replication and repair would be altered. Industries with high cadmium exposure include electroplating, battery making, alloying, and paint manufacturing. In addition, cadmium is found in cigarette smoke (Greco & Kulawiak, 1994). According to Giovannucci (1995), although data from some studies are suggestive, it would be premature to claim an established link between cadmium exposure and increased risk of prostate cancer because the findings are inconsistent and the magnitude of the association appears modest.

Some studies have suggested an increased risk for prostate cancer in men engaged in farming or rubber manufacturing. However, definitive relationships have not been established. Additional research is needed to provide more conclusive evidence.

Tobacco Use

The studies on the relationship between smoking and the development of prostate cancer are inconclusive. Findings from two large cohort studies (Hsing, McLaughlin, Schuman, Bjelke, Gridley, & Wacholder et al., 1990; Hsing, McLaughlin, Hrubgec, Blot, & Fraumeni, 1991) suggest that the relative risk for smokers developing prostate cancer ranges from 1.2 to 2.1. However, two other studies (Fincham, Hill, Hanson, & Wijayasinghe, 1990; Talamini, Franceschi, La Vecchia, Guarneri, & Negri, 1993) found no relationship between tobacco use and an increased risk for prostate cancer. Tobacco use may influence the development of prostate cancer by affecting the metabolism of sex steroid hormones such as testosterone, as well as the adrenal hormones (Matzkin & Soloway, 1993).

Dietary Fat Intake

Epidemiologic studies support the relationship between higher dietary fat intake and the development of prostate cancer. For example, Japanese men who live in Japan have a low incidence of prostate cancer. However, when Japanese men migrate to the United States and adopt a more Western diet, their risk of developing prostate cancer increases (Kolonel, Yoshizawa, & Hankin, 1988). In addition, two large studies (Giovannucci, Rimm, Colditz, Stampfer, Ascherio & Chute et al., 1993; Rose, Boyar, & Wynder, 1986) demonstrated that men consuming diets high in animal fat, particularly red meat, were at increased risk for developing prostate cancer.

The exact mechanism by which dietary fat intake increases the risk of prostate cancer is unknown. One possible explanation is that dietary fat increases the levels of sex steroid hormones, which is proposed to be a risk factor for the development of prostate cancer. Another explanation is that carcinogens are formed when red meat is cooked. An alternative hypothesis is that elevations in a specific fatty acid, namely -linolenic acid, increases the risk for prostate cancer (Giovannucci, 1995).

Summary

While several risk factors associated with the development of prostate cancer (i.e., increasing age, ethnicity, and family history) cannot be modified, other risk factors may be reduced through lifestyle modifications. For example, men can reduce their dietary intake of animal fat. In addition, increased consumption of food sources rich in vitamin A may reduce the risk of prostate cancer (see section on Chemoprevention). Oncology nurses need to design teaching tools and programs to provide men with the most effective strategies for risk factor modification.

CHEMOPREVENTION

Chemoprevention is defined as the administration of natural or synthetic chemical agents to prevent the initiation or promotion of events that occur during carcinogenesis (Boone, Kelloff, & Malone, 1990). Chemoprevention efforts related to prostate cancer have been summarized in two recent papers (Greco & Kulawiak, 1994; Brawer & Ellis, 1995).

Retinoids and Carotenoids

Small-scale trials are underway to evaluate the chemopreventive efficacy of analogs to retinoids in human prostate cancer. Retinoids are natural and synthetic analogs of vitamin A. Vitamin A, a naturally occurring vitamin, is necessary for normal vision, growth, reproduction, and differentiation of epithelial cells. Metaplastic changes in the epithelium, along with increased cell division, occur in the absence of vitamin A. Another substance, beta-carotene, found in orange and yellow vegetables (e.g., carrots, squash) and dark green, leafy vegetables (e.g., spinach, broccoli) is converted to retinol (i.e., vitamin A) in the small intestine (Greco & Kulawiak, 1994).

Retinoids may act directly on non-neoplastic cells to suppress malignant transformation. In a review article, Pienta and Esper (1993) reported that vitamin A intake has been associated with an *increased* risk of prostate cancer in several studies, while other studies reported opposite results. Some work has suggested that beta-carotene may offer some protective effect against prostate cancer.

Additional research is warranted to determine the chemopreventive effects of dietary retinoids and carotenoids. At the present time, data are conflicting about the role that these substances play in the pathogenesis of prostate cancer. Available evidence suggests that vitamin A derived from vegetable sources may offer some protection against the development of prostate cancer. However, vitamin A products derived from animals (e.g., fish oils, liver, egg yolk, whole milk) are also high in dietary fat and may increase the risk of prostate cancer (Greco & Kulawiak, 1994).

Prostate Cancer Prevention Trial

Description. The Prostate Cancer Prevention Trial (PCPT) is a large-scale study funded by the National Cancer Institute that began in October, 1993. Over 18,000 men over 55 years of age will be recruited for this study. The purpose of the study is to determine whether the administration of finasteride (Proscar, Merck & Company, Inc., West Point, PA) reduces the incidence of prostate cancer. Secondary objectives of the PCPT include evaluating the side effects of finasteride; determining the optimal strategy for following men treated with finasteride; determining the incidence of benign prostatic hypertrophy (BPH); determining the effectiveness of prostate specific antigen (PSA) and digital rectal examination (DRE) as screening tools for prostate cancer; determining whether finasteride can prevent the development of the symptoms of BPH, and evaluating other quality-of-life issues (Greco & Kulawiak, 1994; Brawer & Ellis, 1995).

Rationale for the PCPT. In 1974, researchers noted that a group of men diagnosed with a 5-alpha reductase deficiency did not develop BPH or prostate cancer (Imperato-McGinley, Guerrero, Gautier, & Peterson, 1974). A deficiency in the enzyme 5-alpha reductase inhibits the conversion of testosterone to 5-alpha dihydrotestosterone (DHT). Dihydrotestosterone binds to androgen receptors in the cell nuclei of the prostate gland and over time causes prostatic hyperplasia. Evidence exists to suggest that DHT may play a role in the development of prostate cancer (Gormley, 1991).

Results of this study led to the development of finasteride, which inhibits the enzyme 5-alpha reductase. Clinical studies have shown that finasteride reduces prostatic volume, increases urinary flow, decreases serum DHT levels, and does not alter serum testosterone levels (Monda & Osterling, 1993). In 1992, the Food and Drug Administration approved finasteride (5 mg/day) for the treatment of symptomatic BPH.

PCPT procedures. The study design for the PCPT is illustrated in Fig. 68-2. The eligibility criteria for entry into the study are healthy males over 55 years of age with no signs of urinary retention; a normal digital rectal examination (DRE); a prostate-specific antigen (PSA) level less than or equal to 3.0, a life expectancy of 10 years, and absence

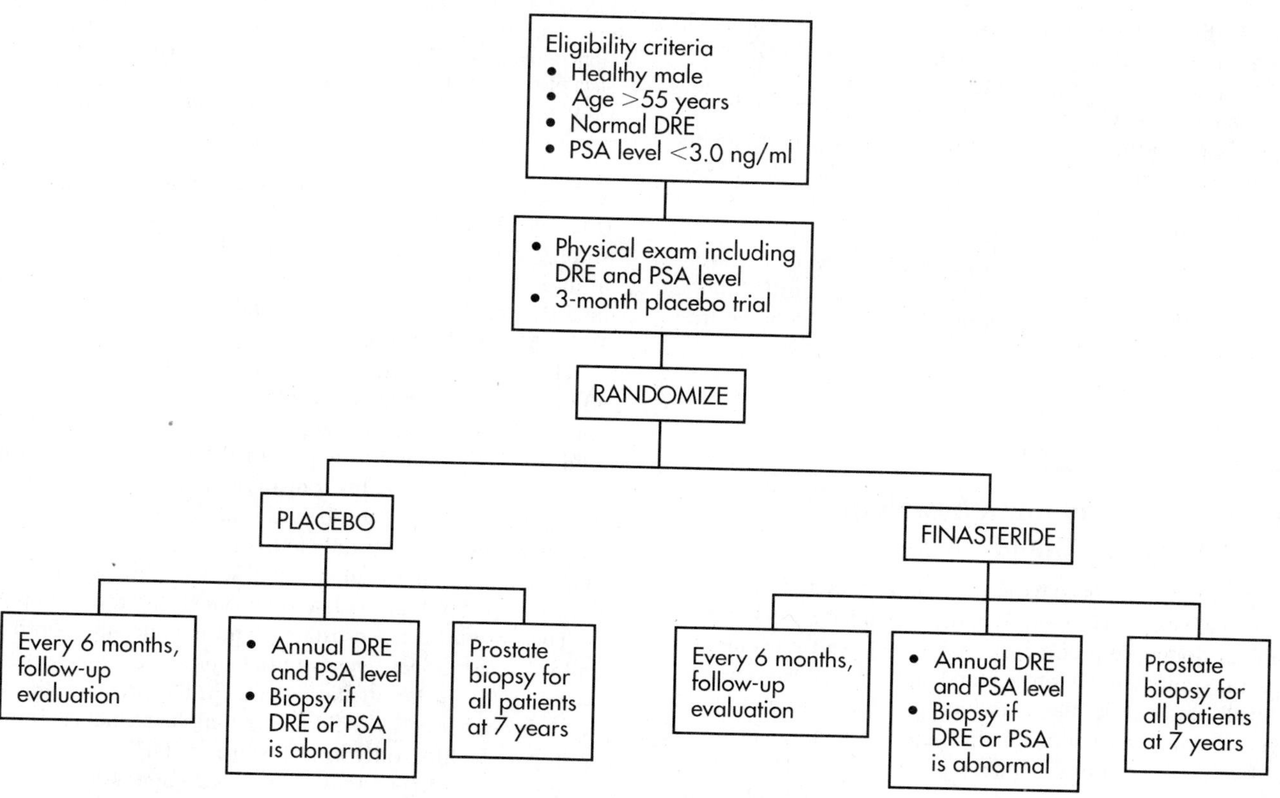

Fig. 68-2 Design of the prostate cancer prevention trial.

Box 68-3
Instructions for Participants in the Prostate Cancer Prevention Trial

1. Inform participants to use barrier contraception.
2. Tell participants that pregnant women should not handle the crushed study tablets because contact with the drug might be harmful to a male fetus.
3. Inform participants that they are not permitted to give blood, because the possibility exists that the blood could be administered to a pregnant woman who is carrying a male fetus.

of other health problems that would interfere with the study.

Prospective participants are given information about the study and asked to sign an informed consent. All participants undergo a physical examination, including a DRE and a PSA blood test. If the physical examination is normal and the participants decide to enter the study, they complete a series of questionnaires, register for the trial, and receive a 3-month supply of placebo medication. In 3 months, participants return for a pill count and a follow-up PSA level. If adherence with the medication regimen occurs and the participants' PSA levels are less than 3.0, participants are randomized to either the placebo arm or the finasteride arm (5 mg, once a day, for 7 years).

Follow-up visits are scheduled for 3, 6, and 9 months and then every 6 months for 7 years. At these visits, adherence with the medication regimen is evaluated, additional medication is dispensed, and study questionnaires are completed. At 6 months and then yearly, participants receive a DRE and a PSA blood test. If abnormalities are found (i.e., elevated PSA, abnormal DRE), a transrectal ultrasound (TRUS) with biopsy is performed. At the end of 7 years, all participants will have a prostate biopsy (Greco & Kulawiak, 1994). Nurses caring for participants in the PCPT should provide them with the information outlined in Box 68-3.

Recruitment for this trial is progressing extremely well. As of August 1994, 14,959 healthy men were enrolled in the PCPT and 9315 had been randomized to the placebo or drug group. Results of this trial should be available sometime in the autumn of 2003.

PATHOPHYSIOLOGY

Normal Anatomy and Physiology of the Prostate Gland

The prostate gland is an exocrine gland located in the depths of the male pelvis (Fig. 68-3) and surrounded by the rectum, bladder, dorsal vein complex, pelvic sidewall musculature, urethral sphincter (which is responsible for passive urinary control), and pelvic plexus (which provides autonomic nervous system innervation to the pelvic organs). The gland lies behind the symphysis pubis, just below the bladder, and in front of the rectum. The prostate gland is pierced by the urethra and the paired ejaculatory ducts.

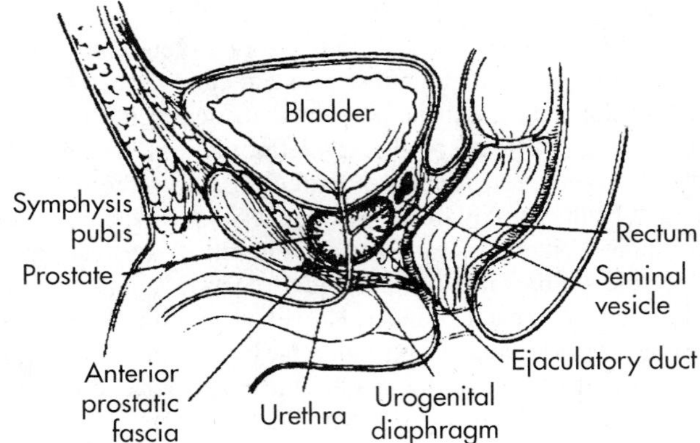

Fig. 68-3 Diagrammatic representation of midsagittal section of the male pelvis showing the relationship of the prostate to nearby structures. (From Maxwell, B. [1993]. Cancer of the prostate. *Seminars in Oncology Nursing, 9*[4], 237-251.)

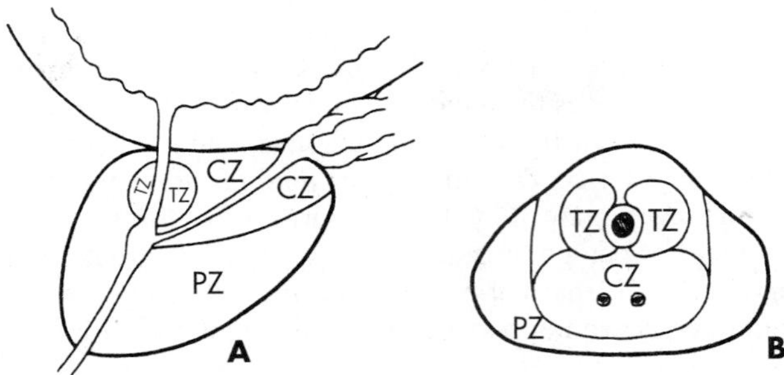

Fig. 68-4 Zonal anatomy of the prostate gland, with **A,** sagittal view, and **B,** transverse view. The outer gland consists of the peripheral zone (PZ) and the central zone (CZ). The inner gland consists of the transition zone (TZ). (From Maxwell, B. [1993]. Cancer of the prostate. *Seminars in Oncology Nursing, 9*[4], 237-251.)

The prostate gland is divided into four anatomic zones (Fig. 68-4), namely a peripheral zone, a central zone, a transition zone, and a periurethral zone. The zones are important in understanding the pattern of spread of cancers that arise in different locations of the gland (Table 68-1) (McNeal, 1988; Maxwell, 1993).

The prostate gland remains small until a male reaches adolescence. At puberty the gland undergoes rapid growth and doubles in size, weighing approximately 20 g in the adult male. The main function of the prostate is to supply the milky fluid that helps transport sperm through the penis during ejaculation. The prostatic fluid also aids conception by providing support and nourishment for the sperm and helping to keep the vaginal canal less acidic. When a male reaches age 50, the prostate gland may begin to enlarge.

The growth of the prostate gland is under the control of androgen hormones. Testosterone, produced in the testes, concentrates in the prostate gland. In the prostate, the hormone is converted by the enzyme 5-alpha reductase into the androgen 5-alpha dihydrotestosterone (DHT). Dihydrotestosterone binds to prostate cell receptors and induces stromal hyperplasia. Androgens regulate the balance between pros-

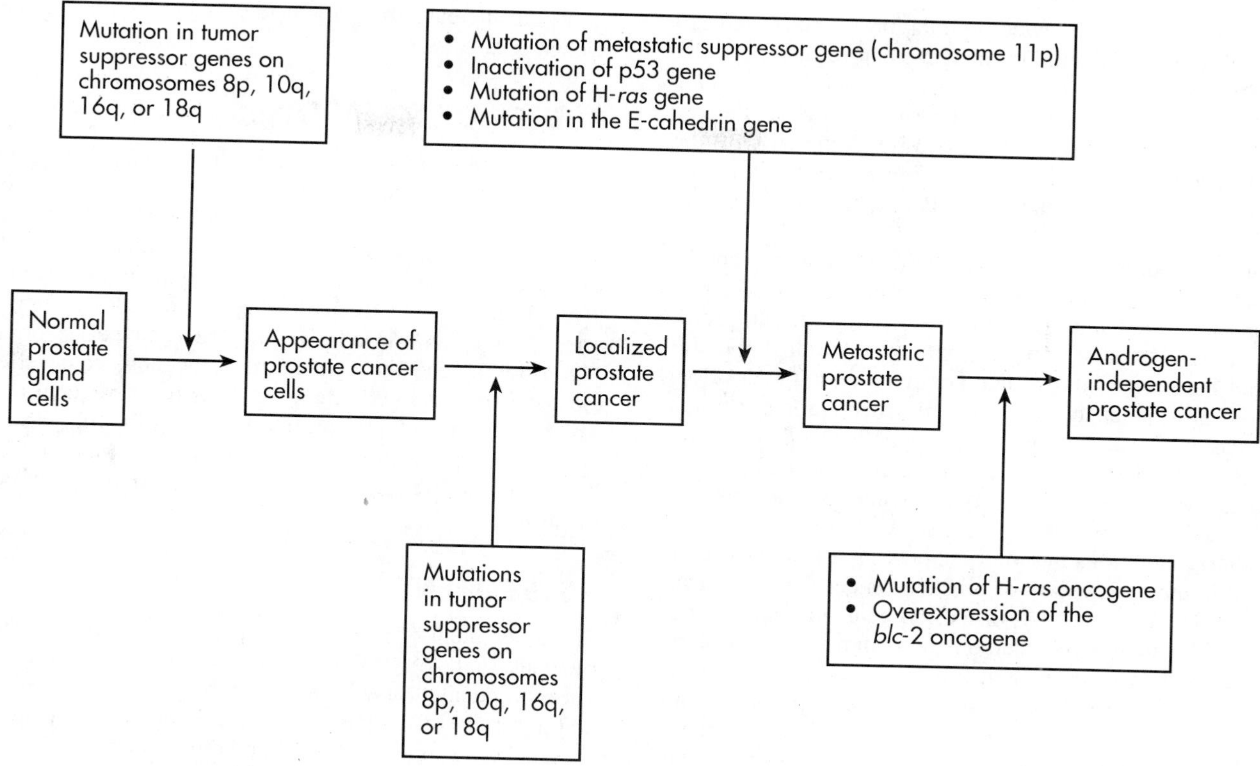

Fig. 68-5 Possible molecular events involved in the development of prostate cancer. (Modified from Scher, H. I., Isaacs, J. T., Fuks, Z., & Walsh, P. C. [1995]. Prostate. In M. D. Abeloff, J. O. Armitage, A. S. Lichter, & J. E. Niederhuber [Eds.], *Clinical oncology.* New York: Churchill Livingstone.)

TABLE 68-1 Zones of the Prostate

Zone	Location	Volume (%) in Normal Adults	% Carcinomas Arising There	Site of Benign Prostatic Hypertrophy
Outer Gland				
Peripheral	Lateral and posterior	75	68	No
Central	Base	25	8	No
Inner Gland				
Transition	Surrounding urethra	5-10	24	Yes
Periurethral	Surrounding urethra	1	–	–

From Maxwell, M. B. (1993). Cancer of the prostate. *Seminars in Oncology Nursing, 9*(4), 237-251.

tatic cell proliferation and death, so that neither overgrowth nor involution of the gland occurs in the normal male.

The Process of Carcinogenesis

Just as with other cancers, development of prostate cancer appears to occur as a multistage process, including initiation, promotion, and progression. The process involved in the development of prostate cancer is illustrated in Fig. 68-5. Because of this multi-step process, the development of prostate cancer may involve various premalignant stages. These premalignant lesions have been termed *prostatic intraepithelial neoplasia* (PIN).

Undoubtedly, changes at the molecular level are involved in the development and progression of prostate cancer. Using sensitive molecular biology methods, the specific genetic (i.e., molecular) changes that occur during the process of carcinogenesis are being identified. A summary of some of the genetic alterations that occur during the multistage process of prostate carcinogenesis is provided in Fig. 68-5.

As with other types of cancers, the molecular events that lead to the development of prostate cancer occur in two types of cellular genes: oncogenes and tumor suppressor genes. Oncogenes are genes that normally function to enhance cell growth and development. The expression of these genes is tightly controlled, so that in normal adult tissues, a balance is maintained between cellular proliferation and cell death. Damage to a cellular oncogene can result in cellular proliferation and the development of prostate cancer. One group of oncogenes that has been well studied is the *ras* family of oncogenes (i.e., H, K, and N). A mutation of the H-*ras* oncogene may be involved in increasing the potential of prostate cancer to metastasize (Partin, Isaacs, Trieger, & Coffey, 1988).

Tumor suppressor genes normally function to prevent the continuous growth of cells. A genetic mutation in a tumor suppressor gene could result in uncontrolled cellular proliferation. As illustrated in Fig. 68-5, several tumor suppressor genes have been identified that are involved in the development of prostate cancer. For example, inactivation of tumor suppressor genes on chromosomes 8p, 10q, 16q, or 18q appear to be involved in the transformation of normal prostate cells to the cancerous phenotype (Scher, Isaacs, Fuks, & Walsh, 1995).

Several mutations in tumor suppressor genes may be involved in the progression of prostate cancer from localized to metastatic disease. Loss of the RB gene and inactivation of the p53 gene has been demonstrated in metastatic lesions from prostate cancer patients. In addition, at least three metastatic suppressor genes (i.e., 10q23, 11p13-p12, and 16q22.1) have been identified. Mutations in these genes are found in metastatic prostate cancer cells but not in nonmetastatic prostate cancer cells. The E-cadherin gene is located on chromosome 16. Expression of the protein product from the gene (i.e., E-cadherin) suppresses, while loss of expression enhances the invasiveness and motility of epithelial cells. A mutation of the E-cadherin gene may increase the metastatic potential of prostate cancer cells (Scher et al., 1995).

The Genetic Basis for Hormonal Independence of Prostate Cancer Cells

Since 1940, clinicians have known that prostate cancers are hormonally responsive tumors. This fact led to the development of treatments aimed at androgen withdrawal. Nearly all men with metastatic prostate cancer treated with surgical or chemical castration experience dramatic effects. While this initial response is beneficial, virtually all patients relapse with androgen-insensitive tumors and tumor progression.

These observations led clinicians to postulate that three types of prostate cancer cells may exist (i.e., androgen-dependent, androgen-sensitive, and androgen-independent cancer cells). These three cell types may exist within the same tumor. Androgen-dependent cancer cells require androgens for continued proliferation. Androgen-sensitive cancer cells do not die if androgen is not present. However, growth rates of these cells are decreased following androgen ablation. Finally, androgen-independent cancer cells do not die in the absence of androgens (i.e., their cellular growth is totally independent of androgen stimulation). Recent evidence suggests that the progression of prostate cancer cells to androgen-independent cells occurs when the *bcl*-2 oncogene is overexpressed. The net effect of *bcl*-2 overexpression is to increase the growth rate of prostate cancer cells (Scher et al., 1995).

ROUTES OF METASTASES

Cancers of the prostate spread by direct extension through the capsule of the gland into the seminal vesicles, the neck of the bladder, and the pelvic lymphatics. Metastatic spread occurs through both lymphatic and hematogenous routes. Lymphatic spread begins in the pelvic lymph nodes near the prostate gland and extends to the lymph nodes around the arteries and veins leading to the legs and pelvic organs. Metastatic spread through the hematogenous route affects the bone and the liver. The bone is the most frequent metastatic site (Maxwell, 1993). In addition, at the time of diagnosis, 6% of patients have lung metastases. Among patients with stage D disease, 25% of the patients have pulmonary metastases.

ASSESSMENT

The assessment of a patient for prostate cancer is summarized in Table 68-2. Clinical evaluation of the patient involves a detailed history, a thorough physical examination, and a variety of diagnostic tests. The signs and symptoms present in the patient often depend on the stage of disease at the time of diagnosis.

History

The patient should be evaluated for all of the identified risk factors for prostate cancer. In addition, a careful history of the genitourinary system should be obtained. When prostate cancer is causing obstruction of the urethra, the patient typically reports symptoms similar to BPH: hesitancy, decreased force of the urinary stream, intermittency, and post-void dribbling. The obstruction produces decreased compliance of the detrusor muscle, which results in the symptoms of urinary frequency, nocturia, and urgency. A report of impotence indicates progression of the disease and tumor invasion of the neurovascular structures. Patients with advanced disease may complain of pain associated with bone metastasis.

Physical Examination

Digital rectal examination (DRE) allows for palpation of the prostate gland through the anterior rectal wall. The normal prostate is a rounded, heart-shaped structure about 2.5 cm in length that projects less than 1 cm into the rectal lumen. The median sulcus can be felt between the two lateral lobes. Only the posterior surface of the prostate is palpable.

Benign prostatic hypertrophy (BPH) presents on DRE as a firm, smooth, symmetric, and slightly elastic enlargement of the gland. The prostate may bulge more than 1 cm into the rectum. The hypertrophied tissue may obliterate the median sulcus. Prostate cancer, on DRE, is associated with the presence of a hard, irregular nodule that produces asymmetry in the gland and a variation in its consistency.

TABLE 68-2 Assessment of the Patient for Prostate Cancer

	Assessment Parameters	Typical Abnormal Findings
History	1. Personal and social history a. Age b. Ethnicity c. Family history 2. Evaluation of genitourinary system 3. Evaluation for pain	1. Personal and social risk factors a. Usually over age 60 b. More prevalent in African Americans than whites than Asians c. Positive family history increases the risk 2. Common symptoms include: hesitancy; intermittency; weak, forceless urinary stream; straining to void; postvoid dribbling, nocturia, urgency, sensation of incomplete voiding; dysuria, incontinence. 3. Patients with metastatic disease frequently complain of bone pain or lumbosacral back pain that radiates to hips or legs.
Physical Examination	1. Digital rectal examination (DRE) 2. Weight 3. Lymph node evaluation 4. Palpation of the bladder	1. With early disease on DRE, the prostate contains firm, nonraised nodules with sharp edges. The prostate may be asymmetric and have an induration. With advanced disease on DRE, the prostate contains hard and stone-like nodule(s) and may have an induration. 2. Weight loss is usually indicative of advanced disease. 3. Presence of supraclavicular or inguinal nodes may indicate metastatic disease. 4. A palpable bladder may indicate urinary outlet obstruction.
Diagnostic Tests	1. Serum PSA level 2. Transrectal ultrasonography (TRUS) 3. Acid phosphatase level 4. Magnetic resonance imaging (MRI) 5. Bone scan 6. Chest x-ray	1. Usually elevated in patients with prostate cancer. Normal range of PSA depends on the patient's age (see Table 68-4). 2. Prostate cancer appears hypoechoic on TRUS in 75% of the cases. 3. Elevated in patients with advanced prostatic cancer. Normal values vary depending on assay method used: Bodansky 0.5 - 2.0 μ/L King-Armstrong 0.1 - 5.0 μ/L Betsy-Lowry-Brock 0.1 - 0.8 μ/L Gutman 0.1 - 2.0 μ/L 4. MRI with an endorectal coil may be useful in the diagnosis and staging of prostate cancer. 5. Bone pain will be positive in patients with metastatic disease to the bone. 6. At the time of diagnosis, 6% of patients have lung metastasis. In patient with stage D disease, 25% of the patients have pulmonary metastasis.

As part of the physical examination, the bladder and lymph nodes should be palpated. The presence of supraclavicular or inguinal nodes may indicate the presence of metastatic disease. A palpable bladder may indicate urinary outlet obstruction. Weight loss in a patient with prostate cancer is usually an indication of advanced disease.

Diagnostic Tests

Prostate-specific antigen level. Prostate-specific antigen is a highly immunogenic glycoprotein, produced only by prostate tissue, that can be assayed from blood serum. The benefits of PSA in the diagnosis and staging of prostate cancer have been reviewed (Oesterling, 1995). Although serum PSA can detect more prostate cancers than DRE, the marker is not perfect. Serum PSA levels can be elevated in patients with acute prostatitis, prostatic ischemia/infarction, and BPH. Therefore its use as a routine screening tool is currently being debated. However, PSA is useful in the staging and follow-up of patients with prostate cancer.

Serum levels of PSA vary, depending on the volume of the cancer, the volume of BPH in the prostate, and the histologic differentiation of the tumor (i.e., more poorly differentiated tissue produces less PSA per gram of tissue). These factors need to be considered when interpreting the results of PSA tests. To correct for the influence of BPH volume on PSA levels, Benson and colleagues (Benson, Whang, Pantuck, Kaplan, Olsson, & Cooper, 1992) introduced the concept of prostate-specific antigen density (PSAD). The PSAD value is calculated by dividing the serum PSA by the estimated weight of the prostate determined by transrectal ultrasonography (TRUS). An additional factor that must be considered when evaluating both PSA and PSAD values is the patient's age. Both of these values increase with age, therefore age-specific normal values have been established (Table 68-3). A recent study (Morgan, Jacobsen, McCarthy,

TABLE 68-3 Age-Specific Normal Ranges for Serum PSA and PSA Density

Age Range (years)	Serum PSA (ng/ml)	PSA Density (ng/ml/ml)
40-49	0.0-2.5	0.0-0.08
50-59	0.0-3.5	0.0-0.10
60-69	0.0-4.5	0.0-0.11
70-79	0.0-6.5	0.0-0.13

From Oesterling, J. E. (1995). Prostate-specific antigen: Its role in the diagnosis and staging of prostate cancer. *Cancer, 75,* 1795-1804.

TABLE 68-4 Age-Specific Reference Ranges for the Prostate-Specific Antigen (PSA) Test, Based on the Fifth Percentile of the Distribution of PSA Levels in the Patients According to Race

	Whites	African Americans
Age (years)	ng of PSA/ml	
40-49	0.0-2.5	0.0-2.0
50-59	0.0-3.5	0.0-4.0
60-69	0.0-3.5	0.0-4.5
70-79	0.0-3.5	0.0-5.5

From Morgan, T. O., Jacobsen, S. J., McCarthy, W. F., Jacobson, M. S., McLeod, D. G., & Moul, J. W. (1996). Age-specific reference ranges for serum prostate-specific antigen in black men. *New England Journal of Medicine, 335,* 304-310.

Jacobsen, McLeod, & Moul et al., 1996) suggests that PSA levels may vary not only by age but also by race. In this study, they determined the distribution of PSA and age-specific reference ranges in African American men, compared with white men, with and without prostate cancer. Serum PSA concentrations in African American men were significantly higher than those in white men. Table 68-4 lists the age-specific reference ranges for the PSA test, based on the fifth percentile of distribution of PSA levels in the study patients according to race (Morgan et al., 1996).

Serum PSA levels are used to follow patients being treated for prostate cancer. Because PSA is under androgen control, PSA levels usually decrease following tumor removal or hormonal deprivation. However, this decrease may not accurately reflect the response of the tumor to treatment. Regardless of this, serum PSA appears to be the single most reliable tumor marker that is available for following patients after definitive therapy. Elevations in serum PSA levels usually precede other clinical evidence of disease progression by at least 6 months (Scher et al., 1995).

Transrectal ultrasonography (TRUS). As illustrated in Fig. 68-6, high-resolution images of the peripheral zone of the prostate can be obtained through the use of transducers. Cancers found in the peripheral zone of the prostate, using TRUS, appear hypoechoic. The procedure has the ability to detect lesions smaller than 5 mm in diameter. However, it cannot detect lesions in the transition zone of the prostate, where approximately 25% of cancers develop.

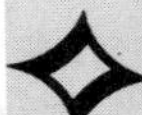

TABLE 68-5 Patient Preparation for Transrectal Ultrasonography

Description of the Procedure: Transrectal ultrasonography (TRUS) creates pictures of the prostate gland from the echoes of high-frequency sound waves passing through the anterior rectal wall.

Patient Preparation: Patient may be instructed to take an enema or a suppository the night before the procedure.

Procedural Considerations

1. Obtain informed consent.
2. Patient needs to disrobe below the waist or wear a gown.
3. Abdominal ultrasound may be done prior to the TRUS to evaluate for kidney distention.
4. Digital rectal examination is performed.
5. Patient is assisted into a knee-elbow or lateral decubitus position.
6. The probe is covered with an air-free, sterile transparent cover or condom; then lubricated and inserted slowly into the rectum.
7. After the probe is inserted, the condom is inflated with 20 ml to 60 ml of deaerated water.
8. The probe is angled anteriorly and the TRUS is performed.

Special Considerations

1. TRUS should be done prior to any intestinal barium tests because barium will interfere with the images.

Modified from Chernecky, C. C., Krech, R. L., & Berger, B. J. (1993). *Laboratory tests and diagnostic procedures.* Philadelphia: W. B. Saunders.

Ultrasound has not been useful in the screening and staging of prostate cancer. However, the technique is valuable in the diagnosis of prostate cancer because it can be used to estimate the volume of the prostate gland (i.e., used to determine PSAD) and in directing prostatic biopsies. The preparation of a patient for a TRUS is outlined in Table 68-5.

Acid phosphatase level. Acid phosphatase is one of a group of enzymes found primarily in the prostate gland and prostatic secretions. Elevations in this enzyme often indicate advanced prostate cancer. Because the development of the assay to measure PSA, serum acid phosphatase measurement is not used to stage the extent of prostate cancer. However, measurement of serum acid phosphatase may be useful in monitoring a patient's response to hormonal therapy.

Bone scan. A bone scan is done to determine if there is evidence of metastatic spread to the bone (Fig. 68-7). Suspicious areas on the bone scan should be evaluated with skeletal radiographs.

Diagnosis of prostate cancer. The diagnosis of prostate cancer is suggested by an abnormal DRE, an el-

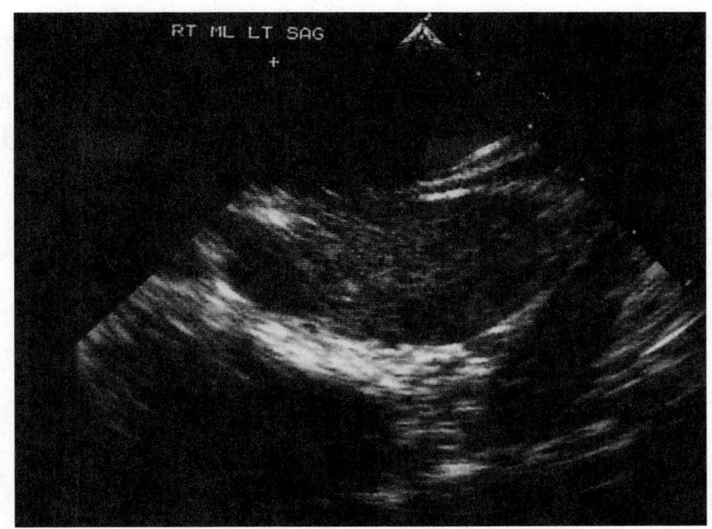

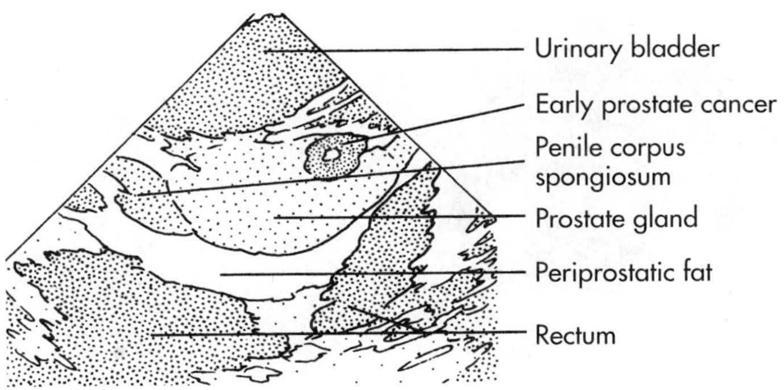

Fig. 68-6 Sagittal section ultrasonogram of prostate cancer. (From Kantoff, P. W., Garnick, M. B., & Corless, C. L. [1996]. Cancer of the genitourinary tract. In A. T. Skarin [Ed.], *Atlas of diagnostic oncology* [2nd ed.]. London: Mosby-Wolfe.)

TABLE 68-6 Diagnostic Algorithm for Using the Results of Age-Specific PSA Levels and DRE to Detect Clinically Significant and Life-Threatening Prostate Cancer

PSA Level*	DRE Findings	Diagnostic Action
Less than age-specific range	Negative →	Annual PSA and DRE
Greater than age-specific range	Negative →	TRUS: biopsy any visible lesions, sextant biopsy of remaining prostate, with two cores containing transition zone tissue
Any value	Positive →	TRUS: biopsy palpable and visible lesions, sextant biopsy of the remaining prostate

From Oesterling, J. E. (1995). Prostate-specific antigen: Its role in the diagnosis and staging of prostate cancer. *Cancer, 75,* 1795-1804.
*Age ranges: 0-49 years = 0-2.5 ng/ml; 50-59 years = 0-3.5 ng/ml; 60-69 years = 0-4.5 ng/ml; 70-79 years = 0-6.5 ng/ml.

evated PSA level, or abnormal findings on TRUS. However, all of these diagnostic tests have pitfalls. For example, only 25% to 50% of men with an abnormal DRE will be found to have cancer. While PSA is prostate-specific, it is not cancer-specific. Approximately one third of men with prostate cancer will have a PSA level below the normal range (PSA <4 ng/ml), and many men with elevated levels of serum PSA do not have cancer. However, cancer is diagnosed in approximately 25% of men with a serum PSA level of 4 to 10 ng/ml and in approximately 60% of men with a PSA level of greater than 10 ng/ml (Scher et al., 1995). A diagnostic algorithm for using the results of age-specific PSA levels and DRE to detect clinically significant and life-threatening prostate cancer is found in Table 68-6 (Oesterling, 1995).

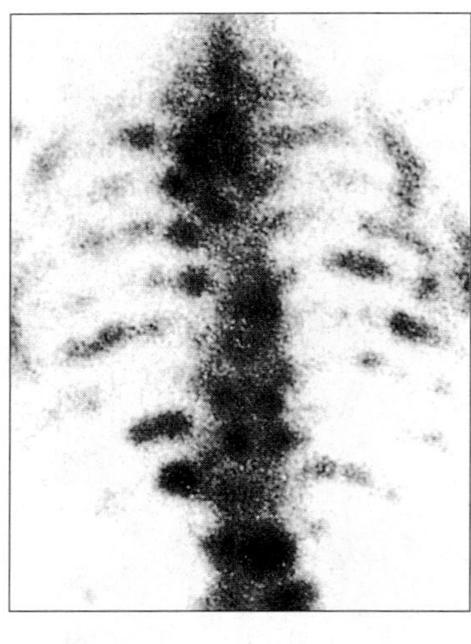

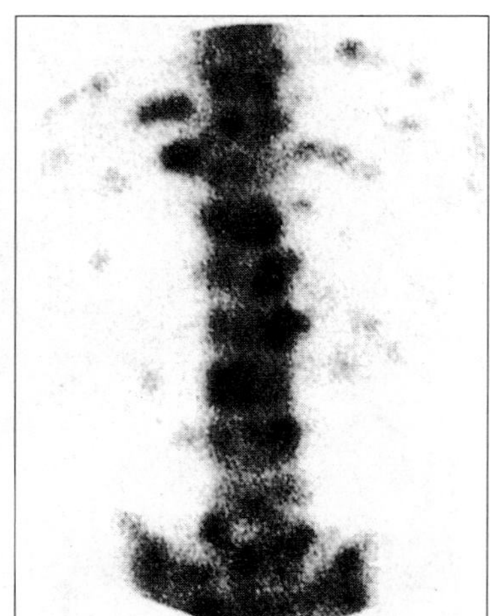

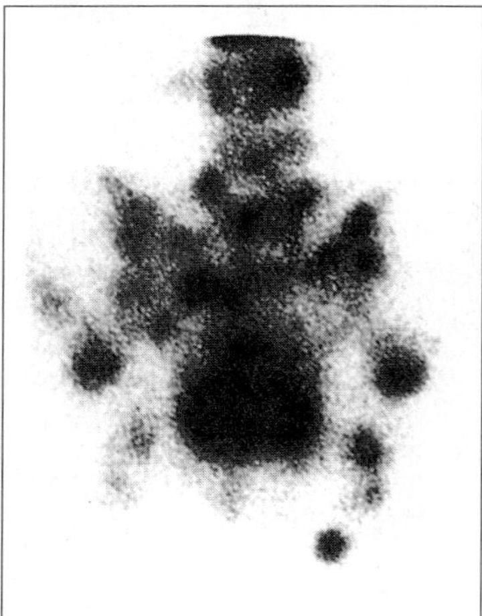

Fig. 68-7 Bone metastases. (From: Kantoff, P. W., Garnick, M. B., & Corless, C. L. [1996]. Cancer of the genitourinary tract. In A. T. Skarin [Ed.], *Atlas of diagnostic oncology* [2nd ed.] London: Mosby-Wolfe.)

STAGING

The staging of prostate cancer involves the use of a histologic staging system (i.e., Gleason grading system) and one of two clinical staging systems (i.e., the 1992 TNM classification system or the American Urological Association [AUA] staging system).

Histologic Staging

Histologic staging refers to the examination of the biopsy specimen(s) by a pathologist after surgery. Surgical removal of the prostate, seminal vesicles, and pelvic lymph nodes is required for complete histologic staging. The purpose of histologic staging is to determine the grade or biologic aggressiveness of the tumor.

The Gleason grading system (Murphy & Whitmore, 1979) has been used since 1979 as the histologic staging system for prostate cancer (i.e., establishes the degree of malignancy of the cancer). The Gleason system assigns a histologic grade to the predominant (i.e., primary) and the lesser (secondary) patterns in the tumor on a scale of 1 to 5 (Fig. 68-8). The grade numbers for the two patterns are added together to obtain the Gleason score, which can range from 2 to 10. The reproducibility of the Gleason score is approximately 80%. Higher scores indicate more aggressive disease.

Clinical Staging

Two systems have been used for the clinical staging of prostate cancer: the 1992 TNM classification system and the AUA system. The TNM staging system was developed by the American Joint Committee on Cancer (AJCC) and the International Union Against Cancer (UICC) (Montie, 1995). The two systems are shown in Table 68-7. Since 1993, TNM staging has been mandatory in all hospitals that are evaluated by the American Joint Commission on Cancer. However, the AUA system is commonly used in the United States because it is less cumbersome than the TNM system (Maxwell, 1993). The clinical staging system defines the extent of the patient's disease.

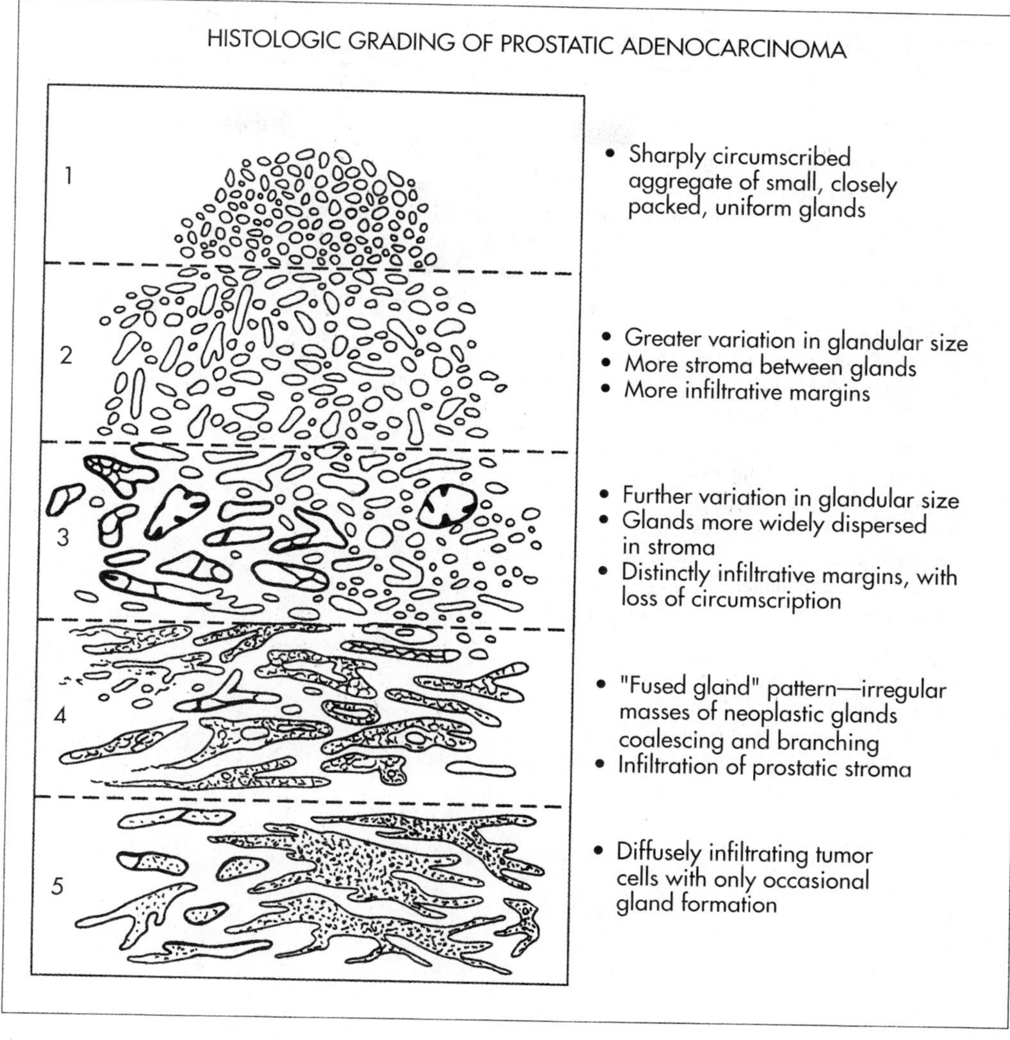

Fig. 68-8 Gleason pattern scores. (From Kantoff, P. W., Garnick, M. B., & Corless, C. L. [1996]. Cancer of the genitourinary tract. In A. T. Skarin [Ed.], *Atlas of diagnostic oncology* [2nd ed.] London: Mosby-Wolfe.)

MEDICAL MANAGEMENT

The treatment of prostate cancer depends on several factors, including the patient's age, the patient's general state of health, the tumor volume, the histologic grade of the tumor, and the stage of the disease (see Table 68-8 for recommendations on the medical management of prostate cancer based on AUA Staging of the disease, and Table 68-9 for recommendations on the medical management based on the TNM staging system). However, the medical management of all stages of prostate cancer remains controversial because data from large-scale, prospective, randomized clinical trials are not available. In general, surgery or radiation therapy are used for localized disease. Hormonal therapy is used for metastatic disease. In some cases, an approach of expectant management or watchful waiting will be used. In addition, new approaches are being developed to manage patients who experience recurrence of their disease following hormonal therapy (Catalano, 1994; Garnick, 1993; Garnick & Fair, 1996a, 1996b; Held, Osborne, Volpe, & Waldman, 1994; Maxwell, 1993; Scher et al., 1995).

Expectant Management

Controversy exists about the aggressive management of patients with stages A and B prostate cancer because the majority of men diagnosed with prostate cancer will die with the disease and not because of it. Because of the relatively low percentage of men who will die from prostate cancer and because of the risks and costs associated with aggressive treatment, some medical professionals are proposing expectant management for patients with early-stage prostate cancer. The use of this option of "watchful waiting" usually depends on the patient's age and the aggressiveness of the tumor (Held et al., 1994; Garnick, 1994).

According to Albertsen (1996), expectant management, or watchful waiting, appears to be most appropriate for

TABLE 68-7 TNM and AUA Staging Systems for Prostate Cancer

TNM Staging System	
Primary tumor (T)	
TX	Primary tumor cannot be assessed
T0	No evidence of primary tumor
T1	Clinically inapparent tumor neither palpable nor visible by imaging
T1a	Tumor incidental histologic finding in 5% or less of tissue resected
T1b	Tumor incidental histologic finding in more than 5% of tissue resected
T1c	Tumor identified by needle biopsy (e.g., because of elevated PSA)
T2	Tumor confined within prostate
T2a	Tumor involves one-half of a lobe or less
T2b	Tumor involves more than one-half of lobe, but not both lobes
T2c	Tumor involves both lobes
T3	Tumor extends through the prostatic capsule
T3a	Unilateral extracapsular extension
T3b	Bilateral extracapsular extension
T3c	Tumor invades seminal vesicle(s)
T4	Tumor is fixed or invades adjacent structures other than seminal vesicles
T4a	Tumor invades bladder neck, external sphincter, or rectum
T4b	Tumor invades levator muscles or is fixed to pelvic wall, or both
Node (N)	
NX	Regional lymph nodes cannot be assessed
N0	No regional node metastasis
N1	Metastasis in a single lymph node, 2 cm or less
N2	Metastasis in a single lymph node, more than 2 cm but not more than 5 cm
N3	Metastasis in a node more than 5 cm
Metastasis (M)	
MX	Presence of metastasis cannot be assessed
M0	No distant metastasis
M1	Distant metastasis
M1a	Nonregional lymph node(s)
M1b	Metastasis in bone(s)
M1c	Metastasis in other site(s)
AUA Staging System	
Stage A	Clinically unsuspected disease
A1	Focal carcinoma, well differentiated
A2	Diffuse carcinoma, usually poorly differentiated
Stage B	Tumor confined to prostate gland
B1	Small, discrete nodule of one lobe of gland
B2	Large or multiple nodules or areas of involvement
Stage C	Tumor localized periprostatic area
C1	Tumor outside prostate capsule, estimated weight less than 70 g, seminal vesicles uninvolved
C2	Tumor outside prostate capsule, estimated weight more than 70 g, seminal vesicles involved
Stage D	Metastatic prostate cancer
D1	Pelvic lymph node metastases or ureteral obstruction causing hydronephrosis or both
D2	Bone, soft tissue, organ, or distant lymph node metastases

older men who face minimal risk of disease progression. Therefore men over 65 years of age with low-grade disease and/or minimal tumor volume and men in their mid-seventies with low-to-moderate-grade disease confined to the prostate may decide that conservative management offers a low probability of death from prostate cancer without treatment-associated morbidity. Expectant management is not appropriate for younger men with modest tumor volumes.

Surgical Management

The two most common surgical procedures for prostate cancer are radical retropubic prostatectomy and radical perineal prostatectomy. A more recent surgical approach for the management of prostate cancer is cryosurgical ablation (Brenner & Krenzer, 1995).

Radical prostatectomy. Radical prostatectomy is usually performed in patients who are in good health under 75 years of age with a normal bone scan, a normal serum

TABLE 68-8 Medical Management of Prostate Cancer Based on the AUA Stage of the Disease

American Urologic Association Stage	Involvement	Therapeutic Options
A_1	Tissue is well-differentiated, often diagnosed as an incidental finding with transurethral resection of the prostate (TURP). Cancer involves less than 5% of resected tissue.	• Periodic observation • Radical prostatectomy • External radiation therapy
A_2	Microscopic disease, diffusely involves prostate gland; moderately to poorly differentiated.	• Radical prostatectomy • External radiation therapy
B_1	Less than 1.5 cm module limited to one prostate lobe.	• Radical prostatectomy • External radiation therapy
B_2	Greater than 1.5 cm nodule or multiple nodules or involving more than one prostate lobe.	• Radical prostatectomy • External or internal radiation therapy
C	Tumor extends through prostatic capsule; tumor involves bladder neck or seminal vesicles.	• External radiation therapy • External radiation therapy plus internal radiation therapy • Prostatectomy with postoperative radiation therapy • Radiation therapy with hormonal therapy • Hormonal therapy
D_1	Metastases to pelvis, pelvic lymph nodes.	• Hormonal therapy, radiation therapy, or both • Investigational drugs
D_2	Distant metastases.	• Hormonal therapy • Chemotherapy including investigational drugs

From Held, J. L., Osborne, D. M., Volpe, H., & Waldman, A. R. (1994). Cancer of the prostate: Treatment and nursing implications. *Oncology Nursing Forum, 21 (9),* 1517-1529.

TABLE 68-9 Recommended Treatment of Prostate Cancer According to the Stage of the Disease and Qualifying Conditions

Stage/Qualifying Condition	Recommended Treatment
T1a	
Projected life expectancy $<$10 yr	Watchful waiting
Projected life expectancy $\leq$ 10 yr	Radical prostatectomy, radiation therapy, watchful waiting
T1b, T1c, T2a, T2b, or T2c	
Projected life expectancy $<$ 10 yr	Radiation therapy, hormonal therapy
Projected life expectancy $\leq$ 10 yr	Radical prostatectomy, radiation therapy, hormonal therapy
Positive Surgical Margins	
Focal and well or moderately differentiated	Watchful waiting
Diffuse and well or moderately differentiated	Radiation therapy
High-grade, diffuse, and poorly differentiated	Hormonal therapy
Lymph-node metastases (with or without prostate removal)	Early or delayed hormonal therapy
Recurrence after Surgery	
Without metastases	Radiation therapy
With metastases	Hormonal therapy
Recurrence after radiation	Hormonal therapy
T3	Radiation therapy
T4	Hormonal therapy
Persistently Elevated Serum Acid Phosphatase	
PSA $\leq$ 20 μg per liter	Hormonal therapy
PSA $<$ 20 μg per liter	Lymphadenectomy and radical prostatectomy, radiation therapy with or without lymphadenectomy, hormonal therapy
Disseminated disease	Hormonal therapy
Hormone-refractory disease	Radiation therapy, corticosteroid therapy, supportive therapy, chemotherapy, suramin

From Catalano, W. J. (1994). Management of cancer of the prostate. *New England Journal of Medicine, 331* (15), 996-1004.

acid phosphatase, and tumors localized to the gland (i.e., stages A_1, A_2, B_1, or B_2 or T1-2N0). According to Nadler and Andriole (1996), the best candidates for radical prostatectomy are men who have a 10-year to 20-year life expectancy with impalpable, clinically organ-confined, low-grade or moderate-grade prostate cancer. Results of a multi-institutional pooled analysis (Gerber et al., 1996) concluded that radical prostatectomy leads to high 10-year disease-specific survival rates in men with all grades of prostate cancer (i.e., 94% with grade 1, 80% with grade 2, and 77% with grade 3).

The approach to radical prostatectomy has changed over the past 15 years. Currently, the surgical approach that is advocated allows for direct intraoperative visualization of the area and the identification of the extent of the disease, with wide excision when necessary.

Radical prostatectomy, using a retropubic or perineal approach, involves the removal of the entire prostate gland, including the prostatic capsule, the seminal vesicles, and a portion of the bladder neck. Prior to removal of the prostate, the pelvic lymph nodes are removed. Before 1982, radical prostatectomy resulted in permanent erectile dysfunction in all patients and urinary incontinence in many. In 1982, Walsh and colleagues theorized that impotence did not have to occur following radical prostatectomy (Walsh & Donker, 1982). They demonstrated that impotence results from injury to the pelvic nerve bundle (or pelvic plexus), which lies between the posterior prostate and the rectum. This observation led to the development of the nerve-sparing technique of radical prostatectomy. Another major advance in prostate cancer surgery is the ability of the surgeon to control bleeding from the dorsal vein complex so that the procedure can be performed in a relatively bloodless field and with minimal blood loss for the patient.

The major complications of radical prostatectomy are impotence and urinary incontinence. Prior to the development of the nerve-sparing procedure, all patients were left impotent. In one study of 600 men between the ages of 34 and 72 years who underwent nerve-sparing radical prostatectomy, 503 were potent preoperatively. After 18 months of follow-up, 68% of the men were potent postoperatively. Three factors correlated with the return of sexual functioning: age, clinical and pathologic stage of the disease, and whether one or both neurovascular bundles remained intact (Quinlan, Epstein, Carter, & Walsh, 1991). Table 68-10 provides data on age differences in the percentage of patients who were potent following radical prostatectomy. In the same study (Quinlan et al., 1991), it was noted that when the relative risk for impotence was adjusted for age, the risk of impotence was two times greater if the cancer had penetrated the capsule of the prostate or invaded the seminal vesicles. Patients who have the best recovery of sexual functioning appear to be those who are younger and have disease that is confined to the prostate.

Table 68-10 Percentage of Patients by Age Who Were Potent Following Radical Prostatectomy

Age (years)	Percent Potent
<50	91
50-60	75
61-70	58
>70	25

From Quinlan, D. M., Epstein, J. I., Carter, B. S., Walsh, P. C. (1991). Sexual function following radical prostatectomy: Influence of preservation of neurovascular bundles. *Journal of Urology, 145*, 998-1002.

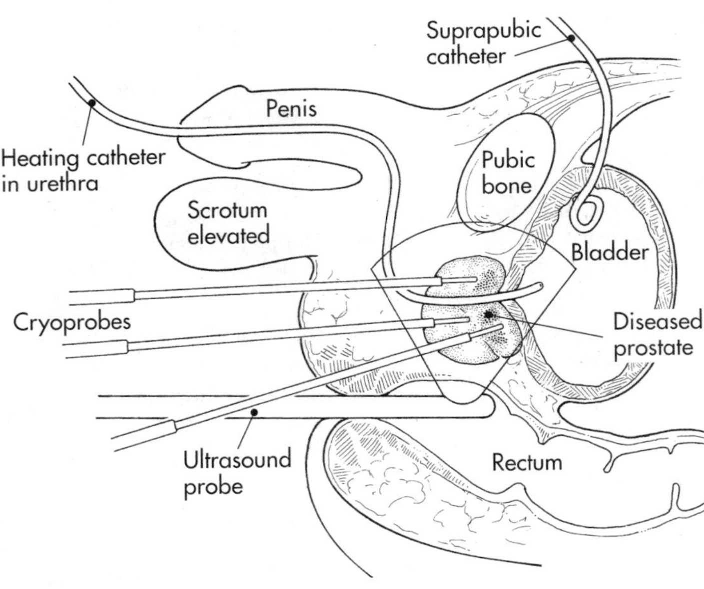

Fig. 68-9 Graphic depiction of perineal cryosurgical ablation of the prostate. (From Long, J. P. [1996]. Is there a role for cryoablation of the prostate in the management of localized prostate carcinoma? *Hematology/Oncology Clinics of North America, 10*[3], 675-690.)

The complication of urinary incontinence has decreased markedly due to improvements in the surgical procedure. This improvement is largely due to better control of intraoperative bleeding, which allows the surgeon better visualization of the juncture between the prostate and the urinary sphincter; preservation of the pelvic plexus, which provides autonomic nervous system innervation to the muscle at the apex of the prostate; and improvements in our understanding of the striated muscle of the urinary sphincter, which enables a more accurate anastomosis of the sphincter to the bladder. Therefore, complete urinary control can be achieved in approximately 92% of patients.

The immediate postoperative complications of radical prostatectomy include bleeding, rectal injury, and pulmonary emboli. Due to new surgical techniques, bleeding is usually minimal following radical prostatectomy. Rectal injury is a rare complication occurring in approximately 1% of patients. Pulmonary emboli occur in approximately 2% of patients following radical prostatectomy (Scher et al., 1995).

Cryosurgical ablation. Cryosurgical ablation of prostate cancer is a surgical procedure that may be considered as an alternative to radiation therapy for patients with localized disease, or as an option for patients in whom radiation therapy was not effective or who are not candidates for radical prostatectomy (Brenner & Krenzer, 1995; Long, 1996; Miller, Cohen, Shuman, & Merlotti, 1996).

The cryosurgical procedure involves freezing the entire prostate gland and portions of the seminal vesicles closest to the prostate. The prostatic urethra is maintained above the patient's core body temperature using an irrigation of water heated to 44° C. The surgeon uses TRUS guidance to pinpoint the places to insert the freezing probes. Generally three to five probes are placed within the prostate (Fig. 68-9). Liquid nitrogen is used to cool the probes, initially down to −70° C (−68.4° F) to fix them in position and then down to −195° C (−293.4° F) (Brenner et al., 1995).

Cryosurgery is believed to cause tumor cell death by a variety of mechanisms (Long, 1996). It is generally believed that the most potent mechanism for cellular destruction involves the creation of intracellular ice crystals. In addition, the creation of extracellular ice crystals appears to destroy cells by inducing intracellular dehydration with the accumulation of toxic concentrations of metabolites. These two mechanisms appear to work in concert to produce cell death. The thawing of the tissue after freezing also appears to contribute to cell death because it produces cell lysis (Long, 1996).

The major complications of the cryosurgical ablation procedure are incontinence, urethrorectal fistula formation, sloughing of urethral tissue, which obstructs urine flow, urethral stricture, numbness of the glans penis, and prostatic abscess. As shown in Table 68-11, these complications are relatively rare.

Radiation Therapy

Radiation therapy is used to treat localized disease in patients who are not good surgical candidates due to age or

TABLE 68-11 Complications Attributable to Cryosurgical Ablation of Prostate (CSAP)

	Shin Ohara et al., 1995	Bahn et al., 1995	Cox et al., 1995	Wieder et al., 1995	Long et al., 1995a Long et al., 1995b			Miller et al., 1994	Onik et al., 1993
					Non-XRT	XRT	Total		
No. patients	65	210	63	83	105	23	128	79	55
Complications (%)									
Urethrorectal fistula	0.8	2.4	3	0	0	13	2.7	0	2.4
Tissue sloughing	NR	NR	19	3.8	3.8	2	4	1.3	4.4
Urethral stricture	NR	NR	3	3.8	0	0	0	1.3	NR
Bladder outlet obstruction	15	3	29	13	8	26	12	1.3	NR
Incontinence (any)	1	9	27	2.5	1	70	16	2.7	NR
Impotence	86	40	NR	80	91	NA	91	NR	65
Perineal pain	NR	NR	11	NR	0	22	4	NR	NR
Urinary tract infection	18	NR	NR	6.3	4	17	5	NR	NR
Epididymitis	3	NR	NR	2.5	3	0	2	NR	NR
Sepsis	NR	NR	3	NR	1.9	0	1.6	NR	NR
Other*	NR	NR	13	2.6	0	0	0	NR	NR
Total complications†	*NR*	*14*	*59*	*NR*	*20*	*75*	*29*	*NA*	*NR*
Operations post-CSAP	NR	NR	43	NR	14	40	18	NR	NR
Any treatment post-CSAP	NR	NR	NR	NR	11	26	13	NR	NR

From Long, J. P. (1996). Is there a role for cryoablation of the prostate in the management of localized prostate carcinoma? *Hematology/Oncology Clinics of North America, 10*(3), 675-690.

*Ureteral obstruction, bladder injury, hematoma, etc.

†Excludes impotence.

XRT, External beam radiation therapy; *NR,* not reported; *NA,* not applicable (all patients impotent pre-CSAP).

concurrent medical illnesses or who refuse surgery. Radiation therapy treatments are administered through an external beam approach or through internal implants.

External beam radiation therapy. The survival rates following external beam radiation are equivalent to radical prostatectomy for patients with localized disease (i.e., stages A_1, A_2, and B, or T1-2a). Radiation treatments are given 5 days a week at doses of 180-200 cGy for 6 to 7 weeks (total dose 6200-7400 cGy). External beam radiation is generally well tolerated by the patient. The acute problems of rectal discomfort, tenesmus, diarrhea, urinary frequency, nocturia, dysuria, and urgency occur in approximately 60% of patients. The symptoms usually occur during the third week of treatment and resolve days to weeks after treatment is completed.

The occurrence of late complications of radiation therapy (i.e., complications that occur 6 or more months after the completion of treatment) are relatively rare. Possible late complications of external beam radiation include cystitis, hematuria, urethral stricture, bladder contracture, chronic diarrhea, proctitis, rectal or anal strictures, rectal bleeding, and rectal ulcers. Sexual function is preserved in 73% to 82% of patients following radiation therapy (Hartford & Zietman, 1996; Scher et al., 1995).

External beam radiation therapy and hormone therapy. Androgen deprivation is an effective method of inhibiting the proliferation of prostate cancer cells and activating the mechanism of aptosis, which results in programmed cell death. Because the likelihood of successful tumor control with radiation therapy increases as the tumor size is reduced, the reduction in tumor bulk induced by androgen deprivation could increase the probability of tumor eradication of a subsequently irradiated tumor (Hartford & Zietman, 1996).

Recently, the Radiation Therapy Oncology Group (RTOG) reported the results of two randomized clinical trials that investigated the effectiveness of androgen suppression used in combination with radiation therapy to radiation therapy alone (i.e., RTOG 85-31 trial, Pilepich, Caplan, & Byhardt, 1995a; RTOG 86-10 trial, Pilepich, Krall, as-Sarraf, John, Doggett, & Sause et al., 1995b). The results of these two RTOG trials are summarized in Table 68-12.

In RTOG 85-31 (Pilepich et al., 1995a), patients with bulky primary tumors (large T_2, T_3, and T_4) were randomized to receive either radiation therapy alone or radiation therapy in combination with 4 months of androgen suppression. The androgen suppression regimen consisted of a total of 4 months of goserelin and flutamide therapy (i.e., 2 months before and 2 months during radiation therapy). With a median potential follow-up of 4.5 years, a significant improvement in progression-free survival was seen at 5 years with combined modality therapy compared with radiation therapy alone (36% vs 15%, $p < 0.001$).

In the second RTOG study, (i.e., RTOG-86), patients with very poor risk but apparently locally or at least regionally confined prostate cancer were randomized to receive either radiation therapy alone or adjuvant androgen suppression following radiation therapy (Pilepich et al., 1995b). At the time the abstract was written, 950 patients were accrued to the study. With a median follow-up on only 3 years, the data show a significant benefit in the prevention of clinical local tumor regrowth (83% irradiation plus ablation vs 68% conventional treatment), and a significant benefit in progression-free survival, using a PSA of greater than 4 ng/ml as the endpoint (53% eradication plus ablation vs 24% conventional treatment, $p < 0.001$).

Internal Radiation Therapy. The exact role for interstitial brachytherapy in the management of prostate cancer has not been determined (D'Amico & Coleman, 1996; Grimm, Blasko, Radge, Sylvester, & Clarke, 1996). The treatment involves the placement of a permanent or temporary radioactive source into the prostate gland. Because of the short range of this form of radiation, high doses can be delivered to the cancer with relative sparing of surrounding tissues. Transperineal permanent seed implantation is typically done as a single outpatient treatment under spinal an-

TABLE 68-12 Results of Two Recently Reported RTOG Comparative Randomized Trials of Radiation Alone versus Combined Modality Treatment with Radiation and Endocrine Therapy in Patients with Advanced Prostate Cancers

	RTOG 85-31 Trial*		RTOG 86-10 Trial‡	
Stage	T3, (+) nodes, (+) margins, or (+) seminal vesicles		T2 ≥ 25 cm², T3-T4	
Median follow-up	3 yrs		4.5 yrs	
Number of patients	950		456	
5-year actuarial data:	XRT alone	XRT + adjuvant androgens*	XRT alone	Androgen ablation with XRT†
Clinical local failures	32%	17% (P < 0.001)	71%	46% (P < 0.001)
Biochemical failures (PSA > 4 ng/mL)	83%	51% (P < 0.001)	85%	64% (P < 0.001)

*Goserelin therapy every 4 weeks, starting after conclusion of radiation therapy.
†Four months of goserelin and flutamide therapy, 2 months before and 2 months during radiation treatment.
XRT, External beam radiation therapy.
‡From Pilepich, M. V., Krall, J. M., as-Sarraf, M., John, M. J., Doggett, R. L., Sause, W. T., Lawton, C. A., Abrams, R. A., Rotman, M., & Rubin, P. (1995). Androgen deprivation with radiation therapy compared with radiation therapy alone for locally advanced prostatic carcinoma: A randomized comparative trial of the Radiation Therapy Oncology Group. *Urology, 45*(4), 616-623.

esthesia. There is no surgical incision. Needles are inserted through a template system into the perineum and directed to their predetermined targets by ultrasound guidance (Fig. 68-10). A typical permanent implant requires 80 to 100 radioactive sources or "seeds." Postoperatively, patients are temporarily placed on antibiotics, anti-inflammatory drugs, and antispasmodic medications (Grimm et al., 1996).

Post-implant evaluations of seed distribution and dose can be performed by use of CT-based dosimetry. PSA levels and digital rectal examinations are typically performed at 3-month intervals, and biopsies are performed at 2 years (Grimm et al., 1996).

Temporary implantation techniques involve the placement of needles into the prostate gland under direct surgical or ultrasound-directed template guidance. The isotope (usually iridium-192) is then inserted into the needle and left in place temporarily. The radioactive source is usually inserted using an afterloading device, while personnel are out of the room, to ensure optimal radiation protection for health care personnel (Grimm et al., 1996).

The most commonly used isotopes for the management of prostate cancer are listed in Table 68-13. The choice of radioisotope depends on the stage of the disease, the use of other concurrent treatments, and the length of time required for the placement. The goal of interstitial brachytherapy is to achieve a predetermined dose of radiation that is effective enough to kill the tumor cells while keeping side effects to a minimum. The potential side effects associated with interstitial brachytherapy include perineal discomfort, difficulty urinating, hematuria, and infection (Held et al., 1994).

Hormonal Therapy

Hormonal therapy is used to manage advanced-stage prostate cancer. Because prostate cancer is a hormonally responsive tumor, treatment is directed at androgen ablation. The major androgen involved in the growth of prostate cancer is testosterone. Approximately 90% to 95% of the circulating testosterone comes from the testes; the remainder is produced by the adrenal gland. Methods used to achieve androgen ablation include orchiectomy or the administration of estrogens, luteinizing hormone–releasing factor (LHRH) agonists, antiandrogens, and adrenal enzyme synthesis inhibitors (e.g., ketoconazole, aminoglutethimide).

Orchiectomy. Orchiectomy, or removal of the testes, is the treatment of choice in severely symptomatic patients and in those with impending or newly diagnosed paralysis secondary to spinal cord compression. The procedure reduces testosterone levels by 90% to 95%. The decrease in the levels of testosterone is extremely rapid, with pain relief

TABLE 68-13 Radioisotopes Used in the Treatment of Prostate Cancer

Radioisotope	Radiation Emission	Method of Administration	Clinical Uses
Iodine-125	Gamma	Permanent interstitial implant	Well to moderately differentiated tumors (Gleason Score 2-6)
Paladium-103	Gamma	Permanent interstitial implant	More poorly differentiated tumors (Gleason Score 7-10)
Iridium-192	Gamma	Temporary implant	Can be used as a low-dose-rate (LDR) or high-dose-rate (HDR) form

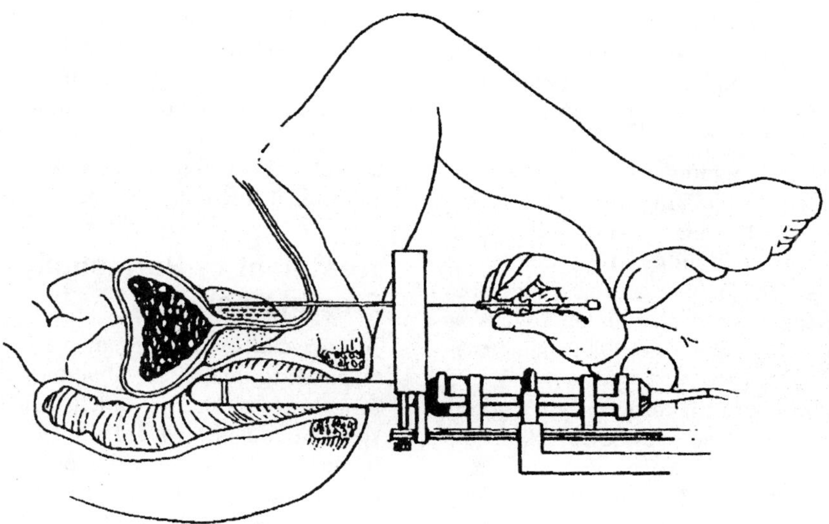

Fig. 68-10 Modern transperineal seed implantation. (From Grimm, P. D., Blasko, J. C., Ragde, H., Sylvester, J., & Clarke, D. [1996]. Does brachytherapy have a role in the treatment of prostate cancer? *Hematology/Oncology Clinics of North America, 10*[3], 653-673.)

occurring in the immediate postoperative period. The major side effects associated with orchiectomy include loss of libido, impotence, and hot flashes (McLeod, 1995; Held et al., 1994).

Estrogen Therapy. Estrogens produce a chemical castration by acting on the hypothalamus to suppress the release of LHRH, which results in the suppression of leutinizing hormone (LH) release from the anterior pituitary. It takes approximately 1 to 2 weeks to achieve castration levels of testosterone. Diethylstilbestrol (DES) is the primary estrogen used in the management of metastatic prostate cancer (McLeod, 1995).

The optimal dose of DES is currently being debated. A daily oral dose of 3 mg of DES appears to be required to obtain a castration level of testosterone. However, in some patients, 1 mg of DES per day will lower testosterone to castration levels. While the cost of DES is negligible, the complications associated with the drug are not. The major complications include fluid retention, angina, ischemic heart disease, venous thrombosis, and stroke. Due to the potential for significant morbidity associated with DES, the drug is seldom used today. However, in some cases, clinicians are prescribing varying doses (1 mg to 3 mg/day) with daily aspirin (McLeod, 1995).

LHRH Agonists. Androgen blockade can be achieved through the use of superpotent LHRH agonists (e.g., leuprolide acetate, goserelin). The LHRH agonists act on the anterior pituitary to decrease the number of receptor sites, which results in complete blockade of LHRH. The complete blockade results in suppression of LH release from the anterior pituitary. In males, LH stimulates the testes to produce testosterone. Ultimately, the LHRH agonists deprive the testes of LH stimulation.

During the first 2 to 4 weeks of therapy, LHRH agonists stimulate the anterior pituitary to produce LH, which stimulates testosterone production. This transitory rise in testosterone may result in the worsening of symptoms or a "flare" reaction during the first several days of therapy. The use of LHRH agonists is contraindicated in patients with severe urethral obstruction or in patients with extensive vertebral metastases where spinal cord compression is imminent. The major side effect of the LHRH agonists is hot flashes (Maxwell, 1993; McLeod, 1995).

Antiandrogens. The antiandrogens are a group of drugs that exert their effects by blocking the uptake of androgens in the target organs. The main mode of action in prostate cancer appears to be their ability to prevent the interaction of testosterone and DHT with androgen receptors on prostate cells. There are two types of antiandrogens or androgen-receptor antagonists, namely steroidal and nonsteroidal compounds.

The two principal steroidal antiandrogens are cyproterone acetate and megestrol acetate. Besides blocking the interaction of testosterone at the androgen receptor, these drugs also suppress LH production. It should be noted that neither compound has been found to suppress androgen production as much as orchiectomy, DES, or LHRH agonists (McLeod, 1995).

The nonsteroidal, or "pure," antiandrogens include flutamide, nilutamide, and bicalutamide. These drugs block the action of testosterone at the androgen receptor but they do not interfere with LH production. Patients taking the nonsteroidal antiandrogens frequently maintain their potency and libido because LH production continues.

Flutamide is the nonsteroidal antiandrogen approved for use in the United States. It is used primarily in conjunction with an LHRH agonist or orchiectomy. The usual dose is 250 mg per day, every 8 hours. The half-life of flutamide is 5.2 hours. The major side effects associated with flutamide are diarrhea, breast tenderness, and hepatotoxicity.

Adrenal Enzyme Synthesis Inhibitors. These agents (i.e., ketoconazole and aminoglutethimide) are commonly used as second-line hormonal agents. Ketoconazole administered at doses of 1200 mg/day produces castration levels of testosterone in 24 hours. This agent may be used in patients with prostate cancer who present with spinal cord compression. The hormonal effects reverse rapidly once the drug is discontinued. Similar effects are seen with the administration of aminoglutethimide (Scher et al., 1995).

Combined Androgen Blockade. Combined androgen blockade (CAB) is the addition of an antiandrogen to either medical (i.e., LHRH agonist, estrogens) or surgical (i.e., orchiectomy) castration. An LHRH agonist or orchiectomy plus flutamide appears to produce better clinical responses. In addition, total androgen blockade appears to delay the time to progression of the disease and improves survival by several months (Crawford & Nabors, 1991). Combined androgen blockade should always be considered when hormonal therapy is indicated (Labrie, Belanger, Simard, Labrie, & Dupont, 1993; Robson & Dawson, 1996; Bubley & Balk, 1996).

Chemotherapy

Metastatic prostate cancer that is refractory to hormone treatment was thought to be unresponsive to chemotherapy. Past reports of the use of cytotoxic chemotherapy demonstrated disappointing response rates of less than 20%. However, recent trials using PSA levels as a surrogate endpoint demonstrate that single agents may actually yield objective responses of up to 60% with minimal side effects. A predictable number of responses are being observed with cyclophosphamide and mitoxantrone (Mani & Vogelzang, 1996). Additional research is needed in this area.

Treatment of Hormonally Refractory Prostate Cancer

Approximately 30% of patients with prostate cancer do not respond to androgen ablation, and almost all patients progress to a state at which their disease is no longer responsive to androgen ablation. This clinical observation led to the hypothesis that within prostate cancers there is a clone of hormone-independent prostate cancer cells. The growth of this clone of cells results in the failure of androgen ablation. The management of hormonally refractory prostate cancer may include the withdrawal of flutamide, the administration of chemotherapy, or the use of suramin (Mani & Vogelzang, 1996).

Flutamide Withdrawal Syndrome. Flutamide withdrawal syndrome refers to a recently described clinical phenomenon seen in prostate cancer patients with progressive disease who are on CAB therapy. In these patients, stopping their flutamide while maintaining their LHRH agonist results in improvement in clinical symptoms and a decrease in their serum PSA levels. The improvement is of short duration (typically 5 months). The mechanism underlying this phenomenon is not completely understood and requires additional investigations (Scher et al., 1995).

Suramin. Suramin is an investigational drug that is currently being tested in patients with hormonally refractory prostate cancer. Suramin produces a wide variety of biologic effects, including inactivating a wide variety of cellular enzymes; inhibiting the binding of growth factors to cell surface receptors; and halting intracellular signalling mechanisms. Although the current clinical trials are promising, the toxicities associated with the administration of suramin are significant. Patients must be monitored for proteinuria, coagulopathies, adrenal insufficiency, immunosuppression, fatigue and malaise, and peripheral neuropathies (Eisenberger, Reyno, Sinibaldi, Sridhara, Carducci, & Egorin, 1995).

ONCOLOGIC EMERGENCIES

The major oncologic emergency associated with prostate cancer is epidural spinal cord compression (SCC). Back pain is the initial symptom in over 95% of the cases. Because the degree of neurologic function following treatment is directly associated with the amount of neurologic function present at the time of diagnosis, prompt recognition and management of SCC is mandatory.

The back pain is usually localized over the site of the SCC but can radiate. The pain exacerbates with coughing, straining, or movement. Progression of symptoms includes motor weakness, sensory deficits (e.g., paresthesias, numbness), and autonomic dysfunction (e.g., urinary retention/incontinence, constipation, or fecal incontinence). Patients with the signs and symptoms of SCC require prompt evaluation and treatment.

NURSING MANAGEMENT

The medical management of prostate cancer is extremely complex and variable depending on the patient's age, clinical condition, and stage of his disease at the time of diagnosis. The nursing management of patients with prostate cancer has been summarized in several publications (Maxwell, 1993; Held et al., 1994; Larkin, 1995). Patients with prostate cancer have numerous problems that require nursing interventions and patient education (Ofman, 1995; Sprouse, 1995; Blaivas, 1995, Kirschenbaum, 1995). While a portion of the patient's care will occur in the inpatient setting, the majority of the patient's care will occur in the outpatient and home care settings.

Early in the course of the patient's disease, the focus of nursing care may be on helping the patient understand the different treatment options. As the disease progresses, patients need information about the rationale for different types of pharmacologic interventions as well as strategies for managing the side effects associated with the disease or treatments. Because each major type of treatment for prostate cancer (i.e., surgery, radiation therapy, and hormonal therapy) poses unique patient problems, the major issues associated with these treatments are discussed below and three standards of care are provided in this chapter.

Surgery

Patients undergoing radical prostatectomy are usually hospitalized for 5 days. The major focus of inpatient nursing care is on the prevention of postoperative complications, including bleeding, thrombophlebitis, infection, and pulmonary emboli. Follow-up care in the outpatient setting requires that nurses evaluate patients for impotence and urinary incontinence. The nursing management of the patient undergoing surgery for prostate cancer is summarized in Table 68-14.

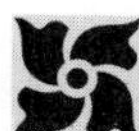

TABLE 68-14 Standard of Care for the Patient Undergoing Radical Prostatectomy

Patient Problem and Outcomes	Nursing Interventions and Rationales	Patient Education Instructions
Anxiety Patient will: • Verbalize an understanding of the surgical procedure. • Express feelings of decreased anxiety. • Identify strategies to cope with anxiety.	1. Assess patient's level of understanding of the surgical procedure. 2. Give patient the opportunity to ask questions or verbalize concerns. 3. Determine which coping strategies the patient has used effectively in the past to decrease anxiety and reinforce the use of these coping strategies. 4. Administer pharmacologic agents to decrease anxiety, if necessary.	1. Utilize a diagram of the anatomy of the male genital tract to explain the radical prostatectomy procedure. 2. Provide patient with information about the preoperative routine: a. Diagnostic tests b. Bowel prep c. Anesthesiology consult d. Use of antiembolism stockings e. NPO after midnight

Continued

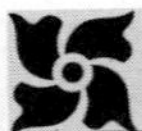

TABLE 68-14 Standard of Care for the Patient Undergoing Radical Prostatectomy—cont'd

Patient Problem and Outcomes	Nursing Interventions and Rationales	Patient Education Instructions
Anxiety—cont'd		3. Teach patient coughing and deep breathing exercises and obtain a return demonstration. 4. Provide patient with information about the postoperative plan of care: a. Pain management b. Management of bladder spasms c. Use of indwelling catheter d. Surgical incision e. Intravenous hydration
Catheter Obstruction Patient will have a urine flow of more than 30 ml/hr.	1. Assess for abdominal distention, which is an indication of catheter obstruction. 2. Measure urine output. 3. Assess catheter for patency and the presence of clots. 4. Irrigate catheter as needed to maintain patency. 5. Keep catheter taped securely to patient's leg or thigh to maintain patency.	1. Teach patient: a. To keep catheter drainage bag below the level of the bladder b. To call the nurse for increased pain or bladder spasms 2. Teach patient how to care for suprapubic tube or Foley catheter at home.
Bladder Spasms Patient will have prompt relief of bladder spasms if they occur.	1. Assess patient for bladder spasms. 2. Administer medications (e.g., belladonna and opium suppositories or oxybutynin) as prescribed.	1. Inform patient that spasms occur as a result of irritation to the bladder during surgery. 2. Tell patient to inform the nurse when spasms occur so that prompt treatment can be initiated.
Pain Patient will experience optimal pain relief with minimal side effects.	1. Assess pain intensity using a 0 to 10 verbal rating scale, every 2-4 hours for the first 48 hours after surgery, then at least once a shift. 2. Administer opioid analgesics around-the-clock for the first 24-48 hours postoperatively. 3. Monitor for analgesic side effects and administer medications to prevent or treat: a. Nausea b. Pruritus c. Constipation	1. Teach patient to inform the nurse if he is experiencing pain. 2. Teach patient the importance of taking pain medication on a regular basis to keep pain under control.
High Risk for Hemorrhage Patient will: • Maintain a normal hemoglobin and hematocrit. • Maintain hemodynamic stability.	1. Assess urinary drainage, including color and the presence of clots. 2. Check hemoglobin, hematocrit, and platelet count. 3. Check surgical incision and dressings for excessive drainage.	1. Teach patient that slight hematuria may occur for up to 2 weeks. 2. Teach patient to avoid strenuous exercises for 2-3 weeks after surgery.
High Risk for Pulmonary Embolism Patient will maintain normal arterial blood gases.	1. Apply antiembolic or compression stockings to both legs. 2. Perform active range-of-motion leg exercises to prevent deep vein thrombophlebitis. 3. Assess for leg pain and signs of thrombophlebitis.	1. Teach patient the importance of wearing antiembolic or compression stockings and the rationale for performing range-of-motion leg exercises.

Radiation Therapy

Patient problems will vary, depending on whether the patient is receiving external beam radiation therapy or interstitial brachytherapy. External beam therapy will be provided on an outpatient basis. The major problems associated with external beam radiation therapy include diarrhea and proctitis as well as cystitis, hematuria, and urethral strictures. Interstitial brachytherapy is done in the inpatient setting. Patients require a great deal of education to understand the precautions that must be instituted while they are receiving their therapy (Table 68-15). The nursing management of the patient with prostate cancer who is receiving external beam radiation therapy is summarized in Table 68-16.

Hormonal Therapy

Most patients receiving hormonal therapy will have advanced disease. Care in most cases is provided in the outpatient setting. Patients must be taught the rationale for the different hormonal treatments. In addition, strategies must be developed with the patient and family to manage the side effects associated with the different hormonal agents. Patients with advanced disease must be taught about the potential complications of the disease, including SCC, urinary tract obstruction, and increased levels of bone pain, which require prompt medical interventions. The management plan for the prostate cancer patient receiving hormonal therapy is summarized in Table 68-17.

Management of Metastatic Bone Pain

The management of pain in patients with prostate cancer has been summarized by Payne (1993). The prevalence of pain in patients with prostate cancer ranges from 55% to 100%.

Table 68-15 Precautions to be Used in Caring for a Patient With Interstitial Brachytherapy

Precautions	Beta Implant	Gamma Implant
Patient must remain in room.	X	X
Avoid contact with pregnant women and children.	X	X
Linen and trash in double plastic bags must remain in room.	X	X
Showers may be taken as desired.	X	X
Limit time in patient's presence (30 minutes per nurse per shift).	X	X
Stay as far away from source as possible	X	X
Use lead shielding.		X
Wear dosimeter film badge.	X	X

Modified from Held, J. L., Osborne, D. M., Volpe, H., & Waldman, A. R. (1994). Cancer of the prostate: Treatment and nursing implications. *Oncology Nursing Forum, 21 (9)*, 1517-1529.

The major causes of pain associated with prostate cancer are bone metastasis, soft tissue metastasis, and pelvic visceral pain. The first-line treatment for bone pain associated with metastatic prostate cancer involves treatment of the tumor. External beam radiation therapy for bone metastasis is usually effective in approximately 80% of patients (Hoskin, 1995; Nielsen, Munro, Tannock, 1991). In addition, hormonal therapies, (e.g., leuprolide) may reduce the pain associated with metastatic prostate cancer.

Another option that may be used in the management of metastatic bone pain is the administration of a radiopharmaceutical (e.g., strontium-89, Samarium SM153 Lexidronam). Partial to complete pain relief following the administration of strontium-89 has been reported to range from 51% to 89%. Within 2 days to 2 weeks after administration of strontium-89, patients may experience an exacerbation of their bone pain. However, pain lessens within 10 to 20 days after the injection, with maximal pain relief occurring within 6 weeks. The major side effects associated with the administration of strontium-89 are anemia, neutropenia, and thrombocytopenia (Strangio & Brudner, 1995).

The most common approaches used in the management of metastatic bone pain are summarized in Box 68-4. Regardless of the approach used to treat metastatic bone pain, patients will require opioid and nonopioid analgesics. These medications should be titrated to achieve optimal pain control with minimal side effects.

HOME CARE ISSUES

Depending on the treatment approaches used to manage prostate cancer, the patient and family caregivers will be faced with several issues in the home care setting. Several sources of patient information on prostate cancer are listed in Box 68-5. Patients recovering from a radical prostatectomy or cryosurgical procedure may need to care for their suprapubic catheter at home and learn how to conduct a voiding trial and monitor their urine output (Table 68-18).

Urinary Incontinence

Another problem patients may need to manage while at home is urinary incontinence. Urinary incontinence is defined as a condition in which involuntary loss of urine is a social or hygiene problem and is objectively demonstrable (Whitehead, Smith-Young, & Lang, 1985). This problem

Box 68-4
Agents Used in the Management of Metastatic Bone Pain

External bean radiation therapy
Hormonal therapy (e.g., leuprolide)
Opioid and nonopioid analgesics
Radiopharmaceuticals (e.g., strontium-89/Samarium SM153 Lexidronan)
Surgical procedures (e.g., hypophysectomy)

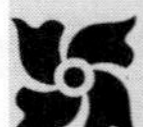

TABLE 68-16 Standard of Care for the Patient Receiving External Beam Radiation Therapy for Prostate Cancer

Patient Problem and Outcomes	Nursing Interventions and Rationales	Patient Education Instructions
Knowledge Deficit Patient will verbalize an understanding of the purpose, benefits, and risks of radiation therapy.	1. Assess patient's level of knowledge about radiation therapy. 2. Assess patient's concerns and fears about radiation therapy.	1. Describe the routine procedures involved in radiation therapy: a. Consultation b. Simulation procedure c. Treatment procedures and routines 2. Describe the major side effects associated with radiation therapy, the importance of notifying the nurse should side effects occur, and self-care measures to manage the side effects of: a. Diarrhea b. Proctitis c. Fatigue d. Cystitis
Fatigue Patient will be able to maintain normal activities of daily living and engage in activities to enhance his quality of life.	1. Assess patient's level of fatigue using a 0 (not at all tired, full of pep) to 10 (total exhaustion) rating scale. 2. Evaluate patient's sleep and activity pattern to be able to teach patient ways to conserve energy.	1. Inform patient that he is likely to experience fatigue toward the end of treatment and for several weeks following treatment. 2. Teach patient energy conservation strategies including: a. Going to bed at a regular time b. Taking short naps during the day c. Exercising at regular intervals during the day
Diarrhea Patient will maintain adequate fluid balance, weight, and energy level.	1. Assess elimination patterns, including frequency, quality, and quantity. 2. Initiate a low-residue diet at the start of treatment, including: a. Limit foods high in roughage b. Limit fried or highly seasoned food c. Avoid uncooked fruits and vegetables d. Limit rich desserts 3. Obtain a consult with a dietitian. 4. Administer antidiarrheal medication (e.g., Lomotil 2.5 mg tablets; 1 to 2 tablets after each loose bowel movement; not to exceed 8 tablets per day). 5. Obtain weights, weekly. 6. Institute a lactose-free diet if diarrhea becomes severe (i.e., greater than 8 bowel movements per day). 7. Administer tincture of opium (0.5 to 1.0 ml every 4 hours until diarrhea is controlled for severe diarrhea.	1. Inform patient that diarrhea occurs within a few weeks of treatment, usually when a dose of 1500-3000cGy is reached. 2. Teach patient to maintain a low-residue diet until bowel patterns return to normal (usually 2 to 6 weeks after the completion of radiation therapy). 3. Teach patient to evaluate for a pattern to the diarrhea and concentrate the administration of antidiarrheal medication to that time of day.
Cystitis Patient will experience relief of urinary symptoms	1. Assess for symptoms of frequency, burning on urination, and urgency. 2. Evaluate for the presence of a urinary tract infection and initiate appropriate antibiotic therapy if an infection is present. 3. Administer urinary antiseptics and antispasmodics: a. Phenazopyridine 200 mg, 3 times a day, after meals b. Oxybutin 5 mg, 2-3 times per day (not to exceed 20 mg/day)	1. Inform patient that urinary symptoms may occur after 3000 cGy have been administered. 2. Teach patient that phenazopyridine (an azo dye with local anesthesia of the urinary mucosa) turns urine an orange-red color. 3. Teach patient that antispasmodics such as oxybutin can cause drowsiness, dry mouth, constipation, and urinary retention.

TABLE 68-17 Standard of Care for the Patient Receiving Hormonal Therapy for Advanced Prostate Cancer

Patient Problem and Outcomes	Nursing Interventions and Rationales	Patient Education Instructions
Impotence		
Patient will be able to engage in alternative forms of sexual expression	1. Obtain a sexual history including: a. Sexual activity b. Effect of previous therapies on sexual functioning c. Onset of the impotency d. Course of the events e. Patient's perception of the problem 2. Encourage alternative methods of sexual expression. 3. Make referrals to appropriate agencies for sexual counseling and rehabilitation for the patient and his partner.	1. Explain to the patient that decrease in the levels of testosterone result in a reduction in sexual desire and impotence.
Hot Flashes		
Patient will experience a reduction in the number of hot flashes	1. Assess for hot flashes in patients who are taking LHRH agonists or who underwent an orchiectomy. Patients complain of a subjective sensation of increased temperature in the upper body and face. The patient sometimes describes a frightening sensation of impending doom. The flashes last a few minutes and may occur 7-50 times per day. 2. Administer megesterol acetate, 20 mg, twice a day, to decrease the number of hot flashes.	1. Teach patient to avoid the following situations that may trigger his hot flashes: a. Warm room b. Hot drinks c. Changing from a standing to a recumbent position d. Alcoholic drinks
Gynecomastia		
Patient will be able to cope with the changes in his body image	1. Assess for the development of gynecomastia. The incidence is reported to be as high as 90% in patients treated with estrogens or flutamide, 8% in those treated with orchiectomy, 3%-15% in those treated with LHRH agonists, and 19% in patients treated with a combination of LHRH agonists and flutamide. 2. Allow patient to discuss feelings about the changes in body image	1. Explain to patient that breast tissue develops because of the increased levels of bioavailable estrogen.
High Risk for the Development of Pathologic Fractures		
Patient will maintain safety precautions to help reduce the risk of pathological fractures	1. Assess for new complaints of pain at each visit. 2. Consult with physical therapist to institute a program of strengthening and reconditioning. 3. Evaluate the need for assistive devices.	1. Explain to the patient that he is at high risk for the development of pathologic fractures due to bone metastasis. 2. Teach measures to reduce the potential for fractures, including: a. Avoid trauma to sites of known metastasis b. Avoid moving/lifting of heavy objects c. Avoid performing the Valsalva maneuver d. Change position gradually e. Use good body mechanics 3. Teach patient methods to safety-proof his home (e.g., remove scatter rugs) to avoid falls.

Box 68-5
Patient Information on Prostate Cancer

Patient Support Organizations

American Cancer Society
Attn: Cancer Control
National Main Office
1599 Clifton Road
Atlanta, GA 30329
(404) 329-7624
http://www.cancer.org
Provider of the largest variety of services and literature on cancer

Cancer Care, Inc.
1180 Avenue of the Americas
New York, NY 10036
(212) 221-3300 or (800) 813-HOPE
http://www.cancercareinc.org
Provides free professional services and counseling to cancer patients and their families

National Prostate Cancer Coalition
3709 West Jetton Avenue
Tampa, FL 33629
(813) 253-0541, ext. 458
Emphasizes advocacy for increased prostate cancer research; a subgroup of the American Cancer Society

Patient Advocates for Advanced Cancer Treatments (PAACT)
1143 Parmalee NW
Grand Rapids, MI 49504
(616) 453-1477
http://www.rattler.cameron.edu/strum/
A cancer support and information network

Prostate Cancer Network
American Foundation for Urologic Disease
300 West Pratt Street, Suite 401
Baltimore, MD 21201
(800) 828-7866; (410) 727-2908
http://www.access.digex.net/~afud
National provider of prostate cancer education, awareness and advocacy information

Prostate Forum
1136 West Fern Drive
Fullerton, CA 92833
(714) 526-3793
An information exchange for cancer patients

US TOO! International, Inc.
930 North York Road, Suite 50
Hinsdale, IL 60521
(800) 80-US TOO
http://www.ustoo.com
Provides survivor support, fellowship and counseling to prostate cancer patients and their families

Disease Education and Research Organizations

American Cancer Society
(see previous information)

American Foundation for Urologic Disease
300 West Pratt Street, Suite 401
Baltimore, MD 21201
(410) 727-2908
http://www.access.digex.net/~afud
Professional society comprised of eight regional physician groups that provide continuing cancer education through seminars and literature

American Urological Association
1120 North Charles Street
Baltimore, MD 21201
(410) 727-1100
http://www.auanet.org
Professional society of physicians specializing in urology, including diseases of the prostate

Cancer Research Institute
"Prostate Cancer Initiative"
681 Fifth Avenue
New York, NY 10022
(212) 688-7515
http://www.cancerresearch.org or cancerres%aol.com
The Prostate Cancer Initiative, developed in partnership with the American Cancer Society, offers a three-pronged approach to prostate cancer, including research, education and a nationwide support network

National Cancer Institute
Cancer Information Service
Patient Guide: "Managing Cancer Pain"
Cancer Pain Guidelines
AHCPR Publications Clearinghouse
PO Box 8547
Silver Spring, MD 20907
(800) 4-CANCER
http://wwwicic.nci.nih.gov.
Twenty-one page brochure for cancer patients on pain management, including types of pain medicines, side effects, pain control diary and non-drug treatments

Prostate Cancer Education Council
UCHSC - Urology - C323
4200 East Ninth Avenue
Denver, CO 80262
(303) 315-MALE
Formed in 1988, this support group initiated Prostate Cancer Awareness Week, the largest cancer screening program in the United States

can occur in patients following radical prostatectomy or radiation therapy.

Patients should be taught that in most instances urinary incontinence is a transitory phenomenon that resolves after several months. Urinary incontinence may be caused by sphincter malfunction, detrusor abnormalities, or urinary retention with overflow. Approximately one third of men with incontinence have only sphincter abnormalities, one-third have both detrusor and sphincter abnormalities, and two-fifths have only detrusor abnormalities (Blaivas, 1995).

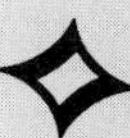

TABLE 68-18 Patient Preparation for Home Care of a Suprapubic Catheter and an Evaluation of Urinary Output

Description of the Procedure: A suprapubic catheter is a tube that has been inserted through your abdominal wall into your bladder to drain urine. This procedure will tell you how to care for your suprapubic catheter and how to get ready to have the catheter removed.

Procedural Considerations

1. Wash your hands with soap and water before you handle your suprapubic catheter.
2. Each morning, clamp your catheter with the clamp you were given.
3. Separate the catheter from the drainage bag tubing and put the plug into the end of the suprapubic catheter.
4. Clean your drainage bag by washing it out with cool water at least once a week.
5. Try to keep your catheter clamped for 3 to 4 hours at a time. If you need to urinate, try to urinate through your penis. When you urinate through your penis, collect the urine and measure the amount. Write down the amount of urine. This urine is called your "voided urine."
6. Immediately after you measure your voided urine, unplug and then unclamp your suprapubic catheter and collect, measure, and record how much urine comes out of your suprapubic catheter. This urine is called your "residual urine." These amounts are important in evaluating when to remove your suprapubic catheter.
7. If during the 3 to 4 hours that your catheter is clamped you feel full and are not able to urinate, unplug and then unclamp your suprapubic catheter and empty your bladder by draining urine from your catheter. Measure and record the amount of urine.
8. At bedtime, unplug your suprapubic catheter and connect it to the urinary drainage bag. Then unclamp your catheter for the night. Secure the drainage bag to a place lower than your mattress.
9. Clean the plug for your catheter with alcohol or soap and water each day. Place the plug in a plastic bag to keep it clean when not in use.
10. Keep the skin around your suprapubic catheter clean and dry. You may shower but be sure to pat the skin dry around the tube and apply a new dressing.

Modified from Brenner, Z. R. & Krenzer, M. E. (1995). Update on cryosurgical ablation for prostate cancer. *American Journal of Nursing, 95* (4), 44-48.

Patients who complain of a constant dribbling and gravitational or stress incontinence most likely have a sphincter abnormality. Men who complain of urinary frequency, urgency, and urge incontinence probably have a detrusor abnormality. Treatment is dictated by the underlying pathophysiology. Ongoing management requires men to use incontinence pads, condom catheters, penile clamps, or an indwelling catheter. Some patients may benefit from biofeedback and behavioral exercises (e.g., bladder training, habit training, timed voiding, prompted voiding, and pelvic muscle exercises). An excellent resource about the management of urinary incontinence is the recently published clinical practice guideline titled Urinary Incontinence in Adults: Acute and Chronic Management (Fantl, Newman, Colling, et al., 1996). Definitive therapy for sphincter incontinence involves the placement of a sphincter prosthesis. Some patients may benefit from periurethral injections. Detrusor abnormalities are usually managed with anticholinergic medications or behavior modification techniques (Blaivas, 1995; Held et al., 1994).

Sexual Dysfunction

Sexual dysfunction involves not only the patient but also the patient's sexual partner. Recent estimates suggest that erectile dysfunction occurs in approximately 85% of patients who have undergone prostate surgery and 40% of patients treated with radiation therapy. The changes in erectile function may be temporary or permanent. Nurses should feel comfortable obtaining a sexual history from a patient to determine if impotence is a problem for the patient and the effects of the problem on the patient's relationship with his partner. Patients may require referral to a sexual counselor or a psychologist or psychiatrist. Treatment options for erectile dysfunction include education and counseling, the use of a vacuum tumescence device, injection of pharmacologic agents (e.g., a mixture of papaverine, phentolamine, and prostaglandin E_1), or the insertion of a penile prosthesis (Sprouse, 1995).

The Cost of Hormonal Therapy

Patients with prostate cancer are generally older men who may be living on a fixed income. Maxwell compared the costs associated with the different forms of hormonal therapy for metastatic prostate cancer (Table 68-19). Costs for a 30-month course of treatment ranged from $300 to $17,250. Patients should be advised about the costs as well as the risks and benefits of the different hormonal agents so that they can make informed decisions about the most appropriate option for them.

PROGNOSIS

The prognosis for patients with prostate cancer varies depending on the stage of the disease at the time of diagnosis, the patient's age, and coexistent medical problems. Other factors that influence a patient's prognosis are hormone status, serum acid phosphatase levels, regional lymph node involvement, Gleason grade of the tumor, and bone scan results. In general, when prostate cancer is confined to the gland, the disease is curable. In fact, most patients will survive 5 years whether or not the disease is treated. With locally advanced disease, patients survive up to 5 years after diagnosis. The median survival time for patients with metastatic disease is one 1 to 3 years (Maxwell, 1993).

TABLE 68-19 The Costs of Hormonal Therapy for Metastatic Prostate Cancer

Modality	Drug	Dose	Cost*	Untoward Effects
Primary Therapy				
Surgical orchiectomy			$4,500	May be unacceptable to some men
LHRH superagonist analogs	Leuprolide acetate depot	7.5 mg intramuscular monthly	$10,500	Hot flashes (30%-50%), gynecomastia (3%), nausea (5%), cardiovascular (1%), flare phenomenon (8%-30%)
	Goserelin acetate	3.6 mg subcutaneous monthly	$10,500	Same as above
Estrogen	Diethylstilbestrol (DES)	1-3 mg orally daily	$300	Gynecomastia (49%), nausea/vomiting (16%), edema (16%), thrombosis, phlebitis, pulmonary embolism
Androgen	Flutamide	250 mg orally 3 times/daily	$6,750	Diarrhea (12%, gynecomastia, nausea, methemoglobinemia)
Secondary Therapy				
Antiandrogen	Flutamide	See above	See above	See above
Androgen synthesis inhibitors	Ketoconazole	400 mg orally 3 times/daily or 4 times daily		Liver toxicity, adrenal suppression
	Aminoglutethimide plus hydrocortisone	250 mg orally twice daily or 4 times daily plus 20 mg hydrocortisone twice daily		Lethargy, skin rash
Total androgen blockade	Castration plus flutamide	Flutamide as above	$11,250	See above
	LHRH superagonist plus flutamide	Leuprolide or goserelin acetate as above, flutamide as above	$17,250	

From Maxwell, M. B. (1993). Cancer of the prostate. *Seminars in Oncology Nursing, 9*(4), 237-251.
*Costs on projected 30-month median survival

EVALUATION OF THE QUALITY OF CARE

Accreditation organizations, such as the Joint Commission for the Accreditation of Health Care Organizations, require that the quality of care provided to patients be evaluated. Because the care provided to patients with prostate cancer requires input from a multidisciplinary team, an evaluation of the quality of care provided to these patients should include aspects of care provided by various members of the team. Tables 68-20 and 68-21 provide examples of quality of care evaluation tools that can be used in the inpatient and outpatient settings, respectively.

RESEARCH ISSUES

Numerous research issues surrounding the diagnosis and management of prostate cancer require further investigations. The genetic basis for the disease and the risk factors associated with the development of prostate cancer remained to be identified. The optimal approach to early detection remains to be determined. Currently, the American Cancer Society recommends a DRE for all men over age 50 years. However, the role of PSA and TRUS in the early detection of prostate cancer remains to be determined. Additional research is needed to determine the risks and benefits associated with the administration of chemopreventive agents such as finasteride.

Numerous randomized, clinical trials are needed to determine the most effective treatments for the various stages of prostate cancer. Additional research is warranted to determine better methods to treat androgen-insensitive prostate cancer cells. All of these research studies need to consider not only the effectiveness of the treatment in improving patients' survival but also the costs of the treatment, the morbidities associated with the treatments, and the effects of the treatments on the patient's quality of life.

TABLE 68-20 Quality of Care Evaluation for a Patient Undergoing Radical Prostatectomy

Disciplines participating in the quality of care evaluation:
☐ Nursing ☐ Surgery
☐ Physical Therapy ☐ Social Services

I. Postoperative Management Evaluation
Data from:
☐ Medical Record Review ☐ Patient/Family Interview

Criteria	Yes	No
1. Patient provided with preoperative information about:		
a. Diagnostic tests	☐	☐
b. Bowel preparation	☐	☐
c. Use of antiembolic stockings	☐	☐
2. Hemoglobin and hematocrit evaluated postoperatively	☐	☐
3. Patient experienced the following complications:		
a. Catheter obstruction	☐	☐
b. Pulmonary embolism	☐	☐

II. Patient/Family Satisfaction
Data from:
☐ Patient Interview ☐ Family Interview

Criteria	Yes	No
1. On a scale of 0 to 10, with 0 being totally dissatisfied and 10 being totally satisfied, how satisfied were you with the pain management you received? ______________		
2. Were you told to call the nurse if you experienced bladder spasms?	☐	☐
3. Were you taught to avoid strenuous exercise for 2-3 weeks after surgery?	☐	☐

TABLE 68-21 Quality of Care Evaluation for a Patient Receiving an LHRH Agonist and an Antiandrogen

Disciplines participating in the quality of care evaluation:
☐ Nursing ☐ Surgery
☐ Physical Therapy ☐ Social Services

Data from:
☐ Mailed Questionnaire ☐ Patient Interview

Criteria	Yes	No
1. Did the doctor or nurse explain to you that you might experience some of the following side effects from your hormone medication?		
a. Impotence	☐	☐
b. Hot flashes	☐	☐
c. Enlarged breasts (gynecomastia)	☐	☐
2. Were you asked if you wanted to see a sex counselor?	☐	☐
3. Were your taught to report any new pain problems to your doctor or nurse?	☐	☐
4. Were your taught how to prevent your bones from breaking accidentally?	☐	☐

REFERENCES

Adolfsson, J., Cartensen, J., Lowhagen, T. (1992). Deferred treatment in clinically localized prostate carcinoma. *British Journal of Urology, 69,* 183-187.

Albertsen, P. C. (1996). Early-stage prostate cancer: When is observation appropriate? *Hematology/Oncology Clinics of North America, 10*(3), 611-625.

Bahn, D. K., Lee, F., Solomon, M. H., Gontina, H., Klionsky, D. L., & Lee, F. T., Jr. (1995). Prostate cancer: US-guided percutaneous cryoablation. *Radiology, 194(2),* 551-556.

Benson, M. C., Whang, I. S., Pantuck, A., Ring, K., Kaplan, S. A., Olsson, C. A., Cooper, W. H. (1992). Prostate specific antigen density: A means of distinguishing benign prostatic hypertrophy and prostate cancer. *Journal of Urology, 147,* 815-816.

Blaivas, J. G. (1995). Urinary incontinence after radical prostatectomy. *Cancer, 75,* 1978-1982.

Boone, C., Kelloff, G., & Malone, W. (1990). Identification of candidate cancer chemoprevention agents and their evaluation on animal models and human critical trials: A review. *Cancer Research, 50,* 2-9.

Brawer, M. K. & Ellis, W. J. (1995). Chemoprevention for prostate cancer. *Cancer, 75,* 1783-1789.

Brenner, Z. R. & Krenzer, M. E. (1995). Update on cryosurgical ablation for prostate cancer. *American Journal of Nursing, 95* (4), 44-48.

Bubley, G. J. & Balk, S. P. (1996). Treatment of metastatic prostate cancer: Lessons from the androgen receptor. *Hematology/Oncology Clinics of North America, 10*(3), 713-725.

Catalano, W. J. (1994). Management of cancer of the prostate. *New England Journal of Medicine, 331*(15), 996-1004.

Chernecky, C. C., Krech, R. L., & Berger, B. J. (1993). *Laboratory tests and diagnostic procedures.* Philadelphia: W. B. Saunders.

Cox, R. L. & Crawford, E. D. (1995). Complications of cryosurgical ablation of the prostate to treat localized adenocarcinoma of the prostate. *Urology, 45,* 932.

Crawford, E. & Nabors, W. (1991). Total androgen oblation: American experience. *Urologic Clinics of North America, 18,* 55-63.

D'Amico, A. V. & Coleman, C. N. (1996). Role of interstitial radiotherapy in the management of clinically organ-confined prostate cancer: The jury is still out. *Journal of Clinical Oncology, 14,* 304-315.

Eisenberger, M. A., Reyno, L., Sinibaldi, V., Sridhara, R., Carducci, M., & Egorin, M. (1995). The experience with suramin in advanced prostate cancer. *Cancer, 75,* 1927-1934.

Fantl, J. A., Newman, D. K., Colling, J., et al. (1996). *Urinary incontinence in adults: Acute and chronic management. Clinical Practice Guideline, No. 2,* 1996 Update. Rockville, MD: U. S. Department of Health and Human Services. Public Health Service, Agency for Health Care Policy and Research.

Finchman, S. M., Hill, G. B., Hanson, J., & Wijayasinghe, C. (1990). Epidemiology of prostate cancer: A case-control study. *Prostate, 17,* 189-206.

Garnick, M. B. (1993). Prostate cancer: Screening, diagnosis, and management. *Annals of Internal Medicine, 118,* 804-818.

Garnick, M. (1994). The dilemmas of prostate cancer. *Scientific American, April,* 72-81.

Garnick, M. B. & Fair, W. R. (1996a). Prostate cancer: Emerging concepts-Part I. *Annals of Internal Medicine, 125,* 118-125.

Garnick, M. B. & Fair, W. R. (1996b). Prostate cancer: Emerging concepts - Part II. *Annals of Internal Medicine,* 125, 205-212.

Gerber, G. S., Thisted, R. A., Scardino, P. T., Frohmuller, H. G. W., Schroeder, F. H., Paulson, D. F., Middleton, A. W., Rukstalis, D. B., Smith, J. A., Schellhammer, P. F., Ohori, M., & Chodak, G. W. (1996). Results of radical prostatectomy in men with clinically localized prostate cancer: Multi-institutional pooled analysis. *Journal of the American Medical Association, 276*(8), 615-619.

Giovannucci, E. (1995). Epidemiological characteristics of prostate cancer. *Cancer, 75,* 1766-1777.

Giovannucci, E., Ascherio, A., Rimm, E. B., Colditz, G. A., Stampfer, M. J., & Willett, W. C. (1993). A prospective cohort study of vasectomy and prostate cancer in U.S. men. *Journal of the American Medical Association, 269,* 873-877.

Giovannucci, E., Rimm, E. B., Colditz, G. A., Stampfer, M. J., Ascherio, A., Chute, C. C., & Willet, W. C. (1993). A prospective study of dietary fat and risk of prostate cancer. *Journal of the National Cancer Institute, 85,* 1571-1579.

Giovannucci, E., Tosteson, T. D., Speizer, F. E., Ascherio, A., Vessey, M. P., & Colditz, G. A. (1993). A retrospective cohort study of vasectomy and prostate cancer in U.S. men. *Journal of the American Medical Association, 269,* 878-882.

Gormley, G. J. (1991). Role of 5-alpha reductase inhibitors in the treatment of advanced prostatic carcinoma. *Urologic Clinics of North America, 18,* 93-97.

Greco, K. E. & Kulawiak, L. (1994). Prostate cancer prevention: Risk reduction through lifestyle, diet, and chemoprevention. *Oncology Nursing Forum, 21(9),* 1504-1511.

Grimm, P. D., Blasko, J. C., Ragde, H., Sylvester, J., & Clarke, D. (1996). Does brachytherapy have a role in the treatment of prostate cancer? *Hematology/Oncology Clinics of North America, 10*(3), 653-673.

Hartford, A. C. & Zietman, A. L. (1996). Prostate cancer: Who is best benefited by external beam radiation therapy? *Hematology/Oncology Clinics of North America, 10*(3), 595-610.

Hayes, R. B., Pottern, L. M., Greenberg, R., Schoenberg, J., Swanson, G. M., Liff, J., Schwartz, A. G., Brown, L. M., & Hoover, R. N. (1993). Vasectomy and prostate cancer in U.S. blacks and whites. *American Journal of Epidemiology, 137,* 263-269.

Held, J. L., Osborne, D. M., Volpe, H., & Waldman, A. R. (1994). Cancer of the prostate: Treatment and nursing implications. *Oncology Nursing Forum, 21(9),* 1517-1529.

Henderson, B. E., Berstein, L., Ross, R. K., Depue, H., & Judd, H. L. (1988). The early in utero oestrogen and testosterone environment of blacks and whites: Potential effects on male offspring. *British Journal of Cancer, 57,* 216-218.

Hoskin, P. J. (1995). Radiotherapy in the management of bone pain. *Clinical Orthopaedics and Related Research, 312,* 105-119.

Hsing, A. W., McLaughlin, J. K., Hrubgec, Z., Blot, W. J., & Fraumeni, J. F. (1991). Tobacco use and prostate cancer: 26-year follow-up of U.S. veterans. *American Journal of Epidemiology, 133,* 437-441.

Hsing, A. W., McLaughlin, J. K., Schuman, L. M., Bjelke, E., Gridley, G., Wacholder, S., Chien, H. T., & Blot, W. J. (1990). Diet, tobacco use, and fatal prostate cancer: Results from the Lutheran Brotherhood cohort study. *Cancer Research, 50,* 6836-6840.

Imperato-McGinley, J., Guerrero, L., Gautier, T., & Peterson, R. (1974). Steroid 5-alpha reductase deficiency in man: An inherited form of male pseudohermaphroditism. *Science, 186,* 1213-1215.

Kantoff, P. W., Garnick, M. B., & Corless, C. L. (1996). Cancer of the genitourinary tract. In A. T. Skarin (Ed.), *Atlas of diagnostic oncology* (2nd ed.). London: Mosby-Wolfe.

Kirschenbaum, A. (1995). Management of hormonal treatment effects. *Cancer, 75,* 1983-1986.

Kolonel, L. N., Yoshizawa, C. N., & Hankin, J. H. (1988). Diet and prostate cancer: A case-control study in Hawaii. *American Journal of Epidemiology, 127,* 999-1012.

Labrie, F., Belanger, A., Simard, J., Labrie, C., & Dupont, A. (1993). Combination therapy for prostate cancer. *Cancer, 71*(Suppl. 3), 1059-1067.

Larkin, M. (1995). Prostate cancer. In Miaskowski, C., *Oncology nursing: Plans of nare for specialty practice.* New York: Delmar.

Long, J. P. (1996). Is there a role for cryoablation of the prostate in the management of localized prostate carcinoma? *Hematology/Oncology Clinics of North America, 10*(3), 675-690.

Long, J. P., Fallick, M. L., & Layne, J. (1995). Cryoablation of the prostate in the treatment of patients with localized disease following radiotherapy. In *Proceedings of the American Urology Association, New England Section.* (October).

Mahon, S. M. (1995). Using brochures to educate the public about the early detection of prostate and colorectal cancer. *Oncology Nursing Forum 22(9),* 1413-1420.

Mani, S. & Vogelzang, N. J. (1996). Is "off-protocol" chemotherapy for androgen-independent carcinoma of prostate warranted? *Hematology/Oncology Clinics of North America, 10*(3), 749-768.

Matzkin, H. & Soloway, M. S. (1993). Cigarette smoking: A review of possible associations with benign prostatic hyperplasia and prostate cancer. *Prostate, 22,* 277-290.

Maxwell, M. B. (1993). Cancer of the prostate. *Seminars in Oncology Nursing, 9*(4), 237-251.

McLeod, D. G. (1995). Hormonal therapy in the treatment of carcinoma of the prostate. *Cancer, 75,* 1914-1919.

McNeal, J. E. (1988). Normal histology of the prostate. *American Journal of Surgical Pathology, 12,* 619-663.

Mettlin, C. J., Murphy, G. P., Ho, R., & Menck, H. R. (1996). The national cancer data base report on longitudinal observations on prostate cancer. *Cancer, 77,* 2162-2166.

Mettlin, C., Natarajan, N., Huben, R. (1990). Vasectomy and prostate cancer risk. *American Journal of Epidemiology, 132,* 1056-1061.

Miller, R. J., Cohen, J. K., Shuman, B., & Merlotti, L. A. (1995). Percutaneous, transperineal cryosurgery of the prostate as salvage therapy for post radiation recurrence of adenocarcinoma. *Cancer, 77,* 1510-1514.

Miller, R. J., Cohen, J. K., Tiffany, K., & Shulman, B. A. (1995). Percutaneous transperineal cryosurgical ablation of prostate (CSAP) as primary treatment for clinical stage adenocarcinoma: Update. *Urology, 153,* 385.

Monda, J. M. & Osterling, J. E. (1993). Medical treatment for benign prostatic hyperplasia: 5 alpha-reductase inhibitors and alpha-adrenergic antagonists. *Mayo Clinic Proceedings, 68*(7), 670-679.

Montie, J. E. (1995). Staging of prostate cancer: Current TNM classification and future prospects for prognostic factors. *Cancer, 75,* 1814-1818.

Moon, T. D. (1992). Prostate cancer. *Journal of the American Geriatric Society, 40,* 622-627.

Morgan, T. O., Jacobsen, S. J., McCarthy, W. F., Jacobson, M. S., McLeod, D. G., & Moul, J. W. (1996). Age-specific reference ranges for serum prostate-specific antigen in black men. *New England Journal of Medicine, 335,* 304-310.

Murphy, G. P. & Whitmore, W. F. (1979). A report of the workshops on the current status of the histologic grading of prostate cancer. *Cancer, 44,* 1490-1494.

Nadler, R. B. & Andriole, G. L. (1996). Who is best benefitted by radical prostatectomy? *Hematology/Oncology Clinics of North America, 10*(3), 581-593.

Nielsen, O., Munro, A. J., & Tannock, I. F. (1991). Bone metastases: Pathophysiology and management policy. *Journal of Clinical Oncology, 9,* 509-524.

Nienhaus, H., Goldacre, M., Seagroatt, V., Gill, L., & Vessey, M. (1992). Incidence of disease after vasectomy: A record linkage retrospective cohort study. *British Medical Journal, 304,* 743-746.

Noble, R. L. (1977). The development of prostatic adenocarcinoma in Nb rats following prolonged sex hormone administration. *Cancer Research, 37,*1929-1933.

Oesterling, J. E. (1995). Prostate specific antigen: Its role in the diagnosis and staging of prostate cancer. *Cancer, 75,* 1795-1804.

Ofman, U. S. (1995). Sexual quality of life in men with prostate cancer. *Cancer, 75,* 1949-1953.

Onik, G., Porterfield, B., Rubinsky, B., & Cohen, J. (1991). Percutaneous transperineal prostate cryosurgery using transrectal ultrasound guidance: Animal model. *Urology, 37,* 227.

Parker, S. L., Tong, T., Bolden, S., & Wingo, P. A. (1996). Cancer statistics 1996. *CA-A Cancer Journal for Clinicians, 65,* 5-27.

Partin, A. W., Isaacs, J. T., Treiger, B., & Coffey, D. S. (1988). Early cell motility changes associated with an increase in metastatic ability in prostate cancer cells transfected with the V-Harvey-*ras*-oncogene. *Cancer Research, 48,* 6050-6053.

Payne, R. (1993). Pain management in the patient with prostate cancer. *Cancer, 71*(Suppl. 3), 1131-1137.

Pienta, K. & Esper, P. (1993). Risk for prostate cancer. *Annals of Internal Medicine, 118,* 793-802.

Pilepich, M. V., Caplan, R., & Byhardt, R. W. (1995a). A Phase III trial of adjuvant androgen suppression using goserelin in patients with carcinoma of the prostate treated with definitive radiotherapy (results of RTOG 85-31) [abstract]. *International Journal of Radiation Oncology, Biology, Physics, 32*(Suppl. 1), 188.

Pilepich, M. V., Krall, J. M., as-Sarraf, M., John, M. J., Doggett, R. L., Sause, W. T., Lawton, C. A., Abrams, R. A., Rotman, M., & Rubin, P. (1995b). Androgen deprivation with radiation therapy compared with radiation therapy alone for locally advanced prostatic carcinoma: A randomized comparative trial of the Radiation Therapy Oncology Group. *Urology, 45*(4), 616-623.

Powell, I. J., Gelfand, D. E., Parzuchowski, J., Heilbrun, L., & Franklin, A. (1995). A successful recruitment process of African American men for early detection of prostate cancer. *Cancer, 75,* 1880-1884.

Quinlan, D. M., Epstein, J. I., Carter, B. S., Walsh, P. C. (1991). Sexual function following radical prostatectomy: Influence of preservation of neurovascular bundles. *Journal of Urology, 145,* 998-1002.

Robson, M. & Dawson, N. (1996). How is androgen-dependent metastatic prostate cancer best treated? *Hematology/Oncology Clinics of North America, 10(3),* 727-747.

Rose, D. P., Boyar, A. P., & Wynder, E. L. (1986). International comparisons of mortality rates for cancer of the breast, ovary, prostate, and colon, and per capita food consumption. *Cancer, 58,* 2363-2371.

Rosenberg, L., Palmer, J. R., Zauber, A. G., Warshaeur, M. E., Stolley, P. D., & Shapiro, S. (1990). Vasectomy and the risk for prostate cancer. *American Journal of Epidemiology, 132,* 1051-1055.

Ross, R. K., Bernstein, L., Judd, H., Hanisch, R., Pike, M. C., & Henderson, B. E. (1986). Serum testosterone levels in young black and white men. *Journal of the National Cancer Institute, 76,* 45-48.

Ross, R. K., Coetzee, G. A., Reichardt, J., Skinner, E., & Henderson, B. E. (1995). Does the racial-ethnic variation in prostate cancer risk have a hormonal basis? *Cancer, 75,* 1778-1782.

Ross, R. K., Paganini-Hill, A., & Henderson B. E. (1983). The etiology of prostate cancer: What does the epidemiology suggest? *Prostate, 4,* 333-344.

Scher, H. I., Isaacs, J. T., Fuks, Z., & Walsh, P.C. (1995). Prostate. In Abeloff, M. D., Armitage, J. O., Lichter, A. S., & Niederhuber, J. E., (Eds.) *Clinical Oncology.* New York: Churchill Livingstone.

Shinohara, K. & Carroll, P. R. (1995). Improved results of cryosurgical ablation of the prostate. *Urology, 153,* 385.

Sidney, S., Queensberry, C. P., Sadler, M. C., Guess, H. A., Lydick, E. G., & Cattolica, E. V. (1991). Vasectomy and the risk of prostate cancer in a cohort of multi-phasic health-checkup examinees: A second report. *Cancer Causes Control, 2,* 113-116.

Smith, J. R., Freije, D., Carpten, J. D., Grönberg, H., Xu, J., Isaacs, S. D., Brownstein, M. J., Bova, G. S., Guo, H., Bujnovsky, P., Nusskern, D. R., Damber, J-E, Bergh, A., Emanuelsson, M., Kallioniemi, O. P., Walker-Daniels, J., Bailey-Wilson, J. E., Beaty, T. H., Meyers, D. A., Walsh, P. C., Collins, F. S., Trent, J. M., & Isaacs, W. B. (1996). Major susceptibility locus for prostate cancer on chromosome 1 suggested by a genome-wide search. *Science, 274,* 1371-1374.

Spitz, M. R., Fueger, J. J., Babaian, R. J., Newell, G. R. (1991). Re: Vasectomy and risk of prostate cancer [Letter]. *American Journal of Epidemiology, 134,* 108-109.

Sprouse, D. (1995). Sexual rehabilitation of the prostate cancer patient. *Cancer, 75,* 1954-1956.

Strangio, L. & Brudner, C. (1995). When pain cuts to the bone. *American Journal of Nursing, 58(6),* 26-29.

Talamini, R., Franceschi, S., La Vecchia, C., Guarneri, S., & Negri, E. (1993). Smoking habits and prostate cancer: A case-control study in northern Italy. *Prevention Medicine, 22,* 400-408.

Walsh, P. C. & Donker, P. J. (1982). Impotence following radical prostatectomy: Insights into etiology and prevention. *Journal of Urology, 128*(3), 492-497.

Whitehead, E., Smith-Young, A., & Lang, P. (1985). Urinary incontinence: Types, etiologies, diagnostic evaluation. *Journal of Urologic Nursing, 4,* 297-305.

Wieder, J., Schmidt, J. D., Casola, G., vanSonnenberg, E., Stainken, B. F., & Parsons, C. L. (1995). Transrectal ultrasound-guided transperineal cryoablation in the treatment of prostate carcinoma: Preliminary results. *Journal of Urology, 154*(2 Pt. 1), 435-441.

Wolf, C. M. (1960). An investigation of the familial aspects of carcinoma of the prostate. *Cancer, 13,* 739-744.

Testicular Cancer

Edithe C. Garvey, RN, MN, OCN

EPIDEMIOLOGY

In 1998 there was an estimated 7600 new cases of testicular cancer. The highest incidence occurred (11.6 per 100,000) in ages 25 to 34 years (Landis, Murray, Bolden, & Wingo, 1998). Deaths resulting from this disease are estimated at around 6000. Despite these figures, testicular cancer is a relatively uncommon disease and accounts for only 1% of all male malignancies (Einhorn, Richie, Shipley, Loehrer, & Williams, 1993; Lind, Kravitz, & Greig, 1993).

Testicular cancer is an interesting disease because its incidence has been increasing over the last several decades in the white male population, yet the incidence in the African-American male population remains low. Testicular cancer is a potentially curable malignancy of young males and is one of the few malignancies with accurate serum markers: human chorionic gonadotropin (HCG) and alphafetoprotein (AFP).

Testicular cancer has been shown to be curable even in the human immunosuppressive virus (HIV) population. This was demonstrated in a retrospective study of 26 men infected with human immunosuppressive disease with a median follow-up of 33 months. Despite the fact that severe hematologic toxicity was observed in 7 of 15 patients, the investigators concluded that patients with HIV who have testicular cancer be offered standard therapies, regardless of their HIV status, because most can be cured of their tumor and have an acceptable quality of life. Special attention should be given to concomitant prophylaxis for opportunistic infection (Bernardi, Salvioni, Vaccher, Repetto, Piersoantelli, & Marini, et al., 1995). Generally, it is thought that testicular cancer has become the model for a curable neoplasm (Einhorn et al., 1993).

RISK FACTORS

Although the risk factors for the development of testicular cancer remain unknown, there is a 10- to 40-fold higher incidence in males with undescended (cryptorchid) testes (Gilbert & Hamilton, 1940). Box 69-1 lists possible risk factors. The effects of orchitis and testicular trauma remain unknown (Carlsen, Giwercman, Keiding, & Skakebaek, 1992), whereas others propose that exogenous estrogens given to women for birth control or as diethylstilbestrol to prevent spontaneous abortions may influence the incidence of testicular cancer in subsequent male children (Hendersen, Bernstein, Ross, Depve, & Judd, 1988).

Signs and symptoms of testicular cancer are listed in Box 69-2. Although these signs are not definitive of cancer, patients should seek medical evaluation if symptoms continue more than 2 weeks to diminish the possibility of metastasis.

PATHOPHYSIOLOGY

Anatomy and Physiology of the Testis

The normal testis is approximately 4 × 3 × 2.5 cm and weighs 10 to 15 g (0.35 to 0.53 oz). The testes hang within the scrotum (Fig. 69-1). During fetal development the testes form inside the abdominal cavity adjacent to the kidneys. As the fetus continues to develop, the testes descend through the abdominal musculature, accompanied by small pockets of peritoneal cavity. Each testis is accompanied by the ductus deferens and the testicular blood vessels, nerves, and lymphatics. Together these form the body of the spermatic cord.

Each testis is located in a separate compartment of the scrotum called the *scrotal cavity.* A narrow space separates the inner surface of the scrotum from the outer surface of the testis. A serous membrane (tunica vaginalis) lines the scrotal cavity and reduces friction between these two surfaces. The tunica vaginalis is a portion of the peritoneum that lost its connection to the peritoneal cavity during descent of the testes.

Beneath the serous membranacea, which covers the testis, is the tunica albuginea, which is a dense layer of connective tissue with collagen fibers. These fibers form a continuous network with those that surround the adjacent epididymis. These collagen fibers also extend into the substance of the testis, forming septae, which converge toward the area next to the proximal portion of the epididymis. This region is called the *mediastinum* of the testis. This mediastinum supports the blood vessels and the lymphatics of the testis and the ducts that transport sperm to the epididymis.

The fluid current helps direct the maturing sperm into the epididymis, which has a head, body, and tail (Fig. 69-2). The tail curves, and, as it ascends, its histology changes until it greatly resembles the ductus deferens. This region is mainly involved in sperm storage.

The ductus deferens, or vas deferens, is 40 to 45 cm long. It begins at the tail of the epididymis and ascends into the spermatic cord (see Fig. 69-2). When it reaches into the abdominal cavity (see Fig. 69-1), the vas deferens passes posteriorly, curving along the lateral surface of the urinary bladder toward the posterior and superior aspect of the prostate gland. The vas deferens not only transports sperm but also can store spermatozoa for several months.

As the vas deferens meets with the seminal vesicle, the ejaculatory duct is formed. This duct enters the muscular prostate gland and empties into the urethra. Secretions of the seminal vesicle mix with those of the prostate due to peristaltic contractions of the ductus deferens, seminal vesicle, and prostate gland. The secretions are then ejected into the prostatic urethra and then through the urethra by further peristaltic contractions. These peristaltic contractions are

Box 69-1

Risk Factors for the Development of Testicular Cancers

- Middle-age men between the ages of 25 and 35.
- Geographic variation: highest incidence rates are recorded in Denmark, Switzerland, and New Zealand.
- In the United States, rates are four to five times higher in whites than African Americans.

Box 69-2

Signs and Symptoms of Testicular Tumor

- A painless mass or lump in either testicle
- Feeling of heaviness in the scrotum
- Any enlargement of a testicle
- A dull ache in the lower abdomen or the groin
- A collection of fluid in the scrotum
- Pain or discomfort in the testicle or scrotum
- Enlargement or tenderness of the breasts

From Einhorn, L.H., Richie, J.P., Shipley, W.U., Loehrer, P.J., & Williams, S.D. (1993). Cancer of the testes. In V.T. DeVita, S. Hellmann, & S.A. Rosenberg (Eds.): *Cancer: Principles and practice in oncology (4th ed.). Philadelphia: J.B. Lippincott.*

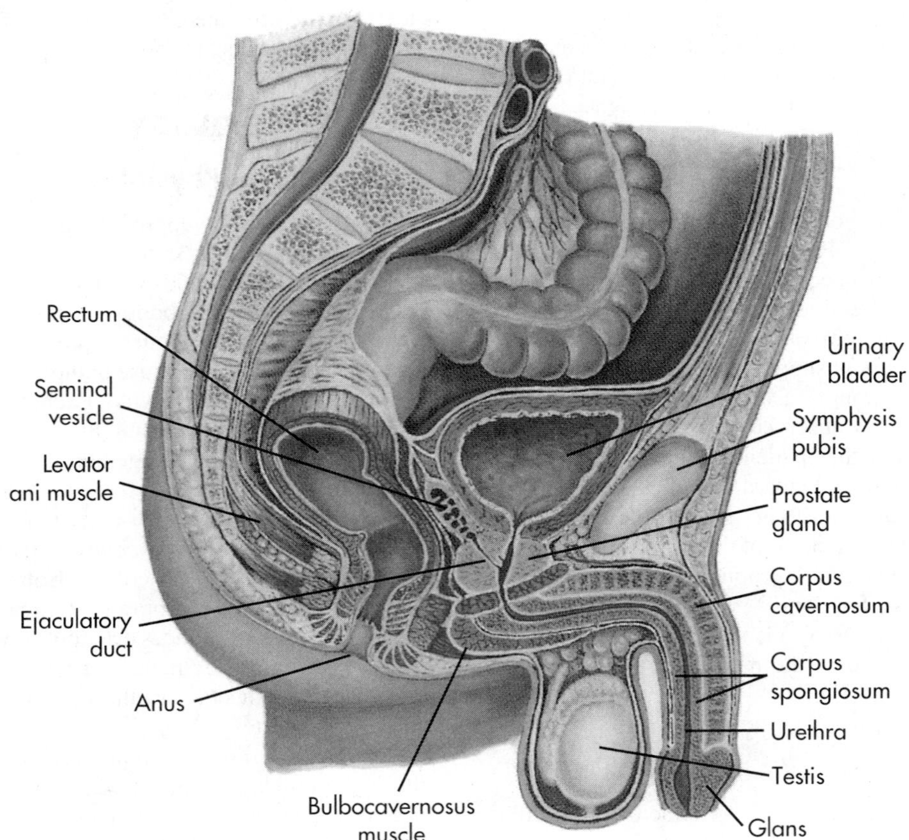

Fig. 69-1 Male reproductive organs. Sagittal section of pelvis showing placement of male reproductive organs. (From Thibodeau, G. A. [1996]. *Anthony's textbook of anatomy and physiology,* [15th ed]. St. Louis: Mosby.)

under the control of the sympathetic nervous system (Einhorn, Richie, Shipley, Loehrer, & Williams, 1993).

Carcinogenesis

Carcinogenesis of testicular cancer is thought to be complex and due to many factors (Moller, 1993); however, only about 4% to 5% of testicular tumors are of nongerminal cell origin, whereas the remaining 95% arise from germinal cells (Einhorn et al., 1993). Several changes occur during carcinogenesis. First are the deoxyribonucleic acid (DNA) changes in a dysplastic cell precursor. This results in carcinoma in situ. Cytogenetic analysis of germ cell tumors have shown an abnormality of the short arm of chromosome 12 in more than 80% of the tumors (Maher, 1994). Some investigators hypothesize that the first carcinogenic event occurs in utero in response to free estrogen. Events combined throughout the male's life may culminate in the abnormal cell producing the neoplastic cell line (Hendersen et al., 1988).

Oncogenes have just begun to be explored in testicular cancer, and much research is still needed. The *ras* oncogene is mutated in certain neoplasms, especially those associated with carcinogenesis. However, a low incidence of *ras* mutation is noted in testicular cancers. Another oncogene, the *hst*-1 oncogene, is found to be overexpressed in nonseminomatous germ cell tumor (NSGCT), especially those with metastatic disease. The *myc* oncogene has also been indicated in testicular cancer. This oncogene encodes nuclear cell growth and differentiation of proteins. The most recent oncogene implicated in testicular carcinogenesis is the *bcl*-2 oncogene. Conversely, the known retinoblastoma gene is a tumor suppressor gene that is found to be underexpressed in testicular cancer (Moul & Heidenreich, 1996). It has been demonstrated that high levels of p53 can be detected in testicular germ cell tumor (Bartkova, Bartek, Lukas, Vojtesek, Staskova, & Rejthar et al., 1991). This p53 gene is an important and well-known cancer-suppressor gene and is altered in cancer. This altered p53 cancer suppressor gene looses its suppressor ability and often becomes a promotor of the cancer cell line (Tominaga, Hamelin, Remvikos, Salmon, & Thomas, 1992). Testicular cancers generally overexpress p53 protein even in the absence of p53 gene mutations, which may be rare (Moul & Heidenreich, 1996).

Carcinogenic transformation of the cell is generally not seen until adulthood for testicular cancer, and thus it is thought that the tumor may develop and grow in the presence of sex hormones or gonadotrophins after pubescence (Moller, 1993). This area is uncharted territory that needs continued investigation.

HISTOLOGIC CLASSIFICATION AND ROUTES OF METASTASES

Testicular cancers can be classified into two main histologic classes, as shown in Table 69-1, the most common being germ cell tumors (GCTs) and the less common nongerm cell tumors (4% to 5%) (Roth, Nichols, & Einhorn, 1993). GCTs are then subclassified as noted in Table 69-1 into seminomatous tumors, or NSGCTs.

Seminomas

Approximately 40% of GCTs are seminomas. These are then subclassified into three histologic types: classic seminoma, spermatocytic seminoma, and anaplastic seminoma. *Anaplastic seminoma* is defined as five mitotic figures per

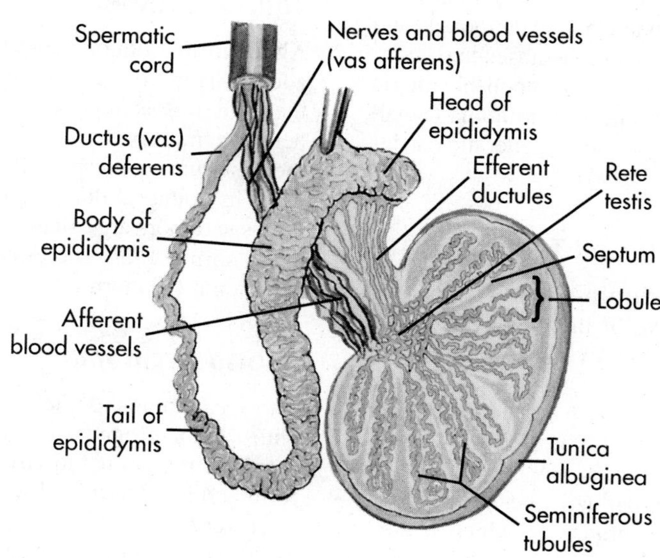

Fig. 69-2 Tubules of the testis and epididymis. Illustration showing epididymis lifted free of testis. The ducts and tubules are exaggerated in size. (From Thibodeau, G. A. [1996]. *Anthony's textbook of anatomy and physiology,* [15th ed]. St. Louis: Mosby.)

TABLE 69-1 Types of Testicular Tumors

Germ Cell Tumors (95%)		
Seminomatous Tumors (40%)	**Nonseminomatous Germ Cell Tumors (NSGCT)**	**Non–Germ Cell Tumors (4%-5%)**
Classic	Embryonal cell (60%)	Leydig cell
Anaplastic	Yolk sac	Sertoli cell
Spermatocytic (5%)	Teratocarcinoma	
	Teratoma	
	Choriocarcinoma	

From Einhorn, L.H., Richie, J.P., Shipley, W.U., Loehrer, P.J., & Williams, S.D. (1993). Cancer of the testes. In V.T. DeVita, S. Hellman, & S.A. Rosenberg (Eds.). *Cancer: Principles and practice of oncology* (4th ed.). Philadelphia: J.B. Lippincott.

high-power field, cellular anaplasia, and tissue disruption; however, this subclassification is of interest only from the histologic point of view because anaplasia does not influence survival or response to therapy (Small & Torti, 1995). Classic seminomas generally present in the fourth to fifth decade of life and represent approximately 40% of testicular tumors (Einhorn et al., 1993). In about 70% of patients it is localized to the testes (stage I) but it may be metastatic to lymph nodes (usually stage II) in 25% (Horwich, 1992). At clinical presentation, only 5% of patients present with visceral metastases; this represents a late phase of the disease. Lymph node metastases presents in an orderly fashion along draining lymph node chains (Small & Torti, 1995). The regional lymph node chains are detailed in Box 69-3. Significance of lymph node metastases in staging testicular cancer relies on the number and size of the nodes and not whether the metastases is unilateral or contralateral.

Spermatocytic seminomas are rare, representing about 5% of all seminomas, and usually occur in the sixth decade. These tend to be more bilateral than classic seminomas and more indolent with less metastases and the absence of lymphatic infiltration or granuloma formation upon histologic examination, as would be seen in classic seminoma (Small & Torti, 1995). Thus this type of seminoma generally carries a good prognosis (Einhorn et al., 1993).

Non-Seminomatous Germ Cell Tumors

Teratoma and Teratocarcinoma. Adult (mature) teratomas are the least aggressive of the NSGCTs (Stoter, Sleijfer, & Scjhornagael, 1993). However, these tumors are not considered biologically benign because they can metastasize and lead to death in 25% of those patients treated with orchiectomy alone (Einhorn et al., 1993; Skinner & Lieskovsky, 1988). Pathologic staging is important for this reason in the adult. In children under age 2 years, such teratomas are considered immature teratomas, which behave unlike the mature teratoma in the adult.

Teratocarcinoma. Teratocarcinoma is a germinal tumor with histologic elements of the mature teratoma. It behaves in part as the mature teratoma and in part as the malignant embryonal carcinoma. Histologically, it has cystic spaces, often containing hemorrhagic or necrotic material, and a definite presence of malignant tissue such as is present in embryonal carcinoma. Trophoblastic cells and fully detectable cartilage, muscle, or epithelial tissue may be seen (Einhorn et al., 1993).

Box 69-3
Regional Lymph Node Chains

- Aortic
- Para-aortic
- External iliac
- Paracaval
- Intrapelvic
- Inguinal

Embryonal Carcinoma

This highly malignant tumor presents with an anaplastic cellular structure, with embryoid features such as immature tubular, papillary, or reticular cells. The adult type varies in its histologic pattern, with the polyembryonic type containing embryonal bodies that resemble its ovarian counterpart. Infantile embryonal carcinomas usually present as yolk sac tumors (Einhorn et al., 1993).

Embryonal carcinoma represents approximately 60% of all NSGCTs and usually occurs in 20- to 30-year-olds. It is malignant, rapid growing, and bulky. It metastasizes via lymphatic and hematogenous spread, particularly to the lungs and liver. More than 60% of patients have already metastasized at clinical presentation (Small & Torti, 1995). Embryonal cells can secrete HCG, AFP, or both.

Yolk Sac Tumor

Although this tumor may present as a distinct form in the adult, it is more common in infants and young children. In the adult, it is an aggressive tumor that metastasizes early by hematogenous route. If it presents as a primary tumor of the mediastinum, it is especially aggressive and virulent. However, in young children it is much less aggressive. These yolk sac tumors are usually associated with an elevated AFP and a normal HCG and often can be mixed with embryonal carcinoma (Einhorn et al., 1993).

Choriocarcinoma

Choriocarcinoma is the most aggressive of the NSGCTs, with a poor prognosis resulting from early hematogenous spread to the brain and viscera. It rarely presents in its pure form and is often mixed with other GCTs, such as embryonal carcinoma and/or teratocarcinoma. Grossly, it is recognized by hemorrhages on its surface. HCG is a diagnostic marker, as are the beta subunits of HCG. Monitoring of these markers is now an indispensable tool in the management of these patients (Lange & Fraley, 1977).

Benign Stromal Cell Tumors (Non–Germ Cell Tumors)

As shown previously in Table 69-1, these are either Leydig cell or Sertoli cell tumors. Only approximately 4% to 5% of testicular tumors are benign tumors of the stromal cells in the adult. They may represent approximately 20% of childhood testicular tumors (Holtz & Abell, 1963). Their behavior is usually benign, with less than 10% having malignant potential. Treatment is with orchiectomy and clinical staging and generally does not necessitate lymph node dissection if the workup is negative. Gynecomastia occurs in 15% of patients with Leydig cell tumors and in 30% of those with Sertoli cell tumors (Small & Torti, 1995; Einhorn et al., 1993).

Extragonadal Germ Cell Tumors

Primary extragonadal GCTs generally arise from midline structures such as the mediastinum, retroperitoneum, pineal gland, prostate, thymus, or stomach. This occurs during embryogenesis, when germinal epithelium, which arises from the yolk sac, undergoes midline migration. This eventually forms the testicular tissue and scrotum. However, during the migration of the germinal epithelial cells, cells may remain along the migration route and later undergo the malignant transformation process.

When this tumor is found a complete workup must be done to search for occult primary tumor of the testes. This is important because the testis serves as a sanctuary for cancer cells, which then would impair the potential for cure from chemotherapy. Response rates range from 56% to 65% despite the GCT chemotherapy protocol used (Einhorn et al., 1993).

ASSESSMENT

Physical Assessment

The most common symptom of testicular cancer is a painless enlargement or palpable nodule, which may be accidentally discovered or be noticed along with a heaviness or dull ache in the scrotum, inguinal area, or lower abdomen. In addition to the firm, diffuse enlargement, there may be an inability to transilluminate the testis and a lack of pain on palpation (Table 69-2). Approximately 25% of patients with advanced disease present with symptoms attributed to their metastases, such as back pain, shortness of breath, chest pain, or hemoptysis (Small & Torti, 1995).

Assessment of the patient includes clinical examination, radiologic studies, laboratory studies, and biopsy (Table 69-3). Physical assessment of the patient includes palpation of the testes (Fig. 69-3), inguinal lymph nodes, abdomen, and supraclavicular lymph nodes to assess for bulky disease. Bilateral ultrasonography of the testes is also done along with transillumination to differentially diagnose testicular torsion, hydroceles, varicoceles, spermatoceles, and epididymitis.

A high inguinal orchiectomy is performed with removal of the entire mass for biopsy purposes. A transcortical testicular biopsy should not be done due to risk of tumor seeding (Presti & Herr, 1992). Histologic confirmation is needed for proper diagnosis.

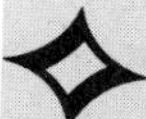

TABLE 69-2 Patient Preparation for Transillumination of a Scrotal Mass

Description of the Procedure: As part of your physical examination, your physician will examine the testicles for a possible mass. The test is not invasive. Fluid masses such as cysts "light up" when examined. Masses that contain blood or solid tissue do not.

Patient Preparation: The room will be darkened to allow the physician to examine the scrotal area using a flash light beam.

The physician will illuminate the scrotum to determine if a scrotal mass exists.

If a scrotal mass that is suspicious for a solid mass is present, your physician will do further testing.

Bates, B., Bickley, B., & Hoekelman, R. (1995). *A pocket guide to physical examination and history taking.* Philadelphia: J.B. Lippincott.

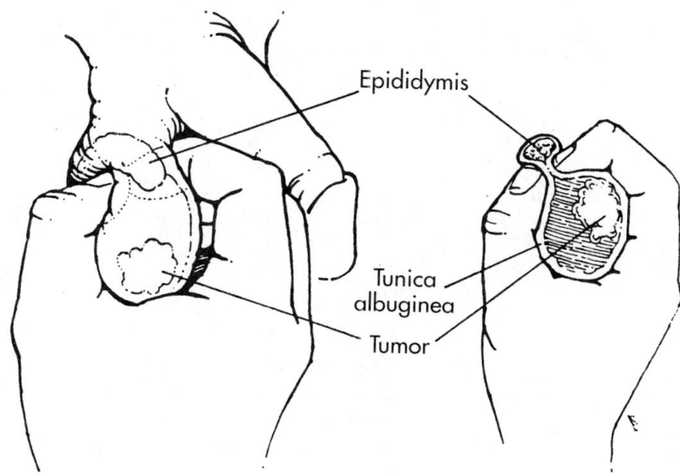

Fig. 69-3 Male scrotal examination. (Einhorn, L.H., Donohue, J.P., & Peckham, M.J. [1985]. Cancer of the testis. In V. T. DeVita, S. Hellman, & S. A. Rosenberg (Eds). *Cancer: Principles and practice of oncology* [2nd ed]. Philadelphia: J.B. Lippincott.)

Radiologic Studies

Radiologic studies include chest radiographs with full-lung computed tomography (CT) to evaluate the patient for pulmonary metastases. Abdominal CT scans are used to evaluate lymph node involvement of the retroperitoneal area. magnetic resonance imaging (MRI) may also be used to confirm or further investigate findings. The results of these tests assist in the evaluation of the patient for staging purposes, for response to therapy, and to plan for retroperitoneal lymph node dissection.

Lymphangiograms were performed in the past and demonstrated a 25% false-negative and a 5% to 10% false-positive rate (Barzell & Whitmore, 1979); lymphangiography is no longer considered necessary for staging purposes (Einhorn et al., 1993). Intravenous pyelograms are done to determine if displacement of the ureters or kidneys exists as a result of tumor or ureteral stenosis or obstruction.

Laboratory Studies

Laboratory studies of serum AFP and beta-HCG have become important tumor markers in determining whether a GCT is present, to evaluate a patient's response to therapy, to detect residual tumor, and possibly to differentiate between seminomatous and nonseminomatous tumors. Both HCG and AFP are glycoproteins. Normal adult levels of AFP are less than 16 to 30 ng/ml and are generally (75%) elevated in nonseminomatous germ cell tumors. High levels of AFP may be indicative of an aggressive tumor (Messing, 1987). AFP is generally never elevated in pure seminomas.

HCG is normally produced by pregnant women. The subunit beta is associated with testicular tumors. Elevated beta-HCG is seen in approximately 60% of patients with nonseminomatous germ cell tumors (Higgs, 1990). Less than 7% of pure seminomas demonstrate an elevated beta-HCG (Presti & Herr, 1992); however, 50% of patients with stage III seminomas have elevated HCG. Modest elevation of HCG is also seen in patients with recent use of marijuana and in those with low serum testosterone levels due to atrophy of the remaining testis secondary to chemotherapy. In

TABLE 69-3 Assessment of the Patient for Testicular Cancer

	Assessment Parameters	Typical Abnormal Findings
History	A. Personal and social history	A. Personal and social factors 1. Undescended testicles. 2. Noted mass on self-examination or by sexual partner. 3. History of trauma, mumps, orchitis. 4. Infertility rare (10%).
	B. Evaluate for pain	B. Complaints of episodic testicular pain, low back pain, groin pain, or abdominal aching or gynecomastia with or without tenderness. Acute pain is presenting symptom in 10% of patients.
Physical Examination	A. Examine scrotal area, breasts, palpate abdomen. Palpation of the scrotal mass includes separation of the anterior testis within the tunica albuginea from the posterior adnexal elements, including the epididymis and cord	A. Common symptoms include a mass or hardness of the testes, with complaints of occasional heaviness or a dull aching sensation in the lower abdomen or scrotum. Infertility is rare. Rule out epididymitis, spermatocele, hydrocele, torsion, testicular trauma, or infarction. Gynecomastia.
	B. Perform transluminal scrotal examination	B. Dense lesions indicating tumor mass will not be translucent.
	C. Assess supraclavicular axillae and inguinal areas to determine possible nodal involvement	C. Some suspicious lymph nodes can be palpated.
Diagnostic Tests	A. Posterior and lateral chest radiograph	A. Determine metastasis to lungs.
	B. MRI Imaging	B. Rule out epididymitis, spermatocele, hydrocele, torsion, testicular trauma, or infarction.
	C. Abdominal CT	C. Determine possible lymph node involvement.
	D. Testicular ultrasound	D. Used for differential diagnosis for testicular torsion, hydroceles, cytoceles, spermatoceles, and epididymitis.
	E. Intravenous pyelogram	E. Detect urinary tract metastases.
	F. Laboratory studies 1. alpha-fetoprotein 2. Serum beta human chorionic gonadotropin 3. Lactic acid dehydrogenase	F. Tumor markers 1. Laboratory values of >16-30 ng/ml may indicate nonseminomatous germ cell tumor or an aggressive tumor. 2. Never found in healthy men and indicates malignancy. 3. Nonspecific marker most likely elevated in the presence of bulky metastases of germ cell tumors.

From Bosl, G.J., Sheinfeld, J., Bajorin, D., & Motzer, R.J. (1997). Testicular cancer. In V.T. DeVita, S. Hellman, & S.A. Rosenberg (Eds). *Cancer: Principles and practice of oncology* (5th ed.). Philadelphia: Lippincott-Raven.

this latter instance, it is recommended to administer an injection of 300 mg of depo-testosterone and repeat the HCG assay in 2 weeks (Einhorn et al., 1993).

Lactic dehydrogenase (LDH) is a nonspecific marker that is most likely to be elevated with bulky metastases of germ cell tumors. Recently, Ki-67 (MIB-1), an immunohistochemical proliferation marker, has been analyzed as a prognostic marker in stage I NSGCT. It has been proposed that MIB-1 staining is superior to the p53 and neovascularity as prognostic indicators (Albers, Orazi, Ulbright, Miller, Haidar, & Donohue et al., 1995); however, others have not been able to reproduce the same results (McLeod, Heidenreich, & Moul, 1996).

STAGING

Histologic verification of the orchiectomy specimen must be used for staging both the primary tumor and the nodal status for testicular cancer. The staging schema is based on the TNM system (Table 69-4). These TNM definitions are grouped into stages as summarized in Table 69-5. Another staging system for NGCTs is noted in Table 69-6. The Royal Marsden schema to stage seminomas is illustrated in Table 69-7. Depicted are two schemas: stage III (C) with supradiaphragmatic lymph node involvement and stage IV with extranodal metastases such as pulmonary, bone, or brain metastases.

Table 69-4 TNM Classification for Testicular Cancer

Definition of TNM

Primary Tumor (T)

The extent of primary tumor is classified after radical orchiectomy.

pTX	Primary tumor cannot be assessed (If no radical orchiectomy has been performed, TX is used.)
pT0	No evidence of primary tumor (e.g., histologic scar in testis)
pTis	Intratubular tumor: preinvasive cancer
pT1	Tumor limited to the testis, including the rete testis
pT2	Tumor invades beyond the tunica albuginea or into the epididymis
pT3	Tumor invades the spermatic cord
pT4	Tumor invades the scrotum

Regional Lymph Nodes (N)

NX	Regional lymph nodes cannot be assessed
N0	No regional lymph node metastasis
N1	Metastasis in a single lymph node, 2 cm or less in greatest dimension
N2	Metastasis in a single lymph node, more than 2 cm but not more than 5 cm in greatest dimension; or multiple lymph nodes, none more than 5 cm in greatest dimension
N3	Metastasis in a lymph node more than 5 cm in greatest dimension

Distant Metastasis (M)

MX	Presence of distant metastasis cannot be assessed
M0	No distant metastasis
M1	Distant metastasis

From Beahrs, O. H., Henson, D. E., Hutter, R. V. (Eds.). (1993). *American Joint Committee on Cancer manual for staging of cancer* (4th ed), Philadelphia: J.B. Lippincott.

Table 69-5 TNM Stage Grouping

Stage 0	pTis	N0	M0
Stage I	Any pT	N0	M0
Stage II	Any pT	N1	M0
	Any pT	N2	M0
	Any pT	N3	M0
Stage III	Any pT	Any N	M1

From Beahrs, O. H., Henson, D. E., Hutter, R. V. (Eds.). (1993). *American Joint Committee on Cancer manual for staging of cancer* (4th ed.). Philadelphia: J.B. Lippincott.

Table 69-6 Pathologic Staging Schema for Non-Seminomatous Germ Cell Tumors

MSKCC Stage	Walter Reed Stage	Definition
A	I	Tumor confined to testis
B1	IIA	Minimal retroperitoneal nodal spread: microscopic and <6 nodes
B2	IIB	Moderate retroperitoneal nodal spread: grossly positive, or >6 lymph nodes
B3	IIC	Bulky retroperitoneal nodal disease: includes palpable nodes
C	III	Metastases above the diaphragm or to extranodal sites.

From Beahrs, O. H., Henson, D. E., Hutter, R. V. (Eds.). (1993). *American Joint Committee on Cancer manual for staging of cancer* (4th ed.). Philadelphia: J.B. Lippincott.

Table 69-7 Royal Marsden Clinical Staging Schema for Seminomatous Tumors

Stage	Definition
I	Confined to testis
IIA	Abdominal nodal disease: <2 cm
IIB	Abdominal nodal disease: 2-5 cm
IIC	Abdominal nodal disease: >5 cm
III	Supradiaphragmatic nodal disease
IV	Extranodal disease

From Beahrs, O. H., Henson, D. E., Hutter, R. V. (Eds.). (1993). *American Joint Committee on Cancer manual for staging of cancer* (4th ed.), Philadelphia: J.B. Lippincott.

MEDICAL MANAGEMENT

Treatment of testicular cancer is dependent on the histology of the tumor and the pathologic staging. Medical management options for diagnosis for stage I testicular cancers are summarized in Fig. 69-4. Possible medical management for advanced GCT is summarized in Fig. 69-5.

Surgery

The surgical procedure of choice for both pathologic diagnosis and control of the primary tumor is an inguinal orchiectomy (Greist, Einhorn, Williams, Donohue, & Rowland, 1984). This approach is the preferred method because it allows the removal of the paratesticular fascial layers as well as surgical control of both the vascular and lymphatic sup-

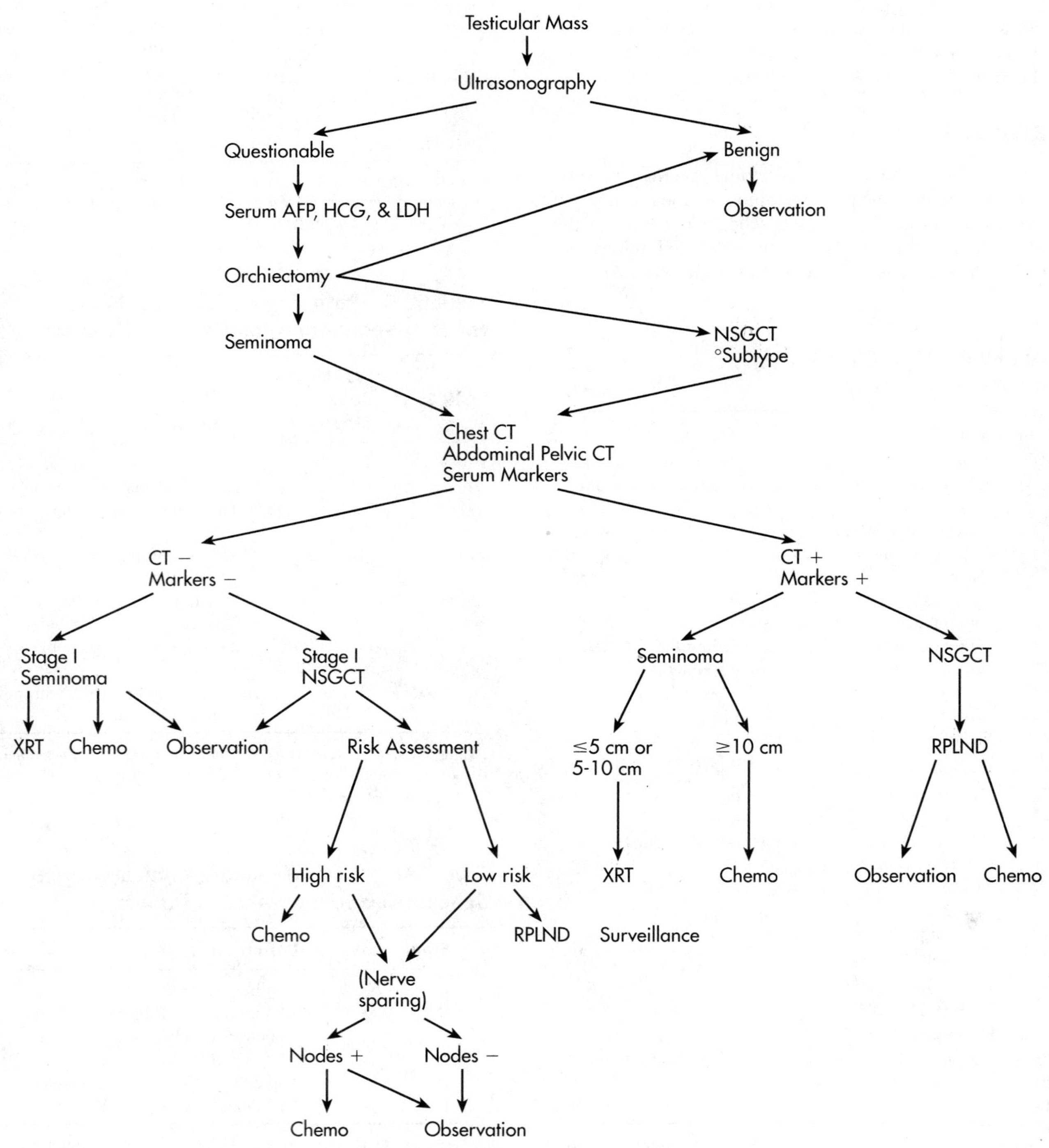

Fig. 69-4 Schema for the diagnosis and treatment of stage I testicular cancer.

ply to the testis. Additionally, a retroperitoneal lymph node dissection (RPLND) (lymphadenectomy) may be performed. RPLND allows for cure without need for chemotherapy in early stages, for accurate staging, for potential decrease in the risk for retroperitoneal metastases, and for removal of residual disease after chemotherapy.

The radical RPLND has been used and is a full, bilateral dissection in which all lymphatic, neural, and connective tissue is removed from the field, from the crux of the diaphragm by the renal arteries and veins superiorly to the bifurcation of the common iliac arteries inferiorly, and by the ureters laterally (Foster & Donohue, 1992). Mortality and morbidity are low in the hands of a surgeon experienced in this procedure; however, loss of ejaculatory function occurs in about 90% to 100% of patients as a result of the removal of the lumbarsympathetic efferent fibers. This can result in retrograde ejaculation but does not influence libido or ability to have an orgasm (Foster, 1992).

This high incidence of ejaculatory dysfunction and the pattern of nodal involvement in the low-risk testicular cancer patient has led many to modify the dissection and salvage the nerves. The areas of dissection are noted in Fig. 69-6. This modification has resulted in the preservation of normal ejaculatory function in 100% of patients while not compromising the necessary pathologic staging or treatment benefit offered by the more radical RPLND. Additional studies have supported these findings (Richie, 1990). Thus the nerve-sparing RPLND is considered to be as effective both diagnostically and therapeutically as the more morbid radical or modified RPLND (Einhorn et al., 1993; Small & Torti, 1995).

Radiation Therapy

The treatment of testicular cancer is dependent on the histologic staging. Doses of radiation therapy may vary from 10 to 35 Gy. These doses are determined by the clinical stage of the seminoma despite the presence of elevated serum HCG or the anaplastic histologic appearance in stages I and IIA patients. Radiation therapy may be administered to the supraclavicular, mediastinal, iliac, inguinal, or paraaortic node groups. Often the iliac, inguinal, or paraaortic nodes are those of the ipsilateral area. Since the 1970s, postorchiectomy radiation in seminoma has yielded excellent 5-year survival rates (Table 69-8) with prophylactic mediastinal irradiation being discontinued as standard therapy (Einhorn et al., 1993).

In NSGCTs, radiation is used with patients demonstrating an incomplete response to postsurgical therapy such as chemotherapy. Doses given are approximately 36 Gy over 4 weeks, but higher doses may be considered in heart or central nervous system (CNS) metastases.

Embryonal carcinoma and teratocarcinoma are sensitive to radiation therapy. This sensitivity is often not fully appreciated due to the high success rate with orchiectomy and chemotherapy. In a study of stage I patients with either em-

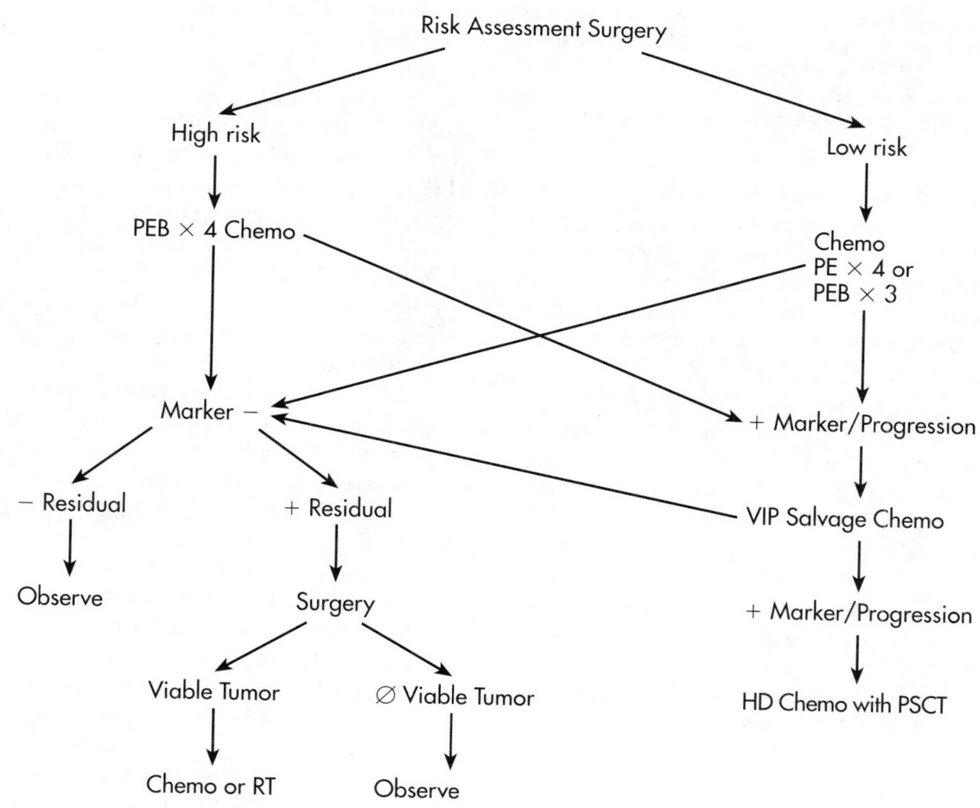

Fig. 69-5 Schema for treatment of advanced germ cell tumors.

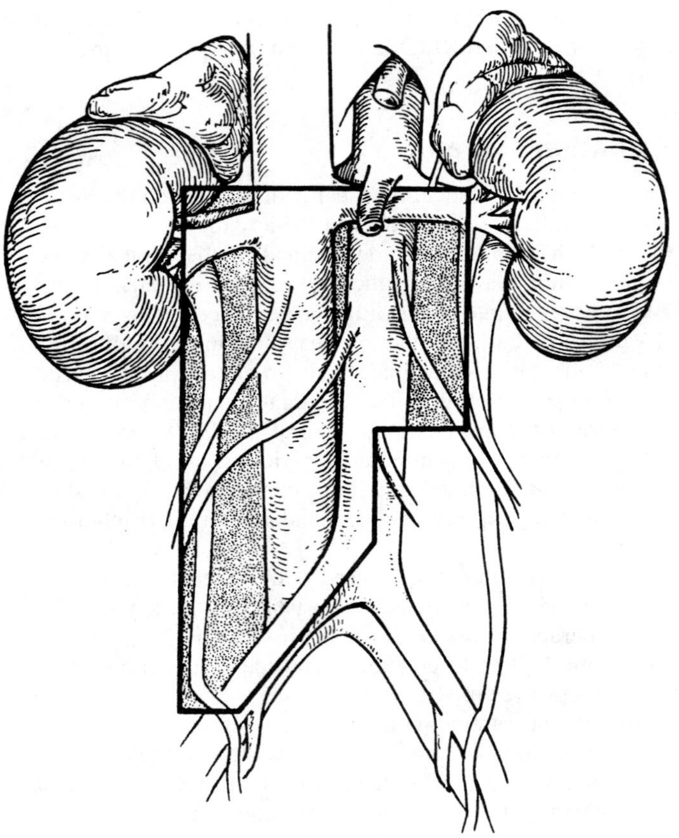

Fig. 69-6 Modified nerve-sparing retroperitoneal lymph node dissection. (Einhorn, L. H., Richie, J. P., Shipley, W. U., Loehrer, P. J., & Williams, S. D. [1993]. Cancer of the testes. In V. T. DeVita, S. Helman, & S. A. Rosenberg [Eds]. *Cancer: Principles and practice of oncology* [4th ed]. Philadelphia: J.B. Lippincott.)

bryonal carcinoma or teratocarcinoma, only two in 84 (2.4%) developed retroperitoneal recurrence after external beam radiation. It was also found that radiation sterilized 93% of the metastases of 2 cm or smaller in the stage II population. Yet when bulky retroperitoneal metastases were treated, radiation sterilized these deposits in only 31% of the patients (Tyrell & Mettler, 1976).

In stages I and IIA seminomas, radiation therapy is used postorchiectomy and includes the treatment fields of the ipsilateral iliac, common iliac, and paraaortic nodes. Extreme care is taken to exactly localize the kidneys in relationship to the treatment fields so that radiation-induced renal complications and damage are eliminated. The areas radiated usually receive approximately 15 Gy. Sperm production is adversely effected by radiation therapy, from a decrease in total sperm count (oligospermia or scant numbers of sperm) to complete abscence of sperm production (azoospermia). Recovery may be from 9 months to 5 years, depending on the dose administered (Bracken, 1988).

Surveillance

In surveillance trials, relapse rates for stage I NSGCT were 35% (Read, Stenning, Cullen, Parkinson, Horwich, & Kaye et al., 1992), 43% (Freedman, Parkinson, Jones, Oliver, Peckham, & Read et al., 1987), and 65% (Klepp, Olsson, Henrickson, Aass, Dahl, & Stenwig et al., 1990). In resected stage II NSGCT, surveillance vs adjuvant chemotherapy has been studied in "good risk" patients. Ninety-eight patients were randomized to an observation group and 97 to an adjuvant group. There was no difference in recurrence or survival rates between the two groups (96% overall), with the median follow-up of 4 years. In this study, N1 and N2a disease was present in 51% of the patients in the surveillance arm. Only 5% in this arm had N3 nodal disease, which has a relapse rate as high as 90% when no chemotherapy is given (Fraley, Naryan, Vogelzang, Kennedy, & Lange, 1985). Thus the results of this study may be somewhat skewed.

It was also noted that 25% of the patients in the surveillance arm failed to keep at least half of their monthly follow-up appointments in the first year. Patients must adhere to a rigorous surveillance follow-up regimen; therefore noncompliant patients are definitely not candidates for surveillance. If recurrence occurs, chemotherapy/treatment would then quickly be instituted (Motzer, Sheinfeld, Mazumdar, Bajorin, Bosl, & Herr et al., 1995).

Chemotherapy

Chemotherapy is recommended when bulky disease is present or relapse is known. Specifically in seminoma, patients with bulky disease or with an elevated AFP or high-stage seminoma IIB or III receive primary chemotherapy. These are generally sensitive to the cisplatin-based regimens such as cisplatinum, vincristine, and bleomycin (PVB); cisplatinum, vinblastine, bleomycin, cyclophosphamide, dactinomycin (VAB-6); or cisplatin and etoposide (PE or EP) (Loehrer, Johnson, Elson, Kinhorn, & Trump, 1995; Mertens & Taylor, 1995). The number of optimal cycles of chemotherapy to be given in an adjuvant setting is related to the quality of the primary surgical resection (Culine, 1996; Motzer et al., 1995) but ranges from 2 to 6 cycles. It is exciting to know that 93% of patients with stage III disease will achieve a complete response with chemotherapy (Presti & Herr 1992).

In NSGCTs, the most recent treatment for early-stage disease is retroperitoneal lymphadenectomy followed by postoperative chemotherapy. Standard therapy (Table 69-9) includes cisplatinum, etoposide, and bleomycin (PEB or PVP16B) (Einhorn, 1988; Williams, Birch, Einhorn, Irwin, Greco, & Loehrer, 1987).

In a study of NSGCT patients who were considered high risk (having a 50% chance of relapse after observation), patients on RPLND, had two cycles of therapy 21 days apart with 100mg/m^2 of etoposide and 20 mg/m^2 cisplatinum per day on days 1 through 5. Patients were eligible for this therapy if they had a lymph node with a tumor greater than 2 cm (N2b), more than six lymph nodes involved with an N2b tumor, or extranodal extension (N3). It was concluded that this regimen can be a therapeutic option in the adjuvant setting after complete resection of N2b and N3 NSGCT and is preferable to observation alone for this group (Motzer et

TABLE 69-8 Results of Postorchiectomy Radiation Therapy in Stage I and IIA Seminoma

Treatment Center	Stage I Seminoma		Stage IIA Seminoma	
	Total Patients	5-year Survival (%)	Total Patients	5-year Survival (%)
Walter Reed Army Hospital	284	97	—	—
Royal Marsden Hospital	232	98	39	95
M.D. Anderson Hospital	161	98	37	95
Massachusetts General Hospital	135	98	18	100
Cross Cancer Institute	147	98	20	85
Johns Hopkins University Hospital	42	100	16	100
Stanford University Hospital	71	100	—	—
U.S. Patterns of Care Study	229	98	—	—
Total	1301	98	130	95

Modified from Einhorn, L. H., Crawford, E. D., Shipley, W. U., Loehrer, P. J., and Williams, S. D. (1993). Cancer of the testes. In V. T. DeVita, S. Hellman, & S. A. Rosenberg, (Eds.). *Cancer: principles and practice of oncology* (4th ed.). Philadelphia: J.B. Lippincott.

TABLE 69-9 PEB (PVP-16B) Chemotherapy

Cisplatin	20 mg/m^2 days 1-5
Etoposide (VP16)	100 mg/m^2 days 1-5
Bleomycin	30 units weekly
Administer 3 to 4 courses at 3-week intervals	

TABLE 69-10 PVB Chemotherapy

Cisplatin	20mg/m^2 days 1-5
Vinblastine	0.15-0.2 mg/kg days 1 & 2
Bleomycin	30 units every week × 2
(Maintenance vinblastine	0.3 mg/kg monthly × 21 months)
Administer for 4 cycles on 3-week intervals	

al., 1995). The investigators contend that this is preferable to vinblastine-based regimens due to better tolerance with elimination of stomatitis, dermatologic toxicity, and ileus, which has been reported (Vugrin, Whitmore, Cvitkovic, Grabstald, Sogani, & Golbey, 1981; Vugrin, Whitmore, Herr, Sogani, & Golbey, 1983). Others support the use of two-cycle EP to prevent relapse in N2b and N3 NSGCT versus PEB (Motzer et al., 1995). This remains under debate (Nichols, Gonin, & Foster, 1995).

For patients with retroperitoneal or visceral metastases (stages B3 and C), chemotherapy with cisplatin, vinblastine, and with or without doxorubicin may be used (Table 69-10) (Smith, 1988). Others have used ifosfamide, cisplatin, and etoposide/vinblastine (Table 69-11). Generally, lymph node dissection is done if residual lymph node involvement is known after completion of chemotherapy (Einhorn, 1988).

Salvage chemotherapy for persistent disease despite therapy is anticipated in the 30% of patients who have metastatic disseminated germ cell tumors. Clinical observation has confirmed that synergy exists between cisplatin and ifosfamide (Woodman, 1971; Goldin, 1982; Roth, 1996).

TABLE 69-11 Salvage Chemotherapy

Cisplatin	20 mg/m^2 days 1-5
Vinblastine	0.22 mg/kg day 1
Ifosfamide	1.2 G/m^2 days 1-5
Administer for 4 cycles at 3-week intervals	
Cisplatin	20 mg/m^2 days 1-5
Etoposide	75 mg/m^2 days 1-5
Ifosfamide	1.2 G/m^2 days 1-5
Administer for 4 cycles at 3-week intervals	

Studies using cisplatin, ifosfamide, and vinblastine (VIP) vs. PEB as first-line therapy in poor-risk disease, consistently showed no difference in response rates; yet VIP produced more significant acute toxicity, especially myelosuppression (Kaye, Mead, Fossa et al., 1995; Loehrer, Einhorn, & Elson 1993; Nichols, Loehrer, Einhorn et al., 1995). Therefore at present cisplatin, ifosfamide, and vinblastine (VIP) are considered salvage chemotherapy (Saxman, 1992). Mesna is dosed at 120 mg/m^2 per day by pretreatment infusion and postchemotherapy administration every 4 hours × 2 for the 5 days of therapy (Table 69-11) (Einhorn et al., 1993).

VIP has demonstrated a 34% complete response (CR), with 24% of patients in continuous CR at a median follow-up of 13 months (Motzer, Cooper, Geller, Bajorin, Dmitrovsky, & Herr et al., 1990; Motzer, Bajorin, & Bosl, 1992). Similar results have been reported by others concerning the ifosfamide-based salvage treatment.

High-dose/dose-escalation protocols with autologous bone marrow/peripheral stem cell transplantation are also being explored for patients with persistent recurrent disease. High-dose carboplatin plus etoposide is being investigated. Carboplatin has been shown to be as active as cisplatin with myelosuppression as its dose-limiting toxicity, making it the best agent for peripheral stem cell transplantation. In addition, it is highly synergistic with etoposide (VP16). At present these two agents are used in high-dose therapy for testicular cancer with peripheral stem cell transplant, and results are still being investigated (Einhorn et al., 1993).

Follow-Up Care

Complete physical examination with emphasis on the remaining testis, the lymph nodes, and the abdomen is necessary. AFP, HCG, and LDH are needed laboratory tests, as are chest CT and radiograph and abdominal CT, or MRI if CT results necessitate further investigation and differential diagnosis.

ONCOLOGIC EMERGENCIES

The most common oncologic emergencies for patients with testicular cancer are those resulting from chemotherapy with subsequent immunosuppression and related sepsis. Surgical intervention may include orchiectomy, and patients are at risk for bleeding, wound infections, and pulmonary problems. Chapter 3 discusses oncologic surgical emergencies, and Chapter 11 discusses oncologic emergencies.

NURSING MANAGEMENT

As shown in Figs. 69-4 and 69-5, medical management depends on the histology and stage of disease. Nursing management derives many of its interventions from the medical treatment plan to be instituted.

Detection

Early detection of testicular cancer can be achieved by testicular self-examination (TSE). An educational brochure often used for patients concerning TSE is shown in Fig. 69-7. However, research into the TSE practices of young men has shown that a small percentage of men regularly perform TSE. One study found that a mere 13% of the 126 college-age male subjects had even heard about TSE (Reno, 1988). Another study found that only 9.5% of the 233 subjects practiced TSE (Blesch, 1986). Vague heaviness or slight discomfort most likely would not cause a male to seek medical attention. This is substantiated by the fact that a good percentage of testicular cancers have already metastasized at the time of clinical diagnosis (Lind, Kravitz, & Greig, 1993).

It is clear that education of the teenage to young adult male population is warranted. This education needs to stress the reason for the need and technique for TSE. Open discussions on the topic can best help the young male overcome inhibitions, discomfort, or cultural barriers to performing the TSE.

As health issues of males are discussed in educational arenas addressing general sexuality, such as pregnancy and parenting, sexuality transmitted diseases and AIDS, and other such issues, TSE must become an integral part of such programs. Depending on the beliefs and values of the patient, the male nurse or physician may prove to be more effective in increasing TSE performance among males.

Box 69-4
The PLISSIT Model

P Permission
L Limited information
S Specific
S Suggestions
I Intensive
T Therapy

Surgical Management

Preoperative and Postoperative Nursing Care. Preoperative care of the patient includes considerable education concerning the diagnostic tests being performed; that is, their rationale as well as what the patient may expect. In addition, education on the actual surgical procedure planned must complement and expand on the information given by the physician. This may include information on incision care, management of postoperative pain, and pulmonary toilet, and anticipating questions the patient or partner may have.

Just before surgery, the patient is administered intravenous fluids such as dextrose 5.5 normal saline. Mannitol may be administered at the time of dissection of the renal hilum to prevent arterial thrombosis and renal ischemia. Broad-spectrum antibiotics are administered empirically preoperatively and perioperatively, and general anesthesia is standard. Postoperative hemodynamic monitoring may be done, especially in patients at high risk for bleeding or other complications.

Orchiectomy. The patient may view orchiectomy as castration, sterility, impotence, or impairment of masculinity, self-worth, and life. He may need time to grieve. Furthermore, he may be embarrassed to discuss this and fear the effects these problems may have on present or future relationships. The patient may not fully understand the normal anatomy and physiology of his reproductive system and may misunderstand basic terms health care professionals normally use. For example, a patient may think that removal of the testis or decreased sperm count is the same as impotence. The nurse needs to open the topic as an acceptable one and offer psychosocial support. Discussion of the patient's desire for a testicular prosthesis for cosmesis should take place. The nurse should be knowledgeable on such topics or on the resources available to address such concerns and follow the PLISSIT model to approach topics on sexuality as noted in Box 69-4. A standard of care for the patient undergoing surgery is described in Table 69-12. The patient is hospitalized postsurgery for 5 days, followed by outpatient and home care support.

Nursing Care of the Patient Receiving Radiation Therapy

Retroperitoneal irradiation is generally tolerated fairly well. Some side effects include fatigue, mild nausea and possible vomiting, myelosuppression, possible diarrhea, and azo-

Testicular Self-Examination

Testicular cancer is the most common type of cancer in men ages 20 to 35. Yet, because it accounts for only about 1 percent of all cancers in men, many people have never heard of this type of cancer.

Testicular cancer is of special concern to young men. It can occur anytime after age 15. It is less common in middle-aged and older men. White men are four times more likely to develop testicular cancer than black men. The rate among Hispanic men lies between those of blacks and whites.

Two groups of men have a greater risk of developing testicular cancer—those whose testicles have not descended into the scrotum and those whose testicles descended after age 6. Testicular cancer is 3 to 17 times more likely to develop in these men.

Testicles are male reproductive organs. They produce and store sperm. They also produce testosterone, a hormone that causes such male traits as facial hair and lower voice pitch. Testicles are smooth, oval-shaped, and somewhat firm to the touch. They are below the penis in a sac of skin called the scrotum.

The testicles normally descend into the scrotum before birth. Parents should have their infant sons examined by a doctor to be sure that the testicles have properly descended. If they have not, this can be easily corrected with surgery.

Fifteen years ago, testicular cancer was often fatal because it spread quickly to vital organs such as the lungs. Today, due to advances in treatment, testicular cancer is one of the most curable cancers, especially if detected and treated promptly.

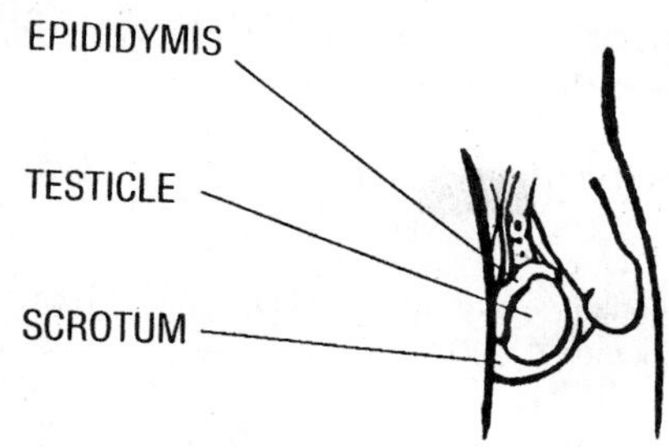

Symptoms

The most common symptom of testicular cancer is a small, painless lump in a testicle or a slightly enlarged testicle. It is important for men to become familiar with the size and feeling of their normal testicles, so that they can detect changes if they occur.

Other possible symptoms include a feeling of heaviness in the scrotum, a dull ache in the lower stomach or groin, a change in the way a testicle feels, or a sudden accumulation of blood or fluid in the scrotum. These symptoms can also be caused by infections or other conditions that are not cancer. A doctor can tell you if you have cancer and what the proper treatment should be.

How To Do TSE

A simple procedure called testicular self-exam (TSE) can increase the chances of finding a tumor early.

Men should perform TSE once a month—after a warm bath or shower. The heat causes the scrotal skin to relax, making it easier to find anything unusual. TSE is simple and only takes a few minutes:

- Examine each testicle gently with both hands. The index and middle fingers should be placed underneath the testicle while the thumbs are placed on the top. Roll the testicle gently between the thumbs and fingers. One testicle may be larger than the other. This is normal.

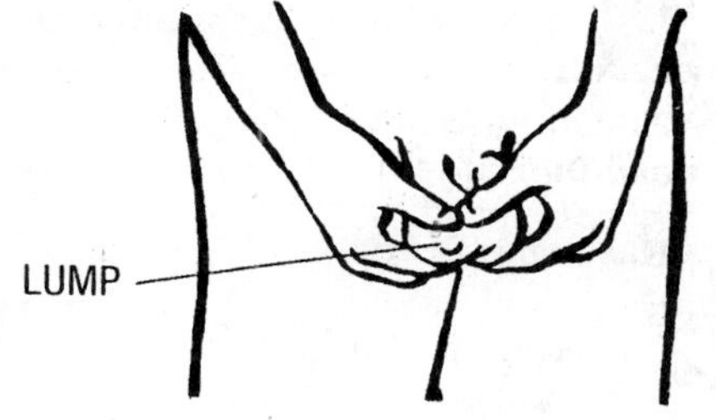

- The epididymis is a cord-like structure on the top and back of the testicle that stores and transports the sperm. Do not confuse the epididymis with an abnormal lump.

- Feel for any abnormal lumps—about the size of a pea—on the front or the side of the testicle. These lumps are usually painless.

If you do find a lump, you should contact your doctor right away. The lump may be due to an infection, and a doctor can decide the proper treatment. If the lump is not an infection, it is likely to be cancer. Remember that testicular cancer is highly curable, especially when detected and treated early. Testicular cancer almost always occurs in only one testicle, and the other testicle is all that is needed for full sexual function.

Routine testicular self-exams are important, but they cannot substitute for a doctor's examination. Your doctor should examine your testicles when you have a physical exam. You also can ask your doctor to check the way you do TSE.

Fig. 69-7 Patient education brochure on testicular self-examination. (From U.S. Department of Health and Human Services, Public Health Services, National Institutes of Health, National Cancer Institute [1994]. NIH Publication No. 94-2636.)

ospermia. Table 69-13 delineates common nursing interventions appropriate for care of the patient.

Nursing Care of the Patient Receiving Chemotherapy

Chemotherapy regimens include a number of agents, and the nursing interventions are specific to those agents' side effects. Table 69-14 addresses some of the side effects of these agents and the nursing interventions appropriate to each side effect. Hawkins and Miaskowski (1996) developed a nursing plan of care that offers excellent information (Table 69-15).

The late sequelae of PEB have been documented as presence of cardiovascular and pulmonary disease, fertility problems, and secondary neoplasms such as leukemia (Bajorin, Motzer, Rodriquez, Murphy, & Bosl, 1993). Studies in the testicular patient, however, do not demonstrate these long-term effects. As seen in Table 69-16, Pont, Albrecht, Postner, Sellner, Angel, & Holtl (1996) reported results of a seven-item questionnaire that showed there was no difference in the patient's report of psychosexual components between those who received PEB chemotherapy versus surveillance. However, this questionnaire is far from comprehensive, lacking both reliability and validity; thus, this aspect needs further investigation. They also investigated sperm counts in pa-

TABLE 69-12 Standard of Care for the Patient Undergoing Surgery for Testicular Cancer

Patient Problems and Outcomes	Nursing Interventions	Patient Education
Knowledge Deficit Patient will verbalize understanding of the purpose and protocol of operative course and immediate postoperative regimen.	1. Assess patient's level of knowledge of the operative procedure and routine. 2. Assess patient's concerns and fears of the operative procedure.	1. Instruct on the usual operative course involving: a. Preoperative workup and preparation. b. Nothing by mouth after midnight. c. Early A.M. admission. d. Preoperative holding area and regimen. e. Perioperative routine. f. Anesthesia recovery and PACU regimen. g. Immediate postoperative care. 2. Instruct on methods to cope with areas of concern.
Postoperative Pain Patient will have postoperative pain maintained within a tolerable level.	1. Assess patient's level of pain on pain scale. 2. Administer pain medication ATC or adjust PCA basal rate and bolus dose to control pain. 3. Institute alternative methods to control pain (e.g., positioning, music).	1. Instruct patient on need to report pain and appropriately control level to maximize recovery. 2. Instruct patient on pain medication dose, rate, frequency, and untoward side effects. 3. Instruct patient on methods to enhance comfort postoperatively.

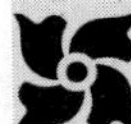

TABLE 69-13 Standard of Care for the Patient Receiving Radiation Therapy for Testicular Cancer

Patient Problems and Outcomes	Nursing Interventions	Patient Education
Knowledge Deficit Patient will verbalize understanding of radiation therapy, purpose, rationale, routines and side effects.	1. Assess patient knowledge of radiation therapy. 2. Assess patient's fears and concerns about radiation therapy.	1. Instruct in the routine procedures of radiation therapy. a. Consultation b. Simulation c. Treatment routines d. Follow-up visits and treatment frequency 2. Instruct on side effects of radiation therapy in accordance with the fields being treated, self-care, methods to minimize side effects, and need to report occurrence. 3. Instruct patient on side effects in need of immediate follow-up by nurse/physician.

tients receiving PEB adjuvant chemotherapy for NSGCT vs those on surveillance (Table 69-17) and found no significant difference between the two groups. The investigator reported that eight children were fathered at least 2 years after completion of adjuvant chemotherapy (as instructed) and are alive and well (Pont et al., 1996). Stephenson, Shelly, Rubin, and Einhorn (1995) studied 30 patients who had 2 to 4 cycles of PEB with semen analysis after at least 24 months. Oligospermia (less than 40×10^6) total sperm count was found in 13 patients (43%) including 6 (20%) who were azoospermic. Only 13 patients (43%) had sperm motility greater than 50%; yet 8 patients fathered children, including 3 with persistent oligospermia. Clearly, the data demonstrate effects on reproductive capacity yet fail to truly define the breath of the difficulties and adjustments of patients or their partners regarding sexuality and self concept.

HOME CARE ISSUES

Much of the therapy for the testicular patient is performed in outpatient settings, except for surgery and immediate post-surgical care. Home care can greatly aid in assisting the patient to returning to his state of health in optimal time. As managed care continues to challenge health providers with shortened hospitalizations, outpatient and home care nurses are challenged to meet desired care outcomes. Home care

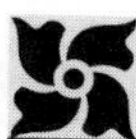

TABLE 69-14 Standard of Care for the Patient Receiving Chemotherapy for Testicular Cancer

Patient Problems and Outcomes	Nursing Interventions	Patient Education
Knowledge Deficit Patient will verbalize understanding of chemotherapy treatment plan, rationale, and side effects.	1. Assess patient knowledge of chemotherapy plan and agents used. 2. Assess patient fears and concerns regarding therapy planned.	1. Instruct on agents being used, rationale, dose, frequency, and side effects. 2. Instruct on side effects and need of follow-up.
Nausea and/or Vomiting Patient will experience no/tolerable nausea and no vomiting.	1. Assess nausea on a scale of 0 to 5 and frequency of emesis. 2. Institute antiemetic regimen prior to treatment and several days after courses on around-the-clock basis. 3. Institute alternative methods to control nausea/vomiting (e.g., music, imagery).	1. Instruct on antiemetic(s) being used, method of administration, frequency, and side effects. 2. Instruct on meal preparation and dietary adjustments needed to maximize patient intake. 3. Instruct on side effects in need of follow-up.
Nutrition Patient will maintain adequate nutrition and hydration during treatment course.	1. Monitor diet and hydration. 2. Assess patient nausea on scale of 0 to 5 and frequency of emesis. 3. Administer antiemetics as ordered around-the-clock during and several days following treatment. 4. Administer IV antiemetics and fluids as indicated. 5. Institute community food/financial resources if indicated (e.g., Meals on Wheels, food stamps). 6. Obtain dietary consult if indicated.	1. Instruct on methods to enhance appeal for food. 2. Instruct on need to maintain diet and hydration. 3. Instruct on rationale and regimen for antiemetic therapy. 4. Instruct on untoward effects in need of follow-up.
Mucositis Patient will remain free of mucositis and oral infection.	1. Assess mucous membranes for signs of breakdown and/or infection. 2. Institute oral care regimen preventively and on a frequent basis. 3. Institute antibiotic/antifungal agents as ordered.	1. Instruct patient on signs and symptoms of mucositis. 2. Instruct on oral care regimen, frequency, and rationale. 3. Instruct on side effects in need of follow-up. 4. Instruct on antiinfectives ordered, rationale, regimen, and side effects.
Myelosuppression Patient will have no morbid side effects due to low counts (e.g., infection).	1. Assess CBC and differential 2. Administer colony stimulating factors (CSFs). 3. Assess degree of physical symptoms exhibited relating to degree of myelosuppression (e.g., fatigue, dizziness).	1. Instruct patient on self care technique in administering CSFs. 2. Instruct on methods to adjust ADLs in accordance with degree of myelosuppression. a. Neutropenic precautions. b. Thrombocytopenic precautions. c. Frequent rest periods for anemia. 3. Instruct on methods to manage side effects of CSFs.
Role Function Patient will verbalize coping with role function(s).	1. Assess patient fears and perceptions on effect of therapy on roles, functions (e.g., "bread winner," husband, sexual partner). 2. Assess patient's response to actual changes in role function. 3. Provide psychosexual support.	1. Discuss methods to adjust to role changes and its effects on self-esteem. 2. Instruct patient on actual effects of the therapy on sexual and reproductive functions.

CBC, complete blood count; *ADL*, activities of daily living.

TABLE 69-15 Nursing Care Plan for the Treatment of Testicular Cancer

Nursing Diagnosis	Indications	Patient Outcomes	Nursing Interventions	Rationales
Body image disturbance related to orchiectomy; cutaneous skin reactions from chemotherapy; alopecia	Expression of negative feelings about body Fear of rejection Change in skin color Hair loss	Patient will describe strategies to cope with changes in body image. Patient will adapt to hair loss by using wigs or head coverings.	1. Encourage patient to verbalize feelings about hair loss and changes in appearance. 2. Assess previous coping strategies and determine which were more effective. 3. Teach patient self-care activities related to body image disturbance. 4. Reinforce any attempts to attend to the body part. 5. Reinforce any verbalizations of feelings about actual or perceived loss. 6. Provide a consultation with hair stylist or barber.	1. Indicates the meaning of the loss for the individual. 2. Knowledge of previously effective coping strategies can be used to assist the patient to cope with these strategies. 3. & 4. Involvement in self-care activities enables adaptation to the changes in body image. 5. Acknowledging thoughts and feelings enables the patient to move through the grieving process.
Sexual dysfunction related to orchiectomy with retroperitoneal lymph node dissection (sterility) related to chemotherapy, radiation therapy	Retrograde ejaculation Failure to ejaculate Decreased libido Azoospermia	Patient will explore ways to enhance sexual satisfaction. Patient will resume previous level of satisfactory sexual activity. Patient will describe sperm banking opportunities	1. Assess patient's knowledge of the cause(s) of the sexual dysfunction and perception of the present problem. Include significant other in the therapeutic discussions of altered sexual activities. 2. Conduct a sexual assessment in privacy. 3. Discuss alternative sexual activities that are compatible with changes in life-style. Refer the patient to a sexual counselor if appropriate. 4. Discuss the advantages and disadvantages of sperm banking.	1. Retrograde ejaculation, or failure to ejaculate because of severing of the sympathetic plexus, occurs in almost all patients undergoing an extended, bilateral retroperitoneal lymph node dissection. The dissection does not affect the patient's ability to have an erection or experience an orgasm. 2. Providing privacy fosters communication. 3. Knowledge that alternatives to sexual intercourse (e.g., hugging, kissing, massage, single or mutual masturbation, sexual aids) are available helps to decrease anxiety and increase sexual satisfaction.
Risk of infection associated with surgery or chemotherapy administration	Decreased white blood cell count Fever Vascular access device	Patient will remain free of infection.	1. Assess for signs and symptoms of acute infection including fever, rashes, and changes in vital signs and white blood cell count. 2. Monitor incisions, wounds, and indwelling catheter site for infection. 3. Obtain blood and urine cultures and chest radiograph prior to administering antibiotics.	1. Temperature elevation (101° F or 38.3° C) may be the only sign of infection. Note that if a patient is receiving bleomycin as part of the chemotherapy regimen, he may experience fever and chills approximately 4 to 6 hours after the infusion. This transient side effect does not require a fever workup. The bleomycin fever usually lasts 2 hours and can be treated with acetaminophen.

			4. Teach patient to: • Avoid contact with sick people • Notify a healthcare professional if a temperature occurs • Maintain a well-balanced diet • Use good hand-washing techniques 5. Administer antibiotics as prescribed or instruct patient to take the full course of the antibiotics.	2. Patients who are immunosuppressed may not exhibit the normal signs and symptoms of wound infection (e.g., swelling, redness). The only clue to an infectious process may be pain at the site of infection when the site is palpated. 3. Fever workup should be completed prior to starting antibiotics.
Constipation related to chemotherapy administration	Abdominal distention Cramping abdominal pain Decreased frequency of defecation Hard, formed, dry stools Palpable fecal mass in rectum Sensation of pressure in rectum Straining during defecation	Patient will maintain a normal bowel elimination pattern.	1. Assess usual bowel pattern, including frequency, size, shape, and consistency. 2. Perform abdominal assessment and auscultate bowel sounds. 3. Institute a high-fiber diet, and teach patient about foods that are high in fiber (e.g., whole grains [breads and cereals], fruits, vegetables, nuts, bran, and bran-containing cereals). 4. Encourage fluid intake of greater than 3 L/day. 5. Administer stool softeners and laxatives, as prescribed. 6. Encourage patient not to avoid the urge to defecate. The defecation reflex is weakened or lost if repeatedly ignored. The strongest urge occurs after meals, especially breakfast, because of increased peristalsis secondary to gastrocolic and duodenocolic reflexes.	1. Constipation can occur in patients being treated with vinca alkaloids. Patients receiving chemotherapy within 6 weeks of retroperitoneal lymphadenectomy seem to be at higher risk of developing chemotherapy-induced constipation. 2. Auscultation of decreased bowel sounds helps to detect early indications of obstipation. Early detection may help to prevent more serious complications, such as paralytic ileus.
Risk of altered renal tissue perfusion associated with cisplatin administration	Increasing serum blood urea nitrogen (BUN) Increasing serum creatinine Dehydration Administration of chemotherapy	Patient will maintain normal renal tissue perfusion.	1. Monitor serum electrolytes, BUN, and creatinine. 2. Maintain strict recordings of intake and output. 3. Weigh patient daily. 4. Administer IV hydration as prescribed.	1. Dose-related nephrotoxicity is a potential complication of cisplatin. 2. Maintaining adequate renal perfusion reduces the risk of nephrotoxicity.

From Hawkins, C. & Miaskowski, C. (1996). Testicular cancer: A review. *Oncology Nursing Forum. 23*(8), 1208-1209.
NOTE: From *Plans of care for specialty practice—Oncology nursing* by C. Miaskowski (Ed.) 1995. Albany, NY: Delmar Publishers. Copyright 1995 by Delmar Publishers. Modified with permission.

clinicians can support the patient who is discharged postsurgery yet continues to require nursing care. Availability of a family caregiver and the patient's age, clinical condition, and ability and motivation for self-care are important considerations for setting realistic outcome measures for home care. Skilled oncology trained nurses must also be available to see patients consistently and to case manage their care to achieve appropriate care outcomes.

Home care support for management of wound care postoperatively or of side effects of radiation and chemotherapy can be extremely beneficial. Hydration prior to and after chemotherapy, intravenous administration of antiemetics, administration of colony stimulating factors, and skilled assessment and intervention by a nurse for other side effects of therapy can be done on an intermittent basis between physician visits to enhance the care rendered to the patient and assist in his adjustment to care. One of the major goals of home care teams is to divert inappropriate readmissions or emergency room visits. Examples of home care treatments are listed in Box 69-5. In the case of the patient needing to flush his IV catheter, the patient will receive instruction such as those in Box 69-6.

PROGNOSIS

Generally, 95% of patients with nonseminoma survive at a higher percentage than those with seminoma. About 80% of patients with metastatic disease can be cured of their disease. There remains a very small group of patients with extensive visceral involvement who are at risk for disease-related death.

More recently, long-term side effects of treatment are being explored. Cardiovascular disease related to cisplatin have been reported. However, when investigated further in a trial of patients receiving no chemotherapy or two or four courses of chemotherapy with cisplatin, there was no difference in the development of hypertension or cardiovascular disease. It was noted that paresthesias or Raynaud's syndrome was more likely in patients who received more che-

TABLE 69-16 Replies to Psychosocial and Psychosexual Self-report Questionnaire

	Chemotherapy (n = 22)		Surveillance (n = 16)		
Question	Yes	No	Yes	No	P
a. Diseases or impairment of well-being: more often?	3	19	2	14	NS
b. Libido: weaker?	3	19	0	16	NS
c. Sexual potency: worse?	2	20	2	14	NS
d. Interference with schooling/training or professional career?	6	16	1	15	NS
e. Loss of job or change of employment?	3	19	2	14	NS
f. Loss or change of sexual partner?	2	20	0	16	NS
g. Unfulfilled desire to have children?	1	19	2	14	NS

From Pont, J., Albrecht, W., Postner, G., Sellner, F., Angel, K., & Holtl, W. (1996) Adjuvant chemotherapy for high-risk clinical stage I nonseminomatous testicular germ cell cancer: Long-term results of a prospective trial. *Journal of Clinical Oncology, 14*(2), 444.
NS, not significant.

Box 69-5
Treatment Available to be Done in the Home

- Postoperative wound care
- Antibiotic therapy
- Antiemetic therapy
- Skilled clinical assessment of side effects of radiation or chemotherapy
- Hydration and electrolyte replacement
- Pain management: postoperative, therapy, or disease-related, terminal pain
- Catheter-related care
- Instruction on self-care needs
- Terminal care–related interventions
- Blood work and laboratory specimens, including culture and sensitivity of blood

TABLE 69-17 Comparison of Sperm Counts in Patients Treated by Adjuvant Chemotherapy and Patients on Surveillance

	Postchemotherapy (n = 18)		Surveillance (n = 15)		
Variable	Mean ± SD	Range	Mean ± SD	Range	P
Sperm concentration (× 10^6/mL)	55 ± 47.6	0-141	21 ± 18.3	1-67	0.01
Motile sperms (%)	46 ± 21.3	0-80	47 ± 21.5	12-81	NS
Abnormal sperms (%)	49 ± 20.7	30-70	57 ± 21.9	20-90	NS

From Pont, J., Albrecht, W., Postner, G., Sellner, F., Angel, K., & Holtl, W. (1996) Adjuvant chemotherapy for high-risk clinical stage I nonseminomatous testicular germ cell cancer: Long-term results of a prospective trial. *Journal of Clinical Oncology, 14*(2), 446.
NS, not significant.

motherapy (Nichols, Ruth, Williams, Gill, Muggia, & Stablein et al., 1992). Symptoms of Raynaud's phenomenon abate in about 50% of the patients (Small & Torti, 1995).

There is also an observation that etoposide may cause secondary leukemia. This seems to be related to dosage and is rarely seen in patients who received less than 2000 mg/m^2 as a total dose and in whom the leukemia had been diagnosed 2 to 4 years posttherapy (Nichols, Breeden, Loehrer, Williams, & Einhorn, 1993).

Azoospermia or oligospermia has been a concern but has been shown to be dose-related as to the length of time it may take to resume normal spermatogenesis. Approximately 25% will remain azoospermic. Most will achieve nearly, if not total, spermatogenesis, and many (about 33%) have been known to father normal children.

EVALUATION OF QUALITY CARE

Outcome-based evaluation of the care given by the multidisciplinary team is necessary and is required for critical accreditation purposes such as the Joint Commission. Collaboration of the various team members participating in the care and successful treatment of the patient with testicular cancer is required to achieve such evaluation. Accordingly, most institutions desiring accrediations develop multidisciplinary work groups to develop processes to evaluate care outcomes. Table 69-18 is an example of a quality evaluation tool.

Box 69-6
Home Care Instructions to Flush a Groshong Catheter

Reason: Your catheter is placed to allow the nurse or doctor an easier way to give you your medicines into your vein(s) and to get blood for tests. Between using it (weekly) and just after using it, the catheter needs to be flushed with fluid so that it remains open and functioning.

Steps to do:

1. Wash your hands well.
2. Take a 12-cc syringe with needle and remove casing.
3. Draw up 10 cc of air.
4. Scrub top of normal saline vial with alcohol pad.
5. Insert needle into vial and push in air, holding the syringe upright.
6. Draw back 10 ml of saline. Remember to keep the needle in the fluid.
7. Remove needle from vial.
8. Remove air or air bubbles from syringe. Hints: tap on the syringe and remember air rises! Put protective cap back on.
9. With nonsterile gloves on, scrub the connection between the catheter hub and the end cap very well with povidone iodine (Betadine) pad. Allow to dry at least 1 minute.
10. Remove end cap and discard. Keep hub from touching anything.
11. Remove needle with screwing motion and attach syringe to catheter hub.
12. Flush catheter with 10 cc of saline.
13. Remove syringe from hub and attach new end cap. You may clean the Betadine off with alcohol pad.
14. Discard your used supplies into the container given to you by your nurse.

TABLE 69-18 Quality of Care Evaluation for Patients Undergoing Chemotherapy for Testicular Cancer

Disciplines participating in the quality of care evaluation:
☐ Nursing ☐ Medical
☐ Medical Social Worker ☐ Pharmacy

Data from:
☐ Patient and family interview
☐ Documentation in medical record

I. Therapy and Side Effects

Criteria	Yes	No
1. Patient verbalized knowledge of:		
a. Rationale for chemotherapy	☐	☐
b. Names of the agents used	☐	☐
c. At least three of the more frequent side effects experienced with:		
(1) Agent ________	☐	☐
(2) Agent ________	☐	☐
(3) Agent ________	☐	☐
d. Three interventions to manage side effects of therapy:		
(1) Nausea and/or vomiting		
(2) Lack of appetite		
(3) Low blood count		
2. Patient remained free of fever and signs and symptoms of infection	☐	☐
3. Complications experienced were rated 2.5 or less on 0 to 5 scale	☐	☐

II. Patient/Caregiver Satisfaction

Data from:
☐ Interview with ☐ Patient
☐ Family/caregiver
☐ Questionnaire

Criteria	Yes	No
1. On a scale of 0 to 10, 0 being totally dissatisfied and 10 being totally satisfied, how satisfied were you with the information given you regarding the drugs and their side effects?	________	
2. Were you taught the signs and symptoms of infection?	☐	☐
3. On a scale of 0 to 5, 0 being very tolerable side effects experienced and 5 being very untolerable side effects, how would you rate your experience with side effects of chemotherapy?	________	

RESEARCH ISSUES

Testicular cancer and its treatment present both physiologic and psychologic sequelae. Further research to determine optimal dosages of chemotherapy with minimal sequelae needs to be continued. Oncogene investigations as they relate to testicular cancers also merit continued exploration. Nursing research aimed at barriers for males to performing TSE, and strategies to increase compliance, is important in the overall preventive health care of males. Comprehensive research delving into patient's alteration in self-concept and sexuality related to diagnosis and treatment of testicular cancer can suggest strategies to enhance the quality of life for the patient and his partner. Nursing research in the area of home care and outcome of care must be innovative and reliable. Nursing needs to embrace challenges of working within the constraints of today's health care environment to establish standards and outcome-based criteria. The discipline of nursing, in concert with other members of the interdisicplinary clinical team, has the ability to ensure that quality care is given to patients with cancer.

REFERENCES

Albers, P., Orazi, A., Ulbright, T. M., Miller, G. A., Haidar, J. H., Donohue, J. P., & Foster, R. S. (1995). Prognostic significance of immunohistochemical proliferation markers (KI-67/MIB-1 and proliferation-associated nuclear antigen), p53 protein accumulation, and neovascularization in clinical stage A nonseminomatous testicular germ cell tumors. *Modern Pathology, 8,* 492-497.

Bajorin, D. F., Motzer, R. J., Rodriquez, E., Murphy, B., & Bosl, G. J. (1993). Acute nonlymphocytic leukemia in germ cell tumor patients treated with etoposide-containing chemotherapy. *Journal of National Cancer Institute, 85,* 60-62.

Barzell, W. & Whitmore, W. F. (1979). Neoplasm of the testis. In J. H. Harrison, R. F. Gittes, A. D. Perlmutter et al. (Eds.), *Campbell's Urology* (4th ed.). Philadelphia: W. B. Saunders.

Bartkova, J., Bartek, J., Lukas, J., Vojtesek, B., Staskova, Z., Rejthar, A., Kovarik, J., Midgley, C. A., & Lane, D. P. (1991). p53 protein alterations in human testicular cancer including pre-invasive intratubular germ-cell neoplasia. *International Journal of Cancer, 49,* 196-202.

Beahrs, O. H., Henson, D. E., Hutter, R. V. P., & Kennedy, B. J. (1993). *American Joint Committee on Cancer manual for staging cancer* (4th ed.). Philadelphia: J. B. Lippincott.

Bernardi, D., Salvioni, R., Vaccher, E., Repetto, L, Piersoantelli, N., Marini, B., Talamini, R., & Tirelli, U. (1995). Testicular germ cell tumors and human immunodeficiency virus infection: A report of 26 cases. *Journal of Clinical Oncology, 13*(11), 2705-2711.

Blesch, K.S. (1986). Health beliefs about testicular cancer and self-examination among professional men. *Oncology Nursing Forum, 13,* 29-33.

Bosl, G.J., Sheinfeld, J., Bajorin, D., & Motzer, R.J. (1997). Testicular cancer. In V.T. DeVita, S. Hellman, & S.A. Rosenberg (Eds). *Cancer: Principles and practice of oncology* (5th ed.). Philadelphia: Lippincott-Raven.

Bracken, R.B. (1988). Cancer of the testis, penis and urethra: The impact of therapy on sexual function. In A. VonEschenbach & D. Rodriquez (Eds.), *Sexual rehabilitation of the urologic cancer patient.* Boston: Hall.

Carlsen, E., Giwercman, A., Keiding, N., & Skakkebaek, N. E. (1992). Evidence for decreasing quality of semen during past 50 years. *British Medical Journal, 305,* 609-613.

Culine, S. (1996). Adjuvant chemotherapy in pathologic stage II nonseminomatous testicular cancer: Are two cycles of etoposide-ciplatin a standard option? [Letter]. *Journal of Clinical Oncology, 14*(7), 2187-2188.

Einhorn, L. H. (1988). Chemotherapy of disseminated testicular cancer. In D. Skinner & G. Lieskovsky (Eds.). *Diagnosis and management of genitourinary cancer.* Philadelphia: W. B. Saunders.

Einhorn, L. H., Richie, J. P., Shipley, W. U., Loehrer, P. J. & Williams, S. D. (1993). Cancer of the testis. In V. T. DeVita, S. Hellman, & S. A. Rosenberg (Eds.). *Cancer: Principles and practice in oncology* (4th ed.). Philadelphia: J. B. Lippincott.

Einhorn, L. H., Donohue, J. P., & Peckham, M. J. (1985.) In V. T. DeVita, S. Hellman, & S. A. Rosenberg (Eds.). *Cancer: Principles and practice in oncology* (2nd ed.). Philadelphia: J. B. Lippincott.

Foster, R. S. & Donohue, J. P. (1992). Surgical treatment of clinical stage nonseminomatus testis cancer. *Seminars in Oncology, 19,* 166.

Fraley, E. E., Naryan, P., Vogelzang, N. J., Kennedy, B. J., & Lange, P. H. (1985). Surgical treatment of patients with stages I and II nonseminomatous testicular cancer. *Journal of Urology, 134,* 70-73.

Freedman, L. S., Parkinson, M. C., Jones, W. G., Oliver, R. T., Peckham, M. J., Read, G., Newlands, E. S., & Williams, C. J. (1987). Histopathology in the prediction of relapse of patients with stage I testicular teratoma treated by orchidectomy alone. *Lancet, 2,* 294-298.

Ghosn, M., Droz, J. P., Theodore, C., Pico, J. L., Baume, D., Spielmann, M., Ostronoff, M., Moran, A., Salloum, E., & Kramar, A., (1988). Salvage chemotherapy in refractory germ cell tumors with etoposide (VP-16) plus ifosfamide plus high-dose cisplatin. *Cancer, 62,* 24-27.

Gilbert, J. B. & Hamilton, J. B. (1940). Incidence and nature of tumors in ectopic testes. *Surgery, Gynecology & Obstetrics, 71,* 731.

Goldin, A. (1982). Ifosfamide in experimental tumor systems. *Seminars in Oncology, 9,* 14-23.

Greist, A., Einhorn, L. H., Williams, S. D., Donohue, J. P., & Rowland, R. G. (1984). Pathologic findings at orchiectomy following chemotherapy for disseminated testicular cancer. *Journal of Clinical Oncology, 2,* 1025-1027.

Hawkins, C. & Miaskowski, C. (1996). Testicular cancer: A review. *Oncology Nursing Forum, 23*(8), 1203-1211.

Henderson, B. E., Bernstein, L., Ross, R. K., Depue, R. H., & Judd, H. L. (1988). The early in-utero oestrogen and testosterone environment of blacks and whites: Potential effects on male offspring. *British Journal of Cancer, 57,* 216-218.

Henderson, B. E., Ross, R. K., & Pike, M. C. (1988). Epidemiology of testicular cancer. In D. Skinner & G. Lieskovshy (Eds.), *Diagnosis and management of genitourinary cancer.* Philadelphia: W. B. Saunders.

Higgs, D. J. (1990). The patient with testicular cancer: Nursing management of chemotherapy. *Oncology Nursing Forum, 17,* 243-249.

Holtz, F. & Abell, M. R. (1963). Testicular neoplasms in infants and children: Tumors of non-germ cell origin. *Cancer, 16,* 982-986.

Horwich, A., Alsanjari, N., Ahern, R., Nicholls, J., Dearnaley, D. P., & Fisher, C. (1992). Surveillance following orchidectomy for stage I testicular seminoma. *British Journal of Cancer, 65,* 775-778.

Horwich, A. & Dearnaley, D. P. (1992). Treatment of seminoma. *Seminars in Oncology, 19,* 171.

Kaye, S. B., Mead, G. M., Fossa, S., et al. (1995). An MRC/EORTC randomized trial in poor prognosis metastatic teratoma, comparing BEP with BOP-VIP. *Proceeding from the American Society of Clinical Oncology, 14,* 246.

Klepp, O., Olsson, A., Henrickson, J., Aass, N., Dahl, O., Stenwig, A. E., Persson, B. E., Cavallin-Stahl, E., Fossa, S. D., & Wahlqvist, L. (1990). Prognostic factors in clinical stage I nonseminomatous germ cell tumors of the testis: Multivariate analysis of a prospective multicenter study. *Journal of Clinical Oncology, 8,* 509-518.

Lange, P. H. & Fraley, E. E. (1977). Serum alpha-fetoprotein and human chorionic gonadotropin in the treatment of patients with testicular tumors. *Urological Clinics of North America, 4,* 393-406.

Landis, S. H., Murray, T., Bolden, S., & Wingo (1998). Cancer statistics, 1998. *CA: A Cancer Journal For Clinicians, 48*(1), 6-29.

Lind, J., Kravitz, K., & Greig, B. (1993). Urologic and male genital malignancies. In S. L. Groenwald, M. H. Frogge, M. Goodman, & C. H. Yarbro (Eds.), *Cancer nursing: Principles and practice* (3rd ed.). Boston: Jones & Bartlett.

Loehrer, P. J., Einhorn, L. H., & Elson, P. (1993). Phase III study of ciplatin plus etoposide with either bleomycin or ifosfamide in advanced stage germ cell tumors: An Intergroup trial [Abstract]. *Proceedings from the American Society of Clinical Oncology, 12,* 261.

Loehrer, P., Johnson, D., Elson, P., Kinhorn, L. H., & Trump, D. (1995). Importance of bleomycin in favorable prognosis disseminated germ cell tumors: An Eastern Cooperative Oncology Group trial. *Journal of Clinical Oncology, 13,* 470-476.

Maher, E. R. (1994). Genetics of urological cancers. *British Medical Bulletin, 50,* 698-707.

Martini, F. H. (1995). *Fundamentals of anatomy and physiology.* Englewood Cliffs, New Jersey: Prentice Hall.

McLeod, D. G., Heidenreich, A., Moul, J. W., (1996). Do cell proliferation markers better predict pathological stage in clinical stage I nonseminomas than quantitative histology? [Abstract]. *Journal of Urology, 155,* 547A.

Mertens, W. C. & Taylor, M. J. (1995). Salvage therapy with ifosfamide, cisplatin and vinblastine or etoposide for germ cell carcinoma patients initially treated with PEB: A tumor marker analysis [Abstract]. *Proceeding from American Society of Clinical Oncology, 14,* 248.

Messing, E. M. (1987). Tumor antigens in the diagnosis, staging, and prognosis of urologic cancer. In R. D. Williams (Ed.), *Advances in urologic oncology*: Vol. 1. New York: MacMillan.

Moller, H. (1993). Clues to the aetiology of testicular germ cell tumours from descriptive epidemiology. *European Urology, 23,* 8-15.

Motzer, R. J. (1995). Adjuvant chemotherapy for patients with stage II nonseminomatous testis cancer. *Seminars in Oncology, 22*(6), 641-646.

Motzer, R. J., Bajorin, D. F., Bosl, G. J. (1992). "Poor-risk" germ cell tumors: Current progress and future directions. *Seminars in Oncology, 19,* 206-214.

Motzer, R. J., Cooper, K., Geller, N. L., Bajorin, D. F., Dmitrovsky, E., Herr, H. Morse, M., Fair, W., Sogani, P., & Russo, P. (1990). The role of ifosfamide plus ciplatin based chemotherapy as salvage therapy for patients with refractory germ cell tumors. *Cancer, 66,* 2476-2481.

Motzer, R. J., Sheinfeld, J., Mazumdar, M., Bajorin, D. F., Bosl, G. H., Herr, H., Lyn, P., & Vlamis, V. (1995). Etoposide and ciplatin adjuvant therapy for patients with pathologic stage II germ cell tumors. *Journal of Clinical Oncology, 13*(11), 2700-2704.

Moul, J. W. & Heidenreich, A. (1996). Prognostic factors in low-stage nonseminomatous testicular cancer. *Oncology, 10*(9), 1359-1374.

Nichols, C., Breeden, E., Loehrer, P., Williams, S., & Einhorn, L. H. (1993). Secondary leukemia associated with a conventional dose of etoposide: Review of serial germ cell tumor protocols. *Journal of National Cancer Institute, 85,* 36-40.

Nichols, C. R., Gonin, R., & Foster, R. (1995). Defining new standards for adjuvant therapy of testis cancer. *Journal of Clinical Oncology, 13*(11), 2681-2683.

Nichols, C. R., Loehrer, P. J., Einhorn, L. H., et al. (1995). Phase III study of cisplatin, etoposide and bleomycin or etoposide, ifosfamide and cisplatin in advanced stage germ cell tumors [Abstract]. *Proceedings from the American Society of Clinical Oncology, 14,* 239.

Nichols, E. R., Ruth, B. J., Williams, S. O., Gill, I., Muggia, F. M., Stablein, D. M., Weiss, R. B., & Einhorn, L. H. (1992). No evidence of acute cardiovascular complications of chemotherapy for testicular cancer: An analysis of the Testicular Cancer Intergroup Study. *Journal of Clinical Oncology, 10,* 760-765.

Pizzocaro, G., Salvioni, R., Piva, L., Faustini, M., Nicolai, N., & Gianni, L. (1992). Modified cisplatin, etoposide (or vinblastine) and ifosfamide salvage therapy for male germ-cell tumors. Long term results. *Annals of Oncology, 3,* 211-216.

Pizzocaro, G., Salvioni, R., & Sperandio, P. (1993). Cisplatin, low-dose vinblastine, bleomycin with salvage cisplatin, etoposide, ifosfamide versus cisplatin, etoposide, bleomycin with salvage cisplatin, vinblastine, ifosfamide in good prognosis metastatic germ-cell testicular tumors [Abstract]. *Proceedings from American Society of Clinical Oncology, 12,* 232.

Pont, J., Albrecht, W., Postner, G., Sellner, F., Angel, K., & Holtl, W. (1996) Adjuvant chemotherapy for high-risk clinical stage I nonseminomatous testicular germ cell cancer: Long-term results of a prospective trial. *Journal of Clinical Oncology, 14*(2), 441-448.

Presti, J. C. & Herr, H. W. (1992). Genital tumors. In E. A. Tanagho, & J. W. McAninch (Eds.), *Smith's general urology* (13th ed.). Norwalk, CT: Appleton, Lange.

Read, G., Stenning, S. P., Cullen, M. H., Parkinson, M. C., Horwich, A., Kaye, S. B., & Cook, P. A. (1992). Medical Research Council prospective study of surveillance for stage I testicular teratoma. *Journal of Clinical Oncology, 10,* 1762-1768.

Reno, D. R. (1988). Men's knowledge and health beliefs about testicular cancer and testicular self-examination. *Cancer Nursing, 15,* 9-15.

Richie, J. P. (1990). Clinical stage I testicular cancer: The role of modified retroperitoneal lymphadenectomy. *Journal of Urology, 144,* 1160-1163.

Roth, B. J. (1996). The role of ifosfamide in the treatment of testicular and urothelial malignancies. *Seminars in Oncology, 23*(3 suppl 7), 19-27.

Roth, B. J., Nichols, C. R., & Einhorn, L. H. (1993). Neoplasms of the testis. In J. F. Holland (Ed.), *Cancer medicine.* Philadelphia: Lea & Febiger.

Saxman, S. (1992). Salvage therapy in testicular cancer: A new and improved model. *Journal of Clinical Oncology, 8,* 1777-1781.

Skinner, D. G. & Lieskovsky, G. (1988). Management of early stage nonseminomatous germ cell tumors of testis. In D. Skinner, & G. Lieskovsky (Eds.). *Diagnosis and management of genitourinary cancer.* Philadelphia: W. B. Saunders.

Small, E. J. & Torti, F. M. (1995). Testes. In M. D. Abeloff, J. O. Armitage, A. S. Lichter, & J. E. Niederhuber (Eds.), *Clinical oncology.* New York: Churchill Livingstone.

Smith, R. B. (1988). Testicular seminoma. In D. Skinner, & G. Lieskovsky (Eds.), *Diagnosis and management of genitourinary cancer.* Philadelphia: W. B. Saunders.

Stephenson, W. T., Shelly, M., Rubin L., & Einhorn, L. H. (1995). Evaluation of reproductive capacity in germ cell tumor patients following treatment with cisplatin, etoposide, and bleomycin. *Journal of Clinical Oncology, 13*(9), 2278-2280.

Stoter, G., Sleijfer, D. T., & Schornagael, J. H. (1993). BEP versus VIP in intermediate risk patients with disseminated nonseminomatous testicular cancer [Abstract]. *Proceeding from the American Society of Clinical Oncology, 12,* 232.

Thibodeau, G. A. (1996). *Anthony's textbook of anatomy and physiology,* (15th ed). St. Louis: Mosby.

Tominaga, O., Hamelin, R., Remvikos, Y., Salmon, R. J., & Thomas, G. (1992). p53 from basic research to clinical applications. *Critical Reviews in Oncogenesis, 3,* 257-282.

Tyrell, E. D. & Mettler, M. J. (1976). The response of lymph nodes metastases of testicular teratoma to radiation therapy. *British Journal of Urology, 48,* 363-370.

Vugrin, D., Whitmore, W., Cvitkovic, E., Grabstald, H., Sogani, P., & Golbey, R. B. (1981). Adjuvant chemotherapy with VAB-3 of stage II-B testicular cancer. *Cancer, 48,* 233-237.

Vugrin, D., Whitmore, W. F., Herr, H. W., Sogani, P., & Golbey, R. B. (1983). VAB-6 combination chemotherapy in resected stage II-B testis cancer, *Cancer, 51,* 5-8.

Williams, S. D. (1994). Testis. In J. F. Foley, J. M. Vose, & J. O. Armitage (Eds.), *Current therapy in cancer.* Philadelphia: W. B. Saunders.

Williams, S. D., Birch, R., Einhorn, L. H., Irwin, L., Greco, F. A., & Loehrer, P. J. (1987). Treatment of disseminated germ cell tumors with cisplatin, bleomycin, and either vinblastine or etoposide. *New England Journal of Medicine, 316,* 1435-1440.

Woodman, R. J. (1971). Effects of combination treatment with CIS-PT(II) and other agents on survival of mice with leukemia L1210 [Abstract]. *Proceedings of American Association of Cancer Research, 12,* 24.

Pediatric Cancers

Deborah B. Crom, RN, PhD
Theresa Bredereck Boggs, PAC, MHS
Belinda N. Mandrell, RN, CPNP, MSN
Robbie Norville, RN, MSN, CPON, OCN

INTRODUCTION

Each year, approximately 10,000 of the 3 million children and adolescents in the United States are diagnosed with cancer (Miller, Young, & Novakovic, 1995). Aggressive multimodality therapy comprising surgery, chemotherapy, and/or radiotherapy cures most patients with childhood cancers. From 1973 to 1988, the overall mortality rate associated with childhood cancers decreased by more than 38% (Ries, Hankey, Miller, Hartman, & Edwards, 1991). Because of this remarkable improvement in survival, it is estimated that 1 of every 900 young adults in the year 2000 will be a survivor of childhood cancer (Meadows & Hobbie, 1986).

Despite dramatic increases in survival rates, cancer remains the third leading cause of death (after accidents and diseases of infancy) among persons younger than 15 years, accounting for 2200 deaths annually (Parker, Tong, Bolden, & Wingo, 1996). However, mortality rates fail to adequately characterize the consequences of childhood cancer. Because of the early onset of these diseases, pediatric and adolescent cancer patients have more years of life at risk than do adults with cancer, in whom the median age at diagnosis is 67 years. Despite recent advances in therapy, more than 100,000 person-years of life are lost each year among children who die of cancer (Bleyer, 1993).

EPIDEMIOLOGY

Definition

The exact age that defines childhood cancer is controversial. The American Cancer Society's Department of Epidemiology and Statistics considers childhood cancers as those occurring in persons younger than 15 years (Parker et al., 1996). However, the National Cancer Institute's Surveillance, Epidemiology, and End Results (SEER) analysis also includes data from patients 15 through 19 years of age. Pediatric and adolescent cancers account for 2% of the cancers diagnosed among residents of the United States (Robison, Mertens, & Neglia, 1991).

Differences Between Childhood and Adult Cancers

The differences between childhood and adult cancers are dramatic and diverse. Compared with its incidence in adults, cancer occurs rarely during childhood. The primary sites, clinical presentation, histology, stage at diagnosis, and response to and outcome of therapy also differ between adult and pediatric cancers (Table 70-1) (Fernbach & Vietti, 1991). Unlike adult forms of cancer, most childhood malignancies are disseminated at the time of diagnosis, and few screening tests are available. Also, in contrast to its presentation in adults, cancers occur more frequently among Caucasian than African-American children; this bias is especially prevalent among patients 0 through 5 years of age (Gurney, Severson, Davis, & Robison, 1995). Carcinomas are rare in patients younger than 15 years of age but account for almost 90% of adult cancers.

Perhaps the most dramatic characteristic of childhood cancers is their response to and outcome of therapy. Overall, about 75% of children treated for cancer are alive 5 years after diagnosis, and many of these survivors live much longer. In contrast, only 50% of adult cancer patients are alive 5 years after diagnosis. Survival rates are poorest among children diagnosed with acute nonlymphocytic leukemia (23%) and best among those treated for retinoblastoma (98%) (Miller, Young, & Novakovic, 1995).

Age, Gender, and Racial Distribution

Fig. 70-1 illustrates the marked diversity in the age distribution of pediatric cancers (Ries, Miller, Hankey, Kosary, Harras, & Edwards, 1994). The incidence of acute leukemia, brain tumors, retinoblastoma, neuroblastoma, and

TABLE 70-1 Differences Between Pediatric and Adult Cancers

	Pediatric Cancer	Adult Cancer
Histology	Sarcomas common (mesodermal/ectodermal origin)	Carcinomas common (epithelial origin)
Primary sites	Involves tissues (blood, lymphatics, central nervous system, muscle, bone)	Involves organs (lung, colon, uterus, breast, prostate)
Stage at diagnosis	80% are disseminated	Only local, regional spread
Response	Responsive to multimodality therapy	Poorly responsive to treatment
Survival rate	>75% 5-year survival	<50% 5-year survival

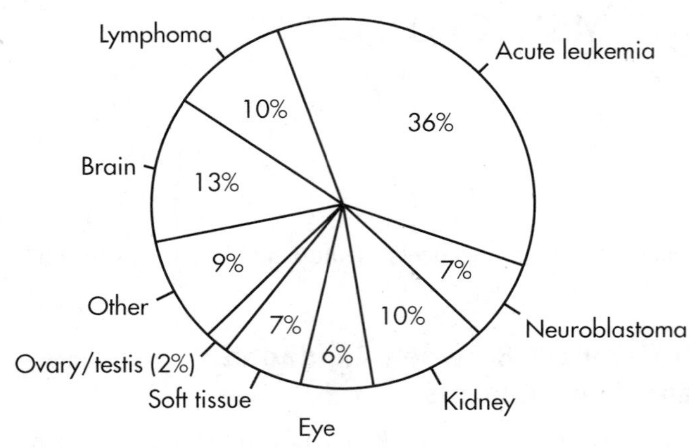

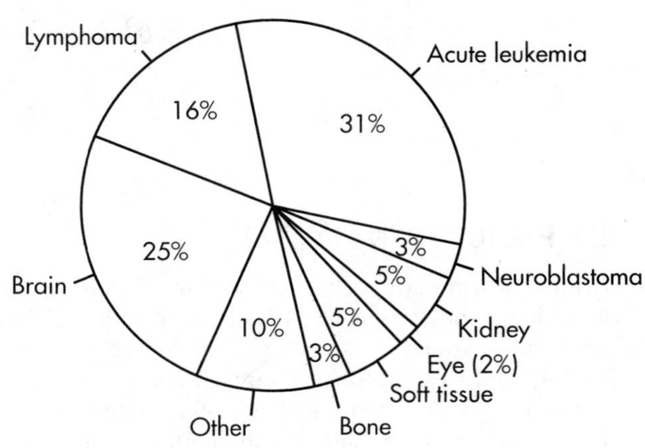

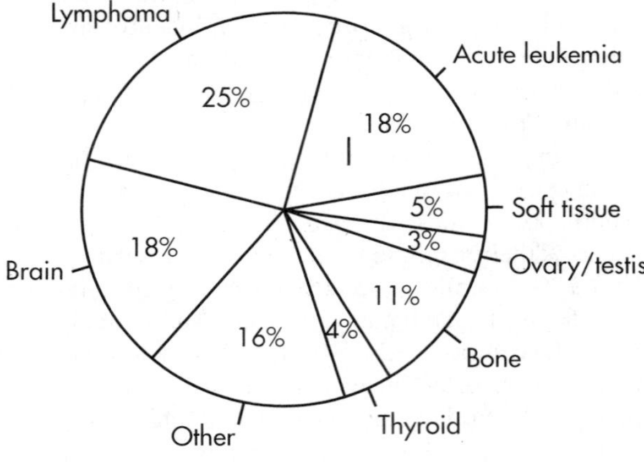

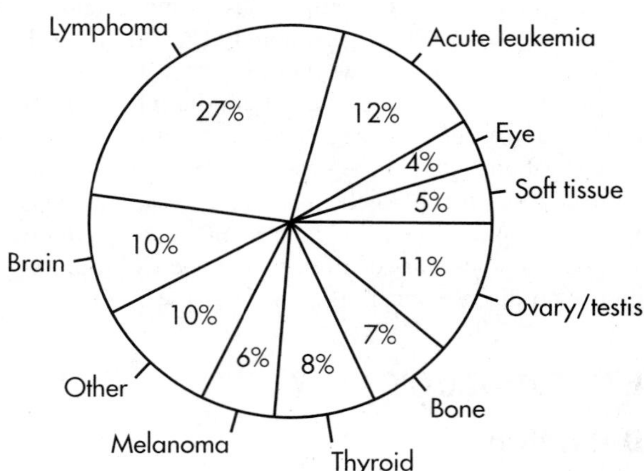

Fig. 70-1 Percentage of primary tumors by site of origin for different age groups.

Wilms' tumor peaks in children younger than 5 years. In contrast, the incidence of lymphomas, bone sarcomas, and ovarian and testicular malignancies generally increases with the age of the patient.

The ratio of male-to-female patients with childhood cancer also varies by age and diagnosis. The overall gender ratio in childhood cancers for boys versus girls is 1 : 1.3. However, according to the 1974-1989 SEER data, the number of cases of retinoblastoma, Wilms' tumor, or osteosarcoma among girls equaled or exceeded that among boys (Miller, Young, & Novakovic, 1995).

Overall survival is better for female patients with childhood cancers than for male patients, but the mechanism of this gender disparity is unknown. Purtilo and Sullivan (1979) suggested that genetic differences in immune function may suppress B cell lymphoproliferative diseases in females, ultimately influencing survival.

In addition to the age- and gender-associated biases among childhood cancers, race influences their incidence. The overall likelihood of cancer is 29% higher among Caucasian children, who are more frequently diagnosed with hematopoietic neoplasms (including acute lymphocytic leukemia, non–Hodgkin's lymphoma, and Hodgkin's disease) than are children of other races. Gurney and colleagues (1995) estimated that the incidence rate of Ewing sarcoma is 11 times higher among Caucasians. In addition, racial differences may be specific to certain geographic areas. For example, the incidence of Burkitt's lymphoma is highest among African children (Magrath, 1991), and tumors of the central nervous system are most frequently seen in Caucasian children from the United States.

Changing Incidence

According to the most recent data from SEER, the overall incidence of cancer increased by 4% from 1972 to 1988 among children younger than 15 years of age in the United States. In this age group, the cases accounting for this increase were distributed equally among males and females, and there was no racial bias. However, cases among children younger than 5 years excessively contributed to this increased incidence. Bleyer (1993) attributed this escalation to an increased incidence in the three most common cancers of childhood: acute lymphoblastic leukemia, central nervous system tumors, and non–Hodgkin's lymphoma. The incidence of central nervous system (CNS) tumors changed most dramatically, showing an increase of 30% between 1972 and 1988.

Despite the increased incidence of childhood cancer from 1972 to 1988, associated mortality rates plummeted 38%. This decline is similarly prominent among boys and girls of all races. Overall survival after pediatric cancer has significantly improved as well, and the following factors have contributed to this improvement. Advances in molecular biology have facilitated the identification of favorable prognostic factors, thereby enabling individualized tailoring of therapy based on the extent of disease. Improvements in diagnostic technology, such as those in magnetic resonance imaging (MRI), have led to more accurate staging and more appropriate therapy. The use of high-energy radiation, which is less toxic and more effective than its conventional counterpart, has limited the morbidity and mortality associated with aggressive multimodality regimens. Finally, enhanced supportive care, including the use of cytokines and better nutritional support, have helped improve the outlook for pediatric cancer patients (Levi, LaVecchia, Lucchini, Negri, & Boyle, 1995).

RISK FACTORS FOR CHILDHOOD CANCERS

Historically, the risk factors associated with the development of childhood cancer have been assigned to one of two broad categories. Intrinsic (host) factors arise because of the child's genetic makeup, whereas extrinsic factors are found in the environment. However, regarding these types of risk factors as mutually exclusive fails to acknowledge that pediatric cancer most likely results from the complex interaction of diverse environmental factors with various genetic states.

Intrinsic risk factors include inherited genetic conditions. Some genetic conditions are not neoplastic in and of themselves but are associated with an increased risk of childhood cancer. For example, children with Down syndrome have a fifteen-fold increased risk of developing leukemia. Also, children with Beckwith-Wiedemann or Drash syndrome are more likely to develop Wilms' tumor (Miller, Fraumeni, & Manning, 1964). A striking example of the association between genetics and childhood cancer is familial (heritable) retinoblastoma. The familial pattern of inheritance is a Mendelian autosomal dominant trait with almost complete (80% to 100%) penetrance. The family history of these patients, who usually have bilateral disease at about 7 months of age, is almost invariably positive for retinoblastoma (Grundy, Wilson, Telzerow, Zhou, & Paterson, 1994).

Other intrinsic factors, such as birth characteristics, have been implicated in the development of childhood cancer. Several studies have suggested a link between acute lymphocytic leukemia and a maternal history of fetal loss or increased birth weight and Wilms' tumor. The influence of advanced paternal age on the development of childhood brain tumors or retinoblastoma has not been conclusively established (Stiller, 1991).

Another risk factor is the development of cancer in siblings, which approximately doubles the likelihood of childhood malignancies (Draper, Sanders, Lennox, & Brownbill, 1996). The cause of this increased risk is thought to be genetic, but common environmental exposures cannot be ruled out (Mulvihill, 1993). Li and Fraumeni (1969) first described a familial neoplastic syndrome in which multiple cases of various cancers were observed among family members. The original report focused on children with rhabdomyosarcoma and correlated the occurrence of sarcomas and carcinomas among many members of their families.

The latency and toxicity of environmental carcinogenic agents vary. However, because most childhood cancers are diagnosed in young children (i.e., during the first decade of life), the potential effect of environmental exposure to most of these agents is likely to be minimal. Perhaps the most notable environmental carcinogen is diethylstilbestrol, which was used during the 1930s to treat diabetes and spontaneous abortion in pregnant women. Transplacental exposure resulted in an increased incidence of vaginal adenocarcinoma in the 1960s among the daughters of these women (Melnick, Cole, Anderson, & Herbst, 1987).

The influence of several other environmental carcinogens on the development of childhood cancer has been proven. The use of anabolic androgenic steroids by adolescents increases their incidence of hepatocellular carcinoma, and asbestos has been implicated as a cause of mesothelioma. Infection by Epstein-Barr virus is an important etiologic factor in Burkitt's lymphoma (Robison, Mertens, & Neglia, 1991). The effects of dietary factors such as an increased intake of nitrosamine or artificial sweeteners, as well as the influence of obesity, are less well established, as are those of exposure to or ingestion of fertilizers or pesticides and exposure to electromagnetic radiation (Heath, 1996).

Exposure to ionizing radiation is a well-documented environmental risk factor for childhood cancer. For example, an unusually high incidence of childhood leukemia was demonstrated 3 to 10 years after the atomic explosions in Hiroshima (Beebe, 1979). The carcinogenic potential of prenatal radiation is uncertain. Stewart, Webb, Giles, and Hewitt (1956) first suggested an association between the exposure of a mother to diagnostic radiation late in pregnancy and the development of childhood cancer by the exposed children. However, subsequent investigations have not conclusively confirmed their hypothesis. In addition, radiation received in utero or later during childhood may not result in neoplasms until adulthood. Radiation carcinogenesis in children varies with the age at exposure and the site and type of exposure.

One event that illustrates the complex interplay of genetic predisposition and environmental exposure to known carcinogens is the development of a second malignancy in survivors of pediatric cancer. Both chemotherapy and radiation therapy have marked carcinogenic potential. Children who survive cancer have a twenty-fold increased risk of developing a second cancer. These data suggest a probable genetic origin of neoplasms in childhood. However, many survivors of childhood malignancies were treated with multimodality therapy, which may iatrogenically induce second malignancies (Hudson, Hancock, & Pui, 1994; Li, Myers, Heise, & Jaffee, 1978).

Although rare, childhood cancer has a significant effect because of its early onset. Many intrinsic and extrinsic factors influence the observed incidence patterns. The relative importance of these factors will be reviewed as the various forms of childhood cancer are presented.

PEDIATRIC BRAIN TUMORS

Even though brain tumors account for 20% of all malignancies diagnosed in children younger than 15 years of age, they are rare malignancies, occurring in 2 to 3 children per 100,000. Although this incidence does not represent a major public health threat, the diagnosis of a brain tumor in children exacts a devastating emotional and financial toll on patients and their families. Any health care provider in the field of pediatrics should have a general understanding of the scope of this disease and its challenges.

Pediatric brain cancers, which differ greatly from CNS tumors in adults, comprise a heterogeneous spectrum of tumor types. The limited number of pediatric patients with a specific tumor type can hamper efforts to accrue reliable data regarding etiology and treatment; this goal requires large, cooperative, multicenter studies. However, fewer than half of the children with CNS cancers are referred to tertiary care centers that conduct such studies. In addition, pediatric brain tumors often go undetected until late in their development because many patients initially have symptoms that mimic other more common pediatric illnesses. Most pediatricians see only one or two patients with pediatric brain tumors during their career. Therefore, this disease is low on their list of differential diagnoses. Finally, it remains a particular challenge to develop aggressive therapies that spare the immature CNS from excessive toxic effects. Overall cure rates for pediatric brain tumors have improved modestly since 1970 because of advances in diagnosis and management, as well as an increased understanding of the biology and genetics of these malignancies (Albright, 1993; Mueller & Gurney, 1992; Shiminski-Maher & Shields, 1995).

Epidemiology of Pediatric Brain Tumors

Brain tumors are the second most common pediatric malignancy (after leukemias) and are the most frequent solid tumor of childhood. Epidemiologic patterns suggest that they differ from adult brain tumors in etiology and biologic behavior. Peak incidence occurs during the school-age years (between ages 5 and 9 years); most of these tumors are of embryonal origin (i.e., medulloblastoma and primitive neuroectodermal tumor [PNET]). The overall incidence of pediatric brain tumors is slightly increased in males and Caucasians. Incidence rates have been stable to slightly increased (particularly in children younger than 5 years) over the last several decades. The overall survival rate associated with childhood brain tumors is 50% to 55%, although this figure varies with individual factors (Gurney, Davis, Severson, Fang, Ross, & Robison, 1996; Heideman, Packer, Albright, Freeman, & Rorke, 1997; Leviton, 1994; Mueller & Gurney, 1992) (Fig. 70-2).

Risk Factors for Pediatric Brain Tumors

Several factors, summarized below, are linked repeatedly with a higher risk for the development of pediatric brain tumors (Boice, 1996; Bondy, Wiencke, Wrensch, & Kyritsis, 1994; Gonzales, 1995; Mueller & Gurney, 1992).

Heredity. Of all of the children diagnosed with brain tumors, 15% have a family history that is positive for cancer. Familial clusters of colon, breast, brain, lung, and hematologic cancers (Li-Fraumeni syndrome) have been tied to a mutation in the tumor suppressor gene p53, and the po-

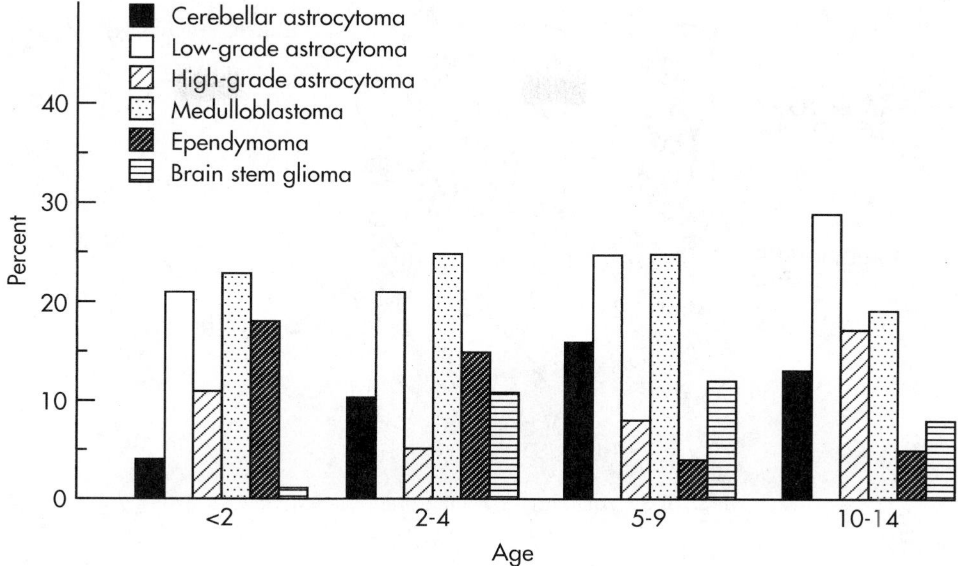

Fig. 70-2 Brain tumor type distribution by age: SEER Registries, 1973-1990.

tential association of this gene with pediatric brain tumors is actively being studied. Children with hereditary neurocutaneous syndromes (phakomatoses), including neurofibromatosis, Von Hippel–Lindau disease, basal cell nevus syndrome (Gorlin syndrome), and tuberous sclerosis, are at risk for brain tumors. Case reports have associated congenital conditions such as anomalies of the genitourinary or gastrointestinal systems, arteriovenous malformations, and Down syndrome (trisomy 21) with an increased potential for developing tumors of the CNS.

Radiation. Exposure to radiation (whether in utero or postnatally) has consistently been implicated in the development of brain tumors. At one time, childhood tinea capitis was treated with low-dose radiation to the scalp, and those patients had an increased incidence of brain tumors. In addition, treatment of other childhood malignancies with CNS radiation (e.g., for CNS prophylaxis of leukemia) increases the risk of subsequent brain tumors. The timing of the exposure and the type of brain tumor induced varies with the dose of radiation received.

Environmental Factors. Both in utero and childhood exposure to environmental and chemical factors seem to influence the development of pediatric brain tumors. In particular, nitrosamines and nitrosamides, which are widespread in the diet, drinking water, passive cigarette smoke, and rubber products found in developed societies are potent carcinogens in laboratory animals. Maternal use of barbiturates during pregnancy may increase the likelihood of brain tumors in her children. Exposure to various viruses during the prenatal and perinatal periods has been associated with increased risk of developing CNS tumors. One example is that of mothers who received polio vaccines that were contaminated with the virus SV-40. Finally, head trauma during early childhood may predispose children to the development of brain tumors.

Much public attention has focused on the potential association between exposures to electromagnetic fields (EMFs) and the development of cancer. Exposure to low-level electric fields may alter deoxyribonucleic acid (DNA) synthesis and transcription, thereby stimulating tumorigenesis. Although children who lived close to electric power lines (within 40 feet) showed an increased risk of brain tumors, this association has not yet been substantiated and continues to be the subject of debate.

Pathophysiology of Pediatric Brain Tumors

Neuroanatomy and Physiology. The CNS develops from the embryologic neural tube and neural crest. Early developing cells migrate and differentiate within these structures to give rise to specific regions: the forebrain, midbrain, hindbrain, and spinal cord. Further differentiation of these progenitor cells leads to precise characteristics that dedicate the cell to architectural or functional duties. The microstructure of the developed brain is composed primarily of two major cell types: glial cells and neurons. Glial cells provide nutritive and supportive functions and include oligodendroglia, astrocytes, ependyma, and Schwann cells. The neurons actually convey the nerve impulse.

The macrostructure of the CNS can be divided into four components: the cerebrum (the telencephalon); the midline, which includes the thalamus and hypothalamus (the diencephalon); the posterior fossa, housing the brain stem and cerebellum; and the spinal cord. The cerebrospinal fluid (CSF), which is made by the choroid plexus in the ventricular system, circulates throughout this closed system. The meninges, a triple-layered membrane covering the outer surface of the CNS, protects the brain and spinal cord and maintains the integrity of the CSF pathways (Fig. 70-3). The cerebrum and the midline structures are separated from the

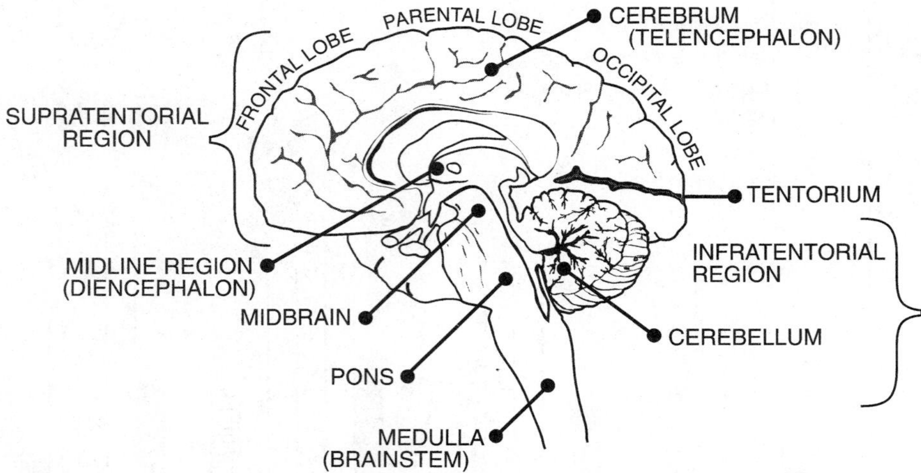

Fig. 70-3 Anatomy of mature brain, sagital view.

posterior fossa by a tough fibrous membrane called the *tentorium*. Structures above this membrane are supratentorial in location; structures below are infratentorial.

The cerebrum itself is made up of two halves, or hemispheres, each of which consists of four lobes: frontal, parietal, temporal, and occipital. Each of these lobes controls specific functions of the opposite side of the body. The frontal lobe is responsible for personality, higher mental functions such as thought processes, and voluntary motor movement. The parietal lobe processes sensation and provides spatial abilities such as depth perception and judging distances. The temporal lobes are the locations for the speech and hearing centers, as well as the centers for behavior and emotion. The occipital lobes are involved in visual perception.

The midline structures (the thalamus, hypothalamus, pineal body, and surrounding structures) regulate involuntary motor movements, metabolism, hormone production, and memory. The cerebellum controls balance and coordination. The brain stem regulates vital functions such as respiration, heart rate, and blood pressure; the cranial nerves originate here as well. The CSF delivers nutrients to the brain and spinal cord and acts as a cushion and shock absorber. In light of the diverse functions of the various components of the CNS, it is easy to appreciate that the signs and symptoms manifested by a particular brain tumor would reflect its location.

Carcinogenesis. The complex process of carcinogenesis results (at least in part) from genetic alterations that abolish normal controls on cell division and differentiation, thereby leading to anaplasia, or disordered and unregulated cell growth. These genetic alterations can involve mutations, rearrangements, or deletions of DNA segments. The gene most often implicated in the development of cancer is the tumor suppressor gene p53, which is located on chromosome 17p. Mutations in this gene subsequently impair its growth-inhibitory capacity. These mutations can be random, inherited, or induced by environmental factors. The potential influence of p53 mutants on the development of pediatric brain tumors (particularly astrocytomas and medulloblastomas) is currently under investigation. Other genes may play a role in the development of pediatric brain tumors. Many of the genetic alterations and processes characteristic of pediatric brain tumors differ from those associated with adult CNS malignancies.

Cellular anaplasia leads to neoplastic growth and malignancy. Progenitor (blast) cells may arrest in a primitive embryologic stage and become neoplastic. Medulloblastomas and PNETs arise through this mechanism. In contrast, anaplastic changes in mature cells lead to neoplasms that resemble the differentiated cell type. Astrocytomas, oligodendrogliomas, and ependymomas are examples of these types of tumors (Agamanolis & Malone, 1995; Bondy et al., 1994; Bronstein, 1995; Cogen & McDonald 1996; Mangiardi, 1995; Moore, 1995).

Classification, Grading, and Staging of Pediatric Brain Tumors

Classification Schema. Developing a logical system for categorizing pediatric brain tumors is complicated by their relative rarity, the diversity in their biologic characteristics, and the limitations in tissue sampling. Current classification systems are descriptive and focus on the histopathologic appearance of the tumor or its anatomic location. The comprehensive classification scheme from the World Health Organization (WHO) recognizes nine categories of brain tumors that are based on the identifiable cell or tissue of origin (Box 70-1). Other systems categorize tumors as embryonal (manifested by disordered embryogenesis) or glial (mutated mature cells). Often, brain tumors are grouped by location (supratentorial, infratentorial, and midline) because clinical course, prognosis, and treatment are intimately correlated with the anatomic function of the area involved (Albright, 1993; Gonzales, 1995; Heffner, 1994; Shiminski-Maher & Shields, 1995).

Box 70-1
World Health Organization Classification of Central Nervous System Tumors

I. Tumors of neuroepithelial tissue
  A. Astrocytic tumor
  B. Oligodendroglial tumor
  C. Ependymal tumor
  D. Mixed glioma
  E. Choroid plexus tumor
  F. Neuroepithelial tumor of uncertain origin
  G. Neuronal and mixed neuronal-glial tumor
  H. Pineal tumor
  I. Embryonal tumor
II. Tumors of cranial and spinal nerves
  A. Schwannoma (synonyms: neurilemmoma, neurinoma)
  B. Neurofibroma
  C. Malignant peripheral nerve sheath tumor (MPNST; synonyms: neurogenic sarcoma, anaplastic neurofibroma, malignant schwannoma)
III. Tumors of the meninges
  A. Tumor of meningothelial cells
  B. Mesenchymal, nonmeningothelial tumors
  C. Primary melanocytic lesions
  D. Tumor of uncertain origin
IV. Hemopoietic neoplasms
V. Germ cell tumors
VI. Cysts and tumorlike lesions
VII. Tumors of the anterior pituitary
VIII. Local extensions from regional tumors
IX. Metastatic tumors

Grading of Pediatric Brain Tumors. Describing the aggressiveness (i.e., malignancy) of a tumor is the purpose of grading systems, with the goal of predicting biologic behavior on the basis of microscopic features. The microscopic appearance of tissue is graded according to four main characteristics: (1) cellular pleomorphism (number and heterogeneity of cells); (2) nuclear atypia (abnormal nuclear morphology); (3) increased mitotic activity (correlates with rapid cellular growth and division); and (4) the presence of areas of necrosis. Many pathologists also believe that endothelial proliferation in a tumor is indicative of malignancy.

This grading system pertains almost exclusively to the astrocytomas, and the grade of a tumor increases with its aggressiveness. Examples of low-grade tumors are pilocystic astrocytomas and oligodendrogliomas. High-grade tumors include anaplastic astrocytomas and glioblastoma multiforme. A tumor may have areas of mixed characteristics, and a relatively low-grade tumor may further degenerate and become more malignant. Because of these properties, a tumor is identified according to its most malignant component, and this assignment influences prognosis and treatment. The results of laboratory assays, such as flow cytometry (which assesses the DNA content of tumor cells) and a determination of the mitotic index with Ki-67 labeling, add information to that gained through microscopic evaluation (Bronstein, 1995; Lanzkowski, 1995; Thapar, Fukuyma, & Rutka, 1995).

Table 70-2 Chang Staging System for Posterior Fossa Medulloblastoma

Stage	Definition
Primary Tumor	
T_1	Tumor less than 3 cm in diameter and limited to the midline position in the vermis, the roof of the fourth ventricle, and (less frequently) to the cerebellar hemispheres.
T_2	Tumor more than 3 cm in diameter that invades one adjacent structure or partially fills the fourth ventricle.
T_3	
T_{3a}	Tumor invading two adjacent structures or completely filling the fourth ventricle with extension into the aqueduct of Sylvius, foramen of Magendie, or foramen of Luschka, thus producing marked internal hydrocephalus.
T_{3b}	Tumor arising from the floor of the fourth ventricle or brain stem and filling the fourth ventricle.
T_4	Tumor further spreading through the aqueduct of Sylvius to involve the third ventricle or midbrain, or tumor extending to the upper cervical cord.
Metastases	
M_0	No gross evidence of subarachnoid or hematogenous metastasis.
M_1	Microscopic tumor cells found in cerebrospinal fluid.
M_2	Gross nodule seedings demonstrated in the cerebellar cerebral subarachnoid space or in the third or lateral ventricles.
M_3	Gross nodule seedings in the spinal subarachnoid space.
M_4	Extra neuraxial metastasis.

Staging of Pediatric Brain Tumors. Tumor staging is a clinical summary of the extent of disease (i.e., tumor size, extent of local spread, and sites of metastases) that aids in predicting outcomes and planning therapy. Staging of brain tumors incorporates observations obtained during surgery and results from diagnostic tests, including magnetic resonance imaging (MRI), computed tomography (CT), and CSF cytology studies. Currently, medulloblastoma is the only pediatric brain tumor that is formally staged because it is the tumor most often associated with distant metastasis. The Chang staging system shown in Table 70-2 is the most widely used system (Albright, 1993; Cohen & Duffner, 1994).

The concept of malignant versus benign becomes moot in the context of brain tumors that grow in an unforgiving, confined space (the skull) and impinge on vital structures. Even a histologically benign tumor can be malignant in effect by virtue of its location; a slow-growing tumor in the

TABLE 70-3 Assessment of the Pediatric Patient for a Suspected CNS Tumor

	Assessment Parameters	Typical Abnormal Findings
History	A. History of past illness 1. Onset, duration, progression, and pattern of current neurologic symptoms	A. Symptoms are progressive and include headache, morning emesis, mental status changes, unilateral weakness, imbalance, and seizures.
	B. Developmental and psychosocial history 1. Growth and development, feeding habits, and academic performance	B. Infants often show a delay or a loss of developmental milestones and failure to thrive. Older children often exhibit a decline in school performance.
	C. Risk factors 1. Past medical history and family history	C. Positive family history, congenital or hereditary conditions, or exposure to radiation may increase risk.
Neurologic Examination	A. Mental status 1. Is child alert and oriented? Observe ability to respond to and follow directions.	A. The child may exhibit lethargy, unresponsiveness, or confusion.
	B. Cranial nerves 1. Assess pupillary reaction to light and ability to visually follow objects; ask child to shut eyes tightly, wrinkle forehead, smile, puff out cheeks, and protrude tongue. 2. Test gag reflex. 3. Note quality of voice and speech.	B. Cranial nerves 3, 6, and 7 are most commonly impaired by posterior fossa tumors. Signs include loss of pupillary reflex, impaired ocular movements, deviated gaze, and unilateral facial paralysis. Loss of gag reflex, tongue deviation, hoarseness, or thick slurred speech may indicate additional cranial nerve involvement. Papilledema is often observed in the presence of increased intracranial pressure.
	C. Motor function 1. Ask child to squeeze your fingers, push palms and soles of feet against your hands, and push away pressure you exert against his arms and legs. 2. Place all joints through range of motion. 3. Note deep tendon reflexes at antecubital spaces, knees, and ankles.	C. Supratentorial tumors may produce signs of hemiparesis, extremity contractures, and increased deep tendon reflexes. Spinal cord tumors may produce flaccid paralysis and decreased deep tendon reflexes.

surgically inaccessible brainstem may affect morbidity and mortality much more than does a high-grade tumor in the temporal lobe. Therefore efforts to characterize brain tumors as benign or malignant must weigh both histopathologic appearance and anatomic location (Bronstein, 1995).

Patterns of Metastasis of Pediatric Brain Tumors

With few exceptions, pediatric brain tumors are unlikely to disseminate outside the CNS. However, spread of tumor in the neural axis is common and can occur by many routes. Direct extension into surrounding tissue is the most frequent pattern, either by infiltrating brain parenchyma or by displacing adjacent structures. Seeding of tumor occurs throughout the subarachnoid space through transport in the CSF; tumor cells can deposit anywhere along the spinal cord or noncontiguous surfaces of the brain. Rarely, tumors can metastasize to the abdomen through ventriculoperitoneal (VP) shunts (a special catheter that has been placed to relieve intracranial pressure by rerouting the CSF).

Systemic metastasis of pediatric brain tumors is rare and generally associated with medulloblastoma. Approximately 15% to 20% of patients with medulloblastoma develop metastases, which occur primarily in the bone and bone marrow. On average, this metastasis occurs about 2 years after the initial diagnosis and is usually accompanied by a CNS recurrence. In addition, ependymomas, glioblastomas, astrocytomas, pineoblastomas, and choroid plexus tumors can disseminate beyond the neuraxis (Cohen & Duffner, 1994).

Assessment of the Patient for a Pediatric Brain Tumor

Table 70-3 summarizes the clinical and diagnostic assessment of the pediatric patient with a suspected CNS tumor. In general, patients have the classic triad of symptoms associated with increased intracranial pressure (ICP): headache, vomiting, and behavioral changes. Further signs and symptoms reflect the specific location of the tumor and its rate of growth and include seizures and focal neurologic deficits. Infants most often have irritability, failure to thrive, and in-

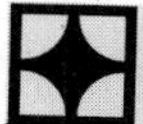

TABLE 70-3 Assessment of the Pediatric Patient for a Suspected CNS Tumor—cont'd

	Assessment Parameters	Typical Abnormal Findings
Neurologic Examination—cont'd	D. Sensory function 1. Distribution of sensation to light touch and pinprick.	D. There may be a segmental loss of sensation or increased paresthesias with a spinal cord tumor.
	E. Coordination/gait 1. Perform finger-to-nose test. 2. Ask child to walk across the room and to hop, skip, or walk heel-to-toe. 3. Romberg test: Ask child to stand still with feet together and eyes closed.	E. There may be a segmental loss of sensation or increased paresthesias with a spinal cord tumor.
Diagnostic Tests	A. Magnetic resonance imaging (MRI)	A. Either a discreet enhancing lesion or diffuse change in signal intensity on MRI may indicate the presence of a neoplasm.
	B. Computed tomography (CT)	B. On CT, a discreet enhancing lesion, areas of calcification, diffuse changes in signal intensity, and enlarged ventricles all indicate abnormalities.
	C. MRI spectroscopy and positron emission tomography (PET)	C. Increased or decreased metabolic activity, measured by either the ratio of chemical elements or the level of glucose, may aid in differentiating normal tissue from abnormal tissue.
	D. MRI angiography	D. Areas of narrowing or constricted blood flow may indicate vessel compression or infiltration by tumor.
	E. Cerebrospinal fluid (CSF) 1. Cell count, chemistries, and pathology, with CSF hormonal markers, if indicated.	E. Increased numbers of white blood cells may indicate infection, whereas increased protein may indicate the presence of tumor. Pathology will demonstrate the presence of tumor cells. β-human chorionic gonadotropin (β-HCG) and alpha fetaprotein (AFP) are increased in a germ cell tumor.
	F. Blood tests 1. Serum hormonal markers, if indicated.	F. Serum β-HCG and AFP may be increased in the presence of a germ cell tumor.
	G. Bone scan	G. Areas of increased uptake may indicate metastatic bony disease.
	H. Bone marrow biopsy	H. The presence of tumor cells indicates metastatic bone marrow disease.

creased head circumference with a bulging fontanelle. Overall, the most characteristic clinical feature of intracranial neoplasms is progressive neurologic dysfunction. When assessing the patient who has neurologic symptoms, the pattern of findings in the history and physical examination is important to the localization of the lesion and the characterization of its biologic behavior (Albright, 1993; Shapiro & Shapiro, 1992; Weiner & Levitt, 1994).

History and Physical Examination. For children with suspected brain tumors, the history of present illness needs to include the onset, duration, progression, temporal pattern, and relieving or exacerbating factors of all complaints. The nurse should be especially persistent in clarifying patterns of headache, emesis, visual disturbances, unilateral extremity weakness, and any other signs and symptoms. Regarding the past medical history, the nurse should obtain information about the patient's gestational and birth history, growth and development, feeding history, and school performance. General questions about all areas of neurologic function are used to screen for the review of systems; where positive, the nurse should further characterize the complaints by performing a focused neurologic examination (Bates, 1991; Engel, 1993).

The focused neurologic examination encompasses five functional categories (Bates, 1991; Goldberg, 1988):

1. Mental Status—The patient's level of consciousness and awareness of his or her surroundings, as well as his or her attention, concentration, and memory, are assessed by evaluating responses to simple and complex commands.
2. Cranial Nerves—The cranial nerves are assessed, and both patterns and symmetry of deficits are noted.
3. Motor—The innervation of major muscle groups is evaluated for signs of asymmetric weakness and/or asymmetric reflexes, thereby providing important clues to the location of a lesion.
4. Sensory—Patterns of paresthesias or anesthesia and altered responses to light touch, pain (pinprick), and heat and cold illuminate the segmental distribution of deficits.
5. Coordination and Gait—The focus here is on the patient's spatial awareness and balance, which can be

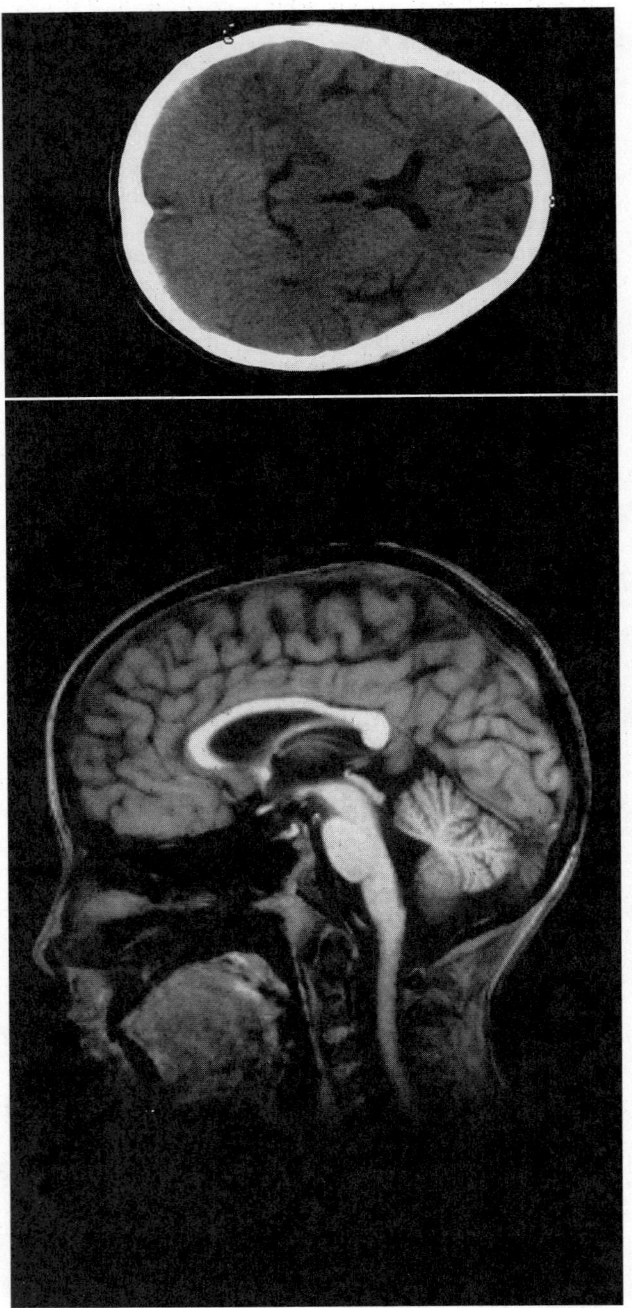

Fig. 70-4 Magnetic resonance imaging of a normal brain.

measured by observing the symmetry and smoothness of maneuvers such as touching the finger to the nose, rapid alternating hand and finger movements, gait, tandem walking, and the Romberg test.

Diagnostic Tests. Several imaging and laboratory studies support the histopathologic diagnosis of a brain tumor and provide staging information. MRI with gadolinium enhancement is the most sensitive method for imaging a brain tumor (especially those occurring in the posterior fossa) and is particularly useful in demonstrating leptomeningeal disease. This modality has virtually replaced myelography in the detection of spinal cord involvement. Advantages of MRI include superior definition of anatomic structures, the elimination of potential risks of radiation (MRI uses high frequency radio waves as its energy source), and the provision of information in three dimensions (Fig. 70-4).

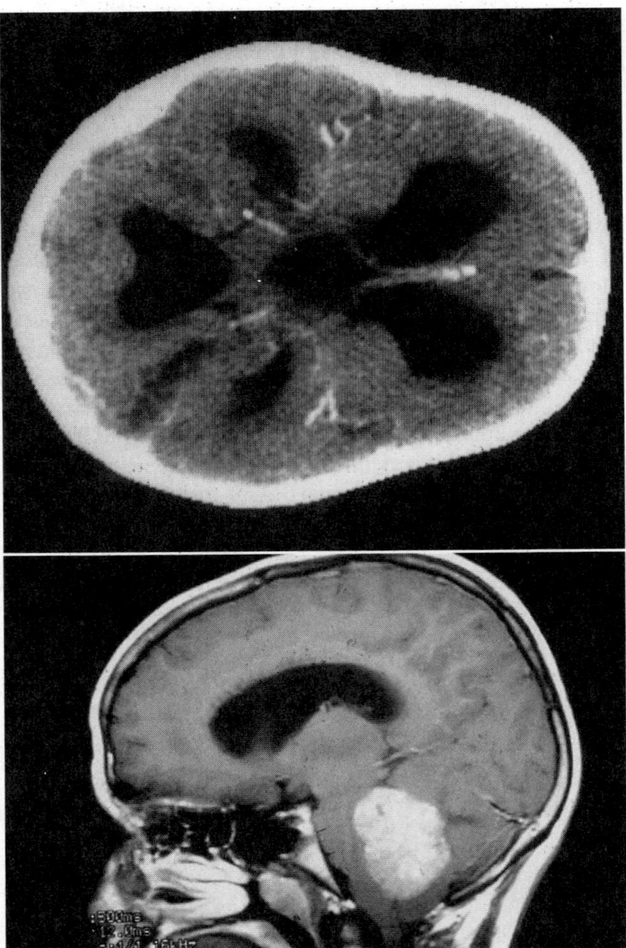

Fig. 70-5 Computed tomography images of a normal brain.

CT is a rapid and accurate study that is especially useful in demonstrating calcified areas in the tumor, the extent of cerebral edema, and ventricular enlargement. Because of its relatively short imaging time, CT is the study of choice for evaluating unstable patients (Fig. 70-5). Magnetic resonance spectroscopy and positron emission tomography (PET) measure the rates of metabolism in various tissues and may aid in differentiating viable tumor from necrotic tumor or normal brain. Magnetic resonance angiography is a noninvasive technique that assesses the distribution of intracranial vessels, that may be compromised due to tumor compression or treatment. To reduce artifacts caused by motion, young patients usually need to be sedated for most imaging studies (Albright, 1993; Kun, 1994; Shiminski-Maher & Shields, 1995; Weiner & Levitt, 1994).

Cerebrospinal fluid can be collected from the lumbar cistern (at the L4-L5 interspace, located at the level of the iliac crest) or VP shunt (if present). The CSF is evaluated for total cell count and differential, protein and glucose levels, and cytology for any tumor cells. Lumbar puncture should not be performed without first verifying the presence of a mass lesion or increased pressure, and it should never be attempted when papilledema is present. If a germ cell tumor is suspected, serum and CSF levels of hormonal markers such as β-human chorionic gonadotropin (β-HCG) and α-fetoprotein (AFP) should be obtained. Additional studies (e.g., bone scan and evaluation of bone marrow aspirates) are completed if the suspected tumor is one that is likely to metastasize systemically.

Principles of Therapy for Pediatric Brain Tumors

The goal of all brain tumor therapy is to reduce the tumor burden to the point that further growth can be suppressed by host immunity. Although very small tumors (because of their location) can lead to clinical signs (e.g., seizures), most lesions are fairly large (30 to 60 g) before they cause overt symptoms. Therefore multimodal therapy regimens offer the best chance of survival (Shapiro & Shapiro, 1992).

Surgery. Complete resection is the treatment of choice for pediatric brain tumors that are discreet and surgically accessible. Other goals of surgical intervention include histopathologic confirmation of the diagnosis, reduction in the volume of the tumor (making it more susceptible to radiation and chemotherapy), and palliation by relieving symptoms caused by increased pressure. Although natural factors will always place practical limits on the extent of surgery, technologic advances are improving the accessibility to previously inaccessible tumors and reducing postoperative sequelae (Mamelak & Edwards, 1994; Shapiro & Shapiro, 1994).

Surgical techniques vary from open biopsy and resection to the more conservative stereotaxic surgery, which is accomplished with the aid of a computer to localize deep tumors. When a tumor involves critical areas such as the speech centers or motor strip, cortical mapping techniques enable the surgeon to avoid damage to these functional areas. One such mapping technique uses intraoperative neurophysiologic monitoring of functional brain tissue; another superimposes (through the surgical microscope) functional MRI or PET scans on the operative field. Continued refinement of surgical techniques leads to the safe resection of tumor from critical or previously inaccessible areas while reducing the risk of damage to adjacent tissues (Chapman, Buchbinder, Cosgrave, & Jiang, 1995; Mamelak & Edwards, 1994).

Potentially necessitating postoperative support through tracheostomy or gastrostomy, surgical sequelae are site-specific and include hemorrhage, hemiplegia, and damage to vital cranial nerves. In particular, aggressive posterior fossa surgery (for medulloblastoma or ependymoma in particular) may cause speech disturbances, cranial nerve dysfunction, and emotional lability. This constellation of postoperative sequelae is termed *posterior fossa syndrome.* Typically these symptoms are manifested 24 hours or more after waking from surgery. However, the syndrome is self-limiting, and symptoms resolve within weeks to months. Attempts to define the underlying cause of this syndrome are as yet inconclusive (Al-Jarallah, Cook, Gascon, Kannan, & Sigueira, 1994; Kirk, Howard, & Scott, 1995; van Dongen, Catsman-Berrevoets, & van Mourik, 1994).

Radiation Therapy. Because it provides additional focal therapy, radiation therapy is a powerful adjunct to surgical intervention. Ionizing radiation kills cells by producing electrons and free radicals that cause breaks in one or both strands of DNA. The level of damage depends on the presence of oxygen (the electron carrier) in the tumor system. Transfusions of packed red blood cells are often given during a prolonged course of therapy because most radiotherapists request that a patient's hemoglobin level be maintained at 10 g/dL or higher to ensure adequate tissue oxygenation.

Conventional external beam radiation (EBR) is given as single daily fractions over 4 to 6 weeks to a defined total dose. In some settings, equivalent or higher total doses of radiation can be delivered with fewer side effects by giving multiple daily (hyperfractionated) doses. The volume treated includes the tumor or operative bed and a surrounding, well-defined margin. In the case of pediatric brain tumors that can spread or disseminate, the whole brain and/or the entire neural axis is treated. The total dose delivered depends on the tolerance of the treated organ, the specific disease, and the treatment goals. In the CNS, because the spine is more radiosensitive than the cerebral hemispheres, total doses to the spine are generally higher than those to the brain. Furthermore, astrocytic and glial tumors are more radioresistant than embryonal tumors (i.e., medulloblastoma and PNET). Therefore the total dose administered and the volume of tissue treated differ between these tumor types.

In addition to conventional EBR, several new delivery techniques offer unique advantages. Three-dimensional conformal techniques use a fixed, multiplanar delivery of radiation, creating a treatment field that closely conforms in shape to the volume to be treated and that spares irradiation of the surrounding normal tissue. Stereotactic radiosurgery and stereotactic radiotherapy use a computer-guided system to focus multiple noncoplanar radiation beams, which are generated by a dedicated machine (e.g., the gamma knife or linear accelerator), on a specific target (Lew & LaVally, 1995). This approach effectively concentrates a maximum amount of radiation to a precisely defined volume while reducing the overall exposure to normal tissue.

Stereotactic radiosurgery denotes a large, one-time radiation dose, whereas stereotactic radiotherapy is given through multiple treatments. These techniques are useful for small, discreet lesions that are centrally located and thus inoperable, as well as for lesions adjacent to critical areas. Another new technique is brachytherapy, the direct interstitial implantation of radioactive seeds (usually I-125) into the tumor volume. This modality is usually reserved for small tumors (<5 cm) in peripheral, easily accessible locations. All of these newer techniques have improved the safety and specificity of treatment and increase the options available for treating younger children (Dunbar, Tarbell,

Kooy, Alexander, Black, & Barnes et al., 1994; Fontanesi, Heideman, Muhlbauer, Mulhern, Sanford, & Douglass et al., 1995; Kun, 1994; Rabb & Apuzzo, 1995; Shapiro & Shapiro, 1992).

These radiation therapy modalities are used either alone, in combination with each other, or in combination with other therapeutic modalities to maximize initial disease management and to treat recurrences. How radiotherapy is used is contingent on the type of tumor, the age of the patient, and the volume of brain or spinal cord that needs to be treated. The accurate delivery of irradiation depends on precise field planning and immobilization of the patient. Elaborate stabilization devices such as molds and head frames are necessary, and often young children require sedation (Dunbar et al., 1994; Saleman, 1995).

Sequelae of radiation treatment are categorized as acute, subacute, and delayed. Acute side effects occur during or immediately after the course of therapy and include fatigue, nausea, vomiting, anorexia, alopecia, and skin changes in the treated field. Subacute toxicity usually develops 6 to 8 weeks after completion of therapy and is primarily manifested as a somnolence syndrome, a self-limiting period of malaise and anorexia.

Delayed consequences occur more than 12 months after therapy and can include neuropsychological impairment, hearing loss, a seizure disorder, endocrine dysfunction, and second malignancies. In addition, radiation necrosis with areas of increased cerebral edema can develop and may be symptomatic. On imaging, such sequelae often mimic recurrent or progressive disease. Studies such as magnetic resonance (MR) spectroscopy or PET scans may facilitate differentiation between delayed consequences and disease recurrence (Bakardjiev, Barnes, Goumnerova, Black, Scott, & Pomeroy et al., 1996; Dunbar et al., 1994; Freeman, Bourgouin, Sanford, Cohen, Friedman, & Kun, 1996; Moore, 1995). Every effort is made to delay the use of radiation therapy in very young children (4 to 5 years of age) to avoid adverse consequences in a developing central nervous system. Particular outcomes of radiation therapy during the early years include endocrine dysfunction (arrested growth and thyroid deficiency), limited cognitive capacity, dysplastic growth of the spine (if treated), and second malignancies.

Chemotherapy. The rationale for the use of chemotherapy to treat pediatric brain tumors is multifold. It allows the delay of radiation therapy to spare the developing brain in infants and very young children. Chemotherapy is a useful adjunct to other modalities, thereby maximizing tumoricidal efforts. It is often given either before radiation (neoadjuvant chemotherapy), to achieve tumor reduction and investigate new agents or drug combinations, or afterward (adjuvant chemotherapy) for an additive or consolidative treatment effect. When used in conjunction with radiation therapy, some chemotherapeutic agents act as radiosensitizers, increasing the efficacy of radiation. Finally, in some circumstances, chemotherapy provides systemic control of disease.

The blood-brain barrier has long been thought to impair the delivery of chemical agents to the CNS. Although the tight cellular junctions of CNS capillaries serve this function in the healthy brain, this barrier is disrupted in most tumor systems and therefore probably has only a minor role in the resistance of CNS tumors to chemotherapy. Intrathecal (IT) administration of chemotherapy is under active investigation because theoretically this route provides the most direct delivery of drugs to the CNS and in potentially higher concentrations than does intravascular delivery. However, because IT chemotherapy penetrates only a few millimeters, this technique is only applicable to tumors with meningeal or CSF spread and is unlikely to eradicate large or deep-seated tumors (Brecher, 1994).

Chemotherapeutic agents are designed to interrupt cellular replication at many different stages. Therefore they tend to be most effective when used in combination and against rapidly growing high-grade tumors. Recent reports suggest that chemotherapy may have a role in the treatment of low-grade tumors as well, both in achieving long-term disease stability and enabling the delay of radiation. Several classes of drugs have confirmed activity against pediatric brain tumors. These drugs include alkylating agents (cyclophosphamide, thiotepa, melphalan), platinum-based compounds (cisplatin, carboplatin), vinca alkaloids (vincristine), and topoisomerase inhibitors (etoposide). At present, the clinical utility of the nitrosoureas (CCNU, BCNU) remains uncertain (Castello, Schiavetti, Padula, Varrasso, Properzi, & Trasimeni et al., 1995; Gajjar, Heideman, Kovnar, Langston, Sanford, & Douglass et al., 1993).

Because all chemotherapy uses tumoricidal agents that poison any rapidly dividing cell, normal tissues that have high mitotic activity (e.g., epithelial mucous membranes, bone marrow, and hair follicles) are often damaged. Consequently, emesis, myelosuppression, and alopecia are commonly seen. The concurrent use of some chemotherapeutic agents and aggressive hydration may lead to increased ICP in the patient with a brain tumor, with the inherent potential for seizures or herniation (compression or displacement of vital brain tissue). Other acute and delayed side effects of the drugs used to treat pediatric brain tumors include peripheral neuropathies, hemorrhagic cystitis, syndrome of inappropriate antidiuretic hormone, nephrotoxicity, ototoxicity, and pulmonary fibrosis. Late development of myelodysplastic syndromes can also occur, although this is rare.

Description of Specific Brain Tumors

Supratentorial Tumors. As a group, the supratentorial tumors comprise about 35% of pediatric CNS neoplasms. These malignancies tend to be astrocytic/glial in histology. Roughly 80% of hemispheric glial tumors are low-grade astrocytomas. Low-grade (grade I and II) tumors typically present with a long history of site-dependent and often nonspecific symptoms. Surgical excision is the primary treatment, followed by surveillance alone if resection is complete. Depending on the patient's age, radiation and/or chemotherapy may be added if residual tumor remains.

The use of chemotherapy in the treatment of low-grade astrocytomas is still somewhat controversial. However, recent studies have demonstrated at least containment of disease if not objective diminution in tumor size. The biggest advantage of this modality may be the opportunity to delay radiation in young children. The survival rate is about 90% at 5 years among patients whose tumors are totally resected and may be as high as 60% for those with an incomplete resection. As always, tumor location and specific histology affect these survival rates (Castello et al., 1995; Gajjar et al., 1996; Heideman et al., 1997).

About 20% of astrocytomas are considered to be high grade or malignant (anaplastic astrocytoma and glioblastoma multiforme) and are some of the pediatric brain tumors with the poorest prognosis. At diagnosis, these infiltrative tumors have spread to the contralateral hemisphere in 25% of the cases. Depending on the area of involvement, patients typically have a short history of focal or nonspecific complaints. Surgery for maximal tumor reduction followed by high-volume irradiation is the preferred initial treatment. Children younger than 5 years of age receive reduced doses of limited-field radiation. In the last decade the addition of conventional chemotherapy has not significantly improved disease-free survival. A new investigational approach includes dose-intensive chemotherapy with autologous bone marrow or stem cell rescue. The efficacy of this approach remains uncertain (Heideman et al., 1997; Lanzkowski, 1995; Shiminski-Maher & Shields, 1995).

Midline Tumors. The common pediatric brain tumors of the midline include hypothalamic/optic chiasm glioma, pineal region tumors, and craniopharyngioma. Gliomas of the hypothalamus and optic chiasm and/or optic nerves account for 2% to 5% of CNS neoplasms in childhood and are associated with neurofibromatosis in 50% to 70% of the patients. Diagnosis is usually made by 5 years of age. The clinical presentation often includes precocious puberty (sudden growth spurt and onset of secondary sexual characteristics in a young child) and visual pathway disturbances. In addition, these patients may have signs and symptoms of increased ICP (due to obstructed outflow of CSF from the third ventricle) that can be alleviated by surgical placement of a VP shunt.

Aside from the possible debulking of a large hypothalamic/optic chiasm glioma, surgical resection is not an effective option due to the deep, central location and the potential for further compromise of vision. Biopsy by stereotactic methods may aid in establishing an accurate diagnosis. Because hypothalamic/optic chiasm gliomas are slow-growing tumors, patients are usually followed for signs of progression (clinical or imaging), at which time radiation therapy or chemotherapy is instituted. Survival is good and may be as high as 80% at 5 years. However, significant neurologic and neuroendocrine morbidity are not uncommon (Heideman et al., 1997; Wisoff, 1992).

Accounting for 3% to 8% of childhood brain tumors, those of the pineal region are derived from germ cell tissue or the pineal parenchyma. The peak incidence occurs during the teenage years and the male-to-female ratio is at least 4:1. Patients have the classic symptoms of impaired upward gaze and pupils that are nonreactive to light (Parinaud's syndrome). Hydrocephalus (due to compression of the Aqueduct of Sylvius) is commonly present. Because pineal tumors are of variable histology, surgery is required to establish the diagnosis, and it may be curative in the low-grade tumors. The higher-grade lesions are extremely radiosensitive and chemosensitive and are treated accordingly. Hormonal markers (e.g., AFP, β-HCG) in both serum and CSF are measured to identify a tumor of germ cell origin and are used in follow-up surveillance of the patient. Prognosis depends on tumor histology (Baumgartner & Edwards, 1992).

Craniopharyngiomas are usually thought to be congenital tumors that arise from embryonal squamous cells of the hypophyseal-pharyngeal duct. These tumors account for 6% to 9% of CNS tumors in children. The incidence of diagnosis peaks in 5- to 10-year-olds. Although benign and indolent by nature, craniopharyngiomas can impinge on critical structures, causing dramatic neuroendocrine dysfunction. These patients often have growth abnormalities, thyroid dysfunction, and diabetes insipidus.

Treatment of craniopharyngiomas consists of radical resection (which can leave the patient with severe endocrine deficits), modified resection followed by radiation therapy, or radiation therapy alone. The last two approaches yield similar results and are associated with less neuroendocrine and neuropsychological morbidity than radical resection. Chemotherapy does not have a role in the treatment of craniopharyngiomas. The associated long-term disease-free survival rate is 60% to 80% (Cohen & Duffner, 1994; Rutka, Hoffman, Drake, & Humphreys, 1992).

Infratentorial/Posterior Fossa Tumors. At least half of all pediatric brain tumors (including medulloblastoma, cerebellar astrocytoma, and brain stem glioma) occur in the posterior fossa. It is also the most common site for ependymoma, which can occur in any location. Derived from undifferentiated neuroepithelial embryonal tissue, medulloblastoma is the most common brain tumor among children, comprising nearly 20% of pediatric CNS tumors. Peak incidence occurs at 5 years of age and shows a slight male predominance. Many posterior fossa tumors have deletions in chromosome 17 that include but are not limited to the p53 gene. These genetic alterations remain an area of active research to elucidate potential etiologies and predict prognosis.

Infratentorial lesions typically arise in the cerebellar midline and may grow to fill the fourth ventricle. They often invade the brain stem and cerebellum and can disseminate throughout the neural axis through the CSF. Posterior fossa tumors are the pediatric brain neoplasms most frequently associated with systemic metastasis. Bone, bone marrow, lymph node, and lung involvement have been observed. The Chang staging system is used to denote the extent of the disease at the time of diagnosis. The typical clinical presentation is a short history (4 months or less) of symptoms of increased ICP (due to obstruction of the fourth ventricle), ataxia, and (often) cranial nerve dysfunction.

Surgery is the frontline therapy, and the extent of resection has important prognostic significance even though surgery alone is not curative. Infratentorial tumors are remarkably radiosensitive; beyond the tumor bed, the whole brain and spinal cord are treated prophylactically. Chemotherapy is used adjunctively and in an effort to delay radiation in infants and young children. Survival for patients with complete resection and limited disease is as high as 80% at 5 years but is closer to 40% for those with disseminated disease (Berger, Magrassi, & Geyer, 1995; Cogen & McDonald, 1996; Heideman et al., 1997).

Ependymomas arise from the ependymal cells that line the ventricular system. These lesions account for 5% to 10% of all primary childhood CNS tumors. Although most ependymomas develop in the fourth ventricle, they can also develop in the supratentorial region and spinal cord. More than half of all ependymomas are diagnosed in children younger than 5 years. A histologic grading system similar to that used with the astrocytomas is often applied to ependymomas, although its prognostic significance in this setting remains controversial. Clinical presentation is that of obstructive hydrocephalus. The initial management is surgical resection, the extent of which (as with medulloblastoma) is an important prognostic factor. Ependymomas are difficult to remove completely because they can encase the brain stem and wrap around the lower cranial nerves (VII through X). Postoperative sequelae are not uncommon and frequently require transient support with tracheostomy and gastrostomy feeding tubes. After surgery, additional therapeutic options are contingent on the age of the patient and grade of the tumor. These options include observation only and craniospinal irradiation with or without chemotherapy. The overall survival rate is 45% at 5 years (Albright, 1993; Bronstein, 1995; Chiu, Woo, Ater, Connelly, Bruner, & Maor et al., 1992).

Astrocytomas account for 10% to 20% of childhood CNS tumors, with the highest incidence occurring during the first decade of life. The pilocystic histologic variant is well-circumscribed and considered benign, whereas diffuse (or fibrillary) tumors are infiltrative and likely to undergo anaplastic degeneration. Neither histologic subtype is likely to exhibit neural axis dissemination. Clinical signs and symptoms include those of obstructive hydrocephalus and ataxia.

In the setting of pilocystic astrocytoma, surgical resection is often curative and can be achieved in nearly 90% of patients. When unresectable residual tumor remains, radiotherapy may be beneficial. Overall survival for pilocystic astrocytoma is as high as 90% at 10 years. In contrast, the fibrillary tumors are rarely resectable and are treated according to the same regimens used with their malignant supratentorial counterparts. Overall survival for fibrillary astrocytoma can approach 80% at 5 years (Albright, 1993; Lanzkowski, 1995; Shapiro & Shapiro, 1992).

Brain stem gliomas comprise 10% to 20% of pediatric brain tumors. The peak incidence occurs during the latter half of the first decade with an equal male-to-female ratio. Most of these infiltrative lesions arise intrinsically in the brain stem (usually in the pons) and may spread into the adjacent brain stem and diencephalon or distal into the cervical spinal cord. Most brain stem gliomas contain low-grade and high-grade features. At autopsy, 60% to 80% of these lesions demonstrate clear evidence of anaplasia, and nearly 50% are consistent with glioblastoma multiforme. The characteristic clinical presentation of brain stem glioma is the recent onset of ataxia, ipsilateral cranial neuropathies, and contralateral hemiparesis. Headache and behavioral changes may accompany these symptoms. However, frank hydrocephalus is uncommon. The diagnostic tool of choice is MRI.

Surgical management is not a viable treatment option for brain stem gliomas, although stereotaxic biopsy may play a role in establishing the histopathology in some cases. Focal radiation therapy is the principal treatment modality for most children. High total doses are associated with increased short-term survival and can be delivered by a hyperfractionated scheme. Chemotherapy may have a palliative benefit in some patients. However, more aggressive treatment with radiation and/or chemotherapy has not affected overall survival rates, which remain dismal. Most patients with brain stem gliomas die of their disease within 2 years of diagnosis (Cohen & Duffner, 1994; Freeman et al., 1996; Packer, Nicholson, Vezina, & Johnson, 1992).

Spinal Cord Tumors. Several tumor types can occur as primary intramedullary lesions of the spinal cord. Overall, these tumors account for approximately 10% of childhood CNS neoplasms. Spinal cord malignancies include astrocytomas, glioblastomas, and ependymomas, as well as developmental tumors such as teratomas and dermoid cysts. The insidious symptoms associated with these lesions most often include back pain and gait disturbances due to lower limb weakness. Sphincter disturbances, numbness, and torticollis may be present as well. Optimal treatment regimens for tumors in the spinal cord are not yet well-defined and remain largely dependent on the tumor biology, extent of the disease, and surgical accessibility (Steinbok, Cochrane, & Poskitt, 1992).

Miscellaneous Brain Tumors. Although they occur infrequently, choroid plexus tumors, oligodendrogliomas, and supratentorial PNETs deserve mention in this section on pediatric brain tumors. Choroid plexus tumors represent 2% to 3% of all brain tumors in children. About 10% to 20% of choroid plexus tumors are diagnosed before the patient is 1 year of age. These lesions arise in the ventricular system, with the lateral ventricles being the most common site. Two histologic types are identified: the slow-growing papilloma and the anaplastic carcinoma. Because these tumors tend to overproduce CSF, hydrocephalus and signs of increased ICP are the predominant symptoms. Surgery is the primary therapeutic intervention and has a critical effect on survival. Complete resection is possible in more than 75% of patients. Adjuvant chemotherapy may be beneficial. The value of radiotherapy remains unclear (Cohen & Duffner, 1994; Heideman et al., 1997; Packer et al., 1992).

Oligodendrogliomas derive from the oligodendrocyte and represent fewer than 1% of childhood CNS tumors. Although they can resemble astrocytomas, oligodendrogliomas can be differentiated on CT scan by the presence of calcifications. Both benign and malignant variants occur, which are graded similarly to the astrocytomas. Most oligodendrogliomas develop in the cerebral hemispheres, and seizures are the primary presenting problem. Treatment depends on tumor biology (Bronstein, 1995; Cohen & Duffner, 1994).

Primitive neuroectodermal tumors are undifferentiated lesions that histologically resemble medulloblastomas. The term *PNET* is reserved for supratentorial, hemispheric lesions. These malignancies constitute 2% to 3% of pediatric brain tumors and typically occur in children younger than 5 years of age. Clinically, PNETs are malignant, with a propensity to disseminate throughout the neural axis. Presentation can include hemiparesis, seizures, and signs of increased ICP. However, it is not uncommon for patients to be relatively asymptomatic, showing only nonspecific signs of behavioral changes. Surgical resection followed by cranial irradiation (with or without the inclusion of the neural axis) is the initial treatment of choice. The role of chemotherapy in the treatment of PNETs has not yet been established. The 5-year overall survival rate is only 20% (Berger, Magrassi, & Geyer, 1995; Heideman et al., 1997).

Overall Prognosis with Pediatric Brain Tumors

The prognosis for a pediatric patient with a brain tumor is highly individual and depends on the specific tumor histology, grade, and location. For the most part, the younger the age at diagnosis, the poorer the outcome. However, this correlation may be confounded by the treatment options available for young children. In addition, survival and extent of surgical resection generally parallel each other. Fig. 70-6 summarizes the overall survival rates associated with various pediatric tumors (Cohen & Duffner, 1994).

Oncologic Emergencies Associated with Pediatric Brain Tumors

Potential oncologic emergencies specific to the CNS include hydrocephalus, increased ICP (with the risk of herniation), seizures, and spinal cord compression. Hydrocephalus is the presence of increased amounts of CSF under elevated pressure and results from overproduction, underabsorption, or obstruction of the natural flow of CSF (due to malfunction of a shunt or mass effect). Subacute hydrocephalus is managed most often by the placement of a shunt system that reroutes the CSF out of the central nervous system. The shunt catheter is placed into the lateral ventricle through a burr hole in the skull and travels under the skin to terminate in either the peritoneal cavity, the pleural cavity, or the right atrium, where the CSF is reabsorbed (Fig. 70-7). Most shunt systems have a reservoir that enables the collection of CSF, the instillation of chemotherapeutic agents, and the assessment of shunt function.

Shunt systems can malfunction because of blockage (due to tumor burden or increased protein in the CSF) or infection. The sudden onset of headache, emesis, or lethargy in a previously well patient who has a shunt should alert the clinician to a potential shunt failure. The signs and symptoms of a shunt malfunction are listed in Table 70-4. Occasionally, hydrocephalus can be corrected by a procedure known as *third ventriculostomy,* in which an opening in the floor of the third ventricle is created surgically. As a result of this procedure, CSF drains directly into the subarachnoid space, where it is absorbed. Third ventriculostomy can obviate the need for an artificial shunt system (Ryan & Shiminski-Maher, 1995).

An acute increase in ICP is potentially fatal and is caused by a growing tumor, intracranial bleeding, or progressive hydrocephalus. The symptoms of increased ICP include headache, emesis, visual disturbances, and changes in mental status. Clinical findings are papilledema and cranial nerve palsies. If left unchecked, increased ICP can lead to herniation (in which brain tissue is compressed and displaced), brain stem compression, secondary vascular compromise, and death. Signs of impending herniation can include increasing unresponsiveness, incontinence, postur-

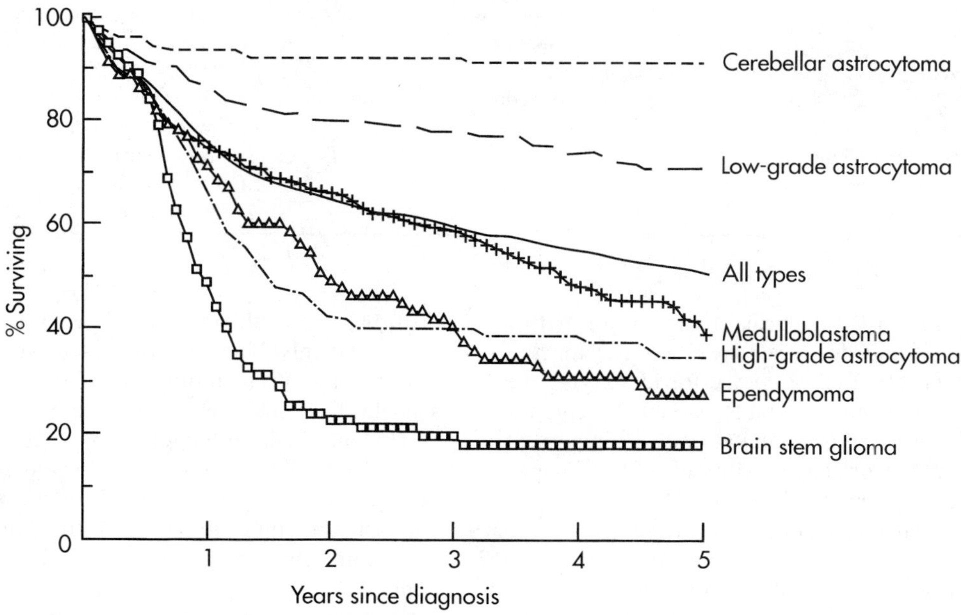

Fig. 70-6 Survival rates of children according to tumor type.

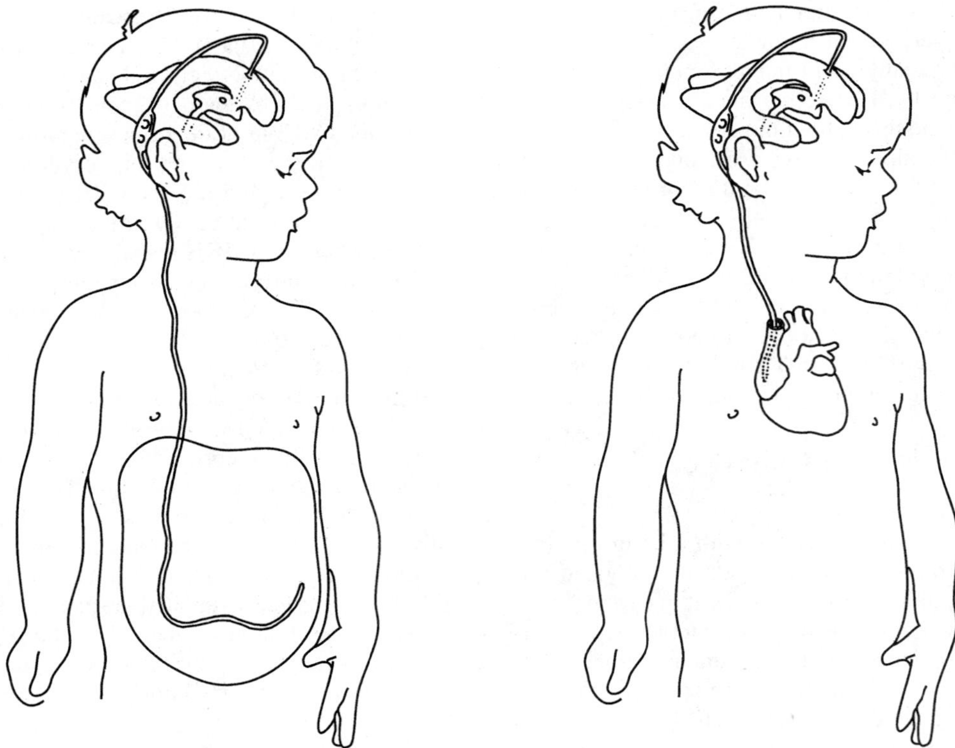

Fig. 70-7 Ventriculoperitoneal and ventriculoaortic shunt systems.

Table 70-4 The Signs and Symptoms of Shunt Malfunction

Infants	Toddlers	Children and Adults
Downward deviation of eyes Enlargement of baby's head Fever Fontanell is full and tense when infant is upright and quiet Irritability Prominent scalp veins Seizures Sleepiness Swelling or redness along shunt tract Vomiting	Fever Head enlargement Headache Irritability and/or sleepiness Loss of previous abilities (sensory or motor function) Seizures Swelling or redness along shunt tract Vomiting	Decline in academic performance Difficulty in waking up or staying awake Fever Headache Irritability and/or tiredness Loss of coordination or balance Personality change Seizures Swelling or redness along shunt tract (infrequent) Vision problems Vomiting

ing, and Cushing's triad (bradycardia, hypertension with a wide pulse pressure, and decreased respiration). Noncontrast CT is the diagnostic tool of choice for identifying the cause of increased ICP in an unstable patient. Emergency management includes steroids, mannitol diuresis, hyperventilation, and ventricular drainage (Albright, 1993; Thapar, Rutka, & Laws, 1995; Weiner & Levitt, 1994).

Symptomatic of an underlying etiology, seizures are a clinical manifestation of excessive neuronal discharge. They can manifest as episodes of disordered consciousness, tonic or clonic movements of the body, or sensory or behavioral disturbances. In the context of pediatric brain tumors, seizures may also indicate increased irritability of cortical brain tissue due to infiltration of or pressure from tumor, scarring from treatment, or pressure from hydrocephalus.

Uncontrolled, prolonged seizure activity (status epilepticus) can lead to hypoxia and hypercapnia. This medical emergency can eventually result in cardiovascular collapse and ischemic injury to the brain. In addition, the associated early compensatory rise in arterial blood pressure and concomitant increase in cerebral blood flow markedly increases intracranial pressure, which may persist as long as 20 minutes after seizure activity has ceased. Immediate intervention is necessary and consists of intravenous boluses of anticonvulsants or benzodiazepines, in addition to the routine emergency management of airway and perfusion (Brill, 1988; Hogan & Ryan, 1989).

Tumor-associated epidural compression and intramedullary expansion cause acute compression of the spinal cord. Favorable outcome of acute spinal compression depends on early intervention. The clinical manifestations include progressive symptoms of back pain with or without a radicular pattern, lower limb weakness, paresthesia, and sphincter disturbances. Diagnostic workup comprises careful neurologic examination and MRI to locate the level of the lesion. Management may include steroids, emergent radiotherapy, and surgical decompression (Weiner & Levitt, 1994).

LEUKEMIA

Leukemia is a malignant process of the bone marrow and lymphatic system that may affect any of the blood-producing cells of the bone marrow. Leukemia is now known to be a very heterogeneous disease with many different subsets. After the subset has been identified, therapy is tailored accordingly so that the focus of current therapy is to cure while minimizing toxicity in relation to disease risk.

Epidemiology of Childhood Leukemia

Acute lymphoblastic leukemia (ALL), also called *acute lymphocytic leukemia,* is the most common childhood cancer. In the United States, approximately 2000 children are diagnosed with ALL each year, and this figure represents 75% of all cases of childhood leukemia. Acute lymphoblastic leukemia occurs most commonly in Caucasian children 2 through 6 years of age, with a peak incidence at 4 years of age. There is no peak incidence in non-Caucasian patients. Acute lymphoblastic leukemia occurs more frequently in boys than girls, with a significant increase in pubertal male children (Poplack, 1993). Some explanations for this increase include improved detection and reporting, more frequent exposure to environmental factors, and the development of second malignancies among childhood cancer survivors.

The treatment of ALL is a success story of Pediatric Oncology, which is reiterated in a review of the St. Jude Children's Research Hospital experience from 1962 through 1988. The review found that in the 1960s, only 8% of the children with ALL were long-term survivors. Today, with intensification and use of multiple agents, the long-term event-free survival rate is 71% in newly diagnosed patients (Rivera, Pinkel, Simone, Hancock, & Crist, 1993).

Among children, acute myeloid leukemia (AML) is much less frequent than ALL. Approximately 500 cases of childhood AML are diagnosed in the United States each year, representing 15% to 20% of the cases of pediatric leukemia. The prevalence of AML exceeds that of ALL only during the first through the fourth weeks after birth. The incidence of AML is stable with a slight increase during adolescence, then plateaus again until the fifth decade, when another increase is seen. The frequency of AML is similar between Caucasian and non-Caucasian children and between the genders. However, girls are typically diagnosed at 5 years of age or younger, whereas males generally develop AML after they are 15 years of age (Poplack, Kun, Magrath, & Pizzo, 1993). Intensive therapy and supportive care lead to remission in approximately 85% to 90% of AML patients (Pui, 1996), but only 30% to 40% achieve long-term remission and cure (Pui, 1995).

Chronic myeloid leukemia (CML) has an occurrence rate of 100 cases per year in the United States, and its incidence is similar between Caucasian children and other ethnic groups. The median age at diagnosis of the juvenile form of CML is 2 years, whereas Philadelphia chromosome–positive [Ph-positive, demonstrating the t(9;22)] CML occurs in older children. Allogeneic bone marrow transplant is the only curative therapy for CML. Chronic lymphocytic leukemia (CLL), a leukemia seen frequently in adults, is rare in children (Pui, 1995).

Risk Factors for Childhood Leukemia

Several factors have been proposed to increase the risk of leukemia. The risk factors most frequently associated with leukemia are genetics, environmental exposure, viral infection, and immunodeficiency. Despite these proposed associations, predisposing risk factors cannot be identified for approximately 90% of children with leukemia (Pui, 1995).

Genetics play an important role in the development of leukemia in children. It is well documented that children with constitutional chromosomal defects have a higher incidence of leukemia. Children with Down syndrome (trisomy 21) are approximately 15 times more likely than the general population to develop leukemia (Poplack, 1993). Children with Down syndrome who are younger than 3 years of age most frequently develop the megakaryoblastic subset of AML, whereas ALL is more common in the older patient with Down syndrome.

Several other syndromes have been associated with the development of leukemia. Fanconi anemia, a constitutional aplasia, is frequently associated with the development of AML. Children with Bloom syndrome, a recessive chromosomal fragility disorder, may develop AML and less frequently, ALL. Patients with ataxia-telangiectasia, an abnormality affecting chromosomes 14 and 7, have a higher incidence of lymphoid malignancies such as ALL. Other syndromes associated with leukemia include Klinefelter syndrome, trisomy G syndrome, Rubinstein-Taybi syndrome, Schwachman syndrome, Poland syndrome, and neurofibromatosis (Poplack, 1993).

A genetic predisposition to leukemia has been observed among families. Siblings of children with leukemia are at a two- to four-fold greater risk of developing the disease. There is also a high rate of concordance for leukemia in identical twins, especially during the first year after birth; if one twin is affected, the other twin has a 25% chance of developing leukemia. This "twins risk" may result from a prepregnancy event, an intrauterine event, or metastases disseminated through the shared placenta (Pui, 1995). The twins risk decreases with age and, by the age of 7 years, is equal that of the general population (Poplack, 1993).

Environmental factors have long been implicated in the development of leukemia. One example is the rate of leukemia among those exposed to the atomic bomb during World War II. The incidence of leukemia among these people increased as their proximity to the explosion decreased (Poplack, 1993). Exposure to diagnostic radiation in utero during the first trimester has been suggested to increase the risk of leukemia. Even though the child's risk of developing leukemia remains low, a study by the National Academy of Science estimated the risk to be increased five-fold after diagnostic radiation (Poplack, 1993). Ionizing radiation in the emissions from nuclear power plants and the electromagnetic field around high-power lines may also contribute to development of leukemia.

Other environmental risk factors are exposure to various chemicals and viral infection. Benzene is associated with the development of AML, and chemotherapeutic treatments with alkylating agents and epipodophyllotoxins may lead to the development of secondary AML (Pui Behm, Raimondi, Dodge, George, & Rivera et al., 1989). Epstein-Barr virus (EBV) is well associated with the development of B-cell leukemia and lymphoma, and patients infected with the human T-cell lymphotropic virus type 1 (HTLV-1) are at risk of developing T cell hairy cell leukemia (Poplack et al., 1993).

Pathophysiology of Childhood Leukemia

The normal bone marrow supports the growth and differentiation of stem cells into mature, functioning blood cells, which enter the circulation as needed. Leukemia occurs when the hematologic progenitor cell (lymphoid, myeloid, or uncommitted) has arrested at a particular stage of development. If lymphocytic progenitor cells are affected, the child develops ALL. The two types of lymphocytic white blood cells are T cells, which provide cell-mediated immunity, and B cells, which form antibodies for humoral immunity.

If the myeloid progenitor cells are affected, the patient develops AML or CML. Acute myeloid leukemia may be a malignancy of the myelocyte (with or without differentiation), promyelocyte, myelocyte and monocyte, monocyte, erythrocyte, or megakaryocyte. Chronic myeloid leukemia in children occurs in two forms: Philadelphia chromosome-positive and juvenile. The Ph-positive form demonstrates granulocytic hyperplasia, eosinophilia, and basophilia, whereas juvenile CML occurs as myelomonocytic leukemia.

The malignant process of leukemia leads to phenotypes and genotypes that may have specific biologic characteristics. For this reason the immunophenotype, as well as the morphologic and cytochemical characteristics, of the leukemia must be established at the time of diagnosis. In addition, any chromosomal abnormalities of the leukemic cells should be identified because these may have prognostic importance (Pui, 1997).

Clinical Presentation of Childhood Leukemia

The symptomatic presentation of leukemia depends on the subset of leukemia and results from malignant replication of the specific blood cell. These malignant cells then compete for nutrients, resulting in hypermetabolism and starvation of normal cells (Fig. 70-8). After this malignant process begins, the child develops symptoms within weeks to months. The most common symptoms and physical findings at the time of diagnosis include anemia, thrombocytopenia, neutropenia, pallor, fatigue, anorexia, petechiae, bleeding, and infection.

At the time of diagnosis, the child with ALL typically has extramedullary disease, as well as infiltration of the bone marrow. Extramedullary spread of the disease outside the bone marrow may produce generalized or localized lymphadenopathy, hepatomegaly, splenomegaly, bone pain, bone fracture, parotid gland infiltration, and testicular infiltration. At the time of diagnosis, only a few boys have overt testicular involvement, although 25% have occult infiltration (Poplack, 1993). A mediastinal mass may be present and is associated with T cell disease.

The child with ALL may also have spread of the leukemia to the CNS system. Only 5% of patients with CNS leukemia have overt neurologic symptoms at the time of diagnosis of ALL. Leukemia of the CNS is thought to occur from seeding into the spinal fluid or from infiltration of cranial marrow. Symptoms of CNS leukemia include increased intracranial pressure, headaches, vomiting, lethargy, nuchal rigidity, and papilledema. Cranial nerve palsies at the time of diagnosis indicate CNS leukemia and typically involve the sixth or seventh cranial nerve (Poplack et al., 1993). Pronounced CNS events have been associated with hyperleukocytosis at the time of diagnosis.

For the child with AML, clinical presentation may be very similar to that of ALL. However, CNS involvement occurs more frequently in cases of AML, with 20% of patients having overt disease. In addition, coagulopathies are more frequent with AML, especially with cases of the M3 subset (Grier & Weinstein, 1993).

Assessment of the Patient for Childhood Leukemia

The child who may have leukemia should be transferred to an institution that treats childhood cancers, where a thorough history and physical examination should be completed (Table 70-5). The history should document the symptoms manifested and their duration. The most important symptoms to document are fever and infection. With this history the child may require immediate hospitalization for antibiotic therapy.

The physical examination should concentrate on the degree of lymphadenopathy and the focus of infection. The child's lymph nodes should be palpated for cervical, axillary, and inguinal adenopathy. The examiner should also perform complete neurologic and fundoscopic evaluations. Palpation of the abdomen should identify any hepatic, splenic, or renal enlargement and abdominal tenderness.

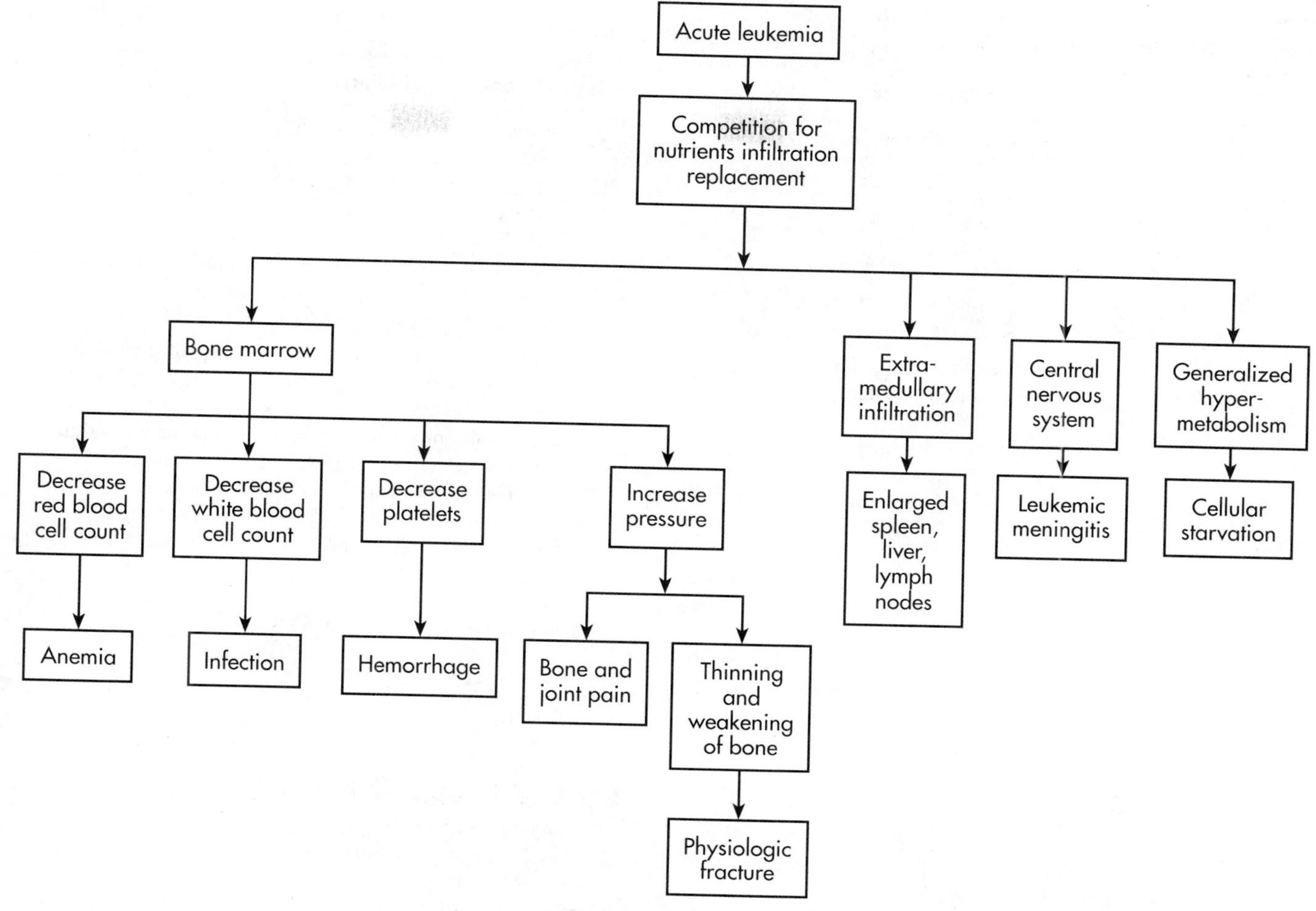

Fig. 70-8 The symptomatic presentation of leukemia.

Male children should have a careful testicular examination, and suspicion of testicular disease may require follow-up with ultrasonography of the testes. The most difficult diagnostic procedures to perform are bone marrow aspirations and lumbar punctures. Patient and parental anxiety is greatly relieved if the child is anesthetized for these procedures. If anesthesia cannot be administered, the child should receive intravenous or oral sedation and a local anesthetic.

Staging of Childhood Leukemia

For the purpose of diagnosing leukemia, samples of bone marrow and spinal fluid must be analyzed cytochemically and morphologically. Cytochemical staining is used to distinguish ALL from AML. The French-American-British (FAB) system is used to assign a case of ALL to one of three subsets (L1, L2, and L3) according to morphologic features. The L1 subset accounts for approximately 85% of the children with ALL. These lymphoblasts are small, with little cytoplasm. L2 lymphoblasts are larger, with abundant cytoplasm and prominent nuclei. Lymphoblasts of the L3 subset are identical to Burkitt lymphoma cells and represent B cell leukemia (Bennett, Catovsky, Daniel, Flandrin, Galton, & Gralnick et al., 1976). Although all cases of ALL are assigned to one of these subsets, this process has not affected the clinical management of ALL (Pui, 1995).

The immunophenotype is determined based on the reactivity of the leukemic cells to lineage-associated antibodies. The antigen expression then correlates with the type of lymphoid progenitor. Approximately 80% of ALL cases have the immunophenotype of early pre-B or pre-B disease. The transitional pre-B immunophenotype is thought to have a favorable prognosis. Further classification of pre-B leukemias reveals that 80% of these cases share a common leukemia associated antigen (CALLA), and expression of CALLA is a favorable feature (Poplack, 1993). About 1% to 2% of children with ALL have mature B cell disease and the T cell immunophenotype is identified in 15% of patients (Pui, 1995). Expression of lymphoid and myeloid antigens leads to the classification of mixed lineage leukemia, more specifically described as myeloid antigen–positive or lymphoid antigen–positive AML.

Analysis of the cytogenetic and molecular features of bone marrow cells establishes both the prognosis and treatment plan. Two important prognostic factors are ploidy and the DNA index. Ploidy is the number of chromosomes in the leukemia cells, whereas the DNA index is the ratio of the DNA content of the leukemia cells to that of normal cells.

TABLE 70-5 Assessment of the Pediatric Patient with Leukemia

	Assessment Parameters	Typical Abnormal Findings
History	A. Personal, family, and social history 1. Age 2. Ethnicity 3. Family history	A. Personal and social risk factors: 1. ALL—peaks at 4 years of age. Prognosis improved if age between 1 and 9 years. AML—incidence does not vary with age. 2. ALL—more prevalent in Caucasians. AML—equal prevalence in Caucasian versus non-Caucasian patients. 3. Increased risk if sibling has had leukemia.
Physical Examination	A. Examination with emphasis on lymphadenopathy, with testicular examination in boys	A. Generalized lymphadenopathy with hepatosplenomegaly; testicular enlargement indicative of infiltration is not common.
	B. Evaluation of associated symptoms	B. Anemia, thrombocytopenia, neutropenia, pallor, fatigue, anorexia, petechiae, bleeding, and/or infection.
	C. Evaluation for disseminated disease	C. Lymphadenopathy, splenomegaly, hepatomegaly, bone pain, bone fracture, parotid gland enlargement, testicular enlargement, cough, shortness of breath, headaches, vomiting.
	D. Examination to rule out clinical evidence of CNS leukemic involvement 1. Complete neurologic examination with emphasis on cranial nerves. 2. Complete funduscopic examination. 3. Rule out leukemia infiltrate, especially in patient with relapsed disease.	D. Abnormal findings on review of cranial nerves (unilateral weakness, other deficits).
Diagnostic Tests	A. Laboratory evaluation 1. Complete blood count 2. Chemistry panel 3. Coagulation 4. Chest x-ray examination 5. Lumbar puncture 6. Bone marrow aspiration	A. Typically, white blood cell (WBC) count is <10,000/cu mm at presentation. 1. Prognosis improved if WBC count <50,000/cu mm. Anemia. Thrombocytopenia. 2. ↑ Uric acid. ↑ AST, ALT, bilirubin with secondary liver involvement. ↑ LDH. ↑ or ↓ Ca. ↑ K. ↑ Phos. 3. Usually normal. Abnormal with AML (i.e., M3). 4. Mediastinal mass associated with T cell leukemia. 5. Few patients have overt leukemia in spinal fluid. 6. Leukemia infiltrate of bone marrow >25% blasts.

AST, aspartate aminotransferase; *ALT,* alanine aminotransferase; *LDH,* lactate dehydrogenase; *AML,* acute myelogenous leukemia.

One type of hyperdiploid leukemic cells has more than 50 chromosomes (DNA index = 1.16 to 1.6); another subset is characterized by leukemic cells that contain 47 to 50 chromosomes. Hyperdiploidy occurs in 30% of ALL cases and denotes a good prognosis. Approximately 42% of ALL patients have pseudodiploid (46 chromosomes) leukemia. Hypodiploidy (<46 chromosomes) is a poor prognostic feature and occurs in 7% of ALL cases in children (Trueworthy, Shuster, Look, Crist, Borowitz, & Carroll et al., 1992).

Because cytogenetic assays of ploidy and DNA index do not reveal the molecular defects of leukemia cases, molecular analyses are important (Pui & Crist, 1994). Occurring in 22% of the cases, the translocation TEL/AML1, found only through molecular analysis, is the most common abnormality in pediatric ALL. It also denotes an excellent prognosis (Shurtleff, Buijs, Behm, Rubnitz, Raimondi, & Hancock et al., 1995).

Morphologic and cytochemical analyses also play a role in the diagnosis of AML. The FAB system is used to classify cases of AML into morphologic subsets M0-M7 (Table 70-6). Immunophenotypic studies help to further diagnose morphologically undifferentiated AML cases, such as those in the M0 subset (Pui, 1995), and cytochemical and molecular studies then provide added prognostic information.

After the diagnostic analysis is completed, the patient is classified according to risk for relapse, and the appropriate therapy is prescribed. The uniform system of risk classification for B-lineage ALL is based on age and initial white

TABLE 70-6 The French-American-British (FAB) Classification of Acute Myeloid Leukemia

AML
Morphology
- M0—Minimal myeloid differentiation
- M1—Poorly differentiated myeloblasts
- M2—Myeloblastic with differentiation
- M3—Promyelocytic
- M4—Myeloblastic and monoblastic
- M5—Monoblastic
- M6—Erythroleukemic
- M7—Megakaryoblastic

TABLE 70-7 Risk Group Classification Criteria for Acute Lymphoblastic Leukemia Patients (St. Jude Children's Research Hospital)

Risk Group	Features
Low risk	DNA index ≥1.16 and ≤1.60 **or** age between 1 and 9 years and WBC < 50 × 10^9/L **AND** Absence of the following: t(9;22) (*BCR-ABL* fusion) t(4;11) (*MLL-AF4* fusion) t(1119) (*E2A-PBS1* fusion) *MLL* rearrangement T-cell phenotype CNS leukemia Testicular leukemia **Or** >5% bone marrow blasts on day 15 of induction therapy
High risk	Those excluded from the low-risk and very high-risk groups
Very high risk	t(9;22) (*BCR-ABL* fusion) with a leukocyte count ≥25 × 10^9/L Age ≤12 months with *MLL* rearrangement Age ≥10 years with *MLL-AF4* fusion **Or** induction failure

blood cell count. High-risk patients are those younger than 1 year or older than 10 years of age whose leukocyte counts exceed 50,000/ul. However, this system fails to take into consideration the importance of results from cytogenetic and molecular analyses. Table 70-7 summarizes the risk group classification currently used at St. Jude Children's Research Hospital (Pui, 1996).

Medical Management of Childhood Leukemia

As soon as the diagnosis is confirmed, the child should begin treatment immediately. All current therapy regimens have four major elements: induction of remission, intensification or consolidation therapy, treatment to prevent CNS relapse, and continuation therapy. Induction therapy consists of asparaginase, vincristine, and a glucocorticoid (prednisone or dexamethasone); daunomycin may also be included. Together, these agents lead to remission in more than 95% of cases (Pui, 1995). Remission has been achieved when a sample of CSF is negative for leukemic cells and when a bone marrow aspirate contains fewer than 5% blasts. After the patient has achieved remission, residual blast cells are destroyed with a brief, intensive treatment. The drugs used may be increased doses of those used previously or may be new agents. One consolidation regimen currently used is high-dose methotrexate and 6-mercaptopurine.

Treatment directed at CNS disease and its prevention significantly improved the long-term survival of leukemia patients during the mid-1960s (Rivera et al., 1993). Currently, most patients receive intrathecal methotrexate, hydrocortisone, and cytarabine at various intervals. Patients with significant CNS disease, leucocytosis at the time of diagnosis, T-cell ALL with leucocytosis, or Philadelphia chromosome–positive leukemia must also receive cranial radiation, which is given over 2 to 3 weeks during chemotherapy (Pui, 1995).

The goal of continuation therapy is to maintain remission. Treatment must continue for 2 to 3 years after remission is achieved, because without continuation therapy the patient would likely relapse within 2 months (Poplack, 1993). Two drugs that frequently are included in continuation regimens are methotrexate and 6-mercaptopurine. These drugs produce an 80% cure rate in low-risk patients (Pui, 1995), and the addition of intermittent pulses of vincristine and prednisone in addition to this antimetabolite therapy further improves outcome. The high-risk patient requires more intense chemotherapy. This therapy is typically given in a rotational combination and may include drugs such as cyclophosphamide, cytarabine, or teniposide (Pui, 1996). Many studies are now including a second induction phase during consolidation. This modification has improved long-term survival among high-risk patients (Poplack, 1993).

Approximately 25% of ALL patients develop relapsed disease, which typically occurs during or within 2 years after treatment. The primary objective after relapse is to obtain a second remission, which is accomplished in 90% of the patients. An allogeneic transplant is the treatment of choice for patients who relapse during therapy. For patients who relapse more than 6 months off therapy, intensified chemotherapy may be a treatment option (Pui, 1996).

Intensive CNS-directed therapy has markedly decreased the number of patients with CNS relapse. Patients who develop relapsed disease in the CNS should receive intensive intrathecal, reinduction, and continuation chemotherapy, as well as cranial radiation therapy. Bone marrow transplantation can be considered for patients previously treated for CNS leukemia or who develop CNS and bone marrow relapse. Improved chemotherapeutic regimens have decreased the incidence of testicular relapse to only 1% of male leukemia patients, and these boys have a good prognosis when treated with intensive chemotherapy and bilateral radiation (Pui, 1996).

Cytarabine and an anthracycline, with or without thioguanine or etoposide, lead to remission in 70% to 85% of patients with AML (Pui, 1995). This induction regimen is typically followed by consolidation therapy comprising additional high-dose chemotherapy or bone marrow transplantation. Alternatively, remission in patients with promyelocytic (M3) AML can be induced with all-transretinoic acid; these patients then receive consolidation chemotherapy as described previously. Patients with M7 leukemia and Down syndrome often achieve remission after receiving chemotherapy alone.

The only curative therapy available to patients with CML is an allogeneic bone marrow transplant. The estimated long-term survival after transplantation is 80% to 90% for patients with Ph-positive CML and 40% to 50% for those with the juvenile form of the disease. Interferon-alpha has prolonged survival and delayed progression of the disease in children for whom allogeneic bone marrow transplantation is not an option (Pui, 1995).

Prognosis for Childhood Leukemia

Most of the children diagnosed with leukemia can now be cured of their disease, and the overall long-term survival rate for ALL is 70%. Advances in therapy, improvements in supportive care, and the option of bone marrow transplantation contribute to this success. Although patients with relapsed ALL have a guarded prognosis, those who achieve a second remission through bone marrow transplantation have a 40% to 50% long-term survival rate. Leukemia of the mature B cell immunophenotype was once associated with a dismal prognosis. Today, these patients are treated with intensive rotational therapy for 6 to 8 months and achieve a long-term survival rate of 80% (Pui, 1995; Pui & Crist, 1994). Unfortunately, patients with AML continue to have a poor prognosis (estimated long-term survival, 40%) despite intensive chemotherapy and bone marrow transplantation (Grier & Weinstein, 1993).

The goal of future therapy is to improve cure rates while minimizing toxicities and the late effects of therapy. An increased understanding of the cell biology of leukemia will enable physicians to better assess the risk status of their patients and to refine risk-adapted treatment, thereby achieving this goal.

NON–HODGKIN'S LYMPHOMA

Lymphoma is the third most common malignancy of childhood. In children younger than 15 years, non–Hodgkin's lymphoma (NHL) occurs slightly more frequently than does Hodgkin's disease (Ries et al., 1994). Non–Hodgkin's lymphomas are heterogeneous and differ markedly from adult lymphomas. Unlike adults with lymphoma, 90% of pediatric patients have extranodal, high-grade tumors belonging to one of three histologic subtypes: small noncleaved cell (34%), lymphoblastic (29%), and large cell lymphoma (27%) (Sandlund, Downing, & Crist, 1996).

Epidemiology of Non–Hodgkin's Lymphoma

About 500 cases of NHL occur each year in children in the United States. The incidence of NHL in the United States rose by almost 30% between 1973 and 1991. The reason for this increase is unclear. Overall, the incidence of lymphoma increases with age (Sandlund, Downing, & Crist, 1996). Among patients younger than 15 years of age, pediatric lymphoma is more frequent in Caucasians and is two to three times more common in males.

Risk Factors for Non–Hodgkin's Lymphoma

Several factors influence the development of NHL. As with leukemia, children with congenital immunodeficiency syndromes such as ataxia-telangiectasia, Wiskott-Aldrich syndrome, and X-linked lymphoproliferative disease are at an increased risk of developing lymphomas. In addition, acquired immunodeficiency secondary to immunosuppressive therapy or infection with the human immunodeficiency virus (HIV) is strongly associated with the development of lymphoma. Patients with acquired immunosuppression have a predisposition for CNS lymphomas, which are seldom seen in immunocompetent individuals. Many of the lymphomas associated with congenital and acquired immunodeficiency have also been associated with the Epstein-Barr virus (Poplack et al., 1993).

Epstein-Barr virus is a topic of significant interest in the discussion of lymphoma. In Africa, Burkitt's lymphoma is endemic and accounts for 50% of all childhood cancers. This high incidence rate is attributed to malaria and the Epstein-Barr virus (Poplack et al., 1993). The sporadic form of Burkitt's lymphoma, seen in the United States, traditionally was not thought to be related to Epstein-Barr virus. However, improved detection methods are identifying the viral genome even in cases of sporadic Burkitt's lymphoma, strongly suggesting a role of the virus in the pathogenesis of this disease (Sandlund, Downing, & Crist, 1996).

Pathogenesis of the Non–Hodgkin's Lymphoma

The lymphatic system is an accessory route for the flow of fluids from interstitial spaces to the blood. In the pathogenesis of NHL, chromosomal translocation, point mutations, deletions, or amplifications give rise to the malignant process and lead to cellular dysfunction in the lymphatic system. This cellular dysfunction results in the local or generalized enlargement of the lymph nodes, which typically is the initial presenting sign of NHL (Magrath, 1993).

Clinical Presentation of Non–Hodgkin's Lymphoma

The clinical course of NHL is insidious, with the development of painless nodal enlargement. As the nodal enlargement continues, tumors become clinically evident. At the time of presentation, most children have locally advanced or metastatic disease. Childhood lymphomas typically occur as extranodal disease, with the most common sites being the mediastinum (26%), abdomen (31%), and head and neck (29%). Other sites of malignancy may include the oropharynx, bone marrow, and skin. Lymphoblastic lymphoma typically occurs as a mediastinal mass, with or without pleural effusion, or as a mass in the head and neck region. Burkitt's lymphoma usually occurs in the abdomen or head and neck, whereas large cell lymphoma may involve the mediastinum, abdomen, head and neck, bone, or skin (Sandlund, Downing, & Crist, 1996).

Symptoms of mediastinal disease include dysphagia, dyspnea, and orthopnea. The child may also have swelling of the upper torso and face due to superior vena cava syndrome secondary to tumor compression. Patients with head and neck disease typically have painless enlargement of the cervical lymph nodes or tonsils. The clinical manifestations of abdominal tumors include abdominal pain, nausea, vomiting, and appendicitis. In addition, the patient may experience a bowel obstruction secondary to tumor compression or intussusception. The patient who has generalized adenopathy and pancytopenia is likely to have bone marrow disease.

Assessment of the Patient for Non–Hodgkin's Lymphoma

The patient who is referred for treatment of lymphoma requires a complete evaluation, beginning with a detailed history and physical examination. The diagnostic workup should be completed promptly due to the rapid growth of lymphomas, especially the β cell neoplasms (Magrath, 1993). To determine the extent of disease, chest radiographs and CT scans of the neck, chest, abdomen, and pelvis should be completed. Bone and gallium scans may be included in the diagnostic workup. Laboratory evaluation should include a complete blood count with differential, chemistry analysis (uric acid, calcium, phosphorus, and lactate dehydrogenase), and viral studies for Epstein-Barr virus and HIV.

To diagnose NHL, biopsy tissue must be obtained for morphologic, immunophenotypic, cytogenetic, and molecular studies. A sample of cerebrospinal fluid and bilateral bone marrow biopsies should be evaluated for patients with a suspected lymphoma. If the child has a mediastinal mass with a pleural effusion, a thoracentesis may yield diagnostic material. The diagnosis becomes T-cell or B-cell leukemia for patients with lymphoblastic or Burkitt's lymphoma, respectively, in whom the bone marrow contains more than 25% blast cells.

Small noncleaved cell lymphoma in children is a subset of Burkitt's lymphoma, a B-cell malignancy. This tumor is made up of monomorphic lymphoid cells that have prominent nucleoli and a classic "starry sky" appearance to the cytoplasm. In 95% of cases, lymphoblastic lymphoma is a T-cell malignancy of the nodal system that is otherwise morphologically identical to T-cell leukemia. The lymphoblasts have round nuclei, distinct membranes, and a small rim of basophilic cytoplasm. This disease is rapidly progressive and can disseminate quickly. Large-cell lymphomas can have a T-cell, B-cell, or indeterminate immunophenotype. Morphologically, most of these lymphomas are classified as immunoblastic or diffuse, and 30% have anaplastic features. Large-cell lymphoma seldom involves the bone marrow or spinal fluid (Sandlund, Downing, & Crist, 1996). Table 70-8 details the clinical and biologic characteristics of NHLs in children and the genetic translocations associated with each type of lymphoma.

Staging of Non–Hodgkin's Lymphoma

After the lymphoma subset has been identified, the staging process begins and involves the same assessment process that was described in the leukemia section. As with leukemia, the stage of the lymphoma determines the chemotherapeutic agents used, the length of time, and the intensity of treatment (Table 70-9) (Murphy, 1980).

TABLE 70-8 Clinical and Biologic Characteristics of Non–Hodgkin's Lymphoma in Children

Subtype	Proportion of Cases (%)	Typical Phenotype	Frequent Sites of Primary Disease	Characteristic Translocation
Small noncleaved cell (Burkitt's)	34	B cell	Abdomen or head and neck	t(8;14)(q24;q32) t(2;8)(p11;q24) t(8;22)(q24;q11)
Lymphoblastic	29	T cells	Mediastinum or head and neck	t(1;14)(p32;q11) t(11;14)(p13;q11) t(11;14)(p15;q11) t(10;14)(q24;q11) t(7;19)(q35;p13) t(8;14)(q24;q11) t(1;7)(p34;q34)
Large cell	27	B cell, T cell, indeterminant	Mediastinum, abdomen, head and neck, or skin	t(2;5)(p23;q35)

TABLE 70-9 Stages of Non–Hodgkin's Lymphoma

Stage	Description
Stage I	A single tumor (extranodal) or involvement of a single anatomic area (nodal), except of the mediastinum and abdomen
Stage II	A single tumor (extranodal) with regional lymph node involvement
	Involvement of two or more anatomic areas on the same side of the diaphragm
	Involvement of two single (extranodal) tumors, with or without regional lymph node involvement, on the same side of the diaphragm
	A primary gastrointestinal tract tumor (usually in the ileocecal area), with or without involvement of associated mesenteric lymph nodes, that is completely resectable
Stage III	Two single tumors (extranodal) on opposite sides of the diaphragm
	Involvement of two or more nodal areas above and below the diaphragm
	Any primary intrathoracic tumor (mediastinal, pleural, or thymic)
	Extensive primary intraabdominal disease
	Any paraspinal or epidural tumor, regardless of involvement of other sites
Stage IV	Any of the above findings with involvement of the central nervous system, bone marrow, or both at diagnosis.

From Murphy, S. B. (1980). Classification, staging and end results of treatment of childhood and non-Hodgkin's lymphomas: Dissimilarities from lymphomas in adults. *Seminars in Oncology, 3,* 332-339.

Medical Management of Non–Hodgkin's Lymphoma

Treatment should be started as soon as possible after the diagnosis of lymphoma has been established. Due to rapid tumor growth, it may even be necessary to begin treatment before completion of the staging workup. Multiagent chemotherapy is indicated for all lymphomas and is curative alone. Surgery has little benefit, except in cases where gross total resection is possible and leads to down-staging of the disease. Radiation may be given in emergency situations (e.g., airway compression) or as palliative therapy.

For limited-stage NHL, therapy consists of 2 to 6 months of multiagent chemotherapy. The chemotherapeutic agents most frequently used are cyclophosphamide, vincristine, and prednisone. For lymphoblastic lymphoma, therapy must be given over a longer period of time. Many current regimens treat lymphoblastic lymphoma in the same way as T-cell lymphoblastic leukemia. For advanced Burkitt's lymphoma (as with B-cell leukemia), current therapy consists of cyclophosphamide, high-dose methotrexate, and cytarabine, sometimes with the addition of ifosfamide and etoposide. This intensive therapy is given over a 2- to 8-month period. Large cell lymphoma continues to be the most difficult lymphoma to treat. Recent studies now suggest that the efficacy of therapy may depend on the tumor immunophenotype. For example, large cell lymphoma of B-cell origin may respond best to intensive therapy administered over a short period of time, whereas the T-cell subtype may require long-term therapy. Table 70-10 details the outcomes associated with stage-directed chemotherapy of childhood NHL (Sandlund, Downing, & Crist, 1996).

Prognosis for Non–Hodgkin's Lymphoma

In the pediatric population, NHL is usually a curable disease. Current therapy leads to a 75% event-free survival rate for advanced cases of Burkitt's or lymphoblastic lymphoma. However, advanced large cell lymphoma is associated with an estimated 5-year event-free survival rate of 50% to 70%. Outcome is generally poor for patients with relapsed lymphoma. In an attempt to achieve a second remission, relapse therapy consists of high-dose chemotherapy with or without bone marrow transplantation.

HODGKIN'S DISEASE

Hodgkin's disease (HD) is a lymphoma that affects children and adults. Approximately 10% to 15% of cases of HD occur in children younger than 16 years of age (Poplack et al., 1993). Today, most of these children become long-term survivors. Therefore management of these patients must consider long-term complications.

Epidemiology of Hodgkin's Disease

In the United States, HD demonstrates two age peaks, the first during the middle to late 20s and the second after the age of 50 years. Hodgkin's disease occurs more frequently in Caucasians. Overall, the incidence of HD is greater in males, although this bias is not apparent among adolescents (Hudson & Donaldson, 1997).

Risk Factors for Hodgkin's Disease

As with other lymphomas, patients who have immunodeficiencies, including those due to ataxia telangiectasia, HIV infection, and iatrogenic agents, have an increased incidence of HD. Infectious agents, including herpesvirus 6, cytomegalovirus, and Epstein-Barr virus, have been implicated in the etiology of HD. Patients with HD have a high incidence of elevated EBV titers, and many have a history of EBV infection (e.g., infectious mononucleosis). Epstein-Barr viral genomes have been identified in cells from patients with HD and are most frequently associated with the

TABLE 70-10 Outcomes of Stage-Directed Chemotherapy in Children with Non–Hodgkin's Lymphoma*

Stage	Chemotherapeutic Agents	Duration of Therapy	Long-term Survival (%)	Comments
I or II (limited)				
Burkitt's or large cell lymphoma	Cyclophosphamide, vincristine, and prednisone, with or without doxorubicin or methotrexate	9-26 wk	85-95	Expected late effects of therapy are minimal.
Lymphoblastic lymphoma	Cyclophosphamide, vincristine, and prednisone, with or without doxorubicin, methotrexate, mercaptopurine, asparaginase, thioguanine, cytarabine, or carmustine	33 wk-24 mo	85-90	With a shorter duration of therapy, retreatment is required in approximately one third of cases.
III or IV (Advanced)				
Burkitt's lymphoma	Cyclophosphamide, vincristine, prednisone, and high-dose methotrexate, with or without etoposide, ifosfamide, doxorubicin, cytarabine, or cisplatin	2-8 mo	75-85	Relapses are rare more than 1 year after diagnosis.
Lymphoblastic lymphoma	Vincristine, prednisone, daunorubicin or doxorubicin, and asparaginase, with or without methotrexate, cyclophosphamide, mercaptopurine, thioguanine, teniposide, hydroxyurea, or carmustine	15-32 mo	65-75	Relapses can occur more than 3 years after diagnosis.
Large cell lymphoma	Vincristine, prednisone, and methotrexate, with or without high-dose methotrexate, cyclophosphamide, mercaptopurine, thioguanine, hydroxyurea, asparaginase, daunorubicin or doxorubicin, carmustine, or bleomycin	3-24 mo	50-70	Among patients with relapses after therapy, the survival rate is approximately 40% with high-dose chemotherapy and autologous bone marrow transplantation.

*Estimates are for survival at 3 to 5 years, without retreatment (event-free survival). For limited-stage lymphoblastic disease, the estimates reflect event-free survival and successful treatment of refractory disease.

mixed cellularity subset of HD. Environmental or genetic-risk factors for HD may exist. The disease has been noted in families, especially among same-gender siblings; there have also been reports of parent-child occurrence (Hudson & Donaldson, 1997).

Pathogenesis of Hodgkin's Disease

Hodgkin's disease is a malignancy of the lymphatic system. The malignant cell of HD is the Reed-Sternberg cell, which appears to develop from B and T lymphocytes in response to many pathologic processes that facilitate the development of HD. After the diagnosis of HD, the histologic subset is defined. According to the Rye classification system, these subtypes are lymphocyte predominant, mixed cellularity, lymphocyte depleted, and nodular sclerosing. Lymphocyte-predominant HD affects 10% to 15% of pediatric patients, is usually localized, and is more common in males and younger patients. Lymphocyte-depleted disease is rare in children with HD, whereas 30% of these patients have mixed cellularity disease. These children are typically 10 years of age or younger and have advanced disease. Nodular sclerosing HD, the most common subset, occurs in 40% of young HD patients and 70% of adolescents (Hudson & Donaldson, 1997).

Clinical Presentation of Hodgkin's Disease

Patients with HD typically have painless cervical and/or supraclavicular adenopathy. Approximately 75% have mediastinal involvement. A nonproductive cough or shortness of breath may be present in children with airway compromise.

Disease of the axillary or inguinal nodes is an uncommon presenting symptom. Primary abdominal disease in children is also rare. Disease outside the lymphatic system is present in 10% to 15% of patients at the time of diagnosis of HD. Extralymphatic disease most frequently involves the lung, pleura, or pericardium. Infrequently, the patient may have anemia, thrombocytopenia, or neutropenia secondary to bone marrow involvement. Approximately 20% to 30% of patients present with systemic "B" symptoms, which include fever, drenching night sweats, and weight loss greater than 10%. Other systemic symptoms include fatigue, pruritus, and pain after the ingestion of alcohol (Hudson & Donaldson, 1997).

Assessment of the Patient for Hodgkin's Disease

The patient who has adenopathy requires a thorough evaluation, including a detailed history and complete physical examination. The physical examination should be done by an experienced examiner familiar with the signs and symptoms of HD. All abnormal nodes should be measured to determine a baseline for subsequent monitoring of a response to treatment.

The diagnostic workup for HD begins with chest radiographs. When a mediastinal mass is present, measurement of the intrathoracic diameter is important, because if the mass is greater than 33% of the chest diameter, the child has a poor prognosis. The hematologic workup should include a complete blood count and chemistry profile. Nonspecific measures such as the erythrocyte sedimentation rate, serum copper concentration, or ferritin levels may be elevated. These tests reflect changes in the reticuloendothelial system and may be used as disease markers.

Imaging studies should include CT scans of the neck, chest, abdomen, and pelvis. Because of the limits of infradiaphragmatic CT imaging, many centers are using lymphangiography to assess abdominal and pelvic lymph nodes. This test has been most helpful in evaluating whether the retroperitoneal lymph nodes have disease involvement. Another method of assessing infradiaphragmatic disease involves pathologic evaluation through nodal dissection and splenectomy. This process is becoming less popular because of the immunosuppressive effects of splenectomy and the morbidity of the surgical procedure.

Nuclear gallium imaging is especially beneficial for evaluating supradiaphragmatic disease. Gallium is also useful in assessing responses to therapy, and persistent avidity is indicative of residual disease. Obtained less frequently than gallium scans, bone scans are useful for assessing skeletal lesions in children with bone pain, elevated alkaline phosphatase levels, and advanced disease. Bilateral bone marrow biopsies should be obtained from the patient with systemic symptoms or recurrent or stage III to IV disease.

Staging of Hodgkin's Disease

After the histologic subset of HD has been determined and the areas of disease involvement have been identified, the stage is defined according to the Ann Arbor staging classification (Table 70-11) (Carbone, Kaplan, Husshoff, Smithers, & Tubiana, 1971). The substage classification "A" denotes that the patient has no systemic symptoms, whereas "B" is indicative of systemic symptoms. The substage "S" indicates splenic disease, whereas "E" denotes extralymphatic disease.

TABLE 70-11 Staging Classification for Hodgkin's Disease (Ann Arbor)

Stage	Definition
I	Involvement of a single lymph node region or site
I_E	Involvement of a single extralymphatic organ or site
II	Involvement of two or more lymph node regions on the same side of the diaphragm
II_E	Localized involvement of an extralymphatic organ or site and one or more lymph node regions on the same side of the diaphragm
III	Involvement of lymph node regions on both sides of the diaphragm,
III_S	which may be accompanied by involvement of the spleen
III_E	or by localized involvement of an extralymphatic organ site
III_{SE}	or both
IV	Diffuse or disseminated involvement of one or more extralymphatic organs or tissues with or without associated lymph node involvement
A	The absence of fever over 100.4° F (38° C) for 3 consecutive days, drenching night sweats, or unexplained loss of 10% or more of body weight in the 6 months preceding admission
B	The presence of above symptoms

Medical Management of Hodgkin's Disease

Selection of appropriate therapy follows the completion of HD staging. Radiation was the first effective therapy used in the treatment of HD and was succeeded by the use of combination chemotherapy; MOPP (mechlorethamine [nitrogen mustard], vincristine, procarbazine, and prednisone) was the first chemotherapeutic regimen used to treat HD. The ABVD (doxorubicin, bleomycin, vinblastine, and dacarbazine) regimen was developed for resistant disease. This addition led to the combination of MOPP/ABVD, which is now the standard chemotherapy for HD. Many treatment protocols now substitute cyclophosphamide for mechlorethamine to reduce the risk of secondary leukemia.

For stages I and IIA disease, radiation alone (total dose, 35 to 44 Gy to involved or extended fields) is the standard therapy. Because this dose may impair growth and development in young children, many institutions are now administering lower doses of radiation (25 Gy) with combination chemotherapy. This therapy is especially recommended for stage II patients with bulky mediastinal disease (>33% maximal intrathoracic diameter) or systemic B symptoms. Combination chemotherapy and radiation are also recommended for patients with stage IIIA disease, whereas chemotherapy is the cornerstone of therapy for patients with stages IIIB and IV disease (Hudson & Donaldson, 1997).

The risk of relapsed HD is greatest during the first 3 years after therapy. For patients who have limited disease at relapse after primary therapy with radiation alone, intensive chemotherapy leads to long-term survival in 50% to 80% of patients. Patients treated with chemotherapy and/or radiation who relapse less than 12 months off therapy and those with multiple sites of relapsed disease have a poor prognosis. Long-term survival is achieved in 20% to 30% of these patients with autologous bone marrow or stem cell transplantation. Chemotherapy is associated with a 40% to 50% estimated 5-year survival rate in patients who relapse after prolonged initial remissions. Further, long-term survival after intensive therapy plus transplantation may be as high as 80% in patients who develop relapsed HD more than 12 months after completing therapy. However, studies comparing outcome after conventional therapy versus high-dose salvage transplant therapy have not been done (Hudson & Donaldson, 1997).

Complications of Therapy for Hodgkin's Disease

The goal of current HD therapy is to minimize the late effects of standard radiation and chemotherapy without compromising cure rates. Late effects of radiation therapy include defects of bony and soft tissue development. Because of the hypersensitivity of the preadolescent thyroid to irradiation, another common sequelae is hypothyroidism. Pelvic radiation in female patients may lead to ovarian failure. However, oophoropexy before initiation of therapy may preserve ovarian function. For males, radiation or chemotherapy may lead to sterility.

Chemotherapy and radiation may also affect cardiac and pulmonary function. Although lung irradiation and bleomycin chemotherapy may lead to pulmonary compromise, patients regain function over time. Because the degree of radiation-induced cardiac injury is directly related to dosage, low-dose mantle therapy leads to fewer problems than high-dose mantle radiation, which can cause vascular injury and accelerated atherosclerosis. Doxorubicin chemotherapy may result in cardiac dysfunction, and this effect is thought to be potentiated by adjuvant radiation. Patients who receive this treatment combination should be monitored closely with echocardiography. However, studies have shown that the incidence of symptomatic disease is low (Hudson & Donaldson, 1997).

The most disturbing late effect of HD therapy is the development of second malignancies, the most common of which is acute nonlymphocytic leukemia (ANLL). Secondary ANLL after HD is associated with MOPP chemotherapy and peaks in incidence 5 to 10 years after therapy. In addition, the incidence of NHL in HD survivors ranges from 0.9% to 5.9% (Hudson & Donaldson, 1997). Other secondary malignancies related to radiation therapy for HD include tumors of the lung, gastrointestinal tract, breast, and thyroid.

Prognosis for Hodgkin's Disease

Overall, current therapy for HD, which typically comprises low-dose radiation and combination chemotherapy, leads to long-term survival in 70% to 90% of pediatric and adolescent patients. This percentage is most dependent on the stage of the disease at the time of diagnosis. Therefore therapy is stage adapted to minimize long-term sequelae in growing children who become cancer survivors.

Oncologic Emergencies Associated with Leukemia and Lymphoma

The child with leukemia or lymphoma may have one of several clinical situations that require immediate attention. Patients with leukemia who have hyperleucocytosis (white blood cell count >200,000) may require immediate hydration and hemapheresis. After tumoricidal therapy is initiated, the child with leucocytosis may develop tumor lysis syndrome because of electrolyte abnormalities caused by the rapid destruction of leukemic cells. Before therapy is initiated, the patient with leukocytosis may require hospitalization for vigorous hydration, alkalization, and administration of allopurinol or urate oxidase; if urate oxidase is available, alkalization is unnecessary.

Prompt treatment of the lymphoblastic leukemia or lymphoma patient who has a mediastinal mass prevents further respiratory distress or respiratory arrest. In addition, all patients with leukemia or lymphoma are at risk for infection and sepsis. If febrile, these patients must be immediately hospitalized to receive intravenous antibiotics. With the recent improvements in supportive care, these disease sequelae no longer have a significant effect on long-term outcome.

RETINOBLASTOMA

Anatomy and Physiology of the Eye

The eye is composed of several anatomically and physiologically distinct structures (Fig. 70-9). The sclera gives shape to the eye. The cornea is the eye's major refractive component, bending light rays as they pass through the lens so that they are focused on the retina. The transparent crystalline lens enables accommodation (i.e., the ability to adjust for distance). The vitreous humor and aqueous humor are gelatinous, delicate connective tissues that fill the posterior and anterior chambers, respectively.

The pigmented part of the eye consists of the iris and the ciliary body, which contain circular and smooth muscle fibers to assist in accommodation, as well as the highly vascular choroidal layer, which nourishes and oxygenates the retina. The retina is the light-sensitive portion of the eye. It contains the cones, which are responsible for color vision, and the rods, which enable sight under low-light conditions. Visual images are transmitted from neurons in the retina

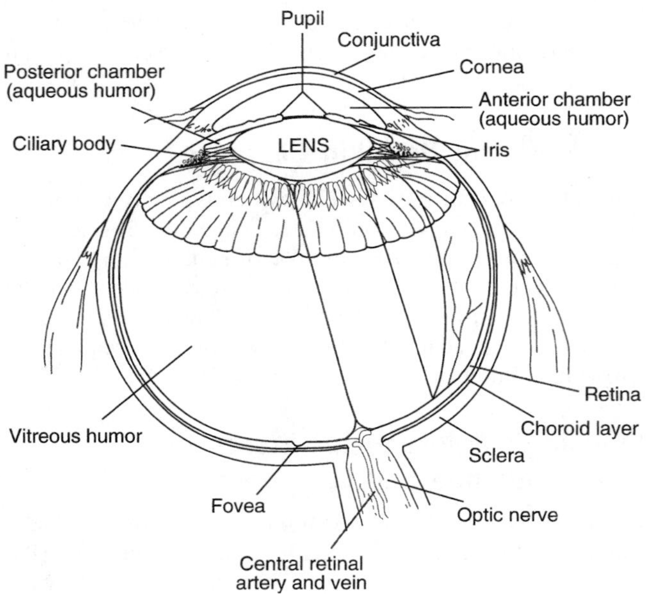

Fig. 70-9 The anatomy of the eye.

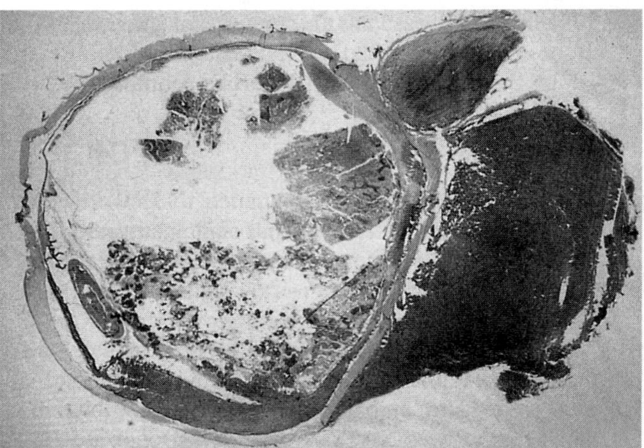

Fig. 70-10 Photomicrograph of endophytic and exophytic tumor arising from the retina.

to the optic nerve and cerebral cortex (Klintworth, & Eagle, 1996).

Epidemiology and Risk Factors for Retinoblastoma

Retinoblastoma is the most common ocular tumor of children, occurring in 1 in 14,000 live births and leading to approximately 250 new cases of cancer in the United States annually. One or both eyes may be affected. Bilateral disease usually results from multicentric tumor development rather than from the spread of tumor to the opposite eye (Kingston & Hungerford, 1992).

Retinoblastoma predominantly affects young children; the median age at the time of diagnosis is 2 years, and 80% of the tumors are diagnosed before age 4. With early diagnosis and prompt treatment, the mortality rate from retinoblastoma is 8%. However, significant morbidity, including facial asymmetry and blindness, can occur. Although the frequency of retinoblastoma is similar between the genders, the overall incidence of this neoplasm is increasing slightly. Improved survival and an increase in retinoblastoma among children born to adult survivors of the malignancy account for the overall increased incidence. Having a family history of retinoblastoma is the most prominent risk factor for developing the disease (Kingston & Hungerford, 1992).

Genetic factors play an important role in the pathogenesis of retinoblastoma. Ellsworth (1969) described two forms of retinoblastoma: a heritable, familial form and a spontaneous form. There are important clinical differences between these two forms of the disease. Familial retinoblastoma occurs in 40% of patients who have bilateral or multifocal unilateral disease (Knudson, 1971). These patients are diagnosed at a median age of 7 months, and many are thought to be born with the tumor. Patients with familial retinoblastoma have an increased risk of developing other malignant neoplasms. Moll, Imhof, Bouter, Kuik, Den Otter, and Bezemer et al. (1996) found that the cumulative incidence of second primary tumors in patients with hereditary disease was 3.7% at 10 years of age and 17.7% at 35 years of age. Melanoma was the most frequent second malignancy among the patients in this series.

Patients with familial bilateral retinoblastoma may have an ectopic focus of the disease in the pineal gland. Retinoblastoma of the pineal gland occurs exclusively in patients with the familial form of the disease. Because the ectopic presentation involves a third area of disease rather than metastatic extension, this tumor pattern has been termed *trilateral retinoblastoma* (Amoaku, Willshaw, Parkes, Shah, & Mann, 1996; Kingston, Plowman, & Hungerford, 1985).

In contrast to patients with familial retinoblastoma, those with the spontaneous, nonhereditary form of the disease are diagnosed at a later age (median age is 24 months). These patients often have a single tumor in one eye, have little increased risk of passing retinoblastoma on to their children, and are unlikely to develop other malignancies.

Pathophysiology of Retinoblastoma

The natural history, histologic features, and routes of metastases of retinoblastoma affect its clinical presentation and management. Retinoblastomas usually occur as chalky, cauliflower-like intraocular masses that often have calcified foci and large areas of necrosis. Most tumors originate in the posterior retina. The tumor may extend from the inner layers of the retina into the vitreous humor (endophytic growth) or may arise from the outer layers of the retina and grow toward the subretinal space (exophytic), causing a retinal detachment. Many tumors have both endophytic and exophytic components (Fig. 70-10).

Histologically, the tumor is characterized by cells with scant cytoplasm and hyperchromic nuclei of various sizes.

Retinoblastoma cells have numerous mitotic figures and are arranged in tight bouquetlike clusters called *rosettes* (Wang, Jenkins, Cu-Unjieng, Meyer, & Donoso, 1996).

Retinoblastoma has become a model for understanding the mechanism of genetic mutations in childhood cancer. In 1971, Knudson suggested that the clinical differences between the hereditary and spontaneous forms of retinoblastoma could only be explained by two independent mutational events (i.e., Knudson's two-hit theory). The first mutation occurs in a copy of the retinoblastoma gene that is inherited from one parent; this event occurs before conception. The second mutation occurs after conception and affects a somatic retinal cell (Knudson, 1971). The retinoblastoma gene is recessive, and the loss of one allele of the gene is insufficient to cause the disease. However, the disease is inherited in a dominant manner. Among children who inherit the germline mutation from an affected parent, 90% acquire the second retinoblastoma mutation and develop the tumor (Vogel, 1979).

The genetic alteration in retinoblastoma has been mapped to chromosome 13q14 and can occur by deletion, translocation, or errors in transcription. A syndrome associated with the partial deletion of 13q14 occurs in 5% of retinoblastoma patients and results in microcephaly, mental retardation, facial asymmetry, and hypoplastic digits. Some of the gene rearrangements observed in cases of retinoblastoma are common to many tumors (Gallie, Dunn, Chan, Hamel, & Phillips, 1991; Horowitz, 1993).

Two studies have suggested that errors during transcription of the retinoblastoma gene (leading to its mutation) occur more frequently in the paternal rather than maternal allele (Dryja, Mukai, Peterson, Rapaport, Walton, & Yandell, 1989; Zhu, Dunn, Phillips, Goddard, Paton, & Becker et al., 1989). This finding suggests that germline mutations occur more frequently during spermatogenesis than oogenesis (Kingston & Hungerford, 1992). The product of the retinoblastoma gene has recently been characterized as an underphosphorylated protein that alters transcription in the cell cycle.

Routes of Metastases for Retinoblastoma

Although infrequent, metastasis of retinoblastoma can result from local extension, distal spread, or hematogenous dissemination of the tumor. Local extension (intraocular spread) of disease can occur through several mechanisms (e.g., when cells detach from the main tumor mass and seed the vitreous humor). Eruption through the retina distant from the initial mass is characteristic of masses that arise after seeding of the vitreous humor; the lesions of multifocal retinoblastoma lack this attribute. Enlargement of the tumor mass also may cause intraocular spread, ultimately obliterating the internal architecture of the eye. In advanced disease, eruption of the mass through the sclera can lead to local extension of retinoblastoma to the surrounding orbit (MacKay, Abramson, & Ellsworth, 1984).

Distal and hematogenous metastases of retinoblastoma are much more infrequent than local extension. Because most lesions involve the posterior retina, distal spread of the disease tends to involve extension into the optic nerve. From the optic nerve, tumor cells may breach the subarachnoid space and metastasize to the brain; a lesion in the optic nerve beyond the enucleation resection site is an ominous prognostic sign. Hematogenous spread may occur secondary to tumor invasion of the vascular choroid layer; lymphatic spread of retinoblastoma occurs rarely.

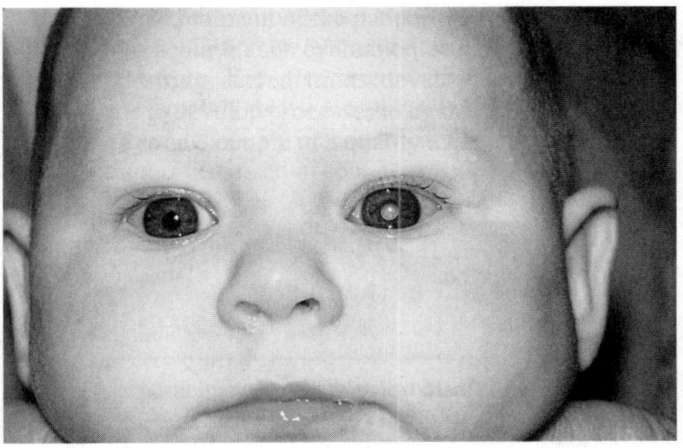

Fig. 70-11 Child with leukocoria.

Assessment of the Patient for Retinoblastoma

The assessment of a child for retinoblastoma (Table 70-12) must address the extent of intraocular disease, distal spread, CNS involvement, and blood-borne metastatic disease. Soon after birth, infants with a positive family history should be anesthetized and evaluated for retinoblastoma by dilated direct and indirect fundoscopic examinations.

In developed countries, most patients are diagnosed while the disease involves only the eye. Leukocoria ("cat's eye reflex") is the most common presenting symptom; strabismus and painful, red eyes may also occur (Fig. 70-11). The leukocoria of retinoblastoma must be differentiated from that of other childhood conditions, such as Coat disease and toxocariasis. Parents of toddlers with sporadic retinoblastoma often bring them to the pediatrician after noticing esotropia or exotropia, or after suspecting decreased vision in one eye.

Staging of Retinoblastoma

The Reese-Ellsworth classification system (Table 70-13) is the current standard for categorizing retinoblastomas (Ellsworth, 1969). Although the number, location, and size of intraocular masses are criteria of this schema, it fails to weigh the contributions of orbital and metastatic disease. In contrast, the pathologic staging schema for retinoblastoma used at St. Jude Children's Research Hospital (Table 70-14) accommodates for all of these factors (Pratt, Fontanesi, Luo, Parham, Elfervig, & Meyer, 1997).

Medical Management of Retinoblastoma

The medical management of retinoblastoma depends on the form (familial versus spontaneous) and stage of disease. Be-

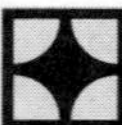

TABLE 70-12 Assessment of the Child for Retinoblastoma

	Assessment Parameters	Typical Abnormal Findings
History	A. Personal and social history 1. Age 2. Detailed family history for relatives with retinoblastoma or ocular loss due to unknown reasons 3. Examination of family photographs 4. Developmental history of child, with emphasis on acquisition of or alterations in visual developmental milestones	A. Personal and social risk factor 1. Median age 2 years (unilateral disease) 7 months (bilateral disease) 2. Family history positive for retinoblastoma 3. White "cat's eye reflex" in affected eye on photographs taken with flash attachment 4. Strabismus, visual loss
Physical Examination	A. Age-appropriate neurologic examination, with funduscopic examination and emphasis on visual motor skills	A. Visual field limitations, failure to track bright object, alteration in pupillary reflex
	B. Dilated direct and indirect funduscopic examination of anesthetized patient by an ophthalmologist	B. Chalky white intraocular tumor mass
Diagnostic Tests	A. Ultrasonography to assess intraglobular extent of disease and location	A. Single or multiple masses
	B. Computed tomography of the orbits to assess extent, location, and clacification of tumors	B. Foci of necrosis and/or calcification
	C. Magnetic resonance imaging of brain to assess extent of disease in central nervous system and involvement of optic nerve head	C. Rarely abnormal in retinoblastoma; intracranial lesions usually occur only in advanced retinoblastoma
	D. Histologic evaluation of cerebrospinal fluid to assess central nervous system spread of disease	D. Rarely abnormal in retinoblastoma
	E. Histologic evaluation of bone marrow to assess hematogenous spread of disease	E. Rarely abnormal in retinoblastoma

TABLE 70-13 Reese-Ellsworth Classification of Retinoblastoma

Group	Description
Group I	Solitary tumor, ≥4 disc diameters,* at or behind equator Multiple masses, <4 disc diameters, all at or behind equator
Group II	Solitary lesion, 4-10 disc diameters, at or behind equator Multiple tumors, all 4-10 disc diameters and at or behind equator
Group III	Any lesion anterior to the equator Solitary mass, >10 disc diameters behind equator
Group IV	Multiple tumors at or behind equator, some >10 disc diameters Any lesion extending to the ora serrata
Group V	Massive tumor (involving over half of the retina) Vitreous seeding

*Disc diameter = 1.5 to 1.75.

cause bilateral disease may occur asynchronously (Fontanesi et al., 1995), every effort must be made to preserve sight without compromising survival. The treatment plan of retinoblastoma may include one or more of the following: xenon laser photocoagulation, cryotherapy, radiotherapy (external beam or plaque brachytherapy), enucleation of the affected eye, and chemotherapy. The specific indications for each of these interventions are detailed elsewhere (Lanzkowski, 1995) and are discussed briefly in this section. Xenon laser photocoagulation is used to obliterate the retinal blood vessels that supply the tumor. This modality is especially valuable in treating the small tumors that may reoccur after radiation therapy. Cryotherapy interrupts the intracellular functions of the treated masses, thereby halting their growth. Photocoagulation and cryotherapy are most effective on small lesions (tumor diameter <4 optic disc diameters) near the sclera. For larger tumors, radiotherapy is the treatment of choice for cases in which there is potential for useful vision after treatment.

Enucleation is indicated when retinal damage is so extensive that useful vision is unlikely regardless of the success or modality of treatment. Further, bilateral enucleation is justified when advanced disease has eliminated the potential for useful vision. Chemotherapy currently offers limited benefits to patients with intraocular disease; it is usually reserved for those with metastatic disease. However, Chan, DeBoer, Thiessen, Budning, Kingston, & O'Brien et al. (1996) found that infants with bilateral familial retinoblastoma benefited from chemotherapy including vincristine,

TABLE 70-14 St. Jude Children's Research Hospital Staging Schema for Retinoblastoma

Stage	Definition	Description
Stage I	Tumor confined to the retina	A. Solitary lesion, <6 D. D. B. Multiple lesions, all <6 D. D. C. Solitary or multiple lesions involving <50% of retinal surface behind equator D. ≥50% of retina involved, all tumor behind equator E. ≥50% retinal involvement, with at least one lesion at or anterior to equator
Stage II	Tumor confined to globe (extraretinal)	A. Extends to optic nerve head B. Extends to choroid Extends to choroid, with replacement of choroid C. Anterior chamber involved D. Extends to choroid and optic nerve
Stage III	Extrachoroidal extension	A. Extends to emissaries B. Extends beyond resected end of optic nerve and subarachnoid space C. Extends through sclera into orbit D. Extends to choroid and beyond resected end of optic nerve E. Extends through sclera and beyond resected end of optic nerve
Stage IV	Distant disease	A. Extends through optic nerve into brain and/or cerebrospinal fluid positive for tumor cells B. Blood-borne metastases of soft tissue, lymph node, or bone C. Bone marrow metastases

D. D. (optic disk diameter) = 1.5 mm.

carboplatin, teniposide, and cyclosporin. Regardless of the treatment regimen, all patients who have completed therapy must receive frequent fundoscopic examinations to enable early detection of recurrent or new disease.

Prognosis for Retinoblastoma

The overall prognosis of retinoblastoma is excellent. Approximately 96% of treated patients remain free of disease 5 years after diagnosis (Miller, Young, & Novakovic, 1995). The potential for the preservation of vision depends on the stage of the disease at the time of diagnosis and the treatment received.

WILMS' TUMOR

Epidemiology and Risk Factors for Wilms' Tumor

Wilms' tumor is the most common childhood renal tumor. The incidence of this neoplasm is similar between boys and girls but is slightly higher (53%) in the left kidney (Nemes & Donahue, 1994). The median age at the time of diagnosis is 3 years, and 75% of patients are diagnosed before 5 years of age. African Americans and Asian Americans have a lower incidence of Wilms' tumor than Caucasian children in the United States (DeKraker, 1992; Wingo, Bolden, Tong, Parker, Martin, & Heath, 1996). Bilateral disease occurs in 5% to 10% of patients; although the bilateral lesions usually occur simultaneously, they may develop sequentially. Like retinoblastoma, bilateral Wilms' tumor usually has a familial genetic component (Coppes, deKraker, van Dijken, Perry, Delemarre, & Tournade et al., 1989). In addition, 1% of Wilms' tumors are associated with congenital conditions (e.g., hemihypertrophy, aniridia, urinary defects) and syndromes such as the Beckwith-Wiedemann syndrome.

The genetics of Wilms' tumor have been studied extensively. Knudson (1993) proposed that, like retinoblastoma, Wilms' tumor develops because of two genetic mutational events, one of which occurs prezygotically in the germinal cell and the other postzygotically in the differentiated cell. Most Wilms' tumors have normal cytogenetics, but about 33% to 50% have loss of genetic material involving chromosome 11p. There are at least two loci, an 11p(11p13) associated with WAGR syndrome (Wilms' tumor, aniridia, genital abnormalities, and mental retardation) and 11p15 associated with Beckwith-Wiedemann syndrome. There may be other important, as yet unidentified, tumor suppressor genes on chromosomes 16q and 1p. These tumor suppressor genes involved in Wilms' tumor are located on chromosomes 11p13, 11p15.5, and 16q (Cohen, 1995).

Several nongenetic factors have been implicated in the development of Wilms' tumor. Advanced paternal age and paternal employment in a metal industry (e.g., as a welder or autobody repairman) increase the risk of Wilms' tumor among their children (Olshan, Breslow, Daling, Falletta, Grufferman, & Robison, et al., 1990). In addition, the birth weights of patients enrolled on the National Wilms' Tumor Study were increased over those of the general population, suggesting that growth factor excess may be an underlying etiology of this malignancy (Beckwith, 1993; Birch & Breslow, 1995; Leisenring, Breslow, Evans, Beckwith, & Grundy, 1994).

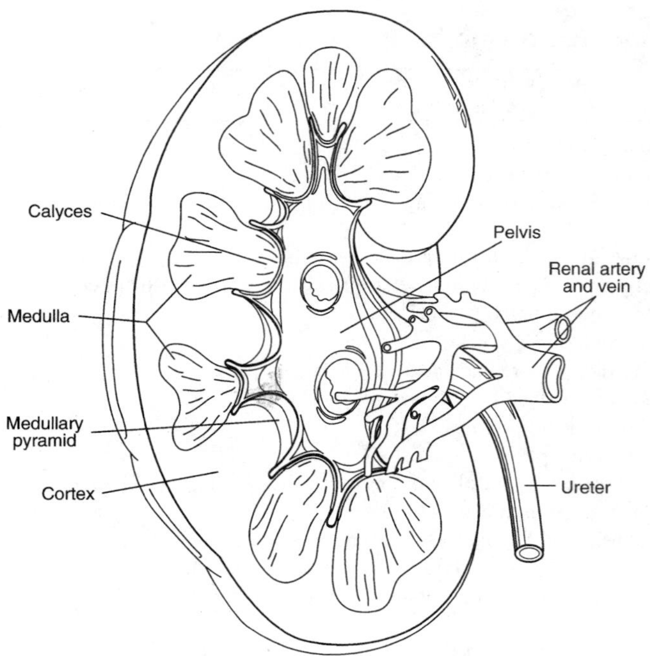

Fig. 70-12 The anatomy of the kidney.

Anatomy of the Kidney and Pathophysiology of Wilms' Tumor

The kidneys are bean-shaped paired organs in the retroperitoneum that have important filtration, reabsorption, and endocrine functions (Fig. 70-12). The renal capsule, a layer of adipose tissue, and a sheet of fascia surround each kidney. These structures protect the kidneys from trauma and infection as they anchor the organs to the abdominal wall and other structures.

The kidneys have three major internal components: the cortex, the medulla, and the collecting system. The functional unit of the kidney is the nephron, which is composed of a glomerulus and tubules. The primary function of cortical nephrons is the reabsorption of water, electrolytes, proteins, and glucose. The medullary nephrons govern the secretion of renin, a hormone important for maintaining normal blood volume and pressure. Together, the cortex and medulla comprise the parenchyma. The collecting system in the renal pelvis is composed of the major and minor calyces, which collect urine from the renal (or medullary) pyramids and divert it to the ureter for excretion (Cohen & Nast, 1996).

Macroscopically, Wilms' tumor is usually a large, multilobulated, friable tumor that arises from the periphery of the renal cortex. Often, a fibrous pseudocapsule separates the tumor mass from the rest of the kidney. The lesion may extend internally or externally and frequently contains large areas of hemorrhage and necrosis (Kirks, Kaufman, & Babcock, 1987).

Microscopically, Wilms' tumor is "triphasic" (i.e., composed of three principal cell types: undifferentiated blastoid cells, differentiated epithelial tissue, and tumor connective tissue or stroma). Beckwith and Palmer (1978) first proposed using histologic features to categorize Wilms' tumors as favorable versus anaplastic. Rhabdoid tumors and clear cell sarcoma are no longer considered Wilms' tumors, but are distinct entities (Schmidt & Beckwith, 1995).

Routes of Metastases for Wilms' Tumor

The child with a Wilms' tumor may have local or distant metastases. The disease may spread locally after breakdown of the tumor's pseudocapsule and direct extension into the kidney, the intrarenal blood vessels, or the lymphatics. Local metastasis often occurs after the tumor erodes the renal capsule (Parham, 1996). Distant metastases develop through hematogenous spread of the tumor to the lung, liver, or regional lymph nodes. The lungs are the most common sites of distant metastases. As reported by the second National Wilms' Tumor Study, the lungs were the only site of metastasis in 80% of patients who had metastatic disease (Grundy, Breslow, Green, Sharples, Evans, & D'Angio, 1989).

Assessment of the Patient for Wilms' Tumor

The assessment of the patient for Wilms' tumor is summarized in Table 70-15. An upper abdominal, one-sided, protuberant mass is frequently the first sign of Wilms' tumor (see Table 70-15). Such a mass is often noted by parents while bathing their young child or by a pediatrician during a well-child examination. Because of tumor-cell–induced increased secretion of renin, hypertension is also a potential sign. Fever and abdominal pain are rare but may occur because of hemorrhage or necrosis in the tumor. Hematuria is rare (Nemes & Donahue, 1994).

Staging of Wilms' Tumor

The staging system for Wilms' tumor is presented in Table 70-16. This staging stratification was developed through the cooperative efforts of two large multicenter clinical trials, the National Wilms' Tumor Study, and the International Society of Pediatric Oncology (Grundy et al., 1989). Residual intraabdominal disease and lymph node involvement are criteria for the diagnosis of advanced-stage disease.

Medical Management of Wilms' Tumor

The medical management of Wilms' tumor includes multimodality therapy, the components of which may depend on the age of the patient and the stage of disease. All patients must have exploratory abdominal surgery, with examination of the contralateral kidney, liver, and regional lymph nodes. Radical nephrectomy is indicated for patients with unilateral disease, and partial nephrectomy is appropriate in cases of bilateral tumor. Additional treatment comprises chemotherapy for nearly all affected children. Radiotherapy is included for patients with advanced disease or adverse prognostic features. Infants younger than 1 year require reduced dosages of chemotherapy and radiotherapy. The doses and schedules of chemotherapy and radiotherapy according to the disease stage are summarized in Table 70-17. Infants less than 24 months with favorable histology and stage I tumors weighing less than 550 g may be cured with nephrec-

TABLE 70-15 Assessment of the Child for Wilms' Tumor

	Assessment Parameters	Typical Abnormal Findings
History	A. Personal, family, and social history 1. Age of child 2. Employment of parent 3. Perinatal history	A. Personal and social risk factors 1. Less than 5 years 2. Often in a metal industry 3. Medications taken by mother during pregnancy, patient's birth weight abnormal, patient has recent weight loss
	B. Evaluation of genitourinary status	B. Recent trauma or infection, abdominal pain
Physical Examination	A. Abdominal inspection and gentle examination by palpation	A. Large, movable abdominal mass; hepatomegaly
	B. Examination of child for associated physical features	B. Presence of aniridia, hemihypertrophy, or characteristic congenital syndromes associated with Wilms' tumor
Diagnostic Tests	A. Laboratory assessment 1. Complete blood count 2. Urinalysis 3. Serum chemistry profile including SGOT, SGPT, BUN, creatinine	A. Laboratory results 1. Anemia secondary to hemorrhage into tumor 2. Hematuria present in 20% of cases 3. Elevated in the presence of extensive disease or hepatic metastasis
	B. Ultrasonography of the abdomen	B. Initially, localized renal tumor; provides dimensions of tumor and information on the integrity of the contralateral kidney and the liver
	C. Computed tomography of the abdomen or magnetic resonance imaging	C. Improved localization of intraabdominal tumors; detects bilateral tumors and presence of tumor in the inferior vena cava
	D. Computed tomography of the chest to assess pulmonary metastatic disease	D. Presence of metastatic tumor nodules in the lungs
	E. Chromosome analysis	E. Rare abnormalities of 11p13 or 11p15.5
	F. Echocardiogram	F. Presence of tumor in right atrium from vena caval extension or for predoxorubicin assessment

SGOT, serum glutamic oxaloacetic transaminase; *SGPT,* serum glutamic pyruvic transaminase; *BUN,* blood urea nitrogen.

TABLE 70-16 Staging System for Wilms' Tumor

Stage	Description
Stage I	Tumor limited to the kidney and is completely excised
Stage II	Tumor extends beyond the kidney but is completely excised
Stage III	Residual tumor is confined to abdomen, nodal involvement, diffuse spillage of tumor
Stage IV	Distant metastases to lung, liver, bone, or brain
Stage V	Bilateral disease at diagnosis

tomy alone. This issue is currently under investigation (Wilimas, Greenwald, & Rao, 1996).

Prognosis for Wilms' Tumor

Overall, the prognosis of disease-free survival is excellent for patients with Wilms' tumor but varies with the stage of the disease. The third National Wilms' Tumor Study documented a 96% 4-year overall survival rate for patients with stage I, favorable histology disease. In contrast, the survival rate for children with stage IV disease and a favorable histology is 55%. Patients with stage IV disease and diffuse and anaplastic histology had only a 20% 4-year survival rate (D'Angio, Breslow, Beckwith, Evans, Baum, & deLorimier et al., 1989). Patients who develop metastatic lesions during initial therapy have poorer prognoses than those who do not, but those who complete chemotherapy before developing recurrent disease have a reasonably favorable prognosis.

Late effects are largely predictable and manageable. These complications include scoliosis in patients treated prior to 1970 (when hemiabdominal radiotherapy was given), anthracycline cardiotoxicity, infertility, and rare benign or malignant second tumors. Long-term treatment-associated morbidity may be reduced when patients are treated in the multidisciplinary setting of a pediatric oncology center.

RHABDOMYOSARCOMA

Epidemiology and Risk Factors for Rhabdomyosarcoma

Approximately 250 children in the United States are diagnosed each year with rhabdomyosarcoma, making it the most common soft tissue sarcoma of childhood. Ragab and colleagues (1986) reported that 80% of the patients with rhabdomyosarcoma in the United States are Caucasian, 12% are African American, and 8% are of other races. Boys develop this neoplasm slightly more frequently than girls (1.4:1) (Miller, Young, & Novakovic, 1995). During the last 10 years, the frequency of childhood rhabdomyosarcoma has increased (Crist, Gehan, Ragab, Dickman, Donaldson, & Fryer et al., 1995). However, this change seems to reflect better case reporting and improved histologic differentiation rather than an actual increase in the incidence of the disease.

Although the mean age at the time of diagnosis for rhabdomyosarcoma is 6 years, two distinct peaks of incidence occur: in children 2 to 6 years of age and in adolescents 15 to 19 years of age. Young children tend to have embryonal tumors of the head and neck or genitourinary system. In contrast, alveolar tumors of the trunk and extremities often occur during adolescence.

Several genetic and environmental risk features have been associated with rhabdomyosarcoma. Li and Fraumeni (1969) first described a familial multiple malignancy syndrome characterized by cases of breast cancer, brain tumors, adrenocortical tumors, osteogenic sarcoma, and soft tissue sarcomas including rhabdomyosarcoma. This syndrome is associated with germline mutations of the p53 tumor suppressor gene. A 1988 review of 115 cases of rhabdomyosarcoma revealed that 32% were associated with congenital anomalies (Ruymann, Maddux, Ragab, Soule, Palmer, & Beltangady et al., 1988), including genitourinary, gastrointestinal, and cardiovascular lesions. Low socioeconomic status, exposure to certain chemicals, and parental age over 30 years have historically been implicated as potential risk factors for rhabdomyosarcoma. However; the most recent report of the Intergroup Rhabdomyosarcoma Study III failed to confirm the carcinogenic influence of these environmental factors (Crist et al., 1995).

Pathophysiology of Rhabdomyosarcoma

Although rhabdomyosarcoma is a malignancy of striated muscle, it can arise in any anatomical location, even in those in which there is little striated muscle. The four most common sites for a primary tumor are the head and neck region (40%), the genitourinary tract (20%), the extremities (20%), and the trunk (10%) (Lanzkowsky, 1995).

Childhood rhabdomyosarcoma is histologically divided into two morphologically distinct subtypes: embryonal and alveolar. The less aggressive embryonal rhabdomyosarcoma represents 75% of all cases and generally affects children younger than 6 years (Rosenberg, 1994). Embryonal rhabdomyosarcomas typically arise in the urogenital tract (bladder, prostate, paratesticular tissues) and in the head and neck area (orbit, middle ear). Grossly, embryonal rhabdomyosarcoma is characterized as a gray-white mass. Microscopically, the tumor cells resemble early fetal striated muscle cells (Miettinen & Weiss, 1996).

The relatively common botryoid subtype of embryonal rhabdomyosarcoma (sarcoma botryoides) is usually found in the walls of hollow mucosa-lined organs such as the nasopharynx, bladder, and vaginal canal. Sarcoma botryoides occurs as a polypoid exophytic mass resembling a bunch of grapes (Parham, 1996). With appropriate treatment, botryoid lesions are associated with an excellent prognosis.

Alveolar rhabdomyosarcoma typically arises in the distal extremities or the head and neck of adolescents. This highly malignant lesion, unlike other sarcomas, tends to metastasize to regional lymph nodes. Small primary lesions may go undetected until dissemination has occurred. Histologically, alveolar rhabdomyosarcoma occurs as nests of undifferentiated round cells; because of poor intercellular cohesion and tumor cell degeneration, small saclike dilatations resembling alveoli are seen (Parham, 1996).

Recently, there has been great progress in clarifying the complex genetic mechanisms that control the normal development of skeletal muscle and in the molecular mapping of tumor-specific chromosomal alterations. These findings have improved our understanding of the pathogenesis of rhabdomyosarcoma (Pappo, Crist, Kuttesch, Rowe, Anhmun, & Maurer et al., 1993). Although rhabdomyosarcoma cells are quite similar in structure to those of normal striated muscle, genetic mutations result in their altered growth and behavior.

TABLE 70-17 Summary of Chemotherapy and Radiotherapy for Wilms' Tumor by Stage and Histology

Disease Stage	Chemotherapy	Radiotherapy
I	Vincristine Dactinomycin	None
II—Favorable histology	Vincristine Dactinomycin	None
III—Favorable histology	Vincristine Dactinomycin Adriamycin	Approximately 12-18 Gy to abdomen
III—Anaplastic histology and IV—Favorable and anaplastic histology	Vincristine Dactinomycin Adriamycin ±Ifosfamide ±Carboplatin ±Etoposide	Doses of 10.8 Gy or above to areas of residual disease

Chromosomal abnormalities have been identified in embryonal and alveolar tumors (Pappo, Shapiro, Crist, & Maurer, 1995; Whang-Peng, Triche, Knutsen, Miser, Kao-Shan, & Tsai et al., 1986). However, the results of cytogenetic studies indicate distinct karyotypic differences. Embryonal tumors are characterized by a loss of heterozygosity in the short arm of chromosome 11. This characteristic is a feature of several pediatric malignancies, including embryonal rhabdomyosarcoma, Wilms' tumor, and neuroblastoma. In contrast to embryonal lesions, alveolar tumors are characterized by a balanced translocation between chromosomes 2 and 13 (Douglass, Valentine, Ectubanas, Parham, Webber, & Houghton et al., 1987). The molecular biology of rhabdomyosarcoma is described in greater detail elsewhere (Parham, 1994).

Routes of Metastases for Rhabdomyosarcoma

Rhabdomyosarcoma is an aggressive malignancy that can extend into adjacent tissues or disseminate through hematogenous or lymphatic vessels. The Intergroup Rhabdomyosarcoma Studies I and II found that one fourth of children with rhabdomyosarcoma have metastases (Crist et al., 1995). The lung was the most common site of metastatic disease. The frequency of metastasis to lymph nodes is not known precisely because the regional lymph nodes are not sampled in all patients. However, the Intergroup Rhabdomyosarcoma studies suggest that metastasis to retroperitoneal lymph nodes occurs in 20% of genitourinary lesions (Maurer, Beltangady, Gehan, Crist, Hammond, & Hayes et al., 1988). Alveolar rhabdomyosarcoma of the extremities, which is particularly aggressive, tends to extend along fascial planes into the surrounding tissue and metastasizes to regional lymph nodes in 15% of the cases (Maurer & Ragab, 1991).

Assessment of the Patient for Rhabdomyosarcoma

Table 70-18 summarizes key factors in the assessment of the child for rhabdomyosarcoma. Rhabdomyosarcoma frequently occurs as a mass lesion or as an interruption of a normal bodily function. Lesions in the head and neck region are usually diagnosed before dissemination occurs. Orbital tumors occur with ptosis or proptosis (Wharam, Beltangady, Heyn, Lawrence, Newton, & Raney et al., 1985). Nasopharyngeal, sinus, or middle-ear rhabdomyosarcomas often produce swelling, pain, or obstruction with or without mucopurulent discharge. Cranial nerve palsy may also occur.

Tumors of the trunk and extremities occur as swellings or masses. Often the diagnosis of these lesions as rhabdomyosarcomas is delayed because such masses frequently are attributed to sports-related trauma. Genitourinary tumors may be accompanied by urinary retention, hematuria, or constipation. Rhabdomyosarcomas of the urinary bladder tend to remain localized, but prostatic and retroperitoneal tumors rapidly metastasize because of the large number of lymph nodes in the retroperitoneum (Carli, Guglielmi, Sotti, Cecchetto, & Ninfo, 1992).

Staging of Rhabdomyosarcoma

Most rhabdomyosarcomas in children are staged according to the surgical and pathologic system developed by the Intergroup Rhabdomyosarcoma Study summarized in Table 70-19 (Lawrence, Gehan, Hays, Beltangady, & Maurer, 1987). In this schema, patients are stratified into clinical groups based on the amount of residual tumor present after initial surgical excision. Because the aggressiveness of rhabdomyosarcoma is multifactorial, many institutions also use a tumor-node-metastasis (TNM) staging system (Table 70-20). To incorporate a variety of clinical risk features in the tailoring, this staging method stratifies patients according to the extent of the tumor (size of the lesion and presence of metastases) at the time of diagnosis. Staging according to the TNM system does not depend on the efficacy of the initial surgery (Pappo, Shapiro, Crist, & Maurer, 1995).

Medical Management of Rhabdomyosarcoma

The optimal medical management of rhabdomyosarcoma incorporates multimodality therapy comprising surgical resection, radiotherapy, and chemotherapy. The goal of surgical resection is the removal of all of the tumor with an adequate margin of uninvolved tissue without major functional or cosmetic impairment. If a lesion cannot be removed completely, a biopsy is obtained. These patients then receive chemotherapy and radiation therapy to shrink the tumor followed by second-look surgery to resect any remaining disease. Because regional lymph nodes frequently contain metastatic rhabdomyosarcoma, routine biopsies of these nodes are recommended (Lawrence, Hays, Heyn, Tefft, Crist, & Beltangady et al., 1987). Mutilating procedures (e.g., pelvic exenteration) are rarely indicated in pediatric cancer care.

All patients with rhabdomyosarcoma, except those with localized, completely resected disease, receive radiotherapy. Because this neoplasm is only moderately sensitive to radiation, high doses are used and the doses are not modified based on the patient's age or the size of the tumor (Lanzkowski, 1995). Doses of 40 Gy are sufficient in cases of microscopic residual tumor after surgical resection. However, even 50 to 60 Gy fail to eliminate macroscopic residual disease, especially in patients with large tumors. Doses in excess of 60 Gy can be associated with the unacceptable toxicities of severe fibrosis and reduced function in irradiated sites (D'Angio, Clatworthy, Evana, Newton, & Tefft, 1978). In addition, high doses of radiation predispose survivors of childhood cancer to secondary malignancies in the radiation ports.

To deliver a tumorcidal dose of radiation while maintaining a safety margin for normal tissues, Eifel (1988) suggested hyperfractionation, dividing the daily dose of radiation therapy into two or more smaller fractions. A 1984-1986 Memorial Sloan Kettering Cancer Center study confirmed the benefit of hyperfractionated radiation in 12 children with gross residual disease (Mandell, Ghavimi, Exelby, & Fuks, 1988). A pilot study of the Intergroup Rhabdomyosarcoma Study IV is investigating

TABLE 70-18 Assessment of the Pediatric Patient for Rhabdomyosarcoma

	Assessment Parameters	Typical Abnormal Findings
History	A. Personal, family, and social history 1. History of progression, sequence of symptoms	A. Family cancer constellation 1. Diagnosis delayed (often by weeks to months)
Physical Examination	A. All patients should have a detailed physical examination and assessment of cranial nerves B. Examination of patient specific to primary site of tumor	
	1. Head and neck area	1. Asymptomatic mass, proptosis, epistaxis, cranial nerve palsy, swelling, sinusitis, hoarse or nasal speech, strabismus
	2. Genitourinary tract	2. Painless abdominal or genitourinary mass, urinary retention, vaginal bleeding, dysuria
	3. Trunk	3. Asymptomatic mass, ascites, gastrointestinal obstruction, hepatomegaly, constipation
	4. Extremity	4. Painless mass of swelling, regional lymph node enlargement, ecchymoses
Diagnostic Tests	A. Laboratory assessment	A. Typical laboratory findings
	1. Complete blood count	1. Anemia; pancytopenia in patients with advanced disease
	2. Urinalysis	2. Hematuria in patients with genitourinary involvement
	3. Serum chemistry profile, electrolytes, BUN, creatinine, LDH, SGOT, SGPT, alkaline phosphatase	3. Abnormal values in patients with obstruction
	4. Histologic examination of bone marrow	4. Abnormal cells in patients with metastatic disease; also cytogenic abnormalities
	5. Histologic examination of the cerebrospinal fluid	5. Pleocytosis, increased protein, and decreased glucose of the cerebrospinal fluid indicative of metastatic disease in patients with meningeal seeding
	B. Diagnostic imaging	B. Typical abnormal findings
	1. Magnetic resonance imaging of primary lesion	1. Especially valuable in determining extent and resectability of disease
	2. Computed tomography of primary lesion and lungs	2. Pulmonary nodules, bone erosion secondary to tumor
	3. Ultrasonography of abdomen and retroperitoneum	3. Retroperitoneal lymph node enlargement in patients with advanced-stage disease
Surgical Evaluation	A. Biopsy	
	1. Primary tumor	1. Pathology consistent with small round cell tumor
	2. Suspicious lymph nodes	2. Determination of metastatic spread of disease

BUN, blood urea nitrogen; *LDH*, lactate dehydrogenase; *SGOT*, serum glutamic oxaloacetic transaminase; *SGPT*, serum glutamic pyruvic transaminase.

the efficacy of 5490 cGy delivered in 54 fractions over 27 days.

In contrast to its response to radiation, childhood rhabdomyosarcoma is a chemosensitive tumor. Effective single agents include cyclophosphamide, actinomycin-D, vincristine, cisplatin, high-dose methotrexate, doxorubicin, melphlan, ifosfamide, and etoposide. The single-agent efficacy of these drugs is enhanced when they are given in sequential combinations; the exact protocol depends on the stage and clinical group of the lesion. Children who have small, completely resected, favorable histology tumors (Clinical Group I) typically are treated with vincristine and actinomycin-D for 1 year. Patients with advanced-stage or refractory rhabdomyosarcoma (Clinical Group IV) often receive high-dose carboplatin, ifosfamide, and etoposide followed by autologous bone marrow transplantation. The chemotherapy of children with rhabdomyosarcoma is reviewed in detail elsewhere (Raney, Tefft, Hays, & Triche, 1993).

Prognosis for Rhabdomyosarcoma

The relative weight of various prognostic factors in rhabdomyosarcoma is unknown. The stage or extent of disease, histology, and location of the tumor are all important prognostic factors that cannot be evaluated independently. The Intergroup Rhabdomyosarcoma Group

TABLE 70-19 Classification System of the Intergroup Rhabdomyosarcoma Study

Group	Description
Clinical Group I	A. Localized, completely resected tumor B. Localized tumor extends beyond site of origin but is completely resected
Clinical Group II	A. Localized tumor is grossly resected, with microscopic residual disease B. Regional disease (involving lymph nodes), completely resected C. Regional disease (involving lymph nodes), grossly resected, with microscopic residual disease
Clinical Group III	A. Gross residual local or regional disease after biopsy only B. Gross residual disease after ≥50% resection of primary tumor
Clinical Group IV	Distant metastases present at diagnosis

TABLE 70-20 Tumor–Lymph Node Metastasis Staging Scheme from the Intergroup Rhabdomyosarcoma Study

A	Localized tumor with favorable histology and clinically negative nodes
B	Locally extensive tumor with favorable histology and clinically negative lymph nodes
C	Tumor with clinically involved regional lymph nodes and/or unfavorable histology
D	Distant metastasis
Tumor:	
T_{site1}*	Confined to anatomic site or origin (a) Maximum diameter <5 cm (b) Maximum diameter ≥5 cm
T_{site2}	Extension or fixation to surrounding tissues (a) Maximum diameter <5 cm (b) Maximum diameter ≥5 cm
Regional lymph nodes:	
N0	Regional nodes not clinically involved
N1	Regional nodes clinically involved by neoplasm
NX	Clinical status of regional nodes unknown
Metastasis:	
M0	No distant metastasis
$M1_{site}$*	Metastases present

*Subscript for T_{site} indicates location of primary tumor; subscript for M_{site} indicates location of metastatic disease.

analyzed the prognostic features of different subgroups of patients in three consecutive clinical trials: IRS-I (1972-1978, n = 686), IRS-II (1978-1984, n = 999), and IRS-III (1984-1991, n = 1062) (Crist et al., 1995; Maurer et al., 1988; Maurer, Gehan, Beltangady, Crist, Dickman, & Donaldson et al., 1993). In each of these studies, patients were assigned based on their presenting signs and symptoms to one of three clinical groups. The prognostic factors associated with each clinical group were evaluated by multivariate analysis.

Overall, these Intergroup Rhabdomyosarcoma Studies confirmed that the extent of disease, tumor histology, and size of the lesion are important prognostic factors (Crist et al., 1995). Children who had localized disease and no detectable metastases had a better outcome than those with widespread disease. Patients whose disease was completely resected fared better than children with gross residual disease after surgical resection who, in turn, had a better outcome than those with metastatic disease.

The histology of the rhabdomyosarcoma tumor also influences prognosis. Patients with embryonal lesions have better survival rates than those with alveolar masses. However, uncertainty remains regarding the relative importance of histology and site of the primary tumor. In 1991, Rodary, Gehan, Flamant, Treuner, Carli, & Auquier et al. suggested that the primary site was the most important predictor of survival. In that series, children with orbital tumors fared better than those with trunk or extremity lesions. The genitourinary site was a favorable prognostic feature in the Intergroup Rhabdomyosarcoma Study I (Crist et al., 1995). The size of the lesion is an important prognostic factor. Among 951 children with rhabdomyosarcoma, those with lesions smaller than 5 cm in diameter had a better prognosis than patients whose tumor diameters were at least 5 cm (Rodary et al., 1991). The prognostic significance of the various genetic markers of rhabdomyosarcoma is currently unknown.

OSTEOSARCOMA

Epidemiology and Risk Factors for Osteosarcoma

Osteosarcoma accounts for 60% of the malignant bone neoplasms diagnosed during the first two decades of life. Most series report a few more male than female patients with this neoplasm (Dahlin, & Coventry, 1967; Huvos, 1991), and the child with osteosarcoma is slightly more likely to be Caucasian than African American, Hispanic, or Asian. Osteosarcomas predominantly arise in the long bones of the body; 50% of these lesions occur in the femur, 26% in the tibia, and 10% in the humerus. About 10% of osteosarcomas affect flat bones (e.g., the pelvis and skull; Huvos, 1991).

The etiology of osteosarcoma is obscure. Various genetic factors have been implicated. Bilateral retinoblastoma is a potential risk factor for the development of osteosarcoma. In addition, cases of osteosarcoma have been reported among patients with familial cancer constellations, such as Li-Fraumeni syndrome (Li & Fraumeni, 1969).

The development of osteosarcoma is associated with several clinical observations. The peak incidence of osteosarcoma occurs at about the same time as the adolescent growth spurt, and this malignancy frequently develops in patients who are taller than average. Therefore rapid bone growth may play a role in the development of this tumor (Link & Eilber, 1993). In addition, osteosarcoma arises almost exclusively in the metaphysis of the long, weight-bearing bones (e.g., the distal femur and the proximal tibia). Chronic bone injury secondary to weight-bearing trauma is a possible etiology for this neoplasm (Tjalma, 1966). Frequently, adolescent patients have a history of acute trauma in an area of osteosarcoma. However, this trauma only serves to call attention to a preexisting lesion and is not believed to be a risk factor in this malignancy.

Finally, 3% of osteosarcomas arise in previously irradiated bone after a latency period of 4 to 40 years. Dahlin and Coventry (1967) associated this incidence with high doses of orthovoltage irradiation. Recent data show that secondary osteosarcomas can also occur after megavoltage irradiation. Treatment with high doses of alkylating agents may potentiate the development of secondary osteosarcoma or may cause osseous malignancies independent of treatment with radiation (Tucker, D'Angio, Boice, Strong, Li, & Stovall et al., 1987). Osteosarcoma was the most common second malignancy among more than 300 survivors of childhood cancer reported in 1991 by the Late Effects Study Group (Newton, Meadows, Shimada, Bunin, & Vawter, 1991).

Pathophysiology of Osteosarcoma

Osteosarcoma cells produce bone matrix, as do several normal bone cells. The osteoprogenitor cells, osteoblasts, and osteocytes are involved in the formation and maintenance of normal bones. Osteoprogenitor cells are multipotential stem cells that produce the precursors of osteoblasts. Osteoblasts are located on the surface of a bone and are responsible for mineralizing bone and producing the bone matrix. After osteoblasts are surrounded with bone matrix, they become osteocytes. Osteocytes are not as metabolically active as osteoblasts, but they have many important regulatory functions, such as the resorption of bone (Rosenberg, 1994).

Based on their shapes, the bones of the body are divided into four types: irregular bones, short bones, flat bones, and long bones. The anatomy of a long bone (Fig. 70-13) comprises the diaphysis (the shaft of the bone), epiphysis (the end of a bone), metaphysis (where the diaphysis joins the epiphysis), periosteum (a dense fibrous membrane surrounding the bone), a medullary (marrow) cavity, and the endosteum (the lining of the medullary cavity). Osteosarcoma may develop in any area of any bone of the body.

The pathology, histologic features, genetics, and routes of metastases of osteosarcoma are important in understanding the clinical presentation and treatment of osteosarcoma. Childhood osteosarcoma is classified into two major categories: intramedullary (occurring in the bone) or juxtacortical (occurring on the surface of the bone).

There are several histologic subtypes of osteosarcoma. The form most frequently diagnosed during childhood and adolescence, classic osteoblastic osteosarcoma, is an intramedullary tumor that is characterized by abundant osteoid tissue. Osteoblastic osteosarcomas may contain chondroblastic (cartilagineous) and fibroblastic (fibrous tissue) elements in various proportions. Historically, telangiectatic osteosarcoma (in which the tumor has a cystic appearance) has been associated with pathologic fractures and poor outcomes (Matsuno, Unni, McLeod, & Dahlin, 1976).

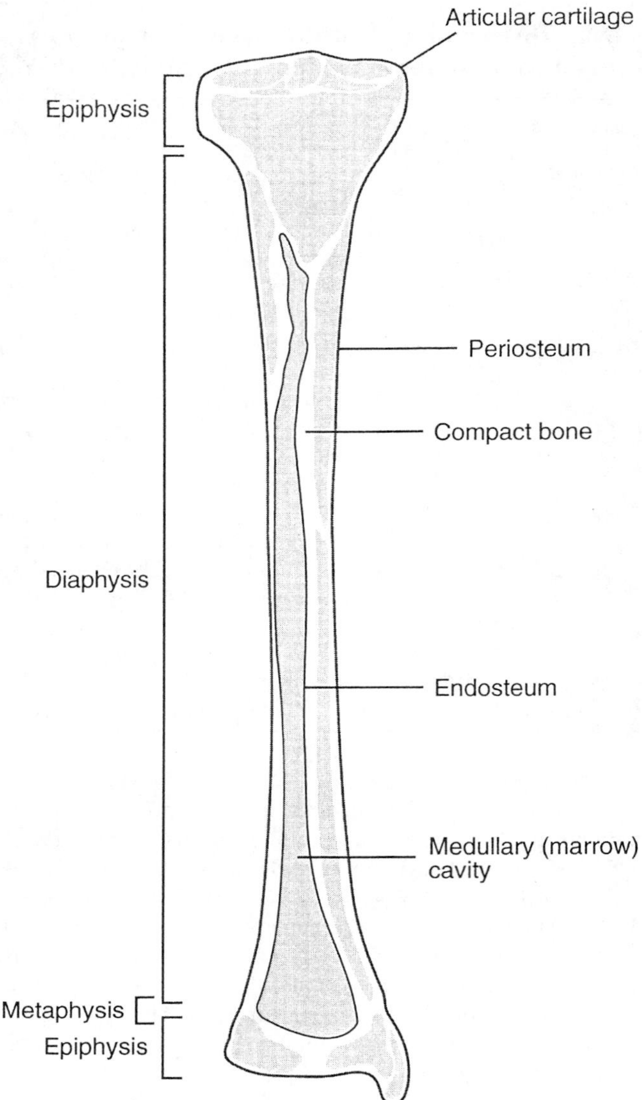

Fig. 70-13 The anatomy of a long bone.

Juxtacortical osteosarcomas include those on and in the periosteum. These parosteal and periosteal lesions arise from the cortex of a bone, rarely involve the medullary cavity, and tend to reoccur locally. In addition, distant metastases are rare (Webber & Parham, 1996). A few patients have multifocal osteosarcoma, in which multicentric tumors of equivalent size can develop synchronously or asynchronously. Unfortunately, such patients have a dismal prognosis.

Grossly, osteosarcomas resemble cumulus clouds. Tumors characteristically erode through the periosteum and

TABLE 70-21 Assessment of the Pediatric Patient for Osteosarcoma

	Assessment Parameters	Typical Abnormal Findings
History	A. Personal and social history	A. Personal and social risk factors
	1. Age	1. Adolescent; development of osteosarcoma associated with rapid growth
	2. Duration of symptoms	2. Prolonged symptoms may indicate indolent tumor
	3. Pain in other bony sites	3. Pain may indicate metastatic disease
Physical Examination	A. Examination of affected area	A. Soft tissue mass at the site of primary tumor; ecchymoses in patients with pathologic fractures
	B. Weight, lymph node evaluation	B. Systemic symptoms only prominent in advanced disease
Diagnostic Tests	A. Diagnostic imaging	A. Key to diagnosis of osteosarcoma
	1. Posterior-anterior and lateral views of the affected bone	1. Lytic to sclerotic destruction of normal bone, indistinct margins (radial "starburst" pattern), no endosteal bone response, soft tissue mass
	2. Computed tomography of the involved bone	2. Reveals local extent of tumor
	3. Magnetic resonance imaging of the involved bone	3. Addresses local extent of tumor, especially intraosseous extent and extent to muscles, fat, joints, or neurovascular structures
	4. Chest radiographs (four views)	4. Metastatic lesions in advanced disease
	5. Computed tomography of the chest	5. Improved identification of metastatic nodules, especially pleura-based lesions
	6. Technetium-99m bone scan	6. Metastasis to other bones in 10% of cases; baseline assessment of vascularity of the primary lesion
	B. Laboratory tests	
	1. Serum chemistry evaluation	1. Alkaline phosphatase and lactic dehydrogenase levels elevated in some patients; abnormal liver functions in patients with advanced metastatic disease; provides baseline for pretreatment status of renal and hepatic function
	2. Coagulation studies (PT, PTT, fibrinogen)	2. Abnormalities in patients with advanced disease
	C. Cardiac evaluation: echocardiogram and electrocardiogram	C. Baseline, pretreatment data
	D. Surgical biopsy	D. Histologically proven osteosarcoma

PT, prothrombin time; *PTT*, partial thromboplastin time.

invade soft tissues. The tumor may also extend into the medullary cavity, and as many as 20% of patients have "skip" lesions (foci of tumor separate from the primary lesion) (Enneking & Kagan, 1975). Depending on the amount of tumorous bone produced, the lesions appear sclerotic, lytic, or mixed in character upon histologic examination.

Genetic mutations are important factors in the etiology of osteosarcoma. Children with familial retinoblastoma have a 500 times increased risk of developing osteosarcoma in an extremity and a 2000 times increased risk of developing osteosarcoma in a previously irradiated bone of the skull (Smith, Donaldson, & Egbert, Link, & Bagshaw, 1989). These patients have a mutated allele of the retinoblastoma gene (RB1, on chromosome 13), a tumor suppressor gene. Somatic inactivation of the normal allele then leads to uncontrolled cell proliferation. Rearrangements in another tumor suppressor, the p53 gene, are also associated with osteosarcoma (Wadayama, Toguchida, Yamaguchi, Saski, & Yamamuro, 1993). Radiation can lead to mutation of the RB1 or p53 locus and secondary osteosarcoma. Finally, osteosarcoma may occur as the result of abnormal expression of growth factors (e.g., CDK4) or the over-expression of c-*fos* (Parham, 1996).

Routes of Metastases for Osteosarcoma

Osteosarcoma metastasizes hematogenously to the lungs, and 20% of patients have pulmonary metastases. Historically, 80% of patients treated with amputation alone developed lung metastases. Metastatic disease to other bones of the body occurs in 10% of patients. Bloem and Kroon (1993) found that metastatic osteosarcoma in less common sites (e.g., liver and kidney) increased with survival.

Assessment of the Patient for Osteosarcoma

The earliest symptoms in patients with osteosarcoma include progressive pain in the involved bone, development of a firm mass, and decreased range of motion in the affected extremity. Although rare, pathologic fractures can occur at the site. Osteosarcoma must be differentiated from other benign conditions that can mimic the malignancy, such as stress fractures and osteoblastomas. The assessment of a pediatric patient for osteosarcoma (Table 70-21) must address the extent of the primary lesions, as well as the presence of metastatic disease.

Staging of Osteosarcoma

Patients with osteosarcoma are categorized only with regard to the presence or absence of metastatic disease at the time of diagnosis. No specific clinical staging system is currently available, despite evidence showing that the size and local extent of the primary tumor influences prognosis (Spanier, Shuster, & Vender Griend, 1990).

Medical Management of Osteosarcoma

The medical management of osteosarcoma (National Comprehensive Cancer Network, 1996) includes multiagent chemotherapy and surgical resection of the tumor. This current therapeutic plan is based on the early work of Jaffe (1972) and Rosen, Caparros, Huvos, Kosloff, Nirenberg, & Cacavio et al. (1982), who used "neoadjuvant" (preoperative) chemotherapy to destroy micrometastatic disease and facilitate limb-sparing procedures (en bloc resection of tumor-involved bones and insertion of a synthetic prosthesis). These and other studies showed that presurgical chemotherapy does not increase the risk of relapse, facilitates the prediction of outcome, and may sufficiently reduce the size of the primary lesion to allow limb-sparing procedures.

Chemotherapeutic regimens used to treat osteosarcoma usually include high-dose methotrexate, doxorubicin, cisplatin or carboplatin, and ifosfamide or cyclophosphamide. Several centers add bleomycin, vincristine, or dactinomycin to the treatment regimen. Patients receive up to 3 months of chemotherapy before surgery and an additional 9 to 10 months of treatment afterward.

The primary osteosarcoma lesion may require amputation or en bloc resection (a limb-sparing procedure). Eligibility criteria for limb-sparing procedures in pediatric patients include the following: no neurovascular involvement by the tumor, adequate disease-free distal and proximal surgical margins, and acceptable preservation of function. Limb-sparing measures are most often successful in patients who have achieved most of their linear growth. However, Lewis (1986) proposed the use of an expandable prosthesis that can "grow" with the child.

Patients with resectable lung disease should be treated with thoracotomy and removal of all masses. Bilateral disease is not a contraindication to surgical resection of pulmonary metastases. Many pulmonary lesions can be removed by wedge resection, thereby preserving the maximum possible amount of normal lung tissue (Meyer, Schell, Kumar, Rao, Green, & Champion et al., 1987).

Osteosarcoma is a radioresistant tumor. Only transient tumor control is achieved, even with radiation doses exceeding 60 Gy. However, high-dose radiotherapy is sometimes used palliatively in children with advanced, unresectable disease.

Immunotherapy for osteosarcoma has not yielded promising results. Green, Pratt, Webster, & Smith (1976) found that, even when given in conjunction with adjuvant chemotherapy, nonspecific immune stimulation with bacillus Calmette-Guerin (BCG) vaccine did not improve patient survival. Although interferon inhibited the growth of osteosarcoma cells in vitro, it failed to increase the relapse-free survival of patients (Strander & Einhorn, 1977).

Prognosis for Osteosarcoma

Several clinical factors associated with osteosarcoma have prognostic significance. The most important factor is the extent of disease at the time of diagnosis—patients with metastatic lesions have a less favorable outcome. Some histologic subtypes (e.g., parosteal osteosarcoma) have a relatively favorable prognosis. Secondary osteosarcomas in survivors of familial retinoblastoma or in areas of previous radiation are associated with a poor prognosis (Webber & Parham, 1996). In addition, the site and size of the primary tumor are important prognostic factors.

Finally, the response of the primary osteosarcoma lesion to preoperative chemotherapy is an important prognostic factor. In fact, Rosen and colleagues (1982) contend that response to chemotherapy is the best prognostic factor. In their review of the Memorial Sloan-Kettering experience, female gender was also associated with a favorable outcome. Poor risk features included patient age younger than 10 years at the time of diagnosis, an elevated alkaline phosphatase level, and a tumor with telangiectatic characteristics.

BONE MARROW TRANSPLANTATION FOR CHILDHOOD CANCERS

Over the last three decades, bone marrow transplantation (BMT) has evolved to become an accepted treatment modality for several pediatric malignancies. Children with acute or chronic leukemia, lymphoma, neuroblastoma, and a variety of other solid tumors have been successfully treated with a bone marrow transplant. As in adults, the type of transplant used depends on the disease being treated, stage of disease, patient's age, and the donor source available. Autologous and allogeneic marrow transplants are used in the pediatric setting. The use of peripheral blood stem cells (PBSCs) to restore hematopoiesis is increasing. However, harvesting PBSCs from children remains problematic, both physiologically and psychologically. Another approach under investigation is the use of stem cells that are obtained from the umbilical cord at delivery and stored for future use. The small quantity of cord blood that can be harvested limits the applicability of this approach (Abramovitz & Senner, 1995).

Bone Marrow Transplantation for Leukemia and Lymphoma

Of the 5500 allogeneic BMTs performed in 1990 and reported to the International Bone Marrow Transplant Registry, approximately 40% were in children younger than 16 years. About 60% of those transplants were performed for the treatment of leukemia, primarily ALL (Horowitz & Bortin, 1993). Allogeneic BMT is an effective treatment for many stages of leukemia and often has curative potential. Disease-free survival (DFS) rates of 63% to 84% have been reported for children with ALL who received an allogeneic BMT during their first remission. This statistic drops to 40% to 60% for those receiving transplants during the second remission of ALL. The results are less favorable (DFS, 10% to 30%) for children with ALL who receive transplants during the third or later remission or during relapse (Balduzzi, Gooley, Anasetti, Sanders, Martin, & Petersdoff et al., 1995; Chao & Forman, 1994; Horowitz & Bortin, 1993).

Several published studies have demonstrated that allogeneic BMT is superior to conventional chemotherapy for children with AML. The best results (DFS, 50% to 80%) are reported for allogeneic transplants performed during the first remission of AML. Children in second remission or with advanced disease have done significantly worse, with associated DFS rates of 10% to 45%.

Allogeneic BMT is the treatment of choice for children with CML because conventional chemotherapy typically is not curative. The best posttransplantation results have been achieved in patients with CML who receive transplants during the chronic phase of the disease and within 1 year of diagnosis. For these patients, DFS rates of 50% to 85% have been reported. The reported DFS estimates for patients receiving transplants after their leukemia has progressed to the accelerated or blast phase are 12% to 40% (Abramovitz & Senner, 1995; Champlin & McGlave, 1994; Horowitz & Bortin, 1993).

The selection of the conditioning regimen is influenced by the type of transplant and the patient's disease and age. Most conditioning regimens for allogeneic transplants to leukemia patients prescribe a combination of chemotherapeutic agents and total body irradiation (TBI). The most commonly used chemotherapeutic agents include busulfan, cyclophosphamide, and cytosine arabinoside (Abramovitz, 1991; Abramovitz & Senner, 1995; Frederick & Hanigan, 1993).

The benefit of autologous BMT is unclear for children with AML. A variety of conditioning regimens containing multiple drug combinations, with and without TBI, have been used. The role of marrow purging remains controversial, and limited data are available from cases of pediatric AML that were treated with autologous BMT. The estimate of event-free survival is 50% to 70% for patients who receive autologous BMT during their first remission of AML. This figure drops to 30% to 40% for those receiving transplants during the second remission (Horowitz & Bortin, 1993).

Bone marrow transplantation is reserved for patients with aggressive or relapsed HD or NHL because combined modality therapy (multiagent chemotherapy and radiotherapy) is highly effective in cases of malignant lymphoma. Because bone marrow involvement is less frequent in lymphoma than leukemia, patients with HD or NHL typically undergo autologous BMT. Estimated DFS rates of 30% to 40% are reported after autologous BMT for relapsed HD and NHL, whereas the few small studies of allogeneic BMT for relapsed lymphomas demonstrate a DFS rate of approximately 20%. Conditioning regimens for autologous BMT in patients with HD or NHL usually consist of combination chemotherapy alone, and cytarabine, carmustine, cyclophosphamide, melphalan, and etoposide are the most frequently used agents (Bierman & Armitage, 1994; Jones, 1994; Phillips, 1994).

Bone Marrow Transplantation for Solid Tumors

Some pediatric solid tumors are very sensitive to chemotherapy, which can effectively result in remission and cure of the primary disease. Unfortunately, metastatic disease at the time of diagnosis or relapse is very common. Consequently, autologous BMT has been used in a variety of pediatric solid tumors to improve complete remission rates and long-term survival. Neuroblastoma continues to have an extremely poor prognosis, with about two thirds of patients having metastatic disease. High-dose chemotherapy and autologous BMT may improve the treatment outcome for these patients. The most effective use of autotransplant is in children with advanced-stage disease who have obtained a partial or complete response with combination chemotherapy with surgery and local radiation therapy and before disease progression. The most common drugs used in the conditioning regimen include melphalan, cisplatin, carmustine, teniposide, carboplatin, and etoposide. The role of purged marrow remains unclear. To date, purged marrow has not had a significant effect on long-term survival. Studies conducted over the last 10 years suggest that long-term DFS can be achieved in 20% to 40% of patients treated with intensive therapy and autologous BMT (Johnson, & Goldman, 1993; Ladenstein, Hartmann, & Pinkerton, 1993; Seeger & Reynolds, 1994).

In children with other solid tumors, such as rhabdomyosarcoma, Ewing sarcoma, Wilms' tumor, and brain tumors, autologous BMT may have a role. However, interpretation of the findings from existing studies is difficult due to the heterogeneity of patients, conditioning regimens, disease stage, and short follow-up. Encouraging results are reported in the treatment of medulloblastoma, but the effect on survival has been minimal. As in neuroblastoma, autologous BMT may be considered for high-grade or relapsed chemosensitive solid tumors such as rhabdomyosarcoma, with varied results reported (Abramovitz & Senner, 1995; Ladenstein, Hartmann, & Pinkerton, 1993).

Nursing Management of Children Undergoing Bone Marrow Transplantation

The complications and many aspects of the nursing care of patients who receive a BMT are similar in the pediatric and adult populations. The complications associated with allogeneic and autologous transplants include pancytopenia, immune suppression, mucositis, nausea and vomiting, diarrhea, fluid and electrolyte imbalance, nutritional deficits, renal insufficiency, skin breakdown, and pain. Additional complications most often associated with allogeneic transplantation are veno-occlusive disease, hemorrhagic cystitis, and graft-versus-host disease (GVHD). The incidence and severity of GVHD and of organ damage from the conditioning regimen may be reduced in children, who may better tolerate the procedure and have better outcomes than adult patients (Abramovitz, 1991; Frederick & Hanigan, 1993).

The psychosocial issues associated with pediatric BMT are dramatically different than those in adult patients. Understanding normal growth and development, as well as family-centered care, is essential to the pediatric BMT nurse. Behaviors commonly observed in hospitalized children include anxiety, fear of death, anger, regression, dependence, and lack of cooperation. Understanding the major developmental milestones for each age group serves as a foundation for patient care and nursing interventions.

During the pretransplant period, nurses play a key role in coordinating services and education. Financial concerns and care of siblings at home are a constant worry for families, and the welfare of the sibling donor is a great concern for parents. All pediatric donors and recipients must be adequately informed and prepared at the age-appropriate level. Participation in the consent process often depends on the child's age and level of cognitive development.

During the transplant and posttransplant period, the role of the nurse includes direct physical care of the child and the emotional support of the child, family, and extended family members, such as grandparents. Infants and toddlers may require sedation or general anesthesia to ensure that the child remains still during radiation therapy. The day of marrow infusion is highly emotional, charged with anticipation and expectation. Parents of sibling donors are especially stressed with the care of two children. While the child and parents await engraftment and recovery from complications, the nurse provides education regarding daily care needs, medication, infection control, and symptoms warranting medical supervision in anticipation of discharge.

Most pediatric transplant units encourage parental participation in the child's care and a liberal visiting policy; many allow parents to stay overnight with the child. Discharge criteria vary, depending on the type of transplant performed and the institution. Each transplant center develops specific posttransplant guidelines and discharge instructions, including the length of time the child and family must remain in close proximity to the transplant center. School, the work of the child, is continued throughout the transplant process by hospital-based or home teachers.

Common home care issues include avoiding infections, managing posttransplant complications (GVHD, nausea, vomiting, or diarrhea), meeting nutritional needs, and facilitating normal growth and development. Late effects of BMT require long-term follow-up in pediatric patients. Children experience many of the same late effects seen in adults, such as infections, chronic GVHD, cataracts, restrictive lung disease, secondary malignancies, and relapse. The late effects involving growth and development, as well as endocrine function, are of special concern in children. The likelihood of long-term sequelae are greater with the more toxic conditioning regimens. For example, a combination of chemotherapy and radiation increases the incidence of growth retardation, gonadal failure, hypothyroidism, and developmental delays (Abramovitz, 1991; Abramovitz & Senner, 1995).

Bone marrow transplantation offers hope and a chance of cure for many children with pediatric cancers. Nurses play an important role in the success of BMT with their involvement in the care of the patients, as well as research. Future areas for attention and research include minimizing acute complications and late effects, developing creative and cost-effective strategies to deliver care, and exploring survivor issues. The challenge of BMT nursing is to remain abreast of evolving therapy and technology changes. The joy of BMT nursing is to see children grow and live healthy, productive lives.

NURSING MANAGEMENT OF CHILDREN WITH CANCER

The practice of pediatric oncology nursing spans a long continuum of care—from primary prevention through early detection of disease to palliative care. At any point along the continuum, care can be provided in a variety of settings, which include the inpatient clinic, the outpatient clinic, hospices, and the patient's home. In these settings, the pediatric oncology nurse may be a caregiver, educator, coordinator, collaborator, researcher, or community activist; these roles are not mutually exclusive.

Beginning at the time of diagnosis, one of the pediatric oncology nurse's primary functions is to interpret medical information for the child and family. The patient's specific plan of care varies with the child's diagnosis, the stage of the disease, and the child's age. Specific details about the pathogenesis of the disease and the planned therapy help families understand treatment options and anticipate toxicities of therapy. Four management issues common to all pediatric patients (pain, nausea and vomiting, nutrition, and fever and neutropenia) are discussed below.

Pain

Little information is available on the prevalence and severity of pain in pediatric cancer patients, even though managing pain in these children poses a prominent challenge for nurses. In a research review of the problem of pain in children with cancer, Sutters and Miaskowski (1992) identified 31 reports on pediatric cancer pain. Most of the studies were descriptive reports of small numbers of patients and focused on the pain and distress associated with medical procedures (e.g., bone marrow aspiration and lumbar puncture). However, in one study, 50% of the children who were hospitalized and 25% of the outpatients had pain that was not due to a diagnostic procedure (Miser, Dothage, Wesley, & Miser, 1987).

In the pediatric oncology setting, pain must be differentiated as procedure related (short duration usually related to treatments or diagnostic tests), continuing (related to disease or surgery or a side-effect of treatment that occurs over time), or phantom (itching, burning, or stabbing sensations that persist or develop after an amputation). The plan of care for each child depends on the type and intensity of the pain experienced. In addition, pain in children is often compounded by other clinical symptoms such as nausea, fatigue, weakness, and dyspnea, which must be managed.

To identify clinically useful and accurate measurements for assessing pain in pediatric oncology patients, West, Oakes, Hinds, Sanders, Holden, & Williams et al. (1994) asked patients, parents, and staff members to evaluate three frequently used pediatric pain rating scales: the Faces Pain Scale, the Poker Chip Tool, and the Oective Pain Scale. Most of the study population preferred the Faces Pain Scale, a scale of five faces reflecting emotions from happy to crying. However, this instrument is limited to patients who can participate in a self-report measurement.

As a prelude to managing pain according to the standard of care developed at St. Jude's Children's Research Hospital (Table 70-22), children older than 3 years are asked to score their pain intensity by using the Faces Pain Scale. Pain in children under 3 is assessed by observing behavioral or

TABLE 70-22 Standard of Care for Pain Management in Pediatric Cancer Patients

Patient Outcomes	Nursing Intervention and Rationales	Patient Education Instructions
The patient will: • Experience an optimal level of pain relief and can expect his or her report of pain to be accepted and analyzed (assessed) and interventions taken (acted on). The patient and family (when applicable) will: • Understand pain and pain-prevention measures. • Participate in pain-management interventions. • Indicate the presence and intensity of pain. • Express pain relief. • Rest/sleep and participate in activities of daily living.	1. Know about the definition and types of pain. 2. Know about effective pain management, including the following: a. Preventing pain by (1) decreasing pain stimuli and (2) administering analgesia on a regular or continuous basis (versus PRN) b. Pharmacologic methods of pain control, such as opioid and nonopioid medications and EMLA cream c. Nonpharmacologic methods 3. Know about fears and myths associated with use of analgesics (fear of addiction and drug-seeking behaviors). 4. Appropriately assess pain in patients of all developmental stages by doing the following: a. Asking the patient (self-report method) if he or she is having any pain. This is done by the nurse at the time of each outpatient visit or as part of the initial assessment of each shift of inpatient care b. Writing "0" if the patient expresses no pain c. Asking the patient to score pain intensity, location, and quality (shooting, sharp, stabbing, cramping, aching). To measure intensity, do the following: (1) Use Faces Pain Scale for patients who are at least 5 years old (use may be attempted for younger children). (2) If unable to use a scale, document patient's own words or behaviors. d. Obtaining other assessment information as appropriate, including the following: (1) Timing and pattern of pain (2) Associated symptoms (3) Patient perceptions (what the patient thinks causes the pain and what measures relieve it) 5. Reassess and document the effectiveness of interventions performed. 6. Evaluate and document readiness for discharge as evidenced by the patient's and family's understanding of the pharmacologic measures and nonpharmacologic interventions used to control pain.	1. Provide information to the patient and family about pain management. a. General materials (e.g., "Do You Know About Pain Control?" and "Making Cancer Less Painful") b. Specific materials on agents (e.g., "Do You Know . . . EMLA?") 2. Encourage families to assist in planning interventions to prevent patient's pain by doing the following: a. Incorporating measures the patient finds effective in minimizing pain b. Timing administration of pharmacologic and nonpharmacologic methods to provide maximum effect 3. Assist in administering the appropriate pharmacologic and nonpharmacologic methods on a timely or continuous basis. 4. Reassess pain intensity after a pain intervention is given.

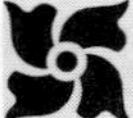

Table 70-23 Standard of Care for the Management of Nausea and Vomiting in Pediatric Cancer Patients

Patient Outcomes	Nursing Intervention and Rationales	Patient Education Instructions
The patient will: • Have adequate hydration and nutritional status with minimal episodes of nausea/vomiting. The patient and family (when applicable) will: • Describe and implement measures to prevent, alleviate, or minimize nausea and vomiting. • Maintain hydration and weight within normal range for height and range. • Maintain electrolyte balance.	1. Assess the patient for factors that may contribute to episodes of nausea/vomiting: a. Chemotherapy b. Radiation therapy c. Tumors of the stomach, intestinal tract, or brain; renal diseases; electrolyte abnormalities (hypercalcemia); and diabetes. 2. Assess the patient for nausea/vomiting prior to the beginning chemotherapy or radiation, at the beginning of each shift, and in response to patient complaints. 3. Assess the patient's past history and pattern of nausea/vomiting, including contributing factors, time of onset, duration, severity, and precipitating factors of nausea/vomiting. 4. Evaluate past and current measures used to control nausea/vomiting. 5. Review chemotherapeutic protocols for indications of electrolyte imbalance and/or compromised function of major organs such as liver and kidneys. 6. Minimize environmental triggers (food, smells, odors) for nausea/vomiting. 7. Institute measures to promote comfort, individualizing the approach to accommodate patient needs: a. Administer antiemetics before administration of chemotherapy/radiotherapy and every 4 hours around the clock. b. Provide patient safety when administering medications. c. Evaluate effectiveness of antiemetic regimen to help the patient find the most effective combinations of drugs. d. Perform mouth care after vomiting, meals, and as needed. e. Test methods (such as those below) to reduce or alleviate nausea and/or vomiting until an effective method for this patient is identified: (1) Withhold food and fluids from the patient for 4 to 6 hours before chemotherapy/radiotherapy. (2) Withhold only food from the patient for 4 to 6 hours before chemotherapy/radiotherapy. (3) Eat only dry foods for 4 hours before chemotherapy/radiotherapy. 8. Monitor intake and output. 9. Maintain hydration fluids as ordered. 10. Weigh the patient three times a week or as indicated/ordered. 11. Document the effectiveness of interventions. 12. Assess for clinical signs/symptoms of dehydration and/or electrolyte imbalances.	1. Assist the patient/family in planning for effective control of nausea and vomiting. 2. Instruct the patient and family regarding measures to minimize nausea/vomiting. 3. Instruct the patient and family to report the following: a. Continuous vomiting for 24 hours without food or fluid intake. b. Signs and symptoms of dehydration. c. Feeling of extreme stomach fullness and/or abdominal pain relieved by vomiting. 4. Instruct the patient/family regarding antiemetic medications, dosage, frequency of administration, and side effects. 5. Encourage the patient to take an oral antiemetic before the trip home (especially if car is mode of transportation) to reduce motion sickness or movement as a trigger for nausea and vomiting.

physiologic responses. Nurses then classify the pain as nociceptive (somatic or visceral; due to tissue damage, mucositis, surgery, or associated with bone metastasis) or neuropathic (pain resulting from damaged or inflamed nerves). Pharmacologic therapy, a mainstay in the management of pain in children with cancer, is titrated to the type and intensity of the pain. Medications vary from acetaminophen, naproxen, ibuprofen, or choline magnesium trisalicylate for mild pain to morphine plus amitriptyline for severe pain. Patient-controlled analgesia pumps permit a patient to self-administer a preset bolus of pain medication as it is required. Continuous morphine infusions are used when prolonged pain is expected (e.g., with early mucositis); a common starting dose is an initial bolus of 0.05 mg/kg followed by 0.01 to 0.04 mg/kg hourly. Hudzinski (1995) developed an algorithm outlining the decisions that must be made when progressing to another level of pharmacologic pain relief.

Two recently developed pharmacologic strategies also contribute to pain management in pediatric cancer patients. The use of a topical mixture of local anesthetics of lidocaine and prilocaine (EMLA) reduces procedure-related pain. Lidocaine and prilocaine concentrate at dermal pain receptors and nerve endings. These drugs prevent pain by inhibiting the ionic alterations required for stimulus initiation (Goede & Betcher, 1994). In addition, the use of indwelling epidural catheters to relieve intense pain has improved symptom control in some patients. This technique, which can be used during home care, provides regional analgesia in children who are recovering from extensive surgery (e.g., limb-salvage procedures). Adjuvant medications may be useful in specific situations. These include nonsteroidal antiinflammatory medications for managing bone pain due to metastases, moderate doses of corticosteroids for compressed nerves, and belladonna and opium (B & O) suppositories to control rectal or bladder spasms (Levy, 1996).

Attention must be given to treating the side effects associated with many pain relief preparations. Patients should have a bowel movement every 2 to 3 days. Bulk plus stimulant (senna or lactulose) laxatives, which are available in liquid forms for young children, help prevent the constipation that can accompany opioid medications. Sole use of stool softeners is inadequate in this situation. Morphine-associated pruritus can be managed by using diphenhydramine (1 mg/kg) or an alternative preparation. After a primary, tumor-related cause is ruled out, nausea and vomiting can be controlled through the use of promethazine or ondansetron.

Nonpharmacologic interventions have an important role in pain management. These include maintaining correct body alignment in the bed-confined child, the supportive presence of the nurse, and comfort-providing actions (e.g., back rubs). Such measures are vital to providing long-term relief of pain (Jacox, Carr, Payne, et al., 1994).

Nausea and Vomiting

Nausea and vomiting are two of the side effects of therapy that pediatric patients and their families find most distressing. In young patients, severe vomiting can lead to fluid and electrolyte imbalances. This situation can delay the timely delivery of therapy, thereby potentially limiting the child's response to treatment. Recent advances in antiemetic research have greatly improved the management of nausea and vomiting in children with cancer.

TABLE 70-24 Emetic Potential of Selected Chemotherapeutic Drugs

High	Moderate	Low
Cisplatin	Carboplatin	5-Flurouracil
Cyclophosphamide	Cytarabine (ara-C)	Bleomycin
Dactinomycin	Daunorubicin	Methotrexate
	Doxorubicin	Vinblastine
	Ifosfamide	Vincristine
	Procarbazine	Etoposide

First described by Wang and Borison in 1952, the central mechanism for nausea and vomiting comprises the chemoreceptor trigger zone (in the fourth ventricle of the medulla) and the vomiting center (in the mid-brain). Chemotherapy induces the release of neurotransmitters (e.g., serotonin [5-hydroxytryptamine], prostanoids, and free radicals) that activate the vomiting center. Autonomic functions are disrupted, leading to vasoconstriction, pupillary dilation, increased salivation, increased secretion of gastric acid, increased gut motility, and emesis. Elevated intracranial pressure or vagal stimulation may also induce emesis.

Rhodes, Johnson, and McDaniel (1995) identified several preexisting factors (e.g., premorbid personality, past experience, ability to understand, and the availability of socioeconomic resources) that influence the responses of pediatric patients and their families to the toxicities of cancer therapy. The nursing management of nausea and vomiting (Table 70-23) begins with knowledge of these factors. Frequent evaluation of symptoms and an intervention scheme that comprises pharmacologic and nonpharmacologic strategies are central to effectively managing nausea and vomiting in children with cancer.

The cause and timing of nausea and vomiting affect the plan for the management of these symptoms. Progression of the tumor or its spread to the CNS can cause nausea and vomiting. These symptoms can also be treatment induced. Table 70-24 classifies frequently prescribed pediatric chemotherapeutic agents by their emetic potential. Posttherapy nausea and vomiting may be acute (occurring within 24 hours after therapy) or delayed (arising after more than 24 hours).

Although therapy related, anticipatory nausea and vomiting occur *before* chemotherapeutic agents are administered. In contrast to induced symptoms, anticipatory nausea and vomiting have little direct relation to the emetic potential of the agents used. Because the problem usually develops after the patient has received one or more cycles of therapy, anticipatory symptoms seem to be conditioned responses.

Many pharmacologic preparations are available to alleviate therapy-induced nausea and vomiting. These medications include phenothiazines (e.g., chlorpromazine), corticosteroids (e.g., dexamethasone), benzodiazepines (e.g., lorazepam and diazepam), and antihistamines (e.g., diphenhydramine). However, because of their associated sedative and extrapyramidal effects, these agents have been largely replaced by serotonin antagonists (e.g., ondansetron).

Ondansetron hydrochloride was the first of a new class of serotonin antagonists to be approved by the Federal Drug Administration for the management of nausea and vomiting. These agents are especially effective in the treatment of anticipatory and acute therapy-induced symptoms. The mechanisms of action include central and peripheral antagonism of serotonin, thereby inhibiting the chemoreceptor trigger zone and intestinal activity (Betcher & Burnham, 1991). The recommended dosage of ondansetron is an infusion of 0.15 mg/kg over 15 minutes, given at least 30 minutes before chemotherapy. At our center, patients receive additional doses 4 and 8 hours after the initial dose. In the event of breakthrough nausea and vomiting, lorazepam is added to the regimen. At our institution, lorazepam, diphenhydramine, and ondansetron are used in combination for patients with refractory anticipatory nausea and vomiting.

Nonpharmacologic interventions for nausea and vomiting in children with cancer include oral hygiene and avoidance of irritating odors. Music therapy has been used successfully in many patients. Also effective, relaxation and visualization skills can be taught to even young children.

Nutrition

Changes in the nutritional status of children with cancer may be associated with the disease process itself, or with toxicity secondary to treatment. Poor nutrition in these patients is often associated with anorexia, an increased metabolic rate, mechanical gastrointestinal problems, malabsorption, nausea and vomiting, and alterations in taste. Anorexia and weight loss occur in up to 60% of pediatric cancer patients but lead to cachexia only in a minority of these individuals. Children differ from adults metabolically, and continued growth and development is desired throughout a course of therapy that often spans years.

Malnutrition is rare in a newly diagnosed patient but is a frequent complication in children with advanced disease. The undesirable consequences of malnutrition include poor disease-free survival, reduced tolerance to therapy, and decreased cell-mediated immunity, resulting in an increased susceptibility to infection. About 8% to 32% of pediatric cancer patients show some evidence of malnutrition during their therapy. In a review of the special nutritional needs of children with malignancies, Mauer, Burgess, Donaldson, Rickard, Stallings, & van Eys et al. (1990) found malnutrition occurs more frequently in patients diagnosed as having Ewing's Sarcoma, Wilms' tumor, head and neck tumors, advanced lymphomas, and neuroblastoma. Work by several investigators has suggested that malnutrition is a critical adverse factor affecting the duration of disease-free survival (Pui, Boyett, Hancock, Pratt, Meyer, & Crist, 1995; Tyc, Vallelunga, Mahoney, Smith, & Mulhern, 1995; Viana, Murao, Ramos, Oliveira, de Carvalho, & de Bastos et al., 1994).

The criteria for nutritional intervention at our institution is a total body weight loss of greater than 10% of preillness weight or a serum albumin of less than 3.2 mg/dl. When assessing nutritional status, the nurse should ask the child and family not only about weight loss, but also about specific food intolerances, altered taste sensations, and whether the current sleep schedule interferes with meal hours. In general, when the gastrointestinal tract is malfunctional for greater than 10 days, or when voluntary food intake decreases to less than 70% of the amount estimated to provide normal growth, nutritional intervention should be initiated.

Fever and Neutropenia

Neutropenia in children with cancer results from the underlying disease process, as well as from their treatment with myelosupressive therapies. Neutropenia is the most prominent factor that predisposes pediatric cancer patients to infection. This risk is greatest at low neutrophil counts and increases with the duration of the insufficiency. Because neutropenia is associated with profound impairment of the inflammatory response, customary signs and symptoms of infection (e.g., erythema, swelling, heat, and pain) may be minimal or absent.

Neutropenia is defined as an abnormally low absolute neutrophil count (ANC), which is calculated by multiplying the total white blood cell count by the sum of the percentages of segmented and band cells. Patients with ANCs between 500/uL and 1000/uL are at moderate risk of infection. If the ANC drops to between 100/uL and 500/uL, the risk of infection is severe. Patients whose ANCs are less than 100/uL are at extreme risk for life-threatening infections. Sources of infectious microbes include the people and objects exposed to the child, as well as the patient's own skin, mouth, nasopharynx, and gastrointestinal tract.

Frequently a harbinger of life-threatening infection, fever in a neutropenic child is a medical emergency. *Fever* is defined as a single oral temperature of at least 100.94° F (38.3° C) or two oral temperatures of at least 100.4° F (38.0° C) taken 1 hour apart. To convert axillary temperature measurements to oral temperatures, add 0.6° C to the axillary value; subtract 0.6° C from rectal temperatures to convert them to oral values.

The standards for nursing management of febrile patients are listed in Table 70-25. Figure 70-14 presents one algorithm used in the medical management of neutropenic pediatric cancer patients with unexplained fever. In addition to the agents noted, granulocyte colony-stimulating factor (G-CSF) and granulocyte-macrophage colony-stimulating factor (GM-CSF) have effectively decreased the incidence of fever and neutropenia among children receiving intensive chemotherapy. These recombinant human cytokines stimulate the proliferation of myeloid precursor cells, activate the differentiated progeny (granulocytes and macrophages) of these precursors, and prolong the life of neutrophils.

Although advances in the treatment of childhood cancer have improved survival rates, serious infections continue to

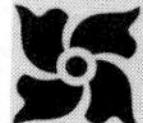

TABLE 70-25 Standard of Care for the Management of Fever and Neutropenia in Pediatric Cancer Patients

Patient Outcomes	Nursing Interventions and Rationales	Patient Education Instructions
The patient will: • Experience minimal complications during periods of neutropenia. The patient will: • Be medically stable throughout periods of neutropenia/infection. a. The patient will not experience infection/sepsis. b. The patient's onset of infection will be identified as soon as the presence of defining signs and symptoms appear. c. The patient will not experience a nosocomial infection. • Perform self-care activities to prevent complications of neutropenia. • The patient/family will demonstrate or describe an understanding of activities, daily care, and measures to prevent infection. • The patient/family will tell the nurse when signs and/or symptoms of infection arise.	1. Know the type of patient at risk for infection (immunosuppressed/neutropenic, postleukopheresis). 2. Know the definition of fever as a single oral temperature $\geq$100.94° F (38.3° C) or two oral temperatures (taken 1 hour apart) $\geq$100.4° F (38.0° C). 3. Assess the patient for specific signs and symptoms of infection: a. Fever b. Flushed appearance, diaphoresis c. Chills, shaking d. White patches on the mouth e. Redness, swelling, heat, pain of any body part (especially joints) f. Cough, tachypnea, dyspnea, rales, rhonchi, decreased breath sounds g. Changes in character and/or color of sputum, urine, or stool h. Urinary frequency or burning, malaise, rash 4. Inspect all sites at risk for infection at the beginning of each shift, including oral and anal areas, intravenous sites, and wound/puncture sites. 5. Report to the physician any evidence of infection and all elevated temperatures that reflect fever. 6. Anticipate medical orders for surface and blood cultures: a. Culture urine, throat, anterior nares, rectum, and any available lesion for bacteria and fungi. b. Obtain blood culture from peripheral vein and all lumen(s) of vascular access devices for bacteria and fungi. 7. Initiate ordered antibiotic therapy according to these guidelines: a. If stat, administer antibiotics within 30 minutes of receiving orders; administer the antibiotic with the broadest spectrum first. b. If routine, sequence first doses into schedules if routine administration time has passed; administer subsequent doses of antibiotics within ordered intervals; obtain samples for pharmacokinetics levels as ordered. c. Antibiotics will be administered in such a manner as to obtain a therapeutic blood level: (1) Doses scheduled every 6 hours will be administered within a 2-hour window that is 1 hour before and 1 hour after the designated time. (2) Doses scheduled every 8 or 12 hours will be administered within a 1-hour window that is 30 minutes before or after 30 minutes	1. Instruct the patient/family about the signs, symptoms, and prevention of infection, including the following: a. Method for oral/axillary temperature monitoring b. Who and when to call for elevated temperature c. Avoid people/crowds with recent/current infection d. Need to enhance personal hygiene (daily shower or bath, oral care, perineal care) e. Need to inspect skin and mucous membranes for signs and symptoms of infection f. Need to wash hands after bowel or bladder elimination g. Definition/cause of neutropenia h. Function of white blood cell count; ranges and values i. Usual periods of neutropenia j. Need to avoid sharing eating utensils or cups k. Importance of adequate rest and sleep l. Need to avoid activities that may compromise skin integrity (e.g., shaving, rough play, sharp toys, use of safety pins or diapers) m. Importance of adequate diet and fluid intake, avoiding raw fish or meat, and washing all fruits and vegetables before eating n. Need to avoid constipation o. Use of only sanitary napkins by female patients

Continued

TABLE 70-25 Standard of Care for the Management of Fever and Neutropenia in Pediatric Cancer Patients—cont'd

Patient Outcomes	Nursing Interventions and Rationales	Patient Education Instructions
	8. Maintain patient comfort level during febrile episodes by encouraging patient to drink cool liquids, administering ordered antipyretics, and applying cool compresses. 9. Prevent exposure of patient to known sources of infection: a. Avoid visiting of patient by persons with communicable diseases or current/recent infections. b. Ensure meticulous handwashing. c. Encourage daily baths, oral care after meals, perineal care, and handwashing. d. Avoid obtaining rectal temperatures and using enemas and suppositories. 10. Minimize risk of infection associated with venous access devices: a. Assess device(s) each shift. b. Change all intravenous tubing every 48 hours. c. Clean external surface of the connection site with alcohol to ensure aseptic technique when "breaks" in the line are needed. d. Inspect and change central line dressings.	

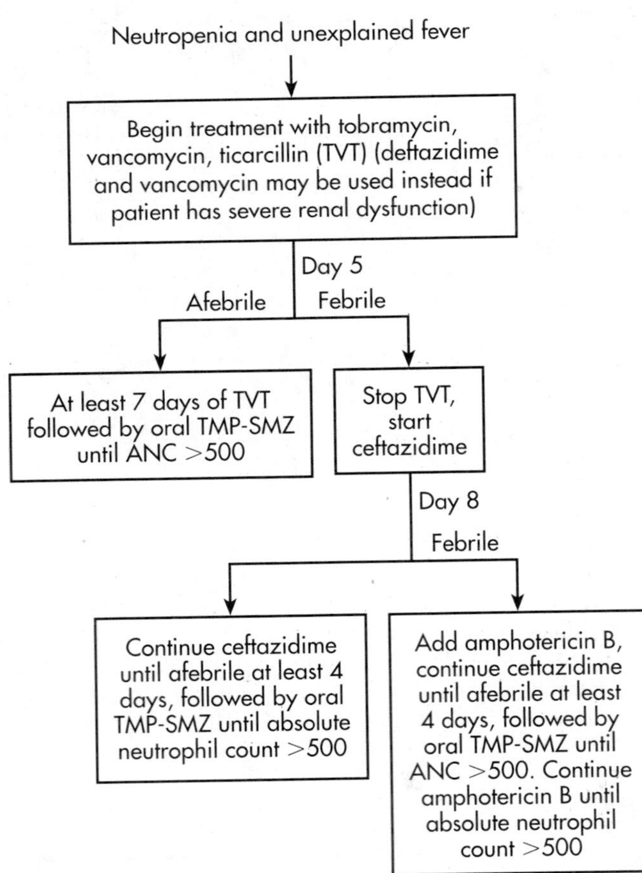

Fig. 70-14 Medical management of neutropenia in pediatric cancer patients with unexplained fever.

be a major cause of suffering and death among these patients. Therefore the prevention, early detection, and prompt treatment of infection are paramount. The pediatric oncology nurse is in a key position to help patients and their families avoid, recognize, and combat episodes of fever, neutropenia, and infection.

HOME CARE ISSUES

Pediatric oncology nurses increasingly assist families in making the transition from hospital-based to home-based care. The use of economical, family-supported, home-based care of children with cancer is escalating at a time when traditional extended-family support systems are declining. To allocate available resources efficiently, identifying the specific needs of patients and their families is essential.

The transition from hospital- to home-based care presents unique problems for the family whose child is being treated or needs terminal care. Children who receive therapy at home may require high-technology care, including antifungal medications, maintenance of venous access devices, chemotherapy, or total parenteral and/or enteral nutrition. These support services can be obtained through public health agencies, Medicare-certified home health agencies, private duty nursing agencies, or companies specializing in the rental of durable medical equipment (e.g., infusion pumps). Many of the issues central to the home care of these patients are discussed in the previous section, Nursing Management of Children with Cancer. In addition, Fig. 70-15 and Table 70-26 detail instructions for parents for flushing Hickman and Broviac single-lumen catheters. These instructions were developed at St. Jude Children's Research Hospital.

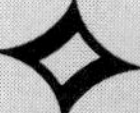

TABLE 70-26 Patient Preparation for Home Care of Hickman and Broviac Catheters

1. Wash your hands with antibacterial soap for 1 full minute. Use paper towels to dry your hands, then use the towel to turn off the water faucet before throwing it away.
2. Pop off the plastic top from the Heparin Lock Flush bottle. Open the alcohol pads, and clean the bottle's rubber top with an untouched part of the alcohol pad. Allow the top to dry.
3. Peel open the syringe package and take out the syringe that has the attached needle. Keep the clear part of the package to put the syringe and needle cover on. Turn the needle clockwise to twist it on tight.
4. Pull the syringe plunger back to the 5-cc mark. The top edge of the black rubber stopper is on the number 5. Take the cover off the needle by pulling it straight off. Put the cover in the clear syringe package. Do not discard the needle cover.
5. Look to see that the bottle's rubber top is dry, and push the needle into it. Turn the bottle upside down and push 5 cc of air into it (Fig. 70-15, *A*).
6. Pull the plunger until the solution comes to the 5-cc mark. Keep the air of the needle below the fluid level. Before removing the needle from the bottle, look for big "air pockets" in the syringe. Push any air pockets back into the bottle, and finish pulling the solution to the 5-cc mark. Pull out the needle from the bottle. Put the cover back on the needle. Push the cover on until you feel it snap.
7. If there are air bubbles in the syringe, do the following:
   - Hold the syringe straight up, with the needle pointing to the ceiling. Tap the syringe with your finger to release air bubbles from the bottom or the sides, or tap the syringe on a hard surface (Fig. 70-15, *B*).
   - Continue to tap all the bubbles until they are in the center of the needle at the top.
   - Push the plunger until a drop of fluid starts out of the needle.
8. Put the syringe down in the clear part of the syringe package while you get the catheter ready to flush. Take off the tape that holds the looped catheter on top of the Coverlet-O.R. dressing. You only need to uncover the injection cap and clamp. Remove the bandage over the injection cap and catheter end. Change this bandage each time you flush.
9. Remove another alcohol pad from the package. Clean the rubber port end of the injection cap with an untouched part of the alcohol pad. Make sure the alcohol completely cleans the rubber port. After the cap is cleaned, you cannot put it down.
10. Hold the syringe and catheter in the same hand, then pull the needle cover off with your other hand. Do not jerk on the catheter as you remove the needle cover (Fig. 70-15, *C*).
11. Push the needle into the rubber port of the injection cap. Stop when you feel resistance, and unclamp the catheter.
12. Push the 5 cc of Heparin Lock Flush solution into the catheter using a steady and moderately firm pressure to "flush" the catheter. It should flush easily. Do not force the solution. If the catheter will not flush, check to make sure the clamp is opened and the catheter is not kinked anywhere. If you still cannot flush the catheter, please call your physician.
13. When the plunger reaches the 1-cc mark on the syringe, reclamp the catheter. Close the clamp while you are still pushing in the solution. This leaves a positive pressure inside the catheter.
14. After the catheter is clamped, remove the needle from the syringe by turning the needle counterclockwise. Throw the needle away into a hard-sided container.
15. Cover the injection cap with a bandage to protect the catheter from germs, and fasten the catheter in place with silk tape.

Although many children are cured of their malignancies, care of the dying is unavoidable in pediatric oncology. Hospice programs and palliative care agencies provide individualized, multidisciplinary, family-centered care to maximize quality of life for children with cancer and their families. Hospice programs are designed to meet the physical and emotional needs of patients whose predicted life span is less than 6 months or whose plan of care contains a "do not resuscitate" order. Often the broad range of services required by many children who eventually die of cancer are unavailable through hospice programs that serve only families of children with very limited life. However, many home health and hospice agencies have expanded their services to include palliative care measures.

According to the World Health Organization, palliative care is the active comprehensive care of patients whose disease is refractory to curative treatment. Palliative care may include chemotherapy, radiation therapy, nutritional support, blood transfusions, and medications for pain and symptom management. Because staff members and parents frequently equate hospice care with abandonment of hope and acceptance of the inevitability of death, palliative care has gained broad acceptance in pediatric oncology. Pediatric hospice/palliative care differs in several aspects from that for adults. Many of these differences are related to the family as the unit of care, to an individual child's developmental stage, or to reimbursement. Managed care organizations and Medicare reimburse the expenses of hospice care on a per diem basis. A designated fee (currently $90.00 per day in Tennessee) must cover both skilled nursing services and the cost of necessary medical equipment, such as a hospital bed or oxygen.

Children's Hospice International has developed standards of practice that focus on pediatric patients. Working closely with this organization, Brenner and Zarbock (1996) developed methods for applying hospice philosophy and systems of care to pediatric patients. Their book, *Implementation Manual: Establishing Hospice Programs to Serve Children and Their Families,* addresses program organization, provides models of care, and contains resource guides. It is available from Children's Hospice International (2202 Mt. Vernon Avenue, Suite 3c, Alexandria, VA 22310).

To provide effective and sensitive palliative care to

A

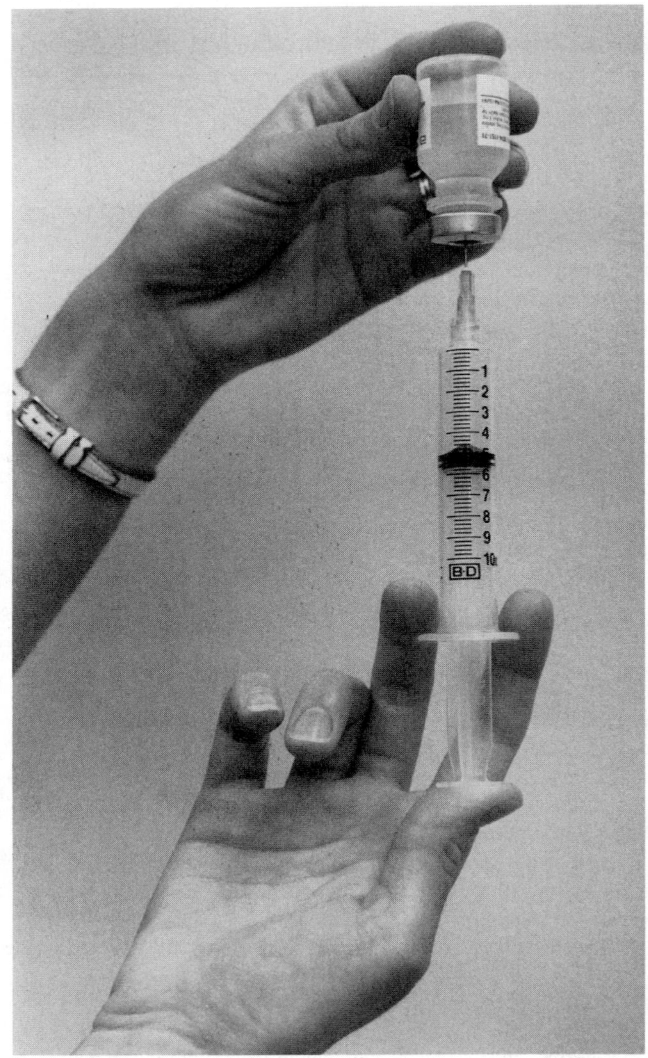

B

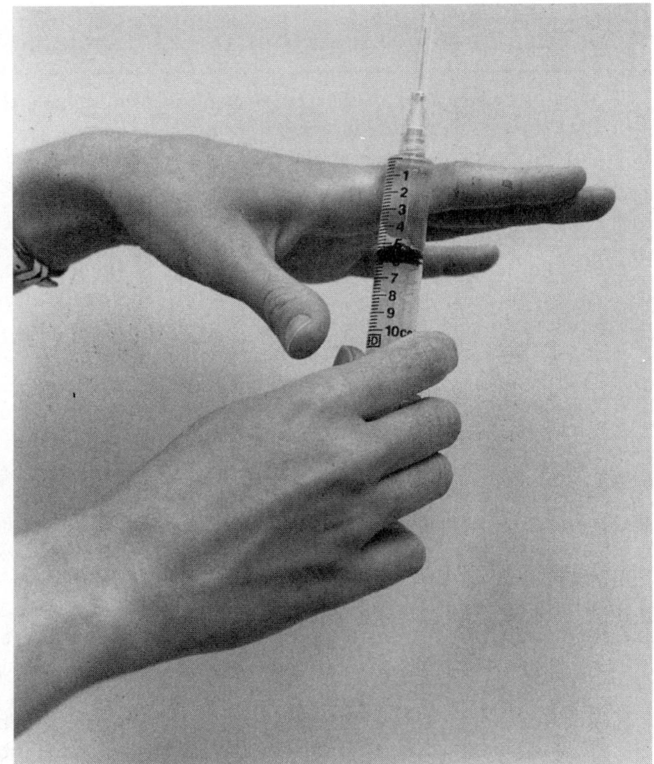

C

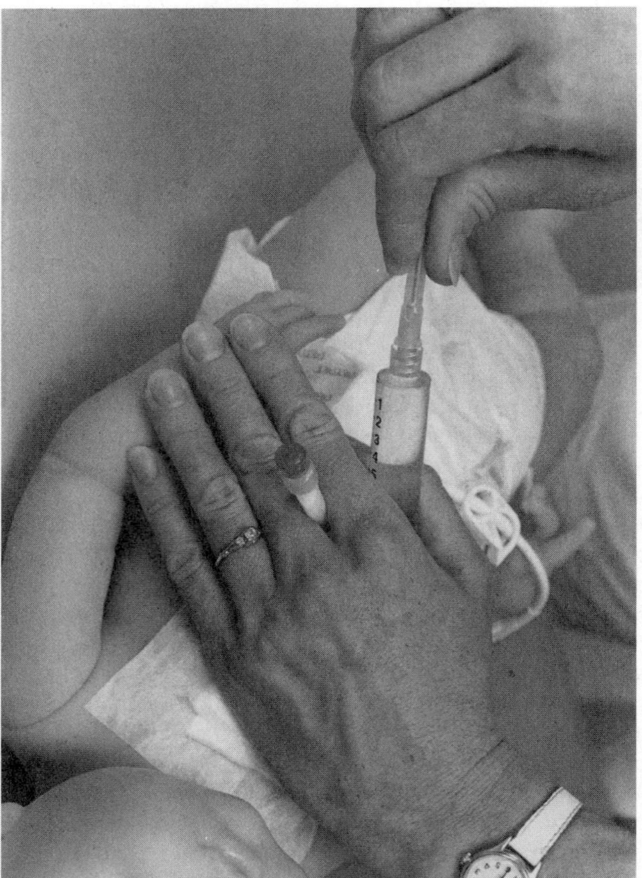

Fig. 70-15 Instructions for flushing a Hickman and Broviac catheter. See Table 70-26 for a more detailed discussion.

pediatric patients and their families, caregivers must realize that children are in developmental evolution, which influences their perceptions of health, illness, life, and death. In addition, the family, rather than the patient, is the basic unit of care in pediatric oncology nursing. Although denial is a normal part of it, the grief process is especially trying for families whose hope for a cure rests on investigational therapy. Further, although losing any family member is emotionally devastating, it is even more so when that person is a child. Not pursuing aggressive therapy is excruciatingly difficult for parents, who typically feel that they are supposed to help their children, to make them better if they are ill. No family should have to carry such a heavy burden unassisted. Although honesty and support are key to dealing with families of terminally ill children, parents also need to feel "hugged" by those caring for them. Palliative care is a crucial part of the patient-family-nurse support matrix that must bridge the gap between hope for cure in the face of advanced disease and acceptance of the reality of impending loss.

EVALUATION OF THE QUALITY OF CARE

In today's health care delivery system, pediatric oncology nurses are increasingly accountable for monitoring the quality of patient care. The development of a sound quality improvement program is central to effective and appropriate standards of care. In pediatric oncology nursing, analysis of quality of care has recently evolved from the exclusive use of predefined monitors to evaluate concrete items (e.g., blood usage and chemotherapy documentation) to a comprehensive assessment that is achieved by total quality and pain management (Table 70-27).

Widely implemented in Japanese industry, total quality management is based on concepts developed after World War II (Deming, 1986). The underlying philosophy focuses on outcomes rather than on people or processes. A basic tenant of total quality management is that the quality of any service is definable and measurable.

In this system a multidisciplinary team addresses a common concern. Evaluation of that issue is facilitated by the use of flow charts, root cause analysis, and brainstorming. Flow charts are constructed to pictorially represent all steps of a process. Root cause analysis helps to identify the underlying problems (rather than symptoms of those problems) that reduce the efficiency of an activity, and brainstorming seeks to quickly generate many potential solutions to the identified problems.

Recently, at St. Jude Children's Research Hospital, the nursing department used total quality management practices to evaluate the efficacy of our metabolic and infusion support service. This service provides parenteral and enteral nutritional support to children with cancer. Problems identified by the multidisciplinary team included sporadic intervention (with some patients "falling through the cracks"), no central place for documentation, lack of communication between primary caregivers and metabolic support staff, and difficulty with outpatient follow-up. Flow charting revealed insufficient communication between the metabolic support team, psychology department, and primary physician. Root cause analysis (Table 70-28) disclosed a lack of consistent evaluation during initial anticancer therapy.

TABLE 70-27 Quality of Care Evaluation of Pediatric Pain Management

Disciplines participating in the quality of care evaluation:
Nursing ☐ Surgery ☐
Medical Oncology ☐ Other ☐

Data from:
Medical Record Review ☐ Patient/Family Interview ☐

Criteria	Yes	No
1. Determination is made of the word the child uses for pain.	☐	☐
2. Determination is made of the behaviors the child exhibits when in pain (especially if the child is preverbal).	☐	☐
3. Pain intensity is evaluated on a routine basis using a standardized pain assessment tool.	☐	☐
4. Pain relief is evaluated after the use of a pain-management intervention.	☐	☐
5. When appropriate, nonpharmacologic strategies are used to manage the child's pain.	☐	☐
6. Child/parent's satisfaction with pain management is evaluated on a regular basis.	☐	☐

The clinical staff adopted several corrective measures that addressed the identified problems. First, a nutritional support patient risk analysis and referral stratification algorithm was constructed (Fig. 70-16). Second, a consistent format for the analysis of nutritional support cases was developed. Third, fact sheets that summarized alternative methods of nutritional support were written for families and staff members. Finally, a procedure was developed through which social work and psychological support can be provided to vulnerable families. The interdisciplinary quality management team evaluates the effectiveness of these measures after they have been in place for 3 months. In addition, the measures and their effectiveness are documented for review by accreditation agencies. The use of performance improvement teams like the one described above contributes to a dynamic environment that ensures optimal patient care.

RESEARCH ISSUES

The Oncology Nursing Society and the Association of Pediatric Oncology Nurses have jointly delineated a preliminary agenda that defines topics central to research in pediatric oncology nursing. The Oncology Nursing Society has re-

TABLE 70-28 Problems/Root Causes Analysis: For Nutritional Support Quality Assurance Patients "Fell Through Cracks"; Early Intervention Lacking; No Criteria to Determine Patient Needs; No Registered Dietitian Available to Routinely Assess All Patients

Risk Assessment Criteria Implementation Steps	Benefits	Costs	Responsibility and Approval	When Initiated (Time to Complete)
1. Establish working group (representatives from pharmacy, clinical nutrition, nursing, social work, and physicians). 2. Gather information regarding historical patients. 3. Survey physicians (personal interview) about perceptions of nutritional needs associated with various protocols; of all patients on front-line protocols. 4. Analyze data. 5. Develop algorithm (incorporate high-risk patients, high-risk portion of protocol, strategies for interventions, automatic checkpoints). 6. Get feedback from clinical staff members (circulate, present, and discuss at quarterly meeting). 7. Finalize algorithm. 8. Incorporate into annual update. 9. Educate staff members: • Clinical staff members • Grand rounds • New personnel 10. Continue ongoing education through some type of circulation (e.g., booklet or other hospital channels).	Improve patient care by increasing the nutrition status of patients on high-risk protocols. Prevent patients from "falling through cracks." Increase the consistency of patient care. Improve the continuity of care. May reduce the cost of nutritional support (reduced aggressiveness of intervention because of earlier intervention; easier integration into plan of care; reduced inpatient loss). Increase the efficiency of staff members through the use of automatic checkpoints.	Staff time Minimal fees associated with education materials: • Printing • Word processing • Distribution	Chief Medical Officer and Director of Nursing	1. 4/1/96 (1 wk) 2. 7/1/93 (3 mo) 3. 7/1/96 (3 mo) 4. 8/1/96 (1 mo) 5. 10/1/96 (2 mo) 6. 1/1/97 (3 mo) 7. 1/1/97 (3 mo) 8. 1/8/97 (1 wk) 9. At first 1997 meeting 10. Dependent on other channels

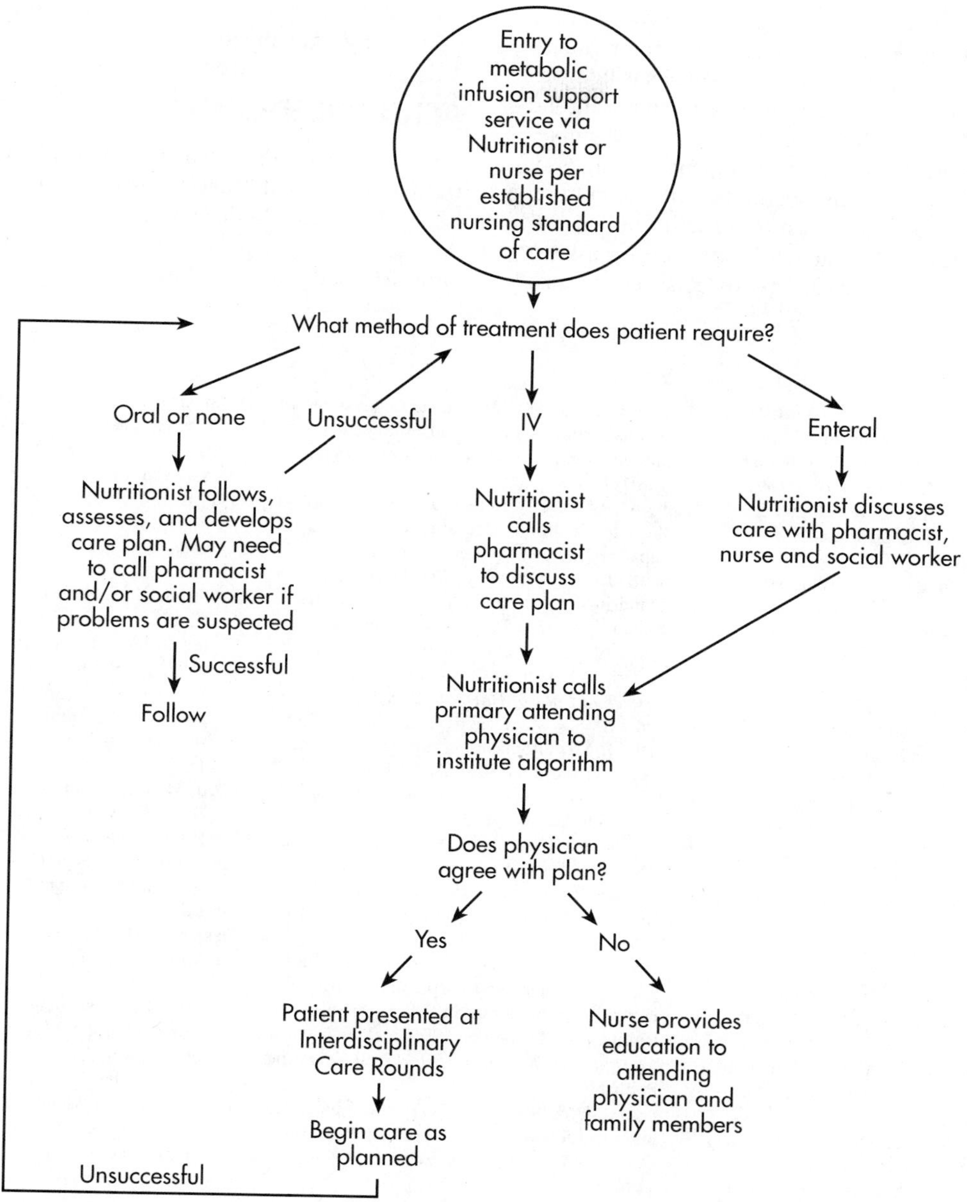

Fig. 70-16 Nutritional support patients risk analysis referral stratification algorithm.

cently funded a multiinstitutional grant that addresses the influence of fatigue on the cancer experience. Future research in pediatric oncology nursing must address strategies to increase access to care, symptom management, quality of life in pediatric patients, and the molecular genetics of childhood cancer.

Although diagnosis and treatment are likely to affect the quality of life of survivors of pediatric cancer, current research in this area is insufficient. Available publications are limited to conceptual articles (Ferrans, 1990b; Meeberg, 1993), methodologic papers (Grant, Padilla, Ferrell, & Rhiner, 1990; Testa & Simonson, 1996), anecdotal accounts (Rougraff, Simon, Kneisl, Greenberg, & Mankin, 1994; Stearns, 1993), and small, descriptive, disease- or toxicity-specific studies (Aaronson, Meyerowitz, Bard, Bloom, Fawzy, & Feldstein et al., 1991; Garre, Gandus, Cesana, Haupt, DeBernardi, & Comelli et al., 1994; Greenberg, Goorin, Gebhardt, Gupta, Stier, & Harmon et al., 1994). None of these studies explores the cumulative, potentially synergistic effects of multiple toxicities on the health or quality of life of survivors. Functional scales, such as the Karnofsky Index (Karnofsky, Abelman, Craver, and Burchenal, 1948) and multivariate health utility scales fail to adequately discriminate even moderate toxicity in cancer survivors. Even though multidimensional scales such as the Ferrans and Powers Quality of Life Index—Cancer (Ferrans, 1990a) and Padilla's Quality of Life Index (Padilla, Ferrell, Grant, & Rhiner, 1990) yield a richer description of the many aspects of quality of life, the challenge of applying such results to quality of life research in pediatric patients remains.

The mechanisms and molecular genetics of childhood malignancies need to be better defined. A clearer understanding of the causes of childhood malignancies is likely to lead to improved targeted therapy, increased survival, and decreased morbidity. Finally, pediatric oncology nurses must be leaders in the efforts to identify better methods of care for vulnerable populations, including various cultural groups, the economically disadvantaged, and adult survivors of childhood cancer. A systematic approach for assessing the special needs of these groups (e.g., access to care and coordination of therapy in a managed care environment) is currently unavailable.

ACKNOWLEDGEMENTS

This work was supported in part by PHS grant CA21765 from the National Cancer Institute and by the American Lebanese Syrian Associated Charities (ALSAC). We thank Amy L. B. Frazier for expert editorial assistance and Vicki Gray for manuscript preparation.

REFERENCES

Aaronson, N. K., Meyerowitz, B. E., Bard, M., Bloom, J. R., Fawzy, F. I., Feldstein, M., Fink, D., Holland, J. C., Johnson, J. E., Lowman, J. T., Patterson, B., & Ware, J. E. (1991). Quality of life research in oncology: Past achievements and future priorities, *Cancer, 67*(Suppl. 3), 839-843.

Abramovitz, L. Z. (1991). Perspectives on pediatric bone marrow transplantation. In M. B. Whedon (Ed.), *Bone marrow transplantation: Principles, practice and nursing insights.* Boston: Jones and Bartlett Publishers.

Abramovitz, L. Z. & Senner, A. M. (1995). Pediatric bone marrow transplantation update. *Oncology Nursing Forum, 22,* 107-115.

Agamanolis, D. P. & Malone, J. M. (1995). Chromosomal abnormalities in 47 pediatric brain tumors. *Cancer Genetics and Cytogenetics, 81,* 125-134.

Albright, A. L. (1993). Pediatric brain tumors. *CA: A Cancer Journal for Clinicians, 43,* 272-288.

Al-Jarallah, A., Cook, J. D., Gascon, G., Kanaan, I., & Sigueira, E. (1994). Transient mutism following posterior fossa surgery in children. *Journal of Surgical Oncology, 55,* 126-131.

Amoaku, W. M., Willshaw, H. E., Parkes, S. E., Shah, K. J., & Mann, J. R. (1996). Trilateral retinoblastoma. A report of five patients. *Cancer, 78,* 858-863.

Bakardjiev, A. I., Barnes, P. D., Goumnerova, L. C., Black, P. M., Scott, R. M., Pomeroy, S. L., Billett, A., Loeffler, J. S., & Tarbell, N. J. (1996). Magnetic resonance imaging changes after stereotactic radiation therapy for childhood low grade astrocytoma. *Cancer, 78,* 864-873.

Balduzzi, A., Gooley, T., Anasetti, C., Sanders, J. E., Martin, P. J., Petersdorf, E. W., Applebaum, F. R., Buckner, C. D., Matthews, D., Storb, R., Sullivan, K. M., & Hansen, J. A. (1995). Unrelated donor marrow transplantation in children. *Blood, 86,* 3247-3256.

Bates, B. A. (1991). *A pocket guide to physical examination.* Philadelphia: J. B. Lippincott.

Baumgartner, J. E. & Edwards, M. S. B. (1992). Pineal tumors. *Neurosurgery Clinics of North America, 3,* 853-862.

Beckwith, J. B. & Palmer, N. F. (1978). Histopathology and prognosis of Wilms' tumor. Results from the First National Wilms' Tumor Study. *Cancer, 41,* 1937-1948.

Beckwith, J. B. (1993). Precursor lesions of Wilms' tumor: Clinical and biological implications. *Medical and Pediatric Oncology, 21,* 158-168.

Beebe, G. W. (1979). Reflections on the work of the Atomic Bomb Causality Commission in Japan. *Epidemiology Review, 1,* 184-210.

Bennett, J. M., Catovsky, D., Daniel, M. T., Flandrin, G., Galton, D. A., Gralnick, H. R., & Sultan, C. (1976). Proposals for the classification of the acute leukemias. French-American-British (FAB) Cooperative Group. *British Journal of Haematology, 33,* 451-458.

Berger, M. S., Magrassi, L., & Geyer, J. R. (1995). Medulloblastoma and primitive neuroectodermal tumors. In A. H. Kaye & E. R. Laws (Eds.), *Brain tumors: An encyclopedic approach.* Edinburgh: Churchill Livingstone.

Betcher, D. L. & Burnham, N. (1991). Ondansetron . . . for the prevention of nausea and vomiting associated with chemotherapy. *Journal of Pediatric Oncology Nursing, 8,* 183-185.

Bierman, P. J. & Armitage, J. O. (1994). Autologous bone marrow transplantation for non-Hodgkin's lymphoma. In S. J. Forman, K. G. Blume, & E. D. Thomas (Eds.), *Bone marrow transplantation.* Boston: Blackwell Scientific Publishers.

Birch, J. M. & Breslow, N. (1995). Epidemiologic features of Wilms' Tumor. *Hematology/Oncology Clinics of North America, 9,* 1157-1178.

Bleyer, W. A. (1993). What can be learned about childhood cancer from "Cancer Statistics Review 1973-1988." *Cancer, 71*(Suppl.), 3229-3236.

Bloem, J. L. & Kroon, H. M. (1993). Osseous lesions. *Radiology Clinics of North America, 31,* 261-278.

Boice, J. D. (1996). Cancer following irradiation in childhood and adolescence. *Medical and Pediatric Oncology, 1*(Suppl.), 29-34.

Bondy, M., Wiencke, J., Wrensch, M., & Kyritsis, A. P. (1994). Genetics of primary brain tumors: A review. *Journal of Neuro-Oncology, 18,* 69-81.

Brecher, M. L. (1994). Principles of chemotherapy. In M. E. Cohen & P. K. Duffner (Eds.), *Brain tumors in children.* New York: Raven Press.

Brenner, P. & Zarbock, S. (1996). *Implementation manual: Establishing hospice programs to serve children and their families.* Alexandria, VA: Children's Hospice International.

Brill, C. B. (1988). Seizure disorders. In R. Kaye, F. A. Oski, & L. A. Barness (Eds.), *Core textbook of pediatrics.* Philadelphia: J. B. Lippincott.

Bronstein, K. S. (1995). Epidemiology and classification of brain tumors. *Critical Care Nursing Clinics of North America, 7,* 79-88.

Carbone, P. P., Kaplan, H. S., Husshoff, K., Smithers, D. W., & Tubiana, M. (1971). Report of the committee on Hodgkin's disease staging classification. *Cancer Research, 31,* 1860-1861.

Carli, M., Guglielmi, M., Sotti, G., Cecchetto, G., & Ninfo, V. (1992). Soft tissue sarcomas. In P. N. Plowman & C. R. Pinkerton (Eds.), *Paediatric oncology: Clinical practice and controversies.* London: Chapman and Hall Medical.

Castello, M. A., Schiavetti, A., Padula, A., Varrasso, G., Properzi, E., Trasimeni, G., Operamolla, P., Gualdi, G. F., & Clerico, A. (1995). Does chemotherapy have a role in low-grade astrocytoma management? A report of 13 cases. *Medical and Pediatric Oncology, 25,* 102-108.

Champlin, R. & McGlave, P. (1994). Allogeneic bone marrow transplantation for chronic myeloid leukemia. In S. J. Forman, K. G. Blume, & E. D. Thomas (Eds.), *Bone marrow transplantation.* Boston: Blackwell Scientific Publications.

Chan, H. S. L., DeBoer, G., Thiessen, J. J., Budning, A., Kingston, J. E., O'Brien, J. M., Koren, G., Giesprecht, E., Haddad, G., Verjee, Z., Hungerford, J. L., Ling, V., & Gallie, B. L. (1996). Combining cyclosporin with chemotherapy controls intraocular retinoblastoma with out requiring radiation. *Clinical Cancer Research, 2,* 1499-1508.

Chao, N. J. & Forman, S. J. (1994). Allogeneic bone marrow transplantation for acute lymphoblastic leukemia. In S. J. Forman, K. G. Blume, & E. D. Thomas (Eds.), *Bone marrow transplantation.* Boston: Blackwell Scientific Publishers.

Chapman, P. H., Buchbinder, B. R., Cosgrove, G. R., & Jiang, J. H. (1995). Functional magnetic resonance imaging for cortical mapping in pediatric neurosurgery. *Pediatric Neurosurgery, 23,* 122-126.

Chiu, J. K., Woo, S. Y., Ater, J., Connelly, J., Bruner, J. M., Maor, M. H., van Eys, J., Oswald, M. J., & Shallenberger, R. (1992). Intracranial ependymoma in children: Analysis of prognostic factors. *Journal of Neuro-Oncology, 13,* 283-290.

Cogen, P. H. & McDonald, J. D. (1996). Tumor suppressor genes and medulloblastoma. *Journal of Neuro-Oncology, 29,* 103-112.

Cohen, A. H. & Nast, C. C. (1996). Kidney. In I. Damjanov & J. Linder (Eds.), *Anderson's pathology.* St. Louis: Mosby.

Cohen, A. H. & Nast, C. C. (1996). Kidney. In I. Damjanov & J. Linder (Eds.), *Anderson's pathology.* St. Louis: Mosby.

Cohen, H. T. (1995). Wilms' tumor. In R. Kurzrock & M. Talpaz (Eds.), *Molecular biology in cancer medicine.* New York: Oxford University Press.

Cohen, M. E. & Duffner, P. K. (1994). Diagnosis and management of common intracranial tumors of childhood. In M. E. Cohen & P. K. Duffner (Eds.), *Brain tumors in children.* New York: Raven Press.

Coppes, M. J., deKraker, J., van Dijken, P. J., Perry, H. J., Delemarre, J. F., Tournade, M. F., Lemerle, J., & Voute, P. A. (1989). Bilateral Wilms' tumor: Long-term survival and some epidemiological features. *Journal of Clinical Oncology, 7,* 310-315.

Crist, W., Gehan, E. A., Ragab, A. H., Dickman, P. S., Donaldson, S. S., Fryer, C., Hammond, D., Hays, D. M., Herrmann, J., Heyn, R., Morris Jones, P., Lawrence, W., Newton, W., Ortega, J., Raney, B., Ruymann, F. B., Tefft, M., Webber, B., Wiener, E., Wharam, M., Vietti, T. J., & Maurer, H. M. (1995). The Intergroup Rhabdomyosarcoma Study III. *Journal of Clinical Oncology, 13,* 610-630.

Dahlin, D. & Coventry, M. (1967). Osteogenic sarcoma: A study of six hundred cases. *American Journal of Bone and Joint Surgery, 49,* 101-110.

D'Angio, G. J., Breslow, N., Beckwith, J. B., Evans, A., Baum, E., deLorimier, A., Fernbach, D., Hrabovsky, E., Jones, B., Kelalis, P., Othersen, B., Tefft, M., & Thomas, R. P. M. (1989). Treatment of Wilms' tumor: Results of the Third National Wilms' Tumor Study. *Cancer 64,* 349-360.

D'Angio, G. J., Clatworthy, H. W., Evena, A. E., Newton, W. A., & Tefft, M. (1978). Is the risk of morbidity and rare mortality worth the cure? *Cancer, 41,* 377-380.

DeKraker, J. (1992). Wilms' tumor and renal carcinoma. In P. N. Plowman & C. R. Pinkerton (Eds.), *Paediatric oncology: Clinical practice and controversies.* London: Chapman and Hall Medical.

Deming, W. E. (1986). *Out of the crisis.* Cambridge, MA: Massachusetts Institute of Technology, Center for Advanced Engineering Study.

Douglass, E. C., Valentine, M., Ectubanas, E., Parham, D., Webber, B. L., Houghton, P. J., Houghton, J. A., & Green, A. A. (1987). A specific chromosomal abnormality in rhabdomyosarcoma. *Cytogenetics and Cell Genetics, 45,* 148-155.

Draper, G. J., Sanders, B. M., Lennox, E. L., & Brownbill, P. A. (1996). Patterns of childhood cancer among siblings. *British Journal of Cancer, 74,* 152-158.

Dryja, T. P., Mukai, S., Peterson, R., Rapaport, J. M., Walton, D., & Yandell, D. W. (1989). Parental origin of mutations of the retinoblastoma gene. *Nature, 339,* 556-558.

Dunbar, S. F., Tarbell, N. J., Kooy, H. M., Alexander, E., III, Black, P. M., Barnes, P. D., Goumnerova, L., Scott, R. M., Pomeroy, S. L., LaVally, B., Sallan, S. E., & Loeffler, J. S. (1994). Stereotactic radiotherapy for pediatric and adult brain tumors: Preliminary report. *International Journal of Radiation Oncology, Biology, Physics, 30,* 531-539.

Eifel, P. J. (1988). Decreased bone growth arrest in weanling rats with multiple radiation fractions per day. *International Journal of Radiation Biology Physics, 15,* 141-145.

Ellsworth, R. M. (1969). The practical management of retinoblastoma. *Transactions of the American Ophthalmological Society, 67,* 462-534.

Engel, J. (1993). *The pocket guide to pediatric assessment.* St. Louis: Mosby.

Enneking, W. F. & Kagan, A. (1975). "Skip" metastasis in osteosarcoma. *Cancer, 36,* 2192-2205.

Fernbach, D. J. & Vietti, T. J. (1991). General aspects of childhood cancer. In D. J. Fernback & T. J. Vietti (Eds.), *Clinical pediatric oncology.* St. Louis: Mosby.

Ferrans, C. E. (1990a). Development of a quality of life index for patients with cancer. *Oncology Nursing Forum, 17*(Suppl. 3), 15-21.

Ferrans, C. E. (1990b). Quality of life: Conceptual issues. *Seminars in Oncology Nursing, 6,* 248-254.

Fontanesi, J. F., Heideman, R. L., Muhlbauer, M., Mulhern, R. K., Sanford, R. A., Douglass, E. C., Kovnar, E., Ochs, J. J., Kuttesch, J. F., Tai, D., & Kun, L. E. (1995). High-activity 125-I interstitial irradiation in the treatment of pediatric central nervous system tumors: A pilot study. *Pediatric Neurosurgery, 22,* 289-297.

Frederick, B. & Hanigan, M. J. (1993). Bone marrow transplantation. In G. V. Foley, D. Fochtman, & K. H. Mooney (Eds.), *Nursing care of the child with cancer.* Philadelphia: W. B. Saunders.

Freeman, C. R., Bourgouin, P. M., Sanford, R. A., Cohen, M. E., Friedman, H. S., & Kun, L. E. (1996). Long term survivors of childhood brain stem gliomas treated with hyperfractionated radiotherapy. Clinical characteristics and treatment related toxicities: The Pediatric Oncology Group. *Cancer, 77,* 555-562.

Gajjar, A., Heideman, R. L., Kovnar, E. H., Langston, J. A., Sanford, R. A., Douglass, E. C., Jenkins, J. J., Horowitz, M. E., & Kun, L. E. (1993). Response of pediatric low grade gliomas to chemotherapy. *Pediatric Neurosurgery, 19,* 113-118.

Gallie, B. L., Dunn, J. M., Chan, H. S., Hamel, P. A., & Phillips, R. A. (1991). The genetics of retinoblastoma. Relevance to the patient. *Pediatric Clinics of North America, 38,* 299-315.

Garre, M. L., Gandus, S., Cesana, B., Haupt, R., DeBernardi, B., Comelli, A., Ferrando, A., Stella, G., Vitali, M. L., Picoo, P., Nantron, M., Dallorso, S., Boni, L., & Massimo, L. (1994). Health status of long-term survivors after cancer in childhood. *American Journal of Pediatric Hematology Oncology, 16,* 143-152.

Goede, I. A. & Betcher, D. L. (1994). EMLA. *Journal of Pediatric Oncology Nursing, 11,* 38-41.

Goldberg, S. (1988). *The four-minute neurological examination.* Miami: MedMaster.

Gonzales, M. F. (1995). Classification and pathogenesis of brain tumors. In A. H. Kaye & E. R. Laws (Eds.), *Brain tumors: An encyclopedia approach.* Edinburgh: Churchill Livingstone.

Grant, M., Padilla, G. V., Ferrell, B. R., & Rhiner, M. (1990). Assessment of quality of life with a single instrument. *Seminars in Oncology Nursing, 6,* 260-270.

Green, A. A., Pratt, C., Webster, R. G., & Smith, K. (1976). Immunotherapy of osteosarcoma patients virus-modified tumor cells. *Annals of the New York Academy of Science, 277,* 396-411.

Greenberg, D. B., Goorin, A., Gebhardt, M. C., Gupta, L., Stier, N., Harmon, D., Mankin, H. (1994). Quality of life in osteosarcoma survivors. *Oncology, 8,* 19-25.

Grier, H. E. & Weinstein, H. J. (1993). Acute myelogenous leukemia. In P. A. Pizzo & D. G. Poplack (Eds.), *Principles and practice of pediatric oncology.* Philadelphia: J. B. Lippincott.

Grundy, P., Breslow, N., Green, D. M., Sharples, K., Evans, A., & D'Angio, G. J. (1989). Prognostic factors for children with recurrent Wilms' tumor: Results from the Second and Third National Wilms' Tumor Study. *Journal of Clinical Oncology, 7,* 638-647.

Grundy, P., Wilson, B., Telzerow, P., Zhou, W., & Paterson, M. C. (1994). Uniparental disomy occurs infrequently in Wilms' tumor patients. *American Journal of Human Genetics, 54,* 282-289.

Gurney, J. G., Davis, S., Severson, R. K., Fang, J. Y., Ross, J. A., & Robison, L. L. (1996). Trends in cancer incidence among children in the U.S. *Cancer, 78,* 532-541.

Gurney, J. G., Severson, R. K., Davis, S., & Robison, L. L. (1995). Incidence of cancer in children in the United States. *Cancer 75,* 2186-2195.

Heath, C. W. (1996). Electromagnetic field exposure and cancer: A review of epidemiologic evidence. *CA: A Cancer Journal for Clinicians, 46,* 29-43.

Heffner, R. R. (1994). Principles of neuropathology. In M. E. Cohen & P. K. Duffner (Eds.), *Brain tumors in children.* New York: Raven Press.

Heideman, R. L., Packer, R. J., Albright, L. A., Freeman, C. R., & Rorke, L. B. (1997). Tumors of the central nervous system. In P. A. Pizzo & D. G. Poplack (Eds.), *Principles and practice of pediatric oncology.* Philadelphia: J. B. Lippincott.

Hogan, G. R. & Ryan, N. J. (1989). Infantile hydrocephalus. In J. P. Mohr (Ed.), *Manual of clinical problems in neurology.* Boston: Little, Brown & Company.

Horowitz, J. M. (1993). Regulation of transcription by the retinoblastoma protein. *Genes, Chromosomes, and Cancer, 6,* 124-131.

Horowitz, M. M. & Bortin, M. M. (1993). Results of bone marrow transplants from human leukocyte antigen-identical sibling donors for treatment of childhood leukemias: A report from the International Bone Marrow Transplant Registry. *American Journal of Pediatric Hematology-Oncology, 15,* 56-64.

Hudson, M. M. & Donaldson, S. S. (1997). Hodgkin's disease. In P. A. Pizzo & D. G. Poplack (Eds.), *Principles and practice of pediatric oncology.* Philadelphia: Lippincott-Raven.

Hudson, M. M., Hancock, M., & Pui, C. H. (1994). Late deaths after treatment for childhood cancer. *Medical and Pediatric Oncology, 23,* 184.

Hudzinski, D. M. (1995). An algorithmic approach to cancer pain management. *Nursing Clinics of North America, 30,* 711-723.

Huvos, A. (1991). *Bone tumors: Diagnosis, treatment, and prognosis.* Philadelphia: W. B. Saunders.

Jacox, A., Carr, D. B., Payne, R., et al. (1994). *Management of Cancer Pain Clinical Practice Guideline No. 9.* AHCPR Publication No. 94-0592. Rockville, MD: Agency for Health Care Policy and Research, U.S. Department of Health and Human Services, Public Health Service.

Jaffe, N. (1972). Recent advances in the chemotherapy of metastatic osteogenic sarcoma. *Cancer, 30,* 1627-1631.

Johnson, F. L. & Goldman, S. (1993). Role of autotransplantation in neuroblastoma. *Hematology-Oncology Clinics of North America, 7,* 647-662.

Jones, R. J. (1994). Allogeneic bone marrow transplantation for lymphomas. In S. J. Forman, K. G. Blume, & E. D. Thomas (Eds.), *Bone marrow transplantation.* Boston: Blackwell Scientific Publications.

Karnofsky, D. A., Abelman, W. H., Craver, L. F., & Burchenal, J. H. (1948). The use of nitrogen mustards in palliative treatment of carcinoma. *Cancer, 1,* 634-656.

Kingston, J. E. & Hungerford, J. L. (1992). Retinoblastoma. In P. N. Plowman & C. R. Pinkerton (Eds.), *Paediatric oncology: Clinical practice and controversies.* London: Chapman and Hall Medical.

Kingston, J. E., Plowman, P. N., & Hungerford, J. L. (1985). Ectopic intracranial retinoblastoma in childhood. *British Journal of Ophthalmology, 69,* 742-748.

Kirk, E. A., Howard, V. C., & Scott, C. A. (1995). Description of posterior fossa syndrome in children after posterior fossa brain tumor surgery. *Journal of Pediatric Oncology Nursing, 12,* 181-187.

Kirks, D. R., Kaufman, R. A., & Babcock, D. S. (1987). Renal neoplasms in infants and children. *Seminars in Roentgenology, 22,* 292-302.

Klintworth, G. K. & Eagle, R. C. (1996). Eye and ocular adnexa. In I. Damjanov & J. Linder (Eds.), *Anderson's pathology.* St. Louis: Mosby.

Knudson, A. G. (1971). Mutation and cancer: Statistical study of retinoblastoma. *Proceedings of the National Academy of Science USA, 68,* 820-823.

Knudson, A. G. (1993). Introduction to the genetics of primary renal tumors in children. *Medical and Pediatric Oncology, 21,* 193-198.

Kun, L. E. (1994). Principles of radiation therapy. In M. E. Cohen & P. K. Duffner (Eds.), *Brain tumors in children.* New York: Raven Press.

Ladenstein, R., Hartmann, O., & Pinkerton, C. R. (1993). The role of megatherapy with autologous bone marrow rescue in solid tumors of childhood. *Annals of Oncology, 4*(Suppl. 1), 45-58.

Lanzkowski, P. (1995). Central nervous system malignancies. *Manual of pediatric hematology and oncology.* New York: Churchill Livingstone.

Lawrence, Jr., W., Gehan, E. A., Hays, D. M., Beltangady, M., & Maurer, H. M. (1987). Prognostic significance of staging factors of the UICC staging system in childhood rhabdomyosarcoma: A report from the Intergroup Rhabdomyosarcoma Study (IRS-II). *Journal of Clinical Oncology, 17,* 46-54.

Lawrence, W., Hays, D. M., Heyn, R., Tefft, M., Crist, W., Beltangady, M., Newton, W., & Wharam, M. (1987). Lymphatic metastases with childhood rhabdomyosarcoma: A report from the Intergroup Rhabdomyosarcoma Study. *Cancer, 60,* 910-915.

Leisenring, W. M., Breslow, N. E., Evans, I. E., Beckwith, J. B., & Grundy, P. (1994). Increased birth weights of National Wilm's Tumor Study patients suggest a growth factor excess. *Cancer Research, 54,* 4680-4683.

Levi, F., LaVecchia, C., Lucchini, F., Negri, E., & Boyle, P. (1995). Patterns of childhood cancer mortality: America, Asia and Oceania. *European Journal of Cancer, 31A,* 771-782.

Leviton, A. (1994). Principles of epidemiology. In M. E. Cohen & P. K. Duffner (Eds.), *Brain tumors in children.* New York: Raven Press.

Levy, M. H. (1996). Pharmacologic treatment of cancer pain. *The New England Journal of Medicine, 335,* 1124-1132.

Lew, C. M. & LaVally, B. (1995). The role of stereotactic radiation therapy in the management of children with brain tumors. *Journal of Pediatric Oncology Nursing, 12,* 212-222.

Lewis, M. M. (1986). The use of an expandable and adjustable prosthesis in the treatment of childhood malignant bone tumors of the extremity. *Cancer, 57,* 499-502.

Li, F. P. & Fraumeni, J. F. (1969). Rhabdomyosarcoma in children: Epidemiologic study and identification of a familial cancer syndrome. *Journal of the National Cancer Institute, 43,* 1365-1373.

Li, F. P., Myers, M. H., Heise, H. W., & Jaffee, N. (1978). The course of five-year survivors of cancer in childhood. *Journal of Pediatrics, 93,* 185-187.

Link, M. P. & Eilber, F. (1993). Osteosarcoma. In P. A. Pizzo & D. G. Poplack (Eds.), *Principles and practice of pediatric oncology.* Philadelphia: J. B. Lippincott.

MacKay, C. J., Abramson, D. H., & Ellsworth, R. M. (1984). Metastatic patterns of retinoblastoma. *Archives of Ophthalmology, 102,* 391-396.

Magrath, I. T. (1991). African Burkitt's lymphoma: History, biology, clinical features, and treatment. *American Journal of Pediatric Hematology Oncology, 13,* 222-246.

Magrath, I. (1993). Malignant non-Hodgkin's lymphomas in children. In P. A. Pizzo & D. G. Poplack (Eds.), *Principles and practice of pediatric oncology.* Philadelphia: J. B. Lippincott.

Mamelak, A. N., & Edwards, M. S. B. (1994). Principles of neurosurgery. In M. E. Cohen & P. K. Duffner (Eds.), *Brain tumors in children.* New York: Raven Press.

Mandell, L. R., Ghavimi, F., Exelby, P., & Fuks, Z. (1988). Preliminary results of alternating combination chemotherapy and hyperfractionated radiotherapy in advanced rhabdomyosarcoma. *International Journal of Radiation Biology Physics, 15,* 197-203.

Mangiardi, J. R. (1995). Biochemistry and metabolism of brain tumors. In A. H. Kaye & E. R. Laws (Eds.), *Brain tumors: An encyclopedic approach.* Edinburgh: Churchill Livingstone.

Matsuno, T., Unni, K. K., McLeod, R. A., & Dahlin, D. C. (1976). Telangiectatic osteogenic sarcoma. *Cancer, 38,* 2538-2547.

Mauer, A. M., Burgess, J. B., Donaldson, S. S., Rickard, K. A., Stallings, V. A., van Eys, J., & Winick, M. (1990). Special nutritional needs of children with malignancies: A review. *Journal of Parenteral and Enteral Nutrition, 14,* 315-324.

Maurer, H. M., Beltangady, M., Gehan, E. A., Crist, W., Hammond, D., Hayes, D. M., Heyn, R., Lawrence, W., Newton, W., & Ortega, J. (1988). The Intergroup Rhabdomoysarcoma Study-I. A final report. *Cancer, 61,* 209-220.

Maurer, H. M. & Ragab, A. H. (1991). Rhabdomyosarcoma. In D. J. Fernbach & T. J. Vietti (Eds.), *Clinical pediatric oncology.* St. Louis: Mosby.

Maurer, H. M., Gehan, E. A., Beltangady, M., Crist, W., Dickman, P. S., Donaldson, S. S., Fryer, C., Hammond, D., Hays, D. M., Herrmann, J., Heyn, R., Morris Jones, P., Lawrence, W., Newton, W., Ortega, J., Ragab, A. H., Raney, B., Ruymann, F. B., Soule, E., Tefft, M., Webber, B., Weiner, E., Wharam, M., & Vietti, T. J. (1993). The Intergroup Rhabdomyosarcoma Study-II. *Cancer, 71,* 1904-1922.

Meadows, A. T. & Hobbie, W. L. (1986). The medical consequences of cure. *Cancer, 58,* 524-528.

Meeberg, G. A. (1993). Quality of life: A concept analysis. *Journal of Advanced Nursing, 18,* 32-38.

Melnick, S., Cole, P., Anderson, D., & Herbst, A. (1987). Rates and risks of diethylstilbestrol-related clear-cell adenocarcinoma of the vagina and cervix: An update. *New England Journal of Medicine, 316,* 514-516.

Meyer, W. H., Schell, M. J., Kumar, A. P. M., Rao, B. N., Green, A. A., Champion, J., & Pratt, C. B. (1987). Thoracotomy for pulmonary metastatic osteosarcoma. An analysis of prognostic indicators of survival. *Cancer, 59,* 374-379.

Miettinen, M. & Weiss, S. W. (1996). Soft-tissue tumors. In I. Damjanov & J. Linder (Eds.), *Anderson's pathology.* St. Louis: Mosby.

Miller, R. W., Fraumeni, J. F., & Manning, M. D. (1964). Association of Wilms' tumor with aniridia, hemihypertrophy, and other congenital malformations. *New England Journal of Medicine, 270,* 922-927.

Miller, R. W., Young, J. L., & Novakovic, B. (1995). Childhood cancer. *Cancer, 75*(Suppl 1), 395-405.

Miser, A. W., Dothage, J. A., Wesley, R. A., & Miser, J. S. (1987). The prevalence of pain in a pediatric and young adult cancer population. *Pain, 29,* 73-83.

Moll, A. C., Imhof, S. M., Bouter, L. M., Kuik, D. J., Den Otter, W., Bezemer, P. D., Koten, J. W., & Tan, K. E. (1996). Second primary tumors in patients with hereditary retinoblastoma: A register-based follow-up study, 1945-1994. *International Journal of Cancer, 67,* 515-519.

Moore, I. M. (1995). Central nervous system toxicity of cancer therapy in children. *Journal of Pediatric Oncology Nursing, 12,* 203-210.

Mueller, B. A. & Gurney, J. G. (1992). Epidemiology of pediatric brain tumors. *Neurosurgery Clinics of North America, 3,* 715-721.

Mulvihill, J. J. (1993). Childhood cancer, the environment and heredity. In P. A. Pizzo & D. G. Poplack (Eds.), *Principles and practice of pediatric oncology.* Philadelphia: J. B. Lippincott.

Murphy, S. B. (1980). Classification, staging and end results of treatment of childhood and non-Hodgkin's lymphomas: Dissimilarities from lymphomas in adults. *Seminars in Oncology, 3,* 332-339.

National Comprehensive Cancer Network. (1996). Osteosarcoma. *Oncology, 10,* 1799-1806.

Nemes, J. & Donahue, M. C. (1994). Solid tumors in children. *Nursing Clinics of North America, 29,* 585-598.

Newton, W. A., Meadows, A. T., Shimada, H., Bunin, G. R., & Vawter, G. F. (1991). Bone sarcomas as second malignant neoplasms following childhood cancer. *Cancer, 67,* 193-201.

Olshan, A. F., Breslow, N. E., Daling, J. R., Falletta, J. M., Grufferman, S., Robison, L. L., Waskerwitz, M., & Hammond, G. D. (1990). Wilms' tumor and parental occupation. *Cancer Research, 50,* 3212-3217.

Packer, R. J., Nicholson, H. S., Vezina, L. G., & Johnson, D. L. (1992). Brainstem gliomas. *Neurosurgery Clinics of North America, 3,* 863-879.

Padilla, G. V., Ferrell, B., Grant, M. M., & Rhiner, M. (1990). Defining the content domain of quality of life for cancer patients with pain. *Cancer Nursing, 13,* 108-115.

Pappo, A. S., Crist, W. M., Kuttesch, J., Rowe, S., Anhmun, R. A., Maurer, H. M., Newton, W. A., Asmar, L., Luo, X., & Shapiro, D. N. (1993). Tumor-cell DNA content predicts outcome in children and adolescents with clinical group III embryonal rhabdomyosarcoma. *Journal of Clinical Oncology, 11,* 1901-1905.

Pappo, A. S., Shapiro, D. N., Crist, W. M., & Maurer, H. M. (1995). Biology and therapy of pediatric rhabdomyosarcoma. *Journal of Clinical Oncology, 13,* 2123-2139.

Parham, D. M. (1994). The molecular biology of childhood rhabdomyosarcoma. *Seminars in Diagnostic Pathology, 11,* 39-46.

Parham, D. M. (1996). Renal Neoplasms. In D. M. Parham (Ed.), *Pediatric neoplasia: Morphology and biology.* Philadelphia: Lippincott-Raven.

Parker, S. L., Tong, T., Bolden, S., & Wingo, P. A. (1996). Cancer statistics, 1996. *CA: A Cancer Journal for Clinicians, 46,* 5-27.

Phillips, G. L. (1994). Transplantation for Hodgkin's disease. In S. J. Forman, K. G. Blume, & E. D. Thomas (Eds.), *Bone marrow transplantation.* Boston: Blackwell Scientific Publishers.

Poplack, D. (1993). Acute lymphoblastic leukemia. In P. A. Pizzo & D. G. Poplack (Eds.), *Principles and practice of pediatric oncology.* Philadelphia: J. B. Lippincott.

Poplack, D. G., Kun, L., Magrath, I., & Pizzo, P. (1993). Leukemia and lymphoma of childhood. In V. T. DeVita, Jr., S. Hellman, & S. A. Rosenberg (Eds.), *Cancer: Principles and practice of oncology.* Philadelphia: J. B. Lippincott.

Pratt, C. B., Fontanesi, J., Luo, X., Parham, D. M., Elfervig, J., & Meyer, D. (1997). Proposal for a new staging scheme for intraocular and extraocular retinoblastoma based on an analysis of 103 globes. *The Oncologist, 2,* 1-2.

Pui, C. H. (1995). Childhood leukemias. *New England Journal of Medicine, 332,* 1618-1630.

Pui, C. H. (1996). Acute leukemia in children. *Current Opinions in Hematology, 3,* 249-258.

Pui, C. H. (1997). The clinical management of childhood leukemia. *Helix, Amgen's Magazine of Biotechnology, 1,* 18-25.

Pui, C. H., Behm, F. G., Raimondi, S. C., Dodge, R. K., George, S. L., Rivera, G. K., Mirro, J., Jr., Kalwinsky, D. K., Dahl, G. V., & Murphy, S. B. (1989). Secondary acute myeloid leukemia in children treated for acute lymphoid leukemia. *New England Journal of Medicine, 321,* 136-142.

Pui, C. H., Boyett, J. M., Hancock, M. L., Pratt, C. B., Meyer, W. H., & Crist, W. M. (1995). Outcome of treatment for childhood cancer in black as compared with white children. The St. Jude Children's Research Hospital experience, 1962 through 1992. *Journal of the American Medical Association, 273,* 633-637.

Pui, C. H. & Crist, W. M. (1994). Biology and treatment of acute lymphoblastic leukemia. *The Journal of Pediatrics, 124,* 491-503.

Purtilo, D. T. & Sullivan, J. L. (1979). Immunological bases for superior survival of females. *American Journal of Diseases of Children, 133,* 1251-1253.

Rabb, C. H. & Apuzzo, M. L. J. (1995). Stereotaxis in the diagnosis and management of brain tumors. In A. H. Kaye & E. R. Laws (Eds.), *Brain tumors: An encyclopedic approach.* Edinburgh: Churchill Livingstone.

Raney, R. B., Tefft, M., Hayes, D. M., & Triche, T. J. (1993) Rhabdomyosarcoma and the undifferentiated sarcomas. In P. A. Pizzo & D. G. Poplack (Eds.), *Principles and practice of pediatric oncology.* Philadelphia: J. B. Lippincott.

Rhodes, V. A., Johnson, M. H., & McDaniel, R. W. (1995). Nausea, vomiting and retching: The management of the symptom experience. *Seminars in Oncology Nursing, 11,* 256-265.

Ries, L. A. G., Hankey, B. F., Miller, R. W., Hartman, A. M., & Edwards, B. K. (1991). *Cancer statistics review 1973-88.* (NIH Publication No. 91-2789). Bethesda: National Cancer Institute.

Ries, L. A. G., Miller, B. A., Hankey, B. F., Kosary, C. L., Harras, A., & Edwards, B. K. (1994). *SEER cancer statistics review 1973-1991: Tables and graphs.* (NIH Publication No. 94-2789). Bethesda: National Cancer Institute.

Rivera, G. K., Pinkel, D., Simone, J. V., Hancock, M. L., & Crist, W. M. (1993). Treatment of acute lymphoblastic leukemia: 30 years' experience at St. Jude Children's Research Hospital. *New England Journal of Medicine, 329,* 1289-1295.

Robison, L. L., Mertens, A., & Neglia, J. P. (1991). Epidemiology and etiology of childhood cancer. In D. J. Fernbach & T. J. Vietti (Eds.), *Clinical pediatric oncology.* St. Louis: Mosby.

Rodary, C., Gehan, E. A., Flamant, F., Treuner, J., Carli, M., Auquier, A., & Maurer, H. (1991). Prognostic factors in 951 nonmetastatic rhabdomyosarcoma in children: A report from the International Rhabdomyosarcoma Workshop. *Medical and Pediatric Oncology, 19,* 89-95.

Rosen, G., Caparros, B., Huvos, A. G., Kosloff, C., Nirenberg, A., Cacavio, A., Marcove, R. C., Lane, J. M., Mehta, B., & Urban, C. (1982). Preoperative chemotherapy for osteosarcoma: Selection of postoperative adjuvant chemotherapy based on the response of the primary tumor to preoperative chemotherapy. *Cancer, 49,* 1221-1230.

Rosenberg, A. E. (1994). Skeletal system and soft tissue tumors. In R. S. Coltran, V. Kumar, & S. L. Robbins (Eds.), *Pathologic basis of disease.* Philadelphia: W. B. Saunders.

Rougraff, B. T., Simon, M. A., Kneisl, J. S., Greenberg, D. B., & Mankin, H. J. (1994). Limb salvage compared with amputation for osteosarcoma of the distal end of the femur: A long-term oncological, functional, and quality of life study. *American Journal of Bone and Joint Surgery, 76,* 649-656.

Rutka, J. T., Hoffman, H. J., Drake, J. M., & Humphreys, R. P. (1992). Suprasellar and sellar tumors in childhood and adolescence. *Neurosurgery Clinics of North America, 3,* 803-820.

Ruymann, F. B., Maddux, H. R., Ragab, A., Soule, E. H., Palmer, N., Beltangady, M., Gehan, E. A., & Newton, W. A. (1988). Congenital anomalies associated with rhabdomyosarcoma: An autopsy study of 115 cases. A report from the Intergroup Rhabdomyosarcoma Study Committee. *Medical and Pediatric Oncology, 16,* 33-39.

Ryan, J. A. & Shiminski-Maher, T. (1995). Hydrocephalus and shunts in children with brain tumors. *Journal of Pediatric Oncology Nursing, 12,* 223-229.

Saleman, M. (1995). Glioblastoma and malignant astrocytoma. In A. H. Kaye & E. R. Laws (Eds.), *Brain tumors: An encyclopedic approach.* Edinburgh: Churchill Livingstone.

Sandlund, J. T., Downing, J. R., & Crist, W. M. (1996). Non-Hodgkin's lymphoma in childhood. *New England Journal of Medicine, 334,* 1238-1248.

Schmidt, D. & Beckwith, J. B. (1995). Histopathology of childhood renal tumors. *Hematology/Oncology Clinics of North America, 9,* 1179-1200.

Seeger, R. C. & Reynolds, C. P. (1994). Neuroblastoma. In S. J. Forman, K. G. Blume, & E. D. Thomas (Eds.), *Bone marrow transplantation.* Boston: Blackwell Scientific Publishers.

Shapiro, W. R. & Shapiro, J. R. (1992). Primary brain tumors. In A. K. Asbury, G. M. McKhann, & W. I. McDonald (Eds.), *Diseases of the nervous system: Clinical neurobiology.* Philadelphia: W. B. Saunders.

Shiminski-Maher, T. & Shields, M. (1995). Pediatric brain tumors: Diagnosis and management. *Journal of Pediatric Oncology Nursing, 12,* 188-198.

Shurtleff, S. A., Buijs, A., Behm, F. G., Rubnitz, J. E., Raimondi, S. C., Hancock, M. L., Chan, G. G., Pui, C. H., Grosveld, G., & Downing, J. R. (1995). TEL/AML1 fusion resulting from a cryptic t(12;21) is the most common genetic lesion in pediatric ALL and defines a subgroup of patients with an excellent prognosis. *Leukemia, 9,* 1985-1989.

Smith, L. M., Donaldson, S. S., Egbert, P. R., Link, M., & Bagshaw, M. A. (1989). Aggressive management of second primary tumors in survivors of hereditary retinoblastoma. *International Journal of Radiation Oncology Biology Physics, 17,* 499-505.

Spanier, S. S., Shuster, J. J., & Vender Griend, R. A. (1990). The effect of local extent of the tumor on prognosis in osteosarcoma. *American Journal of Bone and Joint Surgery, 72,* 643-653.

Stearns, N. M. (1993). Celebrating life: Lessons learned from a bone marrow transplant reunion. *Cancer Practice, 1,* 42-48.

Steinbok, P., Cochrane, D. D., & Poskitt, K. (1992). Intramedullary spinal cord tumors in children. *Neurosurgery Clinics of North America, 3,* 931-943.

Stewart, A., Webb, J., Giles, D., & Hewitt, D. (1956). Malignant disease in childhood and diagnostic radiation in utero. *Lancet, 2,* 447-451.

Stiller, C. A. (1991). Aetiology and epidemiology. In P. N. Plowman & C. R. Pinkerton (Eds.), *Paediatric oncology: Clinical practice and controversies.* London: Chapman and Hall Medical.

Strander, H. & Einhorn, S. (1977). Effect of human leukocyte interferon on the growth of human osteosarcoma cells in tissue culture. *International Journal of Cancer, 19,* 468-473.

Sutters, K. A. & Miaskowski, C. (1992). The problem of pain in children with cancer: A research review. *Oncology Nursing Forum, 19,* 465-471.

Testa, M. A. & Simonson, D. C. (1996). Assessment of quality-of-life outcomes. *The New England Journal of Medicine, 334,* 835-840.

Thapar, K., Fukuyma, K., & Rutka, J. T. (1995). Neurogenetics and the molecular biology of human brain tumors. In A. H. Kaye & E. R. Laws (Eds.), *Brain tumors: An encyclopedic approach.* Edinburgh: Churchill Livingstone.

Thapar, K., Rutka, J. T., & Laws, E. R. (1995). Brain edema, increased intracranial pressure, vascular effects, and other epiphenomena of human brain tumors. In A. H. Kaye & E. R. Laws (Eds.), *Brain tumors: An encyclopedic approach.* Edinburgh: Churchill Livingstone.

Tjalma, R. A. (1966). Canine bone sarcoma: Estimation of relative risk as a function of body size. *Journal of the National Cancer Institute, 36,* 1137-1150.

Trueworthy, J., Shuster, T., Look, W., Crist, M., Borowitz, M., Carroll, A., Frankel, L., Harris, M., Wagner, H., & Haggard, M. (1992). Ploidy of lymphoblasts is the strongest predictor of treatment outcome in B-progenitor cell acute lymphoblastic leukemia of childhood: A Pediatric Oncology Group study. *Journal of Clinical Oncology, 10,* 606-613.

Tucker, M. A., D'Angio, G. J., Boice, J. D., Strong, L. C., Li, F. P., Stovall, M., Stone, B. J., Green, D. M., Lombardi, F., & Newton, W. (1987). Bone sarcomas linked to radiotherapy and chemotherapy in children. *New England Journal of Medicine, 317,* 588-593.

Tyc, V. L., Vallelunga, L., Mahoney, S., Smith, B. F., & Mulhern, R. K. (1995). Nutritional and treatment related characteristics of pediatric oncology patients referred or not referred for nutritional support. *Medical and Pediatric Oncology, 25,* 379-388.

van Dongen, H. R., Catsman-Berrevoets, C. E., & van Mourik, M. (1994). The syndrome of "cerebellar" mutism and subsequent dysarthra. *Neurology, 44,* 22040-22046.

Viana, M. B., Murao, M., Ramos, G., Oliveira, H. M., de Carvalho, R. I., de Bastos, M., Colosimo, E. A., & Silvestrini, W. S. (1994). Malnutrition as a prognostic factor in lymphoblastic leukaemia: A multivariate analysis. *Archives of the Diseases of Children, 71,* 304-310.

Vogel, F. (1979). Genetics of retinoblastoma. *Human Genetics, 52,* 1-54.

Wadayama, B., Toguchida, J., Yamaguchi, T., Saski, M. S., & Yamamuro, T. (1993). p53 expression and its relationship to DNA alterations in bone and soft tissue sarcomas. *British Journal of Cancer, 68,* 1134-1139.

Wang, M. X., Jenkins, J. J., Cu-Unjieng, A. B., Meyer, D., & Donoso, L. A. (1996). Eye tumors. In D. M. Parham (Ed.), *Pediatric neoplasia: Morphology and biology.* Philadelphia: Lippincott-Raven.

Wang, S. C. & Borison, H. L. (1952). A new concept of organization of the central emetic mechanism. Recent studies on the sites of action of apomorphine, copper sulphate and cardiac glycosides. *Gastroenterology, 22,* 1-12.

Webber, B. L. & Parham, D. M. (1996). Bone tumors other than Ewing's sarcoma. In D. M. Parham (Ed.), *Pediatric neoplasia: Morphology and biology.* Philadelphia: Lippincott-Raven.

Weiner, H. L. & Levitt, L. P. (1994). *Neurology.* Baltimore: Williams & Wilkins.

West, N., Oakes, L., Hinds, P. S., Sanders, L., Holden, R., Williams, S., Fairclough, D., & Bozeman, P. (1994). Measuring pain in pediatric oncology ICU patients. *Journal of Pediatric Oncology Nursing, 11,* 64-70.

Whang-Peng, J., Triche, T. J., Knutsen, T., Miser, J., Kao-Shan, S., Tsai, S., & Israel, M. A. (1986). Cytogenetic characterization of selected small round cell tumors of childhood. *Cancer Genetics and Cytogenetics, 21,* 185-208.

Wharam, M., Beltangady M., Heyn, R., Lawrence, W., Newton, W., Raney, R., Ruymann, F., Tefft, M., & Maurer, H. (1985). Localized orbital rhabdomyosarcoma: A report of the Intergroup Rhabdomyosarcoma Study (Abstract C514). *Proceedings of the American Society of Clinical Oncology, 4,* 132.

Wilimas, J. A., Greenwald, C. A., & Rao, B. K. (1996). Wilms' tumor. In N. J. Vogelzang, P. T. Scardino, W. U. Shipley, & D. S. Coffey (Eds.), *Comprehensive textbook of genitourinary oncology.* Baltimore: Williams and Wilkins.

Wingo, P. A., Bolden, S., Tong, T., Parker, S. L., Martin, L. M., & Heath, C. W. (1996). Cancer statistics for African Americans, 1996. *CA: A Cancer Journal for Clinicians, 46,* 113-125.

Wisoff, J. H. (1992). Management of optic pathway tumors of childhood. *Neurosurgery Clinics of North America, 3,* 791-802.

Zhu, X. P., Dunn, J. M., Phillips, R. A., Goddard, A. D., Paton, K. E., Becker, A., & Gallie, B. L. (1989). Preferential germline mutation of the parental allele in retinoblastoma. *Nature, 340,* 312-313.

Osteogenic Sarcoma

Catherine H. Kelley, MSN, RN, OCN
Robbie Thomas, RN, MS, OCN

According to Huvos (1991), osteogenic sarcoma is a malignant bone tumor in which the proliferating spindle cell stroma directly produces osteoid (immature bone). The term *osteogenic* actually has two meanings: one that it is derived from bone, and the other that it is bone producing. Sarcomas of the bone are referred to synonymously as *osteogenic sarcomas* or *osteosarcomas*. A discussion of the histologic types of osteosarcoma and its variants, treatment, and nursing care are discussed in this chapter.

EPIDEMIOLOGY

Osteosarcoma is a relatively rare malignancy. According to Malawer, Link, and Donaldson (1997), malignant tumors from the skeletal system accounted for only 0.2% of all new cancers. It is estimated that in 1998 there were 2400 new cases of bone cancers in the United States, with 1400 estimated deaths (Landis, Taylor, Bolden, & Wingo, 1998). Conventional osteosarcoma, the most common primary bone malignancy (outside of myeloma), has only 1000 new cases diagnosed yearly in the United States (Ayala, Ro, & Raymond, 1996). The two most common bone tumors are Ewing's sarcoma and osteosarcoma. Both are tumors that are seen mainly during childhood, adolescence, and early adulthood (Malawer, Link, & Donaldson, 1993; Vander Griend, 1996). The incidence of osteosarcoma is slightly higher in men than women (Rosen, Forscher, Mankin, & Selch, 1997), although this varies, depending upon the specific variant of the bone disease. It is more common to osteosarcoma in the long bones of the body, primarily those that have the greatest potential for growth. This includes the distal femur, proximal tibia, and proximal humerus, with the majority of osteosarcomas occurring around the knee (Vander Griend, 1996).

RISK FACTORS

Primary Osteosarcoma

As mentioned above, osteosarcoma generally is seen in children, adolescents, and young adults. Primary osteosarcoma is often diagnosed when a patient seeks medical attention after trauma to the area, although trauma has not been found to cause primary osteosarcoma. A history of recent trauma to the knee, in particular, is common when obtaining a diagnosis of osteogenic sarcoma. It is thought that the trauma merely brings the patient's attention to the afflicted area. There are no known risk factors for primary osteosarcoma, other than the diagnosis of retinoblastoma, which will be discussed later.

Secondary Osteosarcoma

Unlike primary osteosarcoma, secondary osteosarcoma is a malignant bone tumor that is seen in older patients. According to one source (Vander Griend, 1996), 25% of osteosarcomas seen in patients over the age of 60 years are secondary. Secondary osteosarcoma is a malignant tumor that arises from a preexisting bone lesion. As seen in Table 71-1, it can also occur in bone that has been irradiated (Vander Griend, 1996; Malawer, Link, & Donaldson, 1997). Paget's disease (of bone), fibrous dysplasia, enchondromatosis, chronic osteomyelitis, and bone infarction are all diseases that have been known to be risk factors for secondary osteosarcoma (Enneking & Conrad, 1989; Vander Griend, 1996; Malawer, Link, & Donaldson, 1997).

Postirradiation may be a risk factor for secondary osteosarcoma if at least 30 Gy of radiation has been directed to the bone. Also, a period of at least 3 years should have elapsed between the radiation and the onset of the tumor (Vander Griend, 1996).

Molecular and Biologic Factors

Molecular genetics and biology have been increasingly studied in recent years. Scientists have found that people with retinoblastoma have greater than a hundred-fold tendency to develop osteosarcoma (Piasecki, 1992).

It was also found that the loss of alleles of chromosome 17, especially 17p13, is seen in over 75% of patients diagnosed with osteosarcoma (Grundmann, Roessner, Ueda, Schneider-Stock, & Radig, 1995). Although the clinical sig-

TABLE 71-1 Risk Factors for Osteosarcoma

Primary Osteosarcoma	Secondary Osteosarcoma
Diagnosis of retinoblastoma	Radiation therapy History of Paget's disease of bone History of fibrous dysplasia History of enchondromatosis Chronic osteomyelitis Prior bone infarction

From Malawer, M., Link, M., Donaldson, S. (1997). Sarcomas of bone. In V. T. DeVita, S. Hellman, & S. A. Rosenberg (Eds.) *Cancer: Principles & Practice of Oncology* (5th ed.). Philadelphia: Lippincott-Raven.

nificance of this is still unknown, it is known that tumor suppressor genes lie along chromosome 17.

PATHOPHYSIOLOGY

Anatomy and Physiology of Normal Bone

To gain a clear understanding of the pathophysiology of osteosarcoma, one must understand the anatomy and physiology of the human bone. Because most osteosarcomas present in the long bones, these bones will be the emphasis of the discussion.

Bone is a kind of connective tissue in which organic matter called *collagen* has mineralized. Collagen's role in bone formation is that of forming fibers in the bone. It is this collagen that forms the matrix of bone, along with other proteins that function in forming and maintaining bone.

Bone tissue can be either compact (cortical) or cancellous (spongy). Cancellous bone has open spaces between bone tissue networks, whereas in compact bone the structure is fitted closely together, giving it a very dense structural appearance. Both types of tissue contain the same structural elements, the major difference being how the elements are organized (Mourad, 1994).

Long bones consist of the epiphysis, diaphysis, and metaphysis, as well as the articular cartilage, periosteum, and medullary canal or cavity. In children, there is also an epiphyseal plate, which disappears once growth has ended. Long bones are composed of cancellous bone and compact bone. The epiphysis, which is composed of cancellous bone, is the end of long bones and is where muscles are attached. The epiphysis provides joint stability. The articular cartilage covers the epiphysis and enables the bones to move smoothly against each other (see Fig. 70-13).

The diaphysis is the main area of the bone, and its function is to provide structural support. It is composed of compact bone. The metaphysis is the area between the epiphysis and diaphysis. It is the metaphysis that contains the growth zones as bones develop. In children and adolescents, the epiphyseal plate is a cartilaginous area of bone that actively produces bone, resulting in longitudinal bone growth. As the child reaches maturity, the epiphyseal plate becomes mature bone, and growth ceases.

Within the diaphysis is the medullary canal. This is the area that consists of bone marrow. In children the marrow produced in this canal is red. In adults the marrow is yellow. The red marrow in the child's medullary canal is involved in hematopoiesis. The periosteum covers the bone. It is composed of fibrous connective tissue. The inner layers of the periosteum contain osteoblasts, which are bone-forming cells. These cells are essential for bone growth and repair of fractures.

Microscopically, compact bone is composed of calcified collagen. The collagen matrix encloses a long canal, called the *haversian canal.* This canal functions to transport blood to the bone tissue. Osteocytes (bone cells) lie in small spaces between the collagen layers in the matrix. Tiny canals, called *canaculi,* connect the osteocytes to one another and to the haversian canal. In cancellous (spongy) bone, bone marrow fills large spaces between the collagen matrix. It is the bone marrow that gives the bone its spongy appearance.

Pathophysiology

According to Enneking and Conrad (1989), bone tumors, both malignant and benign, are categorized by their biologic behavior as well as their histology. The biologic behavior is how the tumors are able to grow and extend beyond their natural barriers. These barriers include the capsule and the reactive zone, as well as compartmental barriers of cortical bone, periosteum, and articular cartilage.

The capsule is a shell of bone or fibrous tissue that surrounds the tumor, and the reactive zone is an area composed of tissue that forms between the capsule and the normal bone (Enneking & Conrad, 1989; Malawer, Link, & Donaldson, 1997). The elements that form the reactive zone include reactive bone or fibrous tissue, called *mesenchymal tissue,* and inflammatory tissue. Tumors that are intracapsulated are those that stay in an intact capsule, while those that extend outside the capsule are classified as extracapsular. Similarly, lesions that are intracompartmental are those that remain within the compartment of origin (and don't penetrate the bone cortex), whereas the lesions that destroy bone cortex are classified as extracompartmental.

Tumors of the bone can be divided into three areas—the osteosarcomas (classic and its variants), chondrosarcomas, and fibrohistiocytomas. (Box 71-1). The emphasis of this chapter will be on osteosarcomas, but the other tumors of the bone will also be discussed briefly.

Classic Osteosarcoma. Classic osteogenic sarcoma (also called *conventional osteosarcoma* or *intramedullary high-grade osteosarcoma*) is a malignant tumor in which the osteoid produced is neoplastic, and the neoplasm is produced by a spindle-cell stroma (Enneking & Conrad, 1989). This form of osteosarcoma accounts for 75% of all osteosarcomas (Vander Griend, 1996). The amount of osteoid substance produced within a tumor may vary, and it is important to study the bone matrix because it is that area that differentiates osteosarcoma from other similar tumors (Inwards & Unni, 1995). Variants of classic osteosarcoma in-

Box 71-1
Osteosarcomas of the Musculoskeletal System

Classic Osteosarcoma (High-grade intramedullary)

Histologic subtypes

- Osteoblastic
- Chondroblastic
- Fibroblastic
- Telangiectatic
- Small cell
- Low-grade intramedullary

Juxtacortical (Surface)

Parosteal
Periosteal
High-grade surface

Unknown Origin

Giant cell

Secondary Osteosarcoma

Osteosarcoma from Paget's disease of the bone
Postradiation osteosarcoma
Secondary osteosarcoma from other benign bone diseases

Modified from Vander Griend, R. (1996). Osteosarcoma and its variants. *Orthopedics of North America, 27,* 575-581.

clude parosteal, periosteal, and telangiectatic osteosarcoma. Osteosarcoma can occur anywhere throughout the skeleton, but the most common site is around the knee (Vander Griend, 1996). Other common sites include the proximal humerus, proximal femur, and pelvis. Most osteosarcomas originate in the metaphysis area of the long bones, which is the region of highest growth (Enneking & Conrad, 1989).

The clinical course of high-grade osteosarcoma can vary, but the tumor usually begins in the metaphyseal area of the long bone, extending up through the medullary canal toward the epiphysis (Vander Griend, 1996). Although the epiphyseal plate (commonly called the *growth plate*) in children is not an effective barrier to the tumor, invasion of the tumor through the subchondral bone and articular cartilage into the joint is rare, unless a pathologic fracture occurs. Given time, the tumor can invade the cortex, periosteum, and the surrounding soft tissues (Fig. 71-1).

Variants of Classic Osteosarcoma. Variants of conventional osteosarcoma include telangiectatic osteosarcoma, small-cell osteosarcoma, low-grade intramedullary osteosarcoma, and the surface, or juxtacortical, osteosarcomas.

Telangiectatic Osteosarcoma. Clinically, this variant of high-grade osteosarcoma is similar to its conventional counterpart (Vander Griend, 1996; Inwards & Unni; 1995; Ayala, Ro, & Raymond, 1996). It is often found in the metaphyseal location of the long bone, but can also occur in the diaphysis. It has a history of extensive bone destruction, and pathologic fractures are commonly found in patients with telangiectatic osteosarcomas (Vander Griend, 1996).

Histologically, this tumor has minimal osteoid production, but is found to have spaces filled with blood or tumor cells, separated by septae filled with malignant tumor cells. On gross examination, the tumor has a "bag of blood" consistency. Historically, this variant was thought to have had a poor prognosis, but recent evidence shows that part of the poor prognosis was due to inaccurate diagnoses (Vander Griend, 1996).

Small Cell Osteosarcoma. This variant of high-grade osteosarcoma is rarely seen. The incidence has been reported to range from 1.1% to 4.0% (Ayala, Ro, & Raymond, 1996). It usually affects people in their twenties. Its small round cells are similar to those seen in Ewing's sarcoma, although they may also resemble those found in large-cell lymphomas. Although the tumor must produce osteoid, in approximately half of the cases there was scant production found (Inwards & Unni, 1995). Prognosis of small-cell osteosarcomas is approximately the same as classic osteosarcoma, but may be slightly worse (Ayala, Ro, & Raymond, 1996).

Low-grade Intramedullary Osteosarcoma. Low-grade medullary osteosarcoma (also called *low-grade central osteosarcoma*) is a rare form of osteosarcoma. It differs from the classic osteosarcoma in its better prognosis. The tumor usually occurs in young adults. Although it has been seen to occur, low-grade central osteosarcomas rarely metastasize. They do have a tendency to recur locally (Inwards & Unni, 1995).

Juxtacortical Osteosarcomas. Juxtacortical, or surface, osteosarcomas are those that originate extracortically. Juxtacortical osteosarcomas are divided into three tumor types: the parosteal, periosteal, and high-grade surface osteosarcomas. These tumors are rare—approximately 6% of all osteosarcomas can be categorized as juxtacortical osteosarcomas (Inwards & Unni, 1995).

Parosteal Osteosarcoma. Parosteal osteosarcomas arise from between the cortex and the muscle (Enneking & Conrad, 1989). They are most commonly seen in young adults, often occurring in the third and fourth decades (Grundmann et al., 1995) and are more common in women than in men (Ayala Ro, & Raymond, 1996). They are usually found on the posterior aspect of the distal femur or on the medial aspect of the proximal humerus (Enneking & Conrad, 1989), although they can be found in other areas. Parosteal osteosarcomas are the most common type of juxtacortical osteosarcomas, their frequency being reported as high as 4% of all osteosarcomas (Inwards & Unni, 1995).

Parosteal osteosarcoma is less aggressive than the conventional osteosarcoma (Enneking & Conrad, 1989) and may have an indolent course for a long time. During this indolent period, the tumor may remain separated from the normal bone by a small amount of soft tissue. However, when the tumor does extend into the underlying bone, the disease becomes classified as more aggressive and often metastasizes to the lungs (Enneking & Conrad, 1989). Radiographs show the tumor to be a dense mass that may circle the metaphysis, separated by a narrow radiolucent zone of reactive tissue. Often, nodules that are separate from the main mass may be seen in the peripheral reactive zone. Late stages of the disease find the tumor invading the medullary canal. Histologically, parosteal

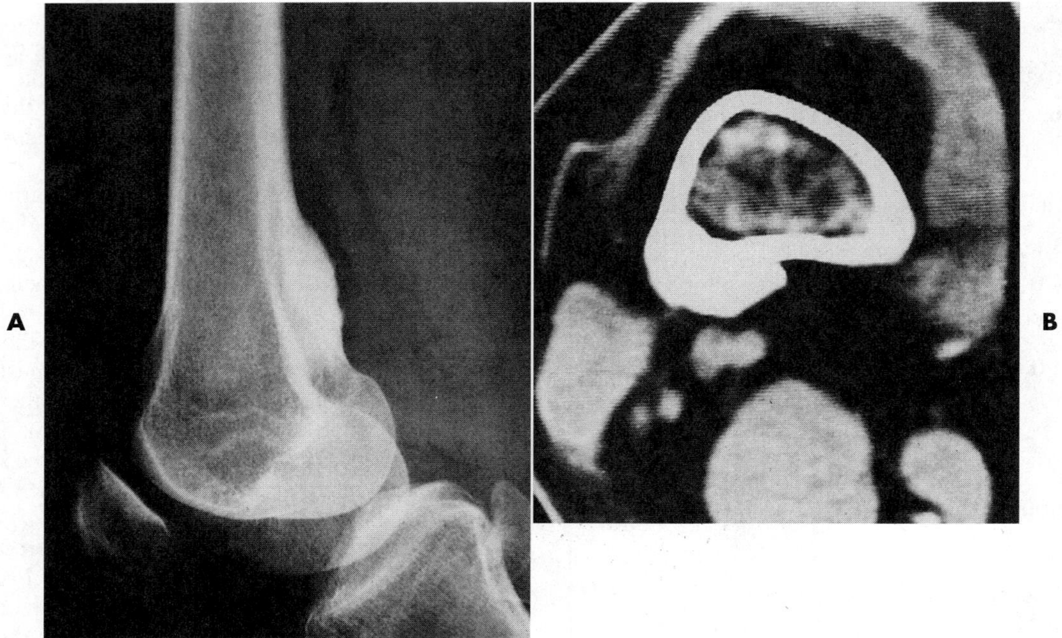

Fig. 71-1 Parosteal osteosarcoma. **A,** Lateral radiograph of the knee of a 37-year-old woman shows an ossific mass attached to the posterior cortex of the distal femur. Its location and appearance are typical of parosteal osteosarcoma. **B,** CT section demonstrates lack of invasion of the medullary portion of the bone. (From Skarin, S. A. [1996]. *Atlas of diagnostic oncology.* [2nd ed.]. London: Mosby-Wolfe.)

osteosarcomas are well-differentiated (Inwards & Unni, 1995). Prognosis is relatively good, although there is a chance of local recurrence.

Periosteal Sarcoma. This variant of high-grade osteosarcoma is most commonly seen in the second and third decades of life. It affects men more frequently than women (Ayala, Ro, & Raymond, 1996). Periosteal osteosarcoma affects the diaphysis or metadiaphysis of long bones and is most commonly seen along the femur and tibia. It often presents as a painless mass that grows from the external surface of the bone into the soft tissue that overlies the area (Enneking & Conrad, 1989). Histologically, these tumors are moderately well-differentiated and consist of predominantly cartilaginous materials with a focal malignant osteoid (Inwards & Unni, 1995). By radiograph, it usually appears as an external mass that is poorly mineralized within a crater-like area or bone erosion with an irregular margin. A spiculated sunburst appearance is often found on radiograph (Ayala, Ro, & Raymond, 1996). Periosteal osteosarcomas may extend through the bone cortex into the medullary canal earlier in the disease course than parosteal osteosarcoma. The prognosis is worse when this occurs, and the incidence of pulmonary metastases is higher (Enneking & Conrad, 1989). However, if the disease is found prior to medullary invasion, prognosis is good.

High-grade Surface Osteosarcoma. This variant of osteosarcoma is very rare (Inwards & Unni, 1995). Medullary involvement is unusual. By radiograph, the tumors' appearance may mimic parosteal or periosteal sarcoma. Histologically, the tumors are high-grade spindle cell neoplasms. Microscopically, their features are identical to the classical osteosarcomas, and the prognosis of this category of osteosarcomas is poorer than other surface osteosarcomas (Inwards & Unni, 1995). Most tumors have been located in the diaphyseal region of the bone, with the femur being the most common site (Malawer, Link, & Donaldson, 1993).

Cartilaginous Tumors. Cartilaginous tumors are lesions in which cartilage is produced, rather than osteoid as in the osteosarcomas. These lesions are categorized as chondromas. The most common is osteochondroma, which is a benign tumor, although in 1% to 2% of cases they transform into a malignant tumor. Likewise, an endochondroma is a benign tumor in adolescents and children, but in adults it usually transforms into a malignant tumor. A chondrosarcoma is the most common malignant tumor to produce cartilage. Most of these tumors are primary, although 10% of them are secondary tumors (Malawer, Link, & Donaldson, 1997). The majority of chondrosarcomas are low-grade lesions, but a small percentage of them are high-grade tumors.

Fibrous Tumors. These are very rare tumors and actually are similar to their counterparts in soft tissue sarcomas. The two most commonly seen are the fibrosarcoma and the malignant fibrous histiocytoma.

Giant Cell Tumors. Giant cell tumors have an unknown origin and until recently were thought to be benign tumors (Malawer, Link, & Donaldson, 1997). However, they are now classified as malignant tumors due to their tendency to have high rates of recurrence locally and malignant transformation. They are considered to be a low-grade sarcoma rather than a high grade.

TABLE 71-2 Assessment of the Patient for Osteosarcoma

	Assessment Parameters	Typical Abnormal Findings
History	A. Patient symptoms 1. Age 2. History of retinoblastoma a. Benign bone disease b. Radiation c. Coughing, dyspnea, or chest pain	A. Personal and social risk factors 1. Osteosarcomas are more prevalent in adolescents and young adults a. Higher risk for osteosarcoma b. Increased risk for secondary osteosarcoma c. Increased risk for secondary osteosarcoma d. May indicate pulmonary metastasis
Physical Examination	A. Inspect, palpate area in question, note location of area B. Coughing, ayspnea, prior irradiation	A. Majority of osteosarcomas involve the knee B. Possible lung metastasis
Diagnostic Examination	A. Radiograph B. Lab work C. CT D. MRI E. Bone scan F. Bone biopsy	A. Often able to provide diagnosis B. Elevated alkaline phosphatase often seen in osteosarcoma C. Used to diagnose lesion, also for pulmonary metastasis D. Good for noting medullary and soft tissue involvement E. Notes metastases F. Provides history of disease, ability to grade tumor

ROUTES OF METASTASES

Because bones lack a lymphatic system, most bone tumors metastasize via blood (Malawer, Link, & Donaldson, 1993). Lymph node involvement is very rare and is found in approximately 10% of all cases at diagnosis. Lymph node involvement is considered to be a poor prognostic indicator (Enneking & Conrad, 1989; Malawer, Link, & Donaldson, 1993). Hematogenous spread is manifested by pulmonary involvement (Malawer, Link, & Donaldson, 1993). A phenomenon known as *skip metastasis* has been noted in osteogenic sarcoma. Skip metastasis is a tumor nodule that is in the same bone as the primary tumor but not connected to the primary tumor. Skip metastases are often seen in high-grade sarcomas rather than in low grade.

Skip metastases develop when the tumor cells embolize within sinusoids in the bone marrow. Technically, they are local metastases that have not yet gone through the circulation. Skip metastases are a sign of poor prognosis and have a significant on local recurrence (Malawer, Link, & Donaldson, 1993).

According to Vander Griend (1996), metastatic disease is still the survival-limiting factor in high-grade osteosarcoma. Although the overall incidence of pulmonary metastasis appears to have decreased with the advent of neoadjuvant treatment, the prognosis for patients who present with pulmonary disease continues to be poor (Vander Griend, 1996).

The risk of metastasis has been found to correlate with positive surgical margins, a large tumor mass, local recurrence, poor response to preoperative chemotherapy, and inadequate number of courses of chemotherapy (Vander Griend, 1996; Enneking & Conrad, 1989). Osteosarcoma can also metastasize to bone and soft tissue. Metastases in these areas are not often seen and are considered to be poor prognostic indicators.

ASSESSMENT

History and Physical

Accurate patient assessment plays a critical role in optimizing the management and survival of patients with osteosarcoma. A thorough history and physical assessment are the mainstays in good patient management. Table 71-2 lists the key elements in a physical examination, and the rationale behind each part of the examination.

Most patients initially present to a physician with a history of pain (Piasecki, 1992). As mentioned previously, this pain may be associated with trauma, although the trauma will not necessarily be associated with the malignancy. It has been noted that pain that is acute enough to wake a patient during the night is usually indicative of a bone lesion (Ayala, Ro, & Raymond, 1996).

It is not unusual for a pathologic fracture to be the first manifestation of a bone malignancy (Ayala, Ro, & Raymond, 1996) However, a history of repeated trauma, including jogging, may lead the clinician toward a diagnosis of a stress fracture rather than a pathologic fracture. Enneking and Conrad (1989) state that the most important clues to an accurate diagnosis of osteogenic sarcoma include the age of the patient, the site of the lesion, and the presence of conditions known to be associated with bone tumors. Most osteosarcomas present in areas associated with high growth (Enneking & Conrad, 1989; Vander Griend, 1996).

Along with the history of unrelenting pain, a patient with osteosarcoma may present with tenderness in the affected area, localized warmth, and complaints of difficulty performing routine motions with the affected area (Ayala, Ro, & Raymond, 1996).

Radiographic Examinations

After obtaining a complete history and physical examination, a plain radiograph of the affected area should be ordered. This very basic tool is probably the most important diagnostic test and, in this day of cost consciousness, should be ordered before other more costly tests. The plain radiograph often can suggest the correct diagnosis, demonstrate the presence of a pathologic fracture, and give some suggestion of the extraosseous extent of the lesion (Meyer & Malawer, 1991). The radiograph may show lytic, or mixed, lesions with or without calcification. There may also be some evidence of new bone formation and extensive periosteal reaction (Himelstein & Dormans, 1996).

There are three patterns of bone destruction often seen radiologically: permeative, moth-eaten, and geographic (Ayala, Ro, & Raymond, 1996). A *geographic pattern* refers to the presence of holes that may reveal sclerosis and well-demarcated margins. This pattern is typical of slow-growing lesions. A *moth-eaten pattern* is indicated by the presence of multiple holes in the bone that may merge. This pattern is seen in moderately aggressive lesions. The *permeative pattern* seen radiographically is manifest by many small, ill-defined areas best visualized in the bone cortex. This pattern is usually indicative of aggressive, infiltrating lesions (Ayala, Ro, & Raymond, 1996).

Classic, or conventional, osteosarcoma often appears radiographically as highly destructive and aggressive. It may appear as completely radiopaque or purely radiolucent. Most cases present as a mixture and show cortical destruction and extension into the soft tissue. Periosteal reactive bone formation and periosteal elevation, known as *Codman's triangle,* may be present (Ayala, Ro, & Raymond, 1996).

Laboratory Tests

Along with the ordering of a plain radiograph, or after attaining the results of it, laboratory tests will also be ordered. These will include a complete blood count, including a sedimentation rate, and serum levels of calcium, phosphorus, and alkaline phosphatase levels, as well as BUN and creatinine assays to assess renal function. A CEA or PSA may be ordered if the practitioner is considering metastatic disease (Rosen, Forscher, Manken, & Selch, 1997). Findings of the alkaline phosphatase level are controversial. Some studies have shown that increased levels have a poorer prognosis (Damron & Pritchard, 1995), but all levels resume to normal after surgical intervention. However, it may be worthwhile to monitor the levels serially.

More scans should be ordered once the radiographs suggest the presence of a malignant tumor. It is important to note that the additional scans should be completed before a biopsy is performed (Meyer & Malawer, 1991). Bone scans, skeletal surveys, Computed tomography (CT), and magnetic resonance imaging (MRI) all play useful roles not only in diagnosing the malignancy but also in providing information that can help the team plan treatment that will optimize survival.

Computed Tomography Scans

Both CT scans and MRI provide information needed for analyzing classic osteosarcoma. The CT scan, introduced in the late 1970s, can provide detailed information about the interaction between the tumor, normal cortex, mineralized structures, cancellous bone, and reactive bone (Ayala, Ro, & Raymond, 1996; Fishman, 1997). It has been suggested that the CT scan is better for bony lesions involving the cortex, without a soft tissue mass, whereas an MRI is more valuable in determining the extent of the marrow involvement as well as soft tissue masses outside the bone (Rosen, et al. 1997). CT scanning should include the entire bone and the joint adjacent to it. It is also the most sensitive technique in detecting pulmonary metastases (Meyer & Malawer, 1991). As seen in Table 71-3, the procedure is relatively simple, although it is important that the patient be adequately prepared to ensure adequate results.

Magnetic Resonance Imaging

An MRI is also useful in assisting the surgical team in making preoperative decisions. It can help visualize the involvement of the tumor and can facilitate limb-salvage therapy (Piasecki, 1992). MRI shows better contrast discrimination than any other imaging modality, and imaging can be performed in any plane. MRI is also useful in detecting skip metastases (Meyer & Malawer, 1991).

Bone Scans

Bone scans also can locate skip metastases, as well as the unusual occurrence of bone metastases (Himelstein & Dormans, 1996). They can also assess tumor activity by the amount of radioisotope uptake in and around the tumor. The greater the uptake, the more aggressive and malignant the tumor usually is (Enneking & Conrad, 1989).

Angiography

Angiography plays an important role when limb-sparing surgery is being considered (Meyer & Malawer, 1991). This procedure provides information regarding the neovascularity of a tumor as well as the involvement of major neurovascular bundles (Enneking & Conrad, 1989). Angiography is considered the most reliable method of determining vascular anatomy (Malawer, Link, & Donaldson, 1993).

Biopsy

A biopsy should be performed after the above-mentioned scans are completed. It is essential that the surgeon or radiologist be provided with the information obtained from the scans to facilitate an optimal biopsy. Biopsy is considered the most important procedure performed in the management of pediatric osteosarcomas, short of the operation for definitive local tumor control (Himelstein & Dormans, 1996). An improperly obtained biopsy may preclude a limb-sparing surgery, leaving the patient and surgeon with no alternative

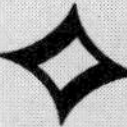

TABLE 71-3 Patient Preparation for Computed Tomography (CT)

Patient Preparation: Tell your doctor or the CT technologist if:

You are or may be pregnant
You are allergic to iodine
You are undergoing radiation therapy

1. Depending on what part of the body will be scanned, you may be asked to fast for 4 to 6 hours before the scan.
2. If the scan is to be performed with contrast, you will be asked to drink some liquid that enhances the effectiveness of the CT scan. You may pour the liquid over ice to make it more palatable, and you may drink it slowly, a few sips at a time. Drink as much as you can approximately 4 to 6 hours before the scan.
3. Do not wear jewelry or eye make-up because metallics may interfere with the accuracy of the image.

At the Time of the Scan:

1. You will most likely have an IV started so that additional contrast material may be injected. It is not unusual to feel warm or flushed as the contrast dye goes through your body.
2. You will be positioned on the scanning table.
3. You will be asked not to move throughout the scan so that the images are not blurred.
4. You will go through the scanner, which is small but air conditioned. The technologist will be watching you at all times, and you can communicate through a microphone in the scanner.
5. Don't be alarmed if you hear some humming noises during the scan—they are from the machine and are normal.
6. The scan normally takes between 30 and 60 minutes, including preparation time.

After the Scan Is Completed:

1. Drink a lot of fluids because the liquid contrast you drank may cause constipation.
2. You may drive home and resume normal activities.
3. Your physician will be able to explain the results of the scan to you after it has been reviewed by a radiologist.

other than amputation (Malawer, Link, & Donaldson, 1993). Preferably, the biopsy should be performed by the surgeon who will make the definitive decision about the operative procedure.

There are different types of biopsies that can be performed. A core, or trephine, biopsy is one in which the site is punctured with a trocar, and multiple samples can be obtained from the same puncture site by altering the position of the approaching angle (Malawer, Link, & Donaldson, 1993). Radiographs should be obtained to document the correct positioning of the trocar. Advantages of this type of biopsy include the following: there is less risk of local contamination than with open biopsy, thus making it an attractive alternative for limb-sparing surgeries, and this procedure is easier to perform in difficult areas, such as the spine, pelvis and hips (Malawer, Link, & Donaldson, 1993). Disadvantages include not obtaining an adequate specimen.

An open biopsy, or incisional biopsy, is one in which a small incision is made in the skin. The obvious advantage of this technique is that an adequate amount of tissue can be obtained to ensure reliable diagnosis and pathologic study (Enneking & Conrad, 1989). However, the disadvantages include contamination of the tumor, as well as the normal risks of infection.

STAGING

Staging studies are based on the progressive changes in the natural history of the lesion (Enneking, Spanier, & Goodman, 1980). Staging studies are valuable for the clinician because they are used to select appropriate treatment and to predict prognosis, response to treatment, and the risks of local recurrence or metastasis (Enneking & Conrad, 1989). Osteosarcomas can be accurately staged after clinical, radiographic, and histologic studies have been performed. It is important to remember that all clinical and radiographic studies should be performed prior to biopsy attainment.

Musculoskeletal Tumor Society's Surgical Staging System

The Musculoskeletal Tumor Society adopted a surgical staging system for bone sarcomas in 1980. The staging system was developed by Enneking and his colleagues and is based on the fact that mesenchymal sarcomas of the bone behave similarly, regardless of histiogenic type (Malawer, Link, & Donaldson, 1993).

The stage of a lesion represents an interrelationship among three factors: the grade (G), which is the assessment of biologic aggressiveness of the tumor; the presence or absence of metastasis (M); and the anatomic site or extent of the tumor (T)—in the case of osteogenic sarcoma, intracapsular or extracapsular, or intracompartmental or extracompartmental (Enneking, Spanier, & Goodman, 1980).

The Enneking and colleagues staging system (Box 71-2) considers G1 (grade 1) to be a low-grade tumor and G2 to be a high-grade tumor. Similarly, T1 is considered to be intracompartmentally located and T2 extracompartmentally located.

Grading

Inwards and Unni (1995) describe bone sarcomas according to grade instead of stage. The grade is based on the histology of the tumor. Those tumor cells that have minimal or moderate anaplasia receive a grade of 1 or 2. The cells with more severe anaplasia are graded 3 or 4. Generally, the lower-grade tumors are associated with a better prognosis than the higher-grade tumors.

Classical, or conventional, osteosaracomas are high-grade tumors (Inwards & Unni, 1995). They are classified as either grade 3 or 4 and represent the majority of osteosarco-

Box 71-2
Musculoskeletal Tumor Society's Surgical Staging System for Osteosarcoma
Stage 1-3 (Grade 0)—Benign Tumors

Malignant

Stage I

- Grade 1 (G1)—Histologically low grade. Cells are well differentiated. Recurrence tends to be local.
  G1-IA—Intraosseous (intracompartmental)
  G1-IB—Extraosseous (extracompartmental; lesions penetrate the bone cortex)

Stage II

- Grade 2 (G2)—Histologically high grade. Cells are poorly differentiated. Tumor is more destructive, nuclei are atypical. There is a higher incidence of metastases.
  G2-IIA—Intraosseous (intracompartmental)
  G2-IIB—Extraosseous (extracompartmental- lesions penetrate bone cortex)

Stage III

- Metastases

From Enneking, W., Spanier, S., & Goodman, M. (1980). A system for the surgical staging of musculoskeletal sarcoma. *Clinical Orthopaedics and Related Research, 153,* 106-119.

mas. The cells are described as having atypical nuclei, a high mitotic rate, and are hyperchromasia (Inwards & Unni, 1995).

It is unusual to identify a low-grade osteosarcoma. These tumors are well-differentiated and intraosseous, with hypocellular stroma and very slight cytologic anaplasia. They are usually graded as a grade 1. Parosteal osteosarcomas are examples of low-grade osteosarcomas.

Periosteal osteosarcomas and osteosarcomas of the jawbones, are usually grade 2 or 3. They have a better prognosis than classical osteosarcoma. They also have a lower metastatic rate than their higher-grade counterparts.

MEDICAL MANAGEMENT

History

Before 1970, the major management of osteosarcoma was amputation of the affected area (Malawer, Link, & Donaldson, 1993). Survival statistics based on this method of managing the disease were dim—patients who were treated with surgical intervention alone had only 8 months (median) before the onset of pulmonary metastases. The 5-year survival was less than 25% (Vander Griend, 1996), with the majority of patients dying with disease 9 months after pulmonary metastases were discovered (Jaffe, Patel, & Benjamin, 1995).

Neoadjuvant and Adjuvant Chemotherapy. Neoadjuvant (preoperatively administered) chemotherapy actually began as an attempt to provide some type of therapy while custom prostheses were being formed. This resulted in improvement in patient survival (Vander Griend, 1996). Surgeons also found that chemotherapy administered prior to surgery actually aided limb-salvage therapy. This was primarily due to the tumor necrosis caused by chemotherapy, but in some patients the tumor actually decreased in size by chemotherapy alone (Vander Griend, 1996; Yasko & Johnson, 1995; Damron & Pritchard, 1995).

Other results of neoadjuvant chemotherapy include a decrease in the zone of neovascularity, inflammation, and the ossification of the unmineralized tumor osteoid (Damron & Pritchard, 1995; Vander Griend, 1996; Yasko & Johnson, 1995).

The responsiveness of the tumor to chemotherapy administered preoperatively became a prognostic indicator—a good response to the chemotherapeutic agents was associated with higher survival rates than a lesser response. A good response was determined to be greater than 90% tumor necrosis (Jaffe, Patel, & Benjamin, 1995; Vander Griend, 1996; Ayala, Ro, & Raymond, 1996).

Other prognostic factors were also identified: tumor size, the extent of the tumor, and location of the tumor, along with the patient's age and sex and the duration of symptoms (Vander Griend, 1996; Ayala, Ro, & Raymond, 1996).

Due to the positive responses seen from neoadjuvant chemotherapy, physicians began including adjuvant chemotherapy as part of their treatment of osteosarcoma. The goal of this was to control the micrometastases that physicians believed were present in the majority of patients (Rodriguez, 1996). The use of chemotherapy after surgical ablation of the tumor produced a 3-year disease-free survival rate of 50% to 80%—much higher than the historical rate of 20% (Jaffe, Patel, & Benjamin, 1995; Cortes, Holland, & Glidewell, 1981).

This led to great controversy, because major medical centers began producing conflicting data concerning the efficacy of adjuvant chemotherapy (Jaffe, Patel, & Benjamin, 1995). The Mayo Clinic provided documentation that stated that between 1972 and 1974, survival rates of patients with osteogenic sarcoma who underwent amputation alone was 50%. Trying to resolve the argument, physicians enrolled patients in a randomized study, comparing the results of patients treated with surgery alone with patients treated with high-dose methotrexate and leucovorin rescue. Results of the study showed no advantage in either arm, with survival in both arms being approximately 40% (Edmonson, Green, & Ivins, 1984).

This led to a multi-institutional clinical trial, known as the Multi-institutional Osteosarcoma Trial (MIOS). The objective was to determine whether adjuvant chemotherapy, utilizing multi-agents after ablative surgery, showed a significant improvement in disease-free survival in patients with nonmetastatic osteosarcoma. The results of the trial showed that those patients who had adjuvant chemotherapy and surgery had a 66% 2-year disease-free survival status, compared with a 20% disease-free survival rate for those patients who had surgery alone, thus effectively resolving the question of the efficacy of adjuvant chemotherapy.

Box 71-3
Treatment Plan for Osteosarcoma

Diagnosis and staging, with biopsy performed after other staging completed
- Neoadjuvant chemotherapy
- Repeat scans to assess response of chemotherapy
- Surgery
- Adjuvant chemotherapy
- Repeat check-ups and evaluations

From Vander Griend, R. (1996). Osteosarcoma and its variants. *Orthopedics of North America, 27,* 575-581.

Current Chemotherapy Use

The current standard of care for treatment of high-grade (conventional) osteosarcoma is the utilization of chemotherapy neoadjuvantly as well as adjuvantly (Box 71-3). A variety of agents are used, including the standards of high-dose methotrexate, adriamycin, cisplatin, cyclophosphamide, ifosfamide, as well as bleomycin, etoposide, and mitomycin C, and dacarbazine (Jaffe, Patel, & Benjamin, 1995; Damron & Pritchard, 1995; Rosen et al., 1997; Ayala, Ro, & Raymond, 1996).

Chemotherapy may be administered systemically as well as intra-arterially (Jaffe, Patel, & Benjamin, 1995). When chemotherapy is administered directly into the vascular supply of the tumor, it is hoped that necrosis will occur (Malawer, Link, & Donaldson, 1997). Doxorubicin and cisplatin are the most frequently used agents. Intra-arterial chemotherapy may have its optimal usage as a neoadjuvant chemotherapy, to facilitate limb-sparing surgery instead of amputation.

Due to the accepted use of neoplastic agents, coordination between the medical oncologists and the surgeons is of great importance. The timing of surgery should be coordinated with the chemotherapy schedule, so that surgery coincides with bone marrow recovery. Surgery is usually not performed until the patient has a neutrophil count of at least 1500 and a platelet count of at least 70,000. Optimal planning should eliminate a long delay in chemotherapy. Patients can usually resume chemotherapy within 2 to 3 weeks after surgical ablation of the tumor (Yasko & Johnson, 1995).

Biologic Response Modifiers

Although recent improvements in surgical and chemotherapeutic methods have improved the disease-free survival of patients with osteosarcoma, pulmonary metastases still remains as a problem. A rationale for this is drug-resistant malignant cells (Kleinerman, 1995). Consequently, treatment is now focused at eliminating those cells. Using biologic response modifiers is one method of doing this.

One such agent, liposomal muramyl tripeptide phosphatidylethanolamine (L-MTP-PE) has been in research trials to determine its efficacy in treating pulmonary metastases in osteosarcoma patients. The drug has been used in conjunction with chemotherapeutic agents in newly diagnosed patients.

The liposomal formulation of the drug allows for the agent to selectively be delivered to the macrophages in the pulmonary system as well as the circulating monocytes. The goal is for the L-MTP-PE to stimulate the pulmonary macrophages' tumoricidal properties. The systemic chemotherapeutic agents would kill the majority of tumor cells, and the pulmonary macrophages would then eliminate the remaining drug-resistant cells (Kleinerman, 1995).

Box 71-4
Indications for Amputation for Osteosarcoma

1. It is the only possible way to remove all the malignant tissue.
2. Amputation and the use of a prosthesis would make the limb more functional than a limb-sparing resection.
3. The patient has a poor prognosis for survival and doesn't have the physical or emotional capacity to undergo rehabilitation after the limb-sparing procedure.
4. The predicted morbidity from the limb-sparing resection is higher than that of amputative surgery.

From Malawer, M., Link, M., & Donaldson, S. (1997). Sarcomas of bone. In V. T. DeVita, S. Hellman, & S. A. Rosenberg (Eds.). *Cancer: Principles and practice of oncology* (5th ed.). Philadelphia: Lippincott-Raven.

Surgical Intervention

Prior to the early 1970s, the standard method of treatment for osteogenic sarcoma was amputation of the affected extremity (Malawer, Link, & Donaldson,1993). However, in the 1970s, surgeons began developing effective limb-sparing (also known as *limb salvage*) techniques. Since that time, limb-salvage procedures have become the primary method used to eradicate local osteosarcoma without compromising local tumor control or patient survival (Yasko & Johnson, 1995).

Amputation is still used when necessary and, as seen in Box 71-4, there are four major indications for selecting amputation instead of a limb-sparing procedure. Obviously, the location of the tumor is a major factor when surgical options are being considered. If the section of bone involved, with or without soft-tissue involvement, is in an area of the body that is not amenable to resection, amputation may be the only choice the patient and surgeon has. Also, if there is major neurovascular involvement, the surgeon may elect to amputate the affected extremity rather than attempt a vascular graft. Although vascular grafting can be successfully performed, the adjacent nerves may be at risk for damage (Malawer, Link, & Donaldson, 1993; Rodriquez, 1996).

The limb-sparing resection obviously should only be performed if the limb would be at least as functional as a prosthetic device. This is of particular importance when the patient's growth potential has not been reached (Rodriquez, 1996; Yasko & Johnson, 1995). Because the tumor usually affects at least one growth plate, and sometimes two, a limb-sparing resection can result in length disparity of the limbs, thus requiring repeated surgeries as the patient matures (Piasecki, 1991).

Patients who have an anticipated poor prognosis for survival and those who do not have the functional and/or psychologic capacity for the rehabilitation process following a limb-salvage procedure, may elect for amputation of the extremity. This would also be the procedure of choice for patients who develop pathologic fractures. Those patients are at great risk of uncontrolled metastases because the fracture may have spread tumor cells throughout the area (Rodriguez, 1996). Another factor leading to the decision to amputate is if the biopsy performed for histologic diagnosis was improperly executed, again contaminating the area with tumor cells (Malawer, Link, & Donaldson, 1993; Rodriquez, 1996).

Finally, if the patient did not show a good response to neoadjuvant chemotherapy, the choice of amputation may increase the patient's chance of survival, due to the resistance of the tumor to chemotherapy.

A last factor to be evaluated is the predicted morbidity of the limb-salvage procedure. Neither procedure is without risks, but because of the individual patient's health and risk factors, the morbidity of amputation may be far less than that associated with a limb-sparing operation (Rodriguez, 1996).

Amputation. The level of amputation is usually determined by the location of the tumor and the extent of the disease. Amputating the involved extremity should be performed judiciously, preserving as much length as possible. This will enhance the use of a prosthetic device. The residual joints should also have good range of motion to enhance the use of the prosthetic device (Rodriguez, 1996). Obviously, if possible, a below-the-knee amputation is preferred to an above-the-knee amputation. A below-the-knee amputation not only preserves the knee joint, making the prosthetic device easier to manipulate, but also enables the patient to expend less energy when ambulating. As will be discussed later in the chapter, energy saving techniques and devices play an important role in the rehabilitation and quality of life for the patient with a lower extremity amputation.

Limb-Sparing Procedures. There are a variety of types of bone resections that the orthopedic oncologist can perform (Yasko & Johnson, 1995). The selection of the resection procedure depends on the anatomic site as well as the extent of the bone involvement. Other factors than can influence the type of reconstruction performed include the integrity of the structures surrounding the tumor-invaded bone, the extent of the resection being considered, the risk and type of potential early and late complications, and the patient's age, expectations, and anticipated functional demands. A young adult would very likely have a different lifestyle than an elderly patient who had a variety of medical problems that often accompany advancing age.

Regardless of the type of reconstructive procedure that is performed, a wide excision (also called an *en bloc incision*) is desired. This type of procedure is one in which the entire tumor, as well as the reactive zone and a cuff of normal tissue, is removed (Malawer, Link, & Donaldson, 1997; Enneking & Conrad, 1989; Enneking, Spanier, & Goodman, 1980). The advantages of this are obvious—by removing the entire tumor, the area surrounding it, and the normal tissue outside, the surgeon has minimized the chance of malignant cells remaining. It is also desirable that the site of the original biopsy be removed, again to reduce the risk of malignant cell spread as well as weakened bone.

There are three phases to any limb-sparing procedure—resection of the tumor, reconstruction of the skeletal area involved, and, finally, the soft tissue and muscle transfer needed to complete the reconstruction (Mawler, Link, & Donaldson, 1997).

Most osteosarcomas arise in the metaphysis of the long bone, usually near a joint. Because of this, the majority of surgical procedures involve the resection of both the segment of tumor-bearing bone and the adjacent joint. This type of bone resection is called an *osteoarticular resection* (Yasko & Johnson, 1995). Most surgical resections are performed through the adjacent joint (an intra-articular resection).

When the bone tumor extends along the capsule of the joint or the ligamentous structures, and/or invades the joint, the entire joint is then resected (extra-articular resection). An intercalary resection is performed when the tumor remains within the diaphysis of the long bone. This occurs in less than 10% of osteosarcomas, but, when it does occur, only the tumor-bearing section of bone is resected, leaving the remainder of the bone intact.

Osteoarticular allografts. The use of donated bone is termed an *allograft.* This type of reconstruction restores the bone stock and adjacent bone surface (Yasko & Johnson, 1995). It provides an area of attachment for the host soft tissues and, optimally, restores active movement at the affected joint. An allograft is especially advantageous when the knee joint is involved because many complications with prosthetic devices occur at the knee joint.

The donor bone is attached to the host bone and secured with a rod or metal plate and screws. The length of this procedure usually is from 3 to 6 hours, but it can take up to 2 years for the host body to incorporate the allograft and to have new host bone start growing. At this time, the donor bone would be at least partially resorbed (Dealy, Pazola, & Heislein, 1995).

Cryosurgery

Cryosurgery is the use of liquid nitrogen in the tumor cavity after the tumor has been removed. The purpose of this is to kill any remaining malignant cells and cause necrosis to occur (Malawer, Link, & Donaldson, 1997). Optimally, after cryosurgery, there will be no need for bone resection. Currently, this approach is being used for low-grade osteosarcomas only (Malawer, Link, & Donaldson, 1997).

Radiation Therapy

Radiation therapy has been used to treat osteogenic sarcomas since the late 1950s and 1960s (Malawer, Link, &

Donaldson, 1997). Results showed that radiation therapy did not have a role in treating these tumors as a primary treatment, although patients with Ewing's sarcoma are treated with radiation therapy and surgery with good results. Radiation therapy is currently used for palliative care for patients with osteosarcoma and for patients who have disease that is unresectable at the axial sites. It is also used to treat those patients who have advanced inoperable tumors in the pelvis or extremities (Malawer, Link, & Donaldson, 1997).

The complications of radiation therapy are related to the dose used and the total volume. Reactions can be divided into early or late reactions. Early reactions are usually minor and can be reversible, whereas the late complications are more serious. Early reactions involve skin problems—usually erythema, epilation, or dry desquamation of the skin. Later complications include fibrosis, contractures, atrophy, impaired growth, secondary fractures, and radiation-induced sarcomas (Malawer, Link, & Donaldson, 1997).

NURSING MANAGEMENT

Although there are no true oncologic emergencies associated with osteosarcoma, a number of acute and long-term complications can arise. The type of surgery used to treat the patient often plays a role in the complications—limb-sparing surgery takes much longer than amputation, and the morbidity of limb-sparing surgery is often higher. Also, the type of limb-sparing procedure employed may alert the nurse as to what type of complications to be aware of, as well as how to tailor the nursing care to meet the patient's needs. Table 71-4 shows a care plan for patients with osteosarcoma. Depending upon the type of surgical procedure used on the patient, the care plan may be modified to fit individual needs.

Diagnostic Nursing Care

Nursing care of the patient with osteosarcoma actually begins at diagnosis. The nurse needs to ensure that the patient and his/her family understand the reasons for the tests ordered for the diagnostic evaluation. The nurse should provide the patient and family with information regarding what is expected of the patient and what the patient can expect during each of the tests for the diagnostic evaluation. The nurse can also provide emotional support, education, and comfort to the patient and family when the diagnosis is made. Because the treatment of osteosarcoma involves a wide range of specialists—the orthopedic oncologist, medical oncologist, and radiation oncologist, as well as the prosthetist—the patient and family may be confused and intimidated. The nurse can be the healthcare team member who can effectively answer questions regarding the different treatment modalities and, if there are questions the nurse cannot answer, then he/she can refer the patient to the appropriate source.

Surgical Nursing Care

Acute nursing care often occurs when the patient is admitted into the hospital for surgery, whether it be amputation or limb salvage. Because most patients now receive some form of neoadjuvant chemotherapy or radiation (Vander Griend, 1996; Malawer, Link, & Donaldson, 1997), the patient will have received education from the medical oncology nurses and the nurses in radiation oncology about those treatments. However, surgery, unless the patient had a pathologic fracture that needed to be repaired, will be a new and stressful experience for the patient and family.

As part of the nursing care of the patient, the nurse should provide the patient and family with information regarding the surgical procedure. The orthopedic oncologist will have discussed the risks of the surgical procedures with the patient when the treatment alternatives were discussed. However, many patients are under so much stress at the time of diagnosis that much of what is explained to them is forgotten, if it was comprehended at all. Thus the nurse has a major role in helping the patient and family anticipate the postoperative care and in how the patient will look and feel after surgery (Dealy, Pazola, & Heislein, 1995) (see Table 71-3).

It may help the patient if another patient (preferably of similar age) who has experienced the procedure and treatment is contacted. Support groups are also an option for the patient and/or family. Because osteosarcoma frequently affects adolescents, the probability of young siblings misunderstanding the attention the patient is receiving is high. Social workers or psychologists associated with the hospital may be able to assist the entire family in adapting to the stressful situation. If those resources are not available, the nurse may be able to provide referrals to outside organizations.

Acute Postoperative Care. Limb-sparing procedures are often more complicated and lengthy than amputations (Piasecki, 1992), and the complications from those procedures are often more severe than those arising from amputations. Regardless of the type of procedure, some of the acute postoperative nursing care is standard.

Infection. All patients are at risk for infection, either superficial skin infections or deep wound infections (Piasecki, 1991; Piasecki, 1992; Dealy, Pazola, & Heislein, 1995; Yasko & Johnson, 1995). The use of laminar air-flow operating rooms as well as prophylactic intravenous antibiotics (Dealy, Pazola, & Heislein, 1995; Piasecki, 1991) reduces the risk of infection but cannot eliminate it totally. Consequently, the nurse must assess the patient's wound frequently for erythema, purulent drainage, and an increase in edema. Monitoring the patient's vital signs, particularly the temperature, and complete blood count (CBC), especially the white blood cell count, will also assist the nurse in monitoring for infection (Piasecki, 1991). An elevated white blood cell count is often a sign of infection, and although many patients may have a low-grade fever after the surgical procedure, a high temperature or a steadily climbing temperature may also be signs of infection. Although all patients will have pain postoperatively, persistent postoperative pain

Text continues on p. 1600

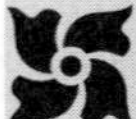

TABLE 71-4 Standard of Care for the Patient Undergoing Surgical Treatment for Osteosarcoma

Patient Problem and Outcomes	Nursing Interventions and Rationales	Patient Education Instructions
Knowledge Deficit Patient/family will: • Verbalize an understanding of the surgical procedure. • Verbalize an understanding of the preoperative teaching (e.g., turn, cough, deep breathe [TCDB], pain management techniques, incentive spirameter, drain function and routines, wound care). • Identify health care team members and their role in the patient's recovery (e.g., physical therapist, social worker, dietitian, radiation and medical oncologist, oncology nurse). • List signs and symptoms of conditions that are to be reported to the medical team, (e.g., signs and symptoms of infection, increased pain, poor wound healing, inability to participate in prescribed care routines).	1. Assess the patient's level of understanding of the surgical procedure. 2. Determine if the patient understands the difference between limb sparing and amputation. 3. Assess the family's understanding of the surgical procedure, including potential complications and outcomes. 4. Give the patient/family the opportunity to ask questions or verbalize concerns. 5. Have patient repeat/demonstrate postoperative care such as deep breathing; use of spirometer; use of trapeze, immobilization of the affected extremity (as appropriate). 6. Identify for the patient possible postoperative complications of wound healing. 7. Demonstrate the use of prosthetic equipment as appropriate. 8. Discuss psychosocial and rehabilitative resources available postoperatively.	1. Use a diagram of the surgical procedure relevant to the anatomic site. 2. If the planned procedure is limb sparing, discuss and review the possibility of amputation. 3. Provide information about the preoperative routines: anesthesiology consult; diagnostic tests; anti-embolism stockings; nothing by mouth (NPO) after midnight. 4. Provide the patient with pertinent information related to postoperative care: pain management; surgical incision; fluid and nutrition management; restrictions in self-care and mobility. 5. Provide information about phantom limb sensation in the case of planned amputation. 6. Review the plan for adjuvant therapy as appropriate. 7. Provide appropriate discharge information relevant to reportable signs and symptoms of potential postoperative problems.
Anxiety Patient will: • Express feelings related to the diagnosis of soft tissue sarcoma. • Express feelings related to the surgical procedure. • Identify strategies to cope with anxiety. • Experience a decrease in symptoms of anxiety and an increase of psychologic and physiologic comfort.	1. Determine which coping strategies the patient has used effectively in the past to decrease anxiety. 2. Identify those individuals that the patient feels are supportive. 3. Assess patient's problem-solving ability, level of concentration, rate of speech, flow of thought, and nonverbal behaviors (gestures, facial grimaces, posture, overall appearance). 4. Note patient's interactions with the health care team and family. 5. Observe patient for signs of anxiety: restlessness, increased heart rate and respiratory rate, purposeless activity, agitation, diaphoresis, or repetitive questioning. 6. Note patient's complaints of physical symptoms that may be related to anxiety: diarrhea, nausea, vomiting, body aches and pains, fatigue, shortness of breath, dry mouth. 7. Reinforce the use of effective coping strategies. 8. Administer pharmacologic agents to decrease anxiety if necessary.	1. Explain all procedures, including potential pain and sensations likely to be experienced. 2. Teach relaxation techniques, visualization, and the use of music therapy to decrease anxiety. 3. Suggest diversional activities for patient and family. 4. Review and reinforce all patient education activities.

From Webb, K., Lewis, S., & Collier, I. (1983). Nursing assessment: Musculoskeletal system. In S. Lewis & I. Collier (Eds.), *Medical-surgical nursing: Assessment and management of clinical problems.* New York: McGraw Hill.

TABLE 71-4 Standard of Care for the Patient Undergoing Surgical Treatment for Osteosarcoma—cont'd

Patient Problem and Outcomes	Nursing Interventions and Rationales	Patient Education Instructions
Pain Patient will: • Rate pain on a standard scale to more effectively evaluate response to pain management efforts. • Experience effective pain management by verbalizing pain relief. • Describe phantom limb sensations and identify ways to manage the symptoms. • Verbalize the importance of reporting changes in perception of pain (e.g., sudden increase in pain experienced; change in characteristics of pain). • Identify nonpharmacologic methods of achieving pain relief.	1. Assess patient's history related to previous pain experiences (e.g., dentistry, accidents, surgery). 2. Assess patient's psychosocial history as related to drug or alcohol abuse and allergies. 3. Identify concerns patient or family may have related to the use of pain medications (particularly narcotics). 4. Explain that most acute surgical pain can be controlled to an acceptable level (defined by the patient) to allow the patient to fully participate in expected postoperative care routines as appropriate.	1. Teach that the experience of pain is very individual and that perceptions of pain are influenced by the patient's anxiety level, past experiences, and expectations. 2. Teach the patient to use a pain rating scale to evaluate pain. 3. Teach the patient to report symptoms of pain early on so that medications will be more effective. 4. Teach the patient how to operate the patient-controlled analgesic (PCA) pump for pain management. 5. Teach the patient and family nonpharmacologic methods of pain management: progressive muscle relaxation, guided imagery, music therapy, massage, diversional activities. 6. Teach the patient to expect phantom limb pain if an amputation is anticipated.
Self-Care Deficit Patient will: • Resume activities of daily living (ADL) within appropriate time frame without assistance. • Resume previous lifestyle after treatment and rehabilitation are completed.	1. Determine expected self-care deficit as it relates to the treatment plan. 2. Allow patient input into the schedule of ADL. 3. Assess the patient for factors that may interfere with self-care: attitude, depression, impaired memory, fatigue level and tolerance of activity, pain. 4. Assess competency of caregivers to assist the patient with self-care activities until the patient becomes independent. 5. Assess effects on family system (roles and responsibilities) with additional care for patient in the home setting. 6. Assess home environment with the help of the patient/family and the home care nurse to identify any potential barriers to successful self-care. 7. Consult occupational therapy preoperatively as appropriate.	1. Teach the patient new skills to enable him or her to manage ADL independently 2. Teach family safe techniques to assist the patient 3. Review with patient and family community resources as appropriate (e.g., respite care, adult day care). 4. Reinforce self-care routines recommended by physical or occupational therapy.

Continued

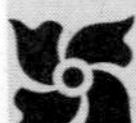

TABLE 71-4 Standard of Care for the Patient Undergoing Surgical Treatment for Osteosarcoma—cont'd

Patient Problem and Outcomes	Nursing Interventions and Rationales	Patient Education Instructions
Impaired Physical Mobility Patient will: • Identify anticipated limitations in physical mobility. • Demonstrate active participation in the rehabilitation plan. • Identify community resources that aid in rehabilitation and recovery. • Set realistic goals with the help of the health care team, to aid in rehabilitation and recovery process.	1. Assess the patient's expectations of his or her physical abilities related to potential loss of physical mobility or body part. 2. Assess the patient's view of his or her physical limitations and potential effects on his or her roles and relationships. 3. Consult physical therapy and occupational therapy preoperatively. 4. Arrange for preoperative or postoperative visit from an individual with similar challenges as appropriate. 5. Assess the patient for signs of impaired mobility such as skin breakdown, atelectasis, constipation, anorexia, or embolism. 6. Supervise ambulation if lower limb is involved in limb-sparing or amputative procedure. 7. Begin discharge planning early with a complete assessment of the home environment as it pertains to the patient's limitations (e.g., need for wheelchair ramp, presence of steps).	1. Teach range-of-motion activities. 2. Explain the importance of early ambulation and good nutrition during recovery. 3. Teach patient and family proper care of the stump in the case of amputation. 4. Teach proper assessment of the stump and the use of the prosthetic device. 5. Teach patient proper care of the stump, including daily cleaning and dressing change or wrapping technique. 6. Teach patient and family to regularly assess the prosthetic device for wear.
Body Image Disturbance Patient will: • Discuss changes in his or her feelings about self as related to his or her diagnosis and surgical treatment. • Develop confidence in his or her ability to accomplish goals. • Identify four positive characteristics related to himself or herself.	1. Assess the patient's view of himself or herself. 2. Clarify misconceptions regarding perception of self. 3. Avoid negative reactions to the surgical site (verbal or nonverbal). 4. Encourage open communication between the patient, his or her family, and the health care team. 5. Promote social interaction and self-care activities. 6. Make appropriate referrals for counseling and support; encourage the use of support groups composed of patients undergoing similar treatment; arrange for pre- or postoperative visits from other patients experiencing similar concerns as appropriate.	1. Teach patient to set realistic goals to accomplish within a particular time frame related to self-care and activities. 2. Have patient identify peers and family members that he or she can share feelings about his condition. 3. Help patient develop a strategy to return to normal routines and activities.
Infection Patient will: • Report signs and symptoms of infection such as tenderness or increased pain at surgical site, discoloration, or drainage. • Along with caregiver, demonstrate proper care of the surgical site and administration of any anti-infective therapies.	1. Assess patient vital signs and temperature q 4 h for signs of fever or infection. Assess fluctuations in temperature. 2. Assess wound for evidence of infection. 3. Assess for evidence of systemic infection: chills, vital sign changes.	1. Review with patient and family reportable signs and symptoms of infection. 2. Demonstrate thorough handwashing and have patient/caregiver return demonstrate.

From Webb, K., Lewis, S., & Collier, I. (1983). Nursing assessment: Musculoskeletal system. In S. Lewis & I. Collier (Eds.), *Medical-surgical nursing: Assessment and management of clinical problems.* New York: McGraw Hill.

Table 71-4 Standard of Care for the Patient Undergoing Surgical Treatment for Osteosarcoma—cont'd

Patient Problem and Outcomes	Nursing Interventions and Rationales	Patient Education Instructions
Infection—cont'd	4. Obtain culture and sensitivities of wound drainage before initiation of antibiotics. 5. Monitor culture results and administer antimicrobial therapy as ordered. 6. Maintain adequate nutrition and hydration. 7. Implement measures to control fever; monitor side effects of antimicrobial drugs.	3. Teach aseptic technique when changing dressing or administrating other care. 4. Help patient and caregiver identify a place within the home that is appropriate for storage of medications and supplies. 5. Teach administration of antimicrobial therapy and related side effects prior to hospital discharge.
Skin Integrity Patient will: • Comply with wound care, which may include immobilization, compression dressings, drain and wound care, and restrictions in self-care routines. • Maintain adequate nutritional intake as noted by calorie count, compliance to dietary advances.	1. Assess surgical wound for edema, hematoma, seroma, and infection q 4 h. 2. Maintain adherent dressing as ordered. 3. Assess for signs and symptoms of decreased perfusion of wound; necrosis of wound edges or flap; and flap/wound edge viability. 1. Avoid excessive pressure on surgical incision that may interfere with tissue perfusion (compression dressing may be appropriate). 2. Assess integrity of suture line q 4 h for evidence of wound dehiscence. 3. Assess nutritional status preoperatively and monitor for nutritional deficits throughout treatment course. 4. Maintain proper body alignment for affected body part.	1. Teach proper wound/stump care. 2. Review information regarding adequate nutrition necessary for wound healing.
Grief Patient will: • Identify areas of perceived loss related to a diagnosis of sarcoma. • Identify actual loss related to physical mobility or body image as a result of therapy.	1. Assess patient's and family's previous experience with loss (e.g., death, illness, job). 2. Assess the effects of the previous loss to individuals and the family system as a whole. 3. Assess current coping strategies and their effectiveness. 4. Assess significance of loss to patient and family (loss of function, mobility, or of a limb) 5. Allow patient/family to verbalize feelings. 6. Acknowledge grief and provide support to patient/family. 7. Refer patient to appropriate professional for counseling. 8. Encourage patient to contact community support groups (amputee, cancer patient).	1. Discuss the normal responses that occur with experience loss. 2. Discuss that grief is a personal experience and that expression of grief varies with individuals. 3. Help the patient and family identify appropriate ways to express caring and concern for each other.

Continued

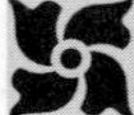

TABLE 71-4 Standard of Care for the Patient Undergoing Surgical Treatment for Osteosarcoma—cont'd

Patient Problem and Outcomes	Nursing Interventions and Rationales	Patient Education Instructions
Fear Patient will: • Discuss concerns about outcome of therapy and disease recurrence. • Identify concrete plan for follow-up care during the next 24 months. • Identify community organizations for cancer survivors.	1. Allow patient to verbalize concerns and fears related to his or her future and potential for disease recurrence. 2. Assist patient in obtaining appropriate information related to his or her disease, treatment plan, and prognosis.	1. Provide patient with follow-up schedule of care over the next 24 months. 2. Teach patient to examine surgical area for signs of local tumor recurrence: new pain, ulceration, lumps, nodules. 3. Discuss issues related to long-term effects of treatment (e.g., effect on growth and development, potential for secondary malignancies with radiation and chemotherapy). 4. Provide information on community/national organizations relevant to cancer survivors (e.g., American Cancer Society's CanSurmount, National Coalition of Cancer Survivorship).
Ineffective Individual Coping Patient will demonstrate successful positive coping and adaptation to diagnosis and treatment through: verbalizing negative feelings appropriately and demonstrates less frequent occurrences; utilizing appropriate resources; participating appropriately in self-care routines and treatment plan.	1. Explain each new diagnostic test and review expected routines (pre- and post-operative) with patient. 2. Assess patient's acknowledgment of the disease process and treatment plan. 3. Allow time for patient to express feelings with family and significant others. 4. Help patient set realistic goals through the recovery process. 5. Assess effect that diagnosis and subsequent therapy may have on sexuality. 6. Discuss how others may cope with the patient's diagnosis and treatment. 7. Encourage and assist patient in efforts to seek more information related to his or her disease, treatment, and resources.	1. Teach patient strategies to enhance positive coping (e.g., clarification of life values; focus on realistic goals; positive affirmation techniques; relaxation techniques). 2. Teach patient methods of problem-solving effectively (e.g., identify positive and negative aspects of a situation and fantasize potential outcomes). 3. Provide information on the relationship between coping and perceived stress. 4. Teach the benefits of emotional release of tension (e.g., crying, exercise, play, talk, humor).

From Webb, K., Lewis, S., & Collier, I. (1983). Nursing assessment: Musculoskeletal system. In S. Lewis & I. Collier (Eds.), *Medical-surgical nursing: Assessment and management of clinical problems.* New York: McGraw Hill.

may also be a sign of a superficial wound infection (Dealy, Pazola, & Heislein, 1995).

Depending on the type of surgical procedure and the length of time the patient is bedfast, infections in the urinary tract from an indwelling catheter and respiratory tract infections from inadequate lung expansion may also occur. The nurse should provide good catheter care and assess the urine for cloudiness, as well as the amount of urine output the patient has on each shift. Again, unexplained changes or trends should be noted and questioned.

Upper respiratory tract infections may be prevalent for patients who had osteoallograft reconstructions because these patients are often in surgery for 6 hours and are kept in bed for approximately 1 week. Prior to the surgical procedure, the nurse should teach the patient how to use an incentive spirometer and ensure that the patient understands the risks associated with pneumonia. Although the use of the incentive spirometer can be monotonous, the nurse can provide incentives and rewards for the younger patient to encourage the use of the spirometer. Involving family members may also encourage patients to use the spirometer—and ensuring that it is within reach of the patient is a simple but important task.

Elderly patients, or those who have an extensive history of tobacco use, also need close monitoring for respiratory infections. For patients who are suspected of being at high risk for a respiratory infection, respiratory therapists may be consulted prior to surgery to inform them of the potential risk. They can then follow the patient as needed postoperatively.

TABLE 71-4 Standard of Care for the Patient Undergoing Surgical Treatment for Osteosarcoma—cont'd

Patient Problem and Outcomes	Nursing Interventions and Rationales	Patient Education Instructions
Ineffective Family Coping Family will: • Identify and utilize appropriate resources to enhance positive coping. • Acknowledge and deal realistically with the situation. • Plan and initiate appropriate changes in family roles and responsibilities.	1. Assess family composition; including extended family and their roles and responsibilities. 2. Identify family strengths and weaknesses in the areas of communication with each other and patient; decision-making processes; family values; problem-solving skills; cultural or ethnic influences. 3. Assess, with the help of the home care nurse, the physical environment of the home; access to facilities; general living conditions. Identify additional current stressors for the family (e.g., other illness, loss of occupation, family member conflicts). 4. Encourage family to interact and communicate openly with patient. 5. Encourage family to share feelings and information with all members of the family. 6. Refer family for financial assistance as appropriate as determined by insurance coverage, out-of-pocket expenses, other family expenses, and expressed needs.	1. Teach family strategies to enhance positive coping (e.g., clarification of life values; focus on realistic goals; positive affirmation techniques; relaxation techniques). 2. Teach family methods of problem-solving effectively (e.g., identify positive and negative aspects of a situation and fantasize potential outcomes). 3. Provide information on the relationship between coping and perceived stress. 4. Teach the benefits of emotional release of tension (e.g., crying, exercise, play, talk, humor).

Pain. All patients will experience pain postoperatively. Pain is typically managed either by epidural analgesics or by patient-controlled analgesic (PCA) pumps (Dealy, Pazola, & Heislein, 1995; Piasecki, 1992). It is important that pain medication is administered around the clock to keep the patient sufficiently comfortable. PCA pumps are useful not only in providing relief from pain, but also in also giving the patient a sense of control. These pumps can be programmed to deliver analgesia continually with added doses delivered when needed, or to deliver the pain medication only when needed. It is easy for the nurse to monitor the patient's need for pain medication by noting how frequently the patient used the PCA. It is also easy to titrate the patient from intravenous narcotics to oral medication when needed.

Patients may need reassurance that they will not become addicted to the pain medication. It is important that they understand the need for them to be comfortable so that they may rest adequately. Family members also will need to understand that the patients will be in pain postoperatively and will require medication.

As a result of the use of narcotic analgesia for the relief of pain, as well as being immobile, the patient may experience constipation. To prevent this, the patient may be administered stool softeners on a regular schedule. The nurse should monitor the patient's bowel habits to prevent an unnecessary complication.

Patients may also experience muscle spasms postoperatively, and the narcotics used for the surgical pain will not be effective in controlling the spasms. Valium may be required to decrease the spasms, or the patient may need to be repositioned.

Phantom limb pain will not be alleviated by narcotics (Piasecki, 1991; Engstrand, 1976; Slye, 1991). This phenomenon is not entirely understood. Melzack (1971) studied the characteristics of phantom limb pain and identified four major characteristics: the pain is chronic, usually lasting longer than 1 year; patients who had a history of limb pain prior to amputation are more likely to experience phantom limb pain; somatic input can either increase or decrease the sensation; and the patient may have trigger zones on healthy areas of the body that when touched can cause phantom limb pain.

Treatment of phantom limb pain consists of mixed modalities. Psychotherapy may be of some help, as well as mental imagery. Having the patient visualize the affected extremity being moved or stroked may help. Behavioral therapy, as well as biofeedback, may also be employed to assist in relieving the pain.

Regardless of the treatment used to relieve the pain, it is important that the patient be aware of phantom limb pain, as well as phantom limb sensation, preoperatively. The patient will need reassurance that this is not "all in his or her head," but a documented phenomenon associated with amputation.

Blood Loss. It is not unusual for the patient to experience a large amount of blood loss during the surgical procedure (Dealy, Pazola, & Heislein, 1995). Nurses should monitor the patient's CBC to note the patient's hemoglobin and hematocrit values. It is common for patients to experience a decline in their hemoglobin and hematocrit levels the first few days postoperatively (Dealy, Pazola, & Heislein, 1995; Piasecki, 1992). Nurses should be prepared to administer packed red blood cell (PRBC) transfusions to the patient if necessary. Patients who received neoadjuvant chemotherapy may be at increased risk for anemia, due to the myelosuppressive side effects of the chemotherapy. Again, education for both the patient and the family is important—many people are still afraid to receive transfusions for fear of receiving blood contaminated with HIV. The nurse can play an important role in educating the patient and family about the risks of infection from blood transfusions, as well as the complications the patient may encounter from not receiving blood when necessary.

Often, the patient will leave the operating room with one or two surgical drains. These drains will be quite bloody the first day postoperatively, but, as time passes, the amount of drainage will be less, and the fluid will become more serosanguinous rather than bloody. It is important that the patient and family are aware of the drains before the patient has the surgery, so that they will not surprise or scare the patient, particularly if the patient is young. Once drainage is limited to approximately 10 ml or less in a 24-hour period, the drains will be pulled. Again, nursing assessment of the amount of drainage each shift, as well as the type of drainage, is important.

Nerve Injury. Nerve damage is a relatively common complication of limb-sparing surgery (Piasecki, 1991; Dealy, Pazola, & Heislein, 1995; Rodriguez, 1996). As part of the acute postoperative nursing care, the nurse should frequently (often hourly immediately postoperatively) assess the sensation and mobility of the toes of the patient (Dealy, Pazola, & Heislein, 1995). It will be important that a baseline sensory assessment be made prior to surgery because the patient may have some deficits unrelated to the surgical procedure (i.e., peripheral neuropathies from diabetes or from chemotherapy). As will be discussed later, the peripheral nerves are the first to be affected in compartment syndrome (Slye, 1991). In a retrospective study of 100 patients who received limb-salvage procedures for osteosarcoma and soft tissue sarcoma (Quill, Gitelis, Morton, & Piasecki, 1990), only two patients experienced nerve palsies. One patient fully recovered from the nerve damage, and the other experienced partial recovery.

Deep Vein Thrombosis. All patients who undergo lengthy surgical procedures are at risk for deep vein thrombosis (DVT). However, those patients who have cancer are at increased risk due to the hypercoagulability of their body due to disease (Slye, 1991; Piasecki, 1991). DVTs are often a result of venous stasis and vein wall injury as well as hypercoagulability. Most occur in veins distal to the surgical site, and they tend to occur within 48 to 72 hours postoperatively (Slye, 1991). To assess for deep vein thrombosis, the nurse should monitor the patients' legs—particularly the calf—for edema and erythema, as well as instruct the patient to report any calf pain experienced. The patient may or may not have a positive Homan's sign with the deep vein thrombosis (Slye, 1991). The patient may be on anticoagulants prophylactically, as well as having intermittent compression boots or TED stockings on. The patient on anticoagulants (usually heparin or warfarin [Coumadin]) will need to have partial prothombin times (PT/PTT) monitored to ensure that the correct dose is administered.

Again, many of the patients may have abnormal CBCs secondary to chemotherapy received neoadjuvantly. If this is so, and the patient is thrombocytopenic, the nurse should also assess the patient for any signs and symptoms of bleeding while the patient is being anticoagulated. Because the patient may go home on anticoagulants, the nurse may want to involve the patient and/or family in learning how to administer heparin subcutaneously as preparation for discharge.

The danger of deep vein thromboses lies in the risk of the patient experiencing a pulmonary embolism as a result of a clot leaving the embolism and traveling to the lungs.

If the patient is complaining of dyspnea, chest pain, feelings of apprehension that are unexplainable, coughing, tachypnea and tachycardia, a pulmonary embolism should be suspected (Slye, 1991). A chest radiograph, electrocardiogram (ECG), and arterial blood gas assay should be performed, as well as a lung scan, to determine if the patient does have a pulmonary embolism.

Prevention of pulmonary embolism is similar to prevention of deep vein thrombosis—have the patient wear elastic stockings or intermittent pneumatic compression boots if the surgical procedure performed requires the patient to have bedrest for an extended time. Otherwise, early ambulation, leg exercises, and prophylactic anticoagulants can be prescribed.

If the patient is diagnosed with a pulmonary embolism, the treatment consists of anticoagulant therapy or surgical intervention.

Soft Tissue Injury. Skin and soft tissue injuries are complications of both limb-sparing procedures and amputations (Rodriguez, 1996; Piasecki, 1992; Yasko & Johnson, 1995). The orthopedic surgeon should assess the condition of the patient's skin and circulation while deciding which surgical procedure would best serve the patient. If a patient with an amputation has an inadequate amount of soft tissue covering the bone, surgical revision may be necessary, requiring an amputation of a higher level (Rodriguez, 1996). Again, the neoadjuvant chemotherapy the patient may have had before surgery, as well as presurgical radiation therapy, may delay healing at the incision site. Other reasons for compromised soft tissue healing may have been the surgical elevation of extensive soft tissue flaps, a prolonged surgical time, or the insertion of a large prosthesis or allograft (Yasko & Johnson, 1995).

In a retrospective study (Quills et al., 1990), wound necrosis was the most common complication observed. This was most frequently experienced by the patient who had radiation therapy prior to surgery.

Again, nursing assessment is of vital importance. The nurse should frequently assess the wound site and monitor healing, reporting any adverse or questionable changes. The nurse should also instruct the patient to assess the wound and monitor the healing process.

The most severe complication associated with compromised soft tissue involvement (other than necrosis, which may cause amputation of the extremity) is compartment syndrome. This is a condition in which increasing pressure within a confined space compromises both the circulation and the function of the tissues within the space (Slye, 1991).

The "compartment" in compartment syndrome is composed of bone, blood vessels, nerves, muscles, and soft tissue. They reside within a fascial envelope. The dressing, splint, or cast can serve as a space-limiting envelope, causing increased tissue pressure. The postsurgical edema commonly causes ischemia, which then affects tissue function. Peripheral nerves and skeletal muscle are particularly susceptible to this, while skin and subcutaneous tissue are better able to survive hypoxia (Slye, 1991).

Nursing assessment for compartment syndrome would include assessing the sensory status of peripheral nerves. Assessment and monitoring of the patient's hydration status is also important. Compartmental pressures normally increase approximately 20% in the first 24 hours after surgery. However, if the patient is given diuretics, the pressures may increase to 25% (Slye, 1991).

Arteriograms, venograms, or Dopplers may be used to diagnose compartment syndrome. There are also devices available to measure tissue pressure in patients at risk of compartment syndrome. If the patient is diagnosed with compartment syndrome, surgical intervention may be necessary. The goals are to decrease the pressure of the tissues, restore blood flow to prevent ischemia, and make the functional loss as minimal as possible.

Fat Embolism. The final complication to be discussed that may occur during the acute phase postoperatively is fat embolism. This is most frequently seen in patients who have pathologic fractures of the pelvis, femur, tibia, and ribs (Slye, 1991).

Fat embolism occurs when globules of fat are released from the bone marrow into the circulation. Following the route of venous flow, they will eventually travel to the lung, where they can cause pulmonary insufficiency and/or adult respiratory distress syndrome (ARDS).

Signs and symptoms associated with a fat embolism include restlessness, dyspnea, tachypnea, tachycardia, fever, and sometimes a petechial skin rash. If fat embolism is suspected, arterial blood gasses should be drawn, and a CBC (which may show thrombocytopenia and anemia), chest radiograph, and electrocardiogram should be ordered.

A fat embolism often occurs within 24 to 48 hours postoperatively. Treatment includes supplemental oxygen, fluid replacement, possible use of corticosteroids and, at times, mechanical ventilation. Prevention of a fat embolism is similar to the treatment—ensuring the patient has adequate hydration, administering supplemental oxygen if needed, possible administration of corticosteroids, and immobilization of the fracture.

Late Complications of Surgery. The major late complications of surgery include deep infection, nonunion, and degenerative arthritis.

Deep Infections. Deep infections of the surgical wound can occur as late as 6 months to 2 years after surgery (Dealy, Pazola, & Heislein, 1995). To prevent them, patients are often discharged from the hospital on oral antibiotics. Patients who received some type of hardware to support their bone as part of the surgical procedure are more at risk than other patients for later infections. They should be instructed to inform their dentists and any other physicians they may see for the need of prophylactic antibiotics for invasive procedures.

Sites prone to infection include the body of the allograft, if an allograft was used, the area of the allograft/host bone interface, the osteosynthesis site of a rotationplasty, and the end of the endoprosthesis stem (Rodriguez, 1996). If the patient is receiving adjuvant chemotherapy after surgery, additional risk of infection is a problem, due to delayed healing. Also, if the chemotherapeutic agents are myelosuppressive, the patient may be unable to fight infection adequately.

Treatment for deep infection includes systemic antibiotics, debridement of the wound, and revision of the surgical procedure with possible amputation (Yasko & Johnson, 1995). The patient should be instructed to inform the physician of pain, erythema, drainage, and edema.

Nonunion. Nonunion is the inability of the bone to bond with the allograft or the hardware implanted to support the injured bone. For patients who had allografts, it may take up to 2 years for the body to incorporate the allograft and replace it with host bone (Dealy, Pazola, & Heislein, 1995).

Nonunion can occur at the site of the allograft-host interface or at the osteosynthesis site in rotationplasty (Rodriguez, 1996). A related problem seen in prosthetic arthroplasty is the loosening of the prosthesis at the area where the bone and cement interface. This usually occurs from the stress caused to the area by repetitive movements during activities of daily living (ADLs).

Nonunions usually occur 1 year after surgery (Piasecki, 1991). The main symptom of a nonunion is pain at the junction site. Treatment consists of an autogenous bone graft and, at times, new internal fixation.

Degenerative Arthritis. Degenerative arthritis is a late complication that is diagnosed with yearly radiographs of the affected extremity. The patient may complain of pain or stiffness at the location. It can be treated with corticosteroids or surgical revision of the affected limb (Piasecki, 1991).

Psychologic Complications

The diagnosis of cancer certainly causes stress to patients, but the additional fear of losing a limb can increase the stress drastically. All patients should have an assessment of their strengths, weaknesses, and coping skills performed preoperatively, to enable the healthcare team to adequately support the patient and family throughout the treatment process. Areas of potential weakness should be identified, and the patient and family should be assisted in adequately coping with the problem. Before a surgical decision is made, an assessment of the patient's lifestyle should be performed and the patient should be able to state his or her goals of the surgical procedure. The nurse should work with the patient to enable him or her to meet those goals or to set realistic ones.

Patients who have limb-sparing procedures performed recuperate more slowly than those with amputations. Although the fact that the patient will be able to keep his or her limb is a bonus, the lengthy recuperation and rehabilitation period cannot be overemphasized. Patients must also be informed of the possible changes in their lifestyles—with limb-sparing surgeries, they may not be able to participate in aerobic exercise and participate in sports activities that they were active in prior to surgery. Alternative activities such as swimming should be suggested to the patient.

Body image is also something that needs to be considered. If at all possible, patients should be able to see pictures prior to surgery, to help prepare them in making a treatment choice, as well as prepare the patient and family for what the affected extremity will look like. Patients who are having amputations performed should meet with their prosthetist prior to treatment to discuss and see prosthetic devices. When discussing rotationplasty as a surgical option, it is important for the patient to see a picture—if not a patient—of a rotationplasty. All members of the healthcare team, both inpatient and outpatient, should be informed of the patient's treatment goals, as well as maintain a unified plan for the patient and family to achieve those goals.

Chemotherapy

Many patients will receive adjuvant chemotherapy after surgery. Due to the desire to not delay chemotherapeutic treatment, chemotherapy is usually begun within 2 to 3 weeks of surgery. Although the patient may have received chemotherapy neoadjuvantly, the nurse should monitor the patient for delayed healing of the wound and for infection. Chemotherapy may continue for as long as 1 year postoperatively (Dealy, Pazola, & Heislein, 1995).

Side effects of chemotherapy may include impaired sexual maturity or fertility, and this should be discussed with the patient and family. If the patient is a child or adolescent, decreased growth may be a side effect and, again, the nurse and medical oncologist should inform the patient of this potentially serious toxicity (Himelstein & Dormans, 1996). Schwart, Hobbie, and Constine (1994) developed an algorithm for healthcare team members to follow. It addresses how adolescent patients should be followed postchemotherapy, depending on the type of chemotherapeutic agent the patient received (Fig. 71-2).

The nurse should also monitor the patient's cardiac and renal status. Doxorubicin has cardiac toxicity as the dose-limiting toxicity, and many regimens include doxorubicin. Renal damage can also occur from chemotherapy, and if the patient has been on aminoglycoside antibiotics, the risk of renal toxicity can be enhanced. The nurse should monitor the patient's fluid status, and electrolytes and chemistry panels should be ordered periodically.

A recent development regarding a side effect of chemotherapy, as well as radiation, is the risk of secondary malignancies. As mentioned previously in this chapter, osteosarcomas can be related to radiation of a body part (Himelstein & Dormans, 1996). However, patients are now developing leukemia from receiving chemotherapeutic agents, in particular the alkylating agents. Even though many patients may choose to risk the occurrence of cancer, this should be discussed.

HOME CARE ISSUES

Home care nursing over the years has evolved from traditional home health care to very high technologically advanced care of high-acuity patients. This focus applies to the osteosarcoma patients, as the hospital length of stay has been significantly reduced, and the emphasis of care continues to revolve around the need for extensive rehabilitation and the management of adjuvant therapy. The goal of the home care nurse is to design a plan of care that optimizes the patient's functional status while integrating the strengths and involvement of appropriate external resources (McEnroe, 1996).

As discussed under medical management, home care management of this patient also involves the collaborative efforts of a multidisciplinary health team. Often, the team members are those that the patient has met during the hospital stay—the physical therapist, nutritionist, social worker, occupational therapist, counselor, and oncology nurse. In addition, the team at this point includes the home care nurse as well as home health aides or homemaker services. Volunteers from the community or family friends may also have a more active role for activities such as transportation, child care, delivery of meals, and other aspects of care in the home (Blesch, 1996).

The home care nurse (HCN) for the patient with sarcoma is the pivotal point in the team approach. The HCN main-

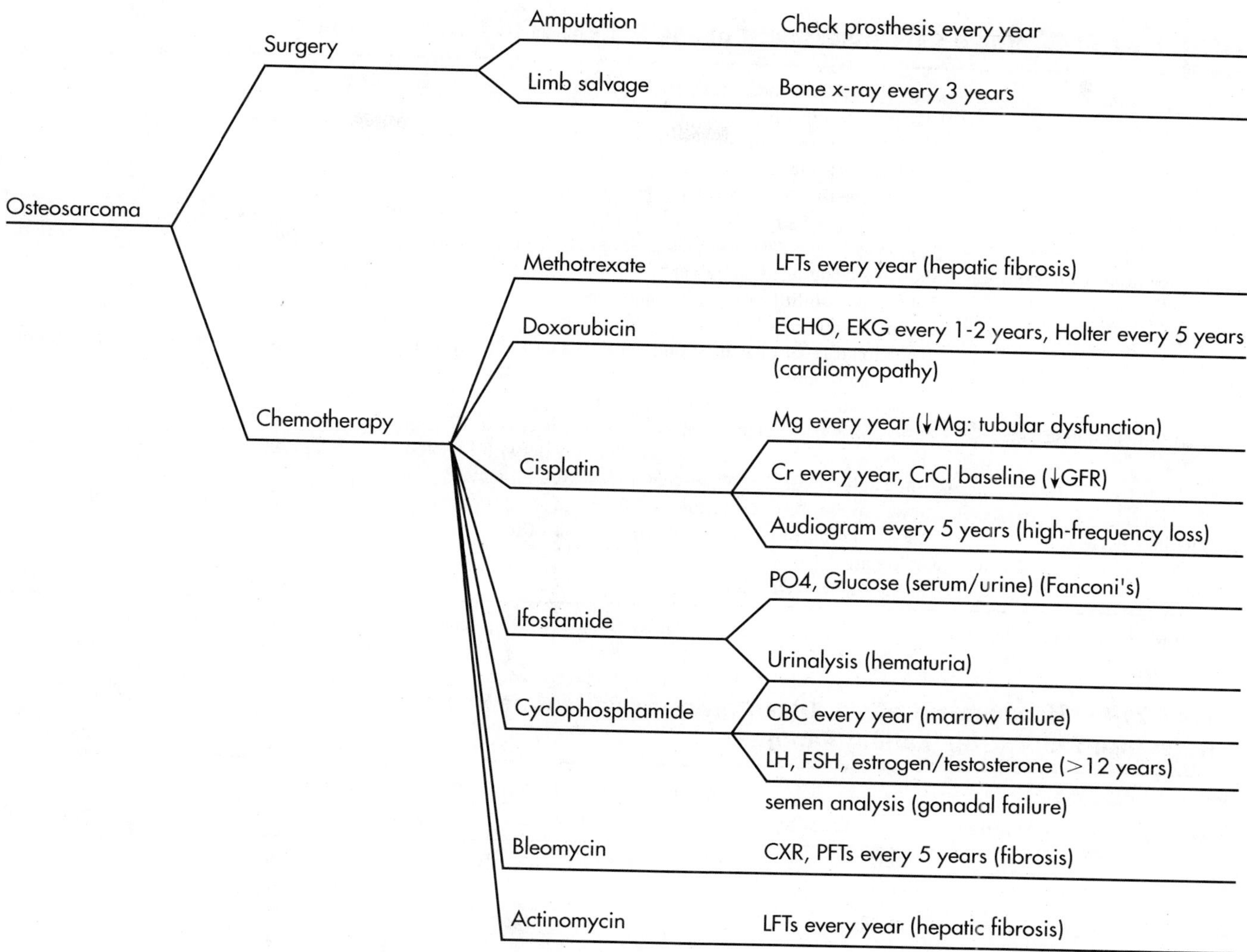

Fig. 71-2 Algorithm for follow-up assessment for young patients receiving chemotherapy for osteosarcoma. (From Jaffe, N., Patel, S., & Benjamin, R. [1995]. Chemotherapy in osteosarcoma: Basis for application and antagonism to implementation. Early controversies surrounding implementation. *Hematology/Oncology Clinics of North America, 9,* 825-839.)

tains a focus of acute care needs while the patient completes adjuvant therapy. The HCN is instrumental in the coordination and planning of the rehabilitative plan of care. The home care nurse's understanding of the effects of a diagnosis such as osteosarcoma, the extent of surgical resection necessary, the use of adjuvant chemotherapy, reconstructive and rehabilitative needs, and overall prognosis is essential for care planning and delivery.

One of the key activities for the home care nurse is the initial assessment of the patient, the family, and the home environment (Table 71-5). Although the inpatient team has usually completed a psychosocial evaluation of the patient and family, the HCN is able to provide an in-depth assessment because the nurse meets the patient and family in the actual home setting. It may be valuable for the HCN to meet the family in the home prior to patient discharge from the hospital, so that the physical environment can be evaluated for ease of access, safety, and infection prevention. Room for maneuvering of wheelchairs, ramps, stair negotiation, and access to a bathroom are some of the issues to consider in the physical environment. A clean environment and education on hygiene may be a part of infection control, particularly when providing wound care and managing the patient during adjuvant therapy. Any necessary adjustments to the environment may be made in a more timely fashion using this approach.

As mentioned earlier, assessment of the family system includes identifying the decision makers in the family; determining the roles and responsibilities of each family member and the effects that role change has on the family; noting patterns of communication and interactions that indicate effective or ineffective coping among family members; and determining the competency of the designated care givers. It is more common and realistic that patients have "rotating" caregivers due to child care and job-related issues. The home care nurse must plan adequate access to all the caregivers to educate each individual.

Assessment of the caregiver competency and availability

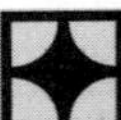

TABLE 71-5 Home Care Assessment of the Patient with Osteosarcoma

History	Compliance with medical therapy Experience with illness
Functional assessment of the patient	Ability to perform self-care activities (ADL) Need for assistance from others Use of assistive devices (brace, prosthesis, cane)
Psychosocial assessment	Coping mechanisms of patient/family Ability to understand and manage patient's physical and psychologic needs
Composition of the family	Status of designated caregiver Role/responsibilities of family members Age of family members Educational level of patient and caregiver and educational needs related to care of the patient at home Health and competency of caregiver Stressors and their effects on the family
Environmental assessment	Basic needs (e.g., electricity, heat, phone, access to EMS [911]) Physical layout (e.g., stairs, room to navigate with assistive device, ramp for wheelchair) Home safety (e.g., smoke detector, assistive rails in bathroom) Infection control (e.g., clean area for storage of supplies and medications, cleaning needs, pets, pests)
Ancillary needs	Transportation to medical center/physician office Child care Grocery delivery/food preparation

From McEnroe, L. E. (1996). Role of the oncology nurse in home care: Family-centered practice. *Seminars in Oncology, 12,* 188-192.

TABLE 71-6 Management of the Osteosaracoma Patient at Home: Reference Tool for the Patient/Caregiver

			Appointment Calendar			
Sunday	**Monday**	**Tuesday**	**Wednesday**	**Thursday**	**Friday**	**Saturday**

Name	**Phone**	**Address**
Surgeon:		
Medical oncologist:		
Radiation therapist:		
Physical therapist:		
Occupational therapist:		
Prosthetist:		
Oncology nurse:		
Home care nurse:		
Social worker:		
Nutritionist:		
Other:		

may also uncover additional family stressors that will interfere with the care of the patient. Financial stress, out-of-pocket expenses (parking, hotel accommodations, child care), or other family care burdens, such as elderly parent care, may alter the discharge plans for the patient.

Care at home is intermittent and episodic. Initially, the patient/caregiver may be taught how to care for the wound (dressing care, stump wrap). The ability of the patient and caregiver to learn proper techniques of care is essential. In addition, much of the teaching revolves around reporting signs and symptoms of wound complications. Helping the patient and family set realistic goals of care is also necessary to provide a smooth transition of care in the home. Promotion of self-care, good nutrition, and symptom management is necessary to prevent re-hospitalization or failure on the part of the patient and family.

Administration of intravenous therapy may also be part of the home care nurse's responsibilities. Completion of antibiotic therapy may be necessary, as well as administration of supportive therapies related to adjuvant chemotherapy.

The success of the patient in the home environment ultimately relies on patient motivation and caregiver support. Assessment, problem identification, and interventions in the care of the patient are an essential part of this process and result in positive clinical outcomes. Adequate, early support of the patient and caregiver provides positive experiences with self-care and helps build the confidence necessary for independent functioning. Table 71-6 is an example of a reference tool for the patient and caregiver. It enables the patient and family to keep track of the multiple appointments the patient will have and also provides the home health nurse, as well as physical therapist or any other healthcare team member, with appointment information with other members of the health care team.

PROGNOSIS

As mentioned previously in this chapter, the survival rate of patients with osteosarcoma has greatly improved during the past 20 years (Damron & Pritchard, 1995, Jaffe, Patel, & Benjamin, 1995). In the 1970s, the 5-year survival rate was only 20%. Patients at that time were not being treated with a combined program including chemotherapy, and the surgical procedure of choice was amputation.

Now, with the advent of chemotherapy for osteosarcoma and improved surgical techniques, the survival rate of patients with osteosarcoma is 80% (Damron & Pritchard, 1995; Jaffe , Patel, & Benjamin, 1995). Also, the majority of surgical procedures performed are limb sparing-procedures rather than amputations, with no noticeable difference in survival (Rodriguez, 1996).

However, there is obviously room for improvement. Today, approximately 30% to 40% of patients with high-grade osteosarcoma still relapse (Saeter, Hoie, Stenwig, Johansson, Hannisdal, & Solheim, 1995). Most of the metastatic disease is in the form of pulmonary metastases.

EVALUATION OF THE QUALITY OF CARE

Much of the nursing care related to the patient with soft tissue sarcoma involves rehabilitation, psychosocial support, and continuity of care between healthcare professionals. In a study by Arzouman, Dudas, Ferrans, & Holm (1991) that evaluated quality of life for patients with sarcomas receiving adjuvant chemotherapy, the need for involvement of support systems in the plan of care was essential. It was emphasized that the nurse's responsibility was to include significant others in patient teaching and to encourage their involvement in the patient's care. The study also emphasized the importance of continuity of care between different settings, for example inpatient, clinic, and home (Arzouman et al., 1991).

To ensure quality of care for this complex patient, a tool such as the one shown in Table 71-7 may help health care professionals track essential information related to continuity of care and provide a method to document involvement of all appropriate care givers.

TABLE 71-7 Quality of Care Evaluation of a Patient with Osteoarcoma

Disciplines participating in the quality of care evaluation:

A. Surgeon ☐	B. Medical Oncologist ☐
C. Radiation Therapy ☐	D. Physical Therapy ☐
E. Occupational Therapist ☐	F. Prosthetist ☐
G. Oncology Nurse ☐	H. Social Worker ☐
I. Nutritionist ☐	J. Other ☐

Data from

☐ Medical Record Review ☐ Patient Family Interview

Criteria	Yes	No
1. Did you and a family member attend a planning conference before you were discharged?	☐	☐
2. Were you given follow-up appointments by: Surgeon ☐, Medical oncologist ☐, Radiation therapy ☐, Physical therapy ☐, Occupational therapist ☐, Prosthetist ☐, Oncology nurse ☐, Social worker ☐, Nutritionist ☐, Other ☐?		
3. Did the nurse provide you with education materials?	☐	☐
4. Were education materials helpful to you?	☐	☐
5. Did you receive information about after-hours care, the phone number to call, and what symptoms to report?	☐	☐
6. Were you given dietary information?	☐	☐
7. Did pharmacists fill your prescriptions promptly and give you medication instructions?	☐	☐
8. What, if anything, would you like to see changed?	☐	☐
9. Were there things about the care you received that you did not like?	☐	☐

RESEARCH ISSUES

Areas of future research include the use of liposomal agents to assist in defeating drug-resistant tumors and improve the survival rates of patients with osteosarcoma. Clinically, nurses can play a role in future research in finding methods to safely discharge patients from the hospital in a timely fashion, as the era of managed care dictates.

Improvements in methods of reconstruction are ongoing and will continue as children with metal plates and rods mature and physicians are able to determine the life span of the hardware. Chemotherapeutic regimens will undoubtedly be changed as additional agents are discovered.

REFERENCES

Arzouman, J., Dudas, S., Ferrans, C. E., & Holm, K. (1991). Quality of life of patients with sarcoma postchemotherapy. *Oncology Nursing Forum, 18,* 889-894.

Ayala, A., Ro, J., & Raymond, A. (1996). Bone tumors. In I. Damjanov & J. Linder (Eds.), *Anderson's pathology* (10th ed.). St. Louis: Mosby.

Blesch, K.S. (1996). Rehabilitation of the cancer patient at home. *Seminars in Oncology Nursing, 12,* 219-225.

Cordon-Cardo, C. (1997). Molecular biology of sarcomas. In V. T. DeVita, S. Hellman, & S. A. Rosenberg (Eds.), *Cancer: Principles & practice of oncology* (5th ed.). Philadelphia: Lippincott-Raven.

Cortes, E. P., Holland, J. F., & Glidewell, O. (1981). Osteogenic sarcoma studies by the cancer and leukemia group B. *National Cancer Institute Monograph, 56,* 207-209.

Damron, T. & Pritchard, D. (1995). Current combined treatment of high grade osteosarcoma. *Oncology, 9,* 327-340.

Dealy, M., Pazola, K., & Heislein, D. (1995). Care of the adolescent undergoing an allograft procedure. *Cancer Nursing, 18,* 130-137.

Edmonson, J. H., Green, S. J., & Ivins, J. C. (1984). A controlled pilot study of high dose methotrexate as postsurgical adjuvant therapy for primary osteosarcoma. *Journal of Clinical Oncology, 2,* 152-156.

Engstrand, J. (1976). Rehabilitation of the patient with a lower extremity amputation. *Nursing Clinics of North America, 11,* 659-669.

Enneking, W., Spanier, S., & Goodman, M. (1980). A system for the surgical staging of musculoskeletal sarcoma. *Clinical Orthopaedics and Related Research, 153,* 106-119.

Enneking, W. & Conrad, E. (1989). Common bone tumors. *Clinical Symposia, 41,* 2-35.

Fishman, E. (1997). Computed tomography. In V. T. DeVita, S. Hellman, & S. A. Rosenberg (Eds.), *Cancer: Principles & practice of oncology* (5th ed.). Philadelphia: Lippincott-Raven.

Grundmann, E., Roessner, A., Ueda, Y., Schneider-Stock, R., & Radig, K. (1995). Current aspects of the pathology of osteosarcoma. *Anticancer Research, 15,* 1023-1033.

Himelstein, B. & Dormans, J. (1996). Malignant bone tumors of childhood. *Pediatric Clinics of North America, 43,* 967-984.

Inwards, C. & Unni, K. (1995). Classification and grading of bone sarcomas. *Hematology/Oncology Clinics of North America, 9,* 545-569.

Huvos, A. (1991). *Bone tumors: Diagnosis, treatment and prognosis* (2nd ed.). Philadelphia: W.B. Saunders.

Jaffe, N., Patel, S., & Benjamin, R. (1995). Chemotherapy in osteosarcoma: basis for application and antagonism to implementation; early controversies surrounding its implementation. *Hematology/Oncology Clinics of North America, 9,* 825-839.

Kleinerman, E. (1995). Biologic therapy for osteosarcoma using liposome-encapsulated muramyl tripeptide. *Hematology/Oncology Clinics of North America, 9,* 927-938.

Landis, S. H., Taylor, M., Bolden, S., & Wingo, P. A. (1998). Cancer statistics, 1998. *CA: A Cancer Journal for Clinicians, 48,* 6-29.

Malawer, M., Link, M., & Donaldson, S. (1993). Sarcomas of bone. In V. T. DeVita, S. Hellman, & S. A. Rosenberg (Eds.), *Cancer: Principles & practice of oncology* (4th ed.). Philadelphia: Lippincott-Raven.

Malawer, M., Link, M., & Donaldson, S. (1997). Sarcomas of bone. In V. T. DeVita, S. Hellman, & S. A. Rosenberg (Eds.), *Cancer: Principles & practice of oncology* (5th ed.). Philadelphia: Lippincott-Raven.

McEnroe, L. E. (1996). Role of the oncology nurse in home care: Family-centered practice. *Seminars in Oncology Nursing, 12,* 188-192.

Melzack, R. (1971). Phantom limb pain: Implications for treatment of pathological pain. *Anesthesiology, 35,* 409-419.

Meyer, W. & Malawer, M. (1991). Osteosarcoma-clinical features and evolving surgical and chemotherapeutic strategies. *Pediatric Clinics of North America, 38,* 317- 348.

Mourad, L. (1994). Structure and function of the musculoskeletal system. In K. McCance & S. Huether (Eds.), *Pathophysiology: The biologic basis for disease in adults and children.* St. Louis: Mosby.

Piasecki, P. (1991). The nursing role in limb salvage surgery. *Nursing Clinics of North America, 26,* 33-41.

Piasecki, P. (1992). Update in orthopaedic oncology. *Orthopaedic Nursing, 11,* 36-43.

Quill, G., Gitelis, S., Morton, T., & Piasecki, P. (1990). Complications associated with limb salvage for extremity sarcomas and their management. *Clinical Orthopaedics and Related Research, 260,* 242-250.

Rodriguez, R. (1996). Amputation surgery and prostheses. *Orthopedic Clinics of North America, 9,* 927-938.

Rosen, G., Forscher, C., Manken, H., & Selch, M. (1997). Bone tumors. In J. Holland, R. Blast, Jr., D. Morton, E. Frei, III, & D. Kufe (Eds.), *Cancer medicine* (4th ed.). Baltimore: Williams & Wilkins.

Saeter, G., Hoie, J., Stenwig, A., Johnansson, A., Hannisdal, E., & Solheim, O. (1995). Systemic relapse of patient with osteogenic sarcoma: Prognostic factors for long term survival. *Cancer, 75,* 242-250.

Skarin, S. A. (1996). *Atlas of diagnostic oncology.* (2nd ed.). London: Mosby-Wolfe.

Slye, D. (1991). Orthopedic complications—compartment syndrome, fat embolism syndrome, and venous-thrombo-embolism. *Nursing Clinics of North America. 26,* 113-132.

Thibodeau, G. A. & Patton, K. T. (1996). *Anatomy & physiology* (3rd ed.). St. Louis: Mosby.

Vander Griend, R. (1996). Osteosarcoma and its variants. *Orthopedics of North America, 27,* 575-581.

Webb, K., Lewis, S., & Collier, I. (1983). Nursing assessment: Musculoskeletal system. In S. Lewis & I. Collier (Eds.), *Medical-surgical nursing: Assessment and management of clinical problems.* New York: McGraw Hill.

Yasko, A. & Johnson, M. (1995). Surgical management of primary bone sarcomas. *Hematology/Oncology Clinics of North America, 9,* 719-731.

Soft Tissue Sarcomas

Catherine H. Kelley, MSN, RN, OCN
Robbie Thomas, RN, MS, OCN

Soft tissue is the nonskeletal connective tissue that makes up more than 50% of the weight of the human body. The term *sarcoma* was derived from the Greek word that means "fleshy tumor." The ancient Greeks were the first to distinguish between soft tissue sarcomas and carcinomas.

Most sarcomas arise from the embryologic mesoderm, which is made up of uncommitted mesenchymal cells that have the potential to differentiate into a specific cell line. However, the tumor cells in sarcomas may vary in morphologic structure from a given area within the tumor, and these cells may be differentiated or undifferentiated. Sarcomas are a very heterogenous group of tumors, resulting in difficulty for the pathologist to diagnose and classify them. Classification of these tumors is based on histogenetic analysis according to the adult tissues they resemble (Miettinen & Weiss, 1996).

Most sarcomas develop deep in soft tissue, expanding along the anatomic tissue planes and creating a pseudocapsule as normal tissue is pushed away. The pseudocapsule does not provide a protective barrier from spread of tumor cells. Very often the pseudocapsule is infiltrated by tumor cells, and extension of tumor results well beyond the palpable mass (Miettinen & Weiss, 1996).

Management of soft tissue sarcomas requires a multidisciplinary approach. Diagnosis and treatment need advanced and informed planning on the part of the surgeon, radiation oncologist, medical oncologist, pathologist, oncology nurse, patient and family, physical therapist, and other support disciplines.

EPIDEMIOLOGY

Soft tissue sarcomas are very rare. The American Cancer Society estimated approximately 6400 new cases of "connective tissue" malignant tumors for 1998; of these new cases, 3700 patients will die of their disease. Incidence of sarcomas by gender shows a slight male predominance; of the 6400 new cases, 3500 occur in men and 2900 in women (American Cancer Society, 1998). The annual incidence is approximately 300 per 100,000 of the general population (Enzinger & Weiss, 1995c). There is no racial predominance in adults or children with sarcomas. Soft tissue sarcomas occur in all age groups, but the overall incidence increases with advancing age. The annual age-adjusted incidence rates are slightly higher for African Americans than for Caucasians in the United States. Sarcomas make up approximately 6.5% of all malignant tumors found in children younger than 15 years (Frable, 1994). Approximately 40% of these tumors are found in adults older than 55 (Enzinger & Weiss, 1995c). Certain types of sarcomas are more prevalent in children between the ages of 5 and 14 years, such as rhabdomyosarcoma and small round cell sarcomas. Approximately three fourths of all sarcomas in infants and toddlers are neuroblastomas. Others, such as synovial and clear cell sarcoma, are seen more frequently in young adults. Liposarcomas and leiomyosarcomas are more common in middle-age adults. The most common type of sarcoma, malignant fibrous histiocytoma, is usually found in older adults. Overall, sarcomas make up about 1% of all malignant tumors. In recent years there has been an increased incidence of soft tissue sarcomas, which some think is explained by acquired immunodeficiency syndrome (AIDS)–associated Kaposi's sarcoma (Mack, 1995; Miettinen & Weiss, 1996; Morton, 1997). Other authors note that the increase may be related to better diagnosis and greater attention to this rare cancer (Enzinger & Weiss, 1995c).

Soft tissue sarcomas can occur throughout the body, although approximately 60% develop in the extremities. Site distribution has been described as approximately 46% in the lower extremities, 13% in the upper extremities, 19% in the trunk, 13% in the retroperitoneum, and 9% in the head and neck (Brennan, Casper, & Harrison, 1997; Morton, 1997).

The prognosis for patients with soft tissue sarcoma is most favorable when the patient is young and has a peripherally located tumor of <5 cm that is superficial rather than deep (Frable, 1994).

RISK FACTORS

The etiologic basis of soft tissue sarcoma is unclear. However, several factors have been shown to be associated with the development of sarcoma in a small number of persons (Table 72-1).

Hereditary Predisposition

Hereditary predisposition has been noted to occur in families with familial cancer syndrome. These families exhibit a high incidence of various cancers in the relatives of children with soft tissue sarcoma. Deletion of the tumor suppressor gene p53 has been identified in these families. Individuals with genetically transmitted diseases such as Werner's syndrome, intestinal polyposis, and Gardner's syndrome also have a slightly higher incidence of sarcoma. In addition, the development of nerve sheath sarcomas in patients with neurofibromatosis type 1 and type 2 (von Recklinghausen's disease) has been well documented, occurring in 1% to 5% of this group of individuals. There is also evidence that chromosomal translocation is responsible for the development of some sarcomas, such as alveolar rhabdomyosarcoma and Ewing's sarcoma. It is thought that these translocations are of etiologic significance (Cordon-Cardo, 1997; Dirix & Van Oosterom, 1995; Enzinger et al., 1995c; Miettinen & Weiss, 1996; Yang, Rosenberg, Glatstein, & Altman, 1993).

Ionizing Radiation

Ionizing radiation is an important external etiologic factor linked to the development of soft tissue sarcomas. It has been noted that approximately 1% to 3% of patients undergoing radiation therapy are at risk for developing a sarcoma 5 to 15 years after therapy. The most common types of sarcoma associated with prior radiation therapy are malignant fibrous histiocytoma, fibrosarcoma, and extraskeletal osteosarcoma (Miettinen & Weiss, 1996). Most sarcomas that have been associated with previous radiation therapy tend to appear as high-grade lesions and have poorer survival rates. Survival rates after radiation-associated sarcoma range from 5% to 26% at 5 years (Brennan, Casper, & Harrison, 1997; Enzinger & Weiss, 1995c).

TABLE 72-1 Risk Factors Associated with Soft Tissue Sarcoma

Risk Factor	Type of Soft Tissue
Hereditary predisposition Werner's syndrome Intestinal polyposis Gardner's syndrome von Recklinghausen's disease	Increased in all types; alveolar rhabdomyosarcoma associated with chromosomal translocations
Ionizing radiation	Associated with malignant fibrous histiocytoma, fibrosarcoma, and extraskeletal osteosarcoma
Chemical exposure Vinyl chloride Asbestos Dioxin, hydrocarbons, hydroxyquinolines	Angiosarcoma Mesothelioma Soft tissue sarcoma and lymphoma
Virus	Possible association with Kaposi's sarcoma
Chronic lymphedema	Angiosarcoma

Chemical Exposure

Some chemicals have also been associated with an increased risk for sarcoma development. Vinyl chloride, used in the manufacture of rubber, has been linked to angiosarcoma of the liver, and asbestos has been associated with the development of mesothelioma. Sarcoma development in animal models has been seen with carcinogens such as hydrocarbons and hydroxyquinolines. Exposure to dioxin, a component in the toxic herbicide "agent orange," has been suspected to increase risk for the development of soft tissue sarcoma and lymphomas. However, the evidence of such risk noted in studies involving agriculturists and Vietnam veterans has failed to show a link between dioxin exposure and sarcoma development. Some think that the follow-up periods in these studies have been relatively short and the level of exposure may have been low (Brennan, Casper, & Harrison, 1997; Enzinger & Weiss, 1995c; Miettinen & Weiss, 1996; Yang et al., 1993). In studies of factory workers exposed to much higher doses of dioxin, there is some evidence that this chemical is a human carcinogen (Enzinger & Weiss, 1995).

Viral Association

Viruses may be associated with sarcoma. Although the viral origin of chicken fibrosarcoma was noted by Rous in 1910, no viruses have been isolated from human sarcomas. The most recent association of a herpes-like virus in AIDS-associated Kaposi's sarcoma is still under investigation (Miettinen & Weiss, 1996). Cytomegalovirus has also been suspect, but no conclusive evidence has been found. Although there has not been strong evidence associated with sarcoma development and viral origin, electron microscopy has frequently identified viral particles within soft tissue sarcoma specimens (Enzinger & Weiss, 1995c).

Long-Term Immunosuppression

Long-term immunosuppression associated with organ transplantation is known to influence the development of soft tissue sarcomas. This has been a risk factor for kidney and liver recipients in particular (Enzinger & Weiss, 1995c).

Chronic Lymphedema

Chronic lymphedema has been noted to precede the development of angiosarcoma. In patients with poor flow of the lymphatics (e.g., postmastectomy for breast cancer), it has been theorized that the normal mechanism for immune surveillance may be impaired, leading to the development of malignancy. It has also been suggested that retention of malignant cells in the area of lymphatic obstruction may lead to the development of a malignancy such as sarcoma (Brennan, Casper, & Harrison, 1997; Enzinger & Weiss, 1995c; Miettinen & Weiss, 1996).

Trauma history has often been reported with the diagnosis of soft tissue sarcoma, but in most cases it probably is coincidental, with the trauma event drawing attention to the new finding of a preexisting tumor (Miettinen & Weiss, 1996). Latent development of sarcomas has been associated with scar tissue from previous surgery, thermal or acid burns, old fracture sites, or the area near a metal implant. Reports of this nature are very rare, and it is difficult to demonstrate a clear relationship between the presence of a metal device, for example, and the development of sarcoma (Enzinger & Weiss, 1995c).

PATHOPHYSIOLOGY

Normal Development of Soft Tissue

Soft tissue sarcomas arise from a common embryonic source of cells, the primitive mesoderm. Approximately 9 to 13 days after fertilization, the human embryo is in transition from the simple division of cells to a more complex phase of morphologic organization. The cells transform into the primary germ layers known as *ectoderm, mesoderm,* and *endoderm.* Each layer develops into specific systems. The outer layer (ectoderm) is the one from which the nervous system, skin, and various glands are formed. The middle layer (mesoderm) develops into connective tissue, muscle, bone, fat, blood, vasculature, lymphatics, and some of the urogenital organs. The innermost layer (endoderm) forms the mucous membranes lining the respiratory and gastrointestinal tracts and the epithelium of the bladder, uretha, and prostate. These germ layers become arranged as two primary types of tissue—epithelial and mesenchymal.

The primitive mesenchyma, which is a network of cells and intercellular matrix within the mesoderm, provides the basis for the development of connective tissues. Soft tissue sarcomas are composed of malignant cells that resemble the different types of connective tissue, such as fibroblasts, lipocytes (fat), synovioblasts (joint capsule and tendons), leiomyosarcoma (smooth muscle), rhabdomyoblasts (striated muscle), and angioblasts (lymph and blood vessels) (Kruzelock & Hansen, 1995; Yang et al., 1993).

There are also similar characteristics, such as anatomic site of origin, clinical presentation, and clinical behavior, found in tumors that arise is Schwann cells. These are cells that surround peripheral nerves. In the embryonic stage they are found in the neural tube of the primitive ectoderm. Schwann cell tumors also are categorized as soft tissue sarcomas.

Soft tissue sarcomas can also be found in tissues that fit the morphologic criteria of epithelium. Historically, tumors that arise from epithelial tissue have been categorized as carcinomas rather than sarcomas, which are associated with connective tissue. *Epithelium* is a morphologic term, not an embryonic one, and it describes cells that line or cover surfaces on or in the body. The epithelial cells can arise from the ectoderm, endoderm, or mesoderm. Endothelium, which lines the lymphatic channels and the vascular structures, and mesothelium, which lines body cavities and visceral organs, are the two types of cellular structures that originate from the mesoderm. These structures can develop malignant tumors that are similar to those that arise in connective tissue. Therefore tumors that develop in the endothelium and the mesothelium are included in the category of sarcomas.

In summary, most sarcomas develop from mesodermal structures and connective tissue. Some arise from the ectodermal structures, and others originate in the epithelium (Fig. 72-1).

Pathogenesis

The process of carcinogenesis in soft tissue sarcomas is unclear. It has been determined that sarcomas do not develop from preexisting benign lesions, as do many other tumors during the typical stage of tumor progression. The development of in situ sarcomas has not been observed. The area of mutation for many of these malignant tumors appears to be molecules in several key regulatory mechanisms. For example, *pRB* (retinoblastoma gene) is thought to participate in cell cycle control and differentation. Altered *pRB* expression has been identified in several sarcomas. Other sarcomas have alteration in p53, which is thought to participate in growth arrest mechanisms. Alteration of this key gene may be a critical factor in the development of sarcomas and may lead to tumor progression (Cordon-Cardo, 1997; Demetri & Elian, 1995).

ROUTES OF METASTASES

Sarcomas spread by hematogenous routes rather than through the lymphatics. The most common site of metastases for patients with extremity sarcomas is the lungs. Metastasis to this organ occurs more than 88% of the time (Brennan, Casper, & Harrison, 1997). Liver and bone are the next most common sites for metastatic spread, especially for patients with retroperitoneal tumors (Miettinen & Weiss, 1996). Patients diagnosed with soft tissue sarcomas have an approximately 50% chance of local recurrence since these tumors spread along tissue planes and involve adjacent tissue.

Lymph node involvement is uncommon and is often associated with a poor prognosis. The subtypes of soft tissue sarcomas most often associated with lymph node involvement are synovial (17%), epitheloid (20%), and rhabdomyosarcomatoid (12%).

Patients with a retroperitoneal soft tissue sarcoma at presentation have a high incidence (75%) of developing a local recurrence. Approximately one third of these patients will develop metastatic disease, which most frequently occurs in the lung or liver. The median time to recurrence in these tumors is 15 months (McGrath, Sloan, & Kennedy, 1994).

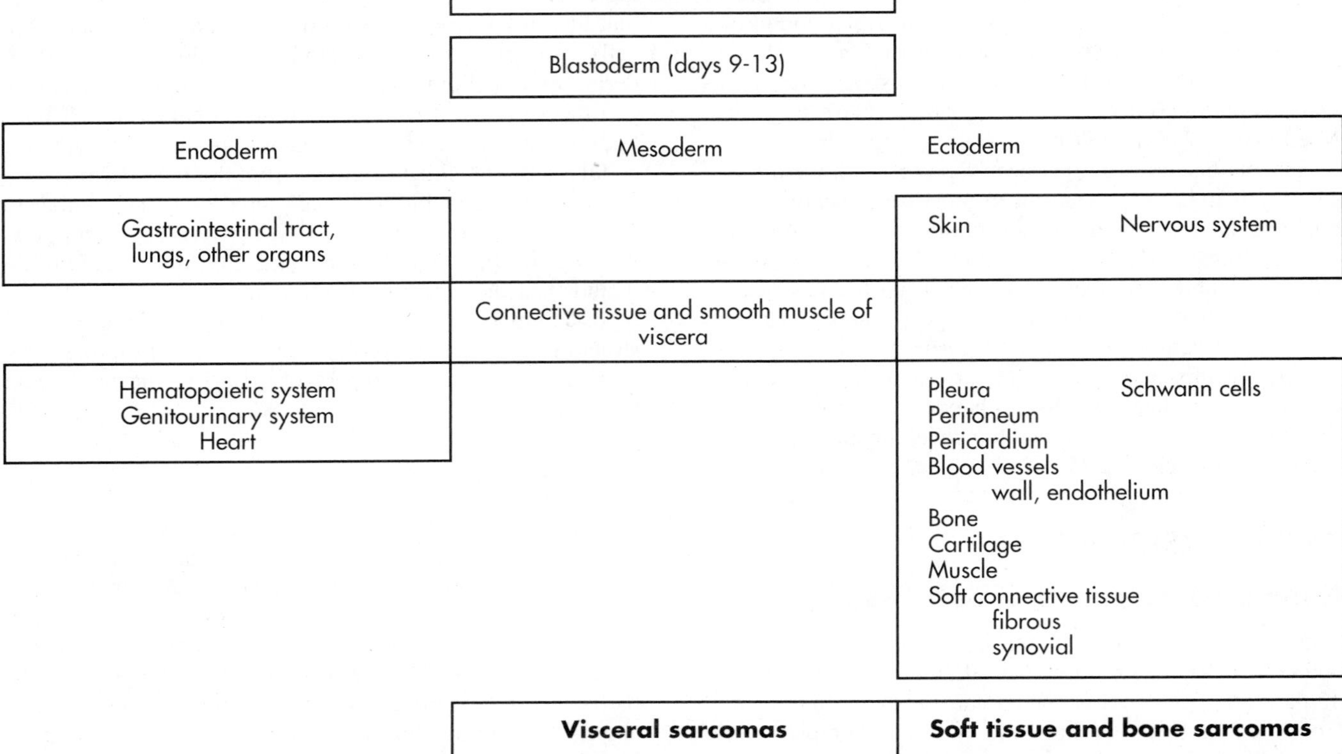

Fig. 72-1 Cells of origin of sarcomas. (Modified from Yang, J. C., Rosenberg, S. A., Glatstein, E. J., & Antman, K. H. [1993]. Sarcomas of soft tissue. In V. T. DeVita, S. Hellman, & S. A. Rosenberg [Eds.], *Cancer: Principles and practice of oncology* [4th ed.]. Philadelphia: Lippincott-Raven.)

ASSESSMENT

The purpose of any clinical staging of sarcomas is to determine tumor size, pattern of local spread, and presence of metastasis. Sarcomas are assessed in a variety of ways.

The diagnostic evaluation includes a complete history and physical examination. A psychosocial assessment should be included when soft tissue sarcoma is first suspected. Since treatment will affect the patient's functional ability and body image, the patient and family coping patterns and support systems should be identified early in this process (Piasecki, 1993). Pertinent questions related to the patient's history are summarized in Table 72-2.

History and Physical Assessment

The complete physical examination should include a detailed description of the size and location of the mass, its degree of firmness, and the level of associated pain. The impact on functional status of the area involved should also be evaluated. Signs of lymph node involvement and symptoms of metastatic disease are also included in the initial physical examination.

Soft tissue sarcomas often first appear as asymptomatic masses in an area of soft tissue. In one survey of more than 5800 patients with sarcoma, the average time that individuals waited to report symptoms was approximately 4 months. A notable 20% of patients had delays of 6 months after seeking treatment before a correct diagnosis was made. Patients may minimize their symptoms (e.g., describing a "pulled muscle"), which may contribute to delays in evaluation. In general, if a soft tissue mass occurs in a patient and there is no trauma associated with the mass, biopsy is indicated. If trauma is present and there is no resolution of the mass in 6 weeks, a biopsy of the lesion should be performed (Chang & Sondak, 1995).

Some sarcomas may be quite large compared to the anatomic structure. For example, a sarcoma in the buttocks may be 8 to 15 cm at first presentation. Symptoms such as pain result from pressure on adjacent nerves or muscles and are commonly associated with sarcomas of the retroperitoneum (Yang et al., 1993). Patients with retroperitoneal sarcomas may have very subtle symptoms at presentation, and diagnosis is frequently delayed up to 5 months from the onset of symptoms. The most common complaint is abdominal or flank pain associated with a palpable mass and weight loss. Patients with this presentation may also complain of nausea, vomiting, abdominal fullness, or back pain (McGrath, 1994). Patients with a complaint of pain at presentation require a thorough assessment of the characteristics of the symptoms. Information related to the location, onset, duration, and quality of pain may assist in the diagnosis of sarcoma (Piasecki, 1993).

TABLE 72-2 Assessment of the Patient with Soft Tissue Sarcoma

	Assessment Parameters	Typical Abnormal Findings
History • Personal and family history	1. Has the patient experienced recent trauma to the area?	1. Rule out hematoma and seroma; trauma itself is coincidental
	2. Does the patient have a history of cancer and cancer treatment?	2. Association with previous radiation therapy
	3. What is the patient's occupation?	3. Association with herbicides, dioxin, vinyl chloride, hydrocarbons, hydroxyquinolines, asbestos
	4. Is the patient a war veteran from Vietnam or the Gulf War?	4. Unproven association
	5. Has the patient been treated for chronic lymphedema?	5. Reported association, particularly with angiosarcoma
	6. Does the patient or family have a history of genetically transmitted disease such as von Recklinghausen's disease, Werner's syndrome, or Gardner's syndrome?	6. Reported association
	7. Is there any pain associated with the area?	7. Usually soft tissue sarcomas first appear as painless masses; however, pain may occur with neural or organ involvement
	8. Does the patient complain of weight loss, fatigue, hemoptosis, cough, or chest pain?	8. May indicate symptoms of metastatic disease
Physical Examination	1. Inspection and palpation of the mass; measure dimensions of the mass; note texture, pain with palpation, temperature to touch of affected area	1. No way to distinguish benign from malignant lesion on physical examination
	2. Note adenopathy	2. Seldom found with soft tissue sarcomas; usually suggests poorer prognosis
	3. Hepatomegaly; note any pulmonary symptoms	3. May suggest metastatic disease
Diagnostic Tests • Local lesion evaluation	1. Plain roentgenogram	1. May determine if lesion involves bone
	2. Magnetic resonance imaging (MRI)	2. Superior soft tissue contrast; determines size and extent of lesion
	3. Arteriography	3. May be used to determine anatomic variations before surgery
	4. Ultrasonography	4. Noninvasive; may be used to differentiate lesion from edema or cyst
• Metastatic disease evaluation	5. Computed tomography (CT) for lung	5. Evaluation of lungs; most frequent site of metastasis; 10% to 20% of patients will have metastatic disease on initial workup
	6. Bone scan	6. Detection of skeletal metastasis
• Tissue evaluation	7. Routine histologic study	7. Determine benign vs malignant; assists in classification and grading
	8. Immunohistochemical studies	8. Identifies common antigens associated with certain types of soft tissue sarcomas
	9. Electron microscopy	9. Shows intracellular relationships to further determine cell type
	10. Deoxyribonucleic acid flow cytometry	10. Provides prognostic information; aneuploidy is a negative prognostic factor
	11. Cytogenic and molecular studies	11. Clonal chromosomal translocations and genetic abnormalities aid in classification of soft tissue sarcoma and help with prognostic information

Rarely does a patient with soft tissue sarcoma have clinical symptoms, such as fever, sweating, or weight loss, at presentation. This is more common in tumors such as Ewing's sarcoma or in metastatic disease (Conrad, Bradford, & Chansky, 1996). There is no way to differentiate a benign lesion from a malignant one based on symptoms.

Diagnostic Tests

Radiographic Evaluation and Magnetic Resonance Imaging. Plain radiography is often the first step as a noninvasive method of determining if the lesion involves bone. Magnetic resonance imaging (MRI) is the next step in providing information for staging and treatment planning. MRI is currently widely accepted as a preferred method over computed tomography (CT) because of its excellent capability of imaging lesions in the axial, coronal, sagittal, and oblique planes. MRI also provides superior soft tissue contrast. Soft tissue, depending on the type, will appear differently with this imaging technique. Intravenous contrast agents used with MRI have not been particularly helpful for the evaluation of soft tissue lesions (Brennan, Casper, & Harrison, 1997; Chang & Sondak, 1995). Table 72-3 presents a sample of patient preparation information for MRI.

Computed Tomography Scan and Bone Scan. During the initial workup an evaluation for metastatic disease is warranted. Approximately 10% to 20% of patients with primary soft tissue sarcoma will have metastatic disease (Arca, Sondak, & Chang, 1994). CT scanning is usually incorporated in the evaluation as the best method for evaluating the lungs for metastasis. Liver involvement is usually rare, with the exception of patients having intraabdominal or retroperitoneal sarcomas at presentation. A CT scan of the liver is indicated in those patients. Bone scans are used to detect skeletal metastases. Other types of imaging, such as positron emission tomography (PET), are being evaluated for clinical importance and cost-effectiveness (Arca, Sondak, & Chang, 1994; Kransdorf, Jelinek, & Moser, 1993; Massengill, Seeger, & Eckardt, 1995; Podoloff, 1995).

Arteriography. Occasionally arteriography may be used in providing normal anatomic variations before surgery, particularly for retroperitoneal sarcomas. It may also be used to establish intraarterial access for subsequent chemotherapy (Kransdorf, Jelinek, & Moser, 1993).

Ultrasonography. Ultrasonography is a noninvasive imaging method that can be used to determine the size and consistency of a soft tissue mass. It can help to distinguish a solid lesion from edema or a cystic lesion (Kransdorf, Jelinek, & Moser, 1993).

Surgical Biopsy. Adequate tissue for a definitive diagnosis is essential for suspected sarcoma tissue. In general, cytologic matter collected from aspiration does not provide enough tissue for immunohistochemical and other studies that need to be conducted. Core-needle or fine-needle biopsies may be appropriate in some situations (Ayala, Ro, Fanning, Flores, & Yasko, 1995), although usually tissue is obtained through an incisional or excisional biopsy. The exception may be the case of a child when there is evidence that fine-needle aspiration may be appropriate for diagnosing metastatic tumor (Brennan, Casper, & Harrison, 1997; Craver, 1996).

Incisional biopsy technique is preferred since the bulk of the mass is left in place, which permits multidisciplinary planning for subsequent treatment. With excision of the tumor at the time of biopsy, there is concern that the physical boundaries of the tumor will be lost (Lawrence, 1994).

The biopsy site requires astute placement because the entire site needs to be removed during definitive resection of the tumor. For biopsy of soft tissue sarcomas of <3 cm in diameter, an excisional biopsy is performed with care taken not to spread tumor cells into surrounding tissue. Because the pseudocapsule is infiltrated with tumor extension, "shelling out" the tumor is never curative. Excision through the capsule can lead to contamination of the surrounding tissue with tumor cells. Tumors τ3 cm in diameter require an incisional biopsy. The biopsy incision should be placed in a location that will facilitate subsequent wide excision of the tumor mass. This technique is preferred because adequate tissue can be obtained without disruption of the surrounding tissue (Arca, Sondak, & Chang, 1994; Yang et al., 1993).

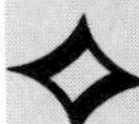

TABLE 72-3 Patient Preparation for Magnetic Resonance Imaging

Magnetic resonance imaging, or MRI, is a test used to diagnose a variety of medical conditions that affect the soft tissues of the body as well as other different organs. The MRI unit uses radio waves and a magnetic field to provide detailed images of body parts. This method of imaging *does not use radiation.*

The MRI produces crosssectional views of the body structures, similar to the slices of a loaf of bread. These different "slices," or views, of your body are transmitted to a computer, which organizes the information and creates views of your body from different angles. These different views give your doctor a very detailed view of your body that allows him or her to diagnose a medical condition more accurately.

The MRI is a painless procedure. You will be asked to lie down on a padded table. You may have a special receiver next to the body part that is to be imaged. The table will slide forward to position your body part at the center of the magnetic field. When the machine begins, you will hear banging sounds and tapping noises. The noise lasts several minutes with some pauses in between. The noise is a normal part of the operation of the machine. During the test you will be asked to lie very still because movement can blur the picture. Children may require a mild sedative. Sometimes the only part of the procedure that may cause some people concern is the closeness of the center of the machine to you. If this bothers you, you can take some deep breaths to relax and think of some pleasant experiences. The technician is always monitoring you via an intercom or through a glass window. You are never left alone while in the machine.

The day of the test, you should allow for spending at least 2 hours at the facility. Usually the test itself takes about 45 minutes. However, you will be asked some health-related questions and may be asked to change into a hospital gown for the procedure. You can usually eat a normal diet the day of the procedure and take your daily medications. However, ask your doctor or the facility to be sure.

Occasionally, your doctor may want the contrast agent injected into your vein during the procedure. This can improve the quality of the images of some organs and structures that may be difficult to see clearly. Most people do not experience any discomfort with the injection, except for a brief needle stick.

When you leave the facility, you may continue with your normal routines. Children who received mild sedation may need to remain at the facility until the sedation wears off. Your doctor will receive the results of the MRI and will review that information with you.

TABLE 72-4 Selected Common Antigens Used to Diagnose Soft Tissue Sarcomas

Antigen	Normal Cell Association	Soft Tissue Sarcoma
Vimentin	Mesenchymal Fibroblasts Chondroblasts Smooth muscle Mesothelium Endothelium	All types of soft tissue sarcomas Adenocarcinoma Some squamous cell carcinomas Melanoma
Cytokeratin	Mesothelium Epithelium	Mesothelioma Adenocarcinoma Synovial sarcoma Epitheloid sarcoma Extrarenal rhabdomyosarcoma
Epithelial membrane	Epithelium Perineurium Meningothelial	Synovial sarcoma Epitheloid sarcoma
Desmin	Skeletal Cardiac Smooth muscle	Leiomyosarcoma Rhabdomyosarcoma
Factor VII	Vascular endothelium	Some angiosarcoma
p53 gene product	Negatively regulates cell division	Malignant fibrous histiocytoma Liposarcoma Synovial sarcoma Carcinomas

Modified from Enzinger, F. M. & Weiss, S. W. (Eds.). (1995a). *Soft tissue tumors* (3rd ed.). St. Louis: Mosby.

Tests of the Surgical Specimen

Histologic Evaluation. Soft tissue sarcomas are very difficult to classify. The initial evaluation by the pathologist is a valuable part of the process. Information related to the size and depth of the tumor; its relationship to overlying skin and fascia; the nature of the borders; and the architectural pattern and overall appearance of the cells help the pathologist begin to classify these tumors. The degree of differentiation and the mitotic counts can provide grading information that is associated with prognosis (Enzinger & Weiss, 1995a).

Immunohistochemical Studies. Immunohistochemical tests are studies performed with antigens that are to some degree specific for epithelial, endothelial, muscle, and neural cells. These studies are the most useful markers for evaluation of soft tissue sarcoma. Table 72-4 gives several examples of the antigens used in diagnosing soft tissue sarcomas (Miettinen & Weiss, 1996).

Electron Microscopy. Electron microscopy can show intercellular relationships to help further identify cell type. Cytoplasmic structures such as specific granules, filaments, or accumulation of glycogen can help to identify sarcomas such as neuroblastomas, rhabdomyosarcomas, and Ewing's sarcoma, respectively (Craver, 1996; Enzinger & Weiss, 1995a).

DNA Flow Cytometry. DNA flow cytometry is used to provide prognostic information related to the sarcoma. In the case of high-grade sarcomas, aneuploidy (greater or lesser than normal amounts of DNA in the tissue) is a negative prognostic factor. DNA aneuploidy is an independent prognostic indicator for increased risk of development of metastatic disease (Zarbo, 1995). One of the drawbacks of DNA flow cytometry is that it does not differentiate between benign and malignant soft tissue tumors (Miettinen & Weiss, 1996).

Cytogenic and Molecular Studies. Cytogenetics has been used to identify clonal chromosomal translocations in many soft tissue sarcomas. A few of these deviations are significant enough to be diagnostic. For example, the translocation of *t(12;16)* indicates a type of liposarcoma (myxoid). Molecular genetics can provide diagnostic information for some sarcomas, such as Ewing's sarcoma, alveolar rhabdomyosarcoma, and synovial sarcoma (Craver, 1996; Dirix & Van Oosterom, 1995; Miettinen & Weiss, 1996; van Unnik, 1995).

Molecular studies may also provide prognostic information. For example, some tumors result from the loss of tumor suppressor genes such as p53, which is an example of a gene that normally inhibits growth and promotes cell differentiation (Dirix & Van Oosterom, 1995). Examples of sarcomas with gene alterations are malignant fibrous histiocytoma, leiomyosarcoma, and rhabdomyosarcoma (Meltzer, 1995). Other types of abnormalities of genes that are found in sarcomas include the retinoblastoma susceptibility gene *(RBI),* the p53 gene, and the neurofibromatosis gene *(NF1)* (Kruzelock & Hansen, 1995). Unrestrained cell growth results in an accumulation of abnormal proteins that can be detected through other studies and may lead to diagnosis of sarcoma. Other tumors exhibit duplication or amplification of genes. Amplified genes have also been associated with several types of sarcoma and often reflect outcome (Craver, 1996).

CLASSIFICATION, GRADING, AND STAGING

Classification

Soft tissue sarcomas are difficult to classify, and there is no universally accepted system of classification of these tumors to date. The ratio of benign tumors to malignant sarcomas is 100:1 (Brennan, Casper, & Harrison, 1997). Often the histiogenesis of a particular sarcoma is difficult to determine. Some sarcomas may contain several cell types; others may have very different histologic portions in one tumor; others may be highly undifferentiated and classified as such.

The American Joint Committee on Cancer Staging (AJCCS) has recommended the classification system developed by the World Health Organization (WHO). This system describes the cell of origin and the intracellular material it produces. The classification system described in Table 72-5 is similar to that of the WHO. In the system presented in the table, the histologic categories are divided into benign

TABLE 72-5 Histologic Classification of Soft Tissue Tumors

I. Fibrous tumors
   A. Benign tumors
      1. Nodular fasciitis
      2. Proliferative fasciitis and myositis
      3. Atypical decubital fibroplasia
      4. Fibroma
      5. Keloid
      6. Elastofibroma
      7. Calcifying aponeurotic fibroma
      8. Fibrous hamartoma of infancy
      9. Fibromatosis cells
      10. Infantile digital fibromatosis
      11. Myofibromatosis
      12. Hyalin fibromatosis
      13. Calcifying fibrous pseudotumor
   B. Fibromatoses
      1. Superficial fibromatoses
      2. Deep fibromatoses
   C. Malignant tumors
      1. Fibrosarcoma
         a. Adult fibrosarcoma
         b. Congenital fibrosarcoma
         c. Inflammatory fibrosarcoma
II. Fibrohistiocytic tumors
   A. Benign tumors
      1. Fibrous histiocytoma
   B. Intermediate tumors
      1. Atypical fibroxanthoma
      2. Dermatofibrosarcoma protuberans
      3. Giant cell fibroblastoma
      4. Plexiform fibrohistiocytic tumor
      5. Angiomatoid fibrous histiocytoma
   C. Malignant tumors
      1. Malignant fibrous histiocytoma
         a. Storiform-pleomorphic fibrous histiocytoma
         b. Myxoid fibrous histiocytoma
         c. Giant cell fibrous histiocytoma
         d. Xanthomatous
III. Lipomatous tumors
   A. Benign tumors
      1. Lipoma
      2. Angiolipoma
      3. Spindle cell or pleomorphic
      4. Myolipoma
      5. Angiomyolipoma
      6. Myelolipoma
      7. Chondroid lipoma
      8. Hibernoma
      9. Lipoblastoma
      10. Lipomatosis
      11. Atypical lipoma
   B. Malignant tumors
      1. Liposarcoma
         a. Well-differentiated
         b. Myxoid
         c. Round cell
         d. Pleomorphic
         e. De-differentiated
IV. Smooth muscle tumors
   A. Benign tumors
      1. Leiomyoma
      2. Angiomyoma
      3. Epitheloid leiomyoma
      4. Intravenous leiomyomatosis
      5. Leiomyomatosis peritonealis disseminata
   B. Malignant tumors
      1. Leiomyosarcoma
      2. Epithelioid leiomyosarcoma
V. Skeletal muscle tumors
   A. Benign tumors
      1. Adult rhabdomyoma
      2. Genital rhabdomyoma
      3. Fetal rhabdomyoma
      4. Intermediate rhabdomyoma
   B. Malignant tumors
      1. Rhabdomyosarcoma
      2. Rhabdomyosarcoma with ganglionic differentiation
VI. Tumors of blood and lymph vessels
   A. Benign tumors
      1. Papillary endothelial hyperplasia
      2. Hemangioma
      3. Deep hemangioma
      4. Lymphangioma
      5. Lymphangiomyoma
      6. Angiomatosis
      7. Lymphangiomatosis
   B. Intermediate tumors
      1. Hemangioendothelioma
   C. Malignant tumors
      1. Angiosarcoma and lymphangiosarcoma
      2. Kaposi's sarcoma
VII. Perivascular tumors
   A. Benign tumors
      1. Glomus tumor
      2. Glomangiomyoma
      3. Hemangiopericytoma

Modified from Enzinger, F. M. & Weiss, S. W. (Eds.). (1995d). *Soft tissue tumors.* (3rd ed.). Mosby: St. Louis.

and malignant, which describes the predominant cell of origin or the association to the embryonal cell (Beahrs, Henson, Hutter, & Kennedy, 1993; Enzinger & Weiss, 1995d).

In a large retrospective study by Kransdorf (1995), 12,370 malignant sarcomas were classified according to histologic study. More than 80% of the tumors reviewed were placed in the following categories: malignant fibrous histiocytoma (24%), liposarcoma (14%), leiomyosarcoma (8%), malignant schwannoma (6%), dermatofibrosarcoma protuberans (6%), synovial sarcoma (5%), fibrosarcoma (5%), and sarcomas of unknown histogenesis (12%). Rhabdomyosarcoma, neuroblastoma, and extraskeletal Ewing's sarcoma are the most common soft tissue sarcomas found in children (Enzinger & Weiss, 1995d).

TABLE 72-5 Histologic Classification of Soft Tissue Tumors—cont'd

- B. Malignant tumors
  1. Malignant glomus tumor
  2. Malignant hemangiopericytoma

VIII. Synovial tumors
- A. Benign tumors
  1. Tenosynovial giant cell tumor
- B. Malignant tumors
  1. Synovial sarcoma
     - a. Biphasic
     - b. Monophasic
  2. Malignant giant cell tumor of tendon sheath

IX. Mesothelial tumors
- A. Benign tumors
  1. Solitary fibrous tumor of pleura and peritoneum
  2. Multicystic mesothelioma
  3. Adenomatoid tumor
  4. Well-differentiated papillary mesothelioma
- B. Malignant tumors
  1. Malignant solitary fibrous tumor of pleura and peritoneum
  2. Diffuse mesothelioma
     - a. Epithelial diffuse mesothelioma
     - b. Fibrous diffuse mesothelioma
     - c. Biphasic diffuse mesothelioma

X. Neural tumors
- A. Benign tumors
  1. Traumatic neuroma
  2. Morton's neuroma
  3. Multiple mucosal neuroma
  4. Neuromuscular hamartoma
  5. Nerve sheath ganglion
  6. Schwannoma
  7. Neurotheleoma
  8. Neurofibroma
  9. Granular cell tumor
  10. Melanocytic schwannoma
  11. Ectopic meningioma
  12. Ectopic ependymoma
  13. Ganglioneuroma
  14. Pigmented neuroectodermal tumor of infancy
- B. Malignant tumors
  1. Malignant peripheral nerve sheath tumor (MPNST)
     - a. Malignant triton tumor
     - b. Glandular MPNST
     - c. Epithelioid MPNST
  2. Malignant granular cell tumor
  3. Clear cell sarcoma
  4. Malignant melanocytic schwannoma
  5. Gastrointestinal autonomous nerve tumor
  6. Primitive neuroectodermal tumor

XI. Paraganglionic tumors
- A. Benign tumors
  1. Paraganglioma
- B. Malignant tumors
  1. Malignant paraganglioma

XII. Extraskeletal cartilaginous and osseous tumors
- A. Benign tumors
  1. Panniculitis ossificans and myositis ossificans
  2. Fibro-osseous pseudotumor of the digits
  3. Fibrodysplasia ossificans progressiva
  4. Extraskeletal chondroma
  5. Extraskeletal osteoma
- B. Malignant tumors
  1. Extraskeletal chondrosarcoma
     - a. Well-differentiated
     - b. Myxoid
     - c. Mesenchymal
  2. Extraskeletal osteosarcoma

XIII. Pluripotential mesenchymal tumors
- A. Benign tumors
  1. Mesenchymoma
- B. Malignant tumors
  1. Malignant mesenchymoma

XIV. Miscellaneous tumors
- A. Benign tumors
  1. Congenital granular cell tumor
  2. Tumoral calcinosis
  3. Myxoma
  4. Angiomyxoma
  5. Amyloid tumor
  6. Parachordoma
  7. Ossifying and nonossifying fibromyxoid
  8. Palisaded myofibroblastoma of lymph node
- B. Malignant tumors
  1. Alveolar soft part sarcoma
  2. Epithelioid sarcoma
  3. Malignant extrarenal rhabdoid tumor
  4. Desmoplastic small cell tumor

XV. Unclassified tumors

Grading

Grading and staging of sarcomas is necessary for consistency of data collection, for determining prognostic information, and for treatment planning. Grading determines the degree of malignancy, and staging refers to the extent of disease.

Grading of soft tissue sarcomas has also been difficult. Most groups agree that the most significant factors to evaluate when grading these malignancies are the number of mitotic figures, the extent of necrosis within the lesion, and the degree of differentiation. The AJCC describes four different grades of sarcomas: G1, well-differentiated; G2, moderately differentiated; G3, poorly differentiated; and G4, undifferentiated. G1 is considered a low-grade tumor that is less likely to metastasize to distant sites (Arca, Sondak, & Chang, 1994; Frable, 1994) (Table 72-6). Examples of high-

TABLE 72-6 American Joint Committee on Cancer Staging System for Soft Tissue Sarcomas

Histopathologic Grade (G)				
Gx	Grade cannot be determined			
G1	Well differentiated			
G2	Moderately differentiated			
G3	Poorly differentiated			
G4	Undifferentiated			
Primary Tumor (T)				
Tx	Primary tumor cannot be assessed			
T0	No evidence of primary tumor			
T1	Tumor 5 cm or less in greatest diameter			
T2	Tumor more than 5 cm in greatest dimension			
Regional Lymph Nodes (N)				
NX	Regional lymph nodes cannot be assessed			
N0	No regional lymph node metastasis			
N1	Regional lymph node metastasis			
Distant Metastasis (M)				
MX	Presence of distant metastasis cannot be assessed			
M0	No distant metastasis			
M1	Distant metastasis			
Stage Grouping				
Stage IA	G1	T1	N0	M0
Stage IB	G1	T2	N0	M0
Stage IIA	G2	T1	N0	M0
Stage IIB	G2	T2	N0	M0
Stage IIIA	G3,4	T1	N0	M0
Stage IIIB	G3,4	T2	N0	M0
Stage IVA	Any G	Any T	N1	M0
Stage IVB	Any G	Any T	Any N	M1

Modified from American Joint Committee on Cancer. (1993). Handbook for staging of cancer. In *Manual for staging of cancer,* (4th ed.). Philadelphia: J. B. Lippincott.

TABLE 72-7 Enneking System for Surgical Staging of Sarcomas

Stage	Grade	Site
IA	Low (G1)	Intracompartmental (T1)
IB	Low (G1)	Extracompartmental (T2)
IIA	High (G2)	Intracompartmental (T1)
IIB	High (G2)	Extracompartmental (T2)
III	Any (G) Regional or distant metastasis	Any (T)

Modified from Enneking, W. F., Spanier, S. S., & Goodman, M. A. (1980). A system for surgical staging of musculoskeletal sarcoma. *Clinical Orthopaedics and Related Research, 153,* 106-120.

TABLE 72-8 Surgical Procedure Based on Surgical Stage for Soft Tissue Sarcomas

Stage	Procedure
IA	Wide excision
IIB	Wide amputation
IIA	Radical resection
IIB	Radical disarticulation

Modified from Enneking, W. F., Spanier, S. S., & Goodman, M. A. (1980). A system for surgical staging of musculoskeletal sarcoma. *Clinical Orthopaedics and Related Research, 153,* 106-120.

grade soft tissue sarcomas include alveolar and embryonal rhabdomyosarcomas, neuroblastoma, and extraskeletal Ewing's sarcoma. Well-differentiated and myxoid liposarcomas are examples of low-grade sarcomas (Enzinger & Weiss, 1995d).

Staging

The AJCCS system is based on the TNM system. It uses the size and extension of the primary tumor (T), the involvement of lymph nodes (N), the presence of metastasis (M), and the type and grade of the sarcoma. This staging system is based on the review of 1215 cases from 13 institutions. Staging for childhood tumors is essentially the same as that for adults (see Table 72-6) (AJCCS, 1993).

Enneking also developed a popular staging system based on anatomic settings (T1 or T2); grade (G1 or G2); and metastasis (M0 or M1). This system describes the lesion as to whether or not it is within a well-delineated surgical area, how aggressive is it by clinical behavior, and the presence of metastasis. Enneking believed strongly that the main factor influencing the extent of the surgical procedure is whether the lesion remained intracompartmentally (confined entirely) in the anatomic site or extended extracompartmentally, beyond the tissue planes and spaces (Enneking, Spanier, & Goodman, 1980) (Table 72-7). He then identified the extent of surgery needed based on the stage of the sarcoma. For example, stage IA would require a wide excision since it is a low-grade intracompartmental tumor. On the other hand, stage II A, which is a high-grade intracompartmental tumor, requires a radical resection (Table 72-8).

Both staging systems provide a useful guide to therapy and offer prognostic information. Some sources think that the Enneking system is best used for sarcomas of the extremities and that the AJCCS system is more applicable to all sites (Enzinger & Weiss, 1995d).

The most common subtypes of soft tissue sarcomas are malignant fibrous histiocytoma, liposarcoma, and leiomyosarcoma. Most of the retroperitoneal sarcomas tend to be liposarcomas or leiomyosarcomas. Sarcomas of the extremities tend to be liposarcomas, multiple fibrous histiocytomas, synovial sarcomas, or fibrosarcomas. Chest wall sarcomas are most frequently desmoids, liposarcomas, and myogenic sarcomas (Brennan, Casper, & Harrison, 1997). Some of the more common soft tissue sarcomas representing different cellular types are described in the following section.

Malignant Fibrous Histiocytoma. A malignant fibrous histiocytoma (MFH) is made up of fibroblasts and histiocyte-like cells. MFH is the most common type of soft tissue sarcoma and tends to be found in deep tissue of the extremities and retroperitoneum. It is associated with older adults between the ages of 50 and 70 years. Approximately two thirds of these tumors occur in men, and this tumor type is more prevalent in Caucasians than in African Americans or Hispanics (Enzinger & Weiss, 1995b). MFH cells show a primitive mesenchymal cell differentiation. Immunohistochemically MFH is diagnosed through the exclusion of other sarcomas. MFH is further classified into subtypes: storiform-pleomorphic, myxoid, giant cell, inflammatory, and angiomatoid. Both myxoid and angiomatoid types are associated with a more favorable prognosis and are less likely to metastasize (Enzinger & Weiss, 1995b; Miettinen & Weiss, 1996; van Unnik, 1995). MFH is commonly found in the lower extremities, followed by the upper extremities and retroperitoneum. Patients with tumors of an extremity report a painless mass that begins to enlarge after several months. Patients with retroperitoneal presentation tend to have initial symptoms that include anorexia, malaise, weight loss, and a sense of abdominal pressure. Some cytogenetic abnormalities have been associated with MFH but not with any reliability (Enzinger & Weiss, 1995b).

Fibrosarcoma. Fibrosarcoma is a rare soft tissue sarcoma composed of malignant fibroblast-like spindle cells. It accounts for <10% of the sarcomas. This type of tumor is found at sites of scars, in subcutaneous fibrous tissue, and in deep connective tissue, around tendons or nerve sheath, muscle fascia, or periosteum. Fibrosarcomas usually appear as a single palpable mass ranging from 3 to 8 cm in diameter. The skin is usually intact, unless the area has been traumatized or a significant delay in diagnosis has occurred. Fibrosarcomas are most commonly diagnosed in patients between the ages of 30 and 55 years (Enzinger & Weiss, 1995b).

Fibrosarcomas may be found in any area of the body that contains fibrous tissue. The majority are found in the thigh and knee, followed in frequency by the trunk, forearms, and lower legs. Because of the nature of their cell of origin, fibrosarcomas are found deep in structures and may surround bone (Enzinger & Weiss, 1995b).

The development of some fibrosarcomas is associated with radiation therapy used to treat lymphoma and breast cancer. These sarcomas may appear 5 to 15 years after the therapy has been completed. The median time is approximately 10 years. Radiation-associated fibrosarcomas are usually high-grade malignancies with a poor prognosis. The overall 5-year survival for patients with this type of sarcoma is 40% to 50%. Grading of the tumor is based on mitotic activity and cellularity. There are no immunohistochemical markers specific for fibrosarcoma (Enzinger & Weiss, 1995d; Miettinen & Weiss, 1996).

The association of fibrosarcoma development with areas of previous thermal burns has been reported. Athough uncommon, such tumors have occurred in patients who were burned severely as children and developed the tumor approximately 30 years after that event (Enzinger & Weiss, 1995b). The 5-year survival rates for patients with fibrosarcomas range from 39% to 54%. As with most soft tissue sarcomas, survival is associated with the grade of the tumor (Enzinger & Weiss, 1995b).

Liposarcoma. Liposarcomas are malignant tumors made up of cells that resemble those of adipose tissue. They are one of the most common types of soft tissue sarcoma and generally occur in adults between the ages of 40 and 60 years. The incidence of this type of soft tissue sarcoma compared to all sarcomas is between 9.8% and 16%. There are five common types of liposarcomas: well-differentiated, myxoid, round cell, pleomorphic (irregular cells containing multiple nuclei), and de-differentiated (Enzinger & Weiss, 1995f).

Liposarcomas often present as a very large tumor. Well-differentiated types closely resemble normal fat. Because of their size, they may push other organs, such as the kidney, out of the way or cause obstruction of the ureters. The major sites of presentation are the thigh and retroperitoneum. There are no classic symptoms reported by patients. However, at presentation, approximately 10% to 15% of patients have pain, tenderness, or functional impairment when the tumor is very large and impinges on other structures. Approximately 50% of these tumors are found in the lower extremities. Almost 20% are found intraabdominally. Lesions found in the extremities recur locally in 50% of cases. Intra-abdominal tumors recur in 90% of patients and lead to death in one third of cases. Overall, recurrence rates of these tumors range from 46% to 57%. Less well differentiated tumors have a greater propensity to metastasize, and the 5-year survival rate may be as low as 20% after surgical resection of these aggressive tumors. The better differentiated liposarcomas have a 5-year survival rate of approximately 80%. Enzinger & Weiss, 1995f; Miettinen & Weiss, 1996).

Angiosarcoma. Angiosarcomas are a group of tumors that originate from two cells within the vascular and lymph systems: the endothelial cells, which line the lumina of blood and lymph vessels, and pericytes, which are found surrounding the outside of capillaries (van Unnik, 1995). They are very rare sarcomas, comprising <1% of sarcomas. Angiosarcomas are usually found in the skin and superficial soft tissue as purple lesions. Additional sites include the breast, liver, bone, and spleen. These tumors are categorized in five groups: (1) cutaneous tumors without preexisting lymphedema, (2) cutaneous tumors arising in lymphadematous extremities, (3) angiosarcoma of the breast, (4) angiosarcoma of deep soft tissue (e.g., liver), and (5) radiation-induced angiosarcoma. The diagnosis of angiosarcoma usually requires immunohistochemical testing (Mark, Poen, Tran, Fu, & Juillard, 1995; Miettinen & Weiss, 1996; van Unnik, 1995).

Chronic lymphedema is a well-recognized predisposing factor for angiosarcoma. Ninety percent of cases tend to be postmastectomy patients who have severe chronic lymphedema (Enzinger & Weiss, 1995i).

Radiation-induced angiosarcoma that is not associated with chronic lymphedema has been observed to occur 12 years posttreatment in patients treated for a variety of solid tumors, as in cervical, ovarian, endometrial, and breast cancer and Hodgkin's disease (Enzinger & Weiss, 1995i).

There have also been reports of angiosarcomas occurring at sites of foreign material, such as shrapnel, steel, plastic or dacron graft material, and surgical sponges. It is theorized that the body's response to such objects is to enclose the foreign material in fibrous tissue. This may be an intermediate step before the development of angiosarcoma (Enzinger & Weiss, 1995i).

Cutaneous angiosarcoma is common in older patients who have a lesion in the scalp at presentation. Prognosis is related to the size of the lesion. Patients with lesions >5 cm have the worst prognosis (Enzinger & Weiss, 1995i).

Angiosarcoma of the breast is very rare and tends to occur in premenopausal women between ages 30 and 40. These tumors are more aggressive that most breast cancers, with overall survival <2 years (Enzinger & Weiss, 1995i).

Angiosarcoma of soft tissue comprises approximately 25% of this category of tumors. These tumors occur at all ages and tend to arise in the extremities or the abdominal cavity, where it appears as a large hemorrhagic mass. In young children with large tumors, serious symptoms include thrombocytopenia, cardiac failure, and exsanguination (Enzinger & Weiss, 1995i).

Leiomyosarcomas. Leiomyosarcomas are tumors originating from smooth muscle differentiation. They are usually found in the skin, the deep soft tissues of the extremities, and the retroperitoneum. This type is the most common soft tissue sarcoma in the gastrointestinal tract and uterus and accounts for 5% to 10% of all soft tissue sarcomas. Leiomyosarcomas are divided into three major groups: (1) deep soft tissue; (2) cutaneous and subcutaneous tissue; and (3) vascular origin (Enzinger & Weiss, 1995e).

Leiomyosarcomas found in the retroperitoneal and abdominal cavities occur more frequently in women, with a median age of 60. At presentation, patients often have nonspecific complaints, such as weight loss, pain, nausea and vomiting, and abdominal swelling. Leiomyosarcomas tend to be very aggressive and are difficult to resect because of their large size and location. The 5-year survival is approximately 29% (Enzinger & Weiss, 1995e).

Cutaneous leiomyosarcomas generally have a good prognosis. Since these tumors are superficial, they are usually detected early in their course. Cutaneous leiomyosarcomas are common between the fifth and seventh decade (Enzinger & Weiss, 1995e; Miettinen & Weiss, 1996; Morton, 1997).

Vascular leiomyosarcomas are very rare and tend to develop in major vessels such as the vena cava. They are seldom seen in the pulmonary artery. At presentation, they are associated with life-threatening symptoms caused by direct extension of the tumor and impairment of circulation. Leiomyosarcomas of the vena cava occur primarily in women over the age of 50 (Enzinger & Weiss, 1995e).

Rhabdomyosarcoma. This type of tumor exhibits striated muscle–like differentiation and occurs mainly in children and adolescents. Overall survival ranges from 80% to 90% in patients with the more favorable types (Miettinen & Weiss, 1996). There are three commonly recognized rhabdomyosarcomas: embryonal, alveolar, and pleomorphic.

Embryonal rhabdomyosarcomas commonly occur in the ocular orbit or genitourinary tract in children. Although these tumors tend to metastasize, they are very responsive to chemotherapy. The worst prognosis is for older patients with this disease (Brennan, Casper, & Harrison, 1997).

Extremity rhabdomyosarcoma in adolescents and young adults has an alveolar histologic basis. Genetic translocation is a common feature. This group of tumors tends to have a worse prognosis that that of embryonal rhabdomyosarcoma (Brennan, Casper, & Harrison, 1997).

Pleomorphic rhabdomyosarcoma is the most common type in adults. It tends to be a high-grade tumor that is similar to other high-grade sarcomas in adults (Brennan, Casper, & Harrison, 1997).

Malignant Peripheral Nerve Sheath Tumors. Occasionally, peripheral nerves are the site of sarcomas. These tumors are difficult to classify since their cell of origin is neuroectoderm rather than mesenchyma. Malignant peripheral nerve sheath tumors (MPNSTs) resemble cells of the nerve sheath, such as Schwann cells, perineural fibroblasts, and fibroblasts. These tumors make up approximately 10% of all soft tissue sarcomas, and 50% of them are associated with patients who have von Recklinghausen's disease (neurofibromatosis type 1). These tumors often appear as lesions that enlarge over the course of several months and may result in pain and paresthesia as they extend along the nerve sheath. MPNSTs occur in adults between age 20 and 50. The majority of these tumors are high grade, resulting in local recurrence and distant metastasis (Enzinger & Weiss, 1995h).

In addition to the association with genetic conditions, approximately 10% of these tumors are attributed to therapeutic or occupational radiation. The period of time from exposure to tumor development is an average of 15 years (Enzinger & Weiss, 1995h).

Chemical carcinogens may be a contributing factor in the development of MPNSTs since these tumors have been chemically induced in laboratory animals (Enzinger & Weiss, 1995h).

Small Round Cell Tumors. These tumors usually occur in children and include rhabdomyosarcoma, Ewing's sarcoma, neuroblastoma and other neuroepithelial tumors, and desmoplastic small round cell tumors. Ewing's sarcoma, which can be present without bone involvement (extraskeletal), appears as a deep soft tissue mass, occurring primarily in adolescents and young adults. Desmoplastic small round cell tumor (DSRCT) is a high-grade malignancy found in the abdomen of boys younger than 15 years. The prognosis for this tumor is quite poor (Miettinen & Weiss, 1996).

Synovial Sarcoma. Synovial sarcoma is an example of the difficult challenge of categorizing soft tissue sarcomas. Some authors classify this type of tumor as being of unknown histogenesis since there is no clear evidence of synovial differentiation.

Synovial sarcoma accounts for about 10% of all soft tissue sarcomas. It generally occurs in adolescents and young adults, between the ages of 15 and 40 years. The median age is 26.5 years. Synovial sarcomas are more common in men than women (Enzinger & Weiss, 1995k).

The most common sites of this tumor are the deep soft

tissues of the popliteal area, knee, thigh, feet, hands, and forearm, but it is uncommon in joint cavities. The 5-year survival rate is 50%, with the most common sites of metastasis being the lungs and pleura. Since synovial sarcoma is associated with latent metastasis, the 10-year survival is only about 20% (Miettinen & Weiss, 1996; Enzinger & Weiss, 1995k).

Mesothelioma. A strong association between mesothelioma and asbestos was first reported in 1960 in South Africa among workers in the asbestos industry. A 20- to 40-year time lag exists between exposure to the carcinogen and the development of mesothelioma. The incidence of this tumor is expected to decline in the next century because of the decrease in use of asbestos (Enzinger & Weiss, 1995j).

This tumor arises from mesothelial cells or mesenchymal cells of serosal surfaces. Most often it appears in men over age 50. The most common site of presentation is the pleural cavity, but it often extends into the peritoneal cavity. Mesothelioma also appears as a primary tumor of the pericardium. The prognosis is associated by type; however, most patients die of complications from this tumor within 12 to 18 months of diagnosis (Enzinger & Weiss, 1995j).

MEDICAL MANAGEMENT

The Role of Surgery

Multidisciplinary management is key to successful treatment of the patient with soft tissue sarcoma. The surgeon, radiation oncologist, medical oncologist, pathologist, oncology nurse, physical therapist, occupational therapist, and social worker represent only some of the essential disciplines involved in the care of the patient.

Wide surgical resection is the most common method of surgical management of the patient. This approach includes the tumor, all previous scars from the biopsy site, and a 2 to 3 cm margin of normal tissue. Since lymph node involvement occurs in only about 3% of soft tissue sarcomas, lymph node dissection is usually not required (Beech & Pollock, 1995; Lawrence, 1994). Wide local excision alone has a local recurrence rate of approximately 49%. With radical excision, such as amputation of muscle compartmental excisions, there is a local recurrence rate of 14%. However, since the 1984 National Institutes of Health consensus conference, limb-sparing procedures combined with additional treatment modalities make up a viable treatment plan for many patients with soft tissue sarcoma (Consensus Conference, 1985).

Successful surgical resection implies that enough margin of normal tissue is included in the excision. Wolf and Enneking (1996) describe four levels of margin around the tumor (Fig. 72-2). As the tumor grows, it encounters natural anatomic barriers. Initially, lesions extend into the pseudocapsule, passing into a reactive zone. Eventually sarcomas extend beyond the boundary of the musculoskeletal compartment.

Many areas of the body do not allow adequate wide resection, and therefore amputation becomes the plan of care. Common sites that preclude wide excision are the groin; knee; portions of the leg, ankle, and foot; forearm; wrist and

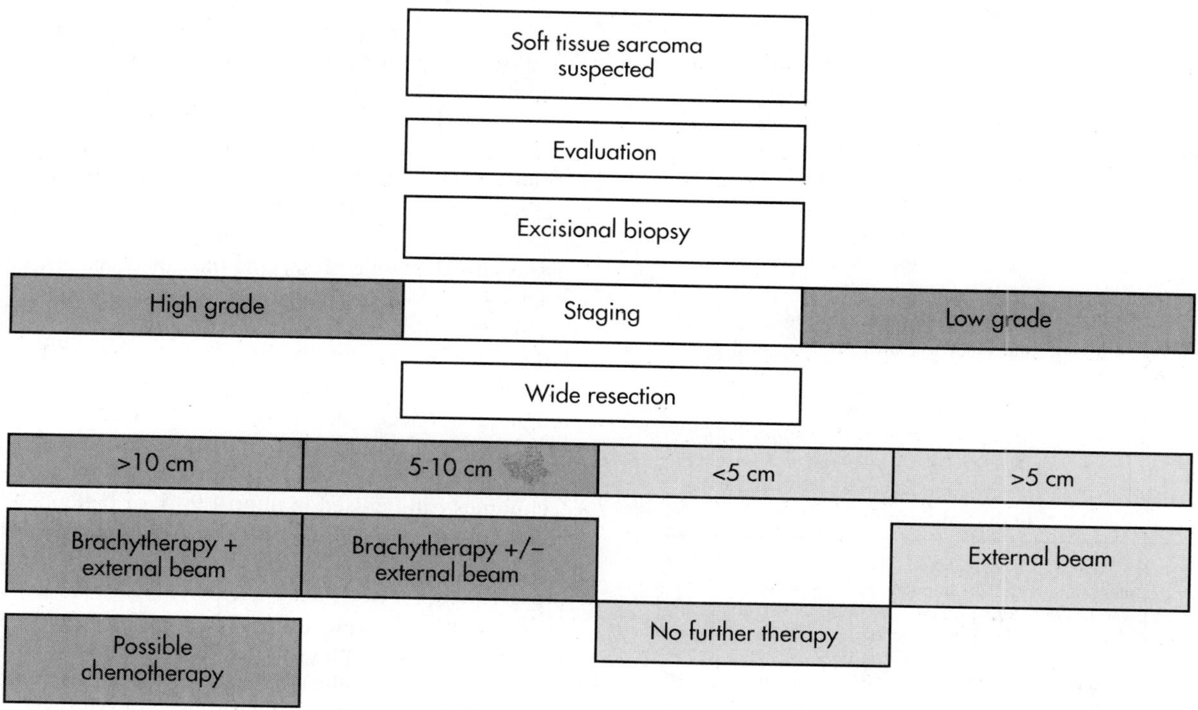

Fig. 72-2 Decision tree for medical management of soft tissue sarcomas. (Modified from Brennan, M. F., Casper, E. S., & Harrison, L. B. [1997]. Soft tissue sarcoma. In V. T. DeVita, S. Hellman, & S. A. Rosenberg [Eds.], *Cancer: Principles and practice of oncology* [5th ed.]. Philadelphia: Lippincott-Raven.)

hand; parts of the head and neck; and various axillary sites. When amputation is the surgical plan, the level of amputation is above the proximal joint (Yang et al., 1993).

There are four major types of surgery performed for soft tissue sarcomas, as described in Table 72-9. Each of the techniques presented has been applied to both limb-sparing procedures and amputation (Nichter & Menendez, 1993; Yang et al., 1993). Wide excision is probably the most common procedure performed for sarcomas. The surgeon often places metal clips to mark the resected margins as a guide for subsequent radiation therapy. With sarcomas located in the trunk or retroperitoneum, wide excision may not be possible. In that setting all gross tumor is resected, sometimes including adjacent organs such as the kidney (Yang et al., 1993).

TABLE 72-9 Definition of Surgical Techniques Used for Soft Tissue Sarcomas

Technique	Description
Intracapsular excision	This procedure is used only for tissue diagnosis since the majority of the tumor is left in place. Local recurrence is 100% with this procedure.
Marginal excision	All gross tumor is removed with the pseudocapsule; however, local recurrence of tumor is 90%.
Wide excision	Tumor is removed en bloc with a margin (2-3 cm) of normal tissue within the muscular compartment of origin. Local recurrence rates are as high as 50% unless combined with adjuvant radiation therapy. Preservation of limb function is possible with this approach.
Radical excision	Tumor is removed in continuity with the entire compartment of origin in the anatomic area. The surgery includes dissecting along tissue planes that are separated from the tumor and its tissues of origin by at least one uninvolved anatomic plane in all directions. The resected tissue includes the origin and insertion of all muscle and any bones or joints involved in that anatomic compartment. This surgery has a local recurrence rate of approximately 10% to 14%. However, this surgery reduces the functional ability of the limb significantly.

Modified from Chang, A. E. & Sondak, V. K. (1995). Clinical evaluation and treatment of soft tissue sarcomas. In F. M. Enzinger & S. W. Weiss (Eds.), *Soft tissue tumors* (3rd ed.). St. Louis: Mosby; Nichter, L. S., & Menendez, L. R. (1993). Reconstructive considerations for limb salvage surgery. *Orthopedic Clinics of North America, 24*(3), 511-521; Wolf, R. E., & Enneking, W. F. (1996). The staging and surgery of musculoskeletal neoplasms. *Orthopedic Clinics of North America, 27*(3), 473-481; Yang, J. C., Rosenberg, S. A., Glatstein, E. J., & Antman, K. H. (1993). Sarcomas of soft tissue. In V. T. DeVita, S. Hellman, & S. A. Rosenberg (Eds.), *Cancer: Principles and practice of oncology* (4th ed.). Philadelphia: Lippincott-Raven.

There are several types of amputative procedures that have been used for soft tissue sarcomas. It is common that amputation includes the joint above the tumor site. Sarcomas that are adjacent to joints or bone or that adhere to major neurovascular structures may require amputation. It has been reported that in 1960 60% to 70% of patients with soft tissue sarcomas underwent amputation. However, because of the success of combining limb-sparing procedures with radiation therapy, the use of amputation has declined to 5% to 7% (Suit & Spiro, 1995).

In general, most procedures for amputation of the foot do not provide adequate margin for soft tissue sarcomas, and surgical treatment is usually combined with adjuvant radiation therapy. Below-knee amputation is usually performed for any large soft tissue sarcoma of the foot. Above-knee amputation is indicated for tumors of the leg found below the knee level.

Hip disarticulation involves amputation or separation of the hip with complete removal of the femur. This procedure may be used for patients with sarcomas located in the middle or distal thigh.

Hemipelvectomy involves removal of the entire lower extremity and hemipelvis with disarticulation of the sacroiliac joint and pubic symphysis. A more conservative version of this surgery, modified hemipelvectomy, allows preservation of the iliac wing, which improves patient rehabilitation. Extended hemipelvectomy is used if lesions in the iliac wing are too close to the sacroiliac joint for disarticulation. In that situation, extension of the normal margin includes removal of the sacral ala at the level of lateral vertebral bodies.

Amputations of the upper extremities are similar to the previously described procedures. Disarticulation of the shoulder joint or forequarter amputation with removal of the scapula and clavicle are reserved for tumors of the upper arm or shoulder.

Since the 1985 Consensus Conference, the National Institutes of Health has supported the use of limb-sparing techniques as the preferred surgical plan when possible. Limb-sparing surgery is a technique that removes the soft tissue sarcoma while preserving the functional and cosmetic appearance of the extremity (Consensus Conference, 1985). When combined with other treatment modalities, particularly radiation therapy, limb-sparing procedures have demonstrated overall survival rates that are equal to those of amputation (Beech & Pollock, 1995; Consensus Conference, 1985). Limb-sparing techniques are very useful for soft tissue sarcomas of the scapular area and buttocks. These techniques can be used in almost 90% of patients with soft tissue sarcomas of the extremities (Lawrence, 1994). Wide excision is the most common procedure performed for limb preservation.

Treatment planning for limb-sparing procedures should include three major phases. The first is evaluation of the patient from an oncologic perspective. The tumor must be removed with adequate margin of normal tissue, and the role of adjuvant therapy must be considered. Second, plans for reconstruction of the soft tissue deficit, which may also include a skeletal defect, are determined. Third, plans for the patient's rehabilitation should be discussed before the resection is done (Nichter & Menendez, 1993) (Fig. 72-3).

Contraindications to limb-sparing surgery include (1) involvement of major vessels or nerves within the primary lesion; (2) poor surgical margins, which will lead to increased radiation toxicity of nearby structures; (3) reconstructive outcomes that are not equal to or superior to results achieved with a prosthetic device; and (4) resection into growth plates, which causes limb length discrepancy in children (Consensus Conference, 1985).

The need for reconstructive surgery after wide resection of soft tissue sarcomas is determined by the site and anatomic position of the tumor in the affected extremity. Soft tissue reconstruction allows for re-establishment of mobility and joint function; stabilization of a joint; coverage of the surgical wound; and filling of dead space, which can lead to seromas and hematomas, thus increasing the patient's risk for serious infection (Nichter & Menendez, 1993).

Wound complications are the most common problems associated with limb-sparing procedures. The incidence of flap necrosis ranges from 15% to 40%. Infection rates have been noted to be as high as 10% to 15%. To minimize these problems, reconstructive techniques often include vascularized tissue transfer and tension-free wound closure. Microvascular reconstruction allows for one-stage procedures. Immediate bone reconstruction with prosthetic implantation or autograft is also possible by using techniques for immediate coverage of the surgical defect. Flaps originating from the gastrocnemius, latissimus dorsi, rectus abdominis, and serratus anterior muscles are frequently used. Pedicle muscle flaps are well vascularized, but their use increases the risk of spread of the primary tumor through tissue planes and may further compromise muscle strength in the area (Beech & Pollock, 1995; Drake, 1995; Lane & Healey, 1993). As with sarcomas of the trunk, reconstruction following resection of the abdominal wall may require the use of prosthetic material or a fascial autograft to obtain closure of the site. Reconstructive techniques following resection of sarcomas of the head and neck are similar to those used for epithelial cancers in that region (Lawrence, 1994).

Suit has offered several suggestions for reducing wound complications after limb-sparing surgery and reconstruction. These include gentle handling of tissue during the surgery; elimination of all dead space with attention to hemostasis before wound closure; use of compression dressings; leaving of drains in the wound until drainage is <10 ml/day; and immobilization of the part for 7 to 10 days (Suit, 1994).

The patient's nutritional status before surgery is also known to affect surgical recovery and outcomes. Nutritional deficiency before surgical resection is associated with poor wound healing after amputation. Other factors that are thought to interfere with wound healing are preoperative chemotherapy, with its associated immunosuppression, and allogeneic blood transfusions, which may also depress immune functioning (Chmell & Schwarz, 1996).

A series of 88 patients were reviewed for functional outcome after limb-sparing surgery combined with either preoperative or postoperative adjuvant radiation therapy. Overall, 68 patients had acceptable functional results, with 61 of these patients returning to work. Patients with poor outcomes tended to have large tumors, neural involvement within the resection, proximal thigh tumors, and postoperative complications (Bell, O'Sullivan, Davis, Langer, Cum-

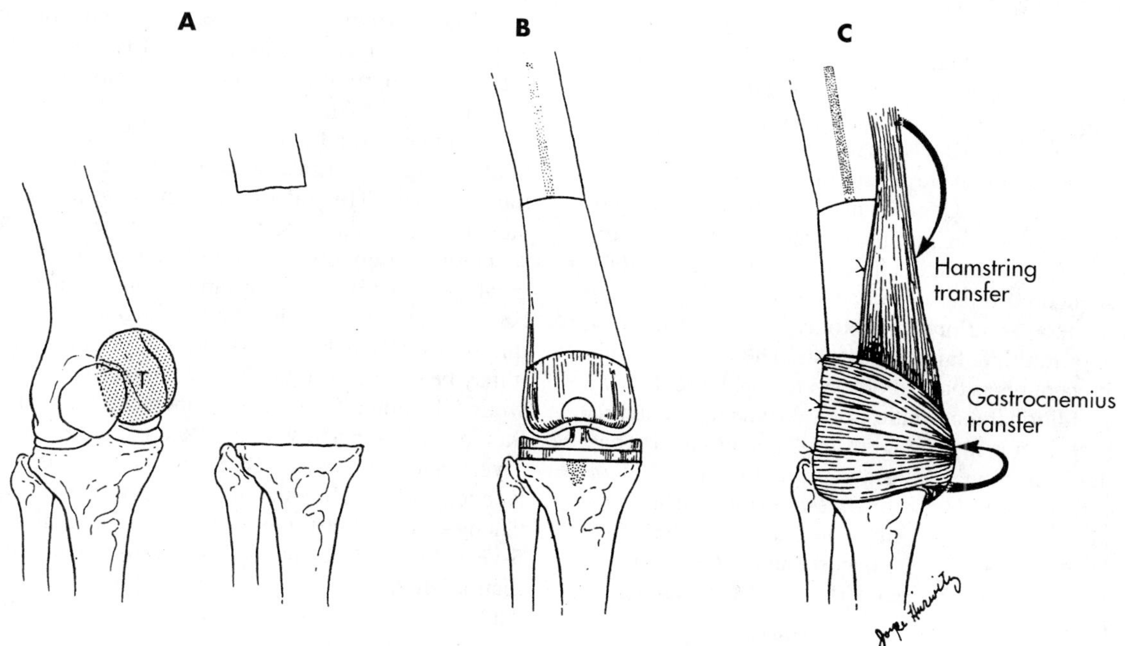

Fig. 72-3 Diagram of the three phases of a limb-sparing procedure. **A,** Tumor resection. **B,** Skeletal reconstruction. **C,** Motor and soft tissue reconstruction. (From DeVita, V. T., Hellman, S., & Rosenberg, S. A. [Eds.]. [1997]. *Cancer: Principles and practice of oncology* [5th ed.]. Philadelphia: Lippincott-Raven.)

mings, & Fornasier, 1991). Radiation therapy has also been associated with reduced muscle power and decreased range of motion when compared to the use of surgery alone. In addition, higher doses of radiation have increased the chance of poor outcomes because of an increased incidence of fibrosis (Suit & Spiro, 1995).

The National Cancer Institute reviewed the long-term complications of patients who had been treated with limb-sparing procedures and radiation therapy. The incidence of bone fracture was 6%; contracture development occurred in 20% of patients; 19% were observed to have 2+ or greater edema of the affected part with induration in 57%; and 20% of patients reported a moderate or severe decrease in muscle strength. However, despite these problems, 84% of patients were ambulating without assistive devices and had minimal, if any, pain associated with their outcomes (Suit & Spiro, 1995).

Adequate resection of soft tissue sarcoma in the retroperitoneum and head and neck region is challenging since achieving wide resection with adequate margins is difficult because of the surrounding structures. In addition, tumors found in the retroperitoneal region are often very large at diagnosis and may involve organs such as the bowel, pancreas, and kidney. Radiation therapy efforts may also be limited because of dose-limiting tissue adjacent to the tumor bed. For these reasons retroperitoneal and head and neck sarcomas tend to have a higher recurrence rate than sarcomas found in the extremities (Suit, 1994).

Metastatic disease presents its own unique challenges in the treatment of soft tissue sarcomas. In a survey done by the American College of Surgeons, more than 52% of patients with recurrent disease had isolated local or regional disease. Approximately 18% had isolated lung metastasis. Most of the patients developed recurrent disease within 5 years from diagnosis (Lawrence, 1994; Yang et al., 1993). Surgical resection of a single site of recurrent disease may be appropriate. The American College of Surgeons survey showed the 5-year survival rate after salvage resection for local recurrences to be 61% (Lawrence, 1994).

Equally good results have been noted after resection of pulmonary recurrences. Overall survival in patients who had complete resection of pulmonary metastases has been reported as 26% at 5 years. Techniques such as single thoracotomy, sequential bilateral thoracotomy, median sternotomy, and bilateral anterior thoracotomy have been used to resect single or multiple lung metastases. The mortality rate with these procedures is only about 1% to 3%. Patients who do not have additional metastatic disease (outside the lung), patients whose tumor is less aggressive histologically, patients with unilateral lung metastatis presenting as less than three nodules, patients whose disease-free interval is >12 months, and patients whose lung metastasis can be completely resected are considered the best candidates for surgical resection of metastatic disease (Frost, 1995; Putnam & Roth, 1995).

Re-excision of the primary tumor before adjuvant therapy was noted by Zornig and colleagues to be valuable for patients with positive margins. These authors reviewed the surgical margins in 189 patients and found that 67 patients did not have adequate clear margins. These patients received re-excision between postoperative days 9 and 28. Zornig and colleagues found that, in comparison to the historical data, the prognosis was improved in the patients who underwent the additional surgery (Zornig, Peiper, & Schroder, 1995).

The Role of Radiation Therapy

Radiation used as a single treatment modality is limited to those patients with extensive, recurrent, or metastatic disease. Local control requires high doses of radiation, and an increased rate of side effects is associated with such aggressive treatment. Radiation complications include soft tissue necrosis, bone fractures, fibrosis, limitation of range of motion, nerve and vascular injury, and edema (McGrath, Sloan, & Kennedy, 1995).

Adjuvant radiation therapy is commonly used with surgical excision (Brennan, Casper, & Harrison, 1997). Radiation is used to treat the remaining microscopic disease. Patients with combined therapy have superior local control of disease compared to patients who have had surgery alone. Radiation not only enhances local control of the tumor, but also results in improved functional and cosmetic outcomes. The sequencing of therapy is controversial. Preoperative radiation therapy may decrease the risk of tumor cell spread during the surgical resection and allow for a smaller treatment portal. Radiation administered before surgery often reduces the tumor volume, permitting more conservative resection. However, there is also concern that preoperative radiation therapy may delay the plan for surgical resection and lead to a higher incidence of wound complications in 30% to 50% of patients (Beech & Pollock, 1995; Cheng, Dusenbery, Winters, & Thompson, 1996; McGrath, Sloan, & Kennedy, 1996). Data suggest that preoperative radiation therapy has a local failure rate of 13% and a disease-free survival of approximately 68% at 5 years (McGrath, Sloan, & Kennedy, 1995).

Postoperative adjuvant radiation therapy allows the patient to undergo surgical resection immediately after the initial diagnosis. This may be a significant psychological advantage for some patients. In general, postoperative radiation therapy does not interfere with healing of the surgical incision. However, a larger volume of radiation may be used to treat the entire surgical area adequately. Also, radiation usually is begun 10 to 20 days postoperatively, but it may be delayed for 2 to 3 weeks if there are problems with wound healing. Overall, postoperative adjuvant radiation therapy is associated with a 17% local recurrence rate and a 5-year survival rate of 60% to 68% (McGrath, Sloan, & Kennedy, 1995). In an additional review of 112 patients by Cheng et al. (1996), there was no significant difference in 5-year disease-free survival between patients receiving radiation therapy preoperatively vs postoperatively. In this study local control at 5 years was found to be 12% vs 8% in the respective groups of patients. Wound complications again showed superior results, with the postoperative radiation group experiencing 8% vs 31% for the preoperative group (Cheng et al., 1996).

Brachytherapy has some additional advantages over preoperative or postoperative radiation therapy. With brachytherapy, afterloading catheters are placed 1 cm apart after the immediate surgical excision is completed. Five days later the catheters are loaded with iridium-192 wires. The treatment is completed in an additional 5 days, with the dose of radiation to the site totaling 4200 to 4500 cGy. After treatment the catheters are removed and the patient is discharged. When this method of treatment is used, the treatment time is significantly less (5 days vs 6 weeks), and there is no delay in surgical excision. Brachytherapy also results in less radiation scatter to other structures than external-beam therapy (Beech & Pollock, 1995; Brennan, Casper, & Harrison, 1997). It is also suggested that the patients who benefit the most from this approach are those with high-grade soft tissue sarcomas, particularly of the extremities or the superficial trunk (Harrison & Janjan, 1995; McGrath, Sloan, & Kennedy, 1995). However, this improved local control does not seem to correlate with the incidence of metastasis or the overall survival (Pisters, Harrison, Leung, Woodruff, Casper, & Brennan, 1996). Harrison and Janjan (1995) reported the wound complication rate for patients undergoing brachytherapy to be approximately 26%, compared to 35% for patients having preoperative radiation therapy. The major or moderate wound complication rate was 16%, but it rose to 27% with the addition of supplemental external beam therapy. According to Harrison and Janjan, major and moderate complications include infection, persistent seroma, hematoma, and wound dehiscence.

Investigational techniques such as intraoperative radiation therapy have been used without demonstrating any survival advantage over standard therapy. Fast-neutron beam therapy has also been used at some centers. Initial results suggest that this method may be appropriate for patients with inoperable soft tissue sarcomas (McGrath, Sloan, & Kennedy, 1995; Yang et al., 1993). Other investigational studies have included radiation sensitizers in the plan of care. Data suggest that further trials should be undertaken, particularly in patients with nonresectable tumors (Suit, 1994).

Scully and colleagues reported the results of a study of 44 patients with high-grade soft tissue sarcomas who completed a neoadjuvant program of hyperthermia and external-beam radiation therapy. After completion of this plan, the patients underwent wide surgical resection of the tumors. The local control rate was very good (97.5%), and survival at 36 months was 72% overall, with disease-free survival at 58%. The conclusion of the study was that the overall survival was comparable to that of patients who received adjuvant therapy with radiation alone (Scully, Oleson, Leopold, Samulski, Dodge, & Harrison, 1994).

A summary of the advantages and disadvantages of several methods of radiation therapy is presented in Table 72-10. In general, for low-grade soft tissue sarcomas <5 cm, wide resection is often used alone unless the site (e.g., hand, foot, neck) precludes adequate resection. In that situation adjuvant external-beam therapy is given. For low-grade soft tissue sarcomas >5 cm, surgical resection is routinely followed by external-beam radiation therapy with doses up to 6000 cGy. For high-grade tumors brachytherapy may be done after surgical resection. If the tumor margins

Table 72-10 Advantages and Disadvantages of Radiation Therapy Based on Type and Timing

Treatment Method	Advantages	Disadvantages
Postoperative radiotherapy	Surgery is immediate; psychological advantage Entire specimen is available for pathologic study Less incidence of wound complications	Larger treatment volumes delivered to tissue Delay in start of radiation because of wound healing
Preoperative radiotherapy	Smaller treatment portal Radiation starts immediately No spread of tumor cells into surgical bed Smaller surgical procedure needed	Delays plan for surgical excision Diagnosis based on small biopsy specimen Cannot use histologic specimen to assess response to chemotherapy when it has been used Higher wound complication rate
Intraoperative brachytherapy	Greatly reduced overall treatment time Radiation may be given at lower dose rate; less scatter of radiation to adjacent organs No delay in surgical plan Lower costs compared to external beam therapy	Treatment volume is limited to direct tumor bed Radiation exposure to hospital staff
Intraoperative electron beam therapy	Radiation is applied directly to tumor bed	Radiation is given as a single large dose
Hyperthermia and limb perfusion chemotherapy	Combined effect of drugs and radiation may be greater than radiation alone	Local toxicity of drugs and radiation

Modified from Brennan, M. F., Casper, E. S., & Harrison, L. B. (1997). Soft tissue sarcoma. In V. T. DeVita, S. Hellman, & S. A. Rosenberg (Eds.), *Cancer: Principles and practice of oncology* (5th ed.). Philadelphia: Lippincott-Raven; Suit, H., & Spiro, I. (1995). Radiation as a therapeutic modality in sarcomas of the soft tissue. *Hematology/Oncology Clinics of North America, 9*(4), 733-745.

are questionable, external beam therapy may be added to the treatment plan (Brennan, Casper, & Harrison, 1997).

The Role of Chemotherapy

Adjuvant chemotherapy for soft tissue sarcomas has been an important addition to the multidisciplinary treatment program for patients. More than 50% of patients who achieve good local control of the disease will develop lung metastasis. Adjuvant chemotherapy, with the use of drugs such as doxorubicin, dacarbazine, vinca alkaloids, and (high-dose) methotrexate, suggests improved outcomes. However, because of the small number of patients with soft tissue sarcomas in any given study and the differences between the types of sarcomas and their anatomic location, it is difficult to demonstrate clearly a survival advantage with adjuvant chemotherapy (Chang & Sondak, 1995; Mertens & Bramwell, 1995).

Doxorubicin has been the most commonly used chemotherapeutic agent used in the management of patients with metastatic disease. This drug had also been used in a number of trials in the adjuvant setting. Currently, randomized trials have not shown improvement in overall survival when postoperative adjuvant doxorubicin is used (as compared to survival after surgery alone). Either doxorubicin combined with cyclophosphamide or methotrexate alone given after surgery resulted in improvement in disease-free survival for patients with high-grade sarcoma of an extremity. There was no additional benefit for patients with sarcoma in the trunk or retroperitoneum. In fact, in light of other studies in which adjuvant chemotherapy was used for nonextremity soft tissue sarcomas, there has not been adequate evidence of benefit for this group of patients (Chang & Sondak, 1995).

The benefit of preoperative chemotherapy, also known as *neoadjuvant chemotherapy,* has also been evaluated in several studies. Although this approach is frequently used for patients with bone sarcomas, it has not shown superior results for soft tissue sarcomas (Chang & Sondak, 1995). For high-risk patients with chemotherapy-sensitive sarcomas, preoperative adjuvant chemotherapy demonstrated improved disease-free survival in comparison with that of patients with nonresponding tumors (McGrath, Sloan, & Kennedy, 1995).

Treatment combining radiation therapy with intraarterial doxorubicin chemotherapy followed by surgical resection was also evaluated (Wanebo, Temple, Popp, Constable, Aron, & Cunningham, 1995). Of 66 patients, 60 were able to undergo limb-sparing surgical resection. Wound complications occurred in 41% of patients. The overall survival and disease-free survival rates at 5 years were 59% and 49%, respectively. The local control rate for patients was 98.5%. Patients who failed to demonstrate local control developed distant metastasis (Wanebo et al., 1995). Intraarterial chemotherapy plus radiation given preoperatively may also increase the percentage of patients who can undergo limb salvage therapy (McGrath, Sloan, & Kennedy, 1995).

The combination of preoperative radiation therapy and continuous infusion of doxorubicin has also been used with hyperthermia for patients who were not candidates for surgical resection. In a small study by Uno, Itami, and Kato (1995), the eight patients treated achieved good local palliation without increased treatment morbidity.

Several studies have compared isolated limb perfusion involving chemotherapy to conventional limb salvage treatment. The results showed no significant difference in local recurrence rates or overall survival (McGrath, Sloan, & Kennedy, 1995).

Currently, limb-sparing surgical resection and radiation therapy are standard in the care of patients with soft tissue sarcomas. Adjuvant chemotherapy should be investigated in the format of clinical trials. Adjuvant chemotherapy may be appropriate for those patients with tumors >5 cm at presentation and those with pathologic evidence of high-grade aggressive tumor (McGrath, Sloan, & Kennedy, 1995).

Many chemotherapy trials of patients with disseminated disease have been evaluated. The results have been variable, depending on the type of sarcoma included in the trial, the dose and schedule of the chemotherapy, the presence or absence of prior therapy, and the number of patients included. In general, chemotherapy for metastatic soft tissue sarcomas is palliative therapy, and it has been associated with lower response rates than those seen with metastatic, osteogenic, and Ewing's sarcoma and with childhood rhabdomyosarcoma (Chang & Sondak, 1995). Both single-agent therapy and combination therapy have been evaluated. The chemotherapy agents used for metastatic soft tissue sarcoma are doxorubicin, cyclophosphamide, ifosfamide, methotrexate, vincristine, cisplatin, dactinomycin, and dacarbazine. The drugs with the most activity are doxorubicin and ifosfamide (Chang & Sondak, 1995). Doxorubicin, used as a single agent at a dose of 60 to 70 mg/m^2, has demonstrated response rates from 15% to 35%. Ifosfamide has been the most effective salvage drug for patients who have failed with doxorubicin. Dacarbazine has a response rate of 18% when used as a single agent, particularly for leiomyosarcomas (Demetri & Elian, 1995; McGrath, Sloan, & Kennedy, 1995; Yang et al., 1993).

Platinum-derived alkylating agents such as cisplatin and carboplatin have been used often for children with bone sarcomas. In adults with soft tissue sarcomas, the single-agent response rate with these drugs is <20% (Demetri & Elian, 1995).

Methotrexate is commonly used with osteogenic sarcoma and has also been applied to soft tissue sarcoma. The single-agent response rate in soft tissue sarcoma is variable, with investigators reporting a range of 0% to 37%. The median response rate is 17%. High-dose therapy with methotrexate is investigational for treatment of soft tissue sarcoma (Demetri & Elian, 1995).

Paclitaxel has been evaluated in a single-agent trial by Balcerzak and colleagues. The drug was given at a dose of 250 mg/m^2 with granulocyte colony stimulating factor (G-CSF) administered to reduce myelosuppression. A modest response to this therapy was reported that was similar to previous responses from agents such as dacarbacine, flurouracil (5-FU), cisplatin, and methotrexate (Balcerzak, Benedetti, Weiss, & Natale, 1995).

Randomized trials through cooperative groups have reported response rates from 17% to 30%. The median survival for patients in many of these studies has been 12 months. Single-agent effective drugs have been evaluated in various combinations. The chemotherapy combination that has shown the highest response rate (51%) and a complete response rate of 10% is doxorubicin (60 mg/m^2) and ifosfamide (7.5 g/m^2), with or without dacarbazine (1 g/m^2) (mesna, adriamycin, ifosfamide, dicarbazine [MAID]). Both doxorubicin and dacarbazine are given by continuous infusion over 4 days to decrease cardiotoxicity and nausea and vomiting (McGrath, Sloan, & Kennedy, 1995; Yang et al., 1993).

Another multidrug program for metastatic disease is CY-VA-DIC, which includes cyclophosphamide (500 mg/m^2), vincristine (1.4 mg/m^2), doxorubicin (50 mg/m^2), and dacarbazine (400 mg/m^2). The effects of myelosuppression were reduced with supportive care, including colony-stimulating factors and antibiotics. Patient tolerance has been improved with the aggressive use of antiemetics (Zalupski & Baker, 1995). However, this same protocol used in an adjuvant trial by Rouesse and colleagues demonstrated a reduction in local recurrence rates for patients with head, neck, and trunk sarcomas, but it did not have the same benefit for patients with extremity sarcomas. Of the 317 patients evaluated in the study, the results failed to demonstrate improved overall survival in any of the groups (Bramwell, Rouesse, Steward, Santoro, Schraffordt-Koops, & Buesa et al., 1994).

Autologous bone marrow transplant for soft tissue sarcomas is a new area of clinical trial development. Two studies from the European Bone Marrow Transplant Group reported the results of two groups—43 patients (group 1) and 49 patients (group 2) with soft tissue sarcoma who received high-dose therapy. Group 1 received high-dose melphalan, and group 2 received various chemotherapy regimens. The overall 5-year disease-free survival was 44% for group 1 and 20% for the group 2. Other studies evaluating patients with soft tissue sarcoma after high-dose therapy have included small numbers of patients with relatively short duration of response (Antman, Elias, & Fine, 1994).

Other forms of dose-intensive chemotherapy have been used in protocols supported by colony-stimulating factors and in protocols for autologous bone marrow transplant. The tumors that have shown to be most responsive in these settings are Ewing's sarcoma, rhabdomyosarcoma, and osteosarcoma (Yang et al., 1993).

In a trial reported by Le Cesne and colleagues, high-dose ifosfamide (4 g/m^2/ day over 3 days) was used for patients with advanced soft tissue sarcoma who were pretreated with doxorubicin. The overall response was 33% (partial and complete response), with 22% having stabilization of disease, which suggested that there was a dose-response effect. Toxicity in this trial was severe but still manageable with routine supportive care. The median duration of response was 8 months, and overall survival was 12 months (Le Cesne, Spielmann, Le Chevalier, Brain, Toussaint, & Janin et al., 1995).

Biologic response modifications have also been applied to soft tissue sarcomas. Agents such as monoclonal antibodies, cytokines, interferons, tumor necrosis factor, M-CSF, and adoptive cellular therapies have shown no benefit for patients with metastatic soft tissue sarcoma (Chang & Sondak, 1995; van Oosterom, & Verweij, 1995).

It is clear that multimodality therapy for soft tissue sarcoma results in improved patient survival and, often, improved quality of life. Since there is no standard treatment plan for all patients, it essential to balance overall survival with the patient's idea of what constitutes a good outcome.

ONCOLOGIC EMERGENCIES

Many of the presenting symptoms of soft tissue sarcomas are subtle. Therefore many times patients may be unaware of the presence of a tumor. However, depending on the location, these tumors can contribute to true oncologic emergencies.

Soft tissue sarcomas are the most common primary malignant tumors of the heart and pericardium. Tumors such as mesothelioma or angiosarcoma spread through the pericardium and encase the heart. Symptoms are dramatic because they reflect constriction of the heart muscle. Patients experience chest pain, hypotension, tachycardia, and malaise. Pericardial effusion, which is often hemorrhagic, can develop into cardiac tamponade and lead to cardiac failure. Tumor infiltration to the heart muscle results in symptoms such as angina, arrhythmia, heart block, heart failure, and myocardial infarction. Sudden death caused by tumor invasion is a possibility (Raaf, 1994).

Other serious symptoms, such as superior vena cava syndrome, hemoptysis, or dysphonia, can been seen with tumor invasion of structures near the heart. Intracavitary left-sided tumors of the heart and aortic tumors may lead to cerebral infarction or cerebral metastasis. Right-sided cardiac tumors and tumors in the pulmonary artery may result in symptoms from tumor emboli. Patients with exertional dyspnea, chest or back pain, or hemoptysis and those who do not respond to thrombolytic therapy should be evaluated for soft tissue sarcomas of these structures (Raaf, 1994).

Other oncologic emergencies may been seen with some retroperitoneal soft tissue sarcomas. Compression of the lumbar or sacral plexus can occur in 27% of these patients. Related symptoms, such as dysuria, hematuria, or urinary tract obstruction, have been reported. Hypoglycemia has been noted with large, poorly differentiated sarcomas that produce an insulin-like substance (McGrath, 1994). See Chapter 11 for a complete discussion of these oncologic emergencies.

NURSING MANAGEMENT

Nursing care of the patient with soft tissue sarcoma often revolves around understanding the patient's risk for acute and long-term complications. The type of surgery used to treat the patient often plays a role in the risk for complications. For example, limb-sparing surgery takes much longer than amputation, and the morbidity associated with the procedure is often higher. The nurse should be knowledgeable of the potential complications, have astute assessment skills, and provide education to the patient and family about prevention and treatment of complications. See Table 72-11 for

Text continues on p. 1632

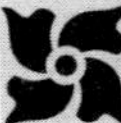

TABLE 72-11 Standard of Care for the Patient Undergoing Surgical Treatment for Soft Tissue Sarcoma

Patient Problem and Outcomes	Nursing Interventions and Rationales	Patient Education Instructions
Knowledge Deficit Patient/family will: • Verbalize an understanding of the surgical procedure • Verbalize an understanding of the preoperative teaching (e.g., turn, cough, deep breathe [TCDB], pain management techniques, incentive spirameter, drain function and routines, wound care) • Identify health care team members and their role in the patient's recovery (e.g., physical therapist, social worker, dietitian, radiation and medical oncologist, oncology nurse) • List signs and symptoms of conditions to be reported to the medical team (e.g., signs and symptoms of infection, increased pain, poor wound healing, inability to participate in prescribed care routines)	1. Assess the patient's level of understanding of the surgical procedure. Determine if the patient understands the difference between limb sparing and amputation. 2. Assess the family's understanding of the surgical procedure, including potential complications and outcomes. 3. Give the patient/family the opportunity to ask questions or verbalize concerns. Have patient repeat/demonstrate postoperative care, such as deep breathing, spirometer, use of trapeze, immobilization of the affected extremity (as appropriate). 4. Identify for the patient possible postoperative complications of wound healing. 5. Demonstrate the use of prosthetic equipment as appropriate. 6. Discuss psychosocial and rehabilitative resources available postoperatively.	1. Use a diagram of the surgical procedure relevant to the anatomic site. 2. If the planned procedure is limb sparing, discuss and review the possibility of amputation. 3. Provide information about the preoperative routines: anesthesiology consult; diagnostic tests; antiembolism stockings; nothing by mouth (NPO) after midnight. 4. Provide the patient with pertinent information related to postoperative care: pain management, surgical incision, fluid and nutrition management, restrictions in self-care and mobility. 5. Provide information about phantom limb sensation in the case of planned amputation. 6. Review the plan for adjuvant therapy as appropriate. 7. Provide appropriate discharge information relevant to reportable signs and symptoms of potential postoperative problems.
Anxiety Patient will: • Express feelings related to the diagnosis of soft tissue sarcoma • Express feelings related to the surgical procedure • Identify strategies to cope with anxiety • Experience a decrease in symptoms of anxiety and an increase of psychological and physiologic comfort	1. Determine which coping strategies the patient has used effectively in the past to decrease anxiety. 2. Identify those individuals whom the patient feels are supportive to him or her. 3. Assess patient's problem-solving ability, level of concentration, rate of speech, flow of thought, and nonverbal behaviors (gestures, facial grimaces, posture, overall appearance). 4. Note patient's interactions with the health team and family. 5. Observe patient for signs of anxiety: restlessness, increased heart rate and respiratory rate, purposeless activity, agitation, diaphoresis, or repetitive questioning. 6. Note patient's complaints of physical symptoms, which may be related to anxiety: diarrhea, nausea, vomiting, body aches and pains, fatigue, shortness of breath, dry mouth. 7. Reinforce the use of effective coping strategies. 8. Administer pharmacologic agents to decrease anxiety if necessary.	1. Explain all procedures, including potential pain and sensations likely to be experienced. 2. Teach relaxation techniques, visualization, and the use of music therapy to decrease anxiety. 3. Suggest diversional activities for patient and family. 4. Review and reinforce all patient education activities.

TABLE 72-11 Standard of Care for the Patient Undergoing Surgical Treatment for Soft Tissue Sarcoma—cont'd

Patient Problem and Outcomes	Nursing Interventions and Rationales	Patient Education Instructions
Pain Patient will: • Rate his or her pain on a standard scale in order to evaluate response to pain management efforts more effectively • Experience effective pain management by verbalizing pain relief • Describe phantom limb sensations and identify ways to manage the symptoms • Verbalize the importance of reporting changes in perception of pain (e.g., sudden increase in pain experienced, change in characteristics of pain) • Identify nonpharmacologic methods of achieving pain relief	1. Assess patient's history related to previous pain experiences (e.g., dentistry, accidents, surgery). 2. Assess patient's psychosocial history as related to drug or alcohol abuse; assess allergies. 3. Identify concerns patient or family may have related to the use of pain medications (particularly narcotics). 4. Explain that most acute surgical pain can be controlled to an acceptable level (defined by the patient) to allow the patient to participate fully in expected postoperative care routines as appropriate.	1. Teach that the experience of pain is very individual and that perceptions of pain are influenced by the patient's anxiety level, past experiences, and expectations. 2. Teach the patient to use a pain rating scale to evaluate pain. 3. Teach the patient to report symptoms of pain early so that medications will be more effective. 4. Teach the patient how to operate the patient-controlled analgesia (PCA) pump for pain management. 5. Teach the patient and family nonpharmacologic methods of pain management: progressive muscle relaxation, guided imagery, music therapy, message, diversional activities. 6. Teach the patient to expect phantom limb pain if an amputation is anticipated.
Self-Care Deficit Patient will: • Resume activities of daily living (ADL) within appropriate time frame without assistance • Resume previous lifestyle after treatment and rehabilitation are completed	1. Determine expected self-care deficit as it relates to the treatment plan. 2. Allow patient input for the schedule of ADL. 3. Assess the patient for factors that may interfere with self-care: attitude, depression, impaired memory, fatigue level and tolerance of activity, pain. 4. Assess competency of caregivers to assist the patient with self-care activities until the patient becomes independent. 5. Assess impact on family system (roles and responsibilities) with additional care for patient in the home setting. 6. Assess home environment with the help of the patient/family and the home care nurse to identify any potential barriers to successful self-care. 7. Consult occupational therapy preoperatively as appropriate.	1. Teach the patient new skills to enable him or her to manage ADL independently. 2. Teach family safe techniques to assist the patient. 3. Review with patient and family community resources as appropriate (e.g., respite care, adult day care). 4. Reinforce self-care routines recommended by physical or occupational therapy.

Continued

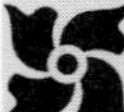

TABLE 72-11 Standard of Care for the Patient Undergoing Surgical Treatment for Soft Tissue Sarcoma—cont'd

Patient Problem and Outcomes	Nursing Interventions and Rationales	Patient Education Instructions
Impaired Physical Mobility Patient will: • Identify anticipated limitations in physical mobility • Demonstrate active participation in the rehabilitation plan • Identify community resources that aid in rehabilitation and recovery • Set realistic goals, with the help of the health care team, to aid in rehabilitation and recovery process	1. Assess the patient's expectations of his or her physical abilities related to potential loss of physical mobility or body part. 2. Assess the patient's view of his or her physical limitations and potential impact on roles and relationships. 3. Consult physical therapy and occupational therapy preoperatively. 4. Arrange for preoperative or postoperative visit from an individual with similar challenges as appropriate. 5. Assess the patient for signs of impaired mobility, such as skin breakdown, atelectasis, constipation, anorexia, or embolism. 6. Supervise ambulation if lower limb is involved in limb-sparing or amputative procedure. 7. Begin discharge planning early with a complete assessment of the home environment as it pertains to the patient's limitations (e.g., need for wheelchair ramp, presence of steps).	1. Teach range of motion activities. 2. Explain the importance of early ambulation and good nutrition during recovery. 3. Teach patient and family proper care of the stump in the case of amputation. 4. Teach proper assessment of the stump and the use of the prosthetic device. 5. Teach patient proper care of the stump, including daily cleaning and dressing change or wrapping technique. 6. Teach patient and family to assess the prosthetic device for wear regularly.
Body Image Disturbance Patient will: • Discuss changes in feelings about self as related to diagnosis and surgical treatment • Develop confidence in ability to accomplish goals • Identify four positive characteristics related to self	1. Assess the patient's view of self. 2. Clarify misconceptions about perception of self. 3. Avoid negative reactions to the surgical site (verbal or nonverbal). 4. Encourage open communication between patient, family, and health care team. 5. Promote social interaction and self-care activities. 6. Make appropriate referrals for counseling and support; encourage the use of support groups composed of patients undergoing similar treatment; arrange for preoperative or postoperative visits from other patients experiencing similar concerns as appropriate.	1. Teach patient to set realistic goals to accomplish within a particular time frame related to self-care and activities. 2. Have patient identify peers and family members with whom he or she can share feelings about condition. 3. Help patient develop a strategy to return to normal routines and activities.
Infection Patient will: • Report signs and symptoms of infection, such as tenderness or increased pain at surgical site, discoloration, or drainage • Along with caregiver, demonstrate proper care of the surgical site and administration of any antiinfective therapies	1. Assess patient's vital signs and temperature every 4 hours for signs of fever or infection. Assess fluctuations in temperature. 2. Assess wound for evidence of infection. 3. Assess for evidence of systemic infection; chills, vital sign changes.	1. Review with patient and family reportable signs and symptoms of infection. 2. Demonstrate thorough handwashing and have patient/caregiver return demonstrate. 3. Teach aseptic technique when changing dressing or administering other care.

TABLE 72-11 Standard of Care for the Patient Undergoing Surgical Treatment for Soft Tissue Sarcoma—cont'd

Patient Problem and Outcomes	Nursing Interventions and Rationales	Patient Education Instructions
Infection—cont'd		
	4. Obtain culture and sensitivities of wound drainage before initiation of antibiotics. 5. Monitor culture results and administer antimicrobial therapy as ordered. 6. Maintain adequate nutrition and hydration. 7. Implement measures to control fever; monitor side effects of antimicrobial drugs.	4. Help patient and caregiver to identify a place within the home that is appropriate for storage of medications and supplies. 5. Teach administration of antimicrobial therapy and related side effects before hospital discharge.
Skin Integrity Patient will: • Comply with wound care, which may include immobilization, compression dressings, drain and wound care, and restrictions in self-care routines • Maintain adequate nutritional intake as noted by calorie count, compliance to dietary advances	1. Assess surgical wound for edema, hematoma, seroma, and infection every 4 hours. 2. Maintain adherent dressing as ordered. 3. Assess for signs and symptoms of decreased perfusion of wound; necrosis of wound edges or flap; and flap/wound edge viability. 4. Avoid excessive pressure on surgical incision, which may interfere with tissue perfusion (compression dressing may be appropriate). 5. Assess integrity of suture line every 4 hours for evidence of wound dehiscence. 6. Assess nutritional status preoperatively, and monitor for nutritional deficits throughout treatment course. 7. Maintain proper body alignment for affected body part.	1. Teach proper wound/stump care. 2. Review information regarding adequate nutrition necessary for wound healing.
Grief Patient will: • Identify areas of perceived loss related to a diagnosis of sarcoma • Identify actual loss related to physical mobility or body image as a result of therapy	1. Assess patient's and family's previous experience with loss (e.g., death, illness, job). 2. Assess the impact of the previous loss to individuals and the family system as a whole. 3. Assess current coping strategies and their effectiveness. 4. Assess significance of loss to patient and family (loss of function, mobility, or a limb). 5. Allow patient/family to verbalize feelings. 6. Acknowledge grief and provide support to patient/family. 7. Refer patient to appropriate professional for counseling. 8. Encourage patient to contact community support groups (amputee, cancer patient).	1. Discuss the normal responses that occur experienced with loss. 2. Discuss that grief is a personal experience and that expression of grief varies with individuals. 3. Help the patient and family identify appropriate ways to express caring and concern for each other.

Continued

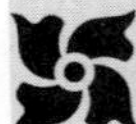

TABLE 72-11 Standard of Care for the Patient Undergoing Surgical Treatment for Soft Tissue Sarcoma—cont'd

Patient Problem and Outcomes	Nursing Interventions and Rationales	Patient Education Instructions
Fear Patient will: • Discuss concerns about outcome of therapy and disease recurrence • Identify concrete plan for follow-up care during the next 24 months • Identify community organizations for cancer survivors	1. Allow patient to verbalize concerns and fears related to his or her future and potential for disease recurrence. 2. Assist patient in obtaining appropriate information related to the disease, treatment plan, and prognosis.	1. Provide patient with follow-up schedule of care over the next 24 months. 2. Teach patient to examine surgical area for signs of local tumor recurrence: new pain, ulceration, lumps, nodules. 3. Discuss issues related to long-term effects of treatment (e.g., effect on growth and development, potential for secondary malignancies with radiation and chemotherapy). 4. Provide information on community/national organizations relevant to cancer survivors (e.g., American Cancer Society's CanSurmount, National Coalition of Cancer Survivorship).
Ineffective Individual Coping Patient will demonstrate successful positive coping and adaptation to diagnosis and treatment by: (1) verbalizing negative feelings appropriately and demonstrating less frequent occurrences; (2) utilizing appropriate resources; participating appropriately in self-care routines and treatment plan	1. Explain each new diagnostic test and review expected routines (preoperatively and postoperatively) with patient. 2. Assess patient's acknowledgment of the disease process and treatment plan. 3. Allow time for patient to express feelings with family and significant others. 4. Help patient set realistic goals throughout the recovery process. 5. Assess impact that diagnosis and subsequent therapy may have on sexuality. 6. Discuss how others may cope with the patient's diagnosis and treatment. 7. Encourage and assist patient in efforts to seek more information related to his or her disease, treatment, and resources.	1. Teach patient strategies to enhance positive coping (e.g., clarification of life values, focus on realistic goals, positive affirmation techniques, relaxation techniques). 2. Teach patient methods of problem solving effectively (e.g., identify positive and negative aspects of a situation and fantasize potential outcomes). 3. Provide information on the relationship between coping and perceived stress. 4. Teach the benefits of emotional release of tension (e.g., crying, exercise, play, talk, humor).

the nursing care plan, which reviews several key nursing problems.

Nursing Care During the Diagnostic Phase

Nursing care of the patient with soft tissue sarcoma actually begins with the initial diagnosis. The nurse needs to ensure that the patient and family understand the specific reasons for diagnostic evaluation. The nurse should provide the patient and family with information about what is expected of the patient and what the patient can expect during each of the tests for diagnostic evaluation. The nurse can also provide emotional support, education, and comfort to the patient and family when the diagnosis is made. Because the treatment of soft tissue sarcoma involves a wide range of specialists—surgical oncologists, medical oncologists, radiation therapists, and the prosthetist—the patient and family may be confused and intimidated. The nurse can be the health care team member who can effectively answer questions about the different treatment modalities. If there are questions that the nurse cannot answer, he or she can refer the patient to the appropriate source.

Surgical Nursing Care

Nursing care of the patient with soft tissue sarcoma continues when the patient is admitted to the hospital for surgery, whether it be amputation or limb salvage (see Chapter 3). Since most patients currently receive some form of adjuvant therapy, they may need education related to the plan of care. In addition, surgery is often a new and stressful experience for the patient and family. As part of the nursing care of the patient, the nurse should provide the patient and family with information about the surgical procedure. Although the sur-

TABLE 72-11 Standard of Care for the Patient Undergoing Surgical Treatment for Soft Tissue Sarcoma—cont'd

Patient Problem and Outcomes	Nursing Interventions and Rationales	Patient Education Instructions
Ineffective Family Coping Family will: • Identify and use appropriate resources to enhance positive coping • Acknowledge and deal with the situation realistically • Plan and initiate appropriate changes in family roles and responsibilities	1. Assess family composition, including extended family and their roles and responsibilities. 2. Identify family strengths and weaknesses in the areas of communication with each other and patient: decision-making processes, family values, problem-solving skills, cultural or ethnic influences. 3. Assess, with the help of the home care nurse, the physical environment of the home; assess facilities, general living conditions. 4. Identify additional current stressors for the family (e.g., other illness, loss of occupation, family member conflicts). 5. Encourage family to interact and communicate openly with patient. 6. Encourage family to share feelings and information with all members of the family. 7. Refer family for financial assistance if appropriate as determined by insurance coverage, out-of-pocket expenses, other family expenses, and expressed needs.	1. Teach family strategies to enhance positive coping (e.g., clarification of life values; focus on realistic goals; positive affirmation techniques; relaxation techniques). 2. Teach family methods of problem solving effectively (e.g., identify positive and negative aspects of a situation and fantasize potential outcomes). 3. Provide information on the relationship between coping and perceived stress. 4. Teach the benefits of emotional release of tension (e.g., crying, exercise, play, talk, humor).

gical oncologist discusses the risks of the surgical procedure with the patient when the treatment alternatives are examined, many patients are severely stressed at the time of diagnosis, and much of what is explained to them is often forgotten or not understood. Thus the nurse has a major role in helping the patient and family anticipate the postoperative care and how the patient will look and feel after surgery (Dealy, Pazola, & Heislein, 1995).

It may help the patient to contact another person (preferably of similar age) who has undergone the surgical procedure and treatment. Support groups are also an option for both the patient and family. Since soft tissue sarcomas may occur in adolescents or young adults, the probability of young siblings misunderstanding the attention that the patient receives is high. Social workers or psychologists associated with the hospital may be able to assist the entire family in adapting to the stressful situation. If such resources are not available, the nurse may be able to provide referrals to outside organizations.

Acute Postoperative Complications. Limb-sparing procedures are often more complicated and lengthy than amputations (Piasecki, 1992), and the complications are often more severe than those arising from amputation. Regardless of the type of procedure, some of the acute postoperative nursing care is standard to surgical nursing.

Infection. All immunosuppressed patients are at risk for infection, either superficial skin infections or deep wound infections. The use of laminar air-flow in operating rooms and prophylactic intravenous antibiotics reduces the risk of infection, but it cannot totally eliminate this risk (Dealy, Pazola, & Heislein, 1995; Piasecki, 1991; Piasecki, 1992). Consequently, the nurse must assess the patient's wound frequently for erythema, purulent drainage, and increased edema. Monitoring the patient's vital signs (particularly body temperature) and the complete blood count (CBC) and white blood cell count will assist the nurse in monitoring for infection (Piasecki, 1993). An elevated white blood cell count is often a sign of infection. Even though many patients may have a low-grade fever after the surgical procedure, a high temperature or a steadily climbing temperature may also be a sign of infection. Although all patients will have pain postoperatively, persistent postoperative pain may be a sign of superficial wound infection (Dealy, Pazola, & Heislein, 1995).

Depending on the type of surgical procedure and the length of time the patient is bedfast, infections of the urinary tract (from an indwelling catheter) and respiratory tract (from inadequate lung expansion) may also occur. The nurse should provide good catheter care, assess the urine for cloudiness, and check urine output at each shift. Again, unexplained changes or trends should be noted and reported.

Upper respiratory tract infections may be prevalent for patients who had allograft reconstruction because these patients are often in surgery for at least 6 hours and are kept in bed for approximately 1 week. Before the surgical procedure, the nurse should teach the patient how to use the incentive spirometer and ensure that the patient understands the risks associated with pneumonia. Although using the incentive spirometer can be monotonous, the nurse can provide incentives and rewards for younger patients to encourage its use. Ensuring that the spirometer is within reach of the patient is a simple but important task.

Older patients or those who have an extensive history of tobacco use also need close monitoring for respiratory infections. For patients who are suspected of being at high risk for respiratory infection, respiratory therapists may be consulted before surgery to inform the patients of the potential risks and to follow up postoperatively as appropriate.

Pain. All patients experience pain postoperatively. Pain is typically managed with epidural analgesics or by a patient-controlled analgesic (PCA) pump (Dealy, Pazola, & Heislein, 1995; Piasecki, 1992).

It is important that pain medication be administered around the clock to keep the patient sufficiently comfortable. PCA pumps are useful not only in providing relief from pain, but also in giving the patient a sense of control. The pump can be programmed to deliver the analgesic continually, with added doses delivered when needed, or to deliver the pain medication only when needed. It is easy for the nurse to monitor the patient's need for pain medication by noting how frequently the patient uses the PCA. It is also easy to titrate the dose of the intravenous narcotics and switch to oral medication when needed.

Patients may need reassurance that they will not become addicted to the pain medication. It is important that they understand that they need to be comfortable so that they can rest adequately. Family members also must understand that the patient will be in pain postoperatively and will require pain medication.

As a result of the use of narcotic pain medication combined with immobility after surgery, the patient may experience constipation. To prevent this occurrence, the patient may be administered stool softeners on a regular schedule. The nurse should monitor the patient's bowel habits to prevent an unnecessary complication.

Patients may experience muscle spasms postoperatively. The narcotics used to control pain are not effective in controlling the spasms. Diazepam (or a related drug) along with repositioning of the body may be required to decrease the spasms.

Phantom limb pain will not be alleviated by narcotics (Piasecki, 1993; Slye, 1991). This phenomenon is not entirely understood. Melzack (1971) studied the characteristics of phantom limb pain and identified four major characteristics: (1) the pain is chronic, usually lasting longer than 1 year; (2) patients with a prior history of limb pain before amputation are more likely to experience phantom limb pain; (3) somatic input can either increase or decrease the sensation; and (4) the patient may have trigger zones on healthy areas of the body that, when touched, can cause phantom limb pain.

Treatment of phantom limb pain consists of mixed modalities. Psychotherapy is one method that may be helpful. Mental imagery also may be useful: for example, having the patient visualize the affected extremity being touched (moved or stroked) may help. In addition, behavioral therapy and biofeedback may be used to assist in relieving the pain.

Regardless of the treatment used to relieve the pain, it is important that the patient be aware of phantom limb pain and the possibility of preoperative phantom limb sensation. The patient will need reassurance that such a sensation is not "all in his head" but a documented phenomenon associated with amputation.

Blood Loss. It is not unusual for the patient to experience a large amount of blood loss during the surgical procedure (Dealy, Pazola, & Heislein, 1995). The nurse should monitor the patient's CBC and note the hemoglobin and hematocrit values. It is common for patients to experience a decrease in these laboratory values the first few days postoperatively (Dealy, Pazola, & Heislein, 1995; Piasecki, 1992). The nurse should be prepared to administer packed red blood cell (PRBC) transfusions to the patient if necessary. Patients who receive neoadjuvant therapy may be at additional risk for anemia because of the myelosuppressive side effects of therapy. Again, education for both the patient and the family is important; many people are still afraid to receive transfusions for fear of receiving blood contaminated with human immunodeficiency virus (HIV). The nurse can provide information about the actual risks of transmitting infection and the complications that the patient may encounter if blood is not received when necessary. Some patients may benefit from the use of recombinant growth factor epoetin alpha.

Often the patient leaves the operating room with one or two surgical drains. On the first postoperative day these drains are bloody, but as time progresses the amount of drainage is less and the fluid becomes more serosanguinous. It is important that the patient and family be told about the drains before the surgery is performed so that they will not be surprised. Once drainage is limited to 10 ml (or less) in a 24-hour period, the drains are removed. Nursing assessment of the amount and type of drainage noted at each shift is important.

Nerve Injury. Nerve damage is a relatively common complication of limb-sparing surgery (Dealy, Pazola, & Heislein, 1995; Piasecki, 1991; Rodriguez, 1996). As part of acute postoperative nursing care, the nurse's frequent (often hourly) assessment of the patient's affected limb for sensation and mobility (e.g., of toes) is necessary (Dealy, Pazola, & Heislein, 1995). Establishing a baseline sensory assessment before surgery, since the patient may have some deficits unrelated to the surgical procedure (e.g., peripheral neuropathies from diabetes or chemotherapy), can help to distinguish surgery-related problems. As discussed later, the peripheral nerves are the first to be affected in compartmental syndrome (Slye, 1991). In a retrospective study of 100 patients who received limb-salvage procedures for sarcoma, only two patients experienced nerve palsies (Quill, Gitelis, Morton, & Piasecki, 1990). One patient fully recovered from the nerve damage, and the other had a partial recovery.

Deep Vein Thrombosis. All patients who undergo lengthy surgical procedures are at risk for the development of deep vein thrombosis (DVT). However, those patients who have cancer are at increased risk because of the hypercoagulability resulting from the disease (Piasecki, 1991; Slye, 1991). In addition, DVT is often a result of venous stasis or vein wall injury. It commonly is located in the vein distal to the surgical site and tends to occur within 48 to 72 hours of surgery (Slye, 1991). To assess for DVT, the nurse monitors the condition of the patient's legs (particularly the calf) for edema and erythema and instructs the patient to report any calf pain. The patient may have a positive Homans's sign with the DVT (Slye, 1991). Prophylactic anticoagulant therapy and the use of intermittent compression boots or antiembolism stockings (TED) may be used to prevent DVT. Patients who are administered anticoagulant therapy (usually heparin or warfarin [Coumadin]) need to have partial prothombin times (PT/PTT) monitored to ensure that the dosages are correct. The nurse should also assess for symptoms of bleeding while the patient is undergoing anticoagulation therapy. If the patient is discharged while this therapy is required, the nurse may assist the patient and family by teaching them how to administer heparin subcutaneously as necessary.

The danger of DVT is that the patient may develop pulmonary embolism as a result of a clot traveling to the lungs. If the patient complains of dyspnea, chest pain, unexplainable feelings of apprehension, coughing, tachypnea, and tachycardia, pulmonary embolism should be suspected (Slye, 1991). A chest radiograph, electrocardiogram (ECG), arterial blood gas measurement, and lung scan should be done for accurate diagnosis of embolism.

Prevention of pulmonary embolism is similar to prevention of DVT. The patient should wear elastic stockings or intermittent pneumatic compression boots if he or she must remain on bed rest for an extended period. Otherwise, early ambulation or leg exercises and prophylactic anticoagulants are prescribed. If the patient is diagnosed with pulmonary embolism, treatment consists of anticoagulant therapy or surgical intervention.

Soft Tissue Injury. Skin and soft tissue injuries are complications of both limb-sparing procedures and amputation (Piasecki, 1992; Rodriguez, 1996). Assessment of the patient's skin and circulation assists the surgeon in deciding on the optimal surgical procedure. If a patient with an amputation has an inadequate amount of soft tissue covering the bone, surgical revision may be necessary, requiring amputation at a higher level (Rodriguez, 1996). Also, neoadjuvant therapy may delay healing at the incision site. Other possible reasons for compromised soft tissue healing include the surgical elevation of extensive soft tissue flaps, a prolonged surgical time, and the insertion of a large prosthesis or allograft (Yarbo & Johnson, 1995).

In a retrospective study Quill and colleagues (1990) noted that wound necrosis was the most common complication observed, particularly in patients having radiation therapy before surgery. Wound necrosis after a limb-sparing procedure can lead to amputation of the extremity.

Nursing observation is of vital importance to assess the wound site, monitor healing, and report any questionable changes. Instructing the patient in self-reporting is helpful.

The most severe complication associated with compromised soft tissue is compartment syndrome, a condition in which increasing pressure within a confined space compromises both the circulation and the function of the tissues within the space (Slye, 1991). The "compartment" in this syndrome is composed of bone, blood vessels, nerves, muscle, and soft tissue. The dressing, splint, or cast serves as a space-limiting envelope, causing increased tissue pressure. The postsurgical edema commonly causes ischemia, which then affects tissue function. Peripheral nerves and skeletal muscle are particularly susceptible to this situation, whereas skin and subcutaneous tissue are able to survive hypoxia better (Slye, 1991).

Nursing assessment for compartment syndrome includes assessing the sensory status of peripheral nerves and the patient's hydration status. Compartmental pressures normally increase approximately 20% in the first 24 hours after surgery. However, if the patient is given diuretics before or during surgery, the pressure may increase to 25% (Slye, 1991).

Arteriograms, venograms, or Doppler findings may be used to diagnose compartment syndrome. Devices are also available to measure tissue pressure in patients at risk for this problem. If the patient is diagnosed with compartment syndrome, surgical intervention may be necessary. The goal is to decrease the pressure of the tissues, restore blood flow to prevent ischemia, and make the functional loss as minimal as possible.

Fat Embolism. The final complication that may occur during the acute phase postoperatively is fat embolism. It is most frequently seen in patients who have pathologic fractures of the pelvis, femur, tibia, or ribs (Slye, 1991).

Fat embolism occurs when globules of fat are released from the bone marrow into the circulation, and, following the route of venous flow, they travel to the lung, where they can cause pulmonary insufficiency and/or adult respiratory distress syndrome.

Signs and symptoms associated with fat embolism include restlessness, dyspnea, tachypnea, tachycardia, fever, and, sometimes, a petechial skin rash. If fat embolism is suspected, arterial blood gases should be measured, and a complete blood count (CBC) (which may show thrombocytopenia and anemia), chest radiograph, and electrocardiogram (ECG) should be done. Fat embolism often occurs within 24 to 48 hours postoperatively.

Treatment includes supplemental oxygen, fluid replacement, possible use of corticosteroids, and, at times, mechanical ventilation. Prevention of fat embolism is similar to its treatment—(1) ensuring that the patient is adequately hydrated and oxygenated and (2) administering corticosteroids.

Late Complications of Surgery

Deep Infection. Deep infections of the surgical wound can occur as late as 6 months to 2 years after surgery (Dealy, Pazola, & Heislein, 1995). To prevent this complication, patients are often discharged from the hospital while continuing antibiotic therapy. Patients who receive some type of hardware to support their bone as part of the surgical procedure are at greater risk for late infections than are other patients They should be instructed to inform their dentists and other physicians about their need for prophylactic antibiotics for invasive procedures. If the patient is receiving adjuvant chemotherapy after surgery, additional risk of infection is a problem because of delayed healing and myelosuppression. Treatment for deep infection includes systemic antibiotic therapy, wound debridement, and revision of the surgical procedure with possible amputation (Yarbro & Johnson, 1995). The patient should be instructed to inform the physician of pain, erythema, drainage, and edema.

Nonunion. Nonunion is the inability of the bone to bond with the allograft or the hardware implanted to support the bone. For patients who have allografts, it may take up to 2 years for the body to incorporate the allograft and replace it with host bone (Dealy, Pazola, & Heislein, 1995). A related problem, seen in prosthetic arthroplasty, is the loosening of the prosthesis where the bone and cement interface. This usually occurs from the stress caused by repetitive movements during activities of daily living. Nonunion usually occurs 1 year after surgery (Piasecki, 1991). The main symptom is pain at the junction site.

Degenerative Arthritis. Degenerative arthritis is a late complication that is diagnosed through yearly radiographs of the affected extremity. The patient may complain of pain or stiffness at the location. This condition can be treated with corticosteroids or by surgical revision of the affected limb (Piasecki, 1991).

Psychological Issues and Nursing Care

The diagnosis of cancer certainly causes stress to patients, but the additional fear of losing a limb or another functional body part can increase the stress dramatically. All patients should have an assessment of their strengths, weaknesses, and coping skills performed preoperatively to enable the health care team to mobilize adequate support for the patient and family throughout the treatment process. Areas of potential weakness should be identified, and the patient and family should be assisted to cope with the problem adequately. Before a surgical decision is made, an assessment of the patient's lifestyle should be performed, and the patient should be able to state his or her goals for the surgical procedure. The nurse should work with the patient to enable him or her to meet those goals or set realistic ones.

Patients who undergo limb-sparing procedures recuperate more slowly than those who have amputation. Although the fact that the patient can keep the limb is positive, the lengthy recuperation and rehabilitation period cannot be overemphasized. Patients must also be informed of changes that may occur in their lifestyles. For example, after limb-sparing surgery, they may not be able to participate in aerobic exercise or sports activities. Alternative activities (e.g., swimming) should be suggested to the patient.

Body image also needs to be considered. If at all possible, before surgery patients should be able to see postoperative photographs to prepare them for how the extremity will look after the procedure. Patients who are scheduled for amputation should meet with the prosthetist before treatment to discuss and view the devices. All members of the health care team, both inpatient and outpatient, should be informed of the patient's treatment goals so that a unified plan of care for the patient and family is developed to meet those goals.

Many patients receive radiation therapy and/or chemotherapy after surgery for soft tissue sarcoma. The nurse should teach the patient to help monitor the wound for signs of delayed healing or infection. Therapy-related toxicity should also be carefully monitored. The side effects of chemotherapy, which may include impaired sexual maturity or fertility, should be discussed with the patient and family before treatment. The risk of treatment-induced secondary malignancies should also be explained, particularly since adjuvant chemotherapy for soft tissue sarcoma is considered investigational.

HOME CARE ISSUES

Over the years home care nursing has evolved from traditional home health care to the highly technical care of oncology patients. As hospitalizations become shorter and the emphasis of care continues to be on the need for extensive rehabilitation and the management of adjuvant therapy, this focus applies to patients with sarcoma. The goal of the home care nurse is to design a plan of care that optimizes the patient's functional status while integrating the strengths and involvement of appropriate external resources (McEnroe, 1996).

As discussed in the section on medical management, home care management of the patient with sarcoma also involves the collaborative efforts of a multidisciplinary team. Often these team members are individuals known to the patient from the hospital stay: physical therapist, nutritionist, social worker, occupational therapist, counselor, and oncology nurse. In addition, at this point the team includes the home care nurse, home health aides, and homemaker services. Volunteers from the community or family friends may also have an active role in home care, participating in activities such as transportation, child care, delivery of meals, and other aspects of home care (Blesch, 1996).

For the patient with sarcoma, the home care nurse is the pivotal person in the team approach. The home care nurse maintains the focus on acute care needs while the patient completes adjuvant therapy, and he or she is instrumental in the coordination and planning of the rehabilitative plan of care. The home care nurse's understanding of the impact of a diagnosis such as soft tissue sarcoma, the extent of surgical resection necessary, the use of adjuvant radiation therapy or chemotherapy, the patient's reconstructive and rehabilitative needs, and the overall prognosis is essential for planning and delivery of care.

One of the key activities for the home care nurse is the initial assessment of the patient, family, and home environment (Table 72-12). Although the inpatient team has usually completed a psychosocial evaluation of the patient and family, the members require the in-depth assessment afforded by the home care nurse, who is able to meet the patient and family in the home setting. It may be valuable for the home care nurse to meet the family in the home before the patient's hospital discharge so that the physical environment can be evaluated for ease of access, safety, and infection prevention. Room for maneuvering a wheelchair, presence or absence of ramps, factors involved in negotiating stairs, and access to a bathroom are some of the issues to consider. Patient education regarding the importance of a clean environment and good hygiene practice may be a part of infection control, particularly when wound care is being provided and during adjuvant therapy. When this type of early assessment approach is used, any necessary adjustments to the environment may be made in a timely manner.

Assessment of the family system includes identifying the decision makers in the family; determining the roles and responsibilities of each member and the impact that role changes may have on the family; identifying patterns of communication and interactions that indicate effective or ineffective coping among family members; and determining the competency of the designated caregivers. It is common for patients to have rotating caregivers because of child care and job-related issues. The home care nurse must plan adequate access to all the caregivers to be able to educate each individual (Jassak, 1992).

Assessment of caregiver competency and availability may also uncover additional family stressors that will interfere with care of the patient. Financial stress, out-of-pocket expenses (e.g., parking, hotel accommodations, child care), or other family care burdens (e.g., elderly parent care) may alter the discharge plans for the patient.

Health care given at home is intermittent and episodic. Initially, the patient or caregiver may be taught how to care for the wound (e.g., dressing care, stump wrap). The ability of the patient and caregiver to learn proper techniques of care is essential. In addition, much of the teaching revolves around reporting signs and symptoms of wound complications. Helping the patient and family to set realistic goals of care is also necessary to provide a smooth transition of care in the home. Promotion of self-care, good nutrition, and symptom management is necessary to prevent rehospitalization or failure on the part of the patient or family.

Administration of intravenous therapies may also be part of the home care nurse's responsibilities. Completion of an-

TABLE 72-12 Home Care Assessment of the Patient with Sarcoma

History	Compliance with medical therapy Experience with illness
Functional assessment	Ability to perform self-care activities Need for assistance from others Use of assistive devices (e.g., brace, prosthesis, cane)
Psychosocial assessment	Coping mechanisms of patient/family Ability to understand and manage patient's physical and psychological needs
Composition of the family	Status of designated caregiver Role/responsibilities of family members Age of family members Educational level of patient and caregiver and educational needs related to care of the patient at home Health and competency of caregiver Stressors and their impact on the family
Environmental assessment	Basic needs (e.g., electricity, heat, phone), access to emergency care services (911) Physical layout (e.g., stairs, room to navigate with assistive device, ramp for wheelchair) Home safety (e.g., smoke detector, assistive rails in bathroom) Infection control (e.g., clean area for storage of supplies and medications, cleaning needs, pets, pests)
Ancillary needs	Transportation to medical center/physician's office Child care Grocery delivery/food preparation

tibiotic therapy may be necessary in addition to the administration of support therapies related to adjuvant therapy.

Whether the patient succeeds in the home environment ultimately depends on patient motivation and caregiver support. Assessment, problem identification, and interventions by the home care nurse are an essential part of this process, resulting in positive clinical outcomes. Adequate early support of the patient and caregiver by the home care nurse provides positive experiences with self-care and helps to build the confidence necessary for independent functioning.

PROGNOSIS

Most experts in the care of patients with soft tissue sarcomas agree that the most important factor in predicting overall survival and the development of distant metastasis is the histologic grading of the tumor. Attempts have also been made to correlate clinical factors with outcome (Brennan, Casper, & Harrison, 1997; Coindre, Terrier, Bui, Bonichon, Collin, & Le Doussal et al., 1996; Dirix & Van Oosterom, 1995).

The French Federation of Cancer Centers reviewed 546 adult patients with locally controlled soft tissue sarcoma to determine which patients were likely to relapse and therefore would be the best candidates for adjuvant therapy. They determined that the patients with grade 3 tumors were the only ones who benefited from adjuvant chemotherapy. Other factors, such as male gender, tumor size of ≥5 cm, grade 3 tumors, and deep location of the lesion, seemed to have a negative impact on overall survival. Patients with poor surgical margins, whose tumors were in a deep location, and who were not given radiation therapy had the highest incidence of local recurrence. Patients with grade 3 tumors that measured ≥10 cm and were located in deep tissue had the highest likelihood of distant metastasis (Coindre et al., 1996).

The AJCCS reported survival results for a series of 1215 patients with soft tissue sarcoma. The overall 5-year survival was 41%. When survival was correlated with tumor stage, the results were as follows: stage 1 patients had a 75% survival; stage 2, a 55% survival; and stage 3, a 29% survival (Zalupski & Baker, 1995).

In a series of 423 patients reviewed by Memorial Sloane-Kettering Cancer Center, the major factors that contributed to prognosis were grade, size, and depth of the tumor. It was noted that grade in particular was predictive of the development of metastatic disease during the first 18 months after initial treatment. Beyond that time frame, tumor size of >5 cm became a more significant factor in predicting relapse. Patients with superficial sarcomas had the most favorable prognosis. Table 72-13 summarizes survival rates based on the number of unfavorable factors (grade, size, and depth) evaluated.

Demetri and Elian (1995) stressed the importance of a multidisciplinary approach to the care of patients with soft tissue sarcoma. They asserted that treatment planning by a surgical oncologist, radiation therapist, and medical oncologist contributed to complete durable responses and therefore improved survival.

EVALUATION OF THE QUALITY OF CARE

Much of the nursing care related to the patient with soft tissue sarcoma involves rehabilitation, psychosocial support, and continuity of care between health care professionals (Table 72-14). In a study by Arzouman and colleagues evaluating the quality of life for patients with soft tissue sar-

TABLE 72-14 Quality of Care and Continuity of Care Between Hospital and Home

Discipline participating in the quality of care evaluation:

☐ Surgeon	☐ Medical oncologist
☐ Radiation therapist	☐ Physical therapist
☐ Occupational therapist	☐ Prosthetist
☐ Oncology nurse	☐ Social worker
☐ Nutritionist	☐ Other

Data from

☐ Mailed questionnaire ☐ Patient interview

Collected by: ____________ Position: ____________

Criteria	Yes	No
1. Were discharge instructions given?	☐	☐
2. Was a follow-up appointment date set?	☐	☐
3. Did you attend a care conference?	☐	☐
4. Were orders sent to your home care agency?	☐	☐

TABLE 72-13 Survival Rates of the Patient with Soft Tissue Sarcomas Based on Number of Unfavorable Factors

Disease-free survival after 12 years with soft tissue sarcomas based on the number of unfavorable factors related to grade, size of tumor, and depth of the lesion.

Number of factors	0	1	2	3
Survival rate	85% (±11)	73% (±7)	58% (±7)	29% (±5)

Modified from Coindre, J. M., Terrier, P., Bui, N. B., Bonichon, F., Collin, F., Le Doussal, V., Mandard, A., Vilain, M., Jacquemier, J., Duplay, H., Sastre, X., Barlier, C., Henry-Amar, M., Mace-Lesech, J., & Contesso, G. (1996). *Journal of Clinical Oncology 14*(3), 869-877.

comas who were receiving adjuvant chemotherapy, the need for involvement of support systems in the plan of care was found to be essential. It was emphasized that the nurse's responsibility was to include significant others in patient teaching and to encourage their involvement in the patient's care. The study also emphasized the importance of continuity of care between different settings (e.g., inpatient, clinic, home) (Arzouman, Dudas, Ferrans, & Holm, 1991).

To ensure quality of care for the complex needs of the patient with sarcoma, a tool such as the one presented in Table 72-15 may help health care professionals to track essential information related to continuity of care and provide a method of documenting the involvement of all appropriate caregivers.

RESEARCH ISSUES

A more thorough understanding and documentation of risk factors will enhance our ability to reduce the risk of soft tissue sarcomas. Gene therapy for patients with gene deletions or translocations may prevent the development of some sarcomas resulting from hereditary predisposition. Others,

TABLE 72-15 Management of the Sarcoma Patient at Home: Reference Tool for the Patient/Caregiver

Appointment Calendar

Sunday	Monday	Tuesday	Wednesday	Thursday	Friday	Saturday

Name	Phone	Address
Surgeon:		
Medical oncologist:		
Radiation therapist:		
Physical therapist:		
Occupational therapist:		
Prosthetist:		
Oncology nurse:		
Home care nurse:		
Social worker:		
Nutritionist:		
Other		

Medications

Drug	Dose	Frequency	Special Comments

____
RN signature/date

Diet Instructions

____
RD signature/date

Special Instructions

Wound care:
RN/Date ____________
Bleeding precautions:
RN/Date ____________
Infection prevention:
RN/Date ____________
Safety instructions:
RN/Date ____________

such as Kaposi's sarcoma, will require continued investigation into the role of viruses in carcinogenesis.

Future chemotherapy trials will continue to optimize the dose-response relationships of both doxorubicin and ifosfamide. Clinical trials with Doxil and paclitaxel are underway. Toxoids seem to have some activity in soft tissue sarcoma (Dirix & Van Oosterom, 1995). All trials will evaluate different protocols related to drug scheduling, dose escalation, and chemotherapy combined with other treatment modalities, such as hyperthermia and limb perfusion.

The use of cardioprotectants may also allow dose escalation of chemotherapeutic drugs (e.g., doxorubicin). Further investigation of chemoresistant disease will also benefit patients with soft tissue sarcoma who relapse. There is some evidence that tumors associated with a poor prognosis express a multidrug-resistant phenotype. Chemosensitizers such as cyclosporine A are being tested with chemotherapy agents such as paclitaxel (Balcerzak, Benedetti, Weiss, & Natale, 1995).

The ability to achieve a consensus in the classification, staging, and grading of soft tissue sarcomas will allow for the collection of more consistent data related to therapy response, prognosis, and quality of life.

REFERENCES

American Cancer Society (1998). *Facts and figures.* Atlanta: American Cancer Society.

American Joint Committee on Cancer Staging. (1993). Handbook for staging of cancer. In *Manual for staging of cancer.* (4th ed.). Philadelphia: J. B. Lippincott.

Antman, K. H., Elias, A., & Fine, H. A. (1994). Dose-intensive therapy with autologous bone marrow transplantation in solid tumors. In S. J. Forman, K. G. Blume, & E. D. Thomas (Eds.), *Bone marrow transplantation.* Boston: Blackwell Scientific Publications.

Arca, M. J., Sondak, V. K., & Chang, A. E. (1994). Diagnostic procedures and pretreatment evaluation of soft tissue sarcomas. *Seminars in Surgical Oncology, 10,* 323-331.

Arzouman, J., Dudas, S., Ferrans, C. E., & Holm, K. (1991). Quality of life of patients with sarcoma postchemotherapy. *Oncology Nursing Forum, 18*(5), 889-894.

Ayala, A. G., Ro, J. Y., Fanning, C. V., Flores, J. P., & Yasko, A. W. (1995). Core needle biopsy and fine-needle aspiration in the diagnosis of bone and soft-tissue lesions. *Hematology/Oncology Clinics of North America, 9*(3), 633-651.

Balcerzak, S. P., Benedetti, J., Weiss, G. R., & Natale, R. B. (1995). A phase II trial of paclitaxel in patients with advanced soft tissue sarcomas. *Cancer, 76*(11), 2248-2252.

Beahrs, O. H., Henson, D. E., Hutter, R. V., & Kennedy, B. J. (1993). Handbook for staging of cancer. In *Manual for staging of cancer* (4th ed.). Philadelphia: J. B. Lippincott.

Beech, D. J. & Pollock, R. E. (1995). Surgical management of primary soft tissue sarcoma. *Hematology/Oncology Clinics of North America, 9*(4), 707-719.

Bell, R. S., O'Sullivan, B., Davis, A., Langer, F., Cummings, B., & Fornasier, V. L. (1991). Functional outcome in patients treated with surgery and irradiation for soft tissue tumors. *Journal of Surgical Oncology, 48,* 224-231.

Blesch, K. S. (1996). Rehabilitation of the cancer patient at home. *Seminars in Oncology Nursing, 12*(3), 219-225.

Bramwell, V., Rouesse, J., Steward, W., Santoro, A., Schraffordt-Koops, H., Buesa, J., Ruka, W., Piario, J., Wagener, T., Burgers, M., van Unnik, J., Contesso, G., Thomas, D., van Glabbeka, M., Markham, D., & Pineda, H. (1994). Adjuvant CYVADIC chemotherapy for adult soft tissue sarcoma: Reduced local recurrence but no improvement in survival: A study of the European Organization for Research and Treatment of Cancer Soft Tissue and Bone Sarcoma Group. *Journal of Clinical Oncology, 12,* 1137-1149.

Brennan, M. F., Casper, E. S., & Harrison, L. B. (1997). Soft tissue sarcoma. In V. T. DeVita, S. Hellman, & S. A. Rosenberg (Eds.), *Cancer: Principles and practice of oncology* (5th ed.). Philadelphia: Lippincott-Raven.

Chang, A. E. & Sondak, V. K. (1995). Clinical evaluation and treatment of soft tissue sarcomas. In F. M. Enzinger & S. W. Weiss (Eds.), *Soft tissue tumors* (3rd ed.). St. Louis: Mosby.

Cheng, E. Y., Dusenbery, K. E., Winters, M. R., & Thompson, R. C. (1996). Soft tissue sarcomas: Preoperative versus postoperative radiotherapy. *Journal of Surgical Oncology, 61,* 90-99.

Chmell, M. J. & Schwarz, H. S. (1996). Analysis of variables affecting wound healing after musculoskeletal sarcoma resections. *Journal of Surgical Oncology, 61,* 185-189.

Coindre, J. M., Terrier, P., Bui, N. B., Bonichon, F., Collin, F., Le Doussal, V., Mandard, A., Vilain, M., Jacquemier, J., Duplay, H., Sastre, X., Barlier, C., Henry-Amar, M., Mace-Lesech, J., & Contesso, G. (1996). Prognostic factors in adult patients with locally controlled soft tissue sarcoma: A study of 546 patients from the French Federation of Cancer Center Sarcoma Group. *Journal of Clinical Oncology 14*(3), 869-877.

Conrad, E. U., Bradford, L., & Chansky, H. A. (1996). Pediatric soft-tissue sarcomas. *Orthopedic Clinics of North America, 27*(3), 655-664.

Consensus Conference. (1985). *Journal of the American Medical Association, 254*(13), 1791-1794.

Cordon-Cardo, C. (1997). Sarcomas of the soft tissue and bone. In V. T. DeVita, S. Hellman, & S. A. Rosenberg (Eds.), *Cancer: Principles and practice of oncology* (5th ed.). Philadelphia: Lippincott-Raven.

Craver, R. D. (1996). Laboratory evaluation of pediatric bone and soft-tissue tumors. *Orthopedic Clinics of North America 27*(3), 461-471.

Dealy, M., Pazola, K., & Heislein, D. (1995). Care of the adolescent undergoing an allograft procedure. *Cancer Nursing, 18,* 130-137.

Demetri, G. D. & Elian, A. D. (1995). Results of single-agent and combination chemotherapy for advanced soft tissue sarcomas. *Hematology/Oncology Clinics of North America, 9*(4), 765-785.

Dirix, L. Y. & Van Oosterom, A. T. (1995). Diagnosis and treatment of soft tissue sarcomas in adults. *Current Opinion in Oncology, 7,* 340-348.

Drake, D. B. (1995). Reconstruction for limb-sparing procedures in soft-tissue sarcomas of the extremities. *Clinics in Plastic Surgery, 22*(1), 123-128.

Enneking, W. F., Spanier, S. S., & Goodman, M. A. (1980). A system for surgical staging of musculoskeletal sarcoma. *Clinical Orthopaedics and Related Research, 153,* 106-120.

Enzinger, F. M. & Weiss, S. W. (1995a). Approach to the diagnosis of soft tissue tumors. In F. M. Enzinger & S. W. Weiss (Eds.), *Soft tissue tumors* (3rd ed.). St. Louis: Mosby.

Enzinger, F. M. & Weiss, S. W. (1995b). Fibrosarcoma. In F. M. Enzinger & S. W. Weiss (Eds.), *Soft tissue tumors* (3rd ed.). St. Louis: Mosby.

Enzinger, F. M. & Weiss, S. W. (1995c). General considerations. In F. M. Enzinger & S. W. Weiss (Eds.), *Soft tissue tumors* (3rd ed.). St. Louis: Mosby.

Enzinger, F. M. & Weiss, S. W. (1995d). Immunohistochemistry of soft tissue lesions. In F. M. Enzinger & S. W. Weiss (Eds.), *Soft tissue tumors* (3rd ed.). St. Louis: Mosby.

Enzinger, F. M. & Weiss, S. W. (1995e). Leiomyosarcoma. In F. M. Enzinger & S. W. Weiss (Eds.), *Soft tissue tumors* (3rd ed.). St. Louis: Mosby.

Enzinger, F. M. & Weiss, S. W. (1995f). Liposarcoma. In F. M. Enzinger & S. W. Weiss (Eds.), *Soft tissue tumors* (3rd ed.). St. Louis: Mosby.

Enzinger, F. M. & Weiss, S. W. (1995g). Malignant fibrohistiocytic tumors. In F. M. Enzinger & S. W. Weiss (Eds.), *Soft tissue tumors* (3rd ed.). St. Louis: Mosby.

Enzinger, F. M. & Weiss, S. W. (1995h). Malignant tumors of the peripheral nerves. In F. M. Enzinger & S. W. Weiss (Eds.), *Soft tissue tumors* (3rd ed.). St. Louis: Mosby.

Enzinger, F. M. & Weiss, S. W. (1995i). Malignant vascular tumors. In F. M. Enzinger & S. W. Weiss (Eds.), *Soft tissue tumors* (3rd ed.). St. Louis: Mosby.

Enzinger, F. M. & Weiss, S. W. (1995j). Mesothelioma. In F. M. Enzinger & S. W. Weiss (Eds.), *Soft tissue tumors* (3rd ed.). St. Louis: Mosby.

Enzinger, F. M. & Weiss, S. W. (1995k). Synovial sarcoma. In F. M. Enzinger & S. W. Weiss (Eds.), *Soft tissue tumors* (3rd ed.). St. Louis: Mosby.

Frable, W. J. (1994). Pathologic classification of soft tissue sarcomas. *Seminars in Surgical Oncology, 10,* 332-339.

Frost, D. B. (1995). Pulmonary metastasectomy for soft tissue sarcomas: Is it justified? *Journal of Surgical Oncology, 59,* 110-115.

Harrison, L. B. & Janjan, N. (1995). Brachytherapy in sarcomas. *Hematology/Oncology Clinics of North America, 9*(4), 747-763.

Jassak, P. F. (1992). Families: An essential element in the care of the patient with cancer. *Oncology Nursing Forum, 19*(6), 871-876.

Kransdorf, M. J. (1995). Malignant soft-tissue tumors in a large referral population: Distribution of diagnoses by age, sex, and location. *American Journal of Radiology, 164,* 129-134.

Kransdorf, M. J., Jelinek, J. S., & Moser, R. P. (1993). Imaging of soft tissue tumors. *Radiologic Clinics of North America, 31*(2), 359-372.

Kruzelock, R. P. & Hansen, M. F. (1995). Molecular genetics and cytogenetics of sarcomas. *Hematology/Oncology Clinics of North America, 9*(3), 513-534.

Lane, J. M. & Healey, J. H. (1993). Orthopedic considerations in limb-sparing surgery. In J. H. Raaf (Ed.), *Soft tissue sarcomas: Diagnosis and treatment.* St. Louis, Mosby.

Lawrence, W. J. (1994). Operative management of soft tissue sarcomas: Impact of anatomic site. *Seminars in Surgical Oncology, 10,* 340-346.

Le Cesne, A., Spielmann, M., Le Chevalier, T., Brain, E., Toussaint, C., Janin, N., Kayitalire, L., Fontaine, F., Genin, J., Vanel, D., Contesso, G., & Tursz, T. (1995). High-dose ifosfamide: Circumvention of resistance to standard-dose ifosfamide in advanced soft tissue sarcomas. *Journal of Clinical Oncology, 13*(7), 1600-1608.

Mack, T. M. (1995). Sarcomas and other malignancies of soft tissue, retroperitoneum, peritoneum, pleura, heart, mediastinum, and spleen. *Cancer, 75*(1), 211-244.

Mark, R. J., Poen, J. C., Tran, L. M., Fu, Y. O., & Juillard, G. F. (1995). Angiosarcoma: A report of 67 patients and a review of the literature. *Cancer, 77*(11), 2400-2406.

Massengill, A. D., Seeger, L., & Eckardt, J. J. (1995). The role of plain radiography, computed tomography, and magnetic resonance imaging in sarcoma evaluation. *Hematology/Oncology Clinics of North America, 9*(3), 571-604.

McEnroe, L. E. (1996). Role of the oncology nurse in home care: Family-centered practice. *Seminars in Oncology Nursing, 12*(3), 188-192.

McGrath, P. C. (1994). Retroperitoneal sarcomas. *Seminars in Surgical Oncology, 10,* 364-368.

McGrath, P. C., Sloan, D. A., & Kennedy, D. E. (1995). Adjuvant therapy of soft-tissue sarcomas. *Clinics in Plastic Surgery, 22*(1), 21-29.

Meltzer, P. S. (1995). Molecular biology of soft tissue tumors. In F. M. Enzinger & S. W. Weiss (Eds.), *Soft tissue tumors* (3rd ed.). St. Louis: Mosby.

Melzack, R. (1971). Phantom limp pain: Implications for treatment of pathological pain. *Anesthesiology, 35,* 409-419.

Mertens, W. C. & Bramwell, V. H. (1995). Adjuvant chemotherapy for soft tissue sarcomas. *Hematology/Oncology Clinics of North America, 9*(4), 801-815.

Miettinen, M. & Weiss, S. W. (1996). Soft-tissue tumors. In I. Damjanov & J. Linder (Eds.), *Anderson's pathology* (10th ed.). St. Louis: Mosby.

Morton, D. L. (1997). Soft-tissue sarcomas. In J. Holland, R. Blast, D. Morton, E. Frei, III, & D. Kufe (Eds.), *Cancer medicine* (4th ed., Vol. 1). Baltimore: Williams & Wilkins.

Nichter, L. S. & Menendez, L. R. (1993). Reconstructive considerations for limb salvage surgery. *Orthopedic Clinics of North America, 24*(3), 511-521.

Parker et al. (1998). Title of article/book. Name of journal/book.

Piasecki, P. A. (1991). The nursing role in limb salvage surgery. *Nursing Clinics of North America, 26*(1), 33-41.

Piasecki, P. A. (1992). Update of orthopaedic oncology. *Orthopaedic Nursing, 11,* 36-43.

Piasecki, P. A. (1993). Bone and soft tissue sarcomas. In S. L. Groenwald, M. H. Frogge, M. Goodman, & C. H. Yarbro (Eds.), *Cancer nursing: Principles and practice* (3rd ed.). Boston: Jones & Bartlett.

Pisters, P., Harrison, L. B., Leung, D., Woodruff, J. M., Casper, E. S., & Brennan, M. F. (1996). *Journal of Clinical Oncology, 14*(3), 859-868.

Podoloff, D. A. (1995). The role of radionuclide scans in sarcoma. *Hematology/Oncology Clinics of North America, 9*(3), 605-626.

Putnam, J. B. & Roth, J. A. (1995). Surgical treatment for pulmonary metastases from sarcoma. *Hematology/Oncology Clinics of North America, 9*(4), 869-886.

Quill, G., Gitelis, S., Morton, T., Piasecki, P. (1990). Complications associated with limb salvage for extremity sarcomas and their management. *Clinical Orthopaedics and Related Research, 260,* 242-250.

Raaf, H. N. (1994). Sarcomas related to the heart and vasculature. *Clinics of North America, 26,* 113-132.

Rodriguez, R. (1996). Amputation surgery and prostheses. *Orthopedic Clinics of North America, 2,* 927-938.

Scully, S. P., Oleson, J. R., Leopold, K. A., Samulski, T. V., Dodge, R., & Harrison, J. M. (1994). Clinical outcome after neoadjuvant thermoradiotherapy in high grade soft tissue sarcomas. *Journal of Surgical Oncology, 57,* 143-151.

Slye, D. (1991). Orthopedic complications: Compartment syndromes, fat embolism syndrome, and venous-thrombo-embolism. *Nursing Clinics of North America, 26,* 113-132.

Suit, H. D. (1994). Role of radiation in the management of adult patients with sarcoma of soft tissue. *Seminars in Surgical Oncology, 10,* 347-356.

Suit, H. & Spiro, I. (1995). Radiation as a therapeutic modality in sarcomas of the soft tissue. *Hematology/Oncology Clinics of North America, 9*(4), 733-745.

Uno, T., Itami, J., & Kato, H. (1995). Combined chemo-radiation and hyperthermia for locally advanced soft tissue sarcoma: Response and toxicity. *Anticancer Research, 15,* 2655-2658.

van Oosterom, A. T., & Verweij, J. (1995). New drugs for the treatment of sarcomas. *Hematology/Oncology Clinics of North America, 9*(4), 909-925.

van Unnik, J. (1995). Classification and grading of soft-tissue sarcomas. *Hematology/Oncology Clinics of North America, 9*(3), 677-699.

Wanebo, H. J., Temple, W. J., Popp, M. B., Constable, W., Aron, B., & Cunningham, S. L. (1995). Preoperative regional therapy for extremity sarcoma. *Cancer, 75*(9), 2299-2306.

Wolf, R. E. & Enneking, W. F. (1996). The staging and surgery of musculoskeletal neoplasms. *Orthopedic Clinics of North America, 27*(3), 473-481.

Yang, J. C., Rosenberg, S. A., Glatstein, E. J., & Antman, K. H. (1993). Sarcomas of soft tissue. In V. T. DeVita, S. Hellman, & S. A. Rosenberg (Eds.), *Cancer: Principles and practice of oncology* (4th ed.). Philadelphia: Lippincott-Raven.

Yarbro, C. & Johnson, M. (1995). Surgical management of primary bone sarcomas. *Hematology/Oncology Clinics of North America, 9,* 719-731.

Zalupski, M. M., & Baker, L. H. (1995). Systemic adjuvant chemotherapy for soft tissue sarcomas. *Hematology/Oncology Clinics of North America, 9*(4), 787-800.

Zarbo, R. (1995). DNA analysis of soft tissue tumors. In F. M. Enzinger & S. W. Weiss (Eds.), *Soft tissue tumors* (3rd ed.). St. Louis: Mosby.

Zornig, C., Peiper, M., & Schroder, S. (1995). Reexcision of soft tissue sarcoma after inadequate initial operation. *British Journal of Surgery, 82,* 278-279.

Malignant Melanoma

Laura Benson, RN, MS, AOCN

EPIDEMIOLOGY

The incidence of melanoma is increasing worldwide faster than any other cancer (Grin, Rigel, & Friedman, 1992). In 1998 an estimated 41,600 new invasive cases of melanoma will be diagnosed, with 24,300 occurring in males and 17,300 in females (Landis, Murray, Bolden, & Wingo, 1998). In addition, 30,000 to 50,000 in situ cases of melanoma will be diagnosed (Salopek, Marghoop, & Slade, 1995). The lifetime risk of an American developing invasive melanoma has now reached 1 in 87 (1 in 70 for Caucasian males) (Rigel, Friedman, & Kopf, 1996). The states with the highest rates of melanoma are California (4300 cases), Florida (2800 cases), and Texas (2500 cases) (Parker et al., 1997). Melanoma rates have been steadily increasing from 1 in 1500 in 1930 to a projected 1 in 75 by the year 2000 (Rigel, 1996). In fact, melanoma rates are rising faster than any other form of cancer in men. In women, melanoma is second only to lung cancer (Glocker-Reis, Miller, & Hankey, 1994). Melanoma of the skin will account for 3% of all new cancer cases in both men and women in the United States in 1997 (Landis et al., 1998).

The estimated death rates from melanoma in 1996 totals 7300; of that number, 4600 are males and 2700 are females. The death rate from melanoma continues to rise about 2% annually. However, survival rates for people with stage I melanoma are increasing. Survival rates for stage I disease have increased from 50% in the 1950s to almost 90% (Rigel, 1996).

The rise in the rates of melanoma is thought to be multifactorial. Reintgen (1995) expresses the belief that a change in attitudes in the 1960s and 1970s, which led Americans to spend more time in the sun and wear less clothing, is one of the reasons for this "undeclared epidemic." Additionally, he believes that the thinning of the ozone layer, along with a concomitant increase in the skin's exposure to ultraviolet radiation are also factors that contribute to the increased incidence of melanoma.

RISK FACTORS

The risk factors for the development of melanoma are summarized in Box 73-1. The evidence supporting these risk factors is summarized in the next sections of this chapter (Balch, Houghton, & Peters, 1993; Cannon-Albright, Kamb, & Skolnick, 1996; Chen, Dubrow, Holford, Zheng, Barnhill, & Fine et al., 1996; Farmer & Naylor, 1996; Friedman, Rigel, Silverman, Kopf, & Vossaert, 1991).

Sun Exposure

The combination of sunlight and fair skin was recognized as early as 50 years ago as being an important risk factor for the development of skin cancer. This observation came as a result of people with Celtic features, from Edwardian England in the 1780s, relocating to an island in the South Pacific that we now call *Australia* (Leffell & Brash, 1996).

The degree and likelihood of sunburn depends on an individual's skin type. The various skin types and the likelihood of developing a sunburn are summarized in Table 73-1.

Ultraviolet Light Exposure

The epidemiologic studies that were performed regarding melanoma suggest that episodic, intense sun exposure (especially in childhood) that causes burns is the most important risk factor for the development of melanoma (Elwood, 1996; Farmer & Naylor, 1996; Seykora & Elder, 1996). There are no animal models for determining which of the sun's rays cause melanoma (Marks, 1996). People with skin types I-III have a higher incidence of melanomas.

There are three types of ultraviolet (UV) rays that are emitted from the sun's surface: UV-A, UV-B, and UV-C rays. UV-A rays (320 to 400 nm) maintain a relatively constant intensity throughout the year. These rays penetrate more deeply into the skin than UV-B rays. Exposure to UV-A rays contributes to premature aging and wrinkling of

Box 73-1
Risk Factors for Melanoma

Exposure to ultraviolet (UV) light
More than 20 congenital nevi
Family history of melanoma
Fair complexion
- Blonde or red hair
- Blue, gray, or green eyes

Personal history of melanoma
History of two or three serious sunburns as a child
Sun sensitivity (skin types I and II)
Inability to tan

TABLE 73-1 Skin Types

Type	Description
I	Never tans, always burns, fair or red hairs, many freckles
II	Burns easily, sometimes tans, freckles, fair hair
III	Tans easily, rarely burns
IV	Always tans, very rarely burns
V	Brown skin, very seldom burns
VI	Black skin, very seldom burns

the skin by damaging collagen and elastin. A study of sunbed and sunlamp users implicated UV-A rays in the development of melanoma (Walter, Marrett, & From, 1990).

UV-B rays (290 to 320 nm) have long been presumed to contribute to the development of melanoma. UV-B rays are stronger than UV-A rays and are more intense during the summer months, at higher altitudes, and at latitudes closer to the equator. UV-B is the most common cause of sunburn and can contribute to premature aging of the skin, can cause cataracts, and contributes to the development of skin cancers.

UV-C rays, although the strongest and the most dangerous, are normally filtered out by the ozone layer.

It is increased exposure to whole sunlight that has caused an increase in the incidence of melanoma worldwide. Protection should be from whole sunlight until there is a clearer understanding of the causative factors involved in the development of malignant melanoma (Marks, 1996).

Some recreational activities appear to carry a higher risk of sunburn. Participation in outdoor water sports results in the highest proportion of people who develop a sunburn. This problem is possibly due to the reflection of ultraviolet radiation off the water and the water's cooling effect (Hill, White, & Marks, 1992; Marks, 1996). In addition, a correlation has been found between air temperature and sunburn levels. When temperatures are low (below 65° F [18° C]), people tend to cover up or stay inside to keep warm; therefore there are fewer sunburns. When the temperature is high (above 83° F [28° C]), people are more likely to think of sun protection. When there are more moderate temperatures (66 to 81° F [19 to 27° C]), including those induced by cloud cover, people are most likely to get sunburned (Hill, White, & Marks, 1992; Marks, 1996).

A positive correlation has been found between the desire for a suntan and an increased risk for a sunburn. In addition, the frequency of sunburns is higher in adolescents and young adults than in older adults. It is also higher in males because sunscreens are more likely to be used by women (Hill, White, & Marks, 1992; Marks, 1996).

PRIMARY PREVENTION ACTIVITIES

The majority of a person's lifetime sun exposure occurs during the first 20 years of life. Primary prevention is aimed at individuals (or their caregivers) who are identified to have one or more risk factors for melanoma or other skin cancers (Koh & Geller, 1995; MacKie, 1995). In addition, recommendations for prevention are made for the general population. Marks (1996) advocates the regular use of sun-protection methods and draws an analogy to the automobile, stating that it would be wrong to suggest that we wear seatbelts only when there is a lot of traffic or when we feel at increased risk of encountering an accident.

Various types of sun-protective activities can be used. First, individuals can reduce their exposure to sun during the peak times of UV radiation exposure. Approximately 60% of the total UV-B is received in the 2 hours on either side of midday (i.e., 10:00 AM to 2:00 PM, or 11:00 AM to 3:00 PM during daylight saving time) (Marks, 1996).

Second, individuals can use sunscreens with a sun protection formula (SPF) of at least 15. This formulation offers protection 15 times greater than no sunscreen before skin erythema is produced (Koh & Geller, 1995). There are also broad-spectrum products, offering both UV-A and UV-B protection. To be effective, these products must be used properly. Application of the sunscreen before exposure to the UV rays is important. It takes approximately 20 minutes for the sunscreen to form a protective barrier. Application of an adequate amount of sunscreen, as well as reapplication after being in the water is recommended. Sunscreen bottles need to be checked for expiration dates to ensure their effectiveness.

In addition, individuals need to use barriers to protect themselves from sun exposure. Sunglasses (with UV protection), wide-brimmed hats (a brim size of 10 cm can lead to a 70% reduction in UV ray exposure to the head and neck), and appropriate clothing (long-sleeved shirts, fabric that is tightly woven and light in color) offer protection (Koh & Geller, 1995; Marks, 1996). In addition, the issue of scatter/reflection radiation must be kept in mind. When exposure is reduced by canopies (e.g., trees), the higher the canopy from the ground, the more opportunity there is for scatter radiation. UV rays are reflected by many surfaces in addition to water, including sand, snow, and white concrete (Marks, 1996).

Finally, individuals need to avoid deliberate tanning, including tanning parlors, tanning beds, and sunlamps (Koh & Geller, 1995; Walter, Marrett, & From, 1990).

Box 73-2
An ABCD Approach to the Early Detection of Melanoma

A = Asymmetry: Melanoma lesions are typically irregular shaped.
B = Border: Melanoma lesions often have uneven, ragged, notched edges, or irregular borders.
C = Color: Melanoma lesions often contain varying shades of blacks and browns.
D = Diameter: Melanoma lesions are often larger than 6 mm (about the size of a pencil eraser).

Awareness Programs

There are a number of programs that are being run in an effort to increase the public's awareness of sun safety. One measure is using newspaper and television announcements to publicize the UV index. This 1-to-10 scale projects the intensity of UV exposure and suggests protective measures. Australia has taken steps to provide shade in public areas, schedule sporting events away from midday, and reduce taxes on sunscreens (Koh & Geller, 1995).

A review article by Elwood (1996) reports the findings of 10 worldwide epidemiologic studies of melanoma. Some studies found that people who "almost always" used sunscreens showed a significant increase in their risk for melanoma. A possible explanation for this finding is that the physical UV blocking properties of the sunscreens may be insufficient to overcome the additional sun exposure encouraged by their use. In addition, numerous other variables, such as the type of sunscreen used, correct application and reapplication of the product, and increased likelihood of people at higher risk to use the sunscreen products, need to be considered when interpreting the findings from epidemiologic studies. Further studies are needed in this area, as well as public education on sun safety and sunscreen use.

In addition to the prevention activities discussed above, efforts are being made to promote early detection. Teaching about self-examination of the skin, as well as public education about the warning signs of melanoma, are ongoing. The use of the ABCD approach to early detection of malignant melanoma is summarized in Box 73-2. In addition, Fig. 73-1 illustrates the ABCD approach to the early detection of melanoma. Table 73-2 provide a framework for the self-examination of the skin.

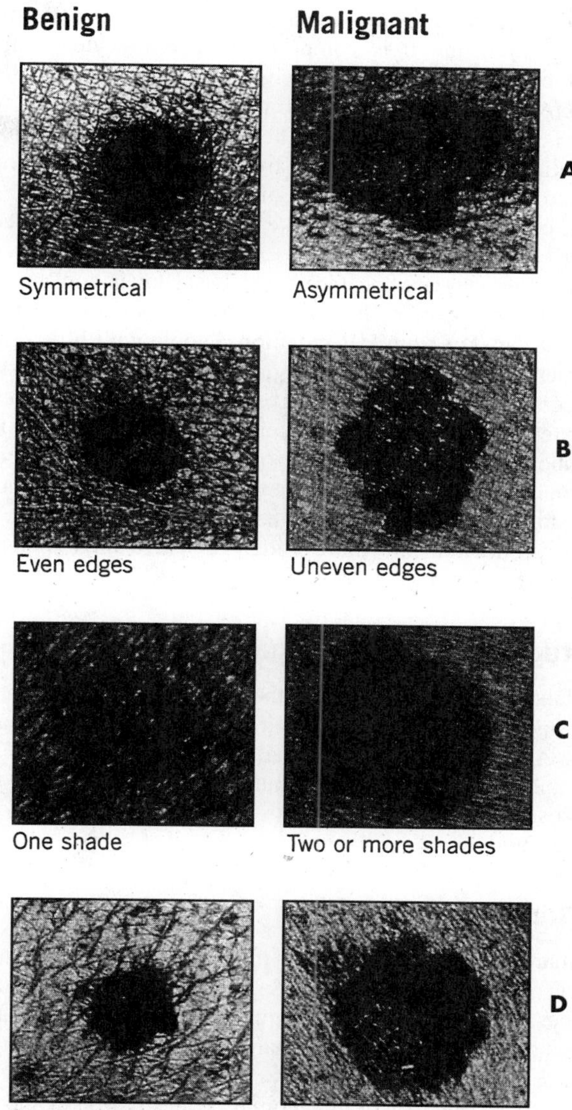

Fig. 73-1 ABCD of melanoma. **A,** Asymmetry; **B,** border; **C,** color; **D,** diameter. (From American Cancer Society. *Understanding melanoma.* Atlanta: American Cancer Society.)

PATHOPHYSIOLOGY

Components of the Skin and Their Function

The skin is a large organ that acts as a barrier to the environment (Table 73-3). As illustrated in Fig. 73-2, the epidermis provides the major barrier. The dermis, which is a vascular layer, is below the epidermis and provides support as well as nutrition for the dividing cells in the epidermis. The dermis also contains nerves and appendages (i.e., sweat glands, hair follicles, and sebaceous glands). The last layer and the deepest is the subcutaneous fat (Lookingbill, 1993).

Normal Anatomy of the Skin

The epidermis is divided into four layers. The outermost, or top, layer is the *stratum corneum,* which contains cells that are large, flat, and filled with keratin. These cells are stacked in vertical layers that range in thickness from 15 to 25 layers on most body surfaces to as many as 100 layers on the palms and soles of the feet. The tightly packed cells provide a semi-impenetrable layer that constitutes the major physical barrier of the skin. In the next layer, the *stratum granulosum,* cells are in the process of differentiation and they are acquiring keratin. The *stratum spinosum* is below the stratum granulosum. It is composed of keratinocytes, which produce keratin, a fibrous protein. The fourth layer is called the *basal cell layer.* "The basal cells can be considered the 'stem cells' of the epidermis. They are undifferentiated, proliferating cells. Daughter cells from the basal layer migrate upward and begin the process of differentiation. In normal skin, cell division does not take place above the basal cell layer" (Lookingbill, 1993).

Melanocytes are located in the basal layer and are the pigment-producing cells. The function of melanocytes is to protect the skin from UV radiation. People with little or no pigment develop notable sun damage and numerous skin cancers. People of all races have similar numbers of melanocytes. The difference in skin pigmentation depends on the number and size of the melanosomes (granules that hold the pigment melanin) and how they are dispersed throughout the skin. Sunlight stimulates melanocytes to increase pigment production and more widely disperse their melanosomes (Lookingbill, 1993).

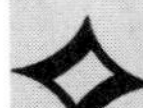

TABLE 73-2 Patient Preparation for Self-Examination of the Skin

Step 1: Make sure room is well-lit and that you have nearby a full-length mirror, a hand-held mirror, a hand-held blow dryer, and two chairs or stools. Undress completely.

Step 2: Hold your hands with the palms face up. Look at your palms, fingers, spaces between the fingers, and forearms. Then turn your hands over, and examine the backs of your hands, fingers, spaces between your fingers, fingernails, and forearms.

Step 3: Now position yourself in front of the full-length mirror. Hold up your arms, bent at the elbows, with your palms facing you. In the mirror, look at the backs of your forearms and elbows.

Step 4: Again using the full-length mirror, observe the entire front of your body. In turn, look at your face, neck and arms. Turn your palms to face the mirror, and look at your upper arms. Then look at your chest and abdomen, pubic area, thighs, and lower legs.

Step 5: Still standing in front of the mirror, lift your arms over your head with the palms facing each other. Turn so that your right side is facing the mirror, and look at the entire side of your body (your hands and arms, underarms, sides of your trunk, thighs, and lower legs). Then turn, and repeat the process with your left side.

Step 6: With your back toward the full-length mirror, look at your buttocks and the backs of your thighs and lower legs.

Step 7: Now pick up the hand-held mirror. With your back still to the full-length mirror, examine the back of your neck, and your back and buttocks. Also examine the backs of your arms in this way. Some areas are hard to see, and you may find it helpful to ask your spouse or a friend to assist you.

Step 8: Use the hand-held mirror and the full-length mirror to look at your scalp. Because the scalp is difficult to examine, we suggest you also use a blow dryer turned to a cool setting to lift the hair from the scalp. While some people find it easy to hold the mirror in one hand and the dryer in the other while looking in the mirror, many do not. For the scalp examination in particular, you might ask your spouse or a friend to assist you.

Step 9: Sit down and prop up one leg on a chair or stool in front of you. Using the hand-held mirror, examine the inside of the propped-up leg, beginning at the groin area and moving the mirror down the leg to your foot. Repeat the procedure for the other leg.

Step 10: Still sitting, cross one leg over the other. Use the hand-held mirror to examine the top of your foot, toes, toenails, and spaces between the toes. Then look at the bottom of your foot. Repeat the procedure for the other foot.

Categories of Melanomas

Melanomas usually arise in the melanocytes. The greatest number of melanocytes are found in the skin and eye. Approximately 9% of melanomas occur in the eye. Melanocytes can also be found in the meninges, the mucosa of the alimentary and respiratory tracts, and the lymph nodes.

Cutaneous Melanomas

Primary melanomas can occur in the meninges, respiratory tract, gallbladder, prostate, and other sites, although occurrences at these sites are rare. Approximately 4% of melanomas have no identifiable primary location (Balch, Houghton, & Peters, 1993).

The vast majority of melanomas occur in the skin and are referred to as *cutaneous melanomas.* Cutaneous melanoma lesions are divided into four main types that are categorized according to their growth patterns: superficial spreading melanoma (SSM), nodular melanoma (NM), lentigo maligna melanoma (LMM), and acral lentiginous melanoma (ALM). The major characteristics of the cutaneous melanomas are summarized in Table 73-4.

Superficial Spreading Melanoma. Superficial spreading melanoma is the most common subtype, accounting for approximately 70% of the cutaneous melanomas (Balch, Houghton, & Peters, 1993; MacKie, 1996; Urist, Miller, & Maddox, 1995). Superficial spreading melanomas can develop at any age after puberty (Balch, Houghton, & Peters, 1993). It is not uncommon for the patient to report a change in an existing lesion. This change may have occurred slowly over a period of 1 to 5 years. The original lesion, which is usually flat, may develop an irregular surface, enlarge, develop irregular borders, and change in color. At an early stage in their development, the lesions may ooze or crust without an obvious ulceration visible (Balch, Houghton, & Peters, 1993; MacKie, 1996; Urist, Miller, & Maddox, 1995). As the lesion enlarges, there is a notching of the borders and the surface becomes glossy (Balch, Houghton, & Peters, 1993). Superficial spreading melanomas occur more commonly in women. Pathologically, SSMs show an upward invasion through the epidermis in a pattern that is similar to Paget's disease. Therefore this

TABLE 73-2 Patient Preparation for Self-Examination of the Skin—cont'd

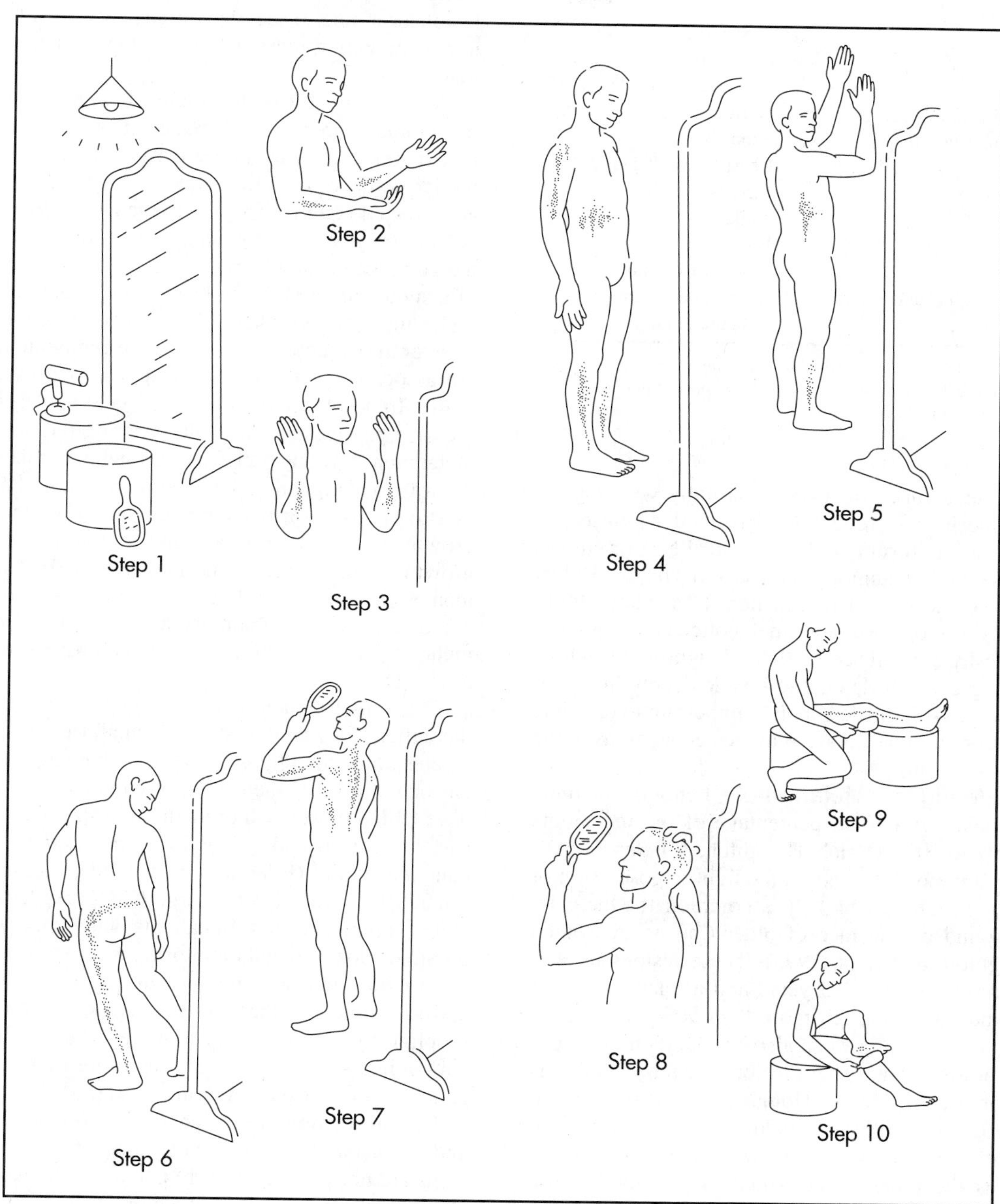

type of lesion is sometimes referred to as *Pagetoid melanoma* (MacKie, 1996).

Nodular Melanoma. Nodular melanomas are the second most common growth pattern, accounting for 15% to 30% of the lesions (Balch, Houghton, & Peters, 1993; Urist, Miller, & Maddox, 1995). They can occur at any age but are seen most commonly in middle age. These lesions are most often located on the trunk or on the head and neck. Men more frequently have NMs than women. Unlike SSMs, which usually are detected by a change in an existing lesion, NMs are associated with the development of a new lesion in an area of previously uninvolved skin. Nodular melanomas

Table 73-3 Functions of the Skin

Function	Responsible Structure
Barrier	Epidermis
Physical	Stratum corneum
Light	Melanocytes
Immunologic	Lagerhans' cells
Tough, flexible foundation	Dermis
Temperature regulation	Blood vessels
	Eccrine sweat glands
Sensation	Nerves
Grasp	Nails
Decorative	Hair
Unknown	Sebaceous glands
Insulation from cold and trauma	Subcutaneous fat
Calorie reservoir	Subcutaneous fat

From Lookingbill, D. P. (1993). Structure and function of the skin. In D. P. Lookingbill & J. G. Marks, Jr. (Eds.), *Principles of dermatology* (2nd ed.). Philadelphia: W. B. Saunders.

are darker in appearance than SSMs, usually with regular borders. The lesion is frequently described as raised or dome shaped and uniform in color. A typical NM resembles a blood blister or hemangioma and is blue black (Balch, Houghton, & Peters, 1993; Urist, Miller, & Maddox, 1995). Approximately 5% of NMs are amelanotic (lack pigment) and have a fleshy appearance (Balch, Houghton, & Peters, 1993). Pathologically, NMs tend to invade deeply in a relatively short time. With this lesion, it is important to examine the specimen for vascular invasion in the deeper areas of the lesion (MacKie, 1996).

Lentigo Maligna Melanoma. Lentigo maligna melanomas make up a small percentage of the melanoma population (4% to 10%) (Balch, Houghton, & Peters, 1993). These lesions are mostly found on the light-exposed skin of older persons (MacKie, 1996). It is common for these lesions to be found on the face of older Caucasian women (Balch, Houghton, & Peters, 1993). These lesions usually have been present for 5 to 15 years and are large (greater than 3 cm) and flat. Although more than 90% of these lesions occur on the face, they can also be found on the backs of the hands or lower legs. These lesions are tan with differing shades of brown (Balch, Houghton, & Peters, 1993; MacKie, 1996; Urist, Miller, & Maddox, 1995). This type of cutaneous melanoma does not have the same inclination to metastasize as the other subclassifications of the disease (Balch, Houghton, & Peters, 1993).

Acral Lentiginous Melanoma. This growth pattern occurs for the most part on the palms, on the soles of the feet, or beneath the nail beds. Just because a lesion is located on the palms or soles does not mean it is exclusively an ALM. There are a small number of NMs and SSMs that begin in these areas. Acral lentiginous melanomas make up 2% to 8% of melanomas in the Caucasian population. In the African-American, Asian, and Hispanic populations, ALMs account for 35% to 60% of the melanoma diagnoses. Acral lentiginous melanomas are most often found on the soles of the feet. They average a diameter of 3 cm. The average age at diagnosis is 60 years. Acral lentiginous melanomas can develop over a period of months to years, with the average development time being 2.5 years. The lesions have a similar appearance to LMMs (tan or brown, flat lesions). It is not surprising to see ulcerations, and when lesions are ignored, fungating masses can develop (Balch, Houghton, & Peters, 1993).

An infrequently seen variant of ALM is the subungual melanoma. These lesions make up only 2% to 3% of the melanoma diagnoses in Caucasian patients but occur in higher numbers in dark-skinned patients. Men and women are affected equally. The age range at the time of diagnosis is 55 to 65 years. Anatomically, most frequently the nails of the great toe or thumb are involved. The most common sign of a subungual melanoma is a brown to black discoloration under the nail bed (Balch, Houghton, & Peters, 1993).

Precursor Lesions. There are pigmented lesions that are associated with an increased risk of developing melanoma. In 1984, Clark, Elder and Guerry described a progressive process that took place during the development of melanoma. Lesions transform through a number of steps on the way to malignancy (i.e., common acquired nevus > dysplastic nevus > primary melanoma [superficial or radical growth phase] > primary melanoma [deep or vertical growth phase] > metastatic melanoma). Two types of pigmented lesions have been identified as "precursors" or "markers" for malignant melanoma. They are congenital melanotic nevi (CMN) and the controversial "dysplastic nevi" (DN).

Congenital melanotic nevi are present at birth or shortly thereafter. They are classified as small (less than 1 cm in diameter), medium (1.5 to 19.9 cm in diameter), and large (20 cm or more in diameter). Approximately 1% of newborns have CMN, most small or medium in size. People with large CMNs have a 6% to 7% increased risk of developing malignant melanoma (Friedman et al., 1991; Ketcham & Loescher, 1993; Koh, 1991). Large CMNs are treated by complete surgical excision. In patients where this excision is not possible, close clinical monitoring is important. A consensus has not been reached on the treatment of small and medium CMNs. Some feel that the lesions should be removed as a prophylactic measure, and some feel that the risk of malignant conversion is small, and therefore lifetime monitoring is acceptable (Friedman et al., 1991).

DN are commonly called *B-K moles* or *atypical moles* and are acquired pigmented lesions of the skin. These lesions are not present at birth. Clinically, an early finding of DN may be an increase in the number of histologically normal moles between the ages of 5 and 8 years. After puberty, dysplastic changes occur within the moles. Patients with DN syndrome are at increased risk of developing melanoma.

According to Seykora and Elder (1996), "dysplastic nevi may be regarded as intermediate lesions of tumor progression, in that approximately 30% of melanomas arise in association with a precursor nevus, which is most commonly dysplastic." DN lesions occur in both familial and nonfamilial settings. Clinically, dysplastic nevi have one or more features of a melanotic lesion (i.e., asymmetry, border ir-

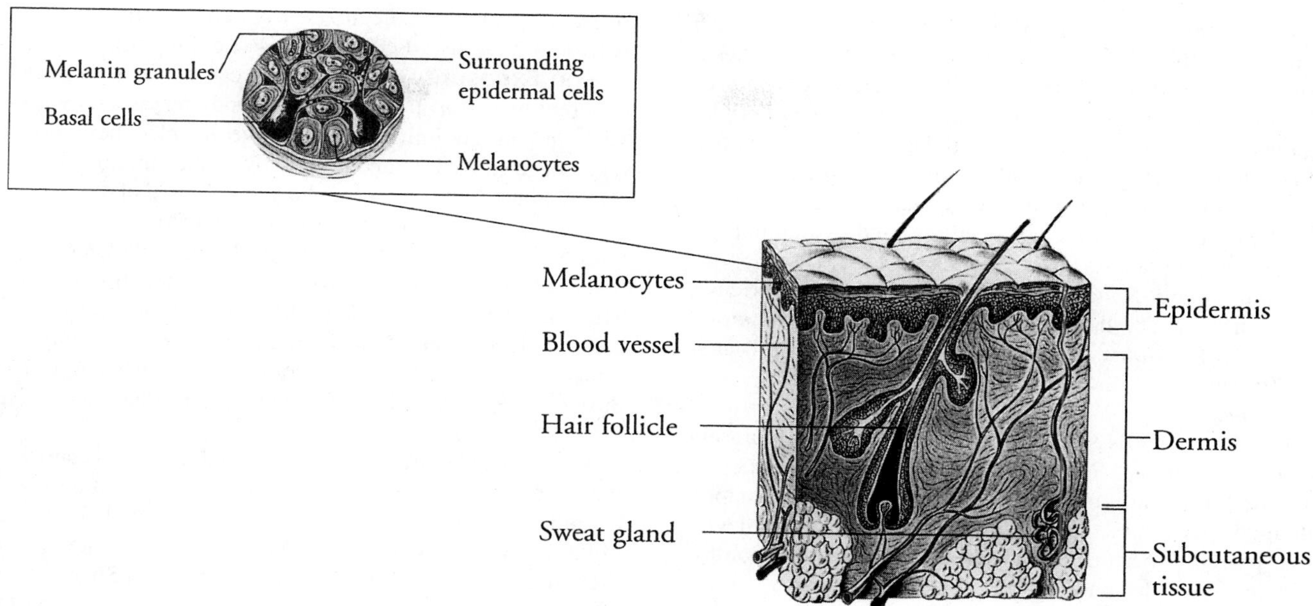

Fig. 73-2 The layers of the skin.

TABLE 73-4 Cutaneous Melanomas

Type	Frequency	Location	Growth	Characteristics
Superficial spreading melanoma (SSM)	Approximately 70%	Women: legs Men: trunk/back	Radial: over 1-5 years Vertical: aggressive	Good prognosis Develops after puberty More common in women
Nodular melanoma (NM)	Approximately 15%-30%	Trunk Head and neck	Vertical: aggressive	Most common in middle age Can occur at any time More common in men Associated with the development of a new lesion Lesions tend to be dark, with regular borders, raised, and dome shaped. Resembles a blood blister
Lentigo maligna melanoma (LMM)	Approximately 4%-10%	Face: mostly women Back of hands Lower legs	Radial: 5-15 years Vertical: aggressive	Older persons Light-exposed areas Tan lesions >3 cm Less likely to metastasize
Acral lentiginous melanoma (ALM)	2%-8% Caucasians 35%-65% darker pigments	Palms, soles of feet Nailbeds	Radial: months-years Average: 2.5 years	>3 cm diameter Average age: 60 years Tan/flat lesion Ulcerations/fungating masses
Subungual variation	2%-3% Caucasians Higher in darker pigments	Nailbeds of great toe or thumb	Radial: months-years Average: 2.5 years	Age 55-65 Black/brown discoloration of nailbeds

regularity, color variation, or a diameter of greater than 6 mm). The patient who has a "classic" DN syndrome has a triad of more than 100 moles, at least one mole 8 mm or larger in diameter, and at least one mole with melanoma-like features. For patients diagnosed with DN syndrome, the risk of developing malignant melanoma increases directly with a personal and/or family history of melanoma (Friedman et al., 1991). This syndrome has been reported in a number of ways in the literature. Clark, Elder, and Guerry (1978) reported it as the *B-K mole syndrome,* whereas Lynch, Frichot, and Lynch (1978) used the term *familial atypical mole-melanoma syndrome (FAMM).* Greene, Clark, and Tucker (1980) suggested the use of the term *dysplastic nevus syndrome.*

Patients with DN syndrome need to be followed closely by a dermatologist. Personal and family histories concerning melanoma are taken. A complete skin examination should be performed. Photographic documentation of the lesions present is performed and repeated every 3 to 6 months. New lesions or lesions that have changed should be examined through biopsy. Clinicians who use documentation photographs have detected more melanomas than the patients themselves (Marks, 1996). Patients and their relatives should be taught to perform a thorough skin examination regularly (Friedman et al., 1991; Ketcham & Loescher, 1993). Marks (1996) reports that individuals with DN and a family history of melanoma are at very high risk of developing malignant melanoma. It is believed that the cumulative lifetime risk approaches 100% for these patients.

Ocular Melanoma

The most common primary ocular melanomas arise in the vascular support structure and uveal tract, and they account for about 80% of primary adult eye tumors (Char, 1994). The uveal tract consists of the iris, ciliary body, and choroid. These patients most often have painless vision loss. Diagnosis is usually made by an ophthalmologist using slip lamp biomicroscopy or indirect ophthalmoscopy (Shields, Shields, DePotter, & Singh, 1996). When this disease metastasizes, it is commonly to the liver and less likely to the lung, skin, and other areas. A number of different modalities are used to treat these uncommon tumors. These therapies include laser photocoagulation, transpupillary thermotherapy, radiotherapy, local resection, enucleation, orbital exenteration, chemotherapy, and immunotherapy. Treatment decisions are made based on the extent and location of disease. The goals of therapy are to decrease ocular morbidity and tumor-related mortality (Char, 1994).

The Process of Carcinogenesis

Growth Phases. Melanomas grow in different phases. The radial (or horizontal) growth phase represents a melanoma that has invaded into the dermis, but the malignant cells in the dermis do not yet form a coherent tumor mass. Tumors in the radial growth phase are believed to carry a better prognosis because it is felt that these tumors have not yet developed metastatic capacity. Vertical growth phase occurs when there are clearly defined large clusters of cells that have invaded the dermis (Lookingbill, 1993).

Sun Exposure. UV radiation can act in a number of different ways: as an initiator, as a promoter, as a cocarcinogen, and as an immunosuppressive agent. These effects take place after UV absorption by deoxyribonucleic acid (DNA), or by other chromophores such as melanin or urocanic acid, and may involve the release of free radicals. UV radiation also stimulates a number of feedback mechanisms that protect the skin against further UV radiation damage. These mechanisms include proliferation of melanocytes, increased deposition of melanin in keratinocytes, and skin thickening, and may involve both direct effects and effects through the melanocyte-stimulating hormone mechanism (Elwood, 1996).

Genetic Alterations. When studying the genetics of melanoma, the disease is usually divided into patients with hereditary disease and patients with sporadic melanoma. Familial or hereditary melanoma has been documented in the literature over the past 150 years. According to Su and Trent (1995), the current estimates of true hereditary melanoma cases range between 5% and 10% of all new patients diagnosed with this disease.

"Human melanoma susceptibility loci have been assigned to three different human chromosomes, namely 1, 6, and 9. The most compelling associations of genetic change with familial occurrence have been the report of genetic linkage to chromosome 9p21 in heredity cases, followed by the identification of a gene termed *p16* (or *multiple tumor suppressor 1, MTS 1*) that frequently is mutated in the germline of patients with hereditary melanoma." (Su & Trent, 1995). The identification of the p16 gene as the germinal change in hereditary melanoma has been controversial. There are studies that indicate p16, which is a cyclin-dependent kinase inhibitor, is mutated in melanoma cell lines.

A study by Fountain, Karayiorgou, and Ernstoff (1992) reported a loss of heterozygosity at 9p16 in multiple melanoma tumors and cell lines. Kamp, Gruis, and Weaver-Feldhaus (1994) published a study that showed the 9p21 locus, previously implicated in melanoma oncogenesis, contains p16, and this gene is mutated in melanoma cell lines. Recently, Koh, Enders, and Dynlacht (1995) showed that mutated tumor derived alleles of p16 found in melanomas are deficient in blocking the G1/S phase transition of the cell cycle. The p16 gene encodes a regulator of the cell cycle that binds to the cyclin-dependent kinase 4 (CDK4), thereby inactivating it. Because cyclines are among the most important determinants of the initiation of DNA synthesis, a mutation in this gene (which serves to control cellular growth) would fail to exert its normal function as an inhibitor of cell division (Su & Trent, 1995).

Multiple chromosomes have been altered in sporadic melanomas. These chromosomes include 1, 6, and 7, followed by 9, 3, 2, 11, and 10. Although no single chromosome abnormality defines melanoma, the locations of recurrent alterations strongly implicate the regions of growth regulatory genes as being important in melanoma biology (Su & Trent, 1995). Some of the band regions that were identified by cytogenetic analysis are 6q16-23 and 9p21.

Chromosome 6 abnormalities are observed in a majority of metastatic melanomas and in a subset of primary melanomas. Alterations involve nonreciprocal translocations or deletions with breakpoints clustering around the midproximal long arm, resulting in the apparent loss of all or part of the distal long arm of this chromosome. This consistent finding (in more than 80% of the cases) involving one or both homologues of 6q suggests that one or more tumor suppressor genes inhabit this location (Su & Trent, 1995).

Chromosome 6, especially the short arm 9p, has been implicated as a recurrent site of abnormalities associated with premalignant nevi and metastatic melanomas. The invasive potential of malignant melanoma has been linked to 10q24-26.

Chromosome 1 is the most frequently altered chromosome in malignant melanoma. The most common abnormality is a translocation and/or deletions clustering around a centromere, 1p11-q22. The significance of this finding is unclear because chromosome 1 is altered in many other human solid tumors (Su & Trent, 1995).

Growth Factors and Melanoma. The transformation of normal melanocytes to melanoma cells is most likely a multistep, multifactorial process. As is seen in other cancers, it is most likely to include a loss of growth-restraining factors (tumor suppressors) and a gain of growth-promoting functions (dominant acting oncogenes). In vitro, normal melanocytes require a number of growth factors, working synergistically, to proliferate (Halaban, 1996; Su & Trent, 1996). These growth factors include several members of the fibroblast growth factor family (FGF), hepatocyte growth factor/scatter factor (HCF/SF), mast/stem cell growth factor (MGF, also known as *KIT ligand, stem cell growth factor,* and *steel factor*), and the neuropeptides endothelin-1, 2, and 3 (ET-1, ET-2, ET-3). Each of these factors by itself is insufficient to elicit proliferation. From this group of peptides, only basic FGF (bFGF/FGF2) appears to play a role in the autonomous growth of melanomas (Halaban, 1996). Basic fibroblast growth factor (bFGF) and transforming growth factor alpha (TGF-α) are expressed in almost all melanoma cell lines examined. They are not detected in normal melanocytes that are cultured (Su & Trent, 1995).

ROUTES OF METASTASES

The process of melanoma metastasis is made up of a number of defined, interrelated steps that depend on a number of variables, including the intrinsic behavior of the melanoma and the host response (Slominski, Ross, & Mihm, 1995). Patients diagnosed with stage III or IV disease have a dramatic decrease in survival. If regional lymph nodes are involved, the 5-year survival rate decreases to about 30% to 40%. The prognosis worsens depending on the number of lymph nodes involved and the presence of extranodal disease (Slominski, Ross, & Mihm, 1995).

Primary lesions located on the trunk versus the extremities have a worse prognosis. When the presence of distant metastasis has been established, the disease is rarely curable. Prognosis worsens with the increasing number of metastatic sites and visceral involvement. It has been suggested that males have a worse prognosis than females (Slominski, Ross, & Mihm, 1995).

The most frequent sites of metastasis for melanoma are the skin, subcutaneous tissue, and lymph nodes. These sites make up approximately 50% of the metastatic lesions. The next most frequent site is the lung (18% to 36%), followed by the liver, brain, and bone (Ho, 1995). After metastatic disease has been identified, cerebral metastases are clinically diagnosed in 40% to 60% of patients. The incidence increases to 70% to 90% at autopsy (Fidler, 1995). The prognosis for stage IV melanoma is grim. The expected 5-year survival rate is less than 10%. Median survival from the time of detection to the development of the first distant metastasis ranges from 6 months to 8.5 months (Ho, 1995).

ASSESSMENT

The assessment of a patient for malignant melanoma is summarized in Table 73-5. Clinical evaluation includes a detailed history and a thorough physical examination with an emphasis on a complete examination of the skin, the suspicious lesion, and draining lymph nodes.

History

The patient should be evaluated for the identified risk factors for melanoma. A history of UV light exposure, both natural and artificial, should be taken. A detailed history of the suspicious lesion should be taken with attention to the length of time it has been present and the changes noted in it (such as itching, tingling, burning, bleeding, and change in size). A family history should also be taken with attention to other melanoma diagnoses, the presence of other skin malignancies, and the presence or absence of dysplastic nevus syndrome.

Physical Examination

Examination of the lesion should be performed, and the lesion should be assessed for the presence of the classic findings associated with melanoma: asymmetry, border irregularity, color change, and an increase in lesion diameter. The lesion should be assessed for ulceration and bleeding. The skin around the lesion should be assessed for other suspicious lesions (i.e., satellite lesions and in-transit metastasis). The entire skin surface should be examined and the location and description of other nevi noted.

Lymph node evaluation by palpation should be performed, especially if the melanotic lesion drains to lymph node beds that are accessible to physical examination (i.e., axilla, groin, popliteal, head, neck, clavicular areas). The remainder of the physical examination should include the heart, lungs, and liver for any signs of the potential presence of metastatic disease.

Diagnostic Tests

The presence of a suspicious lesion usually warrants a biopsy using the appropriate techniques. One form of assess-

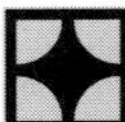

TABLE 73-5 Assessment of the Patient for Melanoma

	Assessment Parameters	**Typical Abnormal Findings**
History	A. Personal and social history 1. Age 2. Gender 3. Family history of melanoma 4. Sun exposure 5. Use of sunscreens 6. Use of tanning beds 7. Personal history of melanoma 8. Nevi history	A. Personal and social risk factors 1. Lentigo maligna melanomas and acral lentiginous melanomas are more common in patients over 60 years. Nodular melanomas are more common in middle-age patients but can occur at any time. Superficial spreading melanomas develop after puberty. 2. Nodular melanomas are more common in men. Superficial spreading melanomas are more common in women. 3. A positive family history increases the risk. 4. A history of two to three serious sunburns increases the risk of melanoma. 5. Intermittent intense exposures to sunlight increase the risk. 6. Use of tanning beds has been implicated as increasing a person's risk. 7. Having a previous melanoma increases the risk. 8. Having more than 20 congenital nevi increases the risk. A history of dysplastic nevi syndrome increases the risk.
	B. Evaluation of the skin	B. Common signs/symptoms include a change in a wart or mole or the development of a new lesion. Lesions are noted for asymmetry, border irregularity, color change, increase in diameter (ABCDs), ulceration, bleeding, or growth of an existing mole. Note the timeline from the time the patient first noted the change until diagnosis. Does the patient perform a self skin examination?
	C. Evaluation for lymph nodes	C. Involved regional lymph nodes can be palpated, especially in the axilla and groin. Evaluate the length of time the patient noted these areas to be involved.
Physical Examination	A. Total body skin assessment	A. A thorough skin examination, with photographic documentation of existing lesions. Note the presence of asymmetry, border irregularity, color changes, and diameters greater than 6 mm. Note the number, condition, and location of nevi. Note bleeding or ulceration of the lesion.
	B. Lymph node evaluation	B. Assess all possible drainage basins accessible to palpation and the involvement of lymph nodes on the prognosis.
Diagnostic Tests	A. Chest x-ray examination	A. Assess the pulmonary status, and observe for a possible metastatic site in the lung.
	B. Complete blood count	B. Assess the hematologic function.
	C. Chemistries	C. Assess for liver function with attention to lactate dehydrogenase (LDH), which may indicate liver metastasis.

ment that may be used before deciding on the need for biopsy is the use of a dermatoscope. This technique is called *epiluminescence microscopy (dermatoscopy).* A health care professional specially trained in this technique performs the examination. Mineral oil is placed on the lesion, which makes the stratum corneum translucent. The lesion is then viewed with the dermatoscope, a hand-held device about the size of an otoscope, which magnifies the lesion (Baron, 1996). The use of this technique can increase positive biopsy results by decreasing the number of unneeded biopsies (Steiner, Pehamberger, & Wolff, 1987). However, the use of this device is not widespread. Additional biopsy procedures are summarized in Table 73-6.

At the initial presentation and staging, a chest x-ray examination should be performed, as well as a complete blood count and chemistries (including lactate dehydrogenase [LDH]). Further workup and testing might be recommended based on the initial findings (Garrison & Nathanson, 1996; Keller & Maize, 1996).

STAGING

The staging of melanoma begins with a biopsy of the suspicious lesion. "A complete pathology report contains a description of the thickness, level of invasion, growth pattern, margin status, dimensions, and presence or absence of ulceration" (Urist, 1996). The vertical thickness of a tumor is the most important pathologic prognostic feature of cutaneous melanoma. There is a strong correlation between tumor thickness, progression of metastasis, and ultimate survival (Garrison & Nathanson, 1996).

TABLE 73-6 Surgical Procedures

Surgical technique	A. Biopsy of lesion	A. A suspicious lesion needs to undergo biopsy appropriately.
	1. Shave biopsy	1. Shave or curette-type biopsies should never be performed on a lesion suspected of being a melanoma. This point is critical because the depth of invasion provides prognostic information.
	2. Excisional biopsy	2. Used if the lesion is small. Excision of the entire lesion is performed. It is appropriate for use on a lesion that is less than 2 cm in diameter and located on a part of the body where the amount of skin removed is not critical. It should not be used over joints or on the face.
	3. Incisional biopsy	3. Reserved for large lesions. The object is to remove the lesion using an elliptical portion of skin that includes the thickest part of the lesion as well as some normal skin from the surrounding area. Normal skin is helpful to the pathologist in determining the depth of invasion. Punch biopsies may be used in some cases.
	B. Dermatoscope	B. A technique known as *epiluminescence microscopy.* This examination requires the use of a dermatoscope and an appropriately trained health care professional. Mineral oil is placed on the lesion to render the stratum corneum translucent. It is then viewed with a dermatoscope, a tool that magnifies the lesion. This procedure can decrease the number of unnecessary biopsies by identifying high-risk lesions.

Box 73-3
Clark's Microstaging System

Clark's Level I: melanoma in situ
Clark's Level II: invading the papillary dermis
Clark's Level III: invading the papillary-reticular dermal interface
Clark's Level IV: invading the reticular dermis
Clark's Level V: invading subcutaneous tissue

Microstaging

Two methods have been used in the microstaging of melanoma. Microstaging describes the depth of invasion of a cutaneous melanoma.

The Clark's Level system classifies the lesion according to the anatomic depth of invasion. The pathologist measures the depth of penetration into the five dermal layers. The Clark's microstaging system is listed in Box 73-3.

The Breslow method uses an ocular micrometer to measure the thickness of the lesion. The vertical height (not exclusively the depth) is measured from the granular layer to the area of deepest penetration (Balch, Houghton, & Peters, 1993). The measurement of an ulcerated lesion starts at the surface of the ulcer and proceeds down to the deepest point of invasion (Fig. 73-3).

If there is a discrepancy between the level of invasion (Clark's) and the tumor thickness (Breslow), microstaging should be based on thickness alone. Analysis of data has shown that if there is excessive emphasis placed on the level of invasion, focus may be shifted from the more important prognostic indicator, which is thickness (Garrison & Nathanson, 1996).

TABLE 73-7 Traditional Staging System

Stage	Extent of Disease
I	Localized primary melanoma
IA	Local recurrence with satellite lesions
II	Regional metastasis (lymph node involvement or in-transit metastasis)
III	Distant metastases

Traditional Staging Systems

The use of the traditional three-stage system (Table 73-7) for melanoma has been replaced by the classification system developed by the American Joint Committee on Cancer (AJCC), shown in Table 73-8 (Beahers, Hensson, & Hutter, 1992; Metcalf, 1996).

MEDICAL MANAGEMENT

Surgical Management

The treatment of malignant melanoma depends on several factors. Accurate staging of the disease determines the need for further therapy. The primary treatment of melanoma is surgical removal of the suspicious lesion (Ball & Thomas, 1995). This removal may be achieved by a number of surgical techniques. Shave or curette-type biopsies should never be performed on a lesion suspected of being melanoma. These techniques do not provide the pathologist with a full-thickness specimen. The full thickness of the specimen is needed to accurately microstage the patient (Baron, 1996) (Fig. 73-4).

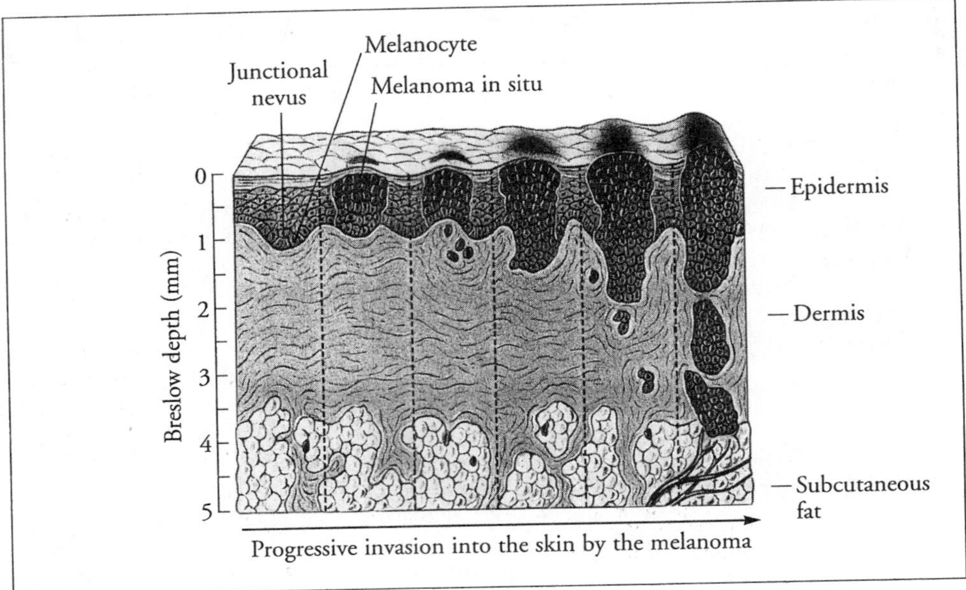

Fig. 73-3 Progressive growth of melanoma.

Excisional Biopsy. Excisional biopsies are used for lesions that are small (usually less than 2 cm in diameter) and located on a body part that can accommodate the loss of skin caused by the procedure. For example, this technique usually is not performed with lesions on the face or joints. If a diagnosis of melanoma is made on the initial biopsy, the patient requires a local wide excision.

The area to be excised is infiltrated with a local anesthetic (lidocaine with or without epinephrine). The incision is made with a scalpel around the lesion in an elliptical shape. The direction of the biopsy incision is important. An excisional biopsy that is *not* oriented properly may require that the patient have a skin graft when an elliptical incision and primary closure might have been possible. The biopsy incision should be oriented so that it can be reexcised with optimal skin margins, as well as minimal skin loss in the event that the biopsy proves to be melanoma (Balch, Houghton, & Peters, 1993). The entire suspicious lesion is removed. The biopsy should penetrate down to the underlying fat when feasible. Punch biopsies (4 to 6 mm) may be used as an alternative to scalpel excision (Baron, 1996; Urist, 1996).

Incisional Biopsy. Incisional biopsies are used for larger lesions. The objective of this technique is to remove an elliptical portion of the skin that includes the thickest part of the lesion. Along with the suspicious area, it is important for the surgeon to include a section of uninvolved skin in the specimen. The normal adjacent skin helps the pathologist determine the depth of invasion. The use of incisional biopsies does not appear to change the prognosis (Urist, 1996).

Surgical Wide Excision. After the diagnosis of melanoma has been confirmed by pathologic examination of the biopsy specimen, the need for wide excision should be addressed. When the term *margin* is used in relationship to melanoma, it is important to realize that the measurement is taken from the edge of the tumor or the scar remaining from a previous biopsy site. Therefore, a 3-cm margin produces a specimen that is 6 cm in diameter. In the 1970s, the standard practice of wide excisions that exceeded a 5-cm radius ceased. Multiple retrospective analyses of surgical techniques led to a change in practice. Currently, the recommended margins of excision are based on the thickness of the excised primary melanoma (Table 73-9). The change in surgical technique, which decreases the margins of wide excision, has lead to fewer functional and cosmetic deficits (Baron, 1996).

Melanomas at Special Sites. The excision guidelines presented in Table 73-9 are appropriate for most melanomas. There are special considerations that need to be taken based on the location of the lesion (Table 73-10). According to Baron (1996), several exceptions to the wide excisional margins need to be considered.

Melanomas of the face are generally treated with a 1-cm margin of resection. Anatomic features such as the eyes, nose, and mouth often prevent larger margins from being taken. Because most of the lesions found on the face are LMMs, there is a low risk of recurrence. Some research has indicated that radiation therapy can be used as a definitive treatment or as an adjuvant to surgery (Baron, 1996).

Lesions of the ear are treated by wedge resection or partial amputation. For patients with extensive disease, the entire ear should be removed.

In the past, mastectomy was used to treat melanoma of the breast. The treatment used should be based on the thickness of the primary biopsy instead of the fact that it is located on the breast.

A subungual lesion of the hands or feet usually requires amputation as the definitive surgery. If a lesion is small and confined to the nailbed, partial amputation may be appropriate. For lesions of the thumb nailbed, amputation can occur just proximal to the interphalangeal joint. For lesions of the finger nailbed, amputation at the distal interphalangeal joint

TABLE 73-8 American Joint Committee on Cancer Staging System for Melanoma

Primary Tumor (pT)	
pTX	Primary tumor cannot be assessed
pT0	No evidence of primary tumor
pTis	Melanoma in situ, not an invasive lesion (Clark's level I)
pT1	Tumor 0.75 mm or less in thickness and invading the papillary dermis (Clark's level II)
pT2	Tumor more than 0.75 mm but not more than 1.5 mm thick, and/or invades to the papillary-reticular dermal interface (Clark's level III)
pT3	Tumor more than 1.5 mm in thickness and/or invades the reticular dermis (Clark's level IV)
pT3a	Tumor more than 1.5 mm but not more than 3 mm in thickness
pT3b	Tumor more than 3 mm but not more than 4 mm in thickness
pT4	Tumor more than 4 mm in thickness and/or invades the subcutaneous tissue (Clark's level V), and/or there are satellite lesions within 2 cm of the primary
pT4a	Tumor more than 4 mm in thickness and/or invades the subcutaneous tissue
pT4b	Satellite(s) within 2 cm of the primary
Regional Lymph Nodes (N)	
NX	Regional lymph nodes cannot be assessed
N0	No regional lymph node metastasis
N1	Metastasis 3 cm or less in greatest dimension in any regional lymph node(s)
N2	Metastasis more than 3 cm in greatest dimension in any regional lymph node(s) and/or in-transit metastasis
N2a	Metastasis more than 3 cm in greatest dimension in any regional lymph nodes
N2b	In-transit metastasis
N2c	Both N2a and N2b
Distant Metastasis	
MX	Presence of distant metastasis cannot be assessed
M0	No distant metastasis
M1	Distant metastasis
M1a	Metastasis in skin or subcutaneous tissue or lymph node(s) beyond the regional lymph nodes
M1b	Visceral metastasis

Stages

Stage	Primary Tumor (T)	Regional Lymph Nodes (N)	Distant Metastasis (M)
Stage IA	pT1	N0	M0
Stage IB	pT2	N0	M0
Stage IIA	pT3	N0	M0
Stage IIB	pT4	N0	M0
Stage III	any pT	N1 or N2	M0
Stage IV	any pT	any N	M1

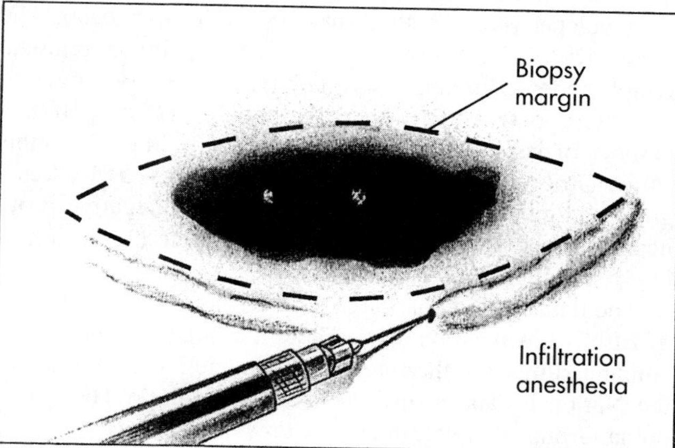

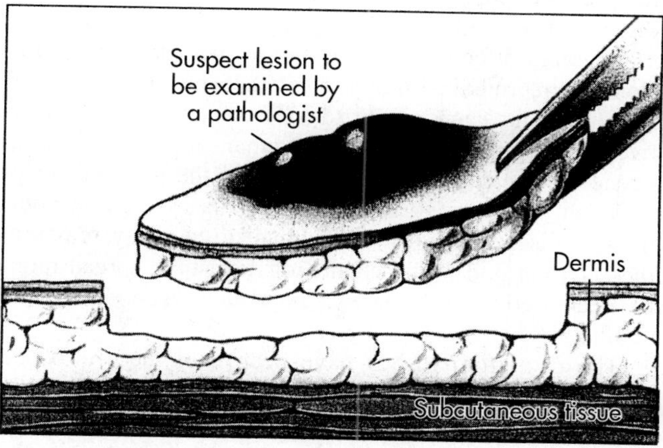

Fig. 73-4 Obtaining a full-thickness specimen for microstaging of malignant melanoma.

TABLE 73-9 Margins of Excision Based on Primary Melanoma Thickness

Thickness	Margin of Excision (cm)	Lymph Node Options
In situ	0.3-0.5	Observation
<1.0 mm	1	Observation
1.0-2.0 mm	2	Observation, SLNBx, ELND
2.01-4.0 mm	2	Observation, SLNBx
>4.0 mm	2-3	Observation, SLNBx

Modified from Urist, M. M. (1996). Surgical management of primary cutaneous melanoma. *CA: A Journal for Clinicians, 46*(4), 222.
SLNBx, Sentinel lymph node biopsy; *ELND,* elective lymph node dissection.

TABLE 73-10 Treatment of Melanoma at Special Sites

Melanoma Site	Treatment
Face	1 cm margin and/or radiotherapy
Ear	Wedge excision
Breast	Excision based on tumor thickness
Subungual	
Fingers	Distal amputation
Toes	Toe amputation
Sole of foot	Excision based on tumor thickness

From Baron, P. L. (1996). The surgical management of melanoma: From diagnosis to local treatment. *Seminars in Oncology, 23*(6), 717.

should occur. These approaches help maximize function without compromising local control. The thickness of a plantar lesion determines the surgical approach just as it would in other anatomic areas. These lesions are often thick, requiring a split-thickness skin graft or local rotational flap.

Lymph Node Evaluation. After the thickness of the primary melanoma has been established, the lymph node status becomes important in predicting the prognosis. For patients with clinically detectable disease, a fine-needle aspiration or complete node dissection may be used to confirm the diagnosis. Controversy persists regarding the use of elective lymph node dissection (ELND). There is a significant amount of morbidity associated with ELND. Multiple prospective and retrospective studies have failed to clearly demonstrate the benefits of this procedure.

Patients with a thin primary melanoma (≤0.75 mm) do not require an ELND. Cure rates from local excision alone are very high (>90%) (Cole & Baron, 1996), and only 2% to 3% of patients have occult positivity on ELND (Garrison & Nathanson, 1996). Patients with thick melanomas (>4.0 mm) have a very high incidence of local, regional, and distant metastasis. These patients do not benefit from ELND because of the probable presence of systemic disease (Garrison & Nathanson, 1996; Urist, 1996). Therapeutic lymph node dissections are performed to improve control of the disease.

The area of controversy occurs in patients that have lesions of intermediate thickness (>0.75 mm to <4.0 mm). These patients carry a 25% to 57% chance of having positive lymph nodes (Garrison & Nathanson, 1996). The sequence of melanoma metastasis places the regional lymph nodes at greatest risk for metastatic disease. These nodes may represent a haven for residual disease. By removing these lymph nodes, the chance of metastatic spread might be decreased. Unfortunately, the data to date have been conflicting.

The data from ELND have been examined retrospectively by a number of different groups. Information from the University of Alabama and the Melanoma Clinic in New South Wales report a survival benefit of 70% to 75% at 5 and 10 years for patients treated with local wide excision and ELND. Patients who were treated with local wide excision alone were reported to have a 55% (Alabama) and a 20% to 40% (Sydney) survival rate. Conflicting retrospective analyses have been reported by other groups, including the University of Pennsylvania and the Lahey Clinic (Cole & Baron, 1996).

Two prospective randomized trials have addressed ELND, one published by the World Health Organization (WHO) Melanoma Group and the second by the Mayo Clinic. The WHO study enrolled 553 patients with clinical stage I malignant melanoma of the extremities. The patients were randomized to receive either local wide excision with lymph node dissection if the regional nodes became clinically apparent, or local wide excision and ELND. The patients were matched for gender, age, histologic type, Clark's level, Breslow depth, and presence of satellite lesions. The mean follow-up was 10.4 years. There was no difference in survival rates between the two groups. The study has been criticized because of a maldistribution of ulcerated lesions (a poor prognostic indicator) and because of a low percentage of males being enrolled (also a poor prognostic indicator).

The Mayo Clinic study enrolled 171 patients who were randomized into three treatment groups. Group I (N = 62) had no lymphadenectomy, Group II (N = 55) had a delayed lymphadenectomy (2 to 3 months after diagnosis), and Group III (N = 54) had an immediate excision of regional lymph nodes. The study reported 10-year survival rates of 85% (Group I), 91% (Group II), and 87% (Group III). A number of issues were raised about the findings from this study. Group I had a higher number of males, as well as a greater number of primary lesions that had negative prognostic factors. Overall, the study had a large proportion of low-risk patients.

The data remain confusing, and no consensus on the use of ELND has been reached. There are ongoing trials being conducted through the Intergroup Melanoma Committee of the National Cancer Institute, as well as the WHO Melanoma Group, that continue to address this issue.

Sentinel Lymph Node Biopsy. Morton, Wen, & Cochran (1992) introduced the concept of sentinel lymph node (SLN) biopsy. The importance of identifying this node is based on the hypothesis that if the SLN is negative for disease, the rest of the nodes in the basin should be negative as well. If the SLN and presence or absence of metastatic disease could be accurately identified, it could lead to screening of regional lymph nodes with minimal morbidity. A directed biopsy of an SLN that was negative for metastatic disease could spare the patient from needing a full lymph node dissection, whereas the confirmation of a positive SLN would justify and appropriately treat the patient with a lymphadenectomy. To achieve this goal, two things must be accomplished: (1) accurate identification of the draining nodal basin and (2) identification and biopsy of the SLN (Cole & Baron, 1996).

This screening uses lymphoscintigraphy to identify the regional lymph node basin for a specific cutaneous melanoma site. Original work in this area showed that an injection of a radionucleotide into the skin at the primary site (before wide excision) could identify the lymph node draining basins. The first draining node (i.e., SLN) is at highest risk for metastatic disease and can be identified.

Further work has been done at the University of Southern Florida College of Medicine by Reintgen and colleagues (1995). They used lymphoscintigraphy to locate the SLN, to identify the presence of in-transit nodal areas (i.e., collections between the primary site and the regional basin), and to estimate the number of SLNs to better direct surgical care.

In one series (N = 82) a preoperative lymphoscintigraphy was performed in patients who were undergoing ELND with intermediate thickness melanomas. Cutaneous drainage patterns identified by lymphoscintigraphy were compared with those predicted by clinical experience or historic and anatomic guidelines. The results were discordant in 63% of patients with head and neck melanomas and 32% of patients with lesions on the trunk. As a result of these findings, surgical intervention was changed in 47% of the patients, with 19% undergoing dissection of nonclassical basins. About 28% of the patients did not have an ELND because of lack of documentation by a scintigram of a predominant drainage basin, or the demonstration of multiple drainage sites. There has been a mean follow-up of these patients after 4 years. There have been no recurrences in basins that were not positive by lymphoscintigraphy. The authors feel that these findings attest to the accuracy of the test in identifying all of the basins at risk for disease. The study concluded that if ELND is based on classic anatomic patterns or clinical experience, the procedure may be misdirected in over 50% of the cases.

Reintgen and colleagues (1995) have updated the initial series to include information on over 500 cases with more than 4 years of mean clinical follow-up. No recurrences have occurred in lymph basins that were not predicted by the scan.

Identification of SLN is a two-step process. First, a preoperative lymphoscintigraphy is performed to define the location and direction of lymph flow. A radionucleotide is injected into the skin around the melanoma lesion or the biopsy scar. This injection should take place before the local wide excision because it is not known if the cutaneous lymphatics are disrupted by local wide excision. After the injection, imaging is performed to identify the SLNs. These nodes are marked with a permanent intradermal tattoo.

Intraoperative lymphatic mapping takes place next. Isosulfan blue, a vital dye, is injected around the primary melanoma site. After 10 minutes, a small incision is made. This incision is directed by the intradermal tattoo made during the preoperative lymphoscintigraphy. The afferent lymphatics are followed to the SLN, which is marked by the blue dye. Success in determining the SLN depends on the surgeon's experience in using this technique.

Intraoperative lymph node mapping provides a substantial amount of information. Melanoma lesions that are metastatic to the SLN are a harbinger of more extensive disease in the lymph bed. In addition, the absence of metastatic disease in the SLN correlates with freedom from disease in other nodes in the basin. No evidence of skip metastasis was found in melanoma patients using intraoperative lymph node mapping. The SLN is not necessarily the lymph node closest to the primary site, and the location of the SLN is variable among patients, even in situations where the primary lesions are located in similar sites (Reintgen et al., 1995).

There has been some difficulty using vital-blue dye alone in identifying the SLN. Technical difficulties in up to 20% of dissections have led to unsuccessful attempts to find the SLN. To address this issue, Reintgen and colleagues (1995) have added the use of intraoperative radiolymphoscintigraphy. A technetium-labeled sulfur colloid is injected around the primary site of the melanoma. A nuclear probe (Neoprobe, Neoprobe Corporation, Columbus, Ohio) is then used to trace the lymphatics from the primary site to the SLN. The neoprobe is a hand-held gamma detector that helps guide the surgeon to the SLN. The SLN is marked by intense radioactivity. After the removal of the SLN, the operative area can be assessed for any further areas of intensity.

Detection of Metastatic Disease in Lymph Node Samples. Lymph nodes can be examined by frozen section at the time of biopsy. Routine histologic examination and immunohistologic staining for the evaluation of metastatic melanoma have a reported sensitivity of approximately 1 tumor cell per 10,000 cells and have enhanced sensitivity if serial sectioning and immunohistochemistry are used. However, this latter methodology requires techniques that are expensive and time consuming, and as a result, serial sectioning and immunohistochemistry are not used routinely in the community hospital (Cole & Baron, 1996).

A new approach to this problem is using a polymerase chain reaction (PCR) to detect messenger ribonucleic acid (mRNA) (reverse transcriptase PCR [RT-PCR]) and to identify melanoma-associated proteins. Transcription of the tyrosinase gene appears to be restricted to cells of melanocytic origin. Applying this technique to lymph node biopsy specimens has a reported sensitivity of 1 melanoma cell per 1,000,000 background lymphocytes. A series reported by Reintgen and colleagues (1995) involved specimens from 29 patients. Routine histopathology and immunohistochemical staining yielded 11/29 pathologically positive specimens. The PCR results yielded 19/29 positive specimens. There were no false negatives. They concluded that the use of the RT-PCR method for the identification of micrometastasis is sensitive, reproducible, efficient, and widely applicable. RT-PCR could become a powerful tool in detecting micrometastasis of melanoma. Clinical trials to confirm sensitivity of this tool are ongoing (Buzaid & Balch, 1996).

Biologic Approaches

An immunologic approach to the treatment of melanoma has been prompted by a number of different observations about this disease. Melanomas are known to spontaneously regress, there is a varying rate of disease progression, there is an increased incidence of melanoma in the immunocompromised patient, and melanoma tumors have an abundance of lymphoid infiltrates, including CD4 and CD8 bearing T cells (Gattoni-Celli & Cole, 1996; Kassas & Kirkwood, 1996; Mastrangelo, Maguire, Sato, Nathan, & Berd, 1996; Morton & Barth, 1996). T-cell–mediated immunity is important for immune recognition and the destruction of growing tumors (Darrow, Abdel-Wahab, & Seigler, 1995).

Adjuvant Therapy with Interferon Alfa 2-b. Interferon (INF) has shown potent immunomodulatory effects on the expression of the major histocompatibility antigens of classes I and II and other tumor-related antigens, as well as showing a host-immune response to tumor cells. Theoretically, interferon would have the greatest benefit in the adjuvant setting (Kassas & Kirkwood, 1996; Kirkwood, Strawderman, Ernstoff, Smith, Borden, & Blum, 1996). There are three types of interferons: alfa (α), beta (β), and gamma (γ). Phase I and II trials of INF-γ have shown minimal antitumor effect against melanoma. Interferon alfa has been tested as a single agent in melanoma. According to Kassas and Kirkwood (1996), the overall response rate in a collected series for interferon alfa in metastatic measurable melanoma is 16.3%. The observation of improved responses in patients with lower tumor burdens, as well as the potential for additive or synergistic effects with other agents, led to interferon alfa being studied in the adjuvant setting. There have been a number of trials that examined different doses and schedules of administration, as well as different types of interferons. Table 73-11 provides a summary of trials. The Eastern Cooperative Oncology Group (ECOG) reported positive results.

In January 1996, Kirkwood and colleagues published the results of the ECOG Trial 1684. This trial was the first randomized, controlled study to demonstrate a significant benefit of adjuvant therapy in melanoma. The patients were randomized to observation or treatment with interferon alfa 2-b. Patients were accrued between 1984 and 1990. The authors reported using high doses of interferon alfa 2-b (Intron-A, Schering Plough, Kenilworth, NJ) at 20 million units per square meter intravenously 5 days a week for an induction period of 4 weeks. This treatment was followed by maintenance dosing of 10 million units per square meter, given subcutaneously, three times per week for 48 weeks. A significant prolongation of relapse-free survival and a prolongation of overall survival were found with this treatment regimen. The increment in median disease-free survival (from 1 to 1.7 years) and overall survival (from 2.8 to 3.8 years) that results from this therapy is associated with a 42% improvement in the fraction of patients who were continuously disease free after treatment with interferon alfa 2-b compared with patients who were observed. Based on the results of this trial, the Food and Drug Administration (FDA) approved the first adjuvant therapy for patients with malignant melanoma at high risk for relapse.

Interferon alfa 2-b therapy was approved for use as an adjuvant to surgical therapy in patients that were free of disease (post surgery) but at high risk for systemic recurrence (Creagen, Dalton, Ahmann, Jung, Morton, & Langdon et al., 1995). These patients were those with lesions of Breslow

TABLE 73-11 Adjuvant INF-α-2 and γ in High-Risk T3-4/Node Plus Resected Melanoma (AJCC Stage IIB/II)

Cooperative Group/PI	Eligible Patients	N	Investigational Treatment	Significant Study Impact on DSF or OS
ECOG 1684/Kirkwood	T4, N1	287	INF-α-2b 20 MU/m2/d IV × 1 mo + 10 MU/m2 SC TIW for 11 mo	DFS (+) OS (+) at 7 years
NCCT 83-7052/Creagan	T3-4, N1	262	INF-α-2a 20 MU/m2/d IM TIW × 3 mo	DFS (−) OS (−) at 7 years
SWOG 8642/Meyskins	T3-4, N1	134	INF-γ 0.2 mg/d SC OD × 1 year	DFS (−) OS (−)
EORTC 18871/Kleeberg	T3-4, N1	800	INF-α-2a 1 MU/d SC OD × 1 year vs. INF-γ 0.2 mg/d SC OD × 1 year	Closed 1996
WHO #16/Casinelli	T3-4, N1	444	INF-α-2a 3 MU/d SC TIW × 3 years	DSF (±) at 22 mo. DFS (−) OS (−) at 39 mo.
ECOG 1690/Kirkwood	T4, N1	642	INF-α-2b 20 MU/m2/d IV × 1 mo + 10 MU/m2 SC TIW × 11 mo vs. 3 MU/d SC TIW × 2 years	Closed 6/1/95

Modified from Kassas, H. E. & Kirkwood, J. M. (1996). Adjuvant application of interferons. *Seminars in Oncology, 23*(6), 737-743.
PI, Principal investigator; *DFS,* disease-free survival; *OS,* overall survival; *SC,* subcutaneous injection; *IV,* intravenously; *OD,* once daily; *TIW,* 3 times a week; *MU,* million units; *mo,* month(s).

thickness >4.0 mm or patients with any Breslow thickness with primary or recurrent nodal involvement.

The toxicity from the regimen was significant, but tolerable, in the majority of study participants. Flulike or constitutional symptoms (i.e., fever, chills, myalgias, headache, malaise) were seen most frequently, but were transient. The myelosuppressive, hematologic, and biochemical hepatic toxicities were largely reversible upon discontinuation of the drug or with dose reduction of the interferon alfa 2-b treatment. Some constitutional and neurologic toxicities were seen that necessitated the discontinuation of therapy. The toxicities from the ECOG 1684 study are summarized in Table 73-12 (Kirkwood et al., 1996).

Although the use of interferon alfa 2-b has demonstrated improvement in relapse-free survival and overall survival, the toxicities experienced with the therapy have caused concern for physicians and patients. An analysis by Cole, Gelber, Kirkwood, Goldhirsch, Barylak, and Borden (1996) used quality-of-life-adjusted survival analysis (Quality-Adjusted Time Without Symptoms and Toxicity [Q-TWiST]) to evaluate the quality-of-life effects of adjuvant high-dose interferon alfa 2-b in patients with high-risk melanoma. The analysis was conducted using data from the ECOG 1684 study (Kirkwood et al., 1996) that randomized patients between high-dose interferon alfa 2-b therapy and observation. The authors reported that patients treated with interferon alfa 2-b had more quality-of-life adjusted time than the observation group. They concluded that, for patients with high-risk melanoma, the clinical benefits of high-dose interferon alfa 2-b can offset the toxic effects.

Other Biologic Approaches. Biologic response modifiers have been active agents in the treatment of melanoma. As previously discussed, interferon alfa 2-b is approved for use in the adjuvant setting. Other agents have been used in patients with melanoma. Interleukin-2 (IL-2), which is produced by lymphocytes, enhances their cytotoxic activity and increases the production of gamma interferon, tumor necrosis factor (TNF), and other cytokines. When IL-2 is incubated with lymphatic cells, they become lymphokine-activated killer (LAK) cells. LAK cells are cytotoxic to tumor cells. These cells are active in melanoma, renal cell carcinoma, and colon carcinoma. The trials by the National Cancer Institute using high-dose IL-2 and LAK cells in malignant melanoma have shown a 4% complete remission rate and an overall response rate of 21% (Ho, 1995). Tumor-infiltrated lymphocytes (TILs) are more potent than LAK cells in animal models. Tumor-infiltrated lymphocytes can be isolated selectively from the patient's tumor, grown in culture with IL-2, and then returned to the patient. There has been an overall response rate of 55% reported from the NCI studies (Dhawan & Kirkwood, 1995; Ho, 1995). Passive transfer immunity has been attempted using monoclonal antibodies against different melanoma surface antigens (Dhawan & Kirkwood, 1995).

TABLE 73-12 Toxic Events from ECOG 1684 N = 143

Type	Grade 1	2	3	4	5
Constitutional*	18	53	64	5	0
Myelosuppression	37	57	34	0	0
Hepatotoxicity	30	39	20	0	2
Neurologic	31	47	33	7	0
Worst grade/ patient	2	30	96	13	2

From Kirkwood, J. M., Strawderman, M. H., Ernstoff, M. S., Smith, T. J., Borden, E. C., & Blum, R. H. (1996). Interferon alfa 2-b adjuvant therapy of high-risk resected cutaneous melanoma: The Eastern Cooperative Oncology Group Trial EST 1684. *Journal of Clinical Oncology, 14*(1), 7-17.

*Worst grade of any constitutional toxicity, including fever, chill, and flulike symptoms: fatigue, malaise, diaphoresis.

Active Specific Immunotherapy. Active specific immunotherapy (ASI) (i.e., the use of tumor "vaccines") has been studied more in melanoma than in any other cancer. Vaccines attempt to stimulate the patient to reject his or her own tumor. The use of vaccines is based on the observation that serum from melanoma patients contained antibodies that reacted with antigens on autologous melanoma cells (Morton & Barth, 1996). Mitchell (1996) advocates the use of the term *therapeutic vaccines* when discussing the use of vaccines for the treatment of established cancers. This approach would help to avoid confusion with the use of prophylactic vaccines that are given to prevent viral infections. Cancer vaccines are made from attenuated whole cells, cell walls, specific antigens, or nonpathologic strains of living organisms (Morton & Barth, 1996). Little toxicity is associated with vaccine therapies, which is one of their biggest advantages. A number of different preparations are under investigation.

Autologous vaccines are made from the patient's own tumor cells. This approach is based on data that melanoma cells have antigens on their cell surface that are unique to the individual and not shared by other melanoma tumors.

A second type of preparation are allogeneic vaccines. A number of different subtypes of allogeneic vaccines have been studied in clinical trials. These subtypes include irradiated whole cells administered with BCG (bacillus *Calmette-Guérin*); viral oncolysates (virally transformed tumor cells); mechanical lysates (mechanically disrupted melanoma cells from two cell lines); extracts that are composed of antigens shed by cultured melanoma cell lines; and defined vaccines that include the use of gangliosides to stimulate IgM and IgG antibodies, as well as antiidiotype vaccines that rely on the property of a subset of antiantibodies to mimic a tumor antigen.

A third group of allogeneic vaccines are genetically engineered vaccines. A number of subtypes of genetically engineered vaccines exist, including cytokines that are genetically inserted into tumor cells. The cytokines with the most promise are GM-CSF, IL-2, IL-4, IL-7, and INF-γ. In addition, melanoma cells can be transduced with accessory molecules, such as B7 (which is normally found on macrophages where it helps with the interactions with helper T cells). Finally, synthetic peptide vaccines against melanoma are currently being developed (Jones & Mitchell, 1996; Mitchell, 1996).

In an attempt to increase the efficacy of melanoma vaccines, nonspecific adjuvants (such as BCG, DETOX, QS-21, or MF-59) or immunomodulators (such as cyclophosphamide, cimetidine, or indomethacin) have been added to the treatment regimen. These agents help counteract the tumor-associated immunosuppression induced by T suppressor cells. Adjuvants can enhance and often modify a patient's immune response to the vaccine by providing carriers, immune stimulants, and antigen targeting to particular cells or organs (Morton & Barth, 1996).

Currently, a number of clinical trials are underway to investigate the benefits of vaccine therapies. In the post-surgical adjuvant setting, the effects of therapeutic vaccines are being compared with high-dose interferon alfa 2-b. For patients with stage IV disease, a number of different vaccine types are being studied alone or in combination with chemotherapy (agents used include dacarbazine, cisplatin, BCNU, and tamoxifen) and other biologic agents such as interferon, GM-CSF, LAK cells, tumor-infiltrated leukocytes, and interleukin (Morton & Barth, 1996). Objective response rates of 20% to 25% have been seen in the vaccine studies. Unfortunately, no evidence of increased survival has emerged from these studies (Dhawan & Kirkwood, 1995; Mastrangelo et al., 1996).

Combination Therapy in the Adjuvant Setting. Interleukin-2 and INF-α-2 have been combined in a number of different doses and schedules. No responses were seen in patients treated with low-dose therapy. High-dose therapy produced responses but was associated with a significant increase in toxicity. Investigations continue into the optimal dose and schedule with acceptable adverse effects. As previously mentioned, studies of the effectiveness of combinations of INF-α-2 and vaccines are ongoing.

Chemotherapy

Single-Agent Therapy. Chemotherapy is used to treat metastatic malignant melanoma. Dacarbazine (DTIC) remains the most active agent used for melanoma to which all other treatment regimens are compared. It has an overall response rate of about 20% (Dhawan & Kirkwood, 1995; Lee, Betticher, & Thatcher, 1995; McClay & McClay, 1996).

Dacarbazine analogues have been synthesized recently. Temozolomide, which is an oral agent, has some advantages over DTIC. It does not depend on metabolic activation by the host. The drug has an excellent oral bioavailability. In a small trial of 60 patients, it produced an overall response rate of 21%, with three complete responses (CRs) and nine partial responses (PRs). All of the CRs were in patients with pulmonary metastasis (Lee, Betticher, & Thatcher, 1995; McClay & McClay, 1996).

Nitrosureas are considered to be the class of drugs used as second-line therapy. These agents include carmustine (BCNU), lomustine (CCNU), and fotemustine. The response rates seen range from 10% to 17%. These drugs are lipid soluble, have the ability to cross into the central nervous system tissue, and were hoped to have an effect on central nervous system metastasis. This hope has not been realized. However, results with fotemustine have been more encouraging, with an overall response rate of 24%.

Platinum analogues including cisplatin and carboplatinum have activity in melanoma. Response rates of up to 15% have been reported. A steep dose-response curve was noted, but even at higher doses, when response rates were better, the results were not durable.

Taxanes, which are derived from the yew tree, have also been used in melanoma. Both paclitaxel (Taxol) and docetaxel (Taxotere) are being investigated. Studies with Taxol, as a single agent, demonstrate response rates of 12% to 18%. Responses have also been seen in patients treated with Taxotere. The vinca alkaloids (i.e., vindesine and vinblastine) are also active in malignant melanoma. Response rates of about 20% have been reported.

Combination Chemotherapeutic Regimens. Combination chemotherapy has been used in a number of different series. It was hoped that synergistic interactions would improve outcomes. Improvements in response rates have been observed, but no improvement in survival has been seen with combination regimens.

The combination of DTIC, BCNU, cisplatin, and tamoxifen (DBDT) produces a 55% response rate. Tamoxifen seems to play a central role in this combination regimen. When it was removed from the combination regimen in a study by McClay, Mastrangelo, Sprandio, Bellet, and Berd (1989) because of the side effects of deep vein thrombosis (DVT) and pulmonary embolism (PE), the response rates fell to 10%. McClay and McClay (1996) reported that tamoxifen can modulate the sensitivity of tumor cells. Tamoxifen has been shown to enhance levels of transforming growth factor beta (TGF beta), which in turn can inhibit the growth of several cancer cell lines (Lee, Betticher, & Thatcher, 1995). A confirmatory study that reintroduced tamoxifen to the regimen saw an improvement in response rates to 52%.

Various combinations of chemotherapy that included tamoxifen have been studied in malignant melanoma. The use of DTIC, cisplatin, and tamoxifen at slightly different doses and schedules has yielded responses ranging from 13% to 28% in small trials of patients. A study of DTIC and tamoxifen, which used higher doses of tamoxifen, yielded mixed results, with responses ranging from 15% to 28%. Nathanson, Meelu, & Losada (1994) added megestrol to DTIC, BCNU, and cisplatin in a small trial of 16 patients and achieved a response rate of 47%.

Chemoimmunotherapy

A number of different studies have added biologic agents to active chemotherapeutic regimes. IL-2 and INF have been added between cycles of DTIC, BCNU, cisplatin, and tamoxifen. The overall response rate was 57%. Toxicities were substantial, requiring extended hospitalizations (18 days) during the treatment cycles.

Interferon alfa was added to DTIC, BCNU, cisplatin, and tamoxifen in three separate trials. Two trials reported no significant benefit with the addition of INF. The third study reported an overall response rate of 42%, with myelosuppression and fatigue being the predominant toxicities (McClay & McClay, 1996).

An analysis of the studies that combine chemotherapy with immunotherapy indicates that the sequence of administration is an important factor in determining response rates. Immunotherapy should be administered after chemotherapy (McClay & McClay, 1996).

Bone Marrow Transplantation

A steep dose-response curve has been noted with the use of alkylating agents. This observation sparked an interest in dose intensification with autologous bone marrow rescue. Trials have been conducted using melphalan, BCNU, thiotepa, DTIC, cyclophosphamide, and cisplatin either alone or in combination. An overall response rate of 53% was seen. However, results were not durable because sustained complete remissions and improvement in long-term survival were rarely seen (Lee, Betticher, & Thatcher, 1995).

Regional Limb Perfusion

Often, locoregional relapses are seen with cutaneous melanomas. Regional (hyperthermic) isolated limb perfusion (HILP) has been used for more than 30 years. The procedure can be done with or without hyperthermia. The rationale for regional treatment is to obtain a high drug concentration limited to the limb for a period of time, without exposing the rest of the body to the drug. This approach attempts to decrease the amount of systemic toxicity (Lee, Betticher, & Thatcher, 1995). The agents used include melphalan with or without biologic agents, TNF, and interferon-α. Hyperthermic isolated limb perfusion is useful in controlling unresectable locoregional recurrence when there is no evidence of systemic spread. Toxicities include the need for skin grafting, temporary paralysis, and leukopenia. A small number of patients have required amputation. Objective responses have been observed, without any increases in survival (Dhawan & Kirkwood, 1995; Lee, Betticher, & Thatcher, 1995).

Gene Therapy

Ho (1995) explains that gene transfer attempts to replace (transfect) defective genes with new genes. The objective is to place a functional new gene into a cell. A working delivery system called a *vector* is required to accomplish this objective. Possible vectors include viruses such as retroviruses and chemicals such as liposomes. These vectors are being investigated. The ultimate goal is to replace the defective oncogene or tumor suppressor gene that caused a benign cell to become a malignant cell. If these cells can be replaced or repaired, the cell might revert to being a normal cell once again. A number of problems stand in the way of the success of gene therapy. It is not likely that a normal gene copy can be delivered to every abnormal cell, and there is evidence to suggest that multiple genetic alterations exist in one malignant process. Currently, research is aimed at changing the genetic structure of the malignant cell so that it can be destroyed by the patient's own immune response, or by a drug or substance that kills the altered cell but spares the rest of the body.

TILs are being studied as vectors. Tumor-infiltrating lymphocytes are lymphoid cells that are found infiltrating a tumor after treatment with IL-2. Because TILs surround and infiltrate tumors, the opportunity to transfect them with genes that are noxious to the tumor cells was seen as a potential new type of cancer treatment. The genes are carried to the tumor to damage the tumor cells.

TNF is a normal human cell product that can destroy tumor cells. It has been used successfully in the laboratory when given to mice. However, humans cannot tolerate the amount of TNF that needs to be given to cause tumor regression (Ho, 1995). The TNF gene has been cloned and can be transfected into TILs with a retroviral vector. This work was begun at the National Institutes of Health by Rosenberg in 1991. The patients were treated with TILs alone or TILs plus IL-2. Patients who received IL-2 plus TILs did better. This study, with less than satisfactory results, demonstrated that it was possible to insert a cytokine gene into a tumor by way of TILs. Since that time, genes for IL-2, IL-4, TNF, and gamma interferon have been inserted into tumor cells and have led to tumor cell death. The research in this area is ongoing (Ho, 1995).

Radiation Therapy

Radiation therapy is used rarely as primary therapy for malignant melanoma. Mostly, it is used in the palliative setting when there is metastasis to the brain, spinal cord, or bones. Radiation therapy produces a 50% response rate for skin lesions and a 30% response rate for brain lesions (Dhawan & Kirkwood, 1995; Ho, 1995; Jenrette, 1996). Radiation may also be used for symptomatic nodal metastasis in sites not accessible to surgery (Dhawan & Kirkwood, 1995). Recent reports suggest that radiation therapy used as an adjuvant to surgery in patients with head and neck lesions produces good locoregional control (Ho, 1995; Jenrette, 1996).

ONCOLOGIC EMERGENCIES

The major oncologic emergency associated with melanoma is spinal cord compression due to epidural metastasis (Dhawan & Kirkwood, 1995). More than 95% of patients with spinal cord compression complain of progressive central or radicular back pain (Deitz & Flaherty, 1993; Glick & Glover, 1995). Pain is often aggravated by lying down, weight bearing, coughing, sneezing, or the Valsalva maneuver. The pain is often relieved by sitting (Glick & Glover, 1995).

Spinal cord compression requires immediate attention to prevent permanent loss of neurologic functioning. Symptoms can progress from mild sensory impairment to full motor loss.

NURSING MANAGEMENT

The medical management of the patient with melanoma varies widely based on the stage of the disease. The initial

TABLE 73-13 Standard of Care for the Patient Undergoing Incisional or Excisional Biopsy for Malignant Melanoma

Patient Problem and Outcomes	Nursing Interventions and Rationales	Patient Education Instructions
Anxiety Patient will: • Verbalize an understanding of the surgical procedure. • Express feelings of decreased anxiety. • Identify strategies to cope with anxiety.	1. Assess the patient's level of understanding of the surgical procedure. 2. Give the patient an opportunity to ask questions and verbalize concerns. 3. Determine which coping strategies the patient has used effectively in the past to decrease anxiety, and reinforce the use of these coping strategies. 4. Administer pharmacologic agents to decrease anxiety, if needed.	1. Use a diagram of the anatomy of the skin to explain the biopsy procedure. 2. Provide the patient with information about the preoperative routine: a. Diagnostic tests b. Anesthesiology consultation (if needed) c. Nothing by mouth after midnight (if needed) 3. Provide the patient with information about the postoperative plan of care: a. Pain management b. Wound care c. Drains, if needed d. Surgical incision
Pain Patient will experience optimal pain relief with minimal side effects.	1. Assess the pain intensity, using a 0-to-10 verbal rating scale, every 2-4 hours for the first 48 after surgery, then every 8 hours. 2. Administer analgesics as needed. Encourage around-the-clock use for the first 24 hours postoperatively. 3. Assess for analgesic side effects, and administer medications to prevent or treat the following: a. Nausea/gastrointestinal distress b. Constipation	1. Teach patients to report pain to their health care provider. 2. Teach the patient the importance of taking pain medication regularly to keep pain under control. 3. Instruct the patient not to drive or operate machinery for 24-48 hours postoperatively (if anesthesia or sedation given) and if taking narcotic/sedating medications.
Knowledge deficit Patient will verbalize an understanding of the purpose, benefits, and risks of the biopsy procedure.	1. Assess the patient's level of knowledge about the surgical procedure. 2. Assess the patient's fears and concerns about the biopsy procedure.	1. Explain the need for the biopsy procedure and associated activities: a. Blood work (if needed) b. Electrocardiogram (EKG), chest x-ray (CXR) (if needed) c. Anesthesia consultation (if needed) d. Intravenous (IV) insertion e. Nothing by mouth (NPO) after midnight 2. Describe postoperative care to the patient, including the following: a. Dressing/wound care b. Pain control c. Signs of wound infection or complications d. Activity level permitted e. Emergency contact phone numbers

biopsy of a suspicious lesion occurs most likely in the physician's office or ambulatory surgical setting. Patients who are undergoing their initial biopsy usually have little or no preoperative preparation, such as maintaining NPO status, blood work, and anesthesia. Biopsies are often performed in the office setting with local anesthesia.

Surgery

Patients with melanoma confirmed by biopsy may, depending on the depth of the lesion, require a local wide excision. This procedure is done to ensure that the surgical margins are free of disease in an attempt to control local recurrences. This procedure is most often

TABLE 73-14 Standard of Care for the Patient Experiencing a Local Wide Excision for Malignant Melanoma

Patient Problem and Outcomes	Nursing Interventions and Rationales	Patient Education Instructions
Anxiety Patient will: • Verbalize an understanding of the surgical procedure. • Express feelings of decreased anxiety. • Identify strategies to cope with anxiety.	1. Assess the patient's level of understanding of the surgical procedure. 2. Give the patient an opportunity to ask questions and verbalize concerns. 3. Determine which coping strategies the patient has used effectively in the past to decrease anxiety, and reinforce the use of these coping strategies. 4. Administer pharmacologic agents to decrease anxiety, if needed.	1. Use a diagram of the anatomy of the skin to explain the biopsy procedure. 2. Provide the patient with information about the preoperative routine: a. Diagnostic tests b. Anesthesiology consultation c. Nothing by mouth (NPO) after midnight d. Skin preparation (if needed) 3. Provide the patient with information about the postoperative plan of care: a. Pain management b. Wound care c. Drains, if needed d. Surgical incision
Pain Patient will experience optimal pain relief with minimal side effects.	1. Assess the pain intensity, using a 0-to-10 verbal rating scale, every 2-4 hours for the first 48 hours after surgery, then every 8 hours. 2. Administer analgesics as needed. Encourage around-the-clock use for the first 24 hours postoperatively. 3. Assess for analgesic side effects, and administer medications to prevent or treat the following: a. Nausea/gastrointestinal distress b. Constipation	1. Teach patients to report pain to their health care provider. 2. Teach the patient/significant other the importance of taking pain medication regularly to keep pain under control. 3. Instruct the patient not to drive or operate machinery for 24-48 hours postoperatively (if anesthesia or sedation given) and if taking narcotic/sedating medications.
Knowledge Deficit Patient will verbalize an understanding of the purpose, benefits, and risks of the surgical procedure.	1. Assess the patient's level of knowledge about the surgical procedure. 2. Assess the patient's fears and concerns about the biopsy procedure.	1. Explain the need for the biopsy procedure and associated activities: a. Blood work b. Electrocardiogram (EKG), chest x-ray (CXR) c. Anesthesia consultation d. Intravenous (IV) insertion e. NPO after midnight 2. Describe postoperative care to the patient, including the following: a. Dressing/wound care b. Pain control c. Signs of wound infection or complications d. Activity level permitted e. Emergency contact phone numbers

performed in the ambulatory surgical setting. This procedure may be performed at the same time as a lymph node dissection, if one is needed. Patients requiring a lymph node evaluation usually require hospitalization, with the length of stay dependent on the extent and location of the lymph node basin that is dissected. The plans of care for patients undergoing surgical procedures are summarized in Tables 73-13 through 73-15 (Miaskowski, 1991; Paice, 1991; Puleo & Luh, 1995).

TABLE 73-15 Standard of Care for the Patient Experiencing a Lymph Node Dissection for Malignant Melanoma

Patient Problem and Outcomes	Nursing Interventions and Rationales	Patient Education Instructions
Anxiety Patient will: • Verbalize an understanding of the surgical procedure. • Express feelings of decreased anxiety. • Identify strategies to cope with anxiety.	1. Assess the patient's level of understanding of the surgical procedure. 2. Give the patient an opportunity to ask questions and verbalize concerns. 3. Determine which coping strategies the patient has used effectively in the past to decrease anxiety, and reinforce the use of these coping strategies. 4. Administer pharmacologic agents to decrease anxiety, if needed. 5. Use nonpharmacologic approaches to reduce anxiety.	1. Use a diagram of the anatomy of the lymph system to explain the biopsy procedure. 2. Provide the patient with information about the preoperative routine: a. Diagnostic tests b. Anesthesiology consultation (if needed) c. Nothing by mouth (NPO) after midnight d. Skin preparation (if needed) 3. Provide the patient with information about the postoperative plan of care: a. Pain management b. Wound care c. Drains, if needed d. Surgical incision 4. Teach the patient alternative methods of anxiety reduction: a. Relaxation techniques b. Medication c. Imagery d. Deep breathing e. Music f. Distraction
Pain Patient will experience optimal pain relief with minimal side effects.	1. Assess pain intensity, using a 0-to-10 verbal rating scale every 2-4 hours for the first 48 hours after surgery, then every 8 hours. 2. Administer analgesics as needed. Encourage around-the-clock use for the first 24 hours postoperatively. 3. Assess for analgesic side effects and administer medications to prevent or treat the following: a. Nausea/gastrointestinal distress b. Constipation	1. Teach patients to report pain to their health care provider. 2. Teach the patient/significant other the importance of taking pain medication on a regular basis to keep pain under control. 3. Instruct the patient not to drive or operate machinery for 24-48 hours postoperatively (if anesthesia or sedation given) and if taking narcotic/sedating medications.

Adjuvant Interferon Therapy

Patients undergoing adjuvant therapy with interferon alfa 2-b are treated in the outpatient setting. The length of the therapy is 1 year, with a daily (5 days/week) induction schedule followed by patient-administered maintenance therapy. Nursing support throughout the course of therapy is crucial. Patients require monitoring on an ongoing basis throughout the year for side-effect management, dose modifications, and adherence issues. In fact, the first 4 months of maintenance therapy hold the highest drop out rate for patients (Kirkwood et al., 1996). It is extremely important to maintain contact with and support patients through this period, as well as through all phases of the treatment.

Patients or family members need to be instructed on the subcutaneous administration of interferon. These instructions need to include reconstitution techniques, drawing up the appropriate dose of medication, injection site selection, injection techniques, and appropriate disposal of needles and syringes.

A plan of care needs to be developed to address the management of side effects associated with adjuvant therapy. This plan of care is summarized in Table 73-16 (Bender, 1994; Haeuber, 1995; Intron A, 1996; Jassak, 1991; Rumsey, 1995).

Some patients/insurance carriers may opt to have the therapy given in the home setting. The same amount of pa-

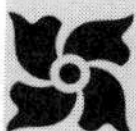

TABLE 73-15 Standard of Care for the Patient Experiencing a Lymph Node Dissection for Malignant Melanoma—cont'd

Patient Problem and Outcomes	Nursing Interventions and Rationales	Patient Education Instructions
Knowledge Deficit		
Patient will verbalize an understanding of the purpose, benefits, and risks of the lymph node dissection.	1. Assess the patient's level of knowledge about the surgical procedure. 2. Assess the patient's fears and concerns about the surgical procedure.	1. Explain the need for a biopsy procedure and associated activities: a. Blood work (if needed) b. Electrocardiogram (EKG), chest x-ray (CXR) (if needed) c. Anesthesia consultation (if needed) d. Intravenous (IV) insertion e. Lymphoscintigraphy f. Other scans g. NPO after midnight 2. Describe postoperative care to the patient and significant other, including the following: a. Dressing/wound care b. Drains c. Pain control d. Signs of wound infection or complications e. Activity level permitted f. Emergency contact phone numbers
High Risk for Lymphedema		
Patient will not experience postoperative lymphedema.	1. Assess the patient's level of knowledge of lymph system structure and function. 2. Assess the baseline condition of the extremity, including the following: a. Color b. Temperature c. Pulses d. Sensation e. Size (circumference measurement) f. Fit of clothing and jewelry g. Range of motion	1. Teach the patient the function of the lymph system. Use a diagram of the lymph system to illustrate. 2. Describe the surgical interruption in lymph flow and potential for lymphedema. 3. Teach the patient to avoid the following on the surgically affected extremity: a. Venipuncture, fingersticks b. Injections (including contrast dyes) c. Blood pressure checks d. Acupuncture e. Liposuction f. Prolonged dependent positioning 4. Instruct the patient to report signs of edema to the health care provider.

tient care is required if the treatment is given at home or in an outpatient setting.

Experimental Therapy

Vaccines are administered on an outpatient basis, in the context of a clinical trial. Follow-up and monitoring schedules are determined by the protocol and/or principal investigator. Other investigational therapies may require hospital stays for observation and monitoring.

Radiation Therapy

Radiation therapy can be administered on an outpatient basis, but because it is usually used in the palliative setting, decisions are made on a per patient basis as to the need for inpatient care.

Chemotherapy

Chemotherapy is administered to patients with stage IV (metastatic) disease or in the context of a clinical trial. The location and side effects of administration depend on the chemotherapeutic agents used, their doses, and their toxicities.

Skin Self-Examination

After a patient has been diagnosed with melanoma, his or her chances of developing additional melanotic lesions in-

Text continues on p. 1672

TABLE 73-16 Standard of Care for the Patient Receiving Adjuvant Interferon Alfa 2-b Therapy for Malignant Melanoma

Patient Problem and Outcomes	Nursing Interventions and Rationales	Patient Education Instructions
Knowledge Deficit Patient will verbalize an understanding of the purpose, benefits, and risks of adjuvant therapy.	1. Assess the patient's level of knowledge of the following: a. Biologic agents (interferon 2-b) b. Adjuvant treatment c. Disease process d. Immune system e. Benefits of therapy 2. Assess and address the patient's concerns and fears about adjuvant interferon therapy. 3. Provide printed materials concerning the planned therapy and to reinforce teaching.	1. Describe the rationale and plan for adjuvant therapy (i.e., induction and maintenance phases). 2. Describe the immune system and its functions. 3. Describe the major side effects associated with interferon alfa 2-b: a. Flulike syndrome b. Change in blood counts (white blood cells and platelets) c. Alteration in liver enzymes d. Depression e. Fatigue f. Alopecia
Knowledge Deficit Patient or family member will be able to administer injections required for maintenance therapy.	1. Assess the patient's/family's knowledge level about subcutaneous injections. 2. Assess the patient's/family's physical and emotional ability to learn and perform subcutaneous injection. 3. Allot adequate time to teach the patient/family. 4. Encourage the patient/family to voice questions and concerns, and address them appropriately. 5. Use video and audiotapes, as well as printed materials, to aide and reinforce teaching. 6. Inquire about/make arrangements for/assist with home drug and equipment procurement. (Patients may benefit from the use of prefilled syringes to decrease anxiety and the amount of teaching required.) 7. Home care consultation, if needed.	1. Explain the need for subcutaneous maintenance therapy. 2. Teach the patient/family member the steps involved in subcutaneous injections: a. Premedication with acetaminophen or ibuprofen b. Aseptic technique c. Reconstitution (interferon alfa 2-b comes in a variety of vial sizes and formulations) d. Drawing up the appropriate dose e. Choosing an appropriate injection site (arms, thighs, abdomen) f. Site preparation g. Injection h. Disposal of needles/syringes i. Monitoring of injection site j. Recording injection and site used k. Proper storage of medication (store at temperatures between 36° and 46° F [2° and 8° C]), keep refrigerated, store away from food, and keep out of reach of children 3. Have patient/family member demonstrate the injection technique.

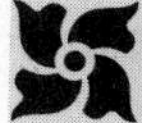

TABLE 73-16 Standard of Care for the Patient Receiving Adjuvant Interferon Alfa 2-b Therapy for Malignant Melanoma—cont'd

Patient Problem and Outcomes	Nursing Interventions and Rationales	Patient Education Instructions
Anxiety Patient will: • Verbalize an understanding of the planned treatment. • Express feelings of decreased anxiety. • Identify strategies to cope with anxiety.	1. Assess the patient's level of understanding of adjuvant therapy. 2. Give the patient an opportunity to ask questions and verbalize concerns. 3. Determine which coping strategies the patient has used effectively in the past to decrease anxiety, and reinforce the use of these coping strategies. 4. Administer pharmacologic agents to decrease anxiety (if needed). 5. Use nonpharmacologic approaches to reduce anxiety.	1. Provide the patient with a schedule for therapy administration and planned evaluations (i.e., blood tests). 2. Provide the patient with information about the administration routine: a. Time of appointments b. Length of infusion and drug administration c. Premedication schedule 3. Teach nonpharmacologic approaches to anxiety management: a. Relaxation techniques b. Deep-breathing exercises c. Imagery d. Distraction e. Music therapy f. Meditation 4. Encourage participation in support group activities.
Flulike Syndrome Patient will verbalize rationale for the occurrence of flulike symptoms, the need to take premedication, and strategies to deal with the syndrome.	1. Assess the baseline vital signs, including the following: a. Blood pressure b. Pulse c. Temperature d. Respirations 2. Administer acetaminophen or ibuprofen 30 minutes before interferon is given, and repeat in 4 hours prn. 3. Ensure adequate hydration is given either by intravenous or oral route. 4. Bedtime administration is suggested for the subcutaneous, maintenance phase. For the induction phase, the administration time should be planned to provide the patient with an opportunity to rest after receiving the infusion. 5. Layering of blankets, use of heating pads, or hot water bottles help to decrease shaking chills. 6. Massage therapy and/or warm baths can help alleviate myalgias. 7. Increase ambient room temperature. 8. Monitor temperature curves.	1. Inform the patient that almost all patients experience some side effects. 2. Teach the patient that side effects will diminish with continued use and time. 3. Explain reasons that flulike symptoms occur. 4. Teach the patient to monitor temperature. 5. Explain the rationale for bedtime administration (maintenance phase). 6. Provide rationale for rest following intravenous administration. 7. Teach the patient rationale for preventing dehydration. 8. Teach the patient that chills and rigors precede the onset of fever. 9. Inform the patient that myalgias and acute fatigue sometimes follow fevers. 10. Teach other techniques to assist the patient: a. Relaxation techniques b. Meditation c. Imagery d. Music e. Deep-breathing exercises f. Distraction

Continued

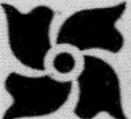

TABLE 73-16 Standard of Care for the Patient Receiving Adjuvant Interferon Alfa 2-b Therapy for Malignant Melanoma—cont'd

Patient Problem and Outcomes	Nursing Interventions and Rationales	Patient Education Instructions
Dehydration (High Risk For) Patient will maintain adequate hydration throughout the course of therapy.	1. Assess the baseline laboratory results: a. Blood urea nitrogen b. Creatinine c. Electrolytes d. Hemoglobin/hematocrit 2. Assess the baseline hydration status by physical examination: a. Mucous membranes b. Skin turgor c. Weight d. Vital signs 3. Encourage oral replacement with the following: a. Decaffeinated fluids b. Water c. Juice d. Sports drinks e. Decaffeinated sodas 4. Perform oral examination daily to assess for signs of dehydration (induction phase).	1. Instruct the patient to drink at least 2 liters of decaffeinated fluids/day. 2. Teach the patient signs/symptoms of dehydration: a. Dry mouth b. Thirst c. Dry skin d. Fatigue e. Lethargy f. Lassitude g. Constipation 3. Inform the patient that dehydration can worsen fatigue and activity intolerance. 4. Teach the rationale for maintaining hydration.
Fatigue (High Risk For) Patient will be able to maintain normal activities of daily living and engage in activities to enhance his/her quality of life.	1. Assess the level of fatigue using a 0 (not at all tired, full of pep) to 10 (total exhaustion) rating scale 2. Evaluate the patient's sleep and activity pattern to be able to teach the patient ways to conserve energy. 3. Provide opportunity for the patient to ask questions and verbalize concerns.	1. Inform the patient that he/she may experience acute fatigue following fevers. 2. Inform the patient that he/she may experience fatigue that may increase in intensity over the 12-month course of therapy. 3. Inform the patient that severe fatigue may require dose modifications, temporary interruptions, or discontinuation of therapy. 4. Suggest bedtime or evening administration (during the maintenance phase) that may allow the patient to sleep during the most severe fatigue. 5. Teach patient energy-conservation strategies, including the following: a. Establish a regular bed time. b. Try to get 8 hours of sleep. c. Take rest periods throughout the day. d. Exercise regularly throughout the day. e. Prioritize activities. f. Plan fewer activities for the day following an injection (maintenance phase). g. Delegate responsibilities to others when feeling fatigued. h. Eliminate nonessential, fatiguing activities. 6. Teach the patient that side effects, including fatigue, resolve with discontinuation of therapy. 7. Encourage adequate hydration. 8. Encourage journal keeping that can help identify the pattern of fatigue.

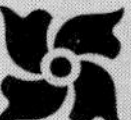

TABLE 73-16 Standard of Care for the Patient Receiving Adjuvant Interferon Alfa 2-b Therapy for Malignant Melanoma—cont'd

Patient Problem and Outcomes	Nursing Interventions and Rationales	Patient Education Instructions
Anorexia (High Risk For) Patient will maintain adequate caloric intake throughout the course of therapy.	1. Evaluate the nutritional status: a. Height/weight b. Laboratory values (serum albumin hemoglobin, hematocrit) c. Anthropometric measurements (arm muscle circumference, triceps skin fold thickness) 2. Obtain a history of food preferences, including the following: a. Lactose and other intolerances b. Cultural and religious preferences c. Allergies 3. Evaluate for coexisting conditions: a. Anxiety b. Depression c. Pain d. Anger e. Fatigue f. Nausea 4. Assess the oral cavity for evidence of the following: a. Poor dentition b. Misfitting dentures c. Stomatitis d. Infection e. Pain 5. Assess the ability to care for self and/or support systems in place for meal preparation and shopping. 6. Provide written and verbal information to the patient regarding nutrition.	1. Teach the patient to report the following: a. Decreased appetite b. Weight change c. Nausea/vomiting d. Diarrhea 2. Teach the patient elements of a nutritious diet. 3. Explain the rationale for the following: a. Routine oral care b. Using different food textures c. Controlling nausea d. Small, frequent meals e. Controlling pain f. Controlling anxiety g. Avoiding fried or fatty foods h. Rest before and after meals i. Adequate hydration j. Avoiding gas-producing foods k. Using high-protein snacks l. Reducing unpleasant environmental stimuli such as odors associated with food preparation, harsh noises, and extremes in temperature because they may interfere with eating 4. Use dietary supplements (if needed).
Nausea (High Risk For) Patient will be free from nausea throughout the course of therapy.	1. Obtain a dietary history, including the following: a. Lactose or other intolerances b. Cultural or religious preferences c. Allergies 2. Administer antiemetics as needed. 3. Consult with a dietitian if needed. 4. Evaluate for coexisting conditions: a. Anxiety b. Depression c. Pain d. Anger e. Fatigue 5. Assess the oral cavity for the following: a. Poor dentition b. Stomatitis c. Infection d. Pain e. Misfitting dentures	1. Explain to the patient that nausea, if it occurs, is usually mild and responds well to treatment. 2. Teach the patient to report nausea if it should occur. 3. Encourage the patient to eat small, frequent meals. 4. Encourage the patient to eat dry foods such as crackers, pretzels, and toast. 5. Encourage the patient to drink cool, decaffeinated fluids. 6. Encourage regular oral hygiene.

Continued

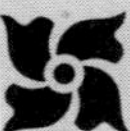

TABLE 73-16 Standard of Care for the Patient Receiving Adjuvant Interferon Alfa 2-b Therapy for Malignant Melanoma—cont'd

Patient Problem and Outcomes	Nursing Interventions and Rationales	Patient Education Instructions
Diarrhea (High Risk For) Patient will maintain adequate fluid balance, weight, and energy levels throughout the course of therapy.	1. Assess an elimination pattern, including the following: a. Frequency of stool b. Quality of stool c. Quantity of stool d. Baseline weight e. Baseline nutritional status 2. Initiate a low-residue diet if diarrhea begins: a. Limit foods high in roughage. b. Limit fried, fatty, or highly seasoned foods. c. Avoid uncooked fruits and vegetables. d. Limit rich foods (like desserts). 3. Administer antidiarrheal agents as needed. 4. Monitor weights. 5. Review current medications being taken by the patient (both prescribed and over the counter) to assess for contributing/coexisting causes of diarrhea.	1. Teach the patient to report any change in bowel habits. 2. Teach the patient to maintain a low-residue diet until diarrhea subsides and bowel habits return to normal. 3. Teach the patient to increase fluid intake (with decaffeinated fluids) to compensate for fluid loss through diarrhea. 4. Teach the patient the correct use of antidiarrheal agents (both over-the-counter and prescription products). 5. Instruct the patient to report weight loss.
Altered Taste (High Risk For) Patient will maintain an adequate caloric intake throughout the course of therapy.	1. Baseline oral examination with attention to the presence of the following: a. Infection b. Stomatitis c. Poor hygiene/dentition d. Obvious caries e. Misfitting denture 2. Baseline nutritional assessment: a. Weight b. Dietary habits c. Anthropomorphic measurements d. Laboratory values (serum albumin, hemoglobin) 3. Monitor weights.	1. Teach the patient to report any change in taste because it might lead to decreased oral intake and weight loss. 2. Encourage experimentation with different seasonings, such as the following: a. Salt b. Lemon c. Vanilla d. Cinnamon e. Marinades 3. Cold foods may be more appealing. 4. Lemon drops, gum, and/or mints may mask the metallic or bitter taste. 5. Teach the patient that side effects resolve with discontinuation of therapy.
Depression (High Risk For) Patient will: • Be able to identify feelings of depression. • Be able to verbalize feelings of depression and seek appropriate care.	1. Assess the baseline mental status and existence of preexisting psychiatric conditions such as depression, which may be a contraindication to adjuvant therapy. 2. Obtain a history concerning the use of the following: a. Tranquilizers b. Sedatives c. Narcotics d. Alcohol As concomitant use may exacerbate depression/altered mental function.	1. Teach the patient that depression and altered mental function can be a side effect of adjuvant interferon alfa 2-b therapy. 2. Encourage the patient/family to be alert for subtle changes in function and mood. 3. Encourage the patient to organize activities, create routines, and keep lists of activities to be performed. 4. Encourage rest periods, with naps as needed.

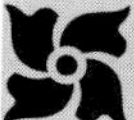

TABLE 73-16 Standard of Care for the Patient Receiving Adjuvant Interferon Alfa 2-b Therapy for Malignant Melanoma—cont'd

Patient Problem and Outcomes	Nursing Interventions and Rationales	Patient Education Instructions
Depression (High Risk For)—cont'd		
	3. Obtain a history of prior antidepressant use. 4. Provide the patient an opportunity to ask questions and verbalize concerns. 5. Administer antidepressants if prescribed. 6. Obtain a psychiatric/counseling consultation as indicated. 7. Establish rapport with the patient/family so that they feel comfortable reporting changes.	5. Encourage the use of antidepressants, if prescribed. 6. Teach the patient the importance of taking antidepressants as prescribed to maintain the proper blood levels, thereby increasing effectiveness. 7. Encourage the patient/family to report changes in mood/affect as they occur. 8. Encourage participation in support group activities. 9. Teach patients that dose modifications may be needed as a result of depression. 10. Teach the patient that side effects resolve with the discontinuation of therapy.
Altered Thought Processes (High Risk For)		
Patient will be able to maintain independence and optimal functioning throughout the course of therapy.	1. Assess the baseline level of functioning. 2. Give the patient the opportunity to ask questions and verbalize concerns. 3. Assess for the use of concomitant medications that can exacerbate altered thought processes: a. Tranquilizers b. Sedatives c. Narcotics d. Alcohol	1. Teach the patient that alteration in thought processes is a side effect of interferon therapy. 2. Encourage the patient to do the following: a. Organize activities b. Create routines c. Make lists of activities to be performed 3. Encourage the patient to identify and consequently seek help with areas identified as problems, for example the following: a. Numeric equations b. Measurements c. Calculations 4. Teach the patient that side effects resolve with discontinuation of therapy. 5. Explain to the patient the importance of reporting these side effects. 6. Teach the patient that dose modifications may be needed to control this side effect.
Leukopenia (High Risk For)		
Patient will: • Remain free from infection for the course of therapy. • Receive appropriate dose reductions for leukopenia throughout the course of therapy.	1. Baseline history, including the following: a. Use of immunosuppressive drugs b. Past use of chemotherapeutic agents c. Past use of radiation therapy 2. Baseline physical examination with attention to possible sites of the following: a. Current infections b. Chronic infections c. Potential infections 3. Obtain a CBC at the following: a. Baseline b. Weekly during induction c. Monthly during maintenance 4. Make appropriate dose modifications for leukopenia.	1. Explain the rationale for monitoring the complete blood count (CBC): a. Weekly during induction phase b. Monthly during maintenance phase 2. Teach the patient the signs and symptoms of infection and to report them if they should occur 3. Teach the patient that a decrease in the white blood cell (WBC) count may require a dose reduction, or temporary interruption, of therapy.

Continued

TABLE 73-16 Standard of Care for the Patient Receiving Adjuvant Interferon Alfa 2-b Therapy for Malignant Melanoma—cont'd

Patient Problem and Outcomes	Nursing Interventions and Rationales	Patient Education Instructions
Elevation in Liver Enzymes (High Risk For)		
Patient will have appropriate dose modifications for altered liver enzymes throughout the course of therapy.	1. Obtain a medication history, including prescription and/or over-the-counter medication and alcohol use. 2. Obtain liver function tests (SGPT/SGOT or ALT/AST) at the following: a. Baseline b. Weekly during induction phase c. Monthly during maintenance phase 3. Make appropriate dose modifications for elevated liver function tests.	1. Teach the patient to report all the medications that he/she takes during the course of therapy. 2. Teach the patient the function of the liver and why it is important to monitor its function on an ongoing basis: a. Weekly during induction phase b. Monthly during maintenance phase 3. Explain to the patient that dose modifications and/or interruptions in therapy may be needed for changes in liver function tests.
Alopecia (High Risk For)		
Patient will verbalize strategies to deal with alopecia (hair thinning) if it occurs.	1. Provide the patient with a list of local establishments that sell cranial prostheses (wigs). 2. Provide information on local American Cancer Society "Look Good Feel Good" programs. 3. Provide time for the patient to ask questions and voice concerns.	1. Teach the patient that alopecia may occur but most patients most often experience a thinning of the hair. 2. Teach patients alternatives to wigs: a. Hats b. Scarves c. Turbans 3. Teach the patient to minimize loss by avoiding the following: a. Excessive brushing b. Dyes c. Permanents d. Hot rollers 4. Inform the patient that hair loss is temporary and that hair will regrow after therapy is completed.

crease. To achieve early detection and treatment of suspicious lesions, patients and families need to be taught to perform skin self-examination regularly. These procedures are summarized in Table 73-17.

HOME CARE ISSUES

Patient care issues in the home care setting depend on the type of surgical management chosen, the type of therapy administered, and the stage of the patient's disease.

Surgical Care

Postoperative patient care is summarized in Tables 73-13 through 73-15. Universally, patients who undergo surgical procedures need nursing care in the areas of pain control, wound care, and education. Some patients might be discharged with drains in place, requiring additional attention.

Adjuvant Interferon Therapy

Some patients and/or their insurance carriers are opting for the induction phase of adjuvant therapy with interferon alfa 2-b to be administered in the home. The nursing care for the patient receiving adjuvant therapy is summarized in Table 73-16.

The maintenance phase of adjuvant therapy requires that patients or a family member learn how to administer a subcutaneous injection. The patients receive subcutaneous injections three times a week for 11 months. Home care agencies may be consulted to continue teaching and monitor the injections in the home. Side effect management and psychosocial support are critical during the maintenance phase of therapy.

Chemotherapy

Chemotherapy is used most often in patients with metastatic disease and has disappointing response rates. The care and

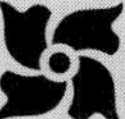

TABLE 73-17 Standard of Care for Patients to Improve Prevention/Early Detection of Malignant Melanoma

Patient Problem and Outcomes	Nursing Interventions and Rationales	Patient Education Instructions
Knowledge Deficit Patient will: • Verbalize an understanding of the purpose and benefits of skin self-examination • Be able to perform skin self-examination independently.	1. Assess the patient's knowledge level about skin self-examination. 2. Assess the patient's fears and concerns surrounding skin self-examination. 3. Allow time for questions, and proceed at the patient's pace. 4. Provide written materials to reinforce teaching. 5. Perform a demonstration skin examination with the patient, and watch a return demonstration.	1. Explain the need to perform skin self-examination. 2. Teach the patient the equipment needed to perform the examination: a. Full-length mirror b. Hand-held mirror c. Hand-held blow dryer d. Two chairs e. Well-lit room 3. Explain the step-by-step procedure to the patient: a. Gather equipment. b. Undress completely. c. Inspect palms, fingers, and spaces between fingers and forearms. Repeat with palms up and palms down. d. In front of a full-length mirror, look at the backs of the forearms and elbows. e. Inspect the entire front, starting at the head, and taking each part in turn, inspect closely. f. Inspect the right side in a full-length mirror, lifting the arm to inspect underneath. Repeat on the left. g. With the back toward the mirror, inspect the buttocks, backs of the thighs, and lower legs. h. Using a hand-held mirror and full-length mirror, inspect the back of the neck, the back, and buttocks. (This can be difficult, and you may ask for the assistance of a spouse or significant other.) i. Use the hand-held mirror and full-length mirror to look at the scalp. You may also use the hand-held dryer, set on cool, to lift hair from the scalp. (This can be difficult, and you may ask for the assistance of a spouse or significant other.) j. Sit on one chair and use the other to prop up your leg. Begin in the groin area, using the hand-held mirror, and inspect all the way down to the foot. Repeat on the opposite leg. k. While sitting, use a hand-mirror to examine the top of your foot, between the toes, the toes, and toenails. Repeat on the other foot. Record findings, and date. 4. Teach patient the ABCDs of early detection: a. Asymmetry: irregular in shape b. Borders: uneven or irregular borders c. Color: contain many shades of brown or black, or a change in color d. Diameter: often larger than 6 mm (about the size of a pencil eraser), a noted change in size of a lesion 5. Encourage regular examinations by a health care professional.

Continued

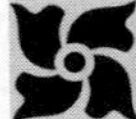

TABLE 73-17 Standard of Care for Patients to Improve Prevention/Early Detection of Malignant Melanoma—cont'd

Patient Problem and Outcomes	Nursing Interventions and Rationales	Patient Education Instructions
Knowledge Deficit Patient will: • Understand the risks of ultraviolet (UV) light exposure in relation to melanoma. • Verbalize five strategies to limit UV light exposure.	1. Examine current UV light exposure patterns and protective mechanisms used. 2. Provide the patient with printed material concerning UV light exposure. 3. Provide adequate teaching time, with an allotted space for questions. 4. Proceed at the patient's pace. 5. Address the patient's fears and concerns.	1. Teach the patient the correlation between UV light and melanoma development. 2. Instruct the patient to limit exposure by doing the following: a. Avoiding the strongest rays in the hours between 10 AM and 3 PM b. Using canopies, such as umbrellas, tents, and trees c. Wearing wide-brimmed hats d. Wearing long-sleeved shirts and long pants e. Always using sunscreens with a sun-protection formula (SPF) of 15 or higher on exposed skin f. Properly using and applying sunscreens: • Apply at least 20 minutes before sun exposure. • Use adequate amounts of sunscreen, and reapply frequently. • Use special preparations for infants and children. g. Avoiding the use of tanning beds and sun lamps h. Being aware that water has a cooling effect and reflective properties that may increase exposure i. Realizing it is possible to burn in the winter and that snow reflects sunlight

issues surrounding this therapy are based on which one of the many drug regimens is chosen for the patient, as well as the sites and extent of metastatic disease. If curative therapy fails, the patient may require palliative radiation for symptom management, as well as supportive care and comfort measures.

Available Resources

A number of organizations have educational and supportive resources available to patients and families.

PROGNOSIS

The prognosis for melanoma varies widely with the stage and extent of the disease. The most important of the prognostic indicators is tumor thickness (Barnhill, Fine, Roush, & Berwick, 1996; Urist, 1996). Table 73-18 shows survival rates based on primary tumor thickness alone. Additional prognostic variables have been identified, but their significance is not always agreed upon. Table 73-19 incorporates a number of different prognostic variables such as ulceration, gender, Clark's level, and anatomic site. A review article by Garrison and Nathanson (1996) addresses several prognostic issues that are identified in Table 73-20.

TABLE 73-18 Survival Rates by Primary Tumor Thickness

Primary Tumor Thickness	5-Year Survival Rates	10-Year Survival Rates
≤0.74 mm	95%	92%
0.75-1.4 mm	85%	76%
1.5-3.9 mm	66%	58%
≥4.0 mm	46%	38%

From Garrison, M. & Nathanson, L. (1996). Prognosis and staging in melanoma. *Seminars in Oncology, 23*(6), 726.

Cutaneous melanoma that has metastasized beyond the confines of regional lymph nodes remains an incurable

TABLE 73-19 Predicted Survival Rates from Initial Diagnosis for Patients with Localized Melanoma as Calculated by a Computerized Model of Multiple Prognostic Factors

Tumor Thickness (mm)	Anatomic Site	Ulceration	Clark's Level	Gender	5-Year Survival Rate (%)	10-Year Survival Rate (%)
<0.76						
	Extremity	—	II	—	99	97
	Extremity	—	other	—	97	94
	Axial	—	II	—	96	92
	Axial	—	other	—	91	84
0.76-1.49						
	Extremity	No	II	—	98	97
	Extremity	No	other	—	93	89
	Extremity	Yes	II	—	94	91
	Extremity	Yes	other	—	82	72
	Axial	No	II	—	95	93
	Axial	No	other	—	85	77
	Axial	Yes	II	—	88	81
	Axial	Yes	other	—	64	49
1.5-2.49						
	Extremity	No	—	—	86	81
	Extremity	Yes	—	—	76	69
	Axial	No	—	—	76	67
	Axial	Yes	—	—	61	49
2.50-3.99						
	Extremity	No	—	Female	80	72
	Extremity	No	—	Male	73	62
	Extremity	Yes	—	Female	74	64
	Extremity	Yes	—	Male	64	51
	Axial	No	—	Female	73	63
	Axial	No	—	Male	63	51
	Axial	Yes	—	Female	65	52
	Axial	Yes	—	Male	53	39
4.0-7.99						
	—	No	II/III	—	80	73
	—	No	IV/V	—	68	58
	—	Yes	II/III	—	67	57
	—	Yes	IV/V	—	51	38
>8.00						
	—	—	—	—	43	25

Modified from Urist, M. (1996). Surgical management of primary cutaneous melanoma. *CA: A Cancer Journal for Clinicians, 46*(4), 219-224.

TABLE 73-20 Other Prognostic Factors for Malignant Melanoma

Prognostic Factor	Outcome
Ulceration	
Present	Poor prognosis
Absent	Better prognosis
Histologic type	
Lentigo maligna (LM)	Best prognosis
Superficial spreading (SSM)	Intermediate prognosis
Nodular melanoma (NM)	Poorer than SSM
Acral lentiginous melanoma (ALM)	Although the least common, it has the poorest outcome
Location of Lesion	
Lower arm, lower leg, and thigh	More favorable prognosis
Thorax, upper arm, scalp, and neck (including ear)	Relatively high risk for death at 10 years
	Especially poor prognosis

Prognostic Factor	Outcome
Lymph Nodes Involvement	
One positive node	40% 10-year survival
Two to four positive nodes	26% 10-year survival
Five or more positive nodes	15% 10-year survival
Age	
Younger age	Better prognosis
Older age	Worse prognosis
Gender	
Females	Better prognosis
Males	Worse prognosis

TABLE 73-21 Quality of Care Evaluation for a Patient Receiving Adjuvant Interferon Therapy for Malignant Melanoma

Disciplines participating in the quality of care evaluation:

☐ Nursing	☐ Social Services
☐ Home Care	☐ Medical Oncology
☐ Surgical Oncology	☐ Other

I. Preadjuvant Therapy Evaluation

Data from:

☐ Medical Record Review ☐ Patient/Family Interview

Criteria	Yes	No
1. Patient provided with information about the following:		
a. Melanoma	☐	☐
b. Treatment plan	☐	☐
c. Risks and benefits of treatment	☐	☐
d. Alternative treatments (experimental therapies/clinical trials)	☐	☐
e. Support available during therapy	☐	☐
2. Pretreatment evaluation:		
a. Complete blood count	☐	☐
b. Blood chemistries (electrolytes, liver function tests, thyroid stimulating hormone (TSH)	☐	☐
c. Electrocardiogram (EKG) (for patients with preexisting cardiac abnormalities)	☐	☐
d. Chest x-ray (CXR)	☐	☐
3. Patient/family taught to self-administer medication through subcutaneous route, including the following:		
a. Aseptic technique	☐	☐
b. Handwashing	☐	☐
c. Premedication	☐	☐
d. Drawing up proper dose of interferon	☐	☐
e. Choosing an injection site	☐	☐
f. Site preparation	☐	☐
g. Rotation of injection site	☐	☐
h. Proper disposal of needle/syringe	☐	☐
i. Recording injection information	☐	☐
j. Proper storage of medication at home and during travel	☐	☐
k. Reporting of side effects to health care professional	☐	☐
l. Emergency phone numbers	☐	☐
4. Ongoing evaluations:		
a. Weekly CBC and chemistries during induction	☐	☐
b. Monthly CBC and chemistries during maintenance	☐	☐
5. Patient experienced the following complications:		
a. Incorrect dosing of interferon	☐	☐
b. Incorrect/no medication regimen	☐	☐
c. Used incorrect/inappropriate injection site	☐	☐
d. Injection site infection	☐	☐
e. Incorrect storage of medication	☐	☐

II. Patient/Family Satisfaction

Data from:

☐ Patient Interview ☐ Family Interview

Criteria	Yes	No
1. On a scale of 0 to 10, with 0 being totally dissatisfied and 10 being totally satisfied, how satisfied were you with the preparation to receive adjuvant interferon therapy? ________		
2. Were you given printed materials concerning the following:		
a. Melanoma	☐	☐
b. Self-injection techniques	☐	☐
c. Side-effect management	☐	☐
d. Proper storage and handling of the interferon	☐	☐
e. Emergency phone numbers	☐	☐

disease (Barth, Wanek, & Morton, 1995; Garrison & Nathanson, 1996). After the disease has metastasized, the prognosis depends on a number of variables such as the initial site of metastasis, disease-free interval before metastasis, and the stage of disease before distant metastasis. The median survival time reported for 1521 patients was 7.5 months (Barth, Wanek, & Morton, 1995).

EVALUATION OF THE QUALITY OF CARE

Accreditation organizations, such as the Joint Commission for the Accreditation of Health Care Organizations, require that the quality of care provided to patients be evaluated. Patients with melanoma who require adjuvant immunotherapy with interferon receive treatment for 1 year. The care that they receive requires input from many different disciplines. Table 73-21 provides an evaluation tool that can be used to assess this aspect of care.

RESEARCH ISSUES

Melanoma is a disease for which research in the medical and nursing fields is ongoing. Many areas are being investigated, including the use of primary prevention techniques before diagnosis and public awareness campaigns. Surgical treatment and the use of sentinel lymph node dissection is an exciting new approach to the surgical management of melanoma patients. As discussed in the medical management section, multiple avenues are being examined as treatment options, such as combination biotherapy, gene transfer therapy, and vaccines. The treatment of metastatic disease continues to be a challenge that is being investigated in a number of different ways, including combination chemotherapy, chemoimmunotherapy, and bone marrow transplantation.

Work is being done to identify tumor markers for malignant melanoma. The ability to detect levels of these markers in the blood would be an advantage when following adjuvant patients for indications of relapse.

As these new therapies emerge, nursing studies are needed to evaluate the most appropriate and beneficial ways to administer cost effective but quality patient care. As new modalities are used, nursing is faced with the investigation of new and unique patient-management techniques. Nursing is challenged with providing quality care with fewer resources. The determination of new intervention techniques should be evaluated in the context of nursing clinical trials.

REFERENCES

American Cancer Society. *Understanding melanoma.* Atlanta: American Cancer Society.

Balch, C. M., Houghton, A. N., & Peters, L. J. (1993). Cutaneous melanoma. In V. T. DeVita, S. Hellman, & S. A. Rosenberg (Eds.), *Cancer: Principles and practice of oncology* (4th ed.). Philadelphia: J. B. Lippincott.

Ball, A. S. & Thomas, J. (1995). Surgical management of malignant melanoma. *British Medical Bulletin, 51*(3), 584-608.

Barnhill, R. L., Fine, J. A., Roush, G. C., & Berwick, M. (1996). Predicting five-year outcome for patients with cutaneous melanoma in a population-based study. *Cancer, 78*(3), 427-432.

Baron, P. L. (1996). The surgical management of melanoma: From diagnosis to local treatment. *Seminars in Oncology, 23*(6), 714-718.

Barth, A., Wanek, L. A., & Morton, D. L. (1995). Prognostic factors in 1,521 melanoma patients with distant metastases. *Journal of the American College of Surgeons, 181*(3), 193-201.

Beahers, O. H., Henson, D. E., & Hutter, R. V. (Eds.). (1992). *American Joint Committee on Cancer: Staging manual for staging cancer* (4th ed.). Philadelphia: J. B. Lippincott.

Bender, C. M. (1994). Cognitive dysfunction associated with biological response modifier therapy. *Oncology Nursing Forum, 21*(3), 515-523.

Buzaid, A. C. & Balch, C. M. (1996). Polymerase chain reaction for detection of melanoma in peripheral blood: Too early to assess clinical value. *Journal of the National Cancer Institute, 88*(9), 569-570.

Cannon-Albright, L. A., Kamb, A., & Skolnick, M. (1996). A review of inherited predisposition to melanoma. *Seminars in Oncology, 23*(6), 667-672.

Char, C. H. (1994). Primary ocular melanomas. In F. J. Lejeune, P. K. Chaudhuri, & T. K. DasGupta (Eds.), *Malignant melanoma: Medical and surgical management.* New York: McGraw-Hill.

Chen, Y., Dubrow, R., Holford, T. R., Zheng, T., Barnhill, R., Fine, J., & Berwick, M. (1996). Malignant melanoma risk factors by anatomic site: A case-control study and polychotomous logistic regression analysis. *International Journal of Cancer, 67,* 636-643.

Clark, W. H., Elder, E. D., & Guerry, D. (1984). The precursor lesions of superficial spreading and nodular melanoma. *Human Pathology, 15,* 1147.

Clark, W. H., Jr., Reimer, R. R., Greene, M., Ainsworth, A. M., & Mastrangelo, M. J. (1978). Origin of familial malignant melanomas from heritable melanocytic lesions. 'The B-K mole syndrome.' *Archives of Dermatology, 114*(5), 732-738.

Cole, B. F., Gelber, R. D., Kirkwood, J. M., Goldhirsch, A., Barylak, E., & Borden, E. (1996). Quality-of-life adjusted survival analysis of interferon alfa-2b adjuvant treatment of high-risk resected cutaneous melanoma: An Eastern Cooperative Oncology Group Study. *Journal of Clinical Oncology, 14*(10), 2666-2673.

Cole, D. J. & Baron, P. J. (1996). Surgical management of patients with intermediate thickness melanoma: Current role of elective lymph node dissection. *Seminars in Oncology, 23*(6), 719-724.

Creagen, E. T., Dalton, R. J., Ahmann, D. L., Jung, S. H., Morton, R. F., Langdon, R. M., Kugler, J., & Rodrigue, L. J. (1995). Randomized, surgical adjuvant clinical trial of recombinant interferon alfa 2-a in selected patients with malignant melanoma. *Journal of Clinical Oncology, 13*(11), 2776-2783.

Darrow, T. L., Abdel-Wahab, Z., & Seigler, H. (1995). Immunotherapy of human melanoma with gene-modified tumor cell vaccines. *Cancer Control,* September/October, 415-421.

Dhawan, M. & Kirkwood, J. M. (1995). Melanoma therapy: A status report. *Contemporary Oncology,* Winter, 16-23.

Dietz, K. A. & Flaherty, A. M. (1993). Oncologic emergencies. In S. L. Groenwald, M. H. Frogge, M. Goodman, & C. H. Yarbro (Eds.), *Cancer nursing principles and practice* (3rd ed.). Boston: Jones and Bartlett.

Elwood, J. M. (1996). Melanoma and sun exposure. *Seminars in Oncology, 23*(6), 650-666.

Farmer, K. C. & Naylor, M. F. (1996). Sun exposure, sunscreens and skin cancer prevention: a year-round concern. *The Annals of Pharmacotherapy, 30,* 662-672.

Fidler, I. J. (1995). Melanoma metastasis. *Cancer Control,* September/October, 398-404.

Fountain, J. W., Karayiorgou, M., & Ernstoff, M. (1992). Homozygous deletions within human chromosome band 9p21 in melanoma. *Proceedings of the National Academy of Science, 89,* 10557-10561.

Friedman, R. J., Rigel, D. S., Silverman, M. K., Kopf, A. W., & Vossaert, K. A. (1991). Malignant melanoma in the 1990s: The continued importance of early detection and the role of physician examination and self-examination of the skin. *CA: A Cancer Journal for Clinicians, 41,* 302-226.

Garrison, M. & Nathanson, L. (1996). Prognosis and staging in melanoma. *Seminars in Oncology, 23*(6), 725-733.

Gattoni-Celli, S. & Cole, D. J. (1996). Melanoma-associated tumor antigens and their clinical relevance to immunotherapy. *Seminars in Oncology, 23*(6), 754-758.

Glick, J. H. & Glover, D. (1995). Oncologic emergencies. In G. P. Murphy, W. Lawrence, & R. E. Lenhard (Eds.), *Clinical oncology* (2nd ed.). Atlanta: American Cancer Society.

Glocker-Reis, L. A., Miller, B. A., & Hankey, B. F. (Eds.). (1994). *SEER cancer statistics review, 1973-1991. Tables and graphs* (NIH Publication No. 94-2789). Bethesda, Maryland: National Cancer Institute.

Greene, M. H., Clark, W. H., & Tucker, M. A. (1980). Precursor naevi in cutaneous malignant melanoma: A proposed nomenclature. *Lancet, 2,* 1024.

Grin, C. S., Rigel, D. S., & Friedman, R. J. (1992). Worldwide incidence of malignant melanoma. In C. M. Balch (Ed.), *Cutaneous melanoma.* Philadelphia: J. B. Lippincott.

Haeuber, D. (1995). The flu-like syndrome. In P. T. Rieger (Ed.), *Biotherapy: A comprehensive overview.* Boston: Jones and Bartlett.

Halaban, R. (1996). Growth factors and melanomas. *Seminars in Oncology, 23*(6), 673-681.

Hill, D., White, V., & Marks, R. (1992). Melanoma prevention: Behavioral and nonbehavioral factors in sunburn among an Australian urban population. *Preventive Medicine, 21,* 654-669.

Ho, R. C. S. (1995). Medical management of stage IV malignant melanoma. *Cancer, 75*(2), 735-741.

Intron A [Interferon alfa 2-b, recombinant] for injection. Product Information Sheet 7/96. Kenilworth, NJ: Schering Corporation.

Jassak, P. F. (1991). Knowledge deficit related to biotherapy. In J. C. McNally, E. T., Somerville, C. Miaskowski, & M. Rostad (Eds.), *Guidelines for oncology nursing practice.* Philadelphia: W. B. Saunders.

Jenrette, J. M. (1996). Malignant melanoma: The role of radiation therapy revisited. *Seminars in Oncology, 23*(6), 759-762.

Jones, V. E. & Mitchell, M. S. (1996). Therapeutic vaccines for melanoma: Progress and problems. *Trends in Biotechnology, 14,* 349-355.

Kamp, A., Gruis, N. A., & Weaver-Feldhaus, J. (1994). A cell cycle regulator potentially involved in genesis of many tumor types. *Science, 264,* 436-440.

Kassas, H. E. & Kirkwood, J. M. (1996). Adjuvant application of interferons. *Seminars in Oncology, 23*(6), 737-743.

Keller, J. M. & Maize, J. C. (1996). The clinical and histological differential diagnosis of malignant melanoma. *Seminars in Oncology, 23*(6), 693-702.

Ketcham, M. & Loescher, L. J. (1993). Skin cancers. In S. L. Groenwald, M. H. Frogge, M. Goodman, & Yarbro, C. H. (Eds.), *Cancer nursing principles and practice.* Boston: Jones and Bartlett.

Kirkwood, J. M., Strawderman, M. H., Ernstoff, M. S., Smith, T. J., Borden, E. C., & Blum, R. H. (1996). Interferon alfa 2-b adjuvant therapy of high-risk resected cutaneous melanoma: The Eastern Cooperative Oncology Group Trial EST 1684. *Journal of Clinical Oncology, 14*(1), 7-17.

Koh, H. J. (1991). Cutaneous melanoma. *New England Journal of Medicine, 325,* 171-182.

Koh, H. K. & Geller, A. C. (1995). Melanoma and skin cancer control: An international perspective. *Cancer Control,* September/October, 385-391.

Koh, J., Enders, G. H., & Dynlacht, B. D. (1995). Tumor derived p16 alleles encoding proteins defective in cell-cycle regulation. *Nature, 375,* 507-510.

Landis, S. H., Murray, T., Bolden, S., & Wingo, P. A. (1998). Cancer statistics, 1998. *CA: A Cancer Journal for Clinicians, 48,* 6-29.

Lee, S. M., Betticher, D. C., & Thatcher, N. (1995). Melanoma: Chemotherapy. *British Medical Bulletin, 51*(3), 609-630.

Leffell, D. J. & Brash, D. E. (1996). Sunlight and skin cancer. *Scientific American, 275*(1), 52-59.

Lookingbill, D. P. (1993). Structure and function of the skin. In D. P. Lookingbill & J. G. Marks, Jr. (Eds.), *Principles of dermatology* (2nd ed.). Philadelphia: W. B. Saunders.

Lynch, H. T., Frichot, B. C., & Lynch, J. F. (1978). Familial atypical multiple mole melanoma syndrome. *Journal of Medical Genetics, 15,* 352-356.

MacKie, R. M. (1995). Melanoma prevention and early detection. *British Medical Bulletin, 51*(3), 570-583.

MacKie, R. M. (1996). Malignant melanoma. In R. M. MacKie, *Skin cancer* (2nd ed.). New York: Mosby.

Marks, R. (1996). Prevention and control of melanoma: The public health approach. *CA: A Cancer Journal for Clinicians, 46*(4), 199-216.

Mastrangelo, M. J., Maguire, H. C., Sato, T., Nathan, F. E., & Berd, D. (1996). Active specific immunization in the treatment of patients with melanoma. *Seminars in Oncology, 23*(6), 773-781.

McClay, E. F., Mastrangelo, M. J., Sprandio, J. D., Bellet, R. E., & Berd, D. (1989). The importance of tamoxifen to a cisplatin-containing regimen in the treatment of metastatic melanoma. *Cancer, 63*(7), 1292-1295.

McClay, E. F. & McClay, M. T. (1996). Systemic chemotherapy for the treatment of metastatic melanoma. *Seminars in Oncology, 23*(6), 744-753.

Metcalf, J. S. (1996). Melanoma: Criteria for histological diagnosis and its reporting. *Seminars in Oncology, 23*(6), 688-692.

Miaskowski, C. (1991). Knowledge deficit related to surgery. In J. C. McNally, E. T. Somerville, C. Miaskowski, & M. Rostad (Eds.), *Guidelines for oncology nursing practice.* Philadelphia: W. B. Saunders.

Mitchell, M. S. (1996). Active specific immunotherapy of melanoma. *British Medical Bulletin, 51*(3), 631-646.

Morton, D. L. & Barth, A. (1996). Vaccine therapy for malignant melanoma. *CA: A Cancer Journal for Clinicians, 46*(4), 225-244.

Morton, D. L., Wen, D. R., & Cochran, A. J. (1992). Management of early stage melanoma by interoperative mapping and selective lymphadenectomy or "Watch and Wait." *Surgical Clinics of North America, 1,* 247-259.

Nathanson, L., Meelu, M. A., & Losada, R. (1994). Chemohormone therapy of metastatic melanoma with megestrol acetate, dacarbazine, carmustine, and cisplatin. *Cancer, 73*(1), 98-102.

Paice, J. (1991). Alteration in comfort: Acute pain. In J. C. McNally, E. T. Somerville, C. Miaskowski, & M. Rostad (Eds.), *Guidelines for oncology nursing practice.* Philadelphia: W. B. Saunders.

Puleo, C. A. & Luh, M. (1995). Management of extremity lymphedema. *Cancer Control,* September/October, 424-431.

Reintgen, D. (1995). Progress in the prevention and management of malignant melanoma. *Cancer Control,* September/October, 377-379.

Reintgen, D., Albertini, J., Berman, C., Cruse, C. W., Fenske, N., Glass, F., Puleo, C., Wang, X., Wells, K., Rapaport, D., DeConti, R., Messina, J., & Heller, R. (1995). Accurate nodal staging of malignant melanoma. *Cancer Control,* September/October, 405-414.

Rigel, D. S. (1996). Malignant melanoma: Perspectives on incidence and its effects on awareness, diagnosis and treatment. *CA: A Cancer Journal for Clinicians, 46*(4), 195-198.

Rigel, D. S. Friedman, R. J., & Kopf, A. W. (1996). The incidence of malignant melanoma in the United States: Issues as we approach the 21st century. *Journal of the American Academy of Dermatology, 34,* 839-847.

Rumsey, K. A. (1995). Patient education. In P. T. Rieger (Ed.), *Biotherapy: A comprehensive overview.* Boston: Jones and Bartlett.

Salopek, T. G., Marghoop, A. A., & Slade, J. M. (1995). An estimate of the incidence of malignant melanoma in the United States: Based on survey of members of the American Academy of Dermatology. *Dermatological Surgery, 21,* 301-305.

Seykora, J. & Elder, D. (1996). Dysplastic nevi and other risk markers for melanoma. *Seminars in Oncology, 23*(6), 682-687.

Shields, J. A., Shields, C. L., DePotter, P., & Singh, A. D. (1996). Diagnosis and treatment of uveal melanoma. *Seminars in Oncology, 23*(6), 763-767.

Slominski, A., Ross, J., & Mihm, M. C. (1995). Cutaneous melanoma: Pathology, relevant prognostic indicators and progression. *British Medical Bulletin, 51*(3), 548-569.

Steiner, A., Pehamberger, H., & Wolff, K. (1987). In vivo epiluminescence microscopy of pigmented skin lesions. *Journal of the American Academy of Dermatology, 17,* 584-591.

Su, Y. A. & Trent, J. M. (1995). Genetics of cutaneous malignant melanoma. *Cancer Control,* September/October, 392-397.

Urist, M. M. (1996). Surgical management of primary cutaneous melanoma. *CA: A Cancer Journal for Clinicians, 46*(4), 217-224.

Urist, M. M., Miller, D. M., & Maddox, W. A. (1995). Malignant melanoma. In G. P. Murphy, W. Lawrence, & R. E. Lenhard (Eds.), *Clinical oncology* (2nd ed.). Atlanta: American Cancer Society.

Walter, S. D., Marrett, L. D., & From, L. (1990). The association of cutaneous malignant melanoma with the use of sunbeds and sunlamps. *American Journal of Epidemiology, 131,* 232-243.

Nonmelanoma Skin Cancers

Georgia Decker, RN, MS, ANP, AOCN

EPIDEMIOLOGY

Nonmelanoma skin cancers (NMSCs) are the most common cancers in Caucasians in the United States (Halder & Bridgemon-Sha, 1995; Kwa, Campana, & Moy, 1992; Smoller & Smoller 1992; Preston & Stern, 1992; Safai, 1997). More than 700,000 cases are diagnosed annually, according to the American Cancer Society. Authors feel this number is extremely conservative because it excludes untreated lesions or lesions treated without biopsy (Preston & Stern, 1992; Gallagher, Hill, Bajdik, Fincham, Coldman, & McLean et al., 1995a; Gallagher, Hill, Bajdik, Fincham, Coldman, & McLean et al., 1995b; Glass & Hoover, 1989; Safai, 1997). NMSCs consist of basal cell carcinoma (BCC) and squamous cell carcinoma (SCC). Skin cancers share common etiologic factors but vary in other ways. Generally, NMSCs have a high incidence but a low metastatic potential and mortality rate. Among African Americans, cancer of the skin is considered to be infrequent. Skin cancer in African Americans has been described as "negligible" (American Cancer Society, 1998). Because data are limited, accurate determination of the incidence of skin cancer in the African-American population is difficult. In fact, BCC in African-Americans is described as a nonentity by some authors (Halder & Bridgeman-Sha, 1995).

Basal Cell Carcinoma

BCC is a malignancy of the epidermis and the most common skin cancer. Approximately 70% to 80% of BCCs occur on the structures of the head and neck. This type of cancer also frequently occurs on the arms, hands, and shoulders. It was once thought to be a disease of the elderly. However, it is seen with increasing frequency in younger populations, including teenagers. The male-to-female ratio is 1.5:1. BCC is seen approximately three times as often as squamous cell carcinoma.

Squamous Cell Carcinoma

Squamous cell carcinoma is the second most common skin cancer, and authors estimate that it represents 20% to 30% of all reported cutaneous malignancies (Safai, 1997; Gantt, 1990; Rosen, Miller, & Schwab, 1996). The greatest number of new cases of SCC are diagnosed in the 65- to 74-year age group, with a male-to-female ratio of 3:1. Squamous cell carcinoma is infrequent in children under age 15 years. This type of skin cancer may develop in areas of chronic scarring or nonhealing wounds, as well as the more commonly known areas such as the structures of the head and neck. It also occurs in sites not exposed to the sun, including genitals and mucous membranes, and for this reason other factors are also recognized. When compared with BCC, SCC has an increased metastatic potential (Gumport, Harris, Roses, & Kopf, 1981). Together, basal cell carcinoma and squamous cell carcinoma are associated with an overall 5-year survival rate of 95% (Enders, Koh, Missero, & Harlow, 1996).

RISK FACTORS

The two major risk factors for the development of skin cancer are skin type and exposure to ultraviolet radiation. Host genetics and immunity play roles in the development of skin cancer, as do ionizing radiation and chronic irritation. Chemical carcinogens and viruses may also play a role in certain types of skin cancer. Factors frequently associated with increased risk of nonmelanoma skin cancers are summarized in Box 74-1.

The risk of skin cancer varies globally. Basal cell carcinoma is more prevalent in northern Europe, the United States, and Australia (i.e., countries with predominantly light-skinned people). The lifetime risk for BCC is at least 50% where light-skinned people are exposed to sunlight (Ziegler, Leffell, Kunala, Sharma, Gailani, & Simon et al., 1993). Squamous cell carcinoma is more prevalent in countries inhabited exclusively by dark-skinned people (e.g.,

Box 74-1
Risk Factors

Increasing age*
Male gender*
Skin that does not tan*
Skin that sunburns easily*
Skin with freckling*
Celtic ancestry*
Red, blond, or light brown hair*
Fair skin*
Genodermatoses*
Scarring dermatoses
Chronic ulceration or inflammation
Chemical carcinogens
Cigarette smoking (squamous cell carcinoma of the lip and mouth)

Modified from Vitaliano, P. P., & Urbach, F. (1980). The relative importance of risk factors in nonmelanoma carcinoma. *Archives of Dermatology, 116,* 454-456; Hunter, D. J., Colditz, G. A., Stampler, M. J., Rosner, B., Willett, W. C., & Speizer, F. E. (1990). Risk factors for basal cell carcinoma in a prospective cohort of women. *Annual Epidemiology, 1,* 12-23.

*The risk for BCC increases two-fold with these factors.

China, Africa, Vietnam) (Whitaker, 1992). There is overwhelming evidence that exposure to ultraviolet radiation (UVR) is the major etiologic factor in the development of nonmelanoma skin cancers (Brash, 1997).

Skin Type

The risk for BCC increases in light-skinned people, those who are freckled, and those who endured repeated sunburn in childhood (Box 74-1). Table 74-1 describes the skin types. The risk for basal cell carcinoma is significantly increased in people who had increased exposure to UVR in childhood and adolescence (Gallagher et al., 1995a). This risk is greatest among individuals who burned rather than tanned when they were exposed to the sun. A study by Kricker and Armstrong (1995) implies increased risk in terms of intense sun exposure endured intermittently by light-skinned individuals who tanned poorly over the same dose of UVR exposure endured consistently over the same time (Chorun, Norris, & Gupta, 1994).

Ultraviolet Radiation Exposure

Squamous cell carcinoma is also clearly related to sun exposure (Safai, 1997). SCC usually develops in the sun-exposed areas of the head and neck. It occurs most frequently in light-skinned individuals and is directly related to UVR exposure. People with outdoor occupations have a higher incidence than those with occupations that are traditionally indoor jobs. Other forms of UV radiation also increase the risk of SCC, as well as other skin cancers.

The types of ultraviolet radiation that are harmful to the skin are UVA and UVB. The amount of exposure, timing of exposure, and skin type determine the risk. Preston and Stern (1992) describe the mechanism by which UVB damages deoxyribonucleic acid (DNA) and its repair system. They suggest that cell-mediated immunity and immune function may be modulated by UVB and thereby participate in tumor development (Nagano, Ueda, & Ischiaski, 1993). Young animals exposed to ultraviolet B light have an increase in the number of suppressor T cells with accompanying decrease in cell-mediated immunity (Fisher & Kripke, 1982). Conversely, Czarnecki, Meehan, McColl, & Kulinskaya (1996) determined that a lymphocyte count is not a reliable way of predicting which patients will have an increased number of skin cancers.

Table 74-1 Skin Types

Skin Type	With UVR Exposure
I	Always burns, never tans
II	Always burns, minimal tan
III	Burns often, tans gradually (light brown)
IV	Burns rarely, tans profusely (dark brown)
V	Never burns, deeply pigmented (black)

Immunosuppression

There is significant increase in the risk of NMSC, especially SCC with immunosuppression. This risk increases with the duration of immunosuppression (Preston & Stern, 1992). Kwa, Campana, and Moy (1992) describe the age of onset of SCC in renal transplant patients as 2 decades younger than the general population. Kinlen (1985) describes a five-fold increase in incidence of SCC in nontransplant patients undergoing immunosuppression. Lymphoproliferative disorders may be important in immunosuppression and skin cancer. It appears that there is an association between the host's immune status and the development of skin cancer (Dinehart, Chu, & Manners, 1990).

Chemical Carcinogens

In 1775 Sir Percival Pott reported an increase in risk of SCC in the genitals of English chimney sweeps. Their exposure to coal-tar products was the first recognized example of chemical carcinogens. The familiar treatment of psoriasis using oral psoralens and UVA photochemotherapy produces an increased risk of developing squamous cell carcinomas. This risk is dose dependent (Preston & Stern, 1992).

Ionizing Radiation

Exposure to ionizing radiation is believed to induce cutaneous malignancies in humans. Radiation-induced skin cancers have been reported in patients receiving ionizing radiation as therapy for tinea capitis, acne, and facial hair (Safai, 1997). In addition to radiodermatitis, telangiectasis, hypopigmentation, or hyperpigmentation, these patients developed large, invasive skin cancers. These uses of x-ray therapy for these conditions have been discontinued, although people continue to be treated with this modality in clinical practice.

Chronic Inflammation or Irritation

Skin cancers can develop in areas of chronic inflammation or irritation. SCC has been noted to occur with long-standing granulomas, venereal granulomas, syphilis, lupus vulgaris, and systemic lupus erythematous (SLE) (Safai, 1997).

Tobacco and Alcohol

Cigarette smoking has a significant role in causing SCC of the lip and mouth and has been implicated in SCC at nonmucosal skin sites. Lip and mouth lesions are associated with chewing tobacco and betel nut. About 20% of patients with the clinical diagnosis of oral leukoplakia have histologic findings consisting of epithelial dysplasia and hyperkeratosis of the mucosa. Approximately 60% of these patients develop invasive squamous cell carcinoma (Safai, 1997). Authors agree that abstinence from tobacco and alcohol are important in decreasing the risk for precancerous oral mucosa leukoplakia.

Viruses

Many malignant neoplasms are caused by viruses in animals. In humans there have been few such associations documented. Certain other human papillomavirus (HPV) types of papillomaviruses appear potentially oncogenic in humans (Ostrow, 1982). Other viruses appear to be potentially oncogenic in humans, but conclusive information is lacking. HPV has been isolated in some skin tumors, especially in immunocompromised patients. For human HTP papillomavirus to induce NMSC, additional factors are probably needed (Preston & Stern, 1992).

Lobo, Chu, Grelan, and Berger (1992) address human immunodeficiency virus (HIV) and nonmelanoma skin cancers. They determined that the major risk factors for developing NMSCs in association with the HIV seems to be the same as in the normal population. Standard treatments were equally effective, except in SCC, which was associated with a 20% recurrence rate.

PATHOPHYSIOLOGY

Normal Anatomy and Physiology

The skin is the largest of the body's organs. It is highly specialized with a wide range of functions. It is waterproof, receives approximately one third of circulating blood, and provides protection from heat, chemicals, light and microorganisms. The skin has multiple functions, which include, but are not limited to, helping to maintain hemostasis, thermoregulation, vitamin D synthesis, production of cytokines, and antigen presentation. The skin has several layers: The epidermis is the uppermost layer, the dermis is the underlying layer, and the hypodermis, or superficial fossa, is the subcutaneous layer. The epidermis is composed primarily of stratified squamous epithelial cells, or keratinocytes, which provide much of the skin's protective properties. Along the basement membrane, separating the dermis from the epidermis, are the basal cells. The single column of basal constitutes the germinative cells responsible for normal epidermal replacement. In the epidermis, between the basal cells, are melanocytes, the cells that produce melanin. The synthesis of keratin, keratinization or carnification, is the main function of the epidermis and provides the body's natural self-regeneration. In the basal layers as cells undergo mitosis, mature cells are displaced, lose their capacity for division, die, and then flake off at the surface.

The dermis, situated between the epidermis and subcutaneous fat, is also known as the *corneum.* Collagen-producing fibroblasts, contained in the dermis, provide the skin with its strength. The vasculature, nerves, lymphatic vessels, sebaceous and sweat glands, and hair follicles are found in the papillary and reticular dermis (Fig. 64-2).

The hypodermis, or subcutis, lies beneath the dermis and is composed primarily of adipose tissue. This layer acts as a cushion to trauma, as well as an insulator. Nerves, blood, and lymph vessels are found in this layer.

Multiple cell and tissue types participate in forming the three layers of the skin. These cell and tissue elements can transform to produce a large number of benign and malignant growths (Thibodeau & Patton, 1996.)

The Process of Carcinogenesis

The two major factors influencing the development of skin cancers are the exposure to ultraviolet radiation and skin type (Table 74-1). Fair complexion, blue eyes, and light hair are important in the development of basal cell carcinoma. This becomes especially true for people with these physical characteristics who live in a sunny region (Rosso, Zanettie, Martinez, Tormo, Schraub, Sancho-Garnier et al., 1996).

UVA and UVB are types of UVR that are harmful to the skin. UVB waves are short and absorbed by the skin. These rays cause sunburn. UVA rays are longer than UVB and are therefore able to penetrate the top layers of the skin, causing damage to the lower layers. The amount of exposure, the timing of exposure, and the skin type being exposed determine the rate of carcinogenesis. As expected, NMSCs are most common on skin sites most often exposed to the sun.

There is increasing concern and controversy regarding the depletion of the ozone layer of the earth's atmosphere. The ozone layer provides protection by absorbing UVR and thereby preventing it from reaching people. The chemicals linked to the depletion of the ozone layer include chlorofluorcarbons (e.g., hair spray). With continued depletion of the ozone there will be an expected increase in skin cancer occurrence. People with light complexions have greater risk of developing skin cancers than those with darker skin. Melanin pigment provides protection from UV radiation. Although skin cancers are infrequently observed in the dark-skinned races, African albinos have a high incidence of skin cancers on sun-exposed areas.

Bajdik, Gallagher, Astrakianakis, Hill, Fincham, and McLean (1996) reported on their case-controlled study of

NMSC, which was conducted among men in the providence of Alberta, Canada. In this study, 226 cases of BCC and 180 cases of SCC were age-matched to 40% controls to provide information, which included skin type, occupational history, recreational history, exposure to sunlight, and sources of nonsolar ultraviolet radiation (NSUVR), as well as other potential risk factors. It is their conclusion, while acknowledging the study's biases, that there was no increase in risk for NMSC with NSUVR exposure. (This is in opposition to the increased risked of melanoma with NSUVR). Table 74-2 reviews recommendations for the prevention of sun damage.

Immunity and Genetics

UV light may influence the development and progression of skin cancers by affecting the host immune system (Safai, 1997; Preston & Stern, 1992). Kripke and Sass (1974) showed that UV-induced cancers in mice are highly antigenic. The cancer was rejected when transplanted into a genetically identical animal. However, the primary host becomes tolerant to the tumor, allowing growth (Kripke & Sass, 1974). Recent studies report a tumor-suppressing protein (p53) is present in very small amounts for short periods of time in normal keratinocytes. Aged p53 may lose the tumor-suppressor ability. Mutants of p53 have been detected in sun-damaged epidermis adjacent to BCC. These tumors also contained a mutant p53 (Shea, McNutt, Volkenandt, Lugo, Prioleau, & Albino, 1992). Mutant p53 has also been identified in SCC (MacGregor, Yu, Dublen, Levinson & MacDonald, 1992; Oran, Orengo, Baer, & Ocal, 1994). Multiple BCCs are seen in these patients identified as having basal cell nevus syndrome. Melanocytes present but do not synthesize melanin in albinism. Patients with xeroderma pigmentosum have an impaired ability to repair ultraviolet-induced DNA damage (Robbins, 1998). When these patients are exposed to ultraviolet light, "hypermutable and hypertransformable cues develop" (Preston & Stern, 1992; Ren, Hendrum, Ponten, Nister, Afshin, Lundeberg et al., 1993). This may suggest an increased risk of skin cancer.

TABLE 74-2 How to Protect Your Skin from Sun Damage

1. Try to avoid being outside when sunlight is most intense: from 10:00 in the morning to 3:00 in the afternoon.
2. Wear a hat, long sleeves, and dry, close-knit clothing while in the sun.
3. Sunscreen products may protect against common skin cancer. Use a sunscreen with an SPF of 15 or higher, and choose a brand that protects against both UVA and UVB radiation (the label will give you this information). Put sunscreen on every part of your body that is exposed, including your ears, lips, nose, neck, and hands. Sunscreen products for your lips are available in tinted (like lipstick) and untinted forms. Don't forget the top of your head if it's bald.
4. Apply sunscreen at least ½ hour before going outside, so the sunscreen has time to work.
5. The risk of sunburn is greater at high altitudes and near snow, sand, or water, so be sure to apply sunscreen before skiing or mountain climbing, even on cloudy days.
6. Sunscreen should be applied every 2 to 3 hours, after each time you swim and after you perspire a lot.
7. Teach your children to use sunscreens. Sun damage begins at an early age.
8. Encourage your children's schools to schedule outdoor events and sports programs at early morning or late afternoon hours.
9. Remember, there is no safe tan. Tanning salons and sun beds should always be avoided.
10. Get into the habit of looking at your skin regularly. If you see a change, ask your physician to look it over.

This information provides a general overview on sun protection and may not apply to everyone. Talk to your family physician to find out if this information applies to you and to get more information on this subject.

Modified from the American Academy of Family Physicians, August, 1984.

Chemical Carcinogens

Arsenic causes palmar and plantar keratoses that are associated with a high risk of SCC. Although the use of arsenic as insecticides has diminished in the United States, it is still found naturally in well water and in isolated areas. Trivalent inorganic arsenic has long been recognized as a cause of BCC and SCC. Arsenic has been the principle compound in preparations used to treat psoriasis, and syphilis (Vargo, 1990).

The risk associated with the use of mustard gas and arsenic as chemical warfare testing conducted by the United States during World War II with subsequent compensation to American servicemen who developed skin cancer as a result of this chemical testing is documented. Table 74-3 describes skin carcinogens for people (Woodhouse, 1960).

TABLE 74-3 Skin Carcinogens for Humans

Agent	Year Recognized
Coal tar	1874
Sunlight	1875
Arsenic	1888
X-rays	1902
Creosote oil	1920
Mineral oil	1870 (shale oil)
	1910 (shale lubricating oil)
Crude paraffin	1930
Cutting oil	1950

Data from Safai, B. (1997). Cancer of the skin. In V. T. DeVita, S. Hellman, & S. A. Rosenberg (Eds.). *Cancer: Principles and practice of oncology (Vol. 2).* (5th ed.). Philadelphia: Lippincott-Raven.

ROUTES OF METASTASES

Basal cell carcinoma tends to occur as a single lesion, has little tendency to metastasize, and usually spreads by direct extension. Domarus and Stevens (1984); Lo, Snow, and Reizner (1991); and Robinson (1987) reported that 36% of 500 BCC patients developed a second BCC within 5 years and 15% developed three or more BCCs during the same period of time. All classifications of BCC can develop under or next to a previous treatment scar. When recurrence occurs, it may appear as modular BCC or as a fullness or lump underneath the scar (Vargo, 1991). Recurrent BCC typically tracks along soft tissue pathways, which are zones of dense connective tissue. The central face, H-zone, is an example of such a zone. Tumor cells are also capable of traveling along nerve sheaths and can infiltrate bone and cartilage. An aggressive tumor or inadequate treatment are associated with recurrence.

Metastases occur in less than 0.1% of basal cell carcinomas, with the greatest number occurring in very large tumors, recurrent tumors, and tumors resistant to radiotherapy. BCC behaves aggressively after metastases occur, with a median survival of approximately 1 year (Cruse, O'Neill, & Rayhack, 1992). Metastasis through lymphatics or blood is extremely rare in BCC, with approximately 70% of metastasis to regional lymph nodes (Vargo, 1991). Hartman, Hartman, and Green (1986) note that metastases usually occurred in patients who had multiple episodes of local recurrence with invasion into underlying structures.

Recurrent squamous cell carcinoma places a patient at risk for developing metastases when invasive. Generally, 2% to 3% of all patients with SCC of the skin develop metastatic disease. Of these patients, 75% die (Lever, 1983). Unlike BCC, metastasis of SCC occurs almost exclusively through lymphatics. Typically, it occurs only after invasion of the subcutaneous lymph nodes, as well as deeper lymphatics of the facial planes, have occurred. Metastatic risk is based on causative factors, morphologic characteristics, and size and depth of the tumor. SCC arising from actinic cheilitis has a higher metastatic potential than SCC arising in solar keratosis on the surface of the skin. Metastasis is most likely to occur within 2 years of diagnosis of the primary tumor and lowers the survival rate (Vargo, 1991). SCC arising in radiation dermatitis and radiation keratosis is highly anaplastic and grows rapidly. Metastasis of squamous cell carcinomas caused by exposure to carcinogens varies, depending on the type of carcinogen, location of the tumor, and length of time from discovery of the lesion to treatment. SCCs arising in burn scars, chronic ulcers, or sinuses are insidious, with a high incidence of metastasis. Increased diameter of cutaneous SCC is associated with increased metastatic potential, with the majority of metastasizing cutaneous SCCs reported in lesions of greater than 2 cm diameter (Dinehart & Pollack, 1989). Other studies found tumor thickness to be a determinant of metastatic potential. Friedman, Cooper, and Wanebo (1985) reviewed 63 patients with cutaneous SCC arising de novo or from actinic lesions and found that all cases recurring or metastasizing were at least 4 mm thick. Breuinger, Black, and Rassner (1990) found no metastasis in 673 cases of SCC with primary lesions less than 2 mm thick. In addition, there was an associated 4.5% rate of metastasis with lesions 2 to 6 mm thick and a 15% rate of metastasis with lesions greater than 6 mm.

Several studies associate a greater depth of invasion with a higher metastatic rate. When SCC invades subcutaneous fat, there is an associated 4.1% rate of metastasis (Breuinger, Black, & Rassner, 1990). Perineural invasion by cutaneous SCC has been associated with metastatic rates of 50% or greater (Frierson & Cooper, 1986). In addition, when cutaneous SCC invades muscle, cartilage, or bone, there is a 12.5% rate of metastasis (Breuinger, Black, & Rassner, 1990). What remains unclear is whether level of invasion and tumor thickness are independent predictors of metastasis.

Risk of metastases has also been associated with altered immune surveillance. Patients with lymphoproliferative disorders have shown an increased risk of metastatic SCC (Frierson, Deutch, & Levine, 1988). Immunosuppressed organ transplant patients are also thought to have increased incidence of metastases (Kinlen, 1985). Dinehart, Chu, and Manners (1990) found that in patients with metastatic cutaneous SCC, 23% had an obvious immunosuppressive condition or were undergoing immunosuppressive therapy. In addition, a study by Kinlen (1985) analyzed cancer incidence in nontransplant patients receiving immunosuppressive therapy for a variety of conditions. Most were receiving azathioprine or cyclophosphamide. There was a five-fold increase in the incidence of cutaneous SCC in these patients compared with the general population. There are less data on the long-term effects of cyclosporine on the incidence of SCC.

ASSESSMENT

Regular skin cancer screenings are worthwhile for any number of reasons (Table 74-4). The screening tool for skin cancers, visual inspection, is noninvasive, inexpensive, and readily available. Skin cancer is common and has the potential to cause significant morbidity and, in some situations, mortality. Early diagnosis has the potential to lessen morbidity and increase survival. Sensitivity of total cutaneous examination (TCE) is high if performed by a health professional who is specifically trained (Marghoob, Slade, Salopek, Kopf, Bart, & Rigel, 1995). A detailed family history and exposure to possible carcinogens should accompany TCE. Screening for any cancer of the skin should be part of a routine physical examination. Primary care providers who can recognize malignant and premalignant lesions of the skin have an important role in improving cure rates, limiting morbidity, and decreasing health care costs (Kibarian & Hruza, 1995).

It is important to examine the entire cutaneous surface for skin cancers. A new basal cell carcinoma develops in approximately 45% of people with BCC within 5 years (Frankel, Hanusa, & Zitelli, 1992; Karagas, Stukel, Greenberg, Baron, Mott, & Stern (1992). Although BCC and SCC are associated with areas of the body exposed to sunlight, approximately 70,000 BCC/SCCs are located on converged anatomic sites (Marghoob et al., 1995). Some authors dis-

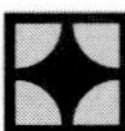

TABLE 74-4 Assessment of the Patient for Nonmelanoma Skin Cancer

	Assessment Parameters	Typical Abnormal Findings
History	A. Personal and social history	A. Personal and social risk factors
	1. Age	1. Usually sun with increasing age but recently with increasing frequency in younger people.
	2. Gender	2. Male-to-female ratio 1.5:1 for BCC and 3:1 in SCC.
	3. Skin type	3. Fair skin, with freckles and light hair, and history of easy sunburn at greatest risk.
	4. Exposure to chemical carcinogens	4. Oral psoralens, arsenic, mustard gas in WWII veterans, tobacco use (Table 74-4).
	5. Exposure to ionizing radiation	5. Patients and others who have been treated with radiation therapy for acne, facial hair, and tinea capitis.
	6. Family history of genetically determined syndromes associated with high risk	6. Xoderma pigmentosum, basal cell nevus syndrome, albinism, epidermodysplasia verruciformis.
	7. Personal history of immunosuppression	7. HIV, s/p transplant, other situations of immunosuppression or compromise. Increased risk for metastasis.
	8. Personal history of certain viruses	8. HIV (increased risk for SCC), HPV, and immunocompromise.
	9. Areas of chronic irritation	9. Increase risk. Especially SCC at sites of long-standing granulomas and others
Physical Examination	Total cutaneous examination (TCE) should be a part of any routine physical examination.	Assessment of all skin areas is best—BCC usually occurs as a single lesion. Any non-healing lesion occurring in a sun-exposed area is of high suspicion. The most common pre-malignant lesion is actinic keratosis—poorly demarcated sun-colored, hyperpigmented or erythematous macules. Usually asymptomatic but patient may report mild itching or burning Any areas of induration, erythema, erosion, pain or change in diameter may represent progression
Diagnostic Tests	A. Biopsy is necessary to confirm diagnosis:	A. Biopsy technique should be appropriate to the lesion and location:
	1. Shave	1. When lesion is superficial
	2. Punch	2. When lesion extends beyond dermis
	3. Incisional	3. When excision biopsy is not possible or there is a risk of spread with punch biopsy
	4. Excisional	4. Recommended when the differential diagnoses include malignant melanoma and pigmented basal cell carcinoma

cuss some perceived disadvantages to total cutaneous examination (Lee, Massa, Welykyj, Choo, & Greaney, 1991). Several of these "disadvantages" are associated with malignant melanoma (MM) and are discussed in Chapter 73. However, TCE detects not only MM, but also BCC, SCC, and premalignant cutaneous lesions. Because of the high prevalence of skin cancers and precancers, regular TCE results in a high number of positive findings of early-stage lesions. Some claim that TCE embarrasses the patient. If this is of concern, an explanation of the importance and avoidance of unnecessary exposure (if done in a proper setting) usually helps avoid embarrassment. For patients who refuse TCE, a compromise can be offered by examining them in undergarments so that a lesion may then be undetected. It has also been argued that TCE is time consuming. For the experienced practitioner, TCE can be done effectively in a few minutes (Marghoob et al., 1995).

Actinic Keratosis

The most common premalignant lesion is actinic keratosis. The solar or actinic keratosis is a precursor and an increased risk for NMSC. They are often poorly demarcated papules, covered by a rough adherent scale. Actinic keratoses may be skin colored, hyperpigmented, or even erythematous macules. Visualization is sometimes difficult but the lesion tends to occur on sun-exposed skin surfaces. Multiple lesions are common findings, but single lesions do occur. The patient may report mild tenderness, itching, or burning, but these lesions are usually asymptomatic.

Actinic keratosis of the lower lip (actinic cheilitis) most often occurs as scaling of the lower lip. Indications of actinic keratosis progression to squamous cell carcinoma include induration, erythema, erosions, pain, hyperkeratosis, and increased lesion diameter (Kibarian & Hruza, 1995).

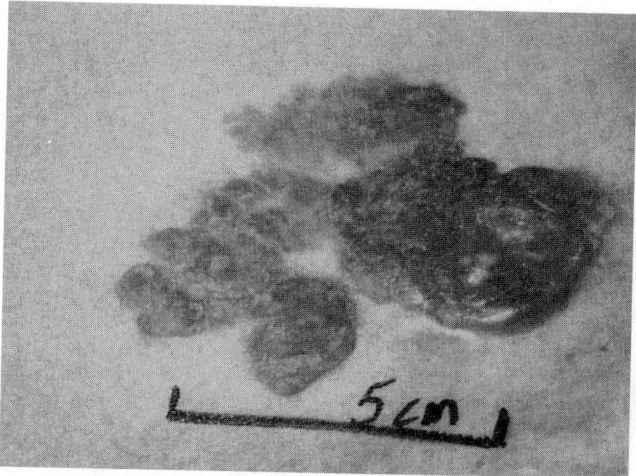

Fig. 74-1 Bowen's disease. This more specific type of premalignant lesion, or intradermal cancer, consists of defined, erythematous, scaly plaques that often resemble psoriasis. In this patient the right side of the lesion has already undergone transformation into an invasive squamous cell carcinoma.

Squamous Cell Carcinoma

A definitive diagnosis of squamous cell carcinoma can be made only through biopsy (Frisch & Melbye, 1995). Differential diagnoses include seborrheic keratosis, basal cell carcinoma, and melanoma. Lesions may appear as plagues or nodules. The lesion of Bowen's disease, or squamous cell carcinoma in situ, develops often, being indolent for a relatively long period of time (Sober & Burstein, 1994). It presents as an erythematous, well-defined, scaly plague which has failed to respond to topical steroids. If Bowen's disease develops in a non–sun-exposed body surface this may be indicative of prior exposure to arsenic. Appropriate risk assessment and follow-up is indicated. Development of Bowen's disease on sun-exposed areas is not associated with an increased risk of arsenic-associated internal malignancy (Sober & Burstein, 1994) (Figs. 74-1, 74-2, and 74-3).

Basal Cell Carcinoma

Basal cell carcinomas appear as round to oval, slow-growing, shiny, skin colored to pink, translucent papules or nodules. An umbilicated center ulcerated with a rolled border is common. The lesions are hard to palpation. There is often telangiectasia in the surrounding skin. Some basal cell carcinomas are pigmented and may exhibit a bluish hue (Maloney, Jones, & Sexton, 1992), as in cystic basal cell carcinoma. Assessment cues include the typical central depression with a rolled border. If trauma occurs at the site of one of these lesions, bleeding may occur. The most common sites for these lesions are the head and neck. Sclerosing basal cell carcinoma is typically a yellow, sclerotic, scarlike patch with indistinct margins. Superficial BCC is flat, erythematous, and scaly with a threadlike border.

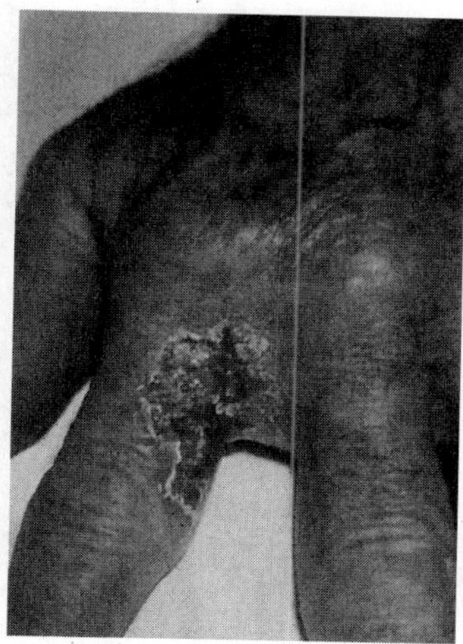

Fig. 74-2 Bowen's disease. Involvement of the hands is quite common and can present diagnostic and therapeutic problems.

Basal Cell Nevus Syndrome

Basal cell nevus syndrome is a rare, inherited disorder in which multiple basal cell carcinomas are associated with characteristic and easily recognizable early manifestations. These manifestations include absent or undescended testes, hydrocephalus, and blindness. The most noteworthy cutaneous characteristic is the early onset of multiple (a few to hundreds) basal cell carcinomas with usual distribution symmetric and bilateral (Fig. 74-4).

Epidermodysplasia Verruciformis

Most warts are not skin cancer precursors. However, a link between warts and skin cancer was first noted for a rare genetic disorder, epidermodysplasia verruciformis. People with this condition develop numerous warts with associated squamous cell carcinoma. HPV types 5 and 8 have been commonly associated with epidermodysplasia verruciformis. HPV has also been associated with Bowen's disease. Viral transformation to SCC has also been noted for giant condyloma acuminata (Buschke-Lowesenstein), which affects anogenital areas (Sober & Burstein, 1994). Lesions are typically 2- to 6-mm wartlike papules. Color varies from tan to red to depigmented. These lesions have been thought to resemble tinea versicolor. When occurring in the elbows and knees, they mimic psoriasis.

Acanthosis Nigricanis

Acanthosis nigricanis is a symmetrically distributed thickening of the skin, characterized by brown pigmentation, hyperkeratosis, and papillomatosis, which results in a velvety appearance. It affects the intertriginous areas, and there may be mucosal involvement (Tong & Fitzpatrick, 1996). The benign type is rare as is the malignant type. The eruption is symmetrical. The earliest sign being an increase in the pigmentation of the skin. This change is caused by hyperkera-

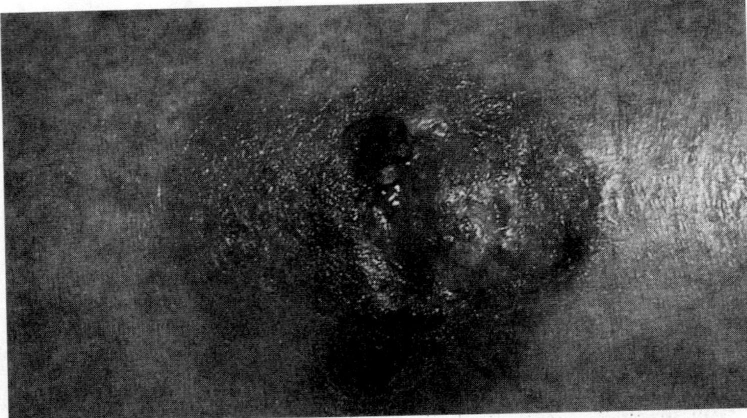

Fig. 74-3 Bowen's disease. The surface of the lesion, seen here in its characteristic presentation as a well-defined, slightly raised, red patch with an adherent scale, may become eroded.

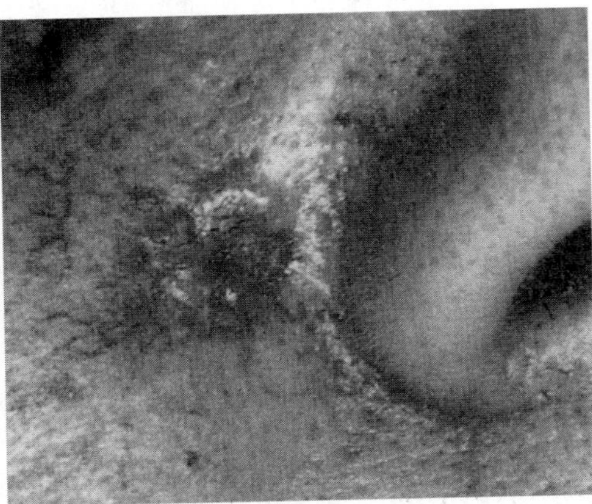

Fig. 74-4 Basal cell carcinoma. This early lesion is beginning to show the translucent, pearly appearance typical of these nodules as they begin to undergo central ulceration.

tosis, not melanin. This is then followed by changes which result in the velvety texture. The onset may be sudden with rapid spread (Tong & Fitzpatrick, 1996).

Seborrheic Keratosis

Seborrheic keratosis (SK) is a benign, pigmented tumor that commonly occurs on the trunk and face. SK may be a solitary lesion, but it is more common to observe multiple lesions on the face, trunk, and upper extremities. Lesions are round to oval in shape and well demarcated. They have a "wacky" quality, and the color may vary from pink to tan to dark brown within a single lesion (Tong & Fitzpatrick, 1996). The vast majority of seborrheic keratoses may be diagnosed clinically with visual inspection. When in doubt, a biopsy specimen taken from the thickest part of the lesion or an excisional biopsy can be obtained. Leser-Trelat sign is described as a sudden onset of multiple seborrheic keratoses in association with internal malignancies. This association of seborrheic keratosis and internal malignancies is not universally accepted (Rampen & Schwengle, 1989). Comprehensive assessment includes the element of risk. Large cell

Table 74-5 Postoperative Care Instructions

Biopsy

1. Remove the surgical dressing (or bandage) the morning after surgery. Leave the wound uncovered, unless it is in an area of friction or rubbing; then apply a loose fitting bandage or gauze pad during the day.
2. Wet a cotton ball with tap water, and apply a few drops of hydrogen peroxide. Gently cleanse the wound site twice a day, rinse, and pat dry.

Signs of Infection

1. Increase in redness (red ring around wound)
2. Irritation
3. Warmth
4. Tender to the touch
5. Excessive drainage, pus (not clear drainage) after 24 hours

If you notice any of these signs, please call the office.

All lesions that are removed are sent to a pathology laboratory, so please call 1 week after your surgery is performed for the results.

Courtesy Judith Mysliorski, MD.

acanthoma can be difficult to distinguish from squamous cell carcinoma. The characteristics that differentiate it include rapid or spontaneous evolution, a dome shape with a central keratin plug, and young age. Generally, keratoacanthoma resolves spontaneously (Fig. 74-5).

Radiation Dermatitis

Radiation dermatitis and *x-ray keratosis* are terms used to describe skin changes due to ionizing radiation, which usually occur many years after exposure. The exposure may have been a result of an occupational hazard or a therapeutic regimen. The skin is dry, scaly, erythematous, thin, sharply demarcated, and discolored, and it corresponds to the field previously irradiated. X-ray keratoses are aggres-

A

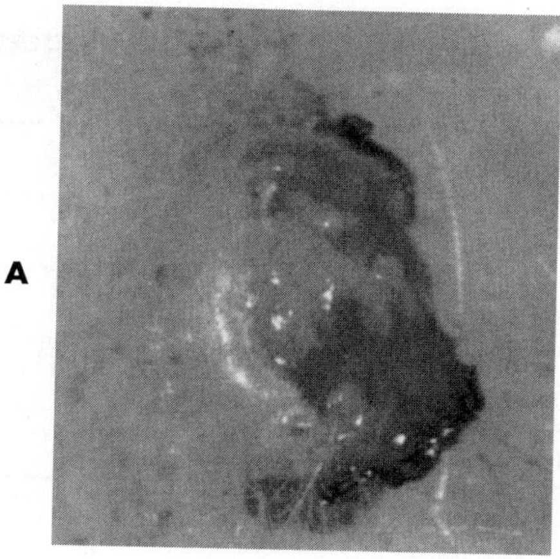

B

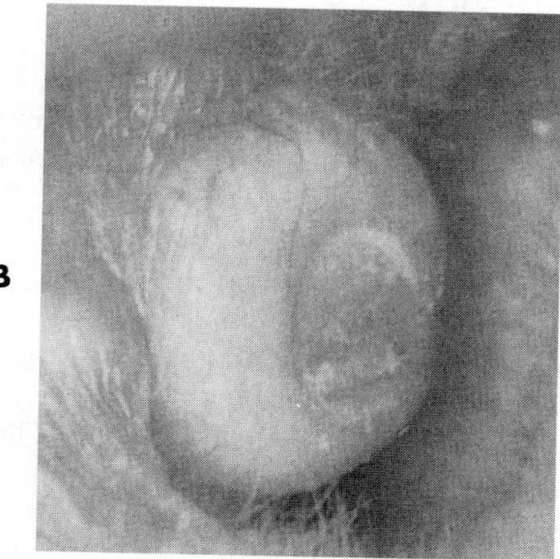

Fig. 74-5 Keratoacanthoma. **A,** A small, early keratoacanthoma has arisen on a sun-exposed portion of the ear. Cuplike hyperplastic epithelium can be seen around the base, and the central crater is granular and friable. **B,** A larger, more mature keratoacanthoma, also in the conchal bowl, shows a central crater filled with keratinous material and a deep surrounding cuff of hyperplastic epithelium.

sive and have a tendency to evolve into SCC or soft tissue sarcomas (Safai, 1997; Tong & Fitzpatrick, 1996).

Epidermal Nevi

Epidermal nevi are benign, congenital, hyperplastic lesions that may have a smoother or hykeratotic surface. They typically appear at birth or in early childhood. These lesions typically vary in color form pale to deeply pigmented. There are rare reported cases of transformation to carcinomas (Safai, 1997) (Table 74-5).

STAGING

A biopsy is needed to confirm a diagnosis of skin cancer and to define the histologic type of skin tumor before specific treatment can be identified and started. The technique selected should be appropriate to the lesion undergoing biopsy. Four types of biopsies may be used for skin lesions when malignancy is suspected. A *shave biopsy* describes a procedure in which a scalpel is used to slice a superficial portion of the tumor. This technique is best used when the lesion is superficial. A *punch biopsy* uses a sharp cylinder to remove a deeper portion of the lesion. The diameter of the cylinder varies from 2 to 8 mm. This technique is used when the lesion extends beyond the dermis. An *incisional biopsy* removes a part of the tumor using a scalpel. This may be used when an excisional biopsy is not possible or the risk of spread with punch biopsy is a consideration. In *excisional biopsy* the entire lesion plus a small portion of normal skin and tissue that surrounds it are removed. Excisional biopsies are recommended when the differential diagnoses include malignant melanoma and pigmented basal cell carcinoma. Some authors recommend specific biopsy procedures based on suspected and differential diagnoses. Postoperative instructions are noted in Table 74-5.

MEDICAL MANAGEMENT

The appropriate treatment choices for cutaneous malignancies are varied. They are curettage, electrodesiccation, excision (with or without frozen section), Mohs' micrographic surgery, and cryotherapy (Table 74-6). Other choices include radiation therapy, topical chemotherapy, and laser. Confirmation of the histology must be made before treatment planning can begin. Other considerations include the size and location of the tumor, as well as the length of time the tumor has been present. Anatomic function and cosmetic appearance should also be considered (Fleming, Amonette, Monaghan, & Flemming, 1995).

The risk for deep invasion is greatest in skin areas located along embryonal fusion planes. Safai (1997) reports that Mohs' micrographic surgery is the treatment of choice in this situation because it provides the highest cure rate with less chance of recurrence (Table 74-7). The chance of deep invasion correlates with how long the tumor has been present. Well-defined borders and slow growth patterns are suggestive of a diminished chance of recurrence compared with ill-defined borders and multicentric, aggressive growth. Basosquamous or morphea histologic patterns have a high rate of recurrence. The typical pattern of spread should also be considered in treatment planning. The general health of the host is pivotal and should be taken into consideration during this process. For example, if a patient is immunocompromised, the risk of infection is great, and therefore Mohs' procedure or excision may be the preferred methods. In the elderly, choosing a procedure that requires fewer office visits may be considered a preferred choice. Tissue preservation is also an important consideration and may indicate radiation therapy as a preferred therapy.

Curettage and Electrodesiccation

Curettage and electrodesiccation are commonly used to treat basal cell carcinoma and precancerous lesions. Differences in the consistency of tumor tissue and normal surrounding tissue are important considerations. A biopsy is recommended before the use of curettage and dissection. Curettage is performed using a curet, which can be round or oval and is sharp on one side. Electrodesiccation is used to de-

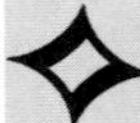

TABLE 74-6 Patient Preparation for Mohs' Micrographic Surgery

Description of the Procedure: A technique developed by Dr. Frederick Mohs, the Mohs' techniques involves removing successive horizontal layers of the skin and surrounding tissue that may be involved. Each layer is microscopically examined, and the section that involves a possible tumor is marked. Subsequent horizontal layers remove the areas of involvement, sparing normal tissue.

Presurgery Teaching

1. Shampoo your hair the night before surgery so that your wound and initial dressing remain dry after your surgery.
   Eat your regular breakfast.
   Wear loose-fitting clothing, and avoid clothes that pull over your head.
   The surgery usually takes 45-50 minutes, but plan to spend at least 4 hours in the clinic after surgery.
   Have a family member or friend drive you home because you may be sedated.

Day of Surgery

2. Sign an informed consent. You will be allowed to ask questions about the procedure.
   The surrounding area of skin to be treated is cleaned, and sterile drapes are placed over you.
   A sticky pad or metal plate is placed in contact with body to provide grounding for the electrosurgical unit that is used to stop any bleeding that occurs during surgery.
   The physician injects the area with an anesthetic so you will not feel pain.
   The visible portion of the growth is removed.
   A thin layer of tissue is removed from the surrounding skin and base.
   The tissue is examined under a microscope to determine that all suspicious cells are removed.
   The procedure is repeated, if necessary.
   You will be given pain medication to take home so you will be comfortable after the effects of local anesthesia diminish.

Special Considerations

3. Most often the surgical area is closed with sutures, but plastic reconstruction may be necessary.

Modified from Dollinger, M., Rosenbaum, E. H., & Cable, G. (1994). *Everyone's guide to cancer therapy.* Kansas City: University Press Syndicate.

stroy residual tumor and produced hemostasis. A shave biopsy before curettage and dissection is preferred over punch or incisional biopsy primarily because of the ease with which the procedure follows a shave procedure. These procedures are used most often as treatment for basal cell carcinoma, superficial squamous cell carcinoma, and hypertrophic actinic keratoses, among others. The cure rate for this procedure is based on appropriate patient selection, as with the other therapies. Long-duration tumors have a high rate of recurrence with this procedure due to the natural tendency of such tumors to be more infiltrative. This technique is not preferred in certain areas due to cosmetic considerations. When performed near the mouth and eyes, there is risk for contracture. There is a risk of excessive tissue destruction and scarring when an excessive current is used in electrodesiccation.

TABLE 74-7 Indications for Mohs' Surgery in Treatment of Nonmelanoma Skin Cancer*

Locally recurrent tumors
Tumors located on the central face, scalp, ear, genitalia, and fingers
Histologically aggressive tumors
Incompletely excised tumors
Tumors in an area previously treated with radiation
Tumors with ill-defined clinical margins
Tumors larger than 2 cm
Tumors in cosmetically important areas

*Basal cell and squamous cell carcinomas.

Cryotherapy

Cryotherapy uses the application of subzero temperature to cause cryonecrosis. Liquid nitrogen (−195.5° C) is used to induce cellular changes that are lethal to cells. The effect of cryotherapy on the microvasculature of the skin and tumor tissue is considered by some to be the more severe effect (Safai, 1997). This procedure is used with patients who are poor surgical risks. It is used for tumors with well-defined margins or recurrent tumors. A 3- to 5-mm tumor-free margin is used to secure the cure rate. This therapy is not indicated when the patient has an abnormal cold intolerance (e.g., Raynaud's disease) for morphea-type basal cell carcinomas or certain anatomic locations (e.g., eyelid, lip). Morbidity includes edema, oozing, erosion, secondary infection, and hemorrhage. Cosmetic results may include hypopigmentation or hyperpigmentation. Hyperpigmentation usually fades within a few months.

Topical Chemotherapy

Topical chemotherapy has been used for precancerous and cancerous lesions of the skin. Many substances have been used, including thiotepa, carmustine, fluorouracil (5-FU), retinoids, salicylic acid, and others. 5-FU is the only agent proven effective. BCNU (carmustine) and nitrogen mustard are used effectively in the treatment of T-cell lymphoma, and retinoids are now being used in clinical trials. 5-FU is effective by inhibiting DNA synthesis. It is applied once or twice a day and causes an inflammatory response in precancerous and malignant areas. Morbidity includes erythema and pigmentary changes. Systemic chemotherapy has not been effective in nonmelanoma skin cancers. Some believe that topical 5-FU is not considered an effective treatment modality for basal cell carcinoma because of the potential for a tumor-free surface with continued tumor growth underneath. Surgical excision is considered to be an effective

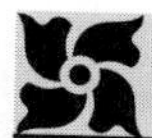

TABLE 74-8 Standard of Care for the Patient Undergoing Mohs' Surgery for Skin Cancer

Patient Problem and Outcomes	Nursing Interventions and Rationales	Patient Education Instructions
Postoperative Pain Patient will experience optimal pain relief.	1. Assess the pain intensity using a 0-10 scale during the immediate postoperative period and by phone after the day of surgery. 2. Administer analgesics during the immediate postoperative area. 3. Provide a prescription and instructions for at-home administration of analgesics. Conform understanding with the caregiver. Provide a copy of postoperative instructions to the home care agency when appropriate.	1. Teach the patient the importance of taking analgesia as ordered to maximize the effect and decrease side effects. 2. Provide written instructions for postoperative pain management.
Risk for Bleeding	1. Assess for signs and symptoms of excessive bleeding during the immediate postoperative period. 2. Provide referral to a home care agency when appropriate.	1. Teach the patient to monitor any drainage or dressing for increasing diameter when at home. 2. Teach the patient to avoid any risk of trauma to the surgical site. 3. Review an emergency phone number if excessive bleeding occurs.
Risk of Recurrence of New Skin Cancer	1. Provide instructions on cutaneous self examination. 2. Demonstrate the proper application of sunscreen. 3. Schedule regular follow-up examinations.	1. Provide written material to support an understanding of skin cancer examination (SCE). 2. Provide written information to support compliance.

treatment modality for these forms of skin cancers. An advantage of this modality is that it allows for microscopic evaluation of the tumor and its margins (Safai, 1997).

Surgical Excision

Surgical excision can be performed under local anesthetic and allows for good cosmetic results. Flaps or grafts are sometimes necessary when the lesion is large or if primary closure may result in an undesirable outcome. An issue is the ability to ensure complete removal before performing a reconstructive procedure. The decision to perform surgical excision must be made within the framework of all other available modalities.

Radiation Therapy

Radiation therapy is often used in the treatment of skin cancer because most skin is radiosensitive. This treatment is commonly indicated when the patients are elderly or frail. Many advantages to radiation therapy are acknowledged, including lack of pain, no required hospitalization, and no change required in the patient's activities of daily living. Another advantage is that radiation therapy allows for normal tissue sparing. A noteworthy disadvantage is the number of visits required to complete treatment. It is the treatment of choice for lesions on the nose, eye, lip, and eyelid. Select tumors along the embryonal fusion planes can also be successfully treated with this modality. Morbidity includes hyperpigmentation or hypopigmentation telangiectasia. Radiation therapy also has the potential to produce precancerous lesions. Before radiation therapy (or any therapy), a histologic diagnosis should be made. Anticipated immediate side effects of radiation therapy include erythema, exudative reaction, mucositis (nose), and loss of eyelashes (eyelid). Although the goal of radiation therapy is to destroy the tumor while sparing normal tissue as much as possible, some effect cannot be avoided (Delaney, 1994).

Electron Beam Irradiation

Electron beam irradiation is used in the treatment of superficial skin tumors. Electron beam irradiation does not affect deep tissue because the depth of penetration is limited. Excellent cosmetic results can be achieved (Greip, Davelaar, Scholteo, Chin, & Leer, 1995).

Chemotherapy and Mohs' Micrographic Surgery

Chemosurgery and Mohs' micrographic surgery is depicted in Table 74-8. This approach was introduced by Frederick Mohs who, when a medical student, noted that injection of 20% zinc chloride into tissues resulted in fixation and preservation. This observation provided the basis of a technique (chemosurgery) for the treatment of skin cancers. In this procedure, zinc chloride paste is serially removed. The excised portion is divided into segments and evaluated using light microscopy. The steps of evaluation are repeated until all margins are clear. The indication for Mohs' microsurgery is in the treatment of tumors that would otherwise be difficult to treat (e.g., difficult basal cell carcinomas and squamous cell carcinomas, Bowen's disease, keratoacanthoma, and others). It is also indicated when recurrence has occurred after conventional surgery and/or treatment modalities (Ratner & Grande, 1994).

Experimental Modalities

Experimental modalities include intralesional injections of interferon. Short-term remissions have been achieved with long-term results pending. Photodynamic therapy has also been used (Lui & Anderson, 1992). An injection of a photosensitizing substance into the tumor (selectively retained by tumor but not normal tissue) is followed by exposure to penetrating light. Tumor cells are destroyed, and normal tissue is spared. Long-term results are not yet available; however, a positive short-term effect has been realized in basal cell carcinoma, squamous cell carcinoma, and Bowen's disease (Safai, 1997; Dachowski & Dalaney, 1992).

NURSING MANAGEMENT

Prevention

Exposure of normal skin to ultraviolet (UV) and visible radiation can alter skin structure and function (Guercio-Hauer, 1994). The most common cutaneous response to solar radiation is an inflammatory response known as *sunburn.* The best treatment for sunburn is prevention (Tangrea, Edwards, Taylor, Hartman, Peck, Salasche et al., 1992). Like sunburn, increased pigmentation of the skin, recognized as suntan, is a response to UV damage. The Western culture has long sought the tan, leading to an increase in radiation exposure and therefore skin damage. Skin that has been repeatedly exposed to the sun shows a wide range of pigmentary changes.

Sunscreens are topical preparations that, if used properly, reduce the harmful effects of UV irradiation. The effectiveness of sunscreens is depicted by the sun protection factor (SPF). SPF represents the ratio of the amount of radiation needed to produce skin redness with the sunscreen, compared with the amount of radiation needed to produce skin redness without sunscreen. Sunscreens are excellent protectors from UVB but are only moderately effective against UVA.

Health care professionals must focus on prevention of skin damage from the sun. Inherent in protecting the skin from the sun is the risk for impaired vitamin D synthesis. Vitamin D supplementation is recommended by some authors for when the skin is effectively protected (Guercio-Hauer, 1994). Sunscreens should be applied at least ½ hour before the person is exposed to the sun and reapplied every 2 to 3 hours and after swimming or perspiring. Reflection of the sun's rays near snow is a frequently overlooked sun-exposure opportunity. Table 74-2 lists key points on sun protection. Loescher, Buller, Emerson, and Taylor (1995) reported that children are a prime target for skin cancer prevention education. The prudent use of sunscreen early in life has the potential to reduce skin cancer incidence.

Screening

Barriers to screening have been discussed by many authors and include, but are not limited to, (1) lack of time (patient needs to disrobe); (2) lack of expertise in examination; (3) disagreement with recommendations; and (4) perception of inadequate reimbursement for time spent on preventive care (Rivers, 1995). These factors contribute to limited screening activity. Strategies to increase skin cancer screening must be addressed. Nurses are uniquely positioned to become the experts in skin cancer screening activities. In the hospital, nursing homes, offices, schools, and in the home a nurse is positioned to be able to assess the patient's skin while providing physical care, help patients to disrobe, and perform other aspects of interviewing, physical assessment, and care. Increased collaboration with dermatologists enhances opportunities. Public education can increase the public's request for total cutaneous examination (TCE) to encourage payor response and encourage primary care–based examinations. Participation in community-based screening programs provides the opportunity to perform mass screenings and enhance the nurse's level of expertise (Kopf, Friedman, & Rigel, 1986).

Posttreatment Management

Because surgical excision remains the most common treatment for skin cancers, postoperative care is determined by the extent of the procedure (Table 74-9). Patients who have had a surgical excision only should be instructed to protect the site against exposure to trauma and irritants and observe for signs of infection. Those who have undergone grafting or flap procedures require more intense observations. Protection against trauma and observing for signs of infection and hemorrhage at the donor and recipient sites is imperative. Education of the patient receiving radiotherapy or laser surgery regarding the expected appearance of the skin and the importance of skin care during treatment should continue throughout therapy. Written instructions in all cases improve compliance and understanding. Patients receiving chemotherapy and immunotherapy require instructions specific to their modality. For all modalities the importance of regular, scheduled follow-up must be stressed. Nursing plays a pivotal role in the preoperative, intraoperative, and postoperative care of the patient with a cutaneous malignancy.

HOME CARE ISSUES

Outpatient surgical procedures for dermatologic diagnoses is not a new concept. However, a significant portion of the patients seen in dermatology practices are greater than age 65 years. Many live alone or have spouses unable to care for them. Because of these reasons, the risk for postoperative complications becomes noteworthy. Fosko and Stecher (1995) describe the positive effect a home care nurse can have on the outcome when a postoperative complication develops. Wound assessment and assessment of patient and/or caregiver understanding are essential to positive outcomes. In some cases, early identification of possible complications can avoid hospitalization.

Although it is not appropriate or necessary for all patients having a dermatologic procedure to have home care visits, it is important to assess for those issues that might contribute to postoperative complications and refer appropriately.

PROGNOSIS

The incidence of nonmelanoma skin cancers is increasing. With early diagnosis and treatment, almost all basal cell and squamous cell cancers can be cured. Patient education regarding the dangers of sun exposure has the potential to reduce the incidence of nonmelanoma skin cancers. To date, however, much effort has been lost to those barriers identified, including the quest for the "perfect tan." Pivotal to a decreased incidence is the appropriate use of sunscreens starting early in life.

The prognosis for procedures improves with early detection of the lesion. The ability to correctly identify and diagnose a skin tumor is essential to provide proper treatment. The treatment modality for BCC and SCC should be made based on the lesion size, anatomic location, depth of invasion, cellular differentiation, and history or previous treatment. Regular follow-up evaluation is important to prevent complications and identify any possible recurrence, as well as reinforce patient education regarding excessive sun exposure and use of sunscreens (Kopf, Salopek, Slade, Marghoob & Bart, 1986).

RESEARCH ISSUES

There is much to be done in the prevention of skin cancer by developing skin cancer education. Loescher and colleagues (1995) suggest that, although children are a prime target for skin cancer prevention education, it has yet to be determined whether structured curricula alone or in combination with others is the best method. In addition, any educational program must be evaluated before general distribution. Controversies regarding the best arena for skin cancer screening (primary care versus large community-based screenings) must be evaluated. The size and depth of skin lesions as independent prognostic indicators require further study. The nurse as expert in skin cancer screening is another research area that is timely as the role of the advanced practice nurse continues to evolve.

TABLE 74-9 Quality of Care Evaluation for Patients Receiving Surgical Excision for Skin Cancer

Disciplines participating in the quality of care evaluation:
☐ Nursing ☐ Physician

Data from:
☐ Medical Record Review ☐ Patient/Family Interview

Criteria	Yes	No
1. Patient provided with information about the following:		
a. Protecting the surgical site from sun exposure, trauma, and irritants such as strong soaps and astringents	☐	☐
b. Guidelines for infection prevention (i.e., washing area with bacteriostatic soaps, washing hands before touching face, washing hands before and after using the bathroom)	☐	☐
c. Signs and symptoms of infection, redness, swelling, pain, pus, fever, or chills	☐	☐
d. An appointment for follow-up care	☐	☐
e. Names, addresses, and phone numbers of support groups in the area	☐	☐
f. Teaching for prevention and early detection of new lesions (i.e., staying out of the sun)	☐	☐

Patient/Family Satisfaction

Data from:
☐ Patient Interview ☐ Family Interview

Criteria	Yes	No
1. On a scale of 0 to 10, with 0 being totally dissatisfied and 10 being totally satisfied, how satisfied were you with the care you received during your surgery? ________		
2. Were you instructed about pain medicine for your biopsy?	☐	☐
3. Were you given prevention and early-detection instructions about cancer?	☐	☐
4. Did you feel you were given adequate instructions about the care of your prosthesis?	☐	☐
5. Did you feel you were given adequate instructions about the surgical procedure?	☐	☐
6. Would you recommend your family and friends to the health care facility?	☐	☐

REFERENCES

American Cancer Society. (1998). *Facts and figures.* Atlanta: American Cancer Society.

Bajdik, C. D., Gallagher, R. P., Astrakianakis, G., Hill, G. B., Fincham, S., & McLean, D. I. (1996). Non-solar ultraviolet radiation and the risk of basal and squamous cell skin cancer. *British Journal of Cancer, 73,* 1612-1614.

Bielan, B. (1995). What's your assessment. *Dermatology Nursing, 6*(4), 254-255.

Brash, D. E. (1997). Cancer of the skin. In V. T. Devita, Jr., S. Hillman, & S. A. Rosenberg (Eds.), *Cancer: Principles and practices of oncology, Vol. 2* (5th ed.). Philadelphia: Lippencott-Raven.

Breuinger, H., Black, G., & Rassner, G. (1990). Microstaging of squamous cell carcinomas. *American Journal of Clinical Pathology, 94,* 624-627.

Chorun, L., Norris, E. C., & Gupta, M. (1994). Basal cell carcinoma in blacks: A report of 15 cases. *Annals of Plastic Surgery, 33*(1), 90-95.

Cruse, C. W., O'Neill, W., & Rayhack, J. (1992). Metastatic basal cell carcinoma of the upper extremity. *Journal of Hand Surgery, 17,* 1093.

Czarnecki, D., Meehan, C. J., McColl, I., & Kulinskaya, E. (1996). Lymphocyte counts of patients who have had skin cancer. *Journal of the American Academy of Dermatology, 34*(5), Part 1, 772-776.

Dachowski, L. J. & Delaney, T. (1992). Photodynamic therapy: The NCI experience and it's nursing implications. *Oncology Nursing Forum, 19*(1), 63-67.

Delaney, T. (1994). Radiation therapy for the treatment of skin cancers of the head and neck. *Dermatology Nursing (CE Series), 6*(2), 104-111.

Dinehart, S. M., Chu, D. Z. J., & Manners, A. W. (1990). Immunosuppression in patients with metastatic squamous cell carcinoma of the skin. *Journal of Dermatologic Surgical Oncology, 16,* 271-274.

Dinehart, S. M. & Pollack, S. V. (1989). Metastases from squamous cell carcinoma of the skin and lip. *Journal of the American Academy of Dermatology, 21,* 241-248.

Dollinger, M., Rosenbaum, E. H., & Cable, G. (1994). *Everyone's guide to cancer therapy.* Kansas City: University Press Syndicate.

Domarus, H. V. & Stevens, P. J. (1984). Metastatic basal cell carcinoma: Report of five cases and review of 170 cases in the literature. *Journal of the American Academy of Dermatology, 10,* 1043-1060.

Enders, G. H., Koh, J., Missero, C., Rustgi, A. K., & Harlow, E. (1996). p16 Inhibition of transformed and primary squamous epithelial cells. *Oncogene, 12,* 1239-1245.

Fisher, M. S. & Kripke, M. L. (1982). Suppressor T lymphocytes control the development of primary skin cancers in ultraviolet-irradiated mice. *Science, 216,* 1133-1134.

Fleming, I. D., Amonette, R., Monaghan, T., & Flemming, M. D. (1995). Principles of management of basal and squamous cell carcinoma of the skin. *CANCER supplement, 75*(2), 699-704.

Fosko, S. W. & Stecher, J. C. (1995). The role of home health nursing: A dermatologic case study. *Dermatology Nursing, 7*(3), 185-187.

Frankel, D. H., Hanusa, B. H., & Zitelli, J. A. (1992). New primary nonmelanoma skin cancer in patients with a history of squamous cell carcinoma of the skin: Implications and recommendations for follow-up. *Journal of the American Academy of Dermatology, 26*(5), Part 1, 720-726.

Friedman, H., Cooper, P. H. & Wanebo, H. J. (1985). Prognostic and therapeutic use of microstaging of cutaneous squamous cell carcinoma of the trunk and extremities. *Cancer, 56,* 1099-2105.

Frierson, H. F. & Cooper, P. H. (1986). Prognostic factors in squamous cell carcinoma of the lower lip. *Human Pathology, 17,* 346-354.

Frierson, H. F., Deutch, B. D., & Levine, P. A. (1988). Clinicopathologic features of cutaneous squamous cell carcinomas of the head and neck in patients with chronic lymphocytic leukemia/small lymphocytic lymphoma. *Human Pathology, 19,* 1397-1402.

Frisch, M. & Melbye, M. (1995). New primary cancers after squamous cell skin cancer. *American Journal of Epidemiology, 141*(10), 916-922.

Gallagher, R. P., Hill, G. B., Bajdik, C. D., Fincham, S., Coldman, A. J., McLean, D. I., & Threlfall, W. J. (1995a). Sunlight exposure, pigmentary factors, and risk of nonmelanocytic skin cancer I: Basal cell carcinoma. *Archives of Dermatology, 131,* 157-163.

Gallagher, R. P., Hill, G. B., Bajdik, C. D., Fincham, S., Coldman, A. J., McLean, D. I., & Threlfall, W. J. (1995b). Sunlight exposure, pigmentation factors, and risk of nonmelanocytic skin cancer II: Squamous cell carcinoma. *Archives of Dermatology, 131,* 157-163.

Gantt, G. (1990). Cutaneous squamous cell carcinoma characteristics. *Dermatology Nursing,* 2(5) 283-287.

Giles, G., Marks, R., & Foly, P. (1988). The incidence of non-melanocytic skin cancer in Australia. *British Medical Journal, 296,* 13-17.

Glass, A. G. & Hoover, R. N. (1989). The emerging epidemic of melanoma and squamous cell skin cancer. *Journal of American Medical Association, 262,* 2097-2100.

Griep, C., Davelaar, J., Scholten, A., Chin, A., & Leer, J. W. H. (1995). Electron beam therapy is not inferior to superficial x-ray therapy in the treatment of skin carcinoma. *International Journal of Radiation Oncology, Biology, and Physiology, 32*(5), 1347-1350.

Guercio-Hauer, C. (1994). Photodamage, photoaging and photoprotection of the skin. *American Family Physician, 50*(2), 327-332.

Gumport, S., Harris, M., Roses, D., & Kopf, A. (1981). The diagnosis and management of common skin cancers. *Ca-A Journal for Clinicians, 31*(2), 8.

Halder, R. M. & Bridgeman-Sha, S. (1995). Skin cancer in African Americans, *CANCER supplement, 75*(2), 667-673.

Hartman, R., Hartman, B., & Green, N. (1986). Long term survival following bony metastases from basal cell carcinoma. *Archives of Dermatology, 122,* 912-914.

Hunter, D. J., Colditz, G. A., Stampfer, M. J., Rosner, B., Willett, W. C., & Speizer, F. E. (1990). Risk factors for basal cell carcinoma in a prospective cohort of women. *Annual Epidemiology, 1,* 12-23.

Karagas, M. R., Stukel, T. A., Greenberg, E. R., Baron, J. A., Mott, L. A., & Stern, R. S. (1992). Risk of subsequent basal cell carcinoma and squamous cell carcinoma of the skin among patients with prior skin cancer. *Journal of the American Medical Association, 267*(24), 3305-3310.

Kibarian, M. A. & Hruza, G. J. (1995). Nonmelanoma skin cancer: Risks treatment options, and tips on prevention. *Postgraduate Medicine, 98*(6), 39-40, 45-48, 55-56.

Kinlen, L. J. (1985). Incidence of cancer in rheumatoid arthritis and other disorders after immunosuppressive treatment. *American Journal of Medicine, 78*(Supplement 1A), 44-49.

Kopf, A., Friedman, R., & Rigel, M. A. (1986). Self examination of the skin. *The Skin Cancer Foundation Journal, 4,* 21-29.

Kopf, A. W., Salopek, T. G., Slade, J., Marghoob, A. A., & Bart, R. S. (1995). Techniques of cutaneous examination for the detection of skin cancer. *CANCER supplement, 75*(2), 685-690.

Kricker, A. & Armstrong, B. K. (1995). Does intermittent sun exposure cause basal cell carcinoma? A case controlled study. *International Journal of Cancer, 60,* 489.

Kripke, M. L. & Sass, E. R. (1974). Antigenicity of murine skin tumors induced by UV light. *Journal of National Cancer Institute, 53,* 1333-1336.

Kwa, R. E., Campana, K., & Moy, R. L. (1992). Continuing medical education—biology of cutaneous squamous cell carcinoma. *Journal of the American Academy of Dermatology, 26*(1), 1-29.

Lee, G., Massa, M. C., Welykyj, S., Choo, J., & Greaney, V. (1991). Yield from total skin examination and effectiveness of skin cancer awareness program: Finding in 874 new dermatology patients. *Cancer, 67,* 202-205.

Lever, W. F. (1983). *Tumors of epidermal appendages in histopathology of the skin.* Philadelphia: J. B. Lippincott.

Lo, J. S., Snow, S. N., & Reizner, G. T. (1991). Metastatic basal cell carcinoma: Report of twelve cases with a review of the literature. *Journal of the American Academy of Dermatology, 24,* 715-730.

Lobo, D. V., Chu, P., Grelan, R. C., & Berger, T. G. (1992). Nonmelanoma skin cancers and infection with the human immunodeficiency virus. *Archives of Dermatology, 126,* 623-627.

Loescher, L. J., Buller, M. K., Buller, D. B., Emerson, J., & Taylor, A. M. (1995). The evolution of skin cancer prevention education for children at a comprehensive cancer center. *CANCER supplement, 75*(2), 651-656.

Lui, H. & Anderson, R. R. (editorial). (1992). Photodynamic therapy in dermatology shedding a different light on skin disease. *Archives of Dermatology, 128,* 1631-1635.

MacGregor, J. K, Yu, C. C., Dublen, E. A., Levinson, D. A., & MacDonald, D. M. (1992). Aberrant expression of p53 tumor-suppressor protein in nonmelanoma skin cancer. *British Journal of Dermatology, 127,* 463.

Maloney, M. E., Jones, D. B., & Sexton, F. M. (1992). Pigmented basal cell carcinoma: Investigation of 70 cases. *Journal of the American Academy of Dermatology, 27,* 74.

Marghoob, A. A., Slade, J., Salopek, T. G., Kopf, A. W., Bart, R. S., & Rigel, D. S. (1995). Screening implications. Basal cell and squamous cell carcinomas are important risk factors for cutaneous malignant melanoma. *Cancer, 75*(2), 707-714.

Nagano, T., Ueda, M., & Ischiaski, M. (1993). Expression of p53 protein is an early event in ultraviolet light-induced cutaneous squamous cell carcinogenesis. *Archives of Dermatology, 128*(9), 1157-1161.

National Cancer Institute. (1988). Non-melanoma skin cancers: Research Report. Bethesda, MD: National Institutes of Health, Publication No. 88-2977.

Oran, Y., Orengo, I., Baer, S. C., & Ocal, T. (1994). p53 Protein expression in squamous cell carcinomas from sun-exposed and non-sun-exposed sites. *Journal of the American Academy of Dermatology,* 417-422.

Ostrow, R. C. (1982). Human papillomavirus DNA in cutaneous primary and metastasized squamous cell carcinomas from patients with epidermodysplasia verruciformis. *Procedure of National Academy of Science United States of America,* 79.

Preston, D. S. & Stern, R. S. (1992). Nonmelanoma cancers of the skin. *New England Journal of Medicine, 327*(23), 1649-1662.

Rampen, H. J. & Schwengle, L. E. (1989). The sign of Leser-Trelat: Does it exist? *Journal of the American Academy of Dermatology,* 21, 50.

Ratner, D. & Grande, D. J. (1994). Mohs' micrographic surgery: An overview. *Dermatology Nursing, 6*(4), 269-273.

Ren, Z. P., Hedrum, A., Ponten, F., Nister, M., Afshin, A., Lundeberg, I., Uhlen, M., & Ponten, J. (1993). Human epidermal cancer and accompanying precursors have identical p53 mutations different from p53 mutations in adjacent areas of clonally expanded non-neoplastic keratinocytes. *Procedure of National Academy of Science United States of America, 90,* 4216-4220.

Rivers, J. K. & Gallagher, R. P. (1995). *CANCER Supplement: Public Education Projects in Skin Cancer, 75*(2), 661-666.

Robbins, J. H. (1988). Xeroderma pigmentosum: Defective DNA repair causes skin cancer and neurodegeneration. *Journal of the American Medical Association, 260,* 384-388.

Robinson, J. K. (1987). Risk of developing another basal cell carcinoma: A 5-year prospective study. *Cancer, 60,* 118-120.

Rosen, M. P., Miller. S. J., & Schwab, D. (1996). Molecular analysis of effectiveness of Mohs' surgical technique. *The Lancet, 347,* 1692-1693.

Rosso, S., Zanettie, R., Martinez, C., Tormo, M. J., Schraub, S., Sancho-Garnier, F. S., Gafa, L., Perea, E., Navarro, C., Laurent, R., Schrameck, C., Talamini, R., Tumino, R., & Wechsler, J. (1996). The multicenter south European study *'Helios'* II: Different sun exposure patterns in the etiology of basal cell and squamous cell carcinomas of the skin. *British Journal of Cancer, 73*(11), 1447-1454.

Safai, B. (1997). Management of skin cancer. In V. T. Devita, S. Hellman, & S. A. Rosenberg (Eds.), *Cancer: Principles and practices of oncology (Vol. 2)* (5th ed.). Philadelphia: Lippincott-Raven.

Schwartz, R. A. (1990). Busche-Lowenstein tumor: Verrucous carcinoma of the penis. *Journal of the American Academy of Dermatology, 23,* 723-727.

Shea, C. R., McNutt, N. S., Volkenandt, M., Lugo, J. Prioleau, P. G., & Albino, A. P. (1992). Over expression of p53 protein in basal cell carcinomas of human skin. *American Journal of Pathology, 141,* 25.

Skarin, A. T. (Ed.) (1996). *Atlas of diagnostic oncology* (2nd ed.). Baltimore: Mosby-Wolfe.

The Skin Cancer Foundation. (1985). *Types and descriptions of skin cancers.* New York: The Foundation.

Smoller, J. & Smoller, B. (1992). Skin malignancies in the elderly, diagnosable, treatable, and potentially curable. *Journal of Gerontological Nursing, 18,* 19-24.

Sober, A. J., & Burstein, J. M. (1994). Precursors to skin cancer. *CANCER supplement, 75*(2), 645-650.

Tangrea, J. A., Edwards, B. K., Taylor, P. R., Hartman, A. M., Peck, G. L., Salasche, S. J., Menon, P. A., Benson, P. M., Melette, J. R., Guill, M. A., Robinson, J. K., Guin, J. D., Stoll, H. L., Grabski, W. J., Winton, G. B., & other members of the Isotretinoin-Basal Cell Carcinoma Study Group. (1992). Long-term therapy with low-dose isotretinoin for prevention of basal cell carcinoma: A multicenter clinical trial. *Journal of the National Cancer Institute, 84*(5), 328-332.

Thibodeau, G. A. & Patton, K. T. (Eds). (1996). *Anatomy & Physiology* (pp. 179-209). St. Louis: Mosby.

Tong, A. K. F. & Fitzpatrick, T. B. (1996). Neoplasms of the skin. In J. F. Holland, R. C. Bast, D. L. Martin, E. Frei, D. W. Kute, & R. R. Weich Selbaum (Eds.), *Cancer medicine* (4th ed.). Philadelphia: J. B. Lippincott.

Vargo, N. (1990). Basal cell carcinoma classifications and characteristics. *Dermatology Nursing, 2*(4), 209-214.

Vargo, N. (1991). Basal and squamous cell carcinomas: An overview. *Seminars in Oncology Nursing, 7*(1), 13-25.

Vitaliano, P. P. & Urbach, F. (1980). The relative importance of risk factors in nonmelanoma carcinoma. *Archives of Dermatology, 116,* 454-456.

Whitaker, D. C. (1992). Unresectable primary facial cutaneous carcinoma. *Journal of Dermatology & Surgical Oncology, 18,* 125-129.

Ziegler, A., Leffell, D. J., Kunala, S., Sharma, H. W., Gailani, M., Simon, J. A., Halperin, A. J., Baden, H. P., Shapiro, P. E., Bale, A. E., & Brash, D. E. (1993). Mutation hotspots due to sunlight in the p53 gene of nonmelanoma skin cancers. *Procedure of National Academy of Science USA, 90,* 4216-4220.

HIV Disease and Related Malignancies

Theresa A. Moran, RN, MS, FNP

EPIDEMIOLOGY

HIV Disease

Acquired immunodeficiency syndrome (AIDS) is the direct result of the havoc wreaked on the immune system by the human immunodeficiency virus (HIV). The constellation of syndromes and diseases known as *AIDS* occurs in the presence of a defective immune system.

The epidemiology of this epidemic has changed since the early years. Originally a disease confined to middle-class homosexual men, injection drug users (IDUs), and recipients of blood products in the Western world, it has since become a heterosexual disease, one of poor and marginalized populations (Ward, Petersen, & Jaffe, 1997).

The scope of this disease is not limited to the Western world. Through June 1995, approximately 1 million AIDS cases were reported to the Global Programme on AIDS of the World Health Organization (WHO) (WHO, 1995). Adjusting for variable health care throughout the world, WHO estimates that the true cumulative case total is 4.5 million adults and children with more than 70% of these cases occurring in Africa. In addition, WHO estimates that 18 million adults and 1.5 million children have the disease worldwide, with the male to female ratio being 3:2 (WHO, 1995).

Seroprevalence data, collected in the United States suggest that the prevalence of HIV among young men and IDUs has stabilized and may be declining in other specific subpopulations. Although the incidence of HIV infection remains relatively stable, the annual incidence of AIDS cases continues to rise with a disproportionate number of those being poor African-American, and Hispanic-American gay or heterosexual individuals living in major urban areas and the rural South of the United States (Ward, Petersen, & Jaffe, 1997).

At the beginning of the epidemic the mortality rate approached 100% within 2 years. However, with the advent of antiretrovirals such as reverse transcriptase and protease inhibitors, as well as the use of prophylaxis, HIV infection and AIDS are thought of less in terms of a rapidly fatal disease and more in terms of a chronic illness (Kaplan & Northfelt, 1997).

Kaposi's Sarcoma

In 1872, Dr. Moritz Kaposi first described the lesions of Kaposi's sarcoma (KS) in seven men of Mediterranean or Jewish ancestry. In 1947 the literature indicated that only 500 cases of KS had been reported, and by 1960 only 1200 total cases had been documented in the 100 years since the disease was first described. The incidence in the general population is estimated to be two to six cases per 100 million people. Thus dermatologists and oncologists were not likely to diagnose this rare malignancy in the course of their professional careers. However, beginning in the 1970s the incidence of KS increased dramatically.

As more sophisticated technologic advances brought on the era of organ transplantation, an increasing number of reports documented the occurrence of this malignancy in patients who were chemically immunosuppressed to prevent organ rejection (Longo, Seis, Lane, Lotze, Rosenberg, & Preble et al., 1984; Steis & Broder 1985). With the development of new drugs, oncologists began seeing KS in patients treated with antineoplastic agents. Reports from Africa in the late 1970s revealed that KS was endemic in certain areas of the continent. In 1981, KS was reported in yet another population, that of previously healthy, young, homosexual men who were neither receiving chemotherapy nor undergoing organ transplantations (Centers for Disease Control [CDC], 1981a, b).

Initially, this outbreak of what was once believed to be a rare skin cancer was considered an isolated anomaly. However, as other cities in the United States began noting the increasing numbers of young men with KS, it became obvious that a new phenomenon was occurring. Some controversy continues to exist over whether KS is a malignancy at all or simply a highly dysplastic phenomenon, although is generally accepted and treated as a malignant disease (Brooks, 1986; Costa & Rabson, 1983). In addition to KS, other opportunistic infections, primarily *Pneumocystis carinii* pneumonia, were diagnosed in this same population (CDC, 1981a, b).

In an effort to determine the cause of this KS outbreak, researchers began evaluating the immune systems of these young homosexual men. All were found to have some degree of immunosuppression (CDC, 1981b). In 1982 these findings led to the clinical definition of a new disease, AIDS, in which the underlying immunodeficiency resulted in the appearance of indicator diseases (CDC, 1982). One of the indicator diseases was the diagnosis of KS in a person younger than 60 years of age. In 1987 the diagnosis of AIDS was expanded to include the advent of KS in a person of any age who is seropositive for HIV antibody (CDC, 1987).

Classic Kaposi's Sarcoma. Before the occurrence of HIV infection, KS was divided into the following categories: classic KS (non-African), endemic KS (African), and KS that occurred in transplant recipients. Cases of classic KS are found in the United States and Europe. Predominantly a disease that occurs in men, it has a male/female ratio of 10 to 15 : 1 and primarily affects men of Mediterranean or Jewish ancestry in the fifth to eighth decades of life. This malignancy is characterized as an indolent, slow-growing cutaneous nodule or plaquelike lesion. In 88% of those diagnosed, lesions are confined to the lower extremities, distal to the knee, without invasive or disseminated disease. Generally, treatment is not indicated because of its indolent nature. It is predictably a chronic, fairly benign malignancy that is rarely fatal (Steis & Broder, 1985).

Endemic Kaposi's Sarcoma. In contrast, endemic KS (African) is a malignant disease that affects persons of all ages, including children, and is found almost exclusively in black Africans. Cases of KS appear to cluster near the equator in the eastern half of the continent. African KS affects men twice as often as women, with a male/female ratio of 2.5 : 1 (Yang, Rosenberg, Glatstein, & Antman, 1993). Clinical presentations range from one similar to that observed in classic KS (nodular and indolent skin lesion) to a florid, infiltrative, and highly aggressive lymphadenopathic form that progresses rapidly and is frequently fatal (Yang et al., 1993).

Transplant Kaposi's Sarcoma. Transplant recipients experience an increased incidence of KS as high as 150 to 200 times the number of cases found in the general population (Krigel & Friedman-Kien, 1985). Transplant KS also affects men at a higher rate than women (2 to 3 : 1), and presentations can range from localized skin lesions to disseminated visceral and mucocutaneous disease. A correlation seems to exist between the degree of immunosuppression and the incidence of KS. The more depressed the immune system, the greater the incidence of KS. Spontaneous remissions have been documented in transplantation patients whose immunosuppression has been reversed (Krigel & Friedman-Kien, 1985).

HIV-Related Kaposi's Sarcoma. The fourth category, AIDS-associated KS, was first described in 1981 and is distinctly different from the other categories of KS (Volberding, 1989). It is 20,000 times more likely to occur in an individual with HIV than in the general population and is 300 times more likely to occur in an individual with HIV than in other immunosuppressed groups (Beral, Peterman, Berkleman, & Jaffe, 1990). Additionally, within the population with HIV, it seems that those patients who acquire HIV through sexual transmission are more likely to develop KS than those whose source is injection drug use. Twenty-one percent of homosexual/bisexual men have an index diagnosis of KS compared with only 1% of hemophiliacs with HIV. Interestingly, women are four times more likely to develop KS if their partners are bisexual. This finding suggests that, in addition to HIV infection, another sexually transmitted organism may play an important role in the development of KS (Beral, Peterman, Berkleman, & Jaffe, 1990).

Systemic Non–Hodgkin's Lymphoma

Beginning in 1982, physicians in San Francisco, Los Angeles, and New York noted an increased incidence of non–Hodgkin's lymphoma (NHL) in homosexual patients. Because they believed that this incidence of NHL was somehow linked to the same immunodeficiency seen in AIDS, they began to prospectively collect blood for evaluation of the immune system. In fact the immune deficiencies found in these patients with NHL were similar to those found in other patients with AIDS. Because cancer in and of itself is immunosuppressive, this finding alone did not establish a diagnosis of AIDS. However, it did initiate further investigation. When the HIV antibody test became available, these patients with NHL were found to be seropositive. Thus the link to HIV disease was demonstrated, and a new category of malignancy was added to the case definition of AIDS. A diagnosis of NHL in a person who is also seropositive for HIV antibody or has positive culture results is considered to affirm a diagnosis of AIDS (Aisenberg, 1973; CDC, 1982; Kaplan, Wofsy, & Volberding, 1987).

It is difficult to determine the impact of HIV-related NHL on cancer statistics. Approximately 52,700 cases of NHL were diagnosed in 1996. However, the percentage of those cases that are HIV-related cannot be determined because statistics concerning tumors do not account for HIV status (American Cancer Society, 1995). Because the reporting of AIDS cases to the CDC is now required by law, the incidence of HIV-related NHL may eventually become known.

It has been estimated that NHL has been diagnosed in 4% to 10% of patients with AIDS. However, it is important to remember that the CDC requires reporting of index diagnosis only and that HIV-testing of all patients with NHL has not become part of the standard workup. In one review by the French Registry of HIV-associated tumors, 33% of NHL occurred in patients already diagnosed with AIDS (56 : 168) (Roithmann, Tourani, & Andrieu, 1991). If the United States statistics parallel the French data, one can assume that there has been a fair amount of underreporting. Of interest in the French review is the histology of the tumors. They reported three distinct categories of AIDS-related NHL: large-cell lymphoma (LCL), immunoblastic lymphoma (IL), and Burkitt's-like lymphoma (BL). They also associated the first two lymphoma histologies with *severe immune suppression,* defined as a median CD4 count of 99 cells/gml compared with BL, which had a median CD4 count of 270 cells/ml. This finding has significance in the pathogenesis of NHL. It is known that LCL and IL are associated with immune suppression, whereas BL is not, suggesting perhaps another reason for the development of BL in persons with HIV (Roithmann, Tourani, & Andrieu, 1991).

A brief mention should be made of the controversy that exists around antiretroviral agents, specifically azidothymidine (AZT) and the development of NHL. The question continues to be asked about whether the use of AZT increases the likelihood of developing NHL. Although AZT has been shown to cause malignancies in laboratory animals, the dosages administered were three to 24 times higher than the recommended human dose. It is now generally recognized that the increased survival attributed to AZT increases the likelihood of developing NHL. Data exist showing that the incidence of developing NHL in long-term survivors of HIV is comparable regardless of whether the patient takes AZT (Chapman & Minor, 1992).

Primary Central Nervous System Non–Hodgkin's Lymphoma

Primary central nervous system (CNS) lymphoma is a rare malignancy, accounting for 0.3% to 2% of all newly diagnosed lymphomas (Henry, Heffner, & Dillard, 1987). Although it can affect immunocompetent hosts, most of those diagnosed with primary CNS lymphoma are immunocompromised. Therefore those patients with primary immunodeficiency, acquired immunodeficiency, and iatrogenic immunologic abnormalities (e.g., organ transplant recipients) are at increased risk for the development of primary CNS lymphoma (Frizzera, Rosai, Dehner, Spector, & Kersey, 1980; Good, Russo, Schnitzer, & Weatherbee, 1978; Levin, Sheline, & Gutin, 1989).

In the case of organ transplant recipients, primary lymphoma involving the brain accounts for 50% of lymphomas in this population. It is common enough to predict its occurrence 28 months after transplantation (Levin, Sheline, & Gutin, 1989). It is not surprising then that primary CNS lymphoma develops in those infected with HIV who have *subsequent severe immune dysfunction,* defined as CD4 counts less than 75/mm^3. Before the AIDS epidemic, primary CNS lymphomas were noted in the 50- to 70-year-old age range with women being affected slightly more than men (So, Beckstead, & Davis, 1986). In the general population, the average time from onset of symptoms to disease is 1 to 2 months. Unfortunately, patients with AIDS are also at risk for the development of infectious CNS disease. Cryptococcosis and toxoplasmosis are AIDS-related opportunistic infections of the CNS. The differential evaluation of these diseases can prolong and complicate the diagnostic process. Yet, in the setting of HIV infection a complete evaluation of all possible pathologic causes is required.

Invasive Squamous Cell Carcinoma of the Cervix

KS, non–Hodgkin's lymphoma, and primary CNS lymphoma account for approximately 95% of all cancers diagnosed in patients with AIDS, but they are not the only malignancies seen in persons who are seropositive for HIV antibody (Friedman, 1988; Levin, 1987). Nor are they the only malignancies that develop in the presence of immune dysfunction. It is reported in the transplant population that there is a 100-fold increase in the development of vulvar and anal cancers and a 14-fold increase in cervical cancer. Therefore it was reasonable to expect that patients who were immunosuppressed as a result of HIV would be at risk of developing anogenital malignancies, in particular, invasive squamous cell cancer (SCC) of the cervix.

Indeed, beginning in 1989, the literature documented an unusually high prevalence of cervical intraepithelial neoplasia (CIN) and human papillomavirus (HPV) in women with HIV. What alarmed researchers was not only the incidence of HPV infection in women who were HIV positive, but also the degree of cervical intraepithelial neoplasia found. Early reports showed an increased HPV positivity in women with HIV (49%) compared with 25% in the general population. In addition, women who are both HIV/HPV infected are 42 times more likely to have cytologic changes (Maiman, Fruchter, Serur, Remy, Feuer, & Boyce, 1990).

In one study, the cervical cytology of 35 women with HIV and 23 women without it was evaluated by one cytologist who was blinded as to the patient's HIV status. Squamous atypia was found in 4% of the seronegative women, whereas 31% of women with HIV had evidence of atypia (Schrager, Friedland, Maude, Schreiber, Adachi, & Pizzuti et al., 1989). In fact, numerous anecdotal reports published over the past 5 to 6 years repeatedly confirmed this phenomenon. Perhaps the most important study in this area was conducted by Maiman and colleagues (1990). They reported on a group of seropositive women in New York with invasive and preinvasive cervical neoplasia. When compared with a group of women with similar characteristics who were seronegative, the researchers found that the women with HIV were more likely to have advanced disease at presentation, recur, have evidence of HPV infection, and have perianal involvement. As evidence mounted for an association between invasive SCC of the cervix and HIV, the CDC in 1993 added this diagnosis to the surveillance definition of AIDS (CDC, 1992).

Before the AIDS epidemic, several characteristics had been identified as risk factors for the development of SCC of the cervix. These characteristics included low socioeconomic status, young age at first sexual experience, multiple sexual partners, multiple pregnancies, prostitution, daughters of mothers who took diethylstilbesterol (DES), and smoking. These risk factors, although well studied and correlated in the general population, appear not to correlate in the HIV population. The only epidemiologic factor of any consequence is merely being a woman infected with HIV (Schrager et al., 1989).

RISK FACTORS

The major risk factors for HIV disease and related malignancies are summarized in Table 75-1.

HIV Disease

HIV is a sexually transmitted disease. The virus has been isolated out of all body secretions, but is most efficiently

TABLE 75-1 Risk Factors

HIV Infection	Kaposi's Sarcoma	Non–Hodgkin's Lymphoma	Primary Central Nervous System Lymphoma	Invasive Squamous Cell Carcinoma of the Cervix
Unsafe sex Injection drug use Vertical transmission mother to child	Homosexual men Women who acquire HIV by sex with a gay or bisexual man ? KSHV	Immunosuppressed	CD4 count $< 75/mm^3$ Epstein-Barr virus positive	Female

transmitted through blood, sexual secretions, and breast milk. Therefore in the adult population, those who practice unsafe sex or share needles without adequately cleaning them are at increased risk of contracting HIV.

In addition to contracting HIV during the birth process, vertical transmission from mother to child through breast milk has been documented. In sub-Saharan Africa, where women with HIV have no choice but to breast feed their infants, Dunn, Newell, Ades, and Peckham (1992) estimated an additional 14% risk of HIV transmission. Breast feeding is a major risk factor for HIV infection in children in developing countries.

Kaposi's Sarcoma

Earlier in the epidemic, there appeared to be a strong link between immunosuppression and KS, even though the degree of immunosuppression provided no predictive ability. In 1990, Friedman-Kien, Saltzman, Cao, Nestor, Mirabile, and Li et al. (1990) reported on the appearance of KS in six gay men who tested negative for HIV. This report supported the hypothesis that a sexually transmitted agent may in fact be responsible for the development of KS and may be expressed more readily in the presence of HIV. There may also exist a large population with this KS-causing agent that remains symptom-free unless they become immunosuppressed.

Human Herpes Virus Type 8. In 1994, Chang and colleagues described an eloquent piece of research they conducted in which representation difference analysis was used to isolate a new viral genome. The result of this research was the identification of a new human herpes virus that has some similarity to the Epstein-Barr virus (EBV) and greatly resembles the Saimiri herpes virus. This new virus is being called both the *Kaposi's sarcoma herpes virus* (KSHV) and *human herpes virus type 8* (HHV8) (Chang, Cesarman, Pessin, Lee, Culpepper, & Knowles et al., 1994).

Since the original paper, further research has demonstrated the presence of this virus in >90% of AIDS-related KS tissue samples. To add credence to the role of this virus in the development of KS, tissue surrounding KS lesions was examined for evidence of this virus, and none has been found. Of interest is the fact that this virus has also been found in tissue samples of classic KS lesions, non–HIV-related KS lesions, as well as in some AIDS-related lymphomas, specifically the body cavity lymphomas. A yet-to-be-answered question is to determine what role this virus plays in the development of KS. Is it merely a passenger virus, or does it directly transform cells or trigger transformations through another mechanism (Cesarman, Chang, Moore, Said, & Knowles, 1995; Cesarman, Moore, Rao, Inghirami, Knowles, & Chang, 1995)?

Other Cofactors. When KS was first reported, it was the initial indicator disease in 30% to 35% of all diagnosed cases of AIDS (Mitsuyasu, 1988a, b). However, a steady decline has been noted in the proportion of AIDS-related KS cases among total AIDS cases. It appears that in the gay population a decline of 20% per year has been noted. In other populations with AIDS-related KS, a 10% decline per year has been reported. It has been suggested that this decline reflects behavior change, as correlated with a decreased risk of developing sexually transmitted diseases (Northfelt, Kahn, & Volberding, 1991). In light of the identification of a new virus, this hypothesis indeed may be the explanation for the decline. However, it is important to keep in mind that a causal relationship has yet to be established between KSHV and the development of KS.

Other possible explanations for this reduction in incidence of KS as the initial diagnosis include medical advancements that enable opportunistic infections to be diagnosed earlier than KS and the elimination of a cofactor that promotes the development of KS. Some researchers link the decreased incidence of KS to the decreased use of "poppers," or amyl nitrate, which is believed to be a cofactor in the development of AIDS-related KS (Haverkos, Pinsky, Drothman, & Bregman, 1985). This connection was suggested in several studies. However, large enough cohorts have not been collected and studied to document a causal relationship. Another group of researchers believes that hereditary or genetic predisposition plays an important role in the development of KS in both immunocompetent and immunodeficient populations. These researchers postulate that men with HIV who carry the human leukocyte antigen (HLA)-DR5 allele may be at increased risk for KS development. Again, a causal relationship has not been established and the postulate remains controversial (Groopman & Broder, 1989).

Homosexual Men. KS is found predominantly in homosexual and bisexual men with AIDS. Other groups diagnosed with AIDS (e.g., women; children; or men who are heterosexual or IDUs, or both) do not have as high an incidence of KS as homosexual men with AIDS (Garrett, Lange, Ashford, & Thomas, 1985; Nissenblatt, 1985). One study found the DNA of cytomegalovirus (CMV) in the nucleus of cells of KS lesions, which suggests a viral cause of KS (Urmacher, Myskowski, Ochoa, Kris, & Safai, 1982; Drew, Mintz, & Miner, 1981). Serologic testing demonstrates that as many as 94% of all homosexual men may have CMV, as evidenced by antibodies to CMV. In addition, CMV has been isolated from the blood, semen, gastrointestinal (GI) tract, CNS, and lungs of patients with AIDS. These findings suggest a possible role of latent CMV infection in AIDS-related KS. In fact, a decline in CMV seroconversion has also been noted in recent years. Together with high CMV antibody seroprevalence, this viral link was once thought to be an explanation for the predominance of KS in homosexual men.

It is also important to remember that statistics for KS are kept only on initial diagnosis of AIDS. Few reports examine the development of KS at any point during the AIDS illness. However, Northfelt and colleagues (1991) reported the San Francisco experience and indeed noted a decline in the reporting of KS at any time during the illness. However, this finding may reflect the expanded definition of AIDS and the increased number of AIDS cases being reported under that expanded definition.

Systemic Non–Hodgkin's Lymphoma and Primary Central Nervous System Lymphoma

The connection between cancers and viruses has not been established fully. However, there are some malignancies in which a causative viral agent has been isolated. One such association exists between the malignancy known as *African lymphoma,* or *Burkitt's lymphoma,* which is a type of high-grade NHL, and EBV. In 1962, Dr. Dennis Burkitt described a malignant lymphoma in African children that was typically extranodal in origin, with an affinity for facial bones. There appeared to be an increased incidence of this malignancy in regions of high temperature and rainfall. This finding suggested to Burkitt some type of insect vector as a method of infection (or transmission). Since then, serologic studies and tissue cultures have established a constant association with the DNA-containing herpes virus known as *EBV* and the development of Burkitt's lymphoma. Although the significance of the geographic distribution remains unclear, it has been hypothesized that malaria or some other insect-borne infection results in a reticuloendothelial hyperplasia that may be a necessary cofactor for the oncogenic virus in the development of the malignancy. In addition, EBV has been implicated as the causative agent in nasopharyngeal carcinoma and in the development of NHL in transplant recipients. It has also been suggested as an important etiologic agent in AIDS-related NHL.

Of interest is that similar research involving patients with AIDS could not causally link EBV to HIV-related NHL. Although the EBV genome has been isolated in 30% to 50% of the DNA of patients with HIV and NHL, a direct relationship is not apparent. The role of EBV in the development of NHL remains unclear (Birx, Redfield, & Tosato, 1986). However, even though the viral link cannot be causally established, it is strongly suspected. Ziegler (1989) hypothesized that once an infection with HIV occurs, EBV may trigger lymphocyte proliferation that remains unchecked as a result of the immune dysfunction caused by HIV. This proliferation, in turn, may allow for the expression of two oncogenes, resulting in a polyclonal or monoclonal NHL.

Confusingly, Kaplan, Abrams, Feigal, McGrath, Kahn, and Neville et al. (1989) reported on EBV-positive serum in a small series of patients with AIDS-related NHL. In the 14 patients whose tissue was tested, four specimens were EBV positive, and in the fifth patient, EBV was recovered from one tumor site but not from the second tumor site. These findings led the researchers to hypothesize that the EBV may be a "passenger" virus and not responsible for malignant transformation. There also seems to be distinct differences in EBV positivity between tumor histology and site of involvement. MacMahon, Glass, and Hayward et al. (1991) reported that large-cell lymphomas were more frequently EBV positive (65%), whereas the small, noncleaved cell (Burkitt's-like) lymphomas were less likely to be EBV positive (20%) in individuals with HIV. They also reported a consistent association between the EBV and primary CNS lymphoma in an individual with HIV. Twenty-one specimens of brain tissue from CNS lymphoma patients with HIV were examined for EBV, and all 21 tested positive, suggesting a different pathogenesis from the systemic form of the disease.

New research by Chang and colleagues (1994) that identified a new viral genome has led to the discovery of this new virus in certain lymphoma tissue specimens, specifically those of body cavity lymphomas. The significance of this finding is unclear and further research is needed.

It is now known that therapeutic immunosuppression increases the risk of lymphoma development. For example, the risk for transplant recipients has been estimated to be between 35 and 200 times greater than that for the general population.

Invasive Squamous Cell Carcinoma of the Cervix

Both HPV16 and HPV18 have been implicated in the development of SCC of the cervix in women without HIV, as has HSV type 2. Mounting evidence suggests that HPV plays a role in the development of invasive SCC of the cervix in women who have HIV, particularly as the immune system deteriorates (Sillman & Sedlis, 1987).

PATHOPHYSIOLOGY

HIV Disease

The immune system is a complicated arrangement of cells and proteins that, when fully functional, protects the host from damage caused by invading microorganisms. In addition to this prime directive, the immune system also plays a role in maintaining homeostasis by removing damaged cells from circulation and providing immune surveillance against the development, growth, and dissemination of abnormal cells. The mechanism through which this is accomplished is complex and finely choreographed so that in the event that one component malfunctions, other components suffer as well.

There are essentially two major arms of the immune system—the humoral arm, made up of predominantly B lymphocytes, and the cell-mediated arm, comprised of T lymphocytes. Through the production and release of cytokines, these two components of the immune system work with one another to maintain a healthy host.

Infection with HIV leads to destruction of cell-mediated immunity. Ironically, HIV seems to use the body's finely tuned immune system against itself. Once inside the body, HIV is recognized as an antigen and the immune system goes to work, capturing the virus and presenting it to helper T lymphocytes (which happen to be CD4 receptor–positive, the primary receptor for HIV) in an effort to amplify the immune response. Instead of amplifying the immune response, this action only results in viral infection of these CD4-positive cells, and the downhill course begins. Since CD4-positive helper T lymphocytes are pivotal in the immune response, their absence is catastrophic, resulting in deficiencies in both cell-mediated and humoral immunity.

Kaposi's Sarcoma

Before discussing the pathogenesis and pathophysiology of KS, it is important to mention several characteristics of the tumor itself. KS is a very unusual tumor that is unlike any other human malignancy. The KS lesions demonstrate a variety of cell types when examined under a microscope. All other human tumors are clonal descendants of a single cell type, but this is not the case with KS. KS is essentially a growth factor disorder. KS cells require exogenous growth factors to proliferate in vitro. In addition, these lesions express a wide variety of cytokines and growth factors, some of which are self-stimulating. The scenario seems to be that spindle cells or their precursors are stimulated to proliferate by exogenous factors produced by other cells in the host. Once activated, these spindle cells then produce cytokines that promote neovascular and inflammatory components. Two additional questions need to be answered in relation to the pathogenesis of KS. The first is what role HIV plays in this process and the second concerns the role of KSHV (Schalling, Ekman, Kaaya, Linde, & Beberfield, 1995).

Numerous attempts have been made to define the role of HIV in the development of KS without much success. However, this problem can be viewed from a different angle. Looking at the epidemiologic data, it is obvious that KS is more prevalent in people with HIV. It is estimated that the risk of developing KS in the presence of HIV is 20,000 times that of the general population. Compare this risk with other types of cancers in which known carcinogens have been linked to their development, as is the case with cigarette smokers. Those individuals who smoke cigarettes have a 20- to 40-fold increased risk of developing lung cancer. For those individuals who are chronic carriers of the hepatitis B virus, the risk of developing liver cancer is 100-fold. In light of these numbers, it becomes clear that HIV does indeed play some role in the development of KS. As for the role of KSHV, that question requires further research to answer, although experts generally believe that a causal relationship will eventually be established.

After the histologic examination, the pathologist has the responsibility of diagnosis. All types of KS (endemic, classic, transplantation-induced, and epidemic) are microscopically similar. Descriptions of lesions include interlacing bands of spindle cells, with vascular structures in a network of reticular and collagen fibers. As the integrity of this network is lost, clefts usually occur among the vascular structures, which allow the extravasation of red blood cells. Lymphatic and blood vessels are present throughout the lesion and on its periphery. The nuclei of the spindle cells are often pleomorphic. Hemosiderin, extravasated red cells, and red cells that phagocytose the hemosiderin may be found between spindle cells. An inflammatory response involving histiocytes, lymphocytes, and plasma cells also may be seen.

Diagnosis can be difficult, especially in early or immature lesions. This stage has been referred to as the *macular stage*. Changes in this stage may be subtle, and the pathologist may observe only abnormally dilated vessels surrounding a normal superficial vasculature. There may be little or no inflammatory response at this stage. Nuclear pleomorphism may be seen in mitosis, with nuclear atypia. As the lesion matures and becomes a plaque, it demonstrates more extensive neoplastic involvement, with proliferation through many layers, including the dermis and occasionally the adipose layers. A marked inflammatory response occurs at this stage, with a corresponding increase in the numbers of spindle cells and the extravasation of red cells. The prominence of hemosiderin deposits also is noted at this time. As the lesion advances toward nodular formation, these effects become more exaggerated. Spindle cells are dense, with considerable reticulum deposition.

Systemic Non–Hodgkin's Lymphoma

Although lymphoma may occur in either the B- or T-cell line of lymphocytes, in persons with HIV the vast majority of disease occurs in the B-cell line. Of those B-cell lymphomas, 70% to 75% have large-cell histology, and 25% to 30% are small, noncleaved or Burkitt's-like lymphomas. The focus of this section is on a discussion of the transformation of B cells. To discuss the transformation that occurs in the B cell resulting in a malignancy, one must first understand the normal maturation of the B cell, immunoglobulin (Ig) formation, and B-cell development.

It is well established that antibody production within the immune system is the purview of B cells and that antibody structure consists of four distinct areas. The N-terminal variable (V) region, the antigen binding site (idiotype), the constant (C) terminal region, and the effector portion (complimen binding) of the antibody. For a B cell to generate an immunoglobulin, several gene rearrangements must occur that result in the production of either heavy or light immunoglobulin chains and that when paired together form a functional antibody. In humans, it is estimated that the naive antibody repertoire encompassing all possible combinations of heavy and light chain pairings and gene rearrangements allows for more than 10 billion antibody specificities.

Increased antibody affinity is possible with several V-region somatic mutations and nucleotide additions. As a result of this specificity, the antigenetically stimulated B cell is essentially fingerprinted. This process makes it virtually impossible for two B cells to develop the exact same combination for antigen specificity. This process becomes important when attempts are made to determine the clonality of a lymphoma (Kocks & Rajewsky, 1989).

The mouse model demonstrates that chronic antigen stimulation produces clonal proliferation of B cells that secrete antibodies specific to the antigens. Hence, with each new daughter cell produced, mutations and gene rearrangements occur that increase antibody affinity and avidity for that specific antigen. Those B cells that do not produce a specific enough antibody are then induced to die through programmed cell death, or apoptosis.

B-Cell Development and B-Cell Lineages. B-cell development has not been well defined in humans, but extrapolating from the murine model, two distinct types of B cells exist, B1 and B2, which are identified by the receptors expressed on their cell surfaces. The exact function of these two distinct types of B cells has not been fully defined. Of interest is the observation that in the individual with HIV, a proportion of B cells appears to increase with disease progression, although absolute numbers of B cells decrease.

B Cells and HIV. A variety of B-cell abnormalities are found in individuals infected with HIV, including polyclonal B-cell activation and aberrant immunoregulation. Additionally, B cells of persons with HIV are different from B cells of individuals without the disease. The former are more likely to secrete high levels of immunoglobulins and produce cytokines that induce B-cell proliferation and differentiation (IL-2 and IL-10). The overproduction of these cytokines in particular is significant in that both IL-6 and IL-10 have been found in the malignant cells of HIV-associated lymphoma. It is hypothesized that this process may result in an autocrine loop necessary for lymphomagenesis. In the most plausible pathogenetic model for lymphoma, lymphomagenesis occurs along a continuum that begins with polyclonal proliferation in response to a macrophage with HIV in an immunocompromised host that lacks the intrinsic controls on this proliferation. Because these cells are proliferating continuously, they are at risk for acquiring additive chromosomal abnormalities, perpetuating these abnormalities, and eventually transforming into an immortalized malignant clone. Reactivation of other mitogenic viruses such as EBV or HIV itself may be a cofactor in the development of the malignant clone.

Lymphomagenesis of Burkitt's-like lymphoma is thought to be somewhat different. In this disorder, c-*myc* translocations are found in more than 76% of cases. Although the location of the chromosomal breakpoint differs. this difference has been attributed to disturbances in normal cellular growth. However, the exact mechanism for the development of this malignancy is not well understood.

The HIV-related NHLs are predominantly B-cell malignancies and are typically intermediate to high grade. However, there have been a few isolated reports of lymphomas that are T cell in origin in men who show HIV seropositivity. The significance of these few cases is unclear; the numbers are small and may simply represent the normal distribution of T-cell lymphoma in the general population. Only through an increase in the frequency of this type of lymphoma can significance be determined. In the meantime, it remains an interesting phenomenon (Kaplan, 1988; Ng & McGrath, 1996).

Most cases of HIV-related NHL have been associated with a previous history of persistent, generalized lymphadenopathy. Benign follicular hyperplasia is a typical histologic finding on biopsy. Current research is under way to determine the role of human T-lymphotropic virus type I as a co-infecting retrovirus in the development of lymphomas in patients with AIDS. Few patients have been identified as being co-infected, and it appears that the course of their disease is determined more by their HIV infection.

If the process of an HIV-related NHL begins in a lymph node, the growing tumor causes structural damage, including effacement of the normal node architecture, replacement of normal cellularity by uniform and/or grossly abnormal cells, and the random extension of cellular proliferations beyond the original structural confines of the node. However, the development of lymphoma, is not limited to lymph nodes or the spleen; all organs have lymphocytes within their boundaries that are capable of transforming and forming tumors. The major characteristics of the HIV-related NHLs are summarized in Table 75-2.

TABLE 75-2 Characteristics of HIV-Related Non–Hodgkin's Lymphoma

	Systemic	Central Nervous System	Body Cavity
Histology	Large cell (60%) Small noncleaved	Large cell	Pleomorphic large cell
Clonal	Monoclonal Polyclonal	Monoclonal	Monoclonal
EBV	Sometimes positive	Positive	Often positive
HHV8	Negative	Negative	100% Positive
Median CD4	100	30	90
Survival	6-8 months	3 months	5 months

Primary Central Nervous System Lymphoma

It is now known that in the patient with a primary CNS lymphoma, the process is similar. However, the early medical literature reflects the confusion encountered in attempting to identify the cell of origin for primary CNS lymphoma. Perithelial sarcoma, reticulum cell sarcoma, and microglioma were a few of the names used to classify primary lymphoma involving the brain. It is now accepted that the cell of origin is the same as that causing NHL elsewhere in the body. The transformed cell, which multiplies in an area that does not allow expansion, is the cause of most presenting symptoms. In approximately 30% of all cases of CNS lymphoma, this neoplasm is multicentric, arising in several different areas of the brain at the same time. This presentation is similar to that described in either spontaneously occurring tumors or in tumors arising in immunodeficient states.

Invasive Squamous Cell Carcinoma of the Cervix

The cervix is the lower part of the uterus. Extending from the isthmus into the vagina, it is divided in two major parts, the endocervix and the exocervix. Where these two parts meet is the *squamocolumnar junction.* This term refers to the area where the squamous epithelium of the exocervix meets the columnar epithelium of the endocervix. This region is the most common area for cervical dysplasia and neoplasia to arise.

Generally, SCC of the cervix is a preventable disease. It is always preceded by dysplasia and squamous intraepithelial lesions (SILs). It arises from the squamocolumnar junction in the cervix, the area referred to as the *transition zone* (T-zone). The lesion is considered invasive when the malignant epithelial cells break through the basement membrane, enter the stroma, and spread by direct extension. In the non-HIV population, this invasion occurs in 10 to 20 years, with 66% of SILs progressing if untreated within 10 years. This process occurs more rapidly in the HIV population.

In addition, HIV itself alters cervical immunity, where both the humoral and cellular components are concerned. Evidence of cervical immunity is demonstrated by the fact that specific immunoglobulin A (IgA) antibodies directed against HIV can be isolated from vaginal secretions. In addition, both subepithelial T cells and Langerhans' cells have been identified within the cervix. Infection of these cells with HIV may lead to decreased immune surveillance and to more rapid replication of HPV or reactivation of latent infection. The exact sequence of events is yet to be defined; it is unclear whether infection with HPV makes the cervix more susceptible to HIV.

ASSESSMENT

HIV Disease

Assessment of an asymptomatic patient with HIV disease is summarized in Table 75-3.

Clinical Presentation. The clinical presentation of a patient with HIV can range from someone who has engaged in unsafe sex and is concerned about seroconversion to someone who has been disenfranchised from the medical system and is acutely ill with an opportunistic infection or malignancy.

History. The history obtained from the patient varies depending on the degree of acuity the patient exhibits. In the relatively well patient, exploring family history, social history, and risk factors, as well as determining the patient's depth of knowledge, may be appropriate. If the patient is presenting acutely ill, a symptom-directed history should be taken, completing the full history when appropriate.

Physical Examination. Assuming the patient is not acutely ill, a complete physical examination should be performed. Inspect the skin closely, looking for signs of KS, folliculitis, eosinophilic folliculitis, seborrheic dermatitis, bacillary angiomatosis, scabies, or molluscum. The buccal mucosa should be examined, again looking for KS, as well as candida, hairy leukoplakia, or aphthous ulcers. Palpate all lymph node chains, noting the size and the number of palpable nodes. Percuss and palpate the abdomen, note the size of both the liver and spleen. A neurologic examination and some basic neuropsychiatric testing should also be performed, noting any psychomotor slowing, mood or affect disorders, or hyperreflexia. A recent study looking at the ability of primary care physicians to diagnose common HIV-related physical findings found that only 25% were able to correctly identify hairy leukoplakia or Kaposi's sarcoma (Paauw, Wenrich, Curtis, Carline, & Ramsey, 1995).

Diagnostic Tests. Blood should be collected on the initial visit. Testing should include a complete blood cell (CBC) count, with white blood cell differential and platelets, serum chemistries, toxoplasmosis titer, syphilis titer, CD4 count, CD8 count, and HIV viral load count. In addition, a purified protein derivative (PPD) test should be placed, and a baseline chest x-ray obtained if there is any suspicion of *Mycobacterium tuberculosis.*

Kaposi's Sarcoma

The assessment of the patient for KS is summarized in Table 75-4.

Clinical Presentation. The clinical presentation of HIV-related KS resembles that of KS in transplant recipients. Multicentric skin lesions may be observed on any part of the body that disseminated mucocutaneous and visceral disease often affects, including the lymphatic, pulmonary, GI, cardiac, renal, biliary, and adrenal systems. There is no characteristic site of initial involvement as with the classic form of the disease. Lesions can be found on almost any skin surface, including the palms of the hands, soles of the feet, genitals, and head and neck. These lesions generally do not metastasize; however, they are multicentric (i.e., each lesion is a primary lesion unto itself). The lesions range in pigmentation from brown, brown-red, purple, dark red, to violet. In rare cases, they may appear to be deep blue-purple, resembling ecchymosis. They may be raised bullous nodules or flat plaquelike lesions. In either presentation, they do not blanch when pressure is applied and are not painful unless they are responsible for structural damage or impinge on vital organs or nerves. African-American patients commonly have nodular lesions, and Caucasian pa-

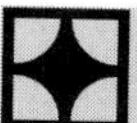

TABLE 75-3 Assessment of the Asymptomatic Patient with HIV Disease

	Assessment Parameters	Typical Abnormal Findings
History	A. Personal and social history 1. Age 2. Ethnicity 3. Risk factors for HIV disease	A. Personal and social risk factors 1. Usually young man or woman age 20 to 45 2. Minority 3. Unprotected sex, injection drug use
	B. Review of systems	B. Fevers, chills, night sweats, weight loss, respiratory symptoms, skin problems, nausea, vomiting, neurological symptoms, peripheral neuropathy
	C. Alternative therapies	C. Ask the patient about any alternative therapies he or she is using including Chinese herbs, megadoses of vitamins, acupuncture, acupressure, medicines obtained through buyers clubs or given to him or her by friends or brought in from other countries.
Physical Examination	A. Skin	A. The HIV patient may have any or all of the following: 1. Seborrheic dermatitis 2. Folliculitis 3. Kaposi's sarcoma 4. Eosinophilic folliculitis 5. Bacillary angiomatosis
	B. Mouth	B. The patient with HIV may demonstrate any of these oral complications 1. Hairy leukoplakia 2. Candida 3. Aphthous ulcers 4. Kaposi's sarcoma
	C. Lymph nodes	C. The following lymph node abnormalities may be seen 1. Localized lymphadenopathy 2. Splenomegaly
	D. Neuropsychiatric	D. Neuropsychiatric may also be present in the form of 1. Mood or affect disorders 2. Psychomotor slowing 3. Hyperreflexia
Diagnostic Tests	A. Complete blood count 1. White blood cell differential 2. Platelet count	A. Generally demonstrates mild anemia, granulocytopenia 1. Mild neutropenia 2. Mild thrombocytopenia
	B. Sedimentation rate	B. Elevated, normal <10 in men, and <15 in women
	C. Serum chemistries	C. Decreased albumin normal 3.4-4.7 g/dL
	D. Liver function tests	D. May see elevations in AST or ALT 1. ALT normal 0-35 U/L 2. AST normal 0-35 U/L
	E. Lactate dehydrogenase	E. May be elevated in the presence of PCP or NHL, normal 80-230 U/L
	F. Toxoplasma titer	F. May be positive and is useful in determining the likelihood of a brain lesion being malignant
	G. CD4/CD8 count	G. CD4 count normal or decreased, normal 359-1725 cells/microliter CD8 normal or elevated, normal 117 1106 cells/microliter
	H. HIV viral load	H. Positive, normal—no detectable virus
	I. VDRL	I. May be positive in the presence of HIV
	J. PPD or chest x-ray	J. May be anergic or positive. CXR indicated if there is a suspicion of mTb and the patient is anergic.

HIV, Human immunodeficiency virus; *AST,* aspartate aminotransferase; *ALT,* alanine aminotransferase; *PCP, Pneumocystis carnii* pneumonia; *NHL,* non–Hodgkin's lymphoma; *VDRL,* Venereal Disease Research Laboratory; *CXR,* chest x-ray.

tients tend to have either nodular or plaquelike lesions. As with HIV infection, the average age range in which HIV-related KS occurs is between 20 to 40 years.

The patient may give a history of the KS lesions developing (i.e., blossoming, exploding) shortly after a bout with an opportunistic infection or treatment with steroids. The reason for this is unclear, but it is an anecdotally observed phenomena. One possible explanation may be the associated deterioration of the immune system in the presence of an opportunistic infection and treatment with steroids.

TABLE 75-4 Assessment of the Patient for Kaposi's Sarcoma

	Assessment Parameters	Typical Abnormal Findings
History	A. Personal and social history 1. HIV positive 2. Prior opportunistic infections 3. Ethnicity	A. Personal and social risk 1. Injection drug use, unprotected sex 2. Not the patient's index diagnosis 3. Classic KS found in older men of Jewish or Mediterranean descent
	B. History of the lesions 1. When did they first appear 2. How often do new ones appear	B. Determining the natural history of the KS helps with treatment decisions. 1. Indicates how long the patient waited before seeking medical attention, also may indicate the amount of knowledge about certain diseases 2. Indicates the pace of disease
	C. Pain	C. Lesions impinging on vital structures may be painful.
Physical Examination	A. Inspect the skin carefully	A. Note the size, color, number, distribution and contour of lesions, important to assess response to therapy.
	B. Mouth	B. Oral-pharyngeal lesions are common
	C. Lymphadenopathy	C. Carefully palpate all lymph node chains and note size and consistency of lymph nodes. Nodal involvement is common. Also note any surrounding edema.
Diagnostic Tests	A. Biopsy	A. There is a differential for violaceous cutaneous lesions that includes bacillary angiomatosis, angiosarcoma, and fungal infections
	B. Labwork 1. HIV test 2. CD4 count	B. Baseline labwork is necessary to determine treatment options 1. Positive 2. Most likely decreased

This tumor can involve in the skin, mucocutaneous surface of the buccal mucosa, hard and soft palate, gums, and sclera of the eyes. In fact, at the time of initial diagnosis of KS, approximately 72% of patients already have involvement of one or more organ systems. Internal organs most commonly affected include the lymph nodes (81%), GI tract (33%), and lungs (11%). KS in these organ systems can cause severe morbidity. In addition, lesions have been found in the liver, pancreas, adrenal glands, spleen, testes, and heart. Symptoms caused by these lesions are usually minimal.

Although the majority of KS found in an organ system remains asymptomatic, one notable exception is pulmonary KS (Brown, Huberman, & Vanley, 1986). KS involves the lungs in 18% to 32% of patients diagnosed with cutaneous disease and may take anywhere from 1 to 36 months to manifest symptoms. These signs and symptoms include a nonproductive cough, fever, and dyspnea. Clinically, it is very difficult to distinguish pulmonary KS from *P. carinii* pneumonia. A chest x-ray often reveals bilateral interstitial or alveolar infiltrates; unilateral or bilateral reticular nodular pattern is less often noted. If the patient is bronchoscoped, violaceous plaques may be found in the tracheobronchial tree. Pulmonary KS lesions are usually not biopsied because they tend to be vascular and submucosal, making biopsy difficult. Visual confirmation of disease is acceptable in this instance (Kaplan, Hopewell, Jaffe, Goodman, Bottles, & Volberding, 1988).

As HIV infection progresses, the immune system becomes increasingly suppressed; with it, the occurrence and severity of KS also increases. Increasing numbers of skin lesions may be found all over the body surface. The multicentric skin lesions continue to enlarge, often coalescing with each other to form one large confluent lesion and encompassing as large an area as the thigh, shin, or forearm. Malignant cells may involve the lymph nodes, thus compromising lymphatic drainage and blood circulation and resulting in severe edema distal to the affected area and stasis ulcers from edematous tissue. The lymph node involvement may be severe enough to cause major shifts in body fluids, limiting the flow of vital proteins from the lymph to the plasma. The patient may succumb to anasarca because of internal coalesced lesions and decreased total serum protein/albumin resulting from the shift of fluid.

Additionally, when the GI tract is involved, the patient may have a protein-losing enteropathy. In this instance, protein is not absorbed from the GI tract, which results in a decreased total serum protein/albumin level. Chronic anemia may also be observed in patients with KS in their GI tract, since the lesions may ooze blood. In cases in which progression of KS involves the lung, symptoms include dyspnea and shortness of breath, eventually culminating in fatal respiratory distress.

History. A complete history is indicated, including the patient's past history of drug use, sexual practices, and ethnic ancestry. Query the patient specifically about pulmonary symptoms. Determine, if possible, the pace of progression of KS. Inquiring about the length of time the lesions have been present, the rate at which new ones appear, the relationship to a prior opportunistic infection, and whether they are causing pain may help with treatment decisions.

Physical Examination. A thorough examination of the integumentary system should be performed. This examination entails having the patient disrobe completely, inspecting the palms of the hands and soles of the feet, as well as the sclera, buccal mucosa, genitalia, and skin folds between the buttocks. If any lesions are found, note the size, color, physical description (nodular vs plaquelike), distribution, and presence of a halo (surrounding yellow/red discoloration). Also examine any areas covered with hair, including beards and the scalp. Palpate all of the lymph node chains and note the size and number of any palpable nodes. Look for edema either surrounding the lesions or distal to them. Auscultate the lungs, noting any rales, rhonchi, or areas of decreased breath sounds. One case of vulvar KS has been reported in the literature, demonstrating the necessity of thorough skin examinations.

Diagnostic Tests. Suspicious lesions must be biopsied before a diagnosis can be established. Visual inspection of lesions alone is insufficient to establish a diagnosis. Experienced physicians who care for patients with AIDS reflect anecdotally on lesions that appear to be symptomatic of KS but are not histologically confirmed. Conversely, examination of tissue from lesions that did not resemble those of KS proved to be diagnostic of KS. A lesion that visually suggests KS may be an immature lesion and does not show the distinctive pathologic changes that are diagnostic of KS. Repeat biopsies of other suspicious lesions at a later date (e.g., in 2 weeks) may in fact yield a diagnosis of KS. Not every lesion that resembles KS is in fact KS. Lesions most often confused with KS are those associated with bacillary angiomatosis. Also KS may not be the only pathology derived from the biopsy. In one biopsy specimen, KS was identified along with bacillary angiomatosis, lymphoma, fungus, and herpes simplex virus (Cole, Cohen, Satra, & Grossman, 1992).

Examination of preparations from a 3-, 4-, or 6-mm punch biopsy of skin lesions is the most common method of diagnosis. Patients with KS involvement of the oral cavity should be referred to an oral surgeon for a diagnostic biopsy. Suspicious lymph nodes are best evaluated by means of an open (excisional) biopsy. Suspected KS involvement of other organs requires more invasive diagnostic procedures. For example, documentation of lung involvement requires a bronchoscopic examination. Similarly, documentation of GI lesions requires endoscopic examination of the upper or lower GI tract. Lesions visualized by means of bronchoscopy or endoscopy may be examined by biopsy, but because of the submucosal and highly vascular nature of the tumor, removal of tissue from these sites may cause bleeding and increased morbidity. For this reason, visual inspection and identification may be adequate for diagnosing lung or GI involvement.

Documenting organ involvement by other means can be difficult. KS involving the lung cannot be diagnosed or distinguished from other causes of respiratory distress by means of chest x-ray (Davis, Henschke, Chamides, & Westcott, 1987). An upper GI series may demonstrate lesions in the gut, but the cause remains unknown without visual inspection by endoscopy or tissue biopsy. Because it appears that the presence or absence of organ involvement, with the exception of the lungs, does not affect survival, documentation of the extent of the disease is not useful in treatment decisions. If treatment of a specific site is to be initiated (e.g., radiation therapy to treat enlarged lymph nodes), then tissue diagnosis must be determined. The literature indicates several reports of patients having both KS and another malignancy in the same lymph node.

Patients with HIV-related KS also may show laboratory abnormalities that probably are more related to HIV infection than to KS. These abnormalities include elevated erythrocyte sedimentation rate (ESR), mild anemia, and leukopenia. Depressed test results with cosyntropin stimulation, elevated serum transaminase levels, and depressed platelet counts may result from KS involvement of the adrenal glands, liver, or spleen respectively.

Systemic Non–Hodgkin's Lymphoma

The assessment of the patient for systemic NHL is summarized in Table 75-5.

Clinical Presentation. In the general population the earliest sign of NHL unrelated to AIDS is usually a painless, enlarged, discrete lymph node located in the neck. Although most patients have no symptoms, approximately 20% may experience "B" symptoms, including fever, night sweats, and weight loss. Patients who do not have AIDS often have a history of intermittent lymphadenopathy that has been present for several months. Although axillary or inguinal lymph nodes may be the first to enlarge, this enlargement is not common. Involvement of Waldeyer's ring, epitrochlear nodes, the testes, and the GI tract is common. The liver and bone marrow may be involved. A higher incidence of CNS involvement occurs in patients with NHL unrelated to AIDS and bone marrow involvement. The disease is localized in fewer than 10% of patients who do not have AIDS. Because of the diffuse presentation of lymphoma, non-AIDS NHL should be included in the differential diagnosis of patients with superior vena cava syndrome, acute spinal cord compression, solitary thyroid nodules, isolated tumor nodules of the skin, bone tumors, unexplained anemia, testicular masses, or solitary brain lesions.

In contrast to the presentation just described, patients with HIV-related NHL have advanced disease, which often involves extranodal sites. In one of the first studies of 90 cases of HIV-related NHL, 19% were classified as intermediate-grade diffuse large cell lymphoma; 28% as high-grade, large-cell immunoblastic lymphoma; and 36% as high-grade, small, noncleaved lymphoma. These presentation rates remain unchanged, with greater than 50% of patients presenting with high-grade lymphoma. Extranodal sites most commonly involved include the CNS, bone marrow, bowel, and anorectum; less commonly involved is the myocardium. In addition, these extranodal sites may be the only site of disease; that is, peripheral lymphadenopathy may be absent. If nodal sites are involved, no predisposition to specific nodes exists. In addition, these patients may have underlying signs and symptoms of HIV infection, AIDS-related complex, or AIDS, including wasting, anorexia, nausea, vomiting, and fever, which confounds the workup and makes diagnosis difficult.

History. Take a thorough history from the patient with suspicious adenopathy, including eliciting the onset of the adenopathy, the pace of disease progression, and the presence or absence of "B" symptoms. Determine the history of HIV infection, and inquire about risk factors and recreational drug use, particularly injection drug use, since lymphadenopathy is common in this patient population.

Physical Examination

On physical examination particular attention should be paid to all lymph node chains, keeping in mind that it is not uncommon for the patient with HIV to have "shotty" adenopathy in the anterior and posterior cervical chains and in the inguinal area. Note the size, number, and characteristics of the enlarged lymph nodes (i.e., hard, fixed, mobile, rubbery, fluctuant). The oral cavity should be inspected thoroughly, noting any tonsillar hyperplasia, and the liver and spleen should be percussed and palpated to detect any hepatosplenomegaly. Auscultating the heart may reveal a murmur, especially in the IDU. Auscultate the lungs, noting any rales, rhonchi, or areas of decreased breath sounds.

Diagnostic Tests. The diagnosis and classification of lymphoma can be made only by means of a biopsy specimen examined by a pathologist. Fine-needle aspirations may be helpful in differentiating a benign vs malignant process; however, because of insufficient tissue yield, they are not useful in classifying the lymphoma. To fully assess HIV-related NHL, the patient's status must be staged and graded. Laboratory tests include CBC, differential cell and platelet count, sedimentation rate, serum chemistries, lactate dehydrogenase, and liver function tests. If a CD4 count has not been done recently, one should be done at this time. These laboratory tests are not specific to lymphoma; they indicate the overall wellness of the patient and are helpful in screening for hypercalcemia, hyperphosphatemia, and hyperuricemia. A chest x-ray and computed tomography (CT) scans of the chest, abdomen, and pelvis also are indicated. These tests usually are not indicated for patients with NHL in the general population, but because of the extensive extranodal involvement characteristic of HIV-related NHL, they are extremely important. Bilateral bone marrow biopsy and aspiration, as well as lumbar puncture, should be performed.

Grading is a histologic assessment of the tumor type, recognizing that different cell types behave differently. Grading a tumor also gives the health care provider some sense of the tumor's aggressiveness.

If AIDS has not been diagnosed previously, an HIV antibody test is indicated. Not all swollen lymph nodes are malignant. Benign reactive lymphadenopathy is a common finding in this HIV-seropositive population and is postulated to be an adaptive physiologic response to the HIV insult. Abdominal masses or lymph nodes in a person who is HIV seropositive could be related to *Mycobacterium avium-intracellulare* infection. Therefore it is essential to obtain a biopsy specimen and compare it with normal tissue before a

TABLE 75-5 Assessment of the Patient for Systemic Non–Hodgkin's Lymphoma

	Assessment Parameters	Typical Abnormal Findings
History	A. Personal and social history 1. HIV history 2. Risk factors 3. CD4 count	A. Typically patient already had a prior AIDS diagnosis: 1. Number and type of prior infections 2. Injection drug use is a negative prognostic factor 3. Prognostic information
	B. Presence or absence of "B" symptoms	B. Offers prognostic information.
Physical Examination	A. Lymph node palpation	A. Carefully palpate all lymph node chains, noting any enlarged, nontender, mobile or fixed rubbery nodes.
	B. Oral cavity	B. Note any tonsillar hyperplasia.
	C. Abdominal examination	C. Assess for splenomegaly.
Diagnostic Tests	A. Biopsy of suspicious lesions	A. Intermediate- to high-grade non–Hodgkin's lymphoma
	B. CT scans	B. Detection of LAN not palpable
	C. Gallium scan	C. The majority of lymphomas are gallium avid, may detect occult sites of disease
	D. Bone marrow biopsy	D. Rule out marrow involvement
	E. Lumbar puncture	E. Rule out CNS involvement
	F. HIV test	F. Ensure that this is an HIV-related lymphoma
	G. CD4 count	G. Offers prognostic information, if $<100/mm^3$ poor prognosis
	H. LDH	H. Often elevated, indicates tumor burden
	I. Serum chemistries	I. If uric acid is elevated the patient may already be experiencing some degree of tumor lysis

diagnosis is made. It is unusual for patients with HIV-related NHL to present at a stage lower than stage III.

Primary Central Nervous System Lymphoma

Assessment of the patient for primary CNS lymphoma is summarized in Table 75-6.

Clinical Presentation. Two retrospective reviews of a total of 26 patients revealed that the most commonly observed symptoms of HIV-related CNS lymphomas included confusion, lethargy, and memory loss (12/26), as well as alterations in personality and behavior (5/26). In the 26 patients, hemiparesis or aphasia was seen in seven, three patients had seizures, two had cranial nerve palsy, one had headache as the only symptom, one had headache associated with a lack of coordination, and one had no symptoms. A further review by So, Beckstead, and Davis (1986) revealed that although only three patients had seizures initially, seizures later developed in four additional patients. More than half of the patients reported more specific symptoms that consisted of focal seizures and progression of focal neurologic symptoms over days or weeks. In another review, all six patients studied had disease within the cranium; four had disease in the frontoparietal region, and two had involvement of the pons and cerebellum (Gill, Levine, Meyer, Boswell, Burlees, & Parker et al., 1985).

History. The patient with a primary CNS lymphoma is often unaware of degenerating neurologic faculties. The history often needs to be obtained from a significant other, friends, or family members. Query the patient regarding onset and duration of altered mental status, seizure activity, and progression of symptoms. The patient may describe a scenario of vague neurologic symptoms such as forgetfulness or mood changes. Since this problem is usually a late manifestation of HIV, it is important to determine during the history whether a durable power of attorney for health care has been designated in the event the patient is unable to make decisions.

Physical Examination. A complete neurologic examination is indicated to find a focal neurologic deficit. Funduscopic examination helps determine the presence of increased intracranial pressure.

Diagnostic Tests. These clinical manifestations are typical of spontaneous primary CNS lymphoma, and are typical symptoms caused by other mass lesions in the CNS. This similarity in symptomatology often makes it difficult to distinguish between CNS lymphoma and vascular and infectious disorders. The most common explanation for a mass lesion in the CNS is toxoplasmosis, which occurs in 10% of patients with AIDS.

Because of the morbidity associated with a brain biopsy, primary CNS lymphoma in most institutions is usually a diagnosis of exclusion; that is, the patient with CNS symptoms and a demonstrated brain mass is generally treated empirically for toxoplasmosis for approximately 2 weeks. Toxoplasmosis in the presence of HIV is almost always a reactivation of infection. This means that if a patient with a mass lesion in the brain has a negative toxoplasmosis titer, the likelihood that the mass lesion is toxoplasmotic is almost nonexistent, and primary CNS lymphoma becomes the most likely diagnosis. If the lesion fails to respond to treatment, then the diagnosis of primary CNS lymphoma is considered. At this point a brain biopsy could yield a definitive diagnosis. However, because of the invasiveness of the procedure, the degree of immunosuppression that is usually present, and the dismal response of primary CNS lymphoma to treatment, a presumptive diagnosis may be established.

In most patients the radiographic findings from the CT and magnetic resonance imaging (MRI) examinations reveal single or multiple discrete lesions. Before the use of a contrast medium on CT scanning, low-density lesions will appear, and a shift of midline structures may be apparent. After the administration of contrast material, the lesion characteristically appears enhanced. Reports differ on the type of enhancement; both uniform and patchy nodular enhancement with varying degrees of surrounding edema have been reported. Primary CNS lymphoma usually appears as single or multiple discrete lesions and exhibits a characteristic pre- and postcontrast appearance. However, some patients with primary CNS lymphoma have demonstrated

TABLE 75-6 Assessment of the Patient for Primary Central Nervous System Lymphoma

	Assessment Parameters	Typical Abnormal Findings
History	A. Personal and social history 1. Home situation 2. Support	A. This is usually a late manifestation of HIV infection, noting the patient's prior history will help determine treatment options. 1. Frequently the patient lives alone 2. May have few family or friends for support
	B. Onset/duration of altered mental status	B. May help determine the pace of disease
Physical Examination	A. Neurologic	A. May have focal deficit, or may have vague neurologic findings
	B. Funduscopic examination	B. If a mass effect is present, signs of increased cranial pressure can be found during a retinal examination
Diagnostic Tests	A. Magnetic resonance imaging of the brain	A. Space-occupying masses are often seen with and without surrounding edema, there may also be a midline shift.

ring-enhancing lesions on CT scan that are often indistinguishable from lesions seen in patients with cerebral toxoplasmosis. It is important to remember that a diagnosis of lymphoma cannot be determined by scans alone. In addition, MRI does not contribute to the differential diagnosis, although MRI may be useful in revealing lesions undetectable by the CT scan and may provide alternative biopsy sites.

Examination of cerebrospinal fluid (CSF) may reveal some abnormalities. However, the results are nonspecific and useful only in that they indicate some abnormality in the CNS. Tests ordered on CSF include toxoplasmosis titers, the Venereal Disease Research Laboratory (VDRL) test, and cytologic examination. Cytologic findings are positive in approximately 50% of patients who have CNS lymphoma. However, this result tends to depend on the volume of CSF obtained. Toxoplasmosis titers and VDRL results can help rule out toxoplasmosis and syphilis as causes for behavioral changes and altered mental status.

Invasive Squamous Cell Carcinoma of the Cervix

The assessment of the patient for invasive squamous cell carcinoma of the cervix is summarized in Table 75-7.

Clinical Presentation. Because so few cases of invasive SCC of the cervix have been reported, any differences between the clinical manifestations in a healthy woman and the woman who is seropositive have not been defined.

History. For the woman with HIV, a complete gynecologic history should be obtained, including menstrual history, birth control history, pregnancies, live births, miscarriages, and abortions (spontaneous or therapeutic). Determining the history of the HIV infection and obtaining an inclusive psychosocial and family history are also important. Since women are often the caretakers of sick children and significant others, it is important to understand the family dynamics and sources of stress that may affect the patient.

Physical Examination. A complete physical examination should be performed, assessing the skin, oral cavity, lymph nodes, heart, lungs, abdominal cavity, and neurologic system. The physical examination should also include a pelvic examination with a Papanicolaou (Pap) test. Current recommendations are that Pap smears be performed every 6 months, and if two negative tests are obtained, then the interval between Pap smears may be extended to annually. However, many of these women do not seek regular health care, so some providers feel that Pap smears should be continued on a biannual basis.

STAGING

HIV Disease

Although there is no formal staging system for HIV disease, it is useful to divide patients into four broad categories (Box 75-1). The first is the initial contact with the patient. At that time, take a baseline history and laboratory work, as well as physical examination. If the patient is a woman, then include a Pap smear as part of the physical examination. Update vaccinations, and assess patient for the need for formal counseling or supportive services. Once the patient's immune status has been determined, the patient can then be further staged as having early (CD4 count >500/mm^3), middle (CD4 count 200 to 500/mm^3), or late (CD4 count <200/mm^3) stage disease. It is important to recognize that these stages may not have any correlation with survival, but function more as a guide to patient care.

Kaposi's Sarcoma

The ability to classify patients with similar stages of the disease would enable researchers to compare data and patient

Box 75-1
Staging of HIV Disease

Early stage (CD4 count > 500/mm^3)
Middle stage (CD4 count 200-500/mm^3)
Late stage (CD4 count < 200/mm^3)

Modified from Hollander, H. (1997). Initiating routine care for the HIV-infected adult. In M. Sande & P. Volberding. *The medical management of AIDS* (5th ed.). Philadelphia: W. B. Saunders.

TABLE 75-7 Assessment of the Patient for Invasive Squamous Cell Carcinoma of the Cervix

	Assessment Parameters	Typical Abnormal Findings
History	A. Personal and social history 1. Risk factors 2. Living situation 3. Family history B. Gynecological history	A. Personal and social risks 1. Unprotected sex, injection drug use 2. May be homeless or living in a shelter 3. May be caring for spouse or child with HIV B. May describe heavy menstrual bleeding, irregular periods
Physical Examination	A. Pelvic examination	A. Abnormal cytology
Diagnostic Tests	A. Pap smear B. Colposcopy	A. Abnormal B. Lesion better visualized

outcomes. To this end, as indicated in Table 75-8, two staging systems for HIV-related KS have been proposed (Laubenstein, 1984; Mitsuyasu, 1988a). These researchers recognized that there are some patients with KS whose prognosis is better than others. The reasons are not clear, and all the variables have not been examined. Some studies have correlated the relationship between the absolute CD4 lymphocyte count and prognosis. For example, if the CD4 value in a patient with KS is lower, then the prognosis is poorer. A person with a helper/suppressor (H:S) ratio of greater than 0.5 and a CD4 lymphocyte count of greater than 300/mm^3 has a relatively good prognosis. A H:S ratio of less than 0.2 and a CD4 lymphocyte count of less than 100/mm^3 indicates a very poor prognosis. The area in between these values is of unclear prognostic value. Other data indicate that patients with head and neck involvement, patients with prior or concomitant opportunistic infections, and patients exhibiting "B" symptoms (e.g., weight loss, fevers, chills, night sweats, diarrhea) all have a shorter life expectancy than those without these factors. With the exception of the lung, organ involvement does not seem to influence prognosis, nor does tumor burden correlate with prognosis.

TABLE 75-8 Staging of Kaposi's Sarcoma

Stage	Characteristics
I	Limited cutaneous lesions (<10 or in one anatomic area)
II	Disseminated cutaneous lesions (>10 or in more than one anatomic area)
III	Visceral lesions only (gastrointestinal lymph node)
IV	Cutaneous and visceral lesions
Subtypes	
A	No systemic signs or symptoms
B	Fevers > 37.8° C unrelated to identifiable infection for >2 weeks or weight loss > 10% of body weight

From Mitsuyasu, R. T. & Groopman, J. E. (1984). Biology and therapy of Kaposi's sarcoma. *Seminars in Oncology, 11,* 53-59.

In 1989 the Oncology Committee of the National Institute of Allergy and Infectious Diseases (NIAID) sponsored the AIDS Clinical Trials Group (ACTG), which developed a proposal for uniform evaluation, response, and staging criteria for KS. This system, similar to the tumor-node-metastasis (TNM) system, used the extent of tumor growth, immune status, and other systemic illnesses (TIS) that are AIDS-related, to determine the stage of disease (Table 75-9). Patients are assigned to either a good-risk or poor-risk category depending on the extent of the tumor, their immune system status, and the presence of other systemic illnesses. In addition to the staging system developed by the NIAID-ACTG, this group also developed criteria for a standardized format of documenting the extent of KS on both initial and subsequent evaluation, as well as response definitions that included assessments of lesion nodularity and tumor-associated edema, supplementing the more traditional method for evaluating tumor response. This new system should allow for more accurate assessment of patients with KS and more meaningful outcomes from research studies.

Systemic Non–Hodgkin's Lymphoma

Staging, or determining the extent of disease involvement, is accomplished by means of the Ann Arbor staging classification system. Once all the tests are complete, the patient is assigned a staging number that can help predict responsiveness to treatment. However, it should be noted that the Ann Arbor staging system was developed specifically for staging Hodgkin's disease, so its predictability with NHL is somewhat diminished.

Primary Central Nervous System Lymphoma

These malignancies are all considered stage IV at presentation because they involve an extranodal organ.

Invasive Squamous Cell Carcinoma of the Cervix

Staging of SCC of the cervix is outlined in Chapter 29.

TABLE 75-9 AIDS Clinical Trials Group Staging of Kaposi's Sarcoma

	Good Risk (0): All of the Following	Poor Risk (1): Any of the Following
Tumor (I)	Confined to the skin and/or lymph nodes and/or minimum oral disease*	Tumor-associated edema or ulceration
Immune status (I)	CD4 cells ≥ 200/microliter	CD4 cells < 200/microliter
Systemic illness (S)	No history of opportunistic infection (OI) or thrush	History of OI or thrush or both
	No "B" symptoms†	"B" symptoms present
	Karnofsky performance status ≥ 70	Karnofsky performance status < 70
		Other HIV related illness (e.g. neurologic disease, lymphoma)

*Minimum oral disease in non-nodular KS confined to the palate
†"B" symptoms are unexplained fever, night sweats, >10% involuntary weight loss, or diarrhea persisting for more than 2 weeks

MEDICAL MANAGEMENT

HIV Disease

There are three main goals for the medical management of a patient with HIV: (1) irradication of the virus to undetectable levels, (2) preventing opportunistic infections through the use of prophylactic medications, and (3) the effective treatment of any opportunistic infections or malignancy the patient may develop.

Irradication of the virus is attempted using three different classifications of medications. Nucleoside analog reverse transcriptase inhibitors were the first class of drugs developed and approved for the treatment of HIV. These agents work by inhibiting the enzyme reverse transcriptase, which is essential for viral replication. Protease inhibitors, a newer class of medications, work by inhibiting the enzyme protease that is responsible for cleaving viral protein into useable lengths for producing new viral particles. Nonnucleoside reverse transcriptase inhibitors are the latest addition to the armamentarium against HIV. Again, these agents inhibit reverse transcriptase (Volberding, 1997).

Providing prophylaxis to a patient is intended to prevent the occurrence of a specific disease known to develop in those with advanced disease. For the patient with HIV, whose immune system is fairly debilitated, two diseases are amenable to prophylaxis: *Pneumocystis carnii* pneumonia (PCP) and *Mycobacterium avium* complex (MAC). The patient with HIV whose CD4 count is $>200/mm^3$ or $>14\%$ of total lymphocytes should receive prophylaxis. The gold standard for PCP prophylaxis is trimethoprim/sulfamethoxazole (Septra, Bactrim)—one double-strength pill once a day. Approximately 40% of patients with AIDS who have advanced disease develop disseminated MAC. Prophylaxis is recommended for those with CD4 counts $>100/mm^3$. Current recommendations are for lifetime prophylaxis with either rifabutin, clarithromycin, or azithromycin.

It is beyond the scope of this chapter to discuss all the possible treatment options for patients with HIV who develop an opportunistic infection.

Kaposi's Sarcoma

Before the epidemic of AIDS and HIV disease, KS seen in the United States was primarily classic KS (i.e., indolent, slow growing, and chronic), which required little or no treatment. In the transplant recipient the reversal of immunosuppression by withdrawing immunosuppressive drugs resolved the problem in 25% to 50% of the cases. In HIV-related KS, treatment of the malignancy provides only temporary remission or stabilization of the disease and does not improve survival rates. The main goal of treatment is to lessen morbidity.

As with other malignancies, three treatment options exist: surgery, radiation therapy, and chemotherapy, either local or systemic. Other than enabling the provider to establish a diagnosis, surgery has almost no role in the treatment of KS. Radiation therapy is highly effective and plays a role in local control of lesions and in cosmetic effects (Chak, Gill Levine, Meyer, Anselmo, & Petrovich, 1988; Hill, 1987). However, this treatment is not free of side effects and affects patients with KS the same way it affects others who receive radiation therapy. For example, irradiation of tonsillar or oral lesions may cause severe stomatitis because of a preexisting *Candida* infection or poor dentition. Response to treatment may be slow, taking up to 1 month after treatment to obtain full results.

Chemotherapeutic agents are useful in the treatment of HIV-related KS when a systemic effect is necessary and the benefits of treatment outweigh the risks to the patient. Guidelines for treatment of HIV-related KS are outlined in Box 75-2. Patients with aggressive or extensive disease who have an absolute neutrophil count greater than $1000/mm^3$ may receive weekly single-agent chemotherapy. Those single agents include doxorubicin, (10 to 15 mg/m^2); vinblastine (0.1 mg/kg); vincristine (2 mg), liposomal doxorubicin (20 mg/m^2), or liposomal daunomycin (40 mg/m^2).

In the recent past a patient with rapidly progressing disease, disease unresponsive to single-agent therapy, or lung

Box 75-2
Algorithm for Treating Patients with Kaposi's Sarcoma

Localized Disease

- Observation
- Local therapy
  - Intralesional treatment
  - Cryotherapy
  - Radiation therapy
- Biologic response modifiers
  - Alpha interferon
- Investigational agents
  - Differentiating agents

Disseminated Disease

- Systemic chemotherapy
  - Vincristine
  - Vinblastine
  - Bleomycin
  - Liposomal agents
    - Doxorubicin
    - Daunomycin
- Investigational agents
  - Topotecan
- Radiation therapy
  - Painful, bulky lesions
  - Oral-pharyngeal lesions

Cytopenic Patients

- Chemotherapy
  - Vincristine
  - Bleomycin
- Radiation therapy

Salvage Treatment

- Chemotherapy
  - Taxol
  - Oral etoposide

involvement would have been offered combination chemotherapy consisting of doxorubicin, bleomycin, and vincristine, administered every other week on the basis of the patient's complete blood count (CBC), or single-agent etoposide, administered either orally or intravenously. Lipsomal agents, either doxorubicin or daunomycin, have all but replaced combination therapy and oral etoposide, being easier to administer with fewer side effects and similar if not superior results. Liposomal daunomycin has been approved as first-line therapy for KS treatment, whereas liposomal doxorubicin has been approved for treatment of those patients with refractory KS (Sturzl, Zietz, Eisenburg, Goebel, Gillitzer, & Hofschneider et al., 1994; Uziely, Jeffers, Isacson, Kutsch, Wei Tsao, & Yehoshau et al., 1995) or those who are intolerant to the side effects of chemotherapy (Harrison, Tomlinson, & Stewart, 1995). Overall, lung involvement is a poor prognostic sign. Patients who are unable to tolerate aggressive chemotherapy because of a low CBC receive a weekly course of either bleomycin or vincristine, alternating with vinblastine every other week.

Interferon has shown efficacy in the treatment of HIV-related KS. Trials of recombinant alpha-interferon began in 1981, and since that time a select group of patients responded favorably to alpha-interferon. Their characteristics include CD4 counts greater than 200/mm^3, no prior AIDS-defining diagnosis, and no "B" symptoms. Objective responses in this group of patients ranged from 42% to 79%. Recommended dosages range from 18 to 30 million units injected subcutaneously once daily, 5 days a week. Because of both subjective (fevers, chills, myalgias) and objective (neutropenia, thrombocytopenia, transient elevated transaminases) side effects, the usual dose tolerated is approximately one quarter to one half the recommended dose (Krown, 1987; Volberding, Gotlieb, & Rothman, 1983).

To minimize systemic side effects, investigators have explored the use of intralesional recombinant tumor necrosis factor, intralesional vinblastine, and intralesional β-HCG for local control. Results from using intralesional recombinant tumor necrosis factor (rTNF) were disappointing. Although 15 of the 16 patients treated with intralesional rTNF showed objective responses, the intense local inflammatory response was thought to be the cause of tumoricidal activity rather than the rTNF (Kahn, Kaplan, Volberding, Ziegler, Crow, & Saks et al., 1989).

Intralesional vinblastine can also be used to treat small, localized lesions. The dosage is 0.4 mg/cc administered directly into the lesion. The patient experiences mild pain on administration, and 3 to 5 days later, the lesion begins to ulcerate. Overall effectiveness is good, with response rates approaching 100% per injected lesion. However, lesions frequently need to be treated more than once, and a hyperpigmented area often remains after treatment (Newman, 1988). Intralesional β-HCG has demonstrated some efficacy in the treatment of KS, but further research is necessary.

The response of KS lesions to chemotherapy can be dramatic. The lesions often decrease in size, flatten and lose their pigmentation. However, they do not completely go away. The area remains pigmented after treatment with chemotherapy and/or radiation therapy.

For the patient who has progressed despite conventional chemotherapy, paclitaxel (Taxol) and oral etoposide are two salvage options. Taxol, given at a dose of 100 mg/m^2, produced response rates of 53% with moderate side effects. Oral etoposide also produced good results and is currently in clinical trials using escalating doses (Laubenstein, Krigel, Odajnk, Hymes, Freedman-Kien, & Muggia, 1984). Topotecan is a topoisomerase agent also being evaluated for efficacy in KS. Studies are being conducted evaluating the effectiveness of differentiating agents on KS. In the form of liarosal and 9-*cis*-retinoic acid, two protocols are currently collecting patients for evaluation. Cytokine manipulation is also being evaluated as a treatment for KS.

Systemic Non–Hodgkin's Lymphoma

Once the disease is staged and graded, treatment for NHL may begin. Treatment options can be determined on the basis of method (e.g., surgery, radiation therapy, and chemotherapy) and grade of tumor. Low-grade tumors are uncommon in persons with HIV. In the general population, tumors are indolent and slow growing, requiring no treatment until they impinge on a vital structure or cause symptoms. At that time, radiation therapy to the affected site usually is sufficient to treat the tumor, although chemotherapy may also be used. Intermediate-grade tumors are more common in persons with HIV and may account for as much as 50% of HIV-related NHL. This grade of tumor in the general population can be treated with either chemotherapy or radiation therapy, depending on the stage of the disease at presentation (Beral, Peterman, Berkleman, & Jaffe, 1991).

The remaining HIV-related NHL occurs as high-grade, advanced-stage disease. Approximately 41% of patients with HIV-related NHL have high-grade disease (DiCarlo, Amberson, Metroka, Ballard, Moore, & Mouradian, 1986). Other investigators found that all patients with HIV-related NHL had either intermediate- or high-grade disease (Ahmed, Wormser, Stahl, Mamtani, Cimino, & Glasser et al., 1987).

The treatment of choice for advanced intermediate- or high-grade lymphoma is combination chemotherapy with CNS prophylaxis. The most active and effective single agent used in the treatment of NHL is cyclophosphamide. Other effective drugs include methotrexate, doxorubicin, vincristine, vinblastine, prednisone, and cytosine arabinoside. Generally, these agents are used in some combination. The most common regimens include M-BACOD (methotrexate, doxorubicin, cyclophosphamide, vincristine, dexamethasone), MACOP-B (methotrexate, doxorubicin, cyclophosphamide, vincristine, prednisone, bleomycin), and CHOP (cyclophosphamide, doxorubicin, vincristine, prednisone).

The patient also receives intrathecal methotrexate or cytosine arabinoside in an effort to prevent a CNS recurrence. Initial responses to chemotherapy usually are dramatic, with shrinkage of the tumor noted within 24 hours; however, the response is usually not long-lived. Typically, patients remain disease-free while receiving chemotherapy. Relapse occurs within 4 to 6 weeks after the discontinuation of chemotherapy. Once chemotherapy is reinstituted, response rates are somewhat diminished. The neutropenia that results from treatment may be severe (attributed to poor bone marrow reserves as a result of either HIV infection or intercurrent opportunistic infection such as *Mycobacterium avium* complex) and sometimes precipitates an opportunistic infection.

Research trials being conducted by the ACTG are examining the use of growth factors to support the bone marrow in patients with HIV-related NHL who are being treated with chemotherapy. Recently, Kaplan, Straus, Testa, Von Roenn, Dezube, and Cooley et al. (1997) reported the results of ACTG 142. This study randomized patients with HIV-related NHL to either low-dose m-BACOD or standard-dose m-BACOD with growth factor support. Little difference was demonstrated between the two arms of the study, and the researchers concluded that low-dose therapy produced equivalent survival with the benefit of reduced toxicity when compared with standard-dose therapy. It is important to remember that these patients have an underlying immune disorder and that whatever the outcome they still have HIV infection and AIDS.

Radiation therapy may be useful for patients with limited bulky disease, for those who are unable to tolerate chemotherapy either because of poor health or low blood counts, for local control, or, in some instances, for CNS prophylaxis. Surgery plays no role in the treatment of NHL other than to obtain a biopsy specimen.

Primary Central Nervous System Lymphoma

Regardless of whether patients with HIV-related CNS lymphoma are treated, the outcome remains the same. In one review (So, Beckstead, & Davis, 1986), six patients experienced a highly aggressive course and died within 2 weeks. In another, seven of 20 patients underwent treatment with radiation therapy. Dosages ranged from 3000 to 6000 cGy. Of the four patients who had CT scans after radiation therapy, three showed dramatic improvement. However, only two of seven patients were alive at 2 months. Most patients die of the concomitant opportunistic infections often experienced in AIDS. In another review (Gill et al., 1985), four patients were treated with subtotal resection of the tumor, followed by whole-brain radiation and systemic chemotherapy. One patient remained alive at 28 months after diagnosis. The diagnosis of this particular patient was based on a pathologic finding of low-grade lymphoma. The other patients survived less than 2 months. An average survival time of 1.7 to 2.7 months has been reported.

A third retrospective review (Baumgartner, Rachlin, Beckstead, Meeker, Levy, Wara, & Rosenblum, 1990) evaluated 55 patients with primary CNS lymphoma who were treated with whole-brain radiation. Complete radiologic responses were reported in 17% of patients, with 52% of the patients achieving a partial response. Clinical improvement was evidenced in 75% of the patients. Although responses were good, they were short-lived. In one group of 29 patients the median survival was 119 days. Cause of death in the majority of patients was an opportunistic infection. No deaths were attributable to unchecked primary CNS lymphoma. Short survival was also reported by Formenti, Gill, Lean, Rarick, Meyer, and Boswell et al. (1989). In this review, six of 10 patients with primary CNS lymphoma had a prior history of opportunistic infections and, when treated with whole-brain irradiation, demonstrated complete responses. Again, the responses were not durable. Median survival in this group of patients was 5.5 months.

Invasive Squamous Cell Carcinoma of the Cervix

Several important pieces of information were obtained from research by Maiman and colleagues (1990). First was the observation that a relationship existed between immune status and CIN. Women with CD4 counts less than 500/mm^3 were at high risk of developing recurrent disease, whereas those with a relatively intact immune system still had twice the risk of recurrence when compared with women who tested negative for HIV. Secondly, the mode of HIV acquisition correlated strongly with recurrent disease, that is, women who acquired HIV through sexual relations were more likely to develop recurrent disease compared with women who acquired HIV through injection drug use. The final result reported that traditional therapy used in the population with HIV produced significantly shorter mean time intervals until disease recurrence and death. Currently, no standard recommendation for treatment is available, and women with invasive SCC should be treated as if they do not have HIV (see Chapter 27).

NURSING MANAGEMENT

HIV Disease

A discussion of the nursing care of patients with HIV at all stages of disease is beyond the scope of this chapter because it can range from providing emotional support for the asymptomatic newly diagnosed patient to aggressive symptom management and intensive intervention for the patient with advanced disease. For more information, please seek specific references regarding HIV care (Hollander, 1997).

HIV-Related Malignancies

Nursing care of the patient with an HIV-related malignancy has many similarities regardless of the type of malignancy, including commonalties among the psychosocial issues, management of treatment-related side effects, and management of symptoms related to other opportunistic infections or malignancies (Jacobson, 1997).

Psychosocial Issues. Determining where the patient is on the continuum of HIV infection helps assess the patient's psychosocial needs. The nursing care of the patient for whom an HIV-related malignancy is the initial diagnosis of AIDS may be different from the nursing care of the patient for whom this diagnosis is but one in a long line of diseases, signaling a steady-but-progressive downhill course. However, similarities may also exist. Basic HIV education, coaching patients to be able to tell friends and families about their HIV status and AIDS diagnosis, as well as helping patients cope with grief and mortality issues, are all aspects of nursing care.

Although great strides have been made to reduce stigmas concerning AIDS and homosexual men, it is important to remember that the patient may be not only explaining his sexual preference to his family for the first time but also informing them that he has a fatal disease. Therefore emotional support is a crucial component of the nursing care of this patient population.

Inquiring about the patient's risk group helps gain insight into how the patient views society and the medical establishment. It may also reflect the patient's ability to follow through with treatment plans. As the disease continues to affect poor minorities, more patients will be disenfranchised from the medical community, will be less able to comply with complicated regimens, and will experience more difficulty with access to care issues. Their living situation may be unstable, they may have no money for their share of cost or copayments, they may have limited access to food, and/or they may be the primary caregiver for another person with HIV (e.g., child or significant other). In fact, for some of these patients, testing positive for HIV or receiving an AIDS diagnosis may be the least of their problems.

If the patient is an IDU, philosophic dilemmas may arise about entering a drug rehabilitation program. Realistic goals are necessary in this patient population because of both drug-seeking and manipulative behavior.

Chemotherapy. Regardless of the type of HIV-related malignancy, the side effects experienced by the patient with HIV are all similar. Mucositis, nausea, vomiting, diarrhea, constipation, myelosuppression, alopecia, fatigue, and anorexia are some of the side effects commonly associated with chemotherapy administration. Patients with HIV experience all these side effects to varying degrees; the differences are in how fast they occur. For this reason, nurses should aggressively assess for potential complications, alert the physician promptly, and implement appropriate nursing interventions. Patients with HIV tend not to have much reserve in the areas of energy, bone marrow, or weight, so side effects cause fatigue, myelosuppression, or weight loss and may be more severe in this patient population. Interventions that are successful in the population without HIV typically work well in this patient population.

These patients have an underlying illness predisposing them to other opportunistic infections and malignancies. Unfortunately, the same side effects induced by chemotherapy may also be a symptom of an opportunistic infection. The patient with HIV is susceptible to other opportunistic infections at any time during the course of the illness. Although the most likely cause of these symptoms may be the chemotherapy, opportunistic infections should be considered as part of the differential diagnosis.

Radiation Therapy. Radiation therapy in the patient with HIV may result in a decrease in CD4 counts and severe side effects, especially if the head and neck, stomach, or bowel are within the radiation port. The patient with cutaneous KS who is receiving superficial electron beam therapy is the exception.

Again, thorough assessments and aggressive interventions are the keys to minimizing symptoms and maximizing quality of life. All symptoms may not be caused by the radiation therapy. Opportunistic infections should be part of the differential diagnosis, especially if a particular intervention is not relieving symptoms.

Issues Specific to Kaposi's Sarcoma

Psychosocial Issues. The disfiguring cutaneous lesions of KS may occur anywhere on the body but occur mostly on the tip of the nose. This problem may cause the patient emotional pain and embarrassment. In addition, privacy is lost. A patient no longer has the right not to disclose his or her diagnosis. Any public appearance announces the disease and may result in social isolation, avoidance, and depression. Providing a safe environment where the patient can voice feelings, anxiety, and concerns is extremely important. Offering concrete solutions such as makeup as camouflage can be useful, too.

Chemotherapy. Patients with HIV-related KS, on receiving the first dose of vinca alkaloids, may experience severe jaw pain. Although this reaction is a reported side effect of treatment with vinca alkaloids, patients with HIV-related KS seem to have an increased incidence of this problem. Treatment with vinca alkaloids should be discontinued in patients with this reaction because the medication may cause irreversible nerve damage. A standard of care for the patient with KS who is receiving intralesional therapy is found in Table 75-10.

Radiation Therapy. Skin care is an important aspect of care of the patient with KS but even more so when the patient is undergoing radiation therapy. Since the skin is the first line of defense against microorganisms, maintaining an intact barrier is essential. Occasionally, radiation therapy to an edematous area causes skin breakdown. If that occurs, then aggressive intervention is necessary because any skin involved with KS is already compromised and the healing process will be very slow. Referral to a wound care specialist may be necessary.

Systemic Non–Hodgkin's Lymphoma

Nursing care of patients with HIV-related NHL is no different from the care of those patients in the general population with non–HIV-related NHL, with the exception of the emotional (psychosocial) aspect.

Chemotherapy. It should be noted that patients with large, bulky, high-grade disease are at high risk for tumor lysis syndrome. The exact number of patients with tumor lysis syndrome is unknown. Some clinicians estimate that it may occur in as many as 10% of patients, regardless of whether or not their NHL is related to HIV. Anecdotally, it appears that patients with HIV-related NHL have a higher incidence of this phenomenon because they tend to present with larger, bulkier tumors.

Tumor lysis syndrome generally occurs when the patient

TABLE 75-10 Standard of Care for the Patient with Kaposi's Sarcoma Receiving Intralesional Therapy

Patient Problem	Nursing Interventions and Rationales	Patient Education Instructions
Knowledge Deficit Patient will verbalize understanding of the pathologic process of KS, treatment options, benefits of treatment, and risks of treatment.	1. Assess patient's level of knowledge of KS. 2. Assess patient's level of knowledge regarding treatment options. 3. Assess patient's level of knowledge of intralesional therapy. 4. Assess patient's concerns and fears about treatment	1. Describe the pathologic process of KS. 2. Describe treatment options to patient: a. Chemotherapy b. Radiation therapy c. Intralesional therapy d. Investigational agents 3. Describe the major side effects associated with intralesional therapy: a. Pain on injection b. Ulceration
Alteration in Protective Barrier Patient will not develop a wound infection. If infection develops it will be evaluated and treated quickly.	1. Assess wound regularly for signs of infection. 2. Assess patient's knowledge of wound care.	1. Describe to patient the appearance of the skin lesion posttreatment: a. Swollen b. Tender c. Slightly erythematous d. Indurated 2. Provide patient with information on proper wound care posttreatment: a. Keep lesion clean and dry b. Note any increasing redness c. Note any excessive warmth d. Note any purulent drainage e. Note any swelling that occurs more than 48 hours after treatment 3. Provide patient with information on how and when to contact primary provider: a. Give patient telephone number b. Give patient specific parameters (e.g. temperature $> 101°$ F, purulent drainage from wound)

is initially treated. It is the result of the lysing of rapidly growing tumor cells that spill their contents into the general circulation, causing a metabolic imbalance. This pathophysiologic process results in hypocalcemia, hyperkalemia, hyperphosphatemia, and hyperuricemia. If left untreated, this condition may result in renal failure and death.

Prevention is the treatment of choice. Therefore any patient suspected of being at high risk for the development of tumor lysis syndrome as determined by elevated uric acid and lactate dehydrogenase levels should receive vigorous hydration (300 to 500 ml/hr) and may receive sodium bicarbonate to alkalinize the urine and prevent hyperuricemia nephropathy. However, sodium bicarbonate interferes with phosphate excretion and should be stopped before administration of chemotherapy. In addition, allopurinol, a drug that blocks the conversion of metabolic wastes to uric acid, should be administered either intravenously or orally. The patient's urine output needs to be monitored every hour, and the physician should be alerted to any sign of urinary insufficiency. Serum chemistry levels are monitored every 6 hours in patients who are at high risk for tumor lysis syndrome, and in some cases the patient may need to be transferred to the intensive care unit. Dialysis may be necessary if the patient's electrolyte levels continue to rise and renal function deteriorates. Generally, there is less morbidity if the patient receives dialysis before renal failure occurs.

Although tumor lysis syndrome occurs in most patients 48 to 72 hours after the initiation of chemotherapy, some patients with HIV-related NHL may develop this phenomenon sooner, usually within 24 hours. However, all patients with HIV-related NHL should be observed for a full 72-hour period for any sign of tumor lysis syndrome. These signs and symptoms include decreased urine output and increased lethargy. If the patient is being monitored by telemetry, arrhythmias may be noted.

Some patients with HIV-related NHL have some form of

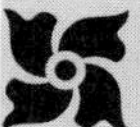

TABLE 75-11 Standard of Care for the Patient with Primary Central Nervous System Lymphoma Undergoing Radiation Therapy

Patient Problem and Outcomes	Nursing Interventions and Rationales	Patient Education Instructions
Anxiety Patient will: • Verbalize an understanding of the surgical procedure if able • Express feelings of decreased anxiety • Identify strategies to cope with anxiety	1. Assess patient's level of understanding of the surgical procedure. Keep in mind that the patient may be incapable of understanding the procedure due to his or her disease. 2. Give patient the opportunity to ask questions or voice concerns. 3. Assess the patient's coping strategies to determine effectiveness in decreasing anxiety, and encourage the patient to continue using these methods. 4. Administer pharmacologic agents to decrease anxiety	1. Use diagrams of the anatomy of the brain to explain the procedure. If possible, visit OR suite where the procedure will be done to familiarize the patient with the equipment used. 2. Provide patient with information about the preoperative surgical procedure: a. Diagnostic tests b. Shaving of a small area c. Anesthesiology consult d. Being conscious during the procedure e. NPO after midnight 3. Provide patient with information about the postoperative plan of care: a. Pain management b. Wound care instructions c. Processing of specimen
Pain Patient will experience optimal pain relief with minimal side effects	1. Assess pain intensity using a 0-10 verbal rating scale every 2-4 hours for the first 48 hours after surgery and then at least once a shift. 2. Administer appropriate analgesics around the clock for the first 24-48 hours postoperatively. 3. Ensure that all analgesics administered do not adversely interact with any medications the patient is already taking.	1. Teach patient to inform the nurse if he is experiencing pain. If the patient is unable to communicate, note physical/nonverbal signs of pain: a. Elevated blood pressure b. Elevated pulse c. Moaning/groaning d. Restlessness 2. Instruct patient of drug incompatibilities, particularly with the protease inhibitors. 3. Teach patient the importance of around the clock dosing.
Safety Patient will be free from injury	1. Assess patient's neurological status at least every 4 hours. 2. Identify patient as a high risk for falls if neurological status is altered or neurological deficit is present.	1. Instruct patient to use call button for assistance to get out of bed. 2. If the patient is unable to cooperate due to altered mental status: a. Instruct family members or significant other that the patient should not be up without assistance b. Keep side rails up c. Keep personal items visible and within reach

tumor lysis syndrome before they receive treatment. This syndrome may be the result of tumor cells replicating and dying at an extraordinary rate, spilling their cellular contents into the general circulation. These patients also may have tumors that produce lactic acid, causing metabolic acidosis before treatment.

Primary Central Nervous System Lymphoma

A standard of care for the patient with primary CNS lymphoma who is undergoing radiation therapy is found in Table 75-11.

Safety Issues. Nursing responsibilities in the care of these patients includes a thorough assessment, paying particular attention to any focal findings, motor incoordination, and cognitive deficits. Safety in the environment must be considered in both the acute care setting and the home. Provisions for activities of daily living also must be anticipated, and a long-term plan must be developed. For example, if the patient cannot be maintained at home, plans should be made for transfer to a skilled nursing care facility. Providing emotional support to the patient and family is essential, regardless of whether this support is through referrals to counselors or given directly by the nurse.

Ethical Issues. Ethical issues may be encountered when treatment is discussed. A determination should be made as to whether the patient is mentally competent to make decisions. If not, it should be determined who is the next of kin or whether someone has been authorized with a power of attorney. If the patient is deemed incompetent, has no next of kin, or has not transferred power of attorney, then a legal guardian needs to be appointed by a court of law to make decisions for the patient.

Invasive Squamous Cell Carcinoma of the Cervix

Perhaps the most important role nurses can play in caring for women infected with HIV is that of a strong advocate for their client. Women are infected at a faster rate than men, and it is estimated that by the year 2004 the number of women infected with HIV will equal the number of infected men (Centers for Disease Control, 1990). While the epidemic in women is thought to lag 5 years behind that in men, research in women is believed to trail closer to 10 years behind. Women have been under studied and under diagnosed. It is known that women will defer receiving care for themselves to care for a sick child or spouse; that women are more likely to be unemployed and on federal assistance programs causing problems with access to care; and that up to 15% of women are unaware of their risk factors for HIV, making screening difficult.

Women are also less likely to receive antiretroviral therapy or prophylactic treatment than men. In addition, in 1990 the CDC reported that 65% of women with HIV died without an AIDS-defining diagnosis. Nurses can have an impact by recognizing two things. First, it is not a label that puts an individual at risk for developing HIV, but rather behavior, as in sexual relations or injection drug use. Second, women with HIV require more time and energy to achieve the same goals as men.

HOME CARE ISSUES

HIV Disease

Issues concerning home care for the patient with HIV disease may range from emotional support to hospice care. It is not within the scope of this chapter to address all home care needs of the patient with HIV. For that information, an HIV-specific reference should be used (Hollander, 1997).

The basic home care issues for the patient with HIV include assessment for safety, access to food, ability to properly store medications, and knowledge of universal body substance precautions. Since this patient population may be receiving growth factors (e.g., erythropoietin or granulocyte colony-stimulating factor) or intravenous treatment for CMV disease at home, it is essential that they have some type of refrigeration to keep these medications at the proper temperature. In addition, saquinavir requires refrigeration. Patients may also need help storing medications safely. For some patients who live in shelters or single-room occupancy hotels, theft is a major problem. If the patient is using narcotics for pain control, then determining a safe storage place may require the nurse's help.

The nurse should be familiar with community resources, including those providing financial assistance (Catholic Charities, AIDS Foundation), food banks, meal delivery resources, shelters, and agencies providing practical support and legal advocates. Providing the patient with this information may ensure adequate access to food, safety, and any legal aid.

Kaposi's Sarcoma

Home care issues specific to the patient with KS include management of treatment-related side effects, skin care, mobility, and pain management. Depending on the type of treatment, the patient may experience nausea, vomiting, diarrhea, constipation, fatigue, or myelosuppression. Reiterating to the patient the side effects of treatment, reinforcing the instructions on the use of antiemetics, antidiarrheal, or laxatives is important. Monitoring for signs and symptoms of myelosuppression is also critical.

If the patient's disease is extensive, he or she may experience mobility problems resulting from pain or functional difficulties. These problems may occur when the lower extremities become edematous due to the coalescing of KS lesions, either cutaneous or lymphatic, blocking lymph drainage. This process can cause throbbing pain and difficulty ambulating. If the circulation is compromised further, stasis ulcers may result. Inspection of these areas should be done on a regular basis. Elevation of the affected areas may provide some relief, but it is usually short-lived, and when the legs are dependent, edema returns quickly. The scrotum and penis may also become edematous, and in the extreme case interfere with urination.

Systemic Non–Hodgkin's Lymphoma

The patient with NHL has home care issues revolving around treatment. Again, continuing to educate the patient about side effects of chemotherapy can help minimize morbidity. If the patient has received therapy as an outpatient, the home care nurse may be asked to observe for signs and symptoms of tumor lysis syndrome. Many of the chemotherapy protocols use steroids orally for several days after the intravenous infusions. Assuring that the patient is taking the medications properly is vital.

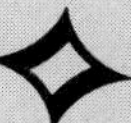

TABLE 75-12 Patient Preparation for Establishing a Safe Home Environment

1. Check for risk factors in the home that pose a threat to safety (e.g., improperly lighted stairways, throw rugs).
2. Install appropriate lighting in hallways and on stairs.
3. Install night-lights in hallways, bedroom, and bathroom.
4. Install handrails to prevent falls.
5. Install guard rails in bathroom near toilet and bathtub.
6. Secure all carpeting, mats, and tile; place nonskid backing under area rugs.
7. Evaluate whether the patient can use electrical appliances and the stove. Consider the need for supportive care services if necessary.
8. Adjust the placement of items in kitchens, bathroom, and bedroom for convenient and easy access.
9. Determine whether the patient can operate a motor vehicle safely.

Primary Central Nervous System Lymphoma

Most of the home care needs for this patient population involve safety issues, especially for the patient with cognitive and functional deficits (Table 75-12). If the patient is unable to remain safely at home, placement will be necessary.

Invasive Squamous Cell Carcinoma of the Cervix

The home care needs for women with HIV and AIDS are many. They range from assessing the family situation and planning child or spousal care to symptom management. Seventy percent of women with AIDS in the United States are women of color. Sexism, racism, poverty and drug use are all very real issues with which the nurse must deal. Education about the disease, contraception, sexually transmitted diseases, and pregnancy options are all home care issues.

PROGNOSIS

HIV Disease

The prognosis for the patient with HIV has improved dramatically over the past decade, in part because of prophylaxis and also antiretroviral therapy. Although HIV was once a fatal disease, patients are now living longer with HIV and with the diagnosis of AIDS.

Kaposi's Sarcoma

Some studies have correlated the relationship between the absolute CD4 lymphocyte count and prognosis (Afrasiabi, Mitsuyasu, Nishanian, Schwartz, & Fahey, 1986; Krigel, 1984, Taylor, Afrasiabi, Fahey, Korns, Weaver, & Mitsuyau, 1986). For example, the lower the CD4 value in a patient with KS, the poorer the prognosis. A person with an H:S ratio of greater than 0.5 and a CD4 lymphocyte count of greater than 300/mm^3 has a relatively good prognosis. A helper/suppressor ratio of less than 0.2 and a CD4 lymphocyte count of less than 100/mm^3 indicates a very poor prognosis. The area in between these values is of unclear prognostic value. Other data indicate that patients with head and neck involvement, patients with prior or concomitant opportunistic infections, and patients exhibiting "B" symptoms (weight loss, fevers, chills, night sweats, diarrhea) all have a shorter life expectancy than those without these factors. With the exception of the lung, organ involvement does not seem to influence prognosis, nor does tumor burden correlate with prognosis. Median survival for the patient with pulmonary involvement is 10 months.

Systemic Non–Hodgkin's Lymphoma

As with other types of cancer, a group of patients can be identified who will respond better to treatment and demonstrate a better prognosis. Kaplan and colleagues (1997) identified a "good" prognosis category that included indicators such as prior AIDS diagnosis, Karnofsky performance status, site of disease, and CD4 count. In addition, they identified a treatment-related indicator, the dose of cyclophosphamide received by the patient. However, they caution that these indicators were not the results of a randomized trial, and that many confounding variables exist.

More recently, a study conducted by the AIDS Clinical Trials Group (ACTG) (Kaplan et al., 1997) found that factors affecting prognosis included age >35, stage of disease (III/IV), injection drug use, and CD4 count $<100/mm^3$. Survival was correlated with the number of factors found in a particular patient. The patient who had two or fewer of these factors survived 45 weeks. Patients with three or more of these factors survived only 18 weeks.

Primary Central Nervous System Lymphoma

Prognosis for the patient with primary CNS lymphoma is dismal. This malignancy is usually a late manifestation of HIV disease, and few patients survive longer than 6 months once the diagnosis is made. In one group of 29 patients, median survival was 119 days. Cause of death in the majority of patients was an opportunistic infection. No deaths were attributable to unchecked primary CNS lymphoma. Short survival was also reported by Formenti and colleagues (1989). In this review, six of 10 patients with primary CNS lymphoma who had a prior history of opportunistic infections and were treated with whole-brain irradiation, demonstrated complete responses. Again, the responses were not durable. Median survival in this group of patients was 5.5 months.

Invasive Squamous Cell Carcinoma of the Cervix

The number of cases of invasive SCC of the cervix reported in women with HIV is small, and as a result the prognosis for these women is not well defined. It is known that the few

TABLE 75-13 Quality of Care Evaluation for the Patient with Kaposi's Sarcoma Undergoing Punch Biopsy

Disciplines participating in the quality of care evaluation:
☐ Nursing ☐ Dermatologist ☐ Social Services

I. Postprocedure Management Evaluation

Data from
☐ Medical Record ☐ Patient/Family Interview

Criteria	Yes	No
1. Patient provided with pre-procedure information regarding:		
a. Use of lidocaine	☐	☐
b. Potential for post-procedure bleeding	☐	☐
c. Potential for post-procedure scarring	☐	☐
d. Processing of specimen	☐	☐
e. Post-procedure wound care	☐	☐
f. Signs and symptoms of wound infection	☐	☐
g. When to contact primary care provider	☐	☐
h. Pain control	☐	☐
2. Allergy profile checked and noted.	☐	☐
3. Patient experienced the following complications:		
a. Excessive bleeding	☐	☐
b. Infection	☐	☐
c. Excessive pain	☐	☐

II. Patient/Family Satisfaction

Data from:
☐ Patient Interview ☐ Family Interview

Criteria	Yes	No
1. On a scale of 0 to 10, with 0 being totally dissatisfied and 10 being totally satisfied, how satisfied were you with the amount of information you were given about the procedure? ____________		
2. Were you told to contact your primary care giver if you had any signs or symptoms of infection?	☐	☐
3. Were you given information about post-procedure wound care?	☐	☐

women who were diagnosed with invasive SCC of the cervix did not respond well to traditional therapy and died quickly when compared with women without HIV. Extrapolating from the experiences of treating other patients with HIV and malignancies, the prognosis is presumed to be poor (Chu, 1990).

EVALUATION OF THE QUALITY OF CARE

Standards of care for the patient with HIV have been proposed by the ACTG and National Institutes of Health. These standards include management of active infections, recommended prophylaxis, and antiretroviral therapy. Standards for the treatment of HIV-related malignancies have not yet been established. Table 75-13 provides an example of a quality of care improvement tool that can be used to monitor care in the outpatient setting.

The Association of Nurses in AIDS Care (ANAC) has also developed standards of nursing care for the patient with HIV. For the patient with HIV-related malignancy, the standards of care developed by the Oncology Nursing Society should be used in conjunction with those developed by ANAC.

RESEARCH ISSUES

Research issues abound for the treatment of HIV and any of the malignancies associated with it. Researchers continue to study the virus, looking for new ways to inhibit its replication and invasion into the cell. Prophylaxis studies are ongoing, specifically targeting CMV and toxoplasmosis. Additionally, research on different treatment options for active infections continues.

With the discovery of HIV-related KS, scientists are focusing on the relationship of this virus with both KS and body cavity lymphomas. Cytokine production and methods of inhibiting its production are also being looked at as a way of treating KS. Topical preparations of some medications and inhaled aerosolized agents are being investigated as local treatment for KS lesions. With NHL, novel approaches to treatment are being considered, including monoclonal antibodies and topoisomerase inhibitors. Researchers are investigating new treatment options for primary CNS lymphoma that include combining chemotherapy and radiation therapy. Clinicians are also studying the role of HPV in the development of anal intraepithelial neoplasia.

REFERENCES

Afrasiabi, A., Mitsuyasu, R., Nishanian, R., Schwartz, K., & Fahey, J. L. (1986). Characteristics of a distinct subgroup of high-risk persons with KS and good prognosis who present with normal T4 cell number and T4:T8 ratio and negative HTLV/LAV serologic test results. *American Journal of Medicine, 81,* 969-973.

Ahmed, T., Wormser, G., Stahl, R. E., Mamtani, R., Cimino, J., Glasser, M., Mittleman, A., Friedland, M., & Arlin, Z. (1987). Malignant lymphomas in a population at risk for acquired immune deficiency syndrome. *Cancer, 60,* 719-723.

Aisenberg, A. (1973). Malignant lymphoma. *New England Journal of Medicine, 288,* 883-890.

American Cancer Society. (1995). *Cancer facts and figures: 1995.* Atlanta: The Society.

Baumgartner, J., Rachlin, J., Beckstead, J., Meeker, T. C., Levy, R. M., Wara, W. M., & Rosenblum, M. L. (1990). Primary central nervous system lymphomas: Natural history and response to radiation therapy in 55 patients with acquired immunodeficiency syndrome. *Journal of Neurosurgery, 73,* 206-211.

Beral, V., Peterman, T., Berkleman, R., & Jaffe, H. W. (1990). Kaposi's sarcoma among persons with AIDS: A sexually transmitted infection. *Lancet, 335,* 123-127.

Beral, V., Peterman, T., Berkleman, R., & Jaffe, H. (1991). AIDS-associated non–Hodgkin lymphoma. *Lancet, 337,* 805-809.

Birx, D., Redfield, R., & Tosato, G. (1986). Defective regulation of Epstein-Barr virus infection in patients with acquired immunodeficiency syndrome (AIDS) or AIDS-related disorders. *New England Journal of Medicine, 314,* 874-879.

Brooks, J. (1986). Kaposi's sarcoma: A reversible hyperplasia. *Lancet, 2,* 1309-1311.

Brown, R., Huberman, R., & Vanley, G. (1986). Pulmonary features of KS. *American Journal of Radiology, 139,* 659-660.

Centers for Disease Control. (1981a). Kaposi's sarcoma and Pneumocystis pneumonia among homosexual men in New York City and California. *Morbidity and Mortality Weekly Report, 30,* 305-308.

Centers for Disease Control. (1981b) Follow-up on Kaposi's sarcoma and Pneumocystis pneumonia. *Morbidity and Mortality Weekly Report, 30,* 409-441.

Centers for Disease Control. (1982). Update on acquired immune deficiency syndrome (AIDS) United States. *Morbidity and Mortality Weekly Report, 31,* 507-514.

Centers for Disease Control. (1987). Revision of the CDC surveillance case definition for acquired immunodeficiency syndrome. *Morbidity and Mortality Weekly Report, 35,* 3S-15S.

Centers for Disease Control. (1990). AIDS in women: United States. *Morbidity and Mortality Weekly Report, 39,* 845-846.

Centers for Disease Control. (1992). 1993 Revised classification system for HIV infection and expanded surveillance case definition for AIDS among adolescents and adults. *Morbidity and Mortality Weekly Report, 41,* 1-19.

Cesarman, E., Chang, Y., Moore, P., Said, J., & Knowles, D. (1995). Kaposi's sarcoma associated herpesvirus-like DNA sequences in AIDS-related body-cavity-based lymphomas. *New England Journal of Medicine, 332,* 1186-1191.

Cesarman, E., Moore, P., Rao, P., Inghirami, G., Knowles, D. M., & Chang, Y. (1995). In vitro establishment and characterization of two acquired immunodeficiency syndrome-related lymphoma cell lines (BC-1 and BC-2) containing Kaposi's sarcoma associated herpesvirus like (KSHV) DNA sequences. *Blood, 86,* 2708-2714.

Chak, L., Gill, P., Levine, A., Meyer, P. R., Anselmo, J. A., & Petrovich, Z. (1988). Radiation therapy for acquired immunodeficiency syndrome-related Kaposi's sarcoma. *Journal of Clinical Oncology, 6,* 863-867.

Chang, Y., Cesarman, E., Pessin, M., Lee, F., Culpepper, J., Knowles, D., & Moore, P. (1994). Identification of herpesvirus-like DNA sequences in AIDS-associated Kaposi's sarcoma. *Science, 266,* 1865-9.

Chapman, M. & Minor, J. (1992). Lymphoma in AIDS patients receiving long-term antiretroviral therapy. *American Journal of Hospital Pharmacy, 49,* 174-175.

Chu, S. (1990). HIV and mortality in women. *Journal of the American Medical Association, 264,* 225-229.

Cole, M., Cohen, P., Satra, E., & Grossman, M. E. (1992). The concurrent presence of systemic disease pathogens and cutaneous Kaposi's sarcoma in the same lesion: Histoplasma capsulatum and Kaposi's sarcoma coexisting in a single skin lesion in a patient with AIDS. *Journal of the American Academy of Dermatology, 26,* 285-287.

Costa, J. & Rabson, A. (1993). Generalized Kaposi's sarcoma is not a neoplasm. *Lancet, 1,* 58.

Davis, S., Henschke, C., Chamides, B., & Westcott, J. (1987). Intrathoracic Kaposi sarcoma in AIDS patients: Radiographic-pathologic correlation. *Radiology, 163,* 495-500.

DiCarlo, E., Amberson, J., Metroka, C., Ballard, P., Moore, A., & Mouradian, J. A. (1986). Malignant lymphomas and the acquired immunodeficiency syndrome. *Archives of Pathology and Laboratory Medicine, 110,* 1012-1026.

Drew, L., Mintz, L., & Miner, R. (1981). Prevalence of cytomegalovirus in homosexual men. *Journal of Infectious Diseases, 143,* 188-192.

Dunn, D., Newell, M., Ades, A., & Peckham, C. (1992). Risk of human immunodeficiency virus type 1 transmission through breast feeding. *Lancet, 340,* 585.

Formenti, S., Gill, P., Lean, E., Rarick, M., Meyer, P. R., Boswell, W., Petrovich, Z., Chak, L., & Levine, A. M. (1989). Primary central nervous system lymphoma in AIDS: Results of radiation therapy. *Cancer, 63,* 1101-1107.

Friedman, S. (1988). Gastrointestinal and hepatobiliary neoplasms in AIDS. *Gastroenterology Clinics fo North America, 17,* 465-486.

Friedman,-Kien, A. E., Saltzman, B. R., Cao, Y., Nestor, M. S., Mirabile, M., Li, J. J., & Peterman, T. A. (1990). Kaposi's sarcoma in HIV-negative homosexual men. *Lancet, 335,* 168-169.

Frizzera, G., Rosai, J., Dehner, L., Spector, B. D., & Kersey, J. H. (1980). Lymphoreticular disorders in primary immunodeficiency: New findings based on an up to date histologic classification of 35 cases. *Cancer, 46,* 692-699.

Garrett, T., Lange, M., Ashford, A., & Thomas, L. (1985). Kaposi's sarcoma in heterosexual intravenous drug users. *Cancer, 55,* 146-1158.

Gill, P. S., Levine, A. M., Meyer, P. R., Boswell, W. D., Burlees, R. L., Parker, J. W., Hofman, F. M., Dworsky, R. L., & Lukes, R. J. (1985). Primary central nervous system lymphoma in homosexual men. *American Journal of Medicine, 78,* 742-748.

Good, A., Russo, R., Schnitzer. B., & Weatherbee, L. (1978). Intercranial histiocytic lymphoma in rheumatoid arthritis. *Journal of Rheumatology, 5,* 75-78.

Groopman, J., & Broder, S. (1989). Cancer in AIDS and other immunodeficiency states. In V. DeVita, S. Hellman, & S. Rosenberg (Eds.), *Cancer: Principles and practice of oncology* (3rd ed.). Philadelphia: Lippincott-Raven.

Harrison, M., Tomlinson, D., & Stewart, S. (1995). Liposomal-entrapped doxorubicin: An active agent in AIDS-related Kaposi's sarcoma. *Journal of Clinical Oncology, 13,* 914-920.

Haverkos, H., Pinsky, P., Drothman, D., & Bregman, D. J. (1985). Disease manifestation and homosexual men with acquired immunodeficiency syndrome: A possible role of nitrites in Kaposi's sarcoma. *Sexually Transmitted Diseases, 23,* 203-208.

Henry, J., Heffner, R., & Dillard, S. (1987). Primary malignant lymphomas of the central nervous system. *Cancer, 34,* 1293-1302.

Hill, D. (1987). The role of radiotherapy for epidemic Kaposi's sarcoma. *Seminars in Oncology, 14*(Suppl.), 1207.

Hollander, H. (1997). Initiating routine care for the HIV-infected adult. In M. Sande & P. Volberding (Eds.), *The medical nanagement of AIDS* (5th ed.). Philadelphia: W. B. Saunders Company.

Jacobson, M. (1997). Disseminated *Mycobacterium avium* complex and other bacterial infections. In M. Sande & P. Volberding (Eds.), *The medical management of AIDS* (5th ed.). Philadelphia: W. B. Saunders.

Kahn, J., Kaplan, L., Volberding, P., Ziegler, J. L., Crowe, S., Saks, S. R., & Abrams, D. I. (1989). Intralesional recombinant tumor necrosis factor for AIDS-associated Kaposi's sarcoma: A randomized double blind trial. *Journal of AIDS, 2,* 217-221.

Kaplan, L. (1988). AIDS-associated lymphomas. In M. Sande & P. Volberding (Eds.), *The medical management of AIDS.* Philadelphia: W. B. Saunders.

Kaplan, L., Abrams, D., Feigal, E., McGrath, M., Kahn, J., Neville, P., Zeigler, J. L., & Volberding, P. (1989). AIDS-associated non-Hodgkin's lymphoma in San Francisco. *Journal of the American Medical Association, 261,* 719-724.

Kaplan, L., Hopewell, P., Jaffe, H., Goodman, P. C., Bottles, K., & Volberding, P. (1988). Kaposi's sarcoma involving the lung in patients with acquired immunodeficiency syndrome. *Journal of AIDS, 1,* 25-31.

Kaplan, L. & Northfelt, D. (1997). Malignancies associated with AIDS. In M. Sande & P. Volberding (Eds.), *The medical management of AIDS* (5th ed.). Philadelphia: W. B. Saunders.

Kaplan, L. D., Straus, D. J., Testa, M. A., Von Roenn, J., Dezube B. J., Cooley, B., Northfelt, D. W., Huang, J., & Tulpule, A. (1997). Low-dose compared with standard-dose m-BACOD chemotherapy for non-Hodgkin's lymphoma associated with human immunodeficiency infection. National Institute of Allergy and Infectious Disease Clinical Trials Group. *New England Journal of Medicine, 336*(23), 1641-1648.

Kaplan, L., Wofsy, C., & Volberding, P. (1987). Treatment of patients with acquired immunodeficiency syndrome and associated manifestations. *Journal of the American Medical Association, 257,* 1367-1372.

Kocks, C. & Rajewsky, K. (1989). Stable expression and somatic hypermutation of antibody V regions in B-cell developmental pathways. *Annual Review of Immunology, 7,* 537-559.

Krigel, R. (1984). Prognostic factors in Kaposi's sarcoma. In A. Friedman-Kien & L. Laubenstein (Eds.), *AIDS: The epidemic of Kaposi's sarcoma and opportunistic infections.* New York: Masson.

Krigel, R. & Friedman-Kien A. (1985). Kaposi's sarcoma in AIDS. In V. DeVita, S. Hellman, & S. A. Rosenberg (Eds.), *AIDS etiology, diagnosis, treatment, and prevention.* Philadelphia: J. B. Lippincott.

Krown, A. (1987). The role of interferon in the therapy of epidemic Kaposi's sarcoma. *Seminars in Oncology, 14* (Suppl. 3), 24-33.

Laubenstein, L. (1984). Staging and treatment of Kaposi's sarcoma in patients with AIDS. In A. Friedman-Kien & L. Laubenstein (Eds.), *AIDS: The epidemic of Kaposi's sarcoma and opportunistic infections.* New York: Masson .

Laubenstein, L., Krigel, R., Odajnk, C., Hymes, K. B., Freedman-Kien, A., & Muggia, F. M. (1984). Treatment of epidemic Kaposi's sarcoma with etoposide or a combination of doxorubicin, bleomycin, and vinblastine. *Journal of Clinical Oncology, 2,* 1115-1120.

Levin, V., Sheline, G., & Gutin, P. (1989). Neoplasms of the central nervous system. In V. T. DeVita, S. Hellman, & S. A. Rosenberg (Eds.), *Cancer: Practice and principles of oncology* (3rd ed.). Philadelphia: Lippincott-Raven.

Levine, A. (1987). Non–Hodgkin's lymphomas and other malignancies in the acquired immune deficiency syndrome. *Seminars in Oncology, 14*(Suppl.), 34-39.

Longo, D. L., Seis, R. G., Lane, H. C., Lotze, M. T., Rosenberg, S. A., Preble, O., Masur, H., Rook, A. H., Fauci, A. S., & Jacob, J. (1984). Malignancies in the AIDS patient: Natural history, treatment strategies, and preliminary results. *Annals of the New York Academy of Sciences, 437,* 421-430.

MacMahon, E., Glass, J., Hayward, S., et al. (1991). Epstein-Barr virus in AIDS-related primary central nervous system lymphoma. *Lancet, 338,* 969-973.

Maiman, M., Fruchter, R., Serur, E., Remy, J. C., Feuer, G., & Boyce, J. (1990). Human immunodeficiency virus infection and cervical neoplasia. *Gynecologic Oncology, 38,* 377-382.

Mitsuyasu, R. (1988a). Kaposi's sarcoma in the acquired immunodeficiency syndrome. *Infectious Disease Clinics of North America, 2,* 511-523.

Mitsuyasu, R. (1988b). Kaposi's sarcoma in the acquired immunodeficiency syndrome. In M. Sande & P. Volberding (Eds.), *The medical management of AIDS.* Philadelphia: W. B. Saunders.

Mitsuyasu, R. T. & Groopman, J. E. (1984). Biology and therapy of Kaposi's sarcoma. *Seminars in Oncology, 11,* 53-59.

Newman, S. (1988). Treatment of epidemic Kaposi's sarcoma (KS) with intralesional vinblastine injection (IL-VLB). *Proceedings of the American Society of Clinical Oncology, 5,* Abstract 19.

Ng, V. & McGrath, M. (1996). Pathogenesis of HIV-associated lymphoma. In S. Gupta (Ed.), *Immunology of HIV infection.* New York: Plenum Press.

Nissenblatt, M. (1985). Cancers and AIDS. In V. Gong (Ed.), *Understanding AIDS.* New Brunswick, NJ: Rutgers University Press.

Northfelt, D., Kahn, J., & Volberding, P. (1991). Treatment of AIDS-related Kaposi's sarcoma. *Hematology/Oncology Clinics of North America, 5,* 297-310.

Paauw, D. S., Wenrich, M. D., Curtis, J. R., Carline, J. D., Ramsey, P. G. (1995). Ability of primary care physicians to recognize physical findings associated with HIV infection. *JAMA, 274*(17), 1380-1382.

Roithmann, S., Tourani, J., & Andrieu, J. (1991). AIDS-associated non-Hodgkin's lymphoma. *Lancet, 338,* 884-445.

Schalling, M., Ekman, M., Kaaya, E., Linde, A., & Beberfield, P. (1995). A role for a new herpesvirus (KSHV) in different forms of Kaposi's sarcoma. *Nature Medicine, 1,* 705-6.

Schrager, L., Friedland, G., Maude, D., Schreiber, K., Adachi, A., Pizzuti, D. J., Koss, L. G., & Klein, R. S. (1989). Cervical and vaginal squamous abnormalities in women infected with human immunodeficiency virus. *Journal of Acquired Immune Deficiency Syndromes, 2,* 570-575.

Sillman, F. & Sedlis, A. (1987). Anogenital papillomavirus infection and neoplasia in immunodeficient women. *Obstetrics and Gynecology Clinics of North America, 14,* 537-558.

So, Y., Beckstead, J., & Davis, R. (1986). Primary central nervous system lymphoma in acquired immunodeficiency syndrome: A clinical and pathological study. *Annals of Neurology, 20,* 566-572.

Steis, R. & Broder, S. (1985). A general overview. In V. T. DeVita, S. Hellman, & S. A. Rosenberg (Eds.), *Etiology, diagnosis, treatment and prevention.* Philadelphia: J. B. Lippincott.

Sturzl, M., Zietz, C., Eisenburg, B., Goebel, F. D., Gillitzer, R., Hofschneider, P. H., & Bogner, J. R. (1994). Liposomal doxorubicin in the treatment of AIDS-associated Kaposi's sarcoma: Clinical, histological and cell biological evaluation. *Research in Virology, 145,* 261-269.

Taylor, J., Afrasiabi, R., Fahey, J. L., Korns, E., Weaver, M., & Mitsuyau, R. (1986). Prognostically significant classification of immune changes in AIDS with Kaposi's sarcoma. *Blood, 76,* 666-671.

Urmacher, C., Myskowski, P., Ochoa, M., Kris, M., & Safai, B. (1982). Outbreak of KS with CMV infection in young homosexual men. *American Journal of Medicine, 74,* 569-575.

Uziely, B., Jeffers, S., Isacson, R., Kutsch, K., Wei Tsao, D., Yehoshau, Z., Muggia, F. M., & Gabizon, A. (1995). Liposomal doxorubicin: antitumor activity and unique toxicities during two complimentary phase I studies. *Journal of Clinical Oncology, 13,* 1777-1785.

Volberding, P. (1989). Kaposi's sarcoma in AIDS. In J. Levy (Ed.), *AIDS, pathogenesis and treatment.* New York: Marcel Dekker.

Volberding, P. (1997). Antiretroviral therapy. In M. Sande & P. Volberding (Eds.), *The medical management of AIDS* (5th ed.). Philadelphia: W. B. Saunders.

Volberding, P., Gotlieb, M., & Rothman, J. (1983). Therapy of Kaposi's sarcoma in acquired immunodeficiency syndrome (AIDS) with alpha-2 recombinant IFN. *Proceedings of the American Society of Clinical Oncology, 2,* 52.

Ward, J., Petersen, L, & Jaffe, H. (1997). Current trends in the epidemiology of HIV/AIDS. In M. Sande & P. Volberding (Eds.), *The medical management of AIDS* (5th ed.). Philadelphia: W.B. Saunders.

World Health Organization. (1995). The current global situation of the HIV/AIDS pandemic. Geneva, Switzerland: World Health Organization.

Yang, J., Rosenberg, S., Glatstein, E., & Antman, K. (1993). Sarcomas of soft tissues. In V. T. DeVita, S. Hellman, & S. A. Rosenberg (Eds.), *Cancer: Principles and practice of oncology* (4th ed.). Philadelphia: Lippincott-Raven.

Ziegler, J. (1989). Lymphomas and other neoplasms associated with AIDS. In J. Levy (Ed.), *AIDS, pathogenesis and treatment.* New York: Marcel Dekker.

Index

A

f indicates illustrations; *t* indicates tables.

B

D

E

F

H

I

J

K

L

M

N

O

P

S

T

U

V

W

X

Y

Z

Internet Address Resource

American Academy of Nurse Practitioners
http://www.aano.org

American Academy of Nursing
http://www.nursingworld.org

The American Academy of Hospice and Palliative Medicine
http://www.aahpm.org/

American Association of Colleges of Nursing
http://www.aacn.nche.edu

American Association of Critical Care Nurses
http://www.aacn.org

American Association for the History of Nursing
http://users.aol.com/NsgHistory/AAHN.html

American Association of Legal Nurse Consultants
http://www.aalnc.org/

American Association of Nurse Attorneys
http://www.taana.org

American Association of Occupational Health Nurses, Inc.
http://www.aaohn.org

American Association of Office Nurses
E-mail to aaofnurs@cyberned.net

American Brain Tumor Association
http://www.abta.org/

American Cancer Society
http://www.cancer.org/

American College of Nurse Practitioners
http://www.nurse.org/acnp

American Holistic Nurses Association
http://www.ahna.org

American Nurses Association
http://www.nursingworld.org

American Organization of Nursing Executives
http://www.aone.org

The American Pain Society
http://www.ampainsoc.org/

American Psychiatric Nurses' Association
http://www.apna.org

American Society for Long-Term Care Nurses
E-mail to padona@epix.net

American Society of Pain Management Nurses
E-mail to aspmn@aol.com

Association of Nurses in AIDS Care
http://www.anacnet.org/aids/

Association of Pediatric Oncology Nurses
http://www.apon.org

Association of Rehabilitation Nurses
http://www.rehabnurse.org/

Brain Tumor Foundation of Canada
http://www.btfc.org/

The Brain Tumor Society
http://www.tbts.org

Breast Cancer Information Clearinghouse
http://nysernet.org/bcic/

Breast Self-Exam—7 Steps
http://www.saintfrancis.com/7step.html

Breast Self-Exam. From *Self* Magazine's Breast Cancer Handbook
http://nysernet.org/bcic/self/breast-exam.html

Cancer Information Network
http://www.cancernetwork.com

Cancer Pain, by Richard Pratt, MD
http://www.mdacc.tmc.edu/~acc/cp/cpinfo.html

Cancer Pain—Myths and Misconceptions, Cancer Care, Inc.
http://www.cacnercareinc.org/clinical/page8.htm

Cancer Research Institute
http://www.cancerresearch.org/

Candlelighters Childhood Cancer Foundation
http://www.candlelighters.org/

Case Management Society of America
http://www.cmsa.org

The Children's Brain Tumor Foundation, Inc.
http://www.childrensneuronet.org/

The Chronic Pain Forum
E-mail to listserv@maelstrom.stjohns.edu